KT-415-978

CANCER

Principles & Practice of Oncology

EDITED BY

Vincent T. DeVita, Jr., M.D.

Physician-in-Chief
Benno C. Schmidt Chair in Clinical Oncology
Memorial Sloan-Kettering Cancer Center
Professor of Medicine
Cornell University Medical College
Visiting Physician
The Rockefeller University Hospital
New York, New York

Samuel Hellman, M.D.

Dean and A. N. Pritzker Professor
Biological Sciences Division
*   and Pritzker School of Medicine*
Vice President for the Medical Center
The University of Chicago
Chicago, Illinois

Steven A. Rosenberg, M.D., Ph.D.

Chief of Surgery
National Cancer Institute
Professor of Surgery
Uniformed Services University of the
*   Health Sciences School of Medicine*
Bethesda, Maryland

161 Contributors

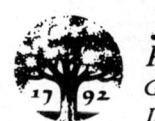

J. B. Lippincott Company
Philadelphia
Grand Rapids New York St. Louis San Francisco
London Sydney Tokyo

CANCER
Principles & Practice of Oncology

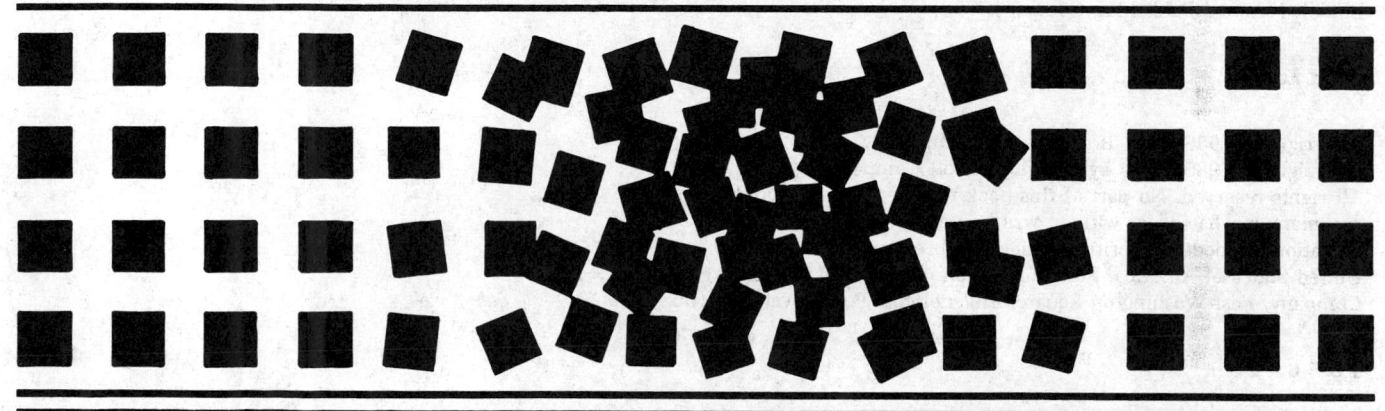

Volume 1

3rd Edition

Sponsoring Editor: Richard Winters
Project Editor: Virginia Barishek
Indexer: Alexandra Weir Nickerson
Design Coordinator: Ellen C. Dawson
Production Manager: Carol A. Florence
Production Supervisor: Charlene Squibb
Production Assistant: Pamela Milcos
Compositor: Digitype, Inc.
Printer: The Murray Printing Company
Binder: National Publishing Company

Third Edition

Copyright © 1989, by J. B. Lippincott Company.
Copyright © 1985, 1982 by J. B. Lippincott Company.
All rights reserved. No part of this book may be used or reproduced in
any manner whatsoever without written permission except for brief
quotations embodied in critical articles and reviews. Printed in the
United States of America. For information write J. B. Lippincott
Company, East Washington Square, Philadelphia, Pennsylvania 19105.

1 3 5 6 4 2

Library of Congress Cataloging-in-Publication Data

Cancer : principles and practice of oncology.

   Also issues in 2 v.
   Includes bibliographies and index.
   1. Cancer. 2. Oncology. I. DeVita, Vincent T. II. Hellman,
Samuel. III. Rosenberg, Steven A. [DNLM: 1. Neoplasms. QZ 200
C21537]
RC261.C274 1989   616.99'4   89-2389
ISBN 0-397-50840-9 (1-vol. ed.)
ISBN 0-397-50843-3 (2-vol. ed. : set)

The authors and publisher have exerted every effort to ensure that
drug selection and dosage set forth in this text are in accord with
current recommendations and practice at the time of publication.
However, in view of ongoing research, changes in government
regulations, and the constant flow of information relating to drug
therapy and drug reactions, the reader is urged to check the package
insert for each drug for any change in indications and dosage and for
added warnings and precautions. This is particularly important when
the recommended agent is a new or infrequently employed drug.

Dedicated to

Mary Kay

Rusty

Alice

Contributors

Daniel A. Albert, M.D.
David G. Cogan Professor of Ophthalmology
Harvard Medical School
Surgeon in Ophthalmology
Director
David G. Cogan Eye Pathology Laboratory
Massachusetts Eye and Ear Infirmary
Boston, Massachusetts

Tom Anderson, M.D.
Professor of Medicine
Chief
Division of Hematology/Oncology
Medical College of Wisconsin
Milwaukee County Medical Complex
Milwaukee, Wisconsin

Karen H. Antman, M.D.
Associate Professor of Medicine
Harvard Medical School
Assistant Physician
Dana Farber Cancer Institute
Boston, Massachusetts

Ehud Arbit, M.D.
Associate Professor of Surgery
Cornell University Medical College
Attending Surgeon and Associate Member
Memorial Sloan-Kettering Cancer Center
New York, New York

Alan R. Baker, M.D.
Senior Investigator
Surgery Branch
National Cancer Institute
Bethesda, Maryland

Charles M. Balch, M.D.
Professor of Surgery
Head
Division of Surgery
University of Texas
M. D. Anderson Cancer Center
Houston, Texas

J. Andrew Billings, M.D.
Assistant Clinical Professor
Harvard Medical School
Assistant Physician
Massachusetts General Hospital
Boston, Massachusetts

Richard S. Bockman, M.D., Ph.D.
Associate Professor of Medicine
Endocrinology Division
Cornell University Medical College
Associate Attending
The Hospital for Special Surgery and New York Hospital
New York, New York

David G. Bragg, M.D.
Professor and Chairman
Department of Radiology
University of Utah School of Medicine
Senior Consultant
Veterans Administration Hospital
Salt Lake City, Utah

Murray F. Brennan, M.D., M.Cb., F.R.A.C.S.
Professor of Surgery
Cornell University Medical College
Alfred P. Sloan Professor and Chairman
Department of Surgery
Memorial Sloan-Kettering Cancer Center
New York, New York

Samuel Broder, M.D.
Director
National Cancer Institute
Bethesda, Maryland

Paul A. Bunn, Jr., M.D.
Director
University of Colorado Cancer Center
Head
Division of Medical Oncology
Professor of Medicine
University of Colorado
Health Sciences Center
University Hospital
Denver, Colorado

J. Robert Cassady, M.D.
Head
Department of Radiation Oncology
University of Arizona
Health Sciences Center
Tucson, Arizona

Nicholas J. Cassisi, D.D.S., M.D.
Professor and Chief
Division of Otolaryngology
Department of Surgery
University of Florida
Shands Hospital
Gainesville, Florida

Bruce A. Chabner, M.D.
Director
Division of Cancer Treatment
National Cancer Institute
Bethesda, Maryland

Alfred E. Chang, M.D.
Associate Professor of Surgery
Chief
Division of Surgical Oncology
University of Michigan Medical Center
Ann Arbor, Michigan

Richard Chang, M.D.
Assistant Professor of Radiology
Georgetown University
Washington, D.C.
Staff Radiologist
Diagnostic Radiology Department
National Institutes of Health
Bethesda, Maryland

Grace Christ, M.A., A.C.S.W.
Director
Program Planning and Project Pending
Department of Social Work
Memorial Hospital
New York, New York

John R. Clark, M.D.
Instructor in Medicine
Harvard Medical School
Clinical Associate in Medicine
Dana Farber Cancer Institute
Boston, Massachusetts

Alfred M. Cohen, M.D.
Associate Professor of Surgery
Cornell University Medical College
Chief
Colorectal Service
Department of Surgery
Memorial Sloan-Kettering Cancer Center
New York, New York

C. Norman Coleman, M.D.
Alvan T. and Viola D. Fuller American Cancer Society Professor
Harvard Medical School
Chairman
Joint Center for Radiation Therapy
Boston, Massachusetts

E. David Crawford, M.D.
Professor and Chairman
Division of Urology
University of Colorado
Health Sciences Center
Denver, Colorado

Joseph W. Cullen, M.D.
Deputy Director
Division of Cancer Prevention and Control
National Cancer Institute
Bethesda, Maryland

Michael Dean, Ph.D.
Program Resources Inc.
NCI–Frederick Cancer Research Facility
Frederick, Maryland

Albert B. Deisseroth, M.D., Ph.D.
Anderson Professor of Cancer Treatment and Research
Chairman
Department of Hematology
University of Texas
M.D. Anderson Cancer Center
Houston, Texas

Thomas F. Delaney, M.D.
Senior Investigator
Radiation Oncology Branch
National Cancer Institute
Bethesda, Maryland

Joel A. DeLisa, M.D.
Professor and Chairman
Department of Rehabilitation Medicine
U.M.D.N.J.–New Jersey Medical School
Medical Director and Chief Medical Officer
Kessler Institute for Rehabilitation
West Orange, New Jersey

Susan S. Devesa, Ph.D.
Epidemiology and Biostatistics Program
Division of Cancer Etiology
National Cancer Institute
Bethesda, Maryland

Sarah A. Donaldson, M.D.
Professor
Department of Radiation Oncology
Stanford University School of Medicine
Stanford University Hospital
Stanford, California

John L. Doppman, M.D.
Chief of Radiology
National Institutes of Health
Professor of Radiology
Georgetown University Medical School
Bethesda, Maryland

Patricia L. Duffey, B.S.N., R.N.
Chemotherapy Research Nurse
Biologic Response Modifier Program
Division of Cancer Treatment
National Cancer Institute
Bethesda, Maryland

John D. Earle, M.D.
Chairman
Division of Radiation Therapy
William H. Donner Professor of Oncology
Mayo Medical School
Rochester, Minnesota

Lawrence H. Einhorn, M.D.
Distinguished Professor of Medicine
Indiana University Medical Center
Department of Medicine
Distinguished Professor of Medicine
University Hospital
Indianapolis, Indiana

William R. Fair, M.D.
Chief
Urology Service
Memorial Sloan-Kettering Cancer Center
Professor of Surgery
Cornell University Medical College
New York Hospital
New York, New York

Geoffrey Falkson, M.B.Ch.B., M.Med.(Int.), M.D.
Professor and Head
Department of Medical Oncology
University of Pretoria
Pretoria, Republic of South Africa

Philip J. Fialkow, M.D.
Professor and Chairman
Department of Medicine
University of Washington
Physician-in-Chief
University Hospital
Seattle, Washington

Kathleen M. Foley, M.D.
Associate Professor of Neurology and Pharmacology
Cornell University Medical College
Chief
Pain Service
Department of Neurology
Attending Neurologist
Memorial Sloan-Kettering Cancer Center
New York, New York

Joseph F. Fraumeni, Jr., M.D.
Associate Director for Epidemiology and Biostatistics
National Cancer Institute
Bethesda, Maryland

Michael A. Friedman, M.D.
National Cancer Institute
Bethesda, Maryland

R. J. Michael Fry, M.D.
Head
Cancer Biology Section
Biology Division
Oak Ridge National Laboratory
Oak Ridge, Tennessee

Zvi Fuks, M.D.
Chairman
Department of Radiation Oncology
Memorial Sloan-Kettering Cancer Center
New York, New York

Lynn H. Gerber, M.D.
Associate Professor of Medicine
George Washington University
Washington, D.C.
Chief
Department of Rehabilitation Medicine
Warren Grant Magnuson Clinical Center
National Institutes of Health
Bethesda, Maryland

Roy Geronemus, M.D.
Assistant Professor of Dermatology
New York University Medical Center
New York, New York

Eli J. Glatstein, M.D.
Professor of Radiology
Uniformed Services University of Health Science
Chief
Radiation Oncology Branch
National Cancer Institute
Bethesda, Maryland

Richard J. Gralla, M.D.
Associate Professor of Medicine
Cornell University Medical College
Head
Section of Thoracic Surgery
Memorial Sloan-Kettering Cancer Center
New York, New York

Peter Greenwald, M.D., Dr.P.H.
Director
Division of Cancer Prevention and Control
National Cancer Institute
Bethesda, Maryland

Thomas W. Griffin, M.D.
Professor of Radiation Oncology
Chairman
Department of Radiation Oncology
Director
University Cancer Center
University of Washington
School of Medicine
Seattle, Washington

Jerome E. Groopman, M.D.
Associate Professor of Medicine
Harvard Medical School
Chief
Division of Hematology/Oncology
New England Deaconess Hospital
Boston, Massachusetts

Leonard L. Gunderson, M.D., M.S.
Professor of Oncology
Mayo Medical School
Consultant in Radiation Oncology
Mayo Clinic
Rochester, Minnesota

Philip H. Gutin, M.D.
Associate Professor
Departments of Neurological Surgery and Radiation Oncology
School of Medicine
University of California
San Francisco, California

H. Ric Harnsberger, M.D.
Associate Professor
ENT/Neuroradiology
University of Utah Medical Center
Cottonwood Hospital
Salt Lake City, Utah

Jay R. Harris, M.D.
Associate Professor
Harvard Medical School
Clinical/Educational Director
Joint Center for Radiation Therapy
Boston, Massachusetts

Daniel M. Hays, M.D.
Professor of Surgery and Pediatrics
University of Southern California
School of Medicine
Attending Physician and Surgeon
Departments of Surgery and Pediatrics
Children's Hospital of Los Angeles
Los Angeles, California

I. Craig Henderson, M.D.
Associate Professor of Medicine
Harvard Medical School
Medical Coordinator
Breast Evaluation Center
Dana Farber Cancer Center
Boston, Massachusetts

Alan D. Hillel, M.D.
Assistant Professor
Department of Otolaryngology/Head and Neck Surgery
University of Washington
Chief
Otolaryngology/Head and Neck Surgery
Veterans Administration Medical Center
Seattle, Washington

Jimmie C. Holland, M.D.
Professor
Department of Psychiatry
Cornell University Medical College
Chief
Psychiatry Service
Memorial Sloan-Kettering Cancer Center
New York, New York

Robert N. Hoover, M.D., Sc.D.
Chief
Environmental Epidemiology Branch
National Cancer Institute
Bethesda, Maryland

Marc E. Horowitz, M.D.
Senior Investigator
Pediatric Branch
National Cancer Institute
Clinical Center
National Institutes of Health
Bethesda, Maryland

William J. Hoskins, M.D.
Associate Professor of Obstetrics and Gynecology
Cornell University Medical College
Associate Chief
Gynecology Service
Memorial Sloan-Kettering Cancer Center
New York, New York

Alan N. Houghton, M.D.
Head
Laboratory of Solid Tumor Immunology
Cornell University Medical College
Head
Melanoma/Sarcoma Section
Department of Medical Oncology
Memorial Sloan-Kettering Cancer Center
New York, New York

Peter M. Howley, M.D.
Chief
Laboratory of Tumor Virus Biology
National Cancer Institute
Bethesda, Maryland

Susan M. Hubbard, R.N.
Associate Director
International Cancer Information Center
National Cancer Institute
Bethesda, Maryland

Daniel C. Ihde, M.D.
Professor of Medicine
Uniformed Services University of the Health Sciences
Head
Clinical Investigations Section
NCI–Navy Medical Oncology Branch
Naval Hospital
Bethesda, Maryland

Elaine S. Jaffe, M.D.
Chief
Hematopathology Section
Deputy Chief
Laboratory of Pathology
National Cancer Institute
Bethesda, Maryland

Robert T. Jensen, M.D.
Senior Investigator
Digestive Diseases Branch
National Institute of Diabetes, Digestive, and Kidney Diseases
National Institutes of Health
Bethesda, Maryland

David Kelsen, M.D.
Associate Professor of Medicine
Cornell University Medical College
Head
Gastrointestinal Section
Division of Medical Oncology
Memorial Sloan-Kettering Cancer Center
New York, New York

Nancy E. Kemeny, M.D.
Associate Professor of Clinical Medicine
Cornell University Medical College
Associate Attending
Memorial Sloan-Kettering Cancer Center
New York, New York

Leo J. Kinlen, M.B., B.S., D.Phil., F.R.C.P.
Director
CRC Cancer Epidemiology Unit
University of Edinburgh
Edinburgh, Scotland

David W. Kinne, M.D.
Associate Professor of Surgery
Cornell University Medical College
Chief
Breast Service
Attending Surgeon
Memorial Sloan-Kettering Cancer Center
New York, New York

Timothy Kinsella, M.D.
Professor and Chairman
Department of Human Oncology
University of Wisconsin School of Medicine
Deputy Director
University of Wisconsin Clinical Cancer Center
University of Wisconsin Hospital and Clinics
Madison, Wisconsin

Libby L. Klein, M.S.W., A.C.S.W.
Social Work Researcher
Memorial Sloan-Kettering Cancer Center
New York, New York

Larry E. Kun, M.D.
Chairman
Department of Radiation Oncology
St. Jude Children's Research Hospital
Professor
Departments of Radiology and Pediatrics
Director
Division of Radiation Oncology
University of Tennessee
Memphis, Tennessee

Marguerite S. Lederberg, M.D.
Clinical Associate Professor of Psychiatry
Cornell University Medical Center
Associate Attending Psychiatrist
Memorial Sloan-Kettering Cancer Center
New York, New York

Lawrence P. Leichman, M.D.
Associate Professor of Medicine
University of Southern California
Associate Director for Medical Oncology
Los Angeles County Hospital
University of Southern California Medical Center
Los Angeles, California

Victor A. Levin, M.D.
Professor and Chairman
Department of Neuro-Oncology
University of Texas
M. D. Anderson Cancer Center
Houston, Texas

Allen S. Lichter, M.D.
Professor and Chairman
University of Michigan Medical School
University of Michigan Hospital
Ann Arbor, Michigan

W. Marston Linehan, M.D.
Head
Urologic Oncology Section
Surgery Branch
National Cancer Institute
Assistant Professor of Surgery
Uniformed Services University of the Health Sciences
School of Medicine
Bethesda, Maryland

Michael P. Link, M.D.
Associate Professor of Pediatrics
Stanford University School of Medicine
Staff Hematologist/Oncologist
Children's Hospital at Stanford
Stanford, California

Lance A. Liotta, M.D., Ph.D.
Chief
Laboratory of Pathology
National Cancer Institute
Bethesda, Maryland

Patrick J. Loehrer, M.D.
Associate Professor of Medicine
Section of Hematology-Oncology
Indiana University School of Medicine
Indiana University Hospital
Indianapolis, Indiana

Dan L. Longo, M.D.
Biological Response Modifiers Program
Division of Cancer Treatment
National Cancer Institute
Bethesda, Maryland

Matthew Loscalzo, A.C.S.W.
Assistant Director
Department of Social Work/Educational Coordinator
Memorial Sloan-Kettering Cancer Center
New York, New York

Michael T. Lotze, M.D.
Assistant Professor
Uniformed Services University of the Health Sciences
Senior Investigator
Surgery Branch
National Cancer Institute
Bethesda, Maryland

Bert L. Lum, Pharm.D.
Associate Professor
University of the Pacific
Stockton, California
Research Associate
Department of Oncology
Palo Alto Veterans Administration Medical Center
Palo Alto, California

John S. Macdonald, M.D.
Professor of Medicine
Director
Division of Hematology and Oncology
Lucille Markey Cancer Center
University of Kentucky Medical Center
Lexington, Kentucky

Martin M. Malawer, M.D.
Associate Professor of Orthopedic Surgery and Child
  Development
Children's Hospital National Medical Center and George
  Washington University School of Medicine
The Washington Hospital Center
Washington, D.C.

Mary Jane Massie, M.D.
Associate Professor of Clinical Psychiatry
Cornell University Medical College
Associate Attending Psychiatrist
Psychiatry Service
Department of Neurology
Memorial Sloan-Kettering Cancer Center
New York, New York

Peter Mauch, M.D.
Associate Professor
Department of Radiation Therapy
Harvard Medical School
Boston, Massachusetts

Rosalie Raps Melnick, Ph.D., M.B.A.
Clinical Assistant Professor
Department of Rehabilitation Medicine
University of Washington
Associate Chief of Staff/Education
Seattle Veterans Administration Medical Center
Seattle, Washington

Joel D. Meyers, M.D.
Professor of Medicine
University of Washington
School of Medicine
Head
Program in Infectious Diseases
Fred Hutchinson Cancer Research Center
Seattle, Washington

Anthony B. Miller, M.B., F.R.C.P.
Professor
Department of Preventive Medicine and Biostatistics
Faculty of Medicine
University of Toronto
Toronto, Ontario, Canada

Donald L. Miller, M.D.
Associate Professor of Radiology
Georgetown University School of Medicine
Associate Professor of Radiology
Uniformed Services University of the Health Sciences
School of Medicine
Director of Vascular/Interventional Radiology
Diagnostic Radiology Department
National Institutes of Health
Bethesda, Maryland

Robert M. Miller, Ph.D.
Clinical Assistant Professor
Speech and Hearing Sciences, Otolaryngology, and
  Rehabilitation Medicine
University of Washington
Chief
Audiology and Speech Pathology Service
Seattle Veterans Administration Medical Center
Seattle, Washington

Rodney R. Million, M.D.
Professor and Chairman
Department of Radiation Oncology
University of Florida
Shands Hospital
Gainesville, Florida

John D. Minna, M.D.
Professor of Medicine
Uniformed Services University of the Health Sciences
Chief
NCI–Navy Medical Oncology Branch
Naval Hospital
Bethesda, Maryland

James B. Mitchell, Ph.D.
Deputy Chief
Radiation Oncology Branch
National Cancer Institute
Bethesda, Maryland

Drogo K. Montague, M.D.
Director
Center for Sexual Function
Head
Section of Urodynamics and Prosthetic Surgery
Department of Urology
Cleveland Clinic Foundation
Cleveland, Ohio

John J. Mulvihill, M.D.
Chief
Clinical Genetics Section
Clinical Epidemiology Branch
National Cancer Institute
Director
Interinstitute Medical Genetics Program
Warren Grant Magnuson Clinical Center
National Institutes of Health
Bethesda, Maryland

Charles E. Myers, M.D.
Chief
Medicine Branch and Clinical Pharmacology Branch
Clinical Center
National Institutes of Health
Bethesda, Maryland

Jeffrey A. Norton, M.D.
Head
Surgical Metabolism Section
Surgery Branch
National Cancer Institute
Bethesda, Maryland

James R. Oleson, M.D., Ph.D.
Associate Professor
Division of Radiation Oncology
Duke University Medical Center
Durham, North Carolina

Stanley E. Order, M.D., Sc.D.
Willard and Lillian Hackerman Professor of Radiation Oncology
The Johns Hopkins Medical Institution
School of Medicine
Director
Radiation Oncology
The Johns Hopkins Hospital
Baltimore, Maryland

Morag Park, Ph.D.
Ludwig Institute for Cancer Research
BRI–Basic Research Program
NCI–Frederick Cancer Research Facility
Frederick, Maryland

Harvey Pass, M.D.
Head
Thoracic Oncology Section
Senior Investigator
Surgery Branch
National Cancer Institute
Bethesda, Maryland

Jennifer A. K. Patterson, M.D.
Assistant Professor
Department of Dermatology
New York University Medical Center
Director of Inpatient and Consultative Services
Department of Dermatology
Bellevue Hospital Center
New York, New York

Carlos A. Perez, M.D.
Director
Radiation Oncology Center
Mallinckrodt Institute of Radiology
Washington University Medical Center
St. Louis, Missouri

Lester J. Peters, M.D.
Professor and Head
Division of Radiotherapy
John G. and Marie Stella Kenedy Chair
University of Texas
M. D. Anderson Hospital Cancer Center
Houston, Texas

Theodore L. Phillips, M.D.
Professor and Chairman
Department of Radiation Oncology
University of California
Attending Physician
Long/Moffitt Hospital
San Francisco, California

Henry C. Pitot, M.D., Ph.D.
Professor of Oncology and Pathology
The Medical School
University of Wisconsin
Pathologist
University Hospitals
Madison, Wisconsin

Philip A. Pizzo, M.D.
Chief of Pediatrics
Head
Infectious Disease Section
National Cancer Institute
Clinical Center
National Institutes of Health
Bethesda, Maryland

David G. Poplack, M.D.
Head
Leukemia Section
Pediatric Branch
National Cancer Institute
Bethesda, Maryland

Abram Recht, M.D.
Assistant Professor
Joint Center for Radiation Therapy
Department of Radiation Therapy
Harvard Medical School
Radiation Therapist
Beth Israel Hospital
Assistant Physician
Dana Farber Cancer Institute
Boston, Massachusetts

Jerome P. Richie, M.D.
Elliott Carr Cutler Professor of
Urological Surgery
Chairman
Harvard Program in Urology
Chief of Urology
Brigham and Women's Hospital
Boston, Massachusetts

E. Chester Ridgway, M.D.
Professor of Medicine
Head
Division of Endocrinology
University of Colorado Health Sciences Center
Denver, Colorado

Anita B. Roberts, Ph.D.
Senior Scientist
Laboratory of Chemoprevention
National Cancer Institute
Bethesda, Maryland

J. C. Rosenberg, M.D., Ph.D.
Professor of Surgery
Wayne State University
Chief of Surgery
Hutzel Hospital
Detroit, Michigan

Jack A. Roth, M.D.
Johnson Professor and Chairman
Department of Thoracic Surgery
Professor of Tumor Biology
M.D. Anderson Cancer Center
Houston, Texas

Janet D. Rowley, M.D.
Professor
Department of Medicine
University of Chicago School of Medicine
Chicago, Illinois

Angelo Russo, M.D., Ph.D.
Head
Experimental Phototherapy
Radiation Oncology Branch
National Institutes of Health
Bethesda, Maryland

Jose Alain Sahel, M.D., Ph.D.
Professor of Ophthalmology
University of Strasbourg
Clinique Ophtalmologique
Centre Hospitalier Regional
Strasbourg, France

Sydney E. Salmon, M.D.
Professor
Internal Medicine
Director
Arizona Cancer Center
University of Arizona College of Medicine
Tucson, Arizona

Wendy S. Schain, Ed.D.
Adjunct Clinical Professor
Georgetown University Medical School
Kensington, Maryland

Claudia A. Seipp, R.N., O.C.N.
Oncology Nurse Clinician
Surgery Branch
National Cancer Institute
Bethesda, Maryland

Brenda Shank, M.D., Ph.D.
Associate Professor of Radiation Oncology in Medicine
Cornell University Medical Center
Associate Member
Memorial Sloan-Kettering Cancer Center
Associate Attending Radiation Oncologist
Memorial Hospital
New York, New York

Glenn E. Sheline, Ph.D., M.D.
Professor of Radiation Oncology
University of California School of Medicine
University of California Hospitals
San Francisco, California

Richard J. Sherins, M.D.
Director
Division of Andrology
Genetics and I.V.F. Institute
Fairfax, Virginia

Moshe Shike, M.D.
Associate Professor of Clinical Medicine
Cornell University Medical College
Associate Attending Physician
Department of Medicine
Memorial Sloan-Kettering Cancer Center
New York, New York

William U. Shipley, M.D.
Associate Professor of Radiation Therapy
Harvard Medical School
Radiation Therapist
Department of Radiation Medicine
Massachusetts General Hospital
Associate Director
Massachusetts General Hospital Cancer Center
Boston, Massachusetts

Edward H. Shortliffe, M.D., Ph.D.
Associate Professor of Medicine and of Computer Science
Stanford University School of Medicine
Attending Physician
Stanford University Medical Center
Stanford, California

Leslie R. Shover, Ph.D.
Head
Section of Psychosexual Disorders
The Center for Sexual Function
The Cleveland Clinic Foundation
Cleveland, Ohio

Richard M. Simon, Ph.D.
Chief
Biometric Branch
National Cancer Institute
Bethesda, Maryland

William F. Sindelar, M.D., Ph.D.
Senior Investigator
Surgery Branch
National Cancer Institute
Bethesda, Maryland

Jack W. Singer, M.D.
Professor of Medicine
University of Washington
Chief of Medical Oncology
Verterans Administration Medical Center
Seattle, Washington

Stephen T. Sonis, D.M.D., D.M.Sc.
Associate Professor of Oral Medicine
Harvard School of Dental Medicine
Chief
Dental Service
Brigham and Women's Hospital
Boston, Massachusetts

Michael B. Sporn, M.D.
Chief
Laboratory of Chemoprevention
National Cancer Institute
Bethesda, Maryland

Glenn Steele, Jr., M.D., Ph.D.
The William McDermott Professor of Surgery
Harvard Medical School
Chairman
Department of Surgery
New England Deaconess Hospital
Boston, Massachusetts

William G. Stetler-Stevenson, M.D., Ph.D.
Senior Staff Fellow
Laboratory of Pathology
National Institutes of Health
Bethesda, Maryland

Rainer Storb, M.D.
Professor of Medicine
University of Washington School of Medicine
Head
Program in Transplant Biology
Fred Hutchinson Cancer Research Center
Seattle, Washington

Diane E. Stover, M.D.
Associate Professor of Medicine
Cornell University Medical College
Chief of Pulmonary Service
Associate Attending Physician
Memorial Sloan-Kettering Cancer Center
New York, New York

Paul H. Sugarbaker, M.D.
Director of Surgical Oncology
Winship Cancer Center
Emory University School of Medicine
Atlanta, Georgia

Ian F. Tannock, M.D., Ph.D.
Associate Professor of Medicine and Medical Biophysics
University of Toronto
Staff Physician/Senior Scientist
Princess Margaret Hospital and Ontario Cancer Institute
Toronto, Ontario, Canada

William M. Thompson, M.D.
Professor and Chairman
Department of Radiology
University of Minnesota
Chairman
Department of Radiology
University of Minnesota Hospital and Clinic
Minneapolis, Minnesota

Frank M. Torti, M.D.
Associate Professor of Medicine
Stanford University
Chief
Oncology Section
Veterans Administration Medical Center
Palo Alto, California

Margaret A. Tucker, M.D.
Chief
Family Studies Section
Environmental Epidemiology Branch
Division of Cancer Etiology
National Cancer Institute
Bethesda, Maryland

John E. Ultmann, M.D.
Professor of Medicine
Director
Cancer Research Center
Division of Biological Science
University of Chicago
Pritzker School of Medicine
Attending Physician
The University of Chicago Hospitals
Chicago, Illinois

George F. Vande Woude, Ph.D.
Director
BRI—Basic Research Program
NCI—Frederick Cancer Research Facility
Frederick, Maryland

Susan Vande Woude, D.V.M.
Post Doctoral Fellow
Division of Comparative Medicine
The Johns Hopkins University
Baltimore, Maryland

Ralph Wallerstein, Jr., M.D.
Assistant Clinical Professor of Medicine
University of California
San Francisco, California

Harold J. Wanebo, M.D.
Professor of Surgery
Director of Surgical Oncology
Brown University
Chief
Department of Surgery
Roger Williams General Hospital
Providence, Rhode Island

Raymond P. Warrell, Jr., M.D.
Assistant Professor of Medicine
Cornell University Medical College
Associate Member
Memorial Sloan-Kettering Cancer Center
New York, New York

Lois L. Weinstein, A.C.S.W.
Department of Social Work
Memorial Sloan-Kettering Cancer Center
New York, New York

Peter H. Wiernik, M.D.
Gutman Professor and Chairman
Department of Oncology
Montefiore Medical Center
Head
Division of Medical Oncology
Albert Einstein College of Medicine
Associate Professor for Clinical Research
Albert Einstein Cancer Center
Bronx, New York

Stephen D. Williams, M.D.
Professor of Medicine
Indiana University
Chief
Hematology-Oncology
Indianapolis Veterans Administration Medical Center
Indianapolis, Indiana

Richard E. Wilson, M.D.
Professor of Surgery
Harvard Medical School
Chief
Surgical Oncology
Brigham and Women's Hospital
Dana Farber Cancer Institute
Boston, Massachusetts

Donald C. Wright, M.D.
Clinical Neurosurgery Section
Surgical Neurology Branch
National Institutes of Neurological and
Communicative Disorders and Stroke
Clinical Center
National Institutes of Health
Bethesda, Maryland

Alan Yagoda, M.D.
Instructor in Medicine
Cornell University Medical College
New York, New York
Assistant Clinical Professor of Medicine
Yale University School of Medicine
New Haven, Connecticut
Attending Physician
Memorial Sloan-Kettering Cancer Center
New York, New York

Joachim Yahalom, M.D.
Assistant Professor
Cornell University Medical Center
Assistant Attending
Department of Radiation Oncology
Memorial Sloan-Kettering Cancer Center
New York, New York

Robert C. Young, M.D.
Associate Director
Centers and Community Oncology Program
National Cancer Institute
Bethesda, Maryland

Preface

Early diagnosis and prompt treatment with carefully integrated, multimodal management continues to provide cancer patients with the best chance of surviving the disease. The integrated, multimodal approach to the treatment of cancer, with a balanced view of how the majority of cancer patients are managed today, was the *raison d'etre* of the first edition of *Cancer: Principles and Practice of Oncology* in 1982 and remains a hallmark of the third edition.

Dramatic changes in cancer research and the management of cancer patients have resulted in a sense of urgency to put the freshest information in the hands of practicing physicians. This sense of urgency has necessitated the timely production of this edition. The first section, "Principles of Oncology," has once again been entirely revised to reflect the rapid accumulation of new information about the etiology and development of cancer at the molecular level. It reflects the need of physicians to have at their disposal a succinct yet comprehensive discussion of the scientific basis of the cancer process. More information has been added on useful aspects of the technology of the molecular biology of cancer and the metastatic process. In addition, the discussions of the increasingly beneficial approaches to cancer prevention have been amplified.

With each passing year, more patients with cancer are curable and treatments are associated with less morbidity than in the past. The second portion of the book, "Practice of Oncology," has been extensively revised to reflect this continued integration of local and systemic treatments and the growing sophistication of multimodality treatments. Since the second edition of this book, new treatments have been developed for the more common visceral tumors. The newest information on the results of these clinical trials is included, where appropriate, as is the latest information on the increasingly widespread benefits of the use of biologics (such as colony-stimulating factors and various lymphokines). The complications of cancer and its treatment, and presentations on approaches to treatments under development, are the main features of the final portion of the book. We have continued to emphasize the need for practicality. The information presented in each chapter is both fresh and usable.

Thus, *Cancer: Principles and Practice of Oncology* continues to be a book for both oncologists and physicians of other specialties whose practices include a significant number of cancer patients. By retaining freshness and practicality without sacrificing comprehensiveness, we have attempted to place at the fingertips of the physician all the necessary data to manage cancer patients within a single book. The pace of discovery in the medical sciences makes this task an increasingly difficult challenge with each edition. We hope that a comprehensive text like *Cancer: Principles and Practice of Oncology* is useful to physicians and their patients.

Vincent T. DeVita, Jr., M.D.,
Samuel Hellman, M.D.
Steven A. Rosenberg, M.D., Ph.D.

Acknowledgments

The editors are especially grateful to those whose excellent help and unflagging enthusiasm contributed to this book.

Alice Rosenberg assumed responsibility for the overall compilation of the contributions to this book and for many of the organizational details involved in its assembly.

Rhanda Steele and Susan Hubbard contributed to the preparation and compilation of many of the manuscripts.

Richard Winters provided valuable editorial assistance in the preparation of the second and third editions.

Stuart Freeman, Editor, Oncology Program, J. B. Lippincott Company, has worked closely with the editors from the book's inception in 1978 through the completion of all three editions. His valuable advice and continuing encouragement have contributed greatly to the preparation of all three.

Contents

3   Principles of Molecular Cell Biology of Cancer: General Aspects of Gene Regulation   31

SUSAN VANDE WOUDE
GEORGE F. VANDE WOUDE

4   Principles of Molecular Cell Biology of Cancer: Oncogenes   45

MORAG PARK
GEORGE F. VANDE WOUDE

60 *Adverse Effects of Treatment* 2135

66 *Newer Methods of Cancer Treatment*   2413

CANCER

*Principles & Practice
of Oncology*

PART 1

Principles of Oncology

IAN F. TANNOCK

CHAPTER 1

Principles of Cell Proliferation: Cell Kinetics

Human tumors have a wide range of growth rates. The introduction of tritiated thymidine and autoradiography in the 1950s allowed the growth of selected human tumors to be analyzed in terms of properties of the constituent cells, and later applications of flow cytometry have allowed more rapid and automated analysis of cell kinetics. These data may provide useful prognostic information, and the ability of flow cytometry to detect aneuploid cell populations makes it an important aid in tumor diagnosis. Many anticancer drugs are selective for proliferating cells, and most drugs, as well as ionizing radiation, vary in their activity around the cell cycle. Tissues containing rapidly proliferating cells such as the bone marrow or intestinal mucosa are frequently dose–limiting in cancer chemotherapy, and an understanding of their cell kinetics provides a basis for the scheduling of anticancer drugs. This chapter describes principles of cell kinetics and uses of flow cytometry, with emphasis on those properties that may have direct application to the diagnosis, prognosis, and treatment of human cancer.

GROWTH OF HUMAN TUMORS

TUMOR DOUBLING TIMES

Determination of the rate of growth of tumors is limited to sites that are accessible to measurement, and most growth curves have been derived from measurements of pulmonary metastases in serial chest radiographs. Steel[1] has reviewed published data on the growth of 780 human tumors in pa-

tients who were not receiving treatment. Many of the investigators made only two or three measurements on each tumor, but in a small number of studies, multiple serial estimates of tumor volume were available. Many of these serial measurements could be fitted by a straight line when tumor volume (on a logarithmic scale) was plotted against time (on a linear scale); that is, the growth curve was exponential (Fig. 1-1). Exponential growth implies that the tumor takes a constant time to double its volume, and representative values of volume doubling time (T_D) for different types of human tumor are shown in Table 1-1.

The following general conclusions can be drawn from the available data on tumor growth rate:

1. Lung metastases derived from many of the more common solid tumors in humans have mean values of T_D in the range of 2 to 3 months. There is, however, a wide range of growth rates among tumors of the same histologic type and tissue of origin.
2. Tumors that are responsive to anticancer drugs (*e.g.*, lymphomas, testicular cancer, and tumors in children) usually grow more rapidly than do less responsive tumors.
3. Lung metastases from tumors of the colon and breast tend to grow more rapidly than do the primary tumors from which they are seeded.

PRECLINICAL GROWTH OF HUMAN TUMORS

The smallest tumor that is likely to be detected by physical or radiologic examination will have a diameter of about 1 cm

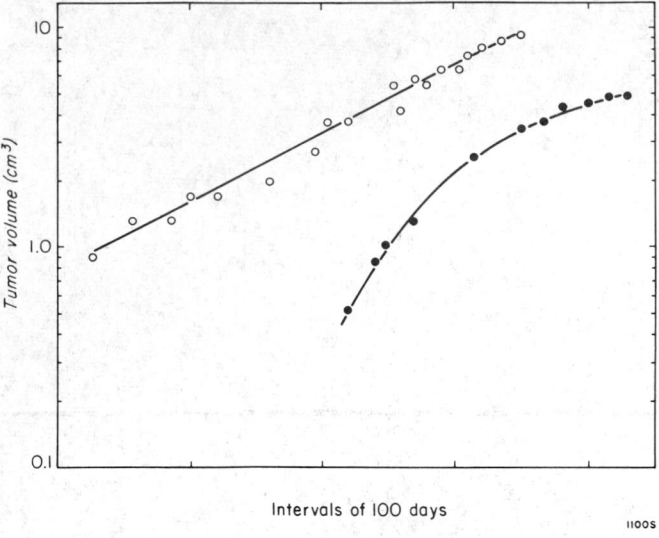

FIG. 1-1. Growth curve for pulmonary metastases from cancer of the breast (*open symbols*) and cancer of the rectum (*closed symbols*). The breast cancer metastasis grew exponentially with a volume doubling time of 3 months, but the rectal cancer metastasis showed decreasing growth rate with increasing size. (Hill RP, Bush RS-Unpublished data)

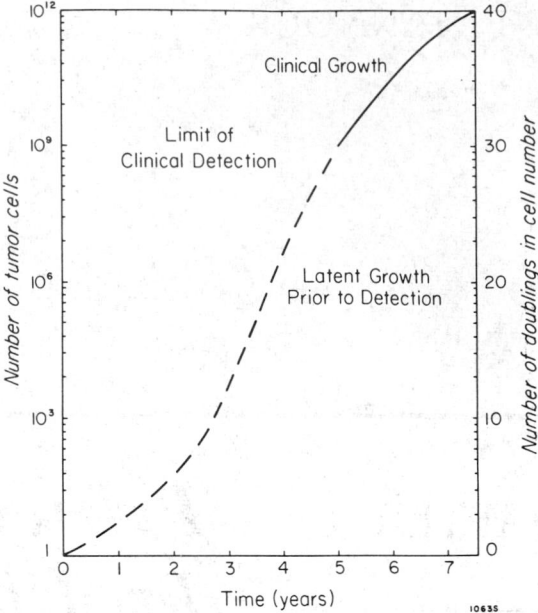

FIG. 1-2. Hypothetical growth curve for a human tumor. Note that the tumor grows for 5 years before attaining a size of ~1 g (~10^9 cells), when it can first be clinically detected. Thereafter, despite some slowing of growth, it attains a lethal mass of ~1 kg (~10^{12} cells) in a further 2.5 years.

and may contain 10^8 to 10^9 tumor cells, depending on the contribution of stroma and other elements to tumor bulk. Such a tumor will have undergone about 30 doublings in cell number if it is clonally derived from a single transformed cell (Fig. 1-2). Growth from a tumor of 1 g (the minimum size detectable) to a potentially lethal mass of 1 kg requires

TABLE 1-1.   Representative Values of Volume Doubling Time for Different Types of Human Tumors

Tumor Type	Number of Tumors	Volume Doubling Time in Weeks (geometric mean value)
Primary lung cancer		
Adenocarcinoma	64	21
Squamous-cell carcinoma	85	12
Anaplastic carcinoma	55	11
Breast cancer		
Primary	17	14
Lung metastases	44	11
Soft-tissue metastases	66	3
Colorectal cancer		
Primary	19	90
Lung metastases	56	14
Lymphoma		
Lymph node lesions	27	4
Lung metastases of:		
Carcinoma of testis	80	4
Childhood tumors	47	4
Adult sarcomas	58	7

Reproduced from Tannock and Hill[2] with permission, and adapted from data reviewed by Steel.[1]

only 10 further doublings of cell number. Thus, the period of tumor growth that is clinically evident represents a rather short period in the total life history of a tumor. There is ample opportunity for seeding of metastases before detection of a primary tumor.

If human tumors grew exponentially from inception to death of the host (or to institution of some form of treatment), the time of origin of the malignancy could be estimated by extrapolating growth curves back to a single cell. If this is done for growth of the lung metastasis of the human breast cancer that is shown in Figure 1-1 (with the assumption that a tumor of volume 1 cm³ contains 10^9 cells), the latency period from a single cell origin of the metastasis would be about 7.5 years.

Although the latency period of slowly growing human tumors is long, some tumors show decelerating growth with time (Fig. 1-1), so the above example may overestimate the latency period. Deceleration of growth is commonly observed for transplantable tumors in animals and probably results in part from decreasing tumor vascularity and cellular nutrition leading to slowing of cell proliferation and increasing cell death.[3] Many human tumors also develop necrosis and are subject to the same processes, so that more rapid growth of small, well-vascularized preclinical tumors seems likely. Mathematical models have been used to fit tumor growth curves that show deceleration of growth, such as the Gompertz equation, but clinical data are insufficient to define a precise model.

Shackney and co-workers[4] have estimated the period of preclinical growth of some human tumors. They studied groups of patients in whom a proportion of tumors were cured by treatment and assumed that tumor recurrence in the remainder was due to proliferation from a small number of residual tumor cells. The time of appearance of recurrent nodules in the chest wall after mastectomy for breast cancer suggested that tumor growth was more rapid during the preclinical phase. In contrast, rapidly progressive tumors such as Burkitt's lymphoma and Wilms' tumor appeared to have grown exponentially at a fairly constant rate.

It is possible that there is a period of slow growth following initiation of some tumors because of the requirement for stimulation of a blood supply[5] and the possibility that the tumor has to escape immunologic and other host defense mechanisms. This effect is observed after transplantation of some tumors in animals, but there are no data for human tumors that allow one to judge the validity of this concept.

Analysis of tumor growth in terms of the proliferation and death of constituent cells will be explored in the following sections.

CELL KINETICS OF HUMAN TUMORS

BASIC CONCEPTS

Must of the available information about cell kinetics of human tumors and normal tissues has been derived from studies using ³H-thymidine and autoradiography. More recently these techniques have been largely superseded by techniques based on flow cytometry, but many of the principles of experimental design are similar.

When ³H-thymidine is injected into animals (including humans), it is incorporated into the DNA that is being synthesized while the remainder is rapidly broken down and excreted as tritiated water. Labeled cells can be recognized in autoradiographs that are prepared by covering tissue sections with photographic emulsion followed by prolonged exposure in the dark (Fig. 1-3); the short range of β-particles released from tritium (mean range $\sim$0.5 μm) exposes only the film immediately overlying the cell nucleus and leads to good resolution of labeled and unlabeled cells.

Classification of the cell cycle into discrete phases followed the demonstration that DNA synthesis took place during a defined time interval, rather than continuously during interphase.[6] The intervals between mitosis (*M*) and DNA synthesis (*S*) were termed the G_1 and G_2 phase (G = gap), thus providing the familiar terminology of Figure 1-4.

In normal renewal tissues such as the bone marrow, small intestine, and skin, cells lose their ability to proliferate as they undergo differentiation, and the production of new cells by mitosis is matched by loss of differentiated cells from the population. Mendelsohn[7] showed that many cells in tumors may also be nonproliferative, and there is evidence that both differentiation and poor nutrition may cause cells to become quiescent. The term growth fraction was applied to the proportion of cells that were in cycle; because most anticancer drugs have greater activity for cycling cells, tumors with high values of growth fraction might be expected to be most responsive to chemotherapy.

The presence of necrosis or pyknotic cells is evidence for cell death in tumors, and the rate of cell death or loss from human tumors can be a high proportion of the rate of cell production.[8] Because of nonproliferating cells and cell loss, the volume doubling time of human tumors is (fortunately) much longer than the mean cell cycle time of the constituent cells. Many tumors may be thought of as analogous to renewal tissues, with only a slight imbalance between production and loss of cells which leads to tumor growth; indeed, tumors have been described as "caricatures" of normal tissue renewal.[9]

The analogy between tumors and renewal tissues may be extended to include the concept of stem cells. In normal renewal populations, there is evidence for the existence of a small population of stem cells whose progeny can proliferate and differentiate to repopulate the tissue. The following evidence suggests that in many tumors there may be only a small subpopulation (also referred to as stem cells) that has the capacity for indefinite proliferation.

1. Tissue-specific differentiation occurs in many human tumors, suggesting the retention of properties of renewal tissues. Studies of thymidine labeling in some animal tumors have shown that differentiated cells (which cannot form tumors on transplantation) are

FIG. 1-3. Autoradiograph of a tumor section. Labeled cells that have taken up ³H-thymidine may be recognized by grains in the photographic emulsion immediately overlying the cell nucleus.

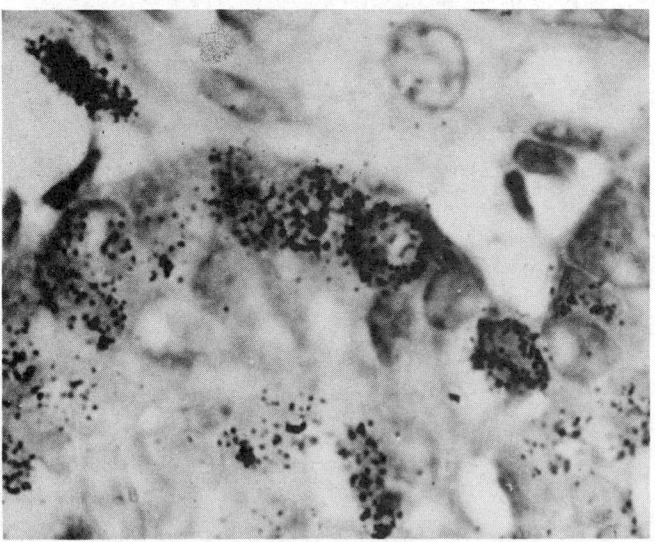

FIG. 1-4. Model of a tumor cell population. The tumor contains proliferating cells (referred to as the growth fraction) and nonproliferating cells. The latter population may include cells that have lost the ability to proliferate (*e.g.*, by differentiation) or cells that can revert to proliferation if factors such as cellular nutrition improve. Most tumors contain a high rate of cell death or loss from the tumor.

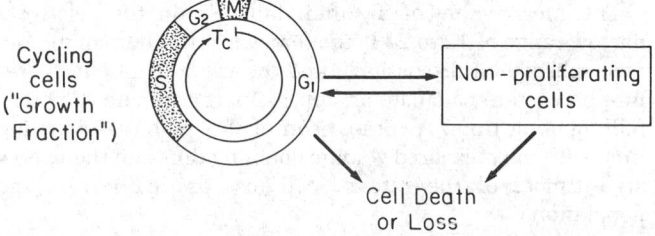

derived from undifferentiated cells that have the ability to generate tumors when implanted into new hosts.[10]

2. The ability to control some human tumors by tolerated doses of radiation is consistent with the radiobiological properties of constituent cells only if one assumes that the target cell population (*i.e.*, stem cells) is much smaller than the total number of cells in the tumor.[11]

3. Growth of colonies from human tumor cells in culture occurs from only a small proportion (usually < 0.1%) of the population.[12,13] Although this property may reflect the imperfect nature of the tissue culture environment, cells from some tumors may be separated by physical means into those with colony-forming potential (*i.e.*, putative stem cells) and those with markers of differentiation.[14]

It is important to distinguish between the proliferative state of a cell and its proliferative potential. There is evidence that pluripotential stem cells in the bone marrow have low frequency of cell division in the absence of stress;[15] in contrast, myeloblasts and myelocytes proliferate rapidly but are not stem cells. Similarly, the proliferative state of a tumor cell gives no information about its ability to produce large numbers of progeny, or its "stemness." Commonly used techniques involving thymidine autoradiography or flow cytometry give information about the proliferative status of the entire cell population. Recognition of cells with large proliferative potential requires an assay of colony formation, and special techniques are required to examine the proliferation kinetics of colony-forming tumor cells.

TRITIATED THYMIDINE AND AUTORADIOGRAPHY

The proportion of cells that is labeled following a short (usually 1 hr) exposure to ^{3}H-thymidine has been termed the labeling index (LI). The LI is often determined by incubation of tissue biopsies with ^{3}H-thymidine in vitro. Provided that the isotope is available to all of the cells, LI represents the proportion of cells in DNA synthesis at the time of ^{3}H-thymidine exposure. LI is thus a measure of the rate of cell production and is related to the duration of DNA synthesis (T_s) and potential doubling time (T) of a tumor population by the formula

$$LI = \lambda \frac{T_s}{T} \qquad (1)$$

Here λ is a factor that is typically about 0.8.[1] The potential doubling time (T) is the doubling time that the tumor would have in the absence of cell loss; it would be equal to mean cell cycle time (T_c) only if all of the cells were in cycle.

The mean value of T_s often falls within the relatively narrow range of 12 to 24 hours for a variety of human tumors (see subsequent discussion), and the value of LI can therefore be used to calculate an approximate estimate of potential doubling time. A comparison of this potential doubling time with the measured volume doubling time can then allow an estimate of the rate of cell loss or death from the population.[8]

Estimation of the duration of individual phases of the cell cycle requires more complex techniques, such as the percent labeled mitoses (PLM) method. The technique requires a single injection of ^{3}H-thymidine followed by the preparation of autoradiographs from sections of serial biopsies; for this reason it is now rarely used in humans, but historically it has provided the most detailed information about the kinetics of selected human tumors.

Percent labeled mitoses curves are generated by plotting the percentage of mitotic cells that are labeled in autoradiographs as a function of time after administration of ^{3}H-thymidine. Under idealized conditions in which there is no variation in the duration of cell cycle phases, the cohort of labeled cells that were initially in S-phase generates successive waves of labeled mitoses as it passes around the cell cycle (Figs. 1-5A and B). These waves of labeled mitoses are of width T_s (*i.e.*, the "width" of the labeled cohort), and of periodicity T_c. In practice, the PLM curve becomes damped because of variability in the duration of cell cycle phases (Fig. 1-5C) but can be analyzed by computer methods to obtain an approximate distribution of cell cycle phase times.

The growth fraction may be estimated from the value of LI

FIG. 1-5. The percent labeled mitoses (PLM) technique. After administration of ^{3}H-thymidine, the cohort of labeled cells moves around the cycle as shown in **A**. Under the idealized conditions in which individual phase times do not vary, the percentage of labeled mitoses varies with time as shown in **B**. Here points a, b, c, d, and e on the curve are derived from the corresponding cycle diagrams of panel **A**. **C** depicts an experimental curve, derived by Shirakawa *et al*[16] for human melanoma. Damping occurs because of variability in cell cycle phase times, but the PLM curve can be analyzed by computer methods to give a distribution of cell cycle times (and of individual phase duration) for the tumor.

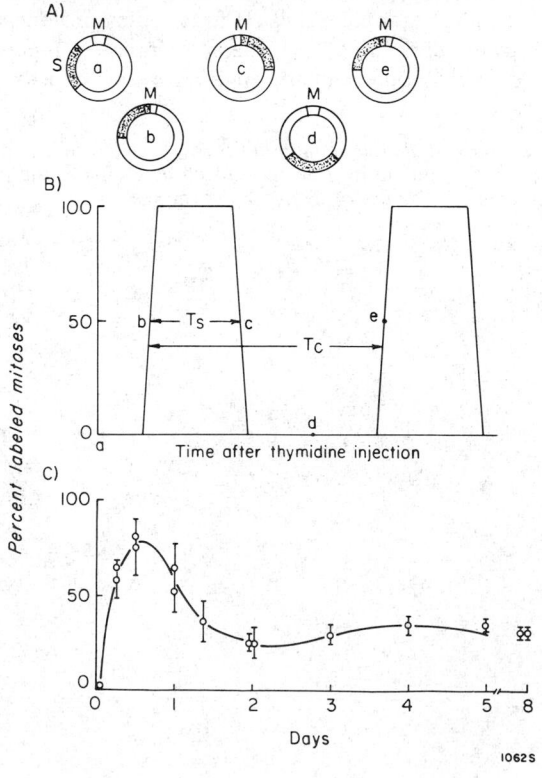

and the distribution of cell cycle phase times. Information about the phase distributions of cycling cells allows calculation of the proportion of proliferating cells that are in S-phase. Since the measured LI is the proportion of total cells in S-phase, the ratio of measured LI to the estimated S-phase fraction of cycling cells is a measure of growth fraction. An alternative method of estimating growth fraction is through determination of the proportion of cells that contain enzymes (*e.g.,* DNA-dependent DNA polymerase) that appear to be induced only in cycling cells.[17] Estimates of growth fraction should be regarded as approximate since techniques are not available to distinguish nonproliferating cells from those with cycle times longer than the mean.

FLOW CYTOMETRY

Techniques using ^{3}H-thymidine have the advantage of preserving tissue geometry, but they are labor-intensive and slow. Newer techniques based on flow cytometry have the major advantages of speed and automation.

The principal features of flow cytometry are the production of a suspension of single cells, their staining with a fluorescent dye, and the derivation of a distribution of fluorescence intensity. The latter is achieved by passing the cells in single file through a laser beam which excites the fluorescence, as shown in Figure 1-6.
An electric charge may be applied to cells of different fluorescence intensity, so that they can be separated in an electrostatic field, allowing their further chemical or biological characterization. This is known as fluorescence-activated cell sorting. Flow cytometry may be used to study a wide variety of cellular properties, depending only on the availability of appropriate fluorescent probes.

For most studies of cell kinetics, fluorescent dyes are used (*e.g.,* acridine orange or propidium iodide) whose binding is proportional to DNA content. The fluorescence intensity thus allows derivation of the distribution of DNA content among the cells of the population (Fig. 1-7). Computer methods are used to estimate the proportion of cells in the G_1, S, and G_2/M phases of the cell cycle from the DNA distribution. Estimates of the proportion of S-phase cells by flow cytometry tend to be slightly higher than estimates of LI determined using ^{3}H-thymidine and autoradiography. By comparison with normal diploid cells as a standard, the flow cytometer also allows detection of aneuploid cells.

Recent innovations have allowed more complex analysis of cell cycle parameters by flow cytometry. Many of these methods have utilized "labeling" of cells by nonradioactive

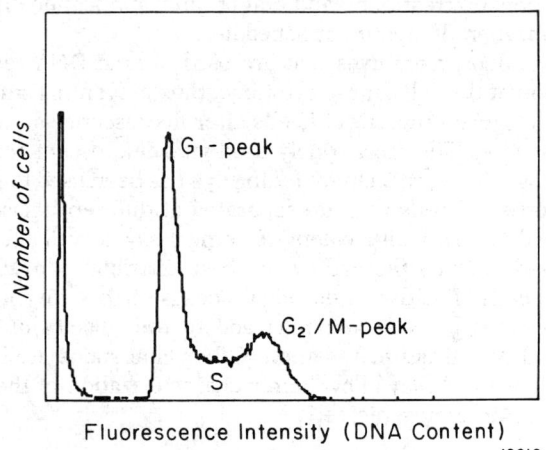

FIG. 1-7. A DNA histogram produced by flow cytometry. Cells of a human bladder cancer cell line were labeled with acridine orange. The peak at the origin represents cellular debris. The DNA distribution may be analyzed by computer methods to estimate the proportion of cells in G_1, S, and G_2/M phases of the cell cycle.

FIG. 1-6. The principal features of a flow cytometer. Single cells are labeled with a fluorescent probe and are directed in single file through a laser beam. Analysis of forward angle light scatter can be used to estimate cell volume. Fluorescence emission from the excited cell then provides a distribution of fluorescence intensity. Electric charge that is related to fluorescence intensity can also be applied to droplets containing single cells, allowing their separation in an electrostatic field. This process is known as fluorescence-activated cell sorting.

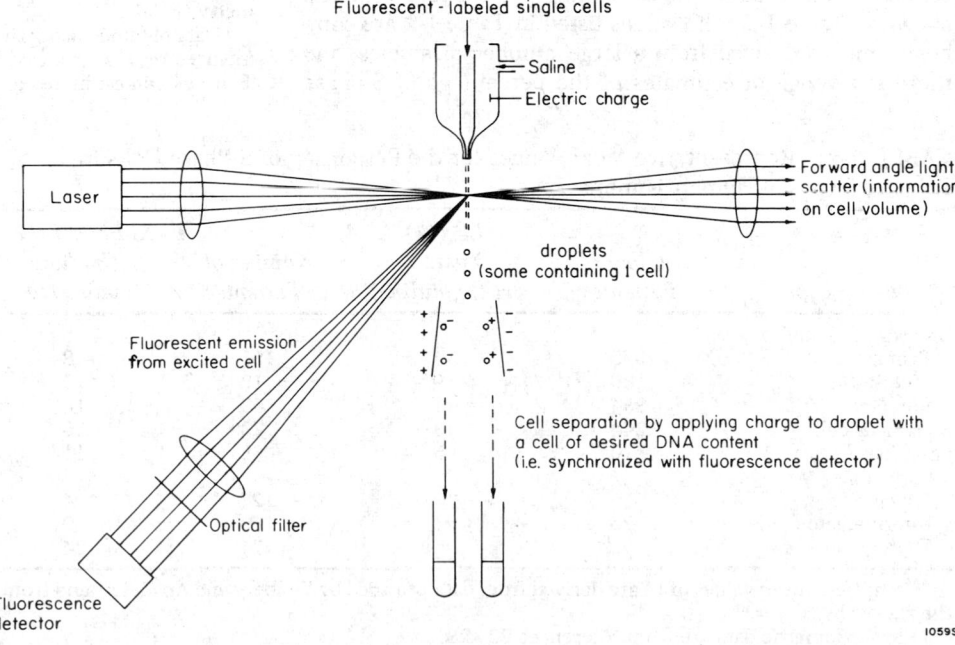

bromodeoxyuridine (BrdUrd), which, like thymidine, is taken up into S-phase cells of the cycle.[18] BrdUrd that is incorporated into DNA may then be detected by flow cytometry, using a fluorescent labeled monoclonal antibody directed against incorporated BrdUrd. A recent application of the BrdUrd method allows estimation of T_s and potential doubling time from a single biopsy.[19] The biopsy is usually taken about 3 hours after i.v. administration of BrdUrd, and two-parameter flow cytometry then allows recognition of the movement of the BrdUrd tagged cells (recognized by the fluorescent monoclonal antibody) through S-phase (defined by their DNA content using propidium iodide or a similar stain). The method is currently being used to determine the potential doubling time of selected human tumors before initiation of treatment and might find application in the optimization of treatment schedules.

Most fluorescent dyes that are used to bind DNA require fixation of the cells or are cytotoxic, thus preventing study of the biological properties of cells after fluorescence-activated cell sorting. The most widely used vital fluorescent stain is Hoechst 33342; this DNA-binding dye has been used to study properties of cells that are separated at different phases of the cell cycle and, if a colony-forming assay is available, can be used to study the cell cycle phase distribution of clonogenic cells. The dye is not ideal because it has toxicity for some types of cells and may add to the toxicity of cells treated with drugs or radiation. Other vital stains are being developed and may allow better characterization of the cell kinetics of clonogenic cells.

KINETIC PROPERTIES OF HUMAN TUMORS

The proportion of tumor cells undergoing DNA synthesis, as measured by thymidine labeling index or from DNA histograms generated by flow cytometry, gives a relatively simple measure of the overall rate of cell proliferation. Data are available for most types of human malignancy, and representative estimates of the percentage of S-phase cells are shown in Table 1-2. The values listed in Table 1-2 are composite means derived from a large number of studies, and there is a range of estimates of the percentage of S-phase

cells for each type of tumor. In general, there is a correlation between the proportion of S-phase cells with increasing tumor grade and with aneuploidy.

The data in Table 1-2 indicate that many solid tumors in humans contain at most 10% cells that are in DNA synthesis, although higher proportions of S-phase cells are found in some rapidly growing tumors such as high-grade lymphomas. Proliferating cells in normal bone marrow and intestinal crypts have values of labeling index in the ranges of 30% to 70% and 12% to 18%, respectively. Thus, tumors do not have a higher proportion of S-phase cells than some normal tissues.

Published information about the duration of the cell cycle and its constituent phases in human tumors has been derived mainly from percent labeled mitoses experiments, and some of these data are summarized in Table 1-3. Recently, flow cytometry after administration of BrdUrd has allowed rapid estimation of the duration of DNA synthesis for several types of human tumor. These studies suggest that the mean duration of DNA synthesis is usually in the range of 12 to 24

TABLE 1-3. Estimates of Mean Duration of DNA Synthesis (T_s) and Cycle Time (T_c) Obtained for Selected Human Tumors

Tumor Type	Mean T_s (h) By FCM*	Mean T_s (h) By PLM†	Mean T_c (days) By PLM†
Melanoma	9	21	2.5
Breast		21	2.5
Squamous cell of head and neck	12	20	2.5
Lung	26	20	4.5
Colon and rectum	25	17	3.0
Lymphomas	16	12	2.0
Acute leukemias	11	22	2.5

*Unpublished data of Wilson GD et al (personal communication) obtained by in vivo administration of BrdUrd followed by flow cytometry (FCM).
†Data obtained using the percent labeled mitoses method (PLM). Includes results reviewed by Steel[1] and Tannock.[29] Mean values of T_c have been estimated to the nearest ½ day.

TABLE 1-2. Representative Mean Values for the Proportion of S-Phase Cells in Selected Types of Human Tumors

Tumor Type	Number of Patients	LI* (%) (using ³H-thymidine)	Number of Patients	S-Phase† (%) (by flow cytometry)
Breast				
Primary	1075	4	151	8
Metastatic	80	9	12	10
Colorectal	284	11	53	18
Squamous cell	244	13	73	19
Sarcomas	70	5	68	11
Lymphomas				
Low grade			127	4
Intermediate grade	79	21	179	9
High grade			74	24

*Composite mean values of LI are derived from data provided by Wolberg and Ansfield[20] and from the review by Meyer.[21]
†Flow cytometric data are from references 22–28.

hours, with mean cell cycle times of 2 to 4 days. The latter estimates must be regarded as approximate because the available techniques are not sufficiently sensitive to distinguish between nonproliferating cells and those with longer cycle times. The mean cycle time of cells within human tumors (typically 2–4 days) is much shorter than the mean volume doubling time of the tumors (typically 2–3 months for common solid tumors). Two factors contribute to this difference: a high proportion of nonproliferating cells and a high rate of cell death.

Estimates of growth fraction obtained by comparing the measured proportion of S-phase cells (by flow cytometry or labeling index) with that predicted from the phase distribution of cycling cells are often consistent with values of growth fraction of the order of 20% to 30%. Tumor cells may be out of cycle because of differentiation or because of limited access to nutrients. There is marked heterogeneity in patterns of thymidine labeling within solid tumors, and the rate of cellular proliferation has been found to decrease rapidly with increasing distance from capillaries in both animal and human tumors.[30,31] This effect may lead to large errors in estimates of LI that are obtained from small biopsies. The observation may also be relevant to therapy in that it defines a population of poorly nourished cells that is known to be resistant to radiation because of hypoxia, and that may be resistant to chemotherapy because of limited drug access and a low rate of cellular proliferation.

The observation of necrosis and pyknotic cells in human tumors is evidence for cell death, and cells may also be lost from the tumor by shedding (e.g., into the bowel) or through blood vessels and lymphatics. Steel[8] has estimated the rate of cell loss in various human tumors by comparing their potential doubling time (see Equation 1), which is the expected doubling time of the tumor in the absence of cell loss, with measured volume doubling times. The rate of cell loss is frequently found to be 80% or more of the rate of cell production. This observation supports the concept that tumors may be regarded as analogues of cell renewal tissues, but where the normal balance between cell production and loss is modified in favor of a slight excess of cell production.

DIAGNOSIS AND PROGNOSIS

FLOW CYTOMETRY AS A DIAGNOSTIC TOOL

Flow cytometry is being used increasingly as an aid in cancer diagnosis and histologic classification. Useful information can be obtained from DNA histograms and from using an increasing array of monoclonal antibodies to detect surface markers or cytoplasmic determinants of cells.

About 70% of all tumors have cells with abnormal DNA content.[32] DNA-specific staining of effusions or tissue biopsies, followed by flow cytometry, can detect a small proportion of aneuploid tumor cells mixed with normal diploid cells. This technique has been used to study the urine of patients who are suspected of having bladder cancer, and in one large study was shown to have a sensitivity of 80%, superior to that of conventional cytology.[33] The technique has also been studied as an alternative to cervical and vaginal cytology; it has the potential advantages of automation and objectivity, but the presence of inflammatory cells and cellular debris and clumps, resulting from imperfect methods for dissociation of tissue into single cells, may complicate the analysis. Future improvements in techniques for cellular dissociation, and simultaneous measurement of DNA content and cellular size by forward-angle light scatter, may allow increased use of flow cytometry in the diagnosis of solid tumors.

Dispersion of cells is not a problem in the study of lymphoma and leukemia, and flow cytometry is used increasingly in their diagnosis and classification. Subtypes of human leukemia and lymphoma may be differentiated by using fluorescence-labeled monoclonal antibodies directed against a variety of cellular antigens, including T-cell antigens, surface or cytoplasmic immunoglobulins, and common acute lymphocytic leukemia antigen (CALLA), among others. These methods not only are useful as a guide to classification but also may influence treatment, since different subtypes of leukemia are optimally treated with different drugs. Similar techniques may provide diagnostic information in the acquired immune deficiency syndrome (AIDS). The ratio of T-helper to T-suppressor cells can be measured by flow cytometry as the ratio of lymphoid cells expressing the T_4 or T_8 antigens, and in healthy individuals is usually in the range of 1.7 to 2.0. In patients with AIDS, the ratio is less than 1.0, although it may also be slightly decreased in homosexual men who are not infected with the AIDS virus.

It is sometimes difficult to diagnose B-cell lymphomas, as compared to reactive hyperplasia, by histologic criteria. B-cells express immunoglobulins on their cell surface, and differential diagnosis can be achieved by using a flow cytometric technique that detects an excess of cells expressing either κ or λ light chains with the aid of fluorescent monoclonal antibodies.[34] The ratio of κ- to λ-expressing cells is normally close to 1.0, and an excess of either cell type indicates clonal proliferation of one type of cell and implies the presence of lymphoma.

An increasing number of monoclonal antibodies are becoming available that react with antigenic determinants that have some degree of specificity for various types of malignant cells. Flow cytometry may allow the detection of a small subpopulation of cells that carry such determinants among a much larger population of normal cells, and it is likely to be used increasingly in cancer diagnosis.

PROGNOSIS

Before the availability of flow cytometry, a number of studies had attempted to correlate values of pretreatment labeling index of human tumors (measured usually by in vitro incubation with ^{3}H-thymidine) and prognosis. Some investigators reported improved prognosis with lower values of labeling index, but others reported the opposite. The probable reason for this discrepancy is that patients with tumors having a lower labeling index were likely to have slowly progressive disease but, because most drugs are more active against proliferating cells, were also less likely to respond to chemotherapy. The technique is time consuming, and most studies were based on small samples of patients with various stages of disease and other prognostic factors.

The ability of flow cytometry to provide rapid, automated analysis of large numbers of cells has prompted a reexamination of the relevance of cell kinetic parameters to prognosis. It is now possible to perform flow cytometry studies using cells dissociated from paraffin-embedded sections.[35] Series of patients who have received uniform treatment in clinical trials and for whom complete clinical follow-up is available can thus be studied retrospectively using archival material obtained from pathology departments. This powerful approach is being applied to large groups of patients with several types of tumors.

Two properties of DNA histograms may be correlated with prognosis: ploidy as measured by the DNA index (the mean DNA content of G_1-cells in the tumor as compared to a DNA index of 1 for normal diploid G_1 cells); and the percentage of S-phase cells. Data from some larger studies are summarized in Table 1-4, and for most (but not all) tumor types, aneuploidy is associated with higher grade and poorer prognosis. In ovarian cancer, for example, aneuploidy was the most critical determinant of prognosis when analyzed with other potential prognostic factors by multivariate analysis.[36] Aneuploid tumors also tended to have a higher proportion of S-phase cells, but in general the correlation of prognosis with S-phase proportion was weak.

Flow cytometry may also provide useful information about hormone receptors in malignant cells. The presence of high estrogen and progestin receptor levels in breast cancer is known to be associated with a more favorable prognosis and is strongly predictive of response to hormonal therapy. Hormone receptors in cells may be detected by flow cytometry with the aid of fluorescence-labeled hormones that recognize the receptors. When perfected, this technique will have the advantage of speed and automation and will allow assessment of heterogeneity of receptor content among the cells of the population, rather than just the average value that is obtained by conventional methods. This information may be of additional prognostic value and might also guide the more appropriate use of hormones in cancer treatment.

CELL KINETICS AND TREATMENT

CYCLE-DEPENDENCE OF THERAPY

Rapidly growing tumors tend to be most sensitive to chemotherapy. Also, damage to normal tissues at short intervals after chemotherapy or wide-field radiation is most often observed in organs such as the bone marrow or the intestine, which are renewal tissues known to contain rapidly proliferating cells. These observations suggest that rapidly proliferating cells may be more susceptible to therapy and have led to several studies of the relationship between cytotoxicity and proliferative rate.

When mammalian cells are cultured, they show a period of exponential growth when all cells are proliferating, followed by slowing of growth as cells become crowded and consume available nutrients. The culture reaches a maximum size in plateau phase, when cell proliferation is very slow (Fig. 1-8A). The effects of a given treatment on rapidly and slowly proliferating cells may therefore be studied by assessing colony formation in new cultures following treatment of cells in exponential and plateau phase. Frequently this type of experiment leads to survival curves similar to those in Figure 1-8B, which show that rapidly proliferating cells are more sensitive to the drug. This technique and others (e.g., the spleen colony assay[38]) have demonstrated that some drugs (e.g., methotrexate, cytarabine, and vinca alkaloids) exert lethal effects only against proliferating cells. Others, including anthracyclines and most alkylating agents, have some activity against slowly proliferating cells but are considerably more toxic to rapidly proliferating cells.[29] Only for a few drugs, including cisplatin, nitrosoureas, and bleomycin, is there little or no selectivity, and this may be cell-line dependent.

Most drugs and ionizing radiation vary in their lethal effects at different phases of the cell cycle. This phenomenon has been studied either by synchronizing cells in a given cell cycle phase[39] or by sorting cells at different phases of the cycle immediately before or after treatment, followed by a cloning assay to assess their viability. Cells may be separated in different phases of the cell cycle by using fluorescence-activated cell sorting, although this technique is currently limited because available nontoxic fluorescent stains for DNA may influence the cytotoxicity of anticancer drugs or radiation.[40] An alternative method, centrifugal elutriation, separates cells on the basis of size in a continuous flow centrifuge and has been useful in obtaining information about treatment effects during the cell cycle. These methods have demonstrated that many drugs exert their maximum lethal effects when cells are synthesizing DNA (Fig. 1-9); this is true for most of the antimetabolites and for anthracyclines. Vinblastine and vincristine also exert their cytotoxic action in the S-phase, although cells may arrest and die when they subsequently attempt to pass through mitosis. For ionizing radiation and many alkylating agents, the pattern of toxicity

TABLE 1-4.   Prognostic Significance of Cellular DNA Content in Selected Human Tumors

Tumor Type	Survival Advantage for Diploid Tumors
Breast*	+
Ovary*	+
Cervix	+
Endometrium	+
Prostate	+
Bladder	+
Kidney	+
Lung	+
Colon	+
Melanoma	−
Brain tumors	−
ALL	−
AML	+
Myeloma*	+
Lymphomas	±

From data reviewed in Friedlander, et al[36] and Cornelisse, et al.[37]
*Ploidy has been shown to be an independent prognostic variable in postmenopausal breast cancer, ovarian cancer, and myeloma.

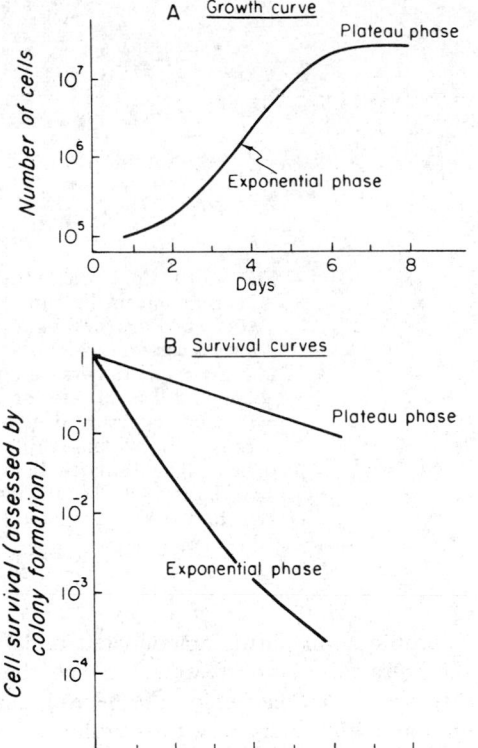

FIG. 1-8. **A.** Cells in tissue culture show a period of rapid proliferation and exponential growth, followed by slowing of growth and a plateau phase as nutrients are depleted and cell concentration increases. **B.** The effect of drugs against slowly and rapidly proliferating cells can be assessed by treatment of cell cultures in exponential and plateau phase. Cells are then replated to assess survival by colony formation. Most drugs show greater toxicity for rapidly proliferating cells in exponential growth phase, as in the example shown.

FIG. 1-9. The position in the cell cycle at which anticancer drugs and radiation most often exert their maximum lethal toxicity. Drugs and radiation may also act to delay progression around the cycle (*e.g.*, vinblastine and vincristine induce mitotic arrest).

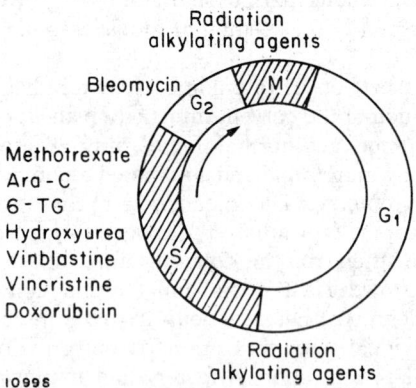

is more complex with two periods of maximum activity, one for cells near the G_1/S transition and one for G_2-phase or mitotic cells.

SCHEDULING OF CHEMOTHERAPY

Because most drugs have varying toxicity for cells in different phases of the cell cycle, immediately after treatment a high proportion of surviving cells will be partially synchronized in a resistant phase. Several investigators have proposed that drug treatment might be scheduled at intervals that allow the synchronized surviving tumor cells to progress to a drug-sensitive phase of the cell cycle, or, conversely, such that cells in critical normal tissues are again in a drug-resistant phase. In practice, the wide heterogeneity of cell cycle parameters among individual cells and of drug distribution makes this difficult to achieve.

It has been demonstrated that therapeutic outcome is markedly dependent on scheduling interval for drug treatment of experimental tumors,[41] but it has been difficult to predict the optimum scheduling interval from knowledge of cell cycle kinetics.[29] It is probable that the interval between injection of cycle-specific drugs within a given course of chemotherapy could have a strong influence on therapeutic outcome in humans, but, at present, any improvements in scheduling are likely to be achieved by empirical means.

Knowledge of the cell population kinetics in critical normal tissues is important in understanding the basis for scheduling of successive courses of chemotherapy. Scheduling is based on a need for recovery between courses of critical normal tissues, most frequently the bone marrow or intestinal mucosa. A schematic illustration of cell proliferation in the bone marrow is shown in Figure 1-10. Pluripotential stem cells normally have a low rate of cell proliferation and are therefore protected from toxicity of cycle-dependent drugs. In contrast, rapidly proliferating granulocyte precursors (myeloblasts, promyelocytes, and myelocytes) are depleted by chemotherapy; this leads to a delayed fall in granulocyte count, since more mature nonproliferating precursors such as metamyelocytes and bands continue to differentiate into mature granulocytes within the first few days after drug treatment. Thereafter, the granulocyte count falls rapidly to a nadir, usually reached at 10 to 14 days after treatment. For some drugs (*e.g.*, vinblastine), the nadir occurs earlier, and there is evidence that many other drugs delay the process of maturation.

Drugs also exert toxic effects against proliferating red cell precursors and megakaryocytes, but the granulocyte count is most susceptible to chemotherapy because mature cells have a short lifespan. When the granulocyte count falls, feedback mechanisms induce stem cells to cycle, leading to recovery that for most drugs is complete within 3 to 4 weeks. This provides the basis for the usual interval between courses of chemotherapy; reinitiation of chemotherapy at earlier intervals may expose stem cells to drugs when they are cycling and cause permanent damage to bone marrow.

The delayed fall in granulocyte count has allowed the development of schedules in which cycle-active drugs are given on days 1 and 8 of a 4-week cycle. This strategy has been used in regimens such as mechlorethamine, vincristine, pro-

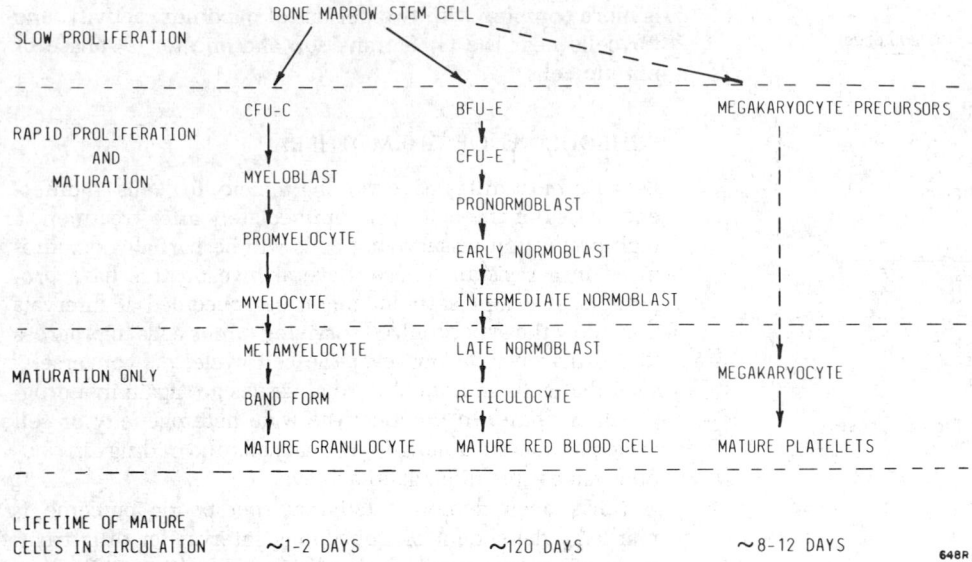

FIG. 1-10. Cell proliferation and differentiation in the bone marrow. Toxicity of drugs for rapidly proliferating precursors leads to a delayed fall in the peripheral granulocyte count. A fall in platelet or erythrocyte count is observed more rarely because of the longer lifetime of these cells. (Tannock IF, Hill RP: The Basic Science of Oncology. Elmsford, NY, Pergamon Press, 1987)

carbazine, and prednisone (MOPP) for Hodgkin's disease and cyclophosphamide, methotrexate, and 5-fluorouracil (CMF) for breast cancer. The second injection of drugs at 1 week after the first is tolerated because the bone marrow stem cells have not yet been stimulated to proliferate, since the second treatment precedes the fall in peripheral granulocyte count.

Some drugs, including melphalan, nitrosoureas, and mitomycin C, cause more prolonged myelosuppression. These drugs show little selectivity for cycling cells and may therefore be expected to damage stem cells. Evidence for damage to stem cells is shown by the decreased ability of murine stem cells to repopulate the marrow following serial treatment with BCNU or melphalan, as compared to treatment with cyclophosphamide, doxorubicin, or 5-fluorouracil.[42,43] These results agree with the clinical experience that cumulative myelosuppression is more common after treatment with BCNU or melphalan.

SCHEDULING OF RADIOTHERAPY

It has been found empirically that radiation treatment may be both effective and tolerated when delivered as a course of small dose fractions (usually 200 cGy or less) over several weeks. Several processes take place between fractions, including repair of sublethal damage, repopulation of surviving cells, redistribution of surviving cells to more radiosensitive phases of the cell cycle, and, in tumors, improvement in cellular oxygenation. Repair and repopulation between fractions are the major processes that allow normal tissues to tolerate protracted fractionated radiation with acceptable levels of damage.

Scheduling of radiotherapy has developed empirically, and most patients are treated daily from Monday to Friday. It is known from animal models that the interval between radiation doses may influence the outcome of therapy, and there has been recent interest in attempting to modify radiation fractionation in an attempt to improve therapeutic index.

Tumor cell proliferation during fractionated radiotherapy may limit the overall success of treatment; hence, there may be therapeutic gain from shortening the overall treatment time for tumors in which surviving cells proliferate rapidly during treatment,[44] provided that dose-limiting normal tissues within the radiation field are slowly proliferating. Several investigators are attempting to measure pretreatment cell cycle parameters, particularly the potential doubling time of constituent cells, using BrdUrd incorporation and flow cytometry. Tumors with rapid proliferation are then treated using accelerated fractionation in which three or more doses are delivered each day, whereas slowly proliferating tumors are treated by conventional fractionation schedules. Data are not yet available to judge the benefits of this approach, but it represents an attempt to improve the outcome of radiotherapy that is based on sound scientific principles.

CONCLUSION

Human tumors often grow exponentially during a period of clinical observation, and typical volume doubling times for common solid tumors are in the range of 2 to 3 months. Tumors have a long period of preclinical growth, offering ample opportunity for seeding of metastases before clinical detection.

Methods based on ^{3}H-thymidine and autoradiography have provided much of the current information about cell kinetics of human tumors and normal tissues, but they are now being supplanted by more rapid and automated techniques employing flow cytometry. The mean cell cycle time of many human tumors is typically in the range of 2 to 4 days, much shorter than their volume doubling time; this is consistent with a low growth fraction and a high rate of cell loss. There is a large degree of heterogeneity in cell kinetic properties within individual tumors. Tumors do not grow because the rate of cell proliferation is faster than in normal tissues;

rather, they grow because the rate of cell production exceeds the rate of cell death.

About 70% of all tumors have abnormal DNA content, and flow cytometry can aid diagnosis by detecting a small proportion of aneuploid tumor cells mixed with normal diploid cells. With the aid of fluorescence-labeled monoclonal antibodies, flow cytometry is used increasingly to characterize the phenotype of malignant cells, especially in the classification of lymphomas and leukemias. DNA histograms have also been generated from paraffin-embedded sections of a variety of tumors, and for many human tumors aneuploidy is associated with poor prognosis.

Most anticancer drugs show greater toxicity for rapidly proliferating cells, and drugs and radiation have variable activity around the cell cycle. It is unlikely that these effects can be used to increase therapeutic index through synchronization of cells because of heterogeneity in cell cycle parameters and drug distribution. The greater sensitivity of rapidly proliferating cells suggests an explanation for the greater responsiveness of rapidly growing tumors to chemotherapy and allows an understanding of the fall and recovery of the granulocyte count following drug treatment. Proliferation of tumor cells during a course of fractionated radiation therapy may limit the success of treatment, and it may be possible to develop accelerated fractionation schedules for tumors with rapid cell proliferation following evaluation of their cycle kinetics by flow cytometry.

REFERENCES

1. Steel GG: Growth Kinetics of Tumours: Cell Population Kinetics in Relation to the Growth and Treatment of Cancer. Oxford, Clarendon Press, 1977
2. Tannock IF, Hill RP: The Basic Science of Oncology. Elmsford, NY, Pergamon Press, 1987
3. Tannock IF: Biology of tumor growth. Hosp Pract [Off] 18:81, 1983
4. Shackney SE, McCormack GW, Cuchural GJ Jr: Growth rate patterns of solid tumors and their relation to responsiveness to therapy. An analytical review. Ann Intern Med 89:107, 1978
5. Folkman J: Tumor angiogenesis: A possible control point in tumor growth. Ann Intern Med 82:96, 1975
6. Howard A, Pelc SR: Nuclear incorporation of P^{32} as demonstrated by autoradiographs. J Exp Cell Res 2:178, 1951
7. Mendelsohn ML: The growth fraction: A new concept applied to tumours. Science 132:1496, 1960
8. Steel GG: Cell loss as a factor in the growth rate of human tumours. Eur J Cancer Clin Oncol 3:381, 1967
9. Pierce GB, Shikes R, Fink LM: Cancer: A Problem of Developmental Biology. Englewood Cliffs, NJ, Prentice-Hall, 1978
10. Pierce GB, Wallace C: Differentiation of malignant to benign cells. Cancer Res 31:127, 1971
11. Bush RS, Hill RP: Biological discussion augmenting radiation effects and model systems. Laryngoscope 85:1119, 1975
12. Hamburger AW, Salmon SE: Primary bioassay of human myeloma stem cells. J Clin Invest 60:846, 1977
13. Courtenay VD, Selby PJ, Smith IE, et al: Growth of human tumour cell colonies from biopsies using two soft-agar techniques. Br J Cancer 38:77, 1978
14. MacKillop WJ, Stewart SS, Buick RN: Density/volume analysis in the study of cellular heterogeneity in human ovarian carcinoma. Br J Cancer 45:812, 1982
15. Fauser AA, Messner HA: Proliferative state of human pluripotent hemopoietic progenitors (CFU-GEMM) in normal individuals and under regenerative conditions after bone marrow transplantation. Blood 54:1197, 1979.
16. Shirakawa S, Luce JK, Tannock I, et al: Cell proliferation in human melanoma. J Clin Invest 49:1188, 1970
17. Nelson JRS, Schiffer LM: Autoradiographic detection of DNA polymerase containing nuclei in sarcoma 180 ascites cells. Cell Tissue Kinet 6:45, 1973
18. Gray JW (ed): Monoclonal antibodies against bromodeoxyuridine. Cytometry 6:499, 1985
19. Begg AC, McNally NJ, Schrieve DC, et al: A method to measure the duration of DNA synthesis and the potential doubling time from a single sample. Cytometry 6:620, 1985
20. Wolberg WH, Ansfield FJ: The relation of thymidine labeling index in human tumors in vitro to the effectivness of 5-fluorouracil chemotherapy. Cancer Res 81:448, 1971
21. Meyer JS: Cell kinetic measurements of human tumors. Hum Pathol 13:874, 1982
22. Frankfurt OS, Greco WR, Slocum HK, et al: Proliferative characteristics of primary and metastatic human solid tumors by DNA flow cytometry. Cytometry 5:629, 1984
23. Johnson TS, Williamson KD, Cramer MM, et al: Flow cytometric analysis of head and neck carcinoma DNA index and S-fraction from paraffin-embedded sections: Comparison with malignancy grading. Cytometry 6:461, 1985
24. McDivitt RW, Stone KR, Craig RB, et al: A comparison of human breast cancer cell kinetics measured by flow cytometry and thymidine labeling. Lab Invest 52:287, 1985
25. Srigley J, Barlogie B, Butler JJ, et al: Heterogeneity of non-Hodgkin's lymphoma probed by nucleic acid cytometry. Blood 65:1090, 1985
26. Christensson B, Tribukait B, Linder I-L, et al: Cell proliferation and DNA content in non-Hodgkin's lymphoma: Flow cytometry in relation to lymphoma classification. Cancer 58:1295, 1986
27. Juneja SK, Cooper IA, Hodgson GS, et al: DNA ploidy patterns and cytokinetics of non-Hodgkin's lymphoma. J Clin Pathol 39:98, 1986
28. Kallioniemi O-P, Hietanen T, Mattila J, et al: Aneuploid DNA content and high S-phase fraction of tumor cells are related to poor prognosis in patients with primary breast cancer. Eur J Cancer Clin Oncol 23:277, 1987
29. Tannock I: Cell kinetics and chemotherapy: A critical review. Cancer Treat Rep 62:1117, 1978
30. Tannock IF: The relation between cell proliferation and the vascular system in a transplanted murine mammary tumour. Br J Cancer 22:258, 1968
31. Moore JV, Hasleton PS, Buckley CH: Tumour cords in 52 human bronchial and cervical squamous cell carcinomas: Inferences for their cellular kinetics and radiobiology. Br J Cancer 51:407, 1985
32. Barlogie B, Raber MN, Schumann J, et al: Flow cytometry in clinical cancer research. Cancer Res 43:3982, 1983
33. Badalament RA, Kimmel M, Gay H, et al: The sensitivity of flow cytometry compared with conventional cytology in the detection of superficial bladder carcinoma. Cancer 59:2078, 1987
34. Ault KA: Detection of small numbers of monoclonal B lymphocytes in the blood of patients with lymphoma. N Engl J Med 300:1401, 1979
35. Hedley DW, Friedlander ML, Taylor IW, et al: Method for analysis of cellular DNA content of paraffin embedded pathological material using flow cytometry. J Histochem Cytochem 31:1333, 1983
36. Friedlander ML, Hedley DW, Taylor IW: Clinical and biological significance of aneuploidy in human tumours. J Clin Pathol 37:961, 1984
37. Cornelisse CJ, Van de Velde CJH, Caspers RJC, et al: DNA ploidy and survival in breast cancer patients. Cytometry 8:225, 1987
38. Till JE, McCulloch EA: A direct measurement of the radiation sensitivity of normal mouse bone marrow cells. Radiat Res 14:213, 1961
38. Nias AH, Fox M: Synchronization of mammalian cells with respect to the mitotic cycle. Cell Tissue Kinet 4:375, 1971
40. Pallavicini MG, Lalande ME, Miller RG, et al: Cell cycle distribution of chronically hypoxic cells and determination of the clonogenic potential of cells accumulated in G_2 and M phases after irradiation of a solid tumor in vivo. Cancer Res 39:1891, 1979
41. Skipper HE, Schabel FM Jr, Wilcox WS: Experimental evaluation of potential anticancer agents. XXI. Scheduling of arabinosylcytosine to take advantage of its S-phase specificity against leukemic cells. Cancer Chemother Rep 54:125, 1967
42. Trainor KJ, Seshadri RS, Morley AA: Residual marrow injury following cytotoxic drugs.Leuk Res 3:205, 1979
43. Botnick LE, Hannon EC, Vigneulle R, et al: Differential effects of cytotoxic agents on hematopoietic progenitors. Cancer Res 41:2338, 1981
44. Denekamp J: Cell kinetics and radiation biology. Int J Radiat Biol 49:357, 1986

MICHAEL DEAN

GEORGE F. VANDE WOUDE

CHAPTER 2 — *Principles of Molecular Cell Biology of Cancer: Introduction to Methods in Molecular Biology*

For a major portion of this century and as recently as 1979, there was considerable controversy over whether viruses cause cancer or whether environmental insults to normal cell genes can initiate the cancer process.[1] Only during the past 4 years have we learned, as a result of extraordinary advances in biotechnology, that both viruses and genetic mutations can mediate neoplastic disease by similar mechanisms. Diverse basic research disciplines, woven together by technological breakthroughs in molecular biology and genetic engineering, have provided new concepts of the molecular basis of neoplastic disease. Absolute measurements in molecular biology and genetic engineering technologies have provided us with our first descriptions of the molecular elements responsible for triggering the events that lead to cancer. The terms DNA sequence, hybridization, molecular cloning, linkage analyses, and pulsed-field gel electrophoresis are part of a growing armamentarium of techniques used to identify, isolate, and characterize the molecular elements that have been implicated in normal and abnormal biological processes in human and animal cells (see Appendix.)

The recent achievements promise important applications of this new information for clinical diagnostics in human diseases and cancer, and for this purpose it is important to understand the technology and how it is used. Certainly, if specific cellular genes are shown to be associated with specific tumor types, like c-*myc* in Burkitt's lymphoma,[2] or c-*abl* in chronic myelogenous leukemia,[3-5] then the molecular biology tools become unambiguous diagnostic reagents. In cancer, we may be relating molecular alterations to types of proliferative growth, and it may be only the temporary lack of technical sophistication that prevents correlation of genetic and molecular changes with benign and preneoplastic (*e.g.*, hyperplasia, metaplasia, dysplasia, anaplasia) or malignant neoplastic cellular changes. The rapidly emerging biotechnology requires familiarization with the specialized terminology of molecular biology, including the key terms mentioned above. It is necessary to introduce the names of molecular structures and techniques used in molecular biology, molecular genetics, and genetic engineering.

GENE EXPRESSION: TRANSCRIPTION TRANSLATION

The flow of information in eukaryotic cells is from DNA to RNA, a process termed RNA transcription, and from RNA into protein, a process termed translation (Fig. 2-1). The

14

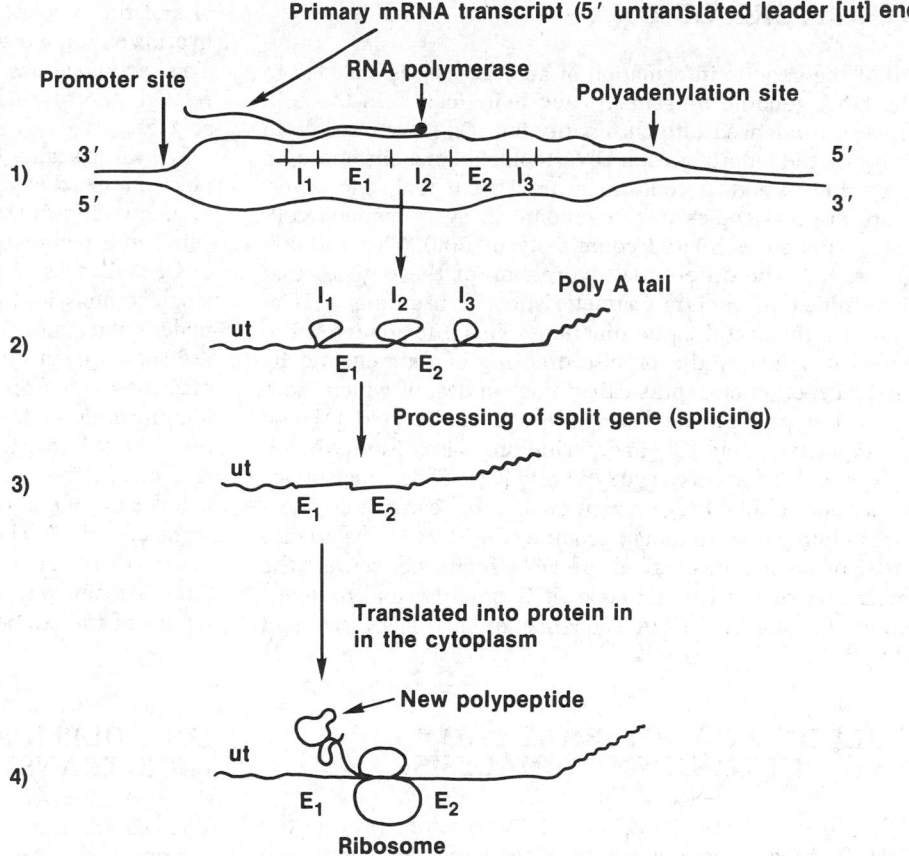

FIG. 2-1. Gene transcription and translation. Messenger RNA synthesis by polymerase II is initiated from a site in the gene called a promoter, and RNA is transcribed from the complementary (nonsense) DNA strand of the structural (protein coding) gene. Thus the 5′ (upstream) end of the RNA is transcribed from a DNA sequence in the 3′ to 5′ orientation (line 1). The first portion usually lacks structural (protein coding) information and is referred to as untranslated (ut) leader. The newly transcribed structural information is interrupted by intervening sequences (introns, I_1 to I_3), which are processed (spliced) from the transcript to leave only structural coding exons (E_1 and E_2) (lines 2 and 3). The transcribed messenger RNA (mRNA) is terminated by the addition of approximately 200 adenine nucleotide bases. The process is called polyadenylation, and the sequence is referred to as the poly A tail. The mRNA is transported to the cytoplasm, where it is translated or decoded into protein. This occurs in cytoplasmic structures called polyribosomes, and the decoding is performed by transfer RNA (tRNA) molecules that recognize the specific nucleotide codon information and provide the appropriate amino acid for linking to the growing polypeptide chain.[93]

enzyme RNA polymerase copies or transcribes genes that encode proteins into RNA[6,7] using monomeric nucleotides similar to, but with subtle differences from, the four nucleotides present in DNA. These monomeric nucleotides are called ribonucleotide bases. The RNA copy of the DNA is referred to as messenger RNA (mRNA) (see Fig. 2-1). Genes that are transcribed into mRNA are translated into the cytoplasm into proteins by a translation system that deciphers the amino acid sequence encoded in the mRNA transcript.[8] RNA synthesis is initiated from a promoter region in the DNA[6,7,9,10] (see Fig. 2-1), and the primary RNA transcript consists of a series of coding and noncoding regions (termed exons and introns, respectively). During processing, introns are removed (spliced out) from the primary transcript and adenylic acid residues added to one end in a process termed polyadenylation. The mature mRNA is then transported to the cytoplasm and subsequently translated into protein on structures termed polyribosomes. The first portion of mRNA usually does not code for a protein sequence and is referred to as untranslated leader. The coding region of the mRNA is dictated by a series of triplets of nucleotide bases called codons, each specifying an amino acid in the translated protein. Thus, the precise order of nucleotides in the DNA sequence determines the precise order of amino acids in a protein chain. The order of the amino acids in a protein chain is responsible for the three-dimensional structure of the protein and its biochemical activity.

The advances in modern biology are paced by the advances in technology which allow the measurements of the various processes, beginning with DNA and its structure and ending with the protein product, its structure and function. Techniques have been developed that allow analysis at each step in the process of information flow from DNA to protein (see Fig. 2-1). For example, the technique first developed by E. Southern and referred to as Southern analysis[11] provides a means for examining DNA structural elements of a single gene in the presence of all the other genes of a eukaryotic organism. Somewhat later, a technique was developed to identify specific mRNA species (transcripts) in the presence of all RNA transcripts expressed within a single cell type.[12] Even though this technique was developed on the west coast of the United States, it has been termed Northern analysis by its founders. Likewise, a technique that detects a single protein species from among all the proteins expressed in a specific cell or tissue has been termed Western blot analysis by its founders.[13] In this chapter we describe the structure and function of DNA and the methods in current use that allow the determination of its primary structure and organization. This will ultimately lead to physical mapping and sequencing of the entire human genome. In the following chapter describing gene regulation, we discuss the methods used for its study and for analysis of the protein products translated from RNA. The descriptions of the methods are coordinated with the presentation of molecular biology of the process.

STRUCTURE OF DNA

All of the genetic information of an organism is encoded in the DNA genome present in each living cell.[14] In the cell, DNA is condensed into chromatin, but if it were possible to measure the length of each DNA molecule in a chromosome from end to end, it could measure 10 cm long. Moreover, there are two copies of the genome in every somatic cell, each with an estimated complexity of 50,000 to 100,000 genes. It is the differential expression of these genes that determines all genetic characteristics from animal speciation to cellular and tissue functions. This information is encoded in DNA by the precise ordering of four chemically distinct monomeric units called nucleotides, of which there are two types: purine bases (deoxyadenylic acid [A] and deoxyguanylic acid [G]) and pyrimidine bases (deoxythymidylic acid [T] and deoxycytidylic acid [C]). These nucleotides or bases are linked together in chains that can number several billion per mammalian genome (Fig. 2-2).[14] The precise order of nucleotides, called the DNA sequence, confers the specificity of the genetic code. It is now possible to determine the absolute DNA sequence of any DNA segment (Fig. 2-3).[15,16]

NUCLEIC ACID HYBRIDIZATION AND HETERODUPLEX ANALYSIS

The properties associated with DNA structure provide the basis for modern genetic engineering technology. First, each DNA molecule consists of two strands (each somatic cell is diploid and therefore possesses four strands) paired together in what is referred to as the Watson-Crick double helix[17] (see Fig. 2-2). Each nucleotide has polarity, and this direction in each DNA strand is indicated by a 5' to 3' notation. Note also that each strand is complementary to the other in the double helix and they run in opposite directions. In the complementary strands, the A nucleotide pairs with T, whereas G always pairs with C (called base pairs).[14] The chemical bonds responsible for base pairing and holding the complementary strands together are weak, and in vitro the two strands can be denatured (separated or melted apart) by temperatures of 70 to 80°C or by alkaline pH conditions. Likewise, the precise order of base pairing between the two strands allows the strands to reanneal at low temperatures in neutral solution because the energy of each base pair is reinforced by that of its neighbors.[18-21] As few as 15 base pairs are sufficient for two strands to anneal.[22-24] The length of the strands can influence annealing efficiency markedly, and very long strands can actually interfere with the process.

The ability to denature or separate the two strands and to allow them to reanneal is the basic principle in the nucleic acid hybridization technique (see Appendix). Annealing can occur between DNA sequences in which fewer than 75% of the bases are complementary (homologous), and the strands will still form base pairs or hybridize.[18] Thus, a DNA sequence from a human gene such as the globin gene, under defined annealing conditions, can form a hybrid with the globin DNA sequences in mouse genomic DNA because the latter share partial homology with the human sequence. If

one of the sequences is first isotopically labeled, then the hybridized sequences can be visualized on autoradiographs. This technique has permitted us to identify the presence of related genes, such as oncogenes, in cells of different species.

We can visualize individual hybrid DNA molecules in the electron microscope (Fig. 2-4). The homologous stretches of sequences in two DNA molecules can be compared and measured in a technique known as heteroduplex analysis. The DNA molecules to be compared are mixed, denatured into single strands, and allowed to form hybrids (double strands) under nondenaturing, annealing conditions.[25] The molecules are then spread on a surface of water, picked up onto an electron microscope grid, and shadowed with metal to allow identification of the DNA single- and complementary double-stranded structures of individual molecules in an electron beam. The example shown is a heteroduplex between a cellular oncogene (c-ras[H], see Chap. 4) and its viral homologue (v-ras[H]).[26] The regions of DNA sequence homology are observed as double-stranded, whereas nonhomologous regions are single-stranded, as revealed by the relative thicknesses of the strands.

DNA DUPLICATION AND NICK TRANSLATION

The DNA molecule is duplicated in vivo by a DNA polymerase enzyme[27,28] that copies the template or parental strand by linking together the individual nucleotides as they base pair with the template DNA (see Fig. 2-2). The new DNA molecules, each consisting of parental strand and a newly synthesized strand, are partitioned to each new daughter cell during cell division.

The DNA polymerase enzyme is used extensively in vitro in the laboratory to copy a DNA sequence that has been treated with the enzyme deoxyribonuclease (DNase) under conditions that cause nicks in single-stranded DNA. The DNA polymerase begins at the nick and replaces (in the 5' to 3' direction) the nucleotides in the nicked strand. When isotopically labeled nucleotides (usually ^{32}P or ^{3}H isotopes) are included in the reaction, the DNA becomes uniformly labeled.[29,30] This reaction is referred to as nick translation (see Appendix). The isotopically labeled DNA sequence can then be used as a probe to detect, by hybridization, its homologous sequence in other DNA fragments. In this manner, a labeled DNA sequence such as a fragment of the globin gene will hybridize only to the unique globin gene copy among the more than 50,000 genes in the DNA molecule of a mammal and is the molecular biologist's tool for finding the proverbial needle in a haystack.

A variation of this technique known as *random priming* uses a randomly generated set of six base-pair oligonucleotides as primers to generate labeled DNA of very high specific activity.[31] A related technique, called the polymerase chain reaction (PCR), uses specific primers to copy and amplify a specific DNA sequence.[32] PCR technology has been used to amplify and then detect or clone selected regions of mammalian DNA.[33] It is possible by this technique

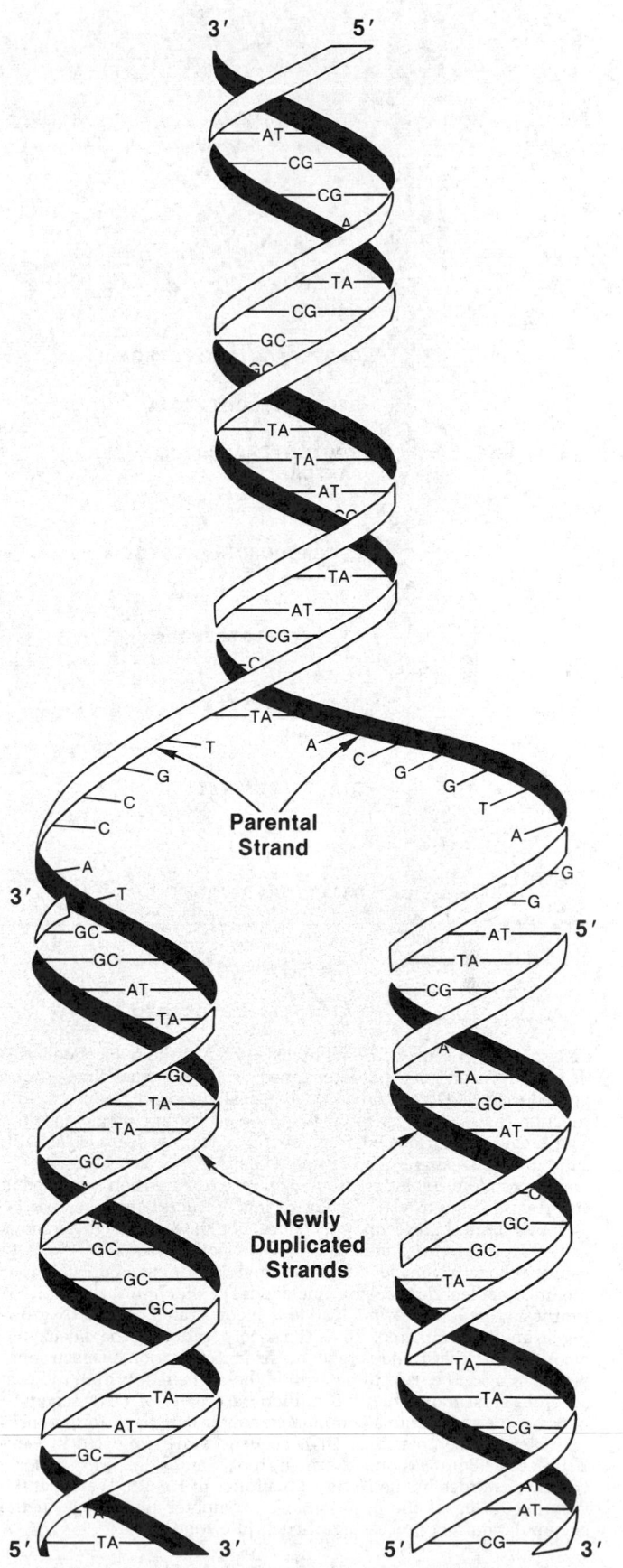

FIG. 2-2. Structure of DNA. The precise order of monomeric deoxyribonucleic acids (adenylic [A], thymidylic [T], guanylic [G], and cytodylic [C] acids) in the DNA molecule encodes all the genetic information for each organism. The DNA molecule consists of two strands in opposite polarity as determined by the orientation of the monomer nucleotide bases and indicated by a 5′ to 3′ notation. The two strands of opposite polarity are held together by weak bonds between pairs of nucleotide bases. Note that A always pairs with T and G with C. When DNA is duplicated by DNA polymerase, the newly synthesized strand is formed by linking the appropriate base pairs as directed by the template of the parental strand.

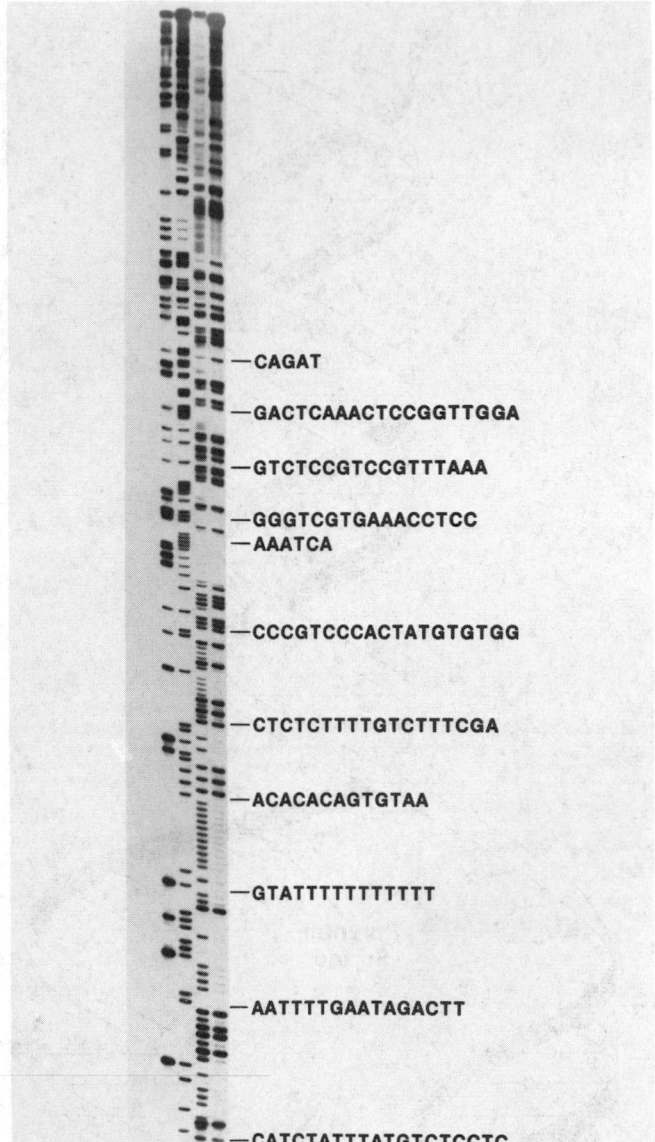

—CAGAT

—GACTCAAACTCCGGTTGGA

—GTCTCCGTCCGTTTAAA

—GGGTCGTGAAACCTCC
—AAATCA

—CCCGTCCCACTATGTGTGG

—CTCTCTTTTGTCTTTCGA

—ACACACAGTGTAA

—GTATTTTTTTTTT

—AATTTTGAATAGACTT

—CATCTATTTATGTCTCCTC

FIG. 2-3. DNA sequence. The precise order of the nucleotide bases in a DNA strand can be determined by DNA sequencing. In one procedure,[15] a DNA strand is labeled at one end by an enzyme reaction that can place isotopically labeled ^{32}P in a single position. The single-strand labeled fragment is randomly degraded chemically in four separate reactions at C, T+C, A+G, and G residues,[15] and the random fragments from each reaction are then subjected to size fractionation by electrophoresis in a polyacrylamide gel matrix, as shown here. In a second procedure, not shown, a single strand is copied from a primer molecule by DNA polymerase (see Fig. 2-1) using radioactive nucleotide bases and limiting amounts of four modified nucleotides (dideoxynucleotides).[16] Each time during DNA synthesis that a dideoxynucleotide is incorporated, the newly growing strand is terminated. Since the incorporation of the dideoxynucleotides into the strand is random, size fractionation by electrophoresis can again be used to determine the sequence. Within the past several years, more than 2.8 million base pairs of DNA sequence have been entered into a common computer data bank for purposes of molecular comparisons. DNA sequences are collected in GenBank (Bolt, Beranek, and Newman, Inc., Cambridge, MA) under a contract awarded by the National Institutes of Health. We are at the very beginning of the application of computer technology in the accumulation and processing of such information.

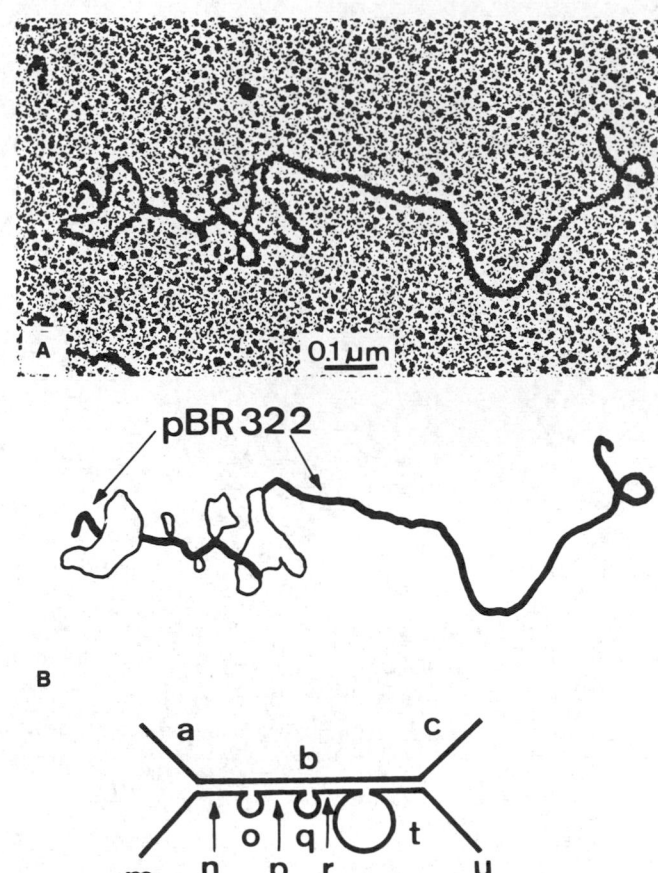

pBR322

FIG. 2-4. Heteroduplex analysis. Two molecularly cloned DNA molecules containing, respectively, the human cellular oncogene locus of ras[H] and the viral oncogene locus of ras[H], were mixed, denatured, and allowed to anneal. The DNA molecules were spread, treated for visualization in the electron microscope,[26] and examined for heteroduplex hybrid molecules. This technique allows individual DNA molecules to be visualized and identifies regions of homology (double-stranded) and nonhomology (single-stranded). In this example, the homologous region represents the human cellular oncogene ras[H] locus in a double-stranded hybrid with the viral ras[H] gene. The magnification is approximately ×100,000. Note that because v-ras[H] is a cDNA copy of the ras[H] gene, the regions o, q, and s, which are introns in c-ras,[H] are deleted in v-ras.[H]

to determine point mutations or DNA rearrangements in very small samples of material.

DNA RESTRICTION ENZYMES

The precise order of nucleotides in the DNA molecules is the basis for the genetic code. If it were possible to reproducibly fragment genomic DNA by cutting at specific nucleotide sequences and to fractionate the fragments by size, we could identify by hybridization (using a radioactive probe prepared as described above) those DNA fragments in the total array of fragments that contain a unique gene.

Restriction Enzyme   **Site**

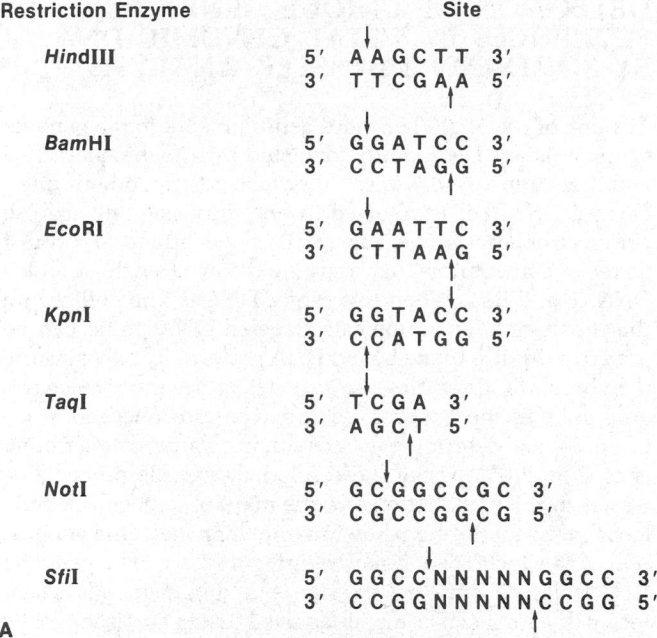

HindIII

5′ A A G C T T 3′
3′ T T C G A A 5′

BamHI

5′ G G A T C C 3′
3′ C C T A G G 5′

EcoRI

5′ G A A T T C 3′
3′ C T T A A G 5′

KpnI

5′ G G T A C C 3′
3′ C C A T G G 5′

TaqI

5′ T C G A 3′
3′ A G C T 5′

NotI

5′ G C G G C C G C 3′
3′ C G C C G G C G 5′

SfiI

5′ G G C C N N N N N G G C C 3′
3′ C C G G N N N N N C C G G 5′

A

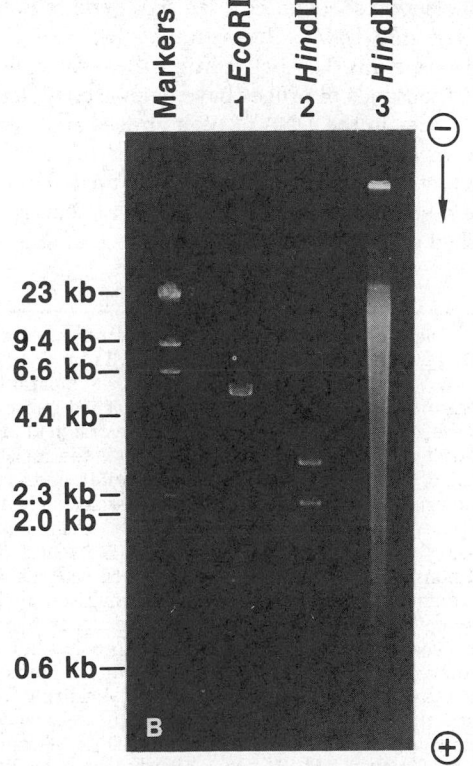

Markers   EcoRI 1   HindIII 2   HindIII 3   ⊖

23 kb—
9.4 kb—
6.6 kb—
4.4 kb—
2.3 kb—
2.0 kb—

0.6 kb—

B   ⊕

FIG. 2-5. **A.** Restriction enzyme recognition sites. The six-base nucleotide sequence recognition sites[35] in double-stranded DNA for HindIII, BamHI, EcoRI, and KpnI are underlined. The orientation 5′ to 3′ is important because with these enzymes the double-strand enzyme cleavage is staggered, leaving a four-base 5′ single-strand overhang (HindIII, BamHI, and EcoRI) or a four-base 3′ overhang (KpnI). Three additional recognition sites for the enzymes TaqI, NotI, and SfiI are shown. These enzymes will cleave double-stranded DNA everywhere in the molecule that the recognition sequence

One of the most important contributions to the study of DNA was the identification of enzymes, known as restriction enzymes, that cut double-stranded DNA at specific nucleotide sequence recognition sites.[34] Several hundred restriction enzymes that recognize more than 150 specific nucleotide sequences in double-stranded DNA have been identified. The recognition sites of several restriction enzymes are shown in Figure 2-5A. These enzymes are produced in bacteria and are part of an elaborate restriction/modification system that protects the bacteria from invasion by foreign DNA.[34-38] Such sites, present in the genome of the bacterial host cell, are protected by a modification enzyme that methylates one of the nucleotide bases in the restriction enzyme recognition site and thereby protects the host DNA from being cleaved.[38] Foreign DNA entering the cell is not modified and is subject to digestion by the restriction enzyme. In vitro, these enzymes provide powerful tools for dissecting DNA genetic information and are fundamental to the principles of recombinant DNA technology.[39]

Most of the restriction enzymes that have been identified, many of which are commercially available, recognize either six, five, or four nucleotide base pairs of DNA sequence.[34] In a DNA molecule of random nucleotide base sequences, a six-base recognition sequence would be expected to occur once in every 4096 base pairs (i.e., once in 4^6 base pairs). In human DNA, which is approximately 3×10^9 base pairs in length, a six-base recognition restriction enzyme would be expected to cut the DNA into several million fragments, whereas the DNA genome of a small DNA tumor virus (e.g., 5300 base pairs in length) would be cut only a few times by the same enzyme. Examples of each are shown in Figure 2-5B. It is possible to fractionate the digested DNA fragments according to size in an agarose gel matrix by electrophoresis. The mobilities of the DNA fragments in this matrix are approximately proportional to the log of their length in base pairs.[40] The DNA fragments can be visualized with ultraviolet light after staining with the fluorescing dye ethidium bromide.[41] Thus, in the example shown in Figure 2-4B, polyoma virus DNA is 5292 base pairs in length,[42] and the HindIII recognition sequence AAGCTT occurs twice in the molecule. Therefore, digestion with the HindIII enzyme yields two fragments, 3030 and 2262 base pairs in length. By comparison, the genomic DNA from human cells is cut several million times by the same enzyme and appears as a smear when resolved by gel electrophoresis and visualized by ethidium bromide staining (Fig. 2-5B).

appears. The overhang allows recombinant DNA gene splicing in the presence of DNA ligase to occur between a heterogeneous population of similarly digested DNA fragments. **B.** Fractionation of restriction fragments by electrophoresis. One microgram of purified polyoma virus DNA is digested with EcoRI (lane 1) or HindIII (lane 2) and subjected to agarose gel electrophoresis. Ten micrograms of human placental DNA is digested with HindIII (lane 3) and likewise subjected to electrophoresis. After being stained with ethidium bromide, the resolved DNA fragments can be visualized by long-wave UV light in the gel. The extreme left lane shows DNA fragments of known size. kb, kilobase pairs in length.

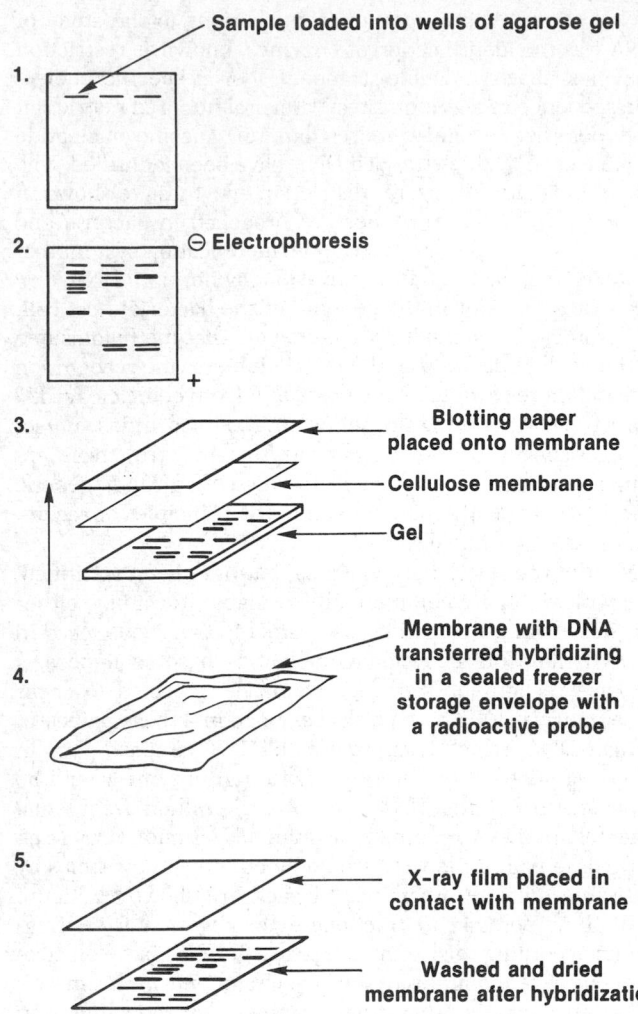

Sample loaded into wells of agarose gel

1.

2. ⊖ Electrophoresis
+

3. Blotting paper placed onto membrane
Cellulose membrane
Gel

4. Membrane with DNA transferred hybridizing in a sealed freezer storage envelope with a radioactive probe

5. X-ray film placed in contact with membrane
Washed and dried membrane after hybridization

Schematic of Steps in the Southern Transfer Analysis

A

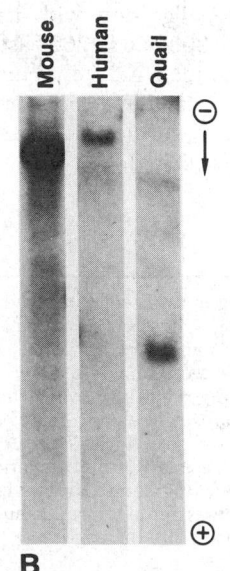

Mouse Human Quail

⊖

⊕

B

DETECTION OF UNIQUE GENE SEQUENCES IN TOTAL GENOMIC DNA BY SOUTHERN TRANSFER ANALYSIS

Any one of the 50,000 or more genes present in the genome of mammalian DNA can be detected by a technique called Southern transfer analysis,[43] in which restriction-enzyme-cleaved DNA that is resolved in one dimension by agarose gel electrophoresis (see Fig. 2-5B) is denatured and transferred to a membrane that traps the resolved single-stranded DNA (Fig. 2-6A). When this target DNA is immobilized on the membrane, an isotopically labeled DNA probe can be used to hybridize to the bound DNA pattern. By exposing the membrane to x-ray film, we can detect a gene that occurs only once in the genome, such as the *mos* oncogene (see Chap. 3), and determine its location in relation to restriction sites (Fig. 2-6B). Using these relatively simple procedures, we can develop restriction enzyme maps of a specific genetic locus in the total genome of a mammalian cell. One application of this technique is shown in Figure 2-6B. The genomic DNA isolated from chicken, mouse, and human cells is subjected to Southern transfer analysis using an isotopically labeled mouse *mos* oncogene probe.[43] The mouse probe detects the homologous sequences in mouse DNA as well as the related nucleotide sequences of the *mos* gene in human and chicken genomic DNA. This result shows that *mos* gene sequences are conserved between all three animal species. Similarly, thousands of probes have been used to detect genomic sequences in the DNA of both viruses and living organisms. A variation of the Southern blot technique is the Northern blot. In this method RNA is run on denaturing gels, blotted to membranes, and hybridized to radioactive probes. This method allows the size and abundance of specific RNA

FIG. 2-6. **A**. Schematic of steps in the Southern transfer analysis.[42] *1.* A 20 cm × 20 cm 0.5% to 1.0% agarose gel, 3 mm or 4 mm thick, is formed in a conventional gel electrophoresis apparatus. *2.* Restriction-enzyme-digested DNA samples are loaded into preformed wells, and the gel is subjected to an electrophoretic field to fractionate the restricted DNA fragments. *3.* For blotting, the gel is placed in a tray on top of absorbent paper wetted with buffer, and a cut-to-size wetted membrane is placed atop the gel and is sandwiched with dry absorbent paper to draw (blot) the resolved DNA fragments onto the DNA-trapping membrane. *4.* After the DNA is fixed to the membrane and nonspecific binding sites are blocked with a special medium, the membrane is sealed in a plastic envelope along with a suitable isotopically labeled probe and placed under hybridization conditions, usually overnight. *5.* The excess isotopic label is washed off and the membrane exposed to x-ray film for 12 hours or more. The film is subsequently developed to reveal hybridizing fragments. **B**. Southern transfer analysis detection of the *mos* oncogene in mouse, quail, and human cellular genomic DNA. Twenty micrograms each of mouse BALB/c DNA digested with *Eco*RI, human placental DNA digested with *Hind*III, and quail QT6 cell line DNA digested with *Bam*HI were subjected to electrophoresis in an agarose gel. The electrophoretically resolved DNA in the gel was then transferred to a cellulose nitrate membrane by the procedure of Southern analysis,[42] and a mouse *mos*-specific isotopically labeled probe[94] was hybridized to the DNA blotted onto the membrane. After hybridization, the membrane was exposed to x-ray film for 12 hours to detect the radioactive fragments containing nucleotide sequences homologous to *mos*. Here we use a radioactive probe to detect the hybrid; a similar hybrid was visualized in the heteroduplex analysis shown in Figure 2-3.

species to be determined. The Western blot involves the electrophoresis and transfer of proteins, which are subsequently detected by antibodies.

PULSED-FIELD GEL ELECTROPHORESIS

The traditional Southern blot technique is useful for a wide variety of applications in the analysis of DNA but suffers from the limitation that fragments larger than 20 kb are poorly resolved on conventional agarose gels. Recent variations of this technique have been described that use alterations in the electrical field applied to the DNA and result in increased resolution of large DNA fragments. Although there are several variations of this method, they all use pulses of current[44] instead of a constant field to increase resolution, hence the name pulsed-field gel electrophoresis (PFGE). Variations of this method involve applying current at different angles to the gel and are referred to as orthogonal field agarose gel electrophoresis (OFAGE).[45]

During conventional electrophoresis, as depicted in Figure 2-5, large DNA fragments run together through the gel. In one version of PFGE, not only are pulses of current applied to the gel, but also the polarity of the field is biased to favor DNA mobility in one direction. This technique is referred to as field-inversion gel electrophoresis (FIGE).[46] This presumably causes large DNA fragments to be oriented in the gel. The size range in which fragments resolve by this method depends on the placement of the electrodes in the gel box and the duration of the pulses, but the separation of fragments as large as 7 million base pairs has been reported.[47] This technique has been made possible by the discovery of restriction enzymes that contain 8 bp recognition sequences (see Fig. 2-5A) (*i.e.*, 4^8 or once in every 65,536 base pairs; yielding ~45,000 fragments per human genome or ~2000–3000 per chromosome). These enzymes generate large DNA fragments 50 to 500 kb long that can be analyzed by PGFE.

With the power to resolve large fragments of DNA, researchers have been able to tackle problems that were previously impossible. The *Escherichia coli* genome is approximately 10 million pairs long, a size too large to map by conventional gel electrophoresis. A complete physical map of the *E. coli* genome was recently reported[48] and will allow the structure of the genome and the organization of its genes to be known in greater detail. The maps of other bacterial genomes, yeast chromosomes, and eventually mammalian chromosomes can now be constructed by PFGE techniques. An example of one application of this technique is shown in Figure 2-7. DNA from a human cell line containing a DNA rearrangement in the *met* oncogene[49,50] is digested with the enzyme Sfi I and subjected to FIGE. The DNA fragments are transferred to and immobilized on a membrane by slight modifications of the conventional procedure described in Figure 2-6. Isotopically labeled DNA probes are again used to detect the sequence homologue on a DNA fragment. In the example shown (see Fig. 2-7) a novel 350-kb DNA fragment is depicted in an Sfi I DNA fragment carrying the rearranged oncogene locus. The normal (allele) fragment, also present in this cell, is revealed on a ~150-kb Sfi I fragment. The oncogene activation event resulted from a DNA rearrange-

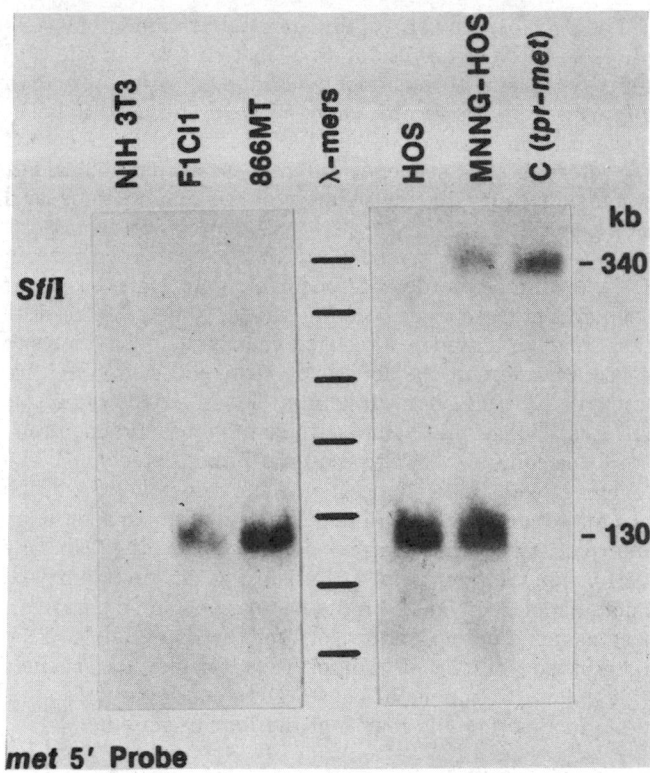

FIG. 2-7. DNA fragments separated by pulsed-field gel electrophoresis. DNA from several human cell lines was digested with the enzyme Sfi I, separated by the pulsed-field technique and Southern blotted. The filter was hybridized with a probe from the *met* oncogene. The appearance of a rearranged allele of the *met* gene can be observed in the DNA from the MNNG-HOS line, a chemically transformed human cell. Note the separation of the fragments between 120 and 340 kb.

ment and generated the new Sfi fragment. By subjecting normal DNA to limited (partial) digestion with these rare cutting enzymes, maps of larger segments of DNA can be generated and used for linking two or more markers, thereby generating a physical restriction map.[51] The size markers often used in these analyses represent the chromosomes of *Saccharomyces cerevisiae*.

RESTRICTION FRAGMENT LENGTH POLYMORPHISMS: DNA-BASED GENETIC MARKERS

In the last few years we have seen dramatic advances in our understanding of several human diseases, including muscular dystrophy, cystic fibrosis, retinoblastoma, and colon and small lung cell cancers. These breakthroughs have been made possible by dramatic developments in the field of human genetics. Genetic analysis of an organism requires the identification of genetic markers that reveal the inherited differences between individuals. Early human genetic markers included ABO blood groups, isozymes, and HLA antigens.[52-54] Progress in linking these markers together was hampered by their small number compared to the size of the human genome.

The development of two-dimensional protein gel electrophoresis allowed the resolution of many more variable proteins, but this method cannot be used to generate more than a few markers per chromosome. However, because all heritable variation is based on DNA sequence variation, a method for detecting DNA sequence differences between individuals would allow virtually any segment of the genome to be used as a genetic marker.

As we have seen, restriction enzymes can recognize in DNA the precise order of specific four to eight base pair segments of a sequence (see Fig. 2-5A). Genetic differences that create or eliminate a restriction enzyme recognition site cause variation in the length of DNA fragments and are known as restriction fragment length polymorphisms (RFLPs).[55] Figure 2-8 shows an example of a unique probe from the long arm of chromosome 7 that detects a 7.5-kb fragment with the enzyme *Taq*I. Approximately 50% of the chromosomes in the white population contain an additional, internal *Taq*I site, creating an additional allele of 4.0 kb.[56] By performing Southern blot analysis using this probe/enzyme combination, individuals in the population can be characterized as being either homozygous for the upper allele (1,1), heterozygous (1,2), or homozygous for the lower allele (2,2). Thus fragments of cloned DNA can be used as a genetic marker for this region of the human genome.

These differences in sequence (between two alleles) occur at a frequency of an estimated 1 per 200 to 500 base pairs[57] and are responsible for the genetic differences between any two individuals. RFLPs can be characterized by both the degree to which they are useful in genetic analysis and their chromosomal location. The frequency of a polymorphism is determined by typing a large number of unrelated individuals and determining the frequency of each allele. For example, if a two allele polymorphism is analyzed in 50 individuals (100 chromosomes) and 60 copies of allele 1 and 40 copies of allele 2 are detected, the frequency is 0.60/0.40. The heterozygosity of an RFLP is related to the frequency and is a measure of the percentage of individuals who are heterozygotes. The polymorphism information content (PIC) is a measure of the percentage of families in which both parents are heterozygous for a given polymorphism.[55]

Probes that detect RFLPs can be mapped to chromosomes by both physical and genetic methods. The physical methods include somatic cell hybridization[58] and in situ hybridization.[59] Briefly, a gene can be assigned to a chromosome by following its segregation in a panel of interspecies hybrids segregating human chromosomes (*i.e.*, human X hamster hybrids). The technique of in situ hybridization is performed by hybridizing an isotopically labeled DNA fragment directly to mitotic phase chromosomes. After the probe is annealed,

A

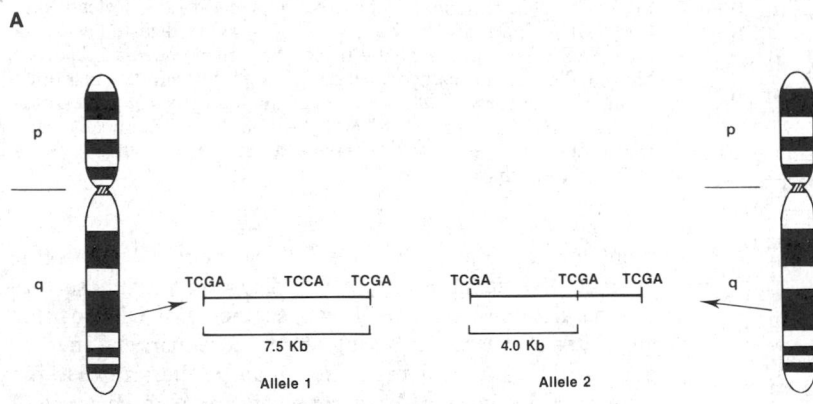

B

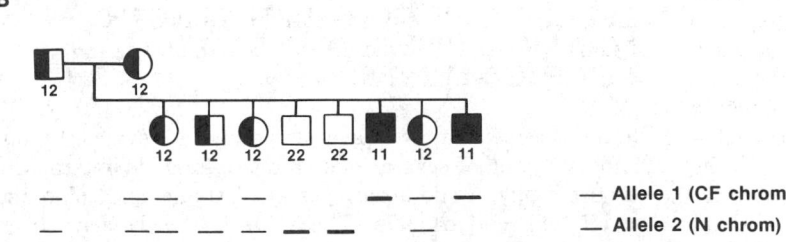

— Allele 1 (CF chrom)

— Allele 2 (N chrom)

C

Normal   Tumor

FIG. 2-8. Use of a DNA-based genetic marker. **A.** An example of an RFLP. A diagram of human chromosome 7 shows the position of the *met* proto-oncogene at 7q31.[95] The sequence TCGA is the recognition sequence of the *Taq*I restriction enzyme, which generates a 7.5-kb fragment. **B.** Use of an RFLP in genetic diagnosis. The *met* gene is tightly linked to the cystic fibrosis (CF) gene,[56] and therefore they are almost always inherited together. In this family, allele 1 is on the CF chromosome and the affected children (*filled symbols*) have a 1,1 genotype. Individuals with a 1,2 genotype are unaffected carriers and 2,2 children are unaffected noncarriers. **C.** RFLP detection of DNA deletion in a tumor. This hypothetical example shows how the deletion of all or part of a chromosome can be detected by comparing tumor and normal DNA from the same patient.

a photographic emulsion is applied, the sample is exposed, and, after developing, the grains are counted over the chromosomes. This technique allows the gene to be assigned not only to a chromosome but also, when combined with chromosome banding techniques, to a band or region on a chromosome (Fig. 2-9). A more precise method for positioning an RFLP is by linking it physically or genetically to another polymorphism. This requires the RFLPs to be typed in the same group of pedigrees. The most efficient families for linking RFLPs have been determined to be three generation families with large sibships.[60] Two RFLPs that are near each other on a chromosome will be inherited together in a family in a meiotic recombination dependent fashion. The genetic distance between two markers is determined by the recombination frequency, the percentage of meioses in which a recombination is detected between two markers. If the recombination is observed in one of 100 meiosis (a frequency of 1%), a genetic distance of 1 centimorgan (cM) occurs between the two markers. In the human genome this is approximately equivalent to one million base pairs in physical distance; for example, ~20 markers spaced 5 cM apart could provide a genetic *linkage map* of a human chromosome (~2.0 /10^8 base pairs).[61]

LINKAGE ANALYSIS

A major use of RFLPs is in the analysis of families that segregate a human disease. DNA from individuals in the

FIG. 2-9. In situ DNA hybridization to a human chromosome. A histogram of human chromosome 7 is displayed showing the results of an in situ hybridization experiment using the *met* oncogene as a probe. In this experiment a radioactive fragment of the gene was hybridized to spreads of human chromosomes. After washing and applying a photographic emulsion, the grains depicting hybridization are recorded. A representation of the number of grains and their location is depicted here, demonstrating that the *met* gene lies on chromosome 7q31.1–31.3.

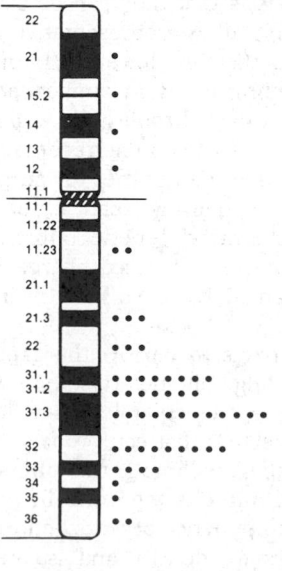

7

pedigree is analyzed by Southern blot using DNA probes that detect RFLPs. The inheritance of the alleles of the genetic marker is correlated with the inheritance of the disease. The data are statistically analyzed by calculating the odds that the association between the marker and the disease occurred by chance. This information is used to calculate a LOD score (the log of the odds), and a LOD score of three (odds of 1000 to 1) is taken as formal proof of linkage.[62] An example of linkage is displayed in Figure 2-8B. RFLP markers that we discovered in the *met* proto-oncogene locus on human chromosome 7 were used by White and co-workers[56] to analyze pedigrees segregating the recessive genetic disease cystic fibrosis. In the first families that could be scored for the inheritance of the marker, there was a perfect correlation between the marker and the disease, generating a LOD score of 8.0. The odds that this situation could occur by chance is greater than 100,000,000 to 1, providing conclusive evidence that the gene responsible for cystic fibrosis lies next to the *met* gene on the long arm of human chromosome 7. These genetic markers were also found to be useful in carrier detection and prenatal diagnosis of families affected by this disease.[63]

CHROMOSOMAL ALTERATIONS IN HUMAN TUMORS

Several human tumor types have been described that contain deletions of specific chromosomal regions. These were first detected by analyzing the karyotypes of the tumor cells in cases such as retinoblastoma[64,65] and Wilms' tumor.[66] More recently, nonrandom deletions have been described for secondary acute nonlymphocytic leukemia, colon, kidney, and lung cancers.[67-70] RFLP markers are a particularly powerful tool for this type of analysis. To analyze tumor samples with RFLPs, samples of the tumor DNA (as free as possible of normal tissue) are compared to DNA obtained from normal tissue or cells from the same patient. The DNA is analyzed with probes that identify polymorphisms. If the normal DNA is heterozygous and the tumor DNA homozygous, this demonstrates that one copy of that gene or chromosomal region has been deleted in the tumor (see Fig. 2-8C). This type of analysis has recently been applied to the analysis of breast tumors, renal cell cancer (see also Chap. 3), lung cancer, and colon cancer. This technique is particularly powerful for analyzing tumors that contain deletions too small to be detected by karyotypic analyses, or for solid tumors in which reliable karyotypic analyses are hard to perform.

CHARACTERIZING THE HUMAN GENOME

Recently much attention has been given to the suggestion that the complete DNA sequence of the human genome be determined, a project that can be described as biology's equivalent to the moon landing. Although few doubt that much valuable information is to be gained from the complete characterization of human genetic material, many worry that such a project would take research money away from other, more productive endeavors.[71] In fact, the idea should be thought of as a series of projects, each with very real promise of benefits to medical research. For example, if a specific genetic locus is identified by RFLP analysis to be linked to a disease, then careful characterization of this locus (*i.e.*, physical mapping and sequence analyses) would serve to assist in the identification of the responsible genetic element. The rest of this chapter will detail the stages and techniques involved characterizing the human genome.

MOLECULAR CLONING

Modern molecular biology is dependent on the technology of molecular cloning—the isolation and propagation of defined DNA fragments. In addition to cutting DNA with restriction enzymes, we also can reseal the cut ends using enzymes called DNA ligases.[72] The combination of restriction and ligation enzymes has provided the basis for recombinant DNA technology.[39] For example, the genome of polyoma virus is a circular double-stranded DNA molecule (see Fig. 2-5B) that is 5292 base pairs in length[42] and contains a single *Bam*HI recognition site (see Fig. 2-5A).[42] Cutting this DNA molecule with *Bam*HI yields a linear fragment. With DNA ligase, the two ends of the linearized, double-stranded DNA can be resealed (covalently linked), and some percentage of the molecules return to the original configuration. However, head-to-head or head-to-tail joining also may occur. The simplest condition for ligation is one in which a single cut has been made in a circular DNA molecule. Obviously, the more unique ends that are introduced into the reaction, the more complex the ligation products become.[39,72]

In bacteria, DNA plasmids carrying drug resistance genes have been used as vectors for cloning DNA fragments. Plasmids are small, circular DNA molecules that replicate as an episome (autonomously from the chromosome). DNA fragments can be inserted into a plasmid vector and thus can replicate with the plasmid. The most commonly used vector for molecular cloning, pBR322,[39,73,74] is a plasmid that replicates episomally in *E. coli*. It consists essentially of three regions that control different genetic functions (Fig. 2-10). One region, the origin of replication (*ori*) where DNA synthesis originates, allows the plasmid to replicate as an episome in *E. coli*. This plasmid also contains two genes (Tet^r and Amp^r) that, when expressed, confer to strains of *E. coli* harboring the plasmid, resistances to the drugs tetracycline and ampicillin, respectively. If a DNA segment is introduced into one of the drug resistance genes, then the gene is rendered inactive and the *E. coli* cell harboring the plasmid becomes sensitive to the drug. In this way, plasmids that contain molecularly cloned fragments can be identified. The procedures for hybridization with bacterial colonies[75] or lambda phage vectors[76] are analogous to the Southern transfer procedure described earlier. DNA from *E. coli* colonies growing on agar in a Petri dish is transferred to a membrane, and a single colony or a single virus plaque in hundreds of thousands can be identified and isolated. DNA from this plasmid or virus vector may contain a single molecularly cloned DNA fragment from the original population of more than one million fragments present in the animal genome. The plasmid or lambda phage vectors are gen-

erally amplified in *E. coli* so that each cell contains many copies of the molecularly cloned fragment.[39] From 1 liter of bacterial culture, 100 μg to 1 mg of purified vector DNA can be recovered. In the example shown in Figure 2-10, the plasmid DNA containing the polyoma viral genome inserted in the pBR322 *Bam*HI site is purified from the transformed *E. coli* cells and subjected to digestion with *Bam*HI to release the polyoma DNA insert from the vector. Here, the insert is recovered after subjecting the digested DNA to gel electrophoresis.[77,78] The desired fragment, isolated and purified in large quantities, can be characterized by DNA sequencing for the determination of absolute genetic information (see Fig. 2-3). *E. coli* host/vector systems have been the most widely applied for molecular cloning, but other cloning vector systems, such as those using mammalian viruses, are also used.[79]

Although well suited for the cloning of small DNA fragments, plasmids are not very suitable for the cloning of DNA fragments larger than 10 kb. Derivatives of the bacteriophage lambda have been developed that allow DNA molecules of up to 20 kb to be cloned (Fig. 2-11). By removing genes that are not essential for the replication of lambda, vectors have been designed to accommodate foreign DNA. By combining the recombinant DNA with the enzymes and proteins required to package lambda DNA into virus particles, recombinant viruses are generated. If the collection of DNA fragments inserted into phage is representative of the entire genome (*i.e.*, at least one or more copies of every region) the collection of lambda phage particles generated is termed a genomic library.[80] Because the packaging of lambda phage is very efficient and the clones can be stably stored, this method is in wide use in molecular biology laboratories.

Researchers have continued to develop vectors that can clone fragments larger than ~20 kb. One such vector (called a cosmid) is a hybrid vector[81] with part plasmid and part phage functions; it contains the phage sequences for packaging DNA into lambda phage particles, but once inside the bacterial cell it replicates using plasmid functions. The advantage of cosmids is that they can be used to clone up to 50 kb of DNA. This allows representative genomic libraries to be constructed that are fewer in number than lambda phage genomic libraries. Both lambda phage and cosmid libraries are useful for "chromosome walking" studies, that is, one end of an insert from one recombinant can serve as probe for rescreening the libraries for purposes of obtaining recombinants that contain adjacent chromosomal DNA sequences.[82] Clearly, more genetic information is spanned when cosmid libraries are used. Large segments of the mouse and human MHC locus have been isolated in this manner.[83]

The recent impetus to narrow the gap between genetic methods of analyzing genomes (distances in the millions of base pairs) and the molecular level has led researchers to develop cloning vectors that can propagate DNA fragments larger than 100 kb. A technique that offers great promise is the generation of minichromosomes in yeast.[84] Analysis of the structural components of yeast chromosomes has allowed researchers to identify and isolate yeast DNA sequences with centromeric and telomeric functions. By add-

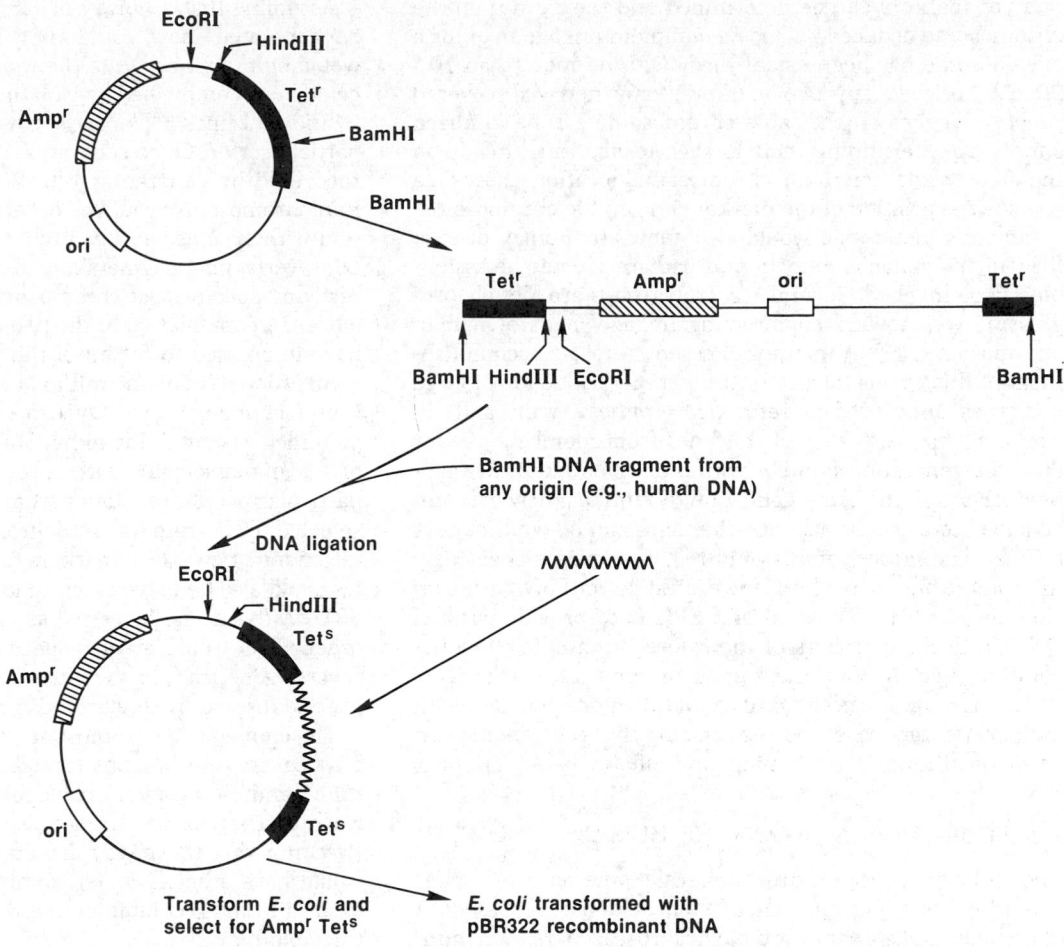

Molecular Cloning Scheme

FIG. 2-10. Molecular cloning scheme. The circular plasmid pBR322 is digested with *Bam*HI restriction enzyme (see Fig. 2-4A) at its single recognition site, which resides in the tetracycline (Tet) gene to yield a linear fragment (*e.g.*, see pBR322, Fig. 2-9, lane 3). This linearized plasmid is mixed with *Bam*HI-digested DNA from any source (*e.g.*, polyoma DNA as in Fig. 2-9, lane 1) and the mixed sample is ligated (see Fig. 2-9, lane 4). A certain fraction of the molecules obtained will have the recombinant structure as shown. The plasmid molecules are transformed into *E. coli* and cells harboring the plasmids are selected by their resistance to the unaltered ampicillin resistance gene. Ampicillin-resistant colonies are tested for resistance to tetracycline; any that are sensitive to tetracycline (Tet) could have new DNA fragments cloned into the *Bam*HI site. Plasmid DNA is prepared from these cells and tested for the presence of the desired insert.

ing these sequences to large fragments of human DNA, large segments of the human chromosomes can be replicated in yeast cells as chromosomes. Recently DNA molecules larger than 125 kb have been successfully cloned into yeast cells.[84] Naturally occurring yeast chromosomes are several million base pairs in length, so there is sufficient reason to believe that recombinant chromosomes of this size can also be generated. This could greatly facilitate human genome analyses by providing a system where genetic markers can be linked to physical restriction maps.

THE HUMAN GENETIC LINKAGE MAP

The first step toward sequencing the human genome is to generate a road map of spaced genetic markers for each chromosome by developing a genetic linkage map.[85] Just as RFLPs are shown to be linked to a gene for a genetic disease, recombination frequencies can be used to link two RFLPs to each other and thereby address whether they are near each other on the same chromosome. By studying the inheritance of RFLPs in the same families, the genetic distance between pairs of markers can be determined and their order on the chromosome deduced.[60] Once a complete linkage map for a chromosome has been established (with no more than 10–20 cM between any two markers), any newly discovered probes or genes on the same chromosome can be localized simply by determining their linkage to markers already on the map. In addition to the chromosomal location, these data provide the position of the marker gene on the chromosome. A human genetic map would also allow any human disease for which a suitable collection of pedigrees could be assembled to be mapped. Several research groups are already progressing well toward constructing linkage maps of human chromosomes.[60,61] A major tool essential to the accomplishment of this goal is the establishment of a collection of large pedigrees to be used as reference families. White and co-workers[60] have established cell lines from members of over 60 three-generation families with 6 to 12 children. By mapping RFLPs in the same collection of families, new data can be added to previous data and the maps can be continuously refined. The success of this venture has been greatly aided by the establishment of the Centre d'Etude du Polymorphism Humain (CEPH). The goal of CEPH is to provide purified DNA from the members of the reference families to collaborating investigators. Each collaborator agrees to analyze RFLP markers in these families and combine the data with the genetic data base, the result being that the genome can be mapped much more rapidly and efficiently.

MOLECULAR CLONING OF THE HUMAN GENOME

The isolation of the entire human genome as a set of ordered, overlapping molecular clones would represent a major accomplishment for biological researchers. At a minimum, this would require 150,000 lambda phage clones, or 60,000 cosmid clones or 3,000 yeast minichromosomes one million base pairs long. Although strategies are being developed to directly link phage or cosmid clones, the task would be much more straightforward with minichromosomes.

Assuming that a library of large minichromosomes could be generated, how could they be ordered? One strategy would be to first separate the individual chromosomes. This could be accomplished by isolating chromosomes in somatic hybrid cell lines[86,87] or by separating them by size using a particle sorter. Once separated, each chromosome could be recovered by generating 1 to 200 minichromosomes. The minichromosomes could be ordered by using DNA hybridization with specific marker probes to detect clones that contain overlapping segments, or by using the DNA probes already mapped on that chromosome to identify and order the clones. A combination of the two approaches would probably have to be used to fill in all the gaps.

An ordered set of one million base pair fragments would be useful in many ways. Once a region of the genome was identified as containing either the gene for a genetic disease or a region associated with chromosomal abnormalities in a particular neoplasm, clones from that region could be easily selected. DNA from the minichromosome could then be used to generate new RFLP markers for that region. Further studies could also be undertaken to identify genes in this stretch of DNA that could be tested as candidate genes for the disorder. This would greatly speed up the process known as reverse genetics[88]; or the cloning of a gene responsible for a genetic disease by its chromosomal location.

The cloning of a chromosome would also allow a complete physical map to be constructed, that is, probes from each minichromosome clone could be used to generate a long-range restriction map using pulse-field gel electrophoresis.[51] By comparing the physical map with the genetic map, we would have a better understanding of the relation between base pairs and recombination distance for specific regions of the genome.

FURTHER DISSECTION OF THE GENOME

To analyze specific regions of the genome in greater detail, the yeast minichromosome DNA fragments could be sub-

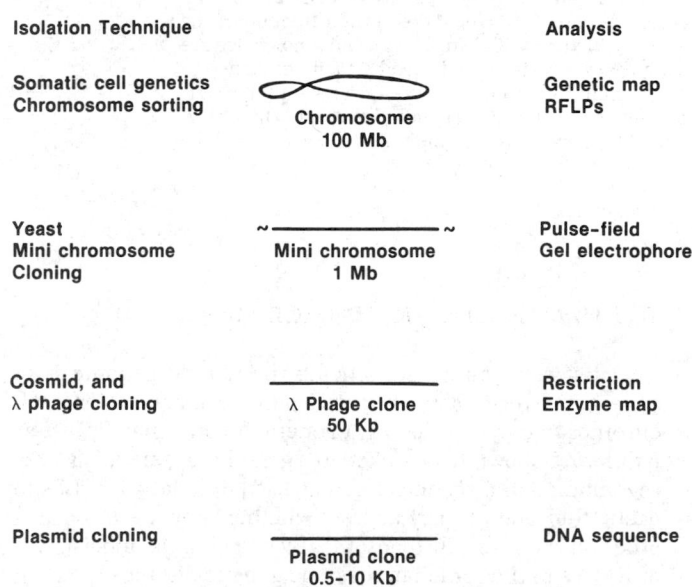

FIG. 2-11. Cloning and analyzing the human genome. A comparison of techniques for capturing portions of genetic information and the types of analyses that they make possible. Somatic cell hybrids and fluorescence-activated cell sorting allow whole chromosomes (50–200 mb) to be isolated.[96] These techniques assist in the construction of genetic lineage maps of chromosomes. Chromosomes can be broken down into 0.1 to 1.0 mb fragments by cloning into yeast minichromosomes.[84] These fragments can be used to generate a physical map using PFGE.[44,45] Minichromosomes can be subdivided by cloning into cosmid and phage vectors,[80,81] and these subclones can then be characterized by conventional restriction curve mapping. Finally, fragments for the phage clones can be inserted into plasmid vectors and the nucleotide sequence determined.

cloned into either cosmid or phage vectors. Restriction mapping and hybridization could be used to order the subcloned DNA by generating a series of overlapping DNA clones spanning the entire minichromosome. The DNA subclones could then be used to generate a detailed restriction map of the region. Having cloned a portion of a gene, a researcher could select the appropriate subclones likely to contain the rest of the gene. This would allow the entire gene and its control sequences to be rapidly characterized.

Once fully automated DNA sequencing procedures are developed,[89,90] the entire genome could be efficiently sequenced. The sequence would allow us to learn a great deal about the organization of the human genome. Gene families would become greatly expanded, allowing researchers to rapidly select new genes that might be of biological and medical importance.

POLYMERASE CHAIN REACTION

A technique has been developed that allows direct analysis of a segment of DNA that is uniquely present in the genome of a single cell in the presence of hundreds of thousands of cells.[32,91,92] This technology is based on a process referred to as the polymerase chain reaction (PCR), and the sensitivity is made possible because the DNA sequence of interest is specifically amplified several hundred thousand times. The PCR can be automated and, because of its extraordinary sensitivity, will have a significant impact in clinical diagnostics. One of the most important applications will be in genetic screening[32] and in detection of minimal residual cells in patients after cancer treatment.[91,92]

AUTOMATION OF MOLECULAR GENETICS

A crucial requirement to determine the sequence of the three billion base pairs of the human genome is the development of machines that automate repetitive tasks. Moreover, it will be necessary to dedicate powerful computers to store the information and to generate the relevant software to process it. Machines have been constructed that extract DNA from cells, synthesize small DNA fragments or oligonucleotides, and determine the DNA sequence of DNA fragments. Cloning and sequencing projects now routinely require the use of oligonucleotides. Oligonucleotides can be used as probes for Southern analysis or for screening genetic libraries; they also can be used to generate specific mutations in the sequence of cloned genes for identifying important sequence elements by altering their function in vitro and in vivo. The first machines able to automatically perform DNA sequence analysis of fragments more than five hundred bases in length are now commercially available. In the near future, then, DNA sequencing will not be the rate-limiting step, but genetic and physical mapping still represent major obstacles. Obviously, the enormous volume of data now being generated by genetic studies and DNA sequencing projects requires the use of increasingly powerful computers and innovative software. More emphasis is being placed on the development of software that predicts molecular structure and facilitates drug design. In 1987, the National Cancer Institute established the first supercomputer facility dedicated totally to biomedical research.

CONCLUSION

The techniques of molecular biology are responsible for many major advances in the biological sciences, especially in genetics, biology, and medicine. By using genetic analyses to identify disease genes, and molecular cloning to determine the structure of genes, complex biological problems can begin to be unraveled. Such advances as the identification of oncogenes and the cloning of the muscular dystrophy and retinoblastoma genes are examples of the power of this approach. There is no doubt that the continued application of molecular methods to biological problems will lead to a greater understanding of normal cellular functions and the mechanisms of abnormal cellular responses.

Research was sponsored by the National Cancer Institute, Department of Health and Human Services, under Contract No. N01-CO-74101 with Bionetics Research, Inc. The contents of this chapter do not necessarily reflect the views or policies of the Department of Health and Human Services, nor does mention of trade names, commercial products, or organizations imply endorsement by the U.S. government.

GLOSSARY OF TERMS USED IN MOLECULAR BIOLOGY AND ONCOGENE RESEARCH

Acute transforming retroviruses: Viruses that have acquired sequences from the host genome that give them the property of causing rapid tumor formation in animals or morphologic transformation in cells in culture. The acquired sequences are termed viral oncogenes.

Antisense: The noncoding strand of the DNA within the RNA-coding region of the gene. It is complementary to the "sense" strand and is used as a template for RNA synthesis.

CAT: Chloramphenicol acetyl transferase, a prokaryotic enzyme that is used in a reporter gene assay to measure protein synthesis in vitro.

cDNA libraries: A collection of clones representative of the mRNA of a given cell type that is formed using the enzyme reverse transcriptase.

Centimorgan (cM): A unit of genetic distance. A centimorgan is equivalent to a meiotic recombination frequency of 1%. In the human genome with approximately 3×10^6 base pairs and 3000 cM, 1 cM is roughly equal to one million base pairs.

cis-acting DNA elements: DNA segments that serve as binding sites for transcriptional activators or repressors; a nondiffusible control element.

Coding sequence: That part of the genome or mRNA that is translated into protein.

Conditional expression: Gene expression that occurs only in response to certain stimuli or specific conditions.

Consensus sequence: A characteristic nucleotide sequence that is identified with a gene regulation function.

Constitutive expression: A gene that is expressed at the same level for most of the cell cycle.

Cosmid: A cloning vector designed to carry large fragments of DNA. The vector contains sequences of lambda bacteriophage that allow the DNA to be packaged as a phage particle. Once inside the bacterium, the cosmid replicates as a plasmid. Cosmid vectors can be used to clone fragments as large as 50 kb.

DNA sequence: The precise order of the four nucleotides, adenine [A], guanine [G], cytosine [C], thymidine [T], as they are linked together to form the DNA chain. This DNA sequence encodes the genetic information of an organism.

DNA transfection: The transfer of DNA into cells in culture. The foreign DNA can associate with the host chromosome and be expressed as an identifiable phenotype.

DNase footprinting: A technique that allows the determination of the specific DNA sequence in the binding sites of a DNA binding protein or protein complex.

Enhancers: DNA elements of varying length that can be located upstream or downstream from a gene in either polarity and enhance gene transcription.

Exon: Gene sequences that are retained in fully mature mRNA. Most often they contain protein coding information.

Gene transcription: Synthesis of an RNA molecule by polymerization of nucleotides complementary to a DNA template. This RNA molecule is a precursor of mRNA and represents a faithful complementary copy of the DNA sequence from which it was transcribed. A specific sequence in front of the gene (promoter) acts to identify the initiation site for transcription. In RNA, uridine (U) occupies positions that thymidine (T) occupies in DNA.

Genomic Library: A collection of clones containing genomic DNA fragments. The library should contain enough clones so that every region of the genome is represented at least once.

Heteroduplex: A double-stranded DNA molecule formed by hybridization of complementary single strands derived from two different sources. Only stretches of homologous or complementary DNA sequences can form double-stranded regions, whereas noncomplementary DNA stretches remain as single strands and are visible as such in the electron microscope.

Hybridization: The annealing or base pairing of two single-stranded DNA or RNA molecules that are homologous or complementary.

Inducible: Capable of being "turned on" in a specific situation; that is, the β-lactamase gene of *E. coli* is "induced" under conditions of low glucose and high galactose concentrations.

Initiation codon: The ribonucleotides "AUG" that translate into the amino acid methionine; is always the first amino acid codon of every mRNA.

Insertional mutagenesis: The process of interrupting the structure —either regulatory elements or protein coding information—of a gene by insertion of foreign genetic information.

Intron: Noncoding DNA sequences that interrupt the coding portions of a gene (exons); it is excised in the fully processed mRNA.

Linkage map: A set of closely spaced genetic markers, generally RFLPs, that have been mapped to the same chromosome. If the linkage map covers the entire chromosome, any gene responsible for an inherited disease can in theory be located.

Linker scanning: A method of in vitro mutagenesis wherein restriction enzyme cleavage sites are inserted at different positions along the gene so that sequences 5' and 3' to the insertions are not altered. Gene function is then assayed to identify functional domains.

Long terminal repeat: A repetitive element of the integrated provirus that is generated during viral DNA synthesis and contains the transcription control elements that regulate virus expression.

Messenger RNA: An RNA molecule that represents a faithful copy of the amino acid–coding sequences of a gene. Noncoding sequences (introns) have been removed. With few exceptions, mRNA possesses a stretch of about 200 adenine bases (poly A tail) attached to its 3' end; this tail is not encoded by DNA.

Minichromosome: A large fragment of DNA that can replicate in yeast cells. Minichromosomes are constructed by adding yeast cen-

tromere and telomere sequences onto foreign DNA fragments. Human DNA fragments as large as 125 kb have been cloned in yeast, and it may be possible to clone one million base pair or longer segments.

Mobility Shift: An assay that allows identification of extracts that contain specific DNA binding proteins.

Molecular cloning: The insertion of a foreign DNA segment of finite length into a vector that replicates in a specific host. The host-vector systems are defined by the NIH "Guidelines for Research Involving Recombinant DNA Molecules" (Federal Register 47:38050–38068, 1982).

Nick translation: A method that replaces nucleotides in double-stranded DNA with the same but isotopically labeled nucleotides after treatment with DNase I and repair with DNA polymerase. Both strands are labeled by this technique.

Null mutations: Mutations that eliminate or inactivate a gene from the genome of an organism.

Polyadenylation: The addition of a stretch of approximately 200 riboadenylic acid residues to the end of an RNA *polII* transcript.

Primer extension: An assay that utilizes mRNA and a complementary oligonucleotide primer to synthesize a DNA antisense copy of the mRNA. It is used to determine mRNA 5' structure.

Promoter: A DNA sequence that signals RNA polymerase to initiate transcription.

Pulsed-field gel electrophoresis (PFGE): A modification of agarose gel electrophoresis of DNA in which fragments several megabases can be resolved. The technique uses pulses of current in either the reverse direction or at angles to the gel to accomplish the increased resolution.

Recombinant DNA: A DNA molecule constructed by joining a fragment of DNA from a different source to a vector, such as a circular bacterial plasmid. The vector is opened at a specific site, a given DNA fragment from another source is inserted, and the circle is closed again. The recombinant DNA is amplified in a host cell that can replicate the vector.

Reporter gene: A gene whose activity can be easily assayed; it is used as a marker of gene expression in transcription or translation systems, or both.

Restriction enzymes: Enzymes made by certain strains of bacteria to protect themselves against invading foreign DNA (*e.g.*, bacteriophage DNA). These enzymes cut DNA at specific recognition sites.

Restriction fragment length polymorphism (RFLP): A variation between individuals in the size of fragments produced by restriction enzyme digestion. The variation is inherited and can be used as a genetic marker in linkage analysis.

Retrovirus: A plus-stranded RNA genome virus that is reverse transcribed into DNA during infection and replication. The DNA copy integrates into the host chromosomal DNA. This DNA template, called a provirus, is transcribed into virion RNA and produces translatable mRNA that codes for virion or oncogene protein products.

Reverse genetics: The use of information on the chromosomal location of a genetic disease gene to clone the gene itself. In some instances chromosomal abnormalities have provided the essential clues, and in other cases genetic linkage data have been used to localize the gene.

Reverse transcriptase: An enzyme produced by retroviruses that makes complementary DNA (cDNA) copies of RNA. The process is called reverse transcription.

S1 nuclease protection analysis: An assay designed to elucidate mRNA structure; it utilizes RNA–DNA hybridization conditions and single-strand specific S1 nuclease enzyme to digest nonannealed RNA or DNA species.

Site-directed mutagenesis: Used to introduce a specific mutation at a specific site in a DNA sequence using DNA techniques.

Southern analysis: A technique for detecting specific sequences in

DNA. A DNA sample is digested with restriction enzymes. The restriction fragments are fractionated by size on agarose gels, transferred to a nitrocellulose membrane, and subjected to hybridization using an isotopically labeled nucleic acid probe.

Subtraction cloning: Use of serial RNA–DNA hybridization reactions with removal of annealed species to enrich for transcripts unique to a particular cell type.

trans-acting factors: Diffusible products that act to regulate transcription at specific sites along the DNA strand.

Transgenic mouse: A mouse generated by the introduction of a recombinant DNA molecule at the one-cell embryo stage. The founder mouse is shown to contain the recombinant DNA molecule by, for example, examining DNA extracted from a segment of the tail, and new strains are developed if the founder mouse is able to transmit the acquired gene in a mendelian fashion.

Tyrosine kinases: Protein enzymes that have specificity for phosphorylating tyrosine residues on target proteins.

Upstream elements: DNA sequences upstream from the RNA start site of a gene that are involved in regulating its expression.

REFERENCES

1. Temin HM: Viral oncogenes. Cold Spring Harbor Symp Quant Biol 44:1, 1979
2. Leder P, Battey J, Lenoir G, et al: Translocations among antibody genes in human cancer. Science 222:765, 1983
3. Groffen J, Stephenson JR, Heisterkamp N, et al: Philadelphia chromosomal breakpoints are clustered within a limited region, *bcr*, on chromosome 22. Cell 36:93, 1984
4. Canaani E, Steiner-Saltz D, Aghai E, et al: Altered transcription of an oncogene in chronic myeloid leukaemia. Lancet 1:593, 1984
5. Collins SJ, Kubonishi I, Miyoshi I, et al: Altered transcription of the c-*abl* oncogene in K-562 and other chronic myelogenous leukemia cells. Science 225:72, 1984
6. Roeder R: Eukaryotic nuclear RNA polymerases. In Losick R, Chamberlin M (eds): RNA Polymerases, pp 285–329. Cold Spring Harbor, NY, Cold Spring Harbor Laboratory, 1986.
7. Corden J, Wasylyk B, Buchwalder A, et al: Expression of cloned genes in new environment. Science 209:1406, 1980
8. Watson JD: Molecular Biology of the Gene, 3rd ed. Menlo Park, NJ, Benjamin/Cummings, 1976
9. Darnell JE Jr: Variety in the level of gene control in eukaryotic cells. Nature 297:365, 1982
10. Ziff E, Evans RM: Coincidence of the promoter and capped 5′ terminus of RNA from the adenovirus 2 major late transcription unit. Cell 15:1463, 1978
11. Southern EM: Detection of specific sequences among DNA fragments separated by gel electrophoresis. J Mol Biol 98:503, 1975
12. Alwine JC, Kemp DJ, Stark GR: Method for detection of specific RNAs in agarose gels by transfer to diazobenzyloxymethyl-paper and hybridization with DNA probes. Proc Natl Acad Sci USA 74:5350, 1977
13. Towbin H, Staehelin T, Gordon J: Proc Natl Acad Sci USA 76:4350, 1986
14. Lewin B: Genes, 3rd ed. New York, John Wiley & Sons, 1987
15. Maxam AM, Gilbert W: A new method for sequencing DNA. Proc Natl Acad Sci USA 74:560, 1977
16. Sanger F, Nicklen S, Coulson AR: DNA sequencing with chain-terminating inhibitors. Proc Natl Acad Sci USA 74:5463, 1977
17. Watson JD, Crick FHC: Molecular structure of nucleic acid. A structure for deoxyribose nucleic acid. Nature 171:737, 1953
18. Bonner TI, Brenner DJ, Beufeld BR, et al: Reduction in the rate of DNA reassociation by sequence divergence. J Mol Biol 81:123, 1973
19. Casey J, Davidson N: Rates of formation and thermal stabilities of RNA:DNA and DNA:DNA duplexes at high concentrations of formamide. Nucleic Acids Res 4:1539, 1977
20. Hutton JR: Renaturation kinetics and thermal stability of DNA in aqueous solutions of formamide and urea. Nucleic Acids Res 4:3537, 1977
21. McConaughy BL, Laird CD, McCarthy BJ: Nucleic acid reassociation in formamide. Biochemistry 8:3289, 1969
22. Suggs, SV, Wallace RB, Hirose T, et al: Use of synthetic oligonucleotides as hybridization probes: Isolation of cloned cDNA sequences for human b2-microglobulin. Proc Natl Acad Sci USA 78:6613, 1981
23. Wallace RB, Shaffer J, Murphy RF, etal: Hybridization of synthetic oligodeoxyribonucleotides to FX174DNA: The effect of single base pair mismatch. Nucleic Acids Res 6:3543, 1979
24. Wallace RB, Johnson MJ, Hirose T, et al: The use of synthetic oligonucleotides as hybridization probes: II. Hybridization of oligonucleotides of mixed sequence to rabbit b-globin DNA. Nucleic Acids Res. 9:879, 1981
25. Tiemeir DC, Tilghman SM, Polsky FI, et al: A comparison of two cloned mouse b-globin genes and their surrounding and intervening sequences. Cell 14:237, 1978
26. Lowy DR, Gonda MA, Furth ME, et al: The human genes homologous to P21 ras viral oncogenes. In Scolnick EM, Levine AJ (eds): Tumor Viruses and Differentiation, p 435. New York, Alan R. Liss, 1983
27. Richardson CC: Enzymes in DNA metabolism. Annu Rev Biochem 38:795, 1969
28. Kornberg A: Aspects of DNA replication. Cold Spring Harbor Symp Quant Biol 43:1, 1980
29. Rigby PWJ, Dieckmann M, Rhodes C, et al: Labeling deoxyribonucleic acid to high specific activity in vitro by nick translation with DNA polymerase I. J Mol Biol 113:237, 1977
30. Maniatis T, Jeffrey A, Kleid DG: Nucleotide sequence of the rightward operator of phagel. Proc Natl Acad Sci USA 72:1184, 1975
31. Feinberg AP, Vogelstein B: A technique for radiolabelling DNA restriction endonuclease fragments to high specific activity. Ann Biochem 132:6, 1983
32. Saiki RK, Scharf S, Faloona KB, et al: Enzymatic amplication of β-globin genomic sequences and restriction site analysis for diagnosis of sickle cell anemia. Science 230:1350, 1985
33. Scharf SJ, Horn GT, Erlich HA: Direct cloning and sequence analysis of enzymatically amplified genomic sequences. Science 233:1076, 1986
34. Roberts R: Restriction and modification enzymes and their recognition sequences. Nucleic Acid Res 10:117, 1982
35. Linn S, Arber W: Host specificity of DNA produced by *Escherichia coli*. X. In vitro restriction of phage fd replicative form. Proc Natl Acad Sci USA 59:1300, 1968
36. Smith HO, Wilcox KW: A restriction enzyme from Hemophilus influenzae. I. Purification and general properties. J Mol Biol 51:379, 1970
37. Kelly TJ Jr, Smith HO: A restriction enzyme from Hemophilus influenzae. II. Base sequence of the recognition site. J Mol Biol 51:393, 1970
38. Roberts RJ: Restriction and modification enzymes and their recognition sequences. Nucleic Acids Res 9:75, 1981
39. Maniatis T, Fritsch, EF, Sambrook J: Molecular Cloning: A Laboratory Manual. Cold Spring Harbor Laboratory, Cold Spring Harbor, NY, 1982
40. Helling RB, Goodman HM, Boyer HW: Analysis of endonuclease RvEcoRI fragments of DNA from lambdoid bacteriophages and other viruses by agarose-gel electrophoresis. J Virol 14:1235, 1974
41. Sharp PA, Sugden B, Sambrook J: Detection of two restriction endonuclease activities in Haemophilus parainfluenzae using analytical agarose-ethidium bromide electrophoresis. Biochemistry 12:3055, 1973
42. Soeda E, Arrand JR, Smolar N, et al: Coding potential and regulatory signals of the polyoma virus genome. Nature 283:445, 1980
43. Southen EM: Detection of specific sequences among DNA fragments separated by gel electrophoresis. J Mol Biol 98:503, 1975
44. Schwartz DC, Cantor CR: Separation of yeast chromosome-sized DNAs by pulsed field gradient gel electrophoresis. Cell 37:67, 1984
45. Carle GF, Olson MV: Separation of chromosomal DNA molecules from yeast by ortiogonalified alternation gel electrophoresis Nucleic Acids Res 12:14, 1984
46. Chu C, Vollrath D, Davis RW: Separation of large DNA molecules by contour-clamped homogeneous electric fields. Science 234:1582, 1986
47. Vollrath D, Davis RW: Resolution of DNA molecules greater than 5 megabases by contour-clamped homogeneous electric fields. Nucleic Acids Res 15:7865, 1987
48. Smith CL, Econome JG, Schutt A, et al: A physical map of the *Escherichia coli* K12 genome. Science 236:1448, 1987
49. Park M, Dean M, Cooper CS, et al: Mechanism of *met* oncogene activation. Cell 45:895, 1986
50. Dean M, Park M, Vande Woude GF: Characterization of the rearranged *tpr-met* oncogene breakpoint. Mol Cell Biol 7:921, 1987
51. Lawrance SK, Smith CL, Srivastava R, et al: Megabase-scale mapping of the HLA gene complex by pulsed field gel electrophoresis. Science 235:1387, 1987
52. Race R, Sadnger R: Blood Groups in Man, 6th ed, p 610. Oxford, Blackwell, 1975
53. Thomas G, Bodmer W, Bodmer J: Karlin S, Nevo E (eds): The HLA system as a model for studying the interaction between selection, migration and linkage. In Population Genetics and Ecology, p 465. New York, Academic Press, 1976
54. Ploegh HL, Orr HT, Strominger JL: Major histocompatibility antigens: The human (HLA-A, -B, -C) and murine (H-LK,-D) class I molecules. Cell 24:287, 1981
55. Botstein D, White R, Skolnick M, et al: Construction of a genetic linkage map in man using restriction fragment length polymorphisms. Am J Hum Genet 32:314, 1980.
56. White R, Woodward S, Leppert M, et al: A closely linked genetic marker for cystic fibrosis. Nature 318:45, 1985
57. White RL, Barker D, Holm T, et al: Approaches to linkage analysis in the human. In Caskey CT, White RL (eds): Banbury Report 14: Recombinant DNA Applications to Human Disease. Cold Spring Harbor, NY, Cold Spring Harbor Laboratory, 1983.
58. O'Brien SJ, Nash WG: Genetic mapping in mammals: Chromosome map of domestic cat. Science 216:257, 1982
59. Harper ME, Saunders GF: Localization of single copy DNA sequences on G-banded human chromosomes by in situ hybridization. Chromosoma 83:431, 1981
60. White R, Leppert M, Bishop DT, et al: Construction of linkage maps with DNA markers for human chromosomes. Nature 101:5, 1985
61. Donis-Keller H, Green P, Helms C, et al: A genetic linkage map of the human genome. Cell 51:319, 1987
62. Morton NE: Sequential tests for the detection of linkage. Am J Hum Genet 7:277, 1955
63. Dean M, O'Connell P, Leppert M, et al: Three additional DNA polymorphisms in the *met* gene and D7S8 locus: Use in prenatal diagnosis of cystic fibrosis. J Pediatr 111:490, 1987

64. Knudson AG, Hethcote HW, Brown BW: Mutation and childhood cancer: A probabilistic model for the incidence of retinoblastoma. Proc Natl Acad Sci USA 72:5116, 1975

65. Francke U: Specific chromosome changes in the human heritable tumors retinoblastoma and nephroblastoma. In Rowley JD, Ultmann JE (eds): Chromosomes and Cancer. Bristol-Myers Symposia Series vol 5, p 99. New York, Academic Press, 1983

66. Cavenee WK, Dryja TP, Phillips RA, et al: Expression of recessive alleles by chromosomal mechanisms in retinoblastoma. Nature 305:779, 1983

67. Bodmer WF, Bailey CJ, Bodmer J, et al: Localization of the gene for familial adenomatous polyposis on chromosome 5. Nature 328: 614, 1987

68. Solomon E, Voss R, Hall V, et al: Chromosome 5 allele loss in human colorectal carcinoma. Nature 328:616, 1987

69. Zbar B, Brauch H, Talmadge C, et al: Loss of alleles of loci on the short arm of chromosome 3 in renal cell carcinoma. Nature 327:721, 1987

70. Rowley JD, Golomb HM, Vardiman JW: Nonrandom chromosome abnormalities in acute leukemia and dysmyelopoietic syndromes in patients with previously treated malignant disease. Blood 58:759, 1981

71. Roberts L: Human genome: Questions of cost. Science 237:1411, 1987

72. Dugaiczyk A, Boyer HW, Goodman HM: Ligation of EcoRI endonuclease-generated DNA fragments into linear and circular structures. J Mol Biol 96:171, 1975

73. Bolivar F, Backman K: Plasmids of *Escherichia coli* as cloning vectors. Methods Enzymol 68:245, 1979

74. Bernard HU, Helinski DR: Bacterial plasmid cloning vehicles. In Setlow JK, Hollaender A (eds): Genetic Engineering, vol 2, p 133. New York, Plenum Press, 1980

75. Grunstein M, Hogness D: Colony hybridization: A method for the isolation of cloned DNAs that contain a specific gene. Proc Natl Acad Sci USA 72:3961, 1975

76. Benton WD, Davis RW: Screen λgt recombinant clones by hybridization to single plagues in situ. Science 196:180, 1977

77. Wu R, Jay E, Roychoudburg R: Nucleotide sequence analysis of DNA. Methods Cancer Res 12:87, 1976

78. Smith HO, Bernstiel ML: A simple method for DNA restriction site mapping. Nucleic Acids Res 3:2387, 1976

79. Gluzman Y: Eukaryotic Viral Vectors. Cold Spring Harbor, NY, Cold Spring Harbor Laboratory, 1982

80. Maniatis T, Hardison RC, Lacy E, et al: The isolation of structural genes from libraries of eucaryotic DNA. Cell 15:687, 1978

81. Saito I, Stark GR: Charomids: Cosmid vectors for efficient cloning and mapping of large or small restriction fragments. Proc Natl Acad Sci USA 83:8664, 1986

82. Watson JD, Tooze J, Kurtz DT: Recombinant DNA: A Short Course. New York, Scientific American Books, 1983

83. Steinmetz M, Moor KW, Frelinger JA, et al: A pseudogene homologous to mouse transplantation antigens: Transplantation antigens are encoded by light exons that correlate with protein domains. Cell 25:683, 1981

84. Steinmetz M, Winoto A, Minard K, et al: Clusters of genes encoding mouse transplantation antigens. Cell 28:489, 1982

85. Burke DT, Carle GF, Olson MV: Cloning of large segments of exogenous DNA into yeast by means of artificial chromosome vectors. Science 236:806, 1987

86. Moore EE, Jones C, Kao FT, et al: Synteny between glycineamide ribonucleotide synthetase and superoxide dismutase soluble. Am J Hum Genet 29:389, 1977

87. Kunkel LM, Tantravahi U, Eisenhard M, et al: Regional localization on the human X of DNA segments cloned from flow sorted chromosomes. Nucleic Acids Res 10:1557, 1982

88. Orkin SH: Reverse genetics and human disease. Cell 47:845, 1986

89. Smith LM, Sanders JZ, Kaiser RJ, etal: Fluorescence detection in automated DNA sequence analysis. Nature 321:674, 1986

90. Prober JM, Trainor GL, Dam RJ, et al: A system for rapid DNA sequencing with fluorescent chain-terminating dideoxynucleotides. Science 238:336, 1987

91. Lee M-S, Chang K-S, Cabanillas F, et al: Detection of minimal residual cells carrying the t(14;18) by DNA sequence amplification. Science 237:175, 1987

92. Crescenzi M, Seta M, Herzig GP, et al: Thermophilic polymerase chain amplification of t(14/18) breakpoints and the detection of minimal residual disease. Proc Natl Acad Sci USA (in press)

93. Watson JD, Tooze J: The DNA Story. San Francisco, WH Freeman, 1981

94. Blair DG, Oskarsson M, Wood TG, et al: Activation of the transforming potential of a normal cell sequence: A molecular model for oncogenesis. Science 212:941, 1981

95. Dean M, Park M, Le Beau MM, et al: The human *met* oncogene is related to the tyrosine kinase oncogenes. Nature 318:385, 1985

96. Gray JW, Dean PN, Fuscoe JC, et al: High-speed chromosome sorting. Science 238:323, 1987

SUSAN VANDE WOUDE

GEORGE F. VANDE WOUDE

CHAPTER 3

Principles of Molecular Cell Biology of Cancer: General Aspects of Gene Regulation

The human genome contains 50,000 to 100,000 genes encoded in its DNA sequence. Each codes for a specific product, either an RNA or a protein, which has a unique function in cellular metabolism. Whether the individual cell is a neuron or hepatocyte, its genetic information is essentially the same. How each cell determines its phenotype and maintains its cellular function throughout its life is a marvelous, albeit complex, achievement.

Genomic DNA is contained in chromosomes as described in a previous chapter. Were it possible to stretch out a DNA molecule, a human chromosome would measure several centimeters in length; in the cell nucleus it is highly coiled in an exquisitely ordered structure to facilitate regulated expression. A myriad of complex protein-nucleotide interactions occur in the process of gene expression that ultimately results in specific protein synthesis. Initially, DNA is copied into RNA in a process called transcription, and the RNA is then used as a template for protein synthesis in a process called translation. The host of events that occur during these processes is discussed in greater detail in the following sections. As will be seen, while some of the particular enzymes and proteins that regulate the actual processes are being characterized, much is yet to be discovered about genes, their control elements, and the protein complexes which control this process. Gene expression, the molecular basis for cell division, specialization, and differentiation, is a vast topic; current molecular biological techniques have just begun to reveal the mechanisms of the detailed cellular processes leading to phenotypic expression. The elucidation of these processes has enormous implications not only for understanding normal cell function, but also for unraveling mechanisms in cell dysfunction.

TRANSCRIPTION

In eukaryotes, the enzyme RNA polymerase II (RNA polII) copies (transcribes) genes (DNA sequences) into messenger RNA (mRNA)[1,2] using monomeric nucleotides similar to the four bases used in DNA. The bases in RNA differ from that of DNA by a single substitution of an alcohol group for a hydrogen at the 2' position of the ribose backbone (hence ribonucleic acid versus deoxyribonucleic acid). Also note that uracil (U) replaces thymidine (T) as one of the four basic subunits of RNA structure. RNA polymerase begins transcription at a promoter initiation site that lies "upstream" of the DNA coding sequence,[1,2] the part of the gene which, once transcribed into RNA, forms a template for protein synthesis.

31

Many eukaryotic promoter regions have been shown to contain characteristic (consensus) nucleic acid sequences. With many genes these regions consist of a TATA box located 25 to 30 nucleotides upstream of the mRNA start site,[3-8] and one or more sites designated as "upstream elements" which lie 20 to 70 bp further upstream.[9] The upstream elements often contain GC rich regions[3,4,10,11] and the sequence CCAAT.[12] The promoter region is responsible for directing the correct initiation point of mRNA transcription; the upstream elements influence frequency of transcription initiation.[3,9,13] Transcription initiation in these regions is mediated or influenced by protein factors in addition to RNA polII that are required as coactivators of initiation. Before transcription initiation, the appropriate regions of DNA must be exposed so that RNA polymerase and transcription activation protein complexes can begin RNA synthesis.[14]

DNA sequences called enhancers are involved in the regulation of transcription. Enhancers are specific DNA sequences that may be 50 to 200 nucleotides in length and are often repeated several times. They are found hundreds to thousands of bases (1000 nucleotides is referred to as a kilobase or kb) on either side (upstream or downstream) of the DNA coding sequence (Fig. 3-1A). These are recognition sequences or targets for DNA binding proteins that participate in enhancing (or suppressing) transcription.[9,13] Enhancers were first identified as control elements of viral transcription and are often constitutively turned on (positively regulated) in host cells to provide the virus access to cell expression systems. In contrast, cellular gene enhancers can be strictly conditional and limit expression to specific cell types. For example, the IgG enhancers only function in lymphoid cells.[15,16] The recognition sequences encoded in the DNA are called cis acting while the factors that bind to these sites act in trans.[17] Thus, gene expression, or transcription, is regulated by cis recognition elements and trans acting factors.

The DNA molecule is double-stranded; one strand is called the sense strand and contains the encoded protein information. The nucleotide sequence is linked via a phosphate backbone in a 5' to 3' direction while the other, complementary DNA strand, contains antisense information and its nucleotide sequence is 3' to 5' in orientation (see Chapter 2). The RNA transcript is transcribed 5' to 3' from the antisense DNA strand. The initial 5' portion of the RNA transcript usually does not encode amino acid sequence information and consequently is known as untranslated (UT) leader. The next segment of the newly synthesized RNA contains coding (exon) and noncoding (intron) information.[18] Most eukaryotic gene primary transcripts contain one or more introns, and during mRNA maturation these introns are removed by processing or splicing to yield the mature mRNA molecule (Fig. 3-1B). The functions of introns are not completely understood,[18] and in most cases, they represent a much greater portion of the genetic locus than the actual coding sequences.

With few exceptions, the protein coding region is followed by noncoding sequences which are referred to as the 3' untranslated region (U). The end of the RNA is terminated by

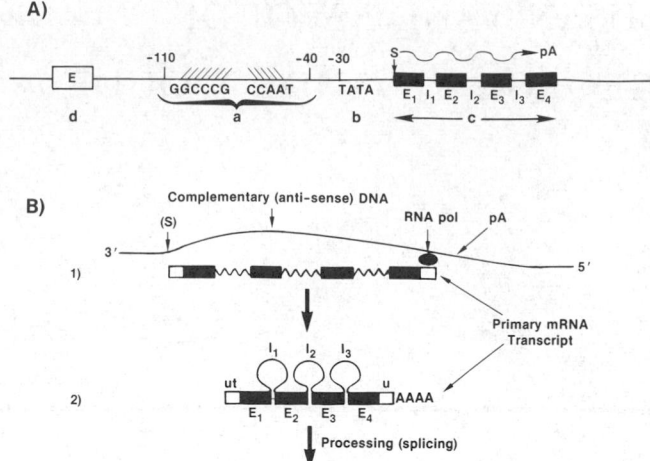

FIG. 3-1. **A.** Diagram of important elements of a eukaryotic transcription unit. *(a)* Upstream elements important for control of transcription initiation. Found 40 to 110 nucleotides upstream from the mRNA start site S, these regions variously contain GC rich and/or CCAAT sequences.[3,9,13] *(b)* The RNA polII binding region or promoter located 30 bp upstream from the mRNA start site and consisting of the sequence TATA. *(c)* The DNA region actually copied into its complementary RNA sequence. S represents the beginning of the untranslated leaders; black (E_1, E_2, E_3, E_4) signifies exons or regions corresponding to amino acid sequences in the corresponding protein product while the introns (I_1, I_2, I_3) represent nonprotein coding regions which are spliced out during mRNA processing. pA signifies the end of the mRNA sequence where polyadenylation occurs. A polyadenylation signal is encoded in the DNA. *(d)* Enhancers are required in cis for efficient transcription to occur from eukaryotic promoters. They can be located hundreds or thousands of bases upstream or downstream or in the DNA coding sequence.[9,13,15,16] **B.** Eukaryotic messenger RNA transcription. mRNA synthesis by polymerase II is initiated from the promoter site described in the text and in **A.** RNA is transcribed from the complementary DNA strand of the structural (protein coding) region of the gene. Thus, the 5' end of the RNA is transcribed from the upstream DNA sequence in the 3' to 5' direction (line 1). Supercoiled DNA must be unwound during this process. For clarity, only the complementary antisense DNA strand is shown. The first portion of the mRNA strand is designated the untranslated (ut) leader as the immediate 5' end of the message usually lacks protein coding information. The newly transcribed mRNA (primary transcript) structural coding information (exons, E_1, E_2, E_3, and E_4) is interrupted by several noncoding regions (introns, I_1, I_2, and I_3), which are processed (spliced) out to form the mature mRNA (lines 2 and 3). The 3' end also often contains untranslatable information (U). Both the 5' and 3' untranslated regions have been implicated in regulating translational efficiency and mRNA stability. The mRNA is terminated by addition of approximately 200 adenine nucleotide bases by the process of polyadenylation.[19] The mature transcript (line 3) is transported to and translated in the cytoplasm.

posttranscriptional modification called polyadenylation. A polymer of adenylic (A) ribonucleotides (poly A tail) approximately 200 bp long[19] is added in response to a cis-acting polyadenylation signal and a specific polyadenylation site usually 20 bases downstream from this signal. Thus, characteristic sequences are identified at the point in mRNA where polyadenylation begins, yet there is not a DNA template for the poly A tail[20,21] (see Fig. 3-1).

CHARACTERIZATION OF SPECIFIC mRNA SPECIES

Central to the study of gene transcription is the ability to isolate mRNA species from the cellular milieu. This process is complicated by the fact that mRNA represents only 1% to 2% of total cellular RNA and because destructive RNases are prevalent in the environment.[22] The other major cellular RNA species are transfer RNA (tRNA), which plays a key role in amino acid polymerization during protein synthesis, and ribosomal RNA (rRNA), which makes up the nucleotide structure of cytoplasmic ribosomes, the structures on which protein translation occurs. mRNA extraction is performed with great care to avoid contamination with RNases, and the unique feature of a poly A tail is used to selectively enrich for the mRNA fraction. Under appropriate salt conditions poly A sequences will anneal (hybridize) to an oligo dT-cellulose column (a polymer of deoxythymidine), while other RNA species and contaminating protein or DNA species are washed through (Fig. 3-2A). The mRNA can then be eluted from the column by lowering the salt concentration and collecting fractions.[23,24]

S1 NUCLEASE PROTECTION AND NORTHERN ANALYSIS

Specific mRNA transcripts from cells can be identified by several methods. One method, S1 nuclease protection analysis, utilizes hybridization (base pairing) between mRNA and a specific DNA probe. An isotopically labeled DNA fragment

FIG. 3-2. mRNA isolation and cDNA cloning. **A**. In order to isolate mRNA from total RNA, the latter is applied to an oligo dt-cellulose column under high salt conditions. Non-poly A sequences wash through as poly A sequences greater than 20 nucleotides can anneal. When a low salt buffer is applied to the column, the bound mRNA will elute off. **B**. To make a cDNA library, the mRNA isolated as described in **A** is incubated with free deoxynucleotides and other cofactors and the enzyme reverse transcriptase (RT) (usually isolated from avian myeloblastosis virus) is added to copy the RNA sequence into DNA. The single-strand DNA copy made from the RNA template ends with a hairpin loop and a 3' double-strand DNA region remains (line 1). The DNA copy of the RNA template is isolated; DNA polymerase is added to complete synthesis of the second DNA strand (line 2). S1 nuclease is then utilized to hydrolyze the single-strand loop (line 3) and the resultant complementary DNAs (cDNAs) are cloned using protocols similar to those discussed in Chapter 2 (line 4).

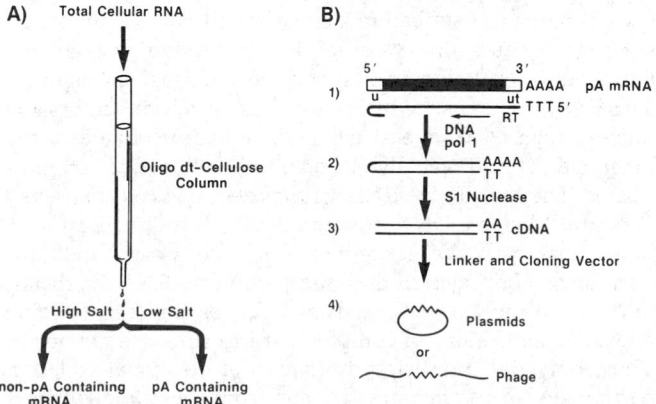

complementary to the specific RNA in question is denatured and mixed with total or poly A-enriched RNA. Conditions are then provided that favor RNA-DNA hybridization. A DNase S1 nuclease reaction is performed that digests all single-stranded RNA and DNA present in the reaction, but not the DNA-RNA hybrids.[25,26] These complexes are then analyzed or resolved by polyacrylamide gel electrophoresis (Fig. 3-3).[25,26] This technique is extremely sensitive because RNA/DNA annealing conditions are very selective. Therefore, genes that are expressed at very low levels can be identified in the presence of very large quantities of "other" RNA because of the sensitivity of single-stranded molecules to S1 nuclease.[27] Recently, procedures have been developed that allow radioisotopically labeled RNA probes with high specific activity to be generated using specific prokaryotic promoter systems. Assays that utilize RNA/RNA hybridization conditions and RNA nuclease enzymes that digest single- but not double-stranded RNA molecules can then be performed.[28]

Perhaps the most widely used technique for detecting mRNA transcripts is a method analogous to the DNA Southern blot analysis (see Chap. 2) and is known as Northern analysis.[29] In this technique, total RNA or poly-A enriched RNA is extracted as described above and subjected to electrophoresis on a gel matrix where it is resolved based on size. The RNA can then be transferred and covalently linked to a membrane filter.[29] Specific mRNA species can then be identified by hybridization with isotopically labeled probes. Northern analyses can reveal quantitative and qualitative information on steady state RNA transcripts and have been useful for identification of amplified gene expression (e.g., c-*myc* in promyelocytic cells, HL60, see Chap. 4) or hybrid RNA transcripts in rearranged genomic loci (e.g., the novel 8.0 kb *bcr-abl* hybrid transcript expressed in chronic myelogenous leukemia that arises from the Philadelphia chromosome 9;22 translocation between *bcr* and *abl*).[30,31]

DETERMINING THE STRUCTURE OF THE mRNA

S1 nuclease protection analysis (see Fig. 3-3) is also useful for identifying RNA transcript structure. For example, if a genomic DNA fragment that overlaps an exon/intron junction is used as probe (*i.e.*, the labeled end is in an exon), hybridization with its homologous RNA will contain a single-stranded region which will be degraded by S1 nuclease. For example, if the -N-N-N- portion of the DNA fragment in Figure 3-3 is intron sequence, this region is processed out of the RNA and the S1 nuclease would truncate the probe corresponding to the exon/intron splice junction, thereby approximating its position in the DNA sequence.[32]

A procedure called primer extension is used to identify the 5' end of an RNA transcript. In this technique, a complementary antisense oligonucleotide primer of finite length (~2–50 bases) which has been isotopically labeled (*e.g.*, at its 5' end) is hybridized with its homologous mRNA. Reverse transcriptase, a retroviral enzyme that promotes DNA synthesis from RNA precursors, is then used to generate a copy of the mRNA toward its 5' end. The product is analyzed by gel electrophoresis for size estimation. It is also possible from this reaction to directly determine the DNA sequence from

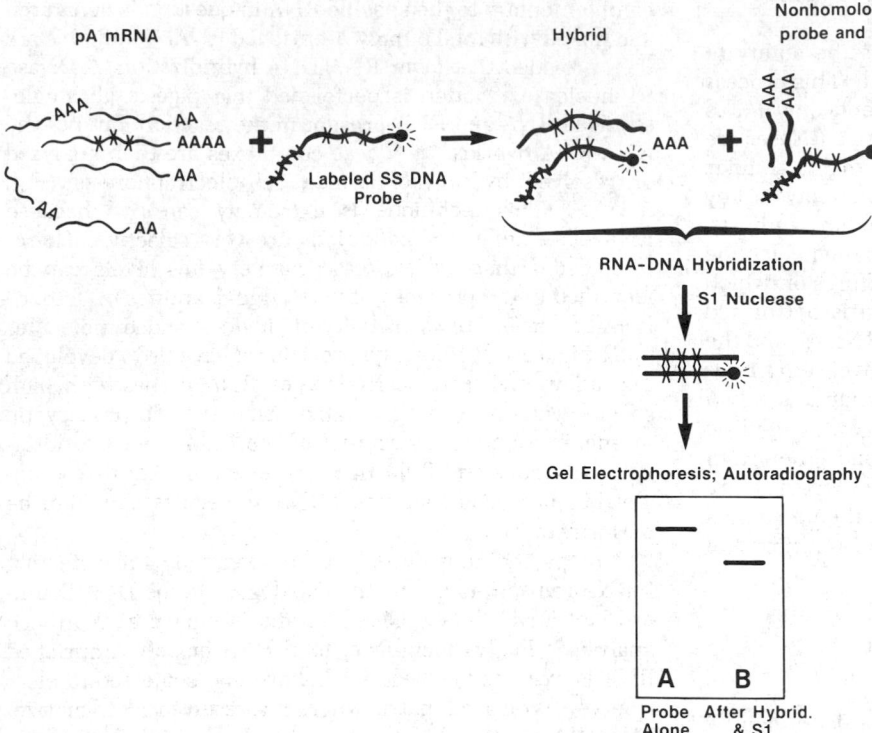

FIG. 3-3. S1 nuclease analysis. S1 nuclease is used to demonstrate that a specific transcript is present in a population of mRNAs. A radioactively labeled single-stranded DNA probe is denatured and mixed with the mRNAs. Buffer and temperature conditions favoring RNA-DNA annealing are provided. S1 nuclease is added, which degrades all single-strand DNA and RNA in the mixture; only the double-strand RNA/DNA product is resistant to digestion. The product is analyzed by gel electrophoresis and autoradiography for size and abundance.

which the RNA was synthesized. This information can be used to localize the transcription initiation site in genomic DNA.[33,34]

COMPLEMENTARY DNA (cDNA) CLONING AND SUBTRACTION CLONING

Techniques to isolate and characterize mRNA provide an important tool for study of gene transcription. Expression of mRNA in various tissues can be identified, quantified, and further studied. In addition, mRNA extraction techniques allow use of a powerful technique called cDNA cloning. mRNAs are isolated from a specific tissue type using oligo dT-cellulose chromatography or a similar method. Reverse transcriptase is used to generate single-stranded DNA copies from the mRNA molecules (see Fig. 3-2B). DNA polymerase is then used to generate double-stranded DNA fragments which can be cloned into conventional prokaryotic vectors as described in Chapter 2 to yield cDNA libraries.[23] cDNA libraries differ from genomic libraries by being limited to only the transcribed portion of genes and therefore are greatly reduced in sequence complexity. These libraries are useful in providing amplified copies of specific sequences; for example, a cDNA library from bone marrow RBC precursors will contain many copies of globin cDNA, whereas this gene occurs only once in a genomic library.

cDNA libraries prepared in a similar manner have been extremely useful for identifying transcripts that are differentially regulated in related cell types in the so-called subtraction cloning technique. For example, to identify novel transcripts specifically expressed in mitogenically stimulated cells compared to resting cells, single-stranded cDNA pre-

pared from the former is annealed with an excess of RNA prepared from the latter. RNA-DNA hybrids representing sequences common to both cell types are removed by chromatographic procedures. After repeating the cycle several times, the remaining noncomplementary single-strand cDNA is recovered. A library is generated from this enriched cDNA fraction and can be screened with isotopically labeled total RNA from each cell type to identify the novel transcripts.[35,36] Obviously, this technique or variation of it can be used to identify transcripts specific for transformed versus normal cell types as well as differentiation specific gene transcripts.

RUN ON, IN VITRO, AND GENE TRANSFER TRANSCRIPTION ASSAYS

Run on transcription is a technique used to study whether a gene is being transcribed in a specific cell type, or in kinetic studies, to determine whether its expression is regulated during differentiation in response to a mitogenic signal.[37] This assay makes use of in situ RNA transcription factors and nuclei prepared from test cells which are incubated in the presence of isotopically labeled ribonucleotide triphosphates. The radioactive RNA synthesized in vitro is extracted and annealed to DNA fragments fixed to nitrocellulose filters that span the genomic locus. The assay conditions only favor continuation and completion of RNA synthesis; initiation of new RNA strands and processing (i.e., splicing and polyadenylation) of completed transcripts will not occur. Thus, only the transcripts initiated before nuclei isolation participate (or run on) in vitro, and from these analyses it is possible to define the kinetics of regulation of gene transcription within a cell cycle and approximate the size of the transcription locus. RNA transcription usually proceeds beyond pA signals, but thus far transcription termination has not been shown to be independent of polyadenylation.[38]

RNA synthesis initiation and characterization of promoters can be studied in vitro (in vitro transcription) by the addition of a DNA substrate to enriched cellular factors containing RNA polymerase and labeled ribonucleotide triphosphates.[37,40-42] The DNA substrate is cleaved by several restriction enzymes downstream from a putative transcription start site, and the size of the RNA products synthesized from the DNA template allows mapping of promoter regions.[25,41-43]

DNA-mediated gene transfer in tissue culture is used to assay gene expression. Under appropriate conditions, recombinant DNA constructs containing a promoter and an appropriate reporter gene can be transferred (transfected) into cells, and expression can be measured by reporter gene activity.[44-47] Analysis of mRNA or a reporter gene product produced by intact cells can be used to reveal cis-acting promoter elements. A sensitive reporter assay has been developed in which a prokaryotic enzyme, chloramphenicol acetyl transferase (CAT), is used as a marker of gene expression.[48] This gene is responsible for inducing chloramphenicol resistance in strains of bacteria. It inactivates chloramphenicol by forming monoacetylated and diacetylated derivatives[49] using acetyl coA as a substrate. If the CAT gene is linked to a eukaryotic transcription control element and these constructs are transfected into mammalian or eukaryotic cells, cell extracts can be readily assayed for CAT activity as a measure of gene expression (Fig. 3-4). Different transcription control elements can reveal quantitative differences in CAT activity and serve to identify tissue-specific enhancers. Mutations introduced into the transcription control element which alter relative CAT activity can identify the responsible cis DNA sequences.

TRANSLATION

The mature processed mRNA (with spliced out introns and a poly A tail) is transported to the cytoplasm where it is pre-

FIG. 3-4. CAT assay for analysis of gene expression in cells. **A**. Constructs are developed using cloning techniques that link an appropriate promoter or enhancer, or both, to the chloramphenicol acetylase gene (CAT). **B**. Tissue culture cells are transfected with the genomic construct. **C**. After an appropriate amount of time, cell extracts containing the CAT protein are mixed with radiolabeled chloramphenicol and acetyl CoA. **D**. Mixtures from **C** are spotted on thin layer silica gels. The separation of chloramphenicol (cm), 1-acetate cm, 3-acetate cm, and 1,3 diacetate cm are rapidly separated by this method of chromatography. Autoradiography subsequently allows visualization of the end products and allows calculation of enzymatic activity and ultimately the level of gene expression.

pared as a substrate for protein synthesis. The 5' sequences of mRNA are methylated or capped[50] during mRNA processing or maturation; this may serve as a protective mechanism by making the mRNA resistant to certain ribonucleases, or may serve a function in ribosomal recognition or transport of the molecule from the nucleus.[51,52] Protein synthesis occurs in the cytosol on large protein-RNA structures known as ribosomes.[53-55] Eukaryotic ribosomes consist of two unequal subunits; they bind mRNA molecules in the presence of appropriate factors and tRNA and direct amino acid polymerization into protein molecules. The mechanism for transport of mRNA from nucleus to cytoplasm and subsequent initiation of ribosomal binding is a complex process where structural features of the mRNA (e.g., 5' and 3' untranslated regions) may play a role.[51,55]

In order for mRNA to be translated into the specific protein for which it encodes, interactions between translation initiation enzymes, cofactors, amino acid charged tRNA, and ribosomes must take place. The protein coding information of mRNA, the series of codons or triplet nucleotides, serve as recognition sites for aminoacyl tRNA (genetic code, Table 3-1). The first amino acid codon of every mRNA is methionine. It is required in all cells for the initiation of translation and therefore AUG is called the initiation codon. Subsequent triplets of nucleotides encode for one of the 20 amino acids found in eukaryotic proteins. The decoding occurs on the surface of the ribosome via the complementary pairing of a specific tRNA, charged with its specific amino acid, to its respective codon. The ribosome translocates from 5' to 3' in an energy-dependent reaction and at each codon the respective charged tRNA contributes its amino acid covalently to a growing peptide chain. Many ribosomes spaced at finite intervals can participate in translation of the same mRNA simultaneously; these structures with multiple growing protein chains are referred to as polyribosomes.[30,54,56,57] The codons UAA, UAG, and UGA are translation termination signals that cause the dissociation of ribosomes from the mRNA and the cessation of the protein synthesis reaction. The protein is released from the ribosome and further processed, transported to its site of action, incorporated into cellular structure, or used as is. Examples of post-translational modifications that can occur and are most often required for biological activity include glycosylation (addition of one or more sugar moieties), phosphorylation (addition of a phosphate group), proteolytic cleavage (e.g., cleavage of proinsulin into C peptide and insulin), or subunit binding (e.g., oligomeric structures such as the adult hemoglobin molecule, which consists of independently synthesized α and β subunits.)[58]

As with transcription, translation can be carried out in vitro in a cell-free extract. Two such systems commonly employed are attained from rabbit reticulocytes[58-60] and wheat germ extract.[58,61,62] Translational activity is studied by uses of radioactively labeled amino acids which are incorporated into protein end products. Gel electrophoresis is then used to separate the synthesized polypeptide; two-dimensional separation can be achieved by subjecting the sample to isoelectric focusing using a pH gradient in the second dimension.[63] Autoradiography then allows visualization of the protein. If antibodies against the protein under study are

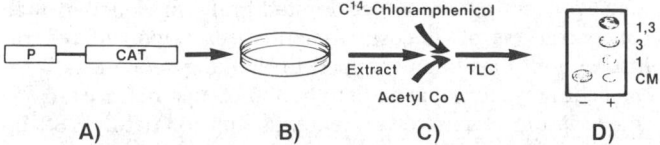

C[14]-Chloramphenicol

P — CAT → (dish) Extract → TLC
Acetyl Co A

1,3
3
1
CM
− +

A)   B)   C)   D)

TABLE 3-1.   The Genetic Code*

First Position in Codon	Second Position in Codon				Third Position in Codon (3' end)
	U	C	A	G	
U	Phe	Ser	Tyr	Cys	U
	Phe	Ser	Tyr	Cys	C
	Leu	Ser	Ter	Ter	A
	Leu	Ser	Ter	Trp	G
C	Leu	Pro	His	Arg	U
	Leu	Pro	His	Arg	C
	Leu	Pro	Gln	Arg	A
	Leu	Pro	Gln	Arg	G
A	Ile	Thr	Asn	Ser	U
	Ile	Thr	Asn	Ser	C
	Ile	Thr	Lys	Arg	A
	Met	Thr	Lys	Arg	G
G	Val	Ala	Asp	Gly	U
	Val	Ala	Asp	Gly	C
	Val	Ala	Glu	Gly	A
	Val	Ala	Glu	Gly	G

*The three RNA nucleotide bases coding for amino acid codons are given in first, second, and third positions in the 5' to 3' notation. For example, the codon 5' AUG 3' on mRNA specifies methionine, whereas CUC specifies leucine. UAA, UAG, and UGA are translational termination signals. AUG codes for methionine and is the first amino acid or initiation signal of every protein, but also codes for internal methionines. Uridine (U), cytidine (C), adenine (A), and guanine (G) are nucleotide bases. Alanine (Ala), arginine (Arg), asparagine (Asn), aspartic (Asp), cysteine (Cys), glutamic (Glu), glutamine (Gln), glycine (Gly), histidine (His), isoleucine (Ilc), leucine (Leu), lysine (Lys), methionine (Met), phenylalanine (Phe), proline (Pro), serine (Ser), threonine (Thr), tyrosine (Tyr), tryptophan (Trp), and valine (Val) are amino acids.

available, immunoprecipitation can be used as an identification method.[64] Tryptic digestion[65-67] and amino acid sequencing[68] are alternative methods of protein analysis and used for comparing one product to another as in a fingerprint (see Chap. 2).

Independent or simultaneous transcription and translation can be performed in *Xenopus laevis* oocytes. These cells have two advantages for use as expression systems; they are extremely large (approximately 1.2 mm in diameter) and contain large stores of gene transcription and mRNA translation machinery. DNA or mRNA can be introduced into the prepared oocyte by microinjection techniques, and protein or RNA end products are assayed as described above.[34,69]

Specific polypeptides and proteins can be detected in cells in culture by in vivo amino acid labeling procedures, followed by immunoprecipitation, gel analysis, and autoradiography as described above. Steady-state levels of polypeptides can be measured by Western blot analysis,[70] in which proteins from either cells or tissues solubilized in ionic detergents are subject to polyacrylamide gel electrophoresis, which fractionates them based on size. The fractionated cell proteins are then transferred to nitrocellulose or nylon membrane,[71] and, following incubation with appropriate antibodies, individual polypeptide bands recognized by the antibody can be visualized by either isotopic or nonisotopic enzymatic labeling procedures.[71]

OVERVIEW

Now that the processes of transcription and translation have been outlined, it may be helpful to discuss the processing of

an expressed gene from start to finish to illustrate some of the aforementioned points (Fig. 3-5). We describe insulin because its synthesis has been fairly well characterized. Insulin is a 5700-dalton protein comprising an A and B chain connected by two disulfide bonds between cysteine residues on each polypeptide.[72] It is synthesized primarily in the beta cells of the islets of Langerhans of the pancreas. Secretion of insulin appears to be mediated by glucose[72,73] and other soluble factors such as amino acids, catecholamines, glucagon, and hormones;[73,74] it is likely that these metabolites play a role both as transcriptional inducers and by increasing posttranscriptional levels of insulin.[75-79]

The human insulin gene is located on chromosome 11 in the terminal band of the short arm (parathyroid hormone, β-globin, and LDH-A genes are also located in this region) and occupies 1.5 kb of the DNA.[80] It contains two introns, an untranslated leader and a noncoding 3' untranslated region.[81,82] As mentioned, glucose is a positive regulator for insulin RNA transcription in the islet cells and increases in cAMP levels seem to correspond to induction of insulin gene expression.[79,83,84] Rising cAMP levels are also induced in islet cells under the influence of glucagon-like peptide with concurrent rise in insulin mRNA transcripts. Thus, insulin gene expression seems to be regulated via cellular second messengers. mRNA stability seems to be increased in high glucose conditions[83] and, as will be discussed later, translational processing is also accelerated in the presence of high concentrations of glucose. An enhancer region of the rat insulin gene has been mapped to flanking sequences 5' of the coding region approximately 330 bp upstream from the transcription start site and extends approximately 130 bp toward the gene. The sequence in this region is highly reiter-

FIG. 3-5. Synthesis of insulin occurs within the β cells of the pancreas. Glucose and other positive regulators likely act through a second messenger intermediate to induce mRNA synthesis. mRNA transcription and processing occur within the nucleus; the initial preproinsulin mRNA is transported through the nuclear membrane to the ribosomes and rough endoplasmic reticulum (RER). The initial translation product (preproinsulin) is 11,500 daltons; a 23 amino acid sequence at the amino terminal end aids transport through the RER, and then is cleaved off. This results in proinsulin, which is subsequently transported to the Golgi apparatus, where it is packaged into vesicles with zinc. While transversing toward the cell membrane, the C peptide is cleaved from the molecule to form mature insulin. The vesicles are released into the pancreatic ducts by emicytosis, an energy-dependent process. ChII, chromosome 11; AAA, poly A tail.

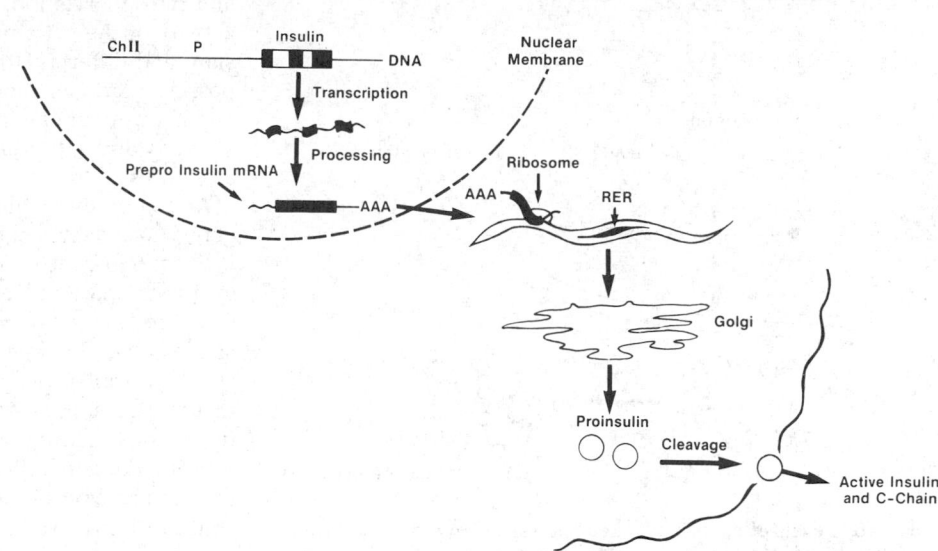

ated and most likely contains several binding sites for various trans-acting factors.[85] A negative regulatory element has also been mapped upstream of the rat insulin gene that seems to suppress enhancer activity.[86]

Once gene activation occurs, the mRNA transcript is synthesized and processed by intron splicing, capping, and polyadenylation. The 600 nucleotide mature transcript is transported from the nucleus to the ribosomes where its initial translation product is an 11,500-dalton protein called preproinsulin. The 23-amino acid sequence at the amino terminus of this polypeptide (a signal peptide) facilitates transport of the molecule through the initial part of the cell secretory apparatus (the endoplasmic reticulum) where it is cleaved to the proinsulin molecule.[72,87] Human proinsulin differs from mature insulin by the presence of an additional 35 amino acid residue referred to as the C chain. This polypeptide links the carboxy terminus of the B chain to the amino terminus of the A chain; it is this form of the molecule that is packaged into secretory granules within the β cell.[72,87]

Recent experimental evidence indicates that at least in vitro, glucose can enhance transcription by stimulating rate of initiation of transcription, increasing elongation rate of the polypeptide (i.e., speeding up synthesis postinitiation of translation), and can increase the rate of transfer of newly synthesized preproinsulin into secretory membranes.[88]

The secretory granules previously alluded to are formed at the Golgi apparatus by pinocytosis. They contain a dense core of insulin within a membranous sac;[89] zinc is also present, most likely in a complex with the insulin molecules, and high concentrations of calcium are also present in the vesicle.[90] The granules move toward the cell membrane via movements of the β cell microtubule microfilament system. As they traverse the cell, the C chain of proinsulin is cleaved from the A and B chains to produce mature insulin molecules. This reaction involves proteolytic cleavage by tryptic and carboxypeptidase enzymes and may be dependent on pH changes occurring within the vesicle.[91-93] The rate of con-

version can also be increased in the presence of glucose.[94] Once at the plasma membrane, fusion of the granules with the β cell membrane occurs and mature insulin is released into the extracellular space.[90] This process, called emicytosis, is an energy dependent process that also requires calcium (see Fig. 3-5).[95] Thus, it is clear that at every level from initiation or induction of gene transcription through release of the biologically active protein product, there are mechanisms that can stoichiometrically influence the amount of gene product expressed.

CONTROL OF GENE EXPRESSION

The preceding sections have described mechanisms of transcription and translation and current techniques being used to elucidate rate and molecular details of these processes for various eukaryotic genes. It is apparent at this point that the production of proteins which alternately determined phenotype and function of a cell can be regulated at many levels. Outlined below are possible sites where various molecular mechanisms could halt or turn on specific gene expression (Fig. 3-6).

REGULATION OF RNA TRANSCRIPTION

This level of gene control is probably the most widely studied by molecular biologists, yet detailed mechanisms of gene regulation at this level remain to be elucidated. Within a specific cell type, certain genes are "switched on" while others are "switched off" and thus inaccessible to the cell's transcriptional machinery. The resultant combination of gene products are responsible for the cell's phenotype (or necessary for expression of the appropriate phenotype). Addition of methyl groups to nucleotide residues, a process termed DNA methylation, is one mechanism that has been proposed as a regulator of gene expression.[51,96] Nuclease

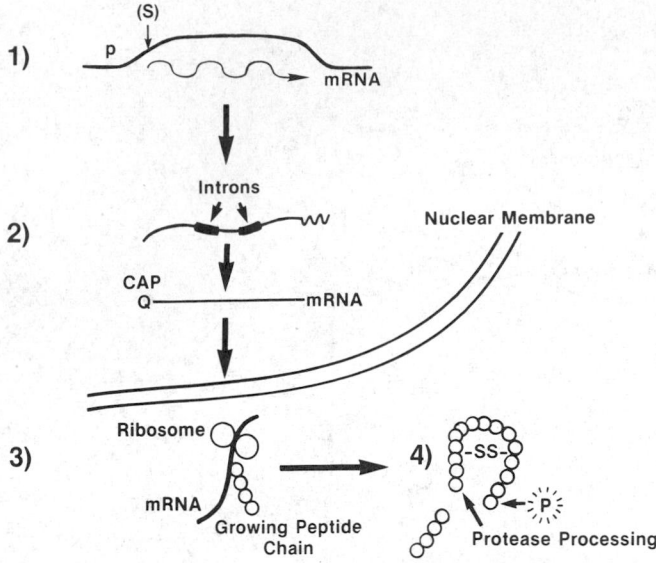

FIG. 3-6. Levels of control of gene expression can exist at (1) transcription of DNA into mRNA; (2) mRNA processing and transport; (3) protein synthesis; and (4) post-translational modification and transport. P, phosphorylation; -SS-, disulfide link; CAP Q, mRNA cap site.

sensitive sites have been mapped in chromatin in important transcription control elements[97] implicating chromosomal unwinding and uncovering of DNA as a possible gene control mechanism. How and when the switching on and off of genes occurs, how the activity of genes may be altered in diseased states and aging, and what outside mechanisms can alter cell behavior via changes in gene regulation are key questions currently being addressed. Considering nature's frugality, it is likely that this level of gene control is the major mechanism for cell diversity.

REGULATION OF mRNA PROCESSING

This level of gene control considers polyadenylation, capping, intron splicing, and transport of mRNA to the ribosome as processes that could alter levels of gene expression. Other factors that regulate mRNA stability may play a role in determining mRNA half-life and utility and thus could conceivably alter levels of transcription products.

REGULATION OF TRANSLATION

Translational initiation and amino acid sequence elongation rate are two areas that can affect product synthesis. In addition, activation of specific ribosome particles may also play a role in rate of protein synthesis.[99,100]

POST-TRANSLATIONAL MODIFICATIONS

Proteins often require cleavage, molecular alterations, or transport before activation. It is evident in some cases that the rate of these processes can be altered to satisfy the changing needs of the cell, tissue, organ, or body. Insulin, for example, can be processed from proinsulin at a faster rate in

the presence of high serum glucose as previously discussed. The most common forms of modification are glycosylation and phosphorylation.[58] The latter modification is a major activity of the gene products that regulate cell growth, division, and differentiation.[101] There are many other types of post-translational modification such as fatty acid acylation and N-terminal glycine myristylation[102] that can apparently serve to direct proteins to the cell membrane and surface structures.

As can be inferred from the above discussion, eukaryotic gene expression is complex to dissect and investigate, and it is likely that gene control exists in multiple levels of protein synthesis and involves complex feedback mechanisms. Because of the relative simplicity of prokaryotes, which are single-celled, haploid, and have no nucleus, the best understood molecular models of gene control have been defined in these organisms. A brief discussion of the simplest and best understood example of gene induction, the lac operon of *Escherichia coli*, follows in order to illustrate some fundamental principles that most likely underlie gene expression control in eukaryotes as well.

The Lac Operon

The bacteria *E. coli* will use glucose as its energy source when it is available. If, however, the disaccharide lactose is presented in lieu of glucose, it too can be utilized via hydrolysis into its constituents, glucose and galactose. This requires production of the enzyme β-galactosidase, which is normally present in minute quantities within the cell. The gene is "induced" or turned on by interaction of lactose with the lac repressor protein. Normally the repressor binds to a specific nucleotide sequence in the operator region of the β-galactosidase gene, thereby blocking its promoter; the repressor has a second binding site for lactose. The lactose-repressor complex is sterically unable to continue to bind the operator, thus the bacterial RNA polymerase can now bind the β-galactosidase promoter and initiate gene transcription (Fig. 3-7A).[103]

Furthermore, high levels of glucose in the presence of lactose has been shown to inhibit β-galactosidase expression. The mechanism for this control operates through the action of cyclic AMP (cAMP). As glucose levels fall, cAMP concentrations rise within the bacterium; cAMP molecules then associate with a bacterial protein called cap that catalyzes RNA polymerase binding to the promoter site of β-galactosidase, thus stimulating its expression (Fig. 3-7B).[104] This simple example of gene control conveys the following points which are relevant to eukaryotic systems:

Certain genes are constitutive, that is, they are produced at constant levels throughout the routine processes of the cell. The constitutively produced proteins generally provide the housekeeping functions of the cell. Other genes are inducible or conditional, that is, the level of their expression can be altered in response to outside stimuli. An example would be the induction of a cascade of host functions in response to a growth factor binding to its receptor. Platelet-derived growth factor (PDGF) and its receptor, a member of the tyrosine

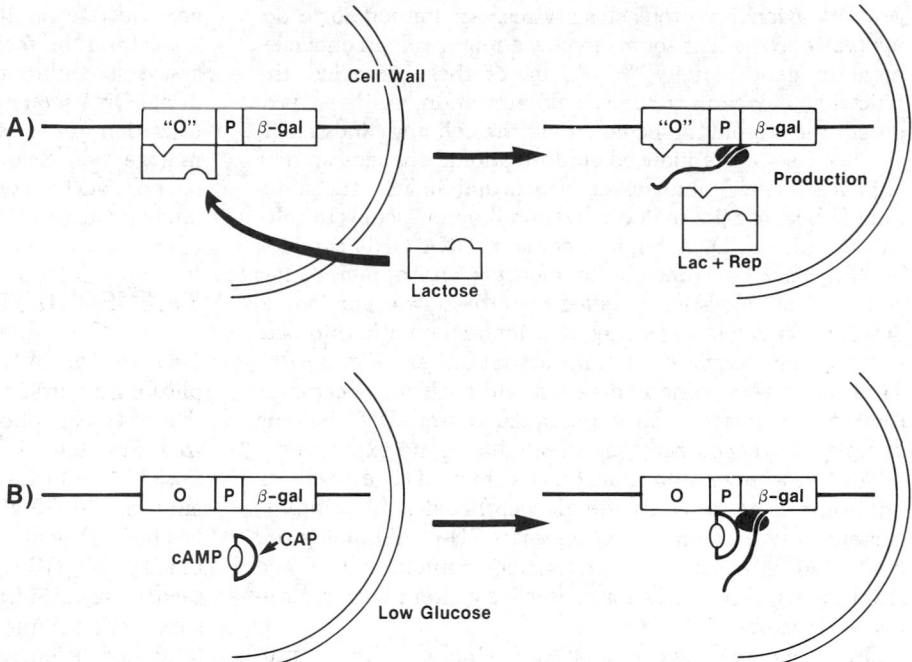

FIG. 3-7. Control of β-galactosidase gene expression of *E. coli*. **A**. A repressor binds to the operator-promoter region of the *E. coli* genome that prevents RNA transcription. Lactose present at high concentration can diffuse through the cell wall, bind a second site on the repressor, and open up the transcription start site for mRNA synthesis. **B**. Cyclic AMP (cAMP) overcomes the catabolite repression exerted over the β-galactosidase gene by high concentrations of glucose. cAMP binds a soluble binding protein (CAP, for catabolite gene activator protein) which subsequently assists the binding of RNA polymerase to the operator-promoter site. cAMP levels are normally inverse of those of glucose in situ. O, operator; p, promoter; β-gal, β-galactosidase gene.

kinase family of growth factor receptors, are examples. PDGF interacts with receptors and induces a cascade of host functions.[105] This occurs via ligand binding with subsequent phosphorylation of specific tyrosine residues on target substrates.

As mentioned earlier, two types of genetic elements are generally identified in control of expression. Cis elements are those DNA segments which serve as binding sites for transcriptional activators or repressors and repress or facilitate transcription. Thus, the operator and promoter regions of the lac operon, and upstream elements, promoters, and enhancers of eukaryotic genes are cis elements. Note that these factors are nondiffusible. Trans elements are diffusible substances which can bind to DNA (at a cis-sequence) and exert control over transcription. Examples in the lac operon model are lactose and cAMP-CAP. Thus, trans elements can activate at multiple sites in the genome.

Some DNA-protein interactions serve to enhance expression and others repress expression. This generalization can be applied to eukaryotic gene expression in many instances, as in the control of DNA expression by the glucocorticoid hormones in eukaryotes.

GLUCOCORTICOID-INDUCED GENE EXPRESSION

It has long been noted that glucocorticoid hormones exert a wide variety of activities such as growth and differentiation of certain eukaryotic cells. It is well accepted that the mechanism for such actions involves diffusion of the hormone into the cytosol with subsequent binding to a soluble receptor (Fig. 3-8). This hormone receptor complex then activates gene expression through a less well-understood mechanism which involves DNA binding at an enhancer sequence. Two human glucocorticoid receptors (HGR) have been fairly well characterized at the molecular level. They consist of chains of 777 (α) and 742 (β) amino acids that have several functional domains as determined by mutant construction. One area of importance is the steroid binding area; surprisingly, deletion of this domain results in constitutive expression of genes induced by the HGR-glucocorticoid complex,[107] indicating that induction may be associated with the removal of a repressor. A second functional domain is responsible for DNA binding and trans-activation of susceptible genes. This domain is a central cysteine-rich region of protein and has sequence homology to several other DNA binding proteins, including the thyroid hormone receptor or the v-*erb*A onco-

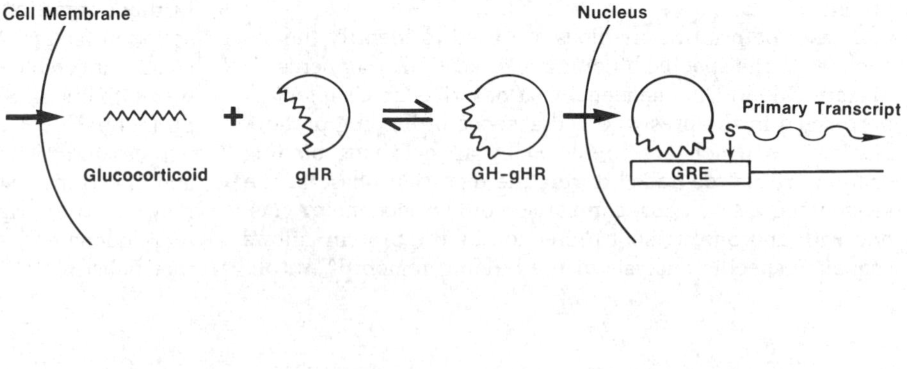

FIG. 3-8. Glucocorticoid binds a soluble cell receptor (*gHR*) upon entering a mammalian cell. This GH-gHR complex then can bind DNA at an enhancer sequence that results in mRNA transcription.

gene of avian erythroblastosis virus. An immunologic domain also exists that seems to play a minor role in enhancement of gene activity.[108] In light of these domains, the following mechanism for steroid activation has been proposed: the steroid molecule enters the cell and binds HGR, and because of the induced conformational change can now bind a specific enhancer sequence and induce transcription.[107] Because the major activation function seems to colocalize with the DNA binding domain, DNA GHR complex binding may be sufficient to induce transcription. Other gene activation systems studied map these two functions to different domains, suggesting that interaction at a third site is sometimes required for trans-activation (see Fig. 3-8).[109] Thus, eukaryotic gene expression, although more complex than in prokaryotes, relies on similar protein-DNA binding complexes (receptor-ligand) which alter gene expression.

The tyrosine amino transferase gene of liver cells is known to be activated by the glucocorticoid-GHR complex; current work in the mouse suggests its GH-GHR binding site lies 2.5 kb upstream of its transcription initiation site, and that binding of the activator causes local alterations in chromatin structure.[110]

One technique used to study functional domains of proteins is that of in vitro mutagenesis. In the case of GHR this was accomplished by linker scanning. Amino acid codons containing restriction enzyme BamHI sites are inserted in such a way that the reading frame for the protein is not disturbed but the amino acid sequence at the site of the insertion is altered. The insertion sites are generated by partial digestion of previously constructed fragments with a frequent cutting restriction enzyme(s). These manipulations result in a series of DNA mutations along the different domains of the plasmid. The constructs are then assayed for various activities to determine the effects of disrupting the DNA sequence in different locations.[109]

MOBILITY SHIFT ASSAYS AND DNASE FOOTPRINTING

Methods commonly used to identify cis-acting sequences and trans-acting factors are known as DNA footprinting and mobility shift assays.[111] In the latter assay, candidate DNA binding sequences (cis elements) are used to identify trans binding proteins present in soluble nuclear-derived cell fractions by mixing isotopically labeled DNA fragments with the protein fraction and subjecting the sample to gel electrophoresis.[112] The protein-DNA complex significantly retards the electrophoretic mobility of the DNA fragment. In this manner, specific-cell types can be screened for trans-acting factors. DNA affinity columns prepared with specific DNA fragments are subsequently used to purify the DNA binding protein.[113]

DNase footprinting methods are used to identify the sequences in the specific binding region of DNA fragments.[114] Maxam-Gilbert DNA sequencing as described in Chapter 2 is performed in the presence and absence of binding protein. Nucleotides which are protected by an overlying binding protein are not degraded during the digestion phase of the sequencing assay. Thus, comparison of two sequencing gels, one with and one without protection by the protein, allows sequence specific analysis of the binding region.[114] An oligonucleotide can then be synthesized with the sequence derived from the footprinting assay and used in mobility shift assays as confirmation of both having identified the appropriate DNA sequence and its protein. More rigorous characterization of the binding sequence is made by site-directed mutagenesis. Search of the DNA sequence in the gene sequence data base can reveal other genes that possess possible binding sites.

TRANSCRIPTIONAL FACTORS

One area currently under intense investigation that may implicate gene dysfunction as a mechanism for oncogenesis is that of transcriptional factors; several have been characterized. For example, Spl has been isolated from HeLa cells, initially as a factor required for optimal function of the Simian virus 40 (SV40) early promoter.[115-117] Subsequently, it has been shown to enhance transcription 10- to 50-fold via binding to a GC-rich sequence.[118] Viral promoters that are responsive to Spl binding besides SV40 include the herpes simplex virus immediate early promoters[119] and the human immunodeficiency virus (HIV) long terminal repeat promoter.[118] Cellular responsive promoters include human metallothionein genes and the mouse dehydrofolate reductase gene.[118] How such a transcription factor operates at the molecular level is not yet understood. Because tandem repeats exist within binding sequences, each with varying affinities to induce transcription, and because multiple transcriptional factors must interact to initiate mRNA transcription, a complex interaction involving DNA-protein binding must occur. Appropriate conformational changes must take place to enhance RNA polII binding initiation and transcription.[118]

jun ONCOGENE, GCN-4 AND AP-1

GCN-4 is a transcriptional control element in yeast that enhances expression of coregulated genes involved in amino acid biosynthesis.[120,121] Its optimal DNA binding sequence is the nearly palindromic oligonucleotide ATGACTCAT.[122] The jun oncogene of avian sarcoma virus[121,123] has no specific sequence homology to other oncogenes or to the tyrosine-specific protein kinases,[123,124] but recently it has been shown that it has considerable sequence homology with GCN-4 in its carboxy terminal region.[124] A chimeric protein containing the amino terminus of GCN-4 and the carboxy terminus of the jun oncogene can induce amino acid biosynthesis in yeast cells in the absence of functional GCN-4, which suggests that the two genes have functional as well as structural homology.[125] A human transcriptional factor, Apl, binds to DNA sequences homologous to GCN-4 binding sites, further suggesting jun is derived from a normal cellular transcription factor.[125] Apl binds to promoter regions of phorbol diester inducible genes (human collagenase, stromelysin, metalothione II, SV40).[126] Phorbol diesters are potent tumor promoters[127-129] and may exert their effect by altering gene expression.[126] The analogies between GCN-4, jun oncogene, and Apl strongly suggest that one mechanism of oncogenesis may be a transcriptional element gone awry; since such factors undoubtedly play a major role in cellular function and metabolism.[130,131]

DNA REARRANGEMENT AS A MECHANISM OF GENE CONTROL

DNA recombination plays a role in diversity of antibody variable regions. Before B cell differentiation, the coding region of the heavy and light chain of the immunoglobulin gene are dispersed throughout multiple sites on the chromosome.[132,133] For example, the promoter region of an unrearranged immunoglobulin gene is located approximately 300 kb upstream from the 3' end of the gene in the germ line configuration. A complex rearrangement event occurs during B cell maturation that draws the various DNA segments of the gene into proximity to form a final transcription unit of 3 kb.[132] The joining sequences in these events are hot spots for imprecise alignment; the resultant reading frame therefore can exhibit enormous diversity in DNA sequence and explains the millions of unique antibody idiotypes produced in a single individual.[132,133]

This example illustrates how genomic rearrangement may be important as a control of gene expression and how such DNA breakage, repair, and mutation may serve as a normal process in certain cellular functions. It has been known for years that chromosomal rearrangements and translocations may also be a common mechanism in neoplastic transformation. For example, translocation of material from chromosome 9 to 22 has long been used as a marker for chronic myelogenous leukemia (the Philadelphia chromosome).[134] It is now known that this rearrangement results in adjoining of two specific genomic regions: breakpoint cluster region (*bcr* of chromosome 9) and the Abelson proto-oncogene (*abl* of chromosome 22).[135,136] The fusion of these genes allows expression of a novel 8.5 kb mRNA[30,31] that encodes for a 210,000 dalton chimeric protein.[137] This protein is a nonintegral tyrosine kinase that may play a role in signal transduction;[138] how it acts to produce a cancer phenotype is not well understood. A more thorough discussion of the phenomenon of genetic rearrangement allowing novel RNA transcripts and protein production which results in neoplasia can be found in Chapter 4.

GENE TRANSFER METHODS IN VITRO AND IN VIVO

GENE TRANSFER/TRANSFECTION

As described earlier, genes and their transcription control elements are now routinely studied by gene transfer methods. These assays are usually performed as transient expression assays, that is, within 48 hours after transfection the cells are disrupted and RNA is extracted and analyzed for quality and quantity of the product that is expressed from the DNA recombinant. In contrast, there has been wide usage of gene transfer technology, where the introduced genes become stably associated with the genetic information of the cell and their influence on the cell phenotype can be monitored in tissue culture. DNA can be introduced into cells by DNA transfection, microinjection,[139] electroporation,[140,141] and the use of specific viral vectors,[142] and have provided biologists with important systems not only for identifying essential regions in promoter transcription control elements but also for studying the properties and phenotype of a gene

product. This technique has been especially important for identifying transforming oncogenes. The DNA transfection assay was actually developed to study and identify the transforming regions of DNA tumor viruses. The assay consists of introducing the DNA to be tested onto recipient nontransformed cell monolayers (described in more detail in Chap. 3). Transformation of cells by DNA is assayed by the appearance of focal areas of morphologically altered cells and by use of less labor intensive modification of the assay in which these cells are injected into nude mice and assayed for tumorigenicity.[143] The major limitations of this assay is that it does not reveal how expression of a specific gene influences normal cell growth and differentiation in the developing embryo and in adult animals. These questions are now being addressed by generating transgenic animals.

TRANSGENIC ANIMALS

The term transgenic was coined to define organisms that carry genetic material that has been introduced into the germ line. The inserted genetic information or transgene can be a segment of genomic DNA from a homologous or a heterologous species or even from viruses complete with its normal regulatory sequences and coding information. Most often, however, genes are introduced into the germ line of these animals using regulatory sequences which direct expression to specific cells or tissue types. Many genes have been introduced into the mouse germ line by direct microinjection into the male pronucleus of a fertilized egg. The egg is then reimplanted into a foster mother to allow normal development.[144] In a fraction of the injected embryos, the recombinant DNA becomes inserted into the germ line at a single chromosomal locus. Most often the newly acquired genetic is transmitted to progeny in mendelian fashion.

Despite the recombinant DNA being arbitrarily localized in the genome, in most cases it is subjected to normal gene regulation.[145] Thus, many new mouse strains have been generated with novel phenotypes that can be traced to the newly inserted genetic information and its expression in specific cells or organs. There have been many examples of the use of tissue-specific upstream regulatory sequences to drive novel structural genetic information. In a number of cases, these promoters have been used to express transforming viral genes and oncogenes in selected tissue types. Regulatory control regions from the elastase[146] or insulin genes have been used to direct SV40 T antigen expression to the pancreas. In these cases, tumors arise in the appropriate target cells. Using the regulatory sequence of a lens crystalline gene, SV40 T antigen expression was confined to the lens of the eye and it was shown that these animals developed heritable lens tumors.[147] Ectopic or increased expression of oncogenes in transgenic animals frequently generates phenotypes that can aid in understanding gene function. A *mos* oncogene transgene expressed at high levels during postnatal eye development caused alterations in lens fiber epithelial cell differentiation (Fig. 3-9). The earliest effect observed because of this ectopic expression was altered polarity in the elongation of lens fiber epithelial cells.[148]

The use of the transgenic mouse provides an exceptional system for studying protocols for gene therapy and several different genetic defects have been corrected using this pro-

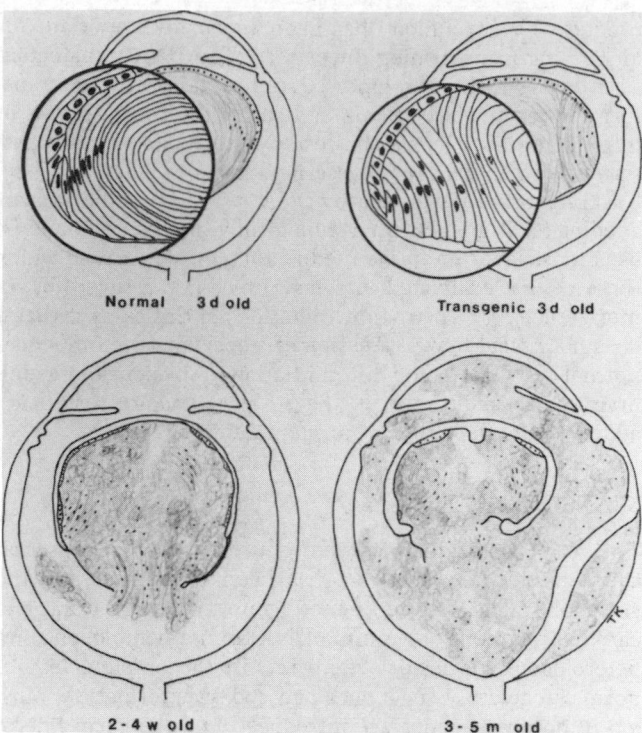

Normal 3 d old · Transgenic 3 d old · 2-4 w old · 3-5 m old

FIG. 3-9. Schematic drawing to summarize histologic findings on lenses of transgenic *mos* mice. In the normal mouse, lens fibers are formed by differentiation of epithelial cells at the equator. Nuclei of concentrically elongating cells form the bow configuration. Abnormality of the transgenic lens becomes apparent on the third postnatal day. The basal ends of the fiber cells extend only a short distance from the equator. The capsule in this area becomes thickened. The posterior capsule is not formed beyond this zone. By 2 to 4 weeks, the attenuated posterior capsule ruptures and lens fiber cells escape into the vitreal cavity. Lens fiber cells become globular in shape. Epithelial cells remain present and newly formed fiber cells are occasionally recognizable. By 3 to 5 months, the anterior capsule becomes very thick and the whole eye cavity, including anterior chamber and subretinal space, fills with globular lens cells.

cedure. For example, a strain of dwarf mice which is defective in growth hormone production was partially corrected by the introduction of a rat growth hormone transgene.[149] Likewise, immune defects have been corrected in mutant animals,[50-152] and most recently, a mutant strain of mice deficient in β-globin synthesis was corrected by introducing β-globin as a transgene. Although this technology raises ethical questions about performing gene therapy in humans, the mouse serves well as an experimental model system for determining the conduct of such procedures. Perhaps the greatest potential of the transgenic system lies in the possibility of introducing mutations into the normal genes of the animal and substituting modifications or mutant genes which will mimic human disease. This is clearly one of the most exciting areas in biology and can provide experimental systems which currently do not exist for studying treatment and therapy modalities for human diseases.

CONCLUSION

It is evident that much is to be learned about specific details of control of gene expression in eukaryotes; it is also being noted with increasing frequency the role that oncogenes play in altering normal cellular activity. For instance, oncogenes may in function resemble cell receptors which conditionally regulate expression of inducible genes, but become constitutively exprssed by the altered oncogene form. Alternatively, mutation of a cis element would alter gene expression and cause subsequent aberrant growth. The rearrangement in a cis regulatory region of the first exon of c-*myc* in Burkitt's lymphoma is an example.[153] Because it is likely that normal gene control relies on a precise sequence of events occurring in a cascade response and often a subsequent diminution reaction, alteration of one important control element could have devastating effects on cell metabolism and growth. It has also been noted that suppressor cancer genes may exist; disruption of the function of these genes can be correlated with the appearance of a neoplastic phenotype.[154] In the ongoing studies of gene expression, it is certain that the current explosion of information will reveal the molecular mechanisms for normal as well as neoplastic processes.

Research sponsored by the National Cancer Institute, Department of Health and Human Services, under Contract No. NO1-CO-74101 with Bionetics Research, Inc. The contents of this chapter do not necessarily reflect the views or policies of the Department of Health and Human Services, nor does mention of trade names, commercial products, or organizations imply endorsement by the U.S. government.

REFERENCES

1. Roeder R: Eukaryotic nuclear RNA polymerases. In Losick R, Chamberlin M (eds): RNA Polymerases, pp 285–329. Cold Spring Harbor, NY, Cold Spring Harbor Laboratory, 1976
2. Corden J, Wasylyk B, Buchwalder A, et al: Expression of cloned genes in new environment. Science 209:1406–1414, 1980
3. Breathnach R, Chambon P: Organization and expression of eukaryotic split genes encoding for proteins. Annu Rev Biochem 50:349–383, 1981
4. Shenk T: Transcriptional control regions: Nucleotide sequence requirements for initiation by RNA polymerase II and III. Curr Top Microbiol Immunol 93:25–40, 1981
5. Benoist C, Chambon P: *In vivo* sequence requirements of the SV40 early promoter region. Nature 290:304–310, 1981
6. Myers RM, Rio DC, Robbins AK, et al: SV40 gene expression is modulated by the cooperative banding of T antigen to DNA. Cell 25:373–384, 1981
7. McKnight SL: Functional relationships between transcriptional control signals of the thymidine kinase gene of herpes simplex virus. Cell 31:355–366, 1982
8. McKnight SL, Kingsbury R: Transcriptional control signals of a eukaryote protein coding gene. Science 217:316–324, 1982
9. Sassone-Corsi P, Borrelli E: Transcriptional regulation by *trans*-acting factors. Trends Genet 2:215–219, 1986
10. Lebowitz P, Ghosh PK: Initiation and regulation of simian virus 40 early transcription *in vitro*. J Virol 41:449–461, 1982
11. Everett R, Baty D, Chambon P: The repeated GC rich motifs upstream from the TATA box are important elements of the SV40 early promoter. Nucleic Acids Res 11:2447–2464, 1983
12. Efstratiadis A, Posakony JW, Maniatis T, et al: The structure and evolution of the human β-globin gene family. Cell 21:653–668, 1980
13. Maniatis T, Goodbourn S, Fisher JA: Regulation of inducible and tissue-specific gene expression. Science 236:1237–1244, 1987
14. Lewin B: RNA polymerase-promoter interactions control initiations. In Genes, Vol 3, p 183. New York, John Wiley & Sons, 1987
15. Voss S, Schlokat U, Gruss P: The role of enhancers in the regulation of cell-type-specific transcriptional control. Trends Biol Sci 11:287–289, 1986
16. Gluzman Y, Shenk T: Current Communications in Molecular Biology: Enhancers and Eukaryotic Gene Expression. Cold Spring Harbor, NY, Cold Spring Harbor Laboratory, 1983
17. Lewin B: The panoply of operons: The lactose paradigm and others. In Genes, Vol 3, p 219. New York, John Wiley & Sons, 1987
18. Gilbert W: Why genes in pieces? Nature 271:501, 1978
19. Adesnik M, Darnell JE: Biogenesis and characterization of histone messenger RNA in HeLa cells. J Mol Biol 67:397–406, 1972

20. Proudfoot NY, Brownlee GG: 3' non-coding region sequences in eukaryotic messenger RNA. Nature 263:211–214, 1976

21. Fitzgerald M, Shenk T: The sequence 5' AAUAAA-3' forms part of the recognition site for polyadenylation of late SV40 mRNAs. Cell 24:251–260, 1981

22. Clemens MJ: Purification of eukaryotic messenger RNA. In Hames BD, Higgins SJ (eds): Transcription and Translation: A Practical Approach, p 211. Oxford, IRC Press, 1984

23. Maniatis T, Fritsch EF, Sambrook J: Molecular Cloning: A Laboratory Manual. Cold Spring Harbor, NY, Cold Spring Harbor Laboratory, 1982

24. Aviv H, Leder P: Purification of biologically active globin messenger RNA by chromatography on oligothymidylic acid cellulose. Proc Natl Acad Sci USA 69:1408–1412, 1972

25. Berk AJ, Sharp PA: Sizing and mapping of early adenovirus mRNAs by gel electrophoresis of S1 endonuclease-digested hybrids. Cell 12:721–732, 1977

26. Favaloro J, Treisman R, Kamen R: Transcriptional maps of polyoma virus-specific RNA: Analysis by two-dimensional nuclease S1 gel mapping. Methods Enzymol 65:718–749, 1980

27. Propst F, Vande Woude G: Expression of c-mos proto-oncogene transcripts in mouse tissues. Nature 315:516–518, 1985

28. Melton DA, Krieg PA, Rebagliati T, et al: Efficient in vitro synthsis of biologically active RNA and RNA hybridization probes from plasmids containing a bacteriophage SP6 promoter. Nucleic Acids Res 12:7035–7056, 1984

29. Alwine JC, Kemp DJ, Stark GR: Method for detection of specific RNAs in agarose gels by transfer to diazobenzyloxymethyl paper and hybridization with DNA probes. Proc Natl Acad Sci USA 74:5340–5354, 1977

30. Shtivelman E, Lifshitz B, Gale RP, et al: Fused transcript of abl and bcr genes in chronic myelogenous leukemia. Nature 315:550–554, 1986

31. Grosveld G, Verwoerd T, Van Agthoven T, et al: The chronic myelocytic cell line k562 contains a breakpoint in bcr and produces a chimeric bcr/c-abl transcript. Mol Cell Biol 6:607–616, 1986

32. Berk AJ, Sharp PA: Sizing and mapping of early adenovirus mRNAs by gel electrophoresis of S1-endonuclease-digested hybrids. Cell 12:721–732, 1977

33. Davies RW: DNA sequencing. In Rickwood D, Hames BD, eds. Gel Electrophoresis of Nucleic Acids: A Practical Approach, pp 117–172. Oxford, IRL Press, 1982

34. Coleman A: Expression of exogenous DNA in Xenopus oocytes. In Hames BD, Higgins SJ (eds): Transcription and Translation: A Practical Approach, pp 49–69. Washington, DC, IRL Press, 1984.

35. Alt FW, Kellems RE, Bertino JR, et al: Selective multiplication of dihydrofolate reductase genes in methotrexate resistant variants of cultured murine cells. J Biol Chem 253:1357–1361, 1978

36. Alt FW, Enea V, Bothwell ALM, et al: Probes for specific mRNAs by subtractive hybridization: anomalous expression of immunoglobulin genes. In Axel R, Maniatis T, Fox CF (eds): Eukaryotic Gene Regulation, pp 407–419. New York, New York Academic Press, 1979

37. Greenberg ME, Ziff EB: Stimulation of 3T3 cells induces transcription of the c-fos proto-oncogene. Nature 311:433–438, 1984

38. McGeady ML, Wood TG, Maizel JV, et al: Sequence upstream to the mouse c-mos oncogene may function as a transcription termination signal. DNA 5:289–298, 1986

39. Dignam JD, Lebovitz RM, Roeder RG: Accurate transcription initiation by RNA polymerase II in a soluble extract from isolated mammalian nuclei, Nucleic Acids Res 11:1475, 1983

40. Manley JL: Analysis of the expression of genes encoding animal mRNA by in vitro techniques. Prog Nucleic Acids Res Mol Biol 30:196–242, 1983

41. McMaster GK, Carmichael GC: Analysis of single- and double-stranded nucleic acids on polyacrylamide and agarose gels by using glyoxal and acridine orange. Proc Natl Acad Sci USA 74:4835–4838, 1977

42. Manley JL: Transcription of eukaryotic genes in a whole cell extract. In Hames BD, Higgins SJ (eds): Transcription and Translation: A Practical Approach, p 74. Oxford, IRL Press, 1984

43. Manley JL: Transcription of eukaryotic genes in a whole cell extract. In Hames BD, Higgins SJ (eds): Transcription and Translation: A Practical Approach, p 79. Oxford, IRL Press, 1984

44. Wigler M, Pellicer A, Silverstein S, et al: DNA-mediated transfer of the adenine phosphoribosyltransferase locus into mammalian cells. Proc Natl Acad Sci USA 76:1373–1376, 1979

45. Lewis WH, Srinivasan PR, Stokoe N, et al: Parameters governing the transfer of genes for thymidine kinase and dihydrofolate reductase into mouse cells using metaphase chromosomes or DNA. Somatic Cell Mol Genet 6:333–347, 1980

46. Graham FL, Bacchetti S, McKinnon R: Transformation of mammalian cells with DNA using the calcium technique. In Baserga R, Croce C, Rovera G (eds): Introduction of Macromolecules into Viable Mammalian Cells. The Wistar Symposium Series 1, pp 3–25. New York, Alan R. Liss, 1980

47. Spandidos DA, Wilkie NM: Expression of exogenous DNA in mammalian cells. In Hames BD, Higgins SJ (eds): Transcription and Translation: A Practical Approach, pp 1–48. Oxford, IRL Press, 1984

48. Gorman C, Moffat L, Howard B: Recombinant genomes which express chloramphenicol acetyltransferase in mammalian cells. Mol Cell Biol 2:1044–1051, 1982

49. Shaw W: The enzymatic acetylation of chloramphenicol by extracts of R factor resistant Escherichia coli. J Biol Chem 242:687–693, 1975

50. Bannerjee AK: 5'-terminal cap structure in eukaryotic messenger ribonucleic acids. Microbiol Rev 44:175–205, 1980

51. Lewin B: Gene Expression-2, Eucaryotic Chromosomes, p 677. New York, John Wiley & Sons, 1980

52. Furiuchi Y, LaFiandra A, Shatkin AF: 5'-terminal structure and mRNA stability. Nature 266:235–239, 1977

53. Lewin B: The ribosome translation factory. In Genes, Vol 3, p 144. New York, John Wiley & Sons, 1987

54. Nomura M, Tissieres A, Lengyel P: Ribosomes. Cold Spring Harbor, NY, Cold Spring Harbor Laboratory, 1974

55. Watson JD, Tooze J: The DNA story. San Francisco, WH Freeman, 1981

56. Lewin B: The messenger RNA template. Genes, Vol 2, p 151. New York, John Wiley & Sons, 1985

57. Wittman HG: Architecture of prokaryotic ribosomes. Annu Rev Biochem 52:35–65, 1983

58. Clemens MJ: Translation of eukaryotic messenger RNA in cell-free extracts. In Hames BD, Higgins SJ (eds): Transcription and Translation: A Practical Approach, pp 231–270. Oxford, IRL Press, 1984

59. McDowell M, Joklik WK, Villa-Komaroff L, et al: Translation of reovirus messenger RNAs synthesized in vitro into reovirus polypeptides by several mammalian cell-free extracts. Proc Natl Acad Sci USA 69:2649–2653, 1972

60. Pelham HRB, Jackson RJ: An efficient mRNA dependent translation system from rabbit reticulocyte lysates. Eur J Biochem 67:247–256, 1976

61. Olliver CL, Grobler-Rabie A, Boyd CD: In vitro translation of messenger RNA in a wheat germ extract cell-free system. In Walker JM (ed): Methods in Molecular Biology, Vol 2, pp 137–144. Clifton, NJ, Humana Press, 1984

62. Roberts BE, Paterson BM: Efficient translation of tobacco mosaic virus RNA and rabbit globin 9S RNA in a cell free system from commercial wheat germ. Proc Natl Acad Sci USA 70:2330–2334, 1973

63. Sinclair J, Rickwood D: Two-dimensional gel electrophoresis. In Hames BD, Rickwood D (eds): Gel Electrophoresis of Proteins: A Practical Approach. Washington, DC, IRL Press, 1981

64. Kessler SW: Use of a protein A bearing staphylococci for the immunoprecipitation and isolation of antigens from cells. Methods Enzymol 73:441–459, 1981

65. Dobos P, Kerr IM, Martin M: Synthesis of capsid and noncapsid viral proteins in response to encephalomyocarditis virus ribonucleic acid in animal cell-free systems. J Virol 8:491, 1971

66. Heywood SM, Rourke AW: Cell free synthesis of myosin. Methods Enzymol 30:699, 1974

67. Woodward WR, Wilairat P, Herbert E: Preparation of reticulocyte aminoacyl-tRNA and the assay of codon recognition properties of isoacceptor tRNA's in a reticulocyte cell-free system. Methods Enzymol 30:740, 1974

68. Devillers-Thiery A, Kindt T, Scheele G, et al: Homology in amino-terminal sequence of precursors to pancreatic secretory proteins. Proc Natl Acad Sci USA 72:5016, 1975

69. Richter JD, Lorenz LJ, Crawford DR, et al: The control of translation by RNA binding proteins in xenopus laevis oocytes. In Matthews MB (ed): Translational Control, Current Communications in Molecular Biology, pp 144–149. Cold Spring Harbor, NY, Cold Spring Harbor Laboratory, 1986

70. Towbin H, Staehelin T, Gordon J: Electrophoretic transfer of proteins from polyacrylamide gels to nitrocellulose sheets: Procedure and some applications. Proc Natl Acad Sci USA 76:4350–4354, 1979

71. Bers G, Garfin D: Protein and nucleic acid blotting and immunobiochemical detection. Bio Tech 3:276–288, 1985

72. Smith DL, Hill RL, Lehman JR, et al: Principles of Biochemistry: Mammalian Biochemistry, pp 474–497. McGraw Hill, New York, 1983

73. Cooperstein SJ, Watkins D: The Islets of Langerhans: Biochemistry, Physiology and Pathology. New York, Academic Press, 1981

74. Drucker DJ, Philippe J, Mojsov S, et al: Glucagon-like peptide I stimulates insulin gene expression and increases cyclic AMP levels in a rat islet cell line. Proc Natl Acad Sci USA 84:3434–3438, 1987

75. Permutt MA, Kipnis DM: Insulin biosynthesis: On the mechanism of glucose stimulation. J Biol Chem 247:1194–1199, 1972

76. Itch N, Okamoto H: Translational control of proinsulin synthesis by glucose. Nature 283:100–102, 1980

77. Brunstead J, Chan SJ: Direct effect of glucose on the prepoinsulin mRNA level in isolated pancreatic islets. Biochem Biophys Methods 106:1383–1389, 1982

78. Giddings SJ, Chirgwin J, Permutt MA: Effects of glucose on proinsulin messenger RNA in rats in vivo. Diabetes 31:624–629, 1982

79. Welsh M, Chirgwin J, Permutt MA: Effects of D-glucose, L-leucine and 2 ketoisocaproate on insulin messenger-RNA levels in mouse pancreatic islets. Diabetes 35:228–231, 1986

79. Lebo RV, Cheung MC, Bruce BD, et al: Mapping parathyroid hormone, β-globin, insulin, and LDH-A genes within the human chromosome 11 short arm by spot blotting sorted chromosomes. Hum Genet 69:316–320, 1985

80. Rotwein P, Naylor SL, Chirgwin JM: Human insulin-related DNA sequences map to chromosomes 2 and 11. Somatic Cell Mol Genet 12:625–631, 1986

81. Lewin B: The organization of interrupted genes. In Genes, Vol 2, p 312. New York, John Wiley & Sons, 1985

82. Lomedico P, Rosenthal N, Efstratiadis A, et al: The structure and evolution of the two nonallelic rat preproinsulin genes. Cell 18:545–558, 1979

83. Welsh M, Nielsen DA, Mackrell AJ, et al: Control of insulin gene expression in pancreatic β-cells and in an insulin-producing cell line, R1N-5F cells. J Biol Chem 260:13590–13594, 1985

84. Ashcroft SJH: Metabolic controls of insulin secretion. In Cooperstein SJ, Watkins D (eds): Islets of Langerhans, pp 117–148. Academic Press, New York, 1981

85. Ohlsson H, Edlund T: Sequence specific interactions of nuclear factors with the insulin gene enhancer. Cell 45:35–44, 1986

86. Laimins L, Holmgren-Konig M, Khoury G, et al: Transcriptional "silencer" element in rat repetitive sequencers associated with the rat insulin 1 gene locus. Proc Natl Acad Sci USA 83:3151–3155, 1986

87. Pemutt MA: Biosynthesis of insulin. In Copperstein SJ, Watkind D (eds): Islets of Langerhans, pp 75–95. New York, Academic Press, 1981

88. Welsh M, Scherberg N, Gilmore R, et al: Translational control of insulin biosynthesis. Biochem J 235:459–467, 1986

89. Howell SL, Lacy PE: In Memoirs of the Society for Endocrinology: Subcellular Organization and Function in Endocrine Tissues. London, Cambridge University Press, 19:469–480, 1970

90. McDaniel ML, Lacy PE: Interactions in cell organelles in insulin secretin. In Cooperstein SJ, Watkins D (eds): Islets of Langerhans, pp 97–115. New York, Academic Press, 1981

91. Docherty K, Steiner DF: Post-translational proteolysis in polypeptide hormone biosynthesis. Annu Rev Physiol 44:625–638, 1982

92. Docherty K, Carrol R, Steiner DF: Conversion of proinsulin to insulin, involvement of a 31,500 molecular weight thiol protease. Proc Natl Acad Sci USA 79:4613–4617, 1982

93. Orci L, Ravazzola M, Amherdt M, et al: Conversion of proinsulin to insulin occurs coordinately with acidification of maturing secretory vesicles. J Cell Biol 103:2273–2281, 1986

94. Bajas JS (ed): Insulin and metabolism, pp 24–28. New York, Excerpta Medica, 1977

95. Grodsky GM: A threshold distribution hypothesis for packet storage of insulin. Diabetes 21:584–593, 1972

96. Rugin R, Riggs AD: DNA methylation and gene function. Science 210:604–610, 1980

97. Groudine M, Weintraub H: Propagation of globin DNAse-1 hypersensitive sites in absence of factors required for induction: A possible mechanism for determination. Cell 30:131–139, 1982

98. Nelson EM, Winkler MM: Regulation of mRNA entry into polysomes. J Biol Chem 262:11501–11506, 1987

99. Hershey JWR, Duncan R, Matthews M: Introduction: Mechanisms of translational control. In Matthews MD (ed): Translational Control, Current Communications in Molecular Biology, pp 1–19. Cold Spring Harbor, NY, Cold Spring Harbor Laboratory, 1986

100. Brown D: Gene expression in eukaryotes. Science 211:667–674, 1981

101. Hunter T: A thousand and one protein kinases. Cell 50:823–829, 1987

102. Towler DA, Gordon JI, Adams SP, et al: The biology and enzymology of eukaryotic protein acylation. Annu Rev Biochem (in press)

103. Jacob F, Monod J: Genetic regulatory mechanisms in the synthesis of proteins. J Mol Biol 3:318–356, 1961

104. Pastan I, Pearlman R: Cyclic AMP in bacteria. Science 169:339–344, 1969

105. Stiles CD, Capone GT, Scher CD, et al: Dual control of cell growth by somatomedins and platelet-derived growth factor. Proc Natl Acad Sci USA 76:1279, 1979

106. Hollenberg SM, Weinberger C, Ong E, et al: Primary structure and expression of a functional human glucocorticoid receptor cDNA. Nature 318:635–641, 1985

107. Hollenberg SM, Giguere V, Segui P, et al: Colocalization of DNA binding and transcriptional activation functions in the human glucocorticoid receptor. Cell 49:39–46, 1987

108. Giguere V, Hollenberg, SM, Rosenfeld MG, et al: Functional domains of the human glucocorticoid receptor. Cell 46:645–652, 1986

109. Keegan L, Gill G, Ptashne M: Separation of DNA binding from the transcription-activating function of a eukaryotic regulatory protein. Science 231:699–704, 1986

110. Jantzen HM, Strahle U, Gloss B, et al: Cooperativity of glucocorticoid response elements located far upstream of the tyrosine aminotransferase gene. Cell 49:29–38, 1987

111. Garner MM, Revzin A: A gell electrophoresis method for quantifying the binding of proteins to specific DNA regions: Application to components of the Escherichia coli lactose operon regulatory system. Nucleic Acids Res 9:3047–3060, 1981

112. Garner MM, Revzin A: The use of gel electrophoresis to detect and study nucleic acid-protein interactions. Trends Biol Sci 11:395–396, 1986

113. Kadonaga JT, Tijian R: Affinity purification of sequence specific DNA binding proteins. Proc Natl Acad Sci USA 83:5589–5893, 1986

114. Galas DJ, Schmitz A: DNAse foot printing: A simple method for the detection of protein-DNA binding specificity. Nucleic Acids Res 5:3157–3170, 1978

115. Short NJ: Are some controlling factors more equal than others? Nature 326:740–741, 1987

116. Briggs MR, Kadonaga JT, Bell SP, et al: Purification and biochemical characterizatin of the promoter-specific transcription factor, Sp1. Science 234:47–52, 1986

117. Dynan WS, Tijian R: Control of eukaryotic messenger RNA synthesis by sequence specific DNA-binding proteins. Nature 316:774–777, 1985

118. Kadonaga JT, Jones KA, Tjian R: Promoter-specific activation of RNA polymerase II transcription by Sp1. Trends Genet 2:20–23, 1986

119. Jones KA, Tjian R: Sp1 binds to promoter sequences and activates herpes simplex virus immediate-early gene transcription in vitro. Nature 317:179–182, 1985

120. Hope IA, Struhl K: GCN4 protein, synthesized in vitro, binds to HIS3 regulatory sequences: Implications for the general control of amino acid biosynthetic genes in yeast. Cell 43:177–188, 1985

121. Arndt K, Fink G: GCN4 protein, a positive transcription factor in yeast, binds general control promoters to all 5′ TGACTC 3′ sequences. Proc Natl Acad Sci USA 83:8516–8520, 1986

122. Hill DE, Hope IA, Macke JP, et al: Saturation mutagenesis of the yeast his3 regulatory site: Requirements for transcriptional induction and for binding by GCN4 activator protein. Science 234:451–457, 1986

123. Maki Y, Bos TJ, Davis C, et al: Avian sarcoma virus 17 carries the jun oncogene. Proc Natl Acad Sci USA 84:2848–2852, 1987

124. Vogt PK, Bos TJ, Doolittle RF: Homology between the DNA-binding domain of the GCN4 regulatory protein of yeast and the carboxyterminal region of a protein coded for by the oncogene jun. Proc Natl Acad Sci USA 84:3316–3319, 1987

125. Struhl K: The DNA-binding domains of the jun oncoprotein and the yeast GCN4 transcriptional activator protein are functionally homologous. Cell 50:841–846, 1987

126. Angel P, Imagawa M, Chiu R, et al: Phorbol ester-inducible genes contain a common cis element recognized by a TPA-medulated trans-acting factor. Cell 49:729–739, 1987

127. Weinstein IB, Lee LS, Fisher PB, et al: Action of phorbol esters in cell culture: Mimicry of transformation, altered differentiation and effects on cell membrane. J Supramol Struct 12:195–208, 1979

128. Blumberg PM: In vitro studies on the mode of action of the phorbol esters, potent tumor promoters. CRC Crit Rev Toxicol 9:153–197, 1981

129. Slaga TJ: Cellular and molecular mechanisms of tumor promotion. Cancer Surv 2:595–612, 1983

130. Bohmann D, Bos TJ, Admon A, et al: Human proto-oncogene c-jun encodes a DNA binding protein with structural and functional properties of transcription factor AP-1. Science 238:1386–1392, 1987

131. Varmus HE: Oncogenes and transcriptional control. Science 238:1337–1339, 1987

132. Tonegawa S: Somatic generation of antibody diversity. Nature 302:575–581, 1983

133. Nossal GJV: Current concepts in immunology: The basic components of the immune system. N Engl J Med 316:1320–1325, 1987

134. Rowley JD: Ph′-positive leukaemia including chronic myelogenous leukaemia. Clin Haematol 9:54, 1980

135. Collins SJ, Kubonishi I, Miyoshi I, et al: Altered transcription of the c-abl oncogene in K-562 and other chronic myelogenous leukemia cells. Science 225:72, 1984

136. Gale RP, Canaani E: An 8-kilobase abl RNA transcript in chronic myelogenous leukemia. Proc Natl Acad Sci USA 81:5648–5652, 1984

137. Konopka JB, Watanabe SM, Witte ON: An alteration of the human c-abl protein in K562 leukemia cells unmasks associated tyrosine kinase activity. Cell 37:1035, 1984

138. Konopka JB, Witte ON: Detection of c-abl tyrosine kinase activity in vitro permits direct comparison of normal and altered abl gene products. Mol Cell Biol 5:3116, 1985

139. Mulcahy LS, Smith MR, Stacey DW: Requirement for ras proto-oncogene function during serum-stimulated growth in NIH 3T3 cells. Nature 313:241–243, 1985

140. Chu G, Hayakawa H, Berg P: Electroporation for the efficient transfection of mammalian cells with DNA. Nucleic Acids Res 15:1311–1325, 1987

141. Toneguzzo F, Keating A: Stable expression of selectable genes introduced into human hematopoietic stem cells by electric field-mediated DNA transfer. Proc Natl Acad Sci USA 83:3496–2499, 1986

142. Gluzman Y: Eukaryotic Viral Vectors. Cold Spring Harbor, NY, Cold Spring Harbor Laboratory, 1982

143. Blair DG, Cooper CS, Oskarsson MK, et al: New method for detecting cellular transforming genes. Science 218:1122–1125, 1982

144. Gordon JW, Scangos GA, Plotkin DJ, et al: Genetic transformation of mouse embryos by microinjection of purified DNA. Proc Natl Acad Sci USA 77:7380–7384, 1980

145. Palmiter RD, Brinster RL: Germ-line transformation of mice. Annu Rev Genet 20:465–499, 1986

146. Ornitz DM, Palmiter RD, Messing A, et al: Elastase 1 promoter directs expression of human growth hormone and SV40 T-antigen genes to pancreatic acinar cells in transgenic mice. Cold Spring Harbor Symp Quant Biol 50:399–409, 1985

147. Mahon KA, Chepelinsky AB, Khillan JS, et al: Oncogenesis of the lens in transgenic mice. Science 235:1622, 1987

148. Khillan JS, Oskarsson MK, Propst F, et al: Defects in lens fiber differentiation are linked to c-mos overexpression in transgenic mice. Genes Dev 1:1327–1335, 1987

149. Hammer RE, Palmiter RD, Brinster RL: Partial correction of murine hereditary disorder by germ-line incorporation of a new gene. Nature 311:65–67, 1987

150. LeMeur M, Gerlinger P, Benoist C, et al: Correcting an immune-response deficiency by creating Eα gene transgenic mice. Nature 316:38–42, 1985

151. Pinkert CA, Widera G, Cowing C, et al: Tissue-specific, inducible and functional expression of the Eαᵈ MHC class II gene in transgenic mice. EMBO J 4:2225–2230, 1985

152. Yamamura K, Kikutani H, Folsom V, et al: Functional expression of microinjected Eαᵈ gene in C57BL/6 transgenic mice. Nature 316:67–69, 1985

153. Cesarman E, Dalla-Favera R, Bentley D, et al: Mutations in the first exon are associated with altered transcription of c-myc in Burkitt lymphoma. Science 238:1272, 1987

154. Klein G: The approaching era of the tumor suppressor genes. Science 238:1539–1545, 1987

155. Park M, Dean M, Cooper CS, et al: Mechanism of met oncogene activation. Cell 45:895–904, 1986

MORAG PARK

GEORGE F. VANDE WOUDE

CHAPTER 4   *Principles of Molecular Cell Biology of Cancer: Oncogenes*

During the past several years we have witnessed extraordinary advances in our understanding of the mechanisms of oncogenesis. This understanding has come about primarily through a synthesis of what were until recently separate cancer research disciplines. The application of the techniques of molecular biology led to the discovery of, in tumor virology, the transforming genes of tumor viruses[1]; in cytogenetics, the genes activated at the breakpoints of nonrandom chromosomal translocations of lymphomas and leukemias[2]; in cell biology, the correlation between growth factors or growth factor receptors and certain transforming genes[3]; and the existence of transforming genes which are activated in vivo and in vitro by direct acting chemical carcinogens.[4] These transforming genes are collectively called oncogenes and their study has elucidated the process of cellular transformation and may ultimately reveal the intricate processes by which cells communicate, grow, divide, and differentiate.

The preceding two chapters describe the advances in technologies that researchers are using to unravel the mysteries of genome order and gene regulation. They provide a useful introduction to this chapter because the genes and their products described herein appear to regulate, at some level, the biological processes of cell division and differentiation. The emerging description of how these biological processes are regulated has far-reaching implications.

All biological systems must faithfully duplicate genetic information and partition it equally among progeny, whether the process is somatic or germ cell division in higher organisms or virus replication in host cells (*i.e.*, amplification and packaging of viral genomes into virions) (Fig. 4-1). These processes are not perfect; errors (mutations) do occur. Such mutations can alter normal physiologic processes, and, indeed, the frequency of chromosomal abnormalities in cancer cells[5] is almost certainly the result of interference with the normal regulation of DNA duplication and chromosome partitioning.

In this chapter we describe oncogenes and their normally functioning cellular counterparts termed proto-oncogenes. Proto-oncogene products are important regulators of biological processes. They are localized in different cell compartments, are expressed at different stages of the cell cycle, and appear to be involved in the cascade of events that serve to maintain the ordered procession through the cell cycle (Fig. 4-2). The cell cycle is regulated by external mitogens (growth factors, peptide and steroid hormones, and lymphokines [Fig. 4-3]) which bind to their specific cell receptors (for example, the insulin, platelet-derived growth factor and epidermal growth factors bind to members of the tyrosine kinase family of growth factor receptors, as shown in Fig. 4-2B.) This activates a process termed signal transduction whereby specific signals are transmitted throughout the cell to the nucleus. The process is also mediated by nonintegral membrane associated proteins belonging to the tyrosine kinase and *ras* gene families (Figs. 4-2C and 4-2D). Signals

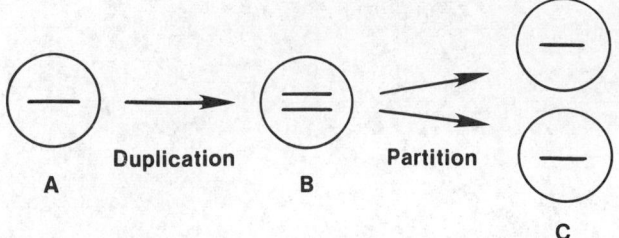

FIG. 4-1. Schematic representation of the process of duplication of genetic information and its partitioning to progeny cells.

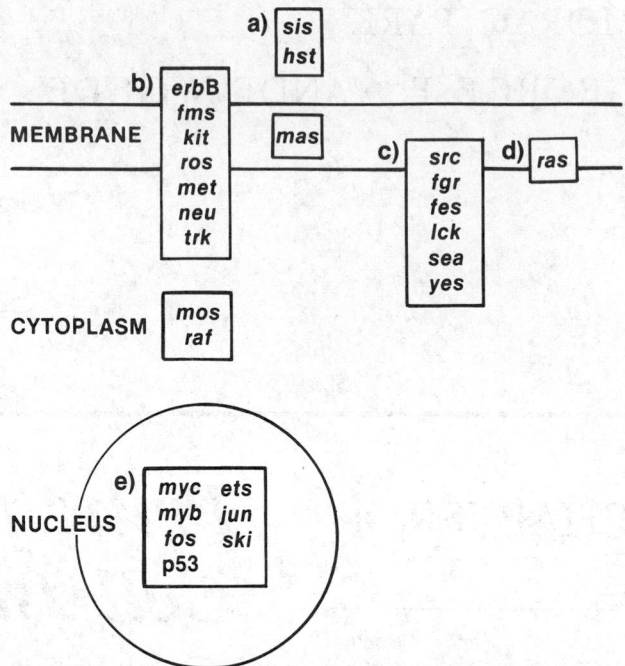

FIG. 4-3. Schematic presentation of the cellular compartments where oncogene or proto-oncogene products are localized. The growth factors (external mitogenic signals) (*a*), transmembrane tyrosine kinase growth factor receptor membranes (*b*), nonintegral membrane associated proteins of the *src* gene family (*c*), and *ras* gene family (*d*) plus oncogenes localized in the nucleus (*e*).

generated by mitogenic stimulation can lead to the expression of specific genes coding for proteins localized to the nucleus (Figs. 4-2E and 4-3). Certain members of the oncogene nuclear protein products have been shown to be transactivators of specific RNA transcripts.

Mutations that alter levels of gene expression or alter the form of the gene products in this pathway have been shown to activate their oncogenic potential (Table 4-1). Indeed, the discovery and study of oncogenes has provided the common link between, for example, a growth factor gene–like platelet derived growth factor (PDGF) and nuclear protein protooncogenes, c-*fos* and c-*myc* (see Fig. 4-2).[6,7] In the cancer cell, this ordered procession (see Fig. 4-2) is partially lost when more than one of these pathway members (see Fig. 4-3) are activated as oncogenes. For example, instead of maintaining conditional regulation at a specific stage in the cell cycle, the oncogene may provide a constitutive signal that perhaps initiates a cascade of subordinate functions out of sync with the normal events.

The term proto-oncogene is misleading because it wrongly implies that these genes latently reside in the genome for the sole purpose of expressing the neoplastic phenotype, when in fact they are essential to the normal biological processes such as cell division. The risk of errors (*e.g.*, chromosomal translocations) which activate their oncogenic potential suggests that numerous safeguards preventing facile activation of oncogenes must exist in the animal genome. The presence of these safeguards is certainly related to the multiple

events (multiple genetic alterations or oncogene activation events occurring in a single cell)[2] believed to occur prior to the onset of neoplastic transformation and tumor progression.

IDENTIFICATION OF ONCOGENES

For a major portion of this century, there was considerable controversy over whether viruses or environmental insults to normal cell genes cause cancer.[8-13] The first oncogenes were identified in studies of cancer-causing retroviruses. An important step in the retrovirus infection cycle is the stable integration of the provirus into the host chromosome.[14,15] By determining the DNA sequence of the integrated retrovirus provirus, researchers learned that these proviruses resemble transposons, or movable genetic elements, which have been studied widely in prokaryotes and lower eukaryotes.[16] These genetic elements move to alternate positions in the chromosomes of a cell. They were first characterized[17] and subsequently studied because of their ability to alter or modify expression of the genetic loci into which they insert.[18] Studies showed that provirus insertion also modifies expression of the region of the host chromosome into which it inserts; when the locus is a proto-oncogene, the provirus insertion can result in tumorigenesis.[19,20] Oncogenes have been isolated also in DNA tumor viruses and in various tumor cells associated with chromosomal breakpoints.

FIG. 4-2. Stimulation of quiescent murine fibroblasts to enter the G1 phase of growth by addition of platelet-derived growth factor (PDGF) or fibroblast growth factor (FGF). A transient increase in the expression of both c-*fos* and c-*myc* follows PDGF or FGF stimulation or treatment of cells with phorbol ester TPA plus a calcium ionophore. Cells rendered competent require epidermal growth factor and insulin-like growth factors to progress through DNA synthesis and the cell cycle.

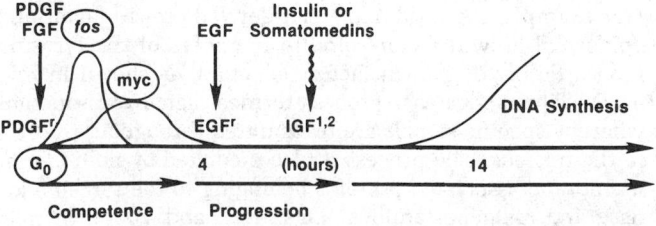

TABLE 4-1.   Oncogenes: Source and Properties

Reference	RNA Tumor Virus	Oncogene	Alternative Method of Identification	Species of Origin	Source	Properties
src Family						Proto-oncogene
Tyrosine Kinases: Integral Membrane						characteristic of growth factor receptors
351	Susan McDonough feline sarcoma virus	v-*fms*		Cat	Sarcoma	From CSF-1 receptor
351	Avian erythroblastosis virus	v-*erb*B		Chicken	Sarcoma/ erythroblastosis	From EGF-receptor
352	HZ4 feline sarcoma virus	v-*kit*		Cat	Sarcoma	
351	UR2 avian sarcoma virus	v-*ros*		Chicken	Sarcoma	
57		*neu*	DNA transfection	Rat	Neuroblastoma	
60		*met*	DNA transfection	Human	MNNG-treated human osteocarcinoma cell line	
61		*trk*	DNA transfection	Human	Colon carcinoma	
Tyrosine Kinases: Membrane Associated						
351	Rous sarcoma virus	v-*src*		Chicken	Sarcoma	
351	Yamaguchi-79 sarcoma virus	v-*yes*		Chicken	Sarcoma	
351	Gardner-Rasheed feline sarcoma virus	v-*fqr*		Cat	Sarcoma	
351	Fujinami sarcoma virus	v-*fps*		Chicken	Sarcoma	
351	Snyder-Theilen feline sarcoma virus	v-*fes*		Cat	Sarcoma	
351	Abelson murine leukemia virus	v-*abl*		Mouse	Leukemia	
351	Hardy Zuckerman 2 feline sarcoma virus	v-*abl*		Cat	Sarcoma	
Serine/Threonine Kinases						
351	Moloney murine sarcoma virus	v-*mos*		Mouse	Sarcoma	
351	3611 murine sarcoma virus	*raf*		Mouse	Sarcoma	
Growth Factor Families						
353	Simian sarcoma virus	v-*sis*		Woolly monkey	Glioma/ fibrosarcoma	B chain PDGF
87		*int*-2	Proviral insertion	Mouse	Mammary carcinoma	Member of FGF family
63		KS3	DNA transfection	Human	Kaposi's sarcoma	Member of FGF family
62		*hst*	DNA transfection	Human	Stomach carcinoma	Member of FGF family
ras Family						
42	Harvey murine sarcoma virus	v-H-*ras*		Rat	Erythroleukemia	GTP binding/ GTPase
43	Kirsten murine sarcoma virus	v-K-*ras*		Rat	Sarcoma	GTP binding/GTPase
47		N-*ras*	DNA transfection	Human DNA	Various	GTP binding/GTPase
Nuclear protein family						
351	Myelocyto-matosis-29 virus	v-*myc*		Chicken	Carcinoma myelocytomtosis	Binds DNA
175		N-*myc*	Gene amplification	Human	Neuroblastoma	?

(continued)

TABLE 4-1. Oncogenes: Source and Properties *(Continued)*

Reference	RNA Tumor Virus	Oncogene	Alternative Method of Identification	Species of Origin	Source	Properties
Nuclear protein family (continued)						
324		L-*myc*	Gene amplification	Human	Small cell lung carcinoma	?
117	Avian myeloblastosis virus	v-*myb*		Chicken	Myeloblastosis	Binds DNA
351	FBJ murine sarcoma virus	v-*fos*		Mouse	Osteosarcoma	Binds DNA
351	Sloan-Kettering avian sarcoma virus	v-*ski*		Chicken	Carcinoma	?
278		v-*jun*		Chicken		Binds DNA
194		P53		Mouse/human	Expressed at high levels in transformed cells	Binds SV40 large T/and adenovirus E1B
Others						
351	Reticulo-endotheliosis virus, strain T	v-*rel*		Turkey	Lymphatic leukemia	
351	E26 avian leukemia virus	v-*ets*		Chicken		
351	Avian erythroblastosis virus	v-*erb*A		Chicken	Erythroblastosis	Derived from steroid receptor for triiodothyronine
33		*mas*	DNA transfection	Human	Mammary carcinoma	Transmembrane protein
118		*int*-1	Proviral insertion	Mouse	Mammary carcinoma	

RETROVIRUSES AND ONCOGENES

Acute transforming retroviruses have been isolated from many avian and mammalian sources and can be divided into two classes based on the latency period between infection and the appearance of a tumor. Leukemia or leukosis viruses[16] produce leukemia or lymphoma in animals after long latent periods (more than 3 months). Acute transforming retroviruses can produce tumors in newborn animals in less than 2 weeks; this characteristic led early investigators to believe that they had identified agents responsible for neoplastic transformation. The difference between the latent periods for disease caused by these two virus classes can be traced to differences in their genetic content. The acute transforming retroviruses possess nucleic acid sequences acquired (transduced) from the genetic information of the host cell, and these gene sequences are responsible for the rapid transforming activity (Fig. 4-4). These host-derived genes are called viral oncogenes (v-*onc*), and many have been identified in acute transforming retroviruses (see Table 4-1). In contrast, the leukemia retroviruses do not contain transduced host oncogenes (see Fig. 4-4). The long latent period for disease caused by these retroviruses is partially the result of the low probability that proviruses will integrate into or adjacent to a host cellular oncogene. The integration activates oncogene expression in the same way as does an acute transforming retrovirus.

Because retroviruses can integrate at many loci in the host chromosome, their insertions can interrupt various normal genetic functions. Provirus insertion can cause mutations by

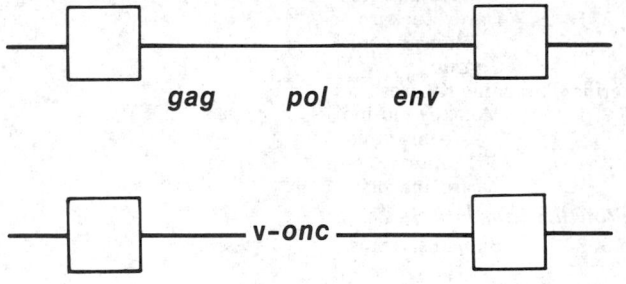

FIG. 4-4. Schematic representation of the general structure of leukemia retroviral and acute transforming retroviral genomes.

interrupting coding sequences or regulatory elements. Expression of adjacent host genes also can be activated or elevated because of enhancer activity (see Chap. 3) of the viral transcription control element or long terminal repeat (LTR) (Fig. 4-5). When integration occurs in a proto-oncogene locus, elevated or unregulated expression of this gene can result in tumor formation. Figure 4-5 shows several models for retroviral activation of oncogene expression and presents a model for provirus acquisition or transduction of a cellular oncogene. There is little question that oncogenes are acquired by retroviruses from the normal genome of the cell.[16]

In the first model (Fig. 4-5, line I), a retrovirus provirus integrates adjacent to a cellular oncogene. In the second model, the transformation/transduction model (Fig. 4-5,

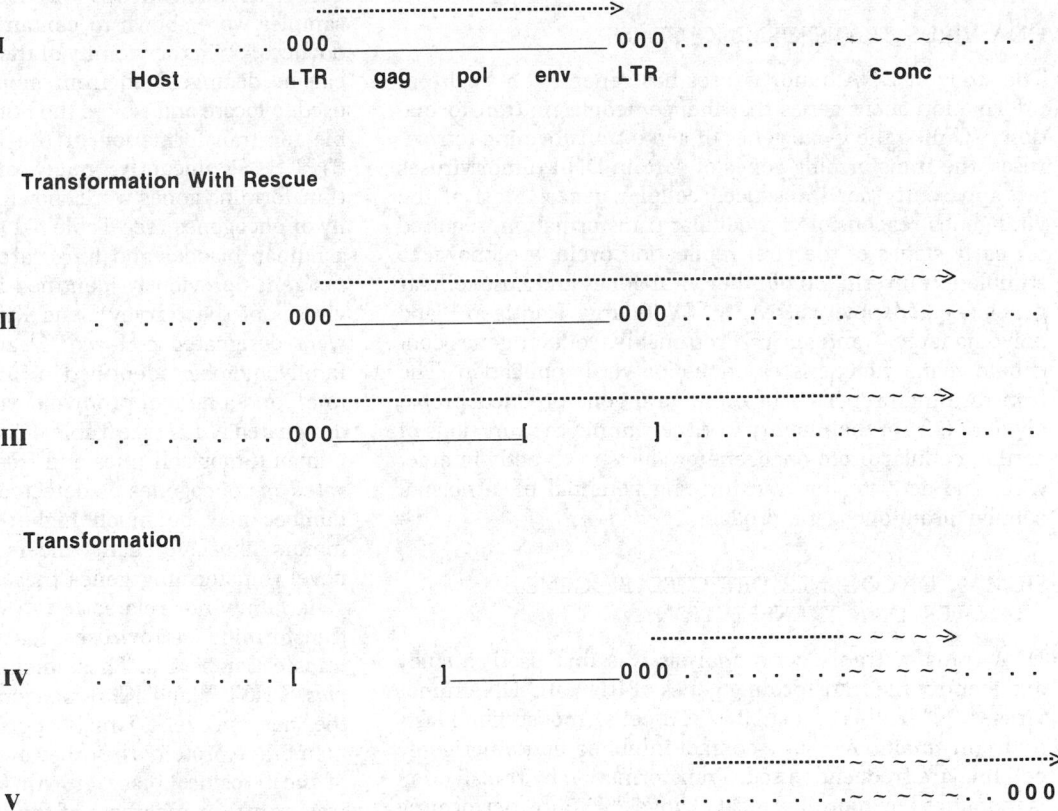

FIG. 4-5. Oncogene activation by provirus insertion. The retrovirus provirus inserts randomly into host chromosomal DNA. If integration occurs adjacent to a cellular oncogene (c-*onc*) and if sufficient levels of RNA are expressed, transformation is possible (lines II and III). However, most LTR-mediated provirus transcripts occur between the LTR elements (line II), and few transcripts proceed into the c-*onc* locus. A DNA rearrangement that results in the loss of the downstream LTR (line III) allows transcription into the c-*onc* locus. With either model the elevated or unregulated LTR-promoted c-*onc* transcription can result in transformation if the c-*onc* portion of the transcript is in the proper configuration to be translated into protein. Neither arrangement (line II or III) may permit transcription of a translatable c-*onc* mRNA, but both could result in transduction of the c-*onc* into a retroviral genome. The viral portion of the transcript can provide the necessary sequences for the entire fused viral c-*onc* transcript to be packaged into virions. As part of the viral genome, the transcript is subject to an enormous increase in genetic rearrangements, and events that generate efficient expression of a c-*onc* transforming product (now as v-*onc*) can result in the generation of an acute transforming retrovirus. The transduced c-*onc* becomes the transforming element or v-*onc* (see Table 4-1). Transformation by provirus insertion is observed more frequently, as shown in lines IV and V with either upstream or downstream insertions.

line II), provirus expression extends beyond the downstream LTR into the cellular oncogene locus. However, most of the transcripts terminate within this LTR element, and it is unlikely that this level of expression would lead to transformation. In the third model (Figure 4-5, line III), the downstream LTR sequences of the provirus have been lost and now proviral transcripts originating in the upstream LTR proceed through into the oncogene locus. This rearrangement can result in a high level of expression of the cellular oncogene and could lead to transformation. These models illustrate the mechanism by which cellular oncogenes can be transduced by retroviruses; c-*onc*-containing transcripts (Fig. 4-5, lines II and III) can be encapsidated into virions and acquired as part of the viral genome. The event is extremely rare.

The transformation models (Fig. 4-5, lines IV and V) show that activation of expression can occur with an LTR either upstream or downstream to the oncogene.[19-22] The activations are, in large part, the result of the transcription enhancer effect which causes unregulated expression of the oncogene from its own promoter (see Chap. 3).

Many novel oncogenes have been discovered on the basis

of the knowledge that provirus insertion causes leukemias and lymphomas after long latent periods by inserting adjacent to proto-oncogene loci (Table 4-2).

DNA VIRUS TRANSFORMING GENES

The study of DNA tumor viruses has generated a wealth of information about genes that induce neoplastic transformation.[23] Unlike the v-onc genes of acute transforming retroviruses, the transforming genes of certain DNA tumor viruses are apparently not transduced cellular genes. Most of the viral genes responsible for cellular transformation, required for early stages of the viral replication cycle, are known to stimulate transcription of other viral genes and host cellular genes (e.g., adenovirus E1A,[24,25] SV40 large T antigen,[26] and polyoma large T antigen.)[27] Presumably, cellular genes contribute many functions essential for viral replication. The transforming properties of these viral gene products probably derive from their ability to either mimic the functions of certain cellular proto-oncogene products or directly interact with, and activate the transforming potential of, a normal cellular proto-oncogene product.

HUMAN ONCOGENES DETECTED BY GENE TRANSFER/DNA TRANSFECTION

DNA transfer/transfection analysis was first used to study and identify the transforming genes of RNA and DNA tumor viruses.[28,29] In this assay, NIH/3T3 cells (mouse fibroblasts in origin) maintained as a contact-inhibited nontumorigenic cell line are frequently used. Transformation by transfection is monitored by morphological changes[30,31] or by performing tumorigenesis assays in nude mice[32,33] (Fig. 4-6A and B). Genomic DNA from mouse and human chemically induced or naturally occurring tumor cell lines were shown to give rise to foci of morphologically altered cells when transfected onto nontransformed mouse cell monolayers.[34,35] DNA from the newly transformed mouse cells can be extracted and cycled again onto nontransformed mouse cell monolayers.

After two or more cycles of DNA transfection, the oncogene is essentially the only foreign DNA detectable in the transformed cells.

Foci obtained in this way from human tumor cell DNA samples were shown to contain human repetitive DNA sequences[36,37] in the vicinity of the oncogene. These sequences can be distinguished from mouse sequences[38] and can be used to locate and isolate the human DNA segment responsible for transformation of the NIH/3T3 cells (see Fig. 4-6).[39-41] Significantly, many of the transfectable human transforming genes were shown to be related to the ras family of oncogenes (see Table 4-1). The transforming genes of a human bladder and lung carcinoma were homologous to ras genes previously identified in acute transforming retroviruses of the Harvey[42] and Kirsten[43] sarcoma viruses and were designated c-H-ras[44-46] and c-K-ras.[44-46] A ras gene family member identified in a human neuroblastoma cell line[47] and a human promyelocytic leukemia cell line[48] were designated N-ras (see Table 4-1).[49-51] Approximately 15% of human tumor cell lines and fresh tumor biopsies have activated ras oncogenes as detected by this assay,[52-54] and this number may be much higher in certain specific human tumors like colorectal cancers.[55,56] A growing number of novel transforming genes that are not members of the ras gene family nor related to the viral oncogenes of the acute transforming retroviruses have been identified by DNA transfection assays. These include the neu,[57-59] met,[60] trk,[61] mas,[33] HST,[62] and KS3 oncogenes.[63] With the exception of the mas oncogene which appears to be a unique integral membrane protein, the other oncogenes are either members of the tyrosine kinase growth factor receptor family (neu, met, or trk) or members of the fibroblast growth factor family (FGF), (HST, KS3).

ONCOGENES IDENTIFIED BY CHROMOSOME ABNORMALITIES

Oncogenes have been associated with the nonrandom chromosomal abnormalities identified by cytogeneticists. Micro-

TABLE 4-2.   Cellular Genes Activated by Insertional Mutagenesis

Gene	Virus	Disease	Animal	Reference
c-myc	ALV, CSV, REV	Bursal lymphoma	Chicken	310,311
	MLV	T cell lymphoma	Mouse	
	FeLV	T cell lymphoma	Cat	312
c-erbB	ALV	Erythroleukemia	Chicken	116
c-myb	MLV	Lymphosarcoma	Mouse	313
c-H-ras	MAV	Nephroblastoma	Chicken	314
c-mos	IAP	Plasmacytoma cell line	Mouse	315
IL-2	GaLV	T cell lymphoma cell line	Ape	124
IL-3	IAP	Myelomonocytic leukemia	Mouse	125
int-1	MMTV	Mammary carcinoma	Mouse	118
int-2	MMTV	Mammary carcinoma	Mouse	87
Pim-1	M-MLV	T-cell lymphoma	Mouse	316
tck(1skT)	M-MLV	Thymoma cell line	Mouse	317
pvt(mis-1)	M-MLV	T or B cell lymphoma	Mouse/rat	318,319
Mlvi-1	M-MLV	T cell lymphoma	Rat	320
Mlvi-2	M-MLV	T cell lymphoma	Rat	320
Mlvi-3	M-MLV	T cell lymphoma	Rat	320
Evi-1	MCF-MLV	Myeloid lymphoma	Mouse	321
Evi-2	MCF-MLV	Myeloid lymphoma	Mouse	322

**DETECTION OF TRANSFORMING HUMAN
DNA SEQUENCES**

Transformed Cells
or Tumor Tissue

High Molecular
Weight DNA

Calcium Phosphate–
DNA Precipitate

Normal Cells

Foci

2nd Cycle

Hybridization
to Human Repeat
Sequences

Tumor

2nd Cycle

A

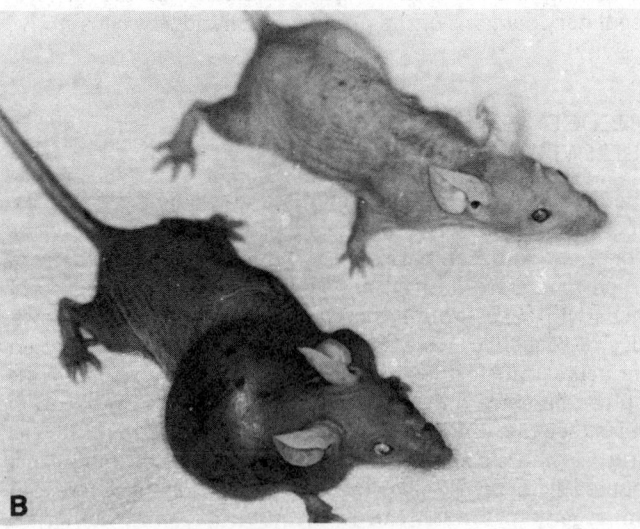

B

scopic structural changes of chromosomes, such as nonrandom chromosomal translocations and homogeneously staining regions (HSR), are associated with mammalian and human tumors.[64-67] This association was the basis for speculation that the chromosome abnormalities were activating oncogenes by mechanisms similar to provirus activation in animal model systems.[65,66] The chromosomal localization of cellular proto-oncogenes determined by in situ hybridization (Table 4-3) revealed proto-oncogenes at or near chromosomal translocation breakpoints.[67,68] Nonrandom chromosomal translocations are consistently associated with some types of leukemias and myelodysplasias.[69,70] In many cases the DNA breakpoints involved in the translocation have been isolated. Oncogenes have been identified at translocation breakpoints in Burkitt's lymphoma (c-*myc*)[71] and chronic myelogenous leukemia (*bcr-abl*).[72] Possible oncogenic loci have been identified by isolating the DNA segments associated with the translocation breakpoints in adult B cell lymphomas, follicular lymphomas, and diffuse histiocytic leukemias (*bcl*I and *bcl*II.)[73,74]

Other oncogenes have been identified in chromosomal abnormalities associated with amplification of specific DNA segments. In human neuroblastomas, up to a 700-fold amplification of a sequence with limited homology to c-*myc*, termed N-*myc*, has been found in homogeneously staining regions of the tumor cells.[75,76]

The loss of DNA from certain regions of chromosomes, thought to unmask recessive mutations present in the remaining allele and often referred to as recessive oncogenes, have been associated with several tumors, especially childhood tumors such as retinoblastoma and Wilms'.[77-79] These chromosomal abnormalities involve deletions of various lengths in portions of chromosomes in different patients; however, analysis of the chromosomes reveals common deleted regions. Patients with retinoblastoma have deletions in chromosome 13 band q14[80] and patients with Wilms' tumor have deletions in chromosome 11 band p13.[81] Recently, a candidate retinoblastoma gene was isolated[82,83] but its function in normal or tumor cells is not yet known.

GROWTH FACTORS AND GROWTH FACTOR RECEPTORS THAT ARE ONCOGENES

The discovery that certain oncogenes (v-*sis* and v-*erb*B) were homologs of a growth factor PDGF[84,85] and growth factor receptor (epidermal growth factor receptor [EGFR])[86] pro-

FIG. 4-6. **A**. DNA transfection. The DNA transfection schemes show the calcium phosphate-dependent protocols used for detecting transforming genes in transformed cells and tumors. The DNA from either primary foci or tumors is recycled in the transfection assay to facilitate the loss of extraneous nontransforming sequences that are carried with the transforming gene in the first transfection. After several cycles, the major portion of the foreign DNA in the focus or tumor is responsible for the transforming activity and can be isolated by conventional recombinant DNA technology. **B**. Nude mouse tumor assay. Both animals received subcutaneous injections of 3×10^6 NIH 3T3 cells that had been transfected 4 days earlier with either normal human DNA or DNA from a pancreatic-carcinoma–derived cell line. Tumor appearance was first noted 6 weeks after the cells had been injected.

TABLE 4-3.   Chromosomal Location of Oncogenes

Chromosome	Location	Proto-Oncogene	Reference
1	1p36	fgr	323
1	1p32	L-myc	324
1	1p11-13	N-ras	325
1	1q22-qter	ski	326
1	1q32	trk	327
2	2p23-24	N-myc	157
2	2p11-12	rel	328
3	3p25	raf	329
5	5q34	fms	330
6	6p21	pim-1	331
6	6q21-22	ros	332
6	6q22-24	myb	333
6	6q24-27	mas	332
7	7p11-13	erbB	334
7	7q31	met	335
8	8q22	mos	336
8	8q24	myc	127
9	9q34.1	abl	142
11	11p14.1	H-ras	337
11	11q13	int-2	338
11	11q23-24	ets-1	339
12	12p12.1	K-ras	340
12	12pter-q14	int-1	341
14	14q21-31	fos	342
15	15q26.1	fes	333
17	17p23	p53	343
17	17q12-22	neu	59
17	17q21-22	erbA	334
18	18q21.3	yes	344
20	20q12-13	src	345
21	21q22	ets-2	346
22	22q11	bcr	72
22	22q13.1	sis	347

vided a direct link with genes responsible for regulating cell division and differentiation, but raised the question whether other members of these families have oncogenic potential. The list has recently expanded to include other growth factors such as members of the fibroblast growth factor family (HST,[62] int-2[87] and KS3[63]) a known hematopoietic growth factor receptor (colony-stimulating factor [CSF-1], v-fms,[88] and v-erbA, the receptor for a thyroid hormone.[89,90] Several oncogenes have been identified that resemble tyrosine kinase growth factor receptor family members (neu,[57] met,[60] and trk[61]), but no candidate ligands are yet known for their products. The increasing number of correlations between oncogenes and growth factors raises the interesting consideration that many growth factors and cell receptors can, under the appropriate circumstances, behave as oncogenes. In the past, oncogenes were identified by a few methods and assays. As their normal functions are revealed, new and better approaches will be developed for their identification; already, it is becoming more common to identify possible oncogenes from structural analyses of genes (Fig. 4-7).

MECHANISMS OF ONCOGENE ACTIVATION

Mechanisms of oncogene activation are best studied by directly comparing the activated oncogene with the proto-on-

cogene from which it was derived. Oncogene activation is always associated with a genetic alteration which can range from a single nucleotide (base) change in the genomic locus (as in ras oncogene activation) to gross changes in DNA structure (as in chromosomal translocations or the extensive changes observed in transduced viral oncogenes).[91,92] In general, however, the changes that activate proto-oncogenes result from an unregulated increase or unscheduled expression of the normal product, or from mutations or deletions in regulatory domains of the protein which induces constitutive activity.

ONCOGENES IN ACUTE TRANSFORMING RETROVIRUSES

The acute transforming retroviruses are, in many respects, laboratory curiosities, but the identification of their v-onc sequences and comparison to the proto-oncogenes from which they were derived have provided a unique source of genes with transforming potential and fundamental knowledge of sequences necessary for their activation. Most often the acute transforming retroviruses are impaired in virus replication since they lack a full complement of replication genes (see Fig. 4-4). However, because they are replicated as viruses, they are subject to a very high mutation rate. This, coupled with investigator-mediated selection for increased tumorigenic potential, can result in viruses with numerous

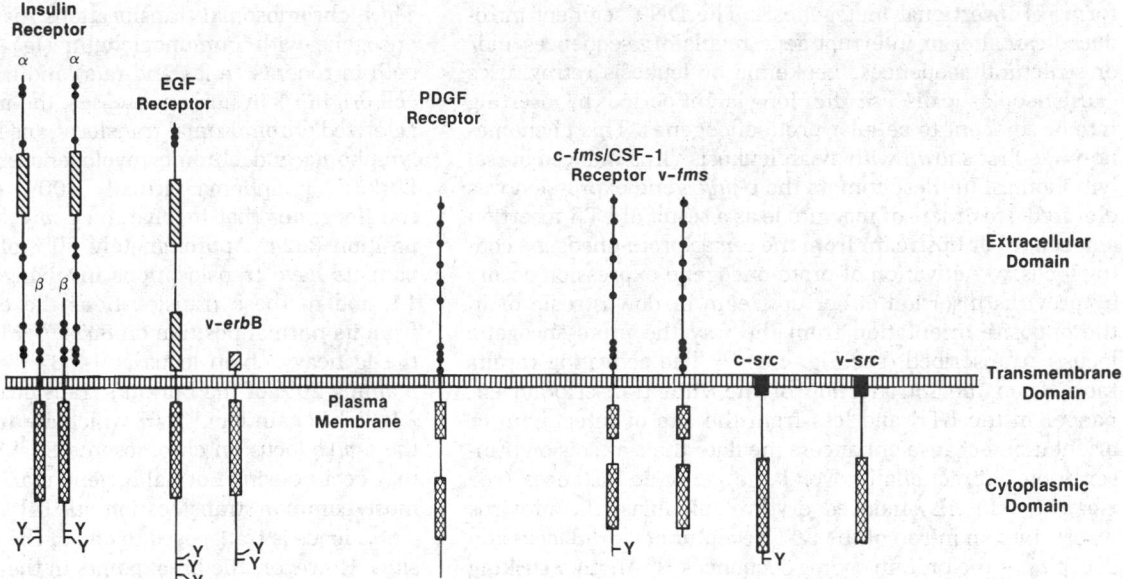

FIG. 4-7. Schematic comparison of structural features of cell surface receptors and tyrosine kinase oncogene products. Regions of high cysteine concentration are shown as hatched boxes and single cysteine residues are filled circles. The tyrosine kinase domain is represented as cross-hatched boxes and the position of carboxy terminal tyrosine residues is shown as Y. The deletions that activate v-erbB, v-fms, and v-src are illustrated. EGF, epidermal growth factor; PDGF, platelet derived growth factor; CSF-1, mononuclear phagocyte colony stimulating factor.

changes in v-*onc* sequences when compared with the proto-oncogene. Thus, mutations can be identified that increase tumorigenic potential. Such mutations include multiple point mutations, deleted upstream or downstream exons, and transcriptional and posttranscriptional regulatory elements. For example, a 3′ noncoding region sequence that normally inhibits c-*fos* expression posttranscriptionally allows v-*fos* to be produced at high levels.[93,94] Many v-*onc* genes are expressed as fusion gene products with viral genes (*gag* and *env*) and at high levels under constitutive control of the retroviral LTR.[95] *gag*- or *env-onc* fusion products may serve to contribute to transforming potential by misdirecting an oncogene product to an improper cellular location. Moreover, the target cell specificity of the retrovirus can result in the expression of the oncogene in an inappropriate cell type. For instance, the presence of *gag* sequences is required for v-*abl* transformation of lymphoid cells.[96] The v-*ras* genes contain point mutations in the same position as in activated c-*ras* genes in human tumors,[97] whereas the v-*src* gene in Rous sarcoma virus contains both point mutations and a C-terminal deletion.[98] The latter deletion has been shown to be essential for activating the *src* proto-oncogene.

The products of the cellular and viral *src* genes possess intrinsic protein tyrosine kinase activity.[99] The tyrosine residue deleted in the v-*src* product (tyr 527)[100,101] may be required for down-regulating the intrinsic *src* kinase activity.[100,102] Other nonintegral tyrosine kinase genes in the *src* family (*yes, fgr, fps, fms*) also have tyrosine residues in their C-terminal amino acid sequences[99] and activated *yes, fgr,* and *fms* oncogenes lack the C-terminal region containing a

tyrosine codon thought to be equivalent in function to the tyrosine 527 in c-*src*.[88,103-106] However, the v-*erb* oncogene, a modified form of the EGF receptor of avian erythroblastosis virus (AEV), in addition to having a C-terminal deletion, has a deletion in its N-terminal ligand-binding domain[107] and is presumed to function as a constitutively activated growth factor receptor.[99,108,109] Thus, as with other members of the *src* family, the truncation of the C terminus may activate the gene. However, a hybrid protein expressed from the EGF receptor locus activated by the insertion of ALV contains the appropriate C-terminal amino acids and, in this case, the deletion of the ligand-binding domain is sufficient for activation.[110] Similarly, the v-*kit* oncogene (see Table 4-1) has both N-terminal and C-terminal deletions and is derived from an oncogene related to the PDGF receptor.[111] However, two oncogenes identified by the DNA transfection assay, *met*[112,113] and *trk*[61] (see Table 4-1), also putative tyrosine kinase receptor genes, appear to be activated by a DNA rearrangement that eliminates the putative ligand-binding domain and substitutes protein domains derived from other genes; this rearrangement may be essential for efficient transformation.[61,113]

ONCOGENE ACTIVATION BY INSERTIONAL MUTAGENESIS

Insertional mutagenesis is an alteration resulting from the insertion of foreign DNA sequences into a defined genetic locus. Provirus insertion or transposition of a movable genetic element that interrupts host genomic sequences are forms of insertional mutagenesis. The DNA segment introduced can alter or interrupt gene regulatory sequences and/or structural sequences. Leukemia or leukosis retroviruses cause neoplastic disease after long latent periods by inserting into or adjacent to cellular proto-oncogenes. This phenomenon was first shown with avian leukosis virus-induced bursal lymphomas. In these tumors the c-*myc* gene expression was elevated two orders of magnitude as a result of LTR insertion adjacent to or upstream from the c-*myc* proto-oncogene coding locus.[114] Activation of proto-oncogene expression occurs by provirus insertion either upstream or downstream or in the opposite orientation from the way the proto-oncogene locus is transcribed (see Fig. 4-5).[115] The activation results more from the introduction of the viral transcription enhancer in the LTR and less from the site of integration or orientation because enhancers mediate their effects on transcription bidirectionally over large genomic distances (see Chap. 3). In ALV-induced erythroleukemias, the provirus inserts into an intron of the EGF receptor or c-*erb*B locus and decapitates the protein coding sequences.[116] Another striking example of activation by truncation occurs in the murine leukemia virus-induced myeloid tumors. In these tumors the provirus insertion occurs in the N-terminal coding domain of the c-*myb* locus.[117]

Leukemia retroviruses can cause many different types of tumors by virtue of the cell types they infect, the genes they integrate adjacent to (and the genes' relevance to the growth properties of that particular cell type), and the influence of the cell-type on the transcriptional enhancement of the LTR. Studies analyzing these variables have identified many oncogenes (see Table 4-2). Specific examples are *int*-1 and *int*-2, which are activated in mouse mammary tumors by provirus insertion.[87,118] Sometimes proviruses are found adjacent to both *int*-1 and *int*-2 in the same tumor.[119] Many times the protein coding domain of oncogenes activated by insertional mutagenesis remain unaltered and in these instances, activation presumably occurs as a result of inappropriate levels of gene expression. *int*-1 and *int*-2 genes are normally only transiently expressed during embryogenesis[120,121] but integration of mouse mammary tumor virus provirus into mammary epithelial cells results in low levels of expression. Although the exact mechanism is unknown, expression of *int*-1 and *int*-2 appears to be required for the development of mammary tumors. Similarly, hematopoietic cell lines that grow in the absence of growth factors have been induced to make their own growth factors as a consequence of proviral insertions adjacent to lymphokine genes IL-2 and IL-3.[122,123] Other studies have shown that when IL-2 or IL-3 genes are introduced by recombinant DNA techniques into retrovirus vectors, the viruses generated render factor-dependent cell lines factor-independent and tumorigenic[124,125] through an autocrine stimulation mechanism.

ONCOGENE ACTIVATION BY CHROMOSOMAL (DNA) REARRANGEMENTS

Nonrandom chromosomal translocations in leukemias and lymphomas of human and animal origin provide some of the most compelling indirect evidence for implicating oncogenes in the formation and progression of neoplastic disease.

Thus, chromosomal translocations that juxtapose the c-*myc* oncogene with immunoglobulin (Ig) sequences are found both in rodents (mice and rats) and humans in tumors of B cell origin.[126] In human diseases, the most extensively characterized chromosomal translocations have been in Burkitt's lymphoma and chronic myelogenous leukemia (CML). In Burkitt's lymphoma virtually 100% of the patients have translocations that involve the c-*myc* locus on chromosome position 8q24. Approximately 80% of Burkitt's lymphoma patients have translocations involving chromosomes 8 and 14, and in these translocations the c-*myc* locus is moved from its normal position on 8q24[127,128] to a position distal to the Ig heavy chain locus at 14q32[129] (Table 4-4). The remaining 20% of the Burkitt's translocations involve the κ or λ Ig light chain loci,[130-132] which are translocated distally to the c-*myc* locus on chromosome 8.[131,133] The translocations may occur during normal Ig gene rearrangement, and in the most common translocation [t8:14] (see Table 4-4), the c-*myc* locus is transposed to one of the Ig heavy chain switch sites. However, the breakpoints in the c-*myc* locus are quite variable.[134] None of the c-*myc* activations can be explained by a single model, although the rearranged c-*myc* gene appears to be expressed constitutively and several mechanisms have been proposed to account for this. First, translocation events appear to alter the first exon of the c-*myc* locus where cis-acting transcription regulatory sequences reside.[135-138] Quite strikingly, even when the translocation breakpoint is quite distant from the first exon, mutations are found in the same first exon cis-acting sequences.[138-140] In some instances, the translocation of the immunoglobulin enhancer cis-acting sequences into the vicinity of c-*myc* has been proposed as a transcriptional activation mechanism for c-*myc* expression.[139-141]

At least 95% of patients with CML possess a typical Philadelphia chromosome resulting from the translocation between chromosome 9 and 22 (9;22) (q34;q11).[167] In this translocation, the c-*abl* proto-oncogene (see Table 4-1) is translocated from chromosome 9 band q34 to chromosome 22 at band q11.[142,143] The breakpoints that occur in chromosome 22q11 are clustered within a 5-kb genomic region, and this region has been referred to as the breakpoint cluster region (*bcr*). In contrast, the breakpoints in the c-*abl* locus on chromosome 9q34 differ considerably from patient to patient with estimated differences of greater than 100 kb. In spite of this, a transcription unit in the *bcr* locus[144] provides the promoter and 5′ end sequences that result in a fused 8.5-kb *bcr-abl* hybrid mRNA[145,146] encoding a novel fusion protein of 210 kilodaltons (kd)[147] (see Table 4-4). Thus, in this disease, DNA rearrangements in the *bcr* locus, the expression of the novel 8.5-kb *bcr-abl* mRNA, and the detection of the novel 210-kd *bcr-abl* protein are all diagnostic for the Philadelphia positive CML.[148] It is not understood how this rearrangement contributes to CML. The normal c-*abl* product is a member of the tyrosine kinase family and may be involved in signal transduction,[56] and it is possible that the *bcr* locus which appears to be expressed in many cell types provides a mechanism for expressing the *abl* tyrosine kinase gene in an unregulated fashion analogous to immunoglobulin rearrangement that results in an enhanced level of c-*myc* expression in Burkitt's lymphoma. However, the *bcr* locus

TABLE 4-4. Chromosomal Translocations in Human Malignancies

Gene Locus	Human Neoplasm	Percentage of Tumors with Translocation or Gene Rearrangement	Chromosome Translocation	Reference
c-myc	Burkitt's lymphoma	80	t(8;14)(q24;q32)	348
		15	t(8;22)(q34;q11)	349
		5	t(2;8)(q11;q24)	141
bcr-abl	Chronic myelogenous leukemia	90–95	t(9;22)(q34;q11)	144
	Acute lymphocytic leukemia	10–15	t(9;22)(q34;q11)	350
bcl-1	Chronic lymphocytic leukemia of B cell type	10–20	t(11;14)(q13;q32)	73
bcl-2	Follicular lymphoma	85–95	t(14;18)(q32;q21)	74

provides N-terminal sequences to the c-abl product; this could either alter protein function or direct the tyrosine kinase to a different cellular location.[149] The acute transforming retroviruses possessing the v-abl oncogene have been shown to render hematopoietic cells growth factor independent after infection.[150] Thus, the bcr-abl rearrangement may stimulate proliferation of certain hematopoietic cells and prevent terminal differentiation. The bcr-abl rearrangement may serve as a paradigm for how other tyrosine kinase gene family members, such as the tropomyosin-trk or tpr-met oncogenes, are activated.

Homogeneously staining chromosomal regions and double minute chromosomes are karyotypes frequently found in tumor cells and tumor cell lines. These atypical chromosome characteristics represent multiple (amplified) copies of a single gene-containing DNA segment, and cellular oncogenes have been found in multiple copies in cells showing this karyotype.[151,152] Even in the absence of these microscopic chromosomal changes, studies using nucleic acid hybridization have shown that cellular oncogenes can be amplified.[151] Gene amplification has been best characterized in studies on the development of cell resistance to cytotoxic drugs[153]; the mechanism of DNA amplification is poorly understood. However, during a single cell cycle, DNA replication must occur repeatedly in a segment of DNA 200 to 2000 kb in size.[154]

Several cellular oncogenes have been found amplified in human tumors (Table 4-5). The c-myc proto-oncogene locus is shown to be amplified in a promyelocytic leukemia both in the primary tumor as well as in the cell line HL-60 derived from the tumor.[155,156] Other oncogenes like c-erbB (EGFR), neu (HER-2), and c-myc family members have been shown to be amplified in specific tumor types (see Table 4-5) and presence of multiple copies have been associated with poor prognosis. Thus, the presence of multiple copies of N-myc (which was first identified as an amplified gene in human neuroblastoma[157]) has been shown to correlate with advanced stages of disease.[158] The presence of multiple copies of myc gene family members in small cell lung carcinoma is also associated with more malignant progression of the disease.[159] Thus the myc family members appear to be associated with the progression of neuroblastomas and small cell lung carcinomas, whereas the c-erbB or EGFR gene has been found amplified in glioblastomas and squamous carcinomas.[160,161] The human homolog of the neu gene, HER-2, is closely related to the EGF receptor or c-erbB gene and is often found amplified in adenocarcinomas and breast tumors.[162] Also, human mammary tumors that have amplified copies of the HER-2 gene are more advanced, are hormone-independent, and have a poor prognosis.[163,164] Tumors with amplified copies of oncogenes express high levels of the oncogene RNA, a finding consistent with experiments showing that overexpression of some of the oncogenes like c-erbB and neu in NIH/3T3 cells results in morphological transformation.[165,166]

ONCOGENE ACTIVATION BY POINT MUTATIONS

The c-H-ras oncogene isolated from a human bladder carcinoma cell line was the first oncogene shown to be activated in a human tumor cell line. This gene was activated by a single point mutation that resulted in a change from a glycine to a valine codon in the 12th amino acid position.[167-169] The ras oncogene has been identified in many animal and

TABLE 4-5. Cellular Oncogenes Amplified in Human Tumors

Tumor	Oncogene	Amplification	Reference
Small-cell lung cancer	c-myc	up to 80×	159
	N-myc	up to 50×	158
	L-myc	up to 20×	324
Neuroblastomas	N-myc	up to 250×	152
Glioblastomas	c-erbB(EGFR)	up to 50×	153
Mammary carcinoma	c-erbB2(HER2)	up to 30×	163,164

human tumor samples[54,96] (see Fig. 4-7). *ras* oncogenes in tumors have been shown to be activated by mutations in the 12th, 13th and the 59th to 61st codons.[96] In addition, studies have shown that mutations created in vitro by site-directed mutagenesis in codons 63, 116, and 119 can also activate *ras* as a transforming gene.[96] Although it is not completely clear how these point mutations or codon changes result in the *ras* protein activation. The normal gene product binds guanidine nucleotides and possesses GTPase activity[170] whereas mutant *ras* oncogene products have greatly reduced GTPase activity, suggesting that this dysfunction may be a factor.

Several studies have shown that *ras* genes are the target of chemical carcinogens in animal tumor model systems. Certain carcinogens cause G to T base transversions or G to A base transitions that are often observed in activated *ras* genes.[171,172] Thus, topical application of the carcinogen dimethylbenzanthracene (DMBA) followed by treatment with tumor promoters, results in benign skin papillomas that contain activated c-H-*ras* genes.[173] In addition, studies using a mammary carcinoma model system showed that treatment of newborn rats with a single dose of nitrosomethylurea (NMU) results in the development of mammary carcinomas 2 to 3 months after animals reach sexual maturity. Eighty-five percent of these tumors contain an activated c-H-*ras* oncogene with the same G to A base transition in the 12th *ras* codon.[174,175] In both of these animal model systems, the *ras* gene participates in a multistep process of carcinogenesis. In the latter case, c-H-*ras* activation must occur as an initiation step since NMU is only active for a few minutes after injection. Thus, although the *ras* gene is the target of the genotoxic chemical carcinogen, expression of the transformed phenotype requires additional steroid dependent promoter activity. Other studies show that *ras* activation can also play a role in tumor progression.[176] With the exception of the *neu* gene in rodents, the *ras* family represent the only known oncogenes thus far that can be activated by a single point mutation. This may explain the predominance of *ras* gene mutations found in animal and human cancers.

ONCOGENE/PROTO-ONCOGENE ACTIVITY

The products of oncogenes presumably display at least a subset of the activities of the proto-oncogene product. Therefore, the functional properties of the proto-oncogene product must be characterized in order to understand the role of an oncogene in tumorigenesis. As was mentioned earlier, proto-oncogenes appear to function in the biological processes of cell division and differentiation (see Figs. 4-2 and 4-3). Because these genes have been conserved in the evolutionary process, they have closely related counterparts in multicellular organisms. Thus, these biological processes can be studied in animal model systems and in genetically well-characterized organisms. Transgenic mouse strains have been developed in which oncogene transgenes have been introduced into the germline so that their in vivo roles in tumorigenesis can be studied. Other techniques are being applied as well and some of these techniques are discussed below.

EVOLUTIONARY CONSERVATION OF PROTO-ONCOGENES

The conservation of proto-oncogenes in different animal species can be studied with the use of nucleic acid hybridization techniques (see Chap. 2). The DNA sequences of certain proto-oncogenes are more highly conserved between species than the DNA sequences of others, a measure that must be related to their function. Some proto-oncogenes have been found in all multicellular organisms studied, indicating that their products have essential biological roles.[177] Of special interest are the proto-oncogene homologs found in organisms that are well suited for classic genetic studies, such as yeast or *Drosophila*. In these organisms, the phenotypic influence of mutated proto-oncogene homologs on cell division or differentiation and embryological development can be tested, and genes can be identified that suppress the mutant phenotype, thereby revealing other members of the biochemical pathway. The nucleotide sequences of most of the oncogenes listed in Table 4-1 have been determined, and in many cases, both their RNA and protein products have been characterized. They have also been compared to the nucleotide or predicted amino acid sequences of the host proto-oncogene from which they were derived and to the proto-oncogene homologs in other species, especially in humans. For instance, recently the *int*-1 oncogene was shown to be a developmentally regulated gene of *Drosophila*.[178] Studies of *ras* genes in yeast are increasing our understanding of what is apparently a highly conserved biochemical pathway of signal transduction.[179-187]

COOPERATING ONCOGENE ASSAY

Oncogenes can be divided into two complementation groups based on their activities in DNA transfection assays performed in rat embryo fibroblast cells (REF cells). Transforming genes of certain DNA tumor viruses display different biological activities in REF cells. REF cells normally undergo a finite number of passages in culture before they become senescent. One class of genes, adenovirus (Ad) E1A and polyoma (Py) large T antigen genes, rescue REF cells from senescence. Thus, the expression of the products of these two DNA tumor virus genes allows cells to be continuously maintained in culture (immortalized). A second class of genes, Ad E1B and Py middle T antigen genes, cause morphological transformation of the rescued cells and render them tumorigenic in nude mice.[188-190] Many of the oncogenes display one or the other of these phenotypes and can be assigned to two complementation groups. For example, foci of transformed cells appear when REF cells are transfected with both v-H-*ras* and v-*myc* oncogenes.[52,53,190,191] Moreover, members from one complementation group, whether a viral gene or an oncogene, can act synergistically with members of the second complementation group. Members of the oncogene group that rescues cells from senescence have products that are localized to the nucleus,[190-194] whereas the genes that morphologically transform the immortalized REF cells are membrane associated and contain members of the *ras* gene family and Py middle T antigen.[52,53,195]

NIH/3T3 cells are similar to REF cells immortalized by a member of the first complementation group. NIH/3T3 cells have been particularly useful for identifying genes that morphologically transform cells in DNA transfection assays. Many of the oncogenes are in the same complementation groups as genes from DNA tumor viruses, suggesting that they may transform cells through similar pathways. For example, the Ad E1A and Py large T antigen gene products bind DNA as shown for some oncogene products located in the nucleus (see Table 4-1) and the DNA tumor virus early genes have been shown to transactivate expression of cellular genes.[26,192] These viral genes are expressed early during DNA tumor virus replication before the onset of viral DNA synthesis. Thus these similarities indicate that the early virus genes may be to virus replication what c-myc is to cell cycle regulation and cell division (see Fig. 4-3). Another interesting correlation has been made among members of the second complementation group. The gene for Py middle T antigen is a membrane-associated phosphoprotein that forms a complex with the c-src protein.[196] In the complex, the kinase activity of the c-src protein is elevated to levels similar to those of the activated v-src product.[53,99,197] Considering the extraordinary differences between these biological systems, that is, between genes that function early during adenovirus or polyomavirus infection and cellular proto-oncogenes, it is striking that they can elicit similar phenotypes. The findings suggest that there are similar gene product requirements for the replication of cells and viruses.

ONCOGENES AND TRANSGENIC MICE

Transgenic mice provide a new and powerful model system for studying the role of oncogenes in tumor development. In this system the expression of foreign genes (transgenes) can be assessed in animals capable of producing normal physiologic responses. As described in Chapter 3, transgenes are introduced into the germ line of mice by microinjection of recombinant DNA molecules into the male pronucleus of fertilized eggs.[198] In this manner, oncogenes under transcriptional regulation of different promoter elements have been studied in transgenic mice.[198-201] A striking finding is that neoplasia or hyperplasia occurs only in clonal populations in specific tissues. For example, mice carrying a c-myc gene coupled with a mouse mammary tumor virus (MMTV) steroid-responsive LTR promoter develop mammary tumors and occasional B cell lymphomas[199] even though myc is expressed at high levels in other tissues. Similarly, mice carrying the v-H-ras gene with the same MMTV LTR promoter develop salivary gland tumors, mammary tumors, and display hyperplasia of the Harderian gland.[202] Long latent periods of 6 to 14 months are required for tumor development in mice bearing the MMTV LTR myc transgene, which clearly indicates that additional changes are required for tumor development.[203] The synergistic action of two oncogenes in vivo has also been tested by crossing the transgenic mouse strain containing the MMTV LTR ras gene with the strain possessing the MMTV LTR myc transgene.[202] Transgenic animals carrying both myc and ras have a higher incidence of tumors (e.g., B cell malignancies were 10-fold higher) with a shorter latent period than found in mouse strains carrying either oncogene alone.[202] However, the tumors, were clonal, and most of the cells expressed both oncogenes without expressing a transformed phenotype.

The best evidence indicating that c-myc-Ig gene rearrangements act as an initiating event in B cell tumors (discussed earlier in Oncogene Activation by Chromosomal Rearrangements and Translocations) was obtained by generating transgenic mice containing a c-myc gene regulated by a lymphoid-specific heavy chain Ig enhancer.[204] The lymphoid cells of these animals expressed high levels of the myc gene regulated by the IgH enhancer and the animals developed lymphoid tumors. However, these tumors were rare and clonal, indicating that additional events are necessary to promote tumorigenesis. These experiments demonstrated, however, that this specific gene rearrangement predisposes the animal to B cell tumors and is indirect evidence supporting the role of similar Ig-c-myc rearrangements in Burkitt's lymphoma in mouse B cell tumors.

These studies fully support the model that tumorigenesis is the result of multiple events in the same cell. One possible explanation for the low incidence of neoplasia in the myc-Ig transgenic mice is that the oncogene may not have been expressed at a critical stage of development or differentiation. It also indicates that oncogenes, as transgenes, are not necessarily dominant transforming genes. It is possible, therefore, that they may require the concomitant loss or alteration of expression of the resident normal gene, which would occur at low frequency, for example, by somatic recombination events as has been described for the retinoblastoma gene.[79] These early transgenic mice experiments demonstrate the power of the technique for addressing specific questions in tumor development and progression.

PROPERTIES OF ONCOGENES/PROTO-ONCOGENES AND THEIR PRODUCTS

GROWTH FACTORS

Growth factors provide the mitogenic signal mediated through their respective receptors that results in the proliferation and/or differentiation of cells.[205,206] In tissue culture, they must be supplied to stimulate proliferation of cell growth and are essential for the propagation of normal, nontransformed cells in culture.[207] However, transformed cells show partial or complete relaxation of requirements for growth factors. Factor dependence is also abrogated by infecting cells with specific acute transforming retroviruses.[208] Thus, viral oncogene products can override factor dependency by perhaps mimicking the action of ligands, their receptors,[209] or some intermediate in the ordered procession of events that follows mitogenic stimulation.

The first correlation of an oncogene with a growth factor was revealed by computer-assisted comparisons showing that the amino acid sequence of the v-sis oncogene was highly related to the beta chain of PDGF.[209-211] PDGF is an important serum mitogen required for mesenchymal cell growth in culture.[212] Connective tissue tumors such as sarcomas and glioblastomas express the c-sis proto-oncogene, whereas their counterparts in normal tissue do not.[212] Presumably, the sarcoma and glial tumor cells synthesize the mitogen to which they respond. Many oncogenes have been shown to be identical to, or related to, polypeptide growth factors. int-2, activated by MMTV proviral insertion in mouse mammary carcinomas,[213,214] the KS3 oncogene identified in gene transfer experiments in genomic DNA from a Kaposi's sarcoma,[63] and HST, a transforming gene identified in a human stomach cancer by DNA transfection[62,215] are all members of the basic or acidic fibroblast growth factor family.[216] The human KS3 and HST oncogenes are identical, but distinct from the closely related mouse int-2 gene. int-2 expression is most abundant in primitive mouse endodermal cells. Its low level of expression activated by proviral insertion in mouse mammary tumors may serve, in an autocrine fashion, to stimulate inappropriate cell proliferation. The fibroblast growth factors exhibit angiogenic properties and are related polypeptide mitogens[217] apparently recognizing different cell-type receptors.

Tumor cells often express transforming growth factors and two, referred to as TGF-α and TGF-β are expressed by rodent cells transformed with acute transforming retroviruses.[218] TGF-α binds to the EGF receptor, and TGF-β binds to a unique cell receptor.[219] TGF-α is normally synthesized only during embryogenesis.[220] It is believed that the transforming growth factors function in an autocrine fashion to stimulate cell proliferation.[221]

TYROSINE PROTEIN KINASES

The tyrosine protein kinases can be subdivided into at least three families. The first is the transmembrane protein tyrosine kinase family to which the growth factor receptors belong. In addition to being homologous in a tyrosine-specific protein kinase domain, these receptor-related molecules traverse the membrane once and have extracellular ligand-binding domains (see Fig. 4-7). It was early shown that the v-erbB oncogene product (see Table 4-1) is a truncated version of the EGF receptor.[222–224] More recently, the v-fms oncogene has been shown to be the activated form of the macrophage colony-stimulating factor receptor (CSF-1).[88] Other members of the tyrosine kinase growth factor receptor family are the ros,[225] kit,[111] met,[113] trk,[61] and neu[57,60] oncogenes (see Table 4-1 and Fig. 4-7). Both N-terminal and C-terminal rearrangements appear to activate the transforming potential of these transmembrane receptor tyrosine kinase family members. These alterations may remove down-modulating domains of the protein and result in the constitutive activation of what is normally a conditionally regulated enzyme activity.

The second family consists of a large number of nonintegral membrane-associated protein tyrosine kinases. The protein product of v-src, the prototype of this family, is associated with the plasma membrane but does not traverse the membrane. Other members of this family are fes, abl, fgr, and yes (see Table 4-1). All of these proto-oncogene products are homologous in the tyrosine kinase domains and each seems to have a myristylated N-terminal glycine residue.[226] The tyrosine kinase domain, as in the growth factor receptor

tyrosine kinase family, is responsible for catalyzing the transfer of phosphate groups from ATP to tyrosine residues during autophosphorylation or transphosphorylation of target molecules. Tyrosine phosphorylation may regulate cell shape with cell growth[227] but it is a rare activity in normal cells and accounts for only a fraction of total protein phosphorylation.[228] Several cellular cytoskeletal proteins are known to be targets of src protein tyrosine kinase phosphorylation. Thus, v-src transforming activity may result from unregulated tyrosine phosphorylation of target molecules present in certain cell lineages.[227] Similarly, although the c-abl proto-oncogene is expressed in many tissues, it only appears to transform cells of the hematopoietic lineage,[229] suggesting that a special target or substrate may be present in these cell lineages.

The members of this subfamily appear to be expressed at high levels and in specific cell types. Thus, the src proto-oncogene product is expressed at low levels in most vertebrate cells but at high levels in platelets and certain neural cell types.[230,231] A similar expression pattern for c-src also is observed in Drosophila where the highest levels are detected in the eye and brain.[232] These findings suggest that src is coupled to a signal transduction system from a cell surface receptor or ion channel specific for neurons.

The third and least understood members of this subtype of proto-oncogenes are the members of the serine kinase family. Certain domains of the proteins of the raf and mos (see Table 4-1) are somewhat homologous to those of src kinase family members, but there is evidence that the phosphorylation specificity of these members is for serine and threonine.[233,234] Curiously, no tyrosine kinase genes have been identified in yeast although many proteins with serine/threonine kinase have. Studies of cell division cycle mutants (cdc) have shown that the serine/threonine kinases are required for movement through the specific point in the yeast cell cycle.[235,236] Several other protein kinase genes have been identified in yeast and some of these genes have also been found in mammals.[237–239] Strikingly, one of the genes isolated from humans complements a mutation in the homologous gene from the yeast strain Schizosaccharomyces pombe indicating that its function is highly conserved during evolution.[237] The study of the serine/threonine kinases in yeast may provide a model for understanding how the serine/threonine kinase genes, such as mos and raf, function in mammalian cells. Recently, the mos gene has been shown to be expressed in male and female germ cells in vertebrates during postmeiotic cell maturation, suggesting that mos gene product may be involved in reductive division.[240–242]

THE RAS FAMILY OF ONCOGENES AND PROTO-ONCOGENES

The ras gene family members are found in human cancers more often than any other oncogene[54] and therefore are among the most intensively studied oncogenes. These investigations have focused primarily on understanding the normal proto-oncogene function and comparing it to the oncogene product activated by point mutations. Because the ras gene is highly conserved,[177] members of this family have been studied in mammals, chickens,[243] fruit flies (Drosophila *melanogaster*),[177] slime molds,[244] and yeast.[245,246] Even in yeast, *ras* is significantly (65%) homologous with the *ras* family members found in humans.

In the mammalian genome, three *ras* gene family members designated c-H-*ras*, c-K-*ras*, and N-*ras* have been characterized (see Table 4-1). The three proto-oncogenes all encode a protein of 21,000 daltons (p21)[247] and are very homologous in amino acid sequence differing primarily at their C termini. The *ras* protein has been shown to bind guanine nucleotides and to possess GTPase activity.[248,249] As with certain members of the *src* kinase family, p21 *ras* is associated with the cytoplasmic surface of the plasma membrane and is a nonintegral membrane-associated product.[250,251] The amino acid sequence of the *ras* gene product is somewhat homologous to α subunit of G proteins that are also involved in guanidine nucleotide binding and signal transduction.[252] The G proteins are effectors of adenylcyclase[253] and include stimulatory G_S and inhibitory G_I effectors. Members of the G protein family also include transducin, a regulator of retinal rod cyclic GMP, phosphodieserase,[254] and cytoskeletal proteins such as tubulin.[255] G proteins are functionally regulated by the binding of guanidine nucleotides after receiving signals from receptors. The regulatory effect is mediated in the GTP-bound state but is transient because of intrinsic G protein GTPase activity. The biochemical activities of p21 *ras* are similar to G proteins; p21 *ras* exists in an equilibrium between an active conformation with bound GTP and an inactive conformation when the GTP is hydrolyzed (Fig. 4-8). Presumably, a receptor-mediated signal results in exchange of GDP for GTP, converting p21 from an inactive to an active form[256,258] and allowing it to interact as an effector with target molecules (see Fig. 4-8).[50] A decrease in the GTPase activity observed in the activated *ras* oncogene product is believed to be responsible for its transforming activity.[259] Thus, the binding of GTP with the diminished capacity to hydrolyze it would maintain the protein in a constitutively active state, thus sending a continuous signal to the cell along the mitogenic pathway.

The mechanism by which the normal p21 product (expressed from the normal allele) and its intrinsic GTPase activity influence the signal transduction properties of the activated oncogene product is not yet understood.

The identification of *ras* genes in yeast has made it possible to study *ras* functions by classical and molecular genetics.[260,261] In *Saccharo-myces cerevisiae*, there are two *ras* genes that are 65% homologous in the N-terminal catalytic domains to mammalian p21 *ras*. [260] The *ras* genes in yeast are necessary for the survival of the organism. In experiments in which yeast *ras* genes were replaced with the human *ras* gene,[262] the yeast survived, demonstrating that the functional activity of *ras* in yeast has been conserved in evolution. In addition, the yeast *ras* gene mutated at the corresponding codon (along with certain other modifications), which activates the mammalian *ras* gene, transforms mouse NIH/3T3 cells.[245,260] These findings are the basis of the remarkable conclusion that the normal activity of p21 must be coupled to its transforming activity. Yeast *ras* genes also bind GTP and have an intrinsic GTPase activity[263,264]; however, in yeast the genes appear to regulate cyclic AMP levels through adenylcyclase,[265,266] and suppressor mutations that rescue *ras*-defective strains of yeast have been shown to map to components of the adenylcyclase pathway.[265,266] In contrast, the *ras* gene in other organisms does not appear to function through adenylcyclase[244,267] and in mammals and higher vertebrates it is probably involved in the second messenger pathways. Its function and its activity in these higher organisms are unknown.

NUCLEAR ONCOGENE/PROTO-ONCOGENE PROTEINS

The nuclear proteins encoded by proto-oncogenes and oncogenes are believed to be directly involved in the regulation of gene expression that leads to cell proliferation, division, and differentiation. Many of these nuclear proteins appear to be able to bind DNA; however, none are as homologous to each other as are the members of the *src* protein kinase or *ras*

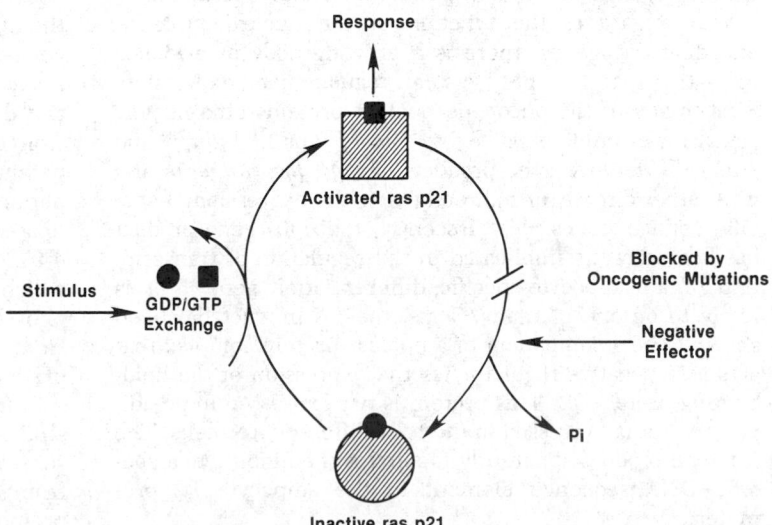

FIG. 4-8. Model for regulation of the *ras* p21 product. The alternating relaxed and activated states of the protein are shown. These are at least in part controlled by the rate of GTP hydrolysis by the intrinsic *ras* GTPase. GTP is diagrammatically represented as the filled small square and GDP as the filled small circle. The putative stimulus that positively regulates and an effector that negatively regulates the activity of p21 *ras* are shown.

gene families, although there are several *myc*-related genes (c-*myc*, N-*myc*, and L-*myc*).[268] Several have been shown to be participate in the same complementation group of the cooperative oncogene assay or have been shown to be transcriptionally activated by mitogenic stimulation (*e.g., myc, fos*, Fig. 4-3).[269] Thus, when quiescent serum-starved (growth-arrested) murine fibroblasts are stimulated with serum or growth factors, the cells immediately enter G_1, and there is a transient increase in the level of c-*myc* and c-*fos*. The induction varies from a peak at 30 minutes for c-*fos*[269-271] to 2 hours for c-*myc*[272] (see Fig. 4-3). p53 RNA expression is also stimulated, but at a much later time; it peaks 18 to 24 hours poststimulation.[273] The induction of the expression of these nuclear protein–encoding proto-oncogenes is observed with either PDGF or fetal calf serum,[271] but the cells only become competent for DNA replication. If PDGF is removed, the cells remain competent, and apparently the expression of a family of genes referred to as competence genes (which includes *fos* and *myc*) has already occurred.[274,275] EGF and insulin-like growth factors are required for cells to progress through G_1 and enter S phase[276] (see Fig. 4-3). These studies suggest that the transient expression of nuclear protein–encoding oncogenes is required for cells to traverse specific points in the cell cycle. The expression of *fos* and *myc* in this system greatly precedes the onset of DNA synthesis and probably is not directly involved in DNA replication. In the cooperative oncogene assay the early genes of DNA tumor viruses are in the same complementation group as *myc*. These early viral genes are not directly involved in viral DNA replication but rather are involved with the transactivation of other viral and host cell genes.

Expression of c-*myb* and c-*myc* decreases dramatically during terminal differentiation, indirect evidence that they play a role in cell proliferation.[277-280] It is also postulated that constitutive expression of c-*myc* prevents differentiation and promotes cell division.[281] Since the expression of these genes appears to occur at specific points in the cell cycle, their expression may either promote proliferation or promote differentiation by being specifically expressed, as shown for c-*fos* where expression is observed during promonocyte differentiation and macrophage proliferation.[282]

With regard to the function of the nuclear protein–encoding oncogenes, there is a growing body of evidence indicating that their products can regulate gene expression. First, many of the oncogene nuclear proteins bind nucleic acids (for example, *myc*,[282] *fos*,[284] *myb*,[285] p53,[194] *jun*,[286] and *erb*A).[287] Moreover, the products of *myc*, *fos*, *jun*, *erb*A and E1A either directly or indirectly alter the expression of specific cellular genes.[288,289] Recently, the c-*fos* gene product has been directly implicated in the regulation of transcription of an adipocyte-specific differentiation gene.[290] It is likely to be one of many. Thus, the *fos* product has been shown to be a component of a nuclear protein complex that acts as a negative regulator for the expression of the lipid-binding protein P2. This protein is not expressed in preadipocytes but is expressed in the fully differentiated cells. The *fos* gene product apparently facilitates the binding to a specific DNA sequence element in the adipocyte P2 promoter.[290]

Perhaps the most dramatic evidence demonstrating the role of nuclear protein–encoding oncogenes as trans-acting factors comes from the studies of the v-*jun* oncogene.[291] DNA sequence analysis revealed that the C terminus of the v-*jun* protein was homologous to the C terminus of the transcriptional activator protein GCN4 from yeast *Saccharomyces cerevisiae*.[292] Furthermore, a chimeric GCN4 gene sequence containing the DNA-binding domain of v-*jun* rescued yeast strains that lacked the GCN4 gene (*null mutations*).[286] The consensus DNA-binding sequence for the yeast GCN4 gene is the same as the mammalian transcription factor AP1. This led to the demonstration that the v-*jun* oncogene clearly is the viral homolog of the normal AP1 transcription factor gene.[293] The AP1 product interacts not only with phorbol ester-inducible promoter elements, but with the enhancer elements found in many viral and cellular transcription control sequences. This finding suggests that the unregulated or ectopic expression of a normal transcription regulator protein contributes to tumor development. Moreover, and most importantly, researchers should be able to identify genes regulated by AP1 or c-*jun* that directly affect growth and expression of a neoplastic phenotype.

A different role has been proposed for the nuclear protein oncogene v-*erb*A, which was first shown to be related to a receptor for steroid hormones[294] and was subsequently identified as a nuclear receptor for thyroid hormones, triiodothyronine, and thyroxin.[295,296] v-*erb*A by itself does not appear to express transforming potential, but its presence potentiates the transforming potential of v-*erb*B by specifically interrupting differentiation of erythryoblasts.[297] The thyroid hormone receptor T3 is known to both positively and negatively regulate the expression of many genes.[298] v-*erb*A arrests expression of genes that play an important role in erythroid differentiation, the anion transporter,[299] and δ aminolevulinic (Ala S),[300] a key enzyme in hemin synthesis. Because of mutations in the v-*erb*A gene, it does not bind T3 or T4 and is therefore ligand independent. As with other nuclear protein–encoding oncogenes, its product probably acts constitutively to either up- or down-regulate expression of target genes, apparently interrupting the regulation of genes that are essential for erythroblast differentiation.

Beginning with mitogenic growth factors and ending with the nuclear proteins encoded by oncogenes and proto-oncogenes, we have described a component of pathways that are involved in the control and regulation of cell proliferation and differentiation and that have been identified primarily from the study of oncogenes. There are, however, additional pathways, the so-called second messages, that are also important in signal transduction. One example is the phospholipase C-mediated cleavage of phosphoinositol[301] (see Fig. 4-9). In this pathway diacylglycerol (DAG) is generated, which activates C kinase and mediates production of phosphorylated inositols.[301] The latter mobilizes calcium stores from the endoplasmic reticulum, increases the cytoplasm pH, and stimulates calcium-dependent protein kinase, resulting in the phosphorylation of specific protein substrates.[302] Protein C kinase also phosphorylates numerous substrates and its implication in mitogenic response stems from its activity as a receptor for phorbol ester tumor promoters.[302]

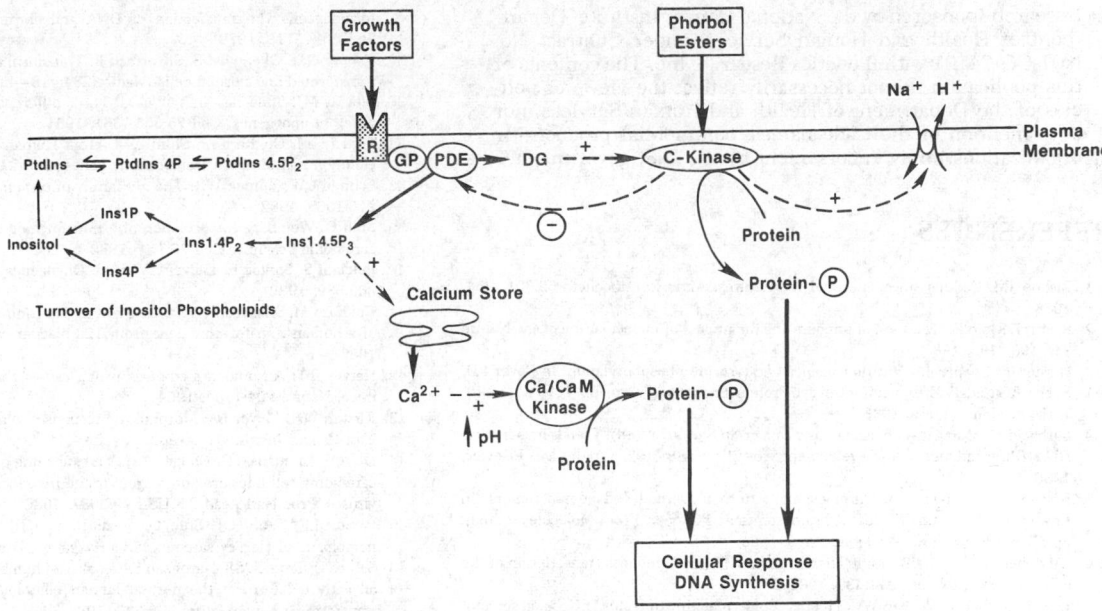

FIG. 4-9. Role of diacylglycerol (DG) and inositol lipid hydrolysis in the control of DNA synthesis. Some growth factors acting on specific receptors (R) uses a GTP-binding protein (GP) to stimulate a phosphodiesterase (PDE) which cleaves phosphatidylinositol (4,5-bi-phosphate) (Ptd Ins 4,5P$_2$) to diacylglycerol (DG) and inositol 1,4,5-triphosphate (Ins 1,45P$_3$). Diacylglycerol has several functions, including the stimulation of the same c-kinase that can be activated by phorbol esters with the subsequent activation of an Na$^+$-H$^+$ exchanger. Ins 1,4,5P$_3$ acts to mobilize intracellular calcium, which results in stimulation of a calmodulin kinase (CaM).
#cf

FUTURE CONSIDERATIONS

Much of our understanding of proto-oncogene function will come from studies using classic and molecular genetics in organisms such as yeast and *Drosophila* since they are well-characterized genetically and can be easily manipulated. However, clearly the new emerging technology for performing studies in molecular genetics directly in higher mammals has enormous promise, as is already evidence for mouse transgenic technology. There is currently a great effort to generate techniques that will produce null mutations in genes of higher organisms,[303,304] which will open new vistas for experimentation.

Numerous techniques already exist in molecular biology to alter the structure of gene products and to express the gene products at very high levels, first in prokaryotic vector systems and more recently in insect and higher eukaryotes, using mammalian viral vector systems. With these techniques, oncogene protein structure and biochemical function can be studied and the three-dimensional structure determined. These studies are the basis for both elucidating the interaction of the protein with its substrate and designing drugs that can perhaps specifically target the activated oncogene product. The three-dimensional protein crystal structure for the *ras* oncogene has recently been described[305] and there is a great effort to determine the three-dimensional structure of other proto-oncogenes products.

We have not described the class of molecules that are referred to as suppressor genes or antioncogenes.[306] The genetic evidence is compelling that such genes exist, but at present it is not understood how these genes function.

Clinical applications of this new information and technology are beginning to emerge. New diagnostic techniques such as the polymerase chain reaction (see Chap. 2) will provide new methods for determining genetic alterations and identifying mutations. For example, with the polymerase chain reaction, which is already automated, it has been possible to identify the breakpoints in the DNA in follicular lymphomas.[307,308] The sensitivity of this technique will allow the detection of one lymphoma cell in the presence of a million normal cells. The procedure is superb for identifying subclinical presence of leukemia cells in patients and for determining the effectiveness of protocols designed to purge malignant cells from bone marrow. It also enables researchers to rapidly sequence chromosomal breakpoints at the DNA level.[308] It will markedly improve the detection of minimal residual disease and improve the ability to assess the stage of cancer in patients and evaluate therapy. We can expect that this is just one of many of the innovations that will have profound impact on the practice of medicine. History demonstrates that improved diagnostic procedures ultimately result in improved therapies. The ability to identify oncogenes associated with a specific tumor type should provide a remarkable way to diagnose disease and improve treatment.[309]

Research sponsored by the National Cancer Institute, Department of Health and Human Services, under Contract No. N01-CO-74101 with Bionetics Research, Inc. The contents of this publication do not necessarily reflect the views or policies of the Department of Health and Human Services, nor does mention of the trade names, commercial products, or organizations imply endorsement by the U.S. government.

REFERENCES

1. Bishop JM: Cellular oncogenes and retroviruses. Annu Rev Biochem 52:301–354, 1983

2. Klein G, Klein E: Evolution of tumours and the impact of molecular oncology. Nature 315:190–195, 1985

3. Hunter T, Cooper JA: Viral oncogenes and tyrosine phosphorylation. In Boyer PD, Krebs EG (eds): Enzyme Control by Protein Phosphorylation, pp 191–246. New York, Academic Press, 1986

4. Barbacid M: Mutagens, oncogenes and cancer. In Stewart A (ed): Trends in Genetics: DNA Differentiation and Development, vol 2, pp 188–192. Cambridge, Elsevier, 1986

5. Rowley JD: Introduction: Chromosome pattern in animal and human tumors. In Rowley JD, Ultmann JE (eds): Chromosomes and Cancer: From Molecules to Man, pp 57–60. New York, Academic Press, 1983

6. Greenberg ME, Ziff EB: Stimulation of mouse 3T3 cells induces transcription of the c-fos oncogene. Nature 311:433, 1984

7. Leof EB, Wharton W, Van Wyk JJ, et al: Epidermal growth factor (EGF) and somatomedin C regulate G1 progression in competent BALB/c-3T3 cells. Exp Cell Res 141:107, 1982

8. Temin HM: On the origin of genes for neoplasia: G.H.A. Clowes Memorial Lecture. Cancer Res 34:2835, 1974

9. Cairns J: Mutation selection and the natural history of cancer. Nature 255:197, 1975

10. Cairns J: The origin of human cancers. Nature 289:353, 1981

11. Klein G: The role of gene dosage and genetic transpositions in carcinogenesis. Nature 294:313, 1981

12. Rous P: A sarcoma of the fowl transmissible by an agent separable from the tumor cells. J Exp Med 13:397, 1911

13. Gross L: Oncogenic Viruses. New York, Pergamon Press, 1970

14. Temin HM: Origin of retroviruses from cellular moveable genetic elements. Cell 21:599, 1980

15. Temin HM: Structure, variation and synthesis of retrovirus long terminal repeat. Cell 27:1, 1981

16. Weiss R, Teich N, Varmus H, et al: RNA Tumor Viruses. Cold Spring Harbor, NY, Cold Spring Harbor Laboratory, 1982

17. McClintock B: Chromosome organization and genic expression. Cold Spring Harbor Symp Quant Biol 16:13–47, 1952

18. Campbell A: Some general questions about movable elements and their implications. Cold Spring Harbor Symp Quant Biol 45:1–9, 1981

19. Hayward WS, Neel BG, Astrin SM: Activation of a cellular onc gene by promoter insertion in ALV-induced lymphoid leukosis. Nature 290:475–479, 1982

20. Blair DG, Oskarsson M, Wood TG, et al: Activation of the transforming potential of a normal cell sequence: A molecular model for oncogenesis. Science 212:941–943, 1981

21. Wood TG, McGeady ML, Blair DG, et al: Long terminal repeat enhancement of v-mos transforming activity: Identification of essential regions. J Virol 46:726–736, 1983

22. Payne GS, Bishop JM, Varmus HE: Multiple arrangements of viral DNA and an activated host oncogene in bursal lymphomas. Nature 295:209–214, 1982

23. Tooze J: Molecular biology of tumor viruses. In DNA tumor viruses, 3rd ed. Cold Spring Harbor, NY, Cold Spring Harbor Laboratory, 1980

24. Berk AJ, Lee F, Harrison T, et al: A pre-early adenovirus 5 gene product regulates synthesis of early viral messenger RNAs. Cell 17:935, 1979

25. Jones N, Shenk T: An adenovirus type 5 early gene function regulates expression of other early viral genes. Proc Natl Acad Sci USA 76:3665, 1979

26. Rigby PWJ, Lane DP: Structure and function of simian virus 40 large T-antigen. In Klein G (ed): Viral Oncology, vol 3, pp 31–57. New York, Raven Press, 1983

27. Green MR, Treisman R, Maniatis T: Transcriptional activation of cloned human B-globin genes by viral immediate-early gene products. Cell 35:137, 1983

28. Hill M, Hillova J: Virus recovery in chicken cells tested with Rous sarcoma cell DNA. Nature 237:35, 1972

29. Graham FL, Van Der Eb AJ: A new technique for the assay of infectivity of human adenovirus 5DNA. Virology 52:456, 1973

30. Weinberg RA: Use of transfection to analyze genetic information and malignant transformation. Biochem Biophys Acta 651:25, 1981

31. Cooper GM, Okenquist S, Silverman L: Transforming activity of DNA of chemically transformed and normal cells. Nature 284:418, 1980

32. Blair DG, Cooper CS, Oskarsson MK, et al: New method for detecting cellular transforming genes. Science 218:1122, 1982

33. Fasano O, Birnbaum D, Edlund L, et al: New human transforming genes detected by a tumorigenicity assay. Mol Cell Biol 4:1695, 1984

34. Shih C, Shilo BZ, Goldfarb MP, et al: Passage of phenotypes of chemically transformed cells via transfection of DNA and chromatin. Proc Natl Acad Sci USA 76:5714–5718, 1979

35. Cooper GM, Okenquist S, Silverman L: Transforming activity of DNA of chemically transformed and normal cells. Nature 284:418–421, 1980

36. Murray MJ, Shilo BZ, Shih C, et al: Three different human tumor cell lines contain different oncogenes. Cell 25:355–361, 1981

37. Perucho M, Goldfarb M, Shimizu K, et al: Human tumor-derived cell lines contain common and different transforming genes. Cell 27:467–476, 1981

38. Schmid CW, Jelinek WR: The alu family of dispersed repetitive sequences. Science 216:1065, 1982

39. Shih C, Weinberg RA: Isolation of a transforming sequence from a human bladder carcinoma cell line. Cell 29:161, 1982

40. Pulciani S, Santos E, Lauver AV, et al: Oncogenes in solid human tumours. Nature 300:539, 1982

41. Goldfarb M, Shimizu K, Perucho M, et al: Isolation and preliminary characterization of a human transforming gene from T24 bladder carcinoma cells. Nature 296:404, 1982

42. Harvey TT: An unidentified virus which causes the rapid production of tumors in mice. Nature 204:1104, 1964

43. Kirsten WH, Meyer LA: Morphologic responses to a murine erythroblastosis virus. J Natl Cancer Inst 39:311, 1967

44. Der CJ, Krontiris TG, Cooper GM: Transforming genes of human bladder and lung carcinoma cell lines are homologous to the ras genes of Harvey and Kirsten sarcoma viruses. Proc Natl Acad Sci USA 79:3637, 1982

45. Parada LF, Tabin CJ, Shih C, et al: Human EJ bladder carcinoma oncogene is homologue of Harvey sarcoma virus ras gene. Nature 297:474, 1982

46. Santos E, Tronick SR, Aaronson SA, et al: T24 human bladder carcinoma oncogene is an activated form of the normal human homologue of BALB- and Harvey -MSV transforming gene. Nature 298:343, 1982

47. Perucho M, Goldfarb M, Shimizu K, et al: Human tumor–derived cell lines contain common and different transforming genes. Cell 27:467, 1981

48. Murray MJ, Shilo B-Z, Shih C, et al: Three different human tumor cell lines contain different oncogenes. Cell 25:355, 1981

49. Hall A, Marshall CJ, Spurr NK, et al: Identification of the transforming gene in two human sarcoma cell lines as a new member of the ras gene family located on chromosome 1. Nature 303:396, 1983

50. Murray MJ, Cunningham JM, Parada LF, et al: The HL-60 transforming sequence: A ras oncogene coexisting with altered myc genes in hematopoietic tumors. Cell 33:749, 1983

51. Shimizu K, Birnbaum D, Ruley MA, et al: Structure of the Ki-ras gene of the human lung carcinoma cell line Calu-1. Nature 304:497, 1983

52. Marshall C: Human oncogenes. In Weiss R, Teich N, Varmus H et al (eds): RNA Tumor Viruses, 2nd ed, pp 487–565. Cold Spring Harbor, NY, Cold Spring Harbor Laboratory, 1984

53. Varmus HE: The molecular genetics of cellular oncogenes. Annu Rev Genet 18:553, 1984

54. Barbacid M: ras genes. Annu Rev Biochem 56:779, 1987

55. Forrester K, Almoguera C, Han K, et al: Detection of high incidence of K-ras oncogenes during human colon tumorigenesis. Nature 327:298, 1987

56. Bos JL, Fearon ER, Hamilton SR, et al: Prevalence of ras gene mutations in human colorectal cancers. Nature 327:293, 1987

57. Bargmann CI, Hung M-C, Weinberg RA: Multiple independent activations of the neu oncogene by a point mutation altering the transmembrane domain of p185. Cell 45:649, 1986

58. Yamamoto T, Ikawa S, Akiyama T: Similarity of protein encoded by the human c-erb-B-2 gene to epidermal growth factor receptor. Nature 319:230, 1986

59. Coussens L, Yang-Feng TL, Liao Y, et al: Tyrosine kinase receptor with extensive homology to EGF receptor shares chromosomal location with neu oncogene. Science 230:1132, 1985

60. Cooper CS, Park M, Blair DG, et al: Molecular cloning of a new transforming gene from a chemically transformed human cell line. Nature 311:29, 1984

61. Martin-Zanca D, Hughes SH, Barbacid M: A human oncogene formed by the fusion of truncated tropomyosin and protein tyrosine kinase sequences. Nature 319:743, 1986

62. Yoshida T, Miyagawa K, Odagiri H, et al: Genomic sequence of hst, a transforming gene encoding a protein homologous to fibroblast growth factors and the int-2-encoded protein. Proc Natl Acad Sci USA 84:7305, 1987

63. Bovi PD, Curatola AM, Kern FG: An oncogene isolated by transfection of Kaposi's sarcoma DNA encodes a growth factor that is a member of the FGF family. Cell 50:729, 1987

64. Yunis JJ: The chromosomal basis of human neoplasia. Science 221:227–236, 1983

65. Klein G: The role of gene dosage and genetic transpositions in carcinogenesis. Nature 294:313–318, 1981

66. Klein G: Specific chromosomal translocations and the genesis of B-cell-derived tumors in mice and men. Cell 32:311–315, 1983

67. Rowley J: Human oncogene locations and chromosome aberrations. Nature 301:290–291, 1983

68. Yunis JJ, Soreng AL, Bowe AE: Fragile sites are targets of diverse mutagens and carcinogens. Oncogene 1:59, 1987

69. Mitelman F: Catalogue of Chromosome Aberrations in Cancer, 2nd ed. New York, Alan R. Liss, 1985

70. Rowley JD, Testa JR: Chromosome abnormalities in malignant hematologic diseases. Adv Cancer Res 36:103, 1982

71. Croce CM, Nowell PC: Molecular basis of human B cell neoplasia. Blood 65:1, 1985

72. Heisterkamp N, Stephenson JR, Groffen J, et al: Localization of the c-abl oncogene adjacent to a translocation break point in chronic myelocytic leukemia. Nature 306:239, 1983

73. Tsujimoto Y, Jorge Y, Onorato-Showe L, et al: Molecular cloning of the chromosomal breakpoint of B-cell lymphomas and leukemias with the t(11;14) chromosome translocation. Science 224:1403, 1984

74. Tsujimoto Y, Finger LR, Yunis J, et al: Cloning of the chromosome breakpoint of neoplastic B cells with the t(14;18) chromosome translocation. Science 226:1097, 1984

75. Kohl NE, Kanda N, Schreck RR, et al: Transposition and amplification of oncogene-related sequences in human neuroblastomas. Cell 35:359–367, 1983

76. Schwab M, Alitalo K, Klempnauer K-H, et al: Amplified DNA with limited homology to myc cellular oncogene is shared by human neuroblastoma cell lines and a neuroblastoma tumor. Nature 305:245–248, 1983

77. Vogel F: Genetics of retinoblastoma. Hum Genet 52:1, 1979

78. Benedict WF, Murphree AL, Banerjee A, et al: Patient with 13 chromosome deletion: Evidence that the retinoblastoma gene is a recessive cancer gene. Science 219:973, 1983

79. Cavenee WK, Dryja TP, Phillips RA, et al: Expression of recessive alleles by chromosomal mechanisms in retinoblastoma. Nature 305:779, 1983

80. Sparkes RS: Cytogenetics of retinoblastoma. Cancer Surv 3:479, 1984

81. Van-Heyningen V, Boyd PA, Searwright A, et al: Molecular analysis of chromosome 11 deletions in aniridia-Wilms' tumor syndrome. Proc Natl Acad Sci USA 82:8592, 1985

82. Friend SH, Bernards R, Rogel S, et al: A human DNA segment with properties of the gene that predisposes to retinoblastoma and osteosarcoma. Nature 323:643, 1986

83. Lee W-H, Bookstein R, Hong F, et al: Human susceptibility gene: Cloning, identification and sequence. Science 235:1394, 1987

84. Waterfield MD, Scaqrce GT, Whittle N, et al: Platelet-derived growth factor is structurally related to the putative transforming protein p28^sis of simian sarcoma virus. Nature 304:35–39, 1983

85. Doolittle RF, Hunkapiller MW, Hood LE, et al: Simian sarcoma virus onc gene, v-sis, is derived from the gene (or genes) encoding a platelet-derived growth factor. Science 221:275–277, 1983

86. Downward J, Yarden Y, Mayes E, et al: Close similarity of epidermal growth factor receptor and v-erb-B oncogene protein sequences. Nature 307:521–527, 1984

87. Peters G, Brookes S, Smith R, et al: Tumorigenesis by mouse mammary tumor virus: Evidence for a common region for provirus integration in mammary tumors. Cell 33:369, 1983

88. Sherr CJ, Rettenmier CW, Sacca R, et al: The c-fms proto-oncogene product is related to the receptor for the mononuclear phagocyte growth factor, CSF-1. Cell 41:665, 1985

89. Sap J, Munoz A, Damm K, et al: The v-erbA protein is a high affinity receptor for thyroid hormone. Nature 324:635, 1986

90. Weinberger C, Thompson C, Ong E, et al: The C-v-erbA gene encodes a thyroid hormone receptor. Nature 324:641, 1986

91. Bishop JM: The molecular genetics of cancer. Science 235:305–311, 1987

92. Coffin JM, Tsichlis PN, Barker CS, et al: Variation in avian retrovirus genomes. Ann NY Acad Sci 354:410, 1980

93. Curran T, Miller Ad, Zokas L, et al: Viral and cellular fos proteins: A comparative analysis. Cell 36:259, 1984

94. Meijlink F, Curran T, Miller AD, et al: Removal of a 67-base-pair sequence in the noncoding region of proto-oncogene fos converts it to a transforming gene. Proc Natl Acad Sci USA 82:4987, 1985

95. Bishop JM: Cellular oncogenes and retroviruses. Annu Rev Biochem 52:301, 1983

96. Levinson AD: Normal and activated ras oncogenes and their encoded products. Trends Genet 2:81, 1986

97. Prywes R, Foulkes JG, Rosenberg N, et al: Sequences of the A-MuLV protein needed for fibroblast and lymphoid cell transformation. Cell 34:569, 1983

98. Takeya T, Hanafusa H: Structure and sequence of the cellular gene homologous to the RSV src gene and the mechanism for generating the transforming virus. Cell 32:881, 1983

99. Hunter T, Cooper JA: Epidermal growth factor induces rapid tyrosine phosphorylation of proteins in A431 human tumor cells. Cell 24:741, 1981

100. Courtneidge SA: Activation of the pp60c-src kinase by middle T antigen binding or by dephosphorylation. EMBO J 4:1471, 1985

101. Cooper JA, Gould KL, Cartwright CA, et al: Tyr527 is phosphorylated in pp60c-src: Implications for regulation. Science 231:1431, 1986

102. Cooper JA, King CS: Dephosphorylation or antibody binding to the carboxy terminus stimulates pp60c-src. Mol Cell Biol 6:4467, 1986

103. Kawakami T, Pennington CY, Robbins KC: Isolation and oncogenic potential of a novel src-like gene. Mol Cell Biol 6:4195, 1986

104. Sukegawa J, Semba K, Yamanashi Y, et al: Characterization of cDNA clones for the human c-yes gene. Mol Cell Biol 7:41, 1987

105. Browning PJ, Bunn HF, Cline A, et al: "Replacement" of COOH-terminal truncation of v-fms with c-fms sequences markedly reduces transformation potential. Proc Natl Acad Sci USA 83:7800, 1986

106. Coussens L, Van Beveren C, Smith D, et al: Structural alteration of viral homologue of receptor proto-oncogene fms at carboxyl terminus. Nature 320:277, 1986

107. Downward J, Yarden Y, Mayes E, et al: Close similarity of epidermal growth factor receptor and v-erb-B oncogene protein sequences. Nature 307:521, 1984

108. Downward J, Parker P, Waterfield MD: Autophosphorylation sites on the epidermal growth factor receptor. Nature 311:483, 1984

109. Schlessinger J: Allosteric regulation of the epidermal growth factor receptor kinase. J Cell Biol 103:2067, 1986

110. Gould KL, Woodgett JR, Cooper JA, et al: Protein kinase C phosphorylates pp60c-src at a novel site. Cell 42:849, 1985

111. Yarden Y, Kuang WJ, Yang-Feng T, et al: Human proto-oncogene c-kit: A new cell surface receptor tyrosine kinase for an unidentified ligand. EMBO J 6:3341, 1987

112. Park M, Dean M, Cooper CS, et al: Mechanism of met oncogene activation. Cell 45:895, 1986

113. Park M, Dean M, Kaul K, et al: Sequence of met proto-oncogene cDNA has features characteristic of the tyrosine kinase family of growth factor receptors. Proc Natl Acad Sci USA, 84:6379, 1987

114. Hayward WS, Neel BG, Astrin SM: Activation of the cellular onc gene by promoter insertion in ALV-induced lymphoid leukosis. Nature 290:475, 1981

115. Payne GS, Bishop JM, Varmus HE: Multiple arrangements of viral DNA and an activated hos oncogene in bursal lymphomas. Nature 295:209, 1982

116. Nilsen TW, Maroney PA, Goodwin RG, et al: c-erbB activation in ALV-induced erythroblastosis: Novel RNA processing and promoter insertion result in expression of an amino-truncated EGF receptor. Cell 41:719, 1985

117. Klempnauer K-H, Ramsay G, Bishop JM: The product of the retroviral transforming gene v-myb is a truncated version of the protein encoded by the cellular oncogene c-myb. Cell 33:345, 1983

118. Nusse R, Varmus HE: Many tumors induced by the mouse mammary tumor virus contain a provirus integrated in the same region of the host genome. Cell 31:99, 1982

119. Peters G, Lee AE, Dickson C: Concerted activation of two potential proto-oncogenes in carcinomas induced by mouse mammary tumor virus. Nature 320:628, 1986

120. Jakobovits A, Shackleford GM, Varmus HE, et al: Two proto-oncogenes implicated in mammary carcinogenesis, int-1 and int-2, are independently regulated during mouse development. Proc Natl Acad Sci USA 83:7806, 1986

121. Wilkinson DG, Bailes JA, McMahon AP: Expression of the proto-oncogene int-1 is restricted to specific neural cells in the developing mouse embryo. Cell 50:79, 1987

122. Metcalf D, Begley CG, Nicola NA, et al: Quantitative responsiveness of murine hemopoietic population in vitro and in vivo to recombinant multi-CSF (IL-3). Exp Hematol 15:288, 1987

123. Hapel AJ, Vande Woude GF, Campbell HD, et al: Generation of an autocrine leukemia using a retroviral expression vector carrying the interleukin-3 gene. Lymphokine Res 5:249, 1986

124. Chen SJ, Holbrook NJ, Mitchell KF, et al: A viral long terminal repeat in the interleukin 2 gene of a cell line that constitutively produces interleukin 2. Proc Natl Acad Sci USA 82:7284, 1985

125. Ymer S, Tucker QJ, Sanderson CJ, et al: Constitutive synthesis of interleukin-3 by leukaemia cell line WEH1-3B is due to retroviral insertion near the gene. Nature 317:255, 1985

126. Klein G, Klein E: Myc/Ig juxtaposition by chromosomal translocations: some new insights, puzzles and paradoxes. Immunol Today 6:208–215, 1985

127. Neel BG, Jhanwar SC, Chaganti RSK, et al: Two human c-onc genes are located on the long arm of chromosome 8. Proc Natl Acad Sci USA 79:7842, 1982

128. Dalla-Favera R, Franchini G, Martinotti S, et al: Chromosomal assignment of the human homologues of feline sarcoma virus and avian myeloblastosis virus onc genes. Proc Natl Acad Sci USA 79:4714, 1982

129. Kirsch IR, Morton CC, Nakahara K, et al: Human immunoglobulin heavy chain genes map to a region of translocations in malignant B lymphocytes. Science 216:301, 1982

130. Erikson J, Martins J, Croce CM: Assignment of the genes for human K immunoglobulin chains to chromosome 22. Nature 294:173, 1981

131. Erikson J, Nishikura K, Ar-Rushdi A, et al: Translocation of an immunoglobulin J locus to a region 3' of an unrearranged c-myc oncogene enhances c-myc transcription. Proc Natl Acad Sci USA 80:7581, 1983

132. McBride OW, Hieter PA, Hollis GF, et al: Chromosomal location of human kappa and lambda immunoglobulin light chain constant region genes. J Exp Med 155:1480, 1982

133. De La Chapelle A, Lenoir G, Boué J, et al: Lambda Ig constant region genes are translocated to chromosome 8 in Burkitt's lymphoma with t(8;22). Nucleic Acids Res 11:1133, 1983

134. Croce CM, Nowell PC: Molecular basis of human B cell neoplasia. Blood 65:1, 1985

135. Piechaczyk M, Yang J-Q, Blanchard J-M, et al: Posttranscriptional mechanisms are responsible for accumulation of truncated c-myc RNAs in murine plasma cell tumors. Cell 42:589, 1985

136. Rabbitts PH, Watson JV, Lamond A, et al: Metabolism of c-myc gene products: c-myc mRNA and protein expression in the cell cycle. EMBO J 4:2009, 1985

137. Remmers EF, Yang J-Q, Marcu KB: A negative transcriptional control element located upstream of the murine c-myc gene. EMBO J 5:899, 1986

138. Cesarman E, Dalla-Favera R, Bentley D, et al: Mutations in the first exon are associated with altered transcription of c-myc in Burkitt lymphoma. Science 238:1272, 1987

139. Leder P, Battey J, Lenoir G, et al: Translocations among antibody genes in human cancer. Science 222:765, 1983

140. Taub R, Moulding C, Battey J, et al: Activation and somatic mutation of the translocated c-myc gene in Burkitt lymphoma cells. Cell 36:339, 1984

141. Croce CM, Thierfelder W, Erickson J, et al: Transcriptional activation of an unrearranged and untranslocated c-*myc* oncogene by translocation of a C K locus in Burkitt lymphoma cells. Proc Natl Acad Sci USA 80:6922, 1983

142. Heisterkamp N, Groffen J, Stephenson JR, et al: Chromosomal localization of human cellular homologues of two viral oncogenes. Nature 299:747, 1982

143. De Klein A, Van Kessel AG, Grosveld G, et al: A cellular oncogene is translocated to the Philadelphia chromosome in chronic myelocytic leukaemia. Nature 300:765, 1982

144. Groffen J, Stephenson JR, Heisterkamp N, et al: Philadelphia chromosomal breakpoints are clustered within a limited region, *bcr*, on chromosome 22. Cell 36:93, 1984

145. Canaani E, Steiner-Saltz D, Aghai E, et al: Altered transcription of an oncogene in chronic myeloid leukaemia. Lancet 1:593, 1984

146. Collins SJ, Kubonishi I, Miyoshi I, et al: Altered transcription of the c-*abl* oncogene in K-562 and other chronic myelogenous leukemia cells. Science 225:72, 1984

147. Konopka, JB, Watanabe SM, Witte ON: An alteration of the human c-*abl* protein in K562 leukemia cells unmasks associated tyrosine kinase activity. Cell 37:1035, 1984

148. Witte ON: Functions of the *abl* oncogene. Cancer Surv 5:183, 1986

149. Konopka JB, Witte ON: Detection of c-*abl* tyrosine kinase activity *in vitro* permits direct comparison of normal and altered *abl* gene products. Mol Cell Biol 5:3116, 1985

150. Pierce JH, Di Fiore PP, Aaronson SA, et al: Neoplastic transformation of mast cells by Abelson-MuLV: Abrogation of IL-3 dependence by a nonautocrine mechanism. Cell 41:685, 1985

151. Alitalo K, Schwab M, Lin CC, et al: Homogeneously staining chromosomal regions contain amplified copies of an abundantly expressed cellular oncogene (c-*myc*) in malignant neuroendocrine cells from a human colon carcinoma. Proc Natl Acad Sci USA 80:1707, 1983

152. Schwab M, Alitalo K, Klempnauer K-H, et al: Amplified DNA with limited homology to *myc* cellular oncogene is shared by human neuroblastoma cell lines and a neuroblastoma tumour. Nature 305:245, 1983

153. Schimke RT: Gene amplification in cultured animal cells. Cell 37:705, 1984

154. Shilo Y, Shipley J, Brodeur GM, et al: Differential amplification, assembly, and relocation of multiple DNA sequences in human neuroblastomas and neuroblastoma cell lines. Proc Natl Acad Sci USA 82:3761, 1985

155. Collins S, Groudine M: Amplification of endogenous *myc*-related DNA sequences in a human myeloid leukaemia cell line. Nature 298:679, 1982

156. Dalla Favera R, Wong-Staal F, Gallo RC: *onc* gene amplification in promyelocytic leukaemia cell line HL-60 and primary leukaemic cells of the same patient. Nature 299:61, 1982

157. Schwab M, Varmus HE, Bishop JM: Chromosome localization in normal cells and neuroblastomas of a gene related to c-*myc*. Nature 308:288, 1984

158. Brodeur GM, Seeger RC, Schwab M, et al: Amplification of N-*myc* in untreated human neuroblastomas correlates with advanced disease stage. Science 224:1121, 1984

159. Little CD, Nau MM, Carney DN, et al: Amplification and expression of the c-*myc* oncogene in human lung cell lines. Nature 306:194, 1983

160. Libermann TA, Nusbaum HR, Razon N, et al: Amplification, enhanced expression and possible rearrangement of EGF receptor gene in primary human brain tumours of glial origin. Nature 313:144, 1985

161. Yamamoto T, Kamat N, Kawano H, et al: High incidence of amplification of the epidermal growth factor receptor gene in human squamous carcinoma cell lines. Cancer Res 46:414, 1986

162. Yokota J, Terada M, Toyoshima K, et al: Amplification of the c-*erb*B-2 oncogene in human adenocarcinomas *in vitro*. Lancet 1:765, 1986

163. Zhou D, Battifora H, Yokota J, et al: Association of multiple copies of the c-*erb*B-2 oncogene with spread of breast cancer. Cancer Res 47:6123, 1987

164. King CR, Kraus MH, Aaronson SA: Amplification of a novel v-*erb*B-related gene in a human mammary carcinoma. Science 229:974, 1985

165. Hudziak RM, Schlessinger J, Ullrich A: Increased expression of the putative growth factor receptor p185 HER2 causes transformation and tumorigenesis of NIH 3T3 cells. Proc Natl Acad Sci USA 84:7159, 1987

166. Di Fiore PP, Pierce JH, Kraus MH, et al: *erb*B-2 is a potent oncogene when overexpressed in NIH/3T3 cells. Science 237:178, 1987

167. Reddy EP, Smith MJ, Srinivasan A: Nucleotide sequence of Abelson murine leukemia virus genome: Structural similarity of its transforming gene product to other *onc* gene products with tyrosine-specific kinase activity. Proc Natl Acad Sci USA 80:3623, 1983

168. Tabin CJ, Bradley SM, Bargmann CI, et al: Mechanism of action of a human oncogene. Nature 300:143, 1982

169. Taparowsky E, Shimizu K, Goldfarb M, et al: Structure and activation of the human N-*ras* gene. Cell 34:581, 1983

170. Shih TY, Weeks MO: Oncogenes and cancer: p21 *ras* genes. Cancer Invest 2:109, 1984

171. Eadie JS, Conrad M, Toorchen D, et al: Mechanism of mutagenesis by 06-methylguanine. Nature 308:201, 1984

172. Loechler EL, Green CL, Essignmann JM: In vivo mutagenesis by 06-methylguanine built into a unique site in a viral genome. Proc Natl Acad Sci USA 81:6271, 1984

173. Balmain A, Pragnell IB: Mouse skin carcinomas induced in vivo by chemical carcinogens have a transforming Harvey-*ras* oncogene. Nature 303:72, 1983

174. Sukumar S, Notario V, Martin-Zanca D, et al: Induction of mammary carcinomas in rats by nitroso-methylurea involves malignant activation of H-*ras*-1 locus by single point mutations. Nature 306:658, 1983

175. Zarbl H, Sukumar S, Arthur AV, et al: Direct mutagenesis of Ha-*ras*-1 oncogenes by N-nitroso-N-methylurea during initiation of mammary carcinogenesis in rats. Nature 315:382, 1985

176. Vousden KH, Marshall CJ: Three different activated *ras* genes in mouse tumours; evidence for oncogene activation during progression of a mouse lymphoma. EMBO J 3:913, 1984

177. Shilo B-Z, Weinberg RA: DNA sequences homologous to vertebrate oncogenes are conserved in Drosophila melanogaster. Proc Natl Acad Sci USA 78:6789, 1981

178. Rijsewijk F, Schuermann M, Wagenaar E, et al: The drosophila homolog of the mouse mammary oncogene int-1 is identical to the segment polarity gene wingless. Cell 50:649–657, 1987

179. Kataoko T, Powers S, Cameron S, et al: Functional homology of mammalian and yeast *ras* genes. Cell 40:19, 1985

180. Defeo-Jones D, Tatchell K, Robinson LC, et al: Mammalian and yeast *ras* gene products: Biological function in their heterologous systems. Science 228:179, 1985

181. Tatchell K, Chaleff DT, Defeo-Jones D, et al: Requirement of either of a pair of *ras*-related genes of Saccharomyces cerevisiae for spore viability. Nature 309:523, 1984

182. Kataoka T, Powers S, McGill C, et al: Genetic analysis of yeast RAS1 and RAS2 genes. Cell 37:437, 1984

183. Tamanoi F, Walsh M, Kataoka T, et al: A product of yeast RAS2 gene is a guanine nucleotide binding protein. Proc Natl Acad Sci USA 81:6924, 1984

184. Temeles GL, Gibbs JB: Yeast and mammalian *ras* proteins have conserved biochemical properties. Nature 313:700, 1985

185. Broek D, Samiy N, Fasano O, et al: Differential activation of yeast adenylate cyclase by wild-type and mutant *ras* proteins. Cell 41:763, 1985

186. Toda T, Uno I, Ishikawa T, et al: In yeast, *ras* proteins are controlling elements of adenylate cyclase. Cell 40:27, 1985

187. Beckner SK, Hattori S, Shih TY: The *ras* oncogene product p21 is not a regulatory component of adenylate cyclase. Nature 317:71, 1985

188. Shiro K, Shimojo H, Swaada Y, et al: Incomplete transformation of rat cells by a small fragment of adenovirus 12 DNA. Virology 95:127, 1979

189. Houweling A, Van Den Elsen PJ, Van Der Eb AJ: Partial transformation of primary rat cells by the left-most 4-5 D fragment of adenovirus 5 DNA. Virology 105:537, 1980

190. Van Den Elsen P, De Pater S, Houweling A, et al: The relationship between region E1a and E1b of human adenoviruses in cell transformation. Gene 18:175, 1982

191. Ruley HE: Adenovirus early region 1A enables viral and cellular transforming primary cells in culture. Nature 304:602, 1982

192. Parada LF, Land H, Weinbert RA, et al: Cooperation between gene encoding P53 tumour antigen and *ras* in cellular transformation. Nature 312:648, 1984

193. Eliyahu D, Raz A, Gruss P, et al: Participation of p53 cellular tumor antigen in transformation of normal embryonic cells. Nature 312:647, 1984

194. Yancopoulos GD, Nisen PD, Tesfaye A, et al: N-*myc* can cooperate with *ras* to transform normal cells in culture. Proc Natl Acad Sci USA 82:5455, 1985

195. Land H, Parada LF, Weinbert RA: Cellular oncogenes and multistep carcinogenesis. Science 222:771–778, 1983

196. Courtneidge SA, Smith AE: Polyoma virus transforming protein associates with the product of the c-*src* cellular gene. Nature 303:435, 1983

197. Bolen JP, Thiele CJ, Israel MA, et al: Enhancement of cellular *src* gene product associated tyrosyl kinase activity following polyoma virus infection and transformation. Cell 38:767, 1984

198. Brinster RL, Chen HV, Trumbauer ME, et al: Factors effecting the efficiency of introducing foreign DNA into mice by microinjecting eggs. Proc Natl Acad Sci USA 82:4438, 1985

199. Stewart TA, Pattengale PK, Leder P: Spontaneous mammary adenocarcinomas in transgenic mice that carry and express MTV/*myc* fusion genes. Cell 38:627, 1984

200. Hanahan D: Heritable formation of pancreatic B cell tumours in transgenic mice expressing recombinant insulin/simian virus 40 oncogenes. Nature 315:115, 1985

201. Messing A, Chen H-Y, Palmiter RD, et al: Peripheral neuropathies, hepatocellular carcinomas and islet cell adenomas in transgenic mice. Nature 316:461, 1985

202. Sinn E, Muller W, Pattengale P, et al: Coexpression of MMTV/v-Ha-*ras* and MMTV/c-*myc* genes in transgenic mice: Synergistic action of oncogenes in vivo. Cell 49:465, 1987

203. Leder A, Pattengale PK, Kuo A, et al: Consequences of widespread deregulation of the c-*myc* gene in transgenic mice: Multiple neoplasms and normal development. Cell 45: 485, 1986

204. Adams JM, Harris AW, Pinkert CA, et al: The c-*myc* oncogene driven by immunoglobin enhancers induces lymphoid malignancy in transgenic mice. Nature 318:533, 1985

205. Robb RJ: Interleukin 2: The molecule and its function. Immunol Today 5:203, 1984

206. Tushinski RJ, Oliver IT, Guilbert LJ, et al: Survival of mononuclear phagocytes depends on a lineage-specific growth factor that the differentiated cells selectively destroy. Cell 28:71, 1982

207. Hamilton JA, Stanley ER, Burgess AW, et al: Stimulation of macrophage plasminogen activator activity by colony-stimulating factors. J Cell Physiol 103:435, 1980

208. Weissman BE, Aaronson SA: Balb and Kirsten murine sarcoma viruses alter growth and differentiation of EGF-dependent Balb/c mouse epidermal keratinocyte lines. Cell 32:599, 1983

209. Doolittle RF, Hunkapiller MW, Hood LE, et al: Simian sarcoma virus *onc* gene, v-*sis*, is derived from the gene (or genes) encoding a platelet-derived growth factor. Science 221:275, 1983

210. Chiu I-M, Reddy EP, Givol D, et al: Nucleotide sequence analysis identifies the human c-*sis* proto-oncogene as a structural gene for platelet-derived growth factor. Cell 37:123, 1984

211. Waterfield MD, Scrace GT, Whittle N, et al: Platelet-derived growth factor is structurally related to the putative transforming protein p28 *sis* of simian sarcoma virus. Nature 304:35, 1983

212. Ross R, Glomset J, Kariya B, et al: A platelet-dependent serum factor that stimulates the proliferation of arterial smooth muscle cells in vitro. Proc Natl Acad Sci USA 71:1207, 1974

213. Dickson C, Smith R, Brookes S, et al: Tumorigenesis by mouse mammary tumor virus: Proviral activation of a cellular gene in the common integration region *int-2*. Cell 37:529, 1984

214. Dickson C, Peters G: Potential oncogene product related to growth factors. Nature 326:833, 1987

215. Taira M, Yoshida T, Miyagawa K, et al: cDNA sequence of human transforming gene *hst* and identification of the coding sequence required for transforming activity. Proc Natl Acad Sci USA 84:2980, 1987

216. Abraham JA, Mergia A, Whang JL, et al: Nucleotide sequence of a bovine clone encoding the angiogenic protein, basic fibroblast growth factor. Science 233:545, 1986

217. Esch F, Baird A, Ling N, et al: Primary structure of bovine pituitary basic fibroblast growth factor (FGF) and comparison with the amino-terminal sequence of bovine brain acidic FGF. Proc Natl Acad Sci USA 82:6507, 1985

218. Delarco JE, Todaro GJ: Growth factors from murine sarcoma virus-transformed cells. Proc Natl Acad Sci USA 75:4001, 1978

219. Roberts AB, Sporn MB: Growth factors and transformation. Cancer Surv 5:405, 1986

220. Twardzik DR, Todaro GJ, Marquardt H, et al: Transformation induced by abelson murine leukemia virus involves production of a polypeptide growth factor. Science 216:894, 1982

221. Kaplan PL, Ozanne B: Cellular responsiveness to growth factors correlates with a cell's ability to express the transformed phenotype. Cell 33:931, 1983

222. Weber W, Gill GN, Spiess J: Production of an epidermal growth factor receptor-related protein. Science 224:294, 1984

223. Merlino GT, Xu Y-H, Ishii S, et al: Amplification and enhanced expression of the epidermal growth factor receptor gene in A431 human carcinoma cells. Science 224:417, 1984

224. Ullrich A, Coussens L, Hayflick JS, et al: Human epidermal growth factor receptor cDNA sequence and aberrant expression of the amplified gene in A431 epidermoid carcinoma cells. Nature 309:418, 1984

225. Ebina Y, Ellis L, Jarnagin K, et al: The human insulin receptor cDNA: The structural basis for hormone-activated transmembrane signalling. Cell 40:747, 1985

226. Hunter T, Cooper JA: Protein-tyrosine kinases. Annu Rev Biochem 54:897–930, 1985

227. Cooper JA, Bowen-Pope DF, Raines E, et al: Similar effects of platelet-derived growth factor and epidermal growth factor on the phosphorylation of tyrosine in cellular proteins. Cell 31:263, 1982

228. Sefton BM, Hunter T, Beemon K, et al: Evidence that the phosphorylation of tyrosine is essential for cellular transformation by Rous sarcoma virus. Cell 20:807, 1980

229. Whitlock CA, Witte ON: The complexity of virus-cell interactions in Abelson virus infection of lymphoid and other hematopoietic cells. In Dixon FJ (ed): Advances in Immunology, vol 37, pp 73–98. New York, Academic Press, 1985

230. Spector DH, Smith K, Padgett T, et al: Uninfected avian cells contain RNA related to the transforming gene of avian sarcoma viruses. Cell 13:371, 1978

231. Brugge JS, Cotton PC, Queral AE, et al: Neurones express high levels of a structurally modified, activated form of pp60c-*src*. Nature 316:554, 1985

232. Simon MA, Drees B, Kornberg T, et al: The nucleotide sequence and tissue-specific expression of Drosophila c-*src*. Cell 42:831, 1985

233. Moelling K, Pfaff E, Beug H, et al: DNA-binding activity is associated with purified *myb* proteins from AMB and E26 viruses and is temperature-sensitive for E26 *ts* mutants. Cell 40:983, 1985

234. Maxwell SA, Arlinghaus RB: Serine kinase activity associated with Moloney murine sarcoma virus-124-encoded p37mos. Virology 143:321, 1985

235. Reed SI, Hadwiger JA, Lorincz AT: Protein kinase activity associated with the product of the yeast cell cycle gene CDC28. Proc Natl Acad Sci USA 82:4055, 1985

236. Simanis V, Nurse PM: The cell cycle control gene *cdc2+* of yeast encodes a protein kinase potentially regulated by phosphorylation. Cell 45:261, 1986

237. Lee MG, Nurse P: Complementation used to clone a human homologue of the fission yeast cell cycle control gene *cdc2*. Nature 327:31, 1987

238. Hanks SK: Homology probing: Identification of cDNA clones encoding members of the protein-serine kinase family. Proc Natl Acad Sci USA 84:388, 1987

239. Draetta G, Brizuela L, Potashkin J, et al: Identification of p34 and p13, human homologs of the cell cycle regulators of fission yeast encoded by *cdc2+* and *suc1+*. Cell 50:319, 1987

240. Propst F, Rosenberg MP, Iyer A, et al: c-*mos* proto-oncogene RNA transcripts in mouse tissues: Structural features, developmental regulation and localization in specific cell types. Mol Cell Biol 7:1629–1637, 1987

241. Propst F, Rosenberg MP, Oskarsson MK, et al: Genetic analysis and developmental regulation of testis-specific RNA expression of Mos, Abl, actin and Hox-1.4. Oncogene 2:227–233, 1988

242. Keshet E, Rosenberg M, Mercer JA, et al: Developmental regulation of ovarian-specific *mos* expression. Oncogene 2:235–240, 1988

243. Westaway D, Papkoff J, Moscovici C, et al: Identification of a provirally activated c-Ha-*ras* oncogene in an avian nephroblastoma via a novel procedure: cDNA cloning of a chimaeric viral-host transcript. EMBO J 5:301, 1986

244. Reymond CD, Gomer RH, Mehdy MC, et al: Developmental regulation of a Dictyostelium gene encoding a protein homologous to mammalian *ras* protein. Cell 39:141, 1984

245. Defeo-Jones D, Skolnick E, Koller R, et al: *ras*-related gene sequences identified and isolated from *Saccharomyces cerevisiae*. Nature 306:707, 1983

246. Powers S, Kataoka T, Fasano O, et al: Genes in *S. cerevisiae* encoding proteins with domains homologous to the mammalian *ras* proteins. Cell 36:607, 1984

247. Shih TY, Weeks MO, Young HA, et al: Identification of a sarcoma virus-coded phosphoprotein in nonproducer cells transformed by Kirsten or Harvey murine sarcoma virus. Virology 96:64, 1979

248. Gibbs JB, Sigal IS, Poe M, et al: Intrinsic GTPase activity distinguishes normal and oncogenic *ras* p21 molecules. Proc Natl Acad Sci USA 81:5704, 1984

249. McGrath JP, Capon DJ, Goeddel DV, et al: Comparative biochemical properties of normal and activated human *ras* p21 protein. Nature 310:644, 1984

250. Willingham MC, Pastan I, Shih TY, et al: Localization of the *src* gene product of the Harvey strain of MSV to plasma membrane of transformed cells by electron microscopic immunocytochemistry. Cell 19:1005, 1980

251. Shih TY, Weeks MO: Oncogenes and cancer: The p21 *ras* genes. Cancer Invest 2:109, 1984

252. Hurley JB, Simon MI, Teplow DB, et al: Homologies between signal transducing G proteins and *ras* gene products. Science 226:860, 1984

253. Gilman AG: G proteins and dual control of adenylate cyclase. Cell 36:577, 1984

254. Stryer L: Cyclic GMP cascade of vision. Annu Rev Neurosci 9:87, 1986

255. Hughes SM: Are guanine nucleotide binding proteins a distinct class of regulatory proteins? FEBS Lett 164:1, 1983

256. McCormick F, Clark BFC, La Cour TFM, et al: A model for the tertiary structure of p21, the product of the *ras* oncogene. Science 228:96, 1985

257. Clanton DJ, Hattori S, Shih TY: Mutations of the *ras* gene product p21 that abolish guanine nucleotide binding. Proc Natl Acad Sci USA 83:5076, 1986

258. Willumsen BM, Christensen A, Hubbert NL, et al: The p21 *ras* C-terminus is required for transformation and membrane association. Nature 310:583, 1984

259. Seeburg PH, Colby WW, Capon DJ, et al: Biological properties of human c-Ha-*ras*1 genes mutated at codon 12. Nature 312:71, 1984

260. Kataoko T, Powers S, Cameron S, et al: Functional homology of mammalian and yeast *ras* genes. Cell 40:19, 1985

261. Defeo-Jones D, Tatchell K, Robinsin LC, et al: Mammalian and yeast *ras* gene products: Biological function in their heterologous systems. Science 228:179, 1985

262. Kataoka T, Powers S, McGill, C, et al: Genetic analysis of yeast RAS1 and RAS2 genes. Cell 37:437, 1984

263. Tamanoi F, Walsh M, Kataoka T, et al: A product of yeast RAS2 gene is a guanine nucleotide binding protein. Proc Natl Acad Sci USA 81:6924, 1984

264. Temeles GL, Gibbs JB: Yeast and mammalian *ras* proteins have conserved biochemical properties. Nature 313:700, 1985

265. Broek D, Samiy N, Fasano O, et al: Differential activation of yeast adenylate cyclase by wild-type and mutant *ras* proteins. Cell 41:763, 1985

266. Toda T, Uno I, Ishikawa T, et al: In yeast, *ras* proteins are controlling elements of adenylate cyclase. Cell 40:27, 1985

267. Beckner SK, Hattori S, Shih TY: The *ras* oncogene product p21 is not a regulatory component of adenylate cyclase. Nature 317:71, 1985

268. Kohl NE, Kanda N, Schreck RR, et al: Transposition and amplification of oncogene-related sequences in human neuroblastomas. Cell 35:359, 1983

269. Greenberg ME, Ziff EB: Stimulation of mouse 3T3 cells induces transcription of the c-*fos* oncogene. Nature 311:433, 1984

270. Kruijer W, Cooper JA, Hunter T, et al: Platelet-derived growth factor induces rapid but transient expression of the c-*fos* gene and protein. Nature 312: 711, 1984

271. Moller R, Bravo R, Burckhardt J, et al: Induction of c-*fos* gene and protein by growth factors precedes activation of c-*myc*. Nature 312:716, 1984

272. Thompson CB, Challoner PB, Neiman PE, et al: Expression of the c-*myb* proto-oncogene during cellular proliferation. Nature 319:374, 1986

273. Reich NC, Levine AJ: Growth regulation of a cellular tumour antigen, p53, in non-transformed cells. Nature 308:199, 1984

274. Leof EB, Wharton W, Van Wyck JJ, et al: Epidermal growth factor (EGF) and somatomedin C regulate G1 progression in competent BALB/c-3T3 cells. Exp Cell Res 141:107, 1982

275. Curran T, Morgan JI: Superinduction of the c-*fos* by nerve growth factor in the presence of peripherally active benzodiazeprines. Science 229:1265, 1985

276. Stiles CD, Capone GT, Scher CD, et al: Dual control of cell growth by somatomedins and platelet-derived growth factor. Proc Natl Acad Sci 76:1279, 1979

277. Eisenman RN, Thompson CB: Oncogenes with potential nuclear function: myc, myb, and fos. Cancer Surv 5:309–327, 1986

278. Westin EH, Gallo RC, Arya SK, et al: Differential expression of the *amv* gene in human hematopoietic cells. Proc Natl Acad Sci USA 79:2194, 1982

279. Campisi J, Gray HE, Parchee AB, et al: Cell-cycle control of c-*myc* but not c-*ras* expression is lost following chemical transformation. Cell 36:241, 1984

280. Torelli G, Selleri L, Donelli A, et al: Activation of c-*myb* expression by phytohemagglutinin stimulation in normal human T lymphocytes. Mol Cell Biol 5:2874, 1985

281. Prochowkni EV, Kukowska J: Deregulated expression of c-*myc* by murine erythroleukemia cells prevents differentiation. Nature 32:848, 1986

282. Mitchell RL, Zokas L, Schreiber RD, et al: Rapid induction of the expression of proto-oncogene *fos* during human monocytic differentiation. Cell 40:209, 1985

283. Donner P, Greiser-Wilke I, Moelling K: Nuclear localization and DNA binding of

the transforming gene product of avian myelocytomatosis virus. Nature 296:262, 1982

284. Sambucetti L, Curran T: The fos protein complex is associated with DNA in isolated nuclei and binds to DNA cellulose. Science 234:1417, 1986

285. Moelling K, Pfaff E, Beug H, et al: DNA-binding activity is associated with purified myb proteins from AMV and E26 viruses and is temperature-sensitive for E26 ts mutants. Cell 40:983, 1985

286. Struhl K: The DNA-binding domains of the jun oncoprotein and the yeast GCN4 transcriptional activator protein are functionally homologous. Cell 50:841, 1987

287. McLeod K, Baxter J: Chromatin receptors for thyroid hormones. J Biol Chem 251:7380, 1976

288. Kingston RE, Baldwin AS, Sharp PA: Transcription control by oncogenes. Cell 41:3, 1985

289. Kaddurah-Daouk R, Greene JM, Baldwin AS Jr, et al: Activation and repression of mammalian gene expression by the c-myc protein. Genes Dev 1:347, 1987

290. Distel RJ, Ro H-S, Rosen BS, et al: Nucleoprotein complexes that regulate gene expression in adipocyte differentiation: Direct participation of c-fos. Cell 49:835, 1987

291. Maki Y, Bos TJ, Davis C, et al: Avian sarcoma virus 17 carries the jun oncogene. Proc Natl Acad Sci USA 84:2848, 1987

292. Vogt PK, Bos TJ, Doolittle RF: Homology between the DNA-binding domain of the GCN4 regulatory protein of yeast and the carboxyl-terminal region of a protein coded for by the oncogene jun. Proc Natl Acad Sci USA 84:3316, 1987

293. Bohmann D, Bos TJ, Admin A, et al: Human proto-oncogene c-jun encodes a DNA binding protein with structural and functional properties of transcription factor AP-1. Science 238:1386, 1987

294. Weinberger C, Hollenberg SM, Rosenfeld MG, et al: Domain structure of the human glucocorticoid receptor and its relationship to the v-erbA oncogene product. Nature 318:670, 1985

295. SAP J, Munoz A, Damm K, et al: The v-erb A protein is a high affinity receptor for thyroid hormone. Nature 324:635, 1986

296. Weinberger C, Thompson C, Ong E, et al: The C-v-erbA gene encodes a thyroid hormone receptor. Nature 324:641, 1986

297. Frykberg L, Palmieri S, Beng H, et al: Transforming capacities of avian erythroblastosis virus mutants deleted in the V-erbA or erbB oncogenes. Cell 32:227, 1983

298. Oppenheimer JH, Samuels HH (eds): Molecular Basis of Thyroid Hormone Action. New York Academic Press, 1983

299. Woods CM, Boyer B, Vogt PK, et al: Asychronous expression of the anion transporter and the peripheral components of the membrane skeleton in AZV- and S13-transformed cells. J Cell Biol 103:1789, 1986

300. Zenke M, Kahn P, Disela C, et al: v-erbA specifically suppresses transcription of the avian erythrocyte anion transporter (band 3) gene. Cell 52:107–119, 1988

301. Nishizuka Y: Studies and perspectives of protein kinase C. Science 233:305, 1986

302. Berridge MJ: Inositol triphosphate and diacylglycerol: Two interacting second messengers. Annu Rev Biochem 56:159, 1987

303. Smithies O, Gregg RG, Boggs SS, et al: Insertion of DNA sequences into the human chromosome β-globin locus by homologous recombination. Nature 317:230–234, 1985

304. Thomas KR, Folger KR, Capecchi MR: High frequency targeting of genes to specific sites in the mammalian genome. Cell 44:419–428, 1986

305. De Vos AM, Tong L, Milburn MV, et al: Three-dimensional structure of an oncogene protein: Catalytic domain of human c-H-ras p21. Science 239:888–893, 1988

306. Klein G: The approaching era of the tumor suppressor genes. Science 238:1539–1545, 1987

307. Lee M-S, Chang K-S, Cabanillas F, et al: Detection of minimal residual cells carrying the t(14;18) by DNA sequence amplification. Science 237:175–178, 1987

308. Crescenzi M, Seto M, Herzig GP, et al: Thermophilic polymerase chain amplification of t(14;18) breakpoints and the detection of minimal residual disease. Proc Natl Acad Sci USA (in press)

309. Miser JS, Kinsella TJ, Triche TJ, et al: Treatment of peripheral neuroepithelioma in children and young adults. J Clin Oncol 5:1752–1758, 1987

310. Hayward WS, Neel BG, Astrin SM: Activation of a cellular onc gene by promoter insertion in ALV-induced lymphoid leukosis. Nature 290:475, 1981

311. Payne GS, Bishop JM, Varmus HE: Multiple arrangements of viral DNA and an activated host oncogene in bursal lymphomas. Nature 295:209, 1982

312. Neil JC, Hughes D, McFarlane R, Wilkie NM: Transduction and rearrangement of the myc gene by feline leukaemia virus in naturally occurring T-cell leukaemias. Nature 308:814, 1984

313. Schen-Ong GLC, Morse HC III, Potter M, et al: Two modes of c-myb activation in virus-induced mouse myeloid tumors. Mol Cell Biol 6:380, 1986

314. Silver J, Kozak C: Common proviral integration region on mouse chromosome in lymphomas and myelogenous leukemias induced by Friend murine leukemia virus. J Virol 57:526, 1986

315. Canaani E, Dreazen O, Klar A, et al: Activation of the c-mos oncogene in a mouse plasmacytoma by insertion of an endogenous intracisternal A-particle genome. Proc Natl Acad Sci USA 80:7118, 1983

316. Voronova AF, Sefton BM: Expression of a new tyrosine protein kinase is stimulated by retrovirus promoter insertion. Nature 319:682, 1986

317. Marth JD, Peet R, Krebs EG, et al: A lymphocyte-specific protein-tyrosine kinase gene is rearranged and overexpressed in the murine T cell lymphoma LSTRA. Cell 43:393, 1985

318. Tsichlis PN, Strauss PG, Hu LF: A common region for proviral DNA integration in MoMuLV-induced rat thymic lymphomas. Nature 302:445, 1983

319. Villeneuve L, Rassart E, Jolicoeur P, et al: Proviral integration site Mis-1 in rat thymomas corresponds to the pvt-1 translocation breakpoint in murine plasmacytomas. Mol Cell Biol 6:1834, 1986

320. Cuypers HT, Selten G, Quint W, et al: Murine leukemia virus-induced T-cell lymphomagenesis: Integration of proviruses in a distinct chromosomal region. Cell 37:141, 1984

321. Mucenski ML, Taylor BA, Ihle JN, et al: Identification of a common ecotropic viral integration site, Evi-1, in the DNA of AKXD murine myeloid tumors. Mol Cell Biol 8:301, 1988

322. Buchberg AM, Bedigian HG, Taylor BA, et al: Localization of Evi-2 to Chromosome 11: Linkage to other proto-oncogene and growth factor loci using interspecific backcross mice. Oncogene Res (in press)

323. Nishizawa M, Semba K, Yoshida MC, et al: Structure, expression and chromosomal location of the human c-fgr gene. Mol Cell Biol 76:511, 1986

324. Nau MM, Brooks BJ, Battey J, et al: L-myc, a new myc-related gene amplified and expressed in human small lung cancer. Nature 318:69, 1985

325. Rabin M, Watson M, Barker PE, et al: N-ras transforming gene maps to region p11-p13 on chromosome 1 by in situ hybridization. Cytogenet Cell Genet 38:70, 1984

326. Rowley JD: Biological implications of consistent chromosome rearrangements in leukemia and lymphoma. Cancer Res 44:3159, 1984

327. Barbacid M: Personal communication

328. Brownell E, Kozak CA, Fowle JR, et al: Comparative genetic mapping of cellular rel sequences in man, mouse, and the domestic cat. Am J Hum Genet 39:194, 1986

329. Bonner T, O'Brien SJ, Nash WG, et al: The human homologous of raf (mil) oncogene are located on human chromosomes 3 and 4. Science 223:71, 1984

330. Roussel MF, Sherr CJ, Barker PE, et al: Molecular cloning of the c-fms locus and its assignment to human chromosome 5. J Virol 48:770, 1983

331. Nagarajan L, Louis E, Twsujimoto Y, et al: Localization of the human pim oncogene (PIM) to a region of chromosome 6 involved in translocations in acute leukemias. Proc Natl Acad Sci USA 83:2556, 1986

332. Rabin M, Birnbaum D, Young D, et al: Human ros1 and mas 1 oncogenes located in regions of chromosome 6 associated with tumor-specific rearrangements. Oncogene Res 1:169, 1987

333. Harper ME, Franchini G, Love J, et al: Chromosomal sublocalization of human c-myb and c-fes cellular onc genes. Nature 304:169, 1983

334. Spurr NK, Solomon E, Jansson M, et al: Chromosomal localization of the human homologues to the oncogenes v-erbA and B. EMBO J 3:159, 1984

335. Park M, Testa JR, Blair DG, et al: Two rearranged met alleles in MMNG-HOS cells reveal the orientation of met on chromosome 7 to other markers tightly linked to the cystic fibrosis locus. Proc Natl Acad Sci USA (in press)

336. Caubet J-F, Mathieu-Mahul D, Berhneim A, et al: Human proto-oncogene c-mos maps to 8q11. EMBO J 4:2245, 1985

337. De Martinville B, Giacalone J, Shih C, et al: Oncogene from human EJ bladder carcinoma is located on the short arm of chromosome 11. Science 219:498, 1983

338. Horn TM, Huebner K, Croce C, et al: Chromosomal locations of members of a family of novel endogenous human retroviral genomes. J Virol 58:955, 1986

339. Detaisne C, Gegonne A, Stehelin D, et al: Chromosomal localization of the human proto-oncogene c-ets. Nature 310:581, 1984

340. McBride OW, Swan DC, Tronick SR, et al: Regional chromosomal location of N-ras, K-ras-1, K-ras-2 and myb oncogenes in human cells. Nucleic Acid Res 11:8221, 1983

341. Van't Veer LJ, Van Kessel AG, Van Heerikhuizen H, et al: Molecular cloning and chromosomal assignment of the human homolog of int-1, a mouse gene implicated in mammary tumorigenesis. Mol Cell Biol 4:2532, 1984

342. Barker PE, Rabin M, Watson M, et al: Human c-fos oncogene mapped within chromosomal region 14q21-q31. Proc Natl Acad Sci USA 81:5826, 1984

343. McBride OW, Merry D, Givol D: The gene for human p53 cellular tumor antigen is located on chromosome 17 short arm (17p13). Proc Natl Acad Sci USA 83:130, 1986

344. Semba K, Yamanashi Y, Nishikawa M, et al: Location of the c-yes gene on the human chromosome and its expression in various tissues. Science 227:1038, 1985

345. Sakaguchi AY, Naylor SL, Shows TB: A sequence homologous to Rous sarcoma virus v-src is on human chromosome 20. Prog Nucleic Acid Res Mol Biol 29:279, 1983

346. Watson DK, Sacchi N, McWilliams-Smith MJ, et al: The avian and mammalian ets genes: Molecular characterization, chromosome mapping and implication in human leukemia. Anticancer Res 6:631–636, 1986

347. Dalla Favera R, Gallo RC, Giallongo A, et al: Chromosomal localization of the human homolog (c-sis) of the simian sarcoma virus onc gene. Science 218:686, 1982

348. Erikson J, Finan J, Nowell PC, et al: Translocation of immunoglobuin VH genes in Burkitt lymphoma. Proc Natl Acad Sci USA 79:5611, 1982

349. Lenoir GM, Preud'Homme JL, Bernheim A, et al: Correlation between immunoglobin light chain expression and variant translocation in Burkitt's lymphoma. Nature 298:474, 1982

350. Sandberg A, Kohno S, Wake N, et al: Chromosome and causation of human cancer and leukemia: XLII. Cancer Genet Cytogenet 2:145, 1980

351. Vande Woude GF, Gilden RV: Principles of cancer biology: The molecular biology of cancer. In DeVita VT Jr, Hellman S, Rosenberg SA (eds): Cancer: Principles and Practices of Oncology, vol 2, pp 23–47. Philadelphia, JB Lippincott, 1985

352. Besmer P, Murphy JE, George PC, et al: A new acute transforming feline retrovirus and relationship of its oncogene v-kit with the protein kinase gene family. Nature 320:415, 1986

353. Robbins KC, Devare SG, Reddy EP, et al: In vivo identification of the transforming gene product of simian sarcoma virus. Science 218:1131, 1982

ANITA B. ROBERTS
MICHAEL B. SPORN

CHAPTER 5

Principles of Molecular Cell Biology of Cancer: Growth Factors Related to Transformation

This chapter reviews the role of peptide growth factors and their receptors in the control of cell differentiation and proliferation. Study of peptide growth factors and their role in malignant transformation is important because it is likely that control of the expression of growth factors eventually will lead to new modalities of cancer prevention or therapy.

In the broadest sense, this approach to prevention or therapy rests on the assumption that cancer is a disease of abnormal cell differentiation, in some cases of arrested cell differentiation.[1-3] Fundamental to this approach are the concepts that neoplasms are caricatures of normal processes of tissue development and renewal[1] and that the malregulated expression of developmentally relevant cellular genes appears to underlie all cancers.[2] It is becoming increasingly clear that many critical developmental phenomena in both normal and malignant tissues are mediated by peptide growth factors and that study of these agents is now of major significance in cancer biology.[4-6]

To understand the role of peptide growth factors in either the genesis of cancer or its prevention and reversal, one must first consider the oncogene concept. Bishop has summarized this concept as follows:[7]

It now appears likely that normal cells bear the seeds of their own destruction in the form of cancer genes, whose anoma-

lous activities mediate tumorigenesis. The term, cancer genes, is a convenience, of course, and is viewed by some as a misnomer: the loci in question may be physiologically essential constituents of the cell's genetic apparatus that become pathogenic only when their structure or control is disturbed by oncogenic agents.

Mintz and Fleischman have suggested that "the gene at issue [may be] any of the numerous "banal" or ordinary genes involved in cell growth and differentiation, rather than special or exotic cancer genes.[2] They have emphasized that

there may be numerous "mundane" genes . . . in normal cells that might cause neoplastic conversion if they were made to function at levels above normal; genes of this sort might promote the growth and proliferation of initially normal stem cells beyond the usual period, thereby "locking" them into the stem-cell mode and making them unresponsive toward stimuli (e.g., specific inducers) to differentiate.

Very recent work has shown that the expression of several different oncogenes within a cell may be needed to achieve tumorigenicity[8,9]; these molecular findings fit very well with classical concepts of initiation-promotion and multistage carcinogenesis.[10] With the above as background, the significance of the peptides growth factors that control cell proliferation and differentiation becomes much clearer because recent discoveries have shown that oncogenes can control expression of certain peptide growth factors and their receptors and can alter their signaling pathways. In a broader sense, it can be considered that the genes for all peptide growth factors, their receptors, and intermediates in their signaling pathways have oncogenic potential.[11] In this chapter we will describe some fundamental properties of peptide growth factors and their receptors before discussing their relationships to oncogenes.

NATURE OF PEPTIDE GROWTH FACTORS AND THEIR RECEPTORS

The term growth factor is difficult to define because there is no consensus as to what properties allow a substance to be considered a growth factor.[12] In general parlance, growth factors are not the typical macronutrients and micronutrients that are well defined in biochemistry textbooks but rather are an ill-defined set of polypeptides that can modulate cell function and exert specific and potent growth regulatory action on target cells. In contrast to micronutrients that act within the cell, growth factors are secreted by cells and interact with specific, membrane-bound glycoprotein receptors that function as transducers of the signal generated by these effector substances. Growth factors are among the most potent known biological substances involved in control of cellular physiology; in many cell culture systems they are active at concentrations as low as 10^{-12}M, and amounts as small as a few picograms (one picogram is one millionth of a microgram) can induce a highly specific biological response. The specificity of the response is believed to reside in the membrane-bound receptor for the growth factor rather than in the growth factor itself. Several different although structurally related polypeptides may bind to the same receptor; for example, insulin and insulin-like growth factors (IGFs) may bind to either the insulin receptor or to IGF receptors.[13,14] The role of the polypeptide growth factor in binding to the receptor is to trigger the receptor to express its program; as Roth has succinctly expressed it, "The receptor has the message."[15]

Receptors for growth factors may be viewed as similar to allosteric enzymes that are in an inactive state until their ligands bind. This binding then triggers the functional activity of the receptor and its intrinsic enzymatic activity. Many of the important receptors for growth factors are now known to have growth factor-dependent tyrosine kinase activity.[6] While many of the polypeptide growth factors are relatively small (5000–25,000 molecular weight), highly stable molecules, typical receptors are much larger (150,000–350,000 molecular weight) and are much less stable, particularly when isolated. For example, during a typical isolation procedure, many growth factors can be subjected to very harsh conditions such as exposure to strong acid, organic solvents such as ethanol, propanol, or acetonitrile, or high temperatures without loss of biological activity. In contrast, receptor molecules, which are integral components of the cell membrane, will often be irreversibly inactivated by such rigorous treatment, and much gentler conditions are required for

their isolation in a physiologically active state. Consequently, because it has been much more difficult to purify receptors than growth factors, knowledge of the molecular properties of receptors is at present much more limited. However, new chemical methods of purification involving affinity chromatography, monoclonal antibodies, and nonionic detergents used to solubilize receptors have recently allowed the purification of the receptors for many of the polypeptide growth factors. Although certain receptors are known to have specific enzymatic activities (such as tyrosine kinase activity),[6,16] very little is known about the mechanism whereby the signal from the receptor is transduced into a specific biological response within the cell itself. Since both the effector and its receptor are often internalized after the binding of the effector, it is possible that the only role of the effector is to translocate the receptor (or a fragment of the receptor) to another compartment of the cell, where its intrinsic enzymatic activity may be manifested.

It is now beginning to be appreciated that most growth factors are multifunctional and can act on a broad range of target cells.[17] Thus not only can they stimulate cell proliferation, but also, under appropriate conditions, they can inhibit cell proliferation or have effects on cell function unrelated to proliferation. Indeed, a specific polypeptide growth factor that may be a potent mitogenic agent in one cellular context may have an entirely different function in another. For example, epidermal growth factor (EGF), a potent mitogen for fibroblasts throughout the body, has recently been identified in the central nervous system of both immature and adult rats, where it has been suggested that it functions as a neurotransmitter substance in the brain.[18] Many other small polypeptides of the gut, which in some contexts may have growth factor activity, likewise may be functioning in the brain as neurotransmitter substances.[19] In a similar vein, transforming growth factor-beta (TGF-beta), which acts synergistically with EGF to enhance mitogenesis of a rat kidney fibroblast cell line (NRK cell line) when grown in soft agar, acts antagonistically to EGF and thus is an antimitogenic agent for the human lung cancer cell line A-549 when it is grown in soft agar.[20]

Another important concept is that the action of any growth factor is not an intrinsic property of that individual peptide but rather a property of a set of conditions that are operant on a cell at a particular time.[17] That set of conditions includes not only the various growth factors to which the cell is exposed but also the extracellular environment of the cell. Thus, in a defined rat fibroblastic cell line (FR3T3, *myc* transfected), TGF-beta synergizes with one growth factor, platelet-derived growth factor (PDGF), to promote anchorage-independent growth but antagonizes the mitogenic effects of a second growth factor (EGF) and suppresses anchorage-independent growth.[20] Moreover, while TGF-beta may be mitogenic for cells growing under anchorage-independent conditions (in soft agar culture), it may be antimitogenic for the same cells (with the same set of added growth factors) growing under anchorage-dependent conditions (in monolayer cultures on a plastic surface).[20] It is difficult, therefore, to be rigid about defining the action of any particular polypeptide growth factor. Rather what appears to have happened during evolution is that polypeptide effectors and their corresponding receptors, which have exquisitely high affinity and specificity for each other and are classic "lock and key" signaling systems, have been used for many different purposes in many different cells throughout the body. Under some circumstances the signal generated by the effector-receptor complex may be mitogenic, whereas under other circumstances the signal may be antimitogenic; the signal may also be used in yet other circumstances for purposes that have nothing to do with the control of the cell cycle.[17]

With an understanding of the multifunctionality of growth factors comes the realization that the names of most growth factors are misnomers. Growth factors have traditionally been named within the context of their original discovery, which may have little to do with their ultimate physiologic role or even with their total tissue distribution. For example, EGF clearly is a highly potent agent for stimulating growth and multiplication of fibroblastic cells, as well as epidermal and other epithelial cells.[21,22] In some situations, EGF can also be a potent antimitogenic agent, as is the case with the A431 human vulvar squamous carcinoma cell line.[23] In another example, polypeptides very similar in structure (perhaps identical) to PDGF have recently been found in cells other than platelets, such as endothelial cells, vascular smooth muscle cells, and many different types of tumor cells.[24] Yet another growth factor that is misnamed is TGF-beta (originally discovered in a phenotypic transformation assay in cell culture), which has been found in high concentration in platelets and would appear to have a physiologic role in promotion of wound healing.[25] It is apparent that the descriptive value of the names of polypeptide growth factors is no greater than the descriptive value of the names of the investigators who discovered them.

AUTOCRINE SECRETION OF GROWTH FACTORS AND CANCER

Autocrine secretion (Fig. 5-1) is an important new concept that is emerging as a unifying theme in studies of the role of polypeptide growth factors in malignancy.[26-28] It has been

FIG. 5-1. Diagrammatic representation of endocrine, paracrine, and autocrine secretion. Peptide growth factors are shown in latent form within the cell. The thickened, semicircular regions of the cell membrane represent receptor sites.[26]

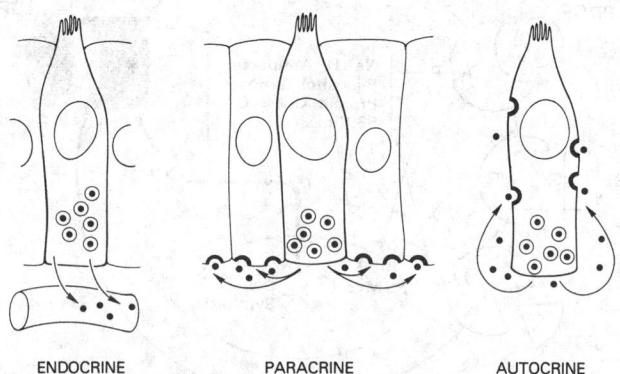

ENDOCRINE   PARACRINE   AUTOCRINE

known for many years that malignant cells in culture require fewer exogenous growth factors for optimal growth and multiplication than do their normal counterparts.[29,30] One explanation is that malignant cells are relatively independent of exogenous growth factors because they are capable of endogenous synthesis of their own growth factors. In 1978, De Larco and Todaro[31] suggested that the endogenous production of polypeptide growth factors, which act on their producer cells via functional external receptors, could be responsible for the malignant transformation of cells. To the extent that a cell is dependent on an exogenous supply of growth factors, provided by endocrine secretion (via the blood) or paracrine secretion (from an adjacent cell), its growth can be controlled by regulating that supply. However, if a cell acquires the ability to produce its own growth factors and has the functional receptors for them (this process has been called autocrine secretion),[26-28] it then is under less-stringent external growth control and has a selective growth advantage over neighboring cells, which are still subject to external regulation.

Autocrine action of growth factors in cancer cells was first shown in rat and mouse cells transformed by Moloney and Kirsten sarcoma viruses.[31] When grown in culture, these tumor cells were found to release polypeptides resembling EGF (originally called "sarcoma growth factor") into the extracellular medium. These polypeptides had the important property of causing reversible, phenotypic transformation (anchorage-independent growth in soft agar) of non-neoplastic indicator cells, and this transformation assay has been used as a primary method for screening and purifying the entire set of "transforming growth factors."[32] It soon became apparent that the EGF-like peptides released by the virally transformed cells were not the same as EGF itself, although their mechanism of action was mediated by binding to the EGF receptor. These EGF-like peptides have subsequently been called type-alpha transforming growth factors (TGF-alpha); their entire amino acid sequences have been determined and their genes cloned from both human and rodent sources. A wide variety of tumor cells, of both human and rodent origin, are now known to synthesize and release TGF-alpha, and it is believed that the autocrine action of this polypeptide growth factor plays an important role in the malignant behavior of these cells.[33]

Other polypeptide growth factors known to have an autocrine action are PDGF[34] and bombesin, the small tetradecapeptide secreted by human small cell lung cancer cells (SCLC).[35] The data on the autocrine action of PDGF are particularly impressive. Several human osteosarcoma and glioma cell lines are known to produce PDGF-like substances that are believed to mediate their abnormal growth. Antisera to PDGF have been shown to block the growth of rodent tumor cells transformed by simian sarcoma virus; these data strongly suggest that the synthesis of PDGF-like molecules is one of the primary factors responsible for the malignant behavior of the transformed cells.[36] Likewise, as illustrated in Figure 5-2, antibodies to bombesin inhibit both the in vitro clonal growth of SCLC cells and the growth of xenografts of these cells in nude mice, suggesting that they have interfered with an essential autocrine pathway responsible for the uncontrolled growth of the tumor cells.[35]

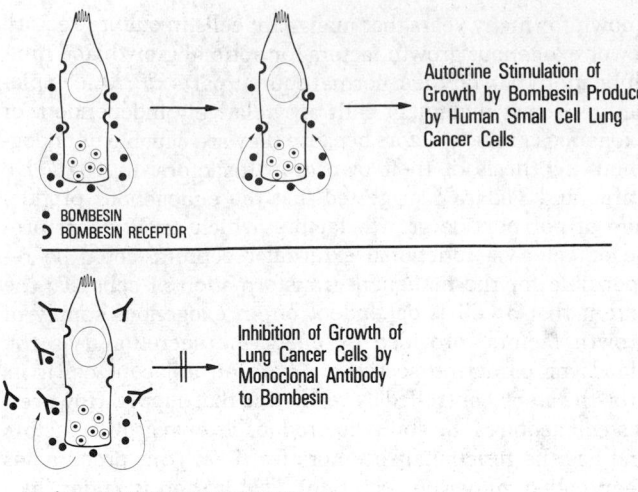

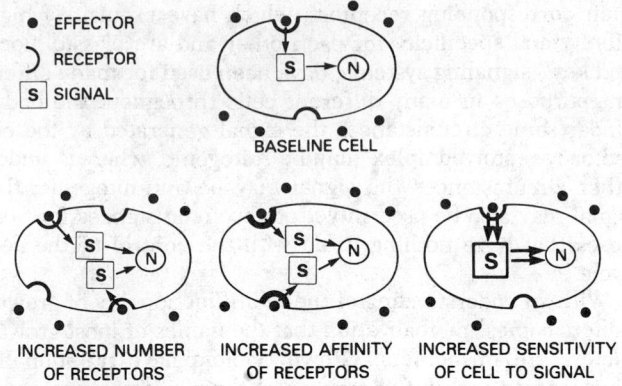

FIG. 5-3. Mechanisms for increasing receptivity of a cell to a peptide growth factor.

FIG. 5-2. Inhibition of growth of human small cell lung cancer cells by monoclonal antibodies to bombesin.[140]

Although we have discussed the importance of autocrine secretion and action of growth factors on the cancer cell, it should not be assumed that autocrine phenomena pertain only to tumor cells. During growth and tissue injury of vascular endothelium and vascular smooth muscle, there is substantial autocrine secretion of PDGF-like molecules.[37] It is likely that embryonic, rapidly growing, or injured tissues are all capable of autocrine secretion of growth factors and that this is an entirely normal physiologic response. The pathologic aspect of autocrine secretion in the cancer cell should be viewed as the continuous inappropriate expression of the polypeptide growth factors or the constant hypersensitivity of the cancer cell to its own growth factors, by mechanisms that will be discussed later.

Although it is apparent that the autocrine concept can be the basis of the uncontrolled growth of tumor cells, paracrine action of tumor growth factors on cellular components of tumor stroma also clearly plays a role in development of the malignancy.[38,39] Thus, for example, fibroblast growth factor (FGF) stimulates the growth of endothelial cells, in that way promoting neovascularization of the tumor,[40] and TGF-beta stimulates fibroblasts to elaborate connective tissue.[25] Such indirect effects of growth factors on tumor growth will be discussed in greater detail later.

Although the original autocrine hypothesis stressed the production of growth factors by tumor cells, it is now clear that the tumor cell may also achieve the same type of autonomy by modification of the synthesis of receptors for growth factors or by alteration of the postreceptor signaling pathway for a particular growth factor rather than by a direct increase in the synthesis and release of the growth factor itself.[27] Thus, as shown in Figure 5-3 (left), increased receptiveness to stimulation by a peptide growth factor may result from either an increased number of receptors on the surface of a cell or an increased affinity of the receptors for the peptide (Fig. 5-3, middle). Either or both of these mechanisms have been shown to be operative in human squamous cell carcinomas of the head and neck or vulva that have been grown in cell culture. These cells have either extremely high numbers

of receptors for EGF[41] or receptors with unusually high affinity for EGF.[42] A third subset of increased sensitivity (Fig. 5-3, right) is the possibility that the availability, number, or affinity of effector or receptor molecules is not altered in a cancer cell but that it becomes more sensitive to the signal generated by the effector-receptor complex (i.e., that there is greater amplification of the signal generated by a peptide growth factor occupying a specific receptor). Signaling cascades are known to involve such intermediates as ion transport channels, phosphoinositol metabolites, protein kinase C, and ribosomal S6 kinase; in addition, activation of nuclear expression of the *myc* and *fos* proto-oncogenes follows mitogenic stimulation of cells (Fig. 5-4). The sequence of events that link the membrane tyrosine kinase activity, the cytoplasmic signals, and the nuclear signals is not yet understood. However, the overlap between activation of these signals by growth factors and by oncogenes suggests that

FIG. 5-4. Diagrammatic representation of intermediates thought to function in intracellular signalling pathways of growth factors. Indicated are cytoplasmic and nuclear elements known to become activated or elevated in concentration following binding of mitogenic peptides to receptors that have tyrosine kinase activity; the sequence of events is not known. In contrast, a growth inhibitor like TGF-beta appears to signal through distinct pathways; treatment of mitogenically stimulated cells with TGF-beta blocks DNA synthesis without interfering with any of the signals generated by the mitogenic growth factors.[25,115,182]

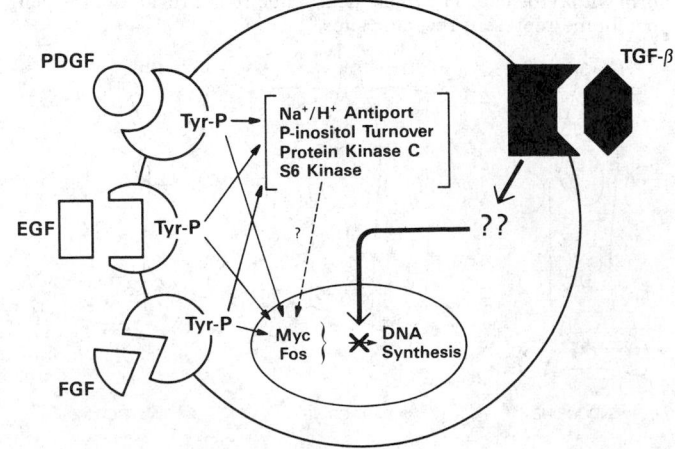

increased sensitivity to signals might result from background oncogene activity; we have already noted that peptide growth factors and oncogene expression may generate similar signals, for example, tyrosine kinase activity. In this way, one can understand how the activities of certain peptide growth factors and oncogenes are permissive for each other.

NEGATIVE GROWTH FACTORS: A REVISED AUTOCRINE HYPOTHESIS

A significant recent finding is that the signaling pathway activated by an autocrine polypeptide may evoke a negative growth response rather than a positive one. The best example of such a negative growth factor is TGF-beta, which has been shown to be a bifunctional regulator of cell growth.[20,25] Interestingly, the signaling pathways of TGF-beta and perhaps of other negative growth regulators appear to be distinct from those of mitogenic peptides whose receptors have intrinsic tyrosine kinase activity; thus, as shown in Figure 5-4, TGF-beta blocks DNA synthesis in cells treated simultaneously with such mitogens without impairing any of the signals they generate.[25] The discovery of the identity of TGF-beta with a growth inhibitor produced by monkey kidney cells demonstrates the existence of negative autocrine pathways, since the monkey kidney cells that produce TGF-beta have receptors for it and respond with an inhibition of cell growth.[43,44] The concept of a cell producing its own growth inhibitory substances is old, but it lacked experimental support until this demonstration of the identity of a growth inhibitor with a homogeneous polypeptide of known amino acid sequence.

Based on these new findings, we have recently suggested that the autocrine hypothesis be extended to include the concept that malignant transformation may be the result not only of excessive production, expression, and action of positive autocrine growth factors, but also of the failure of cells to synthesize, express, or respond to specific negative growth factors that the cells ordinarily release to control their own growth.[27] This loss of negative growth control might be the result of a biochemical lesion in the growth inhibitor, a failure of cells to effectively process and release the inhibitor, a loss or defect of the receptors or the postreceptor signaling pathway for the negative effector, or the failure of cells to activate the release negative growth factor. Examples of two of these mechanisms can be found in the response of transformed cells to TGF-beta. As an example of failure of cells to activate a released negative effector, human lung carcinoma cells (A549) are unable to activate the latent, biologically inactive, TGF-beta that they secrete; however, their growth is inhibited by exogenous active TGF-beta, demonstrating that the receptors and signaling pathways are still functional.[45] An example of alterations in signaling pathways, which have made transformed cells refractory to inhibition by TGF-beta, is found in hepatocytes transformed in vitro by aflatoxin; these cells no longer respond to TGF-beta even though the parental cells, from which they were derived, are exquisitely sensitive to inhibition by TGF-beta.[46] Finally, as an example of cells that have escaped from negative growth control by loss of receptors for TGF-beta, a human squamous cell carcinoma, SCC-25, is not inhibited by TGF-beta and has no detectable cell surface receptors for the factor; in contrast, the growth of normal human prokeratinocytes, which do have TGF-beta receptors, is strongly inhibited by the peptide.[47]

RELATIONSHIPS BETWEEN GROWTH FACTORS AND ONCOGENES

During the past 7 years, two fields of scientific investigation, which had previously been unrelated to each other, have merged into a single domain. As recently as 1980, it was not generally appreciated that there is any significant relationship between polypeptide growth factors and oncogenes. A series of major scientific discoveries has altered this belief, so that it is now almost impossible to discuss the topic of growth factors without immediate reference to oncogenes; conversely, any contemporary review of oncogenes must consider the role of growth factors in their ultimate phenotypic expression. One way to conceptualize the role of oncogenes in causation of cancer is to state that oncogenes confer growth factor autonomy on cells. In this conceptual framework, autocrine secretion and action of growth factors play a central role. The interplay of oncogenes and growth factors occurs at every level: the growth factor itself, the receptor for the growth factor, and the pathways whereby the signal generated by the binding of the growth factor to its receptor is transmitted to the nucleus of the cell. These relationships, some of which will be described in detail, are summarized in Figure 5-5.

The first significant linking of growth factor research and oncogene research came in 1981 when Cohen, Erikson, Hunter, and colleagues[48-50] showed that there is a common enzymatic mechanism shared by the receptor for EGF and the transforming protein, pp60[src], encoded by the Rous sarcoma virus oncogene, src. In this case, it was found that two apparently unrelated phenomena—namely, a biochemical mechanism whereby a receptor for a growth factor causes a signal to be transduced across the plasma membrane of the cell and a biochemical mechanism whereby the unique transforming protein of an oncogenic virus exerts its effects—were one and the same, that is, a mechanism to initiate enzymatic activity with the capacity to phosphorylate a variety of target proteins on tyrosine residues. Subsequently, it has been found that several other important growth factor receptors, including those for insulin,[51] insulin-like growth factor I (IGF-I),[52] and PDGF[53] are also tyrosine kinases (i.e., they induce phosphorylation of tyrosine residues on target proteins). Moreover, it is now known that the gene products of numerous oncogenes other than src, including the fps, yes, ros, abl, and fes genes, are also tyrosine kinases.[6,16]

In 1983, a second major discovery linking growth factors and oncogenes was announced independently by two research groups. They found that the simian sarcoma virus (sis) oncogene codes for the production of a polypeptide that has striking sequence homology with the B chain of PDGF.[54,55] Further studies have confirmed the importance of this work, and it is now known that the N-terminal 109 amino acid residues of the B chain of PDGF are almost identical with the sequence of the transforming protein produced by simian sarcoma virus.[56]

A third important discovery linking growth factors and oncogenes was the 1984 report of major sequence homology

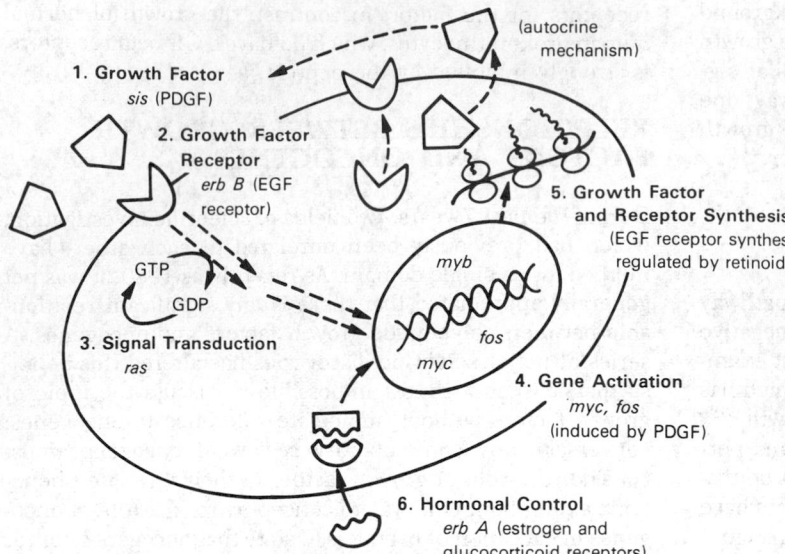

FIG. 5-5. Hierarchic levels of interaction between growth factors and oncogenes. Many oncogenes activate biochemical pathways that facilitate expression of peptide growth factors in an autocrine loop; intermediates include the growth factors (process 1), their receptors (process 2), and signalling pathways (processes 3 and 4). Also shown are mechanisms whereby growth-regulatory molecules such as retinoids and steroids interact with oncogenes and peptide growth factors (processes 5 and 6).

between the receptor for EGF and the viral *erbB* oncogene.[57,58] In this case, the viral oncogene codes for a protein that strikingly resembles the transmembrane and cytoplasmic (tyrosine kinase) domains of the EGF receptor. The protein encoded by *erb*B lacks the portion of the EGF receptor believed to be responsible for the extracellular binding of the ligand, EGF, to the receptor itself. This virally coded "truncated receptor" is believed to be able to generate a mitogenic signal, even in the absence of its natural ligand. It is as if the truncation of the receptor has short-circuited the normal physiologic mechanism for controlling its activity, and the truncated receptor is now permanently turned on, even though no EGF may be present.

A fourth major advance was the demonstration that a specific growth factor, PDGF, can control the expression of specific oncogenes, *myc* and *fos*.[59-61] *Myc* and *fos* both code for nuclear proteins that are believed to have some critical function, as yet unknown, in control of the cell cycle.[62] In particular, the expression of *myc* in turn appears to make a cell more sensitive to the effects of other growth factors, such as EGF.[63] It had been known for some time from the work of Stiles and colleagues[64] that PDGF exerts a permissive action for other growth factors such as EGF or IGF-I. The terms competence and progression have been used to describe this phenomenon, implying that PDGF induces a state of competence in the cell, so that it can respond to a mitogen such as EGF or IGF-I and progress through the cell cycle. The discovery that the action of two oncogenes, *myc* and *fos*, are involved in this process, is yet another example of intimate relationships between growth factors and oncogenes.

These four discoveries have had an overwhelming impact on growth factor and oncogene research. They have made clear that it is no longer possible to separate the two fields conceptually and that the most likely path for future advances will be elucidation of the various mechanisms whereby growth factors control the expression of oncogenes,

and oncogenes in turn control the expression of growth factors.

PROPERTIES OF SPECIFIC GROWTH FACTORS: RELEVANCE TO CANCER

Specific, well-defined polypeptide growth factors play a prominent role in control of cellular proliferation, cellular differentiation, and cellular function.[5,6,12,16] A tumor is a complex tissue composed not only of the tumor cells themselves but also of the stromal elements, including inflammatory cells, fibroblasts, and endothelial cells.[38,39] Therefore, consideration of the roles that these growth factors play in carcinogenesis must take into account which specific cell types are secreting a particular growth factor and which specific cells types can respond to the growth factor. In some instances, stimulation of the proliferation of tumor cells by growth factors may be a direct result of autocrine action of these peptides on the tumor cells; however, in other cases it may be indirect via paracrine stimulation of the supporting stromal elements, as evidenced by increased elaboration of connective tissue and increased neovascularization, or by suppression of immune surveillance. Table 5-1 provides a selected listing of several of the most thoroughly characterized of these peptides that have been demonstrated to play a role in cellular transformation. It is not meant to be comprehensive because peptides such as colony stimulating factors, interleukins, and interferons, which principally control the function of cells of haematopoietic lineages, will not be considered in this chapter. Categorization of polypeptide growth factors into families is based on their chemical structure; receptor and antibody cross-reactivity also may be found within families of growth factors. A brief discussion of each family of growth factors and its mechanistic link to carcinogenesis follows.

TABLE 5-1. Polypeptide Growth Factors Related to Transformation

Growth Factor	Source	Target Tissue	Biological Activity	Molecular Weight (daltons)		Human Chromosomal Location		References (cloning)
				Growth Factor	Membrane Receptor	Growth Factor	Receptor	
Insulin Family								
Insulin	β-Islet cells of pancreas	Liver, adipose, muscle	Supports growth, modulates metabolism of lipids, amino acids, and sugars	5,800	350,000	11	19	(171,172)
IGF-1 and IGF-II	Human plasma	Liver, adipose, muscle, cartilage, fibroblasts	Insulin-like metabolic effects; mitogens; stimulate incorporation of sulfate into cartilage proteoglycans	I:7,600 II:7,500	I:350,000 II:250,000	12 11	15 ?	(173,174) (175,176)
EGF Family								
EGF	Mouse submaxilary gland, human urine	Epidermal cells, fibroblasts, epithelial cells	Mitogen, promotes keratinization, inhibits gastric acid secretion	6,200	180,000	4	7	(86,87)
TGF-alpha	Transformed cells	Identical to EGF	Identical to EGF	5,500	180,000	2	7	(178)
PDGF Family								
Dimers of A and B chains	α-Granules platelets	Fibroblasts, smooth muscle cells, glial	Supports growth of various mesenchymal cells, chemotactic agent	28,000– 35,000	200,000	A: 7 B: 22	5 5	(107) (54,55)
TGF-beta Family								
TGF-beta 1 and 2	α-Granules platelets	All cell types	Often inhibits growth, augments matrix accumulation, chemotactic	25,000	500,000	1: 19 2: ?	? ?	(179) (180*)
MIS	Testis	Müllerian duct	Inhibits growth of cells derived from the Müllerian duct	54,000	?	?	?	(121)
FGF Family								
aFGF	Brain	All cell types	Mitogenic for cells of mesodermal and neuroectodermal origin	17,000	125,000	5	?	(134)
bFGF	Pituitary			17,000	145,000	4	?	(133)

(continued)

TABLE 5-1. Polypeptide Growth Factors Related to Transformation *(Continued)*

Growth Factor	Source	Target Tissue	Biological Activity	Molecular Weight (daltons)		Human Chromosomal Location		References (cloning)
				Growth Factor	Membrane Receptor	Growth Factor	Receptor	
Bombesin/GRP								
Bombesin	Frog skin	Many epithelial and mesenchymal cells	Mitogenic for gastrointestinal, respiratory tract, and 3T3 cells	1,400	?	?	?	(181*)
GRP	Porcine gut			2,700	?	?	?	(139*)

*Reference to amino acid sequence.

INSULIN FAMILY

Several polypeptide growth factors belong to the insulin family, including, in addition to insulin, the insulin-like growth factors IGF-I and IGF-II, nerve growth factor (NGF), and relaxin.[65-68] Human somatomedin C has been shown to be identical with IGF-I.[69] Of these five peptides, all except relaxin have been implicated in carcinogenesis. Insulin and the IGFs have similar biologic activities (generally stimulating growth and cellular metabolism) and a high degree of structural relatedness, including conservation of all three disulfide bonds.[70] The insulin and IGF-I receptors have a similar subunit structure, and the two ligands show a limited degree of receptor cross-reactivity.[13,14] Each receptor has associated with it tyrosine kinase activity that when activated leads to phosphorylation of various cellular proteins including autophosphorylation of the beta subunits of the receptors for both of these peptides (the ligand binding sites are on the alpha subunits). In contrast, the IGF-II receptor has a distinct structure and no associated tyrosine kinase activity[13,14,71]; it cannot bind insulin, even with low affinity. However, treatment of responsive cells with insulin increases expression of IGF-II receptors. Thus the action of these three growth factors on cells is highly cooperative, given the receptor cross-reactivity and the inducibility of the IGF-II receptor by insulin.

There is now substantial evidence suggesting an involvement of IGF-II in a variety of embryonal neoplasms. Wilms' tumor (nephroblastoma), rhabdomyosarcoma, and hepatoblastoma all express significantly elevated levels of IGF-II mRNA relative to nonmalignant adult tissues.[72,73] The level of expression in the tumors is similar to that found in fetal tissues, consistent with the observations that IGF-II plays an important role in embryonic development.[74,75] The IGF-II gene has been localized to chromosome 11p, and loss of heterozygosity for 11p markers has been demonstrated in all three of these tumors that express elevated levels of IGF-II mRNA.[72,73] A human fibrosarcoma cell line that secretes IGF-II has also been described.[76] Whether IGF-II may contribute to the growth of any of these tumors is not known; however, it is to be expected that constitutive synthesis of a mitogenic peptide could provide a cell with significant growth advantage. Exogenous IGF-II can also act as a transforming growth factor in that it can induce phenotypic transformation of untransformed Balb/c cells as measured by their growth as colonies of cells in soft agar medium.[77]

Insulin is permissive for the actions of several polypeptide growth factors on cells in addition to IGF-II.[78,79] Also, both insulin and IGF-I receptors have tyrosine kinase activity that has specific features in common with the tyrosine kinase coded by the Rous sarcoma virus *src* oncogene.[51,52] Thus, in chick heart mesenchymal cells, insulin and EGF, which also stimulates tyrosine kinase activity, synergize to stimulate growth at the same level found in cells infected with Rous sarcoma virus.[80-82]

NGF, a structural homologue of proinsulin, binds to a unique receptor. Although its effects on growth of sympathetic neurons are well understood, the role of its increased secretion by a variety of tumor cells including melanoma, fibrosarcoma, and glioblastoma cells is not currently known.[67]

EPIDERMAL GROWTH FACTOR FAMILY

In addition to EGF (also called urogastrone), this family comprises the TGF-alphas[33,83-85] and possibly other less well-characterized peptides including putative EGF-like molecules encoded in the large messenger RNA transcript for EGF.[86,87] Two protein products of members of the poxvirus family, vaccinia virus protein[88] and a protein encoded by the Shope fibroma virus[89] also have significant homology to EGF and TGF-alpha in their amino acid sequences. Although the various members of this growth factor family share only limited amino acid sequence homology, the positions of all three disulfide bonds are conserved, as was found to be the case in the insulin family of growth factors.

With regard to the EGF family, there has thus far been identified only a single receptor species, the well-characterized EGF receptor, which binds all members of the family with nearly equal affinities[33,88-91]; thus, the infectivity of vaccinia virus can be blocked by pretreatment of the cells with EGF.[92] Like the insulin and IGF-I receptors, this receptor also has intrinsic tyrosine kinase activity that is activated by binding of its ligand; this kinase again has specific features in common with the tyrosine kinase domain of the *src* family of oncogenes.[48-50] All members of the family of tyrosine kinase associated oncogenes, including *src, fes, fps, fgr, abl*, and *erbB*, have in common a region of 250 amino acids which comprise the protein kinase domain. Moreover, the *erbB* oncogene of avian erythroblastosis virus has been shown to specifically represent the transmembrane portions and tyrosine kinase domains of the EGF receptor.[57,93-94] In the case of v-*erbB*, the extracellular ligand binding domain is missing from the receptor, leading to constitutive activation of the receptor in the absence of ligand binding.

Different types of human tumor cells overexpress the EGF receptor; these include glioblastomas and several squamous epidermoid carcinomas, of which the A431 cell line is representative.[41,95,96] In brain tumors of glial origin and in A431 cells there is amplification and rearrangement of the gene encoding the EGF receptor.[97] It is not known whether this plays a role in the development of the malignancy. However, a characteristic feature of human glioblastomas is an increase in the number of copies of chromosome 7, often with rearrangements[98]; since the EGF receptor maps to the short arm of chromosome 7, a relationship between effects on the EGF receptor and the malignant phenotype might be expected.[97]

Both EGF and TGF-alpha usually stimulate proliferation of target cells, and overexpression of either of these peptides has, in certain instances, been correlated with transformation. TGF-alpha was named on the basis of its ability to induce phenotypic transformation of non-neoplastic fibroblasts,[85] and EGF can potentiate the viral and chemical transformation of cultured cells.[99-101] Certain retrovirus-transformed cells and human tumor cell lines synthesize TGF-alpha, whereas their untransformed counterparts do not.[83,85,102] In addition, higher molecular weight peptides related to TGF-alpha are secreted in the urine of patients with tumors but not of controls.[103] However, the original concept that TGF-alpha secretion would be restricted to tumor cells has been disproved; TGF-alpha is secreted by normal bovine anterior pituitary cells in culture,[104,105] and transcriptional activity of TGF-alpha is high in the early mouse embryo.[106]

PLATELET-DERIVED GROWTH FACTOR FAMILY

This family of growth factors appears to be restricted to three homodimeric and heterodimeric combinations (AA,AB,BB) of the A and B chains of PDGF, each of which can cross-react with the same PDGF receptor, and each of which appears to have similar activity in stimulating growth of responsive cells.[24,107] The B chain of PDGF is 96% homologous with the putative transforming protein (p28*sis*) of simian sarcoma virus (SSV),[54,55] and many different lines of evidence show that transformation induced by SSV is mediated by a PDGF-like growth factor.[24,36] To date, the PDGF B chain homodimer is the only growth factor for which there has been identified a corresponding oncogene product. The genes for both the B and the A chains of PDGF are expressed in tumor cells, principally glioma and osteosarcoma cell lines, although some tumor cells express exclusively A chain or B chain transcripts.[107] As with TGF-alpha, elevated urinary levels of proteins antigenically related to PDGF have been associated with some cancer patients.[108] However, secretion of PDGF is not unique to cancer cells; many normal cells also express these transcripts. Thus, activated macrophages express PDGF B chain transcripts, whereas rat skeletal myoblasts and arterial smooth muscle cells express only PDGF A chain transcripts.[109] Interestingly, a different splicing pattern of the A chain RNA has been found in glioma cells, which may lead to preferential secretion of A chain homodimers with markedly enhanced mitogenic activity.[110,111]

Like the other growth factor receptors described thus far, the PDGF receptor also has associated tyrosine kinase activity.[53,112,113] However, in contrast to the receptors for the insulin, EGF, and TGF-beta families of growth factors, which are more or less ubiquitous, PDGF receptor expression is highest in connective tissue cells, vascular smooth muscle cells, and glial cells; it is never found associated with epithelial or endothelial cells.[112] Nonetheless, PDGF secretion by tumor cells is not restricted to PDGF-responsive cells such as glioblastoma and sarcoma cells; certain bladder carcinoma cells, erythroleukemic cells, and leukemia cells, which do not display PDGF receptors, also secrete PDGF-like peptides.[24] This suggests either that secretion of PDGF by these cells is irrelevant to their transformation or that it may support tumor growth indirectly by acting on responsive connective tissue cells in the tumor stroma, as will be discussed in greater detail later.

TRANSFORMING GROWTH FACTOR-BETA FAMILY

The largest growth factor family is that of peptides structurally related to TGF-beta in terms of the homologous positioning of seven to nine cysteine residues, and recent discoveries suggest that yet more family members may be found.[25,114,115] Like PDGF, TGF-beta can exist in both homodimeric and heterodimeric combinations of TGF-beta 1 and 2 chains,[114] and the biologic activity of the dimers is identical in most systems studied[114,116] with only a few exceptions.[117] Other members of the family include the mammalian inhibins[118] and activins,[119,120] mullerian inhibitory substance (MIS),[121] and the predicted products of a pattern gene in *Drosophila* (decapentaplegic gene complex, DPP-C)[122] and of an amphibian gene, Vg1, expressed in oocytes.[123] Thus far, only TGF-beta 1 and 2 and MIS have been implicated in carcinogenesis.

The biologic activities of the TGF-betas are extremely diverse[25,115]; however, unlike the previously described growth factors, TGF-betas often inhibit cell growth and block the action of peptides belonging to the insulin, EGF, and PDGF families. TGF-beta is thought to play an important role in maintaining quiescence in adult tissues, being turned off during specific bursts of growth such as in the pubescent mammary gland[124] or in the regenerating liver.[125] Many of its effects are probably mediated through specific effects on elaboration of extracellular matrix proteins.[25,115]

TGF-beta 1 and 2 react with a unique cell membrane receptor[116,126] that is not yet well characterized like those of the insulin, EGF, and PDGF families, all of which have been cloned and sequenced. However, data suggest that it does not have an associated tyrosine kinase activity[127,128] and therefore probably signals through different intracellular pathways. The TGF-beta receptor is expressed on nearly all cell types, and transformed cells that overexpress the receptor have not been found.[45] Rather, control of TGF-beta activity probably is at the level of activation of the biologically inactive, latent, secreted form of TGF-beta.[45] Many tumors cells exhibit high levels of TGF-beta mRNA,[129] and most tumor cell lines secrete TGF-beta; however, these tumor cells are often refractory to growth control by the TGF-beta they secrete. For example, in human A549 lung carcinoma cells it has been shown that the uncontrolled growth of the cells results from their inability to activate the latent TGF-beta they secrete; growth of the cells is strongly inhibited by activated TGF-beta.[45] Other malignant cells seem to have escaped from the growth-inhibitory actions of TGF-beta by other mechanisms, since they are no longer responsive to active TGF-beta, in contrast to their untransformed counterparts that are inhibited by TGF-beta.[46,47] For these reasons, it has been suggested that TGF-beta secreted by tumor cells may support their growth indirectly by stimulating formation of tumor stroma.[115]

Another member of the TGF-beta family, MIS, a testicular product that causes regression of the mullerian ducts (the anlage of the female reproductive system) in the male embryo,[121] has been found to be inhibitory to the growth of epithelial ovarian carcinomas derived from these tissues.[130,131] Neoplastic progression of the serosal surface of the ovary in the adult recapitulates the development of the embryonic mullerian ducts. This finding suggests that MIS, as well as other yet undiscovered embryonic inhibitors, may herald a new therapeutic approach to tumors derived from their corresponding target tissues.[130]

FIBROBLAST GROWTH FACTOR FAMILY

Basic and acidic fibroblast growth factor (bFGF; aFGF) are two closely related single-chain peptides of approximately 16 kDa that act principally to stimulate mitogenesis in cells of mesodermal and neuroectodermal origin.[40,132] They are probably the most potent known stimulators of the growth of endothelial cells and as such have been postulated to play a role in neovascularization in vivo. Since the cloning and sequencing of the FGFs,[133,134] it has become apparent that many peptides of different cellular origin and ostensibly different biological activities are actually identical to the FGFs.[135] bFGF is synthesized by a wide variety of both normal and transformed cells, including chondrosarcoma, melanoma, rhabdomyosarcoma, hepatoma, retinoblastoma, and osteosarcoma; synthesis of aFGF appears to be more restricted but is also found in both normal and transformed cells. FGFs have high affinity for heparin, a property that has aided significantly in the purification of these peptides.[132] Evidence also suggests that FGF secreted from cells may be integrally associated with extracellular matrix, possibly complexed to heparan sulfate.[136] Both FGFs bind to the same receptors, glycosylated species of 125 and 145 kDa, although there is some evidence for preferential binding of aFGF and bFGF, respectively.[137] These receptors, like those for other mitogenic peptides such as insulin, EGF, and PDGF, are linked to tyrosine kinase activity.[138]

Although direct evidence is lacking, it seems clear that FGF will play a role in tumorigenesis. It is secreted by a wide variety of tumor cells, is a potent mitogen for many cell types of mesenchymal origin, and can stimulate angiogenesis. It may have autocrine effects on proliferation of tumor cells, as well as paracrine effects by stimulation of the neovascularization of the tumor.[40,135,136]

BOMBESIN/GASTRIN-RELEASING PEPTIDE

Bombesin is a tetradecapeptide purified initially from frog skin; it is homologous to the mammalian peptide gastrin-releasing peptide (GRP) that contains 27 amino acids[35,139]; both bind to the same receptor and elicit identical biological activities, including mitogenesis. There is clear evidence that these very small peptides play a pivotal role in control of the growth of human SCLCs.[35] These tumors have long been known to secrete a variety of regulatory peptides, including GRP. The central role of this peptide in autocrine control of tumor growth has been demonstrated by the finding that specific blocking monoclonal antibodies to GRP block both the clonal growth of SCLC in vitro and the growth of SCLC xenografts in vivo (see Fig. 5-2).[140] As in previous examples, it has been postulated that the role of GRP in SCLC reflects its possible role in fetal lung development. This is the first direct evidence that blocking of the autocrine action of a tumor cell mitogen might be useful therapeutically and suggests that peptide antagonists and antibodies that bind to growth factor receptors might be equally useful.

COOPERATIVE INTERACTIONS OF GROWTH FACTORS RELEVANT TO TRANSFORMATION

DIRECT FUNCTIONAL INTERACTIONS OF POLYPEPTIDE GROWTH FACTORS

Many polypeptide growth factors belonging to different structural families are functionally interactive.[141] Thus three distinct peptides—TGF-beta, a peptide related to EGF/TGF-alpha, and PDGF—all found in human platelets, cooperate in inducing phenotypic transformation of nonneoplastic fibroblasts.[142] The transformation response depends on the concentration of each of the three growth factors, and the aberrant expression of any one of them will predispose to transformation.[142] Conversely, as shown by the ability of monoclonal antibodies to bombesin/GRP to block growth of SCLC cells[140] and of monoclonal antibodies to the EGF receptor to block anchorage independent growth of fibroblastic indicator cells induced by the combined actions of EGF and TGF-beta,[143] blocking of one of the obligatory growth factors in a set is sufficient to block the response. Not only are many biological responses the result of the action of a set of growth factors, but also the direction of the response is determined by the particular set of growth factors acting on the cells, not by any intrinsic activity of the individual peptides. Thus, in fibroblasts transfected with a *myc* oncogene, it has been demonstrated that TGF-beta inhibits the formation of colonies of the cells in the presence of EGF but stimulates the formation of colonies of the cells in the presence of PDGF.[20] Finally, there is evidence that functionally interactive growth factors can alter either receptor number or receptor affinity for other members of the set. This inter-receptor communication represents another mechanism for regulation of cellular response patterns.[14,141] Thus TGF-beta can induce the synthesis of cellular receptors for EGF and increase the sensitivity of the cellular response to EGF,[144] and insulin can increase cellular binding of IGF-II.[14] These examples of the obligatory nature of direct cooperative interactions between growth factors suggest possible therapeutic applications.

INDIRECT INTERACTIONS OF GROWTH FACTORS

In addition to cooperative interactions of several growth factors on a particular target cell, the complex nature of tumor tissue suggests that indirect cooperative interactions of several growth factors, each acting on different target cells found within the tumor, can have significant consequences for tumor growth; nontumor target cells include inflammatory cells, fibroblasts, and endothelial cells, all components of tumor stroma.[38,39] Suppression by growth factors of immune surveillance and enhancement of connective tissue and neovascularization can all stimulate tumorigenesis. In this regard, TGF-beta, which is secreted by many tumor cells, has been shown to inhibit growth and expression of differentiated function by all lymphocytic cells, including T-cells,[145] B-cells,[146] cytotoxic killer cells,[147] and lymphokine activated killer cells[148]; to activate fibroblasts to synthesize connective tissue proteins, including type I collagen, fibronectin, and proteoglycans[25,115]; and to stimulate angiogenesis in vivo.[149] Moreover, PDGF and FGF both stimulate proliferation of fibroblasts,[24] while FGF is thought to be the principal endothelial cell mitogen.[136]

The importance of angiogenesis on tumor growth should not be underestimated. It has been known for a long time that tumors implanted into perfused tissues in which mechanisms of neovascularization have degenerated will remain viable but static until reimplanted into an environment in which the tumor can become vascularized.[150] Although FGF is the principal endothelial cell mitogen,[136] TGF-beta has also been shown to stimulate angiogenesis in vivo.[149] Another peptide, angiogenin, isolated from medium conditioned by a human adenocarcinoma cell line, is active in two models of angiogenesis, the chick embryo chorioallantoic membrane assay and the rabbit corneal pocket assay,[151–153] but whether it plays a role in tumor angiogenesis is not known.[154] Control of angiogenesis has been suggested as an alternative therapeutic approach to control of tumor growth.[155,156]

It has been proposed that excessive stimulation of connective tissue by growth factors secreted by tumor cells could contribute to desmoplasia, an increase in connective tissue formation in the immediate vicinity of tumor cells, found most often in malignancies such as melanoma, colorectal carcinoma, and scirrhous carcinoma of the breast.[157] Effects of both TGF-beta[25,115] and PDGF[24] on connective tissue suggest that action of these two growth factors may be found to be associated with desmoplasia. In addition to effects of growth factors, connective tissue proteins themselves may contribute to regulation of tumor cell growth. Thus both collagen fragments and fibronectin are chemotactic for mesenchymal cells,[158] and fibronectin has been shown to stimulate both proliferation and differentiation of certain mesenchymal cells.[159,160] Polymers, too, such as heparin secreted by mast cells, have been suggested to further stimulate neovascularization of tumors.[161]

Yet another aspect of indirect effects of growth factors on tumor growth is their ability to stimulate the migration of different cell types toward a tumor and then activate those cells to produce yet other growth factors. For example, both TGF-beta and PDGF, secreted by tumor cells that themselves might not be responsive to the factors, have chemotactic activity for monocytes, fibroblasts, and smooth muscle cells.[24,25] Both TGF-beta and PDGF, at somewhat higher concentrations, then activate monocytes to secrete other mitogens such as interleukin-1 beta,[162] which acts on fibroblasts. Yet another mechanism for perpetuating growth factor action in tumor stroma is the secretion of growth factors by activated inflammatory cells; thus activated macrophages have been shown to secrete both PDGF and TGF-beta,[163,164] and activated T-lymphocytes also secrete TGF-beta.[145]

In summary, it is clear that growth factors can act at many different levels to modulate carcinogenesis and that understanding of their roles in this process involves consideration of their actions not only on the tumor cells but also on stromal elements of the tumor. Moreover, to understand the complex role of growth factors in this process, it is necessary to consider not only growth factor secretion by the tumor cells but also growth factor secretion by other cell types in the tumor mass.

INHIBITION OF THE ACTION OF POSITIVE GROWTH FACTORS AS A THERAPEUTIC APPROACH TO CANCER

The hope that it will eventually be possible to control growth factor synthesis and expression has given a new rationale to approaching cancer therapy. The autocrine hypothesis provides a conceptual framework for designing new therapeutic agents.[27] One direct new approach to therapy would be to control autocrine growth factor pathways by preventing interactions of the effector polypeptide with its receptor. This could be accomplished in three ways: action of the growth factor could be blocked by use of specific antibodies to the growth factor which bind to its active site; binding of the growth factor to its receptor could be blocked by antibodies to the receptor; or an extracellular antagonist of a presumed autocrine polypeptide, which would compete for receptor binding (but not be functionally active upon binding), could be used. The first approach has recently been accomplished in an experimental model by using monoclonal antibodies to the tetradecapeptide bombesin, which is produced and released by most human small cell lung cancer cells (oat cell cancers). As discussed earlier in this chapter, these highly malignant cells have functional receptors for this peptide and release it in large quantities.[35] Monoclonal antibodies raised against bombesin not only inhibit the binding of bombesin to its receptor but also markedly inhibit both the growth of lung cancer cells in vitro and their ability to form tumors in nude mice (see Fig. 5-2).[140] As an example of the second approach, monoclonal antibodies raised to the EGF receptors of the human epidermoid carcinoma cell line, A431, compete with EGF for receptor binding, and both block the proliferation of the cells in culture and inhibit A431 tumor growth in nude mice.[165] It is clear that these types of experiments provide a paradigm for other growth factors that are presumed to act by an autocrine mechanism and that antibodies against either growth factors or growth factor receptors could potentially prove to be therapeutically useful.

The other approach, that of developing growth factor antagonists, is still untested, but the cloned genes, which are available for many growth factors, should be amenable to methods of in vitro site-directed mutagenesis. In this way, specific amino acid substitutions can be made at any locus in a growth factor molecule. Such mutated growth factors can then be screened for potential antagonist activity. The potential usefulness of such an approach has been demonstrated in several instances with human insulin, where it has been shown that a mutational substitution of a single amino acid in a critical location can convert an agonist to an antagonist. (In these cases the mutations occurred naturally, and the patients with such mutations had clinical diabetes.[166-167]) Thus, although this has not yet been done successfully with other growth factors, recombinant DNA technology has made this a practical laboratory problem.

ENHANCEMENT OF THE ACTION OF NEGATIVE GROWTH FACTORS FOR PREVENTION OF CANCER

In the previous section, we have discussed the possible use of antagonists of positive growth factors as a means to arrest the growth of cancer cells. The discovery of negative autocrine growth factors now opens up a new approach to the cancer problem, particularly for the prevention of cancer. Thus, we would propose that any drug or biological response modifier that could potentially increase the activity of a negative growth factor could represent a practical approach to the prevention of cancer, particularly since preneoplastic cells are more sensitive to the action of negative autocrine factors than their malignant counterparts. One important advance in this regard is the recent demonstration that the estradiol antagonist tamoxifen markedly increases the secretion of TGF-beta in estrogen-sensitive human MCF-7 breast carcinoma cells[168]; this increase in TGF-beta has been linked to a suppression of growth in these cells. These studies demonstrate that increasing the activity of a negative autocrine factor by use of an estrogen analogue is one possible mechanism that can be exploited for control of epithelial cell growth; they are of obvious relevance to animal experiments that have shown that tamoxifen can prevent experimental mammary cancer in rats[169] or to the potential clinical use of tamoxifen to prevent breast cancer in women at high risk.[170]

REFERENCES

1. Pierce GB, Shikes R, Fink LM: Cancer: A Problem of Developmental Biology. Englewood Cliffs, NJ, Prentice-Hall, 1978
2. Mintz BH, Fleischman RA: Teratocarcinomas and other neoplasms as developmental defects in gene expression. Adv Cancer Res 34:211–278, 1981
3. Sachs L: Control of normal cell differentiation and the phenotypic reversion of malignancy in myeloid leukemia. Nature 274:535–539, 1978
4. Sporn MB, Roberts AB: Peptide growth factors and inflammation, tissue repair, and cancer. J Clin Invest 78:329–332, 1986
5. Goustin AS, Leof EB, Shipley GD, et al: Growth factors and cancer. Cancer Res 46:1015–1029, 1986
6. Heldin CH, Westermark B: Growth factors: Mechanism of action and relation to oncogenes. Cell 37:9–20, 1984
7. Bishop JM: Retroviruses and cancer genes. Adv Cancer Res 37:1–32, 1982
8. Land H, Parada LF, Weinberg RA: Tumorigenic conversion of primary embryo fibroblasts requires at least two cooperating oncogenes. Nature 304:596–602, 1983
9. Ruley HE: Adenovirus early region 1A enables viral and cellular transforming genes to transform primary cells in culture. Nature 304:602–606, 1983
10. Land H, Parada LF, Weinberg RA: Cellular oncogenes and multistep carcinogenesis. Science 222:771–778, 1983
11. Roberts AB, Sporn MB: Growth factors and transformation. Cancer Surv 5:405–412, 1986
12. James R, Bradshaw RA: Polypeptide growth factors. Annu Rev Biochem 53:259–292, 1984
13. Rechler MM, Nissley SP: The nature and regulation of the receptors for insulin-like growth factors. Annu Rev Physiol 47:425–442, 1985
14. Czech MP: New perspectives on the mechanisms of insulin action. Recent Prog Hormone Res 40:347–377, 1984
15. Roth J: Insulin binding to its receptor: Is the receptor more important that the hormone? Diabetes Care 4:27–32, 1981
16. Kris RM, Libermann TA, Avivi A, et al: Growth factors, growth-factor receptors and oncogenes. Biotechnol: 1:135–140, 1985
17. Sporn MB, Roberts AB: Peptide growth factors are multifunctional. Nature 332:217–219, 1988
18. Fallon JH, Seroogy KB, Loughlin SE, et al: Epidermal growth factor immunoreactive material in the central nervous system: Location and development. Science 224:1107–1109, 1984
19. Dockray GJ: Evolutionary relationships of the gut hormones. Fed Proc 38:2295–2301, 1979
20. Roberts AB, Anzano MA, Wakefield LM, et al: Type Beta transforming growth factor: A bifunctional regulator of cellular growth. Proc Natl Acad Sci USA 82:119–123, 1985
21. Carpenter G, Cohen S: Epidermal growth factor. Annu Rev Biochem 48:193–216, 1979
22. Hollenberg MD: Epidermal growth factor-urogastrone, a polypeptide acquiring hormonal status. Vitam Horm 37:69–110, 1979
23. Gill GN, Lazar CS: Increased phosphotyrosine content and inhibition of proliferation in EGF-treated A431 cells. Nature 293:305–307, 1981
24. Ross R, Raines EW, Bowen-Pope DF: The biology of platelet-derived growth factor. Cell 46:155–169, 1986
25. Sporn MB, Roberts AB, Wakefield LM, et al: Some recent advances in the chemistry and biology of transforming growth factor-beta. J Cell Biol 105:1039–1045, 1987
26. Sporn MB, Todaro GJ: Autocrine secretion and malignant transformation of cells. New Engl J Med 308:878–880, 1980
27. Sporn MB, Roberts AB: Autocrine growth factors and cancer. Nature 313:747–751, 1985
28. Sporn MB, Roberts AB: Autocrine, paracrine and endocrine mechanisms of growth control. Cancer Surv 4:627–632, 1985
29. Temin HM: Studies on carcinogenesis by avian sarcoma viruses VI. Differential multiplication of uninfected and of converted cells in response to insulin. J Cell Physiol 69:377–384, 1967
30. Holley RW: Control of growth of mammalian cells in cell culture. Nature 258:487–490, 1975
31. De Larco JE, Todaro GJ: Growth factors from murine sarcoma virus-transformed cells. Proc Natl Acad Sci USA 75:4001–4005, 1978
32. Roberts AB, Sporn MB: Transforming growth factors. Cancer Surv 4:683–705, 1985
33. Todaro GJ, Lee DC, Webb NR, et al: Rat type-alpha transforming growth factor: Structure and possible function as a membrane receptor. Cancer Cells 3:51–58, 1985
34. Williams LT: The sis gene and PDGF. Cancer Surv 5:233–241, 1986
35. Cuttitta F, Carney DN, Mulshine J, et al: Autocrine growth factors in human small cell lung cancer. Cancer Surv 4:707–727, 1985
36. Johnsson A, Betsholtz C, Heldin C-H, et al: Antibodies against platelet-derived growth factor inhibit acute transformation by simian sarcoma virus. Nature 317:438–442, 1985
37. Seifert RA, Schwartz SM, Bowen-Pope DF: Developmentally regulated production of platelet derived growth factor-like molecules. Nature 311:669–671, 1984
38. Dvorak HF: Tumors: Wounds that do not heal. New Engl J Med 315:1650–1659, 1986
39. Haddow A: Molecular repair, wound healing, and carcinogenesis: Tumor production a possible overhealing? Adv Cancer Res 16:181–234, 1972
40. Gospodarowicz D, Neufeld G, Schweigerer L: Molecular and biological characterization of fibroblast growth factor: An angiogenic factor which also controls the proliferation and differentiation of mesoderm and neuroectoderm derived cells. Cell Differ 19:1–17, 1986
41. Cowley G, Smith J, Gusterson B, et al: The EGF receptor is expressed at high levels on squamous cell carcinomas. Cancer Cells 1:5–10, 1984
42. Kawamoto T, Sato JD, Le A, et al: Growth stimulation of A431 cells by epidermal growth factor: Identification of high-affinity receptors for epidermal growth factor by an anti-receptor monoclonal antibody. Proc Natl Acad Sci USA 80:1337–1341, 1983
43. Holley RW: Control of animal cell proliferation. J Supramolec Struct 13:191–197, 1980
44. Tucker RF, Shipley GD, Moses HL, et al: Growth inhibitor from BSC-1 cells closely related to those isolated from tumor cells. Science 226:705–707, 1984
45. Wakefield LM, Smith DM, Masui T, et al: Distribution and modulation of the cellular receptor for transforming growth factor-beta. J Cell Biol 105:965–975, 1987
46. McMahon JB, Richards WL, del Campo AA, et al: Differential effects of transforming growth factor-beta on proliferation of normal and malignant rat liver epithelial cells in culture. Cancer Res 46:4665–4671, 1986
47. Shipley GD, Pittelkow MR, Wille JJ Jr, et al: Reversible inhibition of normal human prokeratinocyte proliferation by type beta transforming growth factor-growth inhibitor in serum-free medium. Cancer Res 46:2068–2071, 1986

48. Chinkers M, Cohen S: Purified EGF receptor-kinase interacts specifically with antibodies to Rous sarcoma virus transforming protein. Nature 290:516–519, 1981

49. Erikson E, Shealy DJ, Erikson RL: Evidence that viral transforming gene products and epidermal growth factor stimulate phosphorylation of the same cellular protein with similar specificity. J Biol Chem 256:11381–11384, 1981

50. Cooper JA, Hunter T: Similarities and differences between the effects of epidermal growth factor and Rous sarcoma virus. J Cell Biol 91:878–883, 1981

51. Kasuga M, Fujita-Yamaguchi Y, Blithe M, et al: Characterization of the insulin receptor kinase purified from human placental membranes. J Biol Chem 258:10973–10980, 1983

52. Rubin JB, Shia MA, Pilch PR: Stimulation of tyrosine-specific phosphorylation in vitro by insulinlike growth factor I. Nature 305:438–440, 1983

53. Heldin C-H, Ek B, Ronnstrand L: Characterization of the receptor for platelet-derived growth factor on human fibroblasts. J Biol Chem 258:10054–10061, 1983

54. Doolittle RF, Hunkapiller MW, Hood LE, et al: Simian sarcoma virus onc gene, v-sis, is derived from the gene (genes) encoding a platelet-derived growth factor. Science 221:275–277, 1983

55. Waterfield MD, Scrace GT, Whittle N, et al: Platelet-derived growth factor is structurally related to the putative transforming protein p28^sis of simian sarcoma virus. Nature 304:35–39, 1983

56. Johnsson A, Heldin C-H, Wasteson A, et al: The c-sis gene encodes a precursor of the B chain of platelet-derived growth factor. EMBO J 3:921–928, 1984

57. Downward J, Yarden Y, Mayes E, et al: Close similarity of epidermal growth factor receptor and v-erb-B oncogene protein sequences. Nature 307:521–528, 1984

58. Martin GS: The erbB gene and the EGF receptor. Cancer Surv 5:199–219, 1986

59. Kelly K, Cochran BH, Stiles CD, et al: Cell-specific regulation of the c-myc gene by lymphocyte mitogens and platelet-derived growth factor. Cell 35:603–610, 1983

60. Greenberg ME, Ziff EB: Stimulation of 3T3 cells induces transcription of the c-fos proto-oncogene. Nature 311:433–438, 1984

61. Curran T, Bravo R, Muller R: Transient induction of c-fos and c-myc is an immediate consequence of growth factor stimulation. Cancer Surv 4:655–681, 1985

62. Eisenman RN, Thompson CB: Oncogenes with potential nuclear function: myc, myb and fos. Cancer Surv 5:309–327, 1986

63. Stern DL, Roberts AB, Roche NS, et al: Differential responsiveness of myc- and ras-transfected cells to growth factors: Selective stimulation of myc-transfected cells by EGF. Mol Cell Biol 6:870–877, 1986

64. Stiles CD, Capone GT, Scher CD, et al: Dual control of cell growth by somatomedins and platelet-derived growth factor. Proc Natl Acad Sci USA 76:1279–1283, 1979

65. Humbel RE, Bosshard HR, Zahn H: Chemistry of Insulin. In Greep RO, Astwood EB (eds): Handbook of Physiology, vol 1, pp 311–332. Washington, DC, American Physiological Society, 1972

66. Zapf J, Froesch ER, Humbel RE: The insulin-like growth factors (IGF) of human serum: Chemical and biological characterization and aspects of their possible physiological role. Curr Top Cell Regul 19:257–309, 1981

67. Bradshaw RA: Nerve growth factor. Annu Rev Biochem 47:191–216, 1978

68. Schwage C, Steinetz B, Weiss G, et al: Relaxin. Recent Prog Horm Res 34:123–211, 1978

69. Svoboda ME, Van Wyk JJ, Klapper DG, et al: Purification of somatomedin-C from human plasma: Chemical and biological properties, partial sequence analysis and relationship to other somatomedins. Biochemistry 19:790–797, 1980

70. Blundell TL, Bedarker S, Humbel RE: Teritary structures, receptor binding, and antigenicity of insulin-like growth factors. Fed Proc 42:2592–2597, 1983

71. Morgan DO, Edman JC, Standring DN, et al: Insulin-like growth factor II receptor as a multifunctional binding protein. Nature 329:301–397, 1987

72. Reeve AE, Eccles MR, Wilkins RJ, et al: Expression of insulin-like growth factor-II transcripts in Wilms' tumour. Nature 317:258–260, 1985

73. Scott J, Cowell J, Robertson ME, et al: Insulin-like growth factor-II gene expression in Wilms' tumour and embryonic tissue. Nature 317:260–262, 1985

74. Adams SO, Nissley SP, Handwerger S, et al: Developmental patterns of insulin-like growth factor-I and -II synthesis and regulation in rat fibroblasts. Nature 302:150–153, 1983

75. Han VKM, D'Ercole AJ, Lund PK: Cellular localization of somatomedin (insulin-like growth factor) messenger RNA in the human fetus. Science 236:193–197, 1987

76. Todaro GJ, De Larco JE, Marquardt H, et al: Polypeptide growth factors produced by tumor cells and virus-transformed cells: A possible growth advantage for the producer cells. Cold Spring Harbor Conferences on Cell Proliferation. 6:113–127, 1979

77. Massagué J, Kelly B, Mottola C: Stimulation by insulin-like growth factors is required for cellular transformation by type beta transforming growth factor. J Biol Chem 260:4551–4554, 1985

78. Oppenheimer CL, Pessin JE, Massague J, et al: Insulin action rapidly modulates the apparent affinity of the insulin-like growth factor II receptor. J Biol Chem 258:4824–4830, 1983

79. Rozengurt E: Early signals in the mitogenic response. Science 234:161–166, 1986

80. Carpenter G: The biochemistry and physiology of the receptor-kinase for epidermal growth factor. Mol Cell Endocrinol 31:1–19, 1983

81. Balk SD, Shiu RPC, LaFleur MM, et al: Epidermal growth factor and insulin cause normal chicken heart mesenchymal cells to proliferate like their Rous sarcoma virus-infected counterparts. Proc Natl Acad Sci USA 79:1154–1157, 1982

82. Soderquist AM, Carpenter G: Developments in the mechanism of growth factor action: Activation of protein kinase by epidermal growth factor. Fed Proc 42:2615–2620, 1983

83. Todaro GJ, Fryling C, De Larco JE: Transforming growth factors (TGFs) produced by certain human tumor cells: Polypeptides that interact with epidermal growth factor (EGF) receptors. Proc Natl Acad Sci USA 77:5258–5262, 1980

84. Marquardt H, Hunkapiller MW, Hood LE, et al: Transforming growth factors produced by retrovirus-transformed rodent fibroblasts and human melanoma cells: Amino acid sequence hormology with epidermal growth factor. Proc Natl Acad Sci USA 80:4684–4688, 1983

85. Roberts AB, Frolik CA, Anzano MA, et al: Transforming growth factors from neoplastic and non-neoplastic tissues. Fed Proc 42:2621–2626, 1983

86. Gray A, Dull TJ, Ullrich A: Nucleotide sequence of epidermal growth factor cDNA predicts a 128,000-molecular weight protein precursor. Nature 303:722–725, 1983

87. Scott J, Urdea M, Quiroga M, et al: Structure of a mouse submaxillary messenger RNA encoding epidermal growth factor and seven related proteins. Science 221:236–240, 1983

88. Blomquist MC, Hunt LT, Barker WC: Vaccinia virus 19-kilodalton protein: Relationship to several mammalian proteins, including two growth factors. Proc Natl Acad Sci USA 81:7363–7367, 1984

89. Chang W, Upton C, Hu S-L, et al: The genome of Shope fibroma virus, a tumorigenic poxvirus, contains a growth factor gene with sequence similarity to those encoding epidermal growth factor and transforming growth factor alpha. Mol Cell Biol 7:535–540, 1987

90. Marquardt H, Hunkapiller MW, Hood LE, et al: Rat transforming growth factor type I: Structure and relation to epidermal growth factor. Science 223:1079–1082, 1984

91. Stroobant P, Rice AP, Gullick WJ, et al: Purification and characterization of vaccinia virus growth factor. Cell 42:383–393, 1985

92. Eppstein DA, Marsh YV, Schreiber AB, et al: Epidermal growth factor receptor occupancy inhibits vaccinia virus infection. Nature 318:663–665, 1985

93. Privalsky ML, Ralston R, Bishop JM: The membrane glycoprotein encoded by the retroviral oncogene v-erb-B is structurally related to tyrosine-specific protein kinases. Proc Natl Acad Sci USA 81:704–707, 1984

94. Ullrich A, Coussens L, Hayflick J, et al: Human epidermal growth factor receptor cDNA sequence and aberrant expression of the amplified gene in A431 epidermoid carcinoma cells. Nature 309:418–425, 1984

95. Libermann TA, Rason N, Bartal AD, et al: Expression of epidermal growth factor receptors in human brain tumors. Cancer Res 44:753–760, 1984

96. Thompson DM, Gill GN: The EGF receptor: Structure, regulation and potential role in malignancy. Cancer Surv 4:767–788, 1985

97. Libermann TA, Nusbaum HR, Rason N, et al: Amplification enchances expression and possible rearrangement of the EGF receptor gene in primary human brain tumors of glial origin. Nature 313:144–147, 1985

98. Mark J, Westermark B, Ponten J, et al: Banding patterns in human glioma cell lines. Heredity (Edinburgh) 87:243–260, 1977

99. Fisher PB, Mufson A, Weinstein IB, et al: Epidermal growth factor, like tumor promoters, enhances viral and radiation-induced cell transformation. Carcinogenesis 2:183–187, 1981

100. Harrison J, Auersperg N: Epidermal growth factor enhances viral transformation of granulosa cells. Science 213:218–219, 1981

101. Rose SP, Stahn R, Passovoy DS, et al: Epidermal growth factor enhancement of skin tumor induction in mice. Experientia 32:913–915, 1976

102. De Larco JE, Preston YA, Todaro GJ: Properties of a sarcoma-growth-factor-like peptide from cells transformed by a temperature-sensitive sarcoma virus. J Cell Physiol 109:143–152, 1981

103. Twardzik DR, Sherwin SA, Ranchalis J, et al: Transforming growth factors in the urine of normal, pregnant, and tumor-bearing humans. JNCI 69:793–798, 1982

104. Samsoondar J, Kobrin MS, Kudlow JE: Alpha-transforming growth factor secreted by untransformed bovine anterior pituitary cells in culture. J Biol Chem 261:14408–14413, 1986

105. Kobrin MS, Samsoondar J, Kudlow JE: Alpha-transforming growth factor secreted by untransformed bovine anterior pituitary cells in culture. J Biol Chem 261:14414–14419, 1986

106. Lee D, Rochford R, Todaro GJ, et al: Development expression of rat transforming growth factor-alpha RNA. Mol Cell Biol 5:3644–3646, 1985

107. Betsholtz C, Johnsson A, Heldin C-H, et al: cDNA sequence and chromosomal localization of human platelet-derived growth factor A-chain and its expression in tumor cell lines. Nature 320:695–699, 1986

108. Niman HL, Thompson AMH, Yu A, et al: Anti-peptide antibodies detect oncogene-related proteins in urine. Proc Natl Acad Sci USA 82:7924–7928, 1985

109. Sejersen T, Betsholtz C, Sjolund M, et al: Rat skeletal myoblast and arterial smooth muscle cells express the gene for the A chain but not the gene for the B chain (c-sis) of platelet-derived growth factor (PDGF) and produce a PDGF-like protein. Proc Natl Acad Sci USA 83:6844–6848, 1986

110. Tong BD, Auer DE, Jaye M, et al: cDNA clones reveal differences between human glial and endothelial cell platelet-derived growth factor A-chains. Nature 328:619–621, 1987

111. Collins T, Bonthron DT, Orkin SH: Alternative RNA splicing affects function of encoded platelet-derived growth factor A chain. Nature 328:621–623, 1987

112. Bowen-Pope DF, Ross R: The platelet-derived growth factor receptor. In Birnbaumer L, O'Malley BW (eds): Peptide Hormones. Methods in Enzymology, vol 109, pp 69–101. New York, Academic Press, 1985

113. Yarden Y, Escobedo JA, Kuang WJ, et al: Structure of the receptor for platelet-derived growth factor helps define a family of closely related growth factor receptors. Nature 323:226–232, 1986

114. Cheifetz S, Weatherbee JA, Tsang ML-S, et al: The transforming growth factor-beta

system, a complex pattern of cross-reactive ligands and receptors. Cell 48:409–415, 1987

115. Roberts AB, Flanders KC, Kondaiah P, et al: Transforming growth factor beta: Biochemistry and roles in embryogenesis, tissue repair and remodeling, and carcinogenesis. Recent Prog Horm Res 144:157–197, 1988

116. Segarini PR, Roberts AB, Rosen DM, et al: Membrane binding characterization of two forms of transforming growth factor-beta. J Biol Chem (in press)

117. Ohta M, Greenberger JS, Anklesaria P, et al: Two forms of transforming growth factor-beta distinguished by multipotential haematopoietic progenitor cells. Nature 329:539–541, 1987

118. Mason AJ, Hayflick JS, Ling N, et al: Complementary DNA sequences of ovarian follicular fluid inhibin show precursor structure and homology with transforming growth factor-beta. Nature 318:659–663, 1985

119. Vale W, Rivier J, Vaughan J, et al: Purificiation and characterization of an FSH releasing protein from porcine ovarian follicular fluid. Nature 321:776–779, 1986

120. Ling N, Ying S-Y, Ueno N, et al: Pituitary FSH is released by a heterodimer of the beta-subunits from the two forms of inhibin. Nature 321:779–782, 1986

121. Cate RL, Mattaliano RJ, Hession C, et al: Isolation of the bovine and human genes for müllerian inhibiting substance and expression of the human gene in animal cells. Cell 45:685–698, 1986

122. Padgett RW, St Johnston RD, Gelbart WM: A transcript from a *Drosophila* pattern gene predicts a protein homologous to the transforming growth factor-beta family. Nature 325:81–84, 1987

123. Weeks DL, Melton DA: A maternal messenger RNA localized to the vegetal hemisphere in Xenopus eggs codes for a growth factor related to TGF-beta. Cell 51:861–867, 1987

124. Silberstein GB, Daniel CW: Reversible inhibition of mammary gland growth by transforming growth factor-beta. Science 237:291–293, 1987

125. Fausto N, Mead JE, Braun L, et al: Protooncogene expression and growth factors during liver regeneration. Symp Fundam Cancer Res 39:69–86, 1987

126. Cheifetz S, Like B, Massague J: Cellular distribution of type I and type II receptors for transforming growth factor-beta. J Biol Chem 261:9972–9978, 1986

127. Fanger BO, Wakefield LM, Sporn MB: Structure and properties of the cellular receptor for transforming growth factor type beta. Biochemistry 25:3083–3091, 1986

128. Libby J, Martinez R, Weber MJ: Tyrosine phosphorylation in cells treated with transforming growth factor-beta. J Cell Pysiol 129:159–166, 1986

129. Derynck R, Goeddel DV, Ullrich A, et al: Synthesis of messenger RNAs for transforming growth factors alpha and beta and the epidermal growth factor receptor by human tumors. Cancer Res 47:707–712, 1987

130. Donahoe PK, Fuller Jr, AF, Scully RE, et al: Mullerian inhibiting substance inhibits growth of a human ovarian cancer in nude mice. Ann Surg 194:472–480, 1981

131. Fuller Jr AF, Krane IM, Budzik GP, et al: Mullerian inhibiting substance reduction of colony growth of human gynecologic cancers in a stem cell assay. Gynecol Oncol 22:135–148, 1985

132. Baird A, Esch F, Mormede P, et al: Molecular characterization of fibroblast growth factor: Distribution and biological activities in various tissues. Recent Prog Horm Res 42:143–205, 1986

133. Abraham JA, Mergia A, Whang JL, et al: Nucleotide sequence of a bovine clone encoding the angiogenic protein, basic fibroblast growth factor. Science 233:545–548, 1986

134. Jaye M, Howk R, Burgess W, et al: Human endothelial cell growth factor: cloning, nucleotide sequence, and chromosome localization. Science 233:541–545, 1986

135. Gospodarowicz D: Fibroblast growth factor: Structural and biological properties. Nucl Med Biol 14:421–434, 1987

136. Gospodarowicz D, Ferrara N, Schweigerer L, et al: Structural characterization and biological functions of fibroblast growth factor. Endocr Rev 8:1–20, 1987

137. Neufeld G, Gospodarowicz D: Basic and acidic fibroblast growth factor interact with the same cell surface receptor. J Biol Chem 261:5631–5637, 1986

138. Huang SS, Huang JS: Association of bovine brain-derived growth factor receptor with protein tyrosine kinase activity. J Biol Chem 261:9568–9571, 1986

139. McDonald TJ, Jornvall H, Vagne M, et al: Characterization of a gastrin releasing peptide from porcine non-antral gastric tissue. Biochem Biophys Commun 90:227–233, 1979

140. Cuttitta F, Carney DN, Mulshine J, et al: Bombesin-like peptides can function as autocrine growth factors in human small cell lung cancer. Nature 316:823–826, 1985

141. Zachary I, Rozengurt E: Modulation of the epidermal growth factor receptor by mitogenic ligands: Effects of bombesin and role of protein kinase C. Cancer Surv 4:729–765, 1985

142. Assoian RK, Grotendorst GR, Miller DM, et al: Three growth factors from human platelets coordinating phenotypic transformation. Nature 309:804–806, 1984

143. Carpenter G, Stoscheck CM, Preston YA, et al: Antibodies to the epidermal growth factor receptor block the biological activities of sarcoma growth factor. Proc Natl Acad Sci USA 80:5627–5630, 1983

144. Assoian RK, Frolik CA, Roberts AB, et al: Transforming growth factor-beta controls receptor levels for epidermal growth factor in NRK-fibroblasts. Cell 36:35–41, 1984

145. Kehrl JH, Wakefield LM, Roberts AB, et al: Production of transforming growth factor beta by human T lymphocytes and its potential role in the regulation of T cell growth. J Exp Med 163:1037–1050, 1986

146. Kehrl JH, Roberts AB, Wakefield LM, et al: Transforming growth factor beta is an important immunomodulatory protein for human B lymphocytes. J Immunol 137:3855–3860, 1986

147. Rook AH, Kehrl JH, Wakefield LM, et al: Effects of transforming growth factor beta on the functions of natural killer cells: Depressed cytolytic activity and blunting of interferon responsiveness. J Immunol 136:3916–3920, 1986

148. Mulé JJ, Schwarz SL, Roberts AB, et al: Transforming growth factor-beta inhibits the in vitro generation of lymphokine-activated killer cells and cytotoxic T cells. Cancer Immunol Immunother 26:95–100, 1988

149. Roberts AB, Sporn MB, Assoian RK, et al: Transforming growth factor type beta: Rapid induction of fibrosis and angiogenesis in vivo and stimulation of collagen formation in vitro. Proc Natl Acad Sci USA 83:4167–4171, 1986

150. Folkman J: Toward an understanding of angiogenesis: Search and discovery. Perspect Biol Med 29:10–36, 1985

151. Fett JW, Strydom DJ, Lobb RR, et al: Isolation and characterization of angiogenin, and angiogenic protein from human carcinoma cells. Biochemistry 24:5480–5486, 1985

152. Strydom DJ, Fett JW, Lobb RR, et al: Amino acid sequence of human tumor derived angiogenin. Biochemistry 24:5486–5494, 1985

153. Kurachi K, Davie EW, Strydom DJ, et al: Sequence of cDNA and gene for angiogenin, a human angiogenesis factor. Biochemistry 24:5494–5499, 1985

154. Weiner HL, Weiner LH, Swain JL: Tissue distribution and developmental expression of the messenger RNA encoding angiogenin. Science 237:280–282, 1987

155. Folkman, J: Tumor angiogenesis. Adv Cancer Res 43:175–203, 1985

156. Folkman J: How is blood vessel growth regulated in normal and neoplastic tissue? G.H.A. Clowes Memorial Award Lecture. Cancer Res 46:467–473, 1986

157. Liotta LA, Rao CN, Barsky SH: Tumor invasion and the extracellular matrix. Lab Invest 49:636–649, 1983

158. Yamada KM: Cell surface interactions with extracellular materials. Annu Rev Biochem 52:761–799, 1983

159. Hynes RD: Molecular biology of fibronectin. Annu Rev Cell Biol 1:67–90, 1985

160. Ignotz RA, Massague J: Transforming growth factor-beta stimulates the expression of fibronectin and collagen and their incorporation into the extracellular matrix. J Biol Chem 261:4337–4345, 1986

161. Folkman J: Regulation of angiogenesis: A new function of heparin. Biochem Pharmacol 34:905–909, 1985

162. Wahl SM, Hunt DA, Wong HL, et al: Transforming growth factor beta is a potent immunosuppressive agent which inhibits interleukin 1-dependent lymphocyte proliferation. Immunol 140:3026–3032, 1988

163. Assoian RK, Fleurdelys BF, Stevenson HC, et al: Expression and secretion of type Beta transforming growth factor by activated human macrophages. Proc Natl Acad Sci USA 84:6020–6024, 1987

164. Shimokado K, Raines EW, Madtes DK, et al: A significant part of macrophage-derived growth factor consists of at least two forms of PDGF. Cell 43:277–286, 1985

165. Hamui H, Tomoyuki K, Sato JD, et al: Growth inhibition of human tumor cells in athymic mice by anti-epidermal growth factor receptor monoclonal antibodies. Cancer Res 44:1002–1007, 1984

166. Tager H, Given B, Baldwin D, et al: A structurally abnormal insulin causing human diabetes. Nature 281:122–125, 1979

167. Haneda M, Chan SJ, Kwok CM, et al: Studies on mutant human insulin genes: Identification and sequence analysis of a gene encoding Ser^{B24} insulin. Proc Natl Acad Sci USA 80:6366–6370, 1983

168. Knabbe C, Lippman ME, Wakefield LM, et al: Evidence that transforming growth factor-beta is a hormonally regulated negative growth factor in human breast cancer cells. Cell 48:417–428, 1987

169. McCormick DL, Moon RC: Retinoid-tamoxifen interaction in mammary cancer chemoprevention. Carcinogenesis 7:193–196, 1986

170. Carbone P: In Jordan VC (ed): Estrogen/Antiestrogen Action and Breast Cancer Therapy, p 492. Madison, WI, University of Wisconsin Press, 1986

171. Bell GI, Pictet RL, Rutter WJ, et al: Sequence of the human insulin gene. Nature 284:26–32, 1980

172. Ullrich A, Dull TJ, Gray A, et al: Genetic variation in the human insulin gene. Science 209:612–615, 1980

173. Jansen M, van Schaik FMA, Ricken AT, et al: Sequence of cDNA encoding human insulin-like growth factor I precursor. Nature 306:609–611, 1983

174. Ullrich A, Berman CH, Dull TJ, et al: Isolation of the human insulin-like growth factor I gene using a single synthetic DNA probe. EMBO J 3:361–364, 1984

175. Bell GI, Merryweather JP, Sanchez-Pescador R, et al: Sequence of a cDNA encoding human preproinsulin-like growth factor II. Nature 310:775–777, 1984

176. Dull TJ, Gray A, Hayflick JS, et al: Insulin-like growth factor II precursor gene organization in relation to insulin gene family. Nature 310:777–781, 1984

177. Ullrich A, Gray A, Berman C, et al: Human beta-nerve growth factor gene sequence highly homologous to that of mouse. Nature 303:821–825, 1983

178. Derynck R, Roberts AB, Winkler ME, et al: Human transforming growth factor-alpha: Precursor structure and expression in E. coli. Cell 38:287–297, 1984

179. Derynck R, Jarrett JA, Chen EY, et al: Human transforming growth factor-beta complementary DNA sequence and expression in normal and transformed cells. Nature 316:701–705, 1985

180. Marquardt H, Lioubin MN, Ikeda T: Complete amino acid sequence of human transforming growth factor type beta2. J Biol Chem 262:12127–12131, 1987

181. Anastasi A, Erspamer V, Bucci M: Isolation and structure of bombesin and alytesin, two analogous active peptides from the skin of the European amphibians *Bombina* and *Alytes*. Experientia 27:166–167, 1971

182. Chambard J-C, Pouysségur J: TGF-β inhibits growth factor-induced DNA synthesis in hamster fibroblasts without affecting the early mitogenic events. J Cell Physiol 135:101–107, 1988

JANET D. ROWLEY

CHAPTER 6 *Principles of Molecular Cell Biology of Cancer: Chromosomal Abnormalities*

The close association of specific chromosome abnormalities with particular types of human cancer has been established by a number of investigators in the past decade. A few of the genes involved in consistent chromosome rearrangements, notably translocations, have already been identified, and it is likely that most of the genes affected by these aberrations will be identified within the next decade. Moreover, for several of the rearrangements, some of the changes in gene structure and function have been defined. Therefore, some general principles that may be applicable to all chromosome rearrangements in human malignant disease are beginning to emerge.

Much of the detailed information on the relevant chromosome rearrangements is contained in a number of recent reviews,[1-6] and only a general summary will be presented here. Mitelman has published three editions of his "Catalogue of Chromosome Aberrations in Cancer."[1,7,8] The proportions of abnormal karyotypes listed in the Catalogues

At the Human Gene Mapping 9 (HGM9) meeting in Paris in September 1987, it was decided to identify human genes with capital letters in italics. This change is reflected herein; other chapters may use the formerly accepted convention of lower-cased letters in italics.

according to type of neoplasia are shown in Figure 6-1. Although carcinomas account for the greatest proportion of malignant disease, they represent only about 15% of the karyotypic data; most of the available information concerns leukemia and lymphoma. Only data obtained in untreated patients will be considered here.

From the beginning of the cytogenetic analysis of human malignant disease, it has been clear that virtually all solid tumors, including the non-Hodgkin's lymphomas, have an abnormal karyotype and that some of these abnormalities are limited to a given tumor.[2-6] With regard to the leukemias, it appeared from studies in the 1960s and early 1970s that only about 50% had an abnormal karyotype.[3-5] With improved culture techniques and with the development of processing methods that resulted in longer chromosomes with a larger number of more clearly defined bands, Yunis and associates have provided evidence that a karyotypic abnormality can be detected in virtually all leukemias as well.[6] Some malignant diseases, such as Hodgkin's disease or multiple myeloma, continue to show a high frequency of normal karyotypes. These diseases are characterized by malignant cells with a low mitotic index, and therefore it is likely that the dividing cells studied do not represent the malignant cells. The discussion will be restricted to clonal abnormali-

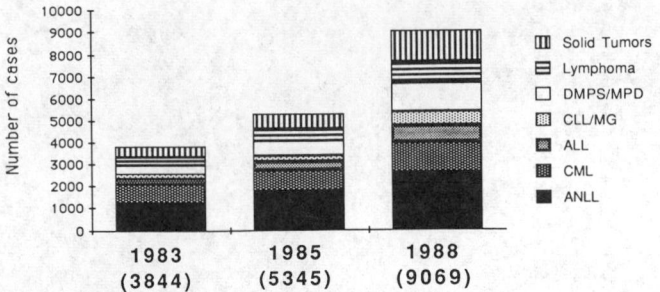

FIG. 6-1. Proportion of abnormal karyotypes by disease type in Mitelman's three catalogs of chromosome aberrations in cancer. The number in parentheses below the date is the total number of abnormal karyotypes in each edition. Patients with CML and only a t(9;22) are not included.

Different chromosome changes have been observed in neoplastic cells, and these often occur in combination. This leads to great difficulty in trying to identify precisely the unique abnormalities in a particular cancer. The simplest change is either a gain or a loss of a whole chromosome. Common structural alterations are *translocations*, with involve the exchange of material between two or more chromosomes, and *deletions*, which involve loss of DNA from a chromosome and thus from the affected cell (Fig. 6-2). In chromosome *inversions* a single chromosome is broken in two places, and the central portion is inverted and rejoined to the ends of the chromosome.

ties, which are defined as at least two cells with the same extra chromosome or structural rearrangement (identified with banding) or three cells with the same missing chromosome.[9] As can be seen from Table 6-1, with the exception of the t(9;22) the chromosome abnormalities in the myeloid leukemias differ from those in the lymphoid leukemias and lymphomas. Molecular analysis of the 9;22 translocation junction has revealed that the break in No. 22 may be different in myeloid and lymphoid leukemia.

A number of international meetings over the last 25 years have led to the establishment of a universally accepted system for chromosome nomenclature; that standard nomenclature will be used here. Each chromosome band is numbered.[10] The total chromosome number is followed by the sex chromosomes, and gains and losses of whole chromosomes are identified by a + or − before the chromosome number. A gain or loss of part of a chromosome is identified by a + or − after the chromosome number; p and q represent the short and long arm, respectively. Translocations are indicated by t; the chromosomes involved are noted in the first set of brackets and the breakpoints in the second set of brackets. Other abnormalities will be defined when they are first described.

TABLE 6-1.   Common Chromosome Changes in Leukemia

Type	Gains	Losses	Rearrangements
Myeloid Leukemia			
CML			
Chronic phase			t(9;22)(q34;q11)
Blast crisis	+8, +Ph[1]	Rare; −7	t(9;22), i(17q)
ANLL			
AML (M2)	+8	−7; less −5	t(8;21)(q22;q22)
APL (M3)			t(15;17)(q22;q11–12)
AMMoL (M4) (abn. eosinophils)	+8	−7	inv(16)(p13q22)
	+22		t(16;16), del(16q)
AMoL (M5)			t(9;11)(p22;q23), t(11q), del (11q)
M2/M4 (incr. basophils)			t(6;9)(p23;q34)
M4 (incr. platelets)			t(3;3)(q21;q26), inv(3)
Lymphoid Leukemia			
CLL			
B-cell	+12		14q+ (q32)
T-cell			t(8;14)(q24;q11) inv(14)(q11q32)
ALL			
Early B-precursor*			t(4;11)(q21;q23)
Common	+21, +6	Rare	t(9;22), del (6q)(q15–q21), near haploid
pre-B			t(1;19)(q23;p13)
B-cell			t(8;14)(q24;q32) t(2;8)(p12;q24) t(8;22)(q24;q11)
Early T-precursor			t(9p), del(9p) (p21–22)
T-cell			t(11;14)(p13;q11), t(8;14)(q24;q11) inv(14)(q11q32)

*CALLA+.

To be relevant to the malignant disease, chromosomes for analysis must be obtained from the tumor cells. Thus, for leukemia, bone marrow cells processed directly or after 1- to 3-day culture are used[11]; lymph nodes or solid tumors are minced to yield a single cell suspension that can be harvested immediately or cultured for a short period of time. The cells are exposed to a hypotonic solution, fixed, and stained according to a variety of protocols.[12]

MYELOID LEUKEMIAS

CHRONIC MYELOID LEUKEMIA

The subtype of leukemia termed *chronic myeloid leukemia* (CML) is important because the first consistent chromosome abnormality in any malignant disease was identified in CML. The abnormality is the Philadelphia or Ph[1] chromosome,[13] which was shown with banding to involve No. 22 (22q−). The correct chromosome defect was shown to be a translocation involving Nos. 9 and 22; this was the first consistent translocation specifically associated with any human or animal disease (Fig. 6-3).[14] The reciprocal nature of the translocation was established only recently, when the Abelson proto-oncogene, *ABL*, normally on No. 9, was identified on the Ph[1] chromosome.[15] Other studies with fluorescent markers or chromosome polymorphisms have shown that, in a particular patient, the same No. 9 and No. 22 are involved in each cell. The karyotypes of many Ph[1]+ patients with CML have been examined with banding techniques by a number of investigators; in a recent review of 1129 Ph[1]

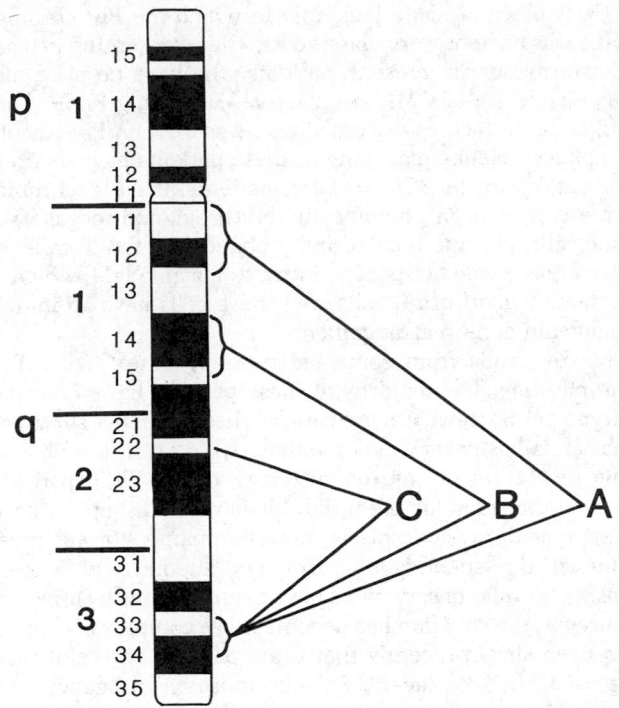

FIG. 6-2. Examples of various deletions of chromosome No. 5. The types are based on the amount of chromosome material missing from the deleted compared with the normal No. 5. Type A is the most extreme example and type C is the least extreme example. The brackets indicate the limits of uncertainty where the band containing the breakpoint has been defined by different staining techniques.

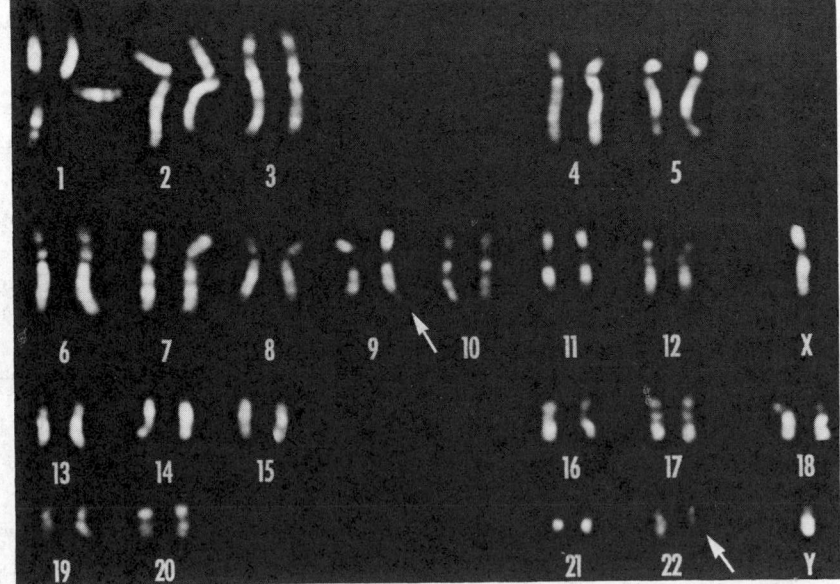

FIG. 6-3. Karyotype of a metaphase cell from a bone marrow aspirate obtained from an untreated male with chronic myeloid leukemia illustrating the t(9;22)(q34;q11). The Philadelphia chromosome (Ph[1]) is the chromosome on the right in pair 22 (↑). The material missing from the long arm of this chromosome (22q−) is translocated to the long arm of chromosome 9 (9q+) (↑), and is the additional pale band that is not present on the normal chromosome 9. Chromosomes were treated with trypsin and stained with Giemsa.

patients, the 9;22 translocation was identified in 1036 (92%).[4] Variant translocations have been discovered, however, in addition to the typical t(9;22). Until very recently, these were thought to be of two kinds: one appeared to be a simple translocation involving No. 22 and some chromosome other than No. 9 (about 4%), and the other was a complex translocation involving three or more different chromosomes, two of which were No. 9 and No. 22 (about 4%). Recent data clearly demonstrate that No. 9 is affected in the simple as well as the complex translocations, and that its involvement had been overlooked.[16] Virtually all chromosomes have been involved in these variant translocations, but No. 17 is affected more often then are other chromosomes. The genetic consequences of the standard t(9;22) or the complex translocation involving at least three chromosomes is to move the *ABL* proto-oncogene on No. 9 next to a gene on No. 22, called *BCR*, whose function is currently unknown. (Fig. 6-4)

When patients with CML enter the terminal acute phase, about 10% to 20% appear to retain the 46, Ph[1]+ cell line unchanged, whereas most patients show additional chromosome abnormalities, resulting in cells with modal chromosome numbers of 47 to 50.[4] During the acute phase of CML, different abnormal chromosomes occur singly or in combination in a distinctly nonrandom pattern. In patients who have only a single new chromosome change, this most commonly involves a second Ph[1], an isochromosome for the long arm of No. 17 [i(17q)], or a +8, in descending order of frequency. Chromosome loss occurs only rarely; that most often seen is −7, which occurs in 3% of patients.[4]

FIG. 6-4. Diagrammatic representation of chromosome translocation that produces the 9q+ and 22q− (Ph[1]) chromosomes. One proto-oncogene, *ABL*, is moved to No. 22 adjacent to a gene of unknown function called *BCR*; the break in No. 22 is distal to the IG lambda locus, which is not involved in the translocation. The *SIS* proto-oncogene is moved to the 9q+ chromosome. It is located some distance from the breakpoint on No. 22 and there is no evidence that it is altered as the result of the translocation.

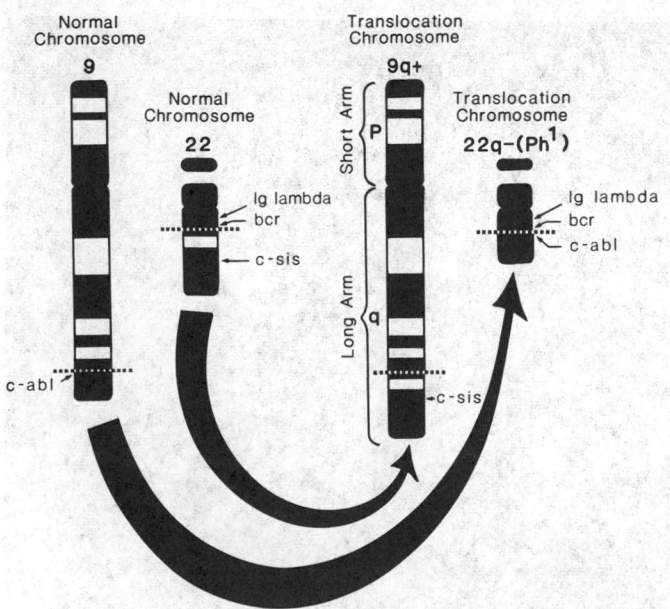

Early cases of acute leukemia in which the Ph[1] chromosome was present were classified as CML presenting in blast transformation; at present, patients who have no prior history suggestive of CML are classified as having Ph[1]+ acute leukemia. In fact, as discussed in the section on Ph[1]+ acute lymphocytic leukemia, some of these patients have a different breakpoint in *BCR*. In CML patients, the Ph[1] chromosome is present in granulocytic, erythroid, and megakaryocytic cells, in some B-cells, and probably in a few T-cells. In blast crisis, some blasts have intracytoplasmic IgM, which is characteristic of pre-B-cells, and these cells have an immunoglobulin gene rearrangement.[17]

Marrow cells from some patients appear to lack a Ph[1] chromosome. The majority of these patients have a normal karyotype. Somewhat surprisingly, these patients survive a substantially shorter time than those whose cells are Ph[1]+.[18] Our recent review of the histology of 25 Ph[1]− patients showed that most of them did not have CML but did have some type of myelodysplasia, most commonly chronic myelomonocytic leukemia or refractory anemia with excess blasts.[19] Similar observations have been reported by others.[20] However, the situation has become more complex because it has been shown recently that some patients with clinically typical CML who lack a Ph[1] chromosome cytogenetically have evidence of the insertion of *ABL* sequences into the *BCR* gene.[21,22] Thus it can be proposed that the sine qua non of CML is the juxtaposition of *BCR* and *ABL*.

ACUTE NONLYMPHOCYTIC LEUKEMIA DE NOVO

With initial banding analysis, clonal chromosome abnormalities were detected in about 50% of patients with acute nonlymphocytic leukemia (ANLL). This percentage has increased with improved banding and culture techniques; many laboratories currently are finding that at least 80% of patients have an abnormal karyotype. The most frequent abnormalities are a gain of No. 8 and loss of No. 7, changes that are seen in most subtypes of ANLL.[3-6,23] Specific rearrangements are closely associated with a particular subtype of ANLL as defined by the French–American–British Cooperative Group (FAB classification).[24] The chromosome abnormalities associated with each subtype are diagrammed in Figure 6-5.

The 8;21 Translocation in ANLL

A translocation between chromosomes 8 and 21 [t(8;21)(q22;q22)] was first identified in 1973.[25] The frequency with which this translocation is detected varies from one laboratory to another; it accounted for 25 (10%) of the 249 abnormal cases reviewed by Rowley and Testa [4] and 12% of the abnormal karyotypes reviewed at the Fourth International Workshop on Chromosomes in Leukemia.[23] The t(8;21) is the most frequent abnormality in children with ANLL, being reported in 10 (17%) of 60 karyotypically abnormal cases.[4] The abnormality initially appeared to be restricted to patients with a diagnosis of M2 (acute myeloblastic leukemia with maturation) according the FAB classification. However, 7% of t(8;21) patients analyzed at the Fourth Workshop had a diagnosis of M4.[23]

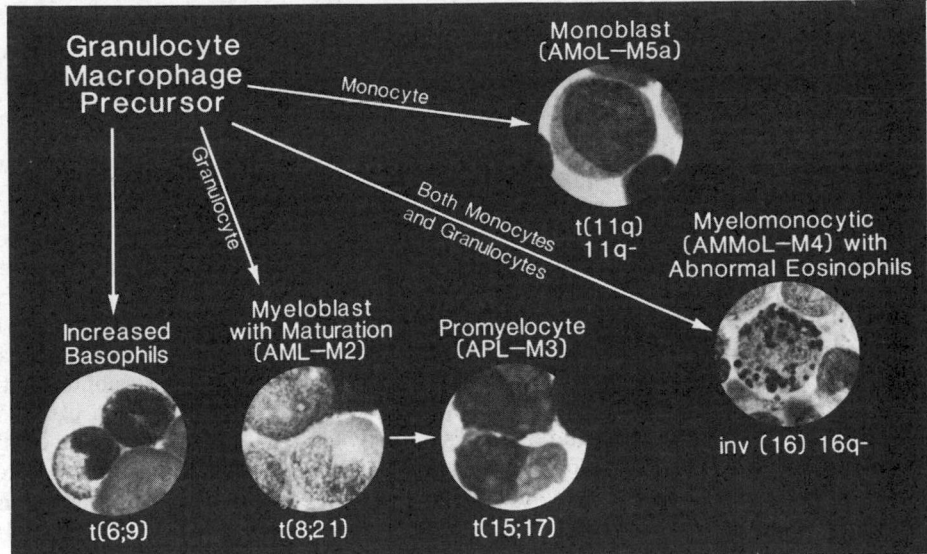

FIG. 6-5. Relationship of the subtypes of ANLL, and particular chromosome abnormality associated with each subtype. Photomicrographs illustrate the special features of the leukemic bone marrow cells obtained from untreated patients; the particular chromosome rearrangements associated with that type of leukemia are listed under the photomicrograph.

The 8;21 translocation is of interest for three other reasons. First, chromosomes 8 and 21 can participate in three-way rearrangements similar to those involving chromosomes 9 and 22 in CML. Second, the t(8;21) is often accompanied by the loss of a sex chromosome; among the cases reviewed at the Fourth Workshop, 28 (85%) of 33 males were −Y and 8 (67%) of 12 females were −X.[23] This association is particularly noteworthy because sex chromosome abnormalities are otherwise rarely observed in ANLL. Third, this translocation has never been reported as a constitutional abnormality or observed in other malignant diseases (Rowley JD: Unpublished observations).

The 15;17 Translocation in Acute Promyelocytic Leukemia

A structural rearrangement involving chromosomes 15 and 17 in acute promyelocytic leukemia was first recognized in 1977.[26] Of the 61 patients whose cases were analyzed at the Fourth Workshop, 43 (70%) had a t(15;17) (q22;q11–12), 3 had other abnormalities, and only 15 (25%) patients had a normal karyotype.[23] This rearrangement is unique to APL. In our recent review, all 44 patients with APL had a t(15;17).[3]

The 6;9 Translocation in ANLL with Increased Basophils

A translocation involving chromosomes 6 and 9 [t(6;9) (p23;q34)] was first described in two patients in 1976, but no common features were detected.[9] Slides from 9 patients with this translocation were recently reviewed; 8 of the 9 patients had an increase in basophils in the bone marrow ranging from 1.5% to 12% (normal value, 0.2%). Similar increases were noted in only 3% of other ANLL de novo patients.[27] Because the marrow in all biopsy specimens was hypercellu-

lar, this represents a marked increase in the total basophil count. The basophils appeared to be morphologically normal. Of the 9 patients, 5 were classified as having M2, 3 as having M4, and 1 as having M1. The breakpoint in No. 9 is in the same band as the t(9;22) in CML, and a marked increase in basophils is a regular feature of Ph[1]+ CML. However, molecular analysis has shown that the breakpoint in chromosome 9 is distal to the *ABL* gene.[28]

Structural Alterations of 11q in Acute Monocytic Leukemia

The close association of translocations, or less often deletions, of the long arm of No. 11 (11q) and acute monoblastic leukemia (M5) was first observed by Berger et al.[29] Abnormalities of 11q occurred most frequently in children with monoblastic leukemia (type *a*) (6 of 8); adults with monoblastic leukemia had the next highest incidence (5 of 16). The incidence in monocytic leukemia type *b* was low (1 of 3 children and 0 of 7 adults). At the Fourth Workshop, 33 patients had some structural rearrangement involving 11q; 21 (63.6%) of the 33 were classified as having M5, 5 as having M4, and 3 as having M2.[23] Of the 21 patients with M5, 15 had the monoblastic type, 3 had the monocytic type, and the slides of 3 could not be subclassified. Five of the patients were less than 1 year old, and 7 others were less than 20 years old. When all patients with M5 leukemia were considered, about 22% had an aberration involving 11q.

Aberrations of 11q differ from the t(8;22) and t(15;17) in two ways. First, the breakpoint in 11q involves band 11q23–24 in about two thirds of patients, but it can also occur in 11q13–14. Second, although translocations are more common (21 of 33 Fourth Workshop patients), 11 patients appeared to have what was identified as a terminal deletion of 11q. Although the other chromosome involved in the translocation is variable, a t(9;11)(p22;q23) is common.[30]

Structural Alterations in No. 16 in Acute Myelomonocytic Leukemia with Abnormal Eosinophils

Another clinical-cytogenetic association recently identified involves myelomonocytic (M4) leukemia with abnormal eosinophils. Arthur and Bloomfield described 5 cases of M2 or M4 in which the bone marrow contained an excess of eosinophils (8%–54%); all 5 patients had a deleted No. 16 [del(16)(q22)].[31] Our group has reported on a related entity, first in 18 patients and then in a larger series of 33 patients.[32] Most of these patients had M4 leukemia with eosinophils that showed unique morphological changes [M4Eo], including large and irregular basophilic granules; one third lacked increased eosinophils because the marrow contained fewer than 5% eosinophils. Twenty-seven patients had an inversion of No. 16, inv(16)(p13q22), and six had a t(16;16) (p13;q22). The strong correlation between abnormal eosinophils and structural rearrangements of No. 16 was confirmed at the Fourth Workshop.[23] In fact, the morphological features of the eosinophils are so specific that our pathologists can accurately predict which patients will have either an inv(16) or a t(16;16) by examining the bone marrow aspirate. It appears that this relatively common (25% of our AMMoL patients have this aberration) but subtle chromosome aberration was undetected in the past, in part because of poor morphology. This chromosome abnormality has clinical implications as well. Among 32 treated patients, 78% achieved a complete remission, compared with 36% of 58 other AMMoL patients. The median survival time was more than 65 weeks for patients with an abnormal No. 16, compared with 29 weeks for those with a normal No. 16.[32] These data confirm an observation reported by Keating that an increase in marrow eosinophils is a good prognostic sign.[33] In fact, at the Fourth Workshop it was clearly shown that the type rather than the presence of a chromosome abnormality has prognostic importance (Table 6-2). Thus, although the projected median survival for all patients was 8 months, those with a t(8;21) had the longest median survival (13

months), while those with abnormalities of chromosomes 5 and 7, t(15;17), or hyperdiploidy had the shortest survivals (3 to 4 months.)

ANLL AND MYELODYSPLASTIC SYNDROME ASSOCIATED WITH TREATMENT

A distinctive disorder of bone marrow morphology and function that terminates in myelodysplastic syndrome (MDS) or in ANLL has been recognized as a late complication of cytotoxic therapy used in the treatment of both malignant and nonmalignant diseases.[34] Characteristic nonrandom chromosome abnormalities are commonly observed in bone marrow cells of patients with t-MDS/t-ANLL. These abnormalities differ in their type and frequency from those noted in ANLL developing de novo. We reported previously that part or all of chromosome Nos. 5 and/or 7 was lost in cells from 23 (86%) of 26 t-MDS/t-ANLL patients.[35] More recently 61 of 63 patients were found to have an abnormal karyotype, and 55 of these had an abnormality of one or both chromosomes 5 and 7.[35] These observations have been confirmed by others.[36,37] After analyzing data in 17 patients with a deletion of the long arm of No. 5 we were able to identify a region, 5q23 to 5q32, that was consistently missing in every patient. In contrast, only about 16% of patients with ANLL de novo have a similar abnormality of chromosome No. 5 or No. 7 or both.[38] Moreover, the latter patients frequently have had significant occupational exposure to potential environmental carcinogens, such as chemicals, solvents, or pesticides.[39,40] Furthermore, one seldom finds the specific rearrangements in t-ANLL that are closely associated with the distinct morphological subsets of ANLL de novo, such as t(8;21), t(15;17), or inv(16).

A number of growth factors or growth factor receptors have been mapped to the region 5q23–32 that is consistently deleted; whether any of them play a role in mutagen-associated leukemia is unknown.[41]

TABLE 6-2.   Correlation of Karyotype and Survival of 660 Patients with ANLL de novo*

Karyotype	Number of Patients	Complete Remission: Median Duration, Months (% of patients)†	Median Survival, Months‡
Normal	307	13 (45)	10
−5 or 5q−	29	4 (28)	4
−7 or 7q−	28	25+ (21)	3
Abn. 5 and 7	21	Too few	3
t(15;17)	43	10 (40)	3
t(8;21)	44	10 (77)	13
llq abn.	29	6 (21)	8
+8	36	8 (22)	6
+21	12	19+ (67)	10
46 abnormal	67	13 (31)	5
>46 chromosomes	31	12 (16)	4
<46 chromosomes	13	6 (46)	5

*Data from Fourth Workshop on Chromosomes in Leukemia. Cancer Genet Cytogenet 11:249–360, 1984.
†Percentage of patients with each karyotype who achieved a complete remission.
‡Difference in survival is significant (p = 0.0002).

MALIGNANT DISEASES AFFECTING LYMPHOCYTES

The chromosome abnormalities in lymphoid disorders, especially in the non-Hodgkin's lymphomas, have been reviewed in considerable detail.[4,42-45] This section reviews the consistent translocations seen in Burkitt's lymphoma and in some cases of B-cell ALL, the other aberrations in ALL, and aberrations in some T-cell disorders.

LYMPHOMA

In 1972, Manolov and Manolova discovered that cells of Burkitt's lymphomas had an additional band at the end of the long arm of the one chromosome No. 14 (14q+).[46] Zech and co-workers in 1976 first observed that the end of the one No. 8 was consistently absent, and they suggested that the missing part of No. 8 was translocated to No. 14 [t(8;14)(q24;q32)].[47] The t(8;14) has also been observed in nonendemic Burkitt's tumors from America, Europe, and Japan that are Epstein-Barr virus negative; thus, it is a highly characteristic chromosome anomaly in Burkitt's tumors. This translocation has also been observed in other lymphomas, particularly those of the diffuse large cell type. Two other, related translocations were later identified in Burkitt's tumors. All three translocations involved No. 8 with a break in the same band, 8q24. One variant translocation involved chromosome No. 2 with a break in the short arm [t(2;8)(p12;q24)], and the other involved No. 22 with a break in the long arm in the band (22q11) that is affected in CML. All three translocations have been identified in patients with B-cell ALL.

The data on Burkitt's lymphoma indicate that No. 8 is the consistently involved chromosome. When the karyotypic aberrations seen in lymphoid disease are considered as a whole, a break in No. 14 at q32, with translocation of material from elsewhere to the broken No. 14, is the single most common change. The only other recurring translocation, t(14;18)(q32;q21), is in fact the most common translocation in lymphoma (Fig. 6-6). This was first identified by Fukuhara and co-workers in 6 of 9 patients with poorly differentiated lymphocytic lymphoma,[48] now called "malignant lymphoma, follicular, predominantly small cleaved cell" (FSC) in the International Classification System.[49] This finding was confirmed by many others.[42-45] The correlation between karyotype and histologic type in 260 cases reviewed at the Fifth International Workshop on Chromosomes in Leukemia and Lymphoma is summarized in Figure 6-7.[45] Fifteen percent of the 260 workshop patients had a normal karyotype. The karyotypic pattern varies greatly among the different subgroups. The t(14;18) is common in follicular lymphomas, whereas the t(8;14) is common in small noncleaved cell lymphoma.

What are the implications of the t(14;18) in tumors with a large cell or diffuse morphology? Analysis of the karyotypic pattern in these tumors shows that certain additional chromosome changes, especially a gain of No. 7 or a deletion of the long arm of No. 6 [(del)6q], appear to correlate with a more malignant phenotype (see Fig. 6-6).[43,44] The translocation junction has been cloned and a gene on No. 18 called

FIG. 6-6. R-banding karyotype of a cell in the leukemic phase illustrating the many complex changes that can occur. There is an extra X and No. 20 and loss of the Y chromosome. Note the deletion of 1q (*left*), 1p (*center*), 2q, 5q (*left*), 6q, 8q, 11q (*right*), and 18q; addition to 4q, 5p (*right*), 10q, 11q (*left*), 13p, and both 14q's; a gain of the abnormal No. 7 (7q+); and four unknown markers (M1 to M4). The 1q— chromosome originates from a translocation with 5p [t(1;5)(q11;p15), and the 1p— chromosome could result from a translocation with No. 17 [t(1;17)(q?21;p?13). The two 14q+ chromosomes result from a 14q translocation with 8q and 18q, [t(8;14)(q24;q32) and [t(14;18)(q32;q21), respectively. The 5q— and the 6q— chromosome each could have an interstitial deletion of the long arm, [del(5)(q13q31)] and [del(6)(q21q23)]. The 11q— chromosome has lost the whole long arm. M4 could be a ring chromosome.

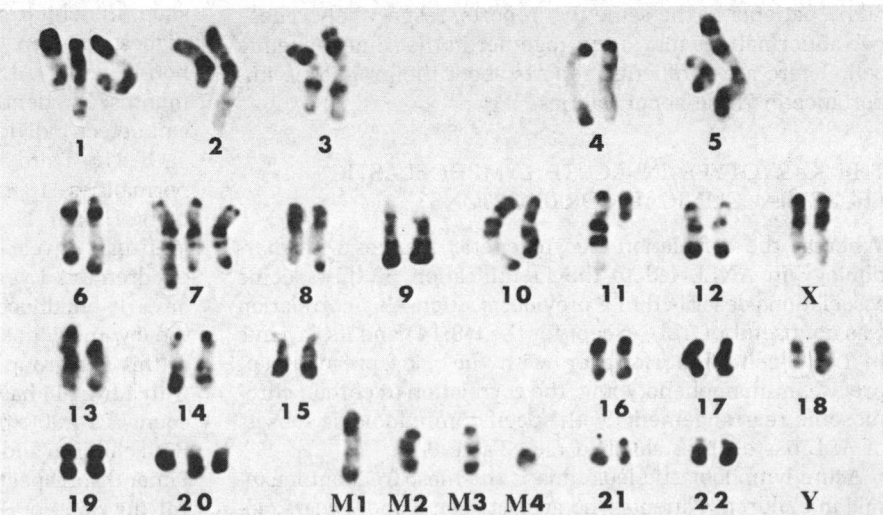

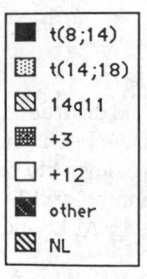

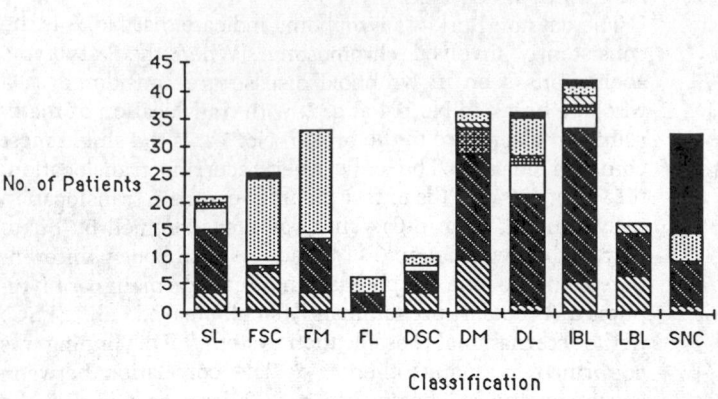

FIG. 6-7. Histogram showing the most common chromosome changes identified in 260 lymphomas studied before treatment and reviewed at the Fifth International Workshop on Chromosomes in Leukemia/Lymphoma; each tumor was classified according to the Working Formulation.

BCL2 (the second B-cell leukemia gene) has been identified.[50] Breakpoints cluster in at least two sites on the gene; the major cluster is in the 3′ untranslated region of the second exon. In the lymphoma cells, the expression of the normal gene is suppressed and an abnormal chimeric *BCL2–IGH* messenger RNA (mRNA) is expressed. This leads to inappropriate expression of a structurally normal protein whose function is unknown.[51]

THE KARYOTYPE IN CHRONIC LYMPHOCYTIC LEUKEMIA

Chronic lymphocytic leukemia (CLL) is the most common leukemia in the United States and Europe, accounting for about 30% of all leukemias. It is considered to be a monoclonal neoplastic proliferation of small lymphocytes which are of B-cell origin in 95% of cases. The early studies of the cytogenetic pattern in CLL showed a normal karyotype in most samples. As better culture and banding methods have been applied to these studies, nonrandom clonal abnormalities have been detected. These include translocations involving 14q32 and trisomy for chromosome 12.[1,52–55] In two reports, translocations of 14q were observed in 17 of 87 patients and in 5 of 16 patients with abnormal karyotypes.[8,54] Trisomy 12 was even more common and was described in 33 and 7 patients in the same two reports, respectively. These two abnormalities may occur together in the same leukemic cell. There are conflicting reports about the prognostic importance of these abnormalities.[53–55]

THE KARYOTYPE IN ACUTE LYMPHOBLASTIC LEUKEMIA: CLINICAL CORRELATIONS

Whereas the correlation of cytogenetic changes with morphology in ANLL led to the identification of the specific associations described in a previous section, this correlation was not useful in ALL, except for the t(8;14) and its variants in L3, B-cell ALL. However, with the widespread use of precise immunophenotyping, the correlation of certain chromosome rearrangements with specific immunologic subsets of ALL has been established (see Table 6-1).

Acute lymphoblastic leukemia is the most frequent leukemia in children. Patients who are between 3 and 7 years old,

who have a white blood cell (WBC) count of less than 10,000/mm³, and whose leukemic cells have non-T, non-B surface markers have the best prognosis. For many years metaphase chromosomes from ALL patients had poor morphology with indistinct bands, making an accurate analysis difficult, and there have been fewer reports of chromosome patterns in ALL than in ANLL. Recent improvements permit correlation of the karyotype with other recognized prognostic factors. It was rigorously demonstrated for the first time at the Third International Workshop on Chromosomes in Leukemia that the karyotype is an important independent prognostic factor in ALL.[56] Of 330 patients whose cases were reviewed at the Third Workshop, 112 appeared to have a normal karyotype; the largest group (39 patients) with a well-defined abnormality had a Ph¹ chromosome. Eighteen patients had a t(4;11), 16 had a t(8;14), and 15 had an abnormality of No. 14 not involving chromosome 8. Other patients with abnormalities were classified by the modal chromosome number.

The Ph¹ chromosome is the most frequent rearrangement, accounting for 17.3% of cases of adult ALL. At the cytogenetic level, the breakpoints appear identical to those in CML; recent molecular analysis indicates that the breakpoint in the *BCR* gene on No. 22 may be more proximal in some patients with Ph¹+ ALL than in CML. At the Third Workshop, the children with a Ph¹ chromosome had the second highest median leukocyte count (75,000/mm³), all had non-B, non-T ALL, and their median survival was only 15 months. By identifying this chromosomal abnormality, one can detect individuals who have a poor prognosis.

Of 216 Third Workshop patients with chromosomal abnormalities, 18 (8.3%) had a t(4;11)(q21;q23) rearrangement. Half of the patients were children, most of whom were less than 1 year old; and the median age of the affected children was 1 year. The association of t(4;11) with neonatal or early childhood ALL is particularly interesting in view of the low incidence of ALL in this age group; acute leukemias in this age group are usually of the myeloid type. Children with a t(4;11) had very high leukocyte counts (median WBC count, 214,000/mm³), which is a poor prognostic factor. Both children and adults had a short median survival—9 and 7 months, respectively. Only patients with abnormalities involving 8q24 or 14q32 had shorter survivals.

Although the morphology of some cells with a t(4;11) often appears lymphoid, other features are more suggestive of monocytic leukemia. A t(4;11) cell line showed rearranged heavy and light chain (κ) genes, although cells lacked cytoplasmic immunoglobulin and thus were probably in a very early stage of B-cell differentiation.[57] However, when cells were cultured with the phorbol ester TPA, a monocytic-like phenotype was induced. Thus these cells appear to be very early precursor cells that have dual lineage capabilities.

Another recurring chromosome abnormality is the t(1;19) (q21;p13), which has been identified in about 25% of patients with a pre-B phenotype, that is, they have cytoplasmic immunoglobulin and are classified as CALLA+.[58-60]

The leukemic cells of some patients with ALL are characterized by a gain of many chromosomes and fewer structural abnormalities.[61-62] Chromosome numbers usually range from 50 to 60, and a few patients have up to 65 chromosomes. Although identical karyotypes are unusual, certain additional chromosomes are commonly seen. Among 31 Third Workshop patients with hyperdiploidy (14% of patients with abnormalities), +21, +6, +18, +14, +4, and +10 in decreasing frequency were seen in 10% to 33%.[56] It is interesting that some of these chromosomes, particularly Nos. 10, 18 and 21, were also seen as additional chromosomes in patients with near-haploidy, with chromosome numbers of 26 to 36 (median, 28). The median age of the 22 children with this abnormality was 3 years, and that of all 31 patients was 5 years, less than that of patients with other abnormalities. The WBC count was low (median, 6,000/mm³). Thus, these patients have all of the previously recognized factors, including age between 3 and 7 years, low WBC count, and non-T, non-B markers, that indicate a good prognosis. In a follow-up study of the Third Workshop patients, the complete remission rate for children was 95%, with a median remission duration that will be greater than 5 years. The median survival of the children with hyperdiploidy is longer than for those with a normal karyotype; for adults, the medial survival for the two groups is comparable. Chromosome losses were less frequent and involved No. 9, 7, 13, 20, or 8 in that order. The three translocations seen in B-cell ALL were described under Burkitt's lymphoma. With regard to karyotype and age, patients with a deletion of 6q and a modal chromosome number greater than 50 were younger, and those with a Ph¹ chromosome or a 14q+ were older than patients with other abnormalities. In summary, the highest remission rates were in patients with a normal karyotype and a modal number greater than 50; the lowest were seen in patients with a Ph¹ chromosome, a 14q+ chromosome, a t(8;14), and a t(4;11).[63]

T-CELL DISORDERS

Although fewer leukemias of T-cell origin have been studied, a distinct pattern of nonrandom karyotypic abnormalities is emerging. Rearrangements involving the proximal bands of chromosome 14 (14q11–q13) are relatively common. Those involving two regions of chromosome 7 (7q35-q36 and 7p15) also occur in T-cell malignancies but have been observed in nonmalignant T-cell disorders as well; breaks involving these regions are very rare in other malignant

diseases. One recurring rearrangement in T-cell neoplasia, particularly CLL, is a paracentric inversion of chromosome 14 with a proximal breakpoint at q11 and a distal breakpoint at q32.[64,65] A closely related rearrangement, t(14;14)(q11;q32), is seen in T-cell neoplasia [64,66] and in phytohemagglutinin-stimulated T-lymphocytes from patients with ataxia-telangiectasia (A-T) as well as in the leukemic cells of A-T patients in whom this disease evolved.[66,67] A number of reports from Japan have described the frequent occurrence of 14q11 breaks in adult T-cell leukemia–lymphoma patients [68,69]; fewer such patients have been described in Western countries, and 14q11 breaks are much less common.[70,71] Williams et al have described a t(11;14)(p13;q13) in the leukemic cells of 4 of 16 patients with T-cell acute lymphoblastic leukemia.[60] Thus, in some of these T-cell diseases, breaks occur in either 14q11 or 14q32, or in both bands in the same patient. In B-cell disorders, however, breaks occur essentially only in 14q32, and they rarely involve 14q11.[54] The data confirm the observation made some time ago that the proximal region of chromosome 14 is important in T-cell neoplasia.[66] More detailed analysis of rearrangements of 7q in T-cell disorders has revealed that a few patients have breaks at 7q32 to 7q36, the location of the β chain for the T-cell receptor.[64,72]

KARYOTYPES OF CANCERS AND OF BENIGN TUMORS

Whereas the karyotype of the leukemic cells has been determined in thousands of patients with either acute or chronic myeloid leukemia, the karyotype has been defined from fewer than 100 samples of any specific cancer. Several reasons account for this discrepancy. First, it is difficult to obtain successful chromosome preparations from solid tumors because of extensive fibrosis or necrosis. Second, until recently, many investigators questioned the relevance of the chromosome changes in malignant cells, and therefore this area of research, was not pursued. Third, the karyotypes of the tumor cells frequently show high modal numbers, often 60 to 90 chromosomes, with many bizarre marker chromosomes, and it is very difficult to distinguish the primary change from changes related to secondary evolution with progression of the malignant phenotype. Those changes that appear to be consistent are summarized in Table 6-3.

TUMORS ORIGINATING IN EMBRYONIC CELLS

Tumors originating in embryonic cells are of particular interest to the cytogeneticist because some of them occur in patients who have specific constitutional chromosome abnormalities. In all preceding sections, the karyotypic changes were somatic mutations in malignant cells and were not present in other unaffected cells. In contrast, some patients at risk of developing retinoblastoma have a variable deletion of chromosome 13 that always includes 13q14, whereas other patients with a deletion of No. 11 (band 11p13) are at risk of developing Wilms' tumor. In general, these deletions also are associated with various phenotypic abnormalities (for review, see refs. 2 and 73). Relatively few

TABLE 6-3. Recurring Chromosome Abnormalities in Solid Tumors

Involving embryonic cells	
Neuroblastoma	Deletion of No. 1 (p32–p36)
Ewing's sarcoma/peripheral neuroepithelioma	t(11;22)(q24;q12)
Wilms' tumor	Deletion of No. 11 (p13)*
	Trisomy 1q
Retinoblastoma	Deletion of No. 13 (q14)*
	Trisomy 1q
Testicular tumors	i(12p)
Adult cancers	
Malignant melanoma	Deletion of No. 1 (p11–p22)
Small cell lung carcinoma	Deletion of No. 3 (p14–p23)
Renal carcinoma	Deletion of No. 3 (p14–p21)
Liposarcoma	t(12;16)(q13;p11)
Synovial sarcoma	t(X;18)(p11.2;q11.2)
Rhabdomyosarcoma (alveolar)	t(2;13)(q37;q14)
Benign tumors	
Pleomorphic adenomas	t(3;8)(p21;q12);
	t(9;12)(p13–22; q13–15)
Meningioma	Loss of No. 22 or deletion (q11)
Lipoma	t(3;12)(q27–q28;q13–q14)

*Observed as a constitutional abnormality as well as in some tumors.

tumors have been analyzed, and deletions of No. 13 or much less often, of No. 11 have been observed in tumor cells from some retinoblastomas or Wilms' tumors, respectively. The most common change that we have observed in Wilms' tumors is trisomy for the long arm of No. 1 (+1q).[74]

Both Wilms' tumors and retinoblastomas have two patterns of inheritance, one as an autosomal dominant and one as a sporadic mutation. The age at tumor detection as well as other observations led Knudsen to propose the two-mutation hypothesis.[75] According to this hypothesis, in patients who inherit the predisposing gene, only one other change is needed for transformation of retinal cells to tumor cells, and in these individuals multiple tumors are diagnosed at a very early age. In sporadic cases, two independent mutations must affect the same cell for transformation to occur; since this event is relatively uncommon, the tumors are unifocal and develop at an older age. Based on the consistent loss of chromosome band, 13q14, this band was thought to be the locus for the retinoblastoma or *RB* gene. Studies confirming that No. 13 was the critical chromosome included the discovery that tumor cells frequently homozygous for DNA markers on chromosome 13 were heterozygous in cells of nontumor tissue from the same patient.[76] Using probes cloned from 13q14, Dryja et al discovered that copies of one of the probes had been deleted from both chromosomes in one of 20 tumors; DNA probes from this region detected mRNA in a retinal cell line that was absent in some retinoblastomas.[77] By making a DNA copy of the mRNA, they identified deletions or mutations in about 30% of retinoblastoma tumors or cell lines.[78] Others have identified mRNA abnormalities in each of six retinoblastomas.[79] Thus, we now have the tools to identify the complete *RB* gene, to understand its function in normal cells, and then to determine why its abnormal function or its absence leads to malignant

transformation of these cells. The current assumption is that the *RB* gene, and the genes that will be identified in the deleted chromosome segments in other tumor cells, function as tumor suppressors or "anti-oncogenes." Presumably these genes inhibit the function of genes stimulating cell proliferation, and their loss allows the growth-promoting genes to function without modulation.[80]

Recurring chromosome abnormalities limited to the malignant cells have also been observed in other childhood tumors. For example, a deletion of some of the long arm of chromosome 1 (1p−) has been noted in neuroblastomas.[81] Neuroblastomas are also of interest because of their proclivity to undergo gene amplification, which is manifested chromosomally as hundreds or thousands of small discrete pieces of chromosomes called *double minutes*, or long unbanded regions on chromosomes called *homogeneously staining regions*, or HSR.[82] In some cell lines, these have been shown to represent amplification of *NMYC*.[83] Amplification of *NMYC* has also been identified in tumor samples; it is highly correlated with advanced stage (III and IV) and with poor survival.[84]

CANCER IN ADULTS

Although karyotypes have been determined for a number of individual tumors, it has been difficult to establish a consistent pattern comparable to that described earlier for ANLL, for reasons already discussed. Loss of chromosomal material may be an important factor in some of the more common tumors in adults, including lung cancer and colon cancer. A deletion of the long arm of No. 1 has been observed in malignant melanoma[85]; the deleted region may be larger than that noted in neuroblastoma. A deletion of the short arm of No. 3 (p14–p23) has been described by Whang-Peng et al[86] in small cell lung carcinoma, and a somewhat different deletion (3p14-p21) has been described in renal cancer.[87,88] Examination of various different types of lung cancers, including small cell, squamous cell, and adenocarcinoma, has revealed the development of homozygosity for DNA markers that are located near 3p21.[89,90] Using the strategies developed for retinoblastoma, a number of laboratories are trying to identify the critical gene within the deletion. Atkin and Baker have noted an isochromosome for the short arm of No. 12 [i(12p)] in testicular tumors.[91]

CHROMOSOME TRANSLOCATIONS IN SARCOMAS

Soft tissue (mesenchymal) tumors are relatively rare, accounting for less than 1% of all human neoplasms. They are very heterogeneous, and may present diagnostic problems. Recently, cytogenetic and molecular analysis of these tumors in their malignant (sarcoma) and benign forms has yielded important clues to the hitherto unsuspected relationship of some of these rare neoplasms and has aided in classifying some of the undifferentiated forms of these tumors. Moreover, the fact that the benign and malignant forms have related karyotypic changes provides an important resource for identifying the additional genetic changes that occur in the malignant compared with the benign form.

Although chromosome translocations have not been a

prominent cytogenetic feature of solid tumors, a number of them have been identified in certain specific tumors, especially sarcomas. One example is the 11;22 translocation [t(11;22)(q24;q12)] in Ewing's sarcoma,[92-93] which has been detected in more than 90% of these tumors. The identity of the genes involved in this translocation has not been established. Cytogeneticists and oncologists were both surprised when it was reported that peripheral neuroepithelial tumors also had the 11;22 translocation.[94] In fact, the neuronal phenotype of Ewing's sarcoma and neuroepithelioma is the same. The similarity is substantiated by molecular analysis: Ewing's sarcoma and neuroepithelioma have identical levels of proto-ocogene expression which differ from those in neuroblastoma.[95] Amplification of NMYC is limited to neuroblastoma. Treatment of neuroepithelial tumors had been disappointing; however, use of therapy for Ewing's sarcoma resulted in a remarkable improvement in response.

Recurring translocations have recently been described in both liposarcoma and synovial sarcoma.[2,96-98] Sandberg and his colleagues have described a t(12;16)(q13;p11) only in the myxoid subgroup of liposarcomas; other abnormalities, including ring chromosome, appeared to be more frequent in well-differentiated sarcomas.[97] The chromosome abnormality in synovial sarcoma [t(X;18)(p11.2;q11.2)] is of interest because it is the first one involving a sex chromosome. This abnormality does not appear to be restricted to a particular histologic pattern.[98]

BENIGN TUMORS

Although much of the discussion in this chapter implies that chromosome aberrations are equivalent to a malignant phenotype, there are a number of exceptions. In the myeloproliferative disorders, patients with clonal chromosome abnormalities in marrow cells have been observed for up to 12 to 15 years without undergoing leukemic transformation.[4,5] Several benign tumors have clonal abnormalities, of which the meningiomas described by Mark et al[99] and by Zankl and Zang[100] have been studied most extensively. Each group has noted either the loss of all of No. 22 or, less commonly, a deletion of the long arm with a break in 22q11. This information led Gusella and his colleagues to examine various neuronal tumors with DNA markers; they discovered the loss of heterozygosity for chromosome 22 probes in acoustic neuromas.[101] Mark et al examined parotid gland tumors and noted a translocation [t(3;8)(p25;q21)] in many of them.[102] Cytogenetic analyses of uterine leiomyomas have only recently been reported; however, it appears that breaks in 14q22–24 and in 12q14–15 are not uncommon.[103,104] An identical translocation, t(12;14)(q14–15;q23–24) was found as the only abnormality in 4 of 34 leiomyomas.[104]

Of special interest with regard to the sarcomas is that many benign neoplasms affect the same cell type. Thus, of 26 lipomas karyotyped, 70% had consistent chromosome rearrangements; 13 of them had a reciprocal translocation involving 12q13–14, the same breakpoint noted in liposarcomas. It may be significant that this region of No. 12 is involved in lipomas–liposarcomas, leiomyomas, and mixed salivary gland tumors.

MOLECULAR ANALYSIS OF CONSISTENT CHROMOSOME ABNORMALITIES, PARTICULARLY TRANSLOCATIONS

HOW AND WHEN CONSISTENT TRANSLOCATIONS OCCUR.

We do not know how consistent structural rearrangements occur, but there are at least two possibilities.[105] The rearrangements may be random, but selection may act to eliminate the vast majority that do not provide the cell with a proliferative advantage. Alternatively, certain changes may occur preferentially and thus may be the ones we see. Some tantalizing data show an association of chromosome rearrangements in tumor cells from patients with fragile sites affecting one of the chromosome bands broken in the tumor cells.[106-108] However, much more research is required to clarify the role of fragile sites as a predisposing factor to malignant transformation.

Croce[109] has proposed that many of the chromosome rearrangements in B- and T-cell tumors involve sequences used in the normal recombination of the V-D-J segments of the immunoglobulin and T-cell receptor genes. The presence of heptamer and nanomer sequences in the nonimmunoglobulin gene at the site of the translocation, namely MYC and BCL2 has been reported. We have no indication at present that the genes involved in the translocations in myeloid leukemias undergo similar DNA rearrangements.

An equally important question is, when in the multistage process of malignant transformation of a particular cell do translocations or other chromosome aberrations occur? Some chromosome changes occur as part of the further evolution of the malignant phenotype (e.g., blast crisis of CML) and they are therefore relatively late events. But what about the occurrence of the t(9;22) in CML, for example? Does the Ph[1] occur in a single normal cell that becomes the progenitor of the leukemic clone, or is there expansion of a clone, possibly a leukemic one, in which a translocation occurs in one of these already abnormal cells? Fialkow et al [110] have presented detailed evidence supporting the latter proposal.

Adams et al[111] have constructed transgenic mice whose cells all have a vector containing the MYC/IgH junction from a murine plasmacytoma. All cells contain this construct; however, the B-cell tumors that occurred in every animal were clonal, indicating that one or more additional charges occurred in one cell, resulting in clonality.

CHROMOSOME LOCATION OF PROTO-ONCOGENES

One of the most surprising revelations in the recent past has involved the cellular oncogenes and their chromosome location. Much of the excitement derives from the observation that many proto-oncogenes are located in the bands that are involved in consistent translocations (Fig. 6-8).[105,111-116] The evidence in Burkitt's lymphoma and in CML clearly points the way for future research in this area. The gene for the proto-oncogene MYC (the cellular homologue of the avian myelocytomatosis virus) is on chromosome 8(q24). The immunoglobulin genes (heavy chain, and κ and λ light chain genes) are located at the breakpoints on the three chromo-

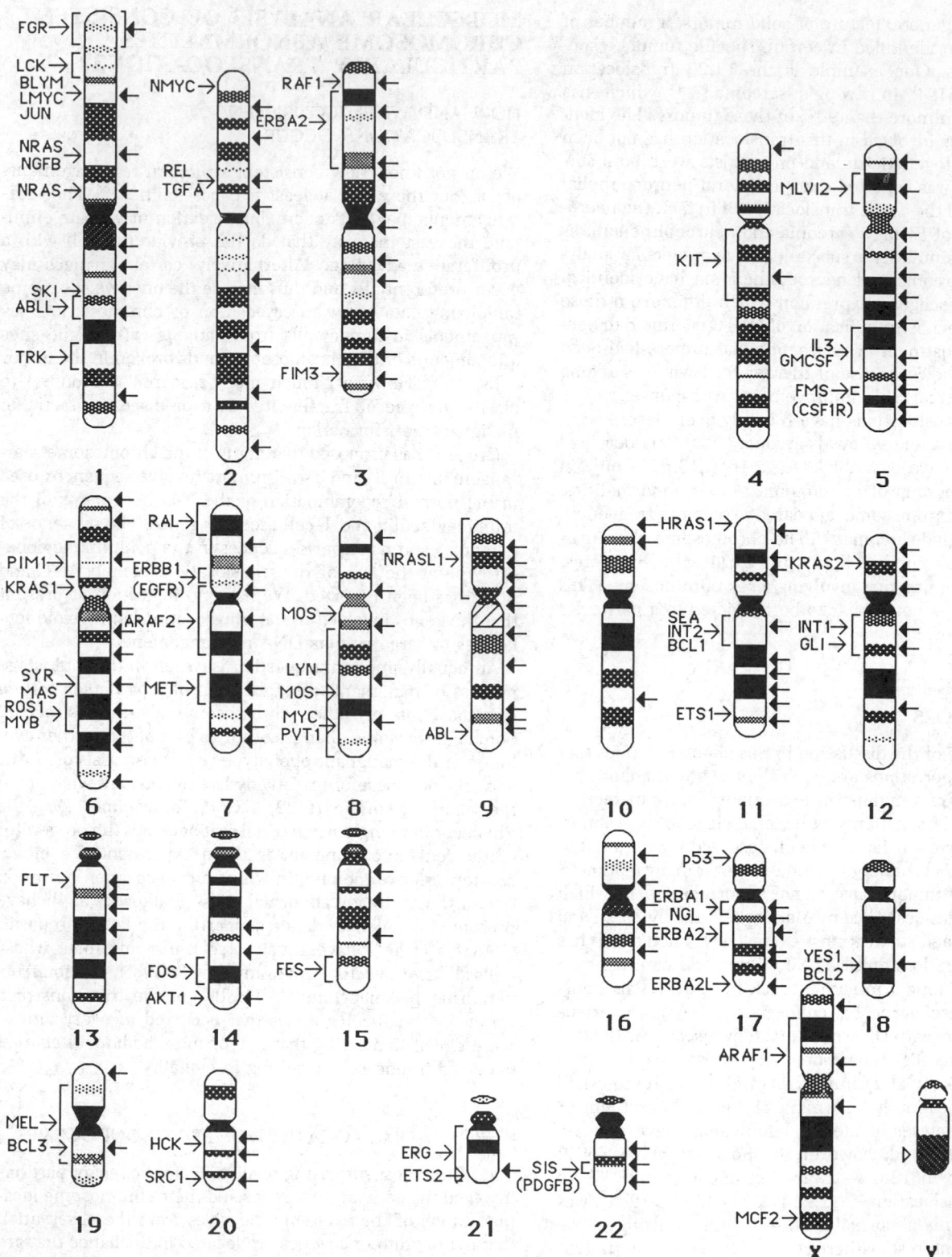

FIG. 6-8. Map of the chromosome location of proto-oncogenes or of genes with transforming properties and the breakpoints observed in recurring chromosome abnormalities in human leukemia, lymphoma, and solid tumors. The proto-oncogenes and their locations are placed to the left of the appropriate chromosome band (*arrow*) or region (indicated by a bracket). The breakpoints in recurring translocations, inversions, deletions, and so forth are indicated with an arrow to the right of the affected chromosome band. The location of the cancer specific breakpoints are based on the Human Gene Mapping 9 report.[5]

somes, other than No. 8, that are involved in the transloca-tions in Burkitt's lymphoma: 14q23, 2p12, and 22q11 re-spectively. These translocations result in the aberrant juxtaposition of MYC and one of the immunoglobulin genes; this in turn leads to abnormal regulation of MYC expression, although the precise nature of the derangement is not pres-ently understood.[113,115] Comparable chromosome transloca-tions and gene rearrangements have been observed in mouse plasmacytomas.[116]

An analogous chromosome abnormality has been defined recently in T-cell leukemia. In this translocation the break-point also involves MYC at 8q24, but the other gene is the α chain for the T-cell receptor (TCRA) which is located at 14q11.[117,118] In SKW3, we and others have shown that the break in MYC is 3' of the third exon and MYC remains on chromosome 8; in TCRA the break is just 5' of a Jα segment (JαD).[119,120] This translocation is similar to these involving the immunoglobulin light chain genes in which MYC also remains on No. 8. The TCRA gene is also involved with translocations affecting 14q32 and the heavy chain gene in the inv(14).[121]

Investigators are now in the process of unraveling the mystery of the Ph[1] translocation in CML and ALL. In the t(9;22) in CML and ALL, the Abelson proto-oncogene (ABL) is translocated to the Ph[1] chromosome.[15] This was an impor-tant observation, because ABL was the first gene known to be on No. 9 that was shown to translocate to No. 22, thus establishing that the translocation was reciprocal. The ABL gene was first identified because of its homology with the viral oncogene that had been isolated from a mouse pre-B-cell leukemia. The breakpoint junction in CML was cloned and the site on the Ph[1] was called bcr, for breakpoint cluster region,[122] since the majority of breaks cluster in a small, 5.8-kilobase (kb) region. In contrast, the breaks on No. 9 occur over an incredible distance of more than 200 kb. We have used pulse field gel electophoresis (PFGE) to great advantage in the study of the ABL proto-oncogene. Southern blotting with standard gel electrophoresis leads to separation of DNA fragments in the size range of 2 to about 25 kb. Since the ABL gene is larger than 200 kb, mapping it in 10- to 20-kb pieces is a formidable task. In contrast, by using PFGE one can separate fragments more than 1,000 kb in size, and this technique is also very effective in the 100-to 600-kb range. A normal chromosome band contains roughly 3000 to 5000 kb, and thus several very large, overlapping fragments could contain a single band. Using many probes for ABL provided by various investigators, Westbrook, Rubin and co-workers have constructed a map of the normal ABL gene.[123] This is a complex gene that normally uses one of two alter-native beginnings, exon Ia or Ib. During transcription, either of these can be spliced at the same point on the remainder of the gene, which is called the common splice acceptor site, or exon II. One of their first discoveries was that the type Ib exon mapped more than 200 kb upstream from exon II. As a result, a very large segment of the RNA transcript is re-moved or spliced out to form the mature mRNA. This is a remarkable feat, not identified before in biologic systems. The breakpoints in the chromosomes of various CML pa-tients and cell lines occur in many locations upstream (5') of exon II. However, the same size (8.5 kb) mRNA is found in all CML patients; this occurs because the bcr exons are spliced to ABL exon II, resulting in a chimeric mRNA that is translated into a chimeric protein (p210 BCR-ABL).[124,125]

With regard to Ph[1]+ ALL, it has always been an enigma why the typical Ph[1] translocation is seen in ALL and in fact is the most common translocation in adults with ALL.[56] One relatively trivial explanation would be that the patients really had CML in lymphoid blast crisis with an undiagnosed chronic phase, and this may occur in some patients. How-ever, analysis of DNA from some Ph[1]+ ALL cells indicates that the breakpoint in the BCR gene on No. 22 differs from that in CML. In one study, the majority of adult patients (13 of 17) appeared to have the BCR rearrangement seen in CML, whereas it was not found in any of 7 children, who presumably had a more 5' breakpoint in the BCR gene.[126]

Data from our laboratory as well as others indicate that the breakpoints on No. 22 are more than 50 kb proximal to the CML break but are still within the BCR gene.[127] The break-points on No. 9 are similar to those in CML. In our studies, 4 of 6 Ph[1]+ (bcr-negative) ALL patients have a rearrangement of BCR detected on PFGE. Several investigators have shown that these Ph[1]+ ALL patients have an abnormal-sized chi-meric BCR-ABL mRNA (7.0–7.4 kb) and ABL protein (p185 BCR-ABL).[128,129] It should be possible to use several DNA probes from the BCR gene and PFGE to distinguish the CML from the ALL breakpoint. In the future, we will understand the role of the BCR and ABL proteins in normal cells and that of the two different chimeric BCR-ABL proteins in CML and in ALL. Thus, the genetic analysis of what appeared to be a simple chromosome change, namely, the 9;22 translocation, has revealed unexpected complexity. An understanding of the altered function of the ABL protein will probably be central to the development of more specific and more effec-tive forms of therapy.

Remarkable progress is being made in the molecular ge-netic analysis of solid tumors. In addition to the amplifica-tion of NMYC in neuroblastoma, Slamon and co-workers have recently reported that amplification of the HER2/neu gene in breast tumor tissue occurred in 40% of patients with positive axillary lymph nodes. This gene amplification showed a more significant correlation with survival than did the extent of lymph node involvement.[130] Bodmer et al re-ported that the gene for familial polyposis coli (FPC) was very closely linked to a DNA marker on the long arm of chromosome 5 near 5q21-q22.[131] The same group found that at least 20% of patients with sporadic colorectal cancers showed loss of heterozygosity for a very polymorphic DNA probe on 5q.[132] These observations, based initially on the identification of an interstitial deletion of chromosome 5 (bands 5q15–q22)[133] in a patient with FPC, will permit cloning of the involved gene using strategies already de-scribed for retinoblastoma. As noted earlier, the observation by Whang-Peng et al[86] of a deletion of the short arm of chromosome 3 in small cell lung cancer provided the essen-tial clue to examining these tumors for loss of heterozygosity for DNA markers on 3p.[89,90]

It is interesting to speculate that the difference in fre-quency of carcinomas compared with leukemia, lymphoma or sarcoma may be related to the difference in size of the target DNA. The latter tumors are associated with relatively specific chromosome rearrangements (translocations or inversions) that lead to the abnormal juxtaposition of two specific genes. Although the breakpoints may show some variability on the DNA level, they must bring together the critical functional elements of the two genes. The identity of the two genes is determined by the cell type within which the rearrangement occurs. These factors lead to the relatively low probability that the critical genetic rearrangement will occur in the appropriate cell type. In contrast, if the preliminary data on the more common cancers (*e.g.*, lung cancer and colon cancer) are confirmed, than a different genetic or cytogenetic mechanism, or both, would be involved in malignant transformation. In these cancers, homozygous chromosome deletion or gene inactivation appears to be a prominent feature, presumably leading to loss of genes that regulate or inhibit cell proliferation. The extent of the detectable deletions is quite variable, the only requirement being that both alleles of the critical gene must be deleted or inactivated. Thus any two chromosome breaks that lead to loss of the critical gene in the appropriate cell type would provide one step in the multistep process of transformation. It is too simplistic to relate the incidence of various neoplasias only to the precision of the DNA changes required, namely, specific translocations versus variable size deletions, but future research may confirm that this difference is a contributing factor.

SPECIFICITY OF CHROMOSOME REARRANGEMENTS

The evidence presented in this chapter clearly demonstrates the remarkable specificity of certain chromosome rearrangements for particular subtypes of tumors, especially leukemia or lymphoma. The mechanisms by which this specificity is achieved are unknown; however, a number of investigators have shown that certain proteins required for promotion of gene expression are synthesized in a very cell-type–specific manner.[134] These proteins are only present in the appropriate cell type, and therefore the particular gene is activated only in that cell type. The chromosome rearrangements affecting *MYC* in B-cell and T-cell tumors strongly support the interpretation that the specificity resides in the gene that is uniquely active in a particular cell type. Thus the immunoglobulin genes are highly regulated in B-cells and they can therefore serve as the switch or activator mechanism for *MYC* in B-cells; on the other hand, *TCRA* is an active gene in T-cells with a strong enhancer/promotor and it clearly is an activator for *MYC* in T-cells. A reasonable paradigm is that translocations bring together in an inappropriate manner a growth factor or growth factor receptor gene (the proto-oncogene in the examples defined to date) adjacent to an active cell specific gene. It should be emphasized that many of the proto-oncogenes were identified in viruses that cause tumors. However, these genes have not been conserved through evolution from yeast and *Drosophila* to the chicken, mouse, and man to cause cancer! Where we have any insight into the function of these genes in normal cells, they are growth factors or growth factor receptors. It is not unexpected that the genes which a virus might coopt if it developed into a tumor-producing virus would be genes that control proliferation, genes that, under viral regulation,

would function abnormally with regard to cell growth. Further support for the concept that oncogenes are growth factors gone wrong is provided by studies performed at the Hall Institute in Melbourne. Investigators inserted the cloned gene for granulocyte–macrophage colony-stimulating factor into a viral vector, transfected mouse myeloid cells with this gene, and injected the cells into mice which developed leukemia.[135] The term "oncogene" is too short and easy for it to be discarded, but it really refers to respectable genes for growth factors or their receptors.

As has been described in this chapter, analysis of various tumors for alterations in proto-oncogenes has revealed that a number are abnormal as a result of translocations, amplification, or mutations. In some situations the relationship of the change in the proto-oncogene to the multistage process of malignant transformation is unclear.[114] Such ambiguity is not a problem with chromosome translocations; the evidence is overwhelming that the t(8;14) in Burkitt's lymphoma and the t(9;22) in CML are an integral component of the cascade of events leading to the transformation of a normal to a malignant cell. The ever-increasing number of translocations reviewed in this chapter provide a potential gold mine for identifying new genes that are unequivocally related to the malignant phenotype of the affected cell. The challenge is to isolate these translocation breakpoint junctions, to identify the genes that are located at these breakpoints, and then to determine the change in gene function that occurs as a consequence of the translocation. The ultimate measure of success, however, will be in the application of these new insights to the development of new, more effective treatments for cancer. In the future, each particular subtype of tumor will be treated in a uniquely defined way that is most appropriate for the specific genetic defect present in that tumor. This should lead to a new era of cancer therapy that is both more effective and less toxic.

GLOSSARY OF CYTOGENETIC TERMINOLOGY

centromere The constriction along the length of the chromosome that is the site of the spindle fiber attachment. The position of the centromere determines whether chromosomes are metacentric (X-shaped, *e.g.*, chromosomes 1, 3, 16, 19, 20) or acrocentric (inverted V-shaped, *e.g.*, chromosomes 13-15, 21, 22, Y). During mitosis the two exact copies of the DNA in each chromosome are separated by shortening of the spindle fibers attached to opposite sides of the dividing cell.

clone In the cytogenetic sense, defined as two cells with the same additional or structurally rearranged chromosome or three cells with loss of the same chromosome.

deletion A segment of a chromosome is missing as the result of two breaks and loss of the intervening piece (see Fig. 6-2).

diploid Normal chromosome number and composition of chromosomes.

haploid Only half the normal complement (*i.e.*, 23 chromosomes).

hyperdiploid Additional chromosomes; therefore the modal number is 47 or greater.

hypodiploid Loss of chromosomes; modal number is 45 or less.

inversion Two breaks occur in the same chromosome with rotation of the intervening segment. If both breaks are on the same side of the centromere, it is called a *paracentric inversion*. If the breaks are on opposite sides it is called a *pericentric inversion*.

isochromosome A chromosome consisting of identical copies of one chromosome arm with loss of the other arm. Thus an isochromosome for the long arm of No. 17 [i(17q)] contains two copies of the long arm (separated by the centromere) with loss of the short arm of the chromosome.

karyotype Arrangement of chromosomes from a particular cell according to a well-established system such that the largest chromosomes are first and the smallest ones are last (see Fig.6-3). Normal female karyotype is 46,XX; normal male karyotype is 46,XY. Karyotype symbols: p = short arm, q = long arm, t = translocation, del = deletion, inv = inversion, i = isochromosome. A + before the chromosome indicates a gain of a whole chromosome (*e.g.*, +8); a + after the chromosome indicates gain of part of the chromosome (*e.g.*, 14q+ denotes added material at the end of the long arm of No. 14). A − before the chromosome indicates a loss of a whole chromosome (*e.g.*, −7); a − after the chromosome indicates loss of part of the chromosome (*e.g.*, 5q− denotes loss of part of the long arm of No. 5). A ? indicates uncertainty about the identity of the chromosome or band listed just after the ?.

translocation A break in at least two chromosomes with exchange of material. In a reciprocal translocation there is no obvious loss of chromosomal material (see Fig. 6-4).

REFERENCES

1. Mitelman F: Catalog of Chromosome Aberrations in Cancer. New York, Alan R Liss, 1988
2. Heim S, Mitelman F: Cancer Cytogenetics. New York, Alan R Liss, 1987
3. Rowley JD: Chromosome abnormalities in leukemia. J Clin Oncol 6:194–202, 1988
4. Rowley JD, Testa JR: Chromosome abnormalities in malignant hematologic diseases. Adv Cancer Res 36:103–148, 1982
5. Bloomfield CD, Trent JM, van den Berghe H: Report of the Committee on Structural Chromosome Changes in Neoplasia. Human Gene Mapping 9. (1987) Cytogenet Cell Genet 46:344–366, 1987
6. Yunis JJ: The chromosomal basis of human neoplasia. Science 221:227–236, 1983
7. Mitelman F: Catalogue of chromosome aberrations in cancer. Cytogenet Cell Genet 36:1–515, 1983
8. Mitelman F: Catalog of chromosome aberrations in cancer. In Sandberg AA (ed): Progress and Topics in Cytogenetics, Vol 5. New York, Alan R Liss, 1985
9. Rowley JD, Potter D: Chromosomal banding patterns in acute nonlymphocytic leukemia. Blood 47:705–721, 1976
10. ISCN: An international system for human cytogenetic nomenclature: High resolution banding. Cytogenet Cell Genet 31:1–23, 1981
11. Testa JR, Rowley JD: Chromosomes in leukemia and lymphoma with special emphasis on methodology. In Catovsky D (ed): The Leukemic Cell, pp 184-202. Edinburgh, Churchill–Livingstone, 1981
12. First International Workshop in Solid Tumors. Cancer Genet Cytogenet 19:3–197, 1986
13. Nowell PC, Hungerford DA: A minute chromosome in human granulocytic leukemia. Science 132:1497, 1960
14. Rowley JD: A new consistent chromosomal abnormality in chronic myelogenous leukemia. Nature 243: 290–293, 1973
15. de Klein A, van Kessel AG, Grosveld G et al: A cellular oncogene is translocated to the Philadelphia chromosome in chronic myelocytic leukemia. Nature 300:765–767, 1982
16. de Klein, Hagemeijer A: Cytogenetic and molecular analysis of the Ph¹ translocation in chronic myeloid leukemia. Cancer Surveys 3:515–529, 1984
17. Bakhshi A, Minowada J, Arnold A et al: Lymphoid blast crises of chronic myelogenous leukemia represent stages in the development of B-cell precursors N Engl J Med 309:826–831, 1983
18. Whang-Peng J, Canellos GP, Carbone PP et al: Clinical implications of cytogenetic variants in chronic myelocytic leukemia (CML). Blood 32:755–766, 1968
19. Pugh WC, Pearson M, Vardiman JW et al: Philadelphia chromosome-negative chronic myelogenous leukaemia: A morphologic reassessment, Br J Haematol 60:457–467, 1985
20. Travis LB, Pierre RV, DeWald GW: Ph¹-negative chronic granulocytic leukemia: A nonentity. Am J Clin Pathol 85:186–193. 1986
21. Morris CM, Reeve AE, Fitzgerald PH et al: Genomic diversity correlates with clinical variation in Ph¹-negative chronic myeloid leukemia. Nature 320:281–283, 1986
22. Bartram CR: Molecular genetic analyses of chronic myelocytic leukemia. In Huhn D, Hellriegel P, Niederle N (eds): Chronic Myelocytic Leukemia and Interferon. New York, Springer-Verlag (in press)
23. Fourth International Workshop on Chromosomes in Leukemia. Cancer Genet Cytogenet 11:249–360, 1984
24. Bennett JM, Catovsky D, Daniel M-T et al: Proposals for the classification of the acute leukemias: French–American–British (FAB) Cooperative Group. BR J Haematol 33: 451–458, 1976
25. Rowley JD: Identification of a translocation with quinacrine fluorescence in a patient with acute leukemia. Ann Genet (Paris) 16:109–112, 1973
26. Rowley JD: Golomb HM, Vardiman J et al: Further evidence for a non-random chromosomal abnormality in acute promyelocytic leukemia. Int J Cancer 20:869–872, 1977
27. Pearson MG, Vardiman JW, Le Beau MM et al: A new cytogenetic subset of acute non-lymphocytic leukemia: t(6;9) associated with bone marrow basophilia. Am J Hematol 18:393-403, 1985
28. Westbrook CA, LeBeau MM, Diaz MO et al: Chromosomal localization and characterization of c-*abl* in the t(6;9) of acute nonlymphocytic leukemia. Proc Natl Acad Sci USA 82:8742–8746, 1985
29. Berger R, Bernheim A, Sigaux F et al: Acute monocytic leukemia chromosome studies. Leuk Res 6:17–26, 1982
30. Hagemeijer A, Hahlen K, Sizoo W et al: Translocation (9;11)(p21;q23) in three cases of acute monoblastic leukemia. Cancer Genet Cytogenet 5:95–105, 1982
31. Arthur DC, Bloomfield CD: Partial deletion of the long arm of chromosome 16 and bone marrow eosinophilia in acute nonlymphocytic leukemia: A new association. Blood 61:994–998, 1983
32. Larson RA, Williams SF, Le Beau MM et al: Acute myelomonocytic leukemia with abnormal eosinophils and inv(16) or t(16;16) has a favorable prognosis. Blood 68:1242–1249, 1986
33. Keating MJ: Early identification of potentially cured patients with acute myelogenous leukemia: A recent challenge. In Bloomfield CD (ed): Adult Leukemias I, pp 237–263. Boston, Martinus Nijhoff, 1982
34. Le Beau MM, Albain KS, Larson RA et al: Clinical and cytogenetic correlations in 63 patients with therapy-related myelodysplastic syndromes and acute nonlymphocytic leukemia: Further evidence for characteristic abnormalities of chromosomes No. 5 and 7. J Clin Oncol 4:325–345, 1986
35. Rowley JD, Golomb HM, Vardiman JW: Nonrandom chromosome abnormalities in acute leukemia and dysmyelopoietic syndromes in patients with previously treated malignant disease. Blood 58:759–767, 1981
36. Arthur DC, Bloomfield CD: Banded chromosome analysis in patients with treatment-associated acute non-lymphocytic leukemia. Cancer Genet Cytogenet 12:189–199, 1984
37. Pedersen-Bjergaad J, Philip P, Pederson NT et al: Acute nonlymphocytic leukemia, preleukemia, and acute myeloproliferative syndrome secondary to treatment of other malignant diseases. Cancer 54:452-462, 1984
38. Larson RA, Le Beau MM, Vardiman JW et al: The predictive value of initial cytogenetic studies in 148 adults with acute nonlymphocytic leukemia. Cancer Genet Cytogenet 10:219–236, 1983
39. Mitelman F, Nilsson PG, Brandt C et al: Chromosome pattern, occupation and clinical features in patients with acute nonlymphocytic leukemia. Cancer Genet Cytogenet 4:187–214, 1981
40. Golomb HM, Alimena G., Rowley JD et al: Correlation of occupation and karyotype in adults with acute nonlymphocytic leukemia. Blood 60:404–411, 1982
41. Le Beau MM, Pettenati MJ, Lemons RS et al: Assignment of the *GM-CSF*, *CSF-1*, and *FMS* genes to human chromosome 5 provides evidence for linkage of a family of genes regulating hematopoiesis and for their involvement in the deletion (5q) in myeloid disorders. In: Molecular Biology of Homo Sapiens. Cold Spring Harbor Symp Quant Biol 51:899–909, 1986
42. Bloomfield CD, Arthur DC, Frizzera G et al: Nonrandom chromosome abnormalities in lymphoma. Cancer Res 43:2975–2984, 1983
43. Koduru PRK, Filippa DA, Richardson ME et al: Cytogenetic and histologic correlations in malignant lymphomas. Blood 69:97–102, 1987
44. Yunis JJ, Frizzera G, Oken MM et al: Multiple recurrent genomic defects in follicular lymphoma: A possible model for cancer. N Engl J Med 316:79–84, 1987
45. Fifth International Workshop on Chromosomes in Leukemia-Lymphoma: Correlation of chromosome abnormalities with histologic and immunologic characteristics in

non-Hodgkin's lymphoma and adult T-cell leukemia–lymphoma. Blood 70:1554–1564, 1987

46. Manolov G, Manolova Y: Marker band in one chromosome 14 from Burkitt lymphomas. Nature 237:33–34, 1972

47. Zech L, Haglund U, Nilsson K et al: Characteristic chromosomal abnormalities in biopsies and lymphoid-cell lines from patients with Burkitt and non-Burkitt lymphomas. Int J Cancer 17:47–56, 1976

48. Fukuhara S, Rowley JD, Variakojis D et al: Chromosome abnormalities in poorly differentiated lymphocytic lymphoma. Cancer Res 39:3119–3128, 1979

49. Working formulation for clinical usage: National Cancer Institute sponsored study of classification of non-Hodgkin's lymphomas. Cancer 49:2112–2135, 1982

50. Tsujimoto Y, Finger LR, Yunis JJ et al: Cloning of the chromosome breakpoint of neoplastic B cells with the t(14;18) chromosome translocation. Science 226:1098–1099, 1984

51. Cleary ML, Sklar J.: Cloning and structural analysis of cDNA's for bcl-2 and a hybrid bcl-2/immunoglobulin transcript resulting from the t(14;18) translocation. Cell 47:19–28, 1986

52. Gahrton G, Robert K-H, Fribert K et al: Nonrandom chromosomal aberrations in chronic lymphocytic leukemia revealed by polyclonal B-cell mitogen stimulation. Blood 56:640-647, 1980

53. Han T, Ozer H, Sadamori N et al: Prognostic importance of cytogenetic abnormalities in patients with chronic lymphocytic leukemia. N Engl J Med 310:288–292, 1984

54. Bird ML, Ueshima Y, Rowley JD et al: Chromosome abnormalities in B-cell chronic lymphocytic leukemia and their clinical correlations. Leukemia (in press)

55. Robert K-H, Gahrton G, Friberg K et al: Extra chromosome 12 and prognosis in chronic lymphocytic leukemia. Scand J Haematol 28:163–168, 1982

56. Third International Workshop on Chromosomes in Leukemia. Cancer Genet Cytogenet 4:95–142, 1981

57. Stong RC, Korsmeyer SJ, Parkin JL et al: Human acute leukemia cell line with the t(4;11) chromosomal rearrangement exhibits B-lineage and monocytic characteristics. Blood 67:391–397, 1986

58. Michael PM, Levin MD, Garson OM et al: Translocation 1;19: A new cytogenetic abnormality in acute lymphocytic leukemia. Cancer Genet Cytogenet 12:333–341, 1984

59. Carroll AJ, Crist WM, Parmley RT et al: Pre-B cell leukemia associated with chromosome translocation 1;19. Blood 63:721–724, 1984

60. Williams DL, Look AT, Melvin SL et al: New chromosomal translocations correlate with specific immunophenotypes of childhood acute lymphoblastic leukemia. Cell 36:101–109, 1984

61. Secker-Walker LM, Swansbury GJ, Hardisty RM et al: Cytogenetics of acute lymphoblastic leukemia in children as a factor in the prediction of long-term survival. Br J Haematol 52:389–399, 1982

62. Williams DL, Tsiatis A, Brodeur GMG et al: Prognostic importance of chromosome number in 136 untreated children with acute lymphoblastic leukemia. Blood 60:864–871, 1982

63. Bloomfield CD, Goldman AI, Alimena G et al: Chromosomal abnormalities identify high-risk and low-risk patients with acute lymphoblastic leukemia. Blood 67:415–420, 1986

64. Ueshima Y, Rowley JD, Variakojis D et al: Cytogenetic studies on patients with chronic T cell leukemia/lymphoma. Blood 63:1028–1038, 1984

65. Zech L, Gahrton G. Hammarstrom L et al: Inversion of chromosome 14 marks human T-cell chronic lymphocytic leukemia. Nature 308:858–860, 1984

66. Kaiser-McCaw B, Hecht F, Harnden DG et al: Somatic rearrangement of chromosome 14 in human lymphocytes. Proc Natl Acad Sci USA 72:2071–2075, 1975

67. Aurias A: Analyse cytogenetique de 21 cas d'ataxie-telangiectase. J Genet Hum 29:235–247, 1981

68. Miyamoto K, Tomita N, Ishii A et al: Chromosome abnormalities of leukemia cells in adult patients with T-cell leukemia. JNCI 73:353–362, 1984

69. Sadamori N, Nishino K, Kusano M et al: Significance of chromosome 14 anomaly at band q11 in Japanese patients with adult T-cell leukemia. Cancer 58:2244–2250, 1986

70. Rowley JD, Haren JM, Wong-Staal F et al: Chromosome pattern in cells from patients positive for human T-cell leukemia virus. In Gallo RC, Essex ME, Gross L (eds): Human T-Cell Leukemia-Lymphoma Viruses; pp 85-89. Cold Spring Harbor, NY, Cold Spring Harbor Laboratory 1984

71. Whang-Peng J, Bunn PA, Knutsen T et al: Cytogenetic studies in human T-cell lymphoma virus (HTLV)-positive leukemia–lymphoma in the United States. JNCI 74:357–369, 1985

72. Raimondi SC, Pui C-H, Behm FG et al: 7q32-q36 translocations in childhood T cell leukemia: Cytogenetic evidence for involvement of the T cell receptor β-chain gene. Blood 69: 131–134, 1987

73. Francke U: Specific chromosome changes in the human heritable tumors retinoblastoma and nephroblastoma. In Rowley JD, Ultmann JE (eds): Chromosomes and Cancer. Bristol–Myers Symposia Series, Vol 5, pp 99–115, New York, Academic Press 1983

74. Kondo K, Chilcote RR, Maurer HS et al: Chromosome abnormalities in tumor cells from patients with sporadic Wilms' tumor. Cancer Res 44:5376–5281, 1984

75. Knudson AG: Mutation and cancer: Statistical study of retinoblastoma. Proc Natl Acad Sci USA 68:800–823, 1971

76. Cavenee WK, Dryja TP, Philllips RA et al: Expression of recessive alleles by chromosomal mechanisms in retinoblastoma. Nature 305:779–784, 1983

77. Dryja TP, Cavenee WK, White R et al: Homozygosity of chromosome 13 in retinoblastoma. N Engl J Med 310:550–553, 1984

78. Friend SH, Bernards R, Rogelj S et al: A human DNA segment with properties of the gene that predisposes to retinoblastoma. Nature 323:643–646, 1986

79. Lee W-H Bookstein R, Hong F et al: Human retinoblastoma susceptibility gene: Cloning, identification, and sequence. Science 235:1394–1399, 1987

80. Murphree AL, Benedict WF: Retinoblastoma: Clues to human oncogenesis. Science 219:1028–1033, 1984

81. Brodeur GM, Green AA, Hayes FA et al: Cytogenetic features of human neuroblastomas and cell lines. Cancer Res 41:4678–4686, 1981

82. Biedler JL, Spengler BA: Metaphase chromosome anomaly: Association with drug resistance and cell-specific products. Science 191:185–187, 1976

83. Schwab M, Alitalo K, Klempnauer K-H et al: Amplified DNA with limited homology to myc cellular oncogene is shared by human neuroblastoma cell lines and a neuroblastoma tumour. Nature 305:245–248, 1983

84. Brodeur GM, Seeger RL, Schwab M: Amplification of N-myc in untreated neuroblastoma correlates with advanced disease stage. Science 224:1121–1124, 1984

85. Balaban G, Herlyn M, Guerry D et al: Cytogenetics of human malignant melanoma and pre-malignant lesions. Cancer Genet Cytogenet 3:243–250, 1981

86. Whang-Peng J, Bunn PA Jr, Kao-Shan CS et al: A nonrandom chromosomal abnormality, del 3p(14-23), in human small cell lung cancer (SCLC). Cancer Genet Cytogenet 6:119–134, 1982

87. Yoshida MA, Ohyashiki K, Ochi K et al: Rearrangement of chromosome 3 in renal cell carcinoma. Cancer Genet Cytogenet 19:351–354, 1986

88. Szucs S, Muller-Brechlin R, DeRiese W, et al: Deletion 3p: The only chromosome loss in a primary renal cell carcinoma. Cancer Genet Cytogenet 26:369–373, 1987

89. Naylor SL, Johnson BE, Minna JD et al: Loss of heterozygosity of chromosome 3p markers in small cell lung cancer. Nature 329:451–454, 1987

90. Kok K, Osinga J, Carritt B et al: Deletion of a DNA sequence at the chromosomal region 3p21 in all major types of lung cancer. Nature 330:578–581, 1987

91. Atkin NB, Baker MC: Specific chromosome change, i(12p), in testicular tumours? Lancet 2:1349, 1982

92. Aurias A, Rimbaut C, Buffe D et al: Chromosomal translocation in Ewing's sarcoma. N Engl J Med 309:496, 1983

93. Turc-Carel C, Philip I, Berger M-P et al: Chromosomal translocation in Ewing's sarcoma. N Engl J Med 309:497–498, 1983

94. Whang-Peng J, Triche TJ, Knutsen T et al: Chromosome translocation in peripheral neuroepithelioma. N Engl J Med 311:584-585, 1984

95. Israel MA, Helman LJ, Miser J: Patterns of proto-oncogene expression: A novel approach to the development of tumor markers. In DeVita VT Jr, Hellman S, Rosenberg SA (eds): Important Advances in Oncology 1987. Philadelphia, JB Lippincott, 1987

96. Dal Cin P, Sandberg AA: Chromosome changes in soft tissue tumors: Benign and malignant. Cancer Invest (in press)

97. Turc-Carel C, Limon J, Dal Cin P et al: Cytogenetic studies of adipose tissue tumors: II. Recurrent reciprocal translocation t(12;16)(q13;p11) in myxoid liposarcomas. Cancer Genet Cytogenet 23: 291–299, 1986

98. Turc-Carel C, Dal Cin P, Limon J et al: Involvement of chromosome X in primary cytogenetic changes in human neoplasia: Nonrandom translocation in synovial sarcoma. Proc Natl Acad Sci USA 84:1981–1985, 1987

99. Mark J, Mitelman F, Levan G: On the specificity of the G abnormality in human meningiomas studied by the fluorescence technique. Acta Pathol Microbiol Immunol Scand [A] 80:812–820, 1972

100. Zankl H, Zang KD: Marker chromosome 20q— does not arise only in bone marrow disorders. Cancer Genet Cytogenet 3:85–87, 1981

101. Seizinger BR, Martuza RL, Gusella JF: Loss of genes on chromosomes 22 in tumorigenesis of human acoustic neuroma. Nature 322:644–647, 1986

102. Mark J, Dahlenfors R, Ekedahl C et al: Cytogenetics of the human mixed salivary gland tumor. Hereditas 99:115–129, 1983

103. Turc-Carel C, Dal Cin P, Boghasian L et al: Consistent breakpoints in region 14q22-q24 in uterine leiomyoma. Cancer Genet Cytogenet 32:25–31, 1988

104. Heim S, Nilbert M, Vanni R et al: A specific translocation, t(12;14)(q14–15;q23–24) characterizes a subgroup of uterine leiomyomas. Cancer Genet Cytogenet 32:13–17, 1988

105. Rowley JD: The biological implications of consistent chromosome rearrangements. Cancer Res 44:3159–3165, 1984

106. Sutherland GR, Hecht F: Fragile Sites on Human Chromosomes. New York, Oxford University Press, 1985

107. Yunis JJ, Soreng AL: Constitutive fragile sites and cancer. Science 226:1199–1204, 1984

108. Le Beau MM: Chromosomal fragile sites and cancer-specific rearrangements. Blood 67:849–858, 1986

109. ar-Rushdi A, Nishikura K, Erickson J: Differential expression of the translocated and the untranslocated c-myc oncogene in Burkitt lymphoma. Science 222:390–393, 1983

110. Fialkow PJ, Singer JW: Tracing development and cell lineages in human hemopoietic neoplasia. In: Weissman IL (ed): Leukemia: Dahlem Konferenzen, pp 203–222. Berlin; Springer-Verlag, 1985

111. Adams JM, Harris AW, Pinkert CA et al: The c-myc oncogene driven by immunoglobulin enhancers induces lymphoid malignancy in transgenic mice. Nature 318:533–538, 1985

112. Bishop JM: The molecular genetics of cancer. Science 235:305–311, 1987

113. Klein G, Klein E: Conditioned tumorigenicity of activated oncogenes. Cancer Res 46:3211–3224, 1986

114. Duesberg PH: Retroviruses as carcinogens and pathogens: Expectations and reality. Cancer Res 47:1199–1220, 1987

115. Leder P, Battey J, Lenoir G et al: Translocations among antibody genes in human cancer. Science 222:765–771, 1983

116. Klein G: Specific chromosomal translocations and the genesis of B-cell derived tumors in mice and men. Cell 32:311–315, 1983

117. Croce CM, Isobe M, Palumbo A et al: Gene for α-chain of human T-cell receptor: Location on chromosome 14 region involved in T-cell neoplasms. Science 227:1044–1047, 1985

118. Caccia N, Bruns GA, Kirsch IR et al: T cell receptor α-chain genes are located on chromosome 14 at 14q11–14q12 in humans. J Exp Med 161:1255–1260, 1985

119. Shima EA, Le Beau MM, McKeithan TW et al: Gene encoding the α chain of the T-cell receptor is moved immediately downstream of c-myc in a chromosomal 8;14 translocation in a cell line from a human T-cell leukemia. Proc Natl Acad Sci USA 83:3439–3443, 1986

120. Mathieu-Mahul D, Caubet JF, Bernheim A: Molecular cloning of a DNA fragment from human chromosome 14(14q11) involved in T cell malignancies. EMBO J 4:3427–3433, 1985

121. Baer R, Chen K-C, Smith SD et al: Fusion of an immunoglobulin variable gene and a T cell receptor constant gene in the chromosome 14 inversion associated with T cell tumors. Cell 44:705–713, 1985

122. Groffen J, Stevenson JR, Heisterkamp N et al: Philadelphia chromosomal breakpoints are clustered within a limited region, bcr, on chromosome 22. Cell 36:93–99, 1984

123. Westbrook CA, Rubin CM, Carrino JJ et al: Long-range mapping of the Philadelphia chromosome by pulsed-field gel electrophoresis. Blood 71:697–702, 1988

124. Konopka JB, Watanabe SM, Witte ON: An alteration of the human c-abl protein in K562 leukemia cells unmasks associate tyrosine kinase activity. Cell 37:1035–1042, 1984

125. Shtivelman E, Lifshitz B, Robert P et al: Fused transcript of abl and bcr genes in chronic myelogenous leukemia. Nature 315:550–554, 1985

126. de Klein A, Hagemeijer A, Bartram CR et al: Rearrangement and translocation of the c-abl oncogene in Philadelphia positive acute lymphoblastic leukemia. Blood 68:1369–1375, 1986

127. Rubin CM, Carrino JJ, Dickler MN et al: Heterogeneity of genomic fusion of BCR and ABL in Philadelphia chromosome–positive acute lymphoblastic leukemia. Proc Natl Acad Sci USA 85:2795–2799, 1988

128. Clark SS, McLaughlin J, Crist WM et al: Unique forms of the abl tyrosine kinase distinguish Ph¹-positive CML from Ph¹-positive ALL. Science 235:85–88, 1987

129. Chan LC, Karhi KK, Rayter SI et al: A novel abl protein expressed in Philadelphia chromosome positive acute lymphoblastic leukemia. Nature 325:635–637, 1987

130. Slamon DJ, Clark GM, Wong SG et al: Human breast cancer: Correlation of relapse and survival with amplification of the HER-2/neu oncogene. Science 235:177–182, 1987

131. Bodmer WF, Bailey CJ, Bodmer J et al: Localization of the gene for familial adenomatous polyposis on chromosome 5. Nature 328:614–616, 1987

132. Solomon E, Voss R, Hall V et al: Chromosome 5 allele loss in human colorectal carcinoma. Nature 328:616–619, 1987

133. Herrera L, Kakati S, Gibas L et al: Gardner syndrome in a man with an interstitial deletion of 5q. Am J Med Genet 25:473–476, 1986

134. Nomiyama H, Fromental C, Xiao JH et al: Cell-specific activity of the constituent elements of the simian virus 40 enhancer. Proc Natl Acad Sci USA 84:7881–7885, 1987

135. Lang RA, Metcalf D, Gough NM et al: Expression of a hemapoietic growth factor cDNA in a factor-dependent cell line results in autonomous growth and tumorigenicity. Cell 43:531–542, 1985

LANCE A. LIOTTA

WILLIAM G. STETLER-STEVENSON

CHAPTER 7 *Principles of Molecular Cell Biology of Cancer: Cancer Metastasis*

CLINICAL SIGNIFICANCE OF INVASION AND METASTASES

Tumor invasion and metastasis is the major cause of treatment failure in cancer patients. Approximately 30% of patients with newly diagnosed solid tumors (excluding skin cancers other than melanoma) already have clinically detectable metastases. Of those 70% of cancer patients who are clinically free of metastases, approximately half can be cured by local tumor therapy alone. The remaining patients have clinically occult micrometastases that ultimately become manifest. Thus, 60% of patients have microscopic or clinically evident metastases at the time of primary tumor treatment. Most patients have multiple metastases. The formation of metastatic colonies is a continuous process that begins early in the growth of the primary tumor and increases with time.[2-9] A few large identifiable metastases in a given organ are frequently accompanied by a greater number of micrometastases that were seeded more recently. The size and age variation in metastases, their dispersed anatomical location, and their heterogeneous composition hinder surgical removal and limit the effective concentration of anticancer drugs that can be delivered to the metastatic colonies.[1-4] The patient with metastatic disease dies of the direct anatomical compromise caused by the metastases or of complications associated with antimetastatic therapy.

Tumors of comparable size can have widely divergent metastatic potential, depending on their intrinsic aggressiveness and histologic type.[3-5] For many common epithelial tumors, tumor cell dissemination begins soon after primary tumor vascularization. It has been calculated that the majority of metastases from breast carcinomas are initiated when the primary tumor is less than 0.125 cm³;[6-8] this is in accord with experimental studies.[9] Indeed, Fidler and Hart have shown that the subpopulation of highly metastatic tumor cells preexists at a very early stage in the development of the heterogeneous primary tumor.[4] These highly aggressive cells may be selected out because they have a higher probability of successfully producing a metastatic colony compared with other subpopulations of primary tumor cells.

HETEROGENEITY OF THE METASTATIC PHENOTYPE

In the last 10 years the biologic heterogeneity of neoplasms has become widely recognized. At the time of diagnosis, most neoplasms consist of different populations of cells with diverse biologic characteristics (Fig. 7-1). Subpopulations differ in immunogenicity, growth rates, karyotype, pigment production, hormone production, receptor content, and susceptibility to cytotoxic drugs. Fidler and Hart have emphasized that neoplasms can be heterogeneous in their propensity to invade and metastasize, and that the aggressive

98

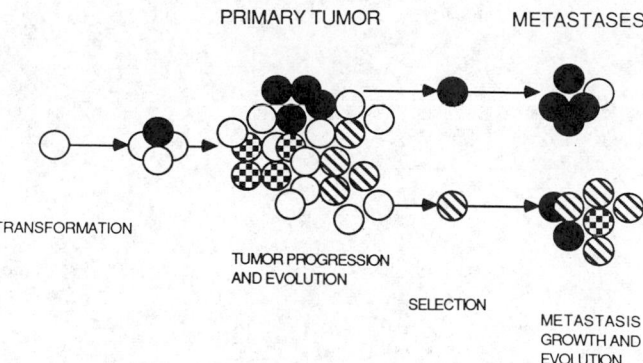

PRIMARY TUMOR   METASTASES

TRANSFORMATION

TUMOR PROGRESSION
AND EVOLUTION

SELECTION

METASTASIS
GROWTH AND
EVOLUTION

FIG. 7-1. Tumor cell heterogeneity. Clinically detectable tumors comprise a variety of subpopulations of tumor cells with diverse biologic characteristics. These subpopulations differ in growth rate, karyotype, immunogenicity, production of hormones or pigments, cell surface receptors, cytotoxic drug susceptibility, and so forth. The generation of cellular diversity within a tumor is attributed to genetic instability, either inherent in malignant cells or acquired during tumor growth. Selective pressures such as the events of the metastatic cascade or chemotherapeutic treatment result in survival of minor subpopulations of cells that preexisted in the primary neoplasm.

subpopulation may be selected out in the formation of metastasis. The first experimental proof of metastatic heterogeneity was provided by Fidler and Kripke in 1977.[10] Working with the murine B16 melanoma, the investigators used a modified fluctuation assay developed by Luria and Delbruck.[11] They discovered that preexisting subpopulations growing in the same tumor exhibit heterogeneous metastatic potential.

The process of metastasis is not random. Instead, it is a cascade of linked sequential steps that must be traversed by tumor cells if a metastasis is to develop. Each step involves multiple tumor–host interactions. A metastatic tumor cell, in order to be successful, must leave the primary tumor and invade local host tissue. It must then enter the circulation, survive in the circulation, arrest at the distant vascular bed, extravasate into the organ interstitium and parenchyma, and multiply to initiate a metastatic colony. Interruption of the metastatic cascade at any of these steps can prevent the production of clinically symptomatic metastasis. A large foundation of experimental work suggests that during each stage of the process of metastasis the rules of survival of the fittest tumor cells apply. Metastasis thus is the end result of a highly selective competition favoring the survival of a minor subpopulation of metastatic cells that preexist within the primary neoplasm.

THE METASTATIC CASCADE

A metastatic colony is the end result of a complicated series of tumor–host interactions (Table 7-1), (Fig. 7-2A). Primary tumor initiation and progression is followed by the transition from in situ to locally invasive cancer, which is accompanied by angiogenesis (Fig. 7-2B).[3,4,12] Newly formed tumor vessels are often defective and easily invaded by tumor cells within the primary mass.[9,13] At the invasion

TABLE 7-1. Tumor-Host Interactions During the Metastatic Cascade

Metastatic Cascade Event	Potential Mechanisms
1. Tumor initiation	Carcinogenic insult, oncogene activation or derepression, chromosome rearrangement
2. Promotion and progression	Karyotypic, genetic, and epigenetic instability; gene amplification; promotion-associated genes and hormones
3. Uncontrolled proliferation	Autocrine growth factors or their receptors, receptors for host hormones such as estrogen
4. Angiogenesis	Multiple angiogenesis factors including known growth factors
5. Invasion of local tissues, blood and lymphatic vessels	Serum chemoattractants, autocrine motility factors, attachment receptors, degradative enzymes
6. Circulating tumor cell arrest and extravasation	Tumor cell homotypic or heterotypic aggregation
a. adherence to endothelium	Tumor cell interaction with fibrin, platelets, and clotting factors; adhesion to RGD-type receptors
b. retraction of endothelium	Platelet factors, tumor cell factors
c. adhesion to basement membrane	Laminin receptor, thrombospondin receptor
d. dissolution of basement membrane	Degradative proteases, type IV collagenase, heparanase, cathepsins
e. locomotion	Autocrine motility factors, chemotaxis factors
7. Colony formation at secondary site	Receptors for local tissue growth factors, angiogenesis factors
8. Evasion of host defenses and resistance to therapy	Resistance to killing by host macrophages, natural killer cells, and activated T-cells; failure to express, or blocking of, tumor-specific antigens; amplification of drug resistance genes

front tumor cells also invade preestablished host blood vessels. Tumor cells are discharged into the venous drainage in single-cell form and in clumps. For rapidly growing tumors 1 cm in size, millions of tumor cells can be shed into the circulation every day.[9] Fortunately for the patient, only a very small percentage (<0.01%) of circulating tumor cells initiate metastatic colonies.[3] Tumors generally lack a well-formed lymphatic network.[14] Therefore, communication of tumor cells with lymphatic channels occurs only at the tumor periphery and not within the tumor mass. Tumor cells entering the lymphatic drainage are carried to regional lymph nodes where they arrest in the large lymphatics of the subcapsular sinus. Within 10 to 60 minutes after initial arrest in the lymph node, a significant fraction of the tumor cells detach and enter the efferent lymphatics. These tumor cells eventually end up in the regional or systemic venous drainage owing to the existence of numerous lymphatic–hematogenous communications. Thus, the regional lymph node does not function as a true mechanical barrier to tumor

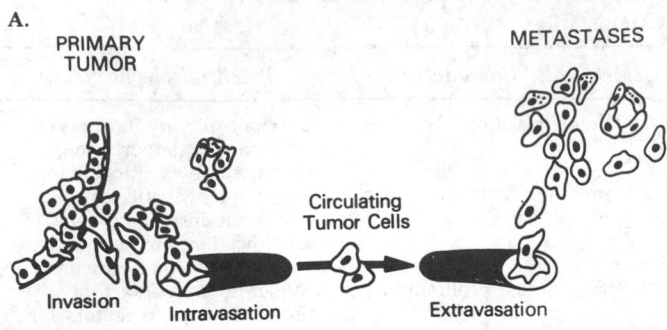

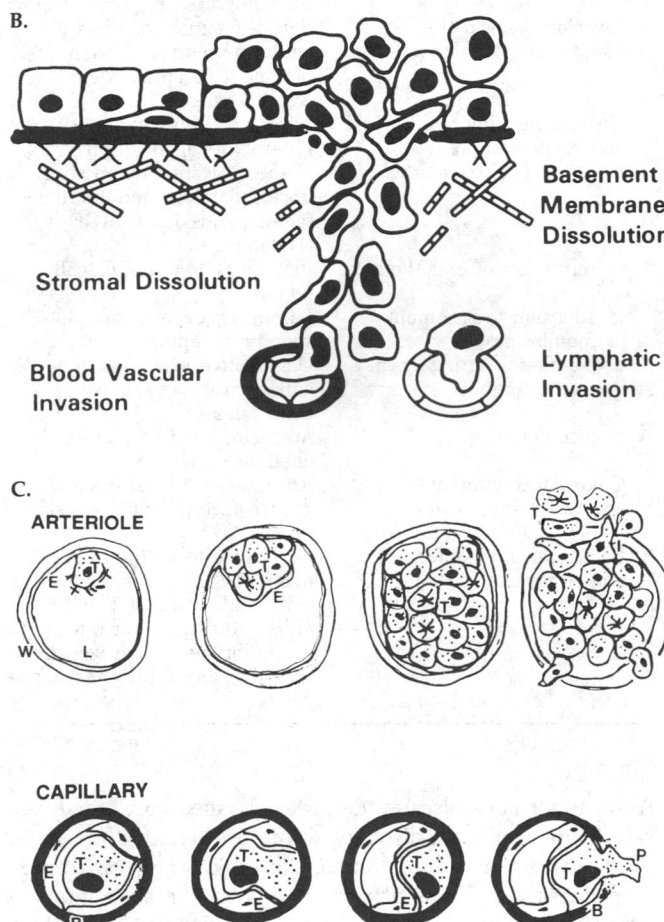

FIG. 7-2. **A**. Overview of the metastatic cascade. Tumor cells invade at the primary tumor site and enter the interstitial stroma, gaining access to blood vessels for further dissemination. Tumor cells invade the vascular wall and are dislodged into the circulation both as single cells and in tumor cell clusters. Circulating tumor cells arrest in the precapillary venules of the target organ by adherence or mechanical trapping. They must then exit the circulation by disrupting the endothelial basement membrane to initiate a metastatic colony. **B**. Early events of the metastatic cascade. The progression from in situ to invasive carcinoma is accompanied by dissolution of the basement membrane (*black line*), penetration of tumor cells into the surrounding stroma, and disruption of the interstitial stroma. Expansion of the primary tumor is accompanied by angiogenesis. Once in the stroma, the tumor cells may invade these newly formed vessels, as well as preexisting host vessels and lymphatics, allowing tumor cell dissemination from the primary tumor site. To enter the bloodstream the tumor cells must penetrate the continuous endothelial basement membrane. This is not the case for lymphatics, which lack a basement membrane. **C**. Late events of the metastatic cascade. Approximately 90% of the circulating tumor cells leave the circulation at the venule or capillary level (lower sequence from left to right). Tumor cells (*T*) arrest by adherence to the luminal surface of endothelial cells. This stimulates retraction of the endothelial cells to expose the underlying basement membrane (*B*). Tumor cells adhere to the basement membrane via cell surface matrix receptors. The retracted endothelial cells migrate over the tumor cell, separating it from the circulation. Over a period of 8 to 24 hours, the tumor cell degrades the basement membrane using a variety of proteases, including type IV collagen–degrading metalloproteinases. The tumor cell then protrudes a pseudopodia (*P*) through the zone of basement membrane lysis; this is followed by migration of the whole tumor cell. Approximately 10% of circulating tumor cells exit at the level of the artery (upper sequence from left to right). Tumor cells (*T*) complexed with fibrin and platelets attach to the artery luminal (*L*) surface. Endothelial cells (*E*) encase the proliferating tumor cell colony, which expands and fills the lumen. Once the lumen is filled (2–4 weeks), individual tumor cells invade the arterial wall (*W*) and exit the circulation.

dissemination. Lymphatic and hematogenous dissemination occur in parallel.

CIRCULATING TUMOR CELL ARREST AND EXTRAVASATION

Circulating tumor cells use a variety of means to arrest in the vessels of the target organ where they will initiate metastatic colonies (Fig. 7-2C). Approximately 80% of the circulating tumor cells are in single-cell form and attach directly to the intact endothelial surface, or to preexisting regions of exposed subendothelial basement membrane. Clumps of circulating tumor cells or tumor cells aggregated with host leuko-

cytes, fibrin, or platelets can directly embolize in the precapillary venules by mechanical impaction (Fig. 7-3A). Tumor cells in single-cell or clump form adhere to the endothelial luminal surface of arterioles. The fate and time course of the arrested tumor cells differ depending on the mechanism and location of lodgement. Tumor cells adherent to the surface of venule or capillary endothelium rapidly (within 1–4 hours) induce the active retraction of the endothelial cells (Figs. 7-3B and C).[3,15–17] The tumor cell then attaches avidly to the exposed basement membrane. Once the tumor cells have attached, the adjacent endothelial cells extend over the tumor cell and separate it from the bloodstream (Figs. 7-3D and E). Tumor cells located between the

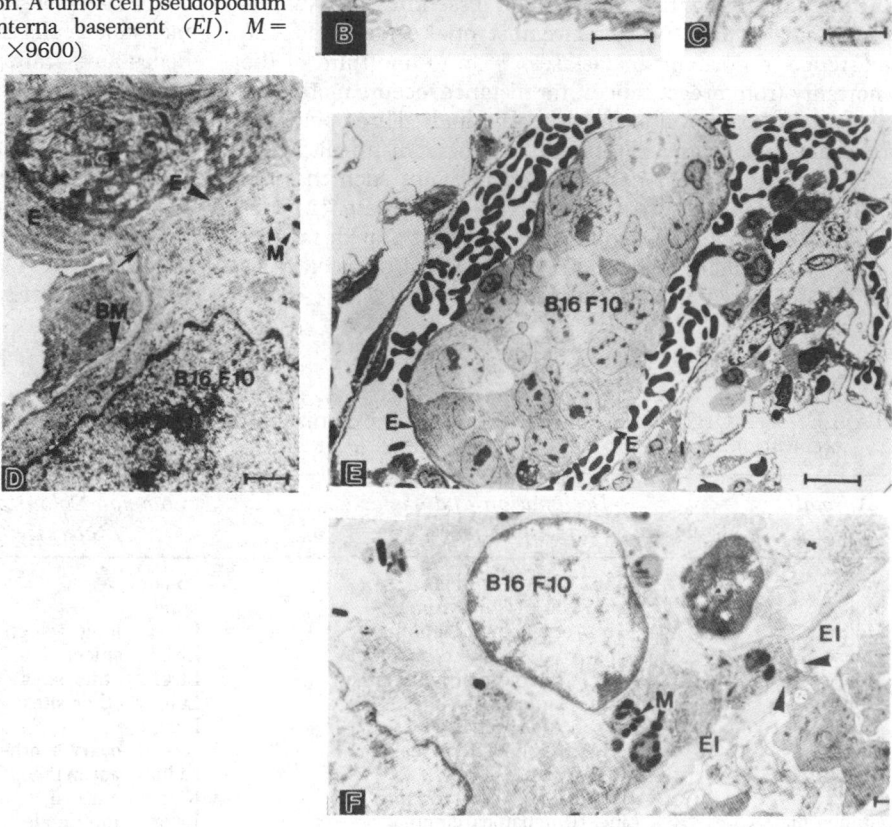

FIG. 7-3. **A**. A B16-F10 tumor cell in a lung capillary 3 hours after IV inoculation. Nonpolymerized fibrin (*F*) and platelets (*P*) are adherent to the tumor
cell. (Scale bar: 1 μm; magnification ×4250) **B**. At 6 hours after IV inoculation, the endothelium (*E*) adjacent to the attached tumor cell is still intact. A
narrow slit can be observed between the tumor cell and the endothelium.
(Scale bar: 1 μm; magnification ×12,800) **C**. A tumor cell in a capillary 12
hours after IV inoculation. Over a small surface area, the tumor cell is tightly
adherent to the basement membrane (*arrowheads*). *E* = endothelium. (Scale
bar: 1 μm; magnification ×12,800) **D**. Tumor cell in a lung capillary 12 hours
after inoculation. The tumor cell is adherent to the basement membrane (*BM*)
over a large surface area. An endothelial cell (*E*) has detached from the
basement membrane (*arrow*) and moved over the tumor cell, separating it
from the fibrin (*F*) deposit. *M* = melanosomes. (Scale bar: 1 μm; magnification ×9600). **E**. A group of tumor cells completely surrounded by an endothelial covering (*E*) in the lumen of an arteriole, 2 weeks after inoculation of
tumor cells. (Scale bar: 10 μm; magnification ×1060) **F**. A portion of a tumor
colony in an arteriole 2 weeks after IV inoculation. A tumor cell pseudopodium
traverses a focal defect of the elastica interna basement (*EI*). *M* =
melanosomes. (Scale bar: 1 μm; magnification ×9600)

endothelium and the basement membrane are held up in this
location for 8 to 24 hours. Local dissolution of the basement
membrane then occurs in association with a tumor cell pseudopodium traversing the basement membrane (Fig. 7-3F).
This step is soon followed by complete extravasation of the
tumor cell and quite often reestablishment of blood flow in
the breached vessel.[15] Tumor cells arrested in the arterial
tree can remain in this location for 2 to 3 weeks. Endothelial
retraction does not occur after arterial arrest. Intra-arterial
tumor cells can actually proliferate and expand as colonies.

As the tumor colonies enlarge, they become covered by a host endothelial surface that lacks a basement membrane. Once the tumor colony fills the arteriole, mechanical damage to the endothelium occurs, and this exposes the basement membrane. Tumor cells at the periphery of the intraarterial colony then invade through the basement membrane and the elastic lamina of the arteriole wall to gain an extravascular position.[15]

At all stages of the metastatic cascade, tumor cells must overcome host defenses.[3–5,18,20] Although tumor-specific antigens have been identified in animal models, it is unclear whether similar antigens play a role in human tumors, and whether recognition of these antigens can be boosted by adjuvant immunotherapy.[18,19] The limited effectiveness of adjuvant immunotherapy for metastases may be due to tumor antigen heterogeneity, tumor antigen shedding, or absence of tumor cell immunogenicity. "Nonspecific" host defenses such as macrophages and natural killer cells may be more effective against heterogeneous tumor cell populations.[20] In animal models these effector cells play an important role in the elimination of circulating tumor cells and destruction of micrometastases.[20]

Extravasated tumor cells proliferate as colonies but require a new vascular supply to grow larger than 0.5 mm.[13] Thus angiogenesis is necessary at the beginning and end of the metastatic cascade. A metastasis can itself metastasize, further amplifying the level of tumor dissemination. Numerous clinical reports provide circumstantial evidence for the existence of dormant metastases.[1,3] Up to one third of the mortality from breast cancer, for instance, occurs more than 5 years after removal of the primary tumor. Three potential mechanisms of tumor dormancy have been distinguished in animal models.[3]: (1) immunologic restraint such that the tumor population death rate equals its growth rate, (2) constitutive dependency of tumor cells on host growth factors, and (3) avascularity, which limits the size of the metastasis due to deficiency in nutrient diffusion.

DISTRIBUTION OF METASTASES BY TARGET ORGAN

The distribution of metastases varies widely, depending on the histologic type and anatomical location of the primary tumor. The most frequent organ location of distant metastasis in many types of cancer appears to be the first capillary bed encountered by the circulating cells. Examples include sarcomas metastasizing to lung, lung cancer metastasizing to brain, and colorectal tumor disseminating to liver.

However, many metastatic sites cannot be predicted from anatomical considerations alone and can be considered examples of organ tropism. For example, clear cell carcinoma of the kidney often metastasizes to bone and thyroid, breast carcinoma to ovaries, and ocular melanoma to the liver.

An increasing number of animal tumor models show preference for metastasizing to one or more distant sites. In many cases, target organ preference in these models cannot be explained based on anatomical considerations. Organ preference of metastatic colonization can be observed in some animal tumors that have not undergone purposeful selection (Table 7-2). In other models, organ selectivity has been experimentally amplified by sequential in vivo passage through the target organ (Table 7-3).

A number of investigators have implanted organ grafts into ectopic sites. The transplanted organ grafts were used as target sites for tumor cell hematogenous colonization. Hart and Fidler[4] observed that intravenously injected B16-F10 melanoma cells colonized the native lung as well as subcutaneous lung grafts. In order to colonize the ectopic site, the tumor cells must have left the first capillary arrest site in the lungs and traveled to the ectopic site. In control mice, ectopic kidney grafts were not colonized by circulating B16-F10 tumor cells, indicating a clear organ selectivity for lung but not kidney.

Theoretical mechanisms for organ tropism include the following[3,17]: (1) Tumor cells disseminate equally in all organs, but preferentially grow only in specific organs. Pref-

TABLE 7-2. Organ Preference of Metastatic Colonization in Animal Tumors Not Purposefully Selected*

Animal Species	Designation and Type of Tumor	Common Colonization Site(s)
Mouse	X5563 plasmacytoma	Spleen
Mouse	Kobayashi plasmacytoma	Bone
Mouse	C198 reticuloendothelioma	Liver > lung, spleen
Mouse	Type A reticulum cell sarcoma	Liver > spleen
Mouse	RAW117 large cell lymphoma	Liver > other sites
Mouse	B16 melanoma	Lung > other sites
Mouse	K-1735 melanoma	Lung
Mouse	M-5076 monocytic sarcoma	Liver > ovary > other sites
Rat	R39 sarcoma	Kidney, adrenal
Rat	Flexner-Jobling carcinoma	Kidney, adrenal
Guinea pig	Line 10 hepatocarcinoma	Liver, lymph node
Chicken	HV-transformed lymphoma	Liver
Rabbit	VX$_2$ carcinoma	Liver, lung

* Modified from Nicolson GL: Organ specificity of tumor metastasis: Role of preferential adhesion, invasion and growth of malignant cells at specific secondary sites. Cancer Metastasis Rev 7:143, 1988.

TABLE 7-3. Organ Preference of Metastases in Some Selected Human and Animal Tumor Models*

Tumor System Subline	Lung	Liver	Brain	Ovary	Spleen	Lymph Node
Murine B16 melanoma (IV or IC)						
B16-F10	++++	±	−	+	±	±
B16-B15b	+++	−	+++	−	−	±
B16-O13	++	−	−	+++	−	±
Murine RAW117 large cell lymphoma (IV or IC)						
RAW117-L17	+++	++++	−	−	++	
Murine Lewis lung carcinoma (IM, IC, or IS)						
HL	++++	−	−	−	−	+
HH	±	++++	±	±	−	+
Chicken MD lymphoma (IV)						
AL-2	−	++++	−	±	−	−
AL-3	−	+	−	+++	−	−
Human A375 melanoma (IV in nude mice)						
A375-SM	++	−	−	−	−	+
A375-L	+	++	−	−	−	−
Human PC-3 prostatic carcinoma (IV in athymic mice)						
PC-3-125-IN	++++	−	−	−	−	−
PC-3-1-LN	++++	+	−	+	±	+++
Human KM12 colon carcinoma (IS or ICM in nude mice)						
KM20C	+	+++	−	−	−	+
KM23C	+	+++	−	−	−	++
Human MeWo melanoma (IV in nude mice)						
MeWo	+	−	−	−	−	−
MeWo-70-W	++	−	++	+	−	−

* Modified from Nicolson GL: Organ specificity of tumor metastasis: Role of preferential adhesion, invasion and growth of malignant cells at specific secondary sites. Cancer Metastasis Rev Cancer Metastasis Rev 7:143, 1988.

Metastases: − = none, ± = sometimes, + = few, ++ = moderate, +++ = many, ++++ = large numbers and heavy tumor burden. IS = intra-splenic, IC = intra-cardia. ICM = intraceum.

erential growth may be induced by local growth factors or hormones present in the target organ for metastasis. (2) Circulating tumor cells may adhere preferentially to the endothelial luminal surface only in the target organ. This hypothesis predicts organ-specific endothelial determinants. (3) Circulating tumor cells may respond to soluble factors diffusing locally out of the target organ. Such factors could act in a chemotactic fashion to attract the tumor cells to extravasate. They could also cause the circulating tumor cells to aggregate and therefore embolize in the target organ. Research with animal models indicates that all of these mechanisms play a role to various degrees, depending on the tumor model system (Table 7-4).[3,17]

BASEMENT MEMBRANE DISRUPTION DURING TRANSITION FROM IN SITU TO INVASIVE TUMORS

The mammalian organism is composed of a series of tissue compartments separated from each other by two types of extracellular matrix: basement membranes and interstitial stroma.[5] The matrix determines tissue architecture, has important biologic functions, and is a mechanical barrier to invasion. During the transition from in situ to invasive carcinoma, tumor cells penetrate the epithelial basement membrane and enter the underlying interstitial stroma. Once the tumor cells enter the stroma they gain access to lymphatics and blood vessels for further dissemination (see Fig. 7-2B). Fibrosarcomas and angiosarcomas, developing from stromal cells, invade surrounding muscle basement membrane and destroy myocytes. Tumor cells must cross basement membranes to invade peripheral nerves and most types of organ parenchyma. During intravasation or extravasation, tumor cells of any histologic origin must penetrate the subendothelial basement membrane.[3,5] In the distant organ where metastatic colonies are initiated, extravasated tumor cells must migrate through the perivascular interstitial stroma before tumor colony growth occurs in the organ parenchyma. Therefore, tumor cell interaction with the extracellular matrix occurs at multiple stages in the metastatic cascade.

General and widespread changes occur in the organization, distribution, and amount of the epithelial basement membrane during the transition from benign to invasive carcinoma.[21,22] The human breast is illustrative. Benign proliferative disorders of the breast such as fibrocystic disease, sclerosing adenosis, intraductal hyperplasia, fibroadenoma, and intraductal papilloma are all characterized by disorganization of the normal epithelial stromal architecture. Extreme forms can mimic the appearance of invasive carcinoma. However, no matter how extensive the architectural disorganization, these benign disorders are always characterized by a continuous basement membrane separating the epithelium from the stroma.[21] In contrast, invasive ductal carcinoma, invasive lobular carcinoma, and tubular carcinoma consistently possess a defective extracellular basement membrane with zones of basement membrane loss around the invading tumor cells in the stroma.[21] The base-

TABLE 7-4.   Evidence for Some Tumor Cell and Host Properties Important in Organ Preference of Blood-borne Metastases*

Tumor System	Properties Associated with Blood-borne Metastases to Specific Sites								
	Increased Primary Invasion†	Increased Entry into Blood	Increased Homotypic Adhesion	Increased Heterotypic Adhesion‡	Increased Attachment to Organ Endothelial Cells	Increased Attachment to Organ BM§	Increased Invasion of Target Organ	Increased Organ Growth Properties‖	Decreased Sensitivity to Host Responses¶
MuB16 melanoma	Yes	Yes	Yes	Yes	Yes	Yes	Yes	Yes	Yes
Mu RAW117 large cell lymphoma	No	No	No	No	Yes	No	Yes	Yes	Yes
Mu L5178Y T-lymphoma (ESb)	Yes	Yes	No	Yes	Yes	Yes	Yes	Yes	Yes
My 3LL lung carcinoma	Yes	Yes	ND**	Yes	Yes	No	Yes	ND	Yes
Rat 13762NF mammary carcinoma	Yes	Yes	Yes	No	Yes	Yes	Yes	Yes	Yes
Rat RMS 9-4 rhabdomyosarcoma	No	Yes	ND	ND	Yes	Yes	ND	No	No

* Modified from Nicolson GL: Organ specificity of tumor metastasis: Role of preferential adhesion, invasion and growth of malignant cells at specific secondary sites. Cancer Metastasis Rev 7:143, 1988.
† Invasion measured at a SC or IM site.
‡ Adhesion measured with syngeneic or nonsyngeneic platelets, lymphocytes, or other blood cells.
§ Attachment measured to organ-derived subendothelial matrix.
‖ Growth stimulation measured with organ-derived soluble factors.
¶ Sensitivity measured as cytolysis or cytostasis by syngeneic host macrophages, lymphocytes, or natural killer cells.
** ND = not determined.

ment membrane is also markedly defective adjacent to tumor cells in lymph node and organ metastases. In some focal regions of well-differentiated carcinoma, partial basement membrane formation can be identified. These findings are directly applicable to diagnostic problems in surgical pathology such as the differentiation of tangential sections of in situ lesions from true invasion, or the differentiation of severe adenosis from invasive carcinoma. Loss of basement membranes in human rectal carcinomas significantly correlates with an increased incidence of metastasis and a poor 5-year survival.[22]

THREE-STEP THEORY OF INVASION

A three-step hypothesis has been proposed to describe the sequence of biochemical events during tumor cell invasion of the extracellular matrix.[5] The first step is tumor cell attachment to the matrix. This attachment may be mediated through specific glycoproteins such as laminin and fibronectin and through tumor cell plasma membrane receptors. Following attachment, the tumor cell secretes hydrolytic enzymes (or induces host cells to secrete enzymes) that can locally degrade the matrix (including degradation of the attachment glycoproteins). Matrix lysis most likely takes place in a highly localized region close to the tumor cell surface where the amount of active enzyme outbalances the natural protease inhibitors present in the serum and in the matrix itself. In contrast to the invasive tumor cell, when a normal cell or benign tumor cell attaches to the matrix it may respond by shifting into a resting or differentiated state. The third step is tumor cell locomotion into the region of the matrix modified by proteolysis. The direction of the locomotion may be influenced by host-derived chemotactic factors and tumor cell–derived motility factors. The chemotactic factors derived from serum, organ parenchyma, or the matrix itself[3,17] may influence the organ specificity of metastasis. Continued invasion of the matrix may take place by cyclic repetition of these three steps.

LAMININ RECEPTORS

Cell surface receptors for the basement membrane glycoprotein laminin mediate adhesion of tumor cells to the basement membrane prior to invasion.[23,24] Laminin as visualized by rotary shadowing electron microscopy has a distinctive cruciform shape with three short arms (35 nm) and one long arm (75 nm) (Fig. 7-4).[25] All arms have globular end regions. The specialized structure of the laminin molecule may contribute to its multiple biologic functions. Laminin plays a role in cell attachment, cell spreading, mitogenesis, neurite outgrowth, morphogenesis, and cell movement. Many types of neoplastic cells contain high affinity (nM Kd) cell surface binding sites (laminin receptors) for laminin.[23] The molecular weight of the isolated receptor is 65 kDa.[7] The laminin receptor binds to the B chain (short arm) region of the laminin molecule.[26] Laminin receptors may be altered in number or degree of occupancy in human carcinomas. This may be the indirect result of defective basement membrane organization in the carcinomas. Breast carcinoma and colon carcinoma tissue contains a higher number of exposed (unoccupied) receptors than benign lesions. The laminin receptors of normal epithelium may be polarized at the basal surface and occupied by laminin in the basement membrane. In contrast, the laminin receptors on invading carcinoma cells are amplified and may be distributed over the entire surface of the cell (Fig. 7-5). The laminin receptor can be shown experimentally to play a role in hematogenous metastasis.[27] Treating tumor cells with the receptor-binding fragment of laminin at very low concentrations markedly inhibits or abolishes lung metastasis from hematogenously introduced tumor cells. The mechanism of action involves blocking the adhesion of circulating tumor cells to the subendothelial basement membrane.

RGD RECOGNITION RECEPTORS

A family of cell surface glycoproteins termed *integrins* has been identified whose members bind with low affinity to a

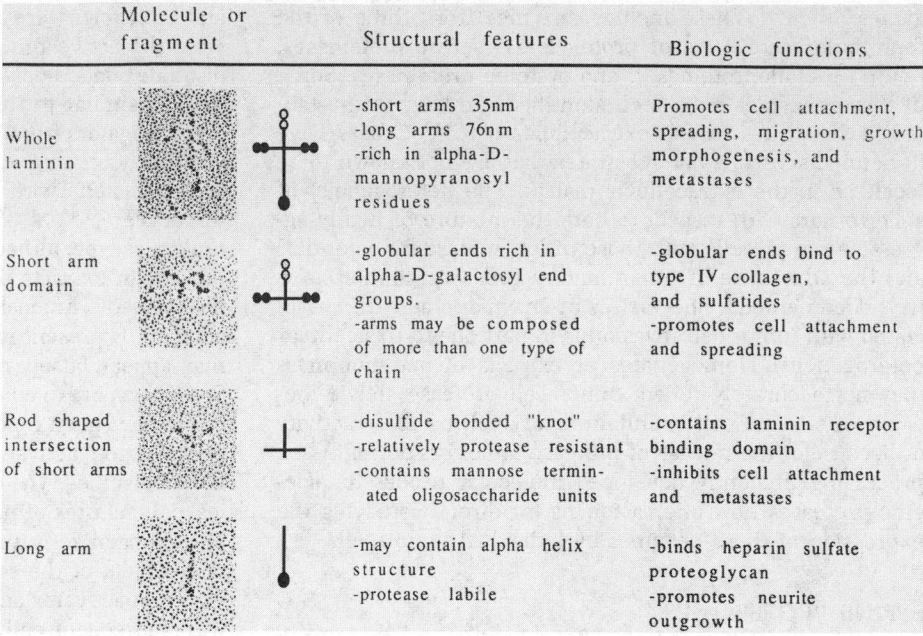

Molecule or fragment			Structural features	Biologic functions
Whole laminin			-short arms 35nm -long arms 76nm -rich in alpha-D-mannopyranosyl residues	Promotes cell attachment, spreading, migration, growth morphogenesis, and metastases
Short arm domain			-globular ends rich in alpha-D-galactosyl end groups. -arms may be composed of more than one type of chain	-globular ends bind to type IV collagen, and sulfatides -promotes cell attachment and spreading
Rod shaped intersection of short arms			-disulfide bonded "knot" -relatively protease resistant -contains mannose terminated oligosaccharide units	-contains laminin receptor binding domain -inhibits cell attachment and metastases
Long arm			-may contain alpha helix structure -protease labile	-binds heparin sulfate proteoglycan -promotes neurite outgrowth

FIG. 7-4. Laminin functional domains. Laminin is a cross-shaped glycoprotein with three short arms and one long arm, all terminating in globular end regions. Electron micrographs of an individual whole laminin molecule or purified fragments are shown; associated structural features and biologic functions are noted.

variety of adhesion proteins including fibronectin, von Willebrand factor, fibrin, vitronectin, type I collagen, and thrombospondin.[28] The integrins are a complex of alpha (140 kDa) and beta (95 kDa) subunit proteins. The functions of several of the integrins are inhibited by peptides related to the Arg-Gly-Asp (RGD) sequence of fibronectin. RGD sequences present on a wide variety of proteins may serve as the recognition site for binding of the integrins. It is likely that specific ligand sequences adjacent to the RGD site may confer preferential recognition of one type of adhesion protein by certain members of the integrin family.[30] Integrin proteins are thought to align adhesion proteins such as fibronectin on the cell surface with cytoskeletal components such as talin and actin, thus altering cell shape.[31] Integrin-type proteins may play an adhesive role in platelet–tumor cell interactions, binding of lymphoid cells to endothelium, and the interaction of circulating tumor cells with endothelial surfaces, fibrin, von Willebrand factor, or thrombospondin. In keeping with this concept, it has been reported that co-injection of tumor cells with large quantities of RGD peptides will inhibit metastasis formation in animal models.[32] The RGD peptides may interfere with the adhesion of tumor cells

to the endothelial surface, which may be mediated directly or indirectly through integrin proteins.

PROTEINASES AND TUMOR CELL INVASION

In vitro studies have shown that tumor cell invasion is not a passive process in response to pressure from excessive cellular proliferation alone but rather is an active process requiring protein synthesis and extracellular proteolysis. Inhibitors of metalloproteinases or protein synthesis, but not of DNA synthesis, block tumor cell invasion into the matrix.[33-35] As outlined earlier, various tissue compartments are separated from each other by interstitial stroma and/or a basement membrane. During the process of invasion, tumor cells must traverse these barriers to cross tissue boundaries. Therefore, it has been suggested that invasive tumor cells secrete matrix-degrading enzymes with activities directed against the major components of these barriers, namely collagens type I, IV, and V, fibronectin, and proteoglycans.[35-38]

Many investigators have explored the possible involvement of proteinases in tumor cell invasion and have proposed a role for a variety of matrix-degrading en-

FIG. 7-5. Immunohistochemistry of laminin receptor distribution. **A**. Normal endometrial gland stained with anti-laminin receptor antibodies. These cells show clear polarization, with the majority of the laminin receptor staining in the basal portion of the cells adjacent to the basement membrane. **B**. Endometrial adenocarcinoma cells stained with anti-laminin receptor antibodies. These cells show an increased staining intensity and lack of polarization when compared with the normal endometrial gland.

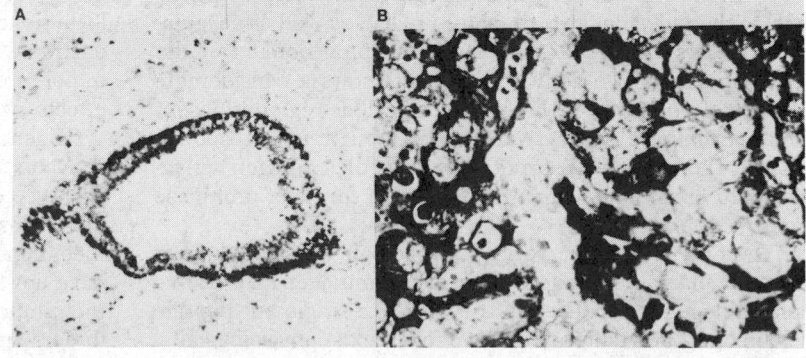

zymes.[35,37,39-41] These include enzymes from three of the four major categories of proteinases—serine proteinases, neutral metalloproteinases, and cysteine proteinases. Some of these enzymes have been identified and have well-established substrates in the extracellular matrix. Others have ill-defined substrates or substrates that are not known to be localized in the extracellular matrix. The heterogeneity of solid tumors with respect to both the mixture of highly aggressive tumor cells with those of low metastatic potential[4] and the admixture of inflammatory cells and fibroblasts is well documented.[3] The variety of enzymatic activities associated with tumor cell invasion is in part due to this cellular heterogeneity. Homogenates or extracts of a tumor mass may not accurately reflect tumor cell protease activity because of stromal cell or inflammatory cell protease activity or because of the release of protease inhibitors during tissue processing. Recently developed molecular probes for specific proteases now offer a means for directly studying the expression of these enzymes by individual tumor cells.

SERINE PROTEINASES

There is considerable experimental evidence documenting increased plasminogen activator and plasmin activity in virally transformed and malignant cells.[36,37] These studies are traced to early observations of the ability of cancer tissue explants to dissolve the plasma clots on which they were grown. Renewed interest in plasminogen activators followed the demonstration that cell transformation by a variety of oncogenic viruses induced a drastic increase in the extracellular release of plasminogen activators. Tumor promoters such as phorbol esters may further potentiate this increase in virally transformed cells.[42,43]

Plasminogen activators exist in at least two forms[36-38,41]: urokinase-type plasminogen activator, so called because it was originally discovered in human urine, and tissue-type plasminogen activator. Tissue-type plasminogen activator is somewhat larger than urokinase and was originally purified from tissue extracts. These forms of plasminogen activators are independent gene products, as has been demonstrated with amino acid sequence analysis and confirmed by cDNA cloning and nucleotide sequencing. In vitro, both enzymes are secreted as single polypeptide, proenzyme forms that are converted to active, disulfide-bonded forms by cleavage at a single proteolytic site. Although the A chains of these forms differ considerably in size, they share structurally conserved regions that are similar to other serine proteinases.[36-38] The A chains contain a cysteine-rich region which shows homology with epidermal growth factor (EGF), as well as coagulation factors IX and X. The amino-terminal domain of the tissue plasminogen activator A chain shows a considerable degree of homology with fibronectin.[37] This region is absent in the urokinase-type activator and is thought to be responsible for the efficient absorption of tissue plasminogen activator onto fibrin clots, an ability that most forms of urokinase lack.

The only well-characterized physiologic substrate known for the plasminogen activators is plasminogen.[36,38] Native plasminogen is produced in the liver as a single polypeptide chain of 92,000 daltons.[44,45] Two forms exist physiologically, and both forms are activated by plasminogen activators to yield the active protease plasmin. Plasmin consists of two disulfide bonded polypeptide chains and its proteolytic specificity is similar to that of trypsin.

Investigators from a number of laboratories have shown by analysis of tumor extracts that plasminogen activator activity is associated with a variety of human and animal tumors.[36,37,41,46-48] Most commonly, this activity is of the urokinase type, although tissue-type plasminogen activator is present in extracts of some tumors. These results must be interpreted cautiously, however, since tissue plasminogen activator is present in endothelial cells and its concentration may appear falsely elevated in highly vascularized tumors. Short-term organ cultures and cell cultures of neoplastic cell origin have been reported to produce urokinase alone, tissue plasminogen activator alone, or both forms, as well as a nondetermined type of plasminogen activator. In other studies, cell cultures of neoplastic tissue have been found to lack plasminogen activator when analyzed immediately after establishment of the cell culture. In still other cell lines plasminogen activator activity, although initially present, is lost with subsequent cell passages.[46,47]

Experiments with several tumor cell lines have indicated that matrix glycoproteins are susceptible to plasmin-mediated proteolytic degradation.[36-38,41,49,50] These lines include human rhabdomyosarcoma cells, human fibrosarcoma cell lines, hamster fibrosarcoma cells, and murine melanoma cell lines. Depending on the cell line, the matrix-degrading activity may or may not become independent of plasminogen conversion to plasmin at high cell density. Human rhabdomyosarcoma cells required the presence of plasminogen at all cell densities in order to effect matrix degradation. For the fibrosarcoma cells and murine melanoma cells, matrix degradation became independent of exogenous plasminogen at high cell densities.[51] This suggests that an additional, as yet unidentified proteolytic activity may be involved in matrix degradation at high cell densities. Metastatic mouse sarcoma cells show laminin-degrading activity that is mostly plasminogen dependent. However, most of the plasminogen-independent laminin degrading activity is removed by inhibitors of metalloproteinases.[38,52]

Studies with the human epidermoid cell line HEP-3 have provided some of the best evidence for the role of plasminogen activators in tumor invasion.[53] Antibodies that specifically inhibit human urokinase activity, but do not cross-react with chicken urokinase, significantly reduced or prevented pulmonary metastases from HEP-3 tumors transplanted onto chick embryo chorioallantoic membranes without reducing local tumor growth. Appropriate immunologic controls demonstrated that this effect was due to inhibition of the human tumor urokinase activity and not secondary immunologic effects.

Evidence for a positive correlation between plasminogen activator activity and tumor invasiveness remains unclear. A positive correlation between plasminogen activator activity and metastatic potential has been established for the murine melanoma cell line B16.[54] Low metastatic cell lines (B16F1) have low plasminogen activator activity, whereas highly metastatic cell lines (B16F10) show high levels in primary tumors and even higher levels in the pulmonary metastases from these primary tumors. The correlation of plasminogen activator activity with metastatic potential has also been observed in the rat mammary adenocarcinoma model.[55] However, in human tumors the situation is not clear-cut. Although there may be some correlation with invasion, plasminogen activator levels certainly do not show a correlation with the metastatic capacity of human tumors when assayed by protein methods. This possibly is a result of a general protease activity that destroys this activity, low levels of active enzyme, or rapid "physiologic" protein turnover of plasminogen activator. A recent report demonstrated a significant (sixfold) elevation of urokinase mRNA levels in human primary lung and breast carcinomas when compared with levels in nonmalignant tissues.[56] Furthermore, a significant correlation between urokinase mRNA levels in lung carcinomas and the presence of regional lymph node metastasis was found. These results need to be confirmed by further studies, but it appears that important prognostic information may be obtained from such investigations. As the investigators suggest, urokinase mRNA content may help identify patients at risk for recurrence or early metastasis. These patients could then be selected for adjuvant therapy.

Metalloproteinases

Tumor cell invasion requires crossing tissue compartment barriers such as basement membranes and interstitial connective tissues. Both of these barriers have various collagen types that compose the structural scaffolding upon which other matrix components such as fibronectin, laminin, and proteoglycans are assembled. In this section we shall consider the metalloenzymes that may be involved in tumor invasion and metastasis.

Tumor-derived collagenases that degrade interstitial collagen types I, II, and III have been purified and characterized by a number of laboratories. The properties of these enzymes are similar to those of the classic collagenase first described by Gross and co-workers.[57] The cDNA for human fibroblast interstitial collagenase has recently been cloned and sequenced.[58,59] The collagenases are calcium- and zinc-dependent metalloproteinases that function at neutral pH. These enzymes produce a single cleavage across all three alpha chains of the native type I collagen molecule, resulting in characteristic fragments corresponding to a cleavage site located 75% of the distance from the amino terminus of the full length substrate. Interstitial collagenase activity has been reported in a number of human tumors and has been correlated with the aggressiveness of human bladder carcinomas.[60,61] Immunohistochemical studies suggest that the tumor cells themselves do not secrete type I collagenase, but instead directly stimulate fibroblast secretion of this enzyme.[60]

Basement membrane collagens types IV and V differ markedly from the interstitial collagenases (types I, II, and III) both in structure and in proteolytic susceptibility. These basement membrane collagens are not susceptible to proteolytic attack by the interstitial collagenases described above. Ultrastructural studies of tumor cell extravasation and invasion demonstrated local dissolution of basement membrane materials and suggested that tumor cells produce a distinct collagenolytic enzyme to degrade basement membranes. In support of this concept, highly metastatic tumor cells, endothelial cells, and polymorphonuclear leukocytes have been found to produce a type IV collagen-specific metalloproteinase.[62] Unique metalloproteinases that degrade type V collagen have also been described.

Type IV collagen–specific metalloproteinase, type IV collagenase, was first identified and purified from a metastatic murine tumor cell line.[63] Type IV collagenase is a neutral metalloproteinase with a pH optimum of 7.6 and is not inhibited by serine protease inhibitors or cysteine protease inhibitors. The enzyme has an apparent molecular weight of approximately 70,000 daltons and generates characteristic cleavage products from native type IV collagen (Fig. 7-6). Human type IV collagenases with similar characteristics have been isolated from fibrosarcoma and melanoma cell lines.[62-65]

Type IV collagenolytic activity correlates with metastatic activity in murine tumor models.[66-68] Highly aggressive human tumors, such as carcinomas, melanomas, hepatomas, fibrosarcomas, and reticulum cell sarcomas, all have elevated levels of type IV collagenase when compared with benign control cells.[66-68] Anti-type IV collagenase antibodies react with invading colon and breast cancer cells as well as lymph node metastases of primary breast cancers on immunohistochemical staining.[21] Furthermore, a quantitative relationship between type IV collagenase activity and in vitro invasion of tumor cells through isolated human amnion membrane has been observed. The penetration of human tumor cells can be inhibited in this assay by metalloproteinase inhibitors.[34] These results suggest that type IV collagenase activity may serve as a useful marker of the invasive capacity and possibly the metastatic potential of some human tumors.

Studies have shown a possible linkage between augmented type IV collagenase activity and the genetic induction of a metastatic phenotype.[68-70] Plasmids containing various Harvey-ras oncogene constructs or cellular proto-oncogene constructs were used to transfect NIH-3T3 cells. A series of transfectants were identified that were nontumorigenic, tumorigenic but nonmetastatic, and tumorigenic, metastatic. This observation allows the tumorigenic and metastatic phenotypes to be separated out for further study. A series of NIH-3T3 cell transfectants that exhibited metastatic capacity in vivo all secreted high levels of type IV collagenase. Spontaneously transformed NIH-3T3 cells that were tumorigenic but not metastatic as well as parental NIH-3T3 cells both produced only very low levels of type IV collagenase. Thus, type IV collagenase may be one of a number of possible metastasis-associated gene products.

A new metalloproteinase activity secreted by phorbol ester–stimulated synovial fibroblasts has been characterized.[71] This enzyme, referred to as stromelysin, is secreted as a 51,000-dalton proenzyme and is capable of degrading a variety of extracellular matrix proteins, including fibronectin, laminin, elastin, IgG, and proteoglycans.[71,72] The enzyme has been cloned from rabbit and human sources, and the amino acid sequences as determined with cDNA sequencing show homology with the rat protein transin, which is a secreted protease.[72,73] This is of interest because the rat

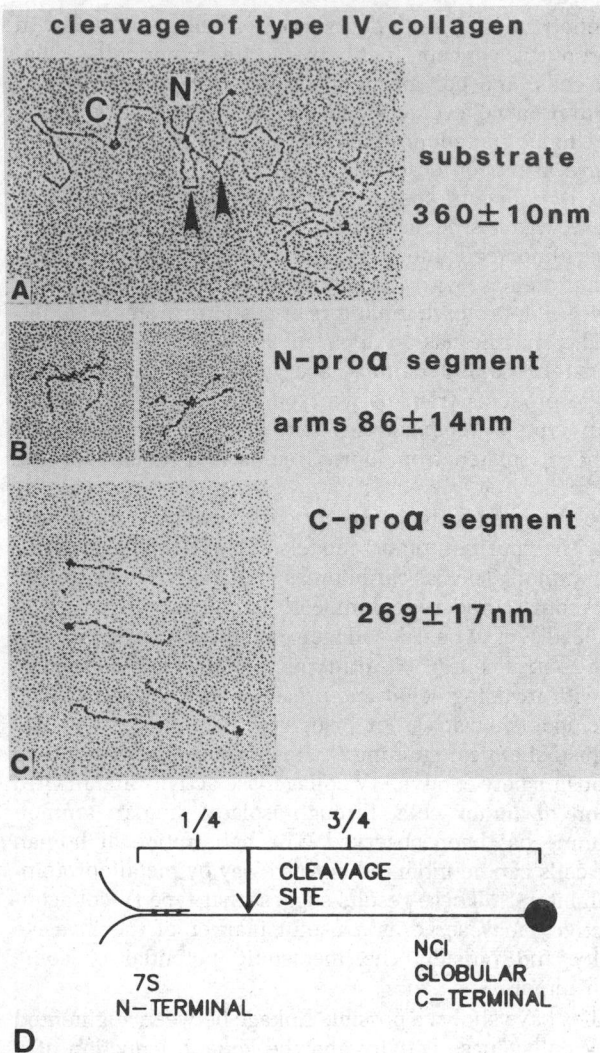

cleavage of type IV collagen

substrate

360±10nm

A

N-proα segment

arms 86±14nm

B

C-proα segment

269±17nm

C

D

FIG. 7-6. Electron micrographs of type IV collagen fragments cleaved by tumor cell–derived type IV collagenolytic metalloproteinase (*CIV*). **Panel A.** Type IV basement membrane collagen molecules (pro-alpha chains) spontaneously link together to form a network with two to four molecules combining at the N-terminus (*N*) and two molecules combining at the globular C-terminus (*C*). Purified tumor cell–derived CIV cleaves the type IV collagen substrate at a location one-fourth the distance from the N-terminus (*arrow*), producing a small cleavage product (**panel B**) and a large C-terminal fragment (**panel C**). **Panel D**. Schematic representation of type IV collagen molecule showing the cleavage site of type IV collagenase.

transin gene is greatly increased in experimentally induced rat carcinomas.[74] In cell lines of fibroblast origin, stromelysin and interstitial collagenase show similar rates of secretion and coordinate gene regulation in response to phorbol ester treatments.[73] Induction was blocked by cycloheximide, which suggests that the signal transduction pathway is indirect and requires new protein synthesis. However, phorbol ester treatment failed to induce stromelysin synthesis in normal human keratinocytes, endothelial cells, or human tumor cell lines, such as melanoma, fibrosarcoma, and *ras*-transformed bronchial epithelial cells.[72] Thus, the possible role of this enzyme in tumor cell invasion awaits further elucidation.

Cysteine Proteinases and Endoglycosidases

As with the other proteases described in this section, there is an accumulating body of correlative evidence that suggests a role for the cysteine protease cathepsin B in tumor cell invasion and metastasis.[39,40] Cathepsin B is a lysosomal acid hydrolase with a broad range of endopeptidase activity against substrates that include myosin, actin, proteoglycans, fibronectin, laminin, and nonhelical portions of type IV collagen.

Cathepsin B activity has been found in association with the plasma membrane fraction of tumor cells, and in the conditioned media from tumor cell cultures.[39] The tumor cell cathepsin B activity isolated from a variety of human tumors appears to be a different enzyme from the lysosomal protease of normal cells, based on *p*H stability profiles. Studies using the murine melanoma cell line B16 have shown a correlation of cathepsin B activity with potential for metastatic colony formation in the mouse lung. Cathepsin B activity in extracts of human tumors has shown a positive correlation with malignant behavior of these tumors.[39,40]

Studies have also focused on enzymatic activities that degrade the proteoglycan components of the extracellular matrix barriers. Nicolson and colleagues have characterized an endoglycosidase activity produced by murine melanoma cells that releases heparan sulfate chains from matrix proteoglycans.[75,76] This heparanase activity correlated with the metastatic potential of the melanoma subline, that is, highly metastatic cells produced greater levels of endoglycosidase activity than cells of low metastatic potential. A similar heparanase activity has been demonstrated in human melanoma cells, and variants of these human cell lines with high metastatic potential produced significantly higher heparanase activities than parental cells of low metastatic potential.[77]

Thus, the increased expression of a variety of enzyme activities, some capable of degrading specific extracellular matrix components (collagenase, heparanase), have been correlated with the invasive or metastatic potential of many different malignant tumor cell types. The malignant cell apparently produces a spectrum of matrix-degrading enzyme activities that varies with cell type, tumor preparation, and cell culture conditions. This finding led investigators to begin dissecting these concerted enzyme activities by using protease-specific inhibitors and activators.[78,79] Results of such studies have suggested the presence of proteolytic activation cascades, such as plasminogen activator–plasmin–collagenase, which may account for the spectrum of enzyme activities associated with malignant cell types. Regulation of proteolysis may occur at many levels, including tumor cell–host cell interactions and protease inhibitors produced by the host or by the tumor cells themselves. Expression of matrix-degrading enzymes is by no means tumor-cell specific. The actively invading tumor cells may merely respond to different regulatory signals than their noninvasive counterparts.

TUMOR CELL MOTILITY FACTORS

Cell motility is necessary for tumor cells to traverse many stages in the complex cascade of invasion. Such stages could include the detachment and subsequent infiltration of cells from the primary tumor into adjacent tissue, the migration of cells through the vascular wall into the circulation (intravasation), and the extravasation of cells to a secondary site. The movement of cells through biologic barriers such as the endothelial basement membranes of the vasculature may well occur by means of chemotactic mechanisms. Indeed, studies on in vitro chemotaxis of some tumor cells indicate that a variety of compounds such as complement-derived materials, collagen peptides, formyl peptides, and certain connective tissue components can act as chemoattractants.[10,80,81] Although these agents may contribute to the directional aspects of a motile response, they are not sufficient to initiate the intrinsic locomotion of tumor cells. The availability of soluble attractants to the tumor cell is greatly dependent on the host, even when the production of attractants is the result of tumor cell–host tissue interaction. At best, it seems that the cell would have access to such motility stimuli at sporadic and irregular intervals. Such conditions are unfavorable to a sustained migration of highly invasive cells. With these considerations in mind, and stimulated by studies of Anzano et al[82] demonstrating autocrine growth factors for transformed cells, the possibility that such cells could elaborate autocrine motility factors was investigated. The action of these substances might, in part, explain both the markedly invasive character and the metastatic property of malignant neoplastic cells. Thus, under the influence of such an autocrine material, a tumor cell might move out into the surrounding host tissue and also exert a "recruiting" effect on adjacent tumor cells in the presence of an attractant gradient. Conceivably, such factors might also attract fibroblastic cells of the host, resulting in the phenomenon of desmoplasia, characteristic of invasive tumors.

It was found that the human melanoma cell line A2058 and human breast carcinoma cells produce in culture a material that markedly stimulates their own motility.[83–85] These cells respond in a dose-dependent manner to various concentrations of conditioned medium obtained by incubating confluent cells in serum-free medium, an indication that the motility factor is derived from the cell. Motility was measured by the modified Boyden chamber procedure. This assay and "checkerboard" analysis,[83] revealed that the conditioned medium factor has both chemotactic (directional) and chemokinetic (randomly motile) properties. The transducer system activated by autocrine motility factor (AMF) involves phospholipase C and phospholipase A_2 (Fig. 7-7).[84]

Early events in migration may involve pseudopodia protrusion.[85] During the course of invasion, the same tumor cell must interact with a variety of extracellular matrix proteins as it traverses each tissue barrier. For example, the tumor cell encounters laminin and type IV collagen when it penetrates the basement membrane, and type I collagen and fibronectin when it crosses the interstitial stroma. It has recently been shown that cells express specific cell surface receptors that recognize extracellular matrix proteins as described above. The first example of such a receptor is the laminin receptor, which binds to laminin with a nanomolar affinity. Laminin receptors have been shown to be augmented in actively invading tumor cells, and may play an important role in tumor cell interaction with the basement membrane. Arg–Gly–Asp (RGD) recognition receptors are another class of cell surface proteins that bind extracellular matrix proteins, which in turn contain the protein sequence

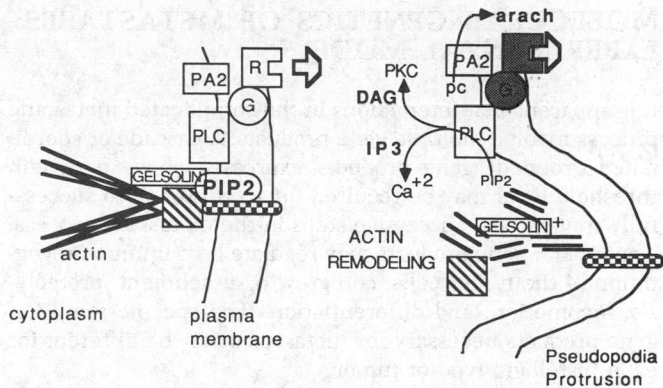

FIG. 7-7. Hypothetical role of membrane lipids in tumor cell motility induced by cytokines such as AMF. Rapid cytoskeleton remodeling may be regulated in part by receptor mediated pathways through guanyl nucleotide–binding proteins (G) coupled to phospholipase C (PLC) and phospholipase A_2 (PA2). Phospholipase C mediates the hydrolysis of phosphatidylinositol 4,5-bisphosphate (PIP2), one of the inositol lipids in the plasma membrane. PIP2 strongly inhibits the actin filament–severing properties of gelsolin, a calcium-dependent actin binding protein. PIP2 is cleaved by PLC to form diacylglycerol (DG) and inositol 1,4,5-triphosphate (IP3). DG stimulates protein kinase C (PKC). IP3 induces a rapid release of calcium (Ca^{2+}) from intracellular stores. The turnover of PIP2 and the increase in local calcium availability could both contribute to an increase in actin depolymerization via gelsolin. Furthermore, PIP2 is known to form a complex with the cytoplasmic domain of transmembrane proteins such as glycophorin, which in turn facilitates binding of membrane skeletal proteins such as protein 4.1, which promotes associations between actin and spectrin. Turnover of PIP2 could therefore uncouple the tethering of the cytoskeleton to the plasma membrane. Phospholipase A_2 cleaves membrane phosphatidylcholine (pc) to generate arachidonic acid (arach). Arachidonic acid and its metabolites contribute to lipid methylation events that alter membrane fluidity. Such a combination of events may affect pseudopodial protrusion.

Arg–Gly–Asp.[28] Such proteins include fibronectin, collagen type I, and vitronectin. The process of cell migration undoubtedly requires a series of adhesion and detachment steps resulting in traction and propulsion. Studies using AMF-stimulated motility as the model system have revealed an important function of pseudopodia protrusion in this process. AMF stimulates motility on a variety of different substrates. Therefore, its action is independent of the mechanism of attachment. Furthermore, AMF induces the rapid protrusion of pseudopodia in both a time- and dose-dependent manner.[83] Isolation of the induced pseudopodia reveals that they are highly enriched in their content of laminin and fibronectin matrix receptors. Since cell pseudopodia formation is known to be a prominent feature of actively motile cells, we can now set forth a working hypothesis to explain the early events in cell motility. Cytokines such as AMF that stimulate intrinsic motility may induce exploratory pseudopodia prior to cell translocation. Such pseudopodia may express augmented levels of matrix receptors (and possibly proteinases). The protruding pseudopodia may serve multiple functions, including (1) acting as "sense organs" to interact with the extracellular matrix proteins and thereby locate directional cues, (2) providing propulsive traction for locomotion, and (3) inducing local matrix proteolysis to assist in the penetration of the matrix.[86,87]

MOLECULAR GENETICS OF METASTASES: EXPERIMENTAL MODELS

It is apparent that interactions in the complicated metastatic process involve multiple gene products. A cascade or coordinated group of gene products expressed above a certain threshold level may be required for a tumor cell to successfully traverse the successive steps in the metastatic process. The crucial gene products may regulate host immune recognition of the tumor cells, cell growth, attachment, proteolysis, locomotion, and differentiation. The specific family of gene products necessary for metastases may be different for each histologic type of tumor.

A growing list of transforming genes or *oncogenes* have been identified that may be involved in the genetic alterations leading to tumor growth, invasion, and metastasis.[88-91] Following introduction into suitable recipient cells, oncogenes confer anchorage-independent colony growth in soft agar, and in many cases, tumorigenicity in animal hosts. Cancer cells must, of course, be tumorigenic in order to grow as a metastatic colony. However, not all tumorigenic cells are necessarily invasive and metastatic. This is because the metastatic phenotype is independent from the tumorigenic phenotype. Most of the past work on oncogene function has emphasized mechanisms related to alteration of growth control. Investigators studying oncogene-transformed cells rarely tested these cells for the ability to produce metastases in animal models.

It is now recognized that some oncogene classes can induce the complete metastatic phenotype in the appropriate recipient cell.[69,92-101] An important example is the H-*ras* oncogene. Transfection of members of the *ras* family oncogene into rat or mouse embryo–derived fibroblasts[69,92,95,100] will lead to full expression of the metastatic phenotype. The mechanism of metastasis induction by *ras* is not related to changes in sensitivity to killing by immune cells. Metastasis induction by *ras* is associated with a cascade of gene expression that elevates the intrinsic aggressiveness of the tumor cells.

Thorgeirsson et al[92] were the first to report the metastatic propensity of murine cells transformed with human tumor genomic DNA. Mouse embryo–derived fibroblasts (NIH-3T3 cells) transfected with AML or bladder cancer tumor DNA produced numerous metastases when injected into immunodeficient nude mice. When the resulting metastatic clones were examined, they were found to have acquired exogenous activated *ras* oncogene sequences. To test whether the *ras* oncogene itself or associated genomic DNA was responsible for the metastatic induction, cloned, defined *ras* oncogenes were transferred into NIH-3T3 cells. The resulting *ras*-transformed cells were fully metastatic but had not become resistant to natural killer cell or macrophage lysis. *ras*-Transfected cells also produce metastases in a nonmammalian system, the chick embryo, as reported by Bondy et al.[93]

Muschel et al.[69,99] transformed NIH-3T3 cells with the viral H-*ras* oncogene or the H-*ras* oncogene from the T24 human bladder carcinoma cell line and isolated multiple independent clones. All of the clones are metastatic following injection into nude mice. Egan et al[95] confirmed these results and found that the number of lung metastases produced was proportional to the level of the *ras* oncogene–encoded P21 protein in each transformant. The rare metastatic variants isolated from cells with barely detectable H-*ras* were found to have high levels of *ras* expression caused by rearrangement or amplification at the DNA level. Egan et al[95] also used a steroid-responsive promoter to show the importance of *ras* oncogene transcript dose on metastasis production. The level of *ras* expression in these experimental models correlates directly with metastatic potential. The H-*ras* oncogene is distinguished from its normal cellular counterpart by one or more point mutations.[89] In the viral and T24 *ras,* the mutation is at the position coding for the 12th amino acid. Transfection of the normal proto-oncogene lacking the mutation will not cause transformation. However, Chang et al[90] demonstrated that the *ras* proto-oncogene joined to a viral promoter and transcriptional enhancer would cause elevated production of the normal P21 protein and could transform NIH-3T3 cells. The cells transformed with elevated levels of the normal *ras* (encoding normal P21 protein) produced tumors at a rate comparable to cells transformed with the mutated *ras.*[90] However, when the same cells were tested for metastatic propensity, the cells transformed by the mutated *ras* were much more efficient in the production of metastases[69,95] than were cells transformed by normal *ras.* Nevertheless, very high levels of the normal P21 could also lead to metastasis production.[95] Taken together, all the results are consistent with a dominant role for *ras*-encoded protein dose in the induction of metastases. Very low levels of the mutated P21 protein will result in poorly metastatic tumors, and moderate to high levels of the mutated P21 protein will result in highly metastatic tumors. In contrast, low or moderate levels of normal P21 will result in tumors and very high levels of P21 will produce metastatic tumors.

The use of NIH-3T3 cells in experimental models of metastasis induction by oncogenes has been criticized because these cells are aneuploid and have a high rate of spontaneous transformation.[94] It was conceivable that *ras* oncogene induction of metastases might require cellular or genetic properties present only in NIH-3T3 cells. Therefore, Muschel et al[69] and Pozzatti et al[100] tested the metastatic propensity of *ras*-transfected diploid primary cells. Muschel et al[69] found that rat skin cells, rat muscle cells, and Chinese hamster lung fibroblasts were induced to become metastatic by transfection of *ras* linked to an enhancer, using a construct of Spandidos and Wilkie. Pozzatti et al[100] examined a series of diploid rat embryo cell clones that had been transformed by H-*ras* alone or H-*ras* linked to an SV-40 enhancer cotransfected with a dominant selectible marker (pRSVneo). These clones were all highly metastatic after intravenous, subcutaneous, or intramuscular injection into nude mice. Thus, the ability of the H-*ras* oncogene to induce metastases is not limited to NIH-3T3 cells but occurs even after transformation of certain diploid primary cells.

The *ras* oncogene can also amplify the metastatic potential in certain poorly metastatic or nonmetastatic established tumor cell lines that were not originally transformed by H-*ras.* Vousden et al[96] transfected H-*ras* into a highly tumorigenic cell line derived from a murine mammary carcinoma.

Although the parent cell line was very weakly metastatic, the subclones transfected with *ras* were all highly metastatic. Multiple clones were isolated from the resulting lung metastases, and most retained the metastatic phenotype. One of the clones was no longer metastatic; it was found to have lost the introduced *ras* oncogene. Collard et al[98] obtained similar results when mutated *ras* oncogenes were inserted into T-lymphoma cells. The lymphoma cells became invasive and metastatic in proportion to the level of H-*ras*-specific mRNA. Kerbel et al[97] had similar results with SP1, a cell line isolated from a nonmetastatic murine mammary carcinoma. Metastatic primary tumors were produced by all clones that incorporated the mutated but not the normal *ras*.

The ability of the H-*ras* oncogene to induce metastases is dependent on the cell type. Transfection of H-*ras* into C127 murine cells will result in highly tumorigenic cells that fail to form metastases after intravenous or subcutaneous injection into nude mice. The carcinogen *N*-nitrosomethylurea will induce skin papillomas and mammary tumors in appropriate strains of mice.[101,102] The vast majority of the induced tumors have an activated *ras* oncogene[102] but are nonmetastatic. Only 10% of DMBA tumors will produce metastases. These results lead to the conclusion that activation of the H-*ras* oncogene is not sufficient to induce metastases in certain cultured cell types or spontaneous tumors. The *ras* oncogene may fail to induce metastases in a particular cell because that cell lacks an appropriate cooperation factor. On the other hand, the resistant cell may possess a means of suppressing the ability of *ras* to induce metastases. The adenovirus 2 E1A is an example of a gene that can suppress metastases caused by H-*ras*. Pozzatti et al[100] showed that cotransfection of E1A with *ras* results in nonmetastatic tumors. The mechanism of inhibition may involve the 12S E1A transcript (Pozzatti, personal communication) and is not related to histocompatibility antigen changes or increased sensitivity to immune cell killing. The results lead us to predict the existence of normal genes that function to suppress the metastatic cascade induced by certain oncogenes such as *ras*.[103]

The mechanism by which the H-*ras* oncogene can induce metastases in the appropriate cell recipient is unknown. It must involve the activation of a multigene cascade since the H-*ras*-transformed cells acquire a large number of new functional properties, including increased adhesiveness, changes in cell surface carbohydrates associated with metastases,[104] motility, and ability to invade tissue barriers.[83,92,104-106] One potential explanation is that H-*ras* transfection leads to genetic or karyotypic instability with the resulting selection of metastatic variants.[91] A second possible mechanism could involve the selected integration of H-*ras* into a specific location in the genome next to metastases-associated genes. Both of these explanations seem unlikely, based on the data obtained so far. Diploid rat embryo fibroblasts transfected with H-*ras* become metastatic as soon as enough cells (four passages) can be grown to inject into nude mice. The resulting metastatic clones do not contain any consistent gross karyotypic alteration and indeed may remain fully diploid.[100] All of the transfectant clones expressing the activated P21 protein are metastatic,[69,95,100] implying that induction of metastases is not a rare event as

would be expected if there were a requirement for *ras* to be integrated into a specific site. The explanation we are left with is that the *ras* P21 protein alters some general pathway in the cell and that this pathway is involved in the metastatic cascade. A likely candidate pathway is the G protein–mediated transducer systems involved in phosphatidylinositol-4,5-bisphosphate and catabolites thereof, as well as the arachidonic acid pathways mediated through phospholipase A_2 (see Fig. 7-4).[83,106,107]

H-*ras* is not the only oncogene that can induce metastatic potential in 3T3 cells. Egan et al[107] recently reported that certain transforming oncogenes encoding protein kinases (*mos, raf, src, fes,* and *fms*) but not nuclear oncogenes such as *myc* or p53 induced 3T3 cells to produce lung metastases after intravenous injection. Whether or not these oncogenes will induce the spontaneous metastatic phenotype in diploid primary cells is unknown. Transformation of cells by *src, fes,* and *fms* may be mediated through a *ras*-dependent mechanism, as Smith et al[108] have shown that transformation by these oncogenes is blocked by antibodies to *ras*-encoded P21. Oncogenes have been found to have multifactorial effects on a variety of general cell pathways.[109,110]

Regardless of the mechanism by which oncogene transfection induces metastases in animal systems, it constitutes a revolutionary model system for studying the biochemical mechanisms of metastases. For example, specific classes of collagenase[70,92] and motility-stimulating cytokines[83] have been shown to be biochemically linked to the induction of metastases by the H-*ras* oncogene. With appropriate combinations of H-*ras* oncogenes with viral enhancers or other oncogenes such as E1A, diploid cells will become either fully tumorigenic but non metastatic or poorly metastatic, or fully metastatic. The metastatic clones are very aggressive, producing more than 200 metastases in the lungs of nude mice after intravenous injection of only 5×10^4 cells. A wide variety of organs are the site of spontaneous metastases produced from primary tumors arising from subcutaneous or intramuscular injection of transfected cells. Virtually unlimited numbers of clones of metastatic or nonmetastatic tumor cells can be produced using transfection methods. The transfection model system has a number of advantages compared to previous metastases models, which were the result of multiple selection steps applied to heterogeneous transplantable tumors.[3,4]

ONCOGENE EXPRESSION CORRELATION WITH HUMAN TUMOR METASTATIC AGGRESSIVENESS

Proto-oncogenes may be activated and may contribute to neoplastic transformation and progression to the metastatic phenotype.[88-90,102,104-114] Activation can occur by multiple pathways, including (1) amplification of the number of copies of the oncogene in the genome of tumor cells, (2) mutation within the coding sequence of the oncogene, (3) chromosomal breaks and translocation with subsequent enhanced expression of the oncogene-encoded protein, and (4) insertion of a retroviral promoter near the proto-oncogene. Yokota et al[115] studied proto-oncogene alteration in 72 samples of tumor tissue and corresponding normal tissue from the same patient. Alterations were frequently found in c-*myc*, c-*ras*, and c-*myb*. No oncogene alterations were observed in the normal tissue. Oncogene alterations may merely be a hallmark of the genetic instability of tumors. On the other hand, if proto-oncogene alterations play an actual functional role in malignant behavior, they might provide a survival advantage and be selected out in the expanding tumor cell population. This could result in increased expression of relevant oncogene products in more aggressive tumors with a higher propensity to metastasize. In fact, oncogene expression does correlate with metastatic behavior in certain classes of human tumors studied to date. However, a different class of oncogene appears to be important for each histologic type of tumor.

Amplification of the HER-2/*neu* oncogene has been correlated with metastases in human breast carcinoma. The HER-2/*neu* (*neu*) oncogene is a member of the *erb*-B–like oncogene family, and is related to, but distinct from, the gene encoding the epidermal growth factor receptor. Slamon et al[112] studied alterations in the gene in 189 primary human breast cancer specimens and found that *neu* was amplified in 30% of the tumors. Amplification was a significant predictor of overall survival, time to relapse, estrogen receptor status, size of primary tumor, and number of axillary lymph nodes positive for metastasis. Van de Vijver et al[114] detected amplification of *neu* in 16 of 95 human breast tumor samples; the amplification was accompanied by overexpression in the tumors from which intact RNA could be isolated. No correlation was found in this study between *neu* amplification and estrogen receptor content, patient age, or clinical stage of disease.

Increased expression of the H-*ras* oncogene has also been correlated with lymph node metastases in human breast carcinoma. Agnantis et al[116] found a significant elevation of H-*ras* transcripts in malignant compared with normal breast tissue, with a higher mean value of expression in cases with lymph node metastases. Horan-Hand et al[117] immunologically assayed the H-*ras* P21 protein in samples of human breast carcinoma and colon carcinoma. Enhanced expression was documented in 66% of breast and 100% of colon carcinomas compared to normal counterparts, with levels in breast carcinoma ranging from 18.4 to 51.7 pg P21/μg protein. Clair et al[118] extended this finding to report a correlation of breast carcinoma P21 expression with advanced-disease stage and positive axillary lymph node metastasis. Lundy et al[119] reported a positive correlation between H-*ras* P21 protein levels and lymph node metastasis, but not between H-*ras* P21 levels and patient age or estrogen receptor status.

N-*myc* amplification is associated with rapid progression of neuroblastomas. Seeger et al[120] studied 89 patients with untreated primary neuroblastoma to determine the relation between the number of copies of the N-*myc* oncogene and survival without disease progression. Analysis of progression-free survival in all patients revealed that amplification of N-*myc* was associated with the worst prognosis. The estimated progression-free survival at 18 months was 70%, 30%, and 5% for patients whose tumors had one, three to ten, or more than ten N-*myc* copies, respectively. It is un-

clear whether or not the poor survival in patients with amplified N-*myc* is due to an increased number of metastases. However, amplified N-*myc* is prevalent in Stage 4 neuroblastomas[121] with distant metastases from hematogenous or lymphatic dissemination. The mechanism by which N-*myc* augments tumor aggressiveness is unknown. Experimental animal studies to date have not shown a significant role for N-*myc* transfection (N-*myc* alone or in combination with H-*ras*[69,107]) in the induction of the metastatic phenotype. However, these experiments have not been conducted with neural cell lines. In patients whose neuroblastoma tumor cells can be grown in vitro as a cell line, there is a very high association with amplified N-*myc* and poor prognosis. Thus, it is conceivable that N-*myc* amplification somehow facilitates the independent growth of neuroblastoma cells in a harsh environment. This would favor the growth of metastatic colonies in distant organ sites. Neuroblastoma cells without N-*myc* amplification may have a greater requirement for cooperating local host factors that support growth.

Tumors other than neuroblastoma have not shown as strong a correlation between N-*myc* amplification and clinical prognosis or extent of metastasis. In contrast to *neu* amplification and H-*ras* overexpression, C-*myc* or N-*myc* oncogene amplification was not correlated with human breast cancer stage of disease, hormonal receptor status, or axillary lymph node metastasis.[111,112] C-*myc* and N-*myc* are amplified in small cell lung cancers and gastrointestinal malignancies, but the level of amplification has not been shown to correlate with metastasis.[122,123] Thus, if oncogenes are indeed important in human tumor progression, the effect of any given oncogene may depend on the genetic background of the host cell.

NEW STRATEGIES FOR METASTASIS DIAGNOSIS AND THERAPY

The elucidation of biochemical and genetic mechanisms that play a role in cancer metastasis (see Table 7-1) has led to new strategies for cancer diagnosis and therapy. Normal host parenchymal cells do not invade and metastasize. Thus, the biochemical changes that are expressed in the malignant phenotype may be a target for strategies that are more selective for the tumor cells than are conventional cytotoxic agents.

The most immediate application of these basic research findings is in the area of tumor diagnosis and prognosis. The clinical aggressiveness of an individual tumor could be more accurately predicted by the measurement of genes or gene products functionally associated with the phenotype of invasion and metastases. These include oncogenes such as *ras*, *myc*, *neu*, newly discovered genes that may be associated with suppression of the metastatic phenotype,[103] and genes that encode receptors, proteinases, and motility factors associated with invasion. The average levels of such metastasis markers could be measured in a sample of the tumor tissue. On the other hand, antibodies or genetic probes for the markers could be applied to a histologic section of the tumor to study the tumor cell population distribution of the marker. In this manner, the proportion of tumor cells reacting with the marker could be used as an index of the aggressive tumor subpopulation. Application of antibodies to metastases-associated antigens by the surgical pathologist may provide increased accuracy in the identification of micrometastases in lymph nodes. Furthermore, immunohistochemical applications are not limited to tumor-associated antigens. Host antigens may also be altered in the vicinity of the tumor. This is the case for host basement membranes which are locally fragmented or lost in the area of tumor cell invasion. Loss of basement membrane antigens has already proved useful in the detection of breast cancer microinvasion and in the grading and staging of colorectal tumors.[21,22]

Some of the proteins associated with invasion and metastasis are secreted by the tumor cell. Examples are degradative enzymes such as type IV collagenase and heparanase, or hormone-like proteins such as tumor autocrine motility factors and growth factors. Following secretion by the tumor cell, the proteins (whole or as fragments), may accumulate in the blood or urine of the patient. Measurement of the level of the proteins by sensitive immunoassay procedures may be a means to (1) detect the existence of occult metastases, (2) estimate the body burden of metastatic disease, and (3) detect local tumor recurrence. Furthermore, in the case of bladder cancer, the level of the marker in the urine may reflect the invasive stage of the transitional cell carcinoma.

Tumor cell proteins functionally associated with the metastatic phenotype may be quantitatively augmented in tumor cells composing the metastatic foci. Systemically administered antibodies or synthetic ligands that bind to the tumor cell proteins may preferentially accumulate in the metastatic foci, compared with other body sites. This could be of use in the radioscintigraphic detection of clinically occult metastases. Furthermore, if the antibody or ligand is coupled to a toxic agent, it may selectively kill the tumor cells in the metastatic foci.

An increased understanding of the mechanisms of tumor cell invasion may lead to the development of pharmacologic agents or strategies that block tumor cell invasion. In theory, blocking any of the necessary steps for invasion listed in Table 7-1 could prevent tumor cell invasion. Tumor angiogenesis may depend on mechanisms similar to cancer invasion, including proteolysis. Consequently, an anti-invasion agent may also block tumor angiogenesis. Chronic systemic treatment or local administration with an anti-invasion agent may be clinically useful in the following settings: (1) preventing the transition from in situ to invasive cancer in high-risk patients, (2) reducing local tumor recurrence and invasion following surgical removal of primary tumors, and (3) inhibiting metastasis formation by circulating tumor cells disseminated by inoperable primary tumors, metastases, or released during surgical manipulation of the primary tumor.

The ultimate goal of metastasis prevention would be the selective eradication of established metastases, perhaps by targeting toxic agents to the metastatic foci. However, actual killing of the tumor cells in the metastatic foci may not be necessary to prevent the usual clinical outcome of metastatic disease. Inhibition of metastatic growth by chronic treatment regimens may achieve the same end. This is a hopeful area for therapy strategies because it has been found that common cellular pathways may be deranged by genetic events,

such as increased *ras* expression, in such a way as to increase both the growth and invasion of tumor cells. An example of a common pathway is the inositol phosphate cascade operating through phospholipase C. This pathway may be altered by a number of oncogenes. Agents that normalize this pathway in tumor cells may act to suppress both growth and invasion.

REFERENCES

1. Sugarbaker EV: Patterns of metastasis in human malignancies. Cancer Biol Rev 2:235, 1981
2. Weiss L, Gilbert HA: Bone Metastases. Boston, GK Hall, 1981
3. Schirrmacher V: Cancer metastasis: Experimental approaches, theoretical concepts, and impacts for treatment strategies. Adv Cancer Res 43:1, 1985
4. Fidler IJ, Hart IR: Biologic diversity in metastatic neoplasms: Origins and implications. Science 217:998, 1982
5. Liotta LA: Tumor invasion and metastases: role of the extracellular matrix. Rhoads Memorial Award Lecture. Cancer Res 46:1, 1986
6. Tubiana M, Chauvel P, Renaud A et al: Vitresse de croissance et histoire naturelle du cancer du sein. Bull Cancer 62:341, 1975
7. Koscielny S, Tubiana M, Valleron A-J: A simulation model of the natural history of human breast cancer. Br J Cancer 52:515, 1985
8. Bauer W, Igot J-P, Le Gal Y: Chronologie du cancer mammaire utilisant un modele de croissance de Gompertz. Ann Anat Pathol (Paris) 25:39, 1980
9. Liotta LA, Kleinerman J, Saidel GM: Quantitative relationships of intravascular tumor cells, tumor vessels, and pulmonary metastases following tumor implantation. Cancer Res 34:997, 1974
10. Fidler IJ, Kripke ML: Metastasis results from pre-existing variant cells within a malignant tumor. Science 197:893, 1977
11. Luria SE, Delbruck M: Mutations of bacteria from virus sensitivity to virus resistance. Genetics 28:491, 1945
12. Furcht LT: Editorial: Critical factors controlling angiogenesis: Cell products, cell matrix, and growth factors. Lab Invest 55:505, 1986
13. Folkman J: Tumor angiogenesis. Adv Cancer Res 43:175, 1985
14. Gullino PM, Grantham F: The vascular space of growing tumors. Cancer Res 24:1727, 1964
15. Lapis K, Paku S, Liotta LA: Endothelialization of embolised tumor cells during metastasis formation. Clin Exp Metastasis 6:73, 1988
16. Wallace AC, Chew E, Jones DS: The arrest and extravasation of cancer cells in the lung. In Weiss L, Gilbert HA (eds): Pulmonary Metastasis, p 26. Boston, GK Hall, 1978
17. Nicolson GL, Dulski K, Basson C et al: Preferential organ attachment and invasion in vitro by B16 melanoma cells selected for differing metastatic colonization and invasive properties. Invasion Metastasis 5:144, 1985
18. Frost P, Kerbel RS: Immunology of metastasis: Can the immune response cope with disseminated tumor? Metastasis Rev 2:239, 1983
19. Old LJ: Cancer immunology: The search for specificity. Cancer Res 41:361, 1981
20. Hanna N, Fidler IJ: Relationship between metastatic potential and resistance to natural killer cell mediated cytotoxicity in three murine tumor systems. JNCI 66:1183, 1981
21. Barsky SH, Siegal GP, Jannotta F et al: Loss of basement membrane components by invasive tumors but not their benign counterparts. Lab Invest 49:140, 1983
22. Forester SJ, Talbot IC, Critshley DR: Laminin and fibronectin in rectal adenocarcinoma: Relationship to tumor grade stage and metastasis. Br J Cancer 50:51, 1984
23. Wewer UM, Liotta LA, Jaye M et al: Altered levels of laminin receptor mRNA in various human carcinoma cells that have different abilities to bind laminin. Proc Natl Acad Sci USA 83:7137, 1986
24. Rao CN, Margulies M, Tralka S et al: Isolation of a subunit of laminin and its role in molecular structure and tumor cell attachment. J Biol Chem 257:9740, 1982
25. Engel J, Odermatt E, Engel A et al: Shapes, domain organization and flexibility of laminin and fibronectin: Two multifunctional proteins of the ECM. Mol Biol 150:97, 1981
26. Wewer UM, Taraboletti G, Sobel ME et al: Laminin receptor: Role in tumor cell migration. Cancer Res 47:5691, 1987
27. Barsky SH, Rao CN, Williams JE et al: Laminin molecular domains which alter metastasis in a murine model. J Clin Invest 74:843, 1984
28. Hynes RO: Integrins: A family of cell surface receptors. Cell 48:549, 1987
29. Ruoslahti E, Pierschbacher MD: Arg-Gly-Asp: A versatile cell recognition signal. Cell 44:517, 1986
30. Yamada KM, Kennedy DW: Dualistic nature of adhesive protein function: Fibronectin and its biologically active peptide fragments can autoinhibit fibronectin function. J Cell Biol 99:29, 1984
31. Horwitz A, Duggan C et al: Binding of fibronectin receptors to talin. Nature 320:531, 1986
32. Humphries MJ, Olden K, Yamada KM: A synthetic peptide from fibronectin inhibits experimental metastasis of murine melanoma cells. Science 233:467, 1986
33. Thorgeirsson UP, Turpeenniemi-Hujanen T, Neckers LM et al: Protein synthesis but

not DNA synthesis is required for tumor cell invasion *in vitro*. Invasion Metastasis 4:73, 1984

34. Thorgeirsson UP, Liotta LA, Kalebic T et al: Effect of natural protease inhibitors and a chemoattractant or tumor cell invasion *in vitro*. JNCI 69:1049, 1982

35. Liotta LA, Thorgeirsson UP, Garbisa S: Role of collagenases in tumor cell invasion. Cancer Metastasis Rev 1:277, 1982

36. Goldfarb RH: Plasminogen activators. Ann Rep Med Chem 18:257, 1983

37. Dano K, Andreasen PA, Grondahl-Hansen J et al: Plasminogen activators, tissue degradation, and cancer. Adv Cancer Res 44:139, 1985

38. Goldfarb RH, Liotta LA: Proteolytic enzymes in cancer invasion and metastasis. Semin Thromb Hemost 12:294, 1986

39. Sloane BF, Rozhin J, Ryan RE et al: Cathepsin B-like cysteine proteinases and metastases. In Honn KV, Powers WE, Sloan BF (eds): Mechanisms of Cancer Metastasis: Potential Therapeutic Implications, p. 377. Boston, Martinus Nijhoff, 1986

40. Sloane BF, Honn KV: Cysteine proteinases and metastasis. Cancer Metastasis Rev 3:249, 1984

41. Markus G: Plasminogen activators in malignant growth. In Davidson JF (ed): Progress in Fibrinolysis, p 587. Edinburgh, Churchill Livingstone, 1983

42. Goldfarb RH, Quigley JP: Purification of plasminogen activator from Rous sarcoma virus transformed chick embryo fibroblasts treated with the tumor promoter phorbol 12-myristate 13-acetate. Biochemistry 19:5463, 1980

43. Goldfarb RH, Quigley JP: Synergistic effect of tumor virus transformation and tumor promoter treatment on the production of plasminogen activator by chick embryo fibroblasts. Cancer Res 38:4601, 1978

44. Lijnen HR, Collen D: Interaction of plasminogen activation and inhibitors with plasminogen and fibrin. Semin Thromb Hemost 8:2, 1982

45. Castellino FJ, Powell SR: Human plasminogen. Methods Enzymol 80:365, 1981

46. Cajot J-F, Sordat B, Kruithof EKO et al: Human primary colon carcinomas xenografted into nude mice: I. Characterization of plasminogen activators expressed by primary tumors and their xenografts. JNCI 77:703, 1986

47. Markus G, Camiolo SM, Kohga S et al: Plasminogen activator secretion of human tumors in short-term organ culture, including a comparison of primary and metabolic tumors. Cancer Res 43:5517, 1983

48. Markus G: The role of hemostasis and fibrinolysis in the metastatic spread of cancer. Semin Thromb Hemost 10:61, 1984

49. Jones PA, DeClerck YA: Extracellular matrix destruction by invasive tumor cells. Cancer Metastasis Rev 1:289, 1982

50. Kramer RH, Bensch KG, Wang J: Invasion of reconstituted basement membrane matrix by metastatic human tumor cells. Cancer Res 46:1980, 1986

51. Bogenman E, Jones PA: Role of plasminogen in matrix degradation by neoplastic cells. JNCI 71:1177, 1983

52. Liotta LA, Goldfarb RH, Brundage R et al: Effect of plasminogen activator (urokinase), plasmin, and thrombin on glycoprotein and collagenous components of basement membrane. Cancer Res 41:4629, 1981

53. Ossowski L, Reich E: Antibodies to plasminogen activator inhibit tumor metastasis. Cell 35:611, 1983

54. Wang BS, McLouglin GA, Richie JP et al: Correlation of the production of plasminogen activator with tumor metastasis in B16 mouse melanoma cell lines. Cancer Res 40:288, 1980

55. Carlsen SA, Ramshaw JA, Warrington RC: Involvement of plasminogen activator production in a rat model. Cancer Res 44:3012, 1984

56. Sappino A-P, Busso N, Belin D et al: Increase of urokinase type plasminogen activator gene expression in human lung and breast carcinomas. Cancer Res 47:4043, 1987

57. Gross J, Nagai Y: Specific degradation of the collagen molecule by tadpole collagenolytic enzyme. Proc Natl Acad Sci USA 54:1197, 1965

58. Goldberg GI, Wilhelm SM, Kronberger A et al: Human fibroblast collagenase: Complete primary structure and homology to an oncogene transformation-induced rat protein. J Biol Chem 261:6600, 1986

59. Fini ME, Plucinska IM, Mayer AS et al: A gene for rabbit synovial cell collagenase: Member of a family of metalloproteinases that degrade the connective tissue matrix. Biochemistry 26:6156, 1987

60. Huang C-C, Blitzer A, Abramson M: Collagenase in human head and neck tumors and rat tumors and fibroblasts in monolayer cultures. Ann Otol Rhinol Laryngol 95:158, 1986

61. Wirl G, Frich J: Collagenase: A marker enzyme in human bladder cancer. Urol Res 7:103, 1979

62. Liotta LA, Rao CN: Role of the extracellular matrix in cancer. Ann NY Acad Sci 460:333, 1985

63. Liotta LA, Abe S, Robey PG et al: Preferential digestion of basement membrane collagen by an enzyme derived from a metastatic murine tumor. Proc Natl Acad Sci USA 76:2268, 1979

64. Salo T, Liotta LA, Tryggvason K: Purification and characterization of a murine basement membrane collagen-degrading enzyme secreted by metastatic tumor cells. J Biol Chem 258:3058, 1983

65. Liotta LA, Rao CN, Barsky SH: Tumor invasion and the extracellular matrix. Lab Invest 49:636, 1983

66. Liotta LA, Tryggvason K, Garbisa S et al: Metastatic potential correlates with enzymatic degradation of basement membrane collagen. Nature 284:67, 1980

67. Nakatsukasa H: Type IV collagen-degrading enzyme activity in hepatocellular carcinoma. Acta Med Okayama 40:83, 1986

68. Turpeenniemi-Hujanen T, Thorgeirsson UP, Hart IR et al: Expression of collagenase IV (basement membrane collagenase) activity in murine tumor cell hybrids that differ in metastatic potential. JNCI 75:99, 1985

69. Muschel R, Williams JE, Lowy DR et al: Harvey *ras* induction of metastatic potential depends upon oncogene activation and type of recipient cell. Am J Pathol 121:1, 1985

70. Garbisa S, Pozzatti R, Muschel RJ et al: Secretion of type IV collagenolytic protease and metastatic phenotype: Induction by transfection with c-Ha-ras but not c-Ha-ras plus Ad2-Ela. Cancer Res 47:1523, 1987

71. Chin JR, Murphy G, Werb Z: Stromelysin, a connective tissue-degrading metalloendopeptidase secreted by stimulated rabbit synovial fibroblasts in parallel with collagenase. J Biol Chem 260:12367, 1985

72. Wilhelm SM, Collier IE, Kronberger A et al: Human skin fibroblast stromelysin: Structure, glycosylation, substrate specificity, and differential expression in normal and tumorigenic cells. Proc Natl Acad Sci USA 84:6725, 1987

73. Frisch SM, Clark EJ, Werb Z: Coordinate regulation of stromelysin and collagenase genes determined with cDNA probes. Proc Natl Acad Sci USA 84:2600, 1987

74. Matrisian LM, Leroy P, Ruhlmann C et al: Isolation of the oncogene and epidermal growth factor-induced transin gene: Complex control in rat fibroblasts. Mol Cell Biol 6:1679, 1986

75. Nakajima M, Irimura T, Di Ferrante D et al: Heparan sulfate degradation: Relation to tumor invasive and metastatic properties of mouse B16 melanoma sublines. Science 220:611, 1983

76. Nakajima M, Irimura T, Di Ferrante N et al: Metastatic melanoma cell heparanase characterization of heparan sulfate degradation fragments produced by B16 melanoma endoglucuronidase. J Biol Chem 259:2283, 1984

77. Nakajima M, Irimura T, Nicolson GL: Tumor metastasis-associated heparanase (heparan sulfate endoglycosidase) activity in human melanoma cells. Cancer Lett 31:277, 1986

78. Mignatti P, Robbins E, Rifkin DB: Tumor invasion through the human amniotic membrane: Requirement for a proteinase cascade. Cell 47:487, 1986

79. Persky B, Ostrowski LE, Pagast P et al: Inhibition of proteolytic enzymes in the *in vitro* amnion model for basement membrane invasion. Cancer Res 16:4129, 1986

80. Lam WC, Delikatny JE, Orr FW et al: The chemotactic response of tumor cells: A model for cancer metastasis. Am J Pathol 104:69, 1981

81. McCarthy JB, Basara ML, Palm SL, et al: Stimulation of haptotaxis and migration of tumor cells by serum spreading factor. Cancer Metastasis Rev 4:125, 1985

82. Anzano MA, Roberts AB, Smith JM et al: Sarcoma growth factors from conditioned media of virally transformed cells composed of both type α and type β growth factors. Proc Natl Acad Sci USA 80:6264, 1983

83. Liotta LA, Mandler R, Murano G et al: Tumor cell autocrine motility factor: Tumor cell autocrine motility factor. Proc Natl Acad Sci USA 83:3302, 1986

84. Stracke ML, Guirguis R, Liotta LA et al: Pertussis toxin inhibits stimulated motility independently of the adenylate cyclase pathway in human melanoma cells. Biochem Biophys Res Commun 146:339, 1987

85. Guirguis R, Margulies IMK, Taraboletti G et al: Cytokine-induced pseudopodial protrusion is coupled to tumour cell migration. Nature 329:261, 1987

86. Bokoch GM, Gilman AG: Inhibition of receptor-mediated release of arachidonic acid by pertussis toxin. Cell 39:301, 1984

87. Smith CD, Cox CC, Snyderman R: Receptor-coupled activation of phosphoinositide-specific phospholipase C by an N protein. Science 232:97, 1986

88. Weinberg RA: Oncogenes of spontaneous and chemically induced tumors. Adv Cancer Res 36:149, 1982

89. Hunter T: Oncogenes and proto-oncogenes: How do they differ? JNCI 73:773, 1984

90. Chang EH, Furth ME, Scolnick EM et al: Tumorigenic transformation of mammalian cells induced by a normal human gene homologous to the oncogene of Harvey murine sarcoma virus. Proc Natl Acad Sci USA 78:3328, 1981

91. Nicolson GL: Tumor cell instability, diversification, and progression to the metastatic phenotype: From oncogene to oncofetal expression. Cancer Res 47:1473, 1987

92. Thorgeirsson UP, Turpeenniemi-Hujanen T, Williams JE et al: NIH/3T3 cells transfected with human tumor DNA containing activated ras oncogenes express the metastatic phenotype in nude mice. Mol Cell Biol 5:259, 1985

93. Bondy GP, Wilson S, Chambers AF: Experimental metastatic ability of H-ras transformed NIH-3T3 cells. Cancer Res 45:6005, 1985

94. Greig RG, Koestler TP, Trainer DL et al: Tumorigenic and metastatic properties of "normal" and ras-transfected NIH/3T3 cells. Proc Natl Acad Sci USA 82:3698, 1985

95. Egan SE, McClarty GA, Jarolim L et al: Expression of H-ras correlates with metastatic potential: Evidence for direct regulation of the metastatic phenotype in 10T1/2 and NIH 3T3 cells. Mol Cell Biol 7:830, 1987

96. Vousden KH, Eccles SA, Purvies H et al: Enhanced spontaneous metastasis of mouse carcinoma cells transfected with an activated c-Ha-ras-1 gene. Int J Cancer 37:425, 1986

97. Kerbel RS, Waghorne C, Man MS et al: Alteration of the tumorigenic and metastatic properties of neoplastic cells is associated with the process of calcium phosphate-mediated DNA transfection. Proc Natl Acad Sci USA 84:1263, 1987

98. Collard JG, Schijven JF, Roos E: Invasive and metastatic potential induced by ras-transfection into mouse BW5147 T-lymphoma cells. Cancer Res 47:754, 1987

99. Muschel RJ, Nakahara K, Chu EW et al: Karyotypic analysis of diploid or near diploid metastatic Harvey ras transformed rat embryo fibroblasts. Cancer Res 46:4104, 1986

100. Pozzatti R, Muschel R, Williams J et al: Primary rat embryo cells transformed by one or two oncogenes show different metastatic potentials. Science 232:223, 1986

101. Gullino PM, Pettigrew NM, Grantham FH: N-nitrosomethylurea as a mammary gland carcinoma in rats. JNCI 54:401, 1975

102. Sukumar S, Notairo V, Martin-Zanca et al: Induction of mammary carcinomas in rats by NMU involves malignant activation of Ha-ras-1 locus by a single point mutation. Nature 306:658, 1983

103. Steeg PS, Bevilacqua G, Kopper L et al: Evidence for a novel gene associated with low tumor metastatic potential. JNCI 80:200, 1988

104. Dennis JW, Laferte S, Waghorne C et al: 1-6 branching of Asn-linked oligosaccharides is directly associated with metastasis. Science 236:582, 1987

105. Stryer L, Bourne HR: G proteins: A family of signal transducers. Annu Rev Cell Biol 2:391, 1986

106. Fleischman LF, Chahwala SB, Cantley L: Ras-transformed cells: Altered levels of phosphatidylinositol-4,5-bisphosphate and catabolites. Science 231:407, 1986

107. Egan SE, Wright JA, Jarolim L et al: Transformation by oncogenes encoding protein kinases induces the metastatic phenotype. Science 238:202, 1987

108. Smith MR, DeGudicibus SJ, Stacey DW: Requirement for c-ras proteins during viral oncogene transformation. Nature 320:540, 1986

109. Jaggi R, Salmons B, Muellener D et al: The v-mos and H-ras oncogene expression represses glucocorticoid hormone-dependent transcription from the mouse mammary tumor virus LTR. EMBO J 5:2609, 1986

110. Rabin MS, Doherty PJ, Gottesman MM: The tumor promoter phorbol 12-myristate 13-acetate induces a program of altered gene expression similar to that induced by platelet-derived growth factor and transforming oncogenes. Proc Natl Acad Sci USA 83:357, 1986

111. Cline MJ, Battifora H, Yokota J: Proto-oncogene abnormalities in human breast cancer: Correlations with anatomic features and clinical course of disease. J Clin Oncol 5:999, 1987

112. Slamon DJ, Clark GM, Wong SG et al: Human breast cancer: Correlation of relapse and survival with amplification of the HER-2/neu oncogene. Science 235:177, 1987

113. Kolata G: Oncogenes give breast cancer prognosis. Science 235:160, 1987

114. van de Vijver M, van de Bersselaar R, Devilee P et al: Amplification of the neu (c-erbB-2) oncogene in human mammary tumors is relatively frequent and is often accompanied by amplification of the linked c-erbA oncogene. Mol Cell Biol 7:2019, 1987

115. Yokota J, Tsunetsugu-Yokota Y, Battifora H et al: Alterations of myc, myb, and ras^ha proto-oncogenes in cancers are frequent and show clinical correlation. Science 231:261, 1986

116. Agnantis NJ, Parissi P, Anagnostakis D et al: Comparative study of Harvey-ras oncogene expression with conventional clinicopathologic parameters of breast cancer. Oncology 43:36, 1986

117. Horan Hand P, Vilasi V, Thor A et al: Quantitation of Harvey ras p21 enhanced expression in human breast and colon carcinomas. JNCI 79:59, 1987

118. Clair T, Miller WR, Cho-Chung YS: Prognostic significance of the expression of a ras protein with a molecular weight of 21,000 by human breast cancer. Cancer Res 47:5290, 1987

119. Lundy J, Grimson R, Mishriki Y et al: Elevated ras oncogene expression correlates with lymph node metastases in breast cancer patients. J Clin Oncol 4:1321, 1986

120. Seeger RC, Brodeur GM, Sather H et al: Association of multiple copies of the N-myc oncogene with rapid progression of neuroblastomas. N Engl J Med 313:1111, 1985

121. Brodeur GM, Seeger RC, Schwab M et al: Amplification of N-myc in untreated human neuroblastomas correlates with advanced disease stage. Science 224:1121, 1984

122. Nau MM, Brooks BJ, Carney DN et al: Human small-cell lung cancers show amplification and expression of the N-myc gene. Proc Natl Acad Sci USA 83:1092, 1986

123. Tsuboi K, Hirayoshi K, Takeuchi K et al: Expression of the c-myc gene in human gastrointestinal malignancies. Biochem Biophys Res Commun 146:699, 1987

HENRY C. PITOT

CHAPTER 8 *Principles of Carcinogenesis: Chemical*

The first source of our knowledge of chemical carcinogenesis was clinical observations in humans. In 1775, Percival Pott, an eminent English physician and surgeon, described the occurrence of cancer of the scrotum in a number of his male patients.[1] The common history of these patients was employment as chimney sweeps when they were young. On the basis of this observation, Dr. Pott, with remarkable insight, concluded that the childhood occupation of these men was directly and causally related to their malignant disease, and that the soot was the causative agent. Strangely enough, Pott did not suggest avoiding the soot as a means of prevention, although his report in 1775 apparently inspired the Danish Chimney Sweepers' Guild to rule 3 years later that its members should bathe daily. It was not until more than a century later that Butlin[2] reported the relative rarity of scrotal cancer in chimney sweeps on the European continent compared with those in England. It appeared that the lower incidence of the disease was the result of frequent bathing and protective clothing.

The lesson from Pott's report took a long time to be learned. One hundred years after its publication, the high incidence of skin cancer among certain German workers finally was traced to their exposure to coal tar, the chief constituent of the chimney sweeps' soot. However, it took another 40 years before the disease was reproduced experimentally, and even today, more than two centuries after Pott's original scientific report on the association of soot and smoke products with the later development of cancer, many

of us still disregard the obvious hazards of the carcinogenic products resulting from the combustion of tobacco in cigarettes and of many of the organic fuels of our industrialized world.

Polycyclic hydrocarbons, soots, and tars, however, were not the only chemicals in the human environment exhibiting a causal relationship with specific human cancers. The chemical dye industry developed and flourished during the last half of the 19th century in Europe. Before World War I, Germany provided more than 80% of the world's supply of aniline, its derivatives, and related aromatic amines, the bases for the synthesis of most dyes used at that time. In 1895 Rehn described the occurrence of bladder cancer in several workers in the aniline dye industry.[3] Other epidemiologic studies incriminated several related aromatic amines, especially naphthylamines and benzidine, as carcinogenic for humans. Although the exact chemical dye responsible for the bladder cancers in workers was not identified in Rehn's report, the distinctly different chemical nature of the crude soots and tars implicated by Pott and Butlin compared with the relatively pure, synthetic aromatic amines used in the dye industry suggested that chemicals of diverse structure were capable of causing cancer in the human. Unfortunately, it took almost another 50 years before experimental proof of the exact nature of the carcinogenic aniline dyes was obtained.[4]

The term *carcinogen* generally has been used by oncologists to indicate an agent that causes cancer. Today such a simplistic definition is not sufficient. We have proposed the following definition to include most instances of agents that are carcinogens.

> A *carcinogen* is an agent whose administration to previously untreated animals leads to a statistically significant increased incidence of neoplasms of one or more histogenetic types as compared with the incidences in appropriate untreated animals, whether the control animals have low or high spontaneous incidences of the neoplasms in question.

This definition includes the induction of neoplasms that are not usually observed, the earlier induction of neoplasms that are usually observed, and the induction of more neoplasms than are usually found. Although it would be important to distinguish between agents that induce neoplasms by direct action on the cells that become neoplastic and those that produce neoplasia by indirect actions in the animal as a whole, at present it is seldom possible to do so. Some agents, such as immune suppressants, can increase the incidence of neoplasms in tissues previously exposed to carcinogens by indirect effects on the host. Agents acting through such effects should not be termed carcinogens.

CHEMICAL CARCINOGENESIS

One hundred forty years after Pott's report of the association of soot from the combustion of coal with skin cancer of the scrotum, an experimental basis for Pott's clinical observation was reported. In 1915, the Japanese pathologists Yamagiwa and Ichikawa reported the first production of skin tumors in animals by the application of coal tar to the skin.[5] These investigators repeatedly applied crude coal tar to the ears of rabbits for a number of months, finally producing both benign and, later, malignant epidermal neoplasms. Later studies demonstrated that the skin of mice was also susceptible to the carcinogenic action of such organic tars. During the next 15 years, extensive attempts were made to determine the nature of the material in the crude tars that caused malignancy. In 1925, Kennaway reported the production of carcinogenic tars by pyrolysis of simple organic compounds comprising only carbon and hydrogen.[6] In the early 1930s, several such polycyclic hydrocarbons were isolated from active crude tar fractions. In 1930, the first synthetic carcinogenic compound was made.[7] This compound, dibenz[a,h]anthracene (1,2,5,6-dibenzanthracene), was tested for carcinogenic activity by being painted on the skin of mice and was found to be a potent carcinogen. The isolation from coal tar and synthesis of the carcinogen, benzo[a]pyrene (3,4-benzpyrene) was achieved in 1932. Polycyclic hydrocarbons vary in their carcinogenic potencies; for example, the isomer of dibenz[a,h]anthracene, dibenz[a,c]anthracene (1,2,3,4-dibenzanthracene), has very little carcinogenic activity. Structures of some polycyclic hydrocarbons are noted in Figure 8-1.

In 1935, Sasaki and Yoshida extended the field of chemical carcinogenesis by demonstrating that the feeding of the azo dye, o-aminoazotoluene, to rats resulted in the development of liver tumors.[8] Kinosita later demonstrated that 4-dimethylaminoazobenzene in the diet also caused neoplasms

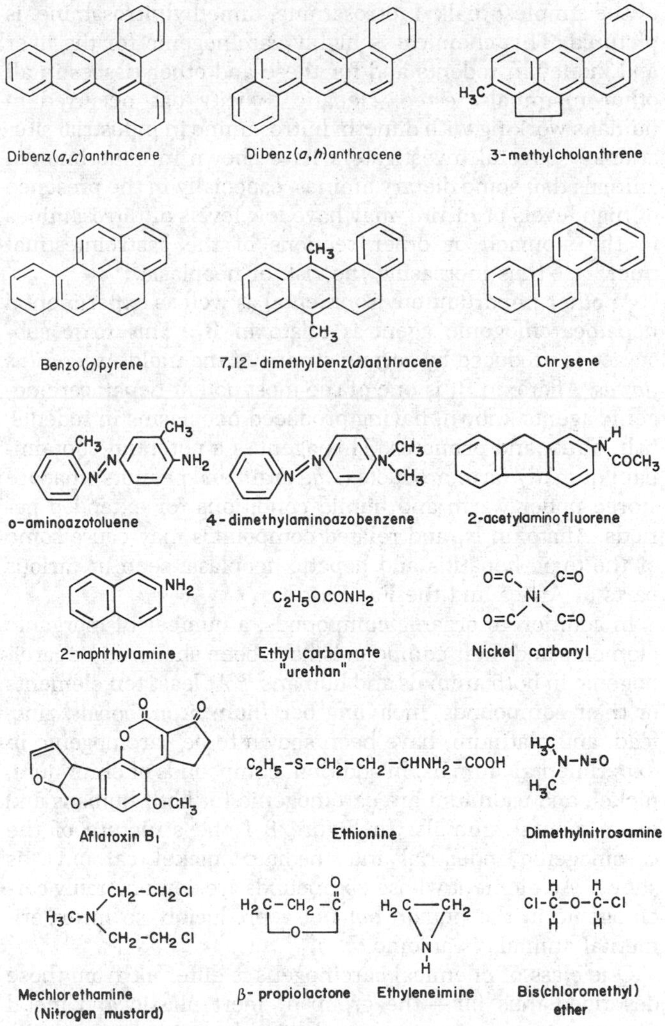

FIG. 8-1. Chemical structures of representative chemical carcinogens. (Adapted from Pitot HC: Fundamentals of Oncology, 3rd ed. New York, Marcel Dekker, 1986)

in the liver.[9] A number of analogues of this compound were also prepared. An interesting correlation arising from these later studies was that the amino group of carcinogenic dyes usually had at least one methyl substituent, although o-aminoazotoluene does not. Unlike the polycyclic hydrocarbons, the azo dyes generally did not act at the site of first contact of the compound with the organism, but rather in a remote area, namely, the liver. Painting of the skin with most azo dyes resulted in few or no tumors, and the ingestion of polycyclic hydrocarbons generally resulted in no hepatomas except in neonates.

2-Acetylaminofluorene, first synthesized as an insecticide but fortunately never used for that purpose, is a model laboratory chemical carcinogen. The best known representative of aromatic amines, carcinogenic for the urinary bladder in humans, is 2-napthylamine, although benzidine and related dyes are equally carcinogenic (see below). The nitrosamines are a class of compounds many members of which are effective chemical carcinogens and of potential importance in the genesis of neoplasia in humans. In Figure 8-1 the structure of the simplest dialkyl nitrosamine, dimethylnitrosamine, is pictured. This chemical is highly carcinogenic for the liver and kidney in rodents and for these and other tissues in all other mammals tested. Hepatic toxicity has occurred in humans working with dimethylnitrosamine in industrial situations.[10] Several investigators have shown in experimental animals that some dietary amines, especially in the presence of high levels of nitrite, may have low levels of nitrosamines in the stomach or other sections of the gastrointestinal tract,[11-13] thus increasing the risk of neoplasia.[14]

Another important environmental as well as experimental hepatocarcinogenic agent is aflatoxin B_1. This toxic substance is produced by certain strains of the mold *Aspergillus flavus*. Aflatoxin B_1 is one of the most potent hepatocarcinogenic agents known, having produced neoplasms in rodents, fish, birds, and primates. This agent is a potential contaminant of many farm products (*e.g.,* grain and peanuts) that are stored under warm and humid conditions for extended periods. Aflatoxin B_1 and related compounds may cause some of the toxic hepatitis and hepatic neoplasia seen in various parts of Africa and the Far East.[15]

In addition to organic compounds, a number of inorganic elements and their compounds have been shown to be carcinogenic in both animals and humans.[16] At least ten elements or their compounds, including beryllium, iron, cobalt, zinc, lead, and platinum, have been shown to be carcinogenic in experimental animals. In addition, compounds of chromium, nickel, and cadmium are carcinogenic for both humans and experimental animals. In Figure 8-1 the structure of the carcinogenic industrial intermediate, nickel carbonyl, is shown. An element whose compounds are demonstrably carcinogenic in the human but not reproducibly so in experimental animals is arsenic.[17]

One class of chemical carcinogens is different from those described thus far—the group of inert plastic and metal films that cause sarcomas at the implantation site, usually subcutaneous, in some rodents.[18] Rats and mice are highly susceptible to this form of carcinogenesis, but guinea pigs appear to be resistant.[19] The carcinogenic properties of the implant are largely dependent on its physical characteristics and surface area. Multiple perforations, pulverization, or roughening of the surface of the implant markedly reduce the incidence of neoplasms.[20]

The chemical nature of the implant is not the critical factor in its ability to transform normal cells to neoplastic cells. Studies by Brand and associates[18] have shown that DNA synthesis occurs in the film-attached cell population throughout the preneoplastic phase and that preneoplastic cells may be identified well before neoplasms develop.[21] These studies may have significance in human neoplasia in view of the recent report that orthopaedic implant materials may induce the same phenomenon in rats.[22]

METABOLISM OF CHEMICAL CARCINOGENS IN RELATION TO CARCINOGENESIS

Although the discovery that polycyclic hydrocarbons and other compounds could induce cancer gave hope that the complete understanding of the nature of neoplasia might follow, we still appear to be far from such an understanding. The principal excretory metabolites of polycyclic hydrocarbons were hydroxylated derivatives, which usually had little or no carcinogenic activity. Similarly, hydroxylation in vivo of the rings of the aromatic amine carcinogens, such as 2-acetylaminofluorene (AAF) and 4-dimethylaminoazobenzene (DAB), usually resulted in a complete loss of activity and facilitated the further metabolism and excretion of the parent compounds.

As is evident from Figure 8-1, the different classes of chemical carcinogens do not have common structural features. The complexity of the various chemicals that can induce cancer posed a striking dilemma in attempts to understand the mechanisms of action of these agents. The beginning of our present-day understanding of the solution to this dilemma was reported in 1947 by the Millers, who first demonstrated that, during the process of hepatocarcinogenesis, carcinogenic azo dyes became covalently bound to proteins of the liver but not to proteins of the resulting neoplasms.[23] The initial studies of the Millers led them to propose that the binding of carcinogens to proteins might lead to the loss or deletion of critical proteins for growth control. At the time this hypothesis was proposed, in 1947, the molecular concept of the gene was in its infancy.

As an extension of this work, Elizabeth Miller[24] demonstrated the covalent binding of benzo[a]pyrene or its metabolite(s) to proteins in the skin of mice treated with the hydrocarbon. This finding strongly suggested that an important step in the induction of cancer by chemicals was the covalent interaction of some form of the chemical with proteins and other macromolecules. Because the parent compound in all cases studied could not bind directly with macromolecules, it was concluded that the interaction of chemicals with macromolecules was the result of the metabolic action of the cell. In 1960 the Millers and Cramer[25] reported that 2-acetylaminofluorene was metabolized not only by ring hydroxylation, but also by hydroxylation of the nitrogen of the acetylamino group. They isolated N-hydroxy-2-acetylaminofluorene (Fig. 8-2) and, in subsequent investigations, found this compound to be more carcinogenic that the parent compound, 2-acetylaminofluorene. N-hydroxy-2-acetylaminofluorene also induced neoplasms not found following administration of the parent compound, such as subcutaneous sarcomas at the site of injection. Further, in animals (such as the guinea pig) that convert little of the 2-acetylaminofluorene to its N-hydroxy derivative in vivo, cancer of the liver was not produced by feeding the parent compound. These studies strongly supported the suggestion that, at least for 2-acetylaminofluorene, the parent compound was not the direct carcinogen, but rather that certain metabolic derivative(s) were the active components in the induction of neoplasia. These studies led to the finding of the activation of carcinogens by means of their metabolism by cellular enzymes.[26]

The Millers continued their investigations of the metabolism of N-hydroxy-2-acetylaminofluorene and demonstrated that the N-hydroxy group could be esterified to yield a highly reactive compound that can react nonenzymatically with nucleophilic sites on proteins and nucleic acids and with specific amino acids and nucleosides. These results led to a

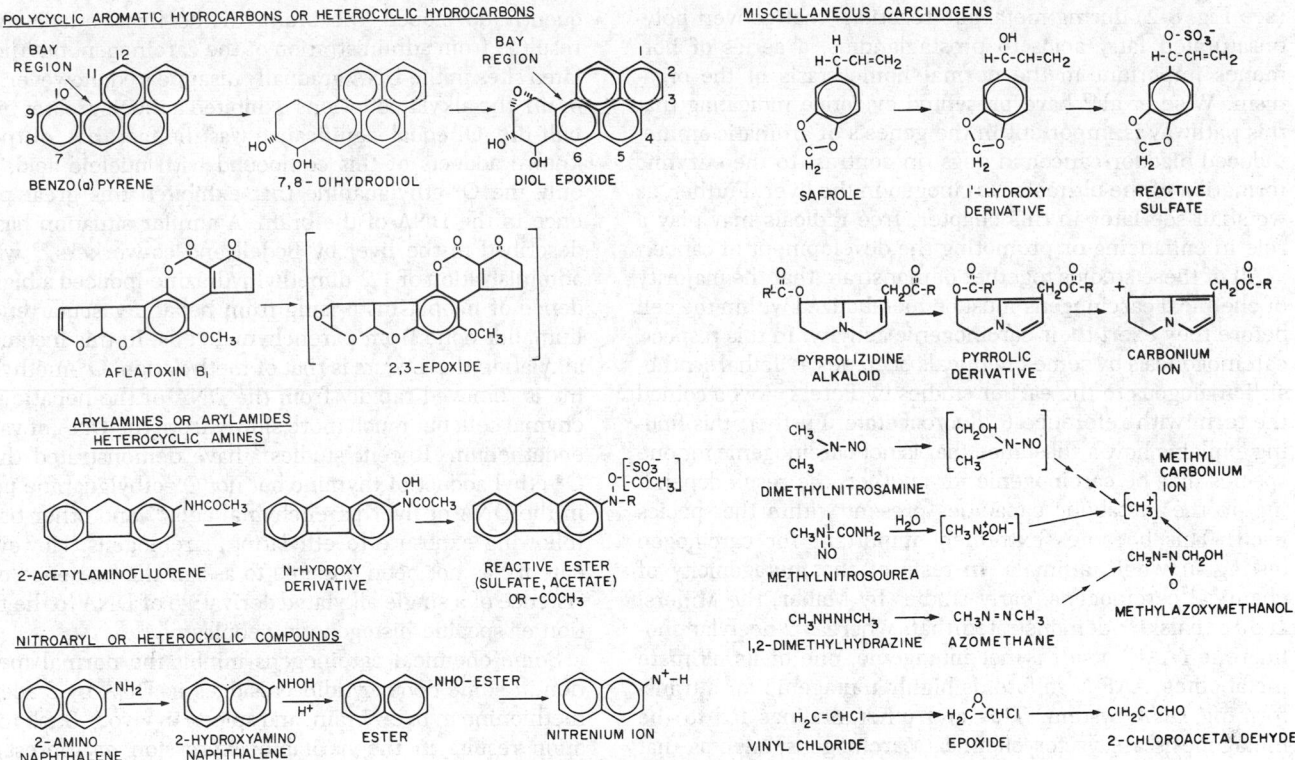

FIG. 8-2. Structures of representative procarcinogens, proximate and ultimate forms of chemical carcinogens. (Adapted from Pitot HC: Fundamentals of Oncology, 3rd ed. New York, Marcel Dekker, 1986)

solution of the dilemma of the variety of structurally unrelated chemical carcinogens. They proposed that chemical carcinogens are, or are converted by metabolism into, electrophilic reactants (chemicals with electron-deficient sites) that exert their biologic effects by covalent interaction with cellular macromolecules. The critical target most probably is DNA.[27]

After the demonstration by the Millers of the critical significance of electrophilic metabolites in chemical carcinogenesis, a number of "proximate" and "ultimate" forms, especially those of aromatic amines, were described (see Fig. 8-2). The ultimate form of the carcinogen, that is, the form that actually interacts with cellular constituents to cause the neoplastic transformation, is the final product shown in most of the pathways in Figure 8-2. However, the carcinogenic polycyclic hydrocarbons still posed a problem. As early as 1950, Boyland[28] had proposed the formation of epoxide intermediates in the metabolism of these chemicals. Later investigations showed that epoxides of polycyclic hydrocarbons could react with nucleic acids and proteins in the absence of any metabolizing system. In 1974, Sims and associates[29] proposed that a diol epoxide of benzo[a]pyrene was the ultimate form of this carcinogen. Subsequent studies by a number of investigators[30,31] have demonstrated that the structure of this ultimate form is (+)-anti-benzo[a]pyrene-7,8-dihydro-9,10-epoxide (see Fig. 8-2).

One of the interesting ramifications of these findings is the importance of oxidation of the carbons of the "bay region" of potentially carcinogenic polycyclic hydrocarbons.

Figure 8-2 shows the bay region of benzo[a]pyrene. Levin and associates[32] as well as others[31] have proposed that epoxidation of a dihydro, angular benzo ring that forms part of a bay region of a polycyclic hydrocarbon is the most likely ultimate carcinogenic form of the hydrocarbon. The bay region is the sterically hindered region formed by the angular benzo ring. Although the bay region concept has not been tested with all known carcinogenic polycyclic hydrocarbons, it appears to be generally applicable thus far.

In addition to the electrophilic intermediates comprising the structures of the ultimate forms of chemical carcinogens, recent evidence also indicates that free radical derivatives of chemical carcinogens may be produced both metabolically and nonenzymatically during their metabolism.[33] Free radicals carry no charge but do possess a single unpaired electron, making the radical extremely reactive. That such forms may be important in the induction of neoplastic transformation by chemicals comes from two lines of evidence. Various molecules that inhibit the formation of free radicals, many of which are termed antioxidants, can inhibit the carcinogenic action of many chemical carcinogens.[34] Although there is no doubt that free radical intermediates are sometimes formed during the metabolism of chemical carcinogens, only recently have relatively specific metabolic reactions of certain chemical carcinogens, particularly polycyclic hydrocarbons, been shown to proceed through free radical intermediates. Marnett[35] has described the co-oxygenation of polyunsaturated fatty acids with polycyclic aromatic hydrocarbons, leading to the formation of the ultimate diol epoxide form (see Fig. 8-2) during metabolic reactions that convert polyunsaturated fatty acids to prostaglandins, a series of hormones important in the normal homeostasis of the organism. Wise et al[36] have presented evidence indicating that this pathway is important in the genesis of aromatic amine-induced bladder cancer in dogs, in contrast to the enzymic formation of the ultimate carcinogen in the liver. Further, as we shall see later in this chapter, free radicals may play a role in enhancing or promoting the development of cancer.

All of these studies together demonstrate that the majority of chemical carcinogens must be metabolized within the cell before they exert their carcinogenic activity. In this respect, carcinogenesis by some chemicals becomes a "lethal synthesis" analogous to the earlier studies by Peters,[37] who coined the term with reference to fluoroacetate. Further, this finding explains how a substance that is not carcinogenic for one species may be carcinogenic for another, the result depending on the metabolic capacities present within the species itself. This becomes extremely important for carcinogen testing in whole animals. In tests of the mutagenicity of chemical carcinogens, early studies by Maher, the Millers, and Szybalski[38] demonstrated that, whereas 2-acetylaminofluorene (AAF) itself is not mutagenic, one of its ultimate metabolites, AAF-N-sulfate, is highly mutagenic for a transforming DNA system. This and other findings led to the mutagenesis assays for chemical carcinogens, such as that developed by Ames and colleagues,[39] which involves the in vitro metabolism of suspected carcinogens by liver microsomal preparations in the presence of a highly mutable strain of bacteria (see below).

Not all chemical carcinogens require intracellular metabolism to become ultimate carcinogens. Examples are the direct alkylating agents β-propiolactone, nitrogen mustard, ethyleneimine, and bis(chloromethyl)ether (see Fig. 8-1), the latter having been shown to be carcinogenic for humans (see below).

One important aspect of chemical carcinogenesis is the nature of the critical molecular interactions between ultimate carcinogens and those components of the cell whose reactions with the carcinogen lead to the neoplastic change. Metabolic studies with labeled carcinogens have investigated the loss of radioactivity from protein, RNA, and DNA and have shown in several instances that adducts are lost almost entirely from the former two components but are retained to a greater or lesser extent in the DNA of cells.[40] These findings have led to the postulation that an interaction critical for the neoplastic transformation occurs between the ultimate form of the carcinogen and DNA. However, not all of the molecular interactions between the ultimate form of a chemical carcinogen and DNA share in the causation of the neoplastic transformation. Goth and Rajewsky[41] emphasized the importance of such an understanding by demonstrating that the presence of *persistent* DNA–carcinogen adducts appeared to be related directly to the susceptibility of a tissue to cancer development. These investigators administered the carcinogen, ethylnitrosourea, to newborn rats and compared the quantitative and qualitative aspects of the ethylation of DNA in a tissue showing no carcinogenic effects of this ethylating agent, the liver, with one in which cancer subsequently developed, the brain. In the liver, ethylated DNA resulted from administration of the carcinogen, but the alkylated sites in the DNA gradually disappeared; however, in the brain, the alkylated lesions exhibited a much greater biologic half-life. Of equal significance was the fact that, of the then known adducts of this compound with nucleic acid, it was only the O^6-ethylguanine that exhibited this great persistence in the DNA of the brain. A similar situation has been described in the liver by Bedell and co-workers,[42] wherein administration of 1,2-dimethylhydrazine induced a high incidence of neoplasms arising from hepatic vascular endothelium, but none from parenchymal cells. In this instance the alkylation that occurs is that of methylation. O^6-methylguanine is removed rapidly from the DNA of the hepatic parenchymal cell, but much more slowly from the DNA of vascular endothelium. Recent studies[43] have demonstrated that the O^4-ethyl adduct of thymine but not O^6-ethylguanine persists in the DNA of liver parenchymal cells[44] and other tissues[45] following exposure to ethylating carcinogens. However, to date it has not been possible to assign the presence or persistence of a single alkylated derivative of DNA to the formation of specific histogenetic neoplasms.[45]

Some chemical carcinogens inhibit the normal methylation of some deoxycytidine residues in DNA by S-adenosylmethionine in liver, brain, and spleen in vivo.[46] Such methylation results in the heritable expression or repression of specific genes in eukaryotic cells. The inhibition of this process appears to occur by several mechanisms, including formation of covalent adducts (see above), single-strand breaks in the DNA, and the direct inactivation of the enzyme, DNA-S-adenosylmethionine methyltransferase, which is responsible for normal methylation.[46] Thus the inhibition of DNA methylation by chemical carcinogens is another potential pathway by which these agents may induce the neoplastic transformation.

A potential application of our knowledge of the presence and persistence of covalent adducts of carcinogenic chemicals in macromolecules is the determination of the amounts of such adducts in human tissues.[47] Immunoassays including the enzyme-linked immunosorbent assay (ELISA)[48] and the radioimmunoassay (RIA)[49] allow the determination of individual specific chemical adducts of DNA with a very high degree of sensitivity and specificity. In addition, a technique of ^{32}P-postlabeling analysis of DNA[50] allows an even greater degree of sensitivity (detection of a single adduct in 10^7–10^8 nucleotides) but without the same specificity as the immunoassays. (For details of the immunoassay method, the reader is referred to Volume 92 of the series *Methods in Enzymology*.[51]) These techniques are indispensable to the new field of "molecular epidemiology."[52] Recent studies have indicated that such techniques can be utilized to detect polycyclic hydrocarbon adducts in DNA of smokers and individuals exposed to high levels of smoke and soot in their work.[52,53] In addition, a marked increase in the form of the aromatic amine carcinogen, 4-aminobiphenyl, covalently bound to hemoglobin in the serum has been reported by use of techniques of gas chromatography and mass spectrometry.[54] Because of DNA excision repair (see below) the levels of DNA adducts found in humans probably represent steady-state levels rather than peak levels, which may be seen shortly after a single exposure. However, these techniques can be used to monitor the risk of individuals exposed to potential environmental carcinogens, allowing the institution of preventive measures to reduce such risk.

The methods by which alkylated lesions in DNA are removed include a number of processes collectively termed DNA repair. Although it is beyond the scope of this chapter to consider the various pathways of DNA repair,[55,56] many features of the processes of DNA repair are important for the process of carcinogenesis. Substantial experimental evidence has demonstrated the existence of chemical damage to DNA after the administration of chemical carcinogens, even at very low doses.[57] Further, there is some evidence that such damage appears to persist, at least in some experimental systems such as murine hepatocarcinogenesis.[58] Although there is some evidence that carcinogenic chemicals and radiation activate some form of "error-prone" mechanism of DNA repair or replication,[59] other evidence suggests that the persistence of unrepaired DNA damage, including DNA-chemical adducts (see above), may be the cause of mutation, resulting in initiation of the affected cell.[60,61] For example, the N-(guan-8-yl)-2-acetylaminofluorene adducts formed in DNA from 2-acetylaminofluorene are repaired rather rapidly with a half-life of 7 days. However, the 3-(guan-N^2-yl)-acetylaminofluorene and N-(guan-8-yl)-2-aminofluorene adducts in DNA are not repaired and thus remain in the cellular genome.[62] The administration of some carcinogens such as dimethylnitrosamine actually stimulates the repair of O^6 alkylation guanines in DNA by such carcinogens given chronically.[63] Perhaps the strongest evidence that faulty DNA repair may lead to carcinogenesis is seen in the high incidence of skin cancer in patients with the autosomal recessive disease, xeroderma pigmentosum.[64] Persons with this condition have a markedly lowered ability to repair damage to DNA caused by ultraviolet light and by certain carcinogenic chemicals. The mechanism for the increased incidence of skin cancer seen in these patients is not known, but several theories have been proposed, including the mismatching of bases in DNA during the process of replicating an unrepaired, damaged DNA template. Sirover and Lobe[65] have suggested that inorganic metallic carcinogens may be carcinogenic by increasing the infidelity of DNA synthesis. With both of these mechanisms, an increase in mutation frequency as well as carcinogenesis would be expected.

Knowledge of both the metabolism of chemical carcinogens and the effects of the reactions of products formed by these metabolic pathways has led to a better understanding not only of the process of chemical carcinogenesis, but also of the relation of the neoplastic transformation by chemicals to the mutagenicity of the same agents. We now know that the vast majority of chemical carcinogens either are themselves mutagens or may be converted in the cell to active mutagens. This fact, coupled with the potential importance of faulty DNA repair associated with an increased incidence of neoplasia in certain genetic conditions, strongly supports the suggestion that chemical carcinogens may exert their effects as both mutagens and carcinogens by direct interaction of their ultimate forms with cellular DNA.

NATURAL HISTORY OF CHEMICAL CARCINOGENESIS: STAGES OF INITIATION, PROMOTION, AND PROGRESSION

One of the ubiquitous characteristics of the natural history of the development of a neoplasm in vivo is the extended time period between the initial application of a carcinogen—be it physical, chemical, or biologic—and the appearance of a neoplasm. Since there is now substantial evidence that neoplasms result from the alteration of a single cell whose progeny develop into the neoplastic lesion which then becomes clinically evident,[66] the latent period preceding cancer development may be simply the result of the continued growth of such clones until one or more are large enough to be called cancer. Foulds proposed such a concept but suggested that changes were continually occurring in this process, which he termed the progression of neoplasia.[67] However, an alternative explanation of this latent period of the development of neoplasia became apparent from studies conducted some four decades ago[68-70] and more recently.[71,72] These studies, carried out principally with mouse epidermis in vivo, suggested that the latent period during epidermal carcinogenesis of the skin of the mouse consisted of at least two stages, now termed *initiation* and *promotion* (Fig. 8-3).

Both Foulds' concept of progression[67] and the concepts of initiation and promotion were developed from model systems in animals, mammary carcinogenesis and epidermal carcinogenesis respectively in the mouse. Today, however, it is apparent that the multistage characteristic of carcinogenesis is not unique to these experimental systems but occurs with the process of carcinogenesis in a number of tissues in

FIG. 8-3. Natural history of neoplastic development, beginning with the initiated cell resulting from administration of an initiating agent with subsequent promotion to a visible lesion, followed by progression of this tumor to metastatic cancer. Euploidy and aneuploidy refer to the karyotypes of the cells during the various stages of neoplastic development. Euploidy indicates a normal complement of chromosomes; aneuploidy denotes abnormalities in the number or structure of one or more chromosomes. (Adapted from Pitot HC: Fundamentals of Oncology, 3rd ed. New York, Marcel Dekker, 1986)

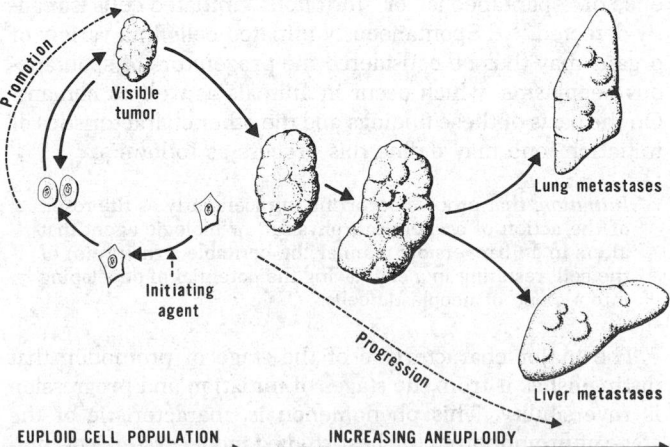

EUPLOID CELL POPULATION   INCREASING ANEUPLOIDY

TABLE 8-1. Morphologic and Biologic Characteristics of the Stages of Initiation, Promotion, and Progression in Hepatocarcinogenesis in the Rat*

Initiation	Promotion	Progression
Irreversible with constant "stem cell" potential; initiated "stem cell" not morphologically identifiable	Reversible	Irreversible Measurable and/or morphologically discernible alteration in cell genome's structure
Efficacy sensitive to xenobiotic and other chemical factors	Promoted cell population existence dependent on continued administration of the promoting agent	
Spontaneous (fortuitous) occurrence of initiated cells can be quantified	Efficacy sensitive to dietary and hormonal factors	Growth of altered cells sensitive to environmental factors during early phase
Requires cell division for "fixation"		
Dose-response does not exhibit a readily measurable threshold	Dose-response exhibits measurable threshold and maximal effect dependent on dose of initiating agent	Benign and/or malignant neoplasms characteristically seen
Relative effect of initiators depends on quantitation of focal lesions following defined period of promotion	Relative effectiveness of promoters depends on time and dose rate to reach maximal effect and on dose rate	"Progressor" agents act to advance promoted cells into this stage but may not be initiating agents

* Adapted from Pitot HC et al: Multistage carcinogenesis: The phenomenon underlying the theories. In Iverson OH (ed): Theories of Carcinogenesis, p. 159. Washington, DC, Hemisphere Publishing, 1987.

several species, including the human.[73] On the basis of such experimental findings, predominantly in the most intensively studied multistage carcinogenesis model systems (those of the skin of the mouse[72] and the liver of the rat[74]), three stages have been characterized (Table 8-1). The irreversibility and "memory" characteristics of the process of initiation are well characterized.[71,75] Evidence of the additivity of initiation comes from numerous investigations of the linearity of the dose-response to carcinogenic agents that initiate cells.[76] As yet it has not been possible to identify unequivocally single initiated cells, but the early clonal progeny of an initiated cell may be recognized in several model multistage carcinogenesis systems, notably that of rat hepatocarcinogenesis.[77] Furthermore, in this system the presence of "spontaneous" or "fortuitous" initiated cells is readily detected.[78,79] Spontaneously initiated cells in a variety of organs may thus be considered the progenitors of spontaneous neoplasms, which occur in animals as well as humans. On the basis of these findings and the other characteristics of initiation, one may define this process as follows:

> Initiation: that process occurring intracellularly as the result of the action of a chemical, physical, or biologic agent that alters in an irreversible manner the heritable structure(s) of the cell, resulting in a cell having the potential of developing into a clone of neoplastic cells.

The major characteristic of the stage of promotion that distinguishes it from the stages of initiation and progression is reversibility. This phenomenon is characteristic of the stage of promotion in the best-studied model systems of multistage carcinogenesis in the rodent[80,81] and in human neoplasia as well.[82] Furthermore, at least in multistage hepatocarcinogenesis in the rat, preneoplastic cells in the stage of promotion that develop from initiated cells are actually dependent on the presence of the promoting agent for their existence in that tissue.[81] Promoting agents by definition cannot initiate but may promote cells that have been initiated by fortuitous events such as background radiation, dietary contaminants, environmental "toxins," and other factors. The existence of fortuitously initiated cells has been discussed above. Therefore, promoting agents are carcinogenic in that they may promote such spontaneously initiated cells to neoplasia. Agents capable of initiation, promotion, and progression to cancer are termed complete carcinogens, but even these, at sufficiently low doses, only initiate cells without subsequent promotion. Under these circumstances, such complete carcinogens may act as "pure" initiating agents or incomplete carcinogens. Some carcinogenic agents, such as urethan, can induce neoplasms in some internal tissues but not in the skin. However, after systemic urethan administration, subsequent treatment of the skin with croton oil results in the appearance of papillomas and carcinomas of the skin.[83] On the basis of these data, urethan was termed an incomplete carcinogen or pure initiating agent for the skin, although this compound is a complete carcinogen for the lung and the liver.

Studies in cell culture[84,85] have demonstrated that initiating agents are most effective at certain stages of the cell cycle, usually at the beginning of DNA synthesis. Further, the ability of a carcinogenic agent to initiate cells may depend on the capacity of the cell to metabolize the agent to its ultimate carcinogenic form. Several studies[86-88] have indicated the importance of one or several rounds of cell division in the presence of the initiating agent in vivo or in vitro for a cell to become initiated. Further, it is possible to inhibit the process of carcinogenesis with agents that have been termed anticarcinogens or to stimulate the process of initiation with agents that have been termed cocarcinogens. Both types of agents usually act during the production of the ultimate form of the carcinogen, although other mechanisms for such processes have also been described.[89,90] On the other hand, tumor promotion may be modulated by various environmental factors, including diet, age, hormonal balance, and sex. Therefore, on the basis of the characteristics of tumor promotion, one may define the process as follows:

> *Promotion:* that stage in the natural history of neoplastic development which, if existent, is characterized by (1) the reversible expansion of the initiated cell population and (2) the reversible alteration of genetic expression.

Boutwell[71] was among the first to propose that promoting agents exert their effects by altering the expression of genetic information within the cell. Since this stage is reversible, these effects of promoting agents during the stage are also reversible. As indicated previously, major characteristics of the process of initiation involve its dose dependency, with the absence of any readily measurable threshold or no-effect dose level and the presence of a maximal effective dose short of lethal cellular toxicity. The existence of a threshold can be predicted from the reversibility characteristic of promotion, whereas a maximal response to the promoting agent, after a single dose of an initiating agent, would be expected if the promoting agent lacked initiating activity. Furthermore, the maximal yield of promoted neoplasms or preneoplastic foci would reflect the number of cells initiated by exposure to the initiating agent.

The diversity of promoting agents can be seen in the structures depicted in Figure 8-4. Several of these compounds act as promoting agents in various tissues and show a relatively high degree of tissue specificity. For example, saccharin is an effective promoting agent in bladder carcinogenesis but not in hepatocarcinogenesis, while phenobarbital, although an effective promoting agent in the liver, was totally ineffective as a promoter for bladder carcinogenesis.[92] Not only estrogens but other hormones have been shown to serve as effective promoting agents in vivo.[93] Not shown in Figure 8-4 is the foreign body or plastic film carcinogenesis discussed previously. Experimental studies[94,95] have indicated that such foreign bodies can act as promoting agents, probably promoting initiated cells already present in normal tissue. Further, Topping and Nettesheim[96] have presented evidence that asbestos acts as a promoting agent in experimental tracheal carcinogenesis. This finding correlates well with the known epidemiologic phenomenon of the marked enhancement of bronchogenic carcinoma in humans exposed to asbestos who are smokers as compared with smokers who were not exposed to abestos (see below).

The reversibility of the stage of tumor promotion makes it an obvious target for some form of regulation of the development of neoplasia in vivo. Paramount among such approaches is that of active chemoprevention by dietary, chemical, or other related mechanisms.[97] Although not all agents

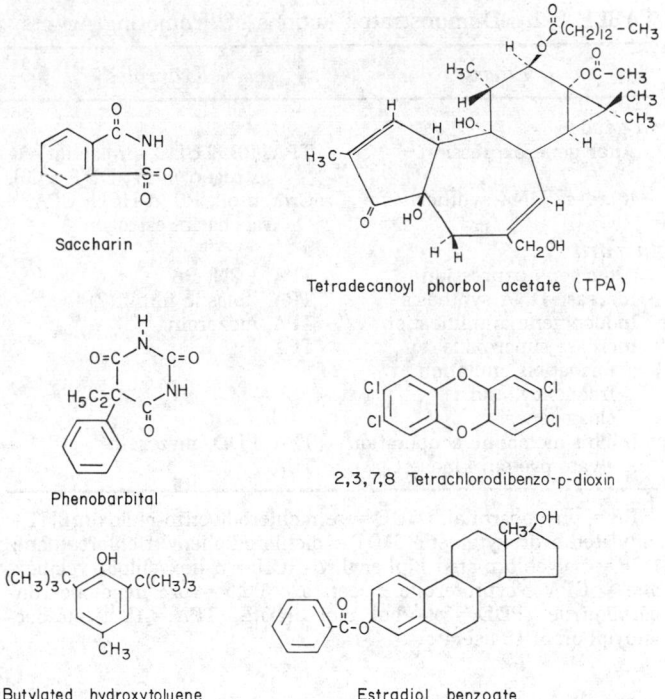

FIG. 8-4. Chemical structures of several promoting agents active in carcinogenesis in several tissues and species. (Adapted from Pitot HC: Fundamentals of Oncology, 3rd ed. New York, Marcel Dekker, 1986)

that have been utilized in such studies specifically inhibit neoplastic development at the stage of promotion, those that have been utilized for potential chemoprevention of cancer in humans, including derivatives of vitamins A, C, and E and selenium, appear to act predominantly at the stage of promotion.[98] This approach is consonant with our knowledge of the importance of promoting agents in the human environment associated with the development of cancer in people (see below).

Our knowledge of the mechanism of action of tumor promotion is still relatively unclear. Unlike the activity of initiating agents, there is little evidence of a major direct role for the metabolism of promoting agents in their mechanism of action. However, various promoting agents do exhibit a variety of actions in vivo and in vitro. Some of these are listed in Table 8-2. In addition to their effects in altering the genetic expression, many tumor-promoting agents have been shown to be mitogenic, at least to certain cell populations. Croton oil, when applied to mouse skin, causes a rapid increase in DNA synthesis in most basal skin cells.[99] Several promoters of hepatocarcinogenesis have been shown to enhance DNA synthesis in early progeny of initiated cells selectively compared with the remaining hepatocytes.[100] Many studies have shown that cell replication is required to "fix" the step of initiation of chemical carcinogenesis, but that such fixation in itself is not sufficient to assure the continuance of the process of promotion and ultimate tumor formation.[91]

Tumor promoters also alter gene expression and increase DNA synthesis in vitro. Several of the phorbol ester promot-

TABLE 8-2. Demonstrated Actions of Promoting Agents

Effect	Examples
In vivo	
Alter gene expression	TPA, PB, TCDD, prolactin, estrogen, BHT, DDT, PCBs
Increase DNA synthesis	Croton oil, PB, α-HCH, CPA, saccharin, estrogen
In vitro	
Alter gene expression	TPA, PCN, PB
Increase DNA synthesis	TPA, "plastic film" (?)
Induce gene amplification	TPA, mezerein
Increase superoxide formation, mutation frequency, and clastogenesis	TPA
Inhibit metabolic cooperation	TPA, PDD, mezerein
Activate protein kinase C	TPA

PB = phenobarbital, TCDD = tetrachlorodibenzo-*p*-dioxin, BHT = butylated hydroxytoluene, DDT = dichlorodiphenyltrichloroethane, PCB = polychlorinated biphenyl, α-HCH = α-hexachlorocyclohexane, CPA = cyproterone acetate, PCN = pregnenolone-16α-carbonitrile, PDD = phorbol didecanoate, TPA = 12-*O*-tetradecanoylphorbol-13-acetate.

ing agents can stimulate the amplification of specific genes within cultured cells.[101,102] Direct effects of tumor promoters on the genome of the cell have not, generally, been considered as a major mechanism of their effects in neoplastic development. However, several studies in vitro[103,104] have demonstrated an indirect effect of 12-*O*-tetradecanoylphorbol-13-acetate (TPA) in the presence of leukocytes, resulting in the formation of DNA strand breaks, chromosomal abnormalities, and structural modification of bases in DNA.[105] Such changes may be the result of action of reactive oxygen metabolites, especially superoxide radicals. Evidence of the importance of such radicals can also be found from the inhibition of tumor promotion by antioxidants, which eliminate the accumulation of oxygen metabolites.[106] Recently, however, Fischer and her associates have reported experiments suggesting that such indirect effects of TPA are not essential for tumor promotion in mouse skin.[107] Another possible mechanism of action of tumor promoters studied extensively by Trosko and his co-workers[108] is the inhibition of intercellular communication (metabolic cooperation) between cells in culture. Although such a phenomenon has not been shown to be a ubiquitous characteristic of promoting agents,[109] a relationship between reactive oxygen species and the inhibition of intercellular communication by promoting agents has been described.[110]

One of the most recent exciting findings in relation to the action of TPA is the demonstration of specific cellular membrane receptors for this tumor promoter in many cells[111] and its identity with the enzyme, protein kinase C.[112,113] This enzyme has been shown to respond to an endogenous ligand, diacylglycerol, and to have multiple effects on a variety of cellular substrates.[113] Several cDNAs for the mRNA of the protein kinase C have been isolated, providing evidence that this important receptor-enzyme consists of a multigene family compatible with its ubiquitous nature and function.[114,115]

However, the relationship of this enzyme to promoting agents other than TPA, if any, remains to be elucidated in the mechanisms of promoting agents.

The stage of progression in the natural history of neoplastic development (see Fig. 8-2) has not yet been clearly defined; however, on the basis of the known action of initiating and promoting agents, irreversible benign and/or malignant neoplasms are characteristic of this stage of neoplastic development. Progression has been defined as that stage of carcinogenesis exhibiting measurable (by recombinant DNA technology or related methods) and/or morphological karyotypic changes in the structure of the cell genome.[116] Furthermore, the karyotypic changes seen in this stage are a reflection of karyotypic instability, which in turn can lead to a variety of other changes characteristically seen in malignant neoplasms, including a less differentiated morphology, increased growth rate, invasion and metastases, gene amplification, and chromosomal translocations and related abnormalities leading to alterations in gene expression. The stage of progression has been identified in both epidermal carcinogenesis in the mouse[117] and in multistage hepatocarcinogenesis in the rat.[118] Although complete carcinogens effectively advance cells through the entire natural history of neoplastic development, agents that act primarily in the final stage of carcinogenesis exist, as evidenced by the effect of benzoyl peroxide in multistage epidermal carcinogenesis in the mouse.[119] Theoretically, such agents should be capable of inducing major genetic changes as defined above for the entrance of a cell into the stage of progression. Protocols exemplified by the initiation–promotion–initiation format[120] have been described both in the mouse skin[121] and rat liver.[122] In the latter case, morphological evidence for the existence of a transition between the stages of promotion and progression is seen with the appearance of "foci within foci." The initial focus results from the clonal expansion of initiated cells, whereas the focus of cells developing within a promoted clone appears to represent further genetic alterations induced by the administration of a second initiating agent during the stage of promotion. Such foci within foci are probably the direct precursors of malignant neoplasms.[123] Furthermore, in multistage epidermal carcinogenesis in the mouse, Aldaz et al have described a systematic study of the karyotypic evolution of mouse skin papillomas to carcinomas, in concert with the stage of progression as defined above.[124]

From the characteristics (see Table 8-1) and definitions of the three stages of neoplastic development, it is obvious that two stages, initiation and progression, appear to involve changes in the structure of the genome of the cell. Initiation probably is the result of multiple point mutations and related subtle genomic alterations, whereas progression results from more major genetic abnormalities, including chromosomal translocation, karyotypic instability, deletions, and so forth. While it is entirely possible that a complete carcinogen, especially at high doses, may directly convert a normal cell to one in the stage of progression, it is likely that most examples of human carcinogenesis do exhibit the reversible stage of promotion (see below). In the concept of the natural history of the development of neoplasia as described here (see Fig. 8-2), there is a clear analogy between the two genetic alterations of initiation and progression and the two-hit theory of Knudson[125] developed from studies of neoplasms in the human that exhibit a clear Mendelian pattern of inheritance.

TARGETS OF CHEMICAL CARCINOGENS

Although the interaction and reaction of chemical carcinogens with DNA appear to be the principal mechanisms for their carcinogenic effects, the probability that such mutational events would occur at one or more specific genetic sites has long been considered. With the demonstration that specific oncogenic viruses, especially retroviruses, contain within their genome genes directly concerned with the oncogenic process, studies in both experimental and human systems have been directed toward investigating the structures and expression of cellular oncogenes (proto-oncogenes) in neoplastic cells as well as normal cells treated with chemical carcinogens.

There is now considerable evidence[126] that a number of proto-oncogenes are expressed at higher levels in many human neoplasms than in their normal tissues of origin. The mechanisms for such increased expression or "activation" have been studied and include genetic mechanisms ranging from base mutations or deletions in sequences to altered expression resulting from enhanced transcription, gene amplification, or changes in gene methylation. Therefore, the mechanism involved in proto-oncogene "activation" may be mutational, transcriptional, or both. Since it is difficult to monitor transcriptional activation during the early stages of neoplastic development, a number of studies have been directed toward determining whether mutational activation of proto-oncogenes occurs during this period. Quintanilla et al[127] have demonstrated that more than 90% of tumors, benign and malignant, exhibit specific mutations in the Harvey-ras proto-oncogene that are related directly to the structural changes in DNA induced by the chemical carcinogen used for initiation. This type of activation was also demonstrated in both adenomas and carcinomas of livers of mice given chemical carcinogens as well as the control animals that received no such agents. While the mutations in control animals were limited to a single codon, those seen in this gene in the livers of mice given chemical carcinogens were found in other codons as well.[128] A more extensive investigation with different chemical carcinogens by Wiseman et al[129] showed quite clearly the correlation between specific mutations at the 61st codon and the chemical agent utilized to induce the neoplasms. In a more direct test of the role of mutationally activated oncogenes in multistage epidermal carcinogenesis in the mouse, Brown et al[130] demonstrated that introduction of viral Harvey-ras genes into epidermal cells in vivo resulted in papillomas and carcinomas when the animals were subsequently treated with TPA, but no lesions occurred in the absence of the promoting agent. Similar correlative studies have been done in the rat mammary gland[131] and liver,[132] but only on examination of resultant carcinomas. These studies suggest that mutational activation of a specific proto-oncogene may be involved in initiation or promotion of carcinogenesis in these systems.

Because it is much more difficult to investigate the early stages of carcinogenesis in humans, most investigations on proto-oncogene activation have been carried out on lesions in the stage of progression. Transcriptional activation of the Harvey-ras proto-oncogene has been described in human gastric carcinoma,[133] prostatic cancer,[134] and pulmonary and pleural neoplasms,[135] the results suggesting that increased progression of the tumor was related to increased expression of the gene. In colorectal tumors this proto-oncogene was expressed at higher levels in primary than in metastatic tumors.[136] Increased expression of the myc proto-oncogene in human carcinomas of the uterine cervix was correlated with a higher incidence of early relapse,[137] while in an extensive study Yokota and his associates[138] demonstrated that amplification of this proto-oncogene occurred in advanced, widespread neoplasms as well as in aggressive primary tumors. Thus, studies in the human suggest an important role for proto-oncogene activation in the stage of progression, and it remains to be determined whether mutational activation of proto-oncogenes during initiation represents the major carcinogen-DNA target that initiates the entire process of chemical carcinogenesis in general.

PROMOTING AGENTS IN THE HUMAN ENVIRONMENT

On the basis of our knowledge of the epidemiology of human neoplasia and the demonstrated promoting action of various agents in the human environment, it is likely that the appearance of cancer in humans is related to the stages of tumor promotion and progression more than to the stage of initiation. Some promoting agents that are a significant part

TABLE 8-3.   Promoting Agents in the Human Environment and Neoplasms Associated with Prolonged Contact with Those Agents*

Agent	Resultant Neoplasm
Dietary fat	Mammary adenocarcinoma
High caloric intake	Increased cancer incidence in general
Cigarette smoke	Bronchogenic carcinoma (esophageal and bladder cancer)
Asbestos	Bronchogenic carcinoma and mesothelioma
Halogenated hydrocarbons (TCDD, PCBs)	Liver cancer†
Phorbol esters	Esophageal cancer
Saccharin	Bladder cancer
Phenobarbital	Liver cancer†
Prolactin	Mammary adenocarcinoma†
Synthetic estrogens	Liver adenomas
Alcoholic beverages	Oral cancer, liver, and esophageal cancer

* Adapted from Pitot HC: The natural history of neoplastic development: The relation of experimental models to human cancer. Cancer 49:1206, 1982.

† Promotion demonstrated in experimental animals but not in humans as yet.

of the human environment[139] are listed in Table 8-3. Although not all of these agents have been shown by epidemiologic studies to be important factors in human cancer, a number clearly are, and others well may be. Doll and Peto[140] reviewed the importance of caloric intake and dietary fat in the genesis of human cancer. In addition, experimental evidence has clearly indicated that dietary fats, especially unsaturated fatty acids, may act as promoting agents in experimental mammary carcinogenesis and possibly in several other histogenetic types of neoplasms.[141] Cigarette smoke is a complete carcinogen but contains many promoting agents, and epidemiologic evidence argues strongly that tumor promotion is an important, if not the major, factor in the final development of pulmonary cancer in humans as a result of smoking.[142] Asbestos fibers have been shown to be promoting agents in experimental systems,[96] and their effects in humans may be explained on the basis of their action as a promoter for both bronchogenic carcinoma and mesothelioma.[143] Although there are numerous controversies over the relation of artificial sweeteners to human bladder cancer and of dioxins in insecticides to human neoplasia, there is ample experimental evidence that both of these agents are potent promoters for bladder and liver cancers in experimental systems.[139] As Berenblum[93] has suggested, all endogenous hormones may be considered to be promoting agents, and the action of synthetic estrogens in inducing liver cell adenomas in humans as well as in rodents argues strongly for a major promoting role of these compounds.[144] Finally, substantial epidemiologic evidence indicates that alcoholic beverages promote esophageal, gastric, and hepatic cancer in humans, although relatively little evidence has been uncovered to demonstrate their promoting action in animals.[145]

CHEMICAL CARCINOGENESIS IN HUMANS

Knowledge of carcinogenesis in humans as a result of the action of specific chemicals has come largely from epidemiologic and statistical investigations on both large and small groups of humans. However, epidemiologic studies can only identify factors that are different between two populations and that are sufficiently important in the etiology of the condition under study to play a determining role under the conditions of exposure. Further, on the basis of epidemiologic studies alone, it is extremely difficult to determine whether a specific chemical is carcinogenic for the human. The reasons for this include the extended lag period between exposure and clinical occurrence of the neoplasm, the high background incidence in the general population, and the relatively imprecise knowledge of the nature of the exposure in most instances. Only under exceptional circumstances is it possible to identify carcinogenic agents solely from epidemiologic studies when the incidence of a cancer induced by an agent is less than 50% greater than the occurrence of that kind of cancer in the total human population. Thus, many negative epidemiologic studies must be considered as inconclusive for indicating the risk factor of relatively weak carcinogens for inducing neoplastic disease in humans.

Because epidemiologic studies in themselves are often insufficient to establish the carcinogenicity of an agent for humans, other techniques involving studies in lower forms of life have been used to complement or, in some cases, supplant existing epidemiologic observations. Later in this chapter we shall consider such methodologies, but at this point our discussion will be restricted to a consideration of epidemiologic data in the determination of the carcinogenicity of agents for humans. One of the pioneer agencies in the establishment of the carcinogenic risk of chemicals for humans has been the International Agency for Research on Cancer (IARC). In a supplement to their monograph series,[146] the IARC has categorized the degrees of evidence of carcinogenicity from studies in humans. Their categorization is as follows:

1. *Sufficient evidence* of carcinogenicity indicates that there is a causal relation between the agent and human cancer.
2. *Limited evidence* of carcinogenicity indicates that a causal interpretation is credible but that alternative explanations, such as chance, bias, or confounding of the data, could not be excluded completely.
3. *Inadequate evidence* indicates that one of three conditions prevailed: (a) there were few pertinent data; (b) the available studies, although showing evidence of association, did not exclude chance, bias, or confounding of the findings; (c) studies were available that did not show evidence of carcinogenicity.

It is evident that epidemiologic studies have many limitations in determining etiologic factors in human cancer. On the other hand, one can never prove that an agent is truly carcinogenic for humans unless epidemiologic evidence in support of such a thesis is forthcoming.

CARCINOGENIC CHEMICAL AGENTS ASSOCIATED WITH LIFE-STYLE

Table 8-4 lists a number of agents, conditions, or processes in our life-styles that are causally related to the development of specific neoplasms in humans on the basis of epidemiologic studies. The carcinogenicity of alcoholic beverages for humans is related almost entirely to their action in association with another known carcinogenic agent. The combination of excessive alcohol ingestion and cigarette smoking markedly increases the risk in men and women of oral and laryngeal cancer, compared with the effect of either of these agents alone or in their absence.[147,148] Cancer of the liver is associated with excessive alcohol consumption,[149] and recent data by Ohnishi and co-workers[150] suggest that habitual alcoholic intake can promote the development of hepatocellular carcinoma in patients infected with the hepatitis B virus, a known oncogenic virus for the human liver. Several recent studies have also indicated an important association between alcohol consumption, even at moderate levels, and a significantly increased risk of breast cancer in women.[151-153] Although some alcoholic beverages contain known chemical carcinogens, including nitrosamines,[154] and different alcoholic beverages may have slightly different influences on the incidence of certain types of human cancer,[155] most evidence suggests that the principal effect is caused by alcohol

CARCINOGENIC CHEMICAL AGENTS ASSOCIATED WITH LIFE-STYLE   127

TABLE 8-4. Chemical Agents Associated with Life-Style and Posing a Carcinogenic Risk to Humans on the Basis of Epidemiologic Studies

Chemical, Physiologic Condition, or Process	Associated Neoplasm	Evidence for Carcinogenicity*
Alcoholic beverages	Esophagus, liver, oropharynx, larynx	Sufficient
Aflatoxins	Liver	Limited
Betel chewing	Mouth	Sufficient
Dietary factors (fat, protein, calories)	Breast, colon, endometrium, gallbladder	Sufficient
Reproductive history:		
Late age at first pregnancy	Breast	Sufficient
Zero or low parity	Ovary	Sufficient
Sexual promiscuity	Cervix uteri	Sufficient
Tobacco smoking	Mouth, pharynx, larynx, lung, esophagus, bladder	Sufficient

* This terminology refers to the IARC categorization and is based on the findings reviewed in the IARC monographs[146] and the review by Doll and Peto.[140]

itself and is largely independent of the form in which it is drunk.[140]

Epidemiologic studies have shown that the geographic regions in which there is extensive contamination of foodstuffs by aflatoxin (see Fig. 8-1 and 8-2) are also the areas where the incidence of human liver cancer is relatively high.[15] Several studies have shown a direct association between the aflatoxin content of food and the frequency of hepatomas in the population. In parts of Africa and East Asia where aflatoxin is found in the diet, levels of 100 to 1000 parts per billion in individual foodstuffs are not unusual. Thus, unlike most other environmental carcinogenic agents for humans, the dose of aflatoxin to which those humans are exposed greatly exceeds that known to produce cancer in experimental animals. Although other mold toxins, such as sterigmatocystin, have been suggested as additional etiologic factors in human liver cancer, their role in this disease has not been proved.

Another example of the induction of cancer in humans by naturally occurring dietary contaminants is that described in several provinces of the People's Republic of China. In these locales, there is a positive correlation between the extremely high incidence of esophageal carcinoma and the consumption of pickled and otherwise moldy foodstuffs,[156] which may contain nitrosamines.[157]

A general association of diet and human cancer incidence has been demonstrated. Doll and Peto[140] have outlined a number of the hypothetical or demonstrable ways in which diet may alter the incidence of human cancer, including carcinogen ingestion (e.g., aflatoxin B_1 and alcoholic beverages). Although food additives, pesticide contaminants, and dietary nitrites are potentially important because of their effects on human carcinogenesis, there is no evidence for a significant role of these factors in human cancer. A major factor in the relation of diet to the incidence of human cancer is caloric intake. There is substantial epidemiologic evidence that the incidence of various human cancers is increased in overweight people.[158] Ample experimental evidence supports such a concept.[159] Thus, although one is unwilling to accept the suggestion that 40% of human cancer is directly related to diet, there is increasing evidence that diet and related factors play a major role in the incidence of human cancer. However, this role is quite complex and, in all likelihood, does not result from the direct conversion of normal to neoplastic cells by dietary constituents, but rather stems from an alteration in the development of cells within the organism that have the potential for cancerous growth, that is, by tumor promotion.

The fact that certain types of reproductive and sexual behavior alter the incidence of human cancer has been known since the time of Ramazzini (see below). Doll and Peto[140] pointed out that pregnancy and childbirth seem to play a significant role in the prevention of cancers of the endometrium, ovary, and breast; all of these conditions are less common in women who have borne children at an early age than in women who have had no children. This relation is most striking in respect to the incidence of breast cancer: parous women become progressively less likely to develop this cancer as the age at the time of the first pregnancy decreases.[160] However, early menarche, late first full-term pregnancy, and late menopause generally have been accepted as the three major factors that increase the risk of breast cancer in the human.[161]

Perhaps the most common single, direct, chemical cause of human cancer is tobacco smoking. Doll and Peto[140] have estimated, from epidemiologic data, that 85% to 90% of the lung cancer cases in the United States annually are the direct result of tobacco smoking. If one adds to this the number of cancers of the bladder and gastrointestinal tract that can be attributed to tobacco smoking, about 30% of all cancer deaths in the United States result from this habit. If all deaths from neoplasms causally related to tobacco smoking are removed from the statistics, there is essentially no annual increase in the overall age-adjusted cancer death rate in men and a continual decreasing cancer death rate in women. Thus, tobacco smoke represents the major known cause of human cancer in our society, and it is the only known factor causing a continual increase in the overall age-adjusted cancer death rate of Americans.

CARCINOGENIC AGENTS ASSOCIATED WITH OCCUPATIONS

In 1713, Bernardino Ramazzini published *De Morbis Artificum [Diseases of Workers],* which was translated in 1964 by Wright. In this text Ramazzini described the high incidence of mammary cancer in nuns and attributed it to their celibate life. Scrotal cancer in one-time chimney sweeps, described by Pott, was another example of occupational cancer. During the 19th century, several reports of the association of specific cancers in the mining, smelting, dye, and lubricating processes industries were published. Unfortunately, in many instances little was done for many years to protect the workers, a neglect from which we are not entirely free today (Table 8-5).

The association of occupational exposure to asbestos and the subsequent development of bronchogenic carcinoma and

mesothelioma has been well established. However, in virtually all of the studies undertaken in this field, the highest incidence of bronchogenic carcinoma was found in those persons exposed to asbestos who also had a history of cigarette smoking. One study of 17,800 asbestos insulation workers in the United States and Canada indicated that the risk of bronchogenic carcinoma in nonsmokers who had been exposed to asbestos was very much lower than in smokers; this suggests the probable requirement for multiple environmental agents in the production of lung cancer in persons exposed to asbestos. On the other hand, there have been several documented cases of people developing mesotheliomas many years after an extremely short exposure to asbestos.[163] Further evidence in support of the direct carcinogenic effect of asbestos is the fact that mesotheliomas can be induced in rodents by appropriate exposure to this material.[164] However, although other fibrous materials such as fiberglass have been shown to be carcinogenic in rodents,[165] there is essentially no evidence to date that fiberglass causes human cancer. Although the mechanism of asbestos induction of cancer is not yet known, the demonstration that the type and size of fiber are important for the carcinogenicity of

TABLE 8-5. Chemical Agents Associated with Occupations and Posing a Carcinogenic Risk to Humans on the Basis of Epidemiologic Studies

Chemical, Process, or Industry	Associated Neoplasm	Evidence for Carcinogenicity*
Acrylonitrile	Lung, colon, prostate	Limited
Arsenic	Lung	Sufficient
Asbestos	Lung, mesothelioma, gastrointestinal tract (?)	Sufficient
Manufacture of auramine	Bladder	Limited
Aromatic amines (aminobiphenyl, benzidine, 2-naphthylamine, 4-nitrobiphenyl)	Bladder	Sufficient
Benzene	Leukemia	Sufficient
Beryllium and its compounds	Lung	Limited
Bis(chloromethyl)ether	Lung	Sufficient
Boot and shoe manufacture and repair	Nasal carcinoma	Sufficient
Cadmium and its compounds	Lung, prostate (?)	Limited
Chromium and some of its compounds	Lung	Sufficient
Furniture manufacture (hardwood)	Nasal carcinoma	Sufficient
Hematite mining (underground)	Lung	Sufficient
Isopropyl alcohol manufacture	Cancer of paranasal sinuses	Sufficient
Nickel refining	Lung, nasal sinuses	Sufficient
Occupational exposure to phenoxyacetic acids and herbicides	Soft tissue sarcoma	Limited
Rubber industry (certain occupations)	Leukemia, bladder	Sufficient
Soots, tars, and oils	Skin, lung, bladder, gastrointestinal tract	Sufficient
Vinyl chloride	Liver (angiosarcoma)	Sufficient

* This terminology refers to the IARC categorization and is based on the findings reviewed in the IARC monographs[146] and the review by Doll and Peto.[140]

this material indicates that its carcinogenic action may be similar to that of the plastic film carcinogenesis discussed earlier in this chapter.

Aromatic amines, especially those used in the dye industry, have long been known to be potential risks for cancer, especially bladder cancer, in humans. Although the severity of the risk to workers in the dye industry varied with the exposure, 100% of the workers who distilled 2-naphthylamine developed bladder cancer.[166] Not until 1938 was verification of the carcinogenicity of these compounds, especially 2-naphthylamine, obtained in experimental animals. Exposure, usually prolonged, to another organic chemical, benzene, has now been linked by epidemiologic studies to the induction of leukemia in persons exposed in an occupational setting.[167]

A review by the IARC in 1975 reported 43 cases of angiosarcoma in ten different countries. All of the patients had a history of working with vinyl chloride. Hepatic angiosarcoma is an extremely rare neoplasm in humans, and the incidence seen in this group is therefore far from what might be expected in the general population. Although the low incidence of these neoplasms suggests that vinyl chloride is a relatively weak carcinogen, the rarity of hepatic angiosarcoma in the general population strongly supports a causal relationship between exposure to the organic monomer and the induction of this mesenchymal neoplasm.

The United States government has sponsored publications that suggest that occupational causes of neoplasia in humans may be responsible for as much as 20% of total cancer mortality, but Doll and Peto[140] have presented compelling arguments that such is not the case. Their review of the currently available statistical and epidemiologic evidence indicates that only about 4% of all cancer deaths in the United States can be attributed to occupational causes. The increasingly strict governmental regulation of actual and potential industrial health hazards promises to decrease this figure to even lower levels in the future.

CARCINOGENIC AGENTS ASSOCIATED WITH MEDICAL THERAPY AND DIAGNOSIS

In modern times, the dictum of Hippocrates that above all a physician should do no harm to his patient has been modified to a consideration of the benefit to the patient in relation to the risk of the procedure or therapy involved. Many times in the past the risk to the patient was unknown or unsuspected, and only later did the risk factor become evident. A good example of such unsuspected risk was the administration of diethylstilbesterol to pregnant women to avert a threatened abortion. The benefit of such a procedure is obvious, but the risk did not become obvious until many years later, when a small percentage of the female offspring of mothers treated with this estrogenic analogue during gestation developed vaginal carcinomas, usually shortly after puberty (Table 8-6).[168] Further evidence of the carcinogenicity of some synthetic estrogen preparations has been obtained as a result of the demonstrated association of liver cell adenomas with the prolonged use of oral contraceptives that contain synthetic steroidal estrogens.[169] In postmenopausal women, the use of estrogens to prevent a variety of symptoms has been clearly documented as associated with an increased risk of endometrial carcinoma, ranging from eightfold to 16-fold.[169]

Although there is no doubt of the association of lung

TABLE 8-6. Chemical Agents Associated with Medical Diagnosis and Treatment That Pose a Carcinogenic Risk to Humans on the Basis of Epidemiologic Studies

Chemical or Drug	Associated Neoplasm	Evidence for Carcinogenicity*
Alkylating agents (cyclophosphamide, melphalan)	Bladder, leukemia	Sufficient
Inorganic arsenicals	Skin, liver	Sufficient
Azathioprine (immunosuppressive drugs)	Lymphoma, reticulum cell sarcoma, skin, Kaposi's sarcoma (?)	Sufficient
Chlornaphazine	Bladder	Sufficient
Chloramphenicol	Leukemia	Limited
Diethylstilbesterol	Vagina (clear cell carcinoma)	Sufficient
Estrogens:		
Premenopausal	Liver cell adenoma	Sufficient
Postmenopausal	Endometrium	Limited
Methoxypsoralen with UV light	Skin	Sufficient
Oxymetholone	Liver	Limited
Phenacetin	Renal pelvis (carcinoma)	Sufficient
Phenytoin (diphenylhydantoin)	Lymphoma, neuroblastoma	Limited
Thorotrast	Liver (angiosarcoma)	Sufficient

* This terminology refers to the IARC categorization and is based on the findings reviewed in the IARC monographs[146] and the review by Doll and Peto.[140]

cancer with chronic exposure to arsenic in industrial situations, arsenic compounds were widely used in the treatment of various diseases in the early 20th century. Organic arsenicals were used to treat syphilis, and there is some evidence of their association with skin cancer in people receiving such treatment for prolonged periods. The association of skin cancer as well as liver cancer with the chronic administration of Fowler's solution has now been well documented.[170] This medicament, in the form of a solution of 1% potassium arsenite in aqueous alcohol, was used to treat dermatitis, arthritis, and other conditions, including chronic leukemia. Since the material was often administered for years, some patients received many grams of arsenic during their period of treatment.

A number of agents known to damage DNA have been used in the diagnosis and treatment of various diseases, especially neoplasia. Alkylating agents are used primarily for the treatment of malignant neoplasms, and a number, including melphalan and cyclophosphamide (Cytoxan), have been causally associated with the induction of carcinoma of the bladder, especially in children receiving intensive therapy for acute leukemia. In addition, the induction of acute non-lymphocytic leukemia in adults receiving such chemotherapy, especially for Hodgkin's disease, has been reported.[171] Methoxypsoralen, which interacts with DNA, has been used in combination with ultraviolet light in the treatment of psoriasis. Definite evidence of the induction of squamous cell carcinoma of the skin by this regimen has been presented.[172]

Of the drugs that have been used in the chemical immunosuppression of patients in preparation for transplantation of organs and tissues from one person to another, azathioprine has been associated with an increased incidence of neoplasia. Although this drug and others used during clinical immunosuppression interact with DNA, it is not clear whether such compounds are actually carcinogenic or act by suppressing the natural resistance of the host. Since the predominant neoplasms appearing in such immunosuppressed patients are those derived from the immune system, it is reasonable to suggest that a major mechanism for the induction of neoplasia in immunosuppressed patients is the loss of host resistance to neoplastic cells already present but normally prevented from expressing their neoplastic potential by immune mechanisms of the host. The recent outbreak of acquired immune deficiency syndrome (AIDS) has further substantiated the role of immunodeficiency in cancer development by the finding of a significant increase in lymphomas and Kaposi's sarcoma in such patients.[173]

The association of leukemia with administration of the antibiotic chloramphenicol may be related to its depressive action on the bone marrow.[171] The association of carcinoma of the renal pelvis with excessive abuse of the analgesic phenacetin is now well known, but the association of lymphomas with the chronic administration of phenytoin for the control of epilepsy is not so well documented.[171] Phenytoin induces lymphoid reactions that are at times difficult to distinguish from neoplasia, but there is limited evidence of its causal association with lymphoma, although the risk is probably much less than the benefit to the epileptic patient. Some forms of medical therapy and diagnosis do present significant carcinogenic risks to the patient, but the total number of cancer cases resulting from such actions is extremely small compared with the incidence of cancer in general in the human population.[174]

PREVENTION OF CHEMICAL CARCINOGENESIS: TESTING OF CHEMICALS FOR CARCINOGENIC ACTIVITY

The prevention of cancer development by active intervention in the natural history of carcinogenesis in the stages of initiation or promotion is a potential reality. Alternatively, cancer may be prevented by eliminating causative agents in the environment. Thus, the identification of chemicals that pose a carcinogenic risk to humans has received major attention in the last two decades. A number of methods have been devised for the bioassay of carcinogenic agents found in the environment. The principal standard for these tests is the induction of neoplasia in experimental animals. Although these studies are tedious and expensive, at present they are the best and most reliable procedures available. However, the mere production of a neoplasm in an experimental animal provides no information about the molecular and biologic processes that precede the appearance of the neoplasm. The induction of neoplasia in animals at a statistically higher level than in controls has been considered indicative of carcinogenicity of the agent under study; however, modern concepts of the natural history of neoplastic development, that is, initiation and promotion, require that this simplistic evaluation of the data be reconsidered.

Although whole-animal bioassay procedures are the basis for determining the potential risk of a chemical for inducing cancer in humans, it became clear some time ago that the testing of all potentially dangerous chemicals by whole-animal bioassays would be physically and financially impossible. Thus, in the last two decades, considerable effort has been directed toward devising "screening" bioassays that may indicate which chemicals can be potentially dangerous and should be selected for whole-animal bioassay. A summary of these short-term tests for carcinogenicity and mutagenicity is given in Table 8-7. The reader is referred to the discussion by Pitot[175] for detailed references to Table 8-7.

One of the most popular screening methods for potential carcinogenicity is the Ames test. Since most carcinogenic chemicals are mutagenic per se or are metabolized in vivo to mutagenic compounds, the Ames assay, which depends on the induced mutation of one or more highly mutable bacterial strains, is a reasonable screening procedure for carcinogenicity. An outline of the Ames test as it is commonly used at present is shown in Figure 8-5. The specifics of the test are given in the legend. If the test agent or its metabolite is mutagenic, a mutation converting the histidine gene back to its normal structure will allow the bacteria to synthesize histidine again de novo, resulting in visible growth of revertant colonies on the Petri dish.

In a study of 300 compounds of known carcinogenic potential, McCann and Ames[176] found that only about 10% of the compounds tested produced false-negative tests. A similar or greater percentage of such false-negative tests occurs

TABLE 8-7.   Short-Term "Screening" Assays for Carcinogenicity and Mutagenicity*

Test	End Point
Prokaryote mutagenesis in vitro (e.g., Ames test)	Back or forward mutations in specific bacterial strains (with added liver homogenate)
Host-mediated prokaryote mutagenesis in vivo	Back or forward mutations in specific bacterial strains
Dominant lethal assay	Death of fertilized egg in mammalian implanted spectra
Sperm abnormality induction	Microscopically abnormal sperm
Mutagenesis in cultured cells	Scoring of dominant or linked mutations
Mutations in Neurospora	Scoring of mutations
Mitotic recombination in yeast alleles to homozygous state	Conversion of heterozygous to homozygous state
Drosophila	Recessive lethal test
Induced chromosomal aberrations	Visible alterations in karyotype
Micronucleus test	Appearance of micronuclei in bone marrow cells in vivo
Sister chromatids differentially exchanged	Visible exchange of labeled sister chromatids
DNA repair in vivo or in vitro	Unscheduled DNA synthesis or DNA strand breaks
Fidelity of DNA polymerases in vitro	Altered fidelity of DNA synthesis in cell-free system

* Adapted from Pitot HC: Relationships of bioassay data on chemicals to their toxic and carcinogenic risk for humans. J Environ Pathol Toxicol 3:431, 1980.

with virtually all of the "screening" bioassay tests that are used. Thus, no single screening procedure is necessarily definitive in identifying a compound that should be subjected to a whole-animal bioassay. In fact, prokaryotic mutagenicity tests have been shown to miss (score negative) from 10%[176] to 23%[177] of known or suspected carcinogenic agents tested.

As indicated in Table 8-7, many of the tests involve the determination of mutations as an end point. Other tests involve the demonstration of DNA repair or changes in the structure of chromosomes of cells in culture. Not shown in Table 8-7 is the use of cell transformation in culture as a method for identifying chemicals that can cause the malignant transformation or a related phenomenon in cells grown in culture. Although this test has the advantage of relative rapidity, not all cells transformed in culture exhibit biologic neoplasia when transplanted in vivo. Further, although human tissues in culture may be used directly as test agents for mutagenesis, certain metabolic activation reactions that must take place for many compounds to be effective as carcinogens do not occur to an appreciable extent in many tissues cultured in vitro. In these cases, some supplementary activating system, such as a feeder layer, is necessary.

Although short-term screening assays for carcinogens and mutagens are relatively convenient and inexpensive, the final proof of carcinogenicity of an agent is its ability to induce neoplasms in mammals. Thus, whole-animal bioassay procedures remain the standard for judging whether an agent is carcinogenic. Many attempts at estimating the risk of environmental agents to humans are based on extrapolations from whole-animal bioassay data to the situation in humans.

Whole-animal bioassay systems, however, are not without problems. One of the most difficult variables found in whole-animal bioassay systems is the "spontaneous" tumor incidence of control animal populations. Neoplasms may appear in test animals, but unless the incidence of such tumors exceeds the spontaneous incidence of neoplasms by a statistically significant margin, the incidence of tumors may be considered as false positive. Most animal tests use 50 control and 50 treated animals. Even when controls have a 0% incidence, at least 10% of the 50 treated animals must exhibit tumors to ensure that the result is statistically significant.[178] By increasing the number of controls, this percentage may be decreased, but even at a tenfold higher number of control animals with 0% incidence, at least a 4% incidence of tumors in the treated animals would be required for statistical significance. Thus it is apparent that the sensitivity of the animal bioassay is markedly limited by statistical considerations.

In addition to the problem of sensitivity of whole-animal bioassays, a number of other problems have arisen, especially in the interpretation of the data obtained. At present it is generally considered, and rather strictly adhered to by regulatory agencies, that chemical carcinogens exert their effects through mechanisms that do not allow the determination of no-effect or threshold levels. This concept is based largely on the extrapolation of data from whole-animal bioassays to very low doses at which no measurements can be obtained by the usual assay procedures. Gehring and Blau[179] discussed various factors related to this problem; a variety of mechanisms tend to invalidate the concept of a no-effect level for various chemicals. Further, promoting agents both theoretically and in practice exhibit no-effect levels, as discussed earlier in this chapter. As Fears and associates[180] have pointed out, false-positive results are much less likely to occur at tissue sites with low spontaneous tumor rates. In fact, even the appearance of a very low

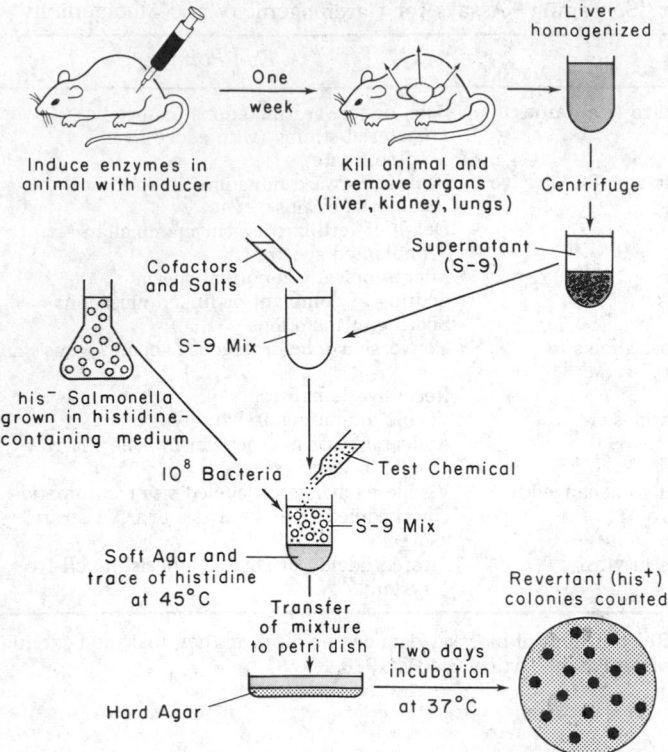

FIG. 8-5. The *Salmonella* (Ames) test to detect mutagenic activity by chemicals requiring metabolic activation. After intraperitoneal drug injection (usually for 1 week) to induce enzyme activity, the liver (and other organs, if desired) of the rodent are removed and homogenized and the mixture is centrifuged. The supernatant (S-9) may be stored frozen, or immediately combined with other biochemicals that promote activation (cofactors and salts). The S-9 mix, the test chemical, and about 10^8 salmonellae unable to synthesize histidine (his⁻) are added to a test tube containing soft agar with a trace of histidine. The trace of histidine is necessary to allow the his⁻ salmonellae to go through at least one or two rounds of replication, allowing "fixation" of any mutations that occur. This entire mixture is then transferred to a Petri dish containing hard agar and incubated for 2 days. If the activated chemical is mutagenic, histidine biosynthesis resumes in the mutated bacterium, and the growth of revertant colonies is later visible on the dish.

incidence of neoplasms at a site that seldom, if ever, exhibits spontaneous tumor formation is considered much more significant in the interpretation of the test results than is a barely statistically significant increase in tumor incidence at a tissue site with a high spontaneous tumor rate. Most bioassays are carried out in at least two different species of rodent, usually rats and mice. A major problem has been in the interpretation of the induction of hepatomas in mice by an agent with no other evidence of carcinogenic effect in either species. Although the whole-animal bioassay, when distinctly positive and exhibiting a reproducible dose-response, is the standard for extrapolation of such data to risk in humans, many, if not most, positive whole-animal bioassays must have other data to support findings of carcinogenicity if an extrapolation to humans is to be meaningful.

Another consideration in the establishment and interpretation of whole-animal bioassays is our increased understanding of the natural history of neoplastic development.[59]

The bioassay most commonly used in determining the carcinogenicity of chemicals is the induction of neoplasms in any tissue of the test animals by chronic administration of the test compound for most of the animal's life span. This test does not distinguish complete carcinogens from promoting agents because the latter may promote cells initiated by incidental environmental factors, such as dietary contaminants, background radiation, and spontaneous mutations. Despite the fact that promoting agents are quite different from complete carcinogens and initiating agents (see Table 8-1), regulatory legislation does not yet distinguish among these types of agents.

CONCLUSIONS

Because we live in an environment permeated with chemicals whose number and diversity increase every year, it is important that we know and understand the mechanisms by which chemicals can induce the neoplastic transformation. Identification of such chemicals and their classification as incomplete or complete carcinogens, promoting agents, or the new class of "progressor" agents is essential for a rational approach to the prevention of chemical carcinogenesis in humans. Although it is the responsibility of all persons to limit their exposure to known cancer-causing chemicals, such as those that occur in cigarette smoke, alcoholic beverages, or in the form of excess calories, the prevention of cancer in the general population ultimately will remain the responsibility of society as a whole through research, education, and, where necessary, regulatory legislation.

REFERENCES

1. Pott P: Chirurgical Observations Relative to the Cataract, the Polypus of the Nose, the Cancer of the Scrotum, the Different Kinds of Ruptures, and the Mortification of the Toes and Feet. London, Hawkes, Clarke and Collins, 1775
2. Butlin HT: Cancer of the scrotum in chimney-sweeps and others: II. Why foreign sweeps do not suffer from scrotal cancer. Br Med J 2:1, 1892
3. Rehn L: Blasengeschwülste bei Fuchsin-Arbeitern. Arch Klin Chir 50:588, 1895
4. Hueper WC, Wiley FH, Wolfe HD: Experimental production of bladder tumors in dogs by administration of beta-naphthylamine. J Indust Hyg Toxicol 20:46, 1938
5. Yamagiwa K, Ichikawa K: Experimentelle Studie Über die Pathogenese der Epithelialgeschwulste. Mitteilungen Med Facultat Kaiserl Univ Tokyo 15:295, 1915
6. Kennaway EL: Experiments on cancer-producing substances. Br Med J 2:1, 1925
7. Kennaway EL, Hieger I: Carcinogenic substances and their fluorescence spectra. Br Med J 1:1044, 1930
8. Sasaki T, Yoshida T: Experimentelle Erzeugung des Lebercarcinoms durch Fütterung mit o-Amidoazotoluol. Virchows Arch Pathol Anat 295:175, 1935
9. Kinosita R: Researches on the cancerogenesis of the various chemical substances. Gann 30:423, 1936
10. Coulston F, Olajos EJ: Toxicology of N-nitroso compounds. Ecotoxicol Environ Safety 6:89, 1982
11. Magee PN, Swann PF: Nitroso compounds. Br Med Bull 25:240, 1969
12. Lijinsky W: Nitrosamines and nitrosamides in the etiology of gastrointestinal cancer. Cancer 40:2446, 1977
13. Matsukura N, Kawachi T, Sasajima K et al: Induction of liver tumors in rats by sodium nitrite and methylguanidine. Z Krebsforsch 90:87, 1977
14. Bartsch H, Montesano R: Relevance of nitrosamines to human cancer. Carcinogenesis 5:1381, 1984
15. Shank RC: Epidemiology of aflatoxin carcinogenesis. In Kraybill HFE, Mehlman MA (eds): Environmental Cancer, p 291. New York, John Wiley & Sons, 1977
16. Martell AE: Chemistry of carcinogenic metals. Environ Health Perspect 40:207, 1981
17. Landrigan PJ: Arsenic: State of the art. Am J Ind Med 2:5, 1981
18. Brand KG, Buoen LC, Johnson KH et al: Etiological factors, stages, and the role of the foreign body in foreign body tumorigenesis: A review. Cancer Res 35:279, 1975
19. Stinson NE: The tissue reaction induced in rats and guinea pigs by polymethylacrylate (acrylic) and stainless steel. Br J Exp Pathol 45:21, 1946
20. Ferguson DJ: Cellular attachment to implanted foreign bodies in relation to tumorigenesis. Cancer Res 37:4367, 1977

21. Thomassen MJ, Buoen LC, Brand I et al: Foreign-body tumorigenesis in mice: DNA synthesis in surface-attached cells during preneoplasia. JNCI 61:359, 1978

22. Memoli VA, Urban RM, Alroy J et al: Malignant neoplasms associated with orthopedic implant materials in rats. J Orthop Res 4:346, 1986

23. Miller EC, Miller JA: The presence and significance of bound amino azo dyes in the livers of rats fed p-dimethylaminoazobenzene. Cancer Res 7:468, 1947

24. Miller EC: Studies on the formation of protein-bound derivatives of 3,4-benzopyrene in the epidermal fraction of mouse skin. Cancer Res 11:100, 1951

25. Miller JA, Cramer JW, Miller EC: The N- and ring-hydroxylation of 2-acetylaminofluorene during carcinogenesis in the rat. Cancer Res 20:950, 1960

26. Miller JA: Carcinogenesis by chemicals: An overview. Cancer Res 30:559, 1970

27. Miller EC: Some current perspectives on chemical carcinogenesis in humans and experimental animals: Presidential Address. Cancer Res 38:1479, 1978

28. Boyland E: The biological significance of metabolism of polycyclic compounds. Biochem Soc Symp 5:40, 1950

29. Sims P, Grover PL, Swaisland A et al: Metabolic activation of benzo(a)pyrene proceeds by a diol-epoxide. Nature 252:326, 1974

30. Harvey RG: Activated metabolites of carcinogenic hydrocarbons. Acc Chem Res 14:218, 1981

31. Conney AH: Induction of microsomal enzymes by foreign chemicals and carcinogenesis by polycyclic aromatic hydrocarbons: GHA Clowes Memorial Lecture. Cancer Res 42:4875, 1982

32. Levin W, Thakker DR, Wood AW et al: Evidence that benzo(a)anthracene 3,4-diol-1,2-epoxide is an ultimate carcinogen on mouse skin. Cancer Res 38:1705, 1978

33. Nagata C, Kodama M, Ioki Y et al: Free radicals produced from chemical carcinogens and their significance in carcinogenesis. In Floyd RA (ed): Free Radicals and Cancer, p 1. New York, Marcel Dekker, 1982

34. Kahl R: Synthetic antioxidants: Biochemical actions and interference with radiation, toxic compounds, chemical mutagens and chemical carcinogens. Toxicology 33:185, 1984

35. Marnett LJ: Peroxyl free radicals: Potential mediators of tumor initiation and promotion. Carcinogenesis 8:1365, 1987

36. Wise RW, Zenser TV, Kadlubar FF et al: Metabolic activation of carcinogenic aromatic amines by dog bladder and kidney prostaglandin H synthase. Cancer Res 44:1893, 1984

37. Peters RA: Mechanism of the toxicity of the active constituent of Dichapetalum cymosum and related compounds. Adv Enzymol 18:113, 1957

38. Maher VM, Miller EC, Miller JA et al: Mutations and decreases in density of transforming DNA produced by derivatives of the carcinogens 2-acetylaminofluorene and N-methyl-4-aminoazobenzene. Mol Pharmacol 4:1, 1968

39. Ames BN, Durston WE, Yamasaki E et al: Carcinogens are mutagens: A simple test system combining liver homogenates for activation and bacteria for detection. Proc Natl Acad Sci USA 70:2281, 1973

40. Bresnick E, Eastman A: Alkylation of mammalian cell DNA, persistence of adducts, and relationship to carcinogenesis. Drug Metab Rev 13:189, 1982

41. Goth R, Rajewsky MF: Persistence of O^6-ethylguanine in rat-brain DNA: Correlation with nervous system-specific carcinogenesis by ethylnitrosourea. Proc Natl Acad Sci USA 71:639, 1974

42. Bedell MA, Lewis JG, Billings KC et al: Cell specificity in hepatocarcinogenesis: Preferential accumulation of O^6-methylguanine in target cell DNA during continuous exposure of rats to 1,2-dimethylhydrazine. Cancer Res 42:3079, 1982

43. Swenberg JA, Dyroff MC, Bedell MA et al: O^4-Ethyldeoxythymidine, but not O^6-ethyldeoxyguanosine, accumulates in hepatocyte DNA of rats exposed continuously to diethylnitrosamine. Proc Natl Acad Sci USA 81:1692, 1984

44. Müller R, Rajewsky MF: Enzymatic removal of O^6-ethylguanine versus stability of O^4-ethylthymine in the DNA of rat tissues exposed to the carcinogen ethylnitrosourea: Possible interference of guanine-O^6 alkylation with 5-cytosine methylation in the DNA of replicating target cells. Z Naturforsch [C] 38:1023, 1983

45. Singer B: In vivo formation and persistence of modified nucleosides resulting from alkylating agents. Environ Health Perspect 62:41, 1985

46. Riggs AD, Jones PA: 5-Methylcytosine, gene regulation, and cancer. Adv Cancer Res 40:1, 1983

47. Farmer PB, Neumann H-G, Henschler D: Estimation of exposure of man to substances reacting covalently with macromolecules. Arch Toxicol 60:251, 1987

48. Oellerich M: Enzyme-immunoassay: A review. J Clin Chem Clin Biochem 22:895, 1984

49. Yalow RS: Radioimmunoassay: A probe for the fine structure of biologic systems. Science 200:1236, 1978

50. Gupta RC, Reddy MV, Randerath K: ^{32}P-postlabeling analysis of non-radioactive aromatic carcinogen-DNA adducts. Carcinogenesis 3:1081, 1982

51. Langone JJ, Van Vunakis H (eds): Methods in Enzymology, Vol 92, Immunochemical Techniques, Part E, Monoclonal Antibodies and General Immunoassay Methods. New York, Academic Press, 1983

52. Perera FP, Weinstein IB: Molecular epidemiology and carcinogen-DNA adduct detection: New approaches to studies of human cancer causation. J Chronic Dis 35:581, 1982

53. Harris CC, Vahakangas K, Newman MJ et al: Detection of benzo[a]pyrene diol epoxide-DNA adducts in peripheral blood lymphocytes and antibodies to the adducts in serum from coke oven workers. Proc Natl Acad Sci USA 82:6672, 1985

54. Bryant MS, Skipper PL, Tannenbaum SR et al: Hemoglobin adducts of 4-aminobiphenyl in smokers and nonsmokers. Cancer Res 47:602, 1987

55. Brash DE, Hart RW: DNA damage and repair in vivo. J Environ Pathol Toxicol 2:79, 1978

56. Teebor GW, Frenkel K: The initiation of DNA excision-repair. Adv Cancer Res 38:23, 1983

57. Brambilla G, Carlo P, Finollo R et al: Viscometric detection of liver DNA fragmentation in rats treated with minimal doses of chemical carcinogens. Cancer Res 43:202, 1983

58. Stout DL, Becker FF: Progressive DNA damage in hepatic nodules during 2-acetylaminofluorene carcinogenesis. Cancer Res 40:1269, 1980

59. Sarasin A, Bourre F, Benoit A: Error-prone replication of ultraviolet-irradiated simian virus 40 in carcinogen-treated monkey kidney cells. Biochimie 64:815, 1982

60. Wintersberger U: Chemical carcinogenesis: The price for DNA repair? Naturwissenschaften 69:107, 1982

61. Stewart BW: Generation and persistence of carcinogen-induced repair intermediates in rat liver DNA in vivo. Cancer Res 41:3238, 1981

62. Neumann H-G: Role of extent and persistence of DNA modifications in chemical carcinogenesis by aromatic amines: Recent results. Cancer Res 84:77, 1983

63. Yarosh DB: The role of O^6-methylguanine-DNA methyltransferase in cell survival, mutagenesis and carcinogenesis. Mutat Res 145:1, 1985

64. Hanawalt PC, Sarasin A: Cancer-prone hereditary diseases with DNA processing abnormalities. Trends Genet 2:124-129, 1900

65. Sirover MA, Lobe LA: Infidelity of DNA synthesis in vitro: Screening for potential metal mutagens or carcinogens. Science 194:1434, 1976

66. Fialkow PJ: Clonal origin of human tumors. Biochim Biophys Acta 458:283, 1976

67. Foulds L: Neoplastic Development. Academic Press, New York, 1969

68. Rous P, Kidd JG: Conditional neoplasms and subthreshold neoplastic states. J Exp Med 73:365, 1941

69. Mottram JC: A developing factor in experimental blastogenesis. J Pathol Bacteriol 56:181, 1944

70. Berenblum I, Shubik P: The role of croton oil applications associated with a single painting of a carcinogen in tumor induction of the mouse's skin. Br J Cancer 1:379, 1947

71. Boutwell RK: Some biological aspects of skin carcinogenesis. Prog Exp Tumor Res 4:207, 1964

72. Slaga TJ: Overview of tumor promotion in animals. Environ Health Perspect 50:3, 1983

73. Pitot HC, Beer D, Hendrich S: Multistage carcinogenesis: The phenomenon underlying the theories. In Iversen OH (ed): Theories of Carcinogenesis, p 159. Washington, DC, Hemisphere Publishing, 1987

74. Goldsworthy TL, Hanigan MH, Pitot HC: Models of hepatocarcinogenesis in the rat: Contrasts and comparisons. CRC Crit Rev Toxicol 17:61, 1986

75. Pitot HC: Drugs as promoters of carcinogenesis. In Estabrook RW, Lindenlaub E (eds): The Induction of Drug Metabolism, p 471. New York, Schattauer Verlag, 1979

76. Port R, Schmähl D, Wahrendorf J: Some examples of dose-response studies in chemical carcinogenesis. Oncology 33:66, 1976

77. Weinberg WC, Berkwits L, Iannaccone PM: The clonal nature of carcinogen-induced altered foci of gamma-glutamyl transpeptidase expression in rat liver. Carcinogenesis 8:565, 1987

78. Schulte-Hermann R, Timmermann-Trosiener I, Schuppler J: Promotion of spontaneous preneoplastic cells in rat liver as a possible explanation of tumor production by nonmutagenic compounds. Cancer Res 43:839, 1983

79. Popp JA, Scortichini BH, Garvey LK: Quantitative evaluation of hepatic foci of cellular alteration occurring spontaneously in Fischer-344 rats. Fundam Appl Toxicol 5:314, 1985

80. Stenbäck F: Tumor persistence and regression in skin carcinogenesis. Z Krebsforsch 91:249, 1978

81. Hendrich S, Glauert HP, Pitot HC: The phenotypic stability of altered hepatic foci: Effects of withdrawal and subsequent readministration of phenobarbital. Carcinogenesis 7:2041, 1986

82. Bühler H, Pirovino M, Akovbiantz A et al: Regression of liver cell adenoma: A follow-up study of three consecutive patients after discontinuation of oral contraceptive use. Gastroenterology 82:775, 1982

83. Berenblum I, Haran-Ghera A: A quantitative study of the systemic initiating action of urethane (ethyl carbamate) in mouse skin carcinogenesis. Br J Cancer 11:77, 1957

84. Grisham JW, Greenberg DS, Kaufman DG et al: Cycle-related toxicity and transformation in 10T1/2 cells treated with N-methyl-N'-nitro-N-nitrosoguanidine. Proc Natl Acad Sci USA 77:4813, 1980

85. McCormick PJ, Bertram JS: Differential cell cycle phase specificity for neoplastic transformation and mutation to ouabain resistance induced by N-methyl-N'-nitro-N-nitrosoguanidine in synchronized C3H10T1/2 C18 cells. Proc Natl Acad Sci USA 79:4342, 1982

86. Columbano A, Rajalakshmi S, Sarma DSR: Requirement of cell proliferation for the initiation of liver carcinogenesis as assayed by three different procedures. Cancer Res 41:2079, 1981

87. Berwald Y, Sachs L: In vitro transformation of normal cells to tumor cells by carcinogenic hydrocarbons. JNCI 35:641, 1965

88. Kakunaga T: The role of cell division in the malignant transformation of mouse cells treated with 3-methylcholanthrene. Cancer Res 35:1637, 1975

89. Lakowicz JR, Englund F, Hidmark A: Particle-enhanced membrane uptake of a polynuclear aromatic hydrocarbon: A possible role in cocarcinogenesis. JNCI 61:1155, 1978

90. Hozumi M, Ogawa M, Sugimura T et al: Inhibition of tumorigenesis in mouse skin by leupeptin, a protease inhibitor from Actinomycetes. Cancer Res 32:1725, 1972

91. Boutwell RK: The function and mechanism of promoters of carcinogenesis. Crit Rev Toxicol 2:419, 1974

92. Nakanishi K, Fukushima S, Hagiwara A et al: Organ-specific promoting effects of phenobarbital sodium and sodium saccharin in the induction of liver and urinary bladder tumors in male F344 rats. JNCI 68:497, 1982

93. Berenblum I: Established principles and unresolved problems in carcinogenesis JNCI 60:723, 1978

94. Brand KG, Buoen LC, Johnson KH et al: Etiological factors, stages, and the role of the foreign body in foreign body tumorigenesis: A review. Cancer Res 35:279, 1975

95. Ryan WL, Stenback F, Curtis GL: Tumor promotion by foreign bodies (IUD). Cancer Lett 13:299, 1981

96. Topping DC, Nettesheim P: Two-stage carcinogenesis studies with asbestos in Fischer 344 rats. JNCI 65:627, 1980

97. Wattenberg LW: Chemoprevention of cancer. Cancer Res 45:1, 1985

98. Bertram JS, Kolonel LN, Meyskens FL Jr: Rationale and strategies for chemoprevention of cancer in humans. Cancer Res 47:3012, 1987

99. Frankfurt OS, Raitcheva E: Fast onset of DNA synthesis stimulated by tumor promoter in mouse epidermis at the initiation stage of carcinogenesis. JNCI 51:1861, 1973

100. Schulte-Hermann R, Schuppler J, Timmermann-Trosiener I et al: The role of growth of normal and preneoplastic cell populations for tumor promotion in rat liver. Environ Health Perspect 50:185, 1983

101. Varshavsky A: Phorbol ester dramatically increases incidence of methotrexate-resistant mouse cells: Possible mechanisms and relevance to tumor promotion. Cell 25:561, 1981

102. Hayashi K, Fujiki H, Sugimura T: Effects of tumor promoters on the frequency of metallothionein I gene amplification in cells exposed to cadmium. Cancer Res 43:5433, 1983

103. Birnboim HC: DNA strand breakage in human leukocytes exposed to a tumor promoter, phorbol myristate acetate. Science 215:1247, 1982

104. Emerit I, Cerutti PA: Tumor promoter phorbol 12-myristate 13-acetate induces a clastogenic factor in human lymphocytes. Proc Natl Acad Sci USA 79:7509, 1982

105. Frenkel K, Chrzan K, Troll W et al: Radiation-like modification of bases in DNA exposed to tumor promoter-activated polymorphonuclear leukocytes. Cancer Res 46:5533, 1986

106. Ito N, Hirose M: The role of antioxidants in chemical carcinogenesis. Jpn J Cancer Res 78:1011, 1987

107. Fischer SM, Baldwin JK, Jasheway DW et al: Possible dissociation of the phorbol ester–induced oxidant response and tumor promotion in the F_1 offspring of SSIN × C57BL/6J mice. Carcinogenesis 8:1521, 1987

108. Loch-Caruso R, Trosko JE: Inhibited intercellular communication as a mechanistic link between teratogenesis and carcinogenesis. CRC Crit Rev Toxicol 16:157, 1985

109. Kinsella AR: Elimination of metabolic co-operation and the induction of sister chromatid exchanges are not properties common to all promoting or co-carcinogenic agents. Carcinogenesis 3:499, 1982

110. Ruch RJ, Klaunig JE: Antioxidant prevention of tumor promoter-induced inhibition of mouse hepatocyte intercellular communication. Cancer Lett 33:137, 1986

111. Leach KL, James ML, Blumberg PM: Characterization of a specific phorbol ester aporeceptor in mouse brain cytosol. Proc Natl Acad Sci USA 80:4208, 1983

112. Ashendel CL: The phorbol ester receptor: A phospholipid-regulated protein kinase. Biochim Biophys Acta 822:219, 1985

113. Nishizuka Y: Studies and perspectives of protein kinase C. Science 233:305, 1986

114. Housey GM, O'Brian CA, Johnson MD et al: Isolation of cDNA clones encoding protein kinase C: Evidence for a protein kinase C-related gene family. Proc Natl Acad Sci USA 84:1065, 1987

115. Knopf JL, Lee M-H, Sultzman LA et al: Cloning and expression of multiple protein kinase C cDNAs. Cell 46:491, 1986

116. Pitot HC: Fundamentals of Oncology, 3rd ed. New York, Marcel Dekker, 1986

117. Weinstein IB, Gattoni-Celli S, Kirschmeier P et al: Multistage carcinogenesis involves multiple genes and multiple mechanisms. J Cell Physiol Suppl 3:127, 1984

118. Schulte-Hermann R: Tumor promotion in the liver. Arch Toxicol 57:147, 1985

119. O'Connell JF, Klein-Szanto AJP, DiGiovanni DM et al: Enhanced malignant progression of mouse skin tumors by the free-radical generator benzoyl peroxide. Cancer Res 46:2863, 1986

120. Potter VR: A new protocol and its rationale for the study of initiation and promotion of carcinogenesis in rat liver. Carcinogenesis 2:1375, 1981

121. Hennings H, Spangler EF, Shores R et al: Malignant conversion and metastasis of mouse skin tumors: A comparison of SENCAR and CD-1 mice. Environ Health Perspect 68:69, 1986

122. Scherer E, Feringa AW, Emmelot P: Initiation-promotion-initiation: Induction of neoplastic foci within islands of precancerous liver cells in the rat. In Börzsönyi M, Lapis K, Day NE et al: (eds): Models, Mechanisms and Etiology of Tumor Promotion, p 57. Lyon, International Agency for Research on Cancer, IARC Scientific Publications, 1984

123. Scherer E: Neoplastic progression in experimental hepatocarcinogenesis. Biochim Biophys Acta 738:219, 1984

124. Aldaz CM, Conti CJ, Klein-Szanto AJP et al: Progressive dysplasia and neuploidy are hallmarks of mouse skin papillomas: Relevance to malignancy. Proc Natl Acad Sci USA 84:2029, 1987

125. Knudson AG Jr: Hereditary cancer, oncogenes, and antioncogenes. Cancer Res 45:1437, 1985

126. Pitot HC: Oncogenes and human neoplasia. Clin Lab Med 6:167, 1986

127. Quintanilla M, Brown K, Ramsden M et al: Carcinogen-specific mutation and amplification of Ha-ras during mouse skin carcinogenesis. Nature 322:78, 1986

128. Reynolds SH, Stowers SJ, Patterson RM et al: Activated oncogenes in B6C3F1 mouse liver tumors: Implications for risk assessment. Science 237:1309, 1987

129. Wiseman RW, Stowers SJ, Miller EC et al: Activating mutations of the c-Ha-ras protooncogene in chemically induced hepatomas of the male B6C3 F_1 mouse. Proc Natl Acad Sci USA 83:5825, 1986

130. Brown K, Qunitanilla M, Ramsden M et al: v-ras genes from Harvey and BALB murine sarcoma viruses can act as initiators of two-stage mouse skin carcinogenesis. Cell 46:445, 1986

131. Zarbl H, Sukumar S, Arthur AV et al: Direct mutagenesis of Ha-ras-1 oncogenes by N-nitroso-N-methylurea during initiation of mammary carcinogenesis in rats. Nature 315:382, 1985

132. McMahon G, Davis E, Wogan GN: Characterization of c-Ki-ras oncogene alleles by direct sequencing of enzymatically amplified DNA from carcinogen-induced tumors. Proc Natl Acad Sci USA 84:4974, 1987

133. Tahara E, Yasui W, Taniyama K et al: Ha-ras oncogene product in human gastric carcinoma: Correlation with invasiveness, metastasis or prognosis. Jpn J Cancer Res 77:517, 1986

134. Viola MV, Fromowitz F, Oravez S et al: Expression of ras oncogene p21 in prostate cancer. N Engl J Med 314:133, 1986

135. Lee I, Gould VE, Radosevich JA et al: Immunohistochemical evaluation of ras oncogene expression in pulmonary and pleural neoplasms. Virchows Arch [Cell Pathol] 53:146, 1987

136. Gallick GE, Kurzrock R, Kloetzer WS et al: Expression of p21^{ras} in fresh primary and metastatic human colorectal tumors. Proc Natl Acad Sci USA 82:1795, 1985

137. Riou G, Le MG, Le Doussal V et al: c-myc- protooncogene expression and prognosis in early carcinoma of the uterine cervix. Lancet 1:761, 1987

138. Yokota J, Tsunetsugu-Yokota Y, Battifora H et al: Alterations of myc, myb, and ras^{Ha} proto-oncogenes in cancers are frequent and show clinical correlation. Science 231:261, 1986

139. Pitot HC: The natural history of neoplastic development: The relation of experimental models to human cancer. Cancer 49:1206, 1982

140. Doll R, Peto R: The Causes of Cancer. New York, Oxford University Press, 1981

141. Carroll KK, Hopkins GJ: Dietary polyunsaturated fat versus saturated fat in relation to mammary carcinogenesis. Lipids 14:155, 1979

142. Hammond EC: Tobacco. In Fraumeni JF Jr (ed): Persons at High Risk of Cancer: An Approach to Cancer Etiology and Control, p 13. New York, Academic Press, 1975

143. Nicholson WJ: Cancer following occupational exposure to asbestos and vinyl chloride. Cancer 39:1792, 1977

144. Ishak KG: Hepatic lesions caused by anabolic and contraceptive steroids. Semin Liver Dis 1:116, 1981

145. Lieber CS, Seitz HK, Garro AJ et al: Alcohol-related diseases and carcinogenesis. Cancer Res 39:2863, 1979

146. Chemicals, Industrial Processes and Industries Associated with Cancer in Humans. IARC Monogr Eval Carcinog Risk Chem Hum [Suppl] 4, 1982

147. Bross IDJ, Coombs J: Early onset of oral cancer among women who drink and smoke. Oncology 33:136, 1976

148. Herity B, Moriarty M, Daly L et al: The role of tobacco and alcohol in the aetiology of lung and larynx cancer. Br J Cancer 46:961, 1982

149. Tuyns AJ: Epidemiology of alcohol and cancer. Cancer Res 39:2840, 1979

150. Ohnishi K, Iida S, Iwama S et al: The effect of chronic habitual alcohol intake on the development of liver cirrhosis and hepatocellular carcinoma: Relation to hepatitis B surface antigen carriage. Cancer 49:672, 1982

151. O'Connell DL, Hulka BS, Chambless LE et al: Cigarette smoking, alcohol consumption, and breast cancer risk. JNCI 78:229, 1987

152. Harvey EB, Schairer C, Brinton LA et al: Alcohol consumption and breast cancer. JNCI 78:657, 1987

153. Willett WC, Stampfer MJ, Colditz GA et al: Moderate alcohol consumption and the risk of breast cancer. N Engl J Med 316:1174, 1987

154. Tuyns AJ, Griciute LL: Carcinogenic substances in alcoholic beverages. In Davis W, Harrap KR, Stathopoulos G (eds): Human Cancer: Its Characterization and Treatment, p 130. Amsterdam, Excerpta Medica, 1980

155. Tuyns AJ, Pequignot G, Abbatucci JS: Oesophageal cancer and alcohol consumption: Importance of type of beverage. Int J Cancer 23:443, 1979

156. Yang CS: Research on esophageal cancer in China: A review. Cancer Res 40:2633, 1980

157. Singer GM, Chuan J, Roman J et al: Nitrosamines and nitrosamine precursors in foods from Linxian, China, a high incidence area for esophageal cancer. Carcinogenesis 7:733, 1986

158. Garfinkel L: Overweight and cancer. Ann Intern Med 103:1034, 1985

159. Birt DF: Fat and calorie effects on carcinogenesis at sites other than the mammary gland. Am J Clin Nutr 45:203, 1987

160. McMahon B, Cole P, Brown J: Etiology of human breast cancer: A review. JNCI 50:21, 1973

161. Pike MC, Krailo MD, Henderson BE et al: "Hormonal" risk factors, "breast tissue age" and the age-incidence of breast cancer. Nature 303:767, 1983

162. Hammond EC, Selikoff IJ: Relation of cigarette smoking to risk of death of asbestos-associated disease among insulation workers in the United States. IARC Sci Publ 8:312, 1973

163. Chen WJ, Karle Mottet N: Malignant mesothelioma with minimal asbestos exposure. Hum Pathol 9:253, 1978

164. Pigott GH, Gaskell BA, Ishmael J: Effects of long term inhalation of alumina fibres in rats. Br J Exp Pathol 62:323, 1981

165. Stanton MF, Layard M, Tegeris A et al: Carcinogenicity of fibrous glass: Pleural response in the rat in relation to fiber dimension. JNCI 58:587, 1977

166. Connolly JG, White EP: Malignant cells in the urine of men exposed to beta-naphthylamine. Can Med Assoc J 100:879, 1969

167. Rinsky RA, Young RJ, Smith AB: Leukemia in benzene workers. Am J Indust Med 2:217, 1981

168. Herbst AL: Clear cell adenocarcinoma and the current status of DES-exposed females. Cancer 48:484, 1981

169. Huggins GR, Zucker PK: Oral contraceptives and neoplasia: 1987 update. Fertil Steril 47:733, 1987

170. Pershagen G: The carcinogenicity of arsenic. Environ Health Perspect 40:93, 1981

171. Hoover R, Fraumeni JF Jr: Drug-induced cancer. Cancer 47:1071, 1981

172. Stern RS, Thibodeau LA, Kleinerman RA: Risk of cutaneous carcinoma in patients treated with oral methoxsalen photochemotherapy for psoriasis. N Engl J Med 300:809, 1979

173. Volberding PA: Kaposi's sarcoma, B-cell lymphoma and other AIDS-associated tumours. Clin Immunol Allergy 6:569, 1986

174. Schmähl D: Iatrogenic carcinogenesis. J Cancer Res Clin Oncol 99:71, 1981

175. Pitot HC: Relationships of bioassay data on chemicals to their toxic and carcinogenic risk for humans. J Environ Pathol Toxicol 3:431, 1980

176. McCann J, Ames BN: Detection of carcinogens as mutagens in the Salmonella/microsome test: Assay of 300 chemicals. Discussion. Proc Natl Acad Sci USA 73:950, 1976

177. Rinkus SJ, Legator MS: Chemical characterization of 465 known or suspected carcinogens and their correlation with mutagenic activity in the Salmonella typhimurium system. Cancer Res 39:3289, 1979

178. Sontag JM: Aspects in carcinogen bioassay. In Hiatt H, Watson J, Winsten J (eds): Origins of Human Cancer, Book C, p 1327. Cold Spring Harbor, New York, Cold Spring Harbor Laboratory, 1977

179. Gehring PJ, Blau GE: Mechanisms of carcinogenesis: Dose response. J Environ Pathol Toxicol 1:163, 1977

180. Fears TR, Tarone RE, Chu KC: False-positive and false-negative rates for carcinogenicity screens. Cancer Res 37:1941, 1977

R. J. MICHAEL FRY

CHAPTER 9 *Principles of Carcinogenesis: Physical*

This chapter discusses the induction of cancer by three types of physical agents: ionizing radiation, ultraviolet radiation, and foreign bodies and fibers. Studies of cancer induction by these agents have two aims: first, the estimate of risk of cancer following exposure, and second, the elucidation of mechanisms of cancer induction. Studies with different agents can help identify features that are independent of the type of carcinogen and those that are agent-specific.

IONIZING RADIATION

Studies of the carcinogenic action of ionizing radiations have been carried out in humans,[1-12] experimental animals,[4,13-17] and in vitro cell systems.[18-21] The ability to determine or calculate absorbed doses of radiation and the knowledge of the effects at the molecular, chromosomal, cellular, tissue, and whole-body levels make ionizing radiation a remarkable tool for investigating the quantitative aspects and mechanisms of cancer induction.

Ionizing radiations have the characteristic of localized release of sufficient energy to break strong chemical bonds. The many types or qualities of radiation usually are divided into electromagnetic radiation, such as x-rays and γ-rays, and particulate radiation, including electrons, protons, neutrons, alpha particles, and heavy ions. Radiation can interact with biologic targets both directly and indirectly. Ionization of the atoms of the target may be caused directly, whereas in the so-called indirect effect radiation interacts with other molecules or atoms in the cell, especially water, producing free radicals that reach critical targets by diffusion. The rate at which energy is deposited is characteristic of the type of radiation and is called the linear energy transfer (LET). LET indicates an average rate of energy deposition at the micron level.

Exposure to sufficient doses of ionizing radiation may result in cancer induction. The susceptibility of tissue varies markedly, but all tissues appear to be at risk,[13,22] although not necessarily in relation to natural incidence. Because we all are exposed to radiation from natural and other sources, the issue of the dose-response relationships and risk estimates is important.

Humans have evolved in a radiation environment, but changes in that environment over time are not known precisely. The latest estimate by the National Council on Radiation Protection Measurements (NCRP) of the average annual effective dose equivalent from all sources in the U.S. population is about 3.6 milli-Sievert* (360 mrem).[23] About 82% of the total dose is from natural sources comprising cosmic rays, radionuclides, terrestrial γ-rays, and radon daughters (Fig. 9-1). About 40% of the total annual dose is considered to be due to radon daughters but with large individual variations. Most soils and rocks contain widely varying concentrations of uranium-238 and radium-226. The decay of radium-226 leads to release of radon into the surrounding water or air. The home is the major source of exposure to radon for the general population. Radon (radon-222) and

---

* Sievert (Sv) is the unit of dose equivalent in International Standard units. $Sv = 1 \, J \cdot kg^{-1} = 100$ rem.

136

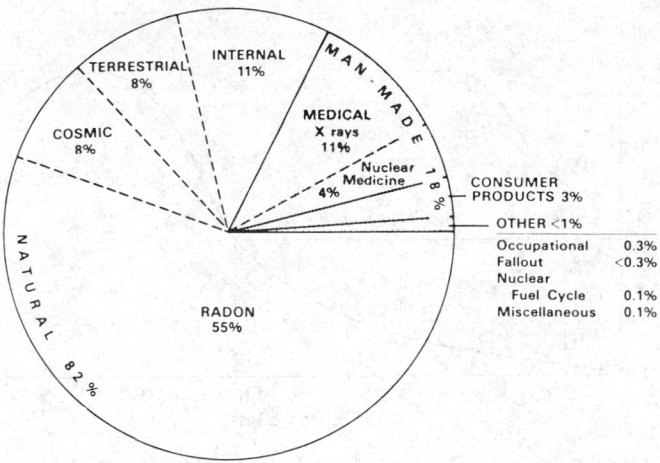

FIG. 9-1. Estimated contribution of various radiation sources to the total average effective dose equivalent in the U.S. population. The estimates of some of the contributing sources, for example, radon, have uncertainties on the order of a factor of two or three. (NCRP Report 93: Ionizing Radiation Exposure of the Population of the United States. Bethesda, MD, NCRP, 1987)

TABLE 9-1. Estimates of Excess Lifetime Risk of Lung Cancer Mortality as a Result of Lifetime Exposure to Radon Daughters

Report, Year (Reference)	Risk Estimate (deaths from lung cancer/ 10^6 person WLM)*
UNSCEAR, 1982 (27)	200–450
National Research Council (BEIR III) 1980 (2)	730
NCRP Report 77, 1984 (24)	130
National Research Council (BEIR IV), 1987 (25)	350

* Working level month (WLM): A unit of exposure to air concentrations of potential alpha energy released from radon daughters. One working level month is defined as the exposure to an average of 1 working level (a unit of air concentration of potential alpha energy released from radon and its daughters which has the energy release of 1.3×10^5 MeV/liter of air or 2.08×10^{-5} J/m³) for a working month of 170 hours or 3.5×10^{-3} Jh/m³.[24] Measurements of radon in homes are expressed in terms of picocuries (pCi) of radon per liter of air. Approximately 4 pCi/liter of radon equals 0.02 WL, and if 12 hours per day is spent in the home, the occupants would be exposed to about 0.5 WLM over a period of a year.

thoron (radon-220) emanate from the ground and building materials, disperse in the air, and decay into short-lived daughters or progeny that are isotopes of polonium, lead, and bismuth. The radon and thoron daughters attach to aerosol particles, and the alpha emitters are deposited with the particles in the tracheobronchial tree.[24,25] The concern is the risk of lung cancer from the high-LET radiation from the decay daughters such as polonium-218 and polonium-214.[24–26]

The potential exposure to radon varies markedly in different parts of the country, depending on geological features. An important variable is the level of thoron daughters, which is not measured separately in most assessments of populations exposure. It has been suggested that thoron can be a significant contributor to the lung dose,[27] but less by a factor of 3 than the exposure due to the progeny of radon-222.[25]

There is as yet no complete survey of indoor radon levels in the United States. Based on the uranium content of rock and soil, locations that have a potential for high indoor radon levels have been mapped and are widespread over the country. Obviously, houses built on reclaimed lands that have been mined and that have ores or soils near the surface may have significant radon levels. But houses in areas with no association of phosphate or uranium mining have also been found with radon at levels that remedial action is considered prudent, for example, in parts of the states of New York, New Jersey, and Pennsylvania.

The estimates of risk of excess lung cancer caused by exposure to radon are shown in Table 9-1. The estimates are based on epidemiologic studies of miners of uranium and of other underground miners.[2,24,25,27] The risk estimates vary with the assumptions made and the models used.

Current epidemiologic studies should establish whether or not living in homes in districts with high radon levels does, in fact, increase the risk of lung cancer. As is the case with some other lung carcinogens, smoking is an important cofactor. It is estimated that smokers exposed to radon have ten times the risk of lung cancer than nonsmokers similarly exposed.

It is estimated that 8% to 12% of houses across the nation may have annual average radon levels greater than 4 pCi/ liter of air, which is considered by the Environmental Protection Agency to be the level at which remedial measures should be considered. A number of different remedial measures are being used, all based on two main principles: (1) stopping the entry of or diverting radon from the house, and (2) removing radon by increasing the rate of ventilation, especially in the basement. For smokers the best advice is to give up smoking. The evidence for an interaction between smoking and irradiation from alpha emitters and the associated increased risk of lung cancer is sufficient to be a warning.

Medical procedures contribute about 15% of the total annual effective dose equivalent, but again, individual doses vary markedly. About 250 million medical radiologic examinations are performed annually in the United States, and the average bone marrow dose has been estimated to be about 1 mSv (100 mrem).[23] With increasing use of techniques that provide more information and involve midplane doses of 1 to 3 rad,[28,29] the average dose may rise.

IONIZING RADIATION AND CANCER

HISTORICAL PERSPECTIVE

A causal relation between the exposure to radiation and cancer was suspected within 6 years of the discovery of roentgen rays.[30] Causal relations between carcinogenic agents and cancer in humans, even if suspected, usually take a long time to establish, mainly because of the long latent period between exposure and the appearance of the cancer.

The cancer that was observed first was skin cancer, not unusual in the early days of radiation, although the dose required to induce cancer of skin is in the hundreds of rads.

An association between radiation and leukemia was suspected some years later.[31] The information about radiation-induced leukemogenesis in humans[2,32-34] and animals is now extensive,[35-40] partly because the latent period for leukemia is shorter than that for solid cancers.

The induction of cancer in humans by radionuclides was suspected first by Martland in radium dial painters in 1931.[41] Osteosarcomas were detected first; later, carcinomas of the mastoid and nasal sinuses were seen.[42] Full accounts have been published of the early radiation workers[43] and of the early studies of radiation-induced cancer in humans and experimental animals.[44]

An increase in our understanding of the risks associated with radiation exposure and the effectiveness of protection[45,46] is underlined by the fact that the maximum permissible lifetime dose for radiation workers has been decreased by a factor of about 10 from 1936, when the level was about 2400 R. The basis of the past, current, and future protection standards has been reviewed recently,[47] and future trends have been outlined.[48] The major factors that influence the estimates of risk are listed in Table 9-2.

PHYSICAL FACTORS

RADIATION QUALITY

X-rays give rise to electrons that are energetic but that have a small mass and are sparsely ionizing. In contrast, alpha particles, with a greater mass and slower velocity, are densely ionizing. Exposures to equal doses of these different radiations do not have the same biologic effect. The relative biologic effectiveness (RBE)† of the high-LET radiations, such as alpha particles and neutrons, is greater than that of the low-LET radiations, such as x-rays and γ- rays. The induction of cancer is no exception. Experimental data suggest that the dose-response relationships are of the forms shown schematically in Figure 9-2. The initial linear slope of the dose-response curve for induction of tumors by high-LET radiation is markedly steeper than that for cobalt-60 γ-rays. The curve for low-LET radiation is initially linear but curves upward as the dose-squared (D^2) component of the response becomes

---

† A ratio of the absorbed dose of a reference radiation, conventionally x-rays but in practice often γ rays, to the absorbed dose of a test radiation to produce the same level of biological effect.

TABLE 9-2.   Factors that Influence the Estimate of Risk for Radiation-Induced Cancer

Physical	Biological	Analytical
Radiation quality	Genetic factors	Choice of:
Dose	Age	Models for dose response
Dose rate	Sex	Projection models
Fractionation	Radionuclide	Absolute risk
	Metabolism	Relative risk

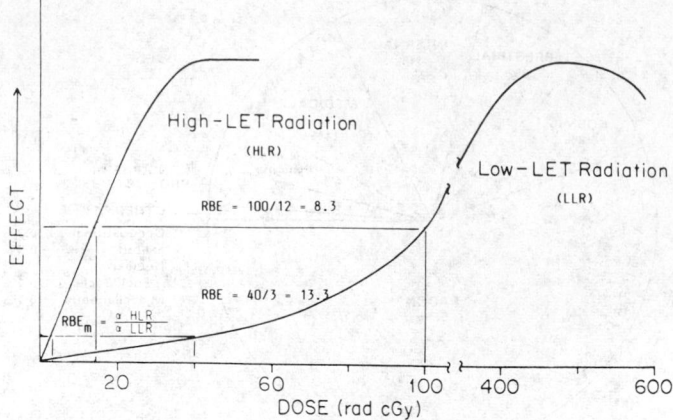

FIG. 9-2. Dose-response relationships for cancer induction by high- and low-LET radiation. Note inverse relationship of RBE to dose and the maximum RBE (RBE$_m$).

predominant. The curves for both high- and low-LET radiation bend over but at very different dose levels. It is suggested that the response curves bend over because cell killing reduces the probability of a cancer. However, especially in the case of high-LET radiation, other factors contribute to the complex shape.

RBE values, which are used to describe quantitatively the differences in effectiveness between different types of radiation, vary with dose, dose rate, fractionation, and the tissue involved. As can be seen from Figure 9-2, the RBE increases with decrease in dose down to dose levels at which both curves become linear and the RBE becomes maximum (RBE$_m$). RBE$_m$ values derived from experimental animal studies are used in the selection of quality factors (Q) for the determination of dose equivalents for different types of radiation because there are no human data for radiations such as neutrons. In 1985 the International Commission on Radiological Protection recommended increasing the Q for neutrons from 10 to 20.[49]

DOSE AND DOSE RESPONSES

The ability to measure the absorbed dose of radiation is a great advantage to both the clinician and the experimenter. However, organ dose becomes a less useful measurement in experimental studies, especially with high-LET radiation at very low doses, because few of the cells will be traversed by particles. The measurement of interest is the absorbed energy in the cell traversed, which is not indicated by the absorbed dose in the tissue. Similarly, at the dimensions of interest in relation to targets (at the micrometer or nanometer level), mean absorbed dose and dose–rate become inappropriate. Another example of the problem is the high dose that is localized in tissue at the sites of deposition of energy from alpha emitters in either the lung or bone. In the case of high-LET particles, both fluence and track structure become essential to the understanding of the relationship of energy deposition and biologic effects. The reader is referred to expert reviews for details of the current concepts of dose and microdosimetry.[50-53]

Three dose-response relationships—linear, quadratic, and linear-quadratic (LQ)—usually are considered relevant, and estimates based on these models have been compared. The aim of protection standards has been well served by the simplest approach, the linear, no-threshold model, but its simplicity ignores the biology. However, the understanding of the dose deposition of radiation and the mechanism of carcinogenesis is not adequate for formulating precise dose-response models. There is not a single form of dose response for carcinogenesis, and the differences reflect differences in the mechanisms. End points, such as chromosomal aberrations that may be associated intimately with carcinogenesis,[54-56] can be described by a linear-quadratic model,[57-59] but radiation-induced cancer involves many factors.[17,60,61] Factors involved in the probability of a cancer being induced include whether or not (1) the targets required for malignant transformation are hit, (2) the transformation events are repaired, (3) the initiated cell survives, and (4) the expression of the initiated cell occurs.

Molecular studies suggest that at least two gene loci on different chromosomes are involved in transformation which is indicative of a large target.[62] A large target is consistent with mechanisms involving chromosome breaks and translocation.[5]

Dose-response curves for incidence of cancer as a function of dose reflect expression as well as initiation. Carcinogenesis usually is considered multistage although there is no obvious requirement for further direct effects on the target cell after initiation, since single exposures to radiation can induce cancer. On the other hand, events involving host factors that in turn alter tissue environment, such as cell–cell interactions,[63] or systemic factors such as hormone levels, or immune capability play an important role and must be considered.[17,60] Models of dose responses should take into account the time-dependent changes in both initiation and expression.[17]

DOSE RATE AND FRACTIONATION

Reductions in dose rate reduce the carcinogenic effect of low-LET radiation both in animals and in in vitro cell systems.[64-67] The reduction may be marked but varies among tumor types, presumably because the mechanisms of carcinogenesis also vary. Reductions in effect are predicted by models of carcinogenesis that involve interaction of lesions or that allow for repair. With low dose rates, the number of tracks per cell does not change, but the probability of interactions between two tracks is diminished. Similarly, with a spatial relationship of two tracks suitable for interaction but separated in time, repair may occur and abrogate interaction. Time is biologically important, and extending the time over which exposure occurs influences a number of responses. With sufficiently low dose rates or low doses, no interactions should occur, and the response will be single track in form and described by $E = \bar{\alpha}D$, where D = dose and $\bar{\alpha}$ is an empirically determined coefficient.

Experimental data for many high dose rate, low-LET radiation-induced tumors can be fitted by a linear-quadratic dose-response model. Such a dose response suggests that the slope of the responses to low dose rates and multiple small fractions will be equivalent to the linear component of the linear-quadratic response. It can be seen from Figure 9-3 that experimental data for two tumors with markedly different dose responses (note the differences in the dose scales) support the basis of the linear-quadratic model. When the dose per fraction is within the dose range over which the linear component of the linear-quadratic response is predominant, the dose response is linear and the slope is equivalent to that after low dose exposures.[68]

Fractionation of doses can take many forms. The simplest, splitting the dose into two fractions (a technique used widely to study repair), reduces the carcinogenic effect in skin.[68,69] On the other hand, suitably spaced multiple fractions at a certain dose level greatly increase the probability that thymic lymphoma will develop. The effects of fractionation on in vitro malignant transformation appear to depend on the choice of dose per fraction.[70-72]

Protraction of exposures over a long period may reduce the effect both because of the reduced dose rate and because, with age, the susceptibility decreases. An exception to the sparing effect of protraction is the apparent requirement for protracted exposures to induce myeloproliferative disease in dogs.[40] It is not known whether protraction allows exposure to the high total doses required without death from marrow damage or whether repeated radiation–induced lesions ensure expression of leukemia.

It has not been possible to establish unequivocally that lowering dose rates reduces the carcinogenic effect in

FIG. 9-3. **A.** Incidence of lung cancer in BALB/c mice as a function of dose after single high dose-rate exposures to γ-rays (●—●), and after 2 × 1 Gy (△), 4 × 0.5 Gy (▲), 20 × 0.1 Gy (■) fractions. Low dose-rate exposures (○—○) are also shown. **B.** Incidence of breast cancer after single high dose–rate exposures to γ rays (●—●) and after 5 × 0.05 Gy (◇) and 25 × 0.01 Gy (□). The low dose-rate data are indicated (○—○). Note that the dose scales vary by a factor of 8. (Adapted from Ullrich RL et al: Radiation carcinogenesis: Time-dose relationships. Radiat Res 111:179–184, 1987)

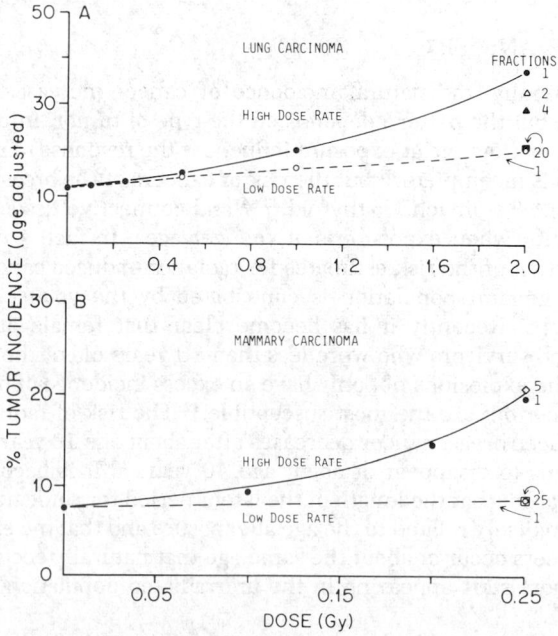

humans, but unless our current understanding of the biophysics and biology of induction of DNA lesions and repair is very wrong, it must be so.

In contrast, not only is the effect of high-LET irradiation not reduced by lowering the dose rate, but, in the case of induction of mammary tumors in mice[73] and malignant transformation in vitro,[74] low dose rate exposures appear to be more effective than single acute exposures.

GENETIC FACTORS

The strain-dependent differences in both natural and radiation-induced incidences of cancer in mice attest to the importance of inherited factors. Evidence has suggested that retroviruses are involved, but it is not clear that the distribution of oncogenes is strain and species dependent. Inherited susceptibility may also be related to host factors that influence expression rather than initiation.

The cells of patients with several human genetic diseases have been shown to be hypersensitive to killing in vitro by ionizing radiation.[75-78] It has been found that cells from individuals with hereditary cutaneous melanoma and familial dysplastic nevus syndrome (FDNS) have an increased sensitivity for induction of chromatid aberrations in G_2.[79] Of particular interest is the finding of the increased sensitivity before clinical expression of the FDNS trait in individuals with FDNS who have increased susceptibility for radiation-induced cancer. The risk of cancer also is elevated in some genetic conditions, for example, ataxia-telangiectasia,[80] but no clear-cut association with an increased susceptibility to induction of cancer by radiation has been established. An important and as yet unanswered question is whether the heterozygotic state of any of the genetic disorders carries an increased risk.

Second cancers in patients treated with radiation for cancer in childhood have a distinct pattern that is related to the type of primary tumor, which suggests a genetically determined susceptibility.

AGE AND SEX

Generally, the natural incidence of cancer increases with age, but the pattern depends on the type of tumor. Information on how age at exposure influences the response to radiation is incomplete,[81] but the risk of cancers of the breast,[10,82] lung,[3,10] stomach,[3,10] thyroid,[83,84] and connective tissues[85] is greater when exposure is at younger ages. In fact, a major fraction of the risk estimates for radiation-induced cancer in the general population is contributed by the younger age groups. Recently it has become clear that female atomic bomb survivors who were less than 10 years old at the time of the explosions not only have an excess incidence of breast cancer but are the most susceptible.[82] The risk of radiation-induced breast cancer decreases after about age 10 years and seems to disappear at about age 40 years.[10] It is becoming apparent that the length of the latent period for some tumors is inversely related to the age at exposure and that the excess cancers occur at about the same age that naturally occurring tumors start appearing in the unirradiated population (Fig. 9-4).[86]

In the case of leukemias in humans, the age dependency of

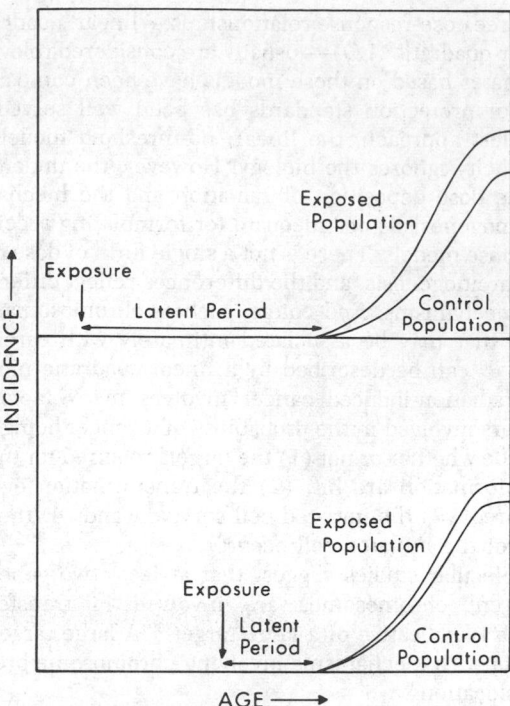

FIG. 9-4. Illustration of inverse relationship of length of latent period with age at exposure found for some cancers, particularly breast cancer. Note greater susceptibility for cancer induction with exposures at a young age compared with exposure at older ages.

susceptibility is more complex.[87] The risk of leukemia was greater in 50-year-old patients with ankylosing spondylitis than in patients less than 25 years old.[87] In the atomic bomb survivors, the risk of acute leukemias was high in those exposed at a young age, less in those exposed at age 20 to 50 years, and again high in those older than 50 years at the time of the explosion.[3,10]

Solid cancers induced by radiation tend not to appear until the age at which the naturally occurring cancer is seen. Therefore, the latent period will be longer when exposure is early in life. This suggests that age-dependent host factors are most important and that the expression of cells initiated in the young is suppressed until the necessary host changes occur. If cancer is a multistage process, then the age dependency of the effect of radiation will depend on whether the early or late stages are the most affected. If the number of cells that have gone through some of the multiple stages of the cancer process increases with age and if radiation acts at a late stage, then the absolute effect would increase with age at exposure.[88] The finding for ankylosing spondylitis is consistent with this idea.

The question of the risk of cancer induction when the exposure is prenatal is still in dispute, although the use of ultrasonography has made it clinically irrelevant.

The risk of radiation-induced cancer is estimated to be 30% to 50% greater in women than men.[1] The difference can be accounted for by sex-specific tumors, particularly those in the breast, which appears to be a susceptible tissue. Thyroid cancer after radiation exposure may also occur with higher frequency in women than in men.[83] On the other hand, male atomic bomb survivors appear to have been at greater risk of leukemia than female survivors.

PROJECTION MODELS

Estimates of risk are expressed either in absolute or relative terms. The absolute risk is the added risk caused by irradiation and is expressed as the number of radiation-related cancers in an exposed population per unit time per unit dose (1 cancer/10^6 persons/year/rad). When such risk estimates are used, the number of years of excess risk should be provided. For persons of similar ages at exposure, absolute risk $= a + bd$, where a is the risk of the specific cancer in the control population, b is the excess risk per rad, and d is the dose in rad. The relative risk is the ratio between the risk in the irradiated population and the risk in the nonirradiated population, and is expressed as a multiple of the natural risk. Such a model assumes that the risk resulting from radiation is determined by the natural incidence and that radiation acts in a multiplicative manner.

The models are illustrated in Figure 9-5. It is apparent that neither model applies to all radiation-induced cancers and that the models are simplistic but useful. The importance of projection models is indicated by the fact that the major source of data for radiation risk estimates is the atomic bomb survivors and that more than 60% of the survivors are still alive. To estimate radiation risks for the U.S. population from such data, projections both in time and across populations must be made.

FIG. 9-5. Absolute and relative risk models used in the estimation and projection of risks. The time between exposure to radiation and the time that the specific cancers appear in excess of the natural incidence is indicated, but for some tumors the length of the latent period is age-dependent.

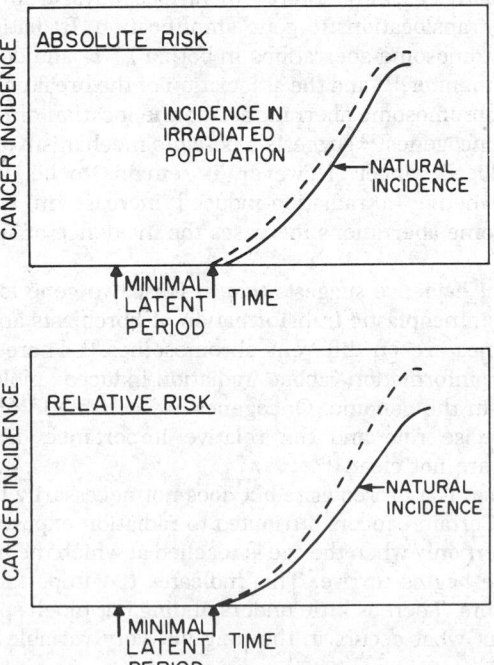

RISK ESTIMATES

Sensible protection standards depend on reliable risk estimates. Despite the breadth of available information, some of the steps in risk estimation still depend on judgment, for example, the choice of a dose-response model and Q values for high-LET radiation. Improvement in the risk estimates will come, as data accumulate and insights develop, from further understanding of mechanisms.

Risk estimates for the induction of cancer by low-LET radiation are based on the human experience. The atomic bomb survivors are the major source of data for high dose-rate whole-body exposure. The doses at Hiroshima and Nagasaki have been reassessed, a major undertaking that is now coming to completion. The new doses indicate that the neutron component was much less than originally thought. The neutron doses are now so low that direct estimates of the effectiveness of neutrons will at best be difficult and at worst impossible to make. The organ doses, except for some surface tissues such as the breast, have not changed markedly. It is likely that any changes in risk estimates will result from the increasing cancer mortality data as the population of atomic bomb survival ages. More than 57,000 of the 91,228 persons in the current Life Span Study are still alive.[11] Almost 7,000 died of cancer between 1950 and 1985. It is estimated that the excess of cancer deaths due to radiation in this population is about 8%.

The estimate of excess risk of radiation-induced leukemia based on the new dosimetry (DS86) and the mortality data for the years 1950 to 1985 is 2.91 per 10^4 person-year Gray (PYGy), compared to 1.75 per 10^4 PYGy with the previous dosimetry (T65D).[11] These estimates are averaged over six categories of sex and age at time of exposure and assume an RBE of 10. The estimates of excess cancer rates for various organs, based on mortality data for 1950 to 1982 and assuming T65D doses, are shown in Figure 9-6.[10]

Risk estimates based on data from all relevant sources were reported in 1985.[8,89] However, the new risk estimates are expected in 1988 when the United Nations Scientific Committee on Effects of Atomic Radiation (UNSCEAR) and the National Academy of Sciences (Biological Effects of Ionizing Radiation V) complete their current deliberations. Not only must the new DS86 dosimetry and updated data from Hiroshima and Nagasaki and other studies be taken into account, but also RBE values, dose-response relationships, and projection models. In the case of the latter, it has become increasingly clear that relative risk is the appropriate model for most solid cancers.[2,90] Not surprisingly, incidence rates are higher and are the appropriate index for tumor induction in organs such as the thyroid.

The recent accidents at Chernobyl in the Soviet Union, Juarez, Mexico, and Goiania, Brazil add impetus to improving estimates of risk.

RADIOLOGIC RISKS

More than 90% of the annual dose received from man-made radiation sources is from medical diagnostic procedures.[23] The differences in the reported organ doses are great and depend on the type of examination and on the techniques; UNSCEAR has reported that doses range from 0.01 to 5 rad

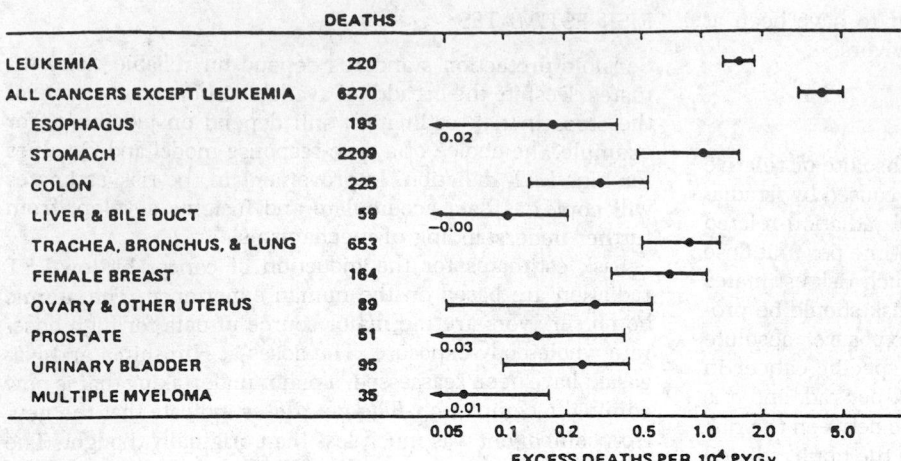

FIG. 9-6. The maximum likelihood estimates and 90% confidence limits for average absolute excess risk of radiation-induced cancer mortality at selected sites in atomic bomb survivors. The estimates are derived from a linear model adjusted for city (Hiroshima or Nagasaki), sex, age at time of exposure, and time since exposure, and are expressed in person-years per Gray (PYGy) (Preston DL et al: Studies of the mortality of A-bomb survivors: 8. Cancer Mortality, 1950–1982. Radiat Res 111:151–178, 1987)

(0.1–50 mGy).[91] The benefit of well-selected procedures is clear, but approaches to reduce exposures make sense.[92] About 250 million diagnostic x-ray examinations are carried out each year, and there has been concern about the risk from routine examinations or methods that result in the accumulation of high doses.[92] There are no direct estimates of cancer induction at very low doses, and the estimates of risk are a matter of judgment. Based on reported radiologic procedures, Harwood and Yaffe estimated the total risk of cancer induction from a diagnostic examination as about $1:10^6$ per year, and small in comparison to the benefit.[93] They exempted barium enema examinations and positive mode mammography from this estimate because of the higher dose with the barium enema examination and the suspected susceptibility of the breast to radiation in positive mode mammography. Evans et al[94] concluded from a study of 75,000 patients that 1% of all cases of leukemia and 0.7% of all cases of breast cancer might be attributed to diagnostic radiography. These figures are probably overestimates. The majority of radiologic examinations are performed on patients who are older than 40 years, and the cancers that the authors considered radiation-induced occurred late in life.

The question of the use of routine x-ray mammography has focused attention on the balance of risk and benefit. In the late 1970s there was concern that the risk of annual mammography in women aged 35 to 49 years might be greater than the benefit. The doses involved in mammography have been reduced since then, and it also has been shown that the risk of radiation-induced breast cancer decreases markedly with age.[82]

Risk estimates of breast cancer have been based on a linear no-threshold dose-response relationship, but this has been questioned recently.[95] If the dose response is, in fact, curvilinear, radiation risk estimates may be adjusted downward. In any case, the current practice of selecting patients for mammography based on age and family history is appropriate.

The use of ultrasonography has made the issue of the risk of exposure in utero of more academic than practical interest. Cancer occurs as a secondary effect of radiation therapy both for benign[7,9,12,96–103] and malignant disease.[5,6,12,104,105] Leukemia is more frequent after chemotherapy than after radiation therapy.[106,107] There are marked differences in susceptibility between organs. For many sites the risk of radiation-induced cancer decreases with age. Conversely, the risk is highest in childhood. Brain tumors have been reported recently in children exposed to 1 Gy.[103] In the case of skin treated with x-rays, subsequent exposure to sunlight[97] or PUVA[108] increases the risk of skin cancer.

The use of magnetic resonance imaging (MRI) has increased and in the future may result in a reduction in the use of diagnostic x-rays. There have been no extensive studies of possible late effects of MRI, but risk of cancer seems unlikely.

MECHANISM OF RADIATION CARCINOGENESIS

A major attraction to the idea that activation of cellular oncogenes is central to initiation of malignant transformation is that it provides a paradigm for explaining a common pathway of effects of very different agents.[109,110]

Gene activity can be altered in various ways, from chromosome translocations to gene amplification. Radiation induces chromosome aberrations in both a LET- and dose-dependent manner,[111] and the association of the breakpoints of specific chromosome aberrations and the location of human cellular oncogenes[112] suggests a possible mechanism of radiation-induced cancer. However, it remains to be demonstrated whether a radiation-induced increase in specific chromosome aberrations increases the incidence of specific cancers.

Current evidence suggests that at least two gene loci are involved in neoplastic transformation of fibroblasts and that these genes are on different chromosomes.[62] There is increasing information about radiation-induced molecular changes in the genome. Oncogenes are activated,[113,114] but their precise role and the relative importance of other changes are not clear.[115]

Initiation is a prerequisite but does not necessarily lead to cancer. Certain cancers attributed to radiation exposure become overt only when the age is reached at which the natural incidence begins to rise. This indicates the importance of host factors. There is little understanding but much speculation about what occurs in the long but very variable latent periods. In some tissues, potential cancer cells may lie dormant for years. In other tissues, cancer may involve a multistep process that includes further mutations and selection. Clearly, different factors are involved in the mechanisms of different types of cancer, especially in the expression stages. In certain tumors, secondary or host factors are the most important determining factors.

ULTRAVIOLET RADIATION CARCINOGENESIS

Skin cancer is by far the most common cancer among whites in the United States. About 400,000 cases of basal cell or squamous cell carcinoma occur each year.[116] Basal cell carcinomas are four times more frequent than squamous cell carcinomas in men; the same ratio in women is 6 : 1.[116] Both types of cancer are found more frequently in men than in women and about 70 times more frequently in whites than in blacks.[116] The cancers usually occur on areas exposed to sunlight, and at higher rates in southern latitudes of the United States. The incidence, mainly of basal cell carcinoma, is increasing, but fortunately the cure rate is above 95%. The marked increase in the incidence of melanoma in developed nations is of greater concern because of the higher mortality rate than in nonmelanoma skin cancer.[117] The evidence for a causal relationship between ultraviolet radiation (UVR) and melanoma is not as watertight as that for nonmelanoma skin cancer but is compelling.[118,119]

Depletion of stratospheric ozone has been a matter of concern for almost 20 years. First, it was feared that supersonic airplanes would inject nitrogen oxides into the stratosphere, resulting in depletion of ozone.[120-122] More recently, the increasing level of chlorofluorocarbons has been suspected as a possible cause of the decrease of ozone in the stratosphere.[123-124] Measurements by the Total Ozone Spectrometer on Nimbus 7 during spring in the Antarctic indicate that the ozone levels have fallen as much as 4%,[125,126] and a "hole" in the ozone layer has appeared. The possibility of a more global reduction has renewed the concern that an increase in skin cancer may result. A recent study of the National Aeronautical and Space Agency concluded that ozone levels have fallen 1% to 3% in the latitudes from Florida to Canada.

The stratospheric ozone layer acts as a highly effective absorbing layer that prevents the most biologically effective wavelengths of UVR, especially UVB (280–320 nm), from reaching humans. Any increase in UVB fluences on Earth would increase the probability of skin cancer. A 1% decrease in stratospheric ozone could result in about a 2% increase in the amount of UVB reaching Earth. It has been estimated that each 1% decrease in ozone might cause about a 4% increase in nonmelanoma cancer. An important question is whether or not the incidence of melanoma would be increased. Scotto et al[127] suggest that there will likely be an increase in the more southern latitudes, and that the increase in melanoma may appear earlier than the predicted increase in nonmelanoma skin cancer. Such a suggestion depends on the validity of the causal relationship between melanoma and UVR. A correlation between the incidence of melanoma and sunspot activity has been claimed,[128] but the study did not take into account the length of the latent period for melanoma induction. The stratospheric changes caused by cyclic changes in sunspot activity are complex and a number of factors, perhaps relevant to skin cancer, vary; for example, galactic cosmic rays can change ozone levels.

Perhaps some comfort may be taken from the report that no increase of UVB was detected between 1974 and 1985 at the various monitoring stations that span the United States from North Dakota to Florida.[127] This finding suggests that ozone depletion may not be as global as feared, or that the attenuation of UVB radiation is more complex than was previously thought. The effect of current levels of chlorofluorocarbons on stratospheric ozone will not be detected for some years. Only time and accurate surveillance will reveal the long-term trend.

HISTORIC PERSPECTIVE

Astute clinical observations were the first stage in understanding the relationship of sunlight to skin cancer in men involved in maritime and outdoor occupations. The association of exposure to greater intensities of sunlight and skin cancer strengthened the evidence that sunlight was a major etiologic factor.[129]

In 1928, it was demonstrated that UVR induced skin cancer in experimental animals[130]; later, the carcinogenic effect was found to be restricted to wavelengths shorter than 320 nm.[131]

MECHANISMS OF UVR CARCINOGENESIS

The evidence that the induction of skin cancer by UVR results in UVR-induced DNA damage is considerable. For example, (1) the action spectra for neoplastic transformation[132] and anchorage-independent growth[133] are similar to those for the induction of cyclobutane pyrimidine dimers; (2) enzymatic photoreactivation of UVR-induced pyrimidine dimers suppresses the induction of in vitro transformation of human fibroblasts,[134] the induction of thyroid neoplasia in fish,[135] and induction of sarcomas in the corneas of opossums[136]; and (3) the cells of patients with Xeroderma pigmentosum, who have a marked susceptibility to melanoma and nonmelanoma skin cancer, lack the ability to repair UVR-induced DNA damage.[137] Although cyclobutane pyrimidine dimers appear to be the pertinent molecular lesion for UVR-induced cancer, the role of other photoproducts, such as pyrimidine-pyrimidine (6-4) photoproduct, may be important.

In humans and experimental animals, protracted or multiple exposures with high total fluences of UVR usually are required to produce carcinomas of the skin. The question is whether the later exposures influence the expression of the changes initiated by the early exposures, and if so, how? It can be seen from Figure 9-7 that the dose–response curve for the experimental induction of skin cancer has an apparent threshold, but that threshold can be altered by treatment with the promoter tissue plasminogen activator (TPA). These results suggest that UVR initiates many cells that do not develop into cancer. There is now a renewed interest in the role of immune surveillance that might explain the apparent suppression of initiated cells.[138,139] It is suggested that

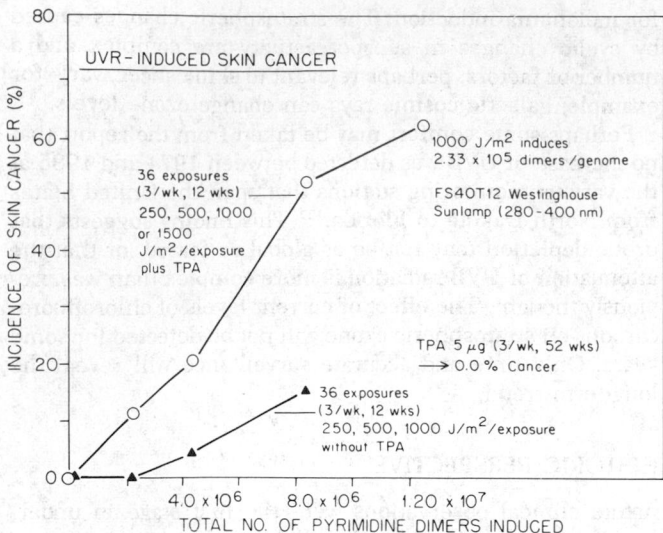

FIG. 9-7. Incidence of squamous cell carcinoma as a function of the number of cyclobutane pyrimidine dimers induced by exposure to UVR (280–400 nm) (▲—▲), and exposure to UVR followed by treatment with 5 μg TPA for 1 year after the end of the UVR regimen (O—O).

UVR affects Langerhans' cells, which are antigen-presenting cells in the epidermis and the most superficial sentinel of the immune system. These effects result in the development of suppressor T-lymphocytes that interfere with the rejection of the tumors.[138]

People are protected from the sequelae of UVR-induced damage by two distinct types of mechanisms. First, pigment, hair, and skin thickness all reduce the absorbed dose. In people of Celtic background, pigmentation is not distributed evenly in the skin, and skin cancer is common. Second, human cells repair UVR-induced DNA damage with great fidelity. This capability is reduced markedly in patients with xeroderma pigmentosum.[137]

XERODERMA PIGMENTOSUM

Xeroderma pigmentosum is a ubiquitous autosomal recessive disease with a frequency of about 1:250,000 in the United States and Europe but reportedly higher in countries such as Egypt and Japan.[140-142] The disease was first described by Hebra and Kaposi 120 years ago.[143] Homozygotes occur more frequently in families of consanguineous marriages, and males and females are equally affected.[140] The disease is characterized by a hypersensitivity to sunlight associated with a marked susceptibility to skin cancer, including melanoma, except in Japan.[141] Almost 50% of patients with xeroderma pigmentosum in the United States, Europe, and Japan also have neurologic abnormalities, but few have all the lesions that are characteristic of the de Sanctis–Cacchione syndrome.[141] Various ocular lesions such as cloudiness of the cornea, pigmentation, and telangiectasia of the conjunctiva have been considered part of the syndrome since the entity was first recognized.[140,141] The description of the early cases concentrated on the degenerative and pigmentation changes as well as telangiectasia,[143,144] and it was not until 1932 that de Sanctis and Cacchione reported the associated neurologic

abnormalities.[145] Both the genetic aspects and the possible role of sunlight in xeroderma pigmentosum were noted by Hebra and Kaposi.[143] As early as 1929, it was suggested that the xeroderma pigmentosum trait might be an essential characteristic of persons who developed skin cancer.[146] The parents of patients with xeroderma pigmentosum are heterozygotes and clinically normal.[141] There has been no consistent evidence that the cells of persons heterozygous for the syndrome were significantly defective in DNA repair. However, although it has been suggested that heterozygotes are at a higher risk for skin cancer,[147] the evidence indicates that the gene for xeroderma pigmentosum must be in the homozygous state to result in the clinical syndrome.

In 1968 Cleaver described the finding of defective excision repair of UVR-induced damage in fibroblasts cultured from the skin of xeroderma pigmentosum patients.[148] Thus began the exciting search for a causal relation between a specific DNA lesion and cancer.

No longer is xeroderma pigmentosum thought to be a disease involving a single defect in DNA repair; rather, there is a complex interrelationship of different repair systems, their genetics, and enzymology. The studies of fusing cells from different xeroderma pigmentosum patients with normal cells have revealed the genetic heterogeneity in the syndrome.[149-151] Seven complementation groups (A to G) have been identified that are deficient in excision repair, which implies the involvement of seven genes. An eighth group, known as variant, shows no CNS abnormalities or the characteristic sensitivity to sunlight.[152-154] However, the cells are more susceptible to UVR-induced mutation than are normal cells.[155]

The important molecular defect of cells of the xeroderma pigmentosum variant is reflected in the interruption of replication forks during semiconservative DNA synthesis after exposure to UVR. An examination of the comparative survival of UV-irradiated cells and the clinical conditions in the eight groups indicated that the occurrence of neurologic abnormalities correlates with the severity of the repair defect.[137] A normal karyotype and normal frequency of sister chromatid exchanges are the usual findings in xeroderma pigmentosum cells,[137,156] although abnormalities have been reported in cells from patients of the complementation groups C and D.[157] However, after exposure to UVR or certain chemical carcinogens, both chromosome aberrations and sister chromatid exchanges are increased more than in similarly exposed normal cells.[158-161]

A new form of xeroderma pigmentosum has been reported recently.[162] A family that demonstrated an apparent dominant inheritance of a DNA repair defect with skin cancer also had two members with defective DNA repair but free of cancers. This family is just one more demonstration that a causal relation between defective DNA repair and cancer is far from clear-cut.

FOREIGN BODY CARCINOGENESIS

NONFIBER FOREIGN BODIES

The introduction of foreign material that is not biodegradable usually stimulates a connective tissue or mesothelial reaction. The characteristics of the reaction depend on the final site of the foreign body. In the case of scars and tissue reactions around schistosomal eggs or tubercular lesions, the foreign body reactions have some probability of neoplastic change. Because the reaction frequently involves connective tissues, sarcomas of various types are the tumors that usually arise, but carcinomas also have been found in relation to foreign bodies. The incidental observation that Bakelite disks[163] and cellophane[164] caused sarcomas opened up an area of research with many facets, reviewed by Bischoff and Bryson[165] and Brand.[166]

Central to sarcomagenesis are the size and shape of the implants: the same materials in a powdered or porous form lose most of their tumorigenicity.[165,166] Within limits, the greater the surface area, the greater is the probability of tumors.[166] The chemical nature of the implants is not a predominant determinant of the development of the capsules and tumors because pure carbon disks produce sarcomas. Perforations, even without a reduction in surface area, reduce the incidence of sarcoma. However, the tumor incidence and latency are influenced by the physicochemical properties of the implants; latency is especially influenced by the smoothness and durability of the surface of the implant.[165,166]

The susceptibility to this form of carcinogenesis is species- and strain-dependent but age-independent.[165-167] Foreign body sarcomas are rare in humans but can be induced easily in some rodents. The events that occur from insertion of disks to the development of sarcomas have been fully documented, but the precise mechanism of neoplastic change is unknown.[168] Because chromosome abnormalities are a consistent finding,[168] the application of the new techniques of molecular biology and chromosome analysis should be rewarding.

When a ^{90}Sr-^{90}Y source is incorporated into laminated mylar disks, the radiation advances the time of appearance and increases the incidence of sarcomas in rats.[169] This type of experiment is an in vivo version of the currently popular in vitro radiation transformation experiments.

FIBER CARCINOGENESIS

Tobacco smoke remains the most important cause of lung cancer, but asbestos exposures account for 4000 to 6000 lung cancers and about 2000 cases of mesothelioma per year in the United States[170] and a comparable number of cancers in Great Britain.[171] Fortunately, in the future the number of cases should decrease because industrial and environmental exposures have been markedly reduced.

Although asbestos has dominated the research in fiber carcinogenesis because of its importance as an industrial and environmental carcinogen,[170,172-173] other types of fibers have biologic effects and have been classified by Leineweber into (1) man-made vitreous fibers, (2) synthetic crystalline fibers, and (3) natural mineral fibers.[174] The group of natural mineral fibers includes zeolites, the cause of a high incidence of cancer in parts of Turkey.[175] Omenn et al provide a detailed classification of fibers, some of which have replaced asbestos.[176] The concern is whether or not fibers that differ chemically from asbestos but are physically similar to it will prove carcinogenic. Reliable bioassays are needed in order to predict and prevent potential risks of the newer fibers.

ASBESTOS

A group of hydrated silicates have a fibrous crystalline structure known commercially as asbestos. There are two major classes of asbestos: the amphiboles, which include crocidolite, and the serpentines, which include chrysotile, the most widely used form of asbestos in the United States.

Because the tissue response to fibers is a fibrous reaction, there is the risk of neoplastic change, and the carcinogenic properties of at least one member of all three classes of fibers listed in the preceding paragraph have been shown. It is thought that chrysotile is less likely to cause pleural mesotheliomas than other asbestiform fibers, and it is not correlated with peritoneal mesothelioma.[176]

Physical characteristics such as length and diameter are more important determinants of carcinogenicity than is the chemical composition.[176-178] Studies have indicated that fibers that are carcinogenic tend to be longer than about 8 μm and less than 1.50 μm in diameter.[178]

Asbestos workers have an increased risk of developing mesothelioma and cancer at a number of sites, especially the lung.[170] Mesothelioma is pathognomonic of fiber carcinogenesis, particularly asbestos.[170,176] These tumors arise from the mesothelial surfaces of the pleura and peritoneum and have a pleomorphic histologic appearance. The tumors spread over the pleural and peritoneal surfaces, do not invade the underlying tissues deeply, but do metastasize.

Large numbers of people have been exposed to asbestos industrially or environmentally. Whether the widespread contamination by small amounts of fibers poses a hazard remains to be determined. It is still not known how the risk of mesothelioma is related to the amount of exposure and the different types of asbestos fiber, but the amount and the route of exposure appear to influence the site at which mesothelioma occurs. The importance of the type of exposure in relation to the occupation is illustrated by the finding that most mesotheliomas were pleural in shipyard workers but were peritoneal in asbestos factory workers. Lung cancer is the most common tumor caused by asbestos. The observed rate of lung cancer in asbestos insulation workers was four times that expected.[170] Chrysotile, amosite, anthophyllite, and crocidolite fibers have been implicated. A multiplicative effect of exposure to tobacco increases the risk of lung cancer in asbestos workers four to five times that of the nonsmoker.[179]

The latent period appears to correlate positively with the level of exposure and negatively with the age at first exposure. There is uncertainty about the appropriate models for risk estimates. It has been assumed that the dose responses for both mesotheliomas and lung cancer are linear. An absolute risk model is appropriate for mesothelioma. Death rates for mesothelioma in asbestos workers with protracted exposures appear to be proportional to the third or fourth power of the time from first exposure "irrespective of age, site, fiber type or dust level."[180] In the case of lung cancer a relative risk model is considered more appropriate.

Although the mechanism of induction of cancer by fibers remains a mystery, some progress has been made. It has been shown that asbestos and glass fibers are phagocytized by cells in culture and accumulate in the perinuclear region of the cytoplasm. Cells appear to selectively phagocytose the longer fibers, with the shorter fibers accumulating on the cell surface.[181] The cellular effects, from cell killing to transformation, depend on the fibers taken up by the cells.[182] In Syrian hamster embryo cells in culture, asbestos fibers induce a dose-dependent increase in micronuclei and chromosome aberrations.[182] Both chromosome aberrations and malignant transformation are induced by decreasing the length of the fibers.[182] This and other evidence suggests a correlation between the induction of chromosome aberrations and malignant transformation.[183-185] Aneuploidy is a consistent finding,[183] as it is in the early stages of other types of tumors. In experiments using the C3H 10T1/2 established cell lines, asbestos fibers were found to be cytotoxic in a dose-dependent manner but were ineffective for the induction of malignant transformation.[186] However, the combined treatment with asbestos fibers and γ radiation had a greater than additive effect on the induction of oncogenic transformation.[186]

This chapter has been authored by a contractor of the U.S. government under contract No. DE-AC05-840R21400. Accordingly, the U.S. government retains a nonexclusive, royalty-free license to publish or reproduce the published form of the contribution, or allow others to do so, for U.S. government purposes.

Research was sponsored by the Office of Health and Environmental Research, U.S. Department of Energy, under contract DE-AC05-840R21400 with the Martin Marietta Energy Systems, Inc.

It is a pleasure to acknowledge the valuable help of Mrs. F. Young.

REFERENCES

1. United Nations Scientific Committee on Effects of Atomic Radiation: Sources and Effects of Ionizing Radiation. 1977 Report to the General Assembly with Annexes, New York, United Nations, 1977
2. National Research Council, Committee on the Biological Effects of Ionizing Radiation (BEIR): The Effects on Populations of Exposure to Low Levels of Ionizing Radiation. Washington, DC, National Academy Press, 1980
3. Wakabayashi T, Kato H, Ikeda T et al: Studies of the mortality of A-bomb survivors: Part III. Incidence of cancer in 1959–78, based on the tumor registry, Nagasaki. Radiat Res 93:112–146, 1983
4. Boice JD Jr, Fraumeni JF Jr (eds): Radiation Carcinogenesis: Epidemiology and Biological Significance. New York, Raven Press, 1984
5. Kohn HI, Fry RJM: Radiation Carcinogenesis. N Engl J Med 310:504–511, 1984
6. Boice JD Jr, Day WE, Andersen A et al: Second cancers following radiation treatment for cervical cancer: An international collaboration among cancer registries. JNCI 74:955–975, 1985
7. Darby SC, Nakashima E, Kato H: A parallel analysis of cancer mortality among atomic bomb survivors and patients with ankylosing spondylitis given x-ray therapy. JNCI 75:1–21, 1985
8. Rall JE, Beebe GW, Hoel DG et al. Report of the National Institutes of Health Ad Hoc Working Group to Develop Radioepidemiological Tables. DHHS publication No. (NIH) 85-2748. Washington, DC, U.S. Government Printing Office, 1985
9. Darby SC, Doll R, Gill SK et al: Long-term mortality after a single treatment course with x-rays in patients treated for ankylosing spondylitis. Br J Cancer 55:179–190, 1987
10. Preston DL, Kato H, Kopecky KJ et al: Studies of the mortality of A-bomb survivors: 8. Cancer mortality, 1950–1982. Radiat Res 111:151–178, 1987
11. Preston DL, Pierce DA: The effects of changes in dosimetry on cancer mortality risk estimates in the atomic bomb survivors. RERF TR 9-87. Hiroshima, Radiation Effects Research Foundation, 1987
12. Boice JD Jr: Carcinogenesis: A synopsis of human experience with external exposure in medicine. JNCI (in press)
13. Storer JB: Radiation carcinogenesis. In Becker FF (ed): Cancer: A Comprehensive Treatise, 2nd ed, vol 1, pp 629–659. New York, Plenum Press, 1982
14. Broerse JJ, Hennen LA, Van Zwieten MJ: Radiation carcinogenesis in experimental animals and its implications for radiation protection. Int J Radiat Biol 48:167–187, 1985
15. Burns FJ, Upton AC, Silini G: Radiation Carcinogenesis and DNA Alterations. NATO ASI Series. New York, Plenum Press, 1986
16. Upton AC, Albert RE, Burns FJ et al: (eds): Radiation Carcinogenesis. New York, Elsevier, 1986
17. Fry RJM, Storer JB: External radiation carcinogenesis. Adv Radiat Biol 13:31–89, 1987
18. Borek C: In vitro transformation. Adv Cancer Res 37:159–231, 1982
19. Hall EJ, Hei TK: Oncogenic transformation of cells in culture: Pragmatic comparisons of oncogenicity, cellular and molecular mechanisms. Int J Radiat Oncol Biol Phys 12:1909–1921, 1986
20. Little JB: The radiobiology of in vitro neoplastic transformation. In Burns FJ, Upton AC, Silini G (eds): Radiation Carcinogenesis and DNA Alterations, pp 163–184. NATO ASI Series. New York, Plenum Press, 1986
21. Hill CK, Han A, Elkind MM: Promotion, dose rate, and repair processes in radiation-induced neoplastic transformation. Radiat Res 109:347–351, 1987
22. Beebe GW: Assessment of health risks from exposure to ionizing radiation. In Prentice RL, Whittemore AS (eds): Environmental Epidemiology: Risk Assessment, pp 3–21. Philadelphia, SIAM, 1982
23. National Council on Radiation Protection and Measurements (NCRP): Ionizing Radiation Exposure of the Population of the United States. NCRP Report No 93. Bethesda, MD, NCRP, 1987
24. National Council on Radiation Protection and Measurements (NCRP): Exposures from the Uranium Series with Emphasis on Radon and its Daughters. NCRP Report No. 77. Bethesda, MD, NCRP, 1984
25. National Research Council: Biological Effects of Ionizing Radiation (BEIR): Health Risks of Radon and Other Internally Deposited Alpha Emitters. Washington, DC, National Academy Press, 1987
26. Harley N, Samet JM, Cross FT et al: Contribution of radon and radon daughters to respiratory cancer. Environ Health Perspect 70:17–21, 1986
27. United Nations Scientific Committee on Effects of Atomic Radiation (UNSCEAR): Ionizing Radiation: Sources and Biological Effects. Report to the General Assembly with Annexes, 1987
28. Schlein B, Tucker TT, Johnson DW: The mean active bone marrow dose to the adult population of the United States from diagnostic radiology. Health Phys 34:587–601, 1978
29. McCullough EC, Payne JT: Patient dosage in computed tomography. Radiology 129:457–463, 1978
30. Frieben A: Demonstration lines cancroids des rechten Handruckens, das sich nach langdauernder Einwirkung von Röntgenstrahlen entwichelt hatte. Fortschr Geb Röntgenstr 6:106, 1902
31. von Jagic N, Scwarz G, von Siebenrock L: Blutbefunde bei Röntgenologon. Berl Klin Wochenschr 48:1220–1222, 1911
32. Ishimaru M, Ishimaru T, Mikami M et al: Incidence of leukemia in a fixed cohort of atomic bomb survivors and controls: Hiroshima and Nagasaki, October 1950–December 1978. RERF TR-13-81. Hiroshima, Radiation Effects Research Foundation, 1982
33. Brodsky JB, Lidell R, Groer PG et al: Temporal analysis of a dose-response relationship: Leukemia mortality in atomic bomb survivors. RERF TR 5-82. Hiroshima, Radiation Effects Research Foundation, 1983
34. Boice JD Jr, Blettner M, Kleinerman RA et al: Radiation dose and leukemia risk in patients treated for cancer of the cervix. JNCI 79:1295–1311, 1987
35. Upton AC, Randolph ML, Conklin JW: Late effects of fast neutrons and gamma rays in mice as influenced by the dose rate of irradiation: Induction of neoplasia. Radiat Res 41:467–491, 1970
36. Kaplan HS: Interaction between radiation and viruses in the induction of murine thymic lymphomas and lymphatic leukemias. In Duplan JF (ed): Radiation-Induced Leukemogenesis and Related Viruses, pp 1–18. Amsterdam, North Holland, 1977
37. Ullrich RL, Storer JB: Influence of gamma radiation on the development of neoplastic disease in mice: I. Reticular tissue tumors. Radiat Res 80:303–316, 1979
38. Mole RH: Radiation-induced myeloid leukemia in the mouse: Experimental observations and in vivo implications for hypotheses about the basis of carcinogenesis. Leuk Res 7:859–865, 1986
39. Ullrich RL, Preston RJ: Myeloid leukemia in male RFM mice following irradiation with fission spectrum neutrons or gamma rays. Radiat Res 109:165–170, 1987
40. Tolle DV, Fritz TE, Seed TM et al: Leukemia induction in beagles exposed continuously to ^{60}Co gamma irradiation: Hematology. In Baum SJ, Ledney GD, Thierfelder S (eds): Experimental Hematology Today 1982, pp 241–249. Basel, S Karger, 1982
41. Martland HS: The occurrence of malignancy in radioactive persons: A general review of data gathered in the study of the radium dial painters with special reference to the occurrence of osteogenic sarcoma and the interrelationship of certain blood diseases. Am J Cancer 15:2435–2516, 1931
42. Rowland RE, Stehney AF, Lucas HF Jr: Dose-response relationships for female radium-dial workers. Radiat Res 76:368–383, 1978
43. Grigg ERN: The Trail of the Invisible Light. Springfield, IL, Charles C Thomas, 1965
44. Upton AC: Physical carcinogenesis: Radiation—history and sources. In Becker FF (ed): Cancer: A Comprehensive Treatise, 2nd ed, pp 551–567. New York, Plenum Press, 1982
45. Stone RS: Maximum permissible exposure standards. In: Protection in Diagnostic Radiology. New Brunswick, Rutgers University Press, 1959

46. Sinclair WK: Radiation Protection: The NCRP Guidelines and some considerations for the future. Yale J Biol Med 54:471–484, 1981

47. Sinclair WK: Risk, research and radiation protection. Radiat Res 112:191–216, 1987

48. National Council on Radiation Protection and Measurements (NCRP): Recommendations on limits for exposure to ionizing radiation. NCRP Report 91. Bethesda, Md, NCRP, 1987

49. International Commission on Radiological Protection (ICRP): Statement from Paris meeting of the ICRP. Phys Med Biol 30:863, 1985

50. Kellerer AM, Rossi HH: A generalized formulation of dual radiation action. Radiat Res 75:471–488, 1978

51. Kellerer AM, Rossi HH: Biophysical aspects of radiation carcinogenesis. In Becker FF (ed): Cancer: A Comprehensive Treatise, 2nd ed, pp 569–616. New York, Plenum Press, 1982

52. Goodhead DT: An assessment of the role of microdosimetry in radiobiology. Radiat Res 91:45–76, 1982

53. Bond VP, Varma MN: A stochastic, weighted hit size theory of cellular biological action. In Booze J, Ebert HG (eds): Radiation Protection: Proceedings of the 8th Symposium on Microdosimetry, pp 423–438, July 1982, Luxemburg 1983

54. Dalla-Favera R, Martinotti S, Gallo RC et al: Translocation and rearrangements of the c-myc oncogene locus in human undifferentiated B-cell lymphomas. Science 219:963–967, 1983

55. Klein G: Chromosomal translocations and the genesis of B-cell-derived tumors in mice and men. Cell 32:311–315, 1983

56. Rowley JD: Biological implications of consistent chromosome rearrangements in leukemia and lymphoma. Cancer Res 44:3159–3168, 1984

57. Sax K: Chromosome aberrations induced by x-rays. Genetics 23:494–516, 1938

58. Lea DE: Actions of Radiations on Living Cells, 2nd ed. Cambridge, University Press, 1955

59. Lloyd DC, Purrott RJ, Dolphin GW et al: The relationship between chromosome aberrations and low-LET radiation dose to human lymphocytes. Int J Radiat Biol 28:75–90, 1975

60. Upton AC: Radiobiological effects of low doses: Implications for radiological protection. Radiat Res 71:51–74, 1977

61. Little JB: Influence of noncarcinogenic secondary factors on radiation carcinogenesis. Radiat Res 87:240–250, 1981

62. Land H, Parada LF, Weinberg RA: Tumorigenic conversion of primary embryo fibroblasts require at least two cooperating oncogenes. Nature 304:596–602, 1983

63. Terzaghi-Howe M: Inhibition of carcinogen-altered rat tracheal epithelial cell proliferation by normal epithelial cells in vivo. Carcinogenesis 8:145–150, 1987

64. Upton AC, Randolph ML, Conklin JW: Late effects of fast neutrons and gamma-rays in mice influenced by the dose rate of irradiation: Induction of neoplasia. Radiat Res 41:467–491, 1970

65. Ullrich RL, Storer JB: Influence of gamma radiation on the development of neoplastic disease in mice: III. Dose-rate effects. Radiat Res 80:325–342, 1979

66. Han A, Hill CK, Elkind MM: Repair of cell killing and neoplastic transformation at reduced dose rates of ^{60}Co gamma rays. Cancer Res 40:3328–3332, 1980

67. National Council on Radiation Protection and Measurements (NCRP): Influence of Dose and Its Distribution in Time and Dose-Response Relationships for Low-LET Radiations. NCRP Report No 64. Washington, DC, NCRP, 1980

68. Ullrich RL, Jernigan MC, Satterfield LC et al: Radiation carcinogenesis: Time-dose relationships. Radiat Res 111:179–184, 1987

69. Burns FJ, Vanderlaan M: Split-dose recovery for radiation-induced tumors in rat skin. Int J Radiat Biol 32:135–144, 1977

70. Terzaghi M, Little JB: Oncogenic transformation in vitro after split-dose X-irradiation. Int J Radiat Biol 29:583–587, 1976

71. Miller R, Hall EJ: X-ray dose fractionation and oncogenic transformation in cultured mouse embryo cells. Nature 272:58–60, 1978

72. Borek C: Neoplastic transformation following split doses of X rays. Br J Radiol 52:845–846, 1979

73. Ullrich RL: Tumor induction in BALB/c mice after fractionated or protracted exposures to fission-spectrum neutrons. Radiat Res 97:587–597, 1984

74. Hill CK, Buonaguro FM, Myers CP et al: Fission-spectrum neutrons at reduced dose rates enhance neoplastic transformation. Nature 298:67–69, 1982

75. Taylor AMR, Harnden DG, Arlett CF et al: Ataxia telangiectasia: A human mutation with abnormal radiation sensitivity. Nature 258:427–429, 1975

76. Arlett CF, Lehmann AR: Human disorders showing increased sensitivity to the induction of genetic damage. Annu Rev Genet 12:95–115, 1978

77. Lewis PD, Carr JB, Arlett CF et al: Increased sensitivity to gamma irradiation of skin fibroblasts in Friedrich's ataxia. Lancet 2:474–475, 1979

78. Smith PJ, Paterson MC, Kraemer KH: In vitro radiosensitivity in a patient with dermatomyositis and cancer. Lancet 1:216–217, 1981

79. Sandford KK, Parshad R, Green MH et al: Hypersensitivity to G_2 chromatid radiation damage in familial dysplastic naevus syndrome. Lancet 2:1111–1116, 1987

80. Kersey JH, Spector BD: Immune deficiency disease. In Fraumeni JF Jr (ed): Persons at High Risk of Cancer: An Approach to Cancer Etiology and Control, pp 55–67. New York, Academic Press, 1975

81. Tucker MA, Meadows AJ, Boice JD Jr et al: Cancer risk following treatment of childhood cancer. In Boice JD, Fraumeni JF Jr (eds): Radiation Carcinogenesis: Epidemiology and Biological Significance, pp 211–224. New York, Raven Press, 1984

82. Tokunaga M, Land CE, Yamamoto T et al: Incidence of female breast cancer among atomic bomb survivors, Hiroshima and Nagasaki 1950–80. Radiation Effects Research Foundation Technical Report 15-84. Hiroshima, RERF, 1985

83. Shore RE, Woodard ED, Hempelmann LH: Radiation-induced thyroid cancer. In Boice JD Jr, Fraumeni JF Jr (eds): Radiation Carcinogenesis: Epidemiology and Biological Significance, pp 131–138. New York, Raven Press, 1984

84. Ron E, Modan B: Thyroid and other neoplasms following childhood scalp irradiation. In Boice JD Jr, Fraumeni JF Jr (eds): Radiation Carcinogenesis: Epidemiology and Biological Significance, pp 139–151. New York, Raven Press, 1984

85. Kim JH, Chu FC, Woodard MR et al: Radiation-induced soft-tissue and bone sarcoma. Radiology 129:501–508, 1978

86. Land CE: Temporal distributions of risk for radiation-induced cancers. J Chronic Dis 40(suppl 2):45S–57S, 1987

87. Smith PG, Doll R: Mortality among patients with ankylosing spondylitis after a single treatment course with x-rays. Br Med J 284:449–460, 1982

88. Day NE: Radiation and multistage carcinogenesis. In Boice JD Jr, Fraumeni JF Jr (eds): Radiation Carcinogenesis: Epidemiology and Biological Significance, pp 437–443. New York, Raven Press, 1984

89. Gilbert E: Health effects model for nuclear power plant accident consequence analysis. In Evans JS, Moeller DW, Cooper DW (eds): NUREG/CR-414. Washington, DC, U.S. Government Printing Office, 1985

90. Storer JB, Mitchell TJ, Fry RJM: Extrapolation of the relative risk of radiogenic neoplasms across mouse strains and to man. Radiat Res 114:331–353, 1988

91. United Nations Scientific Committee on the Effects of Atomic Radiation: 1982 Report to the General Assembly with Annexes, United Nations, 1982

92. Fawkes FGR, Davies ER, Evans KT et al: Multicenter trial of four strategies to reduce use of a radiological test. Lancet 1:367–369, 1986

93. Harwood AR, Yaffe M: Cancer in man after diagnostic or therapeutic irradiation. In Penn I (ed): Cancer Surveys, vol 1, pp 703–731. Oxford, Oxford University Press, 1982

94. Evans JS, Wennberg JE, McNeil BJ: The influence of diagnostic radiography on the incidence of breast cancer and leukemia. N Engl J Med 315:810–815, 1986

95. Howe GR: Epidemiology of radiogenic breast cancer. In Boice JD Jr, Fraumeni JF Jr (eds): Radiation Carcinogenesis: Epidemiology and Biological Significance, pp 119–129. New York, Raven Press, 1984

96. Smith PG, Doll R: Mortality among patients with ankylosing spondylitis after a single treatment course with x rays. Br Med J 284:449–460, 1982

97. Shore RE, Albert RE, Reed M et al: Skin cancer incidence among children irradiated for ringworm of the scalp. Radiat Res 100:192–204, 1984

98. Shore RE, Woodard E, Hildreth N et al: Thyroid tumors following thymus irradiation. JNCI 74:1177–1184, 1985

99. Shore RE, Woodard E, Dvoretsky P et al: Breast cancer among women given x-ray therapy for acute post partum mastitis. JNCI 77:689–696, 1986

100. Schneider AB, Shore RE, Freedman E et al: Radiation-induced thyroid and other head and neck tumors: Occurrence of multiple tumors and analysis of risk factors. J Clin Endocrinol Metab 63:107–112, 1986

101. Lineletof B, Eklund G: Incidence of malignant skin tumors in 14,140 patients after Grenz-ray treatment for benign skin disorders. Arch Dermatol 122:1391–1395, 1986

102. van Vloten WA, Hermans J, van Daal WAJ: Radiation-induced skin cancer and radiodermatitis of the head and neck. Cancer 59:411–414, 1987

103. Ron E, Modan B, Boice JD Jr: Mortality following radiotherapy for ringworm of the scalp. Am J Epidemiol 127:713–725, 1988

104. Tucker MA, D'Angio GJ, Boice JD Jr et al: Bone sarcomas linked to radiotherapy and chemotherapy in children. N Engl J Med 317:588–593, 1987

105. Griem ML, Justman J, Weiss L: The neoplastic potential of gastric irradiation: IV. Risk estimates. Am J Clin Oncol 7:675–677, 1984

106. Coleman CN: Secondary neoplasms in patients treated for cancer: Etiology and perspective. Radiat Res 92:188–200, 1982

107. Tucker MA, Meadows AT, Boice JD Jr et al: Leukemia after therapy with alkylating agents for childhood cancers. JNCI 78:459–464, 1987

108. Stern RS, Thibodeau LA, Kleinerman RA et al: Risk of cutaneous carcinoma in patients treated with oral methoxsalen photochemotherapy for psoriasis. N Engl J Med 300:809–813, 1979

109. Weinberg RA: The action of oncogenes in the cytoplasm and nucleus. Science 230:770–776, 1985

110. Klein G, Klein J: Evolution of tumors and the impact of molecular oncology. Nature (London) 315:190–195, 1985

111. Lloyd DC, Purrott RJ, Dolphin GW: Chromosome aberrations induced in human lymphocytes by neutron irradiation. Int J Radiat Biol 29:169–182, 1976

112. Le Beau MM, Rowley JD: Chromosomal abnormalities in leukemia and lymphoma: Clinical and biological significance. Adv Hum Genet 15:1–54, 1986

113. Guerrero I, Calzava P, Mayer A et al: A molecular approach to leukemogenesis: Mouse lymphomas contain an activated c-ras oncogene. Proc Natl Acad Sci USA 81:202–205, 1984

114. Sawey MJ, Hood AT, Burns FJ et al: Activation of c-myc and c-K-ras oncogenes in primary rat tumors induced by ionizing radiation. Mol Cell Biol 7:932–935, 1987

115. Borek C, Ong A, Mason H: Distinctive transforming genes in x-ray–transformed mammalian cells. Proc Natl Acad Sci USA 84:794–798, 1987

116. Scotto J, Fraumeni JF Jr: Skin (other than melanoma). In Schottenfeld D, Fraumeni JF Jr (eds): Cancer Epidemiology and Prevention, pp 996–1011. Philadelphia, WB Saunders, 1982

117. Magnus K: Incidence of malignant melanoma of the skin in the five Nordic countries: Significance of solar radiation. Int J Cancer 20:477–485, 1977

118. Fitzpatrick TB, Sober AJ: Sunlight and skin cancer. N Engl J Med 313:818–819, 1985
119. Scotto J, Fears TR: The association of solar ultraviolet and skin melanoma incidence among Caucasians in the United States. Cancer Invest 5:275–283, 1987
120. Carter LJ: The global environment: MIT study looks for danger signals. Science 169:660–662, 1970
121. Johnston H: Reduction of stratospheric ozone by nitrogen oxide catalysts from supersonic transport exhaust. Science 173:517–522, 1971
122. Cutchis P: Stratospheric ozone depletion and solar ultraviolet radiation on earth. Science 184:13, 1974
123. National Research Council: Causes and effects of changes in stratospheric ozone: Update 1983. Washington, DC, National Academy Press, 1984
124. Prather MJ, McElroy MB, Wofsy SC: Reductions in ozone at high concentrations of stratospheric halogens. Nature 312:227–231, 1984
125. Farman JC, Gardiner BG, Shanklin JD: Large losses of total ozone in Antarctica reveal seasonal C10$_x$/NO$_x$ interaction. Nature 315:207–210, 1985
126. Solomon S, Garcia RR, Rowland FS et al: On the depletion of Antarctic ozone. Nature 321:755–758, 1986
127. Scotto J, Cotton G, Urbach F et al: Science 239:762–764, 1988
128. Houghton A, Munster EW, Viola MV: Increased incidence of malignant melanoma after peaks of sunspot activity. Lancet 1:759–760, 1978
129. Urbach F (ed): The Biologic Effects of Ultraviolet Radiation. Oxford, Pergamon Press, 1969
130. Findlay GH: Ultraviolet light and skin cancer. Lancet 2:1070–1073, 1928
131. Roffo AH: Cancer et soleil carcinomas provogues par l'action du soleil in toto. Bull Assoc Franc Etude Cancer 23:590–592, 1934
132. Doniger J, Jacobson ED, Krell K et al: Ultraviolet light action spectra for neoplastic transformation and lethality of Syrian hamster embryo cells correlate with spectrum for pyrimidine dimer formation in cellular DNA. Proc Natl Acad Sci USA 78:2378–2382, 1981
133. Sutherland BM, Delihas NC, Oliver RP et al: Action spectra for ultraviolet light-induced transformation of human cells to anchorage-independent growth. Cancer Res 41:2211–2214, 1981
134. Sutherland BM, Cimino JS, Delihas N et al: Ultraviolet light-induced transformation of human cells to anchorage-independent growth. Cancer Res 40:1934–1939, 1980
135. Hart RW, Setlow RB, Woodhead AD: Evidence that pyrimidine dimers in DNA can give rise to tumors. Proc Natl Acad Sci USA 75:5574–5578, 1977
136. Ley RD, Applegate LA, Fry RJM et al: UVA/visible light suppression of ultraviolet radiation-induced skin and eye tumors of the marsupial Monodelphis domestica. Photochem Photobiol 47:45S, 1988
137. Cleaver JE: Xeroderma pigmentosum. In Stanbury JB, Wyngaarden JB, Fredrickson DS et al (eds): The Metabolic Basis of Inherited Disease, pp 1227–1248. New York, McGraw-Hill, 1983
138. Kripke ML: Immunologic mechanisms in UV radiation carcinogenesis. Adv Cancer Res 34:69–106, 1981
139. Parrish JA (ed): The effect of ultraviolet radiation on the immune system. Skillman, NJ, Johnson & Johnson, 1983
140. Robbins JH, Kraemer KH, Lutzner MA et al: Xeroderma pigmentosum: An inherited disease with sun sensitivity, multiple cutaneous neoplasms and abnormal repair. Ann Intern Med 80:221–248, 1974
141. Kraemer K, Lee MM, Scotto J: Xeroderma pigmentosum: Cutaneous, ocular and neurological abnormalities in 830 published cases. Arch Dermatol 123:241–250, 1987
142. Hashem N, Bootsma D, Keijzer W et al: Clinical characteristics, DNA repair, and complementation groups in xeroderma pigmentosum patients from Egypt. Cancer Res 40:13–18, 1980
143. Hebra F, Kaposi M: On Diseases of the Skin Including the Exanthemata, vol 3, pp 252–258 (Tay W, trans). London, New Sydenham Society, 1974
144. Taylor RN: A further contribution to the study of xeroderma of Hebra. Trans Am Dermatol Assoc 37:37–46, 1979
145. de Sanctis C, Cacchione A: L'idiozia xerodermica. Riv Sper Freniatr 56:269–292, 1932
146. Haxthausen H, Hausmann N: Die Lichterkrankugen der Haut. Vienna, Urban und Schwartzenberg, 1929
147. Swift M, Chase C: Cancer in families with xeroderma pigmentosum. JNCI 62:1415–1421, 1979
148. Cleaver JE: Defective repair replication of DNA in xeroderma pigmentosum. Nature 218:652–656, 1968
149. deWeerd-Kastelein EA, Keijzer W, Bootsma D: Genetic heterogeneity of xeroderma pigmentosum demonstrated by somatic cell hybridization. Nature 238:80–83, 1972
150. Kraemer KH, Coon HG, Pettiga RA et al: Genetic heterogeneity in xeroderma pigmentosum complementation groups and their relationship to DNA repair rates. Proc Natl Acad Sci USA 72:59–63, 1975
151. Kraemer KH, deWeerd-Kastelein EA, Robbins JH et al: Five complementation groups in xeroderma pigmentosum. Mutat Res 33:327–340, 1975
152. Jung EG: New form of molecular defect in xeroderma pigmentosum. Nature 228:361–362, 1970
153. Burk PG, Lutzner MA, Clarke DD et al: Ultraviolet-stimulated thymidine incorporation in xeroderma pigmentosum lymphocytes. J Lab Clin Med 77:759–767, 1971
154. Cleaver JE: Xeroderma pigmentosum: Variants with normal DNA repair and normal sensitivity to ultraviolet light. J Invest Dermatol 58:124–128, 1972
155. Maher VM, Ouelette LM, Curren RD et al: Frequency of ultraviolet light–induced mutations is higher in xeroderma pigmentosum variant cells. Nature 261:593–595, 1976
156. Wolff S, Bodycote J, Thomas GH et al: Sister chromatid exchange in xeroderma pigmentosum cells that are defective in DNA excision repair or post-replication repair. Genetics 81:349–355, 1975
157. German J, Gilleran TG, Setlow RB et al: Mutant karyotypes in cultures of cells from a man with xeroderma pigmentosum. Ann Genet 16:23–27, 1973
158. Parrington JM, Delhanty JDA, Baden HP: Unscheduled DNA synthesis: UV-induced chromosome aberrations and SV40 transformation in cultured cells from xeroderma pigmentosum. Ann Hum Genet 35:149–160, 1971
159. Huang CC, Benerjee A, Hou Y: Chromosomal instability in cell lines derived from patients with xeroderma pigmentosum. Proc Soc Exp Biol Med 148:1244–1248, 1975
160. deWeerd-Kastelein EA, Keijzer W, Rainaldi G et al: Induction of sister chromatid exchanges in xeroderma pigmentosum cells after exposure to ultraviolet light. Mutat Res 45:253–261, 1977
161. Wolff S, Rodin B, Cleaver JE: Sister chromatid exchanges induced by mutagenic carcinogens in normal and xeroderma pigmentosum cells. Nature 265:347–349, 1977
162. Kraemer KH, Slor H, Andrews A: A new form of xeroderma pigmentosum: Reduced repair without neoplasia (abstr). J Invest Dermatol 80:331, 1983
163. Turner FC: Sarcomas at sites of subcutaneously implanted Bakelite disks in rats. JNCI 2:81–83, 1941
164. Oppenheimer BS, Oppenheimer ET, Stout AP: Sarcomas induced in rats by implanting cellophane. Proc Soc Exp Biol Med 67:33–34, 1948
165. Bischoff F, Bryson G: Carcinogenesis through solid state surfaces. Prog Exp Tumor Res 5:86–133, 1964
166. Brand KG: Cancer associated with asbestosis and schistosomiasis foreign bodies and scars. In Becker FF (ed): Cancer: A Comprehensive Treatise, 2nd ed, vol 1, pp 661–692. New York, Plenum Press, 1982
167. Brand I, Buoen LC, Brand KG: Foreign body tumors of mice: Strain and sex differences in latency and incidence. JNCI 58:1443–1447, 1977
168. Brand KG: Solid state carcinogenesis. In Butterworth BE, Slaga TJ (eds). Nongenotoxic Mechanisms in Carcinogenesis. Banbury Report 25. Cold Spring Harbor, New York, Cold Spring Harbor Laboratory, 1987
169. Brues AM, Auerbach H, DeRoche GM et al: Mechanisms of carcinogenesis. In: Argonne National Laboratory, Biological and Medical Research Division Annual Report, ANL 7535, pp 28–30. Argonne, IL, ANL, 1968
170. Nicholson WJ, Perbep G, Selikoff IJ: Occupational exposure to asbestos: Population at risk and projected mortality. Am J Ind Med 3:259–311, 1987
171. Doll R, Peto J: Effects on health of exposure to asbestos. Health and Sujet Commission Report. London, Her Majesty's Stationery Office, 1985
172. Wagner JC (ed): Biological Effects of Mineral Fibers, vols. I and II. IARC Scientific Publications No 30. Lyon, World Health Organization, 1980
173. Harrington JS: Fiber carcinogenesis: Epidemiologic observations and the Stanton hypothesis. JNCI 67:977–989, 1981
174. Leineweber JP: Dust chemistry and physics: Mineral and vitreous fibers. In Wagner JC (ed): Biological Effects of Mineral Fibers, vol 2, pp 881–900. IARC Scientific Publications No. 30. Lyon, World Health Organization, 1980
175. Baris YI, Sahin AA, Ozesmi M et al: An outbreak of pleural mesothelioma and chronic fibrosing pleurisy in the village of Karan/Urgup in Anatolia. Thorax 33:181–192, 1978
176. Omenn GS, Merchant J, Boatman E et al: Contribution of environmental fibers to respiratory cancer. Environ Health Perspect 70:51–56, 1986
177. Harrington JS, Allison AC, Badami DV: Mineral fibers: Chemical, physicochemical and biological properties. Adv Pharmacol Chemother 17:291–402, 1975
178. Stanton MF, Layara M, Tegeris A et al: Relation of particle dimension to carcinogenicity in amphibole asbestosis and other fibrous minerals. JNCI 67:965–975, 1981
179. Selikoff IJ (ed): Cancer from Occupational Asbestos Exposure. Projections 1965–2030. Disability Compensation for Asbestos-Associated Disease in the United States. New York, Environmental Sciences Laboratory, Mount Sinai School of Medicine of the City University, 1982
180. Peto J, Seidman H, Selikoff IJ: Mesothelioma mortality in asbestos workers: Implications for models of carcinogenesis and risk assessment. Br J Cancer 45:124, 1982
181. Hesterberg TW, Butterich CJ, Oshimura M et al: Role of phagocytosis in Syrian hamster cell transformation and cytogenetic effects induced by asbestos and short and long glass fibers. Cancer Res 46:5795–5802, 1986
182. Hesterberg TW, Barrett JC: Dependence of asbestos and mineral dust-induced transformation of mammalian cells in culture on fiber dimension. Cancer Res 44:2170–2180, 1984
183. Hesterberg TW, Barrett JC: Induction of asbestos fibers of anaphase abnormalities: Mechanism for aneuploidy induction and possibly carcinogenesis. Carcinogenesis 6:473–475, 1985
184. Oshimura M, Hesterberg TW, Tsutsui T et al: Correlation of asbestos-induced cytogenetic effects with cell transformation of Syrian hamster embryo cells in culture. Cancer Res 44:5017–5022, 1984
185. Oshimura M, Hesterberg TW, Barrett JC: An early nonrandom karyotypic change in immortal Syrian hamster cell lines transformed by asbestos: Trisomy of chromosome 11. Cancer Genet Cytogenet 22:225–237, 1986
186. Hei TK, Geard CR, Osmak RS et al: Correlation of in vitro genotoxicity and oncogenicity induced by radiation and asbestos fibres. Br J Cancer 52:591–597, 1985

PETER M. HOWLEY

CHAPTER 10   *Principles of Carcinogenesis: Viral*

Viral oncology has its foundations in observations made at the turn of the century defining the transmissibility of avian leukemia in Denmark, in 1908, and of an avian sarcoma in chickens, in 1911.[1,2] These important discoveries were not appreciated at the time, and their impact on virology and medicine was not recognized for decades. The work of Peyton Rous,[2] who showed that cell-free extracts from a sarcoma in chickens could induce tumors in injected chickens within a few weeks, even when passed through filters that retained bacteria, was finally recognized and led to a Nobel prize in 1966. Rous's original work demonstrated that the infectious agent was not only capable of inducing tumors, but also imprinted the phenotypic characteristics of the original tumor on the recipient transformed cell. At the time Rous's work was relegated to the ranks of avian curiosities, and its importance was not recognized for several decades.

In the 1930s Richard Shope published a series of papers on cell-free transmission of tumors in rabbits. The first studies involved fibromatous tumors, found in the footpads of wild cottontail rabbits, that could be transmitted by injecting cell-free extracts into either wild or domestic rabbits.[3] Subsequent studies have shown that this virus, now referred to as the Shope fibroma virus, is a pox virus. Additional studies carried out by Shope demonstrated that cutaneous papillomatosis in wild cottontail rabbits could also be transmitted by cell-free extracts. He also observed, as did Peyton Rous, that in a number of cases these benign papillomas would progress spontaneously into squamous cell carcinomas in infected domestic rabbits or in the infected cottontail rabbits.[4,5] In general, however, the field of viral oncology lay stagnant until

the early 1950s with the discovery of the murine leukemia viruses by Ludwig Gross[6] and of the mouse polyomavirus by Gross, Stewart, and Eddy.[7,8] At this point in the 1950s many cancer researchers and virologists turned to the field of viral oncology, hoping that the initial observations in mammals could be extended to humans and that a fair proportion of human tumors might also be found to have a viral etiology. The Special Viral Cancer Program at the National Cancer Institute grew out of this intense interest in viral oncology and the speculation that human tumor viruses would be identified.

Many of the most important developments in modern molecular biology, including the discovery of reverse transcriptase, the development of recombinant DNA technology, the discovery of mRNA splicing, and the discovery of oncogenes, derived directly from studies in viral oncology conducted in the 1960s and 1970s. Oncogenes were first recognized as cellular genes that had been acquired by retroviruses through some type of recombinational process that converted them into acute transforming RNA tumor viruses. It is now known that oncogenes participate in many different types of tumors and can be involved at different stages of tumorigenesis and viral oncology. This has contributed significantly to our concepts of nonviral carcinogenesis. It is likely that the direct transforming, oncogene-transducing retroviruses do not play a major causative role in naturally occurring cancers in animals or in humans, but rather represent laboratory-generated recombinants. A list of human viruses with oncogenic properties is given in Table 10-1. This list includes viruses such as the transforming adenoviruses, which are capable of

TABLE 10-1. Human Viruses with Oncogenic Properties

Virus Family	Type	Human Tumor	Cofactors
Adenovirus	Types 2, 5, 12	None	. . .
Hepadnavirus	Hepatitis B (HBV)	Hepatocellular carcinoma	Aflatoxin, alcohol, smoking
Herpesvirus	Epstein-Barr (EBV)	Burkitt's lymphoma	Marlaria
		Immunoblastic lymphoma	Immunodeficiency
		Nasopharyngeal carcinoma	Nitrosamines, HLA genotype
Papillomaviruses	HPV-16, 18, 33, 39	Cervical neoplasia	Smoking, ?HSV
	HPV-5, 8, 17	Skin cancer	Genetic disorders, sunlight
Polyomavirus	BK, JC	?Neural tumors	
		?Insulinomas	
Retroviruses	HTLV-1	Adult T-cell leukemia-lymphoma	Uncertain
	HTLV-2	Hairy cell leukemia	Unknown

transforming normal cells into malignant cells in the laboratory but have not been associated with any known human tumors. The list also includes viruses such as the papillomaviruses that have been etiologically associated with specific human cancers and have been shown to encode transforming viral oncogenes. Finally, Table 10-1 includes viruses such as the hepatitis B virus that have been closely linked with specific human tumors but have not been shown to encode a viral oncogene. This chapter focuses on viruses that have been associated with specific human cancers and considers their biology and pertinent molecular biology. The evidence for the association of each of these viruses with specific types of human neoplasia is presented, and the mechanisms by which these viruses may contribute to malignant transformation are discussed.

Also listed in Table 10-1 are cofactors believed to be important in the carcinogenic processes associated with the different viruses. It is clear that none of these viruses alone is sufficient for the induction of the specific neoplasias with which it has been associated. Rather, the viruses associated with human cancers are thought to be involved at an early step in carcinogenesis. Subsequent cellular events such as somatic mutations are thought to be important at the subsequent multiple steps involved in malignant progression.

HUMAN RETROVIRUSES

The first tumor viruses described were both retroviruses. These were the avian leukemia virus, described by Ellermann and Bang in 1908,[1] and the avian sarcoma virus, described by Peyton Rous in 1911.[2] Among the tumor viruses, the retroviruses have been a primary subject of research by virologists, oncologists, and molecular biologists. In the past two decades studies with the retroviruses have provided us with reverse transcriptase and oncogenes, and retroviruses have recently been engineered into vectors for the effective delivery of DNA to cells for gene therapy. Interest in viruses as infectious tumor agents was spurred by the findings of Ludwig Gross in the 1950s when he described retroviruses that caused tumors in mice.[6,7] In the early 1960s William

Jarrett discovered the feline leukemia virus (FeLV), which was capable of inducing leukemia as well as aplasia in cats.[9] Subsequent studies established that the leukemia associated with FeLV could be communicated in the natural setting and was not limited to the laboratory. This provided a major impetus to the search for retroviruses as possible tumor viruses causing leukemia in humans. In the retroviruses associated with animal leukemia in chickens, mice, and cats there is extensive viral replication and the virus particles often can be readily visualized with electron microscopy.[10] The studies of the late 1960s through the 1970s that sought human retroviruses in human blood disorders relied heavily on electron microscopy for evidence of such viruses.

As had been shown in 1970 by the Nobel Prize-winning experiments of Howard Temin and David Baltimore, retroviruses contain enzymes called reverse transcriptase which are involved in transcribing the single-stranded RNA copy of the input viral RNA into DNA.[11,12] This enzymatic activity is associated with retrovirus particles and can be readily assayed from infected cells. Thus, assays for reverse transcriptase activities, which are unique to retroviruses, provided an alternative assay for these viruses that was more sensitive to electron microscopy. The first unequivocal evidence of a human retrovirus, HTLV-1, came almost 70 years after Rous's initial description of the avian sarcoma virus.

HUMAN T-CELL LYMPHADENOTROPIC VIRUS TYPE 1

The first substantiated reports of a human retrovirus were published in 1980 and 1981 by Robert Gallo and his colleagues,[13,14] followed in 1982 by reports by Yoshida and his colleagues in Japan.[15] The viral isolates were from T-cell leukemia in humans. The first isolate from Gallo's laboratory was from a patient with a T-cell leukemia and skin abnormalities similar to those seen in mycosis fungoides or Sézary syndrome. Subsequent analysis of other patients with mycosis fungoides and the Sézary syndrome revealed that only a small proportion of such patients had evidence of HTLV-1. The patient studied by Gallo et al was found to have a form of T-cell leukemia known as adult T-cell leukemia (ATL), which differs from mycosis fungoides. ATL, first described in 1977 by Kiyoshi Takatsuki and colleagues of Kyoto University,[16] is endemic in Kyushu and Shikoku, the southernmost islands of Japan; and it was from a case of ATL that the first Japanese isolate of the human retrovirus initially referred to as the adult T-cell leukemia virus was isolated.[15,17] Subsequent studies established that Gallo's initial isolate of HTLV-1 and the ATL virus were identical,[18,19] and by convention the virus is now referred to as HTLV-1.

ATL is a malignancy of mature T4+ lymphocytes.[20] It is endemic in parts of Japan[21] as well as in the Caribbean and in parts of Africa.[22,23] The tumor resembles mycosis fungoides and Sézary syndrome but is more aggressive than these two syndromes. Median survival from the time of diagnosis is only 3 to 4 months. The disease affects visceral organs as well as the skin, and often induces hypercalcemia. The isolation in Gallo's laboratory of HTLV-1 from a leukemia cell line was a consequence and extension of the basic research performed in that laboratory identifying a T-cell growth factor (now referred to as interleukin-2, or IL-2).[24] IL-2 is released by T-cells following stimulation with phytohemagglutinin (PHA), which stimulates T-cells to proliferate. PHA-activated T-cells not only secrete IL-2 but also develop receptor molecules on their surface for the growth factor molecules. With IL-2 bound to its receptor, the cells begin to divide. The characterization and isolation of IL-2 permitted investigators in Gallo's laboratory to grow the human leukemic cells indefinitely and eventually to identify the first human retrovirus.

After the isolation of HTLV-1, immunologic assays were developed to detect antibodies specific for the viral antigens. Such serologic assays became the basis for subsequent epidemiologic and transmission studies. Studies revealed that the viral infection was more common in endemic areas than were malignancies.[21] Less than 1% of seropositive patients ever develop ATL. A preleukemic disease in the form of a chronic lymphocytosis is often seen before the development of acute leukemia or lymphoma.[25]

Although retroviruses are often referred to as leukemia viruses, the spectrum of diseases with which they are associated is not limited to leukemia. Of the animal viruses, the avian leukemia viruses are also associated with an autoimmune wasting disease and osteoporosis. The feline leukemia viruses can be associated with anemia, aplasia, and immunodeficiency. Certain mouse leukemia viruses can induce paralysis and neuropathies. Similarly, HTLV-1 infection in humans has been associated with diseases other than ATL. HTLV-1 has been associated with an increased susceptibility to opportunistic infections as well as with a degenerative neurologic disease. In West Indian patients this disease is referred to as tropical spastic paraparesis,[26,27] and a similar disease in Japan known as HAM (HTLV-I associated myelopathy).[28] Specific risk factors that may be important in determining the development of leukemia, immunodeficiency, or tropical spastic paraparesis in HTLV-1–infected individuals currently are not known.

HUMAN T-CELL LYMPHADENOTROPIC VIRUS TYPE 2

The second human retrovirus, HTLV-2 was described in a cell line established from a patient with an unusual form of hairy cell leukemia.[29] Morphologically the cells of HTLV-2 resemble those of a hairy cell leukemia; however, they contain markers of a T-cell lineage, whereas most hairy cell leukemia cells contain B-cell markers. Unlike HTLV-1, HTLV-2 has not yet been found to be endemic in any specific population of humans. Its association with hairy cell leukemia is somewhat tenuous, although strengthened recently by several other cases of HTLV-2 seropositive T-cell variants of hairy cell leukemia and the isolation of a second HTLV-2 isolate from such a patient.[30] HTLV-2 is distinct from HTLV-1 but shares considerable nucleic acid homology.[31,32]

HUMAN IMMUNODEFICIENCY VIRUS

The human immunodeficiency viruses, HIV-1 and HIV-2, are human retroviruses of the subclass Lentiviridae.[33] Initially referred to as HTLVs, they are now recognized to be distinct viruses. Like HTLV-1 and HTLV-2, the HIVs also infect T4+ cells; in other respects the viruses are not closely related. HIV-1 and HIV-2 are associated with the acquired immune deficiency syndrome (AIDS) but do not appear to directly cause any specific human tumors. However, patients with AIDS have a high incidence of specific tumors.[34] One of the earliest diagnostic features of AIDs in young homosexual men may be Kaposi's sarcoma, which before the AIDs epidemic was regarded as an extremely rare tumor. Other tumors for which AIDS patients are at high relative risk are non-Hodgkin's lymphomas, anogenital warts, and papillomavirus-associated squamous cell carcinomas. In AIDS patients these tumors likely have a viral etiology. The lymphomas may be largely accounted for by the emergence of cells transformed by the Epstein-Barr virus and progressing to malignancy. It is also possible that HTLV-1 may account for some lymphomas in patients with AIDs. The genital warts and perianal squamous cell carcinomas seen in these patients have been shown to harbor specific human papillomavirus DNA types (see below). A viral etiology for Kaposi's sarcoma has been postulated, but no candidate virus has yet been identified.

THE MECHANISM OF TRANSFORMATION

Only a subset of individuals seropositive for HTLV-1 will develop ATL. The virus is not acquired by casual contact but is transmitted through sexual contact, through transfusion of contaminated blood, and possibly from mother to infant through mother's milk.[35-37] The latency period between acquisition of the virus to development of ATL can vary from a few years to as long as 40 years in patients who are destined to develop the malignancy.

How is HTLV-1 involved in leukemogenesis? Several lines of evidence suggest that the virus's role is quite direct. The first is epidemiologic. Infants born in an endemic area who have been infected have the same likelihood of developing ATL if they remain in the endemic area or if they move to an area of low prevalence. Thus it appears that the virus alone is sufficient to initiate the chain of events leading to malignancy, independent of subsequent environmental factors.

Additional evidence supporting the role of HTLV-1 as an etiologic agent in ATL comes from the molecular biology of the virus. In retrovirus-infected cells the provirus (*i.e.,* the double-stranded DNA copy of the viral RNA genome) becomes integrated into the cellular genome. Within HTLV-1–infected cells, the provirus is also randomly integrated into the host chromosome.[38] In the leukemic cells of an ATL patient, however, the viral sequences are found integrated in the same place in each cell, and the site of integration varies from leukemia to leukemia.[39,40] This indicates that ATL is clonal and is derived from a single cell. It also indicates that the viral infection necessarily precedes the origin of the tumor.

HTLV-1 can transform human umbilical cord blood lymphocytes (T-cells) from normal cells into immortalized precancerous cells.[41,42] The mechanism by which HTLV-1 induces leukemogenesis is different from that of the other chronic leukemia retroviruses such as the avian leukosis virus. The combination of the clonality of the tumor cells and the random nature of the integration sites of the provirus from tumor to tumor indicates that HTLV-1 transforms by a novel mechanism for retroviruses. Prior to the detailed studies of HTLV-1, two mechanisms were known by which a retrovirus could induce malignancy. One mechanism involved the transduction of oncogene directly by the retrovirus. Oncogenes are cellular genes often involved in the regulation of cellular growth. For example, the avian sarcoma virus is capable of inducing tumors in chickens because it has acquired extra nucleic acids from a cellular oncogene called *sarc*. Retroviruses containing an oncogene are themselves defective but give rise to a rapidly developing cancer following infection of the appropriate cell. The tumors that result from infection with a retrovirus containing an oncogene are not necessarily monoclonal. The genetic events leading to the recombinational events between the cellular and viral nucleic acids are rare, and these viruses are of importance to the molecular virologist but are of little consequence to the etiology of naturally occurring cancers in humans or animals.

The slow-acting leukemogenic retroviruses such as the feline leukemia virus (FeLV) and the mouse leukemia virus (MuLV) do not contain oncogenes, and they induce leukemia in a manner similar to the HTLV-1–associated human malignancies, in which only a minority of the infected animals develop leukemia. There is also a long latency period between acquisition of the virus and the formation of tumors. In addition, the tumors are clonal. The difference between the mechanisms of leukemogenesis of these slow-acting leukemogenic retroviruses and of HTLV-1 is that although the provirus integrates randomly into the cellular chromosomes in infected cells, it is found preferentially in the vicinity of proto-oncogenes in the tumors that develop. For the slow-acting leukemogenic viruses to induce malignancy, the provirus must integrate in a region of the host genome in a manner that enables the regulatory sequences of the provirus to interact with the nearby oncogene to promote cellular proliferation. The mechanism by which this occurs is referred to as promoter insertion if the proviral long terminal repeat (LTR) acts as a promoter to initiate transcription of the proto-oncogene, or enhancer insertion if it acts as an enhancer to activate the proto-oncogene. In the case of the avian leukosis virus, the integration of the retrovirus occurs in the vicinity of the c-*myc* oncogene, resulting in the deregulation of its expression.[43]

The HTLV-1 provirus can therefore act at a distance. This suggests that the viral genome encodes a factor that is critical in the early stages of leukemogenesis. HTLV-1 and HTLV-2 belong to a distinct group of retroviruses that have been referred to as transregulating retroviruses. This group also includes the bovine leukemia virus, the biology of which is somewhat similar to that of HTLV-1 and HTLV-2.[44] As shown in Figure 10-1, these viruses differ from the chronic leukemia viruses and the acute leukemia viruses in that they contain additional genomic sequences at the 3' end of the genome, originally called the X region by Yoshida et al, who first brought attention to it.[45] Subsequent studies from a number of laboratories have indicated that this region encodes transregulatory factors.[46–49] There appear to be several small regulatory proteins encoded by this region.[50] One gene serves as a master key for activating transcription from the viral LTR and is called the TAT gene, for transactivator of transcription. The TAT gene product acts to increase the transcriptional activity of the viral promoter in the LTR.[48,51,52]

In addition the TAT gene product has been shown to activate transcription of some nonviral genes, including the IL-2 gene and IL-2 receptor.[53] Thus it seems possible that one mechanism by which HTLV-1 could induce cellular prolifer-

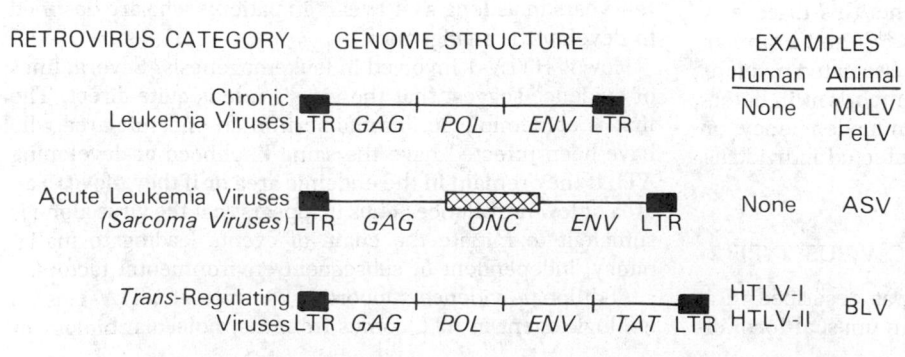

RETROVIRUS CATEGORY   GENOME STRUCTURE

Chronic Leukemia Viruses — LTR GAG POL ENV LTR

Acute Leukemia Viruses (Sarcoma Viruses) — LTR GAG ONC ENV LTR

Trans-Regulating Viruses — LTR GAG POL ENV TAT LTR

EXAMPLES	
Human	Animal
None	MuLV FeLV
None	ASV
HTLV-I HTLV-II	BLV

FIG. 10-1. Genomic organization of different types of retroviruses. The prototype retrovirus represented in the figure by the chronic leukemia viruses contains regulatory sequences at each end derived from the long terminal repeat (LTR) elements of the virus as well as coding sequences for the viral proteins *gag, pol,* and *env*. The acute transforming retroviruses are defective viruses. In addition to losing viral gene segments, they have acquired *onc* sequences from the cellular genome. The transregulatory retroviruses contain sequences, 3' to the *env* gene, that encode regulatory factors. This region has been referred to as the X region and encodes the TAT gene among other regulatory factors.

ation and immortalization could involve the stimulation of both IL-2 and its receptor. The mechanism by which the TAT gene functions is not yet clear. It does not appear to be a direct DNA-binding protein;[54] therefore it does not activate either the viral LTR or the specific cellular genes by direct DNA binding. It most likely acts indirectly by modifying other cellular transcription factors.

HEPATITIS B VIRUS

Hepatitis B virus (HBV) causes hepatitis B infection, a major worldwide public health problem. In endemic parts of the world such as Far East Asia and tropical Africa, approximately 10% of the population are chronic carriers of HBV, and in these areas, chronic active hepatitis and liver cirrhosis associated with HBV infection are the major causes of mortality. Furthermore, HBV has been shown by epidemiologic studies to be of major importance in the etiology of hepatocellular carcinoma (HCC).[55] In China alone, one-half million to one million cases of HCC occur annually.

HBV is a member of a group of animal viruses known as the hepadnaviruses. It is the only member of this group of viruses that has a human reservoir.[56] Other hepadnaviruses include the woodchuck hepatitis virus (WHV), the Beechey ground squirrel hepatitis virus (GSHV), and the Pekin duck hepatitis B virus (DHBV).[57-59] Each of these viruses has a similar structure and each is hepatotropic, leading to persistent viral infections of the liver. Studies of the animal hepatitis viruses have been important in developing our understanding of the molecular biology of the hepadnaviruses. Of the hepadnaviruses, only HBV and WHV have been associated with chronic active hepatitis and HCC.

DISCOVERY

The hepatitis B surface antigen (HBsAg) was discovered in 1963 by Baruch Blumberg and co-workers while studying human serum protein polymorphisms.[60,61] Subsequent studies led to the association of this antigen with acute hepatitis B infection and an intermediate name, hepatitis-associated antigen (HAA), and finally the current name, hepatitis B surface antigen.[62,63] This antigen is the surface or envelope protein of the HBV particle, and its presence in the serum of infected patients remains the most useful marker of active HBV infection.[64] Until recently, HBV had not been successfully grown in tissue culture, and the serum from infected patients became the principal source of viral material for the characterization of the virus.

During an HBV infection, virus particles are present at high titer in the serum: up to 10^5 to 10^9 virions per milliliter are visible by electron microscopy.[65] In addition to the complete virion particles, the serum also contains empty viral envelopes consisting of spherical or filamentous particles 22 nm in diameter.[66] The virion of 42 nm in diameter consists of an envelope and a nucleocapsid containing the double-stranded circular DNA molecule, and the DNA polymerase. This virion particle was first described by Dane[64] and is sometimes referred to as the Dane particle. The outer envelope contains HBsAg, consisting of protein, carbohydrate,

and lipid. The capsid carries the hepatitis B core antigen (HBcAg). The outer envelope of the virion with the HBsAg can be removed by treatment with nonionic detergents such as Nonidet P-40, releasing the free core particles (Fig. 10-2). Treatment of the virion core with a strong detergent such as SDS will then release the double-stranded viral DNA. The serum concentrations of the incomplete viral forms usually greatly exceed the concentrations of the complete virions, and concentrations of up to 10^{13} 22-nm spherical particles have been noted in some human sera.[66] The spectrum of viral forms described for HBV is also found in the serum of animals infected with WHV, GSHV, and DHBV.[57-59]

HBV VIRAL DNA

HBV particles contain small circular DNA molecules that are partially double-stranded.[67,68] The DNA consists of a long strand with a constant length of 3220 bases and a short strand that varies in length from 1700 to 2800 bases in different molecules. A map of the HBV DNA genome is shown in Figure 10-3.[69] The virion particles also contain a DNA polymerase activity that is capable of repairing the single-stranded DNA region to make two fully double-stranded molecules, each approximately 3220 bases long.[70] For this reaction, DNA synthesis initiates at the 3′ end of the short strand, which, as noted earlier, is heterogeneous among different DNA molecules. DNA synthesis terminates when it reaches the uniquely located 5′ end of the short strand. The long strand is not a closed molecule but contains a nick at a unique site approximately 300 base pairs from the 5′ end of the short strand.

Recombinant DNA technology has rapidly advanced our understanding of the biology of HBV. The complete genome

FIG. 10-2. HBV forms in the blood of infected humans (1), the virion core released by nonionic detergent (2), and the viral genome (3). (Redrawn from Robinson.[69])

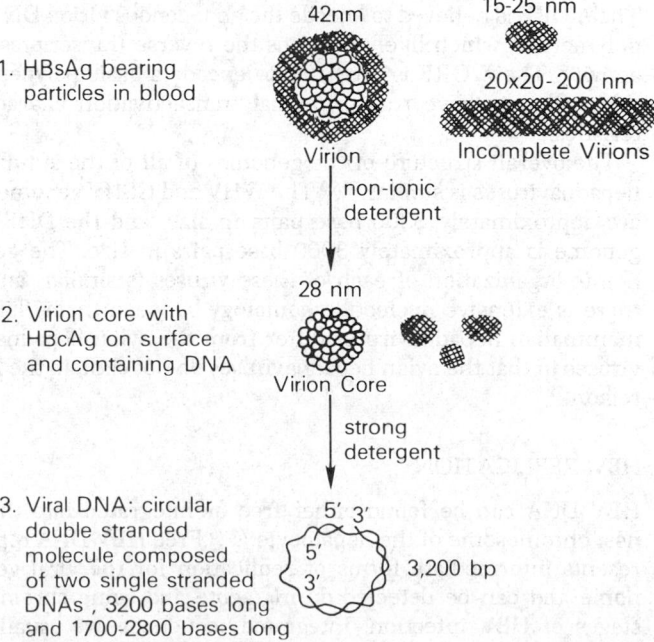

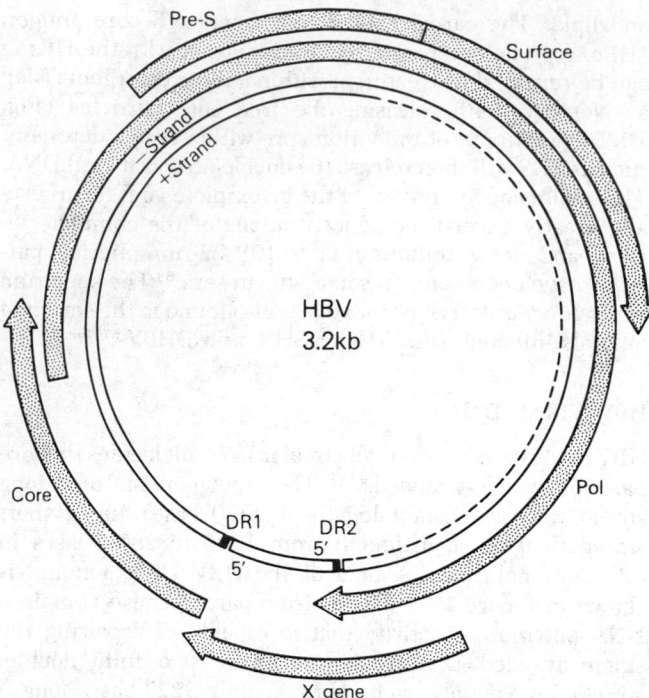

FIG. 10-3. Physical and genetic map of HBV DNA. The arrows surrounding the genome represent the four large open reading frames of the L(−) strand with the genes they encode indicated. The broken line is the S(+) DNA strand. The positions of the 5′ ends of the DNA strands are indicated. The location of the direct repeats (DR1 and DR2) involved in the initiation of DNA replication are also indicated.[72,73]

has been cloned in bacterial cells and the complete nucleotide sequence determined.[71] The viral genome has four open reading frames (ORFs). These ORFs are designated as S and pre-S, C, A, and X.[68,72] S and pre-S represent two contiguous reading frames and code for the HBsAg polypeptides. Region C contains the coding sequences for the core and E antigens. The A ORF is believed to encode the endogenous virion DNA polymerase, which likely contains the reverse transcriptase activity. The X ORF is predicted to encode a basic polypeptide and may have transcriptional transactivation characteristics.

The overall structure of the genomes of all of the animal hepadnaviruses is similar.[72,73] The WHV and GSHV genomes are approximately 3300 base pairs in size, and the DHBV genome is approximately 3000 base pairs in size. The genomic organization of each of these viruses is similar, and there is extensive nucleotide homology between them. The mammalian hepadnaviruses differ from the avian hepadnaviruses in that the avian hepadnaviruses do not contain the X region.[72]

HBV REPLICATION

HBV DNA can be found either free or integrated into the host chromosome of the hepatocyte.[74,75] Free HBV DNA represents intermediate forms of replication for the viral genome and can be detected during acute and some chronic stages of HBV infection. Integrated sequences are usually

found during chronic viral infection and in HCC. The replication mechanism for the hepadnaviruses, first discovered by Summers and Mason for DHBV[76] and later confirmed for HBV, is different from that of other DNA viruses.[73] The replication cycle involves a reverse transcription step resembling that of the retroviruses in that a central feature is the use of an RNA copy of the genome as an intermediate in replication. The hepadnaviruses differ from the retroviruses, however, in that the retrovirus virions contain RNA and the intermediate form of replication is integrated DNA. The virions of the hepadnaviruses contain DNA and the intermediate replication form is RNA. It is thought that integration of the hepadnaviral genome is not a necessary intermediate step for viral genome replication. The similarity between the retroviruses and the hepadnaviruses is also reflected in the genomic organization in which all of the genes are necessarily encoded on only one strand. The order of the genes within the retroviruses (*gag*, *pol*, and *env*) is similar to the order of their counterparts in the hepadnaviruses (core, polymerase, and surface antigen). Other subtle differences in the transcriptional programs utilized to generate the messenger RNAs for these different viruses exist. Of note is that enhancer sequences have been found in both viruses. For the retroviruses, enhancer sequences have been found in the LTRs. For the hepadnavirus, in which no significantly large noncoding region exists, an enhancer element has been found downstream of the S ORF.[77,78] A further similarity between these viruses is the finding that a subset of these viruses encode transcriptional transacting factors. For HTLV-1, described earlier in this chapter, the TAT ORF encodes such a factor. Preliminary evidence from several laboratories indicates that the X gene of the mammalian hepadnaviruses may also encode a factor with transcriptional transactivation functions.

HBV AND HEPATOCELLULAR CARCINOMA

There is considerable evidence of an etiologic involvement of HBV in human HCC. This evidence stems primarily from epidemiologic studies. There is a striking correlation between the worldwide geographic incidence of HCC and the prevalence of HBsAg chronic carriers.[79] Compelling evidence for the role of HBV in HCC comes from the prospective epidemiologic studies performed by Beasley et al in Taiwan and reported in 1981.[55] Those studies revealed that the relative risk for HCC in HBsAg-positive males was 217, compared to the risk in noncarriers. Furthermore, 51% of the deaths in the carriers were caused by cirrhosis of the liver or HCC, compared with only 2% among the control population. Among the noncarriers, 90% had evidence of a prior HBV infection but did not have evidence of HBsAg chronic carrier state. This observation indicated that the high incidence of HCC was clearly related to the carrier state and not to a prior HBV infection per se. The age distribution of HBV infections, which occur at early ages in this Taiwanese population, indicated that the tumors appear after a mean duration of 35 years of HBV infection. Between 60% and 90% of the patients with HCC also had cirrhosis.

These epidemiologic data do not preclude an etiologic role for other factors in HCC, and in fact other factors such as aflatoxin have been recognized as having a role in some cases of liver cancer. However, factors in addition to HBV chronic infection do not need to be implicated in order to explain these striking epidemiologic findings.

HBV infection in humans is not the only hepadnavirus infection associated with HCC in nature. A much higher incidence of hepatoma formation has been observed in woodchucks infected with WHV.[80] Approximately one third of the infected animals held in captivity will develop HCC each year, and no tumors have been observed in noninfected animals. HCC develops in these woodchucks with histologic changes of acute and chronic hepatitis but not in association with cirrhosis.

PAPILLOMAVIRUSES

The viral nature of human warts was first suggested at the turn of the century by Ciuffo, who demonstrated cell-free filtrate transmission.[81] This important group of viruses has remained refractory to standard virologic studies, and no papillomavirus has been successfully propagated in the laboratory in tissue culture. However, advances in basic research through the application of biotechnology have led to a virtual explosion of knowledge concerning the papillomaviruses in the past decade. The molecular cloning of papillomavirus genomic DNA has permitted the generation of sufficient quantities of viral genetic material for systematic investigation of this group of viruses.

BIOLOGY OF HUMAN PAPILLOMAVIRUS INFECTION

The papillomaviruses are widely distributed in nature and infect many higher vertebrate species ranging from birds to man. Although originally classified as papovaviruses because of their icosahedral shape and circular, double-stranded DNA genome, the papillomaviruses are now recognized to be separate from the other papovaviruses such as polyoma and SV40, based on different biologic and genetic characteristics. The papillomaviruses contain a double-stranded circular DNA genome of 8000 base pairs, larger than DNA genome of the polyomaviruses (5000 base pairs), and the virion particles have a correspondingly larger capsid diameter (55 nm versus 40 nm). No papillomavirus has ever been propagated in tissue culture. The development of a permissive cell culture system for papillomavirus replication will be a major step toward elucidating the biology of this virus.

Unlike some other human viruses such as adenoviruses, papillomaviruses cannot be typed by serologic methods because antisera are currently not available that can distinguish among the different HPV types. Consequently, the viruses have been "typed" by DNA hybridization under controlled conditions of stringency.[82] Viruses differing by more than 50% DNA homology when assayed under stringent conditions are considered to be different types. With such methods, a total of 53 types of human papillomavirus have now been categorized, and new types are being recognized on a regular basis. Some of these viruses and the clinical syndromes with which they are associated are listed in Table 10-2.[83-111]

The productive functions of the papillomavirus, including vegetative viral DNA synthesis and the expression of late viral genes, occur only in the fully differentiated squamous epithelial cells of a papilloma. Vegetative viral DNA synthesis has been detected by in situ hybridization techniques only in the squamous epithelial cells of the stratum spinosum and of the granular layer of the epidermis, but not in the basal layer or in the underlying dermal fibroblasts. Viral capsid protein production and virus assembly occur only in the upper stratum spinosum and in the granular layer, where the epithelial cells are terminally differentiated. It is generally believed that the viral genome is present in the epithelial cells of the basal layer and that the expression of specific viral genes in the basal layer and in the lower layers of the epidermis is responsible for cellular proliferation characteristic of a wart. As the cells of the epidermis normally migrate upward through the stratum spinosum into the granular layer, they undergo a program of differentiation. The control of papillomavirus late gene expression is tightly linked to the differentiation state of the squamous epithelial cells.[112] The basis for this transcriptional control is not yet known.

Papillomaviruses are specifically tropic for squamous epithelial cells, and HPV types have specificity for different anatomical sites. HPV-1 has been observed to replicate only in heavily keratinized epithelium such as the palm or the sole, and HPV-16 preferentially replicates in mucosal squamous epithelium. HPV-1 does not replicate in cervical epithelium, and HPV-16 has not been observed in the skin of the hand or foot. Specialized keratinocytes from different anatomical sites may have distinct differentiation patterns, evident from the distinct types of keratin proteins that they synthesize and from the pattern of synthesis of other epithelial specific proteins such as involucrin. The ability of HPV to proliferate at a particular anatomical site may therefore reflect a specific interaction between viral and cellular gene regulatory factors involved in transcription.

HPV GENOMIC ORGANIZATION

All HPV types examined to date have a similar genomic organization. The DNA genomes of each of the HPVs sequenced as well as the other animal papillomaviruses contain approximately 8000 base pairs of genetic information. All of the ORFs that could serve to encode proteins for these viruses are located on only one of the two viral DNA strands. RNA studies have indicated that only one strand, the complementary strand, is transcribed.[113,114]

The HPV genome can be divided into two distinct regions: an "early" region that encodes the viral proteins involved in viral DNA replication, transcription, and cellular transformation, and a "late" region that encodes the viral capsid proteins. This functional division is based on genetic studies carried out with the bovine papillomavirus.[115] The organization of a typical HPV-16 genome is shown in Figure 10-4. The genes located in the early region of the genes are designated as E1, or E2, . . . E7, and the genes located in the late region are designated as L1 and L2. From studies with HPV-1, it is likely that E4 encodes a late gene that is expressed only in productively infected keratinocytes.[116] Thus, although this ORF is located with the early ORFs, its func-

TABLE 10-2.   Human Papillomaviruses

Virus Type*	Clinical Association†	References
HPV-1	Plantar Warts	83,84
HPV-2	Verruca vulgaris	85
HPV-3	Flat warts	86
HPV-4	Plantar warts	87
HPV-5	Macular lesions in EV	88
HPV-6	Genital warts, laryngeal papillomas	89
HPV-7	Common warts in meat handlers	90, 91
HPV-8	Macular lesions in EV[a]	88, 92
HPV-9	Macular lesions in EV	93
HPV-10	Flat warts	94
HPV-11	Laryngeal papillomas, genital warts	95
HPV-12	Macular lesions in EV	94
HPV-13	Oral focal epithelial hyperplasia	96
HPV-14	Macular lesions in EV	97
HPV-15	Macular lesions in EV	98
HPV-16	Cervical dysplasia, Bowenoid papulosis, cervical carcinoma	99
HPV-17	Macular lesions in EV	98
HPV-18	Cervical dysplasia and carcinoma	100
HPV-19	Macular lesions in EV	98, 101
HPV-20	Macular lesions in EV	98, 101
HPV-21	Macular lesions in EV	98
HPV-22	Macular lesions in EV	98
HPV-23	Macular lesions in EV	98
HPV-24	Macular lesions in EV	98
HPV-25	Macular lesions in EV	101
HPV-26	Flat warts	102
HPV-27	Verruca vulgaris	Zachow et al (unpubl.)
HPV-28	Flat warts	Favre et al (unpubl.)
HPV-29	Verruca vulgaris	Favre et al (unpubl.)
HPV-30	Genital warts, laryngeal carcinoma	103
HPV-31	Cervical dysplasia	104
HPV-32	Oral focal epithelial hyperplasia	105
HPV-33	Genital intraepithelial neoplasia, cervical carcinomas	106
HPV-34	Bowenoid papulosis, Bowen's disease	107
HPV-35	Cervical cancer	108
HPV-36	Macular lesions in EV	109
HPV-37	Keratoacanthoma	110
HPV-38	Detected in malignant melanoma	110
HPV-39	Bowenoid papulosis	111
HPV-42	Vulvar papilloma	111

* HPV types 40, 41, and 43 to 53 have been described at meetings but have not yet appeared in the literature.
† EV = epidermodysplasia verruciformis.

tion may only be important in the vegetative replication of the virus.

In productively infected tissue (*i.e.*, tissues in which viral particles are made, such as a wart), mRNA is transcribed from the early *and* late regions of the genome.[114,117] Nonproductive infection of host cells (as seen in the lower cells of the epithelium in a wart) is accompanied by mRNA transcription from only the early region of the genome.[113] Restriction of genomic expression to only the early region involves regulation of transcription at the level of initiation of RNA synthesis and at the level of transcriptional termination.[112]

The functional analysis of the molecular biology of papillomaviruses has been largely limited to the bovine papillomavirus (BPV-1), which can transform a variety of rodent fibroblast cell lines in tissue culture.[118-120] In these transformed cells, the DNA remains as a stable extrachromosomal plasmid, and this system has served as an excellent

model for studying latent infection by papillomavirus.[121] This virus has therefore served as the prototype for unraveling various aspects of the biology of the papillomaviruses over the past decade. Table 10-3 lists the various papillomavirus ORFs and the functions that have been assigned to them in different papillomavirus systems.[122-138] Two independent transforming genes have been mapped to the E5 gene and to the E6 gene of BPV-1 (reviewed in ref. 139). The E2 gene of BPV-1 encodes factors that are involved in the regulation of a conditional transcriptional enhancer located in the viral control region, LCR.[125,128] Mutations in the E2 gene result in decreased transformation efficiency of the BPV-1 and affect DNA replication.[132,133,140] It is believed that this effect may be indirect through the requirement for transcriptional activity of the viral genes that are directly required for transformation (E5 and E6). The E2 genes of other papillomaviruses have also been shown to encode transcriptional regulatory functions.[126,127] In the bovine papillo-

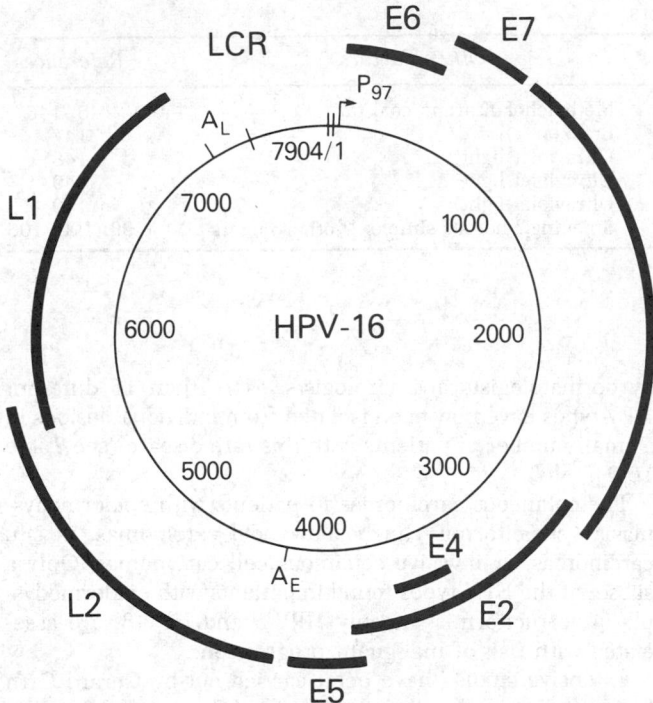

FIG. 10-4. Genomic map of HPV-16 deduced from the DNA sequence. Nucleotide numbers are noted within the circular maps, transcription proceeds clockwise, and the major open reading frames (E1 to E7, L1, and L2) are indicated. The only transcriptional promoter mapped to date for HPV-16 is designated (P_{97}). A_E and A_L represent the putative polyadenylation signals for the early and late transcripts, respectively. The viral long control region (LCR) containing the putative viral transcriptional and replication regulatory elements is noted.

mavirus, the E1 gene is required for extrachromosomal replication.[123,124] The E1 ORF actually encodes at least two genes. The 5' portion encodes a modulator gene (*mod*) that is required for establishing stable plasmid DNA replication but is not required for transient plasmid DNA replication.[122] The 3' portion of the E1 ORF encodes a replication function that is required for transient and stable DNA replication.[124] In the BPV system the E7 gene is also required for high copy num-

ber DNA plasmid maintenance.[136] No function has yet been found for the E3 ORF of BPV-1. The E8 ORF may also be involved in plasmid replication. The L1 ORF of the papillomaviruses encodes the major caption protein, and the L2 ORF encodes a minor caption protein.[137,138] The L1 and L2 ORFs are expressed only in the terminally differentiated keratinocytes.[112,114]

Although papillomavirus transformation studies have been principally carried out with BPV-1 in which the E5 and E6 ORFs have each been shown to encode independent transforming genes,[139] transformation of rodent cells has also been described for HPV-16[140,141] and for HPV-18.[142] This transforming activity has been localized to the E6/E7 ORFs for HPV-16 and HPV-18.[142,143] In addition HPV-16 has been shown to encode a factor capable of cooperating with the activated *ras* oncogene in the transformation of primary rodent cells.[144] This function has also been mapped to the E7 ORF.[143] A transcriptional regulatory function in addition to that of E2 has been mapped to the E7 ORF of HPV-16.[143] This function is similar to the transcriptional regulatory function of the adenovirus E1a gene in that each of these viral proteins can activate the adenovirus E2 promoter. Analysis of the amino acid structure of the adenovirus E1a gene and the E7 genes of several of the genital papillomaviruses has revealed striking similarities mapping to the conserved domains of 1 and 2 of adenovirus E1a and HPV-16 E7.[143] These domains have been shown to be important for the immortalization of primary cells in the adenovirus E1a gene.

PAPILLOMAVIRUSES IN CANCER

A subgroup of papillomaviruses can induce lesions that may progress to squamous cell carcinomas. These viruses and their associated malignancies are listed in Table 10-4.[145-150] The most extensively studied of these viruses has been the Shope papillomavirus, which infects cottontail rabbits in nature (CRPV). Studies with this virus date to the early 1930s, when Shope identified CRPV as the etiologic agent of cutaneous papillomatosis in rabbits.[151] The Shope system has been extensively studied as a model for papillomavirus-induced carcinogenesis.[145,146] One of the features of carcinogenic progression with the papillomaviruses is the synergy

TABLE 10-3.   Papillomavirus Gene Functions

Open Reading Frame	Function(s) Assigned	Virus	References
E1 (5' portion)	Replication modulator	BPV-1	122
E1 (3' portion)	Replication	BPV-1	123, 124
E2 (full)	Transcriptional transactivator	BPV-1, HPV-11, HPV-16	125, 126, 127
E2 (3' portion)	Transcriptional repressor	BPV-1	128
E3	None	. . .	
E4	Cytoplasmic protein in warts	HPV-1	116
E5	Transformation	BPV-1	129–133
E6	Transformation, plasmid copy control	BPV-1	134, 135, 136
E7	Plasmid copy control	BPV-1	136
E8	Possible role in DNA replication	BPV-1	Lusky (unpubl.)
L1	Major capsid protein	BPV-1	137
L2	Minor capsid protein	HPV-1	138

TABLE 10-4. Papillomaviruses and Naturally Occurring Cancers

Papillomaviruses	Cancers	Other Factors	References
CRPV	Skin cancer	Methylcholanthrene coal tar	145, 146
BPV-4	Tongue, esophageal, foregut cancers	Bracken	147
BPV (not typed)	Ocular cancers	Ultraviolet light	148
Ovine papillomavirus	Skin cancer	Ultraviolet light	149
HPV-5, 8 and others	Skin cancer in patients with EV	Ultraviolet light	150
HPV-16, 18, 33	Anogenital cancers, some oral cancers	Smoking,? herpes simplex,? other factors	99, 100, 106

EV = epidermodysplasia verruciformis.

between the virus and carcinogenic external factors (see Table 10-4). In the case of CRPV, carcinomas develop more readily in virally induced papillomas that are painted with coal tar or methylcholanthrene.[152,153] These CRPV-associated carcinomas contain copies of the viral DNA that are transcriptionally active, supporting an active role for these viruses in the cancers that develop.[154,155]

In cattle, BPV-4 has been associated with esophageal papillomatosis and with squamous cell carcinomas of upper alimentary tract.[147,156] Interestingly, however, only those cattle from the highlands of Scotland that are infected with BPV-4 and that also feed on bracken fern, which is known to contain a radiomimetic substance, have a high incidence of squamous cell carcinomas of the esophagus and the foregut.[147] In contrast to the CRPV-associated carcinomas, in which the viral DNA is invariably found, extensive analysis of the squamous cell carcinomas of the upper alimentary tract in cattle infected with BPV-4 has failed to reveal a consistent pattern of viral DNA sequences within the malignant tumors.[157] In the case of these alimentary tract tumors, it is possible that the continued presence of BPV-4 DNA sequences is not required for the maintenance of the carcinogenic stage. However, it is also possible that a different bovine papillomavirus, distinct from BPV-4, may be associated with these carcinomas and that the assays performed to detect the viral DNA sequences have not been sufficiently sensitive.

EPIDERMODYSPLASIA VERRUCIFORMIS

Epidermodysplasia verruciformis is a rare, life-long disease that usually begins in infancy or childhood. The disease is characterized by disseminated polymorphic cutaneous lesions that resemble flat warts, and by reddish macules sometimes referred to as pityriasis-like lesions.[158] Approximately one third of the patients with epidermodysplasia verruciformis develop multiple skin cancers, usually during the third or fourth decade of life. Papillomavirus particles have been detected within the benign lesions but not in the carcinomas. It has been proposed that the disease is linked to a rare, recessive, abnormal allele of an X-linked gene. Patients with epidermodysplasia verruciformis often have impaired cell-mediated immunity, which is believed to play a role in the life-long infection by papillomaviruses. The carcinomas that develop in these patients arise in sun-exposed areas, and ultraviolet radiation is thought to play a cocarcinogenic role with the papillomaviruses in the etiology of these cancers. Epidermodysplasia verruciformis has been intensely studied

by dermatologists and virologists. More than 15 different HPV types have now been isolated from individual lesions in a small number of patients with this rare disease (see Table 10-2).

The cutaneous carcinomas in patients with epidermodysplasia verruciformis can be bowenoid carcinomas, in situ carcinomas, or invasive squamous cell carcinomas. Only a subset of the HPV types found in patients with epidermodysplasia verruciformis, notably HPV-5 and HPV-8, are associated with risk of malignant progression.

Extensive studies have been carried out by Gerard Orth from the Pasteur Institute in Paris and Stephonia Jablonska in Warsaw in analyzing the HPVs in cancers from patients with epidermodysplasia verruciformis. They investigated a total of 28 tumors from 14 patients. HPV genomes were found in 27 of the 28 samples. Twenty-one of these contained HPV-5 DNA, five contained HPV-8 DNA, and one contained HPV-14 DNA.[150] HPV-5 has been found in metastatic squamous cell carcinoma lesions in some patients with epidermodysplasia verruciformis.[159,160] Still other investigators have found additional HPVs in carcinomas in epidermodysplasia verruciformis patients. HPV-3 has been found in an in situ vulvar carcinoma of a patient with epidermodysplasia verruciformis,[161] and HPV-17 has been found in a cutaneous epidermodysplasia verruciformis carcinoma by a group of Japanese investigators.[162] Thus the specific association of carcinomas in patients with epidermodysplasia verruciformis is not strictly limited to HPV-5 and HPV-8. Although metastasis is uncommon in the cancers in these patients, the presence of HPV-5 in the two metastatic lymph node lesions examined strengthens the argument for an etiologic role for HPV.[150,159] Further studies have established that the viral genomes are transcriptionally active within these carcinomas.[163]

GENITAL CARCINOMAS

The epidemiology of genital warts follows a pattern characteristic of a venereally transmitted disease, with a high prevalence in populations of women of high promiscuity.[164,165] Two general types of genital wart viral infections are recognized that can be differentiated by their clinical appearance: condylomata acuminata and flat genital warts. It has been known for many years that condylomata acuminata, which can be localized to the penis, the vulva, the perineum, the anus, and rarely the uterine cervix, are caused by papillomaviruses. Particles have been demonstrated by electron microscopy,[166,167] and in 1980 papillomavirus-specific antigens were detected utilizing antisera to a common papillomavirus antigen.[168] HPV-6 was directly cloned from a condyloma acuminatum, and, using its DNA along with that of the closely related HPV-11, zur Hausen and co-workers in West Germany were able to demonstrate HPV DNA in over 90% of the lesions of condyloma acuminatum that have been examined.[169,170] Less frequently other HPV types can be found in condylomata acuminata. Malignant conversion of condylomata acuminata into squamous cell carcinoma is quite uncommon. Buschke and Lowenstein[171] have described a lesion, designated as a giant condyloma, that has characteristics similar to that of a locally invasive squamous cell carcinoma. These tumors have been associated with HPV-6 and HPV-11.[169,172] The majority of cervical carcinomas and other genital tract carcinomas, however, have been negative when examined for HPV-6 and HPV-11.

Compelling evidence linking an HPV infection with cervical carcinoma came from the recognition that the morphological changes previously interpreted as cervical dysplasia on Papanicolaou-stained smears and tissue sections of the cervix were due to a papillomavirus infection.[173-175] The characteristic cell that is diagnostic for a cervical papillomavirus infection is the koilocyte, found in high association in smears with cervical dysplastic changes.[176] Electron microscopy disclosed papillomavirus particles in the koilocytotic cells, proving the papillomavirus etiology.[177,178] Numerous investigators have found papillomavirus-specific capsid antigens and HPV DNA within cervical dysplastic lesions, confirming the viral etiology of cervical dysplasia.

Epidemiologic studies have implicated an infectious agent in the etiology of human cervical carcinoma.[179,180] Venereal transmission of a carcinogenic factor with a long latency has been suggested by such studies. Sexual promiscuity, early age at onset of sexual activity, and poor sexual hygiene are risk factors for cervical carcinoma. There is a correlation between the incidence rates of cervical cancer and penile carcinoma in different geographic areas, although the incidence rates for penile carcinoma are 20-fold lower than those of cervical carcinoma. A similar incidence ratio of cervical carcinoma and penile carcinoma is maintained in areas of high, medium, or low prevalence, suggesting that the etiologic factors for penile and cervical carcinoma may be the same. The "male factor" also appears to implicate a venereally transmitted agent. Monogamous women are at higher risk for cervical carcinoma if their spouses have multiple sexual partners.

The suggestion of possible involvement of an infectious agent in the etiology of cervical carcinoma has prompted many studies evaluating genital pathogens as potential causative agents. Infections by *Trichomonas*, *Chlamydia*, and bacteria, such as syphilis and gonorrhea, have not been linked to cervical carcinoma. In the late 1960s and early 1970s genital infection by herpes simplex virus (HSV) type 2 was considered a possible etiologic candidate.[181,182] Support for the notion that HSV might be a cancer-associated virus came from studies demonstrating the ability of HSV to transform certain rodent cells in the laboratory in vitro and from serologic studies suggesting a higher frequency of antibodies to HSV-2 in patients with cervical carcinoma. How-

ever, subsequent carefully done molecular studies that sought to demonstrate HSV RNA or HSV DNA in cervical cancer tissues could not provide convincing evidence for a role for HSV in cervical cancer.[183] More recently a large prospective epidemiologic study carried out by Vonka et al has failed to support the involvement of HSV-1 or HSV-2 infections in cervical cancer.[184,185]

The association of an HPV with cervical dysplasia (also referred to as cervical intraepithelial neoplasia, CIN) provided impetus for a close examination of cervical cancer for HPV sequences. The natural history linking CIN to carcinoma in situ and to invasive squamous cell carcinoma of the cervix had already been well established.[186-188] Initial experiments from a number of laboratories revealed HPV sequences in occasional cases of cervical carcinoma and anogenital carcinoma, but no consistent pattern of positivity emerged. Using radioactively labeled HPV-11 DNA under conditions of hybridization of low stringency, zur Hausen and his colleagues at Heidelberg examined human cervical carcinoma DNAs for unknown HPV types and were able to identify two new papillomavirus DNAs, HPV-16 and HPV-18, from two cervical cancer tissues.[99,100] Using HPV-16 and HPV-18 DNA as probes they found these DNAs in approximately 70% of all cervical carcinomas examined.[189] The use of low stringency hybridization techniques has led to the identification of approximately a dozen different HPVs now associated with genital tract lesions. HPV-33, HPV-39, and HPV-42 are each associated with a small percentage of cervical carcinomas.[106,111] Thus, specific HPVs are now regularly found in human cervical carcinoma tissues and in other human genital carcinomas, including penile carcinomas, vulvar carcinomas, and perianal carcinomas. The cloning of this set of HPV DNAs has made available DNA probes that permit extensive analysis of specific lesions for a variety of HPV types. It is now recognized, for instance, that bowenoid papulosis of the penis[190,191] is associated with HPV-16. In general, HPV-16, HPV-18, and HPV-33 are found in cases of moderate to severe dysplasia and in invasive cervical carcinomas; and HPV-6, HPV-11, and HPV-31 are found in cases of condyloma acuminatum and in cases of mild cervical dysplasia. Preliminary epidemiologic studies suggest that lesions associated with HPV-16 and HPV-18 may be at higher risk for progression to cervical carcinoma. More extensive epidemiologic studies with proper controls are now under way to establish these associations more firmly and to identify other risk factors.

HPV infections by themselves are not sufficient for carcinogenic progression. Only a small fraction of individuals infected by a specific HPV will eventually develop cervical carcinoma. Thus the genetic information carried by the virus per se is not sufficient for malignant progression. Other factors must be involved in the progression of viral associated lesions to these genital tract cancers and may work synergistically with papillomavirus infections. For example, epidemiologic studies have suggested that smoking is a risk factor for developing cervical carcinoma.[192-194] The tobacco condensate might accumulate in the vaginal fluids bathing the cervix and act as a cofactor with the papillomavirus infection.[195] It has also been postulated that herpes virus infection could act synergistically with specific papillomaviruses to induce human cervical carcinoma.[196] Specific molecular studies to establish cooperativity between these two viruses have not yet been reported in the literature. The striking association of specific HPV types with genital tract carcinomas has been established. RNA and DNA analyses of biopsy specimens has demonstrated a high correlation of viral transcriptional activity with the presence of viral DNA.[197-199]

In addition, over the years several cell lines have been derived from human cervical carcinomas, including the HeLa, SiHa, and Caski cell lines, which have proved useful in studying the HPVs associated with cervical carcinoma. HeLa cells contain approximately ten incomplete copies of HPV-18 genome integrated and the viral DNA is transcriptionally active.[197,200] In the HeLa cell line, the HPV-18 genome is integrated with 50 kilobases of the c-myc oncogene on chromosome 8.[201] Integration of the HPV genomes in cervical carcinomas within the vicinity of the c-myc locus on chromosome 8 is not a general characteristic of all human cervical carcinomas, however. The SiHa and Caski cell lines contain integrated HPV-16 DNA.[200] The SiHa cell line contains a single copy of HPV-16 and the Caski cell line contains approximately 600 copies of the viral DNA integrated.[200,202] In these cell lines the viral genomes are integrated at other chromosomal sites, indicating that integration is not site specific for the papillomaviruses but apparently can occur at a variety of sites.[201]

Transcriptional analyses of the cervical carcinoma cell lines has shown that a high percentage of these cell lines are positive for HPV transcription and that the E6 and E7 regions of the viral genomes appear to be invariably expressed in the transcriptionally positive lines.[197,200,201] In addition, there is little if any expression of the E2 ORF. In those cell lines in which only a single copy of viral DNA has been integrated, integration appears to be specific for the E1 and E2 ORFs, resulting in disruption of the integrity and expression of the E2 ORF.[197,201] Since the E2 ORF of the human papillomaviruses encodes transcriptional regulatory factors,[126,127] integration resulting in the disruption of the E2 ORF could result in the uncoupling of the control of the HPV promoter in the viral LCR from E2 transregulation. The HPV-16 and HPV-18 control region contains E2-independent enhancer elements that are cell type specific and glucocorticoid responsive.[203,205] Transcription from the LCR promoters leads to expression of the E6 and E7 ORFs, suggesting that expression of the products may be necessary for maintenance of the transformed phenotype. Transformation, immortalization, and transcriptional modulation functions have been mapped to these ORFs in HPV-16 and HPV-18.[140-143]

OTHER HUMAN CANCERS ASSOCIATED WITH PAPILLOMAVIRUSES

The availability of specific HPV DNA probes has allowed investigators to screen a variety of human cancers for HPV sequences. Based on the animal models, it seemed likely that any carcinomas of any squamous epithelium or an epithelium that can undergo squamous metaplasia would be a potential candidate for an HPV association. Studies on oral and upper airway carcinomas have revealed some HPV-positive carcinomas.[103,206,207] HPV DNA has been found in benign oral papillomas,[208-211] and oral focal epithelial hyperplasia has been firmly established as having a papillomavirus etiology.[96,105] In addition, papillomavirus DNA sequences have been found associated with cases of oral leukoplakia.[209,212] HPV-16 sequences have been described in a verrucous carcinoma of the larynx. Recently HPV-11 was found in a squamous cell carcinoma of the lung in a 26-year-old man with a history of laryngotracheobronchial papillomatosis.[213] In this case, HPV-11 DNA was also found within metastatic lesions in the liver and lymph nodes. The viral genome was transcriptionally active, suggesting that expression of the virus may have played an active role in the carcinogenic progression. An association of esophageal carcinomas with HPV has not yet been demonstrated in humans. However there appears to be an excellent candidate for a human cancer that could be associated with an HPV. The esophagus is lined by squamous epithelium, and squamous cell papillomas of the esophagus have been described in humans.[214,215] To date the specific HPVs associated with these papillomas have not been determined, although viral antigens have been detected in several cases.

EPSTEIN-BARR VIRUS

The Epstein-Barr virus (EBV) was the first human tumor virus to be recognized. It was discovered during studies of lymphoma in young children in certain parts of East Africa, which were first described by Dennis Burkitt in 1958.[216] Although this childhood lymphoma had been previously recognized, it had not been clearly defined as a unique entity with characteristic clinical, pathologic, and epidemiologic features. In his early descriptive studies Burkitt suggested that the lymphoma could be due to a virus because its geographic distribution—a belt across equatorial Africa—was similar to that of yellow fever.[216,217] In 1964, Epstein and Barr described virus particles of the herpesvirus family in lymphoblastoid lines cultured from explants of Burkitt's lymphoma.[218,219] The finding of such virus particles in lymphoid lines, however, was not limited to explants of Burkitt's lymphoma tissue since they could also be seen in cell lines established from patients with other malignancies, from patients with infectious mononucleosis, and, occasionally, from normal individuals.

EBV is a double-stranded DNA virus belonging to the herpesvirus family. Other members of the human herpesvirus family include herpes simplex viruses types 1 and 2, varicella zoster virus, cytomegalovirus, and the recently described human B-lymphotropic virus. Morphologically the mature virus is essentially indistinguishable from other members of the herpes family. The viruses are large, 150 to 180 nm in diameter, and contain a large double-stranded DNA genome of approximately 170,000 base pairs. In addition to its central core of genetic material, the virus particle is also composed of a capsid layer made up of capsomeres in an icosahedral shape and an outer lipoprotein envelope. Because of its tropism for lymphoid cells, in vivo and in vitro, EBV is considered a member of the gamma herpesviruses.

Individual members of this group are specific for either B- or T-lymphocytes. EBV and HBLV are the two viruses in this group that cause disease in humans. Other gamma herpesviruses include Marek's disease virus of chickens and two viruses that infect New World monkeys: herpes ateles and herpes saimiri. Our understanding of the biology and clinical importance of HBLV, which was first described in 1986 by investigators at Gallo's laboratory, is still in its infancy.[220,221]

EBV VIRAL GENOME

The EBV viral genome is a double-stranded DNA molecule of approximately 170,000 base pairs.[222] The organization is complex, with regions of repeated DNA sequences and multiple tandem copies (6–12) of a 500-base pair terminal repeat unit at the end of the linear genome. When in one cell nucleus in the latent state, the genome exists in a circular form. Its ability to circularize may involve homologous recombination through the terminal repeated DNA sequences. The EBV genome has now been sequenced in its entirety.[223] The availability of this DNA sequence information has permitted the identification of open reading frames and genes for subsequent genetic and molecular studies.

EBV ANTIGENS

A variety of antigens have been identified in EBV-infected and transformed cells by immunologic methods. The viral capsid antigens and membrane antigens are detected in cells producing EBV particles.[224] The membrane antigens are late antigens; their expression occurs after the onset of vegetative viral DNA synthesis in the life cycle of the virus. The membrane antigens are responsible for eliciting virus-neutralizing antibody.[225] A group of antigens referred to as the EBV-induced early antigens are synthesized early in the virus replication cycle. This group of antigens can be subdivided into diffuse (D) and restricted (R) components based on the distribution of the antigens and the sensitivity of the patterns to fixation.[226] The restricted early antigens are denatured by methanol, whereas the diffuse components are stable. An important complex identified by immunofluorescence procedures is the EBV-induced nuclear antigen (EBNA).[227] This antigen is as an excellent immunologic marker for the presence of the viral DNA because it is expressed in virtually every cell containing the viral genome. EBNA is detected using anticomplement immunofluorescence assays as described by Reedman and Klein in 1973.[227] An additional antigen complex identified in the membranes of EBV-infected cells by lymphocyte cytotoxic assays has been designated LYDMA, for lymphocyte-detected membrane antigen.[228-230] This antigen presumably serves as the target for cytotoxic T-lymphocytes. For the cell biologist and the molecular biologist, the EBNA and LYDMA antigens are the major candidates for transforming proteins because of their expression in transformed cells.

Until recently, the composition and nature of the EBV-induced antigens were unclear because the components of these complexes had not been specifically identified. Monospecific reagents directed against specific constituents of the antigen complex have permitted the definition of specific components. A large amount of data has been generated concerning the EBV proteins over the past few years using monoclonal antibodies.[231,232] The reader is referred to a recent review by Pearson and Luca[233] for a more detailed description of the EBV-determined antigens.

BURKITT'S LYMPHOMA

Burkitt's lymphoma occurs several years after the primary infection with EBV. Studies have indicated that Burkitt's lymphoma is a monoclonal lymphoma,[234] as opposed to infectious mononucleosis, which is a polyclonal disease. African Burkitt's lymphoma is characterized by rapid growth of the tumor at nonlymphoid sites such as the jaw or the retroperitoneum. The tumor is of B-cell origin and is closely related to the small noncleaved cells of normal lymphoid follicles.[235] The biopsy specimens from African Burkitt's lymphoma invariably contain the EBV genome and are positive for EBNA.[236] By contrast, only 15% to 20% of non-African Burkitt's lymphomas contain the EBV genome. EBV has a worldwide distribution and infects most (>90%) individuals by the time they reach adulthood. The clustering of Burkitt's lymphoma in the equatorial belt of East Africa, therefore, remains unexplained. It has been hypothesized that potential alterations of the immune system, possibly due to hyperstimulation by endemic malaria, may play an important role in the outcome of an EBV infection in individuals in this region.[237,238] Individuals from this region have impairment of virus-specific cytotoxic T-cell activity. Normally, it is the T-cell response to EBV infection that limits B-cell proliferation, which is directly stimulated by EBV.[239] It has been postulated that failure of the T-cell immune response to control this proliferation could lead to excessive B-cell proliferation and, as such, provide a suitable background for further mutation, oncogenic transformation, and lymphomogenesis.

Burkitt's lymphomas regularly exhibit abnormalities of the chromosomes that contain the immunoglobulin genes, notably chromosomes 2, 14, and 22. The most common abnormality, observed in more than 90% of Burkitt's lymphomas, is a translocation of the long arm of chromosome 14,[240] which contains the heavy chain immunoglobulin genes, to chromosome 8, which contains the c-myc oncogene. Less frequent translocations involve chromosome 2 (κ light chain) and chromosome 22 (λ light chain).[241] These translocations generally involve reciprocal translocations to the distal arm of chromosome 8 (band 824), which contains the c-myc proto-oncogene.[242] It is believed that Burkitt's lymphomas exhibit abnormal expression of the c-myc oncogene after this translocation, and that the abnormal expression results from proximity of the c-myc oncogene to the transcriptional control elements of the immunoglobulin genes.[242,243] Support for this model is provided by the recent experiments of Dalla-Favera et al, who demonstrated tumorigenic conversion of EBV-infected human B-lymphocytes with the introduction of an activated c-myc oncogene.[244] This study demonstrates that EBV infection and c-myc activation are sufficient for tumorigenic transformation of human B-cells in vitro.

The chromosomal abnormalities noted above are not detected in the peripheral blood lymphocytes of patients with Burkitt's lymphoma, nor are they found in nonmalignant lymphoblastoid cell lines derived from such patients. Thus the translocation appears to be specific for Burkitt's lymphoma and appears to occur at a step following the immortalization by EBV. In 1979 George Klein suggested a scenario for the involvement of EBV in the etiology of African Burkitt's lymphoma.[245] The first step involves the EBV-induced immortalization of B-lymphocytes in a primary infection. The second step involves stimulated proliferation of EBV-positive B-cells. This step is facilitated in the geographic areas where Burkitt's lymphoma is endemic (presumably because of the presence of malaria) through B-cell triggering and the suppression of T-cells involved in the control of the proliferation of EBV-infected cells. This pool of cells thus increases in size as a target cell population for random chromosomal rearrangements. The third and final step is the reciprocal translocation involving a chromosomal locus with an immunoglobulin gene and the c-*myc* gene on chromosome 8. This leads to the deregulation of the c-*myc* gene, the development of the malignant clone, and finally the appearance of a tumor mass.[246] Alternative scenarios have been proposed in which the order of the steps is rearranged such that the B-cell activation by malaria precedes the chromosomal translocation and is followed by EBV infection.[247] Regardless, the components of either of these scenarios account for the geographic distribution of Burkitt's lymphoma, the critical involvement of EBV in lymphomogenesis, and the eventual selection and clonal outgrowth of a population of cells with the critical translocation involving the deregulation of the *myc* gene on chromosome 8.

NASOPHARYNGEAL CARCINOMA

Nasopharyngeal carcinoma has also been linked to EBV (reviewed in ref. 248). Nasopharyngeal carcinoma occurs in adults from ages 20 to 50, although in certain parts of Africa the age distribution extends to children as well. In general, affected males outnumber females in a ratio of 2:1, and although worldwide the annual incidence rates are low, some areas in China (especially the southern province) have a high rate of approximately 10 cases per 100,000 population per year. Since the incidence among individuals of Chinese descent remains high irrespective of where they live, a genetic susceptibility has been proposed. For the Cantonese in Singapore, the annual rates of 29 per 100,000 are higher than for other racial groups living in the same locale. A correlation of certain HLA haplotypes has been noted among the Chinese; however, these associations do not hold true for evaluation of nasopharyngeal carcinoma in Tunisia. Environmental factors that have been implicated as risk factors for nasopharyngeal carcinoma include fumes, chemicals, smoke, and ingestion of salt-cured fish.

EBV genomes are found in nearly all biopsies of undifferentiated NPC specimens from all over the world.[249,250] The genome has been demonstrated to exist in the epithelial cells of the tumors.[251] The EBV genome is transcriptionally active within these tumors, and the regions that are transcribed in the biopsies are the same as those expressed in latently infected lymphocytes.[252] These molecular observations are consistent with an active role for EBV in the neoplastic processes involved in nasopharyngeal carcinoma. Patients with nasopharyngeal carcinoma have elevated levels of IgG antibodies to EBV capsid and early antigens. Furthermore, they have serum IgA antibodies to capsid and early antigen, likely reflecting the local production of such antibodies in the nasopharynx. Characteristic chromosomal translocations have been sought in the nasopharyngeal carcinomas but none have yet been identified. Attempts to identify mutated or activated cellular oncogenes thus far have not been successful.

The presence of immunoglobulin markers for EBV (IgA/ VCA and IgA/EA) has provided the opportunity for early serologic identification of patients with nasopharyngeal carcinoma. The frequency of IgA antibody to the EBV capsid antigen in 150,000 Chinese studied was 1%. About 20% of the patients with elevated IgA antibodies to VCA had nasopharyngeal carcinoma, however, when biopsied. Thus, early detection using serologic tests can be applied in areas where nasopharyngeal carcinoma is prevalent, possibly leading to early therapeutic intervention.[253]

LYMPHOMA IN IMMUNODEFICIENT INDIVIDUALS

EBV is associated with lymphomas in patients with acquired or congenital immunodeficiencies. These lymphomas can be distinguished from the classic Burkitt's lymphomas in that the tumors are often polyclonal. The tumors also do not demonstrate the characteristic chromosomal abnormalities of Burkitt's lymphoma described earlier. The pathogenesis of these lymphomas involves a deficiency in the effector mechanisms needed to control EBV-transformed cells. The prototypic model for this disease has been the X-linked lymphoproliferative syndrome.[254] Patients with X-linked lymphoproliferative syndrome who develop acute infectious mononucleosis exhibit the usual atypical lymphocytosis and polyclonal elevation of serum immunoglobulins as well as increases in specific antibody to VCA and to EA. During these infections, however, patients with X-linked lymphoproliferative syndrome fail to mount and sustain an anti-EBNA response following acute infection. The unique vulnerability of males with X-linked lymphoproliferative syndrome to EBV infection is most likely due to an inherited immune regulatory defect that results in failure to govern the cytotoxic T-cells and natural killer cells required to cope with EBV.

Patients with iatrogenic immunodeficiencies, such as organ transplant recipients, are at increased risk for lymphomas, and these lymphomas often contain EBV DNA and EBNA. Also, patients with AIDS are at a higher risk for developing polyclonal lymphomas that are associated with EBV.

REFERENCES

1. Ellermann V, Bang O: Experimentelle Leukämie bei Huhnern. Zentralbl Bakteriol Abt [I.] 46:595–609, 1908
2. Rous P: A sarcoma of the fowl transmissible by an agent separable from the tumor cells. J Exp Med 13:397–411, 1911

3. Shope RE: A filtrable virus causing a tumor-like condition in rabbits and its relationship to virus myxomatosum. J Exp Med 56:803–1932

4. Shope RE: Infectious papillomatosis of rabbits. J Exp Med 58:607–629, 1933

5. Rous P, Beard JW: The progression to carcinoma of virus-induced rabbit papillomas (Shope). J Exp Med 62:523–548, 1935

6. Gross L: Pathogenic properties, and "vertical" transmission of the mouse leukemia agent. Proc Soc Exp Biol Med 78:342–348, 1951

7. Gross L: A filtrable agent, recovered from Akr leukemia extracts, causing salivary gland carcinomas in C3H mice. Proc Soc Exp Biol Med 83:414–421, 1953

8. Stewart SE: Leukemia in mice produced by a filterable agent present in AKR leukemic tissues with notes on a sarcoma produced by the same agent. Anat Rev 117:532, 1953

9. Jarrett WFH, Martin WB, Crighton GW et al: Transmission experiments with leukemia (lymphosarcoma). Nature 202:566–567, 1964

10. Bernard W: The detection and study of tumor viruses with electron microscopy. Cancer Res 20:712–727, 1960

11. Temin HM, Mizutani S: RNA-dependent DNA polymerase in virions of Rous sarcoma virus. Nature 226:1211–1212, 1970

12. Baltimore D: RNA-dependent DNA polymerase in virions of RNA tumor viruses. Nature 276:1209–1211, 1970

13. Poiesz BJ, Ruscetti FW, Gazdar AF, Bunn PA, Minna JD, Gallo RC: Detection and isolation of type C retrovirus particles from fresh and cultured lymphocytes of a patient with cutaneous T-cell lymphoma. Proc Natl Acad Sci USA 77:7415–7419, 1980

14. Poiesz BJ, Ruscetti FW, Reitz MS, Kalyanaraman VS, Gallo RC: Isolation of a new type C retrovirus (HTLV) in primary uncultured cells of a patient with Sezary T-cell leukemia. Nature 294:268–271, 1981

15. Yoshida M, Miyoshi I, Hinuma Y:Isolation and characterization of retrovirus from cell lines of human adult T-cell leukemia and its implication in disease. Proc Natl Acad Sci USA 79:2031–2035, 1982

16. Uchiyama T, Yodoi J, Sagawa K, Takatsuki K, Uchino H: Adult T-cell leukemia: Clinical and hematological features of 16 cases. Blood 50:481–492, 1977

17. Miyoshi I, Kubonishi I, Yoshimoto S et al: Type C virus particles in a cord T-cell line derived by co-cultivating normal human cord leukocytes and human leukaemic T cells. Nature 294:770–771, 1981

18. Watanabe T, Seiki M, Yoshida M: Retrovirus terminology. Science 222:1178, 1983

19. Watanabe T: HTLV type 1 (US isolate) and ATLV (Japanese isolate) are the same species of human retrovirus. Virology 133:238–241, 1984

20. Hattori T, Uchiyama T, Tibana K, Takatsuki K, Uchino H: Surface phenotype of Japanese adult T-cell leukemia cells characterized by monoclonal antibodies. Blood 58:645–647, 1981

21. Hinuma T, Nagata K, Misoka M et al: Adult T cell leukemia: Antigen in an ATL cell line and detection of antibodies of the antigen in human sera. Proc Natl Acad Sci USA 78:6476–7480, 1981

22. Blattner WA, Kalyanaraman VS, Robert-Guroff M et al: The human type C retrovirus, HTLV, in blacks from the Caribbean region, and relationship to adult T cell leukemia/lymphoma. Int J Cancer 30:257–265, 1982

23. Hunsmann G, Schneider J, Schmitt J et al: Detection of serum antibodies to adult T-cell leukemia virus in non-human primates and in people from Africa. Int J Cancer 32:329–332, 1983

24. Morgan DA, Ruscetti FW, Gallo RC: Selective in vitro growth of T-lymphocytes from normal human bone marrows. Science 193:1007, 1976

25. Yamaguchi K, Nishimura H, Kawano K, Jono M, Miyamoto Y, Takatsuki K: A proposal for smoldering adult T-cell leukemia: Diversity in clinical pictures of adult T-cell leukemia. Jpn J Clin Oncol 13:189–200, 1983

26. Gessain A, Barin F, Vemant JC et al: Antibodies to human lymphotropic virus type-1 in patients with tropical spastic paraparesis. Lancet 2:407–410, 1985

27. Bartholomew C, Cleghorn F, Charles W et al: HTLV-1 and tropical spastic paraparesis. Lancet 2:99–100, 1986

28. Osame M, Usuku K, Izumo S et al: HTLV-I associated myelopathy: A new clinical entity. Lancet 1:1031–1032, 1986

29. Kalyanaraman VS, Sarngadharan MG, Robert-Guroff M et al: A new subtype of human T-cell leukemia virus (HTLV-II) associated with a T-cell variant of hairy cell leukemia. Science 218:571–573, 1982

30. Rosenblatt J, Golde JD, Wachsman W et al: A second isolate of HTLV-II associated with atypical hairy-cell leukemia. N Engl J Med 315:372–377, 1986

31. Gelmann EP, Franchini G, Manzari V, Wong-Staal F, Gallo RC: Molecular cloning of a unique human T-cell leukemia virus (HTLV-II). Proc Natl Acad Sci USA 81:993–997, 1984

32. Shaw GM, Gonda MA, Flickinger GH, Hahn BH, Gallo RC, Wong-Staal F: Genomes of evolutionary divergent members of human T-cell leukemia virus family (HTLV-I and HTLV-II) are highly conserved, especially in pX. Proc Natl Acad Sci USA 81:4544–4548, 1984

33. McClure MO, Weiss RA: Human immunodeficiency virus and related viruses. Curr Top AIDS 1:95–117, 1987

34. Pinching A, Weiss RA: AIDS and the spectrum of HTLV-III/LAV infection. Int Rev Exp Pathol 28:1–44, 1986

35. Tajima K, Tominaga S, Suchi T: Epidemiological analysis of the distribution of antibody to adult T-cell leukemia virus. Gann 73:893–901, 1982

36. Kinoshita K, Hino S, Amagasaki T et al: Demonstration of adult T-cell leukemia virus antigen in milk from three sero-positive mothers. Gann 75:103–105, 1984

37. Okochi K, Sato H, Hinuma Y: A retrospective study on transmission of adult T-cell leukemia virus by blood transfusion: Sero-conversion in recipients. Vox Sang 46:245–253, 1983

38. Seika M, Eddy R, Shows TR, Yoshida H: Non-specific integration of the HTLV provirus genome into adult T-cell leukemia cells. Nature 309:640–642, 1984

39. Yoshida M, Seiki M, Yamaguchi K, Takatsuki K: Monoclonal integration of human T-cell leukemia provirus in all primary tumors of adult T-cell leukemia suggests causative role of human T-cell leukemia virus in the disease. Proc Natl Acad Sci USA 81:2534–2537, 1984

40. Wong-Staal F, Hahn B, Manzari V et al: A survey of human leukemias for sequences of a human retrovirus, HTLV. Nature 302:626–628, 1983

41. Yamamoto N, Okada M, Koyanagi Y et al: Transformation of human leukocytes by cocultivation with an adult T-cell leukemia virus producer cell line. Science 217:737–739, 1982

42. Popovic M, Lange-Wantzin G, Sarin PS, Mann D, Gallo RC: Transformation of human umbilical cord blood T-cells by human T-cell leukemia/lymphoma virus. Proc Natl Acad Sci USA 80:502–506, 1983

43. Hayward WS, Neel BG, Astrin SM: Activation of a cellular onc gene by promoter insertion in ALV-induced lymphoid leukosis. Nature 290:475–480, 1981

44. Burny A, Buck C, Chantrenne H: Bovine leukemia virus: Molecular biology and epidemiology. In Klein G (ed): Viral Oncology, pp 231–280. New York, Raven Press, 1980

45. Seiki M, Hattori S, Hirayama Y, Yoshida M: Human adult T-cell leukemia virus: Complete nucleotide sequence of provirus genome integrated in leukemia cell DNA. Proc Natl Acad Sci USA 80:3618–3622, 1983

46. Sodroski JG, Rosen CA, Haseltine WA: Trans-acting transcriptional activation of the long terminal repeat of human T lymphotropic viruses in infected cells. Science 225:381–385, 1984

47. Fujisawa J, Seiki M, Kiyokawa T, Yoshida M: Functional activation of long terminal repeat of human T-cell leukemia virus type 1 by transacting factor. Proc Natl Acad Sci USA 82:2277–2281, 1985

48. Febler BK, Paskalis H, Klienman-Ewing C et al: The pX protein of HTLV-I is a transcriptional activator of its long terminal repeats. Science 229:675–679, 1985

49. Chen ISY, Slamon DJ, Rosenblatt JD et al: The x gene is essential for HTLV replication. Science 229:54–58, 1985

50. Kiyokawa T, Seiki M, Iwashita S, Imagawa K, Shimizu F, Yoshida M: $p27^{x-III}$ and $p21^{x-III}$, proteins encoded by the pX sequence of human T-cell leukemia virus type I. Proc Natl Acad Sci USA 82:8359–8363, 1985

51. Fujisawa J, Seiki M, Sato M, Yoshida M: A transcriptional enhancer sequence of HTLV-1 is responsible for trans-activation mediated by p40 or HTLV-1. EMBO J 5:713–718, 1986

52. Rosen CA, Sodroski JG, Haseltine WA: Location of cis-acting regulatory sequences in the human T-cell leukemia virus type 1 long terminal repeat. Proc Natl Acad Sci USA 82:6502–6506, 1985

53. Greene WC, Leonard WJ, Wano Y et al: Trans-activator gene of HTLV-II induces IL-2 receptor and IL-2 cellular gene expression. Science 232:877–880, 1986

54. Jeang KT, Brady J, Radonovich M, Duvall J, Khoury G: p4-x trans-activation of the HTLV-I LTR promoter. UCLA Symp Mol Cell Biol 67:181–189, 1988

55. Beasley RP, Lin CC, Hwang L et al: Hepatocellular carcinoma and hepatitis B virus: A prospective study of 22,707 men in Taiwan. Lancet 2:1129–1133, 1981

56. Robinson WS, Marion PL, Feitelson M et al: The hepadna virus group: Hepatitis B and related viruses. In Szmuness W, Alter HJ, Maynard JW (eds): Viral Hepatitis—1981 International Symposium, pp 57–68. Philadelphia, Franklin Institute Press, 1982

57. Summers J, Smolec JM, Snyder R: A virus similar to human hepatitis B virus associated with hepatitis and hepatoma in woodchucks. Proc Natl Acad Sci USA 74:4533–4537, 1978

58. Marion PL, Oshiro L, Regnery DC et al: A virus in Beechey ground squirrels that is related to hepatitis B virus of man. Proc Natl Acad Sci USA 77:2941–2945, 1980

59. Mason WS, Seal G, Summers J: Virus of Pekin ducks with structural and biological relatedness to human hepatitis B virus. J Virol 36:829–836, 1980

60. Blumberg BS, Alter HJ, Visnich S: A "new" antigen in leukemia sera. JAMA 191:541–546, 1965

61. Alter HJ, Blumberg BS: Further studies on a "new" human isoprecipitin system (Australia antigen). Blood 27:297–309, 1966

62. Blumberg BS, Gerstley BJS, Hungerford DA et al: A serum antigen (Australia antigen) in Down's syndrome leukemia and hepatitis. Ann Intern Med 66:924–931, 1967

63. Prince AM: An antigen detected in the blood during the incubation period of serum hepatitis. Proc Natl Acad Sci USA 60:814–821, 1968

64. Dane DS, Cameron CH, Briggs M: Virus-like particles in serum of patients with Australia antigen associated hepatitis. Lancet 2:695–698, 1970

65. Almeida JD: Individual morphological variation seen in Australia antigen positive sera. Am J Dis Child 123:303–309, 1972

66. Kim CY, Tilles JG: Purification and biophysical characterization of hepatitis B antigen. J Clin Invest 52:1176–1186, 1973

67. Summers JA, O'Connell A, Millman I: Genome of hepatitis B virus: Restriction enzyme cleavage and structure of DNA extracted from Dane particles. Proc Natl Acad Sci USA 72:4597–4601, 1975

68. Tiollais P, Pourcel C, Dejean A: The hepatitis B virus. Nature 317:489–495, 1985

69. Robinson WS: Hepatitis B virus. In Fields BN (ed): Virology, pp 1384–1406. New York, Raven Press, 1985

70. Landers TA, Greenberg HB, Robinson WS: Structure of hepatitis B Dane particle DNA and nature of the endogenous DNA polymerase reaction. J Virol 23:368–376, 1977

164   PRINCIPLES OF CARCINOGENESIS: VIRAL

71. Galibert F, Mandart E, Fitoussi F et al: Nucleotide sequence of hepatitis B virus genome (subtype ayw) cloned in E. coli. Nature 281:646–650, 1979
72. Ganem D, Varmus HE: The molecular biology of hepatitis B virus. Annu Rev Biochem 56:651–693, 1987
73. Seeger C, Ganem D, Varmus HE: Biochemical and genetic evidence for the hepatitis B virus replication strategy. Science 232:477–484, 1986
74. Shafritz DA, Shouval D, Sherman H et al: Integration of hepatitis B virus DNA into the genome of liver cells in chronic liver disease and hepatocellular carcinoma. N Engl J Med 305:1067–1073, 1981
75. Brechot C, Pourcel C, Hadchouel M et al: State of hepatitis B virus DNA in liver diseases. Hematology 2:27–34, 1982
76. Summers J, Mason WS: Replication of the genome of a hepatitis B-like virus by reverse transcription of an RNA intermediate. Cell 29:403–415, 1982
77. Shaul Y, Rutter WJ, Laub O: A human hepatitis B viral enhancer element. EMBO J 4:427–430, 1985
78. Jameel S, Siddiqui A: The human hepatitis B virus enhancer requires transacting cellular factor(s) for activity. Mol Cell Biol 6:710–715, 1986
79. Szmuness W: Hepatocellular carcinoma and the hepatitis B virus: Evidence for a causal association. Prog Med Virol 24:40–69, 1978
80. Popper H, Shih JWK, Gerin JL et al: Woodchuck hepatitis and hepatocellular carcinoma: Correlation of histologic with virologic observations. Hematology 1:91–98, 1981
81. Ciuffo G: Imnfesto positivo con filtrato di verruca volgare. Giorn Ital Mal Venereol 48:12–17, 1907
82. Coggins JR, zur Hausen H: Workshop on papillomaviruses and cancer. Cancer Res 39:545–546, 1979
83. Favre M, Orth G, Croissant O et al: Human papillomavirus DNA: Physical map. Proc Natl Acad Sci USA 72:4810–4814, 1975
84. Gissmann L, zur Hausen H: Human papillomaviruses: Physical mapping and genetic heterogenicity. Proc Natl Acad Sci USA 73:1310–1313, 1976
85. Orth G, Favre M, Croissant O: Characterization of a new type of human papillomavirus that causes skin warts. J Virol 24:108–120, 1977
86. Orth G, Jablonska S, Favre M et al: Characterization of two types of human papillomavirus in lesions of epidermodysplasia verruciformis. Proc Natl Acad Sci USA 75:1537–1541, 1978
87. Gissmann L, Pfister H, zur Hausen H: Human papillomaviruses (HPV): Characterization of four different isolates. Virology 7:569–580, 1977
88. Orth G, Favre M, Breitburd F et al: Epidermodysplasia verruciformis: A model for the role of papillomaviruses in human cancer. Cold Spring Harbor Symp Quant Biol [Conference on Cell Proliferation] 7:259–282, 1980
89. Gissmann L, zur Hausen H: Partial characterization of viral DNA from human genital warts (condylomata acuminata). Int J Cancer 25:605–609, 1980
90. Ostrow RS, Kryzyek R, Pass F et al: Identification of a novel human papillomavirus in cutaneous warts of meat handlers. Virology 108:21–27, 1981
91. Orth G, Jablonska S, Favre M et al: Identification of papillomaviruses in butchers' warts. J Invest Dermatol 76:97–102, 1981
92. Pfister H, Nurnberger F, Gissmann L, zur Hausen H: Characterization of a human papillomavirus from epidermodysplasia verruciformis lesions of a patient from Upper Volta. Int J Cancer 27:645–650, 1981
93. Kremsdorf D, Jablonska S, Favre M, Orth G: Biochemical characterization of two types of human papillomaviruses associated with epidermodysplasia verruciformis. J Virol 43:436–447, 1982
94. Kremsdorf D, Jablonska S, Favre M, Orth G: Human papillomaviruses associated with epidermodysplasia verruciformis: II. Molecular cloning and biochemical characterization of human papillomavirus 3a, 8, 10, and 12 genomes. J Virol 48:340–351, 1983
95. Gissmann L, Diehl V, Schultz-Coulon H, zur Hausen H: Molecular cloning and characterization of human papillomavirus DNA derived from a laryngeal papilloma. J Virol 44:393–400, 1982
96. Pfister H, Hettich I, Runne U et al: Characterization of human papillomavirus type 13 from lesions of focal epithelial hyperplasia Heck. J Virol 47:363–366, 1983
97. Tsumori T, Yutsudo M, Nakano Y et al: Molecular cloning of a new human papillomavirus isolated from epidermodysplasia verruciformis lesions. J Gen Virol 64:967–969, 1983
98. Kremsdorf D, Favre M, Jablonska S et al: Molecular cloning and characterization of the genomes of nine newly recognized papillomavirus types associated with epidermodysplasia verruciformis. J Virol 52:1013–1018, 1984
99. Durst M, Gissmann L, Ikenberg H, zur Hausen H: A papillomavirus DNA from a cervical carcinoma and its prevalence in cancer biopsy samples from different geographic regions. Proc Natl Acad Sci USA 80:3812–3815, 1983
100. Boshart M, Gissmann L, Ikenberg H, Kleinheinz A, Scheurlen W, zur Hausen H: A new type of papillomavirus DNA, its presence in genital cancer biopsies and in cell lines derived from cervical cancer. EMBO J 3:1151–1157, 1984
101. Gassermaier A, Lammel M, Pfister H: Molecular cloning and characterization of the DNAs of human papillomaviruses 19, 20, and 25 from a patient with epidermodysplasia verruciformis. J Virol 52:1019–1023, 1984
102. Ostrow RS, Zachow KR, Thompson O, Faras AJ: Molecular cloning and characterization of a unique type of human papillomavirus from an immune deficient patient. J Invest Dermatol 82:362–366, 1984
103. Kahn T, Schwarz E, zur Hausen H: Molecular cloning and characterization of the DNA of a new human papillomavirus from a laryngeal carcinoma. Int J Cancer 37:61–65, 1986
104. Lorincz AT, Lancaster WD, Temple GF: Cloning and characterization of the DNA of a
new human papillomavirus from a woman with dysplasia of the uterine cervix. J Virol 58:225–229, 1986
105. Beaudenon S, Praetorius F, Kremsdorf D et al: A new type of human papillomavirus associated with oral focal epithelial hyperplasia. J Invest Dermatol 88:130–135, 1987
106. Beaudenon S, Kremsdorf D, Croissant O et al: A novel type of human papillomavirus associated with genital neoplasias. Nature 321:246–249, 1986
107. Kawashima M, Jablonska S, Favre M, Obalek S, Croissant O, Orth G: Characterization of a new type of human papillomavirus found in a lesion of Bowen's disease of the skin. J Virol 57:688–692, 1986
108. Lorincz AT, Quinn AP, Lancaster WD, Temple GF: A new type of papillomavirus associated with cancer of the uterine cervix. Virology 159:187–190, 1987
109. Kawashima M, Favre M, Jablonska S, Obalek S, Orth G: Characterization of a new type of human papillomavirus (HPV) related to HPV5 from a case of actinic keratosis. Virology 145:384–389, 1986
110. Scheurlen W, Gissmann L, Gross G, zur Hausen H: Molecular cloning of two new HPV types (HPV37 and HPV38) from a keratoacanthoma and a malignant melanoma. Int J Cancer 37:505–510, 1986
111. Beaudenon S, Kremsdorf D, Obalek S et al: Plurality of genital human papillomaviruses: Characterization of two new types with distinct biological properties. Virology 161:374–384, 1987
112. Baker CC, Howley PM: Differential promoter utilization by the bovine papillomavirus in transformed cells as productively infected wart tissues. EMBO J 6:1027–1035, 1987
113. Heilman CA, Engel L, Lowy DR, Howley PM: Virus-specific transcription in bovine papillomavirus-transformed mouse cells. Virology 119:22–34, 1982
114. Engel LW, Heilman CA, Howley PM: Transcriptional organization of the bovine papillomavirus type 1. J Virol 47:516–528, 1983
115. Lowy DR, Dvoretzky I, Shober R, Law M-F, Engle L, Howley PM: In vitro tumorigenic transformation by a defined subgenomic fragment of bovine papillomavirus DNA. Nature 287:72–74, 1980
116. Doorbar J, Campbell D, Grand RJA et al: Identification of the human papillomavirus type 1a encodes a minor structural protein carrying type-specific antigens. EMBO J 5:355–362, 1986
117. Amtmann E, Sauer G: Bovine papilloma virus transcription: Polyadenylated RNA species and assessment of the direction of transcription. J Virol 43:59–66, 1982
118. Black PH, Hartley JW, Rowe WP, Huebner RJ: Transformation of bovine tissue culture cells by bovine papillomavirus. Nature 199:1016–1018, 1963
119. Thomas M, Boiron M, Tanzer J, Levy JP, Bernard J: In vitro transformation of mice cells by bovine papillomavirus. Nature 202:709–710, 1964
120. Dvoretzky I, Shober R, Lowy DR: Focus assay in mouse cells for bovine papillomavirus. Virology 103:369–375, 1980
121. Law MF, Lowy DR, Dvoretzky I, Howley PM: Mouse cells transformed by bovine papillomavirus contain only extrachromosomal viral DNA sequences. Proc Natl Acad Sci USA 78:2727–2731, 1981
122. Lusky M, Botchan MR: A bovine papillomavirus type 1–encoded modulator function is dispensable for transient viral replication but is required for establishment of the stable plasmid state. J Virol 60:729–742, 1986
123. Sarver N, Rabson MS, Yang Y-C, Bryne JC, Howley PM: Localization and analysis of bovine papillomavirus type 1 transforming functions. J Virol 52:377–388, 1984
124. Lusky M, Botchan MR: Genetic analysis of bovine papillomavirus type-1 trans-acting replication factors. J Virol 53:955–965, 1985
125. Spalholz BA, Yang Y-C, Howley PM: Transactivation of a bovine papillomavirus transcriptional regulatory element by the E2 gene product. Cell 42:183–191, 1985
126. Phelps WC, Howley PM: Transcriptional transactivation by the human papillomavirus E2 gene product. J Virol 61:1630–1638, 1987
127. Hirochika H, Broker TR, Chow LT: Enhancers and trans-acting E2 transcriptional factors of papillomaviruses. J Virol 61:2599–2608, 1987
128. Lambert PF, Spalholz BA, Howley PM: A transcriptional repressor encoded by BPV-1 shares a common carboxy terminal domain with the E2 transactivator. Cell 50:69–78, 1987
129. Yang Y-C, Spalholz BA, Rabson MS, Howley PM: Dissociation of transforming and transactivation functions for bovine papillomavirus type 1. Nature 318:575–577, 1985
130. DiMaio D, Guralski D, Schiller JT: Translation of open reading frame E5 of bovine papillomavirus is required for its transforming activity. Proc Natl Acad Sci USA 83:1797–1801, 1986
131. Schiller J, Vousden K, Vass WC, Lowy DR: The E5 open reading frame of bovine papillomavirus type 1 encodes a transforming gene. J Virol 57:1–6, 1986
132. Groff DE, Lancaster WD: Genetic analysis of the 3' early region transformation and replication functions of bovine papillomavirus type 1. Virology 150:221–230, 1986
133. Rabson MS, Yee C, Yang Y-C, Howley PM: Analysis of the bovine papillomavirus type 1 3' early region transformation and plasmid maintenance functions. J Virol 60:626–634, 1986
134. Yang Y-C, Okayama H, Howley PM: Bovine papillomavirus contains multiple transforming genes. Proc Natl Acad Sci USA 82:1030–1034, 1985
135. Schiller JT, Vass WC, Lowy DR: Identification of a second transforming region in bovine papillomavirus DNA. Proc Natl Acad Sci USA 81:7880–7884, 1984
136. Berg LJ, Singh K, Botchan M: Complementation of a bovine papillomavirus low-copy number mutant: Evidence for a temporal requirement of the complementing gene. Mol Cell Biol 6:859–869, 1986
137. Pilacinski WP, Glassman DL, Krzyzek RA et al: Cloning and expression in Escherichia

coli of the bovine papillomavirus L1 and L2 open reading frames. Biotechnology 1:356–360, 1984

138. Komly CA, Breitburd F, Croissant O et al: The L2 open reading frame of human papillomavirus type 1a encodes a minor structural protein carrying type-specific antigens. J Virol 60:813–816, 1986

139. Howley PM, Schlegel R: Papillomavirus transformation. In Salzman NP, Howley PM (eds): The Papovaviridae: II. The Papillomaviruses, pp 141–163, New York, Plenum Publishing Corp, 1987

140. DiMaio D: Nonsense mutation in open reading frame E2 of bovine papillomavirus DNA. J Virol 57:475–480, 1986

141. Tsunokawa Y, Takebe N, Kasamatsu T et al: Transforming activity of human papillomavirus type 16 DNA sequences in cervical cancer. Proc Natl Acad Sci USA 83:220–223, 1986

142. Bedell MA, Jones KH, Laimins LA: The E6–E7 region of human papillomavirus type 18 is sufficient for transformation of NIH 3T3 and Rat 1 cells. J Virol 61:3635–3640, 1987

143. Phelps WC, Yee CL, Munger K, Howley PM: The human papillomavirus type 16 E7 gene encodes transactivation and transformation functions similar to adenovirus E1a. Cell 53:539–547, 1988

144. Matlashewski G, Schneider J, Banks L et al: Human papillomavirus type 16 DNA cooperates with activated ras in transforming primary cells. EMBO J 6:1741–1746, 1987

145. Rous P, Beard JW: The progression to carcinoma of virus-induced rabbit papillomas (Shope). J Exp Med 62:523–548, 1935

146. Rous P, Kidd JG, Smith WE: Experiments of the cause of the rabbit carcinomas derived from virus-induced papillomas. J Exp Med 96:159–174, 1953

147. Jarrett WFH, McNeil PE, Grimshaw WIR et al: High incidence area of cattle cancer with a possible interaction between an environmental carcinogen and a papillomavirus. Nature 274:215–217, 1978

148. Ford JN, Jennings PA, Spradbrow PB et al: Evidence for papillomaviruses in ocular lesions in cattle. Res Vet Sci 32:257–259, 1982

149. Vanselow BA, Spradbrow PB, Jackson ARB: Papillomaviruses, papillomas and squamous cell carcinomas in sheep. Vet Rec 110:561–562, 1982

150. Orth G: Epidermodysplasia verruciformis: A model for understanding the oncogenicity of human papillomaviruses. In Evered D, Clark S (eds): Papillomaviruses. Ciba Found Symp 120:157–174, 1986

151. Shope RE: Infectious papillomatosis of rabbits. J Exp Med 58:607–624, 1933

152. Rous P, Kidd JG: The carcinogenic effect of a virus upon tarred skin. Science 83:468–469, 1936

153. Kidd JG, Rous P: Effects of the papillomavirus (Shope) upon tar warts of rabbits. Proc Soc Exp Biol Med 37:518–520, 1937

154. Wettstein FO, Stevens JG: Variable sized free episomes of Shope papilloma virus DNA are present in all non-virus-producing neoplasms and integrated genomes are detected in some. Proc Natl Acad Sci USA 79:790–794, 1982

155. Nasseri M, Wettstein FO: Differences exist between viral transcripts in cottontail rabbit papillomavirus-induced benign and malignant tumors as well as non-virus-producing and virus-producing tumors. J Virol 51:706–712, 1984

156. Jarrett WFH, Murphy J, O'Neil BW et al: Virus-induced papillomas of the alimentary tract of cattle. Int J Cancer 22:323–328, 1978

157. Campo MS, Moar MH, Sartirana ML et al: The presence of bovine papillomavirus type 4 DNA is not required for the progression to, or the maintenance of, the malignant state in cancers of the alimentary canal in cattle. EMBO J 4:1819–1825, 1985

158. Lutzner M: Epidermodysplasia verruciformis: An autosomal recessive disease characterized by viral warts and skin cancer. A model for viral oncogenesis. Bull Cancer 65:169–182, 1978

159. Pass F, Faras AJ: Human papillomavirus DNA in cutaneous primary and metastasized squamous cell carcinomas from patients with epidermodysplasia verruciformis. Proc Natl Acad Sci USA 79:1634–1638, 1982

160. Pfister H, Gassenmaier A, Nurnberger F: HPV-5 DNA in a carcinoma of an epidermodysplasia verruciformis patient infected with various human papillomavirus types. Cancer Res 43:1436–1441, 1983

161. Green M, Brackmann KH, Sanders PR et al: Isolation of a human papillomavirus from a patient with epidermodysplasia verruciformis: Presence of related viral DNA genomes in human urogenital tumors. Proc Natl Acad Sci USA 79:4437–4441, 1982

162. Yutsudo M, Shimakage T, Hakura A: Human papillomavirus type 17 DNA in skin carcinoma tissue of a patient with epidermodysplasia verruciformis. Virology 144:295–298, 1985

163. Yutsudo M, Hakura A: Human papillomavirus type 17 transcripts expressed in skin cancer tissue of a patient with epidermodysplasia verruciformis. Int J Cancer 39:586–589, 1987

164. Underwood PB, Hester LL: Diagnosis and treatment of premalignant lesions of the vulva: A review. Am J Obstet Gynecol 110:849–857, 1971

165. Waugh M: Condylomata acuminata. Br Med J 2:527–528, 1972

166. Dunn AE, Ogilvie MM: Intranuclear virus particles in human genital wart tissue: Observation on the ultrastructure of epidermal layer. J Ultrastruct Res 22:282–295, 1968

167. Oriel JD, Almeida JD: Demonstration of virus particles in human genital warts. Br J Vener Dis 46:37–42, 1970

168. Woodruff JD, Braun L, Cavallieri R et al: Immunological identification of papillomavirus antigen in paraffin-processed condyloma tissues from the female genital tract. Obstet Gynecol 56:727–732, 1980

169. Gissmann L, de Villiers EM, zur Hausen H: Analysis of human genital warts (condylomata acuminata) and other genital tumors for human papillomavirus type 6 DNA. Int J Cancer 29:143–146, 1982

170. Gissmann L, Wolnik L, Ikenberg H, Koldovsky U, Schnurch G, zur Hausen H: Human papillomavirus type 6 and 11 DNA sequences in genital and laryngeal papillomas and in some cervical cancers. Proc Natl Acad Sci USA 80:560–563, 1983

171. Buschke A, Lowenstein L: Über carcinomahnlich condylomata acuminata des penis. Arch Dermatol Syph 163:30–46, 1931

172. Boshart M, zur Hausen H: Human papillomaviruses in Buschke-Lowenstein tumors: Physical state of the DNA and identification of a tandem duplication in the non-coding region of a human papillomavirus 6 subtype. J Virol 58:963–966, 1986

173. Meisels A, Fortin R: Condylomatous lesions of the cervix and vagina: I. Cytologic patterns. Acta Cytol 20:505–509, 1976

174. Purola E, Savia E: Cytology of gynecologic condyloma acuminatum. Acta Cytol 21:26–31, 1977

175. Laverty CR, Russell P, Hillis E et al: The significance of noncondylomatous wart virus infection of the cervical transformation zone. Acta Cytol 22:195–201, 1978

176. Koss LG, Durfee GR: Unusual patterns of squamous epithelium of the uterine cervix: Cytologic and pathologic study of koilocytotic atypia. Ann NY Acad Sci 63:1245–1261, 1956

177. Della Torre G, Pilotti S, dePalo G et al: Viral particles in cervical condylomatous lesions. Tumori 64:549–553, 1978

178. Hills E, Laverty CR: Electron microscopic detection of papilloma virus particles in selected koilocytotic cells in a routine cervical smear. Acta Cytol 23:53–56, 1979

179. Kessler IL: Human cervical cancer as a venereal disease. Cancer Res 36:783–791, 1976

180. zur Hausen H: Human papillomaviruses and their possible role in squamous cell carcinomas. Curr Top Microbiol Immunol 78:1–30, 1977

181. Rawls WE, Tompkins WAF, Figueroa ME et al: Herpes simplex virus type 2: Association with carcinoma of the cervix. Science 161:1255–1256, 1968

182. Nahmias AJ, Josey WE, Naib ZM et al: Antibodies to herpes virus hominis types 1 and 2 in humans: II. Women with cervical cancer. Am J Epidemiol 91:548–552, 1970

183. zur Hausen H: Herpes simplex virus in human genital cancer. Int Rev Exp Pathol 25:307–326, 1983

184. Vonka V, Kanda J, Hirsch I et al: Prospective study on the relationship between cervical neoplasia and herpes simplex type-2 virus: II. Herpes simplex type-2 antibody presence in sera taken at enrollment. Int J Cancer 33:61–66, 1984

185. Vonka V, Kanda J, Jelinek J et al: Prospective study on the relationship between cervical neoplasia and herpes simplex type-2 virus: I. Epidemiologic characteristics. Int J Cancer 33:49–60, 1984

186. Peterson O: Spontaneous course of cervical precancerous conditions. Am J Obstet Gynecol 72:1063–1071, 1956

187. Kinlen LJ, Spriggs AI: Women with positive cervical smears but without surgical intervention: A follow up study. Lancet 2:463–465, 1978

188. Richart RM, Barrow BA: A follow-up study of patients with cervical dysplasia. Am J Obstet Gynecol 105:386–393, 1969

189. Gissmann L, Schwarz E: Persistence and expression of human papillomavirus DNA in genital cancer. In Evered D, Clark S (eds): Papillomaviruses. Ciba Found Symp 120:190–197, 1986

190. Ikenberg H, Gissmann L, Gross G, Grussendorf-Conen E-I, zur Hausen H: Human papillomavirus 16 related DNA in genital Bowen's disease and in bowenoid papulosis. Int J Cancer 32:563–565, 1983

191. Gross G, Hagedorn M, Ikenberg H et al: Bowenoid papulosis: Presence of human papillomavirus (HPV) structural antigens and of HPV-16 related DNA sequences. Arch Dermatol 121:858–863, 1985

192. Clarke EA, Morgan RW, Newman AM: Smoking as a risk factor in cancer of the cervix: Additional evidence from a case control study. Am J Epidemiol 115:59–66, 1982

193. Wigle DT: Smoking and cancer of the cervix: Hypothesis. Am J Epidemiol 111:125–127, 1980

194. Winkelstein W Jr: Smoking and cancer of the uterine cervix. Am J Epidemiol 106:257–259, 1977

195. Hoffmann D, Hecht SS, Haley NJ et al: Tumorigenic agents in tobacco products and their uptake by chewers, smokers and nonsmokers. J Cell Biochem 9C:33, 1985

196. zur Hausen H: Human genital cancer: Synergism between two virus infections or synergism between a virus infection and initiating events. Lancet 2:1370–1372, 1982

197. Schwarz E, Freese UK, Gissmann L, Mayer W, Roggenbuck B, Stemlau A, zur Hausen H: Structure and transcription of human papillomavirus sequences in cervical carcinoma cells. Nature 314:111–114, 1985

198. Smotkin D, Wettstein FO: Transcription of human papillomavirus type 16 early genes in cervical cancer and a cancer derived cell line and identification of the E7 protein. Proc Natl Acad Sci USA 83:4680–4684, 1986

199. Shirasawa H, Tomita Y, Kubota K et al: Transcriptional differences of the human papillomavirus type 16 genome between precancerous lesions and invasive carcinomas. J Virol 62:1022–1027, 1988

200. Yee C, Krishnan-Hewlett I, Baker CC et al: Presence and expression of human papillomavirus sequences in human cervical carcinoma cell lines. Am J Pathol 119:361–366, 1985

201. Durst M, Croce CM, Gissmann L et al: Papillomavirus sequences integrate near cellular oncogenes in some cervical carcinomas. Proc Natl Acad Sci USA 84:1070–1074, 1987

202. Baker CC, Phelps WC, Lindgren V et al: Structural and transcriptional analysis of human papillomavirus type 16 sequences in cervical carcinoma cell lines. J Virol 61:962–971, 1987
203. Theirry F, Heard JM, Dartmann K et al: Characterization of a transcriptional promoter of human papillomavirus 18 and the modulation of its expression by simian virus 40 and adenovirus early antigens. J Virol 61:134–142, 1987
204. Gloss B, Bernard HU, Seedorf K et al: The upstream regulatory region of the human papillomavirus 16 contains an E2 protein-independent enhancer which is specific for cervical carcinoma cells and regulated by glucocorticoid hormones. EMBO J 6:3734–3743, 1987
205. Cripe TP, Haugen TH, Turk OP et al: Transcriptional regulation of the human papillomavirus-16 E6-E7 promoter by a keratinocyte-dependent enhancer, and by viral E2 trans-activator and repressor gene products: Implications for cervical carcinogenesis. EMBO J 6:3745–3753, 1987
206. Loning T, Ikenberg H, Becker J et al: Analysis of oral papillomas leukoplakias, and invasive carcinomas for human papillomavirus type related DNA. J Invest Dermatol 84:417–420, 1985
207. Brandsma JL, Steinberg BM, Abramson AL et al: Presence of human papillomavirus type 16 related sequences in verrucous carcinoma of the larynx. Cancer Res 46:2185–2188, 1986
208. Jenson AB, Lancaster WD, Hartman DP et al: Frequency and distribution of papillomavirus structural antigens cerrucae, multiple papillomas, and condylomata of the oral cavity. Am J Pathol 107:212–218, 1982
209. Lind P, Syrjanen K, Koppang HS et al: Immunoreactivity and human papillomavirus (HPV) on oral precancer and cancer lesions. Scand J Dent Res 94:419–426, 1986
210. de Villiers EM, Neumann C, Le JY, Weidauer H, zur Hausen H: Infection of the oral mucosa with defined types of human papillomaviruses. Med Microbiol Immunol 174:287–294, 1986
211. Naghashfar Z, Sawada E, Kutcher MK et al: Identification of genital tract papillomaviruses HPV-6 and HPV-16 in warts of the oral cavity. J Virol 17:313–324, 1985
212. Syrjanen S, Syrjanen K, Lamberg MA: Detection of human papillomavirus DNA in oral mucosal lesions using in situ DNA hybridization applied on paraffin sections. Oral Surg 62:660–667, 1986
213. Byrne JC, Tsao MS, Fraser RS, Howley PM: Human papillomavirus-11 DNA in patient with chronic laryngotracheobronchial papillomatosis and metastatic squamous-cell carcinoma of the lung. N Engl J Med 317:873–878, 1987
214. Syrjanen K, Pyrhonen S, Aukee S et al: Squamous cell papilloma of the esophagus: A tumor probably caused by human papillomavirus (HPV). Diagn Histopathol 5:291–296, 1982
215. Winkler B, Capo V, Reumann W, Ma A et al: Human papillomavirus infection of the esophagus. Cancer 55:149–155, 1985
216. Burkitt D: A sarcoma involving the jaws in African children. Br. J Surg 46:218–223, 1958
217. Burkitt D: Determining the climatic limitations of a children's cancer common in Africa. Br Med J 2:1019–1023, 1962
218. Epstein MA, Barr YM: Cultivation in vitro of human lymphoblasts from Burkitt's malignant lymphoma. Lancet 1:252–253, 1964
219. Epstein MA, Achong BG, Barr YM: Virus particles in cultured lymphoblasts from Burkitt's lymphoma. Lancet 1:702–703, 1964
220. Salahuddin SK, Ablashi DV, Markham PD et al: Isolation of a new virus, HBLV, in patients with lymphoproliferative disorders. Nature 324:596–601, 1986
221. Josephs SF, Salahuddin SK, Ablashi DV et al: Genomic analysis of the human B-lymphotropic virus (HBLV). Nature 324:601–603, 1986
222. Kieff E, Dambaugh T, Heller M et al: The biology and chemistry of Epstein-Barr virus. J Infect Dis 146:506–517, 1982
223. Baer R, Bankier AT, Biggin MD et al: DNA sequence and expression of B95-8 Epstein Barr virus genome. Nature 310:207–211, 1984
224. Hummel M, Kieff E: Mapping of polypeptides encoded by the Epstein-Barr virus genome in productive infection. Proc Natl Acad Sci USA 79:5698–5702, 1982
225. de Schryver A, Klein G, Henle W et al: Comparison of EBV neutralization tests based on abortive infection or transformation of lymphoid cells and their relation to membrane reactive antibodies (anti-MA). Int J Cancer 13:353–362, 1974
226. Henle G, Henle W, Klein G: Demonstration of two distinct components in the early antigen complex of Epstein-Barr virus-infected cells. Int J Cancer 8:272–282, 1971
227. Reedman BM, Klein G: Cellular localization of an Epstein-Barr virus (EBV) associated complement-fixing antigen in producer and non-producer lymphoblastoid cell lines. Int J Cancer 11:499–520, 1973
228. Rickenson AB, Moss DJ, Pope JH: Long-term T-cell mediated immunity to Epstein-Barr virus in man: II. Components necessary for regression in virus-infected leukocyte cultures. Int J Cancer 23:610–617, 1979
229. Rickenson AB, Wallace LE, Epstein MA: HLA-restricted T-cell recognition of Epstein-Barr virus-infected B cells. Nature 283:865–867, 1980
230. Svedmyr E, Jondal M: Cytotoxic effector cells specific for B cell lines transformed by Epstein-Barr virus are present in patients with infectious mononucleosis. Proc Natl Acad Sci USA 72:1622–1626, 1975
231. Thorley-Lawson DA, Geilinger K: Monoclonal antibodies against the major glycoprotein (gp 350/220) of Epstein-Barr virus neutralize infectivity. Proc Natl Acad Sci USA 77:5307–5311, 1980
232. Pearson GR, Vroman B, Chase B et al: Identification of polypeptide components of the Epstein-Barr virus early antigen complex with monoclonal antibodies. J Virol 47:193–201, 1983
233. Pearson GR, Luka J: Characterization of the virus-determined antigens. In Epstein MA, Achong BG (eds): The Epstein-Barr Virus, pp 47–74. New York, John Wiley & Sons, 1986
234. Fialkow PJ, Klein E, Klein G et al: Immunoglobulin and glucose-6-phosphate dehydrogenase as markers of cellular origin in Burkitt lymphoma. J Exp Med 138:89–101, 1973
235. Mann RB, Bernard CW: Burkitts tumor: Lessons from mice, monkeys, and man. Lancet 2:84, 1979
236. Magrath I: Clinical and pathobiological features of Burkitt's lymphoma and their relevance to treatment. In Levine PH, Ablashi DV, Pearson GR et al: Epstein-Barr Virus and Associated Diseases, pp 631–643. Boston, Martinus Nijhoff, 1985
237. Kafuko GW, Burkitt DP: Burkitt's lymphoma and malaria. Int J Cancer 6:1–9, 1970
238. Morrow RH Jr: Epidemiological evidence for the role of falciparum malaria in the pathogenesis of Burkitt's lymphoma. In Lenoir GM, O'Connor G, Olweny CLM (eds): A Human Cancer Model, IARC Sci Publ 60:177–186, 1985
239. Moss DJ, Burrows SR, Catelino DJ et al: A comparison of Epstein-Barr virus-specific T-cell immunity in malaria-endemic and nonendemic regions of Papua New Guinea. Int J Cancer 31:727–732, 1983
240. Manolov G, Manolova Y: Marker band in one chromosome 14 from Burkitt lymphomas. Nature 237:33–34, 1972
241. Lenoir GM, Taub R: Chromosomal translocations and oncogenes in Burkitt's lymphoma. In Goldman JM (ed): Leukaemia and Lymphoma Research: Vol 2. Genetic Rearrangements in Leukaemia and Lymphoma, pp 152–172. London, Harnden, 1986
242. Leder P, Battey J, Lenoir G et al: Translocations among antibody genes in human cancer. Science 222:765–771, 1983
243. Erikson J, Finan J, Nowell PC, Croce CM: Translocation of immunoglobulin V_H genes in Burkitt's lymphoma. Proc Natl Acad Sci USA 79:5611–5615, 1982
244. Lombardi L, Newcomb EW, Della-Favera R: Pathogenesis of Burkitt's lymphoma: Expression of an activated c-myc oncogene causes the tumorigenic conversion of EBV-infected human B-Lymphocytes. Cell 49:161–170, 1987
245. Klein G: Lymphoma development in mice and human: Diversity of initiation is followed by convergent cytogenetic evolution. Proc Natl Acad Sci USA 76:2442–2446, 1979
246. Klein G, Klein E: Evolution of tumors and the impact of molecular oncology. Nature 315:190, 1985
247. Lenoir GM, Bornkamm GW: Burkitt's lymphoma, a human cancer model for the study of multistep development of cancer: Proposal for a new scenario. Adv Viral Oncol 7:173–206, 1987
248. Henle W, Henle G: Epstein-Barr virus and human malignancies. Adv Viral Oncol 5:201–238, 1985
249. zur Hausen H, Schulte-Holthausen H, Klein G et al: EBV DNA in biopsies of Burkitt tumors and anaplastic carcinomas of the nasopharynx. Nature 228:1056–1058, 1970
250. Andersson-Anvret M, Forsby N, Klein G et al: Relationship between the Epstein-Barr virus and undifferentiated nasopharyngeal carcinoma: Correlated nucleic acid hybridization and histopathological examination. Int J Cancer 20:486–494, 1977
251. Raab-Traub N, Flynn K, Pearson G et al: The differentiated form of nasopharyngeal carcinoma contains Epstein-Barr virus DNA. Int J Cancer 39:25–29, 1987
252. Pagano JS: Epstein-Barr virus transcription in nasopharyngeal carcinoma. J Virol 48:580–590, 1983
253. de The G, Zeng Y: Population screening for EBV markers: Toward improvement of nasopharyngeal carcinoma control. In Epstein MA, Achog BG (eds): The Epstein-Barr Virus, pp 237–248. New York, John Wiley & Sons, 1986
254. Purtilo DT, Sakamoto K, Barnabai V et al: Epstein-Barr virus-induced diseases in boys with the X-linked lymphoproliferative syndrome (XLP): Updates on studies of the registry. Am J Med 73:49–56, 1982

PETER GREENWALD

CHAPTER 11 *Principles of Cancer Prevention: Diet and Nutrition*

Laboratory and epidemiologic research findings of the past several decades have converged to provide strong evidence that dietary factors are major determinants for a large proportion of human cancers. Epidemiologists note wide international variations in the occurrence and prevalence of specific types of cancer. For example, death rates from breast cancer are five times higher in certain Western countries than in less developed countries with very different lifestyles. Migration and time trend data coupled with laboratory results implicate several dietary factors in an increased cancer risk; other dietary factors may reduce cancer risk. Although it is clear that the intake of dietary mutagens and carcinogens or poor dietary practices, including inadequate intake of foods high in important nutrients and fiber or an excessive fat and caloric intake, influence certain types of cancer incidence, the exact mechanisms and nutrient interactions are not understood fully.

The concept of diet as a possible etiologic factor has received momentum from basic carcinogenesis studies and population studies and from the recent substantial increase in commitment to research in this field. Cancer prevention through the identification and elimination of dietary components associated with the development of cancer is not feasible. A more logical preventive strategy is to identify factors that act as inhibitors of carcinogenesis and to increase human exposure to them. Two programs at the National Cancer Institute (NCI) focus on nutrient-related research for

cancer prevention: the Chemoprevention Program and the Diet, Nutrition, and Cancer Program. Chemoprevention, a recent area of research emphasis, explores natural and synthetic substances, precisely formulated and measured, that demonstrate the potential to prevent, halt, or reverse carcinogenesis. Particular attention is being directed toward beta-carotene, vitamin A (retinol) and related synthetic retinoids, vitamins C and E, and certain selenium compounds, often in study populations already exposed to cancer-causing agents but before clinical cancer is evident. Many other agents are in preclinical testing. The closely associated Diet, Nutrition, and Cancer Program is looking at less defined macronutrient factors (such as dietary fats or fiber-containing foods) that may affect the risk of cancer development.

The most direct evidence for establishing even a small to moderate causal association for cancer prevention strategies in humans comes from clinical intervention trials. Such trials may provide the only evidence on whether a specific intervention, such as a change in diet, will reduce cancer risk. As data from epidemiologic and carcinogenesis research converged, a sound basis was building for testing hypotheses by initiating human trials. The use of clinical trials to evaluate the efficacy and safety of preventive interventions parallels the earlier work of oncologists who 30 years ago began to set into place a systematic process for clinical testing of new therapies. When the first human cancer prevention trials were begun in the early 1980s, for the most part using specific nutrients thought to have a protective effect, they became the accepted means of proving whether a nutrient or other preventive agent suppresses the carcinogenic process. These studies also began to explore the use of precancerous markers as end points for evaluating the effects of preventive interventions. However, for reasons that will be discussed later in this chapter, clinical trials are not always feasible. When a clinical trial is practical and timely, it should be used. In other instances, we must follow different paths to achieve a scientific consensus on the efficacy and safety of particular interventions for cancer prevention.

This chapter reviews dietary factors associated with the cause and prevention of cancer and addresses the development and potential benefits of diet and cancer research, focusing on the following topics: laboratory studies, epidemiologic studies, specific dietary factors and cancer risk, chemoprevention, prevention research processes, similarities and differences between clinical treatment and prevention trials, an overview of intervention trials completed or in progress, research related to selected diet and cancer hypotheses, the physician's role as a promoter of a healthy diet, and future prospects for cancer prevention research on dietary factors and their impact on carcinogenesis.

OVERVIEW OF DIETARY FACTORS RELATED TO CARCINOGENESIS

Many compounds have been isolated from food sources that can markedly influence the growth and development of cancer in animal models and cell culture systems. These substances represent a structurally diverse group with multiple biologic effects, broad variabilities in efficacy and toxicity, and mechanisms of action as yet not fully elucidated.

Some naturally occurring compounds found to have inhibitory effects on cancer growth are coumarins, phenols, indoles, aromatic isothiocyanates, alkenyl benzenes, methylated flavones, plant sterols, selenium salts, and protease inhibitors. Notable preventive antineoplastic activity also has been demonstrated with pharmacologic amounts of the essential nutrients ascorbic acid (vitamin C), alpha-tocopherol (vitamin E), retinoids (vitamin A and derivatives), and beta-carotene.[1]

Pioneering studies in cancer biology in the early part of the 20th century established that tumors can be chemically induced using coal tar, azo dyes, and polycyclic hydrocarbons. Modifications in study design, particularly the use of oral rather than percutaneous routes of application, led to the observation in 1941 by Kensler that the development of azo dye–induced liver tumors could be retarded by dietary manipulations.[2] Riboflavin (vitamin B_6) was identified as a dietary constituent that expressed a preventive role through enhanced detoxification of the dyes. The macronutrients fiber and fat have been examined for their effect on carcinogenesis in several animal models.[3,4] Restricted caloric intake was found by Tannenbaum and Silverstone to be an important preventive factor in chemical carcinogenesis, with dietary fat tending to augment the carcinogenic process.[5]

A variety of substances have only recently been recognized as major sources of mutagens and carcinogens in the human diet. Large numbers of these substances are synthesized in edible plants, or are produced during the cooking or processing of food, or are used as food additives for preservation or flavor enhancement. Genotoxic, mutagenic, and carcinogenic derivatives, demonstrated in animal models, include dietary phenols, alkaloids and glycoalkaloids, isothiocyanates, alcohol, quinones, and cyclopropenoid fatty acids. Heterocyclic amines isolated from cooked proteins are potent carcinogens. Mycotoxins synthesized by a variety of molds contaminate human food, and several of these toxins are potent carcinogens. Aflatoxin, for example, contaminates grains, peanuts, and other stored foodstuffs and has been shown to be a human carcinogen in animal and epidemiologic studies. Alcohol consumption has been associated with an increased risk of oral, pharyngeal, esophageal, and stomach cancer, especially in smokers. The degree of risk associated with these substances remains largely unknown.[6,7]

Many dietary factors are known to be inhibitors of chemical carcinogenesis. For example, benzyl isothiocyanate (which occurs in cruciferous vegetables) inhibits benzo (a)pyrene-induced forestomach neoplasia in mice and induces glutathione S-transferase activity in the same system.[8] Several classes of compounds that occur naturally in food, such as phenols and lactones, are active in this system as well. Still others act as inhibitors or suppressors of chemical carcinogenesis in other tumor model systems.[9] Associated with this inhibition of carcinogenesis in some cases are elevated levels of certain enzymes involved in the metabolism of a wide range of carcinogens, including benzo(a)pyrene. Elevations in hepatic mixed function oxidase activity and glutathione S-transferase activity are postulated as carcinogen detoxification mechanisms that effectively reduce the intracellular concentration of an ultimate carcinogenic species. However, increased activities of these same enzymes also can enhance the conversion of many procarcinogens to the proximate carcinogen structure.[10]

Other types of biologic activities by dietary factors related to chemoprevention of cancer have been reported. Dietary fiber, which inhibits chemically induced cancer of the colon and small intestine in some studies, may enhance carcinogen excretion.[11] Inhibition of carcinogen formation has been demonstrated with ascorbic acid in both humans and experimental animals. For example, oral administration of ascorbic acid with sodium nitrite or nitrate and amines or amides effectively inhibits N-nitrosamine generation in the stomach under certain conditions.[12]

Inhibition of mutagenesis through the scavenging of potentially mutagenic free radicals (by alpha-tocopherol) and singlet oxygen (by ascorbic acid or beta-carotenes) is also considered to be a potentially plausible preventive mechanism.[9]

There is some suggestion in the epidemiologic literature of an inverse association between ingestion of vitamin C–containing foods and the development of cancer, particularly cancer of the esophagus[13] and stomach.[14] A possible mechanism for the protective effect of vitamin C is inhibition of nitrosamine formation from secondary and higher amines in combination with nitrite.[12,15] However, vitamin A, beta-carotene, and vitamin C are present together in many fruits and vegetables, and the epidemiologic studies in most cases do not allow clear distinction of the dietary factor responsible for potential benefits. Vitamin E is difficult to study epidemiologically because it is present in a wide variety of foods and can vary greatly with individual foodstuffs. Menkes et al[16] found that serum vitamin E (and serum beta-carotene) levels were lower in persons who later developed squamous cell carcinoma of the lung than in controls, an observation different from that reported by Willett et al.[17] Clinical trials are needed to resolve these differences.

Geographic correlation studies suggest a possible benefit from diets high in selenium.[18,19] Such studies cannot be definitive because of the possibility that an undefined covariable is responsible for the results. Ip has reviewed experimental evidence for a chemopreventive role for certain selenium compounds.[20] Among other minerals, calcium (and vitamin D) was reported to be inversely associated with the development of colorectal cancer in a 19-year prospective study in men.[21] This finding is not entirely consistent with data from international studies but merits testing in clinical trials.

The hypothesis that dietary factors can influence cancer risk, particularly in certain high-risk groups, is supported by both descriptive and analytic epidemiologic research. Taken together, results from epidemiologic and laboratory studies provide a rationale for intensive research into the nature of cancer prevention by nutrient components and their synthetic analogues.

DIETARY FACTORS AND CANCER RISK

VITAMIN A/RETINOIDS/CAROTENOIDS

By far the most extensive and clinically applicable research on dietary factors in carcinogenesis relates to the retinoids. The term *retinoids* generally applies to vitamin A (retinol) and its isomers, derivatives (retinal, retinoic acid), and synthetic analogues. These compounds have been found to directly modify the expression of a neoplastic phenotype, in some cases actually arresting the dedifferentiation of a cell. As discussed in more detail below, retinoids are of special interest for use in clinical prevention because they can exert their antineoplastic activity in cells that are already dedifferentiated or initiated into a malignant state.

Vitamin A (or its derivatives) is essential for proper growth and differentiation of epithelial tissue and bone, reproduction, and vision. In experimental animals, vitamin A deficiency is associated with an increased incidence of several types of cancer and with premalignant changes in some tissues.[22] Except for its role in the visual cycle, the mechanism of action of vitamin A in its numerous physiologic roles has not been fully identified. Beta-carotene is a dietary precursor of vitamin A widely distributed in plants. When cleaved enzymatically in the intestine or liver, one molecule of beta-carotene yields two molecules of retinol.

Lasnitzki,[23] using an organ culture system, discovered that vitamin A was able to suppress abnormal differentiation of prostate gland epithelium induced by treatment with 3-methylcholanthrene (3-MC). Later work established that retinoids could inhibit malignant transformation induced by either 3-MC or radiation in tissue culture systems.[24,25] Transformation was suppressed even when the retinoid was added 1 week after 3-MC. Further, it was shown that following removal of the retinoid from the culture medium, full expression of the malignant phenotype occurred.

Examples also exist of retinoids inducing terminal differentiation from neoplastic to a nonneoplastic phenotype. This has been accomplished with murine F9 teratocarcinoma cells[26] and human promyelocytic leukemia cells,[27] among others. In the human leukemia system, malignant cells are terminally differentiated by retinoic acid to a form with the morphological and biochemical characteristics of a mature granulocyte. The extension of these observations to other cell lines (both established and primary cultures), coupled with the observation that some retinoids are active at nanomolar concentrations, suggests that retinoids have a physiological role in normal hematopoiesis.[28]

The study of retinoid activity has been facilitated by the concerted development of synthetic analogues designed to enhance potency and minimize toxicity. One analogue in particular, 13-*cis*-retinoic acid, has undergone extensive study in several organ-specific animal model systems of chemical carcinogenesis. This compound consistently arrests malignant progression in three different rodent bladder cancer systems.[29] A significant inhibitory effect was seen in Fischer rats even when treatment with 13-*cis*-retinoic acid was delayed for 8 weeks following initiation with N-butyl-N-(4-hydroxybutyl)nitrosamine.[30] Other retinoid derivatives have similar inhibitory activity in chemically induced model systems of breast cancer and skin cancer.[29,31] Regression of chemically induced tumors and a delay in the appearance of transplanted tumors have been reported for several other synthetic retinoids.[22]

A number of mechanisms have been suggested to account for the interference by retinoids in the progression of carcinogenesis. In mice, retinoids inhibit the activity of ornithine decarboxylase, an enzyme associated with tumor promotion processes.[31] Retinoids also block cell transformation through inhibition of polypeptide transforming factors, such as sarcoma growth factor.[32] Interference with the synthesis of proteins required for neoplastic progression is another possibility.

Carotenoids are also of interest as chemopreventive agents, although there is little laboratory data to confirm that they have any inherent activity independent of their ultimate conversion to retinoids.[33] Specifically, they do not exhibit any serious toxicity, and blood levels of carotenoids are directly related to dietary intake, unlike the retinoids, which are subject to strict homeostatic control. A direct chemopreventive role for beta-carotene has been suggested because of its very efficient ability to deactivate singlet oxygen and trap organic free radicals.[22] The notable inhibitory effects of retinoids observed in the laboratory are also observed in epidemiologic studies. About 20 reports have evaluated cancer incidence and vitamin A or beta-carotene intake. In nine retrospective studies, a significant increase in cancer risk at various sites was associated with diminished vitamin A intake.[34] Risks reported for the groups with low vitamin A intake were about twice those for the high intake groups.

A retrospective Norwegian study found that cancer patients had an increased risk for colon cancer associated with a vitamin A intake lower than that determined for a healthy control group.[35] Similarly, in a Japanese study, patients with gastric metaplasia had lower vitamin A intakes than a healthy control group.[36] Most other retrospective data confirm the inverse association between ingestion of foods containing vitamin A or beta-carotene and relative cancer risk, with risk levels 2 to 2.5 times higher in the low-intake groups than in the high-intake groups.[37]

The interpretation of retrospective epidemiologic studies is complicated by several factors. Dietary recall information usually is incomplete and imprecise. Cancer induction may take many years, and it is uncertain what time period of dietary intake is most relevant to the process. Also, most studies have tended to focus on food groups rather than specific nutrients. For example, foods high in beta-carotene also are high in other nutrients and may be low in fat. The groups under study may come from populations having wide differences in nutrient status, further complicating the estimation of risk associated with one dietary component.

Two large prospective studies that evaluated vitamin A intake and the risk of lung cancer have yielded consistent findings. In a study of 8,278 Norwegian men, Bjelke found an inverse relationship between lung cancer risk and vitamin A intake, [38] an observation that was confirmed in a study update.[39] The same result was found in a 10-year study of more than 250,000 Japanese adults.[40] In a smaller study, lung cancer incidence was inversely correlated with beta-carotene intake in 2,100 American men.[41]

Both retrospective and prospective studies have been conducted correlating serum retinol levels and relative cancer risk. The results have been contradictory.[34,37] This is not surprising, as retinol levels in serum are not directly influenced by dietary intake and vary only slightly among individuals in developed countries where vitamin A deficiencies are unusual.[33] Further, serum retinol levels may not accurately reflect local retinoid concentration in some tissues. It has been suggested that beta-carotene, if not itself an inherently important chemopreventive agent, could be used as a nontoxic means of increasing the quantity of circulating (pre)retinoids.[37]

FAT AND CALORIC INTAKE

Dietary fat is associated with breast, prostate, and colon cancers in population and animal studies, although not all the reported associations are consistent. Tannenbaum[42] and others in the 1940s demonstrated that high-fat diets enhance the occurrence of both spontaneous and chemically induced mammary tumors in mice.[42] Caloric or fat restriction inhibits spontaneous and chemically induced mammary tumors in animal models.[43,44] The reported cumulative tumor incidence in a review of 82 published experiments was, on average, 42% lower in calorie-restricted mice.[45] These studies demonstrate that dietary fat and caloric intake may differentially modify cancer incidence.

In human population studies, comparisons of the fat intake in the diets of various countries indicate that those populations with the highest per capita fat consumption have the highest breast cancer mortality.[46] A fivefold difference is seen between high-risk countries such as Denmark and low-risk countries such as Japan. A strong positive correlation between the intake of dietary fat and breast cancer mortality is seen in data from 39 countries.[47] Similar but weaker correlations were shown for fat intake and cancer of the colon and prostate.

Most case–control studies support an association between fat intake and breast cancer incidence.[48-52] Cohort studies on dietary fat and breast cancer have been less consistent. Notably, Willett et al found no relationship between dietary fat and breast cancer incidence in a cohort of 90,000 nurses.[53] The lack of correlation may be due to the fact that fat intake in this population varied only marginally, from 32% to 44% of total calories. International studies find broader ranges, with some populations reporting intakes as low as 15%.

International correlation studies find an association between colon cancer incidence and the intake of animal fat.[54] However, correlation studies within countries have not supported this association.[55-57] Case–control studies on colon cancer and fat are also inconsistent.[58] Contradictory data suggest that factors other than fat, such as dietary fiber, may influence colon cancer risk. There is some evidence that dietary fiber modifies the promoting effect of dietary fat and colon cancer incidence.[59] In a recent animal study, fiber moderated the effect of a high-fat diet on chemically induced colon tumors. Tumors developed in 63.7% of rats fed high-fat, low-fiber diets but only in 10.9% of rats fed high-fat, high-fiber diets.[60] Several reports indicate that dietary fat can promote chemically induced intestinal tumors in animal models.[61]

The international correlation data on prostate cancer risk support a positive association with fat intake.[58] Two case–control studies found that prostate cancer risk is correlated with diets high in animal fats, cheeses, cream, and eggs.[62,63]

The type of dietary fat implicated in cancer is a current research topic. There is experimental evidence that high-fat diets rich in linoleic acid, found in corn, safflower, sunflower, and other vegetable oils, may act as tumor promoters. Similar diets rich in oleic acid, from olive oil, and eicosapentaenoic acid, in fish oils, do not promote cancer in animals and may be protective. This may explain the low incidence of breast and colon cancer in Eskimos, whose main fat source is fish, and in people in Greece and Spain, whose main fat source is olive oil.[64]

Currently, Americans consume about 36% to 38% of their total daily calories as fat.[65,66] Numerous health experts have recommended that Americans reduce that figure to 30% or less to reduce risks for heart disease, obesity, and cancer.

FIBER

Since the early 1970s, when Burkitt proposed that dietary fiber may reduce the risk of large bowel cancer,[67] numerous epidemiologic and laboratory studies have explored a possible protective role for fiber. A review of results from 40 epidemiologic studies indicated an inverse relationship between total dietary fiber intake and colon cancer incidence in 32 of the 40 studies.[68]

Most international correlation studies using food availability data find that colon cancer mortality or incidence is inversely associated with fiber-rich food intake. Within-country correlational studies are also consistent. The low colon cancer rates in U.S. Mormons and Seventh-Day Adventists and rural Scandinavians, for example, correlate with higher intakes of fiber-rich foods than in the general population.[69,70]

Results from case–control studies generally reflect an inverse or protective association between dietary fiber and the risk of colon cancer. It should be noted that several studies show no association, and a few studies indicate increased risk.[3] However, inconsistent findings may be explained if one considers that dietary fibers from different food sources are heterogeneous mixtures of specific components, including cellulose, hemicellulose, pectin, gums, and lignin, and thus may have varying physiological effects. In addition, fiber components are difficult to quantify accurately in foods.[68]

More information is needed about which specific fiber components are protective. Laboratory results on chemically induced colon cancers in rodents suggest that inhibitory or enhancing effects are related to the type of fiber, the specific carcinogen, and other experimental variables such as route of administration. For example, cellulose inhibited 1,2-dimethylhydrazine-induced tumors in rats, but pectin had no effect.[71] Watanabe et al[72] noted that pectin was protective but alfalfa and bran were ineffective when azoxymethane and methylnitrosourea were administered parenterally. When administered intrarectally, pectin and bran were ineffective, while alfalfa enhanced carcinogenesis. Wheat bran appears to inhibit colon cancer development in animal models more consistently than other fiber sources.[3]

Several mechanisms have been proposed for the inhibitory effect of fiber on colorectal carcinogenesis. Fiber increases fecal bulk, thus reducing fecal mutagen concentrations. Also, enhanced colonic transit time can reduce the period of exposure of colonic mucosa to fecal mutagens. Finally, mutagen formation may be reduced by fiber-induced changes in colonic *ph* or bacterial metabolism.

The mean dietary fiber intake in the U.S. adult population is about 11 g/day.[73] Because of converging evidence that fiber may moderate the effects of fat, and because epidemiologic data consistently show an inverse association of dietary fiber intake with colon cancer, an increase to 20 to 30 g/day of dietary fiber is currently recommended by the NCI.

MUTAGENS AND CARCINOGENS IN FOOD

A variety of carcinogenic and mutagenic substances occur in our diet. The advent of rapid assays for mutagenicity has spurred the identification of many such compounds in food sources. Some of these substances occur naturally in the diet, whereas others result from food additives, preparation and processing procedures, pesticide residues, environmental pollution, and fungal contamination.[6,11]

Naturally occurring carcinogens include tannins, found in herbal teas,[74] hydrazines, found in edible mushrooms,[75] and safrole and related natural alkenyl benzenes, found in flavorings and spices.[76] Naturally occurring flavonoids, widespread in edible plants and fruits, are mutagenic.[77] Fungal contamination of stored food can produce potent carcinogenic myco-

toxins such as aflatoxin. In some areas of Africa, aflatoxin contamination of grain is implicated in higher than expected rates of liver cancer.[78,79]

Other notable sources of carcinogens in the human diet are the nitrosamines, derived from the interaction of nitrite with secondary or tertiary amines. Both sodium nitrate and its bacterial reduction product, sodium nitrite, occur naturally in plants, meats, and dairy products. They also are widely used as preservatives in smoked meat and salted fish.[11] The nitrosamines, such as dimethylnitrosamine, are potent carcinogens that generate diverse types of cancer in many animal species. Epidemiologic studies conducted in the United States, England, South America, Iran, Japan, and China demonstrate an association between nitrate and nitrite consumption and the incidence of stomach and esophageal cancer.[58] The formation of nitrosamines in humans following oral administration of nitrite and an appropriate substrate amine has been demonstrated.[80] The generation of nitrosamines, in stored food or in the gut, can be reduced by the presence of ascorbic acid or other antioxidants.[81]

Recent research on pyrolysis products formed during cooking led Sugimura and co-workers to identify a series of mutagenic heterocyclic amines in meat and fish. Rodents fed long-term diets containing mutagenic heterocyclic amines consistently developed multiple tumors in the lung, liver, small and large intestine, and colon. Pyrolysates of tryptophan, glutamic acid, and soybean are carcinogenic.[82] Also found in charbroiled meat are polyaromatic hydrocarbons.[83] As a result of environmental contamination, polyaromatic hydrocarbon levels in the range of parts per billion often occur in plants, meat, fish, and refined fats.[84] Other carcinogenic environmental contaminants in food include the growth promoter diethylstilbestrol, pesticides such as DDT and chlordane, and industrial pollutants such as arsenic, asbestos, heavy metals, and polychlorinated biphenyls.[11]

Most food-derived mutagens and carcinogens that have been studied in detail require metabolic activation to reactive electrophilic species. Some, such as the mutagen caffeine, are believed to act through inhibition of DNA repair processes.[6] In evaluating the risk posed to man from exposure to these chemicals, it is important to consider that chemical carcinogenesis is a multistage process that occurs over a relatively long period of time. Many variables can conceivably impinge on and modulate this process. Individual exposures to dietary carcinogens and mutagens are variable in terms of dose, frequency, and duration. Related factors include modification of metabolic activation and detoxification mechanisms, the presence of other protective or inhibitory substances in the diet, and the impact of other life-style–related factors. Although the carcinogenic risk posed to man by dietary carcinogens and mutagens is uncertain, it is no doubt prudent to avoid mycotoxin-contaminated foods and excessive exposure to nitrosamine sources and to minimize the intake of heterocyclic amines produced during cooking.

ALCOHOL

In the United States, alcohol consumption is widespread and represents a significant component of dietary intake for some persons.[85] Epidemiologic research indicates that high alcohol intake is associated with an increased risk of several types of cancer. Cancer of the esophagus, pharynx, larynx, and mouth is observed with high alcohol use in many correlational and case–control studies.[86,87] These cancers are also associated with smoking. Colorectal cancer is associated with excessive beer drinking in several studies,[58] including a recent prospective report.[88]

Of the approximately 17 cohort and case–control studies on alcohol consumption and breast cancer, all but three showed an increased cancer risk.[89] Two recent cohort studies indicated an increase in breast cancer incidence for even moderate drinkers compared with nondrinkers. Willett et al,[53] using a sample of 90,000 nurses, reported a 60% increase in breast cancer risk in women who had one or more alcoholic drinks per day. In a more representative sample, Schatzkin et al found a 40% to 50% increase in risk among women who consumed three alcoholic drinks per week.[90] These studies are limited by the difficulty of obtaining an accurate history of alcohol intake. In a recent case–control study, increased breast cancer risk associated with alcohol consumption was evident only for women who drank at ages less than 30 years, regardless of current consumption.[91]

Based on an analysis of epidemiologic studies, the International Agency for Research on Cancer considers the evidence sufficient for categorizing alcoholic beverages as carcinogenic. The most compelling studies showed enhanced cancer risk when alcohol is present as a cocarcinogen, for example, in combination with cigarette smoking.[92,93]

A more precise evaluation of epidemiologic research on alcohol consumption is hampered by the fact that the ethanol source is variable. Beer, wine, distilled spirits, and locally prepared beverages contain multiple constituents with potential biologic activity. Although not itself a mutagen, the ethanol in fermented preparations is frequently accompanied by mutagenic constituents.[7] Further, excessive alcohol consumption is often associated with impaired nutritional status, which may also influence cancer risk. Stryker et al[94] reported that an intake of 20 g alcohol per day reduced plasma beta-carotene levels 24% in men and 11% in women. Decreased levels of some micronutrients, especially vitamin A and carotenoids, may be linked to cancer development. Finally, the marked hepatoxicity produced by ethanol may interfere with the successful metabolism and excretion of potentially carcinogenic xenobiotics.

DIETARY INTERVENTION: CLINICAL TRIALS

It is estimated that up to 80% of cancer incidence is associated with life-style and environmental factors and, therefore, theoretically subject to prevention efforts.[93] The compelling evidence accumulated from laboratory and population studies on dietary factors associated with lower risk has provided investigators with strong leads for reducing cancer incidence. The NCI, recognizing the need for confirmatory studies, is sponsoring major clinical research efforts directed toward the chemoprevention of cancer.

The Chemoprevention Program, designed to identify and evaluate the efficacy of discrete, well-defined specific mi-

cronutrients, or synthetic analogues, in reducing human cancer, is concerned with questions such as nutrient bioavailability, metabolism, toxicity, and the public health impact of this intervention research. The program depends on the integration of results from epidemiologic and laboratory studies to devise appropriate human intervention trials that test a chemopreventive approach to cancer control. A parallel approach is being used by the Diet, Nutrition, and Cancer Program, which emphasizes the role of macronutrients such as fat and fiber.

The chemoprevention approach to nutrition intervention, defined as the addition of specific micronutrients or synthetic formulations to the diet, has two obvious advantages over the macronutrient approach. First, the biologic effects of chemically defined substances administered in specified dosages are easier to assess than changes associated with the addition or removal of a broadly characterized macronutrient. Second, it usually is much easier to add a dietary supplement than to expect full understanding and compliance with a recommended major dietary change.

RESEARCH STRATEGY

The research and initiation phases of both of the NCI cancer prevention programs follow a prescribed progression of phases designed to systematically and vigorously test a specific proposed intervention strategy. Preclinical investigations select and evaluate candidate substances and determine their efficacy, safety, and pharmacologic parameters in in vitro and in vivo screening systems. Following identification of research leads and method development, controlled intervention trials are used to validate efficacy and safety. Once the value of a preventive intervention has been proved, broad application is targeted to populations at risk or the general population.

In addition to the sequence of cancer control phases within the Chemoprevention Program and the Diet, Nutrition, and Cancer Program at the NCI, "convergence plans," or research flow designs, were developed for assessing the adequacy of pharmacologic, toxicologic, and epidemiologic data. This research flow design, with specified decision and convergence points, is shown for the Chemoprevention Program in Figure 11-1.[95]

If a particular chemoprevention agent or intervention satisfies all of the laboratory and epidemiologic decision points, an evaluation is made as to whether the research data are strong enough to justify intervention in humans. Because of the enormous commitment of resources required for large-scale human intervention trials, studies with the potential for broad public health impact generally have been limited to cancers with the greatest morbidity and mortality. Other studies address populations at very high risk (e.g., asbestos-exposed smokers) or people with precancerous lesions. The research flow designs have been formulated into a series of decision point matrices or stages. Criteria for satisfactory resolutions of the research hypothesis must be met before the research flow is supported for further action. More than 20 human intervention trials sponsored by the NCI Chemoprevention Program are currently in progress. The trials are testing selected chemopreventive agents with

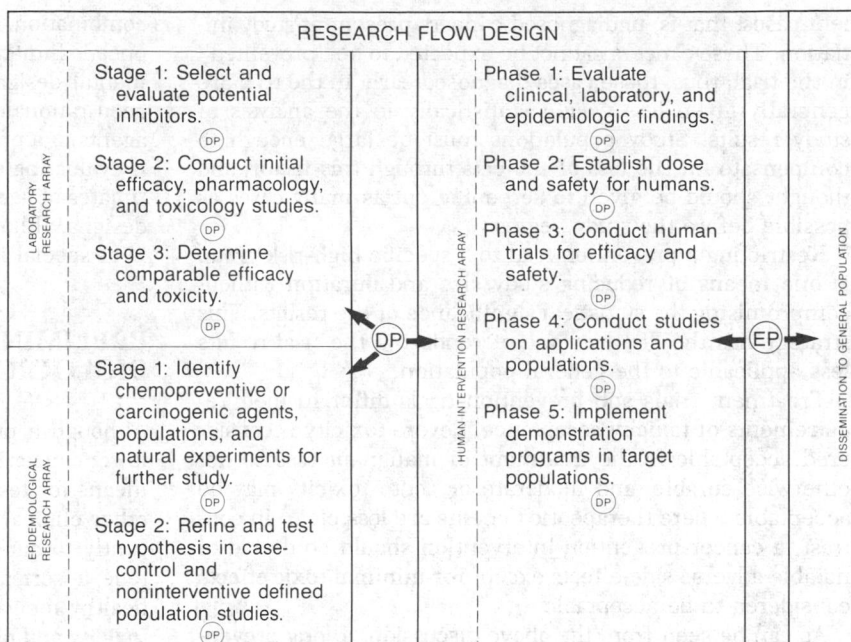

FIG. 11-1. Research flow design of NCI Chemoprevention Program. DP = decision point; EP =
evaluation point.

demonstrated potential for inhibiting lung, breast, colon, esophageal, bladder, and skin cancers—some of the most common cancers in humans.

FEATURES OF PREVENTION TRIALS AND TREATMENT TRIALS

Cancer prevention and cancer treatment trials are both designed to evaluate an intervention strategy for efficacy and toxicity in a clinical setting. Features of a sound research design such as randomization, appropriate controls, blinding when feasible, and an appreciation of statistical considerations are important for both types of trials. They differ significantly, however, with respect to study design and evaluation criteria.

Whereas the goal of a cancer treatment trial is to reduce mortality and morbidity, the intent of a prevention trial is to lower the rate of cancer occurrence. The efficacy of a cancer prevention intervention is based on a decrease in cancer incidence in the test population. Alternatively, the trial end point may measure the occurrence or modification of precursor lesions associated with the eventual appearance of malignant disease. Although no precursor markers have yet been identified as reliable indicators of disease incidence, the evaluation of such parameters in a prevention trial can examine human biologic effects in addition to testing whether or not the intervention will lower the cancer occurrence rate.

A prevention trial may also consider the value of an intervention designed to reduce exposure to a cancer-causing substance, such as cigarettes. The goal in this case would be to reduce the amount of smoking in the intervention group.

The study population in a treatment trial consists of cancer patients, whereas a prevention trial may use as test subjects the general population, persons at high risk for cancer or with precancerous lesions, or currently disease-free subjects previously treated for cancer. The principal investigator and the organizational setting influence the choice and recruitment of a test population. Clinicians are more apt to come in contact with persons requiring medical supervision; thus, it may be easier for them to select patients with precancerous lesions or healthy subjects in screening programs or prepaid health plans. Implementation of a prevention trial using a general or specially defined healthy population requires carefully planned recruitment schemes and an organizational framework to support the effort.

The duration of a prevention trial is usually much longer than that of a treatment trial. The choice of study length is not always obvious because it may take several years before any benefit can be expected, and that benefit may build with time.

Due to statistical considerations, the size of the study population in a prevention trial is usually an order of magnitude greater than that in a treatment trial. Even the most common cancers occur only rarely in a random sampling of several thousand people examined over a 5-year period. Adherence (compliance) to an intervention therapy may be difficult to maintain, requiring a larger test population to compensate for "dropouts." A statistical analysis of expected compliance can be used to help estimate the number of subjects required for a given study, and programs designed to maintain a high level of compliance (including counseling and "recapture" of dropouts) can be implemented. Conversely, some subjects may be "drop-ins," particularly in a study lasting several years. Drop-ins are test subjects in the control group who alter their life-style in such a way as to reflect the intervention plan being tested (e.g., by adopting a low-fat diet or by consuming more carrots).

Another problem associated with the choice of a study population in a prevention trial is the occurrence of prevalent cases, that is, undiagnosed cancers present at study initiation. These cancers cannot be expected to be "prevented" in the trial; thus, those cases diagnosed early in the trial are generally given less weight statistically in the analysis of study results. Study populations must be large enough to compensate for the loss of subjects through this factor, and thought should be given to screening out as many cases as possible before the study begins.

Restricting a prevention trial to a specific high-risk group is one means of reducing study size and duration without compromising the statistical significance of the results. This strategy has the disadvantage of rendering the trial results less applicable to the general population.

Treatment trials and prevention trials differ in their requirements of toxicity acceptance. Severe toxicity is considered acceptable in the treatment of malignant disease not otherwise curable, and moderate or acute toxicity may be acceptable where therapeutic benefits are less clear. In contrast, a cancer prevention intervention should be devoid of notable adverse side-effects except for minimal toxic effects considered to be acceptable.

As can be seen from the above discussion, a long prevention trial in a large population has many potential organizational, logistical, and statistical problems. Pilot studies should be conducted for most prevention trials. The variability in study populations, the size and scope of many trials, and the logistics of study implementation and management all can be tested before a full research effort is initiated. The purpose of a pilot study is rarely to measure outcomes, but rather to test for practical problems in study design.

A useful feature of many prevention trial protocols is the inclusion of a "run-in" period—a period of time, before study initiation and subject randomization, when both the intervention and control groups receive placebos. Because dropouts tend to occur early in a trial, the use of a run-in period can eliminate these cases and strengthen the statistical analysis of the results. This may confound the study interpretation because the remaining subjects represent only those achieving good compliance. To the extent allowed by sample size, a run-in also is useful for determining the rate of reported side-effects to be expected in controls.

Beyond administration of a proposed intervention, investigators in some prevention trials will collect baseline biochemical information to strengthen and expand the analysis of trial results. For example, Hennekens[96] collected blood from a large proportion of physicians in a trial designed to test the efficacy of beta-carotene in reducing cancer risk. In addition to the data on cancer incidence, his group now will be able to determine whether benefits accrued for all subjects, or only for those whose initial blood level of beta-carotene was low.

The study design of a treatment trial generally consists of a treatment group versus a placebo group or an alternate treatment group. More complex, factorial designs are often used for preventive intervention trials. A factorial design[97] allows two or more interventions to be evaluated in one trial, with approximately the same number of study subjects (and expense) as would be required to test a single agent (factor). Prevention trials are well suited for factorial designs because most interventions are nontoxic and can be given safely in combination. The number of agents that can be studied at once is limited by the logistics of managing complex experimental designs rather than by statistical considerations. A good rationale should be provided for inclusion of multiple agents in a prevention trial; the largest trial now in progress is evaluating eight groups of agents (including placebo). Estimates of agent interactions are also possible from factorial designs, although the sample size should be increased if this is of special interest.

PRELIMINARY CLINICAL TRIALS: BIOLOGIC MARKER END POINTS

Although a prospective randomized intervention trial with lower cancer incidence as the end point is the most desirable means for testing the efficacy of a chemopreventive agent, other clinical work preceding such a study can add significantly to our knowledge base. For example, for beta-carotene a series of clinical–metabolic studies performed in healthy men examined the effects of short-term dosing for toxicity and pharmacokinetic factors, generating useful data for the design of testing protocols for larger scale chemoprevention trials.[98]

In many cases, retrospective epidemiologic work and laboratory research combine to establish a strong case for the testing of a chemopreventive regimen. An intervention trial with a selected study population is sometimes used to assess not cancer incidence but a change in the nature of precancerous lesions or other biologic markers thought to be associated with the eventual development of malignant disease. This type of study is less costly than a large randomized trial and likely to provide a statistically significant outcome. A small selective study is also useful for initially establishing the biologic activity of a compound in humans when previous work has been conducted exclusively in the laboratory. In addition, the analysis of efficacy, toxicity, and dosage regimens provides important data for the design of larger randomized trials in the future.

The choice of a precursor or precancerous lesion as the end point for a clinical intervention study should be based on the strength of its association with a specific cancer, the ease with which the end point can be quantitatively evaluated, and the prevalence of this lesion in a study population.[99] It should be emphasized that the use of precursor lesions as predictors of future cancer incidence has not been experimentally validated in large-scale clinical trials. This important step must be taken before we can be fully confident of any marker end point in a clinical trial.

Dietary intervention studies in colon cancer have successfully employed protocols using precursor lesions as the clinical end point of interest. For example, the occurrence of rectal polyps in patients with familial polyposis was reduced by the administration of ascorbic acid (vitamin C).[100] Over a period of 3 to 13 months, rectal polyps disappeared or regressed in five of the eight treated patients. A later randomized trial of ascorbic acid intervention in 49 patients confirmed these results.[101]

Also evaluated in a study of colon cancer has been fecal mutagenicity, possibly associated with colon cancer. Fecal extracts contain mutagenic substances, as assessed by the Ames *Salmonella* test.[102] The occurrence and prevalence of such compounds may be influenced by diet, and therefore, the exposure of colonic epithelium to mutagenic substances may be reduced. Supplemental ascorbic acid and alpha-tocopherol (vitamin E) were used by Dion and colleagues[103] to successfully reduce mutagenic substances in 20 healthy subjects.

Other clinical work related to colon cancer concerns the observation that Seventh-Day Adventist vegetarians have a significantly lower incidence of this cancer than the general population. Lipkin and colleagues[104] found that the proliferation of colonic mucosa epithelial cells was markedly less in these vegetarians than in a control group. Further, Lipkin and Newmark[105] found that calcium carbonate supplementation for 2 to 3 months reduced epithelial cell proliferation in persons at high risk for familial colon cancer. Although the association described is of great interest, equally important is the development of a sensitive assay usable in large populations to measure the proliferation of colonic epithelial cells. When validated to predict cancers, such indices may be used in future trials to quantify the effects of a chemopreventive agent.

Retinoids have been tested clinically for their ability to affect the occurrence and regression of precursor lesions associated with lung and oral cancer. A synthetic retinoid, etretinate, was tested for its ability to reduce bronchial squamous cell metaplasia.[106] This work, conducted in a high-risk population (heavy smokers), suggested that the degree of bronchial metaplasia was reduced in treated subjects. In other work, 13-*cis*-retinoic acid, when applied topically, was found to reduce the severity of oral leukoplakia, an epithelial lesion associated with oral cancer.[107] The study examined several dosages (3, 5, or 10 mg/day for 6 months) and provided a particularly detailed enumeration of adverse side-effects. The leukoplakia recurred after cessation of therapy.

Related work on oral cancer used a test for inhibition of genotoxicity as the clinical end point of interest.[108] Betel nut tobacco chewers, persons at high risk of developing oral cancer, were the test population. The occurrence of micronuclei (a genotoxic marker) in exfoliated oral epithelial cells was assessed after treatment with placebo, vitamin A, beta-carotene, or 4,4'-diketo-beta-carotene. Both vitamin A and beta-carotene notably inhibited the occurrence of micronucleated epithelial cells, but 4,4'-diketo-beta-carotene did not. This beta-carotene derivative is not converted to vitamin A in vivo, suggesting that under these conditions, vitamin A is the active moiety, with beta-carotene an equally effective precursor.

These are a few examples of completed clinical intervention studies that used biologic marker end points. They suggest beneficial effects of chemopreventive agents, adding further impetus to this research field. This type of work can contribute to the overall evaluation of the clinical potential of a chemopreventive agent and supplies valuable information regarding biologic activity in humans, toxicity, dose regimens, and candidate target populations. In some cases, important new technologies are developed that provide research tools helpful not only for prevention research but for other types of cancer research as well. However, before marker end points can be used as a substitute for large-scale trials with cancer incidence end points, the markers will have to be validated in the context of clinical trials. This will take many years to accomplish.

INTERVENTION TRIALS IN PROGRESS

At present, more than two dozen large-scale dietary intervention trials are under way. This research is designed to evaluate the influence of a variety of dietary factors and synthetic retinoids on cancer incidence in specifically defined high-risk populations. Each of these studies is a randomized prospective trial ranging in design from simple to complex factorial. Variations in study designs and protocols are illustrated by the trials described below. Aspects of the research methods are highlighted to help those with an interest in developing this type of research trial.

ISOTRETINOIN–BASAL CELL CARCINOMA PREVENTION TRIAL

The synthetic retinoid isotretinoin (13-*cis*-retinoic acid; Accutane) is currently being evaluated in a long-term low-dosage protocol (10 mg/day for 3 years) for its ability to reduce the incidence of basal cell carcinoma. The subject population is a group of 1000 men and women aged 40 to 75 years who have had two or more biopsy-proven basal cell carcinomas during the 5 years before entry into the study. The trial will include a 2-year postintervention follow-up. The objective is to reduce the incidence of new basal cell carcinomas in persons at high risk because of previous basal cell carcinoma. In addition, information will be gathered regarding the toxicity of isotretinoin when taken for long periods at low doses. This randomized, double-blind, multicenter study is being conducted by the NCI with the collaboration of military medical centers, private medical institutions, and Hoffmann-LaRoche, Inc. The simple randomization into two groups (isotretinoin versus placebo) is similar to many therapeutic trials. This trial had a 6-month pilot phase to monitor patient recruitment and enrollment procedures, test data management and study logistics, and evaluate short-term safety and toxicity. Greenberg and colleagues[109] are using a similar design to determine whether beta-carotene influences the recurrence of nonmelanoma skin cancer in patients who have recently had a nonmelanoma skin cancer removed. The trial will involve 2000 subjects. After a 1-month run-in period to improve trial efficacy, subjects receive either 50 mg beta-carotene or a placebo daily.

U.S.–FINLAND LUNG CANCER PREVENTION TRIAL

A large-scale trial, conducted as a collaborative project by the NCI and the National Public Health Institute of Finland, currently is investigating the efficacy of both beta-carotene and alpha-tocopherol (vitamin E) in reducing lung cancer incidence among 28,000 male cigarette smokers. Reduction in the incidence of other cancers also will be evaluated.

This randomized double-blind 6-year intervention study, begun in March 1984, employs a 2×2 factorial design to evaluate four separate treatment groups: placebo (control), beta-carotene (20 mg/day), vitamin E (alpha-tocopherol, 100 mg/day), and beta-carotene in combination with vitamin E.[110] This design allows estimation of effects associated with the individual agents by comparison of vitamin E or beta-carotene with placebo, as well as estimation of any synergistic effects or inhibitory interaction between beta-carotene and vitamin E with regard to cancer incidence.

An 11-month pilot study in one of five participating clinics was used to evaluate recruitment procedures, clinic staff operations, appropriateness of research forms, compliance, usefulness of a run-in period, and side-effects of the study agents before the full research effort was initiated. Incident cancers will be identified through clinical follow-up procedures and by periodic matching of names of study subjects with the Finnish Cancer Registry.

NUTRITION INTERVENTION TRIALS IN LINXIAN, CHINA

The NCI and the Cancer Institute of the Chinese Academy of Medical Sciences are collaborating in the conduct of two randomized, double-blind, 5-year intervention trials in Linxian, China, an area with a particularly high incidence of esophageal cancer. One study, the General Population Trial, which uses a fractional factorial design, will determine the effect of multiple vitamin/mineral combinations on the incidence of esophageal cancer. The test population is composed of 30,000 men and women, ages 40 to 69, divided into eight intervention groups receiving placebos or specified combinations of vitamin A, beta-carotene, zinc, riboflavin, niacin, vitamin C, molybdenum, selenium, and vitamin E at doses one to four times the U.S. recommended daily allowance (RDA).[111] The fractional factorial design is illustrated in Figure 11-2. This statistical technique allows data to be divided into subsets during analysis to examine specific agent effects or interactions of interest. The Linxian design is a half-repli-

cation of the full 2^4 factorial, testing only 8 of the possible 16 groups. Ability to test the effect of each main factor under study is retained; however, two-way interactions between factors are confounded with each other.[112] Judicious use of a fractional factorial design can reduce a large factorial study, such as the Linxian trial, to practicable size.

A second study, the Dysplasia Trial, will examine the effect of multiple vitamins/minerals on a high-risk population with severe esophageal dysplasia. In a simple study design, 3400 men and women, ages 40 to 69, will receive either a placebo or a multiple vitamin/mineral supplement at levels one to four times the RDA. Participants will be evaluated for disease progression or regression. In both studies, cancer incidence and mortality will be determined through hospital record pathology slides and radiographic reviews in conjunction with the Linxian Esophageal Cancer Registry.

Before initiation of the full-scale trials, a 6-month pilot study indicated that patient recruitment, compliance, and study logistics were feasible. In addition, nutritional assessment data showed that deficiencies were common and that nutritional status could be improved by low-dose vitamin supplementation.

Of the many other cancer prevention trials in progress, 11 are examining the effects of beta-carotene, alone or in combination with other agents, on cancer incidence. For example, a Boston study[96] of 22,000 healthy male physicians, ages 40 to 84, is evaluating the influence of beta-carotene and aspirin on both total cancer incidence and cardiovascular disease, using a factorial study design (Fig. 11-3).

Grouping beta-carotene intervention research by cancer site, seven studies are directed toward reducing the incidence of lung cancer in smoking and other high-risk groups. In one study, the preventive effect of beta-carotene in combination with vitamin A is being tested in a population at high risk for lung cancer and mesothelioma due to occupational exposure to asbestos. Tin miners at high risk for lung cancer are receiving beta-carotene, retinol, vitamin E, and selenium.

Six intervention studies are investigating the prevention of skin cancer in such high-risk groups as albinos in equatorial Africa and subjects with previous skin cancer and precancerous actinic keratosis. The prevention of colon cancer and

FIG. 11-2. The Linxian esophageal cancer prevention trial is a fractional factorial design based on a 2^4 factorial. The asterisks indicate the eight intervention groups included in a half-replicate of the 2^4 factorial design. Thirty thousand participants, 40 to 69 years old, will receive either a daily placebo or one of the seven vitamin/mineral combinations. Treatment agents are (A) vitamin A, beta-carotene, zinc; (B) riboflavin, niacin; (C) vitamin C, molybdenum; (D) selenium, vitamin E.

Intervention Groups

Placebo*	A	B	AB*
C	AC*	BC*	ABC
D	AD*	BD*	ABD
CD*	ACD	BCD	ABCD*

FIG. 11-3. The physicians health study is a 2×2 factorial design in which 22,000 healthy physicians receive, on alternate days, either (A) beta-carotene and aspirin, (B) aspirin and placebo, (C) beta-carotene and placebo, or (D) placebo only.

Intervention Groups

		Beta-carotene	
		Yes	No
Aspirin	Yes	A	B
	No	C	D

cervical cancer is the subject of other dietary intervention trials. Five studies on the prevention of colon cancer are testing vitamin C, vitamin E, beta-carotene, or wheat fiber, alone or in combination, in subjects selected on the basis of familial polyposis or adenotomous polyp diagnosis. Women with cervical dysplasia are being treated with *trans*-retinoic acid or folic acid in two separate trials for the prevention of cervical cancer.[34]

THE PHYSICIAN AS AN EFFECTIVE PROMOTER OF HEALTHY DIET

The clinician involved in primary health care has a leading role in counseling patients on life-style as it affects their overall health. Nutritional science, included in many medical school curricula, is a critical part of effective health promotion education. For the best use of the physician's time, patient education might be seen as a cooperative process involving nurses, dietitians, and others.

A number of studies have examined the potential effectiveness of physicians as agents of health-promoting behavior change in their patients.[113-115] There are several reasons why physicians can be effective. Physicians are often good role models. Physicians are also seen as the most authoritative source of medical and health information. About 70% of Americans make at least one visit a year to their doctor, often because they are ill or otherwise amenable to a suggestion about life-style and behavior change. These visits are often excellent "teachable moments" because of the personal relationship and trust that clinicians are able to establish with their patients.

The following guidelines are ways in which physicians can assist their patients to make positive dietary changes:[116]

1. Discuss risk factors and the benefits associated with dietary modification with patients. The personal communication with the patient and individualized counseling based on the patient's history and situation are key to the success of this effort.
2. Assess the patient's current dietary profile. For example, have the patient fill out a diet history. This will reveal problem areas and allow the physician and patient to discuss the patient's dietary habits more concretely and conceive possible ways of making changes.
3. Have the patient choose several changes to work on until the next visit. Small, incremental steps are easier to make than a total modification of the diet.
4. Provide the patient with information materials to assist him or her in behavior change.
5. On subsequent patient visits, review the diet history questionnaire and recommended behavior changes to monitor compliance and encourage progress.

To assist patients in making dietary changes, some simple strategies may be suggested. One of these is a choose more/choose less approach, developed by NCI for use in its cancer prevention materials.[117] This approach does not preclude the use of any food. Rather, it emphasizes a shift away from high-fat, low-fiber foods that may increase cancer risk toward foods low in fat and rich in fiber and nutrients.

Although not all the answers are fully known about diet and its relationship to disease risks, a number of scientific organizations have issued dietary guidelines for the public. These expert groups believe that sufficient data now exist for the public to be informed and that prudent guidelines based on current evidence are likely to lower risks for major chronic diseases, including cancer, and will do no harm.

In 1980, the U.S. Department of Agriculture and the Department of Health and Human Services jointly published "Nutrition and Your Health: Dietary Guidelines for Americans." A slightly edited version was published in 1985. These guidelines were designed to assist healthy adult Americans in improving their nutritional status and overall health.

Most recently, the NCI has developed for the public a compatible set of dietary guidelines (listed below), adding some specificity to aid in interpretation:[118]

1. Reduce fat intake to 30% of calories or less.
2. Increase fiber intake to 20 to 30 g/day, with an upper limit of 35 g/day.
3. Include a variety of vegetables and fruit in the daily diet.
4. Avoid obesity.
5. Consume alcoholic beverages in moderation, if at all.
6. Minimize consumption of salt-cured, salt-pickled, or smoked foods.

The physician can call on numerous other resources to assist in diet counseling. Effective use of information materials and collaboration with nutrition professionals are critical to the patient's successful change. Qualified professionals, including private-practice registered dietitians and nutritionists and health department or extension nutritionists, can do much to support and complement a physician's efforts. Resources for materials include the Food and Nutrition Information Center of the USDA National Agricultural Library; publications of the USDA and USDHHS; and resources from the American Heart Association, American Cancer Society, American Dietetic Association, and Society for Nutrition Education.

FUTURE PROSPECTS FOR CANCER PREVENTION

Approximately 900,000 new cases of cancer are diagnosed in the United States each year, with 450,000 deaths attributed to this disease annually. The NCI has launched an aggressive effort to control cancer by the year 2000 and to reduce the mortality by 50% between 1985 and 2000.[119] Cancer prevention interventions designed to minimize lifestyle or environmental factors that promote cancer or to maximize exposure to agents that reduce cancer incidence are expected to play a major role in achieving this goal.

The weight of new evidence developed in the second half of this century from laboratory and population studies has focused cancer prevention efforts on two avoidable risks: smoking and dietary factors.[34] The estimated 35% of cancer deaths that may be related to dietary components have stimulated an aggressive effort to explore the roles of diet and nutrition in cancer prevention. Behavior research and nutrition education can contribute much to the success of these prevention efforts and represent major efforts in the prevention programs at the NCI.

The example of retinoids and beta-carotene illustrates how the convergence of basic research and population studies, coupled with developmental research, has led to large prospective clinical intervention trials. The promising clinical work under way with 13-*cis*-retinoic acid emerges from research on the process of carcinogenesis, the development of more active, less toxic retinoid analogues, and epidemiologic research. The specificity of the retinoids in the control of cell function suggests that this group of compounds is a practical tool for the study of several molecular mechanisms of action in cancer prevention. New approaches to the control of cell differentiation are being investigated as a result of the particular interest in the antineoplastic activity of the retinoids. Insights into the expression of oncogenes and modulation of the action of specific peptide growth factors and their membrane-bound receptors have already generated prevention research initiatives.[28]

The identification of human oncogene products and assays for their detection could in the future enable the clinician to screen and intervene before the onset of disease. The development of antisera for the *ras* oncogene product, protein P_{21}, is an example of such a marker under evaluation for the early detection of cancer. The study of tumor suppressor genes that can inhibit the expression of the tumorigenic phenotype is providing evidence, although still fragmentary, of new mechanisms for inhibiting tumor growth potentially more diversified than the oncogenes.[120] Tests such as the micronucleus test[108] for chromosome aberrations may prove useful, when the scoring can be automated, for selecting the most active chemopreventive agents and effective dosages for intervention trials. Further prospects for prevention, although speculative, may be developed with the retroviruses, known to be responsible for animal leukemias and lymphomas and at least one type of human leukemia. It is conceivable that one day there may be an antiviral cancer vaccine available.

In the area of dietary research, all the confounding factors may never be identified; however, this does not preclude testing of specific agents of potential benefit in pilot intervention trials. Thus, literally hundreds of dietary and synthetic agents are under consideration for future study.

Advances in food and agricultural technologies and the development of new dietary synthetic substitutes are contributing to our changing food supply and may have a profound effect on nutritional intake and long-term health effects. Several synthetic fat substitutes such as Simplesse and Olestra are awaiting Food and Drug Administration approval, and if approved, they could have a profound effect on nutritional intake and long-term health effects. Both products are low in calorie and cholesterol content and may appreciably reduce fat intake and chronic disease incidence. Edible plants are now cultivated with specific characteristics that may be nutritionally superior or inferior. This is also true of food production in artificially controlled media such as aquaculture or the rapid multiplication of stock by microculture techniques. Genetic engineering applied to agriculture may revolutionize the production of economically important crops by raising the level of so-called natural pesticides and breeding animals free of genetic or infectious diseases. Obviously, prudence is required in managing the choices of natural and artificial dietary substitutes.

An increasing number of American companies have developed programs aimed at promoting overall health and reducing risk factors for coronary heart disease and cancer. Many major United States employers are participating in cancer education and early detection programs aimed especially at lung, colorectal, breast, and uterine cancers. Diet modification and weight control programs are increasingly found in industry-sponsored wellness programs. In addition, many employers are opting to provide a preventive health care package as part of health insurance benefits, which generally includes a cancer screening schedule that is in accordance with American Cancer Society recommendations. Continued and increased interest in cancer education and prevention in the worksite could contribute greatly to reducing the incidence of certain types of cancer.

The NCI approach to cancer prevention is a rigorous discipline bridging fundamental and applied research that identifies a testable intervention hypothesis by evaluating the scientific evidence, develops intervention methodology, and validates the intervention in clinical trials.

Cancer prevention and control research has intensified in the 1980s, gaining impetus from investigations leading to the recognition that diet and the human nutritional state are linked to the incidence of certain common cancers. To confirm that these correlations directly affect causality, these lines of investigation should be both continued and expanded.

REFERENCES

1. Wattenberg LW: Inhibition of neoplasia by minor dietary constituents. Cancer Res 43:2448–2453, 1983
2. Shimkin MB: Contrary to nature. Washington, DC, Department of Health, Education and Welfare, 1977
3. Pilch SM (ed): Physiological Effects and Health Consequences of Dietary Fiber, pp 118–135. Bethesda, Md, Life Sciences Research Office, FASEB, 1987
4. Ip C, Birt DF, Rogers AE et al (eds): Dietary Fat and Cancer, pp 231–374. New York, Alan R Liss, 1986
5. Tannenbaum A, Silverstone H: Nutrition in relation to cancer. Adv Cancer Res 1:451–501, 1953
6. Ames BN: Dietary carcinogens and anticarcinogens. Science 221:1256–1264, 1983
7. Ames BN, Magaw R, Gold LS: Ranking possible carcinogenic hazards. Science 236:271–280, 1987
8. Sparnins VL, Wattenberg LW: Enhancement of glutathione S-transferase activity of the mouse forestomach by inhibitors of benzo(a)pyrene-induced neoplasia of the forestomach. JNCI 66:769–771, 1981
9. Wattenberg, LW: Chemoprevention of cancer. Cancer Res 45:1–8, 1985
10. Miller EC, Miller JA: Biochemical mechanisms of chemical carcinogenesis. In Busch H (ed): The Molecular Biology of Cancer, pp 342–377. New York, Academic Press, 1974
11. Carr BI: Chemical carcinogens and inhibitors of carcinogenesis in the human diet. Cancer 55:218–224, 1985
12. Krytopoulos SA: Ascorbic acid and the formation of N-nitroso compounds: possible role of ascorbic acid in cancer prevention. Am J Clin Nutr 45:1344–1350, 1987
13. Mettlin C, Graham S, Priore R et al: Diet and cancer of the esophagus. Nutr Cancer 2:143–147, 1981
14. Haenszel W, Correa P: Developments in the epidemiology of stomach cancer over the past decade. Cancer Res 35:3452–3459, 1975
15. Mirvish SS, Wallcave L, Eagen M et al: Ascorbate-nitrite reaction: Possible means of blocking the formation of carcinogenic N-nitroso compounds. Science 177:65–68, 1972
16. Menkes MS, Comstock GW, Vuilleumier JP et al: Serum beta-carotene, vitamins A and E, selenium and the risk of lung cancer. N Engl J Med 315:1250–1254, 1986

17. Willett W, Polk R, Underwood BA et al: Relation of serum vitamins A and E and carotenoids to the risk of cancer. N Engl J Med 310:430–434, 1984
18. Schrauzer GN, White DA, Schneider CJ: Cancer mortality correlation studies: III. Statistical associations with dietary selenium intakes. Bioinorgan Chem 7:23–31, 1977
19. Shamberger RJ, Tylko SA, Willis CE: Antioxidants and cancer: VI. Selenium and age-adjusted human cancer mortality. Arch Environ Health 31:231–235, 1976
20. Ip C: The chemopreventive role of selenium in carcinogenesis. J Am Coll Toxicol 5:7–20, 1986
21. Garland C, Shekelle RB, Barrett-Conner E et al: Dietary vitamin D and calcium and risk of colorectal cancer: A 19-year prospective study in men. Lancet 1:307–309, 1985
22. Hennekens CH, Mayrent SL, Willet W: Vitamin A, carotenoids, and retinoids. Cancer 58:1837–1841, 1986
23. Lasnitzki I: The influence of a hypervitaminosis on the effect of 20-methylcholanthrene on mouse prostate glands grown in vitro. Br J Cancer 9:434–441, 1955
24. Merriman RL, Bertram JS: Reversible inhibition by retinoids of 3-methylcholanthrene-induced neoplastic transformation of C3H/10T-1/2 CL8 cells. Cancer Res 39:1661–1666, 1979
25. Harisiadis L, Miller RC, Hall EJ et al: A vitamin A analogue inhibits radiation-induced oncogenic transformation. Nature 274:486–487, 1978
26. Strickland S, Mahdavi V: The induction of differentiation in teratocarcinoma stem cells by retinoic acid. Cell 15:393–403, 1978
27. Breitman TR, Collins SJ, Keene BR: Terminal differentiation of human promyelocytic leukemia cells in primary culture in response to retinoic acid. Blood 57:1000–1004, 1981
28. Sporn MB, Roberts AB: Role of retinoids in differentiation and carcinogenesis. Cancer Res 43:3034–3040, 1983
29. Sporn MB, Newton DL: Chemoprevention of cancer with retinoids. Fed Proc 38:2528–2534, 1979
30. Becci PJ, Thompson HJ, Grubbs CJ et al: Effect of delay in administration of 13-cis-retinoic acid on the inhibition of urinary bladder carcinogenesis in the rat. Cancer Res 39:3141–3144, 1979
31. Boutwell RK: Retinoids and inhibition of ornithine decarboxylase activity. J Am Acad Dermatol 6:796–798, 1982
32. Todaro GJ, DeLarco JE, Sporn MB: Retinoids block phenotypic cell transformation produced by sarcoma growth factor. Nature 276:272–274, 1978
33. Peto R: The marked differences between carotenoids and retinoids: Methodological implications for biochemical epidemiology. Cancer Surveys 2:327–340, 1983
34. Greenwald P, Sondik E, Lynch BS: Diet and chemoprevention in NCI's research strategy to achieve national cancer control objectives. Annu Rev Public Health 7:267–291, 1986
35. Bjelke E: Epidemiologic studies of cancer of the stomach, colon, and rectum, with special emphasis on the role of diet. Scand J Gastroenterol 9:1–53, 1974
36. Nomura A, Yamakawa H, Ishidate T et al: Intestinal metaplasia in Japan: Association with diet. JNCI 68:401–405, 1982
37. Peto R, Doll R, Buckley JD et al: Can dietary beta-carotene materially reduce human cancer rates? Nature 290:201–208, 1981
38. Bjelke E: Dietary vitamin A and human lung cancer. Int J Cancer 15:561–565, 1975
39. Kvale G, Bjelke E, Gart JJ: Dietary habits and lung cancer risk. Int J Cancer 31:397–405, 1983
40. Hirayama T: Diet and cancer. Nutr Cancer 1:67–81, 1979
41. Shekelle RB, Liu S, Raynor WJ Jr et al: Dietary vitamin A and risk of cancer in the Western Electric Study. Lancet 2:1185–1190, 1981
42. Tannenbaum A: The genesis and growth of tumors: III. Effect of a high fat diet. Cancer Res 2:468–475, 1942
43. Tannenbaum A: The dependence of the genesis of induced skin tumors on the caloric intake during different stages of carcinogenesis. Cancer Res 4:673–677, 1944
44. Kritchevsky D, Weber MM, Buck CL et al: Calories, fat and cancer. Lipids 21:272–274, 1986
45. Albanes D: Total calories, body weight, and tumor incidence in mice. Cancer Res 47:1987–1992, 1987a
46. Wynder EL, MacCormick F, Hill P et al: Nutrition and the etiology and prevention of breast cancer. Cancer Detect Prev 1:293–310, 1976
47. Carroll KK, Hopkins GJ: Dietary polyunsaturated fat versus saturated fat in relation to mammary carcinogenesis. Lipids 14:155, 1979
48. Phillips RL: Role of life-style and dietary habits in risk of cancer among Seventh-Day Adventists. Cancer Res 35:3513–3522, 1975
49. Miller AB, Kelly A, Choi NW et al: A study of diet and breast cancer. Am J Epidemiol 107:499–509, 1978
50. Nomura A, Henderson BE, Lee J: Breast cancer and diet among the Japanese in Hawaii. Am J Clin Nutr 31:2020–2025, 1978
51. Lubin JH, Burns PE, Blot HJ et al: Dietary factors and breast cancer risk. Int J Cancer 28:685–689, 1981
52. Papatestas AE, Knittle J, Lesnick G et al: Diet and human carcinogenesis. In: European Organization for Cooperation in Cancer Prevention Studies: Third Annual Symposium Proceedings, Aarhus, Denmark, June 19–21, 1985; p 66
53. Willett WC, Stampfer MJ, Colditz GA et al: Moderate alcohol consumption and the risk of breast cancer. N Engl J Med 316(19):1174–1180, 1987
54. McKeown-Eyssen G, Bright-See E: Dietary factors in colon cancer: International relationships. Nutr Cancer 6:160, 1984
55. Enstrom JE: Colorectal cancer and consumption of beef and fat. Br J Cancer 32:432–439, 1975
56. Bingham SA, William DR, Cole TJ et al: Dietary fiber and regional large-bowel cancer mortality in Britain. Br J Cancer 40:456–463, 1979
57. Kolonel LN, Nomura AMY, Hinds MW et al: Role of diet in cancer incidence in Hawaii. Cancer Res 43:2397s–2402s, 1983
58. Palmer S: Diet, nutrition, and cancer. Prog Food Nutr Sci 9:283–341, 1985
59. Jensen OM, MacLennan R, Wahrendorf J: Diet, bowel function, fecal characteristics, and large bowel cancer in Denmark and Finland. Nutr Cancer 4(1):5–19, 1982
60. Galloway DJ, Owen RW, Jarrett F et al: Experimental colorectal cancer: The relationship of diet and faecal bile acid concentration to tumour induction. Br J Surg 73:233–237, 1986
61. Reddy BS, Cohen LA, McCoy GD et al: Nutrition and its relationship to cancer. Adv Cancer Res 32:237–345, 1980
62. Graham S, Haughey B, Marshall J et al: Diet in the epidemiology of carcinoma of the prostate gland. JNCI 70:687–692, 1983
63. Kolonel LN, Hankin JH, Lee J et al: Nutrient intakes in relation to cancer incidence in Hawaii. Br J Cancer 44:332–339, 1981
64. Kinsella JE: Food components with potential therapeutic benefits: The n-3 polyunsaturated fatty acids of fish oils. Food Technol 40:89–97, 1986
65. USDA: Nationwide food consumption continuous survey of food intake by individuals: Men 19–50 years, 1 day, 1985. Report No 85-3, pp 1–46, November 1986
66. USDA: Nationwide food consumption continuous survey of food intake by individuals: Women 19–50 years and their children 1–5 years, 1 day, 1986. Report No 86-1, pp 1–46, January 1987
67. Burkitt DP: Epidemiology of cancer of the colon and rectum. Cancer 28:3–13, 1971
68. Greenwald P, Lanza E, Eddy GA: Dietary fiber in the reduction of colon cancer risk. J Am Diet Assoc 87(9):1178–1188, 1987
69. Enstrom JE: Cancer mortality among Mormons in California during 1968–75. JNCI 65:1073, 1980
70. Jensen OM: Cancer risk among Danish male Seventh-Day Adventists and other temperance society members. JNCI 70:1011, 1983
71. Freeman HJ, Spiller GA, Kim YS: A double-blind study on the effect of purified cellulose dietary fiber on 1,2-dimethylhydrazine-induced rat colonic neoplasia. Cancer Res 38:2912–2917, 1978
72. Watanabe K, Reddy BS, Weisburger JH et al: Effect of dietary alfalfa, pectin, and wheat bran on azoxymethane- or methylnitrosourea-induced colon carcinogenesis in rats. JNCI 63(1):141–145, 1979
73. Lanza E, Jones DY, Block G et al: Dietary fiber intake in the U.S. population. Am J Clin Nutr 46:790–797, 1987
74. Korpassy B: Tannins as hepatic carcinogens. Prog Exp Tumor Res 2:245–290, 1961
75. Toth B: Mushroom hydrazines: Occurrence, metabolism, carcinogenesis and environmental implications. In Miller EC et al (eds): Naturally Occurring Carcinogens, Mutagens, and Modulators of Carcinogenesis, pp 57–65. Baltimore, University Park Press, 1979
76. Miller JA, Swanson AB, Miller EC: The metabolic activation of safrole and related naturally occurring alkenylbenzenes in relation to carcinogenesis by these agents. In Miller EC et al (eds): Naturally Occurring Carcinogens, Mutagens, and Modulators of Carcinogenesis, pp 111–125. Baltimore, University Park Press, 1979
77. Brown JP: A review of the genetic effects of naturally occurring flavonoids, anthraquinones and related compounds. Mutat Res 75:243–277, 1980
78. Linsell CA, Peers FG: Aflatoxin and liver cell cancer. Trans R Soc Trop Med Hyg 71:471–473, 1977
79. van Rensburg SJ, van der Watt JJ, Purchase IFH et al: Primary liver cancer rate and aflatoxin intake in a high cancer area. S Afr Med J 48:2508a–d, 1974
80. Magee P (ed): Nitrosamines and Human Cancer. Banbury Report 12. Cold Spring Harbor, New York, Cold Spring Harbor Laboratory, 1982
81. Williams GM, Weisburger JH: Chemical carcinogens. In Klassen CD, Amur MO, Doull J (eds): Casarett and Doull's Toxicology: The Basic Science of Poisons, 3rd ed, pp 99–173. New York, Mcmillan, 1986
82. Sugimura T: Carcinogenicity of mutagenic heterocyclic amines formed during the cooking process. Mutat Res 150:33–41, 1985
83. Lijinsky W, Shubik P: Benzo(a)pyrene and other polynuclear hydrocarbons in charcoal-broiled meat. Science 145:53–55, 1964
84. Howard JW, Fazio T: Review of polycyclic aromatic hydrocarbons in foods: Analytical methodology and reported findings of polycyclic aromatic hydrocarbons in foods. J Assoc Off Anal Chem 63:1077–1104, 1980
85. Vitale JJ, Broitman SA, Gottlieb LS: Alcohol and carcinogenesis. In Newell GR, Ellison NM (eds): Nutrition and Cancer: Etiology and Treatment, pp 291–301. New York, Raven Press, 1981
86. Tuyns AJ: Alcohol. In Schottenfeld D, Fraumeni JF Jr (eds): Cancer Epidemiology and Prevention, pp 293–303. Philadelphia, WB Saunders, 1982
87. Rothman KJ: Alcohol. In Fraumeni JF Jr (ed): Persons at High Risk of Cancer: An Approach to Cancer Etiology and Control, pp 139–148. New York, Academic Press, 1975
88. Pollack ES, Nomura AMY, Heilbrun LK et al: Prospective study of alcohol consumption and cancer. N Engl J Med 310(10):617–621, 1984
89. Graham S: Alcohol and breast cancer. N Engl J Med 316(19):1211–1213, 1987
90. Schatzkin A, Jones DY, Hoover RN et al: Alcohol consumption and breast cancer in the epidemiologic follow-up study of the First National Health and Nutrition Examination Survey. N Engl J Med 316(19):1169–1173, 1987

91. Harvey EB, Schairer C, Brinton LA et al: Alcohol consumption and breast cancer. JNCI 78(4):657–661, 1987

92. International Agency for Research on Cancer: Chemicals, Industrial Processes and Industries Associated with Cancer in Humans. IARC Monogr (Suppl) 4, 1982

93. Doll R, Peto R: The causes of cancer: Quantitative estimates of avoidable risks of cancer in the United States today. JNCI 61:1191–1308, 1981

94. Stryker WS, Kaplan LA, Stein EA et al: The relation of diet, cigarette smoking, and alcohol consumption to plasma beta-carotene and alpha-tocopherol levels. Am J Epidemiol 127(2):283–296, 1988

95. Greenwald P, Dewys WD, Carrese LM et al: Chemoprevention program at the National Cancer Institute. In Prasad (ed): Vitamins, Nutrition, and Cancer, pp 282–291. Basel, S Karger, 1984

96. Hennekens CH: Issues in the design and conduct of clinical trials. JNCI 73:1473–1476, 1984

97. Byar DP, Piantadosi S: Factorial designs for randomized clinical trials. Cancer Treat Rep 69:1055-1062, 1985

98. Dimitrov NV, Boone CW, Hay MB et al: Plasma beta-carotene levels: Kinetic patterns during administration of various doses of beta-carotene. J Nutr Growth Cancer 3:227–237, 1986

99. Bruce WR, McKeown-Eyssen G, Ciampi A et al: Strategies for dietary intervention studies in colon cancer. Cancer 47 (suppl):1121–1125, 1981

100. DeCosse JJ, Adams MB, Kuzma JF et al: Effect of ascorbic acid on rectal polyps of patients with familial polyposis. Surgery 78:608–612, 1975

101. Bussey HJR, DeCosse JJ, Deschner EE et al: A randomized trial of ascorbic acid in polyposis coli. Cancer 50:1434–1439, 1982

102. Bruce WR, Varghese AJ, Furrer R et al: A mutagen in human feces. In Hiatt HH, Watson JD, Winsten JA (eds): Origins of Human Cancer, pp 1641–1644. Cold Spring Harbor, New York, Cold Spring Harbor Laboratory, 1977

103. Dion PW, Bright-See EB, Smith CC et al: The effect of dietary ascorbic acid and alpha-tocopherol on fecal mutagenicity. Mutat Res 102:27–37, 1982

104. Lipkin M, Uehara K, Winawer S et al: Seventh-Day Adventist vegetarians have a quiescent proliferative activity in colonic mucosa. Cancer Lett 26:139–144, 1985

105. Lipkin N, Newmark H: Effect of added dietary calcium on colonic epithelial cell proliferation in subjects at high risk for familial colonic cancer. N Engl J Med 313:1381–1384, 1985

106. Gouveia J, Hercend T, Lemaigre G et al: Degree of bronchial metaplasia in heavy smokers and its regression after treatment with a retinoid. Lancet 1:710–712, 1982

107. Shah JP, Strong EW, DeCosse JJ et al: Effect of retinoids on oral leukoplakia. Am J Surg 146:466–470, 1983

108. Stitch HF, Stitch W, Rosin MP et al: Use of the micronucleus test to monitor the effect of vitamin A, beta-carotene and canthaxanthin on the buccal mucosa of betel nut/tobacco chewers. Int J Cancer 34:745–750, 1984

109. Greenberg ER, Baron JA, Beck JR: Carotenoids and cancer prevention. In Saurat (ed): Retinoids: New Trends in Research and Therapy, pp 360–370. Basel, S Karger, 1985

110. Albanes D, Virtamo J, Rautalahti M et al: Pilot study: The U.S.–Finland lung cancer prevention trial. J Nutr Growth Cancer 3:207–214, 1986

111. Li J-Y, Taylor PR, Li G-Y et al: Intervention studies in Linxian, China: An update. J Nutr Growth Cancer 3:199–206, 1986

112. Blot WJ, Li J-Y: Some considerations in the design of a nutrition intervention trial in Linxian, People's Republic of China. Natl Cancer Inst Monogr 69:29–34, 1985

113. Wechsler H, Levine S, Idelson RC et al: The physician's role in health promotion: A survey of primary care practitioners. N Engl J Med 309(2):97–100, 1983

114. Orleans CT: Understanding and promoting smoking cessation: Overview and guidelines for physician intervention. Annu Rev Med 36:51–61, 1985

115. Valente CM, Sobal J, Muncie HL Jr et al: Health promotion: Physicians' beliefs, attitudes, and practices. Am J Prev Med 2(2):82–88, 1986

116. Glanz K: Nutrition education for risk factor reduction and patient education: A review. Prev Med 14:721–752, 1985

117. US Department of Health and Human Services, Public Health Service: Diet, Nutrition and Cancer Prevention: The Good News. NIH publication No 87-2878, 1986

118. Butram RR, Clifford CK, Lanza E: National Cancer Institute dietary guidelines: Rationale. Am J Clin Nutr (in press)

119. US Department of Health and Human Services, Public Health Service, National Institutes of Health: Cancer Control Objectives for the Nation: 1985–2000. NIH (NCI) publication No 86-2880. Washington, DC, US Government Printing Office, 1986

120. Klein G: The approaching era of the tumor suppressor genes. Science 238:1539–1546, 1987

JOSEPH W. CULLEN

CHAPTER 12 *Principles of Cancer Prevention: Tobacco*

Over the past several decades, our understanding of the cancer process has increased substantially; cancer research has generated an impressive knowledge base related to the fundamental biological mechanisms underlying cell growth and regulation and to the management of cancer in its variety of forms. Of particular note has been the gradual accumulation of scientific evidence linking lifestyle to many cancers and therefore the opportunity to develop strategies to modify lifestyles and thereby prevent what was once regarded as the inevitable consequence of aging.

It is estimated that a large majority of cancers are caused or promoted by lifestyle factors that are controllable at the individual or societal level, or both.[1] That human behavior plays a prominent role in our understanding and control of the nation's second leading cause of mortality has led to a national cancer control agenda with a new emphasis on preventing disease and promoting health whenever possible. Risk factors such as diet, radiation (both actinic and ionizing), some occupational and drug exposures, and excessive alcohol consumption have all been implicated in cancer causation. But the most well-documented risk factor is tobacco use, and particularly smoking. Findings from basic laboratory and epidemiological research clearly indicate that if smoking and tobacco use can be reduced in the United States a marked reduction in cancer incidence and mortality is possible. The objectives of this chapter are to review the knowledge base in tobacco carcinogenesis, tobacco use and trends, particularly for cigarette smoking, and opportunities for cancer prevention. The unique and important role that physicians can play in reducing cancer risk by adopting smoking control interventions will also be discussed.

TOBACCO'S CONTRIBUTION TO CANCER ETIOLOGY AND MORTALITY

Knowledge of the link between tobacco use and cancer is not new. In fact, cancer was the first disease to be linked to tobacco use. For more than two centuries scientific evidence has been accumulating on the cancer consequences of tobacco use. From the earliest observations of John Hill,[2] a London physician who in 1761 reported an association between snuff use and cancer of the nose, to recent studies on the effect of environmental tobacco smoke (ETS) in nonsmokers, countless epidemiological, clinical, and experimental studies have conclusively demonstrated that tobacco use significantly increases the risk of developing cancer.

It is obviously not feasible (that is, ethical) to experiment with humans to prove the cause and effect relationship between the use of tobacco and any disease, cancer included. Scientists and public health specialists have relied on preclinical studies and epidemiological evidence to draw such conclusions. In so doing, they have established a rigorous set of criteria which have been outlined and applied in major scientific reviews[3-5] over the past two decades. These criteria are

Consistency of the association: similar observations by multiple investigators in different locations and situations, at different times, and using different methods of study.

Strength of the association: high ratio of disease rate for the population exposed to the suspected risk factor compared to the population not exposed.

Specificity of the association: associations with the exposure exist for the specific or limited set of diseases, and associations with the disease exist for a specific or limited set of exposures.

Temporal relationship of the association: exposure to the suspected etiologic factor precedes the disease.

Coherence of the association: epidemiologic observations are consonant with all else that is known about the disease.

The first Surgeon General's report on *Smoking and Health* in 1964 may be the most conspicuous document to have used these criteria. In that monograph, if these criteria were judged to be satisfied and pathologic and experimental data were supportive, the term "causal" was applied to the association. The designation "major cause" was used when the relative risk for the cancer in tobacco users was high. The term "contributory factor" was used when the body of evidence was less compelling, the relative risk lower, or the ancillary evidence (pathologic and experimental data) not sufficient for a judgment of causality. The term "association" was used when a relationship between tobacco use and a health consequence existed but the data were inadequate for an assessment of the extent of that relationship.

Thousands of studies detail the numerous and severe health consequences of cigarette smoking, and a succession of Surgeons General have reviewed and summarized the health effects associated with smoking.[3,4,6-21] Smoking is responsible for more than 315,000 deaths per year in the United States.[22] This death toll is greater than all other drug and alcohol abuse deaths combined, seven times more than all automobile fatalities per year, and more than all American military fatalities in World War I, World War II, and Vietnam combined.[23]

Cigarette smoking is a major cause of cancers of the lung, larynx, oral cavity, and esophagus, and is a contributory factor for the development of cancers of the bladder, pancreas, and kidney. A link between smoking and stomach cancer and cancer of the uterine cervix has also been noted.[4] Overall, cigarette smoking has been identified as the chief avoidable cause of cancer death in the United States.[4] In 1984, it was responsible for nearly one million years of potential life lost in the United States population.[22] Table 12-1 provides a recent summary of the deaths attributed to tobacco by cancer site.

LUNG CANCER

According to Tso and Gray,[24] the relationship between tobacco smoke and lung cancer in developed countries may be the most researched subject in medical history. In the United States, conclusive evidence of the association between cigarette smoking and lung cancer was first published in 1950. Wynder and Graham,[25] Doll and Hill,[26] and Levin et al,[27] reported a link between smoking and cancer. Yet the first national reviews were not published until 1962 (Report on Smoking of the Royal College of Surgeons[28]) and 1964 (Report of the Advisory Committee to the Surgeon General of the Public Health Service[3]). Both of these reports included epidemiological studies profiling tobacco consumption, composition, and carcinogenicity in animals and humans. The conclusions reached in these assessments and by a large number of comprehensive reviews since that time are impressively uniform and consistent: cigarette smoking causes lung cancer.[4,15,16,20,29]

Some of the epidemiological evidence in the U.S. Surgeon General's Report of 1964 involved 50 retrospective studies and 8 prospective studies that included more than 17 million person years of data.[4] From the prospective studies, lung cancer mortality ratios were concluded to be substantially greater for smokers than for nonsmokers (Table 12-2). As seen from Table 12-3, these mortality ratios are dose dependent. For men who smoke more than 25 cigarettes a day, the risk of death from lung cancer is 25 times that for the nonsmoker.

Whereas smoking alone has serious lung cancer effects, the morbidity is even greater when there is a concomitant exposure to certain environmental or occupational elements. Cigarette smoking and asbestos exposure, for example, together result in a more than additive increase in lung cancer risk.[14,30-35] The same is true for uranium miners who smoke and are exposed to radon daughters.[36,37]

TABLE 12-1. Total Mortality and Smoking-Attributable Mortality (SAM), by Disease, Cancer Site, and Sex—United States, 1984 (Adults ≥ 20 Years Old)

| Cancer Site | Men | | Women | | Total |
	Deaths	SAM	Deaths	SAM	SAM*
Lip, oral cavity, pharynx	5,754	3,958	2,689	1,110	5,068
Esophagus	6,310	3,717	2,345	1,257	4,974
Stomach	8,463	1,455	5,772	1,467	2,922
Pancreas	11,513	3,459	11,634	1,653	5,112
Larynx	2,959	2,385	664	274	2,660
Trachea, lung, bronchus	82,459	65,659	36,227	27,170	92,829
Cervix uteri	0	0	4,562	1,685	1,685
Urinary bladder	6,597	2,447	3,114	853	3,299
Kidney, other urinary	5,424	1,319	3,403	403	1,722

From the Centers for Disease Control: Smoking-attributable mortality and years of potential life lost—United States, 1984. MMWR 30:42, 1987.

* Sums may not equal total because of rounding.

TABLE 12-2.   Lung Cancer Mortality Ratios—Prospective Studies

Population	Size	Number of Deaths	Cigarette Smokers*
British physicians	34,000 men	441	14.00
	6,194 women	27	5.00
Swedish study	27,000 men	55	7.00
	28,000 women	8	4.50
Japanese study	122,000 men	940	3.76
	143,000 women	304	2.03
ACS 25-state study	358,000 men	2,018	8.53
	483,000 women	439	3.58
U.S. veterans	290,000 men	3,126	11.28
Canadian veterans	78,000 men	331	14.20
ACS 9-state study	188,000 men	448	10.73
California men in nine occupations	68,000 men	368	7.61

From the U.S. Department of Health and Human Services, Office on Smoking and Health: The Health Consequences of Smoking: Cancer. A Report of the Surgeon General, DHHS Pub. No. (PHS) 82–50179, 1982, p 36.
* Ratio of smoker to nonsmoker.

TABLE 12-3.   Lung Cancer Mortality Ratios for Men and Women, by Current Number of Cigarettes Smoked per Day—Prospective Studies

Population	Men		Women	
	Cigarettes Smoked per Day	Mortality Ratios	Cigarettes Smoked per Day	Mortality Ratios
ACS 25-state study	Nonsmoker	1.00	Nonsmoker	1.00
	1–9	4.62	1–9	1.30
	10–19	8.62	10–19	2.40
	20–39	14.69	20–39	4.90
	40+	18.71	40+	7.50
British physicians' study	Nonsmoker	1.00	Nonsmoker	1.00
	1–14	7.80	1–14	1.28
	15–24	12.70	15–24	6.41
	25+	25.10	25+	29.71
Swedish study	Nonsmoker	1.00	Nonsmoker	1.00
	1–7	2.30	1–7	1.80
	8–15	8.80	8–15	11.30
	16+	13.70	16+	
Japanese study: all ages	Nonsmoker	1.00	Nonsmoker	1.0
	1–19	3.49	<20	1.90
	20–39	5.69	20–29	4.20
	40+	6.45		
U.S. veterans study	Nonsmoker	1.00		
	1–9	3.89		
	10–20	9.63		
	21–39	16.70		
	≥40	23.70		
ACS 9-state study	Nonsmoker	1.00		
	1–9	8.00		
	10–20	10.50		
	20+	23.40		
Canadian veterans	Nonsmoker	1.00		
	1–9	9.50		
	10–20	15.80		
	20+	17.30		
California men in nine occupations	Nonsmoker	1.00		
	about ½ pack	3.72		
	about 1 pack	9.05		
	about 1½ packs	9.56		

From the U.S. Department of Health and Human Services, Office on Smoking and Health: The Health Consequences of Smoking: Cancer. A Report of the Surgeon General, DHHS Pub. No. (PHS) 82–50179, 1982, p 38.

Lung cancer is now the leading cause of cancer death for men in the United States.[38] Although breast cancer continues to be the leading cause of cancer death among women, lung cancer is now second in women and in many parts of the United States is the leading cause.[39]

Figure 12-1 presents smoking prevalence in the United States for men and women from 1965 (the year following the first Surgeon General's report on smoking and health) to 1985. Smoking rates for men declined significantly over this period from 51% to 33%.* Smoking rates for women also declined, but not as dramatically, from 31.5% to 28%. In fact, while rates for men had stabilized from the mid 1950s to 1965, rates for women had continued to climb from 24.5% in 1955 to 31.5% in 1965.

Predictably, these divergent smoking profiles have resulted in similar lung cancer rates. As depicted in Figure 12-2, the age-adjusted lung cancer incidence rates for men started to decline in 1983 (for the first time in this century) and continue to decline. Rates for women, on the other hand, continue to increase, and based upon women's smoking prevalence rates since 1955 the rates will continue to incline for some years to come.

Were it not for lung cancer, the overall cancer death rates would actually be decreasing in the United States.[38] As shown in Figure 12-3, there has been a 13% decline in overall mortality rates over the past 35 years for all cancer sites, excluding lung, as compared to a 9% increase in mortality rates for all cancer sites over that same period.

LARYNGEAL CANCER

Cigarette smoking is the major cause of laryngeal cancer.[4] More than 25 retrospective and 6 major prospective studies have examined the relationship between smoking and cancer of the larynx. Cigarette smokers in the prospective studies have up to 13 times more deaths from laryngeal cancer than nonsmokers, and relative risk ratios for the retrospective studies were consistently above 2.0.[4] Cigar and pipe smokers experience a risk for cancer of the larynx similar to that of cigarette smokers.

The risk of developing laryngeal cancer increases with increased exposure to cigarette smoke; heavy smokers have cancer mortality ratios 20 to 30 times greater than nonsmokers.[4] Furthermore, alcohol can act synergistically with cigarette smoking to increase the risk for cancer of the larynx up to 50% more than the sum of the excess risks posed by either behavior alone.[41]

* In 1986 the Public Health Service's Office of Smoking and Health carried out a telephone survey to study the U.S. adult population's knowledge, attitudes, and practices regarding the use of tobacco. This survey collected data from a national probability sample of 13,031 respondents who were at least 17 years old. The results showed the lowest prevalence of current cigarette smoking among adults ever recorded in the United States: 29.5% for men and 23.8% for women.[40] However, the age group in question is not comparable to the age groups for the samples previously collected through the National Health Interview Surveys (at least 20 years old). In addition, telephone surveys tend to underestimate the number of smokers in the age group surveyed because they often miss low socioeconomic status and minority populations that are at higher risk to smoke.

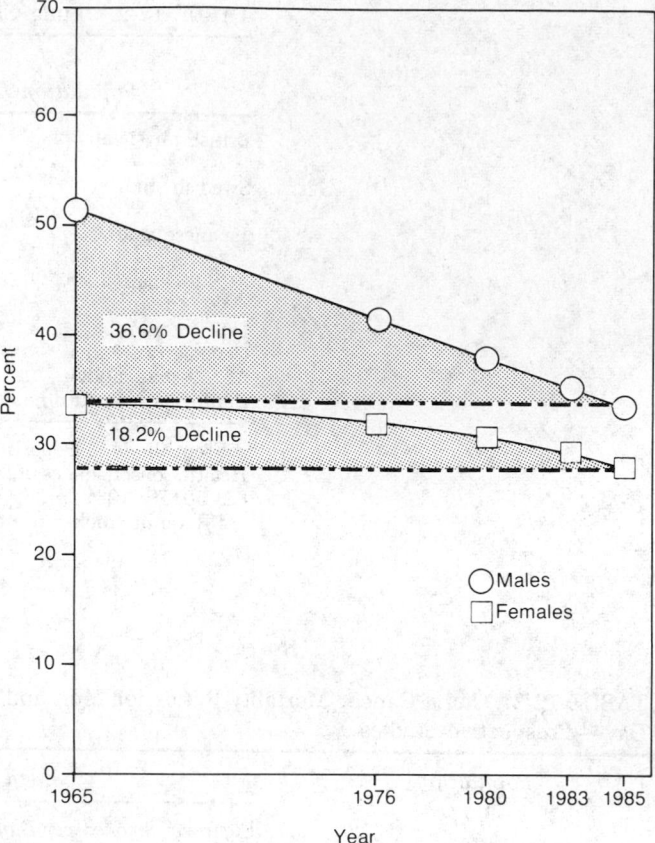

FIG. 12-1. Prevalence of cigarette smoking in the United States. (From the U.S. Department of Health and Human Services, National Center for Health Statistics, National Health Interview Survey)

ORAL CANCER

Cigarette smoking is a major cause of cancers of the oral cavity (including malignant tumors of the lip, tongue, salivary gland, floor of the mouth, mesopharynx, and hypopharynx).[4] A similar risk for oral cancer is posed by pipe and cigar smoking. In studies of U.S. populations, the deaths from oral cancer are from 3 to 14 times greater for smokers than for nonsmokers. This risk is also dose-related. Comparing those who smoke 25 or more cigarettes a day (the standard definition of heavy smokers) to nonsmokers, there is evidence that oral cancer mortality ratios are 5.5 to 33 times greater than in the nonsmoker.

As is true for laryngeal cancer, alcohol synergistically increases the risk of cancer of the oral cavity on a dose-related basis. McLoy and co-workers[42] found that smokers who consumed 7 or more ounces of alcohol per day had a fivefold increase in risk for oral cancer even if they smoked less than half a pack of cigarettes a day. The risk rose to 20-fold for 11 to 20 cigarettes and to 24-fold for more than a pack a day.

ESOPHAGEAL CANCER

Smoking of cigarettes, cigars, and pipes cause carcinoma of the esophagus.[4,22] Death rates for esophageal cancer are up

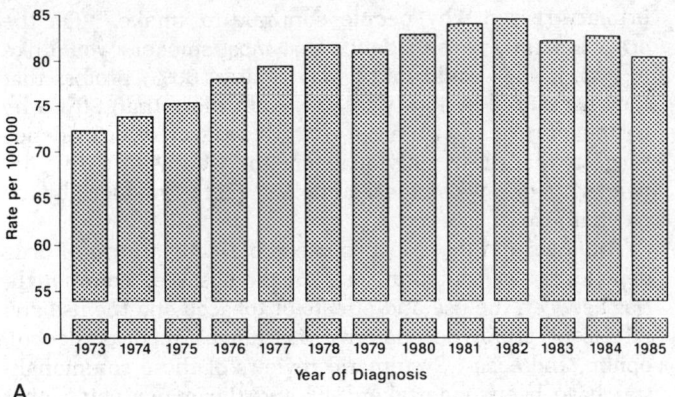

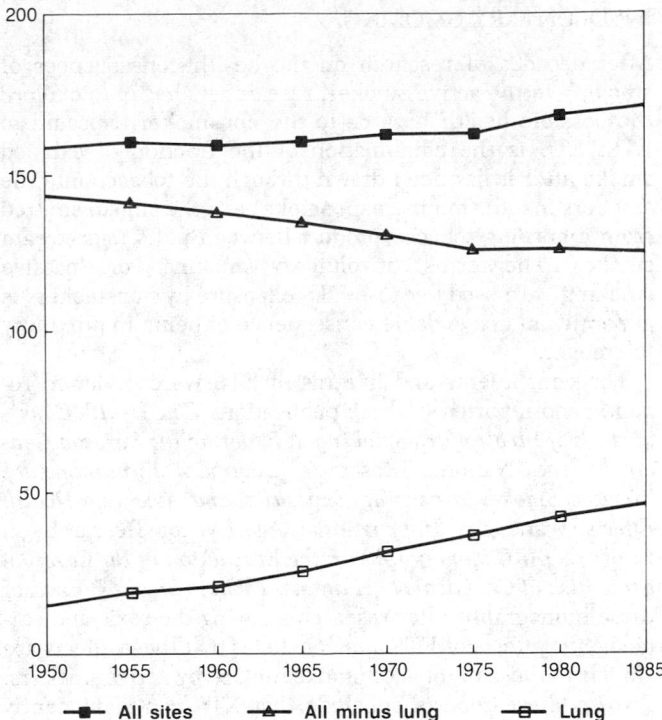

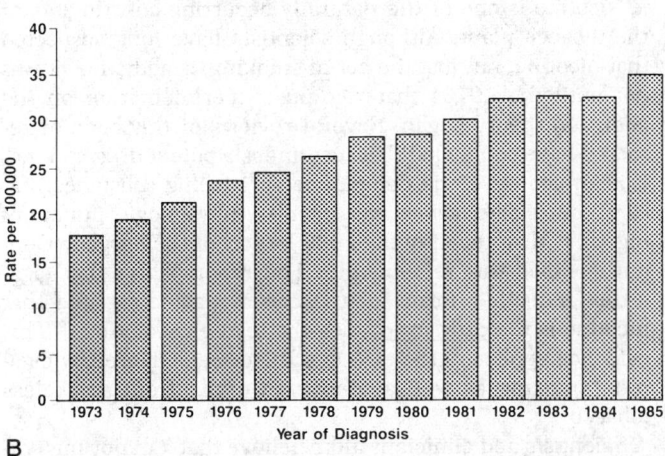

FIG. 12-2. **A**. Age-adjusted lung cancer incidence rates per 100,000, white men, 1973–1985. **B**. Age-adjusted lung cancer incidence rates per 100,000 white women, 1973–1985. Adjusted to the age distribution of the 1970 standard U.S. population. (Data from the SEER program)

FIG. 12-3. Trends in cancer death rates. (From the National Cancer Institute: Annual Cancer Statistics Review including Cancer Trends: 1950–1985. NIH Pub. No. 88–2789, 1988)

to six times greater for smokers than for nonsmokers; the risk is dose-related, and as is true for larynx and oral cancers, a number of studies have found that alcohol consumption acts synergistically with smoking to increase the risk for developing esophageal cancer.[43–51]

OTHER CANCERS

Cigarette smoking is a contributory factor in the development of bladder, kidney, and pancreatic cancers. An association has also been noted between cigarette smoking and cervical and stomach cancers.[4] The attribution of association noted in the 1982 Surgeon General's report between smoking and cervical cancer continues to be strengthened by recent studies providing positive results.[52–54]

SMOKELESS TOBACCO USE

In the United States, smokeless tobacco consists of chewing tobacco and snuff. Experimental investigations have revealed potent carcinogens in these smokeless tobacco products, including nitrosamines, [55–62] polycyclic aromatic hydrocarbons,[63,64] and radiation emitting polonium.[65] The first evidence of cancer among users of snuff or chewing tobacco appeared in case reports during the early 1940s.[66] The first epidemiologic study of smokeless tobacco was not conducted until the early 1950s.[67]

A comprehensive assessment of the available scientific evidence on the health consequences of using smokeless tobacco is now available as a result of recent reviews by three scientific bodies.[5,68,69] The three reviews are consistent in their conclusions. The scientific evidence is strong that the use of snuff causes cancer in humans, with the strongest evidence of causality for oral cancer. Oral cancer has been shown to occur several times more frequently in snuff dippers than in non–tobacco users, and the excess risk of cancers of the cheek and gum may be nearly 50-fold among long-term snuff users.[70] Some investigations suggest that the use of chewing tobacco may also increase the risk of oral cancer, but the evidence is not as strong and the risks have yet to be quantified.

Evidence for an association between smokeless tobacco use and cancer outside of the oral cavity is sparse. There is suggestive evidence that smokeless tobacco users face increased risks of tumors of the upper aerodigestive tract, but results are currently inconclusive.[5]

INVOLUNTARY SMOKING

After decades of research on the health consequences of smoking in the active smoker, researchers began to explore the possible health hazards to the nonsmoker exposure to ETS. ETS is the combination of the fraction of exhaled smoke after it has been drawn through the tobacco into the smokers mouth (mainstream smoke) and the smoke emitted from a burning tobacco product between puffs (sidestream smoke). The terms "involuntary smoking" or "passive smoking" are used because ETS exposure by nonsmokers is generally an unavoidable consequence of being in proximity to smokers.

The constituents and hazards of ETS were reviewed recently and reported in three publications: *The Health Consequences of Involuntary Smoking: A Report of the Surgeon General*,[21] the National Research Council's *Environmental Tobacco Smoke: Measuring Exposures and Assessing Health Effects*,[71] and the International Agency for Research on Cancer's *IARC Monographs on the Evaluation of the Carcinogenic Risk of Chemicals to Humans: Tobacco Smoke*.[28] Each of these monographs cites research showing the toxic and carcinogenic effects of ETS and concludes that these effects are similar to those of tobacco smoke inhaled by active smokers. Two of these reports conclude that ETS can significantly increase the risk of lung cancer in nonsmokers.[21,71] The third report concludes that nonsmokers exposed to ETS have an increased risk of cancer or are not without risk.[28] Although the magnitude of risk is uncertain, an estimate from epidemiological studies of spousal exposure in various populations in Europe, Asia, and North America places the risk of lung cancer in nonsmokers married to smokers at about 34% higher than it is for nonsmoking spouses of nonsmokers.[71]

Although more complete data on the dose and variability of smoke exposure in the nonsmoking population are needed before an accurate quantitative estimate of the number of ETS-induced lung cancers can be made, many experts believe that a meaningful proportion of the lung cancers that occur in nonsmokers are the result of this risk factor.[21] The National Research Council has estimated that ETS is responsible for 20% or 2,400 of the nonsmoker lung cancer deaths per year, with a range of 10% to 50% or 350 to 6,000 deaths.[71] Such an estimate should and does generate a substantial public health concern. With respect to cancers at sites other than the lung, there are insufficient data to evaluate adequately the role of involuntary smoking.

NICOTINE DEPENDENCE: THE LINK BETWEEN TOBACCO AND TOBACCO-RELATED DISEASES

Although there is a growing body of evidence that lifestyle modification affects cancer incidence, this knowledge has yet to be absorbed fully by the public. For example, there are approximately 50 million Americans who continue to smoke. Why individuals persist in this risk-taking behavior despite the knowledge of the serious cancer and other health consequences of tobacco use is curious. On the one hand, tobacco industry representatives cite personal choice as the primary reason why people continue to smoke.[72] On the other hand, there is evidence that most smokers would like to quit, if they could find a way. Many (60%) profess that they have tried seriously to quit,[73] but more than 80% who try to quit relapse within the year. Recent scientific evidence suggests that these individuals are the victims of a drug dependency, or physiological addiction, that is produced by the habitual use of tobacco.

The assertion that tobacco use is basically a form of drug dependence or addiction rests on the observed commonalities between the use and effects of tobacco and the use and effects of prototype addictive substances such as alcohol, opium, and cocas. Systematic reviews of these commonalities have been undertaken[74-78] and the major points that tobacco and addictive substances have in common are summarized in Table 12-4.

The next major question is, what elements of tobacco are critical in controlling the behavior of the user? The conceptual leap from habitual behavior to drug abuse and addiction can be made only on the basis of evidence that a specific psychoactive drug is critical to the behavior.[5]

Nicotine is one of the naturally occurring constituents of the tobacco plant. Although scientists have long suspected that nicotine, not just the act of smoking, is addictive, it was not until the 1970s that rigorous experimentation on the addiction theory began. Several reviews of this body of research have concluded that nicotine is a potent drug and that it is an addictive and dependence-producing substance that can control behavior and modify physiologic functioning.[5,77,78] Most recently the 1988 Report of the Surgeon General codified this relationship. The report states that cigarettes and other forms of tobacco are addicting and that nicotine is the drug in tobacco that causes addiction.[79] This evidence applies to the effects of nicotine delivered by cigarette smoking as well as delivered orally from smokeless tobacco.

Scientists and clinicians alike believe that a major impediment to the reduction of cancer and other tobacco-caused diseases is the nicotine dependence process.[80] Without nicotine dependence, there is no evidence that there would be

TABLE 12-4.   Commonalities Between Tobacco Use and Other Addictive Substances

---

- A centrally (CNS) active substance (drug) is delivered.
- Discriminate (subjective) effects are centrally mediated.
- The substance (drug) is a reinforcer for animals.
- The patterns of acquisition and maintenance of substance ingestion are orderly.
- The patterns of self-administration of the substance are orderly.
- The patterns of self-administration of the substance vary as a function of the dose that is consumed.
- Tolerance to the behavioral and physiologic effects of the substance develops with repeated use (neuroadaptation).
- Therapeutic effects may be produced by the substance.
- The treatment of addiction resulting from the substance (drug) involves similar strategies.

From the U.S. Department of Health and Human Services. The Health Consequences of Using Smokeless Tobacco: A Report of the Advisory Committee to the Surgeon General, pp 146–147. Bethesda, MD, NIH Publication No. 86-2874, 1986.

widespread and compulsive use of tobacco. Nicotine addiction is truly the bridge between tobacco as an environmental toxin and the multitude of diseases that result from repeated exposure.[81]

The significance of this evidence is demonstrated by the inclusion of a specific category for diseases and deaths caused by "tobacco dependence" in the current (ninth) revision of the International Classification of Diseases[82] and the third edition of the Diagnostic and Statistical Manual of Mental Disorders.[83] Tobacco dependence is defined as follows:

> Continuous use of tobacco for at least a month with either (1) unsuccessful attempts to stop or significantly reduce the amount of tobacco use on a permanent basis, (2) the development of tobacco withdrawal, or (3) the presence of a serious physical disorder (*e.g.*, respiratory or cardiovascular disease) that the individual (or the physician) knows is exacerbated by tobacco use. . . . If the individual with a serious case of one of the tobacco-related physical disorders continues to use tobacco, despite awareness of its harmful effects, a reasonable inference can be made that the individual is tobacco dependent.

Although tobacco dependence is the most common of the addictive disorders, most American physicians are believed to be unaware of either the existence or the importance of this diagnostic category.[84] Appropriate use of this category is particularly important because new pharmacotherapy approaches to deal with tobacco are available and are proving to be successful aids in smoking cessation. The most promising of these approaches is discussed later in this chapter.

OPPORTUNITIES FOR TOBACCO USE PREVENTION AND CESSATION

The evidence is clearly positive that quitting smoking decreases the risk for lung cancer. As is evident in Table 12-5, 15 to 20 years after quitting, the ex-smokers' risk of dying from lung cancer declines to a point where it closely approximates the risk of the nonsmoker.[85,86] The magnitude of the residual risk is largely determined by the cumulative exposure to tobacco prior to smoking cessation, that is, the total amount smoked, the age when smoking began, the degree of inhalation, and the tar level of the products used. Similar benefits of smoking cessation have been demonstrated for laryngeal,[87] esophageal,[88] and oral cavity cancers.[88]

The benefits of quitting cigarette smoking are evident. But in themselves they are not sufficient to get people to quit. A comprehensive public health prevention strategy is needed. In the United States, the message about the health consequences of smoking competes with the tobacco industry's multi-billion dollar campaign annually to convince people to smoke and with smokers' own motivations for smoking. In developing a prevention strategy, one must learn more about smokers themselves: Who are they, and what motivates them to smoke or stop smoking? But much more impor-

TABLE 12-5. Lung Cancer Mortality Ratios in Ex-Cigarette Smokers, by Number of Years Stopped Smoking

Study	Years Stopped Smoking	Mortality Ratio	
British physicians	1–4	16.00	
	5–9	5.90	
	10–14	5.30	
	15+	2.00	
	Current smokers	14.00	
U.S. veterans*	1–4	18.83	
	5–9	7.73	
	10–14	4.71	
	15–19	4.81	
	20+	2.10	
	Current smokers	11.28	
Japanese men	1–4	4.65	
	5–9	2.50	
	10+	1.35	
	Current smokers	3.76	
		Number of Cigarettes Smoked per Day	
		1–19	*20+*
ACS 25-state study (men 50–69)	<1	7.20	29.13
	1–4	4.60	12.00
	5–9	1.00	7.20
	10+	0.40	1.06
	Current smokers	6.47	13.67

From the U.S. Department of Health and Human Services, Office on Smoking and Health: The Health Consequences of Smoking: Cancer. A Report of the Surgeon General. DHHS Pub. No. (PHS) 82–50179, 1982, p 46.
* Includes data only for ex-cigarette smokers who stopped for other than physicians' orders.

tantly, there is a need to reduce smoking and tobacco use prevalence by every strategy available that is feasible and effective.

TARGETING HIGH RISK POPULATIONS FOR BEHAVIOR CHANGE

The use of tobacco is an individual decision. As the 1982 Surgeon General's report on smoking and cancer states, "There is no single action an individual can take to reduce the risk of cancer more effectively than quitting smoking, particularly cigarettes."[4] An increasing number of people have heard that message and acted on it. Since the first Surgeon General's report in 1964, approximately 40 million people have quit smoking.[89] Many argue that this immense modification in a society's lifestyle may be the largest socio-cultural change in the history of this country. Within this generally positive profile, however, tobacco use in several population groups warrants special surveillance.

First, approximately 50 million American adults, or about one in three,[89] still smoke, and 2 to 3 million young people aged 12 to 17 are currently cigarette smokers.[90]

Second, ethnic minorities are more likely to smoke than whites, and in particular, black men are more likely to smoke than white men (40.6% versus 33.2%, respectively).[89] Lung cancer incidence rates for blacks already exceed those for whites, and these rate differentials are expected to increase substantially over the next decade. Although smoking prevalence is the same in Hispanic men as in white men (albeit 8% less in women),[89] this advantage may be fast disappearing. Recent data suggest that young Hispanics are smoking as much as, if not more than, their white peers.[91]

Third, there is special concern for the heavy smoker, that is, someone who smokes 25 or more cigarettes a day. There are more heavy smokers today than ever before.[89] A heavy smoker is 15 to 25 times more likely to die of lung cancer than a nonsmoker.[4]

Fourth, numerous surveys and studies have shown that smoking is most often initiated during the junior and senior high school years.[89,92,93] This period provides a prime opportunity for cancer prevention, and a number of smoking prevention programs have been oriented toward that age group. Although it appears that smoking is declining among this group,* the level of cigarette use remains alarmingly high, and female high school seniors continue to smoke at higher rates than their male peers.[94]

Fifth, one of the most disturbing trends in tobacco use by young people is the increasing use of smokeless tobacco — snuff and chewing tobacco. Smokeless tobacco users are the fastest growing group of tobacco users, and the pattern of use is steadily shifting from older to younger users. Currently,

16% of males between the ages of 12 and 25 — over 12 million people — have used smokeless tobacco in the preceding year; 5% to 8%, or about 6 million, are regular users (at least once a week).[95] Use varies widely across the country. Boyd and co-workers in a recent review reported that less than 7% of sixth-grade boys in New York City but more than 68% of sixth-grade boys in rural Montana were users. Use also varies by ethnic group. Hispanics and whites have comparable use rates, whereas use among Native Americans is higher than among whites, and use among blacks and Asians is lower.[96]

Finally, the problem of tobacco use in all these high-risk populations is influenced by current trends in tobacco advertising and marketing. The tobacco industry is spending more than two billion dollars a year on cigarette advertising and promotion. There are also indications that the cigarette market in the United States has become increasingly segmented in response to the decline in cigarette sales and the proliferation of brands.[97] In order to succeed, manufacturers of new cigarette brands must target specific segments of the market. As a result, marketing campaigns have targeted women, minorities, blue-collar workers, and especially children and adolescents. While representatives of the tobacco and advertising industries maintain that the only purpose and effect of cigarette advertising is to promote brand loyalty and brand switching, many health professionals believe that cigarette advertising perpetuates and increases cigarette consumption. Advertising tobacco products may recruit new smokers, induce former smokers to relapse, make it more difficult for smokers to quit, and increase the level of smokers' consumption by acting as an external cue to smoke.[97]

TOBACCO USE INTERVENTIONS

Intervention research programs designed to develop effective methods of reducing cigarette smoking and other forms of tobacco use have proliferated during the past two decades. The results of these studies have been highlighted in several reviews.[98-105]

Much of the initial behavioral research has focused on gaining an understanding of the factors that influence the development and maintenance of smoking and tobacco use behavior. Smoking and cessation are complex behavioral patterns that proceed through a sequence of stages from initiation of smoking to maintenance of cessation. Psychological, social, and demographic factors are strongly associated with smoking initiation; cessation and maintenance of cessation are affected by a combination of physiological and psychosocial variables.

Considerable progress has been made in developing and testing the effectiveness of a variety of intervention methods or techniques to prevent or control tobacco use. These include approaches to decrease physiological addiction[106] and psychological dependence, strategies aimed at maintenance or relapse,[100,107,108] programs that combine physiological, behavioral, aversive, and maintenance techniques,[109,110] self-help techniques,[111,112] mass media,[113] schools,[114] communities as a whole,[115] and interventions involving physicians and dentists.[116]

---

* Because national probability sampling for this age category has not been carried out since 1979, except in high school seniors, the data that are available are in question. High school seniors are a self-selected population. They are under-represented by low socio-economic status and minority populations.

THE PHYSICIAN: AN EFFECTIVE AGENT OF CHANGE

There are a number of reasons physicians can be effective in reducing smoking prevalence. First, physicians are role models for health. Less than 17% smoke, compared with 30% of the general population.[117] Physicians are perceived as the most authoritative source of medical and health information. About 70% of Americans make at least one visit a year to their doctor. Often because they are ill, they may be amenable to a suggestion about lifestyle and behavior change ("the teachable moment"). The personal relationship and trust that clinicians are able to establish with their patients can be used to advantage in counseling patients about cancer prevention habits in general and tobacco use in particular. Some groups, such as smokers, make disproportionately greater use of medical services than other groups, and so there may be more clinical opportunities in which the physician can raise the smoking issue. Table 12-6 illustrates the range of these clinical opportunities.

Many physicians now view health promotion as an important part of their practices. In particular, they consider smoking a serious health hazard and consider it their responsibility to advise their patients to quit.[118] However, recent data indicate that less than 45% of physicians do, in fact, counsel their patients about smoking.[119] Why the disparity between attitude and action? A number of reasons have been cited:[120-122]

1. Lack of time
2. Lack of reimbursement for health promotion counseling
3. Pessimism about their ability to effect behavior change, especially if the patient is there for an unrelated problem
4. Feeling that counseling about lifestyle behaviors, especially if the patient is asymptomatic, is an infringement on the patient's personal freedom
5. Lack of training in health promotion activities and a lack of knowledge about outside health promotion resources
6. Reliance on ineffective health education methods, which then contributes to the sense of pessimism noted earlier

Several of these factors, such as reimbursement and lack of training in health promotion activities, reflect legitimate barriers to effective counseling. Effective ways to eliminate or minimize these barriers must be found to assist physicians in their health promotion efforts. Many of the barriers identified are attitudinal, and a number of studies over the past 20 years belie the belief that physicians are not effective. For example, clinical trial data indicate that even brief advice to the patient from a physician to stop smoking can be effective. A 1979 study by Russell[123] showed that a 1-year quit rate of 5% can be achieved with 1 to 2 minutes of physician counseling supplemented by a four-page brochure and 1- and 12-month telephone follow-up. The seemingly minimal percentage of quitters in this study was achieved with only a very brief intervention by physicians possessing incomplete smoking cessation counseling skills. While the average physician is interested in and accustomed to more successful

TABLE 12-6. Clinical Opportunities to Talk About Smoking with Patients

Symptoms
  Cough
  Sputum production
  Shortness of breath
Tests
  Electrocardiography
  Pulmonary function tests
  Total Leukocyte counts
  Blood pressure measurements
  Hematocrit
  Auscultation of heart and lungs
  Blood lipid studies
  Blood coagulation studies
  Serum alpha$_1$-antiprotease determinations
  Pregnancy tests
  Carboxyhemoglobin determinations
Diagnosis of Disease and Risk Factors
  Coronary heart disease
  Peripheral vascular disease
  Angina pectoris
  Hypertension
  Emphysema
  Chronic bronchitis
  Pneumonia
  Asthma
  Acute bronchitis
  Recurrent respiratory infection
  Diabetes mellitus
  Hypercholesterolemia
  Peptic ulcer
  Allergy
Drug Prescriptions
  Drug and tobacco smoke interactions
  Pharmacologic aids to smoking cessation
    Nicotine chewing gum

From the National Heart, Lung, and Blood Institute: Clinical Opportunity for Smoking Intervention: A Guide for the Busy Physician. National Heart, Lung, and Blood Institute's Smoking Education Program in cooperation with the American Lung Association and the American Thoracic Society. NIH Publication No. 86-2178, 1986.

treatment outcomes than 5%, it is important to note the public health impact of this outcome. Millions of smokers in a decade can be helped to quit, given a success rate of 25 patients per year in the offices of 50,000 physicians (less than 10% of the physicians in the United States). With more commitment and better skills, quit rates could presumably reach much higher levels.

A 1985 study by Goldstein and colleagues[124] also supports the contention that physicians can be effective agents of change. In this study, recently trained family practitioners in Iowa were interviewed about their smoking counseling beliefs, attitudes, and practices. The respondents overwhelmingly expressed strong motivation to counsel their patients who smoked, whether or not they had smoking-related symptoms. They also expressed confidence in their abilities to be effective, particularly if they had received formal training in smoking counseling. Table 12-7 summarizes the attitudes of these physicians[124] and compares them with physicians surveyed in earlier studies.[125]

TABLE 12-7.   Physician Smoking Counseling Studies

	Study Year (%)			
	1978	1981	1984	1985
Respondents who smoke	15		12	2
"Counseling about smoking is important"	85			100
"Quite effective" or "very successful" in counseling	12	3		30
"Physicians have an obligation to counsel"	85	86		99
"I counsel patients whether or not they have a smoking-related illness"	52		89	98
Believed they had influenced patients to stop smoking		14		98

From Goldstein B, et al: Survey of physicians' attitudes and practices in early cancer detection. CA 35:197–213, 1985.

HELPING PATIENTS QUIT SMOKING: A MULTIFACETED APPROACH

A recent consensus conference of smoking intervention researchers reviewed the results from six intervention trials that are testing ways to maximize physician effectiveness in smoking cessation and prevention efforts. The group concluded that physicians can intervene effectively to promote smoking cessation, especially if a specific regimen is followed. The researchers also concluded that an individualized approach to smokers, combined with self-help materials, selected prescriptions of nicotine gum, and follow-up monitoring of a patient's attempt to quit, were more effective than advice alone.[126] Within this consensus, the following program elements, summarized in Table 12-8, were found to be essential in an office-based intervention strategy for physicians.[126]

Conduct Intake and Screening

The physician should determine whether a patient smokes. If the patient does smoke, the physician should assess the smoking history and the patient's motivation to quit. The patient's chart should be flagged, and smoking status should be updated at each subsequent visit.

Recommended Physician Actions

The physician should discuss the hazards of smoking and the benefits of quitting, and should personalize them. A strong recommendation to quit should be given, and if possible, a commitment from the patient to quit by a specific date should be obtained. An individualized quit plan should be outlined, and a pharmacological aid, nicotine gum, should be considered when appropriate. Finally, the physician should assure the patient of support in this effort and state that the office will monitor the patient's progress.

Establish Supportive Office Procedures

The importance of providing an office system that enables a physician-based smoking cessation program to function smoothly and independently of the physician cannot be overstated. Office staff should be involved and their roles should be defined. Office staff activities can include reviewing the

TABLE 12-8.   Essential Elements of a Physician-Guided Smoking Cessation Program

Intake and Screening
- Identify smoking status along with vital signs
- Update tobacco use status regularly (6 months and 12 months).
- Obtain basic data on smoking history and readiness to quit (update regularly if possible).

Physicians Actions
- Assess motivation and risk profile.
- Personalize risk of smoking and benefit of quitting.
- Advise to quit.
- Obtain quit commitment (set quit date).
- Triage (quit plan, including nicotine gum).
- Emphasize that progress will be monitored.

Office Staff Actions
- Define office resources.
- Review quit plan.
- Explain nicotine gum use (as necessary).
- Explain self-help materials (review special sections).
- Facilitate referral to outside resources.
- Schedule follow-up contact (link to quit plan).

Follow-up
- Conduct rapid followup of all patients with plan to change.
- Reassess smoking status at next visit.
- Triage and recycle relapsers at next visit.

Office Environment
- Establish smoke-free office (staff and patients)
- Make smoking education materials available.
- Publicize smoking cessation program.

From the U.S. Department of Health and Human Services: Essential Elements of an HMO-Guided Smoking Cessation Program. NCI Prepublication Edition, June 1987.

quit plan with the patient, reviewing the proper use of nicotine gum, providing self-help materials, assisting with referrals to outside smoking cessation treatments, and scheduling follow-up contacts.

Establish Follow-up Procedures

The physician or office staff should contact the patient soon after the initial visit to check on progress. At each subsequent visit, the patient's smoking status and progress in quitting should be updated and further assistance provided when necessary. If a patient has relapsed, the doctor or staff should assist in identifying an appropriate treatment plan.

Establish an Appropriate Office Environment

The physician and office staff should reinforce nonsmoking message to patients. The most obvious step is a nonsmoking physician and staff and a smoke-free office. Information on the health effects of smoking and smoking cessation programs should be provided in the office. The fact that the physician provides smoking counseling should be publicized.

Numerous resources are available to help physicians establish and maintain smoking cessation efforts in their offices. These aids cover most aspects of quitting and are available in various formats. Table 12-9 lists some existing resources.

PHARMACOLOGIC AIDS FOR SMOKING CESSATION

Because tobacco use is a form of drug dependence, strategies of treatment used with dependence on other drugs have been applied. The most promising treatment and the first recognized as safe and efficacious by the Food and Drug Administration is nicorette, or nicotine gum. It is used in the same way that methadone substitution is used to treat heroin addiction.[127]

It is important to note that the intended use of the gum is unlike ordinary chewing gum. The manufacturer supplies the product buffered to a pH of 8.0 to 8.4. The nicotine component is meant to be absorbed in the mouth transmucosally, and not in the gut from where the chemically active drug will pass through the liver and lose most of its pharmacologic potency. After a small number of chews (approximately 15), the gum should be "parked" between the cheek and the gums for maximum absorption. The gum's effectiveness in aiding cessation has been demonstrated in several placebo-controlled trials.[128-132] Other studies have also shown that under a wide range of conditions the desire to smoke is reduced, although not eliminated, and withdrawal symptoms are lessened.[133-136] Recent work at the Addiction Research Center of the National Institute on Drug Abuse indicates that nicorette not only meets the criteria of therapeutic efficacy and low toxicity but appears to have a relatively low potential for abuse. It is apparently easier for most people to quit using the gum than to quit tobacco use.[79]

There are caveats regarding the use of nicotine gum, however. First, treatment of tobacco dependence is most efficacious when the gum is used in conjunction with a behavioral intervention. Cigarette smoking, like other forms of drug abuse, is only partially mediated by pharmacologic factors. The gum addresses possible physiological dependence, whereas the behavioral program equips the smoker to deal with psychological hurdles.[106] Second, persons who are most effectively treated with the gum thus far are heavily addicted smokers[137] as measured by the Fagerstrom Tolerance Scale.[128] Finally, it has been suggested that the use of the gum would probably be more efficacious if patient and physician compliance were increased.[138] As few as one third of the patients given a prescription for the gum ever fill it and most patients use the gum for less than the recommended 3 months. It is also important to stress that physicians or their staff instruct the patients in proper use of the gum and provide adequate follow-up of the patient to guarantee com-

TABLE 12-9. Smoking Cessation Resources

Title	Available from
Self-Help Manuals	
Clearing the Air—A Guide to Quitting Smoking	Office of Cancer Communications, National Cancer Institute, Bethesda, Maryland 20892
Quit for Good	Office of Cancer Communications, National Cancer Institute, Bethesda, Maryland 20892
Freedom From Smoking in 20 Days	American Lung Association, Local Office
Freedom From Smoking For You and Your Family	American Lung Association, Local Office
The Quitter's Guide—A Seven Day Plan to Help You Stop Smoking	American Cancer Society, Local Office
How to Quit Cigarettes	American Cancer Society, Local Office
Stop Smoking, Stay Trim	American Lung Association, Local Office
Videos	
In Control: A Home Video Freedom From Smoking Program	American Lung Association, Local Office
Why Quit Quiz Video	American Cancer Society, Local Office
Quitting With Nicorette	Minnesota Coalition for a Smoke-Free Society 2000, 2221 University Avenue, S.E., Suite 400, Minneapolis, Minnesota 55414
Motivational Materials	
Fifty Most Often Asked Questions About Smoking and Health and the Answers	American Cancer Society, Local Office
Why Do You Smoke	Office of Cancer Communications, National Cancer Institute, Bethesda, Maryland 20892
Health Hazards Associated With Involuntary Smoking: Cancer Facts	Office of Cancer Communications, National Cancer Institute, Building 31, Room 10A34, Bethesda, Maryland 20892
Second-Hand Smoke: The Fact Series	American Lung Association, Local Office
Physicians/Office Staff Training Guides	
A Physician Talks About Smoking	Office on Smoking and Health, Public Health Service, Rockville, Maryland 20857
Clinical Opportunities for Smoking Intervention—A Guide for the Busy Physician	National Heart, Lung, and Blood Institute in cooperation with the American Lung Association and the American Thoracic Society
The Physicians Guide—How To Help Your Hypertensive Patient Stop Smoking	National High Blood Pressure Education Program, National Heart, Lung, and Blood Institute
Family Physicians' Guide to Smoking Cessation	American Academy of Family Practitioners, 1740 West 92nd Street, Kansas City, Missouri 64114

From the U.S. Department of Health and Human Services: Essential Elements of an HMO-Guided Smoking Cessation Program. NCI Prepublication Edition, June 1987.

pliance and correct usage. When proper instructions are given and compliance is achieved, nicotine gum has a significant effect on short-term cessation and a demonstrable effect on long-term cessation.

PHYSICIAN INTERVENTION OPPORTUNITIES IN THE COMMUNITY

In response to the evidence concerning the health hazards of involuntary smoking, a growing number of states, agencies, and businesses are taking action to restrict smoking in public places. No longer is it solely the smoker's right to smoke if he or she desires. Rather, the nonsmoker has the right to breathe air free of tobacco smoke. As Surgeon General Dr. C. Everett Koop stated in the preface to his report, "The right of smokers to smoke ends where their behavior affects the health and well-being of others."[21]

Physicians have a role to play not only in office practices but also increasingly in the community. As more businesses offer health promotion programs and institute policies to restrict smoking, the need grows for smoking cessation policies and guidelines. Physicians who practice in business and industry can become active in several arenas:[139]

1. They can lay the groundwork for smoking cessation programs by writing articles on smoking in the company newsletter and making presentations to employees and instruction managers.
2. If the company decides to institute a smoking cessation program, the physician can assist in the development of an in-house effort or can assist in selecting a competent professional consultant.
3. They can assist in program implementation through clinical and diagnostic services to screen smoking employees and by advising smokers to participate in smoking cessation programs in the company.
4. They can assist in counseling employees who are either successful (i.e., helping with withdrawal symptoms) or unsuccessful in quitting. They can also prescribe nicotine gum as part of the program.
5. Finally, they can assist in program evaluation and follow-up.

The involvement of physicians in nontraditional roles is also important. These include serving as experts on tobacco control issues to both the lay and medical communities, helping to motivate and mobilize other physicians toward greater involvement, advocating policy and initiatives while sitting on boards of directors for a variety of community organizations, and advocating legislative initiatives while participating in a number of community and state-wide activities.

THE CASE FOR CANCER PREVENTION

The prevention of chronic disease, including cancer, is possible because a modification of lifestyle is possible. A study by Enstrom[140] demonstrates this fact rather dramatically. He showed that the decline in smoking prevalence among California physicians had an important impact on a number of mortality endpoints that included smoking related cancers. Table 12-10 depicts standardized mortality ratios of these physicians compared with other American white men for the periods 1950–1959 and 1970–1979. Reductions in smoking prevalence from 53% in 1950 to about 10% in 1980 resulted in significantly lower death rates from lung cancer. The California physicians' Standard Mortality Ratios (SMR) declined from 62% (already 38% less than the comparison population) in 1950–1959 to 30% in 1970–1979 (70% less than the comparison population). Their SMRs for other smoking-related cancers, ischemic heart disease, and other diseases of the lung and bronchus also declined significantly.

The adoption of risk-reducing behavior patterns is an important element in any effective cancer control strategy. As the first line of authority in health matters, physicians have a critical role to play in a strategy to reduce diseases caused by tobacco use. Helping people to stop smoking and to avoid other forms of tobacco use is one of the greatest challenges facing public health and preventive medicine today. Cancer control authorities recognize that an aggressive, multifaceted strategy to tobacco use prevention and control will be necessary to achieve the National Cancer Institute's mortality reduction goal by the year 2000. An important element of this strategy is the commitment of physicians to actions that will maximize their potential impact as exemplars, authority figures, and interventionists to reduce all tobacco use and cigarette smoking in particular.

TABLE 12-10. Mortality Ratios and Smoking Prevalence

	1950	1950–1959	1970–1979	1980
Standardized mortality rates (%) of California physicians relative to U.S. white men				
Lung cancer		62	30	
Other smoking-related cancers		100	63	
Ischemic heart disease		106	71	
Bronchitis, emphysema, asthma		62	35	
Smoking Prevalence (%)				
California physicians	53			10
U.S. white males	53			38

Enstrom JE: Trends in mortality among California physicians after giving up smoking. Br J Med [Clin Res] 286:1101–1105, 1983.

REFERENCES

1. Doll R, Peto R: The causes of cancer: Quantitative estimates of avoidable risk in cancer in the United States. JNCI 66:1191–1308, 1981
2. Redmond DE: Tobacco and cancer: The first clinical report, 1761. N Engl J Med 282:18–23, 1970
3. US Department of Health, Education, and Welfare, Centers for Disease Control: Smoking and Health: Report of the Advisory Committee to the Surgeon General. PHS Publication No. 1103. Washington, DC, US Government Printing Office, 1964
4. US Department of Health and Human Services, Office on Smoking and Health: The Health Consequences of Smoking: Cancer. A Report of the Surgeon General. Washington, DC, DHHS (PHS) 82–50179, 1982
5. US Department of Health and Human Services, Office on Smoking and Health: The Health Consequences of Using Smokeless Tobacco: A Report of the Advisory Committee to the Surgeon General. Washington, DC, US Government Printing Office, 1986
6. US Department of Health, Education, and Welfare, Public Health Service: The Health Consequences of Smoking: 1967. PHS Publication No. 1696. Washington, DC, US Government Printing Office, 1967
7. US Department of Health, Education, and Welfare, Public Health Service: The Health Consequences of Smoking: 1968. Supplement to the 1967 Public Health Service Review. PHS Publication No. 1696. Washington, DC, US Government Printing Office, 1968
8. US Department of Health, Education, and Welfare, Public Health Service: The Health Consequences of Smoking: 1969. Supplement to the 1967 Public Health Service Review. PHS Publication No. 1696–2. Washington, DC, US Government Printing Office, 1969
9. US Department of Health, Education, and Welfare, Health Services and Mental Health Administration: The Health Consequences of Smoking, A Report to the Surgeon General: 1971. DHEW Publication No. (HSM) 71–7513. Washington, DC, US Government Printing Office, 1972
10. US Department of Health, Education, and Welfare, Health Services and Mental Health Administration: The Health Consequences of Smoking, A Report to the Surgeon General: 1972. DHEW Publication No. (HSM) 71–7516. Washington, DC, US Government Printing Office, 1972
11. US Department of Health, Education, and Welfare, Health Services and Mental Health Administration: The Health Consequences of Smoking: 1973. DHEW Publication No. (HSM) 73–8704. Washington, DC, US Government Printing Office, 1973
12. US Department of Health, Education, and Welfare, Centers for Disease Control: The Health Consequences of Smoking: 1974. DHEW Publication No. (CDC) 74–8704. Washington, DC, US Government Printing Office, 1975
13. US Department of Health, Education, and Welfare, Centers for Disease Control: The Health Consequences of Smoking: 1975. DHEW Publication No. (CDC) 76–8704. Washington, DC, US Government Printing Office, 1976
14. US Department of Health, Education, and Welfare, Public Health Service: Office of the Assistant Secretary for Health, Office on Smoking and Health: The Health Consequences of Smoking: 1977–1978. DHEW Publication No. (PHS) 79–50065. Washington, DC, US Government Printing Office, 1979
15. US Department of Health, Education, and Welfare, Office on Smoking and Health: Smoking and Health: A Report of the Surgeon General. DHEW Publication No. (PHS) 79–50066. Washington, DC, US Government Printing Office, 1979
16. US Department of Health and Human Services, Office on Smoking and Health: The Health Consequences of Smoking for Women: A Report of the Surgeon General. Washington, DC, US Government Printing Office, 1980
17. US Department of Health and Human Services, Office on Smoking and Health: The Health Consequences of Smoking: The Changing Cigarette. A Report of the Surgeon General, 1981. DHHS Publication No. (PHS) 81–50156. Washington, DC, US Government Printing Office, 1981
18. US Department of Health and Human Services, Office on Smoking and Health: The Health Consequences of Smoking: Cardiovascular Disease. A Report of the Surgeon General, 1983. DHHS (PHS) 84–50204. Washington, DC, US Government Printing Office, 1984
19. US Department of Health and Human Services, Office on Smoking and Health: The Health Consequences of Smoking: Chronic Obstructive Lung Disease. A Report of the Surgeon General, 1984. DHHS (PHS) 84–50205. Washington, DC, US Government Printing Office, 1984
20. US Department of Health and Human Services, Office on Smoking and Health: The Health Consequences of Smoking. Cancer and Chronic Lung Disease in the Workplace: A Report of the Surgeon General. Washington, DC, US Government Printing Office, 1985
21. US Department of Health and Human Services, Office on Smoking and Health: The Health Consequences of Involuntary Smoking: A Report of the Surgeon General. Washington, DC, US Government Printing Office, 1986
22. US Department of Health and Human Services, Centers for Disease Control: Smoking-attributable mortality and years of potential life lost. United States, 1984. MMWR 36:693–697, 1987
23. Pollin W: The role of the additive process as a key step in causation of all tobacco-related diseases. JAMA 252:2874–2875, 1984
24. Tso TC, Gray NJ: Personal communication, 1985
25. Wynder EL, Graham EA: Tobacco smoking as a possible etiologic factor in bronchiogenic carcinoma: A study of 684 proved cases. JAMA 143:329–336, 1950
26. Doll R, Hill AB: Smoking and carcinoma of the lung: Preliminary report. Br Med J 2:739–748, 1950
27. Levin ML, Goldstein H, Gerhardt PR: Cancer and tobacco smoking: A preliminary report. JAMA 143:336–338, 1950
28. Royal College of Physicians: Smoking and Health: Summary and Report of the Royal College of Physicians of London on Smoking in Relation to Cancer of the Lung and Other Diseases. New York, Pitman, 1962
29. International Agency for Research on Cancer: IARC Monographs on the Evaluation of the Carcinogenic Risk of Chemicals to Humans: Tobacco Smoking 38:12–20. Geneva, World Health Organization, 1985
30. Berry G, Newhouse ML, Antonis P: Combined effect of asbestos and smoking on mortality from lung cancer and mesothelioma in factory workers. Br J Ind Med 42:12–18, 1985
31. McDonald JC, Liddell FDK, Gibbs GW, et al: Dust exposure and mortality in chrysotile mining, 1910–1975. Br J Ind Med 37:11–24, 1980
32. Liddell FDK, Thomas DC, Gibbs GW, et al: Fibre exposure and mortality from pneumoconiosis, respiratory and abdominal malignancies in chrysotile production in Quebec 1926–1975. Ann Acad Med Singapore (Suppl 2) 13:340–344, 1984
33. Selikoff IJ, Seidman H, Hammond EC: Mortality effects of cigarette smoking among amosite asbestos factory workers. JNCI 65:507–513, 1980
34. Meurman LO, Kiviluoto R, Hakama M: Combined effect of asbestos exposure and tobacco smoking on Finnish anthophyllite miners and millers. Ann NY Acad Sci 330:491–495, 1979
35. Hammond EC, Selikoff IJ, Seidman H: Asbestos exposure, cigarette smoking and death rates. Ann NY Acad Sci 330:473–490, 1979
36. Hornung RW, Samuels S: Survivorship models for lung cancer mortality in uranium mines: Is cumulative dose an appropriate measure of exposure? In Gomez (ed): Radiation Hazards in Mining, pp 363–368. New York, Society of Mining Engineers of the American Institute of Mining, Metallurgical and Petroleum Engineers, 1981
37. Whittemore AS, McMillan A: Lung cancer mortality among US uranium miners: A reappraisal. JNCI 71:489–499, 1983
38. National Cancer Institute: Annual Cancer Statistics Review. NIH Publication No. 87–2789, 1987
39. American Cancer Society: 1987 Cancer Facts and Figures, p 9. New York, American Cancer Society, 1987
40. US Department of Health and Human Services, Centers for Disease Control: Cigarette Smoking in the United States, 1986. MMWR 36:581–585, 1987
41. Flanders WD, Rothman KJ: Interaction of alcohol and tobacco in laryngeal cancer. Am J Epidemiol (in press)
42. McLoy DG, Hecht SS, Wynder EL: The roles of tobacco, alcohol, and diet in the etiology of upper alimentary and respiratory tract cancer. Prev Med 9:622–629, 1980
43. Hirayama T: Prospective studies on cancer epidemiology based on census population in Japan. In Bucalossi P, Veronesi U, Cascinelli N (eds): Cancer Epidemiology, Environmental Factors, Vol 3, pp 26–35. Proceedings of the 11th International Cancer Congress, Florence, Italy, 1974. Amsterdam, Excerpta Medica, 1975
44. Kamionkowski MD, Fleshler B: The role of alcoholic intake in esophageal carcinoma. Am J Med Sci 249:696–700, 1965
45. Kissin B, Kaley MM, Su WH, et al: Head and neck cancer in alcoholics: The relationship to drinking, smoking, and dietary patterns. JAMA 224:1174–1175, 1973
46. Schoenberg BS, Bailar JC III, Fraumeni JF Jr: Certain mortality patterns of esophageal cancer in the United States, 1930–1967. JNCI 46:63–73, 1971
47. Schottenfeld D, Gantt RC, Wynder EL: The role of alcohol and tobacco in multiple primary cancers of the upper digestive system, larynx, and lung: A prospective study. Prev Med 3:277–293, 1974
48. Takano K, Osogoshi K, Kamimura N, et al: [Epidemiology of esophageal cancer—with special reference to the significance of hot food and beverage drinking, smoking, and nutritional deficiency.] Int J Cancer 5:152–156, 1970
49. Williams RR, Horm JW: Association of cancer sites with tobacco and alcohol consumption and socioeconomic status of patients: Interview study from the Third National Cancer Survey. JNCI 58:525–547, 1977
50. Wynder EL, Bross IJ: A study of etiological factors in cancer of the esophagus. Cancer 14:389–413, 1961
51. Wynder EL, Mushinski MH, Spivak JC: Tobacco and alcohol consumption in relation to the development of multiple primary cancers. Cancer 40:1872–1878, 1977
52. Swan S: Smoking and cervical cancer. In Rosenberg MJ (ed): Smoking and Reproductive Health, pp 176–185. Littleton, MA, PSG Publishing, 1987
53. Brinton LA, Schairer C, Haenszel W, et al: Cigarette smoking and invasive cervical cancer. JAMA 255:3265–3269, 1986
54. Baran JA, Byers T, Greenberg ER, et al: Cigarette smoking in women with cancers of the breast and reproductive organs. JNCI 77:677–680, 1986
55. Baumslag N, Keen P, Petering HG: Carcinoma of the maxillary antrum and its relationship to trace and metal content in snuff. Arch Environ Health 23:1–5, 1971
56. Brunnermann KD, Genoble L, Hoffmann D: N-nitrosamines in chewing tobacco: An international comparison. J Agric Food Chem 33:1178–1181, 1985
57. Hoffmann D, Adams JD: Carcinogenic tobacco-specific N-nitrosamines in snuff and in the saliva of snuff dippers. Cancer Res 41:4305–4308, 1981
58. Osterdahl BG, Slorach S: N-nitrosamines in snuff and chewing tobacco on the Swedish market in 1983. Food Addit Contam 1:299–305, 1984
59. Nair J, Ohshima H, Malaveille C, et al: N-nitrosamine compounds (NOC) in saliva and urine of betel quid chewers: studies on occurrence and formation. Carcinogenesis 6:295–303, 1985
60. Hoffmann D, Hecht SS, Ornaf RM, et al: Nitrosonornicotine: Presence in tobacco, formation and carcinogenicity. IARC Sci Publ 14:307–320, 1976

61. Munson JW, Abdine H: Determination of N-nitrosonornicotine in tobacco by gas chromatography/mass spectroscopy. Anal Lett 10:777–786, 1977
62. Adams JD, Brunnemann KD, Hoffman D: Rapid method for the analysis of tobacco-specific N-nitrosamines by gas-liquid chromatography with a thermal energy analyzer. J Chromatogr 256:347–351, 1983
63. Campbell JM, Lindsey AJ: Polycyclic aromatic hydrocarbons in snuff. Chem Ind (Lond) 951, 1957
64. Hoffmann D, Harley NH, Fisenne I, et al: Carcinogenic agents in snuff. JNCI 76:435–437, 1986
65. Harley NH, Cohen BS, Tso TC: Polonium-210: A questionable risk factor in smoking-related carcinogenesis. Banbury Report 3:93–104, 1980
66. Friedell HL, Rosenthal LM: The etiologic role of chewing tobacco in cancer of the mouth. JAMA 116:2130–2135, 1941
67. Moore GE, Bissinger LL, Proehl EC: Tobacco and intraoral cancer. Surg Forum 3:685–688, 1952
68. International Agency for Research on Cancer: Tobacco habits other than smoking: Betel-quid and areca-nut chewing and some related nitrosamines. IARC Monogr Eval Carcinog Risk Chem Hum 37:291, 1986
69. National Institutes of Health: Health implications of smokeless tobacco use. Consensus Development Conference Statement VI 6:1. Bethesda, MD, 1986
70. Winn DM, Blot WJ, Shy CM, et al: Snuff dipping and oral cancer among women in the Southern United States. N Engl J Med 304:745–749, 1981
71. National Research Council, National Academy of Sciences: Environmental Tobacco Smoke: Measuring Exposures and Assessing Health Effects. Washington, DC, National Academy Press, 1986
72. Edwards D: Nicotine: A drug of choice. Sci News 129, 1986
73. US Department of Health and Human Services, National Center for Health Statistics: National Health Interview Survey Smoking Supplement, 1980
74. Jarvik M: The role of nicotine in the smoking habit. In Hunt WA (ed): Learning Mechanisms in Smoking, pp 155–190. Chicago, Aldine, 1970
75. Russell MAH: Cigarette smoking: National history of a dependence disorder. Br J Med Psychol 44:1–16, 1971
76. Jarvik M: Further observations on nicotine as the reinforcing agent in smoking. In Dunn WL (ed): Smoking Behavior: Motives and Incentives, pp 33–49. Washington, DC, Winston, 1973
77. Jaffe JH, Kanzler M: Smoking as an addictive disorder. In Krasnegor NA (ed): Cigarette Smoking as a Dependence Process. NIDA Research Monograph 23, pp 4–23. Washington, DC, US Government Printing Office, 1979
78. Henningfield JE, Griffiths RR, Jasinski DR: Human dependence on tobacco and opioids: Common factors. In Thompson T, Johanson CE (eds): Behavioral Pharmacology of Human Drug Dependence. NIDA Research Monograph. Washington DC, US Government Printing Office, 1981
79. Henningfield JE: Side effects of nicotine dependence. NJ Med 85:108–112, 1988
80. US Department of Health and Human Services, Centers for Disease Control: The Pharmacologic Basis of Tobacco Dependence: A Report of the Surgeon General (in press)
81. Henningfield JE, Nemeth-Costlett R: Nicotine dependence: Interface between tobacco and tobacco-related disease. Chest (in press)
82. World Health Organization: International Classification of Diseases (Ninth Revision). Geneva, World Health Organization, 1978
83. American Psychiatric Association: Diagnostic and Statistical Manual of Mental Disorders, 3rd ed. Washington, DC, American Psychiatric Association, 1979
84. Pollin W, Ravenholt RT: Tobacco addiction and tobacco mortality. JAMA 252:2849–2854, 1984
85. Doll R, Peto R: Mortality in relation to smoking: 20 years' observations on male British doctors. Br Med J 2:1525–1536, 1976
86. Rogot E, Murray JL: Smoking and causes of death among U.S. veterans: 16 years of observation. Public Health Rep 95:213–222, 1980
87. Wynder EL, Stellman SD: Impact of long-term filter cigarette usage on lung and larynx cancer risk: A case-control study. JNCI 62:471–477, 1979
88. Wynder EL, Stellman SD: Comparative epidemiology of tobacco-related cancers. Cancer Res 37:4608–4622, 1977
89. US Department of Health and Human Services, National Center for Health Statistics: National Health Interview Survey, 1985
90. US Department of Health and Human Services, National Institute on Drug Abuse: Drug Abuse Statistics 1985—Population Estimates (based on data from the National Household Survey on Drug Abuse of 1985), November 1986
91. Haynes S: Cigarette smoking among three adolescent Hispanic groups: Results from the Hispanic Health and Nutrition Examination Survey. Presented at the Conference on Tobacco Use Among Blacks and Hispanics, Washington, D.C., March 28–29, 1988
92. Botvin GJ, Eng A, Williams CL: Preventing the onset of cigarette smoking through life skills training. Prev Med 9:135–143, 1983
93. Flay BR, d'Avernas JR, Best JA, et al: Cigarette smoking: Why young people do it and ways of preventing it. In McGrath P, Firestone P (eds): Pediatric and Adolescent Behavioral Medicine, pp 132–183. New York, Springer-Verlag, 1983
94. US Department of Health and Human Services, National Institute on Drug Abuse: Survey of Drug Use Among High School Seniors, 1986
95. US Department of Health and Human Services, National Institute on Drug Abuse: National Household Survey on Drug Abuse, 1985
96. Boyd G, Ary DV, Wirt R, et al: Use of smokeless tobacco among children and adolescents in the United States. Prev Med 16:402–421, 1987

97. Davis R: Current trends in cigarette advertising and marketing. N Engl J Med 316:725–732, 1987
98. Glasgow RE, Bernstein DA: Behavioral treatment of smoking behavior. In Prokop CK, Bradley LA (eds): Medical Psychology: A New Perspective. New York, Academic Press, 1981
99. Glasgow RE, Klesges RC: Smoking intervention programs in the workplace. In US Department of Health and Human Services, The Health Consequences of Smoking: Cancer and Chronic Lung Disease in the Workplace. DHHS Publication No. (PHS) 85-50207. Washington, DC, US Government Printing Office, 1985
100. Lichtenstein E, Brown A: Current trends in the modification of cigarette dependence. In Bellack A, Hersen M, Kazdin AE (eds): International Handbook of Behavior Modification and Therapy, vol 2. New York, Plenum Press, 1983
101. Lichtenstein E, Danaher BG: Modification of smoking behavior: A critical analysis of theory, research, and practice. In Hersen M, Eisler M, Miller PM (eds): Progress in Behavioral Modification. New York, Academic Press, 1976
102. Ockene JK: Changes in cigarette smoking behavior in clinical and community trials. In US Department of Health and Human Services, The Health Consequences of Smoking for Cardiovascular Disease: A Report of the Surgeon General. DHHS Publication No. (PHS) 84-50204. Washington, DC, US Government Printing Office, 1984
103. Pechacek TF: Modification of smoking behavior. In Krasnegor NA (ed): The Behavior Aspects of Smoking, NIDA Research Monograph No. 26. US Department of Health and Human Services, Public Health Service, National Institute on Drug Abuse, DHHS Publication No. (ADM) 79–882, 1979
104. Pechacek TF, Danaher BG: How and why people quit smoking: A cognitive-behavioral analysis. In Kendall PC, Hollen SD (eds): Cognitive-Behavioral Interventions: Theory, Research, and Procedure. New York, Academic Press, 1979
105. US Department of Health and Human Services, Centers for Disease Control: Smoking and health—A national status report: A Report to Congress. DHHS Publication No. (CDC) 87–8396, Rockville, Maryland, 1987
106. Russell MAH: Conceptual framework for nicotine substitution. In Ockene JK (ed): Pharmacologic Treatment of Tobacco Dependence: Proceedings of the World Congress, pp 90–107. Cambridge, MA, Institute for the Study of Smoking Behavior and Policy, Smoking Behavior and Policy Conference Series, 1986
107. Marlatt GA, Gordon JR: Relapse Prevention: Maintenance Strategies in the Treatment of Addiction, New York, Guilford Press, 1985
108. Ockene JK, Broste S, Hymowitz N, et al: For the MRFIT Research Group. Paper presented at Council on Epidemiology, American Heart Association, San Diego, 1983
109. Brown RA, Lichtenstein E, McIntyre KO, et al: The effects of nicotine fading and relapse prevention on smoking cessation. J Consult Clin Psychol 52:307–308, 1984
110. Hall SM, Killen JD: Psychological and pharmacological approaches to smoking relapse prevention. In Grabowski J, Hall SM (eds): Pharmacological Adjuncts in Smoking Cessation. NIDA Research Monograph No. 53, US Department of Health and Human Services, Public Health Service, Alcohol, Drug Abuse and Mental Health Administration, DHHS Publication No. (ADM) 85-1333, 1985
111. Davis AL, Faust R, Ordentilch M: Self-help smoking cessation and maintenance programs: A comparative study with 12-month follow-up by the American Lung Association. Am J Public Health 874:1212–1217, 1984
112. Glasgow RE, Schaeffer L, O'Neil HK: Self-help books and amount of therapist contact in smoking cessation programs. J Consult Clin Psychol 49:659–667, 1981
113. Flay BR: Mass media and smoking cessation. Presented at the International Communication Association Meeting, Chicago, May 1986
114. Snow WH, Gilchrist LD, Schinke SP: A critique of progress in adolescent smoking prevention. Children Youth Serv Rev 7:1–19, 1985
115. Puska P, Koskela K: Community-based strategies to fight smoking: Experiences from the North Karelia Project in Finland. NY State J Med 83:1335–1338, 1983
116. Pederson LL: Compliance with physician advice to quit smoking: A review of the literature. Prev Med 11:71–84, 1982
117. Garfinkel L, Stellman SD: Cigarette smoking among physicians, dentists, and nurses. CA 36:1, 1986
118. Orleans CT: Understanding and promoting smoking cessation: Overview and guidelines for physician intervention. Annu Rev Med 36:51–61, 1985
119. Valente CM, Sobal J, Muncie HL Jr, et al: Health promotion: Physicians' beliefs, attitudes, and practices. Am J Prev Med 2:82–88, 1986
120. Orleans CT, George LK, Houpt JL, et al: Health promotion in primary care: A survey of U.S. family practitioners. Prev Med 14:636–647, 1985
121. Wilson DM, Lindsay-McIntyre E, Best JA, et al: A smoking cessation intervention program for family physicians. Can Med Assoc J 137:613–619, 1987
122. Anda RF, Remington PL, Siento DG, et al: Are physicians advising smokers to quit? A patient's perspective. JAMA 257:14, 1916–1919, 1987
123. Russell MA, Wilson C, Taylor C: The effects of general practitioners' advice against smoking. Br Med J 2:231–235, 1979
124. Goldstein B, Fischer PM, Richards JW, et al: Smoking counseling practices of recently trained family physicians. J Fam Pract 24:195–197, 1987
125. Wechsler H, Levine S, Idelson RK, et al: The physicians's role in health promotion—a survey of primary care practitioners. N Engl J Med 309:97–100, 1983
126. US Department of Health and Human Services, National Cancer Institute: Essential Elements of an HMO-Guided Smoking Cessation Program. Prepublication edition, June 1987
127. Grabowski J, Stitzer ML, Henningfield JE (eds): Behavioral intervention techniques in drug abuse treatment. NIDA Research Monograph Series No. 46. Washington, DC, US Government Printing Office, 1984

128. Fagerstrom K: A comparison of psychological and pharmacological treatment in smoking cessation. J Behav Med 5:343–351, 1982
129. Jarvis MJ, Raw M, Russell MAH, et al: Randomised controlled trial of nicotine chewing-gum. Br Med J 285:337–340, 1982
130. Schneider NG, Jarvik ME, Forsythe AB, et al: Nicotine gum in smoking cessation: A placebo-controlled, double-blind trial. Addict Behav 8:253–261, 1983
131. Hjalmarson AIM: Effect of nicotine chewing gum in smoking cessation: A randomized, placebo-controlled, double-blind study. JAMA 252:2835–2838, 1984
132. Malcolm RE, Sillett RW, Turner JAM, et al: The use of nicotine chewing gum as an aid to stopping smoking. Psychopharmacology (Berlin) 70:295–296, 1980
133. Hughes JR, Hatsukami DK, Pickens RW, et al: Effect of nicotine on the tobacco withdrawal syndrome. Psychopharmacologia 83:82–87, 1984
134. Hughes JR, Hatsukami DK: Short-term effects of nicotine gum. In Grabowski J, Hall SJ (eds): Pharmacological Adjuncts in Smoking Cessation. NIDA Research Monograph No. 53, US Department of Health and Human Services, Public Health Service, Alcohol, Drug Abuse, and Mental Health Administration. DHHS Publication No. (ADM) 85–1333, 1985
135. Schneider NG, Jarvik ME, Forsythe AB: Nicotine versus placebo gum in the alleviation of withdrawal during smoking cessation. Addict Behav 9:149–156, 1984
136. West R, Jarvis MJ, Russell MAH, et al: Effect of nicotine replacement on the cigarette withdrawal syndrome. Br J Addict 79:215–219, 1984
137. Fagerstrom K: Effects of nicotine chewing gum and followup appointment in physician based smoking cessation. Prev Med 13:517–527, 1984
138. Hughes JR: Problems of nicotine gum. In Ockene JK (ed): Pharmacologic Treatment of Tobacco Dependence: Proceedings of the World Congress, pp 141–147. Cambridge MA, Institute for the Study of Smoking Behavior and Policy, Smoking Behavior and Policy Conference Series, 1986
139. Fisher EB, Bishop DB, Mayer JA, et al: The physician's contribution to smoking cessation in the workplace. Chest 93:556–565, 1988
140. Enstrom JE: Health and dietary practices and cancer mortality among California Mormons. In Cairns J, Lyon JL, Skolnick M (eds): Cancer Incidence in Defined Populations, pp 69–92. Cold Spring Harbor, NY, Cold Spring Harbor Laboratory, 1980

Joseph F. Fraumeni, Jr.

Robert N. Hoover

Susan S. Devesa

Leo J. Kinlen

CHAPTER 13 *Epidemiology of Cancer*

Epidemiology is the study of variations in disease frequency among population groups and the factors that influence these variations. Its principal objective is the finding of causes so that, ideally, preventive measures may be applied. By focusing on events that necessarily precede the onset of disease, epidemiology contrasts with clinical medicine in which the primary concern is the diagnosis and treatment of individual patients. In epidemiology, the perennial reference point for individual patients is the population from which they come. This approach encompasses not only unaffected members of the group in question, which may be useful for comparison purposes, but also all affected persons in that population, thereby avoiding the selection factors that can determine the experience of individual clinicians.

Following dramatic improvements in the control of infectious disease during this century, the attention of epidemiologists has increasingly turned toward the study of chronic illnesses. The resulting advances include some of the most important discoveries in the etiology and prevention of cancer. The impact of epidemiology on cancer touches the clinician, experimentalist, policy maker, and even the lay public, whose attention is often drawn to epidemiologic observations and environmental issues by the news media, sometimes in an unbalanced way.

Practicing physicians must often interpret epidemiologic findings for their patients. They have opportunities to use epidemiologic data that will protect high-risk individuals, collaborate in epidemiologic studies, and make clinical observations relevant to etiology. In view of the large volume of current research into the origins of cancer and its prevention, it is increasingly important for the clinical oncologist to understand the principles and methods of epidemiology.

HISTORICAL PERSPECTIVE

Epidemiologic observations in cancer have a long and fascinating history.[1] In 1700, the Italian occupational physician Bernardino Ramazzini noted that breast cancer was more common in nuns than other women, and he suggested the influence of celibacy. In 1775, the British surgeon Percivall Pott reported the first description of occupational carcinogenesis in the form of scrotal cancer among chimney sweeps. In the 18th century there were also reports of cancer risks associated with tobacco, namely snuff taking and nasal cancer by Hill in 1761 and pipe smoking and lip cancer by von Soemmering in 1795. Perhaps the first epidemiologic study of cancer, in any modern sense, was in 1842 by Rigoni-Stern who attempted to quantify the risks of uterine cancer in the city of Verona among nuns and other women and showed that the disease was significantly less common in the former group. Important occupational cancers were also noted in the 19th century: lung cancer (though first described as "mediastinal lymphoma") among the metal miners of Schneeberg and Joachimsthal by Harting and Hesse in 1879, and bladder cancer among aniline dye workers by Rehn in 1895. In 1888 Hutchinson reported the first suggestion of drug-induced cancer with an account of skin cancers in patients treated with an arsenic-containing solution.

These historical observations, and many others that followed,[2,3] illustrate the importance of clinical observations as a source of new discoveries in cancer etiology. They also include an early indication of the long latent interval in human carcinogenesis, for Pott noted that some of the men with scrotal cancer had not worked as chimney sweeps since

196

boyhood. Furthermore, they show how some causes can be detected (and diseases prevented) before specific agents and mechanisms are elucidated by laboratory investigators. Indeed, many decades elapsed before evidence was available to indicate that polycyclic hydrocarbons, radioactive substances, and aromatic amines explained some of the early findings described above.

AIMS OF EPIDEMIOLOGY

It is convenient to stress several key words in the definition of epidemiology, which is the study of the distribution and determinants of disease frequency in human populations.[4] The word "humans" distinguishes the approach from those laboratory disciplines in cancer research that use animals and other test systems in their experiments. The study of "populations" stands in contrast to clinical research, which usually involves investigations at the individual or case series level. The term "frequency" indicates the orientation of epidemiology towards quantifying the occurrence of disease and the risks attributable to various causes. Finally, the phrase "distribution and determinants" points to the two major approaches of epidemiology. In general, descriptive studies examine the distribution of disease frequency in populations that can be useful in generating etiologic hypotheses, while analytical studies test hypotheses by pursuing differences in the personal characteristics or exposures among individuals.

The main contribution of cancer epidemiology is the detection and quantification of the risks associated with specific environmental exposures and host factors. These associations may lead to causal inferences, thus providing the basis for instituting preventive measures. Epidemiologic data support the concept that carcinogenesis is a lengthy multistage process that is affected by a wide variety of factors.[5-7] Some factors appear to act early as initiators, others later as promoters, and still others at both early and late stages. Certain agents act together to accelerate the carcinogenic process, such as the way smoking combines synergistically with asbestos to produce lung cancer or with alcohol to produce oral and esophageal cancers. Furthermore, there is some evidence that the process is retarded by dietary factors, such as certain micronutrients that appear to diminish the risk of various cancer sites including smoking-related lung cancer.

Thus, the aims of epidemiology are to uncover new etiologic leads through peculiarities in the distribution of cancer, quantify the risks associated with different exposures (some of which may be protective), promote insights into the mechanisms of carcinogenesis, and assess the efficacy of preventive measures. While the usual observational methods of epidemiology have succeeded in identifying many causes of cancer, future progress may depend to a considerable degree on innovative strategies that employ laboratory techniques in epidemiologic investigations.

DESCRIPTIVE STUDIES

There is perhaps no disorder that shows a uniform incidence in all human groups. Indeed, cancers are striking in the variations they show according to such factors as age, sex, race, time, socioeconomic class, marital status, and geographic location. Descriptive (or demographic) studies, by revealing the patterns of disease in populations, have provided many clues to cancer etiology. Variations by age, area, and time are often remarkable, even allowing for the fluctuations that might be expected as a result of chance and differences in diagnostic and reporting practices.[6] The descriptive patterns are useful also in monitoring variations and trends that might point to new environmental hazards, in evaluating the effects of cancer prevention, screening, and treatment activities, and in predicting future trends that may help set priorities in various aspects of oncology.[8]

MEASURES OF CANCER FREQUENCY

Descriptive studies measure rates, which are based on three items of information: the number of individuals affected by the disease (numerator), the length of the period covered (time), and the population from which they are derived (denominator). The expression of disease in this manner allows the rates in one population to be compared with the rates in another. Often these rates must be adjusted for such factors as age, race, and social class, which might otherwise spuriously influence the comparison.[9] The rates most often used in cancer epidemiology concern incidence, mortality, and prevalence, with each having its particular uses and limitations. When measures of occurrence are not based on populations at risk, they usually represent proportions, even though sometimes labelled as rates, such as case-fatality rates. Sample calculations of these measures are derived from numbers given in Table 13-1.

The incidence rate provides a direct measure of the probability of developing cancer, and is defined as the

$$\frac{\text{Number of persons developing cancer in a unit of time}}{\text{Total population living at that time}}$$

Most often the unit of time is 1 year, with the mid-year population serving as the denominator. The rates are usually expressed per 100,000 or per million persons. For example, from the data in Table 13-1, the annual occurrence of Hodgkin's disease per 100,000 residents in Connecticut is calculated using the equation on the next page:

TABLE 13-1. Patients with Hodgkin's Disease and Pancreatic Cancer, Connecticut, 1982

Type of Cancer	Patients Alive at Start of Year*	New Cases in Year†	Deaths in Year‡
Hodgkin's disease	1151	120	26
Pancreatic cancer	220	326	297

* Prevalence data estimated from data of Feldman AR, et al: The prevalence of cancer. N Engl J Med 315:1394, 1986.
† Incidence data from Connecticut Tumor Registry.
‡ Mortality data from National Center for Health Statistics.
Estimated populations were 3,112,469 on January 1, 1982 for prevalence and 3,126,488 on July 1, 1982 for incidence and mortality.

$$\text{Incidence rate} = \frac{120}{3{,}126{,}488} \times 100{,}000$$
$$= 3.8 \text{ per } 100{,}000 \text{ per year}$$

Incidence rates may be crude (all ages), as in this example, or age-specific. Because of the great dependence of cancer incidence on age, it is much more informative to use age-specific rates. However, when summary figures are necessary to compare rates between population groups with different age distributions, they should be age-adjusted; this is done by multiplying each age-specific rate by the percent of individuals in a standard population (*e.g.,* the 1970 U.S. population) with the same ages, and then summing to produce a single value. For etiologic studies, incidence rates tend to be more informative than mortality rates, because they cover all diagnosed cases (not merely the fatal ones) at a time which is closer to the point of causation. The information on incident cancers is usually more extensive and reliable, with details often available on histologic type and stage.

The mortality or death rate is defined as the

$$\frac{\text{Number of persons dying of cancer in a unit of time}}{\text{Total population living at that time}}$$

From data in Table 13-1, the mortality rate for Hodgkin's disease is computed as follows:

$$\text{Mortality rate} = \frac{26}{3{,}126{,}488} \times 100{,}000$$
$$= 0.8 \text{ per } 100{,}000 \text{ per year}$$

For etiologic research, mortality rates most clearly reflect the occurrence of those cancer sites with the worst prognosis, and are vulnerable to well-known inaccuracies and variations in death-certificate reporting of diagnoses. However, mortality data are often the only statistics available in certain locations and periods, and they have been especially useful for evaluation of long-term trends and geographic variations on a national or international scale. For several cancers with poor survival, mortality rates nearly equal incidence rates. Even with improvements in survival of many cancers, mortality rates help in clarifying incidence trends for certain cancers (*e.g.,* breast and prostate) that may be distorted by heightened efforts at case finding.[6,8] Mortality rates are also very useful in evaluating the impact of advances in cancer prevention and treatment on the general population. The combined analyses of incidence, mortality, and survival statistics that comprise the Surveillance, Epidemiology, and End Results (SEER) Program of the National Cancer Institute (NCI) provide valuable data on the patterns of cancer in the United States.[10]

The case-fatality rate is a measure of the severity or lethality of disease. A proportion rather than a true rate, it is usually expressed as a percentage and defined as the

$$\frac{\text{Number of deaths from cancer}}{\text{Number of persons developing cancer}} \times 100\%$$

From data in Table 13-1, case-fatality rates are estimated as follows:

$$\text{Case fatality (Hodgkin's disease)} = \frac{26}{120} \times 100\% = 21.7\%$$

$$\text{Case fatality (pancreatic cancer)} = \frac{297}{326} \times 100\% = 91.1\%$$

Because the cases and deaths usually refer to the same period of time, this concept is less meaningful in chronic than in acute diseases, and is generally replaced by survival rates that are discussed below.

The prevalence rate is seldom used in etiologic studies of cancer, but provides a useful measure for planning health services by estimating the burden of disease in the population.[11] Also called point prevalence, it is defined as the

$$\frac{\text{Number of persons with cancer at a given point in time}}{\text{Total population living at that time}}$$

From data in Table 13-1, the prevalence of Hodgkin's disease on January 1, 1982 is calculated as follows:

$$\text{Prevalence} = \frac{1{,}115}{3{,}112{,}469} \times 100{,}000 = 37.0 \text{ per } 100{,}000$$

Table 13-2 summarizes the various kinds of rates for Hodgkin's disease and pancreatic cancer. Hodgkin's disease displays lower incidence and mortality rates than pancreatic cancer, but a higher prevalence rate due to its much lower case-fatality rate (or conversely, higher survival rate).

Proportional rates or relative frequencies are used when details of the population that produce a series of cancer cases or deaths are unknown. This may occur in surveys of hospital patients or death certificates, where the proportions of different cancers may be compared with those in the general population for each sex and age group. Proportional mortality ratios are sometimes used in studies of occupational groups.[12] However, since the denominator refers to total deaths rather than the population at risk, the magnitude of the ratio for a particular cancer may be misleading since it also fluctuates according to the number of deaths from other causes. Thus, positive findings emerging from this type of survey should be interpreted cautiously and pursued by more definitive investigation.

CORRELATIONAL STUDIES

Descriptive studies may use the correlational (or ecological) approach, in which the rates of disease in populations are compared with the geographic or temporal distribution of

TABLE 13-2. Measures of Frequency for Hodgkin's Disease and Pancreatic Cancer, Connecticut, 1982*

Measure	Hodgkin's disease	Pancreatic cancer
Mortality	0.8	9.5
Incidence	3.8	10.4
Prevalence	37.0	7.1

* Crude rates per 100,000 population per year, calculated from data in Table 13-1.

suspected risk factors.[13] The association is often expressed in terms of correlation or regression coefficients. Although a correlational study may be helpful in formulating hypotheses about carcinogenic risks, it falls short of establishing causal relationships. Correlational studies have the advantage of being inexpensive and quick because they often use statistics assembled for other purposes.[13]

The primary weakness of such studies for etiologic research, as with descriptive studies generally, is that they concern populations rather than individuals. Moreover, the exposure measures are usually crude and subject to confounding factors. For example, in early surveys of lung cancer, the temporal increases among men were consistent with the effects of an increasing prevalence of cigarette smoking, but this correlation by itself provided only weak evidence of causation, since other factors such as air pollution and improvements in diagnosis showed a similar pattern. It required analytical studies that pursued these leads to establish the cause-and-effect relationship between smoking and lung cancer. Correlational studies also may provide supporting evidence in evaluating relationships detected by analytical or laboratory studies. This is illustrated by the more recent temporal increases in lung cancer among women, who have lagged about 25 years behind men in their adoption of smoking habits. Another example is the geographic correlation in developing countries between primary liver cancer and intake of foodstuffs contaminated by aflatoxin, a potent hepatocarcinogen in laboratory animals.[6] Nevertheless, while correlational data may provide clues to etiology, one must be careful not to draw a premature or inappropriate conclusion, sometimes referred to as an ecological fallacy.[13]

SOURCES OF DATA

Descriptive studies employ mainly population-based statistics on mortality, incidence, and survival to calculate rates, although clinical series from hospital-based registries or other sources may also provide clues to the etiology and natural history of cancer.

Death Certificates

In many countries, a death certificate is prepared for legal purposes for each person who dies.[14] In addition to a number of demographic variables, the certificate usually includes the underlying and secondary causes of death. Although in 1900 only 11 states in the United States contributed to the national registration system, by 1933 all 48 states were included. Alaska and Hawaii were added in 1959–1960 with their entry into the Union. The National Center for Health Statistics tabulates the deaths annually and calculates rates using population estimates provided by the Census Bureau. The data are also made available on computer magnetic tape for research purposes. A national death registry for the United States was established in 1979. This National Death Index is frequently used to identify persons in epidemiologic studies who have died.

The NCI has examined the national cancer mortality data in several periods. An early tabulation by age, race, sex, and form of cancer included deaths starting in 1930 and continu-

ing through 1955.[15] Geographic variations in cancer mortality at the state level were evaluated for the years 1950–1967.[16] Analyses at the county level for 1950–1969[17] formed the basis for computer-generated color atlases portraying geographic patterns on a small-area scale for whites and nonwhites.[18,19] More recently, cancer mortality was tabulated at the county level by decade from 1950 through 1979.[20] Using data through 1980, maps of cancer mortality were prepared according to state economic area to examine trends in the geographic patterns.[21] Computer graphics have also been used to display national trends by age, race, and sex for 1950–1977.[22] Long-term trends in U.S. cancer mortality and incidence were examined for 1935–1974[23] and more recently for 1947–1984.[24] The geographic and temporal variations of cancer mortality have also been analysed on an international scale.[25]

Despite the value of mortality data for epidemiologic study, reservations are often expressed about the quality of diagnoses reported on death certificates, even though most cancers diagnosed before death are properly recorded on the certificates.[26] However, changes in diagnostic and certification practices as well as in coding rules may produce spurious trends, and it is prudent to consider each observation on its merits. Death certificates are also of great value to epidemiologists in comparing the mortality of a specific group under study with that of the general population. It is important, however, that the death certificates of the study group be coded according to the same rules as for the standard or reference population.

Population-Based Registries

The complete ascertainment of all newly diagnosed cases of cancer in a defined population is a difficult and expensive task. There is no system for gathering incidence data for the entire United States, but such data have been collected for specific areas in different time periods. The longest ongoing population-based resource is the Connecticut Tumor Registry, which has incidence data available from 1935.[27] Several other registries covering states or cities have been in existence for varying time periods.

The NCI has coordinated several periodic surveys of cancer incidence in selected areas of the country. The first survey was in 1937–1939 and the second in 1947–1948,[28] with both covering the same 10 metropolitan areas and referred to as the Ten-Cities Surveys. Information was gathered on cases diagnosed during 1 calendar year in each of the areas, although the specific year varied among the areas. A special survey of cases diagnosed during 1950 was conducted in Iowa to compare cancer incidence patterns among rural and urban residents.[29] The Third National Cancer Survey included cases diagnosed during 1969–1971 in two states and seven cities.[30] Since 1973, the SEER program has included several population-based cancer registries that continuously gather information on cancer incidence, mortality, and survival.[10,31] The SEER registries cover more than 10% of the U.S. population. Although not a probability sample of the entire population, considerable geographic and ethnic variations are represented. It has been possible to evaluate the long-term trends in cancer incidence by focusing on the geographic areas common to the various surveys.[23,24] In other countries a number of cancer reporting systems have been in existence for varying lengths of time, starting with the Danish Cancer Registry in 1942. The International Agency for Research on Cancer has compiled data from many of the registries in five successive volumes of Cancer Incidence in Five Continents. This resource has been immensely valuable for proposing etiologic hypotheses.

In conjunction with the operation of a cancer registry, patients may be followed to ascertain their medical condition and vital status. Such survival data are useful in understanding incidence and mortality trends, and in measuring the dissemination and effect of treatment improvements in the general population. Although not population-based, the End Results Group of the NCI compiled survival data starting in 1950.[32,33] However, since the advent of the SEER program in 1973, it has been possible to continuously monitor population-based survival statistics.[34,35]

Hospital-Based Registries

Although hospital-based cancer registries are valuable for clinical, administrative, and educational purposes, the data have limited use for epidemiologic studies.[36] However, such a registry may be an important component of a population-based cancer reporting system, and provides a means of identifying patients for case-control studies. In addition, a hospital registry may be useful in investigating the natural history of cancer and the risk of developing second primary cancers, and in assembling a clinical series that may provide clues to environmental or genetic factors in cancer etiology.

PATTERNS OF CANCER OCCURRENCE

MAGNITUDE OF THE PROBLEM

In the United States, cancer is second only to heart disease as a cause of death and accounts for 22% of all deaths.[37] Among women aged 35 to 74, it is the leading cause of death. Almost one million newly diagnosed cases of cancer and nearly 500,000 deaths due to cancer are predicted for the United States during 1988 (Table 13-3). Lung cancer is the most common form, accounting for 15% of the cases and 28% of the deaths. Almost as many cases of colorectal cancer occur as lung cancer, but there are more than twice as many deaths from lung cancer. Next most common are cancers of the breast and prostate, so that these four cancers account for 54% and 55% of the total cancer cases and deaths, respectively. The 11 sites shown in Table 13-3 comprise 79% of all cancer cases and 75% of cancer deaths.

Table 13-4 presents the age-adjusted incidence and mortality rates for 44 forms of cancer among white males and females in the United States for the period 1981–1985. Among males the incidence and mortality rates are highest for lung cancer, followed by prostate and colon cancers, whereas among females the rates are highest for breast cancer, followed by cancers of the lung and colon. However, the differential between incidence and mortality is much less for lung cancer than for the other leading cancers, re-

TABLE 13-3.   Estimated New Cases and Deaths in the United States for Major Forms of Cancer—1988

	Number of Cases	Number of Deaths
All sites	985,000	494,000
Lung	152,000	139,000
Colon and rectum	147,000	61,500
Breast	135,900*	42,300
Prostate	99,000	28,000
Urinary tract	68,900	20,000
Uterus	46,900*	10,000
Oral cavity and pharynx	30,200	9,050
Skin	27,300†	7,800‡
Pancreas	27,000	24,500
Leukemia	26,900	18,100
Ovary	19,000	12,000
All other sites	204,900	121,750

From Silverberg E, Lubera JA: Cancer Statistics, 1988. CA 38:5, 1988. Based on incidence data from National Cancer Institute SEER program 1982–1984 and mortality data from the National Center for Health Statistics. All figures are rounded.

* Invasive cancers only; more than 5,000 carcinomas in situ of the breast and 50,000 carcinomas in situ of the cervix are estimated.

† Melanoma only; more than 500,000 nonmelanoma skin cancers are estimated.

‡ Melanoma 5,800; other skin cancers 2,000.

flecting well-known survival differences. All cancers show higher rates among men except for those of the breast, gallbladder, and thyroid.

INTERNATIONAL VARIATION

It has been estimated that about 75% to 80% of all cancer in the United States is due to environmental factors.[6] To obtain this estimate, rates for the lowest-risk countries were subtracted from rates prevailing in the United States. It is convenient to regard the lowest risk as the baseline level for "spontaneous" tumors that in theory cannot be prevented.

Table 13-5 shows in rank form the international variation for a number of cancers based on recent statistics from volume 5 of Cancer Incidence in Five Continents.[38] The variation ranges from 155-fold for melanoma to fivefold for leukemia, and is not believed to be greatly affected by differences in diagnostic and reporting practices between countries.[3,6] Although genetic factors may play some role, as in melanoma, which tends to affect fair-skinned populations, the available evidence suggests that the international differences are mainly due to environmental factors. The patterns observed in Table 13-5 are in fact likely to underestimate the true global variation, since some regions with exceptionally high rates of certain cancers are not covered by registries, such as esophageal cancer in parts of China and Iran, liver cancer in parts of Africa and Asia, and urinary tract cancer in areas endemic with schistosomiasis or Balkan nephropathy.[3] Furthermore, the differences would be more pronounced if data were available for certain subtypes of cancer such as Burkitt's lymphoma and Kaposi's sarcoma, or subsites such as the gingival-buccal mucosa which comes in contact with smokeless tobacco and related products.

TABLE 13-4.   Average Annual Age-Adjusted Incidence and Mortality Rates per 100,000 Among U.S. Whites by Primary Cancer Site, 1981–1985*

	Incidence (SEER)		Mortality (U.S.)	
	Males	Females	Males	Females
All sites	412.1	322.2	211.3	136.2
Lip	3.3	0.3	0.1	0.0
Salivary gland	1.1	0.7	0.3	0.2
Nasopharynx	0.6	0.2	0.4	0.1
Other oral cavity and pharynx	11.9	5.3	4.0	1.4
Esophagus	4.8	1.6	4.6	1.2
Stomach	11.0	4.9	7.1	3.3
Small intestine	1.1	0.8	0.4	0.3
Colon	41.6	32.3	21.2	15.4
Rectum	19.7	12.7	4.1	2.5
Liver	2.8	1.1	2.8	1.3
Gallbladder	0.8	1.6	0.6	1.1
Other biliary	1.6	1.1	1.2	0.9
Pancreas	10.9	8.1	10.1	6.9
Larynx	8.5	1.6	2.5	0.4
Lung and bronchus	82.7	33.8	71.4	24.4
Pleura	1.3	0.2	0.3	0.1
Nasal cavity and sinuses	0.8	0.5	0.3	0.1
Bones and joints	1.0	0.7	0.6	0.3
Soft tissue	2.5	1.7	1.2	1.0
Melanoma of skin	10.7	8.6	3.0	1.7
Other nonepithelial skin	2.5	0.7	1.2	0.3
Breast	0.8	95.7	0.2	27.1
Cervix uteri	—	7.9	—	2.9
Uterus excluding cervix	—	24.2	—	3.7
Ovary	—	14.1	—	8.0
Vagina	—	0.7	—	0.2
Vulva	—	1.6	—	0.3
Prostate	81.3	—	21.4	—
Testis	4.4	—	0.4	—
Penis	0.8	—	0.2	—
Bladder	30.5	7.8	6.4	1.8
Kidney	11.0	4.9	4.7	2.1
Ureter	1.0	0.3	0.2	0.1
Eye and orbit	0.9	0.7	0.1	0.1
Brain and other nervous system	7.5	5.2	5.0	3.5
Thyroid	2.3	5.6	0.3	0.4
Hodgkin's disease	3.5	2.6	1.0	0.6
Non-Hodgkin's lymphoma	14.2	10.2	6.8	4.7
Multiple myeloma	4.5	3.1	3.1	2.1
Acute lymphocytic leukemia	1.6	1.3	0.8	0.5
Chronic lymphocytic leukemia	4.1	2.0	1.7	0.7
Acute myeloid leukemia	3.3	2.2	2.5	1.7
Chronic myeloid leukemia	1.6	0.9	1.0	0.6
Other leukemias	2.6	1.3	2.7	1.6
Miscellaneous	14.8	11.4	15.7	10.8

* Rates age-adjusted based on the 1970 U.S. standard population. Incidence data from the National Cancer Institute SEER program, and national mortality data from the National Center for Health Statistics.

MIGRANT PATTERNS

Further evidence for environmental factors can be found in studies of migrant populations, such as the Japanese who moved to Hawaii and California. After migration, with the adoption of new habits, the risk of various cancers has moved away from the rate prevailing in the country of origin toward that of the new country.[39] Among Japanese migrants, increases in the risk of large bowel cancer were evident within a few decades of migration, whereas changes in breast

cancer continue for generations. In contrast to general environmental exposures, lifestyle practices may change slowly among migrants, depending upon the speed and extent of acculturation.

Migrant patterns have been studied by comparing the cancer mortality rates in the U.S. white population by country of birth with the corresponding rates in the country of origin.[40] Figure 13-1 shows the age-adjusted mortality rates for colorectal and stomach cancers.[41] Stomach cancer rates among migrants are generally lower than in the country of

TABLE 13-5.   International Variation in Cancer Incidence*

	Ratio (H/L)	High (H) Incidence Area	Rate†	Low (L) Incidence Area	Rate†
Melanoma	155	Australia (Queensland)	30.9	Japan (Osaka)	0.2
Lip	151	Canada (Newfoundland)	15.1	Japan (Osaka)	0.1
Nasopharynx	100	Hong Kong	30.0	U.K. (South Western)	0.3
Prostate	70	U.S. (Atlanta, black)	91.2	China (Tianjin)	1.3
Liver	49	China (Shanghai)	34.4	Canada (Nova Scotia)	0.7
Penis	42	Brazil (Recife)	8.3	Israel (Born Eur. and Am.)	0.2
Oral cavity	34	France (Bas-Rhin)	13.5	India (Poona)	0.4
Cervix uteri (F)	28	Brazil (Recife)	83.2	Israel (non-Jews)	3.0
Esophagus	27	France (Calvados)	29.9	Romania (Urban Cluj)	1.1
Stomach	22	Japan (Nagasaki)	82.0	Kuwait (Kuwaitis)	3.7
Thyroid	22	Hawaii (Chinese)	8.8	Poland (Warsaw City)	0.4
Multiple myeloma	22	U.S. (Alameda, black)	8.8	Phillipines (Rural)	0.4
Kidney	21	Canada (NWT and Yukon)	15.0	India (Poona)	0.7
Corpus uteri (F)	21	U.S. (Bay area, white)	25.7	India (Nagpur)	1.2
Lung	19	U.S. (New Orleans, black)	110.0	India (Madras)	5.8
Colon	19	U.S. (Connecticut, white)	34.1	India (Madras)	1.8
Testis	17	Switzerland (Urban Vaud)	10.0	China (Tianjin)	0.6
Bladder	16	Switzerland (Basel)	27.8	India (Nagpur)	1.7
Lymphosarcoma	12	Switzerland (Basel)	9.2	Japan (Rural Miyagi)	0.8
Pancreas	11	U.S. (Los Angeles, Korean)	16.4	India (Poona)	1.5
Hodgkin's disease	10	Canada (Quebec)	4.8	Japan (Miyagi)	0.5
Brain	9	N.Z. (Polynesian Islanders)	9.7	India (Nagpur)	1.1
Larynx	8	Brazil (Sao Paulo)	17.8	Japan (Rural Miyagi)	2.1
Ovary (F)	8	N.Z. (Polynesian Islanders)	25.8	Kuwait (Kuwaitis)	3.3
Rectum	8	Israel (Born Eur. and Am.)	22.6	Kuwait (Kuwaitis)	3.0
Breast (F)	7	Hawaii (Hawaiian)	93.9	Israel (non-Jews)	14.1
Leukemia	5	Canada (Ontario)	11.6	India (Nagpur)	2.2

From C. Muir and M. Parkin, International Agency for Research on Cancer, based on data abstracted from Muir C, Waterhouse J, Mack T, et al (eds): Cancer Incidence in Five Continents, Vol 5. Lyon, International Agency for Research on Cancer, 1987.

*Among males unless specified as females (F); rates based on less than 10 cases are excluded.

†Average annual rate per 100,000, age-adjusted based on the world standard population; rates generally are for the period 1978–1982.

origin, but higher than among U.S.-born whites. In contrast, colorectal cancer mortality in most countries is lower than in the United States, but the rates among migrants not only approach those of the U.S.-born whites but even exceed them in some instances. Those born in Mexico, however, have retained rates that are about 50% those of native-born white Americans. In addition, colorectal cancer mortality among the foreign-born has not reached U.S. rates as frequently for women as for men. When mortality from other cancers among the U.S. foreign-born is compared with statistics in the countries of origin, the rates for breast, corpus uteri, and prostate cancers are generally more closely aligned with those for U.S. native-born whites. Analytical studies among migrants should provide insights into lifestyle factors in cancer causation.

CANCER MAPS

Although variations within countries are not as great as those seen internationally, the computer-generated mapping of cancer death rates in the United States at the county level for the period 1950–1969 revealed a variety of high-risk areas[18,19] that have led to the investigation of environmental exposures. For example, as shown in Figure 13-2, the elevated rates for lung cancer among men along the eastern seaboard drew attention to the unexpected scale and impact of asbestos exposures in shipyards during World War II.[42] Similarly, a clustering of high-risk areas in Louisiana was traced in part to heavy smoking by the Cajun population.[43] Furthermore, studies of the elevated rates for oral cancer among women in the rural south, shown in Figure 13-3, have pointed to the hazards associated with the practice of snuff dipping.[44] A recent update of the cancer maps through the period 1970–1980 has revealed patterns resembling those in the earlier atlas, but with a tendency toward greater uniformity of rates around the country.[21] Yet some new clustering emerged, including elevated rates of lung and oral cancers among women in Florida and along the Pacific coast that seem related to smoking habits and high rates of non-Hodgkin's lymphoma in central regions that may be associated with agricultural exposure to herbicides.[45] The U.S. cancer maps were soon followed by similar atlases from other countries, the total reaching 15 at last count. Most remarkable are the maps from China that have disclosed dramatic variations in mortality and have stimulated a number of analytical studies in areas with exceptionally high rates.[46] In Scandinavian countries that have national cancer registries, atlases based on incidence data have been useful in identifying high-risk communities, particularly for less lethal tumors (e.g., endometrium) that are not measured well by mortality statistics.

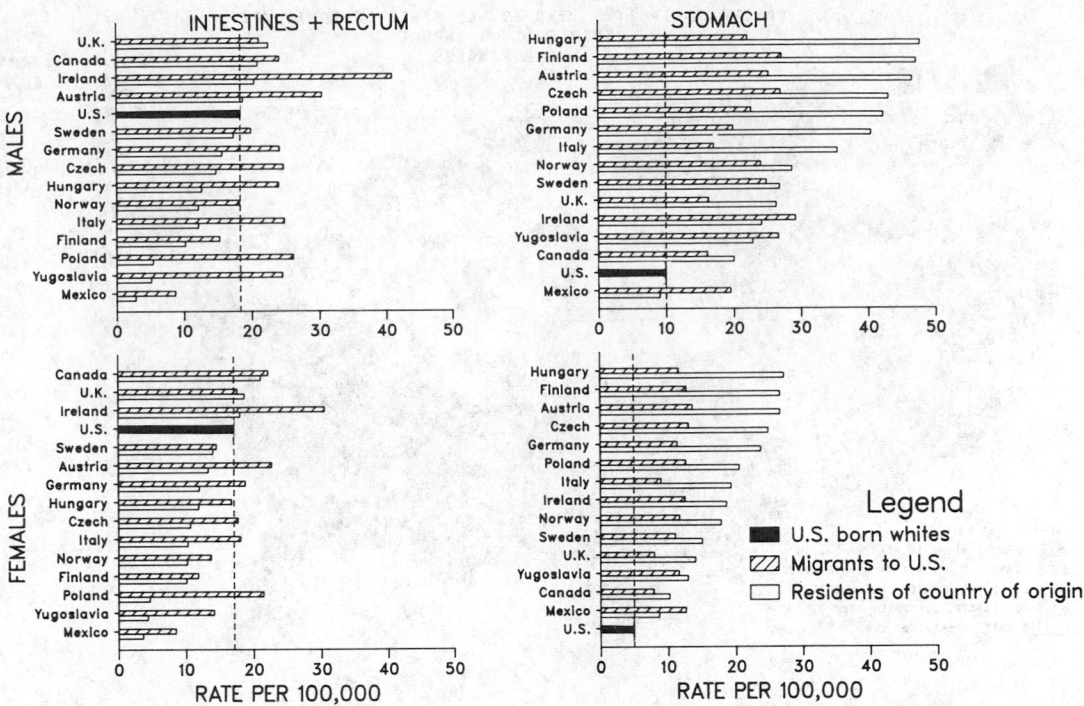

FIG. 13-1. Average annual mortality rates for intestinal and stomach cancers among U.S.-born whites, migrants from selected countries from 1959 to 1961, and residents of the countries of origin, 1960. Rates standardized for age on the 1950 U.S. population. (Data from Lilienfeld AM, Levin ML, Kessler II: Cancer in the United States. Cambridge, MA, Harvard University Press, 1972)

FIG. 13-2. Mapping of lung cancer mortality rates among white males for United States counties, 1950 to 1969. Rates standardized for age on the 1960 U.S. population. (Adapted from Mason TJ, McKay FW, Hoover R, et al: Atlas of Cancer Mortality for U.S. Counties: 1950–1969. DHEW Publication No. [NIH] 75–780. Washington, DC, US Government Printing Office, 1975)

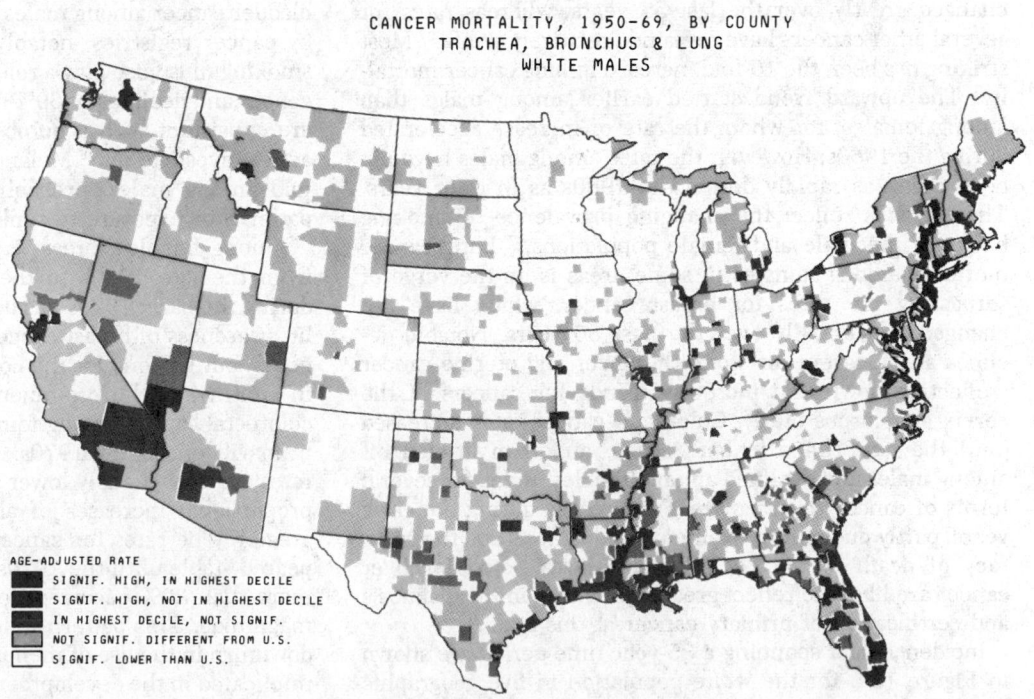

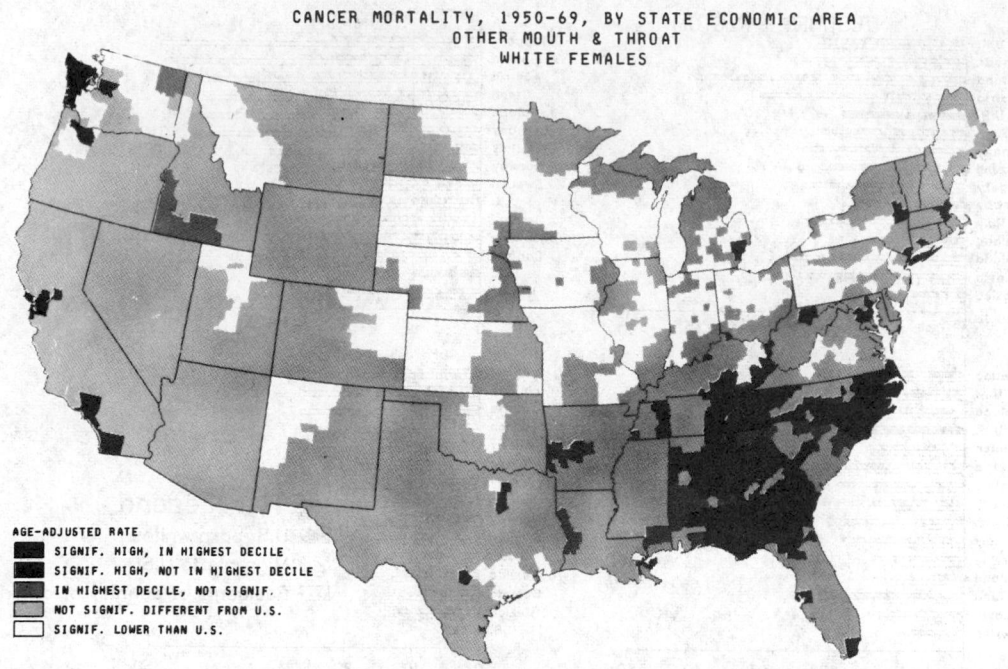

FIG. 13-3. Mapping of oral and pharyngeal cancer mortality rates among white females for United States counties, 1950 to 1969. Rates standardized for age on the 1960 U.S. population. (Adapted from Mason TJ, McKay FW, Hoover R, et al: Atlas of Cancer Mortality for U.S. Counties: 1950–1969. DHEW Publication No. [NIH] 75–780. Washington, DC, US Government Printing Office, 1975)

TIME TRENDS

A major indication of the importance of environmental factors lies in the variation in the mortality and incidence of certain cancers over time. As shown in Figure 13-4, mortality rates for some forms of cancer in the United States have changed greatly over the last 55 years, whereas rates for several other cancers have remained relatively stable.[37] Most striking has been the 10-fold increase in lung cancer mortality. The upward trend started earlier among males than among females, for whom the rate of increase accelerated during the 1960s. However, the rates among males have not been rising as rapidly during the 1980s as in prior years. These trends reflect the changing prevalence of smoking habits in the male and female populations.[47] Lung cancer mortality among females in some areas is on the verge of surpassing the rates for breast cancer, which have not changed substantially over the past 50 years. Notable declines are apparent for stomach cancer and uterine cancer (reflecting downward mortality trends for cancers of the cervix and corpus uteri). Colorectal cancer rates increased until the late 1940s in both sexes, and then leveled off among males and declined among females. Rates for several forms of cancer (*e.g.*, pancreas) increased during the early years, partly due to improvements in diagnosis and the accuracy of death certificates. The decreases noted for liver cancer are likely to reflect greater precision in the diagnosis and certification of primary cancer at this site.

Incidence data spanning a 35-year time period are shown in Figure 13-5 for the white population in five geographic areas of the country.[24] Among males lung cancer incidence

increased almost 3% per year to become the most frequent form of cancer, but the decline in the most recent years may reflect a decrease in smoking prevalence. Prostatic cancer incidence increased substantially, particularly since 1970, which must be due at least partly to the improved detection of early-stage or latent carcinomas. Some of the increases in bladder cancer among males may be due to changing criteria by cancer registries, notably for papillomas, but trends in smoking must also play a role. Increases of 60% in colorectal cancer and declines of 69% in stomach cancer among males are consistent with a number of dietary hypotheses under active investigation.[48] Melanoma incidence rose nearly fourfold among males, probably due in part to the changing patterns of exposure to sunlight.[49]

Among females, breast cancer incidence increased 31% from the late 1940s to the mid-1980s. The striking rise during the early 1970s has been attributed to increased public awareness of breast cancer that precipitated earlier diagnoses, but reasons for the continuing increases are unclear. In contrast to the prominent upward trend among males, colorectal cancer among females increased only about 10%, primarily during the 1970s. Although lung cancer incidence rates are considerably lower among females than males, the proportional increases of almost 6% per year have been greater. The rates for cancer of the body of the uterus appeared stable until the 1970s when a substantial increase of more than 30% occurred, followed by decreases of similar magnitude. This pattern follows the upturn and subsequent downturn in the use of menopausal estrogens that have been implicated in the development of endometrial cancer.[50] Incidence rates for invasive cancer of the cervix uteri declined

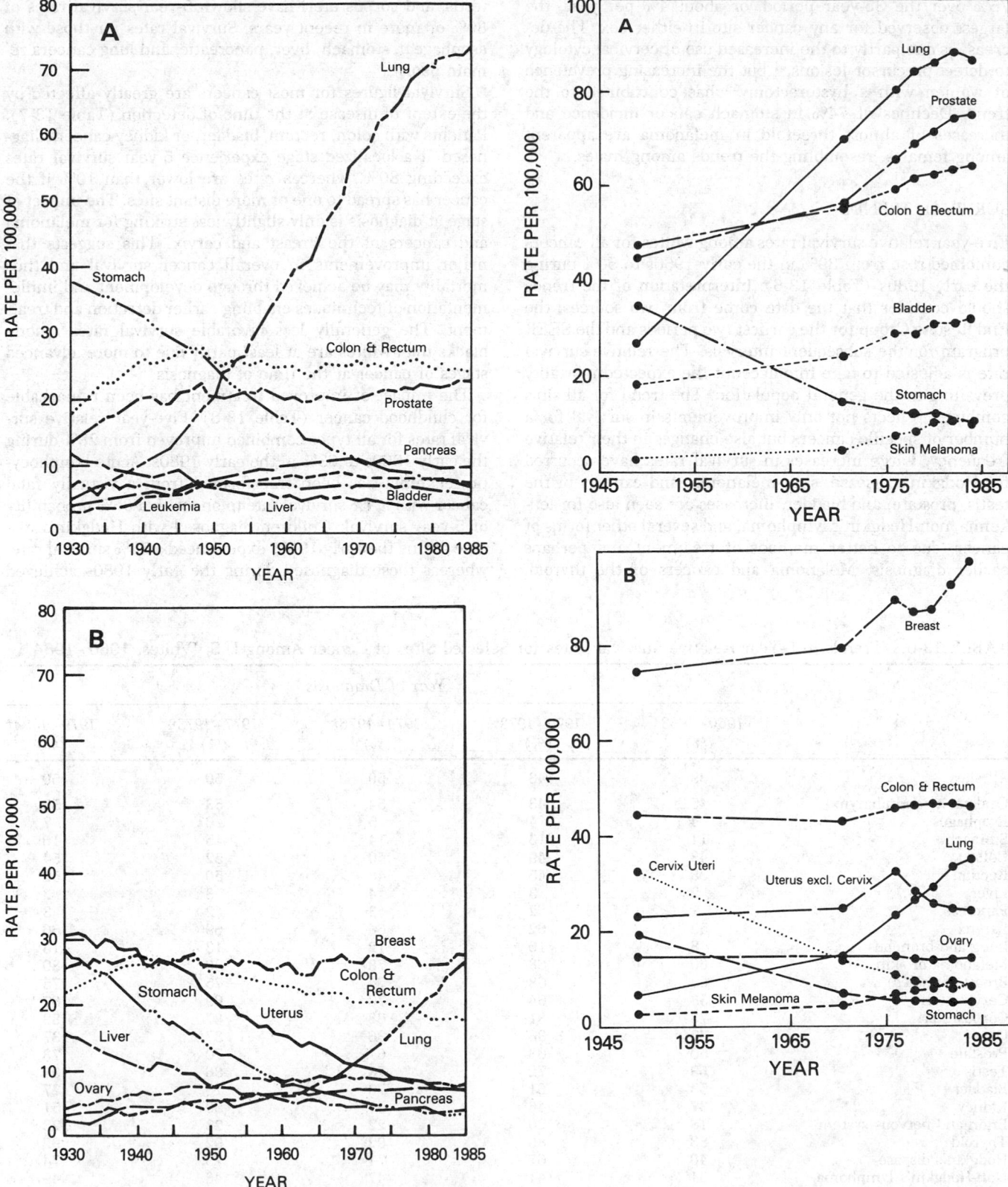

FIG. 13-4. Cancer mortality trends for selected sites in the United States population, 1930 to 1985, among males (**A**) and females (**B**). Rates standardized for age on the 1970 U.S. population. (Data from the National Center for Health Statistics and Bureau of the Census. Modified from Silverberg E, Lubera JA: Cancer Statistics, 1988. CA 38:5, 1988)

FIG. 13-5. Cancer incidence trends for selected sites in five geographic areas of the United States, 1947 to 1984, among white males (**A**) and white females (**B**). Rates standardized for age on the 1970 U.S. population. (Adapted from Devesa SS, Silverman DT, Young JL Jr, et al: Cancer incidence and mortality trends among whites in the United States, 1947–84. JNCI 79:701, 1987)

75% over the 35-year period, or about 4% per year, the largest observed for any cancer site in either sex. The decrease is due partly to the increased use of cervical cytology to detect precursor lesions,[51] but the increasing prevalence of women with a hysterectomy[52] has contributed to the trend. Declines of 74% in stomach cancer incidence and increases of almost threefold in melanoma are apparent among females, resembling the trends among males.

SURVIVAL TRENDS

Five-year relative survival rates among whites for all cancers combined rose from 39% in the early 1960s to 50% during the early 1980s (Table 13-6). Interpretation of the trends should consider that the data come from two sources: the End Results Group for the earliest two periods and the SEER program for the subsequent intervals. The relative survival rate is adjusted to take into account the expected mortality prevailing in the general population. The trend for all sites combined reflects not only improvements in survival for a number of specific cancers but also changes in their relative frequency. Large increases in survival rates have occurred for Hodgkin's disease, skin melanoma, and cancers of the testis, prostate, and bladder. Increases are seen also for leukemia, non-Hodgkin's lymphoma, and several other forms of cancer, due to better methods of treatment and perhaps earlier diagnosis. Melanoma and cancers of the thyroid,

testis, and corpus uteri have shown 5-year survival rates of 80% or more in recent years. Survival rates for those with esophageal, stomach, liver, pancreatic, and lung cancers remain poor.

Survival figures for most cancers are greatly affected by the extent of disease at the time of detection (Table 13-7). Patients with colon, rectum, bladder, or kidney cancers diagnosed at a localized stage experience 5-year survival rates exceeding 80%, whereas rates are lower than 10% if the cancer has spread to one or more distant sites. The impact of stage at diagnosis is only slightly less striking for melanoma and cancers of the breast and cervix. This suggests that major improvements in overall cancer survival and thus mortality may be achieved through development and implementation of techniques enabling earlier detection and treatment. The generally less favorable survival rates among blacks than whites are at least partly due to more advanced stages of cancer at the time of diagnosis.

The impact of improved treatment has been remarkable for childhood cancer (Table 13-8). Five-year relative survival rates for all types combined improved from 28% during the early 1960s to 63% in the early 1980s. Acute lymphocytic leukemia has been transformed from a virtually fatal cancer with a 4% survival rate to one with a 65% probability of 5-year survival. Children diagnosed with Hodgkin's disease during the early 1960s experienced a 52% survival rate, whereas those diagnosed during the early 1980s achieved

TABLE 13-6.   Trends in 5-Year Relative Survival Rates for Selected Sites of Cancer Among U.S. Whites, 1960–1984

	Year of Diagnosis				
	1960–1963* (%)	1970–1973* (%)	1974–1976† (%)	1977–1978† (%)	1979–1984† (%)
All sites	39	43	50	50	50
Oral cavity and pharynx	45	43	54	53	53
Esophagus	4	4	5	6	7
Stomach	11	13	14	15	16
Colon	43	49	50	52	54
Rectum	38	45	48	50	52
Liver	2	3	4	3	3
Pancreas	1	2	3	2	3
Larynx	53	62	66	69	66
Lung and bronchus	8	10	12	13	13
Melanoma of skin	60	68	78	80	80
Breast (females)	63	68	74	75	75
Cervix uteri	58	64	70	69	67
Corpus uteri	73	81	88	87	83
Ovary	32	36	36	37	37
Prostate	50	63	67	70	73
Testis	63	72	78	86	91
Bladder	53	61	73	75	77
Kidney	37	46	51	50	51
Brain and nervous system	18	20	22	23	23
Thyroid	83	86	92	92	92
Hodgkin's disease	40	67	71	73	74
Non-Hodgkin's lymphoma	31	41	47	48	49
Multiple myeloma	12	19	24	24	24
Leukemia	14	22	34	37	32

From National Cancer Institute: Annual Cancer Statistics Review Including Cancer Trends 1950–1985. Bethesda, MD, 1988.
  * Rates based on data from the End Results Group using a series of hospital registries and one population-based registry.
  † Rates based on data from the SEER program, with follow-up of patients through 1985.

TABLE 13-7.   Five-Year Relative Survival Rates Among U.S. Whites for Selected Sites of Cancer According to Stage at Diagnosis, 1979–1984*

	Localized (%)	Regional (%)	Distant (%)
Oral cavity and pharynx	77	42	17
Esophagus	15	5	1
Stomach	57	15	2
Colon	87	58	6
Rectum	81	46	3
Pancreas	6	4	1
Larynx	81	53	24
Lung and bronchus	35	14	1
Melanoma of skin	90	52	12
Breast (females)	90	69	18
Cervix uteri	88	52	15
Corpus uteri	91	71	25
Ovary	84	45	20
Prostate	85	74	31
Testis	97	94	61
Bladder	89	45	8
Kidney	83	53	7
Thyroid	99	91	49

From National Cancer Institute: Annual Cancer Statistics Review Including Cancer Trends 1950–1985. Bethesda, MD 1988.
* Rates based on data from the SEER program, with follow-up of patients through 1985.

rates exceeding 90%. For Wilms' tumor, survival rates increased from 33% to 82% over the same period. The improvements in therapy and survival have resulted in dramatic declines in childhood cancer mortality in recent years.[53]

AGE CURVES

The marked rise in cancer incidence with advancing age has suggested in the past that some aspect of the aging process increases susceptibility to cancer, perhaps by impairing immune function. It is now considered, however, that the relationship of many cancers with increasing age mainly reflects the importance of duration of exposure to carcinogens and of long induction periods.[5] The age-specific incidence rates for cancers of individual sites are reproduced in Appendix Tables 13-1 to 13-4. The rates cover the years 1981 to 1985 for the SEER program of the NCI, and are given by sex and race (whites and blacks).

Figure 13-6 shows the age distribution for selected cancers in the white population, with incidence plotted on a semilog scale. Most epithelial cancers are rare under age 30 but then rise progressively with age (e.g., cancers of the colon and rectum, prostate, and bladder), although at the oldest ages a slight downturn in the curve is probably related to underdiagnosis. For cancers of female reproductive sites, the rates appear to reach a plateau or decline at postmenopausal ages, consistent with an influence of endogenous hormones. Only a few nonepithelial cancers rise sharply with age, notably multiple myeloma and chronic lymphocytic leukemia.[5] Deviations from the usual age trend are illustrated by the cancers plotted in Figure 13-6C. Peaks for leukemia and nervous system cancer occur not only at older ages but also in early childhood, suggesting the influence of prenatal factors. The bimodal age curve for Hodgkin's disease has received much attention and there is some evidence suggesting that the young adult peak may result from an infectious agent.[54] Also intriguing is the pattern of testis cancer, with a peak occurrence among young adult men and a rising incidence over time that remains unexplained.[55] The rates for invasive cervical cancer increase sharply with age among young women, but then level off after age 35.

Table 13-9 shows the incidence rates for the major cancers among white children by age group and sex for the period 1981 to 1985. Except for lymphomas and bone tumors, the highest incidence occurs in children under 5 years of age. In general, boys have somewhat higher rates than girls in all three age groups, especially for the lymphomas.

TABLE 13-8.   Trends in 5-Year Relative Survival Rates for Selected Forms of Cancer Among U.S. White Children Under 15 Years of Age, 1960–1984

	Year of Diagnosis				
	1960–1963* (%)	1970–1973* (%)	1974–1976† (%)	1977–1978† (%)	1979–1984† (%)
All forms	28	45	55	62	63
Acute lymphocytic leukemia	4	34	53	73	65
Acute myeloid leukemia	3	5	16	27	25
Wilms' tumor	33	70	74	80	82
Brain and nervous system	35	45	54	55	56
Neuroblastoma	25	40	48	46	56
Bone	20	30	52	53	48
Hodgkin's disease	52	90	80	82	91
Non-Hodgkin's lymphoma	18	26	43	44	60

From National Cancer Institute: Annual Cancer Statistics Review Including Cancer Trends 1950–1985. Bethesda, MD, 1988.
* Rates based on the End Results Group using a series of hospital registries and one population-based registry.
† Rates based on the SEER program, with follow-up of patients through 1985.

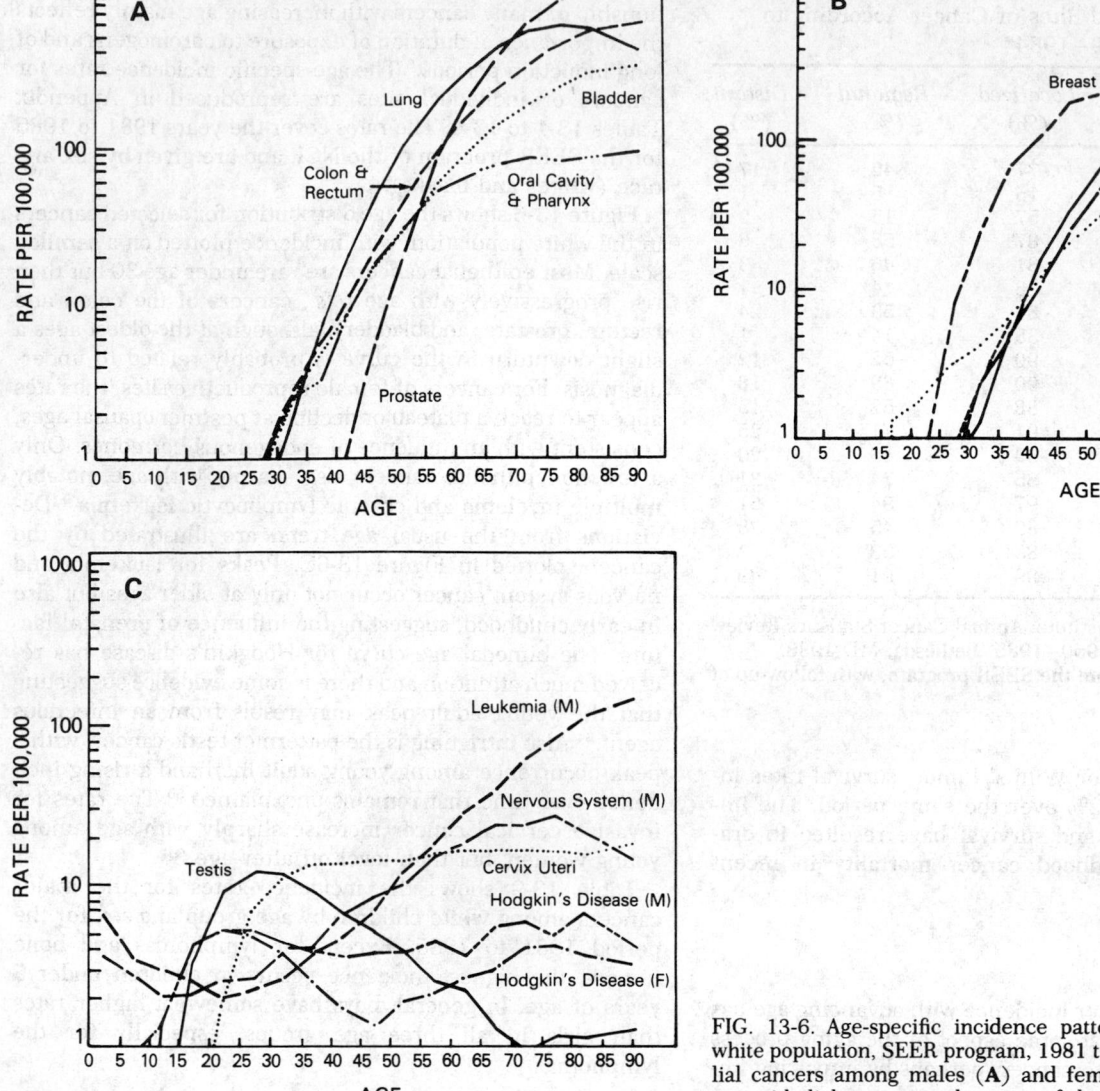

FIG. 13-6. Age-specific incidence patterns in the United States white population, SEER program, 1981 to 1985, for selected epithelial cancers among males (**A**) and females (**B**), and for selected nonepithelial cancers and cancer of the cervix (**C**).

TABLE 13-9. Age-Specific Incidence Rates for Selected Forms of Cancer Among U.S. White Children, 1981–1985*

	Boys			Girls		
	0–4	5–9	10–14	0–4	5–9	10–14
All forms	19.9	11.7	11.8	17.4	9.6	10.7
Leukemia	6.8	3.4	3.0	6.1	3.2	2.3
Brain and central nervous system	3.8	2.8	2.2	2.9	2.6	1.7
Lymphoma	0.8	2.5	3.2	0.3	0.4	1.8
Neuroblastoma	3.3	0.3	0.1	3.0	0.4	0.1
Soft tissue	0.8	0.5	0.6	0.8	0.2	0.6
Wilms' tumor	1.9	0.6	0.2	1.8	0.7	0.1
Bone	0.1	0.7	1.3	0.2	0.7	1.2
Retinoblastoma	1.0	0.1	0.0	1.1	0.1	0.0
All others	2.1	0.9	1.2	2.0	1.4	2.9

* Average annual rates per 100,000 population, based on data from the SEER program.

ETHNIC VARIATION

The SEER program provides data indicating striking racial and ethnic variations in cancer incidence in the United States (Table 13-10). For males, the rates for all cancers combined are highest in blacks, followed by whites and Hawaiians, whereas for females the rates are highest for Hawaiians, followed by whites and blacks. The lowest rates in both sexes are in American Indians. Compared to other groups, whites have especially high rates for melanoma, Hodgkin's disease, non-Hodgkin's lymphoma, leukemia, and cancers of the lip, breast, corpus uteri, ovary, testis, bladder, brain, colon, and rectum. Blacks have elevated rates for multiple myeloma and cancers of the oral cavity, esophagus, colon, pancreas, larynx, lung (males), cervix uteri, and prostate. Hispanics have especially high rates for cervix cancer, and to some extent for cancers of the stomach and biliary tract (females), whereas American Indians have remarkably high rates for cancers of the stomach, biliary tract, cervix, and kidney (females). Chinese experience elevated rates for cancers of the nasopharynx and liver, while Japanese have high rates for stomach cancer and (in males) for cancers of the colon, rectum, and thyroid. Filipinos have high rates for cancers of the thyroid, while Hawaiians show elevated rates for cancers of the lung (notably in females), breast, corpus uteri, stomach, and thyroid. Like migrant populations, the racial and ethnic variations in cancer occurrence within the United States offer special opportunities for studies aimed at clarifying the environmental and host determinants of cancer.

SOCIOECONOMIC PATTERNS

Whereas part of the racial and ethnic variations in rates may reflect genetic influences, many appear strongly influenced by environmental factors, some of which may be associated with socioeconomic status. Data from the Third National Cancer Survey[30] were used to estimate the associations of cancer incidence with median family income and educational achievement as indicated by census tract of residence, and to evaluate the impact of adjustment for socioeconomic disparities on the observed black/white relative risks.[56] Overall, cancer incidence rates among whites were 20% greater in the lowest income group than in the highest, with a continuous gradient in risk (Table 13-11). This pattern varied by primary site, however. Cervix cancer was almost four times as frequent among women in the lowest relative to the highest category, for reasons that are not entirely clear. Rates for esophageal cancer among men varied more than twofold, in line with socioeconomic differences in the use of alcohol and tobacco as well as nutritional status. Striking inverse gradients were also apparent for lung and stomach cancers among males, reflecting smoking and perhaps nutritional patterns. In contrast, positive gradients with income level were apparent for both breast and corpus uteri cancers, which may parallel the distribution of reproductive and menstrual risk factors.

An important question is the extent to which socioeconomic factors account for the black/white differentials in cancer incidence. When adjusted for racial variations in socioeconomic status, the excess risk among blacks is dimin-

TABLE 13-10A. Average Annual Age-Adjusted Incidence Rates per 100,000 for Selected Cancer Sites by Racial and Ethnic Group, 1975–1985, U.S. Males*

	Whites	Blacks	Hispanics	American Indians	Chinese	Japanese	Filipinos	Hawaiians
All sites	404.1	490.2	265.5	184.5	292.7	303.6	242.0	398.9
Lip	3.7	0.2	3.3	0.0	0.1	0.1	0.0	0.0
Nasopharynx	0.6	1.0	0.9	0.5	13.9	1.4	2.9	1.5
Other oral cavity and pharynx	11.8	20.5	5.2	1.7	6.2	6.0	6.8	10.1
Esophagus	4.9	18.4	2.9	1.9	6.1	5.6	4.9	15.1
Stomach	11.5	20.5	20.8	26.1	14.5	38.6	9.6	40.4
Colon	40.3	40.7	17.9	8.4	33.6	42.1	24.0	25.8
Rectum	20.0	14.9	11.5	5.0	19.3	23.4	16.9	18.7
Liver	2.7	5.2	4.3	4.5	19.5	7.1	10.2	9.8
Gallbladder	0.8	0.8	1.5	8.9	1.2	1.5	1.2	1.4
Other biliary	1.6	1.2	2.2	2.8	2.2	3.9	2.1	2.5
Pancreas	11.2	16.9	12.4	9.0	8.7	9.9	7.9	10.6
Larynx	8.6	12.3	4.2	1.1	2.9	3.9	2.8	6.5
Lung and bronchus	82.1	119.6	32.2	14.2	61.2	48.4	39.9	108.2
Melanoma of skin	9.8	0.8	1.6	2.2	0.4	1.5	1.2	1.6
Prostate	77.3	122.8	71.5	45.5	32.5	45.7	47.4	59.6
Testis	4.2	0.8	3.0	1.8	1.9	1.3	0.5	2.6
Bladder	30.2	15.1	10.9	3.6	13.9	12.5	6.0	10.6
Kidney	10.3	9.6	8.7	9.2	4.9	6.1	4.6	6.9
Brain and other nervous system	7.3	4.3	4.9	3.1	3.0	3.1	3.4	3.1
Thyroid	2.3	1.4	2.9	2.3	4.5	6.2	6.8	7.4
Hodgkin's disease	3.5	2.7	3.3	0.7	0.8	0.8	1.7	1.4
Non-Hodgkin's lymphoma	13.0	8.5	6.9	4.7	10.2	9.2	9.8	10.9
Multiple myeloma	4.6	10.3	2.8	2.7	2.2	1.7	4.6	5.9
Leukemia	13.8	11.1	7.8	5.5	7.7	6.9	8.8	9.5
All others	27.8	30.7	21.8	18.7	21.3	16.6	18.0	28.6

* Based on data from the SEER program. Data for Hispanics and American Indians are from New Mexico, whereas those for Chinese, Japanese, and Filipinos are from San Francisco and Hawaii. Rates age-adjusted based on the 1970 U.S. standard population.

TABLE 13-10B.   Average Annual Age-Adjusted Incidence Rates per 100,000 for Selected Cancer Sites by Racial and Ethnic Group 1975–1985, U.S. Females*

	Whites	Blacks	Hispanics	American Indians	Chinese	Japanese	Filipinos	Hawaiians
All sites	316.1	296.6	220.4	168.8	242.2	214.0	202.6	344.1
Lip	0.3	0.1	0.4	0.0	0.0	0.1	0.0	0.0
Nasopharynx	0.3	0.5	0.2	0.0	6.7	0.3	1.6	1.1
Other oral cavity and pharynx	5.2	6.2	1.7	0.6	1.3	2.1	5.3	5.3
Esophagus	1.6	5.0	0.8	0.3	1.2	0.8	1.9	2.2
Stomach	5.1	8.5	10.0	12.3	8.7	19.0	7.2	17.9
Colon	32.3	35.0	16.7	8.1	23.7	25.7	14.9	16.3
Rectum	12.8	10.8	7.6	3.2	10.9	10.9	8.1	8.1
Liver	1.1	1.7	1.9	2.6	4.7	2.4	3.2	2.7
Gallbladder	1.6	1.1	7.1	17.1	1.0	1.7	1.8	1.3
Other biliary	1.1	0.8	1.3	4.4	1.9	2.4	0.7	2.6
Pancreas	7.7	11.5	10.8	4.3	7.8	6.0	4.8	9.2
Larynx	1.5	2.2	0.9	0.0	0.2	0.2	0.7	1.6
Lung and bronchus	29.7	31.2	15.6	4.6	27.6	13.2	17.9	45.8
Melanoma of skin	8.2	0.7	2.2	0.7	0.7	1.0	0.9	1.0
Breast	91.5	76.4	50.9	25.6	58.7	57.1	45.6	104.6
Cervix uteri	8.8	19.7	17.1	20.0	10.5	5.8	10.8	14.5
Uterus excluding cervix	27.1	14.8	11.2	5.2	18.2	17.6	11.0	28.0
Ovary	14.1	9.8	11.3	8.9	10.3	8.5	9.7	13.2
Bladder	7.7	5.5	3.3	0.4	4.0	4.4	3.1	6.0
Kidney	4.7	4.6	4.2	6.2	2.5	2.2	2.2	2.8
Brain and other nervous system	5.1	2.9	2.4	1.8	2.7	2.2	1.3	4.2
Thyroid	5.5	3.5	7.9	6.1	6.9	6.6	17.3	13.7
Hodgkin's disease	2.6	1.2	1.3	0.5	0.8	0.3	1.3	0.9
Non-Hodgkin's lymphoma	9.6	5.7	5.5	4.8	6.5	5.9	7.1	6.6
Multiple myeloma	3.1	6.8	2.8	2.2	1.7	1.3	2.6	5.6
Leukemia	8.0	7.0	6.3	4.5	4.7	5.1	6.4	7.0
All others	20.2	23.6	18.8	24.4	18.1	11.1	15.3	22.2

* Based on data from the SEER program. Data for Hispanics and American Indians are from New Mexico, whereas those for Chinese, Japanese, and Filipinos are from San Francisco and Hawaii. Rates age-adjusted based on the 1970 U.S. standard population.

ished for cancers of the esophagus, stomach, lung, and cervix. Socioeconomic status may also influence cancer survival and mortality patterns by affecting access to diagnosis and treatment.

ANALYTICAL STUDIES

The major contribution of epidemiology has been to test etiologic hypotheses through analytical studies, usually involving cohort or case-control designs. These studies obtain data on suspected risk factors and disease occurrence at the individual instead of at the aggregate (population) level. By using specific methods to select and compare groups of subjects, while controlling for other relevant variables, the risk of disease associated with exposure can be estimated.[4,13,14] In designing these studies, the groups should be sufficiently large and the time intervals between initial exposure and tumor onset sufficiently long to identify the lowest excess risk considered important to detect. Reliable and valid estimates of exposure should be sought, with quantitative measurements to permit dose-response evaluations. Studies must

TABLE 13-11.   Relative Risks (RR) for All Cancers and Selected Sites by Socioeconomic Status (SES) and Race, 1969–1971*

	Income Level Among Whites					Black/White RR	
	Low	2	3	4	High	SES Unadjusted	SES Adjusted†
All sites (males)	1.20	1.09	1.07	1.02	1.00	1.10	1.0
Esophagus (males)	2.13	1.69	1.34	1.20	1.00	3.05	2.3
Stomach (males)	1.39	1.26	1.16	1.02	1.00	1.48	1.2
Lung (males)	1.65	1.44	1.33	1.18	1.00	1.10	0.9
Breast (females)	0.70	0.73	0.80	0.83	1.00	0.85	0.8
Cervix uteri	3.82	2.69	1.95	1.39	1.00	1.74	1.2
Corpus uteri	0.75	0.83	0.88	0.89	1.00	0.70	0.6

* Data derived from the Third National Cancer Survey, 1969–1971. All relative risks adjusted for age and geographic area.
† Also adjusted for income and education.

be designed to minimize potential sources of bias (*i.e.,* systematic error), and to permit the detection and control of confounding (*i.e.,* the distortion of exposure-disease associations by extraneous variables).

COHORT STUDIES

Cohort studies, also referred to as follow-up studies or prospective studies, identify groups of individuals with and without a particular exposure, follow them over time to determine subsequent health outcomes, and compare their mortality or incidence rates of disease.[4,57] An association is suggested when the rates of disease are different in the exposed than in the unexposed group. These investigations may be based on current exposures and future health outcomes, referred to as a prospective cohort study; but more often they use information on exposures collected in the past, termed a retrospective cohort study. Instead of an unexposed comparison group, general population mortality or incidence rates (specific for age, sex, race, geographic area, and calendar time) are often used to estimate an expected number of events. This method assumes that in the absence of the specific exposure of interest the study group would have the same probability of developing the disease as the general population. The cohort approach is used mainly when it is possible to evaluate high exposures in clearly defined subgroups of the population. It has been especially helpful, for example, in assessing the carcinogenic risk from occupational hazards, smoking, or medical exposures such as radiation and certain drugs.

CASE-CONTROL STUDIES

Case-control studies, also called case-referent studies or retrospective studies, identify persons with a particular disease (cases) and a group of similar persons without the disease (controls), and then collect information on past exposures by interview or other methods.[4,57] If the proportion of cases with a certain exposure is greater than that of the controls, an association may be indicated. The case-control approach is especially well-suited for studying uncommon diseases. Although used primarily to test hypotheses, the approach occasionally has taken the form of an exploratory study when a disease is so poorly understood that hypotheses need to be formulated for subsequent investigation. In general, it is desirable that both cases and controls are selected from the same source, which may be either population-based or hospital-based. However, since factors associated with hospitalization may be over-represented among hospital controls, careful consideration should be given to the diagnostic composition of this group. Bias is minimized by selecting hospital controls with a variety of disorders and excluding conditions related to the exposure in question.[58]

COMPARISON OF METHODS

The case-control and cohort methods have different strengths and weaknesses. Case-control studies provide a more efficient means of studying rare diseases, with fewer individuals needed, a shorter study period, and generally lower costs as compared with the cohort approach. In addi-

tion, there are greater opportunities to evaluate more than one risk factor and interactions between them.[59] On the other hand, the case-control approach cannot directly estimate the actual rate associated with a particular exposure, and is subject to recall and other biases that affect the comparability of cases and controls and the precision of past exposure measures.[4] Such studies also are usually limited to evaluating one disease at a time.

The advantages of cohort studies are their capacity to measure directly incidence or mortality rates associated with a particular exposure; to reduce subjective biases by obtaining information before the disease develops; to detect associations between a particular exposure and multiple outcomes; and to evaluate temporal relationships such as latency period and the duration of an effect. However, cohort studies are usually expensive and complex undertakings. They require large numbers of exposed individuals, particularly when uncommon diseases are being investigated, and care in dealing with such problems as persons lost to follow-up or with biased estimates of risk, as produced for example by the healthy worker effect of occupational studies.[4] Moreover, they may not permit as ready an ascertainment of potential confounding factors. To remedy this particular deficiency, case-control studies within defined cohorts, or nested case-control studies, are often initiated.

MEASURES OF ASSOCIATION

For cohort studies, the chief measures of association are based on rates of disease. The relative risk (RR) or risk ratio is the disease rate in the exposed, I_e, divided by the disease rate in the referent (usually nonexposed, I_o) population.[4] As illustrated by Table 13-12, the relative risk from a cohort study is defined as

$$RR = I_e I_o = \frac{a}{n_e} \frac{c}{n_o}$$

This measure gives the relative disease risk between two populations. Thus, an RR of 2.0 would indicate that the exposed group has twice the risk of the unexposed group (*i.e.,* a 100% increase in risk). An important aspect of the calculation is the concept of person-time. Usually individuals are followed for different periods owing to variable times of entry to and exit from observation because of either death or loss to follow-up. In order to accommodate the variable follow-up periods and still preserve the concept of a rate, each person is counted in the denominator only for the interval of time under observation, resulting in measures of person-years or person-months.[4]

An association may also be measured by the risk difference, often referred to as the attributable risk (A_e). This estimate results from the subtraction of the rate among the unexposed from that among the exposed. From Table 13-12, the attributable risk is defined as

$$A_e = I_e - I_o = \frac{a}{n_e} - \frac{c}{n_o}$$

The attributable risk means that if the relationship observed is causal, the difference between the rates of exposed

TABLE 13-12. Measures of Association from a Cohort Study

	Affected Persons (Cases)	Total Persons (Person-Time)
Exposed	a	n_e
Not Exposed	c	n_o
Total	a + c	N

Relative risk (RR) $= \dfrac{a}{n_e} \bigg/ \dfrac{c}{n_o}$

Attributable risk in the exposed $(A_e) = \dfrac{a}{n_e} - \dfrac{c}{n_o}$

Attributable risk percent in the exposed $(A_e\%) = \dfrac{(a/n_e) - (c/n_o)}{a/n_e} = \dfrac{RR-1}{RR} \times 100\%$

Population attributable risk $(A_p) = \dfrac{a+c}{N} - \dfrac{c}{n_o}$

Population attributable risk percent $(A_p\%) = \dfrac{(a+c)/N - (c/n_o)}{(a+c)N} = \dfrac{RR-1}{RR + 1/P-1} \times 100\%$

where P is the proportion of the population that is exposed, or n_e/N

and unexposed groups is the amount of disease attributable to that exposure.[4] When expressed as a percentage of the total disease rate in an exposed group, the attributable risk percent $(A_e\%)$ is the proportion of the exposed group's total risk that is due to the exposure.[60]

The measures of relative risk and attributable risk have somewhat different uses. The magnitude of the RR indicates the strength of a relationship between exposure and disease and the likelihood of causality. The A_e is influenced not only by the magnitude of the difference between the exposed and unexposed but also by the rate of disease in the absence of exposure.

The amount of disease attributable to a particular exposure can be estimated not only among the exposed but also in the population as a whole.[60] This measure would thus reflect the amount of disease that would be eliminated in a definable population if the exposure were removed, and is referred to as the population attributable risk (A_p). It is calculated by subtracting the rate among the unexposed from the rate that exists in the total population. Again, from Table 13-12, the population attributable risk is defined as

$$A_p = I_t - I_o = \frac{a+c}{N} - \frac{c}{n_o}$$

Thus, the magnitude of this estimate is influenced by the size of the relative difference in risk between the exposed and unexposed, by the level of the disease among the unexposed, and by the prevalence of the exposure in the population. When the attributable risk is expressed as a proportion of the total disease rate in population, it is called the population attributable risk percent $(A_p\%)$ or the etiologic fraction.[61]

These measures are illustrated by a recent cohort study involving 1-year survivors of ovarian cancer from five randomized trials.[62] The incidence rates for acute nonlymphocytic leukemia and preleukemia were evaluated among women treated with no chemotherapy, with cyclophosphamide, and with melphalan. The corresponding rates were 0.18, 3.21, and 11.46 cases per 1000 women per year. Com-

pared to those receiving no chemotherapy, the RR of leukemic conditions was 18 (3.21/0.18) for women given cyclophosphamide and 64 (11.46/0.18) for those given melphalan. The magnitude of these risks suggests that the drugs are causally related to leukemia. However, the risk differences obtained by subtracting rates among the exposed from the unexposed groups were not very great. The A_e associated with cyclophosphamide is about 3 per 1000 per year, and with melphalan about 11 per 1000 per year. Given the life-threatening problems posed by ovarian cancer, these risks should not deter physicians from using therapy whose proven benefit outweighs these risks. Also, when the A_e is not large, one can see how difficult it is for an individual clinician, or even a large group practice, to suspect a leukemia risk related to treatment.

If exposure to all alkylating agents were removed, it would have very little impact on the total leukemia rate in the general population, for relatively few persons are exposed to these drugs. However, in the clinical populations under study, the overall rate of leukemic conditions was 2.29 per 1000 patients per year. As shown in Table 13-13, subtracting the rate among those not treated with chemotherapy (.18 per 1000 per year) from the rate for all patients combined yields a population attributable risk of 2.11 cases per 1000 women per year, or an etiologic fraction of 92% in the clinical populations.

For case-control studies, the enumeration of exposed and unexposed populations is not available, as it is in cohort studies, to directly measure rates (or risks). Fortunately, data from cross-classification tables in a case-control study can be used to calculate reasonable estimates of relative and attributable risks. If the sampling fractions for the cases and the controls are known (i.e., the proportion of all the cases in a defined population that is present in the case series, and the proportion of the same population present in the control series), these can be used to estimate the rates among the exposed and unexposed groups and thus to calculate relative and attributable risks. For most case-control studies, however, sampling fractions are unknown. In this circumstance,

TABLE 13-13. Risks of Leukemia and Preleukemia Associated with Chemotherapy

	Cases	Person-Years at Risk	Rate per 1,000
Any Chemotherapy	33	4,295	7.68
No Chemotherapy	2	10,983	0.18
Total	35	15,278	2.29

$$\text{Relative risk (RR)} = \frac{33/4,279}{2/10,983} = \frac{7.68}{0.18} = 42.4$$

$$\text{Attributable risk in the exposed } (A_e) = 33/4,279 - 2/10,983 = 7.40 \text{ per } 1,000$$

$$\text{Attributable risk percent in the exposed } (A_e\%) = \frac{42.4\text{-}1}{42.4} \times 100\% = 98\%$$

$$\text{Population attributable risk } (A_p) = \frac{35}{15,278} - \frac{2}{10,983} = 2.11 \text{ per } 1,000$$

$$\text{Population attributable risk percent } (A_p\%) = \frac{35/15,278\text{-}2/10,983}{35/15,278} \times 100\% = 92\%$$

Adapted from Greene MH, Harris EL, Gershenson DM, et al: Melphalan may be a more potent leukemogen than cyclophosphamide. Ann Intern Med 105:360, 1986.

as shown in Table 13-14, the calculation of relative odds, also termed an odds ratio, usually gives a good approximation of the relative risk.[4] The absolute measures of attributable risk cannot be estimated directly, but algebraic properties of cross-classification tables allow estimations of the attributable risk percent and the etiologic fraction[60] as shown in Table 13-14.

Calculation of these measures is illustrated in Table 13-15, based on a national case-control study of bladder cancer that evaluated the risks associated with smoking.[63] The study estimated a relative risk of 2.2 for cigarette smoking, with 55% of bladder cancer among smokers attributable to their smoking and 43% of bladder cancer in the U.S. population due to smoking. These figures are consistent with the direct estimates of risk from cohort studies.

INTERVENTION STUDIES

Also referred to as experimental studies,[57] controlled intervention trials represent a third strategy of analytical epidemiology that is especially useful for confirming causal relationships suggested by cohort or case-control studies and for directly evaluating the effect of possible preventive measures. This method permits control over extraneous variables and biases that may influence results by the random allocation of subjects to study and control groups. There are no clear guidelines as to when evidence is sufficient to conduct intervention trials, yet when there is a reasonable likelihood of benefit resulting from intervention (as well as any potential for harm), ethical questions may arise. In the field of cancer etiology and prevention, opportunities for inter-

TABLE 13-14. Measures of Association from a Case-Control Study

	Cases	Controls
Exposed	a	b
Not exposed	c	d
Total	a + c	b + d

$$\text{Relative odds (R)} = \frac{ad}{bc}$$

$$\text{Attributable risk percent in the exposed } (A_e\%) = \frac{R\text{-}1}{R} \times 100\%$$

$$\text{Population attributable risk percent } (A_p\%) \text{ or etiologic fraction} = \frac{P_o(R\text{-}1)}{1 + P_o(R\text{-}1)} \times 100\%$$

$$= \frac{(R-1)P_e}{R} \times 100\%$$

where P_o is the exposure rate in the controls, or $\frac{b}{b+d}$ and P_e is the exposure rate in the cases, or $\frac{a}{a+c}$

TABLE 13-15.   Risks of Bladder Cancer Associated with Cigarette Smoking

	Cases	Controls
Smokers	2324	3581
Nonsmokers	657	2198
Total	2981	5779

Relative odds $(R) = \dfrac{(2324)(2198)}{(657)(3581)} = 2.2$

Attributable risk percent in the exposed $(A_e\%) = \dfrac{2.2-1}{2.2} \times 100\% = 55\%$

Population attributable risk percent $(A_p\%)$ or etiologic fraction $= \dfrac{\dfrac{3581}{5779}(2.2-1)}{1 + \dfrac{3581}{5579}(2.2-1)} \times 100\%$

$$= 43\%$$

Alternatively, $\dfrac{(2.2-1)}{2.2} \times \dfrac{2324}{2981} \times 100\% = 43\%$

Adapted from Hartge P, Silverman D, Hoover R, et al: Changing cigarette habits and bladder cancer risk: A case-control study. JNCI 78:1119, 1987.

vention have been limited for various reasons, including the long latency periods that may be involved before an effect is seen. However, intervention studies are now gaining emphasis in the evaluation of diet and nutrition, especially the use of various micronutrient supplements that may inhibit late stages of the carcinogenic process. Also underway are hepatitis-B vaccine trials in endemic areas for liver cancer. After intervention the follow-up and analytical procedures to evaluate outcomes resemble those employed for cohort studies.

STRENGTHS AND LIMITS OF EPIDEMIOLOGY

STRENGTHS

In contrast to laboratory studies, epidemiology directly evaluates the experience of human populations and their response to various environmental exposures and host factors (the risk of disease). Thus, the consequences of an exposure can be measured as it actually occurs in the population. Questionable extrapolations from other species are also avoided. Although positive findings from animal studies may indicate a potential human risk, epidemiology offers the only means of quantifying the risk. Furthermore, even when the specific causal agent cannot be clearly identified (e.g., the precise carcinogens in cigarette smoke), sufficient information can be obtained for the disease to be prevented.

LIMITATIONS

However, cancer epidemiology has certain limitations. First, studies are mainly observational, relying on natural occurrences in human populations, and the opportunities for experiment are rare and limited to efforts at prevention. Second, epidemiology can seldom indicate a cause with great specificity, particularly when the exposures are multiple or

when surrogate measures of exposure are used (e.g., occupation or area of residence), though laboratory techniques may be helpful in such circumstances. Third, study groups chosen on the basis of one characteristic may be distinctive in another, and it may be difficult to disentangle them even with refined analytical methods. Fourth, it is hard to incriminate an agent when there is relative uniformity of exposure in a given population, which may be the case with some dietary factors (e.g., high fat intake). Finally, evidence of an environmental hazard is usually obtained from high or intermediate levels of exposure. As in animal studies, it is difficult to detect causal relationships when the exposure level is low or the excess risk is small compared to the baseline incidence rate. In such situations, the numbers of subjects needed to provide definite results may be virtually impossible to assemble for the purposes of a single study.

BIOCHEMICAL EPIDEMIOLOGY

The power of certain studies may be increased by incorporating laboratory methods into analytical investigations, so-called biochemical or molecular epidemiology.[64,65] The analysis of biological samples in the laboratory can obviously permit the study of exposure to oncogenic viruses. It may also be possible to detect past exposures to chemical and physical agents and to clarify early preneoplastic events, various host factors, and mechanisms of action. At present the approach is providing new opportunities to evaluate carcinogenic risks associated with dietary factors and with markers of genetic predisposition. In view of rapid experimental advances, biochemical epidemiology represents a challenging multidisciplinary approach that should help to elucidate further the causes of cancer. Such studies are complex undertakings that require careful planning and teamwork, including the collaboration of clinicians.

SOURCES OF CLUES

Since an analytical study is designed to evaluate an association between a disease and an antecedent factor, there must be some prior indication or suspicion of such an association. The lead may come from descriptive or correlational studies or from another analytical study. However, the most fruitful source of etiologic clues has been the alert clinician who has uncovered some of the most striking examples of environmental cancer, starting with Pott's discovery of scrotal cancer among chimney sweeps. Usually the clinician recognizes an excessive number of patients with the same tumor and traces the cluster to a particular cultural, occupational, or iatrogenic exposure.[2] Thus, clinical observations have linked asbestos with mesothelioma, vinyl chloride with hepatic angiosarcoma, furniture-making with nasal adenocarcinoma, radium-dial painting with osteosarcoma, and prenatal exposure to diethylstilbestrol with clear-cell adenocarcinoma of the vagina among the offspring. It was possible for clinicians to detect these associations because they involved tumors that are rare in the general population and they also involved exceptionally high risks. In most instances the associations hardly required epidemiologic study for their confirmation, but only to quantify them. Clinicians have also identified a wide variety of heritable conditions associated with susceptibility to cancer.[66] Opportunities for the practicing physician to make significant etiologic discoveries were highlighted recently at a symposium sponsored by the Princess Takamatsu Cancer fund, entitled "Rare Events as Clues to Cancer Etiology."[67] On the other hand, epidemiologists can identify causes of cancer that may seem less dramatic in relative risks but are very important to public health, such as smoking and asbestos in lung cancer.

Another source of leads has been provided by experimental studies, especially those relating chemicals to tumors in laboratory animals. In the case of mustard gas and 4-aminobiphenyl, for example, carcinogenic risks were found in humans after the substances were shown to induce tumors in animal studies.[2] Whatever the sequence of observations, there is no question that clinical, epidemiologic, and experimental data greatly complement one another in determining the risks and mechanisms involved in carcinogenesis. When all approaches are brought to bear on a particular hypothesis, advances in understanding the carcinogenic process may be extraordinary.

INTERPRETATION OF EPIDEMIOLOGIC STUDIES

SAMPLE SIZE AND POWER

A fundamental aspect of planning or evaluating a study is the number of subjects needed to test an etiologic hypothesis.[13] The power of a study is the likelihood of detecting a postulated level of risk. The larger the sample size, the greater the power to detect a specified risk, and conversely, the smaller the sample size, the weaker the power.

The issues of sample size and power are of great concern when evaluating negative results of epidemiologic studies.[68] Only large studies may confidently exclude low to moderate levels of risk, whereas negative results of a small study should be viewed with caution because they usually lack adequate power.

NONCAUSAL ASSOCIATIONS

When interpreting the results of analytical studies, one must ask whether the associations observed between exposure and disease are the result of bias, confounding, chance, or cause-and-effect. Bias or systematic error is usually the result of imperfections in study design or conduct, and often cannot be corrected in the analysis. Many types of bias have been described,[69] but most can be grouped as biases of selection or information.[58] Selection bias involves systematic differences in exposure between those selected and not selected into the study. For example, a case-control study might include only cases referred to a particular institution or only survivors, so that differences observed might reflect factors influencing referral patterns or survival. A similar bias in a cohort study may result from differences in the loss to follow-up between exposed and unexposed groups. Information bias involves differences in measuring the factor in question between groups, and is best illustrated by recall bias or interviewer bias, both of which may affect the outcome of case-control studies. For example, in studies of childhood cancer, parents of cases might provide more reliable or thorough responses than parents of controls because of the soul-searching they had undergone. Also, interviewers might tend to probe more deeply into past events if a subject is known to be a case rather than a control.

Confounding refers to the effect of an extraneous variable that may account, entirely or partly, for an apparent association between exposure and disease, or may obscure a real association.[13,58] Confounding can usually be evaluated and accommodated during analysis by adjustment procedures, including the stratification of subjects on the suspected variable. To be a confounder, a variable must be related to the exposure and related causally to the disease. For example, cigarette smoking could contribute to an excess of lung cancer among some industrial groups if they smoke more heavily than the average. Conversely, a relationship between oral contraceptives and invasive cervical cancer became apparent only after adjustment was made for interval since last Pap smear, because in this study the frequency of screening was found to be related both to pill use and the development of cervical cancer.[70] Whereas analytical methods can control for known confounders, it cannot do this for unknown confounders, which are free to distort observed risk estimates. The advantage of experimental studies, of course, is that the randomization process tends to ensure that the prevalence of all potential confounders is similar among the randomized groups.

The role of chance is evaluated in epidemiologic studies by the use of significance testing and confidence limits. If a risk estimate is statistically significant at a specified level (*e.g.,* 0.05, or 1 in 20) or if the 95% confidence limits exclude 1.0, chance can be assumed to be an unlikely explanation. It does not of course exclude the operation of a chance event, but only indicates that chance would explain a risk estimate of the observed magnitude or greater only 1 out of 20 times. In studies involving multiple comparisons, some significant associations can be anticipated by the play of chance, and each finding should be considered on its own merits.

DETERMINING CAUSALITY

In interpreting associations found in epidemiologic studies, one is influenced by the magnitude of the risk estimates, their statistical significance (likelihood of being due to chance), and especially the rigor of the study design to avoid methodologic pitfalls. If bias, confounding, and chance are excluded as likely explanations for an association, the issue of causality must be considered through a process of scientific judgment that extends beyond any statement of statistical probability.[13,14,58] During the controversy over cigarette smoking and lung cancer, a set of criteria was formulated to assist the epidemiologist in making causal inferences.[71,72] These criteria provide useful guidelines for determining causality, and refer especially to the strength and specificity of an association, the presence of a dose-response gradient, the consistency and reproducibility of results, biological plausibility and coherence, and an appropriate temporal sequence. It may not be possible to satisfy all the criteria in any particular instance, although evidence that the exposure preceded the disease is obviously crucial.[58] With smaller relative risks, especially when interactions between multiple exposures and susceptibility states seem important, the term risk factors is often used instead of causal agents. The finding of small relative risks should not be readily dismissed as due to chance or bias but explored further by examining possible interactions with other risk factors or susceptible subgroups of the population.

Causal inferences from epidemiology usually develop gradually after taking into account all relevant biological information, including laboratory studies. Although epidemiologic observations can accumulate to the point at which causation is virtually inescapable, strictly speaking it is not possible by these means alone to prove causality. Nevertheless, causation can often be shown to be sufficiently probable to provide a compelling basis for preventive and public health action, and certainly so in the case of cigarette smoking and lung cancer.

CAUSES OF CANCER

This section is intended to provide a brief overview of cancer risk factors, based mainly on evidence from analytical epidemiology, including recent observations relevant to the practicing oncologist. The contributions of epidemiology to cancer etiology and prevention are presented elsewhere in greater detail.[6,7,73,74] Best known is the success of the epidemiologic approach in discovering or confirming a number of lifestyle and other environmental exposures as causes of cancer (Table 13-16).

TOBACCO

Among the carcinogenic hazards identified so far, tobacco smoking is the most important in Western countries and increasingly so in developing countries. Smoking has been firmly linked to cancers not only of the lung but also of the larynx, mouth, pharynx, esophagus, bladder, and pancreas.[75] Recent evidence indicates that smokers are also prone to cancers of the kidney parenchyma[76] and pelvis,[77] cervix,[78] nasal passages,[79] and perhaps stomach cancer[80] and leukemia.[81] The wide variety of neoplasms related to smoking is hardly surprising in view of the large number of chemicals detected in cigarette smoke and delivered to a highly vascular and absorptive organ. In the United States it appears that smoking, especially of cigarettes, accounts for about 40% of all cancer deaths in men and about 20% in women, with lung cancers representing the largest proportion. For smokers of two or more packs per day, the risk of lung cancer is about 20 times that of nonsmokers, and is much greater for squamous and small cell carcinomas than for adenocarcinomas.

Epidemiologic studies have demonstrated the benefits of stopping smoking, with lower risks relative to those of continuing smokers appearing within a few years of quitting.[6,75] This is consistent with evidence that smoking exerts an effect at late as well as early stages of carcinogenesis. The introduction of lower tar levels in cigarettes and of filter tips has also reduced the risk of lung cancer, although not nearly to the extent seen with cessation of smoking.[82] The risks of cigar and pipe smokers resemble those of cigarette smokers for cancers of the oral cavity, larynx, and esophagus, but are lower for lung cancer.

Smokeless tobacco is also of concern, since oral cancer has been linked with snuff dipping, a common practice in rural southern parts of the United States.[44] Under suspicion are the high levels of tobacco-specific nitrosamines that have been detected in snuff and in the saliva of snuff users. In parts of Asia, oral cancer is common in people who use tobacco quids often mixed with betel, lime, and other agents.[83] Overall, these findings have prompted recent public health and legislative measures in the United States aimed at discouraging the use of smokeless tobacco, especially among young people.

Passive smoking has been hotly debated as a risk factor for lung cancer. A review of the available evidence suggests that nonsmoking women married to smokers have experienced an excess risk of the order of 30%.[84] There is little question that passive or involuntary smoking is real, since tobacco smoke constituents and metabolites can be detected in the body fluids of exposed nonsmokers. Moreover, a cause-and-effect relationship with lung cancer is suggested by the replication of findings in different populations, by a dose-response effect with excess risks of about 70% among heavily exposed nonsmokers, by cell type patterns resembling those associated with active smoking, and by the similarity in risk estimates between heavy passive smokers and very light active smokers.

ALCOHOL

Consumption of alcoholic beverages has been shown to potentiate the effects of tobacco smoking on cancers of the mouth, pharynx, esophagus, and larynx, and has been estimated to account for about 3% of all cancer deaths.[85,86] It has been difficult to study the effects of alcohol alone and the

TABLE 13-16. Environmental Causes of Human Cancer

Agent	Type of Exposure	Site of Cancer
Alcoholic beverages	Drinking	Mouth, pharynx, esophagus, larynx, liver
Alkylating agents (melphalan, cyclophosphamide, chlorambucil, semustine)	Medication	Leukemia
Androgen-anabolic steroids	Medication	Liver
Aromatic amines (benzidine, 2-naphthylamine, 4-aminobiphenyl)	Manufacturing of dyes and other chemicals	Bladder
Arsenic (inorganic)	Mining and smelting of certain ores, pesticide manufacturing and use, medication, drinking water	Lung, skin, liver (angiosarcoma)
Asbestos	Manufacturing and use	Lung, pleura, peritoneum
Benzene	Leather, petroleum, and other industries	Leukemia
Bis(chloromethyl)ether	Manufacturing	Lung (small cell)
Chlornaphazine	Medication	Bladder
Chromium compounds	Manufacturing	Lung
Estrogens	Medication	
Synthetic (DES)		Cervix, vagina (adenocarcinoma)
Conjugated (Premarin)		Endometrium
Steroid contraceptives		Liver (benign)
Immunosuppressants (azathoprine, cyclosporin)	Medication	Non-Hodgkin's lymphoma, skin (squamous carcinoma and melanoma), soft tissue tumors (including Kaposi's sarcoma)
Ionizing radiation	Atomic bomb explosions, treatment and diagnosis, radium dial painting, uranium and metal mining	Most sites
Isopropyl alcohol production	Manufacturing by strong acid process	Nasal sinuses
Leather industry	Manufacturing and repair (boot and shoe)	Nasal sinuses, bladder
Mustard gas	Manufacturing	Lung, larynx, nasal sinuses
Nickel dust	Refining	Lung, nasal sinuses
Parasites	Infection	
Schistosoma haematobium		Bladder (squamous carcinoma)
Clonorchis sinensis		Liver (cholangiocarcinoma)
Phenacetin-containing analgesics	Medication	Renal pelvis
Polycyclic hydrocarbons	Coal carbonization products and some mineral oils	Lung, skin (squamous carcinoma)
Tobacco chews, including betel nut	Snuff dipping and chewing of tobacco, betel, lime	Mouth
Tobacco smoke	Smoking, especially cigarettes	Lung, larynx, mouth, pharynx, esophagus, bladder, pancreas, kidney
Ultraviolet radiation	Sunlight	Skin (including melanoma), lip
Viruses	Infection	
Epstein-Barr virus		Burkitt's lymphoma; nasopharyngeal carcinoma (?)
Hepatitis-B virus		Hepatocellular carcinoma
Human T-lymphotrophic virus, type I		T-cell leukemia/lymphoma
Vinyl chloride	Manufacturing of polyvinyl chloride	Liver (angiosarcoma)
Wood dusts	Furniture manufacturing (hardwood)	Nasal sinuses (adenocarcinoma)

nature of the interaction with smoking because of small numbers in certain categories of exposure (especially drinkers who abstain from smoking). In a large-scale case-control study of oral cancer, the risks shown in Table 13-17 increased with intake of alcohol among nonsmokers, but in combination with smoking the risks multiplied to 35-fold among heavy consumers of both products.[87] Combined exposures were found to account for about three fourths of all oral and pharyngeal cancers. The risks were not uniform for all forms of alcohol, being higher with hard liquor or beer than with wine. For esophageal cancer, the highest recorded risks from alcohol are those associated with the consumption of home-brewed apple brandies in the northwest part of France. For larynx cancer, the alcohol effect is more prominent for tumors occurring in the supraglottic than in the intrinsic segments. Since ethanol is not carcinogenic in laboratory animals, the mechanism by which alcohol acts is not clear, but it may involve nutritional deficiencies that accompany drinking, contaminants such as nitrosamines and hydrocarbons, or increased permeability of mucous membranes to other carcinogens.

Alcohol is an important cause of hepatic cirrhosis, which is sometimes complicated by hepatocellular carcinoma, although alcohol may also have an independent effect on the risk of this cancer. The role of alcohol in other cancers remains uncertain. Rectal cancer in men has shown positive geographic correlations with beer consumption, but the findings from analytical studies have been inconsistent. For example, cohort studies of brewery workers (who receive a free beer allocation) have revealed an excess risk of rectal cancer in Dublin but not in Copenhagen.[88] Recent interest has centered around the possible relationship of alcohol with breast cancer, with a series of prospective studies showing an excess risk and dose-response gradient.[89,90] Further investigation is needed to determine if this relationship is causal, or if indirect, how it is mediated.

OCCUPATIONAL HAZARDS

The study of occupational groups has identified more carcinogens than any other branch of cancer epidemiology and has led to cancer prevention by reducing or eliminating hazardous exposures in the workplace.[91,92] Occupational exposures may account for about 5% of all cancer deaths, while the proportion is higher in certain areas for particular cancers, such as those of the bladder and lung. Most carcinogenic exposures in the workplace were first detected by clinicians, while others were noted initially by epidemiologists as in the case of asbestos (lung cancer), inorganic arsenic (lung cancer), and the leather industry (nasal cancer), or by experimentalists, as in the case of 4-aminobiphenyl.[2] It is noteworthy that all compounds shown to be carcinogenic in humans have been positive in long-term animal testing, except for arsenic and alcohol. This argues for the importance of bioassay programs, but the exceptions remind us that it may not be prudent to rely solely on laboratory work.

Asbestos represents the major occupational carcinogen in many countries due to its induction of lung cancers rather than mesotheliomas. This is true despite the fact that the relative risk for lung cancer is little more than twofold, whereas that for mesotheliomas is well over 100-fold, the reason being that lung cancer is much more common than mesothelioma in people unexposed to asbestos. A multiplicative relationship exists between asbestos exposure and smoking in the development of lung cancer.[93] As shown in Figure 13-7, American shipyard workers (whose exposure to asbestos was heavy during World War II) have experienced a high incidence, but the far greater excess among smokers than nonsmokers indicates a synergism between the risk factors.[42] The risks also vary according to the type of asbestos fiber and are highest for crocidolite, which is now banned in many countries. Much research is in progress on man-made mineral fibers, but as yet there is no clear evidence of a carcinogenic risk to humans.[92]

Many of the occupational cancers listed in Table 13-16 are characterized by high relative risks and specificity of cell type. A challenge facing epidemiologists is to detect hazards with smaller relative risks that may have a greater impact on the public health when the exposure is widespread and the tumor in question is common. This problem is particularly acute for lung cancer because variations in the prevalence and duration of smoking may mask the detection of occupational risks. The discovery of occupational hazards may also have implications beyond the workplace, since they may point to potential risks experienced at a lower level by the general public.

TABLE 13-17. Relative Risks for Oral and Pharyngeal Cancer Associated with Smoking and Drinking

| Smoking Status | Number of Alcohol Drinks Per Week | | | | |
	<1	1–4	5–14	15–24	30+
Nonsmoker	1.0	1.3	1.6	1.4	5.8
Former smoker	0.7	2.2	1.4	3.2	6.4
Light smoker	1.7	1.5	2.7	5.4	7.9
Moderate smoker	1.9	2.4	4.4	7.2	23.8
Heavy smoker	7.4	0.7	4.4	20.2	37.7

Adapted from Blot WJ, McLaughlin JK, Winn DM, et al: Smoking and drinking in relation to oral and pharyngeal cancer. Cancer Res 48:3282, 1988.
* Light, moderate, and heavy smokers: 1–19, 20–39, and 40+ cigarettes per day for 20+ years, respectively.

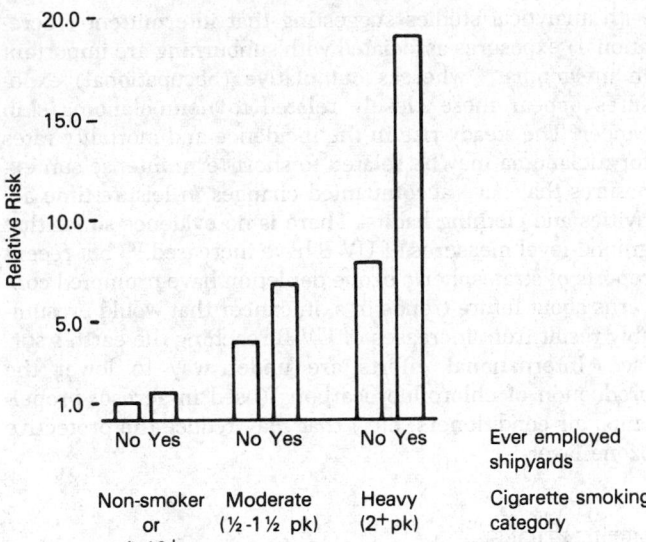

FIG. 13-7. Relative risk of lung cancer according to usual cigarette-smoking category and employment in shipyards during World War II. (Blot WJ, Harrington JM, Toledo A, et al: Lung cancer after employment in shipyards during World War II. N Engl J Med 299:620, 1978)

ENVIRONMENTAL POLLUTION

Pollutants in the urban air have long been suspected in the etiology of lung cancer, with fossil fuel combustion products, especially polycyclic hydrocarbons, being of special concern. The subject has been difficult to study, primarily due to the overpowering effects of smoking, which first became popular in urban areas. Nevertheless, there is suggestive evidence that atmospheric pollution plays a limited role in the causation of lung cancer.[6]

Asbestos bodies and calcified pleural plaques are common in urban populations, but the risks of cancer following non-occupational exposures are uncertain. There are many case reports suggesting that mesotheliomas may result from neighborhood exposures to asbestos industries and from household contact with asbestos dust, perhaps through the laundering of work clothing.[94] A striking example of an environmental carcinogen is the naturally occurring zeolite fiber in parts of Turkey that causes a high mortality from pleural mesothelioma.[95] Another hazard may result from airborne arsenic, because increased mortality rates for lung cancer have been reported in both sexes in the neighborhood of arsenic-emitting smelters that cannot be explained by smoking and occupational exposures.[96]

There is much current interest in the role of indoor air pollution by radon gas and tobacco smoke in lung cancer etiology. In China, the high rates of lung cancer among nonsmoking women have been related to cooking oil vapors generated by wok cooking[97] and to effluents from coal-heating stoves.[98] Also under investigation are contaminants in drinking water, especially since several halogenated organic compounds produced during chlorination are carcinogenic

and mutagenic in laboratory tests. A large case-control study of bladder cancer has found a modest excess risk associated with prolonged use of chlorinated surface water,[99] and studies are underway to see if this risk can be confirmed and whether it extends to other cancers. It has been estimated that only about 2% of cancer deaths are due to environmental pollution,[6] but this estimate is based on limited data and may be modified by the results of future research.

IONIZING RADIATION

Along with tobacco smoking, more is known about the carcinogenic effects of ionizing radiation than about any other human carcinogen.[100] This dates from early observations on radiologists to the comprehensive studies among survivors of the atomic bombs in Japan and among patients receiving radiotherapy for ankylosing spondylitis. It is difficult to measure directly the effects of low doses of ionizing radiation, such as x-rays or gamma rays, and extrapolations have to be made from populations exposed to high and moderate doses for medical, occupational, or military reasons. Although a great deal has been learned about the carcinogenic risks of radiation therapy used for many conditions, there is little firm data about risks from the lower doses of diagnostic radiation, except for a 50% increase of leukemia and other childhood cancers associated with prenatal exposures.

It has been estimated that approximately 3% of all cancer deaths may be attributed to radiation,[101] but the upper limit might be twice as high if certain estimates are confirmed about the risks of lung cancer associated with indoor levels of radon emanating mainly from soils containing uranium deposits. Studies of underground miners exposed to relatively high doses of alpha-radiation have shown excess lung cancer risks, even at levels that might be attained through long-term residential exposure in some parts of the United States.[102] More reliable data should come from ongoing case-control studies of lung cancer that involve careful measurements of indoor radon.

Nearly all sites of the body appear vulnerable to the carcinogenic effects of radiation, with the most radiosensitive tissues being the bone marrow, breast, and thyroid.[103] The patterns of risk provide insights into mechanisms of carcinogenesis and guidelines for radiation protection. For example, radiogenic leukemia shows a distinctive wave-like pattern with the excess risk starting 2 to 4 years after exposure, peaking at 6 to 8 years, and declining to normal within 25 years. In contrast, radiogenic carcinomas have a minimal latent period of 5 to 10 years and a temporal distribution that resembles the natural age-specific incidence curve, suggesting the influence of other factors acting at a later stage of carcinogenesis. The advent of large-scale mammography has renewed interest in the breast cancer experience of atomic bomb survivors and women exposed to medical x-rays. Despite a reasonably linear dose-response curve for breast cancer, the radiation effect is most pronounced among young women and is not evident among those who were exposed after age 40. This finding is reassuring for women in midlife who are most likely to undergo periodic screening with mammography.

SOLAR RADIATION

Ultraviolet (UV) radiation from sunlight is the major risk factor for skin cancer, both squamous and basal cell carcinomas and melanoma.[104] The evidence includes the tendency of tumors to arise on sun-exposed sites, the high incidence associated with outdoor activities, and the predisposition of fair-complexioned people who sunburn easily. Exceptionally high risks of skin cancer occur among persons with genetic diseases exacerbated by sunlight (xeroderma pigmentosum and albinism). Furthermore, in experimental animals, repeated doses of UV radiation, particularly in the UV-B spectral range (290 to 320 nm), can induce skin cancer. In addition, about one half of the melanomas appear to arise from dysplastic nevi, a fairly recently described precursor state that should greatly expand opportunities for early detection and treatment.[105]

Since incidence data for nonmelanoma skin cancer are not collected routinely by most population-based cancer registries, special surveys in the United States were conducted in the 1970s as an adjunct to the SEER program together with measures of UV-B radiation at ground level.[106] The gradient with UV-B levels was steepest for squamous cell carcinoma followed by basal cell carcinoma, and was least apparent for melanoma (Figure 13-8). These differences are consistent

with analytical studies suggesting that intermittent (recreational) exposures associated with sunburning are important in melanoma,[49] whereas cumulative (occupational) exposures appear more closely related to nonmelanoma skin cancer. The steady rise in the incidence and mortality rates for melanoma may be related to short-term intense sun exposures that have accompanied changes in leisure-time activities and clothing habits. There is no evidence so far that ground-level measures of UV-B have increased,[107] but recent reports of stratospheric ozone depletion have prompted concerns about future trends in skin cancer that would presumably result from increases of UV-B reaching the earth's surface. International efforts are under way to lower the production of chlorofluorocarbons (used in aerosol propellants, air conditioners, etc.) that may reduce the protective ozone layer.

MEDICATIONS

Several carcinogens included in Table 13-16 have been detected by studies of patients exposed to medicinal agents that may account for as much as 2% of all cancers. Some drugs have been withdrawn from clinical practice, whereas others are retained because their benefits are judged to outweigh

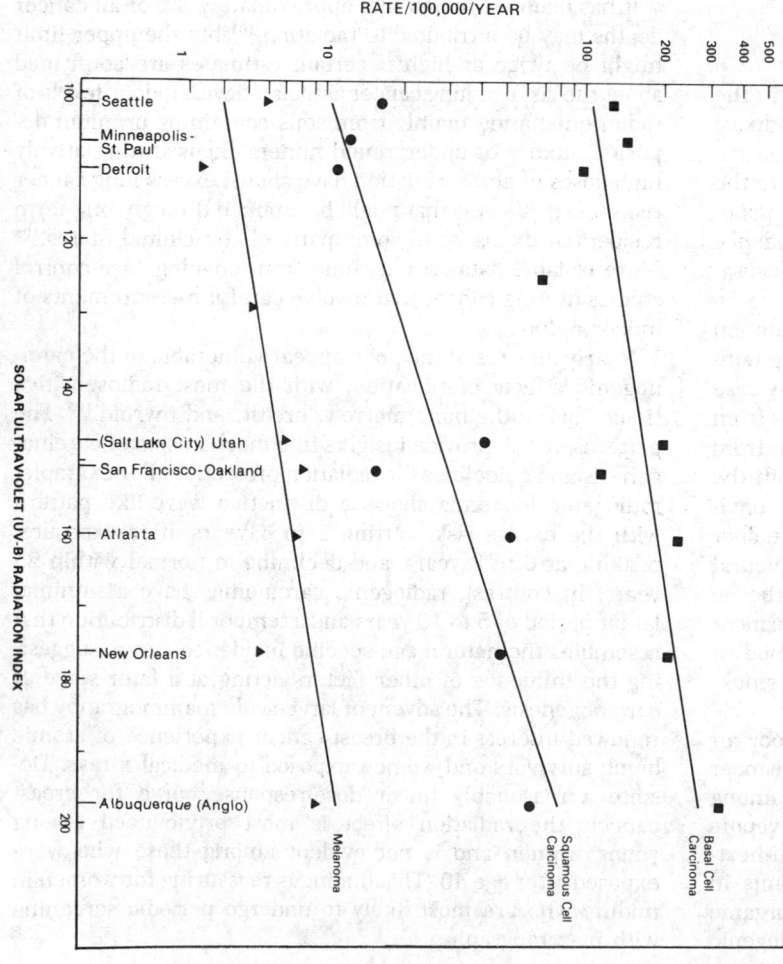

FIG. 13-8. Annual age-adjusted incidence rates for basal and squamous cell carcinomas and melanoma among white females, according to annual UV-B measurements at selected areas of the United States. (Scotto J, Fraumeni JF Jr: Skin (other than melanoma). In Schottenfeld D, Fraumeni JF Jr [eds]: Cancer Epidemiology and Prevention, p 996. Philadelphia, WB Saunders, 1982. Melanoma data are from the SEER program [1973–1976] and nonmelanoma data from a special survey [1977–1978]. Regression lines are based on exponential model.)

their side effects. A major discovery was that synthetic estrogens given during pregnancy produced adenocarcinomas of the vagina and cervix several years later in daughters exposed in utero.[108] This was the first demonstration of transplacental carcinogenesis in humans. Endometrial cancer can result from conjugated estrogens taken for menopausal symptoms, and some studies have suggested an excess of breast cancer in long-term users.[109] Oral contraceptives are still under evaluation, with some studies suggesting an elevated risk of breast cancer when there is early and prolonged use or when there exist predisposing conditions such as familial occurrence or benign breast disease.[110-112] Also, a relationship of pill use to invasive cervical cancer is suggested by recent studies that have controlled carefully for confounding variables such as sexual activity and screening history.[70] It is noteworthy that a reduced risk of endometrial and ovarian cancers has been reported with the combined oral contraceptives, especially following long-term use. The effects of exogenous hormones, along with the relation of female cancers to reproductive and menstrual variables, indicate the importance of investigating endogenous hormones as risk factors.[112,113]

An excess risk of acute nonlymphocytic leukemia has been noted among patients receiving alkylating agents, especially melphalan, cyclophosphamide, and chlorambucil.[62] Thus, the monitoring of carcinogenic risks should be part of randomized therapy trials. For example, when semustine (methyl-CCNU) was evaluated as adjuvant therapy for gastrointestinal cancer, the risks of leukemia and preleukemia were found to be elevated, with a clear dose-response relationship (Table 13-18).[114,115] This finding demonstrates the importance of carefully weighing risks and benefits in designing treatment regimens involving alkylating agents, especially for those cancer patients with a low risk of relapse or for patients with nonmalignant diseases.

Immunosuppressive agents, particularly azathioprine, have been assessed mainly by studies of renal transplant recipients. The risk of non-Hodgkin's lymphoma is very high within a few months of transplantation and remains at about the same level.[116,117] This rapid onset is in marked contrast to the usual behavior of chemical carcinogens and suggests activation of a latent oncogenic virus by immunologic mechanisms. Contrary to the prediction of the "immunosurveil-lance hypothesis" as first proposed, the increase of other cancers is not generalized but is confined to particular types such as squamous carcinoma of the skin, melanoma, Kaposi's sarcoma, and liver cancer (Table 13-19). Although the risk of post-transplant lymphoma might be influenced by antigenic stimulation by the graft, patients treated with azathioprine for other conditions have shown an approximately 10-fold excess of lymphoma.[117] A predominance of lymphomas has been seen also with primary immunodeficiency disorders such as ataxia-telangiectasia, Wiskott-Aldrich syndrome, and the X-linked lymphoproliferative syndrome.[118] For lymphomas in the latter group as well as in transplant patients, there is evidence of causation by the Epstein-Barr virus (EBV).[119] This finding is consistent with animal experiments, indicating that immunosurveillance primarily operates against viral-induced neoplasms.

VIRUSES

The laboratory discovery of many different oncogenic viruses in animals has long suggested that some human cancers have a similar etiology, but convincing evidence in humans was slow to emerge until recently.[120] The proportion of viral-related cancer in the United States has been roughly estimated at 5%,[6] but one can only speculate about upper bounds as rapid advances in molecular virology are made. However, the estimate must surpass 5% in certain developing countries.

EBV is widely considered the necessary cause of endemic Burkitt's lymphoma and perhaps also nasopharyngeal cancer.[121] In Burkitt's lymphoma, holoendemic malaria appears to enhance the oncogenic effect of EBV and produce uneven distribution and occasional clustering of the lymphoma in Africa. EBV appears involved also in the lymphomas that occur in certain immunodeficiency disorders, perhaps by interacting with immunologic and genetic mechanisms. The relation of EBV to nasopharyngeal cancer has been suggested by the higher antibody levels seen in patients than in controls, and the presence of viral genome in epithelial cells from the tumor. The high rates of this cancer in southern China cannot be attributed to EBV infection alone, and other risk factors such as consumption of salted fish or histocompatibility antigens appear to be involved.

TABLE 13-18. Risk of Leukemic Disorders According to Dose of Semustine

	Cumulative Dosage (mg/m²)				
	0	1-	500-	750-	1000+
Number of leukemic disorders	1	3	3	7	5
Number of patients	1,566	714	442	633	278
Relative risk*	1.0	8.7	10.5	18.7	36.9
Five-year cumulative risk (%)†	0.1	0.8	1.2	1.1	2.5

Adapted from Boice JD Jr, Greene MH, Killen JY Jr, et al: Leukemia after adjuvant chemotherapy with semustine (methyl-CCNU)—Evidence of a dose-response effect. N Engl J Med 314:119, 1986.

* The referent category was those who did not receive semustine. Maximum likelihood estimates of relative risk were adjusted for survival times.

† Cumulative probabilities were estimated by the Kaplan-Meier technique (Kaplan EL, Meier P: Nonparametric estimation from incomplete observations. J Am Stat Assoc 53:457, 1958).

TABLE 13-19.   Relative Risk of Certain Cancers in Renal Transplant Recipients in Two Major Studies (with Observed Cancers in Parentheses)

Types of Cancer	United Kingdom-Australasian Study	American College of Surgeons Study*
All types†	2.8 (86)	2.8 (136)
Non-Hodgkin's lymphoma	45.9 (42)	26.9 (53)
Primary liver cancer	37.5 (3)	20.0 (4)
Skin melanoma	8.7 (2)	2.5 (5)
Other cancer‡	1.3 (39)	1.7 (74)

Adapted from Kinlen LJ: Immunosuppressive therapy and cancer. Cancer Surv 1:565, 1982.
* Based on unpublished data from Hoover RN and Fraumeni JF Jr.
† Excludes cervix cancer in situ and nonmelanoma skin cancer, although increases in squamous carcinoma of skin have been reported.
‡ Includes excesses of mesenchymal tumors, notably Kaposi's sarcoma.

Hepatitis-B virus (HBV) infection is an important cause of hepatocellular carcinoma, especially in endemic regions of Asia and Africa. The most convincing evidence comes from a cohort study of 22,707 men in Taiwan in which the risk of liver carcinoma was more than 200 times greater among carriers of hepatitis-B surface antigen than among noncarriers (Table 13-20).[122] It is possible that the oncogenic effects of hepatitis-B are enhanced by early-life infection and dietary exposures to aflatoxin.

The high incidence of adult T-cell leukemia in certain areas, such as Japan and the Caribbean, has been linked to infection with the human T-lymphotrophic virus type I (HTLV-I), the first retrovirus to be detected in humans.[123] In endemic areas the virus appears to be transmitted early in life and may also be spread by sexual activity, drug abuse, and blood transfusions.

Another human retrovirus, now called the human immunodeficiency virus (HIV), has been shown to cause the acquired immunodeficiency syndrome (AIDS).[124] Recognized since 1981, AIDS in the United States affects mainly homosexual men, hemophiliacs, and intravenous drug abusers, and predisposes to Kaposi's sarcoma and non-Hodgkin's lymphoma. The much higher incidence of Kaposi's sarcoma among male homosexuals than other high-risk groups with AIDS suggests that an oncogenic agent is superimposed on HIV infection and is also sexually transmitted. The classic or endemic form of Kaposi's sarcoma in Africa and Mediterranean areas has been associated with cytomegalovirus infection in some studies, but the findings in AIDS patients suggest that it is a passenger virus.

The relationship of cervical cancer to multiple sexual partners has long suggested the venereal transmission of an infectious agent. Although herpes simplex virus type 2 has been a candidate agent for some time, the chief suspect at present is the human papillomavirus (HPV). DNA sequences from certain HPV types, notably HPV-16 and HPV-18, have been found in a high percentage of biopsies from invasive cervical cancer.[125] HPV has been isolated also from many vulvar, penile, and anal cancers, as well as from squamous cell skin cancers associated with the genetic syndrome of epidermodysplasia verruciformis.

Investigations of clusters of leukemia or lymphoma in the community have provided no solid clues to etiology, and statistical studies have not detected any general tendency for space-time clustering of these tumors. A viral origin for Hodgkin's disease in young adults has been suggested by its association with certain childhood environments, such as small family size, that would tend to reduce or delay early-life exposures to infections, such as in paralytic poliomyelitis.[54] EBV has been suspected, since antibody levels tend to be higher in cases than controls and an increased risk of Hodgkin's disease has been reported among persons with infectious mononucleosis. However, molecular viral studies have not been supportive and the relationship with EBV may

TABLE 13-20.   Deaths from Liver Disease According to Hepatitis-B Surface Antigen (HBsAg) Status on Recruitment into Study

HBsAg Status	Cause of Death		Population at Risk	Mortality from Liver Cancer*
	Liver Cancer	Cirrhosis		
Positive	40	17	3,454	1158
Negative	1	2	19,253	5
Total	41	19	22,707	181

Adapted from Beasley RP, Hwang L-Y, Lin C-C, et al: Hepatocellular carcinoma and hepatitis-B virus. Lancet 2:1129, 1981.
* Mortality from primary hepatocellular carcinoma per 100,000 during study period.

be indirect. Despite mounting evidence for oncogenic viruses in humans, there is no indication that any form of cancer is contagious.

DIET AND NUTRITION

When viewed in the light of experimental work showing how dietary manipulation can influence the yield of tumors in laboratory animals, the recent growth of interest in dietary causes of human cancer seems not merely logical but overdue. International correlations and migrant studies also suggest that certain aspects of the affluent Western diet contribute to a sizable but uncertain proportion of all cancers. Various hypotheses about causative and protective factors are under intensive study, but the specific dietary components are elusive and the mechanisms of action appear complex. Problems stem from the inherent limitations of nutritional methods such as dietary recall, but progress may come from cohort studies in which specimens have been stored for subsequent biochemical assay and from intervention studies to determine whether certain dietary modifications and nutrient supplements exert a protective effect against cancer.

Dietary fat has been suggested as a risk factor for certain cancers, especially of the breast and large bowel, by the strongly positive correlations that exist between age-adjusted rates in different countries and per capita consumption of fat.[126] However, the results of case-control and cohort studies have not provided strong support for the fat hypothesis.[48,127,128] Furthermore, no positive relationship has been found between the levels of serum cholesterol, which are influenced by fat intake, and subsequent risk of breast or large bowel cancers. The issue is complicated by methodological difficulties in estimating intake of fat and different types of fat, the limited variation in fat consumption within many countries, problems in evaluating dietary habits in early life (which may be especially important for breast cancer), and difficulties in distinguishing fat per se from calories (since fat is more calorigenic than other nutrients). Calories may influence the risk of breast and other reproductive cancers by increasing body weight or size, for obesity is an established risk factor for certain cancers in women, especially cancer of the endometrium.[50] It is possible that obesity elevates the risk of endometrial and breast cancers by increasing the serum levels of circulating estrogens through a conversion from androstenedione in adipose tissue and perhaps also by a lowering of the sex-hormone binding globulin.[112,113]

Evidence is accumulating that a low intake of certain food groups may predispose to cancer, and indeed a lower consumption of green vegetables and fresh fruit has been one of the more consistent findings in dietary studies of cancer. A protective action for fiber was proposed by Burkitt, who was impressed by the low rates of colon cancer in parts of Africa where fiber intake and stool bulk were high. Correlational studies have indicated that fiber intake, especially when measured as nonstarch polysaccharides, tends to be lower in high-incidence regions.[129] Although the results are less consistent, there is some support from case-control studies that fiber protects against colon cancer.[130] However, the subject is complicated by the relatively crude characterization of fiber and by difficulty in separating the effects of micronutrients found in fiber sources such as fruits and vegetables.

Micronutrients may be responsible for the inverse risks associated with the intake of fruits and vegetables. Several epithelial cancers, especially of the lung, show this negative relationship both in case-control studies and some cohort studies employing serologic tests; the effect has been attributed by some workers to beta-carotene.[48,131] More limited evidence suggests that vitamin C may protect against gastric and certain other cancers, perhaps by blocking the endogenous formation of nitrosamines. However, other components of fruits and vegetables have been suggested as protective factors in experimental and epidemiological studies, for example, indole compounds in cruciferous vegetables that may decrease the risk of colon cancer,[132] and allyl sulfide in garlic and onions that may lower the risk of gastric cancer.[80] The effects of vitamin E, selenium, and calcium are also under study. Furthermore, mixed or multiple deficiencies in the diet may be involved in some tumors, especially among populations with high risks of esophageal cancer.[133] Intervention studies are ideally suited to test the micronutrient hypotheses, and the results of several ongoing trials are awaited with interest.

A variety of other dietary factors, including additives and contaminants, have attracted attention. The consumption of aflatoxin, a carcinogenic metabolite of the fungus *Aspergillus flavus*, has been linked to liver cancer by correlation studies and more recently by a case-control study.[134] A relationship between salted foods and stomach cancer has been claimed in some studies,[80] but this has not been consistently observed. The consumption of salted fish containing high concentrations of nitrosamines has been linked to the high rates of nasopharyngeal cancer in Hong Kong and southern China.[135] Coffee intake has been associated with bladder and pancreatic cancers, but this has not been confirmed in many other studies and there is no evidence for a causal relationship. The artificial sweeteners saccharin and cyclamate cause bladder cancer in laboratory animals, but a large case-control study of bladder cancer indicated that the risk in humans at past levels of consumption is very small if present at all.[136] Cooking practices may generate hydrocarbons or other carcinogens in the food at high temperatures, but no relevant epidemiologic data are available.

GENETIC SUSCEPTIBILITY

Although the geographic and ethnic differentials for most cancers appear largely determined by environmental influences, genetic factors may contribute to some high rates (*e.g.*, nasopharyngeal cancer among Chinese and gallbladder cancer among American Indians) as well as some low rates (*e.g.*, testicular cancer and Ewing's sarcoma among blacks in Africa and the United States). Genetic susceptibility is most evident for skin cancer, with geographic and ethnic variations corresponding to the degree of protective skin pigmentation. The apparently limited evidence for genetic factors based on these patterns, however, does not exclude even large variations in individual susceptibility. Furthermore, the relatively small differences in risk between close relatives of patients with cancer and other people for childhood tumors other than retinoblastoma are in fact consistent with large differences in genetic predisposition. The truth of this perhaps surprising statement can be demonstrated mathematically.[137] Only with advances in biochemical and molecular methods, however, does it seem possible to further define the impact of genetic factors or genetic-environmental interactions in cancer etiology.[138] For example, the phenotype associated with the rapid metabolic oxidation of certain drugs appears to influence the risk of smoking-related lung cancer,[139] supporting the long-held suspicion that certain persons have a higher risk of smoking-induced lung cancer than others because of genetic constitution. The claim is sometimes made that the proportion of people who are susceptible to cancer is limited, with variations only in the specific sites affected (Cramer's hypothesis). This notion has been shown to be false[5] and has given way to mutation models and genetic hypotheses[140] that are stimulating further research into the nature of cancer susceptibility genes.

Although only a small fraction of cancer is inherited in a mendelian fashion, over 200 single-gene disorders have been linked to neoplasia.[141] This does not include several constitutional cytogenetic disorders that predispose to cancer, such as Down's syndrome with leukemia, Klinefelter's syndrome with mediastinal teratoma, gonadal dysgenesis with gonadoblastoma, and aniridia with Wilms' tumor.[66] Table 13-21 lists some cancers that occur as an inherited trait (hereditary neoplasms) and Table 13-22 presents those arising as a complication of inherited precursor lesions (preneoplastic states). Included are several syndromes in which sunlight contributes to multiple skin cancers, including the dysplastic nevus syndrome predisposing to melanoma and xeroderma pigmentosum predisposing to a variety of skin cancers. Genetically determined neoplasms tend to occur earlier in life than other cancers of the same anatomic type and often have a multifocal origin. In addition, several common neoplasms such as breast and colon cancers show small familial risks of the order of twofold to threefold, but among subgroups of patients with onset at young ages and bilateral or multifocal origin, the risks may be as high as 20- to 30-fold.[142] Some families show remarkable aggregations of site-specific cancer that appear consistent with autosomal dominant inheritance. However, because cancer is so common, it is sometimes difficult to know whether familial clusters are simply due to chance, especially if different types of cancer are involved.[143] In this circumstance it can be useful to consider the possibility of a familial multiple-cancer syndrome. A distinct pattern is seen, for example, with a familial aggregation involving several childhood and adult cancers, including soft-tissue and bone sarcomas, breast carcinoma, brain tumors, leukemia, and adrenocortical neoplasms (the Li-Fraumeni cancer family syndrome).[144,145] Family members with this syndrome are prone to multiple primary cancers, including radiogenic sarcomas. Currently, molecular studies including DNA probes are attempting to understand the genetic events and biological mechanisms that may be shared by a variety of neoplasms, including breast cancer.[146,147] Thus, by delineating genetic and familial syndromes of cancer, clinicians have been instrumental not only in helping to identify and protect high-risk individuals but also in pointing experimentalists to new research opportunities. A multidisciplinary approach to genetic susceptibility ranging from clinical observations and epidemiology to molecular biology shows promise in identifying carcinogenic mechanisms, and thus may have consequences in cancer prevention that are at least as important as the detection of environmental carcinogens.

Table 13-21. Hereditary Neoplasms

	Inheritance*	Features
Retinoblastoma	AD	Susceptibility to second primary tumors, including osteosarcoma of leg and radiogenic sarcoma of orbit; chromosome deletion (13q14) in some cases
Nevoid basal cell carcinoma	AD	Basal cell cancers of skin increased by UV and ionizing radiation; medulloblastoma, ovarian fibromas, and developmental defects in some cases
Multiple endocrine neoplasia I	AD	Adenomas of anterior pituitary, parathyroid, pancreatic islet cells, thyroid, and adrenal cortex; carcinoid tumors of intestine and bronchus in some cases
Multiple endocrine neoplasia II	AD	Pheochromocytoma and medullary thyroid carcinoma; parathyroid tumors and neurofibromas in some cases
Polyposis coli	AD	Multiple adenomatous polyps and adenocarcinomas of large bowel; some families exhibit osteomas, fibromas, lipomas, and epidermal cysts (Gardner's syndrome)
Dysplastic nevus syndrome	AD	Hereditary melanomas derived from nevi, especially after sun exposure

* AD, autosomal dominant.

TABLE 13-22. Hereditary Preneoplastic Syndromes

	Inheritance*	Neoplasms
Phacomatoses		
Neurofibromatosis	AD	Sarcomatous change in the neurofibromas of 10% of cases; gliomas of brain and optic nerve, acoustic neuromas, meningiomas, and acute leukemia
Tuberous sclerosis	AD	Hamartomatous growths in several organs; brain tumors, chiefly giant-cell astrocytoma, in 1%–3% of patients
von Hippel-Lindau syndrome	AD	Angiomatosis of retina and cerebellum; renal adenocarcinoma, pheochromocytoma, and ependymoma in some cases
Peutz-Jeghers syndrome	AD	Rare malignant change in hamartomatous polyps of gastrointestinal tract; ovarian neoplasms in 5% of female patients
Cowden's multiple hamartoma syndrome	AD	Oral papillomas, cystic mastopathy and breast cancer, thyroid and colonic neoplasms
Genodermatoses		
Xeroderma pigmentosum	AR	Various skin cancers in all patients exposed to sunlight
Albinism	AR	Skin cancers, chiefly squamous, in sun-exposed areas
Epidermodysplasia verruciformis	AR	Skin cancers, chiefly squamous, in multiple warts induced by papillomavirus
Werner's syndrome (adult progeria)	AR	Soft tissue sarcoma, other tumors
Chromosome instability		
Bloom's syndrome	AR	Acute leukemia, non-Hodgkin's lymphoma, other cancers
Fanconi's anemia	AR	Acute myelomonocytic leukemia and squamous carcinoma of mucous membranes; hepatoma reported after androgen-anabolic steroids
Immune deficiency		
Ataxia-telangiectasia	AR	Non-Hodgkin's lymphoma, acute lymphocytic leukemia, stomach cancer, other tumors; heterozygous carriers prone to cancer, especially of the breast
Common variable immunodeficiency	?AR	Non-Hodgkin's lymphoma, stomach cancer
Wiskott-Aldrich syndrome	XR	Non-Hodgkin's lymphoma, acute leukemia
X-linked (Bruton's) agammaglobulinemia	XR	Non-Hodgkin's lymphoma, acute leukemia
X-linked lymphoproliferative syndrome	XR	Non-Hodgkin's lymphoma, plasmacytoma

* AD, autosomal dominant; AR, autosomal recessive; XR, X-linked recessive.

REFERENCES

1. Shimkin MB: Contrary to Nature. National Institutes of Health (NIH) Report 76–720. Washington, DC, US Government Printing Office, 1977
2. Doll R: Pott and the prospects for prevention. Br J Cancer 32:263, 1975
3. Doll R: The epidemiology of cancer. Cancer 45:2475, 1980
4. MacMahon B, Pugh TF: Epidemiology: Principles and Methods. Boston, Little, Brown, 1970
5. Doll R: An epidemiologic perspective of the biology of cancer. Cancer Res 38:3573, 1978
5. Doll R, Peto R: The causes of cancer. JNCI 66:1191, 1981
7. Schottenfeld D, Fraumeni JF Jr (eds): Cancer Epidemiology and Prevention. Philadelphia, WB Saunders, 1982
8. Muir CS, Malhotra A: Changing patterns of cancer incidence in five continents. Gann Monogr Cancer Res 33:3, 1987
9. Hill AB: Principles of Medical Statistics. New York, Oxford University Press, 1966
10. Young JL Jr, Percy CL, Asire AJ (eds): Surveillance, Epidemiology, and End Results: Incidence and Mortality Data, 1973–77. Natl Cancer Inst Monogr 57, 1981
11. Feldman AR, Kessler L, Myers MH, et al: The prevalence of cancer: Estimates based on the Connecticut Tumor Registry. N Engl J Med 315:1394, 1986
12. Decoufle P, Thomas TL, Pickle LW: Comparison of the proportionate mortality ratio and standardized mortality ratio risk measures. Am J Epidemiol 111:263, 1980
13. Kelsey JL, Thompson WD, Evans AS: Methods in Observational Epidemiology. New York, Oxford University Press, 1986
14. Lilienfeld A, Pederson E, Dowd JE: Cancer Epidemiology: Methods of Study. Baltimore, Johns Hopkins Press, 1967

15. Gordon T, Crittenden M, Haenszel W: Cancer mortality trends in the United States, 1930–1955. Natl Cancer Inst Mongr 6:133, 1961

16. Burbank F: Patterns in Cancer Mortality in the United States: 1950–1967. Natl Cancer Inst Mongr 33, 1971

17. Mason TJ, McKay FW: US Cancer Mortality by County: 1950–1969. DHEW Publication No. (NIH)74–615. Washington, DC, US Government Printing Office, 1974

18. Mason TJ, McKay FW, Hoover R, et al: Atlas of Cancer Mortality for US Counties: 1950–1969. DHEW Publication No. (NIH)75–780. Washington, DC, US Government Printing Office, 1975

19. Mason TJ, McKay FW, Hoover R, et al: Atlas of Cancer Mortality among US Nonwhites: 1950–1969. DHEW Publication No. (NIH)76–1204. Washington, DC, US Government Printing Office, 1976

20. Riggan WB, Van Bruggen J, Acquavella JF, et al: US Cancer Mortality Rates and Trends, 1950–1979, Vols 1–3. Publication No. EPA-600/1–83–015a. Washington, DC, US Government Printing Office, 1983

21. Pickle LW, Mason TJ, Howard N, et al: Atlas of US Cancer Mortality Rates and Trends among Whites, 1950–1980. DHHS Publication No. (NIH)87–2900. Washington, DC, US Government Printing Office, 1987

22. McKay FW, Hanson MR, Miller RW: Cancer Mortality in the United States: 1950–1977. Natl Cancer Inst Monogr 59, 1982

23. Devesa SS, Silverman DT: Cancer incidence and mortality trends in the United States: 1935–74. J Natl Cancer Inst 60:545, 1978

24. Devesa SS, Silverman DT, Young JL Jr, et al: Cancer incidence and mortality trends among whites in the United States, 1947–84. JNCI 79:701, 1987

25. Segi M, Aoki K, Kurihara M: World cancer mortality. Gann Monogr Cancer Res 26:121, 1981

26. Percy C, Stanek E III, Gloeckler L: Accuracy of cancer death certificates and its effect on cancer mortality statistics. Am J Public Health 71:242, 1981

27. Heston JF, Kelly JB, Meigs JW, et al (eds): Forty-five Years of Cancer Incidence in Connecticut: 1935–79. Natl Cancer Inst Monogr 70, 1986

28. Dorn HF, Cutler SJ: Morbidity from Cancer in the United States: Parts I and II. Public Health Monogr 56, 1959

29. Haenszel W, Marcus SC, Zimmerer EG: Cancer morbidity in Urban and Rural Iowa. Public Health Monogr 37, 1956

30. Cutler SJ, Young JL Jr (eds): Third National Cancer Survey: Incidence Data. Natl Cancer Inst Monogr 41, 1975

31. Horm JW, Asire AJ, Young JL Jr, et al (eds): SEER Program. Cancer Incidence and Mortality in the United States, 1973–81. DHHS Publication No. (NIH)85–1837. Bethesda, MD, National Institutes of Health, 1984

32. Axtell LM, Asire AJ, Myers MH: Cancer Patient Survival. Report No. 5. DHEW Publication No. (NIH)77–992. Bethesda, MD, National Institutes of Health, 1976

33. Myers MH, Hankey BF: Cancer Patient Survival Experience. NIH Publication No. (NIH)80–2148. Bethesda, MD, National Institutes of Health, 1980

34. Ries LG, Pollack ES, Young JL Jr: Cancer patient survival: Surveillance, epidemiology, and end results program, 1973–79. JNCI 70:693, 1983

35. Young JL Jr, Ries LG, Pollack ES: Cancer patient survival among ethnic groups in the United States. JNCI 73:341, 1984

36. Newell GR: Hospital- and population-based tumor registries. Cancer Bull 35:283, 1983

37. Silverberg E, Lubera JA: Cancer statistics, 1988. CA 38:5, 1988

38. Muir C, Waterhouse J, Mack T, et al: Cancer Incidence in Five Continents, Vol V. Lyon, International Agency for Research on Cancer, 1987

39. Haenszel W: Migrant studies. In Schottenfeld D, Fraumeni JF Jr (eds): Cancer Epidemiology and Prevention, p 194. Philadelphia, WB Saunders, 1982

40. Lilienfeld AM, Levin ML, Kessler II: Cancer in the United States. Cambridge, MA, Harvard University Press, 1972

41. Ziegler RG, Devesa SS, Fraumeni JF Jr: Epidemiologic patterns of colorectal cancer. In DeVita VT Jr, Hellman S, Rosenberg SA (eds): Important Advances in Oncology 1986, p 209. Philadelphia, JB Lippincott, 1986

42. Blot WJ, Harrington JM, Toledo A, et al: Lung cancer after employment in shipyards during World War II. N Engl J Med 299:620, 1978

43. Pickle LW, Correa P, Fontham E: Recent case-control studies of lung cancer in the United States. In Mizell M, Correa P (eds): Lung Cancer: Causes and Prevention, p 101. Deerfield Beach, FL, Verlag-Chemie International, 1984

44. Winn D, Blot WJ, Shy CM, et al: Snuff dipping and oral cancer among women in the southern United States. N Engl J Med 304:745, 1981

45. Hoar SK, Blair A, Holmes FF, et al: Agricultural herbicide use and risk of lymphoma and soft-tissue sarcoma. JAMA 256:1141, 1986

46. Liu JY, Liu BQ, Li GY, et al: Atlas of cancer mortality in the People's Republic of China: An aid for cancer control and research. Int J Epidemiol 10:127, 1981

47. National Center for Health Statistics: Health: United States, 1985. DHHS Publication No. (PHS)86–1232. Washington, DC, US Government Printing Office, 1985

48. Willett WC, MacMahon B: Diet and cancer—an overview. N Engl J Med 310:633, 697, 1984

49. Elwood JM, Hislop TG: Solar radiation in the etiology of cutaneous malignant melanoma in Caucasians. Natl Cancer Inst Monogr 62:167, 1982

50. Weiss NS: Epidemiology of carcinoma of the endometrium. In Lilienfeld AM (ed): Reviews in Cancer Epidemiology, vol 2, p 46. New York, Elsevier, 1983

51. Cramer DW: Uterine cervix. In Schottenfeld D, Fraumeni JF Jr (eds): Cancer Epidemiology and Prevention, p 881. Philadelphia, WB Saunders, 1982

52. Pokras R, Hufnagel VG: Hysterectomies in the United States, 1965–84. Vital and Health Statistics. Series 13, No. 92. DHHS Publication No. (PHS)88–1753. Washington, DC, US Government Printing Office, 1987

53. Miller RW, McKay FW: Decline in US childhood cancer mortality. JAMA 251:1567, 1984

54. Gutensohn N, Cole P: Epidemiology of Hodgkin's disease. Semin Oncol 7:92, 1980

55. Brown LM, Pottern LM, Hoover RN, et al: Testicular cancer in the United States: Trends in incidence and mortality. Int J Epidemiol 15:164, 1986

56. Devesa SS, Diamond EL: Association of breast cancer and cervical cancer incidences with income and education among whites and blacks. JNCI 65:515, 1980

57. Hutchison GB: The epidemiologic method. In Schottenfeld D, Fraumeni JF Jr (eds): Cancer Epidemiology and Prevention, p 3. Philadelphia, WB Saunders, 1982

58. Rothman KJ: Modern Epidemiology. Boston, Little, Brown, 1986

59. Cole P: The evolving case-control study. J Chronic Dis 32:15, 1979

60. Cole P, MacMahon B: Attributable risk percent in case-control studies. Br J Prev Soc Med 25:242, 1971

61. Miettinen OS: Proportion of disease caused or prevented by a given exposure, trait or intervention. Am J Epidemiol 99:325, 1974

62. Greene MH, Harris EL, Gershenson DM, et al: Melphalan may be a more potent leukemogen than cyclophosphamide. Ann Intern Med 105:360, 1986

63. Hartge P, Silverman D, Hoover R, et al: Changing cigarette habits and bladder cancer risk: A case-control study. JNCI 78:1119, 1987

64. Harris CC (ed): Biochemical and Molecular Epidemiology of Cancer. New York, Alan R. Liss, 1986

65. Perera FP, Weinstein IB: Molecular epidemiology and carcinogen-DNA adduct detection: New approaches to studies of human cancer causation. J Chronic Dis 35:581, 1982

66. Miller RW: Genes, syndromes, and cancer. Pediatr Rev 8:153, 1986

67. Miller RW: Meeting report—Rare events as clues to cancer etiology. Cancer Res 48:3544, 1988

68. Wald NJ, Doll R (eds): Interpretation of Negative Epidemiological Evidence for Carcinogenicity. IARC Scientific Publication No. 65. Lyon, International Agency for Research on Cancer, 1985

69. Sackett DL: Bias in analytic research. J Chronic Dis 32:51, 1979

70. Brinton LA, Huggins GR, Lehman HF, et al: Long-term use of oral contraceptives and risk of invasive cervical cancer. Int J Cancer 38:339, 1986

71. Hill AB: The environment and disease: Association or causation? Proc R Soc Med 58:295, 1965

72. Smoking and Health: Report of the Advisory Committee to the Surgeon General. Public Health Service Publication No. 1103. Washington, DC, US Government Printing Office, 1964

73. Vessey MP, Gray M (eds): Cancer Risks and Prevention. Oxford, Oxford University Press, 1985

74. MacClure KM, MacMahon B: An epidemiologic perspective of environmental carcinogenesis. Epidemiol Rev 2:19, 1980

75. International Agency for Research on Cancer: Tobacco Smoking. IARC Monographs on the Evaluation of the Carcinogenic Risk of Chemicals to Humans, Vol 38. Lyon, International Agency for Research on Cancer, 1986

76. McLaughlin JK, Mandel JS, Blot WJ, et al: A population-based case-control study of renal cell carcinoma. JNCI 72:275, 1984

77. McLaughlin JK, Blot WJ, Mandel JS, et al: Etiology of cancer of the renal pelvis. JNCI 71:287, 1983

78. Brinton LA, Schairer C, Haenszel W, et al: Cigarette smoking and invasive cervical cancer. JAMA 255:3265, 1986

79. Brinton LA, Blot WJ, Becker JA, et al: A case-control study of cancers of the nasal cavity and paranasal sinuses. Am J Epidemiol 119:896, 1984

80. You WC, Blot WJ, Chang YS, et al: Diet and the high risk of stomach cancer in Shandong, China. Cancer Res 48:3518, 1988

81. Kinlen LJ, Rogot E: Leukemia and smoking habits. Br Med J (in press)

82. Lubin JH, Blot WJ, Berino F, et al: Patterns of lung cancer risk according to type of cigarette smoked. Int J Cancer 33:569, 1984

83. International Agency for Research on Cancer: Tobacco Habits Other Than Smoking: Betel-Quid and Areca-Nut Chewing; and Some Related Nitrosamines. IARC Monographs on the Evaluation of the Carcinogenic Risk of Chemicals to Humans, Vol 37. Lyon, International Agency for Research on Cancer, 1985

84. Blot WJ, Fraumeni JF Jr: Passive smoking and lung cancer. JNCI 77:993, 1986

85. Tuyns AJ: Alcohol. In Schottenfeld D, Fraumeni JF Jr (eds): Cancer Epidemiology and Prevention, p 293. Philadelphia, WB Saunders, 1982

86. Rothman KJ: The proportion of cancer attributable to alcohol consumption. Prev Med 9:174, 1980

87. Blot WJ, McLaughlin JK, Winn DM, et al: Smoking and drinking in relation to oral and pharyngeal cancer. Cancer Res 48:3282, 1988

88. Jensen OM: Cancer morbidity and causes of death among Danish brewery workers. Int J Cancer 23:454, 1979

89. Schatzkin A, Jones DY, Hoover RN: Alcohol consumption and breast cancer in the epidemiologic follow-up study of the first National Health and Nutrition Examination Survey. N Engl Med J 316:1169, 1987

90. Willett WC, Stampfer MJ, Colditz GA, et al: Moderate alcohol consumption and the risk of breast cancer. N Engl J Med 316:1174, 1987

91. Decouflé P: Occupation. In Schottenfeld D, Fraumeni JF Jr (eds): Cancer Epidemiology and Prevention, p 318. Philadelphia, WB Saunders, 1982

92. Saracci R: Occupation. In Vessey MP, Gray M (eds): Cancer Risks and Prevention, p 99. Oxford, Oxford University Press, 1985
93. Saracci R: Asbestosis and lung cancer: An analysis of the epidemiological evidence on the asbestos-smoking interaction. Int J Cancer 20:323, 1977
94. Tagnon I, Blot WJ, Stroube RB, et al: Mesothelioma associated with the shipbuilding industry in coastal Virginia. Cancer Res 40:3875, 1980
95. Artvinll M, Baris YI: Malignant mesotheliomas in a small village in the Anatolian region of Turkey: An epidemiologic study. JNCI 63:17, 1979
96. Brown LM, Pottern LM, Blot WJ: Lung cancer in relation to environmental pollutants emitted from industrial sources. Environ Res 34:250, 1984
97. Gao YT, Blot WJ, Zheng W, et al: Lung cancer among Chinese women. Int J Cancer 40:604, 1987
98. Mumford JL, He XZ, Chapman RS, et al: Lung cancer and indoor air pollution in Xuan Wei, China. Science 235:217, 1987
99. Cantor KP, Hoover R, Hartge P, et al: Bladder cancer, drinking water source, and tap water consumption: A case-control study. JNCI 79:1269, 1987
100. Boice JD Jr, Fraumeni JF Jr (eds): Radiation Carcinogenesis: Epidemiology and Biological Significance. Progress in Cancer Research and Therapy, Vol 26. New York, Raven Press, 1984
101. Jablon S, Bailar JC III: The contribution of ionizing radiation to cancer mortality in the United States. Prev Med 9:219, 1980
102. National Research Council, Committee on the Biological Effects of Ionizing Radiations (BEIR) IV: Health Risks of Radon and Other Internally Deposited Alpha-Emitters. Washington, DC, National Academy Press, 1988
103. Boice JD Jr, Land CE: Ionizing radiation. In Schottenfeld D, Fraumeni JF Jr (eds): Cancer Epidemiology and Prevention, p 231. Philadelphia, WB Saunders, 1982
104. Scotto J, Fears TR, Fraumeni JF Jr: Solar radiation. In Schottenfeld D, Fraumeni JF Jr (eds): Cancer Epidemiology and Prevention, p 254. Philadelphia, WB Saunders, 1982
105. Greene MH, Clark WH, Tucker MA, et al: Acquired precursors of cutaneous malignant melanoma: The familial dysplastic nevus syndrome. N Engl J Med 312:91, 1985
106. Scotto J, Fraumeni JF Jr: Skin (other than melanoma). In Schottenfeld D, Fraumeni JF Jr (eds): Cancer Epidemiology and Prevention, p 996. Philadelphia, WB Saunders, 1982
107. Scotto J, Cotton G, Urbach F, et al: Biologically effective ultraviolet radiation: Surface measurements in the United States, 1974 to 1985. Science 239:762, 1988
108. Herbst AL, Cole P, Colton T, et al: Age incidence and risk of diethylstilbestrol-related clear cell carcinoma of the vagina and cervix. Am J Obstet Gynecol 128:43, 1977
109. Brinton LA, Hoover R, Fraumeni JF Jr: Menopausal oestrogens and breast cancer risk: An expanded case-control study. Br J Cancer 54:825, 1986
110. Key TJA, Pike MC: The role of oestrogens and progestogens in the epidemiology and prevention of breast cancer. Eur J Cancer Clin Oncol 24:29, 1988
111. Vessey MP: Exogenous hormones. In Vessey MP, Gray M (eds): Cancer Risks and Prevention, p 166. Oxford, Oxford University Press, 1985
112. Henderson BE, Ross R, Bernstein L: Estrogens as a cause of human cancer. Cancer Res 48:246, 1988
113. Pike MC: Endogenous hormones. In Vessey MP, Gray M (eds): Cancer Risks and Prevention, p 195. Oxford, Oxford University Press, 1985
114. Boice JD Jr, Greene MH, Killen JY Jr, et al: Leukemia and preleukemia after adjuvant treatment of gastrointestinal cancer with semustine (methyl-CCNU). N Engl J Med 309:1079, 1983
115. Boice JD Jr, Greene MH, Killen JY Jr, et al: Leukemia after adjuvant chemotherapy with semustine (methyl-CCNU) — Evidence of a dose-response effect. N Engl J Med 314:119, 1986
116. Hoover R, Fraumeni JF Jr: Risk of cancer in renal-transplant recipients. Lancet 2:55, 1973
117. Kinlen LJ: Immunosuppressive therapy and cancer. Cancer Surv 1:565, 1982
118. Filopovich AH, Spector BD, Kersey J: Immunodeficiency in humans as a risk factor in the development of malignancy. Prev Med 9:252, 1980
119. List AF, Greco FA, Vogler LB: Lymphoproliferative diseases in immunocompromised hosts: The role of the Epstein-Barr virus. J Clin Oncol 5:1673, 1987
120. Evans AS: Viruses. In Schottenfeld D, Fraumeni JF Jr (eds): Cancer Epidemiology and Prevention, p 364. Philadelphia, WB Saunders, 1982
121. Levine PH, Ablashi DV, Nonoyama M, et al (eds): Epstein-Barr Virus and Human Disease. Clifton, NJ, Humana Press, 1987
122. Beasley RP, Hwang LY, Lin CC, et al: Hepatocellular carcinoma and hepatitis B virus: A prospective study of 22,707 men in Taiwan. Lancet 2:1129, 1981
123. Blattner WA: Human retroviruses. In Feigin RD, Cherry JD (eds): Textbook of Pediatric Infectious Diseases, 2nd ed, p 1795. Philadelphia, WB Saunders, 1987
124. Goedert JJ, Blattner WA: The epidemiology and natural history of human immunodeficiency virus. In DeVita VT Jr, Hellman S, Rosenberg SA (eds): AIDS: Etiology, Diagnosis, Treatment and Prevention, 2nd ed. Philadelphia, JB Lippincott, 1988
125. zur Hausen H: Papillomaviruses in human cancer. Cancer 59:1692, 1987
126. Armstrong BK, McMichael AJ, MacLennan R: Diet. In Schottenfeld D, Fraumeni JF Jr (eds): Cancer Epidemiology and Prevention, p 419. Philadelphia, WB Saunders, 1982
127. Graham S: Toward a dietary prevention of cancer. Epidemiol Rev 5:38, 1983
128. Kinlen LJ: Fat and breast cancer. Cancer Surv 6:585, 1987
129. Bingham SA, Williams DRR, Cummings JH: Dietary fibre consumption in Britain: New estimates and their relatin to large bowel cancer mortality. Br J Cancer 52:399, 1985
130. Greenwald P, Lanza E: Role of dietary fiber in the prevention of cancer. In DeVita VT Jr, Hellman S, Rosenberg SA (eds): Important Advances in Oncology, 1986, p 37. Philadelphia, JB Lippincott, 1986
131. Ziegler RG, Mason TJ, Stemhagen A, et al: Carotene intake, vegetables, and the risk of lung cancer among white men in New Jersey. Am J Epidemiol 123:1080, 1986
132. Graham S, Dayal H, Swanson M, et al: Diet in the epidemiology of cancer of the colon and rectum. J Natl Cancer Inst 61:709, 1978
133. Kinlen LJ: Meat and fat consumption and cancer mortality: A study of strict religious orders in Britain. Lancet 1:946, 1982
134. Bulatao-Jayme J, Almero EM, Castro MCA, et al: A case-control dietary study of primary liver cancer risk from aflatoxin exposure. Int J Epidemiol 11:112, 1982
135. Yu MC, Ho JHC, Lai SH, et al: Cantonese-style salted fish as a cause of nasopharyngeal carcinoma: Report of a case-control study in Hong Kong. Cancer Res 46:956, 1986
136. Hoover RN, Strasser PH: Artificial sweeteners and human bladder cancer. Lancet 1:837, 1980
137. Peto J: Genetic predisposition to cancer. Banbury Report 4:203, 1980
138. Chaganti RSK, German JL (eds): Genetics in Clinical Oncology. New York, Oxford University Press, 1985
139. Ayesh R, Idle JR, Ritchie JC, et al: Metabolic oxidation phenotypes as markers for susceptibility to lung cancer. Nature 312:169, 1984
140. Knudson AG: Hereditary cancer, oncogenes, and antioncogenes. Cancer Res 45:1437, 1985
141. Mulvihill JJ: Clinical genetics of pediatric cancer. In Pizzo P, Poplack DP (eds): Principles and Practice of Pediatric Oncology, pp 19–38. Philadelphia, JB Lippincott, 1989
142. Anderson DE: Familial predisposition. In Schottenfeld D, Fraumeni JF Jr (eds): Cancer Epidemiology and Prevention, p 483. Philadelphia, WB Saunders, 1982
143. Mulvihill JJ: Clinical ecogenetics: Cancer in families. N Engl J Med 312:1569, 1985
144. Li FP, Fraumeni JF Jr: Soft-tissue sarcomas, breast cancer, and other neoplasms: A familial syndrome? Ann Intern Med 71:747, 1969
145. Li FP, Fraumeni JF Jr, Mulvihill JJ, et al: A cancer family syndrome in 24 kindreds. Cancer Res (in press)
146. Chang EH, Pirollo KF, Zou ZQ, et al: Oncogenes in radioresistant, noncancerous skin fibroblasts from a cancer-prone family. Science 237:1036, 1987
147. Hansen MF, Cavenee WK: Genetics of cancer predisposition. Cancer Res 47:5518, 1987

APPENDIX TABLE 13-1.   Average Annual Age-Specific Cancer Incidence Rates per 100,000 Population by Site, SEER Program, 1981–1985: White Males

	<5	5–9	10–14	15–19	20–24	25–29	30–34	35–39
All sites	19.9	11.7	11.8	21.2	32.3	43.0	61.9	86.3
Oral cavity and pharynx	—	0.0	0.2	0.2	0.6	0.9	2.5	3.2
Digestive system	1.2	0.2	0.1	0.4	1.1	2.1	4.8	10.0
Esophagus	—	—	—	—	—	0.0	0.1	0.2
Stomach	—	—	0.0	0.1	0.1	0.3	0.5	1.3
Small intestine	0.0	0.0	—	—	—	0.1	0.2	0.2
Colon	—	—	0.0	0.3	0.5	0.8	2.1	4.3
Rectum	—	—	—	—	0.1	0.3	0.8	1.6
Anus and anal canal	—	—	—	—	0.0	0.0	0.2	0.3
Liver	0.6	0.0	—	0.0	0.1	0.1	0.2	0.4
Gallbladder	—	—	—	—	0.0	—	0.0	0.1
Other biliary	0.0	—	—	—	0.0	0.1	0.1	0.1
Pancreas	—	—	—	0.0	0.0	0.1	0.4	1.2
Retroperitoneum	0.6	0.2	—	0.0	0.1	0.1	0.2	0.2
Respiratory system	0.4	0.1	—	0.3	0.6	0.6	2.3	8.0
Nasal cavity, sinuses, ear	0.0	0.0	—	0.0	0.0	0.0	0.1	0.3
Larynx	—	—	—	—	0.0	0.1	0.2	0.9
Lung and bronchus	—	—	—	0.2	0.2	0.4	1.8	6.3
Pleura	—	—	—	—	—	—	0.1	0.2
Bones and joints	0.1	0.7	1.3	2.1	1.0	0.7	0.7	0.5
Soft tissue	1.4	0.5	0.6	0.8	1.1	1.4	1.5	2.0
Melanoma of skin	0.1	0.0	0.1	0.9	2.4	4.6	7.9	11.6
Breast	—	—	—	—	—	0.0	0.1	0.1
Male genital system	0.6	0.2	0.2	3.4	9.5	12.6	12.1	9.9
Prostate gland	0.1	—	—	0.0	0.0	—	0.0	0.1
Testis	0.5	0.1	0.2	3.3	9.3	12.5	12.0	9.5
Penis	—	—	—	—	0.0	0.0	0.1	0.2
Urinary system	2.0	0.6	0.2	0.3	0.9	1.3	3.4	7.1
Urinary bladder	0.0	0.0	—	0.3	0.6	0.9	2.4	4.6
Kidney and renal pelvis	1.9	0.6	0.2	0.1	0.2	0.4	0.9	2.4
Ureter	—	—	—	—	—	—	0.1	0.1
Eye and orbit	1.1	0.2	0.1	0.1	0.1	0.2	0.3	0.3
Brain and nervous system	3.8	2.8	2.1	2.2	2.7	2.8	4.3	4.6
Thyroid	0.0	0.0	0.2	0.8	1.1	1.6	2.7	3.2
Other endocrine	1.3	0.2	0.2	0.3	0.3	0.2	0.2	0.4
Hodgkin's disease	—	0.9	1.4	4.3	5.5	5.3	4.4	4.1
Non-Hodgkin's lymphomas	0.8	1.6	1.8	2.1	2.0	2.7	4.0	7.6
Multiple myeloma	—	—	—	—	0.0	0.0	0.2	0.4
Leukemias	6.7	3.5	3.1	2.6	2.1	2.3	2.8	3.9
Lymphocytic leukemia	5.4	3.0	2.1	1.8	0.9	0.7	0.6	0.7
Acute lymphocytic	5.4	3.0	2.1	1.7	0.8	0.6	0.5	0.4
Chronic lymphocytic	—	—	—	—	0.0	0.0	0.0	0.3
Granulocytic leukemia	0.8	0.3	0.7	0.6	0.9	1.5	1.8	2.6
Acute granulocytic	0.4	0.2	0.4	0.4	0.4	0.9	0.9	1.7
Chronic granulocytic	0.2	—	0.1	0.2	0.4	0.5	0.7	0.8
Monocytic leukemia	0.1	—	0.0	0.1	0.1	0.0	0.1	0.1
Acute monocytic	0.1	—	0.0	0.1	0.1	0.0	0.1	0.1
Chronic monocytic	—	—	—	—	—	—	—	—
Other leukemia	0.4	0.2	0.2	0.1	0.2	0.2	0.4	0.5
Ill-defined/unknown	0.5	0.1	0.2	0.3	0.6	0.7	1.2	1.9

From the National Cancer Institute: Annual Cancer Statistics Review Including Cancer Trends 1950–1985. Bethesda, MD, 1988.

APPENDIX TABLE 13-1 *(continued)*

40-44	45-49	50-54	55-59	60-64	65-69	70-74	75-79	80-84	85+
137.5	239.4	436.4	782.7	1233.0	1830.3	2483.1	3101.1	3576.3	3669.4
8.2	17.9	30.9	51.0	63.8	76.4	83.7	80.5	85.9	90.0
22.6	49.3	97.1	180.9	291.2	432.1	598.6	769.6	926.6	1026.9
1.1	2.6	5.5	12.8	18.8	25.0	29.6	32.2	30.8	32.2
3.1	6.2	11.6	21.1	31.1	50.1	67.2	78.5	116.4	141.8
0.8	1.2	1.6	2.6	3.5	4.7	7.1	6.8	7.3	6.0
8.5	18.2	36.7	66.6	118.6	182.7	268.2	368.7	446.2	513.8
3.9	10.0	21.9	41.6	65.0	93.9	120.6	141.5	162.6	151.1
0.4	0.5	0.9	1.9	2.3	2.7	3.0	4.4	4.5	4.3
0.6	1.3	3.1	5.9	9.4	13.1	17.7	21.3	25.6	21.3
0.1	0.1	0.4	0.9	1.8	3.4	5.0	9.5	8.8	13.9
0.4	0.9	1.2	3.0	4.1	7.5	9.4	14.3	18.7	20.3
3.0	7.3	13.1	22.7	33.9	45.1	66.7	86.0	98.7	111.9
0.5	0.6	0.6	0.8	1.1	1.5	1.7	2.3	3.1	4.0
24.2	57.9	124.7	236.3	347.6	483.9	597.6	641.0	610.4	445.0
0.6	0.9	1.1	2.3	2.6	2.9	3.8	4.4	4.3	5.0
2.8	6.8	16.1	27.2	36.2	43.9	44.4	41.9	36.9	25.2
20.2	48.8	106.0	203.3	303.3	428.9	538.8	582.2	557.4	407.5
0.3	1.1	1.3	2.6	4.5	6.7	9.1	11.6	10.2	6.3
0.6	0.4	0.7	1.1	1.7	1.9	2.3	3.5	1.7	1.0
2.3	2.7	3.8	3.9	4.8	5.8	7.6	12.7	11.1	18.9
14.8	17.9	21.2	25.8	29.0	32.7	33.0	36.2	38.3	42.2
0.5	0.6	1.1	2.0	2.2	3.5	4.2	5.5	5.9	6.3
8.6	12.1	31.7	86.6	203.8	393.9	636.2	873.1	1069.6	1154.1
1.3	5.6	26.4	82.1	199.2	388.7	630.4	865.2	1059.4	1138.8
6.8	5.3	4.0	2.6	2.3	1.3	1.0	1.2	1.2	1.3
0.4	1.0	1.2	1.6	1.8	3.1	3.9	5.2	6.4	10.3
14.8	28.9	49.8	87.0	135.1	190.9	248.5	322.5	384.1	394.9
8.6	16.3	31.7	57.4	92.3	138.5	184.1	240.6	301.1	326.1
5.9	12.3	17.1	27.3	37.8	46.4	54.3	67.5	69.6	56.5
0.1	0.2	0.6	1.7	3.3	4.4	6.9	10.0	9.0	6.0
0.7	0.9	1.2	1.4	2.6	2.2	4.1	4.4	5.4	3.7
6.9	8.9	10.7	15.9	19.3	25.0	24.8	28.1	21.8	14.9
3.5	3.7	4.4	4.7	5.2	6.6	5.0	5.7	5.0	6.0
0.4	0.5	0.7	0.6	1.5	1.8	1.3	0.9	1.2	0.3
3.7	3.9	4.0	4.6	3.8	5.8	6.2	5.1	7.1	4.6
11.1	13.7	22.0	27.2	39.9	52.1	65.7	84.4	101.5	88.0
1.5	2.3	4.5	8.8	14.3	20.3	25.2	40.5	43.3	45.8
5.0	7.3	13.1	19.0	30.4	43.1	65.2	89.2	122.4	151.1
1.4	2.3	5.0	8.6	14.0	17.6	28.3	33.8	48.5	67.4
0.4	0.6	0.6	0.8	1.0	1.1	1.9	1.2	4.0	3.3
1.0	1.6	4.2	7.6	12.6	15.7	25.6	31.3	43.1	60.8
2.4	3.4	5.4	7.0	10.5	17.8	24.5	39.0	53.5	60.1
1.4	2.2	3.3	4.2	6.1	10.7	14.8	23.4	29.6	32.5
0.8	1.1	1.6	2.5	3.3	5.5	8.0	12.2	16.8	21.6
0.1	0.3	0.4	0.4	1.0	1.2	0.8	2.4	4.0	3.3
0.1	0.2	0.3	0.2	0.8	1.1	0.6	1.9	3.1	2.3
—	0.0	—	0.0	0.2	0.1	—	0.3	—	0.3
1.1	1.2	2.2	3.0	4.9	6.4	11.5	13.9	16.3	20.3
3.2	6.2	11.7	23.6	34.1	49.5	69.2	91.1	128.5	164.7

APPENDIX TABLE 13-2.   Average Annual Age-Specific Cancer Incidence Rates per 100,000 Population by Site, SEER Program, 1981–1985: White Females

	<5	5–9	10–14	15–19	20–24	25–29	30–34	35–39
All sites	17.4	9.6	10.7	19.3	28.5	53.5	91.1	154.7
Oral cavity and pharynx	0.0	0.2	0.2	0.5	0.3	0.7	1.4	2.1
Digestive system	1.0	0.0	0.3	0.3	0.8	1.6	4.0	8.7
Esophagus	—	—	—	—	—	0.0	—	0.0
Stomach	—	—	—	0.1	0.0	0.1	0.4	1.1
Small intestine	—	—	—	0.0	0.1	0.0	0.1	0.3
Colon	—	—	0.1	0.1	0.3	0.6	1.7	3.9
Rectum	—	—	—	0.1	0.2	0.2	0.8	1.7
Anus and anal canal	—	—	—	—	—	0.0	0.1	0.2
Liver	0.5	—	0.2	0.1	0.1	0.3	0.2	0.3
Gallbladder	—	—	—	—	—	—	—	0.1
Other biliary	—	—	—	—	—	0.0	0.1	0.1
Pancreas	0.0	—	—	0.0	0.0	0.1	0.4	0.8
Retroperitoneum	0.4	0.0	0.0	—	0.0	0.1	0.1	0.2
Respiratory system	0.4	0.1	0.1	0.2	0.3	0.8	1.6	5.9
Nasal cavity, sinuses, ear	0.1	0.1	—	0.0	0.0	0.1	0.1	0.3
Larynx	—	—	—	—	0.0	0.1	0.1	0.3
Lung and bronchus	—	—	0.1	0.1	0.2	0.6	1.3	5.3
Pleura	—	—	—	—	0.0	—	0.0	—
Bones and joints	0.2	0.7	1.2	1.1	0.5	0.5	0.4	0.3
Soft tissue	1.6	0.3	0.6	1.0	0.8	0.8	1.1	1.4
Melanoma of skin	0.0	0.1	0.1	1.5	3.5	7.8	11.8	14.1
Breast	—	—	—	0.1	0.9	8.0	26.1	66.0
Female genital system	0.1	0.2	0.7	1.9	4.7	12.3	19.8	28.0
Cervix uteri	0.0	—	—	0.3	2.0	7.6	11.8	14.0
Corpus and uterus, NOS	—	0.0	0.0	0.1	0.1	0.6	2.5	5.9
Ovary	—	0.1	0.6	1.3	1.9	3.3	4.3	7.0
Vagina	0.1	—	—	—	0.2	0.2	0.2	0.2
Vulva	0.0	—	0.0	0.0	0.2	0.2	0.5	0.7
Urinary system	1.9	0.7	0.1	0.3	0.2	0.7	1.3	2.9
Urinary bladder	0.0	0.0	—	0.2	0.1	0.4	0.5	1.5
Kidney and renal pelvis	1.9	0.7	0.1	0.1	0.1	0.3	0.7	1.3
Ureter	—	—	—	—	—	—	0.0	—
Eye and orbit	1.3	0.2	0.1	0.0	0.0	0.2	0.3	0.2
Brain and nervous system	2.9	2.7	1.7	1.7	1.6	2.7	3.0	3.7
Thyroid	—	0.2	0.9	2.6	5.9	8.5	9.3	9.1
Other endocrine	1.0	0.3	0.1	0.1	0.1	0.1	0.2	0.2
Hodgkin's disease	—	0.2	1.4	4.6	5.4	4.9	3.8	2.6
Non-Hodgkin's lymphomas	0.2	0.2	0.4	1.0	1.2	1.7	3.0	3.6
Multiple myeloma	—	—	—	—	—	—	0.1	0.4
Leukemias	6.1	3.3	2.3	2.1	1.6	1.5	2.6	3.0
Lymphocytic leukemia	5.2	2.9	1.5	0.9	0.5	0.3	0.4	0.7
Acute lymphocytic	5.2	2.8	1.5	0.9	0.5	0.3	0.4	0.4
Chronic lymphocytic	—	—	—	—	—	—	0.1	0.3
Granulocytic leukemia	0.5	0.3	0.6	0.9	0.9	1.0	1.7	1.9
Acute granulocytic	0.5	0.2	0.4	0.7	0.5	0.7	1.0	1.3
Chronic granulocytic	0.0	—	0.2	0.2	0.2	0.3	0.4	0.5
Monocytic leukemia	0.2	—	0.1	0.1	0.0	0.1	0.2	0.1
Acute monocytic	0.2	—	0.1	0.1	0.0	0.1	0.1	0.1
Chronic monocytic	—	—	—	—	—	—	—	—
Other leukemia	0.2	0.1	0.1	0.2	0.2	0.1	0.3	0.3
Ill-defined/unknown	0.4	0.1	0.2	0.2	0.2	0.2	0.9	1.8

From the National Cancer Institute: Annual Cancer Statistics Review Including Cancer Trends 1950–1985. Bethesda, MD, 1988.

APPENDIX TABLE 13-2 (continued)

40–44	45–49	50–54	55–59	60–64	65–69	70–74	75–79	80–84	85+
247.4	394.4	549.5	761.4	1029.1	1256.6	1475.3	1644.8	1827.9	1876.0
3.3	7.7	11.7	19.6	26.4	30.1	28.1	28.6	27.8	29.5
18.8	39.5	75.3	121.2	185.5	272.7	388.0	524.6	655.2	729.4
0.2	0.6	2.0	4.0	6.5	7.4	8.9	11.1	12.4	13.3
1.5	3.1	5.4	7.6	12.9	17.5	27.8	42.6	54.7	68.1
0.3	1.1	1.4	2.0	2.0	2.8	3.6	4.4	5.8	5.4
8.5	18.3	34.7	57.7	86.7	136.4	193.4	278.7	346.9	390.1
4.0	8.7	16.7	26.2	37.2	50.5	70.8	82.6	97.6	106.0
0.5	0.9	2.0	2.6	3.2	4.0	4.7	4.5	6.7	5.1
0.6	0.5	1.6	2.2	3.1	4.0	6.5	7.9	8.7	10.5
0.4	0.5	1.6	2.3	4.3	6.6	9.7	14.0	19.0	21.8
0.3	0.4	1.5	1.3	3.3	4.3	6.9	9.4	13.7	14.0
2.0	4.4	7.7	13.8	24.2	36.8	52.3	63.5	84.7	88.1
0.2	0.4	0.3	0.6	1.0	0.8	1.1	2.6	1.4	1.2
17.0	37.3	70.5	111.2	153.8	181.2	189.6	159.9	137.6	98.0
0.3	0.5	0.9	0.8	1.8	1.6	1.8	2.5	2.6	1.7
0.8	2.5	3.6	5.1	7.0	8.3	7.3	5.3	3.6	2.5
15.6	33.9	65.7	104.3	144.4	169.6	178.9	150.2	128.7	92.7
0.3	0.1	0.2	0.6	0.5	1.1	1.3	1.6	2.2	0.4
0.3	0.5	0.5	0.5	1.2	1.4	1.5	1.3	2.5	1.7
1.8	1.2	2.1	2.8	3.9	4.5	5.0	5.1	9.3	7.6
14.5	16.7	17.1	18.1	17.7	16.0	18.4	19.3	21.4	22.0
114.5	174.0	201.2	252.0	303.9	344.3	372.0	389.0	400.3	395.0
40.6	65.9	95.1	129.1	184.4	202.7	207.1	190.9	176.9	161.0
14.3	15.0	14.9	16.2	17.2	17.2	17.3	16.8	16.1	19.0
12.1	25.8	47.0	70.9	109.2	123.1	118.9	99.9	82.1	64.1
12.3	21.9	29.3	36.0	49.9	53.2	58.1	55.2	55.6	49.4
0.6	0.8	0.6	1.5	2.2	1.9	2.8	4.0	5.1	5.8
0.8	1.5	2.4	2.6	3.4	5.3	7.7	12.2	15.5	20.1
6.2	11.5	16.6	27.0	43.4	56.6	73.3	89.7	105.3	110.1
2.9	5.9	9.1	14.6	25.6	32.8	46.1	55.1	72.1	82.7
3.4	5.4	7.0	11.5	16.1	21.4	23.4	29.6	28.3	23.0
—	0.1	0.2	0.7	1.0	1.6	2.7	3.4	3.1	2.7
0.6	0.9	0.5	1.7	1.4	2.8	2.5	2.1	2.0	2.1
4.5	4.9	8.8	9.7	13.5	17.0	16.5	16.8	16.1	6.9
9.3	9.4	9.2	8.7	9.3	7.9	9.4	7.0	9.0	6.3
0.3	0.2	0.7	0.7	1.0	0.8	1.3	0.7	0.8	0.3
1.7	1.4	2.0	2.2	2.8	3.1	4.3	4.4	3.9	3.4
6.5	9.6	15.1	22.6	30.1	38.8	53.3	66.0	68.9	66.0
0.7	1.6	3.7	5.2	9.8	14.7	19.2	24.3	29.1	28.5
3.3	5.1	7.5	11.1	15.0	24.1	32.1	41.5	62.3	75.8
0.9	1.3	2.4	3.5	6.3	10.0	14.0	17.7	24.8	32.4
0.6	0.5	0.4	0.3	0.5	0.7	0.6	1.4	1.3	1.7
0.3	0.7	1.9	3.1	5.4	9.2	12.7	15.4	22.0	28.6
1.8	3.1	3.9	5.6	6.5	10.2	14.5	17.7	25.3	28.9
1.0	1.7	2.6	3.8	4.1	6.6	9.2	10.2	14.3	16.1
0.6	1.2	1.2	1.4	1.7	2.5	3.9	5.7	7.6	9.3
0.2	0.2	0.2	0.4	0.4	0.7	0.4	0.8	1.9	2.1
0.1	0.2	0.2	0.3	0.3	0.6	0.4	0.7	1.2	1.0
0.0	—	—	—	0.0	—	—	—	0.5	0.5
0.5	0.5	0.9	1.5	1.9	3.2	3.1	5.4	10.3	12.4
2.8	6.1	11.3	16.9	25.0	36.2	51.6	70.3	94.1	127.2

APPENDIX TABLE 13-3.   Average Annual Age-Specific Cancer Incidence Rates per 100,000 Population by Site, SEER Program, 1981–1985: Black Males

	<5	5–9	10–14	15–19	20–24	25–29	30–34	35–39
All sites	10.7	8.4	9.9	14.4	18.3	22.2	43.8	75.5
Oral cavity and pharynx	0.4	0.2	0.7	0.5	0.9	0.7	3.7	8.7
Digestive system	0.2	0.4	0.2	0.2	0.5	2.9	7.9	14.0
Esophagus	—	—	—	—	—	0.2	0.8	1.1
Stomach	—	—	—	—	—	0.2	0.4	3.4
Small intestine	—	—	—	—	—	0.4	—	0.3
Colon	—	—	0.2	0.2	0.2	0.9	2.9	5.6
Rectum	—	—	—	—	—	0.9	1.2	1.1
Anus and anal canal	—	—	—	—	—	—	—	—
Liver	—	0.2	—	—	0.4	0.4	2.1	0.8
Gallbladder	—	—	—	—	—	—	—	—
Other biliary	—	—	—	—	—	—	—	0.3
Pancreas	—	—	—	—	—	—	0.2	1.4
Retroperitoneum	0.2	0.2	—	—	—	—	0.2	—
Respiratory system	0.6	0.6	0.2	—	0.5	1.1	4.1	11.5
Nasal cavity, sinuses, ear	0.2	0.2	—	—	0.2	—	—	—
Larnyx	—	—	—	—	—	—	0.6	1.1
Lung and bronchus	—	—	0.2	—	0.2	0.9	3.1	9.8
Pleura	—	—	—	—	—	0.2	—	—
Bones and joints	0.2	0.4	0.9	2.3	0.4	0.4	0.4	1.4
Soft tissue	0.7	0.2	0.7	0.5	1.1	1.6	2.3	1.4
Melanoma of skin	—	—	—	—	0.2	—	—	0.6
Breast	—	—	—	—	—	—	—	0.3
Male genital system	0.2	—	0.2	0.7	2.0	2.5	1.7	4.2
Prostate gland	—	—	—	—	—	—	—	1.4
Testis	0.2	—	—	0.5	2.0	2.5	1.4	1.7
Penis	—	—	—	—	—	—	0.2	0.3
Urinary system	2.0	1.2	0.4	0.2	0.5	1.4	2.9	3.6
Urinary bladder	—	—	—	0.2	—	0.5	0.6	1.1
Kidney and renal pelvis	2.0	1.2	0.4	—	0.5	0.7	2.3	2.5
Ureter	—	—	—	—	—	—	—	—
Eye and orbit	1.5	0.2	—	—	—	0.2	0.2	0.6
Brain and nervous system	1.7	2.5	1.4	3.1	1.1	0.7	3.1	1.4
Thyroid	—	—	—	0.4	0.4	0.4	0.6	2.2
Other endocrine	0.6	—	—	—	0.2	—	0.6	0.3
Hodgkin's disease	—	0.4	1.1	2.3	4.4	3.0	3.1	3.4
Non-Hodgkin's lymphomas	0.4	0.8	1.4	1.1	2.0	2.7	5.4	6.7
Multiple myeloma	—	—	—	—	—	—	0.6	2.2
Leukemias	2.0	1.6	2.7	2.7	3.0	2.2	2.5	5.6
Lymphocytic leukemia	1.7	1.2	1.8	1.4	—	0.2	—	1.7
Acute lymphocytic	1.7	1.0	1.8	1.4	—	0.2	—	1.1
Chronic lymphocytic	—	—	—	—	—	—	—	0.6
Granulocytic leukemia	0.2	0.4	0.9	1.1	2.3	1.8	2.5	3.4
Acute granulocytic	0.2	0.4	0.7	0.4	1.2	0.9	0.6	1.4
Chronic granulocytic	—	—	0.2	0.7	1.1	0.7	1.9	2.0
Monocytic leukemia	—	—	—	—	—	0.2	—	0.3
Acute monocytic	—	—	—	—	—	0.2	—	—
Chronic monocytic	—	—	—	—	—	—	—	0.3
Other leukemia	0.2	—	—	0.2	0.7	—	—	0.3
Ill-defined/unknown	0.4	—	—	0.2	0.5	0.5	0.4	4.2

From the National Cancer Institute: Annual Cancer Statistics Review Including Cancer Trends 1950–1985. Bethesda, MD, 1988.

APPENDIX TABLE 13-3 (continued)

40–44	45–49	50–54	55–59	60–64	65–69	70–74	75–79	80–84	85+
185.0	376.0	689.7	1182.5	1739.3	2315.5	3050.3	3294.1	4068.2	3433.6
24.1	49.6	68.3	95.1	86.2	74.7	65.8	44.8	67.9	39.3
47.9	92.1	182.8	283.7	422.4	533.5	707.1	831.6	1078.3	914.5
12.4	24.1	49.0	65.3	86.2	83.8	75.8	73.5	41.5	39.3
5.8	15.6	32.0	40.0	66.3	93.0	114.9	141.6	222.4	151.5
1.1	2.2	2.8	6.3	4.0	4.6	7.8	7.2	—	5.6
13.2	25.5	42.9	77.0	129.8	178.3	262.1	362.0	456.2	381.5
6.9	8.0	19.8	32.2	48.8	61.0	78.1	82.4	147.0	112.2
—	1.3	1.4	2.4	1.7	3.0	3.3	9.0	3.8	11.2
2.2	2.7	8.0	13.2	18.7	33.5	36.8	19.7	26.4	5.6
0.7	—	0.5	1.5	0.6	3.0	6.7	7.2	11.3	11.2
—	0.9	1.4	2.9	4.0	3.0	10.0	10.8	7.5	11.2
5.5	11.6	25.0	39.5	59.5	66.3	109.3	107.5	154.6	168.3
—	—	—	1.0	1.7	0.8	1.1	1.8	3.8	—
52.6	134.6	253.0	444.5	567.5	707.3	801.9	679.3	667.3	460.1
1.1	1.3	1.4	2.9	1.7	1.5	5.6	7.2	11.3	11.2
9.1	16.1	24.5	43.4	59.0	58.7	59.1	48.4	18.9	33.7
41.7	116.7	226.6	393.4	503.4	644.0	733.9	614.7	629.6	403.9
0.4	0.4	0.5	3.9	2.3	3.0	3.3	7.2	7.5	11.2
0.4	0.4	—	1.5	1.1	—	3.3	1.8	—	—
3.7	4.9	1.4	1.9	5.1	9.1	10.0	7.2	3.8	5.6
—	1.8	0.9	0.5	3.4	3.8	—	3.6	11.3	5.6
—	1.8	1.4	5.4	2.3	1.5	7.8	7.2	15.1	5.6
4.8	13.0	52.8	158.4	389.5	644.0	1032.8	1206.2	1583.5	1408.2
2.6	11.2	51.4	155.0	384.9	638.7	1027.2	1197.2	1576.0	1402.6
0.7	0.4	—	0.5	1.1	—	—	—	—	5.6
1.5	0.9	1.4	1.9	2.8	3.8	4.5	9.0	7.5	—
9.9	21.0	40.5	61.4	83.3	133.4	162.8	179.2	192.3	213.2
4.8	9.4	19.3	30.7	44.2	83.1	99.3	114.7	124.4	157.1
4.8	11.6	19.3	28.8	37.4	45.7	53.5	44.8	56.6	50.5
0.4	—	0.5	0.5	0.6	1.5	5.6	5.4	—	5.6
—	0.4	0.5	—	1.1	0.8	—	—	—	11.2
6.9	6.7	8.5	7.3	15.9	11.4	12.3	9.0	11.3	5.6
2.9	3.1	1.4	4.9	4.0	3.8	3.3	3.6	—	5.6
0.4	1.3	0.9	1.0	2.3	—	—	1.8	—	—
2.9	4.0	0.9	1.5	4.0	3.0	4.5	5.4	3.8	22.4
7.3	8.5	15.5	19.5	27.8	38.9	43.5	43.0	49.0	16.8
3.7	9.8	14.1	29.7	34.6	49.5	49.1	93.2	124.4	50.5
7.7	8.9	11.8	19.0	29.5	38.1	55.8	44.8	101.8	84.2
2.2	2.2	5.7	6.8	11.9	13.7	32.3	30.5	49.0	33.7
0.7	—	0.5	—	—	—	1.1	3.6	7.5	—
1.5	1.3	5.2	6.8	11.3	13.0	30.1	26.9	41.5	33.7
4.4	5.8	3.3	8.8	14.2	17.5	15.6	12.5	37.7	39.3
4.0	1.8	0.9	3.4	6.2	9.9	6.7	9.0	22.6	22.4
0.4	3.1	2.4	4.9	7.4	7.6	5.6	3.6	11.3	16.8
—	—	0.9	1.5	0.6	0.8	—	—	—	5.6
—	—	0.9	1.5	1.5	0.6	0.8	—	—	5.6
—	—	—	—	—	—	—	—	—	—
1.1	0.9	1.9	1.9	2.8	6.1	7.8	1.8	15.1	5.6
8.0	10.7	31.6	45.8	55.6	59.4	88.1	125.5	150.8	173.9

234

APPENDIX TABLE 13-4. Average Annual Age-Specific Cancer Incidence Rates per 100,000 Population by Site, SEER Program, 1981–1985: Black Females

	<5	5–9	10–14	15–19	20–24	25–29	30–34	35–39
All sites	17.2	7.7	9.3	12.3	17.1	38.5	88.1	154.3
Oral cavity and pharynx	—	—	0.5	0.7	0.5	0.3	1.1	4.1
Digestive system	1.5	—	0.2	0.5	1.0	2.7	4.8	13.9
Esophagus	—	—	—	—	—	—	0.2	1.2
Stomach	—	—	—	—	—	0.6	0.7	1.7
Small intestine	—	—	—	—	0.2	—	—	0.2
Colon	—	—	—	—	0.3	1.1	2.4	7.3
Rectum	—	—	—	—	—	0.8	0.6	1.9
Anus and anal canal	—	—	—	—	—	—	—	0.5
Liver	0.6	—	0.2	0.4	0.3	—	—	0.2
Gallbladder	—	—	—	—	—	—	—	—
Other biliary	—	—	—	0.2	—	—	—	—
Pancreas	—	—	—	—	0.2	0.2	0.7	0.7
Retroperitoneum	1.0	—	—	—	—	—	—	—
Respiratory system	—	—	—	—	0.2	0.5	1.8	6.3
Nasal cavity, sinuses, ear	—	—	—	—	—	0.2	—	—
Larynx	—	—	—	—	—	—	0.2	1.2
Lung and bronchus	—	—	—	—	—	0.2	1.5	5.1
Pleura	—	—	—	—	—	—	0.2	—
Bones and joints	0.4	0.2	0.9	0.7	0.2	0.5	0.6	0.7
Soft tissue	2.1	0.6	0.9	1.4	0.2	0.8	1.3	0.7
Melanoma of skin	—	0.2	—	—	—	—	0.4	0.5
Breast	—	—	—	—	1.5	12.2	39.8	73.0
Female genital system	0.2	0.6	1.1	2.5	6.1	12.1	21.9	32.1
Cervix uteri	—	—	—	0.7	2.6	7.6	14.7	22.1
Corpus and uterus, NOS	—	—	—	—	—	1.1	1.5	3.9
Ovary	—	0.6	1.1	1.4	2.5	2.3	4.4	4.4
Vagina	0.2	—	—	—	0.2	—	0.2	0.2
Vulva	—	—	—	—	—	0.5	0.6	1.5
Urinary system	3.3	1.0	0.5	0.9	0.8	0.5	1.5	1.2
Urinary bladder	—	—	—	0.4	0.2	0.2	0.4	0.7
Kidney and renal pelvis	3.3	1.0	0.5	0.5	0.7	0.3	0.9	0.5
Ureter	—	—	—	—	—	—	—	—
Eye and orbit	1.1	—	—	—	—	—	—	—
Brain and nervous system	2.5	2.8	1.5	0.5	1.0	1.1	1.3	1.2
Thyroid	—	—	0.2	0.5	1.8	2.7	3.9	3.9
Other endocrine	0.4	0.2	—	0.2	0.2	—	—	0.7
Hodgkin's disease	—	0.2	0.9	1.3	0.8	1.4	1.5	2.4
Non-Hodgkin's lymphomas	0.6	0.4	0.2	0.5	1.3	1.3	2.4	2.9
Multiple myeloma	—	—	—	—	—	—	0.7	1.0
Leukemias	4.8	1.4	2.0	1.6	1.5	1.3	2.0	4.4
Lymphocytic leukemia	4.2	0.8	0.5	0.4	—	0.2	0.2	0.2
Acute lymphocytic	4.2	0.8	0.5	0.4	—	0.2	0.2	—
Chronic lymphocytic	—	—	—	—	—	—	—	0.2
Granulocytic leukemia	0.2	0.4	1.1	1.1	1.3	0.8	1.7	2.9
Acute granulocytic	0.2	0.2	0.5	0.5	1.0	0.6	0.7	1.9
Chronic granulocytic	—	0.2	0.2	0.4	0.3	0.2	0.7	0.7
Monocytic leukemia	0.2	—	0.2	0.2	—	0.2	—	—
Acute monocytic	0.2	—	0.2	0.2	—	0.2	—	—
Chronic monocytic	—	—	—	—	—	—	—	—
Other leukemia	0.2	0.2	0.2	—	0.2	0.2	0.2	1.2
Ill-defined/unknown	0.4	—	0.4	0.2	—	0.3	1.5	3.9

From the National Cancer Institute: Annual Cancer Statistics Review Including Cancer Trends 1950–1985. Bethesda, MD, 1988.

APPENDIX TABLE 13-4 *(continued)*

40–44	45–49	50–54	55–59	60–64	65–69	70–74	75–79	80–84	85+
269.9	389.9	514.1	755.0	925.9	1102.4	1378.6	1514.7	1891.1	1695.3
8.8	17.5	21.0	29.5	22.0	16.7	19.7	16.2	12.8	14.6
31.9	60.1	99.1	162.7	230.5	328.5	466.6	523.7	736.8	697.6
3.3	7.8	15.9	17.9	24.4	21.3	19.7	11.5	19.2	14.6
2.3	7.0	7.1	13.7	19.6	34.0	51.1	61.1	108.6	124.4
1.0	1.6	3.2	2.1	3.3	5.8	9.4	4.6	4.3	4.9
13.4	21.7	37.7	72.4	105.7	156.7	229.0	259.6	347.1	309.8
4.9	7.0	13.1	24.6	28.2	46.7	51.9	70.4	80.9	78.1
2.0	1.6	2.8	3.7	4.3	2.9	5.5	1.2	10.6	7.3
—	1.2	2.4	4.2	4.8	6.9	7.9	13.8	4.3	17.1
0.3	0.8	2.0	3.7	2.9	3.5	4.7	11.5	19.2	7.3
—	—	0.8	0.4	2.4	2.9	5.5	5.8	8.5	14.6
4.2	10.1	13.5	18.3	33.5	46.7	77.9	83.1	129.9	112.2
0.7	1.2	0.4	1.2	1.0	0.6	2.4	—	2.1	—
29.3	58.6	85.6	123.2	158.3	159.1	147.9	151.1	134.2	102.4
0.3	1.2	—	0.8	1.4	0.6	1.6	—	6.4	—
2.0	5.0	8.3	7.9	10.5	8.1	6.3	5.8	6.4	—
27.1	52.0	77.3	114.0	146.3	148.7	140.1	144.2	119.3	97.6
—	0.4	—	—	—	1.7	—	1.2	—	2.4
1.0	0.4	0.4	—	1.0	0.6	—	1.2	2.1	2.4
1.6	1.9	2.8	3.3	4.3	6.9	9.4	12.7	10.6	—
—	1.2	1.2	0.8	2.9	3.5	0.8	4.6	—	9.8
114.8	149.0	158.2	209.3	223.8	244.9	307.7	305.7	389.7	302.5
46.0	53.2	75.7	108.2	141.1	155.0	183.3	205.3	215.1	231.7
31.6	29.1	33.3	34.1	34.0	41.5	51.1	56.5	59.6	87.8
7.2	9.3	19.0	38.3	63.1	68.6	77.9	73.9	89.5	85.4
4.9	11.6	17.4	27.1	35.4	35.7	40.1	56.5	38.3	39.0
0.7	1.2	2.0	3.3	3.8	5.8	8.7	5.8	14.9	9.8
1.3	1.2	2.8	2.9	3.3	—	3.9	8.1	2.1	4.9
5.9	8.5	17.4	30.4	34.9	36.9	47.2	63.4	83.1	73.2
1.0	1.2	5.9	15.0	17.7	24.2	26.8	33.5	49.0	56.1
4.6	5.8	9.5	13.3	13.9	12.1	18.9	25.4	29.8	17.1
—	—	—	—	—	—	1.6	1.2	2.1	—
0.7	—	0.4	—	0.5	—	—	—	—	—
2.6	1.2	5.2	4.2	7.7	9.8	7.9	12.7	14.9	—
6.2	7.8	5.2	8.7	5.7	5.8	8.7	1.2	6.4	12.2
—	0.8	0.4	1.2	1.0	2.3	—	—	—	—
1.0	0.4	1.2	1.7	1.4	2.3	2.4	2.3	2.1	—
3.3	8.9	7.5	13.7	18.7	32.3	30.7	36.9	38.3	34.1
3.3	4.7	11.5	13.7	18.2	26.5	44.1	47.3	63.9	46.3
3.3	4.3	6.7	10.8	21.0	21.3	29.9	48.5	42.6	56.1
—	1.2	1.6	3.7	6.2	7.5	11.8	24.2	19.2	19.5
—	0.4	0.8	0.4	0.5	1.7	0.8	—	—	—
—	0.4	0.8	3.3	5.3	5.2	11.0	23.1	17.0	14.6
2.6	2.3	5.2	5.4	10.5	11.5	13.4	16.2	17.0	22.0
2.0	1.6	3.2	2.9	6.7	5.2	4.7	9.2	10.6	12.2
0.7	0.8	2.0	2.5	3.3	4.6	7.9	5.8	6.4	9.8
—	—	—	0.4	1.0	0.6	1.6	—	—	2.4
—	—	—	0.4	1.0	0.6	1.6	—	—	—
0.7	0.8	—	1.2	3.3	1.7	3.1	8.1	6.4	12.2
9.8	8.5	14.7	31.6	32.5	50.1	70.0	80.8	138.4	112.2

STEVEN A. ROSENBERG

CHAPTER 14 *Principles of Surgical Oncology*

Surgery is the oldest treatment for cancer and, until recently, was the only treatment that could cure patients with cancer. The surgical treatment of cancer has changed dramatically over the last several decades. Advances in surgical techniques and a better understanding of the patterns of spread of individual cancers have allowed surgeons to perform successful resections for an increased number of patients. The development of alternate treatment strategies that can control microscopic disease has prompted surgeons to reassess the magnitude of surgery necessary.

The surgeon who treats cancer must be familiar with the natural history of individual cancers and with the principles and potentialities of surgery, radiation therapy, chemotherapy, immunotherapy, and other new treatment modalities.

The surgeon has a central role in the prevention, diagnosis, definitive treatment, palliation, and rehabilitation of the cancer patient. The principles underlying each of these roles of the surgical oncologist are discussed in this chapter.

HISTORICAL PERSPECTIVE

Although the earliest discussions of the surgical treatment of tumors are found in the Edwin Smith Papyrus from the Egyptian Middle Kingdom (approximately 1600 B.C.), the modern era of elective surgery for visceral tumors began in frontier America in 1809.[1,2] Ephraim MacDowell removed a 22-pound ovarian tumor from a patient, Mrs. Jane Todd Crawford, who survived for 30 years after the operation. This procedure, the first of 13 ovarian resections performed

by MacDowell, was the first elective abdominal operation and provided a great stimulus to the development of elective surgery.

However, the treatment of most tumors depended on two subsequent developments in surgery. The first of these was the introduction of general anesthesia by two dentists, Dr. William Morton and Dr. Crawford Long. The first major operation using general ether anesthesia was an excision of the submaxillary gland and part of the tongue, performed by Dr. John Collins Warren on October 16, 1846, at the Massachusetts General Hospital. The second major development stimulating the widespread application of surgery resulted from the introduction of the principles of antisepsis by Joseph Lister in 1867. Based on the concepts of Pasteur, Lister introduced carbolic acid in 1867 and described the principles of antisepsis in an article in *The Lancet* in that same year.

These developments freed surgery from both pain and sepsis and greatly increased its use for the treatment of tumors. In the decade before the introduction of ether, only 385 operations were performed at the Massachusetts General Hospital. By the last decade of the 19th century, more than 20,000 operations per year were performed at that same hospital.[3]

Table 14-1 lists some selected milestones in the history of surgical oncology. Although this does not include all of the important developments, it does provide the tempo of the application of surgery to cancer treatment.[4] Major figures in the evolution of surgical oncology included Albert Theodore Billroth who, in addition to developing meticulous surgical techniques, performed the first gastrectomy, laryngectomy,

236

TABLE 14-1.   Selected Historical Milestones in Surgical Oncology

Year	Surgeon	Event
1809	Ephraim McDowell	Elective abdominal surgery (excised ovarian tumor)
1846	John Collins Warren	Use of ether anesthesia (excised submaxillary gland)
1867	Joseph Lister	Introduction of antisepsis
1860–1890	Albert Theodore Billroth	First gastrectomy, laryngectomy, and esophagectomy
1878	Richard von Volkmann	Excision of cancerous rectum
1880s	Theodore Kocher	Development of thyroid surgery
1890	William Stewart Halsted	Radical mastectomy
1896	G. T. Beatson	Oophorectomy for breast cancer
1904	Hugh H. Young	Radical prostatectomy
1906	Ernest Wertheim	Radical hysterectomy
1908	W. Ernest Miles	Abdomenoperineal resection for rectal cancer
1912	E. Martin	Cordotomy for the treatment of pain
1910–1930	Harvey Cushing	Development of surgery for brain tumors
1913	Franz Torek	Successful resection of cancer of the thoracic esophagus
1927	G. Divis	Successful resection of pulmonary metastases
1933	Evarts Graham	Pneumonectomy
1935	A. O. Whipple	Pancreaticoduodenectomy
1945	Charles B. Huggins	Adrenalectomy for prostate cancer

and esophagectomy. In the 1890s, William Stewart Halsted elucidated the principles of en bloc resections for cancer, as exemplified by his development of the radical mastectomy. Examples of radical resections for cancers of individual organs include the radical prostatectomy by Hugh Young in 1904, the radical hysterectomy by Ernest Wertheim in 1906, the abdominoperineal resection for cancer of the rectum by W. Ernest Miles in 1908, and the first successful pneumonectomy performed for cancer by Evarts Graham in 1933. Modern technical innovations continue to extend the surgeon's capabilities. Recent examples include the development of microsurgical techniques that enable the performance of free grafts for reconstruction, automatic stapling devices, sophisticated endoscopic equipment that allows for a wide variety of "incisionless" surgery, and major improvements in postoperative management and critical care of patients that have extended the safety of major surgical therapy.

Many critics who feel that the application of surgery has reached a plateau beyond which it will not progress should remember the words of a famous British surgeon, Sir John Erichsen, who in his introductory address to the medical institutions at University College, said,

. . . there must be a final limit to the development of manipulative surgery, the knife cannot always have fresh fields for conquest and although methods of practice may be modified and varied and even improved to some extent, it must be within a certain limit. That this limit has nearly, if not quite, been reached will appear evident if we reflect on the great achievements of modern operative surgery. Very little remains for the boldest to devise or the most dextrous to perform.

These comments, published in *The Lancet* in 1873, preceded the majority of important developments in modern surgical oncology.

THE OPERATION

ANESTHESIA

Modern anesthetic techniques have greatly increased the safety of major oncologic surgery. Both regional and general anesthesia play important roles in a wide variety of diagnostic techniques and local therapeutic maneuvers, as well as in major surgery, and these should be understood by all oncologists.

Anesthetic techniques may be divided into regional and general anesthesia. Regional anesthesia involves a reversible blockade of pain perception by the application of local anesthetic drugs. These agents generally work by preventing the activation of pain receptors or by blocking nerve conduction. A variety of agents commonly used for regional anesthesia are shown in Table 14-2.[5] Topical anesthesia refers to the application of local anesthetics to the skin or mucous membranes. Good surface anesthesia of the conjunctiva and cornea, the oropharynx and nasopharynx, esophagus, larynx, trachea, urethra, and anus can result from the application of these agents.

Local anesthesia involves injecting anesthetic agents directly into the operative field. Field block refers to injection of local anesthetic by circumscribing the operative field with a continuous wall of anesthetic agent. Lidocaine (Xylocaine) in concentrations from 0.5% to 1% is the most common anesthetic agent used for this purpose. Peripheral nerve block results from the deposition of a local anesthetic surrounding major nerve trunks. It can provide local anesthesia to entire anatomic areas.

Major surgical procedures in the lower portion of the body can be performed using either epidural or spinal anesthesia. Epidural anesthesia results from the deposition of a local anesthetic agent into the extradural space within the vertebral canal. Catheters can be left in place in the epidural

TABLE 14-2.   Regional Anesthetic Agents

Technique	Local Anesthetic	Concentration Range (%)	Duration of Action	Maximal Safe Dose (mg)
Topical anesthesia (mucous membranes)	Lidocaine	2–4	15 min	100
	Cocaine	4–10	30 min	100–200
	Tetracaine	1–2	45 min	40
	Benzocaine	2–10	several hours	
Local infiltration	Procaine	0.5	¼–½ h	1000
	Lidocaine	0.5–1	½–1 h	500
	Mepivacaine	0.5–1	½–1 h	500
	Tetracaine	0.025–0.1	2–3 h	75
Major nerve block	Lidocaine	1–2	1–2 h	500
	Mepivacaine	1–2	1–2 h	500
	Tetracaine	0.1–0.25	2–3 h	75

Adapted from Brunner EA, Eckenhoff JE: Anesthesia. In Sabiston DC Jr (ed): Textbook of Surgery. Philadelphia, WB Saunders, 1977.

space, allowing the intermittent injection of local anesthetics for prolonged operations. The major advantage of epidural over spinal anesthesia is that it does not involve puncturing the dura, and thus the injection of foreign substances directly into the cerebrospinal fluid is avoided.

Spinal anesthesia involves the direct injection of a local anesthetic into the cerebrospinal fluid. Puncture of the dural sac generally is performed between the L2 and L4 vertebrae. Spinal anesthesia provides excellent anesthesia for intra-abdominal operations, operations on the pelvis, or procedures involving the lower extremities. Because the patient is awake during spinal anesthesia and is breathing spontaneously, it often has been thought that spinal anesthesia is "safer" than general anesthesia. There is, however, no difference in the incidence of intraoperative hypotension with spinal anesthesia compared with general anesthesia, and thus there is no clear benefit in using spinal anesthesia for patients with ischemic heart disease.[6] Because patients are awake during spinal anesthesia and can become agitated during the surgical procedure, spinal anesthesia actually can cause more myocardial stress than general anesthesia. The health status of patients with preoperative evidence of congestive heart failure is more likely to be worsened by general anesthesia than by spinal anesthesia. In one series, heart failure developed de novo in 4% of adults over the age of 40 years who were undergoing major surgery, and worsened in 22% of patients who had a history of heart failure.[6] Spinal anesthesia was not associated with any new or worsened heart failure. Because of local irritating effects of general anesthesia on the lung, it has been suggested that spinal anesthesia may be safer for patients with severe pulmonary disease.

General anesthesia refers to the reversible state of loss of consciousness produced by a variety of chemical agents that act directly on the brain. Most major oncologic procedures are performed under general anesthesia, which can be induced using either intravenous or inhalational agents. The advantages of intravenous anesthesia are the extremely rapid onset of unconsciousness and improved patient comfort and acceptance. Ultrashort-acting barbiturates, such as sodium thiopental, or tranquilizers, such as the benzodiazepines or droperidol, are the most frequently used intravenous agents for general anesthesia or for sedation during regional anesthesia.

A variety of inhalational anesthetic agents are in clinical use. The most popular is nitrous oxide, usually in combination with narcotics and muscle relaxants. This technique provides a safe form of general anesthesia with the use of nonexplosive agents. Two other agents in widespread use are the fluorinated hydrocarbons, halothane (Fluothane) and enflurane (Ethrane). Although they are used frequently, the fluorinated hydrocarbons have a variety of side-effects. Halothane depresses myocardial function, reduces cardiac output, causes significant vasodilation, and sensitizes the myocardium to both endogenous and administered catecholamines, which can lead to life-threatening cardiac arrhythmias. In rare instances, halothane can cause severe hepatotoxicity, which begins 2 to 5 days after surgery. Enflurane also depresses myocardial function but does not appear to sensitize the myocardium to catecholamines and has not been associated with hepatic toxicity. The newest of the halogenated hydrocarbons is isoflurane, which was introduced in 1980. Isoflurane depresses the myocardium less than halothane or enflurane, but it has more potent vasodilatory properties.

Virtually all general anesthetics affect various biochemical mechanisms, including depression of bone marrow, alteration of the phagocytic activity of macrophages, and exhibition of various immunosuppressive properties. General anesthetic agents, such as cyclopropane and diethyl ether, are rarely used in current practice because of their explosive potential.

Intravenous neuromuscular blocking agents, called muscle relaxants, are commonly used during general anesthesia. These agents are either nondepolarizing (e.g., curare), preventing access of acetylcholine to the receptor site of the myoneural junction, or depolarizing (e.g., succinylcholine) acting in a manner similar to that of acetylcholine by depolarizing the motor end-plate. These agents induce profound muscle relaxation during surgical procedures but have the obvious disadvantage of inhibiting spontaneous respiration because of paralysis of respiratory muscles. Succinylcholine is short acting (3–5 minutes) with a rapid recovery phase. Curare-induced paralysis lasts for 30 to 40 minutes after usual clinical doses of 0.3 to 0.5 mg/kg. Pancuronium is a newer nondepolarizing agent that has fewer side-effects than curare but can induce tachycardia by means of sympathetic stimulation.

DETERMINATION OF OPERATIVE RISK

As with any treatment, the potential benefits of surgical intervention in cancer patients must be weighed against the risks of surgery. The incidence of operative mortality is of major importance in formulating therapeutic decisions and varies greatly in different patient situations (Table 14-3). The incidence of operative mortality is a complex function of the basic disease process that involves surgery, anesthetic technique, operative complications, and, most importantly, the general health status of the patient and his ability to withstand operative trauma.

In an attempt to classify the physical status of patients and their surgical risks, the American Society of Anesthesiologists has formulated a General Classification of Physical Status that appears to correlate well with operative mortality.[7] Patients are classified into five groups depending on their general health status.

Class 1. The patient has no organic, physiologic, biochemical, or psychiatric disturbance. The pathologic process for which the operation is to be performed is localized and does not entail a systemic disturbance. (Examples: a fit patient with a lipoma or an otherwise healthy woman with a fibroid uterus)

Class 2. Mild to moderate systemic disturbance caused by either the condition to be surgically treated or the pathophysiologic processes. The extremes of age are included here, either the neonate or the octogenarian, even though no discernible systemic disease is present. Extreme obesity and chronic bronchitis also are included in this category. (Examples: nonlimiting or only slightly limiting organic heart disease, mild diabetes, essential hypertension, or anemia)

Class 3. Severe systemic disturbance or disease from whatever cause, even though it may not be possible to define firmly the degree of disability. (Examples: severely limiting organic heart disease, severe diabetes with vascular complications, moderate to severe degrees of pulmonary insufficiency, angina pectoris, or healed myocardial infarction)

Class 4. Indicative of the patient with severe systemic disorders that already are life-threatening and not always correctable by an operation. (Examples: severely cachectic patients with metastatic cancer; patients with organic heart disease showing marked signs of cardiac insufficiency, persistent anginal syndrome, or active myocarditis; advanced degrees of pulmonary, hepatic, renal, or endocrine insufficiency; severe neutropenia or thrombocytopenia in cancer patients)

Class 5. The moribund patient who has little chance of survival but who submitted to operation in desperation. Most of these patients require an operation as a resuscitative measure

TABLE 14-3. Determinants of Operative Risk

General health status
Severity of underlying illness
Degree to which surgery disrupts normal physiologic functions
Technical complexity of the procedure (related to incidence of complications)
Type of anesthesia required
Experience of personnel

with little, if any, anesthesia. (Examples: burst abdominal aneurysm with profound shock, major cerebral trauma with rapidly increasing intracranial pressure, massive pulmonary embolus)

Emergency Operation (E). Any patient in classes 1 through 5 who is operated on as an emergency is considered to be in poorer physical condition. The letter *E* is placed beside the numerical classification. (Examples: perforation of a viscus, major hemorrhage from a gastrointestinal mass, or hitherto uncomplicated hernia now incarcerated and associated with nausea and vomiting)

Operative mortality usually is defined as mortality that occurs within 30 days of a major operative procedure. In oncologic patients, the basic disease process will be a major determinant of operative mortality. Patients undergoing palliative surgery for widely metastatic disease have a high operative mortality even if the surgical procedure can alleviate the symptomatic problem. Examples of these situations include surgery for intestinal obstruction in patients with widespread ovarian cancer and surgery for gastric outlet obstruction in patients with cancer of the head of the pancreas. These simple palliative procedures are associated with mortality rates of 20% to 30% in most series because of the debilitated state of the patient and the rapid progression of the basic disease.

Mortality caused by anesthetic administration alone is directly related to the physical status of the patient. In a review of 32,223 operations, Dripps and co-workers determined the mortality thought to be related to anesthetic administration alone (Table 14-4).[8] It is extremely difficult to differentiate the mortality caused by anesthesia from that resulting from other contributors to operative mortality. However, this analysis indicates that operative mortality due to anesthesia in physical status class 1 patients is extremely low, less than 1 in every 16,000 operations. The anesthetic mortality increased with worsened physical status. Most cancer patients

TABLE 14-4. Anesthetic Mortality Related to Physical Status

Physical Status	Number of Patients	Number of Deaths	Anesthetic Mortality (%)
Class I	16,192	0	<.006
Class II	12,154	7	0.058
Class III	4,070	11	0.27
Class IV	720	17	2.4
Class V	87	4	4.6
Total	33,223	39	0.12

(Adapted from Dripps RD, Lamont A, Eckenhoff JE: The role of anesthesia in surgical mortality. JAMA 178:261, 1961)

undergoing elective cancer surgery fall somewhere between physical status 2 and 3. An anesthetic mortality rate of 0.1% to 0.2% is a realistic estimate for this group.

In an attempt to determine the operative mortality from anesthesia alone, similar estimates to that found by Dripps and co-workers have been obtained. For example, Moir found the fatality rate for women undergoing cesarean sections in Great Britain to be 1 in 1250 to 2000 deliveries.[9] The mortality thought to be caused by anesthesia alone was 1 patient in every 6000 to 7500 deliveries. A similar estimate was obtained by Collins and associates, who estimated that the mortality resulting from general anesthesia alone was approximately 1 in 3000 to 5000 in otherwise healthy patients.[10] Several health factors can increase the risks of the operative procedure. If the patient recently had a myocardial infarction, the risk of cardiac death associated with surgery increases significantly.[11] A recurrent myocardial infarction or cardiac death will occur in approximately 30% of patients who have surgery within 3 months after a myocardial infarction and in about 15% of patients who have surgery 3 to 6 months after an infarction. The risk of a recurrent infarction or cardiac death decreases to about 5% after 6 months and remains approximately constant regardless of how much longer the patient survives. Operative risks are similar following either subendocardial and transmural infarctions.

Patients with a preoperative history of pulmonary edema or with clinical evidence of congestive heart failure by preoperative physical examination and chest x-ray films have a markedly increased risk for developing perioperative pulmonary edema. In a study of patients over the age of 40 undergoing major surgery, 23% of patients with a history of pulmonary edema developed cardiogenic pulmonary edema in the postoperative period, compared with 2% of patients with no history of congestive heart failure.[6,11] Because of the complexities of evaluating the general health status of a patient, multivariate analyses have been performed to determine which factors independently predict the development of complications. An example of one such multivariate analysis is presented in Table 14-5.[11] In this series of 1001 patients over the age of 40 years who had major noncardiac surgical procedures performed, nine separate factors were used to group the patients into categories with substantially different risks of cardiac complications. Each factor listed in Table 14-5 was associated with a number of points, and the total number of points determined the risk class. For patients in class I (0–5 points), 0.7% of patients had cardiac complications from the surgical procedure, and 0.2% of patients died of cardiac causes. The risk of cardiac complications and death in class II patients (6–12 points) was 5% and 2%, respectively. In class III patients (13–25 points), the probability of nonfatal complications was 11%, but the risk of death remained at 2%. In class IV risk patients (26 or more points), 56% of patients died of cardiac causes, and an additional 22% had life-threatening, nonfatal complications.

The impact of general health status on operative mortality is seen when operative mortality as a function of age is analyzed. Palmberg and co-workers studied the postoperative mortality of 17,199 patients undergoing general surgical procedures.[12] The overall mortality rate of patients under 70 years old was 0.25%, compared with 9.2% for patients over 70 years of age. In these elderly patients, the operative mortality rate for emergency operations was 36.8%, compared with 7.8% for elective surgical procedures. The four leading causes of operative mortality that accounted for approximately 75% of all postoperative deaths in this age group were pulmonary embolism, pneumonia, cardiovascular collapse, and the primary illness itself.

Reports of most surgical series include an account of oper-

TABLE 14-5. Correlation Between Signs and Symptoms of Preoperative Heart Failure and Risk of Perioperative Pulmonary Edema After Major Surgery in Patients over Age 40

Signs and Symptoms	Total Patients (no.)	Percentage Developing Cardiogenic Pulmonary Edema (%)
No history of congestive heart failure	853	2*
History of left heart failure but not evident on preoperative examination or chest roentgenogram	87	6*
Left heart failure by preoperative physical examination or chest roentgenogram	66	16*
Preoperative NYHA functional class for congestive heart failure		
I	935	
II	15	7
III	34	6
IV	17	25†
History of pulmonary edema	22	23‡
S3 gallop	17	35‡
Jugular venous distention and signs of left heart failure	23	30‡

Goldman L: Cardiac risks and complications of noncardiac surgery. Ann Surg 198:780–791, 1983.

*p < 0.01 for all pairs.
†p < 0.001 for class IV versus all others.
‡p < 0.01 when comparing patients to those without these findings.

ative mortality and operative complications. These results, combined with a consideration of the general health status of the patient, allow a reasonable estimate of the operative mortality for any given surgical intervention in the treatment of cancer.

ROLES FOR SURGERY

PREVENTION OF CANCER

Because the surgeon is often the primary provider of medical care, he is responsible for educating patients about carcinogenic hazards and about direct surgical intervention for the prevention of cancer. All surgical oncologists should be aware of the high-risk situations that require surgery to prevent subsequent malignant disease.

A variety of underlying conditions or congenital or genetic traits are associated with an extremely high incidence of subsequent cancer. When these cancers are likely to occur in nonvital organs, it is necessary to remove the offending organ to prevent subsequent malignancy.[13] Examples of diseases associated with a high incidence of cancer that can be prevented by prophylactic surgery are presented in Table 14-6. An excellent example is presented by patients with the genetic trait for multiple polyposis of the colon. If colectomy is not performed in these patients, approximately half will develop colon cancer by the age of 40. By the age of 70, virtually all patients with multiple polyposis will develop colon cancer.[13] It is therefore advisable for all patients containing the mutant gene for multiple polyposis to undergo prophylactic colectomy before the age of 20 in order to prevent these cancers.

In this situation, as for many of the other familial conditions associated with a high incidence of cancer, the surgeon has a responsibility for alerting the family to the hereditary nature of the disorder and its possible occurrence in other family members. Another disease associated with a high incidence of cancer of the colon is ulcerative colitis. Approximately 40% of patients with total colonic involvement will ultimately die of colon cancer if they survive the ulcerative colitis.[14] Three percent of children with ulcerative colitis will develop cancer of the colon by the age of 10, and 20% will develop cancer during each ensuing decade.[15] Colectomy is

indicated for patients with cancer of the colon if the chronicity of this disease is well established.

Other disorders that require early treatment in order to prevent subsequent cancers include cryptorchidism and multiple endocrine neoplasia. Cryptorchidism is associated with a high incidence of testicular cancer that probably can be prevented by early prophylactic surgery. Patients with multiple endocrine neoplasia (types II and III) should be screened for the presence of C-cell hyperplasia using pentagastrin-stimulation tests. If thyrocalcitonin levels are increased following this provocative test, thyroidectomy should be performed to prevent the subsequent clinical occurrence of medullary cancer of the thyroid gland.

A more complex example of the role of surgery in cancer prevention involves women at high risk for breast cancer. Because the risk of cancer in some women is substantially increased over the normal risk (but does not yet approach 100%), counseling is required. Women in this situation must carefully balance the benefits and risks of prophylactic mastectomy. A careful understanding of the factors involved in increased breast cancer incidence is essential for the surgical oncologist to provide sound advice in this area. Statistical techniques can provide approximations of the risk for patients depending on the frequency of disease in the family history, the age at the first pregnancy, and the presence of fibrocystic disease. For example, a woman with a family history of breast cancer in a sister or mother, who has fibrocystic disease, and either is nulliparous or had a first pregnancy at a late age has an approximately 18% probability of developing breast cancer over a 5-year period.[13] These estimates can be of value in advising women about prophylactic mastectomy.

DIAGNOSIS OF CANCER

The major role of surgery in the diagnosis of cancer lies in the acquisition of tissue for exact histologic diagnosis. The principles underlying the biopsy of malignant lesions vary depending on the natural history of the tumor under consideration. A variety of techniques exist for obtaining tissues suspected of malignancy, including aspiration biopsy, needle biopsy, incisional biopsy, and excisional biopsy.

Aspiration biopsy involves the aspiration of cells and tissue

TABLE 14-6. Surgery That Can Prevent Cancer

Underlying Condition	Associated Cancer	Prophylactic Surgery
Cryptorchidism	Testicular	Orchiopexy
Polyposis coli	Colon	Colectomy
Familial colon cancer	Colon	Colectomy
Ulcerative colitis	Colon	Colectomy
Multiple endocrine neoplasia, types II and III	Medullary cancer of the thyroid	Thyroidectomy
Familial breast cancer	Breast	Mastectomy
Familial ovarian cancer	Ovary	Oophorectomy

Adapted from Mulvihill JJ: Cancer control through genetics. In Arrighi FE, Rao PN. Stubblefield E (eds): Genes, Chromosomes, and Neoplasia. New York, Raven Press, 1980.

fragments through a needle that has been guided into the suspect tissue. Cytologic analysis of this material can provide a tentative diagnosis of the presence of malignant tissue. However, major surgical resections should not be undertaken solely on the basis of the evidence of aspiration biopsy. Even the most experienced cytologist can mistake inflammatory or benign reparative changes for malignant cells. This error is inherent in the uncertainties of individual cell analysis and, even in the best of hands, provides an error rate substantially higher than that of standard histologic diagnosis.

Needle biopsy refers to obtaining a core of tissue through a specially designed needle introduced into the suspect tissue. The core of tissue provided by needle biopsies is sufficient for the diagnosis of most, but not all, tumor types. Soft-tissue and bony sarcomas often present major difficulties in differentiating benign and reparative lesions from malignancies and often cannot be diagnosed accurately. If these latter lesions are considered in the diagnosis, attempts should be made to obtain larger amounts of tissue than are possible from a needle biopsy.

Incisional biopsy refers to removal of a small wedge of tissue from a larger tumor mass. Incisional biopsies often are necessary for diagnosing large masses that require major surgical procedures for even local excision. Incisional biopsies are the preferred method of diagnosing soft-tissue and bony sarcomas because of the magnitude of the surgical procedures necessary to extirpate these lesions definitively. The treatment of many visceral cancers cannot be undertaken without an incisional biopsy, but be aware of opening new tissue planes contaminated with tumor by performing excisional biopsies for large lesions. An inappropriately performed excisional biopsy can compromise subsequent surgical excision. When this is a possibility, incisional biopsies should be performed.

In excisional biopsy, an excision of the entire suspected tumor tissue with little or no margin of surrounding normal tissue is done. Excisional biopsies are the procedure of choice for most tumors if they can be performed without contaminating new tissue planes or further compromising the ultimate surgical procedure.

There is little evidence that differences exist between incisional and excisional biopsies with respect to tumor spread. Several studies comparing incisional and excisional biopsies of suspected melanoma lesions found no differences in ultimate outcome in these patients, but the surgeon should avoid cutting directly into suspected tumor if it is not necessary to do so.[16,17]

The following principles guide the performance of all surgical biopsies.

1. Needle tracts or scars should be placed carefully so that they can be conveniently removed as part of the subsequent definitive surgical procedure. Placement of biopsy incisions is extremely important, and misplacement often can compromise subsequent care. Incisions on the extremity generally should be placed longitudinally so as to make the removal of underlying tissue and subsequent closure easier.

2. Care should be taken not to contaminate new tissue planes during the biopsy. Large hematomas after biopsy can lead to tumor spread and must be scrupulously avoided by securing excellent hemostasis during the biopsy. For biopsies on extremities, the use of a tourniquet may help in controlling bleeding. Instruments used in a biopsy procedure are another potential source of contamination of new tissue planes. It is not uncommon to take biopsy samples from several suspected lesions at one time. Care should be taken not to use instruments that may have come in contact with tumor when obtaining tissue from a potentially uncontaminated area.

3. Choice of biopsy technique should be selected carefully in order to obtain an adequate tissue sample for the needs of the pathologist. For the diagnosis of selected tumors, electron microscopy, tissue culture, or other techniques may be necessary. Sufficient tissue must be obtained for these purposes if diagnostic difficulties are anticipated.

4. Handling of the biopsy tissue by the pathologist is also important. When the orientation of the biopsy specimen is important for subsequent treatment, the surgeon should mark distinctive areas of the tumor carefully in order to facilitate subsequent orientation of the specimen by the pathologist. Different fixatives are best for different types or sizes of tissue. If all biopsy specimens are immediately placed in formalin, the opportunity to perform valuable diagnostic tests may be lost. The handling of excised tissue is the surgeon's responsibility. Biopsy tissue obtained from breast cancer lesions, for example, should be saved for estrogen receptor studies and placed in cold storage until ready for processing.

Surgery also has a role in diagnosing pathologic states in cancer patients that do not directly involve the diagnosis of cancer. Cancer patients often are immunosuppressed by either their disease or their treatment and are subject to a variety of opportunistic infections not commonly seen in most general surgical patients. Open lung or liver biopsies are often important in diagnosing these lesions adequately and in planning suitable therapy.

Oncologists are becoming increasingly aware of the need for precise staging of patients when planning treatment. Lack of proper staging information can lead to poor treatment planning and compromise the ability to cure patients. Staging laparotomy can be important in determining the exact extent of spread of lymphomas. (This is considered in more detail in Chapter 50.)

In performing accurate surgical staging, the surgeon must be familiar with the natural history of the disease under consideration. The development of ovarian cancer treatment is an excellent example. The tendency of ovarian cancer to metastasize to the undersurface of the diaphragm is a good example of the need to biopsy an anatomic site that would not normally be biopsied by most surgeons. Extensive surgical staging may be required before undertaking other major surgical procedures with curative intent. For example, biopsy of the celiac and para-aortic lymph nodes in patients with cancer of the esophagus is often important so that unnecessary esophageal resections can be avoided.

Placement of radio-opaque clips during biopsy and staging

procedures is important in order to delineate areas of known tumor and as a guide to the subsequent delivery of radiation therapy to these areas.

TREATMENT OF CANCER

Surgery can be a simple, safe method to cure patients with solid tumors when the tumor is confined to the anatomic site of origin. Unfortunately, when patients with solid tumors present to the physician for the first time, approximately 70% already will have micrometastases beyond the primary site. The extension of the surgical resection to include areas of regional spread can cure some of these patients, although regional spread often is an indication of undetectable distant micrometastases.

The emergence of effective nonsurgical therapies has had profound impact on the treatment of cancer patients and on the role and responsibilities of the surgeon treating the cancer patient. John Hunter, a brilliant 18th century surgeon, characterized surgery as being "like an armed savage who attempts to get that by force which a civilized man would get by strategem."

Although surgery continues to be the most important aspect of the treatment of most patients presenting with solid tumors, modern clinical research in oncology has been devoted to applying other adjuvant "strategems" to improve the cure rates of those 70% who ultimately will fail surgical therapy alone.

The role of surgery in the treatment of cancer patients can be divided into six separate areas. In each area, interactions with other treatment modalities can be essential for a successful outcome.

1. Definitive surgical treatment for primary cancer, selection of appropriate local therapy, and integration of surgery with other adjuvant modalities
2. Surgery to reduce the bulk of residual disease (Examples: Burkitt's lymphoma, ovarian cancer)
3. Surgical resection of metastatic disease with curative intent (Examples: pulmonary metastases in sarcoma patients, hepatic metastases from colorectal cancer)
4. Surgery for the treatment of oncologic emergencies
5. Surgery for palliation
6. Surgery for reconstruction and rehabilitation

Surgery for Primary Cancer

There are three major challenges confronting the surgical oncologist in the definitive treatment of solid tumors:

1. Accurate identification of patients who can be cured by local treatment alone
2. Development and selection of local treatments that provide the best balance between local cure and the impact of treatment morbidity on the quality of life
3. Development and application of adjuvant treatments that can improve the control of both local and distant invasive and metastatic disease

The selection of the appropriate local therapy to be used in cancer treatment varies with the individual cancer type and the site of involvement. In many instances, definitive surgi-

cal therapy that encompasses a sufficient margin of normal tissue is sufficient local therapy. The treatment of many solid tumors falls into this category. Including the wide excision of primary melanomas in the skin that can be cured locally by surgery alone in approximately 90% of cases. The resection of colon cancers with a 5-cm margin from the tumor results in anastomotic recurrences in less than 5% of cases.

In other instances, surgery is used to obtain histologic confirmation of diagnosis, but primary local therapy is achieved through the use of a nonsurgical modality such as radiation therapy. Examples of this include the treatment of Ewing's sarcoma in long bones and the treatment of selected primary malignancies in the head and neck. In each instance, selection of the definitive local treatment involves careful consideration of the likelihood of cure balanced against the morbidity of the treatment modality.

The magnitude of surgical resection is modified in the treatment of many cancers by the use of adjuvant treatment modalities. Rationally integrating surgery with other treatments requires a careful consideration of all effective treatment options. The surgical oncologist must be thoroughly familiar with adjuncts and alternatives to surgical treatment. It is a knowledge of this rapidly changing field that separates the surgical oncologist from the general surgeon most distinctly.

In some instances, effective adjuvant modalities have led to a decrease in the magnitude of surgery. The evolution of childhood rhabdomyosarcoma treatment is a striking example of the successful integration of adjuvant therapies with surgery in the treatment of cancer (Table 14-7).[18,19]

Childhood rhabdomyosarcoma is the most common soft tissue sarcoma in infants and children. Before 1970, surgery alone was used almost exclusively, and 5-year survivals of from 10% to 20% were commonly reported. Local surgery alone failed in patients with rhabdomyosarcomas of the prostate and extremities because of both extensive invasion of surrounding tissues and the early development of metastatic disease. The failure of surgery alone to control local disease in patients with childhood rhabdomyosarcoma led to the introduction of adjuvant radiation therapy. This resulted in a marked improvement in local control rates that was further improved dramatically by the introduction of combination chemotherapy with vincristine, actinomycin D, and cyclophosphamide. Long-term cure rates are now in the range of 80%. Further consideration of this disease and of the impor-

TABLE 14-7. Treatment of Childhood Rhabdomyosarcoma

Treatment	5-Year Survival (%)
Surgery alone	10–20
Surgery + radiotherapy	40–50
Surgery + radiotherapy + chemotherapy	80–90

Adapted from Kilman JW, Clatworthy HW Jr, Newton WA, et al: Reasonable surgery for rhabdomyosarcoma: A study of 67 cases. Ann Surg 3:346, 1973; and from Heyn RM, Holland R, Newton WA, et al: The role of combined chemotherapy in the treatment of rhabdomyosarcoma in children. Cancer 34:2128–2142, 1974.

tance of adjuvant therapy in its treatment can be found in Chapter 47. Current investigations are exploring the use of preoperative radiation therapy to see if the magnitude of surgery can be reduced further or perhaps even eliminated by using radiation and chemotherapy as the primary treatment modalities, with surgery reserved for elimination of residual disease. This latter approach has been successful in treating Ewing's sarcoma and has largely replaced surgery as the primary therapy. Many other examples of the integration of surgery with other treatment modalities appear throughout this book.

Surgery for Residual Disease

The concept of cytoreductive surgery has received much attention in recent years.[20] In some instances, the extensive local spread of cancer precludes the removal of all gross disease by surgery. The surgical resection of bulk disease in the treatment of selected cancers may well lead to improvements in the ability to control residual gross disease that has not been resected. Studies will be discussed that suggest the merit of this approach in Chapters 48 and 33 (Burkitt's lymphoma and ovarian cancer, respectively).

Enthusiasm for cytoreductive surgery has led to the inappropriate use of surgery for reducing the bulk of tumor in some cases. Clearly, cytoreductive surgery will be of benefit only when other effective treatments are available to control the residual disease that is unresectable. Except in rare palliative settings, there is no role for cytoreductive surgery in patients in whom little other effective therapy currently exists.

Surgery for Metastatic Disease

The value of surgery in the cure of patients with metastatic disease tends to be overlooked. As a general principle, patients with a single site of metastatic disease that can be resected without major morbidity should undergo resection of that metastatic cancer. Many patients with few metastases to lung or liver or brain can be cured by surgical resection (see Chap. 62, sects. 1, 2, and 3). This approach is especially true for cancers that tend not to be highly responsive to systemic chemotherapy. The resection of pulmonary metastases in patients with soft tissue and bony sarcomas can cure up to 30% of patients. As effective systemic therapy is developed for the treatment of these diseases, cure rates may increase. Studies have shown that similar cure rates occur in patients with adenocarcinomas when resected metastatic disease to the lung is the sole clinical site of metastases. Small numbers of pulmonary metastases often are the only clinically apparent metastatic disease in patients with sarcomas. However, this is rare in the natural history of most adenocarcinomas. If solitary metastases to the lung do occur in patients with carcinoma of the colon or other adenocarcinomas, then surgical resection is indicated.

Similarly, there is increasing enthusiasm for the resection of hepatic metastases, especially from colorectal cancer, in patients in whom the liver is the only site of known metastatic disease. In patients with solitary hepatic metastases from colorectal cancer, resection can lead to long-term cure in approximately 25% of patients. This far exceeds the cure rates of any other available treatment.

The resection for cure of solitary brain metastases should also be considered when the brain is the only site of known metastatic disease. The exact location and functional sequelae of resection should be considered when making this treatment decision.

SURGERY FOR ONCOLOGIC EMERGENCIES

As in the treatment of all patients, emergencies arise for oncologic patients that require surgical intervention. These generally involve the treatment of exsanguinating hemorrhage, perforation, drainage of abscesses, or impending destruction of vital organs. Each category of surgical emergency is unique and requires an individual approach. These are considered in detail in Chapter 58, section 4.

The oncologic patient often is neutropenic, thrombocytopenic, and has a high risk of hemorrhage or sepsis. Perforations of an abdominal viscus can result from direct tumor invasion or from tumor lysis resulting from effective systemic treatments. Perforation of the gastrointestinal tract following effective treatment for lymphoma involving the intestine is not uncommon. The ability to identify patients at high risk for perforation may lead to the use of surgery to prevent this problem. Surgery to decompress cancer invading the CNS represents another surgical emergency that can lead to preservation of function.

Surgery for Palliation

Surgical resection often is required for the relief of pain or functional abnormalities. The appropriate use of surgery in these settings can improve the quality of life for cancer patients. Palliative surgery may include the relief of mechanical problems such as intestinal obstruction or the removal of masses that are causing severe pain or disfigurement.

Surgery for Reconstruction and Rehabilitation

Surgical techniques are being refined that aid in the reconstruction and rehabilitation of cancer patients following definitive therapy. The ability to reconstruct anatomic defects can substantially improve both function and cosmetic appearance. The development of free flaps using microvascular anastomotic techniques is having a profound impact on the ability to bring fresh tissue to resected or heavily irradiated areas. Loss of function (especially of extremities) often can be rehabilitated by surgical approaches. This includes lysis of contractures or muscle transposition to restore muscular function that has been damaged by prior surgery or radiation therapy.

THE SURGICAL ONCOLOGIST

Several factors have led to a recent increase in the development of surgical oncology and to the organization of separate sections of surgical oncology in large hospitals and departments of surgery within universities. This enthusiasm derives from the recognition that modern oncologic management requires levels of expertise in cancer surgery, chemotherapy, and radiation therapy that are not common to most general surgeons, as well as a desire to use effectively the resources being committed to cancer care and research by hospitals, private foundations, and the federal government. A sense of urgency has existed because some surgical leaders believe that the surgeon is experiencing a declining intellectual role in modern cancer treatment and research and that steps must be taken to reassert the surgeon's role in modern oncology.

Many surgeons, however, have resisted the development of surgical oncology as a specialty area because of the fear of fragmenting the field of general surgery. A survey of 124 university surgery departments in the United States between January and July, 1985, revealed that 38% had formal divisions of surgical oncology compared with divisions of medical oncology present in 95%, radiation oncology in 94%, pediatric oncology in 76%, and gynecologic oncology in 79% of university medical institutions.[21] Of the 47 divisions of surgical oncology that did exist, only 13 (28%) had formal clinical training programs in surgical oncology.[21] This lack of emphasis on surgical oncology at universities may be a factor in the decreasing success of surgeons in obtaining grant support from the National Cancer Institute. For the six years from 1980 through 1985, an analysis of 6407 applications submitted from clinical departments of medical schools for peer-reviewed grants revealed that 44% were submitted from departments of medicine and only 16% from departments of surgery.[22] Thirty-four percent of applications submitted from departments of medicine were awarded, compared with 25% from departments of surgery.[22]

The development of surgical oncology as a specialty area of surgery depends on a clear delineation of its role. There are six major areas in which the modern surgical oncologist can play a valuable role in the care of cancer patients at major treatment centers:[23]

1. Organize surgical oncology teaching programs for staff, residents, and students
2. Provide expert consultation for unusual or difficult oncologic patient problems
3. Provide unique surgical expertise in surgical cases unfamiliar to general surgeons (*e.g.*, major soft tissue resections, exenterations, head and neck resections, isolation-perfusions)
4. Organize clinical research protocols for surgical oncology patients
5. Coordinate surgical oncology efforts with medical and radiation oncologists
6. Conduct experimental research programs in oncology where possible

The rapid development of new information in surgery, chemotherapy, and medical oncology, in addition to newer disciplines of immunotherapy, hyperthermia, and phototherapy, requires the continuing education of all surgical staff. Surgical oncologists maintain close contact with all of these areas and should be responsible for teaching programs for general surgical staff, residents, and students in these different areas.

Because of the unique training and exposure to oncologic problems, the surgical oncologist has expertise in dealing with unusual or difficult oncologic patient problems, and thus can provide expert consultation in these areas. The surgical oncologist is trained to perform many types of surgical procedures not commonly performed by most general surgeons. Although most surgeons are able to perform many of the standard cancer resections, some operations are not performed frequently by general surgeons and can be performed better by a specialist in surgical oncology.

In most hospital settings, a variety of general surgeons operate on cancer patients. It is often essential, however, that patients receiving care for a variety of cancers enter clinical protocols that will help answer important questions related to the treatment of that cancer. The surgical oncologist can help organize clinical research protocols for surgical oncology patients treated by all surgeons at that institution. A large surgical group should have a surgical specialist capable of coordinating efforts with medical and radiation oncologists. Successful coordination with these nonsurgical specialists requires expertise in medical oncology and radiation therapy that is not common among most general surgeons.

The surgical oncologist can also be involved in administering and defining the need for a variety of adjuvant treatments. Adjuvant chemotherapy commonly is administered by surgeons when the chemotherapy regimens use well-known single or combination agents. The future development of immunotherapies and other new adjuvant treatments can be logically administered by the surgical oncologist to his patient following recovery from the surgical procedure.

Finally, the surgical oncologist, when the situation allows, is in a position to perform experimental research in oncology that can lead to the introduction of new diagnostic and treatment regimens in clinical care. Laboratory research programs that contribute to basic knowledge of cancer biology also provide an important source of stimulation to residents and students.

The emergence of a subspecialty of surgical oncology within general surgery requires that special attention be given to the training of surgeons interested in pursuing this area of clinical care. Although it is generally agreed that all surgical oncologists should be well-trained general surgeons, attempts have been made to define additional areas of expertise that must be studied. In 1978, a group of surgical oncologists met under the sponsorship of the Society of Surgical Oncology and the Division of Cancer Research, Resources, and Centers of the National Cancer Institute to develop guidelines for the training of surgical oncologists.

The guidelines adopted by this meeting included a variety of suggestions for such training.[24,25]

1. Two-year training program on a surgical oncology service after completion of eligibility for general surgical certification by the American Board of Surgery or other surgical specialty board
2. Training at an institution whose cancer program is approved by the Commission on Cancer of the Ameri-

can College of Surgeons and whose clinical resources provide a sufficient variety and volume of clinical material to assure exposure to a broad variety of clinical cancer problems

3. Training at a center with sufficient basic science resources to provide education in these areas, with exposure to both basic and clinical research

4. Training at an institution that will provide adequate operative experience, including standard curative and palliative procedures, with broad exposure to surgical procedures unique to the oncologic patient

5. A full-time assignment during the training period to both radiation oncology and chemotherapy services to allow the trainee to gain confidence and knowledge in these nonsurgical disciplines

These training recommendations are designed to provide general surgeons with the expertise in oncology and nonsurgical disciplines necessary to bring the best aspects of all disciplines of modern oncology to the care of the cancer patient.

REFERENCES

1. Brested JH: The Edwin Smith Surgical Papyrus. Chicago, University of Chicago Press, 1930
2. Thorwald J: Science and the Secrets of Early Medicine. New York, Harcourt, Brace, and World, 1962
3. Wangensteen OH: Has medical history importance for surgeons? Surg Gynecol Obstet 140:434, 1975
4. Hill GJ: Historic milestones in cancer surgery. Semin Oncol 6:409–427, 1979
5. Brunner EA, Eckenhoff JE: Anesthesia. In Sabiston DC Jr (ed): Textbook of Surgery. Philadelphia, WB Saunders, 1977
6. Goldman L, Caldera DL, Nussbaum SR, et al. Multifactorial index of cardiac risk in noncardiac surgical procedures. N Engl J Med 297:845–850, 1977
7. Dripps RD, Eckenhoff JE, Vandam LD: Introduction to Anesthesia. Philadelphia, WB Saunders, 1977
8. Dripps RD, Lamont A, Eckenhoff JE: The role of anesthesia in surgical mortality. JAMA 178:261, 1961
9. Moir DD: Maternal mortality and anesthaesia. Br J Anaesth 52:1–3, 1980
10. Collins VJ: Principles of Anesthesiology. Philadelphia. Lea & Febiger, 1976
11. Goldman L: Cardiac risks and complications of noncardiac surgery. Ann Surg 198:780–791, 1983
12. Palmberg S, Hirsjarvi E: Mortality in geriatric surgery. Gerontology 25:103–112, 1979
13. Mulvihill JJ: Cancer control through genetics. In Arrighi FE, Rao PN, Stubblefield E (eds): Genes, Chromosomes, and Neoplasia. New York, Raven Press, 1980
14. MacDougall IPM: The cancer risk in ulcerative colitis. Lancet 2:655, 1964
15. Devroede GJ, Taylor WF, Sauer WG: Cancer risk and life expectancy of children with ulcerative colitis. N Engl J Med 285:17, 1971
16. Epstein E, Bragg K, Linden GJ: Biopsy and prognosis of malignant melanoma. JAMA 208:1369, 1969
17. Knutson CO, Hori JM, Spratt JS Jr: Melanoma. Curr Probl Surg, Dec 1971
18. Kilman JW, Clatworthy HW Jr, Newton WA, et al: Reasonable surgery for rhabdomyosarcoma: A study of 67 cases. Ann Surg 3:346, 1973
19. Heyn RM, Holland R, Newton WA, et al: The role of combined chemotherapy in the treatment of rhabdomyosarcoma in children. Cancer 34:2128–2142, 1974
20. Silberman AW: Surgical debulking of tumors. Surg Gynecol Obstet 155:577–585, 1982
21. Lawrence W Jr, Wilson RE, Shingleton WW, et al: Surgical oncology in university departments of surgery in the United States. Arch Surg 121:1088–1093, 1986
22. Avis FP, Ellenberg S, Friedman MA: Surgical oncology research—a disappointing status report. Ann Surg 207:262–266, 1988
23. Rosenberg SA: The organization of surgical oncology in university departments of surgery. Surgery 95:632–634, 1984
24. Leffall LD Jr: Presidential address. Surgical oncology—expectations for the future. Cancer 42:2925–2928, 1980
25. Schweitzer RJ, Edwards MH, Lawrence W et al: Training guidelines for surgical oncology. Cancer 48:2336–2340, 1981

SAMUEL HELLMAN

CHAPTER 15 *Principles of Radiation Therapy*

To understand the practice of radiation therapy, one must seek its roots in principles derived from three separate areas. The first is practical radiation physics. This must be understood much as the surgeon understands the use of the equipment available in the operating room and as the internist understands the pharmacologic basis of therapeutics. The basic concepts of physics necessary to consider radiation therapy in the disease-related chapters are introduced in this chapter.

The second important discipline to be understood is cell, tissue, and tumor biology. This chapter describes the fundamental principles of radiation biology and cell kinetics; cell kinetics in relation to both chemotherapy and radiation therapy is discussed in Chapter 1. These two discussions provide the rudiments of cell biology necessary to understand the uses of radiation.

Finally, a large clinical experience in radiation use has resulted in certain principles of treatment. These are discussed separately and related to the physical and biologic concepts that may underlie their success.

PHYSICAL CONSIDERATIONS

Only the most important concepts of the physics of ionizing radiation can be discussed in this chapter. If more detailed information is needed, a standard textbook of radiation physics is a more appropriate source of information.[1]

Ionizing radiation is energy that, during absorption, causes the ejection of an orbital electron. A large amount of energy is associated with ionization. Ionizing radiation can be elec-tromagnetic or particulate, and electromagnetic radiation can be considered both as a wave and as a packet of energy (a photon). It is the particulate nature of electromagnetic radiation that explains much of its biologic activity. The packet of energy is large enough to cause ionizations, and these are distributed unevenly through tissue. Examples of particulate radiation are the subatomic particles: electrons, protons, alpha particles, neutrons, negative pimesons, and atomic nuclei. All of these have been experimentally considered or are being used in radiation therapy.

ELECTROMAGNETIC RADIATION

Electromagnetic radiation consists of roentgen and gamma radiation. They differ only in the way in which they are produced: gamma rays are produced intranuclearly, and roentgen rays are produced extranuclearly. In practice, this means that gamma rays used in radiation therapy are produced by the decay of radioactive isotopes and that almost all of the roentgen rays used in radiation therapy are made by electrical machines. Exceptions are roentgen rays produced by orbital electron rearrangements, as in the decay of ^{125}I, which is a radioactive isotope but produces photons by extranuclear processes. Iodine-125 also emits a small number of gamma rays from the nucleus.

The intensity of electromagnetic radiation dissipates as the inverse square of the distance from the source. Thus, the dose of radiation 2 cm from a point source is 25% of the dose at 1 cm.

The relative prevalence of the three dominant absorption mechanisms of electromagnetic radiation depends on the energy of the radiation. The first is photoelectric absorption, which predominates at lower energies. In this circumstance, the photon interaction results in the ejection of a tightly bound orbital electron. The vacancy left in the atomic shell is then filled by another electron falling from an outer shell of the same atom or from outside the atom. All or most of the photon energy of the transition is lost in this process. Photoelectric absorption varies with the cube of the atomic number (Z^3). This has significant practical implications because it explains why materials with high atomic numbers, such as lead, are such effective shielding materials. It also means that bones will absorb significantly more radiation than soft tissues at lower photon energies, the basis for conventional diagnostic radiology.

The second type of radiation absorption is the Compton type. In this process, the photon interaction is with a distant orbital electron that has a very low binding energy. In this absorptive process, the photon does not give up all its energy to a single electron; an appreciable portion reappears as a secondary photon, which is created in the interaction. In contrast to the photoelectric effect, the probability of Compton absorption does not depend much on atomic number, but rather on electron density. This explains why films made at supervoltage energy to not show much difference between bone and soft tissue, but air cavities are clearly distinguished.

The third type of absorption is the pair production process. This type of absorption requires an incident photon energy greater than 1.02 MeV. In this process, positive and negative electrons are produced at the same time.

The fundamental quantity necessary to describe the interaction of radiation with matter is the amount of energy absorbed per unit mass. This quantity is called *absorbed dose*, and the *rad* was the most commonly used unit. In current nomenclature, absorbed dose is measured in joules per kilogram. Another name for 1 joule/kg is the Gray (1 Gray = 100 rad). This is now the recommended unit. The roentgen (R) is a unit of roentgen rays or gamma rays based on the ability of radiation to ionize air. At the energies used in radiation therapy, 1 R of roentgen rays or gamma rays results in a dose of somewhat less than 1 rad (0.01 Gy) in soft tissue.

The different ranges of electromagnetic radiations used in clinical practice are *superficial radiation* or roentgen rays from approximately 10 to 125 KeV; *orthovoltage* radiation or electromagnetic radiation between 125 and 400 KeV; and *supervoltage* or megavoltage radiation for energies above 400 KeV. There are important differences between these classes. As energy increases, the penetration of the roentgen rays increases, as shown in Figure 15-1, and at supervoltage energies, absorption in bone is not higher than that in surrounding soft tissues, as is the case with lower energies. This is because at supervoltage energies, Compton absorption predominates. Compared with orthovoltage, supervoltage radiation is "skin sparing," meaning that the maximum dose is not reached in the skin, but instead occurs below the surface. The electrons created in the interaction travel some distance and do not attain full intensity until they reach some depth, resulting in a reduced dose to the skin. With orthovoltage radiation, the skin frequently is the dose-limiting normal tissue.

RADIATION TECHNIQUES

Two general types of radiation techniques are used clinically —*brachytherapy* and *teletherapy*. In brachytherapy, the radiation device is placed either within or close to the target volume. Examples of this are interstitial and intracavitary radiation used in the treatment of many gynecologic and oral tumors. Teletherapy uses a device quite removed from the patient, as is the case in most orthovoltage or supervoltage machines.

Because the radiation source is close to or within the target volume with brachytherapy, the dose is determined largely by inverse-square considerations. This means that the geometry of the implant is very important. Spatial arrangements have been determined for different types of applications based on the particular anatomic considerations of the tumor and important normal tissues. An example of isotope distribution around an intracavitary application for carcinoma of the cervix is shown in Figure 15-2. The dose decreases rapidly as the distance from the applicator increases. This emphasizes the importance of proper placement. The applica-

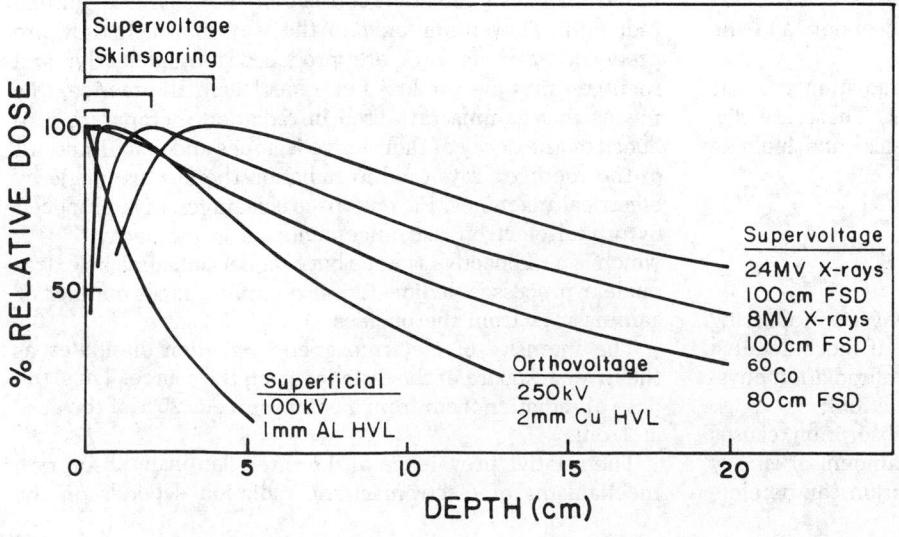

FIG. 15-1. Relative dose at different depths for various types of ionizing radiation.

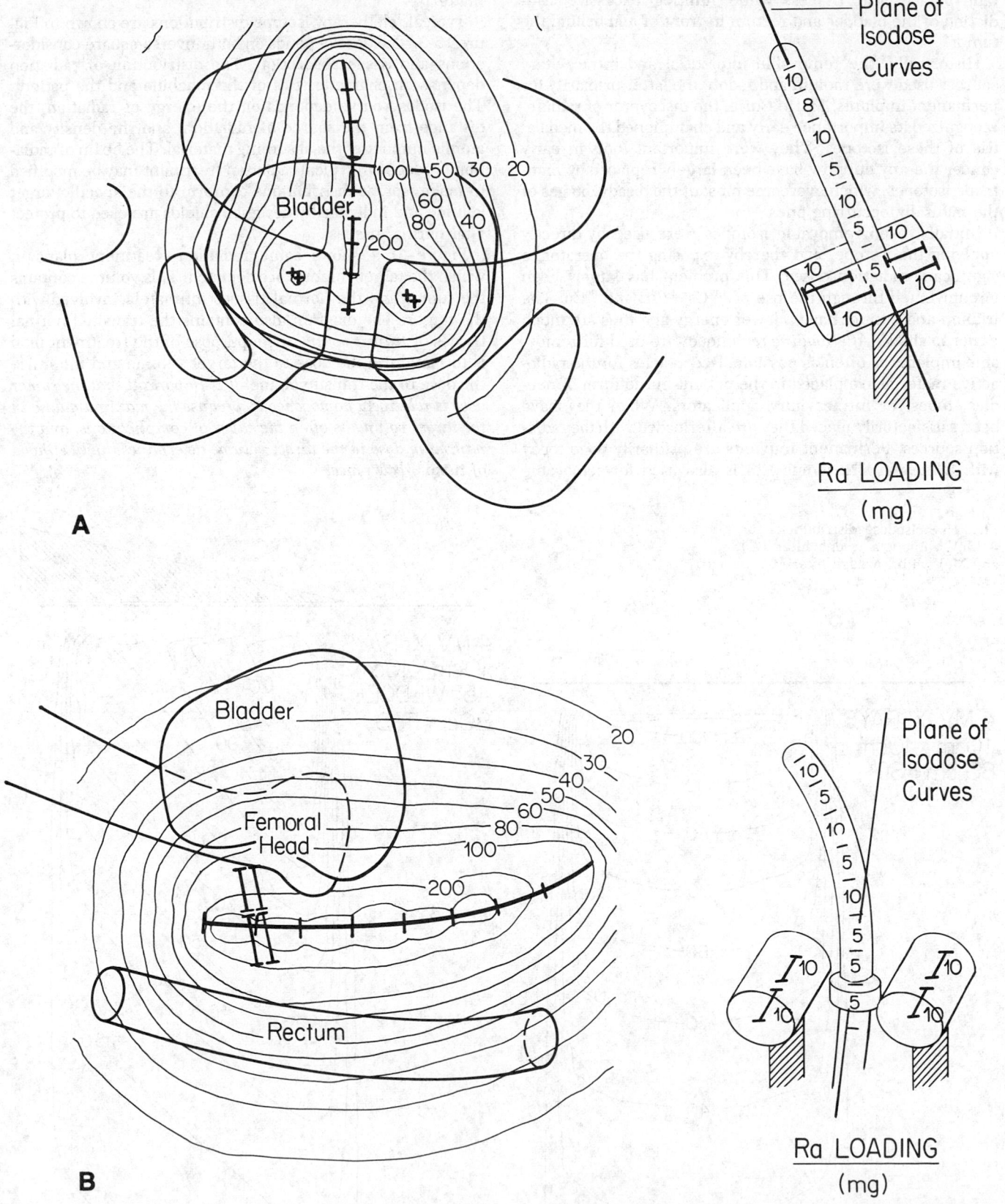

FIG. 15-2. **A**. AP view of isodose distribution around an intrauterine radium applicator. **B**. Lateral view.

tor pictured is used to treat the cervix, uterus, and important paracervical tissues, while limiting excessive irradiation of the bladder and rectum in front of and behind the tumor.

Historically, the removable interstitial and intracavitary sources used were radium and radon, the latter primarily for permanent implants. Marie Curie, the discoverer of radium, recognized its importance early and championed the medical use of these isotopes. They were important tools in early cancer therapy but now have been largely replaced by manmade isotopes, which overcome most of the disadvantages of the naturally occurring ones.

Initially, even removable isotopes were used by directly applying the isotope, and thereby exposing the operator to significant radiation doses. This problem has largely been circumvented through the use of ^{137}Cs, ^{192}Ir, and ^{60}Co. The iridium and cesium have a lower energy and thus are much easier to shield. *Afterloading* techniques are used for removable implants as often as possible. Receptacles for the radioactive material are placed in the patient in the form of needles, tubes, or intracavitary applicators. When they have been satisfactorily placed they are afterloaded with the radiation sources. Permanent implants are primarily done today with ^{198}Au and ^{125}I. Iodine-125 is also used for removable implants. Its very low energy makes shielding a simple matter.

Typical teletherapy isotope distributions are shown in Figure 15-3. The dose depends on both inverse-square considerations and tissue absorption. The distribution of radiation depends on characteristics of the machine and the patient. The isodose curve depends on the energy of radiation, the distance from the source of radiation, and the density and atomic number of the absorbing material. The beam of radiation produced in typical radiation treatment may be modified to make isotope distributions conform to the specific target volume and individually designed shields are used to protect vital normal tissues.

Figure 15-4 shows some radiation treatment plans in which the target volumes are depicted. This volume contains the tumor and the normal tissues intimately involved with the tumor. The diagram also contains the transited normal tissues or *transit volume*. The purpose of the treatment plan is to maximize the dose to the target volume and minimize the dose to the transit volume. *It is important that the tumor dose is relatively homogeneous, because the maximum dose in the target volume is often the cause of complications, and the minimum dose in the target volume determines the likelihood of tumor recurrence.*

FIG. 15-3. Isodose distributions for 4 MeV without a wedge filter (**A**) and MeV with a wedge filter (**B**).

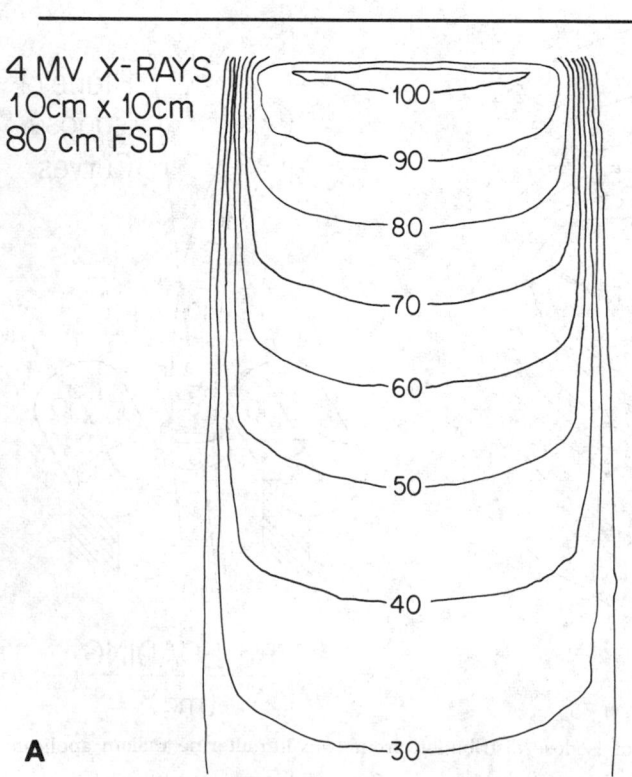

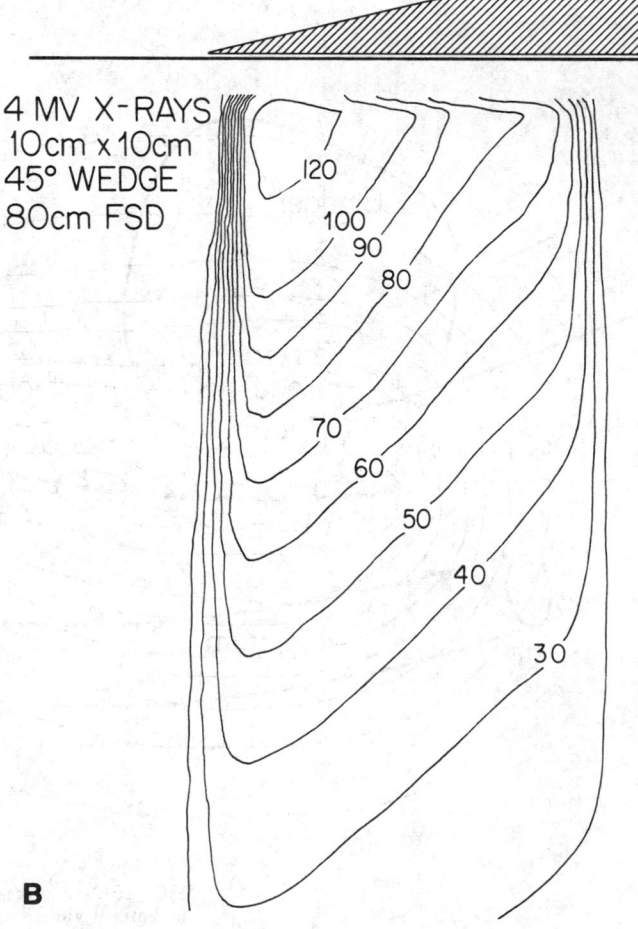

Beam-Modifying Devices

In modern radiation therapy, teletherapy is given almost exclusively with supervoltage equipment. These radiations are produced by the decay of radioactive cobalt or with the production of roentgen rays in the range of 2 to 35 MeV (the most common are 4–8 MeV). Higher-energy photons and electrons can be made by various electrical machines, of which the most common are linear accelerators.

Regardless of the radiation source, the beam must be modified for clinical use. With electrical machines, the beam tends to have a much greater intensity in the center than on the sides. Modification to give a uniform dose of radiation across the beam is done with a *flattening filter* (unnecessary in cobalt units). For the beam to be limited to the designated size, collimators are placed in the head of the machine. These usually are made of materials that have a high Z value and can be varied to conform to the exact rectangular beam dimensions desired.

It is sometimes desirable for the beam to be more intense on one side than the other. This is especially important when fields at angles to each other are to be used. To modify the beam in this fashion, wedge filters are used (Fig. 15-3B). These are literally wedge-shaped pieces of metal that absorb the beam differentially, depending on the thickness that produces the desired angled isodose curves. Depending on the anatomic volume being treated, it is often desirable to outline the beam differently from that which can be constructed by rectangular collimators. In these circumstances, certain areas within the beam should be shielded. To do this, individually fashioned blocks are made to conform to the individual distributions desired for each patient and each beam. They are made of material with a high Z, such as lead or the commercial product Libowitz metal, composed of bismuth, lead, tin, and cadmium.

The primary radiation beam is rectangular. This rectangle may be varied for individual patients, using the secondary collimators in the head of the machine. These can then be further modified by individually constructed blocks made to the contour of the normal tissue, an example of which is shown in Figure 15-5. The newest equipment has multileaf collimators, which permit the collimator to follow closely the desired portal contour, rather than being restricted to a rectangular shape.

RADIATION TREATMENT

Once the decision has been made to treat a patient with radiation, a number of pretreatment procedures must be performed. First, there must be accurate localization of the target volume and determination of the dose-limiting, transited normal tissues. This localization requires physical examination, radiography, ultrasonography, computed tomography (CT), and other diagnostic procedures. Before this, the clinician must understand the natural history of the disease and its patterns of spread. CT has greatly changed the process of tumor localization by allowing much greater accuracy in determining the location of normal tissues, as well as tumor.

Once localization has been completed, the treatment-planning process begins, in which alternative techniques of treatment are considered. The selection of the appropriate treatment plan is made by the clinician consulting with the radiologic physicist and dosimetrist. This team effort must consider the best beam distribution, homogeneity within the target volume, and appropriate minimizing of dose in the transit volume.

Once the appropriate treatment plan has been accepted, the technique is tested using a radiation simulator. This device mimics the treatment machine but produces superficial radiation that can be used for direct imaging with an image intensifier and for producing radiographs that delineate exactly the beam location. Treatment simulation often causes modifications to be made in the treatment plan, thus allowing further sparing of normal tissues. Examples of simulator films are shown in Figure 15-5. These must be compared with the check or portal films made with the supervoltage machine, which confirm the treatment plan (Fig. 15-5). Image quality is poor because they do not distinguish bone from soft tissue. This is because supervoltage radiation is absorbed primarily by the Compton process, which does not depend on Z. In contrast, the simulator films are made with radiations of 80 to 110 KeV, which are in the photoelectric range and therefore dependent on Z^3.

In order for the treatment to be applied as designed on the radiation simulator, proper immobilization and marking techniques must be used. These also ensure that daily treatments are given to the same volume. Markings on the patient's skin may be temporary or permanent. Usually temporary marks are used to supplement the permanent small dots or "tattoos," ensuring that the treatment will be given to the same volume each day. In addition, should the patient require further therapy at a later date, these markings will accurately indicate the location of previous treatment portals. Within the treatment room, light localizers describe the outline of the field, and small laser dots are used to check whether the patient is in the correct position. Immobilization of the patient usually is achieved by devices made of foam, plastic, plaster, and a variety of other materials that can be made to conform to each patient's anatomy. It is most important that the patient be put in a position that is comfortable and easily reproduced from day to day.

Electron Therapy

With the development of betatrons and high-energy accelerators, electron beam therapy has become available for teletherapy. Electrons differ greatly in their characteristic depth-dose distributions (Fig. 15-6). The maximum dose is reached followed by a very prompt fall. There is little skin sparing with electron beam therapy, but it is the most useful radiation in the treatment of superficial tumors because the deeper tissues will be spared by the prompt fall in the radiation dose. With higher electron energy, the penetration is greater and the fall in depth dose is not as steep.

A major problem with electrons is that absorption can be modified greatly by bone or air-containing tissues. Bone will cause the depth dose to be greatly reduced because it will absorb much more of the radiation; the contrary is true for air-containing spaces.

(*Text continues on p. 254.*)

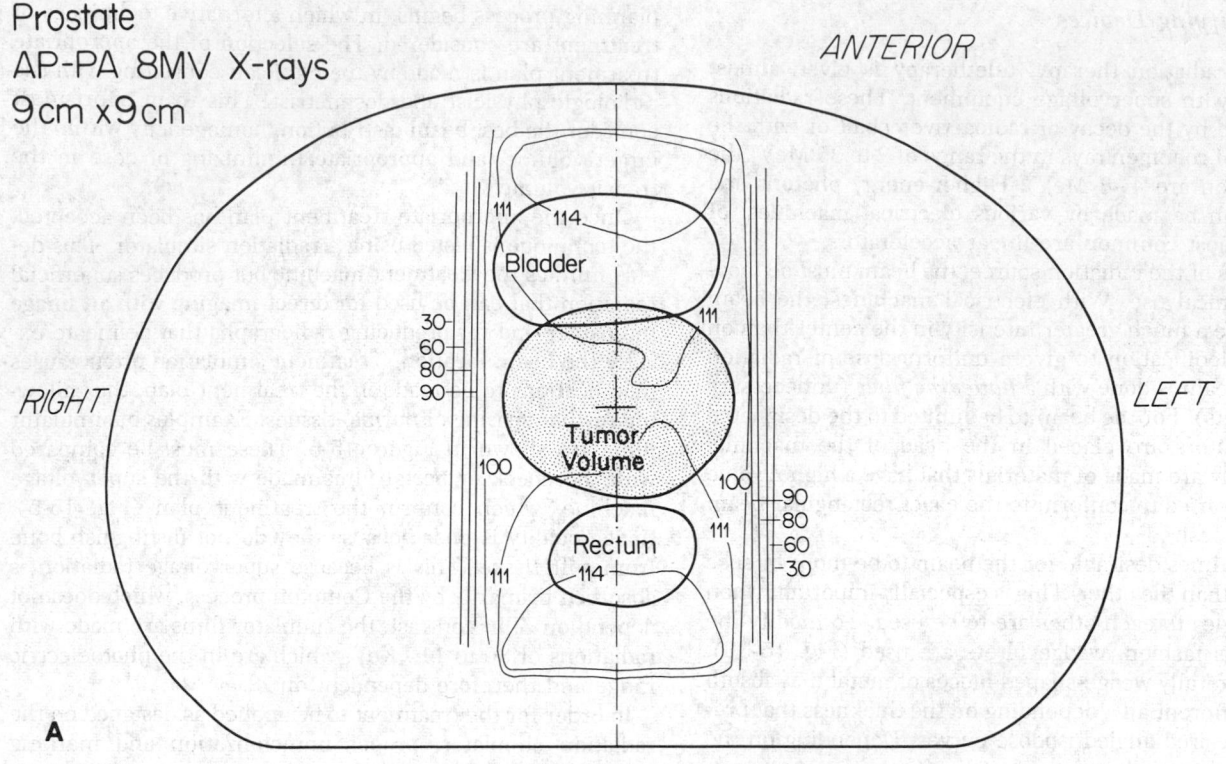

Prostate
AP-PA 8MV X-rays
9cm x9cm

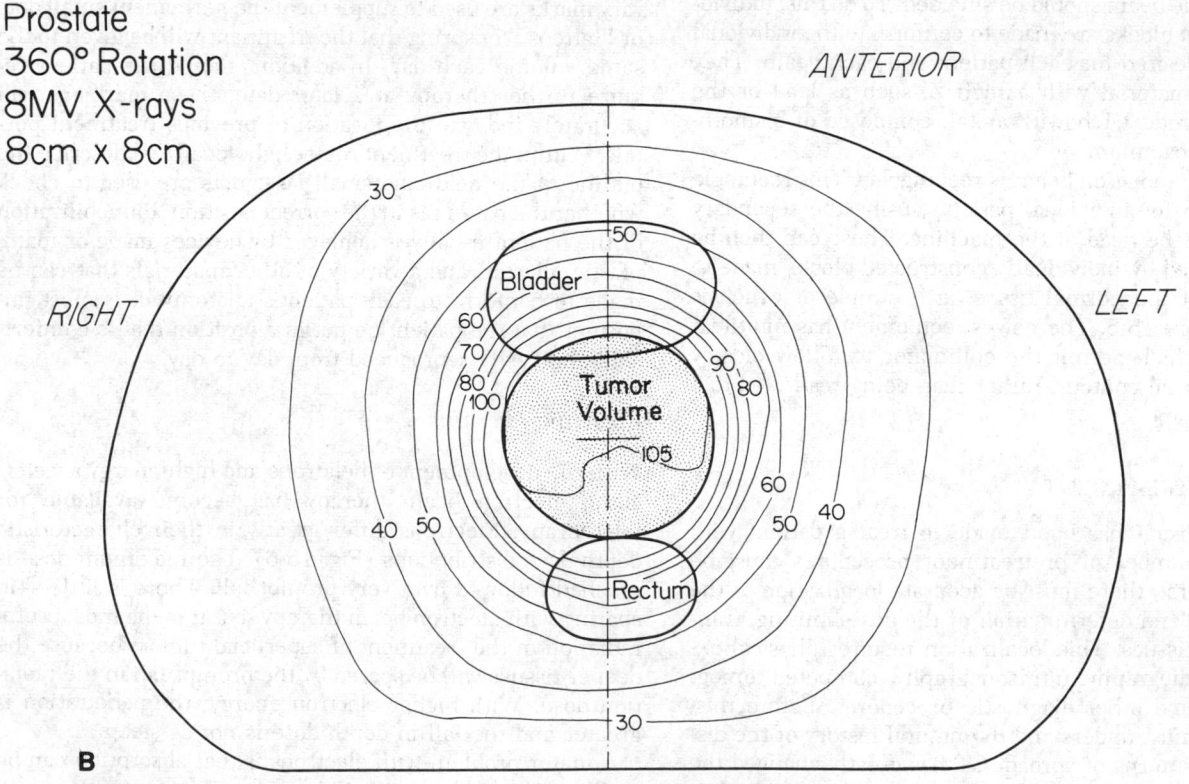

Prostate
360° Rotation
8MV X-rays
8cm x 8cm

FIG. 15-4. Typical supervoltage treatment plans for opposing fields (**A**), rotation (**B**). **C**. Three field. **D**. Wedge rotation.

Esophagus
3-Field Plan   8MV X-rays
Equal Scale
8cm x 8cm

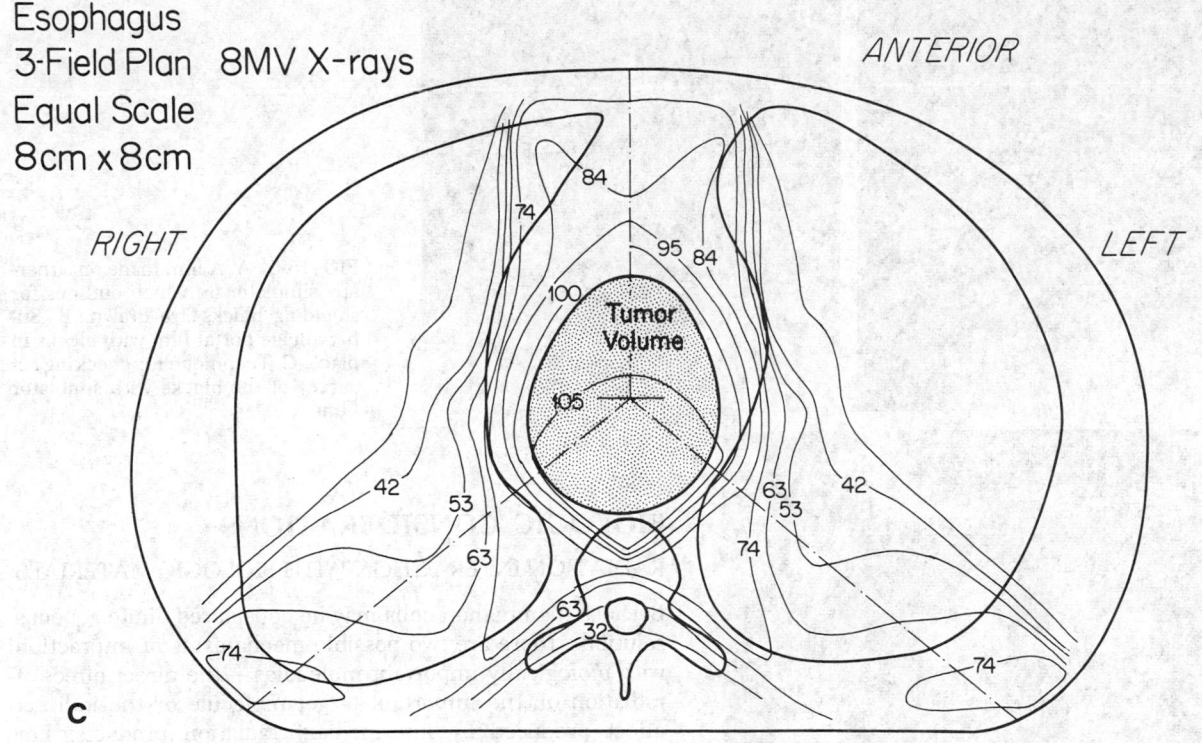

FIG. 15-4. (*continued*). Three field (*C*).

Prostate
270° Rotation with Wedges
8MV X-rays
8cm x 8cm

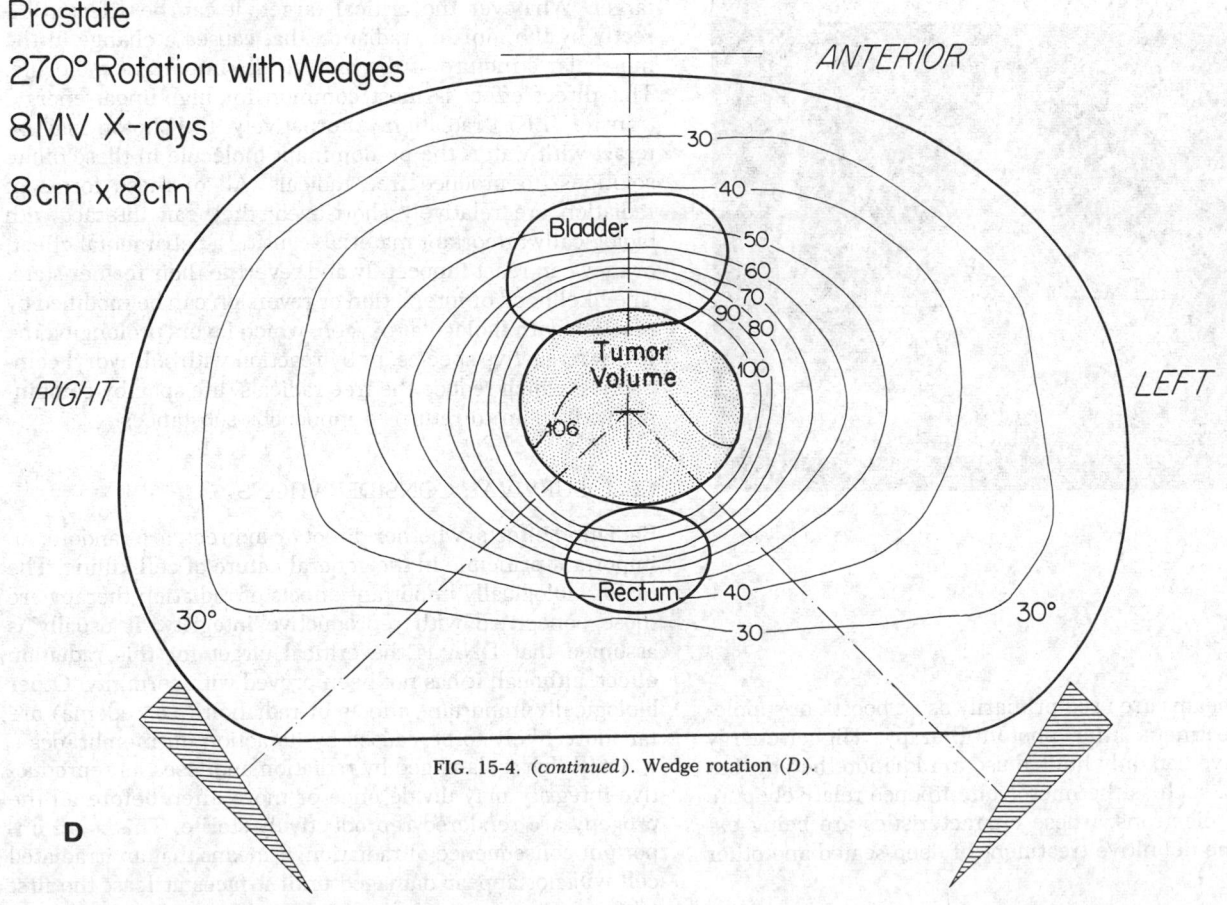

FIG. 15-4. (*continued*). Wedge rotation (*D*).

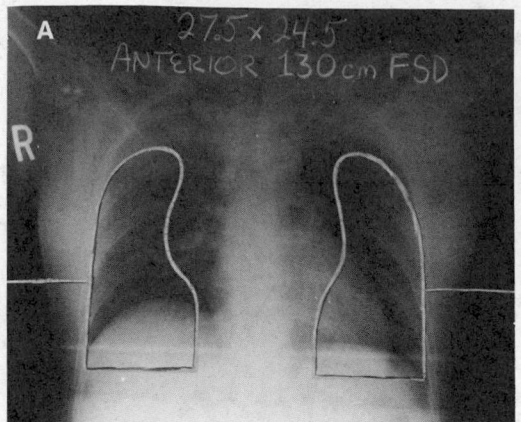

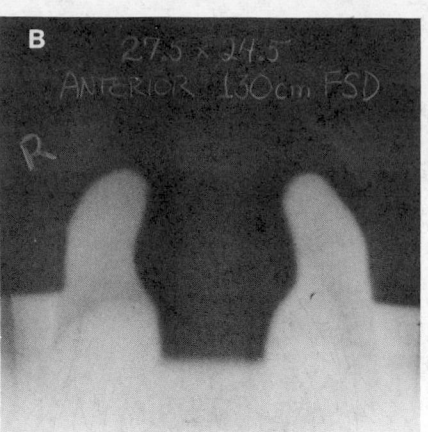

FIG. 15-5. **A.** A film made on a therapy simulator on which outlines for shielding blocks are drawn. **B.** Supervoltage portal film with blocks in place. **C.** Technique for checking accuracy of the blocks with simulator films.

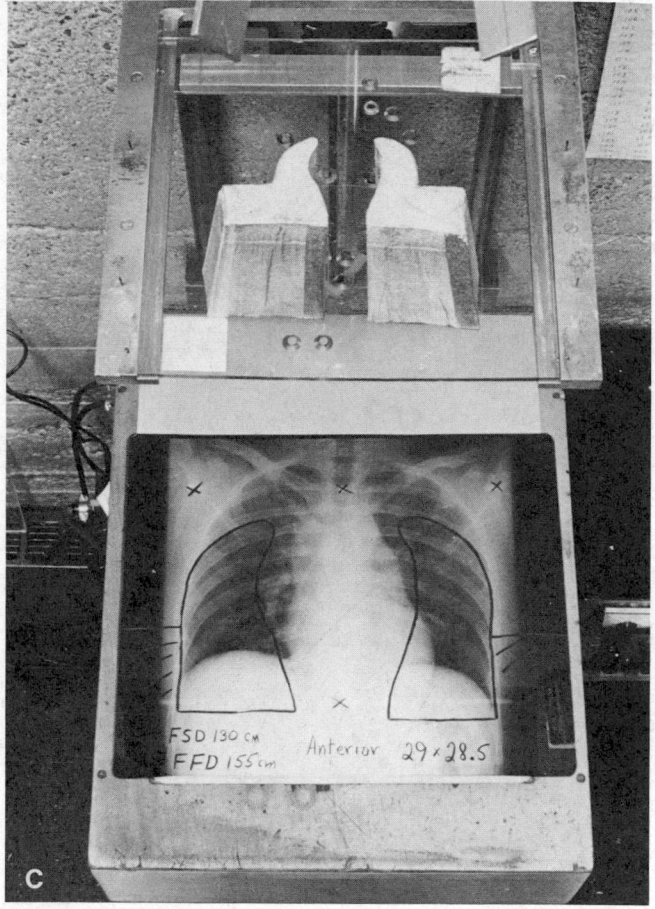

BIOLOGIC CONSIDERATIONS

RADIATION INTERACTION WITH BIOLOGIC MATERIALS

Because mammalian cells may be considered dilute aqueous solutions, there are two possible mechanisms of interaction with biologically important molecules—the direct effect of radiation on the important target molecule or the indirect effect produced by intermediary radiation products. For most events, the important target molecule is thought to be the DNA, and when considering the maintenance of reproductive integrity, it is useful to assume that DNA is the target. Whatever the critical target, it can be affected directly by the ionizing radiation that causes a change in the molecular structure of the biologically important molecule. This direct effect is most common for high-linear-energy-transfer (LET) radiation. Alternatively, the photon may interact with water, the predominant molecule in these dilute solutions, to produce free radicals. All of these forms of radiation are relatively short-lived; they can interact with biologically important material, causing a detrimental effect, or they can react innocently and revert to their former state. The likelihood of interaction or reversion can be modified by reaction with molecular oxygen, which favors prolonging the life of a reactive species, or by reaction with sulfhydryl compounds, which reduce the free radicals' life span by combining with them to return to innocuous substances.

CELL SURVIVAL CONSIDERATIONS

Radiation effects, whether direct or indirect, are random, an important principle in the general nature of cell killing. The major biologically important effects of radiation therapy are those concerned with reproductive integrity. It usually is assumed that DNA is the critical target for this radiation effect, although it has not been proved with certainty. Other biologically important effects of radiation (*e.g.,* edema) are far more likely to be caused by its action on membranes.

A cell that is damaged by radiation and loses its reproductive integrity may divide once or more often before all the progeny are rendered reproductively sterile. This is an important consequence of radiation; it means that an irradiated cell will not appear damaged until it faces at least the first

Electron beams are used primarily as a "boost" or supplementary treatment after photon therapy. Higher-energy electrons have had only limited use in radiation therapy, but new devices, such as the microtron, produce relatively pure high-energy electrons, whose characteristics are being explored for the definitive treatment of deep-seated and other tumors.

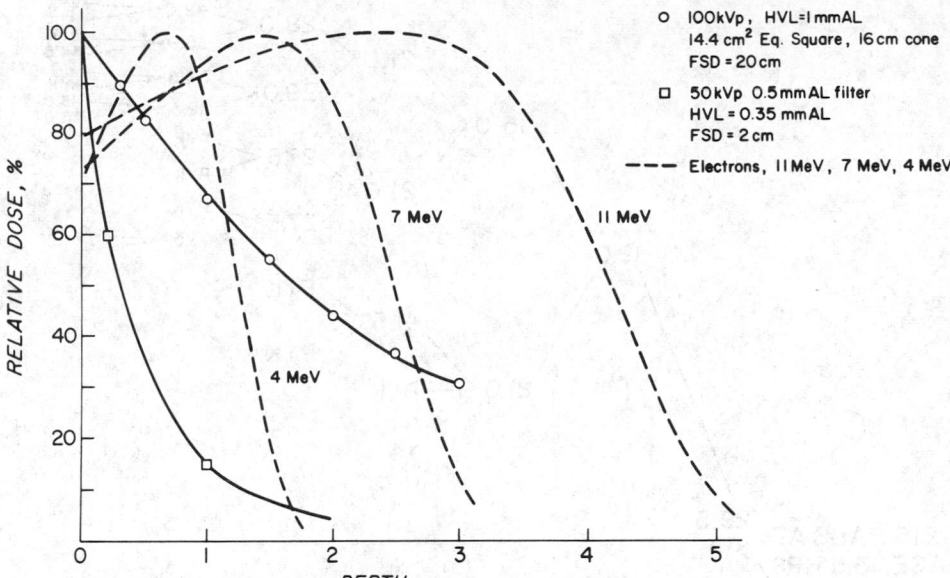

FIG. 15-6. Electron and superficial roentgen ray depth dose curves.

division. At the time of reproduction, there are a number of possible paths for this cell:

1. It may die while trying to divide.
2. It may produce unusual forms as a result of aberrant attempts at division.
3. It may stay as it is, unable to divide, but physiologically functional for a long period of time. Such functional but sterile cells will not appear different from fertile cells.
4. It may divide, giving rise to one or more generations of daughter cells before some or all of the progeny become sterile. Those colonies in which some reproductively viable progeny emerge may then regrow.
5. The cell may suffer no alterations in the divisional process or only minor ones.

Usually some delay in division is produced, even in cells that are not damaged lethally. An example of cellular pedigrees photographed in vitro is shown in Figure 15-7.[2]

Survival Curves

Survival curves plot the fraction of cells surviving radiation against the dose given. Survival is determined by the ability to form a macroscopic colony. The simplest relationship can be seen for bacteria in which survival is a constant exponential function of dose. The importance of this exponential relationship is that for a given dose increment, a constant proportion, rather than a constant number, of cells is killed. Because of the randomness of radiation damage, if there is on average one lethal lesion per cell, some cells will have one lesion, some more than one, and some less than one. Under such circumstances the proportion of cells that have less than one, that is, no lethal events, is e^{-1}, or a survival fraction of 0.37. The dose required to reduce the survival fraction to 37% on the exponential curve is known as the D_0. This term, therefore, is related to the slope of the exponen-

tial survival curve. Thus if a smaller dose is required to reduce the survival fraction to 37%, then the cells are more sensitive to radiation.

Survival curves of most mammalian cells differ from those of bacterial cells by having a "shoulder" in the low-dose region and the exponential relationship at higher doses. This shoulder indicates a reduced efficiency of cell killing. Such an idealized curve is shown in Figure 15-8 with the important shorthand terminology used to describe survival curves. The terminal exponential portion is described by the D_0, whereas the initial shoulder region can be described by the extrapolation number n or the D_q, the quasi-threshold dose. The former is the number on the ordinate found when the exponential portion is extrapolated to 0 dose, whereas D_q is the dose at which the straight portion of the survival curve extrapolated backward intersects the line where the survival fraction is unity. If any two of these are known, the third can be calculated. The survival curve is described as follows: log $e^n = D_q/D_0$. This curve is best described by a linear quadratic model with the formula $S = e^{-(\alpha D + \beta D^2)}$.[3]

Survival curves have been determined for a variety of benign or neoplastic mammalian cells in culture. There are no general characteristics of tumor cells that make them different from normal cells in culture. The survival curves for various human tumors thought to be both sensitive and resistant to radiation were studied by Weichselbaum and co-workers, who failed to show any survival curve characteristics that allow these two to be separated.[4] Therefore, the differences in clinical response cannot be explained by simple acute differences in survival curves.

Normal tissues also have been studied using clonogenic survival as an endpoint, with survival curves determined analogously to those for cells in tissue culture. The simplest clonal system, as originally described by Till and McCulloch, is that used for murine bone marrow stem cells.[5] When bone marrow cells are injected into lethally irradiated recipient animals, colonies are formed in the animals' spleens. These

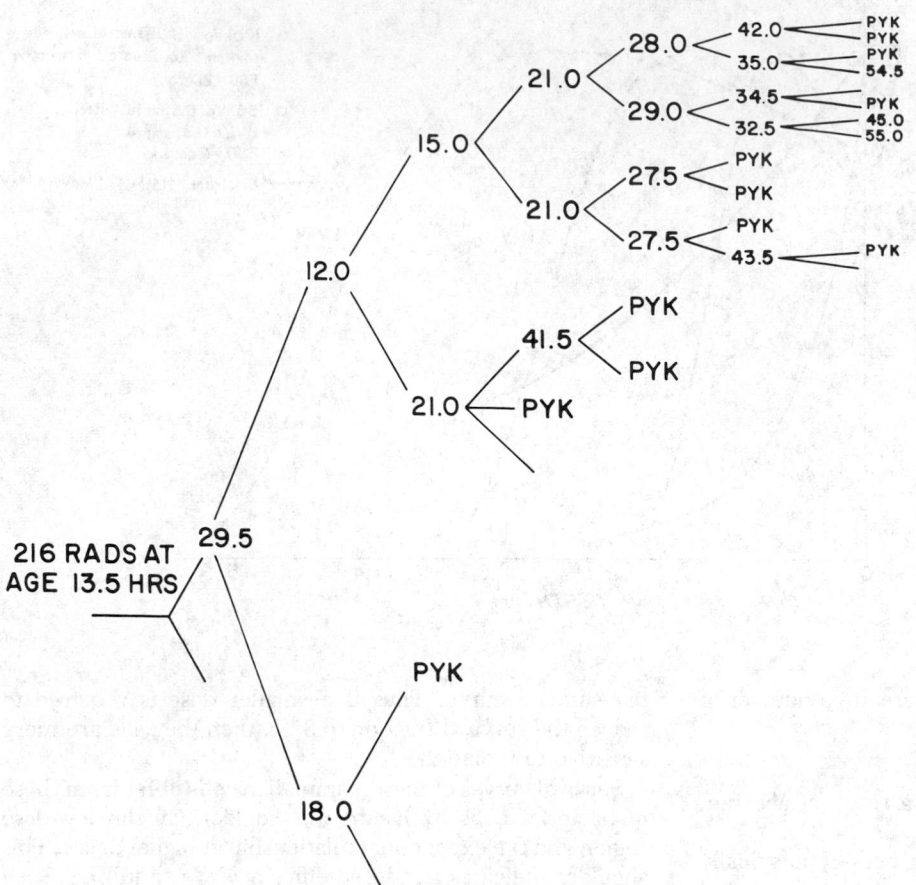

FIG. 15-7. Two cell pedigrees indicating cell cycle times and the outcome of cells irradiated in vitro. *PYK* = pyknosis. (Thompson LH, Suit HD: Proliferation kinetics of x-irradiated mouse L cells studied with time lapse photography: II. Int J Radiat Biol 15:347–362, 1969)

can be used to assess the reproductive integrity of the injected cells. The viability of the small intestinal clonogenic mucosal cells can be assessed by looking at sections of the small intestine at various times after irradiation and determining the appearance of colonies derived from cells surviving this radiation.[6] Using these and other techniques, the general properties of survival curves of both normal and tumor cells are shown in Table 15-1. There are no characteristic differences in survival curves between normal tissues and tumors. Tumors generally resemble their normal tissue of origin in this respect.

Repair of Radiation Damage

When cells are irradiated, lethal damage can occur, or the damage may be modified and not lead irrevocably to cell death. Such amelioration of radiation damage is called repair. Repair can be divided into potentially lethal damage repair and sublethal damage repair.

Potentially lethal damage, under certain circumstances, leads to cell death. However, if postirradiation conditions are modified to allow repair, cells that would have died can be salvaged. In general, postirradiation conditions that suppress

cell division are the ones most favorable to repair of potentially lethal damage. The simplest example of this was shown first in bacteria for both ultraviolet and X-radiation.[7] A similar effect was seen in mammalian cells and persists into the first few postirradiation generations.[8-10] Potentially lethal damage repair may be most important in relating the cell culture studies of human tumors to their clinical response. Weichselbaum and co-workers have shown that osteogenic sarcoma, a tumor characteristically thought to be quite resistant to radiation, has a great capacity for potentially lethal damage repair compared with tumors that may be much more responsive to radiation.[11] After irradiation in the clinical circumstance, the tumor cell may not be faced with the necessity of rapid cell division, and it may have the opportunity for potentially lethal damage repair.

One explanation for the shoulder of the radiation survival curve is that the cell can repair some of the radiation damage, including a great proportion of the damage incurred with low doses of radiation. This is called *sublethal damage*. Elkind and colleagues have studied the shoulder and its return by using divided doses of radiation.[12] They have shown that if the dose of radiation is divided into two fractions and a few hours elapse between radiation doses, the shoulder will

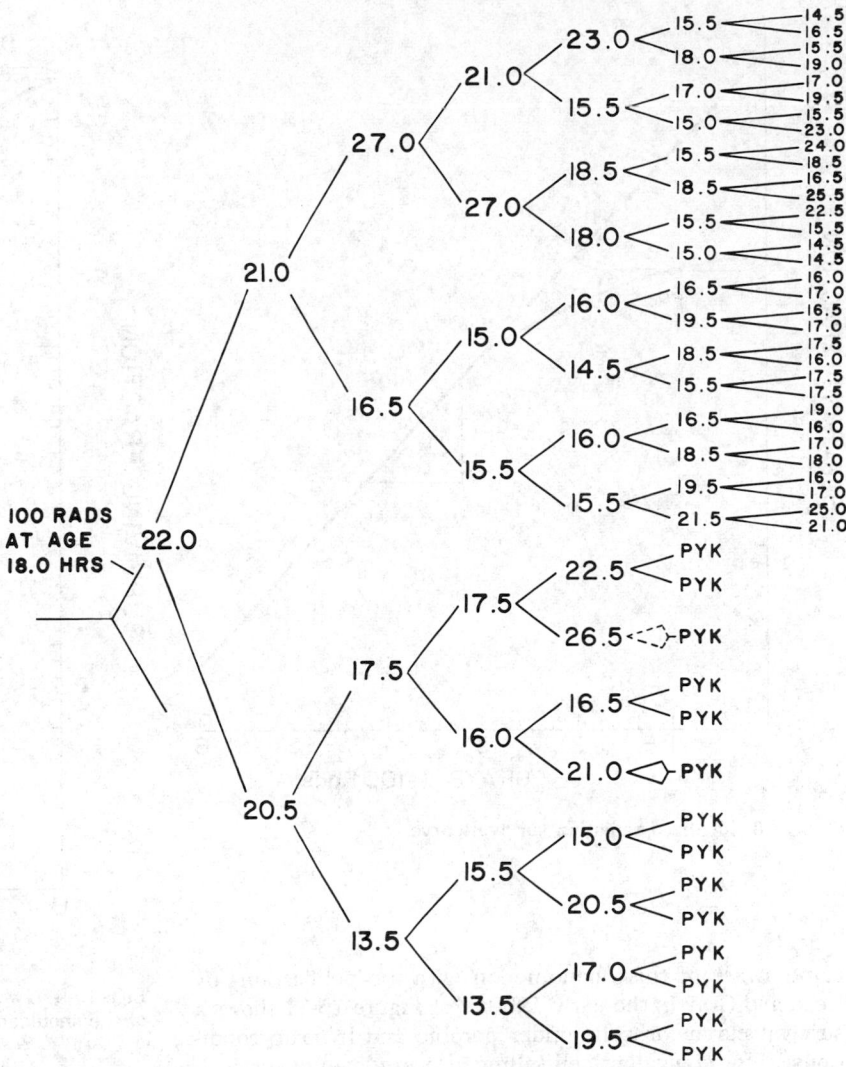

FIG. 15-7. (*continued*)

return. Therefore, two doses of radiation separated in time are less effective than the same total dose given as a single dose. The difference between a single dose and the divided dose that produce equivalent cell kills is the D_q if all the doses are sufficiently large to cause the loss in cell survival to extend to the exponential portion of the survival curve (Fig. 15-9).

The D_q is a measure of sublethal damage repair. Table 15-2 shows the D_q for bone marrow, skin, lung, and gastrointestinal mucosa. The contrast is striking. Bone marrow stem cells have a very small D_q, whereas the others have considerable sublethal damage repair capacity. This suggests that multiple small fractions of radiation can preserve these tissues, but not bone marrow. Radiation fractionation schemes must account for whether or not the fraction size is sufficient to be off the shoulder. If all of the variations are on the shoulder, there will be little difference in cell kill. With such small fractions, essentially all the damage that can be repaired is being repaired already, and fractionation becomes much less important. However, if the fractions are large enough to include a portion of the steeper part of the survival curve, then differences in fraction size are very important, because the proportion of shoulder-to-steep-exponential portion varies for different fraction sizes.

Varying the dose rate of radiation may be considered a form of radiation fractionation. When the dose rate is quite low, such as during interstitial or intracavitary irradiation, it can be considered as a large number of small doses on the shoulder of the survival curve.[12] Therefore, differences between the dose-limiting normal tissues and the tumor in their shoulder characteristics and differences in the break point between shoulder and steep exponential will have great clinical implications for such continuous radiation. An example of this for cells in culture is shown in Figure 15-10.

Importance of Oxygen

The most important modifier of the biologic effect of ionizing irradiation is molecular oxygen. This was noted in the 1920s, but it was not understood, nor was its importance realized, until Mottram and colleagues studied it systematically.[14-16] The general scientific community be-

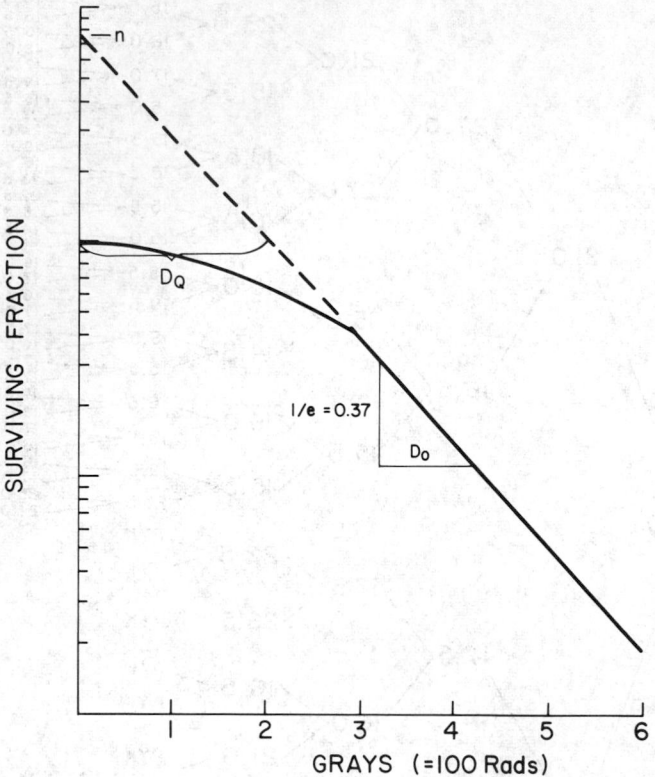

FIG. 15-8. Idealized radiation survival curve.

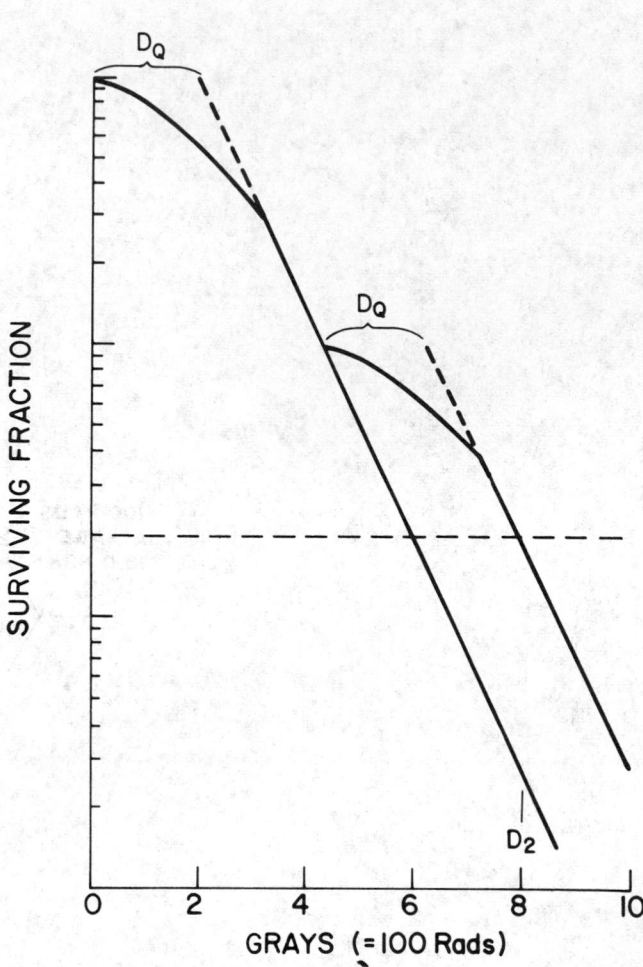

FIG. 15-9. Two dose radiation survival curves demonstrating return of the shoulder.

came aware of this phenomenon with the publications by Read and Gray in the early 1950s.[15,16] Figure 15-11 shows a survival curve for cells under aerobic and hypoxic conditions.[17] For equivalent cell killing at every level of survival, greater doses are required under hypoxic conditions compared with oxic conditions. There is some disagreement in the literature as to whether the dose ratio is the same throughout the survival curve. Most data suggest a smaller difference when low doses are used. A shorthand term, the oxygen enhancement ratio (OER), often is used. OER is the ratio of dose required for equivalent cell killing in the absence compared with the dose required in the presence of oxygen. This term has most relevance on the exponential

TABLE 15-2. D_q Determination for Some Normal Tissues

Normal Tissue	D_q (Gy)*
Mouse skin	~4.00
Mouse intestine	3.50–4.00
Mouse lung	~3.75
Mouse bone marrow	0–0.60

*Average calculated from literature.

TABLE 15-1.   Survival Curve Parameters for Some Mammalian Cells In Vivo or In Vitro

Cell Type	How Determined	D_0 (Rad)	n	D_q (Rad)
Hamster V-79 fibroblast	in vitro	~160	~7	250–300
Chang liver	in vitro	150	2	150
HeLa	in vitro	130	4	180
P 388 leukemia	in vivo	130	8.5	280
Mouse bone marrow	in vivo	90–100	1.5–2.0	~60
Mouse small intestine	in vivo	100	50	390
Mouse chondroblast	in vivo	160	9	350
Rat endothelium	in vivo	170	7	340

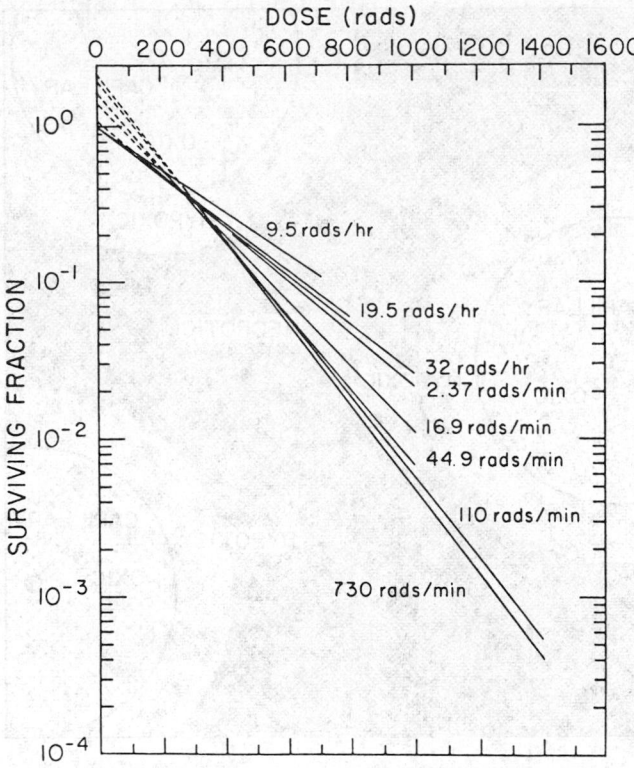

FIG. 15-10. In vitro survival curves for cells irradiated at different dose rates. (Hall EJ: Radiation dose-rate: A factor of importance in radiobiology and radiotherapy. Br J Radiol 45:81–97, 1972)

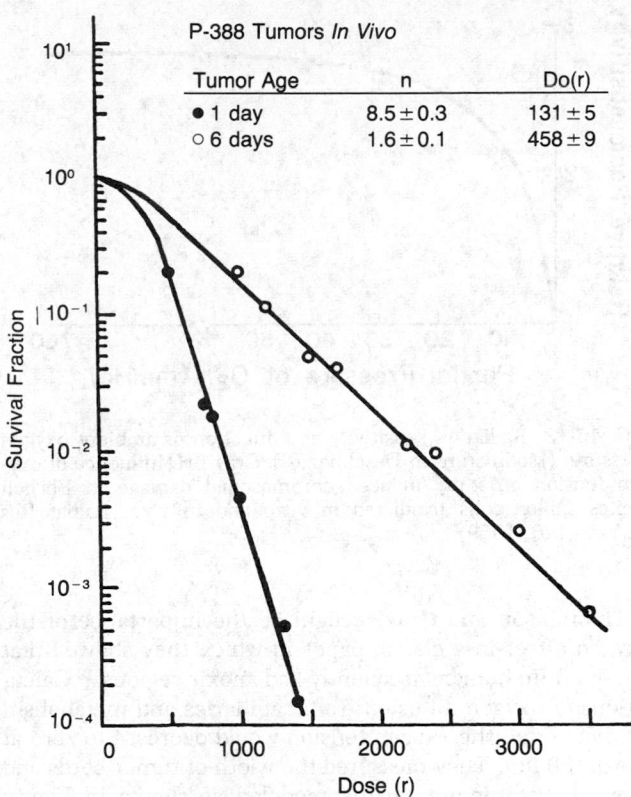

FIG. 15-11. In vivo survival curves for oxic and hypoxic tumor cells. (Belli JA, Dicus GJ, Bonte FJ: Radiation response of mammalian tumor cells: 1. Repair of sublethal damage in vivo. JNCI 38:673–682, 1967).

FIG. 15-12. In vivo curves comparing two dose survival to single dose survival for oxic and hypoxic tumor cells. (Belli JA, Dicus GJ, Bonte FJ: Radiation response of mammalian tumor cells: 1. Repair of sublethal damage in vivo. JNCI 38:673–682, 1967)

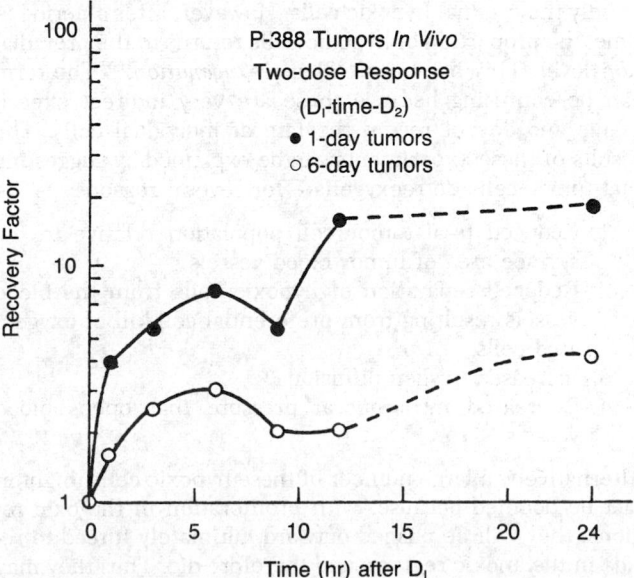

portion of the curve, because there appears to be a reduced shoulder on the survival curve of cells under hypoxic conditions.[17] As shown in Figure 15-12, tumor cells allowed to grow into physiologic hypoxia have reduced capacity to repair sublethal damage.

The OER range for different cells that have been studied varies from about 2.5 to 3.5. This means that for reduction to a given survival level, three times as much radiation is required under hypoxic conditions as under oxic conditions. Because the curves are exponential, the ratio of survival fractions may be much greater at a given dose and will increase with dose. For example, in Figure 15-11, at 1000 rad the ratio of survival is 30.

Study of the phenomenon reveals that oxygen must be present during irradiation. Figure 15-13 shows the relative radiosensitivity of cells as a function of the oxygen tension at the time of irradiation. A very low oxygen tension must be reached before there is a protective effect of hypoxia. The exact mechanism of the oxygen effect has not been determined definitively. It is believed that oxygen affects the initial chemical products of the interaction of radiation with biologic material. The important free radicals have short half-lives. A useful way to think about them is that they may either return to an innocuous state or remain highly reactive molecules. Oxygen appears to favor the latter, whereas the presence of high levels of sulfhydryl compounds favors the former.

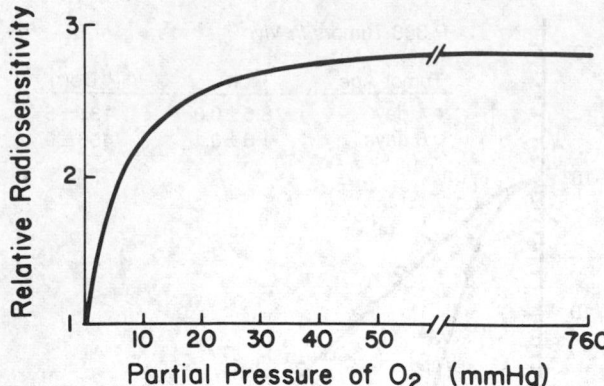

FIG. 15-13. Radiation sensitivity as a function of ambient oxygen pressure. (Modified from Deschner EE, Gray LH: Influence of oxygen tension on x-ray induced chromosomal damage in Ehrlich ascites tumor cells irradiated in vitro and in vivo. Radiat Res 11:115–146, 1959)

Thomlinson and Gray recognized the importance of the oxygen effect in a classic paper in which they showed that tumors from humans frequently had anoxic regions.[19] Calculations of oxygen diffusion from capillaries and metabolism predicted that the oxygen tension would decrease to zero at about 150 μm. They measured the width of tumor cords and showed that tumors can be modeled as shown in Figure 15-14. Those cells within about 100 μm of the capillary are well oxygenated; those beyond 150 μm are anoxic and necrotic; and those between 100 and 150 μm are hypoxic at an oxygen tension that might protect cells from radiation. This model has had a profound influence on radiobiologic and radiotherapeutic thinking. If all tumors look this way and such hypoxic regions contain cells that ultimately could cause tumor regrowth, then no clinically apparent tumor would be cured by radiation therapy. Because this obviously is not the case, this paradox must be explained.

Laboratory experiments have indicated that immediately after a single dose of radiation, the surviving tumor cells are mainly the original hypoxic cells. However, after a period of time, the proportion of hypoxic cells returns to the preradiation level. This has been called *reoxygenation*.[20] The term can be confusing because these are very indirect experiments and do not record the fate of individual cells. The results of these experiments can be explained by suggesting that tumor cells do reoxygenate for several reasons:

1. Reduced total tumor cell population relative to the surface area of tumor blood vessels
2. Reduced separation of hypoxic cells from the blood vessels resulting from preferential cell kill of oxygenated cells
3. Increased oxygen diffusion
4. Decreased intratumoral pressure that opens blood vessels

Alternatively, a large number of these hypoxic cells might in fact be doomed because, with proliferation in the oxic regions, they will be pushed outward, ultimately forced to reside in the anoxic regions, and therefore die. Thus they may

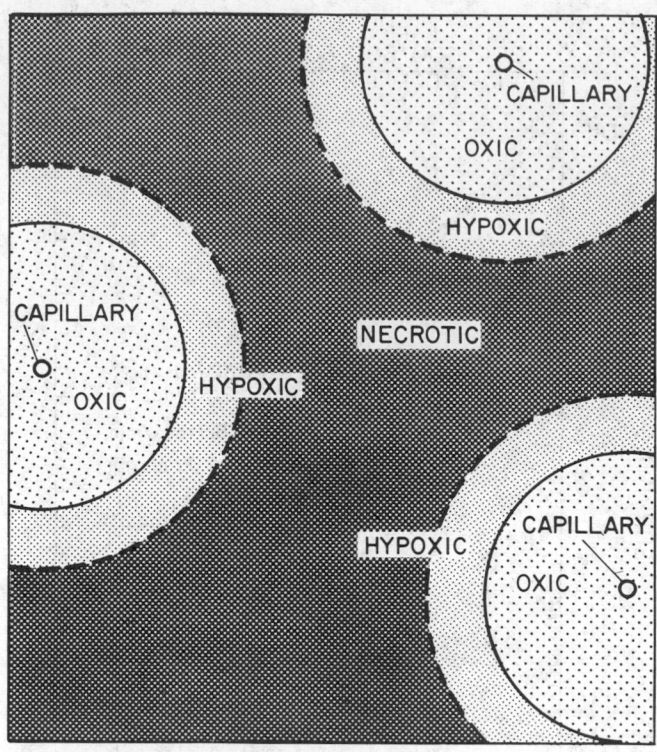

FIG. 15-14. Diagrammatic representation of a tumor.

have only a limited clinical importance in determining tumor curability. It is likely that different mechanisms occur under different circumstances, both in the laboratory and in the clinic.

The obvious clinical importance of the oxygen effect has led to a number of clinical and laboratory experiments, including the use of high-pressure oxygen with radiation therapy to improve results. These studies have indicated that with a small number of radiation fractions, hyperbaric oxygen will increase curability. However, when normal fractionation schemes are used, hyperbaric oxygen often has failed to show an advantage. There are, however, some reports of tumors of the head, neck, and uterine cervix that indicate that hyperbaric oxygen with 10 fractions of radiation results in greater cure than does conventional daily fractionation.[21-23] Table 15-3 depicts the results with head and neck cancers. Despite these promising studies, the hyperbaric oxygen technique is cumbersome, difficult for the

TABLE 15-3. Results of a Randomized Prospective Trial of Hyperbaric Oxygen in the Radiation Treatment of Head and Neck Cancer

	Local Control	Survival at 4 Years
HP O$_2$	61%	56%
Conventional treatment	40%	27%

Henk JM, Kindler PB, Smith CW: Radiotherapy and head and neck cancer: Final report on the first clinical trial. Lancet 2:101–103, 1977.

patient, and prohibits the use of the careful beam definition and beam modification so important in radiation therapy. Thus, the technique has been abandoned in most radiotherapy centers.

A more attractive alternative has been the development of *hypoxic cell sensitizers*. In the 1960s, Adams and colleagues began searching for compounds that would mimic oxygen in its effect.[24,25] They sought agents that would be metabolized slowly and reach all portions of the tumor. This is an important distinction, because high-pressure oxygen increases diffusion only slightly, whereas slowly metabolized sensitizers can reach all areas of the tumor. Although newer methods were based on replacing molecular oxygen, there are other effects of the nitroimidazoles, the most well-studied class of these agents. They appear to be quite cytotoxic to hypoxic cells and may sensitize cells to chemotherapeutic agents.[26,27] How important these last two points are in their use remains to be seen. However, this general class of agents offers a whole new approach to the chemical treatment of tumors based on a known tumor-normal tissue difference (*i.e.*, the presence of hypoxic cells in tumors). These agents and agents designed to protect normal tissue are discussed specifically in Chapter 66, section 3.

A practical clinical concern is whether the presence of anemia affects tumor response to radiation. Historic review and a prospective study from the Princess Margaret Hospital (Table 15-4) appear to indicate that anemia results in an adverse effect on tumor curability by radiation, presumably because it increases the hypoxic component of tumor cells.[28]

A recent review of intercapillary distance and tissue oxygen tension correlates local recurrence with evidence of hypoxia using these parameters in studying carcinoma of the cervix.[29] These studies emphasize the promise of techniques that improve tissue oxygenation in the treatment of epithelial cancers. In vitro measurement of hypoxia using radioactively labelled hypoxic sensitizers may alter selection of appropriate tumors for such therapeutic manipulation.[30,31]

Variable Radiation Response During the Division Cycle

As described in Chapter 1, the cell cycle can be divided into four phases: G1, S, G2, and M. Terasima, Tolmach, and Sinclair studied relatively synchronized populations to determine whether there is a difference in response to radiation as a function of the cell's position in the division cycle.[32,33] They found that generally the mitotic phase (M) is most sensitive and G2 almost as sensitive. G1 is relatively sensi-

tive in cells with a short G1. Cells gradually increase in resistance as they proceed through the late G1 and S phases, reaching a maximum of resistance in the late S phase. In cells with a long G1, there appears to be a peak of resistance early in G1. These findings in vitro seem to be true in vivo as well for both normal and tumor cells.[34,35]

The changes in radiation response are reflected in changes in the shoulder of the survival curve, as well as in the terminal slope. These differences can be quite large. The difference between the most resistant and the most sensitive can show slope ratios equal to that of the oxygen effect. The clinical consequence of a dose of 200 rad is shown in Table 15-5 for two different radiation fractionation schemes: one used in Hodgkin's disease (20 fractions) and one used in epithelial cancer (32 fractions).[36] Note how small differences in survival fractions following a single dose may change the final survival level achieved. All of these fractional survivals are within the range seen for cells in different parts of the cell cycle.

A second consequence of differential cell killing and the mitotic delay induced by radiation is a tendency to partially synchronize the cells. Thus the timing of the second dose of a fractionated scheme may be critical. However, this synchronization is short-lived because cells desynchronize rapidly and redistribute themselves according to the original cell age distribution. This phenomenon, which could pose a clinical problem or a clinical advantage, does not seem to be important unless there is incomplete redistribution between fractions.

CELL PROLIFERATION. During a course of fractionated radiation, the ultimate response of the tumor and normal tissue will depend on whether there has been cell proliferation between the fractions, thereby increasing the number of cells exposed to radiation. This may be caused by cell proliferation within the irradiated volume (*i.e.*, within the tumor or normal cell renewal tissue) or by cells that immigrate from unirradiated adjacent areas. The latter situation is seen in the skin, oral gastrointestinal mucosa, or from great distances, as found with bone marrow and lymph node repopulation. The balance between radiation-induced cell killing and repopulation is responsible for most of the clinical findings seen during fractionated radiotherapy treatment.

TABLE 15-4.   Effect of Anemia on Pelvic Recurrence in Stage IIB–III Cervical Cancer

	Control		Transfused
Hemoglobin (g/dl)	<12	>12	>12
Pelvic recurrence	50%	23%	16%
	(10/20)	(11/48)	(11/67)

Bush RS, Jenkin RP, Allt WE et al: Definitive evidence for hypoxic cells influencing cure in cancer therapy. Br J Cancer 37:302–306, 1978.

TABLE 15-5.   Calculated Cumulative Survival Fraction*

Survival Fraction	X^{32} $X =$	X^{20} $X =$
10^{-11}	0.45	0.28
10^{-10}	0.49	0.32
10^{-9}	0.52	0.35
10^{-8}	0.56	0.40
10^{-7}	0.60	0.45
10^{-6}	0.65	0.50
10^{-5}	0.70	0.56

Hellman S: Cell kinetics, models, and cancer treatment: Some principles for the radiation oncologist. Radiology 114:219–223, 1975.

*Calculated cumulative survival fraction for either 32 or 20 equal fractions when the fractional survival is varied.

In addition to spontaneous repopulation, there may be an induced cell proliferation or *recruitment* of cells.[37,38] Physiologically, many tissues of the body respond to trauma by being recruited into rapid proliferation (*e.g.*, following a wound in the skin, a break of the bone, or a partial hepatectomy). The reparative process requires proliferation of the undamaged cells. Similarly, when the oral mucosa is irradiated, there is strong evidence that the cell cycle time is decreased and that net cell proliferation increases. This also may occur in some tumors but appears to be of less magnitude than that in normal tissues.[39] Part of the differential effect of fractionated radiation may lie in differential recruitment of normal versus tumor cells.

Pharmacologic Modification of Radiation Effects

A number of pharmacologic agents can modify the basic parameters of radiation response. Figure 15-15 shows a radiation survival curve for cells that have semiconservatively incorporated the halogenated pyrimidine, BUDR, into their DNA. Under such circumstances, these cells are

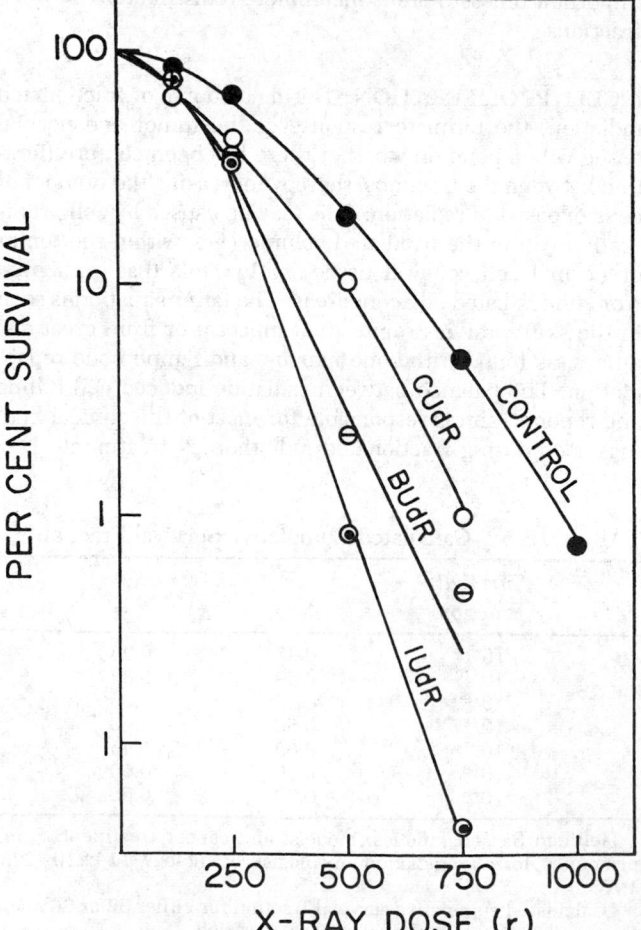

FIG. 15-15. Radiation survival curve for cells incorporating halogenated pyrimidines. (Szybalski W: X-ray sensitization by halopyrimidines. Cancer Chemother Rep 58:539–557, 1974)

more sensitive to radiation, their survival curve having both the slope and the shoulder modified.[40] This occurs only when the halogenated pyrimidines BUDR or IUDR are incorporated into the DNA; their presence at the time of radiation is not sufficient (Fig. 15-15). Sublethal damage repair also is markedly inhibited under these circumstances. Clinical experiments using these agents are discussed in Chapter 66, section 3.

A second class of agents includes those that primarily affect the shoulder and only slightly affect the slope. The two most important agents here are actinomycin D and Adriamycin. Sublethal damage apparently is inhibited by actinomycin D but not by Adriamycin.[41-47] The mechanisms by which these drugs affect radiation response are complicated. From a clinical standpoint, however, there appears to be strong evidence that these drugs can and do modify radiation effects when given simultaneously. Further, when given after radiation therapy, they can "recall" the irradiated volumes by erythema on the skin or by producing pulmonary reactions.[42,45,48,49] It is not known whether this is due to interaction between the damage done by radiation and that by drug or whether it represents only additivity of the effects.

Chemicals may also interact with radiation by preferentially killing cells that are more resistant to radiation. For example, agents that preferentially destroy cells in the most resistant phase of the cell cycle (S), along with radiation, will increase the cell kill; an example of this is hydroxyurea.[50] Hypoxic sensitizers also kill hypoxic cells and therefore act similarly in destroying a population of cells that is resistant to radiation. Radioprotective agents such as sulfhydryl-containing compounds act in the reverse fashion and tend to make cells more resistant.[51]

Agents with dose-limiting normal tissue toxicities different from radiation may be used very effectively with radiation. This is one of the basic principles of multiple-drug chemotherapy—add agents with nonoverlapping toxicities. This also works well with radiation.

The combined effects of drugs and radiation, or of two drugs, can be divided into the following types:

1. Independent—the agents act independently, their mechanisms of action are independent, and their damage is independent.
2. Additivity—the agents act on the same loci, and therefore their sublethal damage and their lethal damage are additive. Because of additive sublethal damage, the lethality of the two together may be greater than the lethality of each alone added together.
3. Synergism—the two agents have a result that is more effective than pure additivity.
4. Antagonism—the cell killing is less than independent action.

The most important parameter for the clinician is the therapeutic index. The sigmoid curve of tumor cure and that of dose-limiting toxicity are portrayed in Figure 15-16. If both curves are moved but their relative place (one to the other) is not changed, then the proportion cured for a given level of toxicity is unchanged. Drug–roentgen-ray interac-

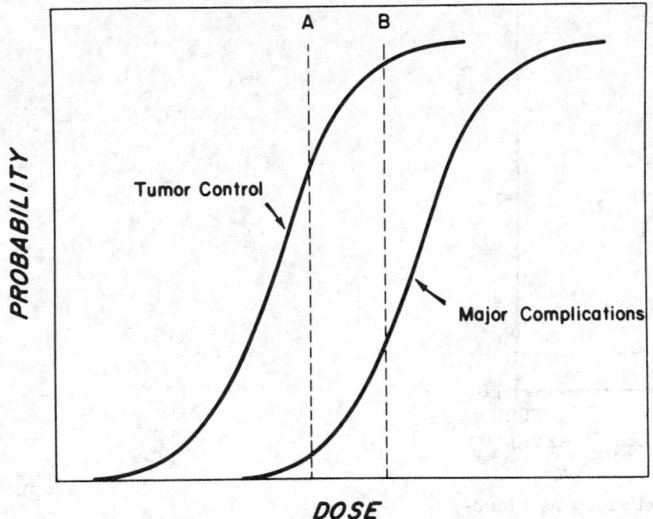

FIG. 15-16. Sigmoid curves of tumor control and complications. **A.** Dose for tumor control with minimum complications. **B.** Maximum tumor dose with significant complications.

tion is useful only when the curves are separated and not merely displaced.

HIGH LINEAR ENERGY TRANSFER RADIATION

Most of the previous discussion has been concerned with sparsely ionizing radiation, such as that produced by photons or high-energy electrons. More densely ionizing radiation is produced by larger atomic particles. The biologic actions of these two types of radiation are quite different and relate to the density of ionization. LET is the rate of energy loss along the path of the particle (de/dl). High LET radiations are very densely ionizing, with de/dl being very high. In general, the density of ionization depends on Z^2/v^2, where Z equals the atomic number and v is the particle velocity. Photons and electrons are characterized by high energy and very low mass. Therefore, the density of ionization will be low until the secondary electrons come to rest at the very end of their path. Particulate radiation ionizes directly. Alpha particles and stripped nuclei have a high LET; neutrons have an intermediate LET due to recoil protons. The Z^2 is quite large for large particles, intermediate for protons, and low for photons.

RELATIVE BIOLOGIC EFFECTIVENESS

Relative biologic effectiveness (RBE) is a commonly used parameter in radiation biology. It is the dose ratio of different average LET beams required to produce the same biologic effect. This term generally is a descriptive one, but its numerical value is fraught with many difficulties because it varies with the biologic endpoint used. High LET radiation differs from low LET radiation in affecting both the shoulder and the slope of the radiation survival curves (Fig. 15-17). If

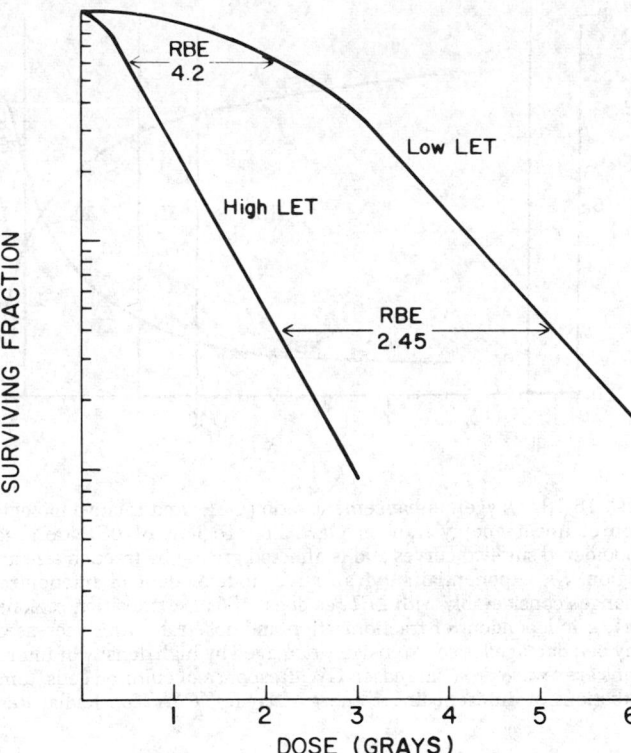

FIG. 15-17. Survival fractions for high and low *LET* radiations.

the biologic endpoint of interest is one associated with a high survival fraction, then the RBE will be large because it considers shoulder differences as well as those of the terminal slope. However, if the biologic endpoint involves a very low survival fraction, the RBE will be less because it primarily considers slope differences. In general, RBE increases as the dose decreases. Not only is the shoulder reduced, but other measures of sublethal damage repair or potentially lethal damage repair are markedly reduced with high LET radiation.

A general explanation is that the ionization is so dense that when a cell is hit, the damage is so great that it cannot be repaired. It is also true that the oxygen effect decreases as the LET increases. With very high LET radiation, there is no oxygen effect. Figure 15-18 plots both RBE and OER as a function of LET.[52] With very high LET radiation, there is a fall in RBE because these very densely ionizing radiations deposit more than one lethal event per cell. Thus, some of the absorbed dose is redundant and becomes less efficient.

Although this obvious advantage in RBE and OER would suggest the possible therapeutic use of these radiations, a cautionary note should be made. Increasing RBE in itself does not afford a therapeutic advantage. It is the therapeutic gain factor that is important—the RBE of the tumor compared with the RBE of the normal tissue. This is quite complicated and greatly depends on the specific tumor and the dose-limiting normal tissue being considered.[53] These forms of radiation will be discussed further in Chapter 66, section 5.)

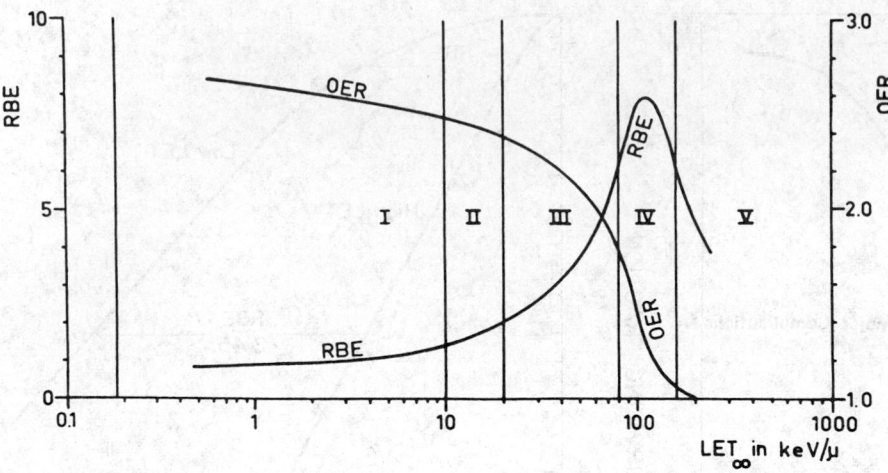

FIG. 15-18. Oxygen enhancement ratio (OER) and relative biologic effectiveness as a function of linear energy transfer OER. Five regions of LET are suggested: I, corresponds to shouldered survival curves and is affected greatly by fraction size and dose rate; II, transition region; III, exponential survival curve, independent of fractionization and dose rate. RBE changes considerably with LET, as does OER; IV, transition region; V, LET in excess of 160 KeV/u independent of fractionization and dose rate. RBE decreases as LET increases, since any cell damaged is so extensively damaged by high density of interactions that some interactions are "wasted." (Barendsen GW: Response of cultured cells, tumors and normal tissues to radiations of different linear energy transfer. Curr Top Radiat Res 4:293–356, 1968)

TUMOR RADIOBIOLOGY

Many experiments have been done using a variety of animal tumors. In general, these tumors are either spontaneous tumors occurring with reasonably high frequency in certain strains of mice (e.g., mammary carcinoma in C3H mice) or tumors induced by carcinogens. Such primary tumors of animals are difficult to use experimentally because their production is time-consuming, and numbers of tumors of the same size and location are limited, restricting some experimental designs. A much more common technique is the use of transplanted tumors. These are tumors that may have occurred spontaneously or from the application of a carcinogen but have now been transplanted from animal to animal. They grow with predictable and known kinetics. Although this is a great advantage in experimental work, it does increase the likelihood that the application of the results may be somewhat limited. Because these tumors are selected for rapid growth and for the ability to transplant serially, they may not represent tumors that occur spontaneously in the host animal.

Tumors can be used in radiobiologic experiments and assayed in a number of ways. The simplest is to study the likelihood for cure. A researcher implants a tumor into animals, allows it to grow to palpable size, treats it with a specific regimen, and then determines how many tumors of this type in various host animals are cured. If the dose of radiation is plotted against the likelihood for cure, a sigmoid curve is generated, as seen in Figure 15.19.[54] There is insufficient cell kill to cause tumor cure at very low doses. However, as the dose is raised (to about one lethal event per cell, the statistics of random cell kill become important. Occa-

FIG. 15-19. Sigmoid curve of tumor control.

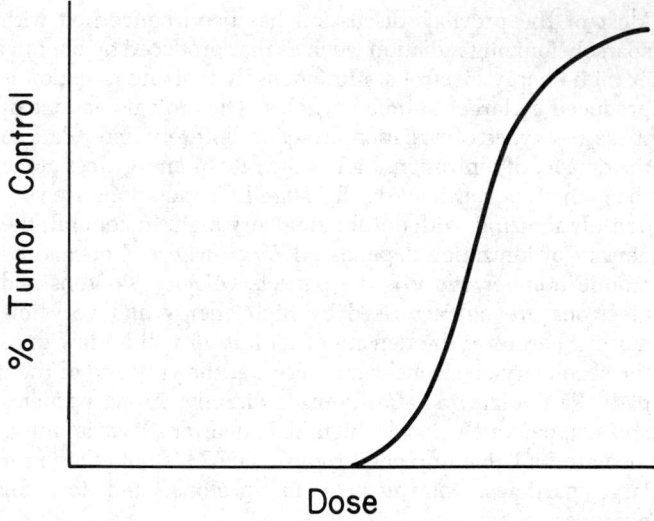

sionally, tumors will have zero viable cells and are cured. The likelihood of cure rises rapidly with dose at this portion of the curve; it starts to plateau when the maximum effect of the particular technique is reached. The dose required to increase a 10% likelihood of tumor control to 90% is about three times the D_0 dose. This sigmoid relationship is very important, because it is true not only for tumors in experimental animals, but also for clinical situations.

The shape and steepness of the sigmoid dose–response relationship for tumors can be affected by many factors. If the radiation survival curve is quite shallow for individual tumor cells (*i.e.*, the D_0 is large), then the dose–response curve will also be shallow. It will also be affected by host defense mechanisms. This curve is quite steep with nonimmunogenic tumors or when the immune response is abrogated, but it is significantly shallower in immunogenic tumors.[55] The shallowness means that there will be occasional cures at low doses and occasional failures at very high doses.

A similar sigmoid relationship is seen when plotting the likelihood for complications against tumor control. Figure 15-16 shows the two sigmoid curves, one for cure and one for complications. This is presented optimistically—the important complication curve is placed to the right of the tumor cure curve. The difference between these curves is a measure of therapeutic gain. Much of clinical medicine and research in cancer treatment is concerned with separating these curves.[53] Once the curves are separated, for a given level of complications, the likelihood of cure can be increased. Or, for a high likelihood of cure, the likelihood of complications can be decreased.

Another method of measuring tumors' response to treatment is to determine their growth delay following treatment. The longer the time for regrowth, the more effective was the treatment. If it is assumed that tumors grow and regrow with the same kinetics when they are at similar sizes, then the separation between the original curve and the regrowth curve is a direct measure of cell kill.[56] A direct measure of tumor cell kill is to remove the tumor after treatment, separate the cells, and score the surviving colony-forming cells, either in vivo or in vitro. Assay techniques include transplantation and measurement in recipient animals of death, tumor growth, or the number of colonies in the lung, liver, or brain. In vitro techniques require tumors to adapt to grow both in vivo and in vitro.

It is important to realize that tumors, like normal tissues, have certain physiologic characteristics. We associate some of these with the definition of malignancy: continued growth and extension into surrounding tissues and the ability to metastasize. In addition, growing tumors must induce a blood supply to meet their increasing metabolic needs. The production of these blood vessels appears to result from the release of a substance described by Folkman and colleagues as "tumor angiogenesis factor." This may have very important clinical implications. If tumors can be prevented from producing such substances, then they could not grow beyond a size supported by diffusion alone.[57-59] From the radiobiologic point of view it also means that when irradiating a tumor, both the radiobiology of the tumor and the vascular endothelial cells are important. Complete destruction of the tumor blood vessels' ability to proliferate will effectively limit tumor growth.

As tumors grow, they often exceed their blood supply and develop areas of necrosis and hypoxia (Fig. 15-14). The proportion of hypoxic cells in a tumor can be determined by studying the radiation survival curves. In Figure 15-20, curve A represents a well-oxygenated cell population, curve B describes hypoxic cells, and curve C represents a mixture of oxic and hypoxic cells (as in a tumor). Extrapolation of the curves to the ordinate gives the proportion of hypoxic cells within a tumor, first described by Powers and Tolmach.[60] In

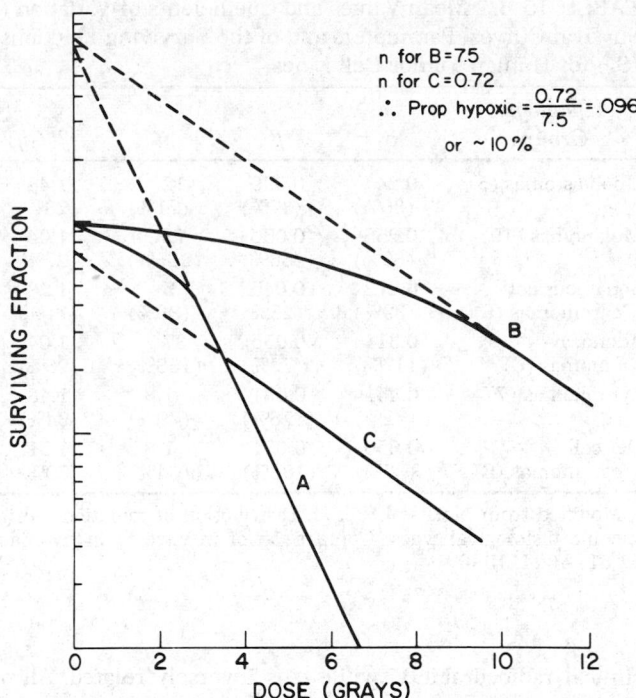

FIG. 15-20. Idealized survival curves for (**A**) oxic tumor cells; (**B**) hypoxic tumor cells; (**C**) a tumor containing both oxic and hypoxic tumor cells.

most experimental tumors studied, the percentage of hypoxic cells is 10% to 20%.

Calculation of the likelihood to cure tumors based on D_0, n, repopulation, repair, and hypoxia indicates that, because each fraction of radiation increases the proportion of hypoxic cells, the currently used treatment regimens should not be effective. Because radiotherapy cures a large number of tumors that have hypoxic components and show necrosis on pathologic examination, then this conclusion must be erroneous. After multiple fractions of radiation, a marked increase in the proportion of the more resistant hypoxic cells could be expected, but in fact, the proportion remained constant when observed 72 hours after the last of five radiation fractions. Kallman has called this *reoxygenation*.[20] Hypoxic cells may not be important in tumors that are cured but may be important in some tumors that are not cured. Clinical evidence that this is significant includes the benefits of correcting anemia, hyperbaric oxygen, and the hypoxic sensitizers. All appear to favorably influence tumor curability in certain clinical circumstances.

There has been a renaissance in trying to determine whether there are appropriate laboratory correlates for clinical radiation treatment.[61,62] Table 15-6 shows a number of important parameters found by in vitro survival determinations for six histologic groups of human tumor cells.[63] The first four parameters have been described earlier. S_2 and S_8 are the survival fractions found with 2 Gy and 8 Gy, respectively. $\overline{D}$ is the mean inactivation dose, a mathematically determined characteristic of the initial portion of the survival curve. It appears that S_2 and $\overline{D}$ correlate directly with

TABLE 15-6.   Mean Values and Coefficients of Variation (in parentheses) of the Survival Curves' Parameters and of the Surviving Fractions at 2 Gy (S_2) and at 8 Gy (S_8) for Human Tumor Cell Lines

Histologic Groups	α	β	n	D_0 (Gy)	S_2 (%)	S_8 (%)	$\overline{D}$ (Gy)
Glioblastomas (5)	0.241 (86%)	0.029 (37%)	12 (71%)	1.44 (28%)	58 (34%)	4.98 (111%)	3.10 (38%)
Melanomas (19)	0.255 (69%)	0.053 (56%)	73 (265%)	1.04 (27%)	51 (28%)	1.11 (109%)	2.43 (25%)
Squamous cell carcinomas (6)	0.273 (39%)	0.045 (25%)	5 (38%)	1.28 (11%)	49 (18%)	0.88 (49%)	2.35 (25%)
Adenocarcinomas (6)	0.311 (117%)	0.055 (79%)	37 (166%)	1.04 (26%)	48 (37%)	0.39 (130%)	2.22 (28%)
Lymphomas (7)	0.451 (42%)	0.051 (126%)	1.8 (79%)	1.48 (34%)	34 (27%)	0.57 (121%)	1.77 (22%)
Oat cell carcinomas (6)	0.650 (37%)	0.081 (183%)	1.8 (104%)	1.51 (70%)	22 (42%)	0.14 (85%)	1.33 (21%)

Modified from Malaise EP et al: Distribution of radiation sensitivities for human tumor cells of specific histological types: Comparison of in vitro to in vivo data. Int J Radiat Oncol Biol Phys 12:617–624, 1986.

clinical radiocurability, while α is inversely related. All of these are measures of the initial portion of the radiation survival curve; S_2 is the most closely correlated with clinical practice, because doses between 1.5 and 2.5 Gy are used most often in patient care.

Because doses are repeated, small differences in S_2 can have very large consequences. Table 15-5 shows that, in a typical 32-fraction radiation treatment, the difference between survival fractions of 0.45 and 0.60 results in an ultimate survival fraction of 10^{-11} compared with 10^{-7}, respectively. Also, certain tumors that are known to be difficult to cure by radiation have been shown to have great capacity to repair radiation damage, as measured by allowing the cells time for repair before plating them for in vitro growth.[64] That these two simple laboratory determinations correlate with clinical results gives hope that in vitro techniques can be used to determine mechanisms of modifying clinical parameters. This does not mean that the other biologic parameters such as oxygenation, position in the cell cycle, and cell proliferation are not important; no doubt all add to the complexity of correlating the clinical response with in vitro determinations.

NORMAL TISSUE RADIATION BIOLOGY

To understand normal tissue radiation biology, an appreciation of the cell kinetics of cell renewal tissues is vital (see Chap. 1). The effects on organ function very much depend on the reproductive requirements of the irradiated cells. Tissues, (e.g., muscle and neurologic tissue) whose functional activity does not require cell renewal are "resistant" to radiation. Both muscle and neurologic tissue also have important vasculoconnective tissue stroma that support them.[65] These stromal cells may be required to divide, and therefore determine the organ response to radiation. The radiation response of endothelial cells demonstrates a D_q = 340 rad, n = 7, and a D_0 = 170 rad, values similar to those of epithelial cells.[66]

Many tissues of the body require continued cellular proliferation for their function, and they promptly demonstrate the effects of radiation. These cell renewal tissues include the skin and its appendages, the gastrointestinal mucosa, bone marrow, reproductive tissues, and many exocrine glands. Clonogenic survival curves for bone marrow stem cells, gastrointestinal epithelial cells, and skin are all available. In slowly proliferating tissues (e.g., lung), the effects of radiation are seen much later, but the effects depend on radiation damage to proliferating cells.

Tissues such as the liver and bone require little or no proliferation during the steady state, and normal function can be maintained despite large doses of radiation. However, both of these respond to injury with rapid cell renewal. If trauma (fracture or partial hepatectomy) occurs, then the cells die when they attempt repair. Irradiation of the liver has few consequences in moderate doses, but if this is followed by a partial hepatectomy, then hepatic failure can occur. This has been of clinical importance in the preoperative irradiation of right-sided Wilms' tumors attached to the liver, in which a significant amount of liver must be removed.[67] Under such circumstances it is far better to operate, allow the liver to regenerate, and then irradiate.

Patients who have received large amounts of radiation to the bone do perfectly well unless the bone is fractured. Such damaged bones will either fail to be reconstituted or will heal slowly, causing a significant deformity and disability to the patient. These examples are included to stress that it is not the different cells that have such great differences in radiation response, but rather that the proliferative requirements of different tissues largely determine the radiation effects. When the proliferative requirements are low, the organ will be considered relatively resistant to radiation. When the proliferative requirements are high, it will be considered very radiosensitive. There may be some common limitations on all systems based on the radiosensitivity of the vascular connective tissue and endothelial cells.[65] Stem cells of the cell renewal tissues may have a limited proliferative capacity, and stem cell exhaustion appears to be a cause of late organ failure following irradiation.[68]

Many other effects of radiation that do not depend on reproductive viability may have clear clinical relevance. For example, radiation is quite damaging to the cell membrane and changes membrane transport. Subsequent radiation-induced edema is seen with moderate doses of radiation. These nonreproductive effects of radiation are far less well understood but may be important in understanding the effects of radiation on nondividing tissue — most importantly, the central nervous system.

Large doses of whole-body irradiation have obvious clinical consequences, which generally are not relevant to conventional radiation therapy. However, because whole-body irradiation has been used in low doses in treating the lymphomas and in high doses in treating metastatic carcinoma, this will be discussed briefly.

Following large doses of radiation, the prodromal syndrome of nausea, vomiting, diarrhea, cramps, fatigue, sweating, fever, and headache occurs. Three distinct modes of death may occur. The first, with very high doses of radiation ($> 10,000$ rad), is seen within hours and appears to result from neurologic and cardiovascular damage. Because this occurs so quickly, it probably is not caused by failure of a proliferating cell system but rather by extranuclear events within these organs. At intermediate doses of radiation ($500-1000$ rad), death occurs within days. It is associated with extensive gastrointestinal mucosal damage, resulting in prolonged, severe, bloody diarrhea, dehydration, and secondary infection occurring as the gastrointestinal mucosa is denuded. At lower doses of radiation (around the LD_{50}), death is caused by hematopoietic failure. This has a latency period because the formed blood elements are nondividing and bone marrow failure does not occur until the progeny of the proliferating cells are required to maintain the patient. The lymphocyte level falls promptly as some of these cells die without dividing. The granulocyte level will fall on about day 5 or 6, and thrombocytopenia will occur later. Anemia does not occur as a direct result of a failure of red cell production because of the long life of the red cell, but it may be caused by hemorrhage.

Whole-body irradiation appears to have significant antitumor activity exceeding that seen when the same dose is given to the tumor alone.[69,70] Very low doses of whole-body radiation in humans ($10-15$ rad, two to three times per week for $6-10$ fractions) may be effective treatment for lymphomas and may cause marked depression of the formed blood elements. The mechanism of action of this type of treatment is not understood. The effects on both tumor and normal tissue are greater than can be explained by the typical survival curve.

ADVERSE EFFECTS OF RADIATION

Some biologic considerations of localized radiation may decrease the likelihood for tumor control. First and most discussed is the effect of radiation on the *immune response.* High-dose, whole-body irradiation has a well-known and profound effect on the immune response. However, this generalized treatment rarely is used in clinical radiation therapy, except as preparation for bone marrow transplantation.

Shortly after the discovery of roentgen rays, whole-body irradiation before the administration of antigens was found to suppress the production of antibodies. After whole-body irradiation, there is a prompt fall in the lymphocyte count. The lymphocytes appear to have two types of radiation response: About 80% die a prompt, intermitotic death, but some lymphocytes survive the radiation. When assayed on the basis of reproductive capacity by either exposure to mitogens after irradiation or other functional endpoints, their radiation survival curves looked similar to that of hematopoietic cells with a D_0 of about 70 to 80 rad and an n of about 1.[71] Response depends on the classes of lymphocytes involved, the extent of cell proliferation required, cell traffic, and the balance between suppressor and helper systems. In general, the following conclusions concerning the effect of radiation on the immune response can be made:[71]

1. B lymphocytes are radiosensitive and undergo both interphase and mitotic death following irradiation.
2. All functional T-cell subpopulations have sensitive precursor cells. Suppressor T-cell precursors may undergo interphase death.
3. The homing potential of cells is affected by radiation.
4. Resting cells are more sensitive to interphase death than are the same cells when stimulated to divide before irradiation. (In the latter case they have an n and D_0 similar to those of hematopoietic stem cells.)
5. The effects of whole-body irradiation are qualitatively and quantitatively different from those caused by localized or regional irradiation.

Whole-body irradiation is more effective in preventing response to new antigens than in modifying response to a previously encountered antigen. Survival of second-set skin grafts are affected much less than are initial grafts. Localized radiation, as used in radiation therapy, affects the immune response by decreasing the number of circulating lymphocytes, presumably by irradiating and destroying them as they pass through the irradiated volume. The consequences of this irradiation appear to be small if the tumor has been in place for a significant time before the irradiation and if the irradiated volume is relatively small. If the animal is irradiated at the time the tumor is implanted, the immune response will be inhibited. However, this rarely is the clinical situation. There have been reports suggesting the deleterious effects of localized radiation on the immune response affecting survival in breast cancer, but this does not appear to be the case in either the original series studied or in subsequent studies.[72-74]

It is clear that localized radiation, despite producing a chronic lymphopenia of both T and B cells, does not affect the immune response to bacterial or viral agents because treated patients do not seem to be more susceptible. This is the case with the immune suppression produced by whole-body irradiation or systemic chemotherapy. Clearly, regional irradiation of the lymph nodes adjacent to tumors has been associated with increased curability in head and neck tumors in adults without adverse effects.[75]

There also may be adverse effects of radiation on the patient other than those on host-defense mechanisms. Radiation-induced *mutagenesis* is of concern for both germ line and somatic cells. If the gonads are irradiated, then there is an increased likelihood of mutation with increasing doses, without any evidence of a threshold dose or of an ameliorating effect of fractionation. At higher doses, however, there is significant cell killing, and the dose–response curve is no longer linear, presumably because the cells that mutated received sufficient radiation to become sterile. Abnormal live births are uncommon after gonadal irradiation because most radiation-induced mutations are recessive. Further, dominant mutations, when they occur, usually are lethal. There is some evidence in the mouse that the risk of mutation decreases with time after ovarian irradiation. Whether this is true in humans and the mechanism by which it occurs in animals are not known. It does not appear to be true for irradiation of the testes.

The mutagenic effects of radiation depend on the type of irradiation. The RBE for high LET radiation can be extremely high for mutations. It is very difficult to quantify the risk because experiments with mice indicate a large difference in the mutation rate for different loci, with as much as a 1000-fold variation in the mutation rate.[76] In general, the prudent figure used is that the mutation rate doubles with approximately every 50 rad.

Perhaps of even greater concern are somatic mutations, especially those that may lead to tumors. A great deal of evidence indicates that low doses of radiation increase the incidence of tumors after significant latent periods. This information comes largely from whole-body exposures to the atomic bomb and experience with patients irradiated for a variety of benign diseases.[77–79] In general, there appears to be a linear increase in tumor incidence with dose until high doses are reached, at which point the incidence reaches a plateau or even falls.[80–81] Presumably, this is true again because of cell killing. Figure 15-21 is an example of this biphasic dose–response curve. Such tumor induction is associated with a latent period of 3 to 5 years for leukemia but is much longer for solid tumors. There are different ages at which tumor induction is most likely. For example, the induction of breast cancer by radiation appears primarily with exposure in the first and second decades of life and decreases with radiation later in life.[82]

Except for irradiation of children, it is difficult to demonstrate a significantly increased incidence of tumors in patients receiving therapeutic radiation for malignant disease. This may be an example of the biphasic nature of the tumor induction curve. For example, long-term studies of patients with carcinoma of the cervix do not show increased incidence of pelvic cancer.[82,83] In contrast, when patients are irradiated to the same volume for benign diseases with much lower doses of radiation, an increased tumor incidence can be seen.[78] Thus there appears to be a difference between the tumorigenicity of radiation doses used for benign disease (200–1000 rad) and that seen when therapeutic doses of radiation are used.

Clearly radiation is a teratogen when a woman is exposed during the rapidly proliferating period of embryogenesis, between weeks 2 and 16.

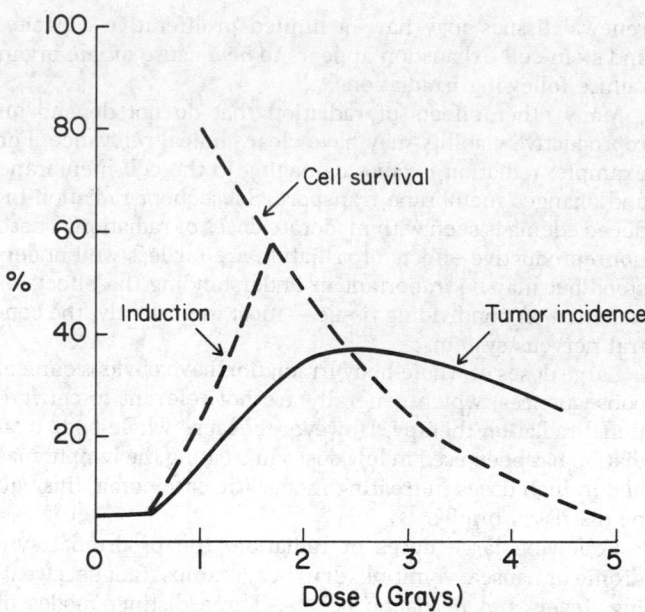

FIG. 15-21. Biphase curve of tumor incidence. (Redrawn from Gray LH: Radiation biology and cancer. In Cellular Radiation Biology, pp 7–25. M. D. Anderson Hospital and Tumor Institute 18th Symposium on Fundamental Cancer Research. Baltimore, Williams & Wilkins, 1965; and Upton AC, Randolph ML, Conklin JW: Late effects of fast neutrons and gamma rays in mice as influenced by the dose rate of irradiation: Induction of neoplasia. Radiat Res 41:467–491, 1970)

CLINICAL CONSIDERATIONS

It is often suggested that the goal of treatment is the greatest probability of uncomplicated cure. Although this is desirable, circumstances actually may dictate a different policy. Consider Figure 15-16, in which the curve for complications is to the right of the sigmoid curve for tumor control. The ideal dose would be that which gives as many cures as possible before the steep portion of the complication curve, as shown by line A. This, however, may not be the optimal dose. It depends very much on the consequences of both tumor failure and the nature of the complications. If tumor failure can be salvaged by subsequent surgery but complications are severe, long-lived, and difficult to manage, then line A is indeed the optimal line.[53] An example of this would be the treatment of T2 and T3 glottic cancer. On the other hand, if complications are either not severe or remediable, but cancer failure is fatal, then line B would be appropriate. This is the case in stage II and III carcinoma of the uterine cervix. Thus, there is no simple answer. Often the worst complication of treatment is tumor recurrence.

There are many clinical examples of sigmoid dose–response curves. An example for tumors of the head and neck is shown in Figure 15-22 and for Hodgkin's disease in Figure 15-23.[84,85] In Figure 15-22, the ordinate is arranged to convert a sigmoid curve to a straight line. These are simple because they do not consider time–dose relationships or tumor volume. An instructive clinical experience is described by Stewart and Jackson in which a consistent ~10% change in dose was used.[86] Figure 15-24 shows the results in

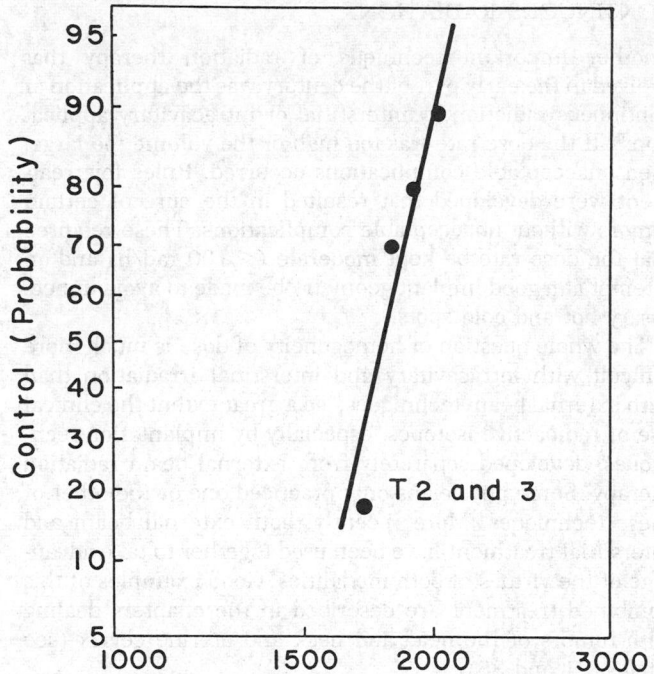

FIG. 15-22. Tumor control versus dose for supraglottic carcinoma. (Shukovsky LJ: Dose, time, volume relationships in squamous cell carcinoma of the supraglottic larynx. Am J Roentgenol Rad Ther Nucl Med 108:27–29, 1970)

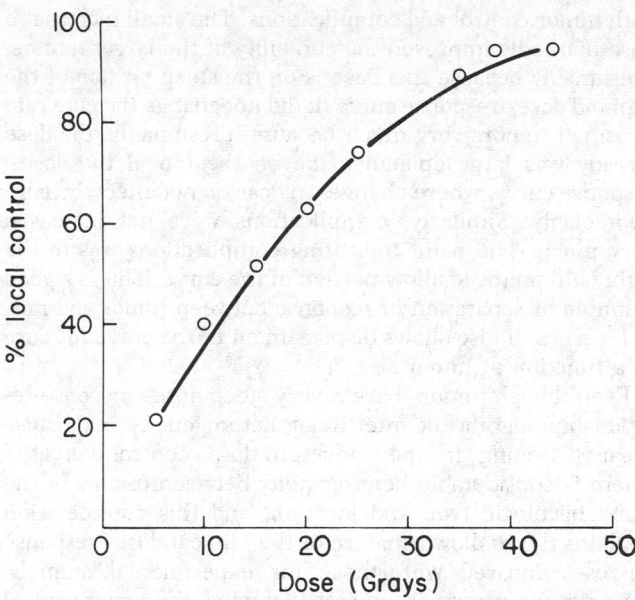

FIG. 15-23. Tumor control versus dose. (Kaplan HS: Evidence for a tumoricidal dose level in the radiotherapy of Hodgkin's disease. Cancer Res 26:1221–1224, 1966)

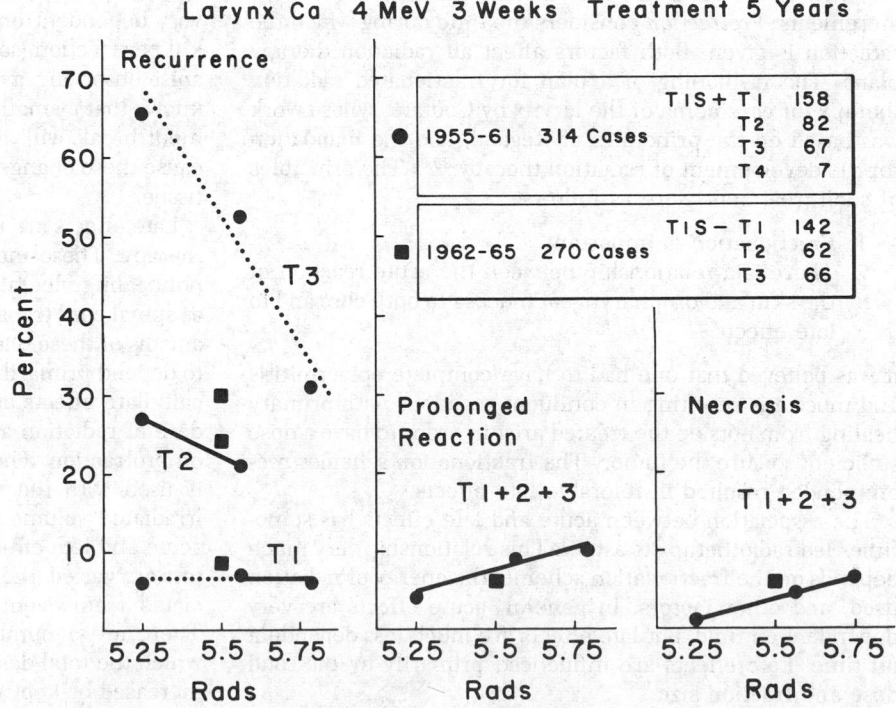

FIG. 15-24. Tumor control versus dose for cancer of the larynx. (Stewart JG, Jackson AW: The steepness of the dose response curve both for tumor and normal tissue injury. Laryngoscope 85:1107–1111, 1975)

both tumor control and complications. The small increase in dose markedly improved the curability of the larger tumors, presumably because this dose is on the steep portion of the sigmoid dose–response curve. It did not change the cure rate for small tumors very much because, presumably, the dose already was large enough to be on the top of the dose–response curve, where changes in dose do not affect the cure appreciably. Similarly, complications were not increased very much. The point indicating complications was to the right, still on the shallow portion of the curve. This is a good example of separation of response between tumor and normal tissues. It also shows displacement of the curve for cure as a function of tumor size.

Even though tumors have a very steep dose–response relationship, significant intertumor heterogeneity may cause great flattening in the radiation dose–control curves.[87] There is considerable heterogeneity between tumors of the same histologic type and location, and this consideration explains the shallower nature of the clinical dose–response curves compared with those for experimental animals. These analyses further indicate that when the tumor control probability is relatively low, the major reason is the high survival fraction associated with the initial fraction, that is, a high S_2. This emphasizes the importance of identifying prospectively tumors that have a high S_2.

FRACTIONATION

Early in this century, as the practice of radiation therapy evolved, the virtues of dividing the radiation into small fractions were noticed. The reasons given were often incorrect, but the clear observation was that fractionation of the dose allowed more effective tumor cure without excessive complications.

Fractionation considers the size and number of radiation increments. *Protraction* considers the time during which the radiation is given. Both factors affect all radiation therapy plans. The fashioning of a plan for fractionated radiation therapy for carcinoma of the larynx by Coutard, whose work was based on the principles of Regaud, laid the foundation for the development of radiation therapy.[88,89] The principles of such treatment were as follows:

1. Fractionation is important.
2. There is a relationship between the acute reaction of the skin and oropharyngeal mucosa to both cure and to late effects.

It was believed that one had to have complete epidermititis and mucositis resulting in confluent reactions with primary healing from outside the treated area in order to have a dose sufficient to cure the tumor. The fractionation schemes recommended resulted in tolerable late effects.

The association between acute and late effects has sometimes led radiotherapists astray. This relationship very much depends on the fractionation scheme, the energy of radiation used, and other factors. In general, acute effects are very dependent on time, but late effects are much less dependent on time. Late effects are influenced primarily by the total dose and fraction size.

CONTINUOUS RADIATION

Another important technique of radiation therapy that evolved in the early part of the century was the application of continuous radiation by interstitial or intracavitary application.[90] If the dose rate was too high or the volume too large, then unacceptable complications occurred. Rules for treatment were developed that resulted in the cure of certain tumors without unacceptable complications. These required that the dose rate be kept moderate (< 100 rad/h) and an attempt at a good implant geometry be made to avoid unnecessary hot and cold spots.

The whole question of homogeneity of dose is much more difficult with intracavitary and interstitial irradiation than with external beam techniques. To a great extent the clinical use of radioactive isotopes, especially by implantation techniques, developed separately from external beam radiation therapy. Some physicians only practiced one or the other of these techniques. More recently, both external beam and interstitial treatment have been used together to take advantage of the virtues of both modalities. Good examples of this combined treatment are described in the chapters dealing with tumors of the head and neck and uterine cervix (see Chaps. 21 and 36).

ACUTE AND LATE NORMAL TISSUE EFFECTS

Acute radiation effects occur largely in renewing tissues, such as skin, oropharyngeal mucosa, small intestine, rectum, bladder mucosa, and vaginal mucosa. These cell-renewing tissues are rapidly proliferating, and as they are confronted with fractionated radiation, the processes of repair, repopulation, and recruitment all obtain. Because the response of rapidly renewing tissues depends on the balance between cell birth and cell death, acute tissue reaction is crucially affected by the time allowed for repopulation, and therefore very dependent on protraction. It also depends on the cell kill per fraction, so fraction size is important. The radiotherapist observing an excessive reaction by the oral mucosa knows that a small decrease in fraction size or a small treatment break will allow rapid resolution of the problem because these changes will permit reconstitution of the normal tissue.

Late effects are really the dose-limiting factor in radiation therapy. These include necrosis, fibrosis, fistula formation, nonhealing ulceration, and damage to specific organs, such as spinal cord transection and blindness. Although the mechanisms of these phenomena are not clear, they do not appear to depend primarily on the rapid proliferation of cells. Clinically late effects appear to depend much more on the total dose of radiation and the size of the radiation fraction than on protraction. Thus, only if the same fractionation scheme is used with the same normal tissue endpoint, the same irradiated volume, and the same treatment technique, can acute and late effects be correlated. If any of these parameters are varied, the acute reactions to radiation may be dissociated from eventual late effects and will be misleading. There are a number of examples in radiation therapy in which the total dose was increased and the fraction size was increased or kept the same, but the time was protracted to minimize acute effects. Such techniques have resulted in unacceptable late complications.

Two hypotheses for late effects are worth discussion. One theory holds that all late effects result from damage to vasculoconnective stroma. Because this is common throughout the body, it would suggest a common mechanism for the late effects in any organ.[65] A variation on this hypothesis is that it is damage to the endothelial cells, ubiquitous throughout the body, that determines late effects.[66] An alternative hypothesis suggests that both the acute and the late effects of radiation and cytotoxic chemotherapy are caused by cell depletion of the targeted cell-renewal tissues. Acute effects depend on the balance between cell killing and compensatory replication of both the stem and proliferative cells. The development of late effects requires that stem cells have only a limited proliferative capacity.[91,92] Compensation for extensive or repeated cell killing may exhaust this capacity, resulting in eventual tissue failure.[64,93]

ALTERING THE THERAPEUTIC INDEX

Goodman and Gilman define the therapeutic index as the relationship between desired and undesired effects of therapy.[94] Clearly for the oncologist, separation of the sigmoid curve of complications from that of local control (Fig. 15-16) is the graphic representation of manipulation of the therapeutic index. Some techniques of time–dose relationships used by the radiotherapist to take advantage of this are fractionation, protraction, split-course technique, interstitial treatment, and manipulation of the target volume. Although fractionation has been discussed, the use of multiple small fractions two, three, or more times a day, *hyperfractionation*, is just beginning to be explored, with some good results.[95-97]

Another technique to reduce complications is the use of normal-sized fractions given more than once a day. This is referred to as multifraction, multiple daily fractions, or *accelerated fractionation*.[98] In the experiments that stimulated the recent interest, the investigators administered two daily fractions of radiation separated by 6 hours, and compared this to daily radiation given as a single fraction.[99] Six hours is believed to be long enough to allow complete sublethal damage repair but not long enough for significant proliferation. Because both methods are daily treatments, repair can be separated from repopulation and recruitment. The general results of the experiments were presented as the recovered radiation, the difference between the dose obtained when the radiation is given in two divided doses separated by 6 hours and that when it is given in one fraction. When the single fraction was 200 rad or less, there was little recovered dose. The recovered dose increased rapidly between 200 and 800 rad; then, with very large fractions, the recovered dose tended to level off. Thus, in clinical situations, when typical radiation doses of about 200 rad are divided into two smaller fractions, only a little more should be given because the recovered dose is small. This has been confirmed in a number of clinics.[100] The use of such hyperfractionation is being tried for several tumors; however, it is too soon to determine whether it will be useful.

When tumor cells are proliferating rapidly, accelerated fractionation makes sense. Waiting 24 hours between each fraction may allow significant proliferation. Perhaps the best example of the changing therapeutic index obtained with accelerated fractionation is the enhanced success in treating Burkitt's lymphoma.[101]

In general, most radiotherapists administer conventional radiation in fractions between 180 and 250 rad each day. This allows tumor control without excessive acute or late effects. The fraction size that is tolerated in terms of acute effects depends on the volume irradiated (the larger the volume, the smaller the fraction size), the amount and type of dose-limiting normal tissue, the age of the patient, and other clinical factors.

Small changes in fraction size will make a big difference in tolerance. Patients often are given small breaks during the treatment. These rest periods usually are caused by weekend interruptions of daily fractionation. This protraction of the treatment allows for repopulation and recruitment. The days of rest also allow amelioration of many acute effects, and they may allow time for tumor regression, resulting in reoxygenation.

An attempt to formalize and extend treatment breaks is the so-called *split course technique*.[102-104] Two to 3 weeks are allowed in the middle of treatment for recovery from the acute effects, as well as to permit tumor regression. When the dose of radiation is not increased, there is some evidence that this treatment (although clearly better tolerated) may be associated with less tumor control.[105] When the split course is administered with an increase in total dose, the results seem to be comparable to conventional fractionation but perhaps with greater late effects.

Interstitial irradiation is administered in radium needle implants, gold and radon seed implants, iridium wire implants, and a variety of other techniques for either permanently or temporarily placing radioactive material into tissues. It requires both biologic and physical considerations. Clearly there is great inhomogeneity in even the most geometrically perfect implant. There is large inhomogeneity of dose and a similar variation in dose rate; the dose rate of radiation is greater in areas of high dose. With temporary implants, the radiologist attempts to administer a calculated dose of between 30 and 100 rad per hour to the minimum tumor location. This is impossible with permanent implants because isotopes decrease their radiation intensity as they decay. The most commonly used isotopes have been radon and [198]Au. More recently, ^{125}I has been used and has created unusual new considerations. The half-life of ^{125}I is quite long (60 days), resulting in a significant amount of the dose being given so slowly that there may be significant cell division occurring in both the tumor and some normal cells. Therefore the important dose may not be the total dose, but rather the dose per cell cycle, which is different for each cell type and different as the isotope decays. Also, ^{125}I irradiates primarily by the emission of very low energy photons, some of which are absorbed by the seeds themselves, leading to even further inhomogeneity.[106]

When implants can be used alone or in combination with external irradiation, the results tend to be better in terms of the therapeutic index than with external beam techniques alone. The high local dose, continuous radiation, and even inhomogeneity allowing normal tissue regrowth all contribute to better cosmetic and functional results and cure of the tumor. Examples are breast cancer and tumors of the tongue and other head and neck sites.[107]

Tumor volume also is quite important in clinical radiotherapy. Although the gross tumor extent can be determined, most clinicians recognize that a characteristic of tumors is to extend far beyond those macroscopically identifiable borders. Determination of the target volume must include this consideration, but if a larger volume must be irradiated, then a smaller dose is tolerated. Conversely, if the volume of the tumor is larger, then a larger dose is required. This dilemma limited the success of early radiotherapy of certain tumors by reducing the target volume, resulting in recurrences at the treatment margins, or by causing significant complications in the treatment of large target volumes. Today, distinctions are made between gross tumor and the subclinical extensions into apparently normal tissues. Subclinical disease means small numbers of cells, perhaps favorable to irradiation (well-oxygenated), which can be controlled with modest doses of radiation (Table 15-7). The large number of cells present in the clinically evidenced tumor requires higher doses, as noted in the curves shown in Figures 15-22 and 15-23. This difference has led to the development of a variety of techniques for administering different doses to microscopic tumor extensions and to the gross tumor. These include shrinking field techniques, boost treatments, and certain strategies of combined surgery and radiotherapy to be described later in this chapter.

Shrinking field technique means giving the largest potential tumor bed a moderate dose of radiation, then reducing the target volume to the tumor and its immediate confines, raising the dose. This can be done by reducing the fields, by changing the treatment technique and target volume, or by using a treatment technique that gives both the desired moderate dose to the larger volume and a higher dose to the smaller volume. A modification of this is the *boost technique*, in which the maximum tolerated dose is given to a volume and then very localized radiation is used to raise the dose to the tumor bed. An implant or an electron boost can be used for this. A number of attempts have been made to consider fractionation, protraction, and even implantation used with external beam in some form of some mathematical formulae, all of which tend to simplify complex clinical circumstances and can be very misleading.

The normal tissues that limit the dose of radiation given may be so close to the tumor that any target volume that includes a tumor must include these normal tissues. Dose-limiting normal tissues are distinguished from these normal tissue transited by the radiation but not in the target volume, although both may contribute to the production of complications and thus be dose-limiting. Radiotherapy with detailed treatment planning, CT scanning, and a variety of techniques, the ultimate of which is computer-controlled radiation therapy, may reduce the dose to the transit volume, possibly changing the therapeutic index.[109] However, it is unlikely that there will be significant physical techniques for reducing the dose to normal tissues in the target volume. This can be done only by some biologic mechanism that distinguishes tumor from normal tissues.

RADIOSENSITIVITY

The term radiosensitivity is used in a number of different ways in the literature and can mean what we define as radiosensitivity, radioresponsiveness, or radiocurability. Each is a somewhat different concept. *Radiosensitivity* means the innate sensitivity of the cells to radiation. For cells that die a reproductive death, this is related to the slope of the survival curve or the D_0.

Radioresponsiveness means the clinical appearance of tumor regression promptly following moderate doses of radiation. This may be a function of the cell's radiosensitivity, but it also may be a function of the active cell kinetics of a tumor. Bergonie and Tribondeau first established an association between the rate of proliferation and the response of normal tissues, although they considered this to be radiosensitivity.[110] A similar relationship was presumed to apply to tumors. Because cells will not die until they face mitosis, some tumors that proliferate rapidly will regress rapidly, but they also may regrow rapidly. This is often confused with radiosensitivity. An excellent example of this is the adenoid-cystic tumor of the salivary gland or cylindroma. Such tumors are quite radioresponsive; however, they require very large doses to be cured.

Radiocurability means that the tumor–normal tissue relationships are such that curative doses of radiation can be applied regularly without excessive damage to normal tissues. Examples of such radiocurable tumors are carcinomas of the cervix, larynx, breast, and prostate, in addition to Hodgkin's disease and seminomas. Some of these are radioresponsive, some are radiosensitive, and some are neither.

RADIATION AND SURGERY

Radiation and surgery can be combined in many different ways. The general rationale for combining surgery and radiation is that the mechanism of failure for the two techniques is quite different. Radiation rarely fails at the periphery of tumors, where cells are small in number and well vascularized. When radiation fails, it usually does so in the center of the tumor where there are large volumes of tumor cells often under hypoxic conditions. Surgery, in contrast, is limited by the required preservation of vital normal tissues adjacent to the tumor. In resectable cancers the gross tumor can be removed, but it is these vital normal tissues that limit the anatomic extent of the dissection. When surgery fails under these circumstances, it is usually due to microscopic tumor

TABLE 15-7.   Control (%) of Subclinical Disease

Dose (Gy)	Adenocarcinoma of the Breast	Carcinoma of Upper Aerodigestive Tract
30–35	60–70%	60–70%
40	80–90%	>90%
50	>90%	>90%

Fletcher GH: Clinical dose–response curves of human malignant epithelial tumours. Br J Radiol 46:1–12, 1973.

cells left behind. It seems logical, therefore, to consider combining the two techniques.

Radiation can be given before or after surgery. Preoperative radiation has the advantages of sterilizing cells at the edges of the resection, sterilizing cells that perhaps would be dislodged and seeded at the time of surgery, and in the special circumstance of unresectable tumors, reducing the tumor volume sufficiently to allow resection. It is not clear how often this really results in a cure, because it may only change gross tumor to microscopic tumor and still result in tumor recurrence. It does seem to benefit selected cases of large unresectable cancers.[111]

There are disadvantages in the use of preoperative irradiation. The pathology reports are not evaluable because, if sufficient time is allowed between the radiation and the surgery, the destruction of tumor caused by preoperative radiation prevents ascertainment of the tumor's initial anatomic extent. In contrast, if the tumor is slow-growing or if the surgery is done shortly after the radiation, the consequences of the radiation will not be represented in the pathologic evaluation of the material because sufficient time was not allowed for tumor destruction and regression.

Another disadvantage is that the patient is irradiated before the careful staging available at surgical exploration, and thus some patients who would not benefit from preoperative radiation are given this treatment (*e.g.*, preoperative radiation to a colorectal carcinoma in a patient with occult liver metastases). Metastases may be found only at the time of surgery.

A disadvantage often mentioned is the delay before surgical resection. This may not be a disadvantage, because as long as the patient's tumor is being treated, the order of treatments should make no difference. The radiation dose usually is moderate (4000–5000 rad) and given in conventional 200-rad fractions 5 days a week or in smaller total doses given more quickly in larger fractions. If the total dose of radiation is kept small (≤ 2000 rad), then the delay between radiation and surgery is small. When the dose reaches approximately 4000 rad, it is valuable to delay the surgery (usually 4–6 weeks) to allow the tissues to recover from the radiation. If the total dose is greater than 5000 rad, then the surgery often will be more difficult. However, with moderate doses of radiation and some time allowed between radiation and surgery, the resection can proceed without difficulty.

The use of smaller doses of radiation over short periods of time, without surgical delay, has many advantages and is becoming the preferred technique. With this technique the pathology is less distorted, tumor reduction does not occur significantly, and the surgeon is not lulled into doing too small an operation. If the major value of the preoperative radiation is to prevent seeding, then large doses of radiation are not necessary. For example, preoperative use of intrauterine radium before surgical treatment of carcinoma of the endometrium is an effective way of preventing seeding. This can be done immediately before surgery.

Postoperative radiation has a number of advantages as well. The subgroup of patients who may be helped by radiation can be defined very accurately as a consequence of the surgical exploration and pathologic review. Unnecessary irradiation to patients who are not likely to benefit can be avoided, and the target volumes are tailored to meet what is found at surgery. Time can be allowed for wound healing so that the radiation will not interfere with this process. A disadvantage of such treatment is that it has no effect on seeding at the time of surgery. Surgery also may alter the physiology of the tumor left behind because of reduction of the vascular supply. Cells that were well-oxygenated may be rendered physiologically hypoxic and thus more resistant to radiation. Another disadvantage in the peritoneal cavity is that the surgery will cause loops of bowel to be fixed in specific positions and thus will increase the likelihood of small intestinal damage by radiation.

There is some uncertainty as to which technique is better for particular clinical circumstances. Both preoperative and postoperative radiation appear to be valuable and the choice of the method, the dose of radiation, and time between radiation and surgery should be considered in terms of the goals planned.

An additional technique for combining surgery with radiation is limited surgical removal of the gross tumor. Because the gross tumor limits the radiotherapeutic treatment, new interest has been raised in using surgery as the boost technique. Full courses of radiation combined with tumorectomy are given. This surgery can be done either before or after the irradiation. An example of this is the "lumpectomy" used in the treatment of breast masses before definitive radiation (see Chap. 38).[112,113] In the latter there appears to be evidence that the removal of gross tumor both displaces the sigmoid curve of cure to lower radiation doses and makes it change more steeply with dose (Fig. 15-25).

FIG. 15-25. Tumor control versus dose for breast cancer Stages II and III. (Hellman S: Improving the therapeutic index in breast cancer treatment. Cancer Res 40:4335–4342, 1980)

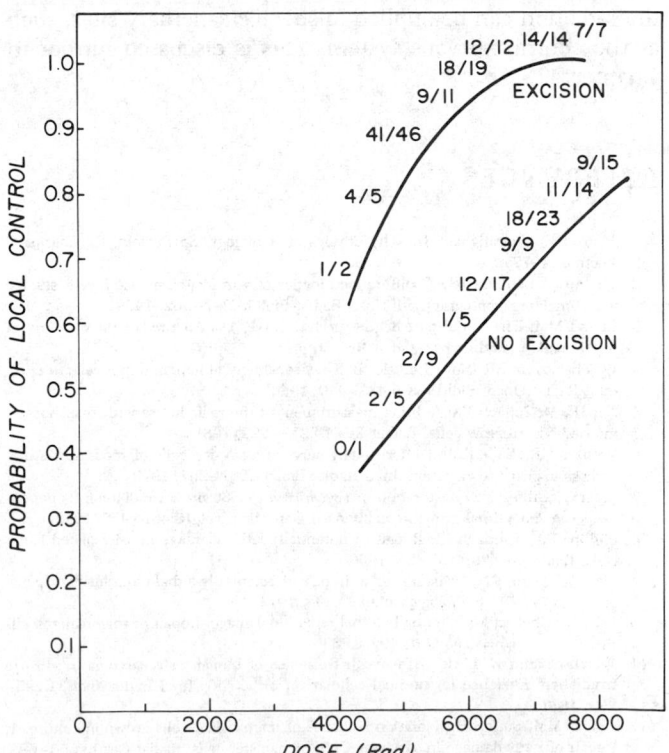

RADIATION AND CHEMOTHERAPY

The principles of combination radiation and chemotherapy were discussed earlier and emphasized that the purpose of such combined treatment is not to decrease the dose of radiation to gain the same effect, but rather to increase the therapeutic index. This may be achieved using a number of techniques that take advantage of the different mechanisms of action of systemic chemotherapy and regional irradiation. Chemotherapeutic agents that directly modify the radiation survival curve may be used. A good example of this is the use of actinomycin D in the treatment of childhood rhabdomyosarcoma or Wilms' tumor. A second way to increase the therapeutic index is to use drugs that specifically affect tumor response to radiation; the most exciting of these are the hypoxic sensitizers because they affect hypoxic cells that usually are restricted to tumors.

A third mechanism is the combination of drugs and roentgen rays with either independent action or additivity. This is just beginning to be explored but appears to be of value in increased local control achieved in head and neck cancer when chemotherapy is given before radiation.[114] Also, enhanced local control is obtained when radiotherapy is followed by or administered concomitantly with adjuvant chemotherapy in locally advanced breast cancer.[115]

Because the major advantage of chemotherapy is that it is distributed widely throughout the body, the combination of radiation and chemotherapy may improve the therapeutic index because, like the combination of surgery and irradiation, the target volumes are different. Adjuvant chemotherapy with radiation for breast cancer, or with surgery and radiation for colon cancer, may improve survival because the chemotherapy is effective against occult micrometastases outside the radiation field. Similarly, radiation may be of value in the treatment of leukemia by chemotherapy because the radiation can be applied to specific sanctuary sites, such as the central nervous system. This is discussed further in Chapter 47.

REFERENCES

1. Johns HE, Cunningham JR: The Physics of Radiology. Springfield, IL, Charles C Thomas, 1977
2. Thompson LH, Suit HD: Proliferation kinetics of x-irradiated mouse L cells studied with timelapse photography: II. Int J Radiat Biol 15:347–362, 1969
3. Elkind MM: The initial part of the survival curve: Does it predict the outcome of fractionated radiotherapy? Radiat Res (in press)
4. Weichselbaum RR, Nove J, Little JB: X-ray sensitivity of human tumor cells in vitro. Int J Radiat Oncol Biol Phys 6:437–440, 1980
5. Till JE, McCulloch EA: A direct measurement of the radiation sensitivity of normal mouse bone marrow cells. Radiat Res 14:213–222, 1961
6. Withers HR, Elkind MM: Microcolony survival assay for cells of mouse intestinal mucosa exposed to radiation. Int J Radiat Biol 17:261–267, 1970
7. Alper T, Gillies NE: Restoration of Escherichia coli Strain B irradiation: Its dependence on suboptimal growth conditions. J Gen Microbiol 18:461–472, 1958
8. Phillips RA, Tolmach LJ: Repair of potentially lethal damage in x-irradiated HeLa cells. Radiat Res 29:413–432, 1966
9. Little JB, Hahn GM, Frindel E et al: Repair of potentially lethal radiation damage in vitro and in vivo. Radiology 106:689–694, 1973
10. Belli JA, Shelton M: Potentially lethal radiation damage: Repair of mammalian cells in culture. Science 165:490–492, 1969
11. Weichselbaum R, Little JB, Nove J: Response of human osteosarcoma in vitro to irradiation: Evidence for unusual cellular repair activity. Int J Radiat Biol 31:295–299, 1977
12. Elkind MM, Sutton H: Radiation response of mammalian cells grown in culture: 1. Repair of x-ray damage in surviving Chinese hamster cells. Radiat Res 13:556–593, 1960
13. Hall EJ: Radiation dose-rate: A factor of importance in radiobiology and radiotherapy. Br J Radiol 45:81–97, 1972
14. Mottram JC: Factors of importance in radiosensitivity of tumors. Br J Radiol 9:606–614, 1936
15. Read J: The effect of ionizing radiation on the broad beam root: The dependence of the x-ray sensitivity on dissolved oxygen. Br J Radiol 25:89–99, 1952
16. Gray LH, Coger AD, Ebert M et al: The concentration of oxygen dissolved in tissues at the time of irradiation as a factor in radiotherapy. Br J Radiol 26:638–648, 1953
17. Belli JA, Dicus GJ, Bonte FJ: Radiation response of mammalian tumor cells: 1. Repair of sublethal damage in vivo. JNCI 38:673–682, 1967
18. Deschner EE, Gray LH: Influence of oxygen tension on x-ray induced chromosomal damage in Ehrlich ascites tumor cells irradiated in vitro and in vivo. Radiat Res 11:115–146, 1959
19. Thomlinson RH, Gray LH: The histological structure of some human lung cancers and possible implications for radiotherapy. Br J Cancer 9:539–549, 1955
20. Kallman RF: The phenomenon of reoxygenation and its implications for fractionated radiotherapy. Radiology 105:135–142, 1972
21. Henk JM, Kindler PB, Smith CW: Radiotherapy and head and neck cancer: Final report of the first clinical trial. Lancet 2:101–103, 1977
22. Henk JM, Smith CW: Radiotherapy and head and neck cancer: Interim report of second clinical trial. Lancet 2:104–105, 1977
23. Watson ER, Halman KE, Dische S et al: Hyperbaric oxygen and radiotherapy: A Medical Research Council trial in carcinoma of the cervix. Br J Radiol 51:879–887, 1978
24. Adams GE, Dewez DL: Hydrated electrons and radiobiological sensitization. Biochem Biophys Res Commun 12:473–477, 1963
25. Adams GE, Ahmed L, Fielden EM et al: The development of some nitromidazoles as hypoxic cell sensitizers. Cancer Clin Trials 3:37–42, 1980
26. Stratford LJ, Adams GE: Effect of hyperthermia on differential cytotoxicity of a hypoxic cell radiosensitizer RO-07-0582 on mammalian cells in vitro. Br J Cancer 35:307–313, 1977
27. Rose CM, Millar JL, Peacock JH et al: Differential enhancement of toxicity in tumors and normal tissues by misonidazole. Proceedings of the Key Biscayne Conference on Hypoxic Cell Sensitizers and Radioprotectors. New York, Masson, 1980
28. Bush RS, Jenkin RP, Allt WE et al: Definitive evidence for hypoxic cells influencing cure in cancer therapy. Br J Cancer 37:302–306, 1978
29. Kolstad P: Intercapillary distance, oxygen tension, and local recurrence in cervix cancer. Scan J Clin Lab Invest [Suppl] 106:145–157, 1968
30. Urtasun RC, Koch CJ, Franko AJ, et al: A novel technique for measuring human tissue pO$_2$ at the cellular level. Br J Cancer 54:453–457, 1986
31. Urtasun RC, Chapman JD, Raleigh JA et al: Binding of ^{3}H-misonidazole to solid human tumors as a measure of tumor hypoxia. Int J Rad Oncol Biol Phys 12:1263–1267, 1986
32. Terasima R, Tolmach LJ: X-ray sensitivity and DNA synthesis in synchronous populations of HeLa cells. Science 140:490–492, 1963
33. Sinclair WK, Morton RA: X-ray sensitivity during the cell generation cycle of cultured Chinese hamster cells. Radiat Res 29:450–474, 1966
34. Chaffey JT, Hellman S: Differing responses to radiation of murine bone marrow stem cells in relation to the cell cycle. Cancer Res 31:1613–1615, 1971
35. Madoc-Jones H, Mauro F: Age response to x-rays vinca alkaloids and hydroxyurea of murine lymphoma cells synchronized in vivo. JNCI 45:1131–1143, 1970
36. Hellman S: Cell kinetics, models, and cancer treatment: Some principles for the radiation oncologist. Radiology 114:219–223, 1975
37. Chaffey JT, Hellman S: Radiation fractionation as applied to murine colony-forming units in differing proliferative states. Radiology 93:1167–1172, 1969
38. Chaffey JT, Hellman S: Studies on dose fractionation as measured by endogenous spleen colonies in the mouse. Radiology 90:363–365, 1968
39. Hermens AF, Barendson GW: Changes in cell proliferation characteristics in a rat rhabdomyosarcoma before and after x-irradiation. Eur J Cancer Clin Oncol 5:173–189, 1969
40. Szybalski W: X-ray sensitization by halopyrimidines. Cancer Chemother Rep 58:539–557, 1974
41. Piro AJ, Taylor CC, Belli JA: Interaction between radiation and drug damage in mammalian cells: 1. Delayed expression of actinomycin D/x-ray effects in exponential and plateau phase cells. Radiat Res 63:346–362, 1975
42. D'Angio GJ, Farber S, Maddock CL: Potentiation of x-ray effects by actinomycin D. Radiology 73:175–177, 1959
43. Bases RE: Modification of the radiation response determined by single-cell techniques: Actinomycin D. Cancer Res 19:1223–1229, 1959
44. Elkind MM, Whitmore GF, Alescio T: Actinomycin D: Suppression of recovery in x-irradiated mammalian cells. Science 143:1454–1456, 1964
45. Pinkel D: Actinomycin D in childhood cancer: A preliminary report. Pediatrics 23:342–347, 1959
46. Hellman S, Hannon E: Effects of adriamycin on the radiation response of murine hematopoietic stem cells. Radiat Res 67:162–167, 1976
47. Belli JA, Piro AJ: The interaction between radiation and adriamycin damage in mammalian cells. Cancer Res 37:1624–1630, 1977
48. Cassady JR, Richter MP, Piro AJ et al: Radiation–adriamycin interactions: Preliminary clinical observations. Cancer 36:946–949, 1975
49. Donaldson SC, Glick JM, Wilbur JR: Adriamycin activating a recall phenomenon after radiation therapy. Ann Intern Med 81:407–408, 1974
50. Sinclair WK: Hydroxyurea: Effects on Chinese hamster cells grown in culture. Cancer Res 27:297–308, 1967

51. Yuhas JM, Yurconic M, Kligerman MM et al: Combined use of radioprotective and radiosensitizing drugs in experimental radiotherapy. Radiat Res 70:433–443, 1977

52. Barendsen GW: Response of cultured cells, tumours, and normal tissues to radiations of different linear energy transfer. Curr Top Radiat Res 4:293–356, 1968

53. Bloomer WD, Hellman S: Normal tissue responses to radiation therapy. N Engl J Med 293:80–83, 1975

54. Holthusen H: Erfahrungen über die Vertaglichkeitsgrenze fur Röntgenstrahler und deren Nutzanwendung zur Verhutung von Schaden. Strahlentherapie 57:254–269, 1936

55. Suit HD, Goitein M: Rationale for use of charged-particle and fast-neutron beams in radiation therapy. In Meyn RE, Withers HR (eds): Radiation Biology in Cancer Research. New York, Raven Press, 1980

56. Thomlinson RH: An experimental method for comparing treatments of intact tumors in animals and its application to the use of oxygen in radiotherapy. Br J Cancer 14:555–576, 1960

57. Folkman J, Tyler K: Tumor angiogenesis: Its possible role in metastasis and invasion. In Day B, Myers WP, Stans Garattini S et al (eds): Cancer Invasion and Metastasis: Mechanisms and Therapy, vol 5, pp 95–103. New York, Raven Press, 1977

58. Folkman J: Tumor angiogenesis: A possible control point in tumor growth. Ann Intern Med 82:96–100, 1975

59. Folkman J, Langer R, Linhardt RJ et al: Angiogenesis inhibition and tumor regression caused by heparin or a heparin fragment in the presence of cortisone. Science 221:719–725, 1983

60. Powers WE, Tolmach LV: A multicomponent x-ray survival curve for mouse lymphosarcoma cells irradiation in vitro. Nature 197:710–711, 1963

61. Fertil B, Malaise EP: Inherent cellular radiosensitivity as a basic concept for human tumor radiotherapy. Int J Radiat Oncol Biol Phys 7:621–629, 1981

62. Deacon J, Peckham MJ, Steel GG: The radioresponsiveness of human tumours and the initial slope of the cell survival curve. Radiother Oncol 2:317–323, 1984

63. Malaise EP, Fertil B, Chavaudra N et al: Distribution of radiation sensitivities for human tumor cells of specific histological types: Comparison of in vitro to in vivo data. Int J Radiat Oncol Biol Phys 12:617–624, 1986

64. Weichselbaum RR, Dahlberg W, Little JB: Inherently radioresistant cells exist in some human tumors. Proc Natl Acad Sci USA 82:4732–4735, 1985

65. Rubin P, Casarett GW: Clinical Radiation Pathology. Philadelphia, WB Saunders, 1968

66. Reinhold HS, Buisman GH: Radiosensitivity of capillary endothelium. Br J Radiol 46:54–57, 1973

67. Filler RM, Tefft M, Vawter GF et al: Hepatic lobectomy in childhood: Effects of x-ray and chemotherapy. J Pediatr Surg 4:31–41, 1969

68. Reincke U, Hannon EC, Rosenblatt M, Hellman S: Proliferative capacity of murine hematopoietic stem cells in vitro. Science 215:1619–1622, 1982

69. Medinger FG, Craver LF: Total-body irradiation. Am J Roentgenol Radium Ther Nucl Med 48:651–671, 1942

70. Hellman S, Chaffey JT, Rosenthal DS et al: Place of radiation therapy in the treatment of non-Hodgkin's lymphomas. Cancer 39:843–851, 1977

71. Anderson RE, Warner NL: Ionizing radiation and the immune response. Adv Immunol 24:215–335, 1976

72. Stjernsward J: Decreased survival related to irradiation postoperatively in early operable breast cancer. Lancet 2:1285–1286, 1974

73. Levitt SH, McHugh RB: Early breast cancer and postoperative irradiation. Lancet 2:1258–1259, 1975

74. Cancer Research Campaign (Kings/Cambridge) Trial for Early Breast Cancer. Lancet 2:55–60, 1980

75. Fletcher GH: Clinical dose–response curves of human malignant epithelial tumours. Br J Radiol 46:1–12, 1973

76. Kohn HI, Melvold RW: Divergent x-ray-induced mutation rates in the mouse for H and "7 locus" groups of loci. Nature 259:209–210, 1976

77. Folley JH, Borges W, Yamawaki T: Incidence of leukemia in survivors of the atomic bomb in Hiroshima and Nagasaki, Japan. Am J Med 13:311–321, 1952

78. Smith PG, Doll R: Late effects of x-irradiation in patients healed for metropathia hemorrhagica. Br J Radiol 49:224–232, 1976

79. Court Brown WM, Doll R: Mortality from cancer and other causes after radiotherapy for ankylosing spondylitis. Br Med J 2:1327–1332, 1965

80. Gray LH: Radiation biology and cancer. In Cellular Radiation Biology, M.D. Anderson Hospital and Tumor Institute 18th Symposium on Fundamental Cancer Research, pp 7–25. Baltimore, Williams & Wilkins, 1965

81. Upton AC, Randolph ML, Conklin JW: Late effects of fast neutrons and gamma rays in mice as influenced by the dose rate of irradiation: Induction of neoplasia. Radiat Res 41:467–491, 1970

82. Boice JD, Hutchinson GB: Leukemia in women following radiotherapy for cervical cancer: Ten-year follow-up of an international study. JNCI 65:115–129, 1980

83. Zippen C, Bailar JC III, Kohn HI et al: Radiation therapy and cervical cancer: Late effects on life span and leukemia incidence. Cancer 28:937–942, 1971

84. Shukovsky LJ: Dose, time, volume relationships in squamous cell carcinoma of the supraglottic larynx. Am J Roentgenol Rad Ther Nucl Med 108:27–29, 1970

85. Kaplan HS: Evidence for a tumoricidal dose level in the radiotherapy of Hodgkin's disease. Cancer Res 26:1221–1224, 1966

86. Stewart JG, Jackson AW: The steepness of the dose–response curve both for tumor and normal tissue injury. Laryngoscope 85:1107–1111, 1975

87. Zagars GK, Schultheiss TE, Peters LJ: Inter-tumor heterogeneity and radiation dose-control curves. Radiother Oncol 8:353–362, 1987

88. Coutard H: Roentgen therapy of epitheliomas of the tonsillar region, hypopharynx, and larynx from 1920 to 1926. Am J Roentgenol 28:313–331, 1932

89. Regaud C, Ferroux R: Discordance des effets des rayons X, d'une part dans la peau, d'autre part dans le testicule par le fractionement de la dose: Diminution de l'efficacite dans le peau, maintien de l'efficacite dans le testicule. Compt Rend Soc Biol 97:431–434, 1927

90. Danlos H: Quelques considerations sur le traitement des dermatoses par le radium. J Physiotherapie (Paris) 3:98–106, 1905

91. Botnick L, Hannon EC, Hellman S: Multisystem stem cell failure after apparent recovery from alkylating agents. Cancer Res 38:1942–1947, 1978

92. Hellman S, Botnick LE: Stem cell depletion: An explanation of the late effects of cytotoxins. Int J Radiat Oncol Biol Phys 2:181–184, 1977

93. Harris JR, Recht A, Almaric R, et al: Time course and prognosis of local recurrence following primary radiation therapy for early breast cancer. J Clin Oncol 2:37–41, 1984

94. Goodman LS, Gilman A: The Pharmacological Basis of Therapeutics, p 21. London, Macmillan, 1970

95. Withers HR, Peters LJ, Thames HD et al: Hyperfractionation. Int J Radiat Oncol Biol Phys 8:1807–1809, 1982

96. Withers HR, Thames HA, Peters LJ: Dose fractionation and volume effects in normal tissues and tumors. Cancer Treat Symp 1:75–83, 1984

97. Shank B, Chu FCH, Dinsmore R et al: Hyperfractionated total body irradiation for bone marrow transplantation. Results in seventy leukemia patients with allogeneic transplants. Int J Radiat Oncol Biol Phys 9:1607–1611, 1983

98. Thames HD Jr, Peters LJ, Withers HR et al: Accelerated fractionation vs hyperfractionation: Rationales for several treatments per day. Int J Radiat Oncol Biol Phys 9:127–138, 1983

99. Dutreix J, Wambersie A, Bounik C: Cellular recovery in human skin reactions: Application to dose, fraction number, overall time relationship in radiotherapy. Eur J Cancer Clin Oncol 9:159–167, 1973

100. Marks RD, Witherspoon BJ, Davis LW et al: Hyperfractionation — where do we stand: A preliminary report. Int J Radiat Oncol Biol Phys 4(suppl):139–140, 1978

101. Norin T, Onyango J: Radiotherapy in Burkitt's lymphoma: Conventional or superfractionated regime — early results. Int J Radiat Oncol Biol Phys 2:399–406, 1977

102. Scanlon P: Split-dose radiotherapy: The original premise. Int J Radiat Oncol Biol Phys 6:527–528, 1980

103. Sambrook DK: Split-course radiation therapy in malignant tumors. Am J Roentgenol 91:37–45, 1964

104. Parsons JT, Thar TL, Bova FJ et al: An evaluation of split-course irradiation for pelvic malignancies. Int J Radiat Oncol Biol Phys 6:175–181, 1980

105. Parsons JT, Bova FJ, Million RR: A re-evaluation of the University of Florida split-course technique for squamous carcinoma of the head and neck. Int J Radiat Oncol Biol Phys 6:1645–1652, 1980

106. Ling CC, Anderson LL, Shipley WU: Dose inhomogeneity in interstitial implants using ^{125}I seeds. Int J Radiat Oncol Biol Phys 5:419–425, 1979

107. Pierquin B, Chassagne D, Baillet F et al: Clinical observations on the time factor in interstitial radiotherapy using iridium-192. Clin Radiol 24:506–509, 1973

108. Beadle GF, Silver B, Botnick L et al: Cosmetic results following primary radiation therapy for early breast cancer. Cancer 54:2911–2918, 1984

109. Levene MB, Kijewski PK, Chin LM et al: Computer controlled radiation therapy. Radiology 129:769–775, 1978

110. Bergonie J, Tribondeau L: Interpretation of some results of radiotherapy and an attempt at determining a logical technique of treatment. Radiat Res 11:587–588, 1959

111. Kligerman MM: Radiotherapy and rectal cancer. Cancer 39:896–900, 1977

112. Harris JR, Beadle GF, Hellman S: Clinical studies on the use of radiation therapy as primary treatment of early breast cancer. Cancer 53:705–711, 1984

113. Hellman S: Improving the therapeutic index in breast cancer treatment. Cancer Res 40:4335–4342, 1980

114. Ervin TJ, Weichselbaum RR, Fabian RL et al: Advanced squamous carcinoma of the head and neck: A preliminary report of neoadjuvant chemotherapy with cisplatin, bleomycin, and methotrexate. Arch Otolaryngol 110:241–245, 1984

115. Harris JR, Sawicka J, Gelman R et al: Management of locally advanced carcinoma of the breast. Int J Radiat Oncol Biol Phys 9:345–349, 1983

VINCENT T. DEVITA, JR.

CHAPTER 16 *Principles of Chemotherapy*

Benign tumors compress tissue in their immediate environment but rarely kill patients unless located in strategic sites, such as the brain. Malignant tumors consist of cells that possess the capability of invading their surrounding stroma, passing through basement membranes, and establishing a metastatic clone even before the primary tumor reaches a clinically detectable level. When localized malignancies are controlled by surgery or radiation therapy, the capacity to cure a patient is limited by the presence of viable micrometastases outside the treatment field, a fact not fully appreciated until the last two decades. The chemotherapy of cancer is thus the treatment of metastases.[1-4]

One of the most important advances in tumor biology in recent years has been the discovery that the metastatic process itself is, in effect, an aberration of normal embryogenesis, and that the steps of this process are under genetic control. This information opens up the possibility of controlling expansion of both the primary tumor and its metastases by interfering with the steps in the metastatic process at the molecular level. A detailed discussion of this subject can be found in Chapter 7.

Systemic treatment had its roots in the work of Paul Ehrlich, who coined the word *chemotherapy*. Ehrlich's use of rodent models of infectious diseases to develop antibiotics led George Clowes, at Roswell Park Memorial Institute in Buffalo, New York, to develop, in the early 1900s, inbred rodent lines that could carry transplanted tumors.[5] These models served as the testing ground for potential cancer chemotherapeutic agents and have only recently been effectively supplemented by human cells grown in culture. Alkylating agents, the first modern chemotherapeutic agents, were a product of the secret war gas program in both world wars. An explosion in Bari Harbor during World War II[6,7] and the exposure of seamen to mustard gas led to the observation that alkylating agents caused marrow and lymphoid hypoplasia and led to their use in humans with Hodgkin's disease and other lymphomas, first attempted at Yale–New Haven Medical Center in 1943. Because of the secret nature of the gas warfare program, this work was not published until 1946.[1,5] The demonstration of dramatic regressions of advanced cancers with chemicals caused much excitement and later much disappointment as the tumors invariably grew back. After Farber's observation on the effects of folic acid on leukemic cell growth in children with lymphoblastic leukemia, and the development of the antifols as cancer drugs, the chemotherapy of cancer began in earnest.

THE RESPONSE TO CHEMOTHERAPY IS AFFECTED BY THE BIOLOGY OF TUMOR GROWTH

In the early 1960s Skipper and his colleagues laid down the guiding principles of present-day chemotherapy, using the rodent leukemia L1210 as a model.[8-10] Applying these principles to the drug treatment of human cancers required an understanding of the differences between the growth characteristics of this rodent leukemia and of human cancers, and the differences in growth rates of normal target tissues in mice and man. For example, L1210 leukemia is a rapidly growing tumor with a high percentage of cells synthesizing DNA (the labeling index) as measured by the uptake of tritiated thymidine (see Chapter 1). Because it has a growth fraction of 100% (that is, all of its cells are actively progressing through the cell cycle), its life cycle is consistent and predictable.[11] On the other hand, the cell cycles of human tumors are heterogeneous and prolonged[12-15]; their growth fraction is small, and many cells contributing to measurable tumor masses are not clonogenic and cannot form metastases.[16-19]

The relationship between cell number and survival in L1210 leukemia is linear, as shown in Figure 16-1. The time to death of animals bearing L1210 leukemia is the interval required to achieve a population size of about one billion (10^9) cells. With a growth fraction of 100% and a doubling

FIG. 16-1. Relationship between size of tumor cell inoculation and time to death of the host in L1210 leukemia in CDF_1 mice.

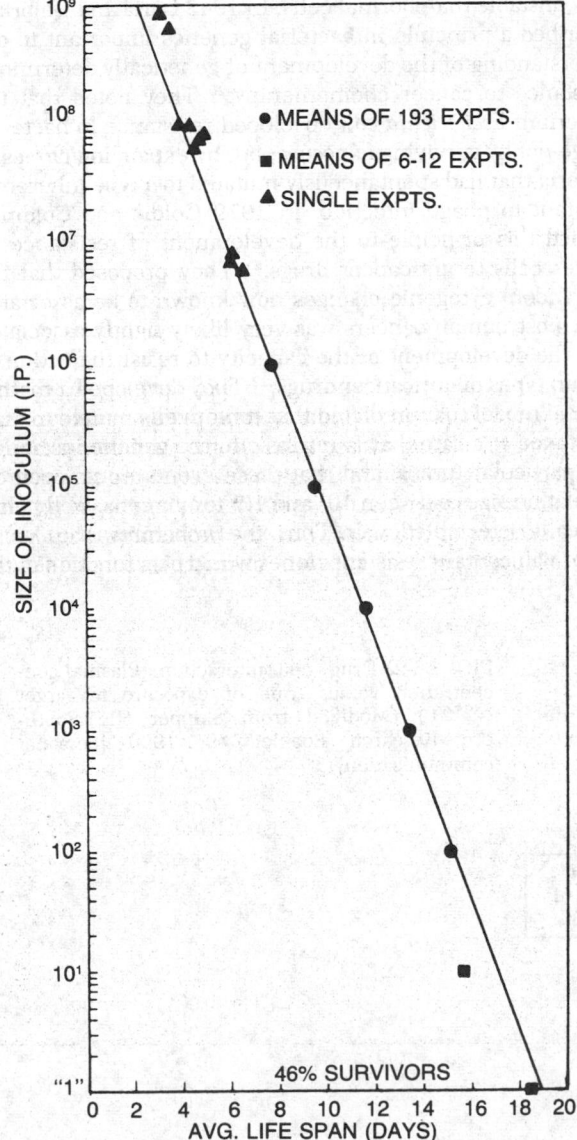

time of 12 hours, 10^9 cells will accumulate by 19 days after the injection of a single cell, by 10 days after the injection of 10^5 cells, and by 5 days after the administration of 10^8 cells. Skipper postulated that the increase in host life span after cytotoxic chemotherapy of L1210 leukemia was largely due to the cytocidal effect of treatment on the tumor cell population. In these early elegant mouse experiments he calculated the residual number of cells after treatment by extrapolating back from the duration of prolongation of life after a single treatment. An increase of 2 days in life would be equivalent to a 90% destruction of tumor cells (a 1-log kill), or a reduction in the cell number from 10^6 to 10^5. A 99.999% destruction of tumor cells, a figure that seems enormous to most clinicians, represents only a 5-log kill and will not cure animals unless the initial inoculum is small, perhaps 10^4 cells or less. If multiple treatments are given, the net tumor cell kill per treatment is the sum of the surviving cells plus the regrowth of the tumor cell population before the next treatment.

The killing effects of cancer drugs thus follow log kill kinetics, that is, if a particular dose of an individual drug kills 3 logs of cells and reduces tumor burden from 10^{10} to 10^7 cells, the same dose used at a tumor burden of 10^5 cells will reduce the tumor mass to 10^2. The cell kill is therefore proportional regardless of tumor burden. This model fits the response of L1210 murine leukemia to chemotherapy. When treatment failed in Skipper's experiments, it was because the initial tumor burden was too high to allow delivery of enough doses of chemotherapy to eradicate the last cell. The cardinal rule of chemotherapy, the invariable inverse relationship between cell number and curability, was established. Skipper went on to show that with an understanding of these basic facts, this rodent leukemia could be cured by specifically designed doses and schedules tied to tumor volume and growth characteristics.[8]

Although murine leukemias seemed to follow exponential kinetics, available data suggested that most human tumors did not appear to grow exponentially. For example, the concept of log kill would have predicted that some large tumors in the clinic should have been more sensitive to treatment than has been experienced. In vitro chemosensitivity studies have shown that the surviving fraction of tumor cells exposed to a particular dose of drug is frequently not constant regardless of the starting population size, as would be expected if the tumor grew exponentially. Larger starting populations have consistently showed a higher surviving fraction. Also, in several studies metastases have been documented to grow faster than primary tumors. In toto, the available data support a Gompertzian model of tumor growth and regression. The critical distinction between Gompertzian and exponential growth is that in Gompertzian kinetics, the growth fraction of the tumor is not constant but decreases exponentially with time (exponential growth is matched by exponential retardation of growth). The growth fraction peaks when the tumor is about 37% of its maximum size. As the tumor enlarges the growth fraction falls exponentially, the growth rate slows, and the tumor volume begins to plateau. In a Gompertzian model, when a patient with advanced cancer is treated the tumor mass is larger, its growth fraction is low, and the fraction of cells killed is therefore small. Gompertzian kinetics also make predictions about the behavior of small tumors, such as tumor burdens that might be present after primary surgical therapy. When the tumor is clinically undetectable, its growth fraction would be at its largest and the fractional cell kill from a "known to be effective" therapeutic dose of chemotherapy would be higher than at later times in the tumor course. Thus, experimental observations imply that there are kinetic reasons for failure of chemotherapy to cure large tumors. This information has been useful in the application of chemotherapy to patients with smaller tumor volume in the clinic since it should be possible to overcome cell kinetic reasons for chemotherapy failure.

BIOCHEMICAL RESISTANCE TO CHEMOTHERAPY IS THE MAJOR IMPEDIMENT TO SUCCESSFUL TREATMENT

Unlike most cellular drug targets, the cancer cell presents a variable and moving target to anticancer drugs. The interrelationship of pharmacokinetics and tumor and normal target cell kinetics is the fulcrum of clinical cancer chemotherapy. The therapeutic and toxic effects of chemotherapeutic agents are related to the time the active principle is exposed in an effective concentration to its target (Fig. 16-2). The same degree of cytotoxicity can be achieved, on different schedules, from the same concentration of drug multiplied by the time of exposure ($C \times T$). This relationship obtains across different species when the drugs are both metabolized and excreted in a similar fashion. This principle has made it possible to translate doses of drugs devised in animals to humans for early clinical testing[23,24] (see Early Clinical Trials of Antitumor Agents, below). A given $C \times T$ will generally be equally cytotoxic in populations of cells with equivalent growth characteristics and sensitivity to the agent(s) in question.

When the active principles of anticancer drugs reach their target, another obstacle to the capacity to kill the cancer cell appears: specific and permanent biochemical resistance to

anticancer drugs. Resistance to drugs either occurs de novo in cancer cells or is concomitant to the process of replication.[21,24-32]

Many specific mechanisms of primary drug resistance have been revealed whereby cancer cells demonstrate the ability to circumvent a well-defined pathway of attack by a given cytotoxic agent. These mechanisms are summarized in Table 16-1 and discussed in detail in Chapter 18. Mechanisms of primary drug resistance include decreased uptake caused by changes in drug-specific transport mechanisms, decreased activation of prodrugs, alteration in the drug's target enzymes, alterations in cellular metabolism and repair mechanisms, and increased inactivation of drugs.[33] Gene amplification of an enzyme target has been documented to occur in a tumor as a result of exposure to the drug[34] with the attendant development of chromosomal homogeneous staining regions or double-minute chromosomes representing an increased copy number of the target gene.

A fundamental property of DNA is spontaneous mutation; there is also evidence that tumor cells may be more genetically unstable than normal cells. In 1943 Luria and Delbruck described a principle in bacterial genetics important to our understanding of the development of genetically determined resistance to cancer chemotherapy.[20] They noted that the bacterium *Escherichia coli* developed resistance to bacteriophage not by surviving exposure, but by expanding clones of bacteria that had spontaneously mutated to a type inherently resistant to phage infection. In 1979 Goldie and Coldman applied this principle to the development of resistance by cancer cells to anticancer drugs.[21] They proposed that the nonrandom cytogenic changes now known to be associated with most human cancers was very likely tightly associated with the development of the capacity to resist the action of certain types of anticancer drugs.[22] They developed a mathematical model that predicted that tumor cells mutate to drug resistance at a rate that is intrinsic to the genetic instability of a particular tumor, and that these events would occur at population sizes between 10^3 and 10^6 tumor cells, well below clinically detectable levels. Thus, the probability that a given tumor will contain resistant clones would be a function of the

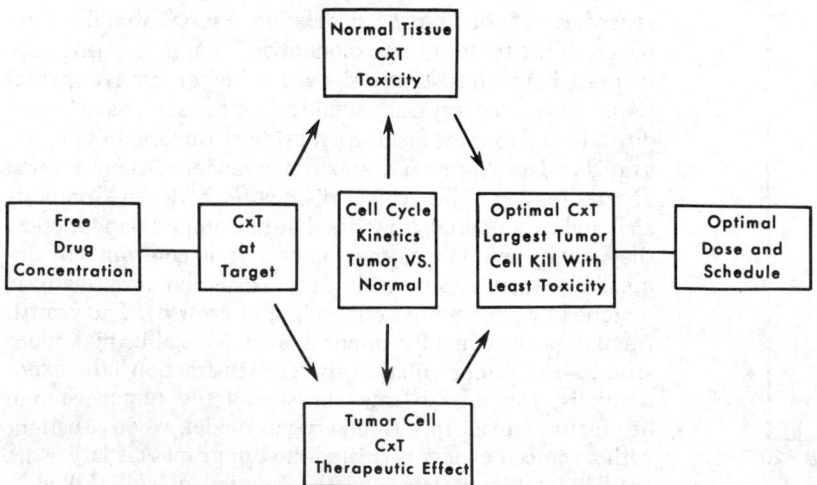

FIG. 16-2. Drug–cell interaction. Plasma concentration versus time of exposure to target ($C \times T$) (Modified from Skipper HE: Southern Research Booklet #9, 1980 [personal communication])

TABLE 16-1.   Mechanisms of Drug Resistance

General Mechanism	Drug	Result
Multidrug resistance	Vinca alkaloids	
	Antitumor antibiotics	Drug actively pumped out
	Etoposide	
Transport defect	Methotrexate	
	Melphalan	Low carrier-mediated uptake
	Nitrogen mustard	
	Cytosine arabinoside	Low membrane binding
Poor activation	Cytosine arabinoside	Low deoxycytidine kinase
	5-Azacytidine	Low uridine-cytidine kinase
	5-Fluorouracil	Low uridine kinase, orotic acid PRT, uridine phosphorylase
	6-Thioguanine	Low hypoxanthine–guanine PRT
	6-Mercaptopurine	
	Methotrexate	Low polyglutamation
	Doxorubicin	Low P-450 enzymes
Drug inactivation	Cytosine arabinoside	High cytidine deaminase
	Alkylating agents	High glutathione
	6-Thioguanine	High alkaline phosphatase
	6-Mercaptopurine	
Improved DNA repair	Alkylating agents	
	Antitumor antibiotics	High efficiency repair of strand breaks, ligase
	Cisplatin	
Gene amplification	Methotrexate	Dihydrofolate reductase
	PALA	Aspartate transcarbamylase
	2-Deoxycoformycin	Adenosine deaminase
	5-Fluorouracil	? Thymidylate synthetase
Alternate pathways	Methotrexate	Increased thymidine salvage
	5-Fluorouracil	Increased thymidine kinase
Altered pools of competing substrate	Cytosine arabinoside	High CTP and dCTP
	5-Fluorouracil	
Target alterations	Vincristine	Tubulin
	Methotrexate	Dihydrofolate reductase
	5-Fluorouracil	Thymidylate synthetase
	Hydroxyurea	Ribonucleotide reductase
	Steroids	Receptor or receptor–DNA binding

PRT = phosphoribosyl transferase, PALP = N-phosphomacetyl-L-aspartic acid, CTP = cytidine triphosphate, dCTP = deoxycytidine triphosphate.

mutation rate and the size of the tumor. If the mutation rate is only around 10^{-6}, a tumor composed of 10^9 cells (a mass only 1 cm in size) would be virtually certain to have at least one drug-resistant clone. However, if the mutation rate is around 10^{-6}, the *absolute number* of resistant cells in a tumor composed of 10^9 cells would be relatively small. In the clinic, such tumors would appear to respond initially to treatment with a complete or partial remission, but then reappear as the resistance clone(s) expanded. Such a pattern is seen with the use of chemotherapy in many cancers in the clinic.

However, some tumors are not responsive to chemotherapeutic agents at all, even when diagnosed with minimal tumor volume, which suggests that they are either inherently resistant or are largely made up of clones that have mutated to resistance. There is a cell kinetic explanation for this phenomenon in some slowly growing visceral tumors. For example, as tumor masses grow, there is considerable cell loss from shedding of cells, say into the lumen of the bowel, or actual cell death, which can amount to 90% of the total tumor volume. In such a setting, a tumor 1 cm in size and

consisting of 10^9 cells, while appearing to be an early tumor, might have gone through 1200 doublings to reach that size to compensate for cell loss, instead of the expected 32 doublings. Such a kinetic history together with the expected genetic instability could well be associated with a very high probability that the entire mass consists of resistant cell lines.

The Goldie–Coldman hypothesis presumed that resistance to drugs occurred in a single step. Another pattern of resistance has emerged. When malignant cell lines are made resistant to a single chemotherapeutic agent by stepwise incubation in increasing amounts of drug, some such lines are curiously found to be resistant to structurally unrelated cytotoxic compounds. This finding has been repeated for many different cell lines initially exposed to many different drugs. This phenomenon of broad resistance was termed *pleiotropic drug resistance,* or *multidrug resistance* (MDR).[35] Cell lines that display the MDR phenotype are generally resistant to natural product cytotoxic agents such as the anthracyclines, vinca alkaloids, epipodophyllotoxins, and actinomycin D.

Since all of these agents are believed to have different mechanisms of action, investigation of MDR has not focused on specific enzymes but rather on the cell's basic defense mechanism against toxic agents found naturally in the environment.

Multidrug resistance was shown to be associated with decreased intracellular drug accumulation and the presence of a 170,000-dalton plasma membrane–associated glycoprotein (P-glycoprotein) that was not detectable in parenteral drug-sensitive lines.[36,37] P-glycoprotein content was shown to directly correlate with both the degree of decrease in intracellular accumulation of the toxins and the degree of drug resistance exhibited by the cell.[38,39] These observations suggested that the P-glycoprotein conferred resistance by regulating transport of toxins in or out of the cell. Most cell lines with the MDR phenotype that have since been established show increased expression of the gene encoding P-glycoprotein, the *mdr* gene.[40-44] A great deal of evidence now suggests that the P-glycoprotein is, in fact, an energy-dependent drug efflux pump. The ability of the P-glycoprotein to bind natural product type drugs has also been demonstrated. It has been shown to bind photoaffinity analogs of vinblastine, a reaction that is competitively inhibited by unlabeled vinblastine as well as by anthracyclines.[45,46] Furthermore, several agents, including the calcium channel blocker verapamil, as well as quinidine and nifedipine, can also bind to the P-glycoprotein and can compete with the vinblastine analogs for binding with the P-glycoprotein.[47] Full-length cDNA sequences encoding the mouse[48] and human[49] P-glycoprotein gene have been isolated and their nucleotide sequences determined. The deduced amino acid sequence of this protein shows structural similarities to a well-characterized bacterial membrane transport protein, diagrammed in Figure 16-3.[48-50a] P-glycoprotein RNA expression has been found in high levels in normal adrenal and kidney tissue and in moderate levels in hepatic and colon tissue.[51] Since colon, kidney, and liver tissues are exposed to naturally occurring environmental toxins, the role of the P-glycoprotein in health may be one of protecting, by facilitating efflux of these toxins. There is evidence that the P-glycoprotein may be a member of a multigene family. At least two different classes of P-glycoprotein cDNAs have been identified in hamster,[52] mouse,[53] and human[54] cells.

In some cell lines the phenomenon of multidrug resistance is associated with more than the production and function of the P-glycoprotein alone. This was suggested by the fact that each MDR cell line displays a slightly different pattern of cross-resistance,[55,56] and the degree of resistance does not always directly correlate with the degree of intracellular accumulation of drugs.[57-59] In addition, despite the relative

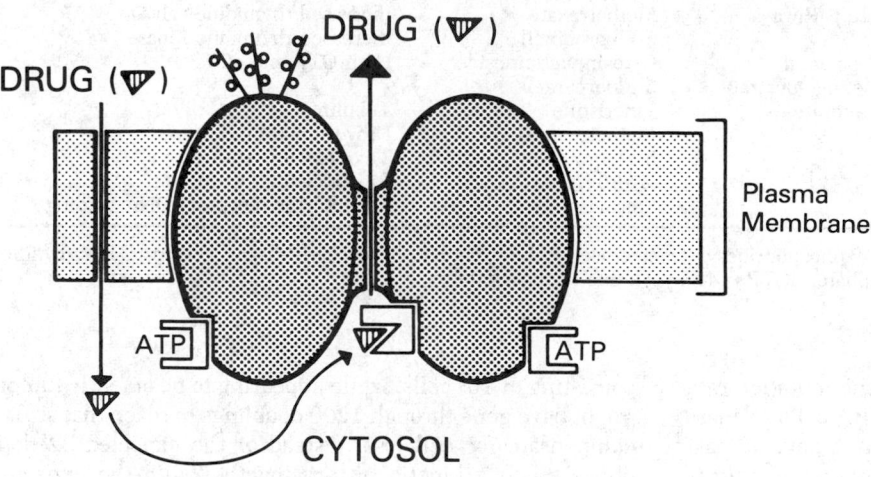

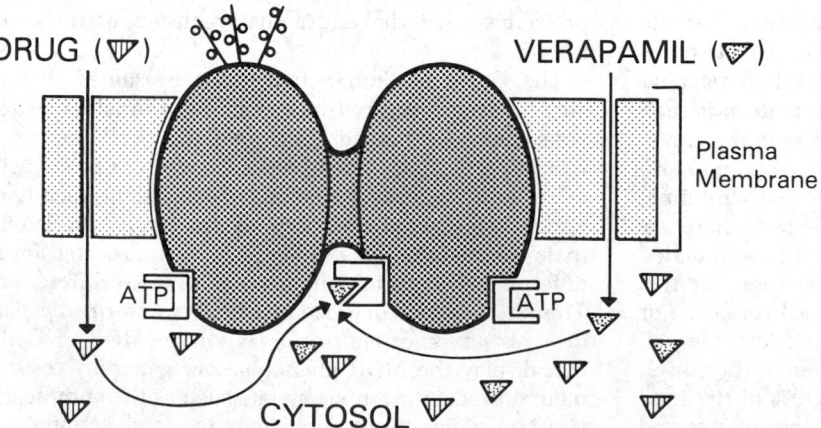

FIG. 16-3. Model of how P-glycoprotein might be involved in transporting cytotoxic drugs, such as vinblastine, out of cells (*top*) and how drugs such as verapamil that reverse multidrug resistance compete with vinblastine to block the pump (*bottom*). (Pastan IH, Gottesman MM: Molecular biology of multidrug resistance in human cells. In DeVita VT Jr, Hellman S, Rosenberg SA [eds]: Important Advances in Oncology 1988, p 9. Philadelphia, JB Lippincott, 1988)

ease with which the *mdr* gene expression is found in resistant cell lines, there have been relatively few reports relating P-glycoprotein expression in vivo to clinical drug resistance.

A model of chemical carcinogenesis proposed by Solt, Medline, and Farber[60] has helped shed some light on a second set of mechanisms associated with MDR. Chemical carcinogenesis is believed to be a two-step process consisting of an irreversible initiation event, followed by exposure to promoting agents. In the Farber model, laboratory rats are exposed to carcinogens and then subjected to partial hepatectomy, which, since it stimulates cell growth in the residual liver, serves as a promoting event. This procedure consistently results in liver nodules, some of which develop into frank hepatocellular carcinomas. The cells in these nodules are found to be more resistant to the toxic effects of the initiating carcinogens than normal hepatocytes,[61] and the hepatocytes in the hepatic nodules are resistant not only to the agent that precipitated their transformation but, like MDR cell lines associated with the P-glycoprotein, also to other structurally dissimilar cytotoxic chemicals.[62] In these nodules, while there is overexpression of the *mdr* gene, there is also decreased activity of several drug-activating microsomal cytochrome P-450 phase I enzymes, including aryl hydrocarbon hydroxylase, increased activities of several drug-conjugating enzymes, including the anionic isoenzyme of glutathione S-transferase, and increased activity of other enzymes involved in drug metabolism, including DT-diaphorase and glucuronyl transferase.[63,64] Each of these changes may play a role in providing the cell with the ability to withstand toxic agents. This complex set of changes, observed in two very different models of broad resistance to xenobiotics, indicates that cells have the capacity to call upon an adaptive, coordinated defense mechanism when assaulted by cytotoxins. Once this program is turned on by one agent, it appears to be effective against others. Such a system may protect normal cells against environmental assault, but in cancer patients it appears to protect neoplastic cells against chemotherapeutic agents, which are also derived from environmental sources.

A third type of MDR has recently been elucidated that is not associated with P-glycoprotein gene expression at all.[65,66] In some cells, drug influx and steady-state intracellular concentrations are no different than in the parenteral drug–sensitive cells; by contrast, cells with the classic MDR phenotype invariably show changes in drug transport. Although the precise defect in the resistant cells that do not show changes in transport is not yet known, there is strong evidence implicating altered topoisomerase activity.[67] Topoisomerases are enzymes necessary for DNA replication that catalyze changes in the secondary and tertiary structures of DNA. Topoisomerase II appears to be the enzyme that is the target of antineoplastic drugs that act as DNA-intercalating agents, such as etoposide and the anthracyclines. An etoposide-resistant Chinese hamster ovary cell line that was cross-resistant to the structurally dissimilar agent m-AMSA, mitoxantrone, and the anthracycline doxorubicin demonstrated altered topoisomerase II activity.[68] In addition, alteration of the topoisomerase I-like activity was found in Chinese hamster cells selected for resistance to ellipticine and cross-resistance to m-AMSA and etoposide.[69] Topoisomerases, therefore, may represent the final common pathway of cytotoxicity of several different classes of antineoplastic agents. However, no studies have been able to show that altered topoisomerase activity plays a role in clinical drug resistance.

As a result of these data there is considerable excitement over the prospect of improving the effectiveness of chemotherapy by preventing the development of MDR or by interfering with the mechanism itself. Drugs that reverse MDR are being tested. The first such drug to reach clinical trial was verapamil, a drug that has reversed acquired drug resistance in a variety of in vitro systems. This calcium channel blocker enhances cytotoxicity by increasing intracellular accumulation of drugs, which suggests that it acts on P-glycoprotein or other transport proteins, as illustrated in Figure 16-3.[47,70] Unfortunately, the verapamil concentrations required to reverse resistance in vitro result in excessive clinical toxicity. Quinidine, a drug that also binds to P-glycoprotein, has also reached clinical trial as an inhibitor of drug resistance, but no definitive results are available. Monoclonal antibodies have also been developed against the P-glycoprotein. In addition to a role in targeting toxins to P-glycoprotein–containing tumor cells,[71] such antibodies should prove useful as a diagnostic tool to identify cells with the MDR phenotype in vivo, and to allow the selection of drugs for treatment that can circumvent the pump.

Buthioninesulphoxamine (BSO) is a synthetic amino acid that inhibits γ-glutamyl-cysteine synthetase, which in turn leads to marked reduction of intracellular concentrations of glutathione, the substrate for the glutathione-S transferase isozymes and glutathione peroxidase involved in some forms of MDR.[72] Several studies of different tumor cell lines have shown reversal of drug resistance after treatment with BSO, corresponding with decreases in intracellular glutathione concentration.[73–75] In vitro toxicity studies on mouse and human bone marrow cells indicate that normal cells may be less susceptible to the toxicity of chemotherapeutic agents than tumor cells when also exposed to BSO. Phase I clinical trials are in progress in which BSO is given with an antineoplastic agent in refractory cancer.

FOR DRUG-SENSITIVE CANCERS IN FAVORABLE KINETIC CIRCUMSTANCES, THE FACTOR LIMITING THE CAPACITY TO CURE IS PROPER DOSING: THE CONCEPT OF DOSE INTENSITY

The dose–response curve in biologic systems is usually sigmoidal in shape with a threshold, a lag phase, a linear phase, and a plateau phase. For both radiation therapy and chemotherapy it is the difference between the dose–response curves of normal and tumor tissue that must be exploited during treatment. In experimental models, the dose–response curve is usually steep in the linear phase. Almost without exception, reduction of doses in the linear phase of the dose–response curve results first in a loss of the capacity to cure the tumor before there is a diminution in the response rate. That is, complete remissions will continue to be observed in animals bearing palpable tumors, but the last few residual cells will not be ablated, and relapse becomes inevitable. There is an extremely important lesson in these animal data for clinicians who, in their daily practice, judge the adequacy of their therapy by measuring response rate of visible or palpable tumor masses. This point is illustrated in Table 16-2, which summarizes data from numerous experiments conducted by Skipper and his colleagues at the Southern Research Institute using the transplantable and palpable Ridgway osteosarcoma tumor model.[76,77] Reduction in the average dose intensity of the two-drug combination of L-phenylalanine mustard (L-PAM) and cyclophosphamide causes a marked decrease in the cure rate *before a significant reduction in the complete remission rate is noted*. On the average, a dose reduction of approximately 20% will lead to a loss in the cure rate in excess of 50%. The converse is also true. In high growth fraction tumors a twofold increase in dose often leads to a tenfold increase (1 log) in tumor cell kill. Although animal models are not the perfect analogue for human cancers, the invariable nature of these data indicate that the general principle is transferable to the clinic and is ignored at great peril. Because anticancer drugs are toxic, it is very appealing to reduce toxicity by diminishing the dose or increasing the intervals between cycles of treatment. This kind of ad hoc adjustment of dosing is probably the main reason for treatment failure in patients with *drug-sensitive human tumors* undergoing their first chemotherapy treatment. If so, the most toxic effect of treatment may be premature death from insufficient dosing.

It has been difficult to compare the impact of different dosing practices in treatment programs. Recently, Hyrniuk and his colleagues analyzed treatment outcome in a number of different tumors as a function of what they have termed dose intensity.[78-83] They defined dose intensity as the amount of drug delivered per unit time, expressed as $mg/m^2/wk$, regardless of the schedule or route of administration. Relative dose intensity (RDI) is the amount of drug delivered per unit time relative to an arbitrarily chosen standard single drug, or, for a combination regimen, the decimal fraction of the ratio of the test regimen to the standard regimen. To compare the dose intensity of combinations of drugs, the average dose intensity of the combination is calculated as the average amount of drugs delivered per unit time compared to an arbitrarily chosen standard. A sample calculation of the RDI for a commonly used regimen, the CMF

combination (cyclophosphamide, methotrexate, 5-fluorouracil) for breast cancer is provided in Table 16-3.[78] To calculate average RDI for a regimen containing fewer drugs than the standard regimen, a dose intensity of zero is assigned to the missing drug(s), and the average RDI of the test regimen is divided by the total number of drugs in the standard.[79] The dose intensity of various programs is compared over whatever time frame the treatment programs are administered. Calculations can be made of intended dose intensity, the dose intensity as described in the treatment protocol, or actual or received dose intensity. Received dose intensity reflects the impact of dose reductions and necessary treatment delays imposed in actual practice because of toxicity and is thus the more important datum.

Since calculations are made on the basis of the amount of drugs given per week regardless of schedule, treatment delays are given equal weight to dose reductions. Calculations of the dose intensity, therefore, require the assumption that scheduling does not determine treatment outcome. While at first this appears to be heretical, close scrutiny of all available data in humans and rodents shows that scheduling influences outcome largely by affecting toxicity, in this way allowing greater doses to be administered over the same time frame. An example can be found in the use of methotrexate both in rodents and in humans. Daily administration of low doses of methotrexate is very toxic and severely limits the dose and duration of therapy with this drug. A twice-weekly schedule, which is much more effective in rodents and in humans, allows much greater doses to be delivered for longer durations, because this schedule is associated with less toxicity. The dose intensity of the twice-weekly schedule is therefore far greater than that of the daily oral schedule when calculated on a basis of $mg/m^2/wk$ of delivered drug. In practice, the impact of scheduling on the calculation of dose intensity can be neutralized by comparing programs in which drugs with toxicities affected by scheduling, such as the antimetabolites, are given in like schedules.

Calculation of an average RDI of a drug combination also assumes equivalency of the affects of all the drugs in the combination. The impact of any single drug, or combinations of two or three drugs in a multidrug combination, can, however, be assessed separately. This has been done by Hyrniuk to show the greater impact of cisplatin in a drug combination for ovarian cancer.[78,84] This kind of analysis can help iden-

TABLE 16-2.   Ridgway Osteogenic Sarcoma: Response to Different Dose Intensity of Two-Drug Combination of Cyclophosphamide and L-PAM*

| CPA | RDI | | % CR | % Cures |
	L-PAM	Average		
0.38	0.82	0.60	100	60
0.75	0.18	0.47	100	44
0.25	0.55	0.44	100	10
0.50	0.12	0.31	10	0
0.17	0.36	0.27	0	0

RDI = relative dose intensity,   CPA = cyclophosphamide,   L-PAM=L-phenylalanine,   CR = complete response. Tumors weighed 2 to 3 g.
* Modified from Skipper HE: Booklet No. 5, Southern Research Institute, 1986.

TABLE 16-3.   Sample Calculations: Dose Intensity, Relative Dose Intensity, and Average Relative Dose Intensity*

	Dose Intensity	Relative Dose Intensity
Calculation of Dose Intensity		
Test Schedule		
Cyclophosphamide 80 mg/m²/day (continuously)	560 mg/m²/wk	
Calculation of Relative Dose Intensity		
Standard		
Cyclophosphamide 80 mg/m²/day (continuously)	560 mg/m²/wk	
Test Schedule		
Cyclophosphamide 100 mg/m²/day (days 1–14, q 28 days)	350 mg/m²/wk	350/560 = 0.62
Calculation of Average Relative Dose Intensity		
Standard†		
Cyclophosphamide 2 mg/kg/day	560 mg/m²/wk	
Methotrexate 0.7 mg/kg/wk	28 mg/m²/wk	
5-Fluorouracil 12 mg/kg/wk	480 mg/m²/wk	
Test Regimen		
Cyclophosphamide 100 mg/m²/day (days 1–14)	350 mg/m²/wk	350/560 = 0.62
Methotrexate 40 mg/m²/days 1, 8	20 mg/m²/wk	20/28 = 0.71
5-Fluorouracil 600 mg/m²/days 1, 8	300 mg/m²/wk	300/480 = 0.62
Repeat cycles every 28 days		*Average* 0.65

* Hryniuk WM: The importance of dose intensity in the outcome of chemotherapy. In DeVita VT, Hellman S, Rosenberg SA (eds): Important Advances in Oncology, pp 121–142. Philadelphia, JB Lippincott, 1988.

† Assume standard regimen to be CMF content of CMFVP regimen of Cooper and associates. To convert mg/kg to mg/m², multiply by 40.

tify the most effective drug in a combination, and it is important because such data can influence how doses and schedules are adjusted to avoid adjustments that radically alter the effectiveness of a program. Alterations in dose intensity of the most effective drug in a combination of drugs has greatest impact, as illustrated in Table 16-4, which displays the effects of the two-drug combination of L-PAM and the antimetabolite 6-mercaptopurine (6-MP) against the Ridgway

osteogenic sarcoma model. In this case, L-PAM is the more effective drug. The relationship of average dose intensity of the two drugs to outcome is erratic, but the relationship of the dose intensity of L-PAM to outcome is linear, as in Table 16-2. Decreases in the dose intensity of L-PAM reduce the effect of the combination even when the dose of 6-MP is increased to compensate for these reductions. In fact, any decrease in the dose intensity of L-PAM below 55% of the

TABLE 16-4.   Ridgway Osteogenic Sarcoma: Effect of Varying Dose Intensity of More Effective Drug, L-PAM*

Relative Dose Intensity				Observed	
L-PAM	6-MP	Ratio (L-PAM/6-MP)	Average	% CR	% Cures
0.82	0.49	1.7	0.66	100	60
0.73	1.3	0.56	1.0	90	50
0.55	1.0	0.55	0.78	90	20
0.55	0.33	1.7	0.44	80	20
0.36	0.67	0.54	0.52	56	0
0.36	0.21	1.7	0.29	30	0
0.27	1.5	0.18	0.89	70	0
0.24	0.44	0.57	0.35	0	0
0.24	0.15	1.6	0.20	0	0
0.18	1.0	0.18	0.59	0	0
0.12	0.67	0.18	0.50	0	0
0.08	0.44	0.18	0.26	0	0

L-PAM = L-phenylalanine mustard; 6-MP = 6-mercaptopurine. Tumors weighed 2 to 3 g. Varying the dose intensity of L-PAM has a greater impact on outcome than can be overcome by increasing the dose of 6-MP.

* Skipper HE: Booklet No. 4, Southern Research Institute, 1986.

optimal single dose schedule results in loss of the capacity of this combination to cure animals, regardless of the dose of 6-MP.

Two additional pieces of information could increase the precision and usefulness of these data: the total dose of each drug administered, and a cumulative dose plot of each drug on a week by week basis for each patient. Collection of such data is not part of routine practice, and these data are not generally available in the literature. It is the opinion of this author, however, that in order to assess the impact of dosing schedules in practice and in clinical trials, such data should be required before papers are accepted for publication. Practicing physicians would also find such data useful in assessing the benefits and limitations of the use of chemotherapy.

A clear-cut relationship between dose intensity and response rate has been demonstrated in advanced ovarian cancer, breast cancer, colon cancer, and in the lymphomas.[77,78,80,81] Hyrniuk is conducting a prospective trial in which the dose intensity of the combination of cyclophosphamide, doxorubicin, and fluorouracil (CAF) used in advanced breast cancer is increased to a point on the dose–response curve calculated to produce response rates superior to the published results with standard CAF.[78] In a preliminary analysis, the data fit on the plotted dose–response curve. This approach has practical implications.

Calculations of the impact of dose intensity on outcome are particularly important in estimating the value and exploring some of the pitfalls of adjuvant chemotherapy. A significant effect of dose intensity on relapse-free survival after the use of drugs or adjuvant therapy has been found for breast cancer (Fig. 16-4). The correlation between dose intensity and outcome is all the more significant since almost all the drugs in the programs shown are used at the low end of their dose–response curve. The invariable inverse relationship between cell number and curability and the steep dose–response curve for anticancer drugs clearly indicate that dose reductions in adjuvant drug treatment programs are likely to be associated with significantly less therapeutic effect. Dose reduction has, however, been the norm in the design of adjuvant trials. An example is given in Table 16-5 for the standard CMF regimen. The model for the regimen was published in 1974 by Canellos et al.[85] It produced an impressive complete remission rate, but its toxicity was considerable. As a result, when it was advanced for use in a cooperative group setting for advanced disease,[84] and later for adjuvant trials by the Milan group,[86] its doses were arbitrarily reduced without pretesting the impact of such reductions on outcome. In addition, further reduction was made, a priori, for patients over the age of 60 years. When the impact of these reductions is related to outcome, there is a strong suggestion of a negative impact. In Table 16-5 dose intensity is compared using the National Cancer Institute (NCI) CMF+P program as the reference standard. A zero is assigned to the value of prednisone in the calculations. In the cooperative group study,[84] the reduced program resulted in a substantial reduction of the complete remission rate; also, the results in women less than 60 years old were significantly better than in women more than 60 years old, which could be the result of the a priori dose reductions, although

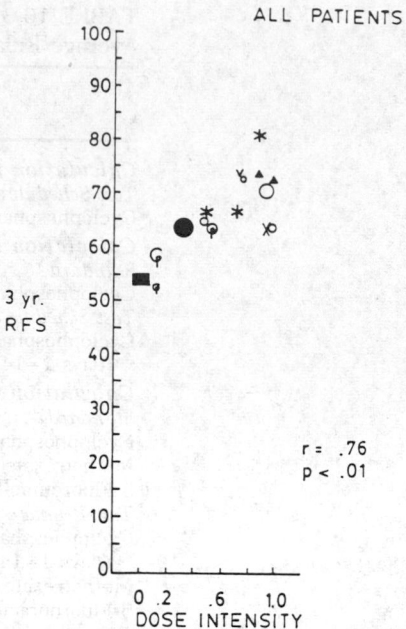

FIG. 16-4. Three-year relapse-free survival (*RFS*) versus average relative dose intensity for adjuvant chemotherapy trials containing all four prognostic subgroups (<50 years; 1–3 or >3 positive nodes; >50 years; 1–3 or >3 positive nodes). The size of the symbols is proportional to the number of cases at each dose intensity. ■, control; ▲, CMFVP; X, CMFP; ●, C_pF; . . , trial with radiotherapy added; *, levels of CMF chemotherapy according to Bonadonna; [25]V, CMFV; O, CMF; ◐, C_pMF; ◑, phenylalanine mustard. (Hryniuk WM: The Importance of dose intensity in the outcome of chemotherapy. In DeVita VT Jr, Hellman S, Rosenberg SA [eds]: Important Advances in Oncology 1988, p 129. Philadelphia, JB Lippincott, 1988)

the dose effect cannot be completely separated from other variables.

In a later analysis of the effect of dose on the outcome in the Milan trial, Bonadonna et al divided the delivered doses of CMF into three levels and determined the impact of dosing at these levels on outcome.[87] The doses at these levels have been converted in Table 16-5 to their dose intensity relative to the NCI CMF+P regimen. In advanced cases, a substantial dose–response effect seems apparent. Since complete responses were not reported, the impact of dose reductions on the quality of response cannot be assessed. In the adjuvant situation, a dose–response effect was also noted. In premenopausal woman the differences in relapse-free survival at the high and low doses are statistically significant. The most important point, however, is that the average dose intensity of CMF as used in clinical trials and in the community is probably only a little more than half the dose intensity of the original program. These dose reductions exceed the levels that animal models predict would lead to a loss in the capacity to cure.

An example of the potential impact dose intensity can have on the design of clinical trials has been provided by Hryniuk in Figure 16-5.[78] The dose intensity of 5-fluorouracil is plotted against response rate for advanced colorectal

TABLE 16-5. Ad Hoc Dose Modifications of the CMF Program Used for Breast Cancer: Impact of Dose Intensity on Outcome

A. Advanced Breast Cancer

Study/Doses*	Intended Dose Intensity	Actual Dose Intensity	Response Rate CR	Response Rate CR + PR
CMF − P (NCI, 1974): 100/60/700	1	. . .	28	68
CMF − P (ECOG, 1976):				
Age < 60 yr: 100/40/600	0.84	. . .	15	53
Age < 60 yr: 100/30/400	0.69	. . .	<60 vs. > 60 yr: p < 0.01	
CMF − P (Milan, 1976)†				
Level I:	>0.71	0.74	. . .	67
Level II:	0.55−0.71	0.58	. . .	53
Level III:	<0.55	0.42	. . .	35

B. Adjuvant Therapy

Study*	Intended Dose Intensity	Actual Dose Intensity	Relapse-Free Survival Premenopausal	Relapse-Free Survival Postmenopausal
CMF − P (Milan, 1976)†				
Level I:	>0.71	0.74	79‡	75§
Level II:	0.55−0.71	0.58	56	56
Level III:	<0.55	0.42	46	49

Intended actual dose intensities are calculated using NCI's CMF − P, the program with the highest dose intensity, as the reference standard according to the method of Hryniuk.[78] ECOG = Eastern Cooperative Oncology Group.

* CMF+P = cyclophosphamide, methotrexate, 5-fluorouracil, +prednisone. Numbers refer to the doses of each drug respectively in mg/m² BSA.

† The Milan trial used the same dose modifications as ECOG, reducing the doses of CMF, a priori, for patients older than 60 years. When reporting results they divided doses into three levels and reported responses by dose level regardless of age. These doses have been recalculated to determine their dose intensity relative to the original NCI CMF+P program.

‡ Differences in RFS of Level I vs. II for premenopausal patients is significant at p < 0.06. Level I vs. Level III is significant at p < 0.05.

§ For postmenopausal patients, p < 0.23, Level I vs. II, p < 0.17, Level I vs. Level III.

cancer in panel A. Points indicated by the asterisks are from a single study in which response was reported for actual delivered doses at three different levels.[88] The steep nature of the dose–response curves should be noted. Panel B of Figure 16-5 plots the same three points from the single study, but adds the doses used in four published adjuvant studies.[88-93] The doses in all of these studies are well below the level that most investigators would consider the threshold for producing useful responses in advanced colorectal cancer.

The effect of dose intensity on the capacity to cure advanced Hodgkin's disease and diffuse large cell lymphomas is also striking and described in detail in Chapters 49 and 50.

Increasing the dose intensity can be a useful way to improve the effect of certain drugs or combinations of drugs, but it is not useful in all clinical circumstances. Large tumor burdens tend to shift the dose–response curve to the right. At the low end of the curability curve (i.e., in the presence of the highest tumor burdens), increasing the dose intensity to unacceptable toxicity, therefore, may not produce more impressive treatment outcomes because the curve is flat. In addition, regimens that are already curing 100% of a subset of patients, such as the combination of platinum, vinblastine, and bleomycin in low-burden testicular cancer and MOPP in Stage IIIA Hodgkin's disease, cannot be expected to be improved upon by augmenting dose intensity. However, for most drugs and most tumors there appears to be a threshold dose that produces responses, and the remarkable success of high-dose chemotherapy programs with marrow support in refractory lymphomas, breast cancer, childhood sarcomas, and neuroblastomas suggests that maximizing dose intensity can improve the chances of cure.

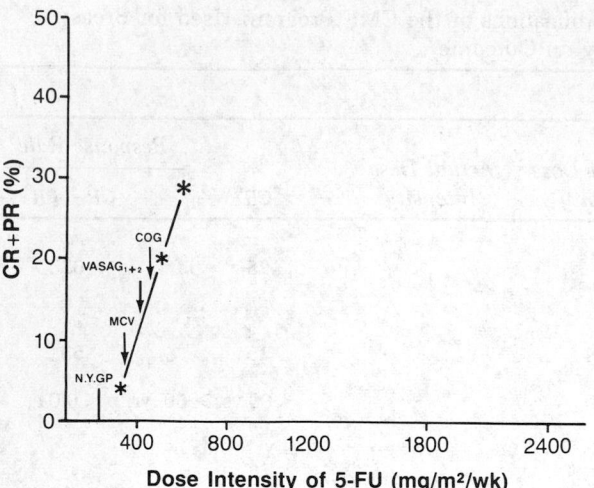

A

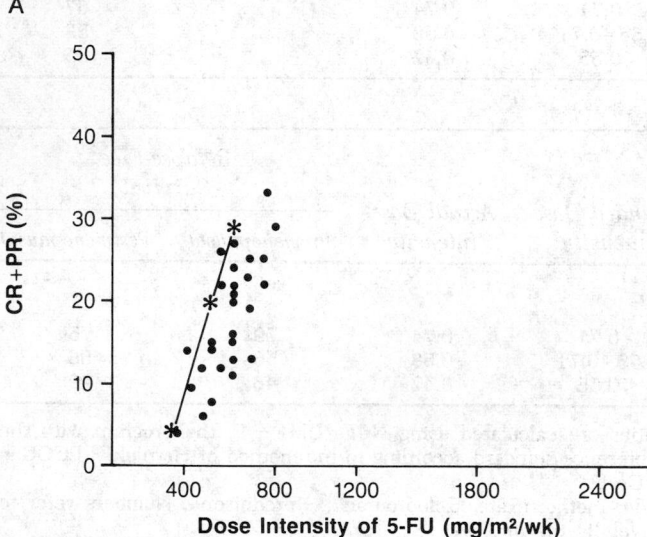

B

FIG. 16-5. **A**. Response rate at various intended dose intensity of 5-fluorouracil in advanced colorectal cancer. Each point represents results from one arm of a randomized trial. Asterisks indicate results of three doses from a single study, and solid circles indicate received dose intensity. **B**. Dose intensities of 5-fluorouracil used in four adjuvant studies of colorectal cancer superimposed on the dose response line for advanced disease shown in panel **A**. Asterisks represent received dose intensity from single study (see text). (Hryniuk WM: The importance of dose intensity in the outcome of chemotherapy. In DeVita VT Jr, Hellman S, Rosenberg SA [eds]: Important Advances in Oncology 1988, p 125. Philadelphia, JB Lippincott, 1988)

PRINCIPLES OF COMBINATION CHEMOTHERAPY

In the early days of chemotherapy, drug combinations were developed based on known biochemical actions of available anticancer drugs rather than on their clinical effectiveness. These programs were largely ineffective.[94-98] The era of effective combination chemotherapy began when an array of effective drugs became available for use in combination in the treatment of leukemias and lymphomas. Combination

chemotherapy has now been extended to the treatment of most other malignancies as described throughout this text.

With the exception of choriocarcinoma and Burkitt's lymphoma, combination chemotherapy is required to cure all drug-sensitive human cancers. The relationship of tumor cell number to the likelihood of the presence of resistant cell lines provides a firm basis for the invariable inverse relationship between cell number and curability and is the most reasonable explanation for the effectiveness of combination chemotherapy. Omission of a drug from a combination may allow overgrowth by a cell line sensitive to that drug alone and resistant to other drugs in the combination. Also, arbitrarily reducing the dose of an effective drug to add other, less effective drugs may reduce the dose below the threshold of effectiveness and destroy the capacity of the combination to cure that particular cancer.

Combination chemotherapy, then, accomplishes three important things not possible with single agent treatment: (1) it provides maximal cell kill within the range of toxicity tolerated by the host for each drug; (2) it provides a broader range of coverage of resistant cell lines in a heterogeneous tumor population; and (3) it prevents or slows the development of new resistant lines.

Several principles have been useful in the selection of drugs in the most effective drug combinations and guide the development of new programs.

1. Only drugs known to be partially effective when used alone should be selected for use in combination. If available, drugs that produce some fraction of complete remission are preferred to those that produce only partial responses.
2. When several drugs of a class are available, a drug should be selected on the basis of toxicity that does not overlap with the toxicity of other drugs used in the combination. Although such selection leads to a wider range of side-effects and greater general discomfort to the patient, it minimizes the risk of a lethal effect caused by multiple insults to the same organ system by different drugs.
3. Drugs should be used in their optimal dose and schedule.
4. Drug combinations should be given at consistent intervals. The treatment-free interval between cycles should be the shortest possible time period necessary for recovery of the most sensitive normal target tissue, which is usually the bone marrow.

Bone marrow has a storage compartment that can supply mature cells to the peripheral blood for 8 to 10 days after the stem cell pool has been damaged by cytotoxic drugs. Thus, events measured in the peripheral blood are usually a week behind events occurring in the bone marrow. In previously untreated patients, leukopenia and thrombocytopenia are discernible on the ninth or tenth day after initial dosing. Nadir blood counts are noted between days 14 to 18, with recovery apparent by day 21 and usually complete by day 28. Prior treatment with drugs or x-irradiation may alter this sequence by depleting the stem cell pool, shortening the time to the appearance of leukopenia and thrombocytopenia, and prolonging the recovery time. Curiously, when the second half of a combination given in the clinic on a day 1, day 8 schedule is omitted, leukopenia and thrombocytopenia comparable to that seen with the full combination usually occur, suggesting that the second set of doses does not cause an equal increment in toxicity, possibly because the stem cell compartment has entered a quiescent state. This also suggests that in most cases, the day 8 doses can be given safely even if leukopenia and thrombocytopenia have already become evident. The cytotoxic effect of greatest importance in the clinic is the duration of the nadir level of white cells and platelets. The highest risk of infection or bleeding occurs with granulocyte counts of less than $500/ml^3$ and platelet counts of less than $20,000/ml^3$. If this nadir lasts only 4 to 7 days it is tolerated by most patients without supplemental support. Increasing doses of most anticancer drugs, within the range of the maximally tolerated dose, usually does not ablate the marrow or even prolong the time to recovery. Repeated dosing during the phase of early recovery of the marrow (days 16–21) may cause more severe toxicity in the second treatment cycle in patients whose marrow is not the source of, or involved with, tumor.

These kinds of data led to the familiar 2-week interval between cycles of the most effective drug combinations (new cycles begin on day 28 after the first dose) to accommodate the recovery time of human bone marrow. Although this treatment schedule is suitable for some tumors, the regrowth characteristics of others, such as diffuse histiocytic lymphoma, Burkitt's lymphoma, and leukemia, often permit the tumor mass to return to pretreatment levels in the interval required for bone marrow recovery, and other approaches to cycling drug combinations are being explored. One approach has been to use non-marrow-toxic chemotherapeutic agents, cycled with marrow-toxic agents, to permit the bone marrow to recover despite continuous treatment. This has been useful in patients with the rapidly growing diffuse large cell lymphomas. It is limited by the sensitivity of the tumor in question to the available non-marrow-toxic agents. The availability of colony-stimulating factors (CSF) as supportive tools (discussed in Chapter 59, Section 4) is altering the design of clinical trials as well. CSF have been coupled with cytotoxic combination chemotherapy, and in the first such report in which G-CSF were used with the combination of methotrexate, vinblastine, Adriamycin, and cisplatin (M-VAC) for treatment of advanced bladder cancer, the nadir leukopenia and thrombocytopenia have been ablated.[99]

The Goldie–Coldman hypothesis also has had a major impact on the design of clinical studies employing combination chemotherapy. Since it suggests that resistance is a problem even with small tumor burdens, it predicts a maximal chance of cure if all available effective drugs are given simultaneously. This approach has not been tested in the clinic because of the fear that the simultaneous use of more than five cytotoxic drugs at full doses would not be possible. Alternatives to using all available effective drugs simultaneously, such as using alternating cycles of equally effective, non-cross-resistant drug combinations, are being tested. Unfortunately, many studies reported to test the Goldie–Coldman hypothesis have been poorly designed. Usually inadequate testing has been done to determine whether the

alternate combination is truly non-cross-resistant and equally effective as the primary treatment, which it must be to fulfill the hypothesis. A more recent approach is the use of half of the drugs of each effective combination on days 1 and 8, respectively (hybrid combinations). This approach is being tried in patients with Hodgkin's disease and diffuse large cell lymphomas. At this juncture, the use of alternating cycles of combination chemotherapy has not yet proved to be more effective than full doses of a single effective combination program.

In reality, no rigid schedule can accommodate all the variables assumed to be important for maximum effectiveness of combination chemotherapy and the requirements of the patients in the practice of medical oncology. Physicians often must adjust doses at intervals to administer drugs safely. The surety that the therapeutic effect of a drug or drug combination can be lost if the dose or schedule is drastically altered should temper these judgments. Reductions in dose rates also often result only in minimal decreases in toxicity. Both the physician and the patient must consider the risk of dying from cancer along with the transient benefits of reducing the side-effects of treatment. Adhering to the standard sliding scale for dose adjustments, usually published with most new treatments, is the most useful approach to follow. In addition to providing guidelines for dose reduction, these sliding scales provide consistency between patients and between studies by preserving both the intervals between cycles and the integrity of the drug combination. These points should be made clear to patients as part of the informed consent process if they are to share intelligently in decisions about dose modifications made by their physicians.[100]

USES OF CHEMOTHERAPY AS PART OF THE INITIAL TREATMENT OF CANCER

There are four ways chemotherapy is generally used[101]: (1) as induction treatment for advanced disease, (2) as an adjunct to the local methods of treatment, (3) as the primary treatment of patients who present with localized cancer, and (4) by direct installation into sanctuaries or by site-directed perfusion of specific regions of the body most affected by the cancer.

INDUCTION CHEMOTHERAPY. The term *induction chemotherapy* has been used to describe the drug therapy given as the primary treatment for patients who present with advanced cancer for which no alternative treatment exists.[102] Selection of treatment is based on the effectiveness of the cancer drugs in rodent models. Combinations of drugs are fashioned based on the effectiveness, level of cross-resistance, and limiting toxicity of the available drugs when used alone in similar patient populations. Patients who fail after one drug treatment and require further chemotherapy pose a particularly difficult treatment problem because of the volume of tumor, their poor general health, and drug resistance. Induction chemotherapy in these patients is referred to as *salvage treatment*.

ADJUVANT CHEMOTHERAPY. Adjuvant chemotherapy denotes the use of systemic treatment after the primary tumor has been removed by an alternative method. The selection of adjuvant treatment program is based on response rates in separate groups of patients with advanced cancers of the same histologic type; the selection of suitable population of patients for adjuvant treatment is based on their risk of recurrence after local treatment alone and on disease variables known to adversely influence prognosis.

PRIMARY CHEMOTHERAPY. Primary chemotherapy denotes the use of chemotherapy as initial treatment for patients who present with localized cancer for which there is an alternative but less than completely effective treatment. This has been described as *neoadjuvant chemotherapy*,[103] but the term *primary chemotherapy*[104] is more accurate. Since the likelihood of development of spontaneous resistant cell lines relates to tumor mass, earlier drug treatment in the form of primary chemotherapy may have the advantage of treatment in the presence of fewer drug-resistant lines, although this point is questionable because the time interval, in practice, between chemotherapy used as adjuvant treatment, after tumor has been removed, or as primary treatment at the time of diagnosis can sometimes be only a few weeks.[105] Primary chemotherapy does have the potential to downstage tumors by decreasing the size and extent of the presenting tumor mass. This can influence both the need for, and radical nature of, the subsequent alternative treatment by influencing operability and/or decreasing tumor hypoxia, and by increasing the effectiveness of a given dose of radiation therapy or decreasing the size of the radiation therapy field. The theoretical disadvantages of primary chemotherapy are that by leaving the primary tumor mass in place, even temporarily, the tumor volume faced by chemotherapy is actually larger than if surgery or radiation therapy were used first and chemotherapy were used as an adjunct. Also, the favorable influence of resection of the primary tumor on the kinetics of proliferation of the residual micrometastases may be lost.[106] In addition, the toxicity of chemotherapy may impair the effectiveness and increase the side-effects of subsequent alternative treatments, and may delay the use of an alternative treatment sufficiently to have an impact on the outcome. As in the case of adjuvant chemotherapy, patients who would otherwise be cured by local treatment alone are exposed to the acute and chronic side-effects of chemotherapy in combined modality programs.

CLINICAL END POINTS IN EVALUATING RESPONSE TO CHEMOTHERAPY

In induction chemotherapy for advanced cancer it is possible to determine the response to drugs on a case by case basis. The partial response rate, usually defined as the fraction of patients who demonstrate a 50% or greater reduction in measurable tumor mass, usually is not of much clinical value because such responses are usually short in duration, but it is useful in the testing of new drug programs to determine whether the particular experimental approach is worth pursuing further. The most important indicator of effectiveness

of chemotherapy is the complete response rate. It is the prerequisite for cure. When new programs consistently produce more than an occasional complete remission, they have invariably later proved of practical value in medical practice. The qualitative and quantitative differences in the clinical value between a complete and partial response is such that complete responses should always be reported separately. The most important indicator of the quality of a complete remission is the relapse-free survival from the time all treatment is discontinued. This is the only clinical counterpart of the quantifiable cytoreductive effect of drugs in rodent systems. The current trend in many clinical protocols to use freedom from progression in complete and partial responders combined as an indicator of the practical potential of a new treatment obscures the value of a relapse-free survival of complete responders as the major determinant of the quality of remission. Other end points such as median response duration or median survival are of little practical value until treatment results have been refined to the point that the complete response rate is over 50%.

There was great excitement concomitant with the move to the use of chemotherapy as an adjunct to local treatments, or adjuvant chemotherapy. The promise was great because tumor volume is at a minimum when adjuvant therapy is initiated, and it was assumed that either a much higher cure rate could be achieved or treatment intensity could be reduced and side-effects thereby diminished. Failure to appreciate the circumstances surrounding the assessment of response to adjuvant chemotherapy is the source of some of the current disillusionment with the positive but less than dramatic results achieved with adjuvant chemotherapy of common tumors such as breast and colorectal cancer.[107,108] The major indicator of effectiveness, the complete remission rate, is lost in the adjuvant setting, since the primary tumor has already been removed. Treatment is selected for individual patients based on response rates in entirely different populations of patients with advanced disease with the same histologic type. While relapse-free survival remains the major end point, the micrometastases in treated patients could consist of tumor cells either sensitive or resistant to chemotherapy. The relapse-free survival in the adjuvant setting, therefore, measures the equivalent of the duration of remission of both complete and partial responders as well as the interval of regrowth in patients who would have been classified as nonresponders, and is similar to the use of freedom from progression in patients with advanced disease. Attempts to use in vitro assays of drug sensitivity from biopsy material of primary tumors (see below) to overcome the shortcomings of the absence of an indicator of individual response have not proved practical.

The unique feature of primary chemotherapy in patients with localized tumor is preservation of the presenting tumor mass as a biologic marker of responsiveness to anticancer drugs. Thus, as with induction chemotherapy, it is possible to determine, on a case by case basis, the potential effectiveness of a new treatment program. By definition, the presenting tumor mass is also the largest aggregate of tumor in the body and historically the oldest, and thus the aggregate mass of tumor cells most likely to contain one or more resistant cell lines.[105] It is also a mass with the least favorable cell kinetics. It is reasonable to assume, then, that whatever the effect of chemotherapy the physician sees on the primary tumor, a similar or greater effect is occurring fairly uniformly in micrometastatic deposits, unless a metastasizing cell line phenotypically is one that spontaneously develops drug resistance. Although there is no direct evidence for the latter occurrence, such an event would explain the clinical observation of control of the primary tumor with chemotherapy, with death resulting from uncontrolled metastases at a distant site. A poor response of the primary tumor to chemotherapy clearly indicates a group of patients for which alternative methods of treatment should be used and used quickly. Another feature of primary chemotherapy is the ability to delineate partial responders with varying degrees of prognosis, as determined by the state of the residual tumor mass after an initial good but partial response. Removal and histologic examination of residual masses allows determination of the viability of remaining tissue. Obviously, the response duration of these categories of responders must be determined separately.

The most important issue facing investigators of primary chemotherapy is whether or not an effective primary chemotherapy treatment, pursued flexibly and intensively to the point of the complete remission, plus two or more additional cycles of treatment, will define a significant fraction of patients whose disease is cured by chemotherapy, with or without the addition of alternative treatments. In carefully selected patients with some stages of the most common tumors for which there is less than satisfactory standard treatment, such studies are ethically and theoretically sound and are being pursued. Such an approach could result in shorter duration, less morbid, and more effective treatment programs. In some tumor types such as localized diffuse large cell lymphomas, limited-stage small cell cancers, some pediatric malignancies, and some subsets of head and neck cancers, primary chemotherapy has already become the standard of treatment.[101]

SPECIAL USES OF CHEMOTHERAPY

Special uses of chemotherapy include the installation of drugs into the spinal fluid, either directly through a lumbar puncture needle or into an implanted Ommaya reservoir, to treat meningeal leukemia and lymphoma; the installation of drugs into the pleural or pericardial space to control effusions; splenic infusion to control spleen size; hepatic artery infusion to treat hepatic metastases selectively; carotid artery infusion to treat head and neck cancers and brain tumors; and the intraperitoneal installation of drugs using dialysis techniques. These uses are discussed throughout this book in relation to specific cancers. In all cases the rationale for directed chemotherapy is based on achieving a greater $C \times T$ against the target tumor tissue, and the sparing of normal tissue. The place of intracerebrospinal fluid and intrapleural administration of drugs is already established. Hepatic infusion of chemotherapy has been simplified and improved by the development of technology for infusion of drugs sufficient to reevaluate these approaches (see Chap. 64). It is now possible to measure both the active principle of

cancer drugs and their targets, within the biologic range, and drugs can be infused in timing with the body's circadian rhythm.

The intraperitoneal administration of drugs to treat ovarian cancer, a disease that kills almost exclusively by local effects in the abdomen, is now commonly used because it allows wide distribution of antitumor drugs in the smallest interstices of the abdominal cavity, and a greater $C \times T$ at the tumor is achieved (see Chaps. 34 and 64).[109-111] The concentration of drug available in the peritoneal cavity for some drugs with this "belly bath" technique far exceeds the plasma level achievable with systemic administration. The effects are particularly marked for drugs like 5-fluorouracil, which is metabolized in the liver as well as excreted by the kidney, and drugs like Adriamycin and cisplatin, which, because of their molecular size, diffuse more slowly across the peritoneal membrane.

Drugs can also be encompassed in lipid bilayer droplets called liposomes.[112-114] The surface characteristics of liposomes can be altered to direct their delivery to specific organ sites or into resistant cell lines. Labile liposomes that dissolve at temperatures of 41°C can deposit drugs selectively in preheated areas.[113] A drawback to liposomes, however, is their failure to leave the vascular system except in the sinusoids of the liver and the spleen, and thus far liposome encapsulation of drugs for targeted delivery has been of limited value.[114]

IN VITRO TESTS TO SELECT CHEMOTHERAPEUTIC AGENTS FOR INDIVIDUALIZED TREATMENT

Short-term assays are not useful for determining the primary treatment for patients for whom a known effective treatment exists. They are of minimal value for the remainder of newly diagnosed patients and for those with drug-sensitive tumors who fail the first trial of chemotherapy. They can be of use to avoid patient exposure to the toxicity of drugs that are unlikely to be effective, but in general, the tests are too cumbersome and expensive for routine practice. No convincing reports in the literature have indicated that short-term assays provide additional benefit over what the clinician can provide by using good judgment and a knowledge of the effectiveness of the limited number of available single agents.

In vitro assays can be divided into three types: (1) clonogenic assays, usually conducted in soft agar media, (2) short-term culture techniques performed in defined media, and (3) short-term biochemical assays, which include histologic, or radioautographic measurements on cells exposed to chemotherapy on a short-term basis.

CLONOGENIC ASSAYS. Clonogenic assays have the advantage that they measure the response of those cells that theoretically have the capacity to reproduce themselves and ultimately kill the host.[115,116] They suffer from the disadvantage that single-cell suspensions are required, with the resulting loss of normal cell–cell interactions. Plating efficiency is also low, and cells already committed to differentiate may also form colonies. In addition, cells in the G_0 growth phase, capable of reentering the growth cycle, are not assayed, and the limited range of clonogenic assays (1- to 2-log kill) is insufficiently sensitive to predict drug sensitivity.[115-118]

In numerous reports the value for true predictions of sensitivity of the clonogenic assay is consistently around 65%, and the figure for true prediction of resistance is consistently about 90%. Two thirds of tumors predicted to be sensitive ultimately respond to the drug selected, and 10% of those predicted to be resistant respond to drugs predicted to be ineffective. An interesting illustration of problems with the use of the clonogenic system has been provided by Twentyman,[119] using data of Von Hoff.[120,121] In Von Hoff's reports, of 8000 tumors cultured, only 2480 (31%) grew enough colonies for testing; therefore, no prediction was possible in 6320 patients whose samples were sent for testing. In only 198 (8%) of the patients whose tissues proved sufficient for testing was the prediction of sensitivity made; of these, 139 responded in vivo but 59 did not. Another 2280 tumors were predicted to be resistant, 228 of these incorrectly so. No survival benefit was found for patients whose tumor cells responded in short-term clonogenic assay over those whose cells did not respond. Therefore, for the vast majority of patients, the assay was of little use in selecting a usable treatment.

DYE EXCLUSION ASSAY. A simple dye exclusion assay has been used by Weisenthal and associates on cells in short-term culture. Cells are stained with the fast green dye and counterstained with hematoxylin–eosin.[122-125] The true response rate is equivalent to that of the clonogenic assay.[124] The major advantages of this assay are its short duration and the fact that relatively unskilled personnel can be trained to read the slides and evaluate the majority of specimens. In a prospective trial it has been used as the assay to determine the potential effectiveness of drugs for small cell lung cancer in permanently derived cell lines.[126] In the experimental arm of this study patients are treated with a predetermined program while cell lines are established, and switched at week 13 of treatment, if response has been less than complete, to three drugs selected on the basis of the dye exclusion assay. Preliminary results suggest some benefit in patients whose continued treatment was selected from results of this in vitro assay.

HUMAN–MURINE XENOGRAFTS. Human xenografts implanted under the renal capsule of athymic mice have been used by Bogden and co-workers as a rapid 6-day screening method.[127] A retrospective and prospective clinical trial has been performed with this assay in 837 patients who contributed 1,000 specimens; 858 (85%) of the specimens resulted in an evaluable assay.[128] The test predicted clinical response in 82% of tumors and clinical resistance in 94%, and thus was comparable to the clonogenic assay. The advantage of this assay is that it retains the spatial relationships of the tumor because cell–cell contact is maintained in the whole fragments that are implanted under the renal capsule. Multiple assays can also be done on tissue from the same patient in 6 days. While this test has a high assay evaluability rate, and allows testing of compounds requiring in vivo activation, it is expensive, particularly since a histologic end point is used, and the testing facility must maintain a very large mouse colony.

Recently, the human–murine xenograft assay was performed with surgical specimens from about 400 patients. In heavily treated patients with drug-resistant, far-advanced cancer, the test identified some active drugs yielding good responses.[129] However, use of surgical specimens for the xenograft assay depends critically on the selection of tumor for implantation and requires long experience.

MICROENCAPSULATION ASSAY. A microencapsulation technique has been recently described[115,130-132] in which human tumor cells encapsulated in 1-mm microcapsules with semipermeable membranes are injected intraperitoneally into nude mice.[130] Chemotherapeutic agents are administered intravenously, and the microcapsules are harvested to determine cell survivability in the treated animals compared to untreated controls. Several properties of the tumor microencapsulation assay make it attractive as a potential future test for drug selection. The antitumor activity of drugs can be tested against human tumor cells under conditions that provide for three-dimensional growth and an in vivo supply of nutrients; the sensitivity of tumor cells can be assessed following exposure to drugs in concentrations achievable in vivo; compounds requiring in vivo metabolic activation can be tested; the effect of each drug injection can be quickly evaluated; the inhibition of tumor cell proliferation versus the cytoreductive effects of drugs can be discriminated; the test is applicable to virtually all histologic types of tumor cells; and the assay is short term, simple, and relatively inexpensive. In the studies reported, the antitumor effects were consistent with the relative therapeutic efficacy or level of resistance to drugs detected by other in vitro and in vivo tests.

OTHER ASSAYS. Other tests have included use of monolayer cultures of cell maintained in short-term cultures in defined medium.[133-135] Further evaluation of newer assays will be required to determine if any of these tests can provide practical assistance to physicians in their choice of treatment, but the usefulness of all tests will likely remain limited as long as the pool of available drugs remains small.

CANCER DRUG DEVELOPMENT

The steps in the development of anticancer drugs are shown in Figure 16-6 and discussed below.

SCREENING

The most important step in the drug selection process is mass screening, the mechanism used to narrow the universe of chemicals potentially useful for the treatment of human cancers to a manageable number of high priority drugs for clinical testing.[136-139]

From its inception in 1955 until 1975, the mainstay of NCI's screening program was the murine L1210 leukemia.

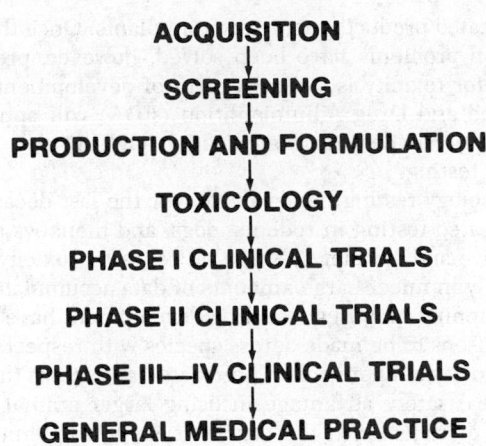

ACQUISITION

↓

SCREENING

↓

PRODUCTION AND FORMULATION

↓

TOXICOLOGY

↓

PHASE I CLINICAL TRIALS

↓

PHASE II CLINICAL TRIALS

↓

PHASE III—IV CLINICAL TRIALS

↓

GENERAL MEDICAL PRACTICE

FIG. 16-6. Steps in cancer drug development.

Drugs found to be active against L1210 were evaluated in other rodent tumors for dose and schedule dependency, but entrance into the clinic was almost exclusively based on the antitumor effect in L1210. Many currently available anticancer drugs active against human leukemias and lymphomas were identified and developed as a result of this system. The input to this type of screening program reached its maximum of 40,000 compounds screened per year in 1975. In 1975 a major change was made in the NCI's screening program because of the availability of new rodent models. More rational selection of compounds was coupled with a panel of transplantable rodent tumor screens designed to match the histologic type of common visceral cancers. These rodent solid tumor screens were matched to human tumor cell lines of the same type grown in nude mice. This panel posed the question of the clinical specificity of the preclinical models. Because of the expense of high volume screening in such a panel, however, a prescreening system was necessary, and prescreening was performed in the rodent P388 mouse leukemia, a leukemia more sensitive to natural products than L1210. An agent shown to have activity against P388 leukemia was passed to the tumor panel where, if antitumor effect was noted, the agent was advanced to clinical trial. The prescreen had the effect of biasing selection of compounds toward those traditionally selected by rodent leukemias. The panel of tumors was changed periodically to pose additional questions to the screening process.[140] Later, human tumors grown in soft agar, and under the renal capsule, were also introduced into the screening program to further test the hypothesis that the use of human tissue in short-term assays could better select compounds more active in the clinic than could simpler rodent tumor models. Problems with the technical details of these in vitro systems led to their discontinuation.[140,143]

As it became possible to maintain human tumor cells in defined media, the screening program was again changed by developing disease-oriented panels of human tumor cell lines grown in defined media.[144,145] The initial selection of cell lines for this screening panel was based on several considerations, including (1) representatives of major histologic subtypes, (2) utilization of multiple cell lines for each tumor type, and (3) utilization of cell lines that retain appropriate features of the tumor of origin. The cell lines now in use include lung, ovarian, and renal cancer, malignant melanoma, brain tumors, and leukemia. Because of the interest in the phenomenon of multidrug resistance and the likelihood that it is one of the factors limiting the effectiveness of chemotherapy, the MCF-7 cell line, a human breast cancer line, and an MDR variant of MCF-7 selected for resistance to Adriamycin are included, along with a P388 murine leukemia and a comparable Adriamycin-induced MDR variant of P388. These cell lines provide the potential for identifying new agents with particular activity against MDR cell populations.

A key element in screening strategy is to maintain the capacity for high volume screening. The most promising assay available to do this is a colorimetric growth inhibition assay that is based on the metabolic reduction of the tetrazolium salt formazan inside viable cells. Under appropriate conditions, a linear relationship is obtained between viable cell number and formazan optical density, measured using a standard ELISA plate reader.[147] Automation of this assay has made it possible to maintain an adequate volume of in vitro screening (10,000 compounds per year) at less expense. Preliminary analysis of screening results indicate that individual cell lines show characteristic degrees of in vitro chemosensitivity to individual test compounds with known patterns of clinical activity. Ease of automation of the colorimetric assay and the stability of the cell lines have largely overcome the technical problems associated with clonogenic or subrenal capsular assays.[143,148] The central goal of the in vitro–based disease-oriented screening program is to identify new antitumor drug candidates that would not have been discovered by the previously available screening program. Clinical testing of these new leads, as with previous versions of preclinical screening, will ultimately be the only way to establish or disprove the validity of the new screen for identifying new drugs active against the common refractory human solid tumors.

In the early days of screening, acquisition of agents was purely random. Random acquisition of chemicals for screening was associated with two major problems: repetitious screening of compounds already tested, and screening of analogs of drugs already known to be active, rather than the identification of new structures. Modern molecular biologic techniques present an unusual opportunity to select materials, defined at the molecular level, that might prove useful in inhibition of vital cell functions. To take advantage of new technology and to reduce the randomness of screening, the NCI has established drug discovery groups, consortia of investigators in academia, government, and industry funded to deal with the development of potential new types of chemicals such as those that inhibit polyamine biosynthesis, oncogene products, the sense message of DNA (antisense message compounds), and inhibitors of topoisomerase II. Still, some collection of compounds on a random basis is required, and the NCI's chemical collection program for screening also emphasizes the collection of natural products from a wide variety of terrestrial and marine sources over collection of synthetic chemicals. This emphasis follows directly from the realization that many of the most useful agents in the therapy of human diseases of all kinds are natural products and that the microbial, plant, and marine worlds are a virtually inexhaustible source of biologically active novel compounds that provide important leads for subsequent structural modification. Also, with the introduction of high-speed computers capable of performing 100 million calculations per second and possessing sophisticated graphics capability, the possibility of designing compounds based on known characteristics of presumed targets has now become a realistic goal. These supercomputers can graphically illustrate the nature of chemicals capable of binding to specific receptors, and chemical synthesis can be simulated through computer programs developed to synthesize complex molecules based on known synthetic reactions. The future of the design of new anticancer drugs may lie in the capacity of these high-speed computers to offer compounds designed on a rational basis for later biologic testing.

Inherent in all screening systems is the tenet that biologic activity in some preclinical system must be demonstrated before human testing is performed. To date, no currently marketed, useful anticancer agent is devoid of such preclinical antitumor effect. Workers in cancer drug development often face advocates for various anticancer agents who, by reason of theory or personal interest, believe their material shows great promise as a human cancer treatment. Whether compounds selected for theoretical reasons, without demonstrated biologic activity in rodent systems, might be effective in human tumors has never been adequately tested. Without demonstrated activity in an in vitro system or in one of the many rodent systems available, the decision usually is not to initiate clinical testing of such materials. Given the need to use some selection criteria to narrow the choice of drugs for clinical trials, screening systems are likely to remain the mainstay for decision-making.

FORMULATION AND TOXICOLOGY TESTING

Formulation and production of anticancer drugs, required before anticancer drugs can proceed to toxicology studies and clinical trials, often present formidable obstacles for chemists. Anticancer agents with considerable activity in rodents have been discarded for lack of an adequate formulation for human use. This is particularly true of the more complicated products extracted from plants. Once these formulation problems have been solved, however, preclinical testing for toxicity is a requirement of development. Then, the Food and Drug Administration (FDA) will approve an investigational new drug application (INDA) that permits clinical testing.

Toxicology testing has evolved over the last decade from complicated testing in rodents, dogs, and monkeys to a less expensive and simpler system that relies on toxicity testing primarily in mice. Large amounts of data accumulated since the beginning of anticancer drug development have allowed comparisons to be made across species with respect to common toxicity of chemicals. These data have shown that there is no real safety advantage in using larger animal species instead of rodents. In the current system, implemented in 1980, the dose–response curve of a new drug is first developed in mice. The lethal dose (LD) in 10%, 50%, and 90% of animals is determined and the reproducible lethal dose in 10% of tested animals (LD_{10}) is used as the basis for establishing the initial dose in clinical trials. Usually, 10% of the LD_{10} dose in rodents is selected for the initial human dose; this dose is first tested for toxicity in dogs, prior to use in humans, to minimize the risks associated with administering an unknown compound to humans. Although correlation of toxic effects on rapidly dividing normal tissue among rodents, dogs, monkeys, and humans is good, correlation of other toxic effects is not as consistent.[149] Therefore routine pathologic examination of rodent tissue is not always performed prior to clinical testing.

TRANSLATION OF DOSES ACROSS SPECIES. All drugs should be given in reference to either body weight or surface area. The preferable reference point is body surface area, because better cross-species comparisons can be made and because doses calculated from body surface area allow doses to be determined for adults and children without further adjustment. The assumptions leading to the dose conversion factors have been described in detail by Freireich and co-workers[24] and are shown in Table 16-6, which is useful in converting doses in milligrams per kilogram to the comparable milligram per square meter dose. Table 16-7 shows the procedure for conversion of a milligram per kilogram dose in rodents, monkeys, or dogs to the equivalent dose in man.

TABLE 16-6.   Representative Surface Area to Weight Ratios (km) of Various Species*

Species	Body Weight (kg)	Surface Area	Surface Area to Weight Ratio (km)
Mouse	0.02	0.0066	3.0
Rat	0.15	0.025	5.9
Monkey	3	0.24	12
Dog	8	0.40	20
Human			
Child	20	0.80	25
Adult	60	1.6	37

* To express a mg/kg dose in any given species as the equivalent mg/m² dose, multiply the dose by the appropriate *km*. In the adult human, for example, 100 mg/kg is equivalent to 100 mg/kg× 37 kg/m² = 3700 mg/m².

TABLE 16-7. Equivalent Surface Area Dosage Conversion Factors*

	Mouse, 20 g	*Rat, 150 g*	*Monkey, 3.0 kg*	*Dog, 8 kg*	*Man, 60 kg*
Mouse	1	1/2	1/4	1/6	1/12
Rat	2	1	1/2	1/4	1/7
Monkey	4	2	1	3/5	1/3
Dog	6	4	5/3	1	1/2
Man	12	7	3	2	1

* This table gives approximate factors for converting doses expressed in terms of mg/kg from one species to an equivalent *surface area* dose expressed in the same terms mg/kg in the other species. For example, given a dose of 50 mg/kg in the mouse, what is the appropriate dose in man assuming equivalency on the basis of mg/m^2?

$$50 \text{ mg/kg} \times 1/12 = 4.1 \text{ mg/kg}$$

EARLY CLINICAL TRIALS OF ANTITUMOR AGENTS

Antitumor agents go through four phases of clinical testing before they are accepted for general medical practice, marketed, or discarded (Fig. 16-6).[137,150–153] The average time from discovery of an effective antitumor agent to marketing of that agent is quite long, in the range of 10 to 12 years. To facilitate access to drugs for desperately ill cancer patients before the drugs are marketed, anticancer drugs with known efficacy are made available to physicians by the NCI in the premarketing phase (Tables 16-8 and 16-9).

Table 16-10 details the phases of clinical testing and the main purpose of each step. Phase I trials are done on small groups of patients, usually no more than 15 to 30 per study. Although the main purpose of Phase I trials is to identify a maximally tolerated dose (MTD) in one of several schedules suggested by the preclinical data, patients are entered into Phase I trials with therapeutic intent. For most of the effective anticancer drugs, some therapeutic effect was often seen even in Phase I trials. Because a limited number of patients with a variety of diseases are treated in Phase I trials, and doses may be below the ultimate therapeutic range in a fraction of the patients, the absence of any positive effect in a Phase I trial is not sufficient reason to discontinue testing of a drug. The only reason not to proceed to a Phase II study is prohibitive toxicity in Phase I trials. Escalation of doses in Phase I trials is usually done by a modified Fibonacci system.[150] Doses are first doubled and then increased at decreasing increments of 66%, 50%, and 33% in succeeding groups of patients (usually three at a time) until limiting toxicity is noted. Recently, attempts have been made to rationalize and accelerate dose escalation by the systematic use of preclinical pharmacologic data.[154] This approach has relied on the assumption that the elimination rate of a drug determines its $C \times T$, and further assumes that for agents showing no major differences in target cell sensitivity, schedule dependence, or toxicity between mouse and man, the $C \times T$ at the mouse LD_{10} and the human MTD should be similar. These assumptions lead naturally to a simple algorithm for escalating doses by targeting the human $C \times T$ in a Phase I trial to the mouse $C \times T$ at LD_{10}.[155] The steps are as follows: (1) determine the mouse LD_{10} (part of the routine preclinical toxicology testing discussed earlier), (2) determine the

TABLE 16-8. National Cancer Institute Classification of New Anticancer Drugs in Clinical Testing

Group A Drugs
This group includes drugs in Phase I clinical trials and Phase II clinical trials in specified tumors. Protocol acceptance and drug distribution are limited to clinical investigators.

Group B Drugs
This group includes drugs already tested in initial Phase II studies and of clinical interest. Protocol acceptance and drug distribution are extended more broadly to clinical cooperative groups, NCI contractors, and cancer centers.

*Group C Drugs**
Group C includes drugs that demonstrate efficacy within a tumor type in more than one study, that alter the pattern of care of the disease in question, and that are administered safely by properly trained physicians without requiring specialized supportive care facilities. This group includes the following:

1. Azacytidine (NSC 102816)—for refractory acute myelogenous leukemia
2. Ervinia asparaginase (NSC 106977)—for acute lymphatic leukemia in patients sensitive to *E. coli* L-asparaginase
3. Hexamethylmelamine (NSC 13875)—for ovarian carcinoma
4. Amsacrine (NSE 249992)—for refractory myelogenous leukemia

* Drugs in Group C are available for use by physicians for specific indications.

TABLE 16-9. Procedure for Obtaining Drugs in Group C of the National Cancer Institute New Anticancer Drug Classification

A physician must be registered with the NCI as an investigator having completed an FDA-Form 1573.
A written request for the drug, indicating the disease to be treated, must be submitted.
Use of the drugs shall be limited to indications outlined in the guidelines that will be provided to the physician.
All adverse reactions must be reported to the Investigational Drug Branch, DCT, NCI.
Office of the Chief, Investigational Drug Branch, CTEP*, DCT, National Cancer Institute, 7910 Woodmont Avenue, Landow Building, Room 4A22, Bethesda, MD 20892 (301-496-6138).

* CTEP = Cancer Therapy Evaluation Program.

TABLE 16-10.   Stages in the Clinical Testing of New Anticancer Agents

Stage of Drug Testing	Objectives	Patient Population Studied
PHASE I	*Determine Tolerance* Maximally tolerable dose (MTD) Limiting toxicity Reversibility of toxicity Proper schedule *Pharmacology* Bioavailability Plasma clearance Biotransformation Excretion *Therapeutic Effect* Secondary	Histologically confirmed advanced malignancy No longer amenable to conventional therapy Physiologically well compensated A variety of tumor types per study permissible
PHASE II	*Therapeutic Effect* Determine effectiveness in a panel of human tumors Dose-response relationships *Nontherapeutic Effects* Toxicity in relationship to therapeutic effect	Histologically confirmed advanced malignancy Measurable tumor masses No longer amenable to conventional therapy A variety of tumor types in groups of 15 to 30 Physiologically well compensated
PHASE III	*Therapeutic Effectiveness* Compare experimental therapy to existing standard therapy *Nontherapeutic Effects* Are toxic effects tolerable in the context of observed therapeutic effect and in comparison to standard therapy?	Histologically confirmed malignancy Patient sample must be of adequate size and uniformity Usually previously untreated Controls usually are selected randomly, but on occasion historical controls are used
PHASE IV	*Therapeutic Effectiveness* Integration of drug therapy into primary treatment in combination with surgery or radiation therapy (*e.g.,* postoperative drug treatment in breast cancer) Compared to current standard program *Nontherapeutic Effects* Are toxic effects sufficiently minimal to risk giving drug to patients whose tumor will not necessarily recur? Long-term toxic effects require monitoring (second tumors, sterility, marrow aplasia)	Histologically confirmed malignancy Patient sample must be of adequate size and uniformity Controls usually randomized

mouse $C \times T$ at LD_{10}, (3) begin human testing at a safe starting dose (currently one-tenth of the mouse-equivalent LD_{10}), (4) determine the human $C \times T$ at the starting dose in Phase I, and (5) escalate doses in subsequent patients based on how close the $C \times T$ at the starting dose is to the target $C \times T$. Preliminary studies have suggested that application of this procedure may save 20% to 50% of escalation steps for many agents. This approach is now being tested prospectively in NCI's Phase I testing program.

The definition of a dose as maximally tolerated depends on how much toxicity the patient and physician are willing and able to tolerate. It has been amply demonstrated that for several drugs such as cyclophosphamide, thiotepa, BCNU, and etoposide, the MTD as determined from toxic effects other than bone marrow suppression is 3 to 10 times higher than the conventional MTD determined by granulocytopenia. The fact that the response rates are commonly a function of dose gives strong impetus to further trials exploring the upper end of the dose curve. As a result, an alternative approach to Phase I testing is under consideration, that is, to redefine the MTD as the dose beyond which unacceptable non-marrow-related toxicity supervenes despite deployment of all modern aspects of care. At the moment it seems prudent to delay decisions on escalation of new agents past the conventionally determined MTD until more information about their clinical characteristics is at hand. This approach should be greatly facilitated by the availability of colony-stimulating factors if they succeed in eliminating bone marrow suppression as the rate-limiting step in early testing.

The purpose of Phase II studies is to develop estimates of the response rate of patients with specified tumor types to a particular drug. Phase II studies determine activity, rather than efficacy, and answer a biologic as well as a clinical question. However, since Phase II study results do determine whether a new treatment should be pursued further, the outcome of the Phase II trial is clearly a decisive point in a drug's development. Specifically, a Phase II testing program should be constructed so as to (1) minimize the chance of a false negative result, (2) maximize the chance of benefit to the individual study patient, and (3) minimize the number of patients treated with drugs that turn out to be inactive. During the 1970s the NCI created a clinical Phase II panel to match the preclinical screening panel in histologic types to create a sufficiently large data base to permit validation of the transplantable murine screen as predictive of clinical activity in corresponding tumor types. An analysis of these data is currently in progress but reveals little correlation between murine and clinical activity for corresponding histologies.

When a drug enters Phase II testing in individual diseases, it should be tested in the patient group that is most likely to show a favorable effect, provided it is ethically permissible to do so. Failure to do this increases the chance of missing potentially useful activity. Obviously, this criterion is best fulfilled by enrolling patients with advanced cancer but who have maximum performance status, minimal heterogeneity of metastatic sites, and a minimal amount of prior chemotherapy.[156] This means that for tumors sensitive to chemotherapy, patients who have failed no more than one prior regimen are ideal for study. For the less sensitive epithelial cancers in many cases previously untreated patients can be entered into Phase II studies. In view of the poor track record of the large majority of single agents in heavily pretreated patients with advanced disease, such a strategy seems sensible, since for patients with advanced drug-resistant cancer, the likelihood of toxicity is vastly greater than the likelihood of therapeutic benefit.

The number of patients accrued to Phase II trials should be appropriate for the scientific goals of the study. Under the best of circumstances, a drug that produces no antitumor effect in 14 patients with the same tumor type, particularly if the heterogeneity of the distribution of metastases is minimized, has a greater than 95% chance of being ineffective against that tumor and could reasonably be dropped from further studies against that specific cancer. One or two responses, however, increase the chance of efficacy sufficiently to dictate an expansion of the trial to 30 or more patients, in order not to miss a drug with a response rate in the 20% range. In general, partial response rates in excess of 20% place the agent in a category of potential clinical usefulness to be determined in further studies. Response rates in the range of 5% to 10% are consistent with observer variation in Phase II trials. Response rates below 20% can be meaningful, however, if the quality of the response is good. For example, a few complete remissions, even if the overall frequency of complete response is low, should lead to a decision to proceed with further testing in that disease since complete disappearance of disease, however infrequent, is an important sign of a potentially effective new treatment. Because multiple doses and schedules may be tested, a Phase II trial for each drug, schedule, and tumor type is required before a drug can be disqualified from further clinical use. Given all these confounding variables, a complete Phase II trial often requires 600 or more patients.

At the completion of a Phase II trial, a decision is made to proceed with or discard the agent. This decision is based on lack of efficacy or excessive or intolerable toxicity, given the observed therapeutic effect. Because it is not possible to test each new agent against every tumor type, the potential for discarding agents that might be useful in rare tumors is significant. The early testing results of cisplatin are particularly instructive. Cisplatin showed very little activity against the common tumors in its early testing, its use was associated with considerable toxicity, and it was almost discarded. Incidental testing in patients with testicular cancer, who were not generally part of major Phase II studies, revealed interesting activity, and cisplatin was very quickly advanced to inclusion with other drugs to treat testicular cancer with curative intent. As a result, very little data on its single agent activity was available to the FDA in its appraisal of the new drug application, and marketing was delayed. This drug has now proved to be not only the mainstay of curative treatment of advanced testicular cancer, but an important part of the therapy of bladder cancer, head and neck cancer, ovarian cancer, and other common tumors.

If a drug is found effective in Phase II trials, Phase III and IV testing establishes its place in the therapeutic armamentarium. These clinical trials usually require large numbers of

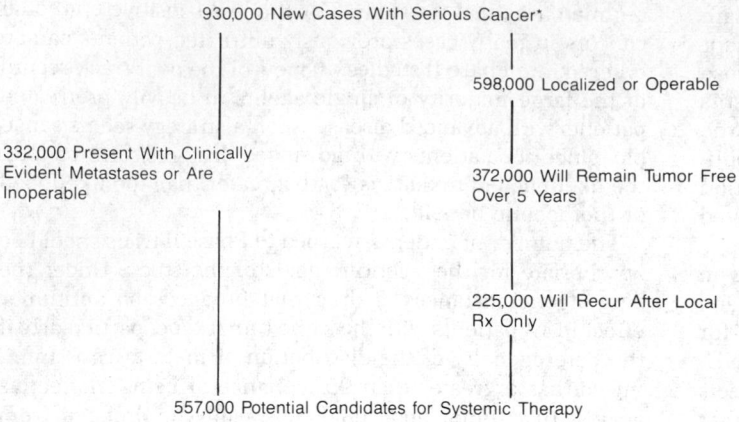

930,000 New Cases With Serious Cancer*

598,000 Localized or Operable

332,000 Present With Clinically
Evident Metastases or Are
Inoperable

372,000 Will Remain Tumor Free
Over 5 Years

225,000 Will Recur After Local
Rx Only

557,000 Potential Candidates for Systemic Therapy

FIG. 16-7. Distribution of cancer patients according to presentation and type of treatment. (Derived from 1986 data from the NCI's Surveillance, Epidemiology and End Results [SEER] Program)

*Total is 1,531,000; 580,000 cases of skin and in situ cervix and breast cancer are excluded.

patients and are difficult to perform. The issue of randomized versus historical controls in Phase III and IV trials is an important one and is discussed in detail in Chapter 19.

THE IMPACT OF CANCER CHEMOTHERAPY

Figure 16-7, using 1986 data, shows an estimate of the distribution of localized and advanced cancers in the United States. The majority of newly diagnosed cancer patients in 1986 (598,000) presented with what appeared to be localized cancers. These patients are primarily managed by surgeons and radiation therapists, with or without the help of medical and pediatric oncologists, and the goal of treatment at this stage is cure. Those who present with either clinically evident metastases (320,000 in 1986) or with recurrences after local treatment for localized tumor (225,000) are usually seen by medical oncologists because the correct treatment is systemic therapy. Thus, the total number of patients per year who might receive systemic therapy (557,000, based on 1986 data) is sizable. In recent years some patients in the latter two groups have also become candidates for treatment with surgery for metastases with curative intent.[157]

Survival rates have improved as new treatments have been introduced into practice, and national mortality has declined. The relative survival rate has been used as an indicator of improvements in management and curability of cancer because it is a comparison of the survival of cancer patients 5 years after diagnosis with survival of an age- and sex-matched control population without cancer.[5] Relative survival rates are good predictors of ultimate outcome since 20-year figures are about 85% of 5-year figures, the decrease largely accounted for by late recurrences in patients with breast, renal, and prostate cancers. Early surgical techniques and crude kilovoltage radiation therapy equipment led to about a 25% 5-year survival rate by the 1930s; this rose to about 33% in the 1950s.[5] Almost all of the improvement was attributable to improvements in surgical techniques and sup-

portive care. The introduction of cobalt radiation therapy units in 1953 and linear accelerators in 1957 gave radiation therapists the proper tools to compete with surgeons in treating some forms of localized cancers. The improvement in relative survival rates from about 33% in the 1950s to 37% by the mid-1960s can be largely attributed to widespread use of improved radiation therapy technology.

The impact of chemotherapy at a national level has appeared only recently. Chemotherapy was not introduced until the late 1950s and was not a consistent part of medical practice until the specialty of medical oncology was established in the early 1970s. By 1973 the U.S. 5-year relative survival rates had risen to 40%, and the most recent figures for the period ending in 1984 (Fig. 16-8) show a relative survival rate of 50% for the white population and 37% for blacks. This 30% improvement in survival rates in the past two decades can be attributed to further improvements in radiation therapy and to the rapid expansion of the use of

FIG. 16-8. Five-year relative survival rates for males and females, with all sites combined. (Data derived from the NCI's SEER Program)

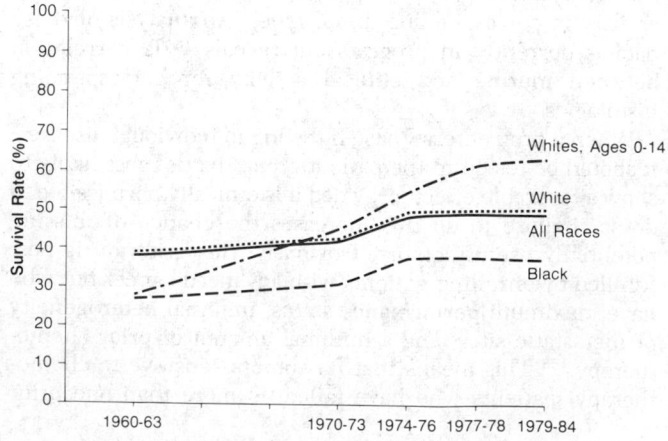

TABLE 16-11. Thirty-five-Year Trends in Cancer Mortality per 100,000 Persons, All Races, Both Sexes

	All Sites			All Sites Minus Lung		
Age	1950	1984	% Change	1950	1984	% Change
0–4	11.1	3.7	−66.7	11.0	3.7	−66.4
5–14	6.7	3.7	−44.8	6.6	3.6	−45.5
15–24	8.6	5.3	−38.4	8.4	5.2	−38.1
25–34	20.0	12.8	−36.0	19.1	12.2	−36.1
35–44	62.7	47.8	−23.8	57.6	39.9	−30.7
45–54	175.1	174.5	−0.3	152.2	121.8	−20.0
55–64	392.9	439.9	12.0	337.7	293.5	−13.1
65–74	692.5	835.9	20.7	623.2	582.6	−6.5
75–84	1,153.3	1,290.9	11.9	1,084.0	1,011.9	−6.7
85+	1,451.0	1,592.1	9.7	1,387.0	1,403.2	1.2
All Ages	157.7	170.7	8.2	144.7	125.1	−13.5

chemotherapy alone or added to surgery and radiation therapy.

A decrease in national mortality rates for cancer for which there is effective treatment also occurred steadily for the period 1950 to 1984 (Table 16-11). National mortality from cancer for patients below the age of 55 decreased most impressively owing to the development of successful treatment in younger patients with lymphomas, ovarian cancer, leukemias, and an array of childhood cancers. One point in Table 16-11 is worthy of emphasis. The impact of lung cancer, a disease that is not effectively treated but is almost totally preventable, is clearly demonstrated by the observation that a decrease in mortality from other cancers occurs up to age 85 when lung cancer mortality rates are examined separately.

Chemotherapy can cure some fraction of patients with advanced cancer of the types listed in Table 16-12. These cancers make up approximately 12% of human tumors. The impact in person-years of life saved is, however, disproportionately large because the younger average age at diagnosis results in a highly significant salvage of person-years of productive life. Other tumor types shown in Table 16-12 are treated for metastatic cancer with chemotherapy with substantial benefit, and in many cases, new treatments described elsewhere in this text offer the prospect of cure.

Systemic treatment bears a special burden of fear of toxicity in the minds of both doctors and patients, beyond that associated with surgery or radiation therapy, because its effects cannot be limited precisely to the region involved by tumor. Even though more sophisticated techniques of delivering systemic therapy to target organs have been developed, systemic toxicity is always a concomitant of systemic treatment. The same is true of biologicals. The promise of diminished side-effects with the use of biologic materials because they were natural products has not been fulfilled. A general principle is that all chemicals, natural or xenobiotic, when used in pharmacologic doses will produce significant side-effects. Patients cured of cancer by any modality generally find the toxicity associated with the treatment a justifiable expe-

TABLE 16-12. Tumors Responsive to Chemotherapy

Tumors Curable in Advanced Stages by Chemotherapy

Choriocarcinoma	Wilms' tumor
Acute lymphocytic leukemia (in children and adults)	Burkitt's lymphoma
Hodgkin's disease	Embryonal rhabdomyosarcoma
Diffuse large cell lymphoma	Ewing's sarcoma
Lymphoblastic lymphoma (in children and adults)	Peripheral neuroepithelioma
Follicular mixed lymphoma	Neuroblastoma
Testicular cancer	Small cell cancer of the lung
Acute myelogenous leukemia	Ovarian cancer

Tumors Curable in the Adjuvant Setting by Chemotherapy

Breast cancer	Soft tissue sarcoma
Osteogenic sarcoma	Colorectal cancer

Tumors Responsive in Advanced States But Not Yet Curable by Chemotherapy

Bladder cancer	Head and neck cancer
Chronic myelogenous leukemia	Endometrial cancer
Chronic lymphocytic leukemia	Adrenocortical carcinoma
Hairy cell leukemia	Medulloblastoma
Multiple myeloma	Polycythemia rubra vera
Follicular small-cleaved cell lymphoma	Prostate cancer
Gastric carcinoma	Glioblastoma multiforme
Cervical carcinoma	Insulinoma
Soft tissue sarcoma	Breast cancer
	Carcinoid tumors

Tumors Poorly Responsive in Advanced Stages to Chemotherapy

Osteogenic sarcoma	Colorectal cancer
Pancreatic cancer	Non-small cell lung cancer
Renal cancer	Melanoma
Thyroid cancer	Hepatocellular carcinoma
Carcinoma of the vulva or penis	

rience. For those with advanced unresponsive cancers, however, who have the burden of progressive tumor and impending death, the risks and side-effects of treatment should be carefully balanced against the potential benefits. Patients who are offered systemic therapy with a potential for cure should be treated aggressively; those for whom palliation is the only choice should not be overly burdened with very toxic treatments that may prolong life in an uncomfortable fashion. In practice this means that patients with metastatic cancer for whom there is no known effective systemic treatment are best advised to take part in one of the many clinical trials testing new treatments, or should be treated minimally to avoid undue side-effects.

To expand the benefits of chemotherapy, greater use of anticancer drugs before and after surgery and radiotherapy will be required, when tumor burden is at a minimum, kinetic features of cell growth are favorable, and drug resistance is less likely. Because patients sometimes feel themselves free of tumor after surgery, however, they may be less willing to accept the additional trauma of chemotherapy unless the benefits are carefully explained and accurately and honestly balanced against the chances of recurrence.

REFERENCES

1. DeVita VT: The evolution of therapeutic research in cancer. N Engl J Med 298:907–910, 1978
2. DeVita VT, Henney JE, Hubbard SM: Estimation of the numerical and economic impact of chemotherapy in the treatment of cancer. In Bruchenal JH, Oettgen HS (eds): Cancer Achievements, Challenges, and Prospects for the 1980s, pp 857–880. New York, Grune & Stratton, 1981
3. Steel GG: Cell loss from experimental tumors. Cell Tissue Kinet 1:193–207, 1968
4. Tannock IF: Biology of tumor growth. Hosp Pract, pp 81–93, 1983
5. Marshall EK Jr: Historical perspectives in chemotherapy. In Goldin A, Hawking IF (eds): Advances in Chemotherapy, vol 1, pp 1–8. New York, Academic Press, 1964
6. Hersh SM: Chemical and biological warfare: America's hidden arsenal. New York, Bobbs Merrill, 1968
7. Alexander SF: Final report of Bari mustard casualties. Allied Force Headquarters, Office of the Surgeon, APO 512, June 20, 1944
8. Skipper HE, Schabel FM Jr, Wilcox WS: Experimental evaluation of potential anticancer agents: XII. On the criteria and kinetics associated with "curability" of experimental leukemia. Cancer Chemother Rep 35:1–111, 1964
9. Skipper HE: Reasons for success and failure in treatment of murine leukemias with the drugs now employed in treating human leukemias. Cancer Chemotherapy, vol 1, pp 1–166. Ann Arbor, MI, University Microfilms International, 1978
10. Skipper HE, Schabel FM Jr, Mellet LB et al: Implications of biochemical, cytokinetic, pharmacologic, and toxicologic relationships in the design of optimal therapeutic schedules. Cancer Chemother Rep 54:431–450, 1950
11. Yankee RA, DeVita VT, Perry S: The cell cycle of leukemia L1210 cells in vivo. Cancer Res 27:2381–2385, 1968
12. Young RC, DeVita VT: Cell cycle characteristics of human solid tumors in vivo. Cell Tissue Kinet 3:285–295, 1970
13. Clarkson B, Ohkita T, Ota K et al: Studies of the cellular proliferation in human leukemia: I. Estimation of growth rates of leukemia and normal hematopoietic cells in two adults with acute leukemia given single injections of tritiated thymidine. J Clin Invest 46:506–529, 1967
14. Whang-Peng J, Perry S, Knutsen TA et al: Cell cycle characteristics, maturation and phagocytosis in vitro in blast cells from patients with chronic myelocytic leukemia. Blood 38:153–161, 1971
15. Tannock I: Cell kinetics and chemotherapy: A critical review. Cancer Treat Rep 62:1117–1133, 1978
16. Perry S, Moxley JH, Weiss GH et al: Studies of leukocyte function by liquid scintillation counting in normal individuals and in patients with chronic myelocytic leukemia. J Clin Invest 45:1388–1399, 1966
17. DeVita VT, Denham C, Perry S: Relationship of normal CDF_1 mouse leukocyte kinetics to growth characteristics of leukemia L1210. Cancer Res 29:1067–1071, 1969
18. Simpson-Herren L, Sanford AH, Holmquist JP: Cell population kinetics of transplanted Lewis lung carcinoma. Cell Tissue Kinet 7:349–361, 1974
19. Mendelsohn ML: The growth fraction: A new concept applied to tumors. Science 132:1496, 1960
20. Luria SE, Delbruck M: Mutations of bacteria from virus sensitivity to virus resistance. Genetics 28:491–511, 1943
21. Goldie JH, Coldman AJ: A mathematic model for relating the drug sensitivity of tumors to the spontaneous mutation rate. Cancer Treat Rep 63:1727–1733, 1979
22. Yunis J: The chromosomal basis of human neoplasia. Science 221(4607):227–236, 1983
23. Schabel FM Jr, Simpson-Herren L: Some variables in experimental tumor systems which complicate interpretation of data from in vivo kinetic and pharmacologic studies with anticancer drugs. Antibiot Chemother 23:113–127, 1978
24. Freireich EJ et al: Quantitative comparison of toxicity of anticancer agents in mouse, rat, dog, monkey and man. Cancer Chemother Rep 50:219–244, 1966
25. Brockman RW: Circumvention of resistance: Pharmacologic basis of cancer chemotherapy. In Proceedings of the 27th Annual Symposium on Fundamental Research, pp 691–711. Baltimore, Williams & Wilkins, 1975
26. DeVita VT Jr, Young RC, Canellos GP: Combination versus single agent chemotherapy: Review of the basis of selection of drug treatment of cancer. Cancer 35:98, 1975
27. Hutchinson DJ, Schmid FA: Cross-resistance and collateral sensitivity. In Mihich E (ed): Drug-Resistance and Selectivity: Biochemical and Cellular Basis, pp 73–126. New York, Academic Press, 1973
28. Brockman RW: Resistance to therapeutic agents. In Bruchenal JH, Oettgen HS (eds): Cancer Achievements, Challenges, and Prospects for the 1980s. New York, Grune & Stratton (in press)
29. Hutchinson DJ: Cross-resistance and collateral sensitivity studies in cancer chemotherapy. In Haddow A, Weinhouse S (eds): Advances in Cancer Research, vol 7, pp 235–350. New York, Academic Press, 1963
30. Klein M: A mechanism for the development of resistance to streptomycin and penicillin. J Bacteriol 53:463–467, 1947
31. Furth J, Kahn MC: The transmission of leukemia of mice with a single cell. Am J Cancer 31:276–282, 1937
32. Goldin A, Venditti JM, Humphries SR et al: Influences of the concentration of leukemic inoculum on the effectiveness of treatment. Science 123:840, 1956
33. Vickers PJ, Townsend AJ, Cowan KH: Mechanisms of resistance to antineoplastic drugs. CRC Crit Rev Dev Cancer Chemother (in press)
34. Ozols RJ, Cowan KH: New aspects of clinical drug resistance: The role of gene amplification and the reversal of drug refractory cancer. In DeVita VT Jr, Hellman S, Rosenberg SA (eds): Important Advances in Oncology 1986, pp 129–157. Philadelphia, JB Lippincott, 1986
35. Biedler JL, Riehm H: Cellular resistance to actinomycin D in Chinese hamster cells in vitro: Cross-resistance, radioautographic and cytogenic studies. Cancer Res 30:1174–1184, 1970
36. Juliano RL, Ling V: A surface glycoprotein modulating drug permeability in Chinese hamster ovary cell mutants. Biochem Biophys Acta 455:152–162, 1976
37. Bech-Hanson NT, Till JE, Ling V: Pleiotropic phenotype of colchicine-resistant CHO cells: Cross-resistance and collateral sensitivity. J Cell Physiol 88:23–32, 1976
38. Ling V, Thompson LH: Reduced permeability in CHO cells as a mechanism of resistance to colchicine. J Cell Physiol 83:103–116, 1973
39. Kartner N, Riordan JR, Ling V: Cell surface P-glycoprotein as associated with multidrug resistance in mammalian cell lines. Science 221:1285–1288, 1983
40. Fojo AT, Whang-Peng J, Gottesman MM et al: Amplification of DNA sequences in human multidrug resistant KB carcinoma cells. Proc Natl Acad Sci USA 82:7661–7665, 1985
41. Gros P, Croop J, Roninson I et al: Isolation and characterization of DNA sequences amplified in multidrug-resistant hamster cells. Proc Natl Acad Sci USA 83:337–341, 1986
42. Fairchild CR, Ivy SP, Kao-Shan CS et al: Isolation of amplified DNA sequences associated with pleiotropic drug resistance from human breast cancer cells. Cancer Res 47:5141–5148, 1987
43. Scotto KW, Biedler JL, Melera PW: Amplification and expression of genes associated with multidrug resistance in mammalian cells. Science 232:751–755, 1986
44. Roninson IB, Abelson HT, Housman DE et al: Amplification of specific DNA sequences correlates with multidrug resistance in Chinese hamster cells. Nature 309:2070–2076, 1984
45. Corwell MM, Safa AR, Felsted RL et al: Membrane vesicles from multidrug-resistant human cancer cells contain a specific 150 to 170-kDa protein detected by photoaffinity labelling. Proc Natl Acad Sci USA 83:3847–3850, 1986
46. Safa AR, Glover CI, Meyers CB et al: Vinblastine photoaffinity labeling of a high molecular weight surface membrane glycoprotein specific for multidrug-resistant cells. J Biol Chem 261:6137–6140, 1986
47. Cornwell MM, Pastan I, Gottesman MM: Certain calcium channel blockers bind specifically to multidrug-resistant human KB carcinoma membrane vesicles and inhibit drug binding to P-glycoprotein. J Biol Chem 262:2166–2170, 1987
48. Gros P, Croop J, Housman D: Mammalian multidrug-resistance gene: Complete cDNA sequence indicates strong homology to bacterial transport proteins. Cell 47:371–374, 1986
49. Chen C-J, Chin JE, Ueda K et al: Internal duplication and homology to bacterial transport proteins in the mdrl (P-glycoprotein) gene from multidrug-resistant human cells. Cell 47:381–389, 1986
50. Gerlach JH, Endicott JA, Juranka PF et al: Homology between P-glycoprotein and a bacterial haemolysin transport protein suggests a model for multidrug resistance. Nature 324:485–489, 1986
50a. Pasten IH, Gottesman MM: Molecular biology of multidrug resistance in human cells. In DeVita VT, Hellman S, Rosenberg SA (eds): Important Advances in Oncology 1988, pp 3–16. Philadelphia, JB Lippincott, 1988

51. Fojo AT, Ueda K, Slamon DJ et al: Expression of a multidrug-resistant gene in human tumors and tissues. Proc Natl Acad Sci USA 84:265–269, 1987

52. Endicott JA, Juranka PF, Sarangi F et al: Simultaneous expression of two P-glycoprotein genes in drug sensitive Chinese hamster ovary cells. Mol Cell Biol 7:4075–4081, 1987

53. Gros P, Ben Neriah Y, Croop JM et al: Isolation and expression of a complementary cDNA that confers multidrug resistance. Nature 323:728–731, 1986

54. Van Der Bliek AM, Baas F, Ten Houte de Lange T et al: The human mdr3 gene encodes a novel P-glycoprotein homologue and gives rise to alternatively spliced mRNAs in liver. EMBO J 6:3325–3331, 1987

55. Beck WT, Mueller TJ, Tanzer LR: Altered surface membrane glycoproteins in vinca alkaloid–resistant human leukemia lymphoblasts. Cancer Res 39:2070–2076, 1979

56. Riordan JR, Deuchars K, Kartner N et al: Amplification of P-glycoprotein genes in multidrug resistant mammalian cell lines. Nature 316:817–819, 1985

57. Louie KG, Hamilton TC, Winker MA et al: Adriamycin accumulation and metabolism in Adriamycin-sensitive and -resistant human ovarian cancer cell lines. Biochem Pharmacol 35:476–472, 1986

58. Chang BK, Gregory JA: Comparison of cellular pharmacology of doxorubicin in resistant and sensitive models of pancreatic cancer. Cancer Chemother Pharmacol 14:132–134, 1985

59. Seigfried JM, Tritton TR, Sartorelli AC: Comparison of anthracycline concentrations in S180 cell lines of varying sensitivity. Eur J Clin Oncol 19:1133–1141, 1983

60. Solt DB, Medline A, Farber E: Rapid emergence of carcinogen-induced hyperplastic lesions in a new model for the sequential analysis of liver carcinogenesis. Am J Pathol 88:595–618, 1977

61. Farber E, Parker S, Gruenstein M: The resistance of putative premalignant liver cell populations, hyperplastic nodules, to the acute cytotoxic effect of some hepatocarcinogens. Cancer Res 36:3879–3887, 1976

62. Fairchild CR, Ivy SP, Rushmore T et al: Carcinogen-induced mdr overexpression is associated with xenobiotic resistance in rat preneoplastic liver nodules and hepatocellular carcinomas. Proc Natl Acad Sci USA 84:7701–7705, 1987

63. Cowan KH, Batist G, Tulpule A et al: Similar biochemical changes associated with multidrug resistance in human breast cancer cells and carcinogen-induced resistance to xenobiotics in rats. Proc Natl Acad Sci USA 83:9328–9332, 1986

64. Moscow JA, Cowan KH: Multidrug resistance. JNCI 80:14–20, 1988

65. Marsh W, Center MS: Adriamycin resistance in HL60 cells and accompanying modifications of a membrane protein contained in drug-sensitive cells. Cancer Res 47:5080–5086, 1987

66. Danks MK, Yalowich JC, Bech WT: Atypical multiple drug resistance in a human leukemic cell line selected for resistance to teniposide (VM-26). Cancer Res 47:1297–1301, 1987

67. Ross WE, Sullivan DM, Chow KC: Altered function of DNA topoisomerases as a basis for antineoplastic drug action. In DeVita VT, Hellman S, Rosenberg S (eds): Import Advances in Oncology 1988, pp 65–81. Philadelphia, JB Lippincott, 1988

68. Glisson B, Gupta R, Hodges P et al: Cross resistance to intercalating agents in an epipodophyllotoxin-resistant Chinese hamster ovary cell line: Evidence for a common intracellular target. Cancer Res 46:1939–1942, 1986

69. Pommier Y, Kerrigan D, Schwartz RE et al: Altered DNA topoisomerase II activity in Chinese hamster cells resistant to topoisomerase II inhibitors. Cancer Res 46:3075–3081, 1986

70. Tsuruo T, Iida H, Tsukagoshi S et al: Increased accumulation of vincristine and Adriamycin in drug-resistant P388 tumor cells following incubation with calcium antagonists and calmodulin inhibitors. Cancer Res 42:4730–4733, 1982

71. Fitzgerald DJ, Willingham MC, Cardarelli CO et al: A monoclonal antibody-*Pseudomonas* toxin conjugate that specifically kills multidrug resistant cells. Proc Natl Acad Sci USA 84:4288–4292, 1987

72. Meister A: Selective modification of glutathione metabolism. Science 220:472–477, 1983

73. Kramer RA, Greene K, Ahmad S et al: Chemosensitization of L-phenylalanine mustards by the thiol-modulating agent buthionine sulfoximine. Cancer Res 47:1593–1597, 1987

74. Ozols RF, Louie KG, Plowman J et al: Enhanced melphalan toxicity in human ovarian cancer in vitro and in tumor-bearing nude mice by buthionine sulfoximine depletion of glutathione. Biochem Pharmacol 36:147–153, 1987

75. Russo A, Mitchell JB: Potentiation and protection of doxorubicin cytotoxicity by cellular glutathione modulation. Cancer Treat Rep 69:1293–1296, 1985

76. Skipper H: Data and Analyses Having To Do with the Influence of Dose Intensity and Duration of Treatment (Single Drugs and Combinations) on Lethal Toxicity and the Therapeutic Response of Experimental Neoplasms. Southern Research Institute, Booklets 13, 1986, and 2–13, 1987

77. DeVita VT, Hubbard SM, Longo DL: The chemotherapy of lymphomas: looking back, moving forward. The Richard and Hinda Rosenthal Foundation Award Lecture. Cancer Res 47:5810–5824, 1987

78. Hryniuk WM: The importance of dose intensity in the outcome of chemotherapy. In DeVita VT, Hellman S, Rosenberg SA (eds): Important Advances in Oncology 1988, pp 121–142. Philadelphia, JB Lippincott, 1988

79. Hryniuk W, Levine MN: Analysis of dose intensity for adjuvant chemotherapy trials in stage II breast cancer. J Clin Oncol 4:1162–1170, 1986

80. Hryniuk W: Average relative dose intensity and the impact on design on clinical trials. Semin Oncol 14:65–74, 1987

81. Levin L, Hryniuk W: Dose intensity analysis of chemotherapy regimens in ovarian carcinoma. J Clin Oncol 5:756–767, 1987

82. Hryniuk W, Bush H: The importance of dose intensity in chemotherapy of metastatic breast cancer. J Clin Oncol 2:1281–1288, 1984

83. Hryniuk W: Editorial: Is more better? J Clin Oncol 4:621–622, 1986

84. Canellos GP, Pocock SJ, Taylor SG III et al: Combination chemotherapy for metastatic breast cancer: Prospective comparison of multiple drug therapy with L-phenylalanine mustard. Cancer 38:1882–1886, 1976

85. Canellos GP, DeVita VT, Gold GL et al: Cyclical combination chemotherapy for advanced breast cancer. Br Med J 1:218–220, 1974

86. Bonadonna G, Brusamalino MP, Valagussa R et al: Combination chemotherapy as an adjuvant treatment in operable breast cancer. N Engl J Med 298:405–410, 1976

87. Bonadonna G, Valagussa R: Dose response effect of adjuvant chemotherapy in breast cancer. N Engl J Med 304:10–15, 1981

88. Horton J, Olson KB, Sullivan J et al: 5-Fluorouracil in cancer: An improved regimen. Ann Intern Med 78:897–900, 1970

89. Grage TB, Moss SE: Adjuvant chemotherapy in cancer of the colon and rectum: Demonstration of effectiveness of prolonged 5-FU chemotherapy in a prospectively controlled randomized trial. Surg Clin North Am 61:1321–1329, 1981

90. Higgins GA, Dwight RW, Smith JV et al: Fluorouracil as an adjuvant to surgery in carcinoma of the colon. Arch Surg 102:339–343, 1971

91. Higgins GA Jr, Humphrey E, Juler GL et al: Adjuvant chemotherapy in the surgical treatment of large bowel cancer. Cancer 38:1461–1467, 1976

92. Lawrence W Jr, Terz JJ, Horsley JS et al: Chemotherapy as an adjuvant to surgery for colorectal cancer. Arch Surg 113:164–168, 1978

93. Grossi CE, Wolff WI, Nealon TF Jr et al: Intraluminal fluorouracil chemotherapy adjunct to surgical procedures for resectable carcinoma of the colon and rectum. Surg Gynecol Obstet 145:549–554, 1977

94. Nathanson L, Hall TC, Schilling AC et al: Concurrent combination chemotherapy of human solid tumors: Experience with three-drug regimen and review of the literature. Cancer Res 29:419–425, 1969

95. Potter VR: Sequential blocking of metabolic pathways in vivo. Proc Soc Exp Biol Med 76:41–46, 1951

96. Elion GB, Singer S, Hitchings GH: Antagonists of nucleic acid derivatives: VIII. Synergism in combinations of biochemically related antimetabolites. J Biol Chem 208:47–488, 1954

97. Sartorelli AC: Approaches to the combination chemotherapy of transplantable neoplasms. Prog Ext Tumor Res 6:228–288, 1965

98. DeVita VT, Schein PS: The use of drugs in combination for the treatment of cancer: Rationale and results. N Engl J Med 288:998–1006, 1973

99. Yagoda A: Use of M-VAC on colony stimulating factors. In DeVita VT, Hellman S, Rosenberg S (eds): Important Advances in Oncology 1988. Philadelphia, JB Lippincott, 1988

100. DeVita VT: Only if you believe in magic. In Jones SE, Salmon SE (eds): Adjuvant Therapy of Cancer IV, pp 3–16. Orlando, Fla, Grune & Stratton, 1984

101. DeVita VT: On the value of response criteria in therapeutic research. In: Proceedings of the 2nd International Congress on Neoadjuvant Chemotherapy. Bull Cancer Colloque INSERM (in press)

102. Holland JF: Induction chemotherapy: An old term for an old concept. In: Neoadjuvant Chemotherapy. Colloque INSERM 137:45–47, 1986

103. Frei A III, Clark JR, Miller D: The concept of neoadjuvant chemotherapy. In: Adjuvant Therapy of Cancer V, p 67. Orlando, Fla, Grune & Stratton, 1987

104. Muggia FM: Primary chemotherapy: Concepts and issues. In: Primary Chemotherapy in Cancer Medicine, pp 377–383. New York, Alan R Liss, 1985

105. Goldie JH: Scientific basis for adjuvant and primary (neoadjuvant) chemotherapy. Semin Oncol 14:1–7, 1987

106. Simpson-Herron L, Sanford AH, Holmquist JP: Effects of surgery on the cell kinetics of residual tumor. Cancer Treat Rep 60:1749–1760, 1976

107. DeVita VT: The relationship between tumor mass and resistance to treatment of cancer. Cancer 51:1209–1220, 1983

108. Skipper HE: Critical variables in the design of combination chemotherapy regimens to be used alone or in adjuvant setting. In: Neoadjuvant Chemotherapy. Colloque INSERM 137:11–12, 1986

109. Dedrick RL, Myers CE, Bungay PM et al: Pharmacokinetic rationale for peritoneal drug administration in treatment of ovarian cancer. Cancer Treat Rep 62:1–11, 1978

110. Jones RB, Myers CE, Guarino AM et al: High volume intraperitoneal chemotherapy ("belly bath") for ovarian cancer: Pharmacologic basis and early results. Cancer Chemother Pharmacol 1:161–166, 1978

111. Jones RB, Collins JM, Myers CE et al: High volume intraperitoneal chemotherapy with methotrexate in patients with cancer. Cancer Res (in press)

112. Papahadjopoulos D, Poste G, Vail WJ et al: Use of lipid vesicles as carriers to introduce actinomycin D into resistant tumor cells. Cancer Res 36:2988–3012, 1976

113. Weinstein JM, Magin RL, Cysyk RL et al: Treatment of solid L1210 murine tumors with local hyperthermia and temperature-sensitive liposomes containing methotrexate. Cancer Res 40:1388–1396, 1980

114. Weinstein JN: Liposomes as drug carriers in cancer therapy. Cancer Treat Rep 68:127–135, 1984

115. Weisenthal LM, Lippman ME: Clonogenic and non-clonogenic in vitro chemosensitivity assays. Cancer Treat Rep 69:615–632, 1985

116. Von Hoff DD, Weisenthal L: In vitro methods to predict patient response to chemotherapy. Adv Pharmacol Chemother 7:133–156, 1980

117. Von Hoff DD, Clark GM, Stogdill BJ et al: Prospective clinical trial of a human tumor cloning system. Cancer Res 43:1926–1931, 1983

118. Alberts DS, Leigh SA, Moon TE et al: Improved survival for relapsing ovarian cancer

patients using the human clonogenic assay to select chemotherapy, p 31. In: Proceedings of the 4th Conference on Human Tumor Cloning, 1984

119. Twentyman PR: Predictive chemosensitivity testing. J Cancer 51:295–299, 1985

120. Von Hoff DD: "Send this patient's tumor for culture and sensitivity." N Engl J Med 308:154, 1983

121. Von Hoff DD, Clark GM: Drug sensitivity of primary versus metastases. In: Salmon SE, Trent JN (eds): Human Tumor Cloning. Orlando, Fla, Grune & Stratton, 1984

122. Weisenthal LM, Marsden JA, Dill PL et al: A novel dye exclusion method for testing in vitro chemosensitivity of human tumors. Cancer Res 43:749–757, 1983

123. Weisenthal LM, Dill PL, Kurnick NB et al: Comparison of dye exclusion assays with a clonogenic assay in the determination of drug-induced cytotoxicity. Cancer Res 43:258–264, 1983

124. Weisenthal LM, Marsden JA, Macaluso CK et al: In vitro chemosensitivity assay based on the concept of total tumor cell kill. Recent Cancer Res (in press)

125. Bosanquet AG, Bird MC, Price WJP et al: An assessment of a short-term tumour chemosensitivity assay to chronic lymphocytic leukemia. Br J Cancer 74:781–789, 1983

126. Ihde D, Russell E, Oic HK et al: Prospective clinical trial of individualized chemotherapy based on in vitro drug sensitivity testing in extensive stage small cell lung cancer. In: Adjuvant Therapy of Cancer V, pp 201–207. Orlando, Fla, Grune & Stratton, 1987

127. Bodgen AE, Kelton DE, Cobb WR et al: A rapid screening method for testing chemotherapeutic agents against human tumor xenografts. In Houchens DP, Ovejera AA (eds): Proceedings of the Symposium on the Use of Athymic (Nude) Mice in Cancer Research, pp 231–250. New York, Gustav Fisher, 1978

128. Griffin TW, Bodgen AE, Reich SD et al: Initial clinical trials of the subrenal capsule assay as a predictor of tumor response to chemotherapy. Cancer 52:2185–2192, 1983

129. Pihl A: UICC study group on chemosensitivity testing of human tumors: Problems — applications — future prospects. Int J Cancer 37:1–5, 1986

130. Gorelik E, Ovejera A, Shoemaker R et al: Micro-encapsulated tumor assay: New short-term assay for in vivo evaluation of the effects of anticancer drugs on human tumor cell lines. Cancer Res 47:5739–5747, 1987

131. Schroy III PC, Cohen A, Winowar SJ et al: New chemotherapeutic drug sensitivity assay for colon carcinomas in monolayer culture. Cancer Res 48:3236–3244, 1988

132. Ajani JA, Baker FL, Spitzer G et al: Comparison between clinical response and in vitro drug sensitivity of primary human tumors in the adhesive tumor cell culture system. J Clin Oncol 5:1912–1921, 1987

133. Gazdar AF, Carney DN, Russel EK et al: Small cell carcinoma of the lung: Establishment of continuous, clonable cell lines having APUD properties. Cancer Res 40:3502–3507, 1980

134. Carney DN, Mitchell JB, Kinsella TJ: In vitro radiation and chemosensitivity of established cell lines of human small cell lung cancer and its large cell morphological variants. Cancer Res 43:2806–2811, 1983

135. Kornblith PL, Smith BH, Leonard LA: Response of cultured human brain tumors to nitrosourceas: Correlation with clinical data. Cancer 47:255–265, 1981

136. Goldin A, Schepartz SA, Venditti JM et al: Historical development and current strategy of the National Cancer Institute Drug Development Program. In DeVita VT, Busch H (eds): Methods of Cancer Research, vol XVI, Cancer Drug Development, Part A, pp 165–247. New York, Academic Press, 1979

137. DeVita VT, Oliverio VT, Muggia FM et al: The Drug Development Program and Clinical Trials Programs of the Division of Cancer Treatment, National Cancer Institute. Cancer Clin Trials 2:195–216, 1979

138. Zubrod CG, Schepartz S, Leiter J et al: The Chemotherapy Program of the National Cancer Institute: History, analysis, and plans. Cancer Chemother Rep 50:349–540, 1966

139. Hirschberg E: Patterns of response of animal tumors to anticancer agents. Cancer Res 23 (suppl 5, Part 2):521–980, 1963

140. Driscol JS: The preclinical new drug research program of the National Cancer Institute. Cancer Treat Rep 68:63–76, 1984

141. Shoemaker RH, Wolpert-DeFilippes MK, Venditti JM: Potentials and drawbacks of the human tumor stem cell assay. Behring Inst Mitt 74:262–272, 1984

142. Rockwell S: Effects of clumps and clusters on survival measurements with clonogenic assays. Cancer Res 45:1601–1607, 1985

143. Shoemaker RH, Wolpert-DeFilippes MK, Kern DH et al: Application of a human tumor colony-forming assay to new drug screening. Cancer Res 45:2145–2153, 1985

144. Boyd M, Shoemaker R, Alley M et al: New NCI disease-oriented drug screening program. In: Proceedings of the 5th NCI-EORTC Symposium on New Drugs in Cancer Therapy. Amsterdam, 1986

145. Boyd MR, Shoemaker RH, McLemore TL et al: New drug development. In Roth JA, Ruckdescel JC, Weisenburger THE (eds): Thoracic Oncology. Philadelphia, WB Saunders, 1987

146. Alley MC, Scudiero DA, Monks A et al: Feasibility of drug screening with panels of human tumor cell lines using a microculture tetrazolium assay. Cancer Res 48:589–601, 1988

147. Mosmann T: Rapid colorimetric assay for cellular growth and survival: Application to proliferation and cytotoxicity assays. J Immunol Methods 65:55–63, 1983

148. Shoemaker RH: New approaches to antitumor drug screening: The human tumor colony forming assay. Cancer Treat Rep 70:9–12, 1986

149. Rozencweig M, Von Hoff DD, Staquet MJ et al: Predictive value of animal toxicology with anticancer agents prior to early clinical trials (abstr). Clin Res 27(2):391A, 1979

150. Muggia FM, Rozencweig M, Chiuten DF et al: Phase II trials: Use of a clinical tumor panel and overview of current resources and studies. Cancer Treat Rep 64:1–9, 1980

151. Wooley PV, Schein PS: Clinical pharmacology and phase I trial design. In DeVita VT, Busch H (eds): Methods in Cancer Research. XVII. Cancer Drug Development, part B, pp 177–199, 1979

152. Muggia FM, McGuire WP, Rozencweig M: Rationale, design and methodology of phase II clinical trials. In DeVita VT, Busch H (eds): Methods in Cancer Research. XVII. Cancer Drug Development, part B, pp 199–215, 1979

153. Von Hoff DD, Rozencweig M, Soper WT et al: Commentary: Whatever happened to NSC---? An analysis of clinical results of discontinued anticancer agents. Cancer Treat Rep 61:759–768, 1977

154. Collins JM, Zaharko DS, Dedrick RL et al: Potential roles for preclinical pharmacology in phase I clinical trials. Cancer Treat Rep 70:73, 1986

155. Goldin A, Venditti JM: Progress report on the screening program at the Division of Cancer Treatment, National Cancer Institute. Cancer Treat Rev 7:167, 1980

156. Marsoni S, Hoth D, Simon R et al: Clinical drug development: An analysis of phase II trials, 1970–1985. Cancer Treat Rep 71:71, 1987

157. Rosenberg SA (ed): Surgical Treatment of Metastatic Cancer. Philadelphia, JB Lippincott, 1987

STEVEN A. ROSENBERG

DAN L. LONGO

MICHAEL T. LOTZE

CHAPTER 17 *Principles and Applications of Biologic Therapy*

"Biologic therapy" refers to cancer treatment that produces antitumor effects primarily through the action of natural host defense mechanisms or by the administration of natural mammalian substances. Biologic therapy has emerged in the last several years as an important fourth modality for the treatment of cancer. This growth has resulted from an increased understanding of the basic aspects of host defense mechanisms against cancer and the rapid development of biotechnologies that have made molecules, previously obtainable only in minute amounts, available in quantities large enough for use in manipulating in vivo biologic processes. Although this field is still in the infancy of its development, many examples now exist of the successful application of biologic therapy to the treatment of cancer in humans.

BASIC PRINCIPLES OF TUMOR IMMUNOLOGY

Most efforts to utilize biologic therapy for the treatment of cancer have involved attempts to stimulate immune defense mechanisms. The immune system evolved as a means to detect and eliminate substances that are recognized as "nonself" and thus eliminate foreign molecules or pathogens yet not react to host (self) tissues. Thus, many biologic immune

therapies have involved attempts to cause the tumor to appear more "foreign" compared with normal tissues or to find means for magnifying relatively weak host immune reactions to growing tumors.

The immune system differs from most other organ systems because its cells are not in constant contact with each other. Rather, they circulate freely throughout the body both in and out of the circulatory and lymphatic systems. Immune reactivity involves the integrated action of a large number of different cell types, including lymphocytes, monocytes, macrophages, basophils, eosinophils, dendritic cells, endothelial cells, and many others throughout the body. Although separate functions have been assigned to these cell types, it is now clear that they interact in many ways and can regulate each others' activities.

Immune cells secrete two major classes of soluble protein. The first of these lymphocyte products to be recognized was the antibody. Antibodies are a group of proteins composed of one or several units, each of which is composed of two pairs of different polypeptide chains (heavy and light chains). Each unit possesses two recognition sites, which are capable of combining with the immunizing antigen. The unique bond between antigen and antibody is part of the basis for the exquisite specificity that is the hallmark of immunologic reactivity. The existence of circulating antibodies was first demonstrated in 1890, and until recently, scientific studies of antibodies monopolized the study of immune reactions.

301

Over the past two decades, it has become clear that selected subpopulations of lymphoid cells can secrete a second (nonantibody) class of protein molecules. These molecules are not biochemically similar to antibodies, are produced in tiny amounts, and are not normally detectable in the circulation. Collectively called cytokines, they represent a new class of hormones with actions on many different target cells both within and outside the immune system. Increasing knowledge of a wide variety of cytokines has dramatically altered our understanding of the functions of the immune system and has opened new possibilities for the immunotherapy of human cancer.

CELLS OF THE IMMUNE SYSTEM

The central cell in immune function is the lymphocyte. Lymphocytes constitute approximately 20% of blood leukocytes and fall into three major classes—B cells, T cells, and null cells—on the basis of ontogeny and function. Recently, however, analysis of cell-surface molecules, usually using monoclonal antibodies, has revealed substantial heterogeneity in human leukocytes and lymphocytes. In November 1982, the First International Workshop on Human Leukocyte Differentiation Antigens was held in Paris to attempt to codify the proliferating number of cell-surface determinants detected on leukocytes and the antibodies used to detect them. As a result of the testing of large numbers of antibodies on target cells of many different leukocyte types, cluster analysis permitted the definition of groups of antigens that are similar and those that are clearly different on each type of target cell. This workshop led to the definition of "clusters of differentiation" (CD), which are now used to define cell-surface components on leukocytes. A summary of selected CD classifications, the cells on which they are found, and the principal antibodies that are used to detect them is shown in Table 17-1.

In birds, B cells develop in a special organ called the bursa of Fabricius. There is no anatomical counterpart of this bursa in man; instead, it is thought that human B cells develop in the bone marrow and acquire surface immunoglobulin, which acts as their antigen receptor. B cells also develop receptors for lymphokines, which enable their regulation by T-cell products. B cells require both the presence of antigen and help from antigen-specific T cells to produce and secrete antibodies.

The term "T cells" was derived from the role of the thymus in the differentiation of these lymphocytes. Lymphoid cells produced in the bone marrow traffic to the thymus late in fetal life, differentiate there, and then seed secondary lymphoid tissues. In the thymus, T cells are thought to acquire antigen-specific receptors and to differentiate into the various T-cell subpopulations. Death of many lymphocytes occurs in the thymus during ontogeny, which is thought to be, in part, the mechanism for the loss of self-reactive clones. T cells are involved in cellular immune reactions and recognize antigen via receptor molecules quite distinct from the immunoglobulin found on B cells. The T-cell receptor is generated from the recombination of germ-line genes to produce a wide diversity of receptors that can bind antigen together with self-MHC (major histocompatibility complex) molecules. Thus the generation of diversity in T-cell receptors is similar to that of antibodies. The T-cell receptor for antigen is associated with a glycoprotein complex, T3, present on all mature human T cells. Whereas B cells can recognize antigen alone, T cells recognize antigen in association with MHC molecules.

Although T cells were initially subtyped by functions (helper, suppressor, cytotoxic), it has now been possible to identify two major T-cell subsets, each of which is restricted to recognizing one of the two major classes of major histocompatibility molecules. Class I molecules (serologically defined as HLA-A, B, or C) are involved with the presentation of processed antigen to T cells expressing the CD8 molecule. Similarly, Class II molecules (currently recognized as DP, DQ, and DR) present antigen to T cells expressing the CD4 molecule. Interestingly, this molecule is the cellular target for HIV, and the profound immunodepression observed in AIDS is probably related to the destruction of this T-cell subset. Both helper and cytotoxic functions can be ascribed to cells of each lineage, and other antigens have been useful to further delineate functional subsets within each of these T-cell populations.

Recently, a third population of lymphocytes, null cells, has been identified that express neither T nor B cell-surface markers. These cells appear to be a distinct lineage of lymphoid cells that bear some T-cell markers early in differentiation and later acquire markers also present on macrophages and neutrophils. Although the principal function of null cells is not known, recent studies have shown that natural killer (NK) cells and lymphokine-activated killer (LAK) cells are derived from this subpopulation. NK cells are cells that can lyse a select group of cultured cell lines without a known prior exposure to an immunizing stimulus. LAK cells are cells that develop the ability to kill fresh tumor cells following exposure of these lymphoid precursors to the lymphokine interleukin-2 (IL-2). Cells mediating antibody-dependent cellular cytotoxicity (see below) also are found in this null cell population.

Other important cells in the immune system are the reticuloendothelial cells, predominantly monocytes and macrophages. Monocytes are long-lived circulating cells that develop into tissue macrophages. Macrophages are highly phagocytic cells that possess a variety of physiologic protective functions. They are also capable of presenting antigen to lymphocytes and may play a role in carrying antigen from the periphery to other immune sites. A variety of other cell types derived from bone-marrow stem cells play a similar antigen-presenting role, including the Langerhans' cells of the skin, follicular dendritic cells in lymph nodes, B cells, and endothelial cells.

IMMUNE EFFECTOR MECHANISMS RESULTING IN CELL DESTRUCTION

A variety of immune effector mechanisms can cause destruction of vascularized tissue or of circulating tumor cells (Table 17-2).

Antibodies can mediate cell destruction either via the binding of complement or by action as an opsonin to facilitate

TABLE 17-1. Selected CD Classifications of Leukocytes

Cluster of Differentiation (CD)	Antibodies Reactive with CD	Cellular Distribution of Determinant
CD1	OKT6, T6, Leu 6	80% of thymocytes
CD2	LFA-2, OKT11, T11, Leu 5	95% of thymocytes, 100% of T cells, and a variable percentage of LGLs; E-rosette receptor
CD3	OKT3, T3, Leu 4	20–80% of thymocytes and 100% of T cells; associated with T-cell antigen receptor (*T1*)
CD4	OKT4, T4, Leu 3	80% of thymocytes and 65–70% of T cells ("helper/inducer" subset)
CD5	OKT1, T1, Leu 1	Thymocytes, most T cells, and some B cells
CD7	3A1, Leu 9	Thymocytes, 100% of T cells, and some LGLs
CD8	OKT8, T8, Leu 2	50–80% of thymocytes, 30–35% of T cells ("cytotoxic/suppressor"), and some LGLs (low density)
CD9	BA2	Monocytes, pre-B cells, and platelets
CD10	CALLA, J5, BA3	Some bone-marrow pre-B cells and >90% of common ALL
CD11a	LFA-1	T cells, B cells, LGLs, monocytes, and granulocytes
CD11b	CR3 (C3bi), OKM1, Mo1, Leu 15	CD8 T cells, LGLs, monocytes, and granulocytes
CD11c	Leu M5	100% of monocytes and granulocytes
CD14	Leu M3, Mo3	70–93% of monocytes
CD15	Leu M1, My 1	100% of monocytes and >95% of mature granulocytes
CD16	Leu 11a,b,c and Vep 13	LGLs (NK cells) and granulocytes; Fc IgG receptor
CD18	See CD11	T cells, B cells, LGLs, monocytes, and granulocytes
CD19	B4, Leu 12	100% of B cells
CD21	CR-2 (C3d), B2	Mature B cells; EBV receptor
CD22	Leu 14, to 15	B cells
CD25	IL-2R, Tac	T cells, B cells, and LGLs; 9.3-negative T cell appears to function as a suppressor cell
CDw29	4B4	Thymocytes, 40% of T cells (appears to identify helper/inducers); some B cells, LGLs, and monocytes
CD35	CR1 (C3b receptor)	B cells, some T cells, monocytes
CD38	OKT10, T10, Leu 17	LGLs, B cells, some T cells, monocytes, thymocytes, bone marrow cells, and activated T cells
CD45	Antileukocyte	>95% of lymphocytes; monocytes and granulocytes
CD45R	2H4, Leu 18	40% of T cells (appears to identify suppressor/inducers); some B cells, LGLs, monocytes, and granulocytes
Leu 8, TQ 1		7% of thymocytes, >50% of T cells (appears to identify suppressor/inducers), some B cells and monocytes
Transferrin receptor, OKT9		Activated T cells and B cells; found on 10% of thymocytes and monocytes
4F2		Activated T cells, B cells, and monocytes
HNK-1, Leu 7		Some T cells and 50% of LGLs
NKH-1, Leu 19		Small percentage of T cells (cytotoxic), most LGLs and monocytes
LFA 3		T cells (100% CTLs), B cells, LGLs, and monocytes
Class I MHC	HLA A,B,C	Thymocytes, T cells, B cells, LGLs, and monocytes
Class II MHC	HLA DP, DQ, DR (Leu 10, 12)	B cells, monocytes, and activated T cells
Surface Ig		B cells
PCA-1		Plasma cells (weakly positive on monocytes)

phagocytosis by macrophages or by other phagocytic cells bearing Fc receptors.

The direct interaction of an immune cell with a target cell can also result in lysis, and a variety of immune cytotoxic cells have been described. The best-characterized lytic immune cell is the cytotoxic T lymphocyte (CTL). These T cells can interact with specific cell-surface antigens via an interaction with the T-cell receptor and a Class I or II MHC molecule. This lysis appears to involve direct cell contact and can occur quickly, with the initial lytic events initiated within minutes of the adhesion of the target cell to the lymphocyte. Although binding of the CTL to the tumor target occurs via the T-cell receptor, other means for binding lytic cells to targets also can result in lysis. One such mechanism

TABLE 17-2.   Immune Effector Mechanisms Resulting in Cell Destruction

---

Antibody-mediated lysis (plus complement or antibody as an opsonin for macrophages and other Fc-receptor-positive cells).
Direct cell-mediated lysis
    Cytotoxic T lymphocytes (CTL)
    Antibody-dependent cellular cytotoxicity (ADCC)
    Lectin-dependent cellular cytotoxicity (LDCC)
    Natural killer cells (NK)
    Lymphokine-activated killer cells (LAK)
    Macrophage lysis
Release of toxic mediators from lymphocytes and other immune cells

---

has been referred to as antibody-dependent cellular cytotoxicity (ADCC). In this lysis, antibody bound to immune cells serves as a cross-link to a cytolytic cell bearing an Fc receptor. The Fc receptor on the immune effector binds to the free Fc portion of the antibody on the target cell; following this cross-linkage, lysis of the target cell occurs. Similarly, the phenomenon of lectin-dependent cellular cytotoxicity (LDCC) involves the association of a lytic cell with a target using a lectin such as concanavalin A or phytohemagglutinin as the cross-linking agent.

Recently, much has been learned of NK cells. These lymphocytes can lyse selected cultured target cells in the absence of a previous sensitizing stimulus. The most common target for NK cells is the K562 leukemia cell line. NK cells have little, if any, ability to kill fresh tumor cells, and therefore their physiologic role as an antitumor effector mechanism is unclear.

LAK cells are lymphocytes that acquire the ability to lyse a broad array of fresh tumor targets following incubation in IL-2. The precursor of LAK cells is a null lymphocyte, and most mature LAK cells do not bear T- or B-cell markers. A subpopulation of LAK cells, however, has been shown to be CD3 positive, and both precursor and effector LAK cells appear to bear the Leu-19 cell-surface marker. LAK cells can lyse a broad array of malignant, but not normal, fresh target cells in 4-hour chromium-release assays. LAK cells also can lyse both normal and malignant cultured lines. Thus, LAK cells appear capable of lysing most cells that have their membranes perturbed by either malignant transformation, culture, or other activation processes.

Activated macrophages also can recognize and lyse tumor cells. Whereas most lymphocyte-mediated lysis can easily be detected in 4 hours, the measurement of significant macrophage-mediated lysis often requires 48 to 72 hours.

Many of the cytokines secreted by immune cells can mediate toxicity of tissue, either directly or via the recruitment of other inflammatory processes. For example, tumor necrosis factor (TNF) and lymphotoxin are two cytokines capable of direct destruction of tumor cells. Gamma-interferon has an antiproliferative effect against some tumor cells. In addition, a wide variety of chemotactic and vascular permeability factors that are involved in inflammatory responses also can indirectly mediate tumor destruction and may play a role in tumor immune phenomena.

CYTOKINES

Cytokines are soluble proteins produced by mononuclear cells of the immune system (usually lymphocytes or monocytes) that have regulatory actions on other cells of the immune system or target cells involved in immune reactions. Cytokines produced by lymphocytes are referred to as lymphokines and cytokines produced by monocytes are referred to as monokines. Cytokines are true hormones, acting on other cells at a distance from the secreting cells.

For the past 25 years, it has been realized the soluble substances produced by immune cells are involved in immune function and regulation. Until recently, these cytokines were identified by the function they exhibit in in vitro assays. Thus, lymphokines that inhibit the migration of macrophages were known as migration-inhibition factor (MIF), and other factors that activate macrophages were known as macrophage-activation factor (MAF). This identification of cytokines on the basis of function led to a confusing situation in which the same molecules were often described by various investigators using different assays for their detection.

Substantial recent progress in this field resulted from the use of molecular biologic techniques to clone the genes for these cytokines, express them in bacteria, and purify them to homogeneity so that large amounts of homogeneous cytokines were available for detailed study. A new nomenclature referring to cytokines as interleukins (meaning "between leukocytes") has been introduced that supplants the acronyms based on functional properties. A meeting of the Second International Lymphokine Workshop in Ermatingen, Switzerland, in 1979 reached a consensus that a variety of lymphokines that had been referred to as T-cell growth factor (TCGF), thymocyte-stimulating factor (TSF), thymocyte mitogenic factor (TMF), killer-cell helper factor (KHF) costimulator, and secondary cytotoxic T-cell-inducing factor were all the same molecule and should be referred to as IL-2. The term "interleukin-1" was adopted to refer to a monocyte product previously called lymphocyte-activating factor (LAF). Since that time, many cytokines have been described, and a list of some of these is presented in Table 17-3. This list is rapidly expanding as new hormones produced by cells of the immune system are described.

Cytokines are proteins or glycoproteins, mostly with molecular weights in the range of 15,000 to 40,000, and many are glycosylated, although it appears that the glycosylation is often not essential for function. In many cases, the cytokines described in both mouse and man are structurally related. For example, IL-1 alpha shows a 61% to 65% amino acid homology between human, rabbit, and mouse. Some lymphokines exhibit species specificity; for example, IL-1, IL-2, IL-5, and IL-6 derived from man are active on cells from both mouse and man, whereas IL-3, IL-4, and gamma-interferon derived from man are active only on human cells and not on mouse cells.

Each cytokine presumably reacts with receptors specific for that cytokine on the cell surface. Little is known about most cytokine receptors with the exception of the IL-2 receptor, which is present in low-, intermediate-, and high-affinity forms, depending on the specific aggregation of a 55- and a 75-kd polypeptide chain receptor.

TABLE 17-3. Cytokines: Sources and Physiological Effects

Cytokine	Other Names	Sources	Effects

IL-1	Endogenous pyrogen (EP)
	Lymphocyte-activating factor (LAF)
	Leukocyte endogenous mediator (LEM)
	Catabolin
	Mononuclear cell factor (MCF)
		Monocyte and macrophage lines
		Dendritic cells
		Natural killer cells
		B-cell lines
		T-cell lines
		Endothelial cells
		Epithelial cells
		  Fibroblasts
		  Astrocytes
		  Keratinocytes
			Induces
			  Lymphokine release from activated T cells and fibroblasts
			  Growth of fibroblasts, synovial cells, endothelial cells
			  Tissue catabolism
			    Release of PGE_2, collagenase, acute-phase proteins
			  Fever
			  Chemotactic for neutrophils, macrophages, lymphocytes
			  Increases NK cell activity
			  Differentiation of activated B cells with B-cell differentiation factor
			  Proliferation of activated B cells with B-cell growth factor

IL-2	T-cell growth factor (TCGF)
	T-cell maturation/stimulating factor (TMF/TSF)
	Killer helper factor (KHF)
	T-cell replacing factor (TRF)
		Activated T cells	Induces
			  Growth of activated T cells, thymocytes
			  Lymphokine production by T cells
			  Cytotoxic T lymphocyte activity
			  Lymphokine-activated killer-cell activity
			Increases
			  NK cell activity
			  Monocyte cytotoxicity
			  Proliferation of
			    Tonsillar B cells with BCGF
			    SAC-activated splenic, tonsillar, PBLB cells
			    Chronic lymphocytic leukemic B cells
			  Differentiation of
			    Small and large tonsillar B cells

IL-3	Multiple colony-stimulating factor (multi-CSF) Most-cell growth factor (MCGF)	Lectin-stimulated peripheral blood lymphocytes (PBL) Activated T-cell clones Gibbon cell line MLA 144	Gibbon MLA 144 supports growth of erythroid and myeloid progenitor cells Stimulates growth of multipotential stem cells
IL-4	B-cell growth factor (BCGF) B-cell stimulatory factor (BSF1) B-cell stimulatory factor pl (BSFpl)	Activated T cells	Growth factor for T cells Proliferation of tonsillar and splenic activated B cells FceR and HLA DR on B-cell lines FceR on PBL and tonsillar B cells IgE secretion by PBLB cells Induces release of CD23 (FceR) from normal B cells
IL-5	Eosinophil differentiation factor (EDF) B-cell growth factor II (BCGF II) Killer helper factor (KHF)	T cells	Induces differentiation of eosinophils IgM secretion by SAC-stimulated PBL and splenic B cells IgA secretion by SAC-stimulated PBLB cells

IL-6	Hybridoma growth factor (HGF)
	Interferon B_2
	B-cell stimulatory factor-2 (BSF-2)
	B-cell differentiation factor (BCDF)
		Monocytes
		HTLV-transformed T-cell lines
		Fibroblasts
		Bladder carcinoma cells
		Osteosarcoma cells
		Cardiac myxoma cells
		Carcinoma cells
			Induces
			  Class I HLA expression on fibroblasts
			  Production of acute-phase proteins by hepatocytes/hepatoma cells
			  Growth of plasmacytomas and hybridoma
			  Ig secretion by EBV-transformed B cells

(continued)

TABLE 17-3. Cytokines: Sources and Physiological Effects *(continued)*

Cytokine	Other Names	Sources	Effects
Tumor necrosis factor-alpha	TNF-alpha Cachectin	Macrophages T cells Thymocytes Endothelial cells	Cytotoxic or cytostatic for selected cell lines Induces Fever Cachexia Chemotaxis of neutrophils Endothelial cell procoagulant activity Endothelial-cell adhesion molecules Bone resorption In vivo injection can cause necrosis of selected subdermal mouse tumors
Tumor necrosis factor-beta	TNF-beta Lymphotoxin	T cells	Cytotoxic or cytostatic for selected cell lines Increases phagocytosis by neutrophils
Interferon-alpha	INF-alpha Type I interferon	Leukocytes Macrophages	Antiviral Antiproliferative Class I MHC expression Synergizes with other lymphokines
Interferon-beta	IFN-beta Type I interferon	Fibroblasts Epithelial cells	Antiviral Antiproliferative Class I MHC expression Synergizes with other lymphokines
Interferon-gamma	IFN-gamma Type II interferon Macrophage activating factor	T cells LGL	Antiviral Antiproliferative Increases HLA DR on endothelial cells, fibroblasts, myelomonocytic cells Antimicrobial and tumoricidal activity of monocytes/macrophages FcYR on myelomonocytic cells NK cell activity Proliferation of anti-Ig-stimulated tonsillar PBL, splenic B cells Proliferation and differentiation of SAC-activated PBL, splenic, lymph node B cells + IL-2 only

Adapted from O'Garra A: Immunology Today, February 1988.

Most research on cytokines has involved in vitro studies or studies in experimental animals. Many cytokines, such as alpha-, beta- and gamma-interferon, IL-2, tumor necrosis factor, and the colony-stimulating factors, have reached clinical application in patients with cancer. The clinical use of colony-stimulating factors will be presented in depth in Chapter 59, section 3. Clinical application of the interferons and of IL-2 is presented in this chapter in more detail.

TUMOR ANTIGENS

The central tenet of tumor immunology is that there are immunologically recognizable molecules at the tumor-cell surface that are qualitatively or quantitatively different from those on normal cells. Operationally, these immunologically detectable differences or "tumor antigens" are the reciprocal counterparts of what are thought to be highly specific immunologic reagents, namely immunoglobulins and spe-

cific cellular receptors found on T lymphocytes. The ability of the immune system to recognize an immense variety of novel antigens is determined by these unique molecules.

Since the successful demonstration of immunization to bacterial and mycobacterial antigens as protective measures against disease, many attempts have been made in both humans and murine tumor models to immunize the host with tumor. The most convincing evidence of tumor immunity is the ability to reject a subsequent tumor challenge. This has been demonstrated with a variety of animal tumors induced by viruses or chemical carcinogens. However, the ability to demonstrate tumor antigens convincingly in humans has been difficult.

The development of two new approaches has made it possible to demonstrate convincingly the differential expression of certain molecules on human tumor cells in concentrations greater than that found on normal cells. The first of these was the description of murine monoclonal antibodies in 1975 by Kohler and Milstein and, more recently, of similar human monoclonal antibodies that recognize tumor antigens (discussed later in this chapter). In addition, the demonstration that the lymphokine IL-2 could be used to expand polyclonal and monoclonal T-cell populations in the human allowed the production of cellular reagents with both specific and nonspecific antitumor reactivity.

The major antigenic class defined on human tumors using monoclonal antibodies are oncofetal antigens, products normally expressed early in embryonic development and subsequently expressed in normal cells only in small amounts or on the surface of dedifferentiated tumor cells. There are also murine monoclonal antibodies that recognize differentiation antigens unique for cells of an individual tissue. These have perhaps best been defined for B and T cells as well as other hematopoietic cell types and have been useful both in classifying normal differentiation stages and also in allocating cells to separate functional subgroups. A limited number of antibodies have also been developed that recognize tumor antigens unique to an individual tumor and absent from others of identical histology, best exemplified by anti-idiotypic antibodies reactive with B-cell lymphoma. Finally, histocompatibility antigens present on many somatic tissues and initially defined by the ability of inbred strains of animals to reject normal tissues such as skin and kidney allografts, play an important role in immune recognition and are especially important for cell-mediated recognition by T cells.

If one posits the presence of tumor antigens in humans, one must also explain the absence of an immunologic response in the individual tumor-bearing host. It is usually assumed that tumor antigens are "weak," especially when compared to histocompatibility or microbial antigens. The methods to increase the antigenicity of tumors include modification of the tumor-cell surface by chemicals and enzymes (such as neuraminidase treatment to strip sialic acid residues), use of "viral oncolysates," which take advantage of the immunogenicity of associated viral proteins, and more traditional immune adjuvants such as Freund's or attenuated or inactivated organisms such as bacillus Calmette-Guerin (BCG) or *Corynebacterium parvum*.[1] Although many clinical trials have been conducted with such active immunization, the actual identity of many of the constituents of the vaccines has not been well defined. Both serologic and cellular reactivity to tumor antigens have been reported with[2-4] or without[5-10] active immunization.

EVIDENCE FOR THE EXISTENCE OF A HOST RESPONSE TO TUMORS IN HUMANS

Probably the earliest evidence suggesting the existence of an immune response to tumors was the spontaneous regression occasionally observed in a variety of malignancies, most frequently in melanoma and renal cell carcinoma.[11,12] Spontaneous regressions occur in about 1% to 2% of patients with melanoma and renal cell carcinoma. In addition, it has been claimed that during periods of immune activation by an acute bacterial infection, tumor regressions occasionally occur.[13,14] Subsequently, the search for autologous serologic and cellular reactivity was carried out. Many of these studies were done at a time when immunologic techniques were less

sophisticated and the ability to address questions of cross-reactivity was somewhat limited. Still, in many tumors, evidence of a host humoral response, especially to melanoma, neuroblastomas, and osteogenic sarcomas, was claimed.[5,7-10,15-17] Most of the antibodies demonstrated were of relatively low titer and, although sometimes capable of immune reactivity via ADCC or complement-mediated cytotoxicity, were of questionable significance. In large part, the search for autologous serologic reactivity has been supplanted by the development of murine monoclonal antibodies. Recent claims for the development of a host anti-idiotypic response to passively transferred murine monoclonal antitumor antibodies, which themselves evoke a host response to the original antigen, have renewed interest in this area.[18]

The earliest claims of specific cell-mediated immunity to human tumors were made in the early 1970s by the Hellstroms and their collaborators.[19-22] These studies, done before the recognition of natural effectors mediating natural and lymphokine-activated killing, were difficult for other investigators to repeat.[23] Subsequent studies reported by Vanky, Vose, Argov, and Klein[24-26] found that both specific proliferative and cytotoxic reactivity could be demonstrated against fresh tumors. These studies helped to demonstrate cell-mediated recognition of the antigens presumed to exist on tumors in their fresh (noncultured) state. Subsequent studies extended these observations,[27,28] demonstrated correlation of antitumor activity with survival,[29] and introduced the use of IL-2 to culture reactive T cells for long periods.[30,31] The use of autologous controls was suggested by the recognition that T cells capable of reacting with both autologous fibroblasts and lymphocytes could be demonstrated in normal patients as well as in those with cancer.[32-34] Autologous normal cells, such as those derived from normal lung, liver, colon, and bowel, proved capable of stimulating comparable responses in mixed lymphocyte–tumor interactions.[35] Subsequent studies focused on the more restricted antigens recognized by cloned T cells selected by limiting dilution culture.[36-50] In addition, these studies used autologous controls and could demonstrate restricted (and presumably specific) killing of tumor by some clones. The most convincing evidence of restricted recognition came with the use of cloned T cells that could recognize only autologous tumor cells and not autologous normal cells or allogeneic targets.

The possibility that active suppression of an immune response to tumor existed has also been explored using cellular reagents in the human.[51-54] Most recently, cultured T cells, derived directly from human tumors (both lines and clones) or tumor-infiltrating lymphocytes (TIL), have been obtained that have tumor specificity and are entering clinical trials.[55,56] Thus, the demonstration of unique tumor antigens using cellular reagents has progressed gradually (Table 17-4) over the last two decades with further understanding of the processes of natural killing, reactivity to autologous normal cells, and technical advances allowing the long-term culture and cloning of human lymphoid cells. Absolute proof of specific cellular recognition of tumor-cell antigens will require the biochemical isolation of such antigens and the successful adoptive transfer of cells that can mediate specific antitumor responses in humans. One of the apparent requirements for T-cell-mediated recognition of antigen is that

TABLE 17-4.   Evidence for Autologous Cellular Reactivity to Human Tumor Antigens*

Year	Tumor(s)	Source of Cells	Autologous Controls	Tumor Targets	Assay	Reference	Notes
1968–73	Bladder, melanoma, neuroblastoma, colorectal	PBL	Fibroblasts, lymphocytes	C	Colony inhibition assays; MCA	15–22	Activity of "natural effectors" (NK, LAK) not recognized at time of these studies
1977	Lung, sarcoma, nasopharyngeal, renal, melanoma	TIL, LN, PBL	None	F	MLTI; MCA	26	Less activity in tumor than PBL and LN; less activity against allogeneic tumors
1981, 1982	Various	Cultured PBL from MLTI	PHA, IL-2 PBL blasts	F	MCA	24–25 30–31	Modest relative specificity by MCA and cold target studies for autologous tumor
1982	Lung, breast, melanoma	Cultured PBL from MLTI	None	F	MCA, MLTI	27–28	Cultured cells lysed autologous targets preferentially
1983	Sarcoma, lung	PBL	None	F	MCA, MLTI	29	Survival correlated with PBL antitumor reactivity; positive tests in 25%–70% of tumors
1984	Various	PBL	Liver, lung, colon, bladder	F	MLTI	35	19/37 (+) MLT1; in 14 with autologous controls, tumor stimulation was no better
1983	Melanoma	Cloned PBL	None	C	MCA	36	Relative specificity for autologous tumor
1984	B-cell lymphoma	Cloned PBL	None	F	MTLI	37	Relatively specific for B-cell lymphomas. Not restricted by MHC; antibodies to CD3, CD4 could not block
1984	Melanoma	Cloned PBL from MLTI	Fibroblasts, T-cell blasts	C	MCA	38	Cloned lines could kill allogeneic melanoma as well; not inhibited by antibody to Class I MHC
1984	Melanoma	Cultured PBL from MLTI	Fibroblasts, EBV-B cells	C	MCA	39,40	7/13 patients with autologous antimelanoma reactivity; activity lost with prolonged culture; some killing of autologous B-cell line
1985	Ovarian	Cloned cells from ascites	None	F	MCA	41	Relative specificity for autologous tumor with 5/6 clones
1985	Melanoma	Cloned PBL from MLTI	IL-2 PBL blasts	C	MCA	42–45	No clones absolutely restricted to autologous tumor; blocked by Class I MHC-directed antibodies; heterogeneity of lysis of cloned tumor cells
1986	Soft-tissue and osteogenic sarcomas	Cloned PBL from MLTI	PBL blasts, fibroblasts	F,C	MCA	46	Cloned lines could kill allogeneic sarcoma as well; one killed only if HLA-2 shared on target
1986	Melanoma	Cloned PBL from MLTI	EBV-B cells	C	MCA	47	Cold target inhibition studies suggest cross-reactivity with other cells
1986	Lung, breast, ovarian, renal	Cloned PBL from MLTI	None	F	MCA, MLTI	48,49	Restricted killing by some clones to autologous tumor; no restriction in MLTI

(continued)

TABLE 17-4. Evidence for Autologous Cellular Reactivity to Human Tumor Antigens* (continued)

Year	Tumor(s)	Source of Cells	Autologous Controls	Tumor Targets	Assay	Reference	Notes
1987	Melanoma	Cloned PBL from MLTI and after in vivo stimulation	EBV-B cells	C	MCA, cell growth	50	Restricted killing and cell growth by autologous tumor; definition of antigens by cloned reagents
1987	Melanoma	Cultured TIL	EBV-B cells PBL blasts, lung	F	MCA	55	Restricted killing in 3/6 patients with melanoma
1987	Melanoma	Cloned PBL from TIL	EBV-B cells, fibroblasts PBL	F	MCA, MLTI	56	Restricted killing of fresh autologous tumor by cloned TILs

*F, fresh; C, cultured; MCA, microcytotoxicity assay; PBL, peripheral blood lymphocytes; NK, natural killer; LAK, lymphokine activated killer; MTLI, mixed lymphocyte–tumor interaction; EBV-B, Epstein–Barr virus-transformed B cells; TIL, tumor-infiltrating lymphocytes; LN, lymph nodes; MHC, major histocompatibility complex; IL-2, interleukin-2.

it occur in the context of restriction elements encoded for within the MHC.[57] This presumably would restrict the use of immortalized cell lines to the individual from which they were derived or, at best, to a small number of others.

Less restricted and more broadly reactive cells that can mediate lysis of fresh tumor cells but not of normal cells have been defined over the last decade.[58] These cells, which are demonstrable following brief culture with IL-2, have been termed LAK cells and are non-MHC restricted in their cytotoxicity.[59] When adoptively transferred in murine tumor models in conjunction with IL-2, they have mediated the regression of a variety of different tumors.[60] Recently, clinical trials have similarly demonstrated an apparent role in the treatment of human tumors.[61,62] No unique tumor antigen or restricted killing has been noted. The tumor-related determinant that is recognized has not yet been defined, and it has been suggested that destruction of tumor cells follows the recognition of a defect in the expression of some otherwise universally expressed determinant. MHC Class I molecules have been suggested as a candidate.[63]

Finally, the suggestion that transferred immunocompetent allogeneic lymphoid cells might mediate direct antitumor effects (graft versus tumor) was initially tested in animal models. The earliest studies, performed in leukemia models in guinea pigs, demonstrated that allogeneic transfer significantly decreases the development of leukemia in these animals.[64] In addition, protection against subsequent leukemic challenge suggested some long-lived immunologic response. Subsequent studies revealed separable graft-versus-host disease and graft-versus-leukemia effects.[65-69] In addition, the ability to stimulate or produce such effects could be demonstrated with donors that were identical at MHC loci.[70] It was subsequently recognized that graft-versus-host disease also had an antileukemic effect in humans receiving allogeneic bone-marrow grafts.[71,72] Methods to decrease graft-versus-host disease in both animals and humans have been associated with increased relapse rates.[73-75] For example, in a recent prospective, randomized, double-blind trial in which monoclonal anti-T-cell antibody and complement depletion of T lymphocytes from donor bone marrow was carried out

before treatment, only 3 episodes of acute graft-versus-host disease in 20 patients were demonstrated, whereas this reaction appeared in 13 of 20 untreated controls.[75] Marrow in five patients in the T-cell-depleted group failed to engraft, whereas all the control patients had successful transplants. Relapse of leukemia occurred in 7 of 20 in the T-cell-depletion group and in two controls. Although this is not definitive evidence that tumor-specific antigens are recognized, such transplants are currently being done in patients with advanced-stage solid tumors, and the demonstration of specific antitumor reactivity could be sought in that setting.

OTHER TUMOR-CELL PRODUCTS POTENTIALLY APPLICABLE TO IMMUNOLOGIC THERAPY

Histologic and serum markers have been sought for cancer diagnosis and therapy for many years (reviewed in reference 76). It is clear that many of the "tumor" markers such as carcinoembryonic antigen[77,78] (CEA) and alpha-fetoprotein[79] (AFP) initially demonstrated are not tumor specific, as they also are expressed on early embryonic or fetal cells. However, this does not preclude their use as either diagnostic markers or potential targets for immune recognition and destruction. In fact, it is likely that most available "tumor-specific" monoclonal antibodies detect antigens expressed at some point in normal human somatic development but reexpressed only on malignant tissue (see discussion below of monoclonal antibodies). In addition, certain blood group antigens have been found to be deleted on a growing tumor cell population and, conversely, that additional antigens, present on normal epithelial cells, are sometimes expressed. Many of these are likely neoantigens, expressed subsequent to the altered glycosylation of normal proteins on the cell membrane.[80,81]

A variety of tumor markers have been used in the serologic diagnosis of cancer, some of which are expressed at the cell surface and are potentially exploitable for therapy. This subject was extensively reviewed recently.[76] The list includes the classically described oncofetal antigens, CEA[82,83] and AFP,[84-86] and enzymes specific for individual tumors such as prostatic acid phosphatase[87] and lactic dehydrogenase,[88] proteins such as ferritin,[89] hormones such as calcitonin[90] and bombesin,[91] or more recently described oncofetal antigens identified by monoclonal antibody preparation techniques.[92-106] There also appears to be differential expression of more universal antigens such as histocompatibility antigens[107-111] on tumor cells, which may be critical to recognition by cellular reagents. Presumably, virtually every novel cell-surface determinant recognized by monoclonal antibodies could be investigated as a shed antigen useful in serodiagnosis. The most recent examples of this are shed IL-2 receptors, which are released after antigen stimulation.[112] Concentrations are elevated in individuals with T- and B-cell tumors[113] and cancer patients undergoing IL-2 therapy.[114]

Even an antigen that is not necessarily specific for tumor might be targeted with cellular or serologic reagents. Examples of this include antibodies to the IL-2 receptors or epidermal growth factor receptors, which have entered or are being developed for clinical trials.[115-120]

MONOCLONAL ANTIBODIES

Shortly after the demonstration that neutralizing substances exist in the serum that can bind to microbes, a similar notion developed that serologic reactivity to tumor cells might be demonstrated and that such sera might be useful in the treatment of cancer.[121] Although evidence steadily accumulated, both in murine tumor models and in humans, that serologically detectable differences between tumors and normal cells exist, there were multiple problems in exploiting these

observations. Much of the difficulty arose because putative tumor antigens had in most cases not been characterized biochemically. For this reason, the generation of xenogeneic antiserum required the immunization of animals, such as goats or rabbits, with crude membrane digests or whole tumor cells. Most of the reactivity thus generated was against antigenic moieties present on normal human cells, and serologic evidence of specific antitumor reactivity required multiple absorptions against normal human tissues. Similarly, most of the reactivity found in humans to their own tumors was of low titer and difficult to characterize. Also, many xenogeneic sera varied from batch to batch and animal to animal, and this variability inherent in polyclonal antisera representing presumably hundreds, if not thousands, of different antibody molecules frustrated investigators for many years.

The development of techniques to produce monoclonal antibodies in 1975 by Kohler and Milstein[122] allowed the identification, selection, and production of antibodies to specific antigens in theoretically unlimited quantities. Although this monoclonal approach is new, considerable work has already been done in developing these reagents for both diagnostic and therapeutic applications.

Before considering in detail the clinical studies that have been performed, some analysis of the factors important to successful use of monoclonal antibodies will be reviewed.

MOLECULAR BIOLOGY, STRUCTURE, AND FUNCTION OF IMMUNOGLOBULINS

Immunoglobulins are the second most prevalent species in human serum after albumin. These glycoproteins are found in every mammal and in their monomeric form are com-

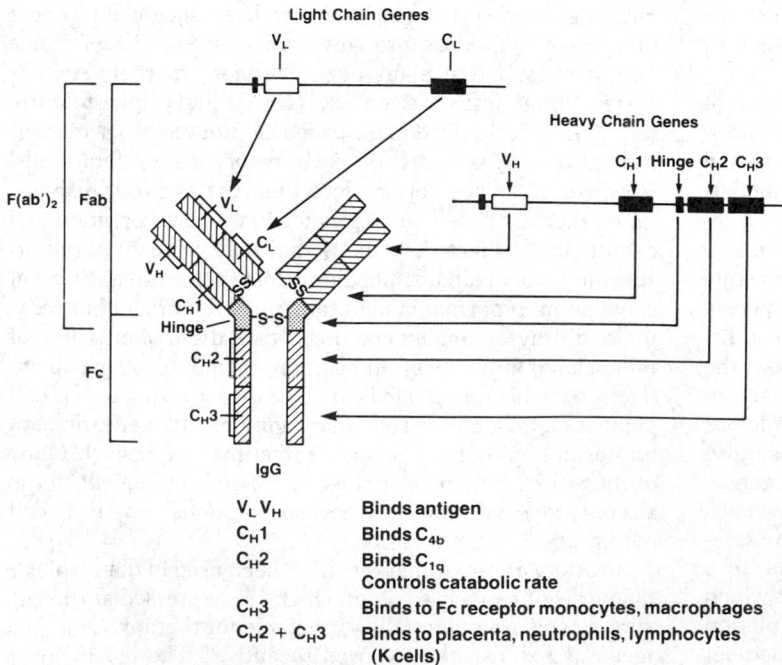

$V_L V_H$	Binds antigen
$C_H 1$	Binds C_{4b}
$C_H 2$	Binds C_{1q}
	Controls catabolic rate
$C_H 3$	Binds to Fc receptor monocytes, macrophages
$C_H 2 + C_H 3$	Binds to placenta, neutrophils, lymphocytes (K cells)

FIG. 17-1. Molecular biology, structure, and functional aspects of an immunoglobulin molecule. The genes for the human bearing chain are located on chromosome 14, the kappa light chain on 2, and the lambda light chain on 22. In mice they are located on chromosomes 12, 6, and 16, respectively. The k : λ ratio in humans is 70 : 30 and in mice 95 : 5. Each chain is encoded for by multiple introns with both variable (V) and constant (C) regions providing the antigen binding and functional domains of the antibody molecule, respectively. Multiple allelic copies of V and J segment genes within the variable region of the light chain and of V, D, and J segment genes of the heavy chain exist. Immunoglobulin diversity occurs by selection and "shuffling" of these genetic elements with varying recombinations, somatic mutations, and association of different heavy and light chains. The hinge region provides some molecular flexibility and serves as the site for disulfhydryl bonds between the heavy chains and with the light chain of IgG1. For the other IgG subclasses the light and heavy chains are joined at the intersection of the variable and constant portions. Enzymatic cleavage by papain will split the molecule into Fab and Fc portions, respectively. Pepsin splits just distal to the hinge heavy chain linkage and maintains a dimeric antigen binding structure [$F(ab')_2$]. The individual constant regions of the heavy chain as shown provide the functional characteristics of the molecule and may become "activated" following antigen binding. Antibody fragments have been used for radioimmunodiagnosis and have been coupled to toxins or radionuclides for therapy.

posed of two heavy and two light chains (Fig. 17-1). The molecular weight of these molecules ranges from 146,000 (IgG) to the 970,000 of the pentameric IgM. The mature molecule consists of globular domains that serve as antigen-binding sites as well as regions involved in antibody effector function.[123,124] The immense diversity within immunoglobulins is generated through variation in isotype (several different subclasses of light and heavy chains), allotype (variability normally encoded in the constant portion of the light or heavy chains), and idiotype (which accounts for most of the heterogeneity in this system). Idiotypic variation has recently been demonstrated to occur through a unique process of gene shuffling, recombination, and somatic mutation.

The predominant immunoglobulin molecule in the serum is IgG, which is represented by four subclasses with somewhat different functions (Table 17-5). Although the earliest molecule to be produced after immunization is usually pentameric IgM, this species cannot bind to effector cells. Consequently, most efforts have been devoted to selecting antibodies of the IgG isotype, and within this isotype, multiple subclasses and enzyme-derived fragments have been prepared from monoclonal sources. For example, the murine IgG3 subclass has been identified as a good mediator in human cells of ADCC, an important effector mechanism in antibody action. Similarly, IgG4 murine antibodies have been selected because of their lack of binding to Fc receptors, making them suitable for use as diagnostic reagents.

Each antibody molecule in its native state is composed of a number of homologous domains which are related to different functions. For example, the $C\gamma1$ and $C\gamma2$ regions bind C4b and C1q (see Fig. 17-1). Complement-mediated lysis of tumor cells is one of the mechanisms by which tumor-cell destruction by antibodies takes place. However, most of the currently available antitumor human monoclonal antibodies interact with human complement components poorly. The terminal domain $C\gamma3$ is important in binding to cellular effectors, such as monocytes, macrophages, neutrophils, and lymphocytes. In addition to its ability to bind antigen, an antibody molecule (because it usually does not subserve an enzymatic function) can also readily dissociate from its target structure without altering it. The relative strength of the interaction between an antibody molecule and the site on a molecule that it recognizes (the epitope) is defined by a dissociation constant or K_d. The K_d of most monoclonal antibodies ranges from 10^{-6} to 10^{-10} M/L. The portions of a molecule that are recognized and bind to an antibody is in a large part determined by the molecular conformation, with regions deep within the three-dimensional structure being less accessible to antigen.[126,127] The ability to engineer an antibody-combining site, or Fab, using molecular biologic techniques to enhance its affinity or specificity[128] or to subserve enzymatic functions[129] is an interesting future direction in the development of antibodies as therapeutic and diagnostic reagents.

PREPARATION OF MONOCLONAL ANTIBODIES

Although others had demonstrated that somatic cells could be fused and that monoclonal antibodies could be produced from murine and human myelomas, it was not until the experiments of Kohler and Milstein[122,130,131] that antibodies of predetermined specificity were obtained. This finding revolutionized biology, and its general application to producing serologic reagents of high affinity, specificity, and reproducibility became widely apparent. It was widely applied to the development of antitumor monoclonal antibodies against melanoma,[132-135] colorectal carcinoma,[136-138] carcinoma of the lung,[139,140] and most other tumors.

The general strategy for the derivation of murine monoclonals[141] is demonstrated in Figure 17-2. In brief, a mouse is immunized with an appropriate antigen, usually whole tumor cells or cell-membrane digests. Reactive B cells are usually obtained from the immunized mouse's spleen or lymph nodes and immortalized by fusing with an enzyme-marked

TABLE 17-5. Human Antibody Subclasses Mediating Biologic Functions

Variable	IgG1	IgG2*	IgG3	IgG4	IgA1	IgA2	sIgA	IgM	IgD	IgE
		IgG				*IgA*				
Allotypes (number)		Gm(20)				Am(2)		Mm(2)		
Molecular weight (kD)	146	146	170	146	160	160	385	970	184	188
Sediment. constant	6.75	6.65	6.65	6.65	75	75	115	195	75	85
Mean serum level (mg/dl)	9	3	1	0.5	3.0	0.5	0.05	1.5	0.03	0.00005
Carbohydrate (%)	2–3	2–3	2–3	2–3	7–11	7–11	7–11	12	9–14	12
Total circulating pool (mg/kg body wt)		494.0			95.0			37.0	1.1	0.019
Half-life (days)		23.0			5.8			5.1	2.8	2.5
Rate of synthesis (mg/kg/day)		33.0			24.0			6.7	0.4	0.016
Placental transfer	+	+	+	+	+	+	–	–	–	–
Monocytes	+	–	+	–	–	–	–	–	–	–
Neutrophils	+	+	+	±	+	+	+	–	–	–
Lymphocytes (K, NK, LAK)	+	+	+	±	–	–	–	–	–	–
Platelets	+	+	+	+	–	–	–	–	–	–
Complement Fixation	++	+	+++	±†	+	+	–	+	+†	–

*Associated with immune response to carbohydrate antigens (in the mouse mediated by IgG3).

†Alternative pathway.

Modified from Roitt I, Brostoff J, Male D: Immunology. St Louis, CV Mosby, 1985, and Jeske DJ, Capra JD: Immunoglobulins: Structure and function. In Paul WE (ed): Fundamental Immunology, pp 131–165. New York, Raven Press, 1984.

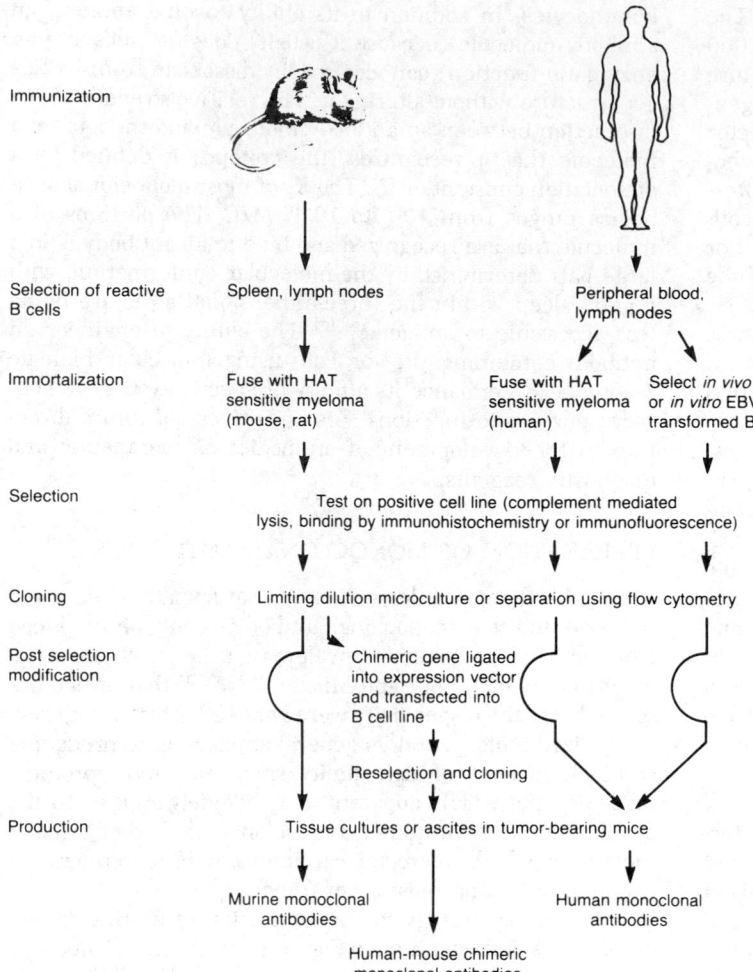

Immunization

Selection of reactive B cells — Spleen, lymph nodes / Peripheral blood, lymph nodes

Immortalization — Fuse with HAT sensitive myeloma (mouse, rat) / Fuse with HAT sensitive myeloma (human) / Select *in vivo* or *in vitro* EBV transformed B cells

Selection — Test on positive cell line (complement mediated lysis, binding by immunohistochemistry or immunofluorescence)

Cloning — Limiting dilution microculture or separation using flow cytometry

Post selection modification — Chimeric gene ligated into expression vector and transfected into B cell line / Reselection and cloning

Production — Tissue cultures or ascites in tumor-bearing mice

Murine monoclonal antibodies / Human-mouse chimeric monoclonal antibodies / Human monoclonal antibodies

FIG. 17-2. Mechanism for preparing monoclonal antibodies. Shown are the usual procedures used to produce monoclonal antibodies from human or murine sources. Human mouse chimeric genes have been produced by ligation of the mouse variable region to a human constant region. They are produced in transfected B-cell lines using conventional molecular biologic techniques. The procurement of large quantities of antibody for clinical trials usually involves production and purification from ascites of hybridoma bearing mice or in tissue culture. The latter produces 10 to 100 μg/ml, whereas ascitic fluid yields as much as 1 to 25 mg/ml.

myeloma. These enzyme-marked cells lack enzymes critical for growth or detoxification of certain compounds. In the usual technique, these myeloma cells lack either thymidine kinase or hypoxanthine guanosine phosphoribosyl transferase (HGPRT). Thus, when the parent and fused cells are grown in hypoxanthine, aminopterine, and thymidine (HAT) medium, the principal synthetic pathway for ribonucleotides is blocked by the aminopterin, and the ability to incorporate these nucleotides is possessed only by hybrid cells, which contain normal levels of HGPRT from the normal B cells derived from the spleen or lymph node. Consequently, the nonfused myeloma cells die, and only the HAT-resistant (fusion) products survive. Individual small groups of cellular supernatant fluids are tested on a tumor cell line either for complement-mediated lysis or for binding (immunohistochemical or immunofluorescence). After identification of an appropriate antibody-secreting hybridoma, limiting-dilution microculture is carried out, and the cloned, immortalized B cell can then be placed either in tissue culture or into the peritoneal cavity of mice to produce large quantities of murine monoclonal antibodies. A similar procedure can be used, although much less successfully, to produce human monoclonal antibodies. Alternatively, Epstein–Barr virus can be used to transform B cells that are making appropriate anti-

body (see below). Most recently, chimeric genes and protein products have been produced using molecular biologic techniques[142] to ligate the genes for the variable portion of both the heavy and light chains to constant portions encoded by human genes. As noted below, such chimeric antibodies are entering clinical trials. The original technique of murine monoclonal antibody preparation, although relatively straightforward, has thus been extended to produce a variety of protein products, some of which differ substantially from the original antibody molecule.

IN VIVO MECHANISMS OF ANTIBODY ACTION

In vivo mechanisms of antibody-mediated tumor inhibition and destruction are listed in Table 17-6. The ability of antibodies to coat targets and, in association with other serum opsonins, to cause phagocytosis or lysis by leukocyte effectors in the human is mediated largely by the IgG1 and IgG3 subclasses.[123,124] The Fc portion of the antibody (Fc: crystallizable fragment) can bind to any one of three different FC receptors that have been defined both in mice and humans. The subset of lymphocytes that expresses Fc receptors with effector function includes large granular lymphocytes, which

TABLE 17-6. Possible in Vivo Mechanisms of Antibody-Mediated Tumor Inhibition and Destruction

Complement-mediated lysis after interaction with antigen
Antibody-dependent cellular cytotoxicity with lymphocytes (K cells), polymorphonuclear leukocytes or monocytes
Organization with normal serum constituents and elimination by reticuloendothelial cells
Radiotoxicity or chemotoxicity secondary to conjugated reagents
Block receptor for autocrine growth products or normal hormones, cytokines
Induction of host antitumor response subsequent to development of anti-idiotypic antibodies (appearing similar to original tumor antigen)

can manifest natural killing, lymphokine-activated killing, and ADCC. The Fc_gRIII Fc receptor, defined by the antibodies 3G8 and Leu 11 (CD16), is a receptor for polymeric IgG and is also present on polymorphonuclear leukocytes (PMNs) and differentiated monocytes.[143,144] This is the major Fc receptor on lymphoid cells. Monocytes express additional receptors known as Fc_gRI and Fc_gRII.[145] Fc_gRI, recognized by the murine monoclonal antibodies 32.2 and 62.2, identifies a receptor with high affinity for monomeric IgG1. This receptor and its mediation of ADCC are increased on monocytes by the lymphokine gamma-interferon, which also causes de novo expression of this molecule on PMNs. The Fc_gRII receptor identified by the antibody IV-3 appears to have relatively low affinity for monomeric antibody and appears to have as its principal role the clearing of heavily opsonized particles. The Fc_gRII has also been identified on human platelets.[146] The identity of Fc receptors on lymphocytes[147] and granulocytes[148] in the human and their susceptibility to modulation by cytokines has now been carefully defined and the genes encoding these molecules cloned in the mouse.[149,150] Other serum proteins, including activated complement components such as C5a and C-reactive protein,[151-155] also appear to have a role in Fc-receptor function and expression. It is presumed that the therapeutic role of native unaltered monoclonal antibodies involves ADCC or opsonization with removal by the reticuloendothelial system.

When various human and murine effector cells are tested for their ability to mediate killing of human tumors using monoclonal antibodies of different isotypes,[138] the cells that can mediate the greatest killing prove to be murine monocytes followed in turn by human lymphocytes and human monocytes. The murine antibody that can mediate the greatest lysis by these cells is IgG3, followed by IgG2a and IgG2b. Other antigens might elicit other isotypes effectively in a different hierarchy. Antibodies recognizing a colorectal antibody and the disialogangliosides GD2 and GD3 effectively target human killer cells.[135,156-158] Certain lymphokines can also activate these lymphoid killers, including alpha- and gamma-interferon and IL-2.[159-161]

ANTIBODY CONJUGATES

The earliest development of antibodies against murine and human tumors was done in the context of using these antibodies coupled to other, more toxic reagents to fashion a magic bullet that would seek out tumor cells and destroy

them uniquely, leaving uninjured the cells to which they did not bind.[162] A large variety of cytotoxic agents have been described for possible conjugation to monoclonal antibodies (Table 17-7) (summarized in Ref. 163). These include different radioisotopes producing alpha and beta emissions.[164] The one used in most clinical trials currently is ^{131}I, employed therapeutically as a beta-particle emittor (Figure 17-4). The limitations of using antibody-coupled radioisotopes include irradiation of adjacent tissues, even in the absence of specific antibody binding.[165] In spite of the great specificity of available antibodies, the maximum tumor-to-normal tissue ratios, in terms of delivered dose, have been only about 10 to 20. One of the advantages, however, associated with the use of such radiolabeled antibodies is that they do not require internalization of the antibody complex as is necessary for toxins or coupled chemotherapeutic agents.

The selection of an individual radionuclide is dependent on a number of factors. Because antibodies require percolation through tissues, it has been estimated that 1 to 3 days will be required for adequate delivery of antibody to tumor sites. This is in large part based on preliminary radiolabeling studies (see below). For that reason, radionuclides with relatively short biologic half-lives—on the order of 24 hours to 5 to 7 days—have been recommended. The range of the toxic-

TABLE 17-7. Cytotoxic Agents for Conjugation to Monoclonal Antibodies

Beta-particle emitters
    Iodine-131
    Scandium-47
    Palladium-109
    Yttrium-90
Alpha-particle emitters
    Bismuth-212
    Astatine-211
Auger electron generators
    Iodine-125
    Bromine-77
Fissionable nuclides
    Boron-10
    Actinides
Protein toxins and cytotoxins
    Ricin
    Diphtheria
    Purothionine
    Pseudomonas exotoxin
    Alpha amanitin
Chemotherapeutic drug
    Vindesine
    Methotrexate
    Daunorubicin
    Doxorubicin
    Cytosine arabinoside
    5-Fluorouridine
Biologic agents
    Interleukin-2
    Interferon
    Cobra venom factor
    Liposomes
    Antibody to lymphocyte surface structures (antibody heteroconjugates)
    Photosensitive agents (hematoporphyrin)

Adapted from Houghton AN, Scheinberg DA: Monoclonal antibodies: Potential applications to the treatment of cancer. Semin Oncol 13:165–179, 1986.

ity of the radionuclides is also important, and it is estimated that up to 0.5 mm will be required for sufficient radiation to penetrate all tumor cells.[166] Radionuclides producing high-energy gamma rays are thus excluded. For example, one of the major deficiencies of ^{131}I as a radiopharmaceutical, in spite of its sufficiently energetic beta ray, is the presence of significant high-energy gamma rays. In addition, iodine radionuclides frequently are stripped from the antibody molecules through a process of dehalogonization. Finally, the radionuclide must be available at reasonable cost and be accessible to clinical centers. Other recently evaluated radionuclides include boron-11([11]B)[162], useful as a neutron target[167], palladium-109 ([109]Pd)[168], Yttrium-90, and Astatine-211.

An alternative to coupling an antibody to a radionuclide is to conjugate it to a chemical toxin, many of which are plant or bacterial products that are extremely toxic at doses of only a few molecules per cell. The antibody–toxin conjugate is presumably endocytosed after binding to the cell surface via coated pits and vesicles and thereafter causes toxicity. For example, the toxins derived from ricin,[118,169-171] diphtheria, and the pseudomonas endotoxin[172] all interrupt ribosomal processes with extremely high efficiency. One of the major problems associated with the use of bacterial or plant toxins is that they can themselves bind directly to the cell surface without antibody coupling. It has therefore been necessary to strip the toxin of this characteristic either by enzyme treatment or by removing a second, B, chain that binds to the cell surface. Most recently, the toxin molecule has been linked to the monoclonal antibody by direct ligation of the antibody gene to the toxin gene using molecular biologic techniques.[142] This same procedure can be used to link toxin molecules to ligands other than antibodies, including hormones and cytokines such as IL-2.[173] These antibody–toxin conjugates have proved active in vitro as toxic molecules and have entered clinical trials. In addition, allogeneic bone marrow has been cleared of T cells using anti-T-cell monoclonal antibody–ricin conjugates.[170] Similarly, other toxins have been developed, including chemotherapeutic agents bound directly to the antibody[174-176] or incorporated into liposomes containing staphylococcal protein A coupled to a chemotherapeutic agent.[177] Hematoporphyrin derivatives have also been coupled directly to antibodies without losing their ability to cause phototoxicity of the relevant target when exposed to light.[178]

Antibodies have been used to block the receptor for autocrine growth products or normal hormones or cytokines. For example, the IL-2 receptor is present on a variety of T-cell leukemias associated with infection by the human T-cell lymphotrophic virus (HTLV-I).[179-181] Antibodies to the IL-2 receptor coupled to diphtheria toxin have been used to treat patients with T-cell leukemia.[182-183] This anti-IL-2 receptor (anti-Tac) has also been coupled to alpha-emitters including [212]bismuth.[184] More recently, antibodies to the epidermal growth factor receptor[120,185,186] have been used in murine models to define human glioma xenografts and to modulate their growth as well as that of epidermal, colorectal, and cervical carcinoma-derived cell lines.[120] An immunotoxin prepared from the monoclonal antibody reactive with the human transferrin receptor coupled with the ricin A chain

has shown tumoricidal activity in an intraperitoneal nude-mouse model.[187]

Finally, it is possible that murine monoclonals act by inducing a host response to the murine antibody or anti-idiotype, which itself bears resemblance to the original tumor antigen and elicits a host response.[188-191] Thus, an initial antibody (antibody-1) may elicit a second host antibody (antibody-2), which in turn elicits a third host antibody (antibody-3), forming a network of interacting antibodies. Antibody-3 and antibody-1 presumably both recognize the same tumor antigen. This network theory, originally proposed by Jerne,[192] has been clearly demonstrated in murine models and has been suggested to be related to the efficacy of murine monoclonal antibodies administered in clinical trials.[188] Administration of anti-idiotypic antibodies has been explored as a means to immunize humans against viruses[193] and to elicit an antitumor response.[194]

ANTIBODY HETEROCONJUGATES

An alternative approach to exploiting the ability of antibodies to target tumor cells is to couple them directly to other antibodies that bind an effector cell.[195] Antibodies directed to cell-surface determinants such as those that bind to T3, associated with the T-cell receptor for antigen or with antibodies to the Fc-gamma receptor, have been effective in vitro. These "heteroaggregates" or "heteroconjugates" will lyse targets such as tumor cells to which one limb of the conjugate is directed.[196-199] These cross-links have been used to lyse murine tumor targets and, more recently, human tumor targets with a demonstration that they can prevent tumor growth in an intraperitoneal nude-mouse model using both anti-T3 and anti-Fc receptor conjugates.[200,201] The utility of such unique heteroconjugates in the treatment of human tumors is now being evaluated. The major advantage of this approach is that it bypasses the requirement for cytolytic T cells or PMNs to interact directly with the tumor through a specific receptor. One of the limitations of such an approach is related to the generation of a host response to these artificial heteroconjugates. Chimeric antibodies could be produced using molecular biologic techniques to overcome this problem in part.

HUMAN ANTIBODIES

Because autologous reactivity in the sera of patients against their own tumor can be demonstrated, attempts have been made to derive human monoclonal antibodies from such individuals. An obvious approach would be to generate a monoclonal antibody from the fusion of human B-cells with a human or murine B-cell fusion partner, which would allow immortalization of this immunoglobulin producing cell. In practice, however, derivation of human monoclonals in this fashion has been extremely difficult.[202] An alternative approach has been to transform cells directly with Epstein–Barr virus to immortalize their secretion of antitumor antibodies. This can be done by transforming them in vitro or by selecting from in vivo sites cells that have already been transformed by endogenous Epstein–Barr virus.[203,204] Most of the antibodies that have been derived from patients with melanoma or colorectal carcinoma have been IgMs, which makes them less suitable for coupling to radionuclides or toxins. Trials have been initiated using these antibodies by injecting them directly into lesions or systemically.[205] Techniques have been developed to select such antigen-specific B-cells using cell-sorting techniques.[206]

An alternative approach to obtaining human antibody molecules with reactivity against human tumors has been to produce genetically engineered antibody molecules combining the variable-region genes for both the heavy and light chain from the mouse, which are in turn directly ligated to the genes encoding the Fc portion of the immunoglobulin molecule from the human[142] (Fig. 17-3). The ability to transfect immunoglobulin genes into lymphoid cells has been demonstrated with production of these unique molecules. Such recombinant monoclonal antibodies have been obtained against the common acute lymphocytic leukemia antigen[207] and three others with broad reactivity against adenocarcinomas 17-1A,[208] L6,[209] and B72.3[210]. These unique molecules can be engineered to be coupled at the genetic level directly to genes encoding other proteins such as toxins or metal-binding proteins. Whether these primary antibodies will be less antigenic is currently unclear, but preliminary human trials are encouraging; both a long half-life and decreased immunogenicity have been noted.

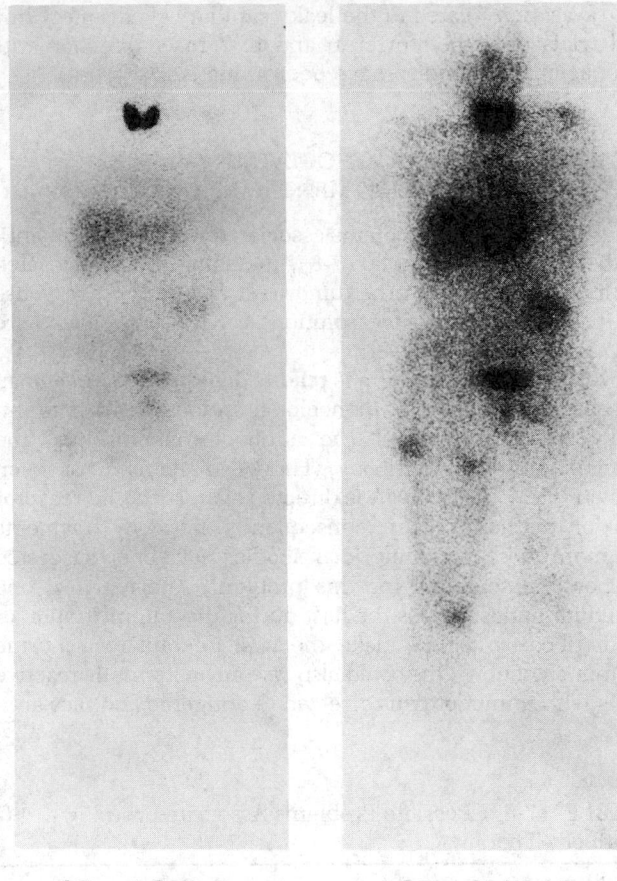

6D, 1ST Rx   6D, 2ND Rx

FIG. 17-4. Radioimaging and therapy with ^{131}I-coupled antimelanoma Fab. Treatment of a patient with 50 mg of antibody labeled with 6.4 mCi of ^{131}I is shown at the end of 6 days following the first and second treatments. Uptake by cutaneous deposits of tumor is apparent, with nonspecific uptake in thyroid, liver, and excretion of radiolabel into the urinary bladder.

FIG. 17-3. Construction of a human–mouse chimeric immunoglobulin. Shown are the steps used to create chimeric L6, an antibody recognizing a variety of adenocarcinomas. The unshaded variable regions from the mouse heavy (V_H) and light chains (V_K) have been ligated to the appropriate constant portion of the human genes in separate plasmids prior to combinational ligation. Alternatively separate plasmids for each chain could be transfected into a B-cell line. Chimeric antibodies such as these have entered clinical trials. (Modified from reference 209)

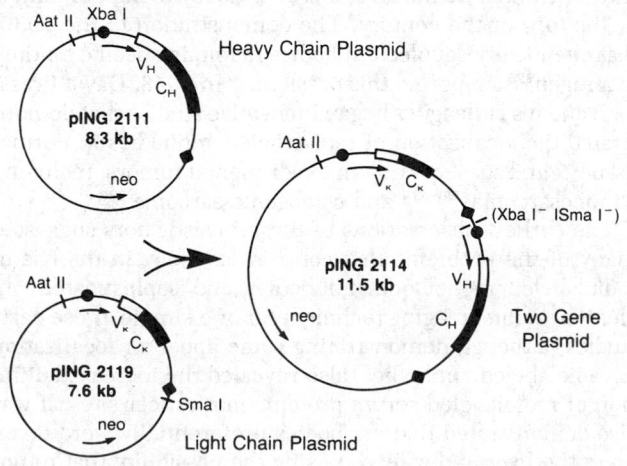

- ● Mouse heavy chain immunoglobulin gene enhancer
- ➔ SV40 early promoter
- ◆ Bidirectional SV40 transcription/polyadenylation signal

ADMINISTRATION IN COMBINATION WITH RECOMBINANT HUMAN CYTOKINES

That cytokines such as interferon could modulate the lysis of tumor cells by immune effectors has been known for some time.[211] Interferon and, more recently, TNF have been demonstrated to markedly increase MHC Class I and Class II antigens and many tumor-associated antigens.[212,213] This ability to augment the expression of MHC antigens is thought to be important in enhancing the therapeutic potential of antibodies in murine models. Anti-idiotypic antibodies in conjunction with alpha-interferon in treatment of murine lymphomas and antibodies to adenocarcinomas in human colon tumor xenograft models have been administered with synergistic effects.[214,215] Recently, IL-2 has been demonstrated to synergize with antitumor antibodies in murine models of melanoma[216] and lymphoma.[217] Presumably, its function is to enhance MHC expression through the secondary elaboration of gamma-interferon, to activate cytolytic effectors with Fc receptors, and to increase the delivery of antibodies to tumor sites secondary to the increased protein extravasation related to the leaky capillary syndrome. Clinical trials of both interferon and IL-2 in conjunction with monoclonal antibodies have been initiated.

POSSIBLE PROBLEMS ASSOCIATED WITH ANTIBODY TREATMENT

There are multiple problems associated with the use of antibodies in therapy (Table 17-8), including those associated with characteristics of the tumor cell and the host response to the antibody. Possible solutions for these problems are also listed in Table 17-8.

Murine immunoglobulin is readily demonstrated in human tissues after infusion of monoclonal antibody,[218] and an immune response against the antibodies themselves, the human antimouse antibody (HAMA) response, has been shown.[219-221] Most HAMA is directed against the Fc receptor portion of the antibody; consequently, antibody fragments or, more recently, chimeric antibodies have been suggested as possible solutions for this problem. Alternatively, one could immunosuppress the host during the administration of an antibody and thus make the host tolerant to a murine immunoglobulin. One could also lyse any potentially reactive cells with immunotoxins directed to antigenic and thus anti-

TABLE 17-8. Possible Problems Associated with Antibody Therapy

Problem	Possible Solutions
Antigenic modulation	Use multiple monoclonal antibodies recognizing same or different antigens; choose nonmodulating antigen
Release of free antigen	Plasmapheresis; varying schedule of monoclonal antibody treatments
Antimouse antibodies	Develop human chimeric antibodies, immunosuppressive drugs, plasmapheresis with immunospecific absorption, large dose of antibody to induce tolerance
Tumor heterogeneity	Treat with multiple antibodies that react with different antigens
Lack of in vivo cytotoxicity of antibody alone	Conjugate monoclonal antibody to drugs, toxins, or radionuclides
Neoplastic cells not accessible to blood supply	Conjugate monoclonal antibody to radionuclides that "emit" radiation beyond a single cell. Produce capillary "leak" with IL-2.
Bone-marrow toxicity from toxin-labeled antibody	Use in association with bone marrow transplantation
Lack of in vivo expression of antigen	Treat with cytokines that induce expression of tumor antigens (interferon, tumor necrosis factor)
Absence of effectors capable of mediating antibody-directed cytotoxicity	In vitro activation and transfer of effectors or direct in vivo activation (Il-2, GM-CSF)

Adapted from Foon KA, Morgan AC: Monoclonal antibody therappy of cancer: Animal models and human trials. In Roth JA (ed): Monoclonal Antibodies in Cancer. Mt Kisco, Futura Publishing, 1986.

idiotypic determinants.[219] The ability to give different antibodies recognizing the same specificity but different idiotypes and potentially different isotypes has also been suggested. Preexisting human antimouse immunoglobulin reactivity has been demonstrated. It appears to be primarily of an IgM type and to be related to polyclonal rheumatoid factors that can be demonstrated in certain cancer patients, in patients with rheumatoid arthritis, and in some normal individuals.[222] Anti-idiotypes and anti-anti-idiotypes have been demonstrated against murine antibodies in mice as well as in humans.[189]

Most, if not all, of the antitumor monoclonals recognize oncofetal antigens, that is, these antibodies recognize products that are normally expressed early in fetal life but which are not expressed, or are expressed only in small amounts, in adults. Consequently, they cannot be considered true tumor-specific transplantation antigens but rather are only preferentially expressed on neoplastic cells. The potential cross-reactivity of these monoclonal reagents is of some concern. For example, several groups of investigators have defined the expression of the melanoma-associated gangliosides (such as G_{D2} and G_{D3}) and have developed antibodies to them.[36-38] These antibodies have antitumor reactivity even though such antigens also can be demonstrated on certain normal cells, such as a subset of human T cells.[223] The administration of antibodies in both murine and human studies has also demonstrated novel findings that were not unexpected, including the ability to induce tolerance by monoclonal antibody therapy[224] and the induction of immunosuppression with immune complexes formed in antibody excess.[225]

IMAGING STUDIES WITH RADIOLABELED ANTIBODIES

EARLY STUDIES

The suggestion that therapy or localization of tumor might be carried out with radiolabeled antibodies was made shortly after the initial demonstrations of antibody to human tumors at the turn of the century. The demonstration in the 1930s that chemically coupled antibodies maintain specific binding to antigen[226] supported this possibility. In 1948, David Pressman and his colleagues began innovative studies that demonstrated the localization of radiolabeled antibodies in normal tissue[227] and subsequently in experimental tumors, including lymphosarcomas[228,229] and osteogenic sarcoma.[230]

The earliest observations of these investigators suggested many of the problems that confront us today in the use of radiolabeled monoclonal antibodies and sophisticated nuclear medicine imaging techniques. For example, these early studies, although demonstrating some apparent localization of radiolabeled antibodies, also revealed the increased diffusion of radiolabeled serum proteins into cancer sites. It was also demonstrated that antibodies preferentially were taken up in the liver and spleen, raising the possibility that tumor antigen existed there or, more likely, that antibody was being cleared by the reticuloendothelial system. Subsequently, Pressman, Day, and Blau developed paired-labeling tech-

(Text continues on page 320.)

TABLE 17-9. Diagnostic Studies with Radiolabeled Antibodies

Year	Institution (ref.)	Route of Injection*	Tumor	No. of Patients	Antigen/ Antibody/ Class	Isotope	Dose mCi	Dose mg	%ID/g	Identification of Lesions
Gliomas										
1965	Duke Univ.[232]	IA	Gliomas	8	Rabbit anti-autologous glioma	[131]I/[125]I	0.1–0.2	0.05	0.001–0.010	11/11 pts and 38/39 clinically positive sites
1968	Duke Univ.[233]	IA	Gliomas	2	Rabbit antimyelin	[125]I	0.170	0.01	–	2/2 glioma pts confirmed higher localization in tumor
Adenocarcinoma										
1974	Tufts Univ.[237]	IV,IA	Colorectal	1	CEA/rabbit Ig	[131]I	0.1–1.59	0.42–480	–	No imaging of lesion, transient drop in CEA with each of three injections
1975	Dalhousie Univ., Nova Scotia[235]	IV	Renal carcinoma	1	Autologous/goat	[131]I	4.2	100	–	1/1 pt and 1/1 lesion; more in tumor, less in liver/spleen at 48 hours
			Melanoma	2	autologous/ rabbit goat Ig		1.95–3.48	100–120		0/2 pt; serum sickness in one patient
			Squamous cell cancer, lung		Autologous/goat		5.6	120		1/1 pt and 1/1 lesions
1978	Dalhousie[236]	IV	Renal carcinoma	6	Renal Ca/goat Ig	[131]I	3.5–4.0	100	–	7/7 lesions observed
1978	Univ. Kentucky[238,240]	IV	Adenocarcinoma	18	CEA/goat Ig	[131]I	0.6–1.6	100–200	–	15/18 pts; 30/40 affinity-purified, hyperimmune goat antisera
1980	Univ. Kentucky[267,268]	IV	Hepatocellular, embryonalca, seminoma, ovarian, Endometrial, adenocarcinoma of lung	16	AFP/goat Ig	[131]I	1.0–2.5	0.13–0.35	–	12/12 pts with AFP-containing tumors; 16/38 lesions image enhancement factor 2.28; required subtraction to enhance differences
1980	Ludwig Inst., Geneva[239]	IV	Colorectal	27	CEA/goat Ig	[131]I	1.0	0.5–1.0	–	11/27 pts; some given F(ab')2 fragments; 4 pts given ^{125}I-labeled goat immunoglobulin concomitantly with ratios of 5–6 less than specific radiolabeled antibody
1981	Ludwig Inst.[241]	IV	Colorectal Pancreatic	28	CEA/VII 23/IgG1 and F(ab')2	[131]I ^{125}I nonspecific	1.0	0.5–1.0	–	14/28 pts positive and six equivocal studies *(continued)*

TABLE 17-9. Diagnostic Studies with Radiolabeled Antibodies (continued)

Year	Institution (ref.)	Route of Injection*	Tumor	No. of Patients	Antigen/ Antibody/ Class	Isotope	Dose mCi	Dose mg	%ID/g	Identification of Lesions
1982	Univ. Nottingham[242]	IV	Colorectal	11	791T/36/IgG2b	^{131}I	1.0	0.2	–	10/11 pts; image enhancement factor 4.4; after subtraction studies and before 1.2–2.0; resected specimens 1.1–5.8 tumor-to-nontumor
1982	Institut Gustave Roussy/ Ludwig Institute[243]	IV	Colorectal and medullary	17	CEA/III-23e, VII-37a/IgG1, IgG2	^{131}I	0.1–0.2 1.0–1.5	0.05–3.33 0.3	0.001–0.010 –	16/17 sites detected; used tomographic techniques to increase visibility of lesions
1983	Ludwig Inst., Cancer Research Centre Rene Gauducheau[244]	IV	Colorectal and others	52 15	/17-1A/IgG2a F(ab')2 and whole Ab	^{131}I	1.0–2.0	0.01–0.5	–	34/63 colorectal tumor sites imaged and 0/20 other tumors; 3.6–6.3-fold higher uptake in tumor compared with normal tissue; specific uptake limited to 2.1–5.1-fold increase
1984	Fox Chase Cancer Center[245]	IV	Colorectal and breast	9	/171A-F(ab')2/IgG2a	^{131}I	NS	NS	0.0047	7/8 pts; 22/32 lesions (69%) detected
1984	Fox Chase Cancer Center[246]	IV	Colorectal	1	/171A-F(ab')2/IgG2a	^{131}I	2.6	0.376	–	1/1 pts; lesion not detected abnormal by CT seen in a lymph node by radiolabeled study
1986	Hammersmith Hospital[247]	IV	GI, breast and ovarian	19	Human milk fat globule protein/ HMFG2/ IgG1 "proliferating cells"/AUA1/ IgG1 L-phenyl-alanine/ placental alkaline phosphatase H317/IgG1	^{131}I specific; ^{125}I nonspecific	0.05–.10	0.01–0.5	0.015	No imaging; maximal tumor:blood ratios 35.8:1 at 12 days 0.026% ID/g in normal lymph nodes
1986	City of Hope[248,249]	IV	Colorectal	45	CEA/T84.66/ NS	^{111}In	2.0	0.20	0.002–0.008	11/16 primary, 10/29 metastatic; increased uptake in liver with liver-to-tumor ratio of 5:6; normal lymph nodes had higher

(continued)

TABLE 17-9. Diagnostic Studies with Radiolabeled Antibodies *(continued)*

Year	Institution (ref.)	Route of Injection*	Tumor	No. of Patients	Antigen/ Antibody/ Class	Isotope	Dose mCi	Dose mg	%ID/g	Identification of Lesions
										uptake (10.8 ± 2.2% ID/kg) than tumor-bearing lymph nodes (3.47 ± 0.54%)
1987	St. Bartholomew's Hospital London[250]	IP,IV	Ovarian	18	Human milk fat globule protein/ HMFG2/ IgG1	$^{123}I/^{125}I/^{131}I$	0.5–2	0.5	0.0001–0.0030	Not examined; 4–71-fold greater localization in ascites when given IP compared with IV
1987	NCI, NIH[251]	IV	Colorectal	27	TAG72/ B72.3/IgG1	^{131}I	0.8–10.0	0.16–20.0	NS	14/27 pts; 17/20 with "specific" uptake in tumor tissue (> × control) 70% of all lesions (99/142)
1987	NCI, NIH[252]	IV,IP	Colorectal	10	TAG72/ B72.3/IgG1	$^{131}I/^{125}I$	5–10	0.76–1.2	0.003–0.017	7/10 pts; peritoneal implants were targeted most efficiently by IP compared with IV injection
Lymphoma										
1986	NIH[253]	IV	Cutaneous T-cell lymphoma	11	CD5/T101/ IgG2a	^{111}In	3.8–5.1	1–50	0.01–0.03	11/11 pts and 38/39 clinically positive sites
Hepatoma										
1982– 1986	Johns Hopkins[254,257]	IV	Hepatoma, cholangio-carcinoma	18	Ferritin/ polyclonal antisera	^{131}I	37–157	NS	NS	6/9 evaluable pts respond to this in combination with radiation and chemo-therapy
Melanoma										
1983	Univ. Washington[258]	IV	Melanoma	6	p97/96.5; 8.2/IgG2a, IgG1	$^{131}I, ^{125}I$ (non-specific)	5	1–10	NS	6/6 specific uptake in 22/25 lesions ≥ 1.5 cm
1983	Univ. Washington[259,260]	IV	Melanoma	33	p97/96.5, 8.2/Fab IgG1, IgG2a	$^{131}I, ^{125}I$ (non-specific)	5	1–10	NS	20/22; specific uptake and clearance correlated with cancer fraction of p97 in tumor; treated 7 pts with high dose Fabs
1985	Univ. Calif., San Diego[261]	IV	Melanoma	21	p97/96.5/ IgG2a	^{111}In	5	1–20	NS	21/21; 56% of lesions ≥ 1.5 cm detected
1986	NCI, NIH[262]	IV, SubQ	Melanoma	59	p97/HMW/ 96.5, 48.7/IgG2a/ IgG1 9.2.27	$^{131}I, ^{111}In$	0.2–12	0.2–50	NS	2/8 pts injected subcutaneously had nodes imaged specifically; 22/38 pts injected systemically had lesions imaged *(continued)*

TABLE 17-9.   Diagnostic Studies with Radiolabeled Antibodies *(continued)*

Year	Institution (ref.)	Route of Injection*	Tumor	No. of Patients	Antigen/ Antibody/ Class	Isotope	Dose mCi	Dose mg	%ID/g	Identification of Lesions
1986	Milan and others[263,264]	IV	Melanoma	254	HMW/225.285/ IgG2a, F(ab')2	[99m]Tc; [111]In	10–30; 2–6	NS	NS	159/191 pts known to have melanoma; 250/412 lesions including 95 occult lesions; Tc had superior characteristics
1986	Univ. Calif., San Francisco[265]	SubQ	Melanoma	6	HMW/ XMMME-01/ IgG2a	[111]In	1	1	NS	6/6 pts imaged whether in the tumor or not; 1/2 pts had proliferative uptake in tumor-bearing nodes
1987	Univ. Utah[266]	IV	Melanoma	12	HMW/ZME-a8/IgG2a	[111]In	5	2.5–10	NS	9/12 pts and 26/33 lesions ≥ 1 cm
Choriocarcinoma										
1980	NCI, NIH; Univ. Kentucky[269]	IV	Choriocarcinoma, embryonal	3	hCG/goat polyclonal	[131]I	1.2–1.8	2–3 g/kg	NS	3/3 pts with (+) hCG
1984	Vancouver Gen. Hospital[270]	IV	Choriocarcinoma, lung	14	hCG/NS/NS, F(ab')$_2$	[99m]Tc	50	0.150	NS	12/14 pts and 15/28 lesions
Thyroid Carcinoma										
1983	Queen Elizabeth Hospital/ Birmingham[271]	IV	Thyroid		Thyroglobulin/ sheep polyclonal IgG	[131]I	0.5–1.0	0.100	NS	12/12 and 34/41 lesions; better than ^{131}I scans
Insulinoma										
1982	Queen Elizabeth Hosp[272]	IV	Insulinoma	3	Insulin, antitumor C peptide/NS	[131]I	1.0	NS	NS	2/3 localized

*IV, intravenous; IP, intraperitoneal; IA, intra-arterial; Subq, subcutaneous; NS, not stated.

niques to demonstrate tumor-specific localization.[231] These investigators speculated that tumors pick up some of the injected antibodies nonspecifically. These studies were also the first to express results as a percentage of injected dose per gram of tissue, terminology that has been widely adopted to express the results in a variety of different trials.

The first reported clinical trials of radiolabeled antibodies were those of Eugene Day and colleagues from Duke University. They initially used xenogeneic antisera from rabbits immunized with a patient's glioma and subsequently absorbed against normal human tissues.[232] It is clear from these and subsequent studies that vascularity and blood flow are of major importance in the localization of antibody in the differential uptake in tumors.

Subsequent studies were performed using antibodies to myelin.[233] Many of the theoretical aspects for these studies were developed by Bales and Spar.[234] Similar studies were carried out using preparations against renal cell carcinoma at Dalhousie University, with successful imaging of this tumor with goat antibodies.[235,236] Subsequently, the demonstration that CEA is recognizable in the serum and on the tumor-cell surface of a large number of adenocarcinomas suggested that such broadly expressed antigens could be targeted. The first attempt at using radiolabeled CEA, involving a rabbit polyclonal immunoglobulin preparation,[237] was unsuccessful. However, using specialized subtraction techniques and a purified goat antiserum to CEA, tumor was clearly imaged, and these studies, performed by Goldenberg and associates at the University of Kentucky,[238] stimulated further development of murine monoclonal antibodies, as well as their use as radiolabeled reagents in cancer diagnosis. These and subsequent studies are summarized in Table 17-9. Much of the information derived from these studies has been helpful in the design of therapeutic protocols using these antibodies and in the evaluation of concepts with regard to better monoclonal antibody preparation.

RADIONUCLIDE SELECTION AND SPECIALIZED NUCLEAR MEDICINE TECHNIQUES

Radioimmunoscintigraphy, or the detection of lesions using antibodies coupled to radionuclides, has been studied for some time. Which radionuclide is selected is dependent on the ease of conjugation and availability to clinical centers. The vast preponderance of studies have used ^{131}I because it has a gamma ray (364 keV) that is readily detectable externally and because it is widely available. On the other hand the high-energy gamma ray that is produced requires specialized collimating devices, which necessarily decreases the sensitivity. In addition, the isotope releases beta particles, which provide additional, unwanted radiation dosing in the setting of radioimaging. For this reason, other radionuclides have been investigated. Iodine-123 has some favorable characteristics (159 keV gamma ray and no production of beta particles). It has a relatively short half-life, however, which has made it difficult to employ in imaging trials, and it is expensive to prepare. Most trials have demonstrated superior imaging 2 to 4 days after injection of the radiolabeled antibody, as clearance of blood pool radiolabel and of nonspecific uptake by nontumor tissues leaves residual radiolabeled antibody at presumably greatest concentrations only in the tumor at these times. Another isotope that has been used is ^{111}In, which has a low-energy gamma ray (173 and 240 keV), is readily detectable by external imaging, and has a short half-life (67 hours). In comparative studies, ^{111}In appears to be superior to ^{131}I but requires specialized chelating agents for its use. Technetium-99m (^{99m}Tc) has been employed only in limited studies because of the problems of coupling it to antibody.

The ability to detect radiolabeled antibodies has been significantly improved by the development of more sophisticated external imaging equipment.[273] Tomographic and computerized gamma detectors have been used to create superior images. Single-photon emission computed tomography (SPECT) has been reported to have greater sensitivity in the detection of lesions. In addition, the ability to subtract images obtained with nonspecific radionuclides, such as technetium, has allowed greater detection of some lesions. As a rule, the sensitivity of external imaging devices is still limited to 1.0 to 1.5 cm, which is well within the range of currently available CT scanning and magnetic resonance imaging techniques.

ROUTES OF ADMINISTRATION OF ANTIBODY

The earliest clinical studies of antibody delivery used intra-arterial administration[232] and subsequently intravenous, intraperitoneal, and intralymphatic routes.[233] Murine and human models have enabled evaluation of therapies[275,276] and suggested the superiority of imaging of nodal metastatic disease after delivery into the lymphatics.[277,278] The high background uptake, probably related to reticuloendothelial-cell processing, even of Fab fragments, has been a significant limitation. In a recent study evaluating these techniques in 20 patients undergoing nodal dissection for melanoma, only two had specific uptake in nodes when radiolabeled antibody was delivered into the subcutaneous tissues.[262] More encouraging has been the delivery of antibodies directly into visceral spaces, such as the peritoneal cavity, which has provided some of the highest tumor-to-normal tissue ratios yet observed.[252,277] In most human studies, the tumor:nontumor ratios with intravenously administered anti-

bodies have ranged from 1 to 10, with most studies reporting ratios between 1 and 4. Very high ratios (greater than 20) have been demonstrated with intraperitoneal administration in a number of studies. This is currently being exploited in the development of specific radiation therapy protocols using highly radiolabeled antibodies delivered directly into the peritoneal cavity.

Great enthusiasm has been generated for the use of radioimaging techniques, and steady improvements have been made in our ability to identify lesions. Most of the lesions that have been identified, however, are those readily apparent using conventional techniques. Improvements would be required to make radioimaging a generally clinically useful technique (which it currently is not). The development of more specific monoclonal antibodies, perhaps chimeric antibodies, used either alone or in combination with radioisotopes with more favorable imaging characteristics coupled with better external detection systems will be required to increase the utility of these techniques.

TREATMENT WITH MONOCLONAL ANTIBODIES

The central problems in using monoclonal antibodies in therapy have been to define the appropriate target structure that is represented uniquely or in a limited fashion on the malignant cells (and to a much lesser extent on normal cells) and to define the conditions under which such antibodies could be made to eradicate tumor.[279] Although some of the earliest imaging studies were conducted with antibodies to CEA, an oncofetal antigen, no major effort has yet been reported in which antibodies to this antigen are used in therapy. To date, most studies of antibody therapy have reported only minor responses and used relatively small amounts of antibody, whereas murine models suggest that gram quantities would be required. Thus, these studies represent very early efforts in the evolution of these treatments. Major efforts in the therapy of cancer with monoclonal antibodies are summarized in Table 17-10.

Some of the first efforts were devoted to producing tumor-specific antibodies unique to an individual's own tumor. This is best represented by B-cell lymphomas. The immunoglobulin molecule expressed on the cell surface of the lymphoma represents a unique target for antibody action with recognition of a specific idiotype. Several studies have been conducted with anti-idiotypic antibodies with up to gram quantities being used.[281-285] The first patient reported to have been given such therapy had a dramatic complete response and remained in complete remission many years later.[281] These innovative studies, begun at Stanford University by Levy, Miller, and colleagues, were continued in a second series of patients, in which only half demonstrated some evidence of an antitumor response.[282] It appears on subsequent analysis that those individuals who "escaped" this therapy did so by developing idiotype-negative tumor variants. Of those who responded partially, most demonstrated an endogenous host T-cell response within residual tumor.

Other studies in the hematologic malignancies used antibodies to differentiation antigens such as CD5 and CD10. Most of the patients obtained only transient reductions in circulating tumor cells. The treatment appeared to have somewhat greater efficacy in some of the cutaneous T-cell lymphomas.[291-295] The most extensively studied antibody to adenocarcinoma has been 17-1A.[292-295] Although minor and partial responses have been reported, long-term follow-up of these individuals has not yet appeared. Combinations of this antibody with autologous lymphocytes or "armed" cells, as well as with gamma-interferon, have also been given. A number of studies have been conducted at the National Institutes of Health (NIH) and the University of Washington using antibodies directed to a transferrin-like molecule, p97, present on 70% to 80% of melanomas and to a similarly prevalent high-molecular weight antigen.[258,259,262,305] These studies, employing relatively low doses of antibody, have not produced significant responses.

Certain gangliosides are expressed at much higher con-

TABLE 17-10.   Therapeutic Studies Using Monoclonal Antibodies*

Year	Institution (Ref.)	Tumor	No. of Patients	Antigen/ Antibody/ Class	Human Antimouse Antibody	Maximum Total Dose (mg)	Tumor Regression
1980	Sidney Farber[280]	B lymphoma	1	AB89/IgG2a	NR	1580	0/1; brief decrease in circulatory cells
1982	Stanford[281]	B lymphoma	1	Anti-idiotype/ IgG2b	0/1	501	1/1; complete remission 60+ months
1984	Dana Farber[282]	B lymphoma	8	CD20/B1/ IgG2a	NR	50	6/8; bone marrow treated ex vivo with antibody
1985	Stanford[283]	B lymphoma	10	Anti-idiotype/ IgG1, IgG2a, IgG2b	5/10	3183	6/10; transient responses
1985	Netherlands Cancer Inst.[284]	B lymphoma	2	Anti-idiotype/ NS	0/2	5800	0/2; no significant response
1984	NCI, NIH[285]	B CLL	1	Anti-idiotype/ IgG2b, IgG1	NR	1500	0/1; transient reduction in circulating tumor cells
1982, 1984	Univ. California San Diego[286,287]	B CLL	4	CD5/T101/ IgG2a	0/4	200	0/4; transient drop in circulating tumor cells
1984	NCI, NIH[288]	B CLL	13	CD5/T101/ IgG2a	0/13	140	0/13; Transient decrease in circulating cells
1981	Dana Farber[289]	ALL	4	CD10/J5/ IgG2a	NR	170	0/4; Transient reduction in circulating cells
1981	Stanford[290]	ALL (T-cell)	1	CD5/L17/F12/ IgG2a	0/1	164	1/1; partial response
1983	Stanford[291]	ALL (T-cell)	8	CD5 & others, IgG2a, IgG1	NR	50	0/8; transient reduction in circulating tumor cells
1981, 1983	Stanford[292,293]	CTCL	6	CD5/L17F12/ IgG2a, IgG1	4/6	100	5/6; minor response
1984	Univ. California San Diego[287,294]	CTCL	4	CD5/T101/ IgG2a	2/4	200	4/12; minor response
1985	NCI, NIH[295]	CTCL	12	CD5/T101/ IgG2a	NR	100	4/4; minor response
1983	Dartmouth[296]	AML	3	Multiple/PMN6/ PMN29/PM8/ AML2-23/ IgG2b and IgM	1/1 tested	930	0/3; transient reduction in circulating tumor cells
1984	Hammersmith Hospital[297]	Squamous and adenocarcinoma	3	HMFG2/IgG1	NR	NR	3/3 (local only); direct injection of radiolabeled (^{131}I) antibody into pericardial, pleural, or peritoneal cavity
1984, 1985	Wistar Inst.[298,299]	Colon, gastrointestinal	40	17-1A/IgG2a	19/38	1000	5/40; minor responses only; some given with cells
1986	NCI, NIH[300]	Pancreas	25	17-1A/IgG2a	23/25	1200	0/25; some minor responses noted; also combined with cells in 15/25 patients

(continued)

TABLE 17-10.   Therapeutic Studies Using Monoclonal Antibodies* *(continued)*

Year	Institution (Ref.)	Tumor	No. of Patients	Antigen/ Antibody/ Class	Human Antimouse Antibody	Maximum Total Dose (mg)	Tumor Regression
1986	Fox Chase[301]	Gastrointestinal	27	171A/IgG2a	8/11 (tested)	400	0/27; gamma-interferon pretreatment
1982	Univ. Calif., San Diego[302]	Melanoma	3	p97,p240/ IgG1, IgG2a	NR	50	0/3
1982	Fred Hutchinson Cancer Center, Veterans Admin.[303]	Melanoma	1	p97/IgG1, Fab	NR	1	0/1; labeled with [131]I
1984	NCI, NIH[304]	Melanoma	8	gp240/9.2.27/ IgG2a	3/8	250	0/8
1985	Fred Hutchinson Cancer Center[305]	Melanoma	5	p97, gp240/96.5, 48.7	4/5	424	0/5
1985	Mainz Universität[306]	Melanoma, apudoma	3	GD3/R24/ IgG3	NR	440	0/3; inflammatory cutaneous responses around lesions noted
1985	Memorial Sloan Kettering[307]	Melanoma	12	GD3/R24/ IgG3	12/12	400	5/12; both partial and mixed responses; inflam- matory responses noted
1987	Children's Hosp., San Francisco[308]	Melanoma	22	p220/XMMME-01/ IgG2a	22/22	300	5/22; ricin-coupled antibody; 1 complete response, 4 mixed responses; significant antibody response to ricin
1987	R.L. Ireland Cancer Center, Case Western Reserve Univ.[309]	Melanoma, neuroblastoma	17	GD2/3F8/ IgG3	17/17	100/m²	7/17 responses with 2 complete responses in patients with neuroblastoma and 2 partial responses in patients with melanoma
1987	Jefferson Univ., Philadelphia[310]	Multiple	20	CD8/Leu 2a/IgG1	20/20	100	0/20; aimed at decreasing "suppressor cells" in cancer patients

*ALL, acute lymphocytic leukemia; G1, gastrointestinal; B-CLL, B-cell chronic lymphocyte leukemia; CTCL, cutaneous T-cell lymphoma; NR, not reported; AML, acute myelogenous leukemia.

centrations on melanoma cells and tumors of neural crest origin. Antibodies to the gangliosides GD_2 and GD_3 have elicited both inflammatory responses within lesions[306,307] and objective antitumor responses at Memorial Sloan-Kettering[307] and, more recently, at Case Western Reserve.[309] Direct injection of a human antibody to GD_2 has been reported to cause regression of cutaneous metastases.[205] Limited responses to a ricin-conjugated antibody to a high-molecular-weight antigen have recently been reported also.[208]

Toxicity associated with the infusion of murine monoclonal antibodies has been tolerable. Fever, chills, pruritus, chest tightness, dyspnea, rash, arthralgia, myalgia, and hypotension have been noted in individual patients and may be related to the rate of infusion of the antibody. Anaphylactoid responses are distinctly unusual. Far more frequent is the subsequent development of a HAMA response, which is associated with more rapid clearance of the antibody and thus presumedly a lesser likelihood of response. Houghton and colleagues at Memorial Sloan-Kettering have administered an anti-GD_3 antibody after the development of significant HAMA and still observed significant antitumor responses.[307] Serum sickness is distinctly uncommon.

It is likely that the immediate future of monoclonal antibodies as cancer treatments will be determined by the success of trials employing large quantities of antitumor antibodies alone or in conjunction with other biologic response modifiers, such as interferon and IL-2. The use of antibodies conjugated to radionuclides or toxins and the further development of anti-idiotypic antibodies will be areas of great interest and clinical activity. Antibodies have also been used to clear bone marrow of malignant cells before reinfusion into the host[310] in transplantation studies. Ex vivo application of these antibodies is being pursued at a number of centers and is suggested by the ability to maximally clear tumor using high doses of chemotherapy in vivo and toxin or complement-mediated lysis of tumor present in the harvested marrow. In addition, the continuous development of novel chimeric antibodies for use either alone or in conjunction with toxins will likely be the major areas of interest over the next decade. The fact that objective antitumor responses have been observed suggests that these approaches will have greater applicability in the future.

IMMUNOTHERAPY

INTRODUCTION

Strategies for the immunotherapy of cancer can be divided into active and passive approaches (Table 17-11). "Active immunotherapy" refers to the immunization of the tumor-bearing host with materials designed to elicit an immune reaction capable of eliminating or retarding tumor growth. Active immunotherapy can be further subdivided into non-specific or specific immunization. Most early attempts at the immunotherapy of cancer utilized nonspecific active approaches to immune stimulation with adjuvants such as BCG, C. parvum, levamisole, and a variety of other substances. Specific attempts at immunotherapy utilized immunization with tumor cells or tumor-cell extracts either alone or in vaccines, often in conjunction with immune stimulators such as BCG. These early approaches were almost uniformly unsuccessful in man and have largely been abandoned. More recently, the advent of recombinant cytokines has provided a more selective means for stimulating the immune system. Treatment with the interferons or with IL-2 is a form of nonspecific active immunotherapy, although the selective action of these purified lymphokines provides a greater ability to manipulate immune responses than was previously possible.

Many studies have demonstrated that the tumor-bearing host is immunosuppressed by growing tumor and thus attempts at active immunotherapy may have intrinsic disadvantages. More recent efforts have concentrated on passive approaches to immunotherapy, which involve the transfer to the tumor-bearing host of previously sensitized immunologic reagents such as cells or antibody that have the ability, either directly or indirectly, to mediate antitumor responses. The term "adoptive immunotherapy" is usually used to denote passive immunotherapy with cells (lymphocytes or macrophages). Recent efforts have been devoted to developing adoptive immunotherapies utilizing LAK cells, TIL, or other

TABLE 17-11.   Classification of Cancer Immunotherapies

Classification	Examples
Active immunotherapy	
Nonspecific	Immune adjuvants such as BCG, C. parvum, levamisole
	Interferon
	IL-2
Specific	Immunization with tumor-cell vaccines
Passive immunotherapy	
Antibodies	Monoclonal or polyclonal antibodies either alone or conjugated with toxins or radiolabels
Cells	LAK cells
	Tumor-infiltrating lymphocytes (TIL)
Indirect	Removal of blocking factors
	Inhibition of growth factors or angiogenic factors

means for in vitro stimulation of cells with antitumor reactivity.

The development of techniques for generating monoclonal antibodies has greatly improved the ability to obtain preparations with specific reactivity to human tumor-associated antigens. Considerable effort is being devoted to the utilization of these antibodies either alone or conjugated with toxins or radiolabels for use in cancer treatment, as discussed earlier.

In addition to these active and passive approaches, the immune system can be used in a variety of indirect ways to mediate antitumor responses. Included in this category are approaches such as the removal of blocking factors from serum or the inhibition of essential tumor growth factors.

ACTIVE NONSPECIFIC IMMUNOTHERAPY

Any agent that can alter host–tumor relationships in favor of the host can be considered a biologic response modifier. Most biologic response modifiers stimulate the immune system.[311] The earliest modifiers were discovered accidentally when clinicians noted rare cases of significant tumor regression after a patient with cancer survived a nearly fatal septic episode with a bacterial organism, or a systemic viral illness such as herpes zoster. Microorganisms are now known to elicit a wide range of host responses that activate neutrophils, macrophages, NK cells, T cells, and B cells and their products, many of which can mediate tumor-cell killing. Thus, initial attempts at boosting the immune system of cancer-bearing humans have used a variety of microorganisms or fractions of microbial products.

Table 17-12 gives a partial list of biologic response modifiers. The largest body of knowledge has been accumulated from the use of microorganisms and their products. Initial experimental use of such reagents in animal tumor models has demonstrated prolongation of survival under certain conditions: the tumor burden is low (immunotherapy given early or used as adjuvant with other cytoreductive treatment; never effective alone against large established tumors), the host is immunocompetent (young animals freshly inoculated with tumor), and the tumor is immunogenic. The immune stimulation appears to work best in the setting where the immunostimulant is in direct contact with the tumor.

There are two implications of these findings. First, the mechanism of tumor-cell killing appears to be an "innocent bystander" effect mediated by a vigorous local immune response; there is little evidence for effective boosting of systemic reactions. Second, it is difficult to relate the conditions for successful experimental immunotherapy in animals to any clinical circumstance in man. Local control of human cancer is rarely an important clinical problem with the judicious application of modern surgical and radiation therapy techniques. Rather, the principal problem in cancer patients is effective treatment of metastatic disease, a setting in which nonspecific active immunotherapies have been largely unsuccessful in animals and are unlikely to be successful in humans. In addition cancer-bearing patients often have demonstrable defects in their immune responses,[312] yet it appears that intact cell-mediated responses are critical to the therapeutic effect of many biologic response modifiers.[2]

TABLE 17-12. Biologic Response Modifiers

Microorganisms

Bacille Calmette-Guerin (BCG)
Corynebacterium parvum
Salmonella typhimurium
Mycobacterium tuberculosis
Viruses (vaccinia, Newcastle disease, influenza)
Brucella abortus
Bordetella pertussis
Listeria monocytogenes
OK-432 (Picibinil)
Mixed bacterial vaccines

Microbial components

Methanol-extractable residue of BCG (MER)
Nocardia rubra cell-wall skeleton
Glucan (from *Saccharomyces*)
Lentinan (from *Basidiomycetes*)
Krestin (from *Basidiomycetes*)
Other glucans
BCG cell walls
Endotoxin
Muramyl dipeptide
Trehalose dimycolate
Schizophillan
Staphylococcal protein A

Immunomodulators from miscellaneous sources

Levamisole
Cyclophosphamide
Polyribonucleotides
Doxorubicin
Alkyl lysophospholipids
Maleic anhydride divinyl ether (MVE-2)
Liposomes
Many natural products
Bestatin
Tuftsin
Flavone acetic acid
Cimetidine
Swainsonine
Prostaglandin inhibitors
Dinitrochlorobenzene (DNCB)

Physiologic mediators

Cytokines
Colony-stimulating factors
Neuropeptides
Antibodies (*e.g.,* anti-CD8)
Complement
LFA 1, LFA 3
Lymphokines (IL1-6, IFNs, NKCF, leukoregulin, etc.)
Endorphins
Thymic hormones
Perforins
Leukocyte dialysates

Finally, as discussed elsewhere in this chapter, spontaneous human tumors may not be very immunogenic. Thus, the application of this animal research to humans was unlikely to be useful, and this has certainly proved to be the case.

Since the 1960s, a large number of clinical studies have attempted to achieve systemic immune stimulation employing BCG or the methanol-extractable residue of BCG (MER); fewer studies have used *C. parvum* or levamisole.[313] Usually, immunotherapy was used in an adjuvant setting after conventional treatment with surgery, radiation, or combination chemotherapy had produced clinical complete remission. In general, initial trials suggested positive results and raised hopes for therapeutic benefit, but such studies often were not properly controlled, involved small numbers of patients, or both. When well-controlled prospective randomized trials were performed with adequate numbers of carefully staged patients, interim analyses of end-points such as disease-free survival at 1 or 2 years of follow-up often demonstrated a trend that favored the immunotherapy arm of the study in a magnitude that was not quite statistically significant. However, when the study matured with reasonable numbers of patients followed for reasonable periods of time, the disease-free or overall survival curves usually were not significantly different. Hersh recently analyzed the more than 175 studies of active nonspecific immunotherapy reported in the literature in the 2-year period 1982–1984.[314] Among 26 studies of BCG-MER administered intravenously or subcutaneously that were either randomized or were thought to have appropriately well-matched historical controls, only six studies (23%) had positive results. Another 150 studies reported results with other agents designed to boost host immunity, but only 60 of these were thought to be analyzable. Twenty-three of the studies (38%) demonstrated therapeutic effects from systemic active nonspecific immunotherapy.

The possible reasons for the failure of so many studies are numerous. Little effort has been devoted to finding a dose and schedule that optimizes in vivo immune responses. Thus, simple inadequate administration of an immunomodulating agent could explain some failures. However, some investigators have carefully documented that the agent, as delivered by them, is capable of boosting host immunity. For example, Hersh and associates demonstrated augmentation of NK activity, monocyte-mediated ADCC, in vitro lymphocyte proliferation, and delayed-type hypersensitivity responses after single or multiple doses of BCG-MER.[315] However, they observed no consistent effects on clinical end-points such as disease-free or overall survival rate. Therefore, it would appear that a significant limitation of systemic immunotherapy is that the available biologic response modifiers do not appear capable of including enough systemic immune augmentation to accomplish clinically significant tumor cytoreduction. This finding does not imply that immune-mediated tumor-cell destruction is not significant in magnitude. However, it must be kept in mind that, like the physiologic mechanisms regulating most organ systems, the immune system is subject to both positive and negative homeostatic influences. Immune stimulation without accompanying downregulation of the immune response would be dangerous, and in the healthy state never occurs. It is clear from the histopathology of the thyroid gland from a patient with Hashimoto's thyroiditis or the pannus of a patient with rheumatoid arthritis that the destructive power of the immune system is enormous. A key limitation to harnessing this power and using it against tumors is our extensive ignorance about the negative control points in an immune response. We intuitively know there are limits on in vivo lymphocyte proliferation and activation (how large was the largest lymph node you have ever seen?); however, the nature of those limits is unknown. We know that lymphocytes become desensitized to stimulation if called upon to act too frequently or if given too much antigen.[316,317] We know that some antigens and some tumors elicit suppression of immune responses.[318] When basic science provides us with an understanding of the physiologic controls of the immune response, we may be able to intervene to remove those controls temporarily so that the nonspecific immune stimulants can turn on the system and it is not turned off until the physician replaces the negative control elements after the therapeutic effect has been achieved. Of course, such a strategy is likely to create a problem similar to that faced in the use of other treatment modalities: how to protect the normal tissues and preserve an appropriate therapeutic index.

Unlike the disappointing results obtained with systemic immunotherapy, the local or regional use of nonspecific immunostimulants more commonly achieves local or regional antitumor responses.[319] The injection of cutaneous metastases of malignant melanoma has been the most common form of local immunotherapy. BCG, MER, and dinitrochlorobenzene (DNCB) have been the agents most commonly injected into tumor masses. The following conclusions can be drawn from the accumulated clinical experience. First, the induction of a local inflammatory–immune response can cause the regression of large tumor masses. Injected lesions regress in 70% to 90% of the cases, and the regressions appear to be clinically useful. Second, histologic study of regressing lesions supports the idea that the tumor is killed as an innocent bystander of a granulomatous inflammatory response. There is the suggestion that local immunity is common, since regrowth of completely regressing injected lesions is rare but recurrence at noninjected sites is common. Third, in about 5% to 15% of cases, noninjected distal cutaneous lesions or, more rarely, organ metastases were documented to regress; therefore, systemic immunity is elicited rarely.[320] However, systemic toxicity was seen and was sometimes fatal.[321] In one series, intralesional injection of BCG followed by surgical excision appeared to result in an unexpectedly large fraction of long-term disease-free survivors.[322] Whether this result was secondary to the elicitation of systemic immunity is unclear; however, it should be noted that successful nonspecific therapy in animal models has followed surgical resection of an injected lesion.[323]

Intralesional injection of primary lung tumors[324] and chest wall recurrences of breast cancer[325] have produced local antitumor responses, but none of the intralesional approaches to the treatment of any cancer has produced long-term disease-free survival of patients with metastatic disease. Intralesional therapy can be palliative in certain instances.

Perhaps the most impressive success of active nonspecific immunotherapy has been in the instillation of agents into tumor-bearing body cavities such as the pleura, the peritoneum, and the bladder. About 75% to 85% of newly identified patients with bladder cancer have superficial tumors, and, even with complete resection, recurrence is common. At least two prospective randomized studies have documented that intravesical BCG results in apparently permanent complete responses in about 70% of patients, including those whose tumors have advanced during intravesical chemotherapy (usually with thiotepa).[326,327] BCG appears to be significantly better than thiotepa in patients with superficial bladder cancer and is viewed as the treatment of choice by many urologists, although the Food and Drug Administration has not yet approved it for routine use. BCG also has been instilled into the pleural cavity to control malignant effusions with some success, but superiority to other methods of effusion control has not been demonstrated. Intrapleural BCG as a surgical adjuvant in the treatment of lung cancer has in some studies been superior to surgery alone;[328] however, the capacity of such therapy to prevent systemic recurrences is unclear. Because the major clinical problem in bladder cancer is local control, the data justify the use of intravesical BCG. Because the major problem in lung cancer is not local control, its role in this disease is less certain.

Corynebacterium parvum is another bacterium that has been used for regional immunotherapy. Unlike BCG, *C. parvum* appears to be able to induce antitumor effects in animals without T cells, a fact that suggests its effects may be more dependent on macrophage-mediated tumor killing. It has been installed into the pleural[329] and peritoneal[330] cavities for the control of malignant ascites and has been used in the treatment of ovarian cancer with some evidence of response.[331,332] Unfortunately, the inflammatory response in the peritoneal cavity can lead to serious medical complications from adhesions compressing the bowel and vasculature. Therefore, the use of *C. parvum* is restricted to palliation of symptoms in these settings.

Another strategy in active nonspecific immunotherapy has been the paring down of bacteria to the smallest subunit capable of eliciting a potent immune response. Trehalose dimycolate (also known as cord factor) is a disaccharide esterified to two long-chain fatty acids that has potent adjuvant effects. However, the smallest structure that retains immune stimulatory capacity is N-acetylmuramyl-L-alanine-D-isoglutamine, also known as muramyl dipeptide. These compounds are undergoing preclinical studies,[333] and a study of muramyl tripeptide enclosed in liposomes is being conducted in man; however, there are not obvious reasons for them to be superior to the organisms from which they were derived in obtaining systemic immune stimulation.

ACTIVE SPECIFIC IMMUNOTHERAPY

The word "immune" is derived from the Greek root meaning memory, the critical attribute of the immune system shared only with the central nervous system. Perhaps the ideal approach to immunologic cancer treatment would be to resect the primary tumor and immunize the patient against his own tumor so that any recurrence in any site at any time thereafter would be remembered, recognized, and rejected. The concept of memory is critical, for it implies the development of *antigen-specific* recognition by cells of the immune system: by B cells that will make tumor-specific antibodies, and by T cells that will make tumor-specific cell-mediated responses. Cells with NK, K, and LAK activity and neutrophils and macrophages can kill tumor cells but have no memory and no antigen-specific tumor recognition capacity.

This principle of vaccination or immunization has ample precedent in infectious diseases and has been pursued for many years in connection with cancer. However, there are several problems that have prohibited a simple direct approach to active specific immunotherapy. First, tumor-associated or tumor-specific antigens are very difficult to demonstrate in man: most of the putative tumor-associated antigens are also expressed to some degree on some normal tissue(s). Second, there is substantial heterogeneity in tumor cells, and there is some evidence that metastatic cells differ antigenically from primary tumors. Thus, the development of immunity to some component of the primary tumor may not be protective against the metastatic deposits. Third, some tumors have managed to escape immune detection by the ingenious mechanism of decreasing or eliminating their expression of MHC antigens, structures that are required for antigen-specific recognition by cytotoxic T lymphocytes. This change renders T cells blind to the tumor. Furthermore, tumors express certain soluble factors that may interfere with or suppress the action of immune cells. Finally, the positive animal models that have been developed have rarely been suitably analyzed to discern what aspect of immunity is critical to the therapeutic effect. Is it critical that the vaccine induce measurable levels of antibody? If so, what antibody class is most important? Does one need to demonstrate delayed-type hypersensitivity to the tumor or its antigens? Are MHC-restricted cytotoxic T cells involved in the effect? What role, if any, is played by antigen-specific helper–inducer-phenotype T cells? What are the critical technical features of vaccine preparation that are associated with the optimal clinical effects?

A variety of strategies have been taken to vaccine development; however, all have employed one or more sources of antigen and an adjuvant of some sort. The antigen source is usually either cells or cell extracts. When cells are used, they may be varied in several ways: autologous or allogeneic tumor cells, living or inactivated by radiation, freeze–thaw alteration, heat alteration, or drug inactivation (e.g., mitomycin C), and often immunogenicity is enhanced in vitro by a process called xenogenation. Xenogenation involves altering the expression of membrane proteins through the use of viruses (xenogenation),[334,335] physical treatment of the cells with, for example, ultraviolet (UV) light or heat (physical xenogenation),[336] or chemical treatment of the cells with enzymes, mutagens, and cancer chemotherapeutic agents (chemical xenogenation).[337] Influenza, Newcastle disease, and vaccinia viruses have all been employed in human clinical trials of tumor vaccines, but study design has not permitted straightforward interpretation of results. Physically altered cells have been examined recently by Edelson and his colleagues.[338] After administering psoralen to 37 patients with cutaneous T-cell lymphoma refractory to local treatments, the investigators leukopheresed the patients and treated the cells with UV light ex vivo before returning the cells to the patients. The psoralen was designed to sensitize any circulating tumor cells to the effects of the UV light. Twenty-seven of these patients with refractory disease experienced clinically significant tumor regressions with this treatment, presumably related to the induction of an antitumor immune response by the UV-damaged infused tumor cells. Chemical xenogenation has been employed in a study in which patients undergoing curative resection of colon cancer were given allogeneic tumor cells treated with neuraminidase before being used as a vaccine.[339] It was said that the vaccinated patients with Dukes' Stage C colon cancer had a significantly increased probability of survival, but the

nature of the immunity induced was not studied. It would be presumed that the immune effector mechanism in this instance, if any, is tumor-specific antibody, because MHC-restricted T-cell responses probably would not be elicited by an allogeneic tumor-cell vaccine. Morton and his colleagues used an allogeneic melanoma cell vaccine plus BCG in a prospective randomized study of patients with Stage II melanoma. Although there were no significant differences in the 5-year survival rates of vaccinated and nonvaccinated patients, among the 37% of vaccinated patients who made IgM antibodies reactive with membrane antigens of cultured melanoma cells there was a highly significant prolongation of survival.[340] Thus, patients who responded to the vaccine appeared to benefit, but most patients made no specific response (although most were alloimmunized to the vaccine's MHC antigens).

Chemical xenogenation appears to have potential clinical applications. The drugs employed to show this effect in animal models are the agents clinicians use to treat patients with cancer. Could our treatments be inducing xenogenation in vivo? It is of interest that at least one membrane change that has been thought to occur in vivo in response to treatment is the expression of the p170 glycoprotein associated with the phenotype of multidrug resistance.[341] Many structurally distinct drugs with different mechanisms of action can elicit this response from tumor cells, which appears to be a stereotyped reaction to xenobiotic toxins. Interestingly, cells induced to express p170 in vitro by drug exposure appear to be more immunogenic. Paired cell lines in which one expresses p170 and the other does not often differ in their capacity to induce tumors in nude mice: the one expressing p170 loses tumorigenicity (because of increased immunogenicity?). Such findings lead to the intriguing notion that cells expressing the multidrug-resistant phenotype may be more susceptible to immune attack. Experiments to test this notion are under way.

Extracts of tumor cells and purified components of tumor-cell membranes given together with immune adjuvants have been explored for their capacity to protect patients from tumor relapse. A series of trials by Hollinshead and her colleagues appear to show consistent therapeutic benefit for patients with Stage I squamous cell carcinoma given a vaccine consisting of membrane proteins from a few primary lung cancer specimens plus Freund's complete adjuvant:[342] The 5-year survival rate for patients receiving the vaccine was 69% compared with 49% for control patients. Vaccinated patients often developed skin-test reactivity to the immunizing proteins. However, there is some variability in the data analysis of a control group that receive Freund's adjuvant alone; sometimes, such patients are considered to have been vaccinated when they undergo repeated skin tests. Furthermore, some surgical series report a 5-year survival rate of 58% in Stage I squamous cell carcinoma of the lung, a result that may not be significantly different from the 69% achieved by vaccinated patients. Thus, it is not clear that patients have benefited specifically from the vaccine.

The most impressive clinical trial to date of active specific immunotherapy was performed by Hoover and Hanna and their colleagues. In this study, patients with Dukes' Stage B2 and C colon cancer were randomized to receive no postoperative treatment or immunization with 10^7 irradiated autologous tumor cells at weekly intervals for 3 weeks with 10^7 BCG organisms given with the first two injections.[3,343,344] The vaccinated group has significantly fewer recurrences and significantly fewer deaths than the control group. About two-thirds of the vaccinated patients made impressive delayed-type hypersensitivity responses upon skin testing with their own tumor. Some patients also made antibody responses, but most of these were the IgM isotype. It is not clear what immune mechanism is responsible for the observed improvement in clinical outcome, but a larger prospective study is under way that will address some of the questions about mechanism. This highly encouraging result obviously hinges on having a primary tumor that can be dispersed to provide adequate numbers of viable tumor cells for the vaccine. If the larger study can shed light on the critical component of the immune response associated with the therapeutic effect, one could imagine further boosting or prolonging cell-mediated mechanisms perhaps by adding IL-2 to the vaccination schedule or by augmenting antibody responses with concomitant administration of some other lymphokines, perhaps IL-4 or IL-6.

There is a suggestion that specific immunity can be obtained in the course of treatment. For example, in the study by Morton and associates of BCG as a nonspecific immunostimulant injected directly into metastatic melanoma lesions, the regression of distant noninjected skin nodules implies that the BCG primed the host immune system to tumor-associated antigens that were recognized at a distance by the cells.[2] Furthermore, it has been proposed that electrosurgery[345] or cryosurgery[346] of primary tumors results in some fraction of patients developing antibodies to the tumor.

Finally, some experimental data have suggested that signals that are normally activation signals for T cells (*e.g.*, antigen, anti-CD3, anti-CD2) can be associated with T-cell tumor regression and the simultaneous development of tumor immunity.[347] The mechanism of this antigen-specific effect is under investigation.

INTERFERONS

BIOLOGIC EFFECTS OF INTERFERONS

Interferon was discovered in 1957 as an activity made in response to viral infection that appeared to protect cells from such infection.[348] In the 30 years since that discovery, much has been learned about the interferon system, and today interferon has been found useful against a number of infectious and immune disorders and is the treatment of choice for at least one malignant disease.[349] There are three types of interferon: alpha, beta, and gamma. Alpha- and beta-interferons are stable to exposure to pH 2 and are sometimes referred to together as type I interferons. Gamma-interferon is labile at pH 2 and is sometimes called type II interferon. There is at least one form of alpha-interferon that is acid-labile, but it has been detected only in the setting of disease (*e.g.*, lupus erythematosus, AIDS).[350] Alpha- and beta-interferons appear to be able to be made by virtually all cells; gamma-interferon is made only by T lymphocytes and

large granular lymphocytes. To date, there have been 15 genes identified that encode for alpha-interferon species, two genes for beta-interferon (although beta-2 interferon appears to be identical to a B-cell differentiation factor), and one gene for gamma-interferon.[351] The human alpha-interferon genes and the beta-1-interferon gene are free of introns, and it appears that their synthesis is induced by release of the genes from repression.[352] A large number of stimuli can induce interferon synthesis, including viruses, double-stranded RNA, synthetic polyribonucleotides (*e.g.*, poly ICLC, poly AU, ampligen), pyran copolymers (*e.g.*, maleic vinyl ether or MVE-2), low-molecular-weight amines, fluorenones (*e.g.*, tilorone), antibiotics (*e.g.*, kanamycin), microorganisms (bacteria [*C. parvum*, mycoplasma, mycobacteria], rickettsiae, fungi, protozoa), microbial components (endotoxin, OK432), drugs (pyrimidinones, flavone acetic acid), and, most recently, certain growth factors and cytokines (*e.g.*, platelet-derived growth factor, TNF, GM-CSF, M-CSF). The best-studied interferon inducer is poly ICLC, a hydrophilic complex formed between poly-1-lysine, carboxymethylcellulose, and the polyribonucleotide composed of inosinic and cytidylic acids. Poly ICLC appears to interact with a cellular gene (a trans-acting factor whose absence from certain cell types limits the inducibility of the interferon gene[353] to release repressors from the control sites of interferon gene transcription. In addition, poly ICLC can stabilize interferon mRNA;[354] thus, inducers act at both the transcriptional and post-transcriptional level.

In contrast to alpha- and beta-interferon genes, the single gamma-interferon gene has four exons and three introns. The mRNA appears to contain an AU-rich region in the 3' untranslated portion of the message, a feature common to lymphokine genes that enhances mRNA stability. The precise mechanisms involved in the tissue-specific expression of gamma-interferon are not yet clear. Recently, some tissues and cells (*e.g.*, placenta) have been found to produce interferons constitutively.[355] The role of such interferons is unknown.

Interferons mediate a wide range of biologic responses: antiviral effects, antiproliferative effects, cytotoxic effects, immunomodulation, gene activation, and differentiation. The individual alpha-interferons differ in their capacity to mediate the various effects and are expressed to different degrees in distinct cell types.[356-358] All the diverse effects of interferons appear to be mediated through distinct receptors: alpha- and beta-interferons can compete with one another for binding to one type of receptor; gamma-interferon has a distinct receptor.[359] The interferon effects on target cells require internalization of the interferon–receptor complex.[360] Interferon appears to enhance the transcription of a large number of genes, at least a few of whose products are responsible for mediating some of the effects attributed to interferon action. Interferon-inducible genes include those encoding for enzymes (*e.g.*, 2',5' oligoadenylate synthetases, RNase L, indoleamine 2,3-dioxygenase, dsRNA-activated initiation factor 2 [eIF2] kinase), proteins with known functions (*e.g.*, Class I and Class II MHC antigens, beta-2 microglobulin, Fc receptors, metallothionein IIA, Mx protein), and a number of proteins whose functions are not yet known. The genes induced by interferons are located all over the genome, but several of them share homologous sequences that may be the target of interferon regulation.[361] The types of interferon vary in their induction of different gene products; for example, the Mx protein is induced only by alpha- or beta-interferon, not by gamma-interferon, and Class II MHC antigens and Fc receptors are more effectively induced by gamma-interferon than by alpha- or beta-interferon.

The mechanisms of some of the effects of interferon have been established. For example, the Mx protein, a 75 kD-protein located in the nucleus of alpha- or beta-interferon-treated cells, is sufficient to mediate resistance to influenza virus and acts by blocking transcription of the viral genome.[362] Furthermore, the gamma-interferon-induced enzyme, indoleamine 2,3-dioxygenase, is responsible for the interferon-related killing of *Toxoplasma gondii* because it breaks down the tryptophan of the host cell, upon which this parasite is exquisitely dependent.[363] The precise mechanisms involved in the effects of interferons on cell proliferation and differentiation are not known, but interferons have been demonstrated to affect the expression of a number of proto-oncogenes including *myc, ras, mos,* and *abl* and growth factor receptors,[364] and certain data suggest that the level of 2′,5′ oligoadenylate synthetase induced by interferon may be inversely related to cell proliferation. For example, levels of the enzyme decrease when liver cells start to regenerate after partial hepatectomy and increase when regeneration is complete.[365] All stages of the cell cycle are lengthened by interferons, but cells in G_0 are the most sensitive to the antiproliferative effects. Thus interferon effects are greater on resting than on dividing cells.

The immunomodulatory effects of the interferons are numerous and affect every cell type involved in host defense including NK cells, T cells, B cells, macrophages, PMNs, and other effector cells derived from the bone marrow. In general, the dominant effect of interferons on the immune system depends on the assay, the timing of interferon administration, the length of exposure, and the type and dose of interferon used. Cell-mediated responses are more affected than are the antibody responses. Even some interferon effects on the tumor cell enhance its susceptibility to cell-mediated lysis; for example, the induction of Class I and II MHC antigens and other cell-surface proteins facilitates the recognition of the tumor by T cells and may also enhance the number of monoclonal antibody molecules that might recognize the tumor. Interferon activates NK cells and can increase NK cell migration into tissues. Interferon can enhance ADCC, mediated by killer (K) cells, that mediate by monocytes by augmenting lytic activity and numbers of Fc receptors expressed on the cell surface, and that mediated by PMNs.

There is a burgeoning literature on the interaction of interferons with other biologic agents. For example, the effects of gamma-interferon on PMN-mediated ADCC is increased when used together with GM-CSF,[366] and the antitumor effects of TNF factor are enhanced when it is used in combination with gamma-interferon.[367] There are no doubt many more salutary interactions among the lymphokines, and it is hoped that some of them will be useful in the treatment of cancer.

Gamma-interferon is much more potent in its effects on the immune system than alpha- or beta-interferon, and most of the changes follow a bell-shaped dose–response curve. This is in contrast to the antiproliferative effects of the interferons, which are directly related to the dose used. Thus, the clinical use of interferons in cancer therapy is complicated. If the primary goal of interferon treatment is to affect tumor proliferation directly, the interferon should be used at the maximal tolerated dose, analogous to any antitumor agent. On the other hand, if the goal of treatment is a maximal boost of an immune response to the tumor, lower doses may be necessary because the optimal immunomodulatory dose can be substantially below the maximum tolerated dose in man.[368]

The mechanisms by which tumors may be affected by the interferons go beyond direct antiproliferative effects on the tumor cells and the manifold effects on the immune system. Interferons also can inhibit tumor angiogenesis.[369] A significant problem with the clinical application of interferons to cancer treatment is that we do not know which of the many effects are the most important for obtaining tumor responses. Because some of the effects occur at disparate doses and most of the effects are not easily assessed or monitored in vivo in man, many of the clinical trials that have been performed over the last 6 years, since an interferon gene was cloned, have been empiric. Despite these difficulties, substantial progress has been made.

CLINICAL APPLICATION OF INTERFERONS

It follows from the above discussion that there are substantial difficulties associated with attempting to use interferons and other biologic response modifiers in humans. The multitude of effects of such agents and the inadequate information about what effects are critical to obtaining in vivo antitumor responses interfere with the development of an optimal dose schedule. Such lack of information minimally interferes with the clinical application of cancer chemotherapeutic agents because the sequence of clinical testing of these drugs is based on the assumption that the agents are poisons with some therapeutic index and that more is better. Thus, clinical trials with drugs seek to establish the therapeutic index by determining the maximum tolerated dose (Phase I), determining the antitumor activity of the maximum tolerated dose in a variety of malignancies (Phase II), and integrating the drug into combinations of drugs and comparing these combinations with standard therapies (Phase III). For biologicals, however, animal models and some human studies[368,370] have suggested that there may be an extraordinarily wide disparity between the maximum tolerated dose and the optimal antitumor dose. Because some of the interferon's effects are direct antiproliferative actions on the tumor, it is conceivable that more is better. However, other interferon effects are immunomodulatory, and when these effects are more important the optimal antitumor does may be closer to the optimal immunomodulatory dose.

Unfortunately, the clinical development of the interferons has proceeded according to the precedent established for cancer chemotherapeutic agents, and at this writing an optimal immunomodulatory dose for alpha- and beta-interferon has not been established. The impact of gamma-interferon on the immune system is greater than that of alpha- and beta-interferon, and an optimal immunomodulatory dose of gamma-interferon has recently been established.[368] Clinical trials of gamma-interferon administered at its optimal immunomodulatory dose are just beginning.

Another factor complicating the use of interferons and other biologic agents, particularly cytokines, is that the physiological role of these agents cannot be easily duplicated by systemic administration in pharmacologic doses. Most of these agents are physiologically elicited in tissues, and they are meant to act locally or over short distances and in concert with a number of other molecules produced by other cells of the immune system. Separating a lymphokine from other mediators, removing it from its physiological compartment, and using it systemically may make it much less effective or even useless. Furthermore, in the process of altering host immunity systemically with these agents, it is possible that the intricate mechanisms that maintain self-tolerance may be altered or broken and deleterious autoimmune phenomena induced. Fortunately, to date, such problems have been rare in the treatment of cancer patients with interferons.

Despite these caveats and concerns, interferons (particularly the alpha species) have been found to be active in patients bearing a variety of tumor types. Table 17-13 lists the tumor types in which alpha-interferons have been most active, the overall response rates, and the doses at which those responses have occurred. The most common solid tumors—lung, colorectal, and breast cancers—have not been highly responsive to alpha-interferon used as a single agent; however, such tumors are refractory to most single-agent treatments. Interferon has been most active in certain hematopoietic tumors. The antitumor activity of interferon in patients with solid tumors is usually obtained with treatment near the maximum tolerated dose. Treatment experience with beta- and gamma-interferon is considerably smaller. As might be expected by the fact that alpha- and beta-interferons share a receptor, it does not appear that they have a different spectrum of single-agent activity. Gamma-interferon is also still under investigation in Phase II studies; however, it seems to differ from the alpha and beta species in that patients with hairy cell leukemia respond poorly to gamma-interferon. However, gamma-interferon appears to have some activity in chronic lymphocytic leuke-

mia, a disease in which alpha- and beta-interferons are inactive.

Because in vitro studies suggest that the antiproliferative effects of interferon are related to the duration of exposure, pharmacokinetics in humans may be an important determinant of response. Interferons are filtered through the glomeruli, but more than 90% of the filtered molecules are reabsorbed and catabolized in the renal tubules.[371] Intravenous infusions result in clearance with a half-life of about 4 to 8 hours, whereas after intramuscular or subcutaneous injection, peak serum levels occur at about 6 to 8 hours with complete clearance by 16 to 24 hours.[372] Thus, longer exposure follows subcutaneous or intramuscular injection, and most responses have been obtained in patients so treated.

The most dramatic clinical antitumor effects from interferon have been seen in patients with hairy cell leukemia, an uncommon tumor of mature B cells characterized by pancytopenia secondary to marrow fibrosis, splenomegaly, and fatigue and associated with serious or fatal infectious and bleeding complications. Before the advent of interferon therapy, the treatment of hairy cell leukemia had been splenectomy, to which 65% to 75% of patients responded. However, for the patients who did not respond and for the one-third to one-half of responding patients whose disease worsened within the first 5 years after splenectomy, there was no effective treatment. Doses of alpha-interferon as low as 3 million units per day have been associated with some evidence of benefit in as much as 95% of patients[370,373] Complete remissions are rare, but 75% or more of patients have partial responses, and it appears that even the patients with apparently stable disease experience a survival advantage, with a dramatic reduction in the incidence of opportunistic infections. There are no differences in the response rates of patients with and without prior splenectomy. Expression of interferon receptors on hairy cells is heterogeneous and does not appear to correlate with responsiveness.[374] The median time to response is 4 to 6 months. Initially, the peripheral blood hairy-cell count falls, and there is often a slight decrease in erythrocyte, platelet, and granulocyte counts before these three cell types begin to increase. Generally, granulocyte counts improve before platelet and erythrocyte counts (within 2 months versus 2–3 months, and 3–6 months, respectively). Monocytopenia is the last peripheral blood abnormality to be corrected. Marrow fibrosis may be slow to clear, and even the patients with the most impressive

TABLE 17-13.   Response Rates and Durations of Tumors Responsive to Alpha-Interferon

Tumor	Dose (mU) and Schedule	Response Rate (%)	Response Duration (mo)
Hairy cell leukemia	3/day or three times weekly	75–90	3–24+
Chronic myelogenous leukemia	5/day	45–85*	6–15+
Cutaneous T-cell lymphoma	50/m²/day × 5 q 3 weeks	45	3–36+
Low-grade lymphocytic lymphoma	50/M² three times weekly	37–40	4–36+
Ovarian cancer	50 IP q week × 3	45	12–30+
Kaposi's sarcoma	20/M²/day	28	4–31+
Glioma	3–54/M²/day	22–35	1–9+
Multiple myeloma	12/M²/day	17	3–26+
Melanoma	12/M² three times weekly	11–17	1–36+
Renal cell carcinoma	20/M²/day	13–15	1–12+

*The 85% response rate includes peripheral blood responses.

clinical responses usually have residual marrow disease detectable morphologically or monoclonal cells detectable by flow cytometry (the tumor cells are the only marrow cells positive for both Leu M5 and Leu 14) or Southern analysis revealing clonal immunoglobulin-gene rearrangements. The concentration of soluble IL-2 receptor in the serum is a reliable noninvasive measure of tumor burden.[375] Responses to alpha-interferon are not sustained for long periods after interferon is stopped; therefore, most patients remain on maintenance doses of interferon (2–3 million units three times a week) essentially indefinitely.

Recently, a study of hairy cell leukemia patients receiving chronic treatment with interferon-alpha 2a (Roferon; Hoffman–LaRoche) revealed that 31 of 51 (59%) developed antibodies to the interferon. In half the patients, the antibodies neutralized the in vitro antiviral effects of alpha-2a-interferon.[376] However, the neutralizing antibodies were specific for the alpha-1-interferon and did not neutralize a mixed preparation of alpha-interferons (Cantell preparation). In this study, nine patients developed clinical resistance to interferon, and all of these patients had antibody to interferon ($p2 < 0.0001$). Whether such patients would respond to higher doses or a different preparation of interferon is under investigation. At the moment, the treatment of choice for interferon-resistant hairy cell leukemia is 2-deoxycoformycin, an adenosine deaminase inhibitor effective in 80% to 90% of patients[377] including those resistant to interferon.[377] Unfortunately, 2-deoxycoformycin is associated with significant depression of CD4+ T cells, similar to the defect in AIDS patients, and some opportunistic infections have been seen in hairy cell leukemia patients receiving the drug.[379] Studies are under way to evaluate the roles of splenectomy, interferon, and 2-deoxycoformycin in the management of hairy cell leukemia.

Remarkably high response rates to low doses of alpha-interferon are also seen in patients with chronic myelogenous leukemia. With the use of 5 million units a day, 75% of patients appear to clear the malignant cells from the peripheral blood, and around 5% have a cytogenetically complete remission in the marrow, a finding extremely rare with any known treatment including aggressive chemotherapy and radiation with bone marrow transplantation.[380] It has not yet been determined whether these responses in patients in the chronic phase of disease will result in either a longer disease-free survival or a longer chronic phase with a survival advantage; however, the remarkable effect of interferon on the expression of the translocated *abl* oncogene is extremely encouraging. Nevertheless, a number of conventional cytotoxic agents can induce transient tumor responses in the chronic phase of the disease; therefore, a cautious interpretation is in order until a survival advantage has been shown for interferon-treated patients.

Another experimental use for interferon in chronic myelogenous leukemia is in conjunction with the chemotherapeutic agent busulfan. This drug usually produces a decrease in the leukemic blood counts, but discontinuation of the drug is usually followed by a slow return of the leukemic cells. A second course of busulfan can result in a second response of similar magnitude, but the interval until the peripheral leukemic cells return to pretreatment levels is shorter and will continue to shorten with each subsequent cycle of busulfan treatment. It is thought that the busulfan increases the tumor growth fraction and causes a recruitment of tumor stem cells into cell cycle. Because interferons decrease the self-renewing capacity of myeloma and acute myeloid leukemia cells, the administration of interferon after busulfan cycles might prolong the busulfan-induced remissions. Preliminary results suggest that interferon is indeed capable of prolonging the effects of busulfan.[381] Further studies are needed to evaluate the role of interferon with and without other treatment modalities in patients with chronic myelogenous leukemia.

Clinically meaningful response rates to alpha-interferon used near the maximum tolerated doses have been obtained in patients with low-grade lymphoma, cutaneous T-cell lymphoma, AIDS-associated Kaposi's sarcoma, melanoma, myeloma, renal cell carcinoma, ovarian cancer, and glioma.[349] By and large, the responses are partial and continue only as long as interferon is administered. However, the fact that any activity has been identified is encouraging. Interferon may be useful in the local setting; for example, in the treatment of bladder cancer or intraepithelial cervical neoplasia. It is still under evaluation in patients with Hodgkin's disease and nasopharyngeal carcinoma, two malignancies with hinted viral contributions to pathogenesis. Interferon is useful in the management of patients with carcinoid tumors and certain secreting malignant endocrine pancreas tumors through its capacity to reduce the secretion of mediators from the tumor, although tumor shrinkage is rare.[382,383]

Efforts to improve response rates to interferon by antagonizing its toxic effects with indomethacin have failed,[384] but it appears that the response rates of renal cell carcinoma to interferon may be significantly augmented by aspirin.[384a] A variety of attempts at integrating interferon into chemotherapy, radiation therapy, and biologic therapy programs have begun,[385] but these are largely empiric combinations with Phase I end-points that have not yet produced dramatic antitumor results. There are myriad ways interferon could be used together with other modalities, and, based on exciting in vitro and in vivo animal model synergy, it seems probable that therapeutic advances will follow.

A major limitation to progress is the lack of methods for measuring the important biologic effects. To date, responses in human tumors have not correlated well with the expression of interferon receptors on the tumor, the induction of NK activity in the peripheral blood, the induction of 2′,5′ oligoadenylate synthetase levels in peripheral blood cells, or any other interferon-related biologic effect. A second significant limitation to progress is the toxicity associated with the use of interferon therapy. Dose-limiting toxicity is usually manifest as fatigue, weakness, anorexia, weight loss, lethargy, and disordered mentation, all symptoms that are difficult to quantitate. Nearly all patients experience flu-like illness, myalgias, fever, and chills, but tachyphylaxis of these symptoms prevents them from becoming dose limiting. Fatigue, inability to concentrate, and depression usually worsen with continued treatment. Table 17-14 lists the toxicities associated with interferon treatment at the maximum tolerated doses.[386] There is anecdotal evidence that administration of interferon at night results in less toxicity,[387] and there are suggestions that biologic response modifiers and other

TABLE 17-14. Toxicities Associated with Alpha-Interferon Treatment

Symptoms	Laboratory Abnormalities
Frequent	
Fever/chills	
Myalgias	
Fatigue/weakness	
Anorexia/weight loss	
Lethargy/lack of concentration	
Neutropenia	
Mild thrombocytopenia	
Elevated transaminases	
Proteinuria	
Less Frequent	
Gastrointestinal	
Nausea/vomiting	
Altered taste	
Diarrhea	
Cardiovascular	
Hypotension	
Hypertension	
Atrial and ventricular	
arrhythmias	
Myocardial infarction	
Neurologic	
Headaches	
Mood alterations	
(depression)	
Dizziness/lightheadedness	
Peripheral neuropathy	
EEG abnormalities	
(including seizures	
rarely)	
Mucocutaneous	
Inflammation at injection	
site	
Urticaria	
Stomatitis	
Reactivation of Herpes	
simplex	
Exacerbation of psoriasis	
Radiation recall	
Mild alopecia	
Increased eyelash growth	
Hematologic	
Normocytic normochromic	
anemia	
Coagulation abnormalities	
Renal/Metabolic	
Hypercalcemia	
Hypocalcemia	
Hyperkalemia	
Hypertriglyceridemia	
Nephrotic syndrome	
Elevated urea nitrogen	
Hepatic	
Elevated alkaline	
phosphatase	
Elevated lactic	
dehydrogenase	

chemotherapeutic agents may have enhanced therapeutic ratios and greater biologic effects if delivered in a fashion that accounts for normal biologic rhythms.[388] Such ideas are only beginning to be carefully studied.

INTERFERON INDUCERS

As noted above, a large number of compounds have been shown to be interferon inducers. The polyribonucleotides, especially poly ICLC, have been the most extensively evaluated in man.[389] The initial clinical trials in the 1970s determined a maximum tolerated dose; however, there was little evidence that interferon was induced. However, it is now clear that lower doses of poly ICLC may be more effective at inducing interferon, as well as other biologic mediators, that interferon-inducible proteins may be detected in the serum even when interferon is not measurable, and that patient-related variables such as age and tumor burden may affect responses. Thus, it is not clear that there is enough information available to evaluate poly ICLC fully as a therapeutic agent. Enthusiasm for taking a closer look at interferon inducers comes from a prospective randomized trial of patients with breast cancer who received either placebo or six weekly intravenous injections of 30 mg of polyadenylic–polyuridylic acid (poly AU) after definitive local therapy.[390] In patients with tumorous axillary lymph nodes, only 19% of controls were alive at 7 years compared with 60% of those receiving poly AU. Such results are similar to those obtained with adjuvant chemotherapy in node-positive breast cancer and suggest that further study is warranted.

Recently, it has been shown that flavone-8-acetic acid, a new agent from the drug development program of the National Cancer Institute, has potent interferon-inducing properties in both animals[391] and humans.[392] In vivo synergy of the drug with IL-2 has been demonstrated in animals,[391] and a clinical trial in humans is under way.

INTERLEUKIN-2 AND ADOPTIVE IMMUNOTHERAPY

BIOLOGIC ASPECTS OF IL-2

Interleukin-2, a lymphokine produced by activated T cells, has a wide variety of actions and plays a central role in immune regulation (reviewed in reference 393). The interaction of antigen in conjunction with IL-1 stimulates T cells to release IL-2, which is the second signal in lymphocyte mitogenesis. The primary action of IL-2 is its ability to stimulate the growth of activated T cells that bear IL-2 receptors,[394] although IL-2 has a variety of other actions on T cells (see Table 17-3),[395-397] B cells,[398,399] macrophages,[400,401] epidermal Langerhans' cells,[402] and oligodendroglial cells.[403] Human IL-2 was first isolated from supernatant fluids of cultured mitogen- or alloantigen-activated T cells.[394] The leukemic cell line Jurkat[404] was found to produce high concentrations of human IL-2,[405] and using this cell line, the gene coding for human IL-2 was isolated and expressed in *E. coli*.[406-408]

Human cells contain a single copy of the IL-2 gene, which consists of four exons and three introns on chromosome 4. The cDNA consists of a single open reading frame coding for 153 amino acids. The first 20 N-terminal amino acids are hydrophobic and are cleaved to give the mature protein, which consists of 133 amino acids and a predicted molecular weight of 15,420. The residue at position 3 of the mature molecule is O-glycosylated, and size and charge heterogeneity are attributable to this post-translational modification. The IL-2 molecule contains a single disulfide bond between residues 58 and 105 that appears to be essential for the full activity of the molecule. One form of IL-2 in clinical use contains a site-specific mutation with a serine-for-cysteine substitution that allows the production of a stable molecule containing the full biologic activity of native IL-2.[407,408]

IL-2 interacts with cells by binding to specific receptors on the cell surface (reviewed in references 117 and 393). High-affinity receptors with a K_d of 10^{-11} M are the principal ones that mediate the physiologic response of T cells to IL-2 and comprise about 10% of the IL-2 receptors. A second group of receptors bind IL-2 with low affinity (K_d 10^{-8} M). It now appears that a 55-kD protein recognized by the anti-Tac monoclonal antibody mediates low-affinity IL-2 binding. A 75-kD IL-2 receptor protein of intermediate affinity has also been identified,[409] and it appears that high-affinity receptors involve the interaction of IL-2 with a combination of the 55-kD and the 75-kD IL-2 receptor molecules.

Many of the actions of IL-2 suggested that this molecule might be of value in cancer therapy.[410] IL-2 causes lymphoid proliferation and, in some cases, reverses immune deficiency both in vitro and in vivo. For example, in vivo administration of IL-2 restores depressed allogeneic responses in cyclophosphamide-treated mice,[411] restores allograft responses in T-depleted rodents,[412] and can restore the cytotoxic response of lymphoid cells from patients with AIDS to cultured NK-sensitive tumor cells.[413] IL-2 also causes proliferation of endogenous and adoptive transferred lymphoid cells in vivo.[414,415]

Lymphoid cells incubated with IL-2 develop a capacity to lyse fresh tumor cells.[59,416-420] This generation of LAK cells occurs both in vitro and in vivo and has served as the basis for the development of adoptive immunotherapies for the treatment of cancer in humans (see section on adoptive immunotherapy below). Moreover, the direct administration of IL-2 to tumor-bearing animals mediates the regression of established hepatic, pulmonary, and subdermal metastases in a variety of murine tumor models.[421-425] Table 17-15 presents some of the characteristics of the effects of IL-2 in these animal studies.

Other actions of IL-2 that suggest an ability to alter tumor growth include its augmentation of the therapeutic effect of the adoptive transfer of lymphoid cells[415,426-430] and its effects on the emigration of lymphoid cells from the peripheral blood.[431] Finally, the administration of IL-2 causes the in vivo release of other lymphokines and hormones that themselves can mediate physiologic effects, often in concert with IL-2.[432]

CLINICAL APPLICATIONS OF IL-2 IN CANCER PATIENTS

The variety of physiologic effects of IL-2 noted above led to explorations of its use for mediating the immunotherapy of advanced cancers in humans. Initial clinical studies used IL-2 derived from the high-producer Jurkat cell line, although only small quantities of purified IL-2 could be obtained. Ex-

TABLE 17-15. Immunotherapy of Murine Tumors with IL-2 Alone

Liver and lung micrometastases (3-day) from a variety of immunogenic and nonimmunogenic sarcomas, melanomas, and adenocarcinomas can be inhibited by IL-2 administration.
Lung macrometastases (10-day) from two immunogenic sarcomas, but not from two nonimmunogenic sarcomas, can be inhibited by IL-2 administration.
A direct relation exists between the dose of IL-2 and the therapeutic effect.
High-dose IL-2 administration leads to in vivo lymphoid proliferation in visceral organs, and these cells have LAK activity in vitro.
The immunotherapeutic effect of IL-2 on 3-day micrometastases is mediated by asialo-GM1-positive LAK cells. In immunogenic tumors, Lyt 2-positive cells also participate.
The immunotherapeutic effect of IL-2 on 10-day macrometastases is mediated by Lyt 2-positive cells.
Immunosuppression with radiation or cyclophosphamide can inhibit IL-2 activity against 3-day metastases but can enhance the effects of IL-2 on 10-day macrometastases.
The sensitivity of macrometastases to therapy with IL-2 appears to be directly related to the expression of MHC antigens (Class I) on the tumor.
The administration of IL-2 can enhance the therapeutic effect of concomitantly administered LAK cells, TIL, and specifically sensitized T lymphocytes.

pression of the gene for IL-2 in *E. coli* has led to the availability of virtually unlimited amounts of recombinant IL-2, and most clinical trials have used this material.

A variety of schedules of IL-2 administration have been explored in humans.[61,62,432-437] Most studies have used the bolus administration of IL-2 at doses between 10,000 and 100,000 U/kg intravenously every 8 hours. IL-2 can also be administered by continuous infusion at doses from 1,000,000 to 7,000,000 U/m²/per day. After the administration of IL-2, a lymphopenia occurs, but the lymphocytes rebound substantially after IL-2 administration is discontinued. If small amounts of IL-2 are administered for more than a week, lymphocytosis may occur as well. There is depletion of LAK precursor cells from the circulation within minutes after IL-2 administration.[431,432] Increases in serum levels of gamma-interferon and other hormones are also seen. After intravenous bolus administration, recombinant IL-2 is cleared from the circulation with an alpha distribution phase of 6.9 minutes and a second beta clearance phase of approximately 70 minutes.[432]

In the treatment of patients with advanced cancer, IL-2 has been used either alone or in conjunction with the adoptive transfer of LAK cells. Clinical results using IL-2 and the toxic side effects of this material will be considered in the next section on adoptive immunotherapy.

ADOPTIVE IMMUNOTHERAPY

Adoptive immunotherapy—the transfer to the tumor-bearing host of cells with antitumor activity—has substantial therapeutic attractiveness as an approach to treating human cancer.[421,438,439] Early cell-transfer experiments in animals demonstrated that the cellular arm of the immune response is crucial in mediating the rejection of allogeneic grafts and syngeneic tumor. In most experimental systems, the transfer of immune cells, but not of antibody directed against cellular antigens, produces immunity to tissue transplants.

The major obstacle to the development of successful adoptive immunotherapies for the treatment of cancer in humans has been the inability to develop immune cells with specific reactivity for human tumors that could be obtained in large enough numbers for transfer to tumor-bearing patients. However, several new approaches have been developed for generating human cells with reactivity to tumor, and the initial clinical experience with the adoptive transfer of these cells has been encouraging.[61,62,421]

Lymphokine-Activated Killer Cells

Beginning in 1980, Rosenberg and colleagues described a technique for generating lymphoid cells from both mice and humans that were capable of lysing fresh tumor but not normal cells.[416-421] The incubation of resting murine splenocytes or human peripheral-blood lymphocytes with the lymphokine IL-2 for 3 to 4 days results in the generation of cells that can lyse fresh tumor but not fresh normal cells. These killer cells have been referred to as lymphokine activated killer (LAK) cells. LAK cells differ from NK cells in their ability to kill fresh human tumor preparations.

The characteristics of LAK cells have been extensively studied.[416-421,440-441] These cells represent a lytic population quite distinct from NK cells or cytolytic T lymphocytes, and their phenotypic surface markers are characteristic of non-MHC-restricted killer cells. LAK cells can be either CD3 positive or negative, are nonadherent and E-rosette negative, and bear NK-like markers such as CD11 and NKH-1 (Leu 19). IL-2 is the sole signal required for the generation of LAK cells, as demonstrated by experiments using purified homogeneous recombinant IL-2.[407] The nature of the determinants recognized on fresh tumor targets by LAK cells is not known, although the determinants appear to be broadly expressed, not only on fresh and cultured tumor cells, but also on cultured normal cells as well. Fresh normal cells, with the possible exception of monocytes, do not appear to bear cell-surface determinants recognized by LAK cells.

Following the description of the LAK cell phenomenon, a variety of studies were undertaken in rodent models to evaluate the use of LAK cells in the adoptive immunotherapy of established tumors. These studies demonstrated that the adoptive transfer of LAK cells in conjunction with IL-2 can mediate the regression of established pulmonary, hepatic, and subdermal metastases from a variety of animal tumor models.[60,423,425,442-445] IL-2 appeared to stimulate the in vivo expansion of LAK cells with maintenance of cellular function.[414,415] A summary of the results of studies in animal models is shown in Table 17-16. In these systems, significant antitumor effects are seen with the administration of IL-2 alone that generally are improved by the adoptive transfer of LAK cells.

Based on these animal models, clinical trials using IL-2 and LAK cells plus IL-2 for the treatment of advanced cancer in humans were developed. A chronology of the development of these studies by Rosenberg and colleagues is shown in

TABLE 17-16. Immunotherapy of Murine Tumors with LAK Cells Plus IL-2

Liver and lung micrometastases (3-day) from a variety of immunogenic and nonimmunogenic sarcomas, melanomas, and adenocarcinomas can be inhibited by treatment with LAK cells plus IL-2.

A direct relation exists between therapeutic effect and the dose of IL-2 and the number of LAK cells.

The precursor of the LAK cell effective in vivo is Thy 1⁻Ig⁻Ia⁻ asialo-GM1.

Three-day incubation of splenocytes appears optimal for the generation of LAK cells effective in vivo.

Immunotherapy of micrometastases with LAK cells and IL-2 is effective in hosts suppressed by total-body irradiation or treatment with cyclophosphamide. Therapy is also effective in "B" mice (thymectomized, lethally irradiated, reconstituted with T-cell-depleted bone marrow).

Immunotherapy of micrometastases with allogeneic LAK cells plus IL-2 is effective.

LAK cells effective in immunotherapy can be generated from the splenocytes of tumor-bearing mice.

Metastases that persist after in vivo therapy with LAK cells plus IL-2 are sensitive to LAK cell lysis both in vitro and in subsequent in vivo experiments. We have been unable to generate LAK-resistant tumor cells.

Administration of IL-2 leads to in vivo proliferation of transferred LAK cells.

Diffuse intraperitoneal carcinomatosis can be treated successfully with intraperitoneal LAK cells plus IL-2.

LAK cells can mediate antibody-dependent cellular cytotoxicity, and administration of IL-2 alone or LAK cells plus IL-2 can enhance the in vivo therapeutic efficiency of monoclonal antibodies with antitumor reactivity.

Table 17-17. Early studies of the use of activated killer cells began with the use of phytohemagglutinin-activated killer (PAK) cells because sufficient amounts of IL-2 were not available to generate LAK cells.[446,447] Similarly, clinical trials of IL-2 alone began with the use of natural Jurkat-derived IL-2.[448] When recombinant IL-2 became available, studies with LAK cells alone or with recombinant IL-2 alone were attempted.[432,447] No antitumor responses were seen in any of these early studies using activated killer cells alone. After these Phase I studies, a combination of LAK cells and recombinant IL-2 was administered to patients with advanced cancer, and regression of tumor was seen in some patients.[61,62]

An outline of the protocol using IL-2 plus LAK cells is shown in Figure 17-5. Patients receiving IL-2 alone received it on a schedule similar to this but without the administration of LAK cells. In the Surgery Branch, National Cancer Institute, 177 patients were treated with IL-2 in conjunction with LAK cells, and 119 patients received IL-2 alone. The results of immunotherapy in these 296 patients are shown in Table 17-18. Most experience with this treatment approach has been obtained in patients with renal cell cancer and melanoma. In these diseases, approximately 10% of patients will obtain a complete regression of metastatic cancer, and about 20% will have objective partial regressions. About 15% of patients with metastatic colorectal cancer will experience an objective regression of tumor. There has been little experience with other tumor types.

Regression of metastatic cancer has been seen at a variety of sites, including lung, liver, bone, skin, subcutaneous tis-

TABLE 17-17. Chronology of Clinical Trials of IL-2 and LAK Cells

Year	Clinical Study	No. of Patients	Findings
1980	Adoptive transfer of long-term-cultured peripheral blood lymphocytes[58]	3	Small numbers (up to 5×10^8) of long-term-cultured PBL can be infused safely
1981	Adoptive transfer of phytohemagglutinin-activated killer (PAK) cells[446]	10	Large numbers (up to 1.7×10^{11}) of activated killer cells, obtained from up to 15 successive leukophoreses, can be infused safely
1982	Adoptive transfer of PAK cells plus cyclophosphamide[447]	6	Activated killer cells can be infused safely in conjunction with high-dose cyclophosphamide (50 mg/kg)
1983	Adoptive transfer of PAK cells plus activated macrophages[447]	5	Activated killer cells plus activated macrophages can be infused safely
1983	Administration of natural (Jurkat-derived) IL-2[448]	16	Natural (Jurkat-derived) IL-2 can be infused safely at doses up to 2 mg
1984	Adoptive transfer of LAK cells[447]	6	LAK cells (activated with recombinant IL-2) can be infused safely
1984	Administration of recombinant IL-2[432]	23	Recombinant IL-2 (from E. coli) can be administered safely, though significant toxicity is seen at high doses
1985	Administration of LAK cells plus recombinant IL-2[61]	25	Regression of metastatic cancer of a variety of types in some patients
1986	Administration of high-dose bolus IL-2 alone[433]	10	Regression of metastatic cancer in 3 patients with melanoma
1987	Administration of IL-2 alone or with LAK cells[62]	157	Complete and partial regression of cancer of several histologic types
1988	Administration of IL-2 alone or with LAK cells*	296	Complete and partial regression of cancer of several histologic types

*Unpublished data.

sue, and circulating tumor cells. When tumor regression is seen at one site, it tends to occur at all sites; mixed responses are unusual. The duration of responses of these patients is shown in Table 17-19. Of 18 patients who achieved complete regression, 10 have remained in complete remission for as long as 42 months follow-up. Examples of patient responses are shown in Figures 17-6 through 17-9. Because these trials began in November 1984, follow-up is short, and the ability of these approaches to cure patients with metastatic cancer has not yet been established.

Because meaningful clinical responses have been seen in patients given high-dose IL-2 and in patients receiving LAK cells and IL-2, Rosenberg and colleagues have conducted a prospective randomized trial in patients with advanced cancer comparing high-dose IL-2 alone and in conjunction with LAK cells. Early results from this trial reveal that both treatments can produce partial and complete responses, although the incidence of complete responses is higher when LAK cells are administered concomitantly with IL-2.

(text continues on page 338)

TABLE 17-18. Results of Immunotherapy in Patients with Advanced Cancer (accrued by 5/1/88)

Diagnosis	LAK/IL-2			IL-2		
	Total Evaluable*	No. of CR†	No. of PR	Total Evaluable‡	No. CR	No. PR
Renal	72	8	17	52	4	7
Melanoma	48	4	6	37	0	9
Colorectal	30	1	4	12	0	0
Non-Hodgkin's lymphoma	5	1	2	6	0	0
Sarcoma	6	0	0	1	0	0
Lung adenocarcinoma	5	0	0	1	0	0
Breast	1	0	0	2	0	0
Brain	1	0	0	2	0	0
Esophageal	1	0	0	0	0	0
Hodgkin's lymphoma	1	0	0	0	0	0
Ovarian	1	0	0	1	0	0
Testicular	1	0	0	0	0	0
Hepatoma	0	0	0	1	0	0
Gastrinoma	1	0	0	0	0	0
Thyroid	1	0	0	0	0	0
Unknown primary	1	0	0	0	0	0
Total	175	14	29	115	4	16

*Two treated patients not included; one (melanoma) died of complications of therapy, and one (breast) was lost to follow-up.
†CR = complete response; PR = partial response.
‡Four treated patients (renal) not included; died of therapy.

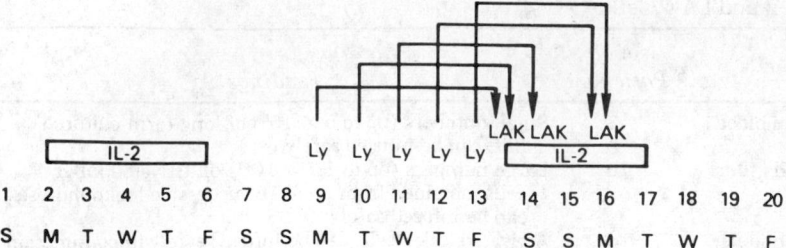

Ly: Lymphocytapheresis
IL-2: 100,000 U/kg I.V. TID
LAK: Infusion of LAK cells I.V.

FIG. 17-5. Clinical protocol for the immunotherapy of human cancer with LAK cells plus recombinant IL-2. IL-2 is administered for 4 to 5 days, resulting in a marked lymphocytosis that increases the yield of lymphocytes obtained from daily lymphocytophereses. Lymphocytes are put into culture to produce LAK cells, and these are then reinfused into patients along with the simultaneous administration of IL-2.

TABLE 17-19. Duration of Response (months) to Immunotherapy

	LAK/IL-2		IL-2	
Diagnosis	CR	PR	CR	PR
Renal	20+,17+,15,13+,13, 11,9,6	26+,17+,13, 11,10+, 10+,10,9,7,7,6,6, 6,6,3,1,1	24+,18+,17+,15+	17+,17+,15+,11+,11, 9+,5+
Melanoma	42+,22+,13,8+	20+,6,5+,3,2,2	–	31+,15,10,8,7+,7,5, 3,2
Non-Hodgkin's lymphoma	10	21+,18+	–	–
Colorectal	21	7+,6,6,2	–	–

Note: 10 of 18 patients achieving CR remain in CR at 11 to 42 months.

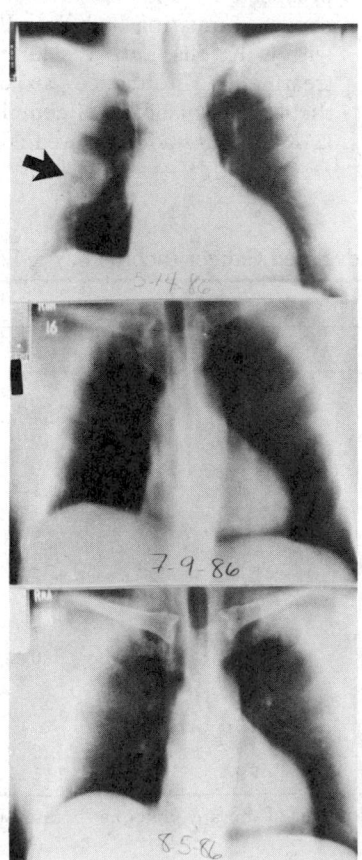

FIG. 17-6. Complete regression of pulmonary metastasis in a patient with renal cell cancer treated with high dose IL-2 alone. **Upper Panel**. Pretreatment. **Middle and Lower Panels**. Post-treatment.

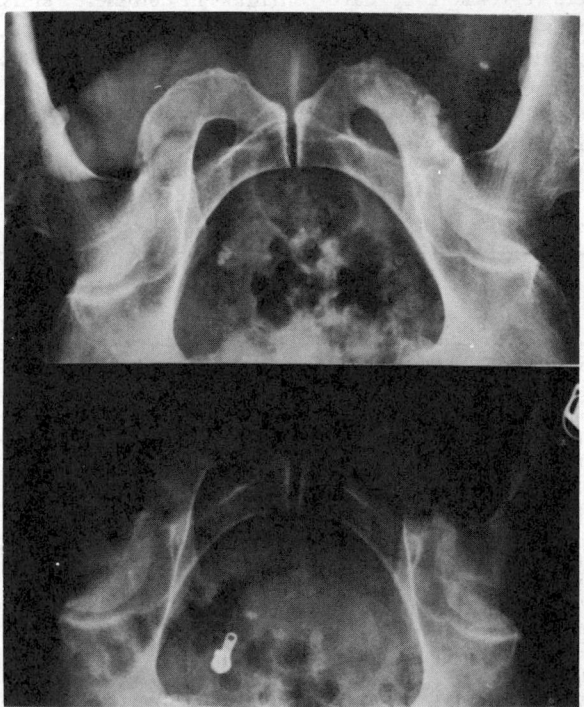

FIG. 17-7. Complete regression of a bony metastasis of the pubic ramus in a patient with renal cell cancer treated with LAK cells and IL-2. **Upper Panel**. Pretreatment. **Lower Panel**. Post-treatment. This patient also underwent complete regression of multiple pulmonary metastases.

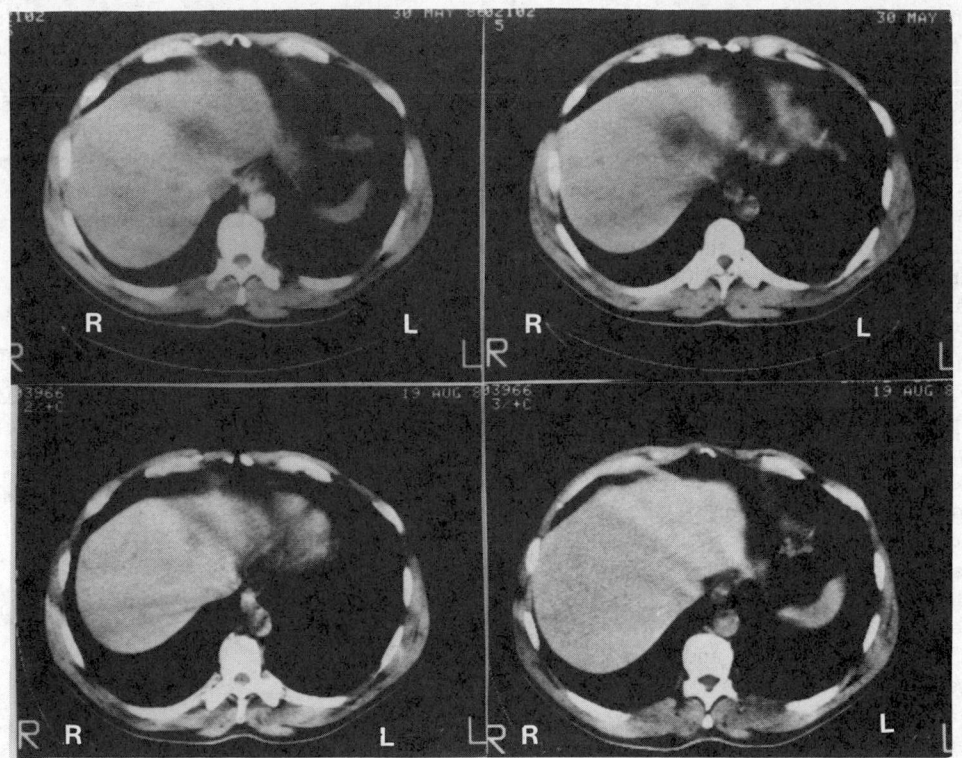

FIG. 17-8. Regression of a liver metastasis in a patient with melanoma treated with high dose IL-2. **Upper Panels**. Pretreatment. **Lower Panels**. Post-treatment.

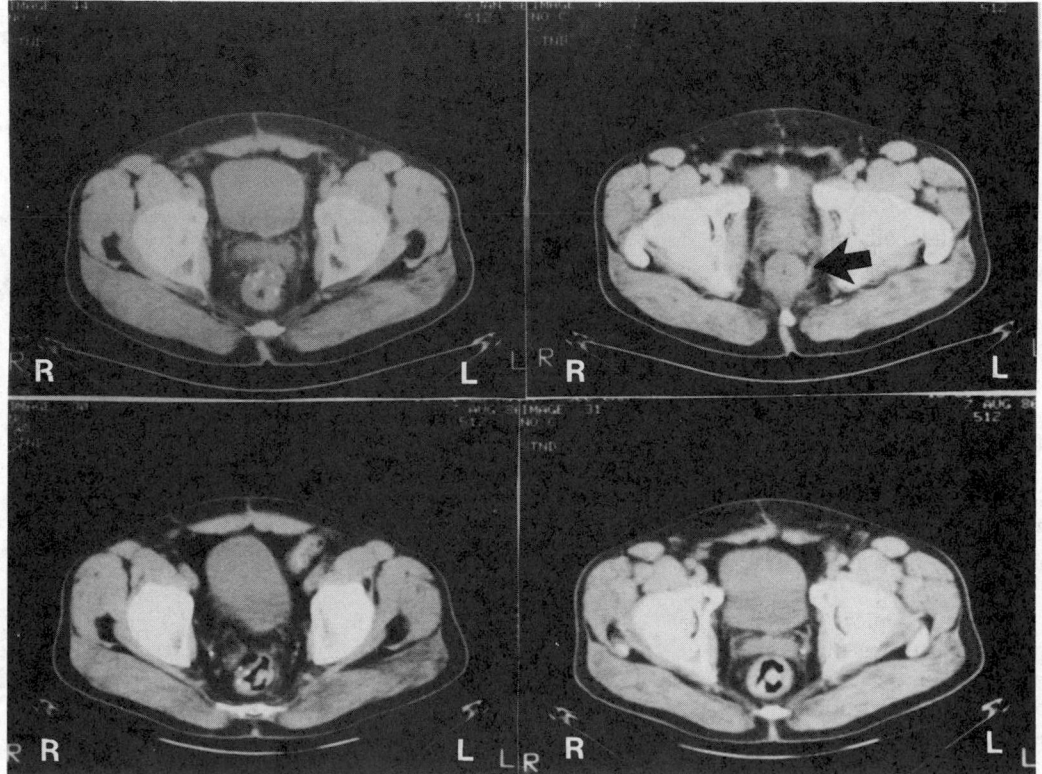

FIG. 17-9. Complete regression of a recurrent tumor mass at the site of a low anterior resection for colorectal cancer in a patient treated with LAK cells and IL-2. **Upper Panels**. Pretreatment. Arrow points to the mass at the site of the anastomosis. **Lower Panels**. Post-treatment. This patient also underwent complete regression of lung and liver metastases.

Other investigators have confirmed both the clinical responses and the toxicities of this treatment regimen. West and co-workers utilized continuous infusion of IL-2 in conjunction with LAK cells and reported 13 partial responses in 40 evaluable patients with advanced cancer.[435] These workers reported that the toxicity resulting from the continuous intravenous infusion of IL-2 was less than that seen with bolus administration, although it is likely that the decreased toxicity was at least in part due to the administration of less IL-2. Using IL-2 bolus administration along with LAK cells, Dutcher and associates saw six partial responses in 32 patients with advanced melanoma, including response of tumor in liver, spleen, kidney, and lymph nodes and of subcutaneous lesions.[449] Similarly, Fisher and colleagues reported five responses in 34 patients with metastatic renal cell cancer.[450] Steiss and co-workers have utilized LAK cells plus IL-2 intraperitoneally to cause partial regression of cancer in patients with intraperitoneal, ovarian, and colorectal cancer.[451] Using a modified procedure for producing LAK cells, Paciucci and co-workers also reported partial responses in patients with advanced cancer.[452]

A variety of questions remain concerning the use of IL-2 and LAK cells in cancer therapy. The dose–response and schedule-dependent characteristics of IL-2 have not been established. Are higher response rates obtained with higher doses? What is the optimal administration schedule of IL-2 and cells? A need exists to test this immunotherapy approach in patients with a variety of cancers at different sites. Are brain metastases affected? A need exists for simpler means of raising more potent cells for use in adoptive immunotherapy. Studies of the pathophysiology of IL-2 toxicities and means for decreasing these toxicities are needed.

Toxicity of Treatment

The adoptive transfer of activated killer cells alone causes little toxicity,[446,447] but the administration of high-dose recombinant IL-2 can be associated with substantial dose-limiting toxic side-effects in a variety of organ systems.[61,62] Many of the side-effects of IL-2 are probably attributable to lymphoid infiltrates in vital organs; to a vascular permeability leak induced by IL-2 that leads to fluid retention and interstitial edema which can compromise organ function,[453] and to the ability of IL-2 to lead to the secretion of other lymphokines such as gamma-interferon, which have a range of physiologic effects and toxicities of their own.[432] The side-effects of IL-2 appear to be completely reversible when administration ceases.

A summary of the clinical course of a typical patient receiving IL-2 and LAK cells, which illustrates many of the physiologic side-effects encountered in these patients, is shown in Figure 17-10.[454] Soon after administration of IL-2, a drop in systemic vascular resistance is seen associated with tachycardia, decreased mean arterial blood pressure, and an increase in cardiac index. As IL-2 administration continues, weight gain occurs secondary to the requisite replacement of fluid lost from the intravascular space by the capillary leak. Urine output drops and serum creatinine rises, probably from prerenal azotemia.[455,456] Vasopressors are often used early in treatment in an attempt to limit the need for fluid

replacement, as exogenous fluid contributes to the interstitial edema, which can lead to respiratory compromise and a decrease in arterial oxygenization. Weight gain, renal dysfunction, and hepatic dysfunction can occur. These toxicities and others seen in 296 patients treated by Rosenberg and associates are summarized in Table 17-20.[61,62,454-458] The treatment-related mortality rate in these 296 patients given high-dose IL-2 either alone or with LAK cells was 2%.

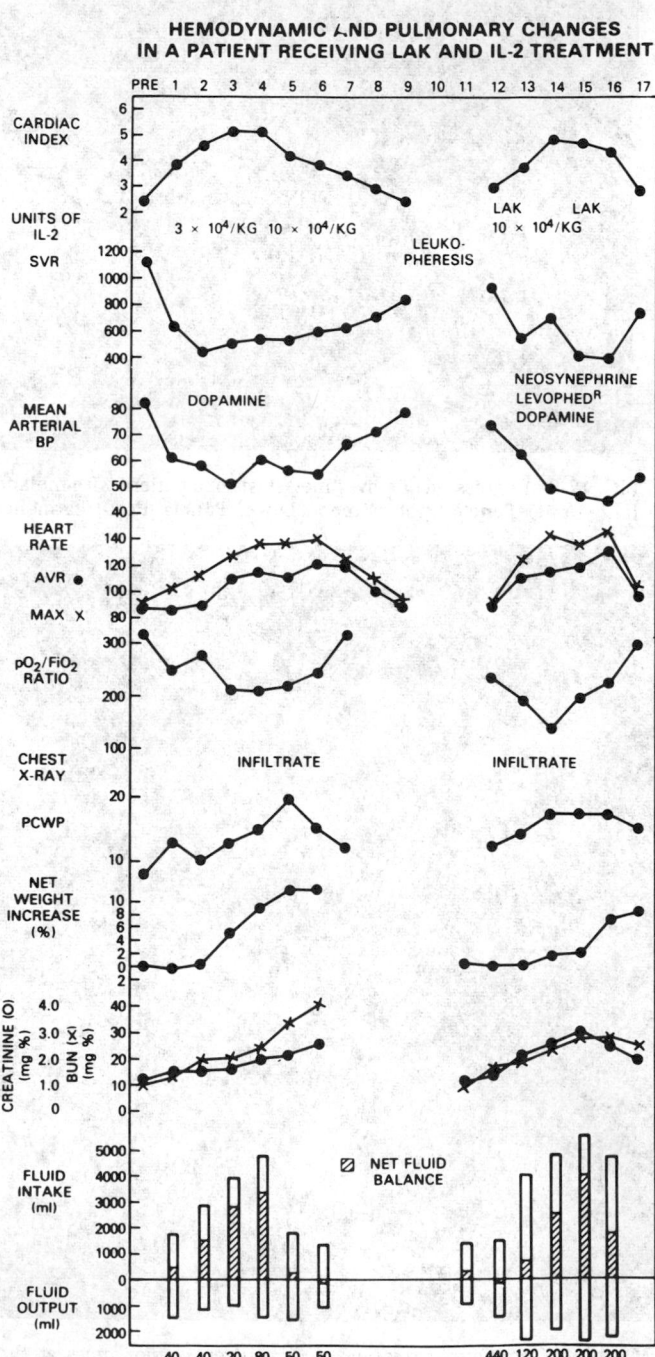

FIG. 17-10. Sequential clinical measurements in a patient receiving treatment with LAK cells and IL-2.

Tumor-Infiltrating Lymphocytes

Considerable efforts are under way to find cells with potent antitumor reactivity for use in adoptive immunotherapy. Rosenberg and colleagues recently described a subpopulation of lymphocytes termed TIL that appear to have far greater efficacy than LAK cells in the treatment of experimental tumors.[429,430] TIL are lymphocytes that infiltrate growing tumors and can be isolated by growing single-cell suspensions from the tumor in IL-2. In experimental animal models, these TIL can be 50 to 100 times as potent as LAK cells in mediating the regression of micrometastases.[429]

TIL have now been isolated from virtually all human tumors.[459-464] The human TIL are T cells and can exhibit specific MHC-restricted lysis of tumor. From approximately half of patients with malignant melanoma, TIL with specific reactivity for the tumor from which they were derived can be obtained. An example of the lytic specificity of TIL is shown in Figure 17-11.[459] Such specificity provides the best available evidence that at least some patients manifest immune reactions to their growing cancers. Clinical trials with TIL are being pursued in the treatment of advanced cancer in humans. Rosenberg and co-workers reported objective remissions in 11 of 20 patients with metastatic melanoma treated with TIL.[465]

TABLE 17-20. Number of Courses in Which Various Toxicities of Treatment with LAK/IL-2 (N = 271) or IL-2 (N = 179) Alone Were Seen

	LAK/IL-2 (177 Pts)	IL-2 (119 Pts)	Total
Chills	160	59	219
Pruritis	74	44	118
Necrosis	0	3	3
Anaphylaxis	0	0	0
Mucositis (requiring liquid diet)	9	4	13
Alimentation not possible	1	1	2
Nausea and vomiting	208	128	336
Diarrhea	197	118	315
Hyperbilirubinemia (maximum mg/dl)			
2.1–6.0	148	89	237
6.1–10.0	51	41	92
≥10.0	32	21	53
Hepatitis A (due to LAK infusion)	5	—	5
Oliguria			
<80 m/8 hours	85	58	143
<240 m/24 hours	11	18	29
Weight gain (% body weight)			
0.0–5.0	85	79	164
5.1–10.0	118	59	177
10.1–15.0	50	32	82
15.1–20.0	14	7	21
20.1+	4	2	6
Elevated creatinine (maximum mg/dl)			
2.1–6.0	188	117	305
6.1–10.0	29	16	45
≥10.0	2	5	7
Hematuria (gross)	2	0	2
Edema (symptomatic nerve or vessel compression)	6	4	10
Tissue ischemia	1	0	1
Respiratory distress			
Not intubated	24	15	39
Intubated	12	14	26
Bronchospasm	4	1	5
Pleural effusion requiring thoracentesis	8	4	12
Somnolence	41	26	65
Coma	8	8	16
Disorientation	76	50	126
Hypotension requiring pressors	196	102	298
Angina	6	4	10
Myocardial infarction	1	4	5
Arrhythmias	29	13	42
Anemia requiring transfusion (No. of units)			
1–5	137	61	198
6–10	49	22	71
11–15	15	4	19
≥16	10	1	11
Thrombocytopenia (minimum per mm³)			
≤20,000	50	24	74
21,000–60,000	110	65	175
61,000–100,000	65	37	102
Central-line sepsis	32	12	44
Death	2	4	6

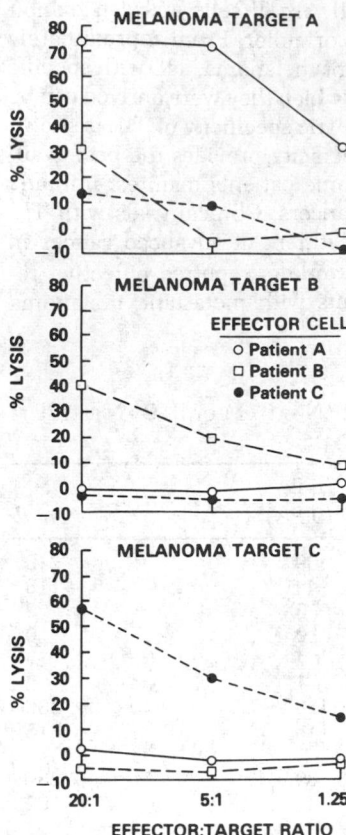

FIG. 17-11. Lytic specificity of TILs from three patients with melanoma tested simultaneously against fresh melanoma cells. Note that TILs exhibit strong preferential lysis for the target from which they were derived (reference 459).

REFERENCES

1. Morton DL: Active immunotherapy against cancer: Present status. Semin Oncol 180–185, 1986
2. Morton DL, Eilber FR, Malmgren RA et al: Immunological factors which influence response to immunotherapy in malignant melanoma. Surgery 68:158–164, 1970
3. Hoover HC Jr, Surdyke MG, Dangel RB et al: Delayed cutaneous hypersensitivity to autologous tumor cells in colorectal cancer patients immunized with an autologous tumor cell: Bacillus Calmette-Guerin vaccine. Cancer Res 44:1671–1676, 1984
4. Morton DL: Active immunotherapy against cancer: Present status. Sem Oncol 13:180–185, 1986
5. Hellstrom I, Hellstrom KE, Warner GA: Increase of lymphocyte-mediated tumor-cell destruction by certain patient sera. Int J Cancer 12:348–353, 1973
6. Roth JA, Holmes EC, Reisfeld RA et al: Isolation of a soluble tumor-associated antigen from human melanoma. Cancer 37:104–110, 1976
7. Ferrone S, Pellegrino MA: Cytotoxic antibodies to cultured melanoma cells in the sera of melanoma patients. J Natl Cancer Inst 58:1201–1204, 1977
8. Brown JM, Thorpe WP, Rosenberg SA: A sensitive assay for the detection of cytotoxic antibodies to mammalian cell surface antigens. J Immunol Meth 30:23–35, 1979
9. Ueda R, Shiku H, Pfreundschuh M et al: Cell surface antigens of human renal cancer defined by autologous typing. J Exp Med 150:564–579, 1979
10. Curry RA, Quaranta V, Pellegrino MA et al: Serologically detectable human melanoma-associated antigens are not genetically linked to HLA-A and B antigens. J Immunol 122:2630–2632, 1979
11. Everson TC, Cole WH: Spontaneous Regression of Cancer. Philadelphia, WB Saunders, 1966
12. Montie JE, Stewart BH, Straffon RA et al: The role of adjunctive nephrectomy in patients with metastatic renal cell carcinoma. J Urol 117:272–275, 1977
13. Coley WB: The treatment of malignant tumors by repeated inoculations of erysipelas: With a report of ten original cases. Am J Med Sci 105:487–511, 1893
14. Gressler I: A. Chekhov and Coley's toxins (letter). N Engl J Med 317:457, 1987
15. Hellstrom I, Hellstrom KE, Pierce GE et al: Demonstration of cell-bound and humoral immunity against neuroblastoma cells. Proc Natl Acad Sci USA 60:1231–1238, 1968
16. Hellstrom I, Hellstrom KE, Pierce GE et al: Cellular and humoral immunity to different types of human neoplasms. Nature 220:1352–1354, 1968
17. Hellstrom I, Hellstrom KE: In vitro demonstration of cell-bound immunity against autologous MCA and plastic disc-induced mouse tumors. Science 156:981–983, 1967
18. Houghton AN, Scheinberg DA: Monoclonal Antibodies: Potential applications to the treatment of cancer. Sem Oncol 13:165–179, 1986
19. Hellstrom I, Hellstrom KE, Bill AH et al: Studies on cellular immunity to human neuroblastoma cells. Int J Cancer 6:172–188, 1970
20. Hellstrom I, Hellstrom KE, Sjogren HO et al: Demonstration of cell-mediated immunity to human neoplasma of various histological types. Int J Cancer 7:1–16, 1971
21. Hellstrom I, Hellstrom KE, Shepard TH: Cell-mediated immunity against antigens common to human colonic carcinomas and fetal gut epithelium. Int J Cancer 6:346–351, 1970
22. Hellstrom I, Hellstrom KE: Some recent studies on cellular immunity to human melanomas. Fed Proc 32:156–159, 1973
23. Hellstrom I, Hellstrom KE: Cell-mediated reactivity to human tumor-type associated antigens: Does it exist? J Biol Response Mod 2:310–320, 1983
24. Vanky F, Argov S, Klein E: Tumor biopsy cells participate in systems in which cytotoxicity of lymphocytes is generated: Autologous and allogeneic studies. Int J Cancer 28:273–280, 1981
25. Vanky F, Klein E: Human T-cell cultures with selective autotumor reactivity. Cancer Immunol Immunother 14:73–77, 1982
26. Vose BM, Vanky F, Klein E: Human tumour–lymphocyte interaction in vitro V: Comparison of the reactivity of tumour-infiltrating, blood and lymphnode lymphocytes with autologous tumour cells. Int J Cancer 20:895–902, 1977
27. Voss BM, Bonnard GD: Human tumour antigens defined by cytotoxicity and proliferative responses of cultured lymphoid cells. Nature 296:359–361, 1982
28. Vose BM, Bonnard GD: Specific cytotoxicity against autologous tumour and proliferative responses of human lymphocytes grown in interleukin-2. Int J Cancer 29:33–39, 1982
29. Vanky F, Willems J, Kreicbergs A et al: Correlation between lymphocyte-mediated auto-tumor reactivities and clinical course. Cancer Immunol Immunother 16:11–16, 1983
30. Vanky F, Gorsky T, Gorsky Y et al: Lysis of tumor biopsy cells by autologous T lymphocytes activated in mixed cultures and propagated with T cell growth factor. J Exp Med 155:83–95, 1982
31. Vanky F, Klein E: Human T-cell cultures with selective autotumor reactivity. Cancer Immunol Immunother 14:73–77, 1982
32. Parkman R, Rosen FS: Identification of a subpopulation of lymphocytes in human peripheral blood cytotoxic to autologous fibroblasts. J Exp Med 144:1520–1530, 1976
33. Tomonari K: Cytotoxic T cells generated in the autologous mixed lymphocyte reaction I: Primary autologous mixed lymphocyte reaction. J Immunol 124:1111–1121, 1980
34. Uchida A, Micksche M: Autologous mixed lymphocyte reaction in the peripheral blood and pleural effusions of cancer patient. J Clin Invest 70:98–104, 1982
35. Grimm EA, Voss BM, Chu EW et al: The human mixed lymphocyte–tumor cell interaction test: I: Positive autologous lymphocyte proliferative responses can be stimulated by tumor cells as well as by cells from normal tissues. Cancer Immunol Immunother 17:83–89, 1983
36. Mukherji B, Guha A, Loomis R et al: Cell-mediated amplification and down regulation of cytotoxic immune response against autologous human cancer. J Immunol 138:1987–1991, 1987
37. Yssel H, Spits H, de Vries JE: A cloned human T cell line cytotoxic for autologous and allogeneic B lymphoma cells. J Exp Med 160:239–254, 1984
38. de Vries JE, Spits H: Cloned human cytotoxic T lymphocyte (CTL) lines reactive with autologous melanoma cells I: In vitro generation, isolation and analysis to phenotype and specificity. J Immunol 132:510–519, 1984
39. Knuth A, Danowski B, Oettgen HF et al: T-cell-mediated cytotoxicity against autologous malignant melanoma: Analysis with interleukin-2 dependent T-cell cultures. Proc Natl Acad Sci USA 81:3511–3515, 1984
40. Knuth A, Dippold W, Meyer zum Bueschenfelde K-H: Target level blocking of T-cell cytotoxicity for human malignant melanoma by monoclonal antibodies. Cell Immunol 83:398–403, 1984
41. Ferrini S, Biassoni R, Moretta A et al: Clonal analysis of T lymphocytes isolated from ovarian carcinoma ascitic fluid: Phenotypic and functional characterization of T-cell clones capable of lysing autologous carcinoma cells. Int J Cancer 36:337–343, 1985
42. Anichini A, Fossati G, Parmiani G: Clonal analysis of cytotoxic T-lymphocyte response to autologous human metastatic melanoma. Int J Cancer 35:683–389, 1985
43. Anichini A, Mortarini R, Fossati G et al: Phenotypic profile of clones from early cultures of human metastatic melanomas and its modulation by recombinant interferon-gamma. Int J Cancer 38:505–511, 1986
44. Anichini A, Fossati G, Parmiani G: Heterogeneity of clones from a human metastatic melanoma detected by autologous cytotoxic T lymphocyte clones. J Exp Med 163:215–220, 1986
45. Fossati G, Anichini A, Parmiani G: Melanoma cell lysis by human CTL clones: Differential involvement of T3, T8, and HLA antigens. Int J Cancer 39:689–694, 1987
46. Slovin SF, Lackman RD, Ferrone S et al: Cellular immune response to human sarcomas: Cytotoxic T cell clones reactive with autologous sarcomas. J Immunol 137:3042–3048, 1986
47. Hersey P, MacDonald M, Schibeci S et al: Clonal analysis of cytotoxic T lymphocytes (CTL) against autologous melanoma. Cancer Immunol Immunother 22:15–23, 1986

48. Roberts TE, Shipton U, Moore M: Proliferative and cytotoxic responses of human peripheral blood lymphocytes to autologous malignant effusions: An analysis at the clonal level. Cancer Immunol Immunother 22:107–113, 1986

49. Roberts TE, Shipton U, Moore M: Role of MHC Class-I antigens and the CD3 complex in the lysis of autologous human tumours by T-cell clones. Int J Cancer 39:436–441, 1987

50. Herin M, Lemoine C, Vessiere F et al: Production of stable cytolytic T-cell clones directed against autologous human melanoma. Int J Cancer 39:390–396, 1987

51. Mukherji B, Guha A, Loomis R et al: Cell-mediated amplification and down regulation of cytotoxic immune response against autologous human cancer. J Immunol 138:1987–1991, 1987

52. Mukherji B, Nashed AL, Guha A et al: Regulation of cellular immune response against autologous human melanoma: II. Mechanism of induction and specificity of suppression. J Immunol 138:1893–1898, 1986

53. Hoon DSB, Bowker RJ, Cochran AJ: Suppressor cell activity in melanoma-draining lymph nodes. Cancer Res 47:1529–1533, 1987

54. Berd D, Mastrangelo MJ: Depletion of suppressor–cytotoxic T-lymphocytes by administration of a murine monoclonal antibody. Cancer Res 47:2727–2732, 1987

55. Muul LM, Spiess PJ, Director EP et al: Identification of specific cytolytic immune responses against autologous tumor in humans bearing malignant melanoma. J Immunol 138:989–995, 1987

56. Tomita S, Lotze MT, Rosenberg SA: Clonal analysis of tumor infiltrating lymphocytes (TIL) against human malignant melanoma. Fed Proc 46:1195, 1987

57. Pellegrino MA, Ferrone S, Reisfeld RA et al: Expression of histocompatibility (HLA) antigens on tumor cells and normal cells from patients with melanoma. Cancer 40:36–41, 1977

58. Lotze MT, Line BR, Mathisen DJ et al: The in vivo distribution of autologous human and murine lymphoid cells grown in T cell growth factor (TCGF): Implications for the adoptive immunotherapy of tumors. J Immunol 125:1487–1493, 1980

59. Grimm EA, Mazumder A, Zhang HZ et al: Lymphokine-activated killer cell phenomenon: Lysis of natural killer-resistant fresh solid tumor cells by interleukin-2-activated autologous human peripheral blood lymphocytes. J Exp Med 155:1823–1841, 1982

60. Mule JJ, Shu S, Schwarz SL et al: Adoptive immunotherapy of established pulmonary metastases with LAK cells and recombinant interleukin-2. Science 225:1487–1489, 1984

61. Rosenberg SA, Lotze MT, Muul LM et al: Observations on the systemic administration of autologous lymphokine-activated killer cells and recombinant interleukin-2 to patients with metastatic cancer. N Engl J Med 313:1485–1492, 1985

62. Rosenberg SA, Lotze MT, Muul LM et al: A progress report on the treatment of 157 patients with advanced cancer using lymphokine-activated killer cells and interleukin-2 or high-dose interleukin-2 alone. N Engl J Med 316:889–897, 1987

63. Wiebke EA, Custer MC, Rosenberg SA, Lotze MT: Cytokines alter target cell susceptibility to lysis I: Evaluation of non-MHC restricted effectors reveals differential effects on natural and lymphokine-activated killing (submitted)

64. Katz DH, Ellman L, Paul WE et al: Resistance of guinea pigs to leukemia following transfer of immunocompetent allogeneic lymphoid cells. Cancer Res 32:133–140, 1972

65. Borton MM, Rimm AA, Saltzstein EC et al: Graft versus leukemia III: Apparent independent antihost and antileukemic activity of transplanted immunocompetent cells. Transplantation 16:182–187, 1973

66. Chester SJ, Esparza AR, Flinton LJ et al: Further development of a successful protocol of graft versus leukemia without fetal graft-versus-host disease in AKR mice. Cancer Res 37:3494–3496, 1977

67. Putman DL, Kind PD, Goldin A et al: Adoptive immunochemotherapy of a transplantable AKR leukemia (K36). Int J Cancer 21:230–233, 1978

68. Bortin MM, Truitt RL, Rimm AA et al: Graft-versus-leukaemia reactivity induced by alloimmunisation without augmentation of graft-versus-host reactivity. Nature 281:490–491, 1979

69. Bortin MM, Truit RL, Shih C-Y et al: Alloimmunization for induction of graft-versus-leukemia reactivity in H-2 compatible donors: Critical role for incompatibility of donor and alloimmunizing strains at non-H-2 loci. Transplant Proc 15:2114–2117, 1983

70. Meredith RF, Okunewick JP: Possibility of graft-vs-leukemia determinants independent of the major histocompatibility complex in allogeneic marrow transplantation. Transplantation 35:378–385, 1983

71. Weiden PL, Flournoy N, Thomas ED, et al: Antileukemic effect of graft-versus-host disease in human recipients of allogeneic-marrow grafts. N Engl J Med 300:1068–1073, 1979

72. Weiden PL, Sullivan KM, Flournoy N et al: Antileukemic effect of chronic graft-versus-host disease. N Engl J Med 304:1529–1532, 1981

73. Denham S, Attridge S, Barfoot RK et al: Effect of cyclosporin A on the anti-leukaemia action associated with graft-versus-host disease. Br J Cancer 47:791–795, 1983

74. Gratama JW, Jansen J, Lipovich RA et al: Treatment of acute graft-versus-host disease with monoclonal antibody OKT3. Transplantation 38:469–473, 1984

75. Mitsuyasu RT, Champlin RE, Gale RP et al: Treatment of donor bone marrow with monoclonal anti-T-cell antibody and complement for the prevention of graft-versus-host disease. Ann Intern Med 105:20–26, 1986

76. Bates SE, Longo DL: Use of serum tumor markers in cancer diagnosis and management. Semin Oncol 14:102–138, 1987

77. Gold P, Freedman SO: Demonstration of tumor specific antigens in human colonic carcinomata by immunologic tolerance and absorption techniques. J Exp Med 121:439–462, 1965

78. Gold P, Freedman SO: Specific carcinoembryonic antigens of the human digestive system. J Exp Med 122:467–481, 1965

79. Braunstein GD, McIntire KR, Waldmann TA: Discordance of human chorionic gonadotropin and alpha-fetoprotein in testicular teratocarcinomas. Cancer 31:1065–1068, 1973

80. Springer GF, Desai P, Murthy M et al: Precursors of the blood group NM antigens as human carcinoma associated antigens. Transfusion 19:233–249, 1979

81. Coon JS, Weinstein RS: Blood group antigens in tumor cell membranes. Biomembranes 11:173–205, 1983

82. Wanebo HJ, Rao B, Pinsky CM et al: Preoperative carcinoembryonic antigen level as a prognostic indicator in colorectal cancer. N Engl J Med 299:448–451, 1978

83. Sugarbaker PH, Zamcheck N, Moore FD: Assessment of serial carcinoembryonic antigen (CEA) assays in postoperative detection of recurrent colorectal cancer. Cancer 38:2310–2315, 1976

84. Waldmann TA, McIntire KR: The use of radioimmunoassay for alpha-fetoprotein in the diagnosis of malignancy. Cancer 34:1510–1515, 1974

85. Heyward WL, Lanier AP, McMahon BJ et al: Early detection of primary hepatocellular carcinoma: Screening for primary hepatocellular carcinoma among persons infected with hepatitis B virus. JAMA 254:3052–3054, 1985

86. Catalona WJ: Tumor markers in testicular cancer. Urol Clin North Am 6:613–628, 1979

87. Gutman AB, Gutman EB: An "acid" phosphatase occurring in the serum of patients with metastasizing carcinoma of the prostate gland. J Clin Invest 17:473–478, 1938

88. Zondag HA, Klein F: Clinical applications of lactate dehydrogenase isozymes: Alterations in malignancy. Ann NY Acad Sci 151:578–586, 1968

89. Jones PAW, Miller FM, Worwood M et al: Ferritinaemia in leukemia and Hodgkin's disease. Br J Cancer 27:212–217, 1973

90. Melvin KEW, Miller HH, Tashjian AH: Early diagnosis of medullary carcinoma of the thyroid gland by means of calcitonin assay. N Engl J Med 285:1115–1120, 1971

91. Said JW, Vimadalal S, Nash G et al: Immunoreactive neuron-specific enolase, bombesin, and chromogranin as markers for neuroendocrine lung tumors. Hum Pathol 16:236–240, 1985

92. Haagensen DE Jr, Kister SF, Panic J et al: Comparative evaluation of carcinoembryonic antigen and gross cystic disease fluid protein as plasma markers for human breast carcinoma. Cancer 42:1646–1652, 1978

93. Foon KA, Schroff RW, Gale RP: Surface markers on leukemia and lymphoma cells: Recent advances. Blood 60:1–19, 1982

94. Koprowski H, Steplewski Z, Mitchell et al: Colorectal carcinoma antigens detected by hybridoma antibodies. Somat Cell Genet 5:957–972, 1979

95. Magnani JL, Steplewski Z, Koprowski H et al: Identification of the gastrointestinal and pancreatic cancer-associated antigen detected by monoclonal antibody 19-9 in the sera of patients as a mucin. Cancer Res 43:5489–5492, 1983

96. Del Villano BC, Brennan S, Brock P et al: Radioimmunometric assay for a monoclonal antibody-defined tumor marker, CA 19-9. Clin Chem 29:549–552, 1983

97. Bast RC Jr, Klug TL, St John E et al: A radioimmunoassay using a monoclonal antibody to monitor the course of epithelial ovarian cancer. N Engl J Med 309:883–887, 1983

98. Greaves MF, Hariri G, Newman RA et al: Selective expression of the common acute lymphoblastic leukemia (gp100) antigen on immature lymphoid cells and their malignant counterparts. Blood 61:628–639, 1983

99. Benson MD, Lurain JR, Newton M: Ovarian tumor antigens. J Reprod Med 28:17–23, 1983

100. Ashall F, Bramwell ME, Harris HJ: A new marker for human cancer cells 1: The Ca antigen and the Ca1 antibody. Lancet 2:1–6, 1982

101. McGee JO'D, Woods JC, Ashall F et al: A new marker for human cancer cells 2: Immunohistochemical detection of the Ca antigen in human tissues with the Ca1 antibody. Lancet 2:7–10, 1982

102. Dippold WG, Lloyd KO, Li LTC et al: Cell surface antigens of human malignant melanoma: Definition of six antigenic systems with mouse monoclonal antibodies. Proc Natl Acad Sci USA 77:6114, 1980

103. Gelder FB, Reese CJ, Moossa AR et al: Purification, partial characterization, and clinical evaluation of pancreatic oncofetal antigen. Cancer Res 38:313–324, 1978

104. Sorenson GD, Bloom SR, Ghatel MA et al: Bombesin production by human small cell carcinoma of the lung. Regul Pept 4:59–66, 1982

105. Staab HJ, Brummendorf T, Hornung A et al: The clinical validity of circulating tumor-associated antigens CEA and CA 19-9 in primary diagnosis and follow-up of patients with gastrointestinal malignancies. Klin Wochenschr 63:106–115, 1985

106. Gupta MK, Arciaga R, Bocci, L: Measurement of a monoclonal-antibody-defined antigen (CA 19-9) in the sera of patients with malignant and nonmalignant diseases. Cancer 56:277–283, 1985

107. Allen CA, Hogg N: Association of colorectal tumor epithelium expressing HLA-D/DR with CD8-positive T-cells and mononuclear phagocytes. Cancer Res 47:2919–2923, 1987

108. van den Ingh HF, Ruiter DJ, Griffioen G et al: HLA antigens in clorectal tumours—Low expression of HLA Class I antigens in mucinous colorectal carcinomas. Br J Cancer 55:125–130, 1987

109. Yamashita K, Nakamura T, Shimizu T et al: Expression of HLA Class I and Class II antigens in human choriocarcinoma cell lines. Int J Gynaecol Obstet 24:301–307, 1986

110. Pesando JM, Graf L: Differential expression of HLA-DR, -DQ, and -DP antigens on malignant B cells. J Immunol 136:4311–4318, 1986

111. Drewinko B, Lichtiger B: Full expression of blood group-related, transplantation-re-

lated, and carcinoembryonic antigens in human colorectal cancer cells with different degrees of phenotypic differentiation. Cancer Res 45:1560–1564, 1985

112. Wagner DK, York–Jolley J, Malek TR et al: Antigen-specific murine T cell clones produce soluble interleukin-2 receptor on stimulation with specific antigens. J Immunol 137:592–596, 1986

113. Medina–Ibarrondo C, Lahuerta–Palacios JJ, Lahuerta–Palacios M: Soluble interleukin-2 receptors in B-cell leukemia and the acquired immunodeficiency syndrome. Ann Intern Med 106:774, 1987

114. Lotze MT, Custer MC, Sharrow SO et al: In vivo administration of purified human interleukin-2 to patients with cancer: Development of interleukin-2 receptor positive cells and circulation soluble interleukin-2 receptors following interleukin-2 administration. Cancer Res 47:2188–2195, 1987

115. Soulillou JP, LeMauff B, Olive D et al: Prevention of rejection of kidney transplants by monoclonal antibody directed against interleukin-2. Lancet 1339–1343, 1987

116. Waldmann TA: The interleukin-2 receptor on malignant cells: A target for diagnosis and therapy. Cell Immunol 99:53–60, 1986

117. Waldmann TA: The structure, function, and expression of interleukin-2 receptors on normal and malignant lymphocytes. Science 232:727–732, 1986

118. Kronke M, Depper JM, Leonard WJ et al.: Adult T cell leukemia: A potential target for ricin A chain immunotoxins. Blood 65:1416–1421, 1985

119. Takahashi H, Herlyn D, Atkinson B et al: Radioimmunodetection of human glioma xenografts by monoclonal antibody to epidermal growth factor receptor. Cancer Res 47:3847–3850, 1987

120. Rodeck U, Herlyn M, Herlyn D et al: Tumor growth modulation by a monoclonal antibody to the epidermal growth factor receptor: Immunologically mediated and effector cell-independent effects. Cancer Res 47:3692–3696, 1987

121. Ranz E: Über Komplimentablenkung durch Serum und Organe. Wien Klin Wochenschr 19:1552–1555, 1906

122. Kohler G, Milstein C: Continuous cultures of fused cells secreting antibodies of predefined specificity. Nature 256:495–497, 1975

123. Jeske DJ, Capra JD: Immunoglobulins: Structure and function. In Paul WE (ed): Fundamental Immunology, pp 131–165. New York, Raven Press, 1984

124. Roitt I, Brostoff J, Male D: Antibody structure and function. In Roitt I, Brostoff J, Male D (eds): pp 5.1–5.8 Immunology, St Louis, CV Mosby, 1986.

125. Berzofsky JA, Berkower IJ: Antigen–antibody interaction. In Paul WE (ed): Fundamental Immunology, pp 595–644. New York, Raven Press, 1984

126. Geysen HM, Tainer JA, Rodda SJ et al: Chemistry of antibody binding to a protein. Science 235:1184–1190, 1987

127. Getzoff ED, Geysen HM, Rodda SJ et al: Mechanisms of antibody binding to a protein. Science 235:1191–1196, 1987

128. Roberts S. Cheetham JC, Reese AR: Generation of an antibody with enhanced affinity and specificity for its antigen by protein engineering. Nature 328:731–734, 1987

129. Massey RJ: Catalytic antibodies catching on. Nature 328:457–458, 1987

130. Kohler G, Howe SC, Milstein C: Fusion between immunoglobulin secreting and non-secreting myeloma cells lines. Eur J Immunol 6:292–298, 1976

131. Kohler G, Howe SC, Milstein C: Derivation of specific antibody producing tissue culture and tumor lines by cell fusion. Eur J Immunol 6:611–617, 1976

132. Brown JP, Woodbury RG, Hart CE et al: Quantitative analysis of melanoma-associated antigen p97 in normal and neoplastic tissues. Proc Natl Acad Sci USA 78:539–543, 1981

133. Morgan AC, Galloway DR, Reisfeld RA: Production and characterization of monoclonal antibody to a melanoma specific glycoprotein. Hybridoma 1:17–36, 1981

134. Hellstrom I, Garrigues HJ, Cabasco L et al: Studies of a high molecular weight human melanoma-associated antigen. J Immunol 130:1467–1472, 1983

135. Hellstrom I, Brankovan V, Hellstrom KE: Strong antitumor activities of IgG3 antibodies to a human melanoma-associated ganglioside. Proc Natl Acad Sci USA 82:1499–1502, 1985

136. Johnson VG, Schlom J, Paterson AJ et al: Analysis of a human tumor-associated glycoprotein (TAG-72) identified by monoclonal antibody B72.3. Cancer Res 46:850–857, 1986

137. Muraro R, Wunderlich D, Thor A et al: Definition by monoclonal antibodies of a repertoire of epitopes on carcinoembryonic antigen differentially expressed in human colon carcinoma versus normal adult tissues. Cancer Res 45:5769–5780, 1985

138. Herlyn D, Herlyn M, Steplewski Z et al: Monoclonal anti-human tumor antibodies of six isotypes in cytotoxic reactions with human and murine effector cells. Cell Immunol 92:105–114, 1985

139. Fargion S, Carney D, Mulshine J et al: Heterogeneity of cell surface antigen expression of human small cell lung cancer detected by monoclonal antibodies. Cancer Res 46:2633–2638, 1986

140. Hellstrom I, Horn D, Linsley P et al: Monoclonal mouse antibodies raised against human lung carcinoma. Cancer Res 46:3917–3923, 1986

141. Kearney JF: Hybridomas and monoclonal antibodies. In Paul WE (ed): Fundamental Immunology, pp 751–766. New York, Raven Press, 1984

142. Morrison SL: Transfectomas provide novel chimeric antibodies. Science 229:1202–1207, 1985

143. Graziano RF, Fanger MW: FcgRI and FcgRII on monocytes and granulocytes are cytoxic trigger molecules for tumor cells. J Immunol 139:3536–3541, 1987

144. Shen L, Guyre PM, Fanger MW: Polymorphonuclear leukocyte function triggered through the high affinity Fc receptor for monomeric IgG. J Immunol 139:534–538, 1987

145. Looney RJ, Abraham GN, Anderson CL: Human monocytes and U937 cells bear two distinct Fc receptors for IgG. J Immunol 136:1641–1647, 1986

146. Rosenfeld SI, Looney RJ, Leddy JP et al: Human platelet Fc receptor for immunoglobulin G: Identification as a 40,000-molecular-weight membrane protein shared by monocytes. J Clin Invest 76:2317–2322, 1985

147. Titus JA, Sharrow SO, Segal DM: Analysis of Fc (IgG) receptors on human peripheral blood leukocytes by dual fluorescence flow microfluorometry II: Quantitation of receptors on cells that express the OKM1, OKT3, OKT4, and OKT8 antigens. J Immunol 130:1152–1158, 1983

148. Perussia B, Kobayashi M, Rossi ME et al: Immune interferon enhances functional properties of human granulocytes: Role of Fc receptors and effect of lymphotoxin, tumor necrosis factor and granulocyte–macrophage colony stimulating factor. J Immunol 138:765–774, 1987

149. Ravetch JV, Luster AD, Weinshank R et al: Structure heterogeneity and functional domains of murine immunoglobulin G Fc receptors. Science 234:718–725, 1986

150. Lewis VA, Koch T, Plutner H et al: A complementary DNA clone for a macrophage–lymphocyte Fc receptor. Nature 324:372–375, 1986

151. Deodhar SD, James K, Chiang T et al: Inhibition of lung metastases in mice bearing a malignant fibrosarcoma by treatment with liposomes containing human C-reactive protein. Cancer Res 42:5084–5088, 1982

152. Muller H, Fehr J: Binding of C-reactive protein to human polymorphonuclear leukocytes: Evidence for association of binding sites with Fc receptors. J Immunol 136:2202–2207, 1986

153. Yancey KB, Hammer CH, Harvath L et al: Studies of human C5a as a mediator of inflammation in normal human skin. J Clin Invest 75:486–495, 1985

154. Yancey KB, O'Shea J, Chused T et al: Human C5a modulates monocytes Fc and C3 receptor expression. J Immunol 135:465–470, 1985

155. Huey R, Hugli TE: Characterization of a C5a receptor on human polymorphonuclear leukocytes (PMN). J Immunol 135:2063–2068, 1985

156. Mujoo K, Cheresh DA, Yang HM et al: Disialoganglioside G_{D_2} on human neuroblastoma cells: Target antigen for monoclonal antibody-mediated cytolysis and suppression of tumor growth. Cancer Res 47:1098–1104, 1987

157. Hersey P, MacDonald M, Burns C et al: Enhancement of cytotoxic and proliferative responses of lymphocytes from melanoma patients by incubation with monoclonal antibodies against ganglioside GD_3. Cancer Immunol Immunother 24:144–150, 1987

158. Thurin J, Thurin M, Kimoto Y et al: Monoclonal antibody-defined correlations in melanoma between levels of GD_2 and GD_3 antigens and antibody-mediated cytotoxicity. Cancer Res 47:1229–1233, 1987

159. Shiloni E, Eisenthal A, Sachs D et al: Antibody-dependent cellular cytotoxicity mediated by murine lymphocytes activated in recombinant interleukin-2. J Immunol 138:1992–1998, 1987

160. Anasetti C, Martin PJ, Morishita Y et al: Human large granular lymphocytes express high affinity receptors for murine monoclonal antibodies of the IgG3 subclass. J Immunol 138:2979–2981, 1987

161. Ortaldo JR, Woodhouse C, Morgan AC et al: Analysis of effector cells in human antibody-dependent cellular cytotoxicity with murine monoclonal antibodies. J Immunol 138:3556–3572, 1987

162. Ghose T, Tai J, Aquino J et al: Tumor localization of ^{131}I-labeled antibodies by radionuclide imaging. Radiology 116:445–448, 1976

163. Houghton AN, Scheinberg DA: Monoclonal antibodies: Potential applications in the treatment of cancer. Semin Oncol 13:165–179, 1986

164. Carrasquillo JA: Radioimmunoscintigraphy with polyclonal or monoclonal antibodies. In Zalutsky M (ed): Antibodies in Radiodiagnosis and Therapy. Boca Raton, FL, CRC Press, 1989

165. Bradwell AR, Fairweather DS, Dykes PW et al: Limiting factors in the localization of tumors with radiolabelled antibodies. Immunol Today 6:163-170, 1985

166. Jungerman JA, Yo K-HP, Zanelli CI: Radiation absorbed dose estimates at the cellular level for some electron-emitting radionuclides for radioimmunotherapy. Int J Appl Radiat Isot 35:883–888, 1984

167. Barth RF, Alan F, Soloway AH et al: Boronated monoclonal antibody 17-1A for potential neutron capture therapy of colorectal cancer. Hybridoma 5:S43–S50, 1986

168. Fawwaz RA, Wang ST, Srivastava SC et al: Potential of palladium-109-labeled antimelanoma monoclonal antibody for tumor therapy. J Nucl Med 25:796–799, 1984

169. Bumol TF, Wang QC, Reisfekd RA et al: Monoclonal antibody and an antibody–toxin conjugate to a cell surface proteoglycan of melanoma cells suppress in vivo tumor growth. Proc Natl Acad Sci USA 80:529–533, 1983

170. Leonard JE, Wang QC, Kaplan NO et al: Kinetics of protein synthesis inactivation in human T-lymphocytes by selective monoclonal antibody–ricin conjugates. Cancer Res 45:5263–5269, 1985

171. Kronke M, Depper JM, Leonard WJ et al: Adult T cell leukemia: A potential target for ricin A chain immunotoxins. Blood 65:1416–1421, 1985

172. Waldmann TA, Tsudo M: Interleukin-2 receptors: Biology and therapeutic potentials. Hosp Pract January 15, 1987, pp 77–94

173. Strom TB: The cellular and molecular basis of allograft rejection: What do we know? Transport Proc 20:143–146, 1988

174. Dillman RO, Shawler DL, Johnson DE et al: Preclinical trials with combinations and conjugats of T101 monoclonal antibody and doxorubicin. Cancer Res 46:4886–4891, 1986

175. Endo N, Kato Y, Takeda Y et al: *In vitro* cytotoxicity of a human serum albumin-mediated conjugate of methotrexate with anti-MM46 monoclonal antibody. Cancer Res 47:1076–1080, 1987

176. Tsukada Y, Ohkawa K, Hibi N: Therapeutic effect of treatment with polyclonal or monoclonal antibodies to alpha-fetoprotein that have been conjugated to duanomycin via a dextran bridge: Studies with an alpha-fetoprotein-producing rat hepatoma tumor model. Cancer Res 47:4293–4295, 1987

177. Matthay KK, Heath TD, Badger CC et al: Antibody-directed liposomes: Comparison of various ligands for association, endocytosis, and drug delivery. Cancer Res 46:4904–4910, 1986

178. Mew D, Lum V, Wat C-K et al: Ability of specific monoclonal antibodies and conventional antisera conjugated to hematoporphyrin to label and kill selected cell lines subsequent to light activation. Cancer Res 45:4380–4386, 1985

179. Waldmann TA: The structure, function, and expression of interleukin-2 receptors on normal and malignant lymphocytes. Science 232:727–732, 1986

180. Waldmann TA, Longo DL, Leonard WJ et al: Interleukin-2 receptor (Tac antigen) expression in HTLV-I-associated adult T-cell leukemia. Cancer Res 45:4559s–4562s, 1985

181. Greene WC, Leonard WJ, Depper JM et al: The human interleukin-2 receptor: Normal and abnormal expression in T cells and in leukemias induced by the human T-lymphotropic retroviruses. Ann Intern Med 105:560–572, 1986

182. Waldmann TA: Use of monoclonal antibody to the interleukin-2 receptor in therapy of patients with adult T-cell leukemia. In Singhal SK, Delovitch (eds): Mediators of Immune Regulation and Immunotherapy, New York, Elsevier Science, 1986

183. Waldmann TA: The interleukin-2 receptor on malignant cells: A target for diagnosis and therapy. Cell Immunol 99:53–60, 1986

184. Kozak RW, Atcher RW, Gansow OA et al: Bismuth-212-labeled anti-Tac monoclonal antibody: Alpha-particle-emitting radionuclides as modalities for radioimmunotherapy. Proc Natl Acad Sci USA 83:474–478, 1986

185. Takahashi H, Herlyn D, Atkinson B et al: Radioimmunodetection of human glioma xenografts by monoclonal antibody to epidermal growth factor receptor. Cancer Res 47:3847–3850, 1987

186. Masui H, Kawamofo T, Sato JD et al: Growth inhibition of human tumor cells in a thymic nude mouse by antiepidermal growth factor receptor monoclonal antibodies. Cancer Res 44: 1002–1007, 1984

187. Griffin TW, Richardson C, Houston LL et al: Antitumor activity of intraperitoneal immunotoxins in a nude mouse model of known malignant mesothelioma. Cancer Res 47:4266–4270, 1987

188. Koprowski H, Herlyn D, Lubeck M et al: Human anti-idiotypic antibodies in cancer patients: Is the modulation of the immune response beneficial for the patient? Proc Natl Acad Sci USA 81:216–219, 1984

189. Herlyn D, Ross AH, Koprowski H: Anti-idiotypic antibodies bear the internal image of a human tumor antigen. Science 232:100–102, 1986

190. DeShambo RM, Krolick KA: Selective in vitro inhibition of an antibody response to purified acetylcholine receptor by using anti-idiotypic antibodies coupled to the A chain of ricin. J Immunol 137:3135–3139, 1986

191. Kusama M, Kageshita T, Tsujisaki M et al: Syngeneic antiidiotypic antisera to murine antihuman high-molecular-weight melanoma-associated antigen monoclonal antibodies. Cancer Res 47:4312–4317, 1987

192. Jerne NK: Towards a network theory of the immune system. Ann Immunol [Paris] 125C:373–389, 1974

193. Burdette S, Schwartz RS: Current concepts: Immunology: Idiotypes and idiotypic networks. N Engl J Med 317:224, 1987

194. Mittelman A, Ferone S, Kageshita T et al: A Phase I clinical trial of murine anti-idiotypic monoclonal antibodies to anti human high molecular weight-melanoma associated antigen monoclonal antibodies in patients with malignant melanoma (abstract). Proc Am Assoc Cancer Res 28:390, 1987

195. Karpovsky B, Titus JA, Stephany DA et al: Production of target-specific effector cells using hetero-cross-linked aggregates containing anti-target cell and anti-Fc receptor antibodies. J Exp Med 160:1686–1701, 1984

196. Staerz UD, Kanagawa O, Bevan MJ: Hybrid antibodies can target sites for attack by T cells. Nature 314:628–631, 1985

197. Staerz UD, Bevan MJ: Use of anti-receptor antibodies to focus T-cell activity. Immunol Today 8:241–245, 1986

198. Perez P, Titus JA, Lotze MT et al: Specific lysis of human tumor cells by T cells coated with anti-T3 cross-linked to anti-tumor antibody. J Immunol 137:2069–2072, 1986

199. Lotze MT, Roberts K, Custer MC et al: Specific binding and lysis of human melanoma by IL-2-activated cells coated with anti-T3 or anti-Fc receptor cross-linked to antimelanoma antibody: A possible approach to the immunotherapy of human tumors. J Surg Res 42:580–589, 1987

200. Titus JA, Garrido MA, Hecht TT et al: Human T cells targeted with anti-T3 cross-linked to antitumor antibody prevent tumor growth in nude mice. J Immunol 138:4018–4022, 1987

201. Titus JA, Perez P, Kaubisch A et al: Human K/natural killer cells targeted with hetero-cross-linked antibodies specifically lyse tumor cells in vitro and prevent tumor growth *in vivo*. J Immunol 139:3153–3158, 1987

202. Yamaguchi H, Furukawa K, Fortunato SR et al: Cell-surface antigens of melanoma recognized by human monoclonal antibodies. Proc Natl Acad Sci USA 84:2416–2420, 1987

203. Watson DB, Burns GF, Mackay IR: *In vitro* growth of B lymphocytes infiltrating human melanoma tissue by transformation with EBV: Evidence for secretion of

204. Haspel MV, McCabe RP, Pomato N et al: Generation of tumor cell-reactive human monoclonal antibodies using peripheral blood lymphocytes from actively immunized colorectal carcinoma patients. Cancer Res 45:3951–3961, 1985

205. Irie RF, Morton DL: Regression of cutaneous metastatic melanoma by intralesional injection with human monoclonal antibody to ganglioside GD2. Proc Natl Acad Sci USA 83:8694–8698, 1986

206. Casali P, Inghirami I, Nakamura M et al: Human monoclonals from antigen-specific selection of B lymphocytes and transformation by EBV. Science 234:476–479, 1987

207. Nishimura Y, Yokoyama M, Araki K et al: Recombinant human–mouse chimeric monoclonal antibody specific for common acute lymphocytic leukemia antigen. Cancer Res 47:999–1005, 1987

208. Shaw DR, Khazaeli MB, Sun LK et al: Characterization of a mouse/human chimeric monoclonal antibody (17-1A) to a colon cancer tumor-associated antigen. J Immunol 138:4534–4538, 1987

209. Liu AY, Robinson RR, Hellstrom KE et al: Chimeric mouse–human IgG1 antibody that can mediate lysis of cancer cells. Proc Natl Acad Sci USA 84:3439–3443, 1987

210. Whittle N, Adair J, Lloyd C et al: Expression in COS cells of a mouse-human chimaeric B72.3 antibody. Protein Engineering 1:499–505, 1987

211. Ng AK, Imai K, Pellegrino A et al: Modulation of immune lysis of tumor cells by interferon. Biomembranes 11:313–339, 1983

212. Houghton AN, Thomson TM, Gross D et al: Surface antigens of melanoma and melanocytes: Specificity of induction of Ia antigens by human gamma-interferon. J Exp Med 160:255–269, 1984

213. Pfizenmaier K, Scheurich P, Schluter C et al: Tumor necrosis factor enhances HLA-A,B,C and HLA-DR gene expression in human tumor cells. J Immunol 138:975–980, 1987

214. Basham TY, Kaminski MS, Kitamura K et al: Synergistic antitumor effect of interferon and anti-idiotype monoclonal antibody in murine lymphoma. J Immunol 137:?3019–3024, 1986

215. Greiner JW, Guadagni F, Noguchi P et al: Recombinant interferon enhances monoclonal antibody-targeting of carcinoma lesions in vivo. Science 235:895–898, 1987

216. Eisenthal A, Lafreniere R, Lefor AT et al: Effect of anti-B16 melanoma monoclonal antibody on established murine B16 melanoma liver metastases. Cancer Res 47:2271–2776, 1987

217. Berinstein N, Levy R: Treatment of a murine B cell lymphoma with monoclonal antibodies and IL 2. J Immunol 139:971–976, 1987

218. Ernst CS, Sears HF, Herlyn M et al: Detection of murine immunoglobulin in human tissues following therapeutic infusion of monoclonal antibody. Hybridoma 5:S79–S85, 1986

219. Chatenoud L, Junker M, Villemain F et al: The human immune response to the OKT3 monoclonal antibody is oligodonal. Science 232:1406–1408, 1986

220. Reynolds JC, Carrasquillo JA, Keenan AM et al: Human antimurine antibodies following immunoscintigraphy or therapy with radiolabeled monoclonal antibodies. J Nucl Med 21:16, 1986

221. Courtenay–Luck NS, Epenetos AA, Moore R et al: Development of primary and secondary immune responses to mouse monoclonal antibodies used in the diagnosis and therapy of malignant neoplasms. Cancer Res 46:6489–6493, 1986

222. Courtenay–Luck NS, Epenetos AA, Winearls CG et al: Preexisting human anti-murine immunoglobulin reactivity due to polyclonal rheumatoid factors. Cancer Res 47:4520–4525, 1987

223. Welte K, Miller G, Chapman PB et al: Stimulation of T lymphocyte proliferation by monoclonal antibodies against GD3 ganglioside. J Immunol 139:1763–1771, 1987

224. Benjamin RJ, Waldmann H: Induction of tolerance by monoclonal antibody therapy. Nature 320:449–451, 1986

225. Caulfield MJ, Shaffer D: Immunoregulation by antigen/antibody complexes I: Specific immunosuppression induced in vivo with immune complexes formed in antibody excess. J Immunol 138:3680–3683, 1987

226. Marrack J: Nature of antibodies. Nature 133:292, 1934

227. Pressman D, Kerghley G: The zone of activity of antibodies as determined by the use of radioactive tracers: The zone of activity of nephritoxic anti-kidney serum. J Immunol 59:140–141, 1948

228. Korngold L, Pressman D: The localization of antilymphosarcoma antibodies in the Murphy lymphosarcoma of the rat. Cancer Res 14:96–99, 1954

229. Day ED: Myelin as a locus for radioantibody absorption *in vivo* in brain tumors. Cancer Res 28:1335–1343, 1968

230. Pressman D, Korngold DL: The in vivo localization of anti-Waagner-osteogenic sarcoma antibodies. Cancer 6:619–623, 1953

231. Pressman D, Day ED, Blau M: The use of paired labeling in the determination of tumor-localizing antibodies. Cancer Res 17:845–850, 1957

232. Day ED, Lassiter S, Woodhall B et al: The localization of radioantibodies in human brain tumors: I. Preliminary exploration. Cancer Res 25:773–778, 1965

233. Day ED, Plannisek J, Korngold L et al: Tumor localizing antibodies purified from antisera against Murphy rat lymphosarcoma. J Natl Cancer Inst 17:517–532, 1956

234. Bale WF, Spar IL: Studies directed toward the use of antibodies as carriers of radioactivity for therapy. Adv Biol Med Phys 5:285–356, 1957

235. Ghose T, Tai J, Aquino J et al: Tumor localization of ^{131}I-labeled antibodies by radionuclide imaging. Radiology 116:445–448, 1975

236. Belitsky P, Ghose T, Aquino J, Tai J et al: Radionuclide imaging of metastases from renal cell carcinoma by ^{131}I-labeled antitumor antibody. Radiology 126:515–517, 1978

237. Reif AE, Curtis LE, Duffield R et al: Trial of radiolabeled antibody localization in metastases of a patient with a tumor containing carcinoembryonic antigen (CEA). J Surg Oncol 6:133–150, 1974

238. Goldenberg DM, Kim EE, DeLand F et al: Clinical studies on the radioimmunodetection of tumors containing alpha-fetoprotein. Cancer 45:2500–2500, 1980

239. Mach J-P, Carrel S, Forni M et al: Tumor localization of radiolabeled antibodies against carcinoembryonic antigens in patients with carcinoma: A critical evaluation. N Engl J Med 303:5–10, 1980

240. Kim EE, DeLand FH, Casper S et al: Radioimmunodetection of colorectal cancer. Cancer 45:1243–1427, 1980

241. Mach J-P, Buchegger F, Forni M et al: Use of radiolabelled monoclonal anti-CEA antibodies for the detection of human carcinomas by external photoscanning and tomoscintigraphy. Immunol Today 2:239–249, 1981

242. Farrands PA, Pimm MV, Embleton MJ et al: Radioimmunodetection of human colorectal cancers by an anti-tumour monoclonal antibody. Lancet 397–400, 1982

243. Berche C, Mach J-P, Lumbruso J-D et al: Tomoscintigraphy for detecting gastrointestinal and medullary thyroid cancers: First clinical results using radiolabelled monoclonal antibodies against carcinoembryonic antigen. Br Med J 285:1447–1451, 1982

244. Mach J-P, Chatal J-F, Lumbroso J-D et al: Tumor localization in patients by radiolabeled monoclonal antibodies against colon carcinoma. Cancer Res 43:5593–5600, 1983

245. Moldofsky PJ, Powe J, Mulhern CB et al: Metastatic colon carcinoma detected with radiolabeled F9ab') monoclonal antibody fragments. Radiology 149:549–555, 1983

246. Moldofsky PJ, Sears HF, Mulhern CB et al: Detection of metastatic tumor in normal-sized retroperitoneal lymph nodes by monoclonal-antibody imaging. N Engl J Med 311:106–107, 1984

247. Epenetos AA, Snook D, Durbin H et al: Limitations of radiolabeled monoclonal antibodies for localization of human neoplasms. Cancer Res 46:3183–3191, 1986

248. Beatty JD, Duda RB, Williams LE et al: Preoperative imaging of colorectal carcinoma with ^{111}In-labeled anticarcinoembryonic antigen monoclonal antibody. Cancer Res 46:6494–6502, 1986

249. Duda RB, Beatty JD, Sheibani K et al: Imaging of human colorectal adenocarcinoma with indium-labeled anticarcinoembryonic antigen monoclonal antibody. Arch Surg 121:131–1319, 1986

250. Ward BG, Mather SJ, Hawkins LR et al: Localization of radioiodine conjugated to the monoclonal antibody HMFG2 in human ovarian carcinoma: Assessment of intravenous and intraperitoneal routes of administration. Cancer Res 47:4719–4723, 1987

251. Colcher D, Esteban J, Carrasquillo JA et al: Quantitative analyses of selective radiolabeled monoclonal antibody localization in metastatic lesions of colorectal cancer patients. Cancer Res 47:1185–1189, 1987

252. Colcher D, Esteban J, Carrasquillo JA et al: Complementation of intracavitary and intravenous administration of a monoclonal antibody (B72.3) in patients with carcinoma. Cancer Res 47:4218–4224, 1987

253. Carrasquillo JA, Bunn PA, Keenan AM et al: Radioimmunodetection of cutaneous T-cell lymphoma with ^{111}In-labeled T101 monoclonal antibody. N Engl J Med 315:673–680, 1986

254. Ettinger DS, Order SE, Wharam MD et al: Phase I–II study of isotopic immunoglobulin therapy for primary liver cancer. Cancer Treat Rep 66:289–297, 1982

255. Leichner PK, Klein JL, Siegelman SS et al: Dosimetry of ^{131}I-labeled antiferritin in hepatoma: Specific activities in the tumor and liver. Cancer Treat Rep 67:647–658, 1983

256. Order SE, Stillwagon GB, Klein JL et al: Iodine 131 antiferritin, a new treatment modality in hepatoma: A Radiation Therapy Oncology Group study. J Clin Oncol 3:1573–1582, 1985

257. Order SE, Klein JL, Leichner PK: Hepatoma: Model for radiolabeled antibody in cancer treatment. NCI Mongr 3:37–41, 1987

258. Larson SM, Brown JP, Wright PW et al: Imaging of melanoma with ^{131}I-labeled monoclonal antibodies. J Nucl Med 24:123–129, 1983

259. Larson SM, Carrasquillo JA, Krohn KA et al: Localization of ^{131}I-labeled p97-specific Fab fragments in human melanoma as a basis for radiotherapy. J Clin Invest 72:2101–2114, 1983

260. Carrasquillo JA, Krohn KA, Beaumler P et al: Diagnosis of and therapy for solid tumors with radiolabeled antibodies and immune fragments. Cancer Treat Rep 68:317–328, 1984

261. Halpern SE, Sillman RO, Witztum KF et al: Radioimmunodetection of melanoma utilizing In-111 96.5 monoclonal antibody: A preliminary report. Radiology 155:493–499, 1985

262. Lotze MT, Carrasquillo JA, Weinstein JN et al: Monoclonal antibody imaging of human melanoma: Radioimmunodetection by subcutaneous or systemic injection. Ann Surg 204:223–235, 1986

263. Siccardi AG, Buraggi GL, Callegaro L et al: Multicenter study of immunoscintigraphy with radiolabeled monoclonal antibodies in patients with melanoma. Cancer Res 46:4817–4822, 1986

264. Buraggi GL, Callegaro L, Mariani G et al: Imaging with ^{131}I-labeled monoclonal antibodies to a high-molecular weight melanoma-associated antigen in patients with melanoma: Efficacy of whole immunoglobulin and its F(ab')$_2$ fragments. Cancer Res 45:3378–3387, 1985

265. Engelstad BL, Spitler LE, Del Rio MJ et al: Phase I immunolymphoscintigraphy with an In-111-labeled antimelanoma monoclonal antibody. Radiology 161:419–422, 1986

266. Taylor Jr A, Milton W, Eyre H et al: Radioimmunodetection of human melanoma with indium-111-labeled monoclonal antibodies. NCI Monogr 3:25–31, 1987

267. Goldenberg DM, DeLand F, Kim E et al: Use of radiolabeled antibodies to carcinoembryonic antigen for the detection and localization of diverse cancers by external photoscanning. N Engl J Med 25:1384–1388, 1978

268. Kim WW, DeLand FH, Nelson MO et al: Radioimmunodetection of cancer with radiolabeled antibodies to alpha-fetoprotein. Cancer Res 40:3008–3012, 1980

269. Goldenberg DM, Kim EE, DeLand FH et al: Radioimmunodetection of cancer using radioactive antibodies to human chorionic gonadotropin. Science 208:1284–1286, 1980

270. Monison RT, Lyster DM, Alcorn L et al: Radioimmunoimaging with ^{99m}Tc monoclonal antibodies: Clinical studies. Int J Nucl Med & Biol 11:184–188, 1984

271. Fairweather DS, Bradwell AR, Watson–James SF: Detection of thyroid tumors using radiolabeled anti-thyroglobulin. Clin Endocrinol 18:563–570, 1983

272. Fairweather DS, Bradwell AR, Dykes PW: Monoclonal antibodies for in vivo localisation. Lancet 2:660, 1982

273. Nimmon CC, Carroll MJ, Flatman W: Partial probability mapping of temporal change: Application to gamma quality control and immunoscintigraphy. Nucl Med Commun 5:231, 1984

274. Order SE, Bloomer WB, Jones AG et al: Radionuclide immunoglobulin lymphangiography: A case report. Cancer 35:1487–1492, 1975

275. Weinstein JN, Steller MA, Covell DG et al: Monoclonal antitumor antibodies in the lymphatics. Cancer Treat Rep 68:257–264, 1984

276. Eger RR, Covell DG, Carrasquillo JA et al: Kinetic model for the biodistribution of an ^{111}In-labeled monoclonal antibody in humans. Cancer Res 47:3328–3336, 1987

277. Parker RJ, Keenan AM, Dower SK et al: Targeting of murine radiolabeled monoclonal antibodies in the lymphatics. Cancer Res 47:2073–2076, 1987

278. Weinstein JN, Black CDV, Barbet J et al: Selected issues in the pharmacology of monoclonal antibodies. In Tomlinson E (ed): Site-Specific Drug Delivery. New York, John Wiley, 1986

279. Schlom J: Basic principles and applications of monoclonal antibodies in the management of carcinomas: The Richard and Hinda Rosenthal Foundation Award Lecture. Cancer Res 46:3225–3238, 1986

280. Nadler LM, Stashenko P, Hardy R et al: Serotherapy of a patient with a monoclonal antibody directed against a human lymphoma-associated antigen. Cancer Res 40:3147–3154, 1980

281. Miller RA, Maloney DG, Warnke R et al: Treatment of B-cell lymphoma with monoclonal anti-idiotype antibody. N Engl J Med 306:517–522, 1982

282. Miller RA, Oseroff AR, Stratte PT et al: Monoclonal antibody therapeutic trails in seven patients with T-cell lymphoma. Blood 62:988, 1983

283. Meeker TC, Lowder JN, Maloney DG et al: A clinical trial of anti-idiotype therapy for B cell malignancy. Blood 65:1349–1363, 1985

284. Rankin EM, Hekman A, Somers R et al: Treatment of two patients with B cell lymphoma with monoclonal anti-idiotypic antibodies. Blood 65:1373–1381, 1985

285. Giardina SL, Schroff RW, Kipps TJ et al: The generation of monoclonal anti-idiotype antibodies to human B cell-derived leukemias and lymphomas. J Immunol 135:653–658, 1985

286. Dillman RO, Shawler DL, Sobel RE et al: Murine monoclonal antibody therapy in two patients with chronic lymphocytic leukemia. Blood 59:1036–1045, 1982

287. Dillman RO, Shawler DL, Dillman JB et al: Therapy of chronic lymphocytic leukemia and cutaneous T-cell lymphoma with T101 monoclonal antibody. J Clin Oncol 2:881–891, 1984

288. Foon KA, Schroff RW, Bunn PA et al: Effects of monoclonal antibody therapy in patients with chronic lymphocytic leukemia. Blood 64:1085–1094, 1984

289. Ritz J, Pesando JM, Sallan SE et al: Serotherapy of acute lymphoblastic leukemia with monoclonal antibody. Blood 58:141–152, 1981

290. Miller RA, Maloney DG, McKillop J et al: In vivo effects of murine hybridoma monoclonal antibody in a patient with T-cell leukemia. Blood 58:78–86, 1981

291. Miller RA, Oseroff AS, Stratte PT et al: Monoclonal antibody therapeutic trials in seven patients with T-cell lymphoma. Blood 62:988–995, 1983

292. Miller RA, Levy R: Response of cutaneous T cell lymphoma to therapy of hybridoma monoclonal antibody. Lancet 2:225–230, 1981

293. Levy R, Miller RA: Tumor therapy with monoclonal antibodies. Fed Proc 42:2650–2656, 1983

294. Foon KA, Schroff RW, Bunn PA: Monoclonal antibody therapy for patients with leukemia and lymphoma. In Foon KA, Morgan AC (eds): Monoclonal Antibody Therapy of Human Cancer, pp 85–101. Boston, Martinus Nijhoff, 1985

295. Rosen ST, Zimmer AM, Goldman-Leikin R et al: Radioimmunodetection and radioimmunotherapy of cutaneous T cell lymphomas using ^{131}I-labeled monoclonal antibody: An Illinois Cancer Council study. J Clin Oncol 5:562–573, 1987

296. Ball ED, Bernier GM, Cornwell GG et al: Monoclonal antibodies to myeloid differentiation antigens: In vivo studies of three patients with acute myelogenous leukemia. Blood 62:1203–1210, 1983

297. Courtenay–Luck N, Epenetos AA: Antibody-guided irradiation of malignant lesions: Three cases illustrating a new method of treatment. Lancet 1:1441–1443, 1984

298. Sears HF, Atkinson B, Mattis J et al: The use of monoclonal antibody in Phase I clinical trial of human gastrointestinal tumors. Lancet 1:762–765, 1982

299. Sears HF, Herlyn D, Steplewski Z et al: Phase II clinical trial of a murine monoclonal antibody cytotoxic for gastrointestinal adenocarcinoma. Cancer Res 45:5910–5913, 1985

300. Sindelar WF, Maher MM, Herlyn D et al: Trial of therapy with monoclonal antibody

17-1A in pancreatic carcinoma: Preliminary results. Hybridoma 5:S125–S132, 1986

301. Weiner LM, Steplewski Z, Koprowski H et al: Biologic effects of gamma interferon pre-treatment followed by monoclonal antibody 17-1A administration in patients with gastrointestinal carcinoma. Hybridoma 5:S65–S77, 1986

302. Sobol RE, Dillman RO, Smith JD: Phase I evaluation of murine monoclonal anti-melanoma antibody in man: Preliminary observations. In Mitchell MS, Oettgen HF (eds): Hybridomas in Cancer Diagnosis and Treatment, pp 199–206, New York, Raven Press, 1982

303. Larson SM, Carrasquillo JA, Krohn KA: Radiotherapy with "anti-p97" iodinated monoclonal antibodies in melanoma. In Raynaud C (ed): Proceedings of the Third World Congress of Nuclear Medicine and Biology, pp 3666–3669. New York, Pergamon Press, 1982

304. Oldham RK, Foon KA, Morgan C et al: Monoclonal antibody therapy of malignant melanoma: In vivo localization in cutaneous metastasis after intravenous administration. J Clin Oncol 2:1235–1244, 1984

305. Goodman GE, Beaumier P, Hellstrom I et al: Pilot trial of murine monoclonal antibodies in patients with advanced melanoma. J Clin Oncol 3:340–352, 1985

306. Dippold WG, Knuth KRK, zum Buschenfelde K-HM: Inflammatory tumor response to monoclonal antibody infusion. Eur J Cancer Clin Oncol 21:907–912, 1985

307. Houghton AN, Mintzer DM, Corden-Cardo C et al: Mouse monoclonal antibody detecting GD3 ganglioside: A phase I trial in patients with malignant melanoma. Proc Natl Acad Sci USA 82:1242–1246, 1985

308. Spitler LE, Del Rio M, Khentigan A et al: Therapy of patients with malignant melanoma using a monoclonal antimelanoma antibody–ricin A chain immunotoxin. Cancer Res 47:1717–1723, 1987

309. Cheung N-KV, Lazarus H, Miraldi FD et al: Ganglioside G_{D2} specific monoclonal antibody 3F8. A Phase I study in patients with neuroblastoma and malignant melanoma. J Clin Oncol 5:1430–1440, 1987

310. Nadler L, Takvorian T, Botnick et al: Anti-B1 monoclonal antibody and complement treatment in autologous bone marrow transplantation for relapsed B cell non-Hodgkin's lymphoma. Lancet 2:427–433, 1984

311. Longo DL: Biological therapy of cancer. In Fortner JG, Rhoads JE (eds): Accomplishments in Cancer Research, p 233. Philadelphia, JB Lippincott, 1986

312. Karavodin LM, Golub SH: Immunocompetence in cancer patients. In Herberman RB (ed): Basic and Clinical Tumor Immunology, p 215. Boston, Martinus Nijhoff, 1983

313. Terry WD, Rosenberg SA (eds): Immunotherapy of Human Cancer. New York, Elsevier-North Holland, 1982

314. Hersh EM: Current status of active non-specific immunotherapy. In Reif AE, Mitchell MS (eds): Immunity to Cancer, p 443. Orlando, Academic Press, 1985

315. Hersh EM, Murphy SG, Quesada JR et al: Effect of immunotherapy with Corynebacterium parvum and methanol extraction residue of BCG administered intravenously on host defense function in cancer patients. JNCI 66:993, 1981

316. Ashwell JD, Fox BS, Schwartz RH: Functional analysis of the interaction of the antigen-specific T cell receptor with its ligands. J Immunol 136:757, 1986

317. Talmadge JE, Herberman RB, Chirigos MA et al: Hyporesponsiveness to augmentation of murine natural killer cell activity in different anatomical compartments by multiple injections of various immunomodulators including recombinant interferons and interleukin-2. J Immunol 135:2483, 1985

318. Rollinghoff M, Starzinski-Powitz A, Pfizenmaier K et al: Cyclophosphamide-sensitive T-lymphocytes suppress the in vitro generation of antigen-specific cytotoxic T lymphocytes. J Exp Med 145:455, 1977

319. Pinsky CM: Local administration of immunomodulators. Semin Oncol 13:141, 1986

320. Bast RC Jr, Zbar B, Borsos T et al: BCG and cancer. N Engl J Med 290:1413, 1974

321. McKhann CF, Hendrickson CG, Spitler LE et al: Immunotherapy of melanoma with BCG: Two fatalities following intralesional injection. Cancer 35:514, 1975

322. Rosenberg SA, Rapp H, Terry W et al: Intralesional BCG therapy of patients with primary stage I melanoma. In Terry WD, Rosenberg SA (eds): Immunotherapy of Human Cancer, p 239. New York, Excerpta Medica, 1982

323. Zbar B, Canti G, Ashley M et al: Eradication by immunization with mycobacterial vaccines and tumor cells of microscopic metastases remaining after surgery. Cancer Res 39:1597, 1979

324. Holmes EC, Ramming KP, Bein ME et al: Intralesional BCG immunotherapy of pulmonary tumors. J Thorac Cardiovasc Surg 77:362, 1979

325. Pardridge DH, Sparks FC, Goodnight JE Jr et al: Intratumor Bacillus Calmette-Guerin therapy for chest wall recurrence of carcinoma of the breast. Surg Gynecol Obstet 148:867, 1979

326. Schellhammer PF, Ladaga LE, Fillion MB: Bacillus Calmette-Guerin for superficial transitional cell carcinoma of the bladder. J Urol 135:261, 1986

327. Herr HW, Pinsky CM, Whitmore WF Jr et al: Long-term effect of intravesical Bacillus Calmette-Guerin on flat carcinoma in situ of the bladder. J Urol 135:265, 1986

328. McKneally MF, Maver C, Kausel HW: Regional immunotherapy of lung cancer with intrapleural BCG. Lancet 1:377, 1976

329. Miller JW, Hunter AM, Horne NW: Intrapleural immunotherapy with Corynebacterium parvum in recurrent malignant pleural effusions. Thorax 35:856, 1980

330. Webb HE, Oaten SE, Pike CP: Treatment of malignant ascitic and pleural effusions with Corynebacterium parvum. Br Med J 1:338, 1978

331. Mantovani A, Sessa C, Peri G et al: Intraperitoneal administration of Corynebacterium parvum in patients with ascitic ovarian tumors resistant to chemotherapy: effects on cytotoxicity of tumor associated macrophages and NK cells. Int J Cancer 27:437, 1981

332. Bast RC Jr, Berek JS, Obrist R et al: Intraperitoneal immunotherapy of human ovarian carcinoma with Corynebacterium parvum. Cancer Res 43:1385, 1983

333. Warren HS, Vogel FR, Chedid LA: Current status of immunological adjuvants. Annu Rev Immunol 4:369, 1986

334. Kobayashi H: Viral xenogenization of intact tumor cells. Adv Cancer Res 30.279, 1979

335. Schirrmacher V, Ahlert T, Heicappell R et al: Successful application of non-oncogenic viruses for antimetastatic cancer immunotherapy. Cancer Rev 5:19, 1986

336. Peppoloni S, Herberman RB, Gorelik E: Induction of highly immunogenic variants of Lewis lung carcinoma tumor by ultraviolet irradiation. Cancer Res 45:2560, 1986

337. Boon T: Antigenic tumor cell variants obtained with mutagens. Adv Cancer Res 39:121, 1983

338. Edelson R, Berger C, Gasparro F et al: Treatment of cutaneous T-cell lymphoma by extracorporeal photochemotherapy: Preliminary results. N Engl J Med 316:297, 1987

339. Wunderlich M, Schiessel R, Rainer H et al: Effect of adjuvant chemo- or immunotherapy on the prognosis of colorectal cancer operated for cure. Br J Surg 72:107, 1985

340. Jones PC, Sze LL, Liu PY et al: Prolonged survival for melanoma patients with elevated IgM antibody to oncofetal antigen. J Natl Cancer Inst 66:249, 1981

341. Bell DR, Gerlach JH, Kartner N et al: Detection of P-glycoprotein in ovarian cancer: A molecular marker associated with multidrug resistance. J Clin Oncol 3:331, 1985

342. Hollinshead A, Stewart THM, Takita H et al: Adjuvant specific active lung cancer immunotherapy trials: Tumor-associated antigens. Cancer 60:1249, 1987

343. Hoover HC Jr, Surdyke MG, Dangel RB et al: Prospectively randomized trial of adjuvant active specific immunotherapy for human colorectal cancer. Cancer 55:1236, 1985

344. Hanna MG, Brandhorst JS, Peter LC: Active specific immunotherapy of residual micrometastasis: An evaluation of sources, doses and ratios of BCG with tumor cells. Cancer Immunol Immunother 7:165–173, 1979

345. Straus AA, Appel M, Saphir J et al: Immunologic resistance to carcinomas produced by electrocoagulation. Surg Gynecol Obstet 121:989, 1965

346. Moore FT, Blackwood J, Sanzenbacker L et al: Hypotherapy for malignant tumors: Immunologic response. Arch Surg 96:527, 1968

347. Ashwell JD, Longo DL, Bridges SH: T-cell tumor elimination as a result of T-cell receptor-mediated activation. Science 237:61, 1987

348. Isaacs A, Lindenmann J: Virus interference. Proc Soc [Biol] 147:258, 1957

349. Clark JW, Longo DL: Interferons in cancer therapy. In DeVita VT Jr, Hellman S, Rosenberg SA (eds): Cancer: Principles and Practice of Oncology Updates, 2nd ed, p 1. Philadelphia, JB Lippincott, 1987

350. Preble OT, Black RJ, Friedman RM et al: Systemic lupus erythematosus: Presence in human serum of an unusual acid-labile leukocyte interferon. Science 216:429, 1982

351. Weissmann C, Weber H: The interferon genes. Prog Nucl Acid Res 33:251, 1986

352. Zinn K, Maniatis T: Detection of factors that interact with the human beta-interferon regulatory region in vivo by DNAase I footprinting. Cell 45:611, 1986

353. Enoch T, Zinn K, Maniatis T: Activation of the human beta-interferon gene requires an interferon-inducible factor. Mol Cell Biol 6:801, 1986

354. Nir U, Cohen B, Chen L et al: A human IFN-beta 1 gene deleted of promoter sequences upstream from the TATA box is controlled post-transcriptionally by dsRNA. Nucl Acid Res 12:6979, 1984

355. Duc-Goiran P, Robert–Galliot B, Lopez J et al: Unusual apparently constitutive interferons and antagonists in human placental blood. Proc Natl Acad Sci USA 82:5010, 1985

356. Week PK, Apperson S, May L et al: Comparison of the antiviral activities of various cloned human interferon-alpha subtypes in mammalian cell cultures. J Gen Virol 57:233, 1981

357. Ortaldo JR, Herberman RB, Harvey C et al: A species of human alpha-interferon that lacks the ability to boost human natural killer activity. Proc Natl Acad Sci USA 81:4926, 1984

358. Hiscott J, Cantell K, Weissmann C: Differential expression of human interferon genes. Nucl Acid Res 12:3727, 1984

359. Branca AA, Faltynek CR, D'Allesandro S et al: Interaction of interferon with cellular receptors. J Biol Chem 257:13291, 1982

360. Faltynek CR, Princler G, Ruscetti FR et al: Lectins modulate the internalization of recombinant interferon alpha and the induction of 2'5'-oligo(A) synthetase (submitted).

361. Friedman RL, Stark GR: Alpha-interferon-induced transcription of HLA and metallothionein genes containing homologous upstream sequences. Nature 314:637, 1985

362. Staeheli P, Maller O, Boll W et al: Mx protein: Constitutive expression in 3T3 cells transformed with cloned Mx cDNA confers selective resistance to influenza virus. Cell 44:147, 1986

363. Pfefferkorn ER: Interferon gamma blocks the growth of Toxoplasma gondii in human fibroblasts by inducing the host cells to degrade tryptophan. Proc Natl Acad Sci USA 81:908, 1984

364. Friedman RM, Merigan T, Sreevalsan T (ed): Interferons as Cell Growth Inhibitors and Antitumor Factors. UCLA Symposia on Molecular and Cellular Biology, New Series Volumn 50, New York, Alan R Liss, 1986

365. Smekens–Etienne M, Goldstein J, Ooms HA et al: Variation of (2'5') oligo (adenylate) synthetase activity during rat liver regeneration. Eur J Biochem 130:209, 1983

366. Perussia B, Kobayashi M, Rossi ME et al: Immune interferon enhances functional properties of human granulocytes: Role of Fc receptors and effect of lymphotoxin,

tumor necrosis factor, and granulocyte–macrophage colony stimulating factor. J Immunol 138:765, 1987

367. Stone–Wolff DS, Yip YK, Kelker HC et al: Interrelationships of human interferon-gamma with lymphotoxin and monocyte cytotoxin. J Exp Med 159:828, 1984

368. Maluish AE, Urba WJ, Longo DL et al: The determination of an immunologically active dose of interferon gamma in patients with melanoma. J Clin Oncol 6:434, 1988

369. Sidky YA, Borden EC: Inhibition of angiogenesis by interferons: effects on tumor- and lymphocyte-induced vascular responses. Cancer Res 47:5155, 1987

370. Quesada JR, Hersh EM, Manning J et al: Treatment of hairy cell leukemia with recombinant alpha interferon. Blood 68:493, 1986

371. Bocci V, Pacini A, Muscetti OM et al: The kidney is the main site of interferon catabolism. J Interferon Res 2:309, 1982

372. Gutterman JU, Fine S, Quesada J et al: Recombinant leukocyte A interferon: Pharmacokinetics, single-dose tolerance, and biologic effects in cancer patients. Ann Intern Med 96:549, 1982

373. Golomb HW, Jacobs A, Fefer A et al: Alpha-2 interferon therapy of hairy cell leukemia: A multicenter study of 64 patients. J Clin Oncol 4:900, 1986

374. Faltynek CR, Princler GL, Rossio JL et al: Relationship of the clinical response and binding of recombinant interferon alpha in patients with lymphproliferative disease. Blood 67:1077, 1986

375. Steis RG, Marcon L, Urba WJ et al: Serum soluble IL2 receptor levels as a tumor marker in patients with hairy cell leukemia. Blood 71:1304, 1988

376. Steis RG, Smith JW, Urba WJ, et al: Resistance to recombinant interferon alpha 1 in hairy cell leukemia associated with neutralizing anti-interferon antibodies. N Engl J Med 318:1409, 1988

377. Spiers ASD, Moore D, Cassileth PA et al: Hairy cell leukemia: Complete remission with pentostatin (2'-deoxycoformycin). N Engl J Med 316:825, 1987

378. Foon KA, Nakano GM, Koller CA et al: Response to 2'-deoxycoformycin after failure to interferon alpha in nonsplenectomized patients with hairy cell leukemia. Blood 68:297, 1986

379. Urba WJ, Steis RG, Clark JW et al: Immune effects of treating hairy cell leukemia patients with deoxycoformycin (submitted)

380. Talpaz M, Kantarjian HM, McCredie K et al: Hematologic remission and cytogenetic improvement induced by recombinant human interferon alpha A in chronic myelogenous leukemia. N Engl J Med 314:1065, 1986

381. Bergsagel DE, Haas RH, Messner HA: Interferon alfa-2b in the treatment of chronic granulocytic leukemia. Semin Oncol 13:29, 1986

382. Oberg K, Funa K, Alm G et al: Effects of leukocyte interferon on clinical symptoms and hormone levels in patients with mid-gut carcinoid tumors and carcinoid syndrome. N Engl J Med 309:129, 1983

383. Anderson JV, Bloom SR: Treatment of malignant endocrine pancreatic tumors with human leukocyte interferon. Lancet 1:97, 1987

384. McKnight J, Clark J, Miller R et al: Randomized trial of recombinant interferon alpha with or without indomethacin in patients with metastatic malignant melanoma (abstr). Proc Am Soc Clin Oncol 6:250, 1987

384a. Creagan ET, Kovach JS, O'Connell MJ et al: Improved response of renal cell carcinoma to alpha interferon by the addition of aspirin. Cancer 61:1787, 1988

385. Borden EC, Hawkins MJ: Biologic response modifiers as adjuncts to other therapeutic modalities. Semin Oncol 13:144, 1986

386. Quesada JR, Talpaz M, Rios A et al: Clinical toxicity of interferons in cancer patients: A review. J Clin Oncol 4:234, 1986

387. Abrams PG, McClamrock E, Foon KA: Evening administration of alpha interferon. N Engl J Med 312:443, 1985

388. Hrushesky WJM: The rationale for non-zero-order drug delivery using automatic, computer-based drug delivery systems (chronotherapy). J Biol Response Mod (in press)

389. Herberman RB, Pinsky CM: Polyribonucleotides for cancer therapy: summary and recommendations for further research. J Biol Response Mod 4:680, 1985

390. Lacour J, Lacour F, Spira A et al: Adjuvant treatment with polyadenylic–polyuridylic acid in operable breast cancer: Updated results of a randomized trial. Br Med J 288:489, 1984

391. Wiltrout RH, Boyd MR, Back TT et al: Flavone-8-acetic acid augments systemic natural killer cell activity and synergizes with interleukin 2 for treatment of murine renal cancer. J Immunol 140:3261, 1988

392. Urba WJ, Longo DL, Lombardo F et al: Flavone acetic acid (NSC 347512) enhances natural killer activity in human peripheral blood. J Natl Cancer Inst 80:521, 1988

393. Smith KA: Interleukin-2: Inception, impact and implications. Science 240:1169–1175, 1988

394. Morgan DA, Ruscetti FW, Gallo RG: Selective in vitro growth of T lymphocytes from normal human bone marrow. Science 193:1007–1008, 1976

395. Stern JB, Smith KA: Interleukin-2 induction of T-cell G_1 progression and c-myb expression. Science 233:203–206, 1986

396. Kornfeld H, Berman JS, Beer DJ et al: Induction of human T lymphocyte motility by interleukin 2. J Immunol 134:3887–3890, 1985

397. Nedwin GE, Svederky LP, Bringman TS et al: Effect of interleukin 2, interferon-x, and mitogens on the production of tumor necrosis factors x and x. J Immunol 135:2492–2497, 1985

398. Waldmann TA, Goldman CK, Robb RJ et al: Expression of interleukin-2 receptors on activated human B cells. J Exp Med 160:1450–1466, 1984

399. Jung LKL, Toshiro H, Fu SM: Detection and functional studies of p60–65 (Tac antigen) on activated human B cells. J Exp Med 160:1597–1602, 1984

400. Malkovsky M, Loveland B, North M et al: Recombinant interleukin-2 directly augments the cytotoxicity of human monocytes. Nature 325:262–264, 1987

401. Hancock WW, Muller WA, Cotran RS: Interleukin 2 receptors are expressed by alveolar macrophages during pulmonary sarcoidosis and are inducible by lymphokine treatment of normal human lung macrophages, blood monocytes, and monocyte cell lines. J Immunol 138:185–191, 1987

402. Steiner G, Tschachler E, Tani M et al: Interleukin 2 receptors on cultured murine epidermal Langerhans cells. J Immunol 137:155–159, 1986

403. Benveniste EN, Merrill JE: Stimulation of oligodendroglial proliferation and maturation by interleukin-2. Nature 321:610–613, 1986

404. Kaplan J, Tilton J, Peterson WD: Identification of T-cell lymphoma tumor antigens on human T-cell lines. Am J Hematol 1:219–226, 1976

405. Gillis S, Watson J: Biochemical and biological characterization of lymphocyte regulatory molecules: V. Identification of an interleukin-2 producing human leukemia T cell line. J Exp Med 152:1709–1715, 1980

406. Taniguchi T, Matsui H, Fujita T et al: Structure and expression of a cloned cDNA for human interleukin-2. Nature 302:305–307, 1983

407. Rosenberg SA, Grimm EA, McGrogan M et al: Biological activity of recombinant human interleukin-2 produced in E. coli. Science 223:1412–1415, 1984

408. Doyle MV, Lee MT, Fong S: Comparison of the biological activities of human recombinant interleukin-2_{125} native interleukin-2. J Biol Response Mod 4:96–109, 1985

409. Sharon M, Klausner RD, Cullen BR et al: Novel interleukin-2 receptor subunit detected by cross-linking under high affinity conditions. Science 234:859–863, 1987

410. Rosenberg SA, Lotze MT, Mule JJ: New approaches to the immunotherapy of cancer. Ann Intern Med 108:853–864, 1988

411. Merluzzi VJ, Walker MM, Fananes RB: Inhibition of cytotoxic T-cell clonal expansion by cyclophosphamide and the recovery of cytotoxic T-lymphocyte precursors by supernatants from mixed lymphocyte cultures. Cancer Res 41:850–853, 1981

412. Clason AE, Duarte AJS, Kupiec–Weglinski JW et al: Restoration of allograft responsiveness in B rats by interleukin-2 and/or adherent cells. J Immunol 129:252–259, 1982

413. Rook AH, Masur H, Lane HC et al: Interleukin-2 enhances the depressed natural killer and cytomegalovirus specific cytotoxic activities of lymphocytes from patients with the acquired immune deficiency syndrome. J Clin Invest 72:398–407, 1983

414. Ettinghausen SE, Lipford EH III, Mule JJ et al: Systemic administration of recombinant interleukin-2 stimulates in vivo lymphoid cell proliferation in tissues. J Immunol 135:1488–1497, 1985

415. Ettinghausen SE, Lipford EH III, Mule JJ et al: Recombinant interleukin-2 stimulates in vivo proliferation of adoptively transferred lymphokine activated killer (LAK) cells. J Immunol 135:3623–3635, 1985

416. Yron I, Wood TA, Spiess P et al: In vitro growth of murine T cells V: The isolation and growth of lymphoid cells infiltrating syngeneic solid tumors. J Immunol 125:238–245, 1980

417. Lotze MT, Grimm E, Mazumder A et al: In vitro growth of cytotoxic human lymphocytes IV: Lysis of fresh and cultured autologous tumor by lymphocytes cultured in T cell growth factor (TCGF). Cancer Res 41:4420–4425, 1981

418. Grimm EA, Ramsey KM, Mazumder A et al: Lymphokine-activated killer cell phenomenon II: The precursor phenotype is serologically distinct from peripheral T lymphocytes, memory CTL, and NK cells. J Exp Med 157:884–897, 1983

419. Rosenstein M, Yron I, Kaufman Y, Rosenberg SA: Lymphokine activated killer cells: Lysis of fresh syngeneic NK-resistant murine tumor cells by lymphocytes cultured in interleukin-2. Cancer Res 44:1946–1953, 1984

420. Rayner AA, Grimm EA, Lotze MT et al: Lymphokine-activated killer (LAK) cell phenomenon: Analysis of factors relevant to the immunotherapy of human cancer. Cancer 55:1327–1333, 1985

421. Rosenberg SA: Adoptive immunotherapy of cancer using lymphokine activated killer cells and recombinant interleukin-2. In DeVita VT Jr, Hellman S, Rosenberg SA (eds): Important Advances in Oncology 1986, pp 55–91. Philadelphia, JB Lippincott, 1986

422. Rosenberg SA, Mule JJ, Speiss PJ et al: Regression of established pulmonary metastases and subcutaneous tumor mediated by the systemic administration of high dose recombinant IL-2. J Exp Med 161:1169–1188, 1985

423. Lafreniere R, Rosenberg SA: Successful immunotherapy of murine experimental hepatic metastases with lymphokine-activated killer cells and recombinant interleukin-2. Cancer Res 45:3735–3741, 1985

424. Mule JJ, Yang JC, Lafreniere R et al: Identification of cellular mechanisms operational in vivo during the regression of established pulmonary metastases by the systemic administration of high-dose recombinant interleukin-2. J Immunol 139:285–294, 1987

425. Papa MZ, Mule JJ, Rosenberg SA: The anti-tumor efficacy of lymphokine-activated killer cells and recombinant interleukin-2 in vivo: Successful immunotherapy of established pulmonary metastases from weakly and non-immunogenic murine tumors of three distinct histologic types. Cancer Res 46:4973–4978, 1986

426. Donohue JH, Rosenstein M, Chang AE et al: The systemic administration of purified interleukin-2 enhances the ability of sensitized murine lymphocyte lines to cure a disseminated syngeneic lymphoma. J Immunol 132:2123–2128, 1984

427. Shu S, Chou T, Rosenberg SA: In vitro sensitization and expansion with viable tumor cells and interleukin-2 in the generation of specific therapeutic effector cells. J Immunol 136:3891–3898, 1986

428. Shu S, Chou T, Rosenberg SA: Generation from tumor-bearing mice of lymphocytes with *in vivo* therapeutic efficacy. J Immunol 139:295–304, 1987

429. Rosenberg SA, Spiess P, Lafreniere R: A new approach to the adoptive immunotherapy of cancer with tumor-infiltrating lymphocytes. Science 223:1318–1321, 1986

430. Spiess PJ, Yang JC, Rosenberg SA: The in vivo anti-tumor activity of tumor infiltrating lymphocytes expanded in recombinant interleukin-2. J Natl Cancer Inst 79:1067–1075, 1987

431. Lotze MT, Custer MC, Rosenberg SA: Interleukin 2 (IL-2) administration to humans results in the rapid emigration of a specific lymphokine subset (CD2$^+$, 3$^-$, 11$^+$, 16$^+$) from the peripheral blood (submitted)

432. Lotze MT, Matory YL, Ettinghausen SE et al: *In vivo* administration of purified human interleukin-2 II: Half life, immunologic effects and expansion of peripheral lymphoid cells in vivo with recombinant IL-2. J Immunol 135:2865–2875, 1985

433. Lotze MT, Chang AE, Seipp CA et al: High-dose recombinant interleukin-2 in the treatment of patients with disseminated cancer: Responses, treatment-related morbidity and histologic findings. JAMA 256:3117–3124, 1986

434. Lotze MT, Custer MC, Rosenberg SA: Intraperitoneal administration of interleukin-2 in patients with cancer. Arch Surg 121:1373–1379, 1986

435. West WH, Tauer KW, Yannelli JR et al: Constant-infusion recombinant interleukin-2 in adoptive immunotherapy of advanced cancer. N Engl J Med 316:898–905, 1987

436. Hank JA, Kohler PC, Weil–Hillman G et al: *In vivo* induction of the lymphokine-activated killer phenomenon: Interleukin-2 dependent human non-major histocompatibility complex-restricted cytotoxicity generated *in vivo* during administration of human recombinant interleukin-2[1]. Cancer Res 48:1965–1971, 1988

437. Thompson JA, Lee DJ, Lindgren CG et al: Influence of dose and duration of infusion of interleukin-2 on toxicity and immunomodulation. J Clin Oncol 6:669–678, 1988

438. Rosenberg SA, Terry W: Passive immunotherapy of cancer in animals and man. Adv Cancer Res 25:323–388, 1977

439. Rosenberg SA: The adoptive immunotherapy of cancer: Accomplishments and prospects. Cancer Treat Rep 68:233–255, 1984

440. Roberts K, Lotze MT, Rosenberg SA: Separation and functional studies of the human lymphokine-activated killer cell. Cancer Res 47:4366–4371, 1987

441. Phillips LL: Dissection of the LAK phenomenon. J Exp Med 164:814–825, 1986

442. Lafreniere R, Rosenberg SA: Adoptive immunotherapy of murine hepatic metastases with lymphokine activated killer (LAK) cells and recombinant interleukin-2 (RIL-2) can mediate the regression of both immunogenic and non-immunogenic sarcomas and an adenocarcinoma. J Immunol 135:4273–4280, 1985

443. Mule JJ, Ettinghausen SE, Spiess PJ et al: The anti-tumor efficacy of lymphokine-activated killer cells and recombinant interleukin-2 in vivo: An analysis of survival benefit and mechanisms of tumor escape in mice undergoing immunotherapy. Cancer Res 46:676–683, 1986

444. Mule JJ, Yang J, Shu S et al: The anti-tumor efficacy of lymphokine-activated killer cells and recombinant interleukin-2 *in vivo*: Direct correlation between reduction of established metastases and cytolytic activity of lymphokine-activated killer cells. J Immunol 136:3899–3909, 1986

445. Shiloni E, Lafreniere R, Mule JJ et al: Effect of immunotherapy with allogeneic lymphokine-activated killer cells and recombinant interleukin-2 on established pulmonary and hepatic metastases in mice. Cancer Res 46:5633–5640, 1986

446. Mazumder A, Eberlein TJ, Grimm EA: Phase I study of the adoptive immunotherapy of human cancer with lectin-activated autologous mononuclear cells, Cancer 53:896–905, 1984

447. Rosenberg SA: Immunotherapy of cancer by the systemic administration of lymphoid cells plus interleukin-2. J Biol Response Mod 3:501–511, 1984

448. Lotze MT, Frana LW, Sharrow SO et al: *In vivo* administration of purified human interleukin-2 I: Half life and immunologic effects of the Jurkat cell line-derived IL-2. J Immunol 134:157–166, 1985

449. Dutcher JP, Creekmore S, Weiss GR et al: Phase II study of high dose interleukin-2 (JIL-2) and lymphokine activated killer (LAK) cells in patients (PTS) with melanoma (abstr). Proc Am Soc Clin Oncol 6:246, 1987

450. Fisher, RI, Coltman CA, Doroshow JH et al: Phase II clinical trial of interleukin II plus lymphokine activated killer cells (IL-2/LAK) in metastatic renal cancer (abstr). Proc Am Soc Clin Oncol 6:244, 1987

451. Steis R, Bookman M, Clark J et al: Intraperitoneal lymphokine activated killer (LAK) cell and interleukin-2 (IL-2) therapy for peritoneal carcinomatosis: Toxicity, efficacy, and laboratory results (abstr). Proc Am Soc Clin Oncol 6:250, 1987

452. Paciucci PA, Konefal R, Ryder J et al: Phase I–II study of adoptive immunotherapy with rIL-2 activated cells and escalating continuous infusion rIL-2 in patients with disseminated cancer (abstr). Proc Am Soc Clin Oncol 6:248, 1987

453. Rosenstein M, Ettinghausen SE, Rosenberg SA: Extravasation of intravascular fluid mediated by the systemic administration of recombinant interleukin-2. J Immunol 137:1735–1742, 1986

454. Lee RE, Lotze MT, Skibber JM et al: Cardiorespiratory effects of immunotherapy with interleukin-2. J Clin Oncol (in press)

455. Belldegrun A, Webb DE, Austin HA et al: Effects of interleukin-2 on renal function in patients receiving immunotherapy for advanced cancer. Ann Intern Med 106:817–822, 1987

456. Webb DE, Austin HA, Belldegrun A, Vaughan E, Linehan WM, Rosenberg SA: Metabolic and renal effects of interleukin-2 immunotherapy for metastatic cancer. Clin Nephrology 30:141–145, 1988

457. Ettinghausen SE, Moore JG, White DE et al: Hematologic effects of immunotherapy with lymphokine-activated killer cells and recombinant interleukin-2 in cancer patients. Blood 69:1654–1660, 1987

458. Denicoff KD, Rubinow DR, Papa MZ et al: The neuropsychiatric effects of interleukin-2/lymphokine activated killer cell treatment. Ann Intern Med 107:293–300, 1987

459. Muul LM, Spiess PJ, Director EP et al: Identification of specific cytolytic immune responses against autologous tumor in humans bearing malignant melanoma. J Immunol 138:989–995, 1987

460. Itoh K, Tilden AB, Balch CM: Interleukin-2 activation of cytotoxic T-lymphocytes infiltrating into human metastatic melanomas. Cancer Res 46:3011–3017, 1986

461. Topalian SL, Muul LM, Rosenberg SA: Growth and immunologic characteristics of lymphocytes infiltrating human tumor. Surg Forum 37:390–391, 1987

462. Kurnick JT, Kradin RL, Blumberg R et al: Functional characterization of T lymphocytes propagated from human lung carcinomas. Clin Immunol Immunopathol 38:367–380, 1986

463. Anderson TM, Ibayashi Y, Holmes EC et al: Enhancement of natural interleukin-2. Surg Forum 37:392–393, 1986

464. Belldegrun A, Muul LM, Rosenberg SA: Interleukin-2 expanded tumor-infiltrating lymphocytes in human renal cell cancer: Isolation, characterization and antitumor activity. Cancer Res 48:206–214, 1988

465. Rosenberg SA, Packard BS, Aebersold PM et al: Immunotherapy of patients with metastatic melanoma using tumor infiltrating lymphocytes and interleukin-2. Preliminary report. N Engl J Med 319:1676–1680, 1988

BRUCE A. CHABNER

CHARLES E. MYERS

CHAPTER 18   *Clinical Pharmacology of Cancer Chemotherapy*

The primary goal of clinical pharmacology is to develop a rational basis for the treatment of disease. Unfortunately, the required information often comes many years after the empirical discovery of active pharmacologic agents, and only then are important drug actions and interactions understood. In dealing with highly toxic agents that possess a narrow therapeutic index, such information is all the more important. The effective use of chemotherapeutic agents in oncology requires a higher level of pharmacologic understanding than in any other subspecialty of internal medicine.

The objective of this chapter is to provide the fundamental information on drug action, metabolism, disposition, and toxicity in humans that will allow optimal clinical use of anticancer drugs. This discussion assumes that the reader has a basic understanding of cell constituents, the general scheme of synthesis of DNA, RNA, and protein, and the fundamental principles of drug transport, metabolism, and excretion. The synthesis of DNA and its precursors is summarized in Figure 18-1. For a review of these latter topics, refer to primary texts in biochemistry and pharmacology.[1,2]

Safe drug use requires a few initial steps: (1) determination of safe dosage range; (2) choice of an appropriate route of administration; (3) awareness of the incidence and course of potentially life-threatening toxicity; (4) awareness of routes of drug elimination and adjustment of dose to accommodate organ dysfunction; and (5) knowledge of drug interactions as influenced by dose and schedule to maximize favorable interactions and minimize toxicity. Each of these points should be considered in developing a new protocol or

in using an unfamiliar protocol for the first time. In addition, each new patient brings unique disease-related or preexisting problems to the therapeutic trial, requiring careful consideration of the choice of drugs and dosage. Every effort should be made to employ the best protocol in full doses, but the oncologist must always be aware of the unique challenges presented by each patient.

A few tables are provided to allow a rapid confirmation of the essential drug characteristics. Dose, toxicity, and pharmacokinetics of the most important agents are summarized in Table 18-1. Table 18-2 provides dose adjustment guidelines for agents affected by organ dysfunction. The indicated dose adjustments, particularly those for hepatic dysfunction, are only approximations, and doses should be calibrated against dose-limiting toxicity, such as myelosuppression. In Table 18-3, a summary of indications for drug-level monitoring of anticancer agents is given. The only routine indication for drug-level monitoring in clinical chemotherapy is for high-dose methotrexate regimens. The other uses indicated are associated with experimental protocols. Table 18-4 contains information on the new drugs that entered clinical trials from 1984 to 1987, under sponsorship of the National Cancer Institute. The reader is referred to Chapter 64 for a practical guide to the administration of chemotherapy and its complications.

Not all agents listed or discussed in this chapter are available commercially. However, a number of "group C" agents are available for specific diseases under protocols of the National Cancer Institute, and upon request for specific pa-

349

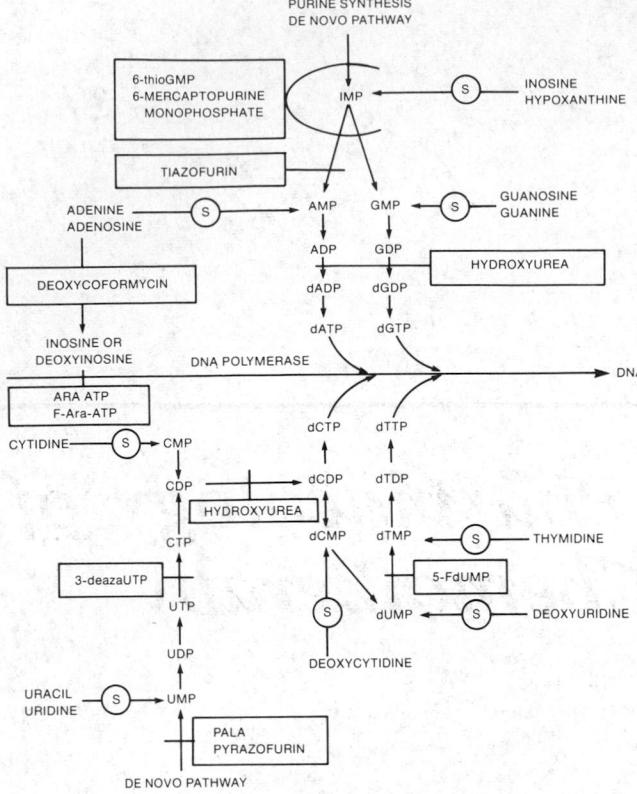

FIG. 18-1. Pathways for synthesis of triphosphate precursors of DNA and site of action of antimetabolites. Salvage pathways of nucleotide biosynthesis are indicated by —(S)→. Agents, or their metabolites, that inhibit specific synthetic reactions are enclosed in box: □. The inhibited pathway is indicated by ┼. d = deoxyribose; MP = monophosphate; DP = diphosphate; TP = triphosphate.

tients, they will be distributed to private physicians in the United States. Limited reporting of side-effects is required in conjunction with group C drug use (Table 18-5).

ANTIMETABOLITES

ANTIFOLATES

Antimetabolites are fraudulent agents that, by virtue of structural similarity with physiologic intermediates, are accepted as substrates for vital biochemical reactions and thus interfere with a required cell process. The first agent in the antifolate class of antimetabolites to find clinical application was aminopterin, a 4-NH_2 analogue of folic acid. Aminopterin has since been replaced in common use by the 4-NH_2,N^{10}-methyl analogue, amethopterin or methotrexate (Fig. 18-2). The latter, although a less-potent antifolate, has more predictable clinical toxicity and at least equal clinical activity.

In the past 20 years, new antifolate compounds such as the diaminopyrimidines and quinazolines have entered clinical trials. The most recent of these is trimetrexate, a more lipid-soluble quinazoline antifolate, which circumvents the requirement of folates and methotrexate for active transport into cells. Trimetrexate has potent antiparasitic activity and antineoplastic effects and is undergoing advanced trials in both clinical subspecialty areas.[3] Another folate of growing interest is 10-EDAM (10-ethyl-5-deaza-aminopterin), a potent inhibitor of dihydrofolate reductase, but with improved transport and polyglutamylation compared with methotrexate.[4] Trimetrexate and 10-EDAM have shown evidence of antitumor activity against carcinomas of the bowel and lung, respectively, in preliminary clinical trials.

Mechanism of Action

Methotrexate exerts its cytotoxic effects through inhibition of the enzyme dihydrofolate reductase (Fig. 18-3). This enzyme is responsible for maintaining the intracellular pool of folates in a reduced state as tetrahydrofolates, which function as carriers of one-carbon groups that are required for synthesis of the purine nucleotides and of thymidylate. In the thymidylate synthesis reaction (catalyzed by thymidylate synthase), N^{5-10} methylene tetrahydrofolate is relieved of its one-carbon methylene group and at the same time is oxidized to dihydrofolate, an inactive form of folic acid. Thus, in the presence of ongoing thymidylate synthesis, an intact dihydrofolate reductase pathway is needed to recycle oxidized folates to their active tetrahydrofolate form.

As a result of inhibition of reductase, methotrexate causes an accumulation of cellular folates in the inactive oxidized form, and a cessation first of thymidylate and then of purine nucleotide synthesis. Thymidylate synthesis inhibition appears to be more sensitive to methotrexate and occurs at free extracellular methotrexate concentrations of 1×10^{-8} M, whereas inhibition of purine synthesis takes place at somewhat higher free drug concentrations (above 1×10^{-7} M).

Cell killing proceeds somewhat more efficiently at higher drug levels, presumably because of the greater lethality of the antipurine effects.[5]

The precise mechanism by which methotrexate produces its toxicity is uncertain. Although inhibition of dihydrofolate reductase would be expected to lead to depletion of intracellular reduced folates, the depletion is only partial. For example, the key folate cofactor for purine biosynthesis, 10-formyl tetrahydrofolate, is present at 60% or more of its baseline concentration at a time when purine biosynthesis is totally inhibited.[6]

Exposure of cells to methotrexate generates a number of toxic metabolites (polyglutamate derivatives) of the parent compound. These compounds have an extended intracellular half-life and have potent, direct inhibitory effects on thymidylate synthase, as well as on the enzymes of de novo purine biosynthesis. In addition, dihydrofolate, which accumulates behind the blocked dihydrofolate reductase, directly inhibits the same distal metabolic sites.[7] Thus, the toxic effects of methotrexate are probably the result of both depletion of reduced folates and direct inhibition of other folate-dependent enzymes (Fig. 18-3).

The requirement for an excess of free (unbound) drug to produce inhibition of nucleotide biosynthesis is thought to result from the reversible nature of methotrexate binding to dihydrofolate reductase. Although methotrexate is bound very tightly in its complex with reductase, a measurable off-rate of inhibitor from enzyme is found in living cells. When there is an excess of dihydrofolate (FH_2), which builds up "behind" the inhibited reaction, an excess of free drug is required to compete for unoccupied binding sites. In addition, the inhibition of thymidylate synthase and inhibition of de novo purine biosynthesis require methotrexate polyglutamates in concentrations ($>10^{-8}$ M) sufficient to compete with intracellular folates.

The biochemical effects of methotrexate can be reversed by administering a reduced folate. The most commonly used rescue agent, leucovorin or DL-N[5]-formyl-tetrahydrofolic acid, effectively prevents methotrexate toxicity to bone marrow and gastrointestinal epithelium if it is administered in sufficient doses following 6-hour to 36-hour infusions of high doses of methotrexate. Longer exposures to methotrexate lead to clinically significant toxicity.

The dose of leucovorin required to reverse methotrexate toxicity depends on the antifolate concentration at the time of antidote administration. The reason for this competitive relationship is unclear, but it may relate to competition between reduced folates and FH_2 or methotrexate polyglutamates at thymidylate synthase, or to competition between FH_2 and methotrexate at dihydrofolate reductase.

Other rescue measures used clinically include administration of thymidine, which restores intracellular pools of thymidine triphosphate (TTP), and administration of carboxypeptidase G_1, an enzyme that hydrolyzes and inactivates methotrexate. These measures are not available for general use.

Methotrexate enters cells by a carrier-mediated, active transport mechanism shared by the physiologic, reduced folates, and it reaches equilibrium concentrations in most cells in less than 30 minutes.[8] The affinity constant of the transport system lies in the range of 1 to 10 μM for most mammalian cells. At higher drug concentrations, methotrexate enters cells by passive diffusion, an inefficient process compared with active transport. Methotrexate efflux is blocked by vincristine in concentrations above those found in clinical use.

Methotrexate undergoes transformation to polyglutamate forms by a process analogous to the polyglutamation of physiologic folates.[9] The methotrexate polyglutamates, consisting of the parent molecule plus one to four additional glutamates in γ-peptide linkage, are formed in tumor cells, bone marrow, and other normal tissues and, in a matter of hours, become the predominant form of drug found intracellularly. The polyglutamates bind to dihydrofolate reductase with the same affinity as the parent drug and inhibit enzymes (thymidylate synthase, GAR, and AICAR transformylase) not affected by the parent compound. After removal of free drug, the polyglutamates of 3 to 5 glutamyl chain length persist intracellularly for a longer period than does the parent compound. Thus, polyglutamate formation may be an important determinant of the duration and site of drug action in both normal and malignant cells.

The kinetic aspects of methotrexate cytotoxicity are important in clinical chemotherapy. For bone marrow granulocyte precursors and for experimental tumors, cell kill is proportional to the duration of exposure to methotrexate. Greater cell kill also is seen with increases in drug concentration above the threshold required for inhibition of DNA synthesis, but in this relationship cell kill is approximately correlated with the log of drug concentration. The dependence on duration of exposure can be explained best by the S-phase specificity of cell kill by antifolates; nonproliferating cells are extremely resistant to this class of compounds. In addition, polyglutamate formation is enhanced by long periods of incubation and may increase toxicity.

In experimental systems, resistance of tumor cells to antifolates results from several different biochemical mechanisms, including deletion of the reduced folate transport system, an increased concentration of dihydrofolate reductase, an altered reductase with decreased affinity for methotrexate, and decreased formation of polyglutamates.[10,11] The increase in enzyme concentration results from amplification of the gene coding for this enzyme. Resistant mutants can be selected by exposing cells to stepwise increases in drug concentrations in cell culture systems. The amplified genes may be present on bits of extrachromosomal material called double minutes or may exist within the chromosome as broad new bands of homogeneously staining genetic material on the long arm of chromosome 10.[12] Gene amplification associated with double-minute chromosomes is unstable and is lost gradually without the selective pressure of methotrexate, but integrated genetic material is heritable and becomes a stable characteristic of the resistant cell lines. Gene amplification has been identified as the cause of increased enzyme levels in resistant human tumor cells from patients treated with methotrexate.[13]

Other clinical studies have yielded examples of resistance
(*Text continues on page 354.*)

TABLE 18-1. Dose, Toxicity, and Pharmacokinetics of Major Antineoplastic Agents

		Acute Toxicity			
Class	Route*	Dose (mg/m^2)	Injection Vehicle	Infusion Duration	Dose Frequency
Plant Alkaloids					
Vincristine	IV	1.0	10 ml NS	1–5 min	qwk
Vinblastine	IV	6.0	10 ml NS	1–5 min	qwk
	IV	2.0	NS	24 h × 5 d	q3wk
Vindesine	IV	2.0	10 ml NS	1–5 min	qwk
VP-16	IV	86	20 ml NS/ml reconstituted drug	1–5 min	2 d qwk
	PO	200			2 d qwk
VM-26	IV	67	20 ml NS/ml reconstituted drug	1–5 min	qwk
Antibiotics					
Actinomycin D	IV	0.6	500 µg/ml SW	1–5 min	qd × 5
Doxorubicin	IV	75	5 mg/ml SW	1–5 min	q3wk
	IV	20	5 µg/ml SW	1–5 min	qwk
Daunorubicin	IV	30	1 mg/ml SW	1–5 min	3d, q3wk
Mithramycin	IV	1.75	500 µg/ml SW, then add to 100 ml D_5W	15–30 min	qod to toxicity
for high Ca++	IV	0.75	500 µg/ml SW	1–5 min bolus	qd × 3–4 d
Mitomycin C	IV	2.0	500 µg/ml SW	1–5 min bolus	qd × 3, q3wk
Bleomycin	IV	10	5 U/ml NS	1-min test dose then IV bolus	qwk
	IM	10	15 U/ml NS		qwk
	SC	10	15 U/ml NS		qwk
Antimetabolites					
Methotrexate (high-dose)	IV	>500	100 ml D_5W or NS	10 min–1 h	q3wk
w/leucovorin	IV	15	In vehicle	Bolus	q6 h × 7 doses
Methotrexate	IV	25	10–25 ml D_5W or NS	Bolus	Twice weekly
	IM	25	2 ml NS		Twice weekly
	IT	12 (total dose)	10 ml Elliott's B	1–5 min	q4 d
5-Fluorouracil	IV	500	Any convenient volume NS	Bolus	qwk or qd × 5
	IV	800–1200	Any convenient volume NS	24 h × 5 d	q 3–4 wk
	IA	800–1200	Any convenient volume NS	24 h	qd × 14–21 d
5-Fluorouracil	IV	375	Any convenient volume NS	Bolus	qwk × 6
w/leucovorin	IV	500	200 ml D_5W	2–h infusion begin 1 h before 5-FU	qwk × 6
5-Fluorodeoxyuridine	IA	5–20	Any convenient volume NS	24 h	qd × 14–21 d
6-Mercaptopurine	PO	100			qd × 5
6-Thioguanine	IV	100	15 mg/ml NS	Bolus	qd × 5
Cytarabine (cytosine arabinoside)	IV	100	20 mg/ml NS	Bolus	q12 h × 5–10 d
	IV	2000–3000	50 mg/ml SW then dilute in 150 ml D_5W	1 h	q12 h × 6 d
5-Azacytidine	IV	200	Reconstitute vial in 20 ml SW, dilute in 150 ml D_5W	15–30 min	qd × 5
Hydroxyurea	IV	1000–1500	100 mg/ml SW	1–5 min	qd × 5
	PO	1000			qd
Deoxycoformycin	IV	4	Any volume NS	Bolus	qowk
Alkylating Agents					
Cyclophosphamide	IV	400	20 mg/ml SW	Bolus	qd × 5
	PO	100			qd × 14
Ifosfamide and	IV	1800–2400	Any volume D_5W or NS	24 h	qd × 5
Mesna	IV	1800–2400	With ifosfamide	24 h	qd × 5.5
Melphalan	PO	4			qd
	IV	8	Reconstituted vial dilute in 100–200 ml D_5W	30–45 min	qd × 5

Plasma WBC	Platelet	Nausea/ Vomiting	Other Toxicity	Elimination†	Plasma Half-Life (h)*
		Acute Toxicity			
Mild	Mild	Mild	Distal neuropathy, inappropriate ADH	M	2.6
Marked	Marked	Mild	Mucositis	M	3.1
Marked	Marked	Mild	Mucositis	M	3.1
Moderate	Mild	Mild	Neurotoxicity	M	1.6
Moderate	Mild	Mild	Distal neuropathy	M, R	6
Moderate	Mild	Moderate			
Moderate	Mild	Mild	Distal neuropathy	M, R	3
Marked	Marked	Moderate	Alopecia, Mucositis	M, R	?
Marked	Marked	Moderate	Alopecia, Cardiomyopathy	M	3/25
Moderate	Moderate	Moderate	Alopecia, less cardiomyopathy	M	3/25
Marked	Marked	Moderate	Alopecia, cardiomyopathy	M	3/?
Mild	Marked	Severe	Renal, hepatic, neurologic, fever, rash	M	?
Mild	Mild	Mild			
Marked	Marked	Moderate	Renal, pulmonary	M	?
Rare	Rare	Mild	Skin, pulmonary fibrosis, fever, allergic reactions	R	0.4/2
Mild	Mild	Moderate	Hepatic dysfunction, renal failure	R M	2/8
Moderate-marked	Moderate-marked	Mild	Stomatitis	R	2/8
Moderate-marked	Moderate-marked	Mild	Stomatitis	R	2/8
Mild	Mild	None	Fever, motor dysfunction	R	12 (CSF)
Moderate-marked	Moderate-marked	Mild	Cerebellar, conjunctivitis	M	0.3
Mild	Mild	Moderate	Mucositis, diarrhea	M	0.3
Mild	Mild	Moderate	Catheter-related	M	0.3
Marked	Marked	Mild	Diarrhea	M	0.3
Mild	Mild	Moderate	Catheter-related	M	0.3
Moderate-marked	Moderate-marked	Mild	Cholestasis	M	0.3–0.6
Moderate-marked	Moderate-marked	Mild	Cholestasis	M	1.5
Marked	Marked	Moderate	Cholestasis, mucositis	M	0.15
Marked	Marked	Marked	Cholestasis, mucositis, sedation, cerebellar, conjunctivitis	M, R	
Marked	Marked	Severe	Neurotoxicity, mucositis	M	Rapid
Marked	Moderate	Moderate	None	R, M	1.7
Marked	Marked	Mild	None	R, M	1.7
Mild	Mild	Mild	None	R	1/10
Marked	Mild	Moderate			
Moderate	Mild	Mild	Cystitis, water retention, alopecia	M	1–4
Moderate	Moderate	Mild	Neurotoxicity, urothelial toxicity	M	5–6
None	None	None	None	M	?
Moderate	Moderate	Mild	Leukemia	M	2
Marked	Marked	Moderate			

*Slash indicates multiple half-lives.

(continued)

TABLE 18-1.   Dose, Toxicity, and Pharmacokinetics of Major Antineoplastic Agents (continued)

Class	Route*	Acute Toxicity Dose (mg/m^2)	Injection Vehicle	Infusion Duration	Dose Frequency
Busulfan	PO	2–6			qd
CCNU	PO	100–150			q6 wk
MeCCNU	PO	150–200			q6 wk
BCNU	IV	200–225	Reconstituted vial diluted to 100 mg/ml D_5W	30–45 min	q6 wk
Streptozotocin	IV	500	Reconstituted vial diluted to 100 mg/ml D_5W	10–15 min	qd × 5 q 3–4 wk
Chlorambucil	PO	1–3			qd
cis-diamminedi-chloroplatinum	IV	50–100	1000 ml/m^2NS‡	6 h	q 3–4 2 wk
		20	150 ml NS	1 h	qd × 5
	IV	40	250 ml 3% saline	1 h	qd × 5
CBDCA (carboplatin)	IV	300	Any volume D_5W	Bolus	qd × 5
Aziridinylbenzoquinone (AZQ)	IV	18–20	150 ml NS	10–15 min	Days 1 and 8 of 28-d cycle
	IV	8	150 ml NS	10–15 min	qd × 5
Miscellaneous					
DTIC (Dacarbazine)	IV	200	10 mg/ml D_5W	10–15 min	qd × 5
mAMSA	IV	120	250 ml D_5W	2 h	qd × 5
Procarbazine	PO	100			qd × 10–14 d
Hexamethylmelamine	PO	150			qd × 14 d
Mitoxantrone	IV	14	10 ml NS	30 min	q3 wk

*IV = intravenous; PO = per os; SC = subcutaneous; IM = intramuscular; IT = intrathecal; IA = intra-arterial; NS = normal saline; D_5W = dextrose (5 g/dl) in water; and SW = sterile water.
†R = renal; M = metabolic; F = fecal.
‡See chapter for details.

related to decreased polyglutamate formation and decreased thymidylate synthase activity (with decreased need for recycling oxidized folates). Two clinical examples of transport deficiency have been reported.[14]

Clinical Pharmacology and Pharmacokinetics

Because of the common use of methotrexate in high-dose regimens and the well-understood relationship between extracellular drug concentration and inhibition of DNA synthesis, monitoring of methotrexate concentrations in plasma has become important for guiding drug dosage, detecting patients at high risk of toxicity, and allowing institution of rescue measures in high-risk situations. At least four methods are available for methotrexate assay, and all provide rapid and sensitive analysis.[15] These include an enzyme inhibition assay using dihydrofolate reductase (most cumbersome assay); a competitive protein-binding assay that uses reductase as the binding protein; a commercial radioimmunoassay that uses an antibody to the methotrexate-albumin conjugate; and an enzyme-linked immunoassay.[16] The competitive protein-binding assay is specific for ligands that bind tightly to the enzyme active site, whereas the immunoassays show degrees of cross-reactivity with a methotrexate metabolite, 2,4-diamino-N^{10} methylpteroic acid (DAMPA).

This metabolite may produce spuriously high assay results. High-pressure liquid chromatographic (HPLC) assay systems can be used to produce clean separation of methotrexate from contaminants and metabolites, with quantitation of the various peaks by spectral or other assay methods, but HPLC is not practical for routine clinical monitoring. Methotrexate undergoes metabolic conversion to 7-OH methotrexate through the action of aldehyde oxidase. The product becomes the predominant compound in plasma within 6 hours, and 7-OH levels exceed the parent compound by tenfold or more at 12 hours.[17] The metabolite weakly inhibits dihydrofolate reductase, but its polyglutamates do inhibit thymidylate synthase and AICAR transformylase and compete for the folate transport mechanism.

Oral methotrexate is well absorbed in doses less than 25 mg/m^2, but bioavailability becomes erratic for larger doses. Except in maintenance regimens, the drug usually is administered intravenously. The plasma pharmacokinetics after intravenous administration vary from patient to patient, but over the clinical dose range of 25 to 1500 mg/m^2, the drug generally follows a three-phase disappearance pattern. A brief distributional phase is followed by a primary elimination half-life of 2 to 3 hours and a final phase of elimination with a half-life of 8 to 10 hours.

Drug excretion occurs primarily through renal elimination. Rapid rates of drug clearance have been correlated with

Plasma WBC	Acute Toxicity		Other Toxicity	Elimination†	Plasma Half-Life (h)*
	Platelet	Nausea/ Vomiting			
Marked	Marked	Mild	Pulmonary fibrosis	M	?
Marked	Marked	Moderate	Leukemia, pulmonary fibrosis, renal failure	M	?
Marked	Marked	Moderate	Leukemia, pulmonary fibrosis, renal failure	M	?
Marked	Marked	Marked	Leukemia, pulmonary fibrosis, renal failure	M	1.0
Mild	Mild	Moderate-marked	Renal failure, hyperglycemia, hepatic enzyme elevation	R	0.25
Moderate	Moderate	Mild	Leukemia	M	1.5
Moderate	Moderate	Severe	Renal failure, Mg** wasting, peripheral neuropathy	R, M	0.3
Mild	Mild	Moderate			
Moderate	Moderate	Marked	Neurotoxicity, ototoxicity	M	0.3
Marked	Marked	Mild		R	
Moderate	Moderate	Moderate	Cumulative myelosuppression	M	0.5
Moderate	Moderate	Moderate	Cumulative myelosuppression	M	0.5
Mild	Mild	Marked	Flulike syndrome	M	0.65
Moderate	Moderate	Mild	Cardiac arrhythmias	M	7
Moderate	Moderate	Mild	Sensitivity to amines	M	?
Mild	Mild	Moderate	Neurotoxicity	M	5
Moderate	Moderate	Mild	Cholestasis	M	0.25/37

*Slash indicates multiple half-lines.

a high risk of relapse in childhood acute lymphocytic leukemia. Methotrexate is filtered by the glomerulus, reabsorbed in the proximal tubule (a process blocked by probenecid), and secreted by the distal tubule. Its clearance equals or exceeds creatinine clearance but is not entirely predictable on the basis of clinical measures of renal function. In patients with compromised renal function or in those receiving potentially lethal doses (above 1000 mg/m²), plasma concentration should be monitored to avoid serious toxicity. In high-dose therapy, small test doses may be used to establish pharmacokinetic characteristics in an individual patient, allowing calculation of a safe dose.[19]

Methotrexate distributes slowly into third-space accumulations of fluid, such as ascites or pleural effusions, but also exists slowly from these spaces. The reentry of the drug into the systemic circulation from these spaces prolongs the terminal phase of plasma drug disappearance and causes unexpected toxicity. It is advisable to evacuate effusions or to monitor drug levels in patients with ascites or massive pleural effusions.

Methotrexate also enters the cerebrospinal fluid (CSF) slowly and produces concentrations that are (during continuous intravenous infusion) approximately 1/30 the concentration found simultaneously in plasma. Cytotoxic drug concentrations can be achieved in the spinal fluid by giving a high dose of methotrexate; peak levels approach 1×10^{-5} M in regimens that use 500 to 1500 mg/m². However, doses of 20 to 30 g/m² are required to achieve the peak concentrations and the concentration × time product resulting from direct installation of small doses of methotrexate into the intrathecal space, and efficacy of systemic high-dose regimens in preventing or treating meningeal leukemia or carcinomatosis is not confirmed.

The pharmacokinetics of trimetrexate are quite different from those of methotrexate. The drug undergoes demethylation and glucuronidation of the O-methoxy groups, with elimination of the glucuronide metabolites in the urine. The primary half-life of the parent compound in plasma is 11 hours.[3] High doses of trimetrexate can be effectively "rescued" with leucovorin, but such regimens have been used only for antiparasitic therapy.[3]

Dose Adjustment

Special emphasis must be given to the rationale, methods, and results of monitoring drug levels during therapy with high doses of methotrexate. These are summarized in Table 18-3. Methotrexate infusions for 6 to 36 hours, in total dosages of 1000 mg/m² or greater, can be given without toxic consequences if preceded by intensive hydration and urinary

TABLE 18-2.   Drugs Requiring Dose Modification for Organ Dysfunction

Agent	Organ Dysfunction	Suggested Dose Modification
Methotrexate	Renal failure or ↓ creatinine clearance	In proportion to ↓ creatinine clearance (normal 60 ml/min/m²)
cis-Platinum (cisplatin)	Renal failure	In proportion to creatinine clearance
Cyclophosphamide	Renal failure (creatinine clearance below 25 ml/min)	50% decrease
Bleomycin	Renal failure (creatinine clearance below 25 ml/min)	50–75% decrease
Streptozotocin	Renal failure (creatinine clearance below 25 ml/min)	50–75% decrease
Carboplatin, Hydroxyurea, VP-16, Deoxycoformycin, mAMSA	Renal failure	In proportion to creatinine clearance
Vincristine, Vinblastine	Hepatic dysfunction	1. Only approximate guidelines can be offered and are probably inaccurate. See text. 2. For bilirubin of >1.5 mg/100 ml, reduce initial dose by 50%. 3. For bilirubin of >3.0 mg/100 ml, reduce initial dose by 75%.

alkalinization and if followed by a series of leucovorin doses. Because of the competitive relationship between leucovorin and methotrexate, the actual dose of leucovorin required to provide rescue depends on the plasma concentration of antifolate at the time of rescue. Doses of leucovorin in the range of 15 to 25 mg/m² usually provide plasma levels of 1×10^{-6} M and are adequate to prevent toxicity of similar concentrations of antifolate. However, in patients with altered renal function, either induced by methotrexate or antedating this treatment, methotrexate excretion is delayed, plasma con-

centrations are higher than anticipated, and conventional doses of leucovorin are inadequate for rescue. Nonsteroidal anti-inflammatory drugs also inhibit renal excretion and the plasma clearance of methotrexate, increasing the risk of inadequate rescue.[20]

Severe myelosuppression and mucositis in patients receiving high dosages of methotrexate have been correlated directly with delayed drug elimination and elevated drug levels in plasma.[21] This relationship has dictated critical guidelines for leucovorin administration based on drug-level monitoring

TABLE 18-3.   Drug Monitoring in Cancer Therapy

Agent	Assay*	Uses
Methotrexate	Competitive binding to enzyme or to antibody HPLC	1. Early detection of patients at high risk of toxicity in high-dose therapy. Drug level >5 × 10⁻⁷ M at 48 h alerts to need for increased and prolonged leucovorin. In toxic patients, tailor leucovorin dosage to plasma methotrexate level. 2. Aid in differential diagnosis of neurotoxicity. High drug level in cerebrospinal fluid favors drug reaction. 3. Predict drug clearance in patients with altered renal function. Allow choice of safe dose.
5-Fluorouracil	HPLC	Design intra-arterial and intraperitoneal chemotherapy regimens with acceptable systemic toxicity. Detect inappropriately elevated (>10⁻⁵ M) venous blood levels.
6-Mercaptopurine, Hexamethylmelamine, L-Phenylalanine mustard	HPLC, HPLC, HPLC	Determine plasma levels after oral therapy to assure adequate bioavailability (experimental).

*See text for references to specific drug assays.

TABLE 18-4.   Drugs in Phase I and II Trials, 1984–1987

Drug	Mechanism of Action	Maximum-Tolerated Dose (mg/m²)	Toxicities
Acodazole		1370, each 3 wk	Cardiac arrhythmias
Amonafide	DNA strand breaks	300, 5 d each 3 wk	Myelosuppression
Curacemide	DNA synthesis inhibition	650 CI, 5 d each 3 wk	Neurotoxicity
Didemnin B	DNA synthesis inhibition	3.5, weekly	Nausea, vomiting, hepatotoxicity
Echinomycin	DNA cross-linker	1.5, each 4 wk	Nausea, vomiting, myelosuppression
Flavone acetic acid	DNA binder	2,300 CI, 1 h weekly (×4)	
		10,000 CI, 3 h each 3 wk	Hypotension neurotoxicity
Menogaril	DNA binder, anthracycline	160, each 4 wk	Myelosuppression
Merbarone	DNA strand breaks	Uncertain	Uncertain
Taxol	Tubulin binder	250 CI, 24 h each 3 wk	Myelosuppression, anaphylaxis, peripheral neuropathy
Trimetrexate	Antifolate	8–12, 5 d each 3 wk	Myelosuppression
Hexamethylene bisacetamide	Differentiation	2400 CI, 5 d	Neurotoxicity
Pibenzimol	DNA binder	15 CI, 5 d each 3 wk	Hyperglycemia
Gallium nitrate	Not known	300, 7 d each 3 wk	
		300, 3 d each 2 wk	Renal, ototoxicity, anemia, neurotoxicity
Dihydro-5-azacytidine	Incorporated into RNA and DNA	2500, 5 d each 3 wk	Chest pain, nausea and vomiting

TABLE 18-5.   Restricted Drugs

Drugs	Indication
Group C Drugs*	
Azacytidine (5-aza)	Refractory acute leukemia single-agent treatment
Amsacrine (mAMSA)	Refractory acute leukemia single-agent treatment
Erwinia asparaginase	Patients allergic to *E. coli* asparaginase
Hexamethylmelamine	Refractory ovarian cancer single-agent treatment
Pentostatin (Deoxycoformycin)	Hairy cell leukemia
Modified Group C Drugs†	
Interleukin-2 (IL-2) with or without lymphokine-activated killer (LAK) cells	Metastatic or unresectable renal cell carcinoma
	Metastatic or unresectable melanoma

*Available as of 1988 to authorized physicians upon request to Investigational Drug Branch, Executive Plaza North, National Cancer Institute, Bethesda, Maryland 20892.
†Restricted for use in cancer centers.

at specific times following infusion and has allowed adjustment of leucovorin dosage to compensate for elevations of plasma methotrexate levels. For the commonly used Jaffe regimen (50–250 mg/kg methotrexate given over 6 hours, followed by eight doses of leucovorin, 15 mg/m² every 6 hours), a plasma methotrexate level above 9×10^{-7} M at 48 hours is associated with a high risk of severe myelosuppression (Table 18-6).[21] Increased leucovorin dosage (100 mg/m² for levels of 10^{-6} M, with proportional increases for higher antifolate concentrations) is effective in preventing myelosuppression.

Alternate high-dose regimens have been used. Infusions of equivalent doses of methotrexate (1.5–7.5 g/m²) over an infusion period of more than 6 hours produce lower plateau concentrations of drug in the range of 10 to 100 μM, but for longer periods. A typical 36-hour regimen used for preoperative chemotherapy of head and neck carcinoma is given in Table 18-6. In this regimen, extreme precautions were taken to assure the adequacy of hydration, urinary alkalinization, and leucovorin rescue in treating a high-risk patient population. A comparison of the pharmacokinetics of high-dose methotrexate given as a 6-hour infusion and 36-hour infusion is shown in Figure 18-4.

There are no known effective means for removing methotrexate from body fluids without normal renal function. Drug can be bound in the intestinal lumen by cholestyramine and removed from the enterohepatic circulation, but the efficacy of this method has not been established.[22] Hemodialysis produces clearance rates of only 35 to 40 ml/min. Circulating drug can be effectively hydrolyzed and inactivated by a bacterial enzyme, carboxypeptidase G_1, but this enzyme is not available for general clinical use.[23]

Only a small fraction of administered drug is metabolized to inactive products. However, two metabolites, DAMPA and 7-OH methotrexate, tend to accumulate in plasma at later

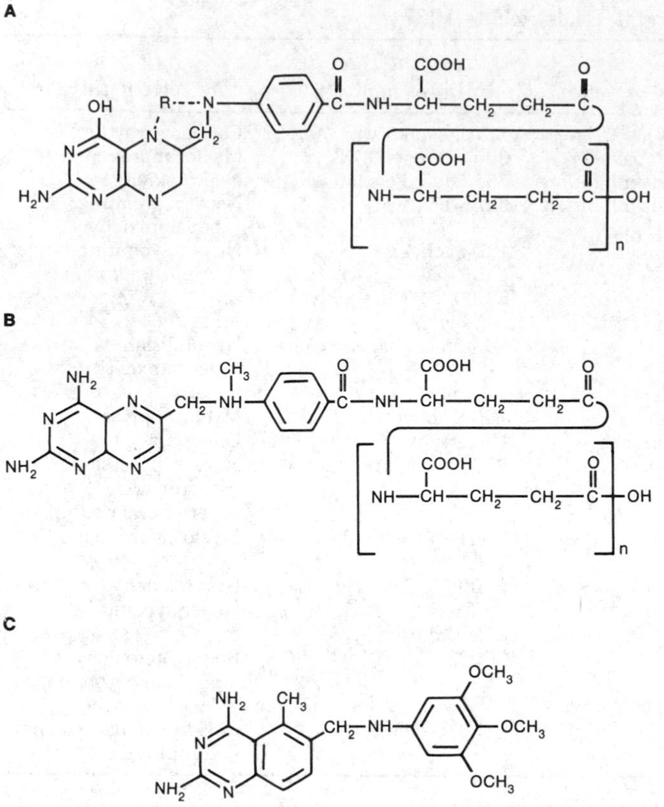

A

B

C

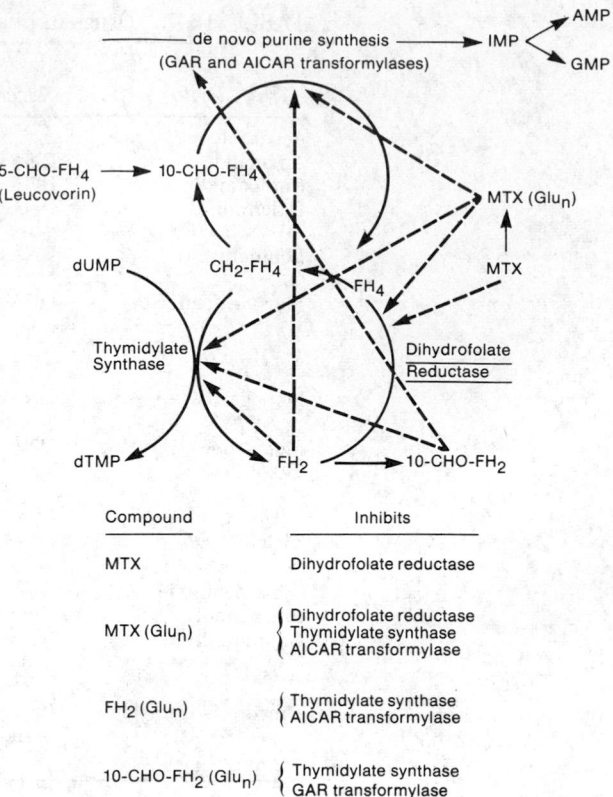

FIG. 18-2. Structure of folic acid (**A**), methotrexate (**B**), and trimetrexate (**C**). Note potential for addition of glutamyl groups to methotrexate and folic acid.

FIG. 18-3. Sites of action of methotrexate (MTX), its polyglutamated metabolites [MTX(Glu$_n$)], and folate byproducts of the inhibition of dihydrofolate reductase, including dihydrofolate (FH$_2$) and 10-formyl-dihydrofolate (10-CHO-FH$_2$). Also shown are 5-10-methylene tetrahydrofolic acid (CH$_2$-FH$_4$), the folate cofactor required for thymidylate synthesis, and 10-formyl-tetrahydrofolate (10-CHO-FH$_4$), the required intermediate in the synthesis of purine precursors. (Other abbreviations as in Figure 18-1.)

Compound	Inhibits
MTX	Dihydrofolate reductase
MTX (Glu$_n$)	Dihydrofolate reductase Thymidylate synthase AICAR transformylase
FH$_2$ (Glu$_n$)	Thymidylate synthase AICAR transformylase
10-CHO-FH$_2$ (Glu$_n$)	Thymidylate synthase GAR transformylase

times in patients receiving high doses of methotrexate. Neither has potent antifolate activity, but both are less soluble than is the parent compound and may contribute to the renal precipitation of methotrexate-derived material observed in high-dose therapy.

The pharmacokinetics of methotrexate in the CSF have an important bearing on both therapeutic and toxic effects. Drug injected in the lumbar intrathecal space is distributed poorly in the ventricular spinal fluid, a factor that may contribute to the high incidence of relapse of meningeal leukemia.[24] For patients with known meningeal leukemia, direct intraventricular injection through an indwelling reservoir is recommended. Peak drug concentrations of approximately 10^{-3} M are reached in the CSF by injection of 12-mg doses; the major half-life in patients without active meningeal disease is approximately 12 hours, but this may be prolonged considerably in patients without active leukemic meningitis. Delayed methotrexate elimination from the CSF is associated with methotrexate neurotoxicity.[25]

Toxicity

The toxicities observed in humans as a consequence of methotrexate therapy fall into two categories: those related to the action of the drug on rapidly proliferating tissues (bone marrow and intestinal and oral epithelium) and those manifested by nondividing tissues, which are less predictable in their incidence. Myelosuppression and mucositis reach

TABLE 18-6.   High-Dose Methotrexate Therapy

1. *Prehydration*
   In 12 h before treatment establish diuresis with 1.5 liters/m^2 D$_5$W with 100 mEq HCO$_3^-$ and 20 mEq KCl per liter. Test urine pH to assure neutrality (pH 7 or >) at time of drug infusion.
2. *Drug Infusion*
   a. Jaffe regimen: 50 to 250 mg/kg methotrexate (MTX) over 6-h infusion. Continue hydration (3 liters/m^2) for 24 h. Begin leucovorin 2 h after end of drug infusion, 15 mg/m^2 1 M q6h × 7 doses.
   b. Alternative: bolus administration of 50 mg/m^2 MTX intravenously followed by infusion of MTX over 36-h period at dose of 1.5 g/m^2. At 36 h, begin leucovorin infusion 200 mg/m^2 for 12 h. At 48 h, give leucovorin 25 mg/m^2 q6h × 6 doses 1 M.
3. *Monitor Points*
   For Jaffe regimen and for 36-h infusion, drug levels above $5 × 10^{-7}$ M at 48 h require additional leucovorin rescue.

Drug Level	Dose Leucovorin
$5 × 10^{-7}$ M	15 mg/m^2 q6h × 8 doses
$1 × 10^{-6}$ M	100 mg/m^2 q6h × 8 doses
$2 × 10^{-6}$ M	200 mg/m^2 q6h × 8 doses

Drug levels should be repeated every 48 h and leucovorin dose adjusted until drug concentration is less than $5 × 10^{-8}$ M.

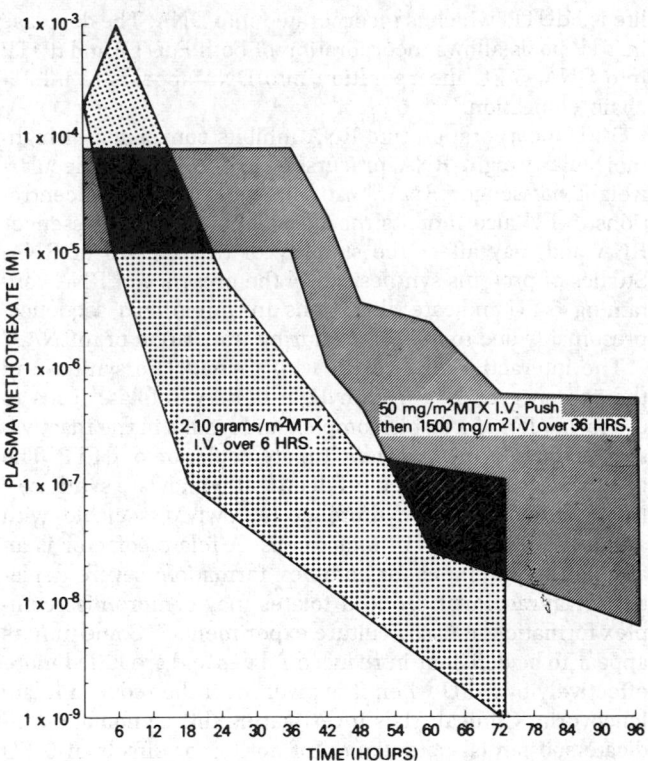

FIG. 18-4. Comparison of methotrexate pharmacokinetics in two high-dose regimens, the first a 6-hour infusion of 50 to 250 mg/kg, the second a bolus dose of 50 mg/m² followed by a 36-hour infusion of 1500 mg/m².

their maximum in 5 to 14 days after a bolus dose or short-term infusion, and recovery usually is rapid thereafter. More prolonged and severe toxicity has been observed in patients who receive high doses of methotrexate and seems to be related to the long exposure (>48 hours) of these sensitive tissues to the circulating drug. These toxicities can be prevented through administration of adequate doses of leucovorin or of thymidine, although the latter form of rescue is less reliable than is rescue with leucovorin.[26] It should be remembered that in patients with renal dysfunction, even small doses of methotrexate may cause serious or fatal myelosuppression.

Renal tubular injury is another serious toxic effect of methotrexate. Conventional doses of methotrexate rarely cause renal injury, but high-dose therapy without adequate hydration (3 liters/m² for 24 h) and urinary alkalinization (pH 7 or higher), is associated with at least a 10% incidence of acute renal injury, as indicated by a rise in BUN and serum creatinine and a decrease in urine volume. In most cases, renal toxicity is believed to be caused by renal precipitation of methotrexate or of methotrexate-derived material; however, other causes of renal damage are suggested by the finding that 30-fold lower doses of aminopterin, a more potent antifolate, cause similar deterioration in renal function.[27,28] These adverse renal effects can be prevented by vigorous pretreatment hydration, by urinary alkalinization, and by dose reduction in patients with underlying renal disease (see Tables 18-2 and 18-3).

Both acute and chronic hepatotoxicity are caused by methotrexate. Acute rises in hepatic enzyme levels often are observed during high-dose therapy, but the levels return to normal within 1 week. Hyperbilirubinemia is occasionally observed in high-dose treatment. Long-term administration of daily oral methotrexate, as used for treatment of psoriasis, is associated with hepatic fibrosis in up to 30% of these patients and with an infrequent occurrence of cirrhosis. The cause of hepatic lesions is unknown. A much lower rate of hepatic fibrosis is seen in patients with rheumatoid arthritis treated with methotrexate on weekly or intermittent schedules.[29] The results of animal experiments suggest impairment of choline synthesis and consequent inhibition of lipid mobilization, which is supported by the finding of fatty infiltration in biopsy material of patients who exhibit acute hepatotoxicity.[30]

Acute pneumonitis is observed occasionally in patients who receive methotrexate.[31] When biopsied, the lung often shows granuloma formation and eosinophilia, suggesting a hypersensitivity reaction. However, retreatment of such patients has not caused a recurrence of this syndrome.

Various manifestations of neurotoxicity are observed in almost 30% of patients receiving intrathecal methotrexate. Symptoms include motor dysfunction of the extremities, cranial nerve palsies, coma, or seizures. This syndrome is different from the acute arachnoiditis often seen during the 48 hours following drug injection. Neurotoxicity usually occurs after the third or fourth course of intrathecal therapy and is found most often in adult patients and in those who have active meningeal leukemia. Symptoms may be accompanied by an increase in spinal fluid pressure, an elevated protein concentration, and a reactive pleocytosis. When the syndrome is recognized, a change in therapy to cytarabine (cytosine arabinoside) or thiotepa is indicated. Continued treatment may be fatal. Chronic brain injury is believed to occur in the many children treated prophylactically with the standard combination of intrathecal methotrexate and cranial irradiation. In these children, computed tomography (CT) reveals intracerebral calcification, thinning of the cerebral cortex, and ventricular dilatation. High-dose systemic methotrexate appears to be an effective alternative to intrathecal methotrexate for prophylaxis of meningeal leukemia in average-risk patients.[32]

FLUOROPYRIMIDINES

Few of the active antitumor agents used clinically have resulted from rational design; rather, most are the product of serendipitous observations or screening. 5-Fluorouracil (5-FU), conceived and synthesized by Dr. Charles Heidelberger at the University of Wisconsin, represents a notable exception (Fig. 18-5).[33] Heidelberger observed that certain malignant cells used the base uracil more efficiently than did rat intestinal mucosa, and he designed a series of uracil analogues with fluorine substitutions at the 5 position. This substitution, after suitable intracellular transformation of the derivative, yields a nucleotide, 5-fluorodeoxyuridylate (5-FdUMP), which inhibits the thymidylate synthase reaction and DNA synthesis (Fig. 18-6).

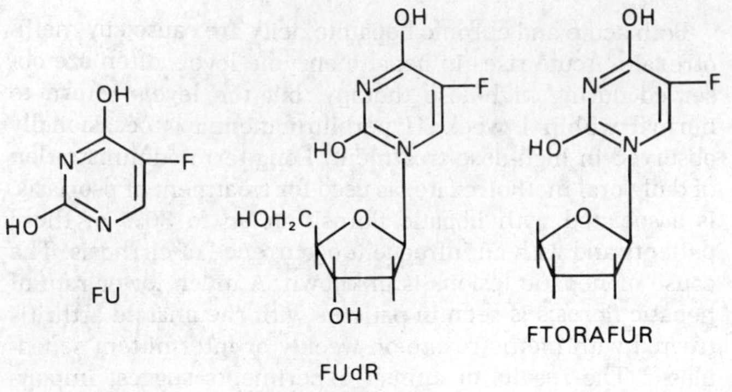

FIG. 18-5. Structures of clinically useful 5-fluoropyrimidines.

5-FU has antitumor activity against many types of solid tumors, including breast, colon, and ovarian carcinomas. In these tumors, the response rates vary from 10% to 40%, but complete remissions are unusual. The drug now is used frequently in combination therapy and has interesting biochemical interactions with methotrexate, physiologic nucleosides like thymidine, and leucovorin, all of which have become the subject of new clinical trials.

Mechanism of Action

5-FU has multiple biochemical actions that may be responsible for its cytotoxicity. It is converted by one of several possible pathways (Fig. 18-6) to the nucleotide fluorouridine monophosphate (FUMP); from this point, two "active" nucleotides may be formed: fluorouridine triphosphate (FUTP), which is incorporated into RNA and inhibits RNA processing and function, and 5-FdUMP, which binds tightly to thymidylate synthase and inhibits the eventual formation of deoxythymidine triphosphate (dTTP), one of the four necessary precursors of DNA. Although interest initially was focused on 5-FdUMP action, evidence from both in vitro and in vivo experiments suggests that the toxicity of 5-FU cannot be accounted for completely by thymidine, a direct precursor of dTMP. Also, manipulations that increase 5-FU incorporation into RNA increase cytotoxicity.[34] A third toxic metabolite is FdUTP, which is incorporated into DNA. The decrease in TTP pools allows incorporation of both FdUTP and dUTP into DNA. 5-FU incorporation into DNA appears to inhibit chain elongation.[35]

5-FU incorporation into RNA inhibits conversion of high-molecular-weight RNA precursors to the lower-molecular-weight messenger RNA.[36] At somewhat higher concentrations, 5-FU also inhibits the polyadenylation of messenger RNA and may affect the stability of this species of RNA. Studies of proteins synthesized in the presence of RNA containing 5-FU indicate alterations in amino acid sequence, presumably due to miscoding during translation of mRNA.[37]

The interaction of FdUMP with thymidylate synthase in the presence of N^{5-10} methylene tetrahydrofolate leads to the formation of a stable complex and results in the inactivation of the enzyme and the ultimate depletion of dTTP. The complex formed between 5-FdUMP–thymidylate synthase–N^{5-10} methylene tetrahydrofolate is slowly dissociable, with a half-life of 6 hours in intact cells. A folate cofactor is an absolute requirement for complex formation; severe depletion of intracellular reduced folates may compromise complex formation in tissue culture experiments.[38] Some tumors appear to be deficient in reduced folates and are killed more effectively by 5-FU when it is given with the reduced folate leucovorin. Clinical trials investigating this combination indicate substantial potentiation of antitumor effects of 5-FU by leucovorin, with some increased gastrointestinal toxicity.

Because the active forms of 5-FU are nucleotides, resistance to 5-FU can develop through deletion of one of the key enzymes required for its activation. In murine tumors, resistance has been associated with deletion of uridine kinase, uridine phosphorylase, or orotic acid phosphoribosyl transferase. In addition, an increase in thymidylate synthase has been seen in resistant cells and is related to amplification of the thymidylate synthase gene.[39]

Resistant mutants have been described that have increased cytidine triphosphate pools, with enhanced feedback inhibition of 5-FU conversion to its active nucleotide forms.[40] It is not known which of these mechanisms is responsible for resistance in humans. Inhibition of tumor thymidylate synthase, a function of the ratio of FdUMP to dUMP, predicted response to therapy in one study of colon cancer patients.[41] In a second clinical study, the drug-activating enzymes were

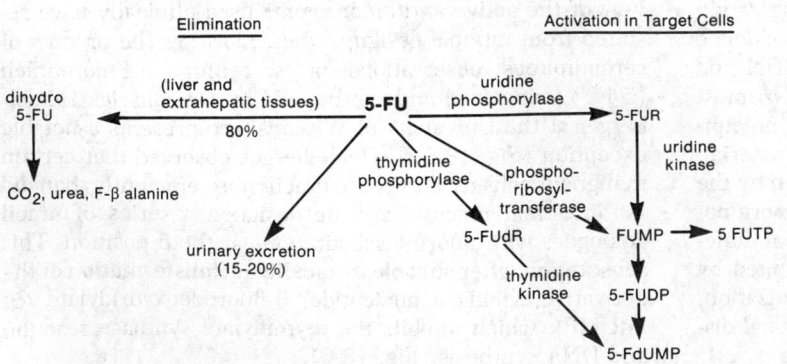

FIG. 18-6. Pathways of 5-fluorouracil elimination and activation.

uniformly high in malignant tissues and did not correlate with response; nor did thymidylate synthase activity, suggesting that fluoropyrimidine incorporation into DNA or RNA might be the important determinant.[42]

In an effort to enhance 5-FU activation and overcome resistance, various antitumor agents and nucleosides have been used in combination with the fluoropyrimidine. When given before 5-FU, methotrexate increases 5-FU nucleotide formation by increasing the intracellular content of phosphoribosylpyrophosphate (PRPP), a substrate required in the orotic acid phosphoribosyltransferase reaction.[43] A metabolite of allopurinol inhibits this enzyme, which appears to be the preferred pathway for 5-FU activation in normal tissues but not in all tumors, and thus improves the therapeutic index of 5-FU against some experimental tumors. However, the combination of 5-FU and allopurinol does not improve antitumor activity in humans.[44] Thymidine and other nucleosides enhance 5-FU incorporation into RNA by unknown mechanisms. In addition, thymidine and uridine delay 5-FU breakdown by the hepatic enzyme dihydrouracil dehydrogenase, and thus prolong 5-FU plasma half-life and increase its toxicity for both normal and malignant cells.[45] The combination of 5-FU and thymidine in humans has not improved clinical results.

Clinical Pharmacology and Pharmacokinetics

A variety of methods may be used to measure 5-FU levels in biologic specimens. The most rapid and sensitive of these methods are those using HPLC, either with anion exchange resins or with reverse-phase columns.[46] The sensitivity of this method, with appropriate sample cleanup, is less than 0.1 μM, or less than the threshold for bone marrow toxicity (probably 1 μM). The sensitivity of HPLC can be enhanced by derivatization of 5-FU with fluorescent conjugates.[47] Gas chromatographic–mass spectrophotometric methods, which are equally sensitive and specific, require derivatization and additional processing time.

An understanding of 5-FU pharmacokinetics is required in order to choose the proper route, schedule, and dose of administration. The alternative routes of administration (oral, intravenous, intraarterial, and intraperitoneal) have unique advantages and disadvantages that determine their usefulness in clinical chemotherapy. The clinical effectiveness and pattern of toxicity seen with each of these routes can be explained largely by pharmacokinetic considerations.

5-FU usually is administered intravenously (IV). Plasma levels vary considerably after oral administration, probably because of erratic absorption and variable first-pass metabolism in the transit from the intestinal tract through the portal system and liver to the systemic circulation.[48] After IV delivery, the drug penetrates well into the CSF and extracellular "third space" fluids, such as ascites or pleural fluid. Following conventional single doses of 10 to 15 mg/kg, peak plasma concentrations reach 0.1 mM to 1.0 mM, but rapid metabolic breakdown to dihydrofluorouracil in the liver and other tissues leads to an abrupt fall in plasma concentrations. The primary plasma half-life of about 10 minutes varies considerably from patient to patient, but its correlation with clinical tests of hepatic function is not clear. Within 6 hours of injection, plasma concentrations of 5-FU fall below 1 μM, the approximate threshold for exerting cytotoxic effects in tissue culture, thereafter they decline more slowly.

Because it is metabolized by the liver, 5-FU can be infused into the hepatic artery or portal vein for treatment of hepatic metastases, and only limited amounts of drug reach the systemic circulation. Preliminary data indicate that infusion of 30 mg/kg/day produces plasma levels of 0.13 to 0.35 μM, although these figures are likely to depend on catheter position and hepatic function.[49] At this infusion rate, more than 50% of the infused drug is cleared in its first pass through the liver.[50] This route is most useful in the treatment of isolated hepatic metastases.

5-FU also has been administered by peritoneal instillation for treatment of ovarian cancer.[51] This route takes advantage of the high intraperitoneal concentration of the drug (4mM), the slow absorption of the drug into the portal circulation, its rapid metabolism in the liver, and the minute amounts of drug that ultimately reach the systemic circulation. Minimal systemic toxicity occurs if drug concentrations are maintained at or below 4 mM in the peritoneal cavity, because a 100:1 to 1000:1 gradient in drug concentration is established between the peritoneal fluid and plasma. The therapeutic effects of this type of regimen have not been evaluated conclusively.

More than 80% of administered 5-FU (by IV or intraarterial route) is eliminated by metabolic conversion to dihydrofluorouracil; the remainder is excreted intact in the urine. The primary metabolite, dihydro-5-FU, is cleaved further to yield α-fluoro-β-ureidoproprionic acid, α-fluoro-β-alanine, and CO_2. The liver, kidney, and gastrointestinal mucosa are the primary sites of metabolism; it is not known whether neoplastic cells also degrade 5-FU. Doses do not have to be modified in the presence of hepatic dysfunction because metabolism occurs in extrahepatic tissues. Cimetidine, the H_2-histamine receptor antagonist, enhances the total drug exposure, as measured by the product of concentration $\times$ time, by inhibiting hepatic blood flow and hepatic drug metabolism.[52]

The active intracellular nucleotides 5-FdUMP and FUTP have prolonged half-lives intracellularly; their decay rates vary among tissues, and their persistence may be an important determinant of the duration and, ultimately, of the magnitude of drug effect.

Clinical Toxicity

The primary clinical toxicity of 5-FU results from its effects on rapidly dividing tissues, specifically intestinal and oral mucosa and bone marrow. After bolus IV administration, using either a 5-day course or single, weekly doses, suppression of the leukocyte and platelet counts occurs in 4 to 7 days, with full recovery within 2 weeks after the last dose. Stomatitis and diarrhea also are frequent side-effects, particularly in patients who receive a 5-day course of treatment. Repeated episodes of watery diarrhea (more than three movements per day) for several days should alert the oncologist to the danger of dehydration, sepsis, and death and should generate dose adjustments in subsequent courses of therapy.

An alternative regimen using continuous IV infusion of

5-FU at doses of 30 mg/kg/day for 5 days gives equivalent therapeutic results but a different pattern of toxicity. Myelosuppression usually is mild, and gastrointestinal symptoms such as stomatitis and diarrhea are the predominant toxicities. Continuous intrahepatic infusion of 5-FU also is a useful alternative to IV therapy in patients with liver metastases. In patients with colonic carcinoma with hepatic metastases, response rates of 50% or greater have been achieved with this mode of therapy. Because at least 50% of the drug is cleared in its first pass through the liver, systemic toxicity is mild, consisting primarily of mucositis and, less frequently, myelosuppression. The primary complications are related to catheter slippage into the gastroduodenal artery, with resultant necrosis of the intestinal epithelium, hemorrhage, or perforation. The physician must be alert to sudden onset of epigastric pain or ileus in the patient as early signs of catheter displacement into a feeding artery of the stomach or small bowel. Thrombosis of the extremity vessel used for insertion of the cannula can be anticipated if the catheter is inserted into a brachial artery. Hepatic portal perfusion is a less favorable form of local therapy because most large hepatic metastases derive their blood supply from the arterial circulation; it may be useful in the adjuvant setting.

Less common adverse effects caused by 5-FU include acute neurologic symptoms (somnolence, ataxia, and upper motor neuron signs) seen primarily in patients receiving intracarotid infusions; this syndrome is thought to be caused by a neurotoxic metabolite, 5-fluorocitrate. A syndrome of chest pain, serum enzyme elevations consistent with myocardial necrosis, and electrocardiographic findings consistent with myocardial ischemia has been described in patients undergoing 5-FU infusion. The reason for these episodes is unclear.

5-FU causes acute and chronic conjunctivitis that may lead to tear-duct stenosis and ectropion. The acute inflammatory response is reversible when the drug is discontinued, but surgical correction of tear-duct stenosis may be required.

Other Fluoropyrimidines

Two other fluoropyrimidines (Fig. 18-5), 5-fluoro-2-deoxyuridine (FUdR) and ftorafur (1-2-tetrahydrofuranyl)-5-fluorouracil, have undergone extensive clinical trials but have not replaced 5-FU in general clinical use. FUdR is converted to 5-FdUMP by a nucleoside kinase and functions primarily as an inhibitor of thymidylate synthase, with lesser effects than 5-FU on RNA. The deoxyribose group is removed readily by the ubiquitous enzyme thymidine phosphorylase, and the resulting 5-FU undergoes metabolic degradation as outlined previously. More than 90% of FUdR is removed in its first pass through the liver.[50] Its pattern of toxicity and the advantages of its use in hepatic perfusion closely parallel the characteristics of 5-FU (Table 18-1).

Ftorafur acts as a depot form of 5-FU and produces little myelosuppression. However, significant diarrhea, nausea, vomiting, and neurotoxicity in the form of altered mental status and ataxia are the usual dose-limiting complaints.[53] It is administered IV in doses of 1.5 g/m²/day for 5 days and is absorbed well orally. The parent compound, ftorafur, has a prolonged plasma half-life of 6 to 16 hours and is eliminated by conversion to hydroxylated metabolites. The circulating concentrations of 5-FU produced are low (less than 0.1 mg/ml), suggesting that conversion to 5-FU may occur predominantly in tumor cells and the liver and that the circulating level of 5-FU may not adequately reflect the extent of this conversion.[54] Another analogue, 5' deoxy-5-fluorouridine, functions as a prodrug, which is cleaved to yield 5-FU in tumor cells by action of the enzyme pyrimidine nucleoside phosphorylase.[55] It has no obvious advantage over 5-FU in clinical practice.

CYTOSINE ARABINOSIDE (CYTARABINE)

Cytosine arabinoside (ara-C) is one of several arabinose nucleosides first isolated from the sponge, *Cryptothethya crypta*, differing from its physiologic counterpart deoxycytidine by the presence of an OH group in the β-configuration at the 2' position (Fig. 18-7). Since this initial discovery, many arabinose nucleosides have been synthesized or isolated from bacterial broths, and a few have been tested as antitumor agents. The most prominent of these are the purine analogues ara-adenine and fludarabine. However, neither of these compounds has as potent clinical activity against human acute myeloblastic leukemia as does ara-C. As a single agent, ara-C induces remission in 50% of patients with acute myeloblastic leukemia (AML) and is the standard agent in combination with anthracyclines for treatment of this disease. It has activity against other human tumors, including the blastic crisis of chronic granulocytic leukemia (CGL), acute lymphoblastic leukemia (ALL), and non-Hodgkin's lymphoma, but its selective activity against rapidly growing tumors and its pharmacokinetic features have

FIG. 18-7. Structure of physiologic cytidine nucleosides and related antimetabolites.

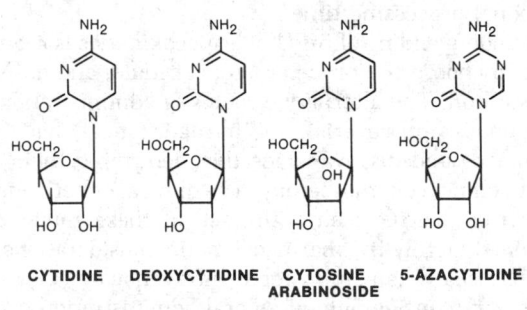

CYTIDINE   DEOXYCYTIDINE   CYTOSINE ARABINOSIDE   5-AZACYTIDINE

5-AZA-2'-DEOXY CYTIDINE   5-AZA-CYTOSINE ARABINOSIDE

rendered this agent less useful in treating most solid malignancies.

Structure and Mechanism of Action

Because of the absence of a 2'-OH group in the α position, ara-C is recognized enzymatically as an analogue of 2'-deoxycytidine and is metabolized by salvage pathway enzymes to its active form, ara-CTP (Fig. 18-8). This nucleotide acts as an inhibitor of DNA polymerase in competition with deoxycytidine triphosphate (dCTP) and has a K_1 of approximately 0.1 μM.[56] Repair of ultraviolet light damage to DNA is inhibited by ara-C—presumably through polymerase inhibition—but not repair of radiation-induced damage.[57] A more important action of ara-C appears to be its incorporation into DNA, leading to a marked slowing of the elongating chain of DNA and a defect in ligation of fragments of newly synthesized DNA.[58] There also is evidence indicating that cells exposed to ara-C during the S, or DNA synthetic, phase of the cell cycle can reinitiate DNA synthesis when ara-CTP levels fall below inhibitory levels, resulting in an abnormal duplication of early portions of the DNA strand.[59]

Ara-C penetrates cells by a carrier-mediated process that allows the rapid achievement of steady-state intracellular drug concentrations.[60] Entry is an important determinant of ara-C sensitivity of human leukemic cells; for example, there is a strong correlation between the number of transport sites and the formation of the ultimate toxic metabolite ara-CTP.[61] At high drug concentrations ($> 100 \mu$M), ara-C enters cells by passive diffusion, a less efficient mechanism.

Intracellular metabolism of ara-C by three sequential phosphorylation reactions, mediated by deoxycytidine kinase, deoxycytidine monophosphate (dCMP) kinase, and nucleoside diphosphate kinase, leads to formation of ara-cytidine triphosphate (CTP). Two inactivating enzymes,

cytidine deaminase and dCMP deaminase, also may act on ara-C or ara-CMP, respectively.[62] These deaminating enzymes are found in high concentrations relative to the activating enzymes and are thought to limit drug action (see Fig. 18-8).

The biochemical changes responsible for resistance to ara-C have not been clearly defined in humans. Deletion of deoxycytidine kinase often is observed in resistant murine leukemia cells and has been implicated by at least one study in AML.[63] A second mechanism of resistance, documented only in preclinical studies, is an increased intracellular pool of dCTP (the nucleotide that competes with ara-CTP). Increased activity of cytidine deaminase has been correlated with resistance in a single study in AML but has not been confirmed subsequently.[64] In separate work, transport capacity of acute nonlymphocytic leukemia cells correlated with achievement of complete remission.[61] All of these changes ultimately decrease ara-CTP concentration. It is possible to predict clinical response to ara-C by a test incubation of leukemic cells with the drug in vitro; the ability of cells to retain ara-CTP after exposure to ara-C can be used to predict the duration of a subsequent remission.[65] These studies require the separation and quantitation of ara-C nucleotides by HPLC and are not adapted easily to routine clinical use.

As an inhibitor of DNA synthesis, ara-C kills cells selectively during the S phase of the cell cycle, although exposure of cells during other phases may lead to chromatid deletions and to a failure to repair strand breaks induced by other agents. The cytotoxicity of ara-C is not only cell-cycle specific, but also depends on the rate of DNA synthesis. Cytotoxic effects are greatest if cells are exposed to ara-C during periods of rapid DNA synthesis, for example, during the recovery phase after treatment with an initial dose of ara-C or another S-phase-specific drug. Thus the timing of the second dose of ara-C may have a critical impact on the therapeutic outcome. Karp and coworkers have demonstrated a marked increase in DNA synthetic rate in residual leukemic cells one week after an initial dose of ara-C and have advocated the use of sequential ara-C doses spaced 1 week apart to take advantage of this change.[66]

In addition to its cytotoxic effects, which are exerted at low concentrations (10 nM maintained continuously in culture will kill 50% of human marrow myeloid progenitors), ara-C is capable of inducing terminal differentiation of leukemic cells. Differentiation is associated in some instances with decreased oncogene (c-myc) expression.[67] Low-dose ara-C regimens induce remission both in leukemic patients and in patients with preleukemic states, and in both instances it has been possible in some cases to demonstrate persistence of chromosomal markers of the leukemic cell line in the mature cells, suggesting differentiation as a mechanism.[68] However, fewer than 20% of preleukemic patients achieve remission, and the dosage of ara-C used (20 mg/m^2/day) achieves cytotoxic concentrations in plasma, leading to severe myelosuppression.

Clinical Pharmacology and Pharmacokinetics

The measurement of ara-C in biologic fluids presents significant problems. Because it is structurally similar to the physi-

FIG. 18-8. Metabolism of cytosine arabinoside by tumor cells. The names of important enzymes are in italics. The conversion of ara-UMP to a triphosphate has not been demonstrated in mammalian cells. d = deoxyribose; MP = monophosphate; DP = diphosphate; TP = triphosphate; NDP = nucleoside diphosphate. See legend to Figure 18-1 for other abbreviations.

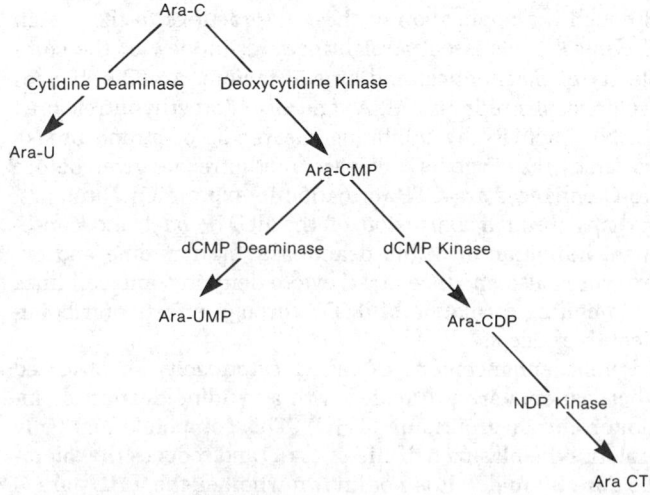

ologic nucleosides (deoxycytidine, cytidine), it is difficult to separate ara-C from these endogenous compounds. Further, ara-C is subject to deamination by cytidine deaminase, an enzyme found in plasma and in granulocytes; thus a deaminase inhibitor, such as tetrahydrouridine, must be included in samples at the time of their collection. Various chemical and microbiologic assays for ara-C have been developed and applied to clinical pharmacokinetic studies. The best of these uses HPLC with a cation-exchange column and cleanly separates ara-C from its primary metabolite ara-U.[69] The sensitivity of this method approaches 0.1 μM in plasma. An easier, more rapid method is the radioimmunoassay based on a sheep antibody to an ara-C conjugate with albumin.[70] This assay, which is more sensitive than HPLC, is highly specific for ara-C (and its nucleotides, which are not found in plasma), takes less than 3 hours to complete, and is applicable to routine pharmacokinetic monitoring and other clinical uses.

Because of the presence of cytidine deaminase in gastrointestinal epithelium and first-pass elimination in the liver, the drug is not given orally. When administered by IV infusion, it distributes rapidly into total-body water; concentrations in the CSF reach 50% of simultaneous plasma levels after 2 hours of continuous IV administration. Peak plasma concentrations reach 1×10^{-5} M after a 100-mg dose and thereafter fall with a primary half-life of 7 to 20 minutes.[71] A second half-life of 0.5 to 2.6 hours has been detected by more sensitive assay procedures but is probably of little clinical significance at standard doses. More than 70% of the clinical dose is excreted in the urine, primarily in the form of the inactive metabolite ara-U. Within minutes of injection, ara-U becomes the predominant form of the drug found in plasma; its formation takes place in the liver, plasma, peripheral granulocytes, and other sites. High-dose ara-C regimens (2–3 g/m² twice daily for 6 days) produce proportionately higher peak plasma concentrations, and ara-C disappears from plasma with a terminal half-life of 6 hours. In high-dose regimens, cerebrospinal fluid concentrations of drug reach a peak of 8 μM and decline with a half-life of 2 hours.[72]

Constant IV infusion of 5 to 10 mg/hour ara-C yields an average plasma concentration of about 3×10^{-7} M; a loading dose of three times the hourly infusion rate should be given before infusion to allow rapid achievement of the steady-state level.

The increases in plasma ara-C are proportional for infusion rates up to 2 g/m²/d, or about 150 mg/hour, but at higher rates of infusion, the deamination capacity is saturated and ara-C levels rise sharply.[73] A maximum-tolerated infusion rate of 2 g/m²/d for 3 days has been recommended and yields steady-state levels of 5 μM.

Schedules of Administration

Because of the rapid inactivation of ara-C by cytidine deaminase and its phase-dependent killing, the drug usually is administered as a continuous infusion or in bolus doses of 100 mg every 8 to 12 hours for 5 to 10 days. Single bolus doses of 4 g/m² produce minimal toxicity because of rapid drug inactivation, whereas the continuous infusion of 2 g/m²/d over a 72-hour period produces severe myelosuppression.

The primary toxic side-effects of ara-C are myelosuppression and gastrointestinal epithelial injury. With the conventional dosage of 200 mg/m²/day for 5 to 7 days, leukopenia and thrombocytopenia reach their maximum in 7 to 14 days. The duration of myelosuppression depends on the dose of ara-C, rate of achievement of remission, the nature of concomitant therapy, and prior treatment experience.

Gastrointestinal toxicity is prominent in patients receiving ara-C. The most frequent complaints include nausea, vomiting, and diarrhea: a spectrum of pathologic changes is observed in the intestinal mucosa, ranging from superficial ulceration to intramural hematoma formation and perforation. Patients receiving ara-C often develop elevated levels of serum enzymes consistent with mild hepatocellular damage, but hepatotoxicity necessitates discontinuation of treatment in fewer than 25% of patients.

High-dose ara-C regimens, using 2 to 3 g/m² given as a 2-hour infusion twice daily for 6 days, have been used to treat patients with refractory forms of acute leukemia. Toxicity in the form of myelosuppression, ataxia, and confusion is tolerable in most patients.

In addition to conventional administration by IV injection or infusion, ara-C may be given by subcutaneous (SC) injection or infusion on an outpatient basis, and total drug exposure (concentration × time) is twofold greater than is achieved by the same doses given by the IV bolus route.[74]

Ara-C also may be administered intrathecally for treatment of meningeal leukemia or carcinomatosis. Because deamination is minimal in the CSF, doses of 50 mg/m² yield peak levels of 1 mM, which decline slowly with a half-life of approximately 2 hours. Cytotoxic concentrations of greater than 0.1 μM are maintained for 24 hours. Ara-C often is used intrathecally as a substitute for methotrexate in patients experiencing antifolate neurotoxicity; however, ara-C also may cause neurotoxic side-effects, including seizures and alteration in mental status.[75]

Drug Interactions

Ara-C has shown synergistic interaction with many other antitumor agents, including alkylating agents, thiopurines, uridine analogues, and antifolates. Each of these interactions has been explained on a biochemical or cellular kinetic basis, although the application of these interactions to the design of clinical trials is not straightforward, in view of the complexity of biochemical and kinetic factors. Ara-C enhances cyclophosphamide, mAMSA, and bischloroethylnitrosourea (BCNU) activity by inhibiting the repair of strand breaks caused by these agents. Likewise, methotrexate given before ara-C enhances ara-CTP formation in experimental tumors, perhaps through expansion of the dUMP pool and consequent inhibition of dCMP deaminase.[76] Thymidine and hydroxyurea also enhance ara-C cytotoxicity in some cell lines by inhibiting formation of dCDP through effects on ribonucleotide reductase.[77]

Potent enhancement of ara-C cytotoxicity is observed when patients are pretreated with a cytidine deaminase inhibitor, tetrahydrouridine (THU). This compound markedly prolongs the plasma half-life of ara-C and reduces the tolerable dose 30-fold.[78] It is not known whether the THU–ara-C combination will have selective toxic effects on human tumor cells, but on the basis of experimental work, this combination would be expected to have synergistic activity only against cells with high deaminase levels, as are found in a fraction of patients with AML.

Other Cytidine Analogues

Because of the rapid metabolism of ara-C, attempts have been made to develop alternate therapies that would resist deamination. Ara-C enclosed in lipid vesicles, or liposomes, has increased potency, probably because of the prolonged half-life of the vesicles in plasma, but this increased potency has not been translated into improved therapeutic efficacy, compared with optimal use of free ara-C.[79] Various conjugates of ara-C, including N^4-acyl analogues, ara-C or ara-CMP esters, and the anhydro compound, cyclocytidine, have shown subject to deamination, but they do not have a superior therapeutic index. Most of these derivatives owe their activity to ara-CTP, and thus have the same mechanism of action as ara-C.

Other nucleosides with distinctly different mechanisms of cytidine antagonism have been developed, and two—5 azacytidine (5-azaC) and 3-deazauridine—have received clinical trial (Fig. 18-7). 5-AzaC has significant activity in the treatment of leukemia. As with ara-C, it is subject to deamination in plasma, in the liver, and in tumor cells, but its activation proceeds by a separate pathway. It is phosphorylated by uridine-cytidine kinase and then follows the same pathways as ara-CMP to reach its active form, 5-azaCTP. The latter is a substrate for RNA polymerase, and when it is incorporated into RNA, it causes defective protein synthesis and polyribosomal degradation.[80] 5-AzaC also is incorporated into DNA and inhibits methylation of DNA; the latter action may explain its ability to induce differentiation of both normal and malignant cells. It has been used clinically to induce fetal hemoglobin synthesis in patients with beta-thalassemia.[81] Resistance to 5-azaC in murine leukemic cells develops through deletion of uridine-cytidine kinase.

The 5-azaC ring system is unstable in solution; this instability may contribute to its lethal effects after incorporation into RNA. The rapid decomposition of 5-azaC in alkaline or neutral solution necessitates either fresh mixing before administration or formulation at a slightly acid pH in Ringer's lactate (pH 6.2), in which it has a half-life of 65 hours at 25°C.

5-AzaC is removed rapidly from the plasma, through both metabolic clearance and chemical decomposition. Less than 2% of an administered dose remains in plasma as the parent compound 30 minutes after administration. The compound is a substrate for cytidine deaminase, but the product, 5-azauridine, is chemically unstable and has not been identified in the urine or plasma of humans.

The primary adverse reactions to 5-azaC are myelosuppression and severe and prolonged nausea and vomiting. The latter symptoms are ameliorated if the drug is administered by prolonged or continuous infusion, which does not change its therapeutic efficacy or myelosuppressive effects. Patients sometimes develop abnormal liver function, myalgias, transient temperature elevation, or rash following 5-azaC therapy.

Other uridine and cytidine analogues have shown antitu-

mor activity. 3-Deaza-uridine, an inhibitor of CTP synthesis, enhances the cytotoxicity of ara-C by diminishing intracellular dCTP. However, clinical trials of this compound as a single agent or in combination with ara-C indicated little antileukemic activity. Two new analogues, 5-azadeoxycytidine and 5-azacytosine arabinoside, are undergoing initial clinical evaluation (Fig. 18-7). The former is incorporated into DNA and, like 5-azacytidine, inhibits DNA methylation. 5-Azacytosine arabinoside acts as a potent inhibitor of DNA synthesis and has a broader spectrum of activity against experimental solid tumors than does either ara-C or 5-azacytidine.

PURINE ANALOGUES

The development of purine analogues for treatment of cancer has been one of the most fruitful endeavors in rational antitumor drug synthesis. Not only have effective antileukemic agents such as 6-mercaptopurine (6-MP) and 6-thioguanine (6-TG) resulted from these efforts, but potent immunosuppressive agents such as azathioprine, the xanthine oxidase inhibitor allopurinol, and the antiviral compounds ara-adenine and acyclovir have proved to be important in nononcologic fields.[82] A new area of great potential has been opened by the discovery of adenosine deaminase inhibitors such as deoxycoformycin, which have selective action against T-lymphocytes and promise to be useful in the treatment of hairy cell leukemia and other lymphoid tumors. This chapter deals with established and potentially important new antipurine agents in cancer chemotherapy.

Structure and Mechanism of Action of 6-Thiopurines

6-MP and 6-TG are used commonly in treating childhood ALL and AML, respectively, but do not have appreciable activity against human solid malignancies. Because of the similarities in their mechanisms of action, pharmacokinetic properties, and patterns of clinical toxicity, these two agents are considered jointly.

The 6-thiopurine analogues have the single substitution of a thiol group in place of the 6-hydroxyl group found in guanine or in the basic purine nucleus (Fig. 18-9). Both 6-MP and 6-TG are inactive compounds in their native state and require activation to the nucleotide level by the enzyme hypoxanthine-guanine phosphoribosyl transferase (HGPRT'ase).

FIG. 18-9. Purine analogues and their physiologic counterparts, hypoxanthine and guanine.

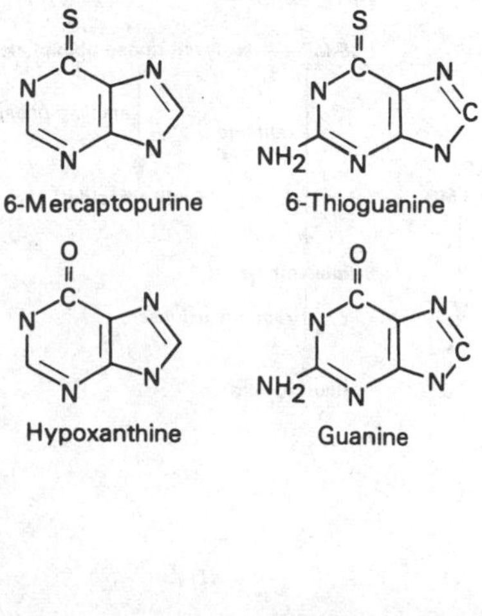

As monophosphate nucleotides, these analogues inhibit *de novo* purine biosynthesis at its first step (phosphoribosylpyrophosphate amidotransferase) and also block the conversion of inosinic acid to adenylic acid or to guanylic acid. The triphosphate nucleotides of 6-TG and 6-MP are incorporated into DNA and produce toxicity that is manifested in a delayed manner after drug exposure.[83] 6-TG incorporation into DNA leads to strand breaks, the frequency of which correlates with cytotoxicity.[84] Incorporation of the nucleophilic 6-TG base also renders DNA more susceptible to alkylation.[85]

Biochemical resistance to these agents has been ascribed to the absence of the activating enzyme (HGPRT'ase) in experimental tumors, but in human leukemic cells, resistance also is associated with increased concentrations of a degrading enzyme, a membrane-bound alkaline phosphatase, and the conjugating enzyme 6-thiopurine methyltransferase.[86,87]

The purine analogues readily penetrate cells. Their intracellular metabolism proceeds in several phases (Fig. 18-10).[88] Substantial quantities are converted to the inactive products 6-thiouric acid and 6-methylmercaptopurine; in the activation pathway, the thiopurines are converted to monophosphate nucleotides, which inhibit de novo purine synthesis, and to the triphosphate nucleotides, which are incorporated into DNA. It is believed that the initial inhibition of purine synthesis allows a buildup of PRPP pools and thus increases conversion of 6-MP and 6-TG to nucleotides. Inhibitors of de novo purine biosynthesis, such as methotrexate, are synergistic with 6-thiopurines because the block in purine synthesis leads to an expansion of the PRPP pool required for thiopurine activation. 6-MP-resistant cells, which lack HGPRT'ase, depend completely on the de novo pathway for purines and are thus highly sensitive to methotrexate.

Clinical Pharmacology and Pharmacokinetics

Although initial information on 6-MP pharmacokinetics came from the use of radiolabeled drug, this approach is impractical for routine monitoring or for repetitive studies in a single patient. Improved analytic techniques using HPLC have been described. The most sensitive of these new methods used derivatization of the thiopurines to phenyl mercury derivatives or oxidation to sulfonates with alkaline permanganate, followed by column separation and fluorometric detection.[89,90] The level of sensitivity of these procedures is approximately 0.1 μM in plasma.

When taken orally, both 6-MP and 6-TG are absorbed erratically; less than 50% of a dose reaches the systemic circulation, but this varies considerably among patients.[91] Both feeding and the antibiotic cotrimoxazole decrease 6-MP absorption.[92,93] The influence of erratic bioavailability on clinical response has not been determined.

The plasma half-lives are approximately 80 to 90 minutes for 6-TG and 20 to 45 minutes for 6-MP. The major determinants of drug elimination are metabolic alteration by several pathways (Fig. 18-10). 6-MP is oxidized to 6-thiouric acid by xanthine oxidase, a reaction sequence inhibited by allopurinol. In the presence of allopurinol, 6-thioxanthine, an intermediate oxidation product, becomes the predominant elimination product of 6-MP.

There is clinical evidence of increased 6-MP toxicity in patients receiving oral 6-MP concomitant with allopurinol but not in those treated with IV 6-MP. A dose reduction of 75% is recommended for patients receiving oral 6-MP and allopurinol. 6-MP also undergoes S-methylation to yield 6-methylmercaptopurine, which on phosphorylation becomes an active antipurine. However, the 6-methylmercaptopurine nucleotides are less cytotoxic than 6-MP nucleotides, and the activity of the methylation enzyme, which is quite variable among patients, has been correlated inversely with 6-MP nucleotide content of erythrocytes.[87] It has been suggested that 6-MP dosage be judged by toxicity (myelosuppression) rather than depend on a fixed dosage.

The catabolism of 6-TG is somewhat different than that of 6-MP. Methylation of the sulfur substituent plays a major role, leading ultimately to oxidation and elimination of the sulfur molecule. 6-TG also is converted to 6-thioxanthine in a reaction catalyzed by the enzyme guanase. This intermediate is oxidized further to 6-thiouric acid by xanthine oxidase, but because the substrate for this reaction, 6-thioxanthine, is inactive, no reduction in 6-TG dosage is required for patients who are also receiving allopurinol.

Dose, Schedule, and Toxicity

6-MP, given orally, and 6-TG, given IV, are well tolerated in doses of approximately 100 mg/m². These doses usually are given for at least 5 days in leukemic induction therapy or, in the case of 6-MP, for longer courses at slightly reduced doses for maintenance of remission. A 6-MP dosage reduction of 75% is indicated for patients also receiving allopurinol. Extremely high doses of 6-MP have been used (up to 1000 mg/m²/day for 5 days by IV infusion) without effectively increasing antitumor activity.[94]

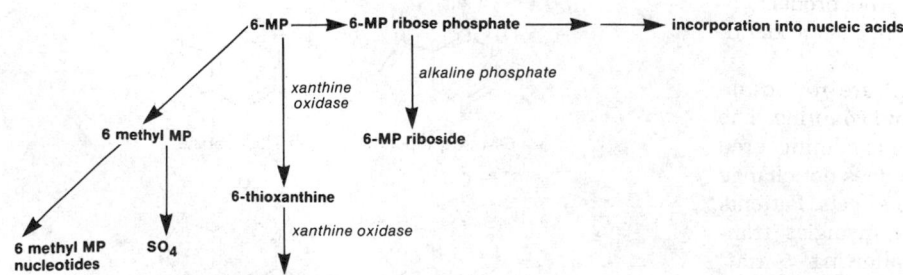

FIG. 18-10. Pathways for activation and degradation of 6-mercaptopurine (6-MP).

Because both 6-MP and 6-TG produce cytotoxicity by virtue of their incorporation into DNA, it follows that their primary toxicity would be exerted against the rapidly dividing precursor cells of the bone marrow and intestinal epithelium. After single doses, myelosuppression is maximal within 7 days of drug administration; the time to recovery is dose-dependent but usually is complete 14 days after the last dose. Reversible hepatotoxicity occasionally is observed after treatment with either thiopurine or, more frequently, after 6-MP. Serum alkaline phosphatase, direct bilirubin, and transaminase levels are elevated during this acute toxicity in a pattern consistent with cholestatic jaundice. Mucositis, esophagitis, and gastrointestinal complaints usually are mild and not a significant hindrance to antipurine therapy.

The 6-thiopurines and the related compound azathioprine, which releases 6-MP through hepatic metabolism following oral administration, are potent suppressors of cell-mediated immunity and are used to suppress rejection of transplanted organs or to treat autoimmune diseases such as Crohn's disease, ulcerative colitis, or rheumatoid arthritis.[95] Therapeutic immunosuppression will occur at doses of 100 mg/day (1.5 mg/kg), which cause only a small decrease in the leukocyte count. Long-term immunosuppressive therapy with azathioprine increases the risk of squamous carcinomas of the skin, histiocytic lymphoma, and Kaposi's sarcoma; these complications have not been reported after chronic 6-MP therapy. Other complications of chronic 6-thiopurine treatment include predispositions to bacterial and parasitic infections.

FIG. 18-11. Adenosine antimetabolites (ara-A and 2-fluoro-ara-AMP) and inhibitors of adenosine deaminase [2'-deoxycoformycin (2'-DCF) and EHNA].

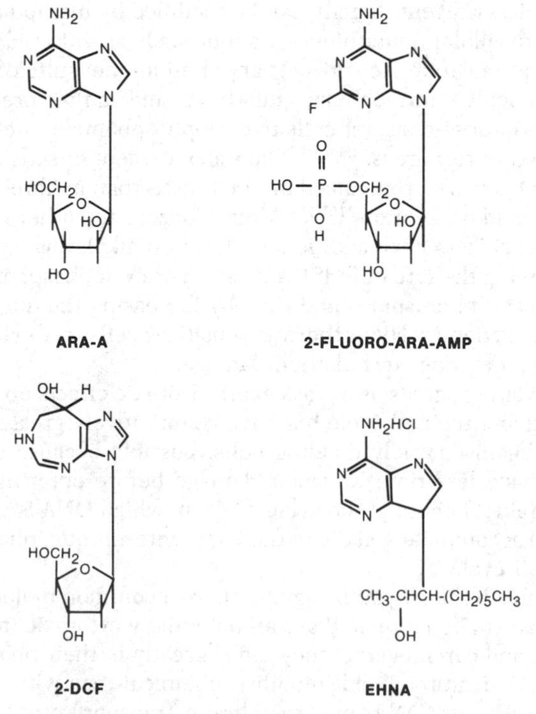

ARA-A   2-FLUORO-ARA-AMP

2'-DCF   EHNA

ADENOSINE ANALOGUES

In addition to the 6-thiopurines which act as guanine analogues, a number of analogues of adenosine have been synthesized or isolated from fermentation broths. The most prominent among these is 9-β-D-arabinofuranosyladenine (ara-A), which, as a triphosphate, inhibits DNA polymerase (Fig. 18-11). This compound has antiviral activity against DNA viruses, particularly those of the herpes group.[96] Although ara-A has shown potent antitumor activity in animal tumors, its clinical usefulness has been hindered by its limited aqueous solubility and its rapid deamination by adenosine deaminase. Its 2-fluoro monophosphate analogue (2-fluoro-AMP) is not susceptible to deamination and is highly toxic to both normal and malignant lymphoid and myeloid cells.[97] Its clinical utility is compromised by severe, late-onset neurotoxicity, including seizures, dementia, coma, and blindness.[98] It is highly active against chronic lymphocytic leukemia.

Inborn deficiency of adenosine deaminase is highly toxic for T-lymphocytes, an observation that has prompted interest in inhibitors of this enzyme for treatment of human T-cell tumors (Fig. 18-11). Two potent inhibitors of adenosine deaminase, 2'-deoxycoformycin and erythro-9-(2-hydroxy-3-nanyl)adenine(EHNA), enhance antitumor potency of ara-A and other adenosine analogues, such as tubercidin, xylosyl adenine, and 3'-deoxyadenosine.[99] The increase in intracellular ara-ATP produced by deoxycoformycin is greatest in tumor cells that contain adenosine deaminase; the decrease is smaller in bone marrow or gastrointestinal epithelium. Deoxycoformycin is highly toxic when given in daily schedules or weekly doses exceeding 10 mg/m² per week; azotemia, confusion, hepatic enzyme elevation, and nausea and vomiting are frequent side-effects. At lower doses (4 mg/m² biweekly), the incidence of side effects is low, but activity against hairy cell leukemia is preserved. Between 30% and 50% of a dose is excreted unchanged in the urine. In patients with normal renal function, sequential plasma half-lives are 1 and 10 hours.[100]

ALKYLATING AGENTS

Two primary classes of cytotoxic compounds have proven useful in the treatment of cancer: those that interfere with the synthesis of DNA precursors and those that chemically interact with DNA itself. Most prominent among the latter compounds are drugs known as alkylating agents because of their ability to form covalent bonds with nucleic acid. It is not fully understood how the alkyl groups that become attached to DNA in this reaction interfere with the integrity or function of DNA, but the alkylation process is known to have significant cytotoxic, mutagenic, and carcinogenic effects.

The biochemical process of alkylation is shown in Figure 18-12. Most alkylating agents form positively charged carbonium ions in aqueous solution. In the cases of the chloroethyl alkylating groups, a preliminary cyclization to form an unstable imonium ion takes place, with spontaneous opening of the three-member ring to yield the alkylating intermediate $R-CH_2-CH_2^+$. This charged group then attacks nucleo-

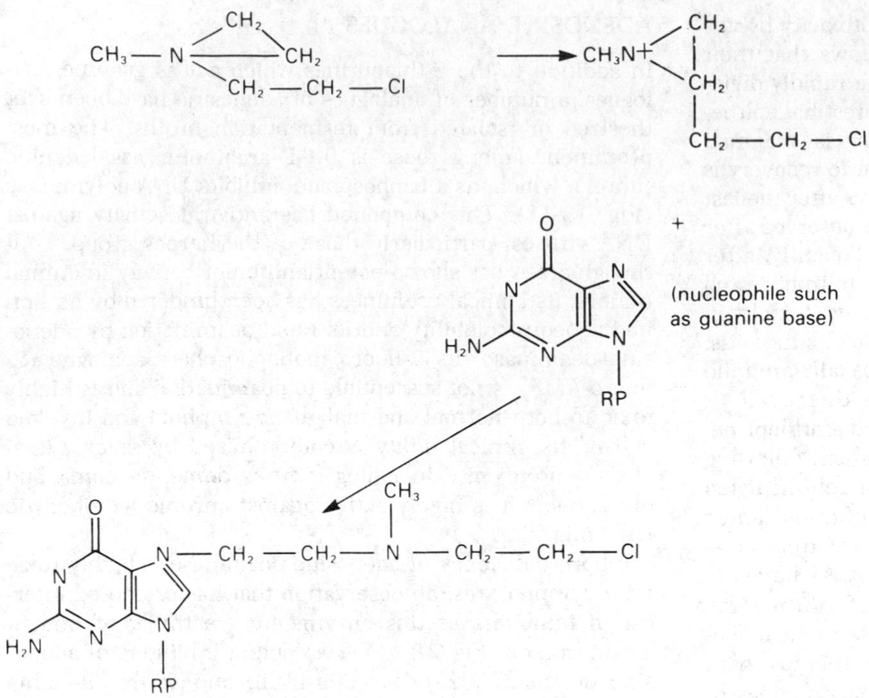

FIG. 18-12. Spontaneous activation of nitrogen mustard to an imonium ion that forms a covalent bond with nucleophilic sites such as the N-7 position of guanine. The remaining free chloroethyl arm of nitrogen mustard can repeat the same sequence of reactions to form DNA cross-links.

philic (electron-rich) sites on nucleic acids, proteins, and small molecules, such as sulfhydryls (glutathione) and amino acids. It seems likely that the primary cytotoxic and mutagenic effects of alkylating agents are caused by their interactions with DNA.[101] The favored sites of DNA attack are the N^7 position of guanine, which accounts for about 90% of alkylated sites; the 1 position of guanine; the 1, 3, and 7 positions of adenine; and the N^3 position of cytosine. It is not clear which of these sites of attack is the most important in producing the pharmacologic action of this class of compounds; alkylation of the N^7 position of guanine has less of an effect on misreading the DNA template than does alteration of the N^3 position of cytidine or the O^6 position of guanine, both of which interfere with accurate base pairing.

The consequences of base alkylation include not only misreading of the DNA code but also cross-linking of DNA and single-strand and double-strand breaks. Additional effects include inhibition of DNA, RNA, and protein synthesis in rapidly dividing tissues. Single-strand breakage occurs primarily as a consequence of the enzymatic processes of repair; the alkylated base is excised by endonuclease enzymes that specifically open the DNA strand at sites of base alkylation. The resulting gap can be repaired by a ligase enzyme if such an enzyme is present in the affected cell. Both alkylation and repair occur preferentially at sites of active DNA transcription.

Cross-linkage of DNA occurs when so-called bifunctional alkylating agents are used. For example, the prototype drug nitrogen mustard possesses two chloroethyl groups, each of which can form a carbonium ion. The establishment of cross-strand covalent binding correlates closely with the lethality of alkylating agents and nitrosourea derivatives.[102]

Repair of alkylated DNA depends on enzymes with highly specific action; for example, the guanine-O-alkyl transferase

that repairs alkylation by nitrosoureas does not remove the alkyl groups fixed to DNA by other agents or platinum-DNA adducts. The intracellular action of alkylating agents may be aborted by their conjugation to glutathione or to thiol-containing proteins such as glutathione transferases (nitrosoureas) or metallothionine (cisplatin). Increased glutathione appears to be a general mechanism of alkylating agent resistance, but mechanisms specific for each agent have also been identified.[103,104]

Alkylating agent toxicity can be modified by manipulation of intracellular glutathione. Agents such as misonidazole (also a radiation sensitizer) and buthionine sulfoximine (BSO) deplete intracellular glutathione and can restore sensitivity of drug-resistant cells to cyclophosphamide, melphalan, and nitrosoureas.[105-107] The enhancement of sensitivity by BSO is more pronounced in tumor cells than in fibroblasts or myeloid progenitors.[108,109] Metronidazole and other radiation sensitizers have additional effects on alkylating agents, depressing the rate of P-450 activation of cyclophosphamide by hepatic microsomes and thereby increasing the duration of drug action.[110] Hyperthermia sensitizes cells to alkylating agents, as it does to radiation damage.

Alkylating agents as a class exert cytotoxic effects on cells throughout the cell cycle but have quantitatively greater activity against rapidly dividing cells, possibly because these cells have less time to repair damage before entering the vulnerable S phase of the cycle. Cells in which DNA is cross-linked accumulate and die in the G_2, or intermitotic, phase of the cell cycle.

Although the alkylating agents share a common molecular mechanism of action and are all potentially cytotoxic, mutagenic, and carcinogenic, they differ greatly in their pharmacokinetic features, lipid solubility, chemical reactivity, alkylation sites on DNA, and membrane transport properties, and thus do not uniformly share cross-resistance in experimental or clinical chemotherapy.[111] Thus the nitrosoureas and cyclophosphamide are not cross-resistant clinically in the treatment of lymphomas. Therefore, a consideration of the pharmacology of individual agents is necessary to understand their unique properties and optimal clinical use. The structures of commonly used alkylating agents are shown in Figure 18-13.

NITROGEN MUSTARD

Nitrogen mustard, or mechlorethamine, was the first alkylating agent to receive clinical trial and was found to produce responses in patients with lymphomas. This agent is highly reactive in aqueous solution and must be administered by IV injection. It also is effective as a topical solution for treatment of mycosis fungoides but produces hypersensitivity to its chloroethyl side-chain when used in this way. Nitrogen mustard penetrates cells through an active transport mechanism shared with the physiologic amine choline.[112] Resistance to the agent is poorly understood; it is believed to result from enhanced ability to repair DNA alkylation, but other mechanisms, such as defective transport or increased inactivation of the carbonium ion by enzymatic conjugation with intracellular sulfhydryl groups, may play a role.[113]

The primary clinical toxicities of nitrogen mustard are shown in Table 18-1 and consist of myelosuppression, nausea, and vomiting. Minor cholinergic side-effects are present at high doses and include lacrimation, diarrhea, and diaphoresis. Because of the high chemical reactivity of this compound, it is a potent vesicant and causes severe local tissue injury when infiltrated into the skin. Thus it is useful for ablating the pleural space in patients with chronic pleural effusion caused by malignant disease. Nitrogen mustard has been replaced to a great extent in clinical use by more stable agents, as described below.

CYCLOPHOSPHAMIDE

In an attempt to improve the selectivity of alkylating agents, cyclophosphamide was designed based on the fact that tumor cells possess a high concentration of enzyme activity that can cleave the P–N bond and liberate the potent phosphoramide mustard. In fact, activation of the drug is a multistep process. The first metabolite, hydroxycyclophosphamide, is produced by hepatic microsomal metabolism (Fig. 18-14).[114] 4-OH cyclophosphamide reenters plasma and is transported to peripheral target tissues, where it crosses the cell membrane and undergoes sequential conversion to aldophosphamide and its ultimate active principles, phosphoramide mustard and acrolein. Aldophosphamide is also subject to inactivation by aldehyde dehydrogenase, an enzyme elevated in some resistant tumor cells.[115] Although phosphoramide mustard is believed to be the primary active product, acrolein is a highly reactive compound capable of depleting gluta-

FIG. 18-13. Structures of commonly used alkylating agents and chloroethylnitrosoureas.

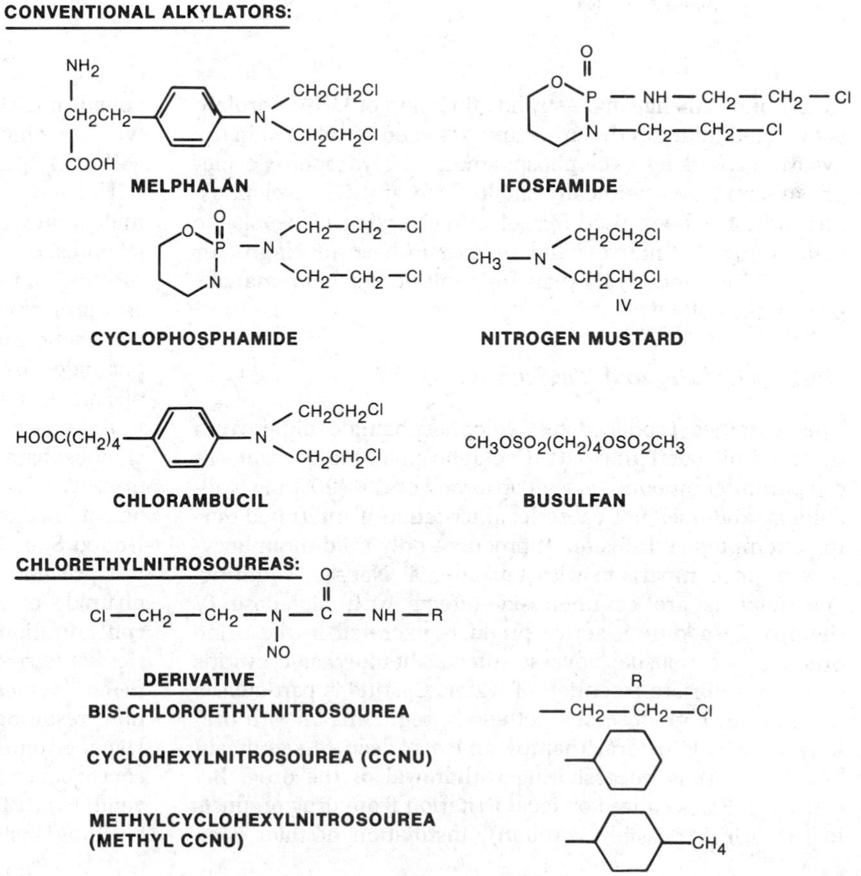

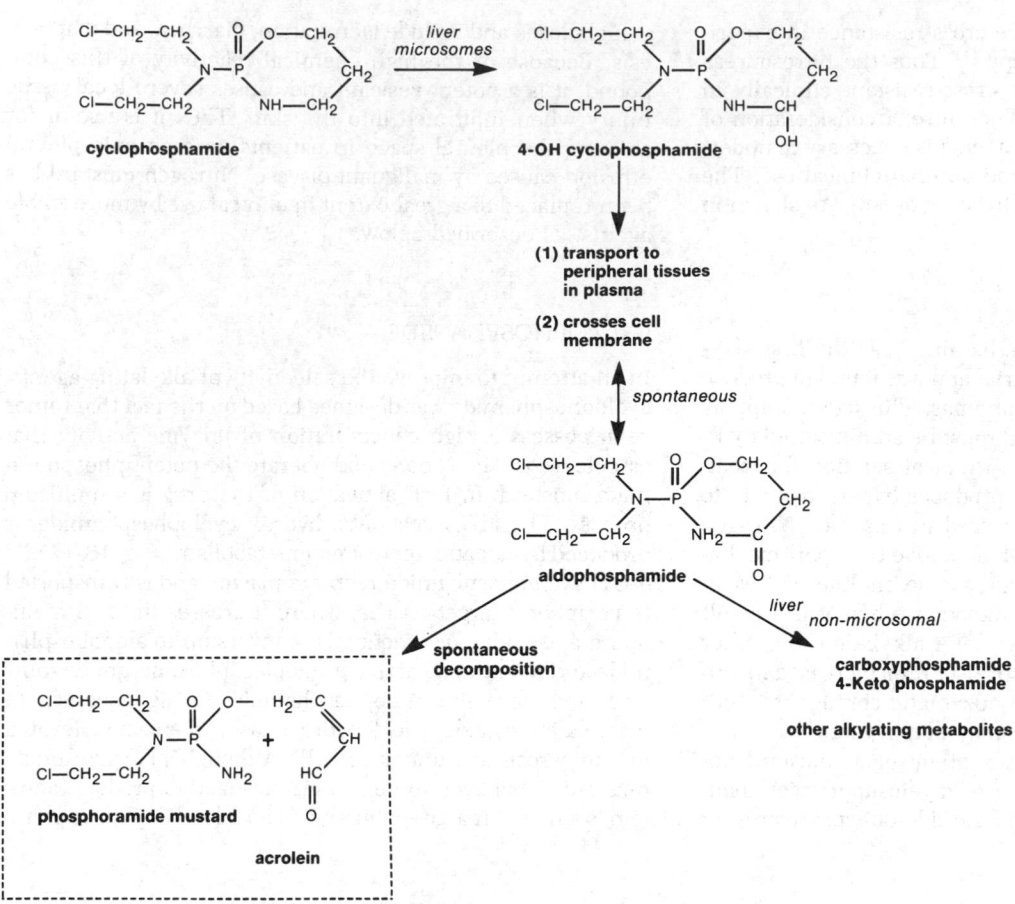

FIG. 18-14. Metabolism of cyclophosphamide by hepatic mixed-function oxidase, and transformation into active intermediates.

thione and causing single-strand alkylation of DNA. Acrolein is excreted intact in the urine and has been implicated in the cystitis caused by cyclophosphamide. 4-Hydroperoxicyclophosphamide, a chemically stable form of 4-OH cyclophosphamide, has been used for selecting purging of neoplastic cells from bone marrow and appears to have much greater toxicity for tumor cells than for multipotent bone marrow progenitor cells.[109]

Dose, Schedule, and Toxicity

The toxicities produced by cyclophosphamide differ from those of nitrogen mustard. Cyclophosphamide is stable as the parent compound, is well absorbed orally (90% bioavailability), and does not cause local irritation if infiltrated during attempted IV infusion. It produces only mild thrombocytopenia in comparison with leukopenia. Nausea, vomiting, and alopecia are common side-effects with high-dose IV therapy. In addition, active products excreted in the urine produce two unusual adverse effects: hemorrhagic cystitis and inappropriate retention of water. Cystitis is particularly common in high-dose chemotherapy regimens or with prolonged periods of oral therapy and may lead to significant blood loss, thus necessitating withdrawal of the drug. Because cystitis is caused by local irritation from drug products in the urine (possibly acrolein), installation of thiol compounds into the bladder or systemic administration of N-acetyl cysteine or sodium-2-mercapto-ethane sulfonate (MESNA) mitigates this toxicity.[116]

The most effective agent for preventing cyclophosphamide urotoxicity is MESNA, which inactivates alkylating metabolites, including acrolein and phosphoramide mustard, by forming an inert thioether. MESNA is particularly attractive as a protectant because it dimerizes in serum to an inactive compound and thus does not inactivate hydroxycyclophosphamide, the essential metabolite of cyclophosphamide, in plasma. Upon excretion into the urine, the dimer hydrolyzes to the parent, mercaptan, which effectively neutralizes cyclophosphamide and ifosfamide alkylating species in the urine. MESNA is available commercially in Europe, but can be obtained only under individual patient exemptions in the United States.

A preventive maneuver for patients receiving cyclophosphamide or ifosfamide is to reduce alkylating metabolite concentration by diuresis.[117] Hydration of such patients carries some risk, however, because in high-dose infusion regimens, cyclophosphamide causes inappropriate water retention resulting from direct effects on the renal tubule. Hyponatremia, seizures, and death have been reported as a consequence of water retention. This toxicity can be prevented with furosemide.[118] In cases of severe or prolonged bleeding, installation of a dilute alum solution (1%) directly into the bladder may be required to stop the hemorrhage; the extreme measure of cystectomy may also be necessary if other measures fail. Chronic bladder inflammation due to cyclophosphamide may ultimately lead to malignant transitional cell tumors of the urothelium.[119]

Other toxicities include potent suppression of both humoral and cell-mediated immunity, although in low doses, cyclophosphamide is preferentially toxic to suppressor cells and thereby enhances cell-mediated immunity.[120] In low-dose schedules, it also enhances natural killer cell activity and macrophage activation and is synergistic with lymphokine-activated killer cells (LAK cells). These effects are highly dependent on dose and schedule of administration.[121]

Cyclophosphamide is carcinogenic in animals and leukemogenic in humans. It causes sterility that is potentially reversible in males and possibly reversible in females, and on rare occasions, it causes interstitial pulmonary fibrosis.[122] Renal and bladder tumors have been reported in patients receiving long-term therapy for both malignant and nonmalignant diseases. Acute myocardial necrosis also has been observed in patients receiving extremely large doses (> 100 mg/kg) of cyclophosphamide before bone marrow transplantation; most instances of cardiac toxicity occur at total doses of greater than 1.55 g/m². Other predisposing factors are age greater than 50 years and prior anthracycline therapy.[123]

Pharmacokinetics

The pharmacokinetics of cyclophosphamide and its metabolites have been studied to a limited extent; because the active metabolites are generated intracellularly from 4-hydroxycyclophosphamide, it is difficult to relate these studies to clinical toxicity. Cyclophosphamide and its 4-OH metabolite can be assayed in plasma by gas chromatography with nitrogen-phosphorous detection.[124] The half-life of the parent compound is 5.3 hours in adults, with somewhat more rapid clearance in children. The half-life for 4-OH cyclophosphamide is 1.5 to 6.0 hours and is primarily a function of its rate of formation in liver.[125] Of possible relevance to the selective action of cyclophosphamide is the longer half-life for repair of phosphoramide mustard adducts to DNA (8.5 hours) compared with 1.6 hours for nitrogen mustard adducts.[126] In patients with renal or hepatic failure, the serum half-life of cyclophosphamide is prolonged and correlates with increased myelosuppression.[127]

IFOSFAMIDE

Ifosfamide, a drug closely related to cyclophosphamide by virtue of its oxazaphosphorine ring structure, differs in its pattern of toxicity, causing less myelosuppression but dose-limiting cystitis. Like cyclophosphamide, it is activated by hepatic P-450 mixed-function oxidase, and alkylating metabolites are excreted in the urine. MESNA effectively prevents cystitis, even in patients with a history of cyclophosphamide-related or ifosfamide-related cystitis.[128] Other significant toxicities include cerebellar dysfunction, seizures, and altered mental status in as many as 30% of patients treated with high doses of ifosfamide (1.6 g/m²/d for 5 days, or >5 g/day as a single dose). The risk of neurotoxicity appears related to hepatic dysfunction.[129] High levels of a potentially neurotoxic metabolite, chloroacetaldehyde, have been detected in patients by gas chromatography.[130]

The drug is well-absorbed orally (100% bioavailability) and has a plasma half-life of 5 to 6 hours after either oral or intravenous administration.[131] It is usually administered as a continuous 5-day infusion in doses up to 2400 mg/m²/day, with equivalent mg doses of MESNA, or in doses up to 3 g/m² daily for two doses every 14 to 28 days, with 600 mg/m² MESNA every 4 hours for 48 hours. Patients should be hydrated, with a urine specific gravity below 1.010 before drug administration.

MELPHALAN

Melphalan, a phenylalanine derivative, was conceived as a compound that would localize preferentially in tumors, such as melanin-producing malignancies, that actively use phenylalanine or tyrosine. The resulting compound has a broad spectrum of antitumor activity similar to that of cyclophosphamide (lymphomas, breast and ovarian cancers, multiple myeloma) but has the added advantage of not causing hemorrhagic cystitis.

Melphalan enters cells by active transport, using a high-affinity carrier—the "L" amino acid transport system, which also transports the amino acids leucine and glutamine. In some tumor cells, a second transport system (which also carries alanine, cysteine, and serine) promotes melphalan uptake but is less effective than the L system at high drug concentrations.[132] High concentrations of leucine and glutamine can reduce melphalan toxicity in both bone marrow colony-forming units in vitro and in tumor cells.[133] Thus, amino acid concentration in plasma or ascitic fluid may influence the uptake and cytotoxicity of melphalan. The antiestrogen tamoxifen inhibits melphalan uptake by breast cancer cells.[134]

The drug shows variable bioavailability when given orally, and thus doses must be adjusted by this route according to bone marrow tolerance.[135] Food slows its absorption. After oral administration, between 20% and 50% of the oral drug is excreted in the stool. After IV administration, the parent compound disappears from plasma with a half-life of approximately 1 to 2 hours, a rate consistent with the rate of hydrolysis of the chloride groups in plasma, with little influence of dose. Monohydroxy and dihydroxy metabolites, as well as alkylated proteins, are found in plasma soon after IV drug administration. About 15% of the drug is excreted intact in the urine.[136] The drug should be used cautiously in patients with severe renal failure, and doses should be reduced initially in patients with greater than 50% reduction in creatinine clearance.

Because the parent compound does not irritate peritoneal surfaces and does not require hepatic activation, melphalan has been employed for treatment of intraperitoneal malignancy by direct intraperitoneal installation.[137] A 100:1 gradient in drug concentration between peritoneal fluid and plasma is achieved by this route, with little systemic toxicity. This schedule produces antitumor responses, but its ultimate usefulness in ovarian cancer and other intraperitoneal tumors has not been established.

Melphalan causes equal suppression of granulocyte and platelet production. These effects are reversed in 10 to 14 days. Alopecia is also common during extended courses of treatment. Melphalan appears to be more carcinogenic than cyclophosphamide. An analysis of acute leukemia in women with ovarian cancer revealed a 93-fold increase in incidence compared with the general, age-matched population and a twofold to threefold increase compared with patients treated with cyclophosphamide.[138]

CHLORAMBUCIL

Chlorambucil, a close structural congener of melphalan, has similar stability in aqueous solution because of the electron-withdrawing properties of its unsaturated ring. Chlorambucil is given orally and is a convenient alkylating agent for treatment of malignancies such as chronic lymphocytic leukemia (CLL), nodular lymphomas, or multiple myeloma, which require long-term management. It has predictable myelosuppressive effects on both granulocytes and platelets but few other side-effects. Like other alkylating agents, chlorambucil has been implicated in late occurrences of AML and in pulmonary fibrosis.[139,140] Its pharmacokinetics are poorly understood, but the drug appears to be eliminated by metabolic transformation.

BUSULFAN

Busulfan consists of two labile methane-sulfonate groups attached at opposite ends of a four-carbon alkyl chain (Fig. 18-13). This compound is stable enough to allow oral administration but rapidly forms carbonium ions after systemic absorption through release of the methane-sulfonate group, leading to alkylation of DNA.[141] Although the potential for interstrand cross-linkage exists in the bifunctional structure of busulfan, such cross-linkage has not been demonstrated.

This agent is used primarily in schedules of daily oral administration for the treatment of chronic granulocytic leukemia, where its strongly myelosuppressive action provides smooth, long-term regulation of the leukocyte count. However, myelosuppression produced by busulfan is not quickly reversible; bone marrow "burn out" may last indefinitely if excessive doses are used, and close monitoring of blood counts is essential. The relationship between drug concentration in plasma and myelotoxicity is not known.

In addition to myelosuppression, busulfan causes two unusual side-effects: diffuse pulmonary fibrosis and an Addisonian-like state characterized by cutaneous hyperpigmentation and weakness, but without abnormalities of adrenal function.

NITROSOUREA

The chloroethylnitrosoureas are highly lipid-soluble and chemically reactive compounds that are clinically active against the lymphomas, malignant melanomas, brain neoplasms, and gastrointestinal carcinomas. Many derivatives that incorporate this basic structure but differ in their lipid solubility, side-group substitution, and aqueous stability have been synthesized in an effort to improve their therapeutic index.[142] Chlorozotocin, streptozotocin, and other glycosylated nitrosoureas (Fig. 18-13) have less bone marrow toxicity but have unproven clinical usefulness.

Chemical decomposition of these agents in aqueous solution (Fig. 18-15) yields two reactive intermediates, a chloroethyldiazohydroxide (II) and an isocyanate group (III). The former decomposes further to yield a reactive chloroethyl carbonium ion (IV) that forms a single-strand adduct with DNA and then, through a dehalogenation step, forms a second reactive site and cross-links DNA. Thus, cross-links are produced by both the monofunctional and bifunctional nitrosoureas.[143]

In distinction to the classic alkylating agents, decomposition of nitrosoureas also yields isocyanates (III) that react with amine groups in a carbamoylation reaction. The isocyanates are believed to deplete glutathione, inhibit DNA repair, and alter maturation of RNA. However, although carbamoylation may contribute to the overall effects of the nitrosoureas, compounds such as chlorozotocin that lack significant carbamoylating activity still preserve antitumor activity. Thus alkylation seems to be a more important feature of nitrosourea action.[144,145]

The nitrosoureas have many of the same features as classical alkylating agents. Their activity is enhanced by nitroimidazoles, hyperthermia, and glutathione depletion. They do not, in many experimental systems, share cross-resistance

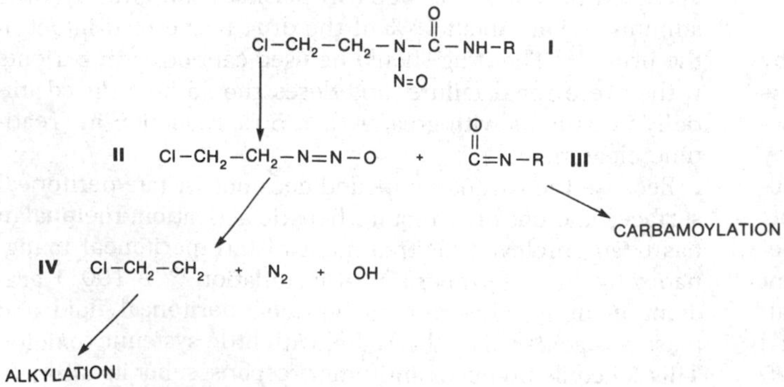

FIG. 18-15. Decomposition of chloroethylnitrosoureas to form chloroethyl carbonium ion and a carbamoylating isocyanate group.

with the classical alkylators. Nitrosourea resistance has been ascribed to increased levels of glutathione-S-transferase and to a specific repair enzyme, guanine-O^6-methyl transferase (found in 80% of tumor cells).

As a result of the extreme clinical reactivity of these compounds in aqueous solution, they disappear rapidly from the blood after absorption or IV infusion. BCNU has a half-life of 22 minutes, while the orally administered CCNU is not detectable as parent drug in plasma.[146] The cyclohexylnitrosoureas undergo ring hydroxylation by hepatic microsomes, resulting in decreased carbamoylating potential but increased alkylating activity.[147] The high lipid solubility of the nitrosoureas may account for their excellent activity against experimental and clinical intracranial tumors; the chloroethyl portion of CCNU crosses readily into the CNS, reaching concentrations that are 30% of those of combined parent and metabolites in plasma.

The toxicities of the clinically useful nitrosoureas are listed in Table 18-1. The most notable and consistent toxicity is delayed myelosuppression, which reaches a nadir 4 to 6 weeks after treatment and prevents the repetition of cyclic therapy at intervals shorter than 6 to 8 weeks. Severe and protracted leukopenia and thrombocytopenia may occur in patients receiving conventional doses of BCNU, CCNU, or methyl-CCNU, particularly in those who have received extensive prior chemotherapy. Prolonged use of these drugs leads to cumulative bone marrow toxicity and, in some patients, to an aplastic bone marrow. AML has been reported following methyl-CCNU treatment.[148]

Prolonged courses of treatment with BCNU and with methyl-CCNU have been associated with pulmonary fibrosis. The total dose of BCNU was 1000 mg/m² or greater in all cases reported and was 2733 mg/m² for the one reported case of pulmonary fibrosis induced by methyl-CCNU.[149] Chronic renal failure has been reported in children receiving methyl-CCNU for the treatment of brain tumor.[150] Azotemia or elevated serum creatinine levels developed after treatment was stopped in five of six patients who received more than 1500 mg/m² methyl-CCNU, and a decrease in kidney size was observed in all six patients. Total doses greater than 1200 mg/m² of either BCNU or methyl-CCNU are associated with an increased risk of renal failure.

CISPLATIN

Cis (II) platinum diamminedichloride (cis-DDP) is the only heavy metal compound used as a cancer chemotherapeutic agent and has a spectrum of unique biologic effects. The biologic activity of platinum coordinate compounds was first recognized in 1965.[151,152] Cis-DDP subsequently entered clinical trials in 1971 and since then has become established as a highly effective drug for treating testicular tumors, ovarian carcinoma, bladder carcinoma, and head and neck cancer.

The antitumor activity of cis-DDP is best understood in terms of its chemical properties in aqueous solution (Fig. 18-16). The tetravalent heavy metal platinum (Pt) binds two potential leaving groups, its chloride ions; in transposition to the chlorides are bound two NH groups in a firm linkage. Only the cis-dichloro structure is an active antitumor agent; the trans-DDP isomer lacks cytotoxic activity, possibly because of its inability to form stable intrastrand DNA cross-links.[153] Both chloride ions undergo a slow displacement by water, a process that may be accelerated in an environment of low chloride concentration (e.g., inside the cell or in urine), generating a positively charged, aquated complex. This activated complex then can interact with a nucleophilic site on DNA, RNA, or protein to form bifunctional covalent links analogous to alkylating reactions. Favored sites of attack are the N^7 position of guanine and the N^3 position of cytosine.[154] A variety of bifunctional and monofunctional covalent bonds are possible, including intrastrand cross-links, interstrand links, and DNA–protein complexes.[155] The formation of intrastrand cross-links, a type of bond not formed by *trans*-DDP, may be an important feature of cis-DDP action, particularly those links that form between the N^7, N^1, or O^6 of one guanine base and the N^3 of a neighboring cytosine.

The consequences of cis-DDP attack on DNA include changes in DNA conformation and inhibition of DNA synthesis.[156] The formation of cross-links is a slow process that continues for hours after drug exposure and is opposed by enzymatic repair processes that excise and rebuild damaged segments of DNA and ultimately determine cytotoxicity.[157,158] DNA cross-links also may be prevented by preincubating the drug with thiourea, which combines readily with the aquated platinum binding sites.[159] Thiourea also can reverse interstrand cross-links in isolated DNA, but the concentrations of thiol required for this reversal cannot be achieved within intact cells.

Other thiols, including sodium thiosulfate, which decreases cis-DDP systemic toxicity, and diethyl dithiocarbamate, which specifically prevents cis-DDP renal toxicity, are potentially of clinical value, particularly in conjunction with

FIG. 18-16. Cis-diamminedichloroplatinum: generation of a reactive complex in aqueous solution.

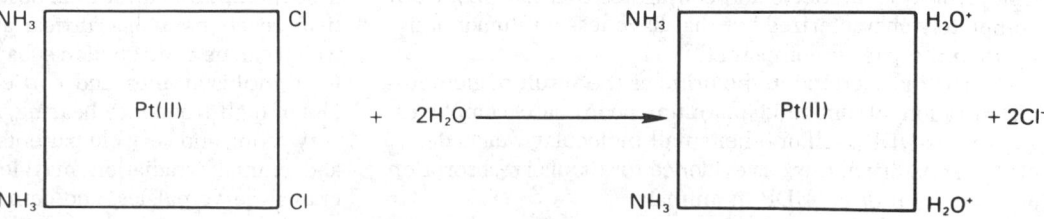

intraperitoneal cis-DDP, or during high-dose cis-DDP therapy.[160] The radioprotector WR2721 also ameliorates platinum toxicity by conjugation with the reactive aquated drug; this combination is undergoing clinical evaluation.[161]

The cell-cycle dependence of cis-DDP is poorly understood. It appears that some cells are most sensitive to cis-DDP when exposed during the G_1 (intermitotic) phase of the cycle, possibly because of the delay in cross-link formation, which would then be maximal during the following S phase.[162] A delay in transit through S phase and the succeeding cell cycle is induced by drug treatment.

Little is known about the mechanisms of resistance to cis-DDP. Resistance to cis-DDP in some experimental studies has been linked to elevated levels of intracellular glutathione or the thiol-rich protein metallothionine.[163] It is likely that the ability to prevent (through sulfhydryl reaction) or repair DNA cross-links plays an important role in determining sensitivity to this drug.[158] Platinum compounds do not share cross-resistance with nitrosoureas or classic alkylating agents in most experimental systems. Although specific processes that repair DNA-platinum adducts have not been identified, it has been possible to quantitate adduct formation with extreme sensitivity and to correlate the level of adducts in peripheral blood leukocytes with the dose of cis-DDP and response to treatment in patients with ovarian cancer.[164] These findings imply that pharmacogenetic or metabolic characteristics common to tumor and peripheral tissues determine response to cis-DDP.

Clinical Pharmacology

Cis-platinum is measured readily in biologic fluids by flameless atomic absorption spectroscopy, a technique that has high sensitivity (about 0.3 μg/ml) and specificity but is not routinely available in pharmacology laboratories.[165] HPLC allows separation and quantitation of the parent drug and its hydrolysis products.[166] Because of the high rate of covalent binding to protein, plasma samples must undergo ultrafiltration to separate the active unbound drug from the inactive protein-bound complex.

The clearance of total platinum from plasma proceeds rapidly during the first 2 hours after injection, but thereafter levels decline very slowly because of covalent binding of the drug to serum proteins.[167] Unbound platinum, presumably the parent drug or the aquated derivative, falls with a half-life of 30 to 40 minutes.[168] Maximum drug concentrations reach approximately 2.5×10^{-5} M for doses of 100 mg/m². Twenty percent to 75% of administered drug is excreted in the urine in the 24 hours after administration, the remainder representing drug bound to tissues or plasma protein.[169] Cis-DDP penetrates poorly into the central nervous system.[170] Even after simple incubation in plasma, the drug forms multiple hydrolysis products and conjugates that have not been completely characterized but that have less antitumor activity than the parent compound.[171]

Cis-DDP is excreted in the urine as the result of glomerular filtration of unbound platinum coordinate complexes, such as cis-DDP itself or other small-molecular-weight derivatives. In addition, there is evidence for tubular reabsorption and secretion of cis-DDP in animals.[172]

Dose, Schedule, and Toxicity

The mode of clinical administration of cis-DDP is determined largely by its primary toxicities. Because of its nephrotoxic potential, cis-DDP usually is administered after a 4-hour to 6-hour period of hydration with 1 liter of fluid and 25 to 50 g of mannitol.[173] Mannitol or furosemide diuresis does not alter the pharmacokinetics of cis-DDP. The total dose administered in most regimens usually is between 40 and 120 mg/m² per cycle of therapy but depends on the frequency of cycles and individual patient tolerance. A common schedule is 20 mg/m²/day for 5 days, a regimen that causes little nephrotoxicity and tolerable nausea.

Renal toxicity of high-dose cis-DDP may be prevented by saline diuresis. The regimen consists of 250 ml normal saline/hour for 12 hours before cis-DDP, continuing for 12 hours after cis-DDP. Furosemide is given with each dose of drug. cis-DDP is administered in 250 ml of 3% hypertonic saline. This regimen allows a dosage as high as 40 mg/m²/day for 5 days with no significant decrease in creatinine clearance.[174]

Without hydration, the incidence of nephrotoxicity reaches 30% in patients treated with 50 to 75 mg/m² per course.[175] Although both the proximal and distal tubules are pathologically affected in animals, in humans the primary finding is coagulative necrosis of the distal tubular epithelium and collecting ducts.[176] A reduction in renal blood flow and glomerular filtration rate occurs within hours of cis-DDP administration, as does a series of changes in tubular function, including magnesium and potassium wasting and the excretion of various high-molecular-weight proteins.[177,178] Asymptomatic hypomagnesemia is a common finding in patients treated with cis-DDP, but magnesium loss may lead to symptomatic tetany. With adequate hydration, repeated cycles of treatment can be tolerated by most patients without clinical impairment of renal function.

Nausea and vomiting are frequent and persistent in patients taking cis-DDP and are relieved only partially by standard antiemetics. The severity of these symptoms can be reduced by dividing the dose into smaller doses given once daily for 5 days. Metoclopramide (3 mg/kg intravenously) with dexamethasone (20 mg intravenously) and diphenhydramine (50 mg intravenously) ameliorate but do not prevent emesis. Myelosuppression is moderate at usual clinical doses but becomes clinically significant in patients who have received prior myelosuppressive treatment or in patients receiving high-dose cis-DDP chemotherapy. Both leukopenia and thrombocytopenia occur; significant anemia, occasionally caused by hemolysis, may develop after extended periods of treatment.

Other toxicities include a distal sensory neuropathy that develops after prolonged treatment, particularly after high-dose therapy and after total doses of 300 mg/m², hypersensitivity reactions such as urticaria, wheezing, and hypotension, which can be controlled in subsequent doses by pretreatment with antihistamines and corticosteroids; and a progressive loss of high-frequency hearing, an effect found most often in very young and very old patients.[179,180] Concomitant cis-DDP and cranial irradiation may lead to enhanced ototoxicity, cranial nerve palsies, and coma in pediatric patients.[181] cis-

DDP is mutagenic to mammalian cells and is carcinogenic in animals.

cis-DDP has been administered by intraperitoneal instillation in patients with intraperitoneal malignancy; 200 mg/m² cis-DDP is diluted in 2 liters of dialysate and instilled in the peritoneal cavity. Residual peritoneal fluid is withdrawn after 4 hours. Systemic toxicity can be prevented by simultaneous administration of sodium thiosulfate (7.5 gm/m² by bolus followed by 2.13 gm/m² over 12 hours). The half-life of intraperitoneal cis-DDP is approximately 1 hour, and most drug is inactivated before it reaches the systemic circulation. Thus, high local concentrations of cis-DDP (approaching 1 mM) can be achieved in the peritoneal cavity with minimal systemic toxicity. A 20:1 gradient in free cis-DDP concentration is established between the peritoneal fluid and plasma. Although responses have been observed in patients with ovarian cancer refractory to systemic cis-DDP, the value of this therapy remains uncertain.[182]

Other experimental approaches to the prevention of cis-DDP toxicity have been considered, including the development of new analogues. Two analogues, CHIP (cis-dichloro-transhydroxy-bis-isopropylamine platinum IV) and CBDCA (carboplatin), produced myelosuppression but little renal toxicity or ototoxicity in initial trials. CBDCA has the most promising antitumor activity (ovarian cancer, testicular cancer, and head and neck cancer). It is less reactive in solution than cis-DDP and is limited by thrombocytopenia and leukopenia, with minimal or no toxicity to the kidneys, hearing, and peripheral nerves. CBDCA is eliminated by renal excretion; dose adjustment should be based on creatinine clearance.[183]

ANTITUMOR ANTIBIOTICS

BLEOMYCIN

One of the most unusual structures that has antitumor activity is bleomycin, a mixture of small-molecular-weight (1500 daltons) peptides isolated from the fungus *Streptomyces verticullus*. Bleomycin is one of a family of antibiotic peptides that possess both antitumor and antimicrobial activity. The bleomycin mixture contains mostly the A_2 peptide, the unique pharmacologic properties of which have been characterized extensively.

The structure of the A_2 compound consists of a DNA-binding fragment and an iron-binding portion located at the opposite end of the molecule. The primary action of bleomycin is to produce single-strand and double-strand breaks in DNA.[184] The sequence of events leading to DNA breakage begins with the binding to DNA, preferentially to G-T or G-C sequences. Ferrous ion (Fe^{2+}), which is bound intimately to the imidazole, pyrimidine, and other nitrogen-containing groups of bleomycin, undergoes spontaneous or enzymatic oxidation to the Fe^{3+} state. The electron that is liberated in this reaction is accepted by oxygen and forms active oxygen intermediates, such as the superoxide or hydroxyl radicals. These radicals, in turn, attack the 4'-H of deoxyribose, leading to cleavage of the sugar and release of its attached base, usually thymine, cytosine, or their propenal adducts.[185] The action of bleomycin is specific for DNA and is not exerted against RNA.

There appears to be some cytokinetic specificity to bleomycin cell kill.[186] Cells in synchronized culture systems are most susceptible during the premitotic or G_2 phase, or in the mitotic phase of the cell cycle. However, cells exposed during G_1, also are killed, and it is not known whether rapid cell division predisposes to cytotoxicity. The possibility of increasing cell kill by exposing cells during the G_2 phase has prompted trials of bleomycin administration by continuous infusion.

The DNA lesions produced by bleomycin are visible as chromosomal breaks and deletions. It seems likely that repair processes play an important role in determining the lethality of these lesions because repair of potentially lethal damage occurs in cultured cells exposed to this agent.[187] There is indirect evidence that the same processes required to repair ionizing radiation damage also are used in bleomycin repair. The repair process is inhibited by calmodulin antagonists such as trifluoperazine.[188] Glutathione enhances bleomycin cytotoxicity, as does misonidazole.[189] Enhancement by glutathione likely relates to the need to recycle the Fe^{3+} ion to its active Fe^{2+} state with each oxidation–reduction cycle.

Little is known about the determinants of bleomycin resistance in tumor cells. A bleomycin-inactivating enzyme has been detected in both normal and malignant cells and is particularly prominent in the liver.[190] The enzyme is found in low concentrations in lung and skin; its concentration in lung varies from one species to another and appears to determine the susceptibility to pulmonary injury.[191] Increased degradative activity has been found in resistant experimental tumors.[192]

Clinical Pharmacology and Pharmacokinetics

The most sensitive and reliable technique for assay of bleomycin is radioimmunoassay; ^{125}I or ^{57}Co-bleomycin is used in this assay.[193]

Bleomycin is administered by parenteral injection, either subcutaneously (SC), intramuscularly (IM), or IV. There are no obvious differences in clinical response rates associated with the different routes, although continuous IV infusion has been used widely in the curative treatment of testicular cancer (see Chap. 35). Bleomycin has a two-phased plasma disappearance curve with half-lives of 24 minutes and 2 to 4 hours. Peak plasma concentrations reach 1 to 10 mU/ml after IV bolus doses of 15 U/m². The postinfusion half-life is approximately 3 hours, a value similar to the β-half-life following bolus administration. Most bleomycin is excreted unchanged in the urine in patients with normal renal function.[194]

Bleomycin pharmacokinetics are altered markedly in patients with abnormal renal function. A half-life of 21 hours has been observed in a patient with a creatinine clearance of 11 ml/min. It thus would be wise to decrease the dosage of bleomycin by 50% to 75% in patients with severely compromised renal function, who are at high risk for pulmonary toxicity, probably because of altered drug-excretion rates.

In addition to conventional routes of administration, bleomycin may be injected into the pleural or peritoneal space to control malignant effusions.[195] Intracavitary doses of 60 mg/m² provide high-effusion concentrations of up to 50 mU/ml, or approximately tenfold higher levels than in plasma. About 50% of an intracavitary dose enters the systemic circulation; the remaining fraction either is metabolized in the pleural or peritoneal cavity or is eliminated in its first pass through the portal circulation.

Clinical Toxicity

In contrast to most antitumor agents, bleomycin has little myelosuppressive toxicity. Only at high doses (> 25 mg/m²) or in patients with severely compromised bone marrow is a decrease in white blood cell count or platelet count observed. The primary toxicity of bleomycin is subacute or chronic pneumonitis that progresses to interstitial fibrosis.

The first signs are cough, dyspnea, and fever. The carbon monoxide diffusion capacity of the lung is decreased progressively with increased total doses of the drug, particularly above 250 mg, and the incidence of clinically significant pulmonary toxicity reaches 10% at total doses of 450 mg or greater.[196] Carbon monoxide diffusion capacity does not appear to be a reliable predictor of impending pulmonary toxicity in asymptomatic patients, most of whom will experience a steady, dose-related decrease of 10% to 15% in this sign over the course of treatment.[197] Toxicity is most frequent in older patients (over 70 years of age), in those with underlying lung disease such as emphysema, and in those previously treated with pulmonary or mediastinal irradiation. Although there appears to be a close relationship between total dose and risk of toxicity, well-documented cases have been observed at total doses below 100 mg.

There are anecdotal cases to suggest that pulmonary fibrosis can be prevented with corticosteroid.

The clinical symptoms and x-ray findings of bleomycin-induced pulmonary toxicity are not distinguished easily from other syndromes commonly found in cancer patients, including progressive metastatic tumor (especially lymphangitic tumor), infectious processes such as *Pneumocystis carinii* or cytomegalovirus, and radiation injury. Radiologic abnormalities, including linear and nodular densities, which may become confluent, are detectable by CT scanning in approximately 40% of asymptomatic patients receiving bleomycin, even though routine chest films are usually negative.[198] Symptomatic patients usually show bibasilar pulmonary infiltrates on chest x-ray film, although symptoms may precede the appearance of obvious radiologic findings. Gallium scans may detect drug-induced effects before routine chest x-ray films. Open lung biopsy often is required, and it reveals an acute inflammatory infiltrate, interstitial and intra-alveolar edema, pulmonary hyaline membrane formation, and intra-alveolar and interstitial fibrosis. In addition, squamous metaplasia of the alveolar lining cells often is found. Radiologic evidence of pulmonary toxicity and abnormalities in carbon monoxide diffusion resolve in most asymptomatic patients after therapy is discontinued. Resolution of abnormalities is often incomplete in symptomatic patients.

Bleomycin frequently produces an unusual cutaneous adverse reaction. Almost 50% of patients develop erythema, induration, thickening, and eventual peeling of the skin on the fingers, palms, and extremity joints. In addition, most patients develop hyperpigmentation of skin creases and a general darkening of the skin. Some patients also may develop Raynaud's phenomenon during bleomycin therapy.

Less frequent side-effects include acute hypertension, primarily in patients receiving doses greater than 25 mg/day, and hyperbilirubinemia. Fever often is observed in the first 48 hours after drug administration, and occasional hypersensitivity reactions, with urticaria and bronchospasm, have been observed. These reactions usually do not necessitate withdrawal of the drug, but pretreatment with antihistamines and corticosteroids is recommended for patients who have a history of allergic reactions to bleomycin.

In addition to its conventional systemic use, bleomycin has been administered by intraarterial infusion and by direct instillation into the urinary bladder.[199,200] The latter route causes a predictable and, at times, severe cystitis. Neither of these routes has proved to be beneficial in the treatment of cancer.

ANTHRACYCLINES

The first anthracyclines in clinical use, daunomycin and doxorubicin, are antibiotics produced from the *Streptomyces* species. These antibodies are, in fact, part of a large group of highly colored bacterial products known as the rhodomycins. There are exhaustive reviews of the structure and properties of the rhodomycins.[201,202] In general, these compounds, like daunomycin and doxorubicin, have a planar anthraquinone nucleus attached to an amino sugar (Fig. 18-17). Within this group, or closely related to it, are compounds that have a wide range of biologic activity, which include antibacterial and antitumor agents.

As antitumor agents, anthracyclines are matched only by alkylating agents in terms of their clinical usefulness. Daunorubicin is one of the most effective agents in the treatment of acute lymphocytic and myelocytic leukemia. Doxorubicin, on the other hand, is used to treat solid tumors, such as carcinomas of the breast, lung, thyroid, and ovary, and soft tissue sarcomas. As a result of this clinical activity, more

FIG. 18-17. Structure of anthracyclines.

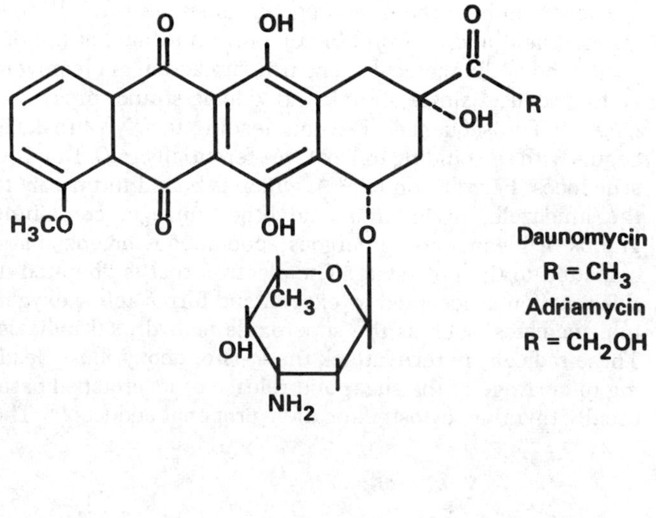

Daunomycin
R = CH₃
Adriamycin
R = CH₂OH

than 500 analogues have been synthesized or isolated from *Streptomyces*. It is likely these will provide the clinician with a number of new anthracyclines with different therapeutic spectra or altered toxicity. For this reason, we shall place some emphasis in this section on pertinent structure–activity relationships.

Mechanism of Action

There is no single, clearly defined mechanism of action for the anthraquinones. Anthraquinones, of which the anthracyclines are a subset, exhibit a wide range of biologic, biochemical, and chemical properties.[203] They are known to chelate divalent cations, especially calcium, and as a result can alter bone metabolism and dissolve kidney stones. Other anthraquinones have laxative effects. Because of the quinone-hydroquinone functionalities characteristic of the anthraquinones, these compounds can participate in oxidation–reduction reactions. Because of the size and planar nature of the anthraquinones, many agents in this group intercalate between strands of the DNA double helix.

Doxorubicin and daunorubicin are known to intercalate DNA, chelate transition metal ions, such as iron or copper, and engage in oxidation–reduction reactions.[204,205] In addition, these agents react directly with cell membranes at low concentrations, with resultant alterations in membrane function.[206,207]

Of these actions, we know most about the interaction with DNA. Both doxorubicin and daunorubicin act as intercalators with the planar anthracycline ring structure that lies perpendicular to the long axis of the DNA double helix. The B and C rings appear to be buried within the helix, with the A and D rings projecting out on either side. The amino sugar appears to add stability to the binding through its interaction with the sugar-phosphate backbone of DNA. DNA intercalation has been shown to block DNA replication and RNA and protein synthesis. However, the drug concentrations required to do so are far greater than those that are clinically relevant. It is now clear that these effects have nothing to do with the clinical utility of these drugs as anticancer agents. DNA intercalation does appear to trigger DNA cleavage by topoisomerase-II, an enzyme critical in the maintenance of DNA tertiary structure.[208] There is now strong circumstantial evidence that supports this topoisomerase-II-mediated antitumor effect in murine cell lines such as L1210.[209] This effect can be demonstrated within a clinically useful drug concentration range.[210]

Another school of thought advocates that the antitumor effect is due to the formation of drug free radicals.[211,212] A wide range of NADPH-dependent reductases, such as cytochrome P-450 reductase, xanthine oxidase, and cytochrome B_5 reductase, are able to reduce doxorubicin and daunomycin to semiquinone free radicals that, in turn, can react with molecular oxygen to yield superoxide, hydrogen peroxide, and the hydroxyl radical.[213] Several workers have shown that this process is the mechanism by which doxorubicin kills human breast cancer cells in vitro. Superoxide dismutase and catalase both protect the MCF-7 human breast cancer cell line at doxorubicin concentrations as low as 10 nM.[211,212]

Doxorubicin may kill tumor cells by either mechanism, depending upon the biochemistry of the tumor being treated. For example, the finding of free-radical formation in breast cancer cells may be conditioned by the high levels of microsomal enzyme activity in that tissue.[212] There are other factors as well. Drug free-radical formation is NADPH-dependent. NADPH is predominantly the product of the pentose phosphate shunt and is also used for such key biochemical processes as fatty acid synthesis. Perhaps because it must produce milk fat, breast tissue is second only to the adrenal gland in the activity of its pentose shunt. This elevated pentose shunt activity is also found in breast cancer cell lines and guarantees adequate NADPH for doxorubicin free-radical formation.[214]

One of the most unusual aspects of the anthracyclines is the ability of these agents to cause cardiomyopathy. Most of the existing evidence supports free-radical formation as the basis for this toxicity. Other hypotheses have been put forward over the years, but none has survived experimental scrutiny for very long. It is now clear that heart tissue is able to activate doxorubicin to a free radical at multiple sites, including the cytosol, mitochondria, and sarcoplasmic reticulum.[215] In addition, cardiac tissue has very low levels of catalase, a key enzyme in the detoxification of hydrogen peroxide.[216] In addition, doxorubicin destroys glutathione peroxidase activity, a second major mechanism of peroxide removal. Thus, doxorubicin stimulates oxygen-radical formation in the heart muscle while simultaneously abrogating the major mechanism by which the heart defends itself against oxygen radicals.

The major criticism of the free-radical hypothesis was that free-radical scavengers, such as tocopherol and N-acetylcysteine, have not been successful in preventing the cardiac toxicity in man. However, at the time these studies were run, the unique involvement of iron in doxorubicin biochemistry was not appreciated.[217] We now know that in most experimental systems involving cells or subcellular organelles, iron must be present for doxorubicin free-radical formation to result in significant damage. Doxorubicin is a remarkably active iron chelator, with measured binding affinities of 10^{28} to 10^{33}. The resulting iron–doxorubicin complex is very reactive in catalyzing a variety of free-radical reactions, such as the conversion of hydrogen peroxide to hydroxyl radical. Neither tocopherol nor thiols such as N-acetylcysteine are very effective in blocking this chemistry.

The logical conclusion of all of this work on doxorubicin chemistry is that the most critical step in the reactions leading up to free-radical-induced cardiac injury is the reaction between doxorubicin, iron, and peroxide. Thus, it is no surprise that the first clinically successful cardioprotective agent is an effective iron chelator, ICRF-187.[218]

This EDTA derivative was originally synthesized as an anticancer agent (Fig. 18-18). The initial phase I clinical trial showed that this drug was a remarkably effective iron chelator, causing a greater than tenfold increase in urinary iron clearance.[219] Preclinical studies had documented that this agent also prevented doxorubicin cardiac toxicity in a wide range of animal species.[220] More recently a randomized clinical trial has demonstrated that ICRF-187 is able to dramatically lessen the cardiac toxicity of doxorubicin in man

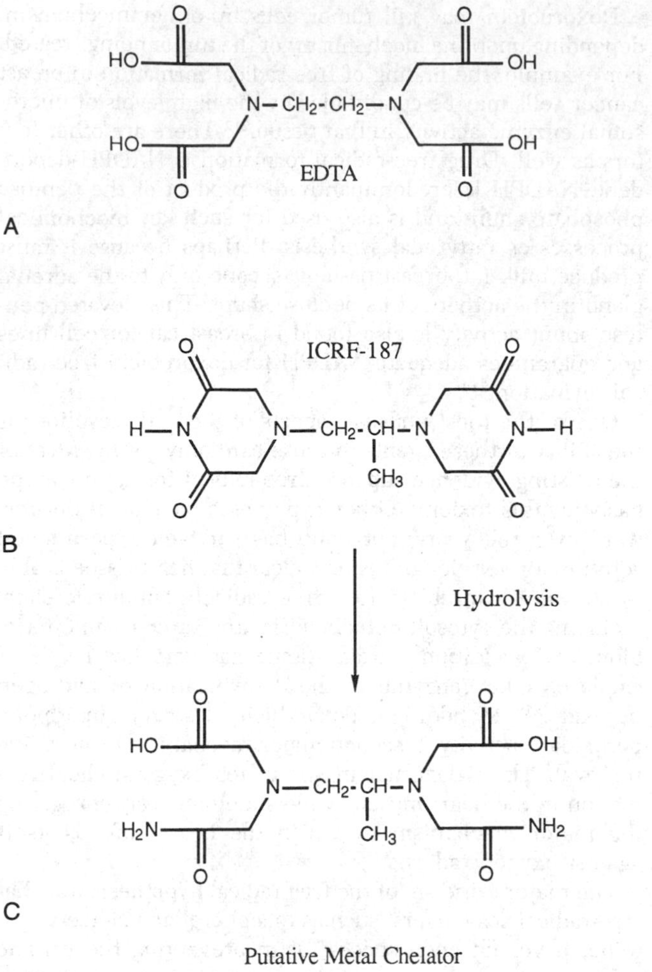

FIG. 18-18. **A**. A strongly charged anion at physiologic pH. Enters cells poorly. **B**. Nonpolar and should enter cells well, but a weak chelator. **C**. A better metal chelator, but will be highly charged like EDTA.

without seriously compromising antitumor activity.[218] While this study obviously needs confirmation, the result is entirely consistent with the biochemistry and preclinical toxicology of the drug.

Clinical Pharmacology and Pharmacokinetics

The clinical pharmacology of the anthracyclines is in its infancy. Only within the past few years has adequate assay methodology become available. For many years, thin-layer chromatography was the method used to separate the parent drug from its metabolites. It now is known that many anthracyclines (*i.e.*, doxorubicin) are unstable on thin-layer chromatographic plates and that significant artifacts resulted from this process. Currently, the only valid assay methodology is with HPLC, which allows rapid resolution of doxorubicin and its metabolites.[221,222]

The major metabolites of daunorubicin and doxorubicin are doxorubicinol and daunorubicinol, the products of reduction by means of aldo-keto reductase. These compounds ex-

hibit antitumor activity, although not as much as the parent drug. The parent drug and these metabolites also predominate in bile and urine. The deoxyalglycones, other metabolites of interest, are one of the by-products of semiquinone radical formation and thus are markers for this process in vivo. Other minor metabolites have been described, the importance of which is not known at present.[223] Although the pharmacokinetics of doxorubicin are undoubtedly complex, its disappearance curves can be fit to a three-compartment model with half-lives of 11 minutes, 3 hours, and 25 to 28 hours.[224] Clearance of doxorubicinol and daunorubicinol does not always parallel that of the parent drug.

The effects of renal and hepatic failure on doxorubicin and daunomycin clearance are important to the clinician because this information may provide a basis for rational modification of drug dosage in cases of malfunction of these organs. Renal clearance of anthracyclines is minor in magnitude, and there is no need to modify drug dosages because of renal failure. Both doxorubicin and daunorubicin are metabolized significantly in the liver. As a result, drug doses often are modified because of abnormal liver function, especially elevated bilirubin. Precise guidelines based on sound pharmacokinetic information, however, are completely lacking, and this subject warrants careful study. Nevertheless, existing information on the pharmacology of doxorubicin suggest that mild-to-moderate liver function abnormalities do not alter the pharmacokinetics of the drug. Furthermore, administration of full doses of doxorubicin in the face of abnormal liver function has not been associated with increased drug toxicity.[225] Because the liver is the major site of doxorubicin clearance, these observations are somewhat surprising. It may be that the prolonged terminal phase of doxorubicin clearance (half-life of 730 hours) is a function of the rate at which the drug dissociates from DNA, rather than a function of liver metabolism.

Toxicity

Both doxorubicin and daunorubicin cause bone marrow suppression and mucositis, which are dose-limiting. Alopecia is a nearly universal adverse effect that, although not life-threatening, often causes significant patient distress. Extravasation of these agents leads to severe local reaction. Erythema and pain usually develop within 24 hours and can progress over weeks, resulting in deep ulceration that can reach tendon and bone. These lesions heal very slowly and are difficult to skin graft. Multiple local measures used to manage this complication include ice packs and local injections of steroids, bicarbonate, or saline solution. Clearly, the best approach is to take all possible precautions to avoid extravasation.

Perhaps the most perplexing reaction these agents cause is cardiac toxicity. Clinically, two aspects are involved. First is an acute syndrome that can be seen for hours to days after a dose of doxorubicin or daunorubicin; it is unrelated to cumulative dose and can manifest as either disturbances in conduction and rhythm or pump failure. Electrocardiographic (ECG) studies have revealed supraventricular arrhythmias, heart block, and ventricular tachycardia. In addition, ECG-gated pool scans have shown major drops in ejection fraction that reach a nadir within 24 to 48 hours after drug administration. In certain patients, this can cause congestive heart failure. Some of these patients develop pericardial effusions, and this whole complex has been called the myocarditis–pericarditis syndrome. It can be severe enough to cause the sudden demise of the patient.

The other aspect of this toxicity is a cumulative, dose-dependent cardiomyopathy that can lead to congestive heart failure in 1% to 10% of the patients who receive a total dose of 550 mg/m² of doxorubicin. The pathologic features of this lesion are unique and can be quantitated readily by endocardial biopsy. This technique is valuable both in diagnosing the cause of congestive heart failure in patients who may have received doxorubicin and in detecting subclinical cardiac damage, which contraindicates further doxorubicin treatment. ECG-gated pool scan measurement of ejection fraction has proved valuable in detecting heart damage. It may be more practical than endocardial biopsy for widespread clinical use.

The mechanism of this cardiac toxicity was discussed in part earlier. It is important to note that three independent investigations suggest that this toxicity may not be related to the antitumor activity of these agents. First, antidotal agents such as ICRF-187 have lessened cardiac toxicity without affecting tumor response in animals. Second, new anthracyclines have been developed that, in animals, possess significantly less cardiac toxicity while preserving antitumor activity.[226,227] Third, alterations in drug schedule affect cardiac toxicity without changing antitumor efficacy.

Importance of Dose and Scheduling

The traditional method of administering doxorubicin was as a bolus at a dosage of 45 to 75 mg/m² every 3 to 4 weeks. It is with this dosage that the risk of cardiac toxicity as a function of total dose was developed. It is now clear that this method of drug administration is not optimal. Repeated small doses (every week) or prolonged infusions (>96 hours) are associated with a much lower risk of cardiac toxicity, without significantly compromising antitumor activity. On these schedules, gastrointestinal toxicity does, however, become a more significant problem.[228] Also, little has been done to work out how prolonged infusions of doxorubicin might be integrated into combination chemotherapy programs.

Analogues

While enormous effort has been expended on anthracycline analogue development, very few agents that have seen clinical trial offer any advantage over daunomycin or doxorubicin (Fig. 18-19). Epirubicin (4′-epidoxorubicin) has been claimed to be less cardiotoxic for equivalent therapeutic doses.[229] However, the advantage is not quantitatively impressive and may merely reflect differences in potency.

Idarubicin (4-demethyoxydaunomycin) has considerable activity in acute leukemia and may find limited use in that disease.[229] In addition, this drug also shows impressive activity in non-Hodgkin's lymphoma, with response rates of 55%, with a median duration of 6 months.[229] This drug has also

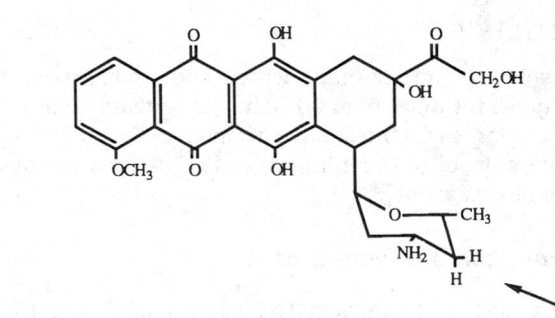
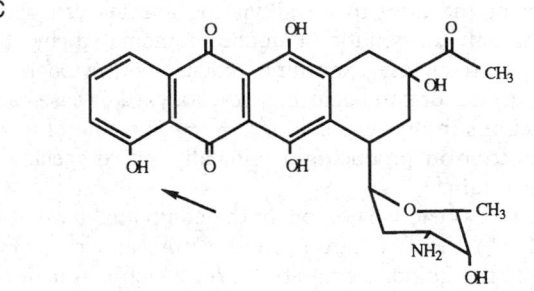

FIG. 18-19. **A**. Doxorubicin. **B**. Epirubicin. **C**. Esorubicin. **D**. Idarubicin.

exhibited very little cardiac toxicity in animal models and in clinical trials.

Esorubicin (4′-deoxydoxorubicin) has shown activity in melanoma, renal cancer and colon cancer. In colon cancer, one complete response and three partial responses occurred in 30 patients.[229] This relatively negative outcome to analogue development may reflect a genuine narrow range of opportunity in this drug class. However, it must be pointed out that several very interesting analogues have never been subjected to clinical trial.

5-Iminodaunomycin is quite inactive in all of the free-radical chemistry described for doxorubicin and is not mutagenic or cardiotoxic.[230] It is, however, quite active in stimulating topoisomerase-II cleavage of DNA. It is less potent than doxorubicin or daunomycin. Nevertheless, it represents the first member of a structural class of anthracyclines in which topoisomerase activity can be clearly separated from free-radical biochemistry and thus could signal a valuable direction for future development.

Mitoxanthrone has a similar ring structure to the anthracyclines in that it is also a hydroxyquinone. However, instead of causing free-radical damage, it appears to actually block doxorubicin-induced free-radical injury.[231] This drug does induce topoisomerase-II-mediated DNA damage, and this appears to be the mechanism of tumor cell kill. This drug does have promising activity in breast cancer.[232] The major controversy surrounding this drug is whether or not it is significantly cardiotoxic. Although this issue has not been resolved, the drug is clearly less cardiotoxic than doxorubicin. In addition, this drug certainly cannot cause cardiac damage by the free-radical-dependent mechanisms that have been invoked for the anthracyclines.

MITOMYCIN C

Mitomycin C is an antibiotic whose antitumor activity has been known for more than 20 years. Its primary clinical use has been for gastrointestinal carcinoma. Several reviews offer more detail of the clinical activity and pharmacologic aspects of this agent.[233,234]

Structure and Mechanism of Action

The structure of mitomycin C is shown in Figure 18-20. Activation of the drug to an alkylating species can occur either through enzymatic reduction, mediated by cytochrome C reductase, xanthine oxidase, or cytochrome P-450 reductase, or can occur in acid-catalyzed or base-catalyzed reactions in aqueous solution.[235,236] The role of enzymatic reduction in producing a clinically active species in vivo is uncertain.[237]

At least three reactive centers of the compound have been identified: (1) the C-1 carbon of the mitosane ring (Fig. 18-20); (2) the quinone ring structure, which can undergo one or two electron reduction to form reactive species; and (3) the urethane group, which can open to form an alkylating site. Once activated, mitomycin C alkylates and crosslinks DNA at the N^6 atom of adenine and the O^6 and N^2 atoms of guanine of DNA.[238] Cross-links result in inhibition of DNA synthesis and cell death. Mitomycin C also induces lipid peroxidation through the intermediate of oxygen radicals.[239]

Although some investigators have found evidence for preferential "bioreductive" activation in hypoxic tumor cells, which have high intracellular NADPH concentrations, a comprehensive examination of human cell lines under hypoxic and euoxic conditions has not substantiated this preferential activity under hypoxic conditions.[240] Resistance to mitomycin C is poorly characterized. In some, but not all, cell lines that demonstrate broad-base multidrug resistance against natural-product drugs, mitomycin C resistance is associated with amplification of the P-170 glycoprotein.[241]

Clinical Pharmacology

After bolus IV administration of 22.5 to 45 mg/m^2, plasma levels peak at an average of 0.4 µg/ml. The drug appears to have a volume of distribution that approaches that of total-body water.

Metabolic activation by reduction appears to occur in all tissues. It does not, therefore, explain the selectivity of this agent for tumor tissue. As a result of this ubiquitous metabolism, clearance of the drug is rapid. As with the anthracyclines, renal clearance is minor, and the role of the liver is defined so poorly that no guidelines can be given for dose modification in the presence of liver or renal disease. The drug may be measured in biological fluids by HPLC. The primary half-life is 54 minutes.[242] The plasma disappearance rate is uniform over the dose range of 15 to 60 mg/m^2.[243] The drug may be used for treatment of carcinoma in situ of the bladder by direct intravesicular installation; after 2 hours, 50% is recoverable in the bladder fluid, but none is measurable in plasma.[244]

Toxicity

The major dose-limiting toxicity of mitomycin C is myelosuppression. This myelosuppression is delayed and cumulative in a fashion similar to that of the nitrosoureas. After a single bolus dose, leukocyte and platelet counts usually reach a nadir between weeks 4 and 6. Typically, by the third course of treatment, doses have to be modified, usually to 50% or less of the initial dose.

Mitomycin C has been implicated as the cause of renal failure, often associated with microangiopathic hemolytic anemia in a syndrome called the hemolytic-uremic syndrome (HUS). Both hemolysis and renal failure appear to be precipitated by renal endothelial injury by the drug, as demonstrated by isolated renal perfusion experiments.[245] Mitomycin-C-induced renal failure is rarely reversible; corticosteroids, plasmapheresis to remove circulating immune complexes, or aspirin are ineffective in patients with HUS. The incidence of renal failure increases strikingly with the total dose of drug administered, being less than 2% at 50 mg/m^2 and rising to 28% at 70 mg/m^2 or higher.[246] The syndrome is exacerbated by blood transfusion, which may precipitate pulmonary edema. Hypertension and neurologic abnormalities frequently supervene in patients with HUS.[247]

Less commonly, this drug has been associated with interstitial pneumonitis and cardiomyopathy. The pneumonitis is uncommon, not dose-related, and exhibits pathologic characteristics similar to those of busulfan lung.[248] The incidence of pneumonitis is higher in patients receiving both mitomycin C and a vinca alkaloid.[249] Pneumonitis is enhanced by raised oxygen tension and appears to be mediated by lipid peroxidation resulting from the generation of reactive oxygen species.[250] It may progress to extensive pulmonary fibrosis. The cardiomyopathy has been reported in patients receiving doxorubicin and mitomycin C in combination and manifests itself as accelerated appearance of cardiac toxicity at doses of doxorubicin that, by themselves, are not associated with significant damage. This phenomenon is not surprising because both doxorubicin and mitomycin C can be activated to radicals by reduction, and in the former case,

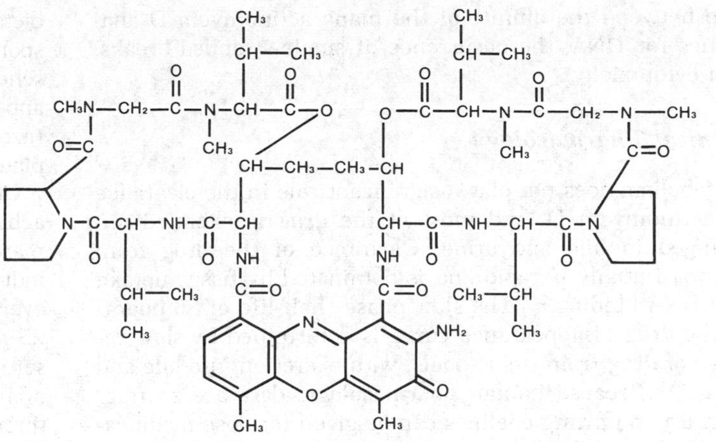

Actinomycin D

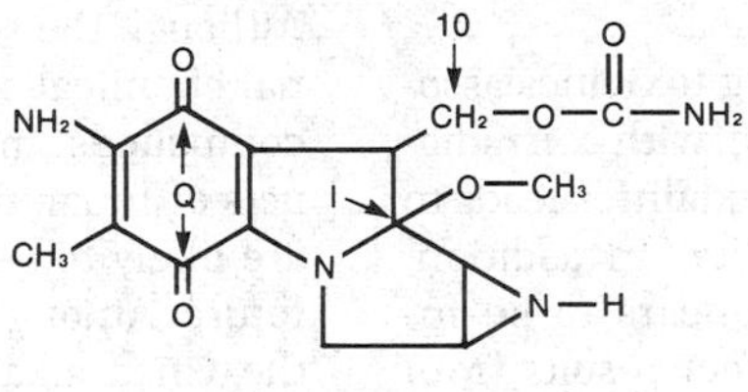

Mitomycin C

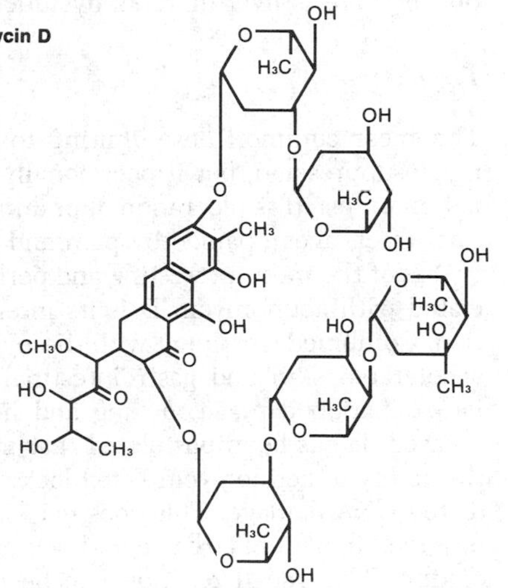

Mithramycin

FIG. 18-20. Antitumor antibiotics. Potential sites of activation of mitomycin C are indicated by arrows and include the carbon linked to a labile methoxy group (1), the C-10 carbon (10), and the quinone ring system (Q).

this radical production has been proposed to be the cause of the cardiac toxicity.[251] Extreme caution should be exercised in preparing for the intravenous infusion of mitomycin C, because extravasation leads to local tissue injury and ulceration.

ACTINOMYCIN D

Actinomycin D is a member of a large class of similar drugs that were first isolated from *Streptomyces* species.[252] It is the only member of the class to achieve significant clinical use. Actinomycin D is effective in the treatment of Wilms' tumor, Ewing's sarcoma, embryonal rhabdomyosarcoma, and gestational choriocarcinoma.[253] Responses also are seen in testicular cancer, Kaposi's sarcoma, and lymphoma.

Structure and Mechanism of Action

Actinomycin D has an interesting structure. It is composed of a phenoxazone ring chromophore that gives a red color to the drug. Two identical cyclic polypeptides are bound to the

chromophore (Fig. 18-20). This antibiotic binds to DNA by intercalation, with the phenoxazone ring inserted perpendicularly to the long axis of the DNA double helix and the polypeptide chains extending along the minor groove. This intercalation depends on a specific interaction between the polypeptide chains and deoxyguanosine and blocks the ability of DNA to act as a template for both RNA and DNA synthesis. At low drug concentrations, inhibition of RNA synthesis predominates, whereas at higher concentrations both RNA and DNA syntheses are affected.[254,255]

In addition to these effects, actinomycin D causes single-stranded DNA breaks in a manner similar to that of doxorubicin.[256] As with doxorubicin, there are several possible explanations for this observation. Actinomycin D can be reduced by means of cytochrome P-450 reductase to a radical intermediate; this has been postulated as the cause of the single-strand breakage. Another hypothesis is that intercalation causes sufficient strain on the three-dimensional topography of the double helix to trigger enzymatic nicking and strand breakage by topoisomerase-II. However, the role of single-strand breaks is unclear because there is no correlation between the affinity of the many actinomycin D analogues for DNA, the occurrence of single-stranded breaks, and cytotoxicity.

Clinical Pharmacology

Metabolism does not play a significant role in the clearance of actinomycin D, and most of the drug is excreted unchanged in bile and urine. Clearance of the drug from plasma initially is rapid and is dominated by tissue uptake and DNA binding.[257] The slow phase (half-life of 36 hours) of the drug disappearance curve is determined by slow release of drug from tissue pools, with excretion into bile and urine.[258] Because human pharmacologic data are so fragmentary, no firm guidelines can be given for dose modification if there is liver or renal dysfunction.

Toxicity

The most common dose-limiting toxicity of this agent is myelosuppression, but it occasionally may be gastrointestinal, manifested as ulceration of oral mucosa and gastrointestinal tract, accompanied by pain and diarrhea.

One of the most interesting and perplexing toxicities associated with actinomycin D is its interaction with x-irradiation. Combined treatment with these two modalities leads to accelerated skin and gastrointestinal toxicity. In addition, late radiation damage to lung and liver appears to be increased. It has been postulated that this effect results from the ability of actinomycin D to block repair of radiation-mediated DNA damage. This does not explain the recall effect observed in patients treated with actinomycin D after x-irradiation. This recall reaction can be observed even after a period of several months between irradiation and drug treatment.

MITHRAMYCIN

Mithramycin, an antibiotic isolated from *Streptomyces plicatus*, not only has antitumor activity against testicular carcinoma, but also has a specific hypocalcemic effect that is valuable in the treatment of malignant hypercalcemia.[259]

Mithramycin is an inhibitor of DNA-directed RNA synthesis. It is administered IV. Little is known about its pharmacokinetics and disposition in humans. There are no suitable assays for this drug at present. It is known to produce differentiation of human myeloid leukemia cells in culture and to produce remissions in the blastic phase of chronic myelogenous leukemia in man, possibly through differentiation.[260] This agent has a number of unusual side-effects in addition to its antitumor activity. It causes acute nausea and vomiting and occasionally diarrhea and stomatitis. More important, a hemorrhagic diathesis often is seen with daily treatment and is manifested as a fall in platelet count, a lengthening of the prothrombin time, and a depression of clotting factors II, V, VII, and X. Deaths resulting from uncontrolled gastrointestinal hemorrhage have been reported with this schedule of administration. Mithramycin also has serious renal and hepatic toxicities, the mechanisms of which are unclear. An alternate-day regimen of 50 μg/kg/day appears to cause predictable and tolerable toxicity and is associated with a response rate of nearly 50% in testicular carcinoma. This schedule is maintained on an alternate-day basis until signs appear that signal hepatic (LDH > 2000 U/100 ml), renal (azotemia), or clotting (prothrombin time > 15 seconds, platelet count < 100,000 cells/mm³) dysfunction.

Other adverse reactions include fever, myalgias, headache, and, uncommonly, vascular thrombosis. Because of its many serious toxic side-effects, mithramycin at present is indicated only for treatment of testicular neoplasms. However, in lower doses and for brief courses of treatment (15–25 μg/kg/day for 3 days), mithramycin effectively lowers serum calcium concentration in patients with hypercalcemia of malignant or nonmalignant origin. Its effects are mediated through decreased bone resorption and last for 7 to 21 days. In most cases, specific therapy directed against the neoplasm in question is required to produce permanent, effective control of the serum calcium level.

PLANT ALKALOIDS

Although the search for new anticancer drugs through rational chemical synthesis of antimetabolites has yielded useful compounds, many more antitumor agents are natural products of fungi, plants, and marine animals, and these sources are likely to be the primary resources for compounds of the future. Among plant products, the most important have been the vinca alkaloids, vincristine and vinblastine, which are derived from the ornamental shrub *Vinca rosea*, and the epipodophyllotoxins, VM-26 and VP-16, derived by modification of a product of the mandrake plant.

The vinca alkaloids are closely related structures composed of two complex multiringed systems linked by a carbon–carbon bridge. A single modification on the catharanthine ring, as shown in Figure 18-21, is the only difference in structure between the two, but the two compounds are significantly different in their spectrum of clinical action and toxicity. A third analogue, vindesine (deacetylvin-

FIG. 18-21. Structure of vinblastine and vincristine.

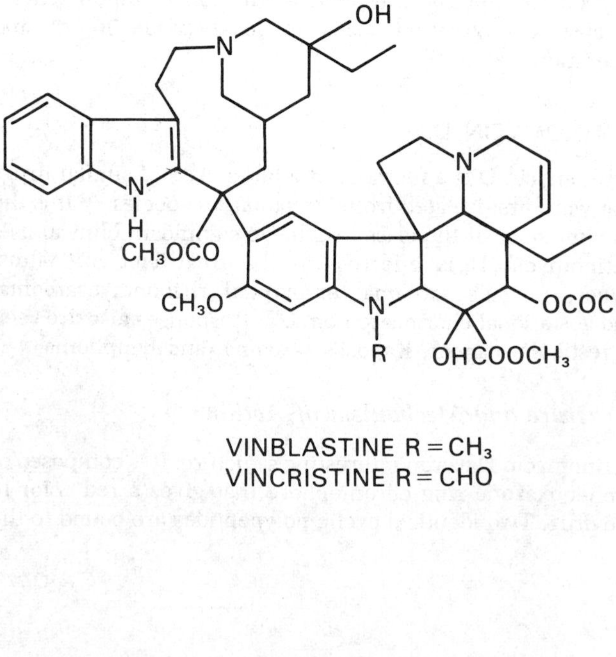

VINBLASTINE R = CH₃
VINCRISTINE R = CHO

blastine), which is also a metabolic product of vinblastine in humans, has activity against lung cancer and hematologic malignancies, but its future clinical development is uncertain.[261]

The vinca alkaloids possess cytotoxic activity by virtue of their binding to tubulin. The latter is a dimeric protein found in the soluble fraction of the cytoplasm of all cells; it exists in equilibrium with a polymerized form, the microtubular apparatus, which forms the spindle along which chromosomes migrate during mitosis. In addition, microtubules play a vital role in maintaining cell structure, providing a conduit for cellular secretions and for neurotransmitter transit along axons. Through their high-affinity binding to tubulin, the vinca alkaloids inhibit the assembly of microtubules and lead to the dissolution of the mitotic spindle.[262] A separate site for binding on tubulin is shared by two other spindle poisons, colchicine and podophyllotoxin.[263] A new spindle poison, taxol (Table 18-4), acts by promoting the assembly of microtubules.[264]

The primary action of the vinca alkaloids is an arrest of cells in the metaphase of mitosis. However, cells in vitro appear to be most sensitive to the cytotoxic effects of these compounds when exposed to drug during the late S phase of the cell cycle.[265] The vinca alkaloids bind strongly to tubulin in their parent form, but evidence is growing that these compounds may undergo oxidative metabolism to potentially reactive intermediates.[266] Ceruloplasmin, a protein found in high concentration in plasma of patients with Hodgkin's disease, can effect this transformation.

The mechanism by which the vinca alkaloids permeate cells is uncertain. There is evidence that they cross the cell membrane by a saturable process.[267] However, these experiments were conducted at drug levels well above those achieved clinically, or those required to kill cells in culture (1×10^{-8} M).[268] Resistance to the vinca alkaloids may result from mutations in tubulin, which leads to decreased drug binding, and from decreased ability of cells to accumulate drug. These latter cells have increased capacity to efflux drug and concomitantly are resistant to taxol, anthracyclines, actinomycin D, and other natural products.[269] This type of pleiotropic drug resistance may be accompanied by amplification of a specific membrane glycoprotein, called the P-170 protein.[270] This protein, an ATP-requiring transport molecule, can be competitively inhibited by calcium channel-blocking drugs, which reverse resistance in culture and animals.[271] There appears to be some specificity in the molecular form of P-170 induced by each vinca alkaloid, in that cells selected for resistance to vincristine, in early passages in culture, may not share complete cross-resistance to vinblastine or taxol.[272] This observation, perhaps explained by the structural heterogeneity of P-170, has its parallel in the lack of cross-resistance of vinca alkaloids in some patients with lymphoma.[273]

CLINICAL PHARMACOLOGY

The development of a comprehensive understanding of the pharmacokinetics of vinca alkaloids has been hindered by the lack of sufficiently sensitive and specific methods for drug assay. Most information has been obtained using radio-labeled drug, supplemented with chromatographic separation of the parent drug from metabolites.[274] Radioimmunoassays for vincristine and vinblastine have been described, although their specificity for parent compound versus metabolites is not known.[275] A highly sensitive immunosorbent assay that can detect as little as 5 pg of vincristine has been developed and may permit more detailed pharmacokinetic studies.[276]

The primary pharmacokinetic characteristics of vincristine and vinblastine are similar and include peak plasma concentrations of approximately 0.4 μM, followed by a multiphasic plasma disappearance with half-lives of 164 minutes for vincristine, and 190 minutes for vinblastine.[274,275,277] A terminal velban half-life of 20 hours has been observed using the radioimmunoassay. Little vincristine permeates into the CSF.[278] A minimal amount of either drug is excreted in the urine. Almost 70% of a vincristine dose is excreted in the feces, primarily as metabolites resulting from hepatic metabolism and biliary excretion.[279,280] The fecal excretion of vinblastine is only 10%, as measured by radioimmunoassay, although drug metabolites may not be measured by this technique.[281]

Vinblastine may also be administered by continuous infusion, in which the cytotoxicity of the spindle poisons is greater for cells in the S phase of the cell cycle and the rapid efflux from tumor cells is faster than with vincristine.[282] Continuous infusion of 2 mg/m²/d for 5 days, a commonly used regimen, produces vinblastine plasma concentrations of 2 ng/ml or about 2 nM, a concentration well within the cytotoxic range for this agent.[283] Serum levels above 1 nM are maintained for 4 days by doses of vinblastine of 6 mg/m² at 0 and 48 hours.

Vincristine and vinblastine are usually administered by IV bolus in doses of 1 to 1.4 mg/m² and 0.1 mg/kg, respectively. Vincristine doses may be repeated at weekly or longer intervals. A progressive and disabling neurotoxicity may occur with vincristine therapy, particularly in older patients, in patients with neuromuscular disorders such as Charcot-Marie-Tooth disease or polio, and in patients receiving weekly treatment.[284,285] The first signs of neuropathy are a decrease in deep tendon reflexes and paresthesias of the fingers and lower extremities. More advanced neurotoxicity may lead to cranial nerve and laryngeal nerve palsy and profound weakness of the dorsiflexors of the foot and extensors of the wrist. At higher doses of vincristine (above a 3-mg total dose), constipation, obstipation, and paralytic ileus may occur because of autonomic neuropathy. Alterations in mental status rarely accompany signs and symptoms of peripheral neuropathy; rarely, seizures may occur.[286] Direct intrathecal injection of vincristine is absolutely contraindicated, and if it occurs by accident, it leads to coma, seizures, and death. There is no effective antidote for vincristine neurotoxicity.[287] Although the motor and sensory changes and reflex changes may improve when vincristine is withdrawn, deficits may be permanent.

Vincristine causes little myelosuppression. As the result of inhibition of mitosis, megakaryocytes undergo endoreduplication, and, at low doses of vincristine, the platelet count actually may rise during treatment. In contrast, the primary toxicity of vinblastine is found in the bone marrow. Leukopenia usually is dose-limiting. Mucositis is another frequent side-effect, and neurotoxicity rarely is observed at conventional doses. Vindesine causes both myelosuppression and mild, but consistent, neurotoxicity similar to that caused by vincristine.[261,288]

In addition to the more common adverse effects, vincristine stimulates the release of antidiuretic hormone and, in rare instances, may lead to symptomatic dilutional hyponatremia.[289] This syndrome is self-limited and, if recognized early, can be treated with simple fluid restriction. Vigorous hydration should be used cautiously in patients receiving high doses of vincristine (> 2-mg total dose).

Although specific pharmacokinetic information is not available as the basis for dose modification in patients with hepatic dysfunction, it is advisable to reduce the dose of either vincristine or vinblastine in these patients. A reduction of 50% is recommended in patients with bilirubin above 3 mg/100 ml. No modification is recommended for patients with impaired renal function. Extravasation of the vinca alkaloids leads to local tissue ulceration and necrosis, a process that can be ameliorated by warming the affected area of drug infiltration.[290] Surgical debridement of affected tissue may be required.

The only well-documented drug interaction of importance is the inhibition of the efflux of methotrexate by the vinca alkaloids. However, this effect requires relatively high concentrations of the vinca alkaloids ($\geq 0.1\ \mu M$), and the combination of methotrexate following vincristine has not been shown to improve treatment results in experiments with murine leukemia.[291]

THE EPIPODOPHYLLOTOXINS

Podophyllotoxin, an extract of the mandrake plant, has been used as a folk remedy for treatment of poisoning, parasites, and warts. Like vincristine and vinblastine, it binds to tubulin and inhibits microtubular assembly, but it failed initial clinical trials because of prohibitive toxicity. However, two glycosidic derivatives, VP-16 and VM-26, have been synthesized and have important clinical activity in the treatment of lymphomas, small-cell carcinoma of the lung, leukemia, and testicular cancer. These derivatives differ only in a single substitution (Fig. 18-22) and have basic similarities in their pharmacodynamics, toxicity, and spectrum of clinical action.[292]

The mechanism of action of these synthetic derivatives is incompletely understood. They have no discernible effect on microtubular assembly and arrest cells in G_2 rather than in mitosis.[293] A more important effect is the production of single-strand and double-strand breaks in DNA.[294] Strand breakage correlates closely with cytotoxicity and may be due to the formation of free-radical derivatives of the parent compound by one-electron oxidation catalyzed by intracellular peroxidases.[295] Unlike the anthracyclines and actinomycins, the epipodophyllotoxins do not intercalate between the DNA strands, but they do form a stable terniary complex with DNA and topoisomerase-II. The enzyme then attaches covalently to DNA, forming single-strand, protein-associated breaks. It is not known which of these mechanisms is most crucial to the cytotoxic action. As with many other agents

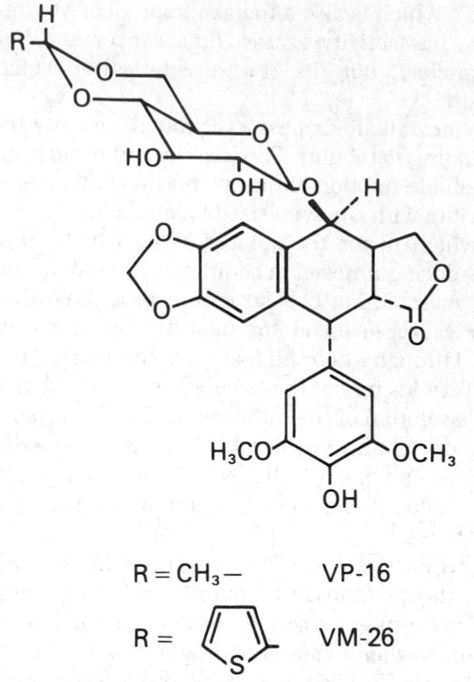

R = CH$_3$—   VP-16

R =   VM-26

FIG. 18-22. Structure of VP-16 and VM-26.

that cause DNA strand breaks, sensitivity to VP-16 is augmented in experimental systems by inhibition of polyamine biosynthesis, by drugs that inhibit DNA repair or synthesis, or by inborn defects in DNA repair, such as in patients with ataxia-telangiectasia.[296]

In experimental studies, resistance to VP-16 and VM-26 develops through amplification of the multidrug resistance exit pump (the P-170 glycoprotein) and through alterations in formation or repair of strand breaks.[297] The epipodophyllotoxins likely undergo significant intracellular metabolism and detoxification, although these processes are poorly understood.

The primary features of epipodophyllotoxin disposition in humans are given in Table 18-7.[298] VP-16 is administered either in the form of capsules or a drinking ampule or by IV infusion, whereas VM-26 is given only IV. VP-16 has a more rapid renal clearance, shorter terminal half-life, and undergoes less metabolism than does VM-26. Both drugs penetrate poorly into the CSF despite their high lipid solubility. The primary route of elimination for VM-26 is metabolic, although the products have not been identified; at least 30% of VP-16 is excreted unchanged. Doses of VP-16 should be modified in proportion to changes in creatinine clearance. Doses of both drugs should not be reduced for patients with hepatic dysfunction.[299,300]

TABLE 18-7.   Pharmacokinetics of VP-16 and VM-26

Characteristics	VM-26	VP-16
Plasma half-life	3.85 h	6 h
Urinary excretion (% dose)	45	45
% excreted as metabolite	79	33

VP-16 has been used in a variety of schedules and administered by both oral and IV routes. At least a twofold increase in dose is required if the drug is given orally in order to compensate for decreased bioavailability. Bioavailability by the oral route varies from 30% to 100% but averages 50% for the drinking ampules.[301] Maximum tolerated IV doses are 45 mg/m²/day for 7 days, 86 mg/m²/day for twice-weekly doses, and 290 mg/m² once weekly. VM-26 usually is given in weekly doses of 67 mg/m².

In standard doses, the dose-limiting toxicity for both drugs is leukopenia. Thrombocytopenia occurs in fewer than 25% of patients. Mild gastrointestinal complaints such as nausea and vomiting are reported by fewer than 20% of patients receiving IV VP-16 or VM-26, but increase to a 55% incidence in those receiving oral VP-16. A mild peripheral neuropathy, usually paresthesias or tenden reflex depression, is observed in fewer than half the patients receiving these drugs but may be severe in patients previously treated with vincristine. High-dose VP-16 (2400 mg/m² over 3 days) has been administered with autologous bone marrow reinfusion 64 hours after the end of chemotherapy infusion and produces severe mucositis and leukopenia.[302]

HEXAMETHYLMELAMINE AND PENTAMETHYLMELAMINE

Hexamethylmelamine (HMM) and pentamethylmelamine (PMM) belong to a unique class of antitumor agents that have uncertain mechanisms of action but significant antineoplastic activity against ovarian cancer, breast cancer, the lymphomas, and small cell carcinoma of the lung. Despite partial elucidation of the complex metabolism of HMM, the active intermediate has not been identified, and the drug has no clear relationship with conventional classes of chemotherapeutic agents. Its relatively mild myelosuppressive effects make this agent a good candidate for combination therapy.

HMM consists of a symmetric, 6-member triazene ring, with three attached dimethylamine groups (Fig. 18-23). PMM, a more water-soluble analogue, has one less methyl side-group. These methyl substitutions are removed readily by microsomal metabolism to yield various possible methyl-

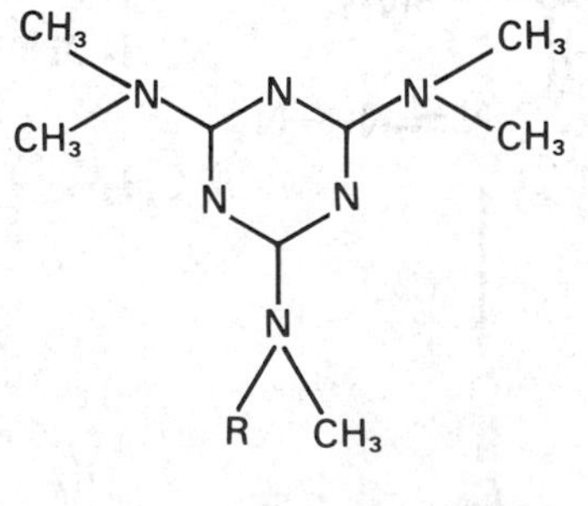

R = CH₃ FOR HEXAMETHYLMELAMINE
R = H FOR PENTAMETHYLMELAMINE

FIG. 18-23. Structure of melamine derivatives.

melamine derivatives, and corresponding quantities of formaldehyde, a weakly cytotoxic compound.[303,304] None of the melamine metabolites is cytotoxic in vitro in the absence of microsomes. HMM and several of its demethyl metabolites can be converted by enzymatic hydroxylation to methylol (R—CH₂OH) analogues, which are cytotoxic in vitro.

Experimental studies with HMM labeled in either the triazene ring or in the methyl groups have demonstrated covalent binding of both types of labeled compound to acid-insoluble material in both tumor cells and normal tissues, indicating possible alkylating action.[305] However, HMM is not consistently cross-resistant with classic alkylating agents in rodent tumors or in human cancer.

As in rodents, both HMM and PMM undergo extensive and rapid N-demethylation in humans. The S-triazene ring is excreted intact, whereas the methyl groups appear as respiratory CO₂, undergo metabolic reuse by the intermediate formaldehyde, or remain attached to the ring system of partially demethylating metabolites.

Following concentration steps, PMM and HMM are best measured by gas chromatography with a nitrogen detector or by gas chromatography–mass spectrometry.[306,307] Both of these methods can detect concentrations as little as 0.1 μM of either compound in plasma.

Because of its limited aqueous solubility, HMM can be given only by the oral route. Usual doses of 4 to 12 mg/kg/day are given for courses of 14 to 21 days. The bioavailability of HMM by this route is highly variable, yielding peak blood levels of 0.2 to 0.8 mg/ml.[308] This variability results from either variable absorption or variable first-pass metabolism in the liver. The parent compound has a half-life of 4.7 to 10.2 hours in plasma. PMM, given IV, has half-lives of 27 and 133 minutes, and therefore is eliminated somewhat faster than HMM.

Both HMM and PMM produce nausea and vomiting as their dose-limiting toxicity. These symptoms, produced by bolus administration of PMM, are particularly severe and have led to the use of more protracted infusion of PMM, which causes less emesis. Oral administration of HMM leads to a gradual increase in these symptoms over a period of days, limiting therapy to 2 to 3 weeks. Higher daily doses of HMM (above 12 mg/kg/day) are tolerated for shorter periods. No standard schedule of PMM dosage has been established in preliminary clinical trials, although single doses of 1500 mg/m² repeated every week produce dose-limiting gastrointestinal symptoms in most patients.

Both PMM and HMM also produce neurotoxic symptoms. HMM treatment may lead to mood alterations, hallucinations, and peripheral neuropathy; these effects appear gradually during a protracted course of treatment and disappear when the drug is withdrawn. PMM has caused convulsive death in preclinical trials and acute coma after rapid IV injection in humans.

DACARBAZINE

Dacarbazine (DTIC) 5-(3,3-dimethyl-1-triazeno)-imidazole-4-carboxamide is the product of a fortuitous misadventure in drug design. This compound resulted from efforts to synthesize analogues of 5-amino-imidazole-4-carboxamide, an intermediate in purine biosynthesis. DTIC actually functions as an alkylating agent. It is active against a broad spectrum of murine solid and ascitic tumors, but its clinical effectiveness is limited to Hodgkin's disease, malignant melanoma, and soft tissue sarcomas.

The probable pathway of metabolic activation of this agent is shown in Figure 18-24 and consists of hepatic microsomal-mediated demethylation, followed by spontaneous rearrangement of the product, which leads to elimination of a methyl diazonium cation ($^{+1}N = NCH_3$). This cation further yields an active methyl cation (CH_3^{1+}) and N_2. Methylation of nucleic acids has been observed in both experimental systems and in urinary excretion products in humans, but the active species of drug and the route of its generation are still not known.[309] In addition to the alkylating activity generated as described above, the metabolite methyltriazinoimidazole carboxamide (MTIC) inhibits purine nucleoside incorporation into DNA.[310]

In addition to its microsomal metabolism, DTIC undergoes spontaneous decomposition when exposed to light, yielding diazoimidazole carboxamide and azahypoxanthine, an active antimetabolite in its own right. This light-activation pathway may account of the antitumor effects of DTIC in vitro in the absence of microsomes, but there is little evidence to support any relevance of this reaction sequence to in vivo toxicity.

The effects of DTIC on cell cycle progression and its cycle specificity are uncertain. It appears to kill cells in all phases of the cell cycle and shows little schedule dependency in experimental studies.

Triazine compounds, in addition to cytotoxicity, induce differentiation of malignant cells at sublethal concentrations.[311]

The parent compound disappears from plasma, with a terminal half-life of 41 minutes. Up to 50% of the parent compound is excreted unchanged in the urine.[312]

Preliminary information indicates that the drug is absorbed adquately when given orally, but a similar dose given IV yields fivefold higher peak blood levels. Its disappearance half-life from plasma is about 3 hours. An ultimate metabolite, aminoimidazolecarboxamide, has been detected in humans.[312]

A variety of schedules of administration are used in humans. Intravenous doses vary from 150 to 300 mg/m²/day for 5 to 10 days, depending on treatment history, concurrent therapy, and patient tolerance. The drug also has been given by intraarterial infusion, but this route lacks rationale because of the likely requirement for hepatic microsomal activation.

The most significant side-effects are nausea and vomiting, which are most severe during the first few days of treatment and which may be lessened by reducing the initial dose and gradually increasing the dose during the course of treatment. Moderate myelosuppression may occur during the second or third week following treatment but usually is not dose-limiting. Other toxicities include a flu-like syndrome and possible enhancement of doxorubicin cardiac toxicity.[313] Fulminant hepatic venoocclusive disease, associated with fever, eosinophilia, and acute hepatic necrosis, has been reported in patients receiving DTIC as adjuvant therapy for malignant melanoma, and it may cause death.[314]

PROCARBAZINE

Procarbazine N-isopropyl-α-(2-methylhydrazino)-p-toluamide hydrochloride was discovered during a search for new monoamine oxidase inhibitors; it also was found to have antitumor activity and has since become an important agent in the treatment of Hodgkin's disease, brain tumors, and lung cancer.

The mechanism of action and metabolism of procarbazine are not understood completely; it is likely, however, that the drug requires microsomal metabolite activation and that the end-product is an alkylating agent, probably a methyldiazonium ion.[315-317]

FIG. 18-24. Metabolic activation of dacarbazine (DTIC). The initial step is enzymatically mediated, but the mechanism of subsequent reactions has not been clarified.

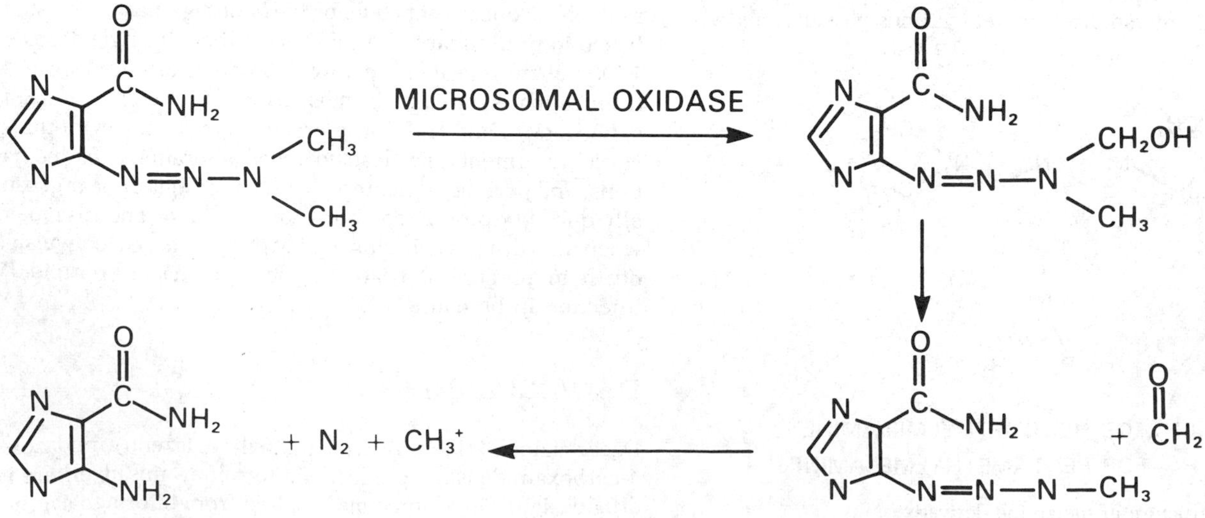

There is no reliable information on the mechanisms of cellular resistance to procarbazine.

The pharmacokinetics of procarbazine in humans have not been characterized completely. The parent drug disappears rapidly from plasma with a half-life of 7 minutes following IV administration. The primary excretion product is N-isopropylterephthalamic acid. Procarbazine-derived radioactivity in the CSF reaches equilibrium with plasma within 15 minutes after injection; the highly lipophilic azoxy metabolites also have been found in rat brains 10 to 30 minutes after IV administration.

The antitumor activity and the rate of microsomal metabolism of procarbazine are increased in rodents by pretreatment with phenobarbital, a microsomal enzyme inducer.[318] However, procarbazine itself inhibits microsomal biotransformation of pentobarbital and aminopyrene, indicating that it may have important interactions with antitumor drugs that undergo microsomal metabolism in humans, such as DTIC and cyclophosphamide.

Procarbazine usually is administered orally in daily doses of 100 mg/m² for 10 to 14 days. When given orally, procarbazine causes moderate nausea and a decrease in appetite, mild-to-moderate leukopenia and thrombocytopenia, and, less frequently, neurotoxicity, which is manifested by paresthesias of the extremities, drowsiness, or depression. These changes in mental status may be related to its inhibition of monoamine oxidase. Patients receiving procarbazine should be warned to avoid foods that contain significant quantities of tyramine, such as wine, bananas, yogurt, and ripe cheese, because these may provoke a hypertensive crisis. Other monoamine oxidase inhibitors such as tricyclic antidepressants and sympathomimetic drugs should not be used concomitantly with procarbazine. Potent hypnotics also should not be used, because procarbazine causes mild hypnotic effects and is known to depress the microsomal inactivation of other agents.

The neurotoxicity of procarbazine is the most prominent and disabling side-effect when the drug is given IV.[319] Total doses of 2 g/m² by this route produce confusion or coma in patients but little myelosuppression. Clinical benefit is uncertain.

Procarbazine has a disulfiram (Antabuse)-like action that may lead to sweating, flushing, and headache after ingestion of alcohol by patients receiving procarbazine. Hypersensitivity reactions also have been observed and frequently include a maculopapular rash and pulmonary infiltrates. In our experience, the development of a rash is not cause for withdrawal of procarbazine. The rash usually abates with concurrent use of corticosteroids, and continued treatment with procarbazine plus corticosteroids does not lead to progressive cutaneous reaction or anaphylaxis.

Procarbazine is a potent immunosuppressant in rodents; it prolongs the survival of the first or second set skin grafts across major histocompatibility barriers.[320] It has been used as an immunosuppressant in patients with lupus erythematosus and for suppression of graft-versus-host disease in bone marrow transplantation. Procarbazine also is a highly teratogenic and carcinogenic agent in rodents.[321] When exposed to the drug in utero, fetal rats acquire a variety of skeletal and nervous system abnormalities. The compound is highly mutagenic in the Ames' assay and produces both adenocarcinomas and AML in rodents and monkeys. An increased incidence of both solid tumors and acute leukemias has been observed in patients receiving MOPP combination chemotherapy with irradiation for Hodgkin's disease (see Chap. 49), and it is believed that procarbazine is the responsible carcinogen. Thus its use in treating nonneoplastic diseases should be considered carefully because of these late toxicities. It also is highly toxic to the reproductive organs, producing azospermia and anovulation.

mAMSA

Amsacrine (mAMSA), a 9-anilino derivative of the DNA binding dye acridine, was synthesized by Bruce Cain and colleagues in New Zealand in 1974 and was found to have potent clinical activity against human acute nonlymphocytic leukemia.[322,323] It is particularly valuable because of its synergy with ara-C, its activity in anthracycline-resistant patients, and its lower incidence of cardiotoxicity than anthracyclines.[324]

MECHANISM OF ACTION

Like other acridine dyes, mAMSA intercalates between strands of DNA and produces single-stranded and double-stranded breaks in DNA. Its cytotoxicity correlates closely with the formation of these breaks.[325] The DNA-cleaving enzyme topoisomerase-II has been implicated in the action of the drug, in that the enzyme forms a tight complex with mAMSA and DNA. Although the normal action of topoisomerase-II is to break and reseal DNA at points of torsion, in the presence of mAMSA, resealing of breaks does not take place and the protein remains bound to the free 5' ends of the broken DNA strand.[326-328] Another hypothesis has been proposed by Crooke and colleagues, who offer evidence that mAMSA in the presence of Cu(II) undergoes oxidation, leading to the formation of oxygen radicals and DNA strand breaks.[329] Evidence from the examination of a number of mAMSA-resistant cell lines supports the role of topoisomerase-II because the enzyme extracted from resistant cells cannot mediate strand breakage in the presence of mAMSA.[330,331]

mAMSA-induced strand breakage and cytotoxicity are greatest during the S phase of the cell cycle, when topoisomerase levels within the cell increase to a maximum.[332] Slowly dividing cells, such as fibroblasts or cells at confluence, are less sensitive to the drug. Resistance to mAMSA has been completely characterized but appears related to altered topoisomerase-II, which no longer cleaves DNA in the presence of mAMSA. Other agents, such as VP-16 and various anthracycline derivatives, that also cleave DNA through activation of topoisomerase-II share cross-resistance with mAMSA in some mAMSA-resistant cell lines.[333-335] There is little evidence to indicate that mAMSA is affected by multidrug resistance related to P-170 amplification, although verapamil, a calcium channel blocker that reverses multidrug resistance, does enhance sensitivity to mAMSA in some cell lines.[336]

CLINICAL PHARMACOLOGY AND PHARMACOKINETICS

mAMSA is administered IV in doses of 100 to 150 mg/m² per day for 5 days. It is concentrated in the liver, where it undergoes conjugation to glutathione and excretion in bile.[337] Its primary plasma half-life is 7.4 hours, but it is prolonged to 17 hours in patients with hepatic dysfunction, leading to recommendation of a 40% dose reduction in patients with serum bilirubin greater than 2 mg/100 ml. Less than 20% of drug is excreted unchanged in urine, and the need to reduce the dose in patients with renal failure is uncertain.[338]

Within liver cells and other tissues, including tumor cells, the parent drug undergoes microsomal metabolism to an oxidized derivative (mAQDI) that may undergo hydrolysis to form mAQI (Fig. 18-25) or may be conjugated to glutathione in a detoxification reaction.[339] Both mAQDI and mAQI are considerably more cytotoxic than the parent compound. Interestingly, the oxidation of mAMSA to mAQDI can also occur in the presence of Cu(II) and may be the mechanism underlying strand breakage mediated by the Cu(II)–mAMSA combination.[329]

mAMSA is highly protein-bound in human plasma, with less than 5% of the drug in its free state in the therapeutic range of 1 to 100 μM.[340] Its ability to penetrate the blood–brain barrier is likely limited by this high degree of protein binding.

The primary toxicity caused by mAMSA is pancytopenia, which reverses within two weeks of drug administration. It also causes acute and chronic cardiac toxicity.[341] The acute effects on the heart are a prolongation in the Q-T interval, atrial and ventricular arrhythmias, and, rarely, acute heart failure, all of which may occur within the first hour after drug administration. Although anecdotal cases suggest that prior anthracycline therapy may predispose to mAMSA-induced cardiac toxicity, the incidence of cardiac events appears to be approximately 1% in both previously treated and previously untreated patients. Toxicity may occur with the first dose of mAMSA, and in most affected patients there is no prior history of cardiac disease. Because of the frequent occurrence of Q-T prolongation with mAMSA therapy, investigators have warned that caution be exercised in treating hypokalemic patients.

In preparing an IV injection of mAMSA, the drug should be diluted in dextrose and water, rather than saline, because free chloride ions lead to mAMSA precipitation.[342]

L-ASPARAGINASE

The growth of malignant and normal cells depends on the availability of specific nutrients used in the synthesis of proteins, nucleic acids, and lipids. Some of these nutrients can

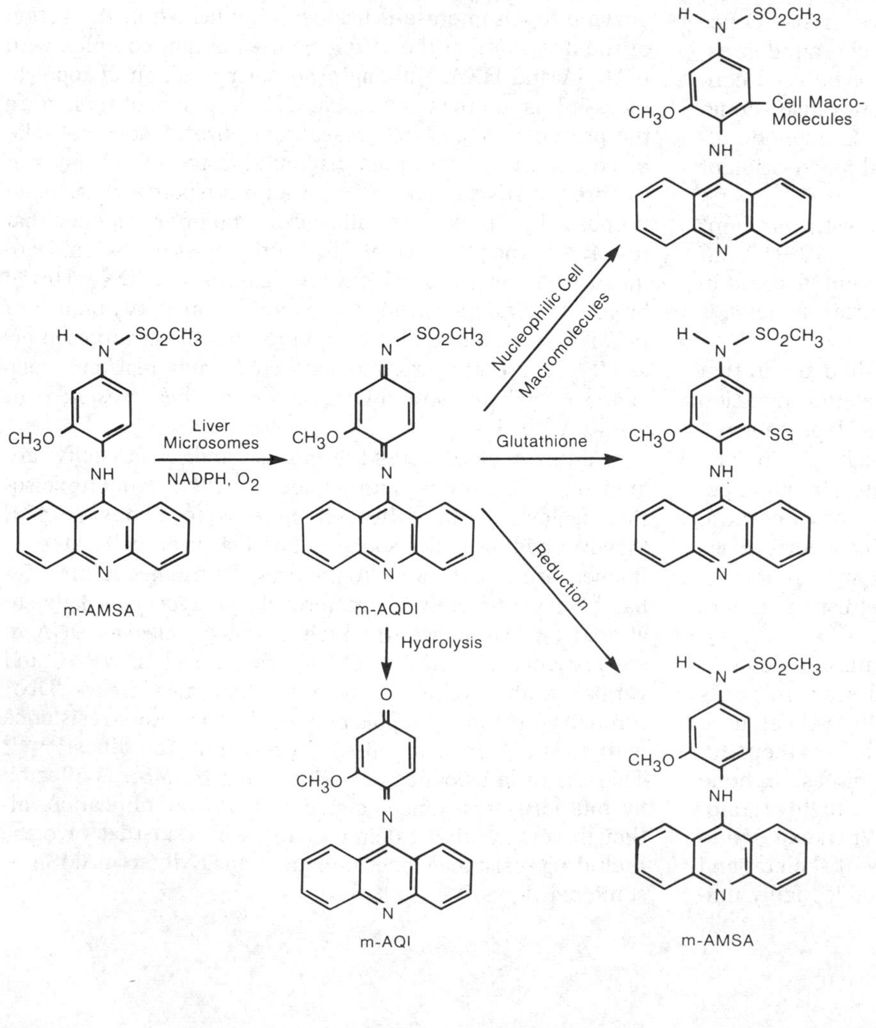

FIG. 18-25. Pathways of microsomal activation of mAMSA to a reactive, alkylating intermediate (mAQDI). mAQDI is inactivated by spontaneous hydrolysis, conjugation with glutathione, or reduction back to the parent compound.

be synthesized within the cell, but others are needed from external sources, such as another organ (liver) or from food sources (essential amino acids). Nutritional therapy of cancer has been directed toward identifying the differences between the host and malignant cells that might be exploited in treatment; these attempts, for the most part, have been unsuccessful because of difficulties in producing a deficiency state by dietary means and a lack of clear differences between the rapidly proliferating host cells and the tumor. The only exception has been the use of L-asparaginase in the treatment of childhood acute leukemia.

L-asparagine is a nonessential amino acid that is synthesized by transamination of L-aspartic acid (Fig. 18-26). The amine group in this reaction is donated by glutamine, and the reaction is catalyzed by the enzyme L-asparagine synthase. This enzyme is constitutive in many tissues, thus accounting for the lack of toxicity of asparagine depletion, but is present in low concentrations in certain human malignancies, particularly lymphocytes. In tumor cells lacking L-asparagine synthase, the amino acid can be obtained only from the circulating pool of amino acids.

In 1953, Kidd observed that the serum of guinea pigs had antileukemic effects when administered to mice.[343] Ten years later, Broome and co-workers demonstrated that the responsible factor copurified with the enzyme L-asparaginase.[344] Subsequently, highly purified preparations of enzyme from E. coli and Erwinia species have shown significant activity against childhood ALL and have become standard components of induction and maintenance regimens in this disease. Their antitumor effects result from the rapid and complete depletion of circulating pools of L-asparagine, whereas resistance to this treatment is caused by an increase in L-asparagine synthase activity in tumor cells. This increase occurs either by a process of mutation or by enzyme induction in response to the fall in intracellular asparagine levels.

Purified L-asparaginase enzyme has a molecular weight of 133,000 daltons and is composed of four subunits that each have one active catalytic site.[345] Enzyme from different bacterial strains have slight differences in specific activity, isoelectric point, and substrate specificity and affinity. Of greater clinical importance, enzymes prepared from Erwinia do not cross-react immunologically with E. coli preparations, and therefore may be used in patients who are hypersensitive to the E. coli L-asparaginase.[346] The clinical preparations have an affinity constant for L-asparagine of approximately 1×10^{-5} M, a figure tenfold higher than the minimum L-asparagine concentration at which the growth of sensitive tumors is retarded in vitro.[347] Thus a considerable excess of enzyme is required to degrade L-asparagine to sufficiently low concentrations.

The cytotoxicity of L-asparaginase results from inhibition of protein synthesis and correlates with effects of the enzyme on the incorporation of an amino acid such as ^{3}H-valine into protein. Inhibition of nucleic acid synthesis also is observed in sensitive cells but is believed to be secondary to the block in protein synthesis. As might be expected, resistant cells have high endogenous activity of asparagine synthase.

Most bacterial L-asparaginase preparations contain low, but significant, L-glutaminase activity (<5% of the L-asparaginase activity). The enzymes from mammalian sources and from certain bacterial sources (Vibrio succinogenes) lack L-glutaminase activity but have lesser affinity for L-asparagine.[348] Evidence suggests that the immunosuppressive properties of E. coli L-asparaginase may be caused by L-glutamine depletion and that cerebral dysfunction observed in patients may be the result of degradation of L-glutamine.[349]

In an effort to circumvent hypersensitivity reactions, bacterial L-asparaginase has been extensively modified by conjugation to dextran or polyethylene glycol; the PEG-modified enzyme has a much prolonged plasma half-life and, based on preliminary clinical results, is active against disease and well-tolerated by patients hypersensitive to unmodified enzyme.[350]

CLINICAL PHARMACOLOGY

L-asparaginase levels are measured easily in biologic fluids by assays that detect ammonia release or by a coupled enzymic assay.[351,352] The drug is given IV or IM; the latter route produces peak drug levels that are 50% lower than the former, but may produce fewer hypersensitivity reactions. The usual doses are 6000 IU/m² every other day for 3 to 4 weeks, or daily doses of 1000 to 20,000 IU/m² for 10 to 20 days. Widely spaced schedules of administration are used infrequently because of the increased risk of anaphylaxis.[353] Blood concentrations of L-asparagine fall below 1 μM within minutes of enzyme injection and cannot be measured for 7 to 10 days after completion of therapy.[354]

The concentration of L-asparaginase in plasma is proportional to the dose for doses up to 200,000 IU/m² and falls with a primary half-life of 14 to 22 hours. L-asparaginase is detectable in blood for 1 to 3 weeks after these doses. (The preparation of L-asparaginase manufactured by Merck & Co. has a somewhat longer half-life than does the preparation made by Bayer.) In patients who are hypersensitive to the enzyme, plasma clearance is accelerated greatly and enzyme activity may be undetectable in plasma as soon as 4 hours

FIG. 18-26. Pathways for synthesis of L-asparagine intracellularly and effect of L-asparaginase on circulating L-asparagine.

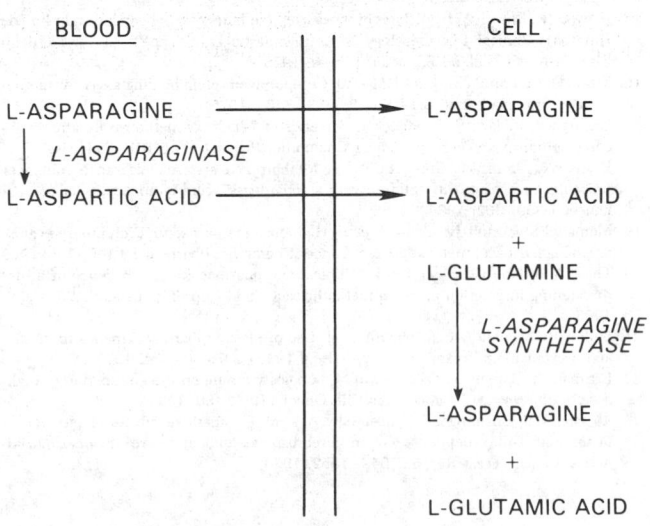

after administration.[355] The enzyme distributes primarily within the intravascular space. However, the concentration of asparagine in CSF falls rapidly, and an antileukemic effect is exerted here despite the poor penetration of enzyme into the CSF. The drug can be given directly into the CSF but exits rapidly from this site, and there appears to be no clear therapeutic advantage for this route.

TOXICITY

The primary toxicities of L-asparaginase fall into two main groups: those related to immunologic sensitization to the foreign protein and those resulting from decreased protein synthesis. Positive skin tests to L-asparaginase rarely are observed before drug administration, but anaphylaxis may occur with the initial dose of drug. More commonly, hypersensitivity phenomena, such as urticaria, laryngeal edema, bronchospasm, hypotension, and abdominal pain, occur after multiple courses of the enzyme. Passive hemagglutinating antibodies are observed in patients who subsequently develop anaphylaxis, and complement-fixing antibodies are found in serum after an anaphylactic episode.[355] The reason for the relatively low incidence of hypersensitivity reactions (< 30%) in patients receiving L-asparaginase may be related to the immunosuppressive properties of the drug itself or to the concomitant administration of other immunosuppressive agents. Patients hypersensitive to the E. coli enzyme can usually tolerate the Erwinia preparation, although about 20% ultimately become sensitive to the second enzyme.[356]

Other adverse effects are related to the inhibition of protein synthesis, the most important being the inhibition of synthesis of clotting factors. Either thrombosis or hemorrhage may result from L-asparaginase therapy, probably resulting from the depletion of vitamin-K-dependent factors, including protein C and its cofactor protein S, which inhibit clotting; antithrombin III, also an inhibitor of clotting; and factors II, VII, IX and X, which are essential for coagulation. Decreases in protein C occur within the first few days of treatment and have been implicated in early thrombotic events.[357,358] Other effects include hypoalbuminemia; decreased serum insulin with hyperglycemia; decreased serum lipoproteins; decreased thyroxin-binding globulin; and in 25% of the patients, cerebral dysfunction with confusion, stupor, or coma.[354] The latter syndrome resembles ammonia toxicity and in some patients correlates with marked elevations in serum ammonia.[359] Alternative explanations include low concentrations of either L-asparagine or L-glutamine in the brain.[354]

Other toxicities are not as easily explained by the mode of action of the drug; the most important of these is acute hyperamylasemia, which occurs in fewer than 15% of patients, but which may progress to severe hemorrhagic pancreatitis. L-asparaginase frequently causes abnormal liver function test findings, including increased serum bilirubin, SGOT, and alkaline phosphatase. Histologic examination reveals fatty metamorphosis.

Approximately two thirds of patients receiving L-asparaginase experience nausea, vomiting, and chills as an immediate reaction, but these side-effects can be mitigated by antiemetics, antihistamines, or, in extreme cases, corticosteroids.

L-asparaginase has no known effects on gastrointestinal mucosa or bone marrow and thus is a favorable agent for combination chemotherapy. The only well-established drug interaction is its ability to terminate methotrexate action, because it inhibits protein synthesis and thus blocks cells in G_1.[360] Polyglutamylation of methotrexate is inhibited by L-asparaginase pretreatment.[361] When the enzyme is given after methotrexate administration, the action of the antifolate is abbreviated. Large doses of the antifolate are well-tolerated if followed by L-asparaginase rescue.

REFERENCES

1. Chabner BA (ed): Pharmacologic principles of cancer treatment. Philadelphia, WB Saunders, 1982
2. Pratt WB, Ruddon RW: The anticancer drugs. New York, Oxford Press, 1979
3. Allegra CJ, Chabner BA, Tuazon CU et al: Trimetrexate, a novel and effective agent for the treatment of Pneumocystis carinii pneumonia in patients with acquired immunodeficiency syndrome. N Engl J Med 79:478–782, 1987
4. Sirotnak FM, DeGraw JI, Schmid FA et al: New folate analogs of the 10-deaza-aminopterin series. Further evidence for markedly increased antitumor efficacy compared to methotrexate in ascites and solid murine tumor models. Cancer Chemother Pharmacol 12:2630, 1984
5. Zaharko DS, Fung W-P, Yang F-H: Relative biochemical aspect of low and high doses of methotrexate in mice. Cancer Res 37:1602–1607, 1977
6. Allegra CJ, Fine RL, Drake JC et al: The effect of methotrexate on intracellular folate pools in human MCF-7 breast cancer cells: evidence for direct inhibition of purine synthesis. J Biol Chem 261:6478–6485, 1986
7. Allegra CJ, Hoang K, Yeh GC et al: Evidence for direct inhibition of de novo purine synthesis in human MCF-7 breast cells as a principal mode of metabolic inhibition by methotrexate. J Biol Chem 262:13520–13526, 1987
8. Kane MA, Portillo RM, Elwood PC et al: The influence of extracellular folate concentration on methotrexate uptake by human KB cells. Partial characterization of a membrane-associated methotrexate-binding protein. J Biol Chem 261:44–49, 1986
9. Schilsky RL, Bailey BD, Chabner BA: Methotrexate polyglutamate synthesis by cultured human breast cancer cells. Proc Natl Acad Sci USA 77:2919–2922, 1980
10. Dedhar S, Hartley D, Goldie JH: Increased dihydrofolate reductase activity in methotrexate-resistant human promyelocyte-leukaemia (HL-60) cells. Biochem J 225:609–617, 1985
11. Curt GA, Jolivet J, Carney DN et al: Determinants of the sensitivity of human small-cell lung cancer cell lines to methotrexate. J Clin Invest 76:1323–1329, 1985
12. Meltzer PS, Cheng YC, Trent JM: Analysis of dihydrofolate reductase gene amplification in a methotrexate-resistant human tumor cell line. Cancer Genet Cytogenet 17:289–300, 1985
13. Curt GA, Carney DN, Cowan KH et al: Unstable methotrexate resistance in human small-cell carcinoma associated with double-minute chromosomes. N Engl J Med 308:199–202, 1983
14. Rodenhuis S, McGuire JJ, Narayanan R et al: Development of an assay system for the detection and classification of methotrexate resistance in fresh human leukemic cells. Cancer Res 46:6513–6519, 1986
15. Bertino JR, Isacoff WH: Methods of measuring methotrexate in body fluids. In Pinedo HM (ed): Clinical Pharmacology of Antineoplastic Drugs, pp 3–11. Amsterdam, Elsevier-North Holland Biomedical Press, 1978
16. Myers CE, Lippman M, Eliot HM et al: Competitive protein binding assay for methotrexate. Proc Natl Acad Sci USA 72:3683–3686, 1975
17. Erttman R, Bielack S, Landbeck G: Kinetics of 7-hydroxy-methotrexate after high-dose methotrexate therapy. Cancer Chemother Pharmacol 15:101–104, 1985
18. Evans WE, Crom WR, Stewart CF et al: Methotrexate systemic clearance influences probability of relapse in children with standard-risk acute lymphocytic leukaemia. Lancet 1:359–362, 1984
19. Monjanel S, Rigault JP, Cano JP et al: High-dose methotrexate: Preliminary evaluation of a pharmacokinetic approach. Cancer Chemother Pharmacol 3:189–196, 1979
20. Thyss A, Milano G, Kubar J et al: Clinical and pharmacokinetic evidence of a life-threatening interaction between methotrexate and ketoprofen. Lancet 1:256–258, 1986
21. Stoller RG, Hande KR, Jacobs SA et al: Use of plasma pharmacokinetics to predict and prevent methotrexate toxicity. N Engl J Med 297:630–634, 1977
22. Erttmann R, Landbeck G: Effect of oral cholestyramine on the elimination of high-dose methotrexate. J Cancer Res Clin Oncol 110:48–50, 1985
23. Abelson HT, Ensminger W, Rosowsky A et al: Competitive effects of citrovorum factor and carboxypeptidase G₁ on cerebrospinal fluid methotrexate pharmacokinetics. Cancer Treat Rep 62:1549–1552, 1978

24. Shapiro WR, Young DG, Mehta BM: Methotrexate distribution in cerebrospinal fluid after intravenous, verticular, and lumbar injection. N Engl J Med 293:161–166, 1975
25. Bleyer WA: The clinical pharmacology of methotrexate. Cancer 41:36–51, 1978
26. Tattersall MHN, Brown B, Frei E III: The reversal of methotrexate toxicity by thymidine with maintenance of antitumor effects. Nature 253:198–200, 1975
27. Jacobs SA, Stoller RG, Chabner BA et al: 7-Hydroxymethotrexate as a urinary metabolite in human subjects and Rhesus monkeys receiving high-dose methotrexate. J Clin Invest 57:534–538, 1976
28. Glode LM, Pitman SW, Ensminger WD et al: A phase I study of high-dose aminopterin with leucovorin rescue in patients with advanced metastatic tumor. Cancer Res 39:3707–3714, 1979
29. Wilke WS, Mackenzie AH: Methotrexate therapy in rheumatoid arthritis: Current status. Drugs 32:103–113, 1986
30. Dahl MGC, Gregory MM, Scheuer PJ: Liver damage due to methotrexate in patients with psoriasis. Br Med J 1:625–630, 1971
31. Sostman HD, Matthay RA, Putman C et al: Methotrexate-induced pneumonitis. Medicine 55:371–388, 1976
32. Brouwers P, Moss H, Reaman G et al: Central nervous system preventive therapy with systemic high-dose methotrexate versus cranial radiation and intrathecal methotrexate: Longitudinal comparison of effects of treatment on intellectual function of children with acute lymphoblastic leukemia. Proc Am Soc Clin Oncol 6:158, 1987
33. Heidelberger C, Chandhari NK, Dannenberg P et al: Fluorinated pyrimidines: A new class of tumor inhibitory compounds. Nature 179:663–666, 1957
34. Mandel HG: Incorporation of 5-fluorouracil into RNA and its molecular consequences. Prog Mol Subcell Biol 1:82–135, 1969
35. Schuetz JD, Collins JM, Wallace HJ et al: Alteration of the secondary structure of newly synthesized DNA from murine bone marrow cells by 5-fluorouracil. Cancer Res 46:119–123, 1986
36. Kanamaru R, Kakuta H, Sato T et al: The inhibitory effects of 5-fluorouracil on the metabolism of peribosomal and ribosomal RNA in L1210 cells in vitro. Cancer Chemother Pharmacol 17:43–46, 1986
37. Dolnick BJ, Pink JJ: Effects of 5-fluorouracil on dihydrofolate reductase and dihydrofolate reductase mRNA from methotrexate-resistant KB cells. J Biol Chem 260:3006–3014, 1985
38. Evans RM, Laskin JD, Hakala MT: Effect of excess folates and deoxyinosine on the activity and site of action of 5-fluorouracil. Cancer Res 41:3288, 1981
39. Jenh CH, Geyer PK, Baskin F et al: Thymidylate synthase gene amplification in fluorodeoxyuridine-resistant mouse cell lines. Mol Pharmacol 28:80–85, 1985
40. Kaufman ER: Resistance to 5-fluorouracil associated with increased cytidine triphosphate levels in V79 Chinese hamster cells. Cancer Res 44:3371–3376, 1984
41. Spears CP, Gustavsson BG, Mitchell MS et al: Thymidylate synthase inhibition in malignant tumors and normal liver of patients given intravenous 5-fluorouracil. Cancer Res 44:4144–4150, 1984
42. Finan PJ, Koklitis PA, Chisholm EM et al: Comparative levels of tissue enzymes concerned in the early metabolism of 5-fluorouracil in normal and malignant colorectal tissue. Br J Cancer 50:711–716, 1984
43. Cadman EC, Heimer R, Davis L: Enhanced 5-fluorouracil nucleotide formation following methotrexate: Biochemical explanation for drug synergism. Science 205:1135–1137, 1979
44. Schwartz PM, Handschumacher RE: Selective antagonism of 5-fluorouracil cytotoxicity by 4-hydroxypyrazolopyrimidine (Allopurinol) in vitro. Cancer Res 39:3095–3101, 1979
45. Vogel SJ, Presant CA, Ratkin GA et al: Phase I study of thymidine plus 5-fluorouracil infusions in advanced colorectal carcinoma. Cancer Treat Rep 63:1–5, 1979
46. Peters GJ, Kraal I, Laurensse E et al: Separation of 5-fluorouracil and uracil by ion pair reversed-phase high-performance liquid chromatography on a column with porous polymeric packing. J Chromatogr 307:464–468, 1984
47. Iwamoto M, Yoshida S, Hirosi S: Fluorescence determination of 5-fluorouracil and 1-(tetrahydro-7-furanyl-5-fluorouracil) in blood serum by high-pressure liquid chromatography. J Chromatogr 310:151–157, 1984
48. Christophidis N, Vajda FJE, Lucas I et al: Fluorouracil therapy in patients with carcinoma of the large bowel: A pharmacokinetic comparison of various rates and routes of administration. Clin Pharmacokinet 3:330–336, 1978
49. Jones RB, Buckpitt AR, Londer H et al: Potential clinical application of a new method for quantitation of plasma levels of 5-fluorouracil and 5-fluorodeoxyuridine. Bull Cancer (Paris) 66:75–78, 1979
50. Ensminger WD, Rosowsky A, Raso V: A clinical pharmacological evaluation of hepatic arterial infusion of 5-fluoro 2'-deoxyuridine and 5-fluorouracil. Cancer Res 38:3784–3792, 1978
51. Speyer JL, Collins JM, Dedrick RL et al: Phase I and pharmacologic studies of intraperitoneal 5-fluorouracil. Cancer Res 40:567–572, 1980
52. Dow RT, Fritz WL: 5-Fluorouracil. In Dow RT, Fritz WL (eds): Cancer Chemotherapy Handbook, pp 435–454. New York, Elsevier-North Holland, 1980
53. Valdivieso M, Bodey GP, Gottlieb JA et al: Clinical evaluation of ftorafur (pyrimidine-deoxyyribose N,-2'-furanidyl-5-fluorouracil). Cancer Res 36:1821–1824, 1976
54. Au JL, Wu AT, Friedman MA et al: Pharmacokinetics and metabolism of ftorafur in man. Cancer Treat Rep 63:343–350
55. Armstrong RD, Diasio RB: Metabolism and biological activity of 5'-deoxy-5-fluorouridine, a novel fluoropyrimidine. Cancer Res 40:3333–3338, 1980
56. Cohen SS: The lethality of ara nucleotides. Med Biol 54:299–326, 1976
57. Fram RJ, Kufe DW: Effect of 1-β-D-arabinofuranosyl cytosine and hydroxyurea on

the repair of x-ray-induced DNA single-strand breaks in human leukemic blasts. Biochem Pharmacol 34:2557–2560, 1985
58. Fridland A: Inhibition of DNA chain initiation by 1-β-D-arabinofuranosylcytosine (ara-C) in human lymphoblasts. J Supramol Struct 771:331, 1978
59. Woodcock DM, Fox RM, Cooper IA: Evidence for a new mechanism of cytotoxity of 1-β-D-arabinofuranosyl cytosine. Cancer Res 39:1418–1424, 1979
60. Wiley JS, Jones SP, Sawyer WH et al: Cytosine arabinoside influx and nucleoside transport sites in acute leukemia. J Clin Invest 69:479, 1982
61. Wiley JS, Taupin J, Jamieson GP et al: Cytosine arabinoside transport and metabolism in acute leukemias and T-cell lymphoblastic lymphoma. J Clin Invest 75:632–642, 1985
62. Chabner BA, Hande KR, Drake JC: Ara-C metabolism: Implications for drug resistance and drug interactions. Bull Cancer 66:89–92, 1979
63. Tattersall MNH, Ganeshagura K, Hoffbrand AV: Mechanisms of resistance of human acute leukaemia cells to cytosine arabinoside. Br J Haematol 27:39–46, 1974
64. Steuart CD, Burke PJ: Cytidine deaminase and the development of resistance to arabinosyl cytosine. Nature 233:109–110, 1971
65. Preisler HD, Rustum Y, Priore RL: Relationship between leukemic cell retention of cytosine arabinoside triphosphate and the duration of remission in patients with acute nonlymphocytic leukemia. Eur J Cancer Clin Oncol 21:23–30, 1985
66. Karp JE, Donehower RC, Dole GB et al: Direct relationship of marrow cell growth and 1-β-D-arabinofuranosylcytosine metabolism. Cancer Res 44:5046–5050, 1984
67. Mitchell T, Sariban E, Kufe D: Effects of 1-β-D-arabinofuranosylcytosine on protooncogene expression in human U-937 cells. Mol Pharmacol 30:398–402, 1986
68. Tilly H, Bastard C, Bizet M et al: Low-dose cytarabine persistance of a clonal abnormality during complete remission of acute nonlymphocytic leukemia (letter). N Engl J Med 314:246–247, 1986
69. Zimm S, Collins JM, Miser J et al: Cytosine arabinoside cerebrospinal fluid kinetics. Clin Pharmacol Ther 35:826–830, 1984
70. Shimada N, Ueda T, Yokoshima T et al: A sensitive and specific radioimmunoassay for 1-β-D-arabinofuranosylcytosine. Cancer Lett 24:173–178, 1984
71. Ho DHW, Frei E III: Clinical pharmacology of 1-β-D-arabinofuranosylcytosine. Clin Pharmacol Ther 12:944–954, 1971
72. Early AP, Preisler HD, Slocum H et al: A pilot study of high-dose 1-beta-D-arabinofuranosylcytosine for acute leukemia and refractory lymphoma: Clinical response and pharmacology. Cancer Res 42:1587, 1982
73. Donehower RC, Karp JE, Burke PJ: Pharmacology and toxicity of high-dose cytarabine by 72-hour continuous infusion. Cancer Treat Rep 70:1059–1065, 1986
74. Moloney WC, Rosenthal DS: Treatment of early acute nonlymphocytic leukemia with low-dose cytosine arabinoside. Haematol Blood Transfus 26:59–62, 1981
75. Aden OB, Goldie W, Wood T et al: Seizures following intrathecal cytosine arabinoside in young children with acute lymphoblastic leukemia. Cancer 42:53–58, 1978
76. Cadman E, Eiferman F: Mechanism of synergistic cell killing when methotrexate precedes cytosine arabinoside. Study of L1210 and human leukemic cell. J Clin Invest 64:788–797, 1979
77. Harris AW, Reynolds EC, Finch LR: Effect of thymidine on the sensitivity of cultured mouse tumor cells to 1-β-D-arabinofuranosylcytosine. Cancer Res 39:538–541, 1979
78. Kreis W, Wokcock TM, Gordon CS et al: Tetrahydrouridine physiologic disposition and effect upon deamination of cytosine arabinoside in man. Cancer Treat Rep 61:1347–1353, 1977
79. Rustum YM, Dave C, Mayhew E et al: Role of liposome type and route of administration in the antitumor activity of liposome-entrapped 1-β-D-arabinofuranosylcytosine against mouse L1210 leukemia. Cancer Res 39:1390–1395, 1979
80. Lu LJW, Randerath K: Effects of 5-azacytidine on transfer RNA methyltransferases. Cancer Res 39:940–948, 1979
81. Ley TJ, DeSimone J, Anagnon NP et al: 5-Azacytidine selectively increases gammaglobin synthesis in a patient with beta-thalassemia. N Engl J Med 307:1469, 1982
82. Elion GB: Biochemistry and pharmacology of purine analogs. Fed Proc 26:898–904, 1967
83. Tidd DM, Paterson ARP: Distinction between inhibition of purine nucleotide synthesis and the delayed cytotoxic reaction of 6-mercaptopurine. Cancer Res 34:733–737, 1974
84. Christie NT, Drake S, Meyn RE et al: 6-Thioguanine-induced DNA damage as a determinant of cytotoxicity in cultured Chinese hamster ovary cells. Cancer Res 44:3665–3672, 1984
85. Bodell WJ, Morgan WF, Rasmussen J et al: Potentiation of 1,3-bis(2-chloroethyl)-1-nitrosourea (BCNU)-induced cytotoxicity in 9L cells by pretreatment with 6-thioguanine. Biochem Pharmacol 34:515–520, 1985
86. Lee MH, Huang Y-M, Sartorelli AC: Alkaline phosphatase activities of 6-thiopurine-sensitive and -resistant sublines of sarcoma 180. Cancer Res 38:2413–2418, 1978
87. Lennard L, Lillyman JS: Are children with lymphoblastic leukemia given enough 6-mercaptopurine? Lancet 2:785–787, 1987
88. Breter HJ, Zahn RK: Quantitation of intracellular metabolites of [35]-6-mercaptopurine in L5178Y cells grown in time-course incubates. Cancer Res 39:3744–3748, 1979
89. Ding TL, Benet LZ: Determination of 6-mercaptopurine and azathioprine in plasma by high-performance liquid chromatography. J Chromatogr 163:281–288, 1979
90. Tidd DM, Dedhar S: Specific and sensitive combined high performance liquid chromatographic-flow fluorometric assay for intracellular-6-thioguanine metabolites of 6-mercaptopurine and 6-thioguanine. J Chromatogr 145:237–246, 1978
91. Zimm S, Collins JM, Riccardi R et al: Variable bioavailability of oral 6-mercaptopur-

ine: Is maintenance chemotherapy in acute lymphoblastic leukemia being optimally delivered. N Engl J Med 308:1005–1009, 1983

92. Burton NK, Barnett MJ, Aherne GW et al: The effect of food on the oral administration of 6-mercaptopurine. Cnacer Chemother Pharmacol 18:90–91, 1986

93. Burton NK, Aherne GW: The effect of cotrimoxazole on the absorption of orally administered 6-mercaptopurine in the rat. Cancer Chemother Pharmacol 16:81–84, 1986

94. Esterhay RJ, Aisner J, Levi JA et al: High-dose 6-mercaptopurine in advanced refractory cancer. Cancer Treat Rep 62:1229–1231, 1978

95. Present DH, Korelitz BI, Wisch N et al: Treatment of Crohn's disease with 6-mercaptopurine. N Engl J Med 302:981–986, 1980

96. Pavan-Langston D, Buchanan RA, Alford CA Jr (eds): Adenine arabinoside: An antiviral agent. New York, Raven Press, 1979

97. Brockman RW, Schabel FM, Montgomery JH: Biologic activity of 9-β-arabinofuranosyl-2-fluoro adenine, a metabolically stable analog of 9-β-D-arabinofuranosyladenine. Biochem Pharmacol 26:2193–2196, 1977

98. Weiss GR, Arteaga CL, Brown TD et al: New anticancer agents. In Pinedo HM, Chabner BA, Longo DL (eds): Cancer chemotherapy, annual 9, pp 93–120. Amsterdam, Elsevier, 1987

99. Plunkett W, Alexander L, Chubb S et al: Biochemical basis of the increased activity of 9-beta-D-arabinofuranosyladenine in the presence of inhibitors of adenosine deaminase. Cancer Res 39:3655–3660, 1979

100. Smyth JF, Paine RM, Jackman AL et al: The clinical pharmacology of the adenosine deaminase inhibitor 2′-deoxycoformycin. Cancer Chemother Pharmacol 5:93–101, 1980

101. Ludlum DB: Alkylating agents and the nitrosoureas. In Becker FF (ed): Cancer: A comprehensive treatise, Vol 5, pp 285–307. New York, Plenum Press, 1977

102. Kohn KW: Interstrand cross-linking of DNA by 1,3-bis(chlorethyl)-1-nitrosourea and other 1-(2-haloethyl)-1-nitroureas. Cancer Res 37:1450–1454, 1977

103. Wang AL, Tew KD: Increased glutathione-S-transferase activity in a cell line with acquired resistance to nitrogen mustards. Cancer Treat Rep 69:677–682, 1985

104. Tobey RA, Tesmer JG: Differential response of cultured human normal and tumor cells to trace-element-induced resistance to the alkylating agent melphalan. Cancer Res 45:2567–2571, 1985

105. Crook TR, Souhami RL, Whyman GD et al: Glutathione depletion as a determinant of sensitivity of human leukemia cells to cyclophosphamide. Cancer Res 46:5035–5038, 1986

106. Somfai-Relle S, Suzukake K, Vistica BP et al: Reduction in cellular glutathione by butathionine sulfoximine and sensitization of murine tumor cells resistant to L-phenylalanine mustard. Biochem Pharmacol 33:485–489, 1984

107. Mulcahy RT, Dembs NL, Ublacker GA: Enhancement of nitrosourea cytotoxicity by misonidazole in vitro: Correlation with carbamoylating potential. Br J Cancer 49:307–313, 1984

108. Henner WD, Peters WP, Eder JP et al: Pharmacokinetics and immediate effects of high-dose carmustine in man. Cancer Treat Rep 70:877–880, 1986

109. DeJong JP, Nikkels PGJ, Brockbank KGM et al: Comparative in vitro effects of cyclophosphamide derivatives on murine bone marrow-derived stromal and hemopoietic progenitor cell classes. Cancer Res 45:4001–4005, 1985

110. Lee FYF, Workman P: Interaction of nitroimidazole sensitizers with drug metabolizing enzymes—spectral and kinetic studies. Int J Radiat Oncol Biol Phys 13:1383–1387, 1986

111. Bergsagel DE: Treatment of plasma cell myeloma with cytotoxic agents. Arch Intern Med 135:172–176, 1975

112. Lyons RM, Goldenberg GJ: Active transport of nitrogen mustard and choline by normal and leukemic human lymphoid cells. Cancer Res 32:1679–1685, 1972

113. Lawley PD, Brookes P: Molecular mechanisms of the cytotoxic action of difunctional alkylating agents and of resistance to this action. Nature 206:480–483, 1965

114. Colvin M: A review of the pharmacology and clinical use of cyclophosphamide. In Pinedo HM (ed): Clinical pharmacology of antineoplastic drugs. pp 245–261. Amsterdam. Elsevier-North Holland, 1978

115. Hilton J: Role of aldehyde dehydrogenase in cyclophosphamide-resistant L1210 leukemia. Cancer Res 44:5156–5160, 1984

116. Brock N, Pohl J, Stekar J: Detoxification of urotoxic oxazaphosphorines by sulfhydryl compounds. J Cancer Res Clin Oncol 100:311, 1981

117. Cox PJ: Cyclophosphamide cystitis. Identification of acrolein as the causative agent. Biochem Pharmacol 28:2045–2049, 1979

118. Green TP, Mirken BL: Prevention of cyclophosphamide-induced antidiuresis by furosemide infusion. Clin Pharmacol Ther 29:634, 1981

119. Manohoran A: Carcinoma of the urinary bladder in patients receiving cyclophosphamide. Aust NZ J Med 14:507–512, 1984

120. Connors TA: Alkylating drugs, nitrosourea and dialkyl triazenes. In Pinedo HM (ed): Cancer chemotherapy, pp 25–55. Amsterdam, Elsevier-North Holland, 1979

121. Hengst JCD, Kempf RA: Immunomodulation by cyclophosphamide. Clin Immunol Allergy 4:199–216, 1984

122. Alvarado CS, Boat TF, Newman AJ: Late onset pulmonary fibrosis and chest deformity in two children treated with cyclophosphamide. J Pediatr 92:443–446, 1978

123. Steinherz LJ, Steinherz PG: Cyclophosphamide cardiotoxicity. Cancer Bull 37:231–234, 1985

124. El-Yazigi A, Martin CR: Improved analysis of cyclophosphamide by capillary gas chromatography with thermionic (nitrogen-phosphorus)-specific detection and silica sample purification. J Chromatogr Biomed Appl 374:177–182, 1986

125. Sladek NE, Powers JF, Grage GM: Half-life of oxazaphosphorines in biological fluids. Drug Metab Dispos 12:553–559, 1984

126. Kallama S, Hemminki K: Stabilities of 7-alkylguanosines and 7-deoxyguanosines formed by phosphoramide mustard and nitrogen mustard. Chem Biol Interact 57:85–96, 1986

127. Juma FD: Effect of liver failure on the pharmacokinetics of cyclophosphamide. Eur J Clin Pharmacol 26:591–593, 1984

128. Andriole GL, Sandlund JT, Miser JS et al: The efficacy of MESNA (2-mercaptoethane sodium sulfonate) as a uroprotectant in patients with hemorrhagic cystitis receiving further oxazaphosphorine chemotherapy. J Clin Oncol 5:799–803, 1987

129. Meanwell CA, Blade AE, Kelly KA et al: Prediction of ifosfamide/MESNA-associated encephalopathy. Eur J Clin Oncol 22:815–819, 1986

130. Goren MP, Wright KR, Pratt CB et al: Dechloroethylation of ifosfamide and neurotoxicity. Lancet 2:1219–1220, 1986

131. Carny T, Margison JM, Thatcher N et al: Bioavailability of ifosfamide in patients with bronchial carcinoma. Cancer Chemother Pharmacol 18:261–264, 1986

132. Vistica DT, Toal JN, Rabinovitz M: Amino-acid-conferred protection against melphalan. Biochem Pharmacol 27:2865–2870, 1978

133. Vistica DT, Toal JN, Rabinovitz M: Amino-acid-conferred protection against melphalan: Interference with leucine protection of melphalan cytotoxicity by the basic amino acids in cultured murine L1210 leukemic cells. Mol Pharmacol 14:1136–1142, 1978

134. Goldenberg GJ, Froese EK: Antagonism of the cytocidal activity and uptake of melphalan by tamoxifen in human breast cancer cells in vitro. Biochem Pharmacol 34:763–770, 1985

135. Tattersall MN, Jarman M, Newlands ES et al: Pharmacokinetics of melphalan following oral or intravenous administration in patients with malignant disease. Eur J Cancer 14:507–514, 1978

136. Alberts DS, Chang SY, Chen HSG et al: Kinetics of intravenous melphalan. Clin Pharmacol Ther 26:73–80, 1979

137. Howell SB, Pfeifle CE, Olshen RA: Intraperitoneal chemotherapy with melphalan. Ann Intern Med 101:14–20, 1984

138. Green MH, Harris EL, Gershenson DM et al: Melphalan may be a more potent leukemogen than cyclophosphamide. Ann Intern Med 105:360–367, 1986

139. Fiere D, Felman P, Vivian H et al: Acute myeloid leukemia following the administration of chlorambucil. Two cases. Nouv Presse Med 7:756, 1978

140. Cole SR, Myers TJ, Klatsky AU: Pulmonary disease with chlorambucil therapy. Cancer 41:455–459, 1978

141. Nedkarni MV, Trams EG, Smith PK: Preliminary studies on the distribution and fate of TEM, TEPA, and myleran in the human. Cancer Res 19:713–718, 1959

142. Heal JM, Franza BR, Schein PS: Pharmacology of nitrosourea antitumor agents. In Pinedo HM (ed): Clinical pharmacology of antineoplastic drugs, pp 263–275. Amsterdam, Elsevier-North Holland, 1978

143. Ewig RAG, Kohn KW: DNA damage and repair in mouse leukemia L1210 cells treated with nitrogen mustard, 1,3-bis(2-chloroethyl)-1-nitrosourea, and other nitrosoureas. Cancer 37:2114–2122, 1977

144. Kann HE Jr: Comparison of biochemical and biological effects of four nitrosoureas with differing carbamoylating activities. Cancer Res 38:2363–2366, 1978

145. Tew KD, Sudhakar S, Schein PS, Smulson ME: Binding of chlorozotocin and 1-(2-chlorethyl)-3-cyclohexyl-1-nitrosourea to chromatin and nucleosomal fractions of HeLa cells. Cancer Res 38:3371–3378, 1978

146. Lee FYF, Workman P, Roberts JT et al: Clinical pharmacokinetics or oral CCNU (Lomustine). Cancer Chemother Pharmacol 14:125–128, 1985

147. Reed DJ, May HE: Cytochrome P-450 interactions with the 2-chloroethylnitrosoureas and procarbazine. Biochimie 60:989–995, 1978

148. Greene MH, Boile JD, Strike TA: Carmustine as a cause of acute nonlymphocytic leukemia. N Engl J Med 313:579, 1985

149. Hundley R, Lukens JN: Nitrosourea-associated pulmonary fibrosis. Cancer Treat Rep 63:2128–2130, 1979

150. Harmon WE, Cohen HJ, Schneeberger EE et al: Chronic renal failure in children treated with methyl CCNU. N Engl J 300:1200–1203, 1979

151. Rosenberg B, Van Camp L, Krigas T: Inhibition of cell division in Escherichia coli by electrolysis products from a platinum electrode. Nature 205:698–699, 1965

152. Rosenberg B, Van Camp L, Trosko JE et al: Platinum compounds: A new class of potent antitumor agents. Nature 222:385–386, 1969

153. Filipski J, Kohn KW, Bonner WM: The nature of inactivating lesions produced by platinum(II) complexes on phage DNA. Chem Biol Interact 32:321–330, 1980

154. Scovell WM, O'Connor T: Interaction of aquated cis-[(NH₃)₂PtII] with nuclei acid constituents: 1. Ribonucleosides. J Am Chem Soc 99:120–126, 1977

155. Zwelling LA, Kohn KW: Mechanism of action of cis-dichlorodiammineplatinum(II). Cancer Treat Rep 63:1439–1444, 1979

156. Cohen GL, Bauer WR, Barton JK, Lippard SJ: Binding of cis- and trans-dichlorodiammineplatinum(II) to DNA: Evidence for unwinding and shortening of the double helix. Science 203:1014–1016, 1979

157. Roberts JJ, Thomson AJ: The mechanism of action of antitumor platinum compounds. Prog Nucleic Acid Res Mol Biol 22:71–133, 1979

158. Meyn RE, Jenkins SF, Thompson LH: Defective removal of DNA cross-links in a repair-deficient mutant of chinese hamster cells. Cancer Res 42:3106, 1982

159. Burchenal JH, Kalaher K, Dew K et al: Studies of cross-resistance, synergistic combination and blocking activity of platinum derivatives. Biochimie 60:961–965, 1978

160. Borch RF, Katz JC, Lieder, PH et al: Effect of diethyldithiocarbamate rescue on tumor

response to cis-platinum in a rat model. Proc Natl Acad Sci USA 77:5441–5444, 1980

161. Glover D, Glick JH, Weiler C et al: Phase I trials of WR-2721 and cis-platinum. Int J Radiat Oncol Biol Phys 10:1781–1784, 1984

162. Fraval HNA, Roberts JJ: G_1 phase Chinese hamster V79-379A cells are inherently more sensitive to platinum bound to their DNA than mid S phase or asynchronously treated cells. Biochem Pharmacol 28:1575–1580, 1979

163. Endressen L, Schjerven L, Rugstad HE: Tumours from a cell strain with a high content of metallothionein show enhanced resistance against cis-dichlorodiammineplatinum. Acta Pharmacol Toxicol 55:183–187, 1984

164. Reed E, Yuspa SH, Zwelling LA et al: Quantitation of cis-diamminedichloroplatinum(II) (cisplatin)-DNA-intrastrand adducts in testicular and ovarian cancer patients receiving cisplatin chemotherapy. J Clin Invest 77:545–550, 1986

165. LeRoy AF, Wehling ML, Sponseller HL et al: Analysis of platinum in biological materials by flameless atomic absorption spectrophotometry. Biochem Med 18:184–191, 1977

166. Marsh KC, Sternson LA, Repta AJ: Post-column reaction detector for platinum(II) antineoplastic agents. Anal Chem 56:491–497, 1984

167. Litterst CL, LeRoy AF, Guarino AM: The disposition and distribution of platinum following parenteral administration to animals of cis-dichlorodiammineplatinum(II). Cancer Treat Rep 63:1485–1492, 1979

168. Vermorken JB, Van der Vijgh WJF, Klein I et al: Pharmacokinetics of free and total platinum species after short-term infusion of cisplatin. Cancer Treat Rep 68:505–513, 1984

169. Patton TF, Himmelstein KJ, Belt R et al: Plasma levels and urinary excretion of filterable platinum species following bolus injection and i.v. infusion of cis-dichlorodiammineplatinum(II) in man. Cancer Treat Rep 63:1359–1361, 1979

170. Gormley P, Poplack D, Pizzo P: The cerebrospinal fluid pharmacokinetics of cis-diamminedichloroplatinum(II) and several platinum analogues. Proc Am Assoc Cancer Res 20:279, 1979

171. Daley-Yates PT, McBrien DCH: Cisplatin metabolites in plasma, a study of their pharmacokinetics and importance in the nephrotoxic and antitumour activity of cisplatin. Biochem Pharmacol 33:3063–3070, 1984

172. Jacobs C, Kalman SM, Tretton M et al: Renal handling of cis-diamminedichloroplatinum(II). Cancer Treat Rep 64(12):1223–1226, 1980

173. Chary KK, Higby DJ, Henderson ES et al: Phase I study of high-dose cis-dichlorodiammineplatinum(II) with forced diversis. Cancer Treat Rep 61:367–370, 1977

174. Ozols RF, Corden BF, Jacob J et al: High-dose cisplatin in hypertonic saline. Ann Intern Med 100:19–24, 1984

175. Madias NE, Harrington JT: PLatinum nephrotoxicity. Am J Med 65:307–314, 1978

176. Gonzalez-Vitale JC, Hayes DM, Cvitkovic E et al: The renal pathology in clinical trials of cis-platinum (II) diamminedichloride. Cancer 39:1362–1371, 1977

177. Schilsky RL, Anderson T: Hypomagnesemia and renal magnesium wasting in patients receiving cis-platin. Ann Intern Med 90:929–931, 1979

178. Jones B, Mladek J, Bhalla R et al: Enzymuria and beta$_2$ microglobulinuria as a sensitive index of cis-platinum nephrotoxicity. Proc Am Soc Clin Oncol 20:336,1979

179. Roelofs RI, Hrushesky W, Rogin J et al: Peripheral sensory neuropathy and cisplatin chemotherapy. Neurology 34:934–938, 1984

180. Wiesenfeld M, Reinders E, Corder M et al: Successful retreatment with cis-DDP after apparent allergic reactions. Cancer Treat Rep 63:219–221, 1979

181. Granowetter L, Rosenstock JG, Packer RJ: Enhanced cis-platinum neurotoxicity in pediatric patients with brain tumors. J Neurooncol 1:293–297, 1983

182. Howell SB, Pfeifle CL, Wang WE et al: Intraperitoneal cisplatin with systemic thiosulfate protection. Ann Intern Med 97:845–851, 1982

183. Egorin MJ, Van Echo DA, Tipping SJ et al: Pharmacokinetics and dosage reduction of cis-diammine(1,1-cyclobutanedicarboxylato) platinum in patients with impaired renal function. Cancer Res 44:5432–5438, 1984

184. Takeshita M, Grollman AP, Ohtsubo E et al: Interaction of bleomycin with DNA. Proc Natl Acad Sci USA 75:5983–5987, 1978

185. Wu JC, Stubbe J, Kozarich JW: Mechanism of bleomycin: evidence for 4'-ketone formation in poly(dA-dU) associated exclusively with free base release. Biochemistry 24:7569–7573, 1985

186. Barranco SC, Humphrey RM: The effects of bleomycin on survival and cell progression in Chinese hamster cells in vitro. Cancer Res 31:1218–1223, 1971

187. Barranco SC, Novak JK, Humphrey RM: Studies on recovery from chemically induced damage in mammalian cells. Cancer Res 35:1194–1204, 1975

188. Chafouleas JG, Bolton WE, Means AR: Potentiation of bleomycin lethality by anticalmodulin drugs: a role for calmodulin in DNA repair. Science 224:1346–1348, 1984

189. Russo A, Mitchell JB, McPherson S et al: Alteration of bleomycin cytotoxicity by glutathione depletion or elevation. Int J Radiat Oncol Biol Phys 10:1675–1678, 1984

190. Umezawa H, Hori S, Sawa T, et al: A bleomycin-inactivating enzyme in mouse liver. J Antibiot 27:419–424, 1974

191. Sehti SM, Lazo JS: Separation of the protective enzyme bleomycin hydrolase from rabbit pulmonary aminopeptidases. Biochemistry 26:432–437, 1987

192. Akiyama S, Kuwano M: Isolation and preliminary characterization of bleomycin-resistant mutants from Chinese hamster ovary cells. J Cell Physiol 107:147, 1981

193. Broughton A, Strong JE: Radioimmunoassay of bleomycin. Cancer Res 36:1418–1421, 1976

194. Alberts DS, Chen HSG, Liu R et al: Bleomycin pharmacokinetics in man: I. Intravenous administration. Cancer Chemother Pharmacol 1:177–181, 1978

195. Alberts DS, Chen HSG, Mayersohn M et al: Bleomycin pharmacokinetics in man: II. Intracavitary administration. Cancer Chemother Pharmacol 2:127–132, 1979

196. Blum RH, Carter SK, Agre K: A clinical review of bleomycin—a new antineoplastic agent. Cancer 31:903–914, 1973

197. Bell MR, Meredith DJ, Gill PG: Role of carbon monoxide diffusing capacity in the early detection of major bleomycin-induced pulmonary toxicity. Auts NZ J Med 15:235–240, 1985

198. Bellamy EA, Husband JE, Blaquiere RM et al: Bleomycin-related lung damage: CT evidence. Radiology 156:155–158, 1985

199. Morrow CP, DiSaia PJ, Mangan CF et al: Continuous pelvic arterial infusion with bleomycin for squamous carcinoma of the cervix recurrent after irradiation therapy. Cancer Treat Rep 61:1403–1405, 1977

200. Bracken RB, Johnson DE, Rodriquez L, Samuels ML, Ayala A: Treatment of multiple superficial tumors of bladder with intravesical bleomycin. Urology 9:161–163, 1977

201. Thompson RH: Naturally Occurring Quinones, pp 536–575. London, Academic Press, 1971

202. DiMarco A, Galtani M, Orezzi PO: Daunomycin, a new antibiotic of the rhodomycin group. Nature 201:706–707, 1964

203. Friedmann CA: Structure–activity relationships of anthraquinones in some pathological conditions. Pharmacology 20:113–122, 1980

204. Handa K, Sato S: Generation of free radicals of quinone group containing anticancer chemicals in NADPH-microsome system as evidenced by initiation of sulfite oxidation. Gann 66:43–47, 1975

205. Pigram WJ, Fuller W, Amilton LDH: Stereochemistry of intercalation: Interaction of daunomycin with DNA. Nature 235:17–19, 1972

206. Murphree SA, Cunningham LS, Hwang KM et al: Effects of adriamycin on surface properties of sarcoma 180 ascites cells. Biochem Pharmacol 25:1227–1231, 1976

207. Mikkelsen RB, Lin PS, Wallach DF: Interaction of adriamycin with human red blood cells: A biochemical and morphologic study. J Mol Med 2:33–40, 1977

208. Liu LF, Rowe TC, Yang L et al: Cleavage of DNA by mammalian DNA topoisomerase-II. J Biol Chem 258:15365–15370, 1983

209. Tewey KM, Chen GL, Nelson EM et al: Intercalative antitumor drugs interfere with the breakage-reunion reaction of mammalian DNA topoisomerase II. J Biol Chem 259:9182–9187, 1984

210. Potmesil M, Kirshenbaum S, Isreal M et al: Relationship of adriamycin concentrations to the DNA lesions induced in hypoxic and euoxic L1210 cells. Cancer Res 43:3528–3532, 1983

211. Doroshow JH: Prevention of doxorubicin-induced killing of MCF-7 human breast tumor cancer cells by oxygen radical scavengers and iron chelating agents. Biochem Biophys Res Commun 135:330–337, 1986

212. Sinha BK, Katki AG, Batist G et al: Differential formation of hydroxyl radicals by adriamycin in sensitive and resistant MCF-7 human breast cells: implication for the mechanism of action. Biochemistry 26:3776–3781, 1987

213. Myers CE, Gianni L, Zweier J et al: The role of iron in adriamycin biochemistry. Fed Proc 45:2792–2797, 1986

214. Yeh GC, Occhipinit SJ, Cowan KH et al: Adriamycin resistance in human tumor cells associated with marked alterations in the regulation of the hexose monophosphate shunt and its response to oxidant stress. Cancer Res 47:5994–5999, 1987

215. Doroshow JH: Role of reactive oxygen production in doxorubicin cardiac toxicity. In Hacker MP, Lazo JS, Tritton TR (eds): Organ directed toxicities of anticancer drugs, pp 31–40. The Hague, Martinus Nijhoff, 1988

216. Doroshow JH, Locker GY, Myers CE: The enzymatic defenses of the mouse heart against reactive oxygen metabolites. J Clin Invest 65:128–135, 1980

217. Myers CE: Role of iron in anthracycline action. In Hacker MP, Lazo JS, Tritton TR (eds): Organ directed toxicities of anticancer drugs, pp 17–30. The Hague, Martinus Nijhoff, 1988

218. Speyer JL, Green MD, Ward C et al: A trial of ICRF-1878 to selectively protect against chronic adriamycin cardiac toxicity: rationale and preliminary result of a clinical trial. In Hacker MP, Lazo JS, Tritton TR (eds): Organ directed toxicities of anticancer drugs, pp 64–76. The Hague, Martinus Nijhoff, 1988

219. Von Hoff DD, Howser D, Lewis BJ et al: Phase I trial of ICRF-187. Cancer Treat Rep 65:249–252, 1981

220. Ferrans VJ, Herman EH, Hamlin RL: Pretreatment with ICRF-187 protects against the chronic cardiac toxicity produced by very large cumulative doses of doxorubicin in beagle dogs. In Hacker MP, Lazo JS, Tritton TR (eds): Organ directed toxicities of anticancer drugs, pp 56–63. The Hague, Martinus Nijhoff, 1988

221. Israel M, Pegg WJ, Wilkinson PM et al: Liquid chromatographic analysis of adriamycin and metabolites in biological fluids. J Liquid Chromatogr 1:795–809, 1978

222. Eksborg S: Reversed-phase liquid chromatography of adriamycin and daunorubicin and their hydroxyl metabolites, adriamycinol, and daunorubicinol. J Chromatogr 149:225–232, 1978

223. Takanashi S, Bachur NR: Adriamycin metabolism in man: Evidence from urinary metabolites. Drug Metab Disp 4:79–87, 1976

224. Benjamin RS: Pharmacokinetics of adriamycin in patients with sarcomas: Cancer Chemother Rep 58:271–273, 1974

225. Sulkes A, Collins JM: Reappraisal of some dosage adjustment guidelines. Cancer Treat Rep 71:229–233, 1987

226. Dantchev D, Slioussantchouk V, Paintrand M et al: Electron microscopic studies of the heart and light microscopic studies of golden hamsters with adriamycin, doxorubicin, AD 32, and aclacinomycin. Cancer Treat Rep 63:875–888, 1979

227. Tong GL, Wu HY, Smith TH et al: Adriamycin analogues: 3. Synthesis of N-alkylated

anthracyclines with enhanced efficacy and reduced cardiotoxicity. J Med Chem 22:912–918, 1979

228. Benjamin RS, Chawla SP, Ewer MS et al: Adriamycin cardiac toxicity—an assessment of approaches to cardiac monitoring and cardioprotection. In Hacker MP, Lazo JS, Tritton TR (eds): Organ directed toxicities of anticancer drugs, pp 41–55. The Hague, Martinus Nijhoff, 1988

229. Myers CE: Anthracyclines. In Pinedo HM, Longo DL, Chabner BA (eds): Cancer chemotherapy and biological response modifiers, annual 9, pp 36–49. Amsterdam, Elsevier, 1987

230. Myers CE, Muindi JR, Zweier J et al: 5-Iminodaunomycin: An anthracycline with unique properties. J Biol Chem 262:11571–11577, 1987

231. Sinha BK, Motten AD, Hanck K: The electrochemical reduction of 1,4-bis-(2-hydroxyethyl)-amino-(ethylamino)-anthracenedione and daunomycin: Biochemical significance of superoxide formation. Chem Biol Inter 43:371–377, 1983

232. Shenkenberg TD, Von Hoff DD et al: Mitoxantrone: A new anticancer drug with significant clinical activity. Ann Intern Med 105:67–70, 1986

233. Crooke ST, Bradner WT: Mitomycin C: A review. Cancer Treat Rev 3:121–139, 1976

234. Reich SD: Clinical pharmacology of mitomycin C. In Carter SK, Crooke ST (eds): Mitomycin C: Current status and new developments, p 243. New York, Academic Press, 1979

235. Keyes SR, Fracasso PM, Heimbrook DC et al: Role of NADPH: cytochrome C reductase and DT-diaphorase in the biotransformation of mitomycin C. Cancer Res 44:5638–5643, 1984

236. Iyengar BS, Remers WA: A comparison of mechanism proposed for the conversion of mitomycins into mitosenes. J Med Chem 28:963–967, 1985

237. den Hartigh J, Verweij J, Pinedo HM: Mitomycin C. In Pinedo HM, Chabner BA (eds): Cancer chemotherapy, annual 7, pp 83–90. Amsterdam, Elsevier, 1985

238. Dorr RT, Bowdan GT, Alberts DS et al: Interactions of mitomycin C with mammalian DNA detected by alkaline elution. Cancer Res 45:3510–3516, 1985

239. Nakano H, Siugoka K, Nakano M et al: Importance of Fe^{2+}-ADP and the relative unimportance of OH in the mechanism of mitomycin C-induced lipid peroxidation. Biochim Biophys Acta 796:285–293, 1984

240. Ludwig CU, Peng YM, Beaudry JN et al: Cytotoxicity of mitomycin C on clonogenic human carcinoma cells is not enhanced by hypoxia. Cancer Chemother Pharmacol 12:146–150, 1984

241. Tsuruo T, Iida-Saito H, Kawabata H et al: Characteristics of resistance to adriamycin in human myelogenous leukemia K562 resistant to adriamycin and in isolated clones. Jpn J Cancer Res 77:682–692, 1986

242. den Hartigh J, McVie JG, Van Oort WJ et al: Pharmacokinetics of mitomycin C in humans. Cancer Res 43:5017–5021, 1983

243. Schilcher RB, Young JD, Ratanatharathorn V et al: Clinical pharmacokinetics of high-dose mitomycin C. Cancer Chemother Pharmacol 13:186–190, 1984

244. Hopkins SC, Robert GB, Matheny R et al: The stability and antitumor activity of recycled (intravesical) mitomycin C. Cancer 53:2063–2068, 1984

245. Cattell V: Mitomycin-induced hemolytic uremic kidney. An experimental model in the rat. Am J Pathol 121:88–95, 1985

246. Valavaara R, Nordman E: Renal complications of mitomycin C therapy with special reference to the total dose. Cancer 55:47–50, 1985

247. Cantrell JE, Phillips TM, Schein PS: Carcinoma-associated hemolytic uremic syndrome: a complication of mitomycin C chemotherapy. J Clin Oncol 3:723–734, 1985

248. Oswoll ES, Kiessling PJ, Patterson JR: Interstitial pneumonia from mitomycin. Ann Intern Med 89:352–355, 1978

249. Kuedee D, McLaughlin TT, Daughaday C et al: Mitomycin C and vindesine associated pulmonary toxicity with variable clinical expression. Cancer 55:542–547, 1985

250. Trush MA, Mimnaugh EG, Ginsburg E et al: Studies on the in vitro interaction of mitomycin C, nitrofuantoin and paraquat with pulmonary microsomes. Stimulation of reactive oxygen-dependent lipid peroxidation. Biochem Pharmacol 31:805, 1982

251. Bachur NR, Gordon SL, Gee RV: A general mechanism for microsomal activation of quinone anticancer agents to free radicals. Cancer Res 38:1745–1750, 1978

252. Selman Waksman Conference on actinomycins: Their potential for cancer chemotherapy. Cancer Chemother Rep 58:1–123, 1974

253. Frei E: The clinical use of actinomycin D. Cancer Chemother Rep 58:49–54, 1974

254. Sobell HM, Jain SC, Sakere TD et al: Stereochemistry of actinomycin-DNA binding. Nature (New Biol) 231:200–205, 1971

255. Reich E, Franklin RM, Shatkin AJ et al: Action of actinomycin D on animal cells and viruses. Proc Natl Acad Sci USA 48:1238–1245, 1962

256. Ross WE, Glaubiger DL, Kohn KW: Quantitative and qualitative aspects of intercalator-induced DNA damage. Biochim Biophys Acta 562:41–50, 1979

257. Galbraith WM, Mellett LB: Tissue disposition of ^{3}H-actinomycin D in rat, monkey and dog. Cancer Chemother Rep 59:1061–1069, 1975

258. Tattersall NHM, Sodergren JE, Segupta SK et al: Pharmacokinetics of actinomycin D in patients with malignant melanoma. Clin Pharmacol Ther 17:701–708, 1975

259. Kennedy BJ: Mithramycin therapy in testicular cancer. J Urol 107:429–433, 1972

260. Koller C, Miller DM: Preliminary observations on the therapy of the myeloid blast phase of chronic granulocytic leukemia with plicamycin and hydroxyurea. N Engl J Med 315:1433–1437, 1986

261. Mathe G, Misset JL, de Vassal F et al: Phase II clinical trial with vindesine for remission induction in acute leukemia, blastic crisis of chronic myeloid leukemia, lymphosarcoma, and Hodgkin's disease: Absence of cross-resistance with vincristine. Cancer Treat Rep 62:805–809, 1978

262. Owellen RJ, Hartke CA, Dickerson RM et al: Inhibition of tubulin-microtubule polymerization by drugs of the vinca alkaloid class. Cancer Res. 36:1499–1502, 1976

263. Lapinjoki SP, Verajankowa HM, Huhtikangas AE et al: An enzyme-linked immunosorbent assay for the antineoplastic agent vincristine. J Immunoassay 7:113, 1986

264. Horwitz SB, Lothstein L, Manfredi JJ et al: Taxol: mechanisms of action and resistance. Ann NY Acad Sci 466:733–744, 1986

265. Madoc-Jones H, Mauro F: Interphase action of vinblastine and vincristine: Differences in their lethal action through the mitotic cycle of cultured mammalian cells. J Cell Physiol 72:185–196, 1968

266. Rosazza JPN, Duffel MW: Metabolic transformation of alkaloids. Alkaloids 27:323–405, 1986

267. Bleyer WA, Frisby SA, Oliverio VT: Uptake and binding of vincristine by murine leukemia cells. Biochem Pharmacol 24:633–639, 1975

268. Jackson DV, Bender RA: Cytotoxic thresholds of vincristine in L1210 murine leukemia and a human lymphoblastic cell line in vitro. Cancer Res 39:4346–4349, 1979

269. Dan K: Development of resistance to daunomycin (NSC 83151) in Ehrlich ascites tumor. Cancer Chemother Rep 55:133–141, 1971

270. Kartner N, Shales M, Riordan JR et al: Daunorubicin-resistant Chinese hamster ovary cells expressing multidrug resistance and a cell-surface P-glycoprotein. Cancer Res 43:4413–4419, 1983

271. Tsuruo T: Reversal of acquired resistance to vinca alkaloids and anthracycline antibiotics. Cancer Treat Rep 67:889–893, 1983

272. Conter V, Beck WT: Acquisition of multiple drug resistance by CCRF-CEM cells selected for different degrees of resistance to vincristine. Cancer Treat Rep 68:831–836, 1984

273. Greenberger LM, Williams SS, Horwitz SB: Biosynthesis of heterogeneous forms of multidrug resistance—associated glycoproteins. J Biol Chem, in press

274. Bender RA, Castle MC, Margileth DA et al: The pharmacokinetics of ^{3}H-vincristine in man. Clin Pharmacol Ther 22:430–438, 1977

275. Owellen RJ, Root MA, Hains FO: Pharmacokinetics of vindesine and vincristine in humans. Cancer Res 37:2603–2607, 1977

276. Lapinjoki SP, Verajankorva HM, Huhtikangas AE et al: An enzyme-linked immunosorbent assay for the antineoplastic agent vincristine. J Immunoassay 7:113–128, 1986

277. Sethi VS, Kimball JC: Pharmacokinetics and vincristine sulfate in children. Cancer Chemother Pharmacol 6:111, 1981

278. Jackson DV, Sethi VS, Spurr CL et al: Pharmacokinetics of vincristine in the cerebrospinal fluid of humans. Cancer Res 41:1466, 1981

279. Castle MC, Margileth DA, Oliverio VT: Distribution and excretion of ^{3}H-vincristine in the rat and the dog. Cancer Res 36:3684–3689, 1976

280. Jackson DV, Castle MC, Bender RA: Biliary excretion of vincristine. Clin Pharmacol Ther 24:101–107, 1978

281. Owellen RJ, Hartke CA, Hains FO: Pharmacokinetics and metabolism of vinblastine in humans. Cancer Res 37:2567–2602, 1977

282. Ferguson PJ, Phillips JR, Selner M et al: Differential activity of vincristine and vinblastine against cultured cells. Cancer Res 44:3307–3312, 1984

283. Zeffren J, Yagoda A, Kelsen D et al: Phase I-II trial of a 5-day continuous infusion of vinblastine sulfate. Anticancer Res 4:411–413, 1984

284. Griffiths JD, Stark RJ, Ding JC et al: Vincristine neurotoxicity in Charcot-Marie-Tooth syndrome. Med J Aust 143:305–306, 1985

285. Miller BR: Neurotoxicity and vincristine. J Am Med Assoc 253:2045, 1985

286. Weiss HD, Walker MD, Wiernik PH: Neurotoxicity of commonly used antineoplastic agents. N Engl J Med 291:127–133, 1974

287. Williams ME, Walker AN, Bracikowski JP et al: Ascending myeloencephalopathy due to intrathecal vincristine sulfate. A fatal chemotherapeutic error. Cancer 51:2041–2047, 1983

288. Dyke RW, Nelson RL: Phase I anticancer agents. Vindesine (desacetyl vinblastine amide sulfate). Cancer Treat Rep 4:135–142, 1977

289. Robertson GL, Bhoopalam N, Zelkowitz LJ: Vincristine neurotoxicity and abnormal secretion of antidiuretic hormone. Arch Intern Med 132:717–720, 1973

290. Dorr RT, Alberts DS: Vinca alkaloid skin toxicity: antidote and drug disposition studies in the mouse. JNCI 74:113–120, 1985

291. Bender RA, Nichols AP, Norton L et al: Lack of therapeutic synergism of vincristine and methotrexate in L1210 murine leukemia in vivo. Cancer Treat Rep 62:997–1003, 1978

292. Radice PA, Bunn PA, Ihde DC: Therapeutic trials with VP-16-213 and VM-26: Active single agents in small cell lung cancer, non-Hodgkin's lymphoma, and other malignancies. Cancer Treat Rep 63:1231–1239, 1979

293. Drewinko B, Barlogie B: Survival and cycle-progression delay of human lymphoma cells in vitro exposed to VP-16-213. Cancer Treat Rep 60:1295–1306, 1976

294. Wozniak AJ, Ross WE: DNA damage as a basis for 4'-demethylepipodophyl-lotoxin-9-(4,6-0-ethylidene-beta-D-glucopyranoside (etoposide) cytoxicity. Cancer Res 43:120, 1983

295. Haim N, Roman J, Nemec J et al: Peroxidative free radical formation and o-demethylation of etoposide (VP-16) and teniposide (VM-26). Biochem Biophys Res Commun 135:215–220, 1986

296. Dorr RT, Liddil JD, Gerner EW: Modulation of etoposide cytotoxicity and DNA strand scission in L1210 and 8226 cells by polyamines. Cancer Res 46:3891–3895, 1986

297. Pommier Y, Schwartz RE, Zwelling LA et al: Reduced formation of protein-associated DNA strand breaks in Chinese hamster cells resistant to topoisomerase II inhibitors. Cancer Res 46:611–616, 1986

298. Allen LM, Creaven PJ: Comparison of the human pharmacokinetics of VM-26 and VP-16, two antineoplastic epipodophylotoxin glucopyranoside derivatives. Eur J Cancer 11:697–707, 1975

299. Cunningham D, McTaggart L, Soukop M et al: Etoposide: a pharmacokinetic profile including an assessment of bioavailability. Med Oncol Tumor Pharmacother 3:95–100, 1986

300. Arbuck SG, Douglass HO, Crom WR et al: Etoposide pharmacokinetics in patients with normal and abnormal organ function. J Clin Oncol 4:1690–1695, 1986

301. D'Incalci M, Farina P, Sessa C et al: Pharmacokinetics of VP16-123 given by different administration methods. Cancer Chemother Pharmacol 7:141, 1982

302. Littlewood TJ, Spragg BP, Bentley DP: When is autologous bone marrow transplantation safe after high-dose treatment with etoposide? Clin Lab Haematol 7:213–218, 1985

303. Worzalla JF, Kaima BD, Johnson BM et al: N-demethylation of the antineoplastic agent hexamethylmelamine by rats and man. Cancer Res 33:2810–2815, 1972

304. Lake LM, Grunden EE, Johnson BM: Toxicity and antitumor activity of hexamethylmelamine and its N-demethylated metabolites in mice with transplantable tumors. Cancer Res 35:2858–2863, 1975

305. Rutty CJ, Connors TA, Nguyen-Hoang-Nam et al: In vivo studies with hexamethylmelamine. Eur J Cancer 14:713–720, 1978

306. Ames MM, Powis G: Determination of pentamethylmelamine and hexamethylmelamine in plasma and urine by nitrogen-phosphorous gas–liquid chromatography. J. Chromatogr 174:245–249, 1979

307. Dutcher JS, Jones RB, Boyd MR: A sensitive and specific assay for pentamethylmelamine in plasma: Applicability to clinical studies. Cancer Treat Rep 64:99–104, 1980

308. D'Incalci M, Bolis G, Mangioni C et al: Variable oral absorption of hexamethylmelamine in man. Cancer Treat Rep 62:2117–2119, 1978

309. Montgomery JA: Experimental studies at Southern Research Institute with DTIC (NSC-45388). Cancer Treat Rep 60:125–134, 1976

310. Hayward IP, Parson PG: Epigenetic effects of the methylating agent 5-(3-methyl-1-triazeno) imidazole-4-carboxamide in human melanoma cells. Austr J Exp Biol Med Sci 62:597–606, 1984

311. Tisdale MJ: Induction of haemoglobin synthesis in the human leukaemia cell line K562 by monomethyltriazenes and imidazotetrazinones. Biochem Pharmacol 34:2077–2082, 1985

312. Breithaupt H, Dammann A, Aigner K: Pharmacokinetics of decarbazine and its metabolite 5-aminoimidazole-4-carboxamide following different dose schedules. Cancer Chemother Pharmacol 9:103, 1982

313. Smith PJ, Ekert H, Waters KD et al: High incidence of cardiomyopathy in children treated with adriamycin and DTIC in combination chemotherapy. Cancer Treat Rep 61:1736–1738, 1977

314. Feaux de Lacroix W, Runne U, Hauk H et al: Acute liver dystrophy with thrombosis of hepatic veins: a fatal complication of dacarbazine treatment. Cancer Treat Rep 67:779–784, 1983

315. Weinkam RJ, Shiba DA: Metabolic activation of procarbazine. Life Sci 22:937–945, 1978

316. Kreis W, Yen Y: An antineoplastic ^{14}C-labeled methyl hydrazine derivative in P815 mouse leukemia. A metabolic study. Experentia 21:284–285, 1965

317. Dost F, Reed D: Methane formation in vivo from N-isopropyl-alpha-(2-methylhydrazino)-p-toulamide hydrochloride, a tumor-inhibiting methyl hydrazine derivative. Biochem Pharmacol 16:1741–1746, 1967

318. Shiba DA, Weinkam RJ: Metabolic activation of procarbazine: Activity of the intermediates and the effects of pretreatment. Proc Am Assoc Cancer Res 20:139, 1979

319. Chabner BA, Sponzo R, Hubbard S et al: High-dose intermittent intravenous infusion of procarbazine. Cancer Chemother Rep 57:361–363, 1973

320. Liske R: A comparative study of the activity of cyclophosphamide and procarbazine on the antibody production in mice. Clin Exp Immunol 15:271–280, 1973

321. Lee IP, Dixon RL: Mutagenicity, carcinogenicity, and teratogenicity of procarbazine. Mutat Res 55:1–14, 1978

322. Cozzarelli NR: DNA topoisomerases. Cell 22:327–328, 1980

323. McCredie KB: Amsacrine: A new drug for hematological malignancies. Eur J Cancer 21:1–3, 1985

324. Minford J, Kerrigan D, Nichols M et al: Enhancement of the DNA breakage and cytotoxic effects of intercalating agents by treatment with sublethal doses of 1-β-D-arabinofuranosylcytosine or hydroxyurea in L1210 cells. Cancer Res 44:5583–5593, 1984

325. Pommier Y, Zwelling LA, Kao-Shan CS et al: Correlations between intercalator-induced DNA strand breaks and sister chromatid exchanges, mutations, and cytotoxicity in Chinese hamster cells. Cancer Res 45:3143–3149, 1985

326. Rowe TC, Chen GL, Hsiang YH et al: DNA damage by antitumor acridines mediated by mammalian DNA topoisomerase-II. Cancer Res 46:2021–2026, 1986

327. Pommier Y, Minford JK, Schwartz RE et al: Effects of the DNA intercalators 4'-(9-acridinylamino)methanesulfon-m-anisidide and 2-methyl-9-hydroxyellipticinium on topoisomerase-II-mediated DNA strand cleavage and strand passage. Biochemistry 24:6410–6416, 1985

328. Zwelling LA, Silberman L, Estey E: Intercalator-induced, topoisomerase-II-mediated DNA cleavage and its modification by antineoplastic antimetabolites. Int J Radiat Oncol Biol Phys 12:1041–1047, 1986

329. Wong A, Huang CH, Crooke ST: Mechanism of deoxyribonucleic acid breakage induced by 4'-(9-acridinylamino)methanesulfon-m-anisidide and copper: role for cuprous ion and oxygen free radicals. Biochemistry 23:2946–2952, 1984

330. Pommier Y, Kerrigan D, Schwartz RE et al: Altered DNA topoisomerase-II activity in Chinese hamster cells resistant to topoisomerase-II inhibitors. Cancer Res 46:3075–3081, 1986

331. Bakic M, Beran M, Anderson BS et al: The production of topoisomerase II-mediated DNA cleavage in human leukemia cells predicts their susceptibility to 4'-(9-acridinylamino)methanesulfon-m-anisidide (m-AMSA). Biochem Biophys Res Commun 134:638–645, 1986

332. Markovits J, Pommier Y, Kerrigan D et al: Topoisomerase-II-mediated DNA breaks and cytotoxicity in relation to cell proliferation and the cell cycle in NIH 3T3 fibroblasts and L1210 leukemia cells. Cancer Res 47:2050–2055, 1987

333. Pommier Y, Schwartz RE, Zwelling LA et al: Reduced formation of protein-associated DNA strand breaks in Chinese hamster cells resistant to topoisomerase-II inhibitors. Cancer Res 46:611–616, 1986

334. Estey EH, Silberman L, Beran M et al: The interaction between nuclear topoisomerase-II activity from human leukemia cells, exogenous DNA, and 4'-(9-acridinylamino)methanesulfon-m-anisidide (m-AMSA) or 4'-(4,6-0-ethylidene-β-D-glucopyranoside) (VP-16) indicates the sensitivity of the cells to the drug. Biochem Biophys Res Commun 144:787–783, 1987

335. Glisson B, Gupta R, Smallwood-Kentro S et al: Characterization of acquired epipodophyllotoxin resistance in a Chinese hamster ovary cell line: loss of drug-stimulated DNA cleavage activity. Cancer Res 46:1934–1938, 1986

336. Darkin S, Ralph RK: Potentiation of 4'-(9-acridinylamino)methanesulphon-m-anisidine) action by verapamil. Cancer Lett 30:25–33, 1986

337. Shoemaker DD, Cysyk RL, Padmanabhan S et al: Identification of the principal biliary metabolite of m-AMSA in rats. Drug Metab Dispos 10:35–39, 1982

338. Hall SW, Friedman J, Legha SS et al: Human pharmacokinetics of a new acridine derivative, 4'-(9-acridinylamino)methanesulfon-m-anisidide (NSC 249992). Cancer Res 43:3422–3426, 1983

339. Shoemaker DD, Cysyk RL, Gormley PE et al: Metabolism of 4'-(9-acridinylamino) methanesulfon-m-anisidide by rat liver microsomes. Cancer Res 44:1939–1945, 1984

340. Paxton JW, Jurlina JL, Foote SE: The binding of amsacrine to human plasma proteins. J Pharm Pharmacol 38:432–438, 1986

341. Weiss RB, Grillo-Lopez AJ, Marsoni S et al: Amsacrine-associated cardiotoxicity: an analysis of 82 cases. J Clin Oncol 4:918–928, 1986

342. Engelking C, Sullivan P, Agoliati G et al: Amsacrine administration: a precautionary note (letter). Cancer Chemother Pharmacol 13:150, 1984

343. Kidd JG: Regression of transplanted lymphomas induced in vivo by means of normal guinea pig serum. I. Course of transplanted cancers of various kinds in mice and rats given guinea pig serum, horse serum, or rabbit serum. J Exp Med 98:565–582, 1953

344. Broome JD: Evidence that the L-asparaginase of guinea pig serum is responsible for its antilymphoma effects. I. Properties of the L-asparaginase of guinea pig serum in relation to those of the antilymphoma substance. J Exp Med 118:99–120, 1963

345. Jackson RC, Handschumacher RE: Escherichia coli L-asparaginase. Catalytic activity and subunit nature. Biochemistry 9:3585–3590, 1970

346. Ohnama T, Holland JF, Meyer P: Erwinia carotovora asparaginase in patients with prior anaphylaxis to asparaginase from E. coli. Cancer 30:376–381, 1972

347. Haley EE, Fischer GA, Welch AD: The requirement for L-asparagine of mouse leukemia cells L5178Y in culture. Cancer Res 21:532–536, 1961

348. Distasio JA, Neederman RA, Kafkewitz D et al: Purification and characterization of L-asparaginase with antilymphoma activity from Vibrio succinogenes. J Biol Chem 251:6929–6933, 1976

349. Haw T, Ohnuma T: L-asparaginase: In vitro inhibition of blastogenesis by enzyme from Erwinia carotovora. Nature 239:50–51, 1972

350. Yoshimoto T, Nishimura H, Saito Y et al: Characterization of polyethylene-glycol-modified L-asparaginase from Escherichia coli and its application to therapy of leukemia. Jpn J Cancer Res 77:1264–1270, 1986

351. Meister A, Levintow L, Greenfield RE et al: Hydrolysis and transfer reactions catalyzed by amidase preparations. J Biol Chem 215:441–460, 1955

352. Cooney DA, Capizzi RI, Handschumacher RE: Evaluation of L-asparagine metabolism in animals and man. Cancer Res 30:929–935, 1970

353. Nesbitt M, Chard R, Evans A et al: Intermittent L-asparaginase therapy for acute childhood leukemia. Proc 10th Int Cancer Cong, p 447, 1970

354. Ohnuma T, Holland JF, Sinks LF: Biochemical and pharmacological studies with L-asparaginase in man. Cancer Res 30:2297–2305, 1970

355. Peterson RC, Handschumacher RF, Mitchell MS: Immunological responses to L-asparaginase. J Clin Invest 50:1080–1090, 1971

356. Clavell LA, Gelber RD, Cohen HJ et al: Four-agent induction and intensive asparaginase therapy for treatment of childhood acute lymphoblastic leukemia. N Engl J Med 315:657–663, 1986

357. Homans AC, Rybak ME, Baglini RL et al: Effect of L-asparaginase administration on coagulation and platelet function in children with leukemia. J Clin Oncol 5:811–817, 1987

358. Bezeaud A, Drouet L, Leverger G et al: Effect of L-asparaginase therapy for acute lymphoblastic leukemia on plasma vitamin-K-dependent coagulation factors and inhibitors. J Pediatr 108:698–701, 1986

359. Leonard JV, Kay JDS: Acute encephalopathy and hyperammonaemia complicating treatment of acute lymphoblastic leukaemia with asparaginase. Lancet 1:162–163, 1986

360. Capizzi R: Improvement in the therapeutic index of L-asparaginase by methotrexate. Cancer Chemother Reps 6 (Pt 3):37–41, 1975

361. Jolivet J, Cole DE, Holcenberg JS et al: Prevention of methotrexate cytotoxicity by asparaginase inhibition of methotrexate polyglutamate formation. Cancer Res 45:217–220, 1985

RICHARD M. SIMON

CHAPTER 19 *Design and Conduct of Clinical Trials*

The purpose of this chapter is to highlight principles for the design and conduct of valuable therapeutic clinical trials in oncology. Many such studies are one of the following types.

1. *Phase I studies*. Determine the relationship between toxicity and dose-schedule of treatment
2. *Phase II studies*. Identify tumor types for which the treatment appears promising
3. *Phase III studies*
   a. Determine the effects of a treatment relative to the natural history of the disease
   b. Determine whether a new treatment is more effective than a standard therapy
   c. Determine whether a new treatment is as effective as a standard therapy but is associated with less morbidity

These classes of studies include evaluation of surgical procedures, radiotherapeutic treatments, chemotherapeutic drugs, immunostimulants, biologic response modifiers, antibiotics, antiemetics, and pain control agents. Each of the objectives stated above is meaningful, however, only within the context of a clearly defined patient population.

The experimental approach plays an important role in clinical oncology today. By the experimental approach, I refer to roughly two components: first, clinical results, rather than deductive reasoning, are required for the evaluation of a treatment[1]; and second, the experimental approach requires that preplanned therapeutic interventions be administered to specified types of patients under conditions that are controlled to enable well-defined medical questions to be answered directly. Comparing the survival rates of breast cancer patients treated with mastectomy to those of patients receiving mastectomy plus postoperative radiotherapy based on regional tumor registry data is an example of a nonexperimental survey. In such surveys, the investigator is a passive observer and abstracts records that he hopes will provide information about the phenomena he wishes to study. Treatment assignments, diagnostic tests, and follow-up procedures are determined by the patients and physicians independently of the investigator. The statistical associations resulting from such studies are in themselves a weak basis for causal inferences about the relationship between treatment administered and results observed. Treatments usually are selected based on subjective assessment of prognosis for the patient, capabilities of the physician, and variable diagnostic evaluations. It is generally impossible to identify and eliminate all the biases inherent in survey data.

Surveys are sometimes called "observational studies," although this is inaccurate because all knowledge is based on observations. Surveys generally are the only feasible mechanisms for epidemiologic assessment of disease etiology, and when performed by highly trained and critical investigators can contribute greatly to public welfare.[2,3] Acute observations in poorly structured therapeutic settings can also lead to immensely valuable ideas to be pursued and tested in the laboratory and planned clinical trials. Surveys are, however, sometimes proposed as an easy alternative to planned clinical trials for the evaluation of treatments.[4,5] For this purpose, the survey is distinctly inferior with regard to inherent reliability of conclusions concerning therapeutic effects. Mac-Mahon and Pugh[3] point out that

Only a minority of statistical associations are causal. . . . Once a statistical association has been demonstrated, how can it be determined whether or not it is causal. . . . The most satisfactory procedure is direct experiment. . . . The evaluation of the causal nature of a relationship, in the absence of direct experiment, is neither easy nor objective. . . . The field of cancer therapy is replete with examples of new modalities that were taken up with enthusiasm and proved worthless only after they had resulted in many years of futile cost and suffering.

The difficult problems in analysis of survey data are discussed elsewhere.[6-8] Improvements in computer technology have increased the ease of conducting medical surveys but have not had a major role in solving the basic weaknesses of this approach.

This chapter addresses principles for the design and conduct of therapeutic clinical trials in oncology. Such studies can be direct and easily interpretable mechanisms for answering important medical questions. To achieve this objective, however, certain principles must be followed in planning the study. The following sections address certain key aspects of this planning process.

The first result of the planning process is a written protocol. Typical subject headings for the protocol are shown in Table 19-1. This document should be self-contained, consistent, and carefully prepared. It should define uniform treatment and evaluation policies for a well-defined set of patients and should not leave important decisions to the discretion of the physician or the study chairperson. The protocol should clearly define the questions to be answered by the study and should directly justify that the number of patients and nature of controls are adequate to answer these questions definitively. It is very easy to embark on a futile or trivial study and to write the protocol merely as a guideline for clinical management supplemented by lofty objectives of no scientific meaning. Rushing the protocol development process and not being sufficiently critical of what is written or omitted contributes to this tendency. From the presentation of scientific background through the definition of data forms, the protocol should show clear, precise, and practical thinking.

STUDY OBJECTIVES

It is important to describe the study objectives specifically in the protocol. This helps orient the protocol to represent a clearly thought-out research plan rather than merely a guide for clinical management. Clearly stated objectives are necessary to ensure that size of the study, nature of controls, and plans for patient management are adequate and unbiased with regard to the questions posed.

Many studies in the social sciences are fishing expeditions that include numerous batteries of tests and result in exhaustive analyses. Such unstructured investigations are likely to result in some erroneous conclusions owing to the multiplicity of the questions addressed.[9] Therapeutic studies in oncology generally have a more specific natural focus. Nevertheless, it is useful to describe the objectives in terms of specific questions to be answered by the study. Some protocols state

---

TABLE 19-1. Subject Headings for a Protocol

1. Introduction and scientific background
2. Objectives
3. Selection of patients
4. Design of study (including schematic diagram)
5. Treatment programs
6. Procedures in event of toxicity
7. Required clinical and laboratory data
8. Criteria for evaluating the effect of treatment
9. Statistical considerations
10. Informed consent
11. Data forms
12. References
13. Study chairperson, collaborating participants, addresses, and telephone numbers

---

that the objective is to "improve treatment" and some list numerous objectives that are not feasible within the size of study planned or for which there are inadequate controls. These characteristics often are an indication that insufficient critical thinking has been done in the planning stage to permit clear interpretation of the results that will be obtained.

The realities of numbers of patients required dictate that most studies should be restricted to one major question. It is best when either positive or negative results are informative for patient management and for developing better treatments. Two examples of such studies are comparison of mastectomy to tumor resection for patients with stage I breast cancer and comparison of high-dose versus conventional-dose therapy with an effective drug. Many current studies provide no leads to build on when the results are negative.

Many current studies also fail to address the most important medical questions. The most important studies are often the most difficult to initiate. They may involve withholding a treatment established by tradition, potential transfer of patient management responsibility across specialties, standardization of procedures among individuals who believe their way is best, and sharing recognition with a large group of collaborators.

PATIENT ELIGIBILITY

Phase I studies generally are conducted with previously treated patients. However, the organ systems that are the expected targets of toxicity should be competent in patients selected for the study. Otherwise, the relationships between dose-schedule and toxicity found in the study will not be relevant to the treatment of less debilitated patients.

Whereas phase I studies need not be performed separately by histologic tumor type, this is not the case for phase II studies. In phase II studies the biologic response of major interest is that of the tumor itself. Because cytosensitivities vary among histologic types, it is important to study enough patients so that evaluation of tumor response can be made separately by type.

Some kinds of advanced cancer have no known therapy that prolongs survival (e.g., melanoma, esophageal, pancreatic). For such sites, phase II studies should consist of nonpreviously treated patients. The chance of tumor response generally decreases with prior treatment. Consequently, the inclusion of previously treated patients in phase II studies of diseases in which treatment does not prolong survival constitutes a decrease in the potential sensitivity of the study and a reduction in the likelihood of patient benefit.[9a]

For phase III studies, determination of eligibility criteria involves a trade-off between broad applicability of conclusions and addressing the study to those patients most likely to benefit from the new treatment. In a study with broad eligibility requirements, a conclusion of no difference between the treatments may result from a positive effect in one subset being cancelled by a negative effect in another or a positive effect in one subset being hidden in the overall comparison by the variability introduced by including patients less likely to benefit. For most studies, the basic analysis should include all patients; thus broad eligibility requirements may entail a loss of sensitivity.

Some statisticians advise that the eligibility criteria be very broad because subset analyses can always be performed later.[10,11] This approach has certain risks, however: misleading conclusions may result from multiple subset analyses, and one must be careful to plan the study so that adequate numbers of patients within each major subset are available for separate analysis.

Studies with relatively narrow eligibility criteria may not yield results that are generalizable to patients of the types excluded. Such studies have been criticized for this.[11a] But if the narrow eligibility criteria provide improved homogeneity of prognosis, then such studies can yield more clearcut answers to therapeutic questions with reasonable numbers of patients of a well-defined type.

In general, clearcut evidence of benefit for a well-defined class of patients is likely to be more valuable than a finding of no effect for a mixed population. Although often it is not obvious which patients are most likely to benefit, some studies of intensive treatment include debilitated patients for whom reduced doses are planned from the outset. Generally, their inclusion is detrimental to the study and not beneficial to the patient. The added numbers they represent are more than compensated for by the increase in variability of response and uncertainty of to whom the conclusions apply. Sir Bradford Hill made this point in discussing a clinical trial of streptomycin for respiratory tuberculosis:[12]

> . . . for it was realized that no two patients have an identical form of the disease and it was desired to eliminate as many of the obvious variations as possible. This planning . . . is a fundamental feature of the successful trial. To start out upon a trial with all and sundry included, and with the hope that the results can be sorted out statistically in the end is to court disaster.

ENDPOINT

The term *endpoint* refers to the criterion by which patient benefit is measured. A meaningful and reliable endpoint is essential for a worthwhile study. In some of the social sciences, lack of an adequate endpoint is a major impediment to progress. For clinical oncology this generally is not a severe problem. Nevertheless, explicit definition of the endpoint(s) is important for determining the size and duration of the trial and for ensuring that the proper measurements are taken and that follow-up evaluations are performed without bias.

The major endpoints of evaluating the effectiveness of a treatment should be measures of patient welfare. Duration of survival and quality of life are two such endpoints. Quality of life is used infrequently because sufficiently simple and reproducible measures of important aspects of quality of life have not been developed. The development of such measures that can be used broadly by clinicians in the conduct of therapeutic evaluations is an important area that warrants research.

Survival generally is the most meaningful measure of benefit for phase III studies. For a variety of reasons, it generally is not the endpoint upon which sample sizes are planned or ultimate therapeutic recommendations are made. The endpoints commonly used instead of or in addition to survival are degree of tumor shrinkage and duration for which the tumor is below the level of clinical detection. These are basically subjective measures. Whether a patient has a partial response depends on who is doing the measuring and what the response criteria are.[13-16]

The more closely one looks, the fewer complete remissions are obtained and the more rapidly recurrent disease is detected. Consequently, it is important that follow-up procedures be standardized in the protocol to ensure that the study is not jeopardized by biased evaluation of response. Lack of standardization of response assessment is a major cause of confusion in communication of results.

It cannot be assumed that response rates, duration of response, or disease-free intervals are proper endpoints for drawing conclusions about therapeutic efficacy because they are not direct measures of patient welfare. There are obvious examples in which survival extensions and cure rates have followed major improvements in complete response rates and complete response durations. The situation is more mixed, however, with regard to partial responses.

A treatment that causes partial responses is not necessarily beneficial to the patient. Even if one demonstrates that partial responders live longer than nonresponders, one cannot conclude that the treatment is beneficial.[17-19] Comparisons of survivals between responders and nonresponders are biased in two ways. First, responders by definition have lived long enough to achieve that status. Second, responders may have more favorable prognostic factors that would result in their living longer than nonresponders even in the absence of any treatment. Finally, one cannot assume that the difference in survival does not result from the treatment's shortening survival for the nonresponders. To demonstrate that treatment extends survival, the comparison of survival between responders and nonresponders is not relevant. One must demonstrate that the treated group as a whole lives longer than an appropriate control group of similar prognosis.

For some kinds of cancer, partial responses are of substantial duration, are clearly associated with improved palliation, and have been demonstrated to represent the effect of treatment on prolonging life by comparison to an appropriate untreated or single agent control group. For other kinds of cancer, however, partial responses are of minimal duration and have not been demonstrated to represent a beneficial therapeutic effect for the patient. Increases in partial response rates without corresponding improvements in survival or palliation for the treated group should not be viewed as therapeutic improvements. However, partial responses are useful indicators of biologic activity for phase II studies, even in diseases where direct patient benefit cannot be demonstrated.

TREATMENT ALLOCATION

PHASE I STUDIES

The simplest phase I studies involve estimation of the relationship between dose and toxicity for a single schedule and mode of administration. Such studies usually are performed by starting with a low dose not expected to produce serious toxicity in any patients and increasing the dose for subsequent patients according to a series of preplanned steps. Several patients are treated at each dosage level, often three patients per step when no toxicity is encountered and six patients per step thereafter.[20,21] The initial dose selection generally is based on animal toxicity data. A starting dose of one tenth the LD_{10} expressed as milligrams per square meter of body surface area in the mouse usually is used.[21a-25]

Dose escalation for subsequent patients occurs only after sufficient time has passed to observe acute toxic effects for patients treated at lower doses. Insufficient attention has been given to quantitative methods of determining dose steps. One commonly used is based on a modified Fibonacci series.[26,27] The second step is twice the starting dose, the third step is 67% greater than the second, the fourth step is 50% greater than the third, the fifth step is 40% greater than the fourth, and each subsequent step is 33% greater than that preceding it. In some cases this procedure may result in an insufficiently rapid escalation,[28] and other methods of dose escalation have been proposed.[29,30]

Escalating doses for subsequent courses in the same patient generally is not carried out except at low doses because it may mask the presence of cumulative toxicity. An escalated second dose for a patient may be toxic because it is a higher dose or because it is a second dose. Many phase I studies that escalate doses within patients are not analyzed in a way that distinguishes patients from courses of therapy.

Some phase I studies evaluate several schedules or modes of administration. If study of the second schedule is begun after evaluation of the first has been completed or is well under way, the accumulated information can be used to establish a starting dose. Otherwise, it may be useful to allocate the schedules randomly to newly eligible patients. This is not crucial but serves to eliminate bias in selecting patients for one schedule or other based upon their condition. Such randomization is not for the purpose of directly comparing the schedules but to better ensure that the maximum tolerable dose determined for one schedule is not misleadingly high or low because of patient selection.

For any phase I study, and particularly for studies of combinations, criteria for dose reductions should be specified clearly in the protocol and monitored closely. Active monitoring of results by the study chairperson is essential for a safe trial.

PHASE II STUDIES

The results of phase II studies can be misleading in two ways.[9a,31] First, little antitumor effect may be seen, but the patients may be so debilitated or extensively pretreated that the results do not reflect true potential usefulness of the agent; and second, because of patient selection or inadequately rigorous response criteria, more favorable results are obtained than will be substantiated by further trials. Both types of results are undesirable.

To deal with these potential problems, it has been suggested that phase II studies involve a randomization between the experimental agent and a treatment known to have antitumor value.[11,32-34] The purpose of randomization would not be for determining which treatment was better, but for having a baseline response rate of similar patients treated with a known therapy. The known therapy would not be a "standard therapy" in the sense of being the treatment of choice. Peto[11] has suggested that two thirds of the patients should be randomized to the new treatment. For phase II studies of previously treated patients, it often is not possible to identify an active control treatment. When it is possible, this design can deal effectively with the false-positivity problem. Adequate standardization of response criteria usually would be just as effective, however. The randomized design appears to have less value for dealing with the false-negativity problem. The control therapy generally will have a low response rate for such patients, and it will not serve as a sensitive control. A better safeguard against false-negative results is to use nonpreviously treated patients in phase II studies when it is ethically possible.

For cooperative groups with sufficient patients to conduct simultaneously several phase II studies in a disease, randomization among the new agents is desirable.[31] There is no question that patient selection can influence results.[35] Such selection can lead to bias in the ranking of new agents. Differences among institutions in evaluation of response can make the problem even more severe. The conduct of one master phase II study with randomized treatment assignment helps alleviate these problems.

Phase II trials may be designed with cross-over to a specified treatment (either another experimental agent or an established drug) when the patient fails the initial therapy. This aspect of the design usually supplies little information because so few patients make it through the secondary treatment, because there are so few responses, and because the condition of the patient has changed.

PHASE III STUDIES

Controls

The interpretation of most phase III studies involves some type of comparison of results. In some cases the basis of comparison will be the natural history of the disease, and in others it will be another treatment. We shall use the term "control" to represent the basis against which a treatment is to be evaluated. Rarely, if ever, do we just want to know whether a treatment is better or worse than the control. We want to estimate the degree of difference. All measurement ultimately is comparative, however, and the categorization of a treatment as "good" or "bad" involves an implicit comparison to the natural history of the disease.

To determine whether a new treatment cures any patients with a disease that is uniformly and rapidly fatal, history is a satisfactory control. In this situation the patient population is completely homogeneous with regard to cure in the absence of the new therapy. If 20% of patients are cured by conventional therapy and we can identify them by patient and tumor characteristics measured at diagnosis, we can restrict a study to the remaining 80% and have complete homogeneity. Once we leave the setting of complete homogeneity with regard to the chosen endpoint, the definition of an adequate nonrandomized control becomes problematical.

In many studies the controls are either numbers determined from publications or patients treated in nonexperimental settings in which the information is abstracted from tumor registries, data banks, or medical records. The meaningfulness of such controls is questionable. Often diagnostic and staging procedures, supportive care, secondary treatments, and methods of evaluation and follow-up are different for the controls and the current treatment group. There generally is differential bias in the selection of patients to be treated resulting from judgments by the physicians, self-selection by the patients, and differences in referral patterns. There may be bias in treatment ineligibility rates.[36] Current patients are sometimes excluded from analysis for not meeting eligibility criteria, not receiving "adequate" treatment, refusing treatment, or a major protocol violation. The controls, on the other hand, generally contain all the patients. There may be differences in the distribution of known and unknown prognostic factors between the controls and the current treatment group. Often there is inadequate information to determine whether such differences are present, and current known prognostic factors may not have been measured or recorded for the controls. It generally is difficult to tell whether the controls would have been eligible for the current study and in what way they represent a selection of all eligible patients.

In the best of circumstances historical controls will be patients treated within the previous few years at the same institution or institutions performing the new study. The controls would be treated on a protocol having exactly the same eligibility requirements, work-up, follow-up, and response evaluation procedures as the current study, referral patterns and accrual rates would be static, no patients in either group would be excluded from analysis because of ineligibility or nonevaluability, and an exhaustive demonstration of similarity in distribution of all suspected prognostic factors would be presented. These circumstances rarely are encountered in practice. Pocock[37] has reported 19 unselected instances under circumstances approaching these where a collaborative group carried one treatment over for two successive studies. Even here, for 4 of the 19 pairs of trials the differences in outcome were statistically significant at the $p < 0.02$ level.

Formation of the control group by random assignment of treatment as an integral part of the planned study can avoid most of the systematic biases mentioned above.[38-41] The random assignment should not be performed until the patient is found eligible, and then a truly random or nondecipherable mechanism should be used. Alternation, day of the week, or other predictable procedures are not adequate because they allow bias in the decision of whether to enter a patient into a study based on knowledge beforehand of what treatment the patient will receive. Randomization does not ensure that the study will include a representative sample of all patients with the disease, but it does help to ensure an unbiased evaluation of the relative merits of the two treatments for the types of patients entered.

Some of the advantages of randomization are subtle and not widely understood. For example, it is sometimes said that randomization is unnecessary because matched historical or concurrent controls can be selected. But one can match only with regard to known prognostic factors, and these generally explain only a minor portion of the heterogeneity in prognosis among patients.[42] Matching with regard to known factors gives no assurance that the distributions of unknown factors are similar between the treatment groups. It also is sometimes said that randomization is not effective in ensuring that the treatment groups are similar with regard to unknown prognostic factors unless the number of patients is large. This is true but reflects a misunderstanding of randomization. Randomization does not ensure that the groups are medically equivalent, but it distributes the unknown biasing factors according to a known random distribution so that their effects can be rigorously allowed for in significance tests and confidence intervals.[43] This is true regardless of the study size. A significance level represents the probability that differences in outcome are due to random fluctuations. Without randomized treatment allocation, a "statistically significant difference" may be due to a nonrandom difference in the distribution of unknown prognostic factors.

Randomization (or stratified randomization, to be discussed later) is inherently the method of treatment assignment that results in the most reliable basis for inference.[44,45] This is not to say that all randomized studies are good or that all nonrandomized studies are bad, but that, everything else being equal, randomization adds considerably to the ease of interpretability of the study since one need not worry about conscious or inadvertent systematic biases in patient selection or treatment assignment. Gehan and Freireich[46] and Pocock[47] have listed conditions under which nonrandomized studies can be considered reliable. The majority of nonrandomized studies do not meet these conditions. The oncology literature is filled with reports of nonrandomized studies in which scant attention is paid to comparability with regard to known prognostic factors. At this point the major advantages of randomization are not the subtle aspects mentioned but avoidance of the major biases of the majority of poorly done, nonrandomized studies. If nonrandomized studies were scrupulously conducted and critically reported under the conditions described above for consecutive trials, the subtle advantages that randomization will always have might be less decisive. Modern alternative approaches based on nonexperimental data bases and tumor registries[4] having concurrent nonrandomized controls are a poor alternative to either method.

Are randomized trials necessary for identifying major advances in treatment? No. There are many examples of therapeutic breakthroughs that were recognized without randomized trials. For the most part, however, these occurred in diseases where the prognosis was 100% predictable before the advent of the new therapy, and hence there was no possibility of bias with regard to patient selection. False innovations are much more numerous than real breakthroughs, however, and it is difficult to distinguish one from the other.[48] There certainly is a role for innovative nonrandomized studies in diseases with uniformly bleak prognoses.

Some physicians are uncomfortable with the notion of randomization, believing that they have an obligation to develop an opinion about the relative merits of alternative possible treatments and to recommend a therapy to their patients accordingly.[49] This position is understandable but must be tempered by the following considerations: different competent physicians often hold widely divergent opinions about the relative merits of alternative treatments for the same patient;[50] the little research done indicates that experienced, well-educated adults are likely to overrate the correctness of their opinions and hunches;[51] and the experimental treatment generally is neither much better nor much worse than the control, and we have little real basis for selecting between the treatments before the trial. As Gilbert, McPeek, and Mosteller point out,[51]

Much of current popular discussion of the ethical issue takes the position that physicians should use their best judgment in prescribing for a patient. To what extent the physician is responsible for the quality of the judgment is not much discussed, except to say that he must keep abreast of the times. Some physicians will feel an obligation to find out that goes beyond the mere holding of an opinion. Such physicians will feel a responsibility to contribute to the research. In similar fashion, some current patients may feel a responsibility to contribute to the better care of future patients. The current model of the passive patient and the active outgoing physician is not the most effective one for a society that not only wants cures rather than sympathy, but insists on them—a society that has been willing to pay both in patient cooperation and material resources for the necessary research.

If randomization is used, it generally should take place as late as possible before effecting treatment of the patient.[10] For example, in evaluating a chemotherapeutic regimen as a postsurgical adjuvant treatment, randomization should take place after the surgery has been completed and the patient has recovered sufficiently to begin receiving chemotherapy.

This approach serves to reduce bias in the surgery administered and possible bias in disqualifications of randomized patients owing to surgical findings, morbidity, or mortality.

Protocols for nonrandomized phase III studies should describe the control group to be used. The control group should consist of patients for whom individual records are available for detailed evaluation of comparability.

Stratified Randomization

When there are known major prognostic factors for patients in a randomized study, it often is advisable to stratify the randomization to assure equal distribution of these factors.[52] This usually is accomplished by preparing a separate randomization list (or set of cards in sealed envelopes) for each distinct subset of patients (stratum). Each list must be balanced so that after each block of four to ten patients within the stratum the treatment groups contain equal numbers of patients. Within the blocks, the sequence of treatment assignments is random. The stratification factors must, of course, be known for each patient at the time of randomization.

For example, as shown in Figure 19-1, in a comparison of treatments for testicular cancer the factors may be histology and stage. These two stratification factors determine six patient strata. For a comparison of two treatments, designated A and B, the sequence of treatment assignments for a stratum can be determined in the following manner. We shall assume that is has been decided that the sequence for each stratum will be balanced in blocks of six patients. One obtains a table of two-digit random numbers and starts reading the table down an arbitrarily selected column. Random numbers in the range 00 to 49 will indicate treatment A, and random numbers in the range 50 to 99 will indicate treatment B. If no more than 30 patients are anticipated in the stratum, the tentative treatment assignments are determined by the first 30 random numbers read. This determines a sequence of a total of 30 As and Bs. This list must be modified in the following way to ensure balance after each block of six patients in the stratum. If the random sequence is

ABAAAABBABABBBBAAAABBAABBAAABB

then it is modified to

ABAABB AABBAB ABBBAA BAAABB ABBAAB.

FIG. 19-1. Example of stratification for a randomized clinical trial.

Histology	Stage	
	II	III
Teratocarcinoma with or without seminoma		
Embryonal carcinoma with or without seminoma		
Either of above with elements of choriocarcinoma		

If three As occur in a block before three Bs, the remainder of the block is automatically filled in with Bs before the random sequence is continued. Similarly, if three Bs occur in a block before three As, the remainder of the block is automatically filled in with As. This procedure is performed separately for each stratum. The sequence of treatment assignments for each stratum is then transferred to a randomization list or to sealed and numbered randomization envelopes. The randomization sequences should be prepared by someone who will not be entering patients into the study. Generally, the blocksize should not be known to the participants, and they should not be permitted to examine the partially used randomization sequences. These procedures are easily generalized to more than two treatments or to block sizes other than six. For unstratified randomizations, the sequence of treatment assignments can be prepared in exactly the same way except that the block size is often larger.

The number of strata increases multiplicatively with the number of stratification factors because the patient subsets are defined by combinations of these factors. Although limited stratification often is desirable, overstratification is detrimental to the trial. If there is extensive stratification, numerous strata will contain very few patients. Consequently, balance with regard to the most important factor or factors may be seriously impaired by the inclusion of factors of secondary importance. Even the total numbers of patients assigned to each of the treatments may be very unequal. Extensive overstratification becomes equivalent to randomization with no stratification at all.[53]

It generally is best to limit stratification to those factors definitely known to have important independent effects on response. If two factors are closely correlated, one, at most, should be included in the stratification. Peto and others[10] believe that stratification is an unnecessary complication because adjustment for imbalances of known factors can be made in the analysis. For small studies, however, such adjustments should not be relied on. Stratification may obviate the chance of gross imbalances that cannot be adjusted for and ensures that the treatment comparisons are not totally dependent on statistical adjustment methods.[54,55] Simon[56] and Kalish and Begg[57] have reviewed the various stratification methods available. Kalish and Begg[57a] studied analytic aspects of adaptive stratification methods.

Cross-over Designs

Cross-over designs have been discussed in the context of phase II studies but also are used in other settings, such as the comparative evaluation of antiemetics and antipain treatments. For example, patients might be randomized to receive either an antiemetic during the first course of chemotherapy and a placebo during the second, or the alternate sequence. This design is motivated by the desire to increase the sensitivity of a study by using each patient as his own control, and thereby to reduce the number of patients required. The usefulness of this approach is limited because the condition of the patient changes with time and the effect of a treatment may be influenced by previous treatments or conditioned by previous responses.

Cross-over designs in which there are more than two treatment episodes per patient are almost always difficult or impossible to interpret clearly. Frequently such studies are analyzed and reported in a manner that fails to distinguish distinct patients from multiple treatment episodes of the same patient.

Useful methods for analyzing a two-period cross-over design are described by Hills and Armitage[58] and by Koch.[59] Use of the cross-over design is controversial and has been discouraged by the Biometric and Epidemiologic Advisory Committee of the Food and Drug Administration.[60] If the relative efficacy of the treatments in the second period differs from that in the first period or is conditioned by first period response, it is not possible to use each patient as his own control. To determine whether such an interaction exists requires as many patients as a non-cross-over design, and one should seriously weigh these considerations before adopting the cross-over design.[61,61a,62]

It is always best to administer a treatment in a clinical trial the way that it would be recommended for administration in general medical practice. The cross-over design is artificial in this regard. Less structured designs that repeatedly rerandomize the same patients are subject to this criticism and suffer from the introduction of additional correlations that generally are impossible to account for properly in the analysis.

Common Control Designs

In randomized multi-institution studies, it is sometimes difficult to obtain agreement among all participants concerning the treatments to be used. A compromise design sometimes suggested is to allow each institution to select between doing randomized study of treatments A and C or doing a randomized study of treatments B and C. These two studies are conducted simultaneously, but at different institutions. It usually is recognized that this design is inferior to a simple randomization among all treatments A, B, and C within each institution, but it is hoped that it is better than a totally nonrandomized design. Schoenfeld and Gelber[63] have shown that unless one can assume that there are no differences among institutions in response to treatment, this design is very inefficient. With three treatments (one being the common control), this design requires twice as many patients as a straightforward three-way randomized design. Makuch and Simon[64] have pointed out that similar results for the common control treatment between the sets of institutions selecting the two options do not ensure that the other two treatments can be validly compared. Systematic differences among the institutions may be manifested only in intensively treated patients. Consequently, the common control design is not a good alternative unless the experimental treatments are minor variants of each other. In general, it is best to standardize the treatments rigorously in order to eliminate extraneous causes of variability and bias.

Factorial Designs

In a 2×2 factorial design there are actually four treatments under study. The first factor represents two alternative treatment interventions, such as amputation or resection. The second factor represents two other alternative interventions superimposed on the first factor, such as adjuvant chemotherapy or no further treatment. Although there are actually four treatment groups (amputation alone, resection alone, amputation plus chemotherapy, resection plus chemotherapy), proponents of such designs[11,45,65] suggest that the effect of each treatment factor can be addressed using all of the patients and pooling with regard to the other factor (or with the influence of the other factor accounted for in the analysis, but not separate analysis for each level of the other factor). The validity of such an analysis depends on the following types of assumptions: if adjuvant chemotherapy is beneficial for amputees, it is also beneficial for resected patients, and the difference in efficacy of the two surgical procedures is either concurrently positive, negative, or zero, both for patients receiving adjuvant chemotherapy and for those not receiving further treatment. If these assumptions are not satisfied, the study must be analyzed by the simultaneous comparison of all four treatment groups. The risk in planning such a study is that the number of patients established will be sufficient only for pooled two-group comparisons, yet the data may suggest that such an analysis is not adequate. Also, the number of patients required to determine whether such an interaction is present is greater than the number required to perform two group comparisons. Thus the factorial design offers the possibility of answering two questions for the price of one, but there is a risk of difficulty in interpretation.[66]

Combining Randomized and Historical Controls

Randomized studies are sometimes conducted weighted 2:1 in favor of the new treatment with the intent of incorporating historical controls in the analysis if their outcomes are similar to those of the randomized controls.[10] This design rarely provides enough randomized controls for an adequate comparison with results for the historical control group.[67] Pocock[47] has investigated other methods of combining controls from two successive studies, but he assumes that the expected difference between outcomes from the control groups is zero. As discussed in the next section, a 2:1 randomization often is reasonable but not for the purpose of including historical controls.

SIZE AND DURATION OF THE STUDY

PHASE I AND PHASE II TRIALS

The size of phase I studies cannot be completely determined in advance. Guidelines that exist for planning the size of such studies have been presented in a previous section.

Simon[68] has recently reviewed the statistical designs that have been developed for phase II trials. With any of the proposed designs, the accrual plan and decision rules are applied seaparately to each subset of patients for whom inferences are to be made (e.g., nonpreviously treated advanced colon cancer patients). The oldest approach is Gehan's two-stage design.[69] If the target activity level of interest is 20%, then 14 patients are accrued in the first

stage. If no responses are obtained, the trial is terminated for such patients and the drug is considered inactive for that subset. The basis for this conclusion is that a drug with a 20% response rate probability has a 95% chance of causing at least 1 response in 14 patients. Thus if we reject the drug for this subset when no responses are seen in the first 14 patients, the rejection error is 5% for a true effectiveness of 20%. Table 19-2 shows the number of patients to be treated in the first stage as a function of the rejection error and true effectiveness proportion. If no responses are seen in the tabulated number of patients, the drug is rejected for this subset.

For a rejection error of 5% and a true activity level of 20%, if at least one response is obtained in the first 14 patients, a second stage of the trial is conducted to better estimate the response rate of the drug. The number of patients required for the second stage depends strongly on the precision desired for the estimated response rate. For a standard error of 10%, about 25 total patients are required (e.g., 14 in the first stage, 11 in the second). For a standard error of 5%, the required total number of patients is generally in the range of 50 to 90. Gehan's design is often applied with 14 patients in the first stage and 25 total if any responses are obtained. A sample of 25 patients, however, generally provides a poor estimate of the true response probability, and a study of 35 to 40 patients is often preferable.

Gehan's plan frequently is misapplied by having too heterogeneous a set of patients in the first stage. If no responses are observed among 14 patients of diverse tumor types or previous treatment experiences, no conclusion can be reached for any single well-defined class of patients. One usually should strive for separate evaluation of results by whether or not the patient has previously received chemotherapy. If nonpreviously treated patients are to be included in order to minimize the number of patients exposed to an ineffective drug, it is advisable to delay entry of previously treated patients until the drug has demonstrated activity.

Gehan's plan also is frequently misapplied by failure to conduct the second stage for strata that exhibit at least one response in the first 14 patients. The second stage usually is essential because even a drug with a 5% response rate has a 51% chance of producing at least one response in 14 patients.

Simon[68] has developed an optimized modification of Gehan's design. It is a two-stage design with n_1 patients in the first stage and n patients total. If the observed response rate at the end of the first stage is $\leq r_1/n_1$, then the trial terminates and the drug is rejected as being of little interest. Otherwise, accrual continues to a total of n patients. At the

TABLE 19-2. Sample Size (n_1) Required for Preliminary Trial of a New Agent for Given Levels of Therapeutic Effectiveness and Rejection Error

Rejection Error (β)	Therapeutic Effectiveness (%)									
	5	10	15	20	25	30	35	40	45	50
5%	59	29	19	14	11	9	7	6	6	5
10%	45	22	15	11	9	7	6	5	4	4

end of the second stage, the drug is rejected if the observed response rate is ≤ r/n.

Table 19-3 shows some of these optimized designs. To select a design one must specify a target activity level p_1 of interest, and also a lower activity level p_0. The optimal designs in Table 19-3 provide probability ≥ 0.90 of rejecting drugs worse than p_0 and probability ≥ 0.90 of not-rejecting drugs better than p_1. Subject to these two constraints the optimal designs minimize the average sample size as functions of n_1, r_1, n, r.

The average sample size is calculated at the activity level p_0. Hence the optimal designs are optimized for screening out poor drugs. Table 19-3 shows for each design the decision criteria, the average sample size, and the probability of stopping after the first stage for a drug with activity level p_0.

Table 19-3 also shows the "minimax" design for each situation. The minimax design is that design with the smallest maximum sample size n that satisfies the two constraints described above. If there are several such designs, the one with the minimum average sample size (calculated at activity level p_0) is shown. Although minimax designs have somewhat larger average sample sizes than optimal designs, in some cases they are preferable because the small increase in average sample size is more than compensated for by a large reduction in maximum sample size.

PHASE III TRIALS

The protocol for a phase III study should specify the number of patients and duration of follow-up planned. These plans should be based on the specific study objectives and endpoints used. In many cases, the same protocol will include plans for treating very distinct subsets of patients (e.g., stage I and stage II breast cancer patients). In such instances, plans should be made for accruing sufficient numbers of patients of each type for separate analyses because the relative merits of the treatments may vary substantially. Because of unforeseen complications or larger than expected treatment differences, patient accrual may have to be terminated prematurely. Nevertheless, target sample sizes are essential to ensure that the study is feasible and to know when to stop in the absence of premature termination. If too few patients are studied, the results may be ambiguous or erroneous, which commonly happens.[70-73] It is equally undesirable to have more patients studied than is necessary to reliably answer the questions posed by the study. The protocol should document that the target sample size can be accrued within a reasonable period of time (usually 3–4 years).

The usual statistical methods of sample size determination in comparative trials are oversimplified as rigid models of the complete analysis but are useful for planning purposes. These methods are based on the assumption that at the conclusion of the trial, a statistical significance test will be performed comparing the treatment groups with regard to the major endpoint(s). A statistical significance level of 0.05 resulting from a treatment comparison has the following meaning: if there is no true difference in treatment efficacy, the probability of obtaining a difference in outcomes as extreme as that observed in the data is 0.05. The significance level does not represent the probability that the null hypothesis is true, it represents a probability of an observed difference, assuming that the null hypothesis is true. Conventional statistical theory ascribes no probabilities to hypotheses, only to data.

With few patients in each of the treatment groups being compared, the difference in observed outcomes must be very extreme in order for the significance level to be as small as 0.05. As the sample size increases, smaller differences in response will be statistically significant at the 0.05 level. In comparing proportions, 10 of 10 compared to 7 of 10 (a difference of 30%) is not statistically significant at the 0.05 level, whereas 40 of 40 compared to 35 of 40 (a difference of 12%) is.

For comparing two proportions, the usual method of sample size determination is as follows. It is assumed that after n patients have been observed on treatment A and n patients have been observed on treatment B, a statistical significance test will be performed. One wishes to determine n to be just large enough so that if the true response rate for A is p_A% (i.e., the response rate that would be observed in an infinite number of patients receiving A) and the true response rate for B is p_B%, 80% of the time the significance level will be no greater than 0.05. The 80% figure is called the power of the test.

If we think of a study resulting in a significance level of less than 0.05 for the major comparison as a positive study, the power represents the probability of getting a true positive result when the actual response rates are p_A and p_B. The power is a design parameter that usually is specified between 80% and 95%. Whereas performing a significance test does not require knowledge of the unknown p_A and p_B, these parameters are an integral part of determining n to achieve a

TABLE 19-3.   Optimum and Minimax Two-Stage Phase II Designs

		Optimum Design				Minimax Design			
p_0	p_1	r_1/n_1*	r/n	PET†	ANP††	r_1/n_1	r/n	PET	ANP
0.05	0.25	0/9	2/24	0.63	14.55	0/13	2.20	0.51	16.41
0.05	0.20	0/12	3/37	0.54	23.50	0/18	3/32	0.40	26.44
0.10	0.25	2/21	7/50	0.65	31.20	2/27	6/40	0.48	33.70
0.20	0.40	3/17	10/37	0.55	26.0	3/19	10/36	0.46	28.26

*Reject drug if observed response rate is ≤ r_1/n_1 or ≤ r/n.
†Probability of early termination, after the first stage, when the true response probability is p_0.
††Average number of patients when the true response probability is p_0.

preplanned power. If treatment A is a standard treatment, p_A is estimated from past data. The absolute magnitude $|p_B - p_A|$ is viewed as a difference that we wish to have a power of 80% (say) for detecting.

For comparing two proportions, Tables 19-4 and 19-5 can be used to determine the number of patients to be assigned each of two treatments in order to achieve a specified power as a function of the true response rates. Table 19-4 is for obtaining one-sided significance levels less than 0.05, and Table 19-5 is for two-sided significance levels of less than 0.05. A two-sided significance level represents the probability by chance alone of obtaining a difference in either direction as large as the one actually observed. A one-sided significance level represents the probability by chance alone of obtaining a difference as large as and in the same direction as that actually observed. Controversy exists over the appropriateness of one-sided or two-sided significance levels. This will be discussed later in the chapter. A conservative approach is to use two-sided significance levels. Suppose that based on past data we estimate the response rate for treatment A to be 30% and that we wish to have 80% power for detecting a true response rate of treatment B of 55%. For a two-sided statistical significance test, we find from Table 19-5 that 68 patients for each of the two treatments are needed (136 patients total). If we wish power of 80% for detecting a true response rate of treatment B of 50%, 103 patients per treatment are needed. The required number of patients increases rapidly as size of the difference to be detected decreases. Almost all phase III studies should be large enough to detect reliably a difference of 20% to 25% in success rate. The "not significantly different" results of smaller comparative studies often are mistakenly interpreted as saying something about the treatments, whereas they may be just a consequence of the inadequate numbers of patients.[70-73]

Tables 19-4 and 19-5 were constructed according to the methods of Casagrande, Pike, and Smith,[74] and are considered more accurate than tables previously published based on other approximations.[75] When the smaller response rate is thought to exceed 50%, the tables given here should be used to compare failure rates (100% minus response rate).

When an unbalanced $K/1$ randomization is contemplated for comparing two treatments, the total sample size obtained from Tables 19-4 and 19-5 should be multiplied by $(K + 1)^2/4K$. For example, a 2:1 randomization requires 12.5% more total patients than an equally weighted design of the same power. Weightings more extreme than 2:1 are rarely desirable.

For comparative trials of proportions using historical controls, appropriate tables are given by Makuch and Simon,[76] and are reproduced here as Tables 19-6, 19-7, and 19-8. These tables are more bulky because the number of patients to be given the experimental treatment depends on the size of the historical control group. Tables 19-6, 19-7, 19-8 are for achieving 80% power with a one-sided significance level of 0.05. If our historical control group of 50 patients showed a response rate of 30% and we want 80% power for detecting a true response rate of 50% for the new treatment, Table

TABLE 19-4. Number of Patients in Each of Two Treatment Groups (One-Sided Test)

Smaller Success Rate	Larger Minus Smaller Success Rate									
	0.05	0.10	0.15	0.20	0.25	0.30	0.35	0.40	0.45	0.50
0.05	512*	172	94	62	45	35	28	23	19	16
	381†	129	72	48	35	27	22	18	15	13
0.10	786	236	121	76	54	40	31	25	21	17
	579	176	91	58	41	31	24	20	16	14
0.15	1026	292	144	88	60	44	34	27	22	18
	752	216	108	66	46	34	26	21	17	14
0.20	1231	339	163	98	66	48	36	29	23	19
	900	250	121	73	50	37	28	22	18	15
0.25	1402	377	178	105	70	50	38	29	23	19
	1024	278	132	79	53	38	29	23	18	15
0.30	1539	407	189	111	73	52	38	30	23	19
	1122	300	141	83	55	39	30	23	18	15
0.35	1642	429	197	114	74	52	38	29	23	18
	1196	315	146	85	56	40	30	23	18	14
0.40	1711	441	201	115	74	52	38	29	22	17
	1246	324	149	86	56	39	29	22	17	14
0.45	1745	446	201	114	73	50	36	27	21	16
	1271	327	149	85	55	38	28	21	16	13
0.50	1745	441	197	111	70	48	34	25	19	15
	1271	324	146	83	53	37	26	20	15	12

*Upper figure: Significance level 0.05, power 0.90.
†Lower figure: significance level 0.05, power 0.80.

TABLE 19-5. Number of Patients in Each of Two Treatment Groups (Two-Sided Test)

Smaller Success Rate	Larger Minus Smaller Success Rate									
	0.05	0.10	0.15	0.20	0.25	0.30	0.35	0.40	0.45	0.50
0.05	620*	206	113	74	54	42	33	27	23	19
	473†	159	88	58	43	33	27	22	18	16
0.10	956	285	146	92	64	48	38	30	25	21
	724	218	112	71	50	38	30	24	20	17
0.15	1250	354	174	106	73	53	41	33	26	22
	944	269	133	82	57	42	32	26	21	18
0.20	1502	411	197	118	79	57	44	34	27	22
	1132	313	151	91	62	45	34	27	22	18
0.25	1712	459	216	127	84	60	45	35	28	23
	1289	348	165	98	65	47	36	28	22	18
0.30	1880	495	230	134	88	62	46	36	28	22
	1414	375	175	103	68	48	36	28	22	18
0.35	2006	522	239	138	89	63	46	35	27	22
	1509	395	182	106	69	49	36	28	22	18
0.40	2090	537	244	139	89	62	45	34	26	21
	1571	407	186	107	69	48	36	27	21	17
0.45	2132	543	244	138	88	60	44	33	25	19
	1603	411	186	106	68	47	34	26	20	16
0.50	2132	537	239	134	84	57	41	30	23	17
	1603	407	182	103	65	45	32	24	18	14

*Upper figure: significance level 0.05, power 0.90.
†Lower figure: significance level 0.05, power 0.80.

19-6 indicates that 69 new patients should be treated with the new experimental therapy. If there were 100 appropriate historical controls, Table 19-7 indicates that 48 new patients should be treated with the experimental therapy. Tables 19-6, 19-7, and 19-8 assume that all new patients will be given the experimental therapy. Mixtures of historical and concurrent controls have not been studied in this way.

Tables for comparing proportions are useful when the endpoint can be dichotomized as success or failure. This can be done for response rate or complete response rate. The tables also can be used when survival or continuous disease-free survival is to be compared. In such cases, the table is used with regard to the proportion of patients who survive (or remain without evidence of disease) for some meaningful time period (e.g., 5 years). The number of patients required must then be observed for this time period. The final analysis of such studies generally will consist of a comparison of the entire survival curves, rather than just the proportions surviving 5 years. It is not possible, however, to produce general tables of required number of patients for comparing survival curves because the results depend on the form of the survival distributions. For example, fewer patients are needed to detect a 50% increase in median survival when the variability in survival time among similarly treated patients is smaller than would be required to detect the same 50% increase if variability were large.

Rubinstein, Gail, and Santner[77] have developed useful methods for determining the required number of patients and duration of follow-up when the survival distributions have an exponential form. Exponential survival corresponds to a constant force of mortality, that is, a constant percentage of the remaining patients die each month. For exponential survivals, the number of deaths required to achieve a specified power depends only on the ratio of median survivals to be detected, not on the actual median values. In using the tables presented here to plan survival studies, it must be remembered that the tabulated entry represents the number of patients per group followed for the specified period of time. George[78] has reviewed methods of sample size planning for phase III studies.

The kinds of methods described are useful for ensuring that sufficient numbers of patients are treated so that an improvement in response is not erroneously missed owing to the random fluctuations of small numbers. For studies comparing a standard treatment to a more conservative or less invasive therapy, it is particularly important that the sample size be large because with few patients it is unlikely that the difference in outcomes will be statistically significant at a level as small as 0.05 even though the conservative treatment may be truly inferior. In the usual statistical formulation, the null hypothesis specifies that the two treatments are equivalent. Acceptance of the null hypothesis may result in erroneous adoption of a new, more conservative therapy. The burden of proof for studies of this type should be on showing that results are similar, not on demonstrating that they are dissimilar. Consequently, accepting the null hypothesis based on a significance test of low power is very inappropriate. Large numbers of patients are required to ensure that

TABLE 19-6. Number of Patients Needed in an Experimental Group for a Given Probability of Obtaining a Significant Result (One-Sided Test) with Significance Level $\alpha = 0.05$ and Power $(1 - \beta) = 0.80$ When $n_c = 20$, 30, 40, and 50 Historical Controls Are Used for Comparison

Proportion of Success for Experimental Patients	Proportion of Success for Historical Control Patients							
	0.1	0.2	0.3	0.4	0.5	0.6	0.7	0.8
0.2	*†							
	*‡							
	>40,000§							
	944||							
0.3	116	*						
	53	*						
	40	*						
	35	*						
0.4	22	385	*					
	17	98	*					
	15	67	*					
	14	55	*					
0.5	11	31	882	*				
	9	23	137	*				
	9	21	87	*				
	8	19	69	*				
0.6	7	13	37	913	*			
	6	12	27	147	*			
	6	11	24	92	*			
	6	10	22	74	*			
0.7	5	8	14	36	455	*		
	4	7	13	27	122	*		
	4	7	12	24	83	*		
	4	7	11	22	68	*		
0.8	4	5	8	14	30	179	*	
	3	5	8	12	24	83	*	
	3	5	7	12	22	63	*	
	3	5	7	11	20	55	*	
0.9	3	4	5	8	12	22	68	*
	3	4	5	7	11	19	47	>40,000
	3	4	5	7	10	17	40	745
	3	4	5	7	10	17	37	355

* No solution.
† Sample size for $n_c = 20$ historical controls.
‡ Sample size for $n_c = 30$ historical controls.
§ Sample size for $n_c = 40$ historical controls.
\|\| Sample size for $n_c = 50$ historical controls.

important differences can be ruled out in the analysis by calculating confidence intervals for the true difference in efficacy. The confidence interval provides a much clearer picture of what differences in efficacy are consistent with the data that does a significance test. Makuch and Simon[65] discuss this approach for planning the size and duration of studies evaluating a conservative therapy.

INTERIM ANALYSES OF PHASE III TRIALS

The methods described above for determining the required number of patients assume that statistical analysis will be performed only at the conclusion of the trial. If statistical significance tests are performed repeatedly throughout the trial, the probability that the difference in outcomes will be statistically significant at the 0.05 level at some point is greater than 5% by chance alone.[79] This probability is called the type 1 error of the design. Fleming et al[80] have shown that the type 1 error can be as great as 26% or more if one performs a significance test every 3 months of a 3-year trial comparing two identical treatments. If the times of the analyses are determined by visual trends in the accumulating data, this error may be even greater. If we think of a study that reports a significance level of less than 0.05 for the major comparison as a positive study, the type 1 error represents the probability of getting a false-positive result.

Interim analyses can be misleading because they may be dominated by differences in treatment efficacy for minor subsets of patients of poorer prognosis and by transient differences in the distribution of prognostic factors.[72] Interim analyses also may influence the types and numbers of patients subsequently entered and even cause undesirable changes in patient management and evaluation of response. For these reasons, it is common in fields other than oncology to review interim results only by a monitoring board rather

TABLE 19-7.   Number of Patients Needed in an Experimental Group for a Given Probability of Obtaining a Significant Result (One-Sided Test) with Significance Level $\alpha = 0.05$ and Power $(1 - \beta) = 0.80$. When $n_c = 75$, 100, 125, and 150 Historical Controls Are Used for Comparison

Proportion of Success for Experimental Patients	Proportion of Success for Historical Control Patients							
	0.1	0.2	0.3	0.4	0.5	0.6	0.7	0.8
0.2	232*							
	156*							
	129‡							
	115§							
0.3	29	907						
	27	383						
	26	271						
	25	223						
0.4	13	44	3373					
	13	40	702					
	12	38	424					
	12	36	327					
0.5	8	18	54	8392				
	8	17	48	949				
	8	16	46	525				
	8	16	44	390				
0.6	5	10	20	58	6016			
	5	10	19	52	893			
	5	10	19	49	511			
	5	9	18	47	385			
0.7	4	7	11	21	55	1944		
	4	6	11	20	50	609		
	4	6	10	19	47	398		
	4	6	10	19	45	316		
0.8	3	5	7	11	19	46	596	
	3	5	7	11	18	42	331	
	3	5	7	10	18	40	253	
	3	5	7	10	18	39	217	
0.9	3	4	5	7	10	16	33	187
	3	4	5	7	10	15	31	146
	3	4	5	6	9	15	30	129
	3	4	5	6	9	15	30	119

*Sample size for $n_c = 75$ historical controls.
†Sample size for $n_c = 100$ historical controls.
‡Sample size for $n_c = 125$ historical controls.
§Sample size for $n_c = 150$ historical controls.

than by the participating physicians. Several cancer cooperative groups blind treatment identification on interim reports. More groups are adopting this or more restrictive policies in response to the potential damage resulting from overinterpretation of interim results. For these same reasons, it generally is inappropriate to present interim results at national meetings.[81]

A number of useful statistical designs have been developed for monitoring and interpreting interim results. Perhaps the simplest is that due to Haybittle[82] and Peto.[11] They suggest that interim differences be discounted unless the difference is statistically significant at the two-sided $p < 0.0025$ level or the one-sided 0.005 level. If the interim differences are not significant at this level, the trial continues until its originally intended size. The final analysis is performed without regard to the interim analyses and the type 1 error is affected little by the monitoring.

Pocock,[83] O'Brien and Fleming,[84] Fleming, Harrington, and Green,[85] and others have developed group-sequential methods for assessing whether one treatment is superior to another based on a prespecified number of interim analyses. The critical p value for determining whether an interim difference should be judged statistically significant depends on the number of analyses that will be performed during the study. For a five-stage trial, four interim analyses and one final analysis, the critical p values are shown in Table 19-9. These designs are further discussed by Geller.[86]

The group-sequential methods are based on the assumption that interim-analyses are performed after equal amounts of information are accumulated during the trial. When survival or disease-free survival is the endpoint, this means that there are equal numbers of "failures" between interim analyses. Simulations by DeMets and Gail[87] have indicated that the boundaries are also valid if the log-rank significance test is used and interim analyses are performed at equal intervals of time.

Extreme treatment differences at an interim analysis are unusual in cancer clinical trials. It is more common to find that interim results do not support the hypothesis that the experimental treatment is substantially better than the con-

TABLE 19-8.   Number of Patients Needed in an Experimental Group for a Given Probability of Obtaining a Significant Result (One-Sided Test) with Significance Level $\mu = 0.05$ and Power $(1 - \beta = 0.80$, When $n_c = 200, 250, 300$, and 500 Historical Controls Are Used for Comparison

Proportion of Success for Experimental Patients	Proportion of Success for Historical Control Patients							
	0.1	0.2	0.3	0.4	0.5	0.6	0.7	0.8
0.2	101*							
	94†							
	90‡							
	82§							
0.3	24	181						
	24	162						
	23	151						
	23	133						
0.4	12	35	250					
	12	34	217					
	12	33	199					
	12	32	170					
0.5	7	16	42	289				
	7	16	41	248				
	7	16	40	226				
	7	15	38	190				
0.6	5	9	18	44	288			
	5	9	18	43	248			
	5	9	18	42	226			
	5	9	17	41	191			
0.7	4	6	10	19	43	248		
	4	6	10	18	42	218		
	4	6	10	18	41	201		
	4	6	10	18	40	174		
0.8	3	5	7	10	17	38	182	
	3	5	7	10	17	37	166	
	3	5	7	10	17	36	156	
	3	5	7	10	17	35	139	
0.9	3	4	5	6	9	15	29	108
	3	3	5	6	9	15	28	102
	3	3	5	6	9	15	28	99
	3	3	5	6	9	14	28	92

*Sample size for $n_c = 200$ historical controls.
†Sample size for $n_c = 250$ historical controls.
‡Sample size for $n_c = 300$ historical controls.
§Sample size for $n_c = 350$ historical controls.

TABLE 19-9.   Some Sequences of Nominal Significance Levels for Two-Sided Five-Stage Group Sequential Trials Maintaining an Overall Significance Level of 0.05

Pocock[7]	Peto et al.[8] and Haybittle[9]	O'Brien nd Fleming[10]	Fleming et al.[11]
0.016	0.001	0.00001	0.0051
0.016	0.001	0.0013	0.0061
0.016	0.001	0.008	0.0073
0.016	0.001	0.023	0.0089
0.016	0.049	0.041	0.0402

trol. The method of stochastic curtailment[88] was developed for evaluating such a circumstance. At any interim analysis one calculates the probability of rejecting the null hypothesis at the end of the trial. This probability is calculated conditional on the data already obtained and on the assumption that the alternative hypothesis of superiority of the experimental treatment, used in designing the trial, is true. If this "conditional power" is less than about 0.20, then the trial may be terminated without rejecting the null hypothesis of treatment equivalence. Stochastic curtailment can also be used as a basis for early rejection of the null hypothesis of equivalence if the probability of rejecting the null hypothesis at the end, conditional on the current data and calculated under the null hypothesis, exceeds 0.80. With stochastic curtailment, interim analyses need not be equally spaced and the number of interim analyses need not be specified in advance; in fact, monitoring may be continuous. Stochastic curtailment is also useful for indicating when the actual failure rate in the control group is so much less than the planned failure rate that the clinical trial is no longer feasible.

DeMets and Ware,[88a] Ellenberg and Eisenberger,[88b] and Thall, Simon and Ellenberg[88c] have also developed designs for early termination of the clinical trial if results are not promising for the experimental treatment. Jennison and

Turnbull[88d] have presented methods for calculating confidence intervals for treatment differences at interim analyses. Such confidence intervals can be very informative.

The sequential designs that have been developed are useful tools for the difficult decisions sometimes presented by interim monitoring. Important clinical trials can be easily ruined by poorly based decisions to terminate early. Such errors are sometimes due to inadequate recognition of the variability of sequentially accumulating data and sometimes due to incomplete or poor quality data. Resulting publications foist unreliable conclusions on the medical community. As discussed above, the protocol should generally specify the target number of patients to be accrued, the duration of follow-up, and an interim monitoring plan that is soundly based statistically. It is usually inappropriate to present interim results at professional meetings or to publish results before accrual is complete and sufficient patient follow-up has occurred to ensure stability of conclusions.

EPIDEMIOLOGY OF CLINICAL TRIALS

Staquet and associates[89] and Zelen[90] have claimed that many of the positive results reported from small trials can be expected to be false-positives. Of the many small trials performed, at least 5% will by chance alone yield differences significant at the 0.05 level when there is no true difference in treatment efficacy. Journal publication policies are biased toward accepting positive results. These individuals believe that there are few true treatment differences of sufficient magnitude to be detected in small clinical trials. Hence they claim that the literature of positive results from small trials is dominated by false-positive claims. For example, Peto states,[11]

> My interpretation is that, having done what resections we can, almost all past claims or hopes of great therapeutic improvements have been mistaken, and so, despite appearances, almost all current therapeutic suggestions will likewise eventually be found to yield either small or no benefits. . . . Because the need is to distinguish between small benefits and no benefits, historically controlled comparisons will not suffice, nor will small randomized trials suffice. . . .

The elimination of moderate sized innovative clinical trials conducted by one or a few cooperating major research centers would eliminate much of the possibility of real breakthrough as well as the false-positive claims.[91] Such studies generally need substantiation, however, on a larger scale.[92] There are so few effective therapies that failure to examine promising intensive treatments may be more troublesome than false-positives. Staquet and associates[89] and Zelen,[90] however, are correct in pointing out that the proportion of false-positive claims in the literature is probably much greater than 5%. For many studies it is clear at the outset that a large number of patients are necessary. Single institutions with inadequate accrual do a disservice by initiating such trials, for misleading results are likely.

DATA MANAGEMENT

Data management is a very important part of the conduct of a clinical trial, particularly for multi-institution studies. Obtaining reliable data requires the same planning and professional expertise as do the other aspects of the study. Some general guidelines for data management follow, although these are not applicable to all situations.

1. Data forms should be as simple and unambiguous as possible.
2. Relatively extensive initial information about patients should be collected, but follow-up information to the major endpoints and acute complications should be limited severely.
3. Details of treatment administration should be reviewed continuously so that errors and misinterpretations can be corrected for future patients quickly.
4. Forms should be filled out only by fully qualified persons. Uniformity of subjective evaluations should be ensured.
5. Epidemiologic, psychosocial, and optional laboratory data should not be included for addressing peripherally related questions. These should be viewed as independent studies to be reviewed critically and requiring additional resource allocation.
6. Whenever possible, an existing computerized data management system should be used rather than hiring programmers to start from scratch.
7. Data management should be treated seriously and problems quickly resolved.

Generally, physicians are tempted to design more elaborate data collection than is really useful. This results in unnecessary complexity in the conduct of the study, increased effort on the part of all involved in data collection, and reduced reliability of the most important data elements. For multi-institution studies, data management can be very complex, expensive, and time consuming. The development of good forms and procedures should occupy a prominent role in the planning process. If it is not treated with due respect by the trial organizers or supported adequately, the consequences are severe. Wright and Haybittle[93] have described specific considerations for the design of data forms.

ETHICS

INFORMED CONSENT

The basic principle of a clinical trial is to give patients the best known treatment in a preplanned manner that allows reliable conclusions to be drawn that can benefit future patients. Medical experiments have been performed by the Nazis and others that were clearly not in the interest of the human subjects. The United States and some other countries have adopted regulations for the protection of human subjects in research.[94] One of the regulations of the U.S. Department of Health and Human Services is that the investigator obtain informed consent of the patient or the patient's legally authorized representative. The three major elements of informed consent are information, comprehension, and voluntariness. The regulation specifies that the consent must be sought under conditions that provide the patient opportunity to consider whether or not to participate and that minimize the possibility of coercion. The information must be in language understandable to the patient. Informed consent must be documented by use of a form signed by the patient. The basic required elements of informed consent are as follows.

1. A statement that the study involves research, an explanation of the purposes and procedures of the research, and identification of experimental procedures to be used
2. A description of reasonably foreseeable risks to the patient
3. A description of any benefits to the patient or others that may result from the research
4. A disclosure of appropriate alternative procedures or treatments
5. A statement concerning confidentiality of records and the possibility that the Food and Drug Administration may inspect the records
6. An explanation of whether compensation or treatment is available if injury occurs
7. An explanation of whom to contact concerning further information on the research or patients' rights and whom to contact in the event of a research-related injury
8. A statement that participation is voluntary and that refusal will involve no loss of benefits to which the patient is otherwise entitled

Informed consent is required today in the United States for clinical trials. Some physicians believe that the process may be detrimental to the mental health of patients who do not want to know all of the potential, although perhaps unlikely, complications of therapy. For randomized studies, informed consent should be sought before the randomization is performed. Consequently, the patient must agree to accept any of the treatments being compared. This makes clear to the patient that the physician does not reliably know which treatment is best. This may be embarrassing to the physician and unsettling to the patient. However, for best reliability of conclusions drawn from a randomized study, the randomization should occur after the patient agrees to receive any of the treatments; otherwise the informed consent process may serve, consciously or unconsciously, to select patients for one treatment or another based on their prognosis. For example, some patients with relatively poor prognosis may refuse to participate in a surgical adjuvant study unless they know beforehand that they will be in the chemotherapy group.

It has been pointed out by many people that informed consent is not really informed because most patients have neither the educational background nor the psychologic composure to be truly informed. Research is being conducted on ways of more effectively informing patients. Some individuals, however, believe that the process of informed consent is "a legalistic trick to devolve what should properly be the doctor's responsibility onto the patient."[11] It is likely that most abuses of good medical treatments today occur outside clinical trials.

PRERANDOMIZATION

Zelen[95] proposed a design in which patients are randomized after being found eligible for the protocol but before consent to participate is sought. With one version of his proposal, consent is sought only for patients randomized to an experimental therapy. This version was controversial with regard to ethical considerations. The other version of Zelen's proposal involves seeking consent for both randomized groups of patients. Since the treatment assignment is known and can be presented at the time consent is sought, it was thought that physicians would approach more patients for participation in the trial and patients would be more likely to participate. To avoid the possibility of bias in analysis of results, patients must be compared "as randomized" rather than "as treated," that is, a patient randomized to treatment A who refuses and received treatment B must be considered in the A group for analysis. Otherwise, the treatment comparison can be biased by a possible relationship between prognosis, treatment, and refusal rate. Since the analysis must be performed "as randomized," refusals dilute the differences in outcome that can be observed. To counteract this effect, the number of patients must be increased compared to a conventional trial in which most refusals occur before randomization and thus can be excluded from analysis. The relationship between refusal rate and increased sample size required for a prerandomization design is dramatic and is shown in Table 19-10. For a 15% refusal rate, the number of patients required is double that of a conventional randomized trial. Even though the informed consent process may be more comfortable for the physician and patient, it seems infrequent that prerandomization would result in a doubling of accrual.

Two other concerns have been expressed about preran-

TABLE 19-10. Sample Size Inflation Factor According to Overall Refusal Rate[96]

Refusal Rate	Inflation Factor
0.02	1.09
0.05	1.23
0.10	1.56
0.15	2.04
0.20	2.78
0.25	4.00
0.30	6.25
0.35	11.11
0.40	25
0.45	100
0.50	*

*If half the patients on each arm refuse and receive the other treatment, determination of differences in treatment effect is impossible regardless of the sample size.

domization.[96] First is the ethical issue of whether patients are really fully informed about possible alternative treatments when randomization has already occurred. The second issue is that there will be demand to analyze results both "as randomized" and "as treated." The results may differ, ruining credibility of the trial.

Prerandomization is attractive to many physicians, although there is a lack of awareness of the above-mentioned problems. The limited experience to date with this design has given mixed results. Refusal rates have ranged from 10% to 30%. Accrual generally has increased but not always by an amount sufficient to compensate for the inefficiency of the design. Prerandomization has been abandoned in one large multicenter trial. The prerandomization design needs to be evaluated more carefully before it can be considered as an acceptable alternative.[96]

ACCUMULATING INFORMATION

Many have struggled with the following question: Although it may be ethical to initiate a randomized clinical trial, does not the accumulation of interim results favoring one treatment make it unethical for a physician to continue entering patients? If the rate of patient entry is rapid compared to the time required to observe the major endpoints (e.g., survival or duration of remission), this problem does not arise. A strong impetus for the development of sequential analysis methods has been to enable a reliable conclusion to be reached as early as possible for trials with slower accrual. Statistical methods of sequential analysis are not in themselves, however, substitutes for the human monitoring of interim results. Chalmers and others[81,97] have suggested that the decision of when a trial should stop should be in the hands of a small monitoring committee that contains individuals who are not themselves entering patients into the study. The physicians entering patients would not see interim results, and hence, in a multi-institution study, their opinions about the relative value of the treatments essentially would remain unchanged. Although the concept of ethical behavior inherent in this plan seems controversial, it is likely that the patients in general would benefit. Clinical trials would not be terminated prematurely or accrual reduced when results remain questionable, causing ambiguity to persist or new trials of the same treatments to be required. This approach is used widely in fields other than oncology.

The focus on ethical problems of accumulating information in randomized clinical trials derives to some extent from an oversimplified view of such studies. Most major trials are complex, requiring long-term follow-up for evaluation of survival and complications and warranting subset analyses to determine which treatment is best for which patients. It is often difficult to evaluate the treatments thoroughly after adequate follow-up and to interpret the results in the context of other studies. This type of reliable evaluation usually is impossible during accrual with limited follow-up on limited numbers of patients. In addition, few randomized studies result in treatments that differ so greatly in efficacy and with such slow accrual as to require early termination.

ANALYSIS

In this section we shall address several general aspects of analysis that are important for interpreting your own results and those of others.

SIGNIFICANCE LEVELS AND HYPOTHESIS TESTS

Medical decision-making is complicated, and clinicians frequently misinterpret statistical significance tests in search of clear-cut answers from ambiguous data. A statistical significance test for comparing outcomes of two treatment groups is performed in the following way. We define a test statistic, for example, difference in response rates, and then calculate the probability of getting a difference as large as that actually obtained if the treatments are actually of equal efficacy and differences occur merely by chance. That probability is called the *significance level*. If we calculate the probability of getting a difference in either direction as large in absolute value as the one we actually obtained, the significance level is called *two-sided*. If the probability is calculated only for differences in the same direction as that actually obtained, the significance level is called *one-sided*. Generally the two-sided significance level is twice the one-sided level.

After significance tests had been used for many years, Neyman and Pearson[98] formalized a mathematical theory of "hypothesis testing." In this theory, before conducting the study you rigidly specify a null statistical hypothesis, an alternative statistical hypothesis, and a decision rule for accepting one hypothesis and rejecting the other, based on the data obtained. The fraction of the time that the null hypothesis will be rejected in hypothetical repetitions of the experiment when it is in fact true is called the *type 1 error*. Similarly, the *type 2 error* is the fraction of the time that the alternative hypothesis would be rejected when it is true. The study involves collecting the data, applying the decision rule, and announcing whether you accept or reject the null hypothesis. This theory had great appeal to mathematical statisticians because its tight structure opened fields of statistical research devoted to finding decision rules having minimum type 2 errors for a given type 1 error and specified probability distribution.

This hypothesis testing framework has dominated introductory statistical courses, in large part because academic statisticians liked its mathematical niceties. The theory also appealed to clinicians because it simplified complex medical decision-making by providing yes or no answers: either the difference is "statistically significant" or it is not, period. With this theory the value of 0.05 for type 1 error has become very special. The distinction between one-sided and two-sided decision rules becomes crucial because a one-sided $p = 0.05$ is simply "nonsignificant" if a type 1 error of 0.05 based on a two-sided decision rule is prespecified (the two-sided $p = 0.10$). Within this theory the interpretation of results critically depends on what was written in the experimental plan, because the specific statistical hypotheses, type 1 and 2 errors, monitoring plan, and decision rules must be prespecified. Consideration of hypotheses suggested by the data is strictly forbidden in this framework.

It is ironic that so many physicians accept the theory of hypothesis testing as the ultimate model of a scientific study, whereas it has been questioned by so many prominent statisticians as a basis for inference in research.[81,88,98–104] Sir Ronald Fisher, a pioneer of modern statistics, dismissed this approach as being applicable only to routine assembly line testing:[99]

> Neyman, thinking that he was correcting and improving my own early work on tests of significance, as a means to the "improvement of natural knowledge," in fact reinterpreted them . . . as an acceptance procedure. . . . I am casting no contempt on acceptance procedures . . . but the logical differences between such an operation and the work of scientific discovery . . . seem to me so wide that the analogy between them is not helpful, and the identification of the two sorts of operations is decidedly misleading. . . . The conclusions drawn by a scientific worker from a test of significance are provisional and involve an intelligent attempt to understand the experimental situation. . . . We have the duty of formulating, of summarising, and of communicating our conclusions, in intelligible form, in recognition of the right of other free minds to utilize them in making their own decisions.

Other prominent statisticians have expressed similar views. Anscombe says of this approach,[101]

> The concept of error probabilities of the first and second kinds . . . has no direct relevance to experimentation. The formation of opinions, decisions concerning further experimentation and other required actions, are not dictated in a simple prearranged way by the formal analysis of the experiment, but call for judgment and imagination. . . . Sequential rules are simultaneously two things, stopping rules and decision rules. . . . When the experiment has been completed, the number of observations taken is an unalterable fact. The verdict, on the other hand, is no better than an opinion of the experimenter, and if anyone considers it to be a mistaken opinion he can form a different opinion of his own. . . . The primary aim of the statistical analysis of the experiment should be to present as clearly and accurately as possible the evidence concerning relative effectiveness. . . .

Cox and Hinkley comment,[102]

> An approach to the analysis of data that confines us to questions and a model laid down in advance would be seriously inhibiting. . . . The relation of the decision problem with significance testing is no more than a crude resemblance.

Greenhouse and colleagues comment,[103]

> . . . the classical precepts of the specifications of the two possible types of error and their relationship to the determination of sample size should serve as a guide . . . in the planning stage of the study. . . . But, it should not bind the investigator or the statistician in the analysis of the data. . . .

It is not the intention here to imply that one should adopt an "anything goes" attitude in the analysis of data. But the hypothesis testing framework is not entirely satisfactory and should not be viewed as a rigid prescription for good science. Significance levels play a prominent role in the reporting of clinical trial results, but they often cannot be interpreted as type 1 errors. Determination of type 1 error is virtually impossible unless a rigid decision rule is used for monitoring interim results. Significance levels can serve as useful aids to interpretation of results, but quibbling about whether a one-sided $p = 0.04$ is significant makes little sense. Significance levels are influenced by sample sizes, and failure to reject the null hypothesis does not mean that the outcomes are not different. In almost all cases, confidence intervals are more informative than significance levels. There is no simple index of truth for interpreting results. Many physicians attempt to use the notion of statistical significance in this way, but the attempt has an unsound basis. Thorough presentation, skeptical evaluation, and cautious interpretation of results are always required.

EXCLUSIONS

Excluding patients from analysis because of treatment deviations, early death, or patient withdrawal for other reasons may seriously bias the results.[10,11] Often, excluded patients have poorer outcomes than those not excluded. One can rationalize that patients not receiving treatment as specified in the protocol did worse because of that fact, but this is just a rationalization, which may be erroneous. The poor prognosis of these patients may have led directly or indirectly to their exclusion. There may be more potential exclusions in one treatment group, or the reasons for potential exclusion may differ among treatments. Excluding patients (or "analyzing them separately," which is equivalent to excluding them) for reasons other than that they did not satisfy the eligibility criteria of the study is a major problem in interpreting many studies. If the conclusions of a study depend on exclusions, then these conclusions are suspect. Eligibility criteria for both patients and collaborators should be established in such a way that there will be few protocol deviations. Generally the treatment plan should be viewed as a policy to be evaluated. This policy cannot be applied completely to all patients, but all patients should generally be evaluable in phase III studies.

PROGNOSTIC FACTORS AND MULTIPLE ANALYSES

The results of a clinical trial are often multifaceted and require analysis with regard to several endpoints. If major prognostic factors are known beforehand, it will frequently be desirable to incorporate these factors into the analysis either to correct for imbalances or to improve the precision of the estimates of treatment differences. Ignoring major prognostic factors in the analysis unnecessarily increases background patient variability and obscures comparisons between the treatments.[105,106] The identification and careful utilization of major prognostic factors can increase the sensitivity of clinical trials considerably. For some major patient or tumor characteristics, it may be desirable to evaluate the treatments separately by the determined subsets.

Multiple analyses can be carried too far, however, and can result in erroneous conclusions caused by ransacking the data. The subsets and adjusting variables preferably should represent characteristics known to be of major prognostic importance before the analysis is begun. They should represent characteristics measurable at the time of patient entry to the protocol and the major subset hypotheses, few in number, should be specified in the protocol. Statistical methodology for performing subset analyses has been described by Simon[106,107] and by Gail and Simon.[108] Generally, it is not valid to subset or to adjust the analysis by characteristics measured after the start of treatment (*e.g.*, treatment compliance, dose delivered or toxicity). Analyses not restricted to the widely recognized endpoints and the few major subset hypotheses specified at the outset should be interpreted generally as hypothesis generation to be tested in a subsequent study.

As mentioned previously, it often is important to perform interim monitoring of results, even though interim results may be misleading and affect the subsequent conduct of the study adversely. In reporting the results of a study, it is desirable to specify whether, when, and on what basis interim analyses were performed, to describe the nature of the interim analyses, and to specify how it was decided to terminate the trial. To some statisticians and clinicians, interpretation of results will be independent of these factors and based solely on the data, which should be summarized clearly and thoroughly. Some readers, however, may wish to revise their assessment of the results based on such information, and adequate information should be presented to permit them to do this. For either type of reader, your conclusions and significance levels are no substitute for extensive data presentations and descriptions of the conduct of the trial.

ESTIMATION OF SURVIVAL FUNCTIONS

Representation of the distribution of survivals for a group of patients is a commonly encountered problem. The problem of representing the distribution of remission duration or time until disease progression is mathematically identical, although we will refer to survivals here. The usual elementary methods of plotting histograms or calculating means and medians generally are not applicable because some patients

will not have died at the time of analysis. Thus the data contain censored observations in the sense that survivals are known only to be at least as great as the observed values for the living patients.

The most satisfactory way of representing such data is to estimate the survival function $S(t)$. This function represents the probability of surviving more than t time units. Time t is measured from diagnosis, start of treatment, or some other meaningful time-point. For randomized studies, it is best to measure time from the date of randomization. There are basically two satisfactory methods for estimating $S(t)$. The first is the life table or actuarial method. It frequently is attributed to Berkson and Gage[109] or Cutler and Ederer[110] and is appropriate when the number of patients is large. The other method is the product limit method of Kaplan and Meier.[111] This method is appropriate for any number of patients, but it involves more effort than the life table method when the number of patients is large.

The first step in the application of either method is the calculation of survival time for all patients. Survival is the duration from the chosen baseline (*e.g.*, date of randomization) until either death or date last known to be alive for patients who are not known to have died. To use the life table method, one determines intervals for the grouping of survival times. The life table, shown in Table 19-11, is then filled out. This sample life table is prepared with yearly intervals in the first column. The number of patients alive at the beginning of the interval is entered in column 2. The number who died in the interval is entered in the fourth column. Patients dying exactly at a time that represents a boundary between two intervals (*e.g.*, 365 days) are considered to have died in the preceding interval (*e.g.*, 0–1 year). The third column contains the number of patients who either are lost to follow-up during the interval or are alive with maximum follow-up duration included in the interval. This last set of patients are referred to as "withdrawn alive" in the conventional life table terminology. The life table method assumes that patients lost to follow-up or withdrawn alive during the interval are at risk of death for half of the

TABLE 19-11. Life Table Method for Estimating a Survival Distribution

(1) Years After Randomization $x - 1$ to x	(2) Number Alive at Beginning of Interval l_x	(3) Number Lost to Follow-up or Withdrawn Alive During Interval w_x	(4) Number Died During Interval d_x	(5) Effective Number Exposed to Risk of Dying During Interval (Col 2 − ½ Col 3) l_x	(6) Proportion Dying (Col 4/Col 5) q_x	(7) Proportion Surviving (1 − Col 6) p_x	(8) Cumulative Proportion Surviving from Randomization Through End of Interval $(p_2 \times p_2 \times \ldots \times p_x)$ S_x
0–1	252	38	94	233	0.40	0.60	0.60
1–2	120	34	10	103	0.10	0.90	0.54
2–3	76	30	4	61	0.07	0.93	0.50
3–4	42	18	4	33	0.12	0.88	0.44
4–5	20	12	0	14	0.00	1.00	0.44
5–6	8	8	0	4	0.00	1.00	0.44

interval. Hence column 5, the number alive at the start of the interval minus half the number lost or withdrawn during the interval, represents an approximate number of patients at risk of death during the interval. Column 6 gives the ratio of the number dying in the interval to the number at risk, which is an estimate of the probability of dying during the interval for patients who are alive at the start of the interval. Column 7 gives the estimated probability of surviving the interval for patients alive at the start of the interval. Column 8 should be studied carefully because it provides the life table estimate of the survival distribution and indicates the logic behind the method. The probability of surviving more than 3 years after randomization, for example, equals the entry in the third row of column 8 (0.50). The logic is as follows. In order to survive 3 full years, you must survive through the first year, and given that you have survived the first year you must survive the second year, and given that you have survived second year you must survive the third year. Consequently, the probability of surviving for at least 3 years is estimated by the product $p_1 \times p_2 \times p_3$ of factors in column 7. By using this product, the life table method takes maximal advantage of the mortality experience of patients with limited follow-up. The entry S_x in column 8, row x, represents the life table estimate of the probability of surviving more than x years from randomization. Computational shortcuts to observe are that for column 8, S_x equals p_x times S_{x-1}, and for column 2, $1_{x+1} = 1_x - w_x - d_x$.

The product limit method of Kaplan and Meier is similar in concept to the life table method. With the Kaplan-Meier approach, however, the intervals are defined by the actual survival times of patients who have died. Suppose, for example, that the survivals are 3, 3, 3+, 5, 6, 8+, 8+, 10, 10, and 12+ months, where a plus follows survivals for patients still alive. Then the intervals are 0 to 3, 3 to 5, 5 to 6, and 6 to 10 months, as shown in Table 19-12. With the Kaplan-Meier method, deaths occur only at the end of intervals. The entry $1'_x$ in column 5 equals $1_x - w_x$ rather than $1_x - \frac{1}{2} w_x$ for the life table method. This is because deaths occur only at the ends of intervals here, and the number of patients at risk of death just before the interval end is $1_x - w_x$. In the entry w_x in column 3 for the Kaplan-Meier method, patients who are lost to follow-up or withdrawn alive at the end of an interval are considered not lost or withdrawn until the following interval. These differences between the Kaplan-Meier and life table methods render the former more appropriate for studies with smaller numbers of patients.

Once the values S_x have been calculated for the Kaplan-Meier method, they may be graphed with time on the horizontal axis. The graph is a step function that starts at time zero and ordinate 1.0. It drops to value S_x at time x, where x is the time at the right end of an interval. The survival curve corresponding to Table 19-11 is shown in Figure 19-2. The tic marks are placed on the curve at 3, 8, and 12 months to represent the follow-up times of living patients. The step function is extended horizontally out to 12 months to represent follow-up of the last patient. The estimator S_x is approximately normally distributed in large samples. If m patients remain alive at time x, the standard error of S_x can be conservatively estimated as

$$S_x \sqrt{(1 - S_x)/m}.^{10}$$

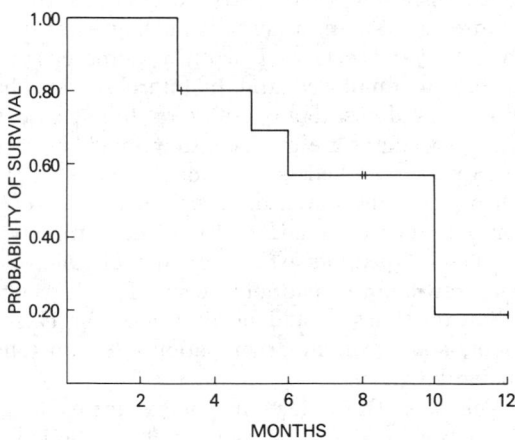

FIG. 19-2. Example of estimated survival distribution.

TABLE 19-12.   Kaplan-Meier Method for Estimating a Survival Distribution

(1) Months After Randomization	(2) Number Alive at Beginning of Interval 1_x	(3) Number Lost to Follow-up or Withdrawn Alive During Interval w_x	(4) Number Died During Interval d_x	(5) Effective Number at Risk of Dying Just Before End of Interval (Col 2 − Col 3) 1_x	(6) Proportion Dying (Col 4/Col 5) q_x	(7) Proportion Surviving (1 − Col 6) p_x	(8) Cumulative Proportion Surviving from Randomization Through End of Interval ($P_1 \times p_2 \times \ldots \times p_x$) S_x
0–3	10	0	2	10	0.2	0.8	0.8
3–5	8	1	1	7	0.14	0.86	0.68
5–6	6	0	1	6	0.17	0.83	0.57
6–10	5	2	2	3	0.67	0.33	0.19

REPORTING RESULTS OF CLINICAL TRIALS

Effective reporting of results is an integral part of good research. Unfortunately numerous surveys have indicated that the quality of reporting of clinical trial results is poor. Simon and Wittes[112] developed a set of methodologic guidelines for reports of clinical trials and these guidelines have been adopted by major cancer journals worldwide. The nine guidelines are listed below with brief comments.

1. Authors should discuss briefly the quality control methods used to ensure that the data are complete and accurate. A reliable procedure should be cited for ensuring that all patients entered on study are actually reported upon. If so such procedures are in place, their absence should be noted. Any procedures employed to ensure that assessment of major endpoints is reliable (*e.g.*, second-party review of responses) should be mentioned or their absence noted.

   Comment: The intent here is that a report make clear the extent to which the major data of the study rest on a firm and verifiable foundation. To ensure that all patients entered on a study are in fact included in the final report, there should be a formal registration mechanism for study entry. Quality control of response assessment requires much greater attention than it usually receives. Currently, numerous response criteria are employed, and the interobserver reliability of these is almost totally unknown. In any case, where such procedures are in place, they should be explicitly cited in the methods section of the manuscript.

2. All patients registered on study should be accounted for. The report should specify for each treatment the number of patients who were not eligible, died, or withdrew before treatment began. The distribution of follow-up times should be described for each treatment, and the number of patients lost to follow-up should be given.

   Comment: Differences in policies for excluding patients from analysis are a source of variation in results among similar studies. Regardless of how response rates are calculated, all patients must be accounted for. This will permit the reader to recalculate rates as he or she wishes.

3. The study should not have an inevaluability rate for major endpoints of greater than 15%. Not more than 15% of eligible patients should be lost to follow-up or considered inevaluable for response due to early death, protocol violation, missing information, or other reasons.

   Comment: The 15% figure is obviously somewhat arbitrary, but inevaluability rates of $\geq$20% usually reflect inappropriate patient selection. For phase III studies, disqualifications are a source of potential bias; when the disqualification rate approaches the magnitude of the difference in outcomes being tested, the results are not sufficiently reliable.

4. In randomized studies, the report should include a comparison of survival and other major endpoints for all eligible patients as randomized, that is, with no exclusions other than those not meeting eligibility criteria.

   Comment: Comparisons of outcomes in randomized studies that exclude eligible randomized patients are subject to potential bias. Patients who refuse further treatment, for example, may be prognostically favorable or unfavorable. This has been clearly demonstrated for placebo patients in major cardiovascular trials. Consequently, the analysis of randomized trials should contain comparisons of all eligible randomized patients. The report may also contain other comparisons.

5. The sample size should be sufficient to either establish or conclusively rule out the existence of effects of clinically meaningful magnitude. For "negative" results in therapeutic comparisons, the adequacy of sample size should be demonstrated by either presenting confidence limits for true treatment differences or calculating statistical power for detecting differences.

   Comment: The point here is basic but frequently not recognized. Small studies that find no statistically significant differences between treatments are generally indeterminate, not negative. Unfortunately, such studies are usually erroneously interpreted as negative. The problem is that the statistical power of small studies (*i.e.*, the probability of obtaining a statistically significant difference if the two treatments are truly different) is low. Reporting confidence limits in addition to or instead of significance levels clarifies the distinction between indeterminate and negative results.[71] For example, suppose the response rate for treatment A is 10 of 20 (50%) and for treatment B is 8 of 20 (40%). This difference is not significant (p = 0.75). But approximate 95% confidence limits for the true differences in response rates are −20.7% to +40.7%. So the data are consistent with both a moderate difference favoring treatment B and a tremendous difference favoring treatment A. The trial is not negative but rather indeterminate; the p value is misleading, and the number of patients is inadequate.

   A sample size that is insufficient to answer the question originally posed by the trial is a serious problem. Oncologists and cancer patients are not well served by the publication of results that are inconclusive because of avoidable flaws in trial execution. The trial that does not accrue an adequate number of patients is a failed experiment; unless the reason for the poor accrual is itself illuminating, the field is no wiser after the trial than before.

6. Authors should state whether there was an initial target sample size and, if so, what it was. They should specify how frequently interim analyses were performed and how the decisions to stop accrual and report results were arrived at.

   Comment: This refers to the sequential analysis of data as they are accumulating. It is not appropriate to interpret significance levels and confidence intervals at face value if one repeatedly analyzes accumulating data. That is, stopping accrual and publishing results as soon as a p value falls below 0.05 is a procedure with a high probability of producing erroneous conclusions. Generally it is necessary to perform interim evaluation of results. But premature termination and reporting of the study should be based upon p values much smaller than 0.05 if unreliable results are to be avoided.

7. All claims of therapeutic efficacy should be based upon explicit comparisons with a specific control group, except in special circumstances where each patient is his own control. If nonrandomized controls are used, the characteristics of the patients should be presented in detail and compared to those of the experimental group. Potential sources of bias should be adequately discussed. Comparison of survival between responders and nonresponders does not establish efficacy and should not generally be included. Reports of phase II trials which draw conclusions about antitumor activity but not therapeutic efficacy generally do not require a control group.

Comment: Controls are generally not required for single agent phase II trials because no claims of therapeutic efficacy are (or should be) made. Such trials attempt to evaluate only antitumor activity. Phase III trials, however, require controls. Nonrandomized studies should be performed as well as possible using explicit controls for which comparability can be thoroughly evaluated on a patient-by-patient basis. Comparison of survival between responders and nonresponders is not a valid way of establishing therapeutic efficacy.[113,114] This comparison can be biased in several ways. First, patients who die quickly are by definition nonresponders. Hence, there is a time bias. Second, responders may have more favorable prognoses regardless of treatment. They may have less disease, less prior treatment, and better performance status. They may also be more favorable with regard to unknown prognostic factors. To evaluate the impact of a treatment on survival or disease-free survival, outcomes for all of the treated patients should be compared to those for an appropriate control group.

8. The patients studied should be adequately described. Applicability of conclusions to other patients should be carefully dealt with. Claims of subset-specific treatment differences must be carefully documented statistically as more than the random results of multiple-subset analyses.

Comment: Care should be employed in extrapolating results to the general population of patients. Only a small fraction of patients enter clinical trials, and they are not a random sample. Proper statistical methodology is necessary to distinguish true subset-specific treatment differences from the random results of multiple-subset analyses. It is not generally recognized that, by chance alone, there is a 40% probability of finding at least one statistically significant false-positive treatment difference in the evaluation of ten disjoint subsets.

9. The methods of statistical analysis should be described in detail sufficient that a knowledgeable reader could reproduce the analysis if the data were available.

META-ANALYSIS

A meta-analysis is a quantitative summary of research in a particular area. It is distinguished from the traditional literature review by its emphasis on quantifying results of individual studies and on combining results across studies. Meta-analysis arose in the social sciences. It has become extremely popular in psychology and education, but the value of the approach remains controversial.[115] A major point of concern is the tendency to combine dissimilar studies and to overemphasize average results. For example, Eysenck[116] objected to the inclusion of all studies on a given topic, regardless of quality: "(Smith and Glass) advocate and practice the abandonment of critical judgments of any kind. A mass of reports—good, bad, and indifferent—are fed into the computer . . . If their abandonment of scholarship were to be taken seriously, a daunting but improbable likelihood, it would mark the beginning of a passage into the dark age of scientific psychology."

Research reviews in medical therapeutics are often limited by unavailability of actual study data to compare, reanalyze, and perhaps combine. Within the past few years a new type of review method has appeared in the medical literature.[117] Key components of this method are to include only randomized clinical trials, include all relevant randomized trials that have been initiated anywhere in the world whether completed, published or not, exclude no randomized patients from analysis, and assess therapeutic effectiveness based upon the average results pooled across trials.

With this approach, attention is restricted to randomized trials because potential bias from nonrandomized comparisons may swamp out small to moderate therapeutic effects. Including all relevant randomized trials that have been initiated anywhere in the world represents an attempt to avoid publication bias and ensures that all relevant evidence is available. Publication bias results from the tendency of journals to accept positive rather than negative studies. Avoiding exclusion of any randomized patient for reasons such as protocol compliance is also to avoid bias because patients excluded from one treatment may be prognostically different than those excluded from another. Assessing therapeutic effectiveness based upon average pooled results is an attempt to make recommendations based on the totality of evidence rather than upon extreme but irreproducible isolated reports. In calculating average results, a measure of difference in outcome between treatments is calculated separately for each study. A weighted average of these study-specific differences is then computed.

A major issue of concern is the reasonableness of the calculation of average effect. When the studies being pooled are similar with regard to the therapy delivered, patient population, and data quality, then averaging of results makes sense. In this situation pooling could be quite valuable for detecting moderate treatment effects and may be essential for examining patient subsets. Often, however, the studies will not be very similar. The studies will differ with regard to the therapeutic interventions compared. In general, even if two studies plan to employ the same interventions, the doses actually delivered may differ grossly. Such differences may be accentuated by including all worldwide studies. Studies may also differ with regard to the kinds of patients included and these differences can influence results. For example, old patients may tolerate intensive chemotherapy less well and have higher rates of death from other causes. Studies may also differ greatly with regard to degree of protocol compliance, adequacy of follow-up and reliability of data.

When the studies differ substantially, one must recognize that the average results may not be representative of the components making up the average. For example, substantial effectiveness of one treatment or one class of patients may be masked by pooling with ineffective treatments or unresponsive types of patients. Peto[118] has argued that although the degree of effectiveness may vary, unanticipated reversals of outcome differences ("qualitative interactions") are unlikely. That is, if one subset of patients benefits from the experimental treatment, then the other subsets may benefit more or less but will not be harmed by the treatment. When dealing with toxic or expensive treatments, however, differences of degree, even without reversals, severely limit the extent to which the results are useful for patient care purposes.

Unfortunately, the database available in an overview will often be insufficient to answer the question of whether different classes of treatments have different levels of effects relative to a control or whether effects differ substantially among subsets of patients. This should not necessarily be viewed as a license to pool results across classes of treatments or patients on grounds of practicality. Although the average result can be of interest in itself, the overview should identify where the data are inadequate as a basis for reaching strong conclusions. For example, in evaluating adjuvant chemotherapy for primary breast cancer, it would seem important to treat intensive CMF (cyclophosphamide, methotrexate, and 5-fluorouracil) combinations separately. If results are inconclusive because of lack of data or substantial interstudy variability, then that should be a primary conclusion.

In reporting a meta-analysis it is important to display the results of individual trials in a manner that permits assessment of whether they are consistent with one another or whether there are outliers that dominate the averages. Although formal interaction tests may not be sufficiently powerful to test homogeneity of results, graphic display is very important. The apparent outliers provide leads to follow-up and may be much more important than the averages in some cases. The overview should attempt to understand major interstudy differences in results, not just average the outcomes. This process requires substantial knowledge of the disease and therapeutic modalities involved.

The overview method described can be very useful in certain circumstances. It may permit one to have sufficiently large samples from randomized trials to identify small to moderate treatment effects and to examine relative treatment efficacy for subsets of patients. Some investigators dismiss this approach as important only for identifying trivial differences. But a 10% difference in long-term survival rate for breast cancer is clinically important yet requires larger sample sizes than are common for even multi-institution phase III clinical trials. For diseases such as primary breast cancer where there are several subsets that warrant separate analysis, the sample size problem is even more severe. Meta-analysis is not a substitute for properly designed and sized clinical trials, but when several very similar major trials have been performed, evaluating and perhaps combining their results in a uniform manner can be quite useful. Some investigators also dismiss pooling results as trivial because even miniscule differences are statistically significant if the sample sizes are large enough. This is a valid criticism of statistical significance testing and emphasizes the importance of focusing attention on the size of the treatment differences found.[71]

Meta-analysis can be a useful tool when several very similar trials have been conducted and methodologic aspects of meta-analysis in medicine have been recently discussed in depth.[117] Often, however, the studies themselves will differ grossly. In such circumstances the average effect only provides an indication of whether or not there is a benefit or detriment of a class of treatments. The ability to answer questions about what treatments are actually effective, how effective they are, and what subsets of patients benefit depends on the existence of well-designed and well-conducted major clinical trials.

REFERENCES

1. Bull JP: The historical development of clinical therapeutic trials. J Chronic Dis 10:218–248, 1959
2. Doll R, Hill AE: A study of the aetiology of carcinoma of the lung. Br Med J 2:1271–1286, 1952
3. MacMahon B, Pugh TF: Epidemiology: Principles and Methods. Boston, Little, Brown & Co, 1970
4. Starmer CF, Rosati RA, McNeer JF: Data bank use in the management of chronic disease. Comput Biomed Res 7:111–116, 1974
5. McShane DJ, Porta J, Fries JF: Comparison of therapy in severe systemic lupus erythematosus employing stratification techniques. J Rheumatol 5:51–58, 1978
6. Cochran WG: The planning of observational studies of human populations. JR Stat Soc A 128:234–250, 1965
7. Byar DP: Why data bases should not replace randomized clinical trials. Biometrics 36:337–342, 1980
8. Dambrosia JM, Ellenberg JH: Statistical considerations for a medical data base. Biometrics 36:323–332, 1980
9. Tukey JW: Some thoughts on clinical trials, especially problems of multiplicity. Science 198:679–684, 1977
9a. Wittes RE, Marsoni S, Simon R, et al: The phase-II trial. Cancer Treat Rep 69:1235–1239, 1985
10. Peto R, Pike MC, Armitage P, et al: Design and analysis of randomized clinical trials requiring prolonged observation of each patient. 1. Introduction and design. Br J Cancer 34:585–612, 1976; 2. Analysis and examples. Br J Cancer 35:1–39, 1977
11. Peto R: Clinical trial methodology. Biomedicine 28:24–36, 1978
11a. Begg CA, Engstrom PF: Eligibility and extrapolation in cancer clinical trials. J Clin Oncol 5:962–968, 1987
12. Hill AB: The clinical trial. Br Med Bull 7:278–282, 1951
13. Schneiderman M: Non-objective art and objective evaluation in cancer chemotherapy. In Brodsky I, Kahn SB, Moyer JH (eds): Cancer Chemotherapy, pp 67–76. New York, Grune & Stratton, 1969
14. Schneiderman MA: The clinical excursion into 5-fluorouracil. Cancer Chemother Rep 16:107–118, 1962
15. Moertel CG, Hanley JA: The effect of measuring error on the results of therapeutic trials in advanced cancer. Cancer 38:388–394, 1976
16. Gurland J, Johnson RO: How reliable are tumor measurements? JAMA 29:973–978, 1965
17. Weiss GB, Bunce H, Hokanson JA: Comparing survival of responders and non-responders after treatment. A potential source of confusion in interpreting cancer clinical trials. Controlled Clin Trials 4:43–52, 1983
18. Anderson JR, Cain KC, Gelber RD: Analysis of survival by tumor response. J Clin Oncol 1:710–719, 1983
19. Simon R, Makuch RW: A non-parametric graphical representation of the relationship between survival and the occurrence of an event: Application to responder versus non-responder bias. Stat Med 3:1–9, 1984

20. Carter SK, Selawry O, Slavik M: Phase I clinical trials. In Saunders JP, Carter SK (eds): Methods of Development of New Anticancer Drugs, pp 75–80. Natl Cancer Inst Monogr 45, Bethesda, US Dept HEW, 1977

21. Woolley PV, Schein PS: Clinical pharmacology and phase I trial design. In DeVita VT Jr, Busch H (eds): Methods in Cancer Research, vol XVII, Cancer Drug Development Part B, pp 177–198. New York, Academic Press, 1979

21a. Freireich EJ, Gehan EA, Rall DP, et al: Quantitative comparison of toxicity of anticancer agents in mouse, rat, hamster, dog, monkey, and man. Cancer Chemother Rep 50:219–244, 1966

22. Shein PS, David RD, Carter S, et al: The evaluation of anticancer drugs in dogs and monkeys for the prediction of qualitative toxicities in man. Clin Pharmacol Ther 11:3–40, 1970

23. Homan ER: Quantitative relationships between toxic doses of antitumor chemotherapeutic agents in animals and man. Cancer Chemother Rep 3:13–19, 1972

24. Shein PS: The prediction of clinical toxicities of anticancer drugs. In The Pharmacologic Basis of Cancer Chemotherapy, pp 383–399. Baltimore, Williams & Wilkins, 1975

25. Guarino AM: Pharmacologic and toxicologic studies of anticancer drugs: of sharks, mice, and men (and dogs and monkeys). In DeVita VT Jr, Busch H (eds): Methods in Cancer Research, vol XVII. Cancer Drug Development Part B, pp 91–174. New York, Academic Press, 1979

26. Schneiderman MA: Mouse to man: Statistical problems in bringing a drug to clinical trial. In Proc Fifth Berkeley Symp Math Statis Prob, Univ of California 4:855–866, 1967

27. Hansen H, Selawry OS, Muggia FM et al: Clinical studies with 1-(2-chloroethyl)-3-cyclohexyl-1-nitrosourea (NSC 79037) Cancer Res 31:223–227, 1971

28. Goldsmith MA, Slavik M, Carter SK: Quantitative prediction of drug toxicity in humans from toxicity in small and large animals. Cancer Res 35:1354–1364, 1975

29. Storer BE: Design and analysis of phase I clinical trials: Preliminary studies using a markov chain representation and monte carlo simulations. Wisconsin Clinical Cancer Center Biostatistics Technical Report # 36, 1986

30. Gottlieb JA: Phase I and II clinical trials: A critical reappraisal. In The Pharmacological Basis of Cancer Chemotherapy, pp 485–498. Baltimore, Williams & Wilkins, 1974

31. Simon R, Wittes RE, Ellenberg SS: Randomized phase II clinical trials. Cancer Treat Rep 69:1375–1381, 1985

32. Herson J, Carter SK: Calibrated phase II clinical trials in oncology. Stat Med 5:441–447, 1986

33. Chalmers TC: Randomization of the first patient. Med Clin North Am 59:1035–1038, 1975

34. Lee YJ, Wesley RA: Statistical considerations to phase II trials in cancer: Interpretation, analysis and design. Semin Oncol 8:403–416, 1981

35. Moertel CG, Schutt AJ, Hahan RG, et al: Effects of patient selection on results of phase II chemotherapy trials in gastrointestinal cancer. Cancer Chemother Rep 59:257, 1974

36. Zelen M: Statistical options in clinical trials. Semin Oncol 4:441–446, 1977

37. Pocock SJ: Randomized clinical trials (letter). Br Med J 1:1161, 1977

38. Lasagna L: The controlled clinical trial: Theory and practice. J Chronic Dis 1:353–367, 1955

39. Ingelfinger FJ: The randomized clinical trial. N Engl J Med 287:100–101, 1972

40. Chalmers TC, Block JB, Lee S: Controlled studies in clinical cancer research. N Engl J Med 287:75–78, 1972

41. Schneiderman MA: Looking backward: Is it worth the crick in the neck? Or: Pitfalls in using retrospective data. Am J Roentgen Rad Ther Nucl Med 96:230–235, 1966

42. Simon R: The importance of prognostic factors in cancer clinical trials. Cancer Treat Rep 68:185–192, 1984

43. Wendel M: Randomization in clinical trials. Science 199:368, 1979

44. Byar DP, Simon RM, Friedewald WT, et al: Randomized clinical trials: perspectives on some recent ideas. N Engl J Med 295:74–80, 1976

45. Pocock SJ: Allocation of patients to treatment in clinical trials. Biometrics 35:183–197, 1979

46. Gehan EA, Freireich EJ: Non-randomized controls in cancer clinical trials. N Engl J Med 290:198–203, 1974

47. Pocock SJ: The combination of randomized and historical controls in clinical trials. J Chronic Dis 29:175–188, 1976

48. Silverman WA: The lesson of retrolental fibroplasia. Sci Am 236(6):100–107, 1977

49. Hellman S: Editorial: Randomized clinical trials and the doctor-patient relationship. Cancer Clin Trials 2:189–193, 1979

50. Shapiro AR: The evaluation of clinical predictions. N Engl J Med 296:1509–1514, 1977

51. Gilbert JP, McPeek B, Mosteller F: Statistics and ethics in surgery and anesthesia. Science 198:684–689, 1977

52. Zelen M: Aspects of the planning and analysis of clinical trials in cancer. In Srivastava JN (ed): A Survey of Statistical Design and Linear Models, pp 629–645. New York, North-Holland, 1975

53. Pocock SJ, Simon R: Sequential treatment assignment with balancing for prognostic factors in the controlled clinical trial. Biometrics 31:103–115, 1975

54. Brown BW Jr: Statistical controversies in the design of clinical trials. Controlled Clin Trials 1:13–27, 1980

55. Simon R: Heterogeneity and standardization in clinical trials. In Tagnon HJ, Staquet MJ (eds): Controversies in Cancer. Design of Trials and Treatment, pp 37–49. New York. Masson Publishing, 1978

56. Simon R: Restricted randomization designs in clinical trials. Biometrics 35:503–512, 1979

57. Kalish LA, Begg CB: Treatment allocation methods in clinical trials: A review. Stat Med 4:129–144, 1985

57a. Kalish LA, Begg CB: The impact of treatment allocation procedures on nominal significance levels and bias. Controlled Clin Trials 8:121–135, 1987

58. Hills M, Armitage P: The two period cross-over clinical trial. Br J Clin Pharmacol 8:7–20, 1979

59. Koch GG: The use of non-parametric methods in the statistical analysis of the two-period change-over design. Biometrics 28:577–584, 1972

60. Brown BW Jr: The crossover experiment for clinical trials. Biometrics 36:69–79, 1980

61. Willan AR, Pater JL: Carryover and the two-period crossover clinical trial. Biometrics 42:593–599, 1986

61a. Olver IN, Simon RM, Aisner J: Antiemetic studies: A methodological discussion. Cancer Treat Rep 70:555–564, 1986

62. Koch GG, Gitomer SL, Skalland L, et al: Some nonparametric and categorical data analyses for a change-over design study and discussion of apparent carry-over effects. Stat Med 2:397–412, 1983

63. Schoenfeld DA, Gelber RD: Designing and analyzing clinical trials which allow institutions to randomize patients to a subset of the treatments under study. Biometrics 35:825–830, 1979

64. Makuch RW, Simon R: A note on the design of multi-institution three-treatment studies. Cancer Clin Trials 1:301-303, 1978

65. Byar DP, Piantadosi S: Factorial designs for randomized clinical trials. Cancer Treat Rep 69:1055–1064, 1985

66. Simon R: A critical assessment of approaches to improving the efficiency of cancer clinical trials. In Baum M, Kay R, Scheurlen H (eds): Recent Results in Cancer Research, vol III. Heidelberg, Springer Verlag, 1988

67. Makuch R, Simon R: Sample size requirements for evaluating a conservative therapy. Cancer Treat Rep 62:1037–1040, 1978

68. Simon R: How large should a phase II trial of a new drug be? Cancer Treat Rep 71:1079–1085, 1987

69. Gehan EA: The determination of the number of patients required in a preliminary and follow-up trial of a new chemotherapeutic agent. J Chronic Dis 13:346–353, 1961

70. Simon R: The size of phase III cancer clinical trials. Cancer Treat Rep 69:1087–1092, 1985

71. Simon R: Confidence intervals for reporting results of clinical trials. Ann Intern Med 105:429–435, 1986

72. Pocock SJ: Size of cancer clinical trials and stopping rules. Br J Cancer 38:757–766, 1978

73. Freiman JA, Chalmers TC, Smith H Jr, et al: The importance of beta, the type II error and sample size in the design and interpretation of the randomized control trial: Survey of 71 "negative" trials. N Engl J Med 299:690–694, 1978

74. Casagrande JT, Pike MC, Smith PG: An improved formula for calculating sample sizes for comparing two binomial distributions. Biometrics 34:483–486, 1978

75. Gehan EA, Schneiderman MD: Experimental design of clinical trials. In Holland JF, Frei E (eds): Cancer Medicine. Philadelphia, Lea & Febiger, 1973

76. Makuch RW, Simon R: Sample size considerations for nonrandomized comparative studies. J Chronic Dis 33:171–175, 1980

77. Rubinstein LV, Gail MH, Santner TJ: Planning the duration of a comparative clinical trial with loss to follow-up and a period of continued observation. J Chronic Dis 34:469–479, 1981

78. George SL: The required size and length of a phase III clinical trial. In Buvse ME, Staquet MJ, Sylvester RJ (eds): Cancer Clinical Trial: Design, Practice and Analysis. New York, Oxford University Press, 1983

79. McPherson K: Statistics: The problem of examining accumulating data more than once. N Engl J Med 290:501–502, 1974

80. Fleming TR, Green SJ, Harrington DP: Considerations of monitoring and evaluating treatment effects in clinical trials. Controlled Clin Trials 5:55–66, 1984

81. Green SJ, Fleming TR, O'Fallon JR: Policies for study monitoring and interim reporting of results. J Clin Oncol 5:1477–1484, 1987

82. Haybittle JL: Repeated assessment of results in clinical trials of cancer treatment. J Radiol 44:793–797, 1971

83. Pocock SJ: Interim analyses for randomized clinical trials: The group sequential approach. Biometrics 38:153–162, 1982

84. O'Brien PC, Fleming TR: A multiple testing procedure for clinical trials. Biometrics 35:549–556, 1979

85. Fleming TR, Harrington DP, O'Brien PC: Designs for group sequential tests. Controlled Clin Trials 5:348–361, 1984

86. Geller N: Planned interim analysis and its role in cancer clinical trials. J Clin Oncol 5:1485–1490, 1987

87. DeMets DL, Gail MH: Use of logrank tests and group sequential methods at fixed calendar times. Biometrics 41:1039–1044, 1985

88. Lan KKG, Simon R, Halperin M: Stochastically curtailed tests in long-term clinical trials. Commun Stat Sequent Anal 1:207–219, 1982

88a. DeMets DL, Ware JH: Group sequential methods in clinical trials with a one-sided hypothesis. Biometrics 67:651–660, 1980

88b. Ellenberg SS, Eisenberger MA: An efficient design for phase III studies of combination chemotherapies. Cancer Treat Rep 10:1147–1152, 1985

88c. Thall PF, Simon R, Ellenberg SS: Optimal two-stage designs for clinical trials with binary response. Stat Med (in press)

88d. Jennison C, Turnbull BW: Repeated confidence intervals for group sequential clinical trials. Controlled Clin Trials 5:33–45, 1984

89. Staquet MJ, Rozencweig M, Von Hoff DD, et al: The delta and epsilon errors in the assessment of cancer clinical trials. Cancer Treat Rep 63:1917–1921, 1979

90. Zelen M: Strategy and alternate randomized designs in cancer clinical trials. Cancer Treat Rep 66:1095–1100, 1982

91. Williams CJ, Whitehouse JMA: Cancer trials. Lancet 2:909, 1979

92. Simon R: Randomized clinical trials and research strategy. Cancer Treat Rep 66:1083–1087, 1982

93. Wright P, Haybittle J: Design of forms for clinical trials. Br Med J 2:529–530, 590–592, 650–651, 1979

94. Fed Register, vol 46, no 17, 8951, January 27, 1981

95. Zelen M: A new design for randomized clinical trials. N Engl J Med 300:1242–1245, 1979

96. Ellenberg SS: Randomization designs in comparative clinical trials. N Engl J Med 310:1404, 1984

97. Chalmers TC, Block JB, Lee S: Controlled studies in clinical cancer research. N Engl J Med 287:75–78, 1972

98. Neyman J, Pearson ES: On the use and interpretation of certain test criteria. Biometrika 20A:175–240, 263–294, 1928

99. Fisher RA: Statistical methods and scientific induction. J R Stat Soc B 17:69–78, 1955

100. Cox DR: Some problems connected with statistical inference. Ann Math Stat 29:357–372, 1958

101. Anscombe F: Sequential medical trials. J Am Stat Assoc 58:365–382, 1963

102. Cox DR, Hinkley DV: Theoretical Statistics. New York. Halsted Press, 1974

103. Cutler SJ, Greenhouse SW, Cornfield J, et al: The role of hypothesis testing in clinical trials. J Chronic Dis 19:857–882, 1966

104. Zelen M: Importance of prognostic factors in planning therapeutic trials. In Staquet MJ (ed): Cancer Therapy: Prognostic Factors and Criteria of Response. New York, Raven Press, 1975

105. Simon R: Importance of prognostic factors in cancer clinical trials. Cancer Treat Rep 68:185–192, 1984

106. Simon R: Patient subsets and variation in therapeutic efficacy. Br J Clin Pharmacol 14:473–482, 1982

107. Simon R: Statistical tools for subset analysis in clinical trials. In Baum M, Kay R, Scheurlen H (eds): Recent Results in Cancer Research, vol III. Heidelberg, Springer-Verlag, 1988

108. Gail M, Simon R: Testing for qualitative interactions between treatment effects and patient subsets. Biometrics 41:361–372, 1985

109. Berkson J, Gage RP: Calculations of survival rates for cancer. Proc Mayo Clin 25:270–286, 1950

110. Cutler SJ, Ederer F: Maximum utilization of the life table method in analyzing survival. J Chronic Dis 8:699–712, 1958

111. Kaplan EL, Meier P: Nonparametric estimation from incomplete observations. J Am Stat Assoc 53:457–481, 1958

112. Simon R, Wittes RE: Methodologic guidelines for reports of clinical trials. Cancer Treat Rep 69:1–3, 1985

113. Anderson JR, Cain KC, Gelber RD: Analysis of survival by tumor response. J Clin Oncol 1:710–719, 1983

114. Simon R, Makuch RW: A nonparametric graphical representation of the relationship between survival and the occurrence of an event. Stat Med 3:35–44, 1984

115. Slavin R: Meta-analysis in education: How has it been used? Educ Res 6–15, 1984

116. Eysenck HJ: An exercise in mega-silliness. Am J Psychol 33:517, 1978

117. Yusuf S, Simon R, Ellenberg S: Proceedings of the workshop on methodologic issues in overviews of randomized clinical trials. Stat Med 6:217–409, 1987

118. Peto R: Statistical aspects of cancer trials. In Halnan KE (ed): Treatment of Cancer, pp 867–871. London, Chapman and Hall, 1982

PART 2 *Practice of Oncology*

CHAPTER 20 *Specialized Techniques of Cancer Management*

SECTION 1

PAUL H. SUGARBAKER
JACK A. ROTH

Endoscopy

Endoscopy is one of the few medical technological advances that has resulted in a simultaneous decrease in patient morbidity and mortality as well as in cost. These advances have been made possible by the delivery of high-intensity cold light and high-resolution images through fiberoptic light bundles. Direct visual inspection of many internal organs and structures is now possible, permitting tissue histologic diagnosis, assessment of operability, and endoscopic surgery without requiring major exploratory procedures. Photography, biopsy, and excision of many pathologic processes are now possible. In this section we shall explore the indications and results, techniques and complications of diagnostic procedures often useful to oncologists. Throughout the discussion we shall emphasize proper techniques, for only with meticulous attention to technical detail can these diagnostic procedures be used repeatedly without appreciable morbidity or mortality. Endoscopic techniques for treatment are discussed in other chapters.

PERITONEOSCOPY (CELIOSCOPY, LAPAROSCOPY)

INDICATIONS AND RESULTS

DETECTION OF PERITONEAL TUMOR IMPLANTS IN PATIENTS WITH ADVANCED CANCER. Peritoneoscopy frequently provides information traditionally obtained only by exploratory laparotomy. It enables the physician to assess operability without making an abdominal incision; consequently, many patients can be spared exploratory surgery. Peritoneal and pelvic tumor implants can be visualized and biopsied to determine the stage of intra-abdominal malignant neoplasms.[1] Suitable candidates include patients with advanced primary gastric and pancreatic cancers, and those with advanced endometrial or rectal cancer. Patients with primary colonic or ovarian cancer do not require preoperative peritoneoscopy, since colonic cancer (and occasionally gastric cancer) requires resection for accurate staging of the disease and to prevent intestinal obstruction and bleeding. Abdominal computed tomography (CT) is notoriously inaccurate in the assessment of low-volume cancer on peritoneal surfaces.[2]

DETECTION OF LIVER METASTASES. Few items of clinical information change patient management more than the presence or absence of hepatic metastases. Several tests can be used to detect hepatic disease; however, all the noninvasive techniques can provide clues only to the presence or absence of hepatitic metastases. Only histologic examination of liver biopsy specimens provides reliable proof of hepatic metastases. Blind percutaneous liver biopsy sometimes can provide this information, but biopsies taken under peritoneoscopic control detect hepatic neoplastic disease nearly twice as frequently.[3-6] In a majority of patients, CT- or ultrasound (US)-guided biopsy is less invasive than biopsy performed under peritoneoscopic control.

STAGING AND FOLLOW-UP OF OVARIAN CANCER. Ozols and co-workers[7] recently reviewed their experience with 159 peritoneoscopic examinations in the management of 99 patients with ovarian cancer. In these patients, all of whom had undergone prior abdominal surgical procedures, peritoneoscopy was reported to be safe and feasible. It could not be technically performed in only 6% of patients. Peritoneoscopy disclosed sites of cancer spread undetected by conventional radiologic and nuclear medicine studies in 64% of examinations and provided the only evidence of followable disease in 38% of patients. Twenty-one percent of patients referred with Stage I or II disease were upstaged to Stage III on the basis of diaphragmatic disease detected at peritoneoscopy. In 66 restaging examinations, residual intra-abdominal disease was found in 33 patients (50%), and peritoneoscopic findings were the only evidence of disease in 24 patients (36%). Twenty-two patients with negative restaging peritoneoscopy went on to exploratory laparotomy; in 12 (55%), residual ovarian cancer was found. Ozols and co-workers urge that a negative peritoneoscopy be followed by a laparotomy before a patient with ovarian cancer can be considered disease free. However, most patients in whom recurrent or persistent intra-abdominal disease was present were spared an exploratory laparotomy by peritoneoscopy.

TECHNIQUES

Examinations are done in the operating room and usually under general anesthesia. In women with an intact uterus and cervix, the legs should be in stirrups, with the buttocks 5 cm off the end of the table. A Cohen-Eder cannula is placed in the uterus and secured with a tenaculum to allow elevation of the uterus out of the pelvis.

A 2- to 3-cm incision is made through the skin only at the lower edge of the umbilicus; the subcutaneous tissue is spread with a large hemostat until the fascia is seen clearly. If a patient has had a midline abdominal incision with possible diffuse fibrous adhesions, the puncture site is made just lateral to the rectus muscle, or the peritoneum is exposed surgically and a Verres needle is introduced under direct vision. After the peritoneum has been punctured, 2 liters of nitrous oxide are introduced into the abdominal cavity under manometric control. Uncontrolled insufflation of gas by syringe or hand pump should not be performed because it exposes patients to a needless risk of air embolism.

The trocar in the sleeve is introduced at an angle of 45° to the abdominal wall. It is passed through the abdominal incision and toward the pouch of Douglas. During penetration, the anterior abdominal wall is stabilized by grasping a fold of skin midway between the umbilicus and the os pubis and pulling upward. As the trocar is removed from its sleeve, a rush of air from the abdominal cavity is noted. The operating peritoneoscope is advanced through the sleeve; and a second puncture can now be made in other parts of the abdomen under direct vision.

When the peritoneal cavity is entered, it is visualized by a standard routine, starting at the pelvis and proceeding clockwise around the abdominal cavity. A percutaneous needle biopsy of most intra-abdominal organs can be performed under direct vision. Biopsy of less stationary lesions or organs is performed with forceps introduced through the peritoneoscope. Irrigation and aspiration for recovery of cytologic specimens frequently is indicated.

We have found it useful to tilt the table to examine different abdominal quadrants; the reverse Trendelenburg position is used to look into the upper part of the abdomen and the Trendelenburg position to look into the pelvis. The spleen is seen only with the patient in a sharp reverse Trendelenburg position and with the right side down. In women, the entire pelvis is visualized if the uterus is moved inward and upward. Rotation and elevation of the uterus with the tenaculum placed to the opposite side of the abdomen improves visualization of a fallopian tube. All gas should be evacuated from the abdomen at the end of the procedure. The skin incision is closed with absorbable subcuticular sutures.[1,6]

COMPLICATIONS

In the study by Ozols and associates,[7] severe complications included bleeding, wound infection, hypotension, and pneumothorax. These complications occurred in only 3% of examinations. Bleeding was most frequently from a biopsy site. If bleeding occurs after a needle biopsy of the liver, there may be hemorrhage into the free peritoneal cavity or into the bile (hemobilia). This blood loss can sometimes be controlled by hepatic angiography and clot embolization. Bleeding from other more accessible biopsy sites usually is controlled easily by electrocoagulation through the peritoneoscope. Bleeding from the anterior abdominal wall as a result of the trocar puncture can be controlled without surgery. A large Foley catheter is inserted into the abdominal cavity through the bleeding puncture wound, the Foley balloon is inflated, and traction is exerted until bleeding stops.

Introduction of the trocar into the abdominal cavity rarely causes bowel perforation. A more common cause of perforation is full-thickness heat necrosis occurring inadvertently during biopsy using electrocautery. Perforations almost always involve small bowel. These are difficult to detect because free air is introduced into the peritoneal cavity by peritoneoscopy, and the onset of symptoms may be delayed. Surgical repair of a perforation immediately after diagnosis is indicated.

The fear of bowel perforation when the trocar is inserted through the abdominal wall has kept peritoneoscopy from being used more widely. Unless the procedure is performed by highly experienced personnel, patients who have had prior abdominal surgery usually do not undergo peritoneoscopy.

COLONOSCOPY

INDICATIONS AND RESULTS

COLONOSCOPIC POLYPECTOMY. Colonoscopy has had its greatest impact in reducing the morbidity, mortality, and cost of medical care by allowing colonic polypectomy without laparotomy.[8,9] All but the largest and most sessile benign lesions can be removed in toto.

DIFFERENTIAL DIAGNOSIS OF DIVERTICULITIS AND CANCER. Not infrequently, diverticulitis and colon cancer produce similar clinical and radiologic findings. Colonoscopy has been found useful in making this differential diagnosis.[10–13] Cancer can be ruled out if the colonoscope can be passed through the entire segment of colon in question and no neoplasm is seen. A diagnosis of cancer is made if biopsy or cytologic brushing reveals malignancy.[11]

DETECTION OF DYSPLASIA IN PATIENTS WITH ULCERATIVE COLITIS. In ulcerative colitis, in situ carcinoma (dysplasia) is thought to precede the development of colon cancer. Several authors have suggested that sampling the colonic mucosa in multiple areas at frequent intervals may enable the clinician to predict when a colitic colon is undergoing malignant degeneration. Prophylactic colectomy may no longer be necessary, since selection of patients for surgery may be based on histopathologic study of biopsy specimens obtained at colonoscopy.[14,15] However, the problems with sampling error in this approach to the long-term management of ulcerative colitis have not yet been determined. Studies to assess the number of cancers that progress to invasive malignancy despite colonoscopic follow-up must be performed. The colitic colon often contains many abnormalities, and proper histopathologic sampling of all lesions may be impossible. In some instances, total colectomy is advisable on clinical grounds even though biopsies may not show dysplasia.

EVALUATION OF SUTURE LINES. Following resection and anastomosis for colon cancer, tumor cells may implant on the suture line and result in recurrent disease (see Chap. 29, section on Natural History of Colon Cancer). These mucosal recurrences are difficult to diagnose by barium enema and often are too far from the anus to visualize by sigmoidoscopy. Colonoscopy and suture line biopsy may lead to a diagnosis of local recurrence and result in a curative repeat resection.

CLARIFICATION OF CONFUSING FINDINGS SEEN ON BARIUM ENEMA. The ileocecal valve and midsigmoid areas often are not defined clearly even with the most meticulous radiologic techniques. Colonoscopy often may complement barium enema, especially if the radiologic findings are confusing.[16–19] Barium enema examination is the indicated procedure after a careful history, physical examination, rectal examination, and stool test for occult blood. The endoscopist should not undertake colonoscopy before a barium enema examination is performed, for several reasons: (1) Colonoscopy with biopsy delays barium enema examination by at least 10 days to allow healing of the mucosal and submucosal damage produced by biopsy. This prevents submucosal dissection of barium or perforation at the time of barium enema. (2) The barium enema examination reveals whether diverticuli are present. If they are, special precautions must be taken so that the colonoscope is not moved into a diverticulum and then through the colon wall, causing perforation. (3) The barium enema examination, by identifying pathology, gives the endoscopist a definite area within the colon to reach and then to inspect and photograph. A narrowed or obstructing lesion presents a serious risk for perforation if not recognized before examination. Sometimes a segment of colon that appears questionable on the barium enema examination may look entirely normal on colonoscopy. Success rates in reaching lesions known to exist are much better than success rates in reaching undefined lesions. (4) A barium enema examination defines the anatomy of the colon so that the endoscopist knows the length and configuration of the bowel. (5) Patients whose barium enema examination suggests inflammatory bowel disease should have multiple biopsies performed.

IDENTIFICATION OF A LESION IN PATIENTS WITH OCCULT RECTAL BLEEDING. Colonoscopy may show a lesion in about 50% of patients with occult blood in the stool and a negative sigmoidoscopy and single contrast barium enema examination.[20]

SURVEILLANCE OF PREMALIGNANT CONDITIONS OF THE LARGE BOWEL IN HIGH-RISK GROUPS AND IN THE NORMAL POPULATION. Shinya[21] has followed patients with serial colonoscopic examinations after resection of a large bowel malignancy or snare polypectomy of an adenomatous polyp or polypoid cancer. These patients have been kept polyp free by subsequent endoscopic follow-up, and second primary large bowel cancers have virtually been eliminated. Apparently the polyp-cancer transition has been eliminated, and therefore invasive malignancy has been prevented. The same type of large bowel cancer surveillance may be applicable in the general population.[22] If individuals are kept polyp free by endoscopy, colorectal cancer can be prevented. The development of self-advancing endoscopy instruments that would allow visualization of the entire large bowel needs to be pursued vigorously.

TECHNIQUES

Advancement of the Colonoscope Tip

The most difficult aspect of colonoscopy is the most fundamental maneuver—advancement of the colonoscope tip up into the colon. Experience indicates that a definite sequence of maneuvers repeated in every patient allows most rapid advancement.[23] A barium enema image is displayed and is used as a road map.

Localization of the Colonoscope Tip

The tip of the colonoscope can be located with fluoroscopy. However, colonoscopy without fluoroscopy is more versatile because examinations can then be performed in the operating room, at the patient's bedside, or in the physician's office, replacing the use of the rigid sigmoidoscope. Guidance for locating the tip of the colonoscope is available from the light transmitted through the abdominal wall, the internal appearance of the colon, and certain gross anatomical landmarks.

EXTERNAL LOCALIZATION BY MEANS OF TRANSMITTED LIGHT. As the colonoscope is passed from the anus to the ileocecal valve, the transilluminated intracolonic light on the abdominal wall can be located at key check points in a darkened room in most patients. The patient initially is positioned in the right lateral decubitus position. As the colonoscope is passed up into the midportion of the sigmoid colon, transmitted light first appears in the left lower quadrant; then the light disappears as the junction of the sigmoid and descending colon is transversed. As the tip of the colonoscope moves up the descending colon, transmitted light appears in the left flank at the level of the splenic flexure. At this point the patient is turned onto his back. Light travels across the abdomen at the level of the umbilicus during navigation of the transverse colon and then disappears behind the liver to reappear at McBurney's point when the cecum is entered.

LOCALIZATION USING INTERNAL APPEARANCE OF COLON. Often the internal appearance of the colon is sufficient to allow the tip of the colonoscope to be located, but overinsufflation of air may distort characteristic anatomical features. The rectum is a smooth-walled cavity partially divided by transverse rectal folds, the valves of Houston. The inferior fold lies left and posterior in the patient; the middle fold lies right and anterior; the superior fold lies left and posterior. The sigmoid colon is characterized by low-profile, irregular mucosal folds, tubular lumen, and, if the colonoscopic examination is prolonged, forceful peristaltic waves. Acute angulations from pelvic adhesions or from overdistention with air may occur upon insertion, for the mesentery allows great mobility of the sigmoid colon within the abdominal cavity. The transverse colon is characterized by a triangular lumen with prominent, repetitive, draperylike mucosal folds, the interhaustral septa. Deep pockets, the haustra, separate triangular interhaustral septa at regular intervals. In the ascending colon and cecum, the lumen is capacious and circular in outline; the folds between irregular haustra are widely separated and deep. Small mucosal lesions may be especially difficult to locate. The appendicular orifice may be patulous, a mere dimple if the lumen of the appendix is scarred shut, or a shallow diverticulum if an appendectomy has been done. When viewed from the ascending colon, the ileocecal valve appears merely as a mound of mucosa projecting from an interhaustral fold. Often it is recognized by a fleck of ileal contents within it. In the terminal ileum the delicate mucosa is arranged in closely spaced folds around the oval lumen. Peristalsis is continuous and makes further advancement of the colonoscope difficult.

LOCALIZATION USING GROSS ANATOMICAL LANDMARKS. A major landmark may be the obstruction to easy advancement encountered at the junction of the sigmoid and descending colons, which may be navigated using the alpha maneuver. At the splenic flexure, respiratory excursions are seen. Beneath the left hemidiaphragm, motion imparted by cardiac contractions is first noted. A darkened indentation caused by the spleen frequently is seen at the splenic flexure, and a similar darkened area is produced by the liver at the hepatic flexure. Both cardiac and respiratory movements disappear as the instrument enters the hepatic flexure. The cecum usually is close enough to the anterior abdominal wall that the application of local pressure at McBurney's point can be seen from within this part of the colon.

Once navigation from anus to cecum is complete, the colonoscope is slowly withdrawn to visualize, biopsy, or remove diseased areas. Usually, locating the lesion seen on barium enema is not difficult. However, certain portions of the colon just beyond acute angulations should be considered blind spots and require special effort to visualize (junction of sigmoid and descending colon, splenic flexure, hepatic flexure).

Biopsy is seldom difficult, although problems in passing the biopsy forceps through the biopsy channel do occur unless this channel is kept well cleaned and lubricated. If difficulty arises during a procedure, 10 to 20 ml of mineral oil injected down the biopsy channel will facilitate passing the biopsy forceps.

TECHNIQUE OF COLONOSCOPIC POLYPECTOMY. Few recent technical advances have had a more favorable impact on the standard of medical practice than colonoscopic polypectomy. Wolff and Shinya developed and popularized the technique in the United States. The technique is basically simple.[24,25] A wire loop is passed over the head of a polyp and secured loosely around the stalk. The loop is pulled into its catheter as electrocautery is applied. However, no two polyps are the same, and multiple technical details must be practiced to keep complications to a minimum (Fig. 20-1). For some very small lesions, excision should not be attempted, since hot biopsy can be used to sample and destroy the lesion simultaneously.[26]

COMPLICATIONS. Complications resulting from diagnostic colonoscopy have been few (0.3%) and usually occur in patients with underlying colorectal pathology that weakens the colon wall.[27] Diverticular disease causes problems because increased intracolonic air pressure can result in a "blowout." In addition, the orifice of a large diverticulum can be mistaken for the colon lumen and the colonoscope passed into the free peritoneal cavity. These problems are magnified greatly in patients with diverticular disease who are taking corticosteroids. Active ulcerative colitis results in a weak colon wall, making examination and biopsy more hazardous. Active granulomatous colitis usually does not weaken the bowel wall, but patients experience severe pain if traction is placed on the involved segment of bowel. A narrowed segment of bowel caused by adenocarcinoma may be extremely friable, and minimal pressure from the colonoscope tip may result in free perforation.

The management of colonoscopic complications rarely requires laparotomy. Bleeding occurs at the time of polypectomy in about 2% of patients; it usually can be controlled with the hot-biopsy forceps. Not infrequently, bleeding may

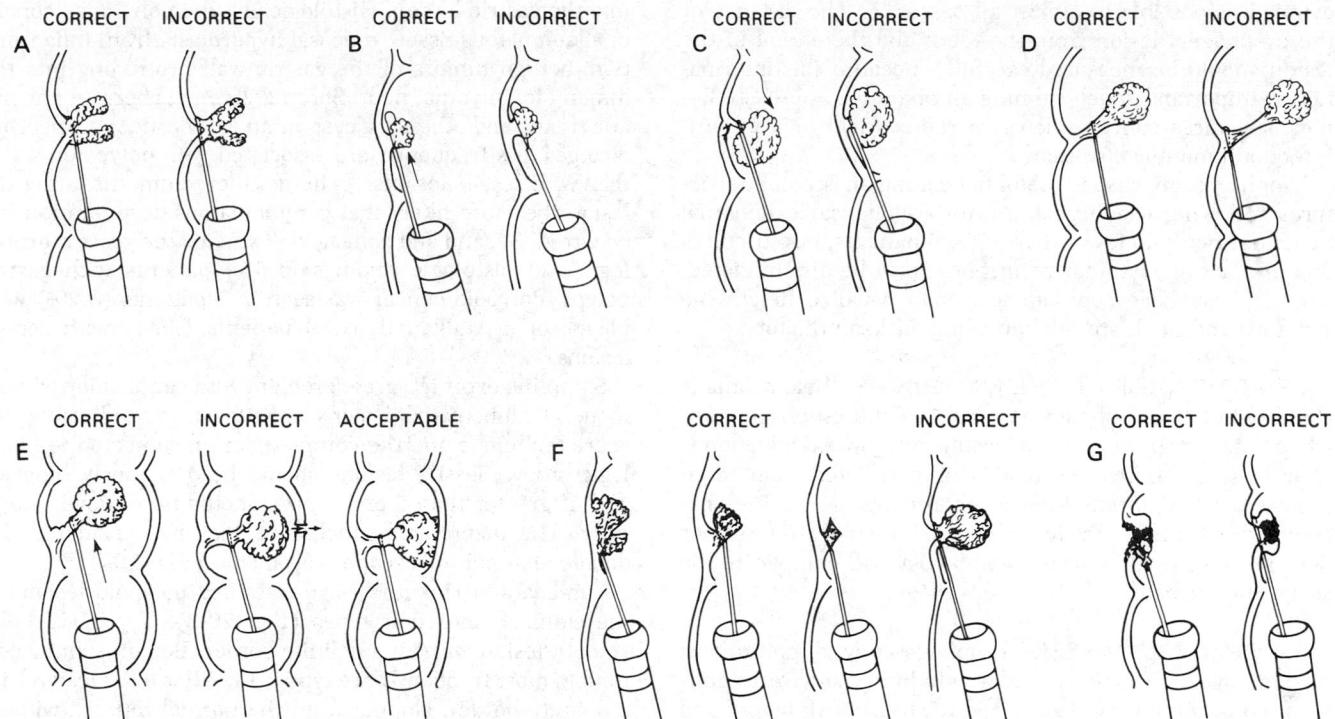

FIG. 20-1. Techniques of colonoscopic polypectomy. **A**. Sessile multilobed polyps. Sessile multilobed polyps should be excised piecemeal. En bloc excision may include bowel wall in the specimen, especially if the polyp occurs on an interhaustral fold. **B**. Excision of small polyps. In excising small sessile or small pedunculated polyps, the catheter should be advanced to the base of the polyp before beginning to even up on the snare wires. If this is not done, the polyp will slip out of the snare as the wires are manipulated to secure the polyp (Shinya maneuver). **C**. Minimally pedunculated polyps. Many polyps that do not appear pedunculated grossly will, on microscopic examination, be shown to be completely excised. Small sessile polyps can be lifted gently away from the colon wall by tenting up the mucosa. **D**. Polyps with long stalks. Excision of polyps with long stalks at their base incurs unnecessary risk of full thickness heat necrosis of the colon wall. Division of the stalk at its midpoint should always be attempted. **E**. Minimizing sparking. Sparking to the bowel wall has caused perforation and should be avoided. The profile of a polyp may be lowered by pushing out on the tightened snare, or sparking may be avoided if a large portion of the opposite colon wall is in contact with the polyp head. **F**. Piecemeal excision of sessile polyps. Sessile polyps, if they are to be removed by colonoscopic polypectomy, should be excised piecemeal. Snare excision of a large tissue mass allows the colon wall to be included in the specimen. If the snare wire is tightened slowly while (not before) electrocautery is applied, hemostasis will be better and the colon wall less likely to be puckered into the resected specimen. **G**. Carcinoma in sessile polyps. Because of distortion and retraction of tissue surrounding invasive cancer, perforation or bleeding has occurred frequently with excision of carcinomatous polyps. A suspicious sessile lesion should be biopsied before excision is attempted.

start 3 to 5 days after polypectomy. Early or late after polypectomy, persistent bleeding usually is controlled by blood replacement and peripheral venous vasopressin infusion, if necessary. If this is unsuccessful, arteriography should be used to identify the bleeding point, and Gelfoam sponge or blood clot should be used to occlude the bleeding vessel.

Perforations occur in about 1% of polypectomies. This is a more serious problem and requires good surgical judgment to prevent a life-endangering situation. Perforations through a segment of diseased bowel or those caused by the colonoscope's being pushed through the colon wall are unlikely to close spontaneously. The danger of bacterial contamination of the peritoneal cavity by bowel flora is great, and laparotomy to close the leak is indicated. If the patient has sus-

pected carcinoma, biopsy confirmation on an emergency basis should be obtained and definitive surgery undertaken. If a small perforation has occurred through a segment of healthy colon, expectant management is indicated. This can be recommended only if the bowel preparation at the time of endoscopy was excellent.

ESOPHAGOSCOPY

INDICATIONS AND RESULTS

ESOPHAGEAL STRICTURES. Differentiation of esophageal strictures as benign or malignant by biopsy and brush cytology is possible in almost all cases.[28,29] The distance of the esophageal lesion from the teeth and the extent of the lesion should be measured carefully, because this information is important in determining an operative approach. Benign strictures can be related to reflux (acid or alkaline), infection (monilia), or scar.

Esophagoscopy also is useful in treating anastomotic strictures following esophagectomy for esophageal carcinoma. Strictures occur in fewer than 10% of patients, but strictures due to scarring or tumor recurrence must be differentiated. The rigid esophagoscope can be used to visualize directly the stricture and facilitate dilation using Jackson dilators.

BENIGN TUMOR OF THE ESOPHAGUS. Leiomyoma is the most common benign neoplasm of the esophagus (see Chap. 24). Its appearance on barium swallow examination is characteristic and can be readily differentiated from carcinoma. It is important for the endoscopist to realize that transmural biopsy of the lesion should be avoided. The tumor does not invade the mucosa, and biopsy will complicate the surgical enucleation.

ESOPHAGEAL CANCER. Esophagoscopy is indicated in all patients with dysphagia and weight loss who have a significant consumption of alcohol and tobacco. With biopsy and cytology added to visual inspection, the accuracy of diagnosis approaches 100%.

Endoscopic ultrasonography is being investigated as a tool for determining the stage and resectability of esophageal carcinoma. In one series, local resectability was correctly demonstrated in five of six patients because a clearly demarcated intramural mass without deep infiltration into surrounding tissues could be identified. Palliative resection was accurately predicted in 11 of 13 patients because abnormal distant lymph nodes were detected with a clearly demarcated tumor mass. However, some difficulty was encountered in distinguishing reactive inflammatory lymph nodes from those infiltrated with tumor.[30]

UPPER GASTROINTESTINAL ENDOSCOPY

Upper gastrointestinal (UGI) endoscopy is a clinical skill shared by the surgeon and gastroenterologist. However, the nature of the disease process usually indicates who should manage a particular patient. The gastroenterologist is asked to consult on those patients whose problems require medical management. On the other hand, cancer patients who are likely to need surgical intervention in the near future usually are directed to the surgeon.

UGI endoscopy is of great use in a preoperative setting. Visualization and biopsy of pathologic lesions allow the surgeon to define better the type and extent of the operation to be performed. Preoperative endoscopy leads to more accurate histopathologic diagnosis and allows the pathophysiology of the lesion to be defined better.

INDICATIONS AND RESULTS

GASTRIC POLYP. A gastric polyp is a local proliferation of abnormal gastric mucosa producing a lesion that protrudes into the gastric lumen. Histologically, the polyp may consist of adenomatous tissue, mucosal hyperplasia from inflammation, benign tumors of the gastric wall protruding into the lumen (leiomyoma, neurofibroma, lipoma, aberrant pancreatic tissue, and others), a cyst, or an early cancer. Cancerous changes less frequently are associated with polyps on stalks than with sessile lesions. As in the colorectum, the larger the lesion the more likely that carcinomatous degeneration has occurred. Sugano and colleagues[31] studied the gross morphologic and histologic findings in 154 patients with gastric polyps. Polypoid cancer was seen in 5 patients (3.2%) with polyps on a stalk and in 39 patients (36%) with sessile lesions.

Sampling error is a great problem with simple biopsy technique. Pedunculated lesions should be excised using the snare technique and the complete lesion subjected to histologic study. Sessile lesions should be generously biopsied and, if greater than 2 cm in size, should be removed surgically. The macrobiopsy technique may be considered if a double-channel endoscope is available (Fig. 20-2).[32]

Yamada and Hukuto[33] have classified polypoid lesions of the stomach into four types (Fig. 20-3). Type I is a flat smooth lesion without a definite border. Benign submucosal tumors most frequently are type I. Type II is a flat lesion with a definite border, sloping from the normal mucosa without indentation. This is the type of lesion frequently seen with early gastric cancer. Type III is a protruding lesion with a definitive indentation at the mucosal margin but not containing a definitive stalk. A Borrmann type II polypoid cancer would have this appearance (see Gastric Cancer, below). A type IV polypoid lesion is a pedunculated polyp with a definitive stalk. This endoscopic classification of gastric polypoid lesions is important because there is a definite relationship between the type of protrusion and the histologic finding.

GASTRIC ULCER. Gastric ulcers usually can be visualized radiologically. Their appearance suggests a benign lesion if mucosal folds radiate into a flat punched-out ulcer. In a malignant ulcer the mucosal folds terminate before they reach a shaggy ulcer bed with raised edges. Other features that tend to differentiate benign and malignant gastric ulcers both radiologically and endoscopically are listed in Table 20-1. However, whether the gross appearance of the ulcer is

FIG. 20-2. Macrobiopsy of gastric mucosa. (Martin TR, Onstad GR, Silvis SE et al: Lift and cut biopsy technique for submucosal sampling. Gastrointest Endosc 23:29–30, 1976)

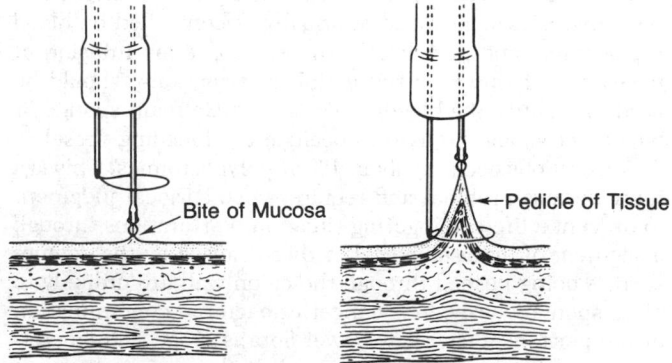

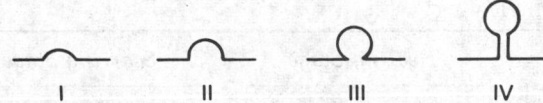

FIG. 20-3. Classification of polypoid lesions of the stomach. Type I lesions are flat; type II appear raised from the surrounding mucosa; type III lesions represent sessile polyps; and type IV lesions are stalked polyps. (Yamada T, Hukuto MI: Gastric polyp. Gastrointest Endosc 7:448–454, 1965)

benign or malignant, multiple biopsies from each quadrant of the ulcer must be secured,[34,35] and specimens from the depths of the ulcer crater may sometimes be helpful. Cytologic brushings from the ulcer and cytology specimens obtained with a water pick are sometimes necessary to confirm the diagnosis of suspected malignancy.[36] Radiologically benign-appearing ulcers can harbor malignancy.[37–40] If the gross appearance of the tumor, the biopsy specimens, and the histologic preparations suggest a benign process, a second endoscopic study 3 to 4 weeks after a medical regimen for ulcer disease should be performed. If, at the second endoscopy, malignancy is not suggested, cancer is highly unlikely; the accuracy of diagnosis approaches 100% when this management plan is followed.[37–39]

A benign gastric ulcer may be seen at different stages of the healing process. Realizing that benign ulcer disease is a dynamic process with expanding or healing lesions may make interpretation of endoscopic findings much clearer.[41] Table 20-2 shows the changes in the endoscopic picture of an ulcer as described by Tsuneoka and colleagues.[41] The irregular appearance of the healing ulcer may cause it to be confused with a malignant process.

GASTRIC CANCER. Gastric cancer has been classified endoscopically according to two different systems that reflect the degree of disease progression at the time of gastroscopy. The macroscopic classification of early gastric carcinoma (mucosal and submucosal malignancy) was agreed on at a meeting of the Japan Gastrointestinal Endoscopy Society in 1962.[42] Early gastric cancer was divided into three main groups and three subgroups on the basis of the macroscopic appearances at endoscopy and in gastrectomy specimens.

Figure 20-4 shows these types. The classification system may become complex when a lesion has features of more than one endoscopic type. Some combinations of types are more common than a single type, and all possible combinations of the five types have been described. The dominant macroscopic feature is placed first; therefore, early gastric cancer can be described as type I plus IIc or type IIc plus III. Combinations of more than two types are not seen often.

The rationale for endoscopic classification of gastric cancer is obvious. Unless one has a high index of suspicion and watches carefully for these subtle lesions, they will be missed. An endoscopically trained eye is needed to detect early gastric cancer. However, the 5-year survival rate after surgical treatment of early gastric carcinoma is about 95%.[43,44] In cases of intramucosal carcinoma, lymph node involvement is exceptionally rare but can occur. In advanced gastric cancer, the frequency of lymph node involvement is 60% to 70%.

In the United States and Europe, gastric cancer rarely is seen endoscopically in its earliest stages. Unfortunately, the Japanese classification of malignancy limited to the gastric mucosa is seldom needed. The endoscopic findings in advanced gastric cancer are described by the Borrmann classification.[45] Type I is a polypoid carcinoma characterized by a localized protuberance of varying size. It is similar in appearance to Yamada's type III polypoid lesion of the stomach (see Fig. 20-3). Type II consists of a noninfiltrating malignant-appearing ulcer. The ulcer's edges are raised and nodular but limited sharply by surrounding mucosa. Type III gastric cancer is an infiltrative carcinomatous ulcer in which the tumor is grossly invading into the surrounding stomach wall. The edge of the ulcer crater is not maintained but is broken down at one or more sites. In type IV cancer, the stomach wall is grossly infiltrated by cancer and becomes rigid. The mucosa may have healed over the cancer in some cases so that deep biopsy may be necessary to make a diagnosis.

The Borrmann classification of gastric cancer endoscopically describes two aspects of this disease: First, the extent of local spread, as suggested by the tumor's endoscopic appearance, indicates that the tumor has been diagnosed early or late in its natural history; second, the biologic nature of the tumor may be reflected in its tendency to grow intraluminally as a polypoid mass or to invade through the gastric wall

TABLE 20-1. Endoscopic and Radiologic Features Useful for Distinguishing Benign from Malignant Gastric Ulcers

Endoscopic Finding	Benign Ulcer	Malignant Ulcer
Ulcer crater	Punched out	Irregular
Base of ulcer crater	Clear	Shaggy
Mucosal folds around ulcer	To edge of crater	Interrupted short of crater
Mucosal surface around ulcer	Smooth and edematous	Heaped up; crater within a mass
Gastric wall surrounding crater	Pliable with peristalsis	Rigid without peristalsis
Depth of crater	Deep, may hold fluid	Shallow with rolled edges
Associated duodenal ulcer or inflammation	Common	Almost never
Evidence of healing with medical management	Rapid healing	Healing slow
Peristalsis in ulcer area	Present	Absent
Size	No indication	No indication
Location	No indication	Greater curvature

TABLE 20-2.   Changes in Endoscopic Picture of a Gastric Ulcer with Healing*

	Acute Active Stage	Regressive Stage	Healing Stage	Scarring Stage
Shape	Round or Oval	Round or Oval	Round, Irregular Linear, or Dumbbell-Shaped	Point, Linear, or Irregular
Edema	++	+	−	−
Diffuse erythema	+	−	−	−
Red halo	−	+	++	+++
Overriding of coating	+(−)	+	−	−
Ulcer bottom	Thick white coating, occasionally mingled with brown or black tint	White or yellow coating	Thin gray or yellowish white coating	No coating
Convergence of folds	−	+	++	+++

* Modified from Tsuneoka K, Tadayoski T, Sotaro F: Fiberoscopy of Gastric Diseases, p 139. Tokyo, Igaku-Shoin, 1973.

as a high-grade malignancy. These correlations of gross pathology and prognosis were noted by Borrmann in 1926 and still have meaning for the UGI endoscopist today.

A not uncommon problem in differential diagnosis occurs in patients seen to have remarkably thickened gastric mucosal folds by UGI radiologic examination. These patients may have hypertrophic gastritis, Menetrier's disease, gastric lymphoma, or superficial spreading carcinoma of the stomach. As shown in Figure 20-2, endoscopy with macrobiology is the procedure of choice to differentiate these entities.

SURVEILLANCE OF PREMALIGNANT CONDITIONS OF THE UPPER GASTROINTESTINAL TRACT

During the last two decades there has been a growing awareness that cancer of the esophagus and stomach may arise in association with several underlying diseases. Definitive guidelines for the use of endoscopy in the long-term management of these diseases cannot be formulated precisely. However, some recommendations can be made that are likely to benefit the patient and yet not lead to untoward medical costs.

ACHALASIA.   In patients with achalasia, esophageal cancer is seen in 2% to 8% of the patients with untreated disease. These cancers occur only after many years of symptomatic disease.[46-51] With effective balloon dilation or myot-

omy, the cancer risk seems to fall to that of the general population. However, in patients who remain symptomatic for many years or in patients treated late in the course of their disease, an increased risk of malignancy may remain for years. A yearly UGI endoscopy is recommended to follow the course of the disease and to rule out the development of esophageal cancer.

BARRETT'S ESOPHAGUS.   With Barrett's esophagus there is a columnar epithelial lining of the lower esophagus. Retrospective studies suggest that the incidence of developing adenocarcinoma may be as high as 10%.[52,53] The cancer may be microinvasive and multifocal in character.[54,55] Although long-term benefits of endoscopic surveillance have not been determined, at least an annual endoscopic examination with biopsies and brushings for cytology in the columnar portion of the esophagus is recommended.

ADENOMATOUS POLYPS.   Adenomatous polyps of the stomach have a well-defined risk for malignancy. As lesions become increasingly sessile and of increasing size, the risk of cancer increases.[56-60] Gastric polyps should be excised endoscopically if possible. Polyps smaller than 2 cm in size may be followed with repeated biopsy. Even if all polyps can be removed, the gastric lining has demonstrated a malignant potential, and endoscopic follow-up is indicated on a yearly basis.

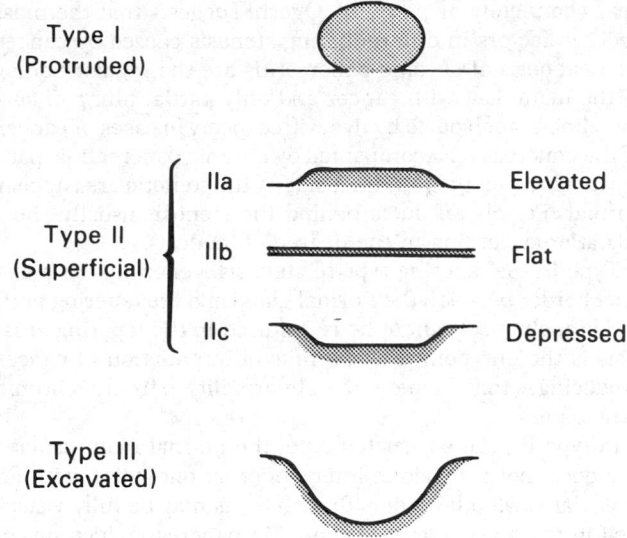

FIG. 20-4. Macroscopic classification of early (mucosal and submucosal) gastric carcinoma.

Type I—the protruded type. The tumor projects clearly into the lumen and includes all polypoid, nodular, and villous tumors. Perhaps the best nomenclature for the English literature would be protuberant or polypoid, rather than protruded.

Type II—the superficial type. This is further subdivided into three subgroups.

Type II(a)—elevated above surrounding mucosa. In carefully prepared gastrectomy specimens, this is seen as a flat, plaque-like lesion, well circumscribed, and raised up above surrounding mucosa only by a few millimeters.

Type II(b)—flat. No abnormality is visible macroscopically, although some color change may be visible endoscopically and in very carefully prepared gastrectomy specimens.

Type II(c)—depressed. The surface is slightly depressed below adjacent mucosa for not more than the thickness of the submucosa. Surface erosion may be apparent from a thin covering of exudate.

Type III—the excavated type. This essentially is ulceration of variable depth into the gastric wall. It rarely is seen in pure form and almost always is combined with any of the other types. (Modified from Morson BC, Dawson IMP: Gastrointestinal Pathology. Oxford, Blackwell Scientific Publications, 1979)

PERNICIOUS ANEMIA. Pernicious anemia and the associated atrophic gastritis were previously thought to be a precursor of gastric malignancy. One recent population study suggests that the incidence of gastric cancer in patients with pernicious anemia is only slightly increased over that of the general population and does not justify the cost of periodic surveillance.[61]

SURGICAL FOLLOW-UP AFTER GASTRIC SURGERY. UGI endoscopy is useful for follow-up after surgery for benign gastric or duodenal ulcer disease. The incidence of gastric cancer in patients who have undergone gastric resection for peptic ulcer may range from 2% to 9%.[62–64] A recent large population base study suggested that the risk of gastric cancer in patients previously operated on for benign disease is no greater than the risk of developing a spontaneous gastric cancer in the same population.[65,66] However, patients with any symptoms deserve annual examination with UGI endoscopy.

After excision of a gastric cancer, frequent repeat endoscopy is indicated. Gastric cancer often may first recur at a previous suture line. Anastomoses traditionally are difficult to evaluate radiologically because postoperative changes distort the normal anatomy. The size and shape of an anastomotic channel, marginal ulceration, and inflammatory changes can be evaluated best with endoscopy. One must be cautioned that endoscopy can detect the presence of recurrent cancer intrinsic to the gut wall, but recurrent disease extrinsic to the intestinal lumen is difficult or impossible to evaluate. Radiologic examination is more accurate than endoscopic examination in assessing progressive recurrent extrinsic disease of a hollow viscus.

UPPER GASTROINTESTINAL BLEEDING. A role for emergency UGI endoscopy in patients with UGI bleeding has not been firmly established as yet. A published summary statement from a National Institutes of Health consensus conference suggested that endoscopy was an excellent tool for the differential diagnosis of UGI bleeding.[67] However, the lack of demonstrated effect on overall morbidity and mortality suggested that the diagnostic information gleaned from emergency UGI endoscopy did not significantly affect the overall prognosis.

ENDOSCOPY IN PATIENTS WITH PANCREATIC CANCER

THE JAUNDICED PATIENT. Obstructive jaundice is likely to be caused by biliary tract stones, pancreatic cancer, or pancreatitis. Percutaneous transhepatic cholangiography with the Chiba needle usually is the simplest procedure that results in a diagnosis in most patients.[68,69] Interventional radiology has the additional advantage of providing temporary preoperative decompression of the obstructed biliary tree by means of percutaneous intubation of the biliary ducts. However, endoscopic retrograde cholangiopancreatography (ERCP) is an additional diagnostic tool in patients in whom the diagnosis cannot be determined from the percutaneous cholangiogram. Duodenoscopy is performed simultaneously with ERCP; this is critical for duodenal cancer and tumors of the ampulla of Vater. Pancreatography and retrograde cholangiography can be performed simultaneously with ERCP and may help greatly in defining the existing pathology accurately.[70,71]

Ogoshi[72] maintains that endoscopic retrograde pancreatography renders a diagnosis of pancreatic cancer in most cases. About 80% of the patients in his experience had pancreatic cancer of ductal orgin that caused some kind of ductal abnormality. Patients with acinar cell carcinoma, which constituted the remaining 20% of cases, had ductal abnormalities less frequently; nevertheless, pancreatography suggested a malignancy in most patients. However, one must always remember that some findings on the pancreatogram strongly suggestive of chronic pancreatitis can be caused by pancreatic cancer.

Changes in the pancreatic duct are extremely varied but can be categorized into three major types (Fig. 20-5). Type I represents a stenotic lesion of the pancreatic duct. In the area of stenosis, the main pancreatic duct is thin and has a beaded border. Branch ducts around the stenotic area disap-

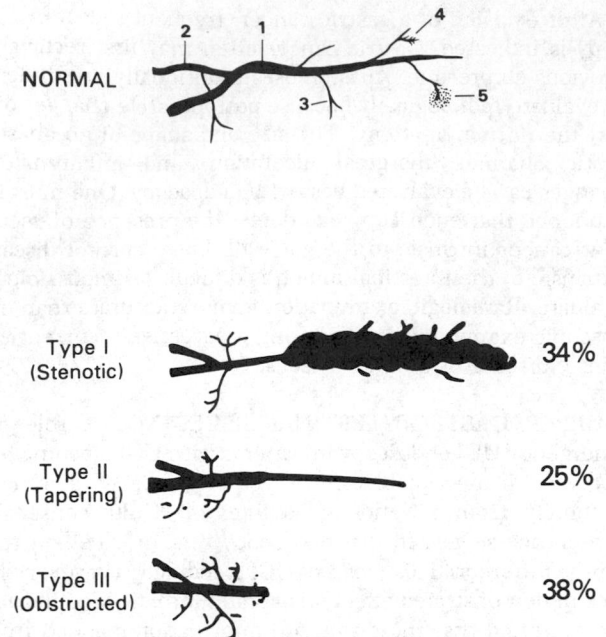

NORMAL

Type I
(Stenotic)   34%

Type II
(Tapering)   25%

Type III
(Obstructed)   38%

FIG. 20-5. Normal and abnormal appearing pancreatic duct radiographs with cancer of the pancreas. The normal pancreatic duct runs a smooth, tapering, slightly wavering course from the ampulla of Vater to the tail of the pancreas (1). The accessory pancreatic duct divides from the main duct in the head of the pancreas and runs superior to the main pancreatic duct, ending at the accessory papilla (2). Branch ducts (3) and fine ducts (4) arise from accessory ducts in an angular fashion. The smallest ducts are called fine pancreatic ducts (5). Pancreatic duct cancer gives four types of pancreatographic findings: type I (stenotic), type II (tapering) and type III (obstructed) include most patterns; type IV or unclassified type of pancreatic duct radiograph represents only 3% of the total. (Modified from Kizu M: Normal endoscopic cholangiopancreatogram. In Takemoto T, Casugai T: Endoscopic Retrograde Cholangiopancreatography. Tokyo, Igaku-Shion, 1979; also modified from Ogoshi K: Diseases of the pancreas and biliary system. In Takemoto T, Casugai T: Endoscopic Retrograde Cholangiopancreatography. Tokyo, Igaku-Shion, 1979)

pear completely or partially. Ogoshi suggests that the most decisive factors in differentiating stenosis caused by cancer from stenosis of chronic pancreatitis are the regular border of the main duct with cancer and only partial filling of surrounding branch ducts by dye with cancer. In cases of cancer of the pancreas unaccompanied by chronic pancreatitis, pancreatic ducts on the proximal side of the stenotic area appear normal. Peripheral ducts behind the stenosis usually show dilatation according to the degree of stenosis.

Type II, the tapering type of stenosis, generally has a distinct border between the normal gland and the tapering part, and branch ducts cannot be recognized in the tapering area. This is the one point that permits differentiation of cancer producing this type of abnormality from chronic pancreatitis.

In type III, the obstructed type, the normal main pancreatic duct shows a sudden interruption at one point, with an irregular sawtooth border. Branch ducts may be fully visualized in the normal area of the main pancreatic duct, but in the obstructed area irregularity in arrangement or interruption usually is observed. In cases of chronic pancreatitis accompanied by a high degree of fibrosis or when a pancreatic calculus exists in the main pancreatic duct, obstruction of the main pancreatic duct in the same manner may be recognized. Differential diagnosis may be obtained by observation of the obstructed main duct and surrounding branch ducts.

Ogoshi[72] reports nearly equal frequency of the three main types of pancreatic duct changes with pancreatic cancer. As shown in Table 20-3, he has summarized the differences that can be used to distinguish pancreatic cancer from chronic pancreatitis. Ogoshi emphasizes that if clear pancreatograms are obtained, differential diagnosis usually is not difficult. However, to obtain such clear radiologic findings in all patients requires extreme skill. He suggests that chronic pancreatitis may overlap with cancer of the pancreas in about 10% of patients, so that in some patients a clear differentiation is impossible. A major problem is that pancreatitis may result in cyst formation. The pancreatic cyst or pseudo-

TABLE 20-3.   Differential Diagnosis of Carcinoma of the Pancreas and Chronic Pancreatitis from Endoscopic Retrograde Pancreatography*

Condition of Main Pancreatic Duct	Carcinoma	Pancreatitis
Strictured	Localized stricture with irregular mucosal pattern within strictural segment	Elongated stricture lined by smooth mucosa
	Irregular pattern of branch ducts	Branch ducts absent
Dilated	Dilatation diffuse and limited to the distal pancreas, main duct distensible	Multiple chain-of-lakes dilation
Tapered	Irregular and rigid tapered segment, irregular pattern to branch ducts	Not seen
Obstructed	Irregular branch ducts in proximal pancreas	Absence of branch ducts

* Modified from Ogoshi K: Diseases of the pancreas and the biliary system. In Takemoto T, Kasugai T (eds): Endoscopic Retrograde Cholangiopancreatography. Tokyo, Igaku-Shoin, 1979.

cyst may cause a mass effect that clearly resembles a cancerous lesion. Conversely, pancreatic cancer may undergo necrosis so that the demonstration of a cyst in or around the pancreas by ERCP does not necessarily rule out the presence of a pancreatic cancer.

Yasuda and colleagues have reported on their experience with endoscopic ultrasonography in the diagnosis of pancreas cancer.[73] They found that small tumors within the pancreas are readily detected with endoscopic ultrasonography. This examination may be superior to conventional radiologic techniques such as CT, ERCP, and extracorporeal ultrasonography. Finally, they suggested that endoscopic ultrasound may help in determining which tumors are operable. The possibility that endoscopes may be used not only to examine the bowel wall, but also, with the aid of ultrasound, to see through it is of great interest.

ENDOSCOPICALLY OBTAINED PANCREATIC DUCT CYTOLOGY AND TUMOR ANTIGENS. In the patient whose radiographs are nondiagnostic, pancreatic duct carcinoembryonic antigen (CEA), pancreatic duct pancreatic oncofetal antigen (OFA), and pancreatic duct cytology may be helpful in differentiating pancreatitis from pancreatic cancer. Estimates of cytology positivity range from 10% to 60%.[72,74,75] More efforts to determine the usefulness of pancreatic duct cytology need to be undertaken.

TECHNIQUES

Rigid esophagoscopy is accomplished most easily under general anesthesia. A small endotracheal tube is used for general anesthesia so that the lumen of the pharynx is not compromised. The eyes must be covered and the upper teeth protected with a moist gauze pad. The scope is held in the right hand and guided by the thumb and index finger of the left hand. Under direct vision, the scope is inserted into the posterior pharynx with the bevel up. The tip is guided into the pharynx where the opening of the esophagus (cricopharyngeal sphincter) is visible. The endoscope is advanced slowly under direct vision down the esophagus. Usually some resistance is met at the seventh cervical vertebra, an area in which perforation commonly occurs. The rigid esophagoscope is useful to visualize and biopsy middle and upper third esophageal tumors. Flexible UGI endoscopy allows better visualization of lower third esophageal tumors and the cardioesophageal junction as well as visualization of the stomach.

Flexible UGI endoscopy is the least technically demanding of the endoscopy procedures discussed thus far. An exception to this is ERCP, which demands meticulous endoscopic technique. For routine UGI endoscopy, the sedated patient is given an anesthetic to the posterior pharynx while seated. Then, with the patient in the right lateral decubitus position, the endoscope tip is passed on the forefinger into the pharynx. Before insertion of the endoscope, the patient is given a generous intravenous dose of meperidine and diazepam. Alternatively, the endoscopist may pass the instrument through the mouth guard and over the tongue to the back of the mouth. Then, with blind tip manipulation, the tip is deflected so that it curls over the back of the tongue and into the midpharynx. While the operator applies slight forward pressure, the patient is asked to swallow to relax the cricopharyngeal sphincter, which lies 15 cm to 18 cm from the teeth. The endoscope passes easily down the esophagus. If the endoscope tip just below the cardioesophageal sphincter is flexed 45° to the patient's left, the greater curvature comes into view. Rotation of the endoscope clockwise scans the anterior surface of the stomach; rotation counterclockwise scans the posterior surface of the stomach. If the endoscope tip is repositioned just below the cardioesophageal sphincter and extended 45° to the patient's right, the lesser curvature is visualized. The cardioesophageal sphincter is visualized from above and then from below by retroflexing the endoscope. The lesser curvature is followed to the antrum and then through the pylorus into the duodenum. Persistent advancement will move the tip to the ligament of Treitz and even beyond.

The techniques involved in UGI endoscopy and colonoscopy are very different. The esophagus, stomach, and duodenum are structures whose positions within the abdominal cavity are fixed; therefore, as the hollow viscus is inflated with air, the endoscope is moved readily ahead under direct vision. This is not so with the colon. The sigmoid, transverse colon, and often ascending colon are free to move nearly anywhere within the abdominal cavity. Therefore, maneuvers to reduce bowel loops by accumulating collapsed colon on the endoscope are required.

COMPLICATIONS

The first rule for esophagoscopy and UGI endoscopy is "Don't push." The incidence of esophageal perforation is reported to be 0.074% with the rigid esophagoscope and 0.093% with the fiberoptic esophagoscope.[76] Treatment should be instituted as soon as the perforation is recognized. If the perforation occurs through a pathologic lesion, surgery must be performed immediately and the lesion resected. If a perforation occurs through normal esophagus, more conservative treatment should be considered. Perforation usually is evidenced by a spiking fever, substernal or upper abdominal pain, subcutaneous emphysema in the neck, and pneumothorax.

A water-soluble contrast esophagogram is indicated but may not demonstrate extravasation. Treatment depends on location of the perforation, time of recognition, status of the esophagus, condition of the patient, and severity of sepsis.[77] Cervical perforations can be managed by no oral feeding, antibiotics, and observation.[78] If an abscess forms, it is easily drained. If a thoracic esophageal perforation is recognized during the first 24 hours and there is evidence of sepsis, closure with adequate chest tube drainage should be attempted. Small perforations or perforations that drain well into the esophagus without sepsis may be managed with pharyngeal suction, antibiotics, and total parenteral alimentation. Perforation proximal to or through an obstructing tumor requires resection of the tumor and perforated segment of esophagus. If recognized very early when inflammation is minimal, a primary gastroesophageal anastomosis may be attempted. Late recognition of perforation in patients with infection requires exclusion of the esophagus by oversewing the esophagogastric junction, creating a diverting cervical esophagostomy and a gastrostomy.[79]

If a perforation occurs through normal stomach or through a benign duodenal ulcer, nasogastric suctioning, intravenous antibiotics, and careful observation usually are enough. However, perforation through a gastric cancer requires immediate surgical intervention. If this occurs, tumor cells are likely to be disseminated throughout the peritoneal cavity, and healing across the perforated malignancy is unlikely to occur.

BRONCHOSCOPY

INDICATIONS AND RESULTS

Bronchoscopy is one of the most useful modalities in the diagnosis and staging of thoracic neoplasms. Bronchoscopy may be indicated for the diagnosis and staging of pulmonary, esophageal, and mediastinal lesions. It is indicated in determining the extent of surgical resection necessary for pulmonary and esophageal tumors. When lung cancer patients have centrally located thoracic masses, bronchoscopy must be performed to assess involvement of mainstem and lobar bronchi. Invasion of tumor into the mainstem bronchi or carina will necessitate pneumonectomy or tracheal reconstruction following resection. Patients with more peripheral lesions generally do not require bronchoscopy before exploration unless there is some indication that the lesions may be multifocal and involve the opposite lung.

Bronchoscopy also may be useful in the localization of hemoptysis that occurs in patients with pulmonary neoplasms, and in the evaluation of diffuse interstitial infiltrates, which are frequently seen in cancer patients undergoing aggressive chemotherapy.

FLEXIBLE VERSUS RIGID BRONCHOSCOPES. Both the flexible and rigid instruments have features that may make one or the other particularly suitable for certain problems (Table 20-4). Thus any physician dealing with thoracic neoplasms must have a working knowledge of both instruments. Different caliber rigid bronchoscopes are available with side arms for ventilation. The Storz model has a fiberoptic optical magnification system and angled lenses that allow direct viewing of all lobar bronchi. Flexible bronchoscopes are available with differing external diameters (3.6–6.5 mm) and interchannel widths (0.8–2.6 mm). The larger flexible bronchoscope requires a minimum of 8 mm of endotracheal tube for convenient passage, whereas the smaller scopes may be passed through small-diameter endotracheal tubes and are useful for pediatric patients and endoscopy through double-lumen endotracheal tubes. The flexible bronchoscope can be used comfortably under local anesthesia and allows direct visualization and biopsy of lesions in subsegmental locations. Peripheral lesions can be biopsied effectively by using either the rigid scope with flexible biopsy forceps and fluoroscopic control or the flexible bronchoscope. The visualization of primary, secondary, and even tertiary bronchi with the fiberoptic instrument is shown in Figure 20-6.

The rigid bronchoscope, especially with the fiberoptic system, provides excellent magnification and clarity. It allows one to obtain larger biopsy specimens than can be obtained through even the largest flexible bronchoscope. In addition, it is considerably more effective in suctioning thick secretions and blood. Finally, use of the rigid instruments allows the operator to judge fixation of the carina, an important prognostic sign indicating advanced unresectable tumor.

BRONCHOSCOPY VERSUS OTHER TECHNIQUES IN THE DIAGNOSIS OF PARENCHYMAL LESIONS. In comparison with other diagnostic techniques, bronchoscopic biopsy will make the diagnosis of malignancy in a lower percentage of cases but with more accurate histologic diagnosis. Payne and co-workers[80] noted that a diagnosis of malignancy was made in 88% of specimens obtained by percutaneous lung biopsy, but the accuracy of the histologic diagnosis was only 48%. Malignant tissue was obtained in 69% of cases with bronchial biopsy, with the correct histologic type predicted in 80% of cases. In the diagnosis of diffuse interstitial pulmonary infiltrates, transbronchial biopsy can be accurate in a high percentage of cases but generally is less accurate than open lung biopsy. Feldman and co-workers[81] achieved 84% accuracy in the diagnosis of

TABLE 20-4.   Comparison of Rigid and Flexible Fiberoptic Bronchoscopy Technique

	Rigid Bronchoscopy	Flexible Fiberoptic Bronchoscopy
Biopsy	Generous specimen	Minute specimen
Visualization of bronchi	Excellent	Excellent
Visualization of segmental bronchi	With angled lenses only	Excellent
Biopsy of peripheral lesions	No	Yes
Anesthesia required	General	Local
Performed through orotracheal tube	No	Yes
Suctioning secretions	Excellent	Good
Complications	Perforation and bleeding reported	Very unusual
Durability of instrument	Durable	Delicate
Training to perform examination	Extensive	Minimal

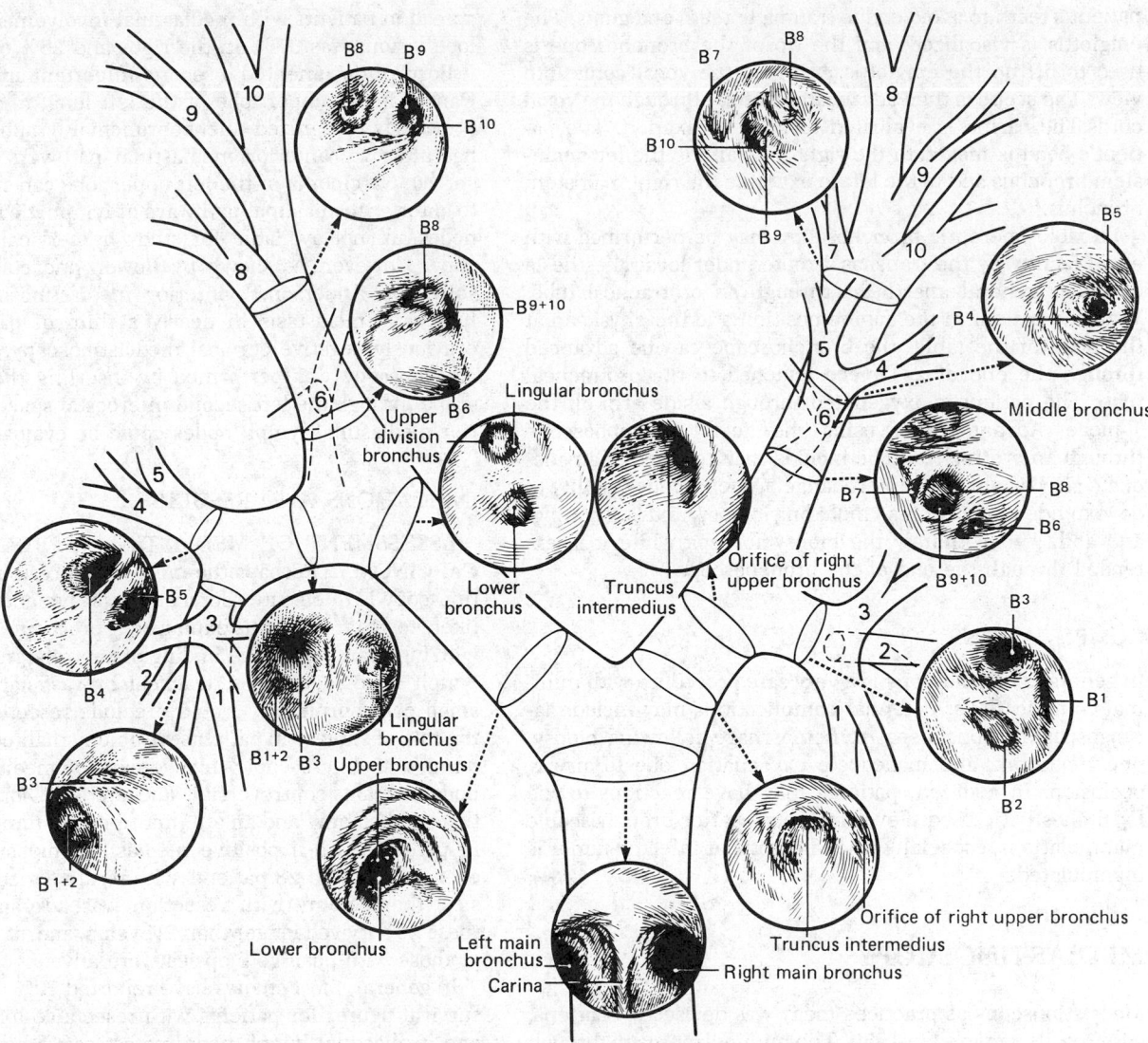

FIG. 20-6. Anatomy of the bronchial tree as seen through the flexible bronchoscope. The diagram shows the tracheobronchial tree; the insets reproduce the bronchoscopic picture obtained at important positions. Checkpoints include the carina and right and left main-stem orifices; major bifurcations on the right into upper, middle, and lower lobes; and major bifurcations on the left into the upper, lingula, and lower lobes. A standard nomenclature for designating tertiary bronchi within lung segments is indicated. Because of variations in the segmental anatomy, endoscopists have found that this simplified nomenclature expedites a thorough description of the endoscopic findings. The letters correspond to the following anatomic segments: Right upper lobe—B^1 apical, B^2 posterior, B^3 anterior; right middle lobe—B^4 lateral, B^5 medial; right lower lobe—B^6 superior segment, B^7 medial basal, B^8 anterior basal, B^9 lateral basal, B^{10} posterior basal; left upper lobe—B^{1+2} apical posterior, B^3 anterior; lingula—B^4 superior, B^5 inferior; left lower lobe—B^6 superior, B^8 anterior basal, B^9 lateral basal, B^{10} posterior basal. (Modified from Ikeda S: Atlas of Flexible Bronchofiberoscopy, p 63. Tokyo, Igaku-Shion, 1974)

diffuse pulmonary infiltrates by transbronchial biopsy compared to only a 43% diagnostic yield in localized infiltrates. In a prospective study, Burt and co-workers[82] compared aspiration needle biopsy, cutting needle biopsy, transbronchial biopsy, and open lung biopsy. They found open lung biopsy to be the most accurate technique, although in two patients a diagnosis was obtained by transbronchial biopsy that could not be obtained by open lung biopsy.

TECHNIQUES

Rigid bronchoscopy can be performed under local anesthesia, but generally the patient is more comfortable and the examination is facilitated when general anesthesia is used. The patient is placed in the supine position with the head extended. The bronchoscope is supported by the examiner's index finger and thumb. A moist gauze is placed over the patient's teeth to avoid undue trauma to teeth and gums. The epiglottis is visualized, and the tip of the bronchoscope is used to lift up the epiglottis, bringing the vocal cords into view. The scope is then advanced carefully through the vocal cords.The carina is evaluated to note its fixation. The patient's head is moved to the right to examine the left mainstem bronchus and to the left to examine the right mainstem bronchus.

Flexible fiberoptic bronchoscopy may be performed with equal facility by the transnasal route under local anesthesia or under general anesthesia through an orotracheal tube. With the patient in the supine position and the physician at the head of the table, the bronchoscope can be advanced through the end of a T-piece attached to the orotracheal tube. The patient is oxygenated through a side arm off the T-piece. Advantages of using the flexible bronchoscope through an orotracheal tube include maintenance of an adequate airway, ability to interchange bronchoscopes, ability to do extended procedures, including biopsy and suctioning, and ability to withdraw the biopsy forceps while it is extended through the end of the bronchoscope.

COMPLICATIONS

In general, bronchoscopy is a very safe procedure with minimal complications. Potential complications may include laryngospasm, bronchospasm, hemorrhage following biopsy, pneumothorax, and inadequate oxygenation due to airway occlusion. In addition, patients may have reactions to the local anesthetic used. Fever may occur after bronchoscopic manipulations, especially when necrotic or infected tumor is manipulated.

MEDIASTINOSCOPY

Mediastinoscopy as practiced today was devised by Carlens, with results reported in 1959. The midline approach through a small, low cervical incision made biopsy of lymph nodes on both sides of the superior mediastinum possible. Through this technique, visualization and biopsy of nearly all paratracheal and hilar lymph nodes in the middle and lower portions of the superior mediastinum were possible. However, Pearson[83] has pointed out that the surgeon is anatomically limited in sampling anterior mediastinal, subaortic, and subcarinal nodes posterior to the trachea. The subcarinal nodes anterior to the tracheal bifurcation are important nodes for visualization and sampling at the lowermost extent of the endoscopic dissection.

Two important anatomical features of the lymphatic drainage of the lung should be noted. First, lymphatic crossover from a lung on one side of the mediastinum to lymph nodes on the opposite side is not unusual. Goldberg and co-workers[84] reported that 28 of 46 patients (60%) with positive mediastinal nodes from lung carcinoma in the right upper lobe had bilateral spread of disease within the mediastinum. One patient (3%) had only contralateral spread. Similarly, 5 of 20 patients (25%) with positive mediastinal nodes from left upper lobe cancer had bilateral mediastinal nodal spread, and 6 (30%) had only contralateral spread. Bilateral

spread in patients with mediastinal involvement from lower lobe lesions was 37% on the right and 25% on the left.

Borrie[85] documented a second important anatomical fact. Cancer in the upper lobe of the left lung, in addition to its previously recognized tracheobronchial lymphatic drainage, has alternate anterior mediastinal pathways of lymphatic spread. Carcinoma of the left upper lobe can spread directly to anterior mediastinal pathways of lymphatic spread. These nodes are not available for study by cervical mediastinoscopy. However, as shown by Bowen and colleagues[86] and Jolly and Anderson,[87] anterior mediastinoscopy revealed lymphatic metastasis in nearly a third of patients having previously negative cervical mediastinoscopy. Anterior mediastinoscopy was performed by inserting the mediastinoscope through the left second intercostal space so that anterior mediastinal lymph nodes could be evaluated.

INDICATIONS AND RESULTS

ASSESSMENT OF MEDIASTINAL SPREAD OF LUNG CARCINOMA. Perhaps the most widespread use of mediastinoscopy is to obviate thoracotomy in patients who are unlikely to profit from this exploratory procedure. For patients with lung carcinoma, the finding of contralateral mediastinal lymph node metastases, tracheal or vascular invasion, or small cell morphology would preclude resection. However, the role of surgery in patients with non-small-cell lung carcinoma with microscopic involvement of mediastinal lymph nodes remains controversial. The study of Gibbons[88] showed that thoracotomy and an attempt to resect tumors curatively in patients with a positive mediastinal biopsy is rarely, if ever, possible. In 28 patients with positive mediastinal biopsies, thoracotomy with resection was attempted; none of these 28 survived longer than 2½ years, and, at 1 year, only 3 of those with positive biopsies were alive.

In general, most studies have reported 10% to 30% 5-year survival figures for patients with resectable lung carcinoma and mediastinal lymph node metastases. Squamous lesions have a better prognosis than other non-small-cell histologic types, but extrapulmonary extension or subcarinal node involvement is a poor prognostic feature. Kirsh and co-workers[89] reported a 34.4% 5-year survival for patients with squamous cell carcinoma and mediastinal lymph node metastases. Martini and co-workers[90] observed a 29% actuarial 5-year survival for patients with non-small-cell lung carcinoma. Thus the presence of mediastinal lymph node metastases alone should not exclude patients from surgery if their disease is otherwise resectable. Mediastinoscopy is therefore useful primarily to determine unresectability in patients with lung carcinoma.

Some authors have presented data to suggest that not all lung cancer patients need mediastinoscopy before thoracotomy; size, location (peripheral versus central), and cell type of the primary tumor influence the incidence of positive mediastinal nodes. Hutchinson and Mills[91] found a high incidence of mediastinal metastases associated with central tumors (63%—100%) of all cell types and with peripheral lesions (63%) of undifferentiated cell types. However, only 8.6% of peripheral carcinomas of adenosquamous or squamous type with a radiographically normal mediastinum were found to have mediastinal metastases. Baker and co-workers[92] found only 3 of 40 patients with T1 lesions (3 cm in size or smaller) to have mediastinal node metastases detected by mediastinoscopy. All 3 patients had large cell undifferentiated tumors. Therefore, in patients with small, peripherally located tumors of well-differentiated histology and a normal mediastinum by radiologic examination, mediastinoscopy need not precede thoracotomy. In this group of patients, the slight risk of mediastinoscopy can be avoided.

The use of CT scans of the chest may eliminate routine mediastinoscopy in patients with lung cancer. The absence of abnormally enlarged mediastinal lymph nodes on CT correlates well with the absence of lymph node metastases and with resectability. However, enlarged lymph nodes detected on CT do not necessarily indicate metastases. Nodal enlargement may be due to inflammatory changes caused by a coexisting infectious process in the lung. Thus, if the presence of nodal metastases would influence the operative decision, histologic confirmation by mediastinoscopy or some other technique is indicated.[93]

DIAGNOSIS OF MEDIASTINAL HODGKIN'S DISEASE.
Vaeth and colleagues[94] reviewed a group of patients with Hodgkin's disease limited to the mediastinum at the time of initial presentation. From their experience, they suggested that if bone marrow biopsy was negative, a tissue diagnosis was best established by mediastinoscopy rather than thoracotomy. An attempt to resect mediastinal Hodgkin's disease is not indicated. However, Redding and co-workers[95] found that the routine use of mediastinoscopy as a staging procedure in all patients with Hodgkin's disease was not indicated.

TECHNIQUES

The patient is placed on his back with the neck hyperextended by a cushion beneath the scapulae (Fig. 20-7). Under general anesthesia, a 4-cm incision is made in the suprasternal notch about 2 cm above the manubrium. The strap muscles are separated in the midline so that the loose areolar tissue anterior to the trachea can be dissected bluntly and bloodlessly using the index finger. The exploring finger

FIG. 20-7. Technique of mediastinoscopy. **A**. Make a 3- to 4-cm incision just above the manubrium. **B**. Use the finger to dissect bluntly the loose fibrofatty tissue in front of the trachea down to the level of the pulmonary artery. **C**. Introduce the endoscope and take biopsies of suspicious tissues. Needle aspiration of structures before biopsy will help to reduce hemorrhagic complications. (Modified from Kerschner PA: Transcervical approach to the superior mediastinum. Hosp Pract, June 1970)

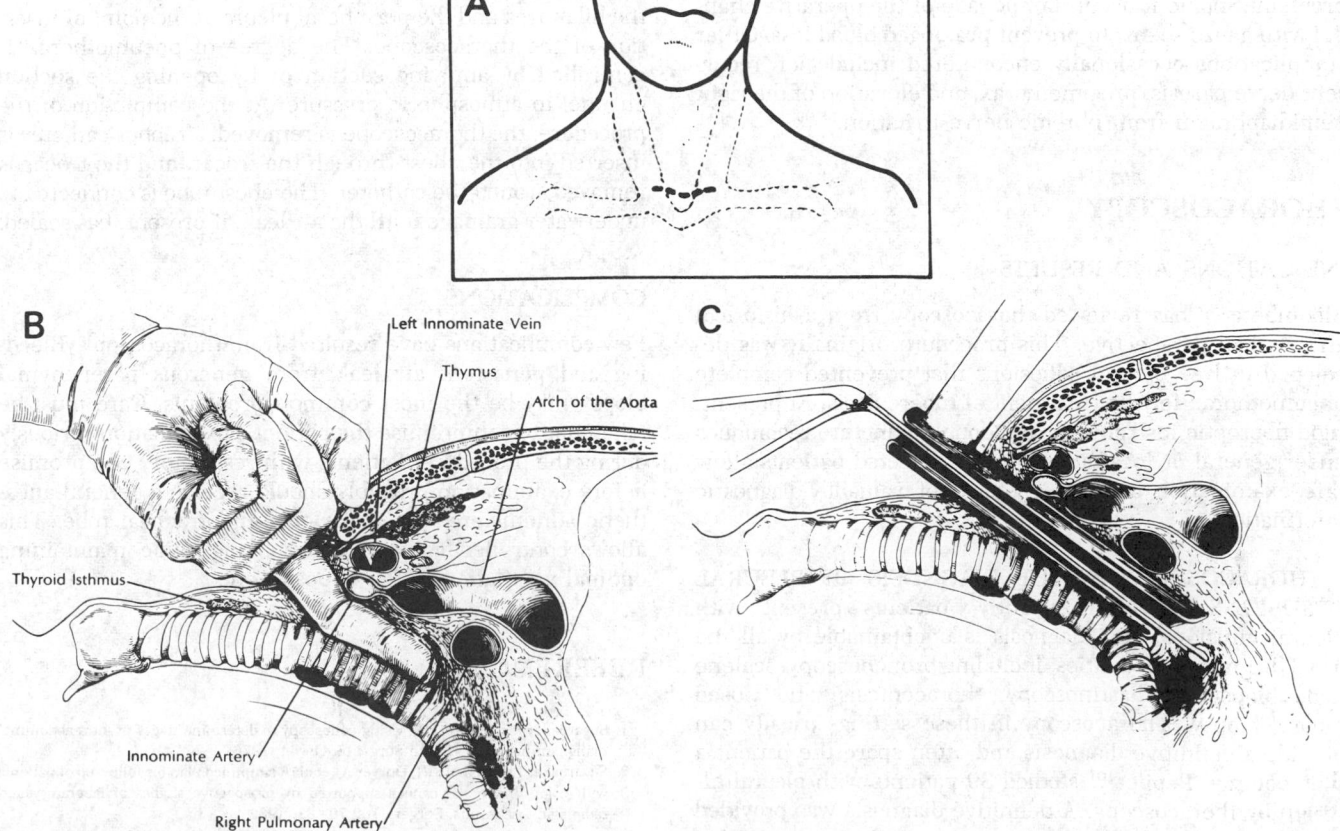

moves along the anterior surface of the trachea beneath the innominate vein, innominate artery, and aortic arch to the level of the tracheal bifurcation. During this dissection, the surgeon should note the position of nodes that feel pathologic for possible later biopsy.[96]

After a tunnel has been prepared, the mediastinoscope is introduced and advanced, with the anterior tracheal wall kept in view. Further dissection is accomplished through the endoscope using a blunt suction apparatus and gauze pledgets. In a complete exploration, which may not be necessary in every patient, both main bronchi, the azygos vein, paratracheal and parabronchial lymph nodes, the right pulmonary artery, the undersurface of the aortic arch, and the left recurrent nerve are visualized.

Biopsy sampling or removal of suspicious lymph nodes is performed; needle aspiration of sutures to be removed may prevent subsequent hemorrhage as a result of damage to vascular channels. Metal clips are useful for hemostasis and to mark biopsy sites. Preparation for emergency thoracotomy should always be made before mediastinoscopy is begun, so that complications may be dealt with quickly.

COMPLICATIONS

Foster and colleagues[97] reviewed 14 mediastinoscopy series published between 1968 and 1970; 3 (0.08%) deaths and 60 (1.6%) complications among 3742 examinations were reported. Postoperative respiratory insufficiency in 2 patients and cardiac arrest in 1 accounted for the 3 deaths. Despite the large number of major vascular structures immediately associated with the dissection, hemorrhage is an unusual problem. Should it occur, tamponade of the operative channel with gauze seems to prevent prolonged blood loss. Other complications occasionally encountered include left recurrent nerve paresis, pneumothorax, and elevation of the right hemidiaphragm from phrenic nerve irritation.[98,99]

THORACOSCOPY

INDICATIONS AND RESULTS

Bloomberg[100] has reviewed thoracoscopy from a historical and clinical perspective. This procedure originally was developed to lyse pleural adhesions that prevented complete pneumothorax for the treatment of tuberculosis. At present, rigid fiberoptic instruments and double-puncture techniques under general or local anesthesia in selected patients allow safe examination and a high yield of valuable diagnostic information.

THORACOSCOPY IN THE DIAGNOSIS OF PLEURAL EFFUSIONS. Not infrequently, patients present with pleural effusions, and diagnosis is unobtainable by all the usual diagnostic modalities, including bronchoscopy, scalene node biopsy, mediastinoscopy, thoracentesis, and closed pleural biopsy. Thoracoscopy in these settings usually can provide a definitive diagnosis and often spare the patient a thoracotomy. Pepper[101] studied 39 patients with pleural effusion by thoracoscopy. A definitive diagnosis was provided

in 31 patients by thoracic endoscopy, and in 22 of these the cause of the pleural effusion was malignancy. Lewis and co-workers[102] reported similarly good results in this group of patients.

PREOPERATIVE SCREENING OF PATIENTS WITH BRONCHIAL CARCINOMA. LeRoux[103] found that 7% of patients with bronchial carcinoma had pleural fluid. Because pulmonary resection is always likely to fail in the presence of pleural metastases, LeRoux recommended preoperative thoracoscopy for patients with pleural fluid. In 82 of 139 patients, pleural metastases were found and a needless thoracotomy was averted.

TECHNIQUES

Oldenburg and Newhouse[104] described the preferred method for performing thoracoscopy. The procedure is performed under local anesthesia in the operating room with adequate premedication. Patients are placed in the lateral decubitus position, the skin is prepared, local anesthesia is administered, and a 1.5-cm incision is made in the midaxillary line of the sixth to eighth intercostal space. The pleural space is entered bluntly, and, after an adequate cavity is ensured, the trocar and sleeve are inserted. A rigid 11-cm-diameter thoracoscope (Stortz) is used for visualization; biopsy, cytologic brushing, and photography of all pleural and some parenchymal lesions are possible. Except where adhesions interfere, the parietal pleura, visceral pleura, mediastinum, and diaphragm are well visualized. Areas difficult to examine are the hilar area and the peripheral pleura at the point of insertion of the thoracoscope. The degree of pneumothorax is controlled by applying suction or by opening the suction channel to atmospheric pressure. At the completion of the procedure, the thoracoscope is removed, a rubber catheter is inserted into the chest through the trocar, and the trocar is removed around the catheter. The chest tube is connected to underwater drainage until the air leak, if present, has sealed.

COMPLICATIONS

Few complications have resulted from thoracoscopy. Bleeding and persistent air leak from generous parenchymal biopsy may be the most common problems. Care must be taken not to compromise the patient's oxygenation seriously during the procedure. Patients with respiratory compromise before examination probably should receive a general anesthetic administered via a Carlen's endotracheal tube. This allows controlled collapse of one lung while maintaining optimal ventilation of the opposite one.

REFERENCES

1. Sugarbaker PH, Wilson RE: Using celioscopy to determine stages of intra-abdominal malignant neoplasms. Arch Surg 111:41–44, 1976
2. Sugarbaker PH, Gianola FJ, Duryer AJ et al: A simplified plan for follow up of patients with colon and rectal cancer supported by prospective studies of laboratory and radiologic test results. Surgery 102:79–83, 1982

3. Jori GP, Peshle C: Combined peritoneoscopy and liver biopsy in the diagnosis of hepatic neoplasm. Gastroenterology 63:1016–1019, 1972

4. Czaja AJ, Steinberg AS, Saldana M et al: Peritoneoscopy: Its value in the diagnosis of liver disease. Gastrointest Endosc 20:23–25, 1973

5. McCallum RW, Berci G: Laparoscopy in hepatic disease. Gastrointest Endosc 23:20–24, 1976

6. Sugarbaker PH: Double peritoneoscopy. Surg Gynecol Obstet 152:655–657, 1981

7. Ozols RF, Fisher RI, Anderson T et al: Peritoneoscopy in the management of ovarian cancer. Am J Obstet Gynecol 140:611–619, 1981

8. Goldhaber Z, Bloom BS, Sugarbaker PH et al: Effects of the fiberoptic laparoscope and colonoscope on morbidity and cost. Ann Surg 179:160–162, 1974

9. Knutson CO, Schrock LG, Polk HC: Polypoid lesions of the proximal colon: Comparison of experiences with removal at laparotomy and by colonoscopy. Ann Surg 179:567–662, 1974

10. Dean ACB, Newell JP: Colonoscopy in the differential diagnosis of carcinoma from diverticulitis of the sigmoid colon. Br J Surg 60:633–635, 1973

11. Sugarbaker PH, Vineyard GC, Lewicki AM et al: Colonoscopy in the management of diseases of the colon and rectum. Surg Gynecol Obstet 139:341–349, 1974

12. Glerum J, Agenant D, Tytgat GN: Value of colonoscopy in the detection of sigmoid malignancy in patients with diverticular disease. Endoscopy 9:228–230, 1977

13. Warwick RRG, Sumerling MD, Gilmour HM et al: Colonoscopy and double contrast barium enema examination in chronic ulcerative colitis. AJR 117:292–296, 1973

14. Dobbins WO, Stock M, Ginsberg AL: Early detection and prevention of carcinoma of the colon in patients with ulcerative colitis. Cancer 40:2542–2548, 1977

15. Riddel RH: Dysplasia in inflammatory bowel disease. Clin Gastroenterol 9:439–458, 1980

16. Wolff WI, Shinya H, Geffen A et al: Comparison of colonoscopy and barium enema in five hundred patients with colorectal disease. Am J Surg 129:181–186, 1975

17. Leinicke JL, Dodds WJ, Hogan WJ et al: A comparison of colonoscopy and roentgenography for detecting polypoid lesions of the colon. Gastrointest Radiol 2:125–128, 1977

18. Amberg JR, Berk RN, Burhenne J et al: Colonic polyp detection: Role of roentgenography and colonoscopy. Radiology 125:255–257, 1977

19. Thoeni RF, Menuck L: Comparison of barium enema and colonoscopy in the detection of small colonic polyps. Radiology 124:631–635, 1977

20. Teague RH, Salmon PR, Read AE: Fiberoptic examination of the colon: A review of 255 cases. Gut 14:139–142, 1973

21. Shinya H: Colonoscopy: Diagnosis and Treatment of Colonic Diseases, pp 163–164. New York, Igaku-Shoin, 1982

22. Gilbertsen VA, Nelms JM: The prevention of invasive cancer of the rectum. Cancer 41:1137–1139, 1978

23. Sugarbaker PH, Vineyard GC, Peterson LM: Anatomic localization and step by step advancement of the fiberoptic colonoscope. Surg Gynecol Obstet 143:457–462, 1976

24. Shinya H, Wolff WI: Colonoscopic polypectomy: Technique and safety. Hosp Pract 10:71–78, 1975

25. Sugarbaker PH, Vineyard GC: Snare polypectomy with the fiberoptic colonoscope. Surg Gynecol Obstet 138:581–583, 1974

26. Williams CB: Diathermy-biopsy—A technique for the endoscopic management of small polyps. Endoscopy 5:215–218, 1973

27. Shamir M, Schuman BM: Complications of fiberoptic endoscopy. Gastrointest Endosc 26:86–91, 1980

28. Kobayashi S, Yoshii Y, Kasugai T: Selective use of brushing cytology in gastrointestinal strictures. Gastrointest Endosc 2:76–77, 1972

29. Winawer S, Posner G, Belladonna J et al: Application of panendoscopic directed brush cytology to the diagnosis of esophageal cancer. Gastrointest Endosc 21:188, 1974

30. Totio TL, Den Hartog Jager CA, Tytgat GNJ: The role of endoscopic ultrasonography in assessing local resectability of oesophagogastric malignancies. Scand J Gastroenterol 21 (suppl 22):78–86, 1900

31. Sugano H, Nakamura K, Takagi K: Pathomorphogical study of polyp, polypogenic cancer and polypoid cancer. Stomach Intest 3:729, 1968

32. Martin TR, Onstad GR, Silvis SE et al: Lift and cut biopsy technique for submucosal sampling. Gastrointest Endosc 23:29–30, 1976

33. Yamada T, Hukuto MI: Gastric polyp. Gastrointest Endosc 7:448–454, 1965

34. Dekker W, Tytgat G: Diagnostic accuracy of fiberendoscopy in the detection of upper intestinal malignancy. Gastroenterology 73:710, 1977

35. Littman A (ed): The VA cooperative study on gastric ulcer. Gastroenterology 61(Part II):567, 1971

36. Kasugai T, Kobayashi S: Evaluation of biopsy and cytology in the diagnosis of gastric cancer. Am J Gastroenterol 62:199, 1974

37. Montgomery R, Richardson B: Gastric ulcer and cancer. Q J Med 44:591, 1975

38. Kukrai JC: Gastric ulcer: An appraisal. Surgery 63:1024, 1968

39. Gear M, Truelove S, Williams G et al: Gastric cancer simulating benign gastric ulcer. Br J Surg 56:739, 1969

40. Myren J, Dybdahl J, Serck-Hanssen A et al: Gastroscopy with directed biopsy and routine x-ray in the diagnosis of malignancies of the stomach. Scand J Gastroenterol 10:193, 1975

41. Tsuneoka K, Tadayoshi T, Sotaro F: Fiberoscopy of Gastric Diseases. Tokyo, Igaku-Shoin, 1973

42. Murakami T: Pathomorphological diagnosis: Definition and gross classification of early gastric cancer. In Murakami T (ed): Early Gastric Cancer, Gann Monograph on Cancer Research II, pp 53–55. Tokyo, University of Tokyo Press, 1971

43. Comfort M, Priestly J, Dockerty M et al: The small benign and malignant gastric lesion. Surg Gynecol Obstet 105:435, 1957

44. Hayashida T, Kidokoro T: End results of early gastric cancer collected from 22 institutions. Stomach Intest 4:1077, 1969

45. Borrmann R: Geschwulste des Magens und Duodenums. Handbuch d. spez. pathol. Anatomie U Histologie 4:812, 1926

46. Just-Viera JO, Haight C: Achalasia and carcinoma of the esophagus. Surg Gynecol Obstet 128:1081–1095, 1969

47. Seliger G, Lee T, Schwartz S. Carcinoma of the proximal esophagus: A complication of longstanding achalasia. Am J Gastroenterol 57:20–25, 1972

48. Pierce WS, MacVaugh III H, Johnson J: Carcinoma of the esophagus arising in patients with achalasia of the cardia. J Thorac Cardiovasc Surg 59:355–359, 1970

49. Hankins JR, McLaughlin JS: The association of carcinoma of the esophagus with achalasia. J Thorac Cardiovasc Surg 69:355–360, 1975

50. Carter R, Brewer III LA: Achalasia and esophageal carcinoma. Am J Surg 130:114–120, 1975

51. Wychulis AR, Woolam GL, Anderson HA et al: Achalasia and carcinoma of the esophagus. JAMA 215:1638–1641, 1971

52. Naef A, Savary M, Ozzello P: Columnar-lined lower esophagus: An acquired lesion with malignant predisposition. J Thorac Cardiovasc Surg 70:826–835, 1975

53. Berenson MM, Riddell RH, Skinner DB et al: Malignant transformation of esophageal columnar epithelium. Cancer 41:554–561, 1978

54. McDonald GB, Brand DL, Thorning DR: Multiple adenomatous neoplasms arising in columnar-lined (Barrett's) esophagus. Gastroenterology 72:1317–1321, 1977

55. Sjogren RW Jr, Johnson LF: Barrett's esophagus: A review. Am J Med 74:313–321, 1983

57. Tomasulo J: Gastric polyps: Histologic types and their relation to gastric carcinoma. Cancer 27:1346–1355, 1971

58. Hay LJ: Surgical management of gastric polyps and adenomas. Surgery 39:114–119, 1956

59. Huppler EG, Priestley JT, Morlock CG et al: Diagnosis and results of treatment in gastric polyps. Surg Gynecol Obstet 110:309–313, 1960

60. Marshak RH, Feldman F: Gastric polyps. Am J Dig Dis 10:909–935, 1965

61. Elsborg L, Mosbech J: Pernicious anemia as a risk factor in gastric cancer. Acta Med Scand 206:315–318, 1979

62. Helsingen N, Hillestad L: Cancer development in the gastric stump after partial gastrectomy for ulcer. Am Surg 143:173–179, 1956

63. Stalsberg H, Taksdal S: Stomach cancer following gastric surgery for benign condition. Lancet 2:1175–1177, 1971

64. Domellof L, Janunger KG: The risk of gastric carcinoma after partial gastrectomy. Am J Surg 134:581–584, 1977

65. Schafer LW, Larson DE, Melton LF III et al: The risk of gastric carcinoma following surgical treatment for benign ulcer disease: A population-based study in Olmsted County, Minnesota. N Engl J Med 309:1210–1213, 1983

66. Ross AHM, Smith MA, Anderson JR et al: Late mortality after surgery for peptic ulcer. N Engl J Med 307:519–522, 1982

67. National Institutes of Health Consensus Development Conference Summary: Endoscopy in upper GI bleeding, Vol 3, No 5, 1980

68. Ferrucci JT, Wittenberg J, Sarns RA et al: Fine needle transhepatic cholangiography: A new approach to obstructive jaundice. AJR 127:403–407, 1976

69. Elias E, Hamlyn AN, Jain S et al: A randomized trial of percutaneous transhepatic cholangiography with the Chiba needle versus endoscopic retrograde cholangiography for bile duct visualization in jaundice. Gastroenterology 71:439–443, 1976

70. Kasugai T, Kuno N, Kobayashi S et al: Endoscopic pancreatocholangiography: I. The normal endoscopic pancreatocholangiogram. Gastroenterology 63:217–226, 1972

71. Kasugai T, Kuno N, Kizu M et al: Endoscopic pancreatocholangiography: II. The pathological endoscopic pancreatocholangiogram. Gastroenterology 63:227–234, 1972

72. Ogoshi K: Diseases of the pancreas and the biliary system. In Takemoto T, Kasugai T (eds): Endoscopic Retrograde Cholangiopancreatography. Tokyo, Igaku-Shoin, 1979

73. Yasuda K, Mukai H, Fujimoto S et al: The diagnosis of pancreatic cancer by endoscopic ultrasonography. Gastrointest Endosc 34:1–8, 1988

74. Mackie CR, Cooper MJ, Lewis MH et al: Non-operative differentiation between pancreatic cancer and chronic pancreatitis. Ann Surg 189:480–487, 1979

75. Cotton PB, Williams CB: Practical Gastrointestinal Endoscopy. Oxford, Blackwell, 1980

76. Katz D: Morbidity and mortality in standard and flexible gastrointestinal endoscopy. Gastrointest Endosc 15:134–138, 1969

77. Michel L, Grillo HC, Malt RA: Esophageal perforation. Ann Thorac Surg 33:203–210, 1982

78. Triggiani E, Belsey R: Oesophageal trauma: Incidence, diagnosis and management. Thorax 32:241–249, 1977

79. Mayer JE Jr, Murray CA, Varco RL: The treatment of esophageal perforation with delayed recognition and continuing sepsis. Ann Thorac Surg 23:568–573, 1977

80. Payne CR, Stovin PGI, Baker V et al: Diagnostic accuracy in primary bronchial carcinoma. Thorax 34:294–299, 1979

81. Feldman NT, Pennington JE, Ehrie MG: Transbronchial lung biopsy in the compromised host. JAMA 238:1377–1379, 1977

82. Burt ME, Flye MW, Webber BL et al: Prospective evaluation of aspiration needle, cutting needle, transbronchial and open lung biopsy in patients with pulmonary infiltrates. Ann Thorac Surg 32:146–153, 1981

83. Pearson FG: An evaluation of mediastinoscopy in the management of presumably operable bronchial carcinoma. J Thorac Cardiovasc Surg 55:617–625, 1968
84. Goldberg EM, Shapiro CM, Glicksman AS: Mediastinoscopy for assessing mediastinal spread in clinical staging of lung carcinoma. Semin Oncol 1:205–215, 1974
85. Borrie J: Lung Cancer Surgery and Survival. New York, Appleton-Century-Crofts, 1965
86. Bowen TE, Zajtchuk R, Green DC et al: Value of anterior mediastinotomy in bronchogenic carcinoma of the left upper lobe. J Thorac Cardiovasc Surg 79:269–271, 1980
87. Jolly PC, Li W, Anderson RP: Anterior and cervical mediastinoscopy for determining operability and predicting resectability in lung cancer. J Thorac Cardiovasc Surg 79:366–371, 1980
88. Gibbons JRP: The value of mediastinoscopy in assessing operability in carcinoma of the lung. Br J Dis Chest 66:162–166, 1972
89. Kirsh MM, Rotman H, Argenta L et al: Carcinoma of the lung: Results of treatment over ten years. Ann Thorac Surg 21:371–377, 1976
90. Martini N, Flehinger BJ, Zaman MB et al: Results of resection in non-oat cell carcinoma of the lung with mediastinal lymph node metastases. Ann Surg 198:386–397, 1983
91. Hutchinson CM, Mills NL: The selection of patients with bronchogenic carcinoma for mediastinoscopy. J Thorac Cardiovasc Surg 71:768–773, 1976
92. Baker RR, Lillemoe KD, Tockman MS: The indications for transcervical mediastinoscopy in patients with small peripheral bronchial carcinoma. Surg Gynecol Obstet 148:860–862, 1979

93. Daily BDT Jr, Failing LJ, Pugatch RD et al: Computed tomography an effective technique for mediastinal staging and lung cancer. J Thorac Cardiovasc Surg 88:486–494, 1900
94. Vaeth JM, Moskowitz SA, Green JP: Mediastinal Hodgkin's disease. AJR 126:123–126, 1976
95. Redding ME, Anagnostopoulos CE, Ultmann JE: The possible value of mediastinoscopy in staging Hodgkin's disease. Cancer Res 31:1741–1745, 1971
96. Kirschner PA: Transcervical approach to the superior mediastinum. Hosp Pract, June 1970
97. Foster ED, Munro DD, Dobell ARC: Mediastinoscopy. A review of anatomical relationships and complications. Ann Thorac Surg 13:273–286, 1972
98. Bacsa S, Czaro Z, Vezendi S: The complications of mediastinoscopy. Panminerva Med 74:402–406, 1974
99. Kliems G, Savic B: Complications of mediastinoscopy. Endoscopy 1:9–12, 1979
100. Bloomberg AE: Thoracoscopy in perspective. Surg Gynecol Obstet 147:433–443, 1978
101. Pepper JR: Thoracoscopy in the diagnosis of pleural effusions and tumors. Br J Dis Chest 72:74–75, 1978
102. Lewis RJ, Kunderman PJ, Sisler GE et al: Direct diagnostic thoracoscopy. Ann Thorac Surg 21:536–539, 1976
103. LeRoux BT: Bronchial Carcinoma, p 127. Edinburgh, E & S Livingston, 1968
104. Oldenburg FA, Newhouse MT: Thoracoscopy: A safe, accurate diagnostic procedure using the rigid thoracoscope and local anesthesia. Chest 75:45–50, 1979

DAVID G. BRAGG
H. RIC HARNSBERGER
WILLIAM M. THOMPSON

SECTION 2

Radiologic Techniques in Cancer

Tumor imaging in its entirety is too broad to cover in the few pages that follow. We have chosen to focus on the controversial anatomical sites, cancers that commonly occur in these sites, and the selection of an appropriate imaging modality for evaluating such cancers. For a more complete discussion of the many challenges and applications for tumor imaging procedures, the reader is referred to the textbook *Oncologic Imaging,* edited by Bragg, Rubin, and Youker.[1]

Tumor imaging has become more complex and controversial as the number of available technologies has increased. In most body sites, imaging is used primarily to detect, stage, and follow the cancer rather than as a screening method. Notable exceptions are certain radiologic screening programs for breast and gastrointestinal tract cancers. One should critically analyze reports concerning the accuracy of imaging procedures in any given tumor site, paying particular attention to the type of equipment used, the date of the report, and the unique challenges posed by each body site. The rapid evolution of imaging technologies has made obsolete many of the earlier reports on the accuracy of various modalities for staging neoplasms, particularly with regard to neoplasms of the central nervous system, chest, and abdomen. The complex changes in magnetic resonance (MR) imaging equipment have further confounded a thoughtful analysis of this technology. The recently completed consensus conference on MR imaging established the dominance of this imaging technique in the central nervous system and reported preliminary advantages in musculoskeletal tumor staging. To date, MR imaging has not been shown to have a clear advantage over computed tomography (CT) in

most other thoracoabdominal sites. MR imaging and CT appear to be nearly equivalent in the detection of most brain tumors; however, because of the absence of bone artifacts, MR imaging is the preferred modality for detecting lesions near the skull vertex, posterior fossa, skull base, and orbit.[2]

DAVID G. BRAGG

Thorax

Current controversies in imaging of thoracic cancer largely focus on the relative accuracy and efficacy of CT versus MR imaging and the appropriate use of these modalities for staging neoplasms and guiding biopsy procedures. This discussion briefly considers the application of these modalities and the use of biopsy procedures in tumors of the chest wall, pleura, lung, and heart.

CHEST WALL

The imaging approach to the individual with a chest wall neoplasm is summarized in Table 20-5. This simplified algorithm does not attempt to consider the variety of different tumor cell types or tumorlike abnormalities that may affect the thoracic cage. The initial step in imaging the chest wall should always be plain radiography, with films showing rib detail. This examination will allow the clinician to determine whether the lesion is destructive or is one of the multitude of traumatic and acquired benign lesions that can mimic tumors. If, based on the plain films, tumor continues to be a diagnostic possibility, a radionuclide bone scan should be the next step to determine whether the lesion is monostotic or polyostotic. If the neoplasm is localized to a single rib or a group of contiguous ribs, consideration of a primary tumor should be paramount. The decision to proceed with CT or

TABLE 20-5. Algorithm of Imaging Approach to Patient with Chest Wall Neoplasm

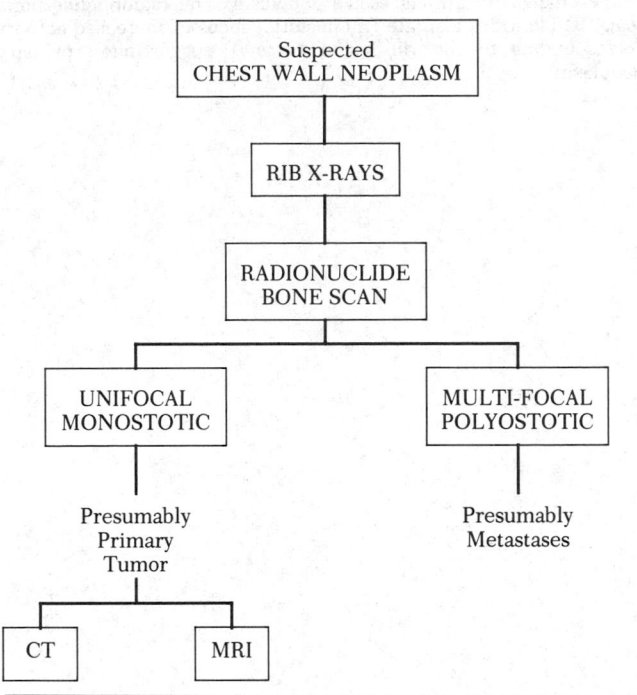

MR imaging to analyze and stage the tumor may be a local option, contingent on the availability of the technology. MR imaging better defines the muscle compartments and provides the surgeon with the information necessary to plan the appropriate surgical procedure and to determine the resectability of the lesion. In addition, T2-weighted MR images are more useful than CT in determining the presence of chest wall invasion with peripheral primary lung cancers.[3,4]

In general, plain radiographs seldom show an associated soft tissue mass with metastatic rib lesions. When a presumed, surrounding soft tissue mass is seen in association with a destructive rib lesion, consideration should be given to multiple myeloma and non-Hodgkin's lymphoma. If MR imaging, CT, or ultrasound is used to further characterize the metastatic rib lesions, a much higher percentage of associated soft tissue masses will be found with metastatic rib lesions, a feature not generally visible on plain radiographs.

MR imaging with both T1- and T2-weighted images is the recommended procedure for staging a variety of primary chest wall neoplasms prior to definitive treatment. Limited post-treatment MR imaging can be used to monitor tumor response to radiation therapy and chemotherapy (Fig. 20-8).

PLEURA

A suspected mesothelioma is often better evaluated by imaging than by microscopic review of the excised tissue. In diffuse malignant mesothelioma the affected pleura exhibits a lobular pleural thickening that often extends into the interlobar fissures, reducing the volume of the hemithorax. The tumor subsequently encases the involved hemithorax, progressively reducing lung volume, yet rarely breaks through the pleura to invade contiguous ribs. Radiographic findings of associated asbestosis are usually lacking. Often, a limited tissue biopsy sample may make a specific pathologic diagnosis very difficult and differentiation from a metastatic adenocarcinoma impossible. Radiographic signs favoring metastatic adenocarcinoma over mesothelioma include bilateral disease, hilar or mediastinal lymphadenopathy, and nodular pulmonary parenchymal disease.[5] Either MR imaging or CT will demonstrate the extent of the mesothelioma before and after treatment. Both of these techniques afford the opportunity to access contiguous invasion, particularly of the mediastinum, pericardium, and diaphragm.[6-8]

Metastatic involvement of the pleural compartment almost invariably manifests as pleural effusion on routine chest radiographs. Rarely are the tumor deposits of sufficient size to be imaged directly by any modality. Neoplasms responsible for secondary pleural involvement represent one of two general categories: either direct extension from primary lung tumors, or metastatic involvement, usually from a primary in the breast or subdiaphragmatic sites. Individuals with ascitic fluid accumulations not infrequently have pleural effusions, due to the communications through the diaphragm with the peritoneum. Pleural effusions in patients with lymphoproliferative disorders are usually secondary manifestations of disease in the mediastinum or lung parenchyma.

LUNG

The three national lung cancer screening trial programs in the United States that used serial chest radiography and sputum cytology to evaluate heavy smokers found an insufficient survival benefit with these procedures to lead to their recommended use in a routine screening protocol. These studies also demonstrated the difficulty in recognizing the low-contrast object represented by a primary lung cancer on a routine chest radiograph. Nearly 90% of the peripheral lung cancers and 75% of the more central lesions could be seen in retrospect on earlier 4-month screening radiographs in one of the trials.[8-11]

It is thought that the majority of primary lung cancers arise distal to a segmental bronchus and undergo approximately 30 doublings before reaching a size of 1.0 cm, the accepted threshold for detection on plain radiographs. Squamous cell carcinomas invariably occur as central lesions and have a tendency to excavate and generally metastasize later than other non-oat cell lung cancers. In contrast, small cell carcinomas have spread outside the thorax in 70% to 90% of patients at the time of diagnosis. These small cell carcinomas often resemble squamous cell cancers on chest radiographs, as both arise as central lesions. Adenocarcinoma, a more frequent peripheral primary lung cancer, tends to metastasize early and has an apparent predilection to spread to the central nervous system and adrenal glands. Large cell carcinomas resemble adenocarcinomas in terms of their peripheral presentation and metastatic characteristics.[12,13] An appreciation of these more common presenting characteris-

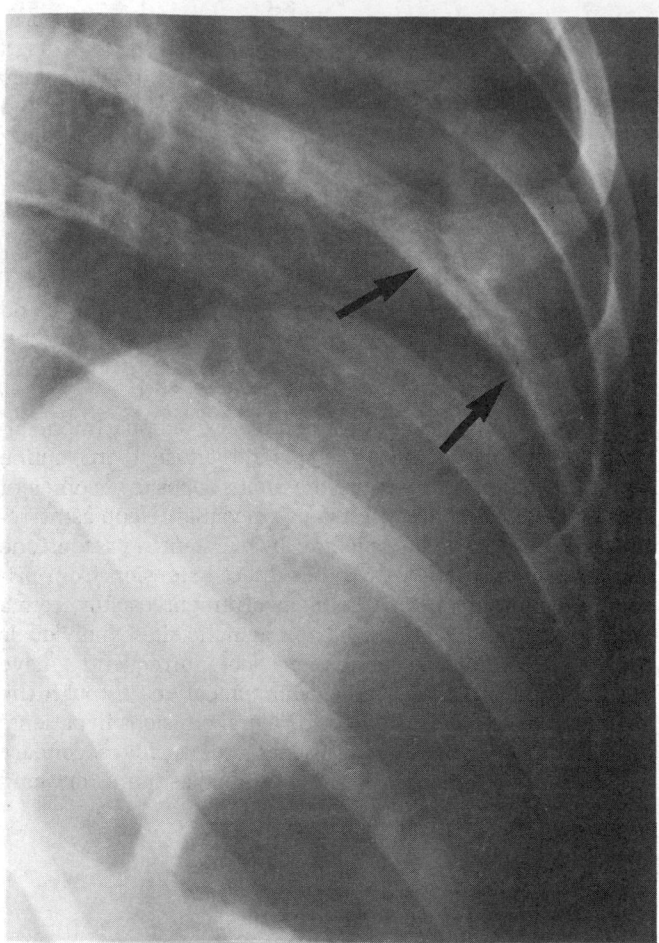

A

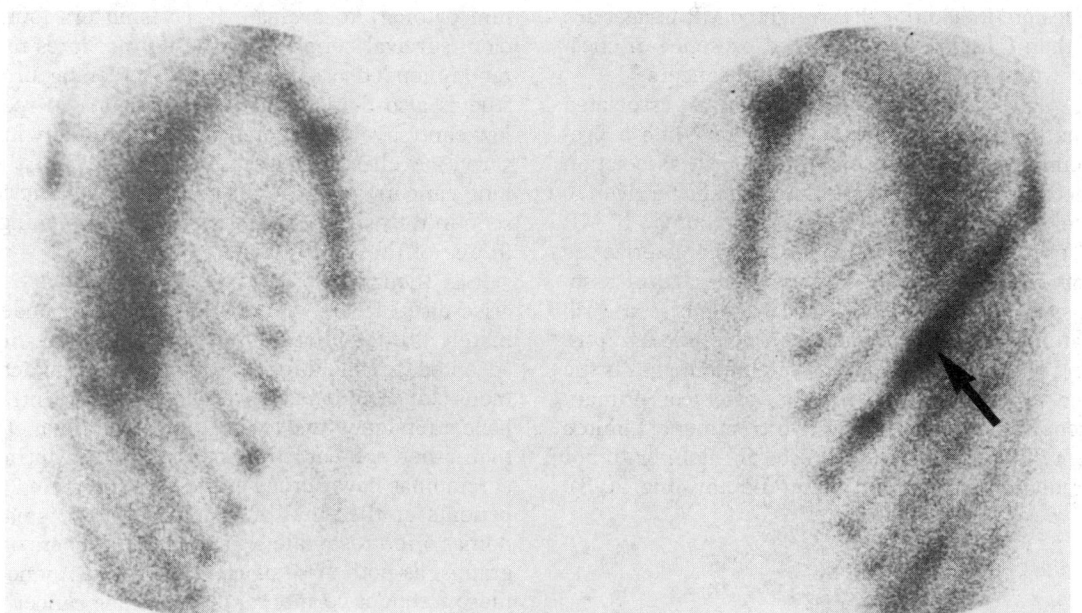

B

FIG. 20-8. An 18-year-old girl had complained of left chest pain for several months but denied a history of trauma. The rib detail films (**A**) show the destructive permeative process (*black arrows*) typical of the changes of an aggressive neoplasm. The radionuclide bone scan (**B**) identifies a single (monostotic) focus of increased activity corresponding to the rib lesion (*arrow*), suggesting a primary neoplasm.

(continued)

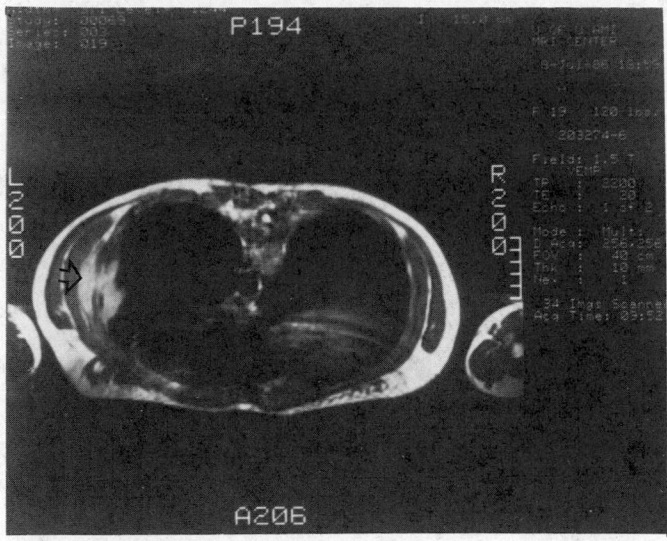

C

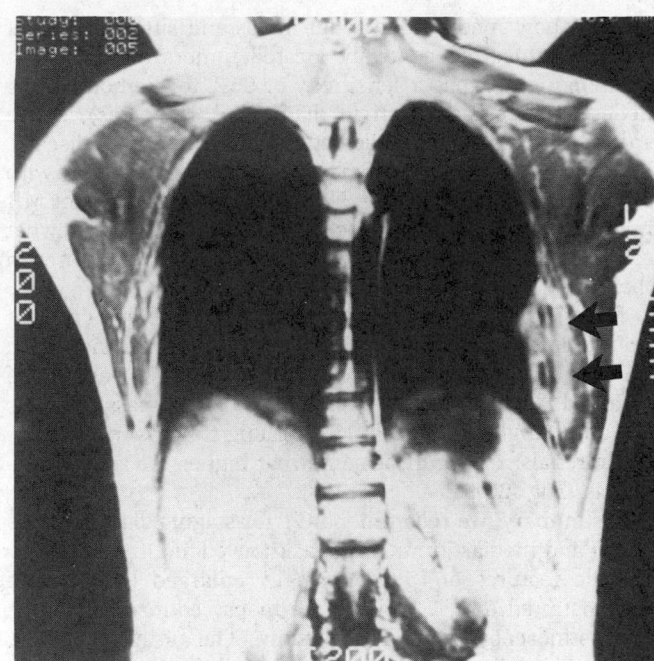

D

(*FIG. 20-8 continued*)
The axial (**C**) and coronal (**D**) MRI scans, T-1 weighted, demonstrate the higher signal, white tumor (*arrows*) displacing but not invading contiguous chest wall musculature. The neoplasm was excised and found to be a high-grade non-Hodgkin's lymphoma.

tics of the primary lung cancers can help the clinician understand both imaging features and radiologic staging protocols.

A CT evaluation of the solitary pulmonary nodule was suggested by Siegelman et al in 1980 as a means of discriminating benign from malignant pulmonary masses. Lesions with high CT numbers in excess of 164 Hounsfield units were presumed to contain calcium and therefore to be benign.[14] Other investigators had difficulty confirming these findings, leading to a multi-institutional trial program in which several different CT scanners and a standardization phantom were used. As a result of these trials it was found that an absolute CT number could not be used as a threshold to separate benign from malignant lesions; however, the characteristics of the tumor margin and its size have helped to unify the recommendations for the potential application of CT in evaluating the solitary pulmonary nodule.[15] In our opinion, the use of CT in this setting will be limited, as it requires an expensive phantom, various imaging procedures, and education of surgeons not familiar with this technique.

The selection of an appropriate imaging procedure to evaluate and further characterize a thoracic neoplasm must be tailored to the anatomical compartment, the presumed or known histology of the neoplasm, and the anticipated treatment. Chest wall invasion cannot be accurately assessed with either CT or MR imaging unless there is frank bone invasion. The mere contact and effacement of fat planes is insufficient evidence from which to infer chest wall invasion. In comparisons of film tomography, CT, and MR imaging in the

evaluation of nodular pulmonary lesions, CT was the most sensitive and accurate; however, it suffers from a lack of specificity. The size threshold for recognition on plain films of the solitary pulmonary nodule representing a primary lung cancer is generally thought to be between 5 and 10 mm.[16] Film tomography is no longer used to screen for lung nodules. Data reported in earlier studies, in which less sophisticated CT instrumentation was used than is currently employed, showed that 35% more pulmonary nodules were detected with CT than with film tomography in a group of 91 patients. CT is considerably more accurate than either plain radiography or film tomography in demonstrating the actual size of pulmonary nodules.[17]

The major controversy in the application of imaging techniques to lung cancer relates to staging. A recent article reported a survey of thoracic surgeons in North America and their opinion regarding the role of CT in the preoperative assessment of the patient with lung cancer. Some 85% of the 329 respondents used CT selectively for the patient with an abnormal hilum or mediastinum on routine chest radiographs, whereas only 10% requested CT in the presence of a "normal" hilum and mediastinum on plain chest radiographs.[18]

Because approximately 50% of patients with lung cancer can be expected to have metastatic nodal involvement at the time of initial presentation, the goal of imaging should be to identify those patients with an abnormal mediastinum who should be further evaluated with mediastinoscopy or mediastinotomy with biopsy prior to thoracotomy. Plain chest radiographs show mediastinal nodal metastatic sites only about half the time; the centrally located tumors are the most challenging. CT has a sensitivity of 95% for demonstrating nodes in excess of 1 cm in diameter (short axis), and a specificity of 65% for nodes containing metastatic disease. The sensitivity and specificity obviously are different with increasing lymph node size. No significant advantage for MR imaging over CT has been shown, other than a somewhat clearer separation of lymph nodes and vascular structures in the hilum with MR imaging.[19,20]

The CT protocol for imaging the mediastinum in a patient prior to initial treatment entails contrast agent infusion, with a bolus injection if sections through the hilum are to be obtained. The examination should also encompass the liver and adrenal glands. Nearly 12% of lung cancers will involve the adrenals; the figure is somewhat higher for adenocarcinomas (Fig. 20-9).

In summary, we recommend CT for staging disease in the hilum and mediastinum, while acknowledging that the nonspecific features of the abnormally enlarged lymph node demonstrated on CT will require biopsy confirmation with mediastinoscopy or mediastinotomy. The ultimate goal of these efforts is to eliminate unnecessary thoracotomies in patients with unresectable disease. MR imaging affords no advantage over CT in the evaluation of the hilum or mediastinum but does appear superior in the assessment of the chest wall and lung apex. Gallium radionuclide scanning, film tomography, and fluoroscopy no longer have a meaningful role in the workup of the patient with primary lung cancer.

The percutaneous biopsy of parenchymal, hilar, or mediastinal abnormalities is a safe and reliable technique for the diagnosis of pulmonary, pleural, or chest wall mass lesions. The technique is firmly based on the experience of both radiologists and pathologists, with accuracies in excess of 95% reported. The incidence of complications is related to patient factors (*e.g.*, his or her ability to cooperate), the location of the lesion (a higher incidence of pneumothorax occurs with apical lesions), and the number of times the needle punctures the pleural surface. In an effort to minimize the latter complication, a "coaxial technique" has been suggested, in which a thin (no. 22 or 23) needle is inserted and a larger 19-gauge needle is passed over the thinner needle. Subsequent biopsies are performed through the larger needle to avoid multiple pleural punctures.[21]

Fluoroscopic guidance is usually all that is required to perform the percutaneous biopsy. Lesions more difficult to biopsy, such as indistinct or central lesions, may require CT guidance, even though complications have been reported to be higher when CT is used, probably due to the longer procedure time and patient characteristics. A postprocedure pneumothorax is usually evident within 4 hours; the vast majority are visible immediately after the biopsy. This complication is reported following approximately 20% of lung biopsies. Local hemorrhage is the only other important complication. Only approximately 10% of these pneumothorax complications require treatment, which often entails the placement of a small, 9-F chest tube attached to a Heimlich valve.[22]

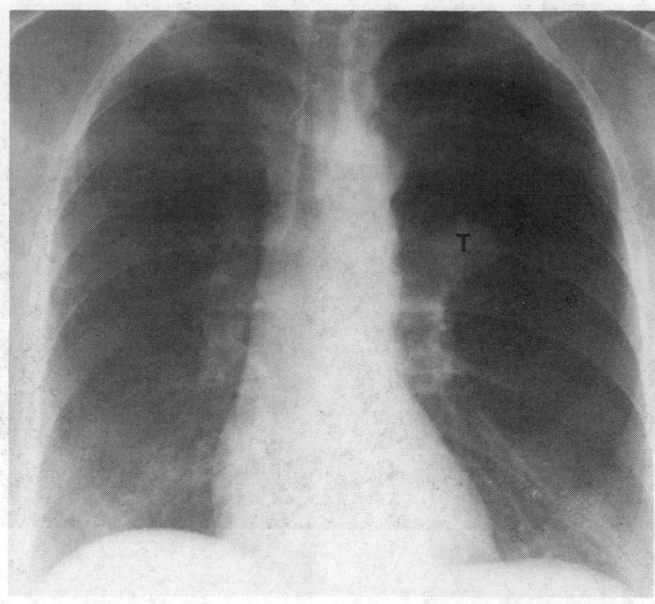

A

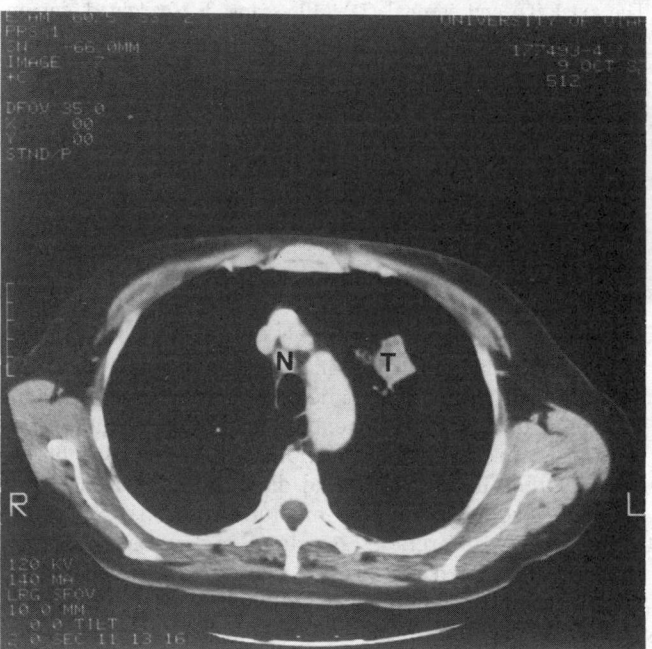

B

FIG. 20-9. A mass lesion was discovered on a routine chest radiograph (**A**) of a 63-year-old female smoker, which was found to be an adenocarcinoma by lung biopsy (labeled T). A staging CT scan (**B**) shows the T-1 tumor (*T*) and pretracheal nodes (*N*), indicating a stage N-2 lung cancer.

HEART

A discussion of the uncommon primary intracardiac tumors is beyond the scope of this chapter. The extension of contiguous mediastinal or lung parenchymal tumors to the heart can now be elegantly imaged with cardiac and respiratory gated MR imaging. The extent of the tumor to or through the pericardium and into the chambers of the heart can be quite accurately assessed with MR imaging. Tumors with a propensity to extend through the great vessels to the heart, such as renal cell cancers, can also be noninvasively imaged with MR imaging techniques, particularly those with reconstruction algorithms that create a positive image of flowing blood

(Fig. 20-10). The MR imaging characteristics of a variety of intracardiac masses have recently been reported, illustrating this potential for cardiac imaging.[23] MR images in coronal projections are useful to the radiation oncologist in treatment planning. Some centers have reported predictable changes on T2-weighted images of mediastinal neoplasms, especially lymphomas, after treatment. A controlled imaging

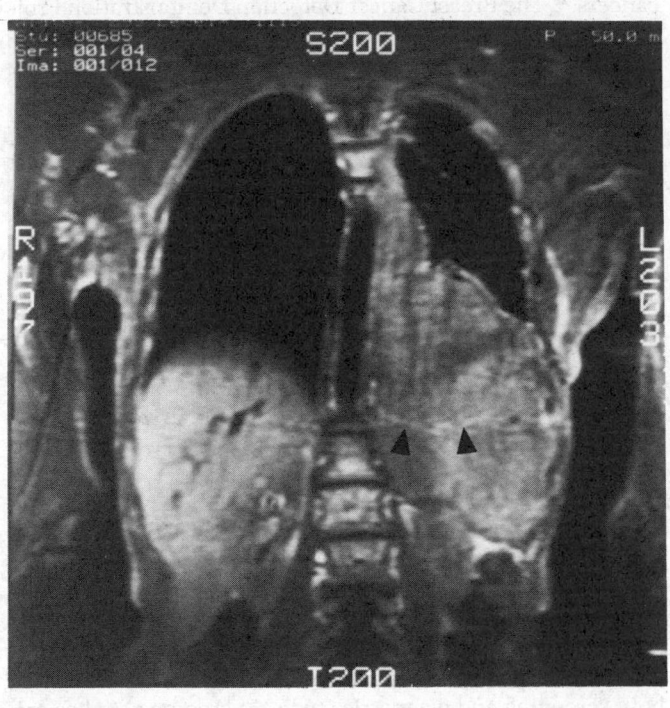

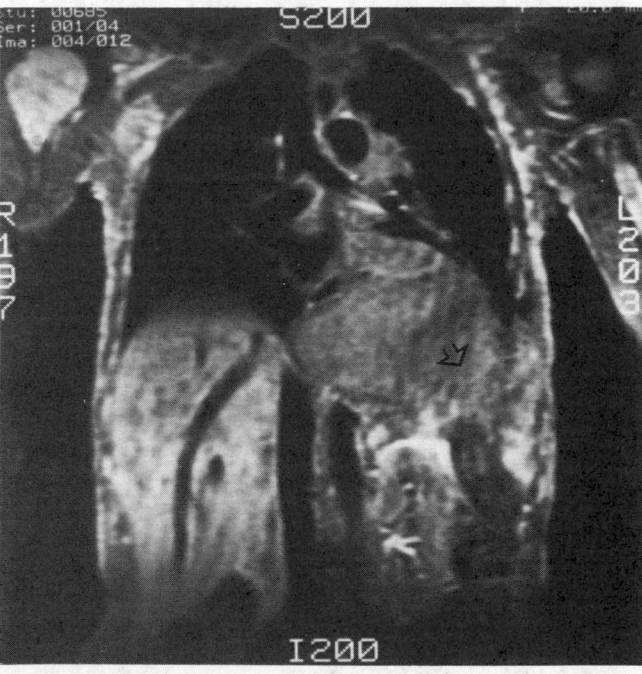

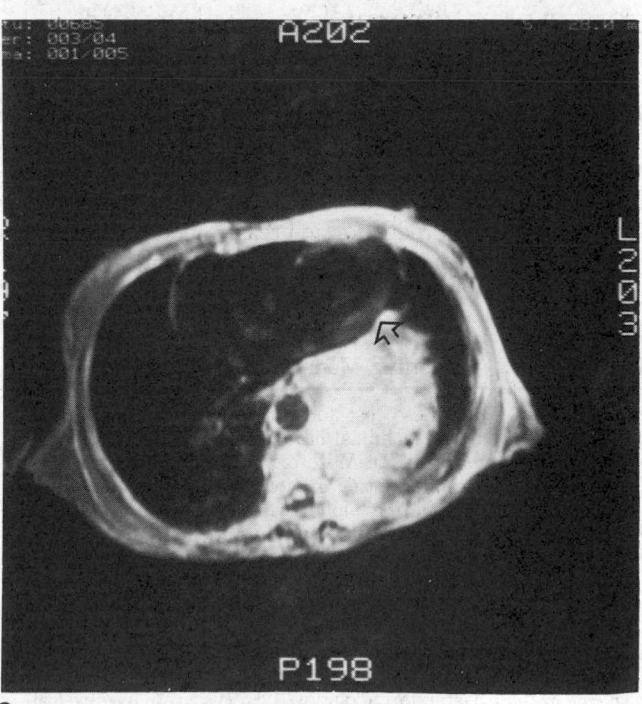

FIG. 20-10. An elderly woman was initially thought to have a mesothelioma because the tumor encased the left chest. Biopsy results revealed a neurosarcoma. Before exploratory surgery, an MR scan was performed and revealed tumor extending through the pericardium (*open arrows* on **B** and **C**). The normal, intact pericardium can be outlined by the white line identified by the arrowheads in **A**.

study of a large number of tumors will be required to confirm these observations, as we have not found these changes to be reliable indicators of disease regression.

DAVID G. BRAGG

Breast

Initial reports on roentgenography of the breast appeared more than 50 years ago, but it was not until the 1960s that dedicated mammographic systems became available and the concept of screening mammography came of age.[24] These initial mammographic studies were flawed by an unacceptably high radiation exposure dose, long exposure times, and less than optimal image quality. Soon after the introduction of dedicated mammographic units in the mid-1960s, alternative imaging techniques were suggested, the first of which was thermography. These alternative screening techniques are summarized in Table 20-6. Xeromammography was introduced in 1972 as a technique to improve breast imaging by providing edge enhancement to structures of differing radiographic contrast density and calcifications.[25]

In the United States, virtually all breast imaging entails either screen-film mammography or xeroradiography. There is no significant difference in the diagnostic yield of these two techniques.[26] Other screening techniques have not proved suitable for stand-alone screening and have a limited role as ancillary diagnostic procedures in certain clinical circumstances.

SCREENING PROGRAMS AND THEIR JUSTIFICATION

The initial study documenting the role of mammography in breast cancer detection was the Health Insurance Plan of New York City (HIP), completed in the 1960s. Long-term follow-up of patients enrolled in these controlled trials has shown a significant reduction in breast cancer mortality that is limited to patients over age 50.[27] Similar results were reported from a controlled, randomized trial in Sweden, with survival advantage also limited to individuals over age 50. The Swedish study used a longer interval of nearly 3 years between screening examinations. The investigators also employed a single oblique mammogram, an imaging strategy that has since been shown to be cost-ineffective and has been discontinued in the United States. The Swedish investigators reported a 31% reduction in breast cancer mortality and a 25% reduction in the incidence of Stage II or more advanced cancers.[28] The Breast Cancer Detection Demonstration Projects (BCDDP) validated the effectiveness of mass mammographic screening through multiple separate screening centers in an uncontrolled trial. Reports from the BCDDP demonstrated the ability of modern mammography to detect early breast cancer before it becomes palpable. In this study, nearly 42% of the proven cancers were seen only with mammography.[29]

The results of these and other mammographic screening programs support a role for screening mammography in the patient over age 50 and suggest the application of this technique as an effective means to detect preclinical breast cancer in the patient under age 50. These data form the basis for the recommendations of the American Cancer Society and American College of Radiology, summarized in Table 20-7.

TECHNICAL ASPECTS, RADIATION DOSES, AND LOCALIZATION PROCEDURES

Dedicated mammography installations using screen-film or xerographic techniques are divided into those facilities dedicated to screening examinations and those which perform both screening and diagnostic studies. Screening studies are limited to the examination of asymptomatic patients in a mass screening setting. In this kind of examination a radiologist is not actively involved; a technician performs the examination, which is subsequently reviewed by a radiologist. A diagnostic study is tailored to the needs of the symptomatic patient and often requires additional views or ancillary studies, such as ultrasound. The characteristics of the more complex, dedicated unit capable of performing diagnostic examinations and a comparison of screen-film versus xerography techniques have been reported.[30,31]

Until recently, screen-film mammography was associated

TABLE 20-6. Screening Modalities

- *Screen-film* (1960): Less cost and lower radiation dose (0.1 rad to midbreast); less technical latitude; misses chest wall
- *Xeromammography* (1972): More expensive, higher radiation dose (0.8 rad to midbreast); greater technical latitude; images chest wall; new toner-developer will decrease dose
- *Digital Mammography:* Early results not encouraging
- *Ultrasound:* Small-part—only for symptomatic patient with dense breast and palpable mass; resolution poor for lesions <1 cm; dedicated—poor with fatty breasts; not adequate for screening
- *Diaphanography* (cancer absorbs more near infrared radiation than benign): Poor for deep lesions
- *Thermography:* Detection accuracy 42% (vs. 57% by physical examination and 91% by mammography)

TABLE 20-7. Screening Mammography Recommendations (1987)

American College of Surgeons, American College of Radiology, American Medical Association:
    Baseline at age 35–40 yr
    Every 1–2 yr at ages 40–50
    Annually for those over age 50
National Cancer Institute, American College of Physicians:
    NCI—before age 50 *only* if at high risk
    ACP—no data to support screening before age 50
American College of Obstetrics and Gynecology:
    Mammography "considered" for high-risk patients aged 40–49 yr

with a considerably lower radiation exposure than xeromammography for a two-view examination. The average mid-breast glandular dose should be less than 0.1 rad with screen-film studies and five to eight times that amount for xeromammography. More recent developments in the xerography technique are claimed to improve image resolution at a reduced radiation dose.

Dedicated ultrasound units have not proved effective as they are incapable of resolving lesions less than 1 cm in diameter and seldom image clinically occult masses. Ultrasound waves do not adequately penetrate fatty breast tissue, making the technique more effective in imaging the dense, nonfatty breast of the premenopausal woman. Small-part ultrasound examination is occasionally useful in characterizing the palpable mass lesion in the symptomatic young patient with dense breasts. Breast transillumination (diaphanography) is based on the principle that cancers absorb more near infrared radiation than benign lesions. This technique is still experimental and has not been shown to be effective as a stand-alone screening technique. It is also not sensitive for the deeper lesions in the breast.

Digital mammography, the registration of mammographic images with a digital rather than an analog technique, shows promise, but at present only prototype systems are available. Digital recording affords the viewer unlimited flexibility in the contrast–recording mode.

Magnetic resonance imaging vividly displays some of the unique characteristics of certain breast neoplasms. Earlier, CT was shown to have a potential ability to discriminate benign and malignant breast cancers. At present MR imaging is of a research rather than a practical interest in the imaging, detection, and characterization of breast cancer. The logistics, cost, and patient numbers make the widespread application of MR imaging or CT to breast diagnosis impractical.

Mammographic signs of cancer are based on the detection of an ill-defined mass, microcalcifications, or one or more indirect signs (Table 20-8). Clusters of microcalcifications less than 0.5 mm in size are visible radiologically in nearly 50% of all breast cancers. "Clustering" refers to a number of these microcalcifications, which should be more than five per square centimeter to qualify as "suspicious." The greater the number of calcifications and the more diverse their

form, the more likely they are to be associated with a cancer. The linear or branching forms are the most suspicious; however, there is an overlap in the appearance of benign and malignant microcalcifications, and biopsy is often needed to distinguish them. These calcifications are presumed to develop within necrotic materials found in the obstructed lumen of ducts in the vicinity of the cancer.[32–34]

The most important of the indirect signs of cancer is asymmetry of the two breasts, with a nonspecific increase in breast tissue density on the abnormal side. Although this sign is nonspecific, it should stimulate additional scrutiny of that involved breast. Architectural distortion is a nonspecific finding in which the normal breast tissue components are distorted or drawn together, in contrast to the usual radial pattern of normal breast tissue oriented toward the nipple. A developing density refers to an area of increased breast tissue density not present in an earlier examination. The breasts should become progressively more atrophic with time, particularly in the postmenopausal patient. The most nonspecific of the indirect signs is a single dilated duct or large vessel, both usually nonspecific and not clinically relevant. A recent review of the mammographic characteristics of 512 consecutive occult mammographic abnormalities showed that the positive predictive value of an ill-defined or stellate mass was 0.75, and that for strongly suspicious microcalcifications, described above, 0.56. An ill-defined mass with poorly defined but not stellate margins had a positive predictive value for cancer of 0.35. None of the other findings had a sufficiently large positive predictive value to warrant a recommendation for biopsy.[35]

LOCALIZATION AND BIOPSY TECHNIQUES

Because nearly 50% of breast cancers will be visible mammographically but not palpable clinically, localization techniques are necessary to identify these abnormalities before biopsy. Many techniques have been proposed; the ideal one remains elusive. Most techniques use a wire placed through a needle, with the coordinates previously established by mammography. Either a visible dye or a hooked wire is introduced through the localizing needle and its placement is confirmed with 90° verification mammograms. The surgeon then excises the lesion that has been localized. If microcalcifications were present, specimen radiographs should be obtained to verify that the abnormality has been excised, and follow-up mammograms should be obtained 4 to 6 months after the procedure (Fig. 20-11).[36]

Localization under radiographic control should enable the radiologist to place the needle–wire system within less than 1 cm from the mammographic abnormality. Newer stereoscopic and computer-aided localization techniques should allow aspiration biopsy and cytologic analysis of mammographic abnormalities in the near future. This should decrease the cost and morbidity associated with breast biopsy procedures.

Galactography is occasionally useful in the patient with persistent nipple discharge, following initial cytologic evalu-

TABLE 20-8. Mammographic Signs of Cancer

Direct
  Microcalcifications
  Mass
Indirect
  Architectural distortion
  Developing density
  Asymmetry
  Large duct or vessel
% Primary Abnormality
  ~40%
  ~40%
  ~20%

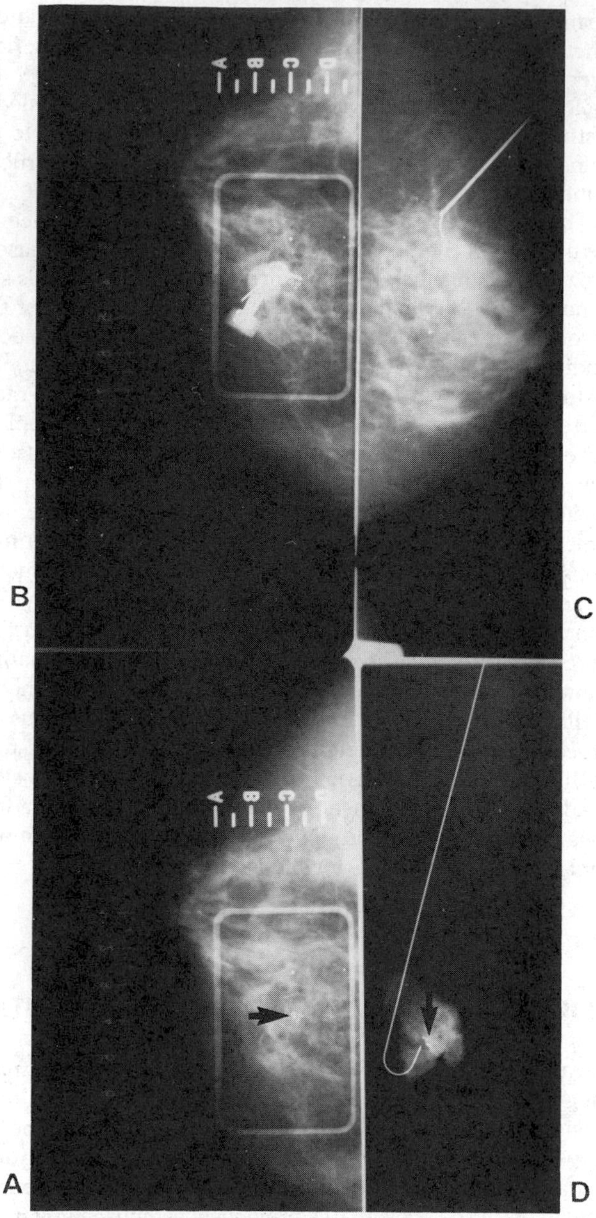

FIG. 20-11. Mammographic localization—homer technique. **A**. The rectangular square is centered on a small cluster of white microcalcifications (*arrow*) which can be localized with the letter and numerical coordinates. A needle with a curved wire is then inserted into the microcalcifications and verification films are obtained (**B** and **C**), showing the curved wire to be surrounding the microcalcifications. **D**. The specimen radiograph with the wire in place identifies that the clustered microcalcifications (*arrow*) indeed have been removed. Verification postbiopsy mammograms should be obtained within 4 to 6 months after the biopsy procedure.

ation of the expressed discharge. Contrast material can be locally instilled and radiographs obtained to analyze the ducts responsible for the discharge, and to help characterize the major duct abnormality. Occasionally, the offending duct can be adequately localized with this technique for surgical biopsy.[37]

H. RIC HARNSBERGER

Head, Neck, and Spine

CENTRAL NERVOUS SYSTEM NEOPLASMS: BRAIN

For most of the last decade, CT has functioned as the principal imaging modality for the detection and follow-up of neoplasms of the central nervous system (CNS).[38-43] Although CT represents a vast improvement over previously available techniques for imaging the CNS, it has multiple blind spots in the search for CNS cancers.[44] In areas of high bone content such as the posterior fossa and the supratentorial brain adjacent to the calvaria, streak artifacts often distort the image and may conceal small neoplasms. Additionally, smaller CNS tumors that lack either significant blood–brain barrier disruption or mass effect often are not visible on CT (Fig. 20-12). Today, MR imaging has emerged as the radiologic method of choice for investigating CNS tumors. MR imaging has inherently greater sensitivity for brain pathology than CT, and it displays the brain in regions adjacent to areas of high bone content with relatively few artifacts.[45-48] This section considers first the advantages of MR imaging over CT for lesions of the head, neck, and spine, and then the profound impact of MR imaging on the diagnosis, treatment, and follow-up of lesions in these areas. The details of MR imaging are beyond the scope of this chapter but are well delineated elsewhere.[49-53] In brief, MR imaging is based on the principle that static tissue protons subjected to an intense external magnetic field will emit a characteristic relaxation signal when perturbed by a specific radiofrequency pulse. This characteristic signal can be spatially localized into an image with the aid of computers. The image may be obtained in the sagittal, coronal, or axial plane. No signal will be detected from moving protons (blood), allowing images to be obtained with clear identification of blood vessels without the use of intravascular contrast medium.[50] Bone generates a weak signal without artifact because of its low proton content; for this reason MR images are superior to CT scans in imaging the skull base, posterior fossa, and cerebellopontine angle.

When MR imaging is compared with CT, several advantages of the former become apparent. The most important advantage of MR imaging is its ability to demonstrate abnormal water content in brain tissue caused by tumor or inflammation, before a blood–brain barrier leak or mass effect is produced. As a result, MR imaging is more sensitive to smaller CNS tumors than CT. MR imaging can display tumors in the range of 3 to 5 mm; these tumors are not visible on CT (see Fig. 20-12). Other advantages of MRI include the use of magnetic fields and radiowaves, rather than x-rays, to produce images; the ability to generate multiplaner (axial, sagittal, and coronal) images without patient repositioning; and no need for intravenous or intrathecal contrast agents in routine screening examinations. Since bone is "proton poor," the bone artifacts ordinarily seen on CT scans are not present on MR images. These qualities of

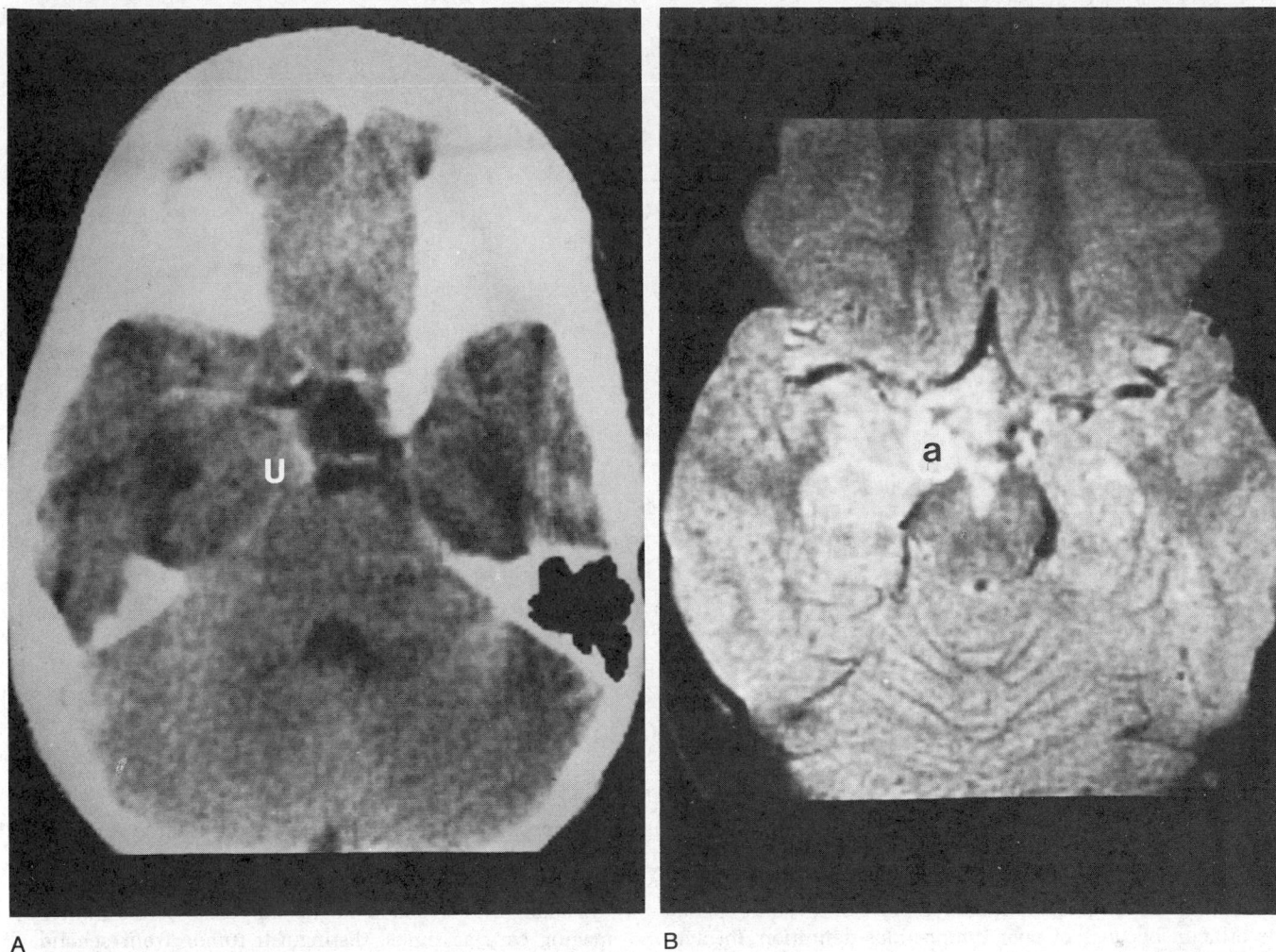

FIG. 20-12. Comparative CT and MR brain images in a patient with a temporal lobe astrocytoma. **A.** Enhanced, axial CT scan through the suprasellar cistern shows an enlarged uncus (*U*) with no evidence for contrast enhancement (blood-brain barrier leak). **B.** T-2 weighted axial MR image through the same level is streak-artifact free and graphically delineates the temporal lobe astrocytoma (*a*).

MR imaging make it a highly sensitive radiologic tool that detects smaller CNS tumors than CT, without subjecting the patient to radiation, iodinated contrast agents, or uncomfortable body positions.

MR imaging has emerged as the examination of choice in the search for CNS mass lesions. Figure 20-13 shows a decision tree for use in imaging patients thought to have brain tumors; the decision tree acknowledges the principal role of this modality in the diagnostic and follow-up phases of brain tumor evaluation.

Because MR imaging can now demonstrate subcentimeter brain lesions that are possibly cancerous but may instead result from demyelination, stroke, or infection, the need for a safe tissue biopsy technique has dramatically increased. Stereotaxic biopsy guided by CT, therefore, has become an important diagnostic and therapeutic technique (Fig. 20-14A).[54-56] The stereotaxic placement of the biopsy needle

has become an extremely accurate technique. Successful biopsies of 5-mm lesions are now routine. Although CT guidance is presently required for stereotaxic biopsy, nonferromagnetic, stereotaxic frames that use MR imaging guidance are being developed (Fig. 20-14B).

MR imaging has also had a major impact on the approach to the treatment of CNS neoplasia with radiation therapy. The superior spatial and contrast resolution and multiplaner capability of MR imaging permit more precise planning of radiation therapy ports than was previously possible with CT. The graphic delineation of tumor margins in sagittal and coronal views allows the information obtained with MR imaging to be translated with high precision onto external beam radiation therapy simulation films. Both the stereotaxic technology and the precise anatomical information available from multiplaner images have greatly improved radiation therapy implant techniques as well.[57]

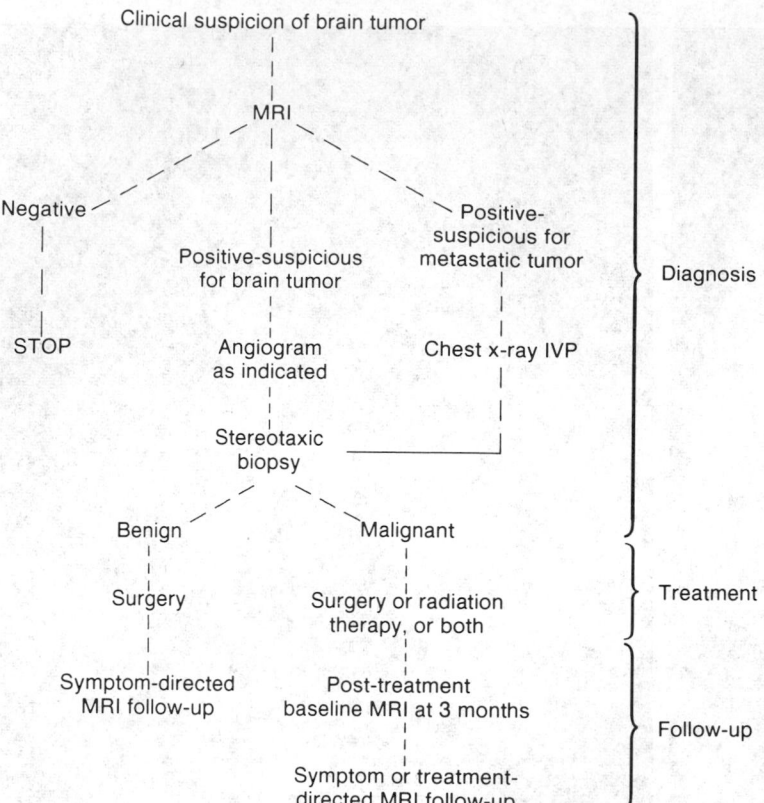

FIG. 20-13. Imaging decision algorithm for patients suspected of having a brain tumor. MRI, magnetic resonance imaging; IVP, intravenous pyelogram.

There are at least three drawbacks to the use of MR imaging for diagnosing CNS tumors. The first drawback becomes evident when the tumor-associated edema is extensive. Planning surgical margins and radiation ports in these cases may be difficult because of poor tumor-nidus definition. Intravenous administration of the paramagnetic contrast agent gadolinium-DTPA, which will be available in the near future, will solve the problem of tumor-nidus identification.[58-60] A second disadvantage is the inability of MR imaging to depict smaller deposits of calcification within the tumor. This shortcoming has proved to be more theoretical than real and has not caused particular problems in clinical practice. A third disadvantage, and one shared by both MR imaging and CT, is that neither modality easily differentiates radiation necrosis from recurrent tumor. Radiation necrosis of the CNS may occur from 1 month to 16 years after treatment, with the peak period of occurrence falling 1 to 3 years after radiation treatment.[61,62] At times, only biopsy can distinguish recurrent CNS tumor from radiation necrosis.

CENTRAL NERVOUS SYSTEM NEOPLASMS: SPINAL CORD

A second anatomical region of the CNS where MR imaging has replaced CT as the preferred method for evaluating suspected tumor is the spinal cord.[63,64] Patients presenting with myelopathy thought to be related to spinal cord neoplasia should now be initially evaluated with MR imaging (Fig. 20-15). This modality directly images the spinal cord, allow-

ing tumors to be detected before an associated mass effect develops. A suggested decision tree for imaging patients with possible spinal cord cancer is given in Figure 20-16.

In addition to its use in diagnosing spinal cord tumors, MR imaging can, at times, distinguish tumor from secondary syringomyelia; this information can be used to plan the surgical margins and radiation therapy ports for each spinal cord tumor. MR imaging also demonstrates the level and extent of encroachment of metastatic epidural tumor on the spinal cord without the need for extensive patient repositioning or intrathecal contrast agent injection.[65] However, drop metastases (tumor deposits within the subarachnoid space of the spine that have spread from more central CNS tumors, such as medulloblastoma and pineal cancers), although occasionally identifiable with MR imaging, usually must still be evaluated with traditional CT/myelographic techniques because of their small size.

EXTRACRANIAL HEAD AND NECK CANCERS

The following discussion considers the issues surrounding the use of CT or MR imaging in the staging of head and neck neoplasms. Additional details on this subject, subdivided by major anatomical areas in the upper aerodigestive tract and neck, can be found in a text by Mancuso and Hanafee.[66]

The introduction of CT vastly expanded the role of radiology in the management of head and neck neoplasms. The radiologist's knowledge of the intricate CT anatomy of

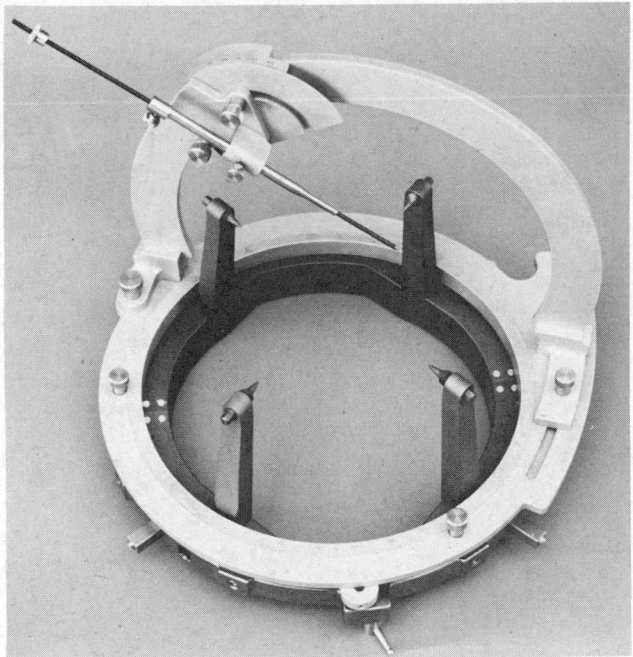

A

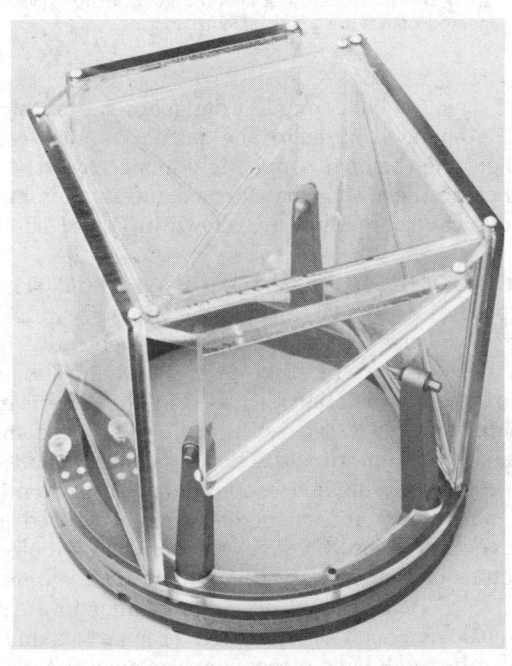

B

FIG. 20-14. Stereotaxic localization frames. **A**. Brown-Roberts-Wells frame, when placed on the patient's head, allows CT coordinates to be defined for placement of a percutaneous biopsy needle or localization of a brain lesion for treatment by interstitial techniques. **B**. Nonferromagnetic MR-compatible frame accomplishes the same goals for lesions identified by magnetic resonance imaging.

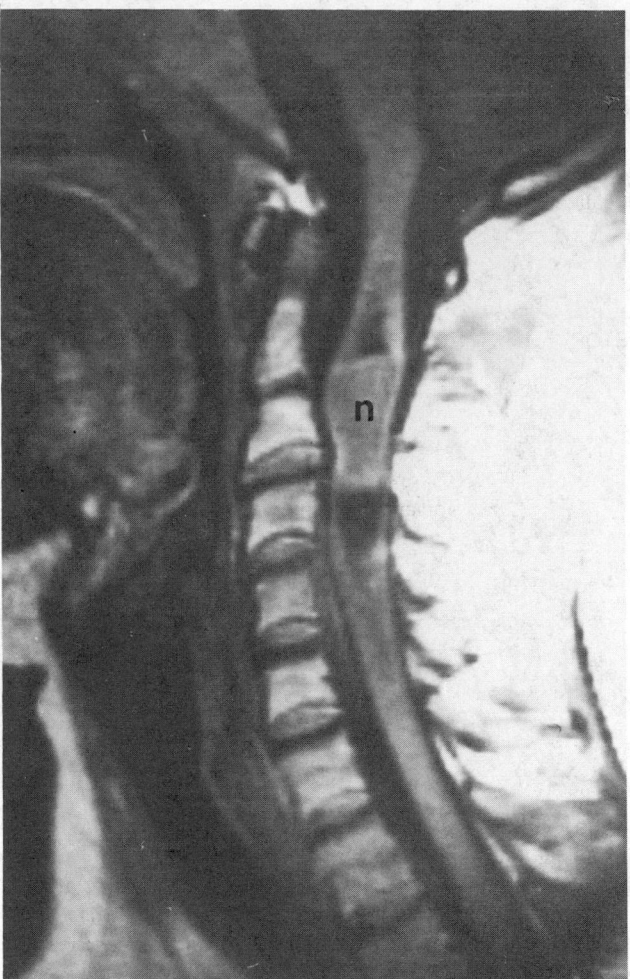

FIG. 20-15. Cervical cord astrocytoma. Sagittal MR image of the spinal cord diagnoses the intramedullary neoplasm (n).

mapping of the deep tissue and regional nodal involvement for a more specific pretreatment assessment of tumor stage.

As in the brain, MR imaging holds great promise for staging tumors of the upper aerodigestive tract and neck.[67-69] Clinical experience with MR imaging of the neck is limited, but the benefits of examining this area without the use of iodinated contrast agent or ionizing radiation are obvious. The routine use of direct sagittal and coronal imaging in tumors with known extensive craniocaudal spread patterns (nasopharynx and tongue base) will allow more complete pretreatment assessment of tumor extent. Early indications suggest that MR imaging will be more sensitive to cartilaginous invasion than will CT, which should prove extremely useful in staging laryngeal carcinoma.[68,70,71] Because of the potential of MR imaging to demonstrate tumor deposits in normal-sized lymph nodes, the detection of malignant lymph nodes may improve, especially with the use of Gd-DTPA. Soft tissue interfaces also are identified better on MR imaging, allowing the primary tumor mass to be differentiated from adjacent nodal involvement.[72]

the head and neck, coupled with his or her understanding of the routes of tumor spread by primary site location, allows tumor stage and extent to be determined accurately. As a result, the endoscopic demonstration of the mucosal extent of primary squamous carcinoma can be combined with CT

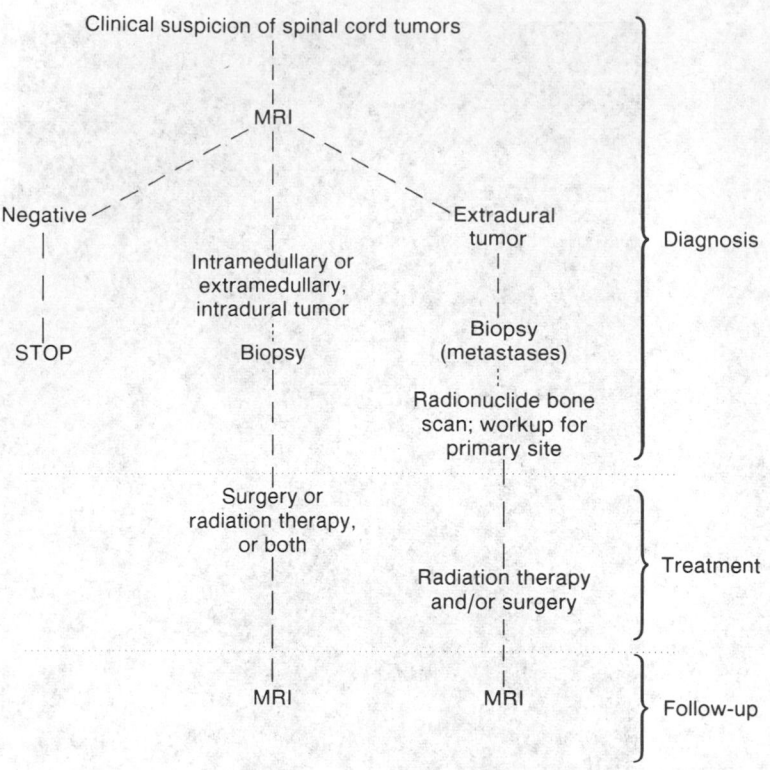

FIG. 20-16. Imaging decision algorithm for patients suspected of having a spinal cord cancer.

The principal disadvantage of MR imaging in the evaluation of head and neck cancer arises from the longer acquisition times necessary. Patients with head and neck squamous cell carcinoma often have obstructive pulmonary disease and an associated exaggerated respiratory motion that degrades MR images. The swallowing motion induced by bulky tumor may also degrade the MR image. Nevertheless, both CT and MR imaging can be effectively applied to this clinical problem.

Although the American Joint Committee's *TNM Staging Manual* currently recommends the use of CT in head and neck cancer only as an adjunctive procedure, extensive clinicopathologic correlation has shown CT to be a powerful imaging modality in evaluating head and neck neoplasms.[70,71,73] CT or MR imaging should be used as the oncologic imaging procedure of choice for the staging and follow-up of nearly all head and neck cancers. The primary role for CT or MR imaging is in staging the primary tumor site and in demonstrating regional nodal disease (Figs. 20-17 and 20-18). CT may also be occasionally helpful when an occult primary tumor of the head and neck is suspected.[74]

GENERAL NECK CT TECHNIQUE. Each CT examination is tailored to the area of the known primary tumor and regional lymphatics. Intravenous contrast agent is administered through a 19-gauge needle in the antecubital fossa vein with an initial 50-ml bolus of 60% meglumine iothalamate, followed by rapid drip infusion of 300 ml of 30% meglumine iothalamate. This rapid drip technique is mandatory for two reasons: (1) it allows neck vessels to be distinguished from lymph nodes (which do not enhance); and (2) extranodal disease and primary tumor extent are delineated best with contrast agent enhancement. Contiguous 5-mm-thick sections are obtained through the primary tumor site and throughout the regional lymphatic drainage routes. General guidelines on the CT format for nodal evaluation based on initial clinical impressions are shown in Figure 20-19.

STAGING THE PRIMARY TUMOR WITH CT. The overall purpose of using CT to stage the primary site of upper aerodigestive tract tumors is to obtain an objective impression of the actual extent of the primary lesion. The primary tumor extent classification (T) used by the American Joint Committee on Cancer is based entirely on size and anatomical extent of the tumor mass. This initial clinical–diagnostic stage is estimated from endoscopic and physical examination results; subsequent treatment decisions are based on this subjective impression. CT gives the clinician a more objective picture of the primary tumor's actual anatomical extent.[70,71,73,75,76] Submucosal tumor and tumor in areas difficult to palpate, such as the high oropharynx and nasopharynx, often will have more extensive deep tissue components on CT examination than are clinically apparent.[77,78] CT findings have been shown to alter treatment planning in up to 35% of patients as a result of changes in primary tumor extent (T) and nodal involvement (N) (Fig. 20-20).[79]

STAGING NECK NODES WITH CT. The reported frequency of cervical nodal metastases from squamous cell carcinoma in the head and neck has a wide variation that relates to the rich system of venous channels and lymphatics at the site of the primary tumor. The detection of cervical nodal metastases, either by clinical examination or with CT, will affect the mode of treatment and the general prognosis.[80]

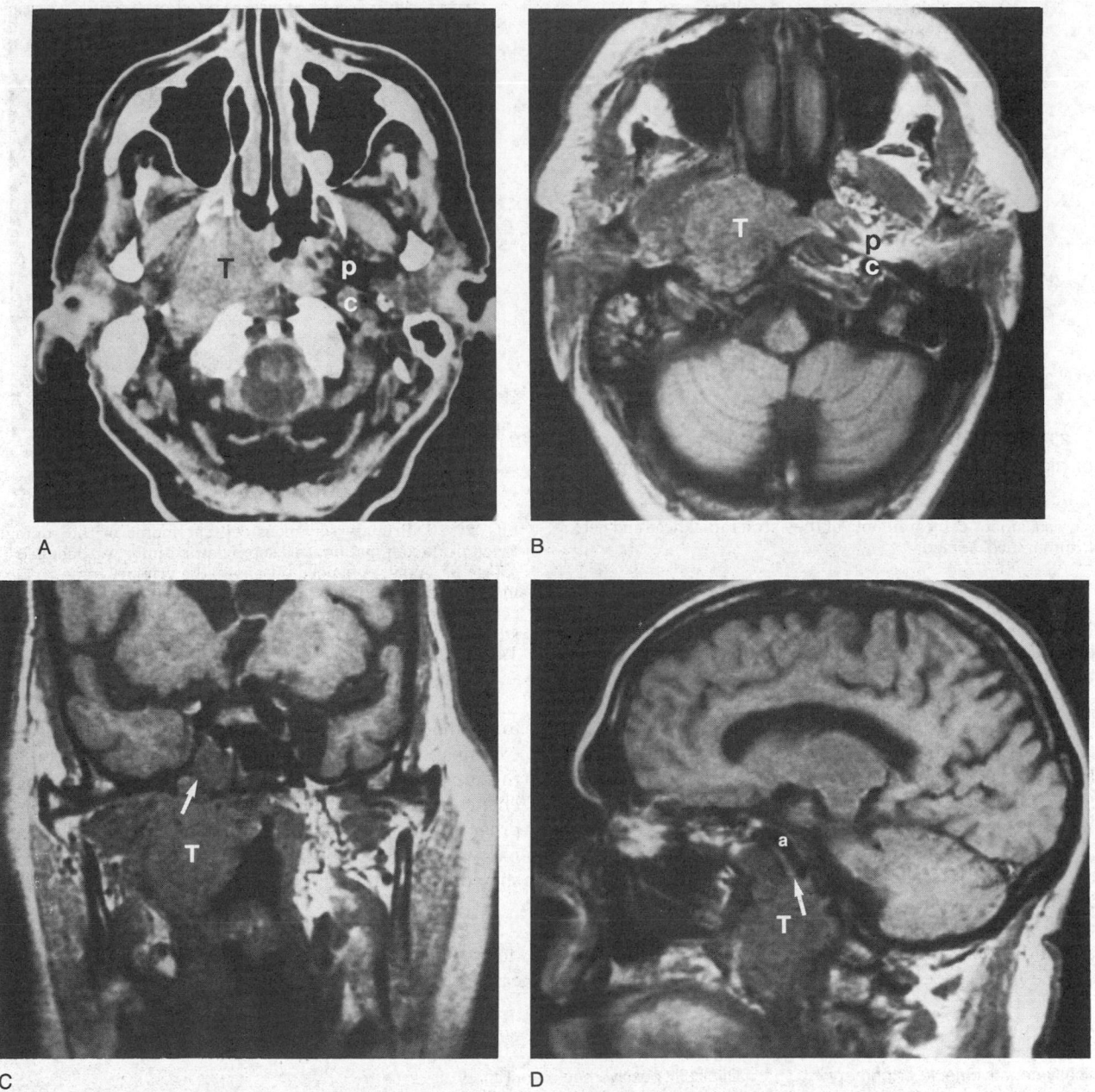

FIG. 20-17. CT and MR staging of nasopharyngeal carcinoma. **A**. Axial, enhanced CT through the nasopharynx shows the tumor (T) invading the parapharyngeal (*p*) and carotid (*c*) spaces. **B**. T-1 weighted axial MR image contains the same information. **C**. Direct sagittal and coronal (**D**) T-1 MR images display the exact craniocaudad extent of the tumor (T). In the sagittal image (**C**), perivascular spread (*arrow*) into the skull base along the internal carotid artery (*a*) is seen. On the coronal image (**D**), the tumor is seen invading (*arrow*) the sphenoid sinus (s).

The overall 5-year survival rate for patients with malignant cervical adenopathy at tumor diagnosis is less than 30%, regardless of primary tumor location.[81] The American Joint Committee's nodal staging criteria are based on the subjective evaluation, by neck palpation, as to the side, size, and extent of nodal disease in the neck. CT can give objectivity to the staging of cervical metastasis if strict criteria are applied.[73] Lymph nodes in the deep cervical chain larger than 1.5 cm, especially those with central necrosis (see Fig. 20-20), should be considered malignant. Extranodal disease is diagnosed when soft tissue planes around the abnormal lymph node are obscured.

The use of CT for tumor staging is limited by its lack of tissue specificity and reliance on size criteria to diagnose malignant adenopathy. Reactive hyperplasia has been shown to enlarge cervical lymph nodes, but generally the nodes will

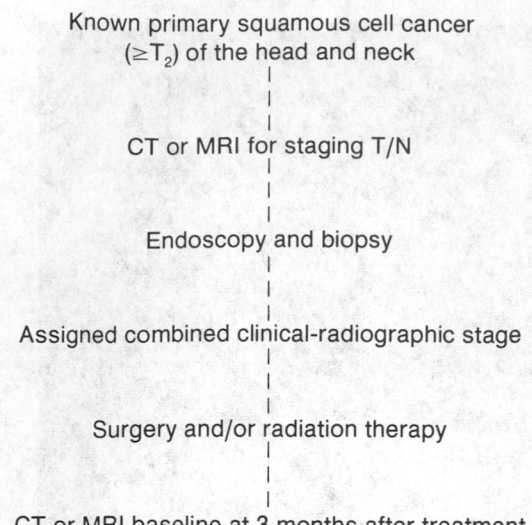

Known primary squamous cell cancer
($\geq T_2$) of the head and neck

|

CT or MRI for staging T/N

|

Endoscopy and biopsy

|

Assigned combined clinical-radiographic stage

|

Surgery and/or radiation therapy

|

CT or MRI baseline at 3 months after treatment
for high-risk tumors or as indicated for low-risk tumors

FIG. 20-18. Imaging decision algorithm for patients with known primary squamous cell carcinoma of the extracranial head and neck. T/N, tumor/nodal stage.

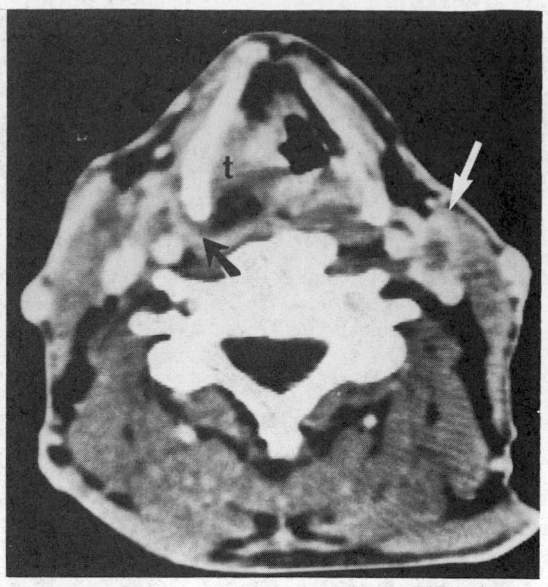

FIG. 20-20. Primary squamous cell carcinoma of the supraglottis. By clinical examination, this supraglottic tumor was labelled T2NO (Stage II). Axial, enhanced CT shows the primary tumor (*t*) extending into the soft tissues of the neck (*dark arrow*) and an 8 mm contralateral nodal metastasis in the middle, deep cervical chain (*white arrow*). CT upgraded this tumor from T2NO (Stage II) to T4N3C (Stage IV).

remain less than 1.5 cm in size.[72] Fine-needle aspiration biopsy in select cases can minimize false-positive results. Small tumor deposits in normal-sized lymph nodes will be missed on both clinical examination and CT.

RECURRENT TUMOR EVALUATION. CT can be a vital tool for evaluating tumor recurrence in the upper aerodigestive tract and neck.[78-82] Because of alterations in the normal deep tissue planes resulting from surgical or radiation therapy, such recurrences often are difficult to evaluate clinically. Subtle symptoms signaling recurrence often remain undiagnosed for months after their onset. In about 25% of cases of suspected tumor recurrence, CT will be the only means of diagnosis (Fig. 20–21). In one third of patients in whom the recurrence is clinically apparent, CT will show it

to be more extensive than was appreciated from physical examination alone.[78] The information available from CT on the presence and extent of recurrent tumor may lead to a change in the radiation therapy ports and the surgical approach.[78] As CT is applied more widely in post-treatment follow-up, delays in the diagnosis of tumor recurrences should be minimized.

THE UNKNOWN PRIMARY TUMOR. CT primarily functions as a staging tool in the workup of head and neck cancers. CT also plays a role in evaluating a small but trou-

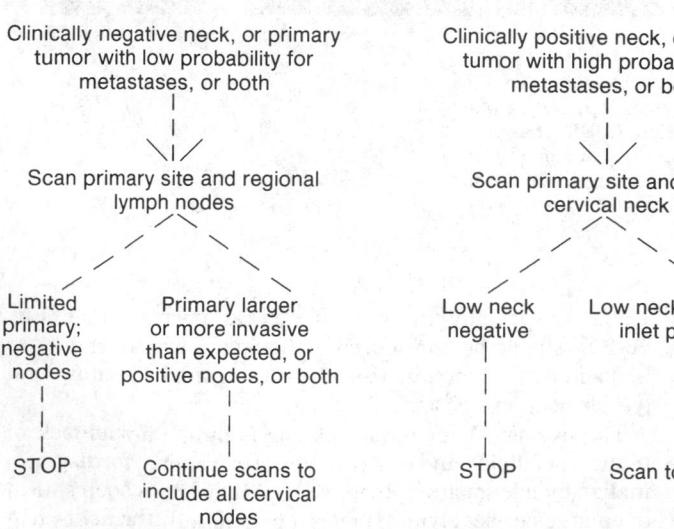

Clinically negative neck, or primary tumor with low probability for metastases, or both

Scan primary site and regional lymph nodes

Limited primary; negative nodes → STOP

Primary larger or more invasive than expected, or positive nodes, or both → Continue scans to include all cervical nodes

Clinically positive neck, or primary tumor with high probability for metastases, or both

Scan primary site and entire cervical neck

Low neck negative → STOP

Low neck, thoracic inlet positive → Scan to carina

FIG. 20-19. CT protocol for studying neck adenopathy in patients with known primary squamous cell carcinoma of the head and neck. (Modified from Mancuso AA: Cervical lymph node metastases. In Bragg DG, Rubin P, Youker JE [eds]: Oncologic Imaging. Elmsford, New York, Pergamon Press, 1985)

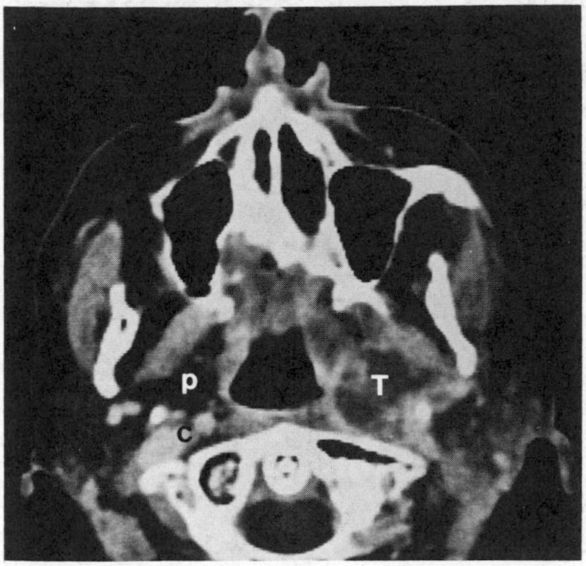

WILLIAM M. THOMPSON

Gastrointestinal and Genitourinary Systems

The newer imaging modalities of ultrasound (US), CT, and MR imaging provide exquisite multiplanar anatomical detail of the gastrointestinal (GI) and genitourinary systems. Based on this detail, specific information about tumor location, size, and extent can be obtained before surgery. This information, coupled with percutaneous biopsy results, provides meaningful staging data not previously available except through surgical and pathologic evaluation.[85,86]

Although not enough experience has accrued to define the advantages and disadvantages of the new imaging modalities in relation to the traditional radiologic techniques, or for that matter in relation to each other, some conclusions can be drawn from current data. Only the more recent and more consequential developments are discussed.

GASTROINTESTINAL TRACT CANCER

Although the cross-sectional imaging modalities play a relatively minor role in the detection of GI cancers, they have a major role in the preoperative staging and follow-up of certain tumors.[87-91] Unfortunately, these new imaging modalities cannot be used to stage GI tumors with the standard tumor–node—metastasis (TNM) system because they are limited in their ability to demonstrate the depth of bowel wall penetration, the T component of the TNM system; accurate demonstration of metastases in lymph nodes, the N criterion, is also beyond their capability.[88,89] Local invasion and distant metastases, especially to the liver, can be demonstrated accurately.

CT has been shown to be accurate in staging squamous cell carcinoma of the esophagus.[87,88,90] Although the barium swallow examination is more precise than CT for determining tumor length, local invasion (Fig. 20-22A) and distant metastases in the liver and subdiaphragmatic lymph nodes can be accurately detected with CT. One group reported poor results using CT for staging,[92] but there were some differences in their study compared with other reports.[87,88,90] CT has been shown to be helpful in evaluating patients who have had an esophagogastrectomy for esophageal cancer.[93]

Although the initial reports were favorable,[87,94] more recent studies[89,95] have shown that CT cannot be reliably used to stage gastric carcinoma (Fig. 20-22B) or colorectal adenocarcinoma (Fig. 20-22C)[89,96,97]; nor does CT accurately demonstrate the exact depth of bowel wall penetration or the presence of metastases in normal-sized lymph nodes, two major criteria in the TNM and Duke's staging systems. Many patients with gastric and colorectal adenocarcinoma have metastases in normal-sized (<1 cm) lymph nodes.[88,89,96,97] Thus, most recent reports do not recommend CT for routine preoperative staging in patients with adenocarcinoma of the stomach, colon, or rectum.[96,97] When indicated, CT can be used to accurately evaluate the liver and can demonstrate the

FIG. 20-21. Recurrent squamous cell carcinoma. Eighteen months after radiotherapy for Stage II (T2) carcinoma of the oropharyngeal tonsil, this patient presented with left ptosis and vocal cord paralysis. No mucosal tumor was seen on physical examination. Axial CT through the superior alveolar ridge demonstrates a deeply invasive recurrent tumor (T) that involves these parapharyngeal (p) and carotid (c) spaces on the left.

blesome group of patients in whom malignant adenopathy is present but the primary tumor is clinically occult. When fine-needle aspiration biopsy reveals a neck mass to be a metastatic squamous cell carcinoma in lymphatic tissue, and no primary source is found on endoscopy, the nodal disease may have originated outside the head and neck region or from an occult primary within the head and neck region.[73,81,84] In the case of an occult head and neck primary tumor, there are three possible explanations for the tumor's apparent absence: the primary tumor site may be very small; the tumor may have regressed after metastasizing to cervical lymph nodes; or the tumor is primarily submucosal in location.[77] In the last case, CT of the upper aerodigestive tract may identify the primary site when endoscopy is negative.[74] Careful attention to the nasopharynx, base of tongue, and piriform sinus is required because these are the areas in which occult carcinoma is commonly found.[83,84] CT is used in this setting to identify the primary tumor (when possible), to locate suspicious areas for deep tissue biopsy at the time of endoscopy, and to help stage the neck for additional nodal disease, extranodal tumor spread, and fixation to critical neck structures, such as the carotid artery. If no primary tumor is found to explain the patient's cervical disease, follow-up CT in 3 to 6 months to reevaluate the upper aerodigestive tract for occult submucosal malignancy is recommended.[74]

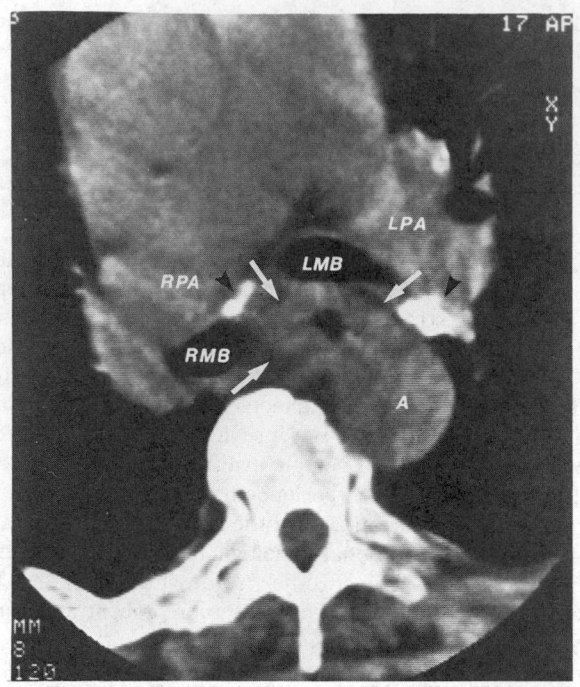

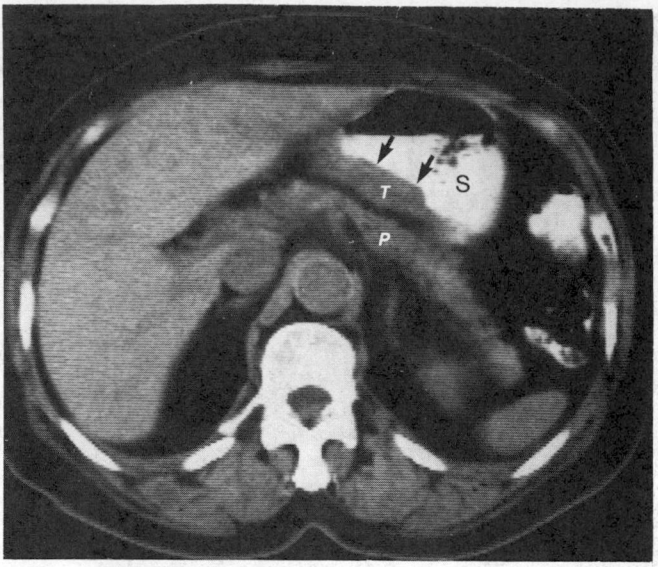

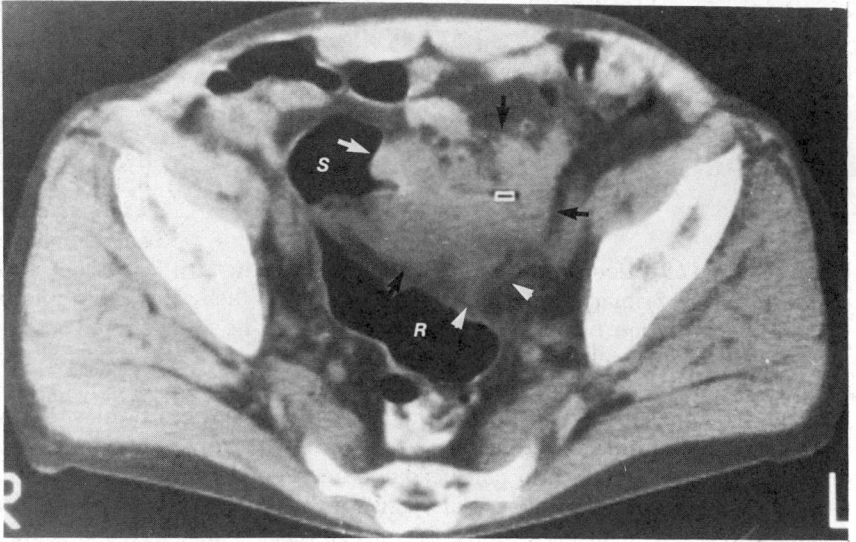

FIG. 20-22. CT imaging gastrointestinal malignancies. **A**. Esophageal carcinoma. CT section through level of carcinoma demonstrating a squamous cell carcinoma (*arrows*) locally invading the left main-stem bronchus (*LMB*) and aorta (*A*). Right main-stem bronchus (*RMB*), right pulmonary artery (*RPA*) and left pulmonary artery (*LPA*). Note calcification in mediastinal lymph nodes (*arrowheads*). **B**. Gastric carcinoma. CT through distal stomach (*S*) showing moderate thickening of posterior gastric wall (*arrows*) because of adenocarcinoma. The fat plane between the tumor (*T*) and the pancreas (*P*) is preserved. At operation the tumor did not extend into the pancreas; however, there were lymph nodes containing metastases in the surgical specimen which were not identified by CT. **C**. Sigmoid carcinoma. Dukes C — CT through level of midpelvis showing air in the rectum (*R*) and sigmoid (*S*). A large adenocarcinoma in the sigmoid (*arrows*) was partially obstructing the bowel lumen (cursor box). The tumor had extended through the bowel wall, which is suggested by the increased density in the pericolic fat (*arrowheads*). A number of lymph nodes in the resected specimen contained metastatic tumor. These were not identified by CT.

(continued)

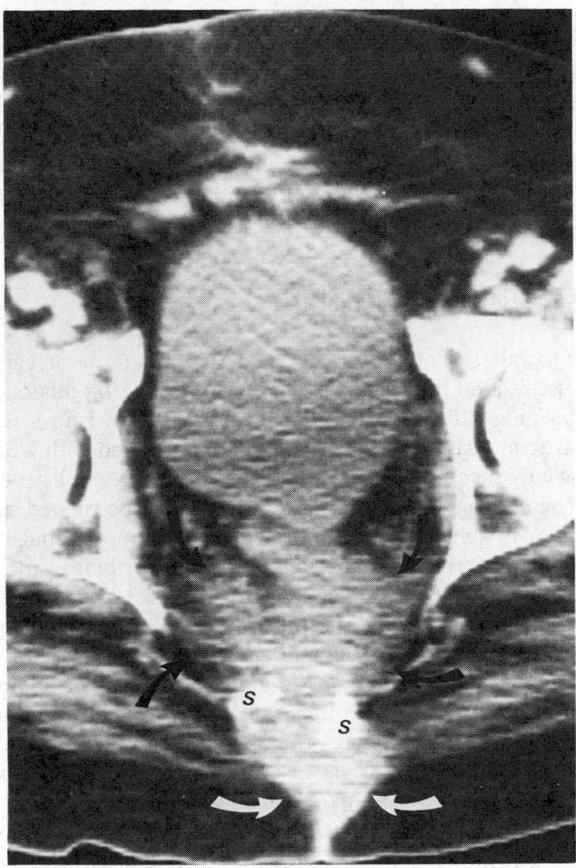

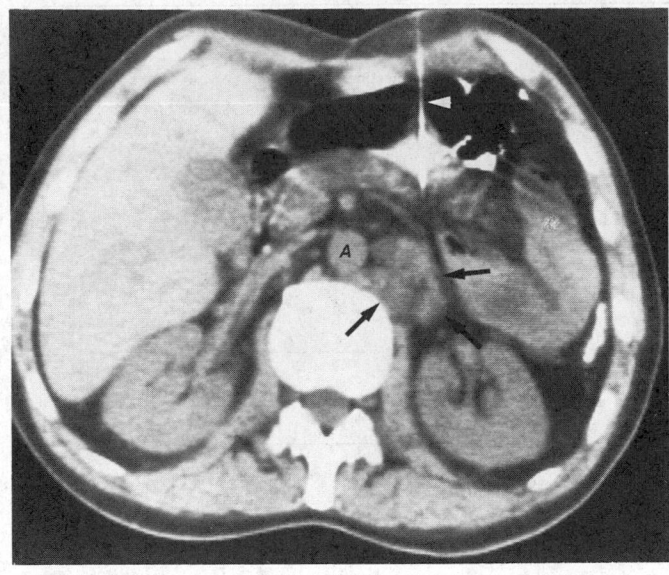

FIG. 20-22. *continued*
D. Recurrent rectal carcinoma. CT through pelvis in a 50-year-old man who had a rectal carcinoma resected 2 years earlier. A large soft tissue mass (*arrows*) is demonstrated in the presacral space and is extending from the bladder through the sacrum (*S*) to the subcutaneous tissues dorsal to the sacrum. The sacrum is being destroyed by the recurrent tumor. **E.** Recurrent rectosigmoid carcinoma in paraaortic lymph nodes. CT through level of kidneys during a percutaneous needle biopsy (needle, *arrowhead*) of enlarged lymph nodes (*arrows*) in the left paraaortic region. Cytologic evaluation confirmed metastatic adenocarcinoma. The patient's primary tumor had been resected 2 years earlier. A, aorta.

amount of extracolonic involvement in large tumors and those that have perforated.

CT has been shown to be effective in monitoring patients who have undergone surgical resection of rectosigmoid carcinoma.[89,96,97] Both postoperative changes and recurrent tumor (Fig. 20-22D) can be detected. In some cases, a percutaneous needle biopsy is required to distinguish between the two.[96] However, if a baseline scan is obtained 3 to 4 months after surgery and the patient is rescanned periodically, postoperative changes can usually be distinguished from recurrent tumor. Since the majority of local rectosigmoid recurrences occur within 2 years of the primary resection, most authors recommend obtaining a postoperative baseline CT scan and then performing CT at 6-month intervals for at least 2 years. After 2 years, annual follow-up CT is adequate. All suspect lesions should be biopsied percutaneously.[85,86,96-98] Metastatic lymph nodes can be biopsied to confirm recurrence (Fig. 20-22E).

The few studies reported to date suggest that MR imaging is not likely to overcome the limitations of CT in evaluating patients with GI carcinoma.[92,99] One preliminary report has suggested that MR imaging may be able to distinguish postoperative fibrosis from recurrent tumor after resection of rectosigmoidal carcinoma.[100] However, no large series has been reported.

Figure 20-23 shows an imaging scheme for the workup of patients with known or suspected GI cancer. This scheme applies primarily to patients with squamous cell carcinoma of the esophagus, and adenocarcinoma of the stomach, small bowel, colon, and rectum. MR imaging is not included because of the current lack of data.

HEPATIC MALIGNANCIES—PRIMARY AND METASTATIC

Several imaging modalities are available to evaluate the liver. CT has been shown to be more sensitive and specific than the radionuclide liver–spleen scan or US for demonstrating both primary and metastatic lesions, especially if CT is coupled with a percutaneous fine-needle aspiration biopsy.[85,86,101,102] The radionuclide liver–spleen scan is still used by some as a screening study because of its lower cost and greater availability. However, it has low spatial resolution, is unable to detect lesions less than 2 cm in diameter, and rarely provides any etiologic information about the space-occupying lesion in the liver. Thus, both the false-negative and the false-positive rates for radionuclide scintigraphy are higher than for US or CT.

US has been shown to be less accurate than CT for detect-

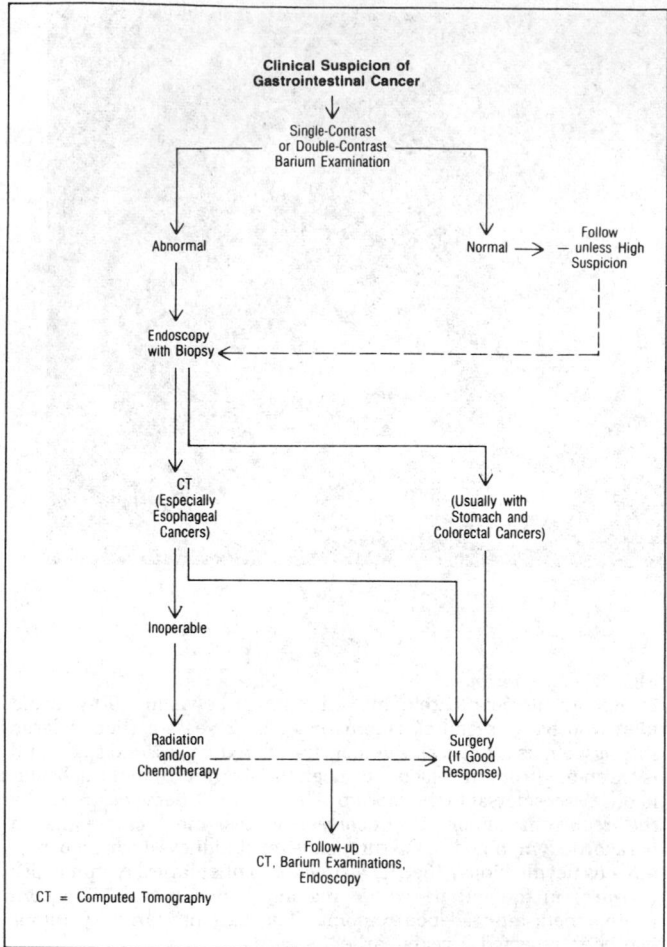

FIG. 20-23. Imaging decision tree for patients with suspected gastrointestinal cancer: Squamous cell carcinoma of the esophagus and adenocarcinoma of the stomach, small bowel, colon, and rectum. Most patients with stomach and colorectal tumors require surgery, so routine preoperative staging with CT is not recommended. CT may help define the extent of small bowel tumors prior to surgery. CT is best for follow-up of GI tumors. (Thompson WM: Imaging strategies for tumors of the gastrointestinal system. CA 37:165–186, 1987)

ing hepatic tumors.[101] Nevertheless, some investigators do advocate the use of US for detecting hepatic masses because of its lower cost and greater availability compared with CT. Also, tumors can be percutaneously biopsied under US guidance. Recently, investigators have used US in the operating room during hepatic resections and have found it is particularly useful for detecting hepatic tumors less than 3 cm in size. Operative US has been found to demonstrate more tumors than preoperative US, CT, or angiography.[103] This technique will be used with increasing frequency, especially in patients undergoing partial hepatectomy for metastatic disease.

Although CT has been the preferred technique for evaluating the liver for the past 6 to 8 years, MR imaging may demonstrate hepatic lesions not shown by even the most advanced CT scanning techniques.[104,105] Some tumors are more easily demonstrated by MR imaging than by CT (Fig. 20-24). MR imaging performed using specific tissue vari-

ables and higher resolution may lead to specific diagnoses and thus may replace CT as the reference standard for detecting and evaluating focal hepatic lesions. Whether percutaneous biopsy of hepatic tumors can be easily performed under MR imaging guidance is unknown at this time. An imaging scheme for hepatic tumors is shown in Figure 20-25. MR imaging is not included due to lack of experience with this modality.

PANCREATIC CANCER

For jaundiced patients thought to have a pancreatic cancer, US is frequently the best modality for detecting dilated bile ducts (Fig. 20-26).[106-108] If the location and cause of the obstruction cannot be adequately demonstrated with US, CT is usually recommended. If the cause and level of obstruction can be determined with CT, the patient can be treated surgically or by percutaneous drainage; endoscopic drainage can also be performed. A fine-needle aspiration biopsy may be needed to confirm the diagnosis. If the level or cause of the obstruction cannot be determined with US or CT, then endoscopic retrograde cholangiopancreatography (ERCP) or percutaneous transhepatic cholangiography (PTC) should be performed to clearly demonstrate the site of obstruction.

The new percutaneous radiologic techniques have had their greatest impact in cases of obstructive jaundice due to malignancy, especially pancreatic carcinoma. Not only can the radiologist confirm the level of obstruction with US and CT[106-108] and establish the diagnosis with a fine-needle aspiration biopsy,[85,86] he or she can now treat the malignant obstruction with percutaneous transhepatic biliary drainage.[109-112] This technique has been used most commonly to decompress the biliary system and allow the serum bilirubin level to decline before operative intervention. Chemotherapeutic agents and local radiation therapy can also be administered through the catheter. In some patients with advanced disease or who refuse an operation, the bile ducts can be permanently drained by converting the external percutaneous transhepatic biliary drainage system to an internal drainage system. Ring and Kerlan have used an endoprosthesis in some patients and have found that the larger endoprosthetic devices remain patent for at least 6 months, thereby functioning beyond the survival of most patients with pancreatic cancer.[111] There is a higher complication rate associated with the endoprosthesis than with the external catheter, and some authors have abandoned its use.[112] Others continue to use an endoprosthesis but take the high complication rate into consideration when deciding what type of drainage should be performed.[111,113]

MR imaging is not included in the imaging scheme in Figure 20-25 because to date it has not been shown to be more accurate than CT.[114]

GENITOURINARY TRACT CANCERS

RENAL CARCINOMA

Despite the greater accuracy of CT, excretory urography, which is more available, costs less, and has an acceptable accuracy, continues to be considered the best imaging mo-

FIG. 20-24. **A.** Contrast-enhanced CT scan through liver in a 30-year-old man with a hepatoma involving left lobe of liver. Note calcification in center of lesion (*arrowhead*), subtle fullness of left lobe of liver (*arrows*), and extension of tumor to local nodes (*curved arrows*). S, stomach containing contrast; SP, spleen; K, left kidney; A, aorta. **B.** MR image of same patient at similar location in liver. This T₁-weighted (TR 2000 MSEC TE 160 MSEC) image shows the hepatoma involving the left lobe of liver. Note fullness of left lobe (*arrows*), tumor extension (*curved arrows*), and no evidence of the calcification (a limitation of MRI). PV, portal veins; IVC, inferior vena cava; A, aorta; S, stomach; SP, spleen. **C.** The tumor (*arrows*) is shown much better on the T₂-weighted (TR 2000 TE 20) image, because it has a stronger signal than the remainder of the liver. (Thompson WM: Imaging strategies for tumors of the gastrointestinal system. 37:165–186, 1987)

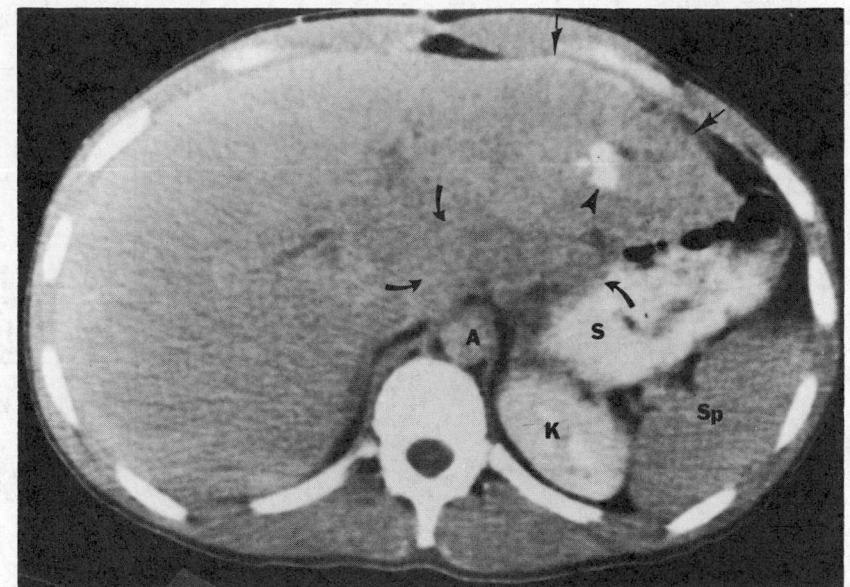

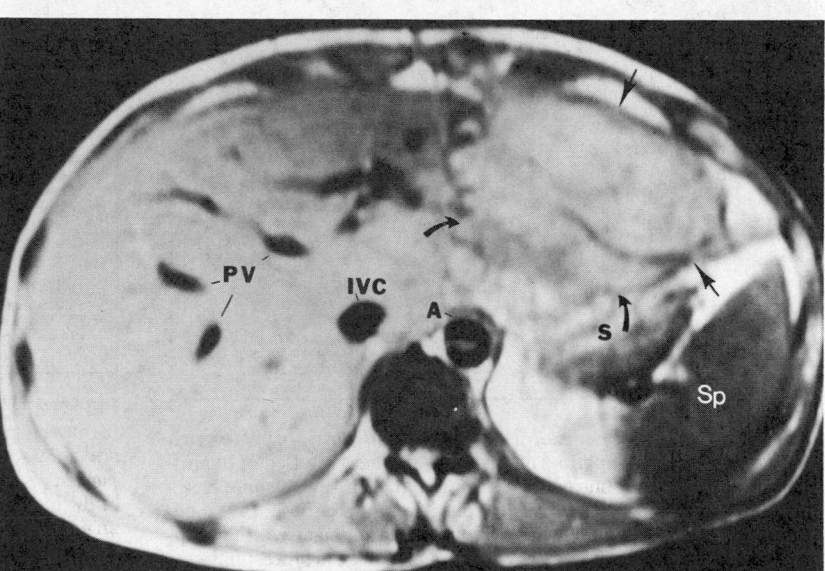

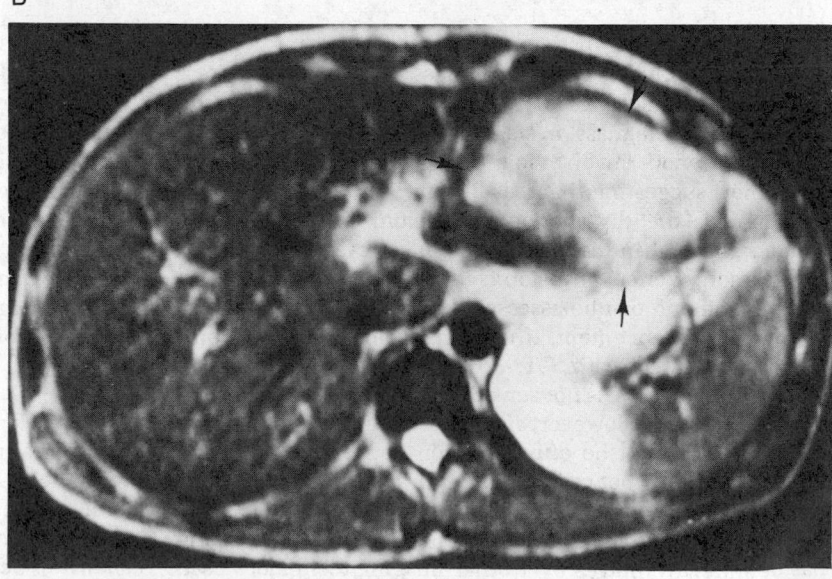

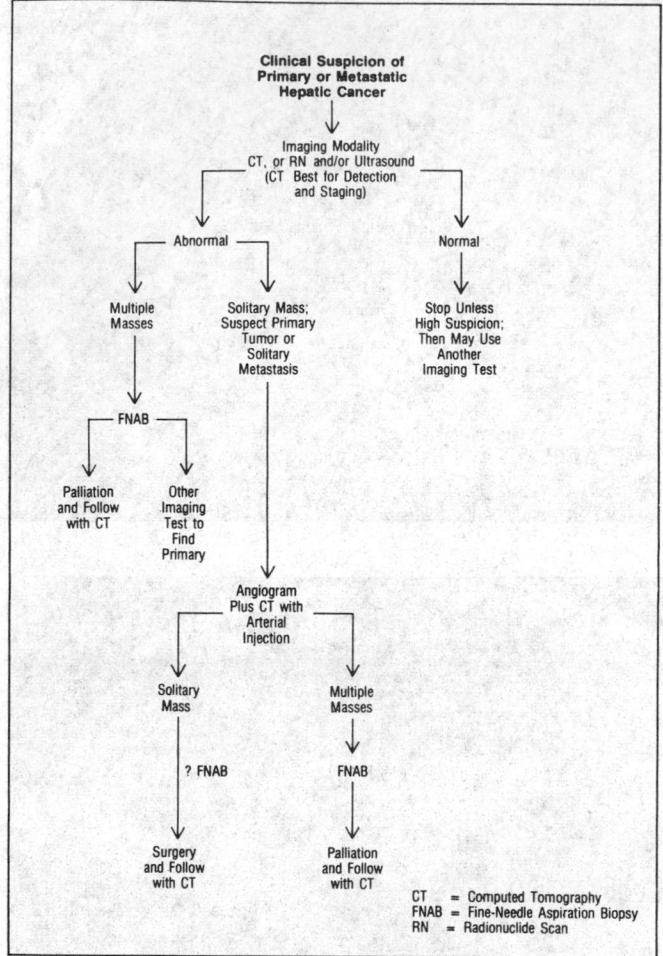

FIG. 20-25. Imaging decision tree for patients with suspected primary or metastatic hepatic cancer. CT is the best method of examination for detection, but cost and limited availability in some cases will dictate use of radionuclide scan or ultrasound, or both. Fine-needle aspiration biopsy is helpful in confirming metastases. (Thompson WM: Imaging strategies for tumors of the gastrointestinal system. CA 37:165–186, 1987)

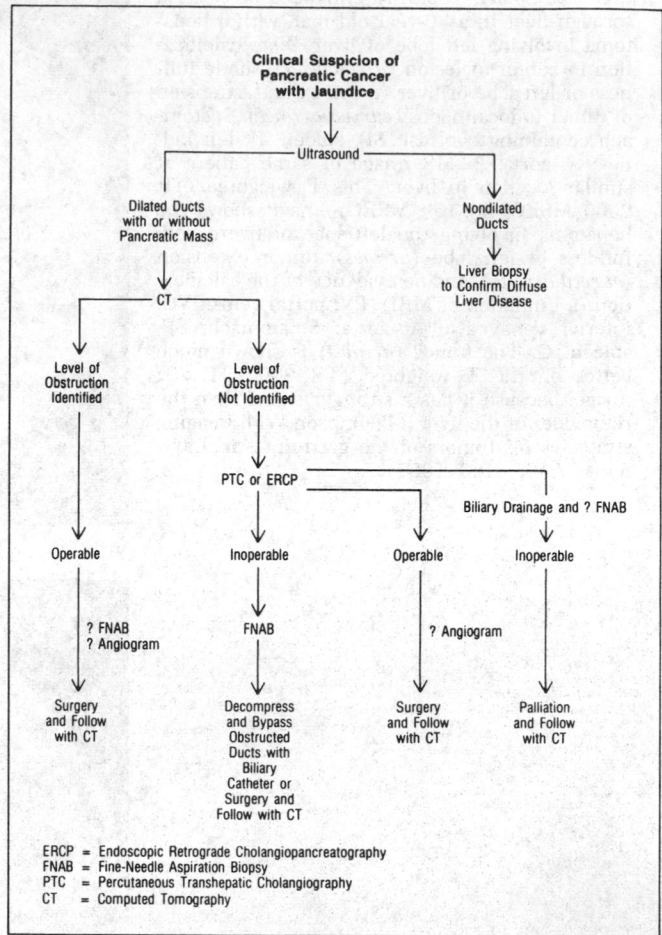

FIG. 20-26. Imaging decision tree for jaundiced patients suspected of having pancreatic cancer. If CT confirms obstructive jaundice and shows the level of obstruction and pancreatic head mass, many patients can go to surgery from CT. Some surgeons may request both fine needle aspiration biopsy to confirm the diagnosis and an angiogram to define the peripancreatic blood vessels. Follow-up of pancreatic tumors is best performed by CT. (Thompson WM: Imaging strategies for tumors of the gastrointestinal system. CA 37:165–186, 1987)

dality for screening patients suspected of having a renal carcinoma.[115] Once a solid renal mass is identified, contrast agent–enhanced CT is of major value in confirming the solid nature of the mass, in staging, in detecting contralateral kidney or venous involvement, and in detecting fat within the tumor, suggesting that it is benign.[115,116] CT is useful in determining the distribution of calcium within a lesion, which is helpful in distinguishing benign cysts from malignant tumors. Venous invasion is of particular importance to the surgeon and can be assessed during CT with bolus contrast agent enhancement. If the renal veins cannot be completely evaluated with CT, US or angiography may be necessary.[115-117] CT is not sensitive in the evaluation of perinephric invasion. However, since most patients undergo radical nephrectomy, the differentiation between Stage I and Stage II tumors is not critical. The overall accuracy of CT for staging renal carcinoma is 90%.[118]

Although much more experience is needed, MR imaging has definite advantages over other imaging techniques used to evaluate renal tumors.[119] MR imaging can differentiate solid masses from benign cystic lesions and can demonstrate major blood vessels and vascular invasion without administration of contrast medium (Fig. 20-27). Limited availability, high cost, long imaging times, inability to demonstrate calcium, and motion artifacts are current disadvantages of MR imaging in the evaluation of renal carcinoma.

Since a number of modalities can identify a solid mass in the kidney, no specific imaging scheme has been developed.[115] Some patients may go directly to surgery after excretory urography. Currently, CT provides the best overall staging information.[118]

PROSTATIC CARCINOMA

The digital rectal examination of the prostate has been the reference standard for the evaluation of prostatic carcinoma with respect to detection, tumor size, prognosis, and response to therapy.[120] However, this examination has been shown to be relatively inaccurate.[121]

The prostate has a central zone and a peripheral zone;

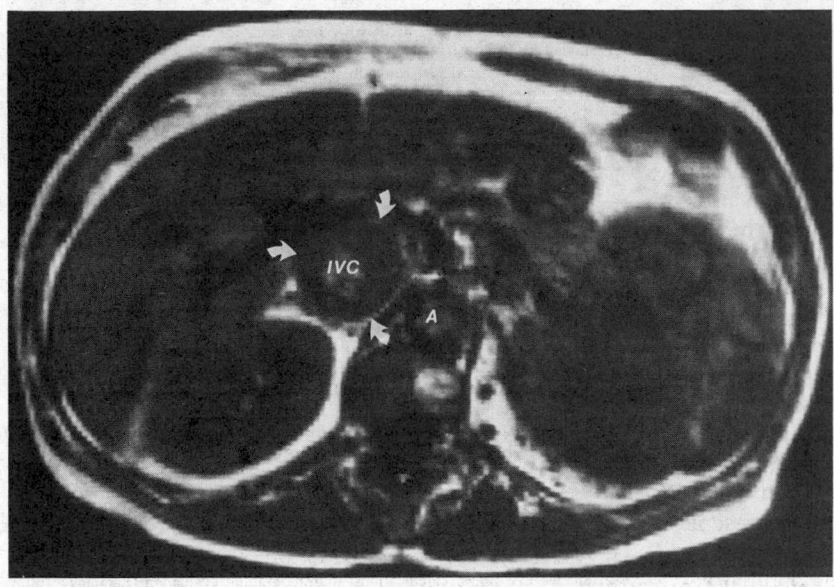

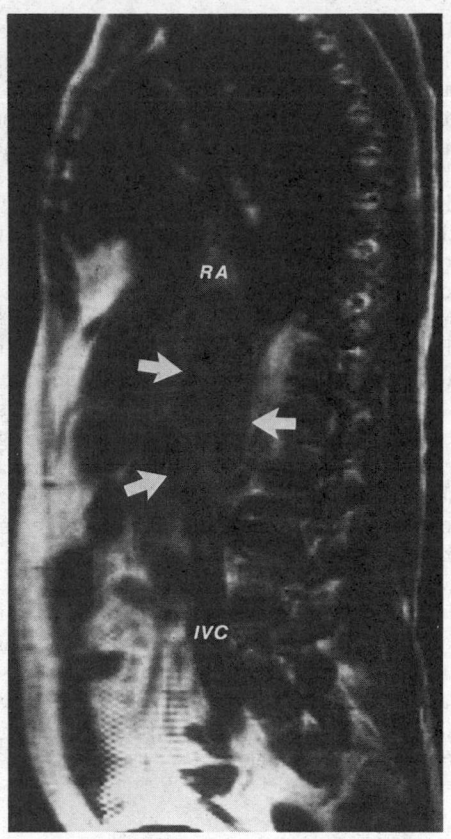

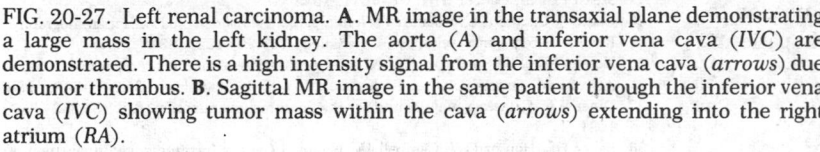

A

B

FIG. 20-27. Left renal carcinoma. **A.** MR image in the transaxial plane demonstrating a large mass in the left kidney. The aorta (A) and inferior vena cava (IVC) are demonstrated. There is a high intensity signal from the inferior vena cava (arrows) due to tumor thrombus. **B.** Sagittal MR image in the same patient through the inferior vena cava (IVC) showing tumor mass within the cava (arrows) extending into the right atrium (RA).

tumors commonly originate in the latter, within a few millimeters of the prostate capsule, and spread by infiltrating adjacent tissue just beneath the capsule and by extending toward the central gland. A variety of imaging techniques have been used to detect and stage prostatic carcinoma.

Transrectal US has recently been developed for evaluating the prostate and has proved more sensitive than digital examination for detecting abnormalities.[122-124] Certain sonographic features suggest benign disease, including areas of increased echogenicity that lie entirely within the prostate.[122] Areas of decreased echogenicity purely within the peripheral zone are highly suggestive of cancer (Fig. 20-28).[122-124] There is some overlap, and most investigators believe that all suspect lesions should be biopsied.[123] Rifkin et al, in the largest series reported to date, found no specific US characteristics that differentiated between many cases of benign prostatic disease and malignancy. Transrectal US may help determine which areas should be biopsied.[123] Also,

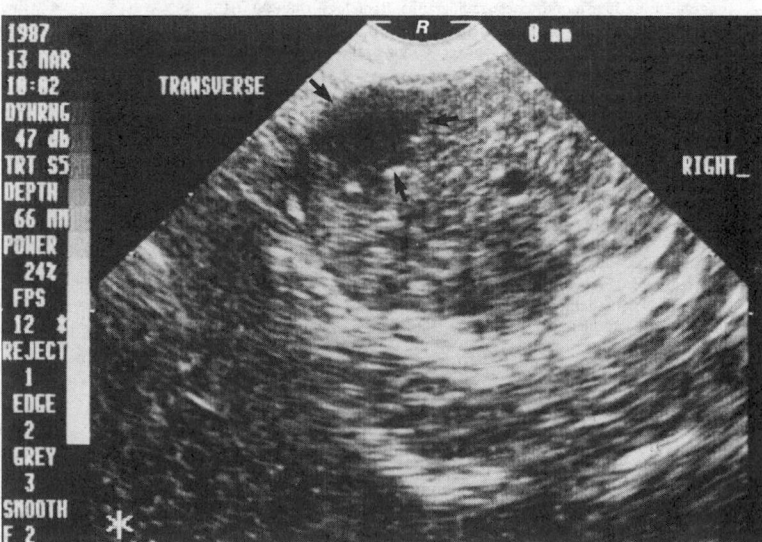

FIG. 20-28. Prostatic cancer: transrectal ultrasound. Transrectal ultrasound through level of prostate, a hypoechoic area is demonstrated in the peripheral zone to the right of midline (arrows), rectal lumen (R). Ultrasound guided needle biopsy of the lesion was positive for adenocarcinoma.

transrectal US can accurately delineate areas that are difficult to palpate, or sonographically abnormal areas that are not palpable. At this time, transrectal US cannot be used alone as a screening technique. In conjunction with US-guided biopsy, however, it allows the detection of many clinically nonpalpable, subtle prostatic cancers.[123]

Initial experience with MR imaging suggested that prostatic carcinoma had a different signal intensity than benign prostatic hypertrophy[125,126]; however, more recent data have shown that MR imaging cannot differentiate prostatic carcinoma from benign prostatic hypertrophy.[127,128]

Both CT and MR imaging have been used to stage prostatic carcinoma. The results with CT have not been favorable. Based on their experience, Platt et al suggest that CT not be used to influence decisions concerning surgical versus nonsurgical treatment in patients with clinically staged local disease. CT has been useful for staging only when unsuspected metastatic nodal disease was detected.[129] At present, MR imaging is the most accurate diagnostic modality for the local staging of carcinoma of the prostate; for optimal results, multiple sequences and at least two of the three orthogonal imaging planes are needed. Using this extensive and time-consuming technique, Hricak et al found that MR imaging had an 83% accuracy.[130] Further work is needed to define the exact role of these imaging techniques in patients with prostatic cancer.

REFERENCES

1. Bragg DG, Rubin P, Youker J (eds): Oncologic Imaging. Elmsford, NY, Pergamon Press, 1985
2. Marx JL: Imaging technique passes muster. Science 238:888–889, 1987
3. Haggar AM, Pearlberg JL, Froelich JW et al: Chest-wall invasion by carcinoma of the lung: Detection by MR imaging. AJR 148:1075–1078, 1987
4. Wetzel LH, Levine E, Murphey MD: A comparison of MR imaging and CT in the evaluation of musculoskeletal masses. RadioGraphics 7:851–874, 1987
5. Adams V, Krishnan KU, Muhm JR et al: Diffuse malignant mesothelioma of pleura: Diagnosis and survival in 92 cases. Cancer 58:1540–1551, 1986
6. Mirvis S, Dutcher JP, Haney PJ et al: CT of malignant pleural mesothelioma. AJR 140:665–670, 1983
7. Dedrick CG, McCloud TC, Shepard JO et al: Computed tomography of localized pleural mesothelioma. AJR 144:275–280, 1985
8. Muhm JR, Miller WE, Fontana RS et al: Lung cancer detected during a screening program using four-month chest radiographs. Radiology 148:609–615, 1983
9. Frost JK, Ball WC, Levin ML et al: Early lung cancer detection: Results of the initial (prevalence) radiologic and cytologic screening in the Johns Hopkins study. Am Rev Respir Dis 130:549–554, 1984
10. Flehinger BJ, Melamed MR, Zaman MB et al: Early lung cancer detection: Results of the initial (prevalence) radiologic and cytologic screening in the Memorial Sloan–Kettering study. Am Rev Respir Dis 130:555–560, 1984
11. Fontana RS, Sanderson DR, Taylor WF et al: Early lung cancer detection: Results of the initial (prevalence) radiologic and cytologic screening in the Mayo Clinic study. Am Rev Respir Dis 130:561–565, 1984
12. Filderman AE, Shaw C, Matthay RA: Lung cancer: Part I. Etiology, pathology, natural history, manifestations and diagnostic techniques. Invest Radiol 21:80–90, 1986
13. Armstrong JD, Bragg DG: Thoracic neoplasms: Imaging requirements for diagnostic and staging. In Bragg DG, Rubin P, Youker J (eds): Oncologic Imaging, chap 10. Elmsford, NY, Pergamon Press, 1985
14. Siegelman SS, Zerhouni EA, Leo FP et al: CT of the solitary pulmonary nodule. AJR 135:1–13, 1980
15. Heitzman ER: The Lung: Radiologic–Pathologic Correlations. St Louis, CV Mosby, 1984
16. Muhm JR, Brown LR, Crowe JK et al: Comparison of whole lung tomography and computed tomography for detecting pulmonary nodules. AJR 131:981–984, 1978
17. Zerhouni EA, Stitik FP, Seigelman SS et al: CT of the pulmonary nodule: Cooperative study. Radiology 160:319–327, 1986
18. Epstein DM, Stephenson LW, Gefter WB et al: Value of CT in the preoperative assessment of lung cancer: A survey of thoracic surgeons. Radiology 161:423–427, 1986
19. Filderman AE, Shaw C, Matthay RA: Lung cancer: Part II. staging and therapy. Invest Radiol 21:173–185, 1986
20. Poon PY, Bronskill MJ, Henkelman RM et al: Mediastinal lymph node metastases from bronchogenic carcinoma: Detection with MR imaging and CT. Radiology 162:651–656, 1987
21. vanSonnenberg E, Lin AS, Deutsch AL et al: Percutaneous biopsy of difficult mediastinal, hilar and pulmonary lesions by computed tomographic guidance and a modified coaxial technique. Radiology 148:300–302, 1983
22. Perlmutt LM, Braun SD, Newman GE: Transthoracic needle aspiration: Use of a small chest tube to treat pneumothorax. AJR 148:849–851, 1987
23. Winkler M, Higgins CB: Suspected intracardiac masses: Evaluation with MR imaging. Radiology 165:117–122, 1987
24. Egan RL: Experience with mammography in a tumor institution: Evaluation of 1,000 studies. Radiology 75:894–900, 1960
25. Wolfe JN: Xerography of the breast. Radiology 91:231–240, 1968
26. Pagani JJ, Bassett LW, Gold RH et al: Efficacy of combined film-screen/xeromammography: Preliminary report. AJR 135:144–146, 1980
27. Shapiro S, Venet W, Strax P et al: Ten to fourteen year effect of screening on breast cancer mortality. JNCI 69:349–355, 1982
28. Tabar L, Gad A, Holmberg LH et al: Reduction in mortality from breast cancer after mass screening with mammography. Lancet 1:829–832, 1985
29. Baker LH: Breast Cancer Detection Demonstration Project: Five-year summary report. CA 32:196–225, 1982
30. Gold RH, Bassett LW, Kimme-Smith C: Breast imaging: State-of-the-art. Invest Radiol 21:298–304, 1986
31. Paulus D: Imaging in breast cancer. CA 37:133–150, 1987
32. Sickles EA: Breast calcifications: Mammographic evaluation. Radiology 160:289–293, 1986
33. Sickles EA: Mammographic features of 300 consecutive non-palpable breast cancers. AJR 146:661–663, 1986
34. Moskowitz M: The predictive value of certain mammographic signs in screening for breast cancer. Cancer 51:1007–1011, 1983
35. Ciatto S, Cataliotti L, Distante V: Nonpalpable lesions detected with mammography: Review of 512 consecutive cases. Radiology 165:99–102, 1987
36. Homer MJ, Pile-Spellman ER: Needle localization of occult breast lesions with a curved-end retractable wire: Technique and pitfalls. Radiology 161:547–548, 1986
37. Diner WC: Galactography: Mammary duct contrast examination. AJR 137:853–856, 1981
38. Baker HL, Houser OW, Cambell JK: National Cancer Institute study: Evaluation of computed tomography in the diagnosis of intracranial neoplasms. I. Overall results. Radiology 136:91–96, 1980
39. Bismar J, Stromblad LG, Stanford LG: Impact of CT in the neurosurgical management of intracranial tumors. Neuroradiology 16:506–509, 1978
40. Davis DO: CT in the diagnosis of supratentorial tumors. Semin Roentgenol 12:97–108, 1977
41. Enzmann DR, Norman D, Levin V et al: Computed tomography in the follow-up of medulloblastomas and ependymomas. Radiology 128:57–63, 1978
42. Marks JE, Gado M: Serial computed tomography of primary brain tumors following surgery, irradiation, and chemotherapy. Radiology 125:119–125, 1977
43. Norman D, Enzmann DR, Levin VA et al: Computed tomography in the evaluation of malignant glioma before and after therapy. Radiology 121:85–88, 1976
44. Anderson R: Brain and spinal cord neoplasms. In Bragg DG, Rubin P (eds): Oncologic Imaging. New York, John Wiley & Sons, 1984
45. Weinstein MA, Modic MT, Pavlicek W et al: Nuclear magnetic resonance for the examination of brain tumors. Semin Roentgenol 19:139–147, 1984
46. Brant-Zawadzki M, Norman D, Newton TH et al: Magnetic resonance of the brain: The optimal screening technique. Radiology 152:71–77, 1984
47. Brant-Zawadzki M, Badami JP, Mills CM et al: Primary intracranial tumor imaging: A comparison of magnetic resonance and CT. Radiology 150:435–440, 1984
48. Zimmerman RA: Magnetic resonance of cerebral neoplasms. Magnetic Resonance Annual, New York, 1985
49. Partain CL, James AE, Rollo FD et al: Nuclear Magnetic Resonance (NMR) Imaging. Philadelphia, WB Saunders, 1983
50. Mills CM et al: Nuclear magnetic resonance: Principles of blood flow imaging. AJNR 4:1161–1166, 1983
51. Brant-Zawadski M: Magnetic resonance imaging principles: The bare necessities. In Brant-Zawadski M, Norman D (eds): Magnetic Resonance Imaging of the Central Nervous System, pp 1–12. New York, Raven, 1987
52. Bradley W, Newton T, Crooks LE: Physical properties of NMR. In Newton TH, Potts DG (eds): Modern Neuroradiology, Vol 2, Advanced Imaging Techniques, pp 15–61. San Francisco, Clavadel Press, 1983
53. Young IR, Burl M, Clarke G et al: Magnetic resonance properties of hydrogen: Imaging the posterior fossa. AJR 137:895–901, 1981
54. Brown RA, Roberts TS, Osborn AG: Simplified CT guided stereotactic biopsy. AJNR 2:181–184, 1981
55. Kelly PJ, Alker GJ: A method for sterotactic laser microsurgery in treatment of deep-seated CNS neoplasms. Appl Neurophysiol 43:210–215, 1980
56. Sheldon CA, McCann G, Jacques S et al: Development of a computerized microsteroetaxic method for localization and removal of minute CNS lesions under direct 3-D vision. J Neurosurg 52:21–27, 1900
57. Sapozink MO, Moeller JH, McDonald DN et al: Improved precision of interstitial brain tumor irradiation using the BRW CT stereotactic guidance system (unpublished)

58. Graif M, Bydder GM, Steiner RE et al: Contrast-enhanced MR imaging of malignant brain tumors. AJNR 6:855–862, 1985

59. Carr DH, Brown J, Bydder GM et al: Gadolinium-DTPA as a contrast agent in MRI: Initial clinical experience in 70 patients. AJR 143:215–224, 1984

60. Claussen C, Laniado M, Schorner W et al: Gadolinium-DTPA in MR imaging of glioblastomas and intracranial metastases. AJNR 6:699–674, 1985

61. Kingsley DP, Kendall BE: CT of the adverse effects of therapeutic radiation of the central nervous system. AJNR 2:453–460, 1981

62. Kramer S, Lee KF: Complications of radiation therapy: The central nervous system. Semin Roentgenol 9:75–83, 1974

63. DiChiro G, Doppman JL, Swyer AJ et al: Tumors and arteriovenous malformations on the spinal cord: Assessment using MR. Radiology 156:689–697, 1985

64. Norman D: The spine. In Brant-Zawadski M, Norman D (eds): Magnetic Resonance Imaging of the Central Nervous System, pp 289–328. New York, Raven, 1987

65. Smoker WRK, Godersky C, Knutson RK et al: The role of MRI in the evaluation of metastatic spinal disease. AJNR 8:901–908, 1987

66. Mancuso AA, Hanafee WN: Computed Tomography of the Head and Neck. Baltimore, Williams & Wilkins, 1982

67. Dillon WP, Mills CM, Kjos B et al: Magnetic resonance imaging of the nasopharynx. Radiology 152:731–738, 1984

68. Lufkin RB, Hanafee WN, Wortham D et al: Larynx and hypopharynx: MR imaging with surface coils. Radiology 158:747–754, 1986

69. Lufkin RB, Larssan SG, Hanafee WN: NMR anatomy of larynx and tongue base. Radiology 148:173–175, 1983

70. Archer CR, Yeager VL: Computed tomography of laryngeal cancer with histopathological correlation. Laryngoscope 92(20):1173–1180, 1982

71. Mafee MF, Schild JA, Valvassori GE et al: Computed tomography of the larynx: Correlation with anatomic and pathologic studies in cases of laryngeal carcinoma. Radiology 147:128, 1983

72. Mancuso AA: Cervical lymph node metastases. In Bragg DG, Rubin P, Youker J (eds): Oncologic Imaging. Elmsford, NY, Pergamon Press, 1985

73. Mancuso AA, Harnsberger HRN et al: Computed tomography of cervical and retropharyngeal lymph nodes: Normal anatomy, variants of normal, and applications in staging head and neck cancer. Parts I and II. Radiology 148:709–714, 1983

74. Muraki AS, Mancuso AA, Harnsberger HR: Metastatic cervical adenopathy from tumors of unknown origin: The role of computed tomography. Radiology 152:749–753, 1984

75. Silver JA, Mawad ME, Hilal SK et al: Computed tomography of the nasopharynx and related spaces: Part II. Pathology. Radiology 147:733–738, 1983

76. Muraki AS, Mancuso AA, Harnsberger HR et al: The upper aerodigestive tract and neck: CT evaluation of recurrent tumors. Radiology 149:725–731, 1983

77. Mancuso AA, Hanafee WN: Elusive head and neck tumors beneath intact mucosa. Laryngoscope 93:133–139, 1983

78. Harnsberger JR, Mancuso AA, Muraki AS et al: The upper aerodigestive tract and neck: CT evaluation of recurrent tumors. Radiology 149:503–509, 1983

79. Gatenby RA, Mulhern CB, Strawitz J et al: Comparison of clinical and CT staging of head and neck tumors. AJNR 6:399–401, 1985

80. Rouvier H: Anatomy of the Human Lymphatic System. Ann Arbor, Edwards Brothers, 1938

81. Blady JV: The present status of treatment of cervical metastases from carcinoma arising in the head and neck region. Am J Surg 111:56, 1971

82. Som PM, Shugar JM, Biller HF: The early detection of antral malignancy in the postmaxillectomy patient. Radiology 143:509–512, 1982

83. Leipsiz B, Winter ML, Hokanson JA: Cervical nodal metastases of unknown origin. Laryngoscope 91:593–598, 1981

84. Templer J, Perry MC, Davis SE: Metastatic cervical adenocarcinoma from unknown primary tumor. Arch Otolaryngol 107:45–47, 1981

85. Ferrucci JT, Wittenburg J, Mueller PR et al: Diagnosis of abdominal malignancy by radiologic fine-needle aspiration biopsy. AJR 134:323–330, 1980

86. Bernadino ME: Percutaneous biopsy. AJR 142:41–45, 1984

87. Moss AA: Computed tomography in the staging of gastrointestinal carcinoma. Radiol Clin North Am 20:761–780, 1982

88. Halvorsen RA Jr, Thompson WM: CT for staging gastrointestinal malignancies: Part I. Esophagus and stomach. Invest Radiol 22:2–16, 1987

89. Thompson WM, Halvorsen RA Jr: CT for staging gastrointestinal malignancies: Part II. Small bowel and colon. Invest Radiol 22:96–105, 1987

90. Thompson WM: Imaging strategies for tumors of the gastrointestinal system. CA 37:165–185, 1987

91. Thompson WM: Esophageal cancer. Int J Radiat Oncol Biol Phys 9:1533–1565, 1983

92. Quint LE, Glazer GM, Orringer MB: Esophageal imaging by MR and CT: Study of normal anatomy and neoplasms. Radiology 156:727–731, 1985

93. Heiken JP, Balfe DM, Roper CL: CT evaluation after esophagogastrectomy. AJR 143:555–560, 1984

94. Moss AA, Schnyder P, Marks WM et al: Gastric adenocarcinoma: A comparison of the accuracy and economics of staging by computed tomography and surgery. Gastroenterology 80:45–50, 1981

95. Sussman SK, Halvorsen RA, Illescas FF et al: Gastric adenocarcinoma: CT vs surgical staging. Radiology 167:335–340, 1988

96. Freeny PC, Marks WM, Ryan JA et al: Colorectal carcinoma evaluation with CT: Preoperative staging and detection of postoperative recurrence. Radiology 158:347–353, 1986

97. Thompson WM, Halvorsen RA, Foster WL Jr et al: Preoperative and postoperative CT staging of rectosigmoid carcinoma. AJR 146:703–710, 1986

98. Butch RJ, Wittenberg J, Muller PR et al: Presacral masses after abdominoperineal resection for colorectal carcinoma: The need for needle biopsy. AJR 144:309–312, 1985

99. Butch RJ, Stark DP, Wittenberg J et al: Staging rectal cancer by MR and CT. AJR 146:1155–1160, 1986

100. Gomberg JS, Friedman AC, Radecki PD et al: MRI differentiation of recurrent colorectal carcinoma from postoperative fibrosis. Gastrointest Radiol 11:361–363, 1986

101. Zeman RK, Paushter DM, Schiebler ML et al: Hepatic imaging: Current status. Radiol Clin North Am 23:473–487, 1985

102. LaBerge JM, Laing FC, Federle MP et al: Hepatocellular carcinoma: Assessment of resectability by computed tomography and ultrasound. Radiology 152:485–490, 1984

103. Castaing D, Emond J, Kunstlinger F et al: Utility of operative ultrasound in the surgical management of liver tumors. Ann Surg 204:600–605, 1986

104. Moss AA, Goldberg HI, Stark DB et al: Hepatic tumors: Magnetic resonance and CT appearance. Radiology 150:141–147, 1984

105. Stark DD, Wittenberg J, Butch RJ et al: Hepatic metastases: Randomized, controlled comparison of detection with MR imaging and CT. Radiology 165:399–406, 1987

106. Freeny PC, Lawson TL: Adenocarcinoma of the pancreas, In Freeney PC, Lawson TL (eds): Radiology of the Pancreas, pp 397–496. New York, Springer-Verlag, 1982

107. Clark LR, Jaffe MH, Choyke PL et al: Pancreatic imaging. Radiol Clin North Am 23:489–501, 1985

108. Ferrucci JT Jr, Adson MA, Mueller PR et al: Advances in the radiology of jaundice: A symposium and review. AJR 141:1–20, 1983

109. Gobien RP, Stanley JH, Soucek CK et al: Routine preoperative biliary drainage: Effect on management of obstructive jaundice. Radiology 152:353–356, 1984

110. Bonnel D, Ferrucci JT Jr, Muller PR et al: Surgical and radiological decompression in malignant biliary obstruction: A retrospective study using multivariate risk factor analysis. Radiology 152:347–351, 1984

111. Ring EJ, Kerlan RK: Interventional biliary radiology. AJR 142:31–34, 1984

112. Mendez G Jr, Russell E, Le Page JR et al: Abandonment of endoprosthetic drainage technique in malignant biliary obstruction. AJR 143:617–622, 1984

113. Mueller PR, Ferrucci JT Jr, Teplick SK et al: Biliary stent and endoprosthesis: Analysis of complications in 113 patients. Radiology 156:637–639, 1985

114. Tashdakoff D, Hricak H, Thoeni R et al: MR imaging in the diagnosis of pancreatic disease. AJR 148:703–709, 1987

115. Davidson AJ, Hartman DS: Imaging strategies for tumor of the kidney, adrenal gland, and retroperitoneum. CA 37:151–164, 1987

116. Cronan JJ, Zeman RK, Rosenfield AT: Comparison of computed tomography, ultrasound and angiography in staging renal cell carcinoma. J Urol 127:712–714, 1982

117. Schwerk WB, Schwerk WN, Rodeck G: Venous renal tumor extension: A prospective US evaluation. Radiology 156:491–495, 1985

118. Johnson CD, Dunnick NR, Cohan RH et al: Renal adenocarcinoma: CT staging of 100 tumors. AJR 148:59–63, 1987

119. Karstaedt N, McCullough DL, Wolfman NT et al: Magnetic resonance imaging of the renal mass. J Urol 136:566–570, 1986

120. Stamey TA: Cancer of the prostate: Analysis of some important contributions and dilemmas. Monogr Urol 4:68–92, 1983

121. Siegelman SS, McNeal JE, Freiha FS et al: Rectal examination in volume determination of carcinoma of the prostate: Clinical and anatomic correlations. J Urol 136:1228–1230, 1986

122. Lee F, Gray JM, McLeary RD et al: Prostatic evaluation by transrectal sonography: Criteria for diagnosis of early carcinoma. Radiology 158:91–95, 1986

123. Rifkin MD, Friedland GW, Shortliffe L: Prostatic evaluation by transrectal endosonography: Detection of carcinoma. Radiology 158:85–90, 1986

124. Lee F, Littrup PJ, McLeary RD et al: Needle aspiration and core biopsy of prostatic cancer: Comparative evaluation with biplanar transrectal US guidance. Radiology 163:515–520, 1987

125. Steyn JH, Smith FW: Nuclear magnetic resonance imaging of the prostate. Br J Urol 54:726–728, 1982

126. Hricak H, Williams RD, Spring DB et al: Anatomy and pathology of the male pelvis by magnetic resonance imaging. AJR 141:1101–1110, 1983

127. Poon PY, McCallum RW, Henkelman MM et al: Magnetic resonance imaging of the prostate. Radiology 154:143–149, 1985

128. Ling D, Lee JKT, Heiken JP et al: Prostatic carcinoma and benign prostatic hyperplasia: Inability of MR imaging to distinguish between the two diseases. Radiology 158:103–107, 1986

129. Platt JF, Bree RL, Schwab RE: The accuracy of CT in the staging of carcinoma of the prostate. AJR 149:315–318, 1987

130. Hricak H, Dooms GC, Jeffrey RB et al: Prostatic carcinoma: Staging by clinical assessment, CT, and MR imaging. Radiology 162:331–336, 1987

DONALD L. MILLER
RICHARD CHANG
JOHN L. DOPPMAN

SECTION 3

Interventional Radiology in Oncology

Interventional radiology may be loosely defined as comprising those procedures in which radiologic guidance is used to direct needles or catheters for the invasive diagnosis or treatment of various disorders. In large measure, interventional radiologic procedures represent an alternative to surgery for either diagnosis or treatment. Whereas the surgeon uses direct vision as a guide, the radiologist relies on indirect vision through the use of a variety of imaging methods.

Interventional radiology is a very young field that essentially began in the 1960s.[1] The term itself was first used by Margolis in 1967.[2] Developments in this area have depended on technological innovations, such as Seldinger's development of a practical method of percutaneous vascular catheterization[3] and Grüntzig and Hopff's development of the balloon dilation catheter,[4] but even more so on the imagination of radiologists such as Dotter, who first conceived of transluminal angioplasty,[5] and Baum and others, who developed catheter techniques for localizing and managing gastrointestinal bleeding.[6]

The techniques of the interventional radiologist can be divided into five categories: diagnostic procedures, performed to obtain material for histologic, cytologic, or other laboratory analysis, and four broad categories of therapeutic intervention (as suggested by White[1]): drainage procedures (biliary, urinary, and abscesses), vascular and nonvascular balloon dilatation, chemotherapy administration, and embolotherapy. All the various paraphernalia and procedures used in modern interventional radiology can be considered as adaptations or applications of these basic concepts.

With regard to the application of interventional radiology to oncology, a simpler classification is more appropriate and will be used in this chapter. Oncologic interventional radiology may be divided into procedures used for cancer diagnosis, procedures used for cancer therapy, and procedures used as adjuncts in the management of cancer patients. This classification excludes several types of procedures, such as stone extraction and transluminal angioplasty, that have no direct application in oncologic practice. This chapter is not intended as a guide to the full extent of interventional radiology, but is narrowly focused on oncologic interventions.

CANCER DIAGNOSIS—PERCUTANEOUS BIOPSY

Percutaneous needle biopsy has become a technique of major importance in the diagnosis and staging of cancer.[7,8] Increased utilization of this technique is a consequence of the availability of safer needles, newer imaging techniques, and advances in cytology.[9]

Technique

Radiologically guided percutaneous needle biopsy is usually performed with thin ("skinny") needles of 20 to 23 gauge, which are designed to yield aspirates of cells for cytologic examination. Some of these needles are also designed to yield small cores of tissue.[10-13] Regardless of which of these needles is used, the technique is usually referred to as fineneedle aspiration biopsy (FNAB).[8,14,15] Larger needles can be used to obtain larger cores of tissue and are most commonly used in the evaluation of bone tumors, hepatic lesions, and lymphomas.[9] In these areas, the larger needles produce more tissue, yield higher accuracy rates, and do not appear to have a higher complication rate.[9,12,16-21] The choice of needle type and size depends on the size, type, and location of the lesion and the preferences of the radiologist and cytopathologist.[22] Pathologists with less experience in cytology may require larger tissue samples for confident diagnosis.

The role of the pathologist is critical, since skill and experience in cytology is the most important factor in reaching an accurate diagnosis. Pathologists vary in their preference for different methods of tissue sampling, tissue fixation, and sample handling.[8,9,23,24] It is wise to follow the pathologist's preferences in this regard. Often it is possible to arrange for the cytologist to be present during the biopsy, and this is extremely helpful: The cytologist can prepare the specimens on the spot and can provide the radiologist with virtually instant information as to their adequacy.[9,25] Although the immediate cytologic assessment of biopsy specimens does not seem to increase accuracy rates or decrease complication rates,[26] it does provide benefits for patient care. This is principally because preliminary results are rapidly available and the selection of further diagnostic tests may be made immediately.

A variety of imaging techniques can be used for needle guidance during biopsy. Fluoroscopy is useful for lesions that are visible on plain films, such as pulmonary nodules, some bone lesions, and lymph nodes opacified by lymphangiography. Ultrasound (US) and computed tomography (CT) have extended our ability to visualize lesions in the mediastinum, abdomen, pelvis, and head and neck and are commonly used to guide biopsies of these areas (Fig. 20-29).[14,15,27,28] It was initially thought that magnetic resonance (MR) imaging would be much less useful to guide percutaneous biopsy, and that nonferrous needles would be required to avoid the creation of the severe artifact commonly seen with ferromagnetic materials and to prevent needle motion due to magnetic field effects. However, Mueller et al have shown that biopsy needles fabricated from a specific stainless steel (SS 316) do not produce artifacts on MR imaging–guided percutaneous biopsies and do not move in a magnetic field. They have performed liver biopsies in humans with these needles.[29] Virtually any imaging technique that provides three-dimensional localization of a lesion can be used to guide a biopsy needle, but the choice of modality is based on lesion size, position, and visibility; equipment availability; and the skills and preference of the individual radiologist. The radiologist who performs the biopsy must be the final arbiter in the choice of imaging modality.

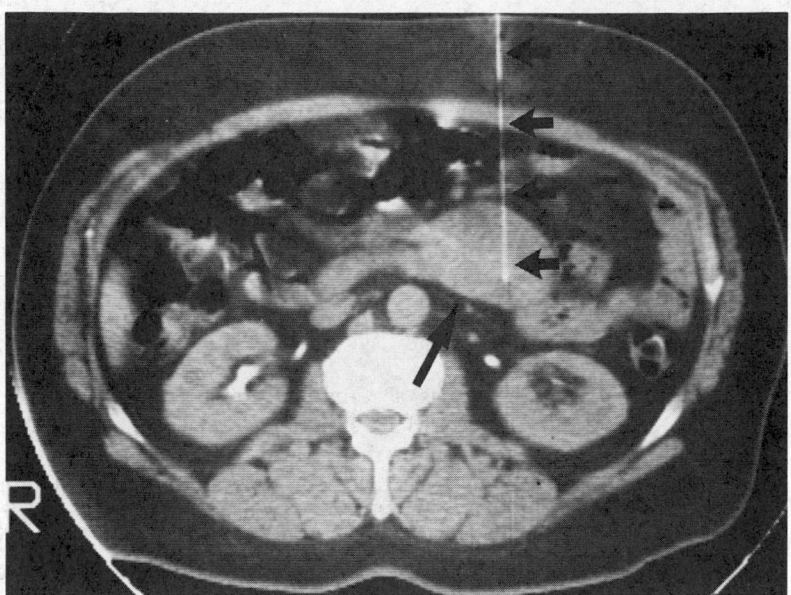

FIG. 20-29. CT-guided biopsy of an abdominal mass. The needle is visible as a thin white line (*short black arrows*) that terminates in the mass (*long black arrow*). Note that the needle passes through gas-containing bowel. With thin needles, this is quite safe. The patient had no complications from the biopsy.

Clinical Advantages

Much of the appeal of percutaneous biopsy is based on the use of this technique as a substitute for surgical biopsy, with an attendant decrease in patient morbidity and decrease in costs.[8,30] In a review of 82 percutaneous biopsies performed in patients with gynecologic malignancies and extrapelvic lesions, biopsy proved highly cost-effective and permitted surgery to be avoided in a number of patients.[31] In 72 patients undergoing percutaneous biopsy of thoracic lesions, biopsy reduced the need for the diagnostic thoracotomy, shortened the time from admission to diagnosis, reduced the total number of thoracotomies, shortened the length of hospital stay, and resulted in a significantly reduced average and total hospitalization charge.[32] In a series of 422 patients with 400 proven pulmonary lesions, Westcott found that percutaneous biopsy established the diagnosis in 191 patients and made mediastinoscopy and/or thoracotomy unnecessary.[33] In 53 patients with a clinical diagnosis of carcinoma of the pancreas, 30 laparotomies were avoided in 37 patients with positive biopsies.[34]

Most biopsies in adults can be performed as outpatient procedures and require only local anesthesia to the skin. Percutaneous biopsy procedures are also appropriate for pediatric patients. Although some form of sedation or regional anesthesia may be necessary, general anesthesia is usually not required in children.[35] In one series of 69 percutaneous diagnostic procedures in children aged 2 days to 17 years, general anesthesia was never necessary.[25] In another series of 14 pediatric patients, general anesthesia was necessary for percutaneous biopsy in three patients.[36]

Accuracy

The accuracy of percutaneous biopsy depends on the radiologist's skill in directing the needle, the size of the specimen, and the cytopathologist's skill in interpreting the specimen. Large masses should be biopsied near their periphery to avoid possible areas of necrosis. Accuracy varies according to the specific biopsy site, as different organs present different problems in terms of access and interpretation. A single needle pass into a malignant lesion will yield a specimen containing malignant cells approximately 75% of the time.[37] Additional needle passes will increase the sensitivity, but more than four passes are rarely necessary.

In general, a negative biopsy report does not necessarily mean that malignancy has been excluded; the wrong site may have been sampled, or the sample may be inadequate. Only positive biopsies should influence therapeutic decisions.

The sensitivity of percutaneous biopsy for the detection of malignancy in lung nodules is as high as 95% to 97%, with accuracies of 96% to 98% reported.[33,38,39] Biopsy of the hila and mediastinum is equally sensitive.[40]

In the abdomen, FNAB of the liver has an accuracy of 84% to 99%.[11,16,23,28] There is some evidence that use of larger needles (14 or 18 gauge) increases sensitivity and accuracy.[12,16,17] Pancreatic biopsy is somewhat less useful, with a sensitivity ranging from 77% to 86% and an accuracy of 80% to 89%.[11,28,34,41] It may be more appropriate to biopsy associated liver metastases or abdominal masses in patients with pancreatic lesions than to biopsy the pancreas directly.[9] Adrenal biopsy is safe in the absence of pheochromocytoma. An adrenal mass in a patient with a malignancy should be biopsied to exclude the presence of a nonfunctioning adenoma, or "incidentaloma." These are seen as serendipitous findings on approximately 1% of abdominal CT scans.[42,43] Adrenal FNAB is successful in 83% to 93% of enlarged glands.[44,45]

The diagnostic accuracy of retroperitoneal and pelvic lymph node biopsy varies from 65% to 90%.[9] Accuracy is higher in patients with nodal metastases from carcinoma than in patients with lymphoma, because the diagnosis of lymphoma requires a much larger tissue sample for accurate evaluation of cell patterns. It was initially thought that biopsy of pelvic nodes that appeared normal on lymphangiography might aid in the staging of prostatic carcinoma, but this appears not to be the case.[46,47]

Percutaneous bone biopsy has an overall accuracy of about 79% in the diagnosis of primary bone tumors and 95% in the diagnosis of osseous metastases.[18,21] Large needles are usually required for the diagnosis of primary bone tumors and for biopsy of blastic lesions.[9] The blood from a bone biopsy specimen should also be sent for cytologic analysis, especially in patients with osseous metastases.[48]

Complications

Fine-needle aspiration biopsy is a remarkably safe technique. The complications of FNAB are summarized in Table 20-9. The risk of hemorrhage is less than 1% and the risk of death is less than 0.01%.[8,49] Deaths have been reported from hemorrhagic pancreatitis following FNAB of the pancreas, and from asphyxiation due to hemoptysis after lung biopsy. Even hepatic hemangiomas can be biopsied with relative impunity using 20- or 22-gauge needles.[50,51] Secondary infection is rare.[52] Despite the theoretical risk of seeding tumor cells along the needle tract, reports of needle tract tumor implants are very uncommon,[53-55] and animal studies have shown the phenomenon to be highly unlikely.[56,57] Further, survival rates for patients with breast, lung, and kidney cancers diagnosed by FNAB have been shown to be similar to those of patients with these cancers diagnosed by open surgical biopsy.[8]

The most common complication of FNAB is pneumothorax, associated with biopsy of lesions in the lung and mediastinum. Pneumothorax occurs in 20% to 41% of these patients, with chest tube drainage required in 5% to 13% of patients undergoing biopsy.[38,40,58-60] The use of a blood patch does not reduce this frequency.[61] In one series of 673 transthoracic needle biopsies, 98% of all pneumothoraces were detected on chest radiographs obtained 1 hour after biopsy, and all pneumothoraces were apparent on chest radiographs obtained 4 hours after biopsy. All pneumothoraces requiring treatment were evident within 1 hour of biopsy, and 88% of these were evident immediately after biopsy.[59] With 4 hours of observation following biopsy, the procedure can be safely performed on an outpatient basis.[58,59] Many pneumothoraces can also be managed on an outpatient basis,

TABLE 20-9. Complications of Fine Needle Aspiration Biopsy (FNAB)

Complication (Refs.)	Frequency
Death* [8,49]	<0.01%
Hemorrhage[49]	<1%
Infection[52]	Rare
Tumor seeding[53-57]	Rare
Pneumothorax (biopsy of lung and mediastinum)[38,40,58-60]	20%–41%
Pneumothorax requiring treatment (biopsy of lung and mediastinum)[38,40,58-60]	5%–13%

* Markedly increased risk with fine-needle aspiration biopsy of pheochromocytoma.[64,65]

with a small, 9-F chest tube placed percutaneously by the radiologist.[58,60,62]

Although biopsy of most adrenal masses is no more dangerous than biopsies of other parts of the body,[44,45,63] inadvertent FNAB of pheochromocytomas is potentially lethal. Several cases of severe hypertension, hypotension, and massive hemorrhage have been reported.[64,65] Since pheochromocytoma is not always clinically evident, caution is in order when adrenal biopsy is performed. Preliminary evidence suggests that MR imaging can distinguish pheochromocytomas from other adrenal masses such as metastases and cortical adenomas.[66]

CANCER TREATMENT

The application of intravascular catheter techniques to the therapy of tumors can be divided into two major modalities, regional chemotherapy delivered through selectively positioned catheters, and infarction of tumor by embolization. Both modalities have benefited from the development of highly selective catheter techniques and suitable embolizing agents. The most recent development is chemoembolization, a combination of both methodologies in which the blood supply to the tumor is occluded with a mixture of embolic material and a chemotherapeutic agent, thereby providing both an ischemic and a chemotherapeutic component to the therapy.

INTRA-ARTERIAL CHEMOTHERAPY

Selective intra-arterial infusion of chemotherapeutic agents is based on the principle that tumor response increases with drug exposure. The narrow therapeutic index of many anticancer drugs limits the systemic dose of chemotherapeutic agent and provides a rationale for selective intra-arterial chemotherapy.[67-69] Infusion of chemotherapeutic agents directly into the arterial supply of a neoplasm can produce higher drug concentrations in the tumor-bearing region without corresponding increases in systemic concentration. The most common target has been metastatic disease in the liver,[70-73] but primary bone sarcomas,[74] pelvic tumors,[75-77] and head and neck tumors[78,79] have all been treated in this way.

Broad experience, meticulous technique, and persistent efforts are required of the angiographer to complete many of these treatment courses. Prior to treatment of hepatic tumors, angiographic occlusion of accessory hepatic arteries or the gastroduodenal artery may be required (Fig. 20-30).[80-83] Occlusion of the hepatic artery frequently complicates prolonged or repeated infusions, and collateral vessels may have to be used for later cycles.[84] Narrowing of the extrahepatic and intrahepatic biliary ducts due to cholangitis induced by the chemotherapeutic agent occurs with distressing frequency.[85-89] In the brain, severe unilateral retinal toxicity complicates internal carotid artery infusions proximal to the ophthalmic artery, and specialized catheters have been designed to permit perfusion distal to the carotid siphon.[90-91]

Because infusion rates for chemotherapeutic agents are

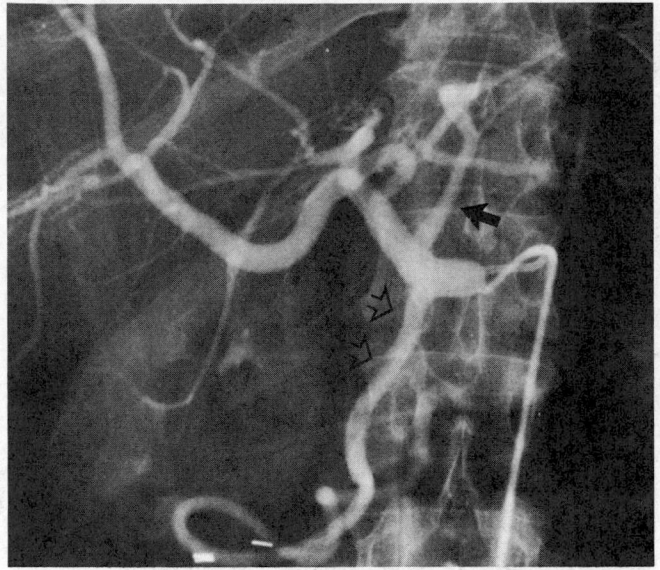

A

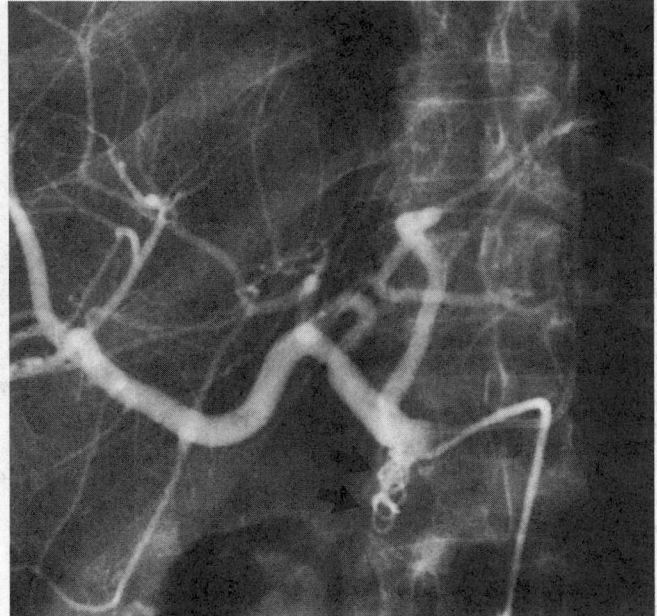

B

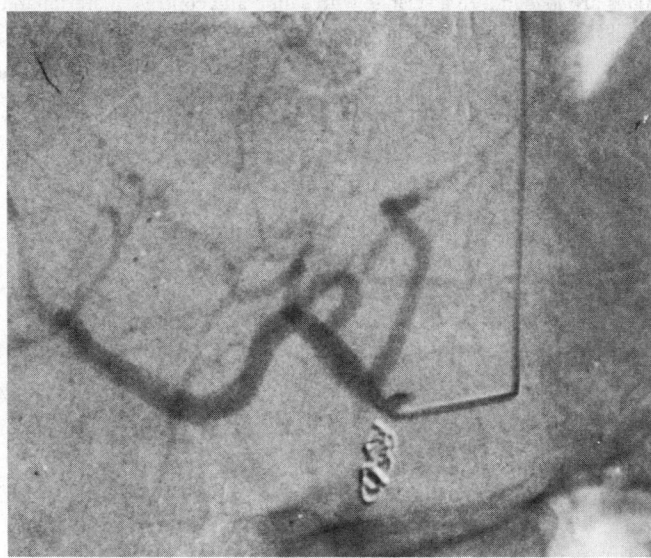

C

FIG. 20-30. Hepatic artery infusion chemotherapy may require the use of interventional radiologic techniques. **A.** A preinfusion, common hepatic artery angiogram reveals that the gastroduodenal artery (*open arrows*) arises nearly opposite the left hepatic artery (*solid arrow*). The origin of the gastroduodenal artery must be blocked or drug will enter its vascular territory and cause gastric, duodenal, and pancreatic toxicity. **B.** The gastroduodenal artery has been occluded at its origin with Gianturco-Wallace-Anderson coils (*arrows*) delivered through the angiographic catheter. Retrograde filling of the gastroduodenal artery from the superior mesenteric artery via the pancreatic arcades will maintain blood supply to the duodenum and pancreas. **C.** Contrast material administered through the infusion catheter fills the right and left hepatic arteries but not the gastroduodenal artery. The effect is equivalent to surgical ligation of the gastroduodenal artery.

invariably very slow, uniform perfusion may not occur, due to the tendency for streaming when slow infusions are performed into a rapidly moving bloodstream.[92,93] Techniques for determining perfusion patterns have been developed, and various pumps have been devised in an attempt to improve the uniformity of distribution of the chemotherapeutic agent.[94–96]

EMBOLIZATION

General Principles

Transcatheter embolization seeks to induce necrosis of tumor by obstructing its arterial supply. This usually entails deliberate sacrifice of the organ of origin, as in embolization of hypernephromas. In the liver, with its dual blood supply, tumor can be embolized via the hepatic artery while the normal hepatic parenchyma is sustained by portal venous inflow.

Embolizing agents can be categorized on the basis of the duration of vascular occlusion (temporary versus long-acting) and site of occlusion (peripheral versus proximal). Temporary agents, such as absorbable gelatin sponge (Gelfoam dental packs) (Fig. 20-31), microfibrillar collagen hemostat (Avitene), and autologous clot, are resorbed over a period of days to weeks. Permanent agents, such as polyvinyl alcohol foam (Ivalon) and Gianturco-Wallace-Anderson coils

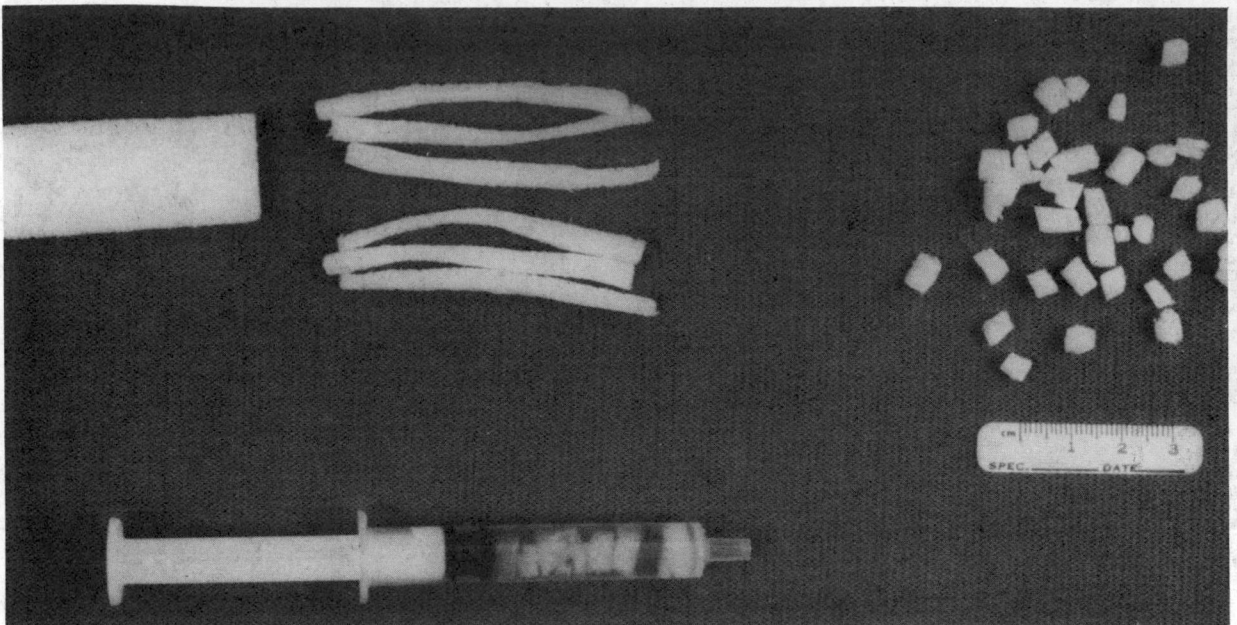

FIG. 20-31. Gelfoam is cut into segments and cubes for arterial embolization. Five to ten cubes are loaded into a syringe with saline and contrast material and injected into the artery for peripheral embolization. They are guided by blood flow in the vessel (flow-guided embolization). (Reprinted from Wallace S, Charnsangavej C, Carrasco CH: Transcatheter management of the cancer patient. In DeVita VT Jr, Hellman S, Rosenberg SA [eds]: Cancer: Principles and Practice of Oncology, 2nd ed, p 2305. Philadelphia, JB Lippincott, 1985)

(Fig. 20-32) are not metabolized, although the embolic effects may not be permanent in all cases.[97]

Even more important than the choice between temporary and permanent agents is the choice between peripheral and proximal occluding agents. Alcohol (dehydrated alcohol injection, USP), which acts as far peripherally as the capillary level, and absorbable gelatin powder (Gelfoam sterile powder), which lodges in arterioles, both cause vascular occlusion at a level distal to any possible collateral anastomoses, and cause necrosis of the embolized territory. Gelfoam pledgets (which are cut into small pieces prior to use, and fragment further as they pass through the angiographic catheter) and Ivalon both cause occlusion proximal to the most distal level of vascular anastomoses. They produce a peripheral embolic effect without infarction. At the most proximal level, coils occlude vessels 2 to 8 mm in diameter. In action and effect they are identical to surgical ligation.

Temporary agents are rarely used as the sole agent for tumor embolization. Also, proximal occlusion of major feeding arteries is generally ineffective in tumor embolization because of the rapidity with which collateral channels develop. Peripheral embolizing agents occlude the arterial bed of a tumor and delay the development of collateral flow. Most angiographers seek to achieve peripheral occlusion of the vascular bed of the tumor with a permanent agent and, if indicated, follow with proximal large-vessel occlusion in an effort to prolong the efficacy of the peripheral occlusion.

Applications

In many respects, tumors of the liver are ideal targets for embolic therapy. The liver has a dual blood supply from the hepatic artery (30%) and the portal vein (70%). Since primary and secondary hepatic neoplasms receive their blood supply exclusively from the hepatic artery with minimal peripheral contributions from the portal vein[98] and since the liver can survive on its portal venous inflow alone, the hepatic artery can be embolized with a great margin of safety. Carrasco et al have listed relative contraindications to hepatic artery embolization.[99] However, the major contraindication is the presence of main portal vein occlusion due to tumor or thrombus.[100] When first- or second-order branches of the portal vein are occluded, hepatic artery embolization increases the risk of segmental hepatic infarction, but there is less risk of hepatic failure. Recently, Nakao et al have sought to produce complete tumor ischemia by deliberately embolizing both the segmental hepatic arterial and portal venous branches leading to a tumor, deliberately infarcting the hepatic segment in an attempt to achieve more complete tumor necrosis.[101]

Embolization of hypernephromas is performed preoperatively to facilitate surgical resection and decrease intraoperative blood loss. It may also be used to control massive hematuria or to reduce the bulk of inoperable tumors, thereby controlling pain. No convincing evidence exists that emboli-

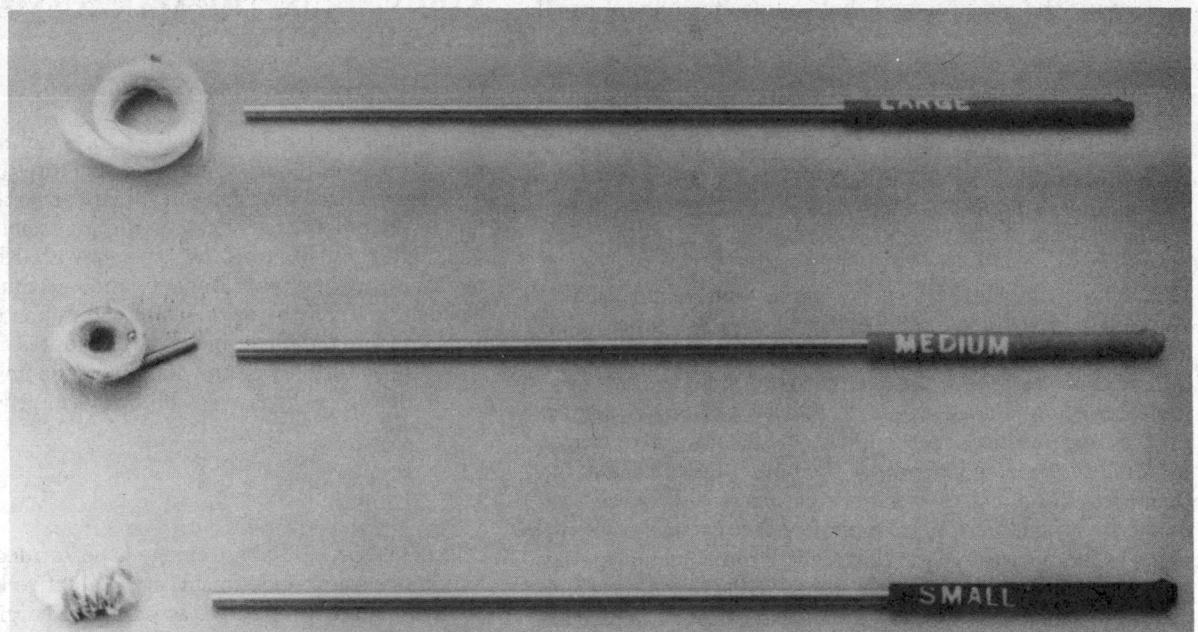

FIG. 20-32. Stainless steel coils are housed inside metal cartridges. When pushed out of the cartridge with a guidewire, the coil resumes a helical configuration. Strands of synthetic fiber are attached to the coil and help promote thrombus formation. The common sizes of coils are 3 mm, 5 mm, and 8 mm. (Reprinted from Wallace S, Charnsangavej C, Carrasco CH: Transcatheter management of the cancer patient. In DeVita VT Jr, Hellman S, Rosenberg SA [eds]: Cancer: Principles and Practice of Oncology, 2nd ed, p 2306. Philadelphia, JB Lippincott, 1985)

zation of renal tumor stimulates an immune response.[102] Infarction with absolute alcohol has replaced particulate embolization in many institutions.[103,104] Reflux of ethanol into the adrenal artery or the aorta may lead to complications.[105,106] Infusion through an occluding balloon catheter in the renal artery is essential.

Control of pain from bony metastases may be achieved with some success with selective embolization.[107,108] Transcatheter embolization has also been recommended to control massive hematuria from radiation cystitis,[109] to reduce vascularity of metastatic renal carcinoma in bone before stabilization operations,[108] and to treat bony tumors of the spine and pelvis, particularly unresectable giant cell tumors or aneurysmal bone cysts.[110]

Complications

All embolization procedures involve the risk of inadvertently embolizing nontargeted, often critical, organs. Cutaneous and mucosal injury during embolization of external carotid or internal iliac arteries has occurred, as has nerve damage, particularly when peripheral occluders such as cyanoacrylate or neurotoxic agents such as alcohol are used. The use of intra-arterial digital subtraction arteriography to monitor the embolic process has reduced the incidence of renal failure associated with excessive doses of contrast agent.

In addition to complications of the embolization procedure itself, about 50% of patients will experience a postemboliza-

tion syndrome consisting of pain, fever, and sometimes nausea and vomiting.[110a] Narcotics will control the pain, and the syndrome is self-limited (24–48 hours). Delayed complications such as abscess formation in the infarcted tumor or organ are surprisingly rare but usually require percutaneous or surgical drainage. Gas within the infarcted tumor or organ, usually demonstrated by CT, occurs routinely either due to tumor necrosis or to air introduced at the time of embolization. In the absence of clinical signs of sepsis, the demonstration of gas is not indicative of infection and antibiotic therapy is not required.[111,112]

CHEMOEMBOLIZATION

Chemoembolization combines the benefits of intra-arterial high-dose chemotherapy with obstruction of the tumor vascular bed.[113] The goal is both to prolong exposure time of the tumor to the chemotherapeutic agent and to add an ischemic component to enhance tumor necrosis.[114] The Japanese have refined this technique and directed it principally at hepatomas, first by incorporating chemotherapeutic agents into ethylcellulose microcapsules[113] and most recently by taking advantage of the prolonged sequestration of intra-arterially injected iodized oil within both primary and secondary hepatic tumors. The iodinated ethyl ester of poppyseed oil (Lipiodol, Ethiodol) is sequestered in both primary and secondary hepatic tumors when injected selectively into the hepatic artery.[115,116] This technique was originally developed to increase the visibility and thus the detectability of small hepatomas and metastases on CT. The mechanism of prolonged retention of these iodized oils within tumors has not been fully explained. Miller et al have demonstrated that in hepatic tumor models in rabbits, iodized oil accumulates within both the tumor vasculature and the abnormal hepatic sinusoids surrounding the tumor.[117]

Regardless of mechanism, the contact time between tumor and chemotherapeutic agent can be increased by combining cytotoxic drugs with iodized oil.[118,119] Takayasu et al[120] mixed Lipiodol with doxorubicin, and Konno et al[121] combined Lipiodol with SMANCS (co-poly[styrene-maleic acid] conjugated neocarzinostatin). In Takayasu's series of 99 patients, the results suggest that iodized oil by itself is an ineffective embolizing agent despite its prolonged persistence in hepatocellular carcinomas.[120] Efficacy was improved by combining iodized oil with a chemotherapeutic agent, but the most promising results were obtained with iodized oil, doxorubicin, and peripheral embolization. Particularly striking was the necrosis of small daughter tumor nodules, seen only when doxorubicin was combined with Gelfoam embolization. Although this therapy is promising, not all hepatocellular carcinomas retain iodized oil.

There is still little experience with chemoembolization in the therapy of liver metastases, although preliminary reports indicate that metastases do retain iodized oil in some instances.[115] If vascularity determines efficacy, as suggested with hepatocellular carcinomas, metastases may prove less susceptible to this interesting new modality.

DIRECT TUMOR ABLATION BY PERCUTANEOUS TECHNIQUES

Several groups[122,122a] have investigated direct intratumoral injections of alcohol. Burgener and Steinmetz injected absolute alcohol percutaneously into adenocarcinomas implanted in the hind leg of rabbits.[123] Local coagulation necrosis was produced with minimal side-effects. Sheu et al treated six patients with hepatocellular carcinomas by direct percutaneous alcohol injection.[124] Serum α-fetoprotein levels decreased in all patients in whom the initial levels were elevated, and returned to normal in two. CT demonstrated necrosis of the tumor, and in five patients follow-up biopsy showed no evidence of viable cancer cells. The role of direct intratumoral injection of alcohol or other cytotoxic agents has not been established. Particularly for avascular tumors that respond poorly to embolization and chemoembolization, such a technique may have application.

Phototherapy of tumors sensitized by the preliminary administration of a photosensitizer (hematoporphyrin derivative — H_pD) is an evolving intervention. Intravesical[125] and transbronchial[126] applications of this technique have been described. Gattenby et al treated a variety of presacral and cervical malignant masses by direct injection of a hematoporphyrin sensitizer (H_pD) followed by laser therapy through a clear plastic sheath percutaneously inserted directly into the tumor under CT control.[127] Reduction of tumor mass was observed.

ADJUNCTS IN THE MANAGEMENT OF CANCER PATIENTS

BILIARY INTERVENTIONS

While interventional radiology has a prominent role in the management of biliary stones and strictures, the major indication for biliary intervention in cancer patients is obstruction of the biliary tree. The obstructing lesion may be proximal in the biliary tree, as is seen with Klatskin tumors, metastases to the porta hepatis, and carcinoma of the gallbladder, or it may be distal, as in carcinoma of the pancreas and carcinoma of the ampulla. The intent is always the same —to relieve the obstruction and divert the flow of bile, either externally or, by bypassing the obstruction with a catheter, internally.

Indications

PALLIATION. Biliary drainage is performed either for palliation or as a prelude to surgery. Palliative biliary drainage procedures are as effective as palliative surgical bypass procedures for the relief of jaundice, and the choice of therapy (surgery versus interventional drainage) does not appear to affect survival. In two large retrospective studies[128,129] and one prospective study[130] there was no difference in mortality at 30 days or in median survival.

Biliary drainage performed as a palliative procedure should be reserved for patients with symptoms related to jaundice (pruritus, anorexia, nausea) and for patients with biliary sepsis, in whom it is a relatively low-risk procedure and potentially lifesaving.[131,132] The procedure is associated with discomfort, and an external catheter, if one is left in place, is a visible reminder to the patient of the underlying malignancy. Some patients find an external catheter psychologically unbearable. For the patient with minimal symptoms due to biliary obstruction, it is wise to remember the maxim that is difficult to make an asymptomatic patient feel better.

PREOPERATIVE DRAINAGE. Guidelines for the use of biliary drainage as a prelude to surgical bypass, rather than as the sole palliative procedure, are much less clear. Two retrospective studies[133,134] report a reduction in surgical mortality and morbidity when preoperative biliary drainage is used, while two prospective studies[132,135] conclude that the addition of preoperative biliary drainage has no effect on mortality and morbidity but does increase hospital costs. In an animal study, external biliary drainage had no effect on mortality in jaundiced rats, but internal drainage did reduce mortality significantly.[136] Another study suggests that preoperative biliary drainage is warranted when the obstructing lesion is located distally in the biliary tree and is inadvisable when the obstructing lesion is proximal.[137] There is no consensus on the appropriateness of preoperative biliary drainage,[138,139] and little guidance can be offered, save to abide by local surgical philosophy. Unfortunately, we are not yet in a position to define subsets of patients who will benefit from preoperative biliary drainage and those who will not.

CHOICE OF TECHNIQUE. The various methods of non-operative therapy of the biliary tree were extensively discussed in a 1987 review by McLean and Burke.[140] Access to the biliary tree may be obtained percutaneously, with percutaneous transhepatic biliary drainage (PTBD), or endoscopically, with endoscopic retrograde biliary drainage (ERBD). The choice of endoscopic versus percutaneous approach to the biliary tree is affected by several factors, not the least of which is the skill and experience of the local radiologist and endoscopist. ERBD requires specialized equipment and is not universally available. In patients with unfavorable anatomy due to previous gastric or duodenal surgery, the endoscopist may be unable to pass the endoscope to the level of the papilla of Vater. Very distal common bile duct obstruction may sometimes prevent cannulation of the biliary tree, and firm proximal lesions in the common hepatic duct may not permit passage of an endoprosthesis.[141] Overall, in experienced hands, ERBD is successful in approximately 90% of patients.[140-142]

PTBD has an initial success rate close to 100%, and the anatomical problems that make ERBD difficult or impossible in some patients are not a factor with PTBD.[128,142] However, ERBD is associated with fewer bleeding complications than PTBD and better patient acceptance.[142] Ascites, coagulopathies, and intrahepatic metastases are relative contraindications to PTBD but not to ERBD.

A final consideration is the use of an endoprosthesis (an entirely internal biliary stent) versus a catheter which extends outside the patient. Endoprostheses can be placed via both PTBD and ERBD, and occasionally both techniques are used simultaneously.[143] Catheters, which can be used for both internal and external drainage, must be placed percutaneously. Endoprostheses have the major advantage of providing relief of obstruction without a protruding external catheter, which may be uncomfortable and psychologically unsettling.[144] However, since access to the biliary tree is lost when the endoprosthesis is placed, ERBD or PTBD must be repeated to remove and replace the endoprosthesis when it becomes occluded.[145,146] Catheters can be irrigated daily to maintain patency, and changing them is a relatively simple matter since access to the biliary tree is available.

An additional factor is that endoprostheses placed endoscopically are usually smaller than those placed by PTBD.[138] While even 6-F catheters permit adequate bile flow in vitro, clinical observation has demonstrated that 10- to 12-F catheters are necessary for adequate drainage in some patients.[147] Endoprostheses of this size often cannot be placed endoscopically, but require a percutaneous approach.[138]

In general, patients with malignant disease and a life expectancy of less than 4 months may be best served by placement of an endoprosthesis with ERBD, if possible.[138,141,144,148] A randomized prospective trial of endoprosthesis placement via ERBD versus PTBD in 75 patients with malignant obstructive jaundice demonstrated a statistically significant higher success rate for relief of jaundice and a significantly lower 30-day mortality for ERBD.[149] In other patients, the choice between endoprosthesis and catheter drainage depends mostly on the individual patient's preference and the technical feasibility and availability of ERBD.

Technique

Before any type of biliary drainage is considered, the diagnosis of biliary obstruction must be made. In patients with an elevated total bilirubin level (>5 mg/dl), dilation of the intrahepatic biliary tree is usually obvious on US. Nonetheless, both obstruction without dilation and dilation without obstruction are well-recognized though uncommon phenomena.[150,151] CT, radionuclide hepatobiliary scintigraphy, and endoscopic retrograde cholangiopancreatography (ERCP) are useful in patients with equivocal US findings.[139,152] Percutaneous transhepatic cholangiography (PTC) with a fine needle is both safe and diagnostic[153] but is more invasive than the other diagnostic studies. When PTC is performed on an obstructed biliary system, an immediate drainage procedure should be considered to prevent leakage of bile along the needle track and into the peritoneum, which may otherwise occur and may cause bile peritonitis.[140]

The first step in biliary drainage is cholangiography, to opacify the biliary tree. Biliary anatomy and the number, location, and appearance of all obstructing lesions must be defined. Cholangiography may be done via either PTC or ERCP, depending on whether drainage is to be performed percutaneously or endoscopically.

For PTBD, a guide wire is then advanced into the biliary tree, and a drainage catheter is placed either proximal to or past the obstruction. If the catheter has not been placed through the obstruction, bile must be drained externally into a collecting bag (external drainage). If the obstruction has been negotiated, bile can pass through proximal sideholes in the catheter and exit distal to the obstruction, reestablishing a physiologically normal bile pathway and draining internally into the duodenum (internal drainage) (Fig. 20-33). If extensive manipulation is required to negotiate the obstruction or if the patient is septic, external drainage is instituted initially, followed 1 to 3 days later by negotiation of the obstruction. The delay permits the ducts to return to normal caliber and allows inflammation in the area of the obstruction to subside.[140] Subsequently, an entirely internal endoprosthesis may be placed across the obstruction, if desired.[148]

With ERBD, the entire procedure is performed endoscopically. Temporary external drainage can be instituted with a nasobiliary catheter, or an endoprosthesis can be placed at the initial sitting. ERBD often requires endoscopic sphincterotomy or papillotomy to ease catheter or endoprosthesis insertion into the common bile duct, but this is not invariably necessary.[140,141,146]

Regardless of the method used to enter the biliary tree, bile samples are obtained for culture and cytology. In the setting of biliary obstruction, Suzuki et al demonstrated infected bile in 89% of patients with fever and 39% of afebrile patients.[154] Escherichia coli and Klebsiella were the most frequent aerobic species. Anaerobes were much less frequent. In another study, Muro et al obtained 10-ml samples of bile during the course of PTBD.[155] Bile cytology was positive in 34% of 100 patients with malignant obstruction of the biliary tree. If desired, brush, screw, and core biopsies of the obstructing lesion can also be obtained via the biliary tree.[156]

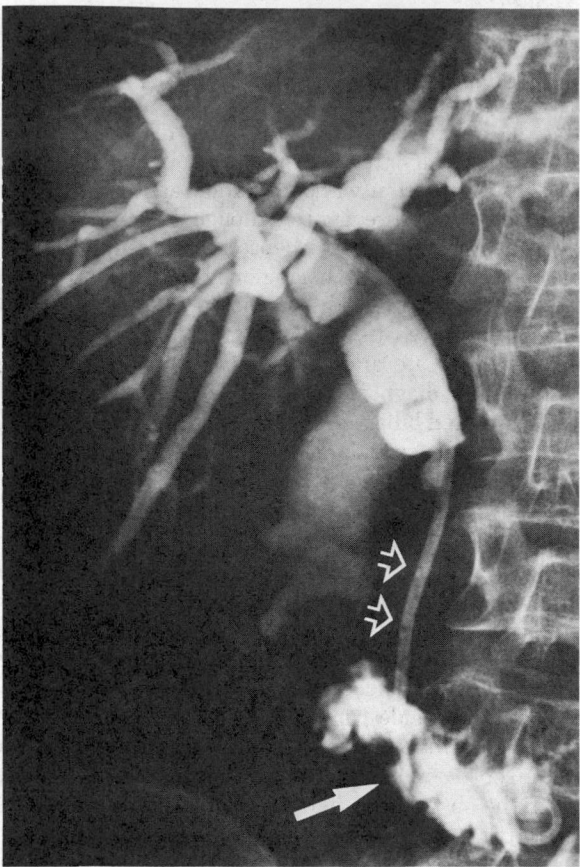

FIG. 20-33. Internal drainage with a percutaneously placed transhepatic biliary drainage catheter. The catheter traverses the area of obstruction in the common bile duct (*open arrows*) and terminates in the duodenum (*long arrow*). Bile enters the catheter through sideholes proximal to the obstruction and exits through sideholes in the duodenum.

Efficacy

Biliary drainage procedures (both PTBD and ERBD) are unquestionably effective for the relief of obstruction and cholestasis. In one series, the mean serum bilirubin level decreased from 15.7 mg/dl before drainage to 4.9 mg/dl 10 days after drainage.[148] In another study, the decrease in bilirubin showed a negative exponential correlation with the duration of drainage.[128] In a third study, the rate of decrease in bilirubin ranged from 0.23 to 4.9 mg/dl/day (mean, 1.4 mg/dl/day) and had no relation to the initial bilirubin value.[157] In patients with proximal obstruction of the biliary tree at or above the level of the bifurcation of the common hepatic duct, relief of jaundice will still occur even if only a portion of the biliary tree is drained. However, cholangitis may develop in the undrained segment, and placement of a second catheter may be required.

Complications

PTBD and ERBD are associated with different types of complications that occur with different frequencies.[142] PTBD results in death in 2% to 9% of patients.[128,158-160] Major complications, including septic shock, pleural effusions, bile peritonitis, hepatic abscess and major hemorrhage, occur in an additional 5% to 17%.[128,158,160] Cholangitis is the most common complication, occurring acutely in approximately 20% of patients. (In debilitated cancer patients, cholangitis may occur, either early or late, in up to 47% of those undergoing PTBD.[159]) Overall, between 20% and 69% of patients will eventually experience some kind of complication.[128,158,159,161] Tumor spread as a result of PTBD has been reported.[161,162]

In contrast, ERBD is considerably safer. Mortality is 4% or less. Major acute complications are seen in 3% to 10% of patients. The overall complication rate is 10% to 18%, and bleeding complications are far less likely with ERBD than with PTBD.[141,142,146] ERBD is safer because it is not necessary to transgress the liver capsule or push catheters through the hepatic parenchyma. The primary risk is that associated with endoscopic sphincterotomy, which has a mortality of 1% to 2% and a major complication rate of 7%.[140]

Intervention in the Gallbladder

In some critically ill, high-risk patients, standard surgical therapy for cholecystitis, gallbladder abscess, and malignant obstruction of the gallbladder may carry high morbidity and mortality.[163] These patients are candidates for percutaneous cholecystostomy. The gallbladder can be punctured percutaneously with a fine needle, and bile obtained for culture.[164] The gallbladder may be opacified with contrast material to diagnose obstruction, and drainage can be instituted for empyema, acute calculous or acalculous cholecystitis, or common bile duct obstruction (Fig. 20-34).[164,165] The procedure may be guided by US or CT. If a portable real-time US unit is used, the entire intervention can be performed as a bedside procedure. The complication rate is low, with no major complications in one series of 17 high-risk patients.[163] Serious vagal reactions have been reported in some patients, especially those with acutely inflamed gallbladders.[164] Although this procedure does not provide access to the entire biliary tree, it is a useful and minimally invasive adjunct in critically ill patients with gallbladder disease.

URINARY TRACT INTERVENTIONS

Since the first report of percutaneous nephrostomy (PCN) in 1955,[166] the number of conditions treated in this fashion has greatly expanded as a result of the development of interventional radiology and endourology.[167-169] Nonetheless, the primary indication for PCN in the oncology patient continues to be urinary diversion, and it has largely replaced operative nephrostomy tube placement for this purpose.

Guidance for PCN can be provided by fluoroscopy, US, CT, or a combination of these methods.[167] Generally, the skin entry site is along the posterior axillary line, below the 12th rib, and the needle is directed toward the posterolateral cortex of the kidney. More cephalad entry sites risk pneumothorax and injury to the spleen or liver. Adjustments in technique are required for splenomegaly, scoliosis, and anomalous rotations and positions of the kidney.

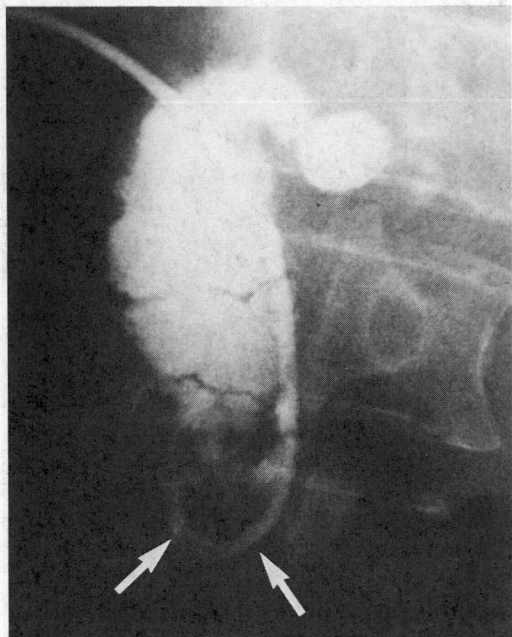

A

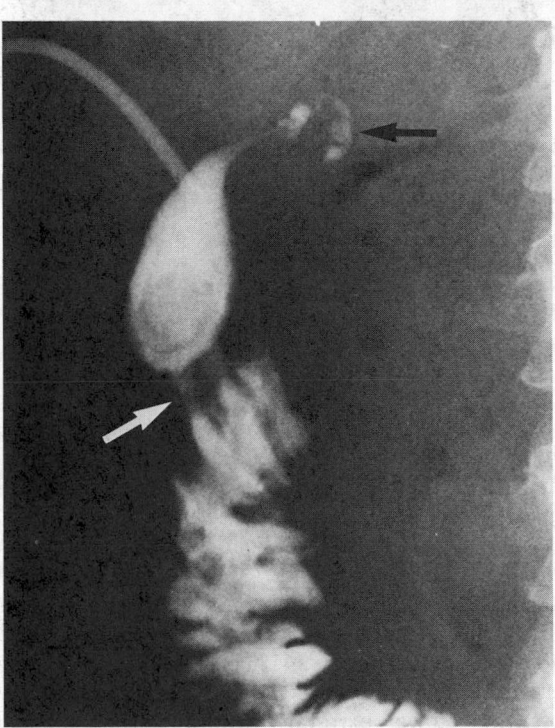

B

FIG. 20-34. Percutaneous cholecystostomy for empyema of the gallbladder. Obstruction of the common bile duct was also present because of a malignant islet cell tumor. **A**. Percutaneous cholecystostomy was performed with ultrasound and fluoroscopic guidance. The catheter tip (*arrows*) is seen in the fundus of the partially opacified gallbladder. **B**. The patient subsequently underwent surgical cholecystoenterostomy as a permanent bypass procedure. The cholecystostomy catheter was left in place in the immediate postoperative period. A contrast study demonstrates the anastomosis (*white arrow*) and reflux of contrast material into the cystic duct (*black arrow*).

Types of Urologic Prostheses

There are three basic types of prostheses for urinary drainage: nephrostomy catheters, internal stents, and external stent catheters. Nephrostomy catheters are short catheters placed in the renal pelvis or upper collecting system to divert urine externally. They do not stent the ureter and cannot be used for internal drainage. They are the simplest devices to place and to change.

Double-J or double-pigtail stents have largely replaced other designs for entirely internal ureteral stents.[170,171] Both the end in the renal pelvis and the end in the bladder have a J or pigtail shape to reduce mucosal irritation and prevent migration (Fig. 20-35). These catheters can be placed using either an antegrade (percutaneous) approach or a retrograde (cystoscopic) approach.[172,173]

The third general type of urologic prosthesis is the ureteral stent with external drainage or access port (nephroureterostomy).[170] In some ways this is the most versatile of the urologic prostheses. The external port may be used for external drainage or can be capped off for internal drainage, and it provides easy accessibility when the catheter needs to be changed.

Each type of urologic prosthesis has advantages and disadvantages. Simple nephrostomy diversion uses a urine collection appliance that requires daily maintenance and is unsuitable for patients who are poorly motivated or who have altered mental status. Some patients find it socially unacceptable. Internal stents obviate many of these inconveniences, but cystoscopy is required for removal or replacement of the stent. Because there is no outward indicator of stent function, stent failure can be insidious and permanent renal damage may occur before it is recognized (see Fig. 20-35). In contrast, nephrostomy tube failure is readily identified by decreased urine volume, leakage around the catheter, fever, or flank pain that leads the patient to seek prompt attention. All urologic prostheses should be changed prophylactically on a regular basis.[171,174,175]

Complications

The mortality associated with PCN is less than 0.2%, and significant complications occur at the rate of only 4% to 5%.[167,176] By contrast, mortality for surgical urinary diversion in the oncology patient is about 3% to 8%, and the complication rate is 25% to 45%.[177,178]

Serious complications associated with PCN are primarily related to septicemia and hemorrhage. Septicemia, including septic shock, occurs in 1% to 2% of patients, most often those with preexisting infection.[179] Minor bleeding is common but clears within a few days. Clinically significant hemorrhage occurs at a rate of 1% to 2%.[167,180] Bleeding may be into the collecting system, the renal parenchyma and subcapsular tissue, or the perinephric space and retroperitoneum.[181,182] Hemorrhage may be delayed rather than immediate, since the nephrostomy tube may initially tamponade the injured vessel.[183]

Permanent injury to the kidney from PCN is rare. In a study of 36 patients 3 years or more after PCN, only one patient had a focal cortical scar that appeared to be related to

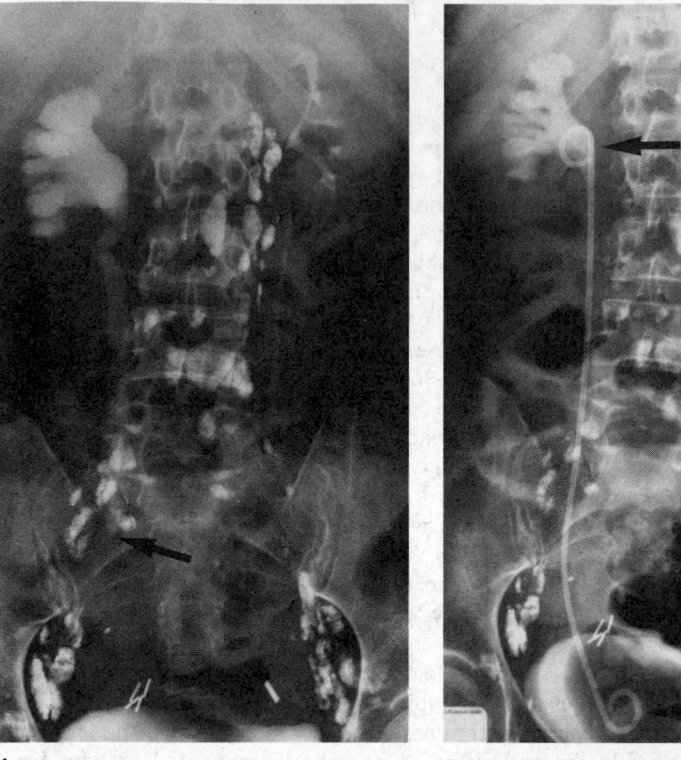
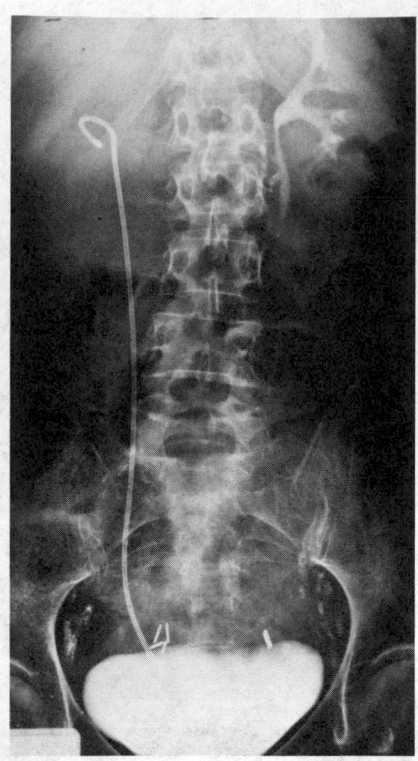

A   B   C

FIG. 20-35. Complete obstruction of the right ureter in a woman with ovarian carcinoma. **A.** The initial intravenous urogram demonstrates hydronephrosis of the right kidney and complete obstruction of the right ureter (*arrow*). **B.** The patient refused any drainage device that was not completely internal. A double pigtail internal ureteral stent was placed percutaneously. One pigtail is in the renal pelvis and the other in the bladder (arrows). **C.** The patient returned for a routine follow-up intravenous urogram 2 months later. She was asymptomatic, but the urogram revealed complete obstruction of the right kidney. The internal stent was removed cystoscopically and a new one placed. The lumen of the original stent was completely blocked by encrustations.

PCN.[184] (For additional information, see Chapter 58, section 5).

OTHER INTERVENTIONS

PERCUTANEOUS PLACEMENT OF INFERIOR VENA CAVA FILTERS. Cancer is a frequent underlying cause of pulmonary embolic disease and a common indication for placement of inferior vena cava (IVC) filters.[185,186] A number of filters have been developed.[187-191] Of these, only two —the Mobin-Uddin filter and the Greenfield filter (Fig. 20-36)— have been in general clinical use. Both can be inserted percutaneously.[192-194] The Mobin-Uddin filter had a high rate of IVC occlusion,[195] and is no longer available.[191]

The Greenfield filter can be inserted surgically or percutaneously through either the femoral vein or the jugular vein, using a carrier system (see Fig. 20-36). Percutaneous insertion avoids the necessity of venotomy and a large surgical incision. The entire procedure can be performed in the radiology department, and much of the discomfort and expense of surgery is avoided. Although metastatic cancer may be a relative contraindication to surgical placement of an IVC

filter,[185] the use of the percutaneous technique eliminates much of this objection since an experienced angiographer can insert a Greenfield filter percutaneously in 10 to 20 minutes with little discomfort to the patient.[193]

In two small series, no complications were observed after percutaneous filter placement.[192,196] In other larger series, the incidence of femoral vein thrombosis after percutaneous filter placement via the femoral route was 2% to 10%.[197-199] In one series of 17 patients, 41% had venographic evidence of femoral vein thrombosis, but only 12% had significant symptoms.[200] Lower extremity swelling, when present, is usually transient.

PERCUTANEOUS ENTEROSTOMY. Percutaneous gastrostomy is a valuable adjunct in patients who require enteral alimentation. It is also occasionally useful for chronic gastrointestinal decompression.[201,202] Percutaneous gastrostomy may be performed by a radiologist, using a trocar or the Seldinger technique,[203-207] or by a surgeon or gastroenterologist using an endoscope.[201,208,209] In either case, local anesthesia is all that is usually required. Fixation and adherence of the stomach to the anterior abdominal wall usually occurs

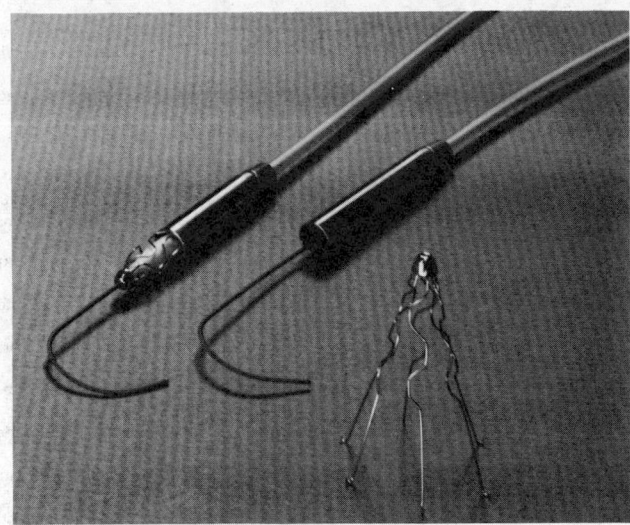

FIG. 20-36. The Greenfield filter (*foreground*) is a conical device designed to be inserted using a special carrier. Different carriers are available for insertion through the femoral vein (*left*) or the jugular vein (*center*). (Courtesy of Medi-tech, Inc., Watertown, MA)

within days.[205,208] In two series totaling 637 endoscopic percutaneous gastrostomies there was a 0.3% to 1.0% mortality and a 3% to 6% rate of major complications.[208,209] There were no major complications in one series of 32 patients who underwent radiologic percutaneous gastrostomy, two major complications in another series of 40 patients, and two major complications in a third series of 72 radiologic procedures.[204,206,207] The endoscopic technique cannot be used in patients with esophageal obstruction, and previous gastric surgery (*e.g.*, Billroth II procedure) may make either approach difficult or impossible.

Percutaneous radiologic techniques can also be used for enterostomy elsewhere in the gastrointestinal tract. There are reports of percutaneous cecostomy for drug instillation and for therapy of Ogilvie's syndrome (adynamic ileus of the colon).[210,211] Leakage of fecal material into the peritoneal cavity does not appear to be a problem. This technique has also been used for nonsurgical relief of a closed-loop small bowel obstruction.[212] As of 1988, these procedures must still be considered experimental.

MISCELLANEOUS PROCEDURES. The patient with cancer often has other medical problems as well, and radiologic interventions of many types may occasionally be useful. New forms of radiologic intervention and new methods for better accomplishing existing interventions are being developed on an almost daily basis. Abscess drainage, management of gastrointestinal bleeding, transluminal angioplasty, intra-arterial and intravenous thrombolysis, treatment of biliary and urinary stones and strictures, and removal of intravascular foreign bodies may all be accomplished by a well-trained radiologist. Radiologic intervention has had and will continue to have a major impact on the practice of oncology.

REFERENCES

1. White RI Jr: Interventional radiology: Reflections and expectations. The 1985 Eugene P. Pendergrass New Horizons Lecture. Radiology 162:593–600, 1987
2. Margolis AR: Interventional diagnostic radiology: A new subspecialty. AJR 99:761–762, 1967
3. Doby T: A tribute to Sven-Ivar Seldinger. AJR 142:1–3, 1984
4. Grüntzig A, Hopff H: Perkutane Rekanalization chronischer Arteriellar verschlüsse mit einem neuen Dilationskatheter: Modification der Dotter-technik. Dtsch Med Wochenschr 99:2502–2505, 1974
5. Dotter CT, Judkins MP: Transluminal treatment of arteriosclerotic obstruction: Description of a new technique and a preliminary report of its application. Circulation 30:654–670, 1964
6. Baum S, Nusbaum, M, Blakemore W: Demonstration of intraabdominal bleeding by selective arteriography. JAMA 191:389–390, 1965
7. Husband JE, Golding SJ: The role of computed-tomography guided needle biopsy in an oncology service. Clin Radiol 34:255–260, 1983
8. Bottles K, Miller TR, Cohen MB et al: Fine needle aspiration biopsy: Has its time come? Am J Med 81:525–531, 1986
9. Bernardino ME: Percutaneous biopsy. AJR 142:41–45, 1984
10. Lieberman RP, Hafez GR, Crummy AB: Histology from aspiration biopsy: Turner needle experience. AJR 138:561–564, 1982
11. Wittenberg J, Mueller PR, Ferrucci JT Jr et al: Percutaneous core biopsy of abdominal tumors using 22 gauge needles: Further observations. AJR 139:75–80, 1982
12. Haaga JR, LiPuma JP, Bryan PJ et al: Clinical comparison of small- and large-caliber cutting needles for biopsy. Radiology 146:665–667, 1983
13. Weisbrod GL, Herman SJ, Tao L-C: Preliminary experience with a dual cutting edge needle in thoracic percutaneous fine-needle aspiration biopsy. Radiology 163:75–78, 1987
14. Grant EG, Richardson JD, Smirniotopoulous JG et al: fine-needle biopsy directed by real-time sonography: Technique and accuracy. AJR 141:29–32, 1983
15. Harter LP, Moss AA, Goldberg HI et al: CT-guided fine-needle aspirations for diagnosis of benign and maligant disease. AJR 140:363–367, 1983
16. Pagani JJ: Biopsy of focal hepatic lesions: Comparison of 18 and 22 gauge needles. Radiology 147:673–675, 1983
17. Martino CR, Haaga JR, Bryan PJ et al: CT-guided liver biopsies: Eight years' experience. Work in progress. Radiology 152:755–757, 1984
18. Ayala AG, Zornosa J: Primary bone tumors: Percutaneous needle biopsy. Radiologic-pathologic study of 222 biopsies. Radiology 149:675–679, 1983
19. Pais MJ, Lightfoote JB, Burnett K et al: Trephine bone biopsy system: A refined needle for radiologists. Radiology 153:253–254, 1984
20. Larédo J-D, Bard M: Thoracic spine: Percutaneous trephine biopsy. Radiology 160:485–489, 1986
21. Mink J: Percutaneous bone biopsy in the patient with known or suspected osseous metastases. Radiology 161:191–194, 1986
22. Hall-Craggs MA, Lees WR: Fine needle biopsy: Cytology, histology, or both? Gut 28:233–236, 1987
23. Kasugai H, Yamamoto R, Tatsuta M et al: Value of heparinized fine-needle aspiration biopsy in liver malignancy. AJR 144:243–244, 1985
24. Zajdela A, Zillhardt P, Voillemot N: Cytological diagnosis by fine needle sampling without aspiration. Cancer 59:1201–1205, 1987
25. vanSonnenberg E, Wittich GR, Edwards DK et al: Percutaneous diagnostic and interventional radiologic procedures in children: Experience in 100 patients. Radiology 162:601–605, 1987
26. Miller DA, Carrasco CH, Katz RL et al: Fine needle aspiration biopsy: The role of immediate cytologic assessment. AJR 147:155–158, 1986
27. Axel L: Simple method for performing oblique CT-guided needle biopsies. AJR 143:341–342, 1984
28. Sundaram M, Wolverson MK, Heiberg E et al: Utility of CT-guided abdominal aspiration procedures. AJR 139:1111–1115, 1982
29. Mueller PR, Stark DD, Simeone JF et al: MR-guided aspiration biopsy: Needle design and clinical trials. Radiology 161:605–609, 1986
30. Bret PM, Fond A, Casola G et al: Abdominal lesions: A prospective study of clinical efficacy of percutaneous fine-needle biopsy. Radiology 159:345–346, 1986
31. Fortier KF, Clarke-Pearson DL, Creasman WT et al: Fine-needle aspiration in gynecology: Evaluation of extrapelvic lesions in patients with gynecologic malignancy. Obstet Gynecol 65:67–73, 1985
32. Gobien RP, Bouchard EA, Gobien BS et al: Thin-needle aspiration biopsy of thoracic lesions: Impact on hospital charges and patterns of patient care. Radiology 148:65–67, 1983
33. Westcott JL: Direct percutaneous needle aspiration of localized pulmonary lesions: Results in 422 patients. Radiology 137:31–35, 1980
34. Mitty HA, Efremidis SC, Yeh H-C: Impact of fine-needle biopsy on management of patients with carcinoma of the pancreas. AJR 137:1119–1121, 1981
35. Diament MJ, Boechat MI, Kangarloo H: Interventional radiology in infants and children: Clinical and technical aspects. Radiology 154:359–361, 1985
36. Towbin RB, Strife JL: Percutaneous aspiration, drainage and biopsies in children. Radiology 157:81–85, 1985
37. Ferrucci JT Jr, Wittenberg J, Mueller PR et al: Diagnosis of abdominal malignancy by radiologic fine-needle aspiration biopsy. AJR 134:323–330, 1980
38. Khouri NF, Stitik FP, Erozan YS et al: Transthoracic needle aspiration biopsy of benign and malignant lung lesions. AJR 144:281–288, 1985

39. Stanley JH, Fish GD, Andriole JG et al: Lung lesions: Cytologic diagnosis by fine-needle biopsy. Radiology 162:389–391, 1987
40. Westcott JL: Percutaneous needle aspiration of hilar and mediastinal masses. Radiology 151:301–304, 1981
41. Hall-Craggs MA, Lees WR: Fine-needle aspiration biopsy: Pancreatic and biliary tumors. AJR 147:399–403, 1986
42. Mitnick JS, Bosniak MA, Megibow AJ et al: Nonfunctioning adrenal adenomas discovered incidentally on computed tomography. Radiology 148:495–499, 1983
43. Belldegrun A, Hussain S, Seltzer SE et al: Incidentally discovered mass of the adrenal gland. Surg Gynecol Obstet 163:203–208, 1986
44. Heaston DK, Handel DB, Ashton PR et al: Narrow gauge needle aspiration of solid adrenal masses. AJR 138:1143–1148, 1982
45. Bernardino ME, Walther MM, Philips VM et al: CT-guided adrenal biopsy: Accuracy, safety, and indications. AJR 144:67–69, 1985
46. Kidd R, Crane RD, Dail DH: Lymphangiography and fine-needle aspiration biopsy: Ineffective for staging early prostate cancer. AJR 141:1007–1012, 1984
47. Kidd R, Correa R Jr: Fine needle aspiration biopsy of lymphangiographically normal lymph nodes: A negative view. AJR 141:1005–1006, 1984
48. Hewes RC, Vigorita VJ, Freiberger RH: Percutaneous bone biopsy: The importance of aspirated osseous blood. Radiology 148:69–72, 1983
49. Rose JS: Invasive Radiology: Risks and Patient Care, p 122. Chicago, Year Book Medical Publishers, 1983
50. Solbiati L, Livraghi T, De Pra L et al: Fine-needle biopsy of hepatic hemangioma with sonographic guidance. AJR 144:471–474, 1985
51. Cronan JJ, Esparza AR, Dorfman GS et al: Cavernous hemangioma of the liver: Role of percutaneous biopsy. Radiology 166:135–138, 1988
52. Martin CR, Haaga JR, Bryan PJ: Secondary infection of an endometrioma following fine-needle aspiration. Radiology 151:53–54, 1984
53. Ferrucci JT Jr, Wittenberg J, Margolies MN et al: Malignant seeding of the tract after thin needle aspiration biopsy. Radiology 130:345–346, 1979
54. Smith FP, MacDonald JS, Schein S et al: Cutaneous seeding of pancreatic cancer by skinny needle aspiration biopsy. Arch Intern Med 140:855, 1980
55. Sinner WN, Zajicek J: Implantation metastasis after percutaneous transthoracic needle aspiration biopsy. Acta Radiol [Diagn] 17:473–480, 1976
56. Eriksson O, Hagmar B, Ryo W: Effects of fine-needle aspiration and other biopsy procedures on tumor dissemination in mice. Cancer 54:73–78, 1984
57. Mühlberger G, Gottschalk A, Gericke D: Needle biopsy and metastasis: Investigations in rats. Radiologe 23:185–188, 1983
58. Stevens GM, Jackman RJ: Outpatient needle biopsy of the lung: Its safety and utility. Radiology 151:301–304, 1984
59. Perlmutt LM, Braun SD, Newman GE et al: Timing of chest film follow-up after transthoracic needle aspiration. AJR 146:1049–1050, 1986
60. Perlmutt LM, Braun SD, Newman GE et al: Transthoracic needle aspiration: Use of a small chest tube to treat pneumothorax. AJR 148:849–851, 1987
61. Bourgouin PM, Shepard J-AO, McCloud TC et al: Transthoracic needle aspiration biopsy: Evaluation of the blood patch technique. Radiology 166:93–95, 1988
62. Casola G, vanSonnenberg E, Keightley A et al: Pneumothorax: Radiologic treatment with small catheters. Radiology 166:89–91, 1988
63. Pagani JJ: Normal adrenal glands in small cell lung carcinoma: CT-guided biopsy. AJR 140:949–951, 1983
64. McCorkell SJ, Niles NL: Fine-needle aspiration of catecholamine-producing adrenal masses: A possibly fatal mistake. AJR 145:113–114, 1985
65. Casola G, Nicolet V, vanSonnenberg E et al: Unsuspected pheochromocytoma: Risk of blood-pressure alterations during percutaneous adrenal biopsy. Radiology 159:733–735, 1986
66. Reining JW, Doppman JL, Dwyer AJ et al: MRI of indeterminate adrenal masses. AJR 147:493–496, 1986
67. Eckman WW, Patlak CS, Fenstermacher JD: Critical evaluation of principles governing the advantages of intra-arterial infusion. J Pharmacokinet Biopharm 102:221–229, 1974
68. Chen HG, Gross JK: Intra-arterial infusion of anticancer drugs: Theoretical aspects of drug delivery and review of response. Cancer Treat Rep 64:31–40, 1980
69. Dedrick RI, Oldfield EH, Collins JM: Arterial drug infusions with extracorporeal removal: I. Theoretical basis with particular reference to brain. Cancer Treat Rep 68:373–380, 1984
70. Sullivan RD, Norcross JW, Watkins E Jr: Chemotherapy of metastatic liver cancer by prolonged hepatic artery infusion. N Engl J Med 270:321, 1964
71. Patt YZ, Chuang VP, Wallace S et al: The palliative role of hepatic artery infusion and arterial occlusion in colorectal carcinoma metastatic to the liver. Lancet 1:349–351, 1981
72. Patt YZ, Peters RE, Chuang VP et al: Effective retreatment of patients with colorectal cancer and liver metastases. Am J Med 75:237–240, 1983
73. Patt YZ, Chuang VP, Wallace S: Hepatic arterial chemotherapy and occlusion for palliation of primary hepatocellular and unknown primary neoplasm in the liver. Cancer 51:1359–1363, 1983
74. Benjamin RS, Murray JA, Wallace S et al: Intra-arterial preoperative chemotherapy for osteosarcoma: A judicious approach to limb salvage. Cancer Bull 36:32–36, 1984
75. Wallace S, Chuang VP, Samuels ML et al: Transcatheter intra-arterial infusion of chemotherapy in advanced bladder cancer. Cancer 49:640–645, 1982
76. Logothetis CJ, Samuels ML, Wallace S et al: Management of pelvic complication of malignant urothelial tumors with combined intra-arterial and IV chemotherapy. Cancer Treat Rep 66:1501–1507, 1982
77. Scarabelli C, Tumolo S, De Paoli A et al: Intermittent pelvic arterial infusion with peptichemo, doxorubicin and cisplatin for locally advanced and recurrent carcinoma of the uterine cervix. Cancer 60:25–30, 1987
78. Molinori R: Present role of intra-arterial regional chemotherapy in head and neck cancer. Drugs Exp Clin Res 7:491–504, 1983
79. Lee YY, Wallace S, Dimery I et al: Intra-arterial chemotherapy of head and neck tumors. AJNR 7:343, 1986
80. Kuribayashi S, Phillips DA, Harrington DP et al: Therapeutic embolization of the gastroduodenal artery in hepatic artery infusion chemotherapy. AJR 137:1169, 1981
81. Granmayeh M, Wallace S, Schwarten D: Catheter occlusion of the gastroduodenal artery. Radiology 131:59–64, 1979
82. Michels NA: Blood Supply and Anatomy of the Upper Abdominal Organs, p 581. Philadelphia, JB Lippincott, 1955
83. Chuang VP, Wallace S: Hepatic arterial redistribution for intra-arterial infusion of hepatic neoplasms. Radiology 135:295–299, 1981
84. Charnsangavej C, Chuang VP, Wallace S et al: Angiographic classification of hepatic arterial collaterals. Radiology 144:485, 1982
85. Makuuchi M, Sukigara M, Mori T et al: Bile duct necrosis: Complication of transcatheter hepatic arterial embolization. Radiology 156:331–334, 1985
86. Botet JF, Watson RC, Kemeny N et al: Cholangitis complicating intra-arterial chemotherapy in liver metastases. Radiology 156:335–337, 1985
87. Pien EH, Zeman RK, Benjamin SB et al: Iatrogenic sclerosing cholangitis following hepatic arterial chemotherapy infusion. Radiology 156:329–330, 1985
88. Shea WJ, Demas BE, Goldberg HI et al: Sclerosing cholangitis associated with hepatic arterial FUDR chemotherapy: Radiographic/histologic correlation. AJR 146:717, 1986
89. Anderson SD, Holley HC, Berland LL et al: Causes of jaundice during hepatic artery infusion chemotherapy. Radiology 161:439, 1986
90. Chrousos G, Oldfield EH, Doppman JL et al: Prevention of ocular toxicity by carmustine (BCNU) with supraophthalmic intracarotid infusion. Ophthalmology 93:1471–1475, 1986
91. Doppman JL, Dedrick RL, Shook DR et al: Glioblastoma catheter techniques for isolated chemotherapy perfusion. Radiology 159:477–483, 1986
92. Blacklock JB, Wright DC, Dedrick R et al: Drug streaming during intra-arterial chemotherapy. J Neurosurg 64:284–291, 1986
93. Lutz RJ, Dedrick RL, Boretos JW et al: Mixing studies during intracarotid artery infusions in an in vitro model. J Neurosurg 64:277–283, 1986
94. Bledin AG, Kim EE, Haynie TP: Technetium Tc 99m macroaggregated albumin angiography and perfusion: Intra-arterial chemotherapy for neoplasms. JAMA 250:941–943, 1983
95. Wright KC, Wallace S, Kim EE et al: Pulsed arterial infusions: Chemotherapeutic considerations. Cancer 57:1952–1956, 1986
96. Shook DR, Beaudet LM, Doppman JL: Uniformity of intracarotid distribution with diastole-phased pulsed infusions. J Neurosurg 67:721–725, 1987
97. Miller DL: Failure of Ivalon to provide permanent hepatic arterial occlusion. Cardiovasc Intervent Radiol 10:111–113, 1987
98. Lin G, Hagerstrand I, Lunderquist A: Portal blood supply of liver metastasis. AJR 143:53, 1984
99. Carrasco CH, Charnsangavej C, Ajani J et al: The carcinoid syndrome: Palliation by hepatic artery embolization. AJR 147:149–154, 1986
100. Yamada R, Sato M, Kawabata M et al: Hepatic artery embolization in 120 patients with unresectable hepatoma. Radiology 148:397–401, 1983
101. Nakao N, Miura K, Takahashi H et al: Hepatocellular carcinoma: combined hepatic arterial and portal venous embolization. Radiology 161:303, 1986
102. Wallace S, Charnsangavej C, Carrasco CH: Transcatheter management of the cancer patient. In DeVita VT, Hellman S, Rosenberg SA (eds): Cancer: Principles and Practice of Oncology, 2nd ed, pp 2304–2320. Philadelphia, JB Lippincott, 1986
103. Ekelund L, Ek A, Forsberg L et al: Occlusion of renal arterial tumor supply with absolute ethanol: Experience with 20 cases. Radiology 155:275, 1985
104. Klinberg I, Hunter P, Hawkins IF et al: Preoperative angioinfarction of localized renal cell carcinoma using absolute ethanol. Radiology 156:271, 1985
105. Fink IJ, Girton M, Doppman JL: Absolute ethanol injection of the adrenal artery: Hypertensive reaction. Radiology 154:357–358, 1985
106. Cox GC, Lee KR, Price HI et al: Colonic infarction following ethanol embolization of renal cell carcinoma. Radiology 145:343, 1982
107. Chuang VP, Wallace S, Swanson D et al: Arterial occlusion in the management of pain from metastatic renal carcinoma. Radiology 133:611–614, 1979
108. Bowers TA, Murray JA, Charnsangavej C et al: Bone metastasis from renal carcinoma. J Bone Joint Surg [AM] 64:749–754, 1982
109. Kobayashi I, Kusano S, Matsubayashi T et al: Selective embolization of the vesical artery in the management of massive bladder hemorrhage. Radiology 136:345–348, 1980
110. Wallace S, Granmayeh M, de Santos LA et al: Arterial occlusion of pelvic bone tumors. Cancer 43:322–328, 1979
110a. Hemingway AP, Allison DJ: Complications of embolization: Analysis of 410 procedures. Radiology 166:669–672, 1988
111. Carroll BA, Walter JF: Gas in embolized tumors: An alternate hypothesis for its origin. Radiology 147:441–444, 1983
112. Rankin RN: Gas formation after renal tumor embolization without abscess: A benign occurrence. Radiology 130:317–320, 1979
113. Kato L, Nemoto R, Mori H et al: Arterial embolization with microencapsulated anticancer drug. JAMA 245:1123–1127, 1981

114. Kerr DJ: Microparticulate drug delivery systems as an adjunct to cancer treatment. Cancer Drug Deliv 4:55–61, 1987

115. Nakakuma K, Tashiro S, Hiraoka T et al: Hepatocellular carcinoma and metastatic cancer detected by iodized oil. Radiology 154:15–17, 1985

116. Yumoto Y, Jino K, Tokuyama K et al: Hepatocellular carcinoma detected by iodized oil. Radiology 154:19–24, 1985

117. Miller DL, O'Leary TJ, Girton M: Distribution of iodized oil within the liver after hepatic arterial injection. Radiology 162:849–852, 1987

118. Ohnishi K, Tsuchiya S, Nakayama T et al: Arterial chemoembolization of hepatocellular carcinoma with mitomycin-C microcapsules. Radiology 152:51–55, 1984

119. Ohishi H, Uchida H, Yoshimura H et al: Hepatocellular carcinoma detected by iodized oil: Use of anti-cancer agents. Radiology 154:25–29, 1985

120. Takayasu K, Shima Y, Muramatsu Y et al: Hepatocellular carcinoma: Treatment with intra-arterial iodized oil with and without chemotherapeutic agents. Radiology 162:345–351, 1987

121. Konno T, Maeda H, Iwai K et al: Effect of arterial administration of high molecular-weight anticancer agent SMANCS with lipid lymphangiographic agent on hepatoma. Eur J Cancer Clin Oncol 19:1053–1065, 1983

122. Livraghi T, Festi D, Monti F et al: US-guided percutaneous alcohol injection of small hepatic and abdominal tumors. Radiology 161:309, 1986

122a. Shiina S, Yasuda H, Muto H et al: Percutaneous ethanol injection in the treatment of liver neoplasms. AJR 149:949–952, 1987

123. Burgener FA, Steinmetz SD: Treatment of experimental adenocarcinomas by percutaneous tumor injection of absolute alcohol. Invest Radiol 22:472–478, 1987

124. Sheu J-C, Huang GT, Chen DS et al. Small hepatocellular carcinoma: Intratumoral ethanol treatment using new needles and guidance system. Radiology 160:43–48, 1987

125. Misaki T, Hizazumi H, Miayoski N: Photoradiation therapy of bladder tumors. In Doiron D, Gomer CJ (eds): Porphyrin Localization and Treatment of Tumors, pp 795–804. New York, Alan R Liss, 1987

126. Hayata Y, Kato H, Konaka C et al: Hematoporphyrin derivative in laser photoradiation and treatment of lung cancer. Chest 81:269–277, 1982

127. Gattenby RA, Hartz WH, Engstrom PF et al: CT-guided laser therapy in resistant tumors: Phase I clinical trials. Radiology 163:172–175, 1987

128. Passariello R, Pavone P, Rossi P et al: Percutaneous biliary drainage in neoplastic jaundice: Statistical data from a computerized multicenter investigation. Acta Radiol [Diagn] 26:681–688, 1985

129. Bonnel D, Ferrucci JT Jr, Mueller PR et al: Surgical and radiological decompression in malignant biliary obstruction: A retrospective study using multivariate risk factor analysis. Radiology 152:347–351, 1984

130. Bornman PC, Harries-Jones EP, Tobias R et al: Prospective controlled trial of transhepatic biliary endoprosthesis versus bypass surgery for incurable carcinoma of the head of the pancreas. Lancet 1:69–71, 1986

131. Pessa ME, Hawkins IF, Vogel SB: The treatment of acute cholangitis: Percutaneous transhepatic biliary drainage before definitive therapy. Ann Surg 205:389–392, 1987

132. Thomas JH, Connor CS, Pierce GE et al: Effect of biliary decompression on morbidity and mortality of pancreaticoduodenectomy. Am J Surg 148:727–731, 1984

133. Gobien RP, Stanley JH, Soucek CD et al: Routine preoperative biliary drainage: Effect on management of obstructive jaundice. Radiology 152:353–356, 1984

134. Gundry SR, Strodel WE, Knol JA et al: Efficacy of preoperative biliary tract decompression in patients with obstructive jaundice. Arch Surg 119:703–708, 1984

135. Pitt HA, Gomes AS, Lots JF et al: Does preoperative percutaneous biliary drainage reduce operative risk or increase hospital cost? Ann Surg 201:545–553, 1985

136. Gouma DJ, Coelho JCU, Schlegal JF et al: The effect of preoperative internal and external biliary drainage on mortality of jaundiced rats. Arch Surg 122:731–734, 1987

137. Lygidakis NJ, Brummelkamp WH, Huibregtse K et al: Different response to preliminary biliary drainage in proximal versus distal malignant biliary obstruction. Surg Gynecol Obstet 164:159–162, 1987

138. McLean GK, Jordan HA: Percutaneous transhepatic biliary drainage: Comments and recommendations. Semin Intervent Radiol 2:69–73, 1985

139. Lokich JJ, Kane RA, Harrison DA et al: Biliary tract obstruction secondary to cancer: Management guidelines and selected literature review. J Clin Oncol 5:969–981, 1987

140. McLean GK, Burke DR: Nonoperative therapy of biliary obstruction. In DeVita VT Jr, Hellman S, Rosenberg SA (eds): Important Advances in Oncology 1987, pp 279–292. Philadelphia, JB Lippincott, 1987

141. Marks WM, Freeny PC, Ball TJ et al: Endoscopic retrograde biliary drainage. Radiology 152:357–360, 1984

142. Stanley J, Gobien RP, Cunningham J et al: Biliary decompression: An institutional comparison of percutaneous and endoscopic methods. Radiology 158:195–197, 1986

143. Tsang T-K, Crampton AR, Bernstein JR et al: Percutaneous-endoscopic bilary stent placement: A preliminary report. Ann Intern Med 106:389–392, 1987

144. Dick R, Platts A, Gilford J et al: The Carey–Coons percutaneous biliary endoprosthesis: A three-centre experience in 87 patients. Clin Radiol 38:175–178, 1987

145. Adam A: Use of the modified Cope introduction set for transhepatic removal of obstructed Carey-Coons biliary endoprosthesis. Clin Radiol 38:171–174, 1987

146. Walta DC, Fausel CS, Brant B: Endoscopic biliary stents and obstructive jaundice. Am J Surg 153:444–447, 1987

147. Kerlan RK Jr, Stimac G, Pogany AC et al: Bile flow through drainage catheters: An in vitro study. AJR 143:1085–1087, 1984

148. Lammer J, Neumayer K: Biliary drainage endoprostheses: Experience with 201 placements. Radiology 159:625–629, 1986

149. Speer AG, Cotton PB, Russel RCG et al: Randomised trial of endoscopic versus percutaneous stent insertion in malignant obstructive jaundice. Lancet 2:57–62, 1987

150. Ferrucci JT Jr, Adson MA, Mueller PR et al: Advances in the radiology of jaundice: A symposium and review. AJR 141:1–20, 1983

151. Beinart C, Efremidis S, Cohen B et al: Obstruction without dilatation: Importance in evaluating jaundice. JAMA 245:353–356, 1981

152. Zeman RK, Lee C, Jaffe MH et al: Hepatobiliary scintigraphy and sonography in early biliary obstruction. Radiology 153:793–798, 1984

153. Pereiras R Jr, Chiprut RO, Greenwald RA et al: Percutaneous transhepatic cholangiography with the "skinny" needle: A rapid, simple and accurate method in the diagnosis of cholestasis. Ann Intern Med 86:562–568, 1977

154. Suzuki Y, Kobayashi A, Ohto M et al: Bacteriological study of transhepatically aspirated bile: Relation to cholangiographic findings in 295 patients. Dig Dis Sci 29:109–115, 1984

155. Muro A, Mueller PR, Ferrucci JT Jr et al: Bile cytology: A routine addition to percutaneous biliary drainage. Radiology 149:846–847, 1983

156. Portner WJ, Koolpe HA: New devices for biliary drainage and biopsy. AJR 138:1191–1195, 1982

157. Clark RA, Mitchell SE, Colley DP et al: Percutaneous catheter biliary decompression. AJR 137:503–509, 1981

158. Yee ACN, Ho C-S: Complications of percutaneous biliary drainage: Benign vs malignant diseases. AJR 148:1207–1209, 1987

159. Carrasco CH, Zornoza J, Becthel WJ: Malignant biliary obstruction: Complications of percutaneous biliary drainage. Radiology 152:343–346, 1984

160. Joseph PK, Bizer LS, Sprayregen SS et al: Percutaneous transhepatic biliary drainage: Results and complications in 81 patients. JAMA 255:2763–2767, 1986

161. Cutherell L, Wanebo HJ, Tegtmeyer CJ: Catheter tract seeding after percutaneous biliary drainage for pancreatic cancer. Cancer 57:2057–2060, 1986

162. Anschuetz SL, Vogelzang RL: Malignant pleural effusion: A complication of transhepatic biliary drainage. AJR 146:1165–1166, 1986

163. Klimberg S, Hawkins I, Vogel SB: Percutaneous cholecystostomy for acute cholecystitis in high-risk patients. Am J Surg 153:125–129, 1987

164. vanSonnenberg E, Wittich GR, Casola G et al: Diagnostic and therapeutic percutaneous gallbladder procedures. Radiology 160:23–26, 1986

165. Teplick SK, Haskin PH, Sammon JK et al: Common bile duct obstruction: Assessment by transcholecystic cholangiography. Radiology 161:135–138, 1986

166. Goodwin WE, Casey WC, Woolf W: Percutaneous trocar (needle) nephrostomy in hydronephrosis. JAMA 157:891–894, 1955

167. Reznek RH, Talner LB: Percutaneous Nephrostomy. Radiol Clin North Am 22:393–406, 1984

168. Coleman CC, Kimura Y, Lange PH et al: Percutaneous nephrostomy: Indications, contraindications, preparation, and complications. Semin Intervent Radiol 1:38–41, 1984

169. Lee WJ, Smith AD, Cubelli V et al: Percutaneous nephrolithotomy: Analysis of 500 consecutive cases. Urol Radiol 8:61–66, 1986

170. Brazzini A, Castaneda-Zuniga WR, Coleman CC et al: Urostent designs. Semin Intervent Radiol 4:26–35, 1987

171. Finney RP: Double-J and diversion stents. Urol Clin North Am 9:89–94, 1982

172. Mazer MJ, LeVeen RF, Call JB: Permanent percutaneous antegrade ureteral stent placement without transurethral assistance. Urology 14:413–419, 1979

173. Rozenblit G, Tarasov E, Srur MF et al: Druy ureteral stent set: Clinical experience in 25 patients. Radiology 160:737–740, 1986

174. Mardis HK: Evaluation of polymeric materials for endourologic devices: Emerging importance of hydrogels. Semin Intervent Radiol 4:36–45, 1987

175. LeRoy AJ, Williams HJ Jr, Segura JW et al: Indwelling ureteral stents: Percutaneous management of complications. Radiology 158:219–222, 1986

176. Stables DP, Ginsberg NJ, Johnson ML: Percutaneous nephrostomy: A series and review of the literature. AJR 130:75–82, 1978

177. Holden S, McPhee M, Grabstald H: The rationale of urinary diversion in cancer patients. J Urol 121:19–21, 1979

178. Sharer W, Grayhack JT, Graham J: Palliative urinary diversion for malignant ureteral obstruction. J Urol 120:162–164, 1978

179. Barbaric ZL: Percutaneous nephrostomy for urinary tract obstruction. AJR 143:803–809, 1984

180. Cope C, Zeit RM: Pseudoaneurysms after nephrostomy. AJR 139:255–261, 1982

181. Cronan JJ, Dorfman GS, Amis ES et al: Retroperitoneal hemorrhage after percutaneous nephrostomy. AJR 144:801–803, 1985

182. Harris RD, Walther PC: Renal arterial injury associated with percutaneous nephrostomy. Urology 23:215–217, 1984

183. Gavant ML, Gold RE, Church JC: Delayed Rupture of renal pseudoaneurysm: Complication of percutaneous nephrostomy. AJR 138:948–949, 1982

184. Hruby W, Marberger M: Late sequelae of percutaneous nephrostomy. Work in progress. Radiology 152:383–385, 1984

185. Walsh DB, Downing S, Nauta R et al: Metastatic cancer: A relative contraindication to vena cava filter placement. Cancer 59:161–163, 1987

186. Maxwell RJ, Greenfield LJ: Effect of pulmonary embolism on survival of patients with Greenfield vena caval filters. Surgery 101:389–394, 1987

187. Günther RW, Schild H, Fries A et al: Vena caval filter to prevent pulmonary embolism: Experimental study. Work in progress. Radiology 156:315–320, 1985
188. Darcy MD, Cardella JF, Hunter DW et al: Experience with the Amplatz Retrievable vena caval filter. Work in progress. Radiology 161:611–614, 1986
189. Günther RW, Schild H, Hollman JP et al: First clinical results with a new caval filter. Cardiovasc intervent Radiol 10:104–108, 1987
190. Burke PE, Michna BA, Harvey CF et al: Experimental comparison of percutaneous vena caval devices: Titanium Greenfield filter versus bird's nest filter. J Vasc Surg 6:66–70, 1987
191. Katsamouris AA, Waltman AC, Delichatsios MA et al: Inferior vena cava filters: In vitro comparison of clot trapping and flow dynamics. Radiology 166:361–366, 1988
192. Denny DF, Cronan JJ, Dorfman GS et al: Percutaneous Kimray-Greenfield filter placement by femoral vein puncture. AJR 145:827–829, 1985
193. Tadavarthy SM, Castaneda-Zuniga W, Salomonowitz E et al: Kimray-Greenfield vena caval filter: Percutaneous introduction. Radiology 151:525–526, 1984
194. Knight L, Rizk G, Amplatz K: Percutaneous introduction of inferior vena caval filter: Human experience. Radiology 111:61–63, 1974
195. Cimochowski GE, Evans RH, Zarins CK et al: Greenfield filter versus Mobin-Uddin umbrella. J Thorac Cardiovasc Surg 79:358–365, 1980
196. Zeit RM: Greenfield filter placement via the femoral vein: Improved technique with extra-long sheath and purse-string suture. Radiology 163:575–576, 1987
197. Pais SO, Mirvis SE, De Orchis DF: Percutaneous insertion of the Kimray-Greenfield filter: Technical considerations and problems. Radiology 165:377–381, 1987
198. Rose BS, Simon DC, Hess ML et al: Percutaneous transfemoral placement of the Kimray-Greenfield vena cava filter. Radiology 165:373–376, 1987
199. Denny DF Jr, Dorfman GS, Cronan JJ et al: Greenfield filter: Percutaneous placement in 50 patients. AJR 50:427–429, 1988
200. Kantor A, Glanz S, Gordon DH et al: Percutaneous insertion of the Kimray-Green-field filter: Incidence of femoral vein thrombosis. AJR 149:1065–1066, 1987
201. Stellato TA, Gauderer MWL: Percutaneous endoscopic gastrostomy for gastrointestinal decompression. Ann Surg 205:119–122, 1987
202. Picus D, Marx MV, Weyman PJ: Chronic intestinal obstruction: Value of percutaneous gastrostomy tube placement. AJR 150:295–297, 1988
203. Wills JS, Oglesby JT: Percutaneous gastrostomy: Further experience. Radiology 154:71–74, 1985
204. Ho C, Gray RR, Goldfinger M et al: Percutaneous gastrostomy for enteral feeding. Radiology 156:349–351, 1985
205. vanSonnenberg E, Wittich GR, Brown LK et al: Percutaneous gastrostomy and gastroenterostomy: 1. Techniques derived from laboratory evaluation. AJR 146:577–580, 1986
206. vanSonnenberg E, Wittich GR, Cabrera OA et al: Percutaneous gastrostomy and gastroenterostomy: 2. Clinical experience. AJR 146:581–586, 1986
207. Gray RR, St Louis EL, Grosman H: Percutaneous gastrostomy and gastro-jejunostomy. Br J Radiol 60:1067–1070, 1987
208. Ponsky JL, Gauderer MWL, Stellato TA et al: Percutaneous approaches to enteral alimentation. Am J Surg 149:102–105, 1985
209. Larson DE, Burton DD, Schroeder KW et al: Percutaneous endoscopic gastrostomy: Indications, success, complications, and mortality in 314 consecutive patients. Gastroenterology 93:48–52, 1987
210. Casola G, Withers C, vanSonnenberg E et al: Percutaneous cecostomy for decompression of the massively distended cecum. Radiology 158:793–794, 1986
211. Haaga JR, Bick RJ, Zollinger RM Jr: CT-guided percutaneous catheter cecostomy. Gastrointest Radiol 12:166–168, 1987
212. Bezreh JS: Percutaneous catheter drainage of closed-loop small-bowel obstruction. AJR 141:797–798, 1983

SECTION 4   ANTHONY B. MILLER

Cancer Screening

Of the approaches to cancer control that can reduce mortality from cancer—prevention, treatment, and screening—screening holds perhaps the greatest promise for a rapid major impact, but for a number of practical and organizational difficulties its potential may not be achieved. Further, there are several scientific reasons why the early detection of cancer does not automatically guarantee reduced cancer mortality.[1] This chapter first reviews the scientific basis for screening and then considers the evidence on screening for a number of major cancer sites.

GENERAL PRINCIPLES OF SCREENING

There are both benefits and disadvantages to screening for cancer.[2] The benefits include an improved prognosis for some patients whose disease is detected by screening, but not for all. Those who benefit are primarily those who in the absence of screening would have died. This is the major benefit sought in screening programs. A second benefit of screening, related to early detection, is that less radical treatment may be needed to cure some cases of disease. This is a potentially important benefit of screening for breast cancer, for example. A third benefit is reassurance for those with negative test results. Indeed, many people participate in screening programs for just this reassurance. A fourth benefit is resource savings, in particular a lower treatment cost if less radical treatment can be instituted, and lower costs for treating patients who otherwise would have died, as these costs for cancer can often be substantial.

The list of disadvantages is somewhat longer. The first is a longer period of morbidity, due to the lead time from screening, for patients whose prognosis is unaltered. A second disadvantage, potentially critical in the case of breast cancer screening, is overtreatment of borderline abnormalities. Many abnormalities brought to light by screening programs might never have been recognized without screening. A third disadvantage is false reassurance for those with false-negative test results. In such cases, the development of symptoms after a false-negative screening test may be ignored, leading to postponement of the diagnosis and consequently a poorer prognosis. A fourth disadvantage is unnecessary morbidity for those with false-positive test results. False-positive results may precipitate a cascade of complex investigations and varying diagnoses, a critical factor influencing the cost-effectiveness of screening for certain cancers, such as colorectal cancer.[3] A fifth disadvantage is the potential hazards of a screening test, a particular concern in mammography,[4] although for several screening tests the concern may be more theoretical than real. Finally, there are resource costs, particularly those resulting from the overtreatment of borderline abnormalities and the investigation and diagnosis of persons with false-positive screening tests.

Because of the potential disadvantages of screening programs, it is appropriate to insist on definitive evaluation of the effectiveness of screening. A number of approaches can be used for evaluating screening programs. These include geographical comparisons, time trends in defined populations, studies in which such trends are correlated with intensity of screening, and quasi-experimental comparisons of trends in different areas based on identification of individuals, but all of these are inferior to the randomized controlled trial.[2] A new approach to which much thought is being devoted is the use of case–control studies to evaluate screening programs.[2,5] Case–control studies should be designed to resemble as far as possible the controlled clinical trial. Thus, cases should be deaths from cancer, or advanced disease as a surrogate for death, and controls should be drawn at random from the same population as the cases and should include living persons (who may or may not have disease, depending on the population sampled) and those without advanced disease.[1]

The preferred evaluation approach, the randomized controlled trial, avoids the biases that are inherent in the assessment of screening if less perfect measures are used. These four screening biases are lead time, or the time by which diagnosis is advanced through screening; length bias, or the tendency of the screening process to detect cases of disease with a more prolonged natural history and thus a better prognosis than normal; selection bias, reflecting the dependence of screening programs on volunteer populations, who inevitably have a different incidence of disease than the general population; and overdiagnosis bias, or the tendency for screening to bring to light and label as disease lesions that might never have been diagnosed in the lifetime of the screenee.[1] These biases must be borne in mind in deciding the end points for evaluation of screening programs. If the screening test used is of any validity, counts of cases, the disease stage distribution of cases, and case fatality (survival) assessments are all influenced by these biases and inevitably result in better indices than for cases detected in the usual fashion in the absence of screening. Disease incidence is appropriate as an end point only if a precursor is removed as a result of using the screening test, as is the case for cancer of the cervix. Mortality is the only absolute measure, although in some circumstances the absolute number of cases of advanced disease could be substituted for deaths.[1]

Once screening programs are in place, continued evaluation is required. Screening programs may fail for many reasons, none of which may necessarily represent an inherent fault in the approach. Such reasons include failure to reach the population at risk, lack of sensitivity of the screening test, too infrequent rescreening to detect rapidly growing disease, and inadequate treatment of the abnormalities detected on screening.[6] Thus, for many cervical cancer screening programs, one should now be concerned with operational issues that could explain relative failure, rather than with the efficacy of the approach itself.

SCREENING FOR CERVICAL CANCER

Several years ago we established a strong correlation between the intensity of screening in Canada and a reduction in mortality from uterine cancer in the 1960s.[7] The correlation was strongest at the census district or county level and persisted when various census-derived socioeconomic status variables were incorporated in a multivariate analysis. This evidence was reviewed by the first Canadian Task Force on the evaluation of screening programs, which concluded that screening for cervical cancer had significantly contributed to the reduced mortality from the disease in Canada.[8] Since then, although mortality has continued to decline in Canada, the correlation has largely disappeared: in practice, screening has not had the anticipated effect of eliminating mortality from the disease, and the areas of country that were less intensely screened in the mid-1960s have largely caught up in terms of screening intensity.[9] There is still some evidence, however, that screening is making an important contribution to the control of cervical disease in Canada.[10] In the meantime, important evidence on the effect of screening on the incidence of and mortality from cervical cancer has come from the Nordic countries.[11] The organized screening programs developed in Iceland and Finland resulted in a fairly rapid and important reduction in incidence; the less organized programs in Sweden and in Denmark have made a delayed but similarly important contribution. Norway, however, which used to have an incidence similar to that of all the other Nordic countries (with the exception of high-incidence Denmark), failed to introduce an organized program, and there was no reduction in incidence.

In Canada, we have noted a reduction in incidence in nearly all age groups until recently, when the incidence appears to have risen in the younger age groups.[12] This change, which reflects differences in expression of risk factors in younger birth cohorts, was regarded with some concern by the second Canadian Task Force on the evaluation of screening programs[12] and resulted in recommendations that more attention should be paid to screening younger women and ensuring that individuals at risk for the disease were brought into screening programs. The second Canadian Task Force's approach to the evaluation of periodicity of rescreening depended rather heavily on mathematical models,[13] as did the American Cancer Society in recommending rescreening at 3-year intervals,[14] based on the model of Eddy.[15] The Canadian Task Force[12] recommended that registers be established to ensure the following: (1) that appropriate follow-up systems were in place so that women with normal test results would be recalled at regular intervals for repeat testing, (2) that action was taken following discovery of an abnormality, and (3) that long-term follow-up was provided for patients treated for an abnormality. In 1982 they reinforced their previous recommendation for centralized registries throughout the country.[8]

This belief in the organization of screening programs to ensure that those at risk enter into the program and that all at risk are rescreened at an appropriate interval was echoed in the deliberations of an International Union Against Cancer (UICC) workshop.[16] This group had available the results of a study coordinated by the International Agency for Research on Cancer (IARC) which documented from a number of screening programs the degree of protection conferred by a negative screening test. Protection was maximal in the first 3 years after a negative test and persisted to some degree for at least 5 years. On the basis of this analysis, it was possible to compute the expected degree of benefit from different intensities of rescreening (Table 20-10). It seems clear that annual schedules are wasteful of resources and that almost as much benefit can be obtained from tests conducted at 3-year intervals, beginning at about age 25 and continuing through age 60.

The UICC group assessed the state of the art of screening for cervical cancer and concluded that the effectiveness of screening programs was established but that within each country a consensual policy was required to ensure that the target population was identified, that individual women were identifiable, that measures were available to guarantee high coverage, that there were adequate field facilities for carry-

TABLE 20-10. Effect of Different Screening Policies for Cervical Cancer, Starting at Age 20

	Screening Schedule	Cumulative Rate per 100,000 Women Aged 20–64	% Reduction in Cancer Rate	Number of Tests
1.	No screening	1575		
2.	Screening every 5 yr, ages 20–64	257.6	83.6	9
2a.	Screening every 5 yr, ages 25–64	286.7	81.8	8
2b.	Screening every 5 yr, ages 35–64	478.8	69.6	6
2c.	Screening every year, ages 20–34, then every 5 yr, ages 35–64	232.3	85.5	21
2d.	Screening at age 25, 26, 30, then every 5 yr	274.5	82.6	9
3.	Screening every 3 yr, ages 20–64	137.8	91.2	15
3a.	Screening every 3 yr, ages 26–64	161.0	89.8	13
3b.	Screening every 3 yr, ages 35–64	352.8	77.6	10
3c.	Screening every year, ages 20–34, then every 3 yr, ages 35–64	131.2	91.7	25
3d.	Screening at age 25, 26, 29 then every 3 yr	156.6	90.1	14
4.	Screening every year, ages 20–64	105.0	93.3	35

ing out cervical cytology examinations, that organized quality control programs were available in the laboratories, and that there were adequate facilities for diagnosis and treatment, with carefully designed referral systems and with an overall program for evaluation and monitoring trends in the population.[16]

Research is still needed on appropriate strategies for screening in developing countries, and on whether or not the natural history in high-incidence areas such as South America and Asia reflects current knowledge of the natural history of the disease from studies in technically advanced countries. Continued research on etiology is desirable to identify markers of high risk, while the long-term effects of therapy for precancerous lesions, especially the use of colposcopically assisted procedures, should be further assessed.

The UICC group recommended that policies be developed for each population, though noting that variation in the rate of progression and in the risk of preinvasive lesions does not currently appear to warrant differences in screening policies.[16] They noted that it appeared cost-effective to start screening at age 25, to rescreen at intervals of 3 years, and to stop after age 60, and that screening only high-risk groups does not seem to have general applicability.

Many of these recommendations were echoed by an expert group convened by the World Health Organization (WHO),[18] though their recommendations were tailored to the lesser resources available in most developing countries. Even a single smear applied to a substantial proportion of the population at an appropriate age (35–40 years) could achieve an important benefit.

Some of the concerns expressed by the Canadian Task Force regarding the changes in disease incidence in younger women[12] were also expressed by many physicians and professional groups in the United States. The working guidelines issued by the National Cancer Institute (NCI) for physicians state that "all women who are, or have been sexually active, or have reached 18 years, [should] have an annual Pap test and pelvic examination. After a women has had three or more consecutive satisfactory normal annual examinations, the Pap test may be performed less frequently at the discretion of her physician."[19] This issue has been addressed by other countries also. European countries, including the United Kingdom,[20] continue to recommend, largely on the grounds of cost-effectiveness, that screening should be offered not more frequently than every 3 years.

The other difference between many recommendations is the age at which women should enter screening programs. This recommendation varies from the age at which a female becomes sexually active, in the Canadian[12] and NCI[19] guidelines, to not before the age of 25, in the UICC guidelines.[16] The recommendation by the Canadian Task Forces that screening should start at age 18 for sexually active girls was based on the premise that those with detectable precancerous lesions and who are less than 25 years old may form an ultra-high-risk group. Thus, if the opportunity presents itself (by their attendance for oral contraceptives or for antenatal or postnatal care) to include them in screening programs, they can be placed on special surveillance if lesions have already developed. However, for countries that have the mechanisms to identify all women potentially at risk from the age of 25, offering screening before that age would not be cost-effective.[16] Clearly more research is needed into the natural history of the disease in younger high-risk birth cohorts; some of this research is ongoing in Canada.

SCREENING FOR BREAST CANCER

United States

Much is known about screening for breast cancer, largely because this is the only entity for which a controlled clinical trial has been completed, that of the Health Insurance Plan of Greater New York (HIP). Other clinical trials are in progress. Although the final report from the HIP study has yet to appear, it is clear that the mortality reduction noted initially at 5 years[21] and confirmed through 14 years[22] for the combination of mammography and physical examination persisted throughout 18 years of follow-up.[23]

The long-term follow-up in the HIP study has emphasized some aspects of breast cancer detection programs that were beginning to be appreciated 4 years earlier.[22] The early lack of a demonstrable effect of screening in women under the age of 50[21] was later replaced by an almost equivalent degree of benefit to that for women aged 50 years or older (Table 20-11). The benefit for those aged 45 to 49 years first became apparent after 5 years of follow-up, and that for women aged 40 to 44 years became apparent after 8 years of follow-up. The early benefit (noted after 3 years) for those aged 50 to 59 years maximized at 5 years and later decreased somewhat. None of the benefits for individual age groups are statistically significant of themselves, but from the results now available it seems likely that screening benefits all ages, with a longer delay in benefit for younger women — perhaps because of a different natural history of breast cancer in premenopausal and postmenopausal women.

The other aspect of the study that deserves emphasis is the question as to which of the two screening modalities used annually for 4 years contributed to the mortality reduction. Again, the design of the HIP study does not allow resolution of this issue, but a clue is derived from the case detection rates (Table 20-12), which emphasize the contributions of both modalities, especially physical examination in younger women.

The HIP study was followed in the United States by the Breast Cancer Detection Demonstration Projects (BCDDP). These projects used mammography, thermography, and physical examination of the breasts in 280,000 women aged 35 years or older, but there was no control group, so the effectiveness of the screening program could not be estab-lished.[24] Further, thermography proved to be of low sensitivity and specificity. Mammography, however, seemed to be of higher sensitivity than physical examination in the BCDDP than in the HIP study, especially in women aged 40 to 49 years.[25]

Recently, survival data have become available on the cancers diagnosed in the BCDDP.[26] These are of considerable interest, as they show almost equivalent survival whether or not the breast cancers were diagnosed by screening, irrespective of age. The data have been interpreted as confirming the benefit of screening in women aged 40 to 49 years, but clearly they do not, as the effects of screening biases related to survival cannot be corrected. However, they do raise the possibility that in self-selected women who attend screening programs, the benefit may not be as great as has been assumed.

The controversy that surrounded the BCDDP[27] resulted in a lack of interest in further large-scale research to evaluate the effects of screening for breast cancer in the United States. The focus therefore shifted to Europe and Canada, where major projects were initiated in the 1970s and 1980s.

The European Studies

Three programs, two in the Netherlands[28,29] and one in Florence,[30] have been assessed by the case–control approach. All three show important reductions in deaths from breast cancer in women over the age of 50, two as a result of programs using mammography alone (in Nijmegen and Florence) and one using the combination of mammography plus physical examination (in Utrecht). The results of the Nijmegen study indicate no benefit so far for women less than 50 years old. There was a nonsignificant reduction in mortality in women less than 50 in the Florence study, possibly reflecting a longer follow-up time.

In the large Swedish WE randomized trial, the initial results again showed no benefit for women aged 40 to 49 years but an important benefit for women more than 50 years old.[31] In this trial, single-oblique-view mammography was used.

In all these studies, the lack of benefit from screening in women less than 50 years old may be explained by the same factors that led to the delayed appearance of benefit in the

TABLE 20-11.   Percentage Reduction in Deaths from Breast Cancer in the HIP Study

Age at Entry (yr)	% Reduction in Breast Cancer Deaths*		Year Reduction Began
	At 5 Years	At 18 Years	
40–44	(18)	36	9
45–49	(0)	16	6
50–54	65	22	3
55–59	(30)	24	3
60–64	(50)	17	3

* Parentheses indicate observations based on 20 or fewer breast cancer deaths in study and control groups combined.

TABLE 20-12.   Breast Cancer Cases Histologically Confirmed in HIP Study, by Screening Modality

Age at Entry (yr)	Total No.	No. Detected by Mammography Alone	% Detected by: Clinical Alone	% Detected by: Mammography and Clinical
40–49	40	25	58	18
50–59	67	39	40	21
60–64	25	32	36	32
All ages	132	33	45	22

HIP study. If so, these studies may all be on the verge of showing mortality reduction in the under 50 age group, although there could be other explanations for a lack of effect in younger women. One possible explanation could be a relative lack of sensitivity of the screen. All of the studies have incorporated mammography, but so far no reported study on European women less than 50 years old has used physical examination. In Utrecht the study was originally planned with objectives other than demonstrating benefit,[32] and therefore women less than 50 years old were not screened initially, as it was expected that little benefit would accrue to them. The absence of physical examination in the European studies could have contributed to a lower sensitivity of the screening program. That the screening was less sensitive in women aged 40 to 49 years than in women over the age of 50 has in fact been demonstrated for the Swedish WE trial,[33] and by a different analysis for the Nijmegen study.[34]

A second possible explanation is that the periodicity of rescreening was too low in women aged 40 to 49 years. There was no difference in the periodicity of rescreening by age in the Nijmegen and Florence studies, but in the Swedish study the younger women were screened every 21 months, compared to every 33 months and then every 24 months in the older cohorts. An attempt to assess the sojourn time of preclinical lesions in the Swedish study (i.e., the total time that a lesion is potentially detectable before clinical presentation) has suggested that this period is not much less in younger women than in older women.[33] Thus, too infrequent a repeat screen in younger women may not be the reason for a lack of demonstrable effect in them.

Ongoing Studies

Three important studies in progress should provide further guidance on screening for breast cancer. The first is the United Kingdom study incorporating women aged 45 to 64; biennial mammography and annual physical examination are used in two centers and breast self-examination (BSE) alone in two more, with four control districts.[35] In one of the mammography screening centers there is randomization by family practices. Time will tell whether this study is sufficiently powerful to provide much additional evidence on the benefits to be expected from this screening approach. For example, it is not clear whether we can expect any elucidation of the age issue, as women aged 40 to 44 were not enrolled in the study. Nor is it clear whether the study will be sufficiently powerful to provide any information on the effectiveness of BSE. Mortality results should be available in 1989–1990.

The National Breast Screening Study in Canada was designed specifically to provide additional information on the benefit of the combination of annual mammography, physical examination, and regular BSE in women aged 40 to 49 years, and the incremental effect of mammography over and above physical examination and BSE in women aged 50 to 59 years.[36] This study should have the power to answer both objectives. So far the women enrolled have had the expected numbers of breast cancers but a much lower mortality from breast cancer than expected. Some of the reduced mortality might reflect a benefit of physical examination in women aged 50 to 59 years and the single physical examination with the teaching of BSE in women aged 40 to 49 years. If the trend continues, follow-up will have to be extended for at least an additional 3 years before mortality results can be reported.

The third ongoing study of critical importance to those countries that have tended to rely on BSE is a randomized trial being conducted in factories in Moscow and polyclinics in Leningrad, evaluating team teaching of BSE in Moscow and individual instruction in Leningrad.[37] This trial will eventually include more than 200,000 women, but results will probably not be available for 8 to 10 years. A geographically controlled comparison of BSE is underway in East Germany, and there are plans to attempt to evaluate the BSE program introduced by Dr. Gastrin in Finland, the "Mama" program, about 14 years ago.[38] Some evidence on effectiveness of BSE could, therefore, become available within the next few years.

The UICC project on screening evaluation concluded that in countries where breast cancer is common and where the necessary resources are available, screening with mammography alone or mammography plus physical examination is applicable as public health policy.[39] However, the greatest initial benefit will be obtained by concentrating screening on women aged 50 to 69 years. The ambiguity of the modality to be used is obvious in this recommendation. Although most people tend to concentrate on mammography, we and others maintain that the benefit of physical examination, either with mammography or in partial substitution for mammography, could be considerable. The experience in Canada, in contradistinction to that of the United Kingdom,[40] is that a policy based on physical examination could be less expensive rather than more (Table 20-13). Whether or not this is

TABLE 20-13. Preliminary Data on Cost-Effectiveness of Mammography Compared to Physical Examination in Detecting Invasive Cancers (NBSS Study), According to Size of Tumor.*

| Size of Tumor | Women Aged 40–49 | | Women Aged 50–59 | |
	Mammography	Physical Examination	Mammography	Physical Examination
All sizes	$18,340	$ 8,290	$ 8,890	$ 5,950
>1 cm	23,390	9,620	11,850	7,380
>2 cm	43,220	19,620	23,130	13,960

* Based on cost per examination of $12 for physical examination and $30 for mammography in Canadian dollars.

confirmed by a full cost-benefit analysis is likely to be resolved by the Canadian trial within the next few years.

POLICIES FOR BREAST CANCER SCREENING

The American Cancer Society[14,41] and the American College of Radiology[42] have both recommended that mammography and physical examination be offered to all women over the age of 40, with a baseline mammogram obtained at ages 35 to 40. The rationale for the baseline mammogram has not been established. Mammography is recommended every 1 or 2 years for women aged 40 to 49 years, and annually for those over age 50. The same periodicity is recommended in the NCI working guidelines.[19] The European studies, however, suggest that these frequencies be reversed.[39] Other countries have recommended policies based on mammography only—such as mammography every 3 years for women more than 50 years old in the United Kingdom.[43] All recognize the need for adequate training and attention to the technical aspects of mammography.[44] This has been confirmed by the experience in the National Breast Screening Study in Canada. Care must be taken in many aspects of technique, including type of machine, appropriate focal spot film distance, processing, positioning of the patient, and adequate compression of the breast.[45] Mammography quality and dosimetry should be monitored on a regular basis. The dosage required for mammography has fallen substantially from the 8-rad surface dose used in the HIP study, to 3 to 1 rad used in the BCDDP, to 0.6 to 0.2 rad used in the National Breast Screening Study with screen-film technology. The low dose achievable in screen-film mammography, better film quality, and the opportunity for batch processing of films make screen-film mammography preferable to xerography for screening. However, these are not the only aspects that must be taken into account when the use of mammography as a screening tool is contemplated. Many lesions can be identified on breast cancer screening, including cysts, mammary dysplasia, benign atypical hyperplasias, borderline abnormalities, in situ cancers with or without microinvasion, and small invasive cancers.[45] For those not palpable, both benign and malignant, considerable care is required for localization, diagnosis, and management. This usually requires specimen radiography and particularly the availability of skilled radiologists, surgeons, and pathologists. For a national program, special training would be required.[44] These

requirements should not be taken lightly. In each Canadian city in which the National Breast Screening Study has been introduced, considerable care has been taken with these aspects of breast screening. The medical profession must be assured it is appropriate to biopsy impalpable abnormalities, and family physicians must be encouraged to refer patients to institutions where the necessary skills are available. Even so, in the National Breast Screening Study currently about one in six biopsies conducted for impalpable abnormalities visible on mammography result in a diagnosis of in situ or invasive cancer. Yet, although mammography is clearly more sensitive than physical examination, the lesions found on mammography alone that potentially have a good prognosis may never surface clinically, whereas the lesions found on physical examination alone tend to be small and infiltrating cancers, possibly with one or two micrometastases, and of a type which, if detected early, might result in better prognosis. Hence, it may be inappropriate to base breast screening policies entirely on considerations of mammography.

BSE as an alternative approach to breast screening may have wider applicability than mammography and physical examination.[46] This conclusion of a WHO-supported meeting reinforces the need for better teaching and more careful evaluation of the effectiveness of BSE. Experience in the National Breast Screening Study shows how women's skills in BSE can be improved by annual reinforcement.[47]

Because only BSE can contribute to the early detection of the interval cancers that occur in all screening programs, BSE reinforcement should be combined with physical examination, whether given by a physician or, as in the Canadian study, by a nurse.

SCREENING FOR COLORECTAL CANCER

Colorectal cancer is an importance cause of morbidity and mortality in both sexes, and its natural history may make it amenable to control by screening.[48] There are two screening tests available, sigmoidoscopy and tests for occult blood in the feces. The American Cancer Society recommends that screening with both should start at age 50, at which time tests for occult blood should be performed annually and sigmoidoscopy every 5 years.[14] The NCI working guidelines call for annual tests for occult blood and sigmoidoscopy every 3 to 5 years from the age of 50.[19]

Unfortunately, the patients at risk are relatively old. Both patients and physicians dislike sigmoidoscopy, and there may have to be major public and professional educational programs to persuade individuals to accept even flexible sigmoidoscopy. However, the scientific basis for recommendations is slight. Gilbertsen et al[49,50] performed annual proctosigmoidoscopy on 21,150 men and women. Of 27 carcinomas found on initial examination, 25 were followed at least 5 years, with a 5-year survival rate of 64%. Though better than usual, this survival rate would be expected from screening biases. Of 13 patients in whom carcinomas were subsequently found, 11 have survived 5 years. Thus, there are 11 known deaths from colorectal cancer over a 5-year period in this population. Although it is difficult to derive an expected survival figure, as the age and sex distribution of the participants is not known, the figure may not be very low: all persons with preexisting colorectal cancers were ineligible for the screen, and it is known that most of the deaths from cancer in any one year occur in people diagnosed in previous years. Once the selective nature of the population screened is considered, it becomes apparent that the survival results may simply reflect a common selection bias in screening.[51]

In the randomized trial reported by Dales et al,[52] digital rectal examination and sigmoidoscopy were included as part of a multiphasic screen provided annually in the study group; the control group was offered "usual care." In an 11-year follow-up period there were 5 deaths from colorectal cancer in the study group and 18 in the control group ($p < 0.05$). However, this study had multiple end points, and thus a p-value of 0.05 cannot be given the usual weight. Further, only 6 cases (out of 20) in the study group were diagnosed after sigmoidoscopy.

The sensitivity of the tests for occult blood in the stool is relatively low, not only for potential precursors of cancer such as adenomatous polyps but also for relatively early, less advanced cancers.[3] The specificity of the tests currently available is also low, increasing costs in terms of the diagnosis and treatment of benign abnormalities and also the potential risk of applying screening tests.

Thus, to date no reduction in the mortality from colorectal cancer has been demonstrated with screening, even though two controlled trials have been in progress for many years in the United States.[53,54] Additional trials have been initiated in the United Kingdom, Denmark, and Sweden.[3] The UICC project on the evaluation of screening[3] concluded that there is as yet no firm evidence that screening for colorectal cancer can result in reduced mortality, and therefore that screening for colorectal cancer or its precursors cannot be recommended as public health policy. This conclusion was largely endorsed by a committee on screening charged to develop the NCI's year 2,000 goals.[55]

SCREENING FOR OTHER CANCERS

The UICC project has evaluated screening programs for cancer in several other sites.[2,3,16] A number of problems have been identified, and no program is currently recommended as public health policy.

LUNG CANCER. Several early studies suggested that screening for lung cancer by means of 6-month chest radiographs with or without sputum cytology did not improve the prognosis of lung cancer in the populations studied.[2] In the 1970s, three randomized trials of lung cancer screening were initiated in the United States, and it now seems clear that although chest radiographs and sputum cytology are capable of detecting cases in high-risk males, sputum cytology at 4-month intervals adds a small proportion of cases to those discovered on annual chest radiographs and does not demonstrably reduce mortality. Further, chest radiographs at 4-month intervals confer no mortality advantage over routine care that includes annual chest radiographs. The UICC group[2] recommended assessing the value of the annual chest radiograph and suggested that case–control studies may have promise in this regard. One such study has since been performed in the German Democratic Republic, evaluating the role of mass miniature radiographs obtained at 2-year intervals, and found no evidence that such radiologic screening reduced the mortality from lung cancer.[56] This may not satisfy those who advocate full-size chest radiographs for screening. However, it seems unlikely that the annual chest radiograph is beneficial when the 4-month chest radiograph conferred no mortality advantage over routine care that included chest radiographs obtained only when symptoms became apparent.

BLADDER CANCER. Urinary cytology is clearly capable of detecting urinary bladder cancers in persons in high-risk occupations, as well as those living in areas where urinary schistosomiasis is endemic. Improved survival of patients with screening-detected bladder cancer has been demonstrated, but it is not known if a reduction in mortality will follow. Screening-detected cases in areas where urinary schistosomiasis is endemic are at an earlier stage and require less extensive therapy than those diagnosed by routine measures. However, if bladder cancer screening is to play a role in cancer control, further research is needed. Critically, the role of urinary cytology in reducing mortality from bladder cancer in high-risk occupational groups and in areas of endemic urinary schistosomiasis must be evaluated. An important prerequisite to such evaluation is to undertake treatment trials of early lesions found by screening.[57]

ORAL CANCER. Visual examination is capable of identifying presymptomatic oral cancers. Exfoliative cytology is less sensitive than visual examination.[2] Neither test has yet been shown to reduce mortality from oral cancer. Thus, research on oral cancer screening programs is clearly needed. In technically advanced countries it will be difficult to evaluate the place of routine dental examinations, as these tend to be restricted to those at low risk, high-risk individuals often avoiding dental care. Evaluation of mortality reduction following screening is needed in areas of high incidence; the role of screening in the primary prevention of oral cancer in persons with oral epithelial dysplasia might be evaluated concurrently. The NCI working guidelines for oral cavity cancer recommend that "oral examination including palpation of the tongue, floor of the mouth, salivary glands and lymph nodes of the neck be performed as part of the periodic health examination," and that "special attention should be given those at high risk due to tobacco and alcoholism."[19]

OVARIAN CANCER. Ovarian cancer is common in Western countries and has a relatively high mortality, often exceeding that for cervical cancer. Several screening tests are under development.[16]

ENDOMETRIAL CANCER. For endometrial cancer, although the disease is relatively common in Western countries, the person-years saved by screening may be limited because it is largely a disease of elderly women. Available screening tests are based on endometrial samples subjected to cytologic analysis. These are not simple tests, requiring considerable care in their application.[16] If endometrial cancer screening is to play a role in cancer control, much further research into its effectiveness is required.

STOMACH CANCER. Considerable mass radiologic screening for stomach cancer has been undertaken in Japan, but its contribution to reduced mortality is unclear. Although Hirayama has demonstrated a correlation between the rate of mass screening for stomach cancer at different ages and the percentage change in death rates from stomach cancer since 1960, he concluded that much of the reduction in mortality has been due to changes in diet rather than to mass screening.[58]

One case–control study performed in Japan provided suggestive evidence that screening reduces mortality from stomach cancer.[59] The UICC group concluded that screening in Japan had contributed to the reduced mortality from stomach cancer, but that its contribution was small in relation to the concomitantly diminishing incidence.[3]

LIVER CANCER. Screening by means of serum α-fetoprotein levels is being evaluated in some parts of China where the risk of liver cancer is very high.[3] There is some evidence that small liver cancers can be successfully treated. However, pending further research, screening for liver cancer cannot be recommended as public health policy.[3]

ESOPHAGUS. A similar conclusion was reached by the UICC group for esophageal cancer screening.[3] Although a possible screening test is available that involves cytologic examination of cells obtained by esophageal intubation and withdrawal, with a scrape obtained with the aid of a balloon, there are difficulties associated with the cytologic diagnosis of esophageal dysplasia (a possible precancerous lesion); another concern is the availability of suitable treatment for any abnormalities found. Research into chemoprevention might provide a solution to the latter problem.

OTHER CANCERS. Screening might be attempted for skin, prostate, and pancreatic cancer, which may potentially benefit from advances in monoclonal antibody technology. The NCI working guidelines recommend that "annual digital rectal examination of the prostate be performed on all males over 40 years of age."[19] Some have advocated screening for melanoma, particularly to search for dysplastic nevi[60]; so far this approach has not been definitively evaluated. However, the NCI working guidelines state that "all individuals should be encouraged to examine their skin thoroughly on a regular basis. That primary care physicians be encouraged to examine the skin as part of the periodic health examination. That further public and professional education be promoted on the early detection of skin cancers and in particular malignant melanoma."[19]

FUTURE PERSPECTIVES

There are many obstacles to a major contribution of screening to cancer control. For some sites, lung cancer being a particular example, the natural history of the disease may make it unamenable to screening. For other sites the potential for screening has so far been poorly evaluated; in this regard it should be noted that case finding is not equivalent to mortality reduction. Poor organization of screening programs has probably prevented the full utilization of cervical cancer screening, yet even for this cancer, the potential for reduction in mortality by screening may be less than assumed.[10] Many screening tests are costly; this seems to be a barrier to accepting mammographic screening in the United States.[61] For other screening programs, persons at risk may be less willing to participate than those not at risk; cervical cancer screening is one example. The cost of and morbidity from treatment consequent on false-positive tests may continue to plague screening for colorectal cancer until new tests are available. Overtreatment in the case of true-positive results may be a psychological barrier to screening for breast cancer, but with increasing support for less radical surgery,[62] mastectomy seems inappropriate unless it is absolutely necessary.

Table 20-14 lists the speculative potential for reduction in mortality from cancer following screening by the year 2000; the figures are mine.[63] Some may find a 60% speculative reduction in mortality from cervical cancer too pessimistic, but this figure is probably realistic, in light of the current epidemiologic situation. Even a 25% reduction in mortality from breast cancer could be overly optimistic, however, un-

TABLE 20-14. Speculative Potential for Reduction in Mortality from Cancer with Screening by Year 2000

Cancer Site	% Reduction in Mortality
Cervix	60
Breast	25
Lung	0
Colon/rectum	20
Bladder	5
Oral	5
Stomach (Japan)	30
Ovary	(10)
Endometrium	0
Other	(5)

less acceptance of screening by women and their physicians improves. For the remaining cancers on the list, the figures are less precisely derived. The NCI has estimated that screening might contribute 11% to 15% to the reduction in cancer mortality by the year 2000, part of the 50% overall reduction in cancer mortality by this time.[55] These figures assume acceptance of breast and cervical cancer screening by a large part of the population.

Screening can be an expensive use of health care resources. There are many barriers to its use, not the least of which is that its mere introduction does not solve the problem. Maintaining some level of effectiveness requires continued application of the screening program. For this reason, screening seems a less optimal approach to cancer control than primary prevention. Nevertheless, primary prevention may require many decades to achieve its full potential, except possibly for cancer of the colon and rectum, and under these circumstances screening appears to offer a fairly rapid return. Wherever it is shown to be effective, it should be included as part of the armamentarium for cancer control.

REFERENCES

1. Miller AB: General principles of evaluation of screening. In Miller AB (ed): Screening for Cancer, pp 3–24. Orlando, Fla, Academic Press, 1985
2. Prorok PC, Chamberlain J, Day NE et al: UICC workshop on the evaluation of screening programmes for cancer. Int J Cancer 34:1–4, 1984
3. Chamberlain J, Day NE, Hakama M et al: UICC workshop of the project on evaluation of screening programmes for gastrointestinal cancer. Int J Cancer 37:329–334, 1986
4. Miller AB: Screening cancer of the breast. In Miller AB (ed): Screening for Cancer, pp 325–345. Orlando, Fla, Academic Press, 1985
5. Morrison AS: Screening in Chronic Disease. Monographs in Epidemiology and Biostatistics, Vol 7. New York, Oxford University Press, 1985
6. Chamberlain J: Reasons that some screening programmes fail to control cervical cancer. In Hakama M, Miller AB, Day NE (eds): Screening for Cancer of the Uterine Cervix. IARC Sc Publ 76:161–168, 1986
7. Miller AB, Lindsay J, Hill GB: Mortality from cancer of the uterus in Canada and its relationship to screening for cancer of the cervix. Int J Cancer 17:602–612, 1976
8. Task Force: Cervical cancer screening programs: The Walton Report. Can Med Assoc J 114:1003–1033, 1976
9. Miller AB, Visentin T, Howe GR: The effect of hysterectomies and screening on mortality from cancer of the uterus in Canada. Int J Cancer 27:651–657, 1981
10. Miller AB: Evaluation of the impact of screening for cancer of the cervix. In Hakama M, Miller AB, Day NE (eds): Screening for Cancer of the Uterine Cervix. IARC Sci Publ 76:149–160, 1986
11. Hakama M: Trends in the incidence of cervical cancer in the Nordic countries. In Magnus K (ed): Trends in Cancer Incidence: Causes and Practical Implications, pp 279–292. New York, Hemisphere, 1982
12. Task Force: Cervical cancer screening programs: Summary of the 1982 Canadian Task Force Report. Can Med Assoc J 127:581–589, 1982
13. Yu SJ, Miller AB, Sherman GJ: Optimising the age, number of tests and test-interval for cervical screening in Canada. J Epidemiol Community Health 36:1–10, 1982
14. American Cancer Society: Guidelines for the cancer-related check-up: Recommendations and rationale. CA 30:193–240, 1980
15. Eddy D: Screening for Cancer: Theory, Analysis, and Design. Englewood Cliffs, NJ, Prentice-Hall, 1980
16. Hakama M, Chamberlain J, Day NE et al: UICC workshop on the evaluation of screening programmes for gynecological cancer. Br J Cancer 52:669–673, 1985
17. IARC Working Group on Cervical Cancer Screening: Summary Chapter. In Hakama M, Miller AB, Day NE (eds): Screening for Cancer of the Uterine Cervix. IARC Sci Publ 76:133–142, 1986
18. Control of cancer of the cervix uteri. Bull WHO 64:607–618, 1986
19. National Cancer Institute, Early Detection Branch: Working guidelines for early cancer detection: Rationale and supporting evidence to decrease mortality. Bethesda, Md, National Cancer Institute, Division of Cancer Prevention and Control, 1987
20. Draper GJ: Screening for cervical cancer: Revised policy. The recommendations of the DHSS committee on gynecological cytology. Br J Family Planning 8:95–100, 1982
21. Shapiro S, Strax P, Venet L: Periodic breast cancer screening in reducing mortality from breast cancer. JAMA 215:1777–1785, 1971
22. Shapiro S, Venet W, Strax P et al: Ten to fourteen year effect of screening on breast cancer mortality. JNCI 69:349–355, 1982
23. Shapiro S, Venet W, Strax P et al: Current results of the breast cancer screening randomized trial: The Health Insurance Plan (HIP) of greater New York study. In Day NE, Miller AB (eds): Screening for Breast Cancer, pp 3–15. Toronto, Hans Huber, 1988
24. Beahrs OH, Shapiro S, Smart C et al: Report of the Working Group to Review the National Cancer Institute-American Cancer Society Breast Cancer Demonstration Projects. JNCI 62:640–709, 1979
25. Baker LH: Breast Cancer Detection Demonstration Project: Five year summary report. CA 32:194–225, 1982
26. Seidman H, Gelb SK, Silverberg E et al: Survival experience in the Breast Cancer Detection Demonstration Project. CA 37:258–290, 1987
27. Thier SO: Breast cancer screening: A view from outside the controversy. N Engl J Med 297:1063–1065, 1977
28. Collette HJA, Day NE, Rombach JJ et al: Evaluation of screening for breast cancer in a non-randomized study (the Dom project) by means of a case–control study. Lancet 1:1224–1226, 1984
29. Verbeek ALM, Hendriks JHCL, Holland R et al: Mammographic screening and breast cancer mortality: Age-specific effects in Nijmegen project, 1975-82. Lancet 1:865–886, 1985
30. Palli D, Del Turco MR, Buiatti E et al: A case–control study of the efficacy of a non-randomized breast cancer screening program in Florence (Italy). Int J Cancer 38:501–504, 1986
31. Tabar L, Fagerberg CJG, Gad A et al: Reduction in mortality from breast cancer after mass screening with mammography. Lancet 1:829–832, 1985
32. de Waard F, Collette HJA, Rombach JJ et al: The DOM project for the early detection of breast cancer, Utrecht, the Netherlands. J Chronic Dis 37:1–44, 1984
33. Day NE, Walter SD, Tabar L et al: The sensitivity and lead time of breast cancer screening: A comparison of the results of different studies. In Day NE, Miller AB (eds): Screening for Breast Cancer, pp 105–109. Toronto, Hans Huber, 1988
34. Verbeek ALM, Straatman H, Hendricks JHCL: Sensitivity of mammography in Nijmegen women under age 50. In Day NE, Miller AB (eds): Screening for Breast Cancer, pp 29–32. Toronto, Hans Huber, 1988
35. U.K. Trial of Early Detection of Breast Cancer Group: Trial of early detection of breast cancer: Description of method. Br J Cancer 44:618–627, 1981
36. Miller AB, Howe GR, Wall C: The national study of breast cancer screening. Clin Invest Med 4:227–258, 1981
37. World Health Organization: The USSR/WHO study: Protocol of the study of the role of breast self-examination in reduction of mortality from breast cancer (in preparation)
38. Gastrin G: Breast Cancer Control. Stockholm, Almqvist & Wiksell, 1981
39. Day NE, Baines CJ, Chamberlain J et al: UICC project on screening for cancer: Report on the workshop on screening for breast cancer. Int J Cancer 38:303–308, 1986
40. Chamberlain J, Clifford RE, Nathan BE et al: Error-rates in screening for breast cancer by clinical examination and mammography. Clin Oncol 5:135–146, 1979
41. American Cancer Society: Mammography guidelines 1983: Background statement and update of cancer related check-up guidelines for breast cancer detection in asymptomatic women age 40–49. CA 33:255, 1983
42. American College of Radiology: New ACR guidelines on mammography. ACR Bull 38:6–7, 1982
43. Working Group: Breast cancer screening: Report to the Health Ministers of England, Wales, Scotland and Northern Ireland. London, Her Majesty's Stationery Office, 1987
44. Miller AB, Tsechovski M: Imaging technologies in breast cancer control: Summary of a World Health Organization meeting. AJR 148:1093–1094, 1987
45. Miller AB, Bulbrook RD: Screening, detection and diagnosis of breast cancer. Lancet 1:1109–1111, 1982
46. Miller AB, Chamberlain J, Tsechkovski M: Self-examination in the early detection of breast cancer: A review of the evidence, with recommendations for further research. J Chronic Dis 38:527–540, 1985
47. Baines CJ, Wall C, Risch HA et al: Changes in breast self-examination behaviour in a cohort of 8214 women in the Canadian National Breast Screening Study. Cancer 57:1209–1216, 1986
48. Winawer SJ, Fath RB, Schottfeld D et al: Screening for colorectal cancer. In Miller AB (ed): Screening for Cancer, pp 347–366. Orlando, Fla, Academic Press, 1985
49. Gibertsen VA: Proctosigmoidoscopy and polypectomy in reducing the incidence of rectal cancer. Cancer 34:936–939, 1974
50. Gilbertsen VA, Nelms JM: The prevention of invasive cancer of the rectum. Cancer 41:1137–1139, 1978
51. Miller AB: Review of sigmoidoscopic screening for colorectal cancer. In Chamberlain J, Miller AB (eds): Screening for Gastro-intestinal Cancer, pp 3–7. Toronto, Hans Huber, 1988
52. Dales LG, Friedman GD, Collen VIF: Evaluating periodic multiphasic health check-ups: A controlled trial. J Chronic Dis 32:385–404, 1979
53. Gilbertsen V, McHugh RB, Schuman LM et al: The colon cancer control study: An interim report. In Winawer SJ, Schottenfeld D, Sherlock P (eds): Colorectal Cancer: Prevention, Epidemiology and Screening, pp 261–266. New York, Raven, 1980
54. Winawer SJ, Andrews M, Flehinger B et al: Progress report on controlled trial of fecal occult blood testing for the detection of colorectal neoplasia. Cancer 43:2959–2964, 1980

55. National Cancer Institute, Division of Cancer Prevention and Control: Cancer Control Objectives for the Nation 1985–2000. NCI Monogr 2, 1986

56. Ebeling K, Nischan P: Screening for lung cancer: results from a case–control study. Int J Cancer 40:141–144, 1987

57. Cartwright RA: Screening for bladder cancer with particular reference to individual groups. In Prorok PC, Miller AB (eds): Screening for Cancer: 1. General Principles on Evaluation of Screening for Cancer and Screening for Lung, Bladder and Oral Cancer, pp 144–160. Geneva, International Union Against Cancer, 1984

58. Hirayama T: Screening for gastric cancer. In Miller AB (ed): Screening for Cancer, pp 367–376. Orlando, Fla, Academic Press, 1985

59. Oshima A, Hirata N, Ubukata T et al: Evaluation of a mass screening program for stomach cancer with a case–control study design. Int J Cancer 38:829–833, 1986

60. National Institutes of Health: Consensus Conference: Precursors to malignant melanoma. JAMA 251:1864–1866, 1984

61. American Cancer Society: Survey of physicians' attitudes and practices in early cancer detection. CA 35:197–213, 1985

62. Fisher B, Bauer M, Margolese R et al: Five-year results of a randomized clinical trial comparing total mastectomy and segmental mastectomy with or without radiation in the treatment of breast cancer. N Engl J Med 312:665–673, 1985

63. Miller AB: Screening for cancer: Issues and future directions. J Chronic Dis 39:1067–1077, 1986

RODNEY R. MILLION

NICHOLAS J. CASSISI

JOHN R. CLARK

CHAPTER 21 *Cancer of the Head and Neck*

EPIDEMIOLOGY OF HEAD AND NECK CANCER

The estimated number of new head and neck cancer cases (excluding skin cancer) in the United States for 1987 is 41,900; this represents 4.3% of the total new cancer cases.[1] The male-to-female ratio is approximately 4:1. The usual time of diagnosis is past the age of 40, except for salivary gland and nasopharyngeal tumors, which may occur in younger age groups. There has been no major change in the incidence of head and neck cancer over the past three decades in either the male or female population, which is somewhat surprising since a common etiologic factor (cigarette smoking) has resulted in a large increase in lung cancer. Cigarette smokers have an increased risk for multiple head and neck primary cancers as well as for lung cancer. Alcohol has also been implicated as a causative factor for certain head and neck cancers, and the effects of alcohol and tobacco seem to be additive. The smoking of marijuana has been reported to be a cause of head and neck cancer; it occurs in a younger age group.[2] We have observed several cases in marijuana users who were in their late 20s or early 30s at the time of diagnosis. Patients with pharyngeal cancer have an increased risk for developing esophageal cancer, and patients with major salivary gland tumors may have an increased risk for breast cancer.

ANATOMY

The regional anatomy is described separately under specific sites.

LYMPHATIC SYSTEM

There are no capillary lymphatics in the epithelium. Tumor must penetrate the lamina propria before lymphatic invasion can occur. One can predict the richness of the capillary network in any given head and neck site by the relative incidence of lymph node metastases at presentation. The nasopharynx and pyriform sinus have the most profuse networks of capillary lymphatics. The paranasal sinuses, middle ear, and vocal cords have few or no capillary lymphatics, based on their low rate of lymph node metastases when tumor is confined to these sites. Muscle and fat contain few capillary lymphatics. Bone and cartilage are thought to have a few capillary lymphatics in the periosteum or perichondrium. There are no capillary lymphatics in the eye, and few in the orbit. The arrangement of the important lymph nodes in the head and neck is shown in Fig. 21-1.[3]

PATHOLOGY

The vast majority of head and neck malignant neoplasms arise from the surface epithelium and are therefore squamous cell carcinoma or one of its many variants, including lymphoepithelioma, spindle cell carcinoma, verrucous carcinoma, and undifferentiated carcinoma. Lymphomas and a wide variety of other malignant and benign neoplasms make up the remaining cases (discussed under the appropriate section or chapter).

Lymphoepithelioma is a carcinoma with a lymphoid stroma. The lymphoid stroma may or may not be present in regional lymph node or distant metastases. Lymphoepithe-

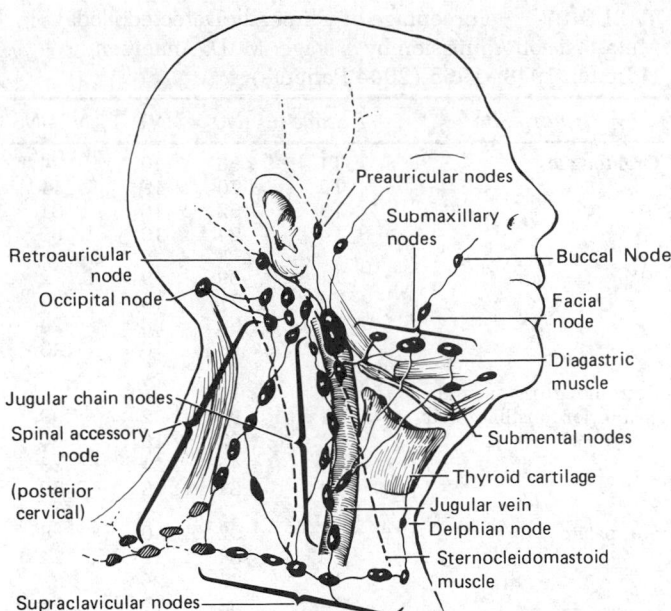

FIG. 21-1. The cervical lymphatics. (Redrawn from Rouvière H: Anatomy of the Human Lymphatic System, p 27. Ann Arbor, Edwards Brothers, 1938)

lioma occurs at anatomical sites with lymphoid aggregates in the submucosa, namely, the nasopharynx, tonsil, and base of tongue; it may also occur in the major salivary glands. This carcinoma has a higher rate of cure by radiation therapy than does squamous cell carcinoma.

In the spindle cell variant, found in 2% to 5% of malignant specimens taken from the upper aerodigestive tract, there is a component of spindle cells that resemble sarcoma intermixed with squamous cell carcinoma. This picture is variously described in the literature as pleomorphic carcinoma, sarcomatoid squamous cell carcinoma, squamous cell carcinoma with spindle cell variant, pseudosarcoma, and spindle cell squamous cell carcinoma, among others. For the most part, these lesions cannot be distinguished grossly from the usual squamous cell carcinoma. In some, the spindle cell component is relatively minor; in others, it dominates the picture and the squamous cell component is difficult to find. The sarcomatoid component may have features that are consistent with malignant fibrous histiocytoma. The lymph node metastases may show only the spindle cell component, only the carcinomatous element, or a mixture of both. This pattern may be seen anywhere that squamous cell carcinoma is found in the head and neck area.

Leventon and Evans reported 20 cases of spindle cell carcinoma.[4] All of the patients with superficially invasive tumors were cured, whereas only 1 of the 10 patients with deep invasion was cured. The tumors responded both to surgery and to radiation therapy, with six of the survivors being treated by operation, three by irradiation only, and two by combined treatment. Six of the tumors were said to have occurred in previously irradiated areas, and five of these patients eventually died. There are no data to compare the effectiveness of surgery and radiation therapy. It is our policy to consider the spindle cell variant as a high-grade carcinoma, but otherwise to disregard the spindle cell element in treatment decisions.

Verrucous carcinoma is a "grade one-half" squamous cell carcinoma found most often in the oral cavity, particularly on the gingiva and buccal mucosa. It usually has an indolent growth pattern and often is associated with the chronic use of snuff or chewing tobacco. Verrucous tumors resemble a wart: white or pink, exophytic, with distinct margins and multiple filiform processes that produce a roughened, cobblestone surface. The lesion may be soft or firm to palpation depending on the degree of keratinization and associated inflammation. The patient with verrucous carcinoma very often has multiple biopsies of an obvious lesion, but the pathologist returns a diagnosis of hyperkeratosis or pseudo-epitheliomatous hyperplasia. Eventually one may recommend cancer therapy based only on the appearance of the lesion and observation of its continued growth. If the pathologist can readily make a diagnosis of invasive carcinoma from histologic examination, the diagnosis of verrucous carcinoma is suspect. De novo verrucous carcinomas rarely develop lymph node metastases.

Small cell carcinoma occurs rarely throughout the head and neck region and is managed by radiation therapy and chemotherapy.

Lymphoma occurring in the upper aerodigestive tract almost always shows a diffuse non-Hodgkin's histologic pattern; nodular non-Hodgkin's lymphoma and Hodgkin's disease rarely involve the mucosal sites. Undifferentiated lymphomas and undifferentiated carcinoma may appear similar under the microscope. If lymphoma is suspected, fresh tissue should be given to the pathologist immediately for preparation for cell membrane studies. Lymphoma cells are quite susceptible to crush artifact, and the specimen should be obtained by sharp dissection rather than with punch biopsy forceps.

NATURAL HISTORY OF SQUAMOUS CELL CARCINOMA

PATTERNS OF SPREAD

Primary Lesion

Epidermoid carcinomas usually begin as surface lesions, but occasionally arise from ducts of minor salivary glands and therefore originate below the surface of the visible mucosa; this latter phenomenon is more likely to occur in the floor of the mouth, base of the tongue, and nasopharynx. The very early surface lesions may show only erythema and a slightly elevated, slightly roughened mucosa. These are the so-called red lesions and always deserve consideration for biopsy.

Spread is dictated by local anatomy, and each anatomical site has its own peculiar spread patterns. Muscle invasion is a common feature, and tumor may spread along muscle or fascial planes for a surprising distance from the palpable or visible lesion. Tumor may attach to periosteum or perichondrium quite early, but actual bone or cartilage invasion is usually a late event.

Bone and cartilage generally act as a barrier to spread, and these structures generally are spared until the neoplasm has explored easier avenues of growth. Tumor that encounters cartilage or bone in its path usually will be diverted and spread along a path of less resistance. Slow-growing neoplasms of the gingiva may produce a smooth pressure defect or saucerization of the underlying bone without actual bone invasion.

Entrance of tumor into the parapharyngeal space allows superior or inferior spread from the base of the skull to the root of the neck.

Spread inside the lumen of the sublingual, submandibular, and parotid gland ducts is not a prevalent pattern. The nasolacrimal duct, however, frequently is invaded in ethmoid sinus and nasal carcinoma.

Perineural spread is an important pathway for tumor spread; no site or histology is immune to this growth pattern. Squamous cell carcinoma and its variants and minor salivary gland tumors, especially adenoid cystic carcinoma, may show this pattern. The presence of perineural invasion predicts a poorer rate of local control when managed by surgery[5]; there are no specific data for success when the management is by radiation therapy. Local recurrence increases the likelihood of perineural involvement, and tumors may track along a nerve to the base of the skull and the central nervous system (CNS). Peripheral perineural spread, that is, growth away from the CNS, is also observed. Patients with perineural invasion often develop neurologic symptoms. Some nerve palsies are probably secondary to compression or entrapment rather than actual nerve invasion.

The risk of perineural spread is related to the anatomic site and diameter of the lesion.[6]

Vascular space invasion is associated with an increased risk for regional and distant metastases.

Lymphatic Spread

The risk of lymph node metastasis may be predicted by the differentiation of the tumor (the more poorly differentiated, the greater the risk), by the size of the primary lesion, by the presence of vascular space invasion, and by the availability of capillary lymphatics. Recurrent lesions likewise have an increased risk.

There is no exclusion of a particular histology from lymphatic spread; mere access to the capillary lymphatics determines the opportunity. In other words, minor salivary gland tumors and sarcomas assume a risk of lymphatic metastasis commensurate with the particular mucosal site.

A patient may present with squamous cell carcinoma in a cervical lymph node, and despite an extensive work-up, the site of origin may remain undetermined. If only the neck is treated, a primary lesion may appear at a later date, but some may never show a primary site.

The risk of subclinical disease in the patient with a clinically negative neck may be obtained either by studying the incidence of positive nodes found in elective neck dissection specimens or by counting the number of necks that become positive when the neck is not treated. The relative incidence of clinically positive lymph nodes on admission by anatomical site and T stage is given in Table 21-1.[7]

Well-lateralized lesions spread to ipsilateral neck lymph nodes. Lesions on or near the midline and lateralized tongue

TABLE 21-1.   Percentage of Clinically Detected Nodal Metastasis on Admission by T stage: M. D. Anderson Hospital, 1948–1965 (2044 Patients)

Primary Site	T Stage	N0	N1	N2–N3
Oral tongue	T1	86	10	4
	T2	70	19	11
	T3	52	16	31
	T4	24	10	66
Floor of mouth	T1	89	9	2
	T2	71	18	10
	T3	56	20	24
	T4	46	10	43
Retromolar trigone and anterior tonsillar pillar	T1	88	2	9
	T2	62	18	20
	T3	46	21	33
	T4	32	18	50
Soft palate	T1	92	0	8
	T2	64	12	24
	T3	35	26	39
	T4	33	11	56
Tonsillar fosa	T1	30	41	30
	T2	32	14	54
	T3	30	18	52
	T4	10	13	76
Base of tongue	T1	30	15	55
	T2	29	14	56
	T3	26	23	52
	T4	16	8	76
Oropharyngeal walls	T1	75	0	25
	T2	70	10	20
	T3	33	22	44
	T4	24	24	52
Supraglottic larynx	T1	61	10	29
	T2	58	16	26
	T3	36	25	40
	T4	41	18	41
Hypopharynx	T1	37	21	42
	T2	30	20	49
	T3	21	26	54
	T4	26	15	58
Nasopharynx	T1	8	11	82
	T2	16	12	72
	T3	12	9	80
	T4	17	6	78

Modified from Lindberg R: Distribution of cervical lymph node metastases from squamous cell carcinoma of the upper respiratory and digestive tracts. Cancer 29:1446–1449, 1972.

and nasopharyngeal lesions may spread to both sides but tend to spread to the side occupied by the bulk of the lesion. Patients with clinically positive lymph nodes in the ipsilateral neck are at risk for contralateral disease, especially if the nodes are large or multiple. Obstruction of the lymphatic pathways by surgery or radiation therapy will also shunt the lymphatic flow to the opposite neck. This shunting is mainly through anastomotic channels that cross through the submental space.[8]

When contralateral metastases occur from well-lateralized lesions, the subdigastric node is the most commonly involved but may be bypassed, with the midjugular or low jugular next affected. When lymph node metastases appear at an unusual site, a careful search must be made for a second primary.

Although there is usually an orderly progression of lymph node involvement, there are examples of skips and random involvement. Rarely one will see retrograde lymph node metastases in the ipsilateral axilla associated with involvement of the lower neck nodes.

Distant Spread

Stage for stage, the risk of distant metastases is the same for patients treated by radiation therapy alone and those treated by surgery alone. The risk of distant metastasis is more related to neck stage than primary stage. The risk is less than 10% for N0–N1 and rises to approximately 30% for N2 and N3.[9,10] Vascular space invasion is associated with an increased risk of distant metastasis. Lung is the most common site, accounting for 52% of the first recognized sites. Mediastinal metastases are uncommon, occurring in only 3%. Almost one half of the metastases are recognized by 9 months, 80% by 2 years, and 90% by 3 years. The risk of distant metastasis doubled in patients developing a recurrence above the clavicles: 16.7% for those having a recurrence, even if salvaged, and 7.9% for those never developing a recurrence.[11]

STAGING

The staging for the primary lesions (T) is given in the appropriate section. The AJCC (1983) neck staging (N) is common to all head and neck sites except the major salivary glands.[12]

NX   Minimum requirements to assess the regional nodes cannot be met

N0   No clinically positive node

N1   Single clinically positive homolateral node 3 cm or less in diameter

N2a   Single clinically positive homolateral node more than 3 cm but not more than 6 cm in diameter or multiple clinically positive homolateral nodes, none more than 6 cm in diameter

N2a   Single clinically positive homolateral node more than 3 cm but not more than 6 cm in diameter

N2b   Multiple clinically positive homolateral nodes, none more than 6 cm in diameter

N3   Massive homolateral node(s), bilateral nodes, or contralateral node(s)

N3a   Clinically positive homolateral node(s), one more than 6 cm in diameter

N3b   Bilateral clinically positive nodes (each side of the neck should be staged separately; e.g., N3b: right, N2a; left, N1)

N3c   Contralateral clinically positive node(s) only

The format for combining T and N stages into a total stage is shown in Figure 21-2.[13] Distant metastasis automatically places the patient into Stage IV. Stage IV represents a wide spectrum of disease. A patient may have a T1, T2, or T3 lesion with treatable N2 or N3A neck disease (Stage IVA) and represent a reasonable candidate for curative therapy, whereas another may have either a far-advanced primary (T4) or far-advanced neck disease (N3B), or both (Stage IVB). The 5-year disease-free survival rate is about twice as high for some sites for Stage IVA as for Stage IVB when radiation therapy is the initial treatment for the primary tumor.[13] A comparison of the results for Stages IVA and IVB when the initial treatment of the primary site is surgical has not been reported.

PRINCIPLES OF TREATMENT

GENERAL PRINCIPLES FOR SELECTION OF TREATMENT

Surgery and radiation therapy are the only curative treatments for carcinoma arising in the head and neck. Chemo-

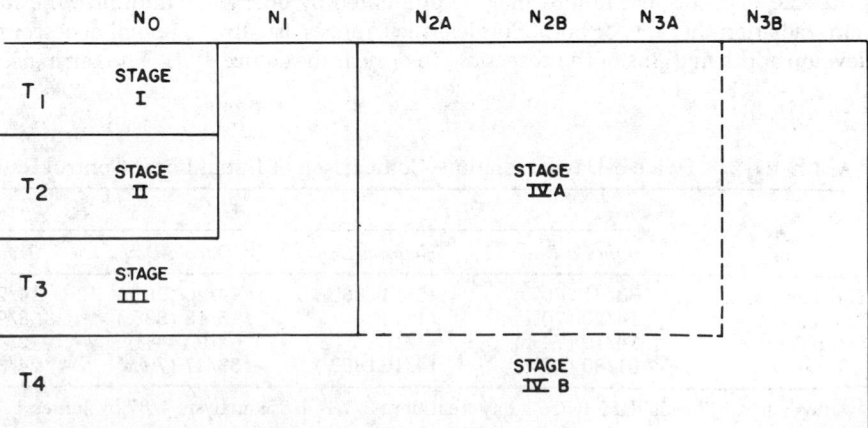

FIG. 21-2. American Joint Committee on Cancer stage grouping, as modified by Mendenhall et al.[12] (Mendenhall WM, Parsons JT, Million RR, et al: A favorable subset of AJCC stage IV squamous cell carcinoma of the head and neck. Int J Radiat Oncol Biol Phys 10:1841–1843, 1984)

therapy must be considered investigational at present; used alone, it is not curative, and its role as an adjunct to surgery, radiation therapy, or both is in a state of flux.

The advantages of an operation compared with radiation therapy, assuming similar cure rates, may include the following:

1. A limited amount of tissue is exposed to treatment.
2. Treatment time is shorter.
3. The risk of immediate and late radiation sequelae is avoided.
4. Irradiation is reserved for a subsequent head and neck primary tumor, which may not be as suitable for an operation.
5. Pathologic examination of tissues permits identification of patients with more extensive disease than originally determined, in whom immediate postoperative irradiation can be added.

The advantages of irradiation may include the following:

1. The threat of the major operation is avoided. An operative mortality of only 1% to 2% may seem high to the patient compared with no immediate threat from radiation therapy.
2. No tissues are removed. Resection of even a relatively small lesion may produce a functional or cosmetic defect. This risk must be weighed against the risk of a radiation necrosis.
3. Elective irradiation of the lymph nodes can be included with little added morbidity, whereas the surgeon either must adopt a "watch and wait" attitude or must proceed with elective neck dissection. This is important for lesions with a high rate of spread to the lymph nodes, especially where there is a high opportunity for bilateral spread (*i.e.*, floor of mouth, base of tongue, soft palate, hypopharynx, and some larynx lesions).
4. The surgical salvage of irradiation failure is more likely than the salvage of a surgical failure. When a primary lesion recurs after irradiation, the recurrence is almost always in the center of the original lesion; marginal failures are uncommon. A rescue operation would be similar in scope had the patient been managed initially by operation, albeit with a greater risk for a serious complication.

Rescue of a surgical failure may be attempted by operation, radiation therapy, or both. Surgical recurrences usually develop at the margins of the resection, in or near the suture line. It is difficult to distinguish the normal surgical scarring from recurrent disease, and diagnosis of recurrence is often delayed. Tumor response to radiation therapy under these circumstances is poor. Small mucosal recurrences and some neck recurrences, however, may be salvaged by an operation, radiation therapy, or both.

MANAGEMENT

PRIMARY SITE

The management of the primary site will be considered separately for each anatomical site. Since radiation therapy has the advantage of preserving anatomical integrity, the local control rates for radiation therapy must be known in order to select either curative radiation therapy with surgery reserved for local failure or initial surgical resection. The initial local control rates with once-a-day treatment and twice-a-day treatment for T2-T4 carcinomas of the oropharynx, larynx, and hypopharynx are compared in Tables 21-2 and 21-3. Patients treated with the twice-a-day scheme have received 120 cGy at each session with a 4-hour gap between treatments.[14] The total dose currently varies between 7440 cGy and 8100 cGy for oropharynx lesions and is limited to 7440 cGy to 7680 cGy when the larynx is in the reduced volume. Local control rates are at least as good or up to 10% to 15% improved with the twice-a-day treatment. Regional control rates are improved and complications fewer.

THE NECK

Management of the neck is closely tied to management of the primary site, but certain general principles may be outlined. Death due only to failure to control neck disease, with the primary tumor controlled, should be an uncommon event if surgery and radiation therapy are used to their maximum advantage.

In a standard *radical neck dissection*, the superficial and deep cervical fascia with its enclosed lymph nodes is removed in continuity with the sternocleidomastoid muscle, the omohyoid muscle, the internal and external jugular veins, the spinal accessory nerve, and the submandibular gland. The incisions used by the surgeon will be governed largely by the primary lesion. Proper physical therapy may minimize the functional changes associated with loss of the spinal accessory nerve and sternocleidomastoid muscle.

The term *modified neck dissection* refers to any neck node

TABLE 21-2.   Twice-a-Day Irradiation: Comparison of Initial Local Control Rates for Oropharynx

Site	T2		T3		T4	
	Once-a-Day	Twice-a-Day	Once-a-Day	Twice-a-Day	Once-a-Day	Twice-a-Day
Tonsillar region	33/41 (80%)	12/14 (86%)	14/20 (70%)	14/21 (67%)	4/11 (36%)	4/9 (44%)
Base of tongue	14/20 (70%)	1/1	15/18 (83%)	8/9 (89%)	2/12 (17%)	3/6 (50%)
Soft palate	14/19 (74%)	1/1	4/9 (44%)	2/4	n.d.	n.d.
Total	61/80 (76%)	14/16 (88%)	33/47 (70%)	24/34 (71%)	6/23 (26%)	7/15 (47%)

University of Florida data; twice-a-day treatment 3/78–4/85; analysis 4/87 by James T. Parsons, M.D. n.d., no data.

TABLE 21-3.   Twice-a Day Irradiation: Comparison of Initial Local Control Rates for Larynx/Hypopharynx

Site	T2 Once-a-Day	T2 Twice-a-Day	T3 Once-a-Day	T3 Twice-a-Day	T4 Once-a-Day	T4 Twice-a-Day
Supraglottic larynx	18/23 (78%)	9/11 (82%)	3/5 (60%)	12/17 (71%)	1/7	0/1
True vocal cord	n.d.	n.d.	7/13 (54%)	10/14 (71%)	n.d.	1/5
Pyriform sinus	12/16	3/3	1/3	1/2	0/2	0/1
Pharyngeal wall	8/17	4/4	8/21 (38%)	5/7 (71%)	1/8	1/2
Total	38/56 (68%)	16/18 (89%)	19/42 (45%)	28/40 (70%)	2/17 (12%)	2/9 (22%)

University of Florida data; twice-a-day treatment 3/78–4/85; analysis 4/87 by James T. Parsons, M.D. n.d., no data.

resection that is less than the radical neck dissection. A modified neck dissection is tailored to remove those groups of lymph nodes at highest risk for metastatic disease while also attempting to reduce the sequelae by selectively preserving certain muscles, nerves, and vessels. A modified neck dissection sparing normal tissues (e.g., the functional neck dissection) is usually recommended for the clinically negative neck, for selected clinically positive necks (mobile, 1–3 cm lymph nodes), and for removing residual disease after radiation therapy when there has been excellent regression of N2 or N3 disease.

Complications after radical neck dissection include hematoma, seroma, lymphedema, wound infections and dehiscence, damage to the 7th, 10th, and 12th cranial nerves, carotid exposure, and carotid rupture. The last-mentioned can be minimized by covering the carotid artery with a dermal graft at the time of surgery.

CLINICALLY NEGATIVE NECK. The risk for subclinical disease for any particular patient may be estimated based on the primary site, the T stage or size of the primary lesion, the differentiation of the neoplasm, and the presence of lymphatic invasion. The incidence of subclinical disease in the regional lymphatics when the neck is clinically negative is presented in Table 21-4.[15] The use of contrast-enhanced CT will improve the diagnostic ability and decrease the chance of underestimating disease in the neck in 5% to 10% of patients.[45] Both irradiation and neck dissection are approximately 90% efficient in eradicating subclinical disease in the neck lymph nodes. A policy of "wait and see" may be adopted for the clinically negative neck to avoid unnecessary treatment, and the neck may then be managed by surgery, radiation therapy, or both only if cervical metastases develop. Even though the salvage neck treatment may be regionally successful, these patients are at an increased risk to develop distant metastasis and therefore have a poorer prognosis compared with patients who have immediate control of neck disease from the beginning. The salvage rate for patients developing clinically positive lymph nodes with the primary lesion controlled is only 60% in the University of Florida experience.[46]

When a neck node does appear, the diagnosis often may be delayed so that the morbidity of the salvage procedure is considerably greater than one would experience with elective treatment.

The physician and patient must adhere to a schedule of very close observation and examination if they choose the policy of observation.

Elective neck treatment has the added advantage of giving complete treatment at the initial point of management and

TABLE 21-4.   Incidence of Lymph Node Metastasis by Site of Primary in Head and Neck Squamous Cell Carcinoma

Site	Percentage N+ at Presentation (Reference)	Percentage N0 Clinically, N+ Pathologically (Reference)	Percentage N0– > N+ with No Neck Treatment (Reference)
Floor of mouth	30–59 (16–18)	40–50 (19, 20)	20–35 (21–23)
Gingiva	18–52 (16, 24–26)	19 (24)	17 (21, 24)
Hard palate	13–24 (26–28)		22 (21)
Buccal mucosa	9–31 (16, 18)		16 (21)
Oral tongue	34–65 (16–18, 29)	25–54 (20, 25, 30–32)	38–52 (23, 29, 31, 33)
Nasopharynx	86–90 (9, 10, 34)		19*–50 (35, 36)
Anterior tonsillar pillar/ retromolar trigone	39–56 (37–39)		10–15 (40)
Soft palate/uvula	37–56 (37–39)		16–25 (39)
Tonsillar fossa	58–76 (9, 10, 17, 34, 38)		22† (41)
Base of tongue	50–83 (34, 38, 40, 42)	22 (42)	
Pharyngeal walls	50–71 (34, 38, 40, 42)	66 (42)	
Supraglottic larynx	31–54 (17, 40)	16–26 (42, 43)	33 (43, 44)
Hypopharynx	52–72 (9, 40, 42)	38 (42)	

Mendenhall WM, Million RR, Cassisi NJ: Elective neck irradiation in squamous cell carcinoma of the head and neck. Head Neck Surg 3:15–20, 1980.
*T1N0 patients only.
†Patients received preoperative irradiation.

simplifying the follow-up neck examinations because of its high success rate. The relative effectiveness of irradiation and surgery in the management of the N0 neck is shown in Tables 21-5, 21-6, and 21-7.[15,48] Partial neck treatment is inefficient for primary lesions of the oropharynx, supraglottic larynx, or hypopharynx (Tables 21-6 and 21-7), and treatment of the entire neck is advised for sites with a high rate of subclinical disease.

When the primary tumor is to be treated surgically, it is our recommendation to add elective neck treatment when the risk of regional lymph node metastasis is 10% to 15% or greater. In some cases elective neck treatment is added when the risk is less; it is relatively easy to add elective neck treatment with either radiation therapy or surgery because of the type of operation or irradiation being delivered to the primary site. If the primary lesion is to be treated with external beam irradiation, then elective neck irradiation adds no cost and, if properly done, little additional morbidity.

When the primary lesion is to be treated surgically, the surgeon has the responsibility to manage the neck unless postoperative irradiation is definitely planned. Most surgeons do not use radical neck dissection for the clinically negative neck so that there are fewer cosmetic or functional problems. Modified neck dissections have as good a rate of disease control as does the radical neck dissection if patients who are found to have multiple positive nodes or disease extending through the capsule are then referred for postoperative irradiation.[49]

Radiation therapy occasionally fails to eradicate subclinical disease. Most of the failures are due to geographic misses with nodes appearing near the edge or just outside the edge of the treatment field. Other causes of failure are low dose, selection of the wrong beam energy (which results in low dose), and failure to detect a clinically positive node.

Elective neck surgery occasionally fails because of a failure to remove all the lymph nodes at risk or because of extranodal extension.

CLINICALLY POSITIVE NECK LYMPH NODES. The rate of neck failure by N stage and therapeutic category reported from M. D. Anderson Hospital is shown in Tables 21-6 and 21-7.[48] The irradiation preceded the operation if the primary site was to be treated by radiation therapy or if the node was fixed. The operation preceded the irradiation if the primary site was to be treated surgically.

TABLE 21-5. Efficacy of Elective Neck Irradiation (ENI) with Primary Tumor Controlled — 125 Patients

Primary Stage	No. of Patients with Neck Controlled/ No. of Patients with Primary Controlled		
	No ENI	Partial ENI	Whole ENI
T1	11/12	17/18	9/10
T2	6/8	17/17	22/22
T3	0/1	10/10	18/18
T4	1/1	5/5	3/3
Total	18/22 (82%)*	49/50 (98%)*	52/53 (98%)*

*Significance level = 0.01, using exact test procedures.[47]
Mendenhall WM, Million RR, Cassisi NJ: Elective neck irradiation in squamous cell carcinoma of the head and neck. Head Neck Surg 3:15–20, 1980.

Radical neck dissection is sufficient treatment for the ipsilateral neck for patients with N1 or N2A disease. Radiation therapy is added for N2B and N3 stages, for control of contralateral subclinical disease (Table 21-7), for invasion through the capsule of the node, and for the finding of multiple positive nodes in the specimen.

When the primary lesion is to be managed by irradiation, then radiation therapy alone is sufficient for patients with N1 (1–3 cm) disease. Neck dissection may be added in selected cases in which the 3 cm node is fixed or fails to regress completely. Radiation therapy is followed by a neck dissection for most N2A and nearly all N3A disease. The decision to add radical neck dissection for N2B and N3B disease is individualized, based on the diameter of the largest node or the multiplicity of palpable nodes. Large, fixed nodes require 6000 cGy to 8000 cGy before neck dissection; some of the specimens will show "no viable tumor," and a substantial number of patients will have the disease controlled in the neck. There will be less fibrosis in the neck by 5 years after treatment when large node masses are managed by radiation therapy followed by neck dissection compared with irradiation alone.

The neck disease control rate in patients managed between 1978 and 1984 with 120 cGy twice daily to doses of 7440 cGy to 8000 cGy to the primary lesion is shown in Table 21-8. At least a part of the upper neck received the same doses. When the primary lesion was controlled by radiation therapy, the rate of control of neck disease was very

TABLE 21-6. Failure of Initial Neck Treatment (596 Patients with Carcinoma of the Tonsillar Fossa, Base of Tongue, Supraglottic Larynx, or Hypopharynx, M. D. Anderson Hospital, 1948–1967)

Treatment	Stage							
	N0			N1	N2A	N2B	N3A	N3B
	No Treatment	Partial	Complete					
Radiation		15%	2%	15%	27%	27%	38%	34%
Surgery	55% (16/29)	35%	7%	11%	8%	23%	42%	41%
Combined		1/5	0/6	0	0	0	23%	25%

Adapted from Barkley HT Jr, Fletcher GH, Jesse RH et al: Management of cervical lymph node metastases in squamous cell carcinoma of the tonsillar fossa, base of tongue, supraglottic larynx, and hypopharynx. Am J Surg 124:462–467, 1972.

TABLE 21-7. Cervical Metastasis Appearing in the Contralateral Neck (596 Patients with Carcinoma of the Tonsillar Fossa, Base of Tongue, Supraglottic Larynx, or Hypopharynx, M. D. Anderson Hospital, 1948–1967)

Treatment	N0	N1	N2A	N2B	N3A
Radiation	2/50	1/52	2/22	2/27	0/21
Surgery	7/28	8/47	3/13	13/30	4/12
Combined	0/6	0/21	0/17	3/28	0/13

Barkley HT Jr, Fletcher GH, Jesse RH et al: Management of cervical lymph node metastases in squamous cell carcinoma of the tonsillar fossa, base of tongue, supraglottic larynx, and hypopharynx. Am J Surg 124:462–467, 1972.

high. There were only four neck failures in 30 patients selected for planned neck dissection; the patients selected for neck dissection were usually those with fixed masses, large masses, or a poor response to radiation therapy. These results have been updated to 1985. Forty-one ipsilateral and 4 bilateral planned neck dissections after twice-a-day therapy have been evaluated for complications. There have been no carotid ruptures and no operative deaths. There were 8 wound complications in 41 unilateral neck dissections and 1 minor wound complication in 4 bilateral neck dissections (JT Parsons, unpublished data, 1986). The average time to discharge was 6 days for non-Veterans Administration patients and 14 days for Veterans Administration patients.

Biopsy of a neck mass for diagnosis by excisional or incisional biopsy has been condemned by many. McGuirt and McCabe[50] compared results with and without open biopsy and concluded that the risks of neck failure, distant metastases, and complications of subsequent neck surgery were all increased. Their patients were managed by operation following open neck biopsy.

Parsons and co-workers[51] studied the results of therapy following incisional or excisional biopsy of a lymph node before treatment. In 25 patients with no gross residual disease after excisional biopsy (NX), the referring surgeons' and pathologists' reports showed that a single, clinically positive lymph node had been totally excised. These patients received irradiation to the primary site and neck. No other clinically positive lymph nodes were found upon referral, and no neck dissections were performed for this group of patients. The rate of control of neck disease was 96%, the absolute 5-year disease-free survival rate was 79%, and the 5-year determinate survival rate was 88%. These results are good, considering that all patients had Stage III or IV disease.

Fifty-five patients had gross residual neck disease after biopsy.[51] In some patients, only an incisional biopsy of a very large mass had been performed; in others, only one of several lymph nodes had been removed. The absolute 5-year disease-free survival rate in this group of patients was 31%, the 5-year determinate survival rate was 38%, and the overall rate of control of neck disease was 64%. All except three had Stage IV disease. The more consistent addition of a neck dissection in recent years had resulted in improved rates of neck disease control and survival in this latter group.

After open biopsy of the neck, it is recommended that radiation therapy be the initial treatment. If the primary tumor is to be managed by radiation therapy, no further neck treatment is needed if the neck node has been removed. If there is residual gross tumor in the neck after open biopsy, a planned neck dissection should be added. If the primary tumor is to be managed by operation, it is recommended that preoperative radiation therapy be used, followed by removal of the primary lesion plus an appropriate neck dissection.

Once the normal lymphatic pathways have been surgically interrupted by the open biopsy procedure, shunting of lymph to the contralateral side of the neck may occur, placing it at risk for lymph node spread when the opposite neck would not normally be at risk.[8,52]

CHEMOTHERAPY

The role of chemotherapy in the management of patients with squamous cell carcinoma of the head and neck has not

TABLE 21-8. Control of Disease in the Neck with Twice-a-Day Fractionation When the Primary Lesion Is Controlled (No. of Heminecks Controlled/No. Treated)

Hemineck Stage	Radiation Therapy Alone	Radiation Therapy plus Neck Dissection	Total
NX	1/1	n.d.	1/1
N0	82/84	n.d.	82/84
N1	21/22	6/7	27/29
N2A	1/1	4/5	5/6
N2B	9/12	11/12	20/24
N3A	0/2*	5/6	5/8
Total		26/30 (87%)	140/152 (92%)

University of Florida data; patients treated 3/78 – 4/84; analysis 4/86 by James T. Parsons, M.D. n.d., no data.
*Lung metastases; neck dissections cancelled.

been adequately defined and remains an area of active investigation. For patients with metastatic or recurrent disease following maximal surgery and radiotherapy, chemotherapy can induce significant tumor regression in 20% to 50% of patients and provide palliation for the patient with symptomatic or life-threatening disease. For patients with potentially curable advanced local–regional disease (M0), the use of chemotherapy as induction, adjuvant, or synchronous treatment with surgery or radiotherapy remains an investigative approach.

Single-Agent Chemotherapy for Advanced Disease

Numerous individual drugs have demonstrable activity against squamous cell carcinoma of the head and neck (Table 21-9). These drugs belong to several major classes of antineoplastic compounds, including bifunctional alkylating agents, antimetabolites, antitumor antibiotics, plant alkaloids, and heavy metal coordination complexes. The response rates recorded in Table 21-9 must be interpreted with caution, as they are derived from pooled data from a large number of individual trials using different criteria for patient entry, variable drug doses and schedules, and often discrepant criteria for response.

Methotrexate was one of the earliest and most thoroughly evaluated single agents in the treatment of squamous cell cancers of the head and neck. By virtue of its documented activity, acceptable toxicity, convenience of administration, and low cost, it remains the standard of therapy for patients with recurrent or metastatic disease. Methotrexate has been given in a wide variety of doses and schedules (Table 21-10). Weekly or twice-weekly conventional dose administration may be more effective than loading doses once every 3 to 4 weeks or daily administration of small doses. Moderate to high doses of methotrexate with leucovorin can be safely administered to patients with head and neck cancer and may limit the myelosuppression, alopecia, nephrotoxicity, and mucositis associated with lower doses of methotrexate without leucovorin. However, the use of moderate to high doses of methotrexate with leucovorin rescue adds cost, inconvenience, and risk of toxicity in noncompliant patients with

TABLE 21-9. Single-Agent Activity in Patients with Recurrent or Metastatic Head and Neck Cancer

Drug	No. of Patients	Response Rate (%)*
Methotrexate[53-65] (doses <200 mg/m²)	447	36
Bleomycin[66-72]	386	26
Cisplatin[73-78]	194	32
5-Fluorouracil[79-87]	115	27
Cyclophosphamide[88]	77	36
Doxorubicin[89-90]	88	13
New or Inadequately Studied Agents		
Hydroxyurea[91]	22	23
Carboplatin[92-95]	115	26
Iproplatin[95]	34	12
Mitozantrone[96-98]	113	4

*Includes subjective, <50%, or unquantified responses.

no apparent increase in antitumor activity, duration of response, or overall survival.[57,59,61,64,65] For palliation of patients with advanced, incurable disease and acceptable renal function, it is appropriate to begin oral or intravenous methotrexate with weekly doses of 40 to 50 mg/m² or biweekly doses of 15 to 20 mg/m² and escalate the dose in weekly increments until either mild toxicity or therapeutic response is achieved. Moderate-dose methotrexate with leucovorin may be appropriate for the patient with treatment-limiting mucositis or myelosuppression on low-dose methotrexate or as a nonmyelosuppressive addition to combination chemotherapy.

Bleomycin is another single agent with activity against squamous cell carcinomas. Response rates from trials in the United States, however, have been consistently lower than those from the initial Japanese studies.[66-72] Experimental data in animals[99,100] support the clinical impression[101-103] that bleomycin's clinical activity and therapeutic index are greater when given by continuous infusion than when administered by intermittent bolus. Despite the potential of skin and mucosal toxicity and severe interstitial pulmonary disease, bleomycin has been employed in many regimens of

TABLE 21-10. Methotrexate Given Parenterally in Doses Less Than 200 mg/m² for Head and Neck Cancer

Investigator	Schedule*	No. of Patients	Percentage of Patients with >50% Tumor Regression
Papac et al.[53]	0.8 mg/kg every 4 days IV	15	53
Lane et al.[54]	25 to 50 mg every 4 to 7 days	27	52
Leone et al.[55]	60 mg/m² weekly IV or 40 mg/m² biweekly IV	35	57
DePalo et al.[56]	40 or 60 mg/m² weekly IV	23	35
Levitt et al.[57]	80 mg/m² for 30 h every 2 wk with escalation to toxicity	16	44
DeConti and Schoenfeld[59]	40 mg/m² weekly IV	81	26
Kirkwood et al.[60]	40 to 200 mg/m² IV on days 1, 4 weekly; leucovorin on days 2, 5	19	63
Woods et al.[61]	50 mg/m² bolus; leucovorin 15 mg PO every 6 h × 12 doses	23	26
Hong et al.[62]	40 to 60 mg/m² IV weekly	17	23
Grose et al.[63]	15 mg/m² IM on days 1 through 3 every 3 wk	44	18
Vogler et al.[64]	60 mg/m² IV weekly	61	35
Total		361	35

*PO, by mouth.

combination chemotherapy for head and neck cancer because of its lack of significant myelosuppression.

The experience with cisplatin suggests that this agent has antitumor activity that is comparable to methotrexate.[73-78] Two relatively small randomized studies comparing cisplatin to methotrexate have shown similar response rates; however, cisplatin produced more nephrotoxicity and emesis, whereas methotrexate resulted in more mucositis and myelosuppression.[62,63] Cisplatin has also been compared to "symptomatic care," infusion bleomycin, or a combination of cisplatin and bleomycin in a randomized trial of patients with recurrent or metastatic disease.[104] In this study, patients treated with cisplatin had significantly prolonged survival in comparison to the control group. In addition, the combination of cisplatin and bleomycin was no more effective than cisplatin alone, and bleomycin offered no benefit over symptomatic care.

Two cisplatin analogues, iproplatin and carboplatin, have recently been evaluated in Phase I and II trials and offer the potential for decreased renal and gastrointestinal toxicity and the advantage of outpatient administration. Both drugs can be administered without prior hydration or mannitol diuresis. Preliminary studies of iproplatin and carboplatin have demonstrated significant antitumor activity with myelosuppression as the principal side-effect. In a single study of 34 patients, a 12% response rate to iproplatin was recorded,[95] and in three studies with 115 total patients, a response rate of 26% to carboplatin was noted.[92-95]

Cyclophosphamide and 5-fluorouracil have also demonstrated substantial antitumor activity as single agents in patients with metastatic or recurrent head and neck cancer. Of particular interest is a recent report of four partial responses in seven such patients treated with infusion 5-fluorouracil.[105]

Numerous other drugs have been evaluated in patients with recurrent or metastatic head and neck cancer. Unfortunately, an encouraging preliminary study of mitoguazone[106] has not been reproduced.[107-109] In addition, clinically significant activity has not been demonstrated in recent studies of mitozantrone,[96-98] m-AMSA,[110-111] dibromodulcitol,[96,112,113] VP-16,[114-116] vindesine,[117-119] and triazinate.[120]

Biologic response modifiers, especially interferon, have also been used in the treatment of patients with advanced head and neck cancer.[121-123] Mendenica and Slack,[122] using human leukocyte interferon, reported 3 complete and 4 partial responses in 12 patients with refractory head and neck cancer. In this study, the duration of response was approximately 10 months. Connors and co-workers[123] similarly evaluated human leukocyte interferon in 12 patients with advanced nasopharyngeal carcinoma and noted measurable responses in 4 patients and stabilization of disease in 3 additional patients.

Combination Chemotherapy for Advanced Disease

Over the past 10 to 15 years, numerous Phase II trials have evaluated combinations of active single agents in patients with advanced head and neck cancer. The majority of published regimens of combination chemotherapy for head and neck cancer have been two- or three-drug schedules of cisplatin, bleomycin, methotrexate, or vincristine. Recent combinations include cisplatin and 5-fluorouracil and sequential methotrexate and 5-fluorouracil. Cisplatin with infusion 5-fluorouracil has been shown to be more effective than cisplatin with bolus 5-fluorouracil.[124] While several studies of patients with recurrent or metastatic disease have suggested modest increases in the rates of complete or total response to combination chemotherapy (Table 21-11), the toxicity of some combinations is formidable, with no obvious therapeutic gain over single-agent cisplatin or methotrexate.

The clinical significance of such Phase II studies is limited by the absence of a control group and the possibility of selection bias. Given the impact of various prognostic factors in treatment outcome, a definitive analysis of combination chemotherapy requires a prospective, randomized study.

To date, six randomized trials have been published that directly compare combination to single-agent chemotherapy in the treatment of patients with metastatic or recurrent squamous cell carcinoma of the head and neck (Table 21-12). As noted, five of the six studies compared combination chemotherapy to single-agent methotrexate. Although combination chemotherapy was associated with a higher total response rate in five of six studies, a statistically significant difference was apparent in only two. More importantly, the use of combination chemotherapy was not associated with an improved duration of response or median survival in any of the six trials.

GENERAL PRINCIPLES OF COMBINING MODALITIES

Surgery Plus Radiation Therapy

Either preoperative or postoperative radiation therapy may be used; there are advocates of each. Analysis of available data suggests that there is no difference in local-regional control or survival rates comparing the two sequences.

Combined modality therapy should be avoided for lesions with a high cure rate (70% or greater) by either surgery or radiation therapy alone. The increased morbidity from combined treatment does not increase the control rate significantly, and many patients with local or regional failure can be salvaged by secondary procedures.

The advantages of postoperative compared with preoperative radiation therapy include less operative morbidity, more meaningful margin checks at the time of the operation, a knowledge of tumor spread for radiation treatment planning, safe use of a higher radiation dose, and no chance that the patient will refuse surgery.

The disadvantages of postoperative radiation therapy include the larger treatment volume necessary to cover surgical dissections and scars, a delay in the start of radiation therapy with possible growth of tumor (especially contralateral neck nodes), and the higher dose required to accomplish the same rate of local-regional control.

PREOPERATIVE RADIATION THERAPY. Preoperative radiation therapy is recommended for the following situations:

1. A trial of radiation therapy (5000 cGy) is given to judge the response of the primary lesion. The patient

TABLE 21-11. Recent Drug Combinations

Investigator	Dosage and Schedule*	No. of Patients†	Response Rate (%)		Duration of Response (mo)
			Total	Complete	
Kish et al.[125]	Cisplatin 100 mg/m² on day 1 5-FU 1000 mg/m²/d on days 1 through 4	30 (5)	70	27	11.3 (if CR) 6.5. (if PR)
Merlano et al.[126]	Cisplatin 20 mg/m²/d on days 1 through 5 5-FU 200 mg/m²/d on days 1 through 5	30 (29)	53	13	6.5 (survival)
Bitran et al.[127]	Doxorubicin 40 mg/m² Cyclophosphamide 750 mg/m²	26 (26)	46	0	6.5
Scherlacher et al.[128]	Methotrexate 250 mg/m² at hour 0 5-FU 600 mg/m² at hour 1	28 (17)	39	18	6.5
Pitman et al.[129]	Methotrexate 250 mg/m² at hour 0 5-FU 600 mg/m² at hour 1	23 (5)	65	13	3.6
Lester et al.[130]	Cisplatin 50 mg/m² on day 1 Bleomycin 7 mg/m² on days 1, 8, 15 Methotrexate 120 mg/m² at hour 0 on days 8, 15, 22 followed by leucovorin 5-FU 600 mg/m² at hour 1 on days 8, 15, 22	74 (19)	52	18	16 (survival CR) 9 (survival PR)
Vogl et al.[131]	Cisplatin 50 mg/m² on day 4 Bleomycin 10 mg/d on days 1, 8, 15 Methotrexate 40 mg/m² at hour 0 on days 1, 15 5-FU 600 mg/m² at hour 1 on days 1, 15	46 (NA)	50	4	3.5
Cognetti et al.[132]	Bleomycin 10 mg/wk Vincristine 2 mg/wk Methotrexate 40 mg/m²/d on days 1, 15 Cisplatin 50 mg/m² on day 4	43 (19)	74	21	6

*5-FU, 5-fluorouracil.
†Number of patients with prior chemotherapy in parentheses; NA, not available.

is reevaluated with the surgeon, and a decision is made to continue for cure by radiation therapy or to stop the irradiation and proceed in 4 to 6 weeks to an operation. This philosophy is selected for moderately advanced lesions that have a reasonable chance of responding favorably to radiation therapy, thereby avoiding a major ablative procedure. The pyriform sinus and larynx are common primary sites for use of this strategy.

2. Solitary neck nodes that are fixed or on the borderline of resectability are a reason to give radiation therapy before surgery. The preoperative dose to the primary lesion is 5000 cGy, but treatment of the major neck mass is continued to a dose of 6000 cGy to 8000 cGy through a reduced tangential portal. Most large nodes will become resectable, and in approximately 50% of the specimens no tumor is seen. A fibrous capsule forms around the neck mass that facilitates dissection from the neurovascular bundles.

3. If the reconstruction and rehabilitation will delay the start of postoperative radiation therapy by more than 6

TABLE 21-12. Chemotherapy for Metastatic or Recurrent Squamous Cell Carcinoma of the Head and Neck—Randomized Trials

Investigator	Drugs Used	No. of Patients	Total Response (%)	Median Survival (mo)
DeConti and Schoenfeld[59]	Methotrexate	81	26	5.0
	Methotrexate/leucovorin	80	24	4.4
	Methotrexate/leucovorin, cyclophosphamide, cytosine arabinoside	76	18	3.2
Kaplan et al.[133]	Methotrexate	61	26*	5.0
	Cisplatin, bleomycin, methotrexate	61	46*	5.5
Jacobs et al.[134]	Cisplatin	41	18	6.2
	Cisplatin, methotrexate	39	33	6.9
Drelichman et al.[135]	Methotrexate	20	33	5.5
	Cisplatin, vincristine, bleomycin	20	41	3.5
Vogl et al.[136]	Methotrexate	83	35†	5.6
	Cisplatin, bleomycin, methotrexate	80	48†	5.6
Williams et al.[137]	Methotrexate	98	16	7.3
	Cisplatin, vinblastine, bleomycin	92	24	6.8

*p = 0.04.
†p = 0.07.

to 12 weeks, then consideration should be given to preoperative radiation therapy.

4. If an operative procedure is planned that includes use of the gastric pull-up for pharyngeal or esophageal reconstruction, preoperative irradiation is preferred because the tolerance limit of the stomach is thought to be 4000 cGy.
5. If a neck mass has been excisionally or incisionally biopsied and the primary lesion is to be resected, preoperative radiation therapy is advised.[50,51]

The dose for preoperative radiation therapy is usually 5000 cGy in 5 to 6 weeks. Short treatment schemes using a few large fractions followed immediately by surgery have shown little or no advantage over surgery alone.[138-141] Moderate-dose schemes, 3000 cGy to 4000 cGy, have not resulted in any great increase in control rates. A dose of 5000 cGy will control a large percentage of subclinical disease in lymph nodes and also reduce the recurrence rates for the primary site. A few venturesome groups have tried higher doses (6000 cGy), but the morbidity may exceed the gain. A reduced volume encompassing a large node may receive a high dose.

POSTOPERATIVE RADIATION THERAPY. Postoperative radiation therapy is considered when the risk of recurrence above the clavicles exceeds 20%. The operative procedure should be one-stage and of such magnitude that irradiation is started no later than 6 to 12 weeks after surgery. The operation should be undertaken only if it is believed to be highly likely that all gross disease will be removed and margins will be negative. It is fashionable to talk about "debulking" operations prior to radiation therapy. This term has no precise meaning and should be avoided because it may imply partial removal of gross disease ("cut-through"), a maneuver that probably reduces the chance of control by radiation therapy rather than enhancing it.

The radiation therapist is frequently called upon to make a decision regarding further treatment based on the pathologist's report following a cancer operation. Positive margins or close margins are an indication for radiation therapy. Looser and co-workers[142] compared the clinical significance of negative and positive margins for 1775 previously untreated squamous cell carcinomas of the head and neck (excluding glottic and skin). Only 3.5% were scored as positive margins. The incidence of recurrence at the primary site was 31.7% for patients with negative margins and 71% for those with positive margins. There was no difference whether the positive margin was due to carcinoma in situ, invasive tumor, or close margin (within 5 mm). Other indications for postoperative irradiation may be cartilage or bone invasion, perineural spread, and high-grade histology.

The findings in the neck dissection frequently are the indication for postoperative radiation therapy. Multiple positive nodes, invasion through the capsule, and high-grade histology predict a high risk of recurrence in both the dissected and the contralateral neck.

Amdur and co-workers[143] analyzed the results of radical surgery and postoperative radiation therapy in 161 patients with advanced, previously untreated squamous cell carcinoma of the oral cavity, oropharynx, hypopharynx, or larynx. Ninety-six percent had Stage III or IV cancer, and none had evidence of gross disease at the start of irradiation. The majority of recurrences above the clavicles occurred in the primary field (84%) as opposed to the posterior neck area (8%) or low neck (8%). Five factors were found to be significantly important for predicting disease control above the clavicles: treatment course (continuous course, 77%, versus split course, 33%; $p < 0.001$), surgical margin (invasive cancer at the margin, 50%, versus margin free of invasive cancer, 81%; $p = 0.01$), primary site (oral cavity, 64%, versus other sites, 83%; $p = 0.029$), multiple positive nodes in the surgical specimen (presence being worse than absence of this finding), and number of indications for irradiation (1-3 indications, 85%, versus ≥ 4 indications, 61%; $p = 0.06$).[144,145] The rate of disease control above the clavicles did not correlate well with AJCC pathologic stage. The interval between surgery and the start of radiation therapy up to 3 months also was not prognostically important.

At 5 years the actuarial survival rate was 33% for the entire group; for patients with invasive cancer at the margin, the survival rate was approximately half that of those whose margins were free of invasive cancer (17% versus 37%). Three factors were found to significantly influence survival rates: course of irradiation (continuous better than split), nodal status (negative better than positive), and extension of the primary tumor into the soft tissues of the neck (absence better than presence of this finding). Overall, 7% of patients experienced a severe complication of combined therapy, including pharyngeal stricture, stomal stenosis, bone or soft tissue necrosis, laryngeal edema, infection, and fistula.

Contrary to an earlier report,[146] there was no obvious dose response (excluding split course) when patients with similar risk factors were compared (Table 21-13). We continue to recommend 6000 cGy in 6 weeks to 6500 cGy in 7 weeks for patients with negative margins and fewer than three indications for radiation therapy. For patients with close (<5 mm) or positive margins we recommend 7000 cGy in 7 to 7.5 weeks or 7440 cGy at 120 cGy twice a day. Oral cavity lesions have a higher failure rate in our experience and may receive the higher doses even with negative margins.

Chemotherapy Plus Local-Regional Treatment

INDUCTION CHEMOTHERAPY. Contrary to the experience with combination chemotherapy for patients with recurrent or metastatic disease, combination chemotherapy may hold special promise for the patients with previously untreated squamous cell carcinoma of the head and neck. Recent studies evaluating combination chemotherapy in this setting have reported significant tumor regression in 70% to 90% of patients, with complete clinical disappearance of tumor in 20% to 50%.[147-172]

Given the apparent sensitivity of previously untreated squamous cell carcinoma of the head and neck to chemotherapy, numerous pilot studies and a few controlled trials have used induction chemotherapy, either single agent or combination, before surgery or radiation therapy with the intent that such treatment will promote tumor regression of primary and nodal disease and enhance local-regional con-

TABLE 21-13.   Squamous Cell Carcinoma of the Head and Neck Treated with Postoperative Radiation Therapy: Control Above the Clavicles by Surgical Margin and Tumor Dose (Continuous-Course Versus Split-Course Irradiation)

	Split Course (19 Patients)	Continuous Course (108 Patients)		p Value[144,145]
Surgical margin				
Invasive cancer	1/4	8/16	(50%)	0.375
CIS or close (≤5 mm)	1/4	19/22	(86%)	0.028
Negative	5/11 (45%)	56/70	(80%)	0.023
Tumor dose (cGy)				
<5000	1/2	0/2		
5000–5900	2/9	17/18	(94%)	<0.001
6000–6500	2/5	48/61	(79%)	0.087
6600–7200	2/3	18/27	(67%)	
All eligible patients	7/19 (37%)	83/108	(77%)	<0.001

Amdur RJ, Parsons JT, Mendenhall WM, et al: Postoperative irradiation for squamous cell carcinoma of the head and neck: An analysis of treatment results and complications. Presented at the 29th Annual Meeting of the American Society for Therapeutic Radiology and Oncology, Boston, 1987

Number controlled/number eligible for analysis of control above the clavicles. CIS, carcinoma in situ.

trol of tumor with subsequent surgery or irradiation; reduce the tumor bulk of initially unresectable lesions and allow eventual surgical resection; identify a patient population for whom, after significant tumor regression by chemotherapy, extensive and radical surgical procedures could be deferred or revised in favor of more conservative procedures; identify a patient population with tumors that responded to induction chemotherapy who may benefit from additional adjuvant chemotherapy following surgery or irradiation; and provide the earliest possible treatment for small foci of subclinical disease (micrometastases), which may be present in 30% to 50% of patients with advanced head and neck cancer.

The experience with induction chemotherapy for patients with squamous cell carcinoma of the head and neck began in the early 1960s when several trials evaluated sequential single-agent chemotherapy and radiation therapy. The earliest trials were uncontrolled and used methotrexate in a variety of doses and schedules before local treatment.[173-176] To date, four randomized trials of single-agent induction chemotherapy have been published, and none has shown that such an approach improves disease-free or overall survival rates.[177-180]

Since the late 1970s, numerous trials of induction chemotherapy for patients with previously untreated, advanced disease have been performed (Table 21-14). Findings from the uncontrolled experience can be summarized:

1. Induction combination chemotherapy causes significant tumor regression in 70% to 90% of patients and complete clinical regression of tumor in 20% to 50% prior to local–regional treatment.[147-156]

2. Tumor regression continues and response rates increase through at least three cycles of induction treatment.[154,157]

3. A complete response to induction chemotherapy is associated with optimal local–regional control of tumor and survival rates.[149,154,155,158,159]

4. Following a complete clinical response to induction chemotherapy, a complete pathologic regression of tumor has been documented in 30% to 70% of patients undergoing subsequent biopsies of the primary site or definitive surgical resection[153,155,159-161]

5. Single-modality radiation therapy or surgery may be sufficient to achieve adequate local–regional control of tumor in selected patients with a complete response to induction chemotherapy.[150,155]

6. An initially unresectable lesion may become resectable after a response to chemotherapy; however, whether such a resection enhances local–regional control rates beyond those achieved with chemotherapy and radiotherapy alone remains uncertain.[149,162]

7. Initial tumor extent as defined by overall stage, T stage, N stage, or resectability predicts for response to chemotherapy and survival.[154,156,159,162,163]

8. The histologic subtype of squamous cell carcinoma of the head and neck does not predict for response to induction chemotherapy or survival when all patients are considered[158,164,165]; however, when only patients achieving a complete response are analyzed, those with poorly differentiated tumors are at greater risk for relapse.[165]

9. The toxicity of local treatment is not significantly increased by initial chemotherapy.[149,150,160,166]

10. Survival rates after induction chemotherapy are improved compared with historical controls treated with conventional surgery or irradiation alone.[149,150,156]

11. The optimal regimen of induction chemotherapy has not been defined, and when the extent of disease and duration of treatment are controlled, the activity of present cisplatin-containing combination chemotherapy regimens may be comparable.[157]

While the results from uncontrolled studies are encouraging and strongly suggest a role for chemotherapy in the treatment of patients with advanced, previously untreated head and neck cancer, the true value of chemotherapy can

TABLE 21-14.   Induction Combination Chemotherapy for Advanced Squamous Cell Carcinoma of the Head and Neck—Uncontrolled Trials

Institution	No. of Patients	Regimen	Response (%) Complete (CR)	Response (%) Partial (PR)	Findings
Boston Veterans Administration[149]	41 (unresectable)	Cisplatin, bleomycin	17	53	Increased survival in CR group; increased resectability without apparent survival advantage if resected; increased disease-free survival compared with institutional controls
Buffalo Veterans Administration[150]	47 (resectable)	Cisplatin, vincristine, bleomycin	22	66	Postoperative radiotherapy deferred in 39 of 43 patients; increased disease-free survival compared with historical controls
Wayne State[153]	61	Cisplatin, 5-fluorouracil	54	39	Increased survival in CR group; pathologic CR in 9 of 13 resected specimens from CR group
Stanford[155]	30 (resectabe)	Cisplatin, 5-fluorouracil	43	40	Increased survival in the CR group; adequate local control with radiotherapy alone in 10 patients with pathologic CR
Dana-Farber[156]	114	Cisplatin, bleomycin, methotrexate, leucovorin	26	52	Increased survival in CR group; increased disease-free survival compared with historical controls; positive randomized study of adjuvant chemotherapy

only be determined by prospective, randomized, controlled trials. To date, the results of five such trials of induction combination chemotherapy have been published. While none has reported an improved survival rate with induction chemotherapy (Table 21-15), critical analysis indicates that these studies cannot be considered definitive.

Stell and co-workers[167] and the Head and Neck Contracts Program[172] utilized only one cycle of induction chemotherapy and recorded complete response rates of only 3% and 5%, respectively. Holoye and co-workers[169] administered either one or two cycles of an induction regimen that did not contain cisplatin, failed to note the percentage of patients

receiving only one course of treatment, and reported a complete response rate of only 10%. Haas and co-workers[170] used up to three cycles of cisplatin with infusion 5-fluorouracil, but reported a complete response rate of only 17%. This low rate of complete response is in sharp contrast to the complete response rate of 54% achieved with an identical induction regimen in an uncontrolled trial at another institution. Martin and co-workers[171] also recorded an unexpectedly low complete response rate of 7% with a four-drug cisplatin-based regimen. Schuller and co-workers[168] evaluated a 9-week, three-course regimen of induction combination chemotherapy in 73 patients with advanced disease. In

TABLE 21-15.   Induction Combination Chemotherapy for Advanced Squamous Cell Carcinoma of the Head and Neck—Controlled Trials

Author	No. of Patients	Regimen	Response (%) Complete (CR)	Response (%) Partial (PR)	Findings
Stell et al.[167]	86	Vincristine, bleomycin, methotrexate, 5-fluorouracil, hydrocortisone			No survival advantage with induction chemotherapy
Schuller et al.[168]	146 (resectable)	Cisplatin, vincristine, methotrexate, bleomycin	20	45	Same
Holoye et al.[169]	83 (resectable)	Bleomycin, cyclophosphamide, methotrexate, 5-fluorouracil	5	64	Same
Haas et al.[170]	50 (resectable)	Cisplatin, 5-fluorouracil	17	70	Same
Martin et al.[171]	60	Bleomycin, methotrexate, 5-fluorouracil, cisplatin	7	57	Same
NCI Head and Neck Contracts Program[172]	462 (resectable)	Cisplatin, bleomycin	3	34	Same

their trial, total and complete response rates of 65% and 20% were achieved, but an improved survival rate was not associated with chemotherapy. This study may have been compromised by the use of less than maximal doses of cisplatin in the induction regimen and the administration of only 5000 cGy of postoperative radiation therapy.

In addition to problems with experimental design, limited follow-up evaluation, and inadequate patient accrual, the inability to document an improved survival rate with induction chemotherapy may relate to attenuations of local–regional treatment delivered to patients receiving chemotherapy. In general, the randomized trials of induction chemotherapy have not reported whether surgery or irradiation was limited in selected patients who had a response to induction chemotherapy. Such reductions were present in the study by Stell and co-workers[167] and may have compromised the survival rate in patients treated with induction chemotherapy.

ADJUVANT CHEMOTHERAPY. Adjuvant chemotherapy after local-regional treatment has been used in relatively few studies of patients with advanced head and neck cancer. The objective of these trials has been to treat subclinical persistent disease after surgery or irradiation and decrease the risk of relapse. Huang and co-workers[181] administered a combination of bleomycin, methotrexate, and CCNU to 31 patients (8 with Stage III, 12 with Stage IV, and 12 with recurrent local–regional disease) after surgery or radiation therapy. With a minimum follow-up of 14 months, only 5 (16%) of 31 patients developed recurrent disease, and none of these 5 patients relapsed prior to 18 months. These survival data were thought to be superior to those of a nonrandomized control group of patients who did not receive adjuvant chemotherapy. In the latter group of 24 patients, 16 patients (67%) relapsed, with most recurrences developing within the first 18 months after treatment.

Johnson and co-workers[182] similarly evaluated a combination of weekly sequential methotrexate and 5-fluorouracil after surgery and irradiation in 50 patients who had histologic evidence of extracapsular spread in cervical lymph nodes at the time of surgical resection. Their regimen of adjuvant chemotherapy was remarkably well tolerated, and the estimated 2-year disease-free survival of 66% was superior to that of a retrospective control group of patients treated with surgery and irradiation alone.

The most remarkable experience with adjuvant chemotherapy was reported by Bitter,[183] who compared postoperative combination chemotherapy to postoperative radiation therapy in a small randomized trial of 33 patients with resectable oral cavity lesions. In this study, significantly improved disease-free and overall survival rates were associated with postoperative chemotherapy.

INDUCTION PLUS ADJUVANT CHEMOTHERAPY. Induction and adjuvant chemotherapy have been administered together in several multidisciplinary studies. Three studies of induction chemotherapy have specifically addressed the use of additional adjuvant treatment by randomized comparison with a control group that received only induction chemotherapy and local–regional treatment. Neither Tejada and Chandler[184] nor the Head and Neck Contracts Program[172]

reported a survival benefit with adjuvant chemotherapy. However, both of these trials reported significant toxicity with adjuvant chemotherapy, which led to periodic interruptions of treatment and poor drug compliance.

Contrasting results have recently been reported by Ervin and co-workers.[156] In a study of 114 patients with advanced disease, 89 patients (78%) responded to induction chemotherapy, and after local–regional treatment, 46 of these patients entered a randomized trial of additional adjuvant cisplatin, bleomycin, and methotrexate. Those patients receiving both induction and adjuvant chemotherapy had an improved disease-free survival rate in comparison with those receiving only induction chemotherapy and local-regional treatment. The apparent success of this trial may have been related to the specific dose-attenuated regimen of adjuvant chemotherapy used, to the acceptable performance status of patients consenting to the randomized trial, or to the fact that patient eligibility was restricted to those who responded to initial chemotherapy.

SYNCHRONOUS CHEMOTHERAPY AND RADIATION THERAPY. The simultaneous administration of chemotherapy and radiation therapy may offer distinct therapeutic advantages over the administration of either modality alone. Potentiation of the cytotoxic effects of radiation by chemotherapy, that is, 5-fluorouracil, cisplatin, bleomycin, and mitomycin-C, has been well documented in preclinical studies. Direct extrapolation of these results to the clinic is impossible, however, given the potential for synergistic enhancement of normal tissue injury by simultaneous chemotherapy and radiation therapy.

Numerous studies of radiation therapy and various single agents have been performed with mixed results. Enhanced mucositis with combined treatment has been a common finding, and many studies have found it necessary to reduce the dose of chemotherapy administered or the use of split-course fractionation schedules of radiation therapy. The majority of randomized trials noting improved local–regional control of disease with synchronous treatment have used bleomycin,[185-188] bolus 5-fluorouracil,[189-190] or mitomycin-C.[191] Randomized trials reporting no advantage with synchronous therapy have frequently employed hydroxyurea[192,193] or methotrexate[178,194-196] with radiation therapy. Several uncontrolled trials of synchronous cisplatin and radiation therapy have been performed and a randomized study has recently been completed by the Radiation Therapy Oncology Group in patients with unresectable advanced head and neck cancer.[197-200]

Synchronous combination chemotherapy and radiation therapy has also been evaluated in patients with advanced head and neck cancer. After a favorable preliminary experience with simultaneous radiation therapy and infusion 5-fluorouracil,[201] the addition of cisplatin[202,203] or mitomycin-C[204] was evaluated. The latter studies utilized split-course fractionation of radiation therapy with chemotherapy, and all reported high initial response rates. Taylor and co-workers[203,205] have reported 34 patients treated "curatively" (5 Stage III, 24 Stage IV, 6 recurrent) with a biweekly regimen of synchronous cisplatin, infusion 5-fluorouracil, and radiation therapy. Initial disease control was achieved in all patients. With a median follow-up of 36 months (range, 24–58 months), four patients have developed recurrent tumor within the field of irradiation and seven additional patients have recurrence at distant sites. Recurrences developed only in those patients with T4 or N3 disease. In addition to the low rate of recurrence, the pattern of recurrence appears affected by this approach. Local–regional failure developed in only 12% of patients and composed only 36% of failures.

REGIONAL CHEMOTHERAPY. Most studies of intra-arterial chemotherapy prior to or with irradiation or surgery may have yielded some short-term control of disease, but randomized trials have not demonstrated a significant increase in long-term survival.[88,196,206,207] Present efforts are directed toward defining the activity of intra-arterial cisplatin and combinations of intra-arterial and systemic therapy against advanced head and neck cancers, as well as toward developing intra-arterial chemoembolization as a therapeutic modality. Further advances await clarification of the pharmacologic advantage of intra-arterial therapy and ultimately the comparison of intra-arterial and systemic chemotherapy by controlled trial.

ORAL CAVITY

The oral cavity consists of the lip, floor of mouth, oral tongue (the anterior two thirds of the tongue), buccal mucosa, upper and lower gingiva, hard palate, and retromolar trigone. Squamous cell carcinomas of the oral cavity mostly occur after the age of 45 and are associated with the use of tobacco and alcohol.

The AJCC staging system for all primary tumors of the oral cavity is as follows:[12]

TX   Minimum requirements to assess the primary tumor cannot be met

T0   No evidence of primary tumor

Tis   Carcinoma in situ

T1   Greatest diameter of primary tumor 2 cm or less

T2   Greatest diameter of primary tumor more than 2 cm but not more than 4 cm

T3   Greatest diameter of primary tumor more than 4 cm

T4   Massive tumor more than 4 cm in diameter with deep invasion to involve antrum, pterygoid muscles, base of tongue, or skin of neck

LIP

The ratio between men and women with cancer of the lip is approximately 15:1.[208] Persons with light-colored skin or with prolonged exposure to sunlight are most prone to develop lip carcinoma; tobacco has not been definitely implicated as a causative agent.

Anatomy

The lips are composed of the orbicular muscle with skin on the external surface and mucous membrane on the internal surface. The transition from skin to mucous membrane of the oral cavity is the lip vermilion, where the muscle is covered by a very thin layer of squamous epithelium that allows the underlying vasculature to show, giving the lips their reddish color. The blood supply is by way of the labial artery, a branch of the facial artery. The motor nerves are branches of the seventh cranial nerve. The sensory nerve to the upper lip is the infraorbital branch of the maxillary nerve, and the lower lip is supplied by the mental nerve.

Pathology

The most common neoplasms are squamous cell carcinomas. Basal cell carcinomas start on the skin of the lip and may secondarily invade the vermilion. Benign lesions such as hemangiomas, fibromas, and cysts may involve the lips. Keratoacanthoma occurs on the skin of the lips and may be mistaken grossly and histologically for squamous cell carcinoma.

Leukoplakia and carcinoma in situ are common problems on the lower lip and may precede the appearance of carcinoma by many years. Primary lesions arising from the moist mucosa of the lip are considered under the section on the buccal mucosa.

Patterns of Spread

Squamous cell carcinoma starts on the vermilion of the lip and invades adjacent skin and the orbicular muscle. Advanced lesions invade the adjacent commissures of the lip, the buccal mucosa, the skin and wet mucosa of the lip, the adjacent mandible, and eventually the mental nerve. Perineural invasion occurred in 2% of the cases reported by Byers and co-workers[209] and was related to recurrent lesions, large tumor size, mandibular invasion, and poorly differentiated histology. Lymphatic spread is to the submental and submandibular lymph nodes and then to the jugular chain. The risk for lymph node metastases is approximately 5% on admission. Bilateral involvement may occur.[210] The risk of lymphatic involvement is increased by high-grade histology, large lesions, spread to involve the wet mucosa of the lip and buccal mucosa, and especially for patients with recurrent disease.

Clinical Picture

The vermilion is the most common site of origin. Squamous cell carcinoma of the red lip may present as an enlarging, discrete lesion that is not tender until it ulcerates and becomes infected. There will be occasional minor bleeding. These lesions are diagnosed easily by their appearance. However, some lesions develop very slowly on a background of leukoplakia and present as superficially ulcerated lesions with little or no bulk and a history of repeated episodes of scab formation without complete healing. These lesions are not so easy to diagnose clinically, and only biopsy provides the answer. An obvious carcinoma is often accompanied by leukoplakia or carcinoma in situ of the remaining lower lip.

Erythema of the adjacent skin suggests dermal lymphatic invasion. Palpation of the lip will reveal the extent of induration. Anesthesia or paresthesias of the skin of the lip indicate nerve invasion.

Methods of Diagnosis and Staging

The diagnosis is readily established by biopsy, or if the lesion is not discrete, a lip shave may be done. Mandible films are requested when bone or mental nerve involvement is suspected.

The AJCC staging for oral cavity cancer includes only those lesions arising from the vermilion.

Treatment

SELECTION OF TREATMENT MODALITY. Early lesions may be cured equally well with surgery or radiation. The length of the relaxed lower lip is approximately 5 cm but tends to be shorter in edentulous patients. Surgical excision is preferred for the majority of lower lip lesions up to 2.0 cm in diameter that do not involve the commissure; the treatment is simple and the cosmetic result quite satisfactory. Removal of more of the lip with simple closure usually results in a poor cosmetic and functional result and therefore requires reconstructive procedures. Irradiation is often preferred for lesions involving the commissure, for lesions over 2.0 cm in length, and for high-grade carcinomas. Upper lip carcinomas may require complex reconstruction and radiation therapy may be preferred. Advanced lesions with bone, nerve, or node involvement frequently require a combined approach. Surgery is preferred for the younger patient who

will have years of climatic exposure and for previously irradiated persons.

The regional lymphatics are not treated electively for early cases. Advanced lesions, high-grade lesions, and especially recurrent lesions should be considered for either elective neck irradiation or elective neck dissection, depending on the treatment selected for the primary lesion. Clinically positive nodes are managed according to policies outlined in "Principles of Treatment."

SURGICAL TREATMENT. Surgical treatment for early lesions (0.5–1.5 cm) involves a W or V excision (see Fig. 21-3). V excisions may be used for very small lesions but do not give as good a margin for the larger tumors. Larger lesions (>1.5 cm) may be closed with an Abbe flap from the upper lip to reconstruct the lower lip defect. If the vermilion is diffusely involved with little or no involvement of the muscle, then a vermilionectomy (lip shave) may be done and the mucosa from the oral cavity advanced to cover the defect. Excision of a carcinoma may be combined with vermilionectomy. If the commissure must be sacrificed, it must be reconstructed to prevent microstomia and to allow the patient to continue to wear dentures.

IRRADIATION TECHNIQUE. Lip cancer may be successfully treated by external beam, interstitial implants, or a combination of both.

Interstitial implants may be accomplished with removable sources such as radium or cesium needles or ^{192}Ir.

External beam techniques use orthovoltage or electrons with lead shields behind the lip to limit exit irradiation. The dose schemes are similar to those used for skin cancer.[174] Fractionation schemes of 4 to 6 weeks are preferred over the shorter regimens for the larger lesions to decrease the normal-tissue effects.

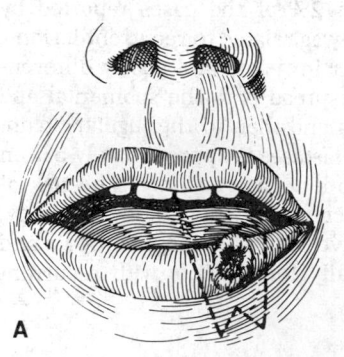
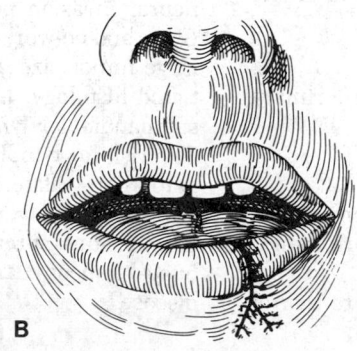
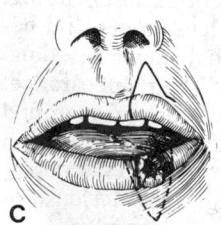
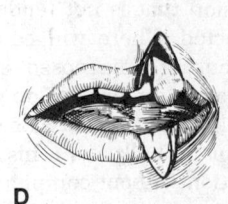
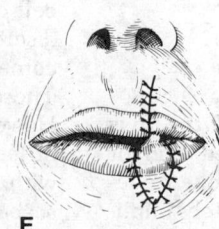

A   B   C   D   E

FIG. 21-3. Small lip lesions that do not involve the oral commissure can be removed using a "W" excision (A) and can be closed primarily (B). Larger lesions of the lip may be removed in a "V" fashion (C), and the defect can be closed using an Abbe flap from the upper lip (D, E). A second procedure to release the flap also can be performed 2 weeks later.

Results of Treatment

MacKay and Sellers[210] reviewed 2854 patients with all stages of lip cancer, of whom 92% were managed initially by radiation therapy. The primary lesion was controlled by the initial treatment in 84% of cases, and an additional 8% were saved by later treatment for an overall local control rate of 92%. Fifty-eight percent of those who presented with clinically involved nodes had control of disease, but only 35% had control of disease when neck nodes appeared later. The determinate 5-year survival rate was 89%; the absolute 5-year survival rate was 65%. Death resulting from intercurrent disease occurred in 17% of patients.

The M.D. Anderson Hospital local control rates for 444 previously untreated patients are shown in Table 21-16.[212] The 3-year and 5-year determinate survival rate was 94%.

Fitzpatrick[208] reviewed the Princess Margaret Hospital results for 361 lip carcinomas seen between 1971 and 1976. Surgery alone (85 patients) controlled 89%, surgery with postoperative radiation therapy (70 patients) controlled 93%, and radiation therapy alone (206 patients) controlled 94%. Regional node metastasis occurred in only 7%. Only 3% of the entire group died of lip cancer. Radiation necrosis of soft tissues requiring surgical intervention occurred in 3%. There were no cases of osteoradionecrosis.

Heller and Shah[213] reported the Memorial Sloan-Kettering Cancer Center results for 171 squamous cell carcinomas treated initially by surgery between 1955 and 1969. The sites of initial recurrence and 5-year determinate survival rates by stage are given in Table 21-17.

Hendricks and co-workers[214] reviewed the Mayo Clinic surgical results for 613 patients seen between 1950 and 1969. The lip recurrence rate was 5% for lesions less than 1 cm, 4% for lesions 1 cm to 3 cm, and 17% for lesions greater than 3 cm.

Mohs[215] reported the results for microscopically controlled surgical treatment for squamous cell carcinomas of the lower lip. Between 1936 and 1976, 1448 patients with squamous cell carcinoma were managed by microscopically controlled surgery. Eighty-three percent had cancers less than 3 cm in diameter, and they had a 5-year cure rate of 96.6%. For patients with cancers that measured 2 cm or greater, the cure rate dropped to 60% for 192 patients. For patients with Grade I or II carcinoma, the 5-year cure rate was 96%, as contrasted with 67% for 81 patients with Grade III or IV carcinoma.

Complications of Treatment

Microstomia and drooling secondary to oral incompetence may occur when a large flap reconstruction is necessary. If the oral opening is too small, the patient may not be able to insert a denture. Speech is not often affected.

There will be some atrophy of the irradiated tissues; this progresses with time. Continued exposure to the elements may result in a soft-tissue necrosis; this problem is reduced by schemes that prolong the treatment. The irradiated lip must be carefully protected from sun exposure by use of hats and UV protectants. Fishermen may wear a surgical face mask while on the water, because the various UV protectants are insufficient.

FLOOR OF THE MOUTH

Anatomy

The floor of mouth is a U-shaped area bounded by the lower gum and the oral tongue; it terminates posteriorly at the insertion of the anterior tonsillar pillar into the tongue. The paired sublingual glands lie immediately below the mucous membrane; they are separated by the paired genioglossus and geniohyoid muscles. Bony protuberances, the genial tubercles, occur at the point of insertion of these two muscle groups at the symphysis. The genial tubercles may be prominent and extend a centimeter or so from the inner rim of the mandible and would interfere with the placement of interstitial sources. The mylohyoid muscle arises from the mylohyoid ridge of the mandible and is the muscular floor for the oral cavity. The mylohyoid muscle ends posteriorly at about the level of the third molars. The normal submandibular gland is about the size of a walnut. Most of the gland rests on the external surface of the mylohyoid muscle in the niche between the mandible and the insertion of the mylohyoid. A tongue-like process wraps around the posterior border of the

TABLE 21-16. Cancer of the Lip in Previously Untreated Patients (M. D. Anderson Hospital)

Size of Lesion	Treatment*	No. of Patients	No. with Local Recurrence	No. Salvaged
0–1 cm	RT	30	0	
	S	239	6	6
1–2 cm	RT	36	2	1
	S	116	3	1
>2 cm	RT	7	0	
	S	7	3	0
Massive	RT	1	0	
	S	8	1	0

MacComb WS, Fletcher GH, Healey JE Jr: Intra-oral cavity. In MacComb WS, Fletcher GH (ed): Cancer of the Head and Neck, pp 89–151. Baltimore, Williams & Wilkins, 1967.
*RT, radiotherapy; S, surgery.

TABLE 21-17. Squamous Cell Carcinoma of the Lip: Sites of Initial Recurrence and 5-Year Determinate Survival (171 Patients Treated at Memorial Sloan-Kettering Cancer Center, 1955–1969)

| | Clinical Stage | | | |
Result	I	II	III	IV
Site of recurrence				
No recurrence	106	24	13	3
Lip	10	1	3	0
Ipsilateral neck	4	1	0	0
Contralateral neck	0	1	1	1
Distant metastasis	0	1	0	0
5-year determinate survival	94%	83%	93%	50%

Modified from Heller KS, Shah JP: Carcinoma of the lip. Am J Surg 138:600–607, 1979.

mylohyoid muscle and extends forward on the internal surface of the mylohyoid. This process is absent in 10% to 20% of cases. The submandibular duct (Wharton's duct) is about 5 cm long. It courses between the sublingual gland and the genioglossus muscle and exits in the anterior floor of mouth near the midline. The relationships of the lingual nerve, hypoglossal nerve, and submandibular duct are shown in Figure 21-4.

Pathology

Most neoplasms are squamous cell carcinoma, usually of moderate grade. Adenoid cystic and mucoepidermoid carcinomas account for about 5% of malignant tumors in this area.

Patterns of Spread

PRIMARY. Approximately 90% of neoplasms originate within 2 cm of the anterior midline floor of the mouth, penetrating quite early beneath the mucosa into the sublingual gland and eventually into the midline genioglossus and geniohyoid muscles. The mylohyoid muscle acts as an effective barrier until the lesion becomes very advanced. Extension toward the gingiva and periosteum of the mandible occurs early and frequently. Even small lesions become attached to the periosteum. The periosteum is an effective barrier to mandibular invasion; when tumor reaches the periosteum, the tumor usually spreads along the periosteum rather than through it. Mandible invasion is usually a late

manifestation. Tumor sometimes will grow over the alveolar ridge before grossly invading bone. The skin of the lower lip may be involved in advanced cases. Posterior extension occurs into the muscles of the root of the tongue; this pattern of extension is usually associated with ulceration of the floor of the mouth and undersurface of the tongue.

One or both submandibular ducts frequently are obstructed by tumor or after biopsy. An enlarged duct may be palpated through the floor of mouth, and it may be difficult to distinguish between tumor extension and low-grade infection in an obstructed duct. Tumor rarely grows inside the duct but may grow along the path of the duct. The submandibular gland frequently will enlarge and become firm and occasionally painful when the duct is obstructed. It is difficult to distinguish between tumor directly invading the gland and chronic infection related to obstruction.

Tumors arising in the lateral floor of the mouth are less common but have the same general spread patterns. Extensive lesions may escape the oral cavity by following the anatomic plane of the mylohyoid muscle to its posterior extremity, emerging in the submandibular space of the neck.

LYMPHATIC. Approximately 30% of patients will have clinically positive nodes on admission; 4% will have bilateral nodes. The reported incidence of conversion from N0 to N+ with no neck treatment varies from 20% to 35%.[21-23] For T1 or superficial T2 lesions, the risk for occult metastasis is probably 10% to 15% (see Table 21-4).[15]

The first nodes involved are the submandibular and the subdigastric nodes (Fig. 21-5). The midline submental nodes

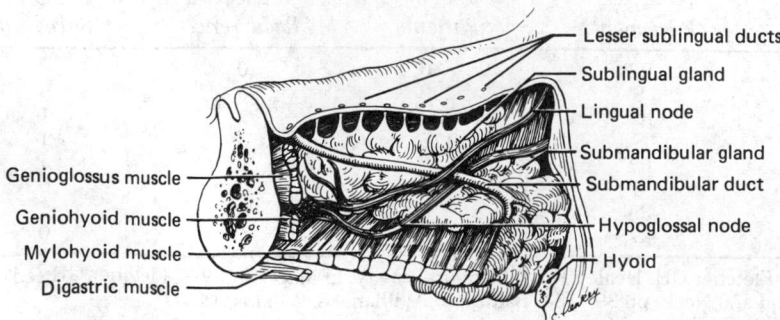

Genioglossus muscle
Geniohyoid muscle
Mylohyoid muscle
Digastric muscle

Lesser sublingual ducts
Sublingual gland
Lingual node
Submandibular gland
Submandibular duct
Hypoglossal node
Hyoid

FIG. 21-4. Anatomic relationships of the floor of the oral cavity.

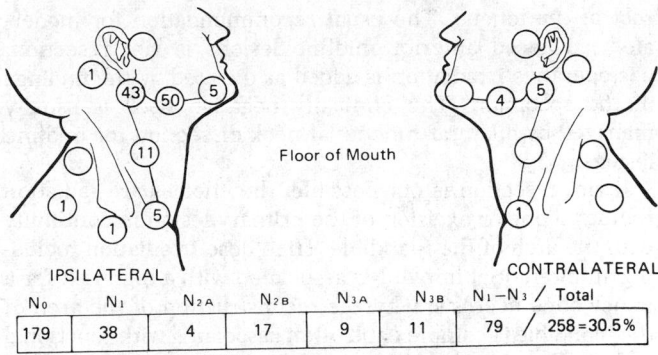

N₀	N₁	N₂ₐ	N₂ᵦ	N₃ₐ	N₃ᵦ	N₁–N₃ / Total
179	38	4	17	9	11	79 / 258 = 30.5%

FIG. 21-5. Floor of mouth cancer: nodal distribution on admission, M.D. Anderson Hospital, 1948–1965. (Lindberg RD: Distribution of cervical lymph node metastases from squamous cell carcinoma of the upper respiratory and digestive tracts. Cancer 29:1446–1450, 1972)

are bypassed; Lindberg[7] reported 2% clinically positive submental nodes in 258 cases. Because most lesions either approach or cross the midline, the risk for bilateral spread is fairly high. Fletcher[44] reported that 47% of patients (9 of 19) with ipsilateral positive necks (N1 or N2) developed contralateral neck disease if no elective neck treatment was given. This rate was reduced to 10% (3 of 28) after 3000 cGy to 4000 cGy to the upper neck.

Clinical Picture

The earliest carcinomas are asymptomatic, red, slightly elevated mucosal lesions with ill-defined borders. A background of leukoplakia may be present. White lesions (leukoplakic) are less likely to be malignant, but 10% eventually become cancer. These lesions are usually diagnosed by the dentist or physician on routine oral examination.

As the carcinoma progresses, the tumor is first noticed when the patient feels a lump in the floor of mouth with the tip of his tongue. There is mild soreness when eating or drinking that is usually thought by the patient (and sometimes the physician) to be due to a canker or denture sore. Dentures may not fit properly. Advanced lesions produce pain, bleeding, foul breath, loose teeth, change in speech owing to fixation of the root of the tongue, and a submandibular mass that is often painful.

On physical examination, the earliest lesions appear as a red area, slightly elevated, with ill-defined borders and very little induration. As the lesion enlarges, the edges of the tumor become distinct, elevated, and "rolled," with a central ulceration and induration. Some lesions start with a background of leukoplakia. If the leukoplakia is extensive, it is difficult to know where or when to biopsy.

Bimanual palpation will determine the extent of the induration and the degree of fixation to the periosteum. Large lesions bulge into the submental space and rarely grow through the mylohyoid muscle into the soft tissues of the neck and even the skin. Gross invasion of the mandible may be detected, especially when the anterior teeth have been removed; tumor may be seen growing through the mandible to involve the gingivolabial sulcus and lip.

The submandibular duct and gland are evaluated by bimanual palpation.

Methods of Diagnosis and Staging

The occlusal view (dental film) of the arch or ramus of the mandible is the best technique for determining early invasion. A Panorex examination of the entire mandible is not useful for determining early bone invasion but may be obtained to evaluate the teeth and to determine the extent of invasion if extensive bony destruction is obviously present. The Panorex also assists the surgeon in evaluating whether enough mandible exists in edentulous patients for a rim resection.

Submandibular gland sialograms are not useful in determining the presence or absence of cancer in the gland. A bone scan will be positive when tumor is attached to the periosteum but is not an accurate method to detect early bone invasion. CT with bone windows is the preferred method for determining bone invasion and extent of local spread in advanced lesions.

Small (5 mm) discrete lesions may be excised. Larger lesions have an incisional or punch forceps biopsy.

Treatment

SELECTION OF TREATMENT MODALITY. *Leukoplakia.* Patches of thin leukoplakia usually are observed. Biopsy is done if the area becomes symptomatic or if the appearance changes and malignancy is suspected. Localized areas of leukoplakia may be excised, but many patients have extensive or scattered areas of leukoplakia that preclude complete excision. Cryotherapy or the laser may be tried in these cases. Radiation therapy is not recommended for treatment of leukoplakia; however, when leukoplakia is inadvertently irradiated along with an adjacent carcinoma, the leukoplakia may disappear. In most cases it will reappear at a later time.

Early Lesions. Operation or radiation therapy is equally effective treatment for T1 or T2 lesions; therefore, treatment decisions are based on rather subtle differences in the expected functional result and on the management of the neck. The status of the teeth and mandible and the age of the patient also enter into the decision.

A few patients are seen after excisional biopsy of a tiny lesion, and the only finding is a surgical scar with varying degrees of induration or nodularity under the scar (TX). The margins are stated to be free, close, or positive. If the excisional biopsy is judged inadequate, these patients are usually treated with an interstitial implant or intraoral cone, because the surgeon has difficulty knowing where to start and stop the reexcision. The use of margin checks is essentially useless under these conditions because there are very few tumor cells present and the pathologist is in effect looking for a needle in a haystack. Additionally, a few tumor cells may be spread at some distance from the excision site by way of the hematoma. The radiation therapist can be generous with the treatment volume and cover potential spread without functional loss. The neck is usually observed. A review of six patients treated in this manner at M.D. Anderson Hospital revealed a 100% local control rate; similar patients treated at the University of Florida had a 100% local control rate.[216] None of the patients developed neck nodes. If the margins of the excisional biopsy are free and there is little or no induration or nodularity, 5500 cGy is delivered. If the margins are positive or if there is slight induration or nodularity, the dose is raised to 6500 cGy. In cases in which gross cut-through is suspected, one may wish to use external beam to a dose of 5000 cGy to include the regional nodes prior to the interstitial implant. A high index of suspicion is important in these cases to avoid undertreatment.

Small lesions (<1 cm) may be excised transorally if there is a margin between the lesion and the gingiva. If the submandibular duct is surgically obstructed, then the submandibular gland also must be removed. A common presentation is an anterior midline lesion, 2 cm to 3 cm in diameter, which abuts the gingiva, with a clinically negative neck; there is a risk for subclinical disease in one or both sides of the neck in 10% to 30% of cases. Most of these lesions are managed by wide local excision with rim resection of the mandible. Either the neck is observed or bilateral elective functional neck dissections are done. If it is necessary to remove one or both salivary ducts, then the submandibular glands are removed or the ducts reimplanted. If the submandibular glands are to be removed, a modified neck dissection is done at the same time. Although radiation therapy produces similar cure rates, there is a lifelong risk of bone and soft tissue necrosis. The ideal candidate for radiation therapy is an edentulous patient in whom the lesion does not approximate the mandible. These patients receive about one third of their dose by an intraoral cone so that the mandible is spared high doses. The primary site and the neck (and thus the mandible) receive 4500 cGy from external beam, which electively treats the lymph nodes. Well-lateralized floor of mouth lesions usually are treated by an operation with an in-continuity ipsilateral neck dissection. These lesions usually abut the mandible and require either a rim resection or a partial mandibulectomy. If the gingiva is uninvolved, radiation therapy is an alternative.

Moderately Advanced Lesions. These lesions usually involve the periosteum and gingiva and frequently involve the root of the tongue. The usual recommendation for moderately advanced anterior midline lesions is rim resection; postoperative irradiation is added as dictated by the findings in the specimen. The clinically negative neck is usually managed by bilateral functional neck dissection for midline lesions.

If rim resection is not possible, the choices are radiation therapy alone or excision of the primary lesion in continuity with the arch of the mandible. High-dose irradiation including an interstitial implant is associated with a high risk for a major bone necrosis, whereas reconstruction of the arch of the mandible is complex and often associated with functional and cosmetic deficits. The local control rate and complications for T2–T3 lesions that extended to the periosteum and gingiva, managed by external beam irradiation plus interstitial implant, are shown in Table 21-18.

Advanced Lesions. Massive lesions are usually associated with bone invasion and extension into the root of the tongue and have a small chance of cure with combined surgery and radiation therapy. The entire arch of the mandible must usually be removed. Only palliation can be offered in some cases.

SURGICAL TREATMENT. *Wide Local Excision.* Small lesions (5 mm or less in size) may be excised transorally with a 1-cm margin with primary closure or a skin graft. If the duct is involved, the submandibular gland and duct are removed in continuity.

Rim Resection. Rim (coronal) resection of the mandible in continuity with excision of the primary lesion preserves the arch and usually gives an adequate surgical margin; the procedure may be combined with postoperative radiation therapy (Figs. 21-6 and 21-7). Invasion of the periosteum is often an indication for this procedure. Patients who have been edentulous for a long time may have a thin, atrophic mandible and are not suitable for rim resection because the mandible is likely to fracture. Rim resection is not recommended for treatment of radiation failures because of the risk of bone necrosis and pathologic fracture. If rim resection is attempted for radiation failure, hyperbaric oxygen should be added before and after the operation.

Mandibulectomy ("Jaw-Neck"). Lateral floor of mouth: a

TABLE 21-18. Floor of Mouth Cancer: Local Control (Radiation Therapy Alone) Related to Gingival Extension (Stage T2–3)

Extent of Disease	Local Control	Surgical Salvage	Ultimate Local Control	Complications Requiring Surgery
Minimal gingiva/periosteal extension	4/8	3/4	7/8	1
Tethered to gingiva/periosteum	4/6	1/2	5/6	0
Fixed to gingiva	6/11	1/2	7/11	4
Total			19/25 (76%)	

University of Florida data: 10/64–12/77; analysis 12/79 by W. M. Mendenhall, M.D.

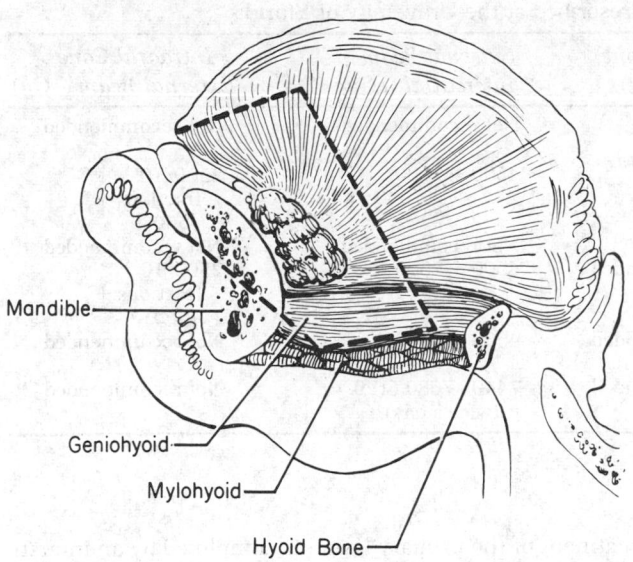

FIG. 21-6. Borders of rim resection for early carcinoma of the floor of the mouth.

radical neck dissection is performed and the specimen remains attached to the mandible. Partial mandibulectomy with resection of the floor of the mouth is done through a lip-splitting incision or by using a visor flap. A cheek flap is elevated to the level of the mandibular condyle to provide exposure. The mandible is separated at the mental foramen anteriorly and the neck of the condyle posteriorly. The primary lesion and neck specimen are then removed in continuity. Primary closure is usually feasible, unless a sizable portion of the oral tongue must be removed, in which case a myocutaneous flap is necessary to repair the defect.

The cosmetic and functional result is acceptable to patients, and very few request mandibular reconstruction. The mandible shifts to the opposite side, and if the patient has teeth, chewing may be impaired but can be corrected with a glide plane. Edentulous patients cannot wear a lower denture.

FIG. 21-7. Schematic for rim resection of the arch of the mandible. **Left**. Anterior view. **Right**. Lateral view.

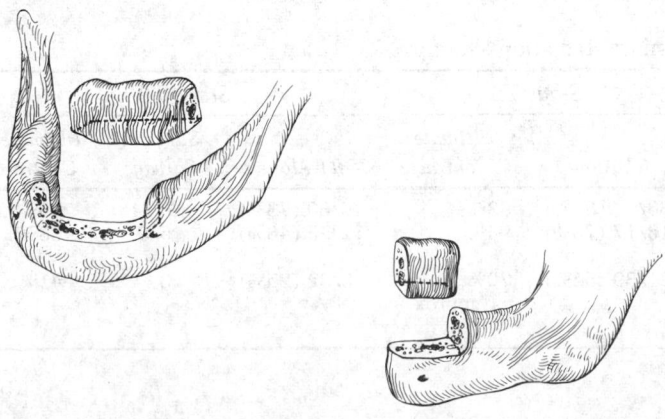

Anterior floor of mouth: a full-thickness resection of the anterior mandible (arch) is required. This operation results in major cosmetic and functional loss and is usually reserved for advanced lesions with bone invasion or for irradiation failures. New techniques for reconstruction include the use of a trapezius myocutaneous flap with a portion of the scapular spine to bridge the bony gap, or the use of a free flap such as the radial forearm flap or the iliac crest flap. The technique currently used at the University of Florida to reconstruct the mandible employs a spacer (such as a cobalt-chromium alloy [Vitallium] tray) for 3 to 6 months. The tray is removed, freeze-dried bone is shaped to fit the defect, and the graft is then packed with bone chips harvested from the iliac crest.

IRRADIATION TECHNIQUE. The current treatment guidelines at the University of Florida are shown in Table 21-19. Prominent geniohyoid tubercles and tori and undesirable teeth should be removed if present prior to radiation therapy. A minimum of 3 weeks for healing is needed before starting treatment.

External Beam Irradiation. External beam portals for anterior floor of mouth carcinoma are opposed lateral portals. The entire width of the mandibular arch is included in the portal. The superior border is shaped to spare part of the parotid and minor salivary glands. The submandibular and subdigastric nodes are included to the level of the thyroid notch if the neck is clinically negative; the lower neck may be electively irradiated on an individual basis. If the neck is clinically positive, the portals are enlarged to include all of the upper neck nodes, and an en face lower neck field is added.

Interstitial Irradiation. The availability of interstitial therapy (or intraoral cone therapy) is essential if maximum local control rates are to be obtained. External beam alone gives inferior local control results even for T1N0 lesions (Table 21-20).[217-219]

Implantation of small lesions confined to the floor of the mouth with minimal extension to the mucosa of the tongue or minimal extension to the gingiva or periosteum can be accomplished with either radium or cesium needles or iridium in the form of ribbons or "hairpins."

A preloaded, custom-designed implant device for radium needles has been in use at the University of Florida since 1976.[220] It holds the radium needles in a fixed position and is used only for T1 or T2 lesions. The arrangement of the needles for early lesions is usually a modified, curved, teardrop-shaped, two-plane implant with a single needle crossing the top of the implant. The arrangement of the needles for an early T2 lesion is shown in Figure 21-8; the needles are shown on a roentgenogram in Figure 21-9.

Implants for late T2 and T3 lesions are usually modified volume or multiplane arrangements. Needles or wires are usually inserted through the tongue.

Intraoral Cone Irradiation. Intraoral cone therapy is preferable to interstitial irradiation since there is little or no irradiation of the mandible. An intraoral cone can be used for

TABLE 21-19.   Floor of Mouth Cancer: Dose Scheme Currently Prescribed at the University of Florida

	Interstitial Only (cGy)	Intraoral Cone Only (cGy)	External Beam + Interstitial (cGy)	Intraoral Cone + External Beam (cGy)
TX— No visible or palpable tumor	5500	5000/4 weeks	Not recommended	Not recommended
TX— Palpable induration or positive margins	6500	5500/4 weeks	4500 + 2500	2500/10 fractions + 4500
Early, superficial	6000–6500	5500/4 weeks	Not recommended	Not recommended
Early, 1–3 cm, induration	Not recommended	Not recommended	4500 + 2500	2500/10 fractions + 4500
Moderately advanced (3–5 cm, induration)	Not recommended	Not recommended	4500 + 3000	Not recommended
Advanced	Not recommended	Not recommended	7440–7680 (120 twice a day)	Not recommended

well-circumscribed anterior superficial lesions; this technique is easiest to perform in the edentulous patient. Minimal extension to the gingiva can sometimes be encompassed with the cone as well as early extension to the undersurface of tongue. The orthovoltage cones in use at the University of Florida are 2 cm to 6 cm in diameter; they are poured from lead and can be trimmed individually to adapt the cone to the anatomy. Electron beam cones can be fabricated individually as described by Tapley.[221] Intraoral cone therapy requires daily positioning by the physician.

Intraoral cone therapy may be used for the entire treatment or as a reduced field treatment in which 2500 cGy is given in conjunction with external beam portals (see Table 21-19). It is preferable to complete the intraoral cone therapy prior to starting the external beam, because the mouth becomes sore and the lesion disappears.

Management of the Neck When the Primary Tumor is Treated by Irradiation Alone. N0: Small superficial lesions are treated by interstitial or intraoral cone irradiation alone; the neck is not treated unless the histology is poorly differentiated. Patients with lesions that are more deeply invasive and have palpable induration received radiation therapy to the primary site and the upper neck lymph nodes on both sides, 4500 cGy to 5000 cGy, to include the submandibular and subdigastric nodes to the level of the thyroid notch.

Treatment of the primary lesion is completed by an interstitial implant or intraoral cone therapy. The lower neck is electively treated through an anteroposterior portal when the risk for occult disease is judged to be significant.

N+: Guidelines for management of the patient with clinically positive neck nodes is outlined in "Principles of Treatment."

COMBINED TREATMENT POLICIES. The results of combined surgery and irradiation may be better than those for single-modality therapy in the large, infiltrative, ulcerative lesions. If rim resection is possible, postoperative irradiation is preferred, since the risk of bone complications and fistulae is higher with preoperative irradiation. Preoperative irradiation may be used if the patient has a large fixed node. The dose for postoperative radiation therapy is 6000 cGy in 6 weeks to 6500 cGy in 7 weeks. If the tongue margins were close or positive, the dose should be 7000 cGy in 7 to 7.5 weeks or 7440 cGy, 120 cGy twice a day, in 6.5 weeks, using reducing fields when possible.

MANAGEMENT OF RECURRENCE. Radiation failures are treated by an operation. The salvage rate is good for patients with early lesions and moderately good for the more advanced lesions (see Tables 21-18 and 21-20). Rim resection may be tried for selected radiation therapy failures, but

TABLE 21-20.   Floor of Mouth Cancer: Local Control with Primary Radiation Therapy

Institution	RT Technique*	Stage T1 RT Alone	Stage T1 Ultimate Control	Stage T2 RT Alone	Stage T2 Ultimate Control	Stage T3 RT Alone	Stage T3 Surgical Salvage	Stage T3 Ultimate Control
M. D. Anderson[217]	Mixed†	48/49 (98%)	100%	68/77 (88%)	93%	46/60 (73%)	11/14	95%
University of Florida[218]	Mixed	14/16 (88%)	88%	13/17 (76%)	94%	12/25 (48%)	5/9	68%
University of California (San Francisco)[219]	External beam	29/38 (76%)	90% (approx.)	21/39 (54%)	70% (approx.)	8/32 (25%)	3	41%

*RT, radiation therapy.
†Mixed, external beam irradiation and interstitial implant.

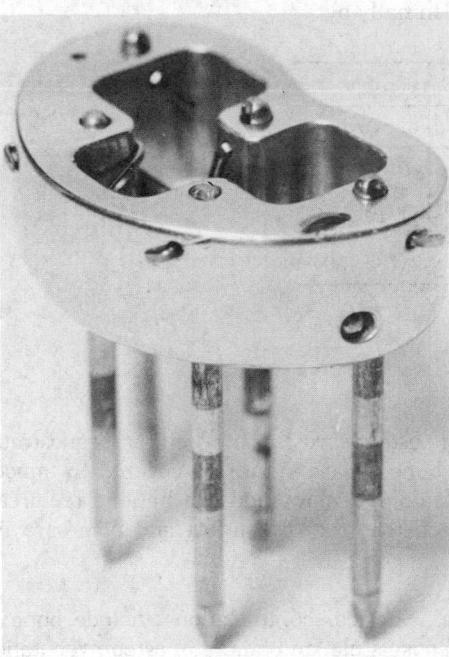

FIG. 21-8. Custom-made implant device for stage T1-T2 carcinoma of the floor of mouth. (Marcus RB Jr, Million RR, Mitchell TP: A preloaded, custom-designed implantation device for stage T1-T2 carcinoma of the floor of mouth. Int J Radiat Oncol Biol Phys 6:111–113, 1980)

the risk of a bone necrosis is significant; hyperbaric oxygen before and after the operation may reduce the risk of necrosis.

Surgical failures may be treated by a repeat operation, radiation therapy, or both on an individual basis. Radiation therapy alone is not likely to succeed.

Results of Treatment

Survival rates at 2 and 5 years for patients initially treated with radiation are shown in Table 21-21.[218] The local control rates for patients with stage III–IV disease treated by combined surgery and radiation therapy are shown in Table 21-22.[218,219,222]

Guillamondegui and Jesse[223] reported 20 patients treated by rim resection. All patients had invasion of the periosteum and 7 had early bone invasion on examination of the specimen. With 1-year follow-up, there was only one local recurrence. Four patients, however, developed recurrence in the neck, and for this reason the authors recommended postoperative radiation therapy.

Atkins and Cassisi[224] reviewed the University of Florida experience for rim resection in 20 patients with squamous cell carcinoma of the floor of the mouth (Table 21-23). Postoperative radiation therapy was added in 3 patients, and preoperative radiation therapy was used in one. Two of the patients had evidence of bone invasion on examination of the specimen, and treatment failed locally in both despite postoperative irradiation. Four rim resections were attempted in patients who had a recurrence after radiation therapy; the disease was controlled in 3 of 4 patients, but all developed a bone complication and loss of mandibular continuity. The local control and salvage rates were nearly identical to those shown in Table 21-12 for irradiation.

Wang and co-workers[225] reported the results for 33 patients with T1–T2 lesions treated by intraoral cone, sometimes combined with external beam radiation therapy. The local control rate was 94% and the 2-year disease-free survival rate was 97%. Soft-tissue ulceration occurred in 23% and osteoradionecrosis occurred in two patients.

FOLLOW-UP POLICY. Patients are seen at 4 to 6 week intervals for the first 2 years. There are two major difficul-

FIG. 21-9. Roentgenograms of an implant in place in the floor of the mouth. (**A**) AP view. (**B**) Lateral view. (Marcus RB Jr, Million RR, Mitchell TP: A preloaded, custom-designed implantation device for Stage T1-T2 carcinoma of the floor of mouth. Int J Radiat Oncol Biol Phys 6:111–113, 1980)

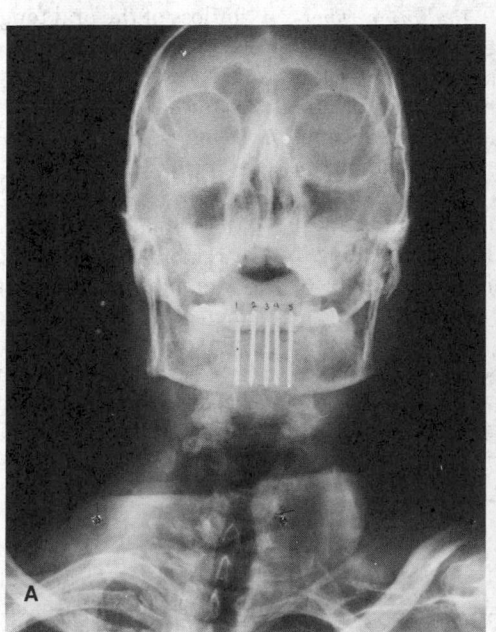
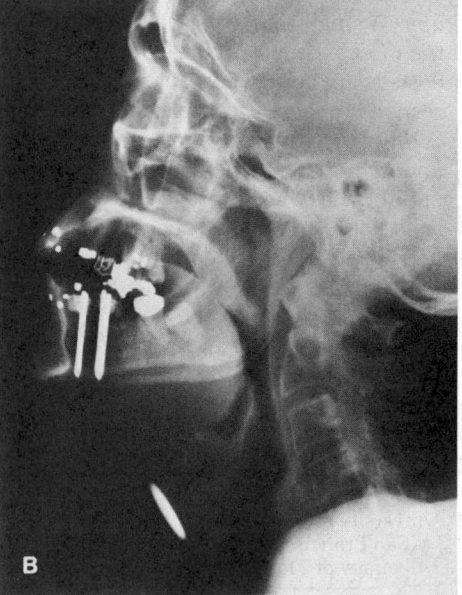

TABLE 21-21.   Floor of Mouth Carcinoma: Survival for Patients Treated Initially by Irradiation ± Radical Neck Dissection with Surgery for Salvage

Stage	Absolute Survival		Determinate Survival*	
	2 Years	5 Years	2 Years	5 Years
I	14/17 (82%)	6/8	14/14 (100%)	6/6
II	11/14 (79%)	4/7	11/13 (85%)	4/4
III	20/28 (71%)	11/27 (41%)	20/24 (83%)	11/19 (58%)
IV	4/14 (29%)	0/7	4/11 (36%)	0/6
Total	49/73 (67%)	21/49 (43%)	49/62 (79%)	21/35 (60%)

University of Florida data.[218] Patients treated 10/64–12/77; analysis 12/79 by W. M. Mendenhall, M.D.
*Excludes patients dead of intercurrent disease.

ties in follow-up after irradiation: soft tissue ulcers and enlarged submandibular glands. An ulcer in the floor of the mouth within 2 years of treatment can be either recurrence or necrosis. If the lesion appears to be soft-tissue necrosis, a trial of conservative therapy and observation at close intervals is adequate. The soft-tissue necroses are notoriously slow to heal. Failure to stabilize or show some indication of healing is an indication for biopsy. A negative biopsy does not rule out recurrence, and if the lesion remains suspicious, repeat deep biopsies are in order.

An enlarged submandibular gland(s) may be a sequel to obstruction of the submandibular duct. The gland may be enlarged on initial examination, or it may enlarge during or after treatment. It is difficult to distinguish between an enlarged submandibular gland and tumor in a lymph node. CT scan with contrast and needle biopsy are useful, but only removal will clarify the situation in most instances.

Follow-up of surgical cases may be difficult if skin grafts or flaps have been used because of the associated induration and thickness of the flaps. If the submandibular ducts have been reimplanted, stenosis may occur with subsequent enlargement of the submandibular glands. This enlargement must be distinguished from cancer metastatic to the neck.

COMPLICATIONS OF TREATMENT.   *Radiation Therapy.* A small soft-tissue necrosis may develop in the floor of the mouth, usually in the site of the original lesion where the dose is highest. These ulcers are moderately painful and respond to local anesthetic, antibiotics, and tincture of time.

If the ulceration develops on the adjacent gingiva, then the underlying mandible is exposed. These areas are mildly painful. They are managed by discontinuing dentures, local anesthetic, antibiotics, and smoothing of the bone by filing if needed. These small bone exposures do not often progress to

TABLE 21-22.   Floor of Mouth Cancer, Stage III–IV: Local Control with Primary Combined Treatment (Surgery + Radiation Therapy)

Institution	Local Control	Ultimate Control
University of Louisville[222]	13/15	13/15 (87%)
University of California (San Francisco)[219]	9/10	9/10 (90%)
University of Florida[218]	5/11	5/11 (46%)

full-blown osteonecrosis. They either sequestrate a small piece of bone or are simply re-covered by mucous membrane. Healing is slow, and the patient requires constant reassurance that the discomfort and ulcer are not due to cancer.

Surgical. Surgical complications include bone exposure, orocutaneous fistula, and failure of osteomyocutaneous flaps. Salvage procedures after radiation therapy are associated with an increased risk of complications.

ORAL TONGUE

Anatomy

The circumvallate papillae locate the division between oral tongue and base of tongue. The papillae foliatae may be recognized as 2 mm to 4 mm, slightly elevated, irregular areas on the dorsum at the junction with the anterior tonsillar pillar.

The arterial supply is mainly by way of paired lingual arteries that are branches of the external carotid. One lingual artery may be sacrificed without danger of necrosis, but sacrifice of both lingual arteries results in an increased risk for loss of the oral tongue and almost certain loss of the base of tongue.

The sensory pathway is by way of the lingual nerve to the gasserian ganglion.

Pathology

More than 95% of oral tongue lesions are squamous cell carcinomas. Coexisting leukoplakia is common. Verrucous carcinoma and minor salivary gland tumors are quite uncommon. Granular cell myoblastoma is a benign tumor of uncertain origin that commonly occurs on the dorsum of the tongue and may be confused histologically with carcinoma because of the associated pseudoepitheliomatous hyperplasia. Granular cell myoblastoma does not respond to radiation therapy.

Patterns of Spread

PRIMARY.   Nearly all oral tongue squamous cell carcinomas occur on the lateral and undersurfaces of the tongue.

TABLE 21-23. Carcinoma of the Floor of the Mouth: Results of Treatment by Rim Resection in 20 Patients*

Stage	No of Patients	Local Recurrence	No. Salvaged/ No. Attempted	Ultimate Control
T2	11	3	1/2	9/11 (81%)
T3	8	4	2/2	6/8 (75%)
T4	1	1	0/0	0/1 (0%)

Million RR, Cassisi NJ: Oral cavity. In Million RR, Cassisi NJ [eds]: Management of Head and Neck Cancer: A Multidisciplinary Approach, p 264. Philadelphhia, JB Lippincott, 1984.

*University of Florida data. Patients treated 6/73–6/81, analysis 3/83 by J. S. Atkins, Jr, M.D., and N. J. Cassisi, D.D.S., M.D.

A few lesions appear on the dorsum. Most of the carcinomas occur on the middle and posterior thirds of the oral tongue. Oral tongue carcinomas tend to remain in the tongue until large unless they originate near the junction with the floor of the mouth. Perineural invasion and vascular space invasion occur.

Anterior third (tip) lesions usually are diagnosed early. Advanced lesions invade the floor of the mouth and root of the tongue, producing ulceration and fixation.

Middle third lesions invade the musculature of the tongue and later invade the lateral floor of the mouth.

Posterior third lesions grow into the musculature of the tongue, the floor of the mouth, anterior tonsillar pillar, base of the tongue, and glossotonsillar sulcus. Posterior third lesions behave more like base of tongue cancer with a higher incidence of lymph node metastasis compared to the anterior two thirds of the oral tongue.

LYMPHATICS. The first-echelon nodes are the subdigastric and submandibular nodes (Fig. 21-10).[7] The submental and spinal accessory lymph nodes are seldom involved. Rouviere[3] describes lymphatic trunks that bypass the subdigastric and submandibular nodes and terminate in the midjugular lymph nodes. One seldom sees this pattern clinically.

The lymphatic vessels of the tongue anastomose freely, allowing contralateral lymph flow. Thirty-five percent of patients with oral tongue cancer have clinically positive nodes on admission; 5% are bilateral. The incidence of occult disease is approximately 30% (see Table 21-4).[15] The incidence of positive nodes increases with T stage (see Table 21-1).[7]

Patients with N1 or N2 ipsilateral nodes have a 27% risk of developing node metastasis in the opposite neck.

Clinical Picture

Mild irritation of the tongue is the most frequent complaint. The patient frequently thinks he has bitten his tongue. The pain may occur only during eating or drinking. As ulceration develops, the pain becomes progressively worse and is referred to the external ear canal. Extensive infiltration of the muscles of the tongue affects speech and deglutition. Patients with advanced lesions have a foul mouth odor.

The extent of disease is determined by visual examination and palpation. The tongue protrudes incompletely and toward the side of the lesion as fixation develops. Posterior oral tongue lesions may grow inferiorly, behind the mylohyoid, and present as a mass in the neck at the angle of the mandible; the mass may be confused with an enlarged lymph

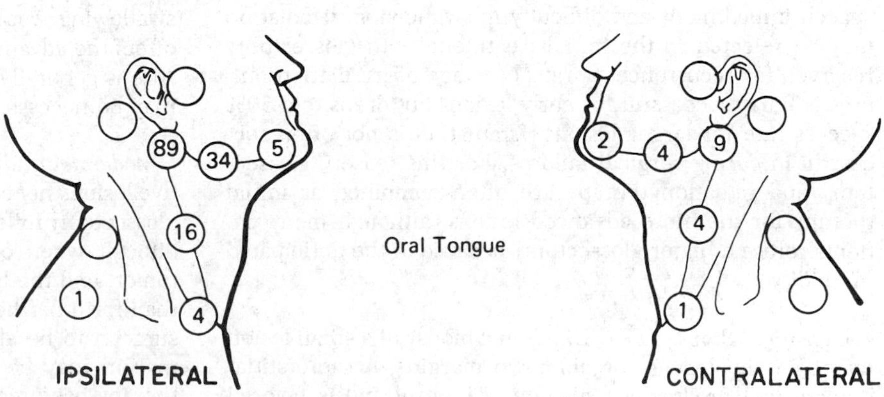

FIG. 21-10. Nodal distribution at admission, M.D. Anderson Hospital, 1948–1965. (Lindberg RD: Distribution of cervical lymph node metastases from squamous cell carcinoma of the upper respiratory and digestive tracts. Cancer 29:1446–1450, 1972)

Oral Tongue

IPSILATERAL   CONTRALATERAL

N_0	N_1	N_{2A}	N_{2B}	N_{3A}	N_{3B}	N_1-N_3	/ Total
197	40	9	32	8	16	105	/ 302 = 35%

node. Invasion of the hypoglossal nerve is rare and may cause atrophy. Posterolateral lesions may be difficult to evaluate because of pain; examination with the patient under anesthesia may be required.

Methods of Diagnosis and Staging

The differential diagnosis includes granular cell myoblastomas, which are usually slow-growing, nontender masses, 0.5 cm to 2.0 cm in size. The lesions are well circumscribed, firm, and slightly raised; they may be multiple. Malignant behavior is either nonexistent or rare, and wide local excision is the treatment of choice. Pyogenic granulomas mimic small exophytic carcinomas. Tuberculous ulcer and syphilitic chancre are rare considerations.

CT scan with contrast is useful to determine the extent of disease in the more advanced lesions and will help define mandible invasion when tumor abuts the jaw; the neck lymph nodes and submandibular gland can also be evaluated when indicated.

A Panorex film may be useful to evaluate dentition and the extent of tumor invasion and to determine if the mandible is large enough for rim resection in edentulous patients. Occlusal dental films are helpful for early bone invasion and dental evaluation. Bone scans are often falsely positive and are not recommended.[226]

Biopsy is by punch forceps or incisional biopsy. Small lesions are excised and margins checked.

Treatment

SELECTION OF TREATMENT MODALITY. Both glossectomy and irradiation are curative for oral tongue cancer, and reported cure rates are similar for similar stages. For this reason, selection of treatment is individualized. The management of the neck may dictate the management of the primary lesion. The disadvantages of surgery include removal of part of the tongue and the decision on whether or not to do a neck dissection for the N0 neck. The disadvantage of radiation therapy is the risk of radiation necrosis. For irradiation to produce satisfactory control rates, the use of interstitial or intraoral cone therapy is essential. When hemiglossectomy is predicted to produce some degree of speech impediment and difficulty in swallowing, irradiation may be selected as the initial treatment, with glossectomy reserved for recurrence. Surgical salvage of irradiation failures is fairly successful for early lesions but drops to a 50% success rate for larger lesions. Irradiation is not often successful in curing surgical failures. For this reason, glossectomy and radiation therapy are often combined as initial therapy for the more advanced lesions, although many patients refuse a major glossectomy because of the anticipated morbidity.

Excisional Biopsy (TX). Excisional biopsy of a small lesion may show inadequate or unknown margins. An interstitial implant will produce a high rate of control and is favored over reexcision.[216]

Early Lesions (T1 or T2). Operation and irradiation pro-

duce similar local control rates, and treatment decisions are based on anticipated functional loss, management of the neck, and patient preference. A limited glossectomy with primary closure may be done transorally in an outpatient setting and is usually the preferred therapy. Postoperative radiation therapy would only be added for positive margins or perineural invasion.

Glossectomy is the treatment of choice for small, well circumscribed, well to moderately differentiated lesions that can be excised transorally, small lesions on the tip of the tongue, and the rare lesion on the dorsum of the tongue. Irradiation may be selected for larger T1 and the T2 lesions in order to preserve speech and swallowing for poorly differentiated carcinomas, and for lesions that have a high risk for bilateral lymph node metastases.

Moderately Advanced Lesions (T2 or T3). Lesions that have a large surface involvement but minimal infiltration are favorable lesions and are managed with radiation therapy alone. Those lesions that are deeply infiltrative will have a higher control rate with combined surgery and radiation therapy, but the patient must be willing to accept glossectomy, possibly mandibulectomy, and flap reconstruction. Postoperative radiation therapy should be considered when the initial margins are microscopically positive even though the margins are ultimately negative.[227] Radical radiation therapy with surgery reserved for salvage is a reasonable alternative.

Advanced Lesions (T4). Combined treatment with surgery and radiation therapy will cure a very few patients, especially those with minimal neck disease. We have never cured a true T4 oral tongue cancer with radiation therapy alone. Operation usually implies total glossectomy, mandibulectomy, neck node dissection on one or both sides, laryngectomy, and postoperative radiation therapy. The chances of cure are slim to none, and the treatment produces major morbidity at enormous cost. Most patients in this category will receive palliative therapy.

SURGICAL TREATMENT. *Early Lesions.* Examples of two lesions and the amount of tongue to be removed are shown in Figure 21-11. Speech impediment and difficulty swallowing would be unlikely in these cases. Glossectomy offers the advantage of a short treatment time. Primary closure is generally done, although with large resections a flap may be necessary.

Moderately Advanced Lesions (T2 or T3). Deeply infiltrative lesions not suitable for irradiation alone are managed by glossectomy followed by postoperative radiation therapy. It is difficult when cutting the tongue to judge projections of tumor, and the likelihood of cutting across tumor is greater than for other head and neck sites. It is an advantage to the surgeon to be able to feel the tumor mass so that a wide margin may be gained, which is not as easy if radiation therapy has preceded the glossectomy. Frozen section control is an essential part of the procedure. Positive margins are an indication for excision of additional tissue. Scholl and co-workers[227] reported that no tumor will be found in 73% of

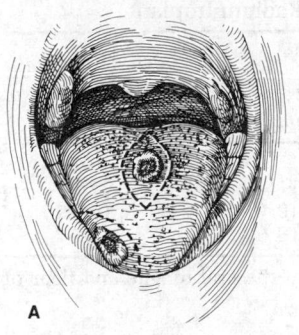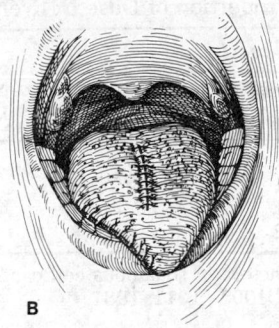

A   B

FIG. 21-11. Small lesions on the anterior free margin of the tongue or in the midline of the tongue can be excised (**A**) and the defect closed primarily (**B**).

cases when the reexcision specimen is examined. Finally, if a mandibulotomy or mandibulectomy is done after preoperative radiation therapy, the likelihood of exposed bone, nonunion, and radionecrosis is increased.

Advanced Lesions (T4). Advanced lesions would require a total glossectomy and usually a laryngectomy combined with postoperative radiation therapy. The procedure would only be offered to patients in good general condition and with minimal neck disease.

IRRADIATION TECHNIQUE. The dose schemes currently prescribed at the University of Florida are given in Table 21-24.

The ability to control the primary lesion is enhanced by giving all or part of the treatment by interstitial radiation therapy or by intraoral cone.[29,217,218,228,229] The time factor is thought to be critical for oral tongue cancer, and the external beam portion of the treatment is shortened to 3000 cGy in 2 weeks in order to increase the proportion of the therapy given by either interstitial or intraoral cone therapy. The interstitial therapy may be given before or after the external beam treatment, but the intraoral cone therapy should be done prior to the external beam treatment. The major advantage of intraoral cone therapy is to avoid irradiation of the adjacent mandible and to avoid the trauma of the implant. The disadvantage of intraoral cone therapy is the technical difficulty in avoiding a geographic miss due to tongue mobility. The local control rate by T stage and the rate of salvage

by operation at the University of Florida are shown in Table 21-25.[218] Treatment of the neck is an integral part of the treatment plan. The authors favor elective neck irradiation for nearly all lesions.

COMBINED TREATMENT POLICIES. When glossectomy is selected for the treatment, postoperative irradiation is considered for positive or close margins, poorly differentiated lesions, vascular space invasion, perineural invasion, and recurrent lesions. If the initial margins (either mucosal or muscular) are positive on frozen section and then become negative on reexcision, radiation therapy is advised.[227] If the indication for postoperative radiation therapy is on account of neck node metastases, the area of primary resection should be included in the fields of irradiation.

Interstitial implants are not used in postoperative radiation therapy because recurrences may appear at any point along the surgical dissection. If the margins in the tongue are positive, the chances of local control are poor; high doses should be tried. Preoperative radiation therapy is advised only when fixed nodes are present.

MANAGEMENT OF RECURRENCE. Most recurrences appear in the first 2 years. Local recurrence after radiation therapy or surgery is heralded by ulceration, pain, or increased induration. A trial of antibiotics such as tetracycline will often reduce the pain of either radiation necrosis or recurrent tumor. Recurrences have a slightly elevated or rolled border, whereas necroses do not. The induration associated with necrosis is usually less than with recurrence. Biopsy should be done as soon as ulceration appears, if the ulcer is within the original tumor site. Ulcers that appear on adjacent normal tissues (*e.g.*, the gingiva) are due to radiation effect and not cancer. Outpatient biopsies with a local anesthetic may miss the tumor. If suspicion remains high for local recurrence after a negative biopsy, generous biopsies with the patient under a general anesthetic are required, and even this maneuver occasionally will miss persistent tumor.

Radiation failure is managed by glossectomy. Surgical failure occasionally is salvaged by radiation therapy or an operation, if the recurrence is limited to the mucosa. Recurrence in soft tissues of the neck is rarely eradicated by any procedure.

Nodes appearing in a previously untreated neck are managed by neck dissection with or without postoperative radiation therapy.

TABLE 21-24.   Irradiation Policies for Oral Tongue Cancer at the University of Florida

	Interstitial Alone (cGy)	*External Beam + Interstitial (cGy)*
TX—No visible or palpable tumor	6000	Not recommended
TX—Palpable induration or nodularity	7000	Not recommended
TX—Tumor at margins; gross residual	7500	5000 + 3000
Early—<1 cm	6500	Not recommended
Early—1–3 cm	Not recommended	3000/2 weeks + 3500
Moderately advanced—3–5 cm	Not recommended	3000/2 weeks + 4000
Advanced	Not recommended	5000 ± 3500
Postoperative radiation therapy, negative margins	Not recommended	6000 to 6500/6 to 7 weeks
Preoperative radiation therapy, fixed nodes	Not recommended	5000/6 weeks

TABLE 21-25.   Oral Tongue Carcinoma: Local Control Versus Proportion of Dose Delivered by Radium Implant

| Stage | No. of Patients with Local Control/No. Treated | | | | No. Salvaged/ No. Attempted | No. Ultimately Controlled/No. Treated |
	Radium or Radium + <3000 cGy	Radium + ≥3000 cGy	External Beam	RT Alone (Total)		
T1	5/5	2/2	0/1	7/8	1/1	8/8
T2	10/11*	7/15*	1/1	18/27	4/7	22/27
T3	0/2	7/20	n.d.	7/22	5/10	12/22
Total	15/18	16/37	1/2	32/57	10/18	42/57

Mendenhall WM, VanCise WS, Bova FJ, et al: Analysis of time-dose factors in squamous cell carcinoma of the oral tongue and floor of mouth treated with radiation therapy alone. Int J Radiat Oncol Biol Phys 7:1005–1011, 1981.
*Significance: p = 0.02, Fisher's exact test.[145]

RESULTS OF TREATMENT. The ultimate control rate above the clavicles (*i.e.,* local plus regional) for a series of 117 patients is shown in Table 21-26. The 2-year survival rate is presented in Table 21-27. Approximately 20% will die of intercurrent disease; 10% will die of distant metastases.

COMPLICATIONS OF TREATMENT.   *Surgical.* Orocutaneous fistula, flap necrosis, and dysphagia are the three most common complications of surgery of the tongue. Damage to the lingual nerve or the hypoglossal nerve during the course of surgery, although rare, increases the difficulty that the patient may have in swallowing and in speaking.

Fistula and flap necrosis must be handled judiciously because the danger of carotid artery hemorrhage increases with either of these complications.

Enunciation difficulties occur whenever the tongue is bound down by scarring. The incidence of complications increases for surgical salvage attempts after radiation failure, and multiple procedures may be necessary to obtain satisfactory healing.

Radiation Therapy. Many patients will complain of a sensitive tongue for many months after completion of treatment, even when the mucosa is well healed. The effect disappears with time.

Taste will reappear from 1 week to several months after treatment. Taste may return to normal, but more frequently it is "not quite as keen" as before. The dryness of the mouth may contribute to the poorer sense of taste.

Return of saliva is variable, depending on the treatment volume and the dose to the salivary glands. Patients treated with interstitial therapy alone eventually will have nearly normal saliva. Patients treated with 4500 cGy external beam therapy plus interstitial therapy will eventually have 25% to 50% return of saliva if one parotid receives 3000 cGy or less.

Soft-Tissue Necrosis. A minor soft-tissue necrosis is fairly common. Once recurrence has been ruled out, considerable patience is required for healing. The patient associates pain with recurrence of the cancer, because the original lesion frequently caused a similar pain. He needs to be reassured constantly that the ulcer will heal slowly and that there is no evidence of recurrence. Patients who develop a necrosis rarely get a recurrence, so in a sense, there is some good news associated with the pain.

There is no good, simple treatment for soft-tissue necrosis. The treatment plan is mainly to rule out recurrent cancer, provide local anesthesia, and reduce local infection. The patient is placed on a biweekly or monthly examination schedule. Broad-spectrum antibiotics (*e.g.,* tetracycline, 1 g/day), local anesthetic to be applied with a cotton-tipped applicator, and analgesics as needed are prescribed. Chewable aspirin (*e.g.,* Aspergum) will give good analgesia if the patient can chew gum. Frequently, pain will be reduced dramatically in 1 to 3 days after starting antibiotics, but sometimes the response is nil. Lidocaine (Xylocaine viscous) can be applied to the ulcer with a cotton swab for local analgesia. The authors have had little success with alcohol nerve blocks. Hyperbaric oxygen treatment may be tried in difficult cases. The authors have tried local fulguration with silver nitrate to attempt pain relief but with little success; they also have a variable experience with cryotherapy. When all else fails, however, and necrosis is persistent and pain uncontrollable, the necrosis must be resected.

TABLE 21-26.   Oral Tongue Carcinoma: Ultimate Control Above the Clavicles by Treatment Technique (117 Patients)

AJCC Stage	Surgery with RT Salvage	RT ± RND with Surgical Salvage*	Postoperative RT	Preoperative RT
I	6/7 (86%)	11/14 (79%)		
II	4/4 (100%)	19/26 (73%)		
III	3/3 (100%)	13/27 (48%)	1/4	1/2
IVA		8/17 (47%)	2/2	0/2
IVB		3/7 (43%)	1/1	0/1

University of Florida data. Patients treated 10/64–3/83; analysis 3/85 by Tim R. Williams, M.D. (2-year minimum follow-up).
*RT, radiation therapy; RND, radical neck dissection.

TABLE 21-27. Oral Tongue Carcinoma: Two-Year Survival Rates by Treatment Technique

AJCC Stage	Surgery with RT Salvage		RT ± RND with Surgical Salvage*		Postoperative RT		Preoperative RT	
	Abs.	Det.	Abs.	Det.	Abs.	Det.	Abs.	Det.
I	56%	71%	72%	93%				
II	67%	80%	70%	78%	0/1	0/1		
III	100%	100%	68%	70%	20%	20%	50%	50%
IVA			55%	65%	100%	100%	50%	50%
IVB			27%	43%	100%	100%	0/1	0/1

University of Florida data. Patients treated 10/64–3/83; analysis 3/85 by Tim R. Williams, M.D. (2-year minimum follow-up).
*RT, radiation therapy; RND, radical neck dissection; Abs., absolute survival; Det., determinate survival.

The key word for management of radiation necroses is patience.

Radiation-Induced Bone Disease. The endentulous person is less likely to develop serious radiation-induced disease of the mandible than is a person with teeth. There are several ways in which the mandible may be affected.

The most frequent problem involving the mandible is termed bone exposure. The gingiva disappears, exposing the underlying bone, with the exposed area or areas usually varying from 2 mm to 2 cm in diameter. If the exposed area is small, the patient is often unaware of the problem. There may be modest discomfort. The bone appears intact. Biopsy is not needed unless there was tumor at that location on the gingiva prior to treatment. If the patient has dentures, they should be discontinued, or in certain cases altered by the dentist to relieve the denture over the exposed bone. If sharp bony edges appear, they are filed to a smooth contour and the bone edge lowered to speed healing. The bone exposure may become more or less stationary at this point. Healing may require months or even years. Healing occurs when the gingiva regrows over the exposed area; a small, superficial piece of bone may sequestrate first, and then the gingiva regrows to cover the exposed area. Again, patience is the major requirement.

In some instances the bone exposure may progress so that a large area of bone is exposed. Pain is usually intermittent, mild to moderate, and occasionally severe. Antibiotics will usually reduce pain when it does occur. Local care is similar to that used for early bone exposures. It is amazing that rampant osteomyelitis rarely develops in the exposed, relatively avascular bone.

In some cases, the bone becomes frankly necrotic with intermittent sequestration. Hyperbaric oxygen treatment has been used with some success. It is a matter of individualization when surgical intervention should be instituted. Conservative measures should be given a fair trial, but if pain becomes a problem an operative procedure must be considered. The dead bone is removed and replaced with tissue such as myocutaneous flap, carrying its own blood supply.

BUCCAL MUCOSA

Epidemiology

Squamous cell carcinoma is relatively uncommon in the United States. In southern India it is common and is related to chewing a combination of tobacco mixed with betel leaves, areca nut, and shell lime.[230]

Anatomy

The buccal mucosa is the mucous membrane covering the inner surface of the cheeks and lips, ending above and below with a transition to the gingiva. It ends posteriorly at the retromolar trigone. The parotid duct opens into the buccal mucosa opposite the second upper molar. The blood supply is a branch of the facial artery. The long buccal nerve, a branch of the mandibular nerve (V), is sensory to the buccal mucosa and the skin of the check that covers the buccinator muscle.

Pathology

Most malignant tumors are low-grade squamous cell carcinoma, frequently appearing on a background of leukoplakia. Verrucous carcinoma occurs and may be particularly difficult to diagnose histologically because of associated inflammatory changes. Minor salivary gland tumors and malignant melanoma occur rarely.

Patterns of Spread

Almost all of the squamous cell carcinomas originate on the mucosa lining the cheeks; primary lesions seldom originate from the wet mucosa of the lips. Early lesions are usually discrete, elevated tumors, often exophytic. As they enlarge, they penetrate the underlying muscles and eventually penetrate to the skin. Peripheral growth occurs into the gingivobuccal gutters and eventually onto the gingiva and underlying bone.

The lymphatic spread is first to the submandibular and subdigastric nodes. The incidence of positive nodes on admission is 9% to 31%, and the risk of occult disease is 16% (see Tables 21-1 and 21-4).[7,15]

Clinical Picture

Early, asymptomatic lesions may be discovered by the dentist or physician. A background of leukoplakia is common and sometimes quite extensive. Small lesions produce the sensation of a lump that is felt with the tongue. Pain is minimal even when the lesion becomes large, unless there is posterior extension to involve the lingual and dental nerves. Pain may be referred to the ear. Obstruction of Stensen's duct will produce parotid enlargement. Extension posteriorly, behind the pterygomandibular raphe or into the buccinator and masseter muscles, eventually will cause trismus. Intermittent bleeding occurs when the lesion is irritated by chewing or is ulcerated by growing against the teeth.

Methods of Diagnosis and Staging

The differential diagnosis includes lues and tuberculosis, both of which are quite uncommon. If the first biopsy report is chronic inflammation or pseudoepitheliomatous hyperplasia and there is an obvious neoplasm present, repeat biopsy is in order. Sometimes multiple repeat biopsies are required to establish the diagnosis and the physician must be persistent.

CT or MRI is used to evaluate the larger lesions.

Treatment

SELECTION OF TREATMENT MODALITY. Small lesions (≤1 cm) may simply be excised with primary closure; small lesions that involve the anterior commissure are best treated by radiation therapy. Lesions 2 cm to 3 cm in size usually are treated by radiation therapy. These lesions can be excised and grafted, but the graft tends to shrink and become irregular and firm; this makes detection of recurrence difficult, and the cheek feels tight and uncomfortable to the patient. Larger lesions are treated by either radical surgical excision, radiation therapy, or a combination of both on an individualized basis. Preference is given to radiation therapy when the tumor invades near the commissure. Preference is given to an operation when there is invasion of the mandible or maxilla.

Surgical Treatment. Lesions that invade the mandible or maxilla require that an appropriate amount of bone be resected along with the soft tissues. Repair may require a maxillary prosthesis. Full-thickness removal of the cheek is repaired by a myocutaneous flap.

Irradiation Technique. Buccal mucosa lesions are suited for treatment with electrons, intraoral cone, and interstitial techniques to spare the contralateral normal tissues. When tumors extend into one of the gingivobuccal gutters or onto bone, treatment must be entirely by external beam. A lead block placed in the mouth will help decrease transit irradiation.

RESULTS OF TREATMENT. MacComb and co-workers[212] reported the results for 115 patients treated between 1947 and 1962. Irradiation was the initial treatment in 69 patients, surgery was used in 44 patients, and combined therapy was used in 2 patients. The local recurrence rate was 10% for Stage I, 12% for Stages II and III, and 38% for Stage IV. The 3-year absolute survival rate was 49% and the 5-year absolute survival rate was 48%. The determinate 3-year and 5-year survival rates were 71% and 70%, respectively. The same authors reported a 35% cure rate for 40 patients referred after failure of initial treatment given elsewhere.

Ash[21] reported 35% absolute 5-year survival for 374 patients with carcinoma of the buccal mucosa for all stages. The primary lesion was controlled initially in 53% of patients with early lesions and in 25% with advanced lesions; salvage raised the ultimate control rates to 69% and 34%. The initial treatment to the primary lesion was radiation therapy in 97% of the patients.

Bloom and Spiro[231] reported the surgical results for 90 patients with buccal mucosal cancer. They reported a 43% local recurrence rate, 37% neck failures, and 22% incidence of distant metastases. The overall failure rate was 42%. The 5-year survival rate by stage was Stage I, 77%; Stage II, 65%; Stage III, 27%; and Stage IV, 18%. The rate of complications was 24%.

Nair and co-workers[230] reported the radiation therapy results for 234 cases of buccal mucosa cancer treated in southern India by radical radiation therapy during a single year, 1982. Treatment was either small-volume external beam (33 patients), single-plane radium implant (45 patients), or single lateral field (106 patients). The disease-free survival rate at 3 years by stage was Stage I, 85%; Stage II, 63%; Stage III, 41%; and Stage IV, 15%. Thirty-two patients had verrucous carcinoma; the 3-year disease-free survival rate was 47%, similar to that for other grades of squamous cell carcinoma.

COMPLICATIONS OF TREATMENT. The buccal mucosa is quite tolerant of high-dose radiation therapy, and complications are uncommon. Bone exposure may appear on the mandible or maxilla. Trismus may develop if the muscles of mastication receive high doses.

Surgical injury of Stensen's duct may cause obstruction and parotitis. The parotid gland will eventually atrophy. Injury to branches of the seventh nerve may occur. Split-thickness skin grafts may shrink and produce partial trismus. Resection of the lip commissure may produce oral incompetence with drooling.

GINGIVA AND HARD PALATE (INCLUDING RETROMOLAR TRIGONE)

Carcinomas arising from the upper and lower gingiva have a similar clinical picture and require a similar approach to diagnosis. Primary squamous cell carcinoma of the hard palate is uncommon, the majority of hard palate neoplasms being minor salivary gland tumors. Some authors include the retromolar trigone with the anterior tonsillar pillar, but in their natural history and management, these lesions are more similar to lesions of the lower gingiva.

Anatomy

The lower gingiva includes the mucosa covering the mandible from the gingivobuccal gutter to the origin of the mobile mucosa on the floor of the mouth. Behind the third molar is a small triangular surface called the retromolar trigone; it is continuous above with the maxillary tuberosity.

Beneath the mucosa of the retromolar trigone is the tendinous pterygomandibular raphe, which is attached to the pterygoid hamulus and the posterior mylohyoid ridge of the mandible and serves as the insertion of the buccinator, orbicular oris, and superior pharyngeal constrictor muscles. Just behind the pterygomandibular raphe and between the medial pterygoid muscle and the ascending ramus is the pterygomandibular space, which contains the lingual and dental nerves. The pterygomandibular space is related posteriorly to the deep lobe of the parotid and the contents of the parapharyngeal space.

There are no minor salivary glands in the attached mucous membrane over the alveolar ridges.

Pathology

Most neoplasms of the lower gum and retromolar trigone are squamous cell carcinoma; squamous cell carcinoma is relatively uncommon on the upper gum and hard palate, where minor salivary gland tumors, usually adenoid cystic carcinoma, are more frequent. Verrucous lesions occur, usually on the lower gingiva. Melanoma is reported. Metastatic lesions to the underlying bone may be confused with primary mucosal tumors.

Epidermoid carcinoma may arise within the body of the mandible or maxilla (intra-alveolar epidermoid carcinoma) either from odontogenic epithelium or from epithelium trapped during embryonic development. It is more frequent in the mandible than the maxilla, and is most common in the molar regions. It must be distinguished from metastatic squamous cell carcinoma and ameloblastoma.

Ameloblastoma is a rare tumor with an incidence of about 1% of all tumors of the maxilla and mandible. Most patients are in the age range of 20 to 50 years. Some 80% of cases of ameloblastoma occur in the mandible with the molar–ramus region most commonly involved. No appreciable differences are found by sex or race.[232] Histologically, the ameloblastoma is an epithelial tumor histologically similar to basal cell carcinoma.[233] The lesion may appear histologically benign, but should be considered a low-grade malignancy.[234] Ameloblastoma may arise in the gingiva without bone involvement.

Patterns of Spread

LOWER GUM. Squamous cell carcinoma invades the periosteum and the adjacent buccal mucosa and floor of the mouth. Slow-growing, low-grade lesions tend to produce atrophy of adjacent bone and produce a smooth, saucerized defect before invading the mandible. Moderate-grade to high-grade lesions invade the bone directly or through recently opened dental sockets and produce a lytic defect.

Lymphatic spread is to the submandibular and subdigastric nodes. Eighteen percent to 52% have clinically positive nodes on admission; occult disease occurs in 17% to 19% (see Tables 21-1 and 21-4).[7,15]

Ameloblastoma is a rather indolent tumor that usually arises in bone, expands, and destroys the bone, slowly extending to adjacent areas by contiguous growth. Regional and even distant metastasis may occur in a few cases, but even when present is compatible with a long natural course. Metastatic disease usually is reported in the lungs, but bone and liver metastases have been reported.[235]

UPPER GUM AND HARD PALATE. Most squamous cell carcinomas originate on the gingiva and spread secondarily to the hard palate, soft palate, buccal mucosa, and underlying bone; the maxillary antrum is invaded quite late unless there are recent extractions that provide an open pathway. Primary carcinoma of the maxillary antrum must be excluded because it frequently presents in the upper gum and hard palate. The risk for positive lymph nodes is 13% to 24% on admission, and the incidence of occult disease is 22% (see Tables 21-1 and 21-4 and "Minor Salivary Gland Tumors").

RETROMOLAR TRIGONE. The retromolar trigone is a small area, and spread to adjacent buccal mucosa, anterior tonsillar pillar, and maxilla occurs early. Posterior spread occurs early into the pterygomandibular space and the medial pterygoid muscle. Posterolateral spread occurs into the buccinator muscle and fat pad.

The submandibular and subdigastric lymph nodes are the first to be involved.

The incidence of clinically positive nodes on presentation is about 30% and the risk for occult disease is about 15% to 25%.[236]

Clinical Picture

The patient with squamous cell carcinoma may present first to the dentist with ill fitting dentures, dental pain, loose teeth, or a sore that will not heal. A history of inappropriate dental extractions or root canal therapy is common. Intermittent bleeding and mild pain occur when the lesion is traumatized. Invasion into the mandible may involve the inferior dental nerve and produce paresthesias or anesthesia of the lower lip. A background of leukoplakia is frequently present.

Retromolar trigone lesions may have pain referred to the external auditory canal and preauricular area. Invasion of the pterygoid muscle produces trismus, usually accompanied by severe pain.

Intra-alveolar epidermoid carcinoma presents with a submucosal mass and dental symptoms. Roentgenograms show a lytic lesion in the mandible.

Ameloblastoma is a slow-growing neoplasm with few symptoms in the early stages. Patients may notice a gradually increasing facial deformity or loosening of teeth in the area of tumor.[237] An intraoral submucosal mass may be present initially. Ulceration occurs as the mass increases in size. On roentgenograms, a radiolucent area is seen with some of the following features: expansion of the overlying cortical plate, a scalloped margin, a multilocular appearance, or resorption of the roots of adjacent teeth.[238]

Minor salivary gland tumors start as a submucosal mass, enlarge slowly, and may present with a central ulceration (see "Minor Salivary Gland Tumors").

Methods of Diagnosis and Staging

The differential diagnosis includes dental disease and underlying bony cysts or tumors, including metastatic tumors.

Dental roentgenograms should be used where fine detail is needed to look for early mandible invasion. It may be difficult to exclude early bone invasion when recent extractions have been done. A CT scan is useful to detect bone invasion, to show posterior extension of retromolar trigone lesions, and to outline the soft-tissue extent of upper gum and hard palate lesions.

The AJCC staging system for oral cavity lesions is difficult to apply to gum lesions. In fact, the presence of mandible invasion is not even included as a staging factor. Evidence of lytic bone invasion should qualify for T4. Because even small lesions (less than 2 cm) may invade bone, there will be a wide prognostic range for T4 tumors. Swearingen and co-workers[239] reported a 56% incidence of mandible involvement for gum lesions and 10% for retromolar trigone lesions.

Treatment

SELECTION OF TREATMENT MODALITY. *Lower Gum.* The majority of lesions are managed by operation. Early lesions may be resected intraorally, removing only soft tissue or a margin of bone (*i.e.,* rim resection) and closing primarily or with a split-thickness skin graft. When bone invasion is present, removal of a segment of mandible is required; a neck dissection is usually included with mandibulectomy since the neck is entered in any event. Irradiation may be used for small lesions or those with only a pressure defect in the bone with good curative results, but the functional results are generally better after operation. Postoperative irradiation may be advised for close or positive margins, nerve involvement, large extensive lesions with bone invasion, recurrent lesions, and multiple node involvement or extracapsular extension.

Ameloblastoma. The initial treatment of ameloblastoma is an operation, but local recurrence is a problem. Sehdev and co-workers[235] reported that curettage was followed by local recurrence in 90% of mandibular and in all maxillary ameloblastomas. Subsequent resection controlled 80% of the mandibular but only 40% of the maxillary tumors. The initial use of segmental mandibular resection controlled 78% (18 of 23) with subsequent resection controlling those that recurred. The use of partial maxillectomy as the first treatment controlled 100% (7 of 7) of maxillary ameloblastomas as opposed to only 40% when partial maxillectomy was performed for recurrence. Hemimandibulectomy controlled 100% of curettage failures in one series.[240]

The lesions respond quite readily to irradiation. However, because radiation therapy has generally been applied to patients only after multiple operative failures and in cases of advanced disease, the curative ability is not clear.

Retromolar Trigone. Small retromolar trigone lesions may appear innocuous and easily cured, but often are more extensive than they seem. For early, well-localized lesions without detectable bone invasion, a rim or marginal resection of mandible may be done to preserve continuity of the mandible. If rim resection is not feasible, consider initial treatment with radiation therapy, reserving partial mandibulectomy for radiation therapy failure. Radiation therapy is recommended for lesions involving a rather large surface area, such as lesions with superficial extension to the anterior tonsillar

pillar, soft palate, and buccal mucosa.[224] Evidence of bone invasion is an indication for partial mandibulectomy. Preference is given to surgical treatment unless the cosmetic and functional result would be unacceptable to the patient, in which case operation is reserved for radiation therapy failure. Moderately advanced lesions usually are managed by resection followed by postoperative radiation therapy.

Upper Gum and Hard Palate. Surgical resection is the usual treatment for most lesions of the upper gum. Postoperative radiation therapy is added as needed. However, if the lesion is superficial and extensively involves the hard palate or involves a significant portion of the soft palate, then radiation should be the initial therapy. If the lesion is small and discrete and there is no bone involvement, the resection includes the periosteum or occasionally some underlying bone. Bone invasion requires a partial maxillectomy. The defect usually is repaired with a prosthesis.

SURGICAL TREATMENT. *Rim Resection (Coronal).* See the section on surgical treatment of floor of mouth lesions.

Segmental Mandibulectomy. For small lesions with minimal bone invasion, a short section of mandible is removed in continuity with the tumor (*e.g.,* removal of the mandible from the angle to the mental foramen).

Partial Mandibulectomy. The mandible and tumor usually are resected from the mental foramen to the coronoid process, usually leaving the head of the condyle. The remaining mandible is stabilized by a cobalt-chromium alloy (Vitallium) mesh spacer if there are teeth; if there are no teeth, no spacer is used. In certain cases, the mandible may be reconstructed at a later date, but few patients actually request the procedure.

Hemimandibulectomy. Extensive lesions may require removal of the mandible from symphysis to condyle on one side. Massive anterior lesions require removal of the mandible from angle to angle. This produces a major cosmetic and functional loss and is reconstructed with flaps and metal trays. A composite osteomyocutaneous flap is also available for reconstruction.

IRRADIATION TECHNIQUE. Small lesions of the lower gum and retromolar trigone may be treated by intraoral cone for all or part of their therapy. Well lateralized lesions of the retromolar trigone and posterior gum may be treated by either an ipsilateral mixed beam or angled wedge portal technique with a lead intraoral stent. Anterior gum lesions are treated by parallel opposed portals.

The usual indication for irradiation of hard palate lesions is a carcinoma that involves nearly the entire hard palate and upper gums with little or no bone invasion. These lesions may be treated by external beam, but an intraoral surface brachytherapy applicator is preferred.

The dose for retromolar trigone lesions is usually 6000 cGy in 6 weeks to 6500 cGy in 7 weeks for T1, 6500 cGy to 7000 cGy for T2, and 7500 cGy in 7.5 weeks for T3. The dose for gum lesions is similar.

TABLE 21-28.   Carcinoma of the Lower Gum: Local Control (26 Patients)*

| Stage | Initial Treatment by Radiation Therapy | | Initial Treatment by Surgery (No. Controlled/ No. Treated) | Initial Treatment by Surgery Plus Radiation Therapy (No. Controlled/ No. Treated) |
	Initial Control (No. Controlled/ No. Treated)	Surgical Salvage (No. Salvaged/ No. Attempted)		
T1	1/1		2/2	0
T2	1/5	0/2	3/5†	0
T3	0		0	0
T4	1/2	0/1	3/4†	4/7†

Million RR, Cassisi NJ: Oral cavity. In Million RR, Cassisi NJ (eds): Management of Head and Neck Cancer: A Multidisciplinary Approach, p 295. Philadelphia, JB Lippincott, 1984).
*University of Florida data. Patients treated 10/64–12/80; analysis 4/83 by G. R. Ayers, M.D.
†Salvage not attempted in any failures.

MANAGEMENT OF RECURRENCE. Radiation therapy failures are managed by operation. Surgical failures may be managed by surgery, radiation therapy, or a combination of both (see Tables 21-28, 21-29, and 21-30).[224] Salvage procedures frequently are not attempted, however, because of the advanced nature of the recurrence.

Results of Treatment

Byers and co-workers[241] reported the results for 61 patients with squamous cell carcinoma of the lower gum managed between 1970 and 1975 at the M. D. Anderson Hospital. Fifty-seven patients were treated by surgical resection and radiation therapy was added in six. The disease was controlled above the clavicles in 96%. There was one operative mortality. The incidence of neck disease was 29%, and the neck disease was controlled in all but two patients. At 2 years, the absolute survival rate was 67% and the determinate rate was 90%.

Byers and co-workers[236] reported the M. D. Anderson Hospital results for 110 previously untreated patients with squamous cell carcinoma of the retromolar trigone treated between 1965 and 1977, with a minimum 5-year follow-up. Surgery was often selected for patients with leukoplakia, poor teeth, mandible invasion, large neck nodes, or trismus.

Radiation therapy was selected for poorly differentiated tumors, for lesions that were mainly exophytic, involved the faucial arch or soft palate, or had ill defined borders, and for poor surgical risk cases. Local control rates by treatment modality are shown in Table 21-31. In spite of the high local and regional control rates, the absolute 5-year survival rate was only 26% due to a high incidence of death due to intercurrent disease, including a 33% risk for second cancers.

Shibuya and co-workers[242] reported the results for 38 cases of carcinoma of the hard palate and 82 cases of carcinoma of the upper gum treated between 1953 and 1982 in Japan. Sixty-six patients were managed initially by radiation therapy alone to the primary lesion, and 54 patients were managed by radiation therapy and surgery. The 5-year actuarial survival rate by stage was Stage I, 56%; Stage II, 41%; Stage III, 32%; and Stage IV, 12%. There was no difference in survival when comparing hard palate versus upper gum, squamous cell carcinoma versus minor salivary gland tumors, or radiation therapy alone versus radiation therapy plus surgery as initial therapy. The overall risk for metastatic lymph nodes was 47% for hard palate and 49% for the upper gum. Thirty patients recorded as having "slight bone invasion" and no metastases had a 5-year survival rate of 75% when treated by radiation therapy. Major bone involvement was an indication for partial maxillectomy.

TABLE 21-29.   Carcinoma of the Retromolar Trigone: Local Control (42 Patients)

| Stage | Initial Treatment by Radiation Therapy | | Initial Treatment by Surgery | | Initial Treatment by Surgery Plus Radiation Therapy |
	Initial Control (No. Controlled/ No. Treated)	Surgical Salvage (No. Salvaged/ No. Attempted)	Initial Control (No. Controlled/ No. Treated)	Radiation Therapy or Surgical Salvage (No. Salvaged/ No. Attempted)	
T1	4/4		1/2	1/1*	0
T2	2/8	0/3	2/2		3/4
T3	2/2		3/4	0/0	2/3†
T4	0/4	0/1	2/3	0/1	3/6†

Million RR, Cassisi NJ: Oral cavity. In Million RR, Cassisi NJ (eds): Management of Head and Neck Cancer: A Multidisciplinary Approach, p 295. Philadelphia, JB Lippincott, 1984.
University of Florida data. Patients treated 10/64–12/80; analysis 4/83 by G. R. Ayers, M.D.
*Follow-up 10 months after salvage by radiation therapy.
†Salvage not attempted in any failures.

TABLE 21-30.   Carcinoma of the Upper Gum: Local Control (Nine Patients)

Stage	Initial Treatment by Radiation Therapy		Initial Treatment by Surgery (No. Controlled/No. Treated)	Initial Treatment by Surgery Plus Radiation Therapy (No. Controlled/No. Treated)
	Initial Control (No. Controlled/ No. Treated)	Surgical Salvage (No. Salvaged/ No. Attempted)		
T1	0		0	1/1
T2	0/2	1/1	0	0
T3	0		0	0
T4	0/1	0	3/5*	0

Million RR, Cassisi NJ: Oral cavity. In Million RR, Cassisi NJ (eds): Management of Head and Neck Cancer: A Multidisciplinary Approach, p 296. Philadelphia, JB Lippincott, 1984.
University of Florida data. Patients treated 10/64 – 12/80; analysis 4/83 by G. R. Ayers, M.D.
*Salvage not attempted in any failures.

The analysis of local control for lower gum, retromolar trigone, and upper gum lesions is shown in Tables 21-28, 21-29, and 21-30.[224] The high rate of local failure for retromolar trigone carcinoma treated with radiation therapy alone (except for T1 lesions) is not explained by low dose or marginal failure. The absolute survival rate for 42 patients was 56% at 2 years and 34% at 5 years.

Fayos[243] reported that local control by radiation therapy alone for lesions with early bone invasion was approximately 50% and for extensive invasion about 25% (Fayos JV: Personal communication, 1973).

Cady and Catlin[24] reported an absolute 5-year survival rate of 43% for patients with lower gum lesions and 40% for upper gum lesions treated by surgery.

Complications of Treatment

Surgical complications include orocutaneous fistula, bone exposure with sequestration, extrusion of a metal tray, and loss of graft or flap. Following hemimandibulectomy, the edentulous patient usually cannot wear dentures and the patient with teeth cannot chew because of shifting of the remaining mandible.

The complications of radiation therapy include soft tissue necrosis with bone exposure and subsequent osteoradionecrosis. The risk is greatest for patients with advanced lesions of the lower gum and retromolar trigone. Byers and co-workers[236] reported that 14% of patients treated by radiation

TABLE 21-31.   Retromolar Trigone Carcinoma: Local Control by Treatment Modality for 110 Patients Treated 1965 – 1977 (No. Controlled/No. Treated)

Stage	Surgery	Radiation Therapy	Surgery + Radiation Therapy	Total
T1	5/5	5/6	2/2	12/13
T2	20/22	26/31	4/4	50/57
T3	10/10	6/7	2/3	18/20
T4	6/9	5/6	4/5	15/20

Data from Byers et al.[236]

therapy for retromolar trigone lesions required a partial mandibulectomy for mandible necrosis. The risk was greatest for patients having preirradiation extraction for poor dentition or impacted molars.

OROPHARYNX

The oropharynx includes four areas: the base of the tongue, the tonsillar region (tonsillar fossa and tonsillar pillars), the soft palate, and that portion of the pharyngeal wall between the pharyngoepiglottic fold and the nasopharynx. The pharyngeal walls will be considered in the section on the hypopharynx.

ANATOMY

The base of the tongue is bounded anteriorly by the circumvallate papillae, laterally by the glossotonsillar sulci, and posteriorly by the epiglottis. The vallecula is a short, smooth strip of mucosa that is the transition from the base of the tongue to the epiglottis; it is considered part of the base of the tongue. The surface of the base of the tongue appears irregular and bumpy due to scattered submucosal lymphoid follicles; the mucous membrane itself is smooth.

The musculature of the base of the tongue is continuous with that of the oral tongue. A midsagittal section through the oropharynx showing important relationships with neighboring sites is presented in Figure 21-12. A cross-section through the oropharynx (Fig. 21-13) shows relationships to the lateral pharyngeal space.

The tonsillar area is a triangular region bounded anteriorly by the anterior tonsillar pillar (palatoglossal muscle), posteriorly by the posterior tonsillar pillar (palatopharyngeal muscle), and inferiorly by the glossotonsillar sulcus and pharyngoepiglottic fold. The palatine tonsil lies within the triangle. The tonsillar region is bounded laterally by the pharyngeal constrictor muscle and its fascia, the mandible, and the lateral pharyngeal space.

The tonsillar area is separated from the base of the tongue by the glossotonsillar sulcus. The sulcus extends from the

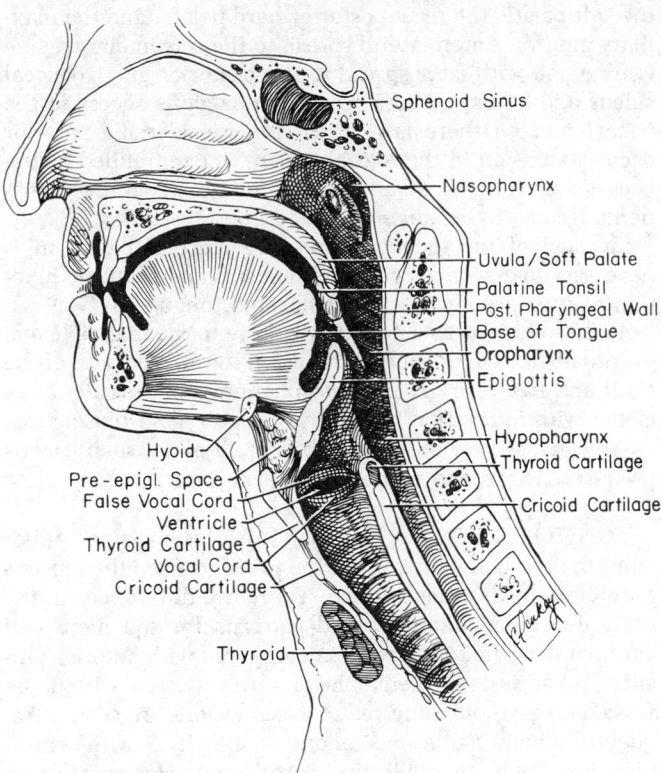

FIG. 21-12. Sagittal section of the upper aerodigestive tract. (Redrawn from Sabotta drawings in Clemente CD: Anatomy: A Regional Atlas of the Human Body. Philadelphia, Lea & Febiger, 1975. Copyright 1975, Urban & Schwarzenburg, Munich, Berliin, Vienna)

anterior tonsillar pillar to the pharyngoepiglottic fold. Beneath the mucous membrane of the sulcus are the styloglossal muscle and the stylohyoid ligament.

The soft palate is a thin, mobile muscle complex that separates the nasopharynx from the oral cavity and oropharynx. The epithelium of the oral side of the soft palate is

squamous and the epithelium of the nasopharyngeal surface is respiratory. The soft palate is continuous laterally with the tonsillar pillars.

PATHOLOGY

Squamous cell carcinoma or one of its variants accounts for 95% of malignant lesions. Lymphoepitheliomas occur in the tonsil and base of tongue. Verrucous carcinomas occur rarely. Malignant lymphomas account for approximately 5% of tonsillar and 1% to 2% of base-of-tongue malignancies. Minor salivary gland malignancies, plasmacytomas, and other rare tumors make up the remainder of the malignancies.

PATTERNS OF SPREAD

Base of the Tongue

PRIMARY. Squamous cell carcinoma of the base of the tongue tends to early, silent, deep infiltration. The tumor tends to remain in the tongue unless it begins at the very peripheral margin. Vallecular lesions spread along the mucosa to the lingual surface of the epiglottis, laterally along the pharyngoepiglottic fold, and then to the lateral pharyngeal wall and anterior wall of the pyriform sinus. Vallecular lesions frequently penetrate through the thin mucous membrane of the vallecula; tumor spread is contained for a while by the hyoepiglottic ligament, but this thin, often incomplete structure eventually is breached and cancer enters the pre-epiglottic space.

Lesions that begin on the lateral base of the tongue may invade the glossotonsillar sulcus. Deep penetration in the glossotonsillar sulcus allows tumor to escape into the neck, because there is no effective muscular barrier at this point. The mylohyoid muscle is an effective barrier for oral tongue lesions, but the mylohyoid terminates near the angle of the mandible. The primary tumor mass may be palpable below

FIG. 21-13. Section at the level of the midoropharynx, depicting relationships in the parapharyngeal area.

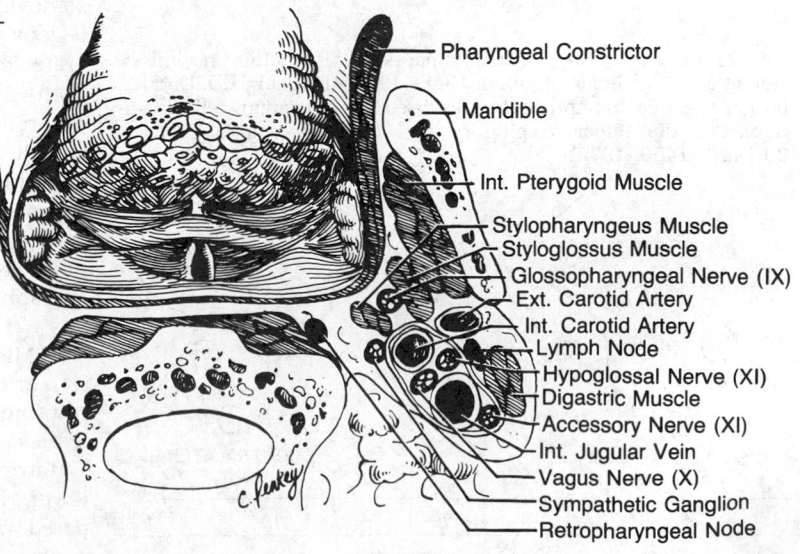

the angle of the mandible and be confused with an involved lymph node.

Advanced lesions tend to spread toward the larynx, oral tongue, and parapharyngeal space. There is a tendency to underestimate the extent of disease.

LYMPHATIC. The first-echelon nodes are the subdigastric; the path of spread is then along the jugular chain to the midjugular and lower jugular nodes. The submandibular nodes may become involved if tumor extends anteriorly into the oral tongue or if massive upper neck disease is present. The posterior cervical nodes are involved often enough to be included in treatment plans.

Approximately 75% of patients with base-of-tongue cancer will have clinically positive neck nodes on admission; 30% will have bilateral nodes (Fig. 21-14).[7] The incidence of occult disease in clinically negative necks is reported at 22% in one series, but this figure is undoubtedly low, considering the selection of these patients for operation and the use of preoperative irradiation.[42] The risk for occult disease is probably 40% to 50%.

Tonsillar Area

The tonsillar area includes the anterior and posterior tonsillar pillars and the tonsillar fossa. Some authors group retromolar trigone lesions with those of the anterior tonsillar pillar. However, the retromolar trigone lesions more appropriately are considered as oral cavity lesions and grouped with the gingival (gum) lesions.

ANTERIOR TONSILLAR PILLAR. Almost all malignant tumors arising on the anterior tonsillar pillar are squamous cell carcinomas. The lesions tend to be early when diagnosed and have relatively little bulk or infiltration and therefore a good prognosis. Asymptomatic lesions are common and may be red lesions, white lesions, or a mixture of both. Their borders are usually indistinct. As the lesions progress they may develop a central ulcer with a rolled margin and infiltrate the palatoglossus. Superior medial spread occurs onto the soft palate, the most posterior hard palate, and the maxillary gingiva. Anterolateral spread to the retromolar trigone is frequent, with later spread to the posterior gingivobuccal sulcus and buccal mucosa. Once tumor gains access to the buccal mucosa there is a threat for considerable anterior occult extension in the buccal pouch, as exemplified by the occasional example of an anterior marginal failure in patients treated by irradiation or operation.

Invasion of the tongue is frequent; careful palpation is necessary to detect the early submucosal nodule at the junction of the anterior tonsillar pillar and tongue.

As these lesions advance, they adhere to the mandible and eventually invade the bone. Extension toward the base of the skull and nasopharynx is a late phenomenon, usually associated with infiltration of the medial pterygoid muscle and possible erosion of the medial pterygoid plate; such lesions produce trismus and marked temporal pain.

TONSILLAR FOSSA. Tonsillar fossa lesions arise either from the remnants of the palatine tonsil or from the mucous membrane within the triangle. There are differences in the early development and spread patterns for squamous cell carcinoma of the tonsillar fossa compared with anterior tonsillar pillar lesions. Leukoplakia rarely occurs within the fossa, and asymptomatic red mucosal lesions are seen infrequently. The initial lesions tend to be exophytic with central ulceration plus an infiltrative component. However, some lesions develop submucosally and present with neck nodes and no obvious tonsillar lesion. Extension to the posterior tonsillar pillar and the oropharyngeal wall occurs early. Invasion into the glossotonsillar sulcus and base of the tongue occurs in approximately 25% of cases. As the lesions advance, they penetrate to the parapharyngeal space and gain access to the base of the skull superiorly. Cranial nerve involvement is uncommon, however. Advanced lesions invade the mandible, nasopharynx, and base of the tongue and may extend below the pharyngoepiglottic fold into the pyriform sinus.

POSTERIOR TONSILLAR PILLAR. Early lesions arising from the posterior tonsillar pillar are uncommon and for some unknown reason have an evil reputation. The only two lesions the authors have seen were 1.0 cm to 1.5 cm, discrete lesions with a raised border and central ulceration. Both were cured by radiation therapy. There are two major differences in their potential spread patterns. They may spread inferiorly along the palatopharyngeal muscle to its insertions into the middle pharyngeal constrictor, the pharyngoepiglottic fold, and the posterior border of the thyroid cartilage. Also, the lymphatic trunks of the posterior tonsillar pillar are theoretically more likely to spread to the junctional (parapharyngeal) and spinal accessory lymph nodes.

LYMPHATIC. The distribution and N staging on admission prior to treatment for previously untreated patients with retromolar trigone/anterior tonsillar pillar and tonsillar fossa squamous cell carcinomas are shown in Figure 21-15.[7]

Retromolar trigone/anterior tonsillar pillar lesions have a lower risk of clinically positive lymph nodes (45%) compared with the tonsillar fossa (76%). The distribution for the

FIG. 21-14. Base-of-tongue carcinoma: nodal distribution on admission at M.D. Anderson Hospital, 1948–1965. (Lindberg RD: Distribution of cervical lymph node metastases from squamous cell carcinoma of the upper respiratory and digestive tracts. Cancer 29:1446–1450, 1972)

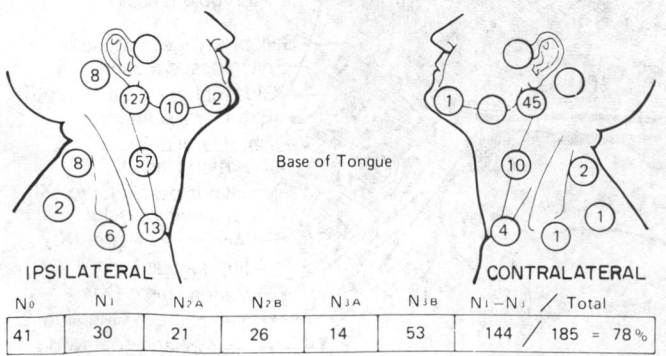

N₀	N₁	N₂A	N₂B	N₃A	N₃B	N₁–N₃ / Total
41	30	21	26	14	53	144 / 185 = 78%

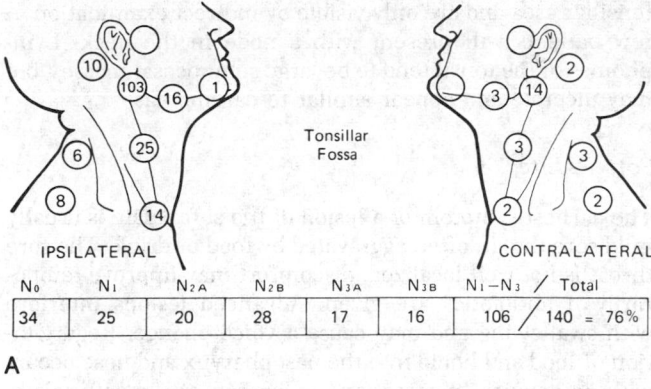

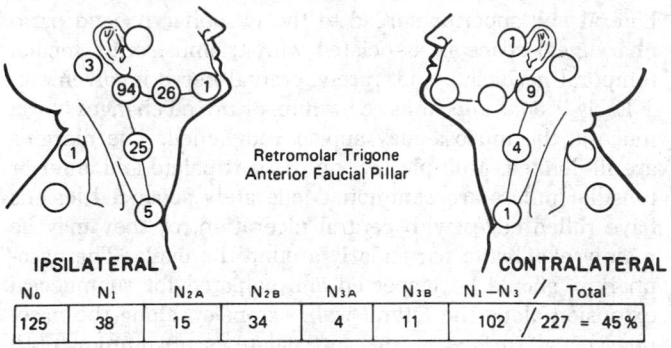

N₀	N₁	N₂ₐ	N₂ᵦ	N₃ₐ	N₃ᵦ	N₁–N₃ / Total
34	25	20	28	17	16	106 / 140 = 76%

A

N₀	N₁	N₂ₐ	N₂ᵦ	N₃ₐ	N₃ᵦ	N₁–N₃ / Total
125	38	15	34	4	11	102 / 227 = 45%

B

FIG. 21-15. Nodal distribution on admission at M.D. Anderson Hospital, 1948–1965. **A**. Carcinoma of the retromolar trigone and anterior tonsillar pillar. **B**. Carcinoma of the tonsillar pillar. (Lindberg RD: Distribution of cervical lymph node metastases from squamous cell carcinoma of the upper respiratory and digestive tracts. Cancer 29:1446–1450, 1972)

retromolar trigone/anterior tonsillar pillar on the ipsilateral side is to the jugular and submandibular lymph nodes with a very low risk for junctional and spinal accessory lymph nodes. Contralateral spread is uncommon (5%) and is confined to the jugular chain. The risk of occult disease in the clinically negative neck (N0) is 10% to 15%.[40] The incidence of positive nodes increases with T stage.

Tonsillar fossa lesions have a high risk of clinically positive lymph nodes (76%) on admission. The lymph node distribution for tonsillar fossa lesions on the ipsilateral side includes the jugular, junctional, spinal accessory, and the more posterior submandibular lymph nodes. Contralateral spread occurs in only 11% of patients and is mainly to the jugular chain lymph nodes, but there is some risk for spinal accessory and submandibular involvement. The risk of contralateral spread is related to invasion of the tongue, spread near or across the midline of the soft palate, and large lymph nodes in the ipsilateral neck that produce lymphatic obstruction; when these features are present, treatment of the opposite neck must be considered. The incidence of occult disease after preoperative irradiation is 22%[41]; the actual risk is probably closer to 50% to 60%.

There is no information about lymphatic spread for posterior tonsillar pillar lesions.

Soft Palate

PRIMARY. Nearly all soft palate squamous cell carcinomas occur on the oral side of the palate. The nasopharyngeal side seems nearly immune to tumor production. Even large tumors of the nasopharynx avoid secondary invasion of the soft palate.

The earliest tumors are red lesions with ill-defined borders. White lesions are common on the soft palate and may be leukoplakia, carcinoma in situ, or early invasive carcinoma. Multiple sites of involvement with normal-appearing intervening mucosa are a common finding, dramatically demonstrated during the first week of radiation therapy when a tumoritis "lights up" the tumor sites, some of which are unsuspected.

The majority of soft palate carcinomas are diagnosed while still confined to the soft palate and adjacent pillars. Spread from the soft palate occurs first to the tonsillar pillars and hard palate. Lateral spread eventually may penetrate the superior constrictor muscle with subsequent invasion of the medial pterygoid muscle and base of skull, and rarely compression or invasion of cranial nerves in the parapharyngeal space. Involvement of the lateral wall(s) of the nasopharynx is common in advanced lesions. Perforation of the palate may occur in advanced cases.

LYMPHATIC. The spread pattern is first to the subdigastric node and then along the jugular chain. The submandibular, submental, and spinal accessory nodes are less commonly involved.

Approximately 56% of patients will have clinically positive nodes on admission; 16% will have bilateral nodes (Figure 21-16).[7] The incidence of occult disease is not well-established because the first-echelon nodes are usually irradiated in all but the earliest lesions. Lindberg and co-workers[39] noted an approximately 20% incidence of occult disease following either no or partial neck irradiation with the primary lesion controlled. The incidence of clinically positive nodes increases with T stage (Table 21-1).

FIG. 21-16. Soft palate carcinoma: nodal distribution on admission at M.D. Anderson Hospital, 1948–1965. (Lindberg RD: Distribution of cervical lymph node metastases from squamous cell carcinoma of the upper respiratory and digestive tracts. Cancer 29:1446–1450, 1972)

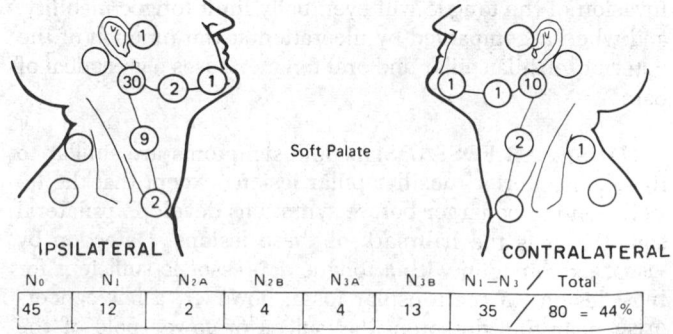

N₀	N₁	N₂ₐ	N₂ᵦ	N₃ₐ	N₃ᵦ	N₁–N₃ / Total
45	12	2	4	4	13	35 / 80 = 44%

CLINICAL PICTURE

Base of the Tongue

Asymptomatic lesions are rarely diagnosed because the base of tongue is visualized only by indirect mirror examination.

Often, the earliest symptom is a mild sore throat. The patient may sense a lump in the back of the tongue and actually feel it by digital palpation; the patient is not amused by the physician who cannot see the lesion with a tongue depressor and fails to palpate the base of tongue. Because many of the early lesions are relatively silent, a subdigastric neck mass, often quite large, is often the first sign. The patient may insist that a 5 cm or larger neck mass "came about overnight." In a sense, the patient is correct. Small clinically positive lymph nodes, 1 cm to 4 cm in diameter, are almost always asymptomatic. Sudden enlargement occurs because of necrosis or internal bleeding with rapid increase in size and mild tenderness. Difficulty swallowing, a nasal voice quality, and deep-seated ear pain occur as the lesion enlarges. Far-advanced lesions fix the tongue. Deep ulceration and necrosis result in foul breath.

Indirect mirror examination, digital palpation, and a high level of suspicion are the ingredients for diagnosis of early lesions of the base of tongue. Because early lesions are often submucosal and relatively soft and the base of tongue is irregular, diagnosis is often a challenge. The rigid fiberoptic telescope will allow examination in some patients not easily examined by indirect mirror examination, and the flexible fiberoptic laryngoscope allows outpatient examination by way of the nose. A small lesion originating in the glossotonsillar sulcus area may ulcerate and produce symptoms quite early; it may be overlooked unless the area is critically examined.

Lymphomas are usually large, mostly submucosal masses, and the diagnosis can be suspected by their appearance. Minor salivary gland tumors are also usually submucosal, but more discrete and firm than lymphomas.

Tonsillar Area

ANTERIOR TONSILLAR PILLAR. Asymptomatic lesions may be found on routine examination by both dentists and physicians. Early symptoms include sore throat, usually aggravated by food or drink. Pain is referred to the ear as soon as ulceration takes place. If the lesion involves the hard palate or posterior upper gum, dentures may fit improperly or cause irritation. Advanced lesions invade the pterygoid or buccinator muscle and produce trismus and temporal pain. Invasion of the tongue will eventually limit tongue mobility, and when accompanied by ulceration at the junction of the anterior tonsillar pillar and oral tongue causes a great deal of pain.

TONSILLAR FOSSA. Signs and symptoms are similar to those for anterior tonsillar pillar lesions except that the lesions tend to be larger before symptoms develop. Ipsilateral sore throat is the hallmark of these lesions. Detection by visual examination with a tongue depressor is sufficient for most lesions of the tonsillar fossa; however, a few cancers arise near the glossotonsillar sulcus or lower pole of the tonsillar area and are only visible by indirect examination. A few patients will present with a node in the neck. Lymphomas of the tonsil tend to be large submucosal masses, but may ulcerate and appear similar to carcinomas.

Soft Palate

The earliest symptom of a lesion of the soft palate is usually mild sore throat, often aggravated by food or drink. The sore throat is not well localized; discomfort may improve temporarily if antibiotics are given. Advanced lesions interfere with swallowing and may cause a voice change. Regurgitation of food and liquid into the nasopharynx and nose occurs with destruction, perforation, or fixation of the soft palate. Lateral and superior spread to the nasopharynx and parapharyngeal space is associated with trismus, otitis media, temporal headache, and, rarely, cranial nerve involvement.

Early lesions appear as red, white, or mixed changes in the mucosa; the mucosa may appear roughened. The margins are ill-defined. Multiple foci on the soft palate and anterior tonsillar pillars are common. Moderately advanced lesions have rolled edges with central ulceration, or they may be mainly exophytic, particularly around the uvula. The nasopharynx should be inspected and palpated for submucosal extension along the lateral wall; extension along the nasopharyngeal surface of the soft palate is uncommon until quite late. Extension to the posterior nasal cavity is seen only in advanced lesions that erode the posterior hard palate.

Carcinoma of the soft palate is associated with an exceptionally high rate of second head and neck primary carcinomas.

METHODS OF DIAGNOSIS AND STAGING

Most lesions of the oropharynx can be biopsied by incisional or punch forceps biopsy under local anesthesia in the outpatient clinic. Base of tongue lesions may require general anesthesia. Frozen section control is helpful in base of tongue lesions since it is sometimes difficult to obtain representative tissue. Fresh tissue is sent to the pathologist if lymphoma is suspected.

Early lesions are staged by physical examination; direct laryngoscopy under general anesthesia may be required for base of tongue or vallecula lesions. CT scan is obtained in the more advanced lesions and used to determine the extent of lymphatic spread.

The AJCC staging system is used:[12]

Tis   Carcinoma in situ
T1   Tumor 2 cm or less in greatest diameter
T2   Tumor more than 2 cm, but not more than 4 cm in greatest diameter
T3   Tumor more than 4 cm in greatest diameter
T4   Massive tumor more than 4 cm in diameter with invasion of bone, soft tissues of neck, or root (deep musculature) of tongue

T1 and T2 are simply measurements of size and are easy to apply. There is a tendency to overestimate the size of lesions in the oropharynx; insertion of a measuring device will help to judge the maximum diameter. The difference between T3 and T4 is not so easily determined. Bone involvement is uncommon but must be seen on roentgenograms to qualify. Invasion of soft tissues of the neck requires some judgment. Tumors of the tonsillar area or base of the tongue that penetrate the glossotonsillar sulcus frequently can be palpated as a deep mass just under the angle of the jaw and qualify as T4 if the mass is larger than 4 cm in diameter. Invasion of the root or deep musculature of the tongue is easy to diagnose if the tongue is partially fixed. If a base-of-tongue cancer can be palpated easily through the floor of mouth or in the submentum, then invasion of deep muscle has probably occurred. Lesions that produce trismus or cranial nerve palsy or grossly invade the nasopharynx usually are classified as T4.

TREATMENT: BASE OF THE TONGUE

Selection of Treatment Modality

Operation and irradiation produce similar cure rates for early (T1) base-of-tongue lesions, but because excision of the base of tongue generally causes greater disability and because of the high risk for bilateral lymphatic involvement, radiation therapy is the treatment of choice for the majority of lesions, with operation reserved for salvage of radiation therapy failures and to help control the neck disease. The local–regional control and survival rates are better for radiation therapy for T2–T4 lesions. Radiation therapy automatically encompasses the neck nodes on both sides of the neck. Extended supraglottic laryngectomy may be used for limited vallecular lesions and lateralized base-of-tongue lesions, but there are definite anatomical criteria that must be satisfied, and this selection limits its usefulness. The following conditions must be met: no gross involvement of the pharyngo-epiglottic fold, preservation of one lingual artery, resection of less than 80% of the base of the tongue, pulmonary function suitable for supraglottic laryngectomy, and medical condition suitable for a major operation. At least an ipsilateral neck dissection is indicated, but with the high risk of bilateral neck disease even in the N0 patient, this represents incomplete treatment. Postoperative irradiation may have to be administered in any event for close margins or for fear of neck failure. Therefore, radiation therapy is usually the treatment of choice for the primary lesion, with neck dissection added as needed (see "Principles of Treatment").

Surgical Treatment

The surgical approach for neoplasms of the base of the tongue is either by splitting the lip, mandible, and tongue in the midline to reach the base of the tongue, or by dividing the horizontal mandible and swinging it outward to expose the tongue base. Suprahyoid, transhyoid, and infrahyoid approaches also can be used to resect small lesions at the base of the tongue. After the tumor has been removed, the mandible is wired together. Only one lingual artery may be sacrificed. A neck dissection is done in continuity with excision of the base-of-tongue lesion. Removal of a large base-of-tongue tumor requires simultaneous removal of part or all of the larynx.

Irradiation Technique

Irradiation of base-of-tongue cancer is accomplished by parallel opposed external beam portals that also encompass the regional nodes on both sides. Interstitial implants may be used for part of the treatment if the lesion is small, discrete, and located in the anterolateral base of the tongue. Implants of posterior lesions are technically difficult; these implants are usually accomplished with a flexible source (e.g., ^{192}Ir ribbons), which allows through-and-through implantation from the base of the tongue to the skin. There is no proven advantage in local control for interstitial boosts as opposed to external beam treatment alone. (For oral tongue cancer, there is no doubt that interstitial treatment significantly improves local control compared with external beam therapy alone.) Base-of-tongue lesions have a good local control rate with external beam therapy alone. The base of the tongue has a good vascular supply and tolerates high doses of radiation without soft-tissue necrosis.

A boost of 1000 cGy to 1500 cGy may be delivered to the base of the tongue by way of the submental route without traversing the mandible. The submental boost may be given with high-energy electrons or a photon beam that is angled superiorly to avoid the previously irradiated spinal cord. The submental boost has proven successful, partly because of the high dose achieved and the relatively small volume irradiated. It is selected for those base-of-tongue lesions that are central and posterior. Large lesions that extend into the oral tongue near the junction with the anterior tonsillar pillar area are not suited for submental boost because the distance from the skin to the tongue surface is several centimeters and the portal is inefficient; an interstitial boost or reduced lateral portals are considered in these cases.

One of the common errors in planning external beam portals is failure to recognize anterior growth of neoplasm as measured by palpation through the lateral floor of the mouth.

The inferior border of the lateral portals is usually the thyroid notch unless tumor has extended into the upper pyriform sinus, lateral pharyngeal wall, or pre-epiglottic space.

The skin and subcutaneous fat in the submental area should be shielded, if possible, because high-dose radiation therapy to this area produces considerable fibrosis. Shielding this area may not be possible if the patient is thin or if tumor is bulging into the mylohyoid muscle.[244]

Management of the lymphatics is critical. One of the major advantages of radiation therapy is the ease of irradiating all the nodes at risk. Even small, well-lateralized base-of-tongue lesions will spread to the opposite neck, and both sides are always treated.

The primary portals include the upper jugular, posterior submandibular, and posterior upper cervical node(s) when the neck is clinically negative. The superior border is approximately 2 cm above the tip of the mastoid even with clinically negative nodes to ensure coverage of the nodes near the base of the skull.

The lower neck nodes on both sides are always treated. If the upper neck is clinically negative, the lower neck portals are carefully tailored to exclude as much normal tissue as possible; the midjugular nodes are the major risk area in this situation. If the upper neck is clinically positive, the lower neck portals become more generous.

The dose for T1 lesions is usually 6000 to 6600 cGy in 6 to 6.5 weeks. Since 1978, T2–T4 lesions have been treated with 120 cGy twice daily with 4 hours between fractions to a total dose of 7440 cGy to 7920 cGy.[245]

Combined Treatment Policies

Combined treatment is seldom selected because an operation for moderately advanced lesions usually implies major functional loss, and few patients are willing to accept the morbidity and possible immediate mortality. The most common indication for offering glossectomy and laryngectomy is a lesion that simply fails to respond to irradiation after 5000 cGy. However, if the patient is offered and accepts a glossectomy-laryngectomy, the authors prefer an operation followed by postoperative radiation therapy.

Management of Recurrence

Radiation failures are treated surgically, but salvage is infrequent except for T1 lesions. Fletcher[246] reported surgical salvage of radiation failure in 2 of 9 patients with T1 disease, 1 of 13 with T3 disease, and 2 of 15 with T4 disease.

Surgical failures are rarely salvaged by either an operation or radiation therapy, except for the early lesion with a discrete local recurrence in the base of tongue.

Recurrence of a small, discrete primary tumor may be managed by a wide local excision. The remaining recurrences require either a jaw-tongue-neck resection or glossectomy-laryngectomy.

RESULTS OF TREATMENT: BASE OF THE TONGUE

Surgical Results

Whicker and co-workers[247] of the Mayo Clinic reported 102 patients selected for curative attempts by operation; 23 received preoperative or postoperative radiation therapy. Eleven were irradiation failures. Some 23% required partial or total laryngectomy; 56% had positive nodes in the specimen. The operative mortality was 4%, with a 27% local recurrence rate and 10% neck failure rate. The 5-year survival rate was 37%.

The Memorial Sloan-Kettering Cancer Center[248] reported the results for 160 squamous cell carcinomas of the base of tongue treated between 1969 and 1978. Radiation therapy alone was used in 33% of cases; radiation therapy was given as an adjunct in 60 patients, but the dose was greater than 5000 cGy in only 14 cases. The 5-year determinate survival for Stages I and II was 33% and for Stages III and IV was 6%.

Irradiation Results

The initial local control rates are shown in Table 21-32 for patients treated for cure with continuous-course external beam irradiation.[245] The actuarial survival curves by stage are shown in Figure 21-17 for a group of 114 patients treated between 1964 and 1981. These survival curves include 24

TABLE 21-32. Base of Tongue Carcinoma: Initial Local Control by Radiation Therapy (Continuous Course)

	One Fraction/Day*	Two Fractions/Day†
T1	2/3	1/1
T2	12/14 (86%)	1/1
T3	12/13 (92%)	8/9
T4	3/12 (25%)	3/6

*Modified from Gardner et al.[245] Excludes split course and radium boost cases.

†Unpublished University of Florida data. Patients treated 3/78–4/85; analysis 4/87 by J. T. Parsons, M.D.

patients managed by the split-course scheme and 24 patients who had an interstitial boost, two treatment schemes that had much poorer results.

FOLLOW-UP POLICY: BASE OF THE TONGUE

Surgical or radiation therapy, or both, will occasionally salvage the failure of an early lesion. Radiation failures may present as an ulcer and must be distinguished from radiation necrosis. Most radiation ulcers will appear in the vallecula or glossotonsillar sulcus, not on the base of tongue proper. Biopsies usually must be done with the patient under general anesthetic to obtain adequate tissue and control of bleeding.

COMPLICATIONS OF TREATMENT: BASE OF THE TONGUE

Surgical Complications

The complications of surgery include an operative mortality of about 5%; fistula, mandibular necrosis, dysphagia, hoarseness, trismus, and carotid rupture are nonfatal complications. Pneumonia is frequent due to aspiration when the glottis is preserved.

FIG. 21-17. Base-of-tongue carcinoma: survival by AJCC stage (actuarial method[249]). University of Florida data; patients treated 10/64 to 9/81. (Analysis 9/83 by K. E. Gardner, M.D.)

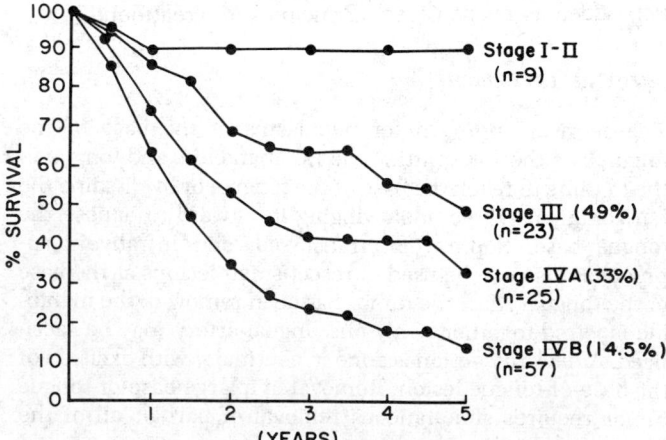

Complications of Irradiation

Bone exposure and osteoradionecrosis are uncommon. Soft-tissue necrosis of mild to moderate degree occurs in approximately 10% and bone exposure of mild to moderate degree occurs in 5% of patients treated solely by external beam irradiation.[245] Severe necroses requiring an operation or hospitalization have not been observed at the University of Florida. The rate of complications has been even less since 1978 with the twice-daily fractionation schedule. Treatment of necrosis requires patience and reassurance to the patient, who assumes the pain is due to cancer. Antibiotics often will reduce pain. The patient will lose weight because of dysphagia and will require nutritional support. Many necroses persist several months. Serious hemorrhage is uncommon.

Hypoglossal nerve palsy occurred in two patients and is reported in other series. It usually is associated with an ulcer in the posterior glossotonsillar sulcus. Unilateral hypoglossal nerve palsy does not produce serious morbidity because the opposite side compensates very nicely.

An occasional patient cured of advanced base-of-tongue cancer by radiation therapy may have difficulty swallowing solid foods. The action of the base of the tongue is to force the bolus of food into the hypopharynx, and loss of full motion impedes swallowing. This is probably a result of some fibrosis of the base of the tongue compounded by a dry mouth. The addition of a radical neck dissection to radiation therapy increases the risk of this problem. Aspiration is unusual, however, even if the tip of the epiglottis has been amputated by tumor.

Complications of Combined Treatment

Preoperative irradiation will increase the risk of fistula, delayed healing, and carotid exposure. Postoperative irradiation increases the amount of fibrosis in the neck. Radiation necrosis of the soft tissues or bone is uncommon. The added effect of xerostomia further worsens the swallowing defect produced by glossectomy.

TREATMENT: TONSILLAR AREA
Selection of Treatment Modality

EARLY (T1 OR T2). Early lesions are generally treated by irradiation with a high rate of success and relatively low morbidity. A small lesion may be cured by wide local excision or tonsillectomy. A surgical attack for larger lesions usually implies removal of the mandible, the tonsillar area including both pillars, a part of the soft palate, and a part of the tongue; additionally, an ipsilateral neck dissection is performed even with a clinically negative neck. The functional loss from this operation is not justified in view of the high success rate with irradiation, which leaves the patient intact; even a dry mouth may be avoided when well-lateralized lesions are treated by techniques that allow at least partial salivary recovery. An operation often will salvage the few radiation treatment failures. The local control, surgical salvage, and ultimate control rates by T stage for tonsillar area lesions treated by continuous-course radiation therapy are shown in Table 21-33. The local control rate is better for T1–T2 tonsillar fossa lesions than for anterior tonsillar pillar lesions.[250-252]

MODERATELY ADVANCED (LATE T2 OR T3). There are advocates of combining surgery and radiation therapy as the initial therapy and advocates of radical radiation therapy with or without neck dissection, with surgery reserved for radiation therapy failure.[250,251,253-257] The local failure rate with radiation therapy is approximately 20% for T2 lesions and 30% for T3 lesions when adequate doses are prescribed; therefore, radiation therapy has been the choice for initial therapy at the University of Florida. Preoperative irradiation followed by an operation has shown better results in some nonrandomized series and no difference in other series compared to radiation therapy with surgical salvage.[258-260] Surgical salvage works better for anterior tonsillar pillar failures than for those of the tonsillar fossa.

ADVANCED (T4). If the lesion is assigned to stage T4 only because of mandible invasion, then combined therapy

TABLE 21-33. Squamous Cell Carcinoma of the Tonsillar Region: Local Control with Radiation Therapy as a Function of Tonsillar Region Site* (No. Controlled/No. Treated)

T Stage	Excluded†	Tonsillar Fossa	Tonsillar Pillars		Overall Control with Irradiation	No. Salvaged/ No. Attempted	Ultimate Control
			Anterior	Posterior			
T1	4	4/4	5/7	1/1	10/12 (83%)	2/2	12/12
T2	9	17/18 (94%)	18/26 (69%)	1/2‡	36/46 (78%)	5/7	41/46 (89%)
T3	8	23/31 (74%)	5/8		28/39 (72%)	0/3	28/39 (72%)
T4	5	3/12 (25%)	2/4		5/16 (31%)	0/1	5/16 (31%)

Mendenhall WM, Parsons JT, Cassisi NJ, et al: Squamous cell carcinoma of the tonsillar area treated with radical irradiation. Radiother Oncol 10:23–30, 1987.

*A total of 136 patients treated 10/64–8/83 with continuous course, once-a-day or twice-a-day fractionation.

†A total of 110 patients eligible for local control analysis with 113 evaluable primary lesions; 26 patients excluded from local control analysis because they died in less than 2 years of intercurrent disease with primary lesion controlled.

‡Failure at 4700 cGy.

should be considered. Mandible invasion usually is associated with extensions that contraindicate surgical removal, however.

Radical irradiation using a hyperfractionation technique will control about 30% of T4 lesions. Combined treatment may be recommended in selected cases.

Surgical Treatment

Surgical treatment for very early cancers of the tonsillar pillars consists of a wide local excision, including tonsillectomy, through a transoral approach. Larger lesions may require removal of the adjacent mandible as well as a portion of the tongue and soft palate. Depending on the size of the defect, a tongue, deltopectoral, or myocutaneous flap may be required to close the defect. Flaps are usually necessary for extensive lesions or after radiation therapy failure. Deglutition is not generally a problem, but some patients remain on liquid diets. Chewing is difficult since a portion of the mandible has been removed and the patient will be unable to wear dentures. Speech may be impaired if a significant portion of the tongue or palate has been removed. A prosthesis may be needed for the palatal defect.

Irradiation Technique

The basic portal arrangement depends to a large degree on the extent of the local lesion and presence or absence of positive lymph nodes. The risk for contralateral lymph node metastases is very small unless there is tongue invasion, invasion of the soft palate within 1 cm to 2 cm of the midline, or clinically positive nodes in the ipsilateral neck. If these risk features are absent, a technique with both photon and electron beams is used to reduce the dose to the contralateral mucosa and salivary glands, if the medial extent of the primary lesion is no more than 4.5 cm from the ipsilateral skin surface. The major advantage of this technique is not a greater cure rate but a lower incidence of xerostomia secondary to partial preservation of minor and major salivary gland function on the contralateral side. An intraoral lead block also may be added, which further protects the minor salivary glands and a portion of the parotid. Because the tonsillar area lesions lie behind the mandible, an extra 1.0 cm to 1.5 cm is added to the depth-dose calculations for the electron portion of the treatment.[244,261]

Lesions with a medial extent greater than 4.5 cm or clinically positive neck nodes are at risk for bilateral neck disease and are treated with parallel opposed photon portals, usually weighted 2:1 or 3:2 to the involved side; if there are positive contralateral nodes or extension across the midline, the portals usually are equally weighted. Small, discrete lesions of the anterior tonsillar pillar may have part of the treatment by intraoral cone.

The dose prescribed for tonsillar area lesions is critical if a high rate of control is to be achieved. An interstitial boost frequently is added to the tongue extension when present; if there is also suspicion of residual tumor in the tonsillar area, the tonsil is implanted at the same time (tongue/pterygoid implant). The local control and complication rates are increased by the implant (Table 21-34).[250]

The dose for tonsillar fossa lesions is 6000 cGy in 6 weeks for T1 lesions, 7440 cGy to 7680 cGy (120 cGy twice a day) with or without an interstitial boost for T2–T3 lesions, and 7920 cGy (120 cGy twice a day) with or without an interstitial boost for T4 lesions. The dose for anterior tonsillar pillar lesions is higher: T1 lesions, 6500 cGy to 7000 cGy with or without an interstitial boost; T2–T3 lesions, 7440 cGy to 7680 cGy (120 cGy twice a day) with or without an interstitial boost; T4 lesions, 7920 cGy to 8160 cGy (120 cGy twice a day) with or without an interstitial boost. Intraoral cone may be substituted for part of the external beam or implant dose for discrete lesions of the anterior tonsillar pillar.

Combined Treatment Policies

Preoperative radiation therapy has been favored by many centers, but surgery followed by radiation therapy is a satisfactory option for those favoring combined therapy.

Management of Recurrence

An operation will salvage a good proportion of T1 or T2 radiation therapy failures, but only an occasional advanced lesion is salvaged (see Table 21-33).

RESULTS OF TREATMENT: TONSILLAR AREA

The results and the complications for 136 patients treated by continuous-course radiation therapy (with planned neck dissection in 32) at the University of Florida are shown in

TABLE 21-34. Carcinoma of the Tonsillar Region: Soft Tissue and/or Bone Complications by Severity (No. Complications/No. Treated)*

T Stage	Mild (1+) E	Mild (1+) E + R	Moderate (2+) E	Moderate (2+) E + R	Severe (3+) E	Severe (3+) E + R
T1	3/15 (20%)		0/15		0/15	
T2	10/41 (24%)	4/12 (33%)	2/41 (5%)	0/12	0/41	0/12
T3	4/23 (17%)	10/24 (42%)	1/23 (4%)	2/24 (8%)	4/23 (17%)	0/24
T4	2/14 (14%)	2/7	0/14	1/7	0/14	1/7

Mendenhall WM, Parsons JT, Cassisi NJ, et al: Squamous cell carcinoma of the tonsillar area treated with radical irradiation. Radiother Oncol 10:23–30, 1987.
*A total of 136 patients.
E, external beam alone; E + R, external beam plus radium needle implant.

TABLE 21-35. Carcinoma of the Tonsillar Region: Control of Neck Disease as a Function of Treatment* (No. Heminecks Controlled/No. Treated)

Hemineck Stage	Radiation Therapy Alone	Ratiation Therapy + Neck Dissection	Overall Control with Initial Treatment	No. Salvaged/ No. Attempted	Overall Ultimate Control
N0†	33/34	0/0	33/34	0/1	33/34
N1	18/18	4/4	22/22		22/22
N2A	1/2	3/4	4/6	0/1	4/6
N2B	9/12	12/12	21/24	1/2	22/24
N3A	0/1	2/3	2/4		2/4

Modified from Mendenhall WM, Parsons JT, Cassisi NJ, et al: Squamous cell carcinoma of the tonsillar area treated with radical irradiation. Radiother Oncol 10:23–30, 1987.

*Primary site continuously disease-free; 43 patients with 56 evaluable heminecks.

†For N0 patients, figures represent the number of patients with neck disease controlled/number of patients treated.

Tables 21-33 through 21-36. The local control rate for T3 lesions was 76% when an interstitial boost was added compared with 56% without the boost.[250] The local control rate for patients treated since 1978 with twice-a-day treatment are given in Table 21-2.

The poorer local control for T1–T2 anterior tonsillar pillar lesions is difficult to explain. An interstitial implant is currently being used as part of the treatment to try to reduce the overall time and increase the local control rates.[262]

Fourteen patients were selected for combined treatment. Eight were treated with preoperative radiation therapy; only one had no evidence of disease over 2 years after treatment. Six were treated by resection and postoperative radiation therapy, and four had no evidence of disease for greater than 2 years.

Dasmahapatra and co-workers[253] compared the results for combined surgery and radiation therapy versus radiation therapy alone for patients with cancer of the tonsil treated between 1962 and 1982. For Stage III, the 5-year survival rate with radiation therapy plus surgery was 31% versus 11% for radiation therapy alone, and for Stage IV, the results for radiation therapy plus surgery were 15% at 5 years compared with 0 for radiation therapy alone.

Shrewsbury[254] compared radiation therapy alone to combined radiation therapy and surgery. The 2-year survival rate for radiation therapy alone by T stage was T1, 78%; T2, 50%; T3, 15%; and T4, 0. The results for combined treatment were T1, 100%; T2, 82%; T3, 76%; and T4, 33%.

Perez and co-workers[257] compared the results of radiation

TABLE 21-36. Carcinoma of the Tonsillar Region: Five-Year Survival by Modified AJCC Stage (No. Alive/No. Treated)*

Modified AJCC Stage	5-Year Survival	
	Absolute	Determinate
I	3/9	3/3
II	13/22 (59%)	13/14 (93%)
III	14/22 (64%)	14/17 (82%)
IVA	6/17 (35%)	6/14 (43%)
IVB	4/24 (17%)	4/19 (21%)

Mendenhall WM, Parsons JT, Cassisi NJ, et al: Squamous cell carcinoma of the tonsillar area treated with radical irradiation. Radiother Oncol 10:23–30, 1987.

*Ninety-four patients eligible for 5-year survival analysis.

therapy alone, preoperative irradiation, and surgery alone for 144 patients with carcinoma of the tonsil. They concluded that combined surgery and radiation treatment produced the same rates of local and regional control and 3- and 5-year survival as radiation therapy alone, and that radiation therapy was the best initial treatment, with surgery reserved for salvage of radiation failures.

COMPLICATIONS OF TREATMENT: TONSILLAR AREA

Radiation Therapy

The rate of bone or soft tissue necrosis following radiation therapy is shown in Table 21-34.[250] The risk for a severe complication requiring surgical intervention was 3%. Improved management of the teeth and use of twice-daily fractionation have reduced the incidence of serious complications. Other complications included laryngeal edema (1), hypoglossal nerve palsy (3), and trismus (2). The complication rate for 83 patients with oropharyngeal tumors (tonsil, base of tongue, soft palate) managed by twice-a-day therapy, of which 28 with tonsil lesions had an interstitial boost after external beam doses of 7440 cGy to 8160 cGy, is shown in Table 21-37.

Surgery

Complications of operation include oropharyngeal dysfunction (limited or no ability to swallow, and drooling), fistula, failure of flaps, complications of neck dissection, and aspiration occasionally leading to laryngectomy.

TREATMENT: SOFT PALATE

Selection of Treatment Modality

Recommendations for management of soft palate cancer must consider the primary lesion and both sides of the neck. Very small (2–5 mm), well-defined lesions may be excised and the neck observed, but the multifocal nature of soft palate lesions predicts marginal recurrence after limited treatment unless patients are very carefully selected. Tiny lesions confined to the uvula may be treated by surgical excision with little morbidity. Irradiation is the modality most often selected for early and advanced soft palate carci-

TABLE 21-37. Oropharynx Cancer: Complications According to Dose for 83 Patients Treated with Twice-a-Day Fractionation

Dose (cGy)	No. of Patients	Complications		
		Mild	Moderate	Severe
≤7440	17	1	0	0
7680	20	3	1	0
7920	11	2	0	2*
8160	7	0	1	0
7440–8160 + 1000–1500 Ra	28	4	1	1*

University of Florida data. Patients treated 3/78–4/85; analysis 4/87 by J. T. Parsons, M.D.
*Severe complications: permanent gastrostomy tube, 1 (7920 cGy); bone necrosis, 2 (7920 cGy; 7800 + 1000 cGy implant).

nomas; neck dissection is added as needed. The initial success rate with irradiation for early lesions is high, leaving the patient functionally intact without the need for a prosthesis or elaborate reconstruction. The local control rate for T3 and T4 lesions treated by radiation therapy is about 50% to 60%, and combined treatment may be considered, but the extent of the surgical resection required usually precludes that option. Elective irradiation of both sides of the neck is included for stage N0, and neck dissection is added in selected patients with clinically positive neck nodes. Fletcher[263] reported a very high rate of success for patients treated by radiation therapy alone.

Surgical Treatment

Small, discrete lesions can be managed by transoral excision and repaired by a pharyngeal flap to prevent any velopharyngeal incompetence. Tonsillectomy may also be necessary in order to obtain an adequate margin. If full-thickness resection is required, however, then a prosthesis generally is required to restore velopharyngeal competence. Operations for salvage after failure of radiation therapy should generally include full-thickness removal of the soft palate.

Irradiation Technique

The basic irradiation technique for early and advanced lesions involves parallel opposed external beam portals that include the primary lesion and the first relay of upper neck nodes on both sides, because even very tiny lesions are at some risk for occult lymph node disease. If the primary lesion is discrete, a portion of the treatment may be given by way of intraoral cone or an interstitial implant. If intraoral cone therapy is to be used, it should be given prior to external beam when the lesion is clearly visible and the mouth is not yet sore from the radiation reaction. Intraoral cone therapy requires meticulous care to avoid geographic miss.

A single-plane implant (e.g., iridium hairpins) is an effective reduced-field technique. The implant is usually done after external beam therapy.[264]

The external beam technique usually is equally weighted, parallel opposed portals. The minimum treatment volume for early lesions includes the entire soft palate and the adjacent tonsillar areas. If the neck is clinically negative, high-energy photons (17–22 MV) will produce an ideal isodose distribution, allowing a tumor dose at the soft palate of 7000 cGy while maintaining the lymph node dose at 5000 cGy. If the lymph nodes are clinically positive, then cobalt-60 or a 4 MV to 6 MV photon beam is preferred on the involved side(s).

Combined Treatment Policies

Combined therapy is seldom planned because of the success rate with radiation therapy and the morbidity associated with resection of the soft palate.

Management of Recurrence

Soft tissue necrosis is uncommon after radiation therapy; thus a persistent ulcer is the hallmark of recurrent disease following irradiation. Recurrence following irradiation is treated by surgical removal when feasible, and a few patients are salvaged.

RESULTS OF TREATMENT: SOFT PALATE

Surgical Results

Ratzer and co-workers[265] reported the Memorial Sloan-Kettering results for 299 patients with squamous cell carcinoma of the soft palate; 112 were treated by surgery, 139 by radiation therapy, and 22 by combined treatment. The 5-year absolute survival rate was 21% and the determinate survival rate was 30%. The determinate survival rate for the group treated by surgery alone was 38%. The main cause of failure was recurrence at the primary site.

Irradiation Results

Weller and co-workers[266] reported a local failure rate of 50% in 30 patients with soft palate lesions. Only 5 of the patients had T1 lesions.

Seydel and Scholl[267] reviewed the results of 41 patients with previously untreated soft palate malignancies, including 4 nonsquamous carcinomas. Thirty-one patients were treated with doses between 6000 cGy and 7000 cGy, and 10 (32%) developed local recurrence.

The local control rate and the 2- and 5-year determinate survival rates for 55 patients treated with radiation therapy at the University of Florida are given in Tables 21-38 and 21-39.[268]

TABLE 21-38. Soft Palate Carcinoma: Control of Disease at the Primary Site with Continuous-Course Irradiation—55 Patients* (No. Controlled/No. Treated)

T Stage	Excluded†	Initial Control	No. Salvaged/ No. Attempted	Ultimate Control
T1	2	8/8		8/8
T2	7	14/19 (74%)	2/5	16/19 (84%)
T3	3	5/11 (45%)	0/2	5/11 (45%)
T4	1	1/4		1/4

Amdur RJ, Mendenhall WM, Parsons JT, et al: Carcinoma of the soft palate treated with irradiation: Analysis of results and complications. Radiother Oncol 9:185–194, 1987.

*Once-a-day or twice-a-day fractionation. Includes two patients who received most or all of their treatment with an interstitial implant.

†Excludes patients who died of other causes <2 years after treatment with no recurrence at primary site.

TABLE 21-39. Soft Palate Carcinoma: Determinate Survival Rates with Continuous-Course Irradiation

Modified AJCC Stage	2-Year Survival	5-Year Survival
I	7/8	5/6
II	13/13	7/9
III	10/12	3/8
IVA	1/2	0/2
IVB	4/10	2/8

Modified from Amdur RJ, Mendenhall WM, Parsons JT, et al: Carcinoma of the soft palate treated with irradiation: Analysis of results and complications. Radiother Oncol 9:185–194, 1987.

Lindberg and Fletcher[269] reported a high rate of control for soft palate lesions (T1, 100%; T2, 88%; T3, 77%; T4, 83%). A few failures were salvaged by operation. A compilation of nine treatment series for squamous cell carcinoma of the soft palate is given in Table 21-40.[268]

COMPLICATIONS OF TREATMENT: SOFT PALATE

Surgical Complications

Nasal speech and regurgitation of food into the nasopharynx are sequelae of full-thickness resection of the soft palate. A prosthesis is only partially successful in correcting the functional defect when the defect is large. Oropharyngeal dysfunction may occur.

Complications of Irradiation

Complications of irradiation are few. Soft-tissue necrosis of the soft palate is uncommon; an ulcer must be considered to be a possible recurrence. The soft palate may become retracted following successful treatment of advanced lesions; this may result in regurgitation into the nasopharynx and slight alteration in speech. Small perforations may persist after successful treatment at sites where tumor has grown through the soft palate. Bone necrosis requiring surgical management occurred in 1 of 55 patients treated at the University of Florida.[268]

LARYNX

Cancer of the larynx represents about 2% of the total cancer risk. The estimated number of new cases in 1987 in the United States was 12,100—9800 in men and 2300 in women, with an estimated 3800 deaths because of laryngeal cancer.

A study of trends in cancer incidence in the United States from 1935 to 1970 showed that cancer of the larynx increased by 33% in white men but was 3.5 times increased in nonwhite men. The incidence in women showed only a very minimal increase in spite of the fact that lung cancer in women quadrupled in the same period.

Cancer of the larynx seems to be related primarily to cigarette smoking. The risk of tobacco-related cancers of the upper alimentary and respiratory tract declines among ex-smokers after 5 years and is said to approach the risk of nonsmokers after 10 years of abstention.[273]

A 12-year American Cancer Society study showed that low-tar and low-nicotine cigarettes (<15 mg of tar and <1 mg of nicotine) resulted in slightly lower death rates from lung cancer, but whether they affect the risk of laryngeal cancer is unknown.

The importance of alcohol in the etiology of laryngeal cancer remains unclear, but it is probably less important than in the other head and neck sites, for which alcohol can be shown to be synergistic to tobacco.[274]

The geographic distribution for laryngeal cancer in the United States shows excess occurrence in the northeast, particularly in northern New Jersey, New York City, and along the Hudson River. The rates are also higher along the southeastern Atlantic Coast and the Gulf Coast, a distribution that closely resembles the high-risk areas for lung cancer.[275]

ANATOMY

The larynx is composed of several cartilages connected by ligaments and muscles, divided anatomically into the supraglottic, glottic, and subglottic regions. The supraglottic larynx consists of the epiglottis, the false vocal cords, the ventricles, the aryepiglottic folds, and the arytenoids; the arytenoids are cartilages that articulate on the cricoid (Fig. 21-18). The glottis includes the true vocal cords and the

TABLE 21-40.   Literature Review for Squamous Cell Carcinoma of the Soft Palate

Series	No. of Patients (Follow-up)	Primary Treatment	Staging System	Ultimate Control of Disease at Primary Site*	5-Year Determinate Survival†
Amdur et al.,[268] University of Florida, 1986	55 (≥2 yr)	RT alone	AJCC	T1, 100%; T2, 84%; T3, 45%; T4, 1/4	I, 83%: II, 78%; III, 38%; IV, 20%
Chung and Constable,[270] University of Virginia, 1979	63 (≥2 yr)	Individualized; RT alone in 51%	AJCC	T1, 100%; T2, 83%; T3, 52%; T4, 2/5	T1–T2, 70%; T3–T4, 25%
Lindberg and Fletcher,[269] M. D. Anderson Hospital, 1978	NS (≥2 yr)	Individualized; RT alone in 70%	AJCC	T1, 100%; T2, 100%; T3, 82%; T4, 83%	NS
Garrett and Beale,[271] Princess Margaret Hospital, 1984	70 (≥2 yr)	RT alone	UICC	T1, 90%; T2, 95%; T3, 56%	T1, 65%; T2, 84%; T3, 28%
Seydel and Scholl,[267] Fox Chase Center, Philadelphia; 1974	41 (NS)	Individualized; RT alone in 73%	AJCC	T1, 83%; T2, 87%; T3, 46%; T4, no data‡	Overall 54%
Eneroth et al.,[28] Karolinska Institute, 1972	112§ (≥5 yr)	Individualized	NS	Overall 86%	Overall 37%
Weller et al.,[266] Stanford, 1976	30 (≥2 yr)	RT alone	UICC	Overall 50%	Overall 38%**
Fee et al.,[272] Stanford and UC(SF), 1979	106 (NS)	Individualized; RT alone in 75%	AJCC	NS	I, 75%; II, 29%; III, 30%; IV, 18%
Ratzer et al.,[265] Memorial Sloan-Kettering, 1970	299†† (≥5 yr)	Individualized; RT alone in 39%	NS	NS	Overall 30%‡‡

Amdur RJ, Mendenhall WM, Parsons JT, et al: Carcinoma of the soft palate treated with irradiation: Analysis of results and complications. Radiother Oncol 9:185–194, 1987.
NS, Not specified; AJCC, American Joint Committee on Cancer; UICC, International Union Against Cancer.
*Includes the results of salvage therapy.
†Excludes deaths from intercurrent disease.
‡Control with initial treatment, not ultimate results. Two additional patients were successfully salvaged with surgery.
§Includes lesions of hard palate as well as soft palate.
**Absolute, not determinate, survival figure.
††Eighteen percent of patients had recurrent lesions following prior treatment at another institution.
‡‡Disease-free survival figure.

anterior commissure. The subglottic area is located below the vocal cords and ends at the upper margin of the first tracheal ring. The transition from the vocal cord to subglottis is ill-defined, but is considered clinically to begin 5 mm below the free margin of the vocal cord. The subglottic larynx is therefore about 2 cm in length.

The preepiglottic space is an important anatomic region because of frequent direct extension to this area.

Anatomically, the preepiglottic space is bounded by the epiglottis posteriorly, the hyoepiglottic ligament and vallecula superiorly, and the thyroid cartilage and thyrohyoid membrane anteriorly and laterally. It can be seen as a low-density area on a CT scan.

The supraglottic structures have a moderately rich capillary lymphatic plexus. The lymphatic trunks pass through the preepiglottic space and the thyrohyoid membrane to the subdigastric nodes. A few trunks drain directly to the middle or lower jugular chain.

There are essentially no capillary lymphatics of the true vocal cords; as a result, lymphatic spread from glottic cancer rarely occurs unless tumor extends to supraglottic or subglottic areas.

The subglottic area has relatively few capillary lymphatics. The lymphatic trunks pass through the thyrocricoid membrane to the pretracheal (Delphian) node(s) in the region of the thyroid isthmus, or the trunks may carry the tumor to the lower jugular nodes. The pretracheal nodes are midline in position and even when clinically positive are small (1–5 mm to rarely >1–2 cm). The subglottic area also drains posteriorly through the cricotracheal membrane with some trunks going to the paratracheal nodes while others pass to the inferior jugular chain.

PATHOLOGY

The laryngeal surfaces of the epiglottis and vocal cords are lined with stratified squamous epithelium and the remainder of the larynx is lined with pseudostratified ciliated columnar epithelium. Nearly all malignant tumors of the larynx arise from the surface epithelium and therefore are squamous cell carcinoma or one of its variants.

Minor salivary gland tumors arise from the mucous glands, but are rare; even more rare is the appearance of a soft-tissue sarcoma, malignant lymphoma, small cell carcinoma, or

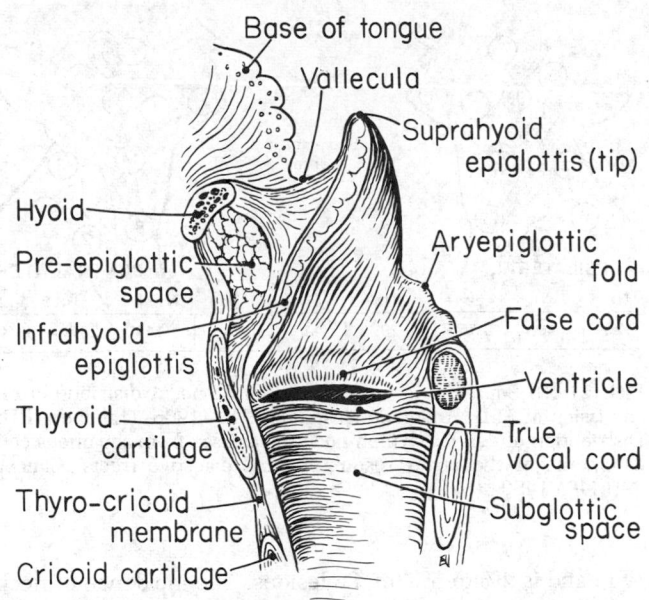

Base of tongue
Vallecula
Suprahyoid
epiglottis (tip)
Hyoid
Aryepiglottic
fold
Pre-epiglottic
space
False cord
Infrahyoid
epiglottis
Ventricle
Thyroid
cartilage
True
vocal cord
Thyro-cricoid
membrane
Subglottic
space
Cricoid cartilage

FIG. 21-18. Diagrammatic sagittal section of the larynx. (Million RR, Cassisi NJ: The management of local and regional laryngeal cancer. In Carter SK, Glatstein E, Livingston RB: Principles of Cancer Treatment. New York, McGraw-Hill, 1981)

plasmacytoma. Benign hemangiomas, chondromas, and osteochondromas are reported, but their malignant counterparts are rare.[276]

Carcinoma in situ is common on the vocal cords. Distinction between dysplasia, carcinoma in situ, squamous cell carcinoma with microinvasion, and true invasive carcinoma is a problem frequently confronting the pathologist and the physician. In patients with minimal lesions, the cord is biopsied by stripping the mucosa; the specimen tends to curl or fold, creating difficulty in orientation of the basement membrane. However, the precise distinction among carcinoma in situ, microinvasion, and invasive carcinoma is a bit academic. The authors recommend treatment, usually irradiation, in most patients. The local recurrence rate after irradiation for carcinoma in situ or microinvasive or invasive carcinoma is, surprisingly, about the same within the T1 category; the recurrences are almost always invasive carcinoma.

Most of the vocal cord carcinomas are either well-differentiated or moderately well-differentiated. In a few cases there is an apparent carcinoma and sarcoma occurring together, but most of these are, in reality, a carcinoma with a spindle cell stroma. The term pseudosarcoma is applied to a rare laryngeal lesion, usually polypoid or pedunculated with a stringlike umbilical cord. It has a favorable prognosis.

Verrucous carcinoma occurs on the vocal cords in about 1% to 2% of patients with carcinoma. The histologic diagnosis is difficult and must correlate with the gross appearance of the lesion.

Supraglottic carcinomas are less differentiated than those of the vocal cord; verrucous lesions are rare. Carcinoma in situ is rarely diagnosed as a distinct entity in the supraglottic larynx, although a zone of carcinoma in situ is seen at the margin between invasive tumor and normal mucosa. Small cell or oat cell carcinomas are reported to occur in the supraglottic larynx and have an aggressive behavior similar to that of oat cell carcinomas of the lungs.

PATTERNS OF SPREAD

Supraglottic Larynx

The majority of lesions are epiglottic in origin. It is difficult to assign a site of origin for advanced lesions.

SUPRAHYOID EPIGLOTTIS. Lesions of the suprahyoid epiglottis may grow like a mushroom, producing a huge exophytic mass with little tendency to destruction of cartilage or spread to adjacent structures. Others may infiltrate the tip and produce destruction of cartilage and eventual amputation of the tip. The latter lesions tend to invade the vallecula and preepiglottic space, the lateral pharyngeal walls, and the remainder of the supraglottic larynx.

INFRAHYOID EPIGLOTTIS. Lesions of the infrahyoid epiglottis tend to produce irregular outgrowths of tumor nodules with simultaneous invasion through the porous epiglottic cartilage into the preepiglottic space. These lesions grow circumferentially to involve the false cords, aryepiglottic folds, and eventually, the medial wall of the pyriform sinus and the pharyngoepiglottic fold. Invasion of the anterior commissure and cords is usually a late phenomenon, and subglottic extension occurs only in advanced lesions. Infrahyoid epiglottic lesions that extend onto or below the vocal cords are at a high risk for cartilage invasion, even if the cords are mobile.[277] Tumor may burrow through the epiglottic cartilage and preepiglottic fat space and present in the vallecula and base of tongue without involving the suprahyoid epiglottis. This anterior and superior extension is difficult to appreciate clinically; CT scan is of assistance in outlining this spread pattern.

FALSE CORD. Early false cord carcinomas usually have the appearance of a submucosal mass and are difficult to delineate accurately by indirect examination. Direct laryngoscopy and CT scan are important for staging. They extend toward the thyroid cartilage and medial wall of the pyriform sinus quite early. Extension to the infrahyoid epiglottis is common. Initial invasion of the vocal cord may occur submucosally and may be difficult to detect at this stage. Gross invasion of the vocal cord is usually associated with thyroid cartilage invasion. Subglottic extension is uncommon until the lesion is advanced.

ARYEPIGLOTTIC FOLD AND ARYTENOID. Early lesions are usually exophytic growths. It is often difficult to decide whether they start on the medial wall of the pyriform sinus or the aryepiglottic fold. As the lesions advance, they extend to adjacent sites and eventually cause fixation of the larynx. Fixation is often secondary to involvement of the cricoarytenoid muscle and joint. It is often impossible to distinguish the cause of fixation at the time therapeutic decisions are made; CT scan may suggest the cause of fixation.

Advanced lesions invade the base of the tongue, pharyngeal wall, and postcricoid pharynx.

Vocal Cord

The majority of lesions begin on the free margin and upper surface of the vocal cord and are easily visible. When diagnosed, about two thirds are confined to one cord. The anterior portion of the cord is the most common site, and extension to the anterior commissure is frequent. Anterior commissure involvement is said to occur when no tumor-free cord can be seen anteriorly; when the lesion crosses to the opposite cord, anterior commissure invasion is certain. Small lesions isolated to the anterior commissure account for only 1% to 2% of all cases.

As vocal cord lesions enlarge, they extend to the ventricle, false cord, vocal process of the arytenoid, and subglottic region. Infiltrative lesions invade the vocal ligament and thyroarytenoid muscles, eventually reaching the thyroid cartilage. As cancers reach the cartilage, they tend at first to grow up or down along the paraglottic fat space rather than attacking the cartilage. The conus elasticus acts initially as a barrier to subglottic penetration. Advanced glottic lesions eventually penetrate through the thyroid cartilage or thyrocricoid membrane to enter the neck and often invade the thyroid gland.

A fixed cord with less than 1 cm of subglottic extension and no false cord involvement does not predict invasion of the thyroid cartilage; if the false cord is also involved, cartilage invasion is likely.[278]

Subglottic Larynx

The epithelium changes from squamous to respiratory about 5 mm below the free margin of the cord, and this is considered the beginning of subglottic area; the inferior border corresponds to the inferior border of the cricoid cartilage.

Subglottic cancers are uncommon. It is difficult to define whether a tumor started on the undersurface of the vocal cord or in the true subglottic larynx with extension to the cord. These lesions involve the cricoid cartilage quite early, because there is no intervening muscle layer. Involvement of the undersurface of the vocal cord is usually present, and fixation of a cord is the rule.

Lymphatic Spread

SUPRAGLOTTIC. The incidence of clinically positive nodes is 55% at the time of diagnosis; 16% are bilateral (Fig. 21-19).[7] Elective neck dissection will show pathologically positive nodes in 16% to 26% of cases; observation of the neck will be followed by the appearance of positive nodes in 33% of cases (see Table 21-4). Extralaryngeal spread to the pyriform sinus and vallecula or base of tongue increases the risk of node metastases. Delphian node involvement is rare and associated with extension to the anterior commissure or subglottic area.

GLOTTIC. The incidence of clinically positive nodes at diagnosis approaches zero for lesions confined to the cords

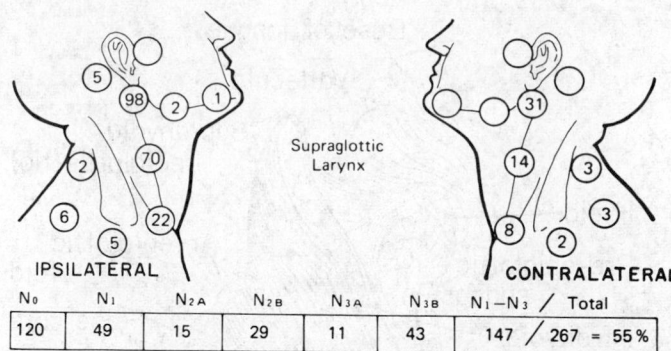

FIG. 21-19. Supraglottic larynx carcinoma: nodal distribution on admission at M.D. Anderson Hospital, 1948–1965. (Lindberg RD: Distribution of cervical lymph node metastases from squamous cell carcinoma of the upper respiratory and digestive tracts. Cancer 29:1446–1450, 1972)

N0	N1	N2A	N2B	N3A	N3B	N1–N3 / Total
120	49	15	29	11	43	147 / 267 = 55%

(T1) and is 2% to 5% for T2 lesions. The incidence of neck metastases increases to 20% to 30% for T3 and T4 lesions. Supraglottic spread is associated with metastasis to the jugulodigastric nodes. Anterior commissure and anterior subglottic invasion is associated with midjugular, lower jugular, and midline pretracheal (Delphian) node involvement. Delphian node involvement is associated with spread to the lower neck nodes on both sides and a high rate of neck failure when treated by surgery alone.[279]

SUBGLOTTIC. Lederman[280] reported a 10% incidence of clinically positive lymph nodes on admission. Spread is primarily to the Delphian nodes and the lower jugular chain.

CLINICAL PICTURE

Presenting Symptoms

VOCAL CORDS. Carcinoma arising on the true vocal cords produces hoarseness at a very early stage. Pain or sore throat is a symptom of advanced lesions. Dysphagia and airway obstruction producing respiratory distress are features of advanced lesions and are rarely seen even with bulky early-stage lesions.

SUPRAGLOTTIC LARYNX. Hoarseness is not a prominent symptom for cancer of the supraglottic larynx until the lesion becomes quite extensive. Changes in voice quality are often subtle and described as having a "hot potato" quality, the voice quality associated with unexpectedly swallowing a bite of very hot food. Pain on swallowing, usually mild, is the most frequent initial symptom. The pain is often described as a mild, persistent irritation or sore throat, and often the patient can point to the area with one finger. Mild difficulty in swallowing is frequent; some patients report a sensation of a lump in the throat. Cancer of the epiglottis may be quite large before symptoms are produced. Pain is referred to the ear by way of the vagus nerve and auricular nerve of Arnold. A mass in the neck may be the first sign of a supraglottic cancer. Late symptoms include weight loss, foul breath, dysphagia, and aspiration.

Physical Examination

In addition to the simple, inexpensive laryngeal mirror, there are rigid and flexible fiberoptic illuminated endoscopes that are now used routinely as a complement to the laryngeal mirror examination. The Hopkins rod with a right-angle lens gives excellent visualization of the infrahyoid epiglottis and anterior commissure, areas that may be difficult, if not impossible, to visualize with the laryngeal mirror. The mirror gives a larger image of the larynx and hypolarynx than that obtained by direct laryngoscopy or by fiberoptic endoscopes. The flexible fiberoptic laryngoscope is inserted through the nose and is useful in the more difficult cases. Sedation with diazepam (Valium) intramuscularly usually will allow outpatient examination of the patient with the most active gag reflex.

A horseshoe-shaped epiglottis may prohibit adequate laryngeal examination for even the most skilled examiner. The tip of the epiglottis may be amputated with a biopsy forceps to facilitate indirect examination of the larynx. Loss of the tip of the epiglottis does not result in functional problems.

Determination of the mobility of the larynx frequently requires multiple examinations because the subtle distinctions between mobile, partially fixed, and fixed cords are often difficult and in fact seem to change from examination to examination. A cord that appeared mobile to the surgeon prior to direct laryngoscopy may show sluggish motion or even fixation after biopsy.

Invasion of the preepiglottic space occurs more frequently than one can diagnose clinically. Early invasion of the preepiglottic space is impossible to diagnose clinically. Ulceration of the infrahyoid epiglottis or fullness of the vallecula is an indirect sign of preepiglottic space invasion. Palpation of diffuse, firm fullness above the thyroid notch with widening of the space between the hyoid and thyroid cartilages signifies invasion of the preepiglottic space. Lateral soft-tissue roentgenograms of the neck may show the presence of irregular air cavities inferior to the vallecula in patients with lesions of the suprahyoid epiglottis that invade into the preepiglottic space by way of the vallecula. CT scan is excellent to show involvement of the prepiglottic space; the hyoepiglottic ligament often causes a shadow, which must not be confused with tumor.[281]

Postcricoid extension may be suspected when the laryngeal "crackle" or "click" disappears on physical examination. The diagnosis is confirmed by direct laryngoscopy and CT scan.

Early invasion of the thyroid cartilage is another difficult clinical diagnosis. Localized pain or tenderness to palpation over one ala of the thyroid cartilage is suggestive. Advanced tumors may actually penetrate through the thyroid ala and be felt as a small bulge on the thyroid ala. Cartilage invasion may be diagnosed by roentgenographic examination, but the cartilage must be calcified to show destructive changes.[282] CT scan of the larynx is of help in detecting catilage invasion, but irregular calcification of the cartilage, coupled with volume-averaging of the CT slice, creates technical problems in interpretation of early cartilage invasion.[281] MRI examination of the larynx has not been helpful as of 1987

due to motion artifact associated with long scanning times (Mancuso AA: Personal communication, 1987).

METHOD OF DIAGNOSIS AND STAGING

The differential diagnosis of laryngeal lesions includes papillomas, polyps, vocal nodules, fibromas, and granulomas. Papillomas can involve the epiglottis or false or true cords and can extend subglottically. They generally occur in children and young adults, possibly persisting into adulthood. Vocal polyps and nodules occur at the junction of the middle and anterior one third of the true vocal cords. There is usually a history of voice abuse followed by hoarseness.

Granulomas of the larynx usually occur as a result of intubation and are located on the posterior one third of the vocal cords, near the posterior commissure. Endoscopic removal is the definitive treatment.

Tuberculosis of the larynx, although rare, still occurs. Generally, the lesion is destructive in nature and occurs at the posterior commissure of the glottis, but the epiglottis and false cords may be involved. The appearance mimics cancer; pulmonary tuberculosis is usually present.

Direct laryngoscopy for biopsy with frozen section is usually performed with the patient under a general anesthetic. A generous biopsy, taken from the bulk of the lesion, will help the pathologist to make the diagnosis. For staging purposes, biopsies should be obtained from suspicious areas as well as areas grossly involved.

Staging

The AJCC staging system for laryngeal primary cancer is as follows:[12]

Supraglottis

Tis Carcinoma in situ
T1   Tumor confined to region of origin with normal mobility
T2   Tumor involving adjacent supraglottic site(s) or glottis without fixation
T3   Tumor limited to the larynx with fixation or extension to involve postcricoid area, medial wall of pyriform sinus, or preepiglottic space
T4   Massive tumor extending beyond the larynx to involve oropharynx, soft tissues of neck, or destruction of thyroid cartilage

Glottis

Tis Carcinoma in situ
T1   Tumor confined to vocal cord(s) with normal mobility (includes involvement of anterior or posterior commissures)
T2   Supraglottic or subglottic extension of tumor with normal or impaired cord mobility, or both
T3   Tumor confined to the larynx with cord fixation
T4   Massive tumor with thyroid cartilage destruction or extension beyond the confines of the larynx, or both

Subglottis

Tis   Carcinoma in situ
T1   Tumor confined to the subglottic region
T2   Tumor extension to vocal cords with normal or impaired cord mobility
T3   Tumor confined to larynx with cord fixation
T4   Massive tumor with cartilage destruction or extension beyond the confines of the larynx, or both

Staging Procedures

Staging procedures for laryngeal cancer include the following:

Indirect laryngoscopy (with photography)
CT scan with contrast prior to biopsy
Direct laryngoscopy with multiple biopsies
Chest roentgenogram

Direct laryngoscopy with multiple biopsies is required to assess extent of tumor and confirm the diagnosis. The ventricles, subglottic area, apex of the pyriform sinus, and postcricoid area must be examined carefully, because these areas are not consistently seen by any other method.

Indirect laryngoscopy actually gives a better panorama and allows better evaluation of function than can be obtained at direct laryngoscopy.

CT scans have replaced conventional tomography and contrast laryngography. CT scan is not useful for early vocal cord lesions.

CT scan may show invasion of the thyroid and cricoid cartilage, cricoarytenoid joint, or preepiglottic fat space, and soft-tissue extension into the neck. CT scan is especially useful for examination of the subglottic space.[45,281,283]

TREATMENT

Vocal Cord Carcinoma

SELECTION OF TREATMENT MODALITY. The goal is cure with the best functional results and the least risk of a serious complication. External beam irradiation and operation are the only curative modalities available.

Dysplasia, Hyperkeratosis, Leukoplakia. Complete stripping of the mucosa of the cord is often curative for lesions classified as leukoplakia, hyperkeratosis, or dysplasia. Careful observation is essential since regrowth often occurs. While repeated stripping may seem a satisfactory plan of management, the cords may become thickened and the voice harsh, and it becomes increasingly difficult to tell whether invasive tumor is present. Irradiation may be recommended when there are repeated recurrences at short intervals.[284]

Carcinoma in situ. Lesions diagnosed as carcinoma in situ may sometimes be controlled by stripping the cord. However, it is difficult to exclude the possibility of microinvasion in these specimens. Recurrence is frequent, and the cord may become thickened and the voice hoarse with repeated stripping.

We recommend irradiation for carcinoma in situ in patients with multiple recurrences that appear in rapid succession.

Many of the patients treated in the past as carcinoma in situ have had obvious residual gross lesions that probably contained invasive carcinoma. We have sometimes proceeded with radiation therapy rather than put the patient through a repeat biopsy.

Early Vocal Cord Lesions (T1, T2). In most centers, irradiation is the initial treatment prescribed for early lesions, with operation reserved for salvage of irradiation failures. While cordectomy or hemilaryngectomy will produce comparable cure rates for selected T1 or T2 vocal cord lesions, irradiation is generally the preferred initial therapy. The major advantages of irradiation compared to cordectomy or hemilaryngectomy are that a major operation is avoided and the voice quality is likely to be better. The voice after hemilaryngectomy remains hoarse; most physicians tell the patient that his voice will be as hoarse as it is now or even worse. After successful irradiation, the voice is usually better than before therapy, but occasional cases are seen in which there is no improvement or, uncommonly, a worsening of voice quality. Hemilaryngectomy may be used as a salvage operation in suitable cases after irradiation failure. Even if the patient has a local recurrence after a salvage hemilaryngectomy, there is a third chance with total laryngectomy, which may still be successful. Hemilaryngectomy is also used in patients who have had prior head and neck irradiation and for the patient who cannot afford 6 weeks away from home or job for the irradiation series.[285]

Although there have been reports that anterior commissure involvement predicts for radiation therapy failure or necrosis, we find no evidence in our data to support this finding.[286]

Currently, there is an increasing use of the carbon dioxide laser in removing benign lesions and very early carcinomas involving the true vocal cords. Although this is being tried in some centers, the experience has not been great enough at this point to determine the long-term results, and the experience of the laserist is most important. If laser is used, it should be used as a cutting instrument rather than to vaporize the tumor. Using this technique, small midcord lesions might be treated with the laser, but the voice would not be as good as expected after radiation therapy.

Verrucous lesions have the reputation of being unresponsive to irradiation and in some instances of losing their verrucous nature to convert into invasive, often anaplastic, metastasizing lesions after unsuccessful irradiation. The authors, however, have observed typical verrucous lesions that have disappeared with radiation therapy and not recurred. Burns and co-workers[287] have also made this observation. The authors favor hemilaryngectomy for early verrucous carcinoma of the glottis, but do not hesitate to use radiation therapy if the alternative is total laryngectomy.

Advanced Vocal Cord Lesions (T3, T4). The mainstay of treatment in most centers is total laryngectomy with or without postoperative irradiation. In some centers, radiation therapy is the initial modality for T3 lesions, with surgery reserved for the failures. The most frequent sites of local failure after total laryngectomy are around the tracheal stoma, in the base of the tongue, and in the neck nodes. If the neck is clinically negative prior to operation and if postoperative irradiation is planned, no neck dissection is done and irradiation is used to treat both sides of the neck. If nodes are clinically positive, a radical neck dissection is done with total laryngectomy. Postoperative irradiation may be used to control subclinical disease in the opposite neck as well as to help prevent recurrence in the dissected neck.

Fixed cord lesions (T3) treated by irradiation fall into two groups. One group consists of patients with fixed, bulky, bilateral, advanced lesions who either refuse laryngectomy or are medically inoperable. Irradiation of these lesions is seldom successful; about 10% to 20% are cured. The second group includes patients with a fixed cord but minimal total tumor bulk. They usually have subglottic extension and minor supraglottic extension confined to one side of the larynx; the airway is adequate and the larynx relatively easy to visualize. An attempt at irradiation in this group is worthwhile. The patient must be willing to return for follow-up every month for the first 2 years and understand that total laryngectomy may be recommended purely on clinical grounds without biopsy-proven recurrence. The reported local control rate for fixed cord lesions (T3N0) varies from 30% to 70%.[14,288,289]

The major difficulty in the use of irradiation for advanced lesions is in distinguishing between radiation edema and local recurrence during follow-up examinations. Progressive edema, increased hoarseness, pain, and immobility of a formerly mobile cord are all signs of recurrence. If the edema is stable or limited to the arytenoids, the patient may be watched, especially if there is no pain. The detection of recurrence is difficult because the surface epithelium may be intact, with tumor growing submucosally. Deep biopsies are necessary, but may aggravate the radiation damage if no tumor is found. The patient must be apprised that total laryngectomy may be recommended if suspicion of recurrence is very high, even without proof of recurrence.

SURGICAL TREATMENT. Stripping of the cord implies transoral removal of the mucosa of the edge of the cord. The operating microscope assists the surgeon in total stripping of the mucosa.

Cordectomy is an excision of the vocal cord. Its use usually is confined to small lesions of the middle one third of the cord. Cordectomy is generally reserved for the uncommon situation in which there is a postirradiation recurrence limited to the middle one third of the cord with normal mobility. Following cordectomy a pseudocord is formed, and the patient has a useful, if somewhat harsh, voice. A portion of the adjacent thyroid cartilage may be removed with the cord.

Hemilaryngectomy is a partial, "vertical" laryngectomy that allows removal of limited cord lesions with voice preservation. There are definite restrictions with this operation. One entire cord plus 5 mm of the opposite cord is the maximum cordal involvement suitable for the operation in men; generally the operation is reserved for lesions involving one cord. Partial fixation of one cord is not a contraindication to hemilaryngectomy, but only a few surgeons have attempted hemilaryngectomy for fixed cord lesions. The maximum subglottic extension allowable is 9 mm to 10 mm anteriorly and 5 mm posteriorly, because the cricoid cartilage must be preserved. Extension to the epiglottis, false cord, or interarytenoid area is a contraindication to hemilaryngectomy. One arytenoid may be sacrificed, but the vocal cord must be fixed in the midline or postoperative aspiration is a possibility, and therefore the patient must have a satisfactory pulmonary status.

The last surgical alternative is total laryngectomy with or without radical neck dissection. Total laryngectomy is used as a salvage procedure for radiation failure in the early lesions that are not suited for conservative operations. It is the operation of choice for advanced lesions. The entire larynx is removed, the pharynx is reconstituted, and a permanent tracheostomy is required.

Artificial speech is created by a number of techniques. Electronic devices may be used immediately after the operation. Esophageal speech is accomplished by belching swallowed air that is used to produce phonation. Only 10% of patients develop satisfactory esophageal speech.

There have been numerous attempts to recreate the larynx after total laryngectomy, with very few producing predictable results. There have been attempts to surgically create a fistula between the trachea and esophagus to shunt air to the pharynx. The problem has been one of aspiration in a large number of cases. Recently, prosthetic devices (e.g., the Singer-Blom valve) have been developed for insertion into a tracheoesophageal fistula; the prosthesis allows the patient to speak without the problem of aspiration.[290-293] This simple innovation has made the impact of total laryngectomy less devastating. Most patients can learn to speak with this technique since it does not require the training and motivation needed for esophageal speech.[294]

IRRADIATION TECHNIQUE. Irradiation for early vocal cord cancer is delivered by small portals covering only the primary lesion. The incidence of lymph node involvement is so small (0–1%) that elective irradiation of nodes usually is recommended only for T3 or T4 lesions or for T2 lesions with poorly differentiated histology.[289] Radiation portals for T1 lesions usually extend from the thyroid notch superiorly to the inferior border of the cricoid; the posterior border depends on posterior extension of the tumor. The field size ranges from 4×4 cm to 5×5 cm. Portals larger than this increase the risk of edema without increasing the cure rate. Because the portals are small and the skin of the neck is mobile, it is the authors' practice to have the physician check the portal on the treatment table each day by palpation of the anatomic landmarks. The portals for T2 lesions are slightly larger, depending on the anatomical extent of the lesion. The dose scheme used at the University of Florida for T1 and T2 lesions is shown in Table 21-41.

Treatment plans for T3 and T4 lesions include the primary lesion and the subdigastric, midjugular, low jugular, and Delphian lymph nodes. The initial treatment with once-a-day fractionation is delivered at 200 cGy/day to a total of 4600 cGy. The portal then is reduced to include only the primary lesion, and the dose per fraction is increased to 225 cGy; the final tumor dose is 6600 cGy to 7000 cGy. The low

TABLE 21-41.   Vocal Cord Cancer: Radiation Treatment Plan at the University of Florida (September 1980)

Stage	Description	External-Beam Irradiation (cGy Tumor Dose)
T1	Early, no visible tumor	5625/25 fractions/5 weeks
T1	Moderate size	6300/28 fractions/5.5 weeks
T2	Early, normal motion	6300/28 fractions/5.5 weeks
T2	Moderate size, reduced motion	6525/29 fractions/6 weeks
T3–T4	Fixed cord	See text

neck is treated through a separate anterior portal.[289] Since 1978, T3 or T4 lesions (and since 1986, T2 lesions) have been managed with 120 cGy twice a day, to a total tumor dose of 7440 cGy to 7680 cGy.[14]

MANAGEMENT OF RECURRENCE. Most recurrences appear within 24 months, but late recurrences may appear after 5 years.[295] Additionally, these patients are prone to develop second primaries in the head and neck area, and 5% to 10% develop lung cancer; for this reason the authors recommend a chest roentgenogram every 6 months.

With careful follow-up, recurrence often is detected before the patient notices return of hoarseness. Edema of the larynx, particularly the false cords and arytenoids, suggests recurrence. Fixation of the cord usually implies local recurrence; the authors have observed two patients who developed a fixed cord with an otherwise normal-appearing larynx and have not shown evidence of recurrence. A paralyzed left vocal cord should also suggest the possibility of lung cancer.

Irradiation failures (T1–T2) are almost always salvaged by cordectomy, hemilaryngectomy, or total laryngectomy. The salvage rate for T3 lesions recurring after radiation therapy is approximately 60%.

Salvage by radiation therapy for recurrences or new tumors that appear after hemilaryngectomy is about 50%. Lee and co-workers[296] reported 7 successes in 12 patients; one lesion subsequently was controlled by total laryngectomy. Isolated recurrences at the trachael stoma may be managed by radiation therapy or surgery. Balm and co-workers[297] reported the results for radiation therapy in conjunction with simultaneous chemotherapy (vincristine, bleomycin, and methotrexate) for 8 patients treated between 1978 and 1985. Three patients had been disease-free for 7, 3, and 2.5 years and 2 patients for less than 1 year after treatment. Only 1 patient developed recurrent disease at the stoma.

A multi-institutional surgical experience in the management of stomal recurrence for the years 1970–1985 was reported by Gluckman and co-workers.[298] Forty-one came to operation. The 2-year determinate survival was 24%. Patients with localized recurrences had a 45% 5-year survival rate.

Supraglottic Larynx Carcinoma

SELECTION OF TREATMENT MODALITY. For purposes of treatment planning, patients may be considered to be in either an early or favorable group suitable for radiation therapy or supraglottic laryngectomy, or a late or unfavorable group managed either by total laryngectomy (with or without radiation therapy) or by radiation therapy with laryngectomy reserved for recurrence at the primary site.

The division of lesions into early and late is arbitrary. T1 and T2 lesions are nearly always early or favorable cases, but T2 lesions, and occasionally T1 lesions, can be quite extensive and still not produce fixation yet not be technically or medically suitable for voice-sparing surgery. Lesions can be staged T3 without fixation and with minimal extension to the postcricoid area, medial wall of the pyriform sinus, preepiglottic space, or base of tongue, and be very suitable for radiation therapy with surgical salvage or extended supraglottic laryngectomy. Fixation and cartilage invasion do not preclude attempted cure with radiation therapy.

EARLY SUPRAGLOTTIC LESIONS. Treatment of the primary lesion is either by external beam irradiation or supraglottic laryngectomy. Total laryngectomy would rarely be indicated as the initial treatment for this group of patients and is reserved for those in whom the initial treatment fails.

Irradiation and supraglottic laryngectomy are both highly successful modes of therapy for the early lesions, and for this reason it is seldom necessary to combine radiation therapy and surgery for initial management of the primary lesions; however, combined treatment may be indicated to control the neck disease. Approximately 50% of patients having a supraglottic laryngectomy at the University of Florida have received postoperative radiation therapy.

The following paragraphs outline our guidelines for selection of either supraglottic laryngectomy or radiation therapy. The patient and family are often instrumental in making the decision, and should be apprised of the alternative modes of therapy.

Approximately one half of the patients seen in our clinic whose lesions are anatomically suitable for treatment by a supraglottic laryngectomy are not suitable for medical reasons (e.g., inadequate pulmonary status or other major medical problems) and are managed by radiation therapy. When the patient is both technically and medically suitable for supraglottic laryngectomy, the patient is apprised of the alternative and makes the decision. The decision process is best described as whimsical most of the time.

The only absolute contraindication to radiation therapy is prior radiation therapy to the laryngeal area. Analysis of local disease control by anatomical subsite within the supraglottic larynx shows no obvious differences in local control by radiation therapy when comparing similar stages (Table 21-42).[301] Similarly, analysis of local control by anatomical subsite shows no obvious difference in local control by supraglottic laryngectomy when comparing similar stages. Transglottic lesions are not suitable for conventional supraglottic laryngectomy, but they may be managed by radiation therapy. Invasion of the preepiglottic space is not a contraindication to supraglottic laryngectomy or radiation therapy.

Lesions that are mainly exophytic are usually suitable for radiation therapy. Extensive submucosal disease predicts a less favorable result; these patients often have partial airway obstruction prior to treatment. Unilateral vocal cord fixation due to invasion of the cricoarytenoid joint is not a contraindication to radiation therapy, but fixation due to extension to the vocal cord or subglottic area predicts a poor result with radiation therapy. Women tend to have a better cure rate than men, and the indications for radiation therapy can be extended.

The status of the neck often determines the selection of treatment for the primary lesion. Patients with clinically negative neck nodes and a high risk for occult bilateral neck disease may be treated by radiation therapy because of the ease of bilateral elective neck irradiation (e.g., poorly differentiated carcinoma of the suprahyoid epiglottis with midline base of tongue extension). Alternatively, supraglottic laryngectomy and bilateral conservative neck dissections may be done.

When a patient presents with an early-stage primary lesion but advanced neck disease (N2B or N3), combined treatment is frequently necessary to produce a high rate of control of the neck disease. In these cases, the primary lesion is preferably treated for cure by irradiation, with neck dissection(s) added to the involved side(s) of the neck. If such a patient is managed with supraglottic laryngectomy followed by a neck dissection and postoperative radiation therapy, the functional result is expected to be poorer, as it is impossible to irradiate both sides of the neck and not irradiate the primary site. This means that the primary site, which was adequately treated by supraglottic laryngectomy, is unnecessarily irradiated, and the resulting edema may produce an unsatisfactory functional result.

If the patient has early, resectable neck disease (N1 or N2A) and surgery is elected for the primary site, postoperative irradiation is only added because of unexpected findings (e.g., positive margin, multiple positive nodes, or extracapsular spread). We prefer to avoid routine high-dose preoperative or postoperative irradiation in conjunction with a supraglottic laryngectomy because the lymphedema of the remaining larynx may be considerable, although it will partially or completely subside with time.

LATE SUPRAGLOTTIC LESIONS (LATE T3, T4). Selected T3 and T4 lesions of the upper supraglottic larynx that are mainly exophytic can be treated by irradiation, since the control rate is fairly high. Borderline lesions are given a trial of irradiation to 4500 cGy to 5000 cGy and if response is good, irradiation is continued for cure. If response is unsatisfactory, irradiation is stopped and total laryngectomy is done 4 to 6 weeks later. There is no proof that one may select patients by this therapeutic trial, but many of the T3 and T4 successes were culled out in this fashion.

Lesions unsuitable for irradiation are managed by total laryngectomy. If the neck disease is resectable, then operation is the initial treatment, and postoperative irradiation is added if needed. If the neck disease is unresectable or borderline, preoperative irradiation is used.

Surgical Treatment

SUPRAGLOTTIC LARYNGECTOMY. Supraglottic laryngectomy is a voice-sparing operation that can be tailored to the individual supraglottic lesion. Because the patient has an increased tendency to aspirate, it is essential that adequate pulmonary reserves be present, as determined by blood gases, pulmonary function tests, chest roentgenogram, and a work test (walking the patient up two flights of stairs to determine tolerance to pulmonary stress). The voice quality is generally good following supraglottic laryngectomy. All patients have some difficulty swallowing in the immediate postoperative period, but almost all learn to swallow in a short time; motivation is the key factor in learning to swallow.

Supraglottic laryngectomy can be used successfully for lesions involving the epiglottis, a single arytenoid, the aryepiglottic fold, and false vocal cords. Extension of the tumor

TABLE 21-42. Supraglottic Larynx Carcinoma: Comparison of Control of Primary Lesion by Irradiation by Subsites in Two Series

	T1		T2		T3		T4	
	MDAH*	UF†	MDAH	UF	MDAH	UF	MDAH	UF
Suprahyoid epiglottis	3/4	4/4	7/7	6/8	13/15	3/3	3/5	2/8
Infrahyoid epiglottis	5/5	2/2	11/12	8/11	3/4	2/3	1/1	0/2
Aryepiglottic folds	5/5	1/1	6/7	2/2	3/4	4/6	3/6	0/1
False cords	2/2	3/4	8/10	4/5		0/2	1/1	
Arytenoids	2/2	1/1	1/1					

Million RR, Cassisi NJ, Parsons JT, et al: Radiation therapy in the management of carcinoma of the larynx. In Fried MP: The Larynx. Boston, Little, Brown (in press)
*MDAH: University of Texas M. D. Anderson Hospital and Tumor Institute (1964–1972); data from Fletcher and Goepfert.[299]
†UF: University of Florida (1964–1981); data from Mendenhall et al.[300]

to the true vocal cords, anterior commissure, or both aryte- noids, fixation, or cartilage invasion excludes supraglottic laryngectomy. The extended supraglottic laryngectomy may be used to include the base of the tongue to the level of the circumvallate papillae as long as one lingual artery is pre- served. A neck dissection on one or both sides may be added as part of the supraglottic laryngectomy; about 35% of pa- tients will have histologically positive nodes even when the neck is negative to clinical appraisal. Postoperative irradia- tion is added only as needed, based on the surgical and patho- logic findings. The incision is usually a modified Schobinger, a half-H, or a hockey stick incision. If the likelihood of a total laryngectomy is high, than an apron flap is used. The neck dissection is completed and left attached to the thyrohyoid membrane. The perichondrium of the larynx is then ele- vated in continuity with the strap muscles. This is very im- portant because it will be used to close the surgical defect. Saw cuts are made through the thyroid cartilage and the hyoid bone so that the preepiglottic space is included in the specimen. The pharynx is entered above the hyoid through the vallecula. The specimen is removed, leaving only the arytenoids and true vocal cords. If one arytenoid has to be sacrificed, the cord must be fixed in the midline to prevent aspiration. The defect is closed by suturing the previously saved perichondrium and muscle into the base of the tongue. After the tracheostomy is removed, usually within seven days, the patient is retrained in the act of swallowing. The patient is then discharged when he can swallow 2000 cc or more without significant coughing.

TOTAL LARYNGECTOMY. The entire larynx and pre- epiglottic space are resected en bloc and a permanent tra- cheostomy is fashioned. A portion of the thyroid gland usu- ally is included with the specimen. The pharynx is sutured to the base of tongue.

Irradiation Technique

The primary lesion and both sides of the neck are included with opposed lateral portals. The dose for T1 lesions is 6000 cGy in 6 weeks to 6500 cGy in 7 weeks. The dose for T2–T3 lesions is 6500 cGy to 7000 cGy in 6.5 to 7 weeks (1 fraction per day). Since 1978 the T2–T3 lesions have been managed with 120 cGy twice a day to a total dose of 7460 cGy to 7680 cGy. The lower neck nodes are irradiated through a separate anterior portal. An anterior "boost" portal may be used for the last 1000 cGy for suprahyoid epiglottic lesions that in- vade the vallecula (see the section on the base of the tongue). It is important to spare a small strip of anterior midline skin, which helps to reduce the degree of lymphedema.[283,300]

Patients develop a sore throat, loss of taste, and moderate dryness during irradiation. Edema of the arytenoids may occur and produce the sensation of a lump in the throat. Tracheostomy is seldom necessary before the start of ther- apy, even for bulky lesions.

Edema of the larynx may persist for several months to a year. Radical neck dissection increases the degree of lymph- edema on the side of the operation. The lymphedema of the larynx and submental space resolves together. Patients who

continue to smoke and drink heighten the side-effects of dryness, dysphagia, and hoarseness.

Combined Treatment Policies

Either surgery or irradiation alone is preferred for the early primary lesions.

If total laryngectomy is required and the lesion is resect- able, postoperative irradiation is preferred, since there is no evidence that preoperative irradiation produces any better local–regional control or survival rates. Radiation therapy is added for close or positive margins, invasion of soft tissues of the neck, cartilage invasion, and N2 or N3 neck disease. The high-risk areas are usually the base of the tongue and neck. The stomal area is at risk only when subglottic extension is present or there is tumor in the low neck lymph nodes. Complications related to postoperative irradiation are rela- tively uncommon in this group.

Irradiation is used prior to total laryngectomy for patients with technically unresectable neck nodes, as a trial of radia- tion therapy prior to deciding on radiation therapy alone or total laryngectomy, or when scheduling problems require a long delay to operation.

A number of patients either refuse laryngectomy or are medically unsuitable for the operation; hence, irradiation is the treatment by default. However, a few of these patients can be cured, and one should not take a hopeless attitude.[295]

MANAGEMENT OF RECURRENCE. Failures after su- praglottic laryngectomy or irradiation frequently can be sal- vaged by further treatment; recognition of recurrence should be pursued vigorously. Salvage of recurrences that develop after total laryngectomy and preoperative or postoperative irradiation is quite uncommon.

Subglottic Larynx Carcinoma

Early lesions are treated with radiation therapy, and ad- vanced lesions are usually managed by total laryngectomy and postoperative radiation therapy.

RESULTS OF TREATMENT

Vocal Cord Cancer

SURGICAL RESULTS. Ogura and co-workers[302] reported a 3-year determinate survival without disease of 86% for patients treated by hemilaryngectomy. The local-regional re- currence rate was 6%. The 3-year determinate survival rate without disease for patients treated by total laryngectomy with or without radical neck dissection was 70%. The local– regional recurrence rate was 22%.

RADIATION THERAPY RESULTS. The results of irradia- tion for 304 patients with T1 and T2 squamous cell carci- noma of the vocal cord treated by irradiation are presented in Table 21-43. The results are grouped by the operation that would have been required as determined by the anatomical extent of disease. Voice preservation for the same group is shown in Table 21-44.[286]

TABLE 21-43. Carcinoma of the Glottic Larynx: Local Control—304 Patients (No. Controlled/No. Treated)

T Stage*	Subgroup	Size	Excluded†	Local Control	No. Salvaged/No. Attempted Hemilaryngectomy	Total Laryngectomy	Ultimate Local Control
T1a	C	<5 mm	1	12/12 (100%)			12/12 (100%)
		5–15 mm	6	73/78 (94%)	3/4	0/1	76/78 (97%)
		>15 mm	2	45/50 (90%)		4/5	49/50 (98%)
T1b	HL	All	0	14/15 (93%)		0/1	14/15 (93%)
	TL	All	2	15/16 (94%)	0/1		15/16 (94%)
T2a	HL	All	5	23/27 (85%)		4/4	27/27 (100%)
	TL	All	2	27/38 (71%)	2/3	7/8	36/38 (95%)
T2b	HL	All	3	13/18 (72%)	1/2	2/3	16/18 (89%)
	TL	All	2	18/25 (72%)		4/6	22/25 (88%)

Mendenhall WM, Parsons JT, Stringer SP, et al: T1–T2 vocal cord carcinoma: A basis for comparing the results of irradiation and surgery. Head Neck Surg 10:373–377, 1988.

C, suitable for cordectomy; HL, suitable for hemilaryngectomy; TL, suitable for total laryngectomy.

*T1 lesions were subdivided as T1a, involvement of one true vocal cord with or without involvement of the anterior commissure; T1b, involvement of both true vocal cords. T2 lesions were subdivided according to mobility of the vocal cord(s): T2a, normal mobility; T2b, reduced mobility.

†Excludes 23 patients who died of intercurrent disease <2 years after treatment with vocal cord cancer controlled.

TABLE 21-44. Glottic Larynx Carcinoma: Voice Preservation in 304 Patients Treated with Radiation Therapy (No. Patients with Voice Preservation/No. Treated)

T Stage	Subgroup	Size	Proportion with Voice Preservation
T1a	C	<5 mm	13/13
		5–15 mm	83/86 (97%)
		>15 mm	47/52 (90%)
T1b	HL	All	14/15 (93%)
	TL	All	17/18 (94%)
T2a	HL	All	28/32 (88%)
	TL	All	31/40 (78%)
T2b	HL	All	17/21 (81%)
	TL	All	20/27 (74%)

Mendenhall WM, Parsons JT, Stringer SP, et al: T1–T2 vocal cord carcinoma: A basis for comparing results of irradiation and surgery. Head Neck Surg 10:373–377, 1988.

C, suitable for cordectomy; HL, suitable for hemilaryngectomy; TL, suitable for total laryngectomy.

A few local failures continue to appear after 5 years of follow-up. Some of these late failures occur on the opposite cord and undoubtedly represent new cancers. The same pattern of late recurrence is also seen after hemilaryngectomy.

The reported results for T3 carcinoma of the vocal cord according to treatment modality are shown in Table 21-45. Irradiation was generally selected for fixed lesions with in-volvement of one vocal cord and with an adequate airway. The current local control rate for T3 lesions managed with 120 cGy twice a day is 70% (10 of 14).[289]

Treatment results for T3 glottic carcinomas for seven series are shown in Table 21-46 and the results for T4 lesions in Table 21-47.

Supraglottic Larynx Cancer

A comparison of irradiation and surgical results for 195 patients managed at the University of Florida over a period of 20 years (1964 to 1984) is presented in Tables 21-48 through 21-54.[315] Selection of therapy was individualized. Supraglottic laryngectomy became a surgical option in 1975. The local control rate for radiation therapy alone, with the use of twice-daily fractionation (since 1978), is 82% for T2 and 71% for T3 lesions.

The absolute survival rates obtained with surgery alone or with combined operation and radiation therapy for stage IV disease are shown in Table 21-55.[299]

COMPLICATIONS OF TREATMENT

Surgical

Repeated stripping of the cord may result in a thickened cord and hoarse voice. Neel and co-workers[316] reported a 26% incidence of nonfatal complications for cordectomy. Imme-

TABLE 21-45. Vocal Cord Carcinoma, Stage T3: Results of Treatment

	No. of Patients	Initial Local Control (%)	Ultimate Local Control (%)	Control Above the Clavicles (%)	5-Year Survival (%) Absolute	Determinate
Irradiation + surgical salvage	22	61	83	79	53	67
Surgery ± irradiation*	46	84	89	87	50	68

Data from Mendenhall et al.[289]

*Preoperative, 7 patients; postoperative, 14 patients.

TABLE 21-46.   T3 Glottic Cancer: Results of Treatment with Irradiation Alone

Reference	No. of Patients	Percentage of All Glottic Cancers Irradiated	Minimum Follow-up (yr)	Local Control (%)		5-Year Survival (%)	
				Initial	Ultimate*	Actuarial	Determinate
Harwood et al.,[288] Toronto, 1980	112	12†	3	51	77	55	74‡
Wang,[303] Mass. General, 1974	56	10	3	52	73		
Mills,[304] University of Cape Town, 1979	18	18	2	44	78	67§	
Fletcher et al.,[305] MDAH, 1969	17	4	2	76			
Stewart et al.,[306] Manchester, 1975	67	23	10	57	69		57
Mendenhall et al.,[289] University of Florida, 1984	22	8**	2	61††	83††	53‡‡	67

Mendenhall WM, Million RR, Sharkey DE, et al: Stage T3 squamous cell carcinoma of the glottic larynx treated with surgery and/or radiation therapy. Int J Radiat Oncol Biol Phys 10:357–363, 1984.

*After surgical salvage of irradiation failures.
†Percentage of glottic cancers treated from 1/65 through 12/74.[307,308]
‡Five-year actuarial determinate survival.
§Crude disease-free survival.
**Percentage of glottic cancers, stage T1–T3, treated from 10/64 through 10/77.[309]
††Excludes 4 patients who were not evaluable for control at the primary site.[289]
††Absolute survival.

diate postoperative complications included atelectasis and pneumonia, severe subcutaneous emphysema in the neck, bleeding from the tracheotomy site or larynx, wound complications, and airway obstruction requiring tracheotomy. Late complications included removal of granulation tissue by direct laryngoscopy to exclude recurrence, extrusion of cartilage, laryngeal stenosis, and obstructing laryngeal web.

The postoperative complications of hemilaryngectomy include aspiration, chondritis, wound slough, inadequate glottic closure, and anterior commissure webs.

The postoperative complications of total laryngectomy may include operative death, hemorrhage, fistula, chondritis, wound slough, carotid rupture, dysphagia, and pharyngeal/esophageal stenosis.

The complication rate following supraglottic laryngectomy is about 10%, including fistula formation, aspiration, chondritis, dysphagia, dyspnea, and carotid rupture.

Radiation Therapy

After irradiation, the quality and volume of the voice tend to diminish at the end of the day. Many patients report changes in voice with changes in weather, upper respiratory infections, and the like. Edema of the larynx is the most common sequela following irradiation for glottic or supraglottic lesions. The rate of clearance of the edema is related to dose of radiation, volume of tissue irradiated, addition of a neck dissection, continued use of alcohol and tobacco, and the size and extent of the original lesion. Edema is accentuated by a radical neck dissection; it may require 6 months to as long as 2 years for the lymphedema to disappear. Steroids (e.g., Decadron) have been used to reduce edema secondary to radiation effect after recurrence has been ruled out by biopsy. If ulceration and pain occur, antibiotics are used.

Soft-tissue necrosis leading to chondritis occurs in about

TABLE 21-47.   T4 Glottic Cancer: Results of Treatment

Author	Stage	No. of Patients	Method of Treatment	Results (NED)
Jesse[310]	T4 N0–N+	48	Laryngectomy	54% at 4 years
Ogura et al.[302]	T4 N0	11	Laryngectomy	45% at 3 years
Skolnick et al.[311]	T4 N0	7	Laryngectomy	30% at 5 years
Vermund[312]	T4 N0	31	Laryngectomy	35% at 5 years
Stewart and Jackson[313]	T4 N0	13	Irradiation with surgery for salvage	38% at 5 years
Harwood et al.[314]	T4 N0	56	Irradiation with surgery for salvage	49% at 5 years*

Modified from Harwood AR, Beale FA, Cummings BJ, et al: T4N0M0 glottic cancer: An analysis of dose-time volume factors. Int J Radiat Oncol Biol Phys 7:1507–1512, 1981.

NED, no evidence of disease.

*Actuarial survival, uncorrected for deaths due to intercurrent disease.

TABLE 21-48. Supraglottic Larynx Carcinoma: Local Control Following Initial Treatment as a Function of T Stage—152 Patients (No. Controlled/No. Treated)

T Stage	Irradiation Alone	Surgery ± Adjuvant Irradiation	Significance Levels[144,145]
T1	12/13 (92%)	9/9	0.591
T2	29/36 (81%)	20/25 (80%)	0.603
T3	12/20 (60%)	17/18 (94%)	0.015
T4	4/13 (31%)	15/18 (83%)	0.005

Weems DH, Mendenhall WM, Parsons JT, et al: Squamous cell carcinoma of the supraglottic larynx treated with surgery and/or radiation therapy. Int J Radiat Oncol Biol Phys 13:1483–1487, 1987.

1% of patients. Soft-tissue and cartilage necroses mimic recurrence with hoarseness, pain, and edema; a laryngectomy may be recommended in desperation for fear of recurrent cancer, even though biopsies show only necrosis.

Mendenhall and co-workers[317] recorded a serious complication rate of 0.54% in 184 T1 lesions and 3.36% in 119 T2 lesions (Table 21-56). Complications were related to use of a single portal, T stage, and high total dose.

Combined Treatment

Most surgeons agree that preoperative irradiation is generally associated with an increased risk of an operative complication and slightly prolonged hospitalization. The increased risk is not prohibitive by any means, but if the same goal can be accomplished by postoperative irradiation, the overall complication rates are reduced. The major late effects of combined treatment are an increased fibrosis of soft tissues, stomal stenosis, and pharyngeal stricture.

HYPOPHARYNX: PHARYNGEAL WALLS, PYRIFORM SINUS, AND POSTCRICOID PHARYNX

Both the oropharyngeal and hypopharyngeal walls will be considered together because there is no distinct difference in the presentation, treatment, or prognosis. The great majority of hypopharyngeal lesions originate in the pyriform sinus. Postcricoid carcinomas fortunately are quite uncommon in the United States.

ANATOMY

The epithelium of the pharyngeal mucous membrane is squamous. It is continuous with the mucous membrane of the nasopharynx; there is no visible point or line of transition. The dividing point between the nasopharynx and posterior pharyngeal wall is actually Passavant's ridge, a muscular ring that contracts to close the nasopharynx during swallowing. The posterior and lateral walls are surrounded by the thin constrictor muscles. Between the constrictor muscle and the prevertebral fascia that covers the longitudinal spine muscles (longus colli and longus capitis) is a thin layer of loose areolar tissue, the retropharyngeal space. The entire thickness of the posterior pharyngeal wall from the mucous membrane to the anterior vertebral body is no more than 1 cm in the midline. Lateral to the pharyngeal wall are the vessels, nerves, and muscles of the parapharyngeal space (see Fig. 21-13). The constrictor muscles are relatively thin, especially the superior constrictor, and do not present much of an obstacle to tumor penetration. There is a variable weak spot in the lateral pharyngeal wall just below the hyoid where the middle and the inferior constrictor muscles fail to overlap. The lateral wall in this area is composed of the thin thyrohyoid membrane, which is penetrated by the vessels, nerves, and lymphatics of the laryngopharynx.

The pharyngeal walls are continuous with the cervical esophagus below. The hypopharyngeal walls are visible by indirect mirror examination; the transition to cervical esophagus is below the arytenoids (C4) and invisible to mirror examination. The transition zone, 3 cm to 4 cm in length, is referred to as the postcricoid pharynx and will be dealt with

TABLE 21-49. Supraglottic Larynx Carcinoma: Ultimate Local Control After Salvage Therapy—152 Patients (No. Controlled/No. Treated)

T Stage	Irradiation Alone	Surgery ± Adjuvant Irradiation	Significance Levels[144,145]
T1	13/13 (100%)	9/9	1.00
T2	32/36 (89%)	21/25 (84%)	0.426
T3	15/20 (75%)	18/18 (100%)	0.031
T4	7/13 (54%)	15/18 (83%)	0.084

Weems DH, Mendenhall WM, Parsons JT, et al: Squamous cell carcinoma of the supraglottic larynx treated with surgery and/or radiation therapy. Int J Radiat Oncol Biol Phys 13:1483–1487, 1987.

TABLE 21-50. Supraglottic Larynx Carcinoma: Ultimate Local Control with Voice Preservation— 195 Patients (No. Controlled with Voice Preservation/No. Treated)

T Stage	Irradiation Alone	Surgery ± Adjuvant Irradiation	Significance Levels[144,145]
T1	15/16 (94%)	8/9	0.600
T2	38/45 (84%)*	12/31 (39%)	<0.001
T3	17/25 (68%)	6/26 (23%)	0.002
T4	14/21 (67%)	3/23 (13%)	<0.001

Weems DH, Mendenhall WM, Parsons JT, et al: Squamous cell carcinoma of the supraglottic larynx treated with surgery and/or radiation therapy. Int J Radiat Oncol Biol Phys 13:1483–1487, 1987.

*One patient had two T2 primary lesions and was thus counted twice.

separately, since tumors of this area present a special clinical picture.

The lateral pharyngeal wall is a rather narrow, ill-defined strip of mucosa. It lies behind the posterior tonsillar pillar in the oropharynx, is partially interrupted by the pharyngoepiglottic fold, and then continues into the hypopharynx, where it becomes the lateral wall of the pyriform sinus. The lateral pharyngeal wall has a maximum width of no more than 2 cm. The posterior cornu of the hyoid bone occasionally will protrude into the lateral pharyngeal wall on one or both sides, producing a submucosal bulge.

The posterior pharyngeal wall is about 4 cm to 5 cm wide and about 6 cm to 7 cm in height. Submucosal bulges, caused by osteophytes on the anterior lips of the cervical vertebrae, may be mistaken for submucosal tumor.

The pyriform sinus is created by the intrusion of the larynx into the anterior aspect of the pharynx, which creates pharyngeal grooves lateral to the larynx. The superior margin of the pyriform sinus is the pharyngoepiglottic fold and the free margin of the aryepiglottic fold. The superolateral margin of the pyriform sinus is considered to be an oblique line along the lateral pharyngeal wall just opposite the aryepiglottic fold. The pyriform sinus is therefore made up of three walls: the anterior, lateral, and medial (there is no posterior wall). The pyriform sinus tapers inferiorly to the apex and usually terminates at the level of the cricoid cartilage. The superior limit of the pyriform sinus is opposite the hyoid. The thyrohyoid membrane is lateral to the upper portion of the pyriform sinus (membranous pyriform sinus), and the thyroid cartilage, cricothyroid membrane, and cricoid cartilage are lateral to the lower portion (cartilaginous pyriform sinus). The internal branch of the superior laryngeal nerve, a branch of the vagus, lies under the mucous membrane on the anterolateral wall of the pyriform sinus. The auricular branch is sensory to the skin of the back of the pinna and the posterior wall of the external auditory canal.

The postcricoid pharynx is funnel-shaped, to direct food into the gullet. There is no discrete superior margin, but it may be considered to begin just below the arytenoids. The anterior wall lies behind the cricoid cartilage and is the posterior wall of the lower larynx; this wall is often called the "party wall." The posterior wall is merely a continuation of the hypopharyngeal walls. The recurrent laryngeal nerve lies between the lateral wall and the deep surface of the thyroid gland.

PATHOLOGY

More than 95% of malignant tumors are squamous cell carcinoma or one of its variants. Carcinoma in situ is commonly seen in surgical specimens at the edge of neoplasms of the pharyngeal wall, and multifocal skip areas of carcinoma in situ may make it difficult to obtain clear margins if excision is done. Minor salivary gland tumors are rare.

TABLE 21-51. Supraglottic Larynx Carcinoma: Control Above the Clavicles Following Initial Treatment— 156 Patients (No. Controlled/No. Treated)

Modified AJCC Stage	Irradiation Alone	Surgery ± Adjuvant Irradiation	Significance Levels[144,145]
I	9/10	9/9	0.526
II	13/17 (76%)	13/15 (87%)	0.392
III	11/18 (61%)	9/10	0.116
IVA	7/10	5/11 (45%)	0.245
IVB	10/28 (36%)	20/28 (71%)	0.008

Weems DH, Mendenhall WM, Parsons JT, et al: Squamous cell carcinoma of the supraglottic larynx treated with surgery and/or radiation therapy. Int J Radiat Oncol Biol Phys 13:1483–1487, 1987.

TABLE 21-52.   Supraglottic Larynx Carcinoma: Ultimate Control Above the Clavicles — 156 Patients (No. Controlled/No. Treated)

Modified AJCC Stage	Irradiation Alone	Surgery ± Adjuvant Irradiation	Significance Levels[144,145]
I	10/10	9/9	1.00
II	16/17 (94%)	14/15 (93%)	0.726
III	15/18 (83%)	10/10	0.249
IVA	8/10	6/11 (55%)	0.221
IVB	14/28 (50%)	23/28 (82%)	0.012

Weems DH, Mendenhall WM, Parsons JT, et al: Squamous cell carcinoma of the supraglottic larynx treated with surgery and/or radiation therapy. Int J Radiat Oncol Biol Phys 13:1483–1487, 1987.

PATTERNS OF SPREAD

Posterior Pharyngeal Wall

Carcinomas of the posterior pharyngeal wall have a strong tendency to remain on the posterior wall, grow up or down the wall, and infiltrate posteriorly; they seldom spread circumferentially to the lateral walls, even when quite advanced. Early lesions are red lesions, sometimes with white areas sprinkled over the involved area. As the lesion progresses, the tumor bulges into the pharyngeal cavity and a ragged, midline, linear ulceration appears. The posterior tonsillar pillars may become involved, and tumor may spread up the pillars, eventually reaching the palate. Advanced lesions tend to terminate inferiorly at the level of the arytenoids without growing into the postcricoid region. Superiorly they may extend into the nasopharynx. Direct invasion of the cervical vertebrae or base of skull is uncommon.

Lateral Pharyngeal Wall

Early tumors may be well-defined exophytic lesions. As they advance, they have a tendency to lateral penetration through the constrictor muscle, thus entering the lateral pharyngeal space or the soft tissue of the neck. A mass may become palpable in the neck just below the hyoid and be confused with a lymph node.

The muscles of the pharynx originate from the base of skull, eustachian tube, styloid process, pterygomandibular raphe, and hyoid bone; tumor may spread along muscle and fascial planes to all muscular points of origin.[318] Tumor also follows a course along cranial nerves IX and X and the sympathetic chain. The thyroid gland is adjacent to the lower walls and often is invaded. Tumor secondarily invades the pharyngoepiglottic fold, the vallecula, and the anterior and lateral walls of the pyriform sinus.

Pyriform Sinus

Early lesions usually appear as nodular mucosal irregularities. Medial wall lesions may grow superficially along the aryepiglottic fold and arytenoids, or invade directly into the false cord and aryepiglottic fold. Medial wall lesions also extend posteriorly to the postcricoid region. Extensive submucosal spread is a characteristic feature. There is frequently an area of central ulceration for lesions larger than 1 cm to 2 cm.

Large bulky exophytic lesions may arise on the upper medial wall and appear similar to primary lesions of the aryepiglottic fold. The vocal cord becomes fixed because of infiltration of the intrinsic muscles of the larynx, the cricoarytenoid joint or muscle, or less commonly, the recurrent laryngeal nerve. These lesions grow posteriorly to involve the postcricoid pharynx and cricoid cartilage and may extend to the opposite pyriform sinus. Spread into the cervical esophagus is a late event.

Lesions arising on the lateral wall tend toward early inva-

TABLE 21-53.   Supraglottic Larynx Carcinoma: Incidence of Severe Complications — 195 Patients

Initial Treatment	No. Patients with Severe Complications/ No. Initially Treated	No. Patients with Severe Complications/No. Attempted Salvage Procedures
Irradiation alone	5/106 (5%)	2/20 (10%)
Surgery alone	6/26 (23%)	1/4
Preoperative irradiation + surgery	6/28 (21%)	0/1
Surgery + postoperative irradiation	6/35 (17%)	1/4

Weems DH, Mendenhall WM, Parsons JT, et al: Squamous cell carcinoma of the supraglottic larynx treated with surgery and/or radiation therapy. Int J Radiat Oncol Biol Phys 13:1483–1487, 1987

TABLE 21-54. Supraglottic Larynx Carcinoma: Determinate 5-Year Survival — 105 Patients (No. Alive/No. Treated)

Modified AJCC Stage	Irradiation Alone	Surgery ± Adjuvant Irradiation	Significance Levels[144,145]
I	6/6	8/8	1.00
II	7/7	8/9	0.562
III	3/6	8/8	0.055
IVA	4/7	3/7	0.500
IVB	5/26 (19%)	11/21 (52%)	0.019

Weems DH, Mendenhall WM, Parsons JT, et al: Squamous cell carcinoma of the supraglottic larynx treated with surgery and/or radiation therapy. Int J. Radiat Oncol Biol Phys 13:1483–1487, 1987.

TABLE 21-55. Squamous Cell Carcinoma of the Supraglottic Larynx: Absolute Survival Rates* in Patients with Stage IV† Disease

Absolute Survival	Surgery Only‡	Surgery and Radiation Therapy
2 years	39.1% (34/87)§	68.5% (37/54)§
5 years	24.4% (19/78)**	42.1% (16/38)**

Fletcher GH, Goepfert H: Larynx and pyriform sinus. In Fletcher GH: Textbook of Radiotherapy, 3rd ed, pp 330–363. Philadelphia, Lea & Febiger, 1980.
  M. D. Anderson Hospital data; patients treated 1954–1972.
  *Living, free of cancer.
  †Stage IV: T4 N0–N1, T1–T4 N2–N3.
  ‡All patients had a total laryngectomy.
  §p < 0.005.
  **p < 0.08.

sion of the posterior thyroid cartilage and the posterior superior cricoid cartilage. The ipsilateral superior lobe of the thyroid gland may be invaded after tumor penetrates the cartilage, but thyroid invasion can occur in cases with no cartilage invasion when tumor penetrates behind the thyroid cartilage or through the cricothyroid membrane. Kirchner[319] reported that thyroid cartilage invasion was associated with involvement of the apex of the pyriform sinus, and the extent of invasion could not be predicted on the extent of visible disease.

Lesions of the lateral walls tend to spread submucosally to the posterior pharyngeal wall. It is often difficult to estimate the extent of posterior pharyngeal wall or postcricoid invasion except at direct laryngoscopy, since these areas are often impossible to visualize indirectly. Even with direct endoscopy, invasion may be underestimated.

Advanced lesions of the pyriform sinus invade all three walls, fix the larynx, involve the ipsilateral posterior pharyngeal wall, invade the thyroid cartilage and thyroid gland, and often escape into the soft tissues of the neck. The preepiglottic space often is involved. Perineural invasion of the recurrent laryngeal nerve may be seen in whole organ sections.

Postcricoid Pharynx

Early lesions of the postcricoid area are rarely diagnosed. Lesions arising from the posterior wall tend to remain on the posterior wall. Lesions arising from the anterior wall tend to invade the posterior cricoarytenoid muscle and the cricoid and arytenoid cartilages. Advanced tumors eventually encircle the lumen. Because the apex of the pyriform sinus terminates in the postcricoid area, some lesions secondarily invade the apex of the pyriform sinus very early.

Lymphatics

PHARYNGEAL WALLS. The lymphatics of the pharyngeal walls terminate primarily in the jugular chain with a secondary avenue by way of the spinal accessory chain. The jugulodigastric node is the most commonly involved node.

TABLE 21-56. T1–T2 Glottic Larynx Carcinoma: Incidence of Serious Complications by Radiation Dose — 303 Patients* (No. Complications/No. Patients Treated)

Total Dose (cGy)	T1 Dose/Fraction 225–255 cGy†	<185–245 cGy	T2 Dose/Fraction 225–245 cGy†	<175–224 cGy	Total Dose/Fraction 225–255 cGy	175–224 cGy
>7000				0/3		0/3
6700–7000		0/2	2/7 (29%)	0/12	2/7 (29%)	0/14
6000–6600	0/86	1/58 (1.7%)	1/61 (1.6%)	1/34 (2.9%)	1/147 (0.7%)	2/92 (2.2%)
5400–5700	0/36	0/2		0/2	0/36	0/4

Mendenhall WM, Parsons JT, Million RR, et al: T1–T2 squamous cell carcinoma of the glottic larynx treated with radiation therapy: Relationship of dose-fractionation factors to local control and complications. Int J Radiat Oncol Biol Phys (in press).
  *Patients treated with once-a-day fractionation.
  †Only one patient was treated at >235 cGy/fraction.

Lindberg[7] reported 59% clinically positive nodes on admission; 17% were bilateral (Fig. 21-20). Wang[320] reported 55% positive nodes for lesions of the posterior pharyngeal wall, of which 10% were bilateral. At the University of Florida, the incidence of clinically positive nodes for posterior pharyngeal wall lesions was 65%.

Retropharyngeal lymph node involvement occurs and is diagnosed by CT or MRI scan.

PYRIFORM SINUS. The capillary lymphatics of the pyriform sinus are profuse. The distribution of lymph node metastases is mainly to the jugular chain with a relatively small proportion to the spinal accessory chain. The subdigastric node is the most commonly involved, but midjugular involvement occurs without subdigastric node involvement.

On admission, 75% of patients have clinically positive nodes and at least 10% have bilateral nodes (see Fig. 21-20). There is no difference in the risk of lymph node metastases by T stage (see Table 21-1). Ogura and co-workers[42] reported a 62% incidence of subclinical disease; some of the patients had 1500 cGy to 3000 cGy of preoperative irradiation. Biller and co-workers[321] reported a 9% incidence of delayed-appearing contralateral nodes after an ipsilateral pathologically positive neck dissection. The risk for late-appearing contralateral lymph nodes was independent of whether the positive ipsilateral lymph nodes were palpable.

FIG. 21-20. Nodal distribution on admission at M.D. Anderson Hospital, 1948–1965. **A.** Oropharyngeal walls. **B.** Hypopharynx. (Lindberg RD: Distribution of cervical lymph node metastases from squamous cell carcinoma of the upper respiratory and digestive tracts. Cancer 29:1446–1450, 1972)

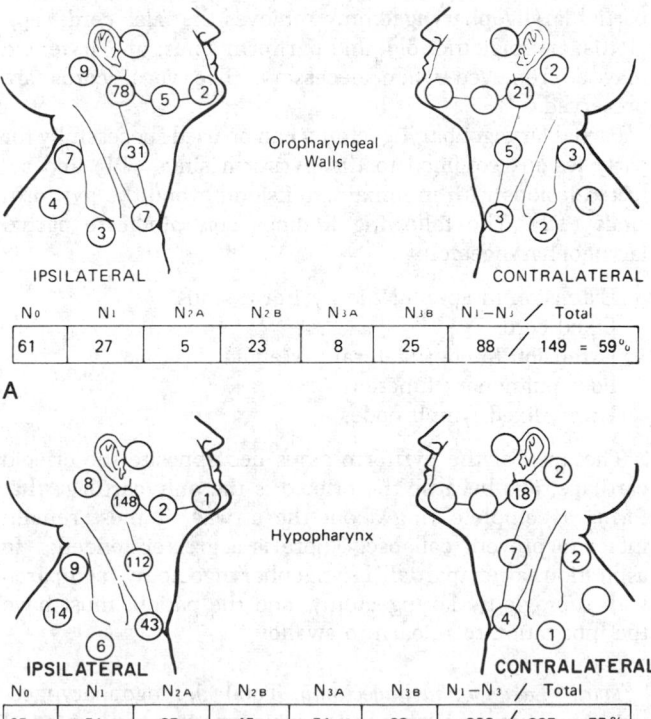

N0	N1	N2A	N2B	N3A	N3B	N1–N3 / Total
61	27	5	23	8	25	88 / 149 = 59%

A

N0	N1	N2A	N2B	N3A	N3B	N1–N3 / Total
65	51	27	45	51	28	202 / 267 = 75%

B

Retropharyngeal lymph node involvement occurs and is diagnosed by CT or MRI scan.

CLINICAL PICTURE

Tumors that are lateralized to the lateral pharyngeal wall or pyriform sinus produce a unilateral sore throat, a symptom rather specific for cancer since infectious sore throat is bilateral. The patient with cancer can point to the painful site with one finger, whereas the patient with inflammatory sore throat cannot. Dysphagia, sensation of foreign body, ear pain, blood-streaked saliva, and voice change occur later. A neck mass may be the presenting complaint.

Lesions of the posterior pharyngeal wall are often overlooked even by competent physicians because of failure to examine the posterior pharyngeal wall routinely during indirect laryngoscopy.

Small lesions of the pyriform sinus are easily missed unless very careful examinations are done. Many of these patients have active gag reflexes, and complete topical anesthesia is required, coupled with patience on the part of the examiner.

Lesions of the apex of the pyriform sinus or postcricoid area produce indirect findings that are clues to tumor not visible by indirect laryngoscopy. Pooling of secretions in the pyriform sinus and arytenoid area indicates obstruction of the upper gullet. Edema of the arytenoids and inability to see into the apex of the pyriform sinus are clues to postcricoid or low-lying pyriform sinus tumors. Invasion of the palatopharyngeal muscle at its insertion into the inferior constrictor can cause shortening of the muscle and asymmetry of the posterior tonsillar pillars. As the postcricoid tumor enlarges it pushes the larynx anteriorly. This produces a full, expanded neck appearance. The thyroid click or crackle is produced by the superior thyroid cornu hitting against the spine while rocking the thyroid cartilage back and forth; this is lost when the larynx and thyroid cartilage protrude anteriorly.

METHODS OF DIAGNOSIS AND STAGING

Lesions of the oropharyngeal wall can sometimes be biopsied in the outpatient clinic with topical anesthetic. Hypopharyngeal lesions usually require general anesthetic and biopsy under direct visualization.

Direct laryngoscopy and esophagoscopy are needed to map the extent of low pharyngeal wall, pyriform sinus, and postcricoid lesions.

CT scans are useful in demonstrating invasion of the pre-epiglottic space, invasion of the thyroid and cricoid cartilages, invasion of the soft tissues of the neck, and the extent of lymph node metastases. CT scan should be done prior to biopsy.

Staging

The AJCC staging for the hypopharynx is satisfactory for the pyriform sinus, but unsatisfactory for the pharyngeal wall.[12]

TX   Minimum requirements to assess the primary tumor cannot be met

T0   No evidence of primary tumor
Tis   Carcinoma in situ
T1   Tumor confined to one site
T2   Extension of tumor to adjacent region or site without fixation of hemilarynx
T3   Extension of tumor to adjacent region or site with fixation of hemilarynx
T4   Massive tumor invading bone or soft tissues of neck

If there is definite decrease in mobility, the lesion should be assigned to the T3 stage.

Lesions of the posterior pharyngeal wall tend to stay on the posterior pharyngeal wall rather than invade the larynx or lateral walls; therefore, fixation does not enter into staging. Posterior pharyngeal wall lesions would be staged more appropriately by tumor diameter.

TREATMENT

Selection of Treatment Modality

POSTERIOR PHARYNGEAL WALL. Most lesions on the posterior pharyngeal wall are treated by radiation therapy, although the results are far from outstanding. Attempts have been made to combine surgery and radiation therapy for selected, moderately advanced lesions, with limited success.

All aspects considered, high-dose radiotherapy will produce cure rates similar to those produced by either surgery alone or combined surgery plus radiation therapy, and with lesser morbidity. A few selected patients who fail to respond to radiation therapy or whose lesions recur after irradiation will be salvaged by pharyngectomy.

LATERAL PHARYNGEAL WALL. There is very little local control information specifically related to the lateral walls. Small lesions (1–2 cm) are usually exophytic and are usually managed by irradiation. Larger lesions tend to be deeply infiltrative, and the control rate by irradiation, surgery, or both is only modest at best. An operation for a large lesion usually implies a laryngectomy in combination with pharyngectomy.

PYRIFORM SINUS. The pyriform sinus is the most common primary site in the hypopharynx. Lesions confined to the pyriform sinus with normal mobility (T1) are locally controlled in 85% to 90% of cases by irradiation or partial laryngopharyngectomy.[322] Irradiation is the preferred choice of the authors because it leaves the patient with nearly normal swallowing and speech while permitting wider coverage of the regional lymphatics. Irradiation is more generally applicable, whereas there are certain anatomical and medical restraints on use of partial laryngopharyngectomy.

Lesions that extend outside the pyriform sinus with normal or reduced mobility (T2–T3) represent the group of cases in which treatment selection is more complex. The local control rate with radiation therapy for selected cases is approximately 60%; some of the failures will be rescued by operation, although the operative mortality and morbidity are considerable after high-dose irradiation.

Invasion of the pyriform sinus apex is a contraindication to partial laryngopharyngectomy, but these same patients do poorly with radiation therapy also; these patients usually are selected for total laryngopharyngectomy plus postoperative radiation therapy, but they may be treated for cure with radiation therapy if apex involvement is minimal. Fixation is a relative indication for total laryngopharyngectomy and postoperative radiation therapy. If the lesion is mainly exophytic and in the upper pyriform sinus, a trial of radiation therapy is offered as an alternative to total laryngopharyngectomy. If the disease disappears at 4500 cGy to 5000 cGy and mobility is returning, radical irradiation is a reasonable choice, with total laryngopharyngectomy reserved for failure. A select group of early T2 lesions with minimal extension beyond the pyriform sinus and a normal apex are also suitable for partial laryngopharyngectomy. However, these are the very patients that do well with radiation therapy only.

The more advanced, infiltrative lesions are best treated with total laryngopharyngectomy, radical neck dissection, and postoperative radiation therapy. Those patients presenting with an extensive primary lesion and extensive neck metastases (and usually accompanied by major medical problems) are frequently offered palliative therapy.

Surgical Treatment

POSTERIOR PHARYNGEAL WALL. If the lesion is high on the posterior wall, then a transoral approach can be used; however, for lower lesions the midline mandibulolabial glossotomy approach may be used. Alternatives are the transhyoid approach or a lateral pharyngotomy approach. The lesion is removed down to the prevertebral fascia, and no skin graft is placed.

PYRIFORM SINUS. *Partial laryngopharyngectomy.* A partial laryngopharyngectomy removes the false cords, epiglottis, aryepiglottic fold, and pyriform sinus; one arytenoid may be removed when necessary. The vocal cords are preserved.

Partial laryngopharyngectomy can be used successfully for early lesions confined to the pyriform sinus (T1) and selected lesions with minimal extension beyond the pyriform sinus (T2). The following findings contraindicate partial laryngopharyngectomy:

Extension to apex of the pyriform sinus
Fixed cord
Extension to contralateral arytenoid
Poor pulmonary function
Large, fixed lymph nodes

The apex of the pyriform sinus lies opposite the cricoid cartilage, and because the cricoid is the only cartilage that forms a complete ring about the airway, it must remain intact to prevent collapse. There is a greater tendency to aspiration after partial laryngopharyngectomy compared with supraglottic laryngectomy, and the patient must have the motivation to relearn to swallow.

Total Laryngopharyngectomy. Total laryngopharyngectomy removes the larynx and varying amounts of pharyngeal wall. Advanced lesions require excision of nearly the entire circumference. The pharynx is reestablished by primary closure after a partial pharyngectomy, but a flap is required after total pharyngectomy. Because almost all these patients received postoperative radiation therapy, the operation should be planned for one-stage reconstruction in order to start radiation therapy within 6 weeks. A planned controlled fistula speeds the healing process and largely eliminates the occurrence of an uncontrolled fistula, which delays healing and the start of radiation therapy. If a myocutaneous flap is used, a controlled fistula is unnecessary.

POSTCRICOID PHARYNX. Postcricoid carcinoma generally requires a total laryngopharyngectomy with immediate reconstruction, generally using a pectoralis major myocutaneous flap. Before undergoing the surgery, however, the patient must undergo direct laryngoscopy and esophagoscopy to determine the extent of the lesion. If the lesion extends into the cervical esophagus, then reconstruction becomes more difficult and often stomach will be used for reconstruction. If irradiation is to be used in conjunction with gastric pull-up, preoperative radiation therapy is preferred.

Irradiation Technique

In selected cases, patients expected to have a poor nutritional status will have placement of a gastrostomy tube prior to irradiation.

POSTERIOR PHARYNGEAL WALL. The irradiation technique for lesions of the posterior pharyngeal wall is opposed lateral fields to include the primary lesion and the regional nodes. Because these lesions tend to have "skip" areas, the entire posterior pharyngeal wall is included initially. If the lesion extends near the arytenoids, the postcricoid pharynx, pyriform sinus, and upper cervical esophagus are included. The retropharyngeal nodes will be included within these fields. The spinal accessory nodes are included even if the neck nodes are negative.

The critical portion of the treatment occurs when the field is reduced at 4500 cGy to 5000 cGy to avoid the spinal cord. The posterior border of the portal is placed just anterior to the spinal cord (*i.e.*, posterior edge of the bodies of the cervical vertebrae).[323] Daily imaging films and precision setups are required.

The dose for T1 lesions (0–2 cm) is 6000 cGy in 6 weeks. The dose for T2–T4 lesions is 7440 cGy to 7680 cGy with 120 cGy twice a day.

PYRIFORM SINUS. Parallel opposed lateral portals are used to encompass the primary lesion and regional nodes on both sides. The superior border is placed 2 cm above the tip of the mastoid to cover the most superior jugular chain and the retropharyngeal lymph nodes. The posterior border encompasses the spinal accessory nodes. Clinically positive nodes behind the plane of the spinal cord require the addition of a neck dissection or electron boosts. The anterior border usually is placed about 1 cm behind the anterior skin edge. When the anterior border is shielded, the radiotherapist checks the setup daily because the margin for error is rather slim. However, protection of this narrow anterior segment reduces irradiation of the anterior arch of the thyroid

and cricoid cartilages, anterior commissure of the glottis, and anterior midline skin. The inferior border is 2 cm below the inferior border of the cricoid. The inferior recess or apex of the pyriform sinus varies, but generally terminates at the upper to middle cricoid. The remaining lower neck lymph nodes are treated through an en face portal.

Dosimetry is individualized, using wedges, compensators, and unequal loadings as needed. The doses are the same as for the posterior pharyngeal wall.

Combined Treatment Policies

POSTERIOR PHARYNGEAL WALL. Operation usually should precede radiation therapy when a combination is selected, unless a gastric pull-up is planned. There is a high incidence of operative mortality and complications with a preoperative dose of 2500 cGy to 3000 cGy.[324] When postoperative irradiation is used, a dose of 6000 cGy to 6500 cGy is used with negative margins.

PYRIFORM SINUS. Following total laryngopharyngectomy with or without radical neck dissection, radiation therapy is recommended if there are close or positive margins, multiple or large positive nodes, extension of nodal disease through the capsule, or cartilage invasion. In short, almost all patients receive postoperative radiation therapy. There is an increased risk of pharyngeal stenosis, especially if the pharyngeal closure is tight.

Irradiation is given before total laryngopharyngectomy in those T2 or T3 patients for whom a trial of radiation therapy is planned; the patients are reevaluated at 4500 cGy with the surgeon. Irradiation is also used prior to operation for patients with a large fixed node to reduce the size of the mass and to help obtain surgical margins. The preoperative dose to the node may be 6000 cGy to 7500 cGy, although the dose to the primary will be only 4000 cGy to 5000 cGy.

Management of Recurrence

POSTERIOR PHARYNGEAL WALL. Recurrence after radiation therapy may be limited to the posterior pharyngeal wall and suitable for surgical excision, with occasional salvage. There is frequently a persistent ulcer at the completion of radiation therapy for the more advanced lesions. If the ulcer does not heal in short order, it should be considered evidence of persistent disease. Surgical excision is limited posteriorly by the prevertebral fascia. Meoz-Mendez and co-workers[325] report 11 irradiation failures salvaged by an operation out of a total of 68 local failures. Irradiation salvage of a surgical failure would be unusual.

PYRIFORM SINUS. The hallmark of local recurrence after radical irradiation is persistent major edema with inability to visualize the pyriform sinus, pain on swallowing, and fixation of laryngeal structures. Direct laryngoscopy is required, but biopsy may be negative and misleading. Eventually a decision may be made to recommend total laryngopharyngectomy for salvage without a positive biopsy.

Recurrence after total laryngopharyngectomy is usually in

the soft tissues of the neck, the untreated opposite neck, the base of the tongue, or the stoma.

Surgical failures after partial laryngopharyngectomy for early lesions may be salvaged by total laryngopharyngectomy. Surgical failures after total laryngopharyngectomy are rarely salvaged.

Radiation failure occasionally may be salvaged by total laryngopharyngectomy with or without radical neck dissection. The risk of an operative mortality or major morbidity is high.

RESULTS OF TREATMENT

Pharyngeal Wall

The treatment policy at the University of Florida primarily has been radical irradiation with neck dissection added as necessary. The local control rates for once-daily versus twice-daily irradiation (external beam treatment only) are given in Table 21-57. The improvement in local control and survival rates with the twice-a-day regimen has been impressive to date.[323]

Wang[320] reported a 25% 3-year survival without recurrence for 36 patients with carcinoma of the posterior pharyngeal wall treated by radiation therapy alone; the 3-year survival rate was 47% for patients with clinically negative nodes. Sixteen of 24 patients (66%) with T1 or T2 lesions had their disease controlled by radiation therapy, as did 3 of 13 patients with T3 lesions.

Meoz-Mendez and co-workers[325] reported the results of radiation therapy alone for 164 patients with lesions arising from the pharyngeal walls. The rates of local control by T stage and salvage of radiation therapy failures are shown in Table 21-58. The cause of death was local failure in 38%, neck recurrence in 6%, distant metastases in 10%, and second primary cancer in 16%.

Marks and co-workers[324] compared low-dose preoperative radiation therapy (2500-3000 cGy) followed by operation to radiation therapy alone (Table 21-59). The local control was slightly better for the combined group, but the 3-year actuarial survival rate was 17%, and the 3-year absolute survival rate was 14%. An operative mortality of 14% and a high risk of major surgical complications offset any gain in local control. M. D. Anderson Hospital reported a group of 25 patients

TABLE 21-57. Pharyngeal Wall Carcinoma: Local Control with Radiation Therapy — External Beam, Continuous Course (No. Controlled/No. Treated)

Stage	Once-a-Day Treatment	Twice-a-Day Treatment
T1 (0–2 cm)	2/3	1/1
T2 (>2–4 cm)	7/12	4/4
T3 (>4–6 cm)	8/19	4/6
T4 (>6 cm)	1/6	1/2

Data from Mendenhall et al.[323]

(5 Stage T2, 10 Stage T3–T4) treated by combined surgery and radiation therapy.[325] Nineteen patients received postoperative radiation therapy, 7 had positive margins, and 3 had close margins. Fifteen patients were dead at 5 years: 6 died of local recurrence or neck recurrence, 5 of distant metastasis, 1 of intercurrent disease, and 3 of uncertain causes. The 5-year absolute survival was 4 of 19 (21%).

Pyriform Sinus

The results of treatment for 80 patients with carcinoma of the pyriform sinus treated at Washington University, St. Louis, by preoperative radiation therapy followed by partial laryngopharyngectomy are given in Table 21-60.[326] Seventy patients had the equivalent of AJCC T1 lesions (disease limited to the pyriform sinus) and 10 patients had disease ex-

TABLE 21-59. Local Control in Carcinoma of the Posterior Pharyngeal Wall (Washington University, St. Louis)

| Treatment | Local Control | | | |
	T1	T2	T3	T4
Surgery (31 patients)*	6/8	7/12	4/12	0/1
Radiation therapy alone	1/1	3/6	0/5	1/1

Adapted from Marks JE, Freeman RB, Lee F, et al: Pharyngeal wall cancer: An analysis of treatment results complications and patterns of failure. Int J Radiat Oncol Biol Phys 4:587–593, 1978.
*Twenty-nine patients had preoperative radiation therapy; 2 patients had postoperative radiation therapy.

TABLE 21-58. Squamous Cell Carcinoma of the Pharyngeal Walls: Local Control (164 Patients: M. D. Anderson Hospital, 1954–1974)

Stage	Local Control with RT* Alone (No. controlled/ No. treated)	Surgical Salvage (No. salvaged)	Ultimate Local Control (No. controlled/ No. treated)
T1 (0–2 cm)	10/11 (91%)	1	11/11 (100%)
T2 (2–4 cm)	33/45 (73%)	2	35/45 (78%)
T3 (>4 cm)	38/62 (61%)	6	44/62 (71%)
T4 (massive)	15/46 (37%)	2	17/46 (41%)

Adapted from Meoz-Mendez RT, Fletcher GH, Guillamondegui OM, et al: Analysis of the results of irradiation in the treatment of squamous cell carcinomas of the pharyngeal walls. Int J Radiat Oncol Biol Phys 4:579–585, 1978.
*RT, radiation therapy.

TABLE 21-60.   Carcinoma of the Pyriform Sinus: Results of Treatment by Low-Dose Radiation Therapy plus Partial Laryngopharyngectomy (PLP) or Low-Dose Radiation Therapy plus Total Laryngectomy and Partial Pharyngectomy (TLP) (Washington University, St. Louis, 1964–1974)

Result	PLP (80 Patients)*	TLP (57 Patients)†
Local recurrence ± neck recurrence	14%‡	14%
Neck recurrence ± distant metastases (primary controlled)	9%	23%
Distant metastases alone	11%	21%
5-year actuarial survival (no evidence of disease)	40%	22%

Data from Marks et al.[326]
*T1, 70 patients; T2–T4, 10 patients (AJC staging).
†T1, 35 patients; T2–T4, 22 patients (AJC staging).
‡Four patients salvaged.

tending beyond the pyriform sinus. None had invasion of the apex of the pyriform sinus, as determined before surgery. The cause of death was cancer in 26%, complications of treatment in 14%, and intercurrent disease in 20%. The 2-year absolute survival rate was 45 of 80 (56%) and the 5-year absolute survival was 25 of 66 (38%) (Marks JE: Personal communication, 1979).

Table 21-60 also shows the results of treatment for 57 patients from the same institution who were treated by preoperative radiation therapy followed by total laryngectomy and partial pharyngectomy.[326] Thirty-five patients had lesions confined to the pyriform sinus (AJCC T1) and the remainder had extension beyond the pyriform sinus (AJCC T2–T4). The cause of death was cancer in 56%, complications of treatment in 11%, and intercurrent disease in 18%.

The results of radiation therapy for carcinoma of the pyriform sinus with neck dissection added in selected cases are shown in Tables 21-61 through 21-64.[327] Most patients with T1 and T2 lesions were selected for radiation therapy; T3 lesions were irradiated if they were exophytic and in the upper pyriform sinus or because the patient refused operation. All T4 lesions were irradiated by default. Patients with stage IVA represent a relatively favorable group with early primary lesions and N2 or N3 neck disease; the neck disease is usually managed by adding a neck dissection after radiation therapy.

El-Badawi and co-workers[328] compared results for 203 pa-

TABLE 21-62.   Pyriform Sinus Carcinoma: Initial Control of the Clinically Positive Hemineck with Radiation Therapy ± Neck Dissection (No. Controlled/No. Treated)*

Stage	Irradiation Alone	Irradiation and Neck Dissection
N1	6/6	1/1
N2A	1/2	3/3
N2B	3/3	5/6
N3A	0/2	1/2

Mendenhall WM, Parsons JT, Cassisi NJ, et al: Squamous cell carcinoma of the pyriform sinus treated with radical radiation therapy. Radiother Oncol 9:201–208, 1987.
*Twenty-three patients, continuously disease-free at the primary site, with 25 evaluable clinically positive heminecks. None of the neck failures were controlled by subsequent treatment.

tients treated by surgery alone, and 125 patients treated by surgery (total laryngopharyngectomy) followed by 6000 cGy of postoperative irradiation or preceded by 4500 cGy to 5000 cGy of preoperative irradiation. The stages of the three groups were comparable. There was a minimum follow-up of 4 years. The patients treated with combined therapy showed approximately a 15% improvement in survival at 5 years (Table 21-65).

The ultimate control rate above the clavicles for 65 patients treated by total laryngopharyngectomy and 2 patients

TABLE 21-61.   Pyriform Sinus Carcinoma: Local Control with Continuous-Course Radiation Therapy ± Neck Dissection (No. Controlled/No. Treated)

Stage	Excluded*	Once-a-Day Fractionation	Twice-a-Day Fractionation†	Total Local Control with Radical Radiation Therapy	No. Salvaged/ No. Attempts	Ultimate Control
T1	2	8/9		8/9	0/0	8/9
T2	10	12/16	3/4	15/20	3/4	18/20
T3	2	1/3	1/2	2/5	1/2	3/5
T4	2	0/2	0/1	0/3	0/1	0/3

Mendenhall WM, Parsons JT, Cassisi NJ, et al: Squamous cell carcinoma of the pyriform sinus treated with radical radiation therapy. Radiother Oncol 9:201–208, 1987.
*Patients were excluded from the local control analysis if they died within 2 years of treatment of other causes with the primary site continuously disease-free.
†University of Florida data. Patients treated 3/78–4/85; analysis 4/87 by J. T. Parsons, M.D.

TABLE 21-63. Pyriform Sinus Carcinoma: Control Above the Clavicles (No. Controlled/No. Treated)

Modified AJCC Stage	Excluded*	Control with Initial Treatment	No. Salvaged/ No. Attempts	Ultimate Control
I	0	1/1	0/0	1/1
II	1	5/6	1/1	6/6
III	3	5/10	1/2	6/10
IVA	6	12/16†	1/2	13/16‡
IVB	2	1/9†	0/2	1/9‡

Mendenhall WM, Parsons JT, Cassisi NJ, et al: Squamous cell carcinoma of the pyriform sinus treated with radical radiation therapy. Radiother Oncol 9:201–208, 1987.

*Patients excluded from analysis of control above the clavicles if they died within 2 years after treatment of other causes, continuously free of disease above the clavicles.

†12/16 versus 1/9, p = 0.003.[145]

‡13/16 versus 1/9, p = 0.001.[145]

TABLE 21-64. Pyriform Sinus Carcinoma: Five-Year Survival (No. Alive/No. Treated)

Modified AJCC Stage	5-Year Survival	
	Absolute	Determinate
I	1/1	1/1
II	3/5	3/3
III	5/13	5/8
IVA	7/17*	7/12†
IVB	2/10*	2/8†

Mendenhall WM, Parsons JT, Cassisi NJ, et al: Squamous cell carcinoma of the pyriform sinus treated with radical radiation therapy. Radiother Oncol 9:201–208, 1987.

*7/17 versus 2/10, p = 0.187.[145]

†7/12 versus 2/8, p = 0.132.[145]

TABLE 21-66. Pyriform Sinus Carcinoma: Ultimate Control Above the Clavicles (Including Salvage) for 67 Patients* Treated by Surgery ± Radiation Therapy (No. Controlled/No. Treated)

Stage	Preoperative Radiation Therapy	Postoperative Radiation Therapy	Surgery Alone
T1	0/1		
T2	1/1	1/1	2/3
T3	8/15	10/15	3/6
T4	1/5	2/2	0/0

Million RR, Cassisi NJ: Hypopharynx: Pharyngeal walls, pyriform sinus, and postcricoid pharynx. In Million RR, Cassisi NJ (eds): Management of Head and Neck Cancer: A Multidisciplinary Approach, pp 373–391. Philadelphia, JB Lippincott, 1984.

University of Florida data. Patients treated 10/64–12/80 (2-year to unlimited follow-up); analysis 2/83 by J. W. Devine, M.D.

*Excludes 16 patients who died of intercurrent disease less than 2 years after treatment with no recurrence above the clavicles.

COMPLICATIONS OF TREATMENT

Posterior Pharyngeal Wall

SURGICAL COMPLICATIONS. Marks and co-workers[324] reported a 14% operative mortality plus major complications

treated by partial laryngopharyngectomy at the University of Florida is presented in Table 21-66.[329] The patients with more advanced lesions in Stages T2 and T3 were selected for an operation. Preoperative or postoperative radiation therapy was added in 54 of the patients. The ultimate control rate above the clavicles for T3 lesions treated by operation was 21 of 36 (58%) and for T4 lesions was 3 of 7. The survival figures are presented in Table 21-67.[329]

TABLE 21-65. Carcinoma of the Pyriform Sinus: Results of Treatment

Treatment Modality	No. of Patients	Failure Above Clavicles (%)	2-Year NED (%)	Cause of Death (>2 Year)
Surgery	203	39*	40†	DM—8 ID—23
Surgery and postoperative irradiation	125	11*	50†	N—1 DM—6 ID—7
Preoperative irradiation and surgery	17	29	47	DM—2 ID—2

Adapted from El-Badawi SA, Goepfert H, Fletcher GH, et al: Squamous cell carcinoma of the pyriform sinus. Laryngoscope 92:357–364, 1982.

M. D. Anderson Hospital data. Patients treated 1949–1976; analysis 1/81.

NED, no evidence of pyriform sinus cancer; DM, distant metastasis; ID, intercurrent disease; N, neck nodes.

*p = <0.001.

†p = 0.04.

TABLE 21-67.   Pyriform Sinus Carcinoma: Survival Free of Disease in 67 Patients
Treated by Surgery ± Radiation Therapy

Modified AJCC Stage	Absolute Survival		Determinate Survival	
	2 Years	5 Years	2 Years	5 Years
I,II	0/2	0/2	0/2	0/2
III	9/14 (64%)	2/9	9/12 (75%)	2/7
IVA	2/4	2/4	2/4	2/4
IVB	18/47 (38%)	7/41 (17%)	18/42 (43%)	7/35 (20%)
Total	29/67 (43%)	11/56 (20%)	29/60 (48%)	11/48 (23%)

Million RR, Cassisi NJ: Hypopharynx: Pharyngeal walls, pyriform sinus, and postcricoid pharynx. In Million RR, Cassisi NJ (eds): Management of Head and Neck Cancer: A Multidisciplinary Approach, pp 373–391. Philadelphia, JB Lippincott, 1984.
University of Florida data. Patients treated 10/64–12/80 (to 12/77 for 5-year figures); analysis 2/83 by J. W. Devine, M.D.

including pharyngocutaneous fistula (31%) and carotid rupture (14%) for patients treated with preoperative radiation therapy, 2500 cGy to 3000 cGy.

RADIATION THERAPY COMPLICATIONS. Meoz-Mendez and co-workers[325] analyzed the complications for 164 patients with carcinoma of the pharyngeal wall treated by radiation therapy alone. There was a 5% incidence of fatal complications. In 7 patients the fatality was secondary to carotid rupture, associated with attempts at surgical salvage. Only 2 patients developed severe laryngeal edema. Radiation myelitis was documented in 2 patients. The overall incidence of radiation therapy–related complications was 12%; the complication rate increased with rising T stage.

Mendenhall and co-workers[323] reported that 8 of 75 patients developed severe complications secondary to radiation therapy. The incidence of severe complications by stage is as follows: Stage I, 0 of 2; Stage II, 1 of 16; Stage III, 2 of 22; Stage IVA, 2 of 14; Stage IVB, 3 of 20. Four patients developed inability to swallow requiring a permanent gastrostomy tube. One patient developed severe laryngeal edema that required a permanent tracheostomy. One patient developed a unilateral vocal cord palsy, Horner's syndrome, brachial plexopathy, and a stricture requiring a permanent gastrostomy; although recurrent disease was initially suspected, she survived for 5 years after treatment without evidence of recurrent cancer before dying of intercurrent disease. Finally, two patients developed severe soft-tissue necrosis of the posterior pharyngeal wall, which was fatal in one case.

Pyriform Sinus

SURGICAL COMPLICATIONS. The complications of partial laryngopharyngectomy include a 12% operative mortality, fistula, aspiration, and dysphagia.[326]

The complications of total laryngopharyngectomy include a treatment-related mortality of 11%, fistula, and pharyngeal stenosis.[326]

The complication rate is increased by the addition of radiation therapy.

RADIATION THERAPY COMPLICATIONS. The major radiation therapy complication is laryngeal necrosis. Laryngeal edema occurs temporarily in most cases and is increased by radical neck dissection.

COMPLICATIONS OF SALVAGE TREATMENT. Attempted surgical salvage of radiation therapy failures has a significant operative morbidity and mortality even in the best of hands, but a few cures are produced.

NASOPHARYNX

Malignant tumors of the nasopharynx are uncommon in the United States. The Chinese have a high frequency; American-born second-generation Chinese maintain the risk of nasopharynx cancer. It is undecided whether the risk is reduced by moving away from China. Nasopharynx cancer has also been shown to have an association with elevated titers of Epstein-Barr virus; this finding is independent of geography.[35]

There is a 3:1 ratio of predominance in men. The age distribution for carcinoma is much younger than for other head and neck sites; about 20% of patients are younger than 30 years of age.

ANATOMY

The nasopharynx is roughly cuboidal in shape. It is in direct continuity with the nasal cavity, inferiorly with the oropharynx, and laterally with the middle ears by way of the eustachian tubes.

The mucosa of the roof and posterior wall is often irregular because of the pharyngeal bursa, pharyngeal tonsil (adenoids), and pharyngeal hypophysis. The mucosa tends to become smooth with age, but many folds may remain in the later years of life, adding to the examiner's confusion as to whether tumor is present. Adenoids may persist well past puberty and may even be present in elderly people. Following successful irradiation, these irregularities are usually replaced by a smooth, atrophic appearance.

The lateral walls include the eustachian openings with the fossa of Rosenmuller (pharyngeal recess) located behind the torus tubarius. The superolateral muscular wall of the nasopharynx is incomplete and provides a meager barrier to tumor spread. Once tumor has penetrated the lateral wall, it enters the lateral pharyngeal space and its contents. The floor of the nasopharynx is incomplete and consists of the upper surface of the soft palate, which is rarely the origin of nasopharyngeal tumors and is invaded infrequently even with the extensive local disease.

Lymphatics

There is an extensive submucosal lymphatic capillary plexus, attested to by the high incidence of neck metastases. Tumor cells spread along three different lymph node pathways: the jugular chain, the spinal accessory chain, and the retropharyngeal pathway.

The lateral retropharyngeal nodes lie in the retropharyngeal space and medial to the carotid artery. Directly behind the nodes are the lateral masses of C1 and C2. Marked nodal enlargement, such as that which occurs in lymphoma, may distort the posterior tonsillar pillar, shifting it medially and anteriorly. Otherwise, diagnosis depends on contrast-enhanced CT or MRI. The involved lymph nodes may have the characteristic CT appearance of metastatic carcinoma: rim enhancement and central necrosis.

Inconstant lymphatic vessels are described as draining directly to the midjugular nodes and to the spinal accessory nodes.[3]

PATHOLOGY

Most histologic varieties of malignant tumor have been reported to arise from the nasopharynx and its immediate supporting structures. Carcinomas compose about 85% and lymphomas about 10% of the malignant lesions. Lymphoepithelioma and transitional cell carcinoma are considered variants within the epithelial group; the incidence of lymphoepithelioma varies from about 30% to 50% in various series. A miscellaneous group of malignant tumors includes melanoma, plasmacytoma, juvenile angiofibroma, carcinosarcoma, sarcomas, nonchromaffin paragangliomas, and unclassified tumors. Minor salivary gland tumors are nearly always adenocarcinomas.

PATTERNS OF SPREAD

Primary

The recognized spread to contiguous structures in 99 patients with epithelial lesions on admission prior to treatment is shown in Table 21-68.[330]

Inferior extension along the lateral pharyngeal walls and tonsillar pillars is recognized in almost one third of patients. Extension into the posterior nasal cavity is frequent but usually limited to <1 cm. Thorough shrinking of the nasal mucosa and examination with a small-diameter fiberoptic nasoscope is the best clinical method for detecting nasal extension. CT scan and MRI are best to determine soft-tissue extension into the nasal cavity, but inflammatory exudates or coagulated blood may give a false impression.

Invasion of the posterior ethmoids, the maxillary antrum, and the orbit occurs fairly often and is important to recog-

TABLE 21-68. Malignant Tumors of the Nasopharynx— Incidence of Spread to Contiguous Structures on Admission (M. D. Anderson Hospital, August 1948–December 1960)

Site of Spread*	No. of Cases
Oropharyngeal wall	29
Base of skull (sphenoid sinus—11)	25
Tonsillar bed	15
Cranial nerves	12
Pterygoid fossa	9
Nasal cavity	5
Maxillary antrum	4
Orbit	3
Soft palate	3
Hard palate	2
Ethmoids	2
Hypopharynx	1

Fletcher GH, Million RR: Malignant tumors of the nasopharynx. AJR 93:44–55, 1965. © 1965, American Roentgen Ray Society.
*In several patients, more than one structure was involved.

nize because it dictates a modification of treatment techniques.

Invasion into or through the base of the skull is recognized roentgenographically or clinically in at least 25% of patients before treatment.[330,331] Early, unrecognized invasion presumably occurs in a far greater number of patients, because the base of the skull, brain, and cranial nerves are frequently the site of local recurrence. The sphenoid sinus frequently is invaded. Tumor may erode through the foramen ovale, the foramen lacerum, and the foramen spinosum. Tumor eventually reaches the cavernous sinus area and has access to cranial nerves II to VI.

The lateral muscular wall of the nasopharynx is incomplete superiorly. This defect, termed the sinus of Morgagni, is traversed by the cartilaginous portion of the eustachian tube and the levator palatine muscle, providing an avenue of egress for cancer of the nasopharynx to the lateral pharyngeal space and base of skull.

Lymphatics

There is an 80% to 90% incidence of metastatic neck node disease on presentation; approximately 50% of patients have bilateral lymph node metastases (Figure 21-21).

Low-grade squamous carcinomas produce fewer metastases (73%) than high-grade carcinomas (92%). There is a curious inverse relationship of neck node metastases relative to T stage (see Table 21-1).

Metastases to submental and occipital nodes may appear when there is blockage of the common lymphatic pathways either by massive neck disease or by an untimely neck dissection.

CLINICAL PICTURE

The most common presenting complaint is a painless upper neck mass or masses, which may be quite large when first discovered. The neck mass may enlarge rapidly owing to necrosis or hemorrhage. A rare patient will report exquisite

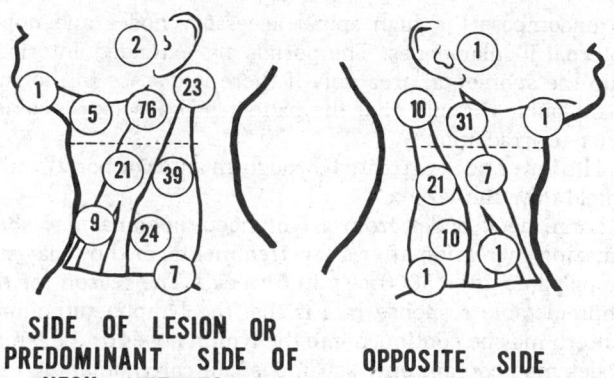

SIDE OF LESION OR
PREDOMINANT SIDE OF   OPPOSITE SIDE
NECK METASTASES

FIG. 21-21. Distribution of metastases to lymph node areas in epithelial tumors of the nasopharynx. The circled numbers indicate the number of times the particular lymph node is involved. Note the high incidence of involvement of the lymph nodes of the spinal accessory chain. Total cases = 99. No lymph nodes were involved in 10 patients (10%); lymph nodes were involved in 89 patients (89%). There was unilateral involvement in 38 patients (39%) and bilateral involvement in 51 patients (51%). (Fletcher GH, Million RR: Malignant tumors of the nasopharynx. Am J Roentgenol Radium Ther Nucl Med 93:44–55, 1965. Copyright © 1965, American Roentgen Ray Society)

tenderness of the nodes and will be unable to tolerate palpation of the masses.

Nasal obstruction, epistaxis, and otitis media are caused by local tumor effect.

Sore throat occurs in about 15% of patients and is related to spread into the oropharyngeal wall. Facial pain may be referred from any of the three divisions of the trigeminal nerve, usually the mandibular division. Occipital or temporal headache frequently is seen. Pain in the scalp over the left mastoid area is related to involvement of a high jugular lymph node that has become fixed to the skull and spine.

Pain in lifting the head and extending the neck is related to posterior infiltration of the prevertebral muscles. Proptosis occurs with posterior orbital invasion and usually displaces the eyeball straight forward. Trismus is related to the invasion of the pterygoid region.

Neurologic symptoms and signs occur in about 25% of patients. Involvement of cranial nerves II to VI indicates intracranial extension into the cavernous sinus and pituitary region. Cranial nerves IX to XII and the sympathetic chain are involved in the lateral pharyngeal space.

Examination of the nasopharynx will show a lesion on the lateral wall or roof; the nasopharyngeal surface of the soft palate is almost never the site of origin and not often invaded secondarily, even by advanced lesions. In early lesions, the findings may be quite subtle—only slight fullness in the fossa of Rosenmuller or a small submucosal bulge in the roof. Lymphomas tend to remain submucosal until quite large.

Nasoscopy may show tumor growing into the posterior and superior nasal cavity.

Tumor may be seen infiltrating submucosally along the posterior tonsillar pillars but infrequently grows very far down the posterior pharyngeal wall. The posterior tonsillar pillars may bulge into the oropharynx if an enlarged node develops in the lateral pharyngeal space.

The cranial nerves should be carefully evaluated; cranial nerve VI is the one most commonly involved. The eyes should be measured for proptosis. Ear examination may show findings of otitis media or, rarely, gross tumor.

METHODS OF DIAGNOSIS AND STAGING

Adults with large, easily visible masses may have a biopsy performed in the outpatient clinic while under local anesthetic. A straight biopsy forceps is placed through the nose and the procedure visualized indirectly from the nasopharynx, or a curved biopsy forceps may be inserted behind the retracted soft palate. Biopsy of a small lesion or random biopsies for suspected lesions require general anesthetic. The palate is retracted with a Yonkers speculum, providing direct visualization of the nasopharynx. Because some of these lesions tend to grow submucosally, random biopsies must be deep to detect an invisible lesion. A mucosal sample is taken and then the biopsy forceps is placed back into the biopsy site and a deeper sample is obtained. If a juvenile angiofibroma is suspected, the work-up should include contrast-enhanced CT.

All patients have a contrast-enhanced CT scan, MRI, or both. MRI has the advantage of obtaining images in sagittal and coronal planes. Involved retropharyngeal lymph nodes can be diagnosed by CT and MRI and are commonly diagnosed.

Staging

The AJCC staging system for nasopharyngeal primary tumors is as follows:[12]

Tis   Carcinoma in situ
T1   Tumor confined to one site of nasopharynx or no tumor visible (positive biopsy only)
T2   Tumor involving two sites (both posterosuperior and lateral walls)
T3   Extension of tumor into nasal cavity or oropharynx
T4   Tumor invasion of skull, cranial nerve involvement, or both

TREATMENT

Selection of Treatment Modality

The treatment of almost all malignancies of the nasopharynx is by radiation therapy since surgical resection is usually not feasible. Neck dissection is used less often in the management of neck disease in nasopharyngeal cancer because of the relatively high success rate with radiation therapy alone, particularly for lymphoepithelioma. Neck dissection should be added for large masses, persistence, or recurrence after irradiation. A small adenocarcinoma or sarcoma may be excised. Juvenile angiofibromas are preferably excised because of the young age of the patient, although the tumors are quite successfully cured by radiation therapy when surgical excision is impossible or dangerous.

Irradiation Technique

The anatomic planning is the same for squamous cell carcinoma, transitional cell carcinoma, and lymphoepithelioma. There is no place for small-volume irradiation even for an early epithelial tumor of the nasopharynx. If after complete clinical and roentgenographic workup the tumor is thought to be limited to the nasopharynx (T1–T2) or to have minimal soft-tissue extension (early T3), the following areas are included in the treatment volume:

1. Nasopharynx proper
2. Posterior 2 cm of the nasal cavity
3. Posterior ethmoid sinuses
4. Entire sphenoid sinus and basioccipital bone
5. Cavernous sinus
6. Base of skull (7–8 cm width encompassing the foramen ovale, carotid canal, and foramen spinosum laterally)
7. Pterygoid fossae
8. Posterior one third of maxillary sinus
9. Oropharyngeal wall to the level of the midtonsillar fossa
10. Retropharyngeal nodes
11. Neck nodes on both sides

Extension to the base of skull or involvement of cranial nerves II to VI requires that the superior border be raised to include all of the pituitary, the base of the brain in the suprasellar area, the adjacent middle cranial fossa, and the posterior portion of the anterior cranial fossa. Patients with anterior invasion into the orbit, ethmoids, or maxillary sinus require an individualized plan to produce a satisfactory volume distribution. The dose specified for the primary lesion is outlined in Table 21-69.[332] Patients are currently managed by irradiation with 120 cGy twice a day, but there are no reportable results to date.[14]

NECK NODES. A comprehensive en bloc plan must be developed to irradiate the neck to the level of the clavicles for both the epithelial lesions and the lymphomas. Even patients with no palpable disease in the neck have full neck irradiation.[9]

The retropharyngeal nodes are included in the treatment of the local lesion. The upper neck nodes are included in the primary fields to the level of the thyroid notch. In the case of no palpable nodes, the posterior margin is placed about 1 to 2 cm behind the posterior border of the sternocleidomastoid to encompass the high spinal accessory nodes and upper internal jugular nodes. The portals are extended anteriorly into the submental area only if there is disease in the submandibular triangle or if the patient had a neck dissection prior to irradiation.

The lower neck is treated through an anterior portal with a shield over the larynx.

Large neck nodes from a lymphoepithelioma may show amazing regression after a few treatments, or they may still be palpable after 5000 cGy in 5 weeks. The reason for the unpredictable response rate is that the lymphoepithelioma pattern may be continued into the lymph nodes or the lymph nodes may contain only squamous cell carcinoma.

ACUTE SEQUELAE. The large volume of mucosa irradiated produces unpleasant side-effects during treatment. Sore throat begins at the end of the second week of therapy and persists for 3 to 4 weeks after the completion of treatment. Dryness is always present and may be quite severe. Loss of taste and appetite is often quite profound, but both return 1 to 6 months after completion of treatment.

The auditory tube is in the high-dose area, and obstruction may occur with secondary otitis media and hearing loss. This condition can be corrected by polyethylene tubes inserted through the eardrums to drain the middle ears. The obstruction often improves or clears completely following mucosal healing of the nasopharynx. Politzerization of the eustachian tubes may reopen the canal.

Although mild nausea may occur, severe nausea and vomiting are uncommon. The overall effect of the treatment is quite wearing on the patient, and a period of several months may be required for successfully irradiated patients to regain a sense of well-being.

Management of Recurrence

The majority of recurrent squamous cell carcinomas are diagnosed within 2 years, but lymphoepithelioma may reappear many years after initial therapy. Recurrence in the base of skull or middle cranial fossa may be difficult to diagnose even with CT scan or MRI. Headache and cranial nerve palsies usually indicate recurrence.

Retreatment for recurrence may be rewarding, particularly in the lymphoepitheliomas. Patients have been kept free of local disease for varying lengths of time by irradiation to a limited portal with a high-energy beam or with brachy-

TABLE 21-69.   Guide to Dosage for Primary Nasopharynx Tumors*

	Squamous Cell Carcinoma (cGy)	Lymphoepithelioma (cGy)	Lymphocytic Lymphoma† (cGy)	Histiocytic Lymphoma† (cGy)
T1, T2, early T3	6500	6000	3000	5000
Late T3, T4	7000	6500	3500	6000

Fletcher GH, Million RR: Nasopharynx. In Fletcher GH (ed): Textbook of Radiotherapy, 3rd ed, pp 364–383. Philadelphia, Lea & Febiger, 1980.
  *850–900 cGy/week.
  †See lymphoma chapter for additional information.

TABLE 21-70. Nasopharynx Cancer: Results of Radiation Therapy

Institution (Dates of Treatment)	No. of Patients	5-Year Survival	Percentage of T4 Lesions	Percentage of Lymphoepithelioma
M. D. Anderson Hospital[333] (1954–1977)	251	52% (actuarial)	30	45
University of Florida* (1964–1984)	69	53% (actuarial)	48	29
Stanford[334] (1956–1973)	74	59% (absolute)	11	36
University of California[36] (1940–1968)	146	37% (absolute)		25

*Analysis 1/87 by A. E. Spangler, M.D.

therapy sources inserted into the nasopharynx by mold technique.

RESULTS OF TREATMENT

The 5-year survival rate has improved considerably over the past 30 years. Survival rates of 10% to 30% were reported before the use of supervoltage techniques. Reports from the supervoltage era give encouraging 5-year survival rates in excess of 50% (Table 21-70).[36,333,334] The gains have not come from earlier diagnosis but from better staging of the primary lesion with tomography or CT scan, use of a larger treatment volume, higher doses, and comprehensive irradiation of the neck.

The actuarial local control curves for 69 patients treated at the University of Florida with a follow-up of 2 to 20 years are displayed in Figure 21-22. Eighty-eight percent of patients were Stage IV. The local control rate was better for lymphoepithelioma compared with similar-stage squamous cell carcinomas; the difference was especially noted for T4 lesions. The disease-free survival rate at 5 and 10 years was similar for lymphoepithelioma and squamous cell carcinoma when comparing similar stages (Figure 21-23). Distant metastasis was most closely related to neck stage and occurred in 18%

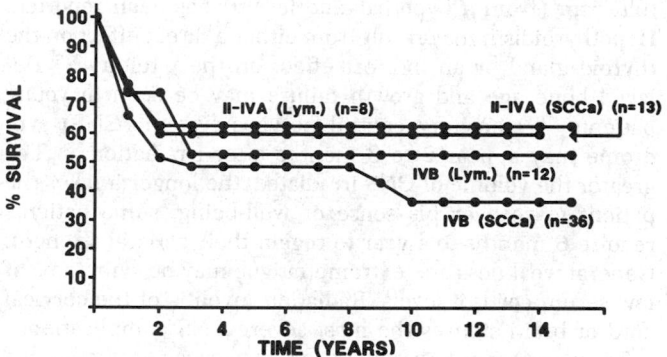

FIG. 21-23. Nasopharynx cancer: disease-free survival by AJCC stage and histology (actuarial method[249]). Lym, lymphoepithelioma; SCCa, squamous cell carcinoma. University of Florida data; patients treated 9/64 to 12/84. (Analysis 1/87 by A.E. Spangler, M.D.)

of N0-N3A patients and 32% of N3B patients. The higher rate of local–regional control for lymphoepithelioma was offset by a higher rate of distant metastasis.

Operative results for juvenile angiofibroma have improved in recent years with the use of arteriography and CT to localize the tumor extent and preoperative arterial occlusion to reduce intraoperative blood loss. Biller and co-workers[335] reported a 93% cure rate with modern techniques.

Briant and co-workers[336] reported the results for irradiation of 45 patients with juvenile angiofibroma treated at the Princess Margaret Hospital. The disease was eventually controlled in all cases. Some 80% of the lesions were controlled by the initial treatment of 3000 cGy to 3500 cGy. Seven patients had their tumors controlled with a second course of radiation therapy and three by operation. No radiation-induced neoplasms have been observed with a follow-up of 2 to 20 years.[337]

FOLLOW-UP POLICY

Follow-up includes careful observation and laboratory testing for possible endocrine hypofunction of the thyroid and pituitary.

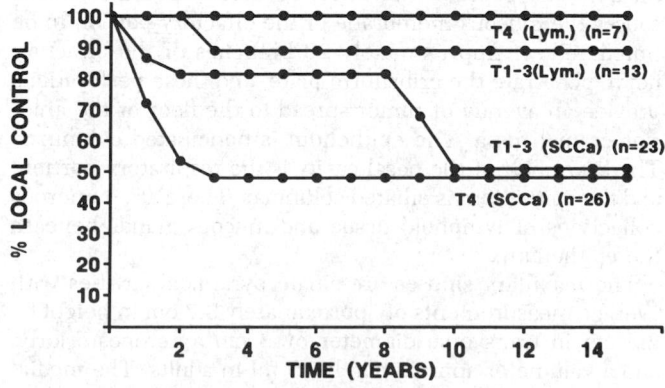

FIG. 21-22. Nasopharynx cancer: local control by stage and histology (actuarial method[249]). Lym, lymphoepithelioma; SCCa, squamous cell carcinoma. University of Florida data; patients treated 9/64 to 12/84. (Analysis 1/87 by A.E. Spangler, M.D.)

Dental care must be closely monitored because of the severe xerostomia.

The neck should be carefully observed because a patient with isolated neck recurrence may be salvaged by neck dissection. Documentation of local recurrence is important, but salvage is rarely possible if high-dose, large-volume treatment has been given initially. Localized recurrence of a lymphoepithelioma may be re-treated, especially if the initial doses were low.

COMPLICATIONS OF TREATMENT

The unavoidable irradiation of part of the brain including the hypothalamus, frontal and temporal lobes, and pituitary to doses between 6000 cGy and 7500 cGy has only rarely been associated with brain necrosis. Primary or secondary hypopituitarism (from a hypothalamic lesion) has been reported. Hypothyroidism may result from either a direct effect on the thyroid gland or an indirect effect on the pituitary.[338] Delayed bone age and growth failure may be seen in young patients. A transitory central nervous system (CNS) syndrome may appear 2 to 3 months after irradiation.[339] The greater the volume of CNS irradiated, the longer it takes the patient to recover his sense of well-being; some patients require 6 months to a year to regain their general strength. General weakness and extreme fatigue may be symptoms of low serum cortisol levels. Radiation myelitis of the cervical cord or brain stem is the most severe CNS complication.

Trismus occurs to varying degrees because of fibrosis and contracture of the pterygoid muscles rather than temporomandibular joint fibrosis. (This complication is more likely in those treated with two opposing portals for the entire course.)

Palsy of cranial nerves IX to XII may occur several years after treatment. This is a problem related to nerve entrapment in the lateral pharyngeal space.

Eye complications (*e.g.*, retrobulbar optic neuritis) may develop owing to irradiation of the optic nerve.

Irradiation of the posterior eyeball to high doses may produce a radiation retinopathy with decreased vision or even total loss of one eye.

NASAL VESTIBULE, NASAL CAVITY, AND PARANASAL SINUSES

Tumors of the nasal vestibule, the anterior entrance to the nasal cavity, are considered separately from nasal cavity tumors because they are essentially skin cancers and have a different natural history.

Primary tumors arising from the nasal cavity and paranasal sinuses are considered together because the lesions are frequently advanced when first seen and it is not always possible to determine the site of origin with certainty. Primary lesions of the lower half of the maxillary sinuses and Stage I lesions of the nasal cavity can be identified as such.

Cancer of the nasal cavity or paranasal sinuses is a relatively rare problem with a yearly risk factor estimated at approximately 1 case for every 100,000 people. These cancers occur more often in men (2:1) and usually appear after the age of 40 except for tumors of minor salivary gland origin or esthesioneuroblastomas, which may even appear before the age of 20.

Nasal cavity and ethmoid sinus adenocarcinomas have been linked to occupations associated with wood dust: the furniture industry, sawmill work, and carpentry. Other occupations with dust-filled work environments such as bootmaking and shoemaking, baking, and the flour milling industry also have been implicated as a cause of adenocarcinomas.[340-343]

Thorotrast, containing the radioactive metal thorium, is a known etiologic agent in maxillary sinus carcinomas. Thorotrast was used in past years as a contrast medium for roentgenographic study of the maxillary sinuses. The Thorotrast was retained in the sinus and was responsible for tumor induction.

Primary carcinomas of the sphenoid sinuses are said to be rare. They mimic nasopharyngeal carcinoma and most often are diagnosed after they penetrate the nasopharynx, at which time they are thought to be advanced nasopharyngeal cancer.

Frontal sinus neoplasms are rare.

ANATOMY

The nasal vestibule is the entrance to the nasal cavity. It is lined by skin in which there are numerous hair follicles and sebaceous glands. The vestibule is a three-sided, pear-shaped cavity about 1.5 cm in diameter that ends posteriorly at the limen nasi. The anterolateral wall is formed by the alar cartilages. The medial wall is the mobile columella, formed by the medial wing of the alar cartilage and the anterior portion of the cartilaginous septum. The floor is the superior surface of the hard palate (maxilla).

The nasal cavity begins at the limen nasi and ends at the posterior nares, where it communicates directly with the nasopharynx. Each lateral wall is composed of thin bony folds that project into the nasal cavity. These are the inferior, medial, and superior nasal turbinates. The nasolacrimal duct enters the nasal cavity beneath the inferior turbinate. The frontal sinus and ethmoid bullae connect to the nasal cavity with openings that lie under the middle turbinate. The sphenoid sinus communicates with the nasal cavity by an opening on the anterior wall of the sphenoid sinus. The olfactory nerves enter the nasal cavity through the cribriform plate and distribute nerve fibers over the upper one third of the septum and superior nasal turbinate, which causes the mucous membrane of the olfactory portion to be tinted yellow. Approximately 20 branches of the olfactory nerve penetrate the cribriform plate, and these perforations provide an avenue of tumor spread to the floor of the anterior cranial fossa. The epithelium is nonciliated columnar. The lower half of the nasal cavity is the respiratory portion, and the epithelium is ciliated columnar. There are numerous collections of lymphoid tissue and mucous glands beneath the epithelium.

The maxillary sinuses are single pyramidal cavities with average measurements of approximately 3.7 cm in height by 2.5 cm in transverse diameter by 3 cm anteroposteriorly, and a volume of approximately 15 ml in adults. The medial wall is the lateral wall of the nasal cavity and has one or two openings that communicate with the middle meatus under the medial turbinate. The inferior wall or floor is the hard palate. The roots of the teeth may penetrate into the cavity. The posterolateral wall is in relation to the zygomatic process and the pterygomaxillary space. The superior wall or roof separates the orbit from the sinus. All walls may be invaded and destroyed by cancer. The medial wall is breached easily by tumor because it is thin, with one or two large natural perforations, and the inferolateral wall may be traversed easily when the roots of the teeth provide partial bone disruption.

The frontal sinuses are two irregular, asymmetrical air cavities separated by a thin bony septum. They connect to the middle meatus of the nasal cavity by the frontonasal duct. Frontal sinus cells may extend far laterally in the orbital process of the frontal bone. They are separated from the anterior ethmoid cells by thin bony walls. The posterior wall separating the frontal sinus from the anterior cranial fossa is quite thick in most patients.

The ethmoid sinuses consist of a number of air cells lying between the medial walls of the orbits and the lateral wall of the nasal cavity. The lateral wall is the lamina papyracea, a very thin, porous bone easily penetrated by tumor. Medially, the ethmoid air cells bulge into the lateral wall of the nasal cavity and form the superior and medial turbinates. The ethmoid cells communicate with the nasal cavity in the middle meatus. These bony walls are thin and easily traversed by tumor. The ethmoid air cells extend quite far anteriorly, and for this reason ethmoid lesions may present as a subcutaneous mass at the inner canthus. The anterior cells actually are covered laterally by the lacrimal bone. The ethmoid bone is porous and presents little resistance to tumor spread. The right and left ethmoid cells are separated anatomically by the midline perpendicular plate of the ethmoid. There is no anatomic barrier between the anterior, middle, and posterior ethmoids.

The sphenoid sinus is a midline structure in the body of the sphenoid bone. The pituitary lies above, the cavernous sinuses laterally, the nasal cavity and ethmoid sinuses in front, and the nasopharynx beneath. The clivus and brain stem lie posteriorly. The pneumatization varies widely and can extend into all portions of the sphenoid bone. The right and left sinuses are partially separated by a septum, but are considered as one in treatment planning as the septum is said to be incomplete and easily penetrated. The sphenoid sinus connects anteriorly with the nasal cavity in the sphenoethmoidal recess.

Lymphatics

NASAL VESTIBULE. The lymphatic trunks run to the submaxillary nodes. There is a small risk for involvement of an intercalated facial node just behind the commissure of the lip along the course of a lymphatic vessel. In addition, preauricular nodes occasionally are involved, especially when tumor invades the lip or skin of the ala nasi.

NASAL CAVITY AND PARANASAL SINUSES. The lymphatics of the nasal cavity are separated into the olfactory group and the respiratory group. According to Rouviere,[3] they do not communicate with each other. There is a connection between the lymphatic network of the olfactory region and the subarachnoid spaces, which allows some absorption of cerebrospinal fluid (CSF) into the lymphatic system.

The lymphatics of the olfactory region of the nasal cavity run posteriorly to terminate in lymph nodes alongside the jugular vein at the base of the skull in the lateral pharyngeal space. The lymphatics of the respiratory nasal cavity also run posteriorly to terminate a bit lower, either in the lateral retropharyngeal node or the subdigastric node. The capillary lymphatic plexus of the nasal mucosa must not be very profuse, judged by the relatively small incidence of metastatic nodes even with advanced disease.

The mucosa of the paranasal sinuses has no capillary lymphatics or a very sparse number of capillary lymphatics. Metastases from carcinoma of the paranasal sinuses are uncommon, even though lesions frequently are quite advanced. It is literally unheard-of for a paranasal sinus tumor to present with cervical lymphadenopathy and an asymptomatic primary lesion confined to a sinus. Metastases probably only occur once tumor has extended beyond the paranasal sinuses to areas containing a supply of capillary lymphatics (e.g., nasopharynx, buccal mucosa, nasal cavity, and skin).

PATHOLOGY

Benign Tumors

Many so-called benign tumors destroy bone and soft tissues and, if uncorrected, cause death. The management of some of these problems is not unlike cancer treatment.

Inflammatory polyps, giant cell reparative granulomas, benign mixed tumors of minor salivary gland origin, benign odontogenic tumors, and necrotizing sialometaplasia are some of the benign lesions appearing in this area.[344]

Malignant Tumors

NASAL VESTIBULE. Almost all malignant tumors arising in the nasal vestibule are squamous cell carcinoma; basal cell carcinoma and adnexal carcinomas are also reported.

NASAL CAVITY AND PARANASAL SINUSES. Squamous cell carcinoma or one of its variants is the most common neoplasm. Minor salivary gland tumors account for about 10% to 15% of neoplasms in this region. Malignant melanoma accounts for less than 1% of all neoplasms of the nasal cavity and paranasal sinuses. Malignant lymphoma, usually histiocytic, occurs in about 5% of cases. It is frequently a locally destructive lesion because it arises more often in bone than in soft tissue.

Esthesioneuroblastoma or olfactory neuroblastoma is a malignant neurogenic tumor that originates from the olfactory mucosa and has a histologic picture resembling adrenal neuroblastoma or retinoblastoma. The normal olfactory epithelium covers the undersurface of the cribriform plate, the upper surface of the middle turbinate, and the superior nasal septum.[276] Histologically, esthesioneuroblastoma may be confused with undifferentiated carcinoma or undifferentiated lymphoma. It occurs at all ages, with cases commonly seen in the second and third decades. A 3-year-old boy with an advanced lesion has been reported; the authors have treated a 12-year-old boy.[345]

A wide range of soft tissue and bone sarcomas is reported for the nasal cavity and paranasal sinus region, including chondrosarcoma, osteosarcoma, Ewing's sarcoma, and most of the soft-tissue sarcomas.

Inverting papilloma of the nasal cavity is a confusing condition often called benign, but for practical reasons it is best classified under malignant because it may have a rather aggressive clinical picture that requires cancer-type management and may be associated with a carcinoma. It is better approached as a "grade ½" neoplasm than as a benign polyp; it may be lethal if uncontrolled. The histologic picture is that of a papilloma that is growing into the stroma rather than growing outward. The histologic appearance does not predict the clinical course. The lesion occurs predominantly in men 40 to 70 years of age. Squamous cell or transitional cell carcinoma is reported in association with inverting papilloma in 5% to 15% of cases and may represent conversion of the papilloma to a more malignant tumor.[346]

Midline lethal granuloma is a rather mysterious, progressively destructive condition that involves the nose, paranasal sinuses, and hard palate, and produces secondary erosion of contiguous structures. Unchecked, the disease is fatal, usually after an extended illness. Death results from extension to the CNS, hemorrhage, sepsis, or inanition. Etiology is debatable. Midline lethal granuloma can be distinguished from Wegener's granulomatosis, which also produces inflammatory and destructive changes in the paranasal sinuses and nasal cavity. Wegener's granulomatosis also involves lung and kidney with a necrotizing vasculitis. Kassel and co-workers[347] subdivide midline lethal granuloma into three different histologic entities: midline malignant reticulosis, malignant lymphoma (usually histocytic lymphoma), and Wegener's granulomatosis.

PATTERNS OF SPREAD

Nasal Vestibule

PRIMARY. Lesions of the nasal vestibule invade the alar and septal cartilages and may extend to the skin surface of the nose. The upper lip is frequently invaded. Posterior growth into the nasal cavity is frequent. Early lesions originating on the columella and anterior septum are often superficial lesions that ulcerate and produce a crust or scab and often present with perforation of the membranous and cartilaginous septum.

LYMPHATIC. Lymph node spread is usually to a solitary ipsilateral submaxillary node, but may be unilateral. The facial, preauricular, and submental nodes are at small risk.

Goepfert and co-workers[348] report only 1 of 26 patients with clinically positive lymph nodes on admission, but 7 patients later developed positive lymph nodes with 4 patients eventually showing bilateral disease. Mendenhall and co-workers[349] reported 2 patients with biopsy-proven lymph nodes out of 22 cases. Another two subsequently developed lymph node metastases. The neck disease was controlled in all 4 cases.

Nasal Cavity and Paranasal Sinuses

NASAL CAVITY. The routes of spread are essentially the same for various histologies, with the exception of esthesioneuroblastoma and minor salivary gland tumors. The latter have a greater propensity for perineural spread, although squamous carcinoma and esthesioneuroblastoma also may follow nerve pathways.

Lesions arising in the olfactory region invade the ethmoids and the orbit, spread through the sievelike cribriform plate to the anterior cranial fossa, and spread between bone and dura. Eventually they penetrate dura and invade the frontal lobes. These lesions also tend to destroy the septum and may invade through nasal bone to the skin. Lesions arising on the lateral wall of the respiratory portion of the nasal cavity invade the medial wall of the maxillary sinus, the ethmoids, and the orbit.

Esthesioneuroblastomas may show submucosal spread and may grow along olfactory nerves and penetrate through an intact dura to the frontal lobe.[350]

The nasopharynx and sphenoid sinus are secondarily invaded in advanced lesions. Tumor may follow the numerous nasal nerves posteriorly and then superiorly toward the sphenopalatine ganglion near the base of the skull or along the maxillary branch of the trigeminal nerve.

MAXILLARY SINUS. All walls of the sinus may be penetrated by tumor. The pattern of spread and bone destruction is largely dependent on site of origin within the sinus. Lesions arising in the anterolateral infrastructure tend to invade through the lateral inferior wall or grow through dental sockets. Cancer presents in the oral cavity when tumor erodes through the maxillary gingiva or into the gingival-buccal sulcus. When tumor erupts through into the oral cavity, the tumor is at first submucosal, causing elevation of the mucosa, loosening of the teeth, or improper seating of a denture. Ulceration follows, with the development of an oral-antral fistula.

Lesions arising on the medial infrastructure readily extend through the thin, porous medial wall into the nasal cavity.

Posterior infrastructure lesions erode through the posterolateral wall and into the infratemporal fossa. The extension is best seen on CT or MRI scan. Recognition of this route of spread is important because tumor escaping posteriorly has immediate access to the base of the skull and may defeat an operative attempt. Extension of lesions to the orbit occurs either directly through the roof of the maxillary sinus, by a circuitous route through the ethmoids and lamina papyracea, or by way of the infratemporal fossa and then through the infraorbital fissure.

Tumors arising in the upper half (suprastructure) of the antrum have two general patterns of development. One group develops laterally, invades the malar bone, and produces a mass just below the lateral floor of the orbit. The soft-tissue mass may become quite large and eventually ulcerate through to the skin, producing an antrocutaneous fistula. The orbit is invaded laterally and displaces the eye inward and upward. The temporal fossa is often involved, as is the zygomatic bone in very advanced lesions.

The suprastructural cancers that develop medially invade the nasal cavity, ethmoid and frontal sinuses, lacrimal apparatus, and medial inferior orbit. It is often impossible to determine whether the origin is maxillary antrum, nasal cavity, or ethmoid.

ETHMOID SINUSES. Lesions of the ethmoid sinuses have many options for local spread because of their location and thin, porous bony walls, none of which offers particular resistance to tumor penetration. The lamina papyracea is the lateral wall for the middle and posterior ethmoid air cells. Invasion through the lamina papyracea into the medial orbit is common. The anterior ethmoid cells are covered laterally by the small, thin lacrimal bone and the frontal process of the maxilla. Thus, the ethmoid air cells extend anteriorly within a centimeter of the inner canthus.[351]

The medial surfaces of the ethmoid labyrinth are the middle and superior nasal conchae, which are formed by thin, convoluted bone; spread into the nasal cavity is common. The more advanced lesions invade the maxillary antrum, nasopharynx, sphenoid sinus, and anterior cranial fossa.

SPHENOID SINUS. There is little information regarding spread patterns for tumors arising in the sphenoid sinus. It is probable that some of the advanced nasopharyngeal lesions are, in reality, primary sphenoid sinus lesions. The fact that a disproportionate number of advanced nasopharynx lesions have no neck metastases is suggestive of their origin in the sphenoid sinus, a site with sparse, if any, capillary lymphatics.

The sphenoid sinus is in close relationship with the cranial nerves in the cavernous sinus: III, IV, and VI, and the ophthalmic and maxillary branches of the trigeminal nerve (Fig. 21-24). Cranial nerve palsies and headache are frequently

FIG. 21-24. Coronal section of the cavernous sinus.

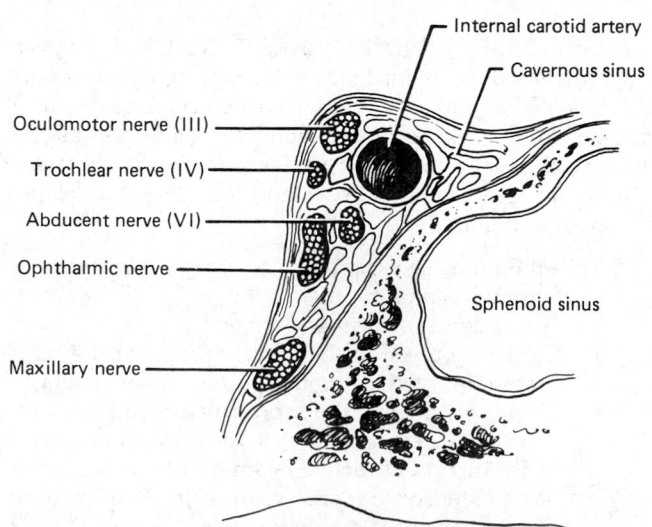

- Internal carotid artery
- Cavernous sinus
- Oculomotor nerve (III)
- Trochlear nerve (IV)
- Abducent nerve (VI)
- Ophthalmic nerve
- Sphenoid sinus
- Maxillary nerve

the first clinical evidence of a sphenoid sinus tumor. Diagnosis is usually made, however, when tumor eventually breaks through into the nasopharynx or nasal cavity where it can be seen and biopsied.

INVERTING PAPILLOMA. A report of 223 cases of inverting papilloma showed that the lateral nasal wall was the most commonly involved site (68%), with ethmoid and maxillary sinus involvement also common (57%), as was involvement of the septum (28%). However, ethmoid and maxillary sinus involvement without tumor of the lateral nasal wall occurred in only 4%. Intracranial extension was usually associated with a carcinoma. Tumor occurred bilaterally when there was spread through the nasal septum; multicentric sites of origin were reported.[352] There are two reports in the literature of cervical metastases from benign-appearing inverted papilloma; the metastases had the microscopic appearance of inverting papilloma.[353,354]

LYMPHATIC. The incidence of lymphatic metastases on admission is 10% to 15% for nasal cavity and ethmoid sinus tumors and probably even lower for antral and sphenoid tumors. The risk of lymphatic metastases is related to extension of tumor outside the sinus to areas with capillary lymphatics. Maxillary sinus tumors that invade the oral cavity and involve the buccal mucosa, maxillary gingiva, or hard palate may spread to the submandibular and jugulodigastric nodes. Lesions that invade the nasal cavity or naropharynx spread posteriorly to the parapharyngeal nodes and then to the jugulodigastric area. Esthesioneuroblastoma, minor salivary gland tumors, melanoma, and sarcomas have an unknown rate of lymph node metastasis.

CLINICAL PICTURE

Nasal Vestibule

These lesions present with symptoms of a slow-growing mass in the entrance to the nose with attendant crusting, scabbing, and occasional minor bleeding. Pain, if it occurs, is usually modest, even with destruction of cartilage or involvement of the lip. Secondary infection may occur, in which case the nose is painful on manipulation. Septal perforation may occur.

Nasal Cavity and Paranasal Sinuses

NASAL CAVITY. The earliest symptoms of nasal cavity neoplasm are a low-grade chronic infection with discharge, obstruction, and minor, intermittent bleeding. The symptoms mimic those associated with nasal polyps; because many of the patients with nasal neoplasms have a previous history of nasal operations for polyps, cancer is often missed in an early stage. The patient often complains of "sinus trouble" and intermittent anterior headache. Subsequent symptoms depend on pattern of growth. Lesions arising in the olfactory region may cause unilateral or bilateral nasal expansion of the bridge of the nose, and a submucosal mass may appear near the inner canthus and eventually ulcerate. Obstruction of the nasolacrimal system may be a presenting complaint, with the patient treated by incision and drainage for a dacryocystitis. Extension through the cribriform plate or onto the ethmoid sinuses is accompanied by frontal headache. Aberration of smell is rare.

Invasion of the medial orbit produces proptosis and diplopia; a mass may be palpated in the orbit. Indirect examination of the nasopharynx may show early submucosal invasion through the posterior nares.

MAXILLARY SINUS. These cancers develop silently when they are confined to the sinus and produce symptoms on extension through the walls. If the tumor invades toward the oral cavity, the presenting symptoms relate to pain associated with the upper teeth; there may be loosening and eventually loss of teeth. The dentist is often the first one consulted, and the patient may have dental extraction without pain relief. Tumor may penetrate into the gingivobuccal sulcus or upper gum and eventually progress to an oral-antral fistula. If the patient wears upper dentures, the first symptom will be an ill-fitting denture. Palpation and observation of the face may show a mass. Early invasion of the floor of the orbit may be detected by feeling both orbits simultaneously with the tips of the index fingers inserted between the bony rim and eyeball. Posterior invasion of the orbit will produce proptosis, diplopia, and edema of the conjunctiva. Invasion of the inferior orbital nerve or its branches in the floor of the orbit may cause paresthesias or anesthesia of the skin of the lower eyelid, side of the nose, and anterior premaxillary skin. Nasal obstruction and bleeding are common complaints, along with "sinus pain" or "fullness" over the involved antrum. Trismus and headache are associated with invasion posteriorly into the pterygopalatine fossa, pterygoid muscles, infratemporal fossa, and base of the skull.

Cancers developing in the medial suprastructure of the antrum present with nasal symptoms of discharge or bleeding, mild infraorbital pain, infected lacrimal sac, and displacement of the eye upward and laterally with proptosis, diplopia, and conjunctival edema.

Cancer developing in the lateral suprastructure produces a mass below the lateral canthus with associated pain. The eye may be deviated medially and upward when orbital invasion occurs. There is edema of the conjunctiva, narrowing of the palpebral opening, diplopia, and proptosis. Tumor may extend to the temporal fossa, producing a diffuse fullness.

ETHMOID SINUSES. Mild to moderate sinus ache or pain referred to the frontal-nasal area is an early symptom. A painless mass may present near the inner canthus; the mass may become infected and be interpreted as a boil or dacryocystitis, at which time an inappropriate incision and drainage procedure is done. Diplopia develops with invasion of the medial orbit. Proptosis is often present, and a mass may be felt by digital palpation of the orbit. Nasal discharge, epistaxis, and obstruction are frequent presenting complaints. Paresthesias may occur over the distribution of sensory nerves.

Physical examination includes anterior and posterior rhinoscopy after thorough shrinking of the nasal mucosa. A fiberoptic nasoscope is a great aid in visualizing the posterior and superior nasal cavity and the nasopharynx. Early inva-

sion of the nasal cavity may produce only submucosal bulging into the superior or medial meatus, which is easily confused with allergic rhinitis, polyps, or inflammatory changes. Pus may be seen coming from beneath the superior, middle, or inferior turbinate.

Eye examination includes palpation of the orbit for masses. Palpation should be carried out simultaneously in both orbits because the changes in the involved orbit are frequently subtle. Extraocular movements are examined and proptosis is measured.

Invasion into the nasopharynx is usually submucosal and appears on the roof and lateral wall. Advanced lesions may obstruct the eustachian canal.

METHODS OF DIAGNOSIS AND STAGING

Biopsy Technique

Tumor in the nasal cavity is biopsied with punch forceps. Biopsy of tumor in the maxillary antrum is usually approached through a Caldwell-Luc procedure, which is an incision through the gingivobuccal sulcus opposite the premolars. The approach allows adequate visualization of the entire antrum.

Biopsy of ethmoid tumors is usually taken from the extension to the nasal cavity or inner canthus area. Tumor confined to the ethmoids may be found unexpectedly at the time of a lateral rhinotomy planned for diagnosis or treatment of benign disease.

An undiagnosed orbital mass occasionally may be the site of biopsy because of incomplete examination of other areas. Sphenoid sinus tumors are biopsied by way of the transnasal route for the rare localized disease, but biopsy is usually made of an extension to the nasopharynx or nasal cavity. Frontal sinus tumors are approached by supraorbital incision and osteotomy.

Staging

NASAL VESTIBULE. The staging used for skin cancer is appropriate for this area. CT and MRI scans are useful for advanced or recurrent lesions.

NASAL CAVITY AND PARANASAL SINUSES. Physical examination alone is inadequate for staging these tumors. CT and MRI scans are essential for determining extent of disease. MRI is particularly helpful to obtain sagittal and coronal planes, to eliminate artifacts from metals, and to distinguish pus from tumor in a sinus. Maxillary sinus cancer is staged as follows:[12]

TX   Minimum requirements to assess the primary tumor cannot be met
T0   No evidence of primary tumor
T1   Tumor confined to the antral mucosa of the infrastructure with no bone erosion or destruction
T2   Tumor confined to the suprastructure mucosa without bone destruction, or to the infrastructure with destruction of medial or inferior bony walls only
T3   More extensive tumor invading skin of cheek, orbit, anterior ethmoid sinuses, or pterygoid muscle

T4   Massive tumor with invasion of cribriform plate, posterior ethmoids, sphenoid, nasopharynx, pterygoid plates, or base of skull

There is no AJCC staging system for nasal cavity or ethmoid, sphenoid, or frontal sinus cancer. The following system, based on prognostic factors that seemed to correlate best with response to treatment, was adopted at the University of Florida:

I   Limited to site of origin
II   Extension to adjacent sites (*e.g.*, orbit, nasopharynx, paranasal sinuses, skin, pterygomaxillary fossa)
III   Base of skull or pterygoid plate destruction, or intracranial extension, or both

TREATMENT

Nasal Vestibule

SELECTION OF TREATMENT MODALITY. Both surgical resection and radiation therapy produce a high degree of success in experienced hands.[348,355,356] Radiation therapy is usually the preferred treatment because of the deformity produced by excision. Excision is preferred for very small lesions, the removal of which will not produce cosmetic deformity or require reconstruction; few lesions fit this description. Radiation therapy is selected for the remainder, with surgery reserved for radiation failure. Radiation therapy has been successful in salvaging surgical failures, but the nasal deformity has already been produced and the value of irradiation lost.

SURGICAL TREATMENT. Excision of lesions in the nasal vestibule usually involves removal of cartilage as well as skin. Depending on the site of the lesion, either the columella, the septum, or the alar cartilages will have to be removed, with a resulting cosmetic deformity that is difficult to reconstruct. If the alar cartilage has been sacrificed, either a composite graft consisting of skin and cartilage from the ear or a nasolabial flap can be used to repair the defect. If the entire external nose is resected, a prosthesis is used.

IRRADIATION TECHNIQUE. External beam, interstitial, or a combination of both may be used.

There are two basic external beam treatment plans: opposed lateral portals and single anterior portal. When the tumor volume can be encompassed by lateral portals, there is an advantage in avoiding unnecessary exit irradiation to the nasal cavity, nasopharynx, and CNS. This technique confines irradiation to the anterior nasal area, but has the disadvantage of full skin reaction because a wax bolus nose block is necessary to ensure homogeneous irradiation. The portals may be angled posteriorly to ensure sufficient posterior coverage; wedges are added to compensate for the angle. Fractionation schemes are those used for orthovoltage because the bolus produces skin reactions comparable to orthovoltage therapy.

The anterior portal technique uses a single anterior portal with a combination of photons and electrons. A wax bolus is used to ensure a homogeneous dose. The advantages of this technique are that the portal may be shaped, it is easier to shield the eyes, and the skin of the tip of the nose and sometimes the bridge of the nose need not be covered by the wax and therefore some of the skin receives a lesser dose of radiation.[349,356]

Interstitial implants of the nasal vestibule and nasal cavity are highly individualized. The basic implant is usually composed of two, three, or four planes of sources inserted through the skin surface of the external nose. The basic arrangement to cover the entire nasal vestibule and upper lip is shown in Figure 21-25. The dose has varied, depending on the size of the lesion.[349,356]

Nasal Cavity

SELECTION OF TREATMENT MODALITY. The histology, extent, and location of the malignant tumor in the nasal cavity are all considered when treatment decisions are made.

Inverting papilloma is treated initially by surgical excision. The local recurrence rate is fairly high, and subsequent excisions may be required. When the lesion begins to act aggressively with rapid recurrences and invasion of the sinuses, orbit, and anterior cranial fossa, it should be considered a low-grade cancer and treated appropriately by more radical removal. Irradiation is recommended for lesions that are surgically unresectable, for patients with multiple recur-

FIG. 21-25. Diagram of interstitial implant for carcinoma of the nasal vestibule.

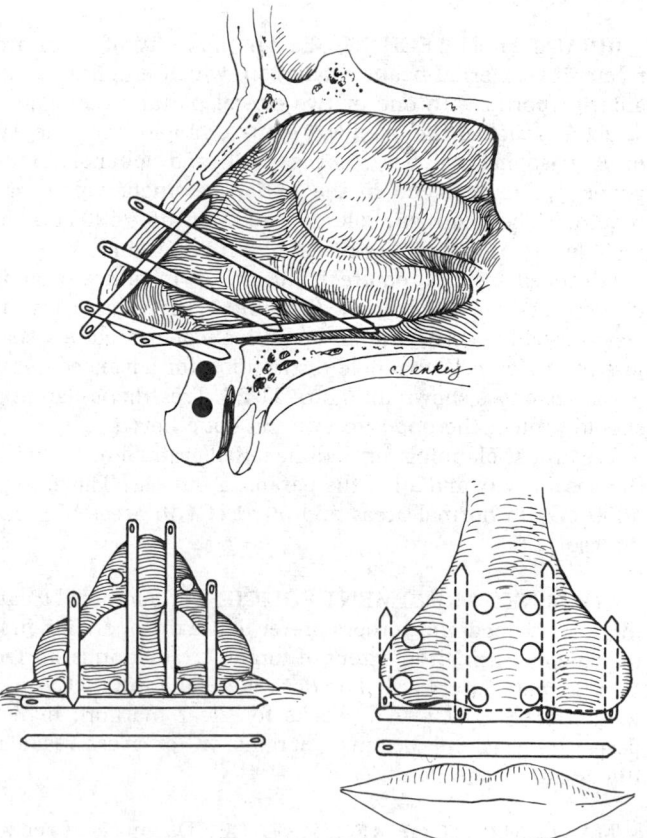

rences, and for those in which carcinoma is found in the specimen.[346,352]

Squamous cell carcinoma and adenocarcinoma of the nasal cavity can be treated with surgery, irradiation, or both. Most analyses of nasal cavity carcinomas are included with paranasal sinus cancer series. Because standardized staging is not applied, it is difficult to compare the results of various therapies. Regional and distant metastases are relatively uncommon, and therefore, local control is tantamount to cure.

Either surgery or radiation therapy is used for discrete early lesions. Operative management may be indicated for early lesions, in which good surgical margins can be expected without cosmetic or functional loss. Excision is also the treatment of choice for melanomas and sarcomas. Radiation therapy is used for the majority of nasal cavity carcinomas because of the difficulty in obtaining en bloc removal of the more advanced lesions and reasonably good results with irradiation. Combined therapy may be recommended in selected cases.

Midline lethal granuloma is treated by radiation therapy to the nasal cavity and all of the paranasal sinuses.

SURGICAL TREATMENT. Lateral rhinotomy provides the best access for resection of lesions of the nasal cavity. Generally reconstruction is not necessary unless the entire cartilaginous septum has been removed, in which case there will be a saddle deformity of the nose. The lateral wall of the nose may be removed by this approach for resection of inverting papilloma and other localized neoplasms. More advanced lesions require removal of involved sinuses and orbit. A craniofacial procedure may be required.

IRRADIATION TECHNIQUE. The majority of cases are treated by external beam irradiation, which emphasizes an anterior portal with one or two lateral portals. Contiguous structures such as the maxillary sinus, ethmoid sinus, medial orbit, nasopharynx, base of the skull, and sphenoid sinus generally are included in the initial treatment volume as required. The treatment volume is reduced after 5000 cGy to include the original gross disease with a margin.

Advanced lesions require inclusion of an entire orbit if tumor grossly invades the medial orbit; in these cases, loss of vision usually occurs, but an operation would require visual loss in any case. A two-field distribution for advanced nasal cavity lesions is shown in Figure 21-26. Treatment planning should protect the opposite eye and optic nerve.

Treatment planning for midline lethal granuloma includes the nasal cavity and all of the paranasal sinuses. The dose is 4000 cGy to normal areas and 5000 cGy to areas of gross disease.

COMBINED TREATMENT POLICIES. If combined treatment is planned, the authors prefer to use the operation first to avoid obscuring the extent of tumor. Irradiation is started 4 to 6 weeks afterward. The dose is usually 6000 cGy in 6 weeks to 6500 cGy in 7 weeks for clear margins; higher doses are used for positive margins or for gross residual tumor after operation.

MANAGEMENT OF RECURRENCE. Diagnosis of recurrent lesions is important because salvage may be possible.

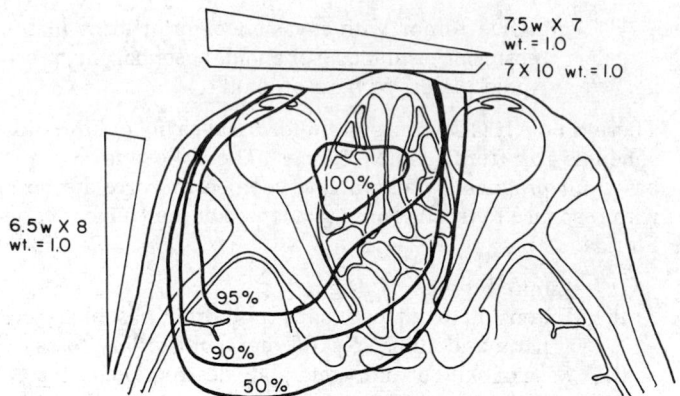

FIG. 21-26. Isodose distribution for carcinoma of the nasal cavity or ethmoid sinus with invasion of the orbit.

Once the patient has had an operation or irradiation, it is difficult to determine the extent of recurrent disease because of changes from the previous therapy. The most common situation for salvage is a radiation or surgical failure that can be treated successfully by a craniofacial resection. Tumor extension to the sphenopalatine fossa with definite destruction of a pterygoid plate is a relative contraindication to a craniofacial procedure. Cranial nerve involvement, invasion posteriorly near the optic chiasm, and sphenoid sinus or cavernous sinus invasion are absolute contraindications to resection. MRI can distinguish between exudate and gross tumor in a sinus, but surgical exploration may be necessary to exclude microscopic extension to the sinuses. The anterior wall of the sphenoid sinus may be removed, but the sinus itself cannot be resected.[357] Postoperative irradiation should be considered whether or not margins are positive. About 25% of patients may be saved by this approach.

Maxillary Sinus

SELECTION OF TREATMENT MODALITY. Surgical resection gives the best results. Early infrastructural lesions may be excised and cured by surgery alone, but for most other cases, irradiation is given postoperatively even if margins are negative. Extension of cancer to the base of the skull, nasopharynx, or sphenoid sinus contraindicates surgical excision. The pterygoid process below the foramen rotundum may be removed along with the attached pterygoid muscles, but destruction of the sphenoid bone above this point is a contraindication to operation. Operations to resect portions of the base of the skull are described for special clinical situations.

SURGICAL TREATMENT. Surgery for carcinoma of the maxillary sinus depends on which walls are involved. If the floor of the orbit is free of disease, then the eye and the orbital rim may be left undisturbed. If, however, there is involvement through the floor of the orbit, then a maxillectomy and orbital exenteration must be performed. If the posterior wall or the pterygoid plates are involved, they too must be included in the resection. A split-thickness skin graft is used to line the cavity, and a dental prosthesis then is used to fill the resulting deformity in the palate. The prosthesis is constructed prior to surgery so that it can be placed at the time of operation and act as a stent. The permanent prosthesis is constructed about 6 months after the operation.

IRRADIATION TECHNIQUE. Irradiation treatment planning includes the entire maxilla, the adjacent nasal cavity, ethmoid sinus, nasopharynx, and pterygopalatine fossa. All or part of the orbit is included in patients with extension into or near the orbital fossa; failure to include the orbital contents is one of the most common causes of failure. The prescribed dose is 6500 cGy to 7000 cGy for irradiation alone. The dose for preoperative irradiation varies from 5000 cGy to 6000 cGy, and the dose for postoperative irradiation varies from 6000 cGy to 7000 cGy. If radiation therapy alone is planned, localized drainage procedures can be done before, during, or after radiation therapy, as dictated by clinical necessity.

COMBINED TREATMENT POLICIES. Except for the early infrastructural lesion, surgical resection is usually followed by external beam radiation therapy.

Ethmoid Sinus

SELECTION OF TREATMENT MODALITY. Ethmoid sinus lesions are usually extensive when first diagnosed. Radiation therapy alone produces better results than surgery alone and is the preferred single treatment.[358] If resection is feasible with acceptable functional and cosmetic results, then the operation is carried out, followed by postoperative radiation therapy even if the margins are clear.

SURGICAL TREATMENT. Localized lesions require resection of the ethmoids and the ipsilateral maxilla and orbit. Extensive lesions are removed by a craniofacial procedure.

IRRADIATION TECHNIQUE. Radiation treatment is entirely by external beam, emphasizing treatment through an anterior field combined with one or two lateral fields. This field arrangement, weighted 2:1 or 3:1 in favor of the anterior field, provides adequate treatment of the tumor volume while avoiding excessive irradiation of the contralateral eye and optic nerve. Wedges are added to achieve a satisfactory dose distribution. Electrons should not be used for the anterior portal.

MANAGEMENT OF RECURRENCE. Recurrent disease is heralded by recurrent pain and cranial nerve palsies. Exploration of the sinuses is necessary for diagnosis.

Localized recurrence after surgery only may be managed by radiation therapy alone or craniofacial resection and postoperative radiation therapy. Radiation therapy failures may be suitable for maxillectomy or craniofacial resection.

Sphenoid Sinus

The treatment is with radiation therapy, and the technique is similar to that for advanced carcinoma of the nasopharynx.

RESULTS OF TREATMENT

Nasal Vestibule

Goepfert and co-workers[348] reviewed the M. D. Anderson Hospital experience of 26 patients with squamous cell carcinoma of the nasal vestibule. The absolute 5-year survival was 78%. Ten patients were treated initially by surgery; one developed a local recurrence and was salvaged by radiation therapy. Sixteen patients were treated by radiation therapy; three developed local recurrence, and two were salvaged by an operation.

Mendenhall and co-workers[349] reviewed 22 patients treated by irradiation at the University of Florida for squamous cell carcinoma of the nasal vestibule; 7 had recurrent disease after one to four previous surgical excisions, and 15 had had no prior treatment. Eleven patients had obvious cartilage invasion, two had bone destruction, and three had massive infiltration of the soft tissues of the face (Table 21-71). Two patients had biopsy-proven lymph node metastases on admission, and both were cured by radiation therapy. Two patients subsequently developed a single submandibular node that was controlled by radical neck dissection; they were alive at 9 and 16 years postsurgery. Radiation therapy complications were minor. There was no example of persistent chondritis or soft-tissue necrosis. The 5-year actuarial determinate survival rate was 95%, and the 10-year and 15-year rate was 82%.

Nasal Cavity and Ethmoid Sinus

INVERTING PAPILLOMA. Weissler and co-workers[352] reported 233 cases of inverting papilloma seen over a 35-year period. One hundred thirty-four patients had at least 1 year of follow-up. The risk of recurrence was 71% in patients who had an intranasal procedure. The recurrence rate was 56% for those having a Caldwell-Luc approach. Patients having a lateral rhinotomy had the smallest incidence of recurrence (29%). Reports from more modern series show an even lower incidence of recurrence when a lateral rhinotomy approach was used.[359]

TABLE 21-71. Nasal Vestibule Carcinoma: Local Control by Radiation Therapy

| | No. Controlled/No. Treated | |
T Stage	De novo	Recurrent
Tx	1/1	
T1	4/4	2/2
T2	1/1	1/1
T3	1/1	1/1*
T4	6/8*†	2/3†
Total	13/15	6/7

Mendenhall NP, Parsons JT, Cassisi NJ, et al: Carcinoma of the nasal vestibule treated with radiation therapy. Laryngoscope 97:626–632, 1987.

University of Florida data. Patients treated 1964 to 1984; minimum 2-year follow-up.

*Two patients had biopsy-proven lymph node metastases on admission.

†None of the 3 failures was salvaged.

Weissler and co-workers[352] also reported 6 patients who received radiation therapy for benign inverting papilloma and 9 for inverting papilloma associated with malignant disease. Twelve of the 15 patients had a complete response to radiation therapy and were free of disease for long periods of follow-up.

Mendenhall and co-workers[346] also reported success with radiation therapy. Their series has been recently updated (Mendenhall WM: Personal communication, 1987), and there are a total of seven patients who received radiation therapy for inverting papilloma. All but one were treated for recurrent disease after one or more operations, and two had foci of carcinoma. Six of the 7 patients remained free of disease at 3, 5, 7, 7, 9, and 14 years. One patient died of persistent disease 17 months after radiation therapy. In one patient treated with preoperative radiation therapy followed by surgery, there was no tumor in the specimen. Two of the patients had surgery followed by immediate irradiation for residual disease and 4 patients were treated with radiation therapy alone.

CARCINOMA. Frazell and Lewis[360] reported a 56% 5-year cure rate for 68 nasal cavity neoplasms treated surgically. The 5-year cure rate by radiation therapy was 18% for 28 patients treated. The selection and stage of patients for each modality were not analyzed. Frazell and Lewis[360] reported that 40% of patients (4 of 10) with ethmoid sinus carcinoma treated by radiation therapy were cured at 5 years, but only 4 of 21 patients treated by an operation were cured. They concluded, however, that the operation was the treatment of choice.

Cheesman and co-workers[361] selected craniofacial resection for 54 patients with a variety of malignant tumors of the nasal cavity and paranasal sinuses; the majority were recurrent after surgery, radiation therapy, or chemotherapy. The operative mortality was 5%. Seven of 25 patients were free of disease with a minimum of 3 years of follow-up.

Bosch and co-workers[362] reported their experience with 40 cases of cancer of the nasal cavity. Eighty-five percent were treated by radiation therapy. The 5-year survival rate was 56% for the entire group and 50% for those treated by radiation therapy alone.

Boone and co-workers[363] reported the M. D. Anderson Hospital experience for 28 patients with nasal cavity carcinoma. The 5-year absolute cure rate was 64%; the local recurrence rate was 21%.

Parsons and co-workers[364] reviewed the results for 48 patients with malignant tumors of the nasal cavity, ethmoid sinus, and sphenoid sinus treated from October 1964 through December 1983 by radiation therapy. Forty-two patients were treated by radiation therapy only and 7 by combined surgery and radiation therapy. Of the 42 patients treated by radical courses of irradiation, 37 had de novo lesions and 5 had postsurgical recurrences. Twenty-one percent presented with clinical evidence of advanced orbital invasion, and 12 others had only radiographic evidence of orbital extension. The actuarial local control results at 5, 10, and 15 years by histology are shown in Table 21-72 and the local control rates[249] by stage are shown in Figure 21-27. Although adenoid cystic carcinomas were initially responsive, late-onset recurrence was the rule. The overall 10-year actuarial local control rate for 42 patients with histologies other than adenoid cystic carcinoma was 52% for all stages combined. Eight patients had evidence of intracranial extension prior to irradiation, and in three the disease remains locally controlled at 3.5, 4, and 9 years following treatment of adenocarcinoma (1 patient) or esthesioneuroblastoma (2 patients). Forty-four patients presented with a clinically neg-

FIG. 21-27. Carcinoma of the nasal cavity and paranasal sinuses: actuarial[249] local control according to tumor stage for all histologies combined. Failures after 5 years are due to minor salivary gland tumors. (Parsons JT, Mendenhall WM, Mancuso AA, et al: Malignant tumors of the nasal cavity and ethmoid and sphenoid sinuses. Int J Radiat Oncol Biol Phys Int J Radiat Oncol Biol Phys 14:11–22, 1988)

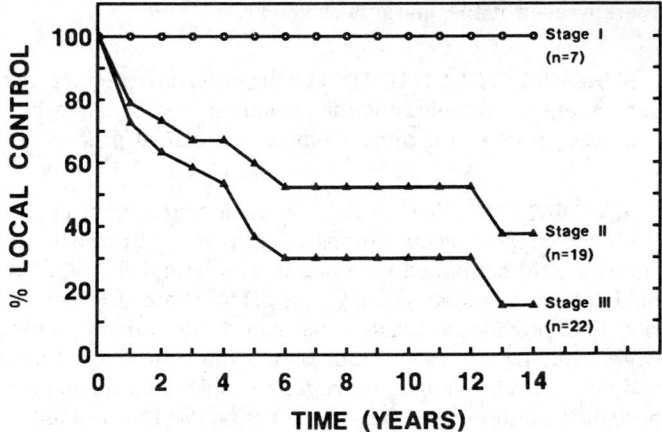

TABLE 21-72.   Actuarial Local Control After Radiation Therapy in Nasal Cavity and Ethmoid/Sphenoid Sinus Cancer (All Stages; 2-Year Minimum Follow-up)

Type of Tumor	No. of Patients	Actuarial Local Control (%)		
		5 Years	10 Years	15 Years
Squamous cell carcinoma	21	45	45	45
Esthesioneuroblastoma	8	43	43	
Minor salivary gland tumors (excluding adenoid cystic)	8	75	75	45
Adenoid cystic	6	65	30	18
Miscellaneous (melanoma, sarcoma)	5	60	60	60

Data from Parsons et al.[364]

ative neck. Elective neck irradiation was given to 22 patients who were thought to be at risk for occult disease in the neck, and none developed recurrence in the neck. Of 22 patients who did not receive elective neck irradiation, 2 developed lymph node metastases in the absence of primary failure, and both were successfully salvaged with a radical neck dissection. Of 4 patients who presented with clinically positive lymph nodes, no neck failures occurred following high-dose radiotherapy alone. Four patients died of distant metastases alone with apparent disease control above the clavicles. Actuarial survival rates for the entire group at 5, 10, 15, and 20 years were 52%, 30%, 22%, and 22%. The 10-year continuously disease-free survival rate for Stage I was 86%, for Stage II, 42%, and for Stage III, 22%. The single failure among the Stage I patients was a submandibular lymph node metastasis at 10 months that was successfully salvaged by radical neck dissection, resulting in 100% survival for Stage I patients. Surgical salvage of local failure was successful in two of eight attempts.

ESTHESIONEUROBLASTOMA. Elkon and co-workers[365] reviewed the world literature on esthesioneuroblastoma and compiled the results of 78 cases (Table 21-73). They concluded that either radiation therapy or surgery was sufficient treatment for early-stage disease, but that combined treatment might be advantageous for late-stage presentations. The 5-year absolute survival rate was 75% for Stage A, 60% for Stage B, and 41% for Stage C.

The Mayo Clinic reviewed 21 cases of esthesioneuroblastoma seen between 1960 and 1980. The 5-year survival rate was 58% with only 4 of 19 patients being continuously free of disease for 7 to 16 years after initial surgery. Local recurrence occurred in 57%. Extension to the brain was noted in 10 patients, 3 at the time of diagnosis and 7 after the initial treatment. The overall rate of cervical metastases was 48%.[350]

Shah and Feghali[366] analyzed the Memorial Sloan-Kettering Cancer Center results for 31 patients seen between 1949 and 1975; there was a 5-year minimum follow-up. The 5-year survival rate was 52% with only 2 patients continuously free of disease. The 5-year survival rates by stage were Stage A, 5 of 6; Stage B, 2 of 6; and Stage C, 9 of 19. Fourteen were

successfully salvaged to date after local or regional recurrence. Late recurrence after 5 years was seen.

Fauci and co-workers[367] reported the results of ten patients with midline lethal granuloma treated by high-dose irradiation. Long-term remissions occurred in seven patients. Four patients developed malignancies at other sites.

Maxillary Sinus

Jesse[368] reviewed 87 patients with squamous cell carcinoma of the maxillary antrum. The 3-year survival rate was about 30% for all cases, including 15 treated for palliation only and 9 that were too advanced for any treatment. Sixty-three were treated for cure with a 3-year survival rate of 44%. Three-year survival after surgery alone for selected lesions was 9 of 20 patients. Patients selected for combined treatment had either preoperative or postoperative irradiation; the results were similar for both techniques. The local recurrence rate with combined treatment was 38%. Patients with infrastructural lesions and superolateral lesions had a 3-year survival rate of 13 of 19 (68%), whereas those with superomedial or superoposterior lesions had a survival rate of only 29%.

Bataini and Ennuyer[369] reported Curie Foundation results for 31 patients with carcinoma of the maxillary antrum treated by supervoltage radiation therapy between 1959 and 1965. Only three patients had limited primary disease; 30% had clinically positive lymph nodes. The 3- and 5-year survival rates were 39% and 32%, respectively.

COMPLICATIONS OF TREATMENT

Surgery

Complications of maxillectomy include failure of the split-thickness skin graft to heal, trismus, cerebrospinal fluid leak, and hemorrhage.

Complications of ethmoid sinus surgery include hemorrhage, meningitis, CSF leak, cellulitis and pansinusitis, brain abscess, and stroke. Complications of the craniofacial procedure are reported by Ketcham and co-workers.[357] About one third of the patients had a life-threatening complication requiring intensive care and prolonged hospitalization. Opera-

TABLE 21-73.   Esthesioneuroblastoma: Results of Treatment to Primary Tumor by Modality and Stage for 78 Patients with Follow-up of 6 Months to 32 Years (No. Controlled/No. Treated)

Modality	Stage A—Confined to Nasal Cavity		Stage B—Confined to Nasal Cavity and Paranasal Sinuses		Stage C—Beyond Nasal Cavity and Paranasal Sinuses	
	Initial Treatment	For Recurrent Disease at Primary Site	Initial Treatment	For Recurrent Disease at Primary Site	Initial Treatment	For Recurrent Disease at Primary Site
Radiation therapy alone	3/5	5/5	6/7	3/4	1/5	1/1
Surgery alone	5/9	2/2	3/6		1/1	0/0
Radiation therapy and surgery	9/10	0/0	15/20	0/1	7/15	0/0
Ultimate local control	24/24 (100%)		27/33 (82%)		10/21 (48%)	

Modified from Elkon D, Hightower SI, Lim ML, et al: Esthesioneuroblastoma. Cancer 44:1087–1094, 1979.

tive mortality was 4%. Complications included meningitis, subdural abscess, CSF leak, diplopia, and hemorrhage. Most of these patients had recurrent or far-advanced disease prior to surgery.

Radiation Therapy

Eye complications are the most frequent and bothersome of the complications of radiation therapy.[370,371] When only a portion of the ipsilateral eyeball is irradiated (medial one third), it is possible to preserve vision in the majority of patients. When there is gross disease in the orbit, however, the entire eyeball is irradiated to a high dose with almost certain loss of vision; however, these same patients would require orbital exenteration if treated by surgery. The actuarial probability of unilateral blindness at 10 years was 65% for 48 patients treated by radiation therapy for carcinomas of the nasal cavity or ethmoid or sphenoid sinus, and the probability of bilateral blindness was about 18% at 10 years.[364] The risk for bilateral blindness can be greatly reduced by use of CT and MRI scans for improved treatment planning and through knowledge of the tolerance of the optic nerve.[371]

A few patients will develop a transitory CNS syndrome that includes vertigo, headaches, decreased cerebration, and lethargy. This syndrome usually appears 2 to 3 months after completion of treatment, but has been seen as late as 12 to 15 months after completion of radiation therapy. The early-appearing CNS syndromes usually last 1 to 2 months, but the late-appearing syndromes last 6 to 12 months before slowly resolving.

Aseptic meningitis, chronic sinusitis, or serous otitis media can occur. High-dose irradiation of the nasal cavity can cause narrowing and synechiae of the nasal cavity. Douching with salt water and daily self-dilations with petrolatum-coated cotton swabs will reduce the problem.

Septal perforations occur when tumor has destroyed part of the septum. These do not usually require treatment and may heal spontaneously.

Destruction of the nasal bone and septum by tumor may result in cosmetic deformity. Two patients had successful reconstructive rhinoplasties after 7000 cGy.

Maxillary necrosis may develop if dental extraction is undertaken, but this can usually be successfully managed because the blood supply is much better than in the mandible.

CHEMODECTOMAS (GLOMUS BODY TUMORS)

Chemodectomas are a fascinating but uncommon group of neoplasms that may originate anywhere glomus bodies are found. The lesions are uncommon before the age of 20, there is a female predominance in some series, and the lesions may occur in multiple sites in about 10% to 20% of cases, especially in families with a history of this tumor. Carotid body tumors are associated with conditions producing chronic hypoxia, such as high altitude habitation, and chronic hypoxemia (as occurs in cyanotic heart disease).

ANATOMY

The normal glomus bodies in the head and neck vary from 0.1 mm to 0.5 mm in diameter. An autopsy study showed a correlation between carotid body size and increased right ventricular weight secondary to emphysema.[372] Because of their small size, the total distribution of glomus bodies in the head and neck remains speculative. Tumors arising in glomus bodies (i.e., chemodectomas or nonchromaffin paragangliomas) arise most often from the carotid and temporal bone glomus bodies, with rare reports of tumors arising in the orbit, nasopharynx, larynx, nasal cavity, paranasal sinuses, tongue, and jaw.

The glomus bodies arising in relation to the temporal bone require special mention in regard to their distribution, because the site of origin of the tumor explains the different clinical pictures. Guild[373] reported an average of 2.82 glomera per temporal bone with a range of 0 to 12. The temporal bone glomus bodies are not found consistently in any location, but vary from person to person. At least one half of the glomus bodies are found in the general region of the jugular fossa and are located in the adventitia of the superior bulb of the internal jugular vein. The remainder are distributed along the course of the nerve of Jacobson (a branch of cranial nerve IX) and the nerve of Arnold (a branch of cranial nerve X). Approximately 20% of all temporal bone glomus bodies lie in the tympanic canaliculus and approximately 10% in relation to the cochlear promontory. A few glomus bodies are located in the descending part of the facial canal.

The carotid bodies are located in relation to the bifurcation of the common carotid. Orbit bodies are in relation to the ciliary nerve, and vagal bodies are adjacent to the ganglion nodosum of the vagus nerve.

PATHOLOGY

Chemodectomas are histologically benign tumors that resemble the parent tissue and consist of nests of epithelioid cells within stroma-containing, thin-walled blood vessels and nonmyelinated nerve fibers. The tumor mass is well circumscribed, but a true capsule is not seen. Dense fibrous bands occur in some tumors and account for the firmness of some masses. The histologic appearance varies, depending upon the relative amounts of epithelioid and vascular tissue present. The criterion of malignancy is based on the clinical progress of the disease rather than the histologic picture. Chemodectomas without cellular atypia may metastasize to regional nodes or to distant organ sites.

PATTERNS OF SPREAD

These lesions usually grow slowly; it is usual to have a history of symptoms for a few years and occasionally for 20 years or longer.

Carotid Body Tumors

Carotid body tumors are usually located at the bifurcation of the common carotid and, as they expand, tend to displace and encircle the internal and external carotid vessels. The tumor begins in the adventitia of the artery and initially derives its blood supply from the vaso vasorum. An accessory blood supply may come from branches of the vertebral artery and the ascending cervical artery.[374] The tumor is usually closely adherent to the wall of the carotid adjacent to the vascular pedicle, and there may be thinning of the arterial wall owing to pressure by the mass. Large masses extend toward the cervical spine, base of the skull, angle of the mandible, and the lateral pharyngeal space and its contents.

Temporal Bone Tumors

Glomus tympanicum lesions tend to be small when diagnosed because they produce symptoms quite early in their course. Tumor may involve the ossicles, tympanic membrane, mastoid, external auditory canal, semicircular canal, and the facial, Jacobson's, and Arnold's nerves.

Glomus jugulare tumors invade the base of skull, petrous apex, jugular vein, middle ear, and middle and posterior cranial fossae. Cranial nerves V to XII may be involved.

Lymphatic

Lymphatic metastases occur in about 5% of carotid body tumors but are very rare for temporal bone tumors. An upper neck mass may be an inferior extension of a jugular fossa or vagal tumor rather than a lymph node metastasis.

Distant Metastases

Distant metastases have been rarely reported for temporal bone tumors; carotid body tumors have a low risk for distant metastases, probably in the range of 5% or less.

CLINICAL PICTURE

Symptoms may be present from a few months to many years before diagnosis; the average is 3 to 4 years. Tumors are reported in children.

Carotid Body Tumors

The most common presenting symptom is an asymptomatic, slow-growing mass in the upper neck near the bifurcation of the carotid. Large masses may encroach on the parapharyngeal space and produce dysphagia, pain, and cranial nerve palsies. A carotid sinus syndrome may occur because of the pressure of the mass.

On examination, the mass usually lies deep to the sternocleidomastoid muscle and is tethered to surrounding structures. Fixation occurs only in large tumors that extend to the spine and base of skull. A submucosal bulge may be seen in the tonsillar area. A bruit may be heard. Steady compression of the mass may reduce its size, which recovers when the pressure is released.

Temporal Bone Tumors

Because glomus bodies are distributed throughout the temporal bone, the initial symptoms and signs depend on the site of origin.

Tumor arising in or near the middle ear presents with an insidious conductive hearing loss, pulsatile tinnitus, vertigo, and headache.

Patients with lesions developing in or around the jugular fossa develop headache, often pulsatile in nature, referred to the orbit or temple. Cranial nerves V to XII and the sympathetic nerves become affected.

Lesions developing in the facial canal present with facial nerve symptoms. Otorrhea and hemorrhage may occur when tumor breaks through into the external auditory canal.

A characteristic blue-red mass may be seen bulging the tympanic membrane or actually occupying the external auditory canal. A mass may be seen or felt in the upper neck between the mandible and mastoid and, at times, may be quite large.

Paralysis of cranial nerves V to XII and sympathetic nerves may occur.

METHODS OF DIAGNOSIS

Carotid Body Tumors

The differential diagnosis includes enlarged lymph nodes, aneurysm of the carotid artery, branchial cleft cyst, benign tumors (e.g., lipoma), and direct extension of a lateral pharyngeal wall or pyriform sinus cancer into the soft tissues of the neck.

Carotid angiography and CT scan with contrast provide the preoperative diagnosis. Biopsy usually produces serious hemorrhage and is not recommended.

Temporal Bone Tumors

The differential diagnosis includes the presentation of an internal carotid artery in the middle ear either as an aberrant vessel or as an aneurysm, and these patients also present with hearing loss, pulsatile tinnitus, and a pulsatile mass behind the eardrum. Needless to say, biopsy may have a disastrous result.[375]

A high jugular bulb may present as a vascular mass in the middle ear and mimic a glomus tumor.[376]

Other diagnoses to be considered include the following:

Polyp of ear canal
Malignant tumor of the nasopharynx with extension to the temporal bone
Acoustic neuroma
Carcinoma of the middle ear
Metastatic carcinoma (especially breast cancer)
Cholesteatoma
Histiocytosis
Chronic serous otitis and mastoiditis

The diagnosis of glomus tumor is established by CT and MRI with contrast enhancement. Biopsy may be associated with serious or even fatal hemorrhage and is not essential if the diagnosis is characteristic by CT and MRI scans. If an operation is planned for a localized lesion of the tympanic cavity, then excision of the lesion is the biopsy.

Staging

There is no accepted staging scheme for chemodectomas. Patients are considered to have an early lesion when there is little or no bone destruction and to have an advanced lesion when there is extensive bone destruction or cranial nerve deficits. Tumors recurring after prior treatment usually are advanced because of the delay in diagnosis.

A 24-hour urine sample may be examined for vanillylmandelic acid (VMA) and metanephrines if hypertension is present, and for 5-hydroxyindoleacetic acid (5-HIAA) if a carcinoid picture is present.

TREATMENT

Selection of Treatment Modality

Although chemodectomas have a low potential for metastatic spread and a slow growth pattern, they can cause major disability and eventually death if unchecked. It may be appropriate to recommend no active treatment in selected cases, but the great majority should be treated.

TEMPORAL BONE TUMORS. Surgical excision is satisfactory for small lesions that can be removed without risk of operative death or damage to normal structures.

Early lesions of the tympanic cavity are managed successfully by excision without loss of hearing or vestibular function. The remainder of the lesions are managed best by irradiation, with a very high success rate and minimal morbidity with modern-day techniques. Partial removal of the tumor prior to irradiation does not improve the results but only increases the overall morbidity and puts the patient at risk for a fatal complication.

There remains a great deal of confusion regarding radiation treatment of chemodectomas.

A recent review by Kim and co-workers[377] of more than 200 patients showed that the recurrence rate after adequate radiation therapy for temporal bone chemodectomas was 2% with doses of 4000 cGy or greater. In some cases, examination of the temporal bone after radiation therapy has shown either no definable tumor or few microscopic residuals. However, in the majority of patients the tumor regresses but stable remnants may be seen for years. Success in these patients is equated with the lack of tumor regrowth and permanent improvement in signs and symptoms. It seems poor judgment to risk any operative resection that carries an operative mortality or morbidity when irradiation has been so successful.

CAROTID BODY TUMORS. Small lesions (1–5 cm) may be successfully removed with little risk to the patient. However, if ligation or replacement of the carotid vessels is anticipated or if a large lesion is fixed or unresectable because of size, radiation therapy is the preferred initial treatment. These lesions are identical histologically to temporal bone chemodectomas, and the response to radiation is similar. It is preferable to use radiation therapy rather than risk the possibility of a stroke or other operative calamity. A radiation dose of 4000 cGy to 4500 cGy does not exclude the possibility of surgical excision.

Surgical Treatment

TEMPORAL BONE TUMORS. Small glomus tympanicum lesions are approached through the eardrum or mastoid area and are removed. Hearing loss may occur from the operation, but if there is conductive hearing loss from the tumor, it may be correctable.

For the glomus jugulare tumors, surgery is reserved for radiation failure, in which case a radical mastoidectomy or a subtotal temporal bone resection would be required. Some surgeons advocate a base-of-skull approach.[378]

CAROTID BODY TUMORS. When an adequate work-up indicates that the most likely diagnosis is a carotid body tumor, hypertension, if present, should be treated. A standard neck incision is made in a skin crease at the level of the carotid bulb, and the carotid sheath and its contents are identified. The tumor mass is usually lying at the crotch of the internal and external carotid arteries, often displacing these vessels. Marked drops in blood pressure and bradycardia can be avoided by injecting the bulb area with lidocaine (Xylocaine). Troublesome bleeding may be avoided by using the bipolar electrode before excising the mass. The mass is then removed, preserving the carotid arteries.

Irradiation Technique

The current treatment plan is 4500 cGy in 5 weeks, 180 cGy/fraction, to the tumor volume. The dose is well below the tolerance of all normal tissues included, even if the brain stem and cord must be included for a large lesion.

Tumor-related symptoms may begin to improve during the first week of treatment, and the tumor mass, if visible, may show a decrease in size during the course of therapy; complete regression would be the exception.

Acute sequelae of treatment should be almost nil at 180 cGy/fraction. The patient will have temporary hair loss in the entrance and exit areas beginning about the third week. Mild nausea may occur.

Late sequelae are few. The hair should regrow over a period of 2 to 4 months but may show a slightly different texture or color. The patient may develop an otitis media, especially if the middle ear is involved with tumor.

Management of Recurrence

The diagnosis of recurrence often is delayed because of the inaccessibility to examination. Therefore, baseline CT or MRI scans should be obtained for reference.

Recurrence after irradiation is so uncommon that the diagnosis must be made only after complete reevaluation and evidence or progression of symptoms or an enlarging mass seen on CT or MRI. Pulsatile tinnitus may persist after irradiation because of incomplete regression of the vascular component of the tumor.[379,380]

Documented recurrence after operation usually is treated by irradiation; the complication rate in this group is higher than for those treated initially by irradiation. Recurrence after irradiation should be treated by operation if feasible; if operation is not possible, reirradiation may be considered. Although there are no reports of reirradiation for this tumor, there is experience with reirradiation of nasopharynx and brain tumors. The potential for a complication would be significant, but, in the face of advancing neoplasm, the risk probably would be acceptable.

RESULTS OF TREATMENT

Temporal Bone Tumors

The local control rates for five irradiation series of temporal bone chemodectomas in which adequate doses were prescribed and the treatment volumes adequate are listed in Table 21-74.[381-385] No patients had documented evidence of disease progression in 71 patients treated. In the University of Florida series, 9 patients have remained free of recurrence for ≥10 years and 5 patients for ≥15 years. Fifty-seven cranial nerve deficits were diagnosed before radiation therapy. Of these, 5 resolved completely, 14 partially improved, 36 were unchanged, and 2 deteriorated. The local control rates for operation for five series are listed in Table 21-75.[386-390]

Carotid Body Tumors

The local recurrence rates after complete excision are low, 0 to 10%.[391-396]

Mendenhall and co-workers[397] surveyed the radiation therapy results for carotid body and ganglion nodosum chemodectomas (Table 21-76). Two carotid body tumors treated at the University of Florida showed complete tumor regression, and the others stabilized with no progression. Five patients treated for de novo lesions remain free of regrowth at 1.5, 1.5, 3.5, 4, and 6 years (Mendenhall WM: Personal communication, 1987).

FOLLOW-UP POLICY

It is not unusual to have a persistent blue-red mass behind the eardrum after irradiation, even though the patient is clinically improved and there is no evidence of progression.

About 5% to 10% of patients will develop a second chemodectoma (often in the head and neck area), either a carotid body tumor or a contralateral temporal bone tumor. Baseline CT and MRI scans are recommended and are usually obtained about 6 months after therapy.

COMPLICATIONS OF TREATMENT

Surgery

Fatalities have been reported from biopsy and resection. The major risks during operation are hemorrhage and injury to cranial nerves. Other complications include hemiparesis, spinal fluid leak, and hearing loss.[376]

Irradiation

There have been isolated reports of brain necrosis; these cases were associated with high doses, high daily fractions, or repeat courses of irradiation. This complication should not occur at a dose of 4500 cGy or less given at 180 cGy a day, 5 days a week. Other complications include cholesteatoma and sequestrum of the mastoid and otitis media. Detectable damage to the hearing mechanism and vestibular apparatus does not occur at 4000 cGy to 4500 cGy to the normal temporal bone. Cranial nerves may regain complete or partial function, especially if the deficit is of recent onset. Cranial nerve palsy due to irradiation should not occur at 4500 cGy. The complication rate is greater when operation and irradiation are combined.

TABLE 21-75. Local Control of Chemodectomas with Surgery

Author	Year	No. of Patients	No. with Recurrence
Newman et al.[386]	1973	14	11
Grubb and Lampe[387]	1965	9	5
Hatfield et al.[388]	1972	16	8
Rosenwasser[389]	1967	8	3
Spector et al.[390]	1975	11 (GT)*	1
		45 (GJ)†	10

Adapted from Tidwell TJ, Montague ED: Chemodectomas involving the temporal bone. Radiology 116:147–149, 1975.
*GT, glomus tympanicum.
†GJ, glomus jugulare.

TABLE 21-74. Local Control of Temporal Bone Chemodectomas with Irradiation

Institution	Tumor Dose (cGy)	Local Control*	Follow-up (yr)
M. D. Anderson Hospital[381]	4250–5000	17/17	4–18
University of Florida[382]	3750–5640	19/19	2–18
Baylor Medical Center[383]	4000–5000	9/9	1–7
Geisinger Medical Center[384]	4000–5000	11/11	1–12
Princess Margaret Hospital[385]	3500	20/20	2–20

*Local control: regression and absence of disease progression.

TABLE 21-76.   Local Control of Carotid Body or Glomus Vagale Chemodectomas with Irradiation

Series	No. of Patients	No. of Lesions	Dose (cGy)	Results
Mitchell and Clyne[398]	6	6	3750–5500	5/6 controlled* at 1.5–8 years
Lybeert et al.[399]	9	11	4000–6000†	9/9 controlled at 1.5–18 years
Krupski et al.[400]	1	1	Not stated	Controlled at 8 years
Wilson[401]	1	1	Not stated	Controlled at 10 years
Endicott and Maniglia[402]	1	1	4500	Controlled at 1 year
Mendenhall et al.[397]	4	6	4000–4800	4/4 controlled at 2–4.5 years

Mendenhall WM, Million RR, Parsons JT, et al: Chemodectoma of the carotid body and ganglion nodosum treated with radiation therapy. Int J Radiat Oncol Biol Phys 12:2175–2178, 1986.
*Controlled = regression or stabilization of local disease; no evidence of lymph node or distant metastasis.
†200 cGy per fraction.

MAJOR SALIVARY GLANDS

Tumors of the major salivary glands account for 3% to 4% of all head and neck neoplasms. The average age of patients with malignant neoplasms is approximately 55 years; for benign tumors, about 40 years. Approximately one fourth of parotid tumors and one half of submandibular tumors are malignant.

ANATOMY

The parotid gland is a relatively simple structure with rather complex anatomic relationships. It is indented and formed by the muscles, bones, vessels, and nerves that come in contact with the gland. The major bulk of the parotid gland is superficial, extending superiorly to the zygomatic arch and anterior aspect of the external auditory canal. The anterior border is variable, but does not continue beyond the opening of the parotid duct into the oral cavity opposite the second molar. Inferiorly, the gland fills the gap between the mastoid and the angle of the mandible. The gland lies in front of and below the external auditory canal. A deep lobe extends into the parapharyngeal area, where it is in relationship to the lateral process of C1, the styloid process, and the contents of the parapharyngeal space.

The parotid gland is encompassed by fascia that is sufficient to contain most parotid infections in addition to benign and low-grade malignant tumors. However, the fascia between the parotid gland and the conchal and tragal cartilages is quite thin; this is a weak spot that tumor quickly traverses. The fascia separating the deep lobe from the parapharyngeal space (stylomandibular fascial membrane) may be sufficiently thin to allow tumor or infection easy access to the parapharyngeal space and pharynx.

The sensory nerve supply to the parotid area and part of the pinna is by way of the greater auricular nerve (C2–3). This nerve is severed in removal of the parotid gland with permanent loss of sensation. The facial nerve penetrates the parotid gland almost immediately upon leaving the stylomastoid canal. The seventh nerve forms an extensive anastomotic network within the gland and gives off branches to the muscles of expression.

The parotid gland is richly supplied from several arteries that freely anastomose and create arteriovenous bleeding during parotidectomy. The external carotid, internal maxillary, and superficial temporal arteries and the posterior facial vein lie deep to the seventh nerve; if these vessels require attention during an operation, the seventh nerve may be damaged.

The superficial preauricular nodes, usually one or two in number, lie outside the fascia of the parotid gland and immediately in front of the tragus. These nodes are important because they drain the skin of the anterior ear, temple, and upper face, including the eye and nose. They are involved most frequently by metastatic skin cancer and lymphoma, but not usually from parotid neoplasms. The preauricular nodes then empty into the superficial cervical nodes along the external jugular vein, or they may communicate with the jugular chain of nodes.

There are two groups of nodes within the fascia of the parotid gland. Within the substance of the parotid gland are numerous lymph follicles and four to ten small lymph nodes scattered along the posterior facial and external jugular veins. Thus, they may lie deep to the seventh nerve. Outside the gland but within the fascia are one or two nodes that lie in front of the tragus and one or two nodes that lie between the inferior aspect of the tail of the parotid and the anterior border of the sternocleidomastoid muscle. These are referred to as the subparotid nodes. When enlarged, the subparotid nodes are difficult to distinguish from a mass in the tail of the parotid gland.

PATHOLOGY

There is a large variety of benign and malignant neoplasms that occur in the major salivary glands. It is not at all unusual to have the diagnosis changed from that given at frozen section; the patient must be made aware of this risk.

Benign Tumors

BENIGN MIXED TUMORS. These slow-growing neoplasms are surrounded by an imperfect pseudocapsule that is traversed by fingers of tumor. Enucleation or removal of a narrow cuff of normal tissue usually results in recurrence. The histologic distinction between benign and malignant mixed tumor is often difficult. The age of appearance begins in the early 20s with a mean age of 40.

PAPILLARY CYSTADENOMA LYMPHOMATOSUM. This benign tumor, also called Warthin's tumor, probably arises from lymphoid elements. It is encased by a thin but complete capsule. It occurs predominantly in older men. It is bilateral in approximately 10% of cases and may be multiple on one or both sides.

BENIGN LYMPHOEPITHELIAL LESIONS. Benign lymphoepithelial lesions (Godwin's tumor) account for about 5% of benign lesions. The tumor may be bilateral and is more common in women. Excision may be followed by recurrence.

ONCOCYTOMA. Oncocytoma is a benign, slow-growing tumor found mostly in the older age group. The encapsulated tumor has a dark appearance similar to melanoma.

BASAL CELL ADENOMA. The basal cell adenoma is an uncommon benign lesion, usually appearing in older people. It is histologically and clinically benign and is cured by simple excision. Basal cell adenoma must be distinguished from basal cell carcinoma of the skin metastatic to parotid lymph nodes.

Malignant Tumors

LOW-GRADE MALIGNANCY. *Acinic Cell Tumor.* Acinic cell tumors typically are slow-growing, low-grade neoplasms that appear in all age groups and are most common in women. They will recur after inadequate removal, sometimes as long as 25 to 30 years after initial treatment. Metastases occur in a small percentage of cases but cannot be predicted by the histologic picture.

Mucoepidermoid Carcinoma, Low Grade. Most mucoepidermoid carcinomas are low-grade lesions readily cured by adequate excision. They may appear in any age group. They grow slowly; there is little or no capsule. They are usually well-circumscribed, but they may widely infiltrate the normal gland or become fixed to skin. The mucin produced by the neoplasm may incite inflammatory changes about the edge of the mass.

HIGH-GRADE MALIGNANCY. *Mucoepidermoid Carcinoma, High Grade.* A few of the mucoepidermoid carcinomas behave in a very aggressive fashion, widely infiltrating the salivary gland and producing lymph node and distant metastases. They may be difficult to distinguish from high-grade epidermoid carcinoma.

Adenocarcinoma; Poorly Differentiated Carcinoma; Anaplastic Carcinoma; Squamous Cell Carcinoma. These histologies tend to appear late in life and have an aggressive behavior. True squamous cell carcinoma arising from the salivary gland occurs rarely. Almost all of the so-called squamous cell carcinomas of the parotid are actually metastatic from skin cancer, especially from the temple area.[403,404]

Malignant Mixed Tumor. A small percentage of benign mixed tumors may develop into frank malignancy.

Adenoid Cystic Carcinoma. This neoplasm is uncommon in the major salivary glands. It varies in growth rate from slow to fast. Metastases to regional lymph nodes and distant sites occur; perineural involvement is characteristic; and recurrences may appear many years after initial treatment.

Lymphoepithelioma (Malignant Lymphoepithelial Lesion, "Eskimoma"). Lymphoepithelioma occurs rarely in the parotid and submandibular gland. Povah and co-workers[405] reported 17 cases from Winnipeg. Fifteen of the patients were Eskimo and 2 were white, with an age range of 17 to 65 years. The histologic picture was that of lymphoepithelioma with varying degrees of nonmalignant lymphoid stroma.

PATTERNS OF SPREAD

Benign Mixed Tumors

Benign mixed tumors of the parotid gland grow by expansion and local infiltration. Most tumors begin in the superficial lobe. Because of their slow growth they rarely cause seventh nerve palsy, although the nerve may be severely stretched by large masses. When incompletely excised, multiple tumor nodules develop within the tumor bed. Skin invasion may occur in recurrent lesions; bone invasion does not occur, but a mass may cause pressure defects of adjacent bone.

Malignant Tumors

The malignant neoplasms infiltrate the parotid gland, invade the seventh nerve and the auriculotemporal nerve, and spread along nerve sheaths. Tumor may invade the adjacent skin, muscles, and bone, depending on the site of origin. Deep lobe lesions invade the parapharyngeal space, infratemporal fossa, and base of skull, and compromise additional cranial nerves.

Malignant tumors of the submandibular gland invade the gland, fix the tumor to the adjacent mandible, and invade the mylohyoid muscle and eventually the tongue, hypoglossal nerve, and oral cavity or oropharynx. Skin invasion occurs in advanced cases.

Sublingual gland neoplasms usually present as a submucosal mass in the floor of the mouth. The advanced lesions show an ulcerated mass in the floor of the mouth with extension to the tongue, mandible, and submental soft tissues.

Lymphatic Spread

Lymph node metastases may occur from all of the malignant neoplasms. Approximately 20% to 25% of patients with malignant tumors will have clinically positive or occult metastases in lymph nodes at the time of diagnosis. Low-grade mucoepidermoid carcinoma and acinic cell adenocarcinoma have a low rate of lymph node metastasis. There is little difference in the rate of lymph node metastasis among the various high-grade lesions. The risk for lymph node metastasis increases with recurrent disease and increased size of the primary lesion.

CLINICAL PICTURE

Parotid Gland

The great majority of patients with either benign or malignant parotid tumors present with a mass that is easily seen and felt. Mild, intermittent pain is associated with a few of the masses, but does not distinguish between benign and malignant. Facial nerve palsy is an infrequent presenting complaint and indicates malignancy, since untreated benign tumors do not cause seventh nerve palsy. Tumors of the deep lobe may produce dysphagia.

The mobility of the mass depends on its size and location. Fixation or reduced mobility may occur in both benign and malignant neoplasms and does not distinguish the two. Tumors presenting in the deep lobe may cause bulging of the palate and tonsillar area.

Advanced malignant lesions may affect cranial nerve VII, and, more rarely, cranial nerves IX to XII and the sympathetic chain if the parapharyngeal space is invaded. The mandibular branch of cranial nerve V may be involved when tumor tracks along the auriculotemporal nerve to the base of the skull; pain is an associated finding.

Submandibular Gland

Both benign and malignant neoplasms present as a mass usually associated with mild pain. Nerve palsy is rarely seen with submandibular gland cases. These lesions may infiltrate the skin in advanced lesions. The tumor mass usually is partially fixed to the mandible unless quite small. Loss of mobility occurs with both benign and malignant lesions.

Sublingual Gland

Sublingual gland lesions are clinically similar to squamous cell carcinomas of the floor of the mouth. They produce a mass, submucosal at first, that may be felt by the tongue; they may displace dentures, and there is mild discomfort, if any, in the early stages.

METHODS OF DIAGNOSIS AND STAGING

Parotid Gland

DIFFERENTIAL DIAGNOSIS. It is often easy to distinguish non-neoplastic from neoplastic conditions by history, physical examination, and simple diagnostic tests. The distinction between benign and malignant neoplasms is more difficult unless there is obvious nerve palsy, pain, or metastatic cervical lymph nodes.

Gallia and Johnson[406] reviewed 140 patients who eventually underwent parotidectomy for diagnoses. Only 11% had malignant masses; the remainder had benign neoplasms (62%) or non-neoplastic conditions (27%).

Conditions that may be confused with a parotid tumor include the following:

Metastatic cancer, lymphoma, or leukemia involving parotid area lymph nodes
Fatty replacement, tail of parotid
Chronic parotitis
Boeck's sarcoid
Stone in duct
Cysts (branchial cleft, dermoid)
Hypertrophy associated with diabetes
Hypertrophy of masseter muscle, unilateral or bilateral
Neoplasms of the mandible
Prominent transverse process of C1 (atlas)
Penetrating foreign bodies
Hemangioma/lymphangioma
Lipoma

RADIOLOGIC EXAMINATION. Radiologic examination of the parotid has progressed to the point that it is an essential tool in the differential diagnosis of parotid conditions and for determining disease extent in neoplastic conditions. MRI is comparable to CT with contrast for examination of the parotid gland; CT with sialography is no longer used. Sialography is reserved for nonacute inflammatory disease. Although one could argue that it is not necessary to perform a CT scan or MRI on every parotid mass (especially discrete, mobile, asymptomatic, slow-growing, superficial masses), observation of numerous diagnostic and surgical errors leads us to advise CT scan with contrast or MRI on a routine basis prior to biopsy or other operative procedures. CT scan and MRI will distinguish between intrinsic and extrinsic parotid masses and show the relationship of the mass to the facial nerve.[45] The characteristics of the mass as seen on CT or MRI scans will often predict for a malignant as opposed to a benign tumor. CT and MRI scans will assist the surgeon with the probable diagnosis, the proper approach to the facial nerve, the probable necessity to remove part or all of the nerve, the degree of invasion of the deep lobe, and the extension outside the parotid to the parapharyngeal space and base of skull. CT and MRI scans prior to surgery also greatly assist in radiation therapy treatment planning if radiation is used in a postoperative setting.

Submandibular Gland

DIFFERENTIAL DIAGNOSIS. The differential diagnosis of a submandibular mass centers around inflammatory disease, squamous cell carcinoma metastatic to a lymph node, and a primary neoplasm of the submandibular gland.

Episodic pain and mass are the hallmark of inflammatory disease, but approximately one third of inflammatory lesions will be asymptomatic.[407]

Obstructive sialadenitis is a common cause of submandibular gland enlargement. It is caused by stricture of the duct or stone in the duct. There is pain and swelling associated with eating that recedes after several hours. There may be erythema over the mass. A stone may be palpated in the duct, and occasionally pus can be stripped from the submandibular duct. A sialogram will show the site of the obstruction. Sialolithiasis may be found, however, in the presence of submandibular carcinoma.

A solitary squamous cell carcinoma metastatic to a submandibular lymph node in the absence of an obvious oral cavity primary lesion is uncommon. A primary submandibular neoplasm, benign or malignant, is a relatively rare event, but failure to recognize the possibility may result in an inappropriate and sometimes disastrous initial step in management.

Gallia and Johnson[406] reviewed 110 submandibular lesions in patients who underwent biopsy. Ninety-three (85%) were non-neoplastic, usually inflamed glands, and 9 (8%) were benign tumors. Eight patients (7%) had malignant lesions, of which 3 were lymphoma, 3 were metastatic carcinoma, and 2 were primary submandibular gland carcinoma.

RADIOLOGIC EXAMINATION. Radiologic examination plays an important part in the differential diagnosis of submandibular space masses of uncertain etiology. CT with contrast is usually the initial imaging procedure, although MRI may be used in selected circumstances. Plain films may reveal an opaque stone, or sialogram may show a nonopaque stone or other benign pathology. In masses that may be either a primary submandibular tumor or possibly a submandibular lymph node metastasis, CT scan with contrast will distinguish intrinsic versus extrinsic mass (*e.g.*, metastatic lymph node) and extent of disease spread to adjacent tissues when neoplasm is present. The diagnosis of malignant neoplasm may be strongly suggested in certain situations.

Biopsy Technique

PAROTID GLAND. The biopsy and the definitive surgical treatment are often the same for parotid masses. Lesions lying in the superficial lobe are biopsied best by performing a superficial parotidectomy. Lesions involving both the superficial and deep lobe or just the deep lobe are "biopsied" by total parotidectomy. This approach avoids contamination of the tumor bed. Incisional or excisional biopsy (*e.g.*, lumpectomy) increases the risk of tumor recurrence and facial nerve damage and increases the definitive surgical procedure by necessitating wide removal of the biopsy site.

There are several advocates of fine-needle aspiration for diagnosis; it is essential that the pathologist be familiar with this method. Fine-needle biopsies, even when correct, do not alter treatment decisions. There is a significant error rate in frozen section diagnoses, so that surgical decisions often rely heavily on clinical and radiographic findings for planning surgical resections. Needle biopsy can be used in the inoperable or recurrent lesion when radiation therapy is planned as the initial treatment.

SUBMANDIBULAR GLAND. Needle biopsy is helpful when positive for tumor, but may delay diagnosis when falsely negative. When needle biopsy is negative, but history, physical examination, and radiographic studies suggest neoplasm, and a careful search of the head and neck area fails to reveal a primary mucosal lesion, the submandibular triangle is dissected as the biopsy procedure. Incisional or excisional biopsy increases the risk of tumor recurrence, even when followed by appropriate treatment, and increases the surgical morbidity by requiring excision of the biopsy site.

Staging

The AJCC staging for salivary gland tumors is as follows:[12]

Primary tumor

TX	Minimum requirements to assess the primary tumor cannot be met
T0	No evidence of primary tumor
T1	Tumor 2.0 cm or less in greatest diameter without significant local extension*
T2	Tumor more than 2.0 cm but not more than 4.0 cm in greatest diameter without significant local extension*
T3	Tumor more than 4.0 cm but not more than 6.0 cm in greatest diameter without significant local extension*
T4a	Tumor over 6.0 cm in greatest diameter without significant local extension*
T4b	Tumor of any size with significant local extension*

Nodal involvement

NX	Minimum requirements to assess the regional nodes cannot be met
N0	No evidence of regional lymph node involvement
N1	Evidence of regional lymph node involvement

TREATMENT

Selection of Treatment Modality

PAROTID GLAND. The initial management of resectable superficial lobe parotid masses is exploration and en bloc superficial lobectomy for diagnosis and treatment. The tumor usually can be dissected free of the facial nerve. If the tumor involves the deep portion of the gland, the nerve is gently retracted and the deep portion excised (*i.e.*, total parotidectomy). If the tumor grossly involves the facial nerve, one or more branches may have to be sacrificed (*i.e.*, radical parotidectomy). Skin, bone, and muscle may also be resected as needed.

Low-grade malignant neoplasms are usually managed by operation only. Radiation therapy is given postoperatively for nearly all high-grade lesions. Radiation therapy is advised for low-grade malignant lesions that are recurrent and those with positive margins or narrow margins on the facial nerve. Tumor spill at the time of operation is a controversial indication for postoperative irradiation.[408] Postoperative radiation therapy is advised for selected benign mixed tumors when there is residual disease after operation, and for nearly all patients operated on for recurrent disease. Inoperable tumors are treated by radiation therapy with occasional success reported.

Chemotherapy has been reserved for patients with incurable disease or planned clinical trials.

SUBMANDIBULAR GLAND. Submandibular triangle dissection is used to make the diagnosis of lesions in this loca-

---

*Significant local extension is defined as evidence of tumor involvement of skin, soft tissues, bone, or the lingual or facial nerves.

tion. If frozen section diagnosis shows a malignant lesion and there is no involvement of nerves, mandible, or soft tissues, the operation is concluded, and postoperative irradiation is given to the submandibular bed and ipsilateral neck. If there is perineural invasion, bone invasion, a clinically positive node, or extension to contiguous soft tissues, then the resection is enlarged to encompass the necessary areas. This may include the mandible, mylohyoid muscle, digastric muscle, adjacent floor of the mouth or tongue, and involved nerves. Postoperative radiation therapy is added in nearly all cases.

Surgical Treatment

SUPERFICIAL PAROTIDECTOMY. The parotid gland is a unilobular gland but is artificially divided into superficial and deep portions by the seventh nerve. A superficial mass in the parotid gland is best approached by a superficial parotidectomy and frozen section diagnosis because this affords the best method of diagnosis and often is the definitive treatment. The facial nerve is not sacrificed unless it is grossly involved with disease.

The incision is made in the preauricular crease and then curves under the earlobe posteriorly and then into the neck. The facial nerve must be identified in all superficial and total parotidectomies. Once this is accomplished, the dissection is carried out between the mass and the facial nerve. A margin of at least 1 cm around the mass is necessary if a benign tumor is suspected, and a larger margin if the mass is malignant. The adequacy of treatment is determined by frozen sections.

TOTAL PAROTIDECTOMY. Total parotidectomy is recommended for tumors in the deep lobe of the parotid gland or for tumors that arise in the superficial lobe and extend into the deep lobe. A superficial parotidectomy generally is performed; then the nerve is dissected free from the underlying deep lobe and the deep lobe and tumor are removed. Occasionally, the mandible must be divided to gain access to the retromandibular portion of the deep lobe of the parotid gland. A partial mandibulectomy is required when the mandible is invaded by tumor. When pain is present, the auriculotemporal nerve should be explored to the base of the skull.

The paraparotid nodes are removed with the primary lesion. If the nodes are positive, a radical neck dissection is added. Radical neck dissection is always included for clinically positive nodes. Elective neck dissection is not done for low-grade lesions.

A radical parotidectomy implies removal of the entire parotid, the facial nerve, and other involved tissues such as skin, bone, or muscle. If a branch of the facial nerve or the entire nerve must be sacrificed, an immediate autologous nerve graft may be done. Postoperative radiation therapy is delayed for 6 weeks, and the chance of successful function is reported to be good.[409]

Radiation Therapy

Radiation therapy plays its major role as an adjunct to surgery and is usually given postoperatively, although preoperative treatment is advised in special situations. Postoperative irradiation is indicated for nearly all high-grade lesions, for low-grade neoplasms with close or positive margins, for tumors of the deep lobe, for perineural invasion, for recurrent tumors, and for multiple regional node metastases. According to Spiro and co-workers,[408] tumor spill at the time of operation may not be a single prognostic factor for recurrence.

The minimum treatment volume for parotid lesions includes the parotid bed and upper neck nodes. Perineural involvement indicates enlargement of the portals to cover the nerve pathways. The entire ipsilateral neck is included for high-grade lesions or for clinically positive nodes in the neck dissection specimen. The tumor dose to the primary area is 6000 cGy to 6500 cGy over 6 to 7 weeks if there is no gross residual disease. Higher doses including interstitial implants are used for gross disease. There are no good data to show a difference in dose required for the various histologies.[410,411]

Submandibular space external beam portals are tailored to the extent of disease found in the surgical dissection. The entire ipsilateral neck is included. The postoperative dose is 6500 cGy to 7000 cGy because the rate of recurrence even with combined treatment is substantial.

RESULTS OF TREATMENT

Parotid Gland

BENIGN MIXED TUMORS. Enucleation or excision with a narrow rim of normal tissue will result eventually in a local recurrence rate of approximately 20% after 10 to 15 years of follow-up.

Rafla[412] reported only a 2.7% recurrence rate when enucleation or excision was followed by postoperative radiation therapy. Superficial parotidectomy (or excision for selected small lesions) will result in a recurrence rate of approximately 5%. Spiro[413] reported a 7% recurrence rate, with a minimum of 10 years of follow-up, for 1342 benign parotid tumors treated by surgery.

The surgical success rate for recurrent lesions depends on the number of previous operations and the size and extent of recurrence. It may be necessary to sacrifice one or several branches of the seventh nerve and to repair the defect with a nerve graft. Postoperative irradiation of 6000 cGy to 6500 cGy is added in selected cases in which there are close margins or residual disease, or in cases in which a subsequent recurrence would be almost impossible to manage surgically or would result in loss of the facial nerve.

Death because of benign mixed tumor should be a rare event.

MALIGNANT TUMORS. Treatment results for parotid tumors have been analyzed by grade or histology, but results have not often been available by stage. The surgical results for low-grade malignant lesions are quite good, and radiation therapy is not often required. The local recurrence rate for operation alone is approximately 50% to 60% for high-grade tumors.[408,414]

McNaney and co-workers[415] reported the M. D. Anderson Hospital experience for 77 patients with malignant parotid tumors who received postoperative radiation therapy. Parotidectomy was performed for a de novo tumor in 70% and for a recurrent tumor in 30%. Patients with a history of more than two surgical procedures for parotid tumor were excluded. There was a minimum follow-up of 3 years; follow-up was greater than 5 years in 81% and greater than 10 years in 27% of the patients. The sites of local–regional failures according to the estimated extent of residual disease after parotidectomy are shown in Table 21-77. The overall incidence of local failure was 8%, and the incidence of neck failure alone was 5%. There were no failures after 4 years of observation. There were no local or regional failures in the 14 patients with low-grade lesions; the local failure rate for high-grade tumors was 10%. Analysis of local recurrence according to the extent of facial nerve sacrifice showed one local failure in 35 cases in which the nerve was preserved, one local failure in 21 cases after partial facial nerve resection, and three local failures in 21 cases after total resection of the nerve. Distant metastasis developed in 23%.

The 5-year absolute survival rate by histology for patients treated with surgery and postoperative radiation therapy added on a selective basis at M. D. Anderson Hospital is shown in Table 21-78.[411]

Theriault and Fitzpatrick[416] reviewed 271 patients with parotid cancer seen at the Princess Margaret Hospital between 1958 and 1980. The minimum follow-up was 5 years and the median follow-up was 10 years. Thirty-five patients had only radiation therapy, 67 had only surgery, and 169 had surgery plus postoperative radiation therapy, 4500 cGy to 5500 cGy in 20 fractions. Relapse-free survival and cause-specific survival (determinate survival) rates are compared to treatment modality in Table 21-79. Local–regional control at 10 years was obtained in 12% by radiation therapy, 22% by surgery, and 71% by surgery plus radiation therapy. Significant prognostic factors for survival were tumor stage, regional metastases, age (young better than old), histology, and facial nerve involvement.

Chemotherapy Results

The development of effective chemotherapy for patients with salivary gland carcinomas has been limited by the heterogeneity of this disease, the relative efficacy of surgery and radiotherapy, and the paucity of patients with recurrent or metastatic disease. Significant tumor regression has been reported with single-agent chlorambucil,[417] hydroxyurea,[418] hexamethylmelamine,[419] daunorubicin,[419] 5-fluoroura-cil,[420,421] doxorubicin,[419,422] and cisplatin.[423,424] The last three drugs appear to be the most active single agents, with partial response rates of 30% to 70% in patients with advanced local–regional or metastatic disease. Responses to single agents, however, are rarely complete or durable.

The experience with combination chemotherapy in this disease is similarly limited. Multiagent chemotherapy has included the aforementioned cytotoxic agents, as well as mitomycin-C, cyclophosphamide, methotrexate, bleomycin, and vincristine.[425-433] Regimens containing doxorubicin have been evaluated in numerous small series. A combination of cyclophosphamide and doxorubicin led to 5 partial but no complete responses in 13 patients with recurrent or metastatic salivary gland tumors.[427] Cisplatin, doxorubicin, and 5-fluorouracil resulted in 2 complete and 4 partial responses in 17 patients with advanced disease.[428] The combination of cyclophosphamide, doxorubicin, and cisplatin (CAP) is the most extensively studied regimen.[430-433] Dreyfuss and co-workers[433] recently summarized the published experience with CAP and noted 10 (28%) complete and 13 (36%) additional partial responses (median duration of response, 5–11 months) to chemotherapy in 36 patients with advanced disease.

The apparent activity of combinations containing cisplatin or doxorubicin in patients with recurrent or metastatic disease suggests a role for chemotherapy as induction or adjuvant treatment in patients with potentially curable lesions

TABLE 21-78. Parotid Cancer: Absolute 5-Year Survival (120 Patients)*

Histology	No. of Patients	5-Year Survival (%)
Acinic cell	12	92
Mucoepidermoid (low grade)	28	76
Adenocarcinoma	12	66
Malignant mixed	27	50
Adenoid cystic	10	50
Squamous cell	6	50
Mucoepidermoid (high grade)	13	46
Undifferentiated	12	33

Guillamondegui OM, Byers RM, Luna MA, et al: Aggressive surgery in treatment for parotid cancer. The role of adjunctive postoperative radiotherapy. AJR 123:49–54, 1975 © 1975, American Roentgen Ray Society.

*M. D. Anderson Hospital, 1944–1965.

TABLE 21-77. Postoperative Radiation Therapy in Malignant Tumors of the Parotid Gland: Local–Regional Failures by Extent of Residual Disease

Residual Disease	No. of Patients	Site of Failure		
		Primary Site	Neck	Primary Site and Neck
Gross (any grade)	14	1	1	0
Microscopic (any grade)	26	2	1	0
High grade (good margin)	16	1	2	0
Unknown grade (good margin)	17	1	0	1
Low grade (questionable margin)	4	0	0	0
Total	77	5	4	1

Adapted from McNaney D, McNeese MD, Guillamondegui OM, et al: Postoperative irradiation in malignant epithelial tumors of the parotid. Int J Radiat Oncol Biol Phys 9:1289–1295, 1983.

TABLE 21-79.   Parotid Carcinoma: Survival in 269 Patients Treated at Princess
Margaret Hospital, 1958–1980 (5-Year Minimum Follow-up)

	Relapse-Free		Cause-Specific (Determinate)	
	5-Year	10-Year	5-Year	10-Year
Surgery plus radiation therapy	69%	63%	78%	72%
Surgery	30%	23%	63%	48%
Radiation therapy	9%	9%	23%	18%

Data from Theriault and Fitzpatrick.[416]

that are at high risk for relapse (*e.g.,* tumors with high-grade histology or base of skull extension). To date, the use of combination chemotherapy in this setting has been anecdotal [427,429,432,433] and its true value awaits definition by multi-institutional cooperative trials.

Submandibular Gland

Byers and co-workers[434] reported the results of treatment for 22 malignant tumors of the submandibular gland with no prior therapy. Treatment was resection followed selectively by postoperative irradiation. The local control rate was 64% and the survival rate was 50%.

Spiro[413] reported the results of surgery for 129 malignant submandibular gland carcinomas seen between 1939 and 1973. All patients had a minimum of 10 years of follow-up. Adenoid cystic carcinoma occurred in 35%, mucoepidermoid carcinoma in 29%, and malignant mixed tumor in 19%. Cervical lymph nodes were malignant in 28%. The local–regional control rate was 40% and the determinate cure rate was 31% at 5 years and 22% at 10 years.

Benign tumors of the submandibular gland were resected in 106 patients; only 2 developed a local recurrence.[413]

COMPLICATIONS OF TREATMENT

Surgery

Temporary facial nerve palsy may occur due to manipulation of the nerve during operation, and function will gradually return over a few months' time. Persistent weakness of the lower lip may occur, even though the remainder of the nerve recovers. Tarsorrhaphy may be required to protect the eye until function returns. Spontaneous return of facial movement has been reported to occur after surgical division of the seventh nerve. Facial nerve palsy may be repaired by a nerve graft. If grafting is not possible, a nerve crossover technique may be used that connects the ipsilateral hypoglossal nerve to branches of the seventh nerve.

Gustatory sweating (Frey's syndrome) occurs in about 10% of patients after parotidectomy. This problem rarely requires treatment.

Persistent salivary fistula is a rare complication.

Radiation Therapy

Xerostomia is avoided by techniques that spare the contralateral salivary tissues.

There may be trismus due to fibrosis of the masseter and pterygoid muscles and the temporomandibular joint. It should be possible to exclude the temporomandibular joint from high doses in most situations.

Otitis media may occur if the ear is irradiated. Localized hair loss may occur with some techniques. Osteoradionecrosis may occur with high doses.

MINOR SALIVARY GLANDS

Tumors of minor salivary gland origin are uncommon, accounting for about 2% to 3% of all malignant neoplasms of the upper aerodigestive tract. They may appear at any age, but are uncommon before age 20 and rare under age 10. There is no known causative agent except for the adenocarcinomas of the nose. They tend to occur most often in the hard palate, nasal cavity, and paranasal sinuses, areas infrequently involved by squamous cell carcinomas. Thus, the site of origin is related more to the population density of the minor salivary glands in a particular tissue than to an environmental factor.

ANATOMY

Minor salivary glands are ubiquitous in the mucosa of the upper aerodigestive tract with the exception of the gingivae and the anterior portion of the hard palate, which are free of minor salivary glands. They are distributed on the undersurface of the anterior and lateral oral tongue and the base of the tongue. Aberrant salivary tissue sometimes is seen in lymph nodes, in the body of the mandible just behind the third molar teeth, in the vestigial remnant of the nasopalatine canal in the anterior maxilla, the middle ear, lower neck, sternoclavicular joint, thyroglossal duct, and other sites.

PATHOLOGY

Approximately one half of minor salivary gland tumors are malignant. The histologic varieties of malignant tumors include adenoid cystic carcinoma, mucoepidermoid carcinoma, adenocarcinoma, malignant mixed, acinic cell, and oncocytic carcinomas. About two thirds are adenoid cystic. The mucoepidermoid carcinoma and adenocarcinomas arise predominantly in the oral cavity.[435]

The benign tumors are benign mixed (pleomorphic adenoma) in the great majority of cases, with a few cases of intraductal papillomas, papillary cystadenomas, basal cell adenomas, and benign oncocytomas.[436]

PATTERNS OF SPREAD

Tongue lesions usually originate from the base of the tongue. There are no minor salivary glands in the anterior one half of the hard palate, so tumors arise on the posterolateral hard palate and all of the soft palate. The site of origin for floor-of-mouth salivary gland tumors is moot — either the sublingual gland or a minor salivary gland. The nasopharynx is an uncommon site of origin.

These tumors grow by local infiltration with eventual invasion of muscle, bone, and cartilage. Perineural spread is a common feature, particularly for adenoid cystic carcinoma. Tumor may track both centrally and peripherally along nerves, but the central spread is the more common event because most lesions arise near the terminations of the nerves. Extension along nerves eventually may traverse the base of skull and surface intracranially, although this spread pattern may not become manifest for several years after the original treatment. Tumor growth along a nerve may be characterized by skipped areas, so that a normal nerve segment is no assurance of free margins. Adenoid cystic carcinoma may grow along the Haversian systems of bone without showing bone destruction.[437]

The risk of positive lymph nodes is related to the site of origin and the histology. Lymph node metastases are most likely from sites with a dense capillary lymphatic network, similar to the pattern for squamous carcinoma. Adenoid cystic carcinoma, low-grade mucoepidermoid carcinoma, and acinic cell carcinoma are at low risk to spread to lymph nodes; about 20% of adenoid cystic carcinomas spread to lymph nodes, but this low incidence is related partly to their frequent site of origin in the hard palate and paranasal sinuses, areas that infrequently produce lymph node metastases. The high-grade tumors (high-grade mucoepidermoid carcinoma, adenocarcinoma, and malignant mixed tumor) have a 30% incidence of lymph node involvement on admission, and eventually 51% showed lymph node metastases. Schell and co-workers[435] reported a 17% incidence of positive nodes on admission for all histologies and grades and subsequent appearance in 11%. Most were staged N1 or N2A and were usually associated with lesions of the tongue or floor of mouth. At least 25% of patients will develop distant metastasis, usually to the lung.

CLINICAL PICTURE

The clinical picture obviously depends on the site of origin. The signs and symptoms differ somewhat from those of squamous cell carcinoma arising in the same area. Many of the lesions are indolent, and the history may go back many months or even years; about 25% will give a history of a mass being present over 10 years. Because the lesions develop under the epithelium, the initial lesion is a submucosal mass that is often painless until ulceration develops. Perineural involvement is expressed as pain or paresthesias. Otherwise, the clinical picture resembles that for squamous cell carcinomas for a given size and site. Lymph node metastases occur at predictable sites. The clinically positive nodes are usually small and mobile, but neck dissection on such a patient may show numerous small, clinically undetectable positive nodes.

METHODS OF DIAGNOSIS AND STAGING

The differential diagnosis includes lesions that produce an enlarging submucosal mass, such as an abscess, a stone in a duct, a cyst of soft tissue or bone, sarcoma, or lymphoma.

Because of the infrequency of these lesions, faulty histologic interpretation is not unusual and often leads to inappropriate therapy.

The same staging systems applied to squamous cell carcinomas may be used, although very few reported series bother to correlate size and extent of tumor with results by various treatment modalities. CT scan and MRI are useful for staging and treatment selection.

TREATMENT

Selection of Treatment Modality

Surgery and radiation therapy are the only curative therapies available. Because radiation therapy has often been used as a last-ditch effort for high-grade, advanced lesions after multiple surgical procedures, it is hardly surprising that results in some reports have been poor. Those series using radiation therapy alone for early lesions or as an immediate postoperative adjunct to surgical removal have had a favorable experience. After all, the histologies of the minor salivary gland tumors are the same as those of parotid tumors, and it is generally accepted that routine postoperative irradiation will decrease the local recurrence rate in high-grade parotid lesions and that irradiation alone will even control a few locally recurrent or inoperable tumors.[410] Similar responses have been observed for mucoepidermoid carcinoma and adenocarcinoma. The complete response rate of malignant minor salivary gland tumors to irradiation is similar to that of squamous cell carcinomas of the same size and same anatomic site, and the doses used are similar.

Benign mixed tumors are managed by operation; postoperative irradiation sometimes is advised in cases in which margins are close or positive. Inoperable lesions are treated with high-dose radiation therapy, and long-term control has been reported.

The low-grade lesions (low-grade mucoepidermoid carcinoma and acinic cell carcinoma) are treated initially by an operation when feasible, but irradiation is sometimes used as the primary treatment for inaccessible lesions or where the functional loss would be considerable. Postoperative irradiation is added for close margins or for those lesions that have recurred more than once. If the patient presents after excisional biopsy of a small lesion, irradiation is an alternative to reexcision, particularly if the procedure would produce significant cosmetic or functional loss.

The treatment of high-grade lesions varies immensely, depending on the site of origin, stage of disease, and willingness of the patient to accept a major cosmetic or functional change subsequent to an operation. Because the philosophy at the University of Florida is to accept radiation therapy as a curative therapy, the authors essentially approach most lesions as they would a squamous cell carcinoma of similar stage and similar anatomic site.

When combined treatment is indicated, the operation should precede radiation therapy to facilitate healing and to gain knowledge of tumor extent for radiation treatment planning.

Chemotherapy

Because of the rarity of these neoplasms, information about chemotherapy is almost entirely anecdotal. Some evidence of antitumor effects has been seen with 5-fluorouracil, hydroxyurea, methotrexate, cisplatin, and bleomycin, but the magnitudes of responses are often difficult to evaluate in the context of broad phase II studies or retrospective review of medical records.[417,419,422,438] Using a combination of methyl-CCNU, doxorubicin, and vincristine, Hayes and co-workers[439] have seen significant responses in adenoid cystic carcinoma.

Surgical Treatment

Benign tumors are removed by wide local excision that includes a cuff of normal tissue. Local excision or enucleation is insufficient treatment due to the high recurrence rate associated with limited procedures.

Small low-grade lesions with a long history of slow growth may be treated with a wide local excision including a shell of normal tissue. Large low-grade lesions and high-grade lesions require a more radical resection. When perineural invasion is present, it is not possible, of course, to remove all the nerves potentially involved, but the nerves that are involved should be sacrificed wherever it is reasonable to do so. As an alternative, postoperative irradiation may be used to cover the perineural routes of spread. Because unsuccessfully treated patients often live many years before they eventually die of the disease, careful planning must go into reconstruction and rehabilitation.

Irradiation Technique

The irradiation techniques are similar to those for squamous cell carcinomas of the same anatomic site and similar tumor size, with the exception that nerve pathways must be covered for adenoid cystic carcinomas. Subclinical perineural spread for adenoid cystic carcinomas must be considered to be present even though not seen on the biopsy or surgical sections. Recurrences frequently are manifested in and about the base of the skull at the termination of the cranial nerves.

A dose of 7000 cGy over 7 to 7.5 weeks to the area of gross disease is recommended for early lesions by radiation ther-apy alone. A dose of 6500 cGy is advised in the postoperative situation.[440] Low doses are inadequate.[440,441]

The regression rate of adenoid cystic carcinoma during treatment is similar to that of squamous cell carcinoma. Successfully treated adenocarcinomas or low-grade muco-epidermoid carcinomas may require several weeks or months to disappear after completion of treatment. The regional lymphatics are irradiated electively, depending on the site of origin and grade of the lesion. The response of benign mixed tumors is predictably slow and usually incomplete.

RESULTS OF TREATMENT

Spiro and co-workers[442] reported the Memorial Sloan–Kettering results for 434 malignant minor salivary gland tumors, of which 90% were treated surgically. The determinate 5-, 10-, and 15-year cure rates were 44%, 32%, and 21%; 51% died of the original cancer. Patients with adenoid cystic carcinoma had the poorest prognosis, with about 20% surviving without recurrence. Those with adenocarcinoma had an intermediate outlook, about 35% surviving without recurrence, and mucoepidermoid carcinomas had the best control rate with about 70% long-term cures. Local control rates differed considerably by site (Table 21-80), but this difference is partly explained by the higher incidence of advanced adenoid cystic carcinoma in the sinuses. Local control was also better for small lesions and those without bone or lymph node involvement. Previous treatment had little effect on cure rate.

Bardwil and co-workers[443] reported a similar series from M. D. Anderson Hospital with shorter follow-up (3–20 years) in which surgery was the sole treatment in 88% of cases (see Table 21-81). Local control was reported to be

TABLE 21-80. Results of Surgical Treatment of Minor Salivary Gland Tumors (267 Patients)*

Site	No. of Patients	Local Control
Oral cavity/oropharynx	198	68%
Sinus/nasal/nasopharynx	58	28%
Larynx	11	55%

Data from Spiro et al.[416]
*Memorial Hospital, 1939–1963. 60%—no prior treatment; 14%—clinically positive nodes on admission; 90%—treated surgically; 5 yr follow-up.

TABLE 21-81. Results of Treatment of Malignant Minor Salivary Gland Tumors (M. D. Anderson Hospital)

	No. of Patients	No Prior Treatment	Follow-Up	Local Control	Distant Metastases	DOD or LWD*	Methods of Treatment†	
1945–1962 Bardwil et al.[443]	87	56%	3–20 years	75%	30%	47%	S	71
							S + RT	10
							RT	6
1970–1978 Schell et al.[435]	118	42%	2–10 years	79%‡	25%	36%	S	11
							S + RT	69
							RT	38

*DOD or LWD, dead of disease or living with disease.
†S, surgery; RT, radiation therapy.
‡Eleven patients salvaged by repeat operations for ultimate control rate of 88%.

TABLE 21-82.   Malignant Minor Salivary Gland Tumors: Primary Recurrence Related to Treatment Modality (No. of Patients with Recurrence After Initial Treatment at M. D. Anderson Hospital/Total Patients Treated)

Histology	Surgery Only	Surgery + Radiation Therapy	Radiation Therapy Only	Total
High grade				
Adenoid cystic	3/4	9/40	0/23	12/67
Mucoepidermoid	0/1	0/6	4/7	4/14
Adenocarcinoma	3/4	3/14	1/4	7/22
Malignant mixed	0/0	0/1	0/0	0/1
Low grade				
Mucoepidermoid	1/2	0/7	1/4	2/13
Acinic cell	0/0	0/1	0/0	0/1
Total	7/11*	12/69†	6/38	25/118

Schell S, Barkley HT Jr, Chiminazzo H Jr: Treatment of malignant minor salivary gland tumors. Unpublished data, 1980.
*Five patients salvaged by repeated surgical resection(s).
†Six patients salvaged by surgery.

75%, but 47% died of their original cancer, a percentage similar to that in the Memorial Sloan–Kettering series.

Schell and co-workers[435] reported a group of 118 malignant salivary gland tumors of which only 10% were treated by operation alone, 58% by surgery plus radiation therapy, and 32% by radiation therapy alone (see Table 21-81). The group treated by radiation therapy alone included 15 early and 23 advanced lesions; follow-up was 2 to 10 years. The initial local control rate for the entire group was 79%; 11 patients were saved by subsequent operation for an ultimate control rate of 88%.

The risk of local recurrence by treatment category and histology is shown in Table 21-82.[432] The low incidence of recurrence with radiation therapy alone for adenoid cystic carcinoma indicates that this histology responds quite consistently to radiation. Surgery plus radiation therapy seems to provide better initial control than surgery alone for high-grade lesions.

Ellis and co-workers[440] compared the University of Florida results of radiation therapy alone versus combined surgery and radiation therapy for 52 patients with malignant minor salivary gland tumors with a follow-up of 2 to 20 years; 80% had a minimum follow-up of 5 years. Control at the primary site is shown in Table 21-83. Although permanent local control was never achieved in 7 patients with advanced adenoid cystic carcinoma treated with radiation therapy, the average time to local recurrence was 5 years and 7 months; in 2 patients the recurrence appeared at 9 and 13 years.

Benign mixed tumors of minor salivary gland origin have a good prognosis. Enucleation, however, is followed by recurrence, and a cuff of normal tissue is required. Spiro[413] reported on 81 benign tumors. Sixty occurred on the palate and 13 on the lip or cheek. With a minimum follow-up of 10 years, the local recurrence rate was 6%.

Bardwill and co-workers[443] reported 13 patients with benign mixed tumors, all of whom were cured, 12 by operation and 1 by radiation therapy alone.

Rafla-Demetrious[444] reported the Royal Marsden experience of 44 cases of benign mixed tumor (see Table 21-84). Eleven patients were treated by radiation therapy alone, and none of the tumors regrew, although not all had complete regression. Several photographs demonstrate the response to radiation therapy. Local recurrence of benign mixed tumor may appear after many, many years, and an occasional patient may eventually die of uncontrolled disease.

TABLE 21-83.   Malignant Minor Salivary Gland Tumors: Initial Local Control at the Primary Site by Histology and Stage and Actuarial Survival Rates at 5 and 10 Years

Histology	Early Stage*		Advanced Stage†		Actuarial Survival	
	RT Alone	RT + Surgery	RT Alone	RT + Surgery	5 Years	10 Years
Adenoid cystic	3/4‡	6/7	0/7§	3/5	63%	43%
Adenocarcinoma		3/3	1/4	3/4	43%	43%
Mucoepidermoid	2/2		1/1	3/3	72%	72%
Malignant mixed	1/1	1/1	0/1	1/1	100%	

Ellis ER, Million RR, Mendenhall WM, et al. The use of radiation therapy in the management of minor salivary gland tumors. Int J Radiat Oncol Biol Phys 15:613–617, 1988.
Follow-up, 2 to 23 years.
*Excludes 1 patient dead of intercurrent disease <2 years after treatment.
†Excludes 7 patients dead of intercurrent disease <2 years after treatment.
‡Ultimate control rate was 4 of 4 after surgical salvage.
§Average time to recurrence was 5 years 7 months.

TABLE 21-84. Incidence of Recurrence of Pleomorphic Adenoma of Minor Salivary Glands in the Royal Marsden Series Distributed According to the Method of Treatment

Method of Treatment	No. of Patients	No. with Recurrence	Length of Follow-up
Radiation alone	11	0	5 for 5+ years
Preoperative radiation and surgery	14	2	9 for 5+ years
Surgery and postoperative radiation	18	0	14 for 5+ years
			9 for 10+ years
Surgery alone	1	0	5 years
Total	44	2	29 for 5+ years

Rafla-Demetrious SF: Mucous and Salivary Gland Tumours, p 118. Springfield, IL, Charles C Thomas, 1970.

REFERENCES

1. Silverberg E, Lubera J: Cancer statistics, 1987. CA 37:2–19, 1987
2. Donald PJ: Marijuana smoking—Possible cause of head and neck carcinoma in young patients. Otolaryngol Head Neck Surg 94:517—521, 1986
3. Rouviere H: Anatomy of the Human Lymphatic System, pp 1–70 (Tobias MJ trans). Ann Arbor, MI, Edwards Brothers, 1938
4. Leventon GS, Evans HL: Sarcomatoid squamous cell carcinoma of the mucous membranes of the head and neck: A clinicopathologic study of 20 cases. Cancer 48:994–1003, 1981
5. O'Brien CJ, Lahr CJ, Soong S-J, et al: Surgical treatment of early-stage carcinoma of the oral tongue: Would adjuvant treatment be beneficial? Head Neck Surg 8:401–408, 1986
6. Carter RL, Foster CS, Dinsdale EA. et al: Perineural spread by squamous carcinomas of the head and neck: A morphological study using antiaxonal and antimyelin monoclonal antibodies. J Clin Pathol 36:269–275, 1983
7. Lindberg RD: Distribution of cervical lymph node metastases from squamous cell carcinoma of the upper respiratory and digestive tracts. Cancer 29:1446–1449, 1972
8. Fisch U: Lymphography of the Cervical Lymphatic System. Philadelphia, WB Saunders, 1968
9. Berger DS, Fletcher GH, Lindberg RD, et al: Elective irradiation of the neck lymphatics for squamous cell carcinomas of the nasopharynx and oropharynx. Am J Roentgenol Radium Ther Nucl Med 111:66–72, 1971
10. Lindberg RD, Jesse RH: Treatment of cervical lymph node metastases from primary lesions of the oropharynx, supraglottic larynx, and hypopharynx. Am J Roentgenol Radium Ther Nucl Med 102:132–137, 1968
11. Merino OR, Lindberg RD, Fletcher GH: An analysis of distant metastases from squamous cell carcinoma of the upper respiratory and digestive tracts. Cancer 40:145–151, 1977
12. American Joint Committee on Cancer: Manual for Staging of Cancer, 2nd ed, pp 25–54. Philadelphia, JB Lippincott, 1983
13. Mendenhall WM, Parsons JT, Million RR: A favorable subset of AJCC stage IV squamous cell carcinoma of the head and neck. Int J Radiat Oncol Biol Phys 10:1841–1843, 1984
14. Parsons JT, Million RR, Cassisi NJ, et al: Hyperfractionation for head and neck cancer. Int J Radiat Oncol Biol Phys 14:649–658, 1988
15. Mendenhall WM, Million RR, Cassisi NJ: Elective neck irradiation in squamous cell carcinoma of the head and neck. Head Neck Surg 3:15–20, 1980
16. Fletcher GH, MacComb WS, Braun EJ: Analysis of sites and causes of treatment failures in squamous cell carcinomas of the oral cavity. Am J Roentgenol Radium Ther Nucl Med 83:405–411, 1960
17. Goffinet DR, Gilbert EH, Weller SA et al: Irradiation of clinically uninvolved cervical lymph nodes. Can J Otolaryngol 4:927–933, 1975
18. Jesse RH, Barkley HT, Lindberg RD et al: Cancer of the oral cavity: Is elective neck dissection beneficial? Am J Surg 120:505–508, 1970
19. Hardingham M, Dalley VM, Shaw HJ: Cancer of the floor of the mouth: Clinical features and results of treatment. Clin Oncol 3:227–246, 1977
20. Southwick HW, Slaughter DP, Trevino ET: Elective neck dissection for intraoral cancer. Arch Surg 80:905–909, 1960
21. Ash CL: Oral cancer: A twenty-five year study. Am J Roentgenol Radium Ther Nucl Med 87:417–430, 1962
22. Campos JL, Lampe I, Fayos JV: Radiotherapy of carcinoma of the floor of the mouth. Radiology 99:677–682, 1971
23. Million RR: Elective neck irradiation for TXN0 squamous carcinoma of the oral tongue and floor of mouth. Cancer 34:149–155, 1974
24. Cady B, Catlin D: Epidermoid carcinoma of the gum: A 20-year survey. Cancer 23:551–569, 1969
25. Del Regato JA, Spjut HJ: Ackerman and del Regato's Cancer: Diagnosis, Treatment, and Prognosis, 5th ed, pp 264, 281, 341, 342, 345. St Louis, CV Mosby, 1977
26. Martin CL, Craffey EJ: Cancer of the gums. Am J Roentgenol Radium Ther Nucl Med 67:420–427, 1952

27. Chung CK, Rahman SM, Lim ML et al: Squamous cell carcinoma of the hard palate. Int J Radiat Oncol Biol Phys 5:191–196, 1979
28. Eneroth CM, Hjertman L, Moberger G: Squamous cell carcinomas of the palate. Acta Otolaryngol (Stockholm) 73:418–427, 1972
29. Horiuchi J, Adachi T: Some considerations on radiation therapy of tongue cancer. Cancer 28:335–339, 1971
30. Beahrs OH, Devine KD, Henson SW Jr: Treatment of carcinoma of the tongue: End-results in one hundred sixty-eight cases. Arch Surg 79:399–403, 1959
31. Frazell EL, Lucas JC Jr: Cancer of the tongue: Report of the management of 1554 patients. Cancer 15:1085–1099, 1962
32. Kremen AJ: Results of surgical treatment of cancer of the tongue. Surgery 39:49–53, 1956
33. Spiro RH, Strong EW: Discontinuous partial glossectomy and radical neck dissection in selected patients with epidermoid carcinoma of the mobile tongue. Am J Surg 126:544–546, 1973
34. Million RR, Fletcher GH, Jesse RH Jr: Evaluation of elective irradiation of the neck for squamous cell carcinoma of the nasopharynx, tonsillar fossa, and base of tongue. Radiology 80:973–988, 1963
35. Ho JHC: An epidemiologic and clinical study of nasopharyngeal carcinoma. Int J Radiat Oncol Biol Phys 4:183–198, 1978
36. Moench HC, Phillips TL: Carcinoma of the nasopharynx: Review of 146 patients with emphasis on radiation dose and time factors. Am J Surg 124:515–518, 1972
37. Barker JL, Fletcher GH: Time, dose, and tumor volume relationships in megavoltage irradiation of squamous cell carcinomas of the retromolar trigone and anterior tonsillar pillar. Int J Radiat Oncol Biol Phys 2:407–414, 1977
38. Jesse RH, Fletcher GH: Metastases in cervical lymph nodes from oropharyngeal carcinoma: Treatment and results. Am J Roentgenol Radium Ther Nucl Med 90:990–996, 1963
39. Lindberg RD, Barkley HT Jr, Jesse RH et al: Evolution of the clinically negative neck in patients with squamous cell carcinoma of the faucial arch. Am J Roentgenol Radium Ther Nucl Med 111:60–65, 1971
40. Southwick HW: Elective neck dissection for intraoral cancer. JAMA 217:454–455, 1971
41. Rolander TL, Everts EC, Shumrick DA: Carcinoma of the tonsil: A planned combined therapy approach. Laryngoscope 81:1199–1207, 1971
42. Ogura JH, Biller HF, Wette R: Elective neck dissection for pharyngeal and laryngeal cancers: An evaluation. Ann Otol Rhinol Laryngol 80:646–651, 1971
43. Putney FJ: Elective versus delayed neck dissection in cancer of the larynx. Surg Gynecol Obstet 112:736–742, 1961
44. Fletcher GH: Elective irradiation of subclinical disease in cancers of the head and neck. Cancer 29:1450–1454, 1972
45. Mancuso AA, Hanafee WN: Computed Tomography and Magnetic Resonance Imaging of the Head and Neck, 2nd ed, pp 16, 139–151, 184. Baltimore, Williams & Wilkins, 1985
46. Mendenhall WM, Million RR: Elective neck irradiation for squamous cell carcinoma of the head and neck: Analysis of time-dose factors and causes of failure. Int J Radiat Oncol Biol Phys 12:741–746, 1986
47. Agresti A, Wackerly D: Some exact conditional tests of independence for T × C cross-classification tables. Psychometrika 42:111–125, 1977
48. Barkley HT Jr, Fletcher GH, Jesse RH et al: Management of cervical lymph node metastases in squamous cell carcinoma of the tonsillar fossa, base of tongue, supraglottic larynx, and hypopharynx. Am J Surg 124:462–467, 1972
49. Byers, RM: Modified neck dissection: A study of 967 cases from 1970 to 1980. Am J Surg 150:414–421, 1985
50. McGuirt WF, McCabe BF: Significance of node biopsy before definitive treatment of cervical metastatic carcinoma. Laryngoscope 88:594–597, 1978
51. Parsons JT, Million RR, Cassisi NJ: The influence of excisional or incisional biopsy of metastatic neck nodes on the management of head and neck cancer. Int J Radiat Oncol Biol Phys 11:1447–1454, 1985
52. Million RR, Cassisi NJ: General principles for treatment of cancers in the head and neck: Selection of treatment for the primary site and for the neck. In Million RR,

Cassisi NJ (eds): Management of Head and Neck Cancer: A Multidisciplinary Approach, pp 43–62. Philadelphia, JB Lippincott, 1984

53. Papac R, Lefkowitz E, Bertino JR: Methotrexate (NSC-740) in squamous cell carcinoma of the head and neck. II. Intermittent intravenous therapy. Cancer Chemother Rep 51:69–72, 1967

54. Lane M, Moore JE, Levin H, et al: Methotrexate therapy for squamous cell carcinoma of the head and neck: Intermittent intravenous dose program. JAMA 204:561–564, 1968

55. Leone LA, Albala MM, Rege VB: Treatment of carcinoma of the head and neck with intravenous methotrexate. Cancer 21:828–837, 1968

56. DePalo GM, DeLena M, Molinari R, et al: Sperimentazione clinica con alte dosi intermittendi di methotrexate nel carcinoma oro-faringeo in fase avanzata. [Clinical evaluation of high weekly intravenous dose of methotrexate in advanced oropharyngeal carcinoma.] Tumori 56:259–268, 1970

57. Levitt M, Mosher MB, DeConti RC, et al: Improved therapeutic index of methotrexate with "leucovorin rescue." Cancer Res 33:1729–1734, 1973

58. Tejada F, Murphy E, Zubrod CG: Proceedings of the International Head and Neck Oncology Conference. Abstract 2.14. National Cancer Institute, 1980

59. DeConti RC, Schoenfeld D: A randomized prospective comparison of intermittent methotrexate, methotrexate with leucovorin, and a methotrexate combination in head and neck cancer. Cancer 48:1061–1072, 1981

60. Kirkwood JM, Canellos GP, Ervin TJ, et al: Increased therapeutic index using moderate dose methotrexate and leucovorin twice weekly vs. weekly high dose methotrexate-leucovorin in patients with advanced squamous cell carcinoma of the head and neck: A safe new effective regimen. Cancer 47:2414–2421, 1981

61. Woods RL, Fox RM, Tattersall MHN: Methotrexate treatment of squamous-cell head and neck cancers: Dose-response evaluation. Br Med J [Clin Res] 282:600–602, 1981

62. Hong WK, Schaefer S, Issell B, et al: A prospective randomized trial of methotrexate versus cisplatin in the treatment of recurrent squamous cell carcinomas of the head and neck (Abstract C-787). Proc Am Soc Clin Oncol 1:202, 1982

63. Grose WE, Lehane DE, Dixon DO, et al: Comparison of methotrexate and cisplatin for patients with advanced squamous cell carcinoma of the head and neck region: A Southwest Oncology Group study. Cancer Treat Rep 69:577–581, 1985

64. Vogler WR, Jacobs J, Moffitt S, et al: Methotrexate therapy with or without citrovorum factor in carcinoma of the head and neck, breast, and colon. Cancer Clin Trials 2:227–236, 1979

65. Taylor SG, McGuire WP, Hauck WW, et al: A randomized comparison of high-dose infusion methotrexate versus standard-dose weekly therapy in head and neck squamous cancer. J Clin Oncol 2:1006–1011, 1984

66. Bonadonna G, Tancini G, Bajetta E: Controlled studies with bleomycin in solid tumors and lymphomas. Prog Biochem Pharmacol 11:172–184, 1976

67. Halnan KE, Bleehen NM, Brewin TB, et al: Early clinical experience with bleomycin in the United Kingdom in series of 105 patients. Br Med J [Clin Res] 4:635–638, 1972

68. Haas CD, Coltman CA, Gottlieb JA, et al: Phase II evaluation of bleomycin: A Southwest Oncology Group Study. Cancer 38:8–12, 1976

69. Yagoda A, Mukherji B, Young C, et al: Bleomycin, an antitumor antibiotic: Clinical experience in 274 patients. Ann Intern Med 77:861–870, 1972

70. Durkin WJ, Pugh RP, Jacobs E, et al: Bleomycin (NSC-125066) therapy of responsive solid tumors. Oncology 33:260–264, 1976

71. EORTC Clinical Screening Co-operative Group: Study of the clinical efficiency of bleomycin in human cancer. Br Med J [Clin Res] 2:643–645, 1970

72. Wasserman TH, Comis RL, Goldsmith M, et al: Tabular analysis of the clinical chemotherapy of solid tumors. Cancer Chemother Rep 6:399–419, 1975

73. Wittes RE, Cvitkovic E, Shah J, et al: Cis-dichlorodiammineplatinum (II) in the treatment of epidermoid carcinoma of the head and neck. Cancer Treat Rep 61:359–366, 1977

74. Jacobs C, Bertino JR, Goffinet DR, et al: 24-hour infusion of cis-platinum in head and neck cancers. Cancer 42:2135–2140, 1978

75. Panettiere FJ, Lehane D, Fletcher WS, et al: Cis-platinum therapy of previously treated head and neck cancer: The Southwest Oncology Group's two-dose-per-month outpatient regimen. Med Pediatr Oncol 8:221–225, 1980

76. Creagan ET, O'Fallon JR, Woods JE, et al: Cis-diamminedichloroplatinum (II) administered by 24-hour infusion in the treatment of patients with advanced upper aerodigestive cancer. Cancer 51:2020–2023, 1983

77. Sako K, Razack MS, Kalnins I: Chemotherapy for advanced and recurrent squamous cell carcinoma of the head and neck with high and low dose cis-diamminedichloroplatinum. Am J Surg 136:529–533, 1978

78. Randolph VL, Wittes RE: Weekly administration of cis-diamminedichloroplatinum (II) without hydration or osmotic diuresis. Eur J Cancer Clin Oncol 14:753–756, 1978

79. Gold GL, Hall TC, Shnider BI, et al: A clinical study of 5-fluorouracil. Cancer Res 19:935–939, 1959

80. Olson KB, Greene JR: Evaluation of 5-fluorouracil in treatment of cancer. JNCI 25:133–140, 1960

81. Weiss AJ, Jackson LG, Carabasi R: An evaluation of 5-fluorouracil in malignant disease. Ann Intern Med 55:731–741, 1961

82. Staley CJ, Kerth JD, Cortes N, et al: Treatment of advanced cancer with 5-fluorouracil. Surg Gynecol Obstet 112:185–190, 1961

83. Ansfield FJ, Schroeder JM, Curreri AR: Five years clinical experience with 5-fluorouracil. JAMA 181:295–299, 1962

84. White JE, Ricketts WN, Strudwick WJ: A clinical study of 5-fluorouracil in a variety of far advanced human malignancies. J Natl Med Assoc 54:315–317, 1962

85. Moore GE, Bross IDJ, Ausman R, et al: Effects of 5-fluorouracil (NSC 19893) in 389 patients with cancer: Eastern Clinical Drug Evaluation Program. Cancer Chemother Rep 52:641–653, 1968

86. Young CW, Ellison RR, Sullivan RD, et al: The clinical evaluation of 5-fluorouracil and 5-fluoro-2'-deoxyuridine in solid tumors in adults: A progress report. Cancer Chemother Rep 6:17–20, 1960

87. Jacobs EM, Luce JK, Wood DA: Treatment of cancer with weekly intravenous 5-fluorouracil. Cancer 22:1233–1238, 1968

88. Carter SK: The chemotherapy of head and neck cancer. Semin Oncol 4:413–424, 1977

89. Krakoff IH: Adriamycin (NSC-123127) studies in adult patients. Cancer Chemother Rep 6:253–257, 1975

90. Blum RH: An overview of studies with Adriamycin (NSC-123127) in the United States. Cancer Chemother Rep 6:247–251, 1975

91. Lee G, Pitman SW, Bertino JR: Weekly hydroxyurea in squamous head and neck cancer (abstract C-572). Proc Am Soc Clin Oncol 4:147, 1985

92. Hornedo-Muguiro J, So M, Spaulding MB, et al: Phase II trial of carboplatin (CBDCA) in aerodigestive malignancies (abstract C-350). Proc Am Soc Clin Oncol 4:136, 1985

93. Basauri L, Pousa AL, Alba E, et al: Carboplatin, an active drug in advanced head and neck cancer. Cancer Treat Rep 70:1173–1176, 1986

94. Eisenberger M, Hornedo J, Silva H, et al: Carboplatin (NSC-241-240): An active platinum analog for the treatment of squamous-cell carcinoma of the head and neck. J Clin Oncol 4:1506–1509, 1986

95. Al-Sarraf M, Metch B, Kish J, et al: Platinum analogs in recurrent and advanced head and neck cancer: A Southwest Oncology Group and Wayne State University Study. Cancer Treat Rep 71:723–726, 1987

96. Vogl SE, Ryan L, Wernz J, et al: Ineffective agents in the chemotherapy (CT) of head and neck cancer (HNCA): Mitoxantrone (DHAD), dibromodulcitol (DBD) and vinblastine (VLB): The Eastern Cooperative Oncology Group (ECOG) experience (abstract 679). Proc Am Assoc Cancer Res 26:171, 1985

97. Williams SD, Birch R, Velez-Garcia E, et al: Phase II study of mitoxantrone in advanced squamous cell carcinoma of the head and neck. A Southeastern Cancer Study Group trial. Invest New Drugs 3:311–313, 1985

98. DeJager R, Cappelaere P, Armand JP, et al: An EORTC phase II study of mitoxantrone in solid tumors and lymphomas. Eur J Cancer Clin Oncol 20:1369–1375, 1984

99. Sikic BT, Collins JM, Mimnaugh EG, et al: Improved therapeutic index of bleomycin when administered by continuous infusion in mice. Cancer Treat Rep 62:2011–2017, 1978

100. Peng Y-M, Alberts DS, Chen H-SG, et al: Antitumour activity and plasma kinetics of bleomycin by continuous and intermittent administration. Br J Cancer 41:644–647, 1980

101. Samuels ML, Johnson DE, Holoye PY: Continuous intravenous bleomycin (NSC-125066) therapy and vinblastine (NSC-49842) in stage III testicular neoplasia. Cancer Chemother Rep 59:563–570, 1975

102. Baker LH, Opipari MI, Wilson H, et al: Mitomycin C, vincristine and bleomycin therapy for advanced cervical cancer. Obstet Gynecol 52:146–150, 1978

103. Carlson RW, Sikic BI: Continuous infusion or bolus injection in cancer chemotherapy. Ann Intern Med 99:823–833, 1983

104. Morton RP, Rugman F, Dorman EB, et al: Cisplatinum and bleomycin for advanced or recurrent squamous cell carcinoma of the head and neck: A randomized factorial phase III controlled trial. Cancer Chemother Pharmacol 15:283–289, 1985

105. Tapazoglou E, Kish J, Ensley J, et al: The activity of a single-agent 5-fluorouracil infusion in advanced and recurrent head and neck cancer. Cancer 57:1105–1109, 1986

106. Perry DJ, Crain SM, Weltz MD, et al: Phase II trial of mitoguazone in patients with advanced squamous cell carcinoma of the head and neck. Cancer Treat Rep 67:91–92, 1983

107. Thongprasert S, Bosl GJ, Geller NL, et al: Phase II trials of mitoguazone in patients with advanced head and neck. Cancer Treat Rep 68:1301–1302, 1984

108. Luedke D, Maddox W, Birch R, et al: Phase II trial of methyl glyoxal bis (guanylhydrazone) (MGBG) in advanced head and neck squamous cell carcinoma (abstract C-506). Proc Am Soc Clin Oncol 4:130, 1985

109. Coninx P, Nasca S, Jezekova D, et al: Essai phase II de mitoguazone chez des patients porteurs de tumeurs cervico-faciales etendues en recidive [Phase II trial of mitoguazone in patients with recurrent head and neck cancer.] Bull Cancer (Paris) 72:153–154, 1985

110. Ratanatharathorn V, Drelichman A, Sexon-Porte M, et al: Phase II evaluation of 4'-(9-acridinylamino)-methanesulfon-m-anisidine (AMSA) in patients with advanced head and neck cancers. Am J Clin Oncol (CCT) 5:29–32, 1982

111. Forastiere AA, Young CW, Wittes RE: A phase II trial of m-AMSA in head and neck cancer. Cancer Chemother Pharmacol 6:145–146, 1981

112. Andrews NC, Weiss AJ, Ansfield FJ, et al: Phase I study of dibromodulcitol (NSC-104800). Cancer Chemother Rep 55:61–65, 1971

113. Andrews NC, Weiss AJ, Wilson W, et al: Phase II study dibromodulcitol. Cancer Chemother Rep 58:653–660, 1974

114. Nissen NI, Pajak TF, Leone LA, et al: Clinical trial of VP 16-213 (NSC 141540) IV twice weekly in advanced neoplastic disease. A study by the Cancer and Leukemia Group B. Cancer 45:232–235, 1980

115. Grunberg SM, Felman IE, Gala KV, et al: Phase II study of etoposide (VP-16) in the treatment of advanced head and neck cancer. Am J Clin Oncol (CCT) 8:393–395, 1985

116. Crivellari D, Veronesi A, Magri MD, et al: Phase II trial of oral VP 16-213 (etoposide) in patients with advanced head and neck cancer. Tumori 71:499–500, 1985

117. Cheng E, Young CW, Wittes RE: Phase II trial of vindesine in advanced head and neck cancer. Cancer Treat Rep 64:1141–1142, 1980
118. Kaplan BH, Vogl SE, Cinberg J, et al: Phase II trial of vindesine in squamous cancer of the head and neck (abstract C-775). Proc Am Soc Clin Oncol 1:199, 1982
119. Sledge GW, Clark GM, Griffin C, et al: Phase II trial of vindesine in patients with squamous cell cancer of the head and neck. Am J Clin Oncol (CCT) 7:209–211, 1984
120. Krasnow S, Eisenberger M, Green M, et al: Phase I–II study of triazinate (TCT) for advanced head and neck cancer (HNC) (abstract 682). Proc Am Assoc Cancer Res 26:172, 1985
121. Ikic D, Padovan I, Brodarec I, et al: Application of human leucocyte interferon in patients with tumours of the head and neck. Lancet 1:1025–1027, 1981
122. Medenica RN, Slack N: Clinical results of leukocytes interferon-induced tumor regression in resistant human metastatic cancer resistant to chemotherapy and/or radiotherapy-pulse therapy schedule. Cancer Drug Deliv 2:53–76, 1985
123. Connors JM, Andiman WA, Howarth CB, et al: Treatment of nasopharyngeal carcinoma with human leukocyte interferon. J Clin Oncol 3:813–817, 1985
124. Kish JA, Ensley JF, Jacobs J, et al: A randomized trial of cisplatin (CACP) + 5-fluorouracil (5-FU) infusion and CACP + 5-FU bolus for recurrent and advanced squamous cell carcinoma of the head and neck. Cancer 56:2740–2744, 1985
125. Kish JA, Weaver A, Jacobs J, et al: Cisplatin and 5-fluorouracil infusion in patients with recurrent and disseminated epidermoid cancer of the head and neck. Cancer 53:1819–1824, 1984
126. Merlano M, Tatarek R, Grimaldi A, et al: Phase I–II trial with cisplatin and 5-FU in recurrent head and neck cancer: An effective outpatient schedule. Cancer Treat Rep 69:961–964, 1985
127. Bitran JD, Goldman M: A phase II trial of cyclophosphamide and Adriamycin in refractory squamous cell carcinoma of the head and neck: An effective salvage regimen. Am J Clin Oncol (CCT) 8:61–64, 1985
128. Scherlacher A, Jaske R, Lehnert M: Therapie rezidivierender Plattenepithelkarzinome (rPECHN) im HNO–Bereich mit einem sequentiellen Methotrexat-(MTX)/5-Fluorouracil (5-FU)-Protokoll. Laryngol Rhinol Otol (Stuttg) 64:58–61, 1985
129. Pitman SW, Kowal CD, Bertino JR: Methotrexate and 5-fluorouracil in sequence in squamous head and neck cancer. Semin Oncol 10 (suppl 2):15–19, 1983
130. Lester EP, Johnson CM, Lester AK, et al: Head and neck advanced squamous carcinoma: Treatment with cis-platinum, bleomycin, and sequential methotrexate/5-fluorouracil (abstract C-707). Proc Am Soc Clin Oncol 3:182, 1984
131. Vogl SE, Komisar A, Kaplan BH, et al: Sequential methotrexate and 5-fluorouracil with bleomycin and cisplatin in the chemotherapy of advanced squamous cancer of the head and neck. Cancer 57:706–710, 1986
132. Cognetti F, Pinnaro P, Carlini P, et al: CABO treatment (cisplatin, methotrexate, bleomycin, vincristine) in advanced or recurrent squamous cell carcinoma of the head and neck. J Exp Clin Cancer Res 3:411–417, 1984
133. Kaplan BH, Schoenfeld D, Vogl SE: Treatment of recurrent (REC) or metastatic (MET) squamous cancer of the head and neck (SCH&N) with methotrexate (M), M plus Corynebacterium parvum (CP) or M plus bleomycin (B) plus diamminedichloroplatinum (D): A prospective randomized trial of the Eastern Cooperative Oncology Group (abstract C-780). Proc Am Assoc Cancer Res 22:532, 1981
134. Jacobs C, Meyers F, Hendrickson C, et al: A randomized phase III study of cisplatin with or without methotrexate for recurrent squamous cell carcinoma of the head and neck. A Northern California Oncology Group study. Cancer 52:1563–1569, 1983
135. Drelichman A, Cummings G, Al-Sarraf M: A randomized trial of the combination of cis-platinum, oncovin, and bleomycin (COB) versus methotrexate in patients with advanced squamous cell carcinoma of the head and neck. Cancer 52:399–403, 1983
136. Vogl SE, Schoenfeld DA, Kaplan BH, et al: A randomized prospective comparison of methotrexate with a combination of methotrexate, bleomycin, and cisplatin in head and neck cancer. Cancer 56:432–442, 1985
137. Williams SD, Velez-Garcia E, Essessee I, et al: Chemotherapy for head and neck cancer: Comparison of cisplatin + vinblastine + bleomycin versus methotrexate. Cancer 57:18–23, 1986
138. Ketcham AS, Hoye RC, Chretien PB, et al: Irradiation twenty-four hours preoperatively. Am J Surg 118:691–697, 1969
139. Lawrence WL, Terz JJ, Rogers C, et al: Preoperative irradiation for head and neck cancer: A prospective study. Cancer 33:318–323, 1974
140. Strong EW: Preoperative radiation and radical neck dissection. Surg Clin North Am 49:271–276, 1969
141. Fletcher GH: Basic principles of the combination of irradiation and surgery. Int J Radiat Oncol Biol Phys 5:2091–2096, 1979
142. Looser KG, Shah JP, Strong EW: The significance of "positive" margins in surgically resected epidermoid carcinomas. Head Neck Surg 1:107–111, 1978
143. Amdur RJ, Parsons JT, Mendenhall WM, et al: Postoperative irradiation for squamous cell carcinoma of the head and neck: An analysis of treatment results and complications. Int J Radiat Oncol Biol Phys (in press)
144. Colton T: Statistics in Medicine, pp 163–167. Boston, Little, Brown, 1974
145. Mendenhall W, Ott L, Larson RF: Statistics: A Tool for the Social Sciences. North Scituate, MA, Duxbury Press, 1974
146. Marcus RB Jr, Million RR, Cassisi NJ: Postoperative irradiation for squamous cell carcinomas of the head and neck: Analysis of time-dose factors related to control above the clavicles. Int J Radiat Oncol Biol Phys 5:1943–1949, 1979
147. Peppard SB, Al-Sarraf M, Powers WE, et al: Combination of cis-platinum, oncovin and bleomycin (COB) prior to surgery and/or radiotherapy in advanced untreated epidermoid cancer of the head and neck. Laryngoscope 90:1273–1280, 1980
148. Elias EG, Chretien PB, Monnard E, et al: Chemotherapy prior to local therapy in advanced squamous cell carcinoma of the head and neck: Preliminary assessment of an intensive drug regimen. Cancer 43:1025–1031, 1979
149. Pennacchio JL, Hong WK, Shapshay S, et al: Combination of cis-platinum and bleomycin prior to surgery and/or radiotherapy compared with radiotherapy alone for the treatment for advanced squamous cell carcinoma of the head and neck. Cancer 50:2795–2801, 1982
150. Spaulding MN, Kahn A, DeLos Santos R, et al: Adjuvant chemotherapy in head and neck cancer: An update. Am J Surg 144:432–436, 1982
151. Randolph VL, Vallejo A, Spiro RH, et al: Combination therapy of advanced head and neck cancer: Induction of remission with diamminedichloroplatinum (II), bleomycin and radiation therapy. Cancer 41:460–467, 1978
152. Brown AW Jr, Blom J, Butler WM, et al: Combination chemotherapy with vinblastine, bleomycin, and cis-diamminedichloroplatinum (II) in squamous cell carcinoma of the head and neck. Cancer 45:2830–2835, 1980
153. Weaver A, Flemming S, Kish J, et al: Cis-platinum and 5-fluorouracil as induction therapy for advanced head and neck cancer. Am J Surg 144:445–448, 1982
154. Rooney M, Kish J, Jacobs J, et al: Improved complete response rate and survival in advanced head and neck cancer after three-course induction therapy with 120-hour 5-FU infusion and cisplatin. Cancer 55:1123–1128, 1985
155. Jacobs C, Goffinet DR, Goffinet L, et al: Chemotherapy as a substitute for surgery in the treatment of advanced resectable head and neck cancer: A report from the Northern California Oncology Group. Cancer 60:1178–1183, 1987
156. Ervin TJ, Clark JR, Weichselbaum RR, et al: An analysis of induction and adjuvant chemotherapy in the multidisciplinary treatment of squamous-cell carcinoma of the head and neck. J Clin Oncol 5:10–20, 1987
157. Clark J, Fallon B, Norris C, et al: A randomized trial of two induction regimens for advanced squamous cell carcinoma of the head and neck (SCCHN): Preliminary results (abstract 515). Proc Am Soc Clin Oncol 5:132, 1986
158. Weichselbaum RR, Clark JR, Miller D, et al: Combined modality treatment of head and neck cancer with cisplatin, bleomycin, methotrexate-leucovorin chemotherapy. Cancer 55:2149–2155, 1985
159. Kies MS, Gordon LI, Hauck WW, et al: Analysis of complete responders after initial treatment with chemotherapy in head and neck cancer. Otolaryngol Head Neck Surg 93:199–205, 1985
160. Norris CM Jr, Clark JR, Frei E III, et al: Pathology of surgery after induction chemotherapy: An analysis of resectability and locoregional control. Laryngoscope 96:292–302, 1986
161. Al-Kourainy K, Kish J, Ensley J, et al: Achievement of superior survival for histologically negative versus histologically positive clinically complete responders to cisplatin combination in patients with locally advanced head and neck cancer. Cancer 59:233–238, 1987
162. Clark J, Fallon B, Weichselbaum R, et al: The influence of resectability on response to induction chemotherapy and survival in advanced squamous cell carcinoma of the head and neck (SCCHN) (abstract C-542). Proc Am Soc Clin Oncol 4:139, 1985
163. Jacobs C, Wolf GT, Makuch RW, et al: Adjuvant chemotherapy for head and neck squamous carcinomas (abstract C-708). Proc Am Soc Clin Oncol 3:182, 1984
164. Fallon B, Clark J, Weichselbaum R, et al: Locoregional control in advanced squamous cell carcinoma of the head and neck after induction chemotherapy (abstract C-541). Proc Am Soc Clin Oncol 4:139, 1985
165. Ensley J, Crissman J, Kish J, et al: The impact of conventional morphologic analysis on response rates and survival in patients with advanced head and neck cancers treated initially with cisplatin-containing combination chemotherapy. Cancer 57:711–717, 1986
166. Posner MR, Weichselbaum RR, Fitzgerald TJ, et al: Treatment complications after sequential combination chemotherapy and radiotherapy with or without surgery in previously untreated squamous cell carcinoma of the head and neck. Int J Radiat Oncol Biol Phys 11:1887–1893, 1985
167. Stell PM, Dalby JE, Strickland P, et al: Sequential chemotherapy and radiotherapy in advanced head and neck cancer. Clin Radiol 34:463–467, 1983
168. Schuller DE, Wilson H, Hodgson S, et al: Preoperative reductive chemotherapy for stage III or IV operative epidermoid carcinoma of the oral cavity, oropharynx, or larynx, phase III: A Southwest Oncology Group study (abstract 185). Presented at the International Conference on Head and Neck Cancer, Baltimore, 1984
169. Holoye PY, Grossman TW, Toohill RJ, et al: Randomized study of adjuvant chemotherapy for head and neck cancer. Otolaryngol Head and Neck Surg 93:712–717, 1985
170. Haas C, Anderson T, Byhardt R, et al: Randomized neo-adjuvant study of 5-fluorouracil (FU) and cis-platinum (DDP) for patients (PTS) with advanced resectable head and neck squamous carcinoma (ARHNSC) (abstract 735). Proc Am Assoc Cancer Res 27:185, 1986
171. Martin M, Mazeron JJ, Glaubiger D, et al: Neo-adjuvant polychemotherapy of head and neck cancer: Preliminary results of a randomized study (abstract 551). Proc Am Soc Clin Oncol 5:141, 1986
172. Adjuvant chemotherapy for advanced head and neck squamous carcinoma: Final report of the Head and Neck Contracts Program. Cancer 60:301–311, 1987
173. Condit PT, Ridings GR, Coin JW, et al: Methotrexate and radiation in the treatment of patients with cancer. Cancer Res 24:1524–1533, 1964
174. Friedman M, DeNarvaes FN, Daly JF: Treatment of squamous cell carcinoma of the head and neck with combined methotrexate and irradiation. Cancer 26:711–721, 1970
175. Tarpley JL, Chretien PB, Alexander JC, et al: High dose methotrexate as a preoperative adjuvant in the treatment of epidermoid carcinoma of the head and neck: A feasibility study and clinical trial. Am J Surg 130:481–486, 1975

176. Ervin TJ, Kirkwood J, Weichselbaum RR, et al: Improved survival for patients with advanced carcinoma of the head and neck treated with methotrexate-leucovorin prior to definitive radiotherapy or surgery. Laryngoscope 91:1181–1190, 1981

177. von Essen CF, Joseph LBM, Simon GT, et al: Sequential chemotherapy and radiation therapy of buccal mucosa carcinoma in South India: Methods and preliminary results. Am J Roentgenol Radium Ther Nucl Med 102:530–540, 1968

178. Knowlton AH, Percarpio B, Bobrow S, et al: Methotrexate and radiation therapy in the treatment of advanced head and neck tumors. Radiology 116:709–712, 1975

179. Fazekas JT, Sommer C, Kramer S: Adjuvant intravenous methotrexate or definitive radiotherapy alone for advanced squamous cancers of the oral cavity, oropharynx, supraglottic larynx or hypopharynx: Concluding report of an RTOG randomized trial on 638 patients. Int J Radiat Oncol Biol Phys 6:533–541, 1980

180. Taylor SG, Applebaum E, Showel JL, et al: A randomized trial of adjuvant chemotherapy in head and neck cancer. J Clin Oncol 3:672–679, 1985

181. Huang AT, Cole TB, Fishburn R, et al: Adjuvant chemotherapy after surgery and radiation for stage III and IV head and neck cancer. Ann Surg 200:195–199, 1984

182. Johnson JT, Myers EN, Schramm VL, et al: Adjuvant chemotherapy for high-risk squamous-cell carcinoma of the head and neck. J Clin Oncol 5:456–458, 1987

183. Bitter K: Postoperative chemotherapy versus postoperative cobalt 60 radiation in patients with advanced oral carcinoma: Report on a randomized study (abst). Head Neck Surg 3:264, 1981

184. Tejada F, Chandler JR: Combined therapy for stage III and IV head and neck cancer (H&N) (abstract C-774). Proc Am Soc Clin Oncol 1:199, 1982

185. Shanta V, Krishramurthi S: The combined therapy of oral cancer. GANN Monogr Cancer Res 19:159–170, 1976

186. Abe M, Shigematsu Y, Kimura S: Combined use of bleomycin with radiation in the treatment of cancer. Recent Results Cancer Res 63:169–178, 1978

187. Kapstad B, Bang G, Rennaes S, et al: Combined preoperative treatment with cobalt and bleomycin in patients with head and neck carcinoma: A controlled clinical study. Int J Radiat Oncol Biol Phys 4:85–89, 1978

188. Fu KK, Phillips TL, Silverberg IJ, et al: Combined radiotherapy and chemotherapy with bleomycin and methotrexate for advanced inoperable head and neck cancer: Update of a Northern California Oncology Group randomized trial. J Clin Oncol 5:1410–1418, 1987

189. Gollin FF, Ansfield FJ, Brandenburg JH, et al: Combined therapy in advanced head and neck cancer: A randomized study. Am J Roentgenol Radium Ther Nucl Med 114:83–88, 1972

190. Ansfield FJ, Ramirez G, Davis HL Jr, et al: Treatment of advanced cancer of the head and neck. Cancer 25:78–82, 1970

191. Papac RJ, Weissberg JB, Son YH, et al: Prospective randomized trial of radiation therapy (RT) ± mitomycin C (MC) in head and neck cancer (abstract 492). Proc Am Soc Clin Oncol 6:126, 1987

192. Stefani S, Eells RW, Abbate J: Hydroxyurea and radiotherapy in head and neck cancer: Results of a prospective controlled study in 126 patients. Radiology 101:391–396, 1971

193. Richards GJ, Chambers RG: Hydoxyurea: A radiosensitizer in the treatment of neoplasms of the head and neck. Am J Roentgenol Radium Ther Nucl Med 105:555–565, 1969

194. Kramer S: Methotrexate and radiation therapy in the treatment of advanced squamous cell carcinoma of the oral cavity, oropharynx, supraglottic larynx, and hypopharynx: Preliminary report of a controlled clinical trial of the Radiation Therapy Oncology Group. Can J Otolaryngol 4:213–218, 1975

195. Condit PT: Treatment of carcinoma with radiation therapy and methotrexate. Mo Med 65:832–835, 1968

196. Bagshaw MA, Doggett RLS: A clinical study of chemical radiosensitization. Front Radiat Ther Oncol 4:164–173, 1969

197. Haselow RE, Adams GS, Oken MM, et al: Simultaneous cis-platinum (DDP) and radiation therapy (RT) for locally advanced unresectable head and neck cancer (Abstract C-780). Proc Am Soc Clin Oncol 1:201, 1982

198. Leipzig B, Wetmore SJ, Klug D, et al: Cis-platinum sensitization to radiotherapy of squamous cell carcinoma in the head and neck. In Vidockler HR (ed): Proceedings of the International Conference on Head and Neck Cancer, p 42. Baltimore, Lancaster Press, 1984

199. Coughlin CT, Grace M, LeMarbre P, et al: Combined modality therapy for advanced head and neck cancer (abstract C-776). Proc Am Soc Clin Oncol 1:200, 1982

200. Al-Sarraf M, Pajak TF, Marcial VA, et al: Concurrent radiotherapy and chemotherapy with cisplatin in inoperable squamous cell carcinoma of the head and neck: An RTOG study. Cancer 59:259–265, 1987

201. Byfield JE, Sharp TR, Frankel SS, et al: Phase I and II trial of five-day infused 5-fluorouracil and radiation in advanced cancer of the head and neck. J Clin Oncol 2:406–413, 1984

202. Adelstein DJ, Sharan VM, Earle AS, et al: Combined modality therapy (CMT) with simultaneous 5-fluorouracil (5FU), cis-platinum (DDP) and radiation therapy (RT) in the treatment of squamous cell cancer of the head and neck (Abstract C-511). Proc Am Soc Clin Oncol 4:131, 1985

203. Taylor SG IV, Murthy AK, Showel JL, et al: Improved control in advanced head and neck cancer with simultaneous radiation and cisplatin/5-FU chemotherapy. Cancer Treat Rep 69:933–939, 1985

204. Kaplan MJ, Hahn SS, Johns ME, et al: Mitomycin and fluorouracil with concomitant radiotherapy in head and neck cancer. Arch Otolaryngol 111:220–222, 1985

205. Taylor SG IV: Integration of chemotherapy into the combined modality therapy of head and neck squamous cancer. Int J Radiat Oncol Biol Phys 13:779–783, 1987

206. Goldsmith MA, Carter SK: The integration of chemotherapy into a combined modal-

ity of approach to cancer therapy. V. Squamous cell cancer of the head and neck. Cancer Treat Rev 2:137–158, 1975

207. Arcangeli G, Nervi C, Righini R, et al: Combined radiation and drugs: The effect of intra-arterial chemotherapy followed by radiotherapy in head and neck cancer. Radiother Oncol 1:101–107, 1983

208. Fitzpatrick PJ: Cancer of the lip. J Otolaryngol 13:32–36, 1984

209. Byers RM, O'Brien J, Waxler J: The therapeutic and prognostic implications of nerve invasion in cancer of the lower lip. Int J Radiat Oncol Biol Phys 4:215–217, 1978

210. Mackay EN, Sellers AH: A statistical review of carcinoma of the lip. Can Med Assoc J 90:670–672, 1964

211. Million RR, Cassisi NJ: Carcinoma of the skin. In Million RR, Cassisi NJ (eds): Management of Head and Neck Cancer: A Multidisciplinary Approach, pp 475–511. Philadelphia, JB Lippincott, 1984

212. MacComb WS, Fletcher GH, Healey JE Jr: Intra-oral cavity. In MacComb WS, Fletcher GH (eds): Cancer of the Head and Neck, pp 89–151. Baltimore, Williams & Wilkins, 1967

213. Heller KS, Shah JP: Carcinoma of the lip. Am J Surg 138:600–603, 1979

214. Hendricks JL, Mendelson BC, Woods JE: Invasive carcinoma of the lower lip. Surg Clin North Am 57:837–844, 1977

215. Mohs FE, Snow SN: Microscopically controlled surgical treatment for squamous cell carcinoma of the lower lip. Surg Gynecol Obstet 160: 37–41, 1985

216. Ange DW, Lindberg RD, Guillamondegui OM: Management of squamous cell carcinoma of the oral tongue and floor of mouth after excisional biopsy. Radiology 116:143–146, 1974

217. Chu A, Fletcher GH: Incidence and causes of failures to control by irradiation the primary lesions in squamous cell carcinomas of the anterior two-thirds of the tongue and floor of mouth. Am J Roentgenol Radium Ther Nucl Med 117:501–508, 1973

218. Mendenhall WM, VanCise WS, Bova FJ, et al: Analysis of time-dose factors in squamous cell carcinoma of the oral tongue and floor of mouth treated with radiation therapy alone. Int J Radiat Oncol Biol Phys 7:1005–1011, 1981

219. Fu KK, Lichter A, Galante M: Carcinoma of the floor of mouth: An analysis of treatment results and the sites and causes of failures. Int J Radiat Oncol Biol Phys 1:829–837, 1976

220. Marcus RB Jr, Million RR, Mitchell TP: A preloaded, custom-designed implantation device for stage T1-T2 carcinoma of the floor of mouth. Int J Radiat Oncol Biol Phys 6:111–113, 1980

221. Tapley N: Clinical Applications of the Electron Beam, pp 125–129. New York, John Wiley & Sons, 1976

222. Flynn MB, Mullins FX, Moore C: Selection of treatment in squamous carcinoma of the floor of the mouth. Am J Surg 126:477–481, 1973

223. Guillamondegui OM, Jesse RH: Surgical treatment of advanced carcinoma of the floor of the mouth. Am J Roentgenol 126:1256–1259, 1976

224. Million RR, Cassisi NJ: Oral cavity. In Million RR, Cassisi NJ (eds): Management of Head and Neck Cancer: A Multidisciplinary Approach, pp 239–297. Philadelphia, JB Lippincott, 1984

225. Wang CC, Doppke KP, Biggs PJ: Intra-oral cone radiation therapy for selected carcinomas of the oral cavity. Int J Radiat Oncol Biol Phys 9:1185–1189, 1983

226. Leipzig, B.: Assessment of mandibular invasion by carcinoma. Cancer 56:1201–1205, 1985

227. Scholl P, Byers RM, Batsakis JG, et al: Microscopic cut-through of cancer in the surgical treatment of squamous carcinoma of the tongue: Prognostic and therapeutic implications. Am J Surg 152:354–360, 1986

228. Fu KK, Ray JW, Chan EK, et al: External and interstitial radiation therapy of carcinoma of the oral tongue: A review of 32 years experience. Am J Roentgenol 126:107–115, 1976

229. Lees AW: The treatment of carcinoma of the anterior two-thirds of the tongue by radiotherapy. Int J Radiat Oncol Biol Phys 1:849–858, 1976

230. Nair MK, Sankaranarayanan R, Padmanabhan TK: Evaluation of the role of radiotherapy in the management of carcinoma of the buccal mucosa. Cancer (in press)

231. Bloom NO, Spiro RH: Carcinoma of the cheek mucosa: A retrospective analysis. Am J Surg 140:556–559, 1980

232. Small IA, Waldron CA: Ameloblastomas of the jaws. Oral Surg Oral Med Oral Path 8:281–297, 1955

233. Sinclair NA: Cysts and ameloblastomas: A relationship. Aust Dent J 22:27–30, 1977

234. Pandya NJ, Stuteville OH: Treatment of ameloblastoma. Plast Reconstr Surg 50:242–248, 1972

235. Sehdev MK, Huvos AG, Strong EW, et al: Proceedings: Ameloblastoma of maxilla and mandible. Cancer 33:324–333, 1974

236. Byers RM, Anderson B, Schwarz EA, et al: Treatment of squamous carcinoma of the retromolar trigone. Am J Clin Oncol 7:647–652, 1984

237. Goldberg SJ, Friedman JM: Ameloblastoma: Review of the literature and report of case. J Am Dent Assoc 90:432–438, 1975

238. McIvor J: The radiological features of ameloblastoma. Clin Radiol 25:237–242, 1974

239. Swearingen AG, McGraw JP, Palumbo VD: Roentgenographic pathologic correlation of carcinoma of the gingiva involving the mandible. Am J Roentgenol Radium Ther Nucl Med 96:15–18, 1966

240. Rankow RM, Hickey MJ: Adamantinoma of the mandible: Analysis of surgical treatment. Surgery 36:713–719, 1954

241. Byers RM, Newman R, Russell N, et al: Results of treatment for squamous carcinoma of the lower gum. Cancer 47:2236–2238, 1981

242. Shibuya H, Horiuchi J-I, Suzuki S, et al: Oral carcinoma of the upper jaw: Results of radiation treatment. Acta Radiol Oncol 23:331–335, 1984

243. Fayos JV: Carcinoma of the mandible: Result of radiation therapy. Acta Radiol Ther Phys Biol 12:378–386, 1973
244. Million RR, Cassisi NJ: Oropharynx. In Million RR, Cassisi NJ (eds): Management of Head and Neck Cancer: A Multidisciplinary Approach, pp 299–314. Philadelphia, JB Lippincott, 1984
245. Gardner KE, Parsons JT, Mendenhall WM, et al: Time-dose relationships for local tumor control and complications following irradiation of squamous cell carcinoma of the base of tongue. Int J Radiat Oncol Biol Phys 13:507–510, 1987
246. Fletcher GH: Oral cavity and oropharynx. In Fletcher GH (ed): Textbook of Radiotherapy, 2nd ed, pp 212–254. Philadelphia, Lea & Febiger, 1973
247. Whicker JH, DeSanto LW, Devine KD: Surgical treatment of squamous cell carcinoma of the base of the tongue. Laryngoscope 82:1853–1860, 1972
248. Callery CD, Spiro RH, Strong EW: Changing trends in the management of squamous carcinoma of the tongue. Am J Surg 148:449–454, 1984
249. Cutler SJ, Ederer F: Maximum utilization of the life table method in analyzing survival. J Chron Dis 8:699–712, 1958
250. Mendenhall WM, Parsons JT, Cassisi NJ, et al: Squamous cell carcinoma of the tonsillar area treated with radical irradiation. Radiother Oncol 10:23–30, 1987
251. Mizono GS, Diaz RF, Fu KK, et al: Carcinoma of the tonsillar region. Laryngoscope 96:240–244, 1986
252. Gelinas M, Fletcher GH: Incidence and causes of local failure of irradiation in squamous cell carcinoma of the faucial arch, tonsillar fossa, and base of tongue. Radiology 108:383–387, 1973
253. Dasmahapatra KS, Mohit-Tabatabai MA, Rush BF, et al: Cancer of the tonsil: Improved survival with combination therapy. Cancer 57:451–455, 1986
254. Shrewsbury D, Adams GL, Duvall AJ, et al: Carcinoma of the tonsillar region: A comparison of radiation therapy with combined preoperative radiation and surgery. Otolaryngol Head Neck Surg 89:979–985, 1981
255. Remmler D, Medina JE, Byers RM, et al: Treatment of choice for squamous carcinoma of the tonsillar fossa. Head Neck Surg 7:206–211, 1985
256. Amornmarn R, Prempree T, Jaiwatana J, et al: Radiation management of carcinoma of the tonsillar region. Cancer 54:1293–1299, 1984
257. Perez CA, Purdy JA, Breaux SR, et al: Carcinoma of the tonsillar fossa: A nonrandomized comparison of preoperative radiation and surgery or irradiation alone: Long-term results. Cancer 50:2314–2322, 1982
258. Weichert KA, Aron BS, Maltz R, et al: Carcinoma of the tonsil: Treatment by a planned combination of radiation and surgery. Int J Radiat Oncol Biol Phys 1:505–508, 1976
259. Perez CA, Lee FA, Ackerman LV, et al: Non-randomized comparison of preoperative irradiation and surgery versus irradiation alone in the management of carcinoma of the tonsil. Am J Roentgenol 126:248–260, 1976
260. Strong MS, Vaughan CW, Kayne HL, et al: A randomized trial of preoperative radiotherapy in cancer of the oropharynx and hypopharynx. Am J Surg 136:494–500, 1978
261. Bova FJ: Treatment planning for irradiation of head and neck cancer. In Million RR, Cassisi NJ (eds): Management of Head and Neck Cancer: A Multidisciplinary Approach, pp 209–230. Philadelphia, JB Lippincott, 1984
262. Mazeron JJ, Marinello G, Leung S, et al: Interstitial radiation therapy for squamous cell carcinoma of the tonsillar region: The Creteil experience (1971–1981). Int J Radiat Oncol Biol Phys 12:895–900, 1986
263. Fletcher GH: The Third Annual Lectureship of the Juan A. del Regato Foundation: Squamous cell carcinomas of the oropharynx. Int J Radiat Oncol Biol Phys 5:2073–2090, 1979
264. Pierquin B, Chassagne DJ, Chahbazian CM, et al: Brachytherapy, pp 104–108. St. Louis, WH Green, 1978
265. Ratzer ER, Schweitzer RJ, Frazell EL: Epidermoid carcinoma of the palate. Am J Surg 119:294–297, 1970
266. Weller SA, Goffinet DR, Goode RL, et al: Carcinoma of the oropharynx: Results of megavoltage radiation therapy in 305 patients. Am J Roentgenol 126:236–247, 1976
267. Seydel HG, Scholl H: Carcinoma of the soft palate and uvula. Am J Roentgenol Radium Ther Nucl Med 120:603–607, 1974
268. Amdur RJ, Mendenhall WM, Parsons JT, et al: Carcinoma of the soft palate treated with irradiation: Analysis of results and complications. Radiother Oncol 9:185–194, 1987
269. Lindberg RD, Fletcher GH: The role of irradiation in the management of head and neck cancer: Analysis of results and causes of failure. Tumori 64:313–325, 1978
270. Chung CK, Constable WC: Squamous cell carcinoma of the soft palate and uvula. Int J Radiat Oncol Biol Phys 5:845–850, 1979
271. Garrett PG, Beale FA: Carcinoma of the oropharynx: Soft palate. J Otolaryngol 13:165–168, 1984
272. Fee WE, Schoeppel SL, Rubenstein R, et al: Squamous cell carcinoma of the soft palate. Arch Otolaryngol 105:710–720, 1979
273. Wynder EL: The epidemiology of cancer of the upper alimentary and upper respiratory tracts. Laryngoscope 88 (suppl 8):50–51, 1978
274. Vincent RG, Marchetta F: The relationship of the use of tobacco and alcohol to cancer of the oral cavity, pharynx or larynx. Am J Surg 105:501–505, 1963
275. Fraumeni JF Jr: Geographic distribution of head and neck cancers in the United States. Laryngoscope 88 (suppl 8):40–44, 1978
276. Batsakis JG: Tumors of the Head and Neck, 2nd ed, pp 219–220, 342. Baltimore, Williams & Wilkins, 1979
277. Pillsbury HRC, Kirchner JA: Clinical vs histopathologic staging in laryngeal cancer. Arch Otolaryngol 105:157–159, 1979
278. Kirchner JA: Staging as seen in serial sections. Laryngoscope 85:1816–1821, 1975
279. Olsen KD, DeSanto LW, Pearson BW: Positive Delphian lymph node: Clinical significance in laryngeal cancer. Laryngoscope 97:1033–1037, 1987
280. Lederman M: Place de la radiotherapie dans le traitment du cancer du larynx [The place of radiotherapy in the treatment of cancer of the larynx.] Ann Radiol 4: 433–454, 1961
281. Mancuso AA, Hanafee WN, Juillard GJF, et al: The role of computed tomography in the management of cancer of the larynx. Radiology 124:243–244, 1977
282. Fletcher GH, Jing B-S: The Head and Neck, p 168. Chicago, Year Book, 1968
283. Million RR, Cassisi NJ: Larynx. In Million RR, Cassisi NJ (eds): Management of Head and Neck Cancer: A Multidisciplinary Approach, pp 315–364. Philadelphia, JB Lippincott, 1984
284. Harwood AR: Cancer of the larynx: The Toronto experience. J Otolaryngol (suppl 11) 3–21, 1982
285. Biller HF, Barnhill FR Jr, Ogura JH, et al: Hemilaryngectomy following radiation failure for carcinoma of the vocal cords. Laryngoscope 80:249–253, 1970
286. Mendenhall WM, Parsons JT, Stringer SP, et al: TI–T2 vocal cord carcinoma: A basis for comparing the results of irradiation and surgery. Head Neck Surg 10:373–377, 1988
287. Burns HP, van Nostrand AWP, Bryce DP: Verrucous carcinoma of the larynx: Management by radiotherapy and surgery. Ann Otol Rhinol Laryngol 85:538–543, 1976
288. Harwood AR, Beale FA, Cummings BJ, et al: T3 glottic cancer: An analysis of dose time-volume factors. Int J Radiat Oncol Biol Phys 6:675–680, 1980
289. Mendenhall WM, Million RR, Sharkey DE, et al: Stage T3 squamous cell carcinoma of the glottic larynx treated with surgery and/or radiation therapy. Int J Radiat Oncol Biol Phys 10:357–363, 1984
290. Singer MI, Blom ED: An endoscopic technique for restoration of voice after laryngectomy. Ann Otol Rhinol Laryngol 89:529–533, 1980
291. Singer MI, Blom ED, Hamaker RC: Further experience with voice restoration after total laryngectomy. Ann Otol Rhinol Laryngol 90:498–502, 1981
292. Panje WR: Prosthetic vocal rehabilitation following laryngectomy: The voice button. Ann Otol Rhinol Laryngol 90:116–120, 1981
293. Panje WR, VanDemark D, McCabe BF: Voice button prosthesis rehabilitation of the laryngectomee: Additional nodes. Ann Otol Rhinol Laryngol 90:503–505, 1981
294. Merwin GE, Goldstein LP: Speech rehabilitation after total laryngectomy. In Million RR, Cassisi NJ (eds): Management of Head and Neck Cancer: A Multidisciplinary Approach, pp 365–372. Philadelphia, JB Lippincott, 1984
295. Fletcher GH, Lindberg RD, Hamberger A, et al: Reasons for irradiation failure in squamous cell carcinoma of the larynx. Laryngoscope 85:987–1003, 1975
296. Lee F, Perlmutter S, Ogura JH: Laryngeal radiation after hemilaryngectomy. Laryngoscope 90:1534–1539, 1980
297. Balm AJM, Snow GB, Karim ABMF, et al: Long-term results of concurrent polychemotherapy and radiotherapy in patients with stomal recurrence after total laryngectomy. Ann Otol Rhinol Laryngol 95:572–575, 1986
298. Gluckman JL, Hamaker RC, Schuller DE, et al: Surgical salvage for stomal recurrence: A multi-institutional experience. Laryngoscope 97:1025–1029, 1987
299. Fletcher GH, Goepfert H: Larynx and pyriform sinus. In Fletcher GH: Textbook of Radiotherapy, 3rd ed, pp 330–363. Philadelphia, Lea & Febiger, 1980
300. Mendenhall WM, Million RR, Cassisi NJ: Squamous cell carcinoma of the supraglottic larynx treated with radical irradiation: Analysis of treatment parameters and results. Int J Radiat Oncol Biol Phys 10:2223–2230, 1984
301. Million RR, Cassisi NJ, Parsons JT, et al: Radiation therapy in the management of carcinoma of the larynx. In Fried MP: The Larynx. Boston, Little, Brown (in press)
302. Ogura JH, Sessions DG, Spector GJ: Analysis of surgical therapy for epidermoid carcinoma of the laryngeal glottis. Laryngoscope 85:1522–1530, 1975
303. Wang CC: Treatment of glottic carcinoma by megavoltage radiation therapy and results. Am J Roentgenol Radium Ther Nucl Med 120:157–163, 1974
304. Mills EED: Early glottic carcinoma: Factors affecting radiation failure, results of treatment and sequelae. Int J Radiat Oncol Biol Phys 5:811–817, 1979
305. Fletcher GH, Lindberg RD, Jesse RH: Radiation therapy for cancer of the larynx and pyriform sinus. EENT Digest 31:58–67, 1969
306. Stewart JG, Brown JR, Palmer MK, et al: The management of glottic carcinoma by primary irradiation with surgery in reserve. Laryngoscope 85:1477–1484, 1975
307. Harwood AR, Hawkins NV, Beale FA, et al: Management of advanced glottic cancer: A 10-year review of the Toronto experience. Int J Radiat Oncol Biol Phys 5:899–904, 1979
308. Harwood AR, Hawkins NV, Rider WD, et al: Radiotherapy of early glottic cancer–I. Int J Radiat Oncol Biol Phys 5:473–476, 1979
309. Dickens WJ, Cassisi NJ, Million RR, et al: Treatment of early vocal cord carcinoma: A comparison of apples and apples. Laryngoscope 93:216–219, 1983
310. Jesse RH: The evaluation of treatment of patients with extensive squamous cancer of the vocal cords. Laryngoscope 85:1424–1429, 1975
311. Skolnik EM, Yee KF, Wheatley MA, et al: Carcinoma of the laryngeal glottis: Therapy and end results. Laryngoscope 85:1453–1466, 1975
312. Vermund H: Role of radiotherapy in cancer of the larynx as related to the TNM system of staging: A review. Cancer 25:485–504, 1970
313. Stewart JG, Jackson AW: The steepness of the dose response curve both for tumor cure and normal tissue injury. Laryngoscope 85:1107–1111, 1975
314. Harwood AR, Beale FA, Cummings BJ, et al: T4N0M0 glottic cancer: An analysis of dose-time volume factors. Int J Radiat Oncol Biol Phys 7:1507–1512, 1981
315. Weems DH, Mendenhall WM, Parsons JT, et al: Squamous cell carcinoma of the

supraglottic larynx treated with surgery and/or radiation therapy. Int J Radiat Oncol Biol Phys 13:1483–1487, 1987

316. Neel H III, Devine KD, Desanto LW: Laryngofissure and cordectomy for early cordal carcinoma: Outcome in 182 patients. Otolaryngol Head Neck Surg 88:79–84, 1980

317. Mendenhall WM, Parson JT, Million RR, et al: T1–T2 squamous cell carcinoma of the glottic larynx treated with radiation therapy: Relationship of dose-fractionation factors to local control and complications. Int J Radiat Oncol Biol Phys (in press)

318. Ballantyne AJ: Principles of surgical management of cancer of the pharyngeal walls. Cancer 20:663–667, 1965

319. Kirchner JA: Pyriform sinus cancer: A clinical and laboratory study. Ann Otol Rhinol Laryngol 84:793–803, 1975

320. Wang CC: Radiotherapeutic management of carcinoma of the posterior pharyngeal wall. Cancer 27:894–896, 1971

321. Biller HF, Davis WH, Ogura JH: Delayed contralateral cervical metastases with laryngeal and laryngopharyngeal cancers. Laryngoscope 81:1499–1502, 1971

322. Million RR, Cassisi NJ: Radical irradiation for carcinoma of the pyriform sinus. Laryngoscope 91:439–450, 1981

323. Mendenhall WM, Parsons JT, Mancuso AA, et al: Squamous cell carcinoma of the pharyngeal wall treated with irradiation. Radiother Oncol 11:205–212, 1988

324. Marks JE, Freeman RB, Lee F, et al: Pharyngeal wall cancer: An analysis of treatment results complications and patterns of failure. Int J Radiat Oncol Biol Phys 4:587–593, 1978

325. Meoz-Mendez RT, Fletcher GH, Guillamondegui OM, et al: Analysis of the results of irradiation in the treatment of squamous cell carcinomas of the pharyngeal walls. Int J Radiat Oncol Biol Phys 4:579–585, 1978

326. Marks JE, Kurnick B, Powers WE, et al: Carcinoma of the pyriform sinus: An analysis of treatment results and patterns of failure. Cancer 41:1008–1015, 1978

327. Mendenhall WM, Parsons JT, Cassisi NJ, et al: Squamous cell carcinoma of the pyriform sinus treated with radical radiation therapy. Radiother Oncol 9:201–208, 1987

328. El-Badawi SA, Goepfert H, Fletcher GH, et al: Squamous cell carcinoma of the pyriform sinus. Laryngoscope 92:357–364, 1982

329. Million RR, Cassisi NJ: Hypopharynx: Pharyngeal walls, pyriform sinus, and postcricoid pharynx. In Million RR, Cassisi NJ (eds): Management of Head and Neck Cancer: A Multidisciplinary Approach, pp 373–391. Philadelphia, JB Lippincott, 1984

330. Fletcher GH, Million RR: Malignant tumors of the nasopharynx. Am J Roentgenol Radium Ther Nucl Med 93:44–55, 1965

331. Chen KY, Fletcher GH: Malignant tumors of the nasopharynx. Radiology 99:165–171, 1971

332. Fletcher GH, Million RR: Nasopharynx. In Fletcher GH (ed): Textbook of Radiotherapy, 3rd ed, pp 364–383. Philadelphia, Lea & Febiger, 1980

333. Mesic JB, Fletcher GH, Goepfert H: Megavoltage irradiation of epithelial tumors of the nasopharynx. Int J Radiat Oncol Biol Phys 7:477–453, 1981

334. Hoppe RT, Goffinet DR, Bagshaw MA: Carcinoma of the nasopharynx: Eighteen years' experience with megavoltage radiation therapy. Cancer 37:2605–2612, 1976

335. Biller HF, Sessions DG, Ogura JH: Angiofibroma: A treatment approach. Laryngoscope 84:695–706, 1974

336. Briant TDR, Fitzpatrick PJ, Berman J: Nasopharynx angiofibroma: A twenty-year study. Laryngoscope 88:1247–1251, 1978

337. Million RR, Cassisi NJ: Juvenile angiofibroma. In Million RR, Cassisi NJ (eds): Management of Head and Neck Cancer: A Multidisciplinary Approach, pp 467–474. Philadelphia, JB Lippincott, 1984

338. Samaan NA, Bakdash MM, Caderao JB, et al: Hypopituitarism after external irradiation: Evidence for both hypothalamic and pituitary origin. Ann Intern Med 83:771–777, 1975

339. Boldrey E, Sheline G: Delayed transitory clinical manifestations after radiation treatment of intracranial tumors. Acta Radiol Ther 5:5–10, 1966

340. Acheson ED, Cowdell RH, Hadfield EH, et al: Nasal cancer in woodworkers in the furniture industry. Br Med J [Clin Res] 2:587–596, 1968

341. Acheson ED, Cowdell RH, Jolles B: Nasal cancer in the Northamptonshire boot and shoe industry. Br Med J [Clin Res]1:385–393, 1970

342. Acheson ED, Hadfield EH, Macbeth RG: Carcinoma of the nasal cavity and accessory sinuses in woodworkers. Lancet 1:311–312, 1967

343. Ironside P, Matthews J: Adenocarcinoma of the nose and paranasal sinuses in woodworkers in the state of Victoria, Australia. Cancer 36:1115–1121, 1975

344. Maisel RH, Johnston WH, Anderson HA, et al: Necrotizing sialometaplasia involving the nasal cavity. Laryngoscope 87:429–434, 1977

345. Kadish S, Goodman M, Wang CC: Olfactory neuroblastoma: A clinical analysis of 17 cases. Cancer 37:1571–1576, 1976

346. Mendenhall WM, Million RR Cassisi NJ, et al: Biologically aggressive papillomas of the nasal cavity: The role of radiation therapy. Laryngoscope 95:344–347, 1985

347. Kassel SH, Echevarria RA, Guzzo FP: Midline malignant reticulosis (so-called lethal midline granuloma). Cancer 23:920–935, 1969

348. Goepfert H, Guillamondegui OM, Jesse RH, et al: Squamous cell carcinoma of the nasal vestibule. Arch Otolaryngol 100:8–10, 1974

349. Mendenhall NP, Parsons JT, Cassisi NJ, et al: Carcinoma of the nasal vestibule treated with radiation therapy. Laryngoscope 97:626–632, 1987

350. Olsen KD, DeSanto LW: Olfactory neuroblastoma. Arch Otolaryngol 109:797–802, 1983

351. Million RR, Cassisi NJ, Hamlin DJ: Nasal vestibule, nasal cavity, and paranasal sinuses. In Million RR, Cassisi NJ (eds): Management of Head and Neck Cancer: A Multidisciplinary Approach, pp 407–444. Philadelphia, JB Lippincott, 1984

352. Weissler MC, Montgomery WW, Turner PA, et al: Inverted papilloma. Ann Otol Rhinol Laryngol 95:215–221, 1986

353. Schoub L, Timme AH, Uys CJ: A well-differentiated inverted papilloma of the nasal space associated with lymph node metastases. S Afr Med J 47:1663–1665, 1973

354. Fechner RE, Sessions RB: Inverted papilloma of the lacrimal sac, paranasal sinus, and cervical region. Cancer 40:2303–2308, 1977

355. Haynes WD, Tapley N: Radiation treatment of carcinoma of the nasal vestibule. Am J Roentgenol Ther Nucl Med 120:595–602, 1974

356. Mendenhall NP, Parsons JT, Cassisi NJ, et al: Carcinoma of the nasal vestibule. Int J Radiat Oncol Biol Phys 10:627–637, 1984

357. Ketcham AS, Chretien PB, VanBuren JM, et al: The ethmoid sinuses: A re-evaluation of surgical resection. Am J Surg 126:469–476, 1973

358. Ellingwood KE, Million RR: Cancer of the nasal cavity and ethmoid/sphenoid sinuses. Cancer 43:1517–1526, 1979

359. Myers EN, Schramm VL, Barnes EL: Management of inverted papilloma of the nose and paranasal sinuses. Laryngoscope 91:2071–2084, 1981

360. Frazell EL, Lewis JS: Cancer of the nasal cavity and accessory sinuses: A report of the management of 416 patients. Cancer 16:1293–1301, 1963

361. Cheesman AD, Lund VJ, Howard DJ: Craniofacial resection for tumors of the nasal cavity and paranasal sinuses. Head Neck Surg 8:429–435, 1986

362. Bosch A, Vallecillo L, Frias Z: Cancer of the nasal cavity. Cancer 37:1458–1463, 1976

363. Boone ML, Harle TS, Highott HW, et al: Malignant disease of the paranasal sinuses and nasal cavity: Importance of precise localization of extent of disease. Am J Roentgenol Radium Ther Nucl Med 102:627–637, 1968

364. Parsons JT, Mendenhall WM, Mancuso AA, et al: Malignant tumors of the nasal cavity and ethmoid and sphenoid sinuses. Int J Radiat Oncol Biol Phys 14:11–22, 1988

365. Elkon D, Hightower SI, Lim ML, et al: Esthesioneuroblastoma. Cancer 44:1087–1094, 1979

366. Shah JP, Feghali J: Esthesioneuroblastoma. Am J Surg 142:456–458, 1981

367. Fauci AS, Johnson RE, Wolff SM: Radiation therapy of midline granuloma. Ann Intern Med 84:140–147, 1976

368. Jesse RH: Preoperative versus postoperative radiation in the treatment of squamous cell carcinoma of the paranasal sinuses. Am J Surg 110:552–556, 1965

369. Bataini J-P, Ennuyer A: Advanced carcinoma of the maxillary antrum treated by cobalt teletherapy and electron beam irradiation. Br J Radiol 44:590–598, 1971

370. Shukovsky LJ, Fletcher GH: Retinal and optic nerve complications in a high dose irradiation technique of ethmoid sinus and nasal cavity. Radiology 104:629–634, 1972

371. Parsons JT, Fitzgerald CR, Hood CI, et al: The effects of irradiation on the eye and optic nerve. Int J Radiat Oncol Biol Phys 9:609–622, 1983

372. Edwards C, Heath D, Harris P: The carotid body in emphysema and left ventricular hypertrophy. J Pathol 104:1–13, 1971

373. Guild SR: The glomus jugulare, a nonchromaffin paraganglion, in man. Ann Otol Rhinol Laryngol 62:1045–1071, 1953

374. Ward PH, Jenkins HA, Hanafee WN: Diagnosis and treatment of carotid body tumors. Ann Otol Rhinol Laryngol 87:614–621, 1978

375. Lapayowker MS, Liebman EP, Ronis ML, et al: Presentation of the internal carotid artery as a tumor of the middle ear. Radiology 98:293–297, 1971

376. Glasscock ME III, Harris PF, Newsome G: Glomus tumors: Diagnosis and treatment. Laryngoscope 84:2006–2032, 1974

377. Kim J-A, Elkon D, Lim M-L, et al: Optimum dose of radiotherapy for chemodectomas of the middle ear. Int J Radiat Oncol Biol Phys 6:815–819, 1980

378. Mischke RE, Balkany TJ: Skull base approach to glomus jugulare. Laryngoscope 90:89–94, 1980

379. Maruyama Y, Gold LHA, Kieffer SA: Clinical and angiographic evaluation of radiotherapeutic response of glomus jugulare tumors. Radiology 101:397–399, 1971

380. Myers EN, Newman J, Kaseff L, et al: Glomus jugulare tumor: A radiographic-histologic correlation. Laryngoscope 81:1838–1851, 1971

381. Tidwell TJ, Montague ED: Chemodectomas involving the temporal bone. Radiology 116:147–149, 1975

382. Friedland JL, Mendenhall WM, Parsons JT, et al: Chemodectomas arising in temporal bone structures. Head Neck Surg (in press)

383. Hudgins PT: Radiotherapy for extensive glomus jugulare tumors. Radiology 103:427–429, 1972

384. Cole JM: Glomus jugulare tumor. Laryngoscope 87:1244–1258, 1977

385. Smith PE: Management of chemodectomas (glomus jugulare). Laryngoscope 80:207–216, 1970

386. Newman H, Rowe JF Jr, Phillips TL: Radiation therapy of the glomus jugulare tumor. Am J Roentgenol Radium Ther Nucl Med 118:663–669, 1973

387. Grubb WB Jr, Lampe I: The role of radiation therapy in the treatment of chemodectomas of the glomus jugulare. Laryngoscope 75:1861–1871, 1965

388. Hatfield PM, James AE, Schulz MD: Chemodectomas of the glomus jugulare. Cancer 30:1164–1168, 1972

389. Rosenwasser H: Current management: Glomus jugulare tumors. Ann Otol Rhinol Laryngol 76:603–610, 1967

390. Spector GH, Fierstein J, Ogura JH: A comparison of therapeutic modalities of glomus tumors in the temporal bone. Laryngoscope 86:690–696, 1976

391. Bergdahl L: Carotid body tumours: A report of twelve cases. Scand J Thorac Cardiovasc Surg 12:275–279, 1978

392. Chambers RG, Mahoney WD: Carotid body tumors. Am J Surg 116:554–558, 1968
393. Farr HW: Carotid body tumors: A thirty year experience at Memorial Hospital. Am J Surg 114:614–619, 1967
394. Morris GC, Balas PE, Cooley DA, et al: Surgical treatment of benign and malignant carotid body tumors: Clinical experience with sixteen tumors in twelve patients. Am Surg 29:429–437, 1963
395. Parry DM, Li FP, Strong LC, et al: Carotid body tumors in humans: Genetics and epidemiology. JNCI 68:573–578, 1982
396. Westbrook KC, Guillamondegui OM, Medellin H, et al: Chemodectomas of the neck: Selective management. Am J Surg 124:760–766, 1972
397. Mendenhall WM, Million RR, Parsons JT, et al: Chemodectoma of the carotid body and ganglion nodosum treated with radiation therapy. Int J Radiat Oncol Biol Phys 12:2175–2178, 1986
398. Mitchell DC, Clyne CAC: Chemodectomas of the neck: The response to radiotherapy. Br J Surg 72:903–905, 1985
399. Lybeert MLM, Van Andel JG, Eijkenboom WMH, et al: Radiotherapy of paragangliomas. Clin Otolaryngol 9:105–109, 1984
400. Krupski WC, Effeney DJ, Stoney RJ, et al: Carotid body tumours. Aust NZ J Surg 53:539–543, 1983
401. Wilson H: Carotid body tumors. Surgery 59:483–493, 1966
402. Endicott JN, Maniglia AJ: Glomus vagale. Laryngoscope 90:1604–1611, 1980
403. Cassisi NJ, Dickerson DR, Million RR: Squamous cell carcinoma of the skin metastatic to parotid nodes. Arch Otolaryngol 104:336–339, 1978
404. Mendenhall NP, Million RR, Cassisi NJ: Parotid area lymph node metastases from carcinoma of the skin. Int J Radiat Oncol Biol Phys 11:707–714, 1985
405. Povah WB, Beecroft W, Hodson I, et al: Malignant lympho-epithelial lesion: The Manitoba experience. J Otolaryngol 13:153–159, 1984
406. Gallia LJ, Johnson JT: Incidence of neoplastic versus inflammatory disease in major salivary gland masses diagnosed by surgery. Laryngoscope 91:512–516, 1981
407. Fee WE Jr, Goffinet DR, Calcaterra TC: Recurrent mixed tumors of the parotid gland: Results of surgical therapy. Laryngoscope 88:265–273, 1978
408. Spiro RH, Huvos AG, Strong EW: Cancer of the parotid gland: A clinicopathologic study of 288 primary cases. Am J Surg 130:452–459, 1975
409. Gullane PJ, Havas TJ: Facial nerve grafts: Effects of postoperative irradiation. J Otolaryngol 16:112–115, 1987
410. King JJ, Fletcher GH: Malignant tumors of the major salivary glands. Radiology 110:381–384, 1971
411. Guillamondegui OM, Byers RM, Luna MA, et al: Aggressive surgery in treatment for parotid cancer: The role of adjunctive postoperative radiotherapy. Am J Roentgenol Radium Ther Nucl Med 123:49–54, 1975
412. Rafla S: Submaxillary gland tumors. Cancer 26:821–826, 1970
413. Spiro RH: Salivary neoplasms: Overview of a 35-year experience with 2,807 patients. Head Neck Surg 8:177–184, 1986
414. Woods JE, Chong GC, Beahrs OH: Experience with 1360 primary parotid tumors. Am J Surg 130:460–462, 1975
415. McNaney D, McNeese MD, Guillamondegui OM, et al: Postoperative irradiation in malignant epithelial tumors of the parotid. Int J Radiat Oncol Biol Phys 9:1289–1295, 1983
416. Theriault C, Fitzpatrick PJ: Malignant parotid tumors: Prognostic factors and optimum treatment. Am J Clin Oncol 9:510–516, 1986
417. Moore GE, Bross IDJ, Ausman R, et al: Effects of chlorambucil (NSC-3088) in 374 patients with advanced cancer: Eastern Clinical Drug Evaluation Program. Cancer Chemother Rep 52:661–666, 1968
418. Richards GJ, Chambers RG: Hydroxyurea in the treatment of neoplasms of the head and neck: A resurvey. Am J Surg 126:513–518, 1973
419. Rentschler R, Burgess MA, Byers R: Chemotherapy of malignant major salivary gland neoplasms: A 25-year review of M. D. Anderson Hospital experience. Cancer 40:619–624, 1977
420. Johnson RO, Lange RD, Kisken WA, et al: Infusion of 5-fluorouracil in cylindroma treatment. Arch Otolaryngol 79:625–627, 1964
421. Tannock IF, Sutherland DJ: Chemotherapy for adenocystic carcinoma. Cancer 46:452–454, 1980
422. Vermeer RJ, Pinedo HM: Partial remission of advanced adenoid cystic carcinoma obtained with Adriamycin: A case report with a review of the literature. Cancer 43:1604–1606, 1979
423. Schramm VL Jr, Srodes C, Myers EN: Cisplatin therapy for adenoid cystic carcinoma. Arch Otolaryngol 107:739–741, 1981
424. Creagan ET, O'Fallon JR, Woods JE, et al: Cis-platinum (P) by 24-hour infusion in advanced upper aerodigestive cancer (ADC) (abstract C-785). Proc Am Soc Clin Oncol 22:533, 1981
425. Skibba JL, Hurley JD, Ravelo HV: Complete response of a metastatic adenoid cystic carcinoma of the parotid gland to chemotherapy. Cancer 47:2543–2548, 1981
426. Budd GT, Groppe CW: Adenoid cystic carcinoma of the salivary gland: Sustained complete response to chemotherapy. Cancer 51:589–590, 1983
427. Posner MR, Ervin TJ, Weichselbaum RR, et al: Chemotherapy of advanced salivary gland neoplasms. Cancer 50:2261–2264, 1982
428. Venook AP, Tseng A Jr, Meyers FJ, et al: Cisplatin, doxorubicin, and 5-fluorouracil chemotherapy for salivary gland malignancies: A pilot study of the Northern California Oncology Group. J Clin Oncol 5:951–955, 1987
429. Triozzi PL, Brantley A, Fisher S, et al: 5-fluorouracil, cyclophosphamide, and vincristine for adenoid cystic carcinoma of the head and neck. Cancer 59:887–890, 1987
430. Alberts DS, Manning MR, Coulthard SW, et al: Adriamycin cis-platinum cyclophosphamide combination chemotherapy for advanced carcinoma of the parotid gland. Cancer 47:645–648, 1981
431. Creagan ET, Woods JE, Schutt AJ, et al: Cyclophosphamide, Adriamycin, and cis-diamminedichloroplatinum (II) in the treatment of advanced nonsquamous cell head and neck cancer. Cancer 52:2007–2010, 1983
432. Eisenberger MA: Supporting evidence for an active treatment program for advanced salivary gland carcinomas. Cancer Treat Rep 69:319–321, 1985
433. Dreyfuss AI, Clark JR, Fallon BG, et al: Cyclophosphamide, Adriamycin and cisplatin combination chemotherapy for advanced carcinomas of salivary gland origin. Cancer (in press)
434. Byers RM, Jesse RH, Guillamondegui OM, et al: Malignant tumors of the submaxillary gland. Am J Surg 126:458–463, 1973
435. Schell S, Barkley HT Jr, Chiminazzo H Jr: Treatment of malignant minor salivary gland tumors (in preparation)
436. Thawley SE, Ward SP, Ogura JH: Basal cell adenoma of the salivary glands. Laryngoscope 84:1756–1766, 1974
437. Ranger D, Thackray AC, Lucas RB: Mucous gland tumors. Br J Cancer 10:1–16, 1956
438. Wittes RE, Brescia F, Young CW, et al: Combination chemotherapy with cis-diamminedichloroplatinum (II) and bleomycin in tumors of the head and neck. Oncology 32:202–207, 1975
439. Hayes DM, Magill GB, Golbey RB, et al: Methyl CCNU, Adriamycin, and vincristine (MAV) chemotherapy of adenoid cystic carcinoma. Proc Soc Surg Oncol 35, 1976
440. Ellis ER, Million RR, Mendenhall WM, et al: The use of radiation therapy in the management of minor salivary gland tumors. Int J Radiat Oncol Biol Phys 15:613–617, 1988
441. Vikram B, Strong EW, Shah JP, et al: Radiation therapy in adenoid-cystic carcinoma. Int J Radiat Oncol Biol Phys 10:221–223, 1984
442. Spiro RH, Koss LG, Jagdu SI, et al: Tumors of minor salivary origin: A clinicopathologic study of 492 cases. Cancer 31:117–129, 1973
443. Bardwil JM, Reynolds CT, Ibanez ML, et al: Report of one hundred tumors of the minor salivary glands. Am J Surg 112:493–497, 1966
444. Rafla-Demetrious S: Mucous and Salivary Gland Tumours, p 118. Springfield, IL, Charles C Thomas, 1970

JOHN D. MINNA,

HARVEY PASS,

ELI GLATSTEIN,

and DANIEL C. IHDE

CHAPTER 22 *Cancer of the Lung*

INCIDENCE AND MORTALITY RATES

Lung cancer is a major cause of death in the United States and throughout the world in both developed and developing countries (Table 22-1; Fig. 22-1). It is the leading cause of cancer death in men 35 years old or older. It also is the second leading cause of cancer deaths in women 35 to 74 years old[1] and if present trends continue will become the leading cancer killer of American women during the 1980s. The majority of cases for both sexes are seen in the age range of 35 to 75 years, with a peak at age 55 to 65 years for each sex. At the time of diagnosis, the disease has spread to regional nodes or distant sites in 70% of patients (Table 22-2).[2] However, even in patients with supposedly localized disease, 5-year survival is the exception rather than the rule. Because of the low rate of cure, the mortality rates are nearly identical to the incidence. In general, women have a better 5-year survival rate than men for as yet unknown reasons.

It is estimated that at current incidence rates, there will be 590,000 new cases of lung cancer each year in the world, of which 80% to 90% are caused by tobacco.[3] Unfortunately, the incidence has, in general, been increasing, contributing significantly to total cancer death rates around the world. In the United States, the age-adjusted incidence in men has increased 225%, from 27 per 100,000 in the 1940s to 89 per 100,000 in 1982, an increase of almost 3% per year.[4] Fortunately, the rate of increase has declined in the United States, and there has actually been a decline in the incidence in white men since 1984,[5] a change that appears to be related to a decrease in cigarette smoking in more recent cohorts of

men. However, the incidence in women rose 400%, from 7 to 35 per 100,000, between 1940 and 1984.[5] Of additional concern, a higher percentage than expected of women than men with lung cancer are clustered in the lower pack-year categories (p <0.0003).[6] Thus, women are developing primary lung cancer at a younger age after smoking for fewer years than men.[6] Also, whereas the rate of beginning to smoke is decreasing in the United States as a whole, there is evidence that smoking onset may be increasing among certain minority groups and in adolescents.[7] This is particularly disturbing because the smoking-attributable years of potential life lost and the mortality rates in blacks are probably twice those among whites.[8]

PREDICTIONS OF FUTURE LUNG CANCER MORTALITY RATES

There have been dramatic decreases in smoking prevalence in the United States over the past 20 years, leading to the expectation of falling lung cancer rates. In fact, declines in age-specific rates of lung cancer for younger persons have been seen as a result of lower smoking prevalence among new cohorts and probably as a result of the lower tar content of cigarettes.[9] Nevertheless, age-adjusted rates of lung cancer mortality have continued to increase for men albeit with a flattening of the curve. However, the incidence and mortality rates for U.S. women continue to increase significantly. Overall, because of the changes in smoking prevalence, the lower tar content of cigarettes, and the increasing

591

TABLE 22-1.   Lung Cancer: Magnitude of the Problem

	Men	Women
Estimated new cases (1988)	100,000	52,000
Estimated proportion of		
Total cancer incidence (1988)	20%	11%
Total cancer deaths (1988)	93,000 (35%)	46,000 (20%)
Deaths by age (1985)		
All	83,854	38,839
35–54	8,926	4,960
55–74	53,756	24,322
75+	20,996	9,279

Data from Silverberg E: Cancer statistics, 1988. CA 38:5–22, 1988.

popularity of low-tar cigarettes, future trends in lung cancer are hard to predict.[9] Brown and Kessler have prepared an age-period-cohort model based on lung cancer mortality data, prevention objectives for smoking behavior established by the National Cancer Institute (NCI), and current smoking consumption data, for projecting lung cancer deaths through the year 2025. If there are no changes in the number of individuals starting or continuing to smoke and no changes in the tar content of cigarettes, those authors project age-adjusted rates in men to be flat through the 1990s and then to decline. The rates for women will peak in 2010, because the age-specific peaks for women lag 5 years behind those for U.S. men. Achieving the reduced smoking objectives will have little impact by the year 2000 but could reduce the male rate by 33% and the female rate by 40% by the period 2023–2027. Brown and Kessler conclude that "recent trends in lung cancer are unlikely to be affected by changes in cigarette composition and consumption in the near term, but increasing the effectiveness of anti-smoking campaigns can have a considerable effect on lung cancer rates in the more distant future."[9]

ETIOLOGY OF LUNG CANCER

Despite application of all our best current diagnostic and treatment modalities, including surgery, radiotherapy, and chemotherapy, the overall cure rate for lung cancer is only about 10%. Thus, any gains made in prevention or new methods of treating this disease, even if they affect only a small percentage of the total cases, would have a large impact in terms of total lives saved. These preventative efforts have to take into account data on the known etiologic factors, including cigarette and other types of smoking, exposures to other carcinogens such as asbestos and radon progeny, and the preventive role of diet. In addition, new approaches to prevention, diagnosis, staging, and treatment ultimately will be based rationally on a firm understanding of the molecular and cellular biology of lung cancer.

PATIENTS WITH LUNG CANCER HAVE BEEN HEAVILY EXPOSED TO CARCINOGENS

It is widely recognized that cigarette smoking (delivering large doses of carcinogens) is causally related to the development of lung cancer. In addition, recent evidence suggests that other carcinogens exist in the workplace and the home, such as alpha-particle-emitting radon daughters, which can increase the risk of lung cancer several-fold and probably act synergistically with cigarette smoke. Thus, there is ample exposure in lung cancer patients to agents that can damage DNA, creating the genetic lesions discussed below. Lowering this exposure provides our first target in preventative efforts.

The identification and characterization of the genetic events caused by this carcinogenic exposure has progressed rapidly over the past decade because of several factors that should have application to many other human tumors as well. These developments include methods to culture lung

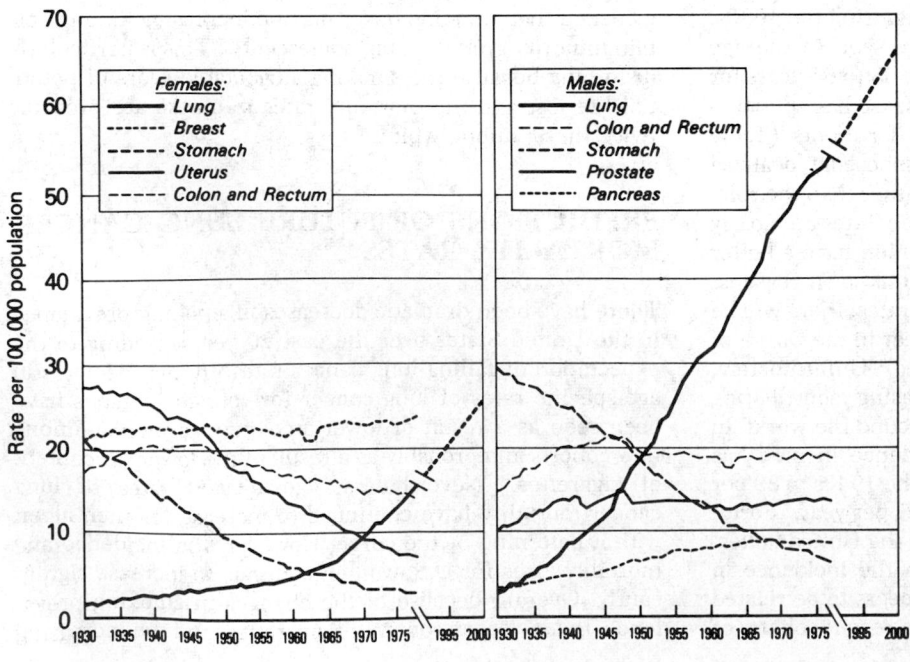

FIG. 22-1. Age-adjusted cancer death rates in the United States for lung cancer and other selected sites, with theoretical projections for lung cancer mortality in the year 2000. (Cancer Bull 32[3], 1980; CA 33[1], 1983. Sources of data cited are the U.S. National Center for Health Statistics and the U.S. Bureau of the Census)

TABLE 22-2.   Extent of Disease at Time of Presentation and Overall 5-Year Survival Rate (%) for Lung Cancer

Stage of Disease (Cases Diagnosed 1970–1973)	%	5-Year Survival % (Cases Diagnosed 1965–1969)	
		Male	Female
Local	17	28	51
Regional spread	22	10	15
Distant metastases	48	(<0.1)†	(<0.1)†
All stages*		8	13

Data from Cancer Patient Survival, Report No. 5, DHEW Publ. No. (NIH) 77-912, 1977.
* Not all patients classified according to stage.
† Not stated, but estimated from data on survival of all stages.

cancer cells in vitro, with the establishment of a large panel of lung cancer cell lines;[10–13] the field of cellular proto-oncogenes and chromosomal deletion analysis; and the identification of autocrine growth factors produced by tumor cells. The lung cancer cell lines have allowed the systematic characterization of cytogenetics, oncogenes, and growth factor production and responses, as well as development of in vitro drug and radiation sensitivity assays for lung cancer cells. As will become clear from the results of lung cancer prevention and treatment efforts, new strategies are urgently needed to approach this disease.

AUTOCRINE GROWTH FACTOR PRODUCTION, CHROMOSOMAL DELETIONS, AND ONCOGENE ACTIVATION IN THE PATHOGENESIS OF LUNG CANCER

Summary of a Current Working Model for the Pathogenesis of Lung Cancer

Evidence from several fronts suggest the following working model for the pathogenesis of lung cancer:[14,15]

1. Carcinogen exposure, probably enhanced by inheritance of a certain debrisoquine metabolic phenotype;
2. Production of gastrin-releasing peptide (GRP; mammalian bombesin) and other growth factors such as insulin-like (IGF) and transferrin-like (TGF) growth factors by neuroendocrine cells of the lung;
3. Autocrine growth stimulation of these neuroendocrine cells and thus increased growth factor production and probable paracrine growth stimulation of other bronchial epithelial cells, with resulting polyclonal proliferation;
4. Continued carcinogen exposure leading to the development of deletions and translocations in the replicating bronchial epithelial cells involving chromosome region 3p(14-23) to give clonal abnormalities exposing recessive oncogenes (which could have developed somatically or been inherited); as well as
5. Other genetic changes, including constitutive activation of myc family oncogenes and other nuclear-acting proto-oncogenes (such as p53 and c-jun) potentially by alterations in oncogene transcription, resulting in locally invasive lesions;
6. Constitutive activation of the nuclear-acting proto-oncogenes, leading to increased transcription of a family of genes providing the malignant phenotype such as that for collagenase type IV by the c-jun (AP-1) transcription factor;
7. Addition of other genetic changes such as mutations of ras family, c-raf-1, and other oncogenes, some of which could involve growth factor or growth factor receptor genes, such as that for the epidermal growth factor receptor (EGFr); other chromosomal deletions (such as of the rb gene on chromosome 13 and other genes on chromosomes 10, 11, and 17); and further deregulation of myc family members by amplification and gene rearrangements to give progressive and metastatic lesions.

Thus, lung cancer cells produce factors capable of promoting their own growth early in pathogenesis, allowing accumulation of a series of genetic lesions involving both the dominant, classic cellular proto-oncogenes[16] and the newly described recessive (chromosomal deletion) or "tumor suppressor" genes,[17] which together account for the transformation to malignancy of lung cells.

Genetic Changes Underlie the Pathogenesis of Human Lung Cancer

Human lung cancer is not generally thought of as a genetic disease. However, a variety of recent experimental evidence (summarized below) leads inextricably to the conclusion that lung cancer cells have accumulated a series of somatic genetic changes that activate the dominantly acting cellular proto-oncogenes on the one hand, while another group of changes would seem to inactivate a second class of genes that appear to be recessive (deletion or tumor suppressor genes), both of which are likely to be necessary for the malignant transformation of lung cells. Experimental systems show that even the dominantly acting oncogenes required the cooperation of more than one oncogene to transform normal cells, (such as a combination of c-myc and a mutated ras gene,[18] and that cancer cells have used many different genetic motifs in activation or inactivation processes. Thus, we expect to find evidence of lesions in more than one of these genes and more than one type of lesion in any given gene in lung cancer cells.

Predisposition to Lung Cancer May Be Inherited

There is mounting circumstantial evidence that some of the genetic changes are inherited in a mendelian fashion.[19,20] Most notably, first-degree relatives of lung cancer probands have a strong (2.4-fold) excess risk for lung cancer[21] or other cancers, many of which are not smoking related.[22] This risk may be through inheritance of a predisposition to chronic obstructive pulmonary disease. In fact, there is a higher risk of lung cancer ($p = 0.024$) in persons with chronic obstructive pulmonary disease, of whom 8.8% develop lung cancer within 10 years.[23] Moreover, lung cancer risk in smokers is modified by characteristics of the smoker and the family history. For example, for smokers with lung cancer, there is a significantly increased frequency of a parent having had lung cancer (6.9%) ($p < 0.001$; odds ratio [OR] = 5.3; range 2.2–12.8), and there is a significantly increased lung cancer risk if there is a personal history of chronic bronchitis or emphysema (OR = 2.0; range 1.4–2.8).[24] The link to chronic obstructive pulmonary disease is strengthened by the finding that smokers with ventilatory obstruction are at greater risk for lung cancer than are smokers without obstruction.[25] Patients with systemic sclerosis carry a significantly increased relative risk (RR = 16.5) of lung cancer.[26] Finally, an abnormal c-Ha-ras allele distribution was found in non-small-cell lung cancer, suggesting a linkage of a chromosome 11p haplotype to this type of cancer.[27]

DEVELOPMENT OF A SECOND MALIGNANCY AFTER LUNG CANCER.

In other inherited disorders, predispositions to multiple tumors are often seen. In lung cancer, it is difficult to sort out whether second cancers are related solely to carcinogen exposure from cigarette smoking or also to some inherited predisposition. Nevertheless, it is important to note that cured lung cancer patients have a very significant risk of a second malignancy such as another lung cancer[28–30] or an acute leukemia.[31–34] Conversely, patients cured of other malignancies outside the respiratory tree can have an increased risk of lung cancer.

Two very large series have looked at the risk of developing a second cancer. In 30,000 persons from Connecticut who had cancer at any site within the respiratory system diagnosed between 1935 and 1982, a 44% excess of all second cancers was seen following cancer of the lung.[35] These second cancers were in the respiratory tract, oral cavity, bladder, and kidney, all sites potentially associated with cigarette smoking. After 10 years of observation, the risk of a second cancer remained high, at 50% above expectation. In another study of 36,000 Danish persons with cancer of the respiratory system diagnosed between 1943 and 1980, there was a 10% increased risk of a second cancer. Elevated rates of second cancers were seen in the lung, buccal cavity, bladder, kidney; surprisingly, excess cancers in the breast and female genital organs, liver, and pancreas were also seen.[36] In both of these series, significant risks of lung cancers were noted after primary laryngeal cancers.

Acute nonlymphocytic leukemia was found in 2 of 377 patients with small cell lung cancer at 22 and 81 months after the start of therapy,[37] representing a highly significant ($p < 0.0001$) increased relative risk value (RR = 154; 95% confidence limit 38–293) for the development of leukemia.

The Kaplan–Meier estimate of the cumulative probability of developing leukemia was $1.9 \pm 1.4\%$ 7 years after the start of treatment.

DEVELOPMENT OF LUNG CANCER AFTER CURE OF ANOTHER MALIGNANCY, PARTICULARLY LARYNGEAL CANCER.

The association of lung cancer with upper aerodigestive cancers such as head and neck cancer is growing very strong, with the highest association being with laryngeal cancers. For example, 26% of 415 patients cured of laryngeal cancer developed lung cancer during the first 14 years of follow-up (RR = 6.73).[38] In another series of 748 laryngeal cancer patients, 9% had second primary lung cancers.[39] In one series of 1373 consecutive patients with head and neck or lung cancer, 2% had multiple primary cancers.[40] In another series of 1450 patients with upper airway cancers, 4% developed a lung cancer, nearly always after the head and neck cancer.[41] The mean interval between the diagnoses of the upper airway and the lung cancers was 6 years. In addition, the lung cancers can be of any histologic type (not only squamous cell cancer), and frequently, they occur in women. The post-thoracotomy management of patients who have had surgery or radiotherapy on their upper airways for head and neck cancer is challenging. If the lung and head and neck cancers occur synchronously, the lung cancer is usually dealt with first, as it appears to be the most life threatening.[41]

Evidence is beginning to accumulate of an increased risk (perhaps twofold to threefold) of lung cancer after treatment for non-Hodgkin's lymphoma or Hodgkin's disease.[42] Six patients among 288 with lymphoma developed lung cancer, suggesting that a lymphoma patient who is a smoker should be investigated thoroughly for lung carcinoma if there are signs or symptoms in the chest.

Correlation of Debrisoquine Metabolic Phenotype with Lung Cancer

There appears to be a strong association between the high metabolic phenotype for 4-debrisoquine hydroxylase and the development of lung cancer.[43] Extensive metabolizers of debrisoquine have a 10-fold increased risk of lung cancer, whereas the extensive metabolizers exposed to asbestos have a 22- to 30-fold increased relative risk, such that within the asbestos-exposed group, there is an approximately 10-fold increase in the risk for lung cancer among extensive metabolizers.[44] *These findings raise the question of whether some people are predisposed to get lung cancer, either by genes that determine how they handle carcinogens or by recessive genes that can also lead to the genesis of other tumors.* Identification of such genes would not only aid in targeting preventive effects for lung cancer but might also provide clues to the genetics of cancer as a whole.

Autocrine Growth Factor Production by Lung Cancer Cells Provides a Mechanism for Accumulation of Genetic Lesions

Lung cancer cells both produce and exhibit a mitogenic response to a variety of growth factors, so that these factors fit the definition of autocrine growth factors.[45,46] In fact, lung cancer cells can grow in medium supplemented with only a few or no added growth factors.[47,49] Other autocrine peptides produced by lung cancer cells include GRP and those with TGF- and IGF-1-like activities.[50-53] In some cases, lung cancer cells express multiple growth factors.[54]

The best-characterized autocrine growth factor in lung cancer is GRP, which is produced by small cell lung cancer[55-58] and acts through high-affinity receptors[59] to stimulate calcium mobilization[60] and phosphatidylinositol turnover, as well as constitutive activation of a protein-tyrosine kinase that phosphorylates a 115 kD protein associated with the GRP–receptor complex[61] and thereby functions as an autocrine growth factor for small cell lung cancer.[62] GRP is produced by the human fetal lung[63] and has known mitogenic effects in vitro and in vivo[64,65] as well as a multiplicity of other effects including induction of anorexia and the release of many other hormones.[66] Thus, it is likely that GRP is an important regulatory peptide for normal lung growth and development and that it may account for some of the paraneoplastic syndromes (see Chap. 55) associated with lung cancer. The complexity of the GRP system is underscored by the production of three mRNA forms from the pre-proGRP gene through alternative mRNA processing[67,68] to give a series of proteins, including three different GRP-gene-associated peptides, which are expressed in small cell lung cancer and human fetal lung.[69] These GRP-gene-associated peptides are further modified by post-translational processing into multiple other peptides,[70] all of which could have biologic activity. In addition to stimulating the growth of small cell lung cancer,[71,72] GRP can stimulate the growth of normal bronchial epithelial cells,[73] implying a role as a paracrine growth factor. Of great interest in this regard is the production of high levels of bombesin-like immunoreactivity detectable in the bronchial lavage fluid of smokers.[74] This observation, if substantiated, would place these growth factor-mediated events very early in the pathogenesis of lung cancer and provide a mechanism for promotion of the genetic lesions caused by carcinogens by allowing the accumulation of multiple lesions in individual cells through cell replication. One could also envision pulmonary neuroendocrine cells undergoing "autocrine" growth and thus expanding the number of cells producing such growth factors without themselves ultimately transforming but rather stimulating other bronchial epithelial cell populations to expand.

Future lines of investigation include testing for such growth factors in the pulmonary tree of smokers and clinical trials seeking to inhibit these growth factors. Antibodies and peptide antagonists against the biologically active portion of GRP inhibit the growth of small cell lung cancer in human tumor xenografts grown in nude mice, as well as in tissue culture.[62,75,76]

Evidence for Genetic Damage (Chromosomal and DNA Deletions) Involving the Recessive or Tumor Suppressor Genes

A variety of cytogenetic studies have indicated many chromosomal changes in lung cancer such as numerical and structural aberrations including deletions and translocations.[77-84] In addition, restriction fragment-length poly-

morphism (RFLP) technology has shown that many of these cytogenetic changes are associated with true loss of DNA from the tumor cell. The most prominent of these losses is deletion of material from chromosome region 3p(14–23), which shortest-region-of-overlap analysis would place at 3p21.[85-88] These changes in 3p21 are found in all types of lung cancer, suggesting they are either a common requirement for the development of lung cancer or an early step in the pathogenesis. Similar deletions have been seen in sporadic renal carcinomas,[89] and there are family pedigrees where the development of renal carcinoma segregates with cytogenetic abnormalities of chromosome region 3p.[90,91] It is of great interest that this region is a fragile site in the human genome, and increased fragility is seen in the normal cells of cigarette smokers.[92] More recently, DNA loss from other chromosomes has been identified, including chromosomes 13, 17, and 11.[93,94] Of great interest, in the case of chromosome 13, the DNA loss has been localized to the rb locus,[95] such that the large majority of small cell lung cancers have absent or dramatically reduced expression of the rb gene product.[96] *All of these changes raise the possibility of recessive mutations on the remaining chromosomal material being uncovered by the deletion.* Supportive evidence for this hypothesis comes from the lack of expression of aminoacylase (a gene assigned to chromosome region 3p21) in some small cell lung cancers.[97] These findings also raise the possibility of correcting the defect by introducing into the lung cancer cell a normal copy of the gene. That this may indeed be possible is suggested by the results of somatic cell hybrid experiments that show suppression of malignancy when a malignant non-small cell lung cancer line is fused to a nonmalignant mouse cell.[98] Candidate genes that reside on chromosome region 3p include a thyroid hormone receptor ErbA β[99] and retinoic acid-receptor-like genes, Hap-1.[100] Thus, one possibility is that the genes that are inactivated code for hormone receptor functions that transmit signals for differentiation.

Evidence for Genetic Damage of Dominant Genes: Oncogene Activation

Oncogenes of several families suffer changes in lung cancer cells (Table 22-3). These changes include point mutations in members of the ras family[101-108] and changes that predispose to the constitutive and often high-level expression of cellular proto-oncogenes that act in the nucleus, including c-myc, N-myc, L-myc, c-myb, and p53.[109-115] The changes in myc family member expression have been associated with gene amplification, gene rearrangement, and loss of intragenic pausing or the "attenuator" function.[116] Experimental studies show that transfecting a mutated ras gene into small cell lung cancer changes its phenotype to one suggesting a non-small cell lung cancer.[117] In addition, constitutive expression of c-raf-1 has been found in all types of lung cancer.[118] This is particularly intriguing because c-raf-1 is assigned to chromosome region 3p25, an area frequently involved in the terminal deletions of chromosome 3 in lung cancer.

The clinical relevance of the c-myc gene has been the first to be explored in any detail. Small cell lung cancer cell lines

TABLE 22-3. Chromosome Regions or Proto-Oncogenes Found to Have Genetic Alterations and/or Alterations of Expression in Human Lung Cancer

Chromosome regions frequently deleted in human lung cancer
(putative recessive or tumor-suppressor genes)
    3p(14–23)
    11p
    13q14 (rb locus)
    17p
Cellular Proto-oncogenes activated in some lung cancers
(dominantly acting genes)
    c-myc
    N-myc
    L-myc
    c-myb
    p53
    c-jun
    H-ras
    K-ras-2
    N-ras
    c-raf-1
    c-fms

with high-level expression of the c-myc gene exhibit faster growth and higher cloning efficiency in vitro[119] and a change in the morphology to that characteristic of the large-cell "variants,"[120] and mark a poor prognosis in extensive-stage patients.[121] In addition, if a c-myc gene is transfected into a classic small cell lung cancer line initially not expressing the gene, the transfected cells take on the growth and morphologic characteristics of the c-myc-amplified small cell lung cancer lines,[122] demonstrating a direct relation between the expression of a particular oncogene and the cellular phenotype.

The L-myc gene was discovered in a small cell lung cancer, where it can be amplified and overexpressed. However, it is of particular interest because it can be expressed in both small cell and non-small cell lung cancer[123]; because it has a restricted pattern of expression during development (especially brain, kidney, and lung)[124]; and because it is associated with GRP-related signal transduction events. In addition, the L-myc gene undergoes a complex series of alternative mRNA processing and polyadenylation site selection to generate four different mRNAs,[125] which in turn generate a series of L-myc protein products.[126] These products transform primary rat embryo cells when cotransfected with a mutated ras gene. However, it is of great interest that they do this with 1% to 10% the efficiency of c-myc,[127] suggesting the need for other genetic lesions such as deletions or other oncogene activation or a more restricted cell type for action. Recently, certain L-myc haplotypes have been implicated in the metastatic behavior of lung cancer of several histologic types.[128]

Recently, another nuclear oncogene product, c-jun, has been found to be expressed at high levels in small cell and non-small cell lung cancer and normal lung.[129] This is of interest because c-jun lies in the same chromosomal region as L-myc (1p31–32),[130] and the c-jun product appears to be a proto-oncogene equivalent of the transcription factor AP-1 and thus intimately involved with regulation of transcription and mediation of tumor promotor effects such as those en-

gendered by phorbol esters.[131] Thus, a scenario is established in normal lung and lung cancer cells where a transcription factor is activated, mimicking chronic stimulation by tumor promoters.

Because of the activation of dominant cellular proto-oncogenes, including those whose products act in the nucleus, as well as GTP-binding oncogene products, and phosphokinases, and because of the presence of the recessive tumor suppressor genes, it appears inescapable that new prevention and treatment strategies for lung cancer must ultimately be directed against the development of deregulated expression or functional outcome of these genes.

SMOKING AND LUNG CANCER

Cigarette smoking is the predominant cause of lung cancer in the United States and around the world (Tables 22-4 and 22-5). International data demonstrate that lung cancer death rates parallel cigarette smoking prevalence rates in both men and women.[132] Moreover, in all studies, there has been a clear dose–response relation between the amount of smoking and the development of lung cancer.[138] In addition, there is a significantly increased risk of lung cancer for pipe and cigar smokers whether or not they also smoke cigarettes (Table 22-4). Thus, effective control of lung cancer and other smoking-associated diseases can only be achieved by reducing smoking prevalence in the developed countries and stopping the increase in smoking in developing countries.[132] Lung cancer in underdeveloped countries is becoming a problem of large economic and political importance, and an epidemic of lung cancer is likely within a decade because of the rapidly increasing cigarette consumption in many of these countries.[138] This is true for blacks in South Africa[139] and Asians in Singapore[140] (67 to 73 cases per 100,000 persons). In China and India, 25% to 33% of all males are addicted to tobacco smoking by the time they are 18 to 20 years old.[138]

The latest in a long series of reports by the U.S. Surgeon General deals directly with cigarette smoking as a drug ad-

TABLE 22-4. Relationship of Smoking to the Development of Lung Cancer*

Cigarette smoking[132–136]
Lung cancer death rates parallel cigarette smoking prevalence[132]
Risk increases with each cigarette smoked per day[133]
Relative risk declines exponentially with duration of smoking cessation
Risk declines 5 years after cessation of smoking
Risk increased for all types of lung cancer,
    Small cell lung cancer (RR = 17.5)
    Adenocarcinoma (RR = 6.7)
        Males OR = 4.49
        Females OR = 3.95
Estimates of risk for other types of smoking[134,137]
    Exclusive cigarette smoking: RR = 13.3
    Exclusive cigar smoking: RR = 5.6
    Exclusive pipe smoking: RR = 1.6
    Mixed cigar and cigarette smoking: RR = 8.5
    Mixed pipe and cigarette smoking: RR = 8.0
    Dose–response relation for cigarette and pipe smoking

*RR = relative risk estimates; OR = odds ratio.

TABLE 22-5.   Total Mortality, Weighted Smoking-Attributable Fractions, and Smoking-Attributable Mortality from Lung Cancer in the United States (1984)

	Males	Females	Total
Smoking-attributable fractions	0.80	0.75	
Smoking-attributable mortality	65,659	27,170	92,829
Total deaths	82,459	36,227	118,686
Involuntary smoking mortality estimate			3825

Data from Oncol Times December 1, 1987, p 8; Centers for Disease Control: Cigarette smoking in the United States, 1986. MMWR 36:581–585, 1987; National Academy of Sciences: Environmental tobacco smoke: Measuring exposures and assessing health effects (Appendix D). Washington, DC, National Academy Press, 1986.

diction.[141] The principal conclusions of this extensive data summary and analysis are:

1. Cigarettes and other forms of tobacco are addicting.
2. Nicotine is the drug in tobacco that causes addiction.
3. The pharmacologic and behavioral processes that determine tobacco addiction are similar to those that determine addiction to drugs such as heroin and cocaine.

This direct confrontation of the addictive properties of nicotine may provide the best method for dealing with the smoking problem.

It is estimated that 54,000,000 Americans smoke cigarettes, including 36% of the total work force or 37,000,000 workers (Table 22-6).[142] Because there appear to be multiple interactions between smoking and workplace carcinogens in the development of lung cancer, as well as effects of smoking on chronic obstructive pulmonary disease and heart disease that influence workplace performance, smoking creates a vast health and financial problem for the U.S. workplace.[143] Thus, there is a confluence of medical, epidemiologic, and economic reasons for focusing antismoking efforts on the workplace. Smoking control strategies include prevention of starting to smoke, efforts to get people to stop smoking, regulatory and legislative measures, and modifications in tobacco product composition. It is not clear how best to achieve a reduction in smoking, and thus the U.S. NCI has initiated intervention research programs to identify and assess the most promising strategies to reduce smoking prevalence in the general public and in high-risk populations (heavy smokers, blacks, Hispanics, women, youth, and smokeless tobacco users).[132]

Although modern cigarettes are usually low in tar and thus presumably in many toxic products and nicotine, epidemiology results have not shown much reduction in the mortality rate that can be attributed to lowering of tar.[143] Public health campaigns have sometimes appeared successful in getting the tobacco industry to reduce tar, but they have also been used by that industry to downplay the dangers of smoking.[143] The delivery of high levels of tar by the smoking products sold in the Third World is another area of serious concern.[143]

Early detection of lung cancer appears not to have a significant impact given current screening methods, as a large number of early detection studies have failed to show a significant impact on lung cancer mortality rates. In fact, analysis of the large population of cigarette smokers periodically screened by the Memorial Sloan-Kettering Cancer Center

TABLE 22-6.   Smoking in the Workplace (United States)*

Group	Estimated Prevalence (%)	Number of Persons Smoking
White males	37	19,864,000
White females	33	13,478,000
Black males	42	2,180,000
Black females	34	1,750,000
Overall	35.6	37,258,000

	Percentage of the Group Smoking the Indicated No. of Cigarettes per Day		
Cigarettes per Day	≤15	15–24	≥24
White males	20	44	36
White females	31	48	22
Black males	49	39	12
Black females	61	34	5

	Smoking Prevalence (%) by Occupational Class and Sex	
	Blue Collar	White Collar
Male	47	33
Female	38	32

Data from LaRosa JH, Haines CM: A Guide to Heart and Lung Health at the Workplace. NIH Publication No. 86-2210, Washington, DC, September 1986.
*Estimated 104,658,000 employed persons in 1985.

(MSKCC) in New York has found, surprisingly, that the mean duration of the early stage of lung cancer is at least 4 years, the detectability less than 0.2, and the curability less than 0.5.[144] Thus, annual radiographic screening between the ages of 45 and 80 might decrease mortality rates from adenocarcinoma of the lung by less than 20%.[144] In contrast, there is significant evidence of a reduced risk of lung cancer beginning 5 years after cessation of smoking.[134]

PASSIVE SMOKING AND INCREASED RISK OF LUNG CANCER

Passive exposure to cigarette smoke and the development of lung cancer is an important issue with many social and political implications. The majority of lung cancers in nonsmoking women are probably related to environmental (passive) tobacco smoke, although passive exposures in utero and very early in life need to be considered.[145] The physicochemical nature of passive smoke (the smoke inhaled by nonsmokers) differs significantly from the mainstream smoke inhaled by the active smoker.[145]

Currently, the best means of assessing exposure to passive smoking is the urinary cotinine level.[145] A summary of 13 studies (10 case-controlled and 3 prospective) showed a highly significant (35% to 53%) increase in the risk of lung cancer among nonsmokers living with smokers compared with nonsmokers living with nonsmokers (RR = 1.35; 95% confidence interval 1.19–1.54, which rose after adjustment to an RR = 1.53, or a 53% increase).[146] Other individual studies confirm this. For example, wives of men who smoke have a twofold to threefold increased risk of lung cancer.[147,148] Also, there is a dose–response relation between the amount of smoking by the spouse and the risk of the nonsmoking spouse getting lung cancer that is significant for squamous cell and small cell lung cancer although not for other histologic types.[148,149] Thus, about one-third of lung cancer in nonsmokers who live with smokers and about 25% of lung cancer in nonsmokers in general comes from passive exposure to cigarette smoke.[146] However, one must beware of bias in passive smoking studies, because there is a strong tendency for smokers to marry smokers and for such "nonsmokers" to give false reports about their own smoking habits (2.5% to 10%).[150]

OTHER ETIOLOGIC AGENTS

Exposure to Asbestos

Mineral fibers, particularly asbestos, represent the greatest cause after cigarette smoking of respiratory cancer attributable to air pollutants.[151] The increased risk in asbestos workers account for about 8 excess cancers per 1000 exposed workers (RR = 1.4–1.7),[152] and for British asbestos workers followed over a long period of time, the relative risk was 1.4 to 2.6.[153] Past asbestos exposure accounts for 2000 mesothelioma deaths per year and 4000 to 6000 lung cancer deaths per year in the United States.[154] However, it is estimated that removal of asbestos from occupational exposure would reduce lung cancers by 23%.[155] All these studies show a strong dose–response effect with asbestos exposure.[156] Of

great importance, the combination of occupational asbestos exposure and smoking further increases lung cancer risk; this association is strongest with small cell lung cancer and weakest with adenocarcinoma.[157,158] All common commercial types of asbestos (crocidolite, amosite, and chrysotile) can cause lung cancer of all histologic types. Most commonly, exposures occur in the workplace (e.g., insulation, cement, shipyard workers). However, nonoccupational exposures are likely to be associated with malignant disease similar to that obtained through occupational exposure.[154]

Exposure to Radon Progeny

URANIUM MINING.[159,160] All underground mining studies show an increased risk of lung cancer with radon (Rn) daughter exposure, and all cell types of lung cancer are increased with Rn exposure. Cumulative exposure to Rn and its alpha-emitting daughters is given by the "working level month" (WLM), which for historical reasons is defined as exposure to approximately 100 pCi of radon per liter of air in 170 hours. Occupational exposure to 4 WLM is estimated to increase lung cancer risk by 60% for the general population of people between 20 and 40 years of age.[161] Smokers are at 10-fold higher risk than nonsmokers of developing lung cancer after this occupational exposure.[160,161] The occupational standard for Rn exposure has been 4 WLM per year, whereas 2 WLM per year had been suggested as a threshold for remedial action in homes. Epidemiologic studies show that miners with cumulative Rn daughter exposures of even 100 WLM have an excess lung cancer mortality, with 3% to 8% of miners followed developing lung cancer attributable to Rn daughters.

A clear dose–response effect (RR increase of 3.3% per WLM) is seen for the development of lung cancer in uranium miners,[162] with an overall increase in relative risk of 2.3 per 100 WLM.[163] The National Institute for Occupational Safety and Health (NIOSH) has developed quantitative risk estimates of lung cancer after exposure to Rn daughters in the follow-up of the U.S. cohort of uranium miners.[164] These figures predict excess relative risks between 0.9 and 1.4 per 100 WLM in the lower cumulative exposure range. Of interest, low exposure rates appear more harmful per unit of cumulative exposure than higher rates. Relative risk increased with age at initial exposure, and the relative risk of lung cancer fell dramatically in the years following cessation of exposure.[164]

^{222}RN GAS PROGENY OUTSIDE THE WORKPLACE.[161,164,166] Many of the general population also may be unknowingly exposed to Rn daughters. In fact, Rn exposure is the most serious cause of human irradiation, and excessive exposures may be readily avoidable. Human exposure to terrestrial gamma rays, cosmic rays, and natural radionuclides in diet is detectable but not highly variable,[166] with a basic background dose of about 1 mSv.[160] In contrast, indoor Rn levels have tremendous variability. In temperate latitudes, the average concentration is about 15 Bq m^{-3} of air, which is the equilibrium equivalent concentration of ^{222}Rn (conversion coefficient 10 Bq m^{-3} = 1 mSv per year).[166] This value can range from as little as one-tenth to 1000-fold higher in otherwise ordinary houses. Thus, annual doses range from 1 mSv or less through an average of 1.5 mSv to 1000 mSv or more.[166]

To relate general population exposure to miners' exposure, the potential risk of lung cancer appears to be between 1 and 2 per 10,000 persons per WLM, which yields a significant number of lung cancers, as some 220 million persons in the United States are exposed on average to 10 to 20 WLM in a life-time.[160] It is estimated that $10 \pm 5\%$ of the lung cancer rate in the general public is attributable to Rn daughters at an exposure rate of 10 to 20 Bq/m^{-3},[167] whereas 25% of lung cancers in nonsmokers and 5% of those in smokers are attributable to exposure to Rn daughters in the home.[168] Some homes have very high levels of Rn. In U.S. homes, the mean level is 1.5 pCi per liter (55 Bq/m^{-3}), but, 1% to 3% of homes exceed 8 pCi per liter. As 1.5 pCi per liter contributes about a 0.3% increased life-time risk of lung cancer, in the million homes with the highest concentrations, where annual exposures approximate or exceed those received by underground uranium miners, long-term occupants suffer an added life-time risk of at least 2%, reaching extraordinary values at the highest concentrations observed.[169]

Steady-state outdoor Rn concentration averages 200 pCi m^{-3}, whereas indoor levels are four times this.[160] The primary source of Rn in homes is the underlying soil, and levels in the homes depend on multiple variables such as reduced ventilation for energy conservation. Thus, high indoor levels are caused by the forced flow of Rn-laden soil gas into buildings.[166] Radon gas itself delivers only a very small dose of irradiation. However, the four immediate daughters of ^{222}Rn are radioactive isotopes of solid elements with short half-lives, two of which transform by emitting alpha particles.[166] The daughters create a radioactive aerosol with small particles in room air, which, inhaled, causes some daughters to be deposited and retained in the respiratory tract, where alpha particles irradiate bronchial epithelial cells, with the most significant result being lung cancer.[166] In addition, there is evidence for radioactive polonium in cigarettes.[170]

The International Commission on Radiological Protection (ICRP) has set the average life-time exposure at equilibrium equivalent concentrations of 15 Bq m^{-3} (to give a relative lifetime risk of lung cancer of 0.1%); the upper acceptable boundary at 100 Bq m^{-3} (to give a relative life-time risk of 0.5%); and the level at which action needs to be taken at 200 Bq m^{-3} (which would give a relative life-time risk of 1%). This action level was chosen because it would be expected to double the life-time risk of lung cancer.[166] This has been studied in Sweden, where women had increased relative risks (RR = 2.2; p = 0.01) for lung cancer associated with living in dwellings close to the ground in areas with an increased risk of Rn emanation. Actual measurements indicated increased Rn daughter concentrations in ground-level dwellings with Rn risk areas where patients had lived, suggesting that this exposure was of etiologic importance.[171]

Other Workplace Carcinogens

In assessing the risk of workplace carcinogens, it is important to estimate and exclude the role that smoking alone would play. However, these carcinogens could interact with smoking to increase lung cancer risk.[172] In the United States, blue collar workers have a higher smoking prevalence than white collar workers (see Table 22-6).[133] The occupations with the highest smoking rates include, for men, painters, construction and maintenance, truck drivers, carpenters, auto mechanics, and guards and watchmen, all of which have a 50% or higher smoking prevalence. For women, waitresses, cashiers, assemblers, nurses' aides, orderlies, machine operatives, practical nurses, packers, and wrappers all have a smoking prevalence exceeding 40%.[133] Thus, when both a high smoking prevalence and a workplace carcinogen exist, the potential for an occupation-associated lung cancer is probably greatly enhanced. In addition to asbestos and radioactive exposure, a variety of other carcinogens and occupations have been identified by epidemiologic studies in the workplace after subtracting the effect of smoking (Table 22-7). These include especially arsenic, cadmium, chromium, and certain chemicals such as chloromethyl ether.

That prevention could play a beneficial role is indicated by the finding of no increased risk of lung cancer in a group of

TABLE 22-7. Chemicals, Metals, Airborne Contaminants, and Occupations Contributing to Lung Cancer Risk[154,175,176]

Chemicals

Chloromethyl ether (chemical workers)[177]
    Obs/Exp = 2.70; p < 0.01; a clear dose–response effect is seen with risk increased more than 10 fold with highest doses; latent period is 10–19 years
Cadmium (nickel–cadmium battery plant)[175,178]
    EPA estimates risk from cadmium at 1.8×10^{-3} cases/μg/m^3, which results in more than 100,000 excess lung cancers (life-time)
Arsenic[175,178,180]
    EPA estimates risk of 4.3 cases/1000 μg/m^3 to give more than 100,000 lung cancers (life-time). Smelter workers exposed to arsenic have lung cancer risk increased 2–9 times. Artesian well water high in arsenic gives 3-fold increased risk of lung cancer and shows dose–response relation (OR = 3.39)
Chromate[181]
Hexavalent chromium (masons)[182,183]
Formaldehyde[184]
Terpenes (wood industry)[185]

Occupations[186,187]

Shipyard workers, truck drivers, plumbers (probably related to asbestos)[188]
Rubber curing and other rubber workers[189,190]
    SMR = 133
Pottery workers[191]
    talc exposure: 3.64 increased risk
Printers (typographers and lithographers in Sweden)[192]
Female cosmetologists[193]
Leather industry[194]
    RR = 2.6; range 1.2–6.0
Building laborers[186]
    RR = 1.7; range 1.0–2.9
Construction workers[186]
    RR = 1.8; range 1.0–3.0
Bakers and pastry cooks[186,195]
    RR = 3.6 range 1.3–10.4
Cooks
    RR = 2.5, range 1.2–5.1
Truck drivers
    Diesel exhaust (possible effect)[196]

iron-ore (hematite) miners where the lack of significant Rn exposure was demonstrated and there was strict smoking prohibition underground, an aggressive silicosis control program, and the absence of underground diesel fuel.[173] In contrast, nowhere has the combined effect of smoking and occupational carcinogen exposure been more dramatic than in the tin miners in the Yunnan province of south central China, who have had the highest lung cancer mortality rate in men in all of China.[174] These miners are exposed to extraordinarily high levels of Rn such that miners with 20 to 30 years of underground service before 1949 would have had 1600 to 2400 WLM of exposure. In addition, most of the miners have smoked, and arsenic trioxide is a by product of the smelting process and contaminates the local food and water supplies. The majority of the cancers have been squamous cell carcinomas, with the remainder mostly small cell carcinoma. The lung cancer incidence in this group of miners is 1% per year and among retired miners 2% to 3% per year.[174] This is some 10-fold greater then the SEER rate for U.S. men age 60 to 64, which is 0.3% per year.

PROTECTIVE EFFECTS OF DIET

Beta-carotene and other constitutents of green and yellow vegetables have strong potential as protective agents (Table 22-8).[197] Selenium also deserves attention as a potential chemopreventive nutrient, however, there are fewer data. Vitamin A intake is inversely associated with lung cancer risk, and this relation is strongest among cigarette smokers.[198] Analyses of index of carotenoids and of individual food items suggest that plant sources of vitamin A may play a more important role in producing the effect than do animal sources.[198] These findings have prompted chemoprevention trials with retinoids in persons at high risk.[199]

TABLE 22-8. Dietary Elements that Epidemiologic Evidence Suggests Decrease the Risk of Lung Cancer

Beta-carotene
    Serum beta-carotene level inversely related to risk of squamous-cell lung cancer (relative odds 4.30; 95% confidence interval 1.38–13.41)[200]
    Intake of dark green and, particularly, dark yellow-orange vegetables (RR = 1.7–2.2 for low intake after adjustment for smoking risk; beneficial effect only noted in current smokers, RR = 1.3 for low intake after adjustment for smoking)[201]
    Current smokers who did not consume carrots showed a threefold risk of lung cancer compared with those who ate them more than once a week (OR = 2.9; p < 0.01); risk was independent of histologic type[202]
Vitamin A
    Intake of vitamin A from fruits and vegetables (carotene) strongly associated with reduced cancer risk, more for males (RR = 1.8) than for females[203]
    Decreased dietary vitamin A intake has increased risk of lung cancer (RR = 1.8)[204]
    Vitamin A-deficient diet increases lung tumorigenesis in rats[205]
Selenium[192]
Vitamin E
    Persons with low serum level had 2.5 times the lung cancer risk[200]

ANATOMICAL CONSIDERATIONS

Because the lungs are paired organs with a large reserve capacity, one lung may be sacrificed with little resultant disability in an otherwise-healthy person. The right lung is composed of three lobes—the upper, middle, and lower—and provides approximately 55% of the ventilatory capacity. The left lung consists of only two lobes—the upper and lower—with the lingular portion of the upper lobe corresponding to the middle lobe on the right. The lobes are separated by fissures that can be identified on roentgenograms, particularly the lateral views. On the right side, usually two fissures are present: the oblique or major fissure that separates the lower lobe from the upper and middle lobes and the horizontal or minor fissure that separates the upper and middle lobes. On the left side, the single fissure separates the upper and lower lobes, running obliquely from the level of the third rib posteriorly and forward, ending in the region of the sixth or seventh costochondral junction.

The bronchopulmonary segment is the basic anatomic unit (Figure 22-2 and Table 22-9). Although the anatomical relations of the pulmonary hilar structures, as well as the arrangement of the bronchopulmonary segments, are relatively constant, variations may be encountered frequently. Therefore, the thoracic surgeon must be alert for these anomalies.

The main structures of the primary pulmonary hilus are the main bronchus, the pulmonary artery, and the superior and inferior pulmonary veins (Fig. 22-2). The relations of these structures differ considerably on the two sides. On the left side, the pulmonary artery curves around the upper lobe bronchus, whereas on the right side, it remains anterior and below the upper lobe bronchus. The segmental arteries follow the segmental bronchi; the veins occupy an intersegmental position, converging to form segmental veins that empty into the superior and inferior pulmonary veins. On the right side, the middle lobe vein empties into the superior pulmonary vein. Variations are common; in order of frequency, they occur in the veins, arteries, and bronchi. The pulmonary arterial tree is a low-pressure system compared with the peripheral arteries, and these vessels are relatively thin-walled and fragile.

The regional lymph nodes and currently used lymph node map are discussed in the section on surgical staging of the mediastinum.

PATHOLOGY OF LUNG CANCER

HISTOLOGIC TYPES

The four major cell types of lung cancer are squamous cell (or epidermoid) carcinoma, small cell (also called oat cell) carcinoma, adenocarcinoma, and large cell (also called large cell anaplastic) carcinoma. However, for the many associated types of pleuropulmonary malignancies, the histologic classification of lung cancer recommended by the World Health Organization (WHO) in 1977 should be used as the current definitive classification (Table 22-10).[206] Carcinomas arising from the bronchial or bronchioloalveolar sur-

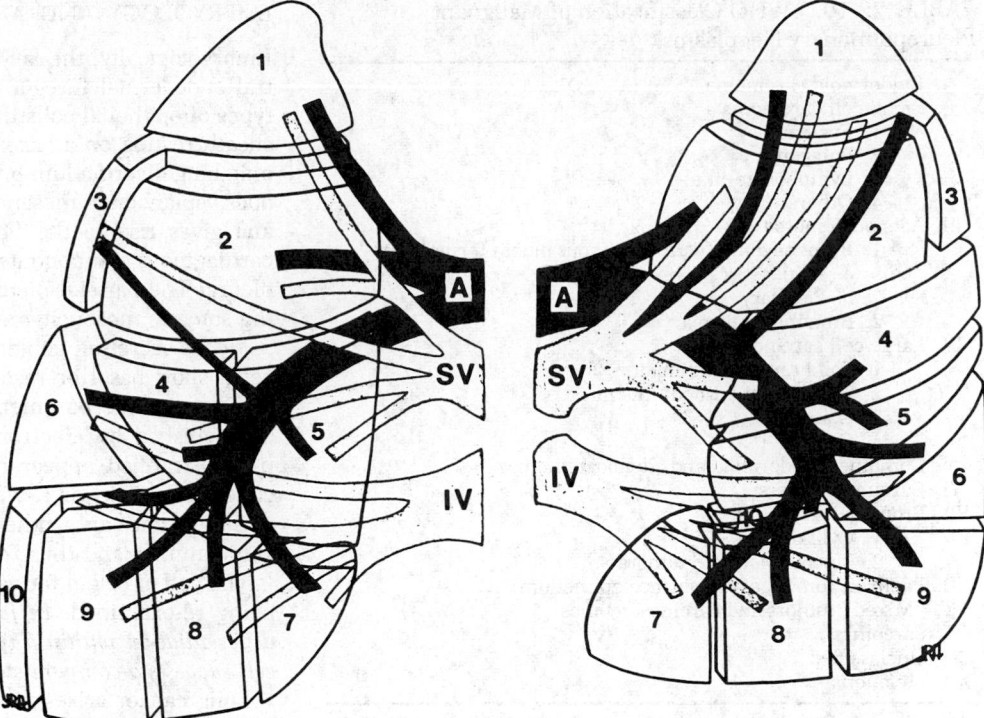

FIG. 22-2. Schematic diagram of segmental and vascular anatomy of the lung. The anatomical distribution of the bronchopulmonary segments is numbered according to the Boyden scheme (see text and Table 22-9 for description of bronchopulmonary segments). A = pulmonary artery; SV = superior pulmonary veins; IV = inferior pulmonary veins. (Redrawn from Sweet RH: Surgical anatomy of the thorax. In Thoracic Surgery. Philadelphia, WB Saunders, 1950)

face epithelium and from the bronchial mucous glands make up 90% to 95% of lung cancers.[207] Approximately 2% to 4% of these tumors will be a combination of squamous and glandular elements and are called adenosquamous cell carcinoma.

These various cell types have different natural histories and responses to therapy. Therefore, correct histologic identification of the cell type is a cornerstone of treatment planning. This is best accomplished by obtaining adequate amounts of tumor material for both histologic and cytologic evaluation. If discrepancies occur in these studies, it is im-

portant to have the material reviewed by a pathologist experienced in the histologic typing of lung cancer.

INCIDENCE OF TYPES

Estimates of the incidence of the four major cell types depend on the source of the pathologic materials reviewed (e.g., biopsy, cytology, surgical resection, or autopsy) (Table 22-11). There appears to have been a shift in incidence of the histologic types over the past 20 years, with a fall in the fraction of cases of epidermoid cancer and a rise in the

TABLE 22-9.   Bronchopulmonary Segments

Right Lung		Left Lung	
Upper Lobe			
Jackson–Huber	Boyden	Jackson–Huber	Boyden
Apical	1	Apical–posterior	1–3
Anterior	2	Anterior	2
Posterior	3		
		Superior lingular	4
		Inferior lingular	5
Middle Lobe			
Lateral	4	Medial	5
Lower Lobe			
Superior	6	Superior	6
Medial basal	7	Anteriomedial	7–8
Anterior basal	8	Lateral basal	9
Lateral basal	9	Posterior basal	10
Posterior basal	10		

Jackson CL, Huber JF: Correlated applied anatomy of bronchial tree and lungs with system nomenclature. Dis Chest 9:319–326, 1943; Boyden EA: Segmental Anatomy of the Lungs.New York, McGraw-Hill, 1955.

TABLE 22-10.   WHO Classification of Malignant Pleuropulmonary Neoplasms

I. Epidermoid carcinoma
II. Small cell carcinoma
    1. Fusiform
    2. Polygonal
    3. Lymphocyte-like
    4. Others
III. Adenocarcinoma
    1. Bronchogenic (with or without mucin formation)
      a. Acinar
      b. Papillary
    2. Bronchioloalveolar
IV. Large cell carcinoma
    1. Solid tumor with mucin
    2. Solid tumor without mucin
    3. Giant cell
    4. Clear cell
V. Combined epidermoid and adenocarcinomas
VI. Carcinoid tumors
VII. Bronchial gland tumors
    1. Cylindromas
    2. Mucoepidermoid tumors
VIII. Papillary tumors of the surface epithelium
IX. "Mixed" tumors and carcinosarcomas
X. Sarcomas
XI. Unclassified
XII. Melanoma

Kreyberg L: Histologic typing of lung tumors. In Kreyberg L (ed): International Histologic Classification of Tumors, No. 1, pp 19–26. Geneva, World Health Organization, 1967; Sobin LH: The World Health Organization's histological classification of lung tumors: A comparison of the first and second editions. Cancer Detect Prev 5:391–406; Yesner R, Gerstl B, Auerbach O: Application of the World Health Organization classification of lung carcinoma to biopsy material. Ann Thorac Surg 1:33–49, 1965; Matthews MJ: Morphologic classification of bronchogenic carcinoma. Cancer Chemother Rep 3:229–302, 1973.

percentage of adenocarcinomas.[208,209] This change is partly a result of the rise in the incidence of lung cancer in women, who have more adenocarcinomas than epidermoid cancers. However, an increase in adenocarcinomas also has been seen in men.

EMBRYOLOGY AND ANATOMY OF PATHOGENESIS

Embryologically, the laryngotracheobronchial tree is a ventral endodermal foregut derivative lined with five or more types of epithelial cells that form a pseudostratified mucosal sheath resting on a basement membrane.[210] As the embryonic lung diverticulum branches to form bronchopulmonary buds, splanchnic mesenchyme surrounds these structures and gives rise to the fibroelastic, vascular muscular, and cartilaginous components of the lung and forms the visceral pleura. The parietal pleura is derived from the corresponding somatic mesenchyme.

Mucus-secreting goblet cells, ciliated cells, brush border cells, short basal or reserve cells, and granular basal cells that rest on the basement membrane, all of which can be distinguished by electron microscopy, give the mucosa a pseudostratified appearance. The granular basal cells are called Kulchitsky or K-type cells. They have neurosecretory granules that can synthesize polypeptide hormones or biogenic amines and thus resemble small cell carcinomas.[211]

The cell of origin for each type of lung cancer is currently being re-examined. *In fact, the finding of several types of differentiation within a tumor or even within a given tumor cell suggests a common stem cell for all types of lung cancer.*

Lung cancer arises most often in segmental and subsegmental bronchi in response to repeated injury and chronic inflammation.[208] At segmental bronchial bifurcations, the epithelium is particularly susceptible to injury, and carcinogens may be deposited in these areas.[212] The carcinogens implicated in this process include the constituents of tobacco smoke, radioisotopes, asbestos, polycyclic hydrocarbons, haloethers, nickel, chromium, inorganic arsenic, iron ore, printing inks, and possibly other occupational and atmospheric pollutants discussed earlier.[213] Initially, basal cells respond to injury by proliferating to generate mucin-secreting goblet cells. When there is added injury, the columnar cells are replaced by orderly metaplastic stratified squamous epithelium. Finally, the epithelium becomes disorganized, and nuclear atypia and mitoses are seen in the basal half of the mucosa, findings that are called atypical metaplasia or

TABLE 22-11.   Incidence of Major Histologic Types of Lung Cancer

Histologic Type	Biopsy Cytology* (n = 4107)	Surgical Specimens† (n = 1,206)	Autopsy‡ (n = 1080)	Mayo Clinic§ (n = 2926)	Johns Hopkins‖ (n = 435)
			% of cases		
Epidermoid carcinoma	45	64	33	34	39
Adenocarcinoma	22	16	25	26	19
Large cell carcinoma	11	9	16	16	20
Small cell carcinoma	19	19	25	22	19
Other (e.g., bronchioloalveolar or mixed)	3	2	1	2	2

*Yesner R et al, Ann Thorac Surg 1:33–49, 1965; Matthews MJ, Gordon PR. In Straus MJ (ed): Lung Cancer Clinical Diagnosis and Treatment. New York: Grune & Stratton, 1977; Mountain CF et al, Am J Roentgenol Rad Ther Nucl Med 120:130–138, 1974; Feinstein AR et al, Chest 66:225–229, 1974.

†Matthews MJ, Gordon PR, In Straus MJ (ed): Lung Cancer Clinical Diagnosis and Treatment. New York: Grune & Stratton, 1977; Hinson KFW, Miller AB, Tall R, Cancer 35:399–405, 1975.

‡Matthews MJ, Gordon PR, In Straus MJ (ed): Lung Cancer Clinical Diagnosis and Treatment. New York: Grune & Stratton, 1977; Auerbach O, Garfinkel L, Parks UR, Chest 67:382–387, 1975.

§Rosenow EC III, Carr DT, CA 29:233–246, 1979.

‖Katlic M, Carter D, Prog Cancer Res Ther 11:143–150, 1979.

dysplasia. When this process occurs throughout the full thickness of the mucosa, a diagnosis of carcinoma *in situ* (intraepithelial carcinoma) is made. Finally, the basement membrane is violated by the neoplastic cells, and frank infiltration of neoplastic cells into the underlying stroma follows.[214-216] This process may take 10 to 20 years and represents the first phase of the natural history of lung cancer. The site of origin of a small cell cancer usually is difficult to identify. These tumors infiltrate the submucosa, while squamous metaplasia or dysplasia is seen in the overlying bronchial mucosa. In many cases, it also is difficult to distinguish whether adenocarcinomas or large cell carcinomas come from bronchial surface epithelium or the underlying mucous glands.

Marked atypia of cells in sputum cytology specimens has been felt to be highly suggestive of later appearances of lung cancer. However, this idea has recently been called into question.[217] Sixteen cases of marked atypia were found in 292 male smoking uranium miners. Four of these men had cells highly suspicious for malignancy, and three of these went on to develop lung cancer. However, the remaining 13 cases all reverted to mild atypia or normal cytologies with follow-up over an average period of 54 months. *These studies suggest that marked atypia will not by itself be useful as a marker in chemoprevention studies or early detection trials.* However, histologic evidence suggests that bronchial epidermoid metaplasia can regress with smoking cessation and retinoid treatment.[218] Forty heavy cigarette smokers had multiple fiberoptic bronchoscopy-directed biospies and were scored for a metaplasia index. They were then treated with a retinoid derivative orally (etretinate 25 mg/day) for 6 months and rebiopsied. Four of the patients stopped smoking, and they had complete regression of their metaplasia, whereas the remaining patients had significant reduction in the metaplasia despite their continuing to smoke.

Epidermoid and small cell carcinomas are usually central in location, whereas *adenocarcinomas and large cell tumors are often peripheral* and associated with pulmonary conditions that cause lung destruction, fibrosis, reconstruction of the airways into nonfunctional spaces, and hyperplasia of pneumocytes. Chronic interstitial lung diseases (*i.e.*, scleroderma, rheumatoid disease, sarcoidosis, interstitial pneumonitis, pulmonary scars and fibrosis from pulmonary infarcts, tuberculosis, chronic abscesses, and other necrotizing pulmonary diseases) have been noted as predisposing factors.[219-223] With progressive pulmonary fibrosis, avascularity, local tissue anoxia, and proliferation of the bronchioloalveolar epithelium are stimulated, resulting in adenomatous foci that frequently become metaplastic and mucus producing.[208] Exogenous agents involved in these processes include asbestos, cadmium, beryllium, gases, mineral oils, viruses, mycobacteria, and pneumoconiotic dusts.[213]

EPIDERMOID CARCINOMA

Epidermoid tumors grow centrally toward the main-stem bronchus and locally invade underlying bronchial cartilage, adjoining lung parenchyma, and lymph nodes. The bronchial mucosa usually shows squamous metaplasia, dysplasia, or frank intraepithelial neoplasia, processes that provide evidence for the primary nature of the tumor in the lung.[208]

ADENOCARCINOMA

Most adenocarcinomas are located peripherally, unrelated to bronchi except by contiguous growth or lymph node metastases. The tumors provoke a desmoplastic response, present as firm, localized, subpleural masses, and tend to invade the overlying pleura. Tumors arising from the bronchial epithelium present as thick, firm, gray–white pipestemmed structures with narrowed lumina. It may be difficult to distinguish the tumors in the lung from cancer of the pancreas, kidney, breast, or colon that metastasize to bronchi.[208] Adenocarcinomas arising from bronchia mucous glands form lobules of neoplastic glands that may produce mucin or exhibit a cribriform pattern.

BRONCHIOLOALVEOLAR CARCINOMA

Bronchioloalveolar carcinoma presents either as single nodules or in a multinodular pattern. The latter presentation has suggested that there are multiple primaries.[224,225] Papillary configurations may be seen in adenocarcinomas arising from bronchial surface epithelium and in tumors associated with scars, as well as in the classic bronchioloalveolar carcinoma. Psammoma bodies are noted in 5% to 15% of papillary tumors. Bronchioloalveolar cancer in the lung may be indistinguishable histologically from metastases to the lung from other adenocarcinomas, such as those of the kidney, ovary, thyroid, uterus, or colon, although ultrastructural studies suggest that the cell of origin is the bronchiolar lining cell, with subcellular features of the Clara and ciliated epithelial cells.[226] Some of these tumors have osmiophilic lamellar bodies and demonstrate surfactant production, relating them to the type II pneumocyte. The tumor is similar to the viral-induced pulmonary carcinoma of sheep.[227] Mice, horses, and guinea pigs have similar diseases as well.

Bronchioloalveolar carcinoma usually is reported to be associated with prior lung disease leading to fibrosis, including repeated pneumonias, idiopathic pulmonary fibrosis, granulomata, inflammation, asbestosis, fibrosing alveolitis, scleroderma, and Hodgkin's disease.[219,228,229] However, in some isolated reports, no antecedent lung damage has been found. The cancer also is found in families with other tumors and has been seen in identical twins.[230,231] Bronchioloalveolar carcinoma is not correlated with smoking.[232] Because of its association with fibrosing lung disease, any new roentgenographic mass or persistent infiltrate in such patients should be suspected of being bronchioloalveolar carcinoma.[233]

LARGE CELL CARCINOMA

Large cell carcinomas present as large peripheral subpleural lesions with necrotic or cavitary surfaces. These tumors usually are unrelated to bronchi except by contiguous growth, and they have a tendency to invade pulmonary parenchyma and the overlying pleura. In small foci, recognizable attempts at differentiation, usually glandular, may be identified, but the predominant anaplastic nature of the tumor is overwhelming. Microscopically, these tumors are a composite of all the anaplastic features of poorly differentiated squamous carcinomas and adenocarcinomas. A subtype of large cell carcinoma, giant cell carcinoma, is composed of bizarre cells with giant nuclei and very large quantities of cytoplasm that often show phagocytic activity or contain mucin vacuoles. Approximately 30% of lung cancers have areas of clear cell changes, whereas more than two-thirds of large cell carcinomas may show these changes, and almost one-third of adenocarcinomas and epidermoid carcinomas also will show these features.[234] The clear cells stain strongly for glycogen but weakly for mucin. However, it is rare to find a tumor composed solely of clear cells. The prognosis of tumors containing large areas of clear cells is no different from that of the other common lung cancer histologic types; the importance of recognizing the clear cell type of primary lung cancer is to differentiate it from metastatic renal carcinoma.

SMALL CELL CARCINOMA

Small cell carcinomas appear as submucosal infiltrates in the early phase of the disease. The mucosa may be normal or slightly lifted by a plaque that obliterates normal bronchial markings. In advanced stages, bronchial lumina may be obstructed by extrinsic compression or endobronchial tumor.[235] Silver stains are focally positive in approximately half the cases, and neurosecretory granules are usually found on electron micrographic studies.[208] However, electron microscopic findings, including absence of neurosecretory granules, do not predict responses to therapy so long as the light microscopic criteria for the diagnosis of small cell lung cancer are fulfilled.[236]

The 1981 WHO classification divides small cell lung cancer into three subtypes, including the oat cell or lymphocytelike, the intermediate, and the combined (oat cell combined with squamous or adenocarcinoma).[237] The classic oat cell type is characterized by small round or oval cells with darkly staining nuclei, indistinct or absent nucleoli, and scanty cytoplasm. The intermediate type is comprised of larger cells with a lower nuclear : cytoplasmic ratio and polygonal or fusiform nuclei. All subtypes of small cell carcinoma consist of cells that are at least two to three times the size of a mature lymphocyte and exhibit the characteristic features of "salt and pepper" distribution of chromatin, nuclear molding, areas of cellular necrosis, and deposition of DNA-derived material on elastic fibrils.[208] Numerous atypical mitoses may be identified. Mixtures of lymphocyte-like and intermediate subtypes of small cell cancer frequently are seen in a single tumor. The histologic distinction between small cell and non-small cell cancers is of great clinical importance. The intermediate subtype of small cell cancer may sometimes be confused with poorly differentiated epidermoid carcinoma, large cell cancer, or poorly differentiated adenocarcinoma, particularly in metastatic sites. Also, some tumors form distinct tubules as well as rosettes and can be confused with adenocarcinomas. In some small cell tumors, prominent clusters of anaplastic large cells may be seen; in others, nests of squamous cells may be found.

Despite their submucosal location, small cell carcinomas often have malignant cells exfoliated into sputa and cytologic washings, and bronchoscopy yields malignant cells in more than 90% of patients with clinically apparent disease.[235] With well-preserved material, cytologic diagnosis appears as accurate as tissue diagnosis.[238] Other features of clinicopathologic interest in small cell cancer include the presence of marked osteoblastic activity in a minority of patients with bony metastases, with new bone formation similar to that in prostate and breast cancer metastases; pancreatic involvement from peripancreatic nodal disease associated focal acute pancreatitis and possibly severe fat necrosis; and a significant number of metastases to endocrine organs (*i.e.*, thyroid in 8%, pituitary in 15%, testes in 7%, and parathyroid in 1%).[208,213,235-242]

CLINICOPATHOLOGIC CORRELATION WITH HISTOLOGIC TYPE

Differences in long-term survival rates according to the histologic type of lung cancer have been analyzed in a large number of patients (Table 22-12). In most instances, these patients have been treated with local modalities (*i.e.*, surgery and radiotherapy). The figures for small cell lung cancer have changed with the advent of intensive combination chemotherapy. At present, patients with epidermoid cancers have the best survival, followed by those with adenocarcinomas and large cell carcinomas. Until recently, it was rare for a patient with small cell carcinoma to survive for 5 years.

Epidermoid cancer is more common in males; adenocarcinoma is more common in females. An equal sex distribution exists for the other cell types. On the whole, females have a better survival rate than do males, independent of the stage of cancer.[243] Epidermoid and small cell cancers have a much higher incidence in smokers than nonsmokers, whereas adenocarcinoma is the predominant type in nonsmokers (Table 22-13). This may be accounted for in part by the inclusion of adenocarcinomas from an "unknown primary" with metastases to the lung in the nonsmoker group. *In any event, in women with a lung adenocarcinoma, it is important to rule out a primary breast or gynecologic tumor that would need different therapy than a primary lung cancer.*

The location of the primary tumor will determine the presenting signs and symptoms and dictate the methods for

TABLE 22-12. Overall 5-Year Survival (%) for Major Histologic Types of Lung Cancer

Histologic Type	All Cases ($n = 2155$)	Resected ($n = 835$)	Per cent Resectable
Epidermoid carcinoma	25	37	60
Adenocarcinoma	12	27	38*
Large cell carcinoma	13	27	38*
Small cell carcinoma	1	0	11

Matthews MJ, Gordon PR: Morphology of pulmonary and pleural malignancies. In Straus MJ (ed): Lung Cancer: Clinical Diagnosis and Treatment. New York: Grune & Stratton, 1977; Mountain CF, Carr DT, Martini N et al: Staging of lung cancer 1979. American Joint Committee for Cancer Staging and End Results Reporting, Task Force on Lung Cancer, Chicago, 1980.

*Combined in AJC report.

TABLE 22-13.   Incidence According to Sex and Smoking Status of Major Histologic Types of Lung Cancer at the Mayo Clinic

Histologic Type	Male (n = 2411)	Female (n = 515)	Smokers (n = 2708)	Never Smoked (n = 218)
	% of cases			
Epidermoid carcinoma	37	18	36	9
Adenocarcinoma	22	44	23	64
Large cell carcinoma	17	12	16	14
Small cell carcinoma	22	20	23	3
Bronchioloalveolar	2	6	2	9

Rosenow EC III, Carr DT: Bronchogenic carcinoma. CA 29:233–246, 1979.

obtaining a histologic diagnosis (Table 22-14). Proximal tumors usually have histologic material obtained by bronchoscopy or sputum cytology, whereas distal lesions usually are detected on screening chest films and thus are diagnosed by transbronchial or percutaneous needle biospy or at the time of resection.

In surgically resected specimens, small cell cancer involves the lymph nodes in most cases, whereas the non-small cell cancers have lymph node involvement in approximately 40% of cases (see Table 22-14). Epidermoid carcinomas (28%) and large cell carcinomas (22%) cavitate more frequently than do adenocarcinomas (12%) or small cell carcinomas (8%).[244] In contrast, adenocarcinomas and large cell carcinomas show visceral pleural invasion more often than do other types of surgically resected tumors because of their peripheral location.

Approximately 20% to 30% of lung cancers studied histologically are associated with scars from other lung injury (called "pulmonary scar carcinoma").[245] The majority of these (58%–88%) are adenocarcinomas or bronchioloalveolar cancers and occur in peripheral locations. Chest roentgenographs often (50% of cases) are negative, and bronchoscopy and sputum cytology are ineffective as initial diagnostic tools. These patients frequently present with nonpulmonary symptoms of metastatic disease, and the chest lesion is clinically undetectable. However, when the primary is resectable, their survival rate is similar to that of other patients of similar postsurgical stage.[246]

The clinicopathologic correlation of therapeutic importance for bronchioloalveolar carcinoma relates to the number of nodules (solitary or multicentric) and the degree of differentiation.[247] Lymph node metastases occur in only 23% of patients with solitary nodules but in more than 77% of patients with multicentric lesions. A majority (84%) of patients with solitary nodules have well-differentiated tumors. In contrast, only 45% of multicentric tumors are as well differentiated. Some 80% of poorly differentiated tumors have lymph node metastases at presentation, whereas only 20% to 30% of the more highly differentiated tumors show this spread.

ACCURACY OF HISTOLOGIC DIAGNOSIS

The first principle of treatment is a correct histologic diagnosis. The quality and quantity of the samples are important for such diagnosis. Common problems for the clinical pathologist are crush artifact, poor fixation, overstaining, or inadequate amounts of materials. Crushing artifact in a needle aspiration must not be mistaken for small cell carcinoma, as sometimes occurs. A diagnosis of malignancy may be based on a cytologic sample, and differentiated malignancies and small cell carcinomas may be diagnosed as readily and as accurately in cytologic specimens as in small biopsies.[248,249] However, a histologic (tissue block) diagnosis is strongly preferred.

A significant problem in the use of histologic criteria when

TABLE 22-14.   Anatomical Location of Primary Tumors in Relation to Histologic Type of Lung Cancer and Frequency of Early Regional Spread

Histologic Type	Proximal Location n	Proximal Location %	Resected Surgical Specimen — Lymph Node Involvement n	Lymph Node Involvement %	Visceral Pleural Involvement n	Visceral Pleural Involvement %
Epidermoid carcinoma	275	81	158	42	109	33
Adenocarcinoma	140	29	109	41	59	59
Large cell carcinoma	113	49	65	42	27	52
Small cell carcinoma	96	83	29	72	13	15
Overall	641	63	631	48	211	41

Vincent RG, Pickren JW, Lane WW et al: The changing histopathology of lung cancer: A review of 1682 cases. Cancer 39:1647–1655, 1977; Rilke F, Carbone A, Clemente C et al: Surgical pathology of resectable lung cancer. Prog Cancer Res Ther 11:129–142, 1979.

determining prognosis and types of treatment is the degree of interobserver and intraobserver variability in reading the same specimens. In addition, there is heterogeneity within the tumor itself in both the primary and metastatic sites.[238,244,250,251] Tumors often show features of several histologic subtypes, suggesting a morphologic continuum. This is a particular problem with small cell carcinoma.[252,253] Some series have reported imperfect correlations between cytologic and subsequent histologic diagnosis of the cell type, and misleading results may be obtained from biopsy of cavitary lesions and necrotic tumors.[254] The distinction between small cell carcinoma and the non-small cell types is consistent in 90% of cases when adequate material is reviewed by well-trained observers experienced in lung cancer pathology.[244] The assignment of tumors to each of the major types of non-small cell cancer is less consistent (approximately 70%). Attempts to subdivide the four major types currently are subject to an even larger degree of interobserver variation.[255,256] This problem is particularly marked in the diagnosis of specimens of small cell carcinoma mixed with other major histologic types, especially large cell carcinoma. It may be necessary to obtain the opinion of several pathologists unless biochemical or immunologic markers of small cell cancer can be assessed. If several pathologists agree that a definite small cell component exists, the patient probably should be considered to have small cell carcinoma. *At present, we believe that the only treatment-related decisions that should be based on histologic type are the distinction between small cell cancer and the other, non-small cell, types and possibly identification of well-differentiated epidermoid lesions, which often appear amenable to aggressive local therapy.*

Epidermoid and adenocarcinoma have been subdivided in the WHO classification into groups that exhibit different degrees of histologic differentiation. Squamous tumors present with about equal frequency as well-, moderately, or poorly differentiated lesions, whereas adenocarcinomas present more frequently as poorly differentiated lesions.[244] At present, there appears to be a 5-year survival advantage for well- and moderately differentiated epidermoid carcinomas (20%–39%) compared with poorly differentiated lesions. There is no difference between well- and moderately differentiated (23%) and poorly differentiated (26%) adenocarcinomas.[256,257]

In studies of small cell carcinoma subtyping, large numbers of patients were evaluated extensively before therapy, then treated with intensive combination chemotherapy or with chemotherapy and radiotherapy. With one exception, no difference was seen between subtypes with respect to stage of disease, sites of metastases, response to therapy or number of complete responses, response duration, or survival.[252,253,258] When histologic subtypes in the primary biopsy specimen were compared with the subtype of other pathologic specimens from the same patient, concordance was present in only 71%, whereas two or three histologic subtypes were present in the remaining 29%.[259] The clinical implications of the combined subtype are unknown. At present, there appears to be no reason to base decisions on the presence of histologic subtypes of small cell carcinoma, with one exception: the mixed small cell–large cell carcinoma variant that occurs in approximately 6% to 14% of

small cell lung cancer cases.[260,261] This type has a lower overall response to combination chemotherapy, a lower complete response rate, and a shorter median survival than small cell carcinoma without large cell components. The oat cell and intermediate subtypes have similar clinical features and prognosis, and because the oat cell subtype (which is never observed in vitro) may be an artifact of tissue fixation, a new subclassification of small cell carcinoma that combines these two subtypes as "classic small cell carcinoma" is in preparation. Cell biology and autopsy studies indicate that a transition can occur between small cell carcinoma and large cell carcinoma accompanied by a loss of expression of differentiated functions by the cells.[262-264] The cells with small cell carcinoma histology express the amine precursor uptake and decarboxylation (APUD) properties of high levels of DOPA decarboxylase (L-aromatic amino decarboxylase), formaldehyde-induced fluorescence after exposure to 5-hydroxytryptophane, and neurosecretory granules, whereas the large cell variants do not.[264] Recent molecular biology studies have shown that many of the large cell variants of small cell carcinoma (SCLC-V cells) have amplification of the c-*myc* oncogene and express large amounts of c-*myc* messenger RNA. Thus one mechanism of producing these histologic and biochemical variants with a poor prognosis may be oncogene amplification. Autopsy studies at Johns Hopkins and the NCI conducted on 131 patients after intensive chemotherapy or chemoradiotherapy for small cell carcinoma showed that 27% of the tumors also had a large cell, giant cell, squamous cell, tubular, or carcinoid component; 4% were pure squamous cell carcinoma without small cell elements; 3% were pure large cell tumors; and 1% were pure adenocarcinoma.[262,263,265] Thus, in a very large percentage of cases, other histologic types of lung cancer are found at autopsy. At the Finsen Institute (Copenhagen), the 13% of small cell carcinoma patients with non-small cell components at autopsy had shorter survival than patients with pure small cell lung cancer on postmortem microscopic examination.[266] The presence of the different histologic types of lung cancer could reflect the presence of separate primary tumors or the presence of a common stem cell that can differentiate along several pathways. These possibilities will have to be resolved by cell biology, cloning, and chromosome studies.

NEWER METHODS OF PATHOLOGIC DIAGNOSIS

New findings in cellular biology should eventually allow pathologists to distinguish small cell from non-small cell lung cancer, as well as subtype lung cancers by tests other than light microscopy. It has been demonstrated clearly that small cell tumors express the peptide hormone GRP, L-DOPA decarboxylase, neuron-specific enolase, and the BB isozyme of creatine kinase, as well as dense core granules by electron microscopy, whereas non-small cell tumors much less frequently express these markers. A list of these and other distinctions is provided in the section on the cellular biology of lung cancer. As biochemical and immunologic reagents become generally available, and as these markers are studied in prospective clinical trials, their utility in diagnosis and patient management can be assessed and documented.

New approaches for the identification of malignant cells

include isolation of antibodies reactive with lung cancer but not with normal respiratory epithelium or with products produced by lung cancer cells. Antisera against lung cancer antigens that react with antigens of apparent endodermal and neural crest derivation have been described.[267] Recently, monoclonal antibodies with specificity for lung cancer cells have been prepared.[268-270] Another approach involves identifying cells with increased DNA content, a condition frequently seen in malignant cells. There appears to be a progressive increase in the amount of DNA per cell in squamous metaplastic cells or in neoplastic cells exhibiting progressive amounts of atypia.[271] Combining DNA staining with new cell-sorting instruments will allow the screening of large numbers of cells by flow cytometry in individual sputum samples. Using flow cytometry, 83% of small cell and 85% of non-small cell patients' tumor specimens from metastatic sites were aneuploid.[272] A recent study utilizing flow cytometry of paraffin-embedded pathologic sections from 100 surgically treated patients with non-small cell lung cancer indicates that patients whose tumors had aneuploid DNA content had shorter survival.[273]

NATURAL HISTORY OF LUNG CANCER

Understanding the natural history of lung cancer is important for prevention, early detection, rationally planned initial curative or palliative therapy, anticipation of possible complications, and the institution of therapy at the time of relapse. The natural history of lung cancer begins with the exposure of a susceptible host to carcinogens, eventually leading to the cytologic changes of cellular atypia identifiable in cells exfoliated into the sputum. These changes progress to carcinoma in situ, then to frank invasion. Accurate definition of these early events is important to plan preventive therapy in future trials and for instituting surgery, radiotherapy, or chemotherapy in the patient with clinically occult disease. Information on early history will be provided from the mass screening program data described later in this chapter.

SIGNS AND SYMPTOMS OF LUNG CANCER

With the onset of local tumor growth and invasion, lung cancer can give rise to signs and symptoms as well as to chest radiograph or sputum cytology abnormalities (Table 22-15).[274] Findings may be the result of local tumor growth,

TABLE 22-15. Common Signs and Symptoms of Lung Cancer

Symptoms secondary to central or endobronchial growth of the primary tumor
  Cough
  Hemoptysis
  Wheeze and stridor
  Dyspnea from obstruction
  Pneumonitis from obstruction (fever, productive cough)
Symptoms secondary to peripheral growth of the primary tumor
  Pain from pleural or chest wall involvement
  Cough
  Dyspnea on a restrictive basis
  Lung abscess syndrome from tumor cavitation
Symptoms related to regional spread of the tumor in the thorax by contiguity or by metastasis to regional lymph nodes
  Tracheal obstruction
  Esophageal compression with dysphagia
  Recurrent laryngeal nerve paralysis with hoarseness
  Phrenic nerve paralysis with hemidiaphragm elevation and dyspnea
  Sympathetic nerve paralysis with Horner's syndrome
  Eighth cervical and first thoracic nerves with ulnar pain and Pancoast's syndrome
  Superior vena cava syndrome from vascular obstruction
  Pericardial and cardiac extension with resultant tamponade, arrhythmia, or cardiac failure
  Lymphatic obstruction with pleural effusion
  Lymphangitic spread through lungs with hypoxemia and dyspnea

Cohen MH: Signs and symptoms of bronchogenic carcinoma. In Straus MJ (ed): Lung Cancer: Clinical Diagnosis and Treatment, pp 85–94. New York, Grune & Stratton, 1977.

invasion of adjacent structures, regional growth (from metastasis to peribronchial, hilar, mediastinal, and supraclavicular nodes) by way of lymphatic spread, growth in distant sites after hematogenous dissemination, or a remote effect of the tumor (paraneoplastic syndromes).

Unfortunately, by the time a sign, symptom, or visible nodule appears, dissemination to regional or distant lymph nodes or distant extranodal sites usually has occurred. This can be seen at autopsy when the patients die of other causes after a supposedly curative resection for lung cancer (Table 22-16). Patients with all histologic types of lung cancer sometimes had microscopic residual disease; these sites were frequently outside the areas where postoperative chest radiotherapy would have been directed. Small cell carcinoma in particular has a high frequency of extrathoracic metas-

TABLE 22-16. Incidence at Autopsy of Persistent Tumor After "Curative" Surgical Therapy for Lung Cancer in Patients Dying of Other Causes Within 30 Days Postoperatively

Cell Type	No. of Patients	Percentage with Persistent Tumor		
		Total	Local Disease Only	Distant Metastases
Epidermoid carcinoma	131	34	17	17
Adenocarcinoma	30	43	3	40
Large cell carcinoma	22	14	0	14
Small cell carcinoma	19	69	6	63

Matthews MJ, Kanhouwa S, Pickner J et al: Frequency of residual and metastatic tumors in patients undergoing curative surgical resection of lung cancer. Cancer Chemother Rep 3:63–67, 1973.

tases, followed by adenocarcinoma and then the other non-small-cell types. Often, these metastases were intra-abdominal.[275] Other data demonstrating the early metastatic behavior of lung cancer have been generated from analysis of surgical specimens. In non-small cell carcinoma, the approximate frequency of lymph node involvement in such specimens is 40%; invasion of veins occurs in 19%, invasion of arteries in 18%, and invasion of the visceral pleura in 44% (see Table 22-14).[244]

Excluding cases found by mass screening programs, most patients present with symptomatic disease. In 678 Yale-New Haven Hospital and Yale Veterans Administration patients, Feinstein found that 6% were asymptomatic, 27% had symptoms related to the primary tumor, 32% had symptoms of metastatic disease, and 34% had systemic symptoms that suggested tumor, such as anorexia, weight loss, and fatigue.[276] There was a significant difference in 5-year surival rate, with 18% of the asymptomatic, 12% of the primary symptomatic, 6% of the systemic symptomatic, and none of the patients with metastatic symptoms surviving 5 years.[276] Patients with a long history of symptoms related to their primary tumor had a better 5-year survival rate (16%) than those with a short duration of symptoms (9%), suggesting that some tumors may have an inherently more indolent course; this, in turn, may be related to their rate of growth. Of great interest was the correlation of symptomatic stage with anatomic stage. Here, there was an effect of symptoms independent of anatomic stage. *Thus, the accurate determination of signs and symptoms can be of prognostic value, and these features should be correlated with clinical and surgical pathologic evidence of disease when planning treatment and determining prognosis for individual patients.*

The frequency of the various presenting signs and symptoms will vary, depending on whether the series represents all patients presenting with lung cancer or the subpopulations selected for more limited disease, advanced disease, or from mass screening series. Recently, a large series of patients undergoing radical radiotherapy for cure contained a high incidence of asymptomatic patients with disease discovered on routine chest films and a lower percentage of patients with symptoms of regional spread or systemic symptoms compared with the Yale study (Table 22-17).[277]

Signs, symptoms, and radiographic findings in the chest are related to the central or peripheral location of the primary tumor, in addition to whether regional spread has occurred, both of which are related to the histologic type (Table 22-18, Fig. 22-3).[278] In general, epidermoid cancers have a central location, with atelectasis, pneumonitis (from bronchial obstruction), hilar adenopathy, and a tendency to cavitate; adenocarcinomas have a defined nodule in a periph-

TABLE 22-17.   Manner of Presentation of Lung Cancer in 170 Patients Referred for Treatment with Radical Radiotherapy

Symptoms or Finding	Percentage of Patients
Routine chest radiograph (asymptomatic)	16
Primary tumor (total)	81
Hemoptysis	30
Cough	25
Dyspnea	11
Pneumonitis	8
Pain	6
Wheeze	2
Regional spread (total)	2
Dysphagia	1
Hoarseness	0.5
Systemic symptoms	
Weight loss	0.5

Coy P, Kennelly GM: The role of curative radiotherapy in the treatment of lung cancer. Cancer 45:698–702, 1980.

TABLE 22-18.   Presenting Chest Roentgenologic Findings in Lung Cancer by T, N, and M Factor

Roentgen Finding	Percentage with Finding			
	Epidermoid Carcinoma	Small Cell Carcinoma	Adenocarcinoma	Large Cell Carcinoma
	(n = 338–585)	(n = 114–252)	(n = 135–301)	(n = 97)
Tumor (T) factor				
Nodule <4 cm	14	21	46	18
Nodule >4 cm	18	8	26	41
Peripheral location	29	26	65	61
Central location	64	74	5	42
Atelectasis	23	31	2	14
Pneumonitis	13	21	14	24
Cavitation	5	0	3	4
Pleural or chest wall	3	5	14	2
Lymph node (N) factor				
Hilar adenopathy	38	61	19 (40)*	32
Mediastinal adenopathy	5	14	9 (27)	10

Cohen MH: Signs and symptoms of bronchogenic carcinoma. In Straus MJ (ed): Lung Cancer: Clinical Diagnosis and Treatment, pp 85–94. New York, Grune & Stratton, 1977; Byrd RB, Carr DT, Miller WE et al: Radiographic abnormalities in carcinoma of the lung as related to histologic cell type. Thorax 24:573–575, 1969; Green N, Kurohara SS, George FW III et al: The biologic behavior of lung cancer according to histologic type. Radiol Clin Biol 41:160–170, 1972.

*Newer evidence suggests a large proportion of adenocarcinomas (numbers in parentheses) can present with hilar or mediastinal masses from involved lymph nodes on plain radiographs. (Woodring JH, Stelling CB, AJR 140:657–664, 1983.)

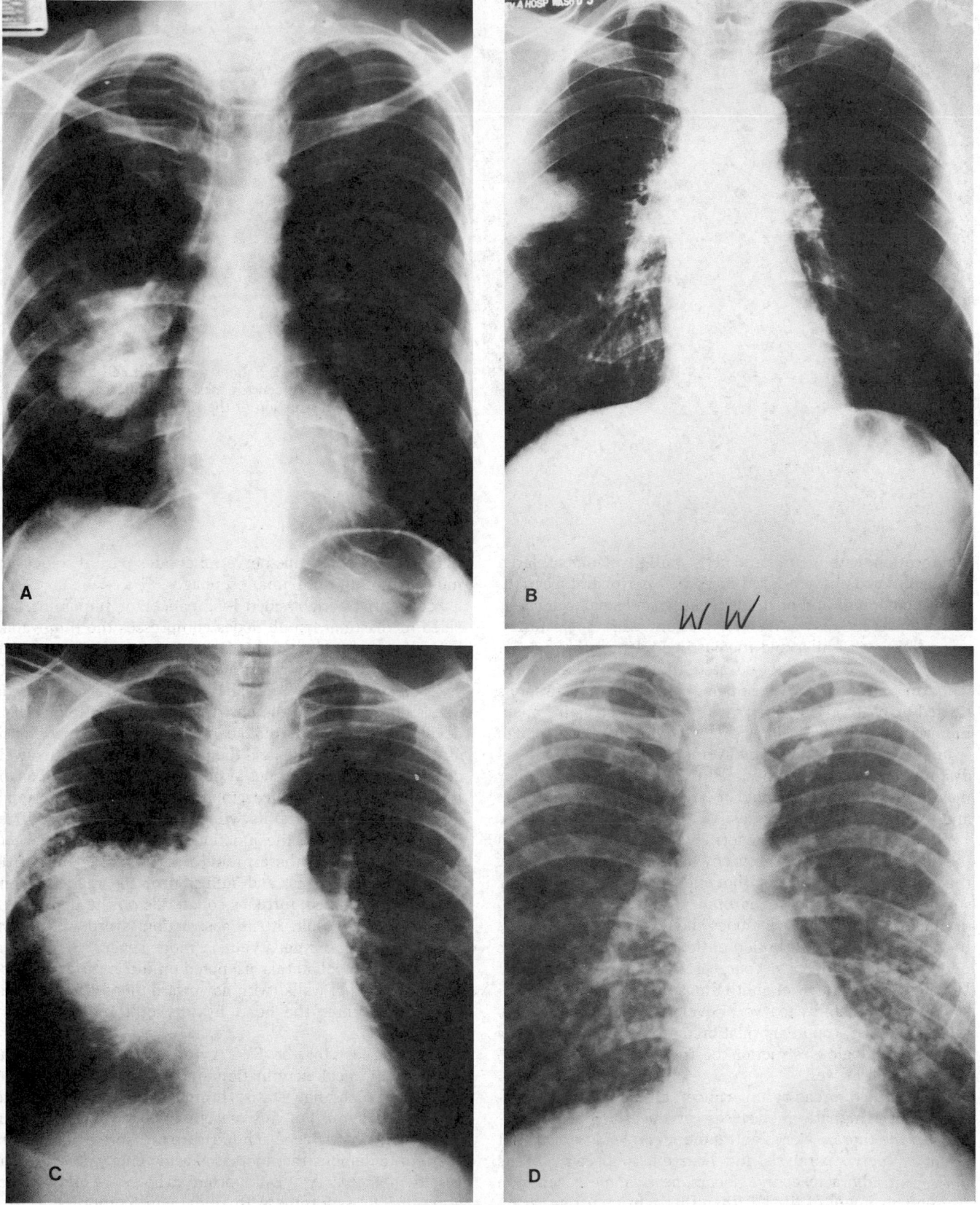

FIG. 22-3. Chest radiographs of patients with different histologic types of lung cancer. **A**. Patient with epidermoid lung cancer in which the tumor mass is centrally located, with beginning pneumonitis from bronchial obstruction, slight volume loss, and central cavitation. **B**. Patient with adenocarcinoma of the lung. The tumor denotes a peripherally located nodule with early pleural thickening suggesting involvement. **C**. Patient with large cell lung cancer containing a large mass with some peripheral pneumonitis. **D**. Patient with bronchioloalveolar carcinoma with multiple bilateral pulmonary nodules present for more than a year. (*Fig. 22-3 continues on p. 610*)

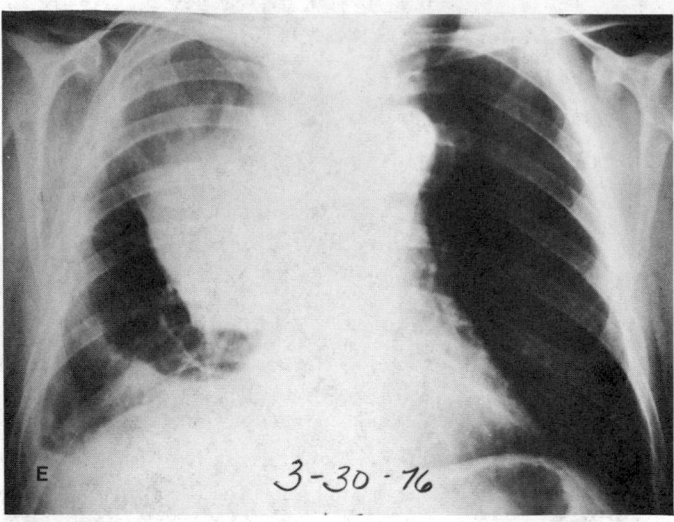

3-30-76

FIG. 22-3. (*continued*) **E** Patient with small cell lung cancer involving a large, bulky central mass with hilar and mediastinal adenopathy and obstruction of the right upper lobe.

eral location, with pleural and chest wall involvement; large cell carcinomas have a large mass in a peripheral location, with pneumonitis and hilar adenopathy; and small cell carcinomas present as a central lesion with atelectasis–pneumonitis and hilar and mediastinal adenopathy.

Symptoms of centrally located tumors include cough, wheezing, stridor, deep chest pain, hemoptysis, and dyspnea caused by obstruction with or without postobstructive pneumonitis. Peripheral lesions present with pain and cough from pleural or chest wall involvement, pleural effusion, and dyspnea on a restrictive basis.[274] Occasionally, large tumor masses, usually of epidermoid or large cell histology, cavitate and present as lung abscesses.

When a tumor (usually epidermoid carcinoma) presents in the apex of the lung and grows by local extension to involve the eighth cervical and first thoracic nerves, the Pancoast or superior sulcus tumor syndrome results.[278-281] The syndrome characteristically includes shoulder pain that radiates in the ulnar nerve distribution of the arm. With sympathetic nerve involvement from paravertebral tumor extension, Horner's syndrome of enophthalmus, ptosis, miosis, and ipsilateral loss of ability to sweat develops. With early involvement, mydriasis (pupillary dilation on the affected side) may result. Radiologic destruction of the first and second rib often is seen as well.

Intrathoracic spread of lung cancer, either by direct extension or by lymphatic metastases, produces regional symptoms in the thorax. Nerve entrapment can lead to recurrent laryngeal nerve paralysis and hoarseness. Because of its longer intrathoracic course, hoarseness is more common from involvement of the left than the right recurrent laryngeal nerve. Involvement of the phrenic nerve can lead to paralysis and elevation of the hemidiaphragm with resulting dyspnea. Compression of the esophagus by the tumor can lead to dysphagia. Also, with recurrent laryngeal nerve paralysis, dysphagia for both solids and liquids (and aspiration)

may result because this nerve innervates part of the cricoid musculature and proximal esophagus.[282]

Frequently, a right-sided lung cancer or tumor in right-sided mediastinal lymph nodes compresses the thin-walled, low-pressure system of the superior vena cava; hence, an obstructive vascular syndrome, *superior vena cava (SVC) syndrome* results.[274,283,284] The type of SVC syndrome depends on the level of the obstruction and the rapidity of its development. In epidermoid carcinoma, the obstruction usually develops gradually, and the patient presents with a well-developed collateral venous system visible on physical examination. With small cell carcinoma, the onset is more rapid, and frequently, collaterals will not have developed. If the obstruction is above the junction of the SVC and azygous veins, distention of the arm and neck veins; edema of the face, neck, and arms; and suffusion of the mucous membranes, with dilated, tortuous collaterals on the upper chest and back, will result. If the obstruction is proximal to the entrance of the azygous vein, a more severe clinical syndrome results: collaterals are noted on the anterior and posterior abdominal walls (with downward blood flow) because blood must enter the heart by way of the inferior vena cava.[284]

The diagnosis of the SVC syndrome usually is obvious from the physical examination and a review of chest films. Because of blood flow stasis, thrombosis occurs as a secondary phenomenon. For this reason, angiographic studies are not useful; although one can measure pressure in an arm and leg vein to demonstrate increased arm venous pressure, this is seldom necessary. It is important to be aware of the association of SVC syndrome with spinal cord compression from tumor extension and possibly vascular congestion.[285] A careful neurologic examination and review of roentgenographic films for bony abnormalities in this area are helpful because myelographic studies can be extremely difficult in these patients. Another association is that of SVC syndrome with tumor extension into the pericardium with resultant tamponade. It probably is useful to perform an echocardiogram in all patients with SVC obstruction as well as in those suspected of having pericardial tamponade. The treatment of SVC obstruction is discussed in Chapter 56, section 1.

Cardiac metastases occur in 15% to 35% of lung cancer patients.[286] Tumor extension into the pericardium and heart can result in pericardial tamponade, arrhythmias, and congestive heart failure. The exact frequency of these symptoms is unknown, largely because cardiac metastases only recently have been sought antemortem. One retrospective review showed that only 4% of patients who were proved pathologically to have cardiac metastases had both absence of clinical signs or symptoms related to the heart and a normal electrocardiogram.[287] Thus, the development of cardiac signs or symptoms in lung cancer patients should prompt consideration of heart involvement by tumor in the differential diagnosis. At autopsy, the pericardium is involved more frequently (88% of heart metastases) than the myocardium (45% of metastases, often by extension) for all cell types.[287] (Diagnosis and management of pericardial tamponade are discussed in Chapter 58). The development of arrhythmias, enlarging cardiac silhouette, increasing venous pressure, or congestive failure all can precede tamponade. The diagnosis is confirmed readily by echocardiography. The absence of the classic signs of tamponade (paradoxical pulse, grossly elevated venous pressure, distant heart sounds, friction rub, Kussmaul's sign, or low voltage on the electrocardiogram) should not stop the physician from obtaining an echocardiogram if there is any clinical reason to suspect cardiac involvement by tumor. The treatment and definitive diagnosis usually are accomplished together in the cardiac catheterization laboratory with pericardiocentesis and decompression followed by cytologic analysis of the pericardial fluid.

Bronchioloalveolar carcinoma can present on chest films as a solitary nodule, multiple nodules, persistent infiltrate, lobar consolidation, or a cavitary lesion.[233] Approximately 60% of cases present as solitary nodules and the remainder as multicentric disease.[225,227,232] However, what appears radiographically to be a single nodule is multifocal disease in 30% of cases. On chest films, 50% of these cancers have a "rabbit ear" or "tail" sign, with one or more fibrotic strands extending from the edge of a nodule toward the pleural surface.[288]

Patients with a persistent, unresolving, soft, fluffy infiltrate on chest films present a diagnostic problem as to whether this is inflammatory or neoplastic disease. Because the fluffy infiltrate represents alveolar involvement, an air bronchogram is seen on the film, and there is no airway obstruction or atelectasis.[233] True cavitation is rare, and what appears as cavities usually is alveolar spaces not involved by tumor.[233] Whereas a true solitary nodule is surgically curable, diffuse multinodular lesions represent an advanced stage of the disease, with survival being less than 1 to 2 years.[224,247]

Although bronchioloalveolar carcinomas can create signs and symptoms similar to those of other types of lung cancer (particularly adenocarcinoma), some findings particularly suggest this cell type. Oxygen transfer across capillary membranes may be impaired by the tumor cells growing along alveolar surfaces; hence, respiratory insufficiency with dyspnea and hypoxemia induces electrolyte disturbances and hypovolemia and predisposes to pneumonia.[233,286] In contrast to adenocarcinoma, pleura and chest wall invasion usually are not seen.[233]

EXTRATHORACIC METASTATIC DISEASE

Autopsy studies have found lung cancer metastases in nearly every organ system (Table 22-19). Again, there are differences in the frequency of metastases to different sites for each of the histologic types. At autopsy, extrathoracic metastases are epidermoid in 25% to 54%, adenocarcinoma in 50% to 82%, large cell carcinoma in 48% to 86%, and small cell carcinoma in 74% to 96%.[208,289] Common clinical problems related to distant metastatic disease are neurologic deficits, bone pain and pathologic fractures, and liver dysfunction and pain. Lymph node metastases usually occur in the supraclavicular region, but occasionally axillary and groin node lesions can be painful and break down and ulcerate if not treated. Except for the relatively small group of patients cured by primary treatment, lung cancer patients often will need therapy to palliate metastatic disease.

PARANEOPLASTIC SYNDROMES

The diagnosis, management, and pathophysiology of paraneoplastic syndromes are discussed in detail in Chapter 55. However, they frequently are encountered in the clinical management of lung cancer patients[290-295] and thus warrant comment here.

Table 22-20 lists the types and approximate frequencies of paraneoplastic syndromes.[296-300] In some cases, the syndrome is associated with a particular histologic type of lung cancer. Reversal of the clinical syndromes associated with successful treatment of the tumor in many cases provides documentation that the tumor caused the syndrome. The peptide hormones produced by lung cancer are the best understood mechanism underlying paraneoplastic syndromes, with classic examples being hyponatremia caused by production of arginine vasopressin and Cushing's syndrome secondary to excessive ACTH, both of which are associated with small cell lung cancer. Hypercalcemia related to the production of parathormone is associated with epidermoid carcinoma. However, some hormones such as GRP, documented in experimental animals to have many effects, as yet do not have a clinically associated syndrome.

Recently, the development of immune responses (best documented by detecting antibodies) in patients with lung cancer against normal tissue antigens that are also present on tumor cells have been described.[301] These include the Lambert–Eaton myasthenic syndrome, retinal blindness, and sensory neuronopathy. In the case of the Lambert–Eaton myasthenic syndrome (LEMS), this appears to be related to an antibody that blocks calcium-dependent voltage channels.[302]

The paraneoplastic syndromes sometimes are the first indication of a tumor's presence. In addition, many of the paraneoplastic syndromes can mimic metastatic disease and,

TABLE 22-19.   Metastatic Patterns Found at Autopsy in Patients with Lung Cancer

Site of Metastasis	Percentage of Patients with Metastasis			
	Epidermoid Carcinoma	Adenocarcinoma	Large Cell Carcinoma	Small Cell Carcinoma
Number of patients studied	126	110	80	102
Hilar, mediastinal lymph nodes	77	80	84	96
Pleura	34	60	67	34
Chest wall	20	20	20	13
Diaphragm	9	11	15	14
Alternate lung	21	60	34	34
Cardiovascular system (total)	21	26	33	21
Pericardium	20	25	25	18
Myocardium	8	11	20	14
Limited to thorax	46	18	14	4
Liver	25	41	48	74
Adrenals	23	50	59	55
Bone	20	36	30	37
Kidney	21	23	28	22
CNS	18	37	25	29
Meninges	0	10	9	3
Dura	0	5	9	1
GI tract	12	5	20	14
Esophagus	13	8	3	14
Pancreas	4	12	22	41
Thyroid	4	2	6	18
Spleen	3	6	13	10
Parathyroid	1	0	0	1
Pituitary	1.6	4.5	3	15
Abdominal lymph nodes	10	24	30	52
Testes	0	0	0	7
Skin	0	0	6	0

Matthews MJ: Problems in morphology and behavior of bronchopulmonary malignant disease. In Israel L. Chahanian P (eds): Lung Cancer: Natural History, Prognosis, and Therapy, pp 23–62. New York, Academic Press, 1976.

unless detected, can lead to inappropriate palliative rather than curative treatment. For example, arterial emboli from *marantic endocarditis* can simulate brain metastases, as can cerebellar or cortical degeneration. *Hypertrophic pulmonary osteoarthropathy* with periostitis, in addition to clubbing, can cause pain, tenderness, and swelling over the affected bones and a positive bone scan, appearing as bone metastases. One of the most distressing syndromes is *weight loss and anorexia*, occurring in nearly one-third of patients and for which no mechanism currently is known. When noncachectic patients with non-small cell lung cancer are studied metabolically, they exhibit increases in protein turnover, glucose production, and muscle catabolism.[303] In addition, severe hypovitaminosis C, with values below the threshold for clinical scurvy, has been found in lung cancer patients.[304] Recent studies have shown that lung cancer patients with mild anemia have lower erythropoietin levels than control patients, supporting the concept of the lack of an appropriate erythropoietin response to anemia in these patients.[305]

OTHER MEDICAL PROBLEMS IN LUNG CANCER PATIENTS

Patients with lung cancer often have other medical problems, most commonly chronic obstructive pulmonary disease related to smoking, chronic bronchitis and emphysema, and cardiac problems related to coronary artery disease and pulmonary

disease. In addition, it is not uncommon to see lung cancer patients in whom the disease is associated with ethanol abuse and related liver damage. All of these and the other medical problems commonly seen in the peak age range of lung cancer (55–65 years) have to be considered when planning and executing treatment. Often, the treatment (surgery, radiotherapy, or chemotherapy) can exacerbate these other medical problems. In addition, although lung cancer can metastasize and cause symptoms in many sites, new symptoms often are related to these nonmalignant medical problems. The challenge to the physician caring for such patients is to sort out these etiologies and institute the proper treatment.

As discussed earlier, multiple cancers frequently are seen in lung cancer patients, complicating treatment planning.[306,307] These cancers can be either synchronous or metachronous with the lung cancer. Common sites of secondary primary tumors include the lung, head and neck, esophagus, bladder, and pancreas (see earlier section for discussion).[306] These secondary neoplasms may have etiologies in common with lung cancer, such as smoking and possibly ethanol abuse.[308] *Because the development of a new primary cancer in a patient previously treated for lung cancer may simulate metastatic disease, it usually is important to document (i.e., biopsy) such a lesion, particularly if the patient could otherwise be cured of the first lung cancer.*

Conversely, a solitary lung shadow may appear either at the same time as or before or after a primary extrathoracic cancer. It should not be assumed automatically that this ab-

TABLE 22-20. Paraneoplastic Syndromes in Lung Cancer and the Histologic Type Predominantly Associated with the Syndrome*

Systemic symptoms
    Anorexia–cachexia (31%)
    Fever (21%)
    Suppressed immunity
Endocrine (12%)
    Ectopic parathyroid hormone: hypercalcemia (epidermoid)
    Inappropriate secretion of antidiuretic hormone: hyponatremia (small cell)
    Ectopic secretion of ACTH: Cushing's syndrome (small cell)
Skeletal
    Clubbing (29%)
    Hypertrophic pulmonary osteoarthropathy: periostitis (1–10%) (adenocarcinoma)
Neurologic–Myopathic (1%)
    Myasthenic syndrome: Eaton–Lambert syndrome (small cell)
    Peripheral neuropathy
    Subacute cerebellar degeneration
    Cortical degeneration
    Polymyositis
    Retinal blindness
Coagulation–Thrombotic (1–4%)
    Migratory thrombophlebitis, Trousseau's syndrome: venous thrombosis
    Nonbacterial thrombotic (marantic) endocarditis: arterial emboli
    Disseminated intravascular coagulation: hemorrhage
Cutaneous (1%)
    Dermatomyositis
    Acanthosis nigricans
Hematologic (8%)
    Anemia
    Granulocytosis
    Leukoerythroblastosis
Renal (<1%)
    Nephrotic syndrome
    Glomerulonephritis

*See Chapter 55 for a detailed discussion.
Odell WD, Wolfsen AR: Humoral syndromes associated with cancer. Ann Rev Med 29:379–406, 1978; Ayvazian LF: Extrapulmonary manifestations of tumors of the lung. Postgrad Med 63:93–99, 1978; Rassam JW, Anderson G: Incidence of paramalignant disorders in bronchogenic carcinoma. Thorax 30:86–90, 1975; Byrd RB, Divertie MB, Spittell JA: Bronchogenic carcinoma and thromboembolic disease JAMA 202:1019–1022, 1967; Greenfield GB, Schorsch HA, Shkolnik A: The various roentgen appearance of pulmonary hypertrophic osteoarthropathy. Am J Roentgenol Rad Ther Nucl Med 101:927–931, 1976; Croft PB, Wilkinson M: Carcinomatous neuromyopathy: its incidence in patients with carcinoma of the lung and breast. Lancet 1:184–188, 1965; Tyler HR: Paraneoplastic syndromes of nerve, muscle and neuromuscular junction. Ann NY Acad Sci 230:348–357, 1974; Heber D, Chlebowski RT, Ishibashi DE, Herrold JN, Block JB: Abnormalities in glucose and protein metabolism in noncachectic lung cancer patients. Cancer Res 42:4815–4819, 1982.

normality resulted from a metastasis from the extrathoracic cancer, because it frequently is a primary lung cancer. Because lung cancer has a worse prognosis than most other primary tumors, it is wise to approach a single pulmonary nodule (particularly in patients over 35 years of age who smoke) as though it were a primary lung cancer. Cahan, at the MSKCC, has studied this problem extensively and collected a large series of patients with multiple primaries, one of which was lung[309] (Table 22-21). Because of these data,

the authors recommend vigorous evaluation for surgical resection of the lung nodule in patients with a single pulmonary nodule in addition to an extrathoracic primary neoplasm. This will establish a firm histologic diagnosis, potentially curing the patients of either the lung cancer or the other neoplasm. For example, after surgical treatment of patients with colon cancer and a single pulmonary nodule, the total 5-year survival rate free of cancer of either type was 22%; the total fraction of patients alive or dead with no evidence of cancer was 31%. Of interest was the fact that all of the primary group who survived later had a third primary tumor.[309]

SCREENING STUDIES FOR THE EARLY DIAGNOSIS OF LUNG CANCER

Although the overall incidence and mortality rates of lung cancer have been rising in parallel, the percentage of localized disease and overall resectability has remained approximately 20% over the past 30 years.[310] Local curative modalities (surgery and radiotherapy) have maintained an overall 5-year survival rate of 8% to 10% during the same period.[311] Staging studies have suggested that in the earlier stage of disease, more patients are likely to be cured of lung cancer, which has led to the hope that screening studies to detect early lung cancer will lead to earlier treatment and increased rates of cure. However, the actual survival benefits must be proved in prospective, controlled clinical trials.[311]

The highest incidence of lung cancer is seen in men over 40 years of age who have smoked 40 or more cigarettes a day for a long period.[308] Several mass roentgenographic screenings of such patients have been done at 4- to 6-month intervals. Early studies suggest that patients discovered by such screening have a 5-year survival rate of 15% to 18%, whereas control unscreened persons developing lung cancer have a 5-year survival rate of less than 10%.[312,313] The Philadelphia Pulmonary Neoplasm Research Project found lung cancer in 1.5% of the high-risk group they screened.[314] However, only 37% of the 94 lung cancers discovered were resectable; the 5-year survival rate for this group was 18% (7% for the entire group of cancers). Chest films and sputum cytology studies complement one another in early lung cancer diagnosis, detecting central tumors while cytologies and radiographs pick up peripheral lesions.[315] Following this lead, Johns Hopkins, the Mayo Foundation, MSKCC, and the University of Cincinnati have undertaken prospective randomized trials using chest films and sputum cytologies when screening men over 45 years of age who smoke one pack or more of cigarettes per day but who initially do not have signs or symptoms of lung cancer.[311,316,317]

The three radomized controlled trials conducted by Johns Hopkins Medical Institutions, the MSKCC, and the Mayo Clinic and sponsored by the NCI involving 31,360 men 45 years or older who smoked at least one pack of cigarettes daily and who were screened for early lung cancer have all shown that intensive screening with sputum cytology and chest films detects early lung cancer. However, this intense screening did not alter the mortality rate from lung cancer compared with standard recommendations for annual testing

TABLE 22-21.   Probable Nature of a Solitary Lung Shadow with Known Cancer Elsewhere, MSKCC 1933–1972

Site of Other Primary Cancer	No. of Cases	Ratio of New Lung Primary: Solitary Metastasis
Head and neck (excluding skin)	168	15.8
Trachea and lung (all types)	51	11.8
Prostate	26	All new lung primaries
Urinary bladder	22	6.3
Stomach	7	All new lung primary
Breast	63	1.7
Colorectal	52	1.4
Kidney	20	1.2
Testicle	18	0.5
Bone sarcoma	23	0.13
Melanoma	36	0.24
Soft tissue sarcoma	37	0.06

Cahan WG: Multiple primary cancers of the lung, esophagus, and other sites. Cancer 40:1954–1960, 1977.

in such patients.[318,319] The Mayo Foundation first screened asymptomatic persons with chest films and sputum cytologies to detect prevalence cases (i.e., cancer already present). They then randomized patients to an intensively screened group (chest film and sputum cytology every 4 months) and "unscreened" persons—those who were advised only to have a yearly chest film and sputum test.[311] The MSKCC group initially screened 10,400 men for signs and symptoms of lung cancer and then randomized patients to annual chest films with sputum cytologies every 4 months or to annual radiographs alone.[316] At the start of the study, the Mayo group found a prevalence of 8.4:1000 persons; MSKCC found a rate of 4 to 7:1000. At the Mayo Foundation, 62% of the prevalence cases were detected by radiographs, 18% by cytology, and 20% by both. For all prevalence cases, the

overall curative resection rate was 57%, and the 5-year survival rate was 40%.[311] At MSKCC in the group screened by radiographs and cytology tests, 60% of the cancers were detected by radiographs, 33% by cytology tests, and 7% by both. The overall curative resection rate was 69%; survival data were not presented.[316]

After the prevalence cases were removed, the Mayo group screening studies identified lung cancer in 1.6% of the persons followed.[311] In the intensively screened group, 72% had lesions detected radiographically, 20% had cytologic detection, and 6% had tumors detected by both procedures (Table 22-22). In the screened group, fewer patients had symptoms at the time of detection than in the control group, and the frequencies of lung cancer cell types were similar in the two groups. More people in the screened group had resectable

TABLE 22-22.   Early Results of the Mayo Foundation Randomized Controlled Trial to Detect Early Lung Cancer*

	Prevalence Cases (n = 87)	Incidence Cases (n = 9223) Screened (n = 87)	Incidence Cases (n = 9223) Control (n = 57)
Cell type (%)			
Epidermoid	47	32	32
Adenocarcinoma	25	21	23
Large cell carcinoma	16	20	12
Small cell carcinoma	11	28	33
Symptoms at detection	?None	11	67
Resectability (%)	57	62	28
AJC postsurgical stage			
Occult	10	Not stated	Not stated
I	39	53	21
II	6	Not stated	Not stated
III	45	37	68
Probability of 5-year survival (rate/1000 persons/year)	40	45	19
Incidences of new cases	Not applicable	4.7	3.0
Deaths from lung cancer		1.8	2.1

Fontana RS: Early diagnosis of lung cancer. Am Rev Respir Dis 116:399–402, 1977; Sanderson D, Fontana R: Results of the Mayo lung project: An interim report. Recent Results Cancer Res 82:179–186, 1982.

*11,001 patients initially screened.

lesions, more had postsurgical Stage I cancer (American Joint Committee system; see below), and there was a greater actuarial 5-year survival rate. Sputum cytology has the added benefit of detecting upper airway (head and neck) cancers. In fact, by early 1978, in the screened group, 18 persons had had an upper airway cancer detected. Of these lesions, 44% were first detected by cytology.[320] Thus, screening a high-risk population with chest films and sputum cytology detects lung cancer at an earlier, more resectable stage than is found in prevalence or control cases. All of the patients detected in these screening studies who were postsurgical Stage I had the excellent 5-year survival expected for Stage I patients (80% plus). However, between 45% and 60% were postsurgical Stage II or III with corresponding inferior survival (5-year rate less than 15%), indicating that even this intensive screening failed to detect lung cancer before it had become incurable by surgery. In addition, all three centers concluded that mortality rates from lung cancer were not significantly different in the screened group than in the control group. Thus, there is no current justification for large-scale application of these screening methods, even in high-risk populations.[321] In considering the individual patient at risk, one approach may be to perform the screening follow-up in heavy smokers who have quit smoking.

BIOCHEMICAL MARKERS FOR EARLY DETECTION

At present, no biochemical markers should be used routinely to screen for lung cancer. However, some plasma or serum markers, such as polypeptide hormones (e.g., ACTH, calcitonin) may be useful clinically. Of 74 patients with lung cancer, 72% had increased ACTH immunoreactivity.[322] In contrast, none of 24 patients with benign chest film abnormalities and 20% of patients with chronic obstructive pulmonary disease (COPD) had elevated levels; 10% of patients with granulomatous lung disease had elevated ACTH levels during an acute exacerbation of their disease, which returned to normal with recovery. Twenty-five percent of COPD patients with elevated ACTH levels and only 2% with normal ACTH levels developed lung cancer within 2 years.[322] Concentrations of the amino terminus of human pro-opiomelanocortin (pro-ACTH) were found to be elevated in 60% of patients with cancer. This immunoassay is simple and does not require plasma extraction before the assay, as does the assay for ACTH.[322]

Recently, a large number of serum markers were studied by radioimmunoassay in patients with localized lung cancer and compared with values from normal controls and patients with benign lung disease.[324] These substances included ferritin, lipid-bound sialic acid, total sialic acid, beta-2-microglobulin, lipotropin, alpha and beta subunits of human chorionic gonadotropin (hCG), calcitonin, parathyroid hormone, and carcinoembryonic antigen (CEA). A series of statistical methods were used to see which could distinguish lung cancer from control patients. Unfortunately, to achieve 95% specificity, the sensitivity rate was less than 40%.[324] It appears that markers with much greater tumor specificity are needed. CEA is not a sensitive indicator in the screening for

lung cancer because 60% of 130 patients who had surgical resection of histologically proved lung cancer had normal levels (i.e., values less than 2.5 ng/ml).[325] However, it may have prognostic value, as a CEA level greater than 15 ng/ml indicated a reduced possibility of a successful resection. In addition, patients who in follow-up appeared to be cured by surgery had significantly fewer elevated CEA measurements postoperatively than did patients who relapsed. Thus, a rising or persistently elevated CEA concentration appears to be a good indicator of relapse or a second primary tumor.[325] An elevated CEA level (720 ng/ml) also appears to be an excellent marker for monitoring the response to chemotherapy and tumor progression for all types of lung cancer.[326]

OCCULT (STAGE 0) LUNG CANCER

Sputum cytology screening has identified patients with cancer who have normal chest radiographs (discussed later as tumor stage Tx). In order for treatment involving surgery or radiotherapy to be instituted, the lesion or lesions must be located. Conversely, lesions detected by chest radiographs are localized, but appropriate treatment requires a histologic diagnosis. Although chemotherapy is the primary treatment for small cell lung cancer, there are as yet no data suggesting that such systematic therapy is appropriate for persons who have only malignant sputum cytology suggestive of small cell cancer but no radiographic or bronchoscopic evidence of the primary tumor and no metastatic lesions visible.

The groups at Johns Hopkins, the Mayo Foundation, and MSKCC have investigated patients with positive sputum cytologies and normal chest radiographs in order to locate their tumors (Table 22-23).[327-329] The method has been pioneered by Marsh at Johns Hopkins.[328,329] Smoking is discontinued before the procedure. In addition, bronchitis is treated, because inflammatory cells can interfere with cytologic interpretation. The patient first has a complete examination of the upper aerodigestive tract, particularly the nasopharynx, the base of the tongue, larynx, and hypopharynx, to detect an asymptomatic tumor by indirect and direct nasopharyngoscopy and laryngoscopy. A detailed fiberoptic bronchoscopic examination lasting up to 2 hours is then performed under general anesthesia with extensive examination of the bronchial tree out to the fifth-generation of bronchi. Suspicious areas, bronchial bifurcations (spurs), and prospective surgical margins are biopsied, and a series of differential brushings is collected. These biopsies are predictive that surgical margins will be clear or involved with in situ cancer.[327]

Additional endobronchial tumor markers are needed for the 10% of tumors that cannot be located bronchoscopically in order to assist in the initial localization and to detect multicentric lesions in patients with a lesion found by radiograph or bronchoscopy. The Johns Hopkins group has used tantalum powder bronchography, an experimental procedure.[327] Tantalum is instilled with a controlled catheter, bronchography is performed followed by a cine examination, and films are taken at 24 and 48 hours to detect delayed clearance of the tantalum. The tantalum bronchogram local-

TABLE 22-23.   Findings and Management of Patients with Positive Sputum Cytology and Radiographically Occult Lung Cancer: Follow-up of ≥3 Years from Johns Hopkins and the Mayo Foundation

Number of patients	62
Age range	30–79 years (all men)
Upper aerodigestive cancer causing positive cytology	11%
In remaining 55 patients	
Fiberoptic bronchoscopic (FOB) localized the lesion	89% (49/55)
Squamous cancer found	98%
FOB gross lesion	48%
Carcinoma in situ found	43% (JH data only)
Multicentric in situ lesions or multiple tumors found	22% (6/27 patients with data)
Of those lesions localized	
Overall patients who had surgery	78% (38/49)
Tumor resected	98%
AJC Stage I	85%
AJC Stage III	15%
Lymph nodes positive	5%
Pneumonectomy required	24% (9/38)
Radiation therapy required instead of surgery for technical or medical reasons	11% (Mayo data only)
No treatment given for medical or technical reasons	13% (Mayo data only)

Baker RR, Ball WC Jr, Carter D et al: Identification and treatment of clinically occult cancer of the lung. Prog Cancer Res Ther 11:243–249, 1979; Sanderson DR, Fontana RS, Woolner LB et al: Bronchoscopic localization of radiographically occult lung cancer. Chest 65:608–612, 1974; Fontana RS: The needle in the haystack editorial. Mayo Clin Proc 53:616–617, 1978; Sanderson DR, Fontana RS: Early lung cancer detection and localization. Ann Otol Rhinol Laryngol 84:583–589, 1975.

ized lesions in more than 90% of cases and thus can direct the fiberoptic bronchoscopic examination.

The Mayo group has pioneered the use of a derivative of hematoporphyrin (an experimental procedure) that involves a photodynamically active dye that concentrates in cancer cells. It then exhibits a salmon-red fluorescence on excitation by ultraviolet (UV) light that is detected photoelectrically with a system that generates an audiosignal for the fiberoptic bronchoscopist.[330,331] Early results show the concentration of dye in areas where no mucosal abnormalities are seen through the fiberoptic bronchoscope, yet, biopsy reveals carcinoma in situ.[332] This method could greatly simplify bronchoscopic location of tumor in patients with occult cancer.

MANAGEMENT AND TREATMENT DECISIONS

Once the radiologically occult lung cancer has been located, treatment decisions can be made. These are complicated because of the multicentric nature of the lesions, the tendency for multiple primary lung cancers to develop, and reports of following patients with in situ lesions for several years without the appearance of invasive cancer.[327–330,333,334] Pathologically, the Johns Hopkins group found in situ carcinomas in only 43% of resected specimens but noted extensive glandular involvement in these cases.[325]

The Johns Hopkins and Mayo experiences in managing patients with radiographically occult lung cancer are similar (see Table 22-23).[327,328,330,333] Of the 55 patients in the combined group, nearly all had squamous carcinoma; 11% of the lesions could not be located. A large fraction had carcinoma in situ (including carcinoma in situ at the bronchial margins)

or multicentric tumors, and new lung primaries already have started to appear in follow-up of resected cases.

Recently, the Mayo group has updated its 10-year experience with occult lung cancer.[335] The cancer eventually was located in all 54 patients studied, but this required three or more bronchoscopies in more than 90% of the patients over intervals of 1 year. Pulmonary resection was performed in all patients, and all tumors were squamous cell. Postsurgical pathologic staging revealed carcinoma in situ in 35% of the cases, Stage I lesions in 56%, Stage II lesions in 7%, and Stage III M0 in 2%. The overall 5-year survival rate was 90%. However, 22% of the patients subsequently developed an additional lung cancer (usually squamous cancer), half of which were again occult. Thus close surveillance is indicated.[336]

Current recommendations are for the most conservative surgical resection permitted to remove the cancer and to conserve lung parenchyma, even if the bronchial margins are positive for carcinoma in situ.[325,328,332,333] Because of the multicentric nature of so many of these tumors, there is a need for a local ablative procedure to deal with the multiple foci. Fontana estimates the projected 5-year survival rate of these patients with occult cancers detected by sputum cytology to be approximately 60% or greater, although follow-up is still short.

ESTABLISHING A TISSUE DIAGNOSIS OF LUNG CANCER

Once the signs and symptoms of lung cancer have developed or an abnormality has been detected on chest film or sputum cytology in a screening study, it is necessary to establish a histologic diagnosis of malignancy, determine the cell type, and stage the disease in order to select appropriate treatment. The procedures used depend on the individual clinical situation. In some cases (*i.e.*, patient with a solitary, asymptomatic pulmonary nodule), the tissue diagnosis will be made at the time of definitive surgical resection, whereas in others, it will be made at the time of bronchial biopsy or biopsy of a metastatic focus. In all cases, it is mandatory that a histologic diagnosis be made and the lung cancer cell type established.

A reasonable approach in the patient suspected of having lung cancer is first to review the patient's history and physical examination, looking specifically for signs or symptoms to direct a search for a tissue diagnosis. This involves careful examination of supraclavicular lymph node areas for palpable masses, the skin for subcutaneous nodules, and the chest for signs and symptoms of endobronchial tumor. If an obvious tumor-bearing lymph node or skin nodule is found, it should be biopsied. If a pleural effusion is present, it should be sampled and cytologic tests performed on a cytocentrifuge-prepared specimen. Also, needle biopsy of the pleura in patients with an effusion is a simple method to obtain a diagnosis and has a moderate positive yield. If the liver is grossly enlarged or if it has nodular lesions on physical examination or radionuclide scan, a biopsy may be done. In unexplained anemia, a bone-marrow biopsy may be performed. Occasionally, lytic or blastic bone lesions on radiograph or localized bone scan abnormalities in sites accessible to needle biopsy by an orthopedic surgeon may be investigated when no other tumor tissue is available. If there are no obvious distant lesions, it is best to proceed to a flexible fiberoptic bronchoscopic study, examining washings, brushing, and biopsies of suspicious lesions.

BRONCHOSCOPIC TECHNIQUES

Flexible Fiberoptic Bronchoscopy

Flexible fiberoptic bronchoscopy has largely replaced rigid bronchoscopy for the evaluation of patients with tracheobronchial disorders.[337-341] A greater area of the tracheobronchial tree can be examined with the fiberoptic instrument, and in several series, 13% to 39% of lesions not seen with the rigid instrument were seen with the fiberoptic one.[342] The efficacy of bronchoscopy in establishing a diagnosis of lung cancer will be influenced by the nature of the cancer itself as well as by the combination of techniques (forceps biopsy, bronchial brushing, washings) used to establish the diagnosis. The false-positive rate of bronchoscopic diagnostic biopsies is very low (0.8%), and most such errors are associated with squamous metaplasia in inflammatory lesions.[338] When a tumor is visible endoscopically, an accurate histologic diagnosis can be made in 71% to 94% of the cases.[338,343] When bronchial brushing and washings are added to forceps biopsy, the diagnostic yield of a centrally located tumor is increased to 94% and that of a peripheral tumor to 86%.[344] For peripheral lesions that cannot be biopsied with forceps, washings and brushing each have a diagnostic rate of about 55%, whereas the yield for central le-

sions from brushing and washing is close to 75%.[345] The estimated probability of obtaining cancer from an endobronchial lesion after one biopsy is 0.89, that after 2 biopsies 0.99, and that after three close to 0.999.[346]

When the lesion is visible endobronchially, forceps biopsy is usually performed. There may be a role, however, for needle biopsy of endobronchial lesions suspected to be excessively vascular or necrotic.[347-349] Submucosal lesions are difficult to biopsy with forceps, and bronchoscopic needle aspiration will increase the diagnostic yield over forceps biopsy alone.[350] By combining forceps with needle aspiration, the submucosal lesion can be diagnosed in 87% of the cases, and when washings and brushings are added, the yield is increased to 97%.[351]

For peripheral lesions not visible endoscopically, the yield of diagnosis for washings, brushings, and biopsy individually are 51%, 52%, and 61%.[352] Transbronchial biopsy and brush combined will have an average yield of 60%.[353-357] The yield of peripheral lesions will vary with the size of the lesion, with the lowest yields seen in tumors less than 2 cm (28%).[340] Bronchiographic mapping has been used with some success to increase the yield of diagnosis with these small lesions.[358]

Peripheral lesions not visible endoscopically merit fluoroscopically guided biopsies, either transbronchial or percutaneous. Brush biopsy under fluoroscopic guidance will produce a diagnosis in 63% to 90% of the cases.[340,344,359] The use of fluoroscopy itself will more than double the diagnostic yield. Transbronchial forceps biopsy of a peripheral lesion under fluoroscopy will be successful in 70% to 75% of the cases,[342,360] although four to six biopsies are necessary to prevent sampling error.[346,355] Recently, transbronchial needle aspiration has been shown to increase the yield of bronchoscopy in the diagnosis of peripheral carcinomas.[361,362] For lesions less than 2 cm, 33% positive biopsies will occur, whereas in lesions greater than 2 cm, the yield increases to 80%.[350] When passage of forceps for transbronchial biopsy is impossible because of extrinsic compression, needle aspiration has been associated with a positive diagnosis in 80% of the cases.[361]

Complications of fiberoptic bronchoscopy and related diagnostic procedures (including pneumothorax, bronchospasm, and hemoptysis) are minimal, with a mortality rate of less than 0.05% and morbidity of less than 0.15%.[363-365] Use of transbronchial biopsy increases the morbidity and mortality rates, with the most common cause of death being cardiac related. Modern-day use of fluoroscopy has decreased the rate of significant pneumothorax to less than 2%. Whereas correction of coagulation disorders prior to bronchoscopy will decrease the chance of bleeding, patients with moderate to severe coagulation disorders are not candidates for endoscopic biopsy. The use of oximetry and supplemental oxygen during the examination has decreased the incidence of hypoxemia and arrhythmia. Washings with large volumes should be avoided, as they have been associated with transient (<24 h) hypoxemia.[366]

Aspiration Biopsy of Mediastinal Lymph Nodes

The use of transcarinal needle biopsy for the evaluation of mediastinal adenopathy has been pioneered by Wang and associates[367] and by Shure.[350] Both flexible plastic and rigid steel needles that can be guided through the biopsy port of the flexible bronchoscope are available. Three aspiration sites are routinely sampled in the carina: anterior, mid portion, and posterior. Peritracheal aspirations are more difficult because of the tracheal rings.[368] In patients with suspicious adenopathy as defined by chest roentgenography or computed tomography (CT), a sensitivity of 50% and a specificity above 90% have been reported.[368] To avoid false-positive biopsies, the mediastinum should be aspirated before examination of the bronchi to prevent contamination of the specimen by bronchial secretions. The highest yield of positive transcarinal biopsies occurs in patients with visible endobronchial tumors or an abnormal-appearing carina, and approximately 15% of patients with lung cancer undergoing routine transcarinal biopsy will have positive aspirates.[369] The complication rate is low (0.3%); the complication is usually pneumomediastinum or pneumothorax.

TRANSTHORACIC PERCUTANEOUS FINE-NEEDLE ASPIRATION BIOPSY (PFNAB)

The ability to locate parenchymal and mediastinal lesions precisely by biplane fluoroscopy or CT has increased the ability to sample abnormalities by percutaneous insertion of a fine-bore needle. The use of PFNAB has been reported to reduce the need for diagnostic and all thoracotomy and to shorten the time from admission to diagnosis as well as the length of hospital stay.[370] Proper use involves coordination of the efforts of the radiologist, pathologist, and primary physician.

A 22-gauge Chiba needle attached to a stopcock and 20-ml syringe is inserted percutaneously into the lung or mediastinal mass with the patient adequately sedated and anesthetized.[371] Most biopsies can be performed with fluoroscopic guidance; CT-guided aspirations are performed in patients having prior unsuccessful fluoroscopic biopsies, for lesions not visible on fluoroscopy, to avoid puncturing necrotic areas of large lesions, or to define the safest route of biopsy in patients with severe pulmonary disease, especially when doing mediastinal biopsies.[371] The PFNAB can also be guided by real-time sonography, especially when lesions are located near the mediastinal, diaphragmatic, or apical lung surfaces. Smears are made for immediate fixation in 95% ethanol and stained by the Papanicolaou method. The remainder of the aspirate is suspended in medium for processing by membrane filters, direct smears, cytocentrifugation, and cell blocks. After rapid Pap staining with a 4% aqueous solution of toluidine blue and examination by the cytopathologist, the radiologist can be notified immediately regarding the diagnostic suitability of the aspirate; if necessary, aspiration can be repeated.

Contraindications to the procedure include unconscious or uncooperative patients, hemorrhagic diathesis, severe respiratory distress, or high fever and uncontrollable cough. Patients with severe emphysema have a higher complication rate. Serious complications include pneumothorax (20%), but only 4% of all patients having PFNAB will require chest tube drainage.[371] Transient hemoptysis (2%–4%) and, rarely, air embolism can occur.[371] Implantation of tumor cells along the needle track has been reported in only two cases,[372,373] and seeding of tumor cells into the blood is similarly rare. Local bleeding around the lesion is seen by chest films in 4% to 11% of patients and usually requires only observation.

Sinner reported on 5300 transthoracic needle biopsies in 2726 patients and Sagel and coworkers reported on 1211 patients.[374,375] Final diagnosis was established in 91% of these patients, with 46% to 71% having cytologic evidence of malignancy (approximately 85% of which were primary lung cancers).[375,376] The false-positive rate was 2.4% and the false-negative rate 23%. One aspiration provided malignant cells in 87% of the patients subsequently proved to have malignant disease; this rose to 96% after two procedures.[375] In a recent series of 1518 PFNAB of the lung from Duke Medical Center, 653 specimens were interpreted as showing a primary malignant neoplasm.[377] Tumor types diagnosed by this method included squamous cell carcinoma in 37.7%, large cell carcinoma 30%, adenocarcinoma 13.2%, small cell carcinoma 11.6%, and adenosquamous carcinoma in 3.5%. No opinion regarding the classification of the malignancy could be reached in 3.8%. Of these 653 patients, 122 had confirmation of the diagnosis by open thoracotomy or biopsy within a week. Nineteen percent of the tissue specimens revealed a cancer that was not detected by PFNAB, and the false-positive rate was 1%. In a similar series of 132 patients whose needle aspiration showed no cancer, 29% ultimately were found to have malignancy.[378]

Agreement between the confirmed histologic diagnosis and the PFNAB diagnosis differs among cell types: squamous cell carcinoma 72%, adenocarcinoma 95%, large cell carcinoma 28%, and small cell carcinoma 98%.[377] In scanty specimens, crushing artifact may sometimes be misread as small cell carcinoma. The low concurrence rate with large cell carcinoma probably reflects the failure of the PFNAB specimen to permit correct recognition of adenomatous differentiation. However, PFNAB, is able to diagnose small cell cancers with high accuracy and should not falsely predict the presence of a carcinoid, atypical carcinoid, or lymphoma. The aspirate is able to confirm the diagnosis of malignancy in 45% of the patients whose preaspirate sputum or bronchoscopic material was suspicious or positive for malignancy, confirming that the diagnostic yield of routine sputa and bronchoscopic evaluations are higher than that of PFNAB, and in most cases the former should be used before resorting to PFNAB.

Although PFNAB is widely used, it does not provide a histologic diagnosis, and it is frequently falsely negative. Thus, the indications need to be carefully defined:

1. Pulmonary masses in the patient unsuitable for curative thoracotomy who needs a definitive tissue diagnosis. These cases would include patients with compromised pulmonary function or a medical contraindication to thoracotomy and those who refuse thoracotomy.
2. Identification of the patient with small cell lung cancer.[276] Although fiberoptic bronchoscopy provides cytologic or biopsy material for definitive diagnosis in a high percentage of proven cases of small cell lung

cancer,[337] recent adjuvant chemotherapy results after resection of small cell carcinoma pulmonary nodules are good enough (discussed later in this chapter) to recommend resection of a single peripheral nodule without mediastinal adenopathy, even if small cell lung cancer is proved.

3. Localized or worsening pneumonic infiltrate in an immunocompromised patient despite standard antibiotic therapy when an etiologic agent is not known.

4. A patient with a history of another malignancy, to allow the differentiation between a new primary, a metastatic lesion, or an inflammatory process.

5. During a thoracotomy, if excisional biopsy is judged to be hazardous or unlikely to yield a definite diagnosis.

6. Other masses identified on chest films or CT scan such as mediastinal masses that need to be evaluated histologically to develop a therapeutic plan.

CORE BIOPSY

Fine-needle or core biopsy with a 20-gauge needle can also be used for the sampling of anterior and central mediastinal lesions, including those in the paratracheal area, to evaluate suspicious lymphadenopathy. The sensitivity of this method in detecting metastatic carcinoma is 71%, and the technique is very accurate (90%) in the diagnosis of small cell carcinoma metastatic to the mediastinal nodes.[371] The subcarinal area, however, remains difficult to biopsy, and this almost always requires CT guidance.

STAGING OF LUNG CANCER

Efficient and appropriate staging can proceed once a tissue diagnosis of lung cancer is obtained. The purpose of staging is to aid in the selection of treatment, estimate the probability of cure and survival, facilitate accurate communication about a patient's status, and compare results from different clinical treatment series. Staging becomes more important with the development of multimodality treatment regimens and in evaluation of experimental clinical trials. For non-small cell lung cancer, only surgery or radiotherapy as single modalities offer the opportunity for long-term survival and cure for a significant number of patients, and selection of patients for a curative attempt by either of these modalities is determined by the anatomic stage of the disease and the technical and physiologic considerations concerning the patient's ability to tolerate the treatment and still be functional. Although there are biological differences between epidermoid carcinoma, adenocarcinoma, and large cell carcinoma, these differences at present probably should not be used in ruling out curative local therapy. However, there are great biologic differences between these non-small cell cancers and small cell carcinoma of the lung. Although anatomic considerations also are important in small cell cancer patients, the total tumor bulk and physiologic ability of the patient to tolerate chemotherapy with or without radiotherapy appear to be more important.

ANATOMICAL STAGING

The two major systems used for the staging of lung cancer have been those proposed by the American Joint Committee on Cancer (AJCC) and the Union Internationale contre Cancer (UICC), both of which use a TNM-based system as originally proposed by Denoix.[379] The TNM system is based on the primary tumor size and extent (*T factor*), regional lymph node involvement (*N factor*), and the presence or absence of distant metastases (*M factor*). Such TNM-based systems can incorporate different types of evidence available for classifying the extent of disease at different sites and at different times in the course of disease and patient evaluation. These types of evidence include (1) *clinical diagnostic staging* (all pretreatment information including that from endoscopy, mediastinoscopy, or other biopsies); (2) *surgical evaluative staging* (findings at exploratory thoracotomy), (3) *postsurgical pathologic staging* (surgical pathology report), (4) *retreatment staging* (staging at relapse), and, finally, (5) *autopsy staging*. Of greatest importance to the patients is the clinical diagnostic staging, which is used to select the mode of primary treatment, and the post-therapy staging, as an early indicator of potential success of therapy and the need for additional treatment.

The AJC system, developed in 1979,[380] was based on the analysis of 2155 cases of lung cancer in the United States and was in use until 1987. Currently, there are discrepancies between the AJC and UICC systems that need reconciliation, including:

1. Patients with N1 positivity (tumor in the peribronchial or the ipsilateral hilar lymph nodes or both including direct extension) and having T1 tumors (less than 3 cm in diameter) were classified as having Stage I disease according to the AJC criteria. This view was challenged by the Japanese Cancer Committee, which noted that the outcome for T1N1 patients was significantly worse than that of T1N0 patients and more closely resembled that of Stage II patients.

2. Subgroups of patients with N2 (mediastinal lymph node positivity) seemed to have different survival patterns.

3. Patients with T3 lesions needed to be reclassified to define those patients who could have complete resection. These patients included those with peripheral tumors invading the chest wall, tumor with direct extension to the mediastinum or pericardium, superior sulcus tumors in patients without a true Pancoast syndrome, and tumor involving the proximal main bronchus and carina that are amenable to sleeve resection.

4. Patients with N3 disease (contralateral and supraclavicular or scalene lymph nodes) needed reclassification with regard to potential radiotherapeutic curability. Nodal positivity at these sites indicated a subset of Stage III disease not amenable to surgical resection. However, tumor involvement of these nodes had been considered "regional disease" by the radiotherapists, and such nodal groups were routinely included in a "curative" radiation field.

5. The need to establish a role in the staging system for cytology-negative pleural effusions.

A new International Staging System (ISS) based on the records of 3753 patients from the M.D. Anderson Hospital and those treated under the auspices of the Lung Cancer Study Group (LCSG) was proposed in 1986[381] (Table 22-24). The ISS classification has been adopted by the LCSG and will, it is hoped, help in the prospective study of survival patterns after treatment with newer multimodality therapies. This system combines the UICC and AJC staging systems into one system consistent with international objectives, and we also recommend its use.

TABLE 22-24.   TNM Definitions

Primary Tumor (T)

TX   Tumor proved by the presence of malignant cells in bronchopulmonary secretions but not visible roentgenographically or bronchoscopically, or any tumor that cannot be assessed as in a retreatment staging

T0   No evidence of primary tumor

TIS   Carcinoma in situ.

T1   A tumor that is 3.0 cm or less in greatest dimension, surrounded by lung or visceral pleura and without evidence of invasion proximal to a lobar bronchus at bronchoscopy*

T2   A tumor more that 3.0 cm in greatest dimension, or a tumor of any size that either invades the visceral pleura or has associated atelectasis or obstructive pneumonitis extending to the hilar region. At bronchoscopy, the proximal extent of demonstrable tumor must be within a lobar bronchus or at least 2.0 cm distal to the carina. Any associated atelectasis or obstructive pneumonitis must involve less than an entire lung

T3   A tumor of any size with direct extension into the chest wall (including superior sulcus tumors), diaphragm, or the mediastinal pleura or pericardium without involving the heart, great vessels, trachea, esophagus, or vertebral body, or a tumor in the main bronchus within 2 cm of the carina without involving the carina

T4   A tumor of any size with invasion of the mediastinum or involving the heart, great vessels, trachea, esophagus, vertebral body, or carina or the presence of malignant pleural effusion.†

Nodal Involvement (N)

N0   No demonstrable metastasis to regional lymph nodes

N1   Metastasis to lymph nodes in the peribronchial or the ipsilateral hilar region, or both, including direct extension

N2   Metastasis to ipsilateral mediastinal lymph nodes and subcarinal lymph nodes

N3   Metastasis to contralateral mediastinal lymph nodes, contralateral hilar lymph nodes, ipsilateral or contralateral scalene or supraclavicular lymph nodes

Distant Metastasis (M)

M0   No (known) distant metastasis

M1   Distant metastasis present—specify sites(s)

Mountain CF: A new international staging system for lung cancer. Chest 89:225s–233s, 1986.

*The uncommon superficial tumor of any size with its invasive component limited to the bronchial wall that may extend proximal to the main bronchus is classified as T1.

†Most pleural effusions associated with lung cancer are secondary to tumor. There are, however, some patients in whom cytopathologic examination of pleural fluid on more than one specimen is negative for tumor and fluid is nonbloody and is not an exudate. In such cases, where these elements and clinical judgment dictate that the effusion is not related to the tumor, the patients should be staged T1, T2, or T3, excluding effusion as a staging element.

NEW TNM DEFINITIONS OF THE 1986 INTERNATIONAL STAGING SYSTEM

T: Primary Tumor

Four specific categories of primary tumors have been classified. The T1 tumor is a parenchymal nodule without invasion of the visceral pleural or proximal to a lobar bronchus. The T2 classification remains the same with the exception that it is now independent of the presence or absence of a pleural effusion. The T3 category is now reserved for operable resectable lesions, in which the areas of invasion to contiguous structures could be encompassed by either standard or tracheobronchial sleeve resection. The T4 category includes a superior sulcus lesion with vertebral body invasion (possibly resectable), lesions that are unresectable secondary to invasion of nonsacrificeable mediastinal contents, and tumors accompanied by a malignant pleural effusion.

N: Regional Lymph Nodes

The N1 category is unchanged from the previous classification. To identify objectively patients with limited mediastinal nodal involvement who could undergo resection, the N2 category has been restricted to ipsilateral mediastinal or subcarinal node involvement. Regional nodal spread outside the confines of the ipsilateral hemithorax (contralateral mediastinal or any supraclavicular scalene or node) is now classified as N3 and is by this definition unresectable.

M: Distant Metastases

Extrathoracic metastases exclusive of cervical regional nodal positivity has been classified as M1.

Stage Grouping

The changes in stage grouping include the reclassification of T1N1 disease as Stage II (Table 22-25) (Fig. 22-4). Stage III disease has been subdivided into Stage IIIa (T3N0N1, or any N2) and Stage IIIb (any N3 or any T4). Thus, Stage IIIa defines subsets of patients who may have a surgical option on

TABLE 22-25.   Stage Grouping of the New International Staging System

Occult carcinoma	TX	N0	M0
Stage 0	TIS	Carcinoma in situ	
Stage I	T1	N0	M0
	T2	N0	M0
Stage II	T1	N1	M0
	T2	N1	M0
Stage IIIa	T3	N0	M0
	T3	N1	M0
	T1–3	N2	M0
Stage IIIb	Any T	N3	M0
	T4	Any N	M0
Stage IV	Any T	Any N	M1

Mountin CF: A new international staging system for lung cancer. Chest 89:225s–233s, 1986.

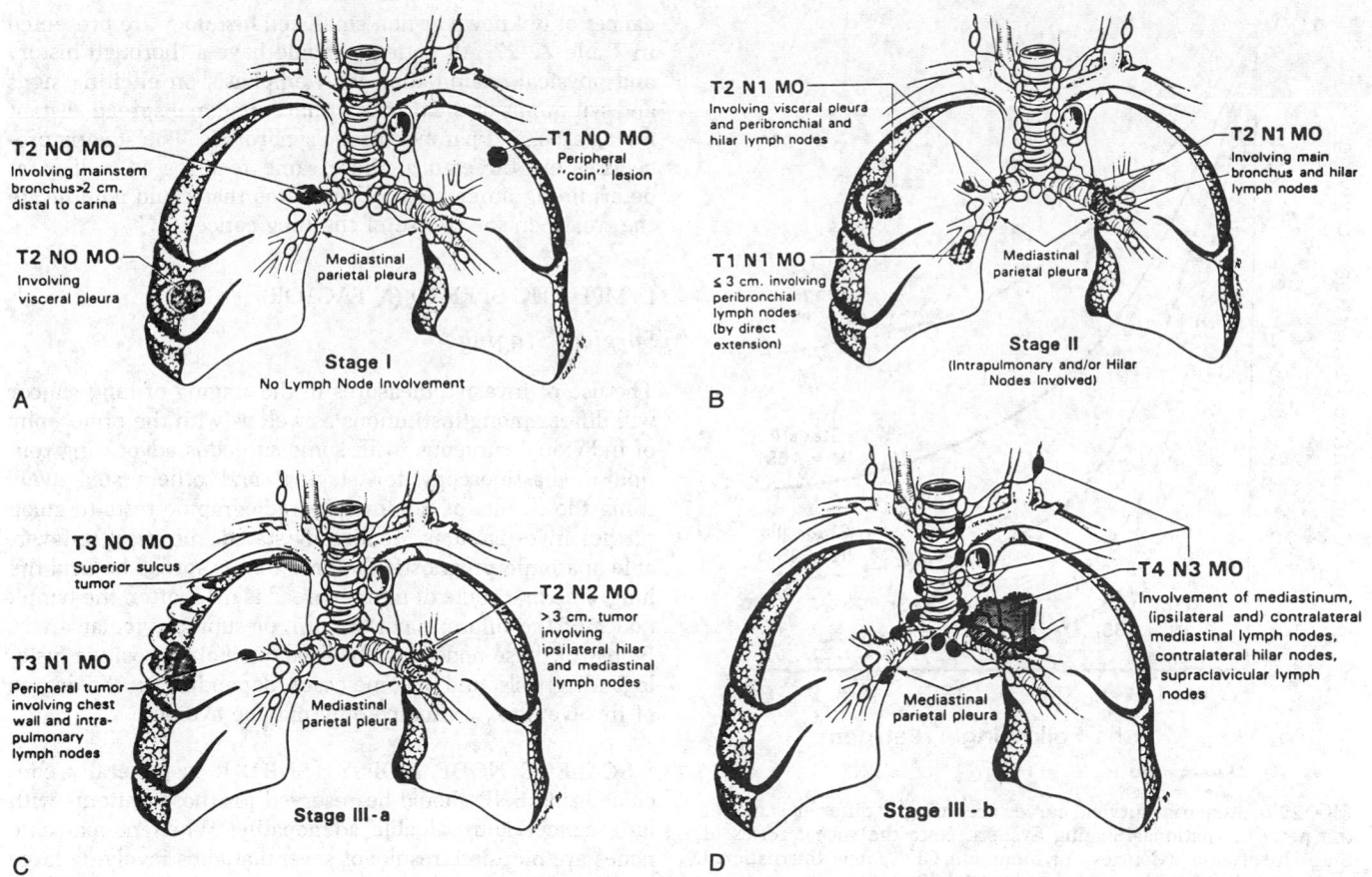

FIG. 22-4. New International Staging System (ISS): **A.** categories of Stage I disease; **B.** categories of Stage II disease; **C.** categories of Stage IIIa disease; **D.** categories of Stage IIIb disease. (Courtesy of Mountain CF: A new international staging system for lung cancer. Chest 89:225S, 1986)

presentation despite mediastinal disease or who may represent the upper limits of resectability for whom preoperative therapy may be indicated. At this time, Stage IIIb patients are considered to have nonresectable disease. The results according to the new staging system demonstrate the significant survival differences in the different stages (Fig. 22-5).

INFLUENCE OF HISTOLOGY AND LYMPHATIC AND BLOOD VESSEL INVASION

For patients with non-small cell cancers who have sufficiently limited disease permitting surgical resection, the overwhelming prognostic factor is whether the cancer has remained localized to the lung or has spread by local extension or metastases to the regional lymph nodes as determined by the postsurgical pathologic review. Histologic subtype has not in the past been of prognostic significance. Recently, however, in a prospective series of 282 patients with non-small cell cancer who were able to undergo a "curative resection," significant differences in survival were noted between those with epidermoid or adenocarcinoma histologies and those with large cell histologies.[382] The absence of lymph node involvement was associated with significantly longer survival, whereas the presence of peribronchial or mediastinal nodal involvement reduced median

survival. Parenchymal lymphatic vessel invasion by itself without lymph node metastases indicated a poor prognosis, whereas blood vessel invasion identified by routine histologic examination did not provide any additional predictive information. When analyzed prospectively, in only patients with T3 lesions had inferior survival after resection when considered independent of lymph node involvement. In patients having a curative resection and in whom microscopic examination revealed no invasion of lymph nodes, lymphatic vessels, or blood vessels, the 3-year survival rate was 61%; with lymphatic vessel invasion and no nodal metastases, 42%; with lymph node invasion alone, 35%; and with both, 34%.

OVERALL APPROACH TO STAGING

By initial clinical diagnostic stage and postsurgical anatomic stage, the chances of a patient being cured by resection can be determined and compared with operative mortality rates and postoperative functional status. However, in practice, most clinicians want to know whether the chance of cure is within the general range of the operative mortality rate. Similar questions should be posed in discussions advocating curative radiotherapy or chemoradiotherapy for small cell lung cancer. The goal, thus, should be to identify that group of patients with non-small cell cancer who most surgeons,

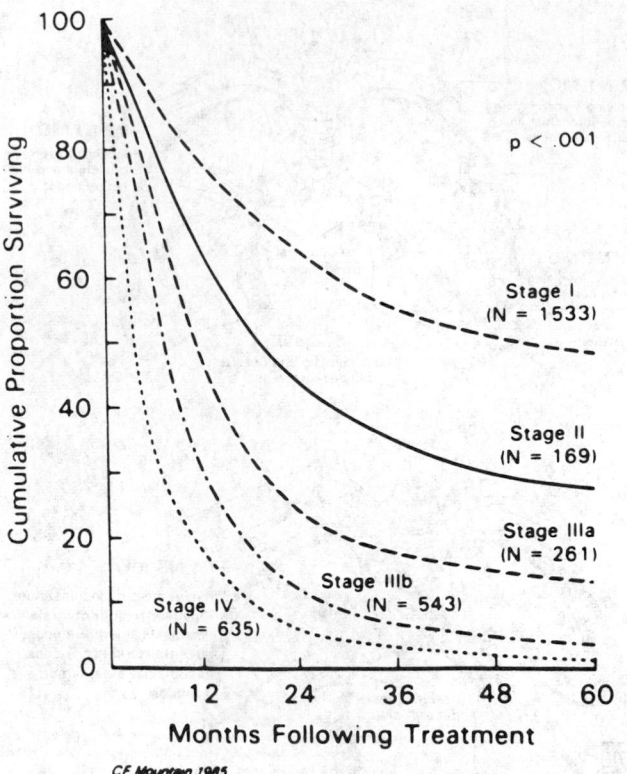

FIG. 22-5. Actuarial survival curves according to different stages of the new International Staging System. Note the subcategories of Stage III disease. (Courtesy of Mountain CF: A new international staging system for lung cancer. Chest 89:225S, 1986)

radiotherapists, and oncologists believe are essentially not curable by surgery or radiotherapy alone and that group with small cell carcinoma who are unlikely to gain long-term survival from intensive chemotherapy. When these patients are identified, the therapeutic approach should be directed at palliation. Because of the greater than 50% long-term survival prospects in patients with Stage I non-small cell cancer, trials of adjuvant therapy must enroll large numbers to detect significant differences. However, the 70% to 90% failure rate for patients with Stage II and Stage III disease means that newer approaches can be tested in fewer patients if cure is the end-point measured.

The first goal of staging is to obtain tumor tissue to confirm the diagnosis of cancer and determine the histologic type, particularly distinguishing non-small cell from small cell cancer. The next goal is to determine if the lesion is surgically resectable or can be encompassed within a tolerable radiotherapy port designed for cure. Obviously, the discovery of extrathoracic metastatic disease removes the curative potential of these local modalities. However, there are features generally agreed to be contraindications to attempts to cure lung cancer with surgery or radiotherapy alone (Table 22-26). Finally, assessment is made of the patients' physiologic status and ability to tolerate the treatment. A sensible plan is to proceed from simple and noninvasive procedures to more complex ones in as economic a fashion as possible.

Pretreatment staging procedures for patients with lung cancer of unknown or non-small cell histology are presented in Table 22-27. All patients should have a thorough history and physical examination with emphasis on eliciting signs and symptoms of the primary tumor, regional spread, distant metastases, and paraneoplastic syndromes. The staging procedures are directed at these same features as well as at determining other medical problems that could complicate the treatment or course of the lung cancer.

LYMPHATIC SPREAD (N FACTOR)

Surgical Staging

The use of invasive measures in the staging of lung cancer will differ among institutions as well as with the philosophy of individual surgeons, with some surgeons advocating routine mediastinoscopy for staging, and others selectively using the results of noninvasive radiographic tests to guide further investigations. As already stated, the most unfavorable anatomic prognostic factor is tumor spread beyond the lung. The first route of tumor spread is most often the lymph nodes of the hilum, mediastinum, or supraclavicular areas. Biopsy of these nodes may be used to obtain a positive histologic diagnosis, and in some cases, depending on the degree of involvement, a thoracotomy may be avoided.

SCALENE NODE BIOPSY (SNB). It is generally concluded that SNB should be reserved for those patients with lung cancer and palpable adenopathy. When nonpalpable nodes are biopsied, results of several studies involving large numbers of patients show positive results in only 4% to 10%.[383,384] Scalene node biopsy is performed under local anesthesia with a 3-cm incision over the lateral edge of the sternocleidomastoid muscle. The fat pad overlying the anterior scalene muscle is located and nodes sampled from this area. A 2% rate of complications is usually reported, including infection, pneumothorax, phrenic nerve injury, recurrent laryngeal nerve damage, and thoracic duct injury.

TABLE 22-26.　Anatomical–Biologic Aspects of Tumor Involvement That Are Major Contraindications to Curative Attempts by Surgery or Radiotherapy Alone with Standard Methods

Extrathoracic distant metastases
Superior vena cava syndrome
Vocal cord paralysis
Malignant pleural effusion
Cardiac tamponade with pericardial involvement
Tumor within 2 cm of the carina*
Metastasis to the contralateral lung
Bilateral endobronchial tumor*
Metastasis to the supraclavicular lymph nodes
Lymph node metastasis in the contralateral mediastinum*
Involvement of mainstem pulmonary artery
Histologic diagnosis of small cell carcinoma†

*Depending on tumor location and physiologic factors, such tumors may be encompassed in a tolerable radiotherapy port and treated for cure.
†When an asymptomatic pulmonary nodule is resected and found to be small cell carcinoma, adjuvant chemotherapy is recommended.

TABLE 22-27. Pretreatment Staging Procedures for Lung Cancer Patients

All Patients

Complete history, physical examination, and evaluation of all medical problems, including determination of performance status and weight loss

Ear, nose, and throat examinations

Chest posterior-anterior and lateral roentgenograms

Complete blood count with platelet determination

Routine blood chemistries, including electrolytes, blood glucose, calcium, phosphorus, and renal and liver function tests

Electrocardiogram (ECG)

Pulmonary function studies and arterial blood-gas measurements if any signs or symptoms of minimal respiratory insufficiency are present

Skin tests for tuberculosis

CT or radionuclide scans of brain, liver, or bone if any of the above studies suggest presence of tumor in these organs; radiographs of any bony lesions suspicious by scan or symptom

Barium swallow radiographic examination if esophageal symptoms are present, followed by esophagoscopy if abnormalities are found

Biopsy of any accessible lesions suspicious for cancer if a histologic diagnosis is not yet made or if treatment or staging decisions would be based on whether or not the lesion contained cancer

Routine medical evaluation of any abnormalities detected in the first part of the screen not related to cancer

Patients Presenting with a Solitary Pulmonary Nodule

All of the above plus

Fiberoptic bronchoscopy with washings, brushings, and biopsy of suspicious areas

Pulmonary function tests, arterial blood-gas measurements

Coagulation tests

Transthoracic fine-needle aspiration biopsy or transbronchial forceps biopsy of peripheral lesions if material from routine fiberoptic bronchoscopy gives negative results and the patient is poor surgical candidate

Patients with a Mass Lesion in the Chest and No Obvious Contraindication to a Curative Local Approach (Surgery or Radiotherapy)

All of the above plus

CT or radionuclide scans of brain, liver, and bone if signs, symptoms, or laboratory abnormalities are detected in these systems

CT scans of areas where regular radionuclide scans are nondiagnostic

Mediastinoscopy or lateral mediastinotomy in individual patients (see text for discussion)

Patients with Disease Confined to the Chest but Not Resectable (Candidate for Curative Radiotherapy)

All of the above except mediastinoscopy plus

Transthoracic fine-needle aspiration biopsy or transbronchial forceps biopsy of peripheral lesion if material from routine fiberoptic bronchoscopy gives negative results

*Patients with Disease Not Curable by Either Surgery or Radiotherapy, Alone or Together**

All under first entry plus

Biopsy of accessible lesions suspicious for tumor to obtain histologic diagnosis or if therapy would be altered by findings of tumor

Fiberoptic bronchoscopy if indicated by hemoptysis, obstruction, pneumonitis, or no histologic diagnosis of cancer

Tap and cytologic examination of pleural effusion

Transthoracic fine-needle aspiration biopsy or transbronchial forceps biopsy of peripheral lesions if material from routine fiberoptic bronchoscopy gives negative results and no other material exists for a histologic diagnosis

---

*Extrathoracic metastatic disease or malignant pleural effusion.

MEDIASTINOSCOPY. Maasen and Greschuchner in 1975 reviewed the results of 1487 mediastinoscopies performed on patients with suspected or proved carcinoma of the lung and found that 36% of the nodes contained metastatic tumor, with central tumors having a higher rate of positivity than peripheral tumors (42% and 30%, respectively).[385] The pattern of mediastinal spread of tumor is not uniformly predictable, however, and thus one must sample the various nodal groups at the time of surgery.

Two recent series are representative of the results of mediastinoscopy in large numbers of patients at institutions where mediastinoscopic evaluation of lung cancer patients prior to surgery is routine.[386,387] Of 2259 mediastinoscopies, 624 (28%) found tumor in lymph nodes. With regard to primary cell type, 22% of the patients with squamous cell carcinomas had positive nodes, whereas 30% of those with large cell and adenocarcinomas had positive lymph node. Of 1510 patients who had negative mediastinoscopic findings, only 151 (10%) were found to have nodal tumor at thoracotomy. In fact, 88% of the patients with negative mediastinoscopic results were able to undergo "curative" resection. Complication rates of mediastinoscopy were lower than in earlier reports (hemorrhage 0.13%, pneumothorax 0.6%, recurrent nerve injury 0.3%, and tracheobronchial injury 0.09%). Both series also analyzed results of the subgroup of patients with metastatic cancer confined to ipsilateral nodes and discovered only by microscopic examination ("intranodal" disease). Only 98 (15%) of the 635 patients with nodal positivity qualified for this subanalysis, of which 81 (83%) had resectable disease with an estimated 5-year survival rate of 18%.

TECHNIQUE OF CERVICAL MEDIASTINOSCOPY. Cervical mediastinoscopy is usually performed under general anesthesia. After making a 2- to 4-cm incision in the suprasternal notch, dissection is continued in the pretracheal plane until the area of the carina is reached (Fig. 22-6). The mediastinoscope is then inserted and the lymph nodes sam-

FIG. 22-6. Transverse view of structures encountered during mediastinoscopy. Note the limited visualization of the left owing to the presence of the aortic arch.

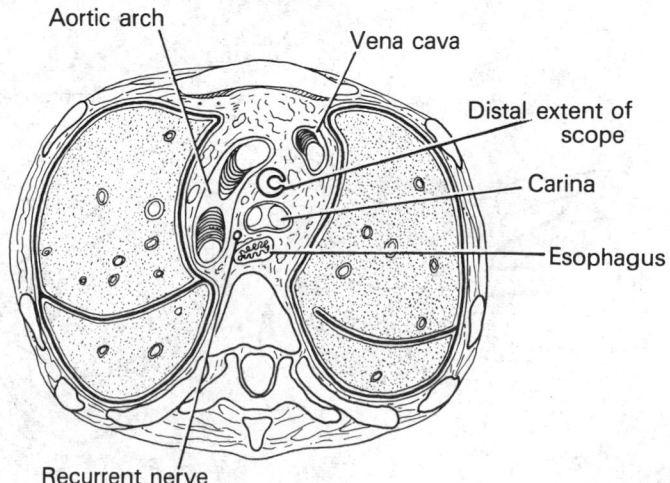

pled after aspiration to distinguish vascular from lymphatic structures.

The complication rate of standard mediastinoscopy is low, with a morbidity rate of 1.6% and a mortality rate of 0.08%.[388] The principal avoidable complication is hemorrhage from inadvertent biopsy of the right pulmonary artery, azygous vein, or aorta, all of which necessitate emergency thoracotomy. Other complications include vocal cord paralysis, esophageal perforation, mediastinitis, bradycardia, tumor seeding, myocardial infarction, stroke, and air embolism. Although SVC obstruction is a relative contraindication to mediastinoscopy, the procedure can be performed in such circumstances without death if there is a pressing clinical need to make a tissue diagnosis. The safety of repeat mediastinoscopy has also been detailed in two series of patients.[389-391]

ANTERIOR PARASTERNAL MEDIASTINOTOMY (CHAMBERLAIN PROCEDURE). Parasternal mediastinotomy is often performed instead of cervical mediastinoscopy when evaluating the left side of the mediastinum, because the subaortic and anterior hilar nodes cannot be evaluated by the suprasternal approach. However, anterior mediastinotomy also can be performed on the right. Other nodal groups inaccessible by cervical mediastinoscopy include those of the anterior mediastinum, subaortic area, and posterior subcarinal region.

A 6-cm incision is made over the second or third intercostal cartilages in a vertical fashion; alternatively, a horizontal incision in the interspace can be performed, obviating cartilage removal. Posterior dissection is carried past the internal mammary vessels, and the pleura can either be retracted or entered directly (Fig. 22-7). The mediastinum in the area of the aorticopulmonary window is thus accessible for biopsy of anterior and left-sided lesions, evaluation of extension of tumor, and biopsy of the aorticopulmonary nodes. Hiloscopy, as described in 1979 by Paris, adds direct mediastinoscopic evaluation of the hilum.[392] Greater access for evaluation of aortic or diaphramatic invasion, pleural metastases, and direct biopsy of the hilar, subaortic, or periaortic nodes is afforded by this technique. The procedure can be performed under the same anesthesia with standard mediastinoscopy.

Mediastinotomy, with or without hiloscopy, is associated with low morbidity and mortality rates.[393]

Roentgenographic Evaluation of the Mediastinum

COMPUTED TOMOGRAPHY. Since the late 1970s, there has been enthusiasm for the use of CT scanning in the preoperative staging of lung cancer patients, particularly to interpret the mediastinal shadows seen on chest roentgenography with regard to nodal positivity. The original hope for the CT scan was that it would be able to predict noninvasively which patients had obvious mediastinal invasion or nodal involvement, rendering operative or other invasive staging unnecessary if its specificity and sensitivity was consistently high. In addition, the cross-sectional imaging, free from overlying shadows, made the mediastinal soft-tissue structures recognizable in their full transverse extent (Fig. 22-8). With the use of intravenous contrast medium, accurate differentiation between malignant deposits, fatty tissue, and vascular structures theoretically could be achieved. Various anatomic structures, specifically bronchial anatomy and lymph nodes, would be mapped, not only for staging purposes, but also to aid the surgeon in subsequent dissection.

In actual practice, there has been a learning process of the limitations of CT in the staging of the mediastinum. Misinterpretations can occur secondary to excessive slice intervals, poor contrast enhancement of vascular structures, and misreading.[394] Direct extension of tumor into the mediastinum is often convincingly demonstrated by CT, yet pitfalls exist, as simple abutment of tumor against mediastinal structures cannot be scored as invasion with great confidence. Circumferential narrowing of bronchovascular structures associated with a mass or the interdigitating of tumor mass with mediastinal fat is confidently recognized as tumor invasion, however.

When trying to evaluate nodal pathology by CT scans, one must measure the relative sizes of the nodes in order to classify them as abnormal. Mediastinal nodes greater than 1.5 cm in diameter in patients with bronchogenic carcinoma will harbor tumor in 94% to 97% of the cases, whereas lymph nodes ranging from 1 to 1.5 cm in diameter are involved with tumor in 50% of the cases and those less than

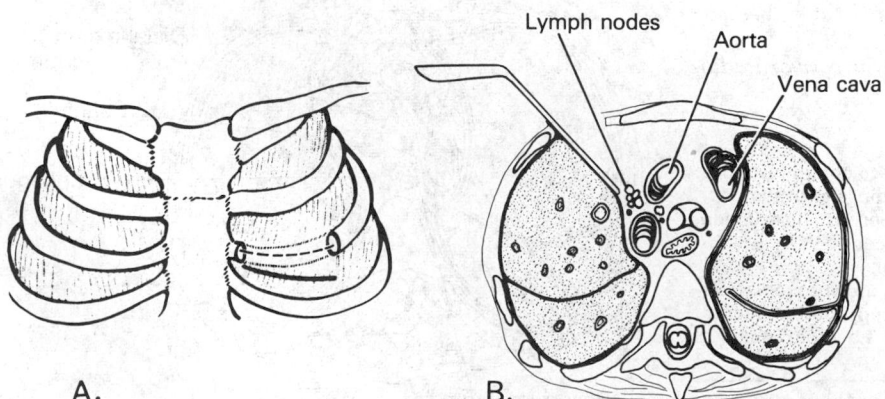

Lymph nodes   Aorta   Vena cava

A.   B.

FIG. 22-7. Parasternal mediastinotomy (Chamberlain procedure). **A.** Transverse incision in second and third intercostal space. A vertical incision can also be used. **B.** Depiction of transverse anatomy encountered for access to anterior mediastinal nodes on the left (see text for description).

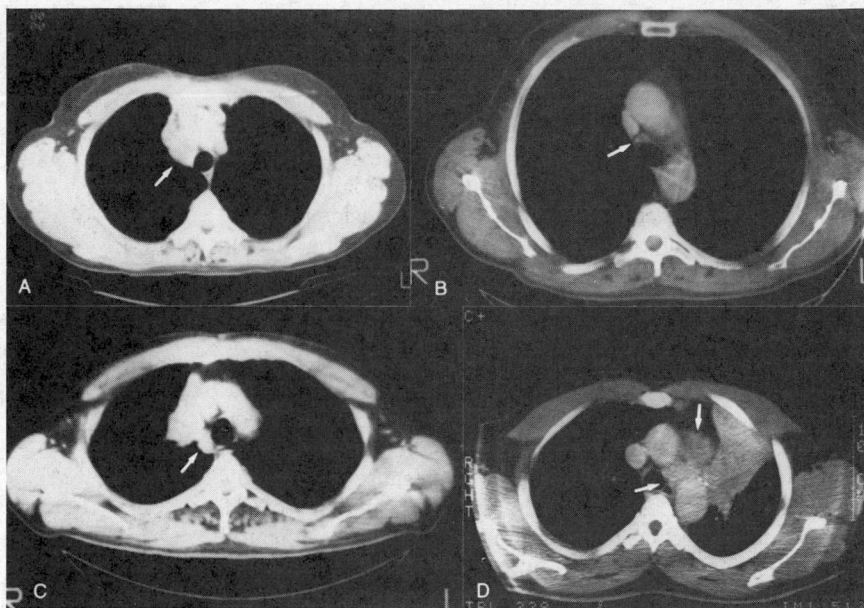

FIG. 22-8. Nodal basins in lung cancer (*arrows*) as visualized on computed tomography. **A**. High bulky tracheal nodes. **B**. Subtle 1.5-cm anterior tracheal node behind the vena cava. **C**. Posterior paratracheal node. **D**. Left-sided anterior mediastinal nodes and aorticopulmonary nodes with left upper lobe atelectasis.

1 cm are usually uninvolved.[395-397] Genereux and Howie found that 99% of normal nodes imaged by CT were less than 16 mm in diameter and 90% of the nodes in the precarinal and subcarinal area were in the 6- to 10-mm range.[398] Normal nodal size is influenced by location, with the largest nodes in the paratracheal regions and smaller nodes in the subcarinal and paraesophageal areas.[398] Nonpathologic lymph nodes in the region of the azygous vein commonly measure up to 1 cm.[397,399] Moreover, the size of the node will depend on the axis through which the node is imaged. Also, reactive nodes secondary to chronic infection accompanying atelectasis are larger than the upper limits of normal.

Usefulness of CT Scans in the Staging of Lung Cancer: Results of Various Series. There have been many conflicting reports regarding the efficacy of CT scans for preoperative staging of bronchogenic carcinoma. Table 22-28 summarizes the results in 1758 patients reported since 1978 correlating CT scan interpretation with histologic confirmation of nodal involvement. Nodes less than 1 cm in diameter have a low probability for tumor involvement, nodes 1 to 1.5 cm have an intermediate probability of tumor involvement, and those greater than 1.5 cm have a high probability of tumor involvement. Overall, those studies that use 1 cm as the upper limit of normal size have high sensitivity but low spec-

TABLE 22-28. Accuracy of CT Scans in Staging Lung Cancer 1978-1987[396,400-423]

Number of patients	1758
Overall sensitivity	73%
Overall specificity	80%
Accuracy	77%
Positive predictive index	72%
Negative predictive index	83%

ificity, whereas the sensitivity is low and specificity high when nodes up to 2 cm are considered normal. The greatest accuracy with the highest specificity was seen with a cut-off size of 1.5 cm, with the positive predictive index, or chance of a CT-called positive being correct, and the negative predictive index reaching 82% and 92%, respectively (Table 22-29).

Implications of CT for Selective Surgical Mediastinal Staging. The present CT studies indicate that patients with intermediate- or high-probability nodal sizes should have operative staging of the mediastinum by transcarinal needle biopsy, mediastinoscopy, or mediastinotomy. In patients with peripheral lesions and a normal-appearing mediastinum on chest roentgenography and CT, the possibility of

TABLE 22-29. Accuracy of CT Scans: Influence of Node Size*

Size (cm)	Sensitivity (%)	Specificity (%)	Accuracy (%)	Prediction Index (%)	
				Positive	Negative
<1	94	70	80	70	94
1.0	78	78	78	67	87
1.5	71	93	85	82	92
2.0	41	95	77	81	76

*Data derived from studies listed in Table 22-28 in which node size was specified.

performing a "curative" resection approaches 100%, obviating invasive preresection mediastinal staging. When an abnormal hilum or mediastinum is seen on routine chest radiography, CT can be used to identify patients with abnormally large nodes for selective mediastinal staging prior to resection, with 80% demonstrating nodal metastases histologically. Patients with obvious bulky bilateral nodal disease in the presence of a documented endobronchial lesion probably can proceed to radiotherapy without further staging studies.

Other Roentgenographic Techniques

[67]GALLIUM SCANNING. Gallium-67 accumulates nonspecifically in lung lesions ranging from neoplasm to inflammation, and the detection of metastases in the hilum and mediastinum with gallium scanning has been investigated extensively with variable results.[424,425] Because of gallium's lack of sensitivity, as well as the greater availability of CT and the decreased cost effectiveness of gallium compared with other techniques, the enthusiasm for using gallium scanning to direct the management of patients with lung carcinoma has subsided. This view is reinforced by the lack of agreement regarding the implications that gallium scanning results have for mediastinoscopy among enthusiasts for the technique.

MAGNETIC RESONANCE IMAGING (MRI). A number of reports have compared MRI with CT (Fig. 22-9) in the staging of lung cancer, and the consensus is that MRI scans have been disappointing. Glazer and associates, comparing CT and MRI for the imaging of the hilum in 35 patients, found that MRI could not distinguish between benign and malignant enlarged nodes.[426] Webb and Levitt and their associates, in similar series of 33 and 37 patients, respectively, could distinguish lymph nodes from surrounding mediastinal tissues, but the imaging sequences could not distinguish lymph nodes that were involved by tumor from those that were uninvolved.[427,428] Similar information regarding the presence and size of lymph nodes was seen with CT or MRI. MRI was superior to CT, however, in distinguishing hilar structures, and in these series, collapsed peripheral lung gave a different image than the offending tumor. Webb and coworkers thought that MRI was qualitatively superior to CT in demonstrating mediastinal invasion. In a prospective study of 34 patients from MSKCC, equal sensitivity (61% and 65%) was seen in the imaging of lymph node metastases by CT and MRI, with equally low specificity (42%).[429] Neither method could distinguish contact from invasion by tumor. Poon and coworkers, in a series of 48 patients, confirmed that MRI was not superior to CT for lymph node staging.[430]

In summary, it is generally thought that further developments to improve tissue characterization will be necessary before MRI can supplant the CT scan in the mediastinal evaluation of bronchogenic carcinoma.

PULMONARY ANGIOGRAPHY. Pulmonary angiography may be able to assess pulmonary artery, pericardial, and arterial involvement in some patients.[431] However, a significant portion of patients with abnormal angiograms have re-

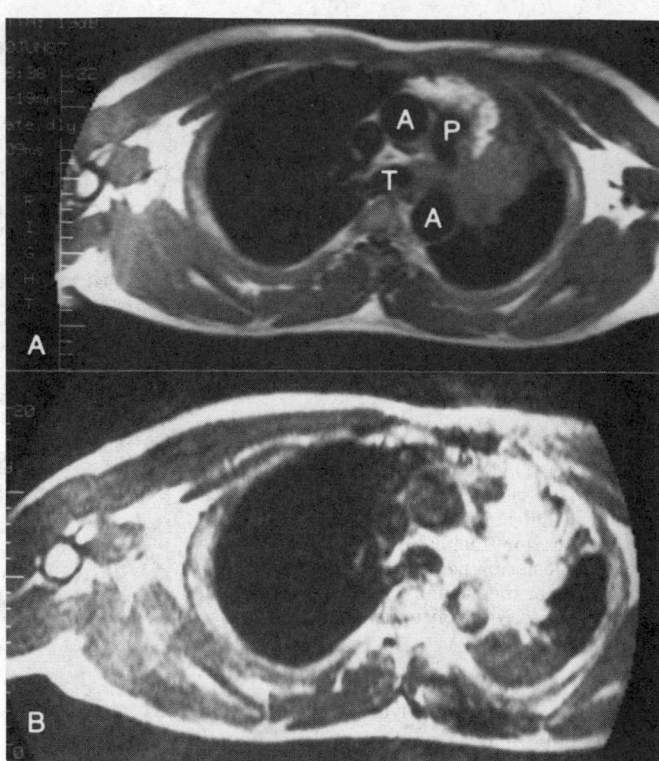

FIG. 22-9. Magnetic resonance image of patient whose CT scan is shown in Figure 22-8D. Image **A** is to be contrasted with Image **B**, which is an inversion recovery sequence that highlights the extent of tumor and the lymph nodes involved (shown in white). A = aorta; P = pulmonary artery; T = trachea.

sectable tumors, and thus an angiogram must always be used in conjunction with mediastinoscopy and CT scanning to make preoperative decisions regarding resectability.

Other Indirect Tests of Mediastinal and Hilar Nodal Involvement

The findings on mediastinal tomograms, esophagrams, azygograms, and perfusion lung scans correlate poorly with mediastinoscopy results, with false-positive and false-negative rates of 30% to 50%.[432-435] B-mode gray-scale sonography is useful in determining whether a large area of radiographic opacification is caused by fluid, tumor, or intrinsic pulmonary disease such as obstruction or consolidation.[436]

Monoclonal Antibody Imaging

Clinical studies of radiolabeled monoclonal antibodies recognizing specific determinants on cancer cells are just beginning in lung cancer (Figs. 22-10 and 22-11). So far, there have been relatively few antibodies shown to localize in lung tumors. Polyclonal anti-CEA antibodies[437] have been studied with mixed successes, as have polyclonal antibodies raised against alpha-fetoprotein.[438] Perkins and coworkers, using antibody 791T/36 labeled with ^{131}I reported imaging of three of eight primary lung tumors after blood pool subtraction and higher success rates (69%) when the antibody was linked

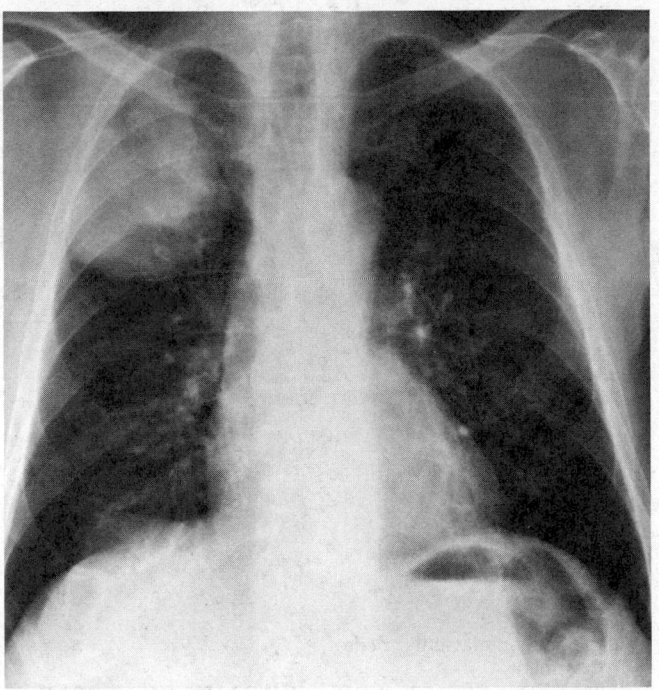

FIG. 22-10. Chest radiograph of a patient with a large right upper lobe mass invading the chest wall. This patient would require chest wall resection and en bloc lobectomy.

with indium-111.[439] Chan and associates, using radiolabeled antibodies directed against a c-*myc* oncogene product, had tumor localization in 12 of 14 patients with lung cancer, but success was dependent on the size of the tumor.[440]

FIG. 22-11. Monoclonal antibody scan performed on patient whose x-ray film is shown in Figure 22-10. Triangular arrows depict posterior and anterior views of the chest wall mass. Some cardiac blood pool is visualized, as is the thyroid.

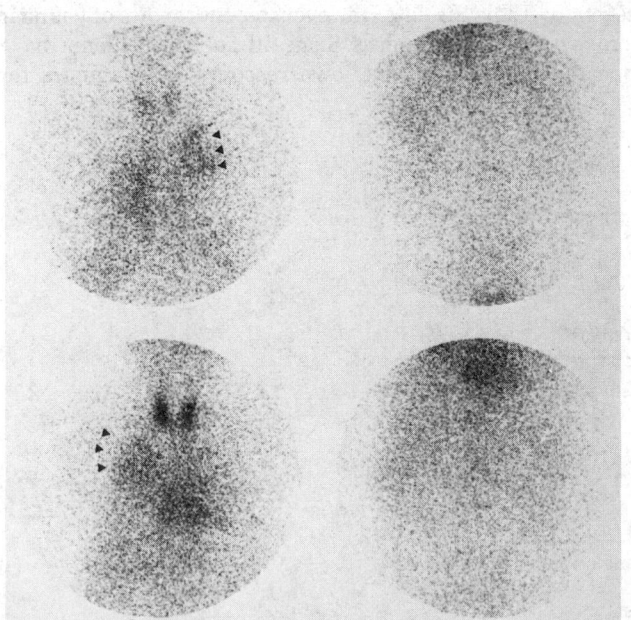

STAGING PROCEDURES FOR DISTANT METASTASES (M FACTOR)

The best screen for extrathoracic spread is a careful history and physical examination along with laboratory data including serum calcium, bilirubin, transaminases, lactate dehydrogenase (LDH), and alkaline phosphatase determination. The liver, bones, central nervous system, adrenal glands, and lymph nodes frequently harbor metastatic disease, yet the routine use of bone, brain, liver, and spleen scans is controversial.[441-447] Positive bone scans or liver scans may in fact represent areas of old inflammation or fracture and thus delay treatment unnecessarily. Moreover, in the absence of symptoms and signs, these tests will be positive in only 5% to 10% of patients. Thus, current recommendations by the authors are to perform brain, liver, and bone scans or skeletal surveys only if there is other clinical evidence that suggests the possibility of metastases. Biopsy of the bone marrow and liver in patients with non-small cell carcinomas and no other clinical evidence of metastases is positive in 10% to 15% or less of cases.[448-450] Therefore, we do not recommend routine biopsy of these sites unless some other clinical evidence suggests the possibility of metastases.

Whereas staging CT scans are vital in the conduct of clinical trials investigating new therapies, their cost effectiveness is low in the management of asymptomatic patients. Nevertheless, it would appear prudent to use head and upper-abdominal CT scans in all candidates for a curative approach with surgery or radiotherapy, as the finding of definitive evidence of brain or abdominal metastases would clearly alter the primary treatment plan. In a recent series of 63 patients screened with EEG, neurologic examination, and brain CT who were asymptomatic from a neurologic standpoint, five had silent brain metastases.[451] More routine use of upper-abdominal CT scanning at the time of chest CT has been advocated to evaluate the liver and adrenal glands. For example, 5 of 38 patients were found to have occult adrenal metastases in a recent series.[452]

PHYSIOLOGIC STAGING OF THE PATIENT

Assessment of the patient's physiologic and performance status is critical in order to determine his or her ability to tolerate thoracotomy and pulmonary resection, aggressive radiotherapy, or intensive chemotherapy. Patients with lung cancer often have cardiopulmonary problems related to chronic pulmonary disease or their age, and many studies have been performed to assess patients' ability to tolerate general anesthesia and pulmonary surgery, including whether pneumonectomy or lobectomy can be undertaken. The essence of preoperative physiologic evaluation is to determine which patients can undergo surgery with a reasonable operative mortality rate and still be functional. It is not always possible to predict whether a lobectomy or a pneumonectomy will be required until the time of surgery; thus, preoperative estimation of tolerance should always consider the possibility of pneumonectomy.

PERFORMANCE STATUS, AGE, AND SEX

Performance status (PS) is an important prognostic factor. Patients who are fully ambulatory and either asymptomatic (PS 0) or symptomatic (PS 1) tolerate surgery or aggressive chemoradiotherapy better than do those who are not fully ambulatory but are out of bed more than 50% of the time (PS 2). These patients, in turn, do better than those who are ambulatory less than 50% of the time (PS 3) and those who are bedridden (PS 4). When other medical problems are identified and corrected (including nutritional deficits, anemia, electrolyte disorders, dehydration, and infection), the performance status may improve and thus also improve prognosis and operability.[453-456]

The combination of a serious reduction in the patient's pulmonary reserve and significant cardiovascular, hepatic, or renal disease or poor performance status is a contraindication to resectional pulmonary surgery.[453,454] Stanley analyzed 77 prognostic factors in more than 5000 patients with lung cancer entered in Veterans Administration Lung Group (VALG) protocols between 1968 and 1978.[456] The most important prognostic factors, in order of importance, were initial performance status, extent of disease, weight loss greater than 10 pounds in the previous 6 months, and the presence of any systemic symptoms (Tables 22-30 and 22-31). In a similar study performed by Finkelstein and associates, looking at those pretreatment predictors of survival in 893 patients on Eastern Cooperative Oncology Group (ECOG) protocols, initial performance status, the absence of metastatic disease, female sex, and absence of weight loss in the previous 6 months all correlated with survival greater than 1 year.[457] The contributions of other factors such as tumor size and histologic type were minor after correction for the major prognostic features, particularly performance status. Interestingly, age does not seem to have a prognostic impact.[456,458] Although the operative mortality rate in general is greater for older patients, the rate in selected patients over 70 years old is no greater than the expected mortality rate for younger patients.[459] Thus, it is important to assess the patient's physiologic rather than chronologic age when making decisions about patients who are on the borderline of operability.

TABLE 22-31. Influence of Various Pretreatment Variables on the Survival of Patients with Inoperable Lung Cancer*

Variable	Median Survival (wk)	% of Patients with Variable
Stage of disease†		
Limited	28	21
Extensive	13	79
Weight loss (lb)		
Less than 10	22	52
More than 10	11	48
Presence of systemic symptoms		
No	28	49
Yes	15	51
Reduced appetite		
No	27	53
Yes	15	47
Initial lymphocyte count/ml		
>2000	16	42
<1000	8	19
Any metastatic disease symptoms		
No	22	64
Yes	15	36
Scalene or supraclavicular node involvement		
No	22	83
Yes	14	17

*Stanley KE: Prognostic factors for survival in patients with inoperable lung cancer. JNCI 65:25–32, 1980.

†Limited-stage disease is defined by VA Lung Group as disease confined to one hemithorax with or without scalene or supraclavicular node involvement; extensive-stage disease in all disease beyond one hemithorax and ipsilateral supraclavicular nodes.

In the United States, female patients with lung cancer tend to have better survival rates than do males. This difference is not explained by age, resectability, operative mortality rate, histopathology, location of the tumor, or differences in tumor stage.[460-462] The difference is particularly marked in female patients with localized disease who undergo surgical resection (Table 22-32). However, recent reports of younger women with bad-prognosis Stage III adenocarcinoma have appeared.[463] Also, for unknown reasons, the prognosis for

TABLE 22-30. Influence of Pretreatment Performance Status On Survival of 5022 Men with Inoperable Lung Cancer*

Performance Status Scale				
ECOG (Zubrod)†	Karnofsky	Definitions	Median Survival (wk)	% of Patients In Group
0	100	Asymptomatic	34	2
1	80–90	Symptomatic, fully ambulatory	24–27	32
2	60–70	Symptomatic, in bed <50% of day	14–21	40
3	40–50	Symptomatic, in bed >50% of day but not bedridden	7–9	22
4	20–30	Bedridden	3–5	5

*Stanley KE: Prognostic factors for survival in patients with inoperable lung cancer. JNCI 65:25–32, 1980.

†Eastern Cooperative Oncology Group (ECOG) or Zubrod performance status score.

TABLE 22-32.   Comparison of Survival Rates of Men and Women with Lung Cancer*

Stage of Disease	Time Period	5-Year Survival (%)	
		Male	Female
NCI SEER Program†			
All	1965–1969	8	13
Localized		28	51
Regional spread		10	15
Localized disease, postsurgical resection‡	1949–1962	29	49
	1950–1959	35	68

*The number of patients in each group is more than 1000.
†Silverberg E: Cancer statistics, 1984. CA 34:7–23, 1984; Cancer Patient Survival, Report No. 5, DHEW Publ. No. (NIH) 77-992, 1977.
‡Watson WLL, Schottenfeld D: Survival in cancer of the bronchus and lung 1949–1962: Comparison of men and women patients. Dis Chest 53:65–72, 1968; Ederer F, Mersheimer WL: Sex differences in the survival of lung cancer patients. Cancer 15:425–432, 1962; Connelly RR, Cutler SJ, Baylis P: End results in cancer of the lung: Comparison of male and female patients. JNCI 36:277–287, 1966.

women is worse than that for men in Wales and England and possibly in France even after surgical resection of localized disease.[464]

The observation that blood transfusion may deleteriously affect the survival of patients undergoing resection for colon cancer, breast cancer, and sarcoma has led to similar investigations in good-risk patients undergoing lung cancer resection. Perioperative blood transfusion was found to be a significant prognostic factor adversely affecting disease-free survival, with the prognosis being worse with intraoperative transfusion than postoperative transfusion.[465] The survival effected was long term and related to cancer recurrence, as patients receiving transfusions had a 62% disease-free rate at 5 years, whereas the other patients' rate was 76%. These findings were confirmed in a retrospective review by Hyman and associates,[466] and further cooperative studies are being analyzed to verify the deleterious survival impact of perioperative transfusion.

CARDIAC STATUS

The signs or symptoms of a myocardial infarction in the past 6 months in the patient with lung cancer should be sought and serial ECGs reviewed. An infarct in this period would be a contraindication to surgery and a documented infarct within the past 3 months an absolute contraindication to thoracic surgery. More than 20% of such patients will die of a complication related to reinfarction alone.[467] About 10% to 15% of all patients evaluated for lung cancer surgery will have ECG abnormalities, and all cardiac arrhythmias should be identified and, if possible, corrected. Serum potassium deficits and calcium excess should be identified and corrected as well, because these can potentiate digitalis toxicity and anesthetic hazard.[455,468] Uncontrolled major arrhythmias, such as multifocal premature ventricular contractions, carry a high risk and usually will contraindicate surgery. Bundle branch block is not a contraindication to surgery. However, in estimating risk, a right bundle-branch block or a left anterior fascicular block carries less risk than does a left posterior fascicular block, whereas combination and bifasci-

cular blocks put the patient at greatest risk.[453] If the patient has a history of angina, cardiology evaluation should be obtained and noninvasive tests of myocardial function such as echocardiography performed. If the angina is progressive and not under treatment, evaluation with radionuclide multigated acquisition (MUGA) scans at rest and exercise may define high-risk groups (i.e., triple coronary vessel disease and left main artery occlusive disease). Positive exercise multigated acquisition (MUGA) scans should be followed by coronary angiography, and if significant coronary occlusion is found, appropriate medical treatment with calcium-channel blockers or beta blockers (if underlying pulmonary disease permits) should be begun. For patients with significant coronary artery stenosis deemed better served by bypass grafting, this should be performed prior to or concomitantly with pulmonary resection. A series of 43 patients undergoing concomitant pulmonary cardiac operations requiring heart-lung bypass has been reported from the Mayo Clinic, of whom 10 had bronchogenic carcinoma.[469] Wedge resection, lobectomy, or pneumonectomy could be performed safely, and the resection was performed before commencing bypass or after the heparin was reversed with protamine to avoid hemorrhage, the cause for the two operative deaths (4.6%). Despite the technical ability to perform the operation via sternotomy, the ability to sample lymph node basins is compromised by this incision.

PULMONARY FUNCTION STATUS

Lung cancer surgery strenuously tests the patients' pulmonary reserve. Thus, patients must have pulmonary function testing to evaluate respiratory reserve before surgery. In lung cancer patients, in addition to chronic lung disease and cigarette abuse, the size of the primary tumor, its proximity to the hilum, and involvement of the ipsilateral hilar lymph nodes determine the extent of functional impairment. Thoracotomy is followed by postoperative chest pain with reduction in the depth of inspiration and inhibition of cough. Postoperative pain and the use of narcotics and other analgesics result in alveolar collapse, possibly leading to pneumonitis and respiratory failure. Postoperative respiratory complications are increased secondary to hypercarbia and ventilatory insufficiency if the patient's postoperative FEV_1 is less than 0.8 liters. Thus, preoperative attempts to improve pulmonary function should be aggressive and include cessation of smoking, bronchodilators, antibiotics in patients with bronchitis, inhalation of humidified air, segmental postural drainage, and chest physiotherapy. Preoperatively, if the FEV_1 is greater than 50% of the FVC and greater than 2.1 liters, the maximum voluntary ventilation is greater than 50% of predicted values, and the ratio of residual volume to total lung capacity is less than 50%, the patient is a reasonable candidate for surgery. If the FEV_1 is 2.5 liters or more, the patient can tolerate pneumonectomy; if the FEV_1 is less than 1 liter, the patient usually cannot tolerate any loss of functional lung tissue. However, if the FEV_1 falls between 1.1 and 2.4 liters of flow, the risk of any resection and the maximum tolerable resection are judgmental and require further study.[453,470–472]

The patient's postoperative pulmonary functional status will depend on the extent of resection and the functional contribution of the resected segments. A number of studies have indicated the ability of quantitative radionuclide ventilation scans to predict lung function following resection in patients with impaired pulmonary function and help plan the extent of resection in lung cancer patients.[473] Scintigraphic ventilation—perfusion studies may also provide serial data regarding radiation-induced changes to guide high-dose radiotherapy. Split function studies are carried out by summing the activity of each lung in the anterior and posterior view, and the postoperative function is predicted by multiplying the preoperative value by the ratio of the counts in the remaining lung to the total lung acitivity. Pneumonectomy is functionally tolerable if the percentage of ventilation to the nontumor-bearing lung when multiplied by the FEV_1 equals 1 liter or more of flow. If the volume of the normal lung exceeds its ventilation by more than 5%, there is a greater chance of postpneumonectomy ventilatory failure.[474] An estimated postoperative FEV_1 of less than 33% of the predicted value, when accompanied by evidence of severe generalized airway obstruction and abnormal V/Q distribution within the nontumor-bearing lung, indicates a high surgical risk.[474,475] The quantitative techniques are limited by the difficulty in predicting segmental or lobar contributions. Krypton scintigraphy and aerosol inhalation studies may provide better quantification of both regional ventilation and lobar ventilation–perfusion ratios.[476]

Preoperative blood gas analysis should also be performed for moderate to high-risk patients, with abnormalities ($PaCO_2$ exceeding 45 Torr or PaO_2 below 55 Torr) indicating a high risk of postoperative pulmonary insufficiency.[453] Abnormalities of CO_2 are more significant than abnormalities of PO_2 because the former can result only from alveolar hypoventilation, whereas the latter may result from an admixture of venous and arterial blood in the tumor area.[472] However, many patients who appear to be marginal surgical risks readily tolerate even extended resection if the burden of the ventilation defect is in the tumor-bearing area. If significant shunting occurs on the affected side, pulmonary function and arterial blood gases may improve after resec-

tion. Although hypoperfusion on the V/Q scan is not a sign of inoperability, a preoperative finding of less than 33% perfusion to the tumor-bearing lung suggests a pneumonectomy will be required for surgical cure.[477,478]

The measurement of preoperative pulmonary artery pressure as an indication of the development of postoperative pulmonary hypertension is rarely performed now, but criteria of mean pulmonary arterial pressure of 30 mm Hg or greater after unilateral occlusion, CO_2 greater than 45 mm Hg, and predicted postpneumonectomy FEV_1 above 0.8 liter still define patients who would not be able to tolerate pneumonectomy.

INFLUENCE OF OTHER FACTORS ON SURVIVAL

Lung Cancer in the Elderly

Lung cancer incidence increases with age in the United States, and analysis of nearly 23,000 cases from the Centralized Cancer Patient Data System showed that the percentage of patients with local-stage disease increases with age and that this is independent of sex, race, and histologic subtype.[479] At age 54 or younger, 15% present with local-stage disease, whereas the figure is 19% for those 55 to 64 years, 22% for those 65 to 74 years, and 25% for those 75 or older.[479] In addition, analysis of 6332 patients who underwent surgical staging showed a greater likelihood of local-stage disease with increasing age.[479]

Although elderly patients (over 70 years of age) with lung cancer do have other medical problems, they do not differ with respect to many presurgical variables such as smoking history, arterial blood gas values, degree of airflow obstruction, or cell type.[480] Although operative mortality rate in the elderly is greater (9% versus 4% in one series), there are no statistically significant differences in postoperative complication rates, length of postoperative hospital stay, or actuarial survival rates. Thus, elderly patients with reasonable cardiopulmonary function should not be denied potentially curative pulmonary resection simply because of concern about possible age-related complications.[480]

Effects of Socioeconomic Status on Lung Cancer Treatment

The role of socioeconomic factors in determining lung cancer treatment is not well defined. Studies conducted on patients treated between 1955 and 1964 found no significant difference between Veterans Administration status, whites, blacks, indigent versus nonindigent, income status, or private versus nonprivate patient status in the percentage of patients with localized disease or in survival.[481] Thus, the biology of the disease appeared to be more important than differences in natural history, detection, or treatment imposed by race or socioeconomic status. Recently, however, these observations have been challenged. Greenberg and associates studied 1403 cases of non-small cell cancer diagnosed between 1973 and 1976 in the regional tumor registries of New Hampshire and Vermont.[482] They found that the probability that patients would undergo potentially curative surgery was enhanced if they were younger, married, had private medical insurance, lived more than 39 km from a specialized center, had localized disease, or had a better functional status. Among the 1137 patients who did not undergo surgery, some form of cancer therapy (such as radiation or chemotherapy) was more frequently offered to patients who were younger, had private medical insurance, had a better functional status, or had no evidence of distant metastatic disease. Significantly, the probability of 3-year survival (about 11% in the 1403 patients) was unrelated to marital status, type of health insurance, or distance from a cancer treatment center. Those authors interpret their data as suggesting that physicians treat married patients and those with adequate medical insurance more aggressively, although these factors could also indicate these patients' better knowledge of the medical care system.[483]

STAGING AND PROGNOSTIC FACTORS IN PATIENTS WITH SMALL CELL LUNG CANCER

In patients who have histologic or cytologic evidence of small cell lung cancer, a different staging system and approach to staging are used because the primary treatment modality will be chemotherapy with or without radiotherapy, and no patients will receive solely locoregional therapy. In the uncommon case of a resected pulmonary nodule that proves to be small cell carcinoma, appropriate staging procedures should be employed postoperatively.

Mountain, in a review of 268 small cell lung cancer patients for the AJC staging system, found no difference in survival rate for small cell lung cancer for more than 40 characteristics, including sex; age; peripheral, central, or apical tumor location; radiographic appearance; size of the lesion (including tumors less than 3 cm in diameter); presence, absence, or degree of atelectasis; pneumonitis; pleural effusion; mediastinal invasion; regional lymph node involvement; or presence or absence of distant metastases (Table 22-33). There was no significant difference in 41 patients according to postsurgical Group (I, II, or III) in survival; none were cured.[484] Because the TNM factors did not appear to be prognostic for survival in small cell cancer patients treated predominantly with surgery or radiotherapy, the AJC initially recommended applying their system to small cell cancer only for purposes of later reference. With the recent recognition that a few small cell lung tumors can be extirpated surgically, detailed TNM staging has proved useful in identifying candidates for an operative approach and in estimating the prognosis in this infrequent clinical setting.[485] However, for the great majority of patients not undergoing thoracotomy for resection, nearly all investigators studying the treatment of small cell lung cancer have adopted the simple two-stage system of the VALG.[484]

In this two-stage system, limited disease is defined as that confined to one hemithorax and to the regional lymph nodes (including mediastinal and contralateral hilar and, usually, ipsilateral supraclavicular), whereas extensive disease is defined as that beyond this area, including distant lymph nodes, brain, liver, bone, bone marrow, and intra-abdominal and soft-tissue metastases. The definition of stage relates to

TABLE 22-33. Frequency of TNM Findings at Diagnosis in the AJC Group of 368 Small Cell Lung Cancer Patients

	% of Patients
Asymptomatic at diagnosis	6
Tumor location	
Hilar	68
Peripheral	12
Apical	2
Mainstem bronchus	17
Tumor size	
<3 cm	20
>3 cm	80
Atelectasis/pneumonitis	
None	35
Segmental	43
Lobar	18
Entire lung	4
Pleural effusion	15
Clinical evidence of	
Mediastinal invasion	30
Metastases outside hemithorax of origin and mediastinum (M1)	48
Scalene or supraclavicular node involvement	30
Regional lymph node involvement clinically by radiography	
N0	27
N1 (hilar)	26
N2 (mediastinal)	47

Mountain CF: Clinical biology of small cell carcinoma: Relationship to surgical therapy. Semin Oncol 5:272–279, 1978.

whether the known tumor can be encompassed within a tolerable radiation port. Thus, ipsilateral pleural effusion, recurrent laryngeal nerve involvement, and SVC obstruction can still be considered limited-stage disease. However, pericardial effusion and bilateral pulmonary parenchymal involvement are scored as extensive-stage disease. Ipsilateral pleural effusion and various degrees of supraclavicular node involvement have been considered consistent with either limited or extensive disease by different authors. Among patients with otherwise limited tumors, neither of these factors appears to influence survival.[486,487]

PROGNOSTIC FACTORS

Limited-stage patients have both higher response rates and longer survival than do extensive-stage patients given identical or similar therapy.[487,488] In trials of combination chemotherapy with or without radiotherapy, patients classified as limited stage had an 86% total objective tumor regression rate, a 60% rate of complete clinical regression of tumor (complete response), and a median survival of 51 weeks. In contrast, patients scored as extensive stage had a 77% total response rate, a 25% complete response rate, and a median survival of 33 weeks.[488] Occasionally, similar response rates have been observed for both stages, with stage predicting only survival differences.[489,490] The durability of partial responses is only modestly affected by stage. However, complete response duration and long-term survival is markedly superior in limited-stage disease.[482,491,492]

Initial performance status strongly influences survival both in untreated patients and in patients receiving combination chemotherapy with or without radiotherapy.[486,493-496] Although more favorable performance status is found more frequently in limited-stage patients, within either stage, performance status is the most important variable.[486,487,491] Also, in extensive-stage patients, a strong correlation exists between worsening performance status and the number of sites of metastatic disease, suggesting that the prognostic effect of performance status may in some part be accounted for by its association with overall tumor burden.[486]

Stage of disease and performance status are the principal prognostic factors in previously untreated small cell lung cancer. In addition to stage (limited versus extensive), other tumor-related factors influence survival. For example, considerable variation in prognosis exists within extensive disease according to the distribution of tumor involvement. In an early review of 106 patients entered on NCI trials, extensive-disease patients with only a single site of metastases (outside areas of involvement included with limited stage) had survival rates that were not statistically distinguishable from those of patients with limited disease.[486] However, metastatic involvement of the liver, the central nervous system (CNS), or three or more extrathoracic organ systems presaged an especially unfavorable outcome. A more recent study of more than 800 patients from the Finsen Institute revealed that bone marrow, brain, and liver metastases, as well as the number of organ systems involved with metastatic cancer, significantly influenced prognosis in univariate analyses. In multivariate analysis, however, after stage of disease and probable "surrogate markers" of tumor burden such as performance status, plasma hemoglobin, and serum LDH were considered, specific sites of metastatic involvement no longer contributed significantly to prognosis.[497] When only 18-month disease-free survival rather than overall survival was the end-point, only stage of disease, and not performance status, hemoglobin, LDH, or specific sites of tumor, significantly influenced outcome.[498] The relatively favorable prognosis of one category of limited-disease patients, those whose tumor has been completely resected prior to initiation of chemotherapy or chemoradiotherapy, should be emphasized.[499-501] Whether this is attributable solely to the tumor resection or to the lesser tumor burden in patients whose cancers can be resected completely is not fully resolved.

In addition to performance status, other host-related factors, some of which correlate with performance status and others of which do not, affect prognosis. In some studies, weight loss is an unfavorable prognostic factor independent of stage and performance status for both untreated patients[493] and those given chemotherapy,[502] particularly for more ambulatory cases with a smaller tumor burden. Impaired immune status, as assessed by delayed hypersensitivity skin testing, also correlates with shorter survival, especially in patients with an otherwise favorable prognosis.[503] Sex and age were formerly thought to have little influence on prognosis,[486,504] but more recent studies of larger numbers of patients suggest that women[505] and younger patients[506] have better outcomes when receiving chemotherapy. A single study suggests that small cell lung cancer patients who discontinue cigarette smoking, particularly those who quit more than a year prior to diagnosis, have a better outcome that is

independent of other prognostic factors.[507] Therefore, all such patients should be encouraged to stop smoking.

Finally, as in all other cancers, patients with small cell lung cancer who suffer tumor progression during or after administration of chemotherapy have an extremely poor prognosis, with a median survival of only 8 weeks in one large cooperative group study.[508]

Virtually all of the information on prognostic factors in small cell lung cancer has been derived from patients entered in prospective clinical trials. Although there is no reason to believe that such factors do not predict prognosis in the majority of patients who do not participate in these studies, survival differences might exist between patients who are and are not entered in clinical trials. In a recent study of 215 consecutive cases of small cell carcinoma, for various reasons, only 20% of patients were placed on available chemotherapy protocols.[509] Survival in extensive-stage patients placed on study was superior to that in patients who were managed "off protocol." In limited-stage patients, however, no survival differences were noted. These results are consistent with conventional wisdom that patients with poor performance status or those with severe non-neoplastic illnesses are less often entered in clinical trials. Because most limited-stage patients have their disease diagnosed while they are still in relatively good medical condition, however, their survival is much less affected by whether they are judged suitable for protocol entry.

CLINICAL PRESENTATION

Signs and symptoms of small cell lung cancer depend on the size and location of the primary tumor and the presence or absence of regional or distant metastases. With the exception of certain paraneoplastic syndromes, which are relatively uncommon, most clinical signs are no more specific for small cell carcinoma than for other types of lung cancer.[510] Because the primary tumor most often arises centrally, patients typically present with cough, dyspnea, wheezing, hemoptysis, chest pain, or postobstructive pneumonitis. The usual submucosal location of small cell carcinoma accounts for the relatively lower frequency of hemoptysis compared with squamous cell cancer.[511] Tumor extension to the mediastinum occurs almost invariably, accounting for the frequent occurrence of regional metastatic symptoms such as SVC syndrome, hoarseness from recurrent laryngeal nerve paralysis, and dysphagia. Almost 10% of patients will have SVC syndrome at diagnosis, and judicious invasive diagnostic procedures can usually be performed safely. Survival is similar to that in patients of the same stage without the syndrome.[512]

Patients may or may not be symptomatic from small cell carcinoma metastases. Radiographically detectable central nervous system (CNS) metastases are symptomatic in more than 90% of cases. Although bone metastases may be painful, they are not in most patients, and pathologic fractures are rare. Liver metastases cause (usually mild) dysfunction detectable by laboratory tests in 50% to 60% of cases with liver involvement, but liver function is impaired seriously in only a few of these cases. Usually, the liver involvement causes problems by its mass and overall contribution to tumor bulk and decreased performance status. In occasional patients, jaundice is secondary to extrahepatic biliary obstruction from pancreatic or nodal metastases rather than to tumor replacement of the liver; the prognosis is not so dire in the former group as in the latter.[513] Anemia, leukopenia, or thrombocytopenia related to bone marrow involvement is uncommon, and hemoglobin and white cell levels are not indicative of marrow involvement.[234,504] During intensive induction chemotherapy, patients with positive bone marrows have more severe infections and require more red blood cell transfusions than do patients without tumor in the marrow. However, leukopenia, thrombocytopenia, and the need for platelet transfusions during induction therapy do not appear to correlate with marrow involvement.[504]

Elevated plasma concentrations of immunologically detected polypeptide hormones are much more frequent in small cell lung cancer than are symptoms from the corresponding paraneoplastic syndromes.[514-516] The syndrome of inappropriate secretion of antidiuretic hormone (SIADH), ectopic Cushing's syndrome, and the Eaton–Lambert or myasthenia-like syndrome are relatively specifically associated with small cell carcinoma. The frequency of SIADH at presentation differs according to definition of the syndrome but in one recent large series was 11%. Only 27% of patients fulfilling the diagnostic criteria for SIADH, however, were symptomatic from hyponatremia. The presence of SIADH was not correlated with stage of disease, tumor involvement of specific metastatic sites, or prognosis.[517]

STAGING PROCEDURES

Staging procedures are of value in selecting individual patients who can benefit from therapy that is efficacious only in certain stages, most commonly patients who can be managed suitably with locoregional treatment alone; in assigning prognosis; and in identifying areas of tumor involvement that can be monitored to determine response. In groups of patients, the staging process documents patterns of failure with a given form of treatment, thus suggesting new therapeutic strategies and, through the use of staging systems derived from these procedures, permits uniform and more easily interpreted reporting of results of clinical trials. Because of overt or covert distant metastases at the time of diagnosis, all patients with small cell lung cancer will receive chemotherapy, and staging procedures do not identify patients who can be given solely locoregional treatment. However, the staging process does divide patients into limited- and extensive-stage disease, which is of clear prognostic significance, and in most cases will lead to the administration of chest radiation in addition to chemotherapy in the former group. In addition, documenting initially involved sites of tumor aids in the later evaluation of response to therapy and diagnosis of eventual tumor progression. Except for the CNS, initial local or metastatic tumor deposits are the areas in which relapse develops in most cases.

The extent of the initial staging evaluation depends on clinical circumstances. Our recommendations are given in Table 22-34. When distant metastases are obvious or treatment will not be affected by stage, simple screening tests followed by only those studies that have an increased likeli-

hood of being positive[518,519] are performed outside a clinical trial setting. In a prospective clinical trial or when stage-specific therapy is to be administered, additional studies are appropriate. If the purpose of the staging is to exclude patients with extensive disease from receiving chest irradiation, then no further procedures need be done after an unequivocal site of distant metastases is documented. Because of the frequent involvement of mediastinal lymph nodes in small cell lung cancer and the poor prognosis of node-positive patients who undergo surgical resection,[485] additional staging tests to evaluate the mediastinum are recommended in patients with known small cell lung cancer in whom surgical removal of the primary tumor is being considered.

The timing of restaging to assess response and the tests that should be performed depend on the cost and availability of specific procedures and the philosophy of the treating physician. Clearly, tumor sites that were initially involved should be reevaluated.

Finally, it should be recognized that any set of staging recommendations is somewhat arbitrary and that individualization of the process in different clinical circumstances is often appropriate. The initial therapy (combination chemotherapy with or without radiotherapy) is, in many respects, as demanding as thoracotomy and pulmonary resection. Thus, physiologic as well as anatomic staging is required. The intensity of the initial therapy and the combined use of chemotherapy and aggressive radiotherapy produced treatment-associated mortality rates of 5% or more in many recent series. The most important risk factor for treatment-related death appears to be the initial performance status. Although there are few data from recent trials, it would appear prudent to submit to extremely aggressive induction therapy only those patients who are ambulatory more than 50% of the time and who have adequate cardiopulmonary, renal, and hepatic function.

The primary tumor and regional nodal spread are evaluated by chest posteroanterior and lateral roentgenograms. In addition, fiberoptic bronchoscopy with bronchial washings and biopsy is essential to document the extent of disease and may be used to determine the degree of tumor response during follow-up. Before treatment, fiberoptic bronchoscopy will reveal evidence of cancer in more than 90% of patients, including approximately 8% to 10% in whom the tumor is not evaluable on chest films.[235] In follow-up, patients with evidence of tumor by bronchoscopy after initial therapy have a much higher relapse rate in the chest within a 6-month period than do patients with normal bronchoscopy findings at this time.[235,520]

Computed tomographic scans of the thorax provide more precise definition of parenchymal, mediastinal, and pleural disease.[521] They are probably most useful in the design of radiotherapy portals and in assessing persistence or early relapse of chest tumor. In our experience, all patients with intrathoracic tumor resolution by chest roentgenography and persistent endobronchial disease on bronchoscopy are identified as not being in complete remission by chest CT scans; additional patients in only partial remission are also detected.

The common sites of extrathoracic metastatic disease detected during pretreatment staging are bone in 38%, liver in

TABLE 22-34. Staging Procedures for Small Cell Lung Cancer

Minimum Survey (Screening Tests)
Complete history and physical examination
Chest roentgenography (with CT to assist in portal design if other than palliative chest irradiation is to be given)
Liver function tests and physical examination of liver (with radionuclide or CT liver scan if results abnormal)
Bone pain/alkaline phosphatase (with radionuclide bone scan if results abnormal)
Neurologic history and examination (with CT scan of brain if results abnormal)
Platelet count or leukoerythroblastic peripheral blood smear (with bone marrow aspiration/biopsy if results abnormal; also recommended if no other unequivocal distant metastatic disease has been documented or if all initial sites of involvement are to be reassessed to determine response)

*Procedures for Patients in Clinical Trials or Receiving Stage-Dependent Therapy**
Complete history and physical examination
Chest roentgenography plus CT scan of chest to assist in portal design if chest irradiation (other than palliative) is to be employed; plus fiberoptic bronchoscopy if no evaluable tumor on chest film)
Liver function tests/radionuclide or CT liver scan
Liver biopsy (peritoneoscopy or ultrasound guided) if either liver function tests or scan abnormal and best information concerning liver status is required to select therapy
Radionuclide bone scan
CT scan of brain in presence or absence of neurologic abnormalities if brain irradiation is to be given to asymptomatic patients
Bone marrow aspiration/biopsy (bilaterally if best information concerning marrow status is required)

Procedures Prior to Attempted Surgical Resection if Patient Is Known to Have Small Cell Cancer
All staging procedures listed for patients in clinical trials
Fiberoptic bronchoscopy
Evaluation of mediastinum
    CT scan of chest
    Mediastinoscopy†

Modified from Ihde DC: Staging evaluation and prognostic factors in small cell lung cancer. In Aisner J (ed): Lung Cancer, pp 241–268. New York, Churchill Livingstone, 1985.
*Evaluation can be stopped after documentation of extensive disease if staging is being used only to identify candidates for stage-specific therapy.
†Unless thought unnecessary by operating surgeon.

22% to 28%, bone marrow in 17% to 23%, and the CNS in 8% to 14% (Table 22-35).[486,505] Radionuclide bone scans are more sensitive than skeletal roentgenograms in identifying osseous metastases; the latter should be employed principally to confirm or exclude potential metastatic sites detected on bone scan.[504,522] The greater the number of bone scan abnormalities, the more likely it is that sites of extraosseous metastatic disease will be found. Improvement or worsening on follow-up scans correlates with the extraosseous tumor response 70% of the time.[522] As in other cancers, however, the principal difficulty with bone scans in small cell lung cancer is false-positive examinations secondary to benign bone and joint disease. Therefore, bone scans should not serve as the sole basis for making therapeutic decisions but rather should alert the clinician to the need for further evaluation. After treatment, osteoblastic changes sometimes can be seen on bone radiographs, probably representing regeneration of bone, not new metastases.[504] Thus, unless some other evidence of tumor progression exists, such changes alone should not be an indication for changing therapy. Bone marrow involvement is found with marrow aspiration and biopsy; often, the two procedures are complementary, and thus aspiration may be positive when the biopsy is not, and vice versa.[504] An additional 10% of patients (30% of all with positive marrows) will be found to have marrow involvement if bilateral biopsies are done.[504]

Fewer than 5% of patients will have bone marrow involvement as the sole site of extensive-stage disease.[523] A positive marrow examination does, however, yield pathologic proof that extensive disease is present, providing assurance of extrathoracic metastases that cannot be obtained with equivocal imaging studies. The results of bone scans and marrow examinations are significantly correlated, but they are complementary as each can be positive when the other is unrevealing.[522,524] Interestingly, in patients receiving chemotherapy, the requirement for transfusion of blood products or drug dosage reductions does not predict that bone marrow metastases will be found at autopsy.[525]

Although liver function tests are abnormal in 93% of patients whose livers are histologically positive for tumor, they also are abnormal in 41% of patients with histologically negative livers.[504] Both false-positive and false-negative liver radionuclide scans are seen in small cell cancer. If patients have a filling defect on liver scan and abnormal liver function tests, histologic proof of liver involvement can be obtained in almost 90% of cases, whereas patients in whom both scan and function tests are negative will have positive liver biopsies less than 10% of the time. If either the scan or

TABLE 22-35.   Results of Pretreatment Staging Procedures in Small Cell Lung Cancer*

	% of Patients with Finding
Final stage†	
Limited stage	31
Extensive stage	69
Chest staging	
Chest film mass‡	90
Fiberoptic bronchoscopy‡	
Visual endobronchial tumor	83
Washings/biopsy pathologically positive	87
Pleural effusion†	9
Ipsilateral supraclavicular node†	6
Contralateral lung†	7
Bilateral endobronchial tumor†	5
Bone (bone scan)†	38
Liver (histologically proven by biopsy)†§	22–28
Bone marrow*‖#**	17–23
Central nervous system†‡‡#	8–14
Brain	10
Spinal	5
Leptomeningeal	2
Retroperitoneal metastases (CT scan)§§	16
Soft tissue biopsy proven†	24

*Each category consists of between 100 and 600 patients.
†Ihde DC, Makuch RW, Carney DN et al, Am Rev Respir Dis 123:500–507, 1981.
‡Ihde DC, Cohen MH, Bernath AM et al, Chest 74:531–536, 1978.
§Dombernowsky P, Hirsch F, Hansen HH et al, Cancer 41:2008–2012, 1978.
‖Ihde DC, Simms EG, Matthews MJ et al, Blood 53:667–686, 1979.
#Hirsch FR, Hansen HH, Hainau B, Acta Pathol Microbiol Scand 87:59–62, 1979.
**Hirsch F, Hansen HH, Dombernowsky P et al, Cancer 39:2463–2567, 1977.
††Hansen HH, Dombernowsky P, Hirsch FR, Semin Oncol 5:280–287, 1978.
‡‡Bunn PA Jr, Nugenet JL, Matthews MJ, Semin Oncol 5:314–322, 1978.
§§Dunnick NR, Ihde DC, Johnston–Early A, AJR 133:1085–1088, 1979.

the function tests, but not both, is abnormal, the probability of liver involvement at biopsy is approximately 20%.[526] If it is deemed essential to prove or disprove liver involvement pathologically, the best method of detecting metastases is with multiple biopsies at peritoneoscopy.[504,526,527] Recent data suggest that ultrasound-guided fine-needle aspiration of the liver is approximately as sensitive as peritoneoscopy in yielding pathologic confirmation of liver involvement.[528] Contraindications to obtaining liver biopsy confirmation are bleeding disorders, a patient unable to cooperate, massive pleural effusion, or respiratory decompensation so that the procedure cannot be tolerated.

Metastases to the CNS are extremely common clinical problems, occurring in approximately 30% of patients at diagnosis or during the subsequent course of the disease.[529] CT scans of the brain are superior to radionuclide scans in documenting brain metastases in patients with neurologic symptoms or signs, but both tests are abnormal in the great majority of cases. As screening examinations in asympto-

matic patients, the yield of both is low, in the range of 5% to 10% for CT scan and less than 5% for radionuclide scan.[518,530,531] However, the CT scan is clearly the examination of choice, with greater sensitivity and positive predictive accuracy.[532] Many clinicians advocate screening CT scans at diagnosis of small cell lung cancer in asymptomatic patients, because brain irradiation would be administered if the test were positive. In one series, however, there was no evidence that detection of brain metastases in asymptomatic patients is associated with survival rates superior to those in patients whose metastases are diagnosed because of neurologic symptoms or signs.[532] Patients with brain metastases as the only site of extensive-stage disease have a median survival not markedly different from that of patients with limited disease, although long-term survival is rare and relapse in the brain after irradiation is frequent.[530,532] At present, in asymptomatic patients with a negative, careful neurologic examination, a clear-cut indication for a head CT scan would be just before administration of prophylactic cranial irradiation. If asymptomatic lesions were discovered, a higher dose of radiotherapy would be delivered.[533,534]

Metastases to the CNS can be intracranial, spinal epidural with spinal cord compression, or leptomeningeal with carcinomatous meningitis.[533–535] Screening asymptomatic patients with cerebrospinal fluid (CSF) cytologies is unrewarding.[535,536] However, it is important to know that once one site of CNS metastatic disease is discovered, the probability of finding disease at other CNS sites is increased greatly. Clinically apparent multiple sites are present in 20% of patients with CNS metastases and are discovered in 73% of such patients at autopsy.[534] Patients suspected of having spinal cord compression should undergo a myelogram promptly. Likewise, patients with signs and symptoms of leptomeningeal involvement should have CSF cytologies performed. Brain imaging studies should also be performed in both situations. Back pain and abnormal spine findings on bone scan or radiographs or minimal neurologic abnormalities suggesting an epidural lesion in the presence of an intracranial metastasis or carcinomatous leptomeningitis should be an indication for a myelogram. Back pain and bone destruction on radiographs are found in most patients whose cord compression is present at diagnosis of small cell lung cancer but less often in patients whose epidural lesion is documented during the subsequent course of disease.[537] Occasional patients with symptoms of spinal cord dysfunction, often manifested as Brown-Sequard syndrome, will prove to have intramedullary rather than epidural tumor.[538]

Because of the high frequency of intra-abdominal metastases found at autopsy in the adrenals, pancreas, kidneys, and lymph nodes, pretreatment staging of these areas would be useful (see Table 22-19).[208] Abdominal CT scanning may be useful for such staging, but its general use in screening currently is not recommended, although CT scans are frequently used instead of radionuclide scans to image the liver. Upper abdominal CT scans performed prospectively reveal metastases in 36% of patients.[539] The most common site is the liver, whereas retroperitoneal metastases are found in 16%. The CT scan has a sensitivity of approximately 88% and a specificity of 94% as judged by biopsy results.[539] Although abdominal CT scans in small cell cancer can demonstrate metastatic dissemination that cannot be evaluated by other means, they provide relatively little therapeutically relevant information beyond that obtained with standard staging procedures,[536,540,541] because most positive studies occur in patients already known to have more extensive tumor dissemination.[536,540] However, in individual patients, CT scans may be excellent indicators of disease extent and response. When 24 patients with normal adrenal glands by CT scan underwent percutaneous thin-needle biopsy, 17% of the 29 glands sampled adequately contained metastases.[542] Thus, metastatic spread had occurred even to CT-negative organs.

POTENTIAL NEW METHODS FOR STAGING AND FOLLOW-UP OF LUNG CANCER PATIENTS

Although imaging studies provide excellent staging and follow-up data, they obviously are expensive and time consuming. Tumor markers that could be followed by blood tests would be highly desirable. Unfortunately, no such tests are as yet available. Potential candidates include neuron-specific enolase (NSE), creatine kinase BB (CK-BB), and chromogranin A (CGA, the matrix protein of neurosecretory granules) in small cell lung cancer and CEA for all types of lung cancer. Small cell lung cancer produces high levels of NSE, CK-BB, and CGA intracellularly, and with tumor cell breakdown, these products are released into the serum where they can be measured by radioimmunoassay.[543-547] Compared with normal adult controls, serum NSE was raised by more than 12 ng/ml in 69% of 94 newly diagnosed cases of small cell lung cancer. This included 39% of limited-stage and 87% of extensive-stage disease, and extensive-stage patients had higher NSE levels (59 ng/ml) than did limited-stage patients (13 ng/ml). Serial measurements in 23 patients receiving combination chemotherapy showed an excellent correlation between serum NSE and clinical response.[542,545,546] Thus, elevated serum NSE levels are associated with tumor cell bulk (and poor prognosis) and mirror tumor response in small cell lung cancer. A small number of reports indicate that the same observations hold for CK-BB and CGA.[544,545] There has been no demonstration, however, that utilization of any of these markers, including CEA (see below), can substitute for more conventional staging procedures or lead to improved therapeutic results.

CEA also is correlated with disease extent and clinical course. In small cell lung cancer, elevated levels (greater than 2.5 ng/ml) occurred in 88% of extensive-stage and 45% of limited-stage cases, whereas all patients with CEA levels exceeding 50 ng/ml had liver involvement.[548] CEA values provide prognostic information that is independent of stage and performance status,[549] and changes over time correlate with response to chemotherapy and relapse.[548,550] In addition, there is a strong correlation between positive staining of the tumor for CEA and plasma CEA elevation.[551] Thus, in the individual patient, an immunohistochemical stain can indicate whether CEA will be a followable marker.

TREATMENT OF LUNG CANCER BY SURGERY OR RADIOTHERAPY WITH CURATIVE INTENT

SURGICAL TREATMENT
Historical

The first successful total pneumonectomy for bronchogenic carcinoma was performed by Graham and Singer in 1933.[552] Up to that time, there were six cases in the literature in which a patient had survived the removal of a carcinoma for 1 year or more.[553] Rienhoff and colleagues described an individual ligation technique for pneumonectomy with improved management of the bronchial stump,[554] paving the way for the modern practice of individual venous, arterial, and bronchial ligation.

Overview

INFLUENCE OF RANDOMIZED TRIALS. Surgical resection currently offers the best hope of cure in non-small cell lung cancer (Tables 22-36 and 22-37). However, the disappointing results of surgical therapy alone in all stages have led to the investigation of multimodal therapies with the hope of improving survival. With historical study designs, it is not possible to establish unequivocally the extent of comparability between the cases investigated and the control groups. The advantage of prospective randomized trials in the investigation of treatment efficacy thus cannot be overemphasized, even in trials that answer only surgically related questions. Moreover, survival of patients participating in prospective randomized trials significantly exceeds that of nonparticipants,[555] and this survival advantage is not explained by differences in pretreatment disease status or factors of known prognostic significance to the extent to which such data are available. In other words, participation in controlled trials of cancer therapy seems to ensure an inherent advantage, regardless of whether trial patients received experimental therapy or standard therapy. Whatever the reason for this benefit, it should provide a strong impetus for patients to enter such trials.

The NCI LCSG was established in 1977 to carry out prospective randomized trials of adjuvant therapy in resectable lung cancer. The multicenter approach has assured that accrual of patients would not be a limiting factor in the performance of these trials. This group has been at the forefront, not only in the design of such protocols, but also in establishing the modern-day statistics on mortality and survival rates of resectional therapy for lung cancer. The LCSG has investigated the differences in the extent of resection with regard to survival and evaluated the extent and location of nodal positivity in relation to survival and treatment options, as well as serving as a source for pathologic evaluation of resected material. Because of the uniformly high quality of data representing nine institutions, we emphasize the current results of the LCSG over those from many other studies reported previously.

TECHNICAL CONSIDERATIONS. The selection of the appropriate surgical procedure in resectable cases is deter-

TABLE 22-36.   Survival After Surgical Resection of Lung Cancer

Histologic Type*	5- and 10-Year Survival (%)				
	5-Year	Range	n	10-Year	n
Epidermoid carcinoma	33	26–43	1643	17	1115
Adenocarcinoma	26	20–34	535	16	352
Large cell carcinoma	28	6–36	278	8	278
Bronchioloalveolar	51	48–61	76	24	76
Small cell carcinoma	1	0–20	125	<0.5	125
Total	30	26–36	2790	15	1946

Mountain CF: Assessment of the role of surgery for control of lung cancer. Ann Thorac Surg 24:365–373, 1977; Paulson DL, Reisch JS: Long-term survival after resection for bronchogenic carcinoma. Ann Surg 184:324–332, 1976; Wilkins WE Jr, Scannell JG, Crauer JG: Four decades of experience with resection for bronchogenic carcinoma at the Massachusetts General Hospital. J Thorac Cardiovasc Surg 76:364–368, 1978; Ashor GL, Kem WH, Meyer BW et al: Long term survival in bronchogenic carcinoma. J Thorac Cardiovasc Surg 70:581–589, 1975; Kirsch MM, Rotman H, Argenta L et al: Carcinoma of the lung: results of treatment over ten years. Ann Thorac Surg 21:371–377, 1976.

*Miscellaneous histologic types (e.g., adenosquamous) had a 10-year survival rate of 14% for 87 patients.

mined by the size of the tumor, its anatomic extent, and the physiologic status of the patient. The actual extent of resection remains a matter of surgical judgment and experience based on the findings at exploration. The surgeon is guided by the principle of performing the procedure that will ensure removal of all known disease with maximum conservation of pulmonary tissue. Two decades ago, it was widely held that pneumonectomy with hilar node dissection should always be performed regardless of the size of the primary lesion. Now, lobectomy is considered the operation of choice by most surgeons when the lesion is confined to one lobe and no nodal positivity is suspected. In a large series of patients followed by the Veterans Administration Surgical Oncology Group, long-term survival was essentially the same after lobectomy as pneumonectomy.[556] The use of segmental resections or large wedge resections combined with lymph node sampling instead of lobectomy (even in patients with good pulmonary function) is now under investigation and will be discussed later in the chapter.

In all cases, the decision to resect for cure is based on the expectation that no gross residual disease would remain at the conclusion of the procedure. Thus, there is general agreement that candidates for curative surgical resection are those with Stage I and Stage II disease. Lobectomy is indicated for lesions totally confined within a lobe so as to permit 1 cm or more of normal lobar bronchus proximally. In addition, there should be no gross lymph node involvement central to the origin of the lobar bronchus. Careful attention is paid to en bloc dissection of the regional lymph nodes with frozen sections reviewed intraoperatively to ensure an adequate resection. It is with the Stage III lesions that controversy has always existed because of the finding of intraoperative mediastinal nodal positivity, which carries an unfavorable prognosis. The considerations for surgical resection in these situations revolve around the surgeon's findings at operation, including the extent and location of nodal positivity; the intactness of nodal capsules; the involvement of contiguous, sacrificeable structures; and the functional outcome predicted for the patient after an extended resection. These factors are discussed individually in a separate section of this chapter.

OTHER TECHNICAL CONSIDERATIONS. Anesthetic considerations for pulmonary resection involve the use of the safest inhalational and narcotic agents, proper airway control, and appropriate cardiovascular and respiratory

TABLE 22-37.   Five-Year Survival (Cumulative %) After Surgical Resection of Lung Cancer by Postsurgical Stage (Old AJC System)*

Histology	Stage I	Stage II	Stage III (M0)	Stage III-N2
Epidermoid	54	35	19	13
	(231)†	(61)	(236)	(62)
Adenocarcinoma and large cell	51	18	10	2‡
	(99)	(42)	(165)	(45)
Small cell (41)	0	0	0	0

Carr DT, Mountain CF: The staging of lung cancer. Semin Oncol 1:229–234, 1974; Carr DT: Is staging of cancer of value? Cancer 51(12 Suppl):2503–2505, 1983.

*Figures in parentheses are numbers of patients.

†The fraction of these patients receiving postoperative radiotherapy is not reported.

‡The large cell cancer group had only a few patients but had an 11% 5-year survival rate.

monitoring. Patients with significant cardiac history or disease documented in the preoperative work-up benefit from on-line continuous arterial blood pressure monitoring as well as selective use of central venous catheterization. Highest-risk patients should have intraoperative Swan-Ganz catheterization, which can be used to optimize preload, afterload, and cardiac output to prevent an undue increase in myocardial oxygen consumption or fluid overload. For operations expected to be longer than 3 to 4 hours, urinary bladder catheterization is advised.

The routine use of disposable double-lumen endotracheal tubes and continuous digital oximetry have greatly facilitated inspection of the operative field for nodal mapping, defining fissures for transection, and permitting lung-sparing options, specifically sleeve lobectomies. Proper positioning of the tube prior to the start of the operation (to avoid upper lobe collapse by improper placement) can be achieved with the use of pediatric fiberoptic intubation bronchoscopes. On-line oximetry and measurement of end tidal PCO_2 will ensure that adequate oxygen tensions are being recorded without the need for multiple blood-gas measurements. The use of high-frequency ventilation, permitting reduced lung movements and lower airway pressures, is being evaluated at present and has been associated with improved oxygenation, increased hemodynamic stability, and better surgical access during major airway reconstruction.[557]

CHOICE OF INCISION. Pulmonary resection can be performed via a number of incisions: posterolateral, anterolateral, prone, or sternal splitting (Fig. 22-12). The most frequently used incision is the posterolateral thoracotomy beginning just below the nipple, curving posteriorly below the tip of the scapula, and extending cephalad to the vertebral column. The latissimus dorsi and serratus anterior muscles are divided and the chest entered usually via the resected fifth rib or through the fifth interspace (Fig. 22-13). This incision gives good visibility of both the bronchus and the blood vessels and improves management with the double-lumen tube by preventing spillage of secretions and blood into the opposite lung, collapsing the lung and expedit-

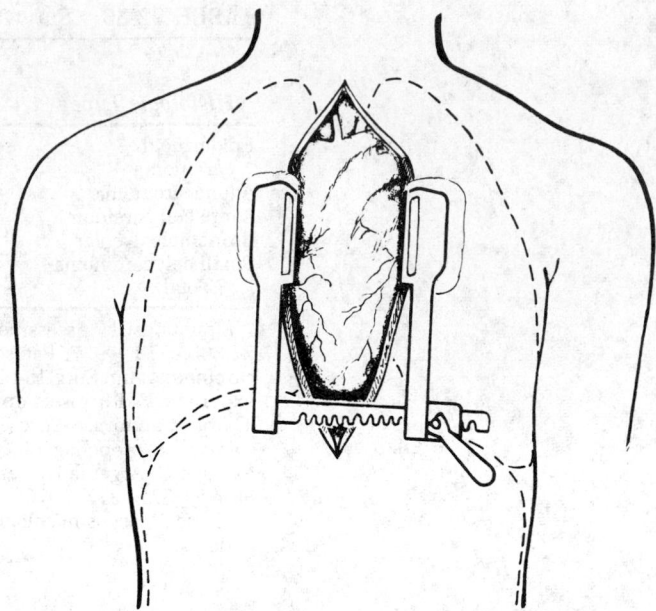

FIG. 22-12. Median sternotomy incision for pulmonary resection, allowing bilateral palpation of the lungs. However, left lower lobe resections are more difficult.

ing the manipulation and resection. However, it is a painful incision postoperatively. The anterolateral incision is less painful but does not provide the access needed for more difficult larger resections (Fig. 22-13). The prone incision, although providing ideal ventilation and drainage, has largely been abandoned because of the difficulty of performing cardiac resuscitation if necessary, inexperience of the anesthesiologists with it, and the resurgence of double-lumen technology. The median sternotomy has been championed by a number of surgeons as the incision of choice, citing decreased postoperative pain, quicker discharge from the hospital, and possible extension of pulmonary resection to patients with reduced pulmonary function who may not tolerate lateral thoracotomy.[558] However, experience with this technique is required to obtain maximum mediastinal

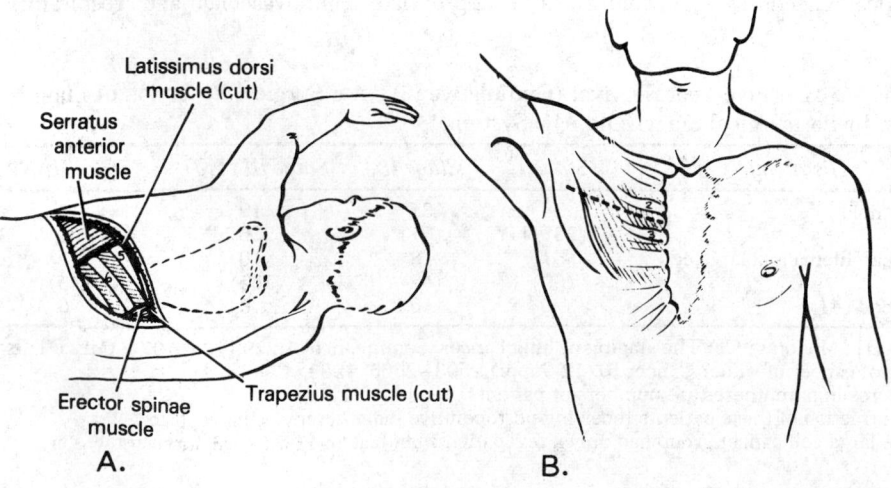

FIG. 22-13. **A.** Posterolateral thoracotomy incision for pulmonary resection. **B.** Anterior thoracotomy incision used for pulmonary resection.

Latissimus dorsi muscle (cut)

Serratus anterior muscle

Erector spinae muscle

Trapezius muscle (cut)

A.

B.

exposure, and left lower-lobe resection may be difficult in obese individuals. Moreover, the median sternotomy incision cannot be used for resection of superior sulcus tumors or of posterior chest wall extensions. Finally, nodal sampling is compromised, especially access to the posterior subcarinal nodes.

DISSECTION, LIGATION, AND DIVISION OF PULMONARY VESSELS. Once the chest has been opened, the tumor and nodal basins must be assessed for resectability. Examination of the tumor will give an idea regarding the need for lobectomy, pneumonectomy, or sleeve resection. Palpation of the lesion should be performed, noting the position of the tumor with regard to the interlobar fissures and its proximity to the bronchovascular structures. Preoperative bronchoscopy will give the surgeon an idea of the proximal extent of the tumor with regard to its nearness to the carina. Intraoperative palpation and direct examination will reveal discrepancies from the preoperative findings if the tumor is densely adherent to the side wall of the main bronchus at a level higher than suspected from the preoperative bronchoscopy. The surgeon must then decide whether this T_3 lesion will require tracheal sleeve resection to remove it in its entirety (if a sleeve option is available) or if pneumonectomy at the level of the carina will suffice. The character and location of the nodal basins must be carefully investigated. Hilar nodes can be examined rapidly by sweeping back the pleura medially; subaortic and anterior mediastinal areas are palpated on the left, whereas paratracheal and azygous nodes are examined on the right.

Contiguous involvement of the pericardium, chest wall, or, rarely, the diaphragm must be assessed with regard to the ability to remove areas of invasion en bloc. When the hilum is difficult to evaluate, the pericardium can be opened for rapid examination of the pulmonary veins as well as the main pulmonary artery. This maneuver is critical when there is initial indecision regarding pulmonary artery involvement with tumor, because dissection without proximal control could lead to uncontrollable hemorrhage.

Once it is determined that the tumor is resectable, resection is accomplished in the most conservative manner that allows total tumor extirpation. The use of the stapling device has revolutionized pulmonary resection in all phases of the operation. Fissure division can be accomplished with the GIA stapling self-dividing device. The use of vascular staples can accomplish secure closure of the main pulmonary artery without suture reinforcement as well as division of the pulmonary veins; arterial division, however, is usually accomplished with the stapling device more easily in pneumonectomies than in lobectomies, necessitating double-ligation techniques for lobar arterial division with nonabsorbable suture ligature. Bronchial closure with the 4.8-mm stapler has been associated with a significantly lower incidence of bronchopleural fistula, yet the basic principle of maintaining a short bronchial stump without devascularization by nodal dissection must be upheld. Most surgeons prefer reinforcing the bronchial stump closure with a flap of mediastinal pleura, pericardium, or intercostal muscle pedicle flap, especially after right-sided pneumonectomy.

Careful intraoperative lymph node dissection and mapping must be performed in any resection for lung cancer and necessitates sampling of (at least) the paratracheal, subcarinal, hilar, and bronchopulmonary nodes. These nodes should be reported using the nomenclature for classification of pulmonary and mediastinal lymph nodes developed by the AJC.[380] Once the resection is completed, including lymph node dissection and sampling, the bronchus should be inspected and tested for air leak by sequentially subjecting it to airway pressures up to 40 cm H_2O. Any air leak should be repaired or the area reinforced.

Intraoperative measures aimed to decrease postoperative pain include intercostal blocks, yet these will last only 6 to 12 hours and will not block visceral pain or pain referred to the shoulder from the diaphragm. Placement of intercostal catheters for drug administration after surgery along four or five interspaces has had favorable results with regard to analgesia and improved pulmonary mechanics.[559] Other analgesic techniques include epidural local anesthetics, cryosurgery of intercostal nerves, or use of transcutaneous electrical nerve stimulation.[560]

The closure of the chest after pneumonectomy is performed without chest drainage; however, the mediastinum and intrathoracic pressures must be balanced by removing just enough air from the chest to establish a negative intrapleural pressure. After lobar or wedge resection, two intrapleural catheters are placed, one anteriorly for drainage of air and the other anteriorly for drainage of fluid. These are connected to closed underwater seal drainage and removed when they are no longer functional or when drainage of pleural fluid is less than 200 ml per 24 hours in the absence of a bronchopleural fistula.

Modern-day Mortality Rates After Pulmonary Resection

The majority of reports on 30-day operative mortality rate for the resection of lung cancer have been based on surgical series over the past 10 to 25 years, reporting rates of 2.1% to 12.4%.[561-566] With improvement in preoperative evaluation as outlined above, along with improvement in anesthetic techniques, the mortality rate for resectional surgery has decreased. Two recent reports, one from the LCSG and the other from a large university experience, have verified the lower death rates.[567,568] Between 1979 and 1981, 2200 resections for lung cancer were performed (1508 lobectomies, 569 pneumonectomies, and 143 lesser procedures) by the LCSG with mortality rates of 2.9%, 6.2%, and 1.4%, respectively. Three strata of risk according to the age of the patients were identified: patients under the age of 60 have a minimal risk (1.3%), those between 60 and 69 have a moderate risk (4.1%), and those 70 or older have a significant risk (7.1%), although in 85 patients over 70 years of age, the operative mortality rate was 5.9%. The most common causes of death following pulmonary resection were postoperative pneumonia and respiratory failure, bronchopleural fistula and empyema, myocardial infarction, and pulmonary embolus. In the university series covering the years 1972 to 1984, 19 of 476 patients (4.0%) died within the 30-day postoperative period. Risk factors included age greater than 60 years (7.4% versus 2.4%), extent of resection with pneumonectomy having an 11.7% mortality rate, and cardiac status as indicated by the presence of premature ventricular contractions. The causes of death were similar to those reported by the LCSG. Because of the greater number of pneumonectomies in the LCSG group, their lower mortality rate is probably more representative of modern-day standards. The causes of death during the immediate postoperative period include pulmonary thromboembolism (20%), myocardial infarction (24%), pneumonia and empyema (18%), bleeding (11%), and respiratory insufficiency (20%).

Specific Surgical Situations and Results

THE SOLITARY PULMONARY NODULE. Any patient in the lung cancer age group, particularly one who is a smoker, with an indeterminant nodular lung lesion, however small, on chest roentgenography that is undiagnosed by other methods should undergo thoracotomy. The Veterans Administration and Armed Services Hospitals (VA-ASH) conducted a combined study of asymptomatic solitary pulmonary nodules less than 6 cm in diameter;[569] considering all ages, 35% of the nodules were proved to be malignant, and 86% of these were primary bronchogenic carcinomas. In patients over 50 years of age, 56% of the nodules were malignant.

This same principle holds true in patients with suspected but unconfirmed pulmonary malignancies appearing different from a nodule. In a series of 303 patients over a 10-year period who did not have a diagnosis prior to thoracotomy but were suspected to have lung carcinoma, 102 had lobectomy, of whom 69% were found to have carcinoma.[570] However, a significant number of patients who appear preoperatively to have only a lung cancer nodule actually have disseminated disease, and the 5-year survival rate in patients with primary cancer in the VA-ASH study was only 38%.

OCCULT LUNG CANCER. "Occult" lung cancer describes the situation where sputum cytology examination is either diagnostic or highly suggestive of cancer but chest roentgenography and ear, nose, and throat examination reveal no lesion, and the patient has no history of aerodigestive cancer. The problem is to localize the lesion for definitive treatment. This is done by repeat bronchoscopic and ear, nose, and throat examinations and, often, selective bronchial washings.

The largest series of patients with roentgenographically occult lung cancer is an outgrowth of the Mayo Lung Project.[571] Fifty-four patients were found to have abnormal findings on sputum cytology, and all tumors were located by bronchoscopy requiring a mean of 1.5 examinations either by direct vision or by selective washings. All patients had complete resection. Nine (17%) were found to have N1 disease, and the overall 5-year survival rate was 74%. The continued follow-up of these patients is as important as the initial localization. In fact, a second cancer developed in 12 patients (22%), of which 11 were second primary lung cancers. Because of the possibility of second lesions, resection of the smallest amount of pulmonary tissue compatible with tumor extirpation should be considered. Interestingly, all of the patients in whom the lung cancer was not visible endoscopically had no evidence of extrabronchial invasion or metastatic involvement of lymph nodes. This subset of patients may be candidates for photodynamic therapy, and, in fact, long term survival has been reported in this situation. Patients in whom the cancer is seen, however, will have a 23% chance of metastatic involvement of regional lymph nodes and should be treated by conventional surgical resection.

T1-2N0M0 AND T1N1M0 DISEASE. To discuss current results of resection, the T1-2N0M0 and T1N1M0 categories should be considered separately, where formerly they were lumped together as Stage I disease. The LCSG has been able to analyze the prognostic factors in 392 patients with resected non-small cell cancer, and comment on freedom from recurrent lung cancer as well as the long-term survival. Patients with T1N0 squamous cell carcinoma had an 89% 3-year survival rate, whereas those with nonsquamous cell disease (adenocarcinoma and large cell carcinoma) in the same stage has a 79% 3-year survival rate.[572] This compares favorably with the 90% 3-year survival rate for 128 T1N0M0 patients from MSKCC.[573] For larger T2 lesions, survival was poorer. From the LCSG series, 73% of T2N0 patients with squamous histology were alive at 3 years compared with 65% of those with non-squamous histology. In the MSKCC series, a similar decrease in survival with T2 lesions (80%) compared with T1N0 lesions was noted. When death rates were compared in patients with N1 disease in the LCSG series, patients with non-squamous T1N1 disease had a significantly poorer 3-year survival rates than those with squamous histologies (55% versus 88%), and the presence of N1 disease seemed to have a greater impact on survival than the size of the primary lesion. A recent prospective analysis of 199 early-stage (T1-2 N0-1) patients also confirms the importance of N1 disease on survival, with no significant difference (72% versus 62%) in 2-year survival rates for T1N0 and T2N0 patients; patients with N1 disease had a 34% 2-year survival rate.[574]

CANCER RECURRENCE AFTER CURATIVE RESECTION. The presence of N1 disease also correlated with a higher risk of recurrence in the LCSG report, as did the presence of visceral pleural invasion.[572] Iascone and associates report that 64% of patients with resected N0 disease will be free of recurrence, compared with 19% of patients with resected N1 disease, at 5 years.[575] This has also been seen in a series from the Mayo Clinic, where the 5-year rates of freedom from recurrence after resection of T1N0, T2N0, and T1N1 disease were 70%, 58%, and 32%, respectively.[576] The overall rate of recurrence of cancer was 8.6% per year of observation and ranged from 15% the first year to 2.3% in the seventh or greater postoperative year. Fifty-six percent of the recurrences were distant metastases, and 26% of the cancers detected represented new primary lung cancers. A similar rate of 32% development of second primary cancers after resection of Stage I disease has been reported from MSKCC.[573] The management of second primary lung cancers should be resection, if possible, and will be discussed in a later section.

Overall Conclusions: Stage I Disease

The following conclusions can be arrived at concerning Stage I disease:

1. Stage I disease (T1-2N0M0) determined by postoperative pathologic staging is associated with 80% to 90% long-term survival rates following surgical resection.
2. Patients with Stage I disease are at great (20% to 30%) risk for the development of second primary lung cancers and need close surveillance.
3. The shift of the T1-2N1M0 category from Stage I to Stage II appears justified because of the poorer survival and increased recurrence rates in this group.

Results of Surgical Resection with Higher-Stage Disease: T3 Lesions and Mediastinal Nodal Positivity (N2 Disease)

The results of surgical resection in patients with Stage III lung cancer are disappointing, and many oncologists and thoracic surgeons feel that patients with such disease, as demonstrated by preoperative studies, are not candidates for surgical resection. In a noninvestigational situation, these patients are referred for radiotherapy or chemotherapy. There are reports in the literature of subsets of Stage III patients who may be curable, but, there is no consensus in the surgical community about how to identify this subset. The following sections represent an attempt by the authors to do this.

T3 DISEASE. The heterogeneous nature of T3 lesions, ranging from contiguous invasion of resectable mediastinal structures to proximity to the carina, makes it difficult for large series of such patients to be identified and analyzed independent of lymph node involvement. Mountain reported a series of 69 patients with either T3N0 or N1 disease who were felt to have had complete resection as defined by the encompassing of all gross disease, negative margins, freedom from tumor of the most distal node, and intact nodal capsules.[577] Although adjuvant chemotherapy was used in certain patients and could have played a role in survival, the 43% 5-year survival rate for squamous cell carcinomas and 23% rate for adenocarcinomas were excellent. Patients with tumor within 2 cm of the carina were treated by tracheobronchial resection and reconstruction, and those with chest wall involvement had en bloc chest wall resection with the tumor. The survival of 25 patients with chest wall resection was 35% at 5 years in this series. Although the majority of recurrences in these patients were distant, the T3 lesion also had a high rate of local recurrence, even without N2 involvement.

TRACHEAL SLEEVE PNEUMONECTOMY. In-continuity tracheal resection for large T3 lesions involving the trachea (tracheal sleeve pneumonectomy) has recently been popularized by various groups. DesLauriers and coworkers have published a large series involving tracheal sleeve pneumonectomies for patients with right and left upper-lobe tumors extending to the lower lateral tracheal wall[578] and thus unresectable by standard definition. Patients with mediastinal nodal positivity were not operated on. Five-year survival rates of 15% to 23% have been reported.[579] These operations were accomplished with jet ventilation via selective bronchial catheter placement. A high operative mortality rate (27%) was seen in these patients but was comparable to that in a similar series of patients with sleeve resection reported by Jensik and associates.[580] The most common cause of death was contralateral lung infection with respiratory failure, and long-term survivors usually had squamous cell tumors.

INTRATHORACIC ORGAN AND CHEST WALL INVOLVEMENT. Recent reports from the Mayo Clinic and MSKCC of the surgical and survival implications of invasion of intrathoracic structures by lung cancer emphasize the efficacy of extended resection and indicate that overall survival is influenced by nodal status, completeness of the resection, and, possibly, the age of the patient.[581-583] The importance of complete resection is stressed. In the absence of lymph node metastases, the depth of chest wall invasion does not significantly affect survival provided a complete resection is performed with negative microscopic margins. The 5-year actuarial survival rate was 54%: 56% in those patients without lymph node metastases and 21% in those with nodal metastases. The Mayo series also noted an improved survival rate for patients younger than 60 years of age. Operative mortality was tolerable at 4% to 12%.

The use of extrapleural versus full-thickness chest wall resection is controversial; however, with the low mortality rate of chest wall removal, as well as better methods of chest wall reconstruction either with muscle or with Marlex or Goretex sheets, the Mayo group urges chest wall resection and in fact found a survival advantage of full-thickness versus extrapleural resection. Despite higher morbidity (25%) than in standard resections, the Mayo group also feels that if complete resection can be performed, extended resection can be applied to other intrathoracic structures including the pericardium, phrenic or vagus nerve, left atrium, superior vena cava, and diaphragm. The role of the adjuvant therapy after chest wall resection is unanswered but is the subject of a LCSG randomized protocol.

MEDIASTINAL NODAL POSITIVITY (N2 DISEASE). The adverse prognostic implications of mediastinal nodal positivity in patients with lung cancer is pronounced, with only 25% of patients with N2 disease who undergo a "curative resection" alive at 5 years (Table 22-38). Resection strategies in this situation differ among surgeons, and several ways have been used to classify N2 disease morphologically, microscopically, and anatomically. It is only recently, with the use of mediastinoscopy for evaluation of disease, that the impact of the timing of the discovery of N2 positivity (i.e., preresection versus at the time of thoracotomy) has become important. A detailed discussion of these subsets of N2 disease is presented in light of the ISS system of lung cancer, which would identify patients with ipsilateral mediastinal node and subcarinal node involvement as N2, placing them in Stage III, a category with a greater likelihood

TABLE 22-38. Five-Year Survival Rate (%) of Lung Cancer Patients with Resected N2 Disease

Year	Histology	No. of Patients	5-Year Survival
1972[584]	Squamous	110	37
	Adenocarcinoma	76	20
1977[585]		56	28.5
1978[586]	Squamous	110	29.5
	Adenocarcinoma	95	16.7
1982[587]		141	24
1983[588]	Squamous	46	26
	Adenocarcinoma	94	34
	Large cell	11	10
1983[589]		181	
	Squamous		24.2
	Adenocarcinoma		14.3
1984[577]	Squamous	36	39
	Adenocarcinoma	51	14
1985[590]	Squamous	43	48
	Adenocarcinoma	51	14
1987[574]		370	25
Overall totals		1741	
	All histologies		26
	Squamous		33
	Nonsquamous		21

of 5-year survival compared with other sites of mediastinal node involvement.[381]

Influence of Primary Neoplasm Histology. In most reports of large series of patients who have had resection in the face of mediastinal node positivity, the importance of the primary tumor's histology has been emphasized, with patients with squamous cancer having better survival rates than those with adenocarcinoma or large cell carcinoma[574,577] (Table 22-38). It is probably reasonable to say that the prognosis after resection of large cell carcinoma in patients with N2 disease is worse than that of epidermoid or adenocarcinoma, whereas squamous histology may be more favorable than adenocarcinoma after resection of mediastinal nodes.

Primary Tumor Status. The size of the primary tumor as well as its location or invasion of contiguous structures seems to influence the long-term survival of patients who have undergone resection with N2 mediastinal nodes. Patients with T1N2 lesions have a greater survival rate than those with T2 or T3N2 disease.[586,591-593] In the study by Martini's group, survival was related to the size of the tumor as assessed after resection:[588] a better survival rate was noted in patients with small tumors (T1; 41% 5-year survival) than in those with large tumors (T2; 32% survival) or with extension outside the lung (T3; 29% survival), yet tumor size did not correlate with the number of levels of nodal involvement or with the location of the involved nodes. Naruke and coworkers likewise found significant decreases in survival as T stage increased with N2 positivity: 27.3% 5-year survival in T1, 18% in T2, and 0 in T4.[586,589]

Location or Level of the N2 Nodes. Naruke and coworkers were among the first to perform extensive lymph node mapping, such that levels of nodal involvement as well as the number of levels involved could be reported consistently.[586] This mapping is now a crucial element for all resections, regardless of the stage of the disease resected. It becomes even more crucial when different institutions belong to a cooperative group such as the LCSG and must standardize the reporting of nodal positivity, levels of nodes involved, and whether multiple levels are involved in any prognostic implications are to be investigated (Fig. 22-14).

Naruke's group found significantly decreased 5-year survival rates in patients who had positive subcarinal nodes compared with those with negative subcarinal nodes (9.1% versus 29%). Those authors found no significant difference in prognosis between patients with and without metastases to the superior mediastinal lymph nodes, tracheobronchial lymph nodes, or subaortic and para-aortic lymph nodes. This poor prognosis of subcarinal lymph node metastases probably stems from the high percentage of contralateral mediastinal node metastases.[586] Pearson and associates noted no

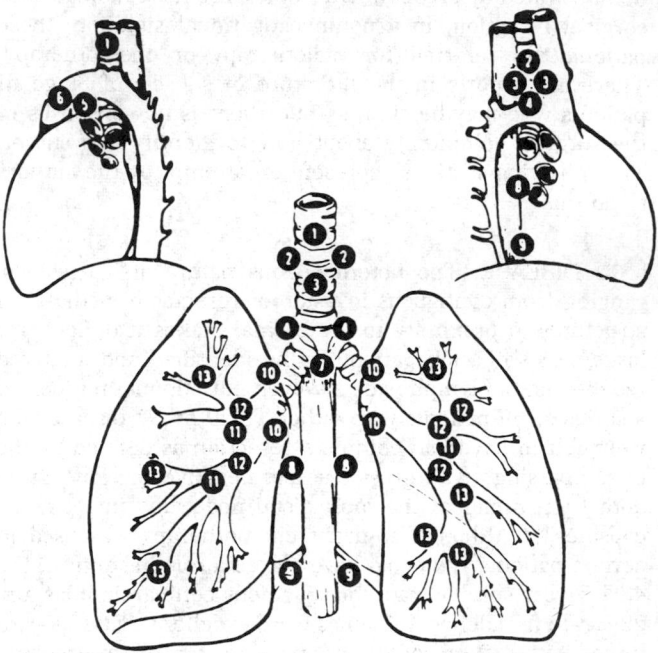

FIG. 22-14. Lymph node map showing mediastinal (N2) and hilar lobar nodes (N1) (see text for details).

N2 Nodes
● Superior Mediastinal Nodes
  1. Highest Mediastinal
  2. Upper Paratracheal
  3. Pre- and Retrotracheal
  4. Lower Paratracheal
    (including Azygos Nodes)

● Aortic Nodes
  5. Subaortic (aortic window)
  6. Para-aortic (ascending aorta or phrenic)

● Inferior Mediastinal Nodes
  7. Subcarinal
  8. Paraesophageal (below carina)
  9. Pulmonary Ligament

N1 Nodes
10. Hilar
11. Interlobar
12. Lobar
13. Segmental

5-year survivors among patients with metastases to the highest paratracheal level.[587-590] Martini and coworkers found that 5-year survival was significantly poorer in patients with subcarinal node positivity compared with those with tumor in other lymph node stations (18% versus 34%, respectively).[588] Contrary to Pearson's findings, patients with involved nodes in the upper paratracheal region had no significant difference in survival from those without upper node positivity (25% versus 30%). The extent of lymph node involvement affected survival, with those patients with involvement at only one level doing better at 3 years than those with more than one positive level. At 5 years, however, the survival advantage of single-level positivity was less pronounced. A recent report from the Toronto group emphasizes the ability to obtain long-term survival in patients with isolated subaortic lymph node positivity (28%), with an even greater survival rate at 5 years if the resection is complete (42%).[594] The report excluded patients with tumor in other nodal sites.

Contralateral nodal positivity at this time is really the only agreed upon objective finding that would contraindicate exploration for resection. Some surgeons, on the basis of the above findings, believe that the presence of any positive mediastinal node, even ipsilateral, is a contraindication to resection, whereas others feel that in the presence of "favorable histology" (squamous) and easily resectable cancer confined to ipsilateral nodes, a resection should be performed. Other groups feel that independent of the level of nodal positivity, N2 positivity detected prior to thoracotomy mandates preoperative adjuvant treatment with resection if the patient has an objective response. This approach, in the authors' opinion, remains investigational.

Intranodal Versus Perinodal Disease. An important prognostic factor that is insufficiently emphasized in the analysis of mediastinal nodal positivity is the implication of microscopic disease confined to the lymph node without breaching of the capsule (intranodal) disease versus that in which tumor cells have escaped from the confines of the lymph node (perinodal or internodal disease). Perinodal involvement can be evident at the time of mediastinoscopy or at thoracotomy and can be subtle or associated with masses of contiguous lymph node groups with fixation and invasion of mediastinal structures. A series of studies show a significant survival advantage for patients with intranodal rather than perinodal mediastinal lymph node involvement.[591,595,596] The relative weight of intracapsular as opposed to extracapsular disease, however, has not been submitted to the necessary multivariate analysis to see if it functions as an independent predictor of survival distinguishable from the level of lymph node involvement, histology of the tumor, or completeness of resection.

Prognostic Implications of Mediastinal Lymph Node Involvement Found at Mediastinoscopy or at Thoracotomy

In patients with suspicious mediastinal lesions on chest roentgenography or CT scan who are otherwise good candidates for thoracotomy with possible resection, the use of mediastinoscopy is gaining popularity. In 1982, Pearson and associates reported a series of 141 mediastinal node-positive patients, all of whom had preoperative mediastinoscopy.[587] Of those, 79 patients were found to have tumorous nodes by mediastinoscopy. In all patients, the mediastinoscopic findings were correlated with thoracotomy findings. In the mediastinoscopy-negative group, 40% were able to undergo operation with curative intent. In contrast, only 15% of the positive-mediastinoscopy group were able to have curative resection. A significant difference in long-term survival was also seen between the two groups, with the 5-year survival rate being 9% for all cases of mediastinoscopy-positive patients and 24% for the patients with positive nodes found at surgery. In total, over 17 years, Pearson's group found that the group of mediastinal lymph node-positive patients able to undergo a complete resection represented only 4% of all patients. Thus, preoperative mediastinoscopy is extremely useful in identifying both those patients able to undergo a potentially curable resection and those likely to be cured by such a procedure.

Intraoperative Decision-making with Regard to Resecting Positive Mediastinal Nodes and Overall Conclusions

If the primary lesion can be extirpated by appropriate resection without impairing postoperative respiratory reserve or performed without undue mortality and morbidity, then the decision becomes limited by the extent of nodal involvement. A conservative approach would be to perform radical lymphadenectomy along with the pulmonary resection if the nodal disease is intranodal, regardless of the number of lymph node levels involved. In contrast, extranodal bulky disease, which might upgrade the necessary resection to a pneumonectomy without assuring curative intent, is associated with higher mortality and complication rates and offers no survival advantage. The real challenge, however, is in the prediction of those patients who will not benefit from thoracotomy prior to having to make these difficult intraoperative decisions. The authors believe that only by performing mediastinoscopy in all patients with the slightest suspicion of preoperative mediastinal abnormalities will such a uniform database be compiled. Once patients are found to have N2 disease on mediastinoscopy, they probably are best served by radiotherapy or enrollment in prospective trials studying multimodality therapy, such as neoadjuvant programs performed in a prospective randomized fashion.

Special Surgical Situations

PARENCHYMA-SPARING PROCEDURES. There has been increasing interest in lung-sparing resections, especially in older patients with compromised pulmonary function, patients with synchronous or second primary lung cancers, and patients whose primary tumors could be removed by a more limited procedure. There are two schools of thought with regard to elective resections in good-risk patients. First, some surgeons believe that the anatomic boundaries of lobectomy are arbitrary and that the patient should have the least amount of parenchyma removed. In their opinion, the removal of excess lung tissue will not affect long-term survival. The other school points to the increase in the local recurrence rate in patients with lesser resections, as well as the reported increase in operative morbidity from segmental resection. Iascone and associates, reviewing a series of patients with N0 and N1 disease who had been treated by lobectomy or pneumonectomy, reported local recurrence rates of 26% and 18%, respectively, arguing for even more aggressive resection in early-stage disease.[575]

The chief proponent of conservative resection is Jensik, who has reported a series of 467 segmental-type resections over a 26-year period, 274 in Stage I or II disease, 123 in Stage III cancer, and 70 in patients with a previous pulmonary resection.[597] Cumulative survival rates for the early-stage patients were 55% at 5 years, 27% at 10 years, and 21% at 15 years, which compare favorably with the results of standard resection. In the patients reoperated on, survival at 5 and 10 years after the second thoracotomy was 33% and 20%, respectively. Various segments were resected, the most frequent of which were the superior segments of the lower lobes, the anterior segment of the right upper lobe, and the superior division of the left upper lobe. The most common complication was persistent air leak (8%), some of which necessitated completion lobectomy, management of empyema, or changing of the chest tubes. The perioperative mortality rate was 1% for patients with Stage I or II disease, 4% for those with Stage III disease, and 6% for those with previous resection. Local recurrence was seen in 12%.

In another series of 197 patients with Stage I disease treated over a 17-year period, 100 received lobectomy, whereas 97 received wedge resection with lymph node sampling because of inferior preoperative pulmonary function.[598] Perioperative mortality (3% versus 2.1%) and morbidity were comparable in the two groups, and differences in 2-year (72% versus 74%) and 6-year survival (69% versus 75%) rates were not statistically significant. Unfortunately, recurrence patterns were not analyzed in detail in this study.

However, McCormack and Martini in a series of 61 patients undergoing segmentectomy or wedge resection for T1N0 or T2N0 lesions, reported a recurrence within the same lobe in 19% of the patients.[599] The perioperative mortality rate was acceptable (3.7%); the 5-year survival rate was lower than in the other series (50%). Their results with the use of lobectomy for Stage I disease (not performed as a prospective, randomized comparison with the wedge/segmentectomy group) were significantly better, with a 5-year survival rate of 72% and no local recurrences except for three patients developing regional lymph node metastases. Of this group of 135 patients who had lobectomies, 15 (11%) developed a second primary lung cancer, which is very close to the figure reported by Jensik. Currently, the LCSG is conducting a prospective randomized comparison of conservative resection and standard lobectomy or pneumonectomy in Stage I disease. Until the results of this trial are completed, either approach appears warranted.

SYNCHRONOUS LUNG CANCERS. If a preoperative evaluation indicates no evidence of an extrapulmonary source of malignancy or of extrapulmonary metastases, the appearance of two lesions strongly suggests synchronous lung cancers, the incidence of which is reported to be 1% to 7%.[600] If the CT evaluation reveals negative mediastinal nodes, evaluation for an extrathoracic primary lesion is indicated, including intravenous urography and a gastrointestinal series. Suspicious CT nodes must be confirmed by mediastinoscopy. If the mediastinal nodes are positive for tumor, the survival rate of the patients is so poor as not to warrant resection. In patients with two lesions on the same side (often located in separate lobes), pneumonectomy is the operation of choice. If pulmonary functions are limiting, lobectomy and wedge resection can be performed. In patients with lesions in both lungs, median sternotomy or staged thoracotomies can be performed. Segmental resection beginning with the most advanced lesion is done; preservation of lung tissue without compromise of the cancer resection is critical, but mediastinal or nodal dissection must be performed. Median survival for patients with resected synchronous Stage I cancers is 25 to 27 months and 11 months for those with Stage II or III cancers.

SECOND AND THIRD PRIMARY LUNG CANCERS. A 10% incidence of second bronchogenic lung cancers has been reported by the Mayo Clinic, which agrees with the reports of Jensik and Martini (see previous section).[597,599] Mathisen and colleagues defined the criteria for a second lung cancer as one of a histologic cell type different from the previous primary, a long interval between resections (metachronous tumors), location of the new lesion in the contralateral lung or a different ipsilateral lobe, or the presence of synchronous bilateral tumor.[601] Over a 23-year period, 90 patients met these criteria in those authors' series, of which 10 were synchronous lung cancers.

The majority of patients with second primary lung cancers will be asymptomatic, and the lesion will be discovered at the time of follow-up for their first cancer. The mean interval between the first and second cancers is 46 months, and the secondary or tertiary lesions can be handled with equal frequency by segmentectomy, lobectomy, sleeve lobectomy, pneumonectomy, or completion pneumonectomy. Survival was the worst in patients with synchronous cancers, whereas the 5- and 10-year survival rates for patients with metachronous tumor are 33% and 20%. Patients whose disease-free interval between separate tumors is greater than 3 years have significantly longer survival than those with shorter intervals. According to the Mathisen's group, the ability to salvage these patients over the long run is related to an initial conservative resection.

SLEEVE LOBECTOMY. The concept of segmental bronchial resection encompassing the involved main bronchial or tracheal segment in continuity with the involved lobe followed by reanastomosis of the bronchus in order to preserve pulmonary tissue is not new. The operation was popularized by Price Thomas,[602] Paulson and Shaw,[603] and Johnston and Jones[604] in the 1950s. The use of the operation in lung cancer resection is based on the anatomic principle that there is lymphatic drainage of the upper lobe to the ipsilateral hilar and low paratracheal areas, and the majority of resections performed involve tumors at the orifice of the right upper lobe. Weisel and coworkers reported 5- and 8-

year survival rates of 43% and 30% in patients with Stage I disease subjected to sleeve resection, with 31% (5-year) and 15% (8-year) survival in Stage II disease.[605] A review by Lowe and colleagues found an overall 5-year survival rate of 33% and a 10-year rate of 21%.[606]

The operation may be considered as an alternative to pneumonectomy if the tumor is centrally located and small and if it is anatomically possible to perform anastomosis with curative intent. Sleeve lobectomy also can serve as a limited resection in a patient with compromised pulmonary function. The procedure has been described with concomitant sleeve or patching of the ipsilateral pulmonary artery, and the presence of positive interlobar nodes is no longer considered a contraindication to its performance.[607] The operative mortality rate ranges from 0 to 7% in modern series,[608] chiefly from hemorrhage and bronchial anastomotic dehiscence. The latter complication can usually be prevented by wrapping the anastomosis with a pleural flap, but the chief factor is a meticulously performed air-tight anastomosis (Fig. 22-15). Postoperative atelectasis requires the liberal use of bronchoscopy to remove secretions, and bronchoscopy should be performed intraoperatively to assure removal of blood from the lung. The advent of double-lumen catheter anesthesia with reliably placed disposable tubes has also increased the use of sleeve lobectomy. Finally, late bronchial anastomotic stricture can usually be prevented with the use of absorbable suture material.

Local recurrence rates remain a problem with sleeve lobectomy, ranging from 7% to 16% in the literature.[605,608,609] This problem is usually related to nodal disease; a high anastomotic recurrence rate should be avoided by the compulsive use of frozen-section evaluation of the bronchial margins to assure completeness of resection (Fig. 22-15).

Complications of Pulmonary Resection

The primary complications of pulmonary resection have already been mentioned in previous sections. *Hemorrhage* is rare but can be from any site in the operative field, including the bronchovascular structures or the incision. Hemorrhage in excess of 100 ml per hour for 4 hours should alert the surgeon to check the patient's coagulation functions; if these are normal, mechanical bleeding necessitating reoperation is suggested. Patency of the pleural tubes must be maintained to prevent intrathoracic clot formation, which, if not drained, increases the chance of empyema or late fibrothorax with lung entrapment.

Pulmonary insufficiency is usually seen in patients with marginal pulmonary function and poor performance status prior to the operation. Positive-pressure ventilation with appropriate diuresis as well as optimizing cardiac output with guidance from a Swan-Ganz catheter is essential to reverse the insufficiency. These patients will also require nutritional support via enteral or intravenous alimentation while receiving respiratory support to try to prevent further muscle catabolism and inability to generate sufficient respiratory mechanics for ventilation. When secretions become a limiting factor and prevent safe extubation, the use of tracheostomy should be considered early in the patient's postoperative course. Vigorous clearing of airway secretions must be performed and cultures taken in order to guide antibiotic management of pneumonitis.

Management of *cardiac arrhythmia* will require treatment of pulmonary resection-induced atrial and ventricular tachyarrhythmias, management of hypokalemia, and digitalization. Patients with a cardiac disease history should have optimization of systemic blood pressure and volume management to prevent undue increases in myocardial oxygen requirements. This may necessitate the use of preload-reducing agents such as nitroglycerin or afterload reduction with nitroprusside.

A postoperative chest roentgenogram is examined to document complete expansion of the residual or contralateral lung, especially after pneumonectomy, to rule out *contralateral pneumothorax* or *inadequate expansion* secondary to the use of double-lumen catheter anesthesia. *Persistent air leakage* after pulmonary resection, either by lobectomy or segmentectomy, will usually respond to tube drainage with underwater seal suction. Expansion of the residual lung with adhesion formation will usually obliterate these peripheral bronchopleural fistulae.

Empyema after lobar resection can be treated with tube

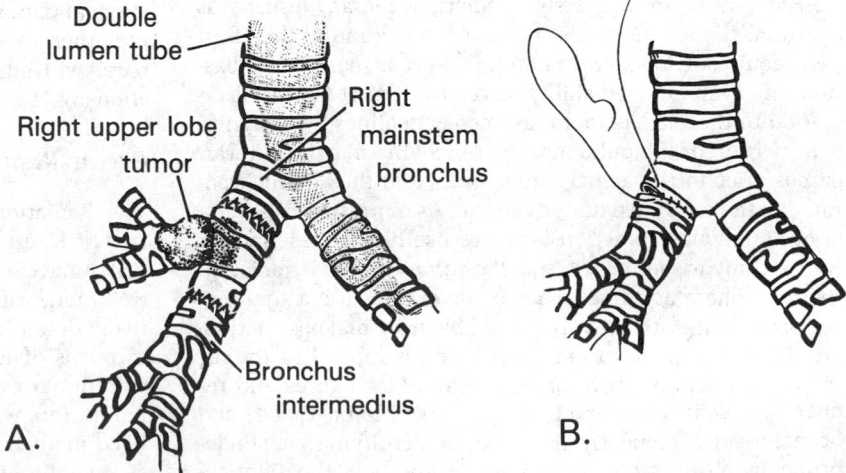

FIG. 22-15. Sleeve lobectomy, right upper lobe. **A.** Double-lumen anesthesia is used and the incision made in the right main-stem bronchus and the bronchus intermedius. **B.** The bronchus intermedius is anastomosed to the right main-stem bronchus after ensuring negative margins by frozen section analysis for tumor during surgery.

Double lumen tube

Right upper lobe tumor

Right mainstem bronchus

Bronchus intermedius

A.

B.

drainage and antibiotics. However, empyema after pneumonectomy, with or without associated bronchopleural fistula, remains the most morbid complication in these patients. Early empyema without associated bronchopleural fistula has been treated successfully with early catheter irrigation of the postpneumonectomy space either with iodine-containing solutions alone or with systemic antibiotics, but success with this technique is the exception rather than the rule. Most postpneumonectomy empyemas must be treated with early tube drainage to evacuate the space, with subsequent rib resection and conversion to open thoracostomy with irrigation of the cavity with bacteriostatic solutions when the mediastinum has stabilized. Closure of the thoracostomy at a later time, when the bacterial colony count is minimal, and institution of triple-antibiotic solution (Clagett's procedure) will succeed approximately 50% of the time. If empyema recurs, space obliteration with either muscle transposition or thoracoplasty will be necessary.

Empyema may signal the presence of a postpneumonectomy bronchopleural fistula and indeed contribute to its development in the early postoperative period. However, the cardinal sign of postpneumonectomy bronchopleural fistula is change in the air–fluid level by chest radiography with increasing amounts of air on the resected side. The acute development of a postpneumonectomy fistula will cause uncontrollable coughing secondary to the flooding of the opposite lung with the contents of the pneumonectomy space. Immediate placement of a chest tube to drain the pneumonectomy space must be performed, and usually the patient also requires tracheal intubation with isolation of the contralateral lung. Early postpneumonectomy fistulas are amenable to repair with a variety of muscle flaps, including those of intercostal muscle, serratus anterior, latissimus dorsi, or pectoralis. These muscle flaps have also made a tremendous impact in the closure of chronic or late-developing fistulae and at the same time can add bulk to the pneumonectomy space to obliterate it further.

RADIOTHERAPEUTIC TREATMENT

Determination of the Ability to Undergo Radical Radiation Therapy for a Cure

Consideration for aggressive radiation therapy usually is based on the extent of disease and the volume of the chest that requires irradiation. Whenever there is massive mediastinal involvement, the ability to restrict the volume of irradiation to the mediastinum and nodes declines, as a significant portion of the pulmonary parenchyma may lie anterior or posterior to the actual tumor mass and thus be incorporated in the irradiated tumor volume. As in presurgical evaluation, pulmonary function tests are useful as a baseline for future comparison, but no specific values preclude radiation therapy. There are times when some of the patient's pulmonary symptoms are actually caused by bronchial obstruction, and in such a patient, radiation therapy applied to the affected area can improve breathing and blood gases and reduce pulmonary symptoms. Midplane tomography and bronchoscopy frequently are useful in identifying such endobronchial obstruction. Unfortunately, the typical patient referred for radiation therapy has extensive disease that requires more than attention to relief of bronchial obstruction. The role of radiotherapy in the treatment of lung cancer has been summarized in several recent reviews.[610–612]

Radiotherapy Administered with Curative Intent

For patients who have non-small cell lung cancer that, after extensive evaluation, appears to be in Stage I or II, surgery is unequivocally the treatment of choice if the patient's underlying pulmonary status and other medical considerations suggest that he or she can tolerate a radical surgical procedure. Unfortunately, Stage I or Stage II disease is seen in only a minority of patients with carcinoma of the lung. In addition, many patients who appear clinically to have Stage I or II disease turn out at surgery to have microscopic involvement of lymph nodes in the mediastinum. Radiation therapy is considered an alternative to surgery for patients who either decline thoracotomy with its attendant risks or those whose underlying pulmonary and other medical problems make surgery excessively risky.[613] There are only limited data on primary radiotherapy in lieu of surgery for resectable disease in operable patients. The reported series from England, in which relatively low (4000–5000-rad) doses were used, suggest that modern high-dose radiotherapy is probably a reasonable approach for patients who decline surgery. Hilton and Smart reported more than 20% of patients surviving more than 5 years after radical radiotherapy for otherwise operable lung cancer.[614,615]

The vast majority of patients with lung cancer of the non-small cell varieties present with Stage III disease that is unresectable. Although it can be debated whether chest radiotherapy should be given to such patients,[615] we believe that in selected patients, it is beneficial in terms of local control (achieved in greater than 60% of patients) and possibility of cure.[616] Stage III patients who have clinically evident mediastinal adenopathy can be considered for curative radiotherapy, with or without surgery, although the long-term survival figures remain poor. Patients with distant metastases or positive supraclavicular nodes generally are not considered for curative radiation treatment. The median survival for patients with unresectable disease undergoing primary radiotherapy is less than 1 year; however, the 5-year survival data show about 6% of patients alive and well with radiotherapy alone (Table 22-39). This should not be compared with surgical results because patients selected for radiation are less favorable cases than those selected for surgery.

Recent Results of Curative Radiotherapy

The Radiation Therapy Oncology Group (RTOG) randomized 551 patients with unresectable or inoperable non-small cell lung cancer to different types of potentially curative treatment with radiation therapy.[617] These studies quantitatively define the limits for state of the art radiation therapy in terms of local tumor control and the need for effective systemic treatment for distant metastases. The intrathoracic failure rate within the irradiated volume varied in a dose-related manner: 48% for 4000 cGy continuous, 38% for 5000 cGy continuous (or 4000 cGy split course), and 27% for

TABLE 22-39. Five-Year Survival Data Following "Curative" Radiotherapy for Patients with Inoperable or Unresectable Lung Cancer

Series	No. of Patients	5-Year Survival (%)
Stanford*	284	6
Columbia†	253	5
Hammersmith‡	513	6
Pennsylvania§	171	6
Finland‖	158	6
Massachusetts General Hospital#	108	7

*Caldwell WL, Bagshaw MA: Cancer 22:999–1004, 1968.

†Guttman RJ: Am J Roentgenol Rad Ther Nucl Med 93:99–103, 1965; Guttman RJ: Carcinoma of the bronchus. In Deeley TJ (ed): Modern Radiotherapy, p 193. New York, Appleton-Century-Crofts, 1971.

‡Deeley TJ, Singh SP: Thorax 22:562–566, 1967.

§Katz HR, Alberts RW: Am J Clin Oncol 6:445–457, 1983.

‖Holsti LR, Mattson K: Int J Rad Oncol Biol Phys 6:977–981, 1980.

#Choi NCH, Doucette JA: Cancer 48:101–109, 1981.

6000 cGy continuous. The failure rate in the nonirradiated lung was 25% to 30% irrespective of the radiation dose. Seventy-five to eighty percent of all the patients developed distant metastases. Brain metastases ultimately occurred in 16% of those with squamous cell carcinomas and 30% of those with adenocarcinoma or large cell carcinoma.

It would clearly be an advantage if chest radiotherapy could be administered more conveniently. Thus, it is of interest that the University of Maryland found no differences in the preliminary analysis of a randomized trial in 100 patients comparing once-a-week radiotherapy (500-rad fractions given to a total dose of 6000 rad) with a 6000-rad total dose administered via 200-rad fractions given conventionally 5 days a week.[618]

When modern results of chest radiotherapy given with or without chemotherapy are compared for elderly (over 70 years) or younger patients, no significant differences are seen,[619] suggesting that older patients should be individually evaluated and, if they have a good performance status, be treated according to physiologic rather than chronologic age.

When curative treatment is planned with radiation, the intention is to take the known tumor volume to midplane doses of 5500 to 6000 rad. If the tumor is relatively small or the location favorable, one may consider boosting a small volume to an even higher dose. The principal concern is the amount of lung parenchyma that will be included within the treatment area. Organs that limit the amount of irradiation that can be applied to the thorax include the lung parenchyma, spinal cord, and heart. The esophagus, although frequently symptomatic from acute desquamation during the course of treatment, usually is not considered a dose-limiting organ in terms of long-term complications. For patients who have no significant degree of COPD, treatment plans may consist of opposing anterior and posterior fields, usually with a 2-cm margin around the entire tumor mass, for approximately 3000 rad before switching to a second treatment plan, which usually consists of an anterior field in conjunction with a posteriorly obliqued field to keep the spinal cord dose well within tolerance limits. In most cases, the entire upper mediastinum is included, whereas the inferior margin typically extends about 6 to 7 cm below the carina in the treatment position. Such treatment plans, which ideally require isocentric planning, have helped to improve dosimetry in these patients (Fig. 22-16). When such tools are available to assist in treatment planning, it is essential not only that the plan be documented at the tumor level, but also that a second treatment plan be obtained at the level of the thoracic inlet, where the chest is comparatively narrow compared with the lower level of the tumor itself. This discrepancy in

FIG. 22-16. **A.** Anterior port used in the treatment. **B.** Response to treatment after 5500 rad. Considerable tumor shrinkage has been achieved with good palliative results in terms of symptoms.

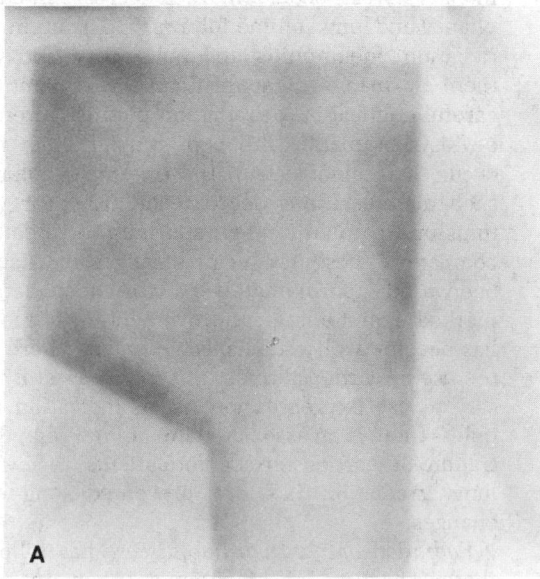

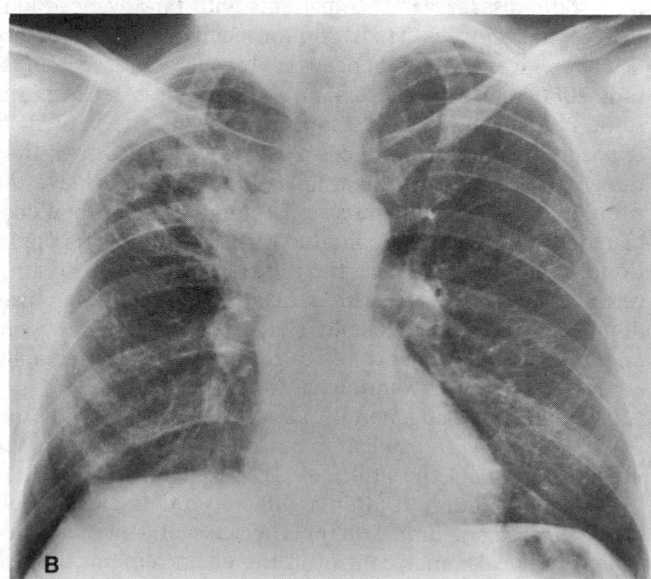

anterior–posterior chest thickness means that the spinal cord dose at the upper level of the treatment volume may be higher than the actual dose being delivered at the tumor level because there is less tissue at the upper level to attenuate the radiation. Knowledge of the exact dose being applied at the upper portion of the chest to the spinal cord will allow appropriate decisions to be made to minimize the dose to the upper thoracic spinal cord. Such consideration and meticulous execution of the dosimetric treatment plan should eliminate any concern about radiation myelitis.

For the patient who has a significant degree of restrictive pulmonary disease, the treatment plan usually is confined to opposing anterior–posterior fields with a spinal cord block inserted posteriorly somewhere between the 3000- and 4000-rad tumor dose to keep the total cord dose below 4500 rad. Such a treatment plan is considered a major compromise from optimal tumor treatment because the block may reduce the tumor dose as well. If possible, it is preferable to reduce the tumor volume at the time of shifting to the obliqued field, but this cannot always be done. Supraclavicular nodes usually are not included within the treatment volume in such patients, in contrast to the more typical patient with unresectable disease, in whom an anterior neck field ordinarily is used to treat the supraclavicular nodes routinely, regardless of their clinical status.

Time, Dose, and Fractionation

With time, dose, and fractionation schemes, the question of split-course treatment versus continuous therapy has been raised. No significant superiority in survival has been achieved by split-course treatment compared with continuous fractionation.[620,621] The case for split-course treatment (approximately 2500 to 3000 rad over 2 weeks followed by 2 to 3 weeks off treatment before a final 2500 to 3000 rad is delivered over 2 to 3 weeks) is predicated on better tolerance, simplicity for integration into combined-modality approaches, and an opportunity to reevaluate patients before their second half of treatment for any new manifestations of metastatic disease.[622-624] In patients with far-advanced lung cancer, once-a-week irradiation for locally advanced disease has been given (500 rad once weekly to a total dose of 6000 rad; 2050 ret) with success. If a tumor mass receives the same number of rad over a longer time with the same daily exposure, biologic differences exist between those two fractionation schemes. In the simplest concept, to achieve the same effect from split-course treatment, a higher total dose of radiation would be required to offset the tumor repopulation that may occur during the time of treatment. The long-term success achieved with radiation therapy alone (predominantly in unresectable Stage III disease or poor operative risks) remains relatively poor with either split-course treatment or continuous fractionation.

The poor survival generally achieved in patients with lung cancer treated with irradiation may have led to unwarranted conclusions about the utility of local control with radiation therapy. In addition, it often is difficult to define accurately the pretreatment tumor volume because of atelectasis and collapse. Local tumor control in the chest remains difficult to determine because of problems in distinguishing subtle differences between radiation changes and tumor on chest films. Inasmuch as metastatic disease has dominated the clinical course of these patients, it has been thought that local recurrence is not a significant problem.[624] This remains to be seen because local recurrence can be slow to manifest itself and certainly would predispose to further metastatic disease.[625]

Clinical Care of Patients During Radiotherapy

Most patients will tolerate daily doses of 200 to 300 rad midplane without significant problems during treatment. Approximately 3 weeks after their treatment has started, dysphagia caused by acute desquamation of the esophageal mucosa appears. This usually will persist (and can be severe in some patients, necessitating an unplanned break) for approximately 2 to 3 weeks after radiation therapy has been completed. Bronchial secretions will be altered by radiation therapy, becoming noticeably more tenacious. A nonproductive cough is common during and after radiation therapy; it may be present for the rest of the patient's life. Frank radiation pneumonitis does not occur during treatment; it is more likely to be seen in the first 1 to 3 months after completion of radiation therapy. Care should be taken to evaluate patients thoroughly before treatment to be sure that incipient obstructive pneumonia is not present. Such a problem may require antibiotics and can delay treatment until it clears, particularly if intensive chemotherapy is planned as part of the treatment.

Long-term Follow-up and Complications

Problems with *radiation pneumonitis* will depend on the dose and volume of lung incorporated within the radiation field.[624] *Pulmonary fibrosis* may take months to years to develop; it can be disabling or even fatal. However, such lethal complications are uncommon. The pathophysiology appears to represent both vascular and parenchymal cell injury. The diffusion capacity is reduced markedly, and interstitial fibrosis of pulmonary septa occurs. Whenever pulmonary fibrosis occurs, marked decrease in pulmonary compliance and lung volume follows.[626] The optimal approach to radiation pneumonitis and pulmonary fibrosis is to avoid them by means of sophisticated treatment planning and careful delineation of radiation portals. Often, patients will be asymptomatic although radiographic manifestations occur that coincide with the treatment volume. Typically, such manifestations decrease or disappear without symptoms or treatment. When shortness of breath or fever accompanies these radiologic changes, corticosteroids have been used; approximately half of the patients will report marked symptomatic improvement.[627] If radiation fibrosis has become well established, however, there is no value in the use of corticosteroids. In severe cases, it may be necessary to use oxygen. There is no indication for antibiotics unless there is an associated infection. Prophylactic administration of corticosteroids to patients receiving large-field lung irradiation has not prevented long-term radiation changes.

Radiation-induced cardiac disease has followed radiation therapy in lung cancer patients. It remains relatively rare, probably because of the short survival times of patients who have this disease. Again, elimination of most of the cardiac silhouette from the high-dose radiation volume avoids this problem for most patients. If the cancer is located close to the heart, this problem may be seen and can be difficult to distinguish from recurrent tumor. Paradoxical pulse may be present if pericardial constriction is present. Echocardiography, cardiac catheterization, and pericardiocentesis may be necessary for diagnostic and therapeutic purposes. Pericardial fluid must be evaluated cytologically to rule out a malignant effusion.

Acute radiation esophagitis usually occurs during treatment but proves self-limited once the mucosa has repopulated. During the acute esophagitis, viscous lidocaine often is helpful. Long-term esophageal problems are relatively rare, although stenosis has been reported occasionally, usually when relatively large (250- to 300-rad) daily fractions have been used. For most patients with this uncommon problem, simple esophageal dilatation will be adequate.

Spinal cord injury should be avoided by careful treatment planning. As noted above, careful delineation of dose distribution within the patient, not only at the level of the tumor but also in the upper thorax, should allow the therapist to avoid this problem. When the patient receives radiation to a posterior oblique field, care must be taken to ensure that the spinal cord is not included within the portal; if the location of the tumor makes the angle of the obliquity such that the spinal cord is included at the upper portion of the portal, an additional block must be inserted to reduce the exposure of the spinal cord.

INTEGRATION OF SURGERY, RADIOTHERAPY, AND CHEMOTHERAPY IN THE PRIMARY TREATMENT OF NON-SMALL CELL LUNG CANCER WITH CURATIVE INTENT

Non-small cell lung cancer accounts for 75% of all lung cancer, and roughly 30% of these patients present with extrathoracic metastatic disease, 30% present with clinical AJC Stage I and II disease and are treated with surgery or radiotherapy as described above, and 40% present clinically or at surgery with N2 (mediastinal) involvement. This group (about 41,000 patients in the United States) represents a significant therapeutic challenge, and many physicians have tried various combinations of surgery and radiotherapy, surgery and chemotherapy, or, recently, all three modalities. Combined-modality treatment appears appropriate for at least some of these patients.

Analysis of the failure patterns of current surgical and radiation treatment of lung cancer has been undertaken.[611,628-630] The results for surgical therapy have been summarized earlier (see Table 22-16).[629] For radiation therapy, 57% of epidermoid cancer patients will have their first failure in the chest area and 44% will have local failure only, whereas 33% will fail distantly and 20% will have distant failure only. For adenocarcinoma and large cell carcinoma, 25% will fail locally (19% local only), and 56% will fail in distant sites (40% distant sites only).[630] These results emphasize the importance of both local control and effective therapy for systemic metastases that are present early in the course of the disease. A significant therapeutic gain in either area would have an immediate impact on the disease.

ADJUVANT THERAPY: PREOPERATIVE, POSTOPERATIVE, AND INTRAOPERATIVE RADIATION THERAPY

Preoperative Radiation Therapy

The use of preoperative radiation therapy in the hope of modifying the survival results in early or locally advanced lung cancer began in the 1950s and has been reviewed by Faber.[631] Bromley and Szur, in a series of 66 patients, found that 47% could be sterilized of tumor, and a minority of patients who were thought to be inoperable could indeed have their disease resected after preoperative radiation therapy.[632] However, a high mortality rate (15%) and excessive rate of empyema and fistula were noted. Bloedorn and associates, in 1960, described similar results in 37 patients, with 46% sterilization of tumor using doses up to 6000 rad.[633] Nevertheless, a prohibitive mortality rate of 22% was noted, with a 5-year survival rate of 20%. Most of the studies that followed were nonrandomized and retrospective and differed in the radiation treatment plans used (Table 22-40). Some of these nonrandomized trials have suggested benefit, whereas others have not.

Randomized trials comparing surgery alone with preoperative radiation therapy followed by surgery have shown no benefit of preoperative radiotherapy (Table 22-40).[640,641] The VA cooperative study, supervised by Shields, randomized more than 300 patients who were all thought to have resectable disease to surgery alone or preoperative irradiation with 4000 to 5000 rad.[640] There was a predominance of squamous cell carcinoma, and most of the patients received pneumonectomy. The 4-year survival rate of the control group was 21% whereas that of the preoperative radiotherapy group was only 13%. Postoperative complications, including bronchopleural fistula, were more frequent in the radiation therapy group. In a 17-hospital collaborative study sponsored by the NCI in 1975 randomizing in excess of 550 patients, similar survival rates were noted for controls (14%) and irradiated patients (16%) at 5 years.[641] Similar smaller studies by Eichorn[642] and Tildon[643] and their coworkers revealed no survival advantage of preoperative radiation therapy in patients with resectable disease, and a randomized trial by Kazem and associates,[644] which revealed a modest survival advantage at 10 years using short-course radiotherapy (2000 rad in 1 week followed by immediate surgical resection) has never been corroborated.

At present, therefore, no study has established a survival benefit with the use of preoperative radiation therapy in patients with operable lung cancer. However, although its value is unconfirmed by prospective randomized studies, preoperative radiation therapy is routinely used in the management of superior sulcus tumors.

Diagnosis and Management of Carcinomas in the Superior Pulmonary Sulcus

Carcinomas in the superior pulmonary sulcus produce a characteristic clinical pattern known as Pancoast's syndrome.[279,281,645,646] The tumor occurs in the sulcus or groove made by the subclavian artery in the cupola of the pleura and apices of the upper lobes of the lungs. It produces pain in the

TABLE 22-40.   Preoperative Radiation Therapy in Non-Small Cell Lung Cancer

Histology	Pretherapy Resectability	Radiation Dose (Gy)	No. of Patients	Survival Advantage	Reference
Nonrandomized Studies					
Mixed	78 yes +173 no	20–45	254	Yes: 45% vs 35% at 5 years	634
Mixed	36 yes +14 no	30–36	50	None apparent	635
Mixed	All no	30	107	None apparent	636
Mixed	54 yes +34 no	30–45	94	Yes: 47% vs 34% at 5 years	637
Mixed	Marginally yes	30	53	18% 5-year for all; 27% if resectable	638
Mixed	41/45 + mediastinoscopy (+20 postoperative)	35	48	18% at 5 years	639
Randomized Studies					
Mixed	Yes	40–50	166 treated; 165 controls	None: 13% vs 21% at 4 years	640
Mixed	Yes	40	290 treated; 278 controls	None: 14% vs 16% at 5 years	641
Mixed	Yes	55	99 treated; 97 controls	None: 28% vs 35% at 5 years	642
Mixed	Yes	45	21 treated; 16 controls	None: 6/21 vs 7/16 alive	643
Squamous	Yes	20	28	None: 58% vs 43% at 5 years	644

distribution of the eighth cervical and first and second thoracic nerve distribution and Horner's syndrome. A shadow is seen on chest films at the extreme apex of the lung; in 40% of patients, it appears only as an apical cap or thickening.[281] The pain is steady, severe, and unrelenting. At first, it is localized in the shoulder and vertebral border of the scapula and later extends down the ulnar distribution of the arm to the elbow (T1 distribution) and finally to the ulnar surface of the forearm and fourth and fifth fingers of the hand (C8 dermatome).[281] The first or second ribs or vertebrae and the related intercostal nerves also may be involved, increasing the pain and, in some cases, leading to spinal cord compression. With involvement of the sympathetic chain and stellate ganglion by direct extension, Horner's syndrome and anhidrosis develop on the same side of the face and arm. However, rib destruction and Horner's syndrome do not have to be present to diagnose a superior sulcus tumor.

Paulson has pioneered an aggressive approach to these patients that includes preoperative irradiation followed by extended resection.[281,646] (A review of results in the management of superior sulcus tumors from the various series is seen in Table 22-41). This approach was prompted by the

TABLE 22-41.   Results of Preoperative Radiation and Resection for Pancoast Tumors

Series	No. of Patients	Survival at 5 Years (%)
Paulson[646]	78	35
Miller et al.[647]	25	40
Wright et al.[648]	21	27
Attar et al.[649]	19	23 (3 years)
Stanford et al.[650]	16	50
Shahian et al.[651]	18	56

observation that these tumors usually grow slowly and metastasize late. Patients should have the usual staging procedures done for any potentially resectable lung cancer lesion. However, there should be special emphasis on radionuclide bone scans, bone and cervical spine roentgenograms, and a CT scan of the area to determine tumor extent, as well as neurologic examination with electromyography. Mediastinoscopy usually is recommended because of the poor survival of patients with superior sulcus tumors even after radical procedures when these nodes are involved. However, scalene node biopsy is done only when palpable nodes are present or when the patient is of borderline operability.[281,647]

In contrast to other situations, a histologic diagnosis often is not made before radiation and surgery because of the inaccessibility of the lesions, even to needle biopsy, and a desire not to violate tissue planes.[281,646] If the precise definition of a tumor mass in the extreme apex of the chest with pain down the ulnar distribution of the arm in T1 and C8 distribution is followed strictly, the diagnostic accuracy for cancer is better than 90%.[281,646] With inoperable or doubtful cases, open biopsy of the cupola of the pleura may be made through a supraclavicular scalenotomy incision if needed for histologic proof.[281]

Preoperative irradiation to a dose of 3000 rad in ten treatments over 12 days is given to the apex of the lung, upper ribs, upper mediastinum, ipsilateral hilum, and lower cervical spine.[646,647] This allows resection 3 to 6 weeks later. Standard higher doses have not been used routinely preoperatively because of the risk of increased radiotherapeutic and operative morbidity.[281] If surgery is not to be performed because of spread or underlying pulmonary risks, the dose to the spinal cord must be carefully limited. In these patients, shrinking-field techniques are used to achieve tumor doses of approximately 6000 rad. Pancoast tumors usually can be treated to high dose precisely because they are peripherally located, away from the midline. In fact, results with high-dose irradiation alone appear similar to those of combined-modality effort in selected patients without rib erosion.[652,653]

An extended en bloc resection of the chest wall often is carried out after radiotherapy and usually involves an extended radical lobectomy or segmental resection. The posterior portions of the first three ribs, portions of the upper thoracic vertebrae (including the transverse processes), the intercostal nerves, the lower trunk of the brachial plexus, the stellate ganglion, and a portion of the dorsal sympathetic chain are resected along with the involved lung.[281] Long-term complications include permanent ulnar nerve neurologic defects and Horner's syndrome, which do not appear to bother patients.[281] Immediate complications are respiratory in nature and include instability of the chest wall. They necessitate endotracheal tube ventilatory support for the first 3 postoperative days, bronchoscopy for removal of secretions in the immediate postoperative period, and Velpeau dressing to stabilize the chest wall.[646] There is debate about the number of patients who achieve pain relief, but at least two-thirds (and probably most long-term survivors) appear to do so.

Contraindications to resection generally include extensive invasion of the brachial plexus, subclavian artery, vertebral bodies, esophagus, or mediastinum and distant metastases.[646,647] Recent reports document successful arterial reconstruction when subclavian vessel resection was necessary.[648] Patients with hilar, mediastinal, or scalene node involvement have such a poor prognosis following the procedure that metastases in these sites also should be considered contraindications.[646,647] Only 50% of superior sulcus tumors are epidermoid; 30% are large cell or giant cell, and 15% are adenocarcinomas[649,650] Although the fraction of 3-year survivors was 42% for the epidermoid cancers and 21% for the large cell and adenocarcinomas, histology alone should not be used to determine resectability.[281] The use of postoperative radiation therapy for these tumors is controversial if complete resection can be accomplished.[651]

Innovative Radiotherapy Techniques

BRACHYTHERAPY. Brachytherapy or interstitial implantation has been championed by the MSKCC group and involves the placement of encapsulated radioactive sources within or close to the tumor or tumor residual at the time of surgical resection.[654-659] The MSKCC indications for brachytherapy include patients with limited pulmonary reserve, patients with hilar tumors adherent to the major vessels or extending to mediastinal structures where resection with negative margins is impossible, or patients with all gross primary or nodal tumor resected but where the margins of resection are involved. Iridium-192, [198]Au, or ^{125}I have been used. In theory, interstitial implantation allows delivery of a higher, more-uniform dose of radiation to the tumor, with less normal-tissue exposure than with external-beam therapy. The radioactive implants can be placed by the thoracic surgeon or afterloaded in intrathoracic catheters placed by the surgeon.[657] The disadvantages of such a technique include the necessity to keep the patient in specialized areas

for radiation precautions and obligatory use of thoracotomy in a patient with potentially unresectable disease.

More than 1000 patients have been accumulated in the MSKCC experience since 1941. In 470 patients with non-small cell cancer treated by brachytherapy and thoracotomy, local control was obtained in 78% of those with Stage I or II disease, 71% with Stage III and negative nodes, and 63% of patients with involved lymph nodes.[657] However, the 5-year survival rate showed no improvement over that with other forms of therapy, with Stage I and II patients having a 33% 5-year survival rate and Stage III patients a 7% rate.

More recently, MSKCC has combined surgery with intraoperative brachytherapy and postoperative external-beam radiation in patients with residual gross disease or close resection margins.[660] A low complication rate, 7%, was observed. Despite good local control (53% for patients with positive margins and 89% for patients made free of disease), the actuarial 5-year survival rate was no different from that with other forms of treatment, and systemic disease accounted for cancer deaths. The absence of randomized comparisons of this therapy with surgery alone or external-beam radiation therapy alone, as well as the lack of survival improvement, currently relegates this unique methodology to an undefined role in the adjunctive management of locally advanced lung cancer. Moreover, it is unclear whether this technique can be applied outside a major cancer center, thus limiting its routine use.

Interstitial therapy has also been performed via bronchoscopic techniques for patients with malignant airway obstruction or hemorrhage or in patients with recurrent local disease such as stump recurrence.[661,662] The flexible or rigid bronchoscope can be used to deliver radon, ^{125}I or [198]Au. A dose of 3000 rad is delivered locally; however, problems include catheter dislodgment, airway obstruction, and hemoptysis. Currently, endobronchial brachytherapy has largely been replaced by the use of lasers.

INTRAOPERATIVE RADIATION THERAPY. Intraoperative radiation therapy delivered as a single large dose while the patient's chest is open has been described as a potentially useful adjunct to operation, external-beam irradiation postoperatively, or both in the treatment of locally advanced tumors.[663-668] Its utility in the treatment of lung cancer must be questioned, as severe toxicities have been noted at 2500 rad.[669] Only through further carefully designed clinical trials using lower doses will intraoperative radiotherapy ever be shown to have an appropriate risk:benefit ratio.

Postoperative Radiotherapy for Non-Small Cell Lung Cancer

RETROSPECTIVE TRIALS. The rationale for using postoperative radiation is to prevent locoregional relapse and hence increase the chance for cure and long-term survival. Unfortunately, there is scant scientific support for improved cure rate or survival despite the continued widespread use of this approach (Table 22-42). The use of postoperative radiation therapy in patients subjected to either curative or incomplete resection had been studied only in a retrospective fashion until the 1980s. Two widely quoted studies, by Green et

TABLE 22-42. Effect of Postoperative Radiation Therapy on Survival in Non-Small
Cell Lung Cancer

Randomized Trials	Control Arm	Radiotherapy Arm
Van Houtte et al. 1980*		
"Completely resected" N2-negative, all histologies		
Number of patients	92	83
Radiation dose	–	60 Gy
5-year survival rate (%)	43	24
Lung Cancer Study Group 1978–1985†		
Stage II and III "completely resected" epidermoid carcinoma (20% N2+)		
Number of patients	108 (120)	102 (110)
Radiation dose	–	50 Gy
5-year survival rate (%)	38	38

Nonrandomized Trials	Surgery Alone	Surgery + Radiation
Green et al. 1954–1966‡		
Epidermoid and Adenocarcinoma		
Number of patients	38	52
Radiation dose	–	50–60 Gy
5-year survival rate (%)		
Epidermoid	6	21
Adenocarcinoma	14	50
Kirsh et al. 1959–1969§		
Epidermoid and Adenocarcinoma		
Number of patients	20	66
Radiation dose	–	Not specified
5-year survival rate (%)		
Epidermoid	0	34
Adenocarcinoma	0	12
Choi et al. 1971–1977‖		
Epidermoid and Adenocarcinoma		
Number of patients	50	86
Radiation dose	–	40–60 Gy
5-year survival rate (%)		
Epidermoid	33	33
Adenocarcinoma	8	43

*Van Houtte PV, Roemans P, Smets P et al: Postoperative radiation therapy in lung cancer: A
controlled trial after resection of curative design. Int J Radiat Oncol Biol Phys 6:983, 1980.
†The Lung Cancer Study Group: Effects of postoperative mediastinal radiation on completely
resected Stage II and Stage III epidermoid cancer of the lung. N Engl J Med 315:1377–1381, 1986.
‡Green N, Kurohara SS, George FW III, Crews QE Jr: Postresection irradiation for primary lung
cancer. Radiology 116:405–407, 1975.
§Kirsh MM, Rotman H, Argenta L, et al. Carcinoma of the lung: Results of treatment over ten
years. Ann Thorac Surg 21:371–377, 1976.
‖Choi NCH, Grillo HC, Gardiello M, Scannell JG, Wilkins EW Jr: Basis for new strategies in
postoperative radiotherapy of bronchogenic carcinoma. Int J Radiat Oncol Biol Phys 6:31–35, 1980.

al[670] (52 patients with non-small cell cancer treated with surgery and postoperative irradiation for hilar and mediastinal nodes) conducted between 1954 and 1966 and Kirsh and associates[671] (66 patients treated with surgery and postoperative irradiation for the mediastinal nodes) conducted between 1959 and 1969, showed 5-year survival rates of 24% to 34% (depending on histology) compared with 0 to 22% with surgery alone (retrospective controls). In contrast, Choi and coworkers,[672] in a study of 86 patients, found 5-year survival rates of 33% to 43% compared with 8% (adenocarcinoma) to 33% (epidermoid carcinoma) historical controls with surgery alone. Thus, Green and Kirsh and their associates found an advantage for postoperative irradiation in both epidermoid carcinoma and adenocarcinoma, whereas Choi et al. found potential benefit only for adenocarcinoma. Both Cox,[673] a radiation oncologist, and Holmes,[674] a thoracic

surgeon and chairman of the LCSG, have summarized the retrospective trials and their inconclusive results.

PROSPECTIVE RANDOMIZED TRIALS. Two randomized trials specifically examining the role of postoperative radiation therapy in resected non-small cell lung cancer have been reported, and both revealed no survival advantage of such adjuvant therapy. Van Houtte and associates randomized 175 patients with completely resected N2-negative disease to postoperative radiation therapy (6000 rad; 83 patients) or to no postoperative radiotherapy (92 patients).[669] The 5-year survival rate was actually lower in the postoperative radiation therapy group (24% versus 43%), although the difference was not statistically significant. Moreover, the radiation therapy group suffered more complications, including lung fibrosis, radiation pneumonitis, esophageal rupture, and constrictive pericarditis. Patients with squamous cell, large cell, and adenocarcinomas did equally poorly. Despite a small decrease in the local relapse rate in the radiation therapy group, this did not affect survival, with most patients dying from metastatic disease.

The LCSG[675] randomized 230 patients with "completely resected" Stage II (T2N1) and III (T3 tumor or any N2 disease) epidermoid lung cancer to receive postoperative adjuvant radiotherapy or no adjuvant treatment. Their patients were carefully staged intraoperatively, and the randomized groups were equally balanced as to prognostic factors. The mean follow-up time was 3.5 years. However, a relatively small fraction of patients had mediastinal node involvement, and this is the group traditionally receiving postoperative irradiation. Their 5-year survival rate was 38%, which was as good as any previously reported and may be related to the strict eligibility requirements and improved preoperative and intraoperative operative staging techniques in this study. The toxic effects of radiation included esophagitis (24%), other gastrointestinal symptoms (20%), dermatologic problems (11%), and neurologic problems (10%); interestingly, pulmonary toxicity was not significantly more common than in the control group (16% versus 9%). Their abstract summarizes the results of this important trial and their conclusions:

> There was no evidence that radiotherapy improved survival, and although recurrence rates appeared to be somewhat reduced among patients assigned to radiotherapy, these decreases were not statistically significant. However, radiotherapy did produce a striking and significant reduction in recurrences to the ipsilateral lung and mediastinum. Moreover, overall recurrence rates were reduced by radiotherapy in patients with N2 disease (p <0.05), although even this subgroup had no evidence of improved survival. We conclude that radiotherapy can reduce local recurrences after resection of epidermoid carcinoma of the lung, but that it does not increase survival rates.

We concur with this analysis and believe that there is no mandated role for postoperative radiation therapy in carefully staged patients who have undergone potentially curative resection for lung cancer, as the reduction in the local recurrence rate does not translate into a survival advantage. However, insufficient patients with mediastinal node involvement (N2)—the group deriving the most benefit in retrospective studies—have been evaluated prospectively to exclude a small survival benefit in this category. No prospective trials to date have examined the efficacy of postoperative radiation therapy in higher-stage resected adenocarcinoma or large cell carcinoma.

POSTOPERATIVE ADJUVANT CHEMOTHERAPY

Studies of Historical Interest

Over the past 20 years, there have been a number of studies, a few of which were randomized, investigating the use of postoperative adjuvant chemotherapy in non-small cell lung cancer. Two large cooperative groups, one composed of VA hospitals and the second of university hospitals, began prospective randomized trials in which nitrogen mustard was administered at the end of the operation and in the immediate postoperative period.[676,677] There were no demonstrable survival benefits. A second trial, performed by the VA group, used chemotherapy administered during and immediately after the operation as well as a second course 5 weeks into the postoperative period. Again, there was no survival benefit compared with controls. A third trial compared postoperative cyclophosphamide with cyclophosphamide and methotrexate, both versus surgery alone.[678] Chemotherapy was given at 5-week intervals for 18 months. Survival was identical in all three arms. A fourth trial compared CCNU and hydroxyurea postoperatively with surgery alone. There was no demonstrable benefit from drug therapy.[679]

During this period, a number of reports from the United States from nonrandomized or partially randomized trials suggested improved survival with adjuvant chemotherapy.[680–682] However, all of the trials reporting beneficial survival figures were uncontrolled and involved small numbers or biased selection of patients. There also were a number of trials reported from outside the United States during this period, all indicating no benefit from adjuvant chemotherapy.[683–685] Some of these reports have been widely cited. Brunner et al.[686] administered cyclophosphamide for a 2-year period following surgical resection, and after a 9-year follow-up, the authors found that the rate of recurrence and death from lung cancer was significantly higher in the group receiving long-term chemotherapy. This finding raised the possibility that cyclophosphamide, a drug with strong immunosuppressive effects, impairs unspecified defense mechanisms against tumor cells. The British Medical Research Council conducted a large randomized trial of busulphan versus cyclophosphamide versus placebo and found no significant difference in survival at 5 years; however, the survival rates of 28%, 27%, and 34%, respectively, suggested a possible slight detriment to the chemotherapy-treated groups.[687] A cooperative group effort studied adjuvant CCNU therapy in postsurgical Stage I and II patients with non-small cell cancers.[688] More pronounced, even life-threatening, complications were found in the CCNU-treated arm, and if anything, the cancer relapse rate was higher, if not significantly so, with the chemotherapy.

Recent Adjuvant Chemotherapy Trials

Only with the recent discovery of drug combinations (many of which contain cisplatin) with better tumor response rates in patients with metastatic non-small cell lung cancer could the question of postoperative adjuvant chemotherapy be reinvestigated. The first evidence of the importance of cisplatin to drug combinations came from Eagan and co-workers, with the report of a 38% response rate with CAP chemotherapy (cyclophosphamide, Adriamycin [doxorubicin], and cisplatin).[689] Combination chemotherapy with cisplatin-containing regimens has produced initial response rates between 28% and 56%,[690–693] whereas in ECOG trials with larger groups of patients, such regimens have produced response rates of 23% to 31%, with the greatest 1-year survival rate (25%) seen with cisplatin and etoposide.[694]

The LCSG recently reported the results of a prospective randomized trial comparing surgery and immunotherapy with surgery and postoperative adjuvant chemotherapy in resected Stage II and Stage III non-small cell cancer.[695] Eligible patients had to undergo a complete resection of tumor with staging on the basis of lymph node mapping. Resection of subcarinal, paratracheal, hilar, and bronchopulmonary lymph nodes was required in all cases. The postoperative chemotherapy was CAP, whereas the control arm received BCG and levamisole immunotherapy. One hundred forty-one patients were randomized, of which 130 were eligible; of these 130, 23 did not receive the assigned treatment. There were no differences in the rates of postoperative complications. The usual side effects—gastrointestinal or hematologic toxicities—were noted with the CAP chemotherapy. Analysis of the data revealed a significantly lower recurrence and death rate in the chemotherapy group. With a mean time since randomization of 4 years and a mean observation period of 1.7 years among the 130 eligible patients, disease-free survival was longer, and deaths from cancer were significantly fewer, in the group receiving chemotherapy, and there was no evidence of a deleterious effect of the immunotherapy. Whether this early survival advantage will persist for 5 years or longer is unknown at this time and should be reported in the near future by the group. Although it appears unlikely that immunotherapy would have a deleterious effect, it would have been more conclusive to have a group treated by surgery alone.

The LCSG study is the first prospective randomized modern trial to show a survival advantage for adjuvant chemotherapy in non-small cell cancer. More trials with newer agents must be performed and carefully scrutinized to confirm the LCSG result before widespread application of such postoperative adjuvant chemotherapy becomes routine. At the present time, therefore, the addition of adjuvant chemotherapy after surgical resection should be considered investigational.

COMBINED-MODALITY TREATMENT WITH RADIATION AND CHEMOTHERAPY IN NON-SMALL CELL CARCINOMA OF THE LUNG WITH CURATIVE INTENT

Early Trials of Chemotherapy Added to Radiation

The addition of chemotherapy to high-dose radiation therapy given with curative intent could, in theory, kill tumor cells outside the treatment field and also act as a radiation sensitizer within the field. Cyclophosphamide, 5-fluorouracil (5-FU), nitrogen mustard, and vinblastine, when used as single drugs along with radiotherapy, have not improved survival over that obtained using radiotherapy alone.[696-704] In some cases, there actually appears to be a decrease in survival associated with radiochemotherapy. There have been several reports of nonrandomized trials that added combination chemotherapy to high-dose radiation with claims of improved median or long-term survival compared with historical controls treated with radiotherapy alone, with response rates in the 30% to 40% range.[705-711] Cox[712] and Cullen[713] and their coworkers, in two uncontrolled series, investigated the efficacy of cisplatin plus etoposide and radiation therapy in patients with limited-stage inoperable squamous cell carcinoma. The objective tumor response rates were 20% and 32%, yet the 1-year survival rates (47% and 40%, respectively) were not significantly different from historical controls given radiation therapy alone. Thus, patients given new drug combinations must be compared in a randomized fashion with a group of patients receiving the best current definitive radiation therapy with curative intent.

Recent Controlled Trials of Combined-Modality Therapy

Two recent controlled studies have evaluated the concomitant administration of cisplatin-containing chemotherapy regimens and high-dose radiotherapy (Table 22-43). Some

TABLE 22-43.   Randomized Studies of Combined-Modality Therapy for Non-Small Cell Lung Cancer*

Series	Patients (No. Evaluable)	Thoracic Irradiation Dose (Gy)	Chemotherapy†	Response Rate (%)	Median Survival (mo)	Statistical Analysis
Radiotherapy With or Without Chemotherapy						
Wils et al.‡	14	60	None	50	5	
	19	60	P + A + VP-16	81	11	Significant
Van Houtte et al.§	32	50	None	55	12	
	27	45	P + VP-16 + VDS	20	9	Not significant
Incomplete Resection + Radiation With or Without Chemotherapy						
LCSG‖	164	40	none		12.7	Significant
		40	C + A + P		20	

*Adapted from Klastersky J: Therapy with cisplatin and etoposide for non-small cell lung cancer. Semin Oncol 13:104–111, 1986.

†C = cyclophosphamide, P = cisplatin, A = doxorubicin, VP-16 = etoposide, VDS = vindesine.

‡Wils JA, Utama I, Naus A, et al: Phase II randomized trial of radiotherapy alone vs the sequential use of chemotherapy and radiotherapy in Stage III non small cell lung cancer: Phase II trial of chemotherapy alone in Stage IV non small cell lung cancer. Eur J Cancer Clin Oncol 20:911–918, 1984.

§Van Houtte P, Klastersky J, Nguyen H et al: Comparative randomized study of chest radiotherapy preceded or not by chemotherapy with cisplatin, etoposide and vindesine for the treatment of non small cell lung cancer (NSCLC) (abstract). Proc Am Assoc Cancer Res 25:795, 1984.

‖Lad T, Rubinstein L, Sadeghi A: The benefit of adjuvant treatment for resected locally advanced non-small-cell lung cancer. J Clin Oncol 6:9–17, 1988.

of the studies showed modest improvement in survival in the patients receiving the combined-modality therapy.[714,715] Thus in the absence of significant numbers of controlled trials, and the lack of large increases in survival, *there remains no convincing evidence that chemotherapy added to appropriately delivered high-dose radiation therapy reproducibly and significantly increases the median survival or the fraction of long-term disease-free survivors.*

COMBINED-MODALITY TREATMENT WITH SURGERY, RADIATION, AND CHEMOTHERAPY OF NON-SMALL CELL LUNG CANCER

The use of both radiation therapy and chemotherapy after either "curative" or marginal resection of higher-stage non-small cell lung cancer has not been vigorously pursued in either controlled or uncontrolled studies. The rationale for such an approach posits radiation sterilization of residual microscopic disease after resection to prevent local recurrence with systemic adjuvant chemotherapy in the hope of preventing distant relapse. A nonrandomized retrospective study was performed by Newman and associates[716] over a 7-year period in which patients having resection of Stage II disease received either no adjuvant therapy, postoperative radiation therapy alone, or postoperative radiation therapy and CAMP (cyclophosphamide, doxorubicin, methotrexate, procarbazine). This study involved small numbers of patients in each subgroup, yet there was a significant survival advantage for those patients treated with postoperative multimodality therapy compared with those treated with surgery alone or surgery with postoperative radiotherapy alone: median survival 72+ months with combined-modality therapy, 12 months with surgery alone, and 37+ months with postoperative radiotherapy. Of note, there was a high rate of CNS relapse. In contrast, the LCSG,[717] in a prospective randomized trial, investigated postoperative chemoradiation therapy in 164 patients with non-small cell carcinoma who were able to have only incomplete resection of tumor. After resection, patients were randomized to receive either radiation therapy or 4000 rad of radiation plus CAP chemotherapy. Both recurrence and death rates were lower in the combined-modality arm. However, this difference was apparent only in the first

year after randomization. Thus, longer follow-up is needed to see if the plateau values between the two arms are significantly different. From the paucity of data, *there seems to be no role at this time for routine chemoradiation therapy after resection of non-small cell cancer*, but future prospective randomized trials with more active agents are warranted in an investigational setting.

NEOADJUVANT (PREOPERATIVE) CHEMOTHERAPY OF NON-SMALL CELL LUNG CANCER

There is renewed interest in preoperative chemotherapy because of the more favorable tumor response rates (exceeding 50%) with the new drug combinations when given preoperatively to patients with disease confined to the ipsilateral hemithorax with lymph node positivity compared with the more typical 25% response rate seen in patients with extrathoracic disease (Table 22-44).[718] Thus, a major thrust of many investigative protocols at present in locally advanced disease involves the use of preoperative (also called neoadjuvant) chemotherapy with or without radiation therapy followed by attempted surgical resection (Table 22-45). The potential advantages of neoadjuvant therapy include increasing the incidence of complete resections by sterilizing local micrometastases, minimizing hematogenous or local seeding of cancer caused by surgical manipulation, and conservation

TABLE 22-44. Response to Combination Chemotherapy in Non-Small Cell Lung Cancer Related to Stage of Disease*

Chemotherapy Regimen	Objective Tumor Response Rate (%)	
	Limited to the Chest	Metastatic
Mitomycin-C + vinblastine + cisplatin	53	28
Cyclophosphamide + doxorubicin + cisplatin	47	23
Etoposide + cisplatin	56	27

*Adapted from Bonomi P: Brief overview of combination chemotherapy in non-small cell lung cancer. Semin Oncol 13:89–94, 1986.

TABLE 22-45. Use of Preoperative (Neoadjuvant) Chemotherapy and Radiotherapy in Non-Small Cell Lung Cancer

Year	Histology/Stage	No. of Patients	Chemotherapy*	No. with Pretherapy Resectability	No. of Responses (%)	No. (%) with Posttherapy Resectability	Survival Rate or Advantage
1987[719]	Mixed/IIIA	41	Mito-C, VDS, P	0	30 (73)	21 (51)	>3.5 year median
1987[720]	Mixed/III	64	P, 5-FU, XRT	0	36 (56)	39 (60)	30% 2 years
1986[721]	Mixed/IIIB	20	V, P, VP16	7	14 (70)	7 (35)	34% 1 year
1984[722]	Squamous/I,II,III	32	P, Bleo, Mito-C	0	24 (75)	29 (91)	58% 1 year
1982[723]	Squamous/III	9	P, Mito-C	0	5 (56)	5 (56)	None
1982[724]	Squamous/I,II,III	16	P, Bleo	3	12 (75)	3 (19)	None
1982[725]	Mixed/III	12	C, A, P, XRT	0	6 (50)	11 (92)	None
1980[726]	Mixed/III	207	P	0	86 (43)	38 (18)	Yes
1979[727]	Squamous/III	27	Bronchial art Mito-C	0	18 (67)	15 (56)	None
1971[728]	Mixed/I,II,III	31	Bronchial art Mito-C	17	13 (42)	17 (55)	Yes

P = cisplatin; Mito-C = mitomycin C; Bleo = bleomycin; C = cyclophosphamide; VDS = vindesine; VP16 = etoposide; 5-FU = 5-fluorouracil; A = doxorubicin; XRT = radiation therapy; Bronchial art = bronchial artery infusion.

of normal lung by permitting less extensive resections. The potential hazards of neoadjuvant therapy include an increase in surgical morbidity or mortality related to the chemotherapy and loss of the surgical option if the tumor progresses during the chemotherapy. The patients for whom this approach seems particularly suited are those defined by the new staging system as having Stage IIIa disease.

The concept of neoadjuvant therapy is not new, with the earliest studies performed in mixed non-small cell histologies of various stages where mitomycin C was infused into the bronchial artery. Several recent studies have documented very high tumor response rates for neoadjuvant therapy and the conversion of unresectable tumors to resectable ones (Table 22-45). The impressive results of Martini and associates[719] have been confirmed in a series of 24 patients by R. Ginsberg (personal communication). In addition, recent reports of four ongoing studies of patients with unresectable Stage III non-small cell cancer who were treated with preoperative chemotherapy and in some cases radiotherapy showed 40 of 74 (54%) able to undergo a resection following the neoadjuvant therapy.[729–732]

NEOADJUVANT CHEMOTHERAPY REGIMENS AND TOXICITY

Three regimens appear to have the most activity in neoadjuvant studies: cisplatin plus etoposide, cisplatin plus 5-FU, and mitomycin C plus vinblastine (or vindesine) plus cisplatin (MVP). The cisplatin–etoposide combination has proved as good as any other regimen and was associated with a 30% overall response rate and the longest survival in metastatic disease in ECOG studies (Table 22-46).[694] However, toxicity in the ECOG studies included 3% deaths in 124 patients treated, with the most significant toxicities being hematologic and gastrointestinal. In fact, chemotherapy in the Martini study was associated with a 5% mortality rate, and the necessity for high-dose platinum required hospitalization.[719] Likewise, the study by Taylor and associates showed an 8% myocardial infarction rate and a 5% mortality rate attributable to the chemotherapy.[720] In investigating various adjuvant programs, it thus will be important to evaluate the ease of delivery, patient compliance, and toxicity in addition to survival and recurrence data. In this regard, the cisplatin plus etoposide combination can be administered in an outpatient setting, and in studies by Klastersky and associates,[733] there was no difference in the response rates between high- and low-dose cisplatin when combined with etoposide (Table 18-46).

Investigation of the role of neoadjuvant therapy in non-small cell lung cancer should be encouraged. However, such trials must be carefully designed with regard to the patient populations studied. The best population for such therapy would be those patients with locally advanced Stage IIIa disease. It is crucial that nodal disease be verified histologically in such patients prior to randomization to eliminate population heterogeneity caused by assumed nodal positivity based on CT scans alone. A neoadjuvant prospective randomized evaluation is in progress at the U.S. NCI comparing preoperative and postoperative cisplatin and etoposide chemotherapy and surgical resection with surgery and postoperative radiotherapy alone in Stage IIIa disease. Only after the completion of such trials can recommendations be made as to the standard use of neoadjuvant therapy for the management of locally advanced lung cancer.

PROPHYLACTIC CRANIAL IRRADIATION IN NON-SMALL CELL LUNG CANCER

The role of prophylactic cranial irradiation (PCI) in non-small cell cancer has not been defined. The frequency of brain metastases is less in this group than in those with small cell carcinoma of the lung both initially and during follow-up. However, patients with Stage III M0 adenocarcinoma of the lung receiving combined-modality therapy have been reported to have a very high rate (38%) of CNS metastases as the first site of relapse.[709] In N1 patients having an apparent complete surgical resection of non-small cell cancer, the brain was the most frequent site of recurrence (39%).[745] Likewise, in patients having a curative surgical resection for N2 disease, the brain was the most common site of distant metastases (19%).[746] In patients with Stage III M0 disease treated with curative radiation,[611,747] a large fraction relapsed with brain metastases, approaching 40% to 50% probability in patients living 3 years or more. In all of these studies, adenocarcinoma and large cell carcinoma spread to the brain more frequently than did epidermoid carcinoma (see also Table 22-19).

All of these studies suggest the possible utility of PCI to treat patients with non-small cell lung cancer (especially adenocarcinoma) potentially cured by surgery or radiotherapy.[611,747] The VALG conducted a prospectively randomized trial of PCI in all types of lung cancer and found a significant reduction in the frequency of clinically detectable brain metastases in those with non-small cell cancer (13% in the unirradiated and 6% in the irradiated group overall, and 29%

TABLE 22-46. Overview of Clinical Trials of Cisplatin plus Etoposide for Metastatic Non-Small Cell Lung Cancer*

Cisplatin Dose (mg/m²)	Etoposide Dose (mg/m²)	No. of Studies	No. of Patients	Response Rate (%) Partial	Response Rate (%) Complete
60	100 or 120 × 3	4	273	27	1.8
80–90	50 × 4, 80 × 3, 100 × 3, 120 × 3	4	158	30	2.5
100	75 × 5, 80 × 3, 100 × 3, 120 × 3	5	158	35	2.5
120	120 × 3	1	93	29	NR†

*Adapted from Klastersky J: Therapy with cisplatin and etoposide for non-small cell lung cancer. Semin Oncol 13:104, 1986. Primary references are 734–744.

†NR = not reported.

versus 0 for adenocarcinoma).[748] Although there was no survival benefit of the PCI for these groups as a whole, patients exhibiting brain metastases had significantly shorter survival than those who did not. In a retrospective analysis of adenocarcinoma of the lung after potentially curative treatment, 5% of patients receiving PCI developed brain metastases compared with 24% of patients not receiving PCI.[749] Because of this information, many radiation oncology departments are starting to use PCI in potentially cured adenocarcinoma, particularly in patients with nodal involvement. Although this therapy must undergo further investigation, we believe it is reasonable to treat patients with adenocarcinoma or large cell carcinoma who are potentially cured but with high risk of relapse (N1, N2, and Stage III M0) with PCI. However, the long-term side-effects of PCI in adults with lung cancer, such as in those with small cell lung cancer, are only now being reported, and patients must be informed that there are potential long-term complications from PCI.[750,751]

LUNG CANCER IN YOUNG PERSONS

Lung cancer in patients under 40 years of age is uncommon and in children is rare.[753,754] The cancers in young adults occur in heavy smokers, and there is a higher frequency in female children. Adenocarcinomas and small cell cancers are much more common than epidermoid cancers. Survival after surgical resection is similar to that of adults; however, a more aggressive surgical resection and combined-modality therapy approach often is used.[752] In patients with unresectable disease, survival is short (6 months or less), and the disease is said to be more virulent than in older patients.[752]

APPROACH TO PATIENTS WITH DISSEMINATED NON-SMALL CELL LUNG CANCER

ALTERNATIVES

Patients with histologically documented, unresectable or inoperable non-small cell lung cancer should be evaluated first for radiotherapy. If it is believed the disease is sufficiently limited that it can be encompassed within a tolerable radiotherapy port and thus treated "for cure," or if there are pressing symptomatic needs for palliation such as, complete bronchial obstruction, hemoptysis, or upper airway or SVC obstruction, the initial treatment should be radiotherapy (with or without chemotherapy or surgery, if part of an experimental protocol). If a patient has more disseminated disease and there is no pressing need for radiotherapy, the approach can involve supportive therapy alone if the patient is reliable for follow-up or consideration of the use of chemotherapy.[493,754]

USE OF RADIOTHERAPY IN PALLIATION

Patients who have AJC Stage III cancer clearly have a poor prognosis, yet there is a small salvage rate with surgery or radiotherapy in those whose disease has not spread beyond the mediastinal nodes. In contrast, the question of whether the primary disease should be irradiated for palliation often arises in asymptomatic patients with poor prognostic features.[755,756] However, the argument is not so much to avoid treatment as to defer it to a time at which the patient becomes symptomatic. The case for palliative treatment of the asymptomatic patient is to prevent serious symptoms from occurring within the thorax. The case for delaying treatment really rests on the reliability of the patient.

The need for palliative chest radiotherapy was studied by following 134 inoperable patients not suitable for curative radiotherapy.[757] Immediate chest radiotherapy was believed to be necessary in 64% of the patients because of significant intrathoracic symptoms. The remaining patients were followed regularly without initial radiotherapy, and 54% of these (30% of the initial group) required radiotherapy within a median of 10 months because of progressive and significant symptoms of intrathoracic disease. Thus, more than 90% of the patients eventually needed to be irradiated.

If the patient can be followed closely, then deferring treatment until symptoms appear may very well be appropriate. However, patients with lung cancer often are followed infrequently, and these patients may present after a long interval with extreme symptoms (e.g., SVC obstruction, obstructive pneumonia, or lobar collapse), all of which represent potentially life-threatening problems to the patient who has COPD in addition to lung cancer. In addition, when obstructive pneumonia complicates the patient's disease, the treatment often must be started with larger radiotherapy fields than would have been used at presentation or under emergency conditions, and sometimes must be delayed until sepsis can be controlled. The authors stress that if a decision is made not to irradiate asymptomatic tumors, *careful follow-up is required to avoid having a patient develop a highly symptomatic total bronchial obstruction that is difficult to relieve.*

When a patient relapses in the chest after primary surgical therapy, there may well be an indication for radiation therapy to the primary lesion. If prior radiation has not been used and the recurrence appears to be within the mediastinum, a course of low-dose palliative radiation (3000 rad in 2 weeks or slightly higher) often is given to the mediastinum to prevent progressive disease from obstructing the SVC or airway or from predisposing to pneumonia or sepsis. If the patient has a local relapse after surgery, careful restaging reveals no distant metastases, and the patient is in good shape physiologically, a course of high-dose radiotherapy can be attempted. However, no data from controlled trials demonstrate benefit in these cases. Retreatment with irradiation after prior palliative radiation also may be considered, depending on the previous volume and dose, the time course of symptoms after the first course, the progression of disease at other sites, and alternative treatment plans. The decision should be made by the radiotherapist in conjunction with other physicians taking care of the patient.

COMMON PROBLEMS IN THE MANAGEMENT OF LUNG CANCER

The general principles of diagnosis and management of metastatic disease, oncologic emergencies, and paraneoplastic syndromes (all common problems in lung cancer patients) are discussed in Chapters 55, 58, and 62. Other approaches to the primary therapy of small-cell lung cancer are discussed later. However, when lung cancer of any cell type presents as a localized problem that manifests symptoms, radiation therapy is frequently used (Table 22-47). A problem such as *SVC obstruction* usually can be relieved with a course of 3000 to 4000 rad over a 2- to 4-week period, with most patients achieving a response.[283,284,758,759] Recently, patients with SVC syndrome responded to radiotherapy in 50% to 70% of cases.[760] About 13% of patients will show a recurrence of the syndrome, and about 17% of those with non-small cell cancer and 24% of those with small cell lung cancer will survive for 1 year after such treatment. *Cardiac tamponade* also can be alleviated in many patients with pericardiocentesis and radiation therapy to the entire cardiac silhouette.[761] Such treatment usually is fractionated more slowly than standard treatment because of the possibility of later cardiac toxicity, interactions with chemotherapeutic agents, and the typically large volume of lung that has to be incorporated into the treatment volume behind the enlarged heart silhouette. Malignant pleural effusion usually does not respond well to radiation because the dose to the entire pleura is limited to about 2000 rad in order to spare the adjacent lung tissue. *Hemoptysis* as a symptom of tumor usually is relieved with radiation therapy.

Atelectasis from tumor obstruction is a common problem that is often difficult to relieve, responding in less than 25% of cases. However, recent data indicate that more than 60% of patients with non-small cell lung cancer presenting with atelectasis can have this problem relieved by appropriate radiotherapy.[762] When an entire lobe or lung has been collapsed by *bronchial obstruction*, radiation therapy frequently is used but with only modest success. In general, a lobe or lung has the greatest probability of being re-expanded if it has been collapsed only a short time (hours to few days); the longer the tissue has been collapsed, the less likely it is that radiation will be able to induce re-expansion.

TABLE 22-47.   Local Symptomatic Relief Achieved by Radiation Therapy in Patients with Bronchogenic Carcinoma (All Cell Types)

Symptom	Relief of Symptom (%)
Hemopytsis*†	84
Cough*	60
Dyspnea*†	60
Atelectasis†‡	23
Superior vena caval obstruction†§‖	70–86
Vocal cord paralysis*	6
Pain*†	66
Brain metastasis#	70–90

*Philips TL, Miller RJ, Am Rev Respir Dis 117:405–410, 1978.
†Slawson RG, Scott RM, Radiology 132:175–176, 1979.
‡Majid OA, Lee S, Khushalani S, Seydel HG, Int J Radiat Oncol Biol Phys 12:231–232, 1986.
§Line D, Deeley TJ: Palliative therapy. In Deeley TJ (ed): Carcinoma of the Bronchus: Modern Radiotherapy, pp 298–306. New York, Appleton-Century-Crofts, 1972.
‖Armstrong BA, Perez CA, Simpson JR, Hederman MA, Int J Radiat Oncol Biol Phys 13:531–539, 1987.
#Perez CA, Presant CA, Van Ambury AL, Semin Oncol 5: 123–134, 1978.

Symptomatic *brain metastases* and *bone metastases* usually respond to palliative doses of radiation therapy (approximately 3000 rad in 2 weeks). Occasionally, such lesions will clear completely with treatment, but usually, careful evaluation of the site will show persistent neoplasm that is asymptomatic. If such a metastasis is the only site of distant spread, physicians occasionally decide to treat the metastasis and the primary with curative doses, hoping that the known sites of involvement can be controlled and that no other involvement exists.

MANAGEMENT OF BRAIN METASTASES IN NON-SMALL CELL LUNG CANCER

The median survival time of patients with brain metastasis is 3 to 4 months.[759] In addition to radiotherapy, dexamethasone is given. Seventy percent or more of patients have some relief of their symptoms; convulsions and headache usually are more thoroughly relieved than is motor loss or impaired mentation.[763] Patients whose CNS metastases respond to radiotherapy live twice as long as do those whose tumors do not respond.

Occasionally, patients are seen with a lung cancer and a solitary cerebral metastasis, which can present after or concurrent with the lung cancer.[764-766] When single brain metastases are found in patients with non-small cell carcinoma, surgical resection followed by radiotherapy may be undertaken when neurologically feasible. After careful staging to exclude other metastatic disease, if the brain lesion is a solitary peripheral (*i.e.*, neurosurgically accessible) lesion, these patients can be approached with surgical resection and then brain radiotherapy along with appropriate therapy of the primary lung cancer. Some 13% of these patients live for more than 1 year.[761] The MSKCC has compared the course of 43 such patients with an isolated brain metastasis treated with neurosurgical resection and radiotherapy with that of 43 patients treated with radiotherapy alone and found superior survival, lower recurrence rates, and fewer neurologically related deaths in the patients treated with surgical resection.[767]

SPINAL CORD COMPRESSION

Spinal cord compression should be suspected in patients complaining of back pain with or without lower-extremity weakness. In general, patients with spinal cord compression represent an emergency in which the best neurologic results are achieved by early diagnosis and treatment. Radiation usually will be the treatment of choice unless symptoms are rapidly progressive. Paralysis of the lower legs, with or without a radicular component of pain and with or without bowel or bladder dysfunction, makes the diagnosis obvious. When a spinal cord compression syndrome is suspected, a myelogram is essential to delineate the extent of the problem. Palliative irradiation usually is successful at alleviating the symptoms unless significant neurologic compromise has already occurred. Because lung cancer is the most common neoplastic cause of spinal cord compression, a low threshold for the diagnosis is the most important variable in achieving a good functional result.[768-770] The more extensive the neurologic deficit at the time of diagnosis, the more difficult it is to restore neurologic normality with radiation therapy.

Spinal cord compression can occur from extension into the spinal canal either from a vertebral metastasis or from a paravertebral mass invading through an intervertebral foramen. Because the compression may be occurring anywhere along the circumference of the spinal cord, decompressive laminectomy usually is reserved for patients whose symptoms are progressing so rapidly that there does not appear to be time for a response to irradiation; for those with recurrent cord compression in whom further irradiation cannot be delivered safely; and for those in whom a tissue diagnosis is not at hand. The more extensive the compression, the more difficult it is to return to normal neurologic function. Moreover, the more extensive the laminectomy, the greater is the instability of the spine that results. Because removal of the lamina only exposes the posterior aspect of the spinal cord, postoperative irradiation still is indicated in these patients because metastatic disease is rarely confined to the posterior aspect of the cord. With or without surgery, doses of 3000 to 4000 rad over 2 to 4 weeks are necessary for palliation, often starting with 300- to 400-rad fractions. Concomitantly, dexamethasone, 25 to 100 mg per day divided into four doses, is given initially and tapered rapidly to the lowest dosage that relieves the symptoms.[770] Again, the more extensive the neurologic deficit before treatment, the less recovery can be expected.

If the patient has had previous radiation therapy to the mediastinum and supraclavicular fossa, it can be difficult to distinguish between a brachial plexus syndrome caused by tumor and one caused by radiation injury. Typically, pain is more likely to be manifestation of tumor than of a radiation injury.[771] The presence of a supraclavicular mass is certainly suggestive of tumor. On the other hand, if the patient had radiation more than 6 months before the development of the brachial plexus syndrome, does not manifest pain, and has induration throughout the supraclavicular fossa without a discrete mass, then the chance of radiation injury is high. Correlation with careful dosimetric reconstruction is necessary, and a clinical diagnosis will often have to be made. When doubt exists and the patient is otherwise in good shape, surgical biopsy of the area may be necessary to plan treatment properly.

SELECTION OF PATIENTS FOR CHEMOTHERAPY OF METASTATIC NON-SMALL CELL LUNG CANCER

Everyone who has treated patients with small cell lung cancer using combination chemotherapy can readily appreciate both the prompt objective shrinkage of tumor and the relief of symptoms associated with the chemotherapy, which, in most cases, far outweigh any chemotherapy toxicity. In addition, many trials have demonstrated the survival benefit of such treatment and the cure of some of these patients (see later section). Such obvious clinical benefit is simply not seen with chemotherapy in the large majority of patients with non-small cell cancers.[772,773] Because of the strong correlation of tumor response with other significant prognostic factors such as performance status and bulk of disease (that is, the "best risk" patients have the best chance

of responding to chemotherapy), there have been very few studies demonstrating a survival benefit from chemotherapy for metastatic non-small cell cancer. The median survival times for all patients treated are 5 to 6 months. Nevertheless, in nearly all studies, patients who show objective responses to chemotherapy have had significantly longer survival than those who do not respond.[772,774,775] Simply put, although response to chemotherapy is a significant prognostic factor in non-small cell cancer, *we do not know if this survival advantage is related to the chemotherapy or to some biologic feature of the disease that would permit increased survival independent of any treatment.* For this reason, it is generally accepted that *there is no "standard" regimen or chemotherapy treatment plan for non-small cell lung cancer.*[776-778]

RESPONSE TO SINGLE-AGENT CHEMOTHERAPY IN NON-SMALL CELL LUNG CANCER

No single-agent chemotherapy has significantly increased overall survival. The objective tumor responses that occur are usually brief, lasting 2 to 4 months, and complete responses are rare. Response rates are almost uniformly higher in patients who have not received prior chemotherapy of any type. Using relatively strict criteria for objective tumor response, Kris, Joss, and Bakowski and their colleagues have reviewed a large number of Phase II single-agent trials (Table 22-48).[776-778] More than 50 drugs were tested, but only six had significant antitumor activity in more than 15% of patients: *cisplatin, ifosfamide, mitomycin C, vindesine, vinblastine,* and *etoposide.* These agents were significantly different from the inactive drugs. For example, in 31% of the trials, no tumor responses of any kind were seen to the inactive drugs. Overall, the three reviews were in general agreement, although Kris et al[776] believed that etoposide was not as active as the other most active drugs. The response rates for these drugs were not related to tumor histology (squamous cell, adenocarcinoma, and large cell carcinoma). However, patients with prior chemotherapy had a lower response rate than did previously untreated patients.

Thus, only a few drugs have significant antitumor effects as single agents in non-small cell lung cancer. One of these drugs, ifosfamide, has been used more widely in European trials than in the United States. One of its serious side effects, urotoxicity, can be lowered by concomitant administration of the drug 2-mercaptoethane sulfonic acid (mesna) at 20% of the ifosfamide dose.[779] In addition to its activity as a single agent, ifosfamide is effective in combination with either etoposide or cisplatin. However, it is not yet clear to the authors whether it is superior to cyclophosphamide.

NEW DRUGS WITH POTENTIAL ACTIVITY AGAINST NON-SMALL CELL LUNG CANCER

The ECOG studied 676 patients in randomized trials comparing various combination chemotherapy regimens involving the platinum analogue *CBDCA* as a single agent.[780] The survival benefits and lesser toxicity of CBDCA led the ECOG to recommend further studies of this agent. A new antifolate, *10-EDAM* (10-ethyl-10-deaza-aminopterin), was found in

TABLE 22-48.   Response Rates of Single-Agent Chemotherapy for Non-Small Cell Lung Cancer*

Drug	No. of Patients	Response Rate (%)†
Most active agents		
Cisplatin	305	16 (15, 20)
Ifosfamide	130	27 (25, 26)
Mitomycin-C	88	17 (17, 20)
Vinblastine	22	27
Vindesine	370	16 (19, 17)
Etoposide‡ (VP-16-213)		18
Agents with less activity		
Cyclophosphamide	405	12
Lomustine (CCNU)	216	10
Doxorubicin	296	12
5-FU	26	8
Methotrexate	105	11

*Data from Kris M, Cohen E, Gralla R: An analysis of 134 Phase II trials in non-small cell lung cancer (NSCLC). Proc. IV World Conference on Lung Cancer Cancer, Toronto 1985. Other agents reviewed with less than 15% response rates included the following commonly available drugs: cyclophosphamide, 5-FU, 6-mercaptopurine, methotrexate, PALA, BCNU, methyl-CCNU, CCNU, vincristine, teniposide, etoposide, L-asparaginase, dacarbazine, hexamethylmelamine, doxorubicin, and bleomycin as well as a series of other agents for a total of 51 drugs in 4340 patients. Note that these authors did not find etoposide to have activity equivalent to that of the other five agents.

†Response rates in parentheses correspond to the values obtained in the literature reviews by Joss RA, Cavalli F, Goldhirsch A et al: New agents in non-small cell lung cancer. Cancer Treat Rev 11:205–237, 1984; and Bakowski MT, Creech JC: Chemotherapy of non-small cell lung cancer: a reappraisal and look to the future. Cancer Treat Rev 10:159–172, 1983.

‡Etoposide (VP-16) data from Bakowski MT, Creech JC: Chemotherapy of non-small cell lung cancer: a reappraisal and look to the future. Cancer Treat Rev 10:159–172, 1983.

preclinical studies to have more selective entry into tumor cells and greater conversion to polyglutamate forms within tumor cells than its sister compound methotrexate.[781] A 33% tumor response rate was seen in 18 previously untreated patients by the MSKCC group, and stomatitis, rather than myelosuppression, was the limiting toxicity. Similarly, a nonclassical antifolate, trimetrexate, was found to have antitumor activity in 55 previously untreated patients.[782]

RESPONSES TO COMBINATION CHEMOTHERAPY IN NON-SMALL CELL LUNG CANCER

Over the past 15 years, several thousand patients with metastatic non-small cell cancer have been entered onto clinical studies testing various chemotherapy combinations (summarized in Tables 22-49 through 22-52) (for recent reviews, see Mulshine and Ruckdeschel[772] and Gralla[774]). Whereas tumor response rates of 50% to 70% are seen in the "neoadjuvant," preoperative setting (representing results in fully ambulatory patients with disease limited to the chest), the rates in patients with extrathoracic metastatic disease are significantly less: 20% to 40% objective response rates, with less than a 5% complete tumor remission rate.[772,774] Most studies have not found a difference in the response rates of the different histologic types of tumor, although occasional trials suggest such differences.[783]

TABLE 22-50.   Pooled Results of Combination Chemotherapy with Cisplatin-Containing Regimens for Non-Small Cell Lung Cancer*

Combination†	No. of Patients (No. of Trials)	Significant Response Rate (%)
C + A + P	432 (5)	29
VDS + P	426 (9)	35
VP16 + P	384 (5)	29
VP16 + P (120 mg/m²)	241 (1)‡	29
vs. P (60 mg/m²)		25
Mito-C + (VBL or VDS) + P	362 (7)	49
Total	1845 (27 trials)	

*Data from Gralla RJ: Issues and agents in the chemotherapy of non-small-cell lung cancer. Mediguide Oncol 5:1–5, 1985 covering randomized and nonrandomized trials.

†C = cyclophosphamide, A = doxorubicin, P = cisplatin, VDS = vindesine, VP16 = etoposide, Mito-C = mitomycin C, VBL = vinblastine.

‡Data on randomized high- vs. standard-dose cisplatin from Klastersky J, Sculier JP, Ravez P et al: A randomized study comparing a high and a standard dose of cisplatin in combination with etoposide in the treatment of advanced non-small-cell lung carcinoma. J Clin Oncol 4:1780–1786, 1986.

TABLE 22-49.   Results of Combination Chemotherapy for Metastatic Non-Small Cell Lung Cancer*

Series	Chemotherapy†	Objective Tumor Response Rate (%)
Bitran et al.[784]	C + doxorubicin + MTX + procarbazine (CAMP)	48
Chahinian et al.[785]	MTX + doxorubicin + C + CCNU (MACC)	46
Vogl et al.[786]	MTX + doxorubicin + C + CCNU (MACC)	12
Eagan et al.[787]	C + doxorubicin + P (CAP)	39
Gralla et al.[788]	Vindesine + P (VP)	43
Longeval & Klastersky[789]	Etoposide + P (EP)	28
Mason & Catalono[790]	Mitomycin C + vinblastine + P (MVP)	53

*Adapted from Bonomi P: Brief overview of combination chemotherapy in non-small cell lung cancer. Semin Oncol 13:89, 1986.

†C = cyclophosphamide; MTX = methotrexate; CCNU = lomustine; P = cisplatin.

TABLE 22-51. Results of Combination Chemotherapy for Metastatic Non-Small Cell Lung Cancer in Eastern Cooperative Oncology Group Trials*

Trial and Regimen†	No. of Patients	Response Rate (%)	Median Survival (wk)
EST 2575 Generation III‡			
HEX + A + MTX vs.	77	13	22
C + A + MTX + PCZ	77	22	20
EST 2575 Generation IV§			
C + A + VP16 vs.	100	14	18
Mito-C + VBL	100	13	18
EST 2575 Generation V¶			
A + 5FU + P vs.	109	17	22
C + A + P vs.	107	23	24
C + Bleo + P vs.	112	20	22
Mito-C + VBL + P	104	26	24
EST 1581**			
C + A + MTX + PCZ	15	17	24
vs. Mito-C + VBL + P vs.	121	31	22
VDS + P vs.	126	26	26
VP16 + P	124	23	26
Total	1272		

*Patients were stratified by histology (squamous, adenocarcinoma, large cell), performance status, and in some cases prior weight loss and randomly assigned to the different regimens. Exclusions included: small cell carcinoma histology, ECOG performance status of 3 or 4 (nonambulatory), prior radiotherapy to areas of evaluable disease, prior chemotherapy, inadequate laboratory values for renal, liver, and bone marrow function, brain metastases, and symptomatic cardiovascular disease.

†HEX = hexamethylmelamine; A = doxorubicin; MTX = methotrexate; C = Cyclophosphamide; PCZ = procarbazine; VP16 etoposide; Mito-C = mitomycin C; 5-FU = 5-fluorouracil; P = cisplatin; Bleo = bleomycin; VDS = vindesine.

‡Ruckdeschel JC, Mehta CR, Salazar OM, Creech RH, Sponzo RW: Chemotherapy for metastatic non-small cell bronchogenic carcinoma: EST-2575, generation III, HAM vs. CAMP. Cancer Treat Rep 65:959–963, 1981.

§Ruckdeschel JC, Day R, Weissman CH et al: Chemotherapy for metastatic non-small cell bronchogenic carcinoma: EST-2575, generation IV, cyclophosphamide, doxorubicin, and etoposide vs. mitomycin–vinblastine. Cancer Treat Rep 68:1325–1329, 1984.

¶Ruckdeschel JC, Finkelstein DM, Mason BA, Creech RH: Chemotherapy for metastatic non-small cell bronchogenic carcinoma: EST-2575, generation V: A randomized comparison of four cisplatin-containing regimens. J Clin Oncol 3:72–79, 1985.

**Ruckdeschel JC, Finkelstein DM, Ettinger DS et al: A randomized trial of the four most active regimens for metastatic non-small cell lung cancer. J Clin Oncol 4:14–22, 1986.

TABLE 22-52. Analysis of Long-Term Survivors in ECOG Combination Chemotherapy Trials for Metastatic Non-Small Cell Lung Cancer*

Total number of patients treated	893
Per cent surviving >1 year (N = 168)	19
Per cent surviving >2 years (N = 36)	4
Per cent suffering lethal complications	2
Overall major tumor response rate (per cent)	22
Overall complete tumor response rate (per cent)	2
Characteristics of patients surviving >1 year	
Major tumor response rate (per cent)	44
Complete tumor response rate (per cent)	8

*Finkelstein DM, Ettinger DS, Ruckdeschel JC: Long-term survivors in metastatic non-small cell lung cancer: An Eastern Cooperative Oncology Group study. J Clin Oncol 4:702–709, 1986.

RANDOMIZED TRIALS OF SINGLE-AGENT VERSUS COMBINATION CHEMOTHERAPY FOR METASTATIC NON-SMALL CELL LUNG CANCER

There have been several recent randomized trials that begin to provide information on the issue of the benefit or lack thereof from combination chemotherapy in non-small cell lung cancer. Overall, it appears that these trials demonstrate clinical benefit for combination chemotherapy. One type of trial randomized patients to single-agent chemotherapy versus a cisplatin combination. Elliot et al.[791] randomized 105 patients with metastatic cancer to treatment with vindesine alone or the combination of vindesine and cisplatin. More than 60% of patients in both treatment arms had tumor limited to the chest and thus had very favorable disease. The major tumor response rate to vindesine was 7%, with a 4-month median survival, whereas that to the combination was 33%, with an 11-month median survival, both highly significant differences. The Umbrian Lung Cancer Group trial also suggested benefits for combination chemotherapy.[792] It randomized 116 patients to cisplatin alone (4% response rate, 12% 1-year survival), cisplatin plus etoposide (38% response rate, 36% 1-year survival), or cisplatin plus etoposide plus mitomycin C (33% response rate, 24% 1-year survival).[792] The FONICAP trial in Italy randomized 124 patients to etoposide alone or etoposide plus cisplatin,[793] while the Southeastern Cooperative Group (SEG) randomized 453 patients to vindesine alone or vindesine plus mitomycin or vindesine plus cisplatin.[794] In the latter two trials, the combination chemotherapy resulted in a higher major tumor response rate, but no survival advantage despite increased toxicity. Indiana University randomized 124 patients with unresectable disease to therapy with vindesine alone (V; 14% response rate, 17 weeks' median survival), vindesine plus cisplatin (VP; 27% response rate, 26 weeks' median survival), or the two drugs plus mitomycin C (MVP; 20% response rate, 17 weeks' median survival).[795] There was no significant difference in overall survival, duration of remission, or survival of responders with the combination chemotherapy regimens compared with those receiving single-agent chemotherapy.

RANDOMIZED TRIALS OF COMBINATION CHEMOTHERAPY VERSUS SUPPORTIVE CARE FOR METASTATIC NON-SMALL CELL LUNG CANCER

Three studies have randomized patients with metastatic disease to treatment with combination chemotherapy and supportive care or supportive care alone, and thus compared survival and quality of life benefits from chemotherapy with those of supportive care alone.[796-798] The National Cancer Institute of Canada randomized 136 eligible patients to "best supportive care" or chemotherapy with vindesine and cisplatin (VP) (25% tumor responses) or CAP (16% tumor responses).[797] Although toxicity on the chemotherapy arms was significant, the median survival of the supportive-care group was 17 weeks, whereas it was 23 weeks for CAP and 31 weeks for VP, the latter being a significant improvement. The UCLA Solid Tumor Study Group randomized 63 patients with metastatic cancer to receive either supportive care, including palliative radiation, psychosocial support, analgesics, and nutritional support alone, or the same supportive care plus chemotherapy with VP.[798] Between 70% and 80% of the patients consented to the trial. The median survival time with supportive care only was 14 weeks compared with 20 weeks for chemotherapy plus supportive care (not significantly different). Differences in quality of life could not be determined because of difficulty in administering the test questionnaire to this population.

OUTPATIENT REGIMENS FOR CISPLATIN-COMBINATION CHEMOTHERAPY

Several chemotherapy regimens used to treat non-small cell lung cancer are described in Table 22-53. Hospitalization for chemotherapy obviously impacts on patients' lives, and it is desirable to keep this to a minimum when there are no curative or dramatic survival gains in sight. Whereas initial cisplatin-based combinations required hospitalization and intensive hydration, recently, programs of cisplatin and oral etoposide have been given safely in the outpatient setting with little toxicity and reasonable response rates.[801] Similarly, the Northern California Oncology Group divided the cisplatin dose between days 1 and 8 instead of administering the drug in the usual 5-day schedule.[802] Although the degree of nephrotoxicity was similar using this approach, the incidence and severity of myelosuppression and peripheral neuropathy were markedly reduced, while a high tumor response rate (47%) was maintained. The Institut Jules Bordet randomized 241 patients with advanced non-small cell lung cancer to chemotherapy with high-dose (120 mg/m² on day

1) or standard-dose (60 mg/m² on day 1) cisplatin therapy, both schedules given in combination with etoposide (120 mg/m² on days 3, 5, and 7). There was no significant response difference (25% versus 29%) or difference in overall survival or survival of responders between the two regimens.[803] As expected, toxicity (predominantly myelosupression), was significantly worse in the high-dose cisplatin arm. These results suggest using "standard-dose" cisplatin regimens.

PROGNOSTIC FEATURES IN THE SELECTION OF PATIENTS FOR CHEMOTHERAPY OF METASTATIC NON-SMALL CELL LUNG CANCER, PARTICULARLY THOSE PREDICTING LONG-TERM SURVIVAL

In many studies, the principal factors predicting a response to chemotherapy and survival in metastatic non-small cell cancer are performance status, disease extent, site of metastases, sex (females do better than males), and age.[772,776] In contrast, the histologic subtype appears to play little role. Quite often, medical oncologists give combination chemotherapy to patients with the hope of producing a dramatic response leading to significant prolongation of life (e.g. for a period of 1 to 2 years). Two large series, one from the ECOG[776] and the other from the MSKCC,[804] provide information on this question.

Eastern Cooperative Oncology Group Studies

The ECOG treated 893 good-performance-status patients using several combination chemotherapy regimens (listed in Table 22-51 and references 691 and 805) and obtained an overall median survival of 23 to 24 weeks, with no significant differences in survival among the seven different chemotherapy regimens. Nineteen percent of the patients survived for more than 1 year, and 4% survived for more than 2 years. The ECOG analyzed their multiple studies to identify characteristics associated with survival of 1 year or more (Table 22-52), finding that pretreatment characteristics most predictive of survival for more than 1 year were initial asymptomatic performance status (PS = 0); no bone, liver, or subcutaneous metastases; female sex; a histology other than large cell carcinoma; a prior weight loss of less than 5%; and no symptoms of shoulder or arm pain.[694] The 1-year survivors had a higher tumor response rate and complete regression rate than the population as a whole. Sixty-two percent of the complete responders and 34% of the partial responders, but only 14% of the nonresponders, lived for more than 1 year. The etoposide plus cisplatin combination had the highest proportion of 1-year survivors (25%), compared with 18% for the other regimens, whereas the mitomycin C plus vinblastine plus cisplatin combination had significantly fewer 1-year survivors (12%) than any of the other regimens despite having the highest tumor response rate (Table 22-51). The ECOG hypothesized that this was attributable to increased toxicity caused by long-term use of mitomycin.

Of interest, the ECOG found that those patients whose tumor took a long time to respond to chemotherapy maintained the response the longest. Thus, patients whose tumors took more than 90 days to exhibit the best response to ther-

TABLE 22-53.   Sample Drug Regimens Used in the Treatment of Non-Small Cell Lung Cancer

CAP*

Cyclophosphamide	400 mg/m² IV
Doxorubicin	40 mg/m² IV
Cisplatin	40 mg/m² IV

All given day 1 and repeated every 4 weeks.

1. Patients must have normal cardiac and renal status (creatinine <1.5 mg/dl).
2. Doses are given by rapid IV, infusion with 1 liter of 5% glucose in half-normal saline over 1 to 2 hours; no special diuresis program is routinely used.
3. Doses are modified to obtain WBC nadirs of 1500–2500/μl or platelet nadirs of 75,000–100,000/μl measured at day 14. Before each subsequent treatment, WBC should be >4,000/μl and platelets >100,000/μl.
4. Stop cisplatin permanently if creatinine rises above 2.0 mg/dl or hearing loss develops.
5. Stop doxorubicin at a maximum cumulative dose of 450 mg/m² or if signs of congestive heart failure or arrythmias develop.

VP-16 + Cisplatin†

VP-16	120 mg/m² IV days 1, 3, 5. Repeat combination every 3 weeks.
Cisplatin	60 mg/ms², IV day 1

1. Patients must have normal renal function.
2. All patients will have nausea, vomiting, and alopecia.
3. Appropriate dose modifications are made for hematologic and renal toxicity. Omit cisplatin if creatinine is 2 mg/dl or higher until creatinine returns to less than 1.5 mg/dl.
4. Patients also should be monitored for hearing loss.
5. Hydration for cisplatin includes furosemide, 20 mg IV, given at the start of 2-hour infusion of 2 liters of 5% glucose in half-normal saline with 10 mEq of KCl/liter. Thirty minutes into infusion, 12.5 g of mannitol is given IV. If diuresis ensues, cisplatin is administered as an IV bolus. If no diuresis by 30 minutes, additional furosemide should be given.‡

Vinblastine + Cisplatin§

Vinblastine	6 mg/m² IV
Cisplatin	120 mg/m² IV or 60 mg/m² IV

1. Follow comments for VP-16 and cisplatin above.
2. In a comparison of cisplatin + vinblastine versus cisplatin + vindesine (3 mg/m²) there was no difference in response rates (41% versus 33%), median response durations (5.6 versus 8.6 months), or median survival times of responding patients (16.2 versus 18.4 months). However, more patients receiving vinblastine + cisplatin had WBC counts below 2100/μl whereas the vindesine-treated patients had more neurotoxicity.
3. Whether 120 mg/m² is better than 60 mg/m² for the cisplatin dose is not yet known. A randomized comparison in 85 patients between the same dose of another vinca alkaloid, vindesine, and either high-dose (120 mg/m²) or low-dose (60 mg/m²) cisplatin showed the same overall response rate of 43%, but the high-dose cisplatin regimen was superior to the low-dose regimen in median duration of response and in median survival for responding patients.[799] Patients receiving the high dose usually are hospitalized for hydration (150 ml/hour of 5% glucose normal saline with 20 mEq of KC1/liter) for 12 hours before therapy. Immediately before treatment, mannitol 12.5 g is given as a rapid IV infusion. The volume of fluid ordinarily requires either a large-bore Angiocath or a central venous line. Just before cisplatin is administered, 20 mg of furosemide is given IV. The high-dose cisplatin is mixed in 250 ml of 3% saline and infused over 30 min.[800] If patients cannot tolerate this fluid load for the full period of hydration despite appropriate medical management

(diuretics), the hydration regimen can be altered to 5% glucose in half-normal saline at 150 ml/hour with KCl supplementation.

*Data from Eagan RT, Ingle JN, Frytak S et al: Platinum based polychemotherapy versus dianhydrogalacticol in advanced non-small cell lung cancer. Cancer Treat Rep 61:1339–1345, 1977; Ruckdeschel JC, Finkelstein DM, Mason BA, Creech RH: Chemotherapy for metastatic non-small cell bronchogeneic carcinoma: EST-2575, generation V: A randomized comparison of four cisplatin-containing regimens. J Clin Oncol 3:72–79, 1985

†Data from Klatersky J, Longeval E, Nicaise C, Weerts D: Etoposide and cisplatinum in non-small-cell bronchogenic carcinoma. Cancer Treat Rev 9(Suppl A):133–138, 1982; Longeval E, Klastersky J: Combination chemotherapy with cisplatin and etoposide in bronchogenic squamous cell carcinoma and adenocarcinoma: A study by the EORTC Lung Cancer Working Party (Belgium). Cancer 50:2751–2756, 1982; Goldhirsch A, Joss R, Cavalli F, Brunner KW: Etoposide as single agent and in combination chemotherapy of bronchogenic carcinoma. Cancer Treat Rev 9(Suppl A):85–90, 1982; Ruckdeschel JC, Finkelstein DM, Ettinger DS, et al: A randomized trial of the four most active regimens for metastatic non-small cell lung cancer J Clin Oncol 4:14–22, 1986.

‡Vogl SE, Zaravinos T, Kaplan BH et al: Safe and effective two hour outpatient regimen of hydration and diuresis for the administration of cis diaminedichloroplatinum(II). Eur J Cancer 17:345–350, 1981.

§Kris GM, Gralla RJ, Kalman LA et al: Randomized trial comparing vindesine plus cisplatin with vinblastine plus cisplatin in patients with non-small cell lung cancer, with an analysis of methods of response assessment. Cancer Treat Rep 69:387–395, 1985.

apy were more likely to be long-term survivors than were those whose tumors responded more quickly (less than 30 days). This result suggested a biologic difference between rapidly and slowly responding tumors.[694] Not surprisingly, long-term survivors were more likely to maintain or improve their performance status and serum albumin concentration during the first 3 months following therapy than patients living less than 1 year. However, the ECOG also noted that the 1-year survivors experienced more intense hematologic and gastrointestinal (vomiting) toxicity that was probably related to the longer duration of chemotherapy.[694]

Memorial Sloan-Kettering Cancer Center Study

The 554 patients with unresectable non-small cell cancer treated by the MSKCC group received cisplatin plus a vinca alkaloid (vindesine or vinblastine) with or without mitomycin C; 9.6% achieved a complete remission.[809] These patients, in general, had excellent pretreatment performance status and no weight loss, and 40% were women. A complete remission was achieved in 5.8% with chemotherapy alone, whereas another 3.8% where able to obtain a complete remission with surgical resection after a significant tumor response to chemotherapy. All of the patients improved or maintained their performance status while in a complete remission and lived a median of 28 to 36 months, compared with a median survival of 11 months for the overall series. In another multivariate analysis of 378 of these patients, the

Memorial group found that a good initial performance status (Karnofsky 80–100) was significantly related to achieving a significant tumor response to chemotherapy and increased survival, whereas bone metastases, elevated serum LDH, and male sex were associated with poorer response rate and shorter remission duration and survival, as was the presence of two or more extrathoracic metastatic organ sites.[775]

TOXICITIES IN THE TREATMENT OF NON-SMALL CELL LUNG CANCER WITH CHEMOTHERAPY

Most of the combination-chemotherapy trials in non-small cell lung cancer have produced significant treatment-related toxicities including death.[773] For example, of 65 consecutive patients treated with intensive induction chemotherapy by a major cancer center skilled in supportive care, more than half experienced an infectious episode, and 5% suffered drug-related infectious death.[806]

In addition, poor performance status patients were at significantly higher risk of developing an infectious complication.[806] Similarly, in trials reporting excellent objective response rates and increased survival for responders compared with nonresponders, significant chemotherapy toxicity was noted in more than half the patients, and both performance status and body weight dropped significantly during chemotherapy among all patients.[807]

Combination chemotherapy regimens that include repeated (more than three cycles) administration of mitomycin C, often with a vinca alkaloid, have been associated with pulmonary toxicity manifested by the clinical triad of progressive dyspnea, rales, and pulmonary infiltrates and associated with hypoxemia and profound reduction in diffusion capacity.[808] Transbronchial biopsy reveals characteristic but nonspecific changes. Treatment involves high-dose glucocorticoids, which have to be tapered gradually, and immediate discontinuation of mitomycin C when pulmonary toxicity is suspected. Most patients respond promptly to this therapy.

PERCEPTION OF RISK: BENEFIT RATIO FOR CHEMOTHERAPY IN THE MANAGEMENT OF NON-SMALL CELL LUNG CANCER

Such results cause many experienced physicians to feel that the deterioration in patients' well-being from chemotherapy offsets any potential survival advantage.[807] A dramatic testament to this clinical experience was provided in a study questionnaire administered to 118 Canadian physicians who treat lung cancer.[809,810] Whereas opinion was divided as to the role of immediate radiotherapy in operable cancer and the role of postoperative radiotherapy after incomplete resection, there was little debate as to the role of chemotherapy. Only 3% would want for themselves adjuvant chemotherapy after surgery for early disease, only 9% would want chemotherapy for advanced disease confined to the chest, and only 15% would want chemotherapy for symptomatic metastatic disease. Thus, experts in the field would not prescribe for themselves treatment currently given in many clinical trials for non-small cell lung cancer.

EXPERIMENTAL TREATMENT APPROACHES TO NON-SMALL CELL LUNG CANCER

Role of Combined-Modality Radiotherapy and Chemotherapy for Advanced Non-Small Cell Lung Cancer

Three trials indicate that combined-modality (chemoradiotherapy), now experimental, may hold some promise. Two hundred sixty-eight patients with localized unresectable epidermoid lung cancer were treated with cisplatin plus bleomycin and either mitomycin, vindesine, or etoposide followed by radiation therapy. There was a 62% objective tumor response rate.[811] The median survival for the group was 9 months. However, there was a 35% 1-year and a 13% 2-year survival rate. Sixty-four patients with Stage III locally unresectable cancer were given cisplatin plus 5-FU chemotherapy with simultaneous radiation therapy (40 Gy) followed by attempted surgical resection. Sixty-one percent underwent the resection, and 14% of the original group were found to have no tumor in the surgical specimens.[812] However, when 81 patients with inoperable cancer were randomized to receive split-dose irradiation alone or with cisplatin-based combination chemotherapy, the survival and quality of life measures were not different in the groups.[813]

New Types of Treatment

Chemoprevention trials using vitamin A (retinol palmitate), retinoids with or without beta-carotene, or N-acetylcysteine are being designed,[814,815] and thus it is of interest that clinically evident lung cancer has shown responses to these agents. A Phase II trial of 13-cis-retinoic acid (100 mg/m² per day) in advanced non-small cell lung cancer produced one significant response among 23 evaluable patients that lasted 5 months,[816] whereas another trial showed one response in 10 patients and minor responses in two others.[817]

The RTOG randomized 117 patients to treatment with radiotherapy alone or with the hypoxic cell sensitizer misonidazole.[818] They found misonidazole did not enhance the effect of radiotherapy on either local tumor control or overall survival in patients with advanced lung cancer. In contrast, the Northern California Oncology Group, in a randomized trial of 100 patients, found that misonidazole did function as a chemosensitizer for the drug L-phenylalanine mustard in non-small cell lung cancer.[819]

Hydrazine sulfate, which is thought to improve the abnormal metabolism and reverse weight loss in patients with advanced cancer, was associated with significantly longer survival then was a placebo in a randomized trial of 65 patients with metastatic lung cancer receiving combination chemotherapy.[820] In a prospective double-blind trial, 12 malnourished lung cancer patients were randomized to receive placebo or hydrazine sulfate (60 mg three times daily). Fasting lysine flux was studied before and after treatment and revealed a significant improvement after 30 days of hydrazine sulfate administration.[821] In contrast, 102 patients with metastatic non-small cell cancer randomized to receive either ad lib diets or specific nutritional intervention during a 12-week period while receiving combination chemotherapy (vindesine and cisplatin) showed no difference in response rates, median time to progression, or overall duration of survival.[822]

Mopidamol (RA-233) is a derivative of dipyridamole (a phosphodiesterase inhibitor) that inhibits the progression of malignancy in experimental animal models. A Veterans Administration Cooperative Group randomized a large number of patients with small cell and non-small cell lung cancer to chemotherapy alone or chemotherapy with RA-233.[823] No significant difference in survival was found for small cell carcinoma patients (limited or extensive stage) or patients with disseminated non-small cell cancer. However, in the 71 patients with non-small cell disease limited to one hemithorax, the patients randomized to RA-233 and chemotherapy (with cyclophosphamide, doxorubicin, and methotrexate) had significantly longer survival than patients treated with chemotherapy and a RA-233 placebo (46 versus 29 weeks). This important trial needs to be confirmed with larger numbers of patients. However, it may be that RA-233 inhibits the breakdown of cyclic AMP and thus promotes the transduction of growth-inhibitory signals in tumor, possibly through effects on the function of the *ras* proto-oncogene.[824]

Immunotherapy

RANDOMIZED CLINICAL TRIALS. There is a large literature on impaired immune function in lung cancer patients, and this has stimulated many clinical trials of immunotherapy. Several randomized studies have evaluated immunotherapy, usually as an adjuvant to surgery, and over the past 10 years, there have been flurries of excitement about the benefits of such adjuvant immunotherapy. However, recent large-scale randomized trials suggest there is no standard role for such therapy at present. The Ludwig Lung Cancer Study Group prospectively randomized 303 patients with resected Stage I and II non-small cell cancer to receive intrapleural *Corynebacterium parvum* (*C. parvum*) and then subsequent intravenous *C. parvum* or a placebo.[825] They found no significant difference between the treatments with respect to disease-free interval or survival. In another trial, the Ludwig group prospectively randomized 441 patients with resected Stage I and II non-small cell cancer to adjuvant treatment with either intrapleural BCG (Tice strain) between postoperative days 6 and 12 or placebo.[826] There was no significant difference between the groups with respect to survival, but there was a high rate of pleural empyema in the BCG-treated group and a significant decrease in the disease-free interval for the patients who had undergone a pneumonectomy. In the Netherlands, the administration of intrapleural BCG actually appeared to enhance tumor growth.[827] Another study found significant survival advantages for patients with resected disease treated with the streptococcal preparation OK-432 and chemotherapy compared with those given chemotherapy alone.[828] However, until these observations are substantiated, these approaches should not be applied outside clinical trials.

RECENT FINDINGS OF IMMUNOLOGIC IMPORTANCE IN LUNG CANCER PATIENTS. The subpopulation of lymphocytes designated natural killer (NK) cells are capable of killing a variety of tumor cell targets. Despite high blood levels of NK cell activity, the NK activity of lymphocytes is significantly lower in lung specimens of patients undergoing a curative resection for lung cancer than in lymphocytes from normal lung specimens obtained from cadavers undergoing medicolegal autopsy.[829] This change appears to result from the release of inhibitors by pulmonary macrophages in lung cancer patients. Interleukin-2 (IL-2)-derived T lymphocytes were grown from explants of tumor tissues and given to lung cancer patients, where they were associated with tumor reduction in five of seven patients and an increase in delayed cutaneous hypersensitivity in three of these patients.[830] Intrapleural instillations of recombinant IL-2 in 11 patients with malignant pleural effusions resulted in clearing of the effusions and cancer cells in the effusions in nine patients, with side effects being fever, eosinophilia, and a transient increase in the effusion.[841]

NEW APPROACHES TO PALLIATIVE THERAPY

Neodynium: YAG Laser and Photodynamic (Hematoporphyrin) Therapy for Bronchial Obstruction

Management of intrabronchial lesions recurrent after surgery and radiotherapy, as well as of such lesions in patients with comprised pulmonary function, and treatment decisions about radiographically occult cancers are challenging. Two new forms of treatment offer promise in these arenas. *Neodynium: YAG (yttrium–aluminum–garnet) laser therapy* has been used increasingly in treating recurrent endotracheal and endobronchial lesions in lung cancer, usually in patients relapsing after several other therapies including surgery and radiotherapy.[832,833] Treatment can often be administered via a flexible fiberoptic bronchoscope, and usually, this is done under general anesthesia. Palliative improvement is seen in 80% to 90% of cases, and many patients have been treated. Serious complications include massive hemorrhage (usually related to high power settings), intrabronchial explosions, and damage to normal tissues.

After administration of *hematoporphyrin*, which may localize in tumors and which sensitizes tissues to light, *bronchoscopic phototherapy* has been administered to intrabronchial lesions.[834] Small, radiographically occult carcinomas treated this way will often regress completely for long periods of follow-up, whereas larger lesions will often show at least a partial response.

Malignant Pleural Effusions

The development of malignant pleural effusion in patients with lung cancer is an ominous sign. These effusions are usually recurrent and can be highly symptomatic, leading to shortness of breath and pain. The key to their management in lung cancer is prompt and complete chest tube drainage of all but the smallest effusions after appropriate physical examination and diagnostic tests to exclude congestive heart failure and infection. Although a variety of other treatments such as intrapleural instillation of tetracycline or chemotherapy, play a role, they are secondary to appropriate chest tube drainage.

666   CANCER OF THE LUNG

Pain Control

Fortunately, severe, unrelenting pain is not a frequent problem in lung cancer compared with such problems as bronchial obstruction or brain metastases. Management of cancer-related pain is discussed in detail in Chapter 59, section 4. In a series of 221 lung cancer patients with intractable pain, the three chief causes were skeletal metastatic disease (34%), Pancoast's tumor (31%), and chest wall disease (21%), together accounting for 78% of the cancer-related pain problems.[835] The median interval between cancer diagnosis and the onset of pain was only 1 month, and the median survival after the onset of the pain was 10 months. A variety of treatment modalities have been employed, including local radiation, percutaneous cordotomy, regional deafferentation, and pharmacotherapy.

THERAPY OF SMALL CELL CARCINOMA OF THE LUNG

Small cell lung cancer differs from the other cell types in its more aggressive clinical course in the absence of treatment and in its superior responsiveness to chemotherapy and thoracic irradiation. Median survival of patients with surgically unresectable disease randomized to supportive care alone in a trial conducted during the 1960s was only 12 weeks for patients with limited-stage and 5 weeks for those with extensive-stage disease.[493] The disease's natural history is characterized by relentless progression and the early development of distant metastatic deposits. When compared with other types of lung cancer with a similar extent of tumor dissemination, a shorter duration of symptoms prior to diagnosis and reduced survival once a diagnosis is established are evident.[493,836] In a study of 19 patients subjected to potentially curative surgical resection and dying within 30 days of operation of noncancer-related causes, 70% had distant metastases at postmortem examination.[837] More than 70% of patients have mediastinal lymph node involvement at diagnosis, which in itself precludes surgical resection.[838,839] Approximately two-thirds of patients will have evidence of metastases beyond the hemithorax of origin.[839] At autopsy of patients managed without surgical extirpation of the primary tumor, only 4% will not demonstrate tumor dissemination beyond the thorax.[840]

These findings of frequent tumor spread to regional lymph nodes and distant extrathoracic sites by the time of initial clinical presentation indicate that small cell carcinoma is a systemic disease process very early after inception in almost all patients. Therefore, it is not surprising that reliance on solely locoregional forms of treatment fails in the vast majority of patients. In a British study performed in the 1960s, patients who were considered candidates for surgical resection by the standards of the time were randomized to thoracotomy with the intent of tumor removal or to definitive irradiation to the primary tumor and regional lymphatics.[841] Although radiotherapy proved superior to attempted surgical removal in terms of survival (Table 22-54), fewer than 4% of these apparently operable patients were alive 5 years after randomization. Today, these patients (if they had been appropriately staged) would represent a very favorable subset of limited-stage disease. Shortly thereafter, a review of the outcome of a large number of American small cell lung cancer patients who were thought to be operable revealed absolutely no differences in survival whether or not a thoracotomy was performed.[842] These data led to the abandonment of surgical therapy by many thoracic surgeons in patients with an established diagnosis of small cell carcinoma until the present decade.

In 1969, an important randomized trial by the Veterans Administration LCSG documented that three courses of cyclophosphamide more than doubled the median survival compared with supportive care alone in extensive-stage small cell lung cancer.[843] This finding sharply contrasted with the results of similar studies of single-agent chemotherapy in other cell types of lung cancer and led to the rapid investigation of the role of chemotherapy in patients with small cell carcinoma. Randomized studies (which employed what would today be considered suboptimal chemotherapy) in most instances demonstrated that adjuvant chemotherapy after surgical resection prolonged survival compared with no further treatment. Because of the small numbers of patients enrolled in most of these trials, this result becomes more obvious when the data are pooled (Table 22-55). Similarly, in most randomized clinical trials, the addition of chemotherapy to chest irradiation in patients with limited-stage small cell lung cancer yielded improved median or longer-term survival compared with a policy of irradiation as the sole initial treatment followed by chemotherapy at the time of tumor progression (Table 22-56). Once again, the chemo-

TABLE 22-54.   Survival in Patients with Operable Small Lung Cancer Randomized to Surgery or Radiotherapy

Group	No. of Patients	Mean Survival (mo)	Survival Rate (%)		
			1-Year	2-Year	5-Year
Surgery	71	6.5	21	4	1†
Radiotherapy	73	10*	22	10	4

*Significant survival difference (p = 0.04) in favor of radiotherapy.
†One patient unable to receive surgery; given irradiation.
Modified from Fox W, Scadding JG: Medical Research Council comparative trial of surgery and radiotherapy for primary treatment of small-celled or oat-celled carcinoma of bronchus. Lancet 2:63–65, 1973.

TABLE 22-55. Pooled Results from Randomized Surgical Adjuvant Studies in Small Cell Lung Cancer

Adjuvant Therapy	No. of Patients	2-Year Survivors (%)
Chemotherapy	92	26
Placebo	61	8

Higgins GA, Shields TW: Experience of the Veterans Administration Surgical Adjuvant Group. Prog Cancer Res Ther 11:433–442, 1979; Shields TW, Humphrey EW, Eastridge CE et al: Adjuvant cancer chemotherapy after resection of carcinoma of the lung. Cancer 5:2057–2062, 1977; Wingfield HV: Combined surgery and chemotherapy for carcinoma of the bronchus. Lancet 1:470–471, 1970; Karrer K, Pridun N, Denck H: Chemotherapy as an adjuvant to surgery in lung cancer. Cancer Chemotherapy Pharmacol 1:145–159, 1978.

therapy used in these early trials, either as single agents or in combinations, was not optimal by current standards. Nevertheless, these early trials of chemotherapy as an adjuvant to locoregional treatments and multiple other studies employing chemotherapy as the sole form of therapy quickly established that small cell carcinoma was by far the most drug-responsive type of lung cancer.

The strategies of chemotherapy administration in small cell lung cancer are similar to the optimal methods of drug treatment in several adult cancers that can sometimes be cured with chemotherapy alone. For example, in small cell carcinoma, testicular carcinoma, Hodgkin's disease, and diffuse aggressive lymphomas, although numerous single agents induce objective responses, combination chemotherapy produces superior survival compared with single-agent treatment; responses to chemotherapy occur relatively quickly; increasing drug doses (up to a point) improves survival rates; and maintenance chemotherapy for responding patients is of little or no value. Over the past two decades, therapeutic research in small cell lung cancer has been built on the assumptions that this is fundamentally a systemic disorder that is usually responsive to chemotherapeutic agents and that combination chemotherapy is therefore the mainstay of treatment. Several detailed reviews summarizing the therapy of this neoplasm and critically evaluating which approaches yield optimal results have been published in the 1980s.[836,844–849]

PRETREATMENT EVALUATION

Several issues must be considered before therapy of the patient with small cell lung cancer is initiated: the pathologic diagnosis must be confirmed, the extent of tumor dissemination determined, and the ability of the patient to tolerate therapy assessed. Because the distinction of small cell carcinoma from other cell types of lung cancer has significant therapeutic implications, an experienced lung cancer pathologist should review the biopsy specimen. Although the oat cell subtype of small cell carcinoma is usually readily recognized, the intermediate subtype may be mistaken for non-small cell lung cancer by the less-experienced pathologist. Difficulties in diagnosis are most likely when the specimen is of poor quality, especially, in our experience, when the only material available for review is a fine-needle aspirate.

Staging procedures have already been discussed in detail. In brief, the purpose of staging is to assign prognosis, to identify tumor lesions that can be monitored to assess the

TABLE 22-56. Selected Randomized Trials of Radiotherapy Alone Versus Chemotherapy plus Radiation Therapy in Limited-Stage Disease*

Series	2 Year Radiotherapy Dose (cGy)	Chemotherapy†	No. of Patients	Survival Median (mo)	Survival 1 Year (%)	Survival 2 Year (%)
Seydel et al.	4500	None	110	10	NR	2
		C + CCNU	107	11‡	NR	8
MRC	3000	None	121	6	18	NR
		C + MTX + CCNU	115	10§	34	NR
Bergsagel	4000–5000	None	14	5	NR	NR
		C	27	10‖	NR	NR
Petrovich	5000–6000	None	33	5	28	12
		CCNU + HU	35	9§	28	5
Perez	4500	None	23	11	36	15
		C + A + DTIC	24	8‡	38	22

*Modified from Bunn PA, Ihde DC: Small cell bronchogenic carcinoma: A review of therapeutic results. In Livingston RB (ed): Lung Cancer 1, pp 169–208. Amsterdam, Martinus Nijhoff, 1981. Data from Seydel HG, Creech R, Pagano M et al: Small-cell carcinoma: Combined modality treatment of regional small cell undifferentiated carcinoma of the lung. Int J Radiat Oncol 9:1135–1141, 1983; Medical Research Council Lung Cancer Working Party et al: Radiotherapy alone or with chemotherapy in the treatment of small-cell carcinoma of the lung: The results at 36 months. Br J Cancer 44:611–617, 1981; Bergsagel D, Jenkin R, Pringle J et al: Lung cancer: Clinical trial of radiotherapy alone vs radiotherapy plus cyclophosphamide. Cancer 30:621–627, 1972; Petrovich Z, Ohanian M, Cox JD: Clinical research on the treatment of locally advanced lung cancer. Cancer 42:1129–1134, 1978; Perez CA, Krauss S, Bartolucci A et al: Thoracic and elective brain irradiation with concomitant or delayed multiagent chemotherapy in the treatment of localized small cell carcinoma of the lung. Cancer 47:2407–2413, 1981

†Abbreviations: NR = not reported, C = cyclophosphamide, CCNU = lomustine, MTX = methotrexate, HU = hydroxyurea, A = doxorubicin, DTIC = dacarbazine.

‡Survival differences between groups not statistically significant.

§Significantly improved survival with chemotherapy.

‖Survival differences not analyzed.

response to therapy, and to determine if treatment in addition to combination chemotherapy is required or desirable. In a clinical investigative setting, additional staging may be mandated. Patients with extensive-stage disease clearly have a worse prognosis, and those with limited-stage tumors or brain metastases will most often receive chest or brain irradiation, respectively. Ambulatory or performance status is not only an important prognostic factor, but bedridden patients and those with other serious illnesses tolerate intensive therapy poorly with increased morbidity and mortality rates. Pulmonary compromise secondary to cigarette abuse, which is often present, may limit the volume of lung that can be irradiated safely or render an otherwise-indicated surgical procedure inadvisable.

SINGLE-AGENT CHEMOTHERAPY

During the 1970s, seven chemotherapeutic agents that produced response rates of at least 30% when given to 30 or more patients with small cell lung cancer were identified (Table 22-57). Only two additional drugs fulfilling these criteria, carboplatin and teniposide, have been discovered since. Complete response rates to single-agent therapy are less than 5%, and the impact on survival is modest.[850,851] Furthermore, only vincristine and hexamethylmelamine among active drugs do not have myelosuppression as their dose-limiting toxicity, making it difficult to construct combination drug programs in which the full single-agent dose of each compound is employed. Cyclophosphamide, doxorubicin, vincristine, etoposide (VP-16), and cisplatin are probably the most commonly utilized agents. Vincristine is usually administered every 3 weeks because of neurotoxicity, although the best evidence for its single-agent activity was obtained with a weekly schedule.[852] In a randomized study comparing three schedules of etoposide as sole therapy, schedules with three or five doses per week produced higher response rates than a weekly schedule.[853] This drug is therefore most commonly administered several times per week,

TABLE 22-57. Chemotherapeutic Agents with Documented Activity Against Small Cell Lung Cancer

Group 1 (Confirmed response rate of >30% in at least 30 patients)
   Cyclophosphamide
   Mechlorethamine (nitrogen mustard)
   Doxorubicin (Adriamycin®)
   Methotrexate
   Hexamethylmelamine†
   Etoposide (VP-16-213)
   Vincristine
   Carboplatin (CBDCA)†
   Teniposide (VM-26)†
Group 2 (Lesser or less well confirmed activity)
   Cisplatin*
   Ifosfamide†
   Lomustine (CCNU)
   Carmustine (BCNU)
   Semustine (methyl-CCNU)†
   Procarbazine
   Vindesine†
   Nimustine (ACNU, nitrosourea)†

*Adequate single-agent data only in previously treated patients.
†Not commercially available in the United States.

although when given with other active agents in combination regimens, a single dose every 3 weeks may be as effective.[854]

Highly active drugs in patients with no prior chemotherapy may exhibit only marginal activity in patients with relapsed small cell lung cancer. For example, etoposide has a response rate of more than 40% in previously untreated patients,[851] but when given to 116 patients relapsing after modern combination chemotherapy, it produced only a 9% response rate.[855] A similar situation is observed with the etoposide analogue teniposide (VM-26), which has a 90% response rate in untreated, and a 15% response rate in previously treated, patients.[856] In one of the few randomized studies designed to evaluate a dose–response relation for a single agent in small cell lung cancer,[857] too few responses to allow analysis were seen with etoposide at any of three dose levels up to 900 mg/m² in 77 previously treated patients.

Only five new drugs have been demonstrated to possess clear activity in Phase II trials in small cell lung cancer during the 1980s, and all of them are analogues of drugs already known to be useful. However, it is quite possible that some active drugs were among the 23 agents deemed inactive during the same era in studies that were conducted principally in previously treated patients. For example, whereas the single-agent response rate to cisplatin is only 15%,[858] placing it in the list of "less active" drugs in Table 22-57, it has been evaluated as a single drug almost exclusively in previously treated patients. Thus, it probably has significantly more activity, comparable to that of its analogue, CBDCA (carboplatin), which produced 60% response rate in 30 previously untreated patients.[859] These considerations have led to the suggestion that Phase II trials should be performed in previously untreated patients with a poor prognosis, that is, patients with extensive disease. If the disease fails to respond after a short time, a standard combination-chemotherapy regimen could be administered. Such a strategy is certainly acceptable when the Phase II agent is active, as already demonstrated with some drugs.[856,859] However, further experience is needed before this approach is generally adopted, as two recent Phase II studies in untreated extensive-stage patients, including one study utilizing a doxorubicin analogue, yielded shorter than anticipated survival.[860-862] Better drugs for the treatment of small cell lung cancer are clearly needed, and new agents, preferably those with novel mechanisms of action, will certainly continue to be tested in the setting of refractory disease. Any treatment that is useful in previously treated cases will immediately be evaluated in untreated patients.

COMBINATION CHEMOTHERAPY

Treatment programs including aggressive combination chemotherapy regimens yield the best response rates (Fig. 22-17) and the highest percentage of long-term survivors.[836,847] In limited disease, optimal current regimens should produce 85% to 95% overall response rates, 50% to 60% complete response rates, median survival times of 12 to 16 months, and 2-year disease-free survival rates of 15% to 20%. Corresponding results in patients with extensive disease are overall response rates of 75% to 85%, complete

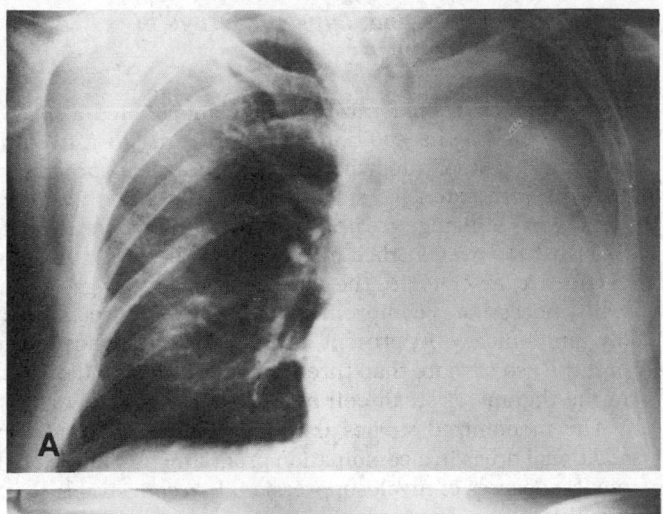

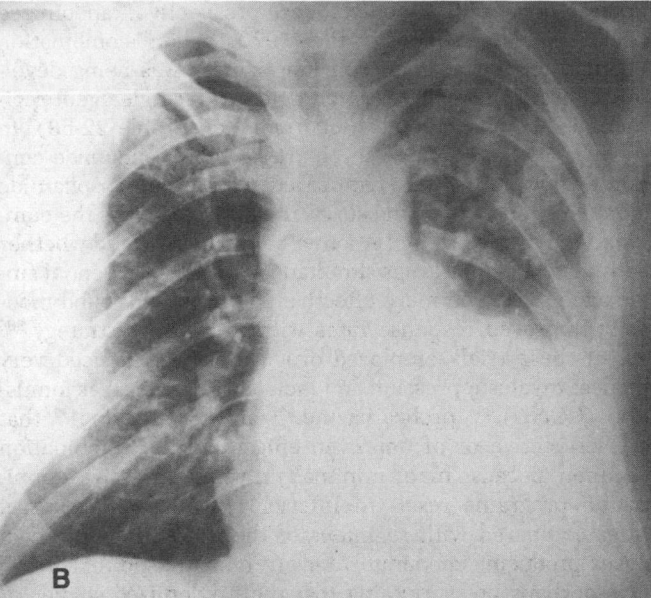

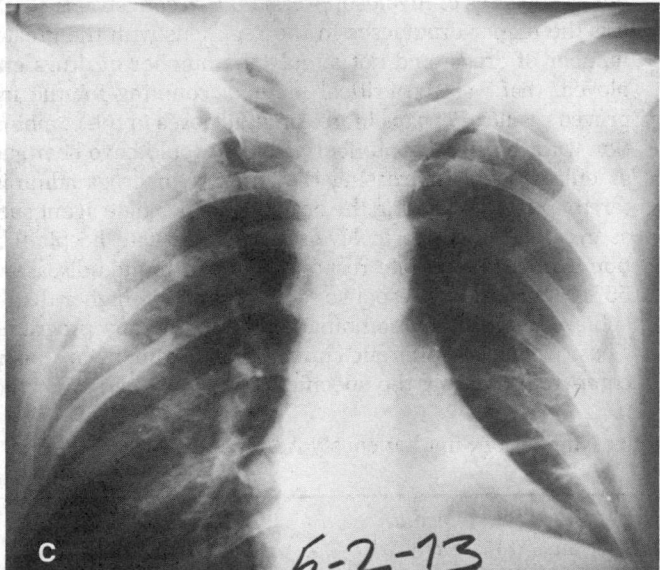

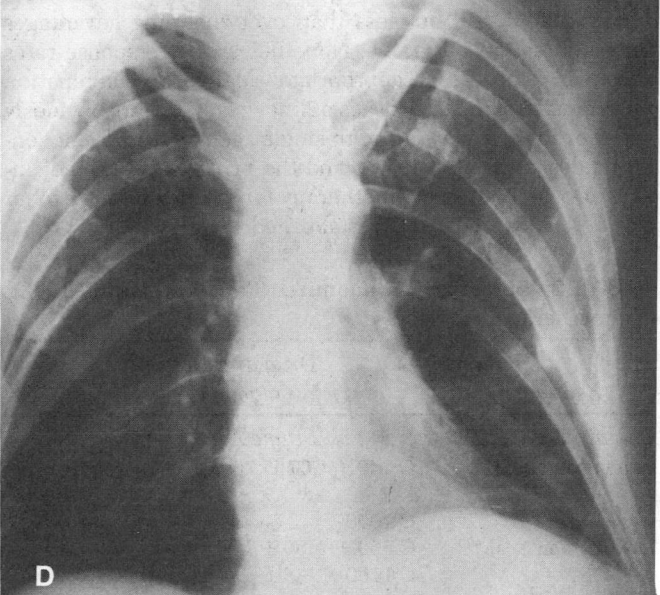

FIG. 22-17. Sequential chest radiographs of a patient with small cell lung cancer treated with intensive combination chemotherapy alone (cyclophosphamide + methotrexate + CCNU regimen). **A.** Pretreatment showing large mass in left chest, with obstruction, collapse of left lower lobe, loss of volume, and tracheal deviation. **B.** One week after the start of therapy showing response of tumor and remaining bulk of tumor in pulmonary parenchyma, hilar, and mediastinal nodes. **C.** Three weeks after the start of therapy. Almost complete resolution of tumor; however, there is still some residual stranding and possible mediastinal adenopathy. **D.** Five weeks after the start of treatment; no tumor visible by chest radiograph. Fiberoptic bronchoscopy with washings and biopsy at 6 weeks revealed no evidence of tumor.

response rates of 15% to 30%, and median survival of 7 to 11 months. Two-year disease-free survival in extensive disease is rare.

Although these therapeutic outcomes obviously leave substantial room for improvement, they do represent a four- to five-fold increase in median survival compared with that of untreated patients and have been made possible only by the effective combination chemotherapy programs. The charac-

teristics of currently optimal combination regimens for small cell lung cancer will be discussed in detail in this section.

Superiority to Single Agents

Although, as just discussed, response rates routinely seen with current combination chemotherapy appear greatly superior to the rates observed with single agents in previously untreated patients,[863] only a few prospective randomized trials, conducted during the 1970s when combination chemotherapy for small cell lung cancer was being developed, directly compared combination with single-agent regimens in the absence of chest irradiation (Table 22-58). In two trials where two- or three-drug cyclophosphamide-containing programs were compared with cyclophosphamide alone, response rates and survival were better with the combination regimens.[490,864] Another study investigated whether administering four drugs simultaneously or as sequential single agents was the more effective approach and found modestly improved response rates with the former strategy.[865] All of these trials employed drug doses that induced very modest myelosuppression and included drugs such as lomustine (CCNU),[864] probcarbazine,[865] and dacarbazine[490] that are less active or of unproven efficacy in the combination regimen. Because many minimally myelosuppressive combination programs result in inferior response and survival rates compared with regimens of the same drugs given in doses producing moderately severe hematologic toxicity,[866] it is perhaps not surprising that the randomized studies of combination versus single-agent chemotherapy sometimes demonstrated real but less than overwhelming advantages for combination programs. Nonetheless, the response rates attained with current appropriately delivered combination programs utilizing only drugs of known activity are obviously superior to the early data with single agents given in conventional doses (Table 22-59), and the principle of the advantage of combination chemotherapy for small cell lung cancer can be considered firmly established.[847]

Optimal Number and Types of Drugs in Combination Regimens

Two prospective randomized trials demonstrated a survival advantage with the addition of a third drug to a two-drug program[867] and of a fourth agent to a three-drug program in patients with extensive stage disease (see Table 22-58).[253] Regimens utilizing greater numbers of agents simultaneously have been studied infrequently. Because most active agents are myelotoxic, the use of too many drugs concurrently necessitates compromises in dosage that would probably limit efficacy. At present, there is little evidence to support the use of more than three or four drugs simultaneously in the therapy of small cell lung cancer.[850]

The randomized studies that support the value of using additional drugs in a combination program[253,867] showed only modest degrees of myelosuppression. It is conceivable that it was the higher drug doses in the regimens with the greater number of drugs, and not simply the number of drugs employed, that was the critical factor accounting for the improved results. Perhaps increasing the doses in the combination with the smaller number of drugs would have been just as efficacious as increasing the number of drugs administered. In fact, escalating the dose of even a single agent such as cyclophosphamide to levels that necessitate hospitalization can yield complete response rates in limited disease of 55%,[868] a complete response rate as high as or higher than is achieved with many combination-chemotherapy programs. Thus, whenever different combination regimens are being compared, not only the specific agents being administered,

TABLE 22-58. Early Randomized Trials Evaluating the Optimum Number of Simultaneously Administered Chemotherapeutic Agents

Reference	Drug and Dose (mg/m²)*	No. of Patients	CR + PR Rate (%)	Median Survival	Comments
Combination Chemotherapy vs. Single Agents					
Edmonson et al.[864]	C 700 + CCNU 70	110	43	20 wk	Combination drugs better, p < 0.01
	C 1000	118	22	17 wk	CR + PR, p = 0.07 survival
Lowenbraun et al.[490]	C 500 + A 50 + DTIC 250	207	57	31 wk	Combination drugs better, p < 0.01
	C 1100				CR + PR, p = 0.01 survival
		34	12	18 wk	
Alberto et al.[865]	MTX 40 + C 420 + VCR 1.2 + PCZ 560†	59	65	NR	Simultaneous drugs better, p = 0.1
	MTX → C → PCZ → VCR‡	14	36	NR	CR + PR; survival not different
Three Drugs vs. Two Drugs					
Hansen et al.[253]	C 500 + MTX 20 + CCNU 50§	33	56	33 wk	3 drugs better, CR + PR not
	C 500 + MTX 20				different, p = 0.17 survival
		29	38	23 wk	
Four Drugs vs. Three Drugs					
Hansen et al.[867]	C 700 + MTX 20 + CCNU 70 + VCR 1.3‖	52	78	7.7 mo	4 drugs better, CR + PR not
	C 700 + MTX 20 + CCNU 70	53	75	6.0 mo	different, p < 0.01 survival

Modified from Ihde DC, Bunn PA: Chemotherapy of small cell bronchogenic carcinoma. In Williams CJ, Whitehouse JMA (eds): Recent Advances in Clinical Oncology, pp 305–323. Edinburgh, Churchill Livingstone, 1982.

*CR = complete response, PR = partial response, VCR = vincristine, PCZ = procarbazine; other drugs as in Table 22-56.

†Weekly doses given for 8 weeks.

‡Sequential single agents each given for 2 weeks.

§C every 3 weeks, MTX twice weekly, CCNU every 6 weeks.

‖C and CCNU every 4 weeks, MTX × 2 in week 3, VCR weekly first cycle.

TABLE 22-59. Summary of Objective Tumor Responses to Single-Agent or Combination Chemotherapy in Previously Untreated Patients with Small Cell Lung Cancer (No Radiation Therapy)

Drug Treatment	No. of Patients	Response (%)	
		All Objective†	Complete
Single agent‡	753	15–20	2.5
Combination	1236	70	31

*Adapted from Bunn PA Jr, Ihde DC: Small cell bronchogenic carcinoma: A review of therapeutic results. In Livingston RB (ed): Lung Cancer: Advances in Research and Treatment, pp 169–208. The Hague, Martinus Nijhoff, 1981.

†Objective tumor responses include partial and complete responses. Complete response rate data available for only 572 patients.

‡Includes only data for cyclophosphamide, nitrogen mustard, doxorubicin, methotrexate, etoposide, hexamethylmelamine, and vincristine.

but also the dose intensity with which they are delivered, must be considered. For example, a randomized study that found significantly improved response rates and survival in extensive-stage patients treated with cyclophosphamide, etoposide, and vincristine compared with those in patients receiving cyclophosphamide and vincristine more convincingly demonstrated the contribution of etoposide to the three-drug program, because the cyclophosphamide dose was doubled in the two-drug combination so that the myelosuppression associated with each regimen was similar.[869]

Although many combination-chemotherapy regimens for small cell lung cancer appear to possess similar efficacy, the CAV program (representative doses: cyclophosphamide 1000 mg/m², doxorubicin 45 mg/m², vincristine 2 mg) has been one of the most commonly used during the 1980s and reproducibly yields the current optimal response rates, median survival, and long-term survival outlined previously in both limited- and extensive-stage disease. It may reasonably be considered a "standard" regimen against which newer approaches can be compared. Etoposide is probably the most actively studied newer agent in recent years, and many randomized trials have attempted to determine whether adding etoposide to or substituting it for one of the components of CAV is of value.

Two studies compared CAV plus etoposide (CAVE) with CAV alone and found significantly greater response rates with CAVE. However, survival was not significantly improved in either study when results were adjusted for differences in pretreatment prognostic factors.[870,871] In an equitoxic comparison of standard-dose CAVE versus higher-dose CAV, there were no differences in response rates or survival.[872] Two other randomized trials addressed the utility of substituting etoposide for one of the drugs in CAV. Median survival in extensive-stage patients was prolonged by only 2 months when etoposide was substituted for either doxorubicin[869] (CEV versus CAV) or vincristine[873] (CAE versus CAV), although myelosuppression, and thus perhaps drug dose intensity, was greater with CAE in the latter trial. In neither study did the etoposide-containing program prove superior in limited-stage patients. In a large randomized study of 269 extensive-stage patients, etoposide was substituted for methotrexate at two different times in a 4-week cycle, four-drug regimen consisting of cyclophosphamide, methotrexate, CCNU, and vincristine.[874] Significantly improved survival was seen when etoposide was given early but not when it was given later in each cycle of chemotherapy. Increased myelosuppression, possibly correlating with increased antitumor effects, was observed with early etoposide. On balance, these studies adding etoposide to or substituting it in a standard combination program cannot be regarded as providing unequivocal evidence that etoposide-containing programs are superior to programs not containing this drug, although etoposide is clearly among the most active agents against small cell lung cancer.

The combination of etoposide and cisplatin exhibits therapeutic synergy in murine leukemia,[875] produces some long-term survivors in refractory testicular cancer,[876] and has recently been evaluated in many types of cancer. In previously treated small cell lung cancer, this two-drug program produced objective response rates of 50% or more in some recent studies,[877,878] which contrasts strikingly with the usual response rate of less than 10% for many other salvage regimens evaluated in the present decade. These encouraging results suggested the use of this combination as first-line therapy, either followed by other drugs[879,880] or as sole chemotherapeutic treatment.[881] The therapeutic results appear as good as or better than those with the standard CAV regimen in both limited and extensive disease, although results directly comparing CAV with etoposide–cisplatin are not yet available. In addition, etoposide–cisplatin is associated with less hematologic toxicity than most other active regimens,[882] suggesting an improved therapeutic index. One trial randomizing limited-stage patients to receive or not receive two cycles of etoposide–cisplatin after six cycles of CAV with or without chest irradiation demonstrated a 30-week improvement in median survival.[883] These data imply that etoposide–cisplatin may be able to eradicate tumor cells resistant to CAV.

Substitution of carboplatin for cisplatin in the etoposide–cisplatin program has yielded an active combination with reduced gastrointestinal toxicity.[884] In previously untreated patients, survival with etoposide–cisplatin was superior to that with etoposide–ifosfamide in a German study,[885] further supporting the value of the etoposide–cisplatin regimen.

Final definition of the role of this promising two-drug combination in the initial therapy of small cell lung cancer must await the results of ongoing clinical trials. Doses and schedules of some active combination regimens currently popular in the treatment of small cell carcinoma are provided in Table 22-60.

Intensity of Initial Chemotherapy

Most current chemotherapeutic programs for small cell lung cancer, with the possible exception of etoposide–cisplatin, are designed to produce moderately severe myelosuppression with leukopenia of 1000 to 2000 cells/μl in the majority of patients. Such regimens do not necessitate hospitalization but do mandate careful monitoring to avoid or ameliorate infectious or bleeding complications. One approach to the problem of drug resistance in this tumor has been to administer more intensive chemotherapeutic regimens, because the tenets of the dose–response relation in chemotherapy of cancer, both in animals and in humans, suggest that the dose rate may be critical to tumor cell kill, particularly in more responsive neoplasms.[886] Although increases in drug doses and frequency of administration might increase the response rate and duration, this approach is limited by toxicity to normal host tissues.

Several randomized (Table 22-61) and nonrandomized trials have studied the concept of dose–response relation in small cell lung cancer. The first randomized trial addressing this question administered two-fold higher doses of the CMC (cyclophosphamide–methotrexate–CCNU) regimen only

for the initial 6-week induction period and demonstrated significantly improved response rates and survival with higher drug doses.[866] A much larger randomized trial of the CMC regimen studied the effects of a higher dose only of the cyclophosphamide component during the first 6 weeks and found modest but significant increases in response rate and survival, particularly in patients with limited-stage disease.[887] Nonrandomized trial results also suggest that extremely high doses of cyclophosphamide (4.8–8.0 g/m^2) as a single agent produce a substantially higher than anticipated fraction of complete responses in both limited[868] and extensive[888] disease.

Increasing the doses of other standard chemotherapy programs or drugs in an outpatient setting has yet to improve results. In two randomized studies of the CAV regimen, the doses of cyclophosphamide were increased 20% to 56% and those of doxorubicin 18% to 75% during the first 9 to 12 weeks of chemotherapy.[889,890] Although the complete response rate was modestly improved in one trial,[889] there was no effect on response duration or survival with higher doses of CAV in either study. Preliminary results of a smaller trial involving administration of 67% higher doses of etoposide and cisplatin for the first 6 weeks of therapy suggest no benefit for the high-dose program.[882] There appears to be no benefit of high-dose methotrexate with leucovorin rescue compared with standard-dose methotrexate when added to the CAV regimen.[891] It is conceivable that CMC is less effective than other regimens such as CAV or etoposide–cisplatin and that higher, more toxic doses of CMC are needed to produce the same therapeutic results that other programs

TABLE 22-60.   Effective Commonly Used Combination Chemotherapy Programs for Small Cell Lung Cancer*

CAV		
Cyclophosphamide	1000	mg/m^2 IV day 1
Doxorubicin (Adriamycin®)	45	mg/m^2 IV day 1
Vincristine	2	mg IV day 1
Repeat cycle every 3 weeks		
CAVP16		
Cyclophosphamide	1000	mg/m^2 IV day 1
Doxorubicin	45	mg/m^2 IV day 1
Etoposide (VP-16)	50	mg/m^2 IV days 1–5
Repeat cycle every 3 weeks		
CAVVP-16		
Cyclophosphamide	1000	mg/m^2 IV day 1
Doxorubicin	50	mg/m^2 IV day 1
Vincristine	1.5	mg/m^2 IV day 1
Etoposide (VP-16)	60	mg/m^2 IV days 1–5
Repeat cycle every 3 weeks		
VP16-P		
Etoposide	100	mg/m^2 IV days 1–3
Cisplatin	25	mg/m^2 IV days 1–3
Repeat cycle every 3 weeks		
CMCcV		
Cyclophosphamide	700	mg/m^2 IV day 1
Methotrexate	20	mg/m^2 PO days 18, 21
Lomustine (CCNU)	70	mg/m^2 PO day 1
Vincristine	1.3	mg/m^2 IV days 1, 8, 15, 22 first cycle and then day 1.
Repeat cycle every 4 weeks		
CAV/VP-16P		
Cycle of CAV as above alternating every 3 weeks with cycle of VP-16P as above		

* Modified from Ihde DC: Chemotherapy in lung cancer. In Brain MC, Carbone PP (eds): Current Therapy in Hematology–Oncology 3, pp 213–217. Toronto, BC Decker, 1988.

TABLE 22-61.   Completed Randomized Studies of Intensity of Initial Combination Chemotherapy in Small Cell Lung Cancer

Series	Drug and Dose (mg/m²)	No. of Patients	CR + PR Rate (%)	Median Survival (mo)	Comments
Cohen et al.[866]	C 1000 + MTX 15 + CCNU 100*	23 9	96	10.5	High doses better: p < 0.05 CR + PR, p < 0.05 survival
	C 500 + MTX 10 + CCNU 50		45	5.0	
Mehta et al.[887]	C 1500 + MTX 15 + CCNU* 700 + MTX 15 + CCNU 70	175†	64	10.25	High dose better: p = 0.04 CR + PR, p = 0.04 survival
		174	54	9	
O'Donnell[888a]	C 2000 + VCR total 2 + MeCCNU 100‡	14	73 (57 CR)	9	High dose better: p < 0.05 CR; CR + PR and survival not different
	C 750 + VCR total 2 + MeCCNU 75	14	43 (21 CR)	10.75	
Johnson et al.[889]	C 1200 + A 70 + VCR 1‡	101	63 (22 CR)	7	High dose better: p = 0.04 CR; CR + PR and survival not different
	C 1000 + A 40 + VCR 1	146	53 (12 CR)	8	
Figueredo et al.[890]	C 1560 + A 59 + VCR 0.9§	52	71 (21 CR LD, 8 ED‖)	14	No differences in CR, response duration, or survival
	C 990 + A 50 + VCR 1.0	51	61 (22 CR LD, 8 ED)	12	

* High-dose regimen for first 6 weeks.
† Approximate number.
‡ High-dose regimen for first 9 weeks.
§ Doses are actual doses given, not intended doses; high dose regimen for first 12 weeks.
‖ LD = limited disease, ED = extensive disease.

achieve with less toxic doses. This could explain why improved antitumor effects can be demonstrated with dose escalation of one or more components of CMC.

Multiple nonrandomized trials involving even higher doses of cyclophosphamide, doxorubicin, etoposide, or cisplatin that necessitate hospitalization of most or all patients and are occasionally given with autologous bone-marrow transplant have been initiated in the hope of obtaining markedly increased tumor-cell kill, most often in patients with extensive-stage disease. Several earlier studies attempted to give higher individual doses or more frequent doses of cyclophosphamide, doxorubicin, and etoposide,[892–894] whereas more recent trials with similar philosophic intent utilized alternating drug combinations or regimens including high doses of etoposide and cisplatin.[895,896] Although high complete response rates sometimes have been observed, response duration and survival time appear similar to those attained with many standard, less intensive programs. Very high doses of initial chemotherapy with available agents have thus far produced substantially increased toxicity with only minimal additional therapeutic benefit. At present, such approaches are appropriate only in the setting of a clinical trial.

Late Intensification

Because most patients with small cell lung cancer ultimately relapse, several groups have proposed treating the smaller tumor burden in maximally responding patients with an intensive approach rather than awaiting overt tumor progression. This strategy would administer intensive treatment only to responders, those most likely to derive benefit; allow treatment to a reduced tumor bulk, which probably would be less resistant to treatment than at time of relapse; and apply intensive therapy only to patients in the best possible medical condition. Nine trials treating at least five patients each

with such "late intensification" have been completed.[897–905] Most included patients with extensive-stage disease and did not restrict entry to patients in complete remission after standard therapy. The proportion of patients beginning standard therapy who received the late intensification ranged from only 18% to 38%. The late intensification programs were diverse and included both single-agent and combination chemotherapy with local field or total body irradiation in some cases. Autologous bone-marrow infusions were given to some or all patients, although this was probably unnecessary in many patients except for those receiving total body irradiation.

Treatment-associated death rates ranged from 15% to 30% in four of the nine trials. Although some patients not having a complete response to standard therapy achieved a complete response with the late intensification, these new complete responses were nearly always brief. The fraction of disease-free survivors among patients receiving late intensification has been small, and most such patients were in complete remission prior to the late intensive therapy. There has been no obvious improvement in the outcome of all patients beginning standard chemotherapy with the intent of administering late intensification compared with patients given standard therapy without late intensification.[900,906] The one randomized trial of late intensification found improved response duration but not survival in patients receiving it, but the 2-year survival rate for all patients beginning standard therapy was 7%, similar to that in many studies of conventional treatment.[899]

Late intensive therapies remain a suitable subject of clinical investigation, particularly in limited-stage patients who attain a complete response to standard therapy. However, because markedly superior results cannot be expected with this approach using currently available drugs, randomized trials will probably be required to demonstrate efficacy.

Cyclic Alternating Combination Chemotherapy

As might be predicted from its relatively rapid growth rate, responses to chemotherapy in small cell lung cancer occur quickly. Symptomatic improvement is usual with the first cycle of treatment, and it is uncommon for tumor masses to demonstrate further regression after 12 or sometimes even 6 weeks.[836,850,879] Thus, introduction of a new noncross-resistant drug program prior to tumor progression is conceptually attractive. Goldie and Coldman have provided a detailed mathematical model of the spontaneous origin of drug-resistant clones in malignant tumors at a mutation rate proportional to the number of actively dividing tumor cells.[907] This model predicts that as many active agents as possible should be given at full doses as quickly as possible to maximize the chance of eradication of the entire tumor cell population. Because myelosuppressive toxicity does not allow all possible drugs to be given simultaneously, another suitable strategy is to alternate the administration of two combination regimens that are equally effective and noncross-resistant.[908] This strategy has become common in the treatment of small cell lung cancer.

Although this point has not been rigorously demonstrated, many chemotherapy programs in small cell carcinoma appear to have approximately equal efficacy. If noncross-resistance is defined such that a second drug combination produces a substantial fraction of complete remissions when administered after tumor progression on a first drug combination, most, if not all, chemotherapy programs in small cell lung cancer are *not* noncross-resistant. Thus, it should not be surprising that there has not been a substantial survival benefit from alternation of two different combination regimes in small cell lung cancer, although new complete responses sometimes occur with initiation of the second combination and the duration of initial remission has been prolonged by this strategy in some randomized trials.[909-912] Occasional randomized studies have shown improved survival with alternating combinations, but the magnitude of the benefit has been extremely modest, requiring randomization of more than 500 patients to be detectable[913] or utilizing combinations that probably had unequal efficacy.[914]

Etoposide–cisplatin has recently been shown to be an active salvage regimen in patients failing CAV treatment and appears at least as efficacious as CAV when used as first-line therapy. Thus, it may be less cross-resistant with CAV than any combination studied to date. Although its complete response rate in CAV failures is still less than 10%,[877,878] several randomized trials alternating CAV and etoposide–cisplatin were recently initiated. A study of 289 patients with extensive-stage disease found an increased response rate, response duration, and survival time with an alternating CAV–etoposide/cisplatin program compared with CAV alone,[915] although the improvement in median survival was only 6 weeks. It is not clear whether the superiority of the cyclic alternating treatment was attributable to the alternating strategy or to the fact that etoposide–cisplatin is superior to CAV. This question should be resolved by ongoing clinical trials. Nonetheless, alternation of CAV and etoposide–cisplatin is an effective treatment program that produced excellent long-term survival results in a study began in 1979.[916]

At present, cyclic alternating administration of two active combination chemotherapy regimens is an acceptable but not mandatory treatment strategy in small cell lung cancer. At a minimum, this approach may reduce the toxicities of chemotherapy that are dependent on the total cumulative dose of a single drug, such as the cardiac toxicity of doxorubicin and the neurotoxicity of cisplatin and vincristine.

Duration of Chemotherapy Administration

Based on treatment strategies for acute lymphoblastic leukemia, chemotherapy in responding small cell lung cancer patients was often continued for up to 2 years in the 1970s. However, several early studies of CAV with chest irradiation for patients with limited-stage disease produced similar survival outcomes despite variations in the planned duration of chemotherapy from 3 or 4 to 24 months (Table 22-62). This suggests that a disproportionate fraction of the antitumor effects of chemotherapy occurs in the early cycles, consistent with the results of some randomized studies comparing

TABLE 22-62.   Early Studies of Combined-Modality Therapy in (CAV + Chest RT) in Limited-Stage Disease with Various Durations of Maintenance Chemotherapy

Series	Duration of Therapy (mo)*	No. of Patients	CR Rate (%)	Median Survival (mo)	2-Year Disease-free Survival Rate (%)
Johnson et al.†	3–4	36	75	18.5	28
Greco et al.‡	14	32	91	16	25
Einhorn et al.§	24	19	89	17	26

Modified from Ihde DC, Bunn PA: Chemotherapy of small cell bronchogenic carcinoma. In Williams CJ, Whitehouse JMA (eds): Recent Advances in Clinical Oncology, pp 305–323. Edinburgh, Churchill Livingstone, 1982.
*Total duration of chemotherapy planned in responding patients.
†Johnson RE, Brereton HD, Kent C, Ann Thorac Surg 25:509–515, 1978.
‡Greco FA, Richardson RL, Snell JD et al, Am J Med 66:625–630, 1979.
§Einhorn LH, Bond WH, Hornback N et al, Semin Oncol 5:309–313, 1978.

higher and lower doses of the same drugs (see Table 22-61) in which higher doses given for only the first 6 or 9 weeks produce superior response rates or survival. If most or all tumor regression is indeed accomplished within the first few cycles of therapy, continuation of chemotherapy (or "maintenance") would obviously be of minimal benefit.

Recently, treatment programs based on CAV and chest irradiation intended to last for 61 and 18 weeks had almost identical outcomes in consecutive large patient groups with respect to response rates and median and 2-year survival.[917] Many chemotherapy programs employed during the 1980s are intended to be discontinued after 4 to 6 months in responding patients, with therapeutic results that are similar to previously utilized 12- and 24-month regimens.

Few randomized trials have addressed the optimal duration of chemotherapy in small cell lung cancer. The results of almost all of them suggest that, as in most other cancers that are potentially curable with chemotherapy, there is very little role for maintenance therapy. A study of ten cycles of CAV following four cycles of etoposide–cisplatin with chest irradiation versus no further therapy showed no survival advantage for continued chemotherapy,[880] nor did another trial, in which complete responders with extensive disease who received maintenance chemotherapy had survival equivalent to that of patients in whom chemotherapy was discontinued.[913] A study that found superior median survival in extensive-stage patients with a complete or good partial response who continued to receive CAV compared to patients not given maintenance treatment also showed precisely the opposite result in limited-stage patients.[918] A preliminary report of a large European trial demonstrated a longer time to tumor progression in patients receiving twelve rather than five cycles of chemotherapy, but survival was modestly improved only in patients with extensive disease or a partial remission, the groups deriving the least benefit from therapy.[919] Administering chemotherapy for only 4 to 6 months in responding patients is recommended, as this approach produces at least similar survival, minimizes the toxicities of chemotherapy, and may be associated with a higher frequency of palliative responses to salvage chemotherapy programs (see below).

Toxicities

The principal acute toxicities produced by all combination chemotherapy programs utilized in small cell lung cancer are those related to myelosuppression, specifically neutropenia-associated fever and infection and, to a much lesser extent, thrombocytopenic bleeding. Patients with poor performance status or extensive-stage disease are at greater risk. Nausea, vomiting, and alopecia are also seen with many drugs. Toxicities peculiar to specific agents, such as cardiomyopathy with doxorubicin, neurotoxicity with vincristine and cisplatin, and hemorrhagic cystitis with cyclophosphamide, can also be observed.

With most currently employed standard chemotherapy programs, the duration of neutropenia is relatively short. Febrile episodes are reported in about 30% of patients, documented infections in about 5%, and infectious deaths in 2%.[920] Even much more intensive chemotherapy programs can be delivered in a hospital setting with a low frequency of treatment-related deaths provided there is strict adherence to meticulous supportive care.[921] In some randomized studies, the administration of prophylactic antibiotics such as trimethoprim–sulfamethoxazole significantly reduced the incidence of infection and time spent on antibiotics,[922] but this is not standard practice. Herpes zoster[923,924] and perirectal abscesses[925] occasionally develop during chemotherapy.

When chemotherapy is combined with chest irradiation, especially when the two modalities are given concurrently, the rate of infectious complications is increased because of the significantly greater myelosuppression.[920,926] The addition of chest radiotherapy to chemotherapy significantly reduces the frequency of circulating granulocyte–monocyte precursor colony-forming units in the peripheral blood,[927] and even the small radiation portals utilized for brain metastases can increase the degree of myelosuppression from concurrent chemotherapy.[928]

Acute myeloblastic leukemia has been reported in 17 long-term survivors who received chemotherapy for small cell lung cancer. The actuarial risk at 2 to 3 years is 2% to 4% in two large series,[929,930] and chromosomal deletions similar to those seen in treatment-associated leukemia after chemotherapy of Hodgkin's disease have been reported.[930,931] The majority of affected patients had received protracted chemotherapy including procarbazine or a nitrosourea or both; the current shorter durations of treatment and lesser utilization of nitrosoureas and procarbazine may reduce the frequency of this uncommon complication. Although several drugs administered to small cell carcinoma patients, including methotrexate, cyclophosphamide, and nitrosoureas, are associated with pulmonary toxicity, this problem occurs infrequently in patients not receiving chest irradiation. Serial pulmonary function studies in patients with tumor regression during chemotherapy alone generally show improvement.[932,933] Although acute tumor lysis syndrome, with hyperkalemia, hyperphosphatemia, and hypocalcemia, has been reported with initiation of chemotherapy in a single patient,[934] routine administration of allopurinol and frequent monitoring of serum electrolytes is not necessary.

Overall treatment-associated death rates of 0 to 4% in limited-stage and 2% to 8% in extensive-stage small cell lung cancer patients can be anticipated with standard chemotherapy regimens given with or without chest irradiation. This potential for major morbidity and occasional death emphasizes that chemotherapy for this neoplasm should be administered only by physicians experienced in avoiding and managing drug-related toxicities. However, the survival benefits of modern therapy greatly exceed the decrements in lifespan produced by its side effects.

COMBINED-MODALITY THERAPY

Chest Irradiation in Limited-Stage Small Cell Lung Cancer

The systemic nature of small cell lung cancer even when it appears localized after careful staging precludes sole reliance on a locoregional form of therapy. Most patients with limited-stage disease given chest irradiation alone rapidly die of distant metastases, emphasizing the need for primary systemic treatment. After combination chemotherapy began to be employed in the management of small cell carcinoma in the 1970s, the high response rates and improved survival led to speculation that chest radiotherapy added toxicities while contributing little or no therapeutic advantage in chemotherapy-treated patients. However, this neoplasm is the most responsive of all cell types of lung cancer to thoracic radiotherapy, with tumor regression in excess of 50% occurring in 90% of patients,[935] which is particularly important in that the primary tumor complex is a site of progression in as many as 80% of relapsing limited-stage patients treated with chemotherapy alone.[845,910] Thus, the premise that chest irradiation in conjunction with chemotherapy may improve therapeutic results, particularly in patients with limited disease, appears logical.

Retrospective review of numerous nonrandomized trials employing chemotherapy with or without chest irradiation for limited-stage disease suggested the following conclusions.[850,936] First, a lower rate of chest relapse is seen with combined-modality therapy, although the frequency of relapse still approaches 33%. Second, hematologic, pulmonary, and esophageal complications are increased with the employment of both modalities. Third, whereas the median survival time appears similar, the 2-year disease-free survival rate was superior for combined-modality therapy compared with that achieved with chemotherapy alone. Retrospective data, however, suffer from a number of deficiencies. Because chemotherapy alone is less toxic than combined-modality treatment, there may have been a consistent bias against giving combined modality therapy to poor-risk patients. If administration of radiotherapy is delayed until chemotherapy is completed, patients with the worst prognosis who suffer early failure are automatically excluded from combined-modality series. Analysis of local relapse rates can also be misleading, since only an isolated chest recurrence in a completely responding patient might be expected to compromise survival, and definitions of local relapse are far from uniform. Variations in dose and schedule of irradiation and specific chemotherapy programs employed further complicate comparison of chest relapse rates in different series. Less effective chemotherapy combined with effective irradiation will reduce the frequency of first failures in the chest (because distant metastases will be more prone to develop), whereas more effective chemotherapy combined with less efficacious irradiation will yield the opposite result. All these factors make it extremely difficult to determine the value of the addition of chest irradiation to combination chemotherapy from retrospective data.

In the past 5 years, this uncertainty has been clarified by the completion of several prospective randomized trials. Seven mature trials in which at least 80 patients with limited disease were randomized to receive chemotherapy alone or the same chemotherapy with chest irradiation are summarized in Table 22-63. The temporal relations between chemotherapy and irradiation have been far from uniform in these studies. In Table 22-63, "concurrent therapy" means combined-modality therapy in which chemotherapy and radiotherapy are given simultaneously. In "alternating therapy," radiotherapy is administered on days of the chemo-

therapy cycle in which no drugs are given, without any delay in the subsequent chemotherapy cycle. "Sequential therapy" is defined as administration of chemotherapy and radiotherapy separately in time, with delay in chemotherapy doses for delivery of irradiation or with one modality begun only after completion of the other. The trials also differed in the chemotherapy regimen employed, the time at which chest radiotherapy was begun, the dose and schedule of irradiation, whether it was given to all patients randomized to receive it or only to responders (or only complete responders) to chemotherapy, and whether PCI was administered.

Four of the seven studies reported significantly improved overall survival rates with combined-modality treatment; two employed concurrent radiotherapy,[926,937] one alternating radiotherapy,[938] and one sequential irradiation during a chemotherapy hiatus.[855] The magnitude of the survival benefit was relatively modest, ranging from 1 to 4 months' improvement in median survival and increases in 2-year survival from 7% to 17%. The two studies with the longest follow-up demonstrate much less advantage beyond 3 to 5 years for patients given radiotherapy,[926,935] at least partially because of intercurrent deaths and second lung cancers in the combined-modality arms. Of the three studies not demonstrating improved survival with added chest irradiation, two[939,940] employed sequential radiotherapy and one[941] a concurrent regimen in which only a single drug was given simultaneously with irradiation. The negative sequential trial conducted exclusively in patients in complete remission from chemotherapy[940] was initiated because of earlier data from uncontrolled trials suggesting marked improvement in disease-free survival when irradiation was given to complete responders at the completion of drug administration.[942] Combined-modality treatment also increased the complete response rate in three of the four trials for which this information was available and significantly reduced chest recurrence rates in five of seven trials.

Whether variables in delivery of the thoracic irradiation component of combined-modality therapy influence its antitumor efficacy is by no means resolved. Concurrent and alternating combined-modality programs that do not incorporate planned delays in chemotherapy for radiotherapy administration appear to possess superior antitumor efficacy. Among the randomized trials in Table 22-63, three of four concurrent or alternating programs yielded improved survival, whereas only one of the three sequential programs did so. The only positive sequential trial was able to demonstrate survival benefit only with multivariate statistical techniques.[943] This apparent superiority of concurrent or alternating programs is consistent with the known dominance of distant metastases as the principal determinant of survival in most patients and suggests that these methods should be employed in standard treatment. However, no randomized comparisons of concurrent or alternating versus sequential strategies have been reported.

The dose of thoracic irradiation needed to control locoregional small cell carcinoma was initially thought to be reduced when chemotherapy was also given.[944] As improved drug treatment allowed longer control of distant metastases, however, a high frequency of local failures with lower-dose schedules such as 3000 cGy (rad) in 2 weeks became appar-

TABLE 22-63. Randomized Prospective Trials of Combined-Modality Therapy Versus Chemotherapy Alone in Limited-Stage Small Cell Lung Cancer

Reference	Drugs*	Chest Radiotherapy	No. of Patients	Median Survival (mo)		Survival Differences	2-Year Disease-free or Overall Survival (actual or projected) (%)	
				CT	CMT		CT	CMT
Bunn et al.[926]	CML/VAP	40Gy/15Fx/wk 1/CONC/Cont	96	11.6	15.0	p = 0.035	12 6	28 (OS) 23 (DFS)
Perry et al.[937]	CAEV	I:50Gy/25Fx/wk 1/CONC/Cont II:50Gy/25Fx/wk 10/CONC/Cont	399	13.6	I: 13.1 II: 14.6	p = 0.009	8	I: 15 (DFS) II: 25
Perez et al.[938]	CAV	40Gy/14Fx/wk 5,8,11/ALT/ Split	291	11.2	14.0	p = 0.030	19	28 (OS)
Fox[855,943]	CAV	40Gy/20Fx/wk10/ SEQ/Cont	84	12.7	16.5	p = 0.003†	2	15 (DFS)
Østerlind et al.[941]	CMVL	40Gy/10Fx/wk 6,10/CONC/ Split	125	11.5	10.5	p = 0.240	8	5 (DFS)
Souhami et al.[939]	AV/CM	40Gy/20Fx/wk 13/SEQ/Cont	130	R: 12.0 NR: 7.0	13.0 8.5	p > 0.05 p > 0.05	12 12	14 (OS) 4
Kies et al.[940]	VMEAC	48Gy/22Fx/wk 13,17/SEQ/ Split/CR only	93	16.0‡	16.0‡	p = 0.860	25‡	35‡ (OS)

Modified from Seifter EJ, Ihde EJ, Ihde DC: Therapy of small cell lung cancer: A perspective on two decades of clinical research. Semin Oncol (in press).

*C = cyclophosphamide, M = methotrexate, L = lomustine, V = vincristine, A = doxorubicin, P = procarbazine, E = etoposide, P = cisplatin, CT = chemotherapy alone, CMT = combined-modality therapy, R = responders, NR = nonresponders, CR = complete responders, CONC = concurrent with chemotherapy, SEQ = sequential administration of two modalities with delay of chemotherapy to administer radiotherapy, ALT = alternating chemotherapy and radiotherapy without delay of chemotherapy, Cont = continuous radiotherapy five fractions per week, Split = split-course radiotherapy, Fx = fractions, wk = week(s), OS = overall survival, DFS = disease-free survival

†Influence of radiotherapy in a multivariate regression analysis.[943]

‡Survival values for complete responders only.

ent.[945] Most authorities now agree on the need for higher doses, in the range of 4500 to 5000 cGy or more with conventional fractionation, for optimal local control. Furthermore, simply because a radiotherapy program reduces local recurrences does not mean it is optimal. Even more effective irradiation might be able to eradicate chest tumor completely in additional patients with intrathoracic neoplasm as their only remaining cancer; this might be evident only if survival is the end-point analyzed. One randomized study by Cancer and Leukemia Group B[937] has evaluated whether radiation should be administered concurrently with the initiation of chemotherapy or given only after three cycles of drugs have been delivered (see Table 22-63). Delaying radiotherapy gave the best results in terms of response, disease-free survival, and overall survival, although these differences were of borderline significance. The delayed radiotherapy was associated with less hematologic toxicity and a greater percentage of projected chemotherapy doses actually administered, perhaps accounting for its greater effectiveness.

The optimal method for combining chemotherapy and chest radiotherapy in limited-stage small cell lung cancer has by no means been settled. Minimizing the toxicities of the approach without compromising therapeutic efficacy is one pertinent objective. Chest irradiation has added to toxicity in most studies. In addition to increased hematologic toxicities, particularly with concurrent regimens, pulmonary and esophageal complications of treatment are clearly increased with combined modality therapy. In the U.S. NCI trial[926,933] 26% of combined-modality recipients suffered severe pulmonary toxicity necessitating hospitalization a median of 2 months after the beginning of treatment, compared with 4% of patients given chemotherapy alone, and five combined-modality patients in complete remission died of this complication. In completely responding patients, pulmonary function tests improved in those given chemotherapy alone but not in combined-modality cases.[933] The Finsen Institute, which also employed concurrent chemotherapy and irradiation, reported a 7% death rate from pulmonary and pericardial complications in complete responders.[941] More than 70% of patients receiving 8.0 g/m² of cyclophosphamide followed by chest irradiation suffered symptomatic radiation pneumonitis.[946] This frequency of pulmonary complications in patients given combined-modality treatment is clearly higher than is seen, not only in patients given solely chemotherapy, but also in patients receiving chest irradiation alone. However, not all concurrent combined modality programs have noted excessive pulmonary toxicity,[934] suggesting that the specific drugs combined with irradiation may be important in this regard. Several trials report high rates of esophagitis (with occasional strictures) and weight loss in patients given combined-modality therapy.[926,934,941] Excess deaths from second malignancies, most often non-small cell lung cancer, have been noted in the combined-modality arm of two randomized trials,[926,941] possibly related to increased time at risk or to the treatment itself.

Although they have been utilized less often, alternating regimens with interdigitating chemotherapy and irradiation appear to have reduced pulmonary toxicity while maintaining a therapeutic advantage from radiotherapy.[938,947] Studies of radiation toxicity in animals suggest that concurrent chemotherapy programs might be expected to be more toxic than alternating or sequential designs, and available clinical data are consistent with this hypothesis, particularly with regard to pulmonary injury. Delivering chest irradiation in multiple daily fractions is another approach, which on experimental grounds might be expected to ameliorate pulmonary toxicity, and preliminary results from one pilot study are promising, with excellent survival rates and minimal pneumonitis.[948]

On balance, some programs incorporating chest irradiation in addition to chemotherapy in limited-stage small cell lung cancer improve survival, particularly when radiotherapy is given in a concurrent or alternating fashion. Combined-modality therapy is a technically complex undertaking requiring close coordination between medical and radiation oncologists. Custom-shaped radiation portals and shrinking field techniques (requiring repeated simulation) as the tumor regresses to attempt to preserve the maximum possible functional pulmonary tissue are recommended. Because not all combined-modality programs increase survival whereas essentially all increase toxicity, chest irradiation need not be considered mandatory in all patients, especially those with impaired pulmonary function or poor performance status. Investigational studies that do not include chest irradiation remain appropriate. Survival gains from greater antitumor efficacy of combined-modality programs are partially compromised by the toxicities of treatment, which can perhaps be modified, and by the tendency of cigarette abusers to develop second smoking-related cancers, which probably cannot. If the results of chemotherapy improve so that more patients have eradication of systemic but not of local tumor, chest radiotherapy could affect survival in larger numbers of cases. At present, however, most patients who are irradiated still die of their small cell carcinoma, and distant metastases remain the predominant cause of failure. Thus, improvements in systemic treatment currently have a much greater potential for producing survival gains in small cell lung cancer than does increased efficacy of locoregional therapy.

Chest Irradiation in Extensive-Stage Small Cell Lung Cancer

In retrospective reviews of the literature, the addition of chest irradiation to chemotherapy for extensive-stage small cell lung cancer reduced the frequency of progressive disease in the thorax but did not alter the overall response rates, median survival, or 2-year disease-free survival rate.[850,936] Because extensive-disease patients have complete response rates of only 15% to 30% with standard chemotherapy regimens and frequently relapse in distant sites, it is logical that a localized form of treatment would have little survival impact. Successive large studies by the Southwest Oncology Group confirm that although thoracic radiotherapy can substantially reduce the frequency of initial relapses at the primary tumor site, there is not apparent effect on survival.[949]

Three clinical trials have randomized patients with extensive disease to chemotherapy alone or chemotherapy with irradiation to the chest tumor and to some or all sites of overt distant metastases. In these studies as well, there were no worthwhile response or survival advantages with the addition of radiotherapy.[945,950,951] At present, other than as part of a clinical trial, there is no role for chest irradiation in extensive-stage small cell lung cancer except for symptomatic palliation.

Wide-Field Radiation Therapy

A number of pilot studies have examined the role of hemibody irradiation and total body irradiation in this radioresponsive malignancy. Hemibody irradiation is an active agent in small cell lung cancer, as it can induce some complete responses in patients in only partial response after combination chemotherapy.[952] The initial treatment is usually given to the upper hemibody, where the bulk of the tumor burden is located; in some studies, treatment of the lower hemibody is administered after hematologic recovery from the upper hemibody dose. In an early study employing what would today be considered suboptimal chemotherapy, patients who had received initial chest irradiation were randomized to receive chemotherapy or sequential upper and lower hemibody radiotherapy. Survival in limited-stage patients was similar, but in extensive disease, the addition of chemotherapy yielded superior results. As an adjunct to combination chemotherapy in both limited- and extensive disease, hemibody irradiation produced substantial toxicity in several pilot studies without obvious benefit in tumor response or survival.[952–955] There is no evidence that low doses of total body irradiation are of benefit as an adjuvant to chest irradiation or chemotherapy in limited- or extensive-stage patients.[952,956,957] In a large randomized trial in patients with limited disease given chemotherapy and chest irradiation,[958] additional radiotherapy to potential upper-abdominal sites of relapse produced no improvement in response duration or survival. Currently, wide field irradiation does not have a proven role in the management of small cell lung cancer.

Prophylactic Cranial Irradiation

Brain metastases are detected in approximately 10% of small cell lung cancer patients at the time of presentation and are subsequently diagnosed during life in another 20% to 25%, with an increasing likelihood of development with lengthening survival.[535,959] In the absence of therapy to the CNS, actuarial analysis reveals a probability of brain metastases of 50% to 80% in 2-year survivors.[535,960] At postmortem examination, such metastases are found in as many as 65% of cases.[961] Because these metastases are sometimes the sole site of clinical relapse from complete remission and are frequently disabling, PCI has been used for the past 10 to 15 years in an effort to curtail their development.

A review of 702 patients entered into seven prospective randomized trials assessed the benefit of PCI given at or within a few months of diagnosis to patients initially free of CNS involvement (Table 22-64). When the results of all these trials are considered together, doses of PCI ranging from 2000 to 4000 cGy reduced the frequency of clinically detected brain metastases from 20% to 6%.[967] In five of the seven trials, this reduced risk of intracranial tumor spread was statistically significant. However, no significant impact of PCI on survival could be appreciated. Retrospective analyses suggested that virtually all benefit in preventing intracranial metastases with PCI was confined to patients with a complete response to systemic therapy.[968,969] In actuarial analyses, partial responders or nonresponders had equivalent likelihoods of recurrence in the brain whether or not PCI was administered.[968] This is not surprising, as residual systemic cancer could readily metastasize to the CNS after completion of PCI.

It is also reasonable to predict that only complete responders could derive any survival benefit from PCI, because in patients without complete response, systemic tumor will likely be the predominant factor influencing survival. However, in both randomized and nonrandomized studies that addressed this question, there is no evidence that PCI influences survival in completely responding patients.[970,971] Thus, some investigators have proposed dispensing with PCI in favor of therapeutic brain irradiation when clinically indicated.[972] This policy assumes that cranial irradiation can effectively control symptoms from overt brain metastases for the duration of the patient's life in most instances. Because the duration of survival is short in most patients who develop brain metastases during therapy, this assumption is not unreasonable. However, other physicians[959,973] have questioned the durability of palliation following therapeutic brain radiotherapy (see below).

Even if survival were not improved, there would be no reason other than patient inconvenience and expense not to offer PCI to completely responding patients if it were free of toxicity. However, with the advent of greater numbers of long-term survivors with small cell lung cancer, it has become evident that some patients have neurologic and intellectual impairment and abnormalities on CT scan of the brain that are potentially related to PCI.[974-977] In one study, both CT scan and clinical CNS abnormalities were significantly more frequent in patients who had received PCI or therapeutic brain irradiation than in those who had not.[975] These findings are especially disturbing because complete responders—those most likely to benefit from PCI—also live longer and are at greater risk for complications. Many deficits on neuropsychologic testing are unsuspected on casual examination, but a few patients have obvious serious impairments. Neurologic abnormalities were most prominent in one series in patients who were given PCI concurrently with high-dose chemotherapy or in large radiation fractions of 400 cGy.[974] Certainly these abnormalities may not be attributable solely to PCI; chemotherapy, possible paraneoplastic syndromes, and the effects of chronic cigarette abuse are but some of the factors that might be contributory. In fact, administration of methotrexate and procarbazine was specifically associated with their occurrence in one study.[975]

Present opinion on whether PCI should be utilized in small cell carcinoma is widely divergent, and no consensus is possible. Current clinical trials randomizing completely responding patients to receive or not receive PCI should provide more conclusive documentation of toxicities and potential survival benefits. Until the results of such trials are available, we recommend the employment of PCI with the following guidelines: (1) only complete responders should be treated; (2) radiotherapy fractions of 200 to 300 cGy should be given over 2 to 3 weeks to a total dose of 2400 to 3000 cGy; and (3) PCI should not be administered on days when chemotherapy is given, and the interval between drug and radiation treatments should be as long as feasible. For patients with less than a complete response, cranial irradiation should be withheld until objective evidence of intracranial relapse supervenes.

TABLE 22-64. Randomized Trials of Prophylactic Cranial Irradiation

Series	No. of Patients	PCI Dose (cGy)	PCI Initiation	% of Patients with Brain Relapse PCI	% of Patients with Brain Relapse No PCI	p Value
Jackson et al.[962]	29	3000	Day 1	0	27	<0.05
Maurer et al.[487]	163	3000	Wks 8–12	4	18	<0.01
Hirsch et al.[963]	111	4000	Week 12	9	13	NS
Beiler et al.[964]	54	2400	Week 3	0	16	<0.05
Cox et al.[965]	45	2000	Day 1	17	24	NS
Seydel et al.[966]	271	3000	Day 1	5	21	<0.005
Aisner et al.[911]	29*	3000	AtCR	0	36	<0.02
Total	702			6	20	

Modified from Bleehan NM, Bunn PA, Cox JD et al: Role of radiation therapy in small cell anaplastic carcinoma of the lung. Cancer Treat Rep 67:11–19, 1983.
*Only those with complete response (CR) randomized.

Therapeutic Brain Irradiation

Brain metastases are a significant source of morbidity in patients with small cell lung cancer.[533] Furthermore, patients with brain metastases are at increased risk for spread to other areas of the CNS, especially for epidural and meningeal metastases.[534] Because the prognoses of patients with brain metastases differ widely, the therapeutic philosophy with which these metastases are approached is dependent on the clinical setting. In general, patients whose lesions are diagnosed at the time of presentation of small cell carcinoma have a relatively better prognosis,[978] with little difference in median survival in some series between patients with limited disease and those with brain metastases as the sole site of extensive disease at diagnosis.[532,979] Median survival is only 3 months, however, when metastases develop during treatment.[958,978] Not surprisingly, the prognosis is better if brain metastases are the only evidence of disease outside the thorax.[978] Two series report that neurologic symptoms at the time brain metastases are discovered have no impact on survival,[959,978] probably because many patients have successful short-term palliation and widespread systemic disease is present in most patients.

Radiotherapy is the treatment of choice for brain metastases in small cell lung cancer. Many radiation oncologists administer steroids (often dexamethasone 4 mg four times daily) with irradiation, especially if neurologic symptoms are present. After completion of irradiation, steroids are tapered to the lowest level that suppresses neurologic symptoms and often can be discontinued. Doses of cranial irradiation differ widely and are usually affected by performance status, life expectancy, extent of tumor dissemination, and the likelihood of meaningful response of systemic tumor. A common palliative dose schedule is 3000 cGy in 10 fractions over 2 weeks. Higher doses are often administered in appropriate clinical settings and are associated with better results, although patient selection factors probably explain much of this association.

Immediate response to brain irradiation is usually reported in terms of relief of neurologic symptoms, and the rate ranges from 60% to 85%.[958,972,978] In one series in which responses were confirmed by brain CT scans, complete and partial response rates were 32% and 31%, respectively.[978] Response duration can be disappointing, however. Brain metastases were said to be symptomatic or to be a continuing cause of death after irradiation in 45% and 54% of patients in two studies.[959,973] In another report,[978] 24 of 37 responding patients had clinical evidence of progressive intracranial tumor prior to death. The actuarial median response duration was 10 months in complete and 5 months in partial responders, with patients who died without evidence of intracranial tumor progression being censored at the time of death. The actuarial likelihood of remaining in response at 12 months for all responding patients was approximately 20%.

Despite these inadequacies in long-term control of brain metastases by irradiation, it remains true that small cell carcinoma is a widely disseminated disease in most patients afflicted with this problem, and that treatment of brain metastases will have little influence on survival in most patients. Therefore, short-term symptomatic control is an appropriate goal in most cases. It is patients with prospects for longer survival in whom the durability of therapeutic effects is relevant. These cases include those who are found to have brain metastases as the only site of disseminated disease at diagnosis and those whose complete response to systemic therapy is terminated solely by brain metastases. Although there is no conclusive evidence of better efficacy, more aggressive radiation dose schedules, such as 4000 to 5000 cGy in 4 to 5 weeks, are recommended in this setting.

Treatment of Spinal Cord and Leptomeningeal Metastases

Patients with small cell lung cancer can experience cancer dissemination throughout the neuraxis, including the spinal cord and leptomeninges.[534] At the time of diagnosis, approximately 2% will have spinal metastases and fewer than 0.5% will have meningeal tumor,[534,537,980] but a clinical diagnosis of spinal or meningeal cancer can be made at some time in the patient's course in an estimated 5% and 2.5% of cases, respectively.[529,534,537,980] As with brain metastases, the actuarial likelihood of developing spinal or meningeal tumor increases with lengthening survival but appears to plateau after approximately 3 years.[534,968,980]

The diagnostic evaluation and management of patients with spinal cord compression are outlined in detail in Chapter 58. In brief, early diagnosis is the key to successful therapy, as patients who are paraplegic by the time the diagnosis is established can only infrequently be restored to an ambulatory status with any form of treatment.[533] This is especially critical in small cell carcinoma, because a relatively high proportion of patients with spinal cord metastases present at initial diagnosis with a life expectancy of at least several months when chemotherapy is given.[534,537] Preservation of ambulation for this length of time is of obvious importance. Because of the increased risk of leptomeningeal carcinomatosis in patients with epidural or intramedullary small cell cancer of the spinal cord, cerebrospinal fluid obtained at myelography should always be submitted for cytologic analysis.

Median survival after the clinical diagnosis of carcinomatous leptomeningitis is less than 2 months. Eighty-six percent of patients have already been treated with chemotherapy and have either progressive or persistent systemic cancer at the time of diagnosis, so treatment has little influence on survival except in the minority of cases with meningeal involvement at initial diagnosis or as the sole site of relapse from complete remission.[981] Intrathecal methotrexate, often accompanied by irradiation to symptomatic areas of the neuraxis, is the most commonly utilized therapy. Patients treated with this combined approach are reported to clear their cerebrospinal fluid of malignant cells approximately 50% of the time but less often have complete resolution of neurologic symptoms and signs.[533,980] However, it is likely that only better-prognosis patients without rapidly advancing systemic tumor undergo this therapy. In the occasional patient with a life expectancy of 3 months or longer, we recommend placement of an Ommaya reservoir for intrathecal chemotherapy and monitoring of cerebrospinal fluid status. Because of the rarity of carcinomatous meningitis as the sole site of initial failure in completely responding patients, prophylactic therapy of the entire meningeal space is not indicated.

SURGICAL RESECTION

More than one-third of the rare patients who present with a solitary pulmonary nodule that upon surgical resection is diagnosed as small cell lung cancer will survive for 5 years or longer.[981] However, the inexorable development of distant metastases in most patients receiving surgical therapy alone, and the similar outcome of patients with apparently operable disease who did and did not undergo surgical resection in the early 1970s,[484] led many thoracic surgeons to forego any attempts at thoracotomy in patients with a confirmed pathologic diagnosis.

Several factors have recently caused this policy to be reappraised. First, patients undergoing resection of the primary tumor have relatively good survival. In 132 patients of the Veterans Administration Surgical Oncology Group surviving 30 days after complete resection, the actuarial 5-year survival rate was 23%; in patients with pathologically confirmed Stage I disease, constituting almost half the group, it was 41%.[982] Although adjuvant chemotherapy, usually with a single agent, was given to approximately half the patients, it had no effect on survival. Thus, these 5-year survival rates may legitimately be attributed to surgical therapy alone. A population-based study confirms the superior outcome of small cell cancer patients receiving initial surgical resection, often without subsequent adjunctive therapy.[983] Second, operative removal of the primary tumor favorably affects local tumor control. Relapse in the primary tumor site still occurs in completely responding limited-stage patients given chemotherapy, either alone or with chest irradiation,[936] whereas after surgical extirpation of the primary tumor, local relapse is infrequent.[984-986] Finally, excellent survival rates are observed in patients with thoroughly staged limited-stage tumor who have undergone surgical resection prior to the administration of chemotherapy (Table 22-65).[984,987,988] With various follow-up times, 42% of retrospectively identified patients who received postoperative combination chemotherapy with standard regimens (with or without chest irradiation) were alive and disease-free, including a small number of pathologically staged Stage I and II patients with an estimated 5-year survival rate of 80%.[989] Interestingly, patients who undergo an incomplete resection have a prognosis similar to that of operable cases who did not receive surgery.[988]

Current practice considers surgery as an adjunct to primary treatment with chemotherapy with or without thoracic radiotherapy. Resection of the primary tumor could be performed either before the initiation of chemotherapy or after response to treatment has been achieved. Fewer than 10% of patients with limited-stage small cell carcinoma have received combination chemotherapy after the primary tumor has been surgically removed.[984,987,988] Little data exist on how often surgical resection at the time of diagnosis is possible. Prospective studies of the feasibility of initial thoracotomy by their nature cannot include cases without a preoperative diagnosis who are discovered only at thoracotomy to have resectable small cell lung cancer. A large retrospective analysis of 435 limited-stage patients by Østerlind and associates[988] indicated that as many as 35% might have been considered operable. Of 96 operable patients actually subjected to thoracotomy, only 38% could have their tumors resected completely. This yields an estimated resectability rate of 13% (35% × 38%) in limited disease.

TABLE 22-65. Disease-Free Survival in Patients Undergoing Surgical Resection for Small Cell Lung Cancer in Conjunction with Chemotherapy or Chemoradiotherapy

Series	No. Surgically Resected	No. Alive and Disease-free (%)	Comment
Surgery Before Chemotherapy			
Friess et al.[987]	15	4 (27)	Retrospective, minimum 4-year follow-up
Shepherd et al.[984]	34	19 (56)	Retrospective, 1-year follow-up; includes 7 patients with chemotherapy before surgery
Meyer[989]	10	8 (80)	Retrospective, 2.5-year follow-up; Stages I and II patients
Østerlind et al.[988]	36	9 (25)	Retrospective, 3.5-year follow-up
Total	95	40 (42)	
Chemotherapy Before Surgery			
Prager et al.[985]	8	4 (50)	Prospective, 1-year follow-up
Johnson et al.[986]	24	4 (17)	Prospective, 1-year follow-up; no resection if biopsy negative
Baker et al.[992]	20	12 (60)	Prospective,† 10-month follow-up
Valdivieso[h]	13	6 (46)	Prospective, short follow-up
Williams et al.*	21	7 (33)	Prospective, 10-month follow-up
Total	86	33 (38)	

Table modified from Williams CJ, McMillan I, Lea R, et al: Surgery after initial chemotherapy for localized small cell carcinoma of the lung. J Clin Oncol 5:1579–1588, 1987.
*Prospectively identified patients from unknown population base.
†Valdivieso M, McMurtrey MJ, Farha P et al, Proc Am Soc Clin Oncol 3:220, 1984.

One important point concerning initial surgical resection of small cell carcinoma remains unresolved: is the superior outcome of limited-stage patients who undergo complete resection prior to initiation of chemotherapy attributable to the resection itself or to an inherently better prognosis for patients with a tumor burden small enough to permit resection? Retrospective data suggest much of the better prognosis of patients who are operated on is attributable to the latter factor. In Toronto, patients with "very limited" disease, defined as no evidence of mediastinal lymph node involvement on chest radiography or at mediastinoscopy, had a median and 5-year actuarial survival rate after chemoradiotherapy alone similar to that of surgically treated patients who then received chemoradiotherapy.[990] Danish patients with operable but nonresected limited-stage tumor had 18-, 30-, and 42-month survival rates of 17%, 13%, and 6%, respectively, compared with survival rates at identical time points of 22%, 18%, and 13% in patients receiving thoracotomy with the intent of complete resection. Although survival is better in operable patients subjected to thoracotomy, this degree of improvement cannot be regarded as conclusive from a retrospective study.[988]

In our opinion, resection of small cell lung cancer, if appropriate according to standard surgical criteria, should be performed in patients in whom the diagnosis is established only at thoracotomy. In patients with a known diagnosis preoperatively, a thoracotomy with intended complete tumor resection if possible is appropriate but not mandatory if complete staging, including evaluation of the mediastinum, reveals clinical Stage I or Stage II tumor. After resection, six cycles of adjuvant chemotherapy with a standard combination regimen should be administered, with or without chest irradiation.

Surgical resection in limited small cell carcinoma might be more effective if performed after initial chemotherapy rather than at diagnosis for several reasons. First, immediate chemotherapy would be given to attempt to eradicate occult distant metastatic disease. Only patients responding to chemotherapy—those most likely to benefit—would undergo thoracotomy. Second, comprehensive initial preoperative staging procedures could be avoided, because chemotherapy would be the first form of treatment. Finally, after response to chemotherapy, a larger fraction of patients might be surgical candidates.

Stringent criteria for operability after chemotherapy have allowed only 18% to 20%[985,986] to 37%[991] of limited-stage patients beginning induction chemotherapy to undergo eventual tumor resection in prospective trials, although this is still a potentially higher fraction than at the time of diagnosis. Among the factors preventing thoracotomy are poor response to chemotherapy, poor pulmonary function or other medical problems, presentation with SVC syndrome, and patient refusal.[991] No excessive operative morbidity or mortality compared with performing thoracotomy prior to chemotherapy is evident from most published series. Local recurrences are probably reduced in these patients.[986] No cancer is present in resected specimens in 5% to 20% of cases,[991,992] and not surprisingly, this patient subset enjoys a better prognosis. However, patients who have a negative biopsy of the primary tumor site and then do not have resec-

tion have a high frequency of local recurrence within a median of 5 months.[986] From 0 to 20% of resected or biopsied tumors after chemotherapy have contained non-small cell lung cancer or mixed small cell–non-small cell elements.[986,987,991–993] This frequency compares with an incidence of 25% of non-small cell components on biopsy of relapsing tumor following chemotherapy in one small series[994] and an incidence of 13% to 30% at autopsy.[266,995] Whether these pathologic findings are attributable to selection of non-small cell elements present in the original tumor, histologic changes induced by chemotherapy, the presence of a second lung cancer, or an incorrect initial diagnosis is not resolved. In any event, it is conceivable that surgery represents optimal treatment for residual non-small cell disease.

Data from the literature, summarized in Table 22-65, indicate that patients whose tumor can be surgically resected after response to modern combination chemotherapy have a better survival rate than all limited-stage patients beginning chemotherapy. In predominantly prospective series with various lengths of follow-up, the disease-free survival rate of patients whose disease was resected is 38%. Patient selection factors cloud interpretation of these results, however, and in the largest series,[991] survival of 38 patients beginning chemotherapy with the intent of performing later tumor resection if possible was no different from the survival of all 59 limited-stage cases seen during the interval of the study. The presence of lymph node involvement at prechemotherapy mediastinoscopy appears to be an especially poor prognostic factor.[996] This pretreatment staging procedure has not been performed in most series; hence, the definition of subsets of patients who may benefit from postchemotherapy surgery is not possible. In the absence of a clear-cut survival advantage for the policy of planned thoracotomy when possible after chemotherapy response, we do not recommend this approach outside the setting of a clinical trial. A current large LCSG trial of chemotherapy followed by surgery with postoperative radiotherapy versus chemotherapy followed by chest irradiation should help to resolve these issues.

TREATMENT OF RELAPSING OR PROGRESSIVE TUMOR

Although response rates to chemotherapy at diagnosis are high in small cell lung cancer, most patients eventually suffer tumor recurrence. The results of salvage therapy for disease relapsing or progressing after initial chemotherapy are poor, with infrequent objective responses and a median survival of 2 to 3 months.[836] Long-term disease-free survival after relapse is virtually nonexistent. Etoposide–cisplatin is currently the most commonly utilized salvage regimen in patients who have not received either of these agents previously. Although several studies have reported objective response rates of 50% or more with this treatment after failure of CAV chemotherapy,[877,878] complete responses are uncommon, and the impact on survival is uncertain. It is possible that the recent practice of administering initial chemotherapy for only 4 to 6 months has allowed the activity of etoposide–cisplatin in the relapse setting to be documented, because patients receiving this program in two studies that reported high response rates had not received any chemotherapy for a median of 3 to 5 months before relapse.[877,878] In contrast, another trial of etoposide–cisplatin in patients who had received six previous drugs with a median time off chemotherapy of only 3 weeks reported a 12% response rate.[997]

Although the usual practice in small cell carcinoma patients with relapsing disease is to administer agents to which the patient's tumor has not been previously exposed, it is important to recognize that patients who relapse after a long response, especially a complete response, demonstrate better response to salvage regimens, including those that consist of the same agents used for initial therapy,[998] than do patients with only a short remission. Similar results are noted in the therapy of relapsing multiple myeloma and Hodgkin's disease.

Radiotherapy is often the most useful palliative agent in patients with progressive symptomatic small cell carcinoma. The objective response rates of 60% or more to chest irradiation[999] are consistently higher than can be obtained with chemotherapeutic agents in this setting. Thoracic radiotherapy should be strongly considered in patients with pulmonary symptoms or in those who relapse solely in the chest. In a small pilot study in highly selected patients with relapse confined to the thorax after administration of chemotherapy alone, twice-daily chest irradiation followed by a new chemotherapy regimen was associated with a 67% complete response rate and a median survival of 6 months.[1000] Radiotherapy is the treatment of choice for SVC syndrome recurrent after chemotherapy, painful bone metastases, spinal cord compression, and brain metastases in patients without previous cranial irradiation and often provides short-term symptomatic relief. Unfortunately, patients with brain metastases following PCI or therapeutic cranial irradiation have an extremely poor prognosis and only occasionally derive palliative benefit.[978]

Relapsed patients frequently undergo testing with investigational chemotherapeutic agents in Phase I or Phase II trials. The difficulties in identifying new active drugs in this setting, in which most patients have poor prognostic factors such as impaired performance status and bulky advanced tumor, have already been discussed. New approaches to the development of useful salvage therapy for small cell carcinoma are sorely needed.

IMMUNOTHERAPY AND OTHER FORMS OF TREATMENT

Chemotherapy, radiotherapy, and, in selected cases, surgical resection are effective forms of therapy for small cell lung cancer. Other treatment modalities have been investigated but are not yet established. In early studies, lung cancer patients sometimes demonstrated both in vitro and in vivo evidence of immunosuppression, as manifested by depressed lymphocyte response to mitogens, low lymphocyte counts, and defective immunologic response to DNCB.[1001,1002] Impaired response to cutaneous delayed hypersensitivity testing has been associated with a poorer survival in small cell carcinoma.[503] These and other considerations led to a series of trials of immunotherapy as an adjunct to standard treatment modalities, beginning in the 1970s.

Nonspecific immunostimulation with both BCG vaccine

and the methanol-extractable residue (MER) of BCG has been evaluated in several prospective randomized studies. In two large Southwest Oncology Group studies,[1003,1004] response rate, response duration, and overall survival were no different in patients given chemotherapy and chest irradiation who were randomized to receive or not receive BCG. There was a suggestion that long-term survival was improved with BCG in limited-stage, but impaired with BCG in extensive-stage, disease. At least three randomized trials demonstrated no benefit of the addition of MER-BCG to various standard treatments.[1005–1007]

Sixty-seven patients with small cell lung cancer were randomized to receive or not to receive calf thymosin fraction V (a modulator of T-cell function capable of correcting some immunologic defects in inherited T-lymphocyte disorders). Doses of 60 mg/m², 20 mg/m², or no thymosin were administered twice weekly during the first 6 weeks of chemotherapy with or without chest irradiation.[1008] Although no differences in complete response rates were noted, patients given thymosin 60 mg/m² had significantly improved survival, even after adjusting for other prognostic factors. However, a recent larger study conducted in 91 patients randomly assigned to thymosin 60 mg/m² twice weekly for 16 weeks or no thymosin during initial combined modality treatment could not confirm these findings.[1009] There was no evidence of effects on response rate, response duration, overall survival, long-term survival, or various serially studied immunologic parameters in the two patient groups. Interferon-alpha has not produced any objective responses in small Phase II trials.[858] In summary, there is no convincing evidence of therapeutic efficacy of any of the various forms of immunotherapy employed in any of these studies.

The nutritional status of small cell carcinoma patients is sometimes abnormal. Prior to treatment, patients can have preferential fat oxidation, ketogenesis, and changes in serum amino acid concentrations.[1010] Weight loss is also a negative prognostic factor in untreated patients.[502] Randomized trials have shown that some of these changes can be reversed with total parenteral nutrition during chemotherapy, but the weight gained with this maneuver is mostly fat or fluid and is not associated with improved total body nitrogen retention.[1011] No improvements in response rate or survival with total parenteral nutrition were noted in a randomized study of 119 patients.[1012]

Another adjunctive therapy evaluated because of antimetastatic effects in some animal tumor systems is systemic anticoagulation. A small randomized trial[1013] studied the effect of the addition of warfarin to combination chemotherapy and radiation and found improved time to tumor progression and survival. Results of larger studies designed to confirm or refute this observation are not yet mature.

SMALL CELL CARCINOMA ARISING IN EXTRAPULMONARY SITES

Four to five percent of small cell carcinoma patients present with no obvious pulmonary or mediastinal lesion on chest radiography and CT scan of the thorax and on bronchoscopy or sputum cytology.[1014,1015] These cases fall into two groups —those with an obvious primary extrapulmonary tumor aris-

CANCER OF THE LUNG

ing in sites such as the larynx, esophagus, or uterine cervix, and a smaller fraction with lymph node or disseminated metastases without a detectable primary tumor in the lung or elsewhere.[1014-1016] These neoplasms resemble small cell lung cancer morphologically, usually contain neurosecretory granules on electron microscopy, and are occasionally associated with the same endocrine paraneoplastic syndromes (ectopic Cushing's syndrome, inappropriate antidiuretic hormone secretion) as pulmonary small cell lung cancer. Although there is some heterogeneity among different primary sites, their clinical behavior is also aggressive, with a median survival time of less than a year and a tendency for development of nodal and disseminated metastatic disease.[1014,1016] These unusual cancers are grouped collectively on morphologic grounds, but they probably represent several different neoplasms with variable biology, as suggested by the deletion of the short arm of chromosome 3 on karyotypic or genetic analysis of tumor cell lines (a finding present in more than 90% of pulmonary small cell carcinomas) in only a minority of extrapulmonary small cell lesions.[1017]

The most common sites of origin of extrapulmonary small cell carcinoma recorded in the literature are the uterine cervix (although many reports do not distinguish between neuroendocrine and squamous variants), esophagus, larynx and pharynx, colon and rectum, prostate, and paranasal sinuses.[1016] Merkel cell carcinoma of the skin, although not strictly a small cell carcinoma, is difficult to distinguish from small cell cancer morphologically, contains neurosecretory granules, and exhibits more aggressive clinical behavior than other skin carcinomas.[1018] Among all carcinomas arising in various organs where extrapulmonary small cell carcinoma has been observed, the frequency of small cell carcinoma is approximately 3.5% in the minor salivary glands, 1% in the pancreas, 0.9% in the esophagus, 0.3% in the larynx and pharynx, 0.2% in the colon and rectum, and extremely variable (from 0.2%–14%) in the uterine cervix, probably because of differing diagnostic criteria with inconsistent inclusion of the squamous cell variant.[1016]

Because of their low incidence and origin in diverse anatomic sites, uniform recommendations for therapy of these cancers cannot be made. In patients with a documented primary site and regional lymph node metastases, the prognosis is clearly worse.[1014] Partial and occasional complete responses to chemotherapy regimens utilized in small cell lung cancer are reported, although experience is insufficient to estimate response rates reliably.[1014-1016,1018] Patients with tumors arising in the esophagus, larynx and pharynx, and prostate have short median survival, and systemic chemotherapy as an adjunct to locoregional treatment should be considered. Although there is no clear documentation of survival benefit, complete responses to chemotherapy alone lasting as long as 12 months have been anecdotally reported in a few cases of esophageal tumors.[1014,1016] Because of the high frequency of nodal metastases, radiation therapy is recommended for tumors of the uterine cervix. There are few data on effects of chemotherapy in proved neuroendocrine small cell cervical carcinoma, but adjuvant chemotherapy in localized disease is sometimes suggested.[1016] Small cell carcinomas of the paranasal sinuses and minor salivary glands

and colorectal tumors without nodal metastases have relatively good prognoses with locoregional therapy, and chemotherapy has not been utilized.[1016] In Merkel cell tumors originating in the skin of the head and neck, elective and therapeutic node dissections have been recommended; response to chemotherapy has been reported in a few cases of metastatic disease.[1018] In patients who present with distant metastatic and perhaps with regionally recurrent extrapulmonary small cell carcinoma, with or without a known primary tumor site, combination chemotherapy utilized for small cell lung cancer should be administered.

SUMMARY OF THE PRINCIPLES OF PRIMARY THERAPY OF SMALL CELL LUNG CANCER

The principles of initial treatment of the patient with small cell lung cancer and our recommendations for their implementation are outlined in Table 22-66. As in any malignant neoplasm, a correct pathologic diagnosis is imperative before therapy is initiated. Review of diagnostic material by an experienced pathologist is always appropriate, but especially so when the sole material available is from a fine-needle aspirate. The number of pretreatment staging procedures needed to determine the extent of tumor dissemination is dependent on the clinical situation, but sufficient procedures to identify tumor lesions to permit response assessment and to separate limited- from extensive-stage disease if therapy is to be affected by stage are required. Determination of the patient's ability to tolerate aggressive chemotherapy or combined-modality treatment is obviously important to avoid excessive morbidity and death in minimally ambulatory and other patients who derive little benefit from more toxic therapy. In patients believed to have Stage I or II tumor after thorough work-up that includes pathologic evaluation of the mediastinum, thoracotomy with attempted surgical resection may be considered. Moderately intensive combination chemotherapy (cyclophosphamide 750–1000 mg/m^2) with a published regimen of two to four drugs that is documented to produce at least 10% to 15% 2-year survival rates in limited-stage disease should be employed. This mandates the

TABLE 22-66. Principles of Initial Therapy for Small Cell Lung Cancer

---

Correct histologic diagnosis on adequate pathologic material

Appropriate initial staging to determine extent of tumor dissemination

Assessment of physiologic status and ability to tolerate therapy

Consideration of surgical resection in fully staged Stages I and II patients

Moderately intensive (cyclophosphamide doses 750–1000 mg/m^2) combination chemotherapy with a published regimen of proved efficacy consisting of two to four drugs

Capacity to provide good supportive care

Incorporation of chest irradiation into management of limited-stage disease

Restaging to assess response

Discontinuation of chemotherapy in responding patients after 4 to 6 months

Use of cyclic alternating combination chemotherapy appropriate but of unproved survival benefit

Consideration of prophylactic cranial irradiation in complete responders

---

capacity to provide supportive care of myelosuppressive complications, particularly infection and bleeding.

In limited-stage patients, concurrent or alternating combined-modality programs of chemotherapy and chest irradiation, preferably a program shown to increase survival in a prospective randomized trial, are recommended. Reevaluation of sites of initial disease to assess response should be performed after 12 to 18 weeks or possibly sooner. We believe that chemotherapy should be discontinued in responding patients after 18 to 24 weeks. Known effective cyclic alternating combination-chemotherapy regimens are certainly appropriate treatment and may well increase initial response duration, but their impact on survival is not clarified. Risk:benefit considerations for prophylactic cranial irradiation are far from defined. If PCI is to be administered, we recommend that it be given to complete responders shortly after documentation of response status, with avoidance of high doses per fraction of irradiation and of concurrent chemotherapy and cranial irradiation.

There is no question that current optimal treatments for small cell lung cancer have had a significant impact on survival (Table 22-67). Major gains in median survival occurred with the introduction of chemotherapy into the management of this disease, and this statistic has been improved fourfold to fivefold in both limited- and extensive-stage disease in comparison with results in patients receiving only supportive care. Furthermore, a fraction of patients with limited, and rare patients with extensive, disease attain 2- to 3-year disease-free survival and potential cure of their original neoplasm (see below). Nonetheless, it is also true that minimal improvement in therapeutic outcome has been documented since the early 1980s despite many modifications, combinations, and permutations of available agents and modalities, and approximately 95% of patients with small cell lung cancer will ultimately die of their affliction. Significant advances in understanding of the biology of this cancer have been forthcoming, however, at the same time that the pace of clinical advances has slowed. These advances may lead to novel and more effective approaches to the prevention, diagnosis, and therapy of small cell lung cancer.

LONG-TERM SURVIVAL AND CURE

Given the intensity and complexity of the staging and therapy of small cell lung cancer, it is reasonable to ask if any patients can be cured by applying the principles outlined in the preceding section. In the original publication describing the TNM staging system for lung cancer by the AJC,[1020] the outcome of small cell lung cancer patients treated during the 1960s at American university medical centers, some of which were centers devoted exclusively to the treatment of cancer patients, was reported. The 5-year survival rate in 368 patients was less than 1%. This figure amply documents the almost completely ineffective management of this neoplasm prior to the introduction of systemic chemotherapy.

In 1984, a compilation of nine reports covering 1343 small cell lung cancer patients treated with combination chemotherapy with or without chest irradiation revealed that 90 patients (7%) were alive and disease-free 2 years or more from the start of therapy.[836] These 2-year disease-free survivors represented 13% of patients presenting with limited, but only 2% of patients with extensive, stage disease. More than 80% of the 2-year survivors had received chest irradiation as part of their treatment, and almost all of the few extensive-stage patients had metastases confined to a single organ system. However, this duration of follow-up is not adequate to assess long-term survival, because relapses can still occur beyond this point.[836]

Sufficient time has now elapsed since the widespread utilization of chemotherapy for small cell lung cancer to permit assessment of survival at 5 years and beyond (Table 22-68). Overall calculations reveal that 72 patients (4%) of 2006 cases beginning what would today be regarded as standard treatment were alive 5 years later. One report excluded pa-

TABLE 22-67. Impact of Treatment on Survival in Small Cell Lung Cancer According to Extent of Disease

Therapy	Median Survival (mo)		2–3 Year Survival (%)	
	LD*	ED	LD	ED
Supportive care	3	1.5	–	–
Surgery	5–6†	–	4–5†	–
	11‡	–	30–35‡	–
Thoracic radiotherapy	10†	–	10†	–
	3–9	–	2–7	–
Single-agent chemotherapy	6	4	–	–
Combination chemotherapy	10–14	7–11	5–15	1–3
Combination chemotherapy with chest irradiation	12–16	7–11	10–25	1–2

Modified from Morstyn G, Ihde DC, Lichter AS et al: Small cell lung cancer 1973–1983: Early progress and recent obstacles. Int J Radiat Oncol Biol Phys 10:515–539, 1984.
*LD = limited disease, ED = extensive disease.
†Operable patients in prechemotherapy era.
‡Selected, carefully evaluated, pathologically staged patients.

TABLE 22-68. Studies Reporting Small Cell Lung Cancer Patients Living 5 Years or Longer*

Series	Stage	5-Year Survivors (%) (no./total)	% of Survivors at 5 Years (both stages)
Smith et al.‡	Limited	417(24)	12
	Extensive	1/25 (4)	
Livingston et al.§	Limited	11/103 (11)	5
	Extensive	6/270 (2)	
Vogelsang et al.‖	Limited	5/94 (5)	2
	Extensive	0/131	
Johnson et al.#	Limited	17/103 (17)	8
	Extensive	4/149 (3)	
Jacobs et al.†**	Limited	2/102 (2)	1
	Extensive	0/138	
Østerlind et al.††	Limited	19/443 (4)	3
	Extensive	3/431 (1)	
Total	Limited	58/862 (7)	
	Extensive	14/1144 (1)	
Overall Total		72/2006 (4)	

*Modified from Seifter EJ, Ihde DC: Therapy of small cell lung cancer: A perspective on two decades of clinical research. Semin Oncol 15:278–299, 1988.

†Excluding patients with Stage I or II carcinomas.

‡Smith IE, Sappino P, Bondy P, Gilby ED: Long-term survival five years or more after combination chemotherapy and radiotherapy for small cell lung carcinoma. Eur J Cancer Clin Oncol 17:1249–1255, 1981.

§Livingston RB, Stephens RL, Bonnet JD et al: Long-term survival and toxicity in small cell lung cancer. Am J Med 77:415–417, 1984.

‖Vogelsang GB, Abeloff MD, Ettinger DS et al: Long-term survivors of small cell carcinoma of the lung. Am J Med 79:49–56, 1985.

#Johnson BE, Ihde DC, Bunn PA et al: Patients with small cell lung cancer treated with combination chemotherapy with or without irradiation: Data on potential cures, chronic toxicities, and late relapses after five- to eleven-year follow-up. Ann Intern Med 103:430–438, 1985.

**Jacobs RH, Greenberg A, Bitran JD et al: A ten-year experience with combined modality therapy for Stage III small cell lung carcinoma. Cancer 58:2177–2184, 1986.

††Østerlind K, Hansen HH, Hansen M et al: Long-term disease-free survival in small cell carcinoma of the lung: A study of clinical determinants. J Clin Oncol 4:1307–1313, 1986; Østerlind K, Hansen HH, Hansen M et al: Mortality and morbidity in long-term surviving patients treated with chemotherapy with or without irradiation for small cell lung cancer. J Clin Oncol 4:1044–1052, 1986.

tients with Stage I and II cancer, a prognostically more favorable group.[1020] The actual 5-year survival for limited-stage patients is 7%, and for extensive stage, it is 1%. These publications confirm that relapses of small cell lung cancer continue to occur between 2 and 5 years. However, approximately two-thirds of patients who are disease-free after 2 years will not relapse,[929,1021] and the likelihood of relapse is 26% and 14%, respectively, in patients who are disease free 30 months and 3 years from the beginning of treatment.[1021] Although a rare relapse can occur after 5 years, in small cell carcinoma, as in other types of lung cancer, 5 years of follow-up appears to be an appropriate time after which the curative potential of a therapy can be estimated.

Given a 5-year survival rate in limited disease of 7% when current treatment principles are applied, there is little question that modern therapy has had a quantitatively greater impact on median survival than on long-term survival. It is of some interest, therefore, to review older data on the long-term survival effects of surgical resection and chest irradiation when given to selected patient groups. In the large series of Shields and associates,[981] actuarial 5-year survival rate of completely surgically resected, pathologically staged patients who received either no or ineffective postoperative chemotherapy was 23%. In the majority with pathologically proved Stage I or II disease, an extremely uncommon presentation among all limited-stage small cell lung cancer, the estimated 5-year survival rate was 29%. In a small recent series of pathologically proved Stage I and II patients given postoperative combination chemotherapy, the 5-year survival rate was 80%.[485] In the 1960s, a Veterans Administration Lung Group study reported only 7% 1-year survival in limited-stage patients randomized to chest irradiation alone.[1022] In the 1960s British study of limited-stage patients who were thought to be operable,[841] 4% randomized to thoracic radiotherapy lived 5 years.

Few trials thereafter involved irradiation as the sole treatment for small cell lung cancer, and long-term survival with chest irradiation in the era of chemotherapy and of improving radiotherapy techniques can be assessed only in studies of patients who received radiotherapy alone, with chemotherapy often being administered when progressive disease developed. In this setting, reported survival rates for patients given radiotherapy as the sole initial treatment include 2% at 2 years,[1023] 7% at 30 months,[1024] 4% at 3 years,[1025] and 3% at

5 years.[1026] Given expected additional relapses up to the 5-year point and the heterogeneity in patient selection factors, the long-term survival results with a policy of chest irradiation alone for those with limited-stage disease at diagnosis must be considered inferior to those with initial chemotherapy or combined-modality therapy. There is no justification for the former policy, even when only potential cure rates are considered and overall survival disregarded.

Even though the original small cell lung cancer can be eradicated in a small fraction of patients, the risk of death from other causes in long-term survivors is far higher than in the age-matched population. Development of second malignancies, most notably non-small cell lung cancer and other smoking-related tumors, represents a significant threat to these patients.[929,1021] In the U.S. NCI series,[1027] non-small cell lung cancers appeared in most instances to be second primary cancers by virtue of their occurrence in pulmonary sites not involved with the initial small cell neoplasm. After 3 years of disease-free survival, subsequent pulmonary cancers were more likely to be of non-small cell than of small cell histology. In long-term survivors who present with a pulmonary mass, confirmation of the pathologic diagnosis is required, because an occasional patient will have a resectable non-small cell tumor. The risk of development of non-small cell lung cancer beyond 2 years from the diagnosis of small cell carcinoma was 4.4% per person–year, approximately 10 times higher than the rate found in screening studies in smoking men over the age of 45.[1027] As already discussed, long-term survivors of small cell lung cancer have a small but definite risk of treatment-associated acute myeloblastic leukemia and myelodysplastic syndromes.[930]

Chronic pulmonary, esophageal, and neurologic complications of treatment can also be present in long-term survivors of small cell lung cancer, as already mentioned. Between 50% and 70% of these patients, however, are able to resume a life-style similar to that which they led prior to the diagnosis of cancer.[929,1021] Although the increased risks of second malignancies and late toxicities can be devastating in individual patients, they clearly do not outweigh the benefits of prolonged survival for most patients and the small but real possibility of cure available with current therapeutic approaches. Nonetheless, it remains sobering that the vast majority of small cell lung cancer patients die of their disease despite the significant advances these approaches represent.

RESULTS OF RECENT STUDIES ON THE BIOLOGY OF LUNG CANCER

IN VITRO CHEMOTHERAPY AND RADIATION SENSITIVITY TESTING

With the advent of new tissue culture techniques and experience, and the identification of growth factor requirements, the past decade has seen rapid advances in the ability to grow lung cancer cells in vitro.[10–12,1028–1031] These cultures have opened up the possibility of drug[1032–1037] and radiation sensitivity testing, as well as testing of biologic response modifiers[1038,1039] and of differentiation-inducing agents[1040,1041] and antigrowth factors to identify new potentially beneficial treatments. It is possible that these tests could be used to select therapy for individual patients. The cell lines also provide material for biochemical analysis of the basis of drug resistance.[1042,1043] In fact, studies with methotrexate and doxorubicin in vitro have shown how complex and multifactorial drug resistance is in lung cancer cells. In the case of doxorubicin resistance, decreased intracellular drug levels, increased DNA repair, and altered drug–topoisomerase interaction were all noted.[1044]

Radiation sensitivity testing has revealed that lung cancer lines differ greatly in their sensitivity, with small cell tumor lines exhibiting greater sensitivity than non-small cell lines or the large cell variants of small cell lung cancer.[1045–1047] However, some of the small cell lines are more resistant, whereas some of the non-small cell lines are dramatically more sensitive. It will be important to know if these radiation response patterns for the individual tumors in vitro are the same as those the tumors exhibited in the patient. The results for the tumor cell lines showing small or no shoulders (low extrapolation numbers; ñ) on their radiation survival curves suggest the use of hyperfraction in treating patients.

Several assays, including tumor cloning, radiometric, and dye exclusion, have been used, and in other tumors, there is a good correlation between a tumor's response in vitro and that in vivo.[1048–1050] One hundred sixty-eight fresh lung cancer specimens were tested in the human tumor clonogenic assay, and 73% grew adequately for chemosensitivity testing. Most of the tumors were resistant to drugs, but the in vitro sensitivity varied markedly between specimens.[1051] The small cell lung cancer specimens were more sensitive than the non-small cell lung cancers, and the untreated patients' tumors were more sensitive than those whose tumors had relapsed during chemotherapy. In addition, primary and metastatic specimens from the same patient gave similar profiles. Recently, a tetrazolium dye-based semiautomated colorimetric assay (MTT assay)[1051] has been developed and applied to lung cancer cells for chemosensitivity and radiation sensitivity testing.[1053,1054] This assay appears to have several advantages over the clonogenic assays and allows the rapid and large-scale testing of large numbers of tumor cell lines against many different drugs, drug combinations, or combined-modality therapy. The assay has been applied to test the chemosensitivity to doxorubicin, melphalan [representing an alkylating drug], vincristine, vinblastine, VP-16, cisplatin, and BCNU [representing the nitrosoureas] of 30 lung cancer cell lines of all histologic types. These included untreated small cell lung cancers as well as those relapsing on chemotherapy and non-small cell lung cancer lines. The tumor lines derived from untreated small cell lung cancer patients were the most chemosensitive, whereas non-small cell and relapsed small cell tumors were significantly more resistant.[1055]

BIOLOGIC CHARACTERIZATION OF LUNG CANCER CELL TYPES AND STEM CELL OF ORIGIN

The development of human lung cancer cell lines has greatly facilitated the study of the cellular biology of lung cancer. Advances have been made in establishing markers that distinguish small cell from non-small cell lung cancer and,

TABLE 22-69.   Comparison of the Biologic Properties of Lung Cancer Types[10-12,1030]

Property	Small Cell[1056]	Small Cell Variant	Non-Small Cell[1057]
L-DOPA decarboxylase activity	High	Absent/low	Absent
Dense core granules	Present	Absent/rare	Absent
Formaldehyde-induced fluoroescence	Present	Absent	Absent
Neuron-specific enolase	Present	Present	Absent
Creatine kinase-BB isozyme	High	High	Low/absent
Gastrin-releasing peptide	Present	Absent/low	Absent
Other peptide hormones	Present	Seldom	Seldom
HLA, B_2-microglobulin[1058,1059]	Absent-low	Absent/low	Present
Neurofilaments[1060,1061]	Present	Present	Absent
Intermediate filament pattern[1062]	"SCLC"	"Variant"	"NSCLC"
Leu-7, HNK-1 antigen[1063,1064]	Present	Present	Absent
Cell-surface protein phenotype[1065]	"SCLC"	"SCLC"	"NSCLC"
Macrophage–myeloid cell antigens[1066]	Present	?	?
Monoclonal antibody (MoAb) reactivity[1067]	"SCLC"		"NSCLC"
MoAb reactivity, epithelial antigens[1068]	Present?	Present	
Opioid peptides and receptors[1069]	Present	?	?
EGF receptors[1070,1071]	Low or absent?	Present	
Levels of high-energy phosphates[1072]	Diphosphodiesterphosphocreatine	Absent	
Glycolipid antigen expression[1073]	Unique	Unique	Unique

more recently, a non-small cell category with neuroendocrine features (Table 22-69). Although these studies have established markers that characterize these major types, nearly all investigators have found considerable heterogeneity in the expression of the markers within a tumor type and, in several cases, overlap of markers between the major divisions (such as some small cell lung cancers' expression of non-small cell lung cancer features, and vice versa). *This overlap suggests that there is a common stem cell for all types of lung cancer or that multiple programs of differentiation can be expressed in lung cancer cells.* Recently, Ruff and Pert proposed that the presence of macrophage and hematopoietic cell-surface markers indicates "that SCLC tumors are hemopoietic cells that arise from macrophages or their precursors . . . ."[1074] Although the expression of these cell-surface markers and their potential role in the pathogenesis of lung cancer has been noted by several investigators the extrapolation of lineage relation does not necessarily follow.

REFERENCES

1. Silverberg E: Cancer statistics, 1988. CA—A Cancer Journal for Clinicians 38:5–22, 1988
2. U.S. Department of Health, Education and Welfare: Cancer Patient Survival, Report Number 5. DHEW No. (NIH) 77-992. Washington, DC, 1977
3. Stanley KE: Lung cancer and tobacco: A global problem. Cancer Detect Prevent 9:83–89, 1986
4. Devesa SS, Silverman DT, Young JL Jr et al: Cancer incidence and mortality trends among whites in the United States, 1947–84. JNCI 79:701–770, 1987
5. Horm JWW, Kessler LG: Falling rates of lung cancer in men in the United States. Lancet 1:425–426, 1986
6. McDuffie HH, Klaassen DJ, Dosman JA: Female–male differences in patients with primary lung cancer. Cancer 59:1825–1830, 1987
7. Anonymous: Report calculates years lost, deaths attributable to smoking. Oncol Times, December 1, 1987, p 8 and Predictors of smoking examined among ethnic adolescent groups, p 10
8. Centers for Disease Control: Cigarette smoking among blacks and other minority populations. MMWR 36:404–407, 1987 and Cigarette smoking in the United States, 1986, pp. 581–585
9. Brown CC, Kessler LG: Projections of lung cancer mortality in the United States: 1985–2025. JNCI 80:43–51, 1988
10. Gazdar AF, Carney DN, Russell EK et al: Establishment of continuous clonable cultures of small-cell carcinoma of the lung which have amine precursor uptake and decarboxylation cell properties. Cancer Res 40:3502–3507, 1980
11. Carney DN, Gazdar AF, Bepler G et al: Establishment and identification of small cell lung cancer cell lines having classic and variant features. Cancer Res 45:2913–2923, 1985
12. Brower M, Carney DN, Oie HK, Gazdar AF, Minna JD: Growth of cell lines and clinical specimens of human non-small cell lung cancer in a serum-free defined medium. Cancer Res 46:798–806, 1986
13. Gazdar AF, Oie HK: Cell culture methods for human lung cancer. Cancer Genet Cytogenet 19:5–10, 1986
14. Minna JD, Battey JF, Brooks BJ et al: Molecular genetic analysis reveals chromosome deletion, gene amplification, and autocrine growth factor production in the pathogenesis of human lung cancer. Cold Spring Harbor Symp Quant Biol 51:843–853, 1986
15. Minna J, Battey J, Birrer M et al: Genetic changes involved in the pathogenesis of human lung cancer including oncogene activation, chromosomal deletions, and autocrine growth factor production. In Accomp Cancer Res—1987. General Motors Cancer Res Found. Fortner JG, Rhoads JE (Eds). Philadelphia: JB Lippincott Co, 155–182, 1988
16. Bishop JM: The molecular genetics of cancer. Science 235:305–311, 1987
17. Klein G: The approaching era of tumor suppressor genes. Science 238:1539–1545, 1987
18. Land H, Parada LF, Weinberg RA: Tumorigenic conversion of primary embryo fibroblasts requires at least two cooperating oncogenes. Nature 304:596–602, 1983
19. Kokuhata GK, Lilienfeld AM: Familial aggregation of lung cancer among hospital patients. Public Health Rep 78:277–283, 1963
20. Tokuhata GK, Lilienfeld AM: Familial aggregation of lung cancer in humans. J Natl Cancer Inst 30:289–312, 1963
21. Ooi WL, Elston RC, Chen VW, Bailey–Wilson JE, Rothschild H: Increased familial risk for lung cancer. JNCI 76:217–222, 1986
22. Lynch HT, Kimberling WJ, Markvicka SE et al: Genetics and smoking-associated cancers: A study of 485 families. Cancer 57:1640–1646, 1986
23. Skillrud DM, Offord KP, Miller RD: Higher risk of lung cancer in chronic obstructive pulmonary disease: A prospective, matched, controlled study. Ann Intern Med 105:503–507, 1986
24. Samet JM, Humble CG, Pathak DR: Personal and family history of respiratory disease and lung cancer risk. Am Rev Respir Dis 134:466–470, 1986
25. Tockman MS, Anthonisen NR, Wright EC, Donithan MG: Airways obstruction and the risk for lung cancer. Ann Intern Med 106:512–518, 1987
26. Peters–Golden M, Wise RA, Hochberg M, Stevens MB, Wigley FM: Incidence of lung cancer in systemic sclerosis. J Rheumatol 12:1136–1139, 1985
27. Heighway J, Thatcher N, Cerny T, Hasleton PS: Genetic predisposition to human lung cancer. Br J Cancer 53:453–457, 1986
28. Rohwedder JJ, Weatherbee L: Multiple primary bronchogenic carcinoma with a review of the literature. Am Rev Respir Dis 109:435–445, 1974
29. Martini N, Melamed MR: Multiple primary lung cancers. J Thorac Cardiovasc Surg 70:606–612, 1975
30. Johnson BE, Ihde DC, Matthews MJ et al: Non-small cell lung cancer: A major cause of late mortality in small cell lung cancer patients. Am J Med 80:1103–1110, 1986
31. Bradley EC, Schechter GP, Matthews MJ et al: Erythroleukemia and other hematologic complications of intensive therapy in long-term survivors of small cell lung cancer. Cancer 49:221–223, 1982
32. Markman M, Pavy MD, Abeloff MD: Acute leukemia following intensive therapy for small-cell carcinoma of the lung. Cancer 50:672–675, 1982

33. Whang-Peng J, Young RC, Lee EC, Longo DL, Schecter GP, DeVita VT Jr: Cytogenetic studies in patients with secondary leukemia/dysmyelopoietic syndrome after different treatment modalities. Blood 71:403–414, 1988

34. Dang SP, Liberman BA, Shepherd FA, Messner H et al: Therapy-related leukemia and myelodysplasia in small-cell lung cancer: Report of a case and results of morphologic, cytogenetic, and bone marrow culture studies in long-term survivors. Arch Intern Med 146:1689–1694, 1986

35. Boice JD Jr, Fraumeni JF Jr: Second cancer following cancer of the respiratory system in Connecticut, 1935–1982. Natl Cancer Inst Monogr 68:83–98, 1985

36. Olsen JH: Second cancer following cancer of the respiratory system in Denmark, 1943–1980. Natl Cancer Inst Monogr 68:309–324, 1985

37. Johnson DH, Porter LL, List AF, Hande KR, Hainsworth JD, Greco FA: Acute nonlymphocytic leukemia after treatment of small cell lung cancer. Am J Med 81:962–968, 1986

38. Christensen PH, Joergensen K, Munk J, Østerlind A: Hyperfrequency of pulmonary cancer in a population of 415 patients treated for laryngeal cancer. Laryngoscope 97:612–614, 1987

39. de Vries N, Snow GB: Multiple primary tumors in laryngeal cancer. J Laryngol Otol 100:915–918, 1986

40. Lyons MF, Redmon JD, Covelli H: Multiple primary neoplasia of the head and neck and lung: The changing histopathology. Cancer 57:2193–2197, 1986

41. Yellin A, Hill LR, Benfield JR: Bronchogenic carcinoma associated with upper aerodigestive cancers. J Thorac Cardiovasc Surg 91:674–683, 1986

42. Abernathy D, Beltran G, Stuckey W: Lung cancer following treatment for lymphoma. Am J Med 81:215–218, 1986

43. Ayesh R, Idle JR, Ritchie JC, Crothers MJ, Hetzel MR: Metabolic oxidation phenotypes as marker for susceptibility to lung cancer. Nature 312:169–170, 1984

44. Caporaso N, Hayes R, Dosemeci M, Hoover R, Idle J, Ayesh R: Debrisoquine metabolic phenotype (MP), asbestos exposure, and lung cancer (abstract). Proc Am Soc Clin Oncol 6:229, 1987

45. Minna JD, Cuttitta F, Battey JF et al: Gastrin-releasing peptide and other autocrine growth factors in lung cancer: Pathogenetic and treatment implications. In: DeVita VT Jr, Hellman S, Rosenberg SA (eds): Important Advances in Oncology 1988, pp 55–64. Philadelphia, JB Lippincott, 1988

46. Minna JD, Carney DN, Oie H, Bunn PA Jr, Gazdar AF: Growth of human small-cell lung cancer in defined medium. Cold Spring Harbor Conf Cell Prolif 9:627–639, 1982

47. Simms E, Gazdar AF, Abrams P, Minna JD: Growth of human small cell (oat cell) carcinoma of the lung in serum-free growth factor-supplemented medium. Cancer Res 40:4356–4363, 1980

48. Carney DN, Bunn PA, Gazdar AF, Pagan JF, Minna JD: Selective growth in serum-free hormone-supplemented medium of tumor cells obtained by biopsy from patients with small cell carcinoma of the lung. Proc Natl Acad Sci USA 78:3185–3189, 1981

49. Cuttitta F, Levitt M, Park J-G et al: Growth of human cancer cell lines in unsupplemented basal media as a means of identifying autocrine growth factors (abstract). Proc Am Assoc Cancer Res 28:27, 1987

50. Sherwin SA, Minna JD, Gazdar AF, Todaro GJ: Expression of epidermal and nerve growth factor receptors and soft agar growth factor production by lung cancer cells. Cancer Res 41:3538–3542, 1981

51. Nakanishi Y, Mulshine J, Kasprzyk PG et al: Small cell lung cancer cells autostimulate their growth via an insulin-like growth factor-1 activity: Evaluation of four cell lines. J Clin Invest 82:354–359, 1988

52. Natale RB, Cuttitta F, Nakanishi Y, Minna J, Gazdar A, Mulshine J: IGF-1 can stimulate proliferation of non-small cell lung cancer cell lines in vitro (abstract). Proc Am Soc Clin Oncol 7:197, 1988

53. Mucaulay V, Teale JD, Everard M, Joshi GP, Smith IE, Millar JL: Somatomedin-C (SM-C)/insulin-like growth factor 1 is a mitogen for human small cell lung cancer (abstract). Proc Am Assoc Cancer Res 28:54, 1987

54. Betsholtz C, Bergh J, Bywater M et al: Expression of multiple growth factors in a human lung cancer cell line. Int J Cancer 39:502–507, 1987

55. Moody TW, Pert CB, Gazdar AF, Carney DN, Minna JD: High levels of intracellular bombesin characterize human small cell lung carcinoma. Science 214:1246–1248, 1981

56. Wood SM, Wood JR, Ghatei MA, Lee YC, O'Shaughnessy D, Bloom SR: Bombesin, somatostatin and neurotensin-like immunoreactivity in bronchial carcinoma. J Clin Endocrinol Metab 53:1310–1312, 1981

57. Erisman MD, Linnoila RI, Hernandez O, DiAugustine RP, Lazarus LH: Human small-cell carcinoma of the lung contains bombesin. Proc Natl Acad Sci USA 79:2379–2383, 1982

58. Sorenson GD, Bloom SR, Ghatei MA, DelPrete SA, Cate CC, Pettengill OS: Bombesin production by human small cell carcinoma of the lung. Regul Pept 4:59–66, 1982

59. Moody TW, Carney DN, Cuttitta F, Quattrocchi K, Minna JD: High affinity receptors for bombesin/GRP-like peptides on human small cell lung cancer. Life Sci 37:105–113, 1985

60. Heikkila R, Trepel JB, Cuttitta F, Neckers LM, Sausville EA: Bombesin-related peptides induce calcium mobilization in a subset of human small cell lung cancer cell lines. J Biol Chem 262:16456–16460, 1987

61. Gaudino G, Cirillo D, Naldini L, Rossino P, Comoglio PM: Activation of the protein-tyrosine kinase associated with the bombesin receptor complex in small cell carcinomas. Proc Natl Acad Sci USA 85:2166–2170, 1988

62. Cuttitta F, Carney DN, Mulshine J, Moody TW, Fedorko J, Fischler A, Minna JD: Bombesin-like peptides can function as autocrine growth factors in human small-cell lung cancer. Nature 316:823–826, 1985

63. Wharton J, Polak JM, Bloom SR et al: Bombesin-like immunoreactivity in the lung. Nature 273:769–770, 1978

64. Rozengurt E, Sinnett–Smith J: Bombesin stimulation of DNA synthesis and cell division in cultures of Swiss 3T3 cells. Proc Natl Acad Sci USA 80:2936–2940, 1983

65. Lehy T, Accary JP, Labeille D, Dubrasquet M: Chronic administration of bombesin stimulates antral gastrin cell proliferation in the rat. Gastroenterology 84:914–919, 1983

66. Lezoche E, Basso N, Speranza V: Action of bombesin in man. In Bloom SR, Polak JM (eds): Gut Hormones, pp 419–424. London, Churchill Livingstone, 1981

67. Spindel ER, Chin WW, Price J, Rees LH, Besser GM, Habener JF: Cloning and characterization of cDNAs encoding human gastrin-releasing peptide. Proc Natl Acad Sci USA 81:5699–5703, 1984

68. Sausville EA, Lebacq–Verheyden A-M, Spindel ER, Cuttitta F, Gazdar AF, Battey JF: Expression of the gastrin-releasing peptide gene in human small cell lung cancer: Evidence for alternative processing resulting in three distinct mRNAs. J Biol Chem 261:2451–2456, 1986

69. Cuttitta F, Fedorko J, Gu J, Lebacq–Verheyden A-M, Linnoila RI, Battey J: Gastrin-releasing peptide gene associated peptide (GGAP) expressed in normal human fetal lung and small cell lung cancer. J Clin Endocrinol Metab 67:576–583, 1988

70. Lebacq–Verheyden AM, Kasprzyk P, Raum MG, Van Wyke, Coelingh K, LeBacq JA, Battey JF: Complex proteolytic processing of baculovirus expressed and of endogenous human gastrin-releasing peptide precursor. Mol Cell Biol 8:3129–3135, 1988

71. Carney DN, Cuttitta F, Moody TW, Minna JD: Selective stimulation of small cell lung cancer clonal growth by bombesin and gastrin-releasing peptide. Cancer Res 47:821–825, 1987

72. Weber S, Zuckerman JE, Bostwick DG, Bensch KG, Sikic BI, Raffin TA: Gastrin releasing hormone is a selective mitogen for small cell lung carcinoma in vitro. J Clin Invest 75:306–309, 1985

73. Willey JC, Lechner JR, Harris CC: Bombesin and the C-terminal tetradecapeptide of gastrin-releasing peptide are growth factors for normal human bronchial epithelial cells. Exp Cell Res 153:245–248, 1984

74. Aguayo SM, Kane M, Schwarz MI et al: Bombesin-like immunoreactivity in bronchoalveolar lavage from smokers and interstitial lung disease (abstract). Clin Res 35:530A, 1987

75. Sienhart D, Grauer L, Miller Y, Kane M, Bunn PA: A monoclonal antibody, BBC353, binds gastrin releasing peptide and inhibits growth of small cell lung cancer in vitro and in vivo (abstract). Clin Res 35:523A, 1987

76. Woll PJ, Rozengurt E: [D-Arg^1,D-Phe^5,D-Trp^{7,9},Leu^{11}] substance P, a potent bombesin antagonist in murine Swiss 3T3 cells, inhibits the growth of human small cell lung cancer cells in vitro. Proc Natl Acad Sci USA 85:1859–1863, 1988

77. Whang-Peng J, Kao-Shan CS, Lee EC et al: A specific chromosome defect associated with human small-cell lung cancer: Deletion 3p(14-23). Science 215:181–182, 1982

78. Whang-Peng J, Punn PA, Kao-Shan CS et al: A non-random chromosomal abnormality, del 3p(14-23), in human small cell lung cancer. Cancer Genet Cytogenet 6:119–134, 1982

79. Zech L, Bergh J, Nilsson K: Karyotypic characterization of established cell lines and short-term cultures of human lung cancers. Cytogenet Cell Genet 15:335–347, 1985

80. Yunis JJ: The chromosomal basis of human neoplasia. Science 221:227–236, 1983

81. Falor WH, Ward–Skinner R, Wegryn S: A 3p deletion in small cell lung carcinoma. Cancer Genet Cytogenet 16:175–177, 1985

82. de Leij L, Postmus PE, Buys CHCM, et al: Characterization of three new variant type cell lines derived from small cell carcinoma of the lung. Cancer Res 45:6024–6033, 1985

83. Graziano SL, Cowan BY, Carney DN et al: Small cell lung cancer cell line derived from a primary tumor with a characteristic deletion of 3p. Cancer Res 47:2148–2155, 1987

84. Morstyn G, Brown J, Novak U, Gardner J, Bishop J, Garson M: Heterogeneous cytogenetic abnormalities in small cell lung cancer cell lines. Cancer Res 47:3322–3327, 1987

85. Naylor SL, Johnson BE, Minna JD, Sakaguchi AY: Loss of heterozygosity of chromosome 3p markers in small-cell lung cancer. Nature 329:451–454, 1987

86. Brauch H, Johnson B, Hovis J et al: Molecular analysis of the short arm of chromosome 3 in small-cell and non-small-cell carcinoma of the lung. N Engl J Med 317:1109–1113, 1987

87. Kik K, Osinga J, Carritt B et al: Deletion of a DNA sequence at the chromosomal region 3p21 in all major types of lung cancer. Nature 330:578–581, 1987

88. Johnson BE, Sakuguchi AY, Gazdar AF et al: Restriction fragment length polymorphism studies show consistent loss of chromosome 3p alleles in small cell lung cancer patients' tumors. J Clin Invest 82:502–507, 1988

89. Zbar B, Brauch H, Talmadge C, Linehan M: Loss of alleles of loci on the short arm of chromosome 3 in renal cell carcinoma. Nature 327:721–724, 1987

90. Pathak S, Strong LC, Ferrell RE, Trindale A: Familial renal cell carcinoma with a 3;11 chromosome translocation limited to tumor cells. Science 217:939–941, 1982

91. Cohen AJ, Li FP, Berg S et al: Hereditary renal-cell carcinoma associated with a chromosomal translocation. N Engl J Med 301:592–595, 1979

92. Kao-Shan C-S, Fine RL, Whang-Peng J, Lee EC, Chabner BA: Increased fragile sites

and sister chromatid exchanges in bone marrow and peripheral blood of young cigarette smokers. Cancer Res 47:6278–6282, 1987

93. Yokota AJ, Wad M, Shimosato Y, Terada M, Sugimura T: Loss of heterozygosity on chromosomes 3, 13, and 17 in small cell carcinoma and on chromosome 3 in adenocarcinoma of the lung. Proc Natl Acad Sci USA 84:9252–9256, 1987

94. Shiraishi M, Morinaga S, Noguchi M, Shimosato Y, Sekiya T: Loss of genes on the short arm of chromosome 11 in human lung carcinomas. Jpn J Cancer Res 78:11302–11308, 1987

95. Friend SH, Bernards R, Rogelj S et al: A human DNA segment with properties of the gene that predisposes to retinoblastoma and osteosarcoma. Nature 323:643–650, 1986

96. Harbour JW, Lai S-L, Whang-Peng J, Gazdar AF, Minna JD, Kaye FJ: Abnormalities in structure and expression of the human retinoblastoma gene in small cell lung cancer. Science 241:353–357, 1988

97. Miller YE, Sullivan N, Kao B, Gazdar AF: Reduced or absent aminoacylase-1 activity in small cell lung cancer: Evidence for inactivation of genes encoded by chromosome 3p (abstract). Clin Res 34:568A, 1986

98. Carney DN, Edgell CJ, Gazdar AF, Minna JD: Suppression of malignancy in human lung cancer (A549/8) × mouse fibroblast (3T3-4E) somatic cell hybrids. JNCI 62:411–415, 1979

99. Weinberger C, Thompson CC, Ong ES, Lebo R, Gruol DJ, Evans RM: The c-erb-A gene encodes a thyroid hormone receptor. Nature 324:641–646, 1986

100. de The H, Marchio A, Tiollais P, Dejean A: A novel steroid thyroid hormone receptor-related gene inappropriately expressed in human hepatocellular carcinoma. Nature 330:667–670, 1987

101. Yuasa Y, Srivastava SK, Dunn CY, Rhim JS, Reddy EP, Aaronson SA: Acquisition of transforming properties by alternative point mutations within c-bas/has human proto-oncogenes. Nature 303:775–779, 1983

102. Capon DJ, Seeburg PH, McGrath JP et al: Activation of Ki-ras 2 gene in human colon and lung carcinomas by two different point mutations. Nature 304:507–513, 1983

103. Shimizu K, Birnbaum D, Ruley MA et al: Structure of the Ki-ras gene of the lung carcinoma cell line Calu-1. Nature 304:497–500, 1983

104. Santos E, Martin–Zanca D, Reddy EP, Pierotti MA, Della Porta G, Barbacid M: Malignant activation of a K-ras oncogene in lung carcinoma but not in normal tissue of the same patient. Science 223:661–664, 1984

105. Slamon DJ, deKernion JB, Verma IM, Cline MJ: Expression of cellular oncogenes in human malignancies. Science 224:256, 1984

106. Winter E, Yamamoto F, Almoguera C, Perucho M: A method to detect and characterize point mutations in transcribed genes: Amplification and overexpression of the mutant c-Ki-ras allele in human tumor cells. Proc Natl Acad Sci USA 82:7575–7579, 1985

107. Kurzrock R, Gallick GE, Gutterman JU: Differential expression of p21 ras gene products among histological subtypes of fresh primary human lung tumors. Cancer Res 46:1530–1534, 1986

108. Rodenhuis S, van de Wetering ML, Mooi WJ, Evers SG, van Zandwijk N, Bos JL: Mutational activation of the K-ras oncogene: A possible pathogenetic factor in adenocarcinoma of the lung. N Engl J Med 317:929–935, 1987

109. Little DC, Nau MM, Carney DN, Gazdar AF, Minna JD: Amplification and expression of the c-myc oncogene in human lung cancer cell lines. Nature 306:194–196, 1983

110. Griffin CA, Baylin SB: Expression of the c-myb oncogene in human small cell lung carcinoma. Cancer Res 45:272–275, 1985

111. Nau MM, Brooks JB, Carney DN et al: Human small-cell lung cancers show amplification and expression of the N-myc gene. Proc Natl Acad Sci USA 83:1092–1096, 1986

112. Nau MM, Brooks BJ, Battey J et al: L-myc: A new myc-related gene amplified and expressed in human small cell lung cancer. Nature 318:69–73, 1985

113. Brooks BJ, Battey J, Nau MM, Gazdar AF, Minna JD: Amplification and expression of the myc gene in small-cell lung cancer. Adv Viral Oncol 7:155–172, 1987

114. Kiefer PE, Bepler G, Kubassch M, Havemann K: Amplification and expression of proto-oncogenes in human small cell lung cancer cell lines. Cancer Res 47:6236–6242, 1987

115. Gu J, Linnoila RI, Seibel NC, Gazdor AF, Minna JD, Brooks BJ, Hollis GF, Kirsch IR: A study of myc-related gene expression in small cell lung cancer by in situ hybridization. Am J Path 132:13–17, 1988

116. Krystal G, Birrer M, Way J, Nau M, Sausville E, Thompson C, Minna J, Battey J: Multiple mechanisms for transcriptional regulation of the myc gene family in small-cell lung cancer. Mol Cell Biol 8:3373–3381, 1988

117. Mabry M, Nakagawak T, Gesell M, Nelkin BD, Eggleston JC, Ihle JN, Baylin SB: Introduction of Harvey murine sarcoma virus (Ha-MSV) into human small cell lung cancer (SCLC) is associated with phenotypic changes (abstract). Proc Am Assoc Cancer Res 28:39, 1987

118. Rapp UR, Huleihel M, Pawson T et al: Role of rat oncogenes in lung carcinogenesis. Lung Cancer (in press)

119. Gazdar AF, Carney DN, Nau MM, Minna JD: Characterization of variant subclasses of cell lines derived from small cell lung cancer having distinctive biochemical, morphological, and growth properties. Cancer Res 45:2924–2930, 1985

120. Radice PA, Matthews MJ, Ihde DC et al: The clinical behavior of "mixed" small cell/large cell bronchogenic carcinoma compared to "pure" small cell subtypes. Cancer 50:2894–2902, 1982

121. Johnson BE, Ihde DC, Makuch RW et al: Myc family oncogene amplification in

122. tumor cell lines established from small cell lung cancer patients and its relationship to clinical status and course. J Clin Invest 79:1629–1634, 1987

122. Johnson BE, Battey J, Linnoila I et al: Changes in the phenotype of human small cell lung cancer cell lines following transfection and expression of the c-myc proto-oncogene. J Clin Invest 78:525–532, 1986

123. Vinocour M, Levitt M, Sausville EA, Nau MM, Seifter E, Minna JD: Expression of myc family members and p53 in human lung cancer cell lines. (in preparation)

124. Zummerman KA, Yancoupoulos GD, Collum RG et al: Differential expression of myc family genes during murine development. Nature 319:780–783, 1986

125. Kaye F, Battey J, Nau M et al: Structure and expression of the human L-myc gene reveal a complex pattern of alternative mRNA processing. Mol Cell Biol 8:186–195, 1988

126. De Greve J, Battey J, Fedorko J et al: The human L-myc gene encodes nuclear phosphoproteins from alternatively processed mRNAs. (submitted)

127. Birrer MJ, Segal S, De Greve JS, Kaye F, Sausville EA, Minna JD: L-myc cooperates with ras to transform primary rat embryo fibroblasts. Mol Cell Biol 8:2668–2673, 1988

128. Kawashima K, Shikama H, Imoto K et al: Close correlation between restriction fragment length polymorphism of the L-myc gene and metastasis of human lung cancer to the lymph nodes and other organs. Proc Natl Acad Sci USA 85:2353–2356, 1988

129. Schütte J, Nau M, Birrer M, Thomas F, Gazdar A, Minna J: Constitutive expression of multiple mRNA forms of the c-jun oncogene in human lung cancer cell lines (abstract). Proc Am Assoc Cancer Res 29:455, 1988

130. Haluska FG, Huebner K, Isobe M, Nishimura T, Croce CM, Vogt PK: Localization of the human JUN protooncogene to chromosome region 1p31-32. Proc Natl Acad Sci USA 85:2215–2218, 1988

131. Bohmann D, Bos TJ, Admon A, Nishimura T, Vogt PK, Tjian R: Human proto-oncogene c-jun encodes a DNA binding protein with structural and functional properties of transcription factor AP-1. Science 238:1386–1392, 1987

132. Cullen JW, McKenna JW, Massey MM: International control of smoking and the US experience. Chest 89(Suppl 4):2206S–2218S, 1986

133. National Academy of Sciences: Environmental Tobacco Smoke: Measuring Exposures and Assessing Health Effects, Appendix D. Washington, DC, National Academy Press, 1986

134. Damber LA, Larsson LG: Smoking and lung cancer with special regard to type of smoking and type of cancer: A case-control study in north Sweden. Br J Cancer 53:673–681, 1986

135. Vena JE, Byers TE, Cookfair D, Swanson M: Occupation and lung cancer risk: An analysis by histologic subtype. Cancer 56:9110–9117, 1985

136. Brownson RC, Reif JS, Keefe TJ, Ferguson SW, Pritzl JA: Risk factors for adenocarcinoma of the lung. Am J Epidemiol 125:25–34, 1987

137. Benhamou S, Benhamou E, Flamant R: Lung cancer risk associated with cigar and pipe smoking. Int J Cancer 37:825–829, 1986

138. Stanley KE: Lung cancer and tobacco: A global problem. Cancer Detect Prevent 9:83–89, 1986

139. McGlashan ND, Harington JS: Lung cancer 1978–1981 in the black peoples of South Africa. Br J Cancer 52:339–346, 1985

140. Lee HP: The epidemiology of lung cancer in Singapore. Ann Acad Med Singapore 14:485–490, 1985.

141. U.S. Department of Health and Human Services: The Health Consequences of Smoking: Nicotine Addiction: A Report of the Surgeon General. Washington, DC, DHHS Office on Smoking and Health, Publication No. (CDC) 88-8406, 1988

142. LaRosa JH, Haines CM: A Guide to Heart and Lung Health at the Workplace. Washington, DC, U.S. National Institutes of Health, Publication No. 86-2210, September 1986

143. Gray N: Low-tar cigarettes: Bane or benefit? Cancer Detect Prevent 10:187–192, 1987

144. Flehinger BJ, Kimmel M: The natural history of lung cancer in a periodically screened population. Biometrics 43:127–144, 1987

145. Kuller LH, Garfinkel L, Correa P et al: Contribution of passive smoking to respiratory cancer. Environ Health Perspect 70:57–69, 1986

146. Wald NJ, Nanchahal K, Thompson SG, Cuckle HS: Does breathing other people's tobacco smoke cause lung cancer? Br Med J 293:1217–1222, 1986

147. Garfinkel L, Auerbach O, Joubert L: Involuntary smoking and lung cancer: A case-control study. JNCI 75:4463–4469, 1985

148. Pershagen G, Hrubec Z, Svensson C: Passive smoking and lung cancer in Swedish women. Am J Epidemiol 125:17–24, 1987

149. Dalager NA, Pickle LW, Mason TJ et al: The relation of passive smoking to lung cancer. Cancer Res 46:4808–4811, 1986

150. Lee PN: Lung cancer and passive smoking: Association or an artefact due to misclassification of smoking habits? Toxicol Lett 35:157–162, 1987

151. Hughes JM, Weill H: Asbestos exposure: Quantitative assessment of risk. Am Rev Respir Dis 133:5–13, 1986

152. Kolonel LN, Yoshizawa CN, Hirohata T, Myers BC: Cancer occurrence in shipyard workers exposed to asbestos in Hawaii. Cancer Res 45:3924–3928, 1985

153. Hodgson JT, Jones RD: Mortality of asbestos workers in England and Wales 1971–1981. Br J Ind Med 43:1158–1164, 1986

154. Omenn GS, Merchant J, Boatman E et al: Contribution of environmental fibers to respiratory cancer. Environ Health Perspect 70:51–56, 1986

155. Kjuus H, Langard S, Skjaerven R: A case-referent study of lung cancer, occupational

exposure and smoking III: Etiologic fraction of occupational exposures. Scand J Work Environ Health 12:210–215, 1986

156. Seidman H, Selikoff IJ, Gelb SK: Mortality experience of amosite asbestos factory workers: Dose–response relationships 5–40 years after onset of short-term work exposure. Am J Ind Med 10:479–514, 1986

157. Kjuus H, Skjaerven R, Langard S, Lien JT, Aamodt T: A case-referent study of lung cancer, occupational exposures and smoking II: Role of asbestos exposure. Scand J Work Environ Health 12:203–209, 1986

158. Kjuus H, Skjaerven R, Langard S, Lien JT, Aamodt T: A case-referent study of lung cancer, occupational exposures and smoking I: Comparison of title-based and exposure-based occupational information. Scand J Work Environ Health 12:193–202, 1986

159. Saccomanno G, Yale C, Dixon W, Auerbach O, Huth GC: An epidemiological analysis of the relationship between exposure to Rn progeny, smoking and bronchogenic carcinoma in the U-mining population of the Colorado plateau—1960–1980. Heath Phys 50:605–618, 1986

160. Harley N, Samet JM, Cross FT, Hess T, Muller J, Thomas D: Contribution of radon and radon daughters to respiratory cancer. Environ Health Perspect 70:17–21, 1986

161. National Research Council: Health Risks of Radon and Other Internally Deposited Alpha-Emitters. Washington, DC, National Academy Press, 1988

162. Howe GR, Nair RC, Newcombe HB, Miller AB, Abbatt JD: Lung cancer mortality (1950–1980) in relation to radon daughter exposure in a cohort of workers at the Eldorado Beaverlodge uranium mine. JNCI 77:3357–3362, 1986

163. Thomas DC, McNeill KG, Gougherty C: Estimates of lifetime lung cancer risks resulting from Rn progeny exposure. Health Phys 49:825–846, 1985

164. Hornung RW, Meinhardt TJ: Quantitative risk assessment of lung cancer in U.S. uranium mines. Health Phys 52:417–430, 1987

165. Ginevan ME, Mills WA: Assessing the risks of Rn exposure. The influence of cigarette smoking. Health Phys 51:163–174, 1986

166. O'Riordan M: Natural radiation: How to live with radon. Nature 331:302, 1988

167. Jacobi W, Paaretzke HG: Risk assessment for indoor exposure to radon daughters. Sci Total Environ 45:551–562, 1985

168. Radford EP: Potential health effects of indoor radon exposure. Environ Health Perspect 62:281–287, 1985

169. Nero AV, Schwehr MB, Nazaaroff WW, Revzan KL: Distribution of airborne radon-22 concentrations in U.S. homes. Science 234:992–997, 1986

170. Marmorstein J: Lung cancer: Is the increasing incidence due to radioactive polonium in cigarettes? South Med J 79:145–150, 1986

171. Svensson C, Eklund G, Pershagen G: Indoor exposure to radon from the ground and bronchial cancer in women. Int Arch Occup Environ Health 59:123–131, 1987

172. Steenland K, Thun M: Interaction between tobacco smoking and occupational exposures in the causation of lung cancer. J Occup Med 28:110–118, 1986

173. Lawler AB, Mandel JS, Schuman LM, Lubin JH: A retrospective cohort mortality study of iron ore (hematite) miners in Minnesota. J Occup Med 27:507–517, 1985

174. Schatzkin A: Lung cancer in Yunnan mines. Cancer Prevention Studies Branch, Division of Cancer Control and Prevention, National Cancer Institute. Personal communication, 1988

175. Peters JM, Thomas D, Falk H, Oberdorster G, Smith TJ: Contribution of metals to respiratory cancer. Environ Health Perspect 70:71–83, 1986

176. Speizer FE: Overview of the risk of respiratory cancer from airborne contaminants. Environ Health Perspect 70:9–15, 1986

177. Maher KV, DeFonso LR: Respiratory cancer among chloromethyl ether workers. JNCI 78:839–843, 1987

178. Elinder CG, Kjellstrom T, Hogstedt C, Andersson K, Spang G: Cancer mortality in cadmium workers. Br J Ind Med 42:651–655, 1985

179. Lee–Feldstein A: Cumulative exposure to arsenic and its relationship to respiratory cancer among copper smelter employees. J Occup Med 28:296–302, 1986

180. Chen CJ, Chuang YCC, You SL, Lin TM, Wu HY: A retrospective study on malignant neoplasms of bladder, lung and liver in Blackfoot disease endemic area in Taiwan. Br J Cancer 53:399–405, 1986

181. Nishiyama H, Yano H, Nishiwaki Y et al: Lung cancer in chromate workers: Analysis of 11 cases. Jpn J Clin Oncol 15:489–497, 1985

182. Braver ER, Infante P, Chu K: An analysis of lung cancer risk from exposure to hexavalent chromium. Teratogen Carcinogen Mutagen 5:365–378, 1985

183. Rafnsson V, Johannesdottir SG: Mortality among masons in Iceland. Br J Ind Med 43:522–525, 1986

184. Nelson N, Levine RJ, Albert RE et al: Contribution of formaldehyde to respiratory cancer. Environ Health Perspect 70:23–35, 1986

185. Kauppinen TP, Partanen TJ, Nurminen MM et al: Respiratory cancers and chemical exposures in the wood industry: A nested case-control study. Br J Ind Med 43:84–90, 1986

186. Coggon D, Pannett B, Osmond C, Acheson ED: A survey of cancer and occupation in young and middle aged men I: Cancers of the respiratory tract. Br J Ind Med 43:332–338, 1986

187. Kvale G, Bjelke E, Heuch I: Occupational exposure and lung cancer risk. Int J Cancer 37:185–193, 1986

188. Blair A, Walrath J, Rogot E: Mortality patterns among U.S. veterans by occupation I: Cancer. JNCI 75:11039–11047, 1985

189. Deizell E, Monson RR: Mortality among rubber workers IX: Curing workers. Am J Ind Med 8:537–544, 1985

190. Sorahan T, Parkes HG, Veys CA, Waterhouse JA: Cancer mortality in the British rubber industry: 1946–1980. Br J Ind Med 43:363–373, 1986

191. Thomas TL, Stewart PA: Mortality from lung cancer and respiratory disease among pottery workers exposed to silica and talc. Am J Epidemiol 125:35–43, 1987

192. Malker HS, Gemmne G: A register-epidemiology study on cancer among Swedish printing industry workers. Arch Environ Health 42:73–82, 1987

193. Osorio AM, Bernstein K, Garabrant DH, Peters JM: Investigation of lung cancer among female cosmetologists. J Occup Med 28:291–295, 1986

195. Tuchsen F, Nordholm L: Respiratory cancer in Danish bakers: A 10 year cohort study. Br J Ind Med 43:516–521, 1986

196. Steenland K: Lung cancer and diesel exhaust: A review. Am J Ind Med 10:177–189, 1986

197. Colditz GA, Stampfer MJ, Willet WC: Diet and lung cancer: A review of the epidemiologic evidence in humans. Arch Intern Med 147:157–160, 1987

198. Bond GG, Thompson FE, Cook RR: Dietary vitamin A and lung cancer: Results of a case-control study among chemical workers. Nutr Cancer 9:109–121, 1987

199. Prentice RL, Omenn GS, Goodman GE et al: Rationale and design of cancer chemoprevention studies in Seattle. Natl Cancer Inst Monogr 69:249–258, 1985

200. Menkes MS, Comstock GW, Vuilleumier JP, Helsing KJ, Rider AA, Brookmeyer R: Serum beta-carotene, vitamins A and E, selenium and the risk of lung cancer. N Engl J Med 315:1250–1254, 1986

201. Ziegler RG, Mason TJ, Stemhagen A et al: Carotenoid intake, vegetables, and the risk of lung cancer among white men in New Jersey. Am J Epidemiol 123:1080–1093, 1986

202. Pisani P, Berrino F, Macaluso M, Pastorino U, Crosignani P, Baldasseroni A: Carrots, green vegetables and lung cancer: A case-controlled study. Int J Epidemiol 15:463–468, 1986

203. Byers TE, Graham S, Haugher BP, Marshall JR, Swanson MK: Diet and lung cancer risk: Findings from the western New York diet study. Am J Epidemiol 125:351–363, 1987

204. Kolonel LN, Hinds MW, Nomura AM, Hankin JH, Lee J: Relationship of dietary vitamin A and ascorbic acid intake to the risk for cancers of the lung, bladder, and prostate in Hawaii. Natl Cancer Inst Monogr 69:137–142, 1985

205. Dogra SC, Khanduja KL, Gupta MP: The effect of vitamin A deficiency on the initiation and postinitiation phases of benzo(a)pyrene-induced lung tumourigenesis in rats. Br J Cancer 52:931–935, 1985

206. Kreyberg L: Histologic typing of lung tumors. In Kreyberg L (ed): International Histologic Classification of Tumors, No. 1, pp 19–26. Geneva, World Health Organization, 1967

207. Yesner R, Gerstl B, Auerbach O: Application of the World Health Organization classification of lung carcinoma to biopsy material. Ann Thorac Surg 1:33–49, 1965

208. Matthews MJ, Gordon PR: Morphology of pulmonary and pleural malignancies. In Strauss MJ (ed): Lung Cancer: Clinical Diagnosis and Treatment. New York, Grune & Stratton, 1977

209. Vincent RG, Pickren JW, Lane WW et al: The changing histopathology of lung cancer: A review of 1682 cases. Cancer 39:1647–1655, 1977

210. Soroken SP: The respiratory system. In Greep RO, Weiss L (eds): Histology, 3rd Ed, pp 675–712. New York, McGraw-Hill, 1973

211. Tischler AS: Small cell carcinoma of the lung: Cellular origin and relationship to other neoplasms. Semin Oncol 5:244–252, 1978

212. Macholda F: Bronchogenic carcinoma: Study of growth and evolutionary dynamics of bronchogenic carcinoma: Its significance for early diagnosis. Acta Univ Carol 41(Suppl):39–62, 1970

213. Fraumeni JF Jr: Respiratory carcinogenesis: An epidemiologic appraisal. J Natl Cancer Inst 55:1039–1046, 1975

214. Auerbach O, Gere JB, Pawlowski JM: Carcinoma in situ and early invasive cancer occurring in the tracheobronchial tree in cases of bronchial carcinoma. J Thorac Surg 34:298–307, 1957

215. Valaitis JN, McGrew EA, Chomet B: Bronchogenic carcinoma in situ in asymptomatic high risk population of smokers. J Thorac Cardiovasc Surg 57:325–332, 1969

216. Auerbach O, Stout AP, Hammond EG et al: Changes in bronchial epithelium in relation to cigarette smoking and in relation to lung cancer. N Engl J Med 265:253–269, 1961

217. Band PR, Feldstein M, Saccomanno G: Reversibility of bronchial marked atypia: Implication for chemoprevention. Cancer Detect Prevent 9:157–160, 1986

218. Misset JL, Mathe G, Santelli G et al: Regression of bronchial metaplasia in heavy smokers with etretinate treatment. Cancer Detect Prevent 9:167–170, 1986

219. Meyer EC, Liebow AA: Relationship of interstitial pneumonia honeycombing and atypical epithelial proliferation to cancer of the lung. Cancer 18:322–350, 1965

220. Batsakis JG, Johnson HA: Generalized scleroderma involving lungs and liver with pulmonary adenocarcinoma. Arch Pathol 69:633–638, 1960

221. Moolten SE: Scar cancer of lung complicating rheumatoid lung disease. Mt Sinai J Med 40:736–743, 1973

222. Brincker H, Wilbek E: The incidence of malignant tumours in patients with respiratory sarcoidosis. Br J Cancer 29:247–251, 1974

223. Carroll R: The influence of lung scars on primary lung cancer. J Bacteriol 83:293–297, 1962

224. Liebow AA: Bronchiolar–alveolar carcinoma. Adv Intern Med 10:329–358, 1960

225. Hewlett TH, Gomez AC, Aronstam EM et al: Bronchiolar carcinoma of the lung: Review of 39 patients. J Thorac Cardiovasc Surg 48:614–624, 1964

226. Greenberg SD, Smith MN, Spjut HG: Bronchiolo–alveolar carcinoma: Cell or origin. Am J Clin Pathol 63:153–167, 1975

227. DeMartini JC, Rosadio RH, Sharp JM, Russell HI, Lairmore MD: Experimental coinduction of Type D retroviral-associated pulmonary carcinoma and lentivirus-associated lymphoid interstitial pneumonia in lambs. J Natl Cancer Inst 79:167–177, 1987

228. Beaver DL, Shapiro JL: A consideration of chronic pulmonary parenchymal inflammation and alveolar cell carcinoma with regard to a possible etiology relationship. Am J Med 21:879–887, 1956

229. Lutwyche VU: Another presentation of fibrosing alveolitis and alveolar cell carcinoma. Chest 70:292–293, 1976

230. Mulvihill JJ: Host factors in human lung tumors: An example of oncology. J Natl Cancer Inst 57:3–7, 1976

231. Joishy SK, Cooper RA, Rowley PT: Alveolar cell carcinoma in twins: Similarity in time of onset, histochemistry, and site of metastasis. Ann Intern Med 87:447–450, 1977

232. Watson WL, Farpour A: Terminal bronchiolar or "alveolar cell" cancer of the lung: Two hundred sixty-five cases. Cancer 19:776–780, 1966

233. Donaldson JC, Kaminsky DB, Elliott RC: Bronchiolar carcinoma: Report of 11 cases and review of the literature. Cancer 41:250–258, 1978

234. Katzenstein AA, Briolequ PG, Askin FG: The histologic spectrum and significance of clear-cell change in lung carcinoma. Cancer 45:943–947, 1980

235. Ihde DC, Cohen MH, Bernath AM et al: Serial fiberoptic bronchoscopy during chemotherapy of small cell carcinoma of the lung. Chest 74:531–536, 1978

236. Copple B, Wright SE, Moatamed E: Electron microscopy in small cell lung carcinoma: Clinical correlation. J Clin Oncol 2:910–916, 1984

237. World Health Organization: The World Health Organization histological typing of lung tumors. Am J Clin Pathol 77:123–136, 1982

238. Yesner R, Gerstl B, Auerbach O: Application of the World Health Organization classification of lung carcinoma to biopsy material. Ann Thorac Surg 1:33–49, 1985

239. Jett JR, Cortese DA, Fontana RS: Lung cancer: Current concepts and prospects. CA—A Cancer Journal for Clinicians 33:74–86, 1983

240. Saccomanno G, Archer VE, Auerbach O et al: Histologic types of lung cancer among uranium miners. Cancer 27:515–523, 1971

241. Gazdar AF, Carney DN, Guccion JE et al: Small cell carcinoma of the lung: Cellular origin and relationship to other tumors. In Greco FA, Oldham RK, Bunn PA (eds): Small Cell Lung Cancer. New York, Grune & Stratton, 1981

242. Ihde DC, Simms EG, Matthews MJ et al: Bone marrow metastases in small cell carcinoma of the lung: Frequency, description, and influence on chemotherapy toxicity and prognosis. Blood 53:667–686, 1979

243. Harley HRS: Cancer of the lung in women. Thorax 31:354–364, 1976

244. Rilke F, Carbone A, Clemente C et al: Surgical pathology of resectable lung cancer. Prog Cancer Res Ther 11:129–142, 1979

245. Bakris GL, Mulopulos GP, Korchik R, Ezdinli EZ, Ro J, Yoon BH: Pulmonary scar carcinoma: A clinicopathologic analysis. Cancer 52:493–497, 1983

246. Ochs RH, Katz AS, Edmunds LH, Miller CL, Epstein DM: Prognosis of pulmonary scar carcinoma. J Thorac Cardiovasc Surg 84:359–366, 1982

247. Tao LC, Delarue NC, Sanders D et al: Bronchiolo-alveolar carcinoma. Cancer 42:2759–2767, 1978

248. Kanhouwa SB, Matthews MJ: Reliability of cytologic typing of lung cancer. Acta Cytol 20:229–232, 1976

249. Cagneten CB, Geller CE, Saenz MDC: Diagnosis of bronchogenic carcinoma through the cytologic examination of sputum, with special reference to tumor typing. Acta Cytol 20:530–536, 1976

250. Hinson KFW, Miller AB, Tall R: An assessment of the World Health Organization classification of histologic typing of lung tumors applied to biopsy and resected material. Cancer 35:399–405, 1975

251. Feinstein AR, Gelfman NA, Yesner R: Observer variability in the histopathologic diagnosis of lung cancer. Am Rev Respir Dis 101:671–684, 1970

252. Burdon JGW, Sinclair RA, Henderson MM: Small cell carcinoma of the lung: Prognosis in relation to histologic subtype. Chest 76:302–304, 1979

253. Hansen HH, Dombernowsky P, Hansen M et al: Chemotherapy of advanced small cell anaplastic carcinoma. Ann Intern Med 89:177–181, 1978

254. Flower CD, Verney GI: Percutaneous needle biopsy of thoracic lesions: An evaluation of 300 biopsies. Clin Radiol 30:215–218, 1979

255. Hirsch FR, Matthews MJ, Yesner R: Histopathologic classification of small cell carcinoma of the lung: Comments based on an interobserver examination. Cancer 50:1360–1366, 1982

256. Yesner R: Observer variability and reliability in lung cancer diagnosis. Cancer Chemother Rep 4:55–57, 1973

257. Katlic M, Carter D: Prognostic implications of histology: Size and location of primary tumors. Prog Cancer Res Ther 11:143–150, 1979

258. Matthews MJ, Gazdar AF: Pathology of small cell carcinoma of the lung and its subtypes: A clinico-pathologic correlation. In Livingston RB (ed): Lung Cancer I, pp. 283–306. The Hague, Martinus Nijhoff, 1981

259. Carney DN, Matthews M, Ihde DC et al: Influence of histologic subtype of small cell carcinoma of the lung on clinical presentation, response to therapy and survival. JNCI 65:1225–1230, 1980

260. Hirsch FR, Østerlind K, Hansen HH: The prognostic significance of histopathologic subtyping of small cell carcinoma of the lung according to the classification of the World Health Organization: A study of 375 consecutive patients. Cancer 52:2144–2150, 1983

261. Radice RA, Matthews MJ, Idhe DC et al: The clinical behavior of "mixed" small cell/large cell bronchogenic carcinoma compared to "pure" small cell subtypes. Cancer 50:2894–2902, 1982

262. Matthews MJ: Effects of therapy on the morphology and behavior of small cell carcinoma of the lung—A clinicopathologic study. Prog Cancer Res Ther 11:155–165, 1979

263. Abeloff MD, Eggleston JC, Mendelsohn G et al: Changes in morphologic and biochemical characteristics of small cell carcinoma of the lung: A clinicopathologic study. Am J Med 66:757–764, 1979

264. Gazdar A, Carney D, Baylin S et al: Small cell carcinoma of the lung: Altered morphological, biologic and biochemical characteristics in long term cultures and heterotransplanted tumors (abstract). Proc Am Assoc Cancer Res Am Soc Clin Oncol 21:51, 1980

265. Little DC, Nau MM, Carney DM, Gazdar AF, Minna JD: Amplification and expression of the c-myc oncogene in human lung cancer cell lines. Nature 306:194–196, 1983

266. Sehested M, Hirsch FR, Østerlind K et al: Morphologic variations of small cell lung cancer: A histopathologic study of pretreatment and posttreatment specimens in 104 patients. Cancer 57:804–807, 1986

267. Bell CE, Seetharam S: Expression of endodermally derived and neural crest derived differentiation antigens by human lung and colon tumors. Cancer 44:13–18, 1979

268. Cuttitta F, Rosen S, Gazdar A et al: Monoclonal antibodies which demonstrate specificity for several types of human lung cancer. Proc Natl Acad Sci USA 78:4591–4595, 1981

269. Minna JD, Cuttitta F, Rosen S et al: Methods for production of monoclonal antibodies with specificity for human lung cancer cells. In Vitro 17:1068–1070, 1981

270. Mulshine JL, Cuttitta F, Bibro M et al: Monoclonal antibodies that distinguish non-small cell from small cell lung cancer. J Immunol 131:497–502, 1983

271. Nasiell MG, Kato H, Auer G et al: Cytomorphological grading and Feulgen DNA-analysis of metaplastic and neoplastic bronchial cells. Cancer 41:1511–1521, 1978

272. Bunn PA, Carney DN, Gazdar AF et al: Diagnostic and biologic implications of flow cytometric DNA content analysis in lung cancer. Cancer Res 43:5026–5032, 1983

273. Zimmerman PV, Bint MH, Hawson GAT et al: Ploidy as a prognostic determinant in surgically treated lung cancer. Lancet 2:530–533, 1987

274. Cohen MH: Signs and symptoms of bronchogenic carcinoma. In Straus MJ (ed): Lung Cancer: Clinical Diagnosis and Treatment, pp 85–94. New York, Grune & Stratton, 1977

275. Matthews MJ, Kanhouwa S, Pickner J et al: Frequency of residual and metastatic tumors in patients undergoing curative surgical resection of lung cancer. Cancer Chemother Rep 3:63–67, 1973

276. Carbone PP, Frost JK, Feinstein AR et al: Lung cancer: Perspectives and prospects. Ann Intern Med 73:1003–1024, 1970

277. Coy P, Kennelly GM: The role of curative radiotherapy in the treatment of lung cancer. Cancer 45:698–702, 1980

278. Paulson DL: Superior sulcus tumors: Results of combined therapy. NY State J Med 71:2050–2052, 1971

279. Pancoast HK: Superior pulmonary sulcus tumor: Tumor characterized by pain, Horner's syndrome, destruction of bone and atrophy of hand muscles. JAMA 99:1391–1396, 1932

280. Doehner GA, Marcus SS, Wolff WI: Pancoast's tumor: Five-year survival after combined radiotherapy and surgery. NY State J Med 67:2378–2380, 1967

281. Paulson DL: Carcinomas of the superior pulmonary sulcus. J Thorac Cardiovasc Surg 70:1095–1104, 1975

282. Henderson RD, Boszko A, Van Nostrand AWP: Pharyngoesophageal dysphagia and recurrent laryngeal nerve palsy. J Thorac Cardiovasc Surg 68:507–512, 1974

283. Salsali M, Cliffton EE: Superior vena cava obstruction with lung cancer. Ann Thorac Surg 6:437–442, 1968

284. Lokich JJ, Goodman R: Superior vena cava syndrome: Clinical management. JAMA 231:58–61, 1975

285. Rubin P, Hicks GL: Biassociation of superior vena cava obstruction and spinal cord compression. NY State J Med 73:2176–2182, 1973

286. Homma H, Kira S, Takahasi Y et al: A case of alveolar cell carcinoma accompanied by fluid and electrolyte depletion through production of voluminous amounts of lung liquid. Am Rev Respir Dis 111:857–862, 1875

287. Strauss BL, Matthews MJ, Cohen MH et al: Cardiac metastases in lung cancer. Chest 71:607–610, 1977

288. Rigler LG: Bronchiolo-alveolar carcinoma of lung with report on new roentgenologic sign. Int Congr Radio 1965

289. Matthews MJ: Problems in morphology and behavior of bronchopulmonary malignant disease. In Israel L, Chahanian P (eds): Lung Cancer: Natural History, Prognosis, and Therapy, pp 23–62. New York, Academic Press, 1976

290. Odell WD, Wolfsen AR: Humoral syndromes associated with cancer. Annu Rev Med 29:379–406, 1978

291. Blackman MR, Rosen SW, Weintraub BD: Ectopic hormones. Adv Intern Med x:85–113, 1978

292. Ayvazian LF: Extrapulmonary manifestations of tumors in the lung. Postgrad Med 63:93–99, 1978

293. Rassam JW, Anderson G: Incidence of paramalignant disorders in bronchogenic carcinoma. Thorax 30:86–90, 1975

294. Goldstraw P, Walbaum PR: Hypertrophic pulmonary osteoarthropathy and its occurrence with pulmonary metastases from renal carcinoma. Thorax 31:205–211, 1976

295. Green N, Kurohara SS, George FW III et al: The biologic behavior of lung cancer according to histologic type. Radiol Clin Biol 41:160–170, 1972

296. Byrd RB, Divertie MB, Spittell JA: Bronchogenic carcinoma and thromboembolic disease. JAMA 202:1019–1022, 1967

297. Sack GH, Levin J, Bell WR: Trousseau's syndrome and other manifestations of

chronic disseminated coagulopathy in patients with neoplasms. Medicine 56:1–37, 1977

298. Greenfield GB, Schorsch HA, Shkolnik A: The various roentgen appearance of pulmonary hypertrophic osteoarthropathy. Am J Roentgenol Rad Ther Nucl Med 101:927–931, 1976

299. Croft RB, Wilkinson M: Carcinomatous neuromyopathy: Its incidence in patients with carcinoma of the lung and breast. Lancet 1:184–188, 1965

300. Tyler HR: Paraneoplastic syndromes of nerve, muscle and neuromuscular junction. Ann NY Acad Sci 230:348–357, 1974

301. Anderson NE, Cunningham JM, Posner JB: Autoimmune pathogenesis of paraneoplastic neurologic syndromes. Crit Rev Clin Neurol 3:245–299, 1987

302. Kim YI, Neher I: IgG from patients with Lambert Eaton syndrome blocks calcium-dependent voltage channels. Science 239:405–408, 1988

303. Heber D, Chlebowski RT, Ishibashi DE, Herrold JN, Block JB: Abnormalities in glucose and protein metabolism in noncachetic lung cancer patients. Cancer Res 42:4815–4819, 1982

304. Anthony HM, Schorah CJ: Severe hypovitaminosis C in lung-cancer patients: The utilization of vitamin C in surgical repair and lymphocyte-related host resistance. Br J Cancer 46:354–367, 1982

305. Cox R, Musial T, Gyde OH: Reduced erythropoietin levels as a cause of anaemia in patients with lung cancer. Eur J Cancer Clin Oncol 22:511–514, 1986

306. Berg JW, Schottenfield D: Multiple primary cancers at Memorial Hospital 1949–1962. Cancer 40:1954–1960, 1977

307. Cahan WG: Multiple primary cancers of the lung, esophagus, and other sites. Cancer 40:1954–1960, 1977

308. Wynder EL, Muskinski MJ, Spivak JC: Tobacco and alcohol consumption in relation to the development of multiple primary cancers. Cancer 40:1872–1878, 1977

309. Cahan WG, Castro EB, Hajdu SI: The significance of solitary lung shadow in patients with colon carcinoma. Cancer 33:414–426, 1974

310. Enstrom JE, Austin DF: Interpreting cancer survival rates. Science 195:847–851, 1977

311. Fontana RS: Early diagnosis of lung cancer. Am Rev Respir Dis 116:399–402, 1977

312. Nash FA, Morgan JM, Tomkin JG: South London Lung Cancer Study. Br Med J 2:715–721, 1968

313. Brett GZ: Earlier diagnosis and survival in lung cancer. Br Med J 4:260–262, 1969

314. Weiss W, Boucot KE, Cooper DA: The Philadelphia Pulmonary Neoplasm Research Project: Survival factors in bronchogenic carcinoma. JAMA 216:2119–2123, 1973

315. Gryzbowski S, Coy P: Early diagnosis of carcinoma of lung: Simultaneous screening with chest x-ray and sputum cytology. Cancer 25:113–120, 1970

316. Melamed M, Flehinger B, Miller D et al: Preliminary report of the Lung Cancer Detection Program in New York. Cancer 39:369–382, 1977

317. Levin ML, Tockman MS, Frost JK, Ball WC: Lung cancer mortality in males screened by chest x-ray and cytologic sputum examination: A preliminary report. Recent Results Cancer Res 82:138–146, 1982

318. Fontana RS, Sanderson DR, Woolner LB, Taylor WF, Miller WE, Muhm JR: Lung cancer screening: The Mayo program. J Occup Med 28:746–750, 1986

319. Fontana RS: Screening for lung cancer: Recent experience in the United States. Cancer Treat Res 28:91–111, 1986

320. Neel HB III, Woolner LB, Sanderson DR: Sputum cytologic diagnosis of upper respiratory tract cancer. Ann Otol Rhinol Laryngol 87:468–473, 1978

321. Anonymous: Lung cancer mortality appears unaffected by roentgenographic and sputum screening in asymptomatic persons: Report from the NIH. JAMA 241:1582, 1979

322. Wolfsen AR, Odell WD: proACTH: Use for early detection of lung cancer. Am J Med 66:765–772, 1979

323. Chan JS, Seidah NG, Chretien M: Human NH2 terminal of pro-opiomelanocortin as a potential marker for pulmonary carcinoma. Cancer Res 43:3066–3069, 1983

324. Gail MH, Muenz L, McIntire KR et al: Multiple markers for lung cancer diagnosis: Validation of models for localized lung cancer. JNCI 80:97–101, 1988

325. Vincent RG, Chu TM, Lane WW et al: Carcinoembryonic antigen as a monitor of successful surgical resection in 130 patients with carcinoma of the lung. Prog Cancer Res Ther 11:191–198, 1979

326. Mountain CF: Surgery of lung cancer including adjunctive therapy. In Hansen HH, Rorth M (eds): Lung Cancer 1980, pp 71–92. Amsterdam, Excerpta Medica, 1980

327. Baker RR, Ball WC Jr, Carter D et al: Identification and treatment of clinically occult cancer of the lung. Prog Cancer Res Ther 11:243–249, 1979

328. Sanderson DR, Fontana RS, Woolner LB et al: Bronchoscopic localization of radiographically occult lung cancer. Chest 65:608–612, 1974

329. Martini N, Beattie EJ, Cliffton EE et al: Radiologically occult lung cancer: Report of 26 cases. Surg Clin North Am 54:811–823, 1974

330. Fontana RS: The needle in the haystack (editorial). Mayo Clin Proc 53:616–617, 1978

331. Kinsey JH, Cortese DA, Sanderson DR: Detection of hematoporphyrin fluorescence during fiberoptic bronchoscopy to localize early bronchogenic carcinoma. Mayo Clin Proc 53:594–600, 1978

332. Cortese DA, Kinsey JH, Woolner LB, Sanderson DR, Fontana RS: Hematoporphyrin derivative in the detection and localization of radiographically occult lung cancer. Am Rev Respir Dis 126:1087–1088, 1982

333. Bell JW: Positive sputum cytology and negative chest roentgenogram: A surgeon's dilemma. Ann Thorac Surg 9:149–157, 1970

334. Sanderson DR, Fontana RS: Early lung cancer detection and localization. Ann Otol Rhinol Laryngol 84:583–589, 1975

335. Cortese DA, Pairolero PC, Bergstrahl EJ et al: Roentgenographically occult lung cancer: A ten-year experience. J Thorac Cardiovasc Surg 86:373–380, 1983

336. Ikeda S, Yanai T, Ishikawa S: Flexible bronchofiberscope. Keio J Med 17:1–18, 1968

337. Ihde DC, Cohen MH, Bernath AM et al: Serial fiberoptic bronchoscopy during chemotherapy of small cell carcinoma of the lung. Chest 74:531–536, 1978

338. Kvale PA, Bode FR, Kini S: Diagnostic accuracy in lung cancer: Comparison of techniques used in association with flexible fiberoptic bronchoscopy. Chest 69:752–757, 1976

339. Saltzstein SL, Harrell JH II, Cameron T: Brushings, washings or biopsy? Obtaining maximum value from flexible fiberoptic bronchoscopy in the diagnosis of cancer. Chest 71:630–632, 1977

340. Radke JR, Conway WA, Eyler WR et al: Diagnostic accuracy in peripheral lung lesions: Factors predicting success with flexible fiberoptic bronchoscopy. Chest 76:176–179, 1979

341. Mohsenifar Z, Chopra SK, Simmons DH: Diagnostic value of fiberoptic bronchoscopy in lung cancer presenting as mediastinal mass(es). Cancer 44:1894–1896, 1979

342. Khan MA, Whitcomb ME, Snider GL: Flexible fiberoptic bronchoscopy. Am J Med 61:151–155, 1976

343. Martini N, McCormack PM: Assessment of endoscopically visible carcinomas. Chest 73:718–720, 1978

344. Richardson RH, Zavala DC, Jukerjee PK et al: The use of fiberoptic bronchoscopy and brush biopsy in the diagnosis of suspected pulmonary malignancy. Am Rev Respir Dis 109:63–66, 1974

345. Zavala DC: Diagnostic fiberoptic bronchoscopy: Techniques and results of biopsy in 600 patients. Chest 68:12–19, 1975

346. Shure D, Astarita RW: Bronchogenic carcinoma presenting as an endobronchial mass: Optimum number of biopsy specimens for diagnosis. Chest 83:865–867, 1983

347. Givens CD Jr, Marini JJ: Transbronchial needle aspiration of a bronchial carcinoid tumor. Chest 88:152–153, 1985

348. Lundgren R, Bergman F, Angstrom T: Comparison of transbronchial fine needle aspiration biopsy, aspiration of bronchial secretion, bronchial washing, brush biopsy and forceps biopsy in the diagnosis of lung cancer. Eur J Respir Dis 64:378–385, 1983

349. Buirski G, Calverley PMA, Douglas NJ et al: Bronchial needle aspiration in the diagnosis of bronchial carcinoma. Thorax 36:508–511, 1981

350. Shure D: Fiberoptic bronchoscopy: Diagnostic applications. Clin Chest Med 8:1–13, 1987

351. Dhillon DP, Haslam PL, Townsend PJ et al: Bronchoalveolar lavage in patients with interstitial lung diseases: Side effects and factors affecting fluid recovery. Eur J Respir Dis 68:342–350, 1986

352. Lam WK, So SY, Hsu C et al: Fiberoptic bronchoscopy in the diagnosis of bronchial cancer: Comparison of washings, brushings and biopsies in central and peripheral tumours. Clin Oncol 9:35–42, 1983

353. Hanson RR, Zavala DC, Rhodes ML et al: Am Rev Respir Dis 114:67–72, 1976

354. Fletcher EC, Levin DC: Flexible fiberoptic bronchoscopy and fluoroscopically guided transbronchial biopsy in the management of solitary pulmonary nodules. West J Med 138:364–370, 1983

355. Popovich J Jr, Kvale PA, Eichenhorn MS et al: Diagnostic accuracy of multiple biopsies from flexible fiberoptic bronchoscopy: A comparison of central versus peripheral carcinoma. Am Rev Respir Dis 125:521–523, 1982

356. Teirstein AS, Chuang MT, Choy AR et al: Flexible bronchoscopy in nonvisualized carcinoma of the lung. Ann Otol 87:318–321, 1978

357. Zavala DC, Richardson RH, Mukerjee PK et al: Use of the bronchofiberscope for bronchial brush biopsy: Diagnostic results and comparisons with other brushing techniques. Chest 63:889–892, 1973

358. Ono R, Loke J, Ikeda S: Bronchofiberscopy with curette biopsy and bronchography in the evaluation of peripheral lung lesions. Chest 79:162–166, 1981

359. Solomon DA, Sollida NH, Gracey DR: Cytology in fiberoptic bronchoscopy: Comparison of bronchial brushings, washings and postbronchoscopy sputum. Chest 65:616–619, 1974

360. Ellis JH: Transbronchial lung biopsy via the fiberoptic bronchoscope: Experience with 107 consecutive cases and comparison with bronchial brushings. Chest 68:524–532, 1975

361. Shure D, Fedullo PF: Transbronchial needle aspiration of peripheral masses. Am Rev Respir Dis 128:1090–1092, 1983

362. Wang KP, Haponik EF, Britt EJ et al: Transbronchial needle aspiration of peripheral pulmonary nodules. Chest 86:819–823, 1984

363. Credle WF, Smiddy JF, Elliott RC: Complications of fiberoptic bronchoscopy. Am Rev Respir Dis 109:67–72, 1974

364. Simpson FG, Arnold AG, Purvis A et al: Postal survey of bronchoscopic practice by physicians in the United Kingdom. Thorax 41:311–317, 1986

365. Suratt PM, Smiddy JF, Gruber B: Deaths and complications associated with fiberoptic bronchoscopy. Chest 69:747–751, 1976

366. Burns DM, Shure D, Francoz R et al: The physiologic consequences of saline lobar lavage in healthy human adults. Am Rev Respir Dis 127:696–701, 1983

367. Wang KP, Haponik EF, Gupta PK et al: Flexible transbronchial needle aspiration: Technical considerations. Ann Otol Rhinol Laryngol 93:233–236, 1984

368. Schenk DA, Bower JH, Bryan CL et al: Transbronchial needle aspiration staging of bronchogenic carcinoma. Am Rev Respir Dis 134:146–148, 1986

369. Shure D, Fedullo PF: The rule of transcranial needle aspiration in the staging of bronchogenic carcinoma. Chest 86:693–696, 1984
370. Gobien RP, Bouchard EA, Gobien BS et al: Thin needle aspiration biopsy of thoracic lesions: Impact on hospital charges and patterns of patients care. Radiology 148:65–67, 1983
371. Weisbrod GL: Percutaneous fine needle aspiratory biopsy of the mediastinum. Clin Chest Med 8:27–41, 1987
372. Ferrucci JT, Wittenberg J, Margolies MN et al: Malignant seeding of the tract after thin needle aspiration biopsy. Radiology 130:345–346, 1979
373. Sinner WN, Zajicek J: Implantation metastases after percutaneous transthoracic needle aspiration biopsy. Acta Radiol [Diagn] 17:473–475, 1976
374. Sinner WN: Pulmonary neoplasms diagnosed with transthoracic needle biopsy. Cancer 43:1533–1540, 1979
375. Sagel SS, Ferguson TB, Forrest JV et al: Percutaneous transthoracic aspiration needle biopsy. Ann Thorac Surg 26:399–405, 1978
376. Sinner WN, Sandstedt B: Small cell carcinoma of the lung: Cytological, roentgenologic, and clinical findings in a consecutive series diagnosed by fine needle aspiration biopsy. Radiology 121:269–274, 1976
377. Johnston WW: Cytologic diagnosis of lung cancer: Principles and problems. Pathol Res Pract 181:1–35, 1986
378. Calhoun P, Feldman PS, Armstrong P et al: The clinical outcome of needle aspirations of the lung when cancer is not diagnosed. Ann Thorac Surg 41:592–596, 1986
379. Denoix PF: Enquete permanente dans les centres anticancereaux. Bull Inst Nat Hyg 1:70–80, 1946
380. Task Force on Lung Cancer: Staging of lung cancer 1979. In American Joint Committee for Cancer Staging and End Results Reporting: Manual for Staging of Cancer. Chicago, American Joint Committee, 1979
381. Mountain CF: A new international staging system for lung cancer. Chest 89:225S–232S, 1986
382. Kayser K, Bulzebruck H, Probst G et al: Retrospective and prospective tumor staging evaluating prognostic factors in operated bronchus carcinoma patients. Cancer 59:355–361, 1987
383. Yee J, Llewellyn GA, Williams PA, May IA, Dugan DJ: Scalene lymph node dissection: A study of 354 consecutive dissections. Am J Surg 118:596–601, 1969
384. Schatzlein MH, McAuliffe SE, Orriner MB, Kirsh MM: Scalene node biopsy in pulmonary carcinoma: When it is indicated? Ann Thorac Surg 31:322–324, 1981
385. Maasen W, Greschuchner D: Die endoskopische und bioptische Untersuchung des Mediastinums. Atem U Lungenkrankheit 3:161–169, 1975
386. Luke WP, Pearson FG, Todd TR et al: Prospective evaluation of mediastinoscopy for assessment of carcinoma of the lung. J Thorac Cardiovasc Surg 91:53–56, 1986
387. Coughlen M, Deslauriers J, Beaulieu M et al: Role of mediastinoscopy in pretreatment staging of patients with primary lung cancer. Ann Thorac Surg 40:556–560, 1985
388. Jepsen O: Mediastinoscopy. Copenhagen, Munksgaard, 1966
389. Lewis RJ, Siskler GE, Mackenzie JW: Mediastinoscopy in advanced superior vena caval obstruction. Ann Thorac Surg 32:458–462, 1981
390. Lewis RJ, Sisler GE, Mackenzie JW: Repeat mediastinoscopy. Ann Thorac Surg 37:147–149, 1984
391. Palva T, Palva A, Karja J: Re mediastinoscopy. Arch Otolaryngol 101:748–750, 1975
392. Paris F, Padilla J, Tarazona V et al: Results of surgical therapy for lung carcinoma. Cancer Clin Trials 2:71–76, 1979
393. Swain J: Surgical techniques in the diagnosis of pulmonary disease. Clin Chest Med 8:43–51, 1987
394. Martini N, Heelan R, Westcott J et al: Comparative merits of conventional, computed tomographic, and magnetic resonance imaging in assessing mediastinal involvement in surgically confirmed lung carcinoma. J Thorac Cardiovasc Surg 90:639–648, 1985
395. Nagaishi C: Functional Anatomy and Histology of the Lung, American Edition, p 102. Baltimore, University Park Press, 1972
396. Rea HH, Shevland JE, House AJ: Accuracy of computed tomographic scanning in assessment of the mediastinum in bronchial carcinoma. J Thorac Cardiovasc Surg 81:825–829, 1981
397. Hutchinson CM, Mills NL: The selection of patients with bronchogenic carcinoma for mediastinoscopy. J Thorac Cardiovasc Surg 71:768–773, 1976
398. Genereux GP, Howie JL: Normal mediastinal lymph node size and number: CT and anatomic study. AJR 142:1095–1100, 1984
399. James EC, Ellwood RA: Mediastinoscopy and mediastinal roentgenology. Ann Thorac Surg 18:531–538, 1974
400. Shevland JE, Chiu LC, Schapiro RL et al: The role of conventional tomography and computed tomography in assessing the resectability of primary lung cancer: A preliminary study. CT 2:1–19, 1978
401. Crowe JK, Brown LR, Muhm JR; Computed tomography of the mediastinum. Radiology 128:75–87, 1978
402. Underwood GH Jr, Hooper RG, Azelbaum SP, Goodwin DW: Computed tomographic scanning of the thorax in the staging of bronchogenic carcinoma. N Engl J Med 300:777–778, 1979
403. Mintzer RA, Malave SR, Neiman HL, Michaelis LL, Vanecko RM, Sanders JH: Computed vs. conventional tomography in evaluation of primary and secondary pulmonary neoplasms. Radiology 132:653–659, 1979
404. Ekholm S, Albrechtsson U, Kugelberg J, Tylen U: Computed tomography in preoperative staging of bronchogenic carcinoma. J Comput Assist Tomogr 4:763–765, 1980
405. Hirleman MT, Yiu-Chiu VS, Chiu LC, Shapiro RL: The resectability of primary lung carcinoma: A diagnostic staging review. CT 4:146–150, 1980
406. Richardson JV, Zenk BA, Rossi NP: Preoperative non invasive mediastinal staging in bronchogenic carcinoma. Surgery 88:382–385, 1980
407. Faling LJ, Pugatch RD, Jung Legg Y et al: Computed tomographic scanning of the mediastinum in the staging of bronchogenic carcinoma. Am Rev Respir Dis 124:690–695, 1981
408. Moak GD, Cockerill EM, Farber MO, Yaw PB, Manfredi F: Computed tomography vs standard radiology in the evaluation of mediastinal adenopathy. Chest 82:69–75, 1982
409. Osborne DR, Korobkin M, Ravin CE et al: Comparison of plain radiography, conventional tomography and computed tomography in detecting intrathoracic lymph node metastases from lung carcinoma. Radiology 142:157–161, 1982
410. Lewis JW, Madrazo BL, Gross St C et al: The value of radiographic and computed tomography in the staging of lung carcinoma. Ann Thorac Surg 34:553–558, 1982
411. Modini C, Passariello R, Jascone C et al: TNM staging in lung cancer: Role of computed tomography. J Thorac Cardiovasc Surg 84:569–574, 1982
412. Baron RL, Levitt RG, Sagel SS, White MJ, Roper CL, Marberger JP: Computed tomography in the preoperative evaluation of bronchogenic carcinoma. Radiology 145:727–732, 1982
413. Goldstraw P, Kurzer M, Edwards D: Preoperative staging of lung cancer: Accuracy of computed tomography versus mediastinoscopy. Thorax 38:10–15, 1983
414. Khan A, Khan FA, Garvey J et al: Oblique hilar tomography and mediastinoscopy. Chest 86:424–429, 1984
415. Richey HM, Matthews JI, Helsel RA, Cable H: Thoracic CT scanning in the staging of bronchogenic carcinoma. Chest 85:218–221, 1984
416. Frederick H, Bernardino ME, Baron M et al: Accuracy of chest computerized tomography in detecting hilar and mediastinal involvement by squamous cell carcinoma of the lung. Cancer 54:2390–2395, 1984
417. Daly DBT, Faling LJ, Pugatch RD et al: Computed tomography: An effective technique for mediastinal staging in lung cancer. J Thorac Cardiovasc Surg 88:486–494, 1984
418. Imhof E, Perruchoud AP, Tan KG et al: Mediastinal staging of bronchial carcinoma: Can computed tomography replace mediastinoscopy? Respiration 48:257–260, 1985
419. McKenna RJ, Libshitz HI, Mountain CE et al: Roentgenographic evaluation of mediastinal nodes for preoperative assessment in lung cancer. Chest 88:206–210, 1985
420. Graves WG, Martinez MJ, Carter PL et al: The value of computed tomography in staging bronchogenic carcinoma: A changing role for mediastinoscopy. Ann Thorac Surg 40:57–59, 1985
421. Doyle PT, Weir J, Robertson EM et al: Role of computed tomography in assessing "operability" of bronchial carcinoma. Br Med J 292:231–233, 1986
422. Ferguson MK, MacMahon H, Little AG et al: Regional accuracy of computed tomography of the mediastinum in staging of lung cancer. J Thorac Cardiovasc Surg 91:498–504, 1986
423. Matthews JI, Richey HM, Helsel RA et al: Thoracic computed tomography in the preoperative evaluation of primary bronchogenic carcinoma. Arch Intern Med 147:449–453, 1987
424. Santiago S, Houston D, Ezer J et al: Gallium scanning and tomography in the preoperative evaluation of lung cancer. Cancer 58:341–343, 1986
425. DeMeester TR, Golomb HM, Kirchner P et al: The role of gallium 67 scanning in the clinical staging and preoperative evaluation of patients with carcinoma of the lung. Ann Thorac Surg 28:451–464, 1979
426. Glazer GM, Gross BH, Aisen AM et al: Imaging of the pulmonary hilum: A prospective comparative study in patients with lung cancer. AJR 145:245–248, 1985
427. Webb WR, Jensen BG, Svelluto R et al: Bronchogenic carcinoma: Staging with MR compared with staging with CT and surgery. Radiology 156:117–124, 1985
428. Levitt RG, Glazer HS, Roper CL et al: Magnetic resonance imaging of mediastinal and hilar metastases: Comparison with CT. AJR 145:9–14, 1985
429. Martini N, Heelan R, Westcott J et al: Comparative merits of conventional computed tomographic and magnetic resonance imaging in assessing mediastinal involvement in surgically confirmed lung carcinoma. J Thorac Cardiovasc Surg 90:639–648, 1985
430. Poon PY, Bunnill MJ, Henkelman RM et al: Mediastinal lymph node metastases from bronchogenic carcinoma: Detection with MR imaging and CT. Radiology 162:651–656, 1987
431. Delarue NC, Sanders DE, Silverberg SA: Complementary role of pulmonary angiography and mediastinoscopy in individualizing treatment for patients with lung cancer. Cancer 26:1370–1378, 1970
432. Fishman NH, Bronstein MJ: Is mediastinoscopy necessary in the evaluation of lung cancer? Ann Thorac Surg 20:578–585, 1975
433. Benfield JE, Bonney H, Crummy AB et al: Azygograms and pulmonary arteriograms in bronchogenic carcinoma. Arch Surg 99:406–409, 1969
434. McLeod RA, Brown LR, Miller WE et al: Evaluation of the pulmonary hila by tomography. Radiol Clin North Am 14:51–83, 1976
435. Macumber HH, Calvin JW: Perfusion lung scan patterns in 100 patients with bronchogenic carcinoma. J Thorac Cardiovasc Surg 72:299–302, 1976
436. Cunningham JJ: Gray scale echocardiography of the lung and pleural space: Current applications of oncologic interest. Cancer 41:1329–1339, 1978

437. Biersach HJ, Bokisch A, Oehr P et al: Clinical results of immunoscintigraphy in a variety of malignant tumors with special reference to immunohistochemistry. Nuklearmedizin 25:167–171, 1986
438. Goldenberg DM, Kim EE, Deland F et al: Clinical studies on the radioimmunodetection of tumors containing alpha-fetoprotein. Cancer 48:2500–2502, 1980
439. Perkins AC, Perom MV, Morgan DAL et al: I¹³¹ and In¹¹¹-labeled monoclonal antibody imaged primary lung carcinoma. Nucl Med Commun 7:729–739, 1986
440. Chan SYT, Evan GI, Ritson A et al: Localisation of lung cancer by a radiolabelled monoclonal antibody against the c-myc oncogene product. Br J Cancer 54:761–769, 1986
441. Hansen HH, Muggia FM: Staging of inoperable patients with bronchogenic carcinoma with special reference to bone marrow examination and peritoneoscopy. Cancer 30:1395–1401, 1972
442. Muggia FM, Chervu LR: Lung cancer: Diagnosis in metastatic sites. Semin Oncol 1:217–228, 1974
443. O'Mara RE: Skeletal scanning in neoplastic disease. Cancer 37:480–486, 1976
444. Hansen HH, Muggia FM, Selawry OS: Bone marrow examination in 100 consecutive patients with bronchogenic carcinoma. Lancet 2:443–445, 1971
445. Newman SJ, Hansen HH: Frequency, diagnosis and treatment of brain metastases in 247 consecutive patients with bronchogenic carcinoma. Cancer 33:492–496, 1974
446. Ransdell JW, Peters RM, Taylor AT et al: Multiorgan scans for staging lung cancer: Correlation with clinical evaluation. J Thorac Cardiovasc Surg 73:653–659, 1977
447. Turner P, Haggith JW: Preoperative radionuclide scanning in bronchogenic carcinoma. Br J Dis Chest 75:291–294, 1981
448. Bell JW: Abdominal exploration in one-hundred lung carcinoma suspects prior to thoracotomy. Ann Surg 167:199–203, 1969
449. Yashar J: Transdiaphragmatic exploration of the upper abdomen during surgery for bronchogenic carcinoma. J Thorac Cardiovasc Surg 52:599–603, 1966
450. Hansen HH, Muggia FM: Staging of inoperable patients with bronchogenic carcinoma with special references to bone marrow examination and peritoneoscopy. Cancer 30:1395–1401, 1972
451. Mintz BJ, Tuhrim S, Alexander S: Intracranial metastases in the initial staging of bronchogenic carcinoma. Chest 86:850–853, 1984
452. Chapman GS, Kumar D, Redmond J et al: Upper abdominal computerized tomography scanning in staging non-small cell lung cancer. Cancer 54:1541–1543, 1984
453. Mountain CF: Biologic, physiologic, and technical determinants in surgical therapy for lung cancer. In Straus MJ (ed): Lung Cancer: Clinical Diagnosis and Treatment, pp 185–198. New York, Grune & Stratton, 1977
454. Mountain CF: Assessment of the role of surgery for control of lung cancer. Ann Thorac Surg 24:365–373, 1977
455. Tarhan S, Moffitt EA: Principles of thoracic anesthesia. Surg Clin North Am 53:813–826, 1973
456. Stanley KE: Prognostic factors for survival in patients with inoperable lung cancer. JNCI 65:25–32, 1980
457. Finkelstein DM, Ettinger DS, Ruckdeschel JC: Long term survivors in metastatic non small cell lung cancer: An Eastern Cooperative Oncology Group study. J Clin Oncol 4:702–709, 1986
458. Lee JY, Marks JE, Simpson JR: Age as a criterion for eligibility in a lung cancer trial. Am J Clin Oncol 5:449–452, 1982
459. Golebiowski A: Pulmonary resection in patients over 70 years of age. J Thorac Cardiovasc Surg 61:265–270, 1971
460. Watson WL, Schottenfeld D: Survival in cancer of the bronchus and lung 1949–1962: Comparison of men and women patients. Dis Chest 53:65–72, 1968
461. Ederer F, Mersheimer WL: Sex differences in the survival of lung cancer patients. Cancer 15:425–432, 1962
462. Connelly RR, Cutler SJ, Baylis P: End results in cancer of the lung: Comparison of male and female patients. JNCI 36:277–287, 1966
463. Kirsh MM, Tashian J, Sloan H: Carcinoma of the lung in women. Ann Thorac Surg 34:34–39, 1982
464. Harley HRS: Cancer of the lung in women. Thorax 31:254–264, 1976
465. Tartler PI, Burrirus L, Kirschner P: Perioperative blood transfusion adversely affects prognosis after resection of Stage I (subset N0) non oat cell lung cancer. J Thorac Cardiovasc Surg 88:659–662, 1984
466. Hyman NH, Fostes RS, DeMeules JE et al: Blood transfusions and survival after lung cancer resection. Am J Surg 149:502–507, 1985
467. Tarhan S, Moffitt EA, Taylor WF: Myocardial infarction after general anesthesia. JAMA 220:1451–1454, 1972
468. Robbins HM, Morrison DA, Sweet ME et al: Biopsy of the main carina: Staging lung cancer with the fiberoptic bronchoscope. Chest 75:484–486, 1979
469. Piehler JM, Trastek FV, Pairolero PL et al: Concomitant cardiac and pulmonary operations. J Thorac Cardiovasc Surg 90:662–667, 1985
470. Parker FB Jr: Surgery in chronic lung disease. Surg Clin North Am 54:1193–1202, 1974
471. Olsen GN, Block AJ, Swenson EW et al: Pulmonary function evaluation of the lung resection candidate: A prospective study. Am Rev Respir Dis 111:379–387, 1975
472. Legge JS, Palmer KN: Effect of lung resection for bronchial carcinoma on pulmonary function in patients with and without chronic obstructive bronchitis. Thorax 30:563–565, 1975
473. Alderson PO: Scintigraphic evaluation of patients with lung carcinoma. Chest 89:2455–2485, 1986
474. Block AJ, Olsen GN: Preoperative pulmonary function testing. JAMA 235:257–258, 1976
475. Ali MK, Mountain CF, Ewer MS et al: Predicting loss of pulmonary function after pulmonary resection for bronchogenic carcinoma. Chest 77:337–342, 1980
476. Ciofetta G, Silverman M, Hughes JMB: Quantitative approach to the study of regional lung function in children using krypton 81m. Br J Radiol 53:950–959, 1980
477. Ali ML, Ewer MS, Atallah MR et al: Regional and overall pulmonary function changes in lung cancer. J Thorac Cardiovasc Surg 86:1–8, 1983
478. Bria WF, Kanarek DJ, Kazemi H: Prediction of postoperative pulmonary function following thoracic operations. J Thorac Cardiovasc Surg 86:186–192, 1983
479. O'Rourke MA, Feussner JR, Feigl P, Laszlo J: Age trends of lung cancer stage at diagnosis: Implications for lung cancer screening in the elderly. JAMA 258:921–926, 1987
480. Sherman S, Guidot CE: The feasibility of thoracotomy for lung cancer in the elderly. JAMA 258:927–930, 1987
481. Page WF, Kuntz AJ: Racial and socioeconomic factors in cancer survival: A comparison of Veterans Administration results with selected studies. Cancer 45:1029–1040, 1980
482. Greenberg ER, Chute CG, Stukel T et al: Social and economic factors in the choice of lung cancer treatment: A population-based study in two rural states. N Engl J Med 318:612–617, 1988
483. Mayer RJ, Patterson WB: How is cancer treatment chosen? N Engl J Med 318:636–638, 1988
484. Mountain CF: Clinical biology of small cell carcinoma: Relationship to surgical therapy. Semi Oncol 5:272–279, 1978
485. Meyer JA: Effect of histologically verified TNM stage on disease control in treated small cell carcinoma of the lung. Cancer 55:1747–1752, 1985
486. Ihde DC, Makuch RW, Carney DN et al: Prognostic implication of sites of metastases in patients with small cell carcinoma of the lung given intensive combination chemotherapy. Am Rev Respir Dis 123:500–507, 1981
487. Maurer LH, Tulloh M, Weiss RB et al: A randomized combined modality trial in small cell carcinoma of the lung: Comparison of combination chemotherapy–radiation therapy versus cyclophosphamide–radiation therapy: Effects of maintenance chemotherapy and prophylactic whole brain irradiation. Cancer 45:30–39, 1980
488. Bunn PA Jr, Cohen MH, Ihde DC et al: Advances in small cell bronchogenic carcinoma. Cancer Treat Rep 61:333–342, 1977
489. Israel L, Depierre A, Choffel C et al: Immunochemotherapy in 34 cases of oat cell carcinoma of the lung with 19 complete remissions. Cancer Treat Rep 61:343–347, 1977
490. Lowenbraun S, Bartolucci A, Smalley RV et al: The superiority of combination chemotherapy over single agent chemotherapy in small cell lung carcinoma. Cancer 44:406–413, 1979
491. Livingston BR, Moore TN, Heilbrun L et al: Small cell carcinoma of the lung: Combined chemotherapy and radiation. Ann Intern Med 88:194–199, 1978
492. Østerlind K, Hansen HH, Dombernowsky P et al: Determinants of complete remission induction and maintenance in chemotherapy with or without irradiation of small cell lung cancer. Cancer Res 47:2733–2736, 1987
493. Zelen M: Keynote address on biostatistics and data retrieval. Cancer Chemother Rep 4:31–42, 1973
494. Einhorn LH, Bond WH, Hornback N et al: Long-term results in combined modality treatment of small cell carcinoma of the lung. Semin Oncol 5:309–313, 1978
495. Eagan RT, Carr DT, Lee RE et al: Phase II studies of polychemotherapy regimens in small cell lung cancer. Cancer Treat Rep 61:93–96, 1977
496. Cohen MH, Ihde C, Bunn PA et al: Cyclic alternating combination chemotherapy of small cell bronchogenic carcinoma. Cancer Treat Rep 63:163–170, 1979
497. Østerlind K, Andersen PK: Prognostic factors in small cell lung cancer: Multivariate model based on 778 patients treated with chemotherapy with or without irradiation. Cancer Res 46:4189–4194, 1986
498. Østerlind K, Hansen HH, Hansen M et al: Long-term disease-free survival in small cell carcinoma of the lung: A study of clinical determinants. J Clin Oncol 4:1307–1313, 1986
499. Østerlind K, Hansen M, Hansen HH et al: Treatment policy of surgery in small cell carcinoma of the lung: Retrospective analysis of a series of 874 consecutive patients. Thorax 40:272–277, 1985
500. Shepherd FA, Ginsburg RJ, Feld R et al: Reduction in local recurrence and improved survival in surgically treated patients with small cell lung cancer. J Thorac Cardiovasc Surg 86:498–506, 1983
501. Friess GG, McCracken JD, Troxell ML et al: Effect of initial resection of small cell carcinoma of the lung: A review of Southwest Oncology Group Study 7628. J Clin Oncol 3:964–968, 1985
502. DeWys WD, Begg C, Lavin PT et al: Prognostic effect of weight loss prior to chemotherapy in cancer patients. Am J Med 69:491–497, 1980
503. Johnston–Early A, Cohen MH, Fossieck BE et al: Delayed hypersensitivity skin testing as a prognostic indicator in patients with small cell lung cancer. Cancer 52:1395–1400, 1983
504. Hansen HH, Dombernowsky P, Hirsch FR: Staging procedures and prognostic features in small cell anaplastic bronchogenic carcinoma. Semin Oncol 5:280–287, 1978
505. Dearing MP, Steinberg SM, Phelps R et al: Women small cell lung cancer patients live longer than men (abstract). Proc Am Soc Clin Oncol 7:199, 1988
506. Poplin E, Thompson B, Whitacre M et al: Small cell carcinoma of the lung: Influ-

ence of age on treatment outcome. Cancer Treat Rep 71:291–296, 1987

507. Johnston-Early A, Cohen MH, Minna JD et al: Smoking abstinence and small cell lung cancer survival: An association. JAMA 244:2175–2179, 1980

508. Livingston RB, Trauth CJ, Greenstreet RL: Small cell carcinoma: Clinical manifestations and behavior with treatment. In Greco FA, Oldham RK, Bunn PA (eds): Small Cell Lung Cancer, pp 285–300. Orlando, Grune & Stratton, 1981

509. Quoix E, Finkelstein H, Wolkove N et al: Treatment of small cell lung cancer on protocol: Potential bias of results. J Clin Oncol 4:1314–1320, 1986

510. Seifter EJ, Ihde DC: Small cell lung cancer: A distant clinicopathologic entity. In Bitran JD, Golumb HM, Little AG, Weichselbaum RR (eds): Lung Cancer: A Comprehensive Treatise, pp 257–279. Chicago, Grune & Stratton, 1988

511. Cohen MH, Matthews MJ: Small cell bronchogenic carcinoma: A distinct clinicopathologic entity. Semin Oncol 5:234–241, 1978

512. Sculier JP, Evans WK, Feld R et al: Superior vena cava syndrome in small cell lung cancer. Cancer 57:847–851, 1986

513. Johnson DH, Hainsworth JD, Greco FA: Extrahepatic biliary obstruction caused by small cell lung cancer. Ann Intern Med 102:487–490, 1985

514. Gropp C, Havemann K, Scheuer A: Ectopic hormones in lung cancer patients at diagnosis and during therapy. Cancer 46:347–354, 1980

515. Hansen M, Hammer M, Hummer L: Diagnostic and therapeutic implications of ectopic hormone production in small cell carcinoma of the lung. Thorax 35:101–106, 1980

516. Hansen M, Hansen HH, Hirsch FR et al: Hormonal polypeptides and amine metabolites in small cell carcinoma of the lung, with special reference to stage and subtypes. Cancer 45:1432–1437, 1980

517. List AF, Hainsworth JD, Davis BW et al: The syndrome of inappropriate secretion of anti-diuretic hormone in small cell lung cancer. J Clin Oncol 4:1191–1198, 1986

518. Wittes RE, Yeh SDJ: Indications for liver and brain scans: Screening tests for patients with oat cell carcinoma of the lung. JAMA 238:506–507, 1977

519. Ihde DC: Staging evaluation and prognostic factors in small cell lung cancer. In Aisner J (ed): Lung Cancer, pp 241–268. New York, Churchill Livingstone, 1985

520. Nakhosteen JA, Niederle N: Small cell lung cancer: Serial bronchofiberscopy and photographic documentation—the bridge sign. Chest 83:12–16, 1983

521. Harper PG, Houang M, Spiro SG, Geddes D, Hodson M, Souhami RL: Computerized axial tomography in the pretreatment assessment of small-cell carcinoma of the bronchus. Cancer 47:1775–1780, 1981

522. Levenson RM, Sauerbrunn BJL, Ihde DC, Bunn PA Jr, Cohen MH, Minna JD: Small cell lung cancer: Radionuclide bone scans for assessment of tumor extent and response. AJR 137:31–35, 1981

523. Campling B, Quirt I, DeBoer G et al: Is bone marrow examination in small cell lung cancer really necessary? Ann Intern Med 105:508–512, 1986

524. Levitan N, Byrne RE, Bromer RH et al: The value of bone scan and bone marrow biopsy in staging small cell lung cancer. Cancer 56:652–654, 1985

525. Kristjansen PEG, Østerlind K, Hansen M: Detection of bone marrow relapse in patients with small cell carcinoma of the lung. Cancer 58:2538–2541, 1986

526. Mulshine JL, Makuch RW, Johnston-Early A et al: Diagnosis and significance of liver metastases in small cell carcinoma of the lung. J Clin Oncol 2:733–741, 1984

527. Dombernowsky P, Hirsch F, Hansen HH et al: Peritoneoscopy in the staging of 190 patients with small-cell anaplastic carcinoma of the lung with special reference to subtyping. Cancer 41:2008–2012, 1978

528. Hansen SW, Jensen F, Pedersen NT et al: Detection of liver metastases in small cell lung cancer: A comparison of peritoneoscopy with liver biopsy and ultrasonography with fine-needle aspiration. J Clin Oncol 5:255–259, 1987

529. Sculier JP, Feld R, Evans WK et al: Neurologic disorders in patients with small cell lung cancer. Cancer 60:2275–2283, 1987

530. Crane JM, Nelson MJ, Ihde DC et al: A comparison of computed tomography and radionuclide scanning for detection of brain metastases in small cell lung cancer. J Clin Oncol 2:1017–1024, 1984

531. Johnson DH, Windham WW, Allen JH, Greco FA: Limited value of CT brain scans in the staging of small cell cancer. AJR 140:37–40, 1983

532. Giannone L, Johnson DH, Hande KR et al: Favorable prognosis of brain metastases in small cell lung cancer. Ann Intern Med 106:386–389, 1987

533. Bunn PA Jr, Nugent JL, Matthews MJ: Central nervous system metastases in small cell bronchogenic carcinoma. Semin Oncol 5:314–322, 1978

534. Nugent JL, Bunn PA Jr, Matthews MJ et al: CNS metastases in small cell bronchogenic carcinoma: Increasing frequency and changing pattern with lengthening survival. Cancer 44:1885–1893, 1979

535. Rosen ST, Aisner J, Makuch RW et al: Carcinomatous leptomeningitis in small cell lung cancer: A clinicopathologic review of the National Cancer Institute experience. Medicine 61:45–53, 1982

536. Ihde DC, Dunnick NR, Johnston-Early A, Bunn PA, Cohen MH, Minna JD: Abdominal computed tomography in small cell lung cancer: Assessment of extent of disease and response to therapy. Cancer 49:1485–1490, 1982

537. Pedersen AG, Bach F, Melgaard B: Frequency, diagnosis, and prognosis of spinal cord compression in small cell bronchogenic carcinoma: A review of 817 consecutive patients. Cancer 55:1818–1822, 1985

538. Murphy KC, Feld R, Evans WK et al: Intramedullary spinal cord metastases from small cell carcinoma of the lung. J Clin Oncol 1:99–106, 1983

539. Dunnick NR, Ihde DC, Johnston-Early A: Abdominal CT in the evaluation of small cell carcinoma of the lung. AJR 133:1085–1088, 1979

540. Poon PY, Feld R, Evans WK, Ege C, Yeoh JL, McLoughlin ML: Computed tomography of the brain, liver, and upper abdomen in the staging of small cell carcinoma of the lung. J Comput Assist Tomogr 6:963–965, 1982

541. Lewis E, Bernardino ME, Valdivieso M, Farha P, Barnes PA, Thomas JL: Computed tomography and routine chest radiography in oat cell carcinoma of the lung. J Comput Assist Tomogr 6:739–745, 1982

542. Pagani JJ: Normal adrenal glands in small cell lung carcinoma: CT-guided biopsy. AJR 140:949–951, 1983

543. Carney DN, Ihde DC, Cohen MH et al: Serum neuron-specific enolase: A marker for disease extent and response to therapy of small-cell lung cancer. Lancet x:583–585, 1982

544. Carney DN, Zweig MH, Ihde DC et al: Elevated serum creatine kinase-BB levels in patients with small cell lung cancer. Cancer Res 44:5399–5403, 1984

545. Sobol RE, O'Connor DT, Addison J et al: Elevated serum chromogranin A concentrations in small cell lung carcinoma. Ann Intern Med 105:698–700, 1986

546. Johnson DH, Marangos PJ, Forbes JT et al: Potential utility of serum neuron-specific enolase in small cell carcinoma of the lung. Cancer Res 44:5409–5414, 1984

547. Ariyoshi Y, Kato K, Ishiguro Y, Ota K, Sato T, Suchi T: Evaluation of serum neuron-specific enolase as a tumor marker for carcinoma of the lung. Gann 74:219–225, 1983

548. Goslin RH, Skarin AT, Zamcheck N: Carcinoembryonic antigen: A useful monitor of therapy of small cell lung cancer. JAMA 246:2173–2176, 1981

549. Sculier JP, Feld R, Evans WK et al: Carcinoembryonic antigen: A useful prognostic marker in small cell lung cancer. J Clin Oncol 3:1349–1354, 1985

550. Woo KB, Waalkes P, Abeloff MD, Ettinger DS, McNutt KL, Gehrke CW: Multiple biologic markers in the monitoring of treatment for patients with small cell carcinoma of the lung: The use of serial levels of plasma CEA and serum carbohydrates. Cancer 48:1633–1642, 1981

551. Goslin RH, O'Brien MJ, Skarin AT, Zamcheck N: Immunocytochemical staining for CEA in small cell carcinoma of the lung predicts clinical usefulness of the plasma assay. Cancer 52:301–306, 1983

552. Graham EA, Singer JJ: Successful removal of an entire lung for carcinoma of the bronchus. JAMA 101:1371–1374, 1933

553. Carlson HA, Ballon HC: The operability of carcinoma of the lung. J Thorac Surg 2:323–340, 1933

554. Reinhoff WE Jr, Gannon J Jr, Sherman I: Closure of the bronchus following pneumonectomy. Ann Surg 116:481–531, 1942

555. Davis S, Wright PW, Schulman SF et al: Participants in prospective randomized trials for resected non small cell lung cancer have improved survival compared with nonparticipants in such trials. Cancer 56:1710–1718, 1985

556. Shields T, Higgins GA: Minimal pulmonary resection in the treatment of carcinomas of the lung. Arch Surg 108:420–422, 1974

557. Hildebrand PJ, Prakash D, Cosgrove J et al: High frequency ventilation: A method for thoracic surgery. Anaesthesia 39:1091–1095, 1984

558. Urschel HC, Razzuk MA: Median sternotomy as a standard approach for pulmonary resection. Ann Thorac Surg 41:130–134, 1986

559. Olivet RT, Nauss LA, Payne WS: A technique for continuous intercostal nerve block analgesia following thoracotomy. J Thorac Cardiovasc Surg 80:308–311, 1980

560. Danielson DR, Nauss LA: Post thoracotomy analgesia. In Grillo HC, Eschapasse H (eds): International Trends in General Thoracic Surgery, Vol 2, pp 189–197. Philadelphia, WB Saunders, 1987

561. Vincent RG, Takita H, Lane WW et al: Surgical therapy of lung cancer. J Thorac Cardiovasc Surg 71:581–591, 1976

562. Fryjordet A, Klevmark B: Lung cancer. Scand J Thorac Cardiovasc Surg 5:92–102, 1971

563. Kirsh MM, Rotman H, Argenta L et al: Carcinoma of the lung: Results of treatment over 10 years. Ann Thorac Surg 21:371–377, 1976

564. Weiss W: Operative mortality and 5 year survival rates in men with bronchogenic carcinoma. Chest 66:483, 1974

565. Naruke T, Suemasu K, Ishikawa S: Lymph node mapping and curability at various levels of metastases in resected lung cancer. J Thorac Cardiovasc Surg 76:832–834, 1978

566. Nagasaki F, Flehinger BJ, Martini N: Complications of surgery in the treatment of carcinoma of the lung. Chest 82:25–29, 1982

567. Ginsberg RJ, Hill LD, Eagan RT et al: Modern thirty day operative mortality for surgical resection in lung cancer. J Thorac Cardiovasc Surg 86:654–658, 1983

568. Kohman LJ, Meyer JA, Ikins PM et al: Random versus predictable risks of mortality after thoracotomy for lung cancer. J Thorac Cardiovasc Surg 91:551–554, 1986

569. Steele JD: The solitary pulmonary nodule. J Thorac Cardiovasc Surg 46:21–39, 1963

570. Keagy BA, Starek PJ, Manay GF et al: Major pulmonary resection for suspected but unconfirmed malignancy. Ann Thorac Surg 38:314–316, 1984

571. Cortese DA, Pairolero PC, Bergstrahl EJ et al: Roentgenographically occult lung cancer. J Thorac Cardiovasc Surg 86:373–380, 1983

572. Gail MH, Eagan RT, Feld R et al: Prognostic factors in patients with resected Stage I non small cell lung cancer. Cancer 54:1802–1813, 1984

573. Martini N, Flehinger BJ, Nagasaki F et al: Prognostic significance of N1 disease in carcinoma of the lung. J Thorac Cardiovasc Surg 86:646–653, 1983

574. Kayser K, Bulzebruch H, Probst G et al: Retrospective and prospective tumor staging evaluating prognostic factors in operated bronchus carcinoma patients. Cancer 59:355–361, 1987

575. Iascone C, DeMeester TR, Albertucci M et al: Local recurrence of resectable non oat cell carcinoma of the lung. Cancer 57:471–476, 1986

576. Pariolero PC, Williams DE, Berstrahl EJ et al: Postsurgical Stage I bronchogenic carcinoma: Marked implications of recurrent disease. Ann Thorac Surg 38:331–338, 1984

577. Mountain CF: The biological operability of Stage II non small cell lung cancer. Ann Thorac Surg 40:60–64, 1985

578. DesLauriers J, Beaulieu M, Benuzera A et al: Sleeve pneumonectomy for bronchogenic carcinoma. Ann Thorac Surg 28:465–474, 1978

579. DesLauriers J: Discussion of survival in patients undergoing tracheal sleeve pneumonectomy for bronchogenic carcinoma. J Thorac Cardiovasc Surg 84:489–496, 1982

580. Jensik RJ, Faber LP, Kittle CF et al: Survival in patients undergoing tracheal sleeve pneumonectomy for bronchogenic carcinoma. J Thorac Cardiovasc Surg 84:489–496, 1982

581. Trastek FF, Pairolero PC, Piehler JM et al: En bloc (non chest wall) resection for bronchogenic carcinoma with parietal fixation. J Thorac Cardiovasc Surg 87:352–358, 1984

582. Piehler JM, Pairolero PC, Weiland LH et al: Bronchogenic carcinoma with chest wall invasion: Factors affecting survival following en bloc resection. Ann Thorac Surg 34:684–691, 1982

583. McCaughan BC, Martini N, Bains MS et al: Chest wall invasion in carcinoma of the lung. J Thorac Cardiovasc Surg 89:836–841, 1985

584. Kirsh MM, Prior M, Gago O et al: The effect of histological cell type on the prognosis of patients with bronchogenic carcinoma. Ann Thorac Surg 13:303–310, 1972

585. Abbey Smith R: The importance of mediastinal lymph node invasion by pulmonary carcinoma in selection of patients for resection. Ann Thorac Surg 25:5–11, 1978

586. Naruke T, Suemasu K, Ishikawa S: Lymph node mapping and curability of various levels of metastases in resected lung cancer. J Thorac Cardiovasc Surg 76:832–839, 1978

587. Pearson FG, Delarue NC, Ilves R et al: Significance of positive superior mediastinal nodes identified at mediastinoscopy in patients with resectable cancer of the lung. J Thorac Cardiovasc Surg 83:1–11, 1982

588. Martini N, Flehinger BJ, Zaman MB et al: Results of resection in non oat cell carcinoma of the lung with mediastinal lymph node metastases. Ann Surg 198:386–397, 1983

589. Naruke T: Staging of N2 disease. Chest 89:338S–339S, 1986

590. Pearson FG: Radical surgery for N2 disease. Chest 89:339S–340S, 1986

591. Bergh NP, Larsson S: The significance of various types of mediastinal lymph node metastases in lung cancer. In Jepsen O, Sorenson HR (eds): Mediastinoscopy: Proceedings of an International Symposium. Odense, Odense University Press, 1971

592. Martini N, Flehinger BJ, Zaman MB et al: Prospective study of 445 lung carcinomas with mediastinal lymph node metastases. J Thorac Cardiovasc Surg 80:390–399, 1980

593. Watanabe Y, Iwa T, Kobayashi H et al: Results of surgical treatment for lung cancer with N2 disease. Presented at the Third World Conference on Lung Cancer, Tokyo, Japan, 1982

594. Patterson GA, Pizza D, Pearson FG et al: Significance of metastatic disease in subaortic lymph nodes. Ann Thorac Surg 43:155–159, 1987

595. Bergh NP, Schersten I: Bronchogenic carcinoma: A follow up study of a surgically treated series with special references to prognostic significance of lymph node metastases. Acta Chir Scand (Suppl) 347:1–42, 1965

596. Larsson S: Pretreatment classification and staging of bronchogenic carcinoma. Scand J Thorac Cardiovasc Surg 7:1–130, 1973

597. Jensik RJ: The extent of resections for localized lung cancer: Segmental resection. In Kulle CF (ed): Current Controversies in Thoracic Surgery, pp 175–182. Philadelphia, WB Saunders, 1986

598. Errett LF, Wilson J, Chiu RC et al: Wedge resection as an alternative procedure for peripheral bronchogenic carcinoma in poor risk patients. J Thorac Cardiovasc Surg 90:656–661, 1985

599. McCormack PM, Martini N: Primary lung cancer: Results with conservative resection in treatment. NY State J Med 80:612–616, 1980

600. Ferguson MK, DeMeester TR, DesLauriers J et al: Diagnosis and management of synchronous lung cancers. J Thorac Cardiovasc Surg 90:378–385, 1985

601. Mathiesen DJ, Jensik RJ, Faber LP et al: Survival following resection for second and third primary lung cancers. J Thorac Cardiovasc Surg 88:502–510, 1984

602. Price Thomas C: Conservative resections of the bronchial tree. J Roy Coll Surg Edinburgh 1:169–171, 1956

603. Paulson DL, Shaw RR: Bronchial anastomosis and bronchoplastic procedures with interest of preservation of lung tissue. J Thorac Surg 29:238–259, 1955

604. Johnston JB, Jones PH: The treatment of bronchial carcinoma by lobectomy and sleeve resection of the main bronchus. Thorax 14:48–54, 1959

605. Weisel RD, Cooper JD, Dalarue NC et al: Sleeve lobectomy for carcinoma of the lung. J Thorac Cardiovasc Surg 78:839–849, 1979

606. Lowe JE, Bridgeman AH, Sabiston DC Jr et al: The role of bronchoplastic procedures in the surgical management of benign and malignant pulmonary lesions. J Thorac Cardiovasc Surg 83:227–234, 1982

607. Vogt Moykopf I, Toomes H, Heinrich ST: Sleeve resection of the bronchus and pulmonary artery for pulmonary lesions. Thorac Cardiovasc Surgeon 31:193–198, 1983

608. Eschapasse H, Gaillard J, Dahan M: Sleeve lobectomy for carcinoma of the lung. Chest 89:335S–336S, 1986

609. Bennett WF, Smith RA: A twenty year analysis of the results of sleeve resection for primary bronchogenic carcinoma. J Thorac Cardiovasc Surg 76:840–845, 1978

610. Kjaer M: Radiotherapy of squamous, adeno- and large cell carcinoma of the lung. Cancer Treat Rev 9:1–20, 1982

611. Cox JD, Byhardt RW, Komaki R: The role of radiotherapy in squamous, large cell, and adenocarcinoma of the lung. Semin Oncol 10:81–94, 1983

612. Choi NC: Curative radiation therapy of unresectable non-small-cell carcinoma of the lung: Indications, techniques, results, and Role of postoperative radiation therapy in lung cancer with either metastases to regional lymph nodes (N1 or unforeseen N2) or direct invasion beyond visceral pleura (T3). In Grillo H, Choi NC (eds): Thoracic Oncology, 163–199. New York, Raven Press, 1983

613. McNeil BJ, Weichselbaum RR, Parker SG: The fallacy of the five year survival in lung cancer. N Engl J Med 299:1397–1400, 1978

614. Hilton G: Present position relating to cancer of the lung: Results with radiotherapy alone. Thorax 15:17–18, 1960

615. Smart J: Can cancer of the lung be cured by radiation alone? JAMA 195:1034–1035, 1966

616. Cox JD, Komaki R, Byhardt RW: Is immediate chest radiotherapy obligatory for any or all patients with limited-stage non-small cell carcinoma of the lung? Yes. Cancer Treat Rep 67:327–331, 1983

617. Perez CA, Pajak TF, Rubin P et al: Long-term observations of the patterns of failure in patients with unresectable non-oat cell carcinoma of the lung treated with definitive radiotherapy: Report by the Radiation Therapy Oncology Group. Cancer 59:1874–1881, 1987

618. Salazar OM, Slawson RG, Poussin–Rosillo H, Amin PP, Sewchard W, Strohl RA: A prospective randomized trial comparing once-a-week vs daily radiation therapy for locally advanced, non-metastatic, lung cancer: A preliminary report. Int J Radiat Oncol Biol Phys 12:779–787, 1986

619. Kusumoto S, Koga K, Tsukino H, Nagamachi S, Nishikawa K, Watanabe K: Comparison of survival of patients with lung cancer between elderly (greater than or equal to 70) and younger age groups. Jpn J Clin Oncol 16:319–323, 1986

620. Katz HR, Alberts RW: A comparison of high-dose continuous and split-course irradiation in non-oat-cell carcinoma of the lung. Am J Clin Oncol 6:445–457, 1983

621. Holsti LR, Mattson K: A randomized study of split-course radiotherapy of lung cancer: Long term results. Int J Radiat Oncol Biol Phys 6:977–981, 1980

622. Caldwell WL, Bagshaw MA: Indications for and results of irradiation of carcinoma of the lung. Cancer 22:999–1004, 1968

623. Abramson N, Cavanaugh PJ: Short course radiation therapy in carcinoma of the lung: A second look. Radiology 108:685–687, 1973

624. Salazar OM, Rubin P, Brown JC et al: The assessment of tumor response to irradiation of the lung cancer. Int J Radiat Oncol Biol Phys 1:1107–1118, 1976

625. Eisert DR, Cox JD, Komaki R: Irradiation for bronchial carcinoma: Reasons for failure: Analysis of local control as a function of dose, time, and fractionation. Cancer 37:2665–2670, 1976

626. Salazar OM, Houtte V, Rubin P: Once-a-week irradiation for locally advanced lung cancer. Int J Radiat Oncol Biol Phys 9:923–930, 1983

627. Moss WT, Haddy FFJ, Sweany SK: Some factors altering the severity of acute radiation pneumonitis: Variation with cortisone, heparin, and antibiotics. Radiology 75:50–54, 1960

628. Stanley K, Cox JD, Petrovich Z et al: Patterns of failure in patients with inoperable carcinoma of the lung. Cancer 47:2725–2729, 1981

629. Shields TW: Treatment failures after surgical resection of thoracic tumors. Cancer Treat Symp 2:69–76, 1983

630. Alsner J. Forastiere A, Aroney R: Patterns of recurrence for cancer of the lung and esophagus. Cancer Treat Symp 2:87–105, 1983

631. Faber LP: Role of radiation and/or chemotherapy combined with surgery in advanced lung cancer. Presented at the 20th Postgraduate Program, Society of Thoracic Surgeons, 1986

632. Bromley LL, Szur L: Combined radiotherapy and resection of carcinoma of the bronchus: Experiences with 66 patients. Lancet 2:937–941, 1955

633. Bloedorn FG, Cowley RA, Cuccia CA et al: Combined therapy: Irradiation and surgery in the treatment of bronchogenic carcinoma. Am J Roentgenol Rad Ther Nucl Med 85:175–181, 1961

634. Perelman MI, Grigr'eva SP, Ivanov AN: [Surgical treatment of lung cancer after preoperative beta irradiation.] (Russ) Vopr Onkol 28:48–52, 1982

635. Klimenko AA, Kharchenko VP, Karibov I et al: [Fractionated operative irradiation in the combination therapy of lung cancer.] (Russ) Med Radiol (Mosk) 27:36–39, 1982

636. Paulson DL: Extended resection of bronchogenic carcinoma in the superior pulmonary sulcus. Surg Rounds 3:10–21, 1980

637. Grigr'eva SP, Ots ON: [Combined treatment of peripheral lung carcinoma.] (Russ) Vestn Rentgenol Radiol 4:80–85, 1980

638. Sherman DM, Neptune W, Weichselbaum RR et al: An aggressive approach to marginally resectable lung cancer. Cancer 41:2040–2045, 1978

639. Kirschner PA: Lung cancer: Preoperative radiation therapy and surgery. NY State J Med 81:339–342, 1981

640. Shields TW: Preoperative radiation therapy in the treatment of bronchial carcinoma. Cancer 30:1388–1393, 1972

641. Collaborative Study: Preoperative irradiation of cancer of the lung: Final report of a therapeutic trial. Cancer 36:914–925, 1975

642. Eichorn AJ, Eule H, Lessel A et al: Results of a controlled clinical trial for evaluation of intensive preoperative irradiation therapy for lung cancer. Arch Geschwulstforsch 45:376–380, 1975

643. Tildon TT, Hughes RK: Complications from preoperative irradiation therapy for lung cancer. Ann Thorac Surg 3:307–326, 1967

644. Kazen I, Jongerius CM, Lacquet LK et al: Evaluation of short course preoperative radiation in the treatment of resectable bronchus carcinoma: Long term analysis of a randomized pilot study. J Radiat Oncol Biol Phys 10:981–985, 1984

645. Paulson DL, Shaw RR, Kee JL et al: Combined preoperative irradiation and resec-

tion for bronchogenic carcinoma. J Thorac Cardiovasc Surg 44:281–294, 1962

646. Paulson DL: Carcinoma in the superior pulmonary sulcus. Ann Thorac Surg 28:3–4, 1979

647. Miller JI, Mansour KA, Hatcher CR: Carcinoma of the superior pulmonary sulcus. Ann Thorac Surg 28:44–47, 1979

648. Wright CD, Moneure AC, Shepherd JO et al: Superior sulcus lung tumors. J Thorac Cardiovasc Surg 94:69–74, 1987

649. Attar S, Miller JE, Satterfield J et al: Pancoast's tumor: Irradiation or surgery? Ann Thorac Surg 28:578–586, 1979

650. Stanford W, Barner RP, Tucker AR: Influence of staging in superior sulcus (Pancoast) tumors of the lung. Ann Thorac Surg 29:406–409, 1980

651. Shahian DM, Neptune WB, Ellis, FH: Pancoast tumors: Improved survival with pre and postoperative radiotherapy. Ann Thorac Surg 43:32–38, 1987

652. Komaki R, Roh J, Cox JD et al: Superior sulcus tumors: Results of irradiation in 36 patients. Cancer 48:1563–1568, 1981

653. Van Houtte P, MacLennon I, Poulter C, Rubin P: External radiation in the management of superior sulcus tumor. Cancer 54:223–227, 1984

654. Hilaris BS, Martini N, Batata M et al: Interstitial irradiation for unresectable carcinoma of the lung. Ann Thorac Surg 20:491–500, 1975

655. Martini N, Hilaris BS, Beattie EJ Jr: Interstitial vs. external irradiation combined with pulmonary resection in lung cancer. Cancer 26:638–641, 1970

656. Hilaris BS, Martini N: Interstitial brachytherapy in cancer of the lung: A 20 year experience. Int J Radiat Oncol Biol Phys 5:1951–1956, 1979

657. Hilaris BS, Nori D, Beattie EJ Jr, Martini N: Value of perioperative brachytherapy in the management of non oat cell carcinoma of the lung. Int J Radiat Oncol Biol Phys 9:1161–1166, 1983

658. Hilaris BS, Luomanen RK, Mahan DG, Henschke UK: Interstitial irradiation of apical lung cancer. Radiology 99:655–660, 1971

659. Hilaris BS, Martini N: Multimodality therapy of superior sulcus tumors. In Bonica JJ et al (eds): The Management of Lung Cancer, pp 113–122. New York, Raven Press, 1982

660. Hilaris BS, Gomez J, Dattatreyudu N et al: Combined surgery, intraoperative brachytherapy, and postoperative external radiation in Stage III non-small cell cancer. Cancer 55:1226–1231, 1985

661. Hilaris BS, Martini N, Luomanen RK: Endobronchial interstitial implantation. Clin Bull 9:17–20, 1979

662. Law MR, Henk JM, Goldstraw P et al: Bronchoscopic implantation of radioactive gold grains into endobronchial carcinomas. Br J Dis Chest 79:147–151, 1985

663. Tepper J, Sindelar W: Summary of the Workshop on Intraoperative Radiation Therapy. Cancer Treat Rep 65:911–930, 1981

664. Abe M, Yabumoto E, Takahashi M et al: Intraoperative radiotherapy of gastric cancer. Cancer 34:2034–2045, 1974

665. Wood WC, Shipley WU, Gunderson LL et al: Intraoperative irradiation for unresectable pancreatic carcinoma. Cancer 49:1271–1276, 1982

666. Cohen AM, Gunderson LL, Wood WC: Intraoperative electron beam radiation therapy boost in the treatment of recurrent rectal carcinoma. Dis Colon Rectum 23:453–458, 1980

667. Sindelar WF, Kinsella TJ, Tepper J et al: Experimental and clinical studies with intraoperative radiotherapy. Surg Gynecol Obstet 156:25–36, 1983

668. Pass HI, Sindelar WF, Kinsella T et al: Delivery of intraoperative radiation therapy after pneumonectomy: Experimental observations and early clinical results. Ann Thorac Surg 44:14–20, 1987

669. Van Houtte PV, Roemans P, Smets P et al: Postoperative radiation therapy in lung cancer: A controlled trial after resection of curative design. Int J Radiat Oncol Biol Phys 6:983–986, 1980

670. Green N, Kurohara SS, George FW III, Crews QE Jr: Postresection irradiation for primary lung cancer. Radiology 116:405–407, 1975

671. Kirsh MM, Rotman H, Argenta L et al: Carcinoma of the lung: Results of treatment over ten years. Ann Thorac Surg 21:371–377, 1976

672. Choi NCH, Grillo HC, Gardiello M, Scannell JG, Wilkins EW Jr: Basis for new strategies in postoperative radiotherapy of bronchogenic carcinoma. Int J Radiat Oncol Biol Phys 6:31–35, 1980

673. Cox JD: Non small cell lung cancer: Role of radiation therapy. Chest 89:284S–288S, 1986

674. Holmes EC: Surgical adjuvant therapy of non-small-cell lung cancer. Chest 89:295(s)–298(s), 1986

675. Lung Cancer Study Group: Effects of postoperative mediastinal radiation on completely resected Stage II and Stage III epidermoid cancer of the lung. N Engl J Med 315:1377–1381, 1986

676. Slack HH: Bronchogenic carcinoma: Nitrogen mustard as a surgical adjuvant and factors influencing survival: University Surgical Adjuvant Lung Cancer Project. Cancer 25:987–1002, 1970

677. Higgins GA, Humphrey EW, Hughes RA et al: Cytoxan as an adjuvant to surgery for lung cancer. Surg Oncol 1:211–228, 1969

678. Higgins GA, Shields TW: Experience of the Veterans Administration Surgical Adjuvant Group. Prog Cancer Res Ther 11:433–442, 1979

679. Shields TW, Higgins GW Jr, Humphrey EW, Matthews MJ, Keehn RJ: Prolonged intermittent adjuvant chemotherapy with CCNU and hydroxyurea after resection of carcinoma of the lung. Cancer 51:1713–1721, 1982

680. Pirogov AI, Trakhtenberg AK: Results and prospects of combined surgery and antitumor chemotherapy for lung cancer. Cancer Treat Rep 60:1489–1491, 1976

681. Wingfield HV: Combined surgery and chemotherapy for carcinoma of the bronchus. Lancet 1:470–471, 1970

682. Katsuki H, Shimada K, Koyama A et al: Long term intermittent adjuvant chemotherapy for primary, resected lung cancer. J Thorac Cardiovasc Surg 70:590–599, 1975

683. Crosbie WA, Kamdar HH, Belcher JR: A controlled trial of vinblastine sulphate in the treatment of cancer of the lung. Br J Dis Chest 60:28–35, 1986

684. Dolton EG: Combined surgery and chemotherapy for carcinoma of the bronchus. Lancet 1:40–41, 1970

685. Buyze EAC, Nelemans FA: A study of postoperative cytostatic medication in patients with operable carcinoma of the lung. Arzneimittelforschung 23:860–862, 1973

686. Brunner KW, Marthaler T, Muller W: Adjuvant chemotherapy with cyclophosphamide (NSC 26271) for radically resected bronchogenic carcinoma: 9 year follow up. Prog Cancer Res Ther 11:411–420, 1979

687. Stott H, Stephens WF, Roy DC: Five year follow up of cytotoxic chemotherapy as an adjuvant to surgery in carcinoma of the bronchus. Br J Cancer 34:167–173, 1976

688. Mountain CF, Vincent RG, Sealy R et al: A clinical trial of CCNU as surgical adjuvant treatment for patients with surgical Stage I and Stage II non small cell lung cancer: Preliminary findings. Prog Cancer Res Ther 11:421–431, 1979

689. Eagan RT, Ingle JN, Frytak S et al: Platinum based poly chemotherapy versus dianhydrogalactitol in advanced non-small cell lung cancer. Cancer Treat Rep 61:1339–1345, 1977

690. Ruckdeschel JC, Finkelstein DM, Ettinger DS: Chemotherapy of metastatic non small cell lung cancer (NSCLC): The Eastern Cooperative Group experience. Proc Fourth World Conference on Lung Cancer, p 39, 1985

691. Ruckdeschel JC, Finkelstein DM, Mason BA, Creech RH: Chemotherapy for metastatic non small cell bronchogenic carcinoma: EST 2575, generation V: A randomized comparison of four cisplatin-containing regimens. J Clin Oncol 3:72–79, 1985

692. Fram R, Skarin A, Balikian J et al: Combination chemotherapy followed by radiation therapy in patients with regional Stage III unresectable non small cell lung cancer. Cancer Treat Rep 69:587–590, 1985

693. Wagner H, Ruckdeschel J, Bonomi P et al: Treatment of locally advanced non small cell lung cancer (NSCLC) with mitomycin C, vinblastine, and cisplatin (MVP) followed by radiation therapy: An ECOG pilot study (abstract). Proc Am Soc Clin Oncol 4:183, 1985

694. Finkelstein DM, Ettinger DS, Ruckdeschel JC: Long term survivors in metastatic non small cell lung cancer: An Eastern Cooperative Group study. J Clin Oncol 4:702–709, 1986

695. Holmes EC, Gail M, Lung Cancer Study Group: Surgical adjuvant therapy for Stage II and Stage III adenocarcinoma and large-cell undifferentiated carcinoma. J Clin Oncol 4:710–715, 1986

696. Brouet D: Results of a trial using radiotherapy and chemotherapy in bronchial cancer. Eur J Cancer 4:437–445, 1968

697. Host H: Cyclophosphamide (NSC 26271) as an adjuvant to radiotherapy in the treatment of unresectable bronchogenic carcinoma. Cancer Chemother Rep 4:161–164, 1973

698. Kaung DT, Wolf J, Hyde L et al: Preliminary report on the treatment of nonresectable cancer of the lung. Cancer Chemother Rep 58:359–364, 1974

699. Holsti LR: Alternative approaches to radiotherapy alone and radiotherapy as part of a combined therapeutic approach for lung cancer. Cancer Chemother Rep 4:165–169, 1973

700. Hall TC, Dederick MM, Chalmers TC et al: A clinical pharmacologic study of chemotherapy and X-ray therapy in lung cancer. Am J Med 43:186–193, 1967

701. Benninghoff DL, Alexander LL: Treatment of lung carcinoma: Radiation versus radiation combined with 5-fluorouracil. NY State J Med 68(Pt 1):532–534, 1967

702. Krant MJ, Chalmers TC, Dederick MM et al: Comparative trial of chemotherapy and radiotherapy in patients with nonresectable cancer of the lung. Am J Med 35:363–373, 1963

703. Durrant KR, Ellis F, Black JM et al: Comparison of treatment policies in inoperable bronchial carcinoma. Lancet 1:715–719, 1971

704. Coy P: A randomized study of irradiation and vinblastine in lung cancer. Cancer 26:803–809, 1970

705. Hansen HH, Muggia FM, Andres R et al: Intensive combined chemotherapy and radiotherapy in patients with non-resectable bronchogenic carcinoma. Cancer 30:315–324, 1972

706. Samuels ML, Barkley HT Jr, Holoye PY et al: Combination chemotherapy with bleomycin (NSC 125066), vincristine (NSC 67574), and methotrexate (NSC 740), plus split course radiotherapy in the treatment of non oat cell bronchogenic carcinoma. Cancer Chemother Rep 59:377–383, 1975

707. Bitran JD, Desser RK, DeMeester T et al: Combined modality therapy for Stage III M0 non oat cell bronchogenic carcinoma. Cancer Treat Rep 62:327–332, 1978

708. Schultz HP, Overgaard M, Sell A: X ray therapy and combination chemotherapy in non small cell carcinoma of the lung: A pilot study. Abstracts Second World Conf Lung Cancer, Copenhagen, p 137. Amsterdam, Excerpta Medica, 1980

709. Bitran J, Golomb H, DeMeester T et al: Combined modality therapy for Stage II M0 non small cell bronchogenic carcinoma (abstract). Proc Am Assoc Cancer Res Am Soc Clin Oncol 21:446, 1980

710. Weshler Z, Sulkes A, Fuks Z et al: Combined modality treatment with radiation and chemotherapy in locally advanced bronchogenic carcinoma. Abstracts Second World Conf Lung Cancer, Copenhagen. Amsterdam, Excerpta Medica, 1980

711. Wils JA: Sequential combination chemotherapy and radiotherapy in metastatic non small cell cancer. Abstracts Second World Conf Lung Cancer, Copenhagen. Amsterdam, Excerpta Medica, 1980

712. Cox JD, Samson MK, Herskovic AM et al: Cisplatin and etoposide before definitive radiation therapy for inoperable carcinoma of the lung: A Phase II study of the RTOG. Cancer Treat Rep 70:1219–1220, 1986

713. Cullen MH, Latief TN, Spooner D et al: Cisplatin, etoposide, and radiotherapy in regional inoperable squamous cell carcinoma of the bronchus. Semin Oncol 12:14–16, 1985

714. Van Houtte P, Klastersky J, Nguyen H et al: Comparative randomized study of chest radiotherapy preceded or not by chemotherapy with cisplatin, etoposide and vindesine for the treatment of non small cell lung cancer (NSCLC) (abstract). Proc Am Assoc Cancer Res 25:795, 1984

715. Wils JA, Utama I, Naus A et al: Phase II randomized trial of radiotherapy alone vs the sequential use of chemotherapy and radiotherapy in Stage III non small cell lung cancer: Phase II trial of chemotherapy alone in Stage IV non small cell lung cancer. Eur J Cancer Clin Oncol 20:911–914, 1984

716. Newman SB, DeMeester TR, Golomb HM et al: The treatment of modified Stage II (T1N1M0, T2N1M0) non small cell bronchogenic carcinoma. J Thorac Cardiovasc Surg 86:180–185, 1983

717. Lung Cancer Study Group, Lad T, Rubinstein L, Sadeghi A: The benefit of adjuvant treatment for resected locally advanced non-small-cell lung cancer. J Clin Oncol 6:9–17, 1988

718. Bonomi P: Brief overview of combination chemotherapy in non small cell lung cancer. Semin Oncol 13:89–90, 1986

719. Martini N, Kris MG, Gralla RJ et al: The effects of preoperative chemotherapy on the resectability of non small cell lung carcinoma with mediastinal lymph node metastases (N2M0)(abstract). Proc Soc Thorac Surg 23:28, 1987

720. Taylor SG, Trybula M, Bonomi PD et al: Simultaneous cisplatin, fluorouracil infusion and radiation followed by surgical resection in regionally localized Stage III, non-small cell lung carcinoma. Ann Thorac Surg 43:87–91, 1987

721. Bitran JD, Golomb HM, Hoffman PC et al: Protochemotherapy in non small cell lung carcinoma. Cancer 57:44–53, 1986

722. Raul Y, Hui N, Claver J et al: Surgery and chemotherapy: A new method of treatment for squamous cell bronchial carcinoma. J Thorac Cardiovasc Surg 88:754–757, 1984

723. Fuller BL, Bonomi P, Reddy SG et al: Cisplatin and mitomycin C preceding local therapy in squamous cell bronchogenic carcinoma (abstract). Proc Am Soc Clin Oncol 1C:560, 1982

724. Israel L, Aquillera J, Breau JL: Potency of continuous infusion over 5 or 6 days of cis platinum and bleomycin on squamous cell carcinoma of the lung. Exerpta Medica Int Congr Ser 558:323, 1982

725. Skarin A, Veeder M, Malcolm A: Chemotherapy (CAP) prior to radiotherapy and surgery in marginally resectable non small cell lung cancer (NSCLC)(abstract). Proc Am Soc Clin Oncol 1C:544, 1982

726. Takita H, Edgerton F, Conway D et al: Reductive surgery of inoperable lung carcinoma (abstract). Proc Am Assoc Cancer Res 21:459, 1980

727. Hellekant C: Bronchial arteriography and intraarterial chemotherapy in bronchogenic carcinoma. Radiologe 19:521–524, 1979

728. Neyazaki T, Suzuki C: Bronchial artery infusion therapy for lung cancer in man. Panminerva Med 13:305–310, 1971

729. Strauss G, Sherman D, Schwartz J et al: Combined modality therapy for regionally advanced Stage III non small cell carcinoma of the lung (NSCLC) employing neoadjuvant chemotherapy (CT), radiotherapy (RT) and surgery (S) (abstract). Proc Fifth Int Conf Adjuvant Ther Cancer, March 1987, p 81

730. Sridhar SK, Thurer RJ, Raskin N, Beattie EJ: Multimodality treatment of non small cell lung cancer: Response to cisplatin, etoposide and 5 FU chemotherapy, surgery and radiation therapy (abstract). Proc Fifth Int Conf Adjuvant Ther Cancer, March 1987, p 81

731. Gralla RJ, Kris MG, Burke MT, Martini N: Adjuvant chemotherapy in non small cell lung cancer (abstract). Fifth Int Conf Adjuvant Ther Cancer, March 1987, p 36

732. Spain R, Jost J, Kircher T: Neoadjuvant mitomycin (M), cisplatin (P), and vinblastine (V) infusion (MPV) for Stage III limited, initially unresectable non small cell lung cancer (NSCLC): An analysis at 37+ month median follow up (abstract). Proc Fifth Int Conf Adjuvant Ther Cancer, March 1987, p 38

733. Klasterksy J, Sculier JP, Ravez P et al: A randomized study comparing a high and a standard dose of cisplatin in combination with etoposide in the treatment of advanced non-small-cell lung carcinoma. J Clin Oncol 4:1780–1786, 1986

734. Klastersky J: Therapy with cisplatin and etoposide for non-small cell lung cancer. Semin Oncol 13:104–114, 1986

735. Dhingra HM, Valdivieso M, Booser DJ et al: Chemotherapy for advanced adenocarcinoma and squamous cell carcinoma of the lung with etoposide and cisplatin. Cancer Treat Rep 68:671–673, 1984

736. Goldhirsch A, Joss RA, Cavalli F et al: Cis-chlorodiaminepaltinum(II) and VP16 213 combination chemotherapy for non small cell lung cancer. Med Pediatr Oncol 9:205–208, 1981

737. Joss RA, Alberto P, Olbrecht JP et al: Combination chemotherapy for non small cell lung cancer with doxorubicin and mitomycin or cisplatin and etoposide. Cancer Treat Rep 68:1079–1084, 1984

738. Giaccone G, Musella R, Bertetto O et al: DDP VP16 combination chemotherapy in unresectable non small cell lung cancer (abstract). Proc Thirteenth Int Congr Chemother, Vienna, 1983

739. Scagliotti G, Lodico D, Gozzelino F: Clinical trial with high dose cisplatin and VP 16 213 in advanced non small cell lung cancer: Results after two years (abstract). Proc Thirteenth Int Congr Chemother, Vienna, 1983

740. Veronesi A, Zagonel V, Sanatarossa M et al: Cisplatinum and etoposide combination chemotherapy of advanced non oat cell bronchogenic carcinoma. Cancer Chemother Pharmacol 11:35–37, 1983

741. Rinaldi M, Venturo J, Tonachella R et al: Chemotherapy with DDP and VP16 213 in non small cell lung cancer: Results and toxicity (abstract). Proc Thirteenth Int Congr Chemother, Vienna, 1983

742. Mitrou PS, Graubner M, Berdel WE et al: Cisplatinum (DDP) and VP16 213 (etoposide) combination chemotherapy for advanced non small cell lung cancer: A Phase II clinical trial. Eur J Clin Oncol 20:347–351, 1984

743. Holsti LR, Mattson K, Grohn P et al: Cis platinum plus vindesine versus VP16 in combination with radiotherapy in the treatment of non small cell carcinoma of the lung (abstract). Proc World Conf Lung Cancer, Tokyo, 1982

744. Paccagnella A, Fiorentino MV, Brandes A et al: Cis platin (DDP) plus vindesine (VDS) versus DDP plus VP16 213 (VP) versus doxorubicin (DXR) plus Cytoxan (CTX): A randomized study in advanced non small cell carcinoma of the lung (NSCLC)(abstract). Proc Thirteenth Int Congr Chemother, Vienna, 1983

745. Martini N, Flehinger BJ, Nagasaki F, Hart B: Prognostic significance of N1 disease in carcinoma of the lung. J Thorac Cardiovasc Surg 86:646–653, 1983

746. Shields TW, Higgins GA Jr, Matthews MJ, Kühn RJ: Surgical resection in the management of small cell carcinoma of the lung. J Thorac Cardiovasc Surg 84:481–488, 1982

747. Komaki R, Cox JD, Stark R: Frequency of brain metastases in adenocarcinoma and large cell carcinoma of the lung: Correlation with survival. Int J Radiat Oncol Biol Phys 9:1467–1470, 1983

748. Cox JD, Stanley K, Petrovich Z et al: Cranial irradiation in cancer of the lung of all cell types. JAMA 245:469–472, 1981

749. Jacobs RH, Awan A, Bitran JD et al: Prophylactic cranial irradiation in adenocarcinoma of the lung: A possible role. Cancer 59:2016–2019, 1987

750. Johnson BE, Ihde DC, Lichter AS et al: Five to 10 year follow-up of small cell lung cancer (SCLC) patients disease free at 30 months: Chronic toxicities and late relapses (abstract). Proc Am Soc Clin Oncol 3:218, 1984

751. Looper JD, Einhorn LH, Garcia SA, Hornbach NB, Vincent B, Williams SD: Severe neurologic problems following successful therapy for small cell lung cancer (abstract). Proc Am Soc Clin Oncol 2:231, 1984

752. DeCaro L, Benfield JR: Lung cancer in young persons. J Thorac Cardiovasc Surg 83:372–376, 1982

753. Hartman GE, Shochart SJ: Primary pulmonary neoplasms of childhood: A review. Ann Thorac Surg 36:108–119, 1983

754. Hyde L, Wolf J, McCracken S et al: Natural course of inoperable lung cancer. Chest 64:309–312, 1973

755. Brashea RE: Should asymptomatic patients with inoperable bronchogenic carcinoma receive immediate radiotherapy? Am Rev Respir Dis 117:411–414, 1978

756. Phillips TL, Miller RJ: Should asymptomatic patients with inoperable bronchogenic carcinoma receive immediate radiotherapy? Yes. Am Rev Respir Dis 117:405–410, 1978

757. Carroll M, Morgan SA, Yarnold JR, Hill JM, Wright NM: Prospective evaluation of a watch policy in patients with inoperable non-small cell lung cancer. Eur J Cancer Clin Oncol 22:1353–1356, 1986

758. Slawson RG, Scott RM: Radiation therapy in bronchogenic carcinoma. Radiology 132:175–176, 1979

759. Perez CA, Presant CA, Van Ambury AL: Management of superior vena cava syndrome. Semin Oncol 5:123–134, 1978

760. Armstrong BA, Perez CA, Simpson JR, Hederman MA: Role of irradiation in the malignancy of superior vena cava syndrome. Int J Radiat Oncol Biol Phys 13:531–539, 1987

761. Katz RJ, Simms EB, DiBianco R et al: Pericardial tamponade in lung cancer: Diagnosis, management and response to treatment. (unpublished)

762. Majid OA, Lee S, Khushalani S, Seydel HG: The response of atelectasis from lung cancer to radiation therapy. Int J Radiat Oncol Biol Phys 12:231–232, 1986

763. Borgelt B, Gelber R, Kramer S et al: The palliation of brain metastases: Final results of the first two studies by the Radiation Therapy Oncology Group. Int J Radiat Oncol Biol Phys 6:1–9, 1980

764. Deviri E, Schachner A, Halevy A, Shalit M, Levy MJ: Carcinoma of lung with a solitary cerebral metastasis: Surgical management and review of the literature. Cancer 52:1507–1509, 1983

765. Sundaresan N, Galicich JH, Beattie EJ Jr: Surgical treatment of brain metastases from lung cancer. J Neurosurg 58:666–671, 1983

766. Hendrickson FR, Lee MS, Larson M, Gelber RD: The influence of surgery and radiation therapy on patients with brain metastases. Int J Radiat Oncol Biol Phys 9:623–627, 1983

767. Patchell RA, Cirrincione C, Thaler HT, Galicich JH, Kim JH, Posner JB: Single brain metastases: Surgery plus radiation or radiation alone. Neurology 36:447–453, 1986

768. Bruckman JE, Bloomer WD: Management of spinal cord compression. Semin Oncol 5:135–140, 1978

769. Raichle ME, Posner JB: The treatment of extradural spinal cord compression. Neurology 20:391–396, 1970

770. Gilbert RW, Kim JH, Posner JB: Epidural spinal cord compression from metastatic tumor: Diagnosis and treatment. Ann Neurol 3:40–51, 1978

771. Thomas JE, Colby MY Jr: Radiation-induced or metastatic brachial plexopathy? A diagnostic dilemma. JAMA 222:1392–1395, 1972

772. Mulshine J, Ruckdeschel JC: The role of chemotherapy in the management of disseminated non-small-cell lung cancer. Roth JA, Ruckdeschel JC, Weisenburger TH (eds): Thoracic Oncology, 220–228. Philadelphia: WB Saunders, 1989

773. Hansen HH: Advanced non-small-cell lung cancer: To treat or not to treat? J Clin Oncol 5:1711–1712, 1987

774. Gralla RJ: Issues and agents in the chemotherapy of non-small-cell lung cancer.

Mediguide Oncol 5:1–5, 1985

775. O'Connell JP, Kris MG, Gralla RJ et al: Frequency and prognostic importance of pretreatment clinical characteristics in patients with advanced non-small-cell lung cancer treated with combination chemotherapy. J Clin Oncol 4:1604–1614, 1986

776. Kris M, Cohen E, Gralla R: An analysis of 134 Phase II trials in non-small cell lung cancer (NSCLC)(abstract). Proc Fourth World Conf Lung Cancer, Toronto, 1985

777. Joss RA, Cavalli F, Goldhirsch A et al: New agents in non-small cell lung cancer. Cancer Treat Rev 11:205–237, 1984

778. Babowski MT, Creech JC: Chemotherapy of non-small cell lung cancer: A reappraisal and look at the future. Cancer Treat Rev 10:159–172, 1983

779. Sakurai M, Saijo N, Shinkai T et al: The protective effect of 2-mercapto-ethane sulfonate (mesna) on hemorrhagic cystitis induced by high-dose ifosfamide treatment tested by a randomized crossover trial. Jpn J Clin Oncol 16:153–156, 1986

780. Bonomi P, Mehta C, Ruckdeschel J, Blum R, Mason B, Greene M: Phase II–III trial of mitomycin–vinblastine–cisplatin (MVP): vinblastine–cisplatin (VP); MVP alternating with cyclophosphamide–Adriamycin–methotrexate–procarbazine (MVP/CAMP); CBDCA followed by MVP; and CHIP followed by MVP in patients with metastatic non-small cell lung cancer (NSCLC): An ECOG study (abstract). Proc Am Soc Clin Oncol 6:A699, 1987

781. Shum KY, Kris MG, Gralla RJ et al: 10-ethyl-10 deaza-aminopterin (10-EDAM) in patients with non-small cell lung cancer (NSCLC): Trial of an active new agent (abstract). Proc Am Soc Clin Oncol 6:A698, 1987

782. Maroun J, Wiernik P, DeConti R et al: Phase 2 efficacy of trimetrexate (CI-898; TMTX) in patients (pts) with non-small cell lung cancer (NSCLC) (abstract). Proc Am Soc Clin Oncol 6:A669, 1987

783. Egan RT, Frytak S, Creagan ET, Richardson RL, Coles DT, Jett JR: Differing response rates and survival between squamous and non-squamous non-small cell lung cancer: Comparison of CAP versus MAP. Am J Clin Oncol 9:249–254, 1986

784. Bitran JD, Desser RK, DeMeester TR et al: Cyclophosphamide, Adriamycin, methotrexate, and procarbazine (CAMP): Effective four drug combination chemotherapy for metastatic non oat cell bronchogenic carcinoma. Cancer Treat Rep 60:1225–1230, 1976

785. Chahinian AP, Arnold DJ, Cohen JM et al: Chemotherapy for bronchogenic carcinoma: Methotrexate, doxorubicin, cyclophosphamide, and lomustine. JAMA 237:2392–2396, 1977

786. Vogl SE, Hemta CR, Cohen MH: MACC chemotherapy for adenocarcinoma and epidermoid carcinoma of the lung. Cancer 44:864–868, 1979

787. Eagan RT, Ingle JN, Frytak S et al: Platinum based poly chemotherapy versus dianhydrogalactictol in advanced non-small cell lung cancer. Cancer Treat Rep 61:1339–1345, 1977

788. Gralla RJ, Casper ES, Kelson DP et al: Cisplatin and vindesine combination chemotherapy for advanced carcinoma of the lung: A randomized trial investigating two dosage schedules. Ann Intern Med 95:414–420, 1981

789. Longeval E, Klastersky J: Combination chemotherapy with cisplatin and etoposide in bronchogenic squamous cell carcinoma and adenocarcinoma: A study for the EORTC Lung Cancer Working Party (Belgium). Cancer 50:2751–2756, 1982

790. Mason BA, Catalano RB: Mitomycin, vinblastine, and cisplatin combination chemotherapy in non small cell lung cancer (abstract). Proc Am Soc Clin Oncol 21:477, 1980

791. Elliot JA, Ahmedozcie S, Hole D et al: Vindesine and cisplatin combination chemotherapy compared with vindesine as a single agent in the management of non-small cell lung cancer: A randomized study. Eur J Cancer Clin Oncol 20:1025–1032, 1984

792. Crino L, Tonato M, Darwish S et al: A randomized trial of three cisplatin (CDDP)-containing chemotherapy regimens in advanced non-small cell lung cancer (NSCLC): A study of the Umbrian Lung Cancer Group (abstract). Proc Am Soc Clin Oncol 6:A716, 1987

793. Rosso R, Salvati F, Ardizzoni A et al: Etoposide (E) vs E plus cisplatin (P) in the treatment of advanced non small cell lung cancer (NSCLC): A FONICAP randomized trial (abstract). Proc Am Soc Clin Oncol 6:A732, 1987

794. Luedke DW, Sarma PR, Greco FA, Birch R, Prestridge K: Preliminary report of a randomized trial of vindesin (V) as V with mitomycin (M) or with cisplatin (C) in non-small cell lung cancer (NSCLC)(abstract). Proc Am Soc Clin Oncol 6:A670, 1987

795. Einhorn LH, Loehrer PJ, Williams SD et al: Random prospective study of vindesine versus vindesine plus high-dose cisplatin versus vindesine plus cisplatin plus mitomycin C in advanced non-small-cell lung cancer. J Clin Oncol 4:1037–1043, 1986

796. Woods RL, Levi JA, Page J et al: Non small cell cancer: A randomized comparison of chemotherapy with no chemotherapy (abstract). Proc Am Soc Clin Oncol 4:177, 1985

797. Rapp E, Pater J, Willan A et al: A comparison of best supportive care to two regimens of combination chemotherapy in the management of advanced non-small cell lung cancer (NSCLC): A report of a Canadian multicentre trial (abstract). Proc Am Soc Clin Oncol 6:168, 1987

798. Ganz PA, Giflin RA, Haskell CM et al: Supportive care (SC) vs supportive care plus chemotherapy (SCC) in advanced metastatic lung cancer: Response, survival, and quality of life (abstract). Proc Am Soc Clin Oncol 6:171, 1987

799. Gralla RJ, Casper ES, Kelsen DP et al: Cisplatin and vindesine combination chemotherapy for advanced carcinoma of the lung: A randomized trial investigating two dosage schedules. Ann Intern Med 95:414–420, 1981

800. Mitrou PS, Fischer M, Weissenfels I et al: Treatment of inoperable non-small-cell bronchogenic carcinoma with etoposide and cis-platinum. Cancer Treat Rep 9(Suppl A):139–142, 1982

801. Focan C, Le Hung S, Frere MH, Schallier D: Ambulatory combination chemotherapy with oral etoposide and cisplatin for advanced non small cell lung carcinoma patients: A Phase II study. Anticancer Res 6:977–981, 1986

802. Gandara DR, DeGregorio MW, Wold H et al: High-dose cisplatin in hypertonic saline: Reduced toxicity of a modified dose schedule and correlation with plasma pharmacokinetics: A Northern California Oncology Group pilot study in non-small-cell lung cancer. J Clin Oncol 4:1787–1793, 1986

803. Klastersky J, Sculier JP, Ravez P et al: A randomized study comparing a high and a standard dose of cisplatin in combination with etoposide in the treatment of advanced non-small-cell lung carcinoma. J Clin Oncol 4:1780–1786, 1986

804. Stampleman LV, Kris MG, Gralla RJ et al: Complete response (CR) in Stage III and IV non-small cell lung cancer (NSCLC) with chemotherapy (chemo) or chemotherapy plus surgery: An analysis of treatment in 554 patients (abstract). Proc Am Soc Clin Oncol 6:A696, 1987

805. Ruckdeschel JC, Finkelstein DM, Ettinger DS et al: A randomized trial of the four most active regimens for metastatic non-small cell lung cancer. J Clin Oncol 4:14–22, 1986

806. Fuks JZ, Patel H, Hornedo J, Van Echo DA, Moody M, Aisner J: Infections in patients with non-small-cell lung cancer treated with intensive induction chemotherapy. Med Pediatr Oncol 14:255–261, 1986

807. Bakker W, van Oosterom AT, Aaronson NK et al: Vindesine, cisplatin, and bleomycin combination chemotherapy in non-small cell lung cancer: Survival and quality of life. Eur J Cancer Clin Oncol 22:963–970, 1986

808. Chang AY, Kuebler JP, Pandya KJ et al: Pulmonary toxicity induced by mitomycin C is highly responsive to glucocorticoids. Cancer 57:2285–2290, 1986

809. Mackillop WJ, Ward GK, O'Sullivan B: The use of expert surrogates to evaluate clinical trials in non-small cell lung cancer. Br J Cancer 54:661–667, 1986

810. Mackillop WJ, O'Sullivan B, Ward GK: Non-small cell lung cancer: How oncologists want to be treated. Int J Radiat Oncol Biol Phys 13:929–934, 1987

811. Breau JL, Morere JF, Israel L: Response rates and survival for 268 unresectable epidermoid lung carcinoma patients treated with a cisplatin bleomycin based chemotherapy (abstract). Proc Am Soc Clin Oncol 6:A703, 1987

812. Taylor SG, Trybula M, Bonomi PD et al: Simultaneous cisplatin fluorouracil infusion and radiation followed by surgical resection in regionally localized Stage III non-small cell lung cancer. Ann Thorac Surg 43:87–91, 1987

813. Minet P, Bartsch P, Chevalier P et al: Quality of life of inoperable non-small cell lung carcinoma: A randomized Phase II clinical study comparing radiotherapy alone and combined radiochemotherapy. Radiother Oncol 8:217–230, 1987

814. Omenn GS, Goodman G, Rosenstock L et al: Cancer chemoprevention with vitamin A and beta-carotene in populations at high risk for lung cancer. In Nygaard OF, Simic M, Cerutti P (eds): Anticarcinogenesis and Radiation Protection. New York, Plenum Publishing, 1988

815. Pastorino U, deVries N, van Zandwijk N (coordinators): EUROSCAN (EORTC 24871, EORTC 08871) study on screening and chemoprevention with vitamin A and or N-acetylcysteine. EORTC Data Center, 125 Boulevard de Waterloo, 1000 Brussels, Belgium. Published October 1987

816. Grunberg SM, Itri L: Treatment of advanced non-small cell lung cancer with 13-cis-retinoic acid (abstract). Proc Fifth Int Conf Adjuvant Ther Cancer, March 1987, p 79

817. Uphouse W, Oishi N, Bernenberg J et al: Treatment of advanced non-small cell lung cancer with 13-cis retinoic acid (abstract). Proc Am Soc Clin Oncol 6:A712, 1987

818. Simpson JR, Bauer M, Wasserman TH et al: Large fraction irradiation with or without misonidazole in advanced non-oat cell carcinoma of the lung: A Phase II randomized trial of the RTOG (Radiation Therapy Oncology Group). Int J Radiat Oncol Biol Phys 13:861–867, 1987

819. Carlson RW, Coleman CN, Kohler M, Gribble MJ, Halsey J: A randomized Phase II study of L-PAM versus L-PAM + the chemosensitizer misonidazole (MISO) for non-small cell lung cancer (NSCLC): A Northern California Oncology Group study (abstract). Proc Am Soc Clin Oncol 6:A106, 1987

820. Chlebowski RT, Bulcavage L, Grosvenor M et al: Influence of hydrazine sulfate on survival in non-small cell lung cancer: A randomized, placebo-controlled trial (abstract). Proc Am Soc Clin Oncol 6:688, 1987

821. Tayek JA, Heber D, Chlebowski RT: Effect of hydrazine sulphate on whole-body protein breakdown measured by ^{14}C-lysine metabolism in lung cancer patients. Lancet 2:241–244, 1987

822. Evans WK, Nixon DW, Daly JM et al: A randomized study of oral nutritional support versus ad lib nutritional intake during chemotherapy for advanced colorectal and non-small-cell lung cancer. J Clin Oncol 5:113–124, 1987

823. Zacharski LR, Moritz TE, Baczek LA et al: Effect of RA-233 (Mopidamol) on survival in carcinoma of the lung and colon: Final report of Veterans Administration Cooperative Study No. 188. JNCI 80:90–96, 1988

824. Livingston RB: Mopidamol in non-small cell lung cancer: Antioncogene or accident? JNCI 80:77–78, 1988

825. Ludwig Lung Cancer Study Group: Intrapleural and intravenous Corynebacterium parvum in patients with resected Stage I and II non-small cell carcinoma of the lung. Cancer Immunol Immunother 23:1–4, 1986

826. Ludwig Lung Cancer Study Group: Immunostimulation with intrapleural BCG as adjuvant therapy in resected non-small cell lung cancer. Cancer 58:2411–2416, 1986

827. Bakker W, Nijhuis–Heddes JM, van der Velde EA: Post-operative intrapleural BCG in lung cancer: A 5-year follow-up report. Cancer Immunol Immunother 22:155–159, 1986

828. Watanabe Y, Iwa T: Clinical value of immunotherapy with the streptococcal prepara-

tion of OK-432 in non-small cell lung cancer. J Biol Response Modif 6:169–180, 1987

829. Weissler JC, Nicod LP, Toews GB: Pulmonary natural killer cell activity is reduced in patients with bronchogenic carcinoma. Am Rev Respir Dis 135:1353–1357, 1987

830. Kradin RL, Boyle LA, Preffer FI et al: Tumor-derived interleukin-2-dependent lymphocytes in adoptive immunotherapy of lung cancer. Cancer Immunol Immunother 24:76–85, 1987

831. Yasumoto K, Mivazaki K, Nagashima A et al: Induction of lymphokine-activated killer cells by intrapleural instillations of recombinant interleukin-2 in patients with malignant pleurisy due to lung cancer. Cancer Res 47:2184–2187, 1987

832. Gelb AF, Epstein JD: Neodymium-yttrium–aluminum–garnet laser in lung cancer. Ann Thorac Surg 43:164–167, 1987

833. Brutinel WM, Cortese DA, McDougall JC, Gillio RG, Bergstrahl EJ: A two-year experience with the neodymium–YAG laser in endobronchial obstruction. Chest 8:159–165, 1987

834. Edell ES, Cortese DA: Bronchoscopic phototherapy with hematoporphyrin derivative for treatment of localized bronchogenic carcinoma: A 5-year experience. Mayo Clin Proc 62:8–14, 1987

835. Watson PN, Evans RJ: Intractable pain with lung cancer. Pain 29:163–173, 1987

836. Morstyn G, Ihde DC, Lichter AS et al: Small cell lung cancer 1973–1983: Early prognosis and recent obstacles. Int J Radiat Oncol Biol Phys 10:515–539, 1984

837. Matthews MJ, Kanhouwa S, Pickner J et al: Frequency of residual and metastatic tumors in patients undergoing curative surgical resection of lung cancer. Cancer Chemother Rep 3:63–67, 1973

838. Hansen HH, Dombernowsky P, Hirsch FR: Staging procedures and prognostic features in small cell anaplastic bronchogenic carcinoma. Semin Oncol 5:280–287, 1978

839. Østerlind K, Ihde DC, Ettinger DS et al: Staging and prognostic factors in small cell carcinoma of the lung. Cancer Treat Rep 67:3–9, 1983

840. Matthews MJ: Problems in morphology and behavior of bronchopulmonary malignant diseases. In Israel L, Chahinian AP (eds): Lung Cancer: Natural History, Prognosis, and Therapy, pp 23–62. New York, Academic Press, 1976

841. Fox W, Scadding JG: Medical Research Council comparative trial of surgery and radiotherapy for primary treatment of small-celled or oat-celled carcinoma of bronchus: Ten-year follow-up. Lancet 2:63–65, 1973

842. Mountain CF: Clinical biology of small cell carcinoma: Relationship to surgical therapy. Semin Oncol 5:272–279, 1978

843. Green RA, Humphrey E, Close H et al: Alkylating agents in bronchogenic carcinoma. Am J Med 46:516–525, 1969

844. Greco FA, Einhorn LH: Small cell lung cancer. Semin Oncol 5:233–235, 1978

845. Johnson DH, Greco FA: Small cell carcinoma of the lung. CRC Crit Rev Oncol/Hematol 4:303–336, 1986

846. Seifter EJ, Ihde DC: Therapy of small cell lung cancer: A perspective on two decades of clinical research. Semin Oncol 15:278–299, 1988

847. Aisner J, Alberto P, Bitran J et al: Role of chemotherapy in small cell lung cancer: A consensus report of the International Association for the Study of Lung Cancer workshop. Cancer Treat Rep 67:37–43, 1983

848. Livingston RB: Small cell carcinoma of the lung. Blood 56:575–584, 1980

849. Comis RL: Small cell carcinoma of the lung. Cancer Treat Rev 9:237–258, 1982

850. Bunn PA Jr, Ihde DC: Small cell bronchogenic carcinoma: A review of therapeutic results. Cancer Treat Res 1:169–208, 1981

851. Ihde DC, Bunn PA Jr: Chemotherapy of small cell bronchogenic carcinoma. In Whitehouse JMA, Williams CJ (eds): Recent Advances in Clinical Oncology, vol 1, pp 305–323. Edinburgh, Churchill Livingstone 1982

852. Dombernowsky P, Hansen HH, Sorenson PG et al: Vincristine in the treatment of small cell anaplastic carcinoma of the lung. Cancer Treat Rep 60:239–242, 1976

852. Cavalli F, Sonntag R, Jungl F et al: VP-16-213 monotherapy for remission induction of small cell lung cancer: A randomized trial using three dosage schedules. Cancer Treat Rep 62:473–475, 1978

854. Mead GM, Thompson J, Sweetenham JW et al: Extensive stage small cell carcinoma of the bronchus: A randomized study of etoposide given orally by one-day or five-day schedule together with intravenous Adriamycin and cyclophosphamide. Cancer Chemother Pharmacol 19:172–174, 1987

855. Issell BF, Einhorn LH, Comis RL et al: Multicenter Phase II trial of etoposide in previously treated small cell carcinoma of the lung. Cancer Treat Rep 69:127–128, 1985

856. Bork E, Hansen M, Dombernowsky P et al: Teniposide (VM-26), an overlooked highly active agent in small cell lung cancer: Results of a Phase II trial in untreated patients. J Clin Oncol 4:524–527, 1986

857. Wolff SN, Birch R, Sarma P et al: Randomized dose–response evaluation of etoposide in small cell carcinoma of the lung. Cancer Treat Rep 70:583–587, 1986

858. Joss RA, Cavalli F, Goldhirsch A et al: New drugs in small cell lung cancer. Cancer Treat Rev 13:157–176, 1986

859. Smith IE, Harland SJ, Robinson BA et al: Carboplatin: A very active new cisplatin analog in the treatment of small cell lung cancer. Cancer Treat Rep 69:43–46, 1985

860. Aisner J: Identification of new drugs in small cell lung cancer: Phase II agents first? Cancer Treat Rep 71:1131–1133, 1987

861. Cullen M, Smith SR, Benfield GFA et al: Testing new drugs in untreated small cell lung cancer may prejudice the results of standard treatment: A Phase II study of oral idarubicin in extensive disease. Cancer Treat Rep 71:1227–1230, 1087

862. Malik STA, Rayner H, Fletcher J et al: Phase II trial of mitoxantrone as first-line chemotherapy for extensive small cell lung cancer. Cancer Treat Rep 71:1291–1292, 1987

863. Broder LE, Cohen MH, Selawry OS: Treatment of bronchogenic carcinoma II: Small cell cancer. Cancer Treat Rev 4:219–260, 1977

864. Edmonson JH, Lagako SW, Selawry OS et al: Cyclophosphamide and CCNU in the treatment of inoperable small cell carcinoma and adenocarcinoma of the lung. Cancer Treat Rep 60:925–932, 1976

865. Alberto P, Brunner KW, Martz G et al: Treatment of bronchogenic carcinoma with simultaneous or sequential combination chemotherapy, including methotrexate, cyclophosphamide, procarbazine, and vincristine. Cancer 38:2208–2216, 1976

866. Cohen MH, Creaven PJ, Fossieck BE et al: Intensive chemotherapy of small cell bronchogenic carcinoma. Cancer Treat Rep 61:349–354, 1977

867. Hansen HH, Selawry OS, Simon R et al: Combination chemotherapy of advanced lung cancer: A randomized trial. Cancer 38:2201–2207, 1976

868. Souhami RL, Finn G, Gregory WM et al: High-dose cyclophosphamide in small cell carcinoma of the lung. J Clin Oncol 3:958–963, 1985

869. Comis RL, Lawson R, Maroun J et al: Cytoxan, etoposide, vincristine versus Cytoxan, Adriamycin, vincristine versus Cytoxan, vincristine in the treatment of small cell lung cancer (abstract). Proc Am Soc Clin Oncol 6:168, 1987

870. Jackson DV, Case DL: Small cell lung cancer: A ten-year perspective. Semin Oncol 13(Suppl 3):63–74, 1986

871. Messieh AA, Schweitzer JM, Lipton A et al: Addition of etoposide to cyclophosphamide, doxorubicin, and vincristine for remission induction and survival in patients with small cell lung cancer. Cancer Treat Rep 71:61–66, 1987

872. Lowenbraun S, Birch R, Buchanan R et al: Combination chemotherapy in small cell lung cancer: A randomized study of two intensive regimens. Cancer 54:2344–2350, 1984

873. Einhorn L, Greco F, Wampler G et al: Cytoxan, Adriamycin, etoposide versus Cytoxan, Adriamycin, vincristine in the treatment of small cell lung cancer (abstract). Proc Am Soc Clin Oncol 6:168, 1987

874. Hirsch FR, Hansen HH, Hansen M et al: The superiority of combination chemotherapy including etoposide based on in vivo cell cycle analysis in the treatment of extensive small cell lung cancer: A randomized trial of 288 consecutive patients. J Clin Oncol 5:585–591, 1987

875. Schabel FM, Trader MW, Laster WK et al: Cisdichlorodiamineplatinum(II): Combination chemotherapy and cross-resistance studies with tumors of mice. Cancer Treat Rep 63:1459–1473, 1979

876. Hainsworth JD, Williams SD, Einhorn LH et al: Successful treatment of resistant germinal neoplasms with VP-16 and cisplatin. J Clin Oncol 3:666–671, 1985

877. Evans WK, Osoba D, Feld R et al: Etoposide (VP-16) and cisplatin: An effective treatment for relapse of small cell lung cancer. J Clin Oncol 3:65–71, 1985

878. Porter LL, Johnson DH, Hainsworth JD et al: Cisplatin and etoposide combination chemotherapy for refractory small cell carcinoma of the lung. Cancer Treat Rep 69:479–481, 1985

879. Sierocki JS, Hilaris BS, Hopfan S et al: cis-Dichlorodiamineplatinum(II) and VP-16-213: An active induction regimen for small cell carcinoma of the lung. Cancer Treat Rep 63:1593–1597, 1979

880. Woods RL, Levi JL: Chemotherapy for small cell lung cancer: A randomized study of maintenance chemotherapy with cyclophosphamide, Adriamycin, and vincristine after remission induction with cis-platinum, VP-16-213 and radiotherapy (abstract). Proc Am Soc Clin Oncol 3:214, 1984

881. Evans WK, Shepherd FA, Feld R et al: VP-16 and cisplatin as first-line therapy for small cell lung cancer. J Clin Oncol 3:1471–1477, 1985

882. Ihde DC, Johnson BE, Mulshine JL et al: Randomized trial of high dose versus standard dose etoposide and cisplatin in extensive stage small cell lung cancer (abstract). Proc Am Soc Clin Oncol 6:181, 1987

883. Einhorn LH, Crawford J, Birch R et al: Cisplatin plus etoposide consolidation following cyclophosphamide, doxorubicin, and vincristine in limited small cell lung cancer. J Clin Oncol 6:451–456, 1988

884. Bishop JF, Raghavan D, Stuart–Harris R et al: Carboplatin (CBDCA, JM-8) and VP-16-213 in previously untreated patients with small cell lung cancer. J Clin Oncol 5:1574–1578, 1987

885. Wolf M, Havemann K, Holle R et al: Cisplatin/etoposide versus isosfamide/etoposide combination chemotherapy in small cell lung cancer: A multicenter German randomized trial. J Clin Oncol 5:1880–1889, 1987

886. Frei E, Canellos GP: Dose: A critical factor in cancer chemotherapy. Am J Med 69:585–591, 1980

887. Mehta C, Vogl SE: High-dose cyclophosphamide in the induction chemotherapy of small cell lung cancer: Minor improvements in rate of remission and survival (abstract). Proc Am Assoc Cancer Res 23:155, 1982

888. Ettinger DS, Karp JE, Abeloff MD et al: Intermittent high-dose cyclophosphamide chemotherapy for small cell carcinoma of the lung. Cancer Treat Rep 62:413–422, 1978

888a. O'Donnell MR, Ruckdeschel JC, Baxter D et al: Intensive induction chemotherapy for small cell anaplastic carcinoma of the lung. Cancer Treat Rep 69:571–575, 1985

889. Johnson DH, Einhorn LH, Birch R et al: A randomized comparison of high-dose versus conventional-dose cyclophosphamide, doxorubicin, and vincristine for extensive stage small cell lung cancer. J Clin Oncol 5:1731–1738, 1987

890. Figueredo AT, Hryniuk WM, Straufmanis I et al: Co-trimoxazole prophylaxis during high-dose chemotherapy of small cell lung cancer. J Clin Oncol 3:54–64, 1985

891. Hande KR, Oldham RK, Fer MF, Richardson RL, Greco FA: Randomized study of high-dose low-dose methotrexate in the treatment of extensive small cell lung cancer. Am J Med 73:413–418, 1982

892. Abeloff MD, Ettinger DS, Order SE et al: Intensive induction chemotherapy with 54

patients with small cell carcinoma of the lung. Cancer Treat Rep 65:639–646, 1981

892a. Valdivieso M, Cabanillas F, Keating M et al: Effects of intensive induction chemotherapy for extensive disease small cell bronchogenic carcinoma in protected environment-prophylactic antibiotic units. Am J Med 76:405–412, 1984

893. Brower M, Ihde DC, Johnston—Early A et al: Treatment of extensive stage small cell bronchogenic carcinoma: Effects of variation in intensity of induction chemotherapy. Am J Med 75:993–998, 1983 and Valdivieso M, Cabanillas F, Keating M et al: Effects of intensive induction chemotherapy for extensive disease small cell bronchogenic carcinoma in protected environment–prophylactic antibiotic units. Am J Med 76:405–412, 1984

894. Farha P, Spitzer G, Valdivieso M et al: High-dose chemotherapy and autologous bone marrow transplantation for the treatment of small cell lung carcinoma. Cancer 52:1351–1355, 1983

895. Johnson DH, DeLeo MJ, Hande KR et al: High-dose induction chemotherapy with cyclophosphamide, etoposide, and cisplatin for extensive stage small cell lung cancer. J Clin Oncol 5:703–709, 1987

896. Markman M, Abeloff MD, Berkman AW et al: Intensive alternating chemotherapy regimen in small cell carcinoma of the lung. Cancer Treat Rep 69:161–166, 1985

897. Klastersky J, Nicaise C, Longeval E et al: Cisplatin, Adriamycin, and etoposide (CAV) for remission induction of small-cell bronchogenic carcinoma: Evaluation of efficacy and toxicity and pilot study of a "late intensification" with autologous bone-marrow rescue. Cancer 50:652–658, 1982

898. Stewart P, Buckner CD, Thomas ED et al: Intensive chemoradiotherapy with autologous bone marrow transplantation for small cell carcinoma of the lung. Cancer Treat Rep 67:1055–1059, 1983

899. Humblet Y, Symann M, Bosly A et al: Late intensification chemotherapy with autologous bone marrow transplantation in selected small cell carcinoma of the lung: A randomized study. J Clin Oncol 5:1864–1873, 1987

900. Ihde DC, Deisseroth AB, Lichter AS et al: Late intensive combined modality therapy followed by autologous bone marrow infusion in extensive stage small cell lung cancer. J Clin Oncol 4:1443–1454, 1986

901. Smith IE, Evans BD, Harland SJ et al: High-dose cyclophosphamide with autologous bone marrow rescue after conventional chemotherapy in the treatment of small cell lung carcinoma. Cancer Chemother Pharmacol 14:120–124, 1985

902. Spitzer G, Farha P, Valdivieso M et al: High-dose intensification therapy with autologous bone marrow support for limited small cell bronchogenic carcinoma. J Clin Oncol 4:4–13, 1986

903. Sculier JP, Klastersky J, Strychkmans P et al: Late intensification in small cell lung cancer: A Phase I study of high doses of cyclophosphamide and etoposide with autologous bone marrow transplantation. J Clin Oncol 3:184–191, 1985

904. Cunningham D, Banham SW, Hutcheon AH et al: High-dose cyclophosphamide and VP-16 as late dosage intensification therapy for small cell carcinoma of the lung. Cancer Chemother Pharmacol 15:303–306, 1985

905. Cornbleet M, Gregor A, Allan S et al: High-dose melphalan as consolidation therapy for good prognosis patients with small cell carcinoma of bronchus (abstract). Proc Am Soc Clin Oncol 3:210, 1984

906. Harper PG, Souhami RL: Intensive chemotherapy with autologous bone marrow transplantation in small cell carcinoma of the lung. Recent Results Cancer Res 97:146–156, 1985

907. Goldie JH, Coldman AJ: A mathematical model for relating drug sensitivity of tumors to their spontaneous mutation rate. Cancer Treat Rep 63:1727–1733, 1979

908. Goldie JH, Coldman AJ: Genetic origins of drug resistance in neoplasms. Cancer Res 44:3743–3653, 1984

909. Østerlind K, Sorenson H, Hansen HH et al: Continuous versus alternating combination chemotherapy for advanced small cell carcinoma of the lung. Cancer Res 43:6085–6089, 1983

910. Cohen MH, Ihde DC, Bunn PA et al: Cyclic alternating combination chemotherapy of small cell bronchogenic carcinoma. Cancer Treat Rep 63:163–170, 1979

911. Aisner J, Whitacre W, Van Echo DA, Wiernik PH: Combination chemotherapy for small cell carcinoma of the lung: Continuous versus alternating non-cross-resistant combinations. Cancer Treat Rep 66:221–230, 1982

912. Elliott JA, Østerlind K, Hansen HH: Cyclic alternating "non-cross resistant" chemotherapy in the management of small cell anaplastic carcinoma of the lung. Cancer Treat Rev 11:103–113, 1984

913. Ettinger DS, Mehta CR, Abeloff MD et al: Maintenance chemotherapy versus no maintenance chemotherapy in complete responders following induction chemotherapy in extensive disease small cell lung cancer (abstract). Proc Am Soc Clin Oncol 6:175, 1987

914. Daniels JR, Chak LY, Sikic BL et al: Chemotherapy of small cell carcinoma of the lung: A randomized comparison of alternating and sequential combination chemotherapy programs. J Clin Oncol 2:1192–1199, 1984

915. Evans WK, Feld R, Murray N et al: Superiority of alternating non-cross resistant chemotherapy in extensive small cell lung cancer. Ann Intern Med 107:451–458, 1987

916. Natale RB, Shank B, Hilaris BS et al: Combination cyclophosphamide, Adriamycin, and vincristine rapidly alternating with combination cisplatin and VP-16 in treatment of small cell lung cancer. Am J Med 79:303–308, 1985

917. Feld R, Evans WK, DeBoer G et al: Combined modality induction therapy without maintenance chemotherapy for small cell carcinoma of the lung. J Clin Oncol 2:294–304, 1984

918. Cullen M, Morgan D, Gregory W et al: Maintenance chemotherapy for anaplastic

small cell carcinoma of the bronchus: A randomized controlled trial. Cancer Chemother Pharmacol 17:157–160, 1986

919. McVie JG, Dalesio O, Kirkpatrick A et al: Induction versus induction plus maintenance therapy in small cell lung cancer (abstract). Proc Am Soc Clin Oncol 5:188, 1986

920. Abeloff MD, Klastersky J, Drings PD et al: Complications of treatment of small cell carcinoma of the lung. Cancer Treat Rep 67:21–26, 1983

921. Markman M, Abeloff MD: Management of hematologic and infectious complications of intensive induction therapy for small cell carcinoma of the lung. Am J Med 74:741–746, 1983

922. De Jongh CA, Wade JC, Finley RS et al: Trimethoprim/sulfamethoxazole versus placebo: A double-blind comparison of infection prophylaxis in patients with small cell carcinoma of the lung. J Clin Oncol 1:302–307, 1983

923. Huberman M, Fossieck BE, Bunn PA Jr, Cohen MH, Ihde DC, Minna JD: Herpes zoster and small cell bronchogenic carcinoma. Am J Med 68:214–218, 1980

924. Feld R, Evans WK, DeBoer G: Herpes zoster in patients with carcinoma of the lung. Am J Med 73:795–801, 1982

925. Earle MF, Fossieck BE, Cohen MH, Ihde DC, Bunn PA Jr, Minna JD: Perirectal infections in patients with small cell lung cancer. JAMA 246:2464–2466, 1981

926. Bunn PA, Lichter AS, Makuch RW et al: Chemotherapy alone or chemotherapy with chest radiation therapy in limited stage small cell lung cancer: A prospective randomized trial. Ann Intern Med 106:655–662, 1987

927. Abrams RA, Lichter AS, Bromer RH et al: The hematopoietic toxicity of regional radiation therapy: Correlations for combined modality therapy with systemic chemotherapy. Cancer 55:1429–1435, 1985

928. Lee JS, Umsawasdi T, Dhingra HM et al: Effects of brain irradiation and chemotherapy on myelosuppression in small cell lung cancer. J Clin Oncol 4:1615–1619, 1986

929. Johnson BE, Ihde DC, Bunn PA et al: Patients with small cell lung cancer treated with combination chemotherapy with or without irradiation: Data on potential cures, chronic toxicities, and late relapses after five- to eleven-year follow-up. Ann Intern Med 103:430–438, 1985

930. Johnson DH, Porter LL, List AF et al: Acute nonlymphocytic leukemia after treatment of small cell lung cancer. Am J Med 81:962–968, 1986

931. Bradley EC, Schechter GP, Matthews MJ et al: Erythroleukemia and other hematologic complications of intensive therapy in long-term survivors of small cell lung cancer. Cancer 49:221–223, 1982

932. Sorensen PG, Østerlind K, Groth S et al: Effects of intensive chemotherapy on respiratory function in patients with small cell carcinoma of the lung. Eur J Cancer Clin Oncol 19:901–906, 1983

933. Brooks BJ, Seifter EJ, Walsh TE et al: Pulmonary toxicity with combined modality therapy for limited stage small cell lung cancer. J Clin Oncol 4:200–209, 1986

934. Vogelzang NJ, Nelimark RA, Nath KA: Tumor lysis syndrome after induction chemotherapy of small cell bronchogenic carcinoma. JAMA 249:513–514, 1983

935. Salazar OM, Rubin P, Brown JC et al: Predictors of radiation response in lung cancer: A clinico-pathobiologic analysis. Cancer 37:2636–2650, 1976

936. Lichter AS, Bunn PA, Ihde DC et al: The role of radiation therapy in the treatment of small cell lung cancer. Cancer 55:2163–2175, 1985

937. Perry MC, Eaton WL, Propert KJ et al: Chemotherapy with or without radiation therapy in limited small cell carcinoma of the lung. N Engl J Med 316:912–918, 1987

938. Perez CA, Einhorn L, Oldham RK et al: Randomized trial of radiotherapy to the thorax in limited small cell carcinoma of the lung treated with multiagent chemotherapy and elective brain irradiation: A preliminary report. J Clin Oncol 2:1200–1208, 1984

939. Souhami RL, Geddes DM, Spiro SG et al: Radiotherapy in small cell cancer of the lung treated with combination chemotherapy: A controlled trial. Br Med J 288:1643–1646, 1984

940. Kies MS, Mira JG, Livingston RB et al: Multimodal therapy for limited small cell lung cancer: A randomized study of induction combination chemotherapy with or without thoracic irradiation in complete responders, and with wide field versus reduced volume radiation in partial responders. J Clin Oncol 5:592–600, 1987

941. Østerlind K, Hansen HH, Hansen HS et al: Chemotherapy versus chemotherapy plus irradiation in limited small cell lung cancer: Results of a controlled trial with five years of follow-up. Br J Cancer 54:7–17, 1986

942. Cox JD, Holoye PY, Libnoch JA: The role of consolidation irradiation in combined modality therapy of small cell carcinoma of the lung. Int J Radiat Oncol Biol Phys 8:1271–1276, 1982

943. Smyth J, Hansen HH: Current status of research into small cell carcinoma of the lung: Summary of the Second Workshop of the International Association for the Study of Lung Cancer (IASLC). Eur J Cancer Clin Oncol 21:1295–1298, 1985

944. Cox JD, Byhardt R, Komaki R et al: Interaction of thoracic irradiation and chemotherapy on local control and survival in small cell carcinoma of the lung. Cancer Treat Rep 63:1251–1255, 1979

945. Williams C, Alexander M, Glatstein EJ et al: The role of radiation therapy in combination with chemotherapy in extensive oat cell cancer of the lung: A randomized study. Cancer Treat Rep 61:142–143, 1977

946. Trask CWL, Joannides T, Harper PG et al: Radiation-induced lung fibrosis after treatment of small cell carcinoma of the lung with very high dose cyclophosphamide. Cancer 55:57–60, 1985

947. Arriagada R, LeChevelier T, Baldeyrou P et al: Alternating radiotherapy and chemo-

therapy schedules in small cell lung cancer, limited disease. Int J Radiat Oncol Biol Phys 11:1461–1467, 1985

948. Turrisi AT, Glover DJ, Mason B et al: Concurrent twice-daily multifield radiotherapy and platinum–etoposide chemotherapy for limited small cell lung cancer: Update 1987 (abstract). Proc Am Soc Clin Oncol 6:172, 1987

949. Livingston RB, Mira JG, Chen TT et al: Combined modality treatment of extensive small cell lung cancer. J Clin Oncol 2:585–590, 1984

950. Wilson HE, Stanley K, Vincent RG et al: Comparison of chemotherapy alone versus chemotherapy and radiation therapy of extensive small cell carcinoma of the lung. J Surg Oncol 23:181–184, 1983

951. Livingston RB, Schulman S, Mira JG et al: Combined alkylators and multiple-site irradiation for extensive small cell lung cancer. Cancer Treat Rep 70:1395–1401, 1986

952. Urtasun RC, Belch A, Bodnar D et al: Radiation as a non-cross resistant systemic agent: Experience with hemibody and total body irradiation in patients with small cell lung cancer. Cancer Treat Symp 2:41–47, 1985

953. Mason BA, Richter MP, Catalano RB, Creech RB: Upper hemibody and local chest irradiation as consolidation following response to high-dose induction chemotherapy for small cell bronchogenic carcinoma: A pilot study. Cancer Treat Rep 66:1609–1612, 1982

954. Powell BL, Jackson DV, Scarantino CW et al: Sequential hemibody irradiation integrated into a chemotherapy–local radiotherapy program for limited disease in small cell lung cancer. Int J Radiat Oncol Biol Phys 12:1951–1956, 1986

955. Salazar OM, Creech RH, Rubin P et al: Half-body and local chest irradiation as consolidation following response to standard induction chemotherapy for disseminated small cell lung cancer. Int J Radiat Oncol Biol Phys 6:1093–1102, 1980

956. Dillman RO, Seagren SL, Taetle R: Failure of low-dose, total-body irradiation to augment combination chemotherapy in extensive-stage small cell carcinoma of the lung. J Clin Oncol 1:242–250, 1983

957. Byhardt RW, Cox JD, Wilson JF et al: Total body irradiation vs. chemotherapy as a systemic adjuvant for small cell carcinoma of the lung. Int J Radiat Oncol Biol Phys 5:2043–2048, 1979

958. Hansen HH, Dombernowsky P, Hirsch FR et al: Prophylactic irradiation in bronchogenic small cell anaplastic carcinoma: A comparative trial of localized versus extensive radiotherapy including prophylactic brain irradiation in patients receiving combination chemotherapy. Cancer 46:279–284, 1980

959. Cox JD, Komaki R, Byhardt RW et al: Results of whole-brain irradiation for metastases from small cell carcinoma of the lung. Cancer Treat Rep 64:957–961, 1980

960. Komaki R, Cox JD, Whitson W: Risk of brain metastases from small cell carcinoma of the lung related to length of survival and prophylactic irradiation. Cancer Treat Rep 65:811–814, 1981

961. Hirsch FR, Paulson OB, Hansen HH, Vraa-Henssen J: Intracranial metastases in small cell carcinoma of the lung: Correlation of clinical and autopsy findings. Cancer 50:2433–2437, 1982

962. Jackson DV, Richards F, Cooper MR et al: Prophylactic cranial irradiation in small cell carcinoma of the lung: A randomized study. JAMA 237:2730–2733, 1977

963. Hirsch HH, Paulson OB et al: Development of brain metastases in small cell anaplastic carcinoma of the lung. In Kay J, Whitehouse J (eds): CNS Complications of Malignant Disease, pp 175–184. London, Macmillan Press, 1979

964. Beiler DD, Kane RC, Bernath AM et al: Low dose elective brain irradiation in small cell carcinoma of the lung. Int J Radiat Oncol Biol Phys 5:944–945, 1979

965. Cox JD, Petrovich Z, Paig C et al: Prophylactic cranial irradiation in patients with inoperable carcinoma of the lung. Cancer 42:1135–1140, 1978

966. Seydel HG, Creech R, Pagano M et al: Small cell carcinoma: Combined modality treatment of regional small cell undifferentiated carcinoma of the lung. Int J Radiat Oncol Biol Phys 9:1135–1141, 1983

967. Bleehen NM, Bunn PA, Cox JD et al: Role of radiation therapy in small cell anaplastic carcinoma of the lung. Cancer Treat Rep 67:11–19, 1983

968. Rosen ST, Makuch RW, Lichter AS et al: Role of prophylactic cranial irradiation in prevention of central nervous system metastases in small cell lung cancer: Potential benefit restricted to patients with complete response. Am J Med 74:615–624, 1983

969. Aroney RS, Aisner J, Wesley MN et al: Value of prophylactic cranial irradiation given at complete remission in small cell lung carcinoma. Cancer Treat Rep 67:675–682, 1983

970. Sargent EN, Turner AF, Gordonson J et al: Percutaneous pulmonary needle biopsy: Report of 350 patients. Am J Roentgenol Rad Ther Nucl Med 122:758–768, 1974

971. Seydel HG, Creech R, Pagano M et al: Prophylactic versus no brain irradiation in regional small cell lung carcinoma. Am J Clin Oncol (CCT) 8:218–223, 1985

972. Baglan JR, Marks JE: Comparison of symptomatic and prophylactic irradiation of brain metastases from oat cell carcinoma of the lung. Cancer 47:41–45, 1981

973. Lucas CF, Robinson B, Hoskin PJ et al: Morbidity of cranial relapse in small cell lung cancer and the impact of radiation therapy. Cancer Treat Rep 70:565–570, 1986

974. Johnson BE, Becker B, Goff WB et al: Neurologic, neuropsychologic, and computed cranial tomography scan abnormalities in 2- to 10-year survivors of small cell lung cancer. J Clin Oncol 3:1659–1667, 1985

975. Lee JS, Umsawasdi T, Lee YY et al: Neurotoxicity in long-term survivors of small cell lung cancer. Int J Radiat Oncol Biol Phys 12:313–321, 1986

976. Livingston RB, Stephens RL, Bonnet JD et al: Long-term survival and toxicity in small cell lung cancer. Am J Med 77:415–417, 1984

977. Licciardello JTW, Cersosimo RJ, Karp DD et al: Disturbing central nervous system complications following combination chemotherapy and prophylactic whole-brain irradiation in patients with small cell lung cancer. Cancer Treat Rep 69:1429–1430, 1985

978. Carmichael J, Crane JM, Bunn PA et al: Results of therapeutic cranial irradiation in small cell lung cancer. Int J Radiat Oncol Biol Phys 14:455–459, 1988

979. Van Hazel G, Scott M, Eagan RT: The effect of CNS metastases on the survival of patients with small cell cancer of the lung. Cancer 51:933–937, 1983

979a. Rosen ST, Aisner J, Makuch RW et al: Carcinomatous leptomeningitis in small cell lung cancer: A clinicopathologic review of the National Cancer Institute experience. Medicine 61:45–53, 1982

980. Van Hazel G, Scott M, Eagan RT: The effect of CNS metastases on the survival of patients with small cell cancer of the lung. Cancer 51:933–937, 1983

981. Higgins GA, Shields TW, Keehn RJ: the solitary pulmonary nodule: Ten-year follow-up of Veterans Administration–Armed Forces Cooperative Study. Arch Surg 110:570–575, 1975

982. Shields TW, Higgins GA, Matthews MJ et al: Surgical resection in the management of small cell carcinoma of the lung. J Thorac Cardiovasc Surg 84:481–488, 1982

983. Davis S, Wright PW, Schulman SF et al: Long-term survival in small cell carcinoma of the lung: A population experience. J Clin Oncol 3:80–91, 1985

984. Shepherd FA, Ginsburg RJ, Feld R et al: Reduction in local recurrence and improved survival in surgically treated patients with small cell lung cancer. J Thorac Cardiovasc Surg 86:498–506, 1983

985. Prager RL, Foster JM, Hainsworth JD et al: The feasibility of adjuvant surgery in limited stage small cell carcinoma: A prospective evaluation. Ann Thorac Surg 38:622–626, 1984

986. Johnson DH, Einhorn LH, Mandelbaum I et al: Postchemotherapy resection of residual tumor in limited stage small cell lung cancer. Chest 92:241–246, 1987

987. Friess GG, McCracken JD, Troxell ML et al: Effect of initial resection of small cell carcinoma of the lung: A review of Southwest Oncology Group Study 7628. J Clin Oncol 3:964–968, 1985

988. Østerlind K, Hansen M, Hansen HH et al: Influence of surgical resection prior to chemotherapy on the long-term results in small cell lung cancer: A study of 150 operable patients. Eur J Cancer Clin Oncol 22:589–593, 1986

989. Meyer JA: Effect of histologically verified TNM stage on disease control in treated small cell carcinoma of the lung. Cancer 55:1747–1752, 1985

990. Shepherd FA, Ginsberg R, Evans WK et al: "Very limited" small cell lung cancer: Results of non-surgical treatment (abstract). Proc Am Soc Clin Oncol 3:223, 1984

991. Williams CJ, McMillan I, Lea R et al: Surgery after initial chemotherapy for localized small cell carcinoma of the lung. J Clin Oncol 5:1579–1588, 1987

992. Baker RR, Ettinger DS, Ruckdeschel JD et al: The role of surgery in the management of selected patients with small cell carcinoma of the lung. J Clin Oncol 5:697–702, 1987

993. Valdivieso M, McMurtrey MJ, Farha P et al: Prospective evaluation of adjuvant surgical resection in small cell lung cancer. (abstract). Proc Am Soc Clin Oncol 3:220, 1984

994. Abeloff MD, Eggleston JC, Mendelsohn G et al: Changes in morphologic and biochemical characteristics of small cell carcinoma of the lung: A clinico-pathologic study. Am J Med 66:757–764, 1977

995. Matthews MJ: Effects of therapy on the morphology and behavior of small cell carcinoma of the lung: A clinicopathologic study. In Muggia F, Rozencweig M (eds): Lung Cancer: Progress in Therapeutic Research, pp 155–165. New York, Raven Press, 1979

996. Meyer JA, Gullo JJ, Ikins PM et al: Adverse prognostic effect of N2 disease in treated small cell carcinoma of the lung. J Thorac Cardiovasc Surg 88:495–501, 1984

997. Batist G, Carney DN, Cowan KH et al: Etoposide (VP-16) and cisplatin in previously treated small cell lung cancer: Clinical trial and in vitro correlates. J Clin Oncol 4:982–986, 1986

998. Batist G, Ihde DC, Zabell A et al: Small-cell carcinoma of lung: Reinduction therapy after late relapse. Ann Intern Med 98:472–474, 1983

999. Ochs JJ, Tester WJ, Cohen MH, Lichter AS, Ihde DC: "Salvage" radiation therapy for intrathoracic small cell carcinoma of the lung progressing on combination chemotherapy. Cancer Treat Rep 67:1123–1126, 1983

1000. Choi NC, Propert K, Carey R et al: Accelerated radiotherapy followed by chemotherapy for locally recurrent small cell carcinoma of the lung. Int J Radiat Oncol Biol Phys 13:263–266, 1987

1001. Holmes EC: Immunology and lung cancer. Ann Thorac Surg 21:250–258, 1976 and Chest 71:643–644, 1977

1002. Price–Evans DA: Immunology of bronchial carcinoma. Thorax 31:493–506, 1978

1003. McCracken JD, Chen T, White J et al: Combination chemotherapy, radiotherapy, and BCG immunotherapy in limited small cell carcinoma of the lung. Cancer 49:2252–2258, 1982

1004. McCracken JD, Heilbrun L, White J et al: Combination chemotherapy, radiotherapy, and BCG immunotherapy in extensive (metastatic) small cell carcinoma of the lung. Cancer 46:2335–2340, 1980

1005. Jackson DV, Paschal BR, Ferree C et al: Combination chemotherapy–radiotherapy with and without the methanol-extraction residue of Bacillus Calmette-Guerin (MER) in small cell carcinoma of the lung: A prospective randomized trial of the Piedmont Oncology Association. Cancer 50:48–52, 1982

1006. Maurer LH, Pajak T, Eaton W et al: Combined modality therapy with radiotherapy, chemotherapy, and immunotherapy in limited small cell carcinoma of the lung. J Clin Oncol 3:969–976, 1985

1007. Aisner J, Wiernik PH: Chemotherapy versus chemoimmunotherapy for small cell undifferentiated carcinoma of the lung. Cancer 46:2543–2549, 1980

1008. Cohen MH, Chretien PB, Ihde DC et al: Thymosin fraction V and intensive combination chemotherapy: Prolonging the survival of patients with small cell lung cancer. JAMA 241:1813–1815, 1979, and Cohen MH, Chretien PB, Early AJ et al: Thymosin fraction V prolongs survival of intensively treated small cell lung cancer patients. In Terry W, Windhorst D (eds): Immunotherapy of Cancer: Present Status of Trials in Man, Second International Conference. New York, Raven Press, 1980

1009. Scher HJ, Shank B, Chapman R et al: Randomized trial of combined modality therapy with and without thymosin fraction V in the treatment of small cell lung cancer. Cancer Res 48:1663–1670, 1988

1010. Evans WK, Russell DM, Shepherd FA et al: Changes in substrate–hormone profiles and amino acid metabolism in small cell lung cancer (abstract). Proc Am Assoc Cancer Res 24:651, 1983

1011. Shike M, Russell DM, Detsky As et al: Changes in body composition in patients with small cell lung cancer: The effect of total parenteral nutrition as an adjunct to chemotherapy. Ann Intern Med 101:303–309, 1984

1012. Clamon GH, Feld R, Evans WK et al: Effect of adjuvant central IV hyperalimentation on the survival and response to treatment of patients with small cell lung cancer: A randomized trial. Cancer Treat Rep 69:167–177, 1985

1013. Zacharski LR, Henderson WG, Rickles FR et al: Effect of warfarin on survival in small cell carcinoma of the lung: Veterans Administration Study No. 75. JAMA 245:831–834, 1981

1014. Levenson RM, Ihde DC, Matthews MJ et al: Small cell carcinoma arising in extrapulmonary sites: Response to chemotherapy. JNCI 67:607–612, 1981

1015. Fer MF, Levenson RM, Cohen MH et al: Extrapulmonary small cell carcinoma. In Greco FA, Oldham RK, Bunn PA (eds): Small Cell Lung Cancer, pp 301–325. New York, Grune & Stratton, 1981

1016. Remick SC, Hafez GR, Carbone PP: Extrapulmonary small cell carcinoma: A review of the literature with emphasis on therapy and outcome. Medicine 66:457–471, 1987

1017. Johnson BE, Naylor SL, Zbar B et al: Restriction fragment length polymorphism studies show loss of chromosome 3 alleles in small cell lung cancer but not in extrapulmonary small cell cancer (abstract). Proc Am Soc Clin Oncol 7:199, 1988

1018. Goepfert H, Remmler D, Silva E et al: Merkel cell carcinoma (endocrine carcinoma of the skin) of the head and neck. Arch Otolaryngol 110:707–712, 1984

1019. Mountain CF, Carr DT, Anderson WA: A system for the clinical staging of lung cancer. Am J Roentgenol Rad Ther Nucl Med 120:130–138, 1974

1020. Jacobs RH, Greenberg A, Bitran JD et al: A ten-year experience with combined modality therapy for Stage III small cell lung carcinoma. Cancer 58:2177–2184, 1986

1021. Østerlind K, Hansen HH, Hansen M et al: Mortality and morbidity in long-term surviving patients treated with chemotherapy with or without irradiation for small cell lung cancer. J Clin Oncol 4:1044–1052, 1986

1022. Roswit B, Patno ME, Rapp R et al: The survival of patients with inoperable lung cancer: A large-scale randomized study of radiation therapy versus placebo. Radiology 80:688–697, 1968

1023. Seydel HG, Creech R, Pagano M et al: Small cell carcinoma: Combined modality treatment of regional and small cell undifferentiated carcinoma of the lung. Int J Radiat Oncol Biol Phys 9:1135–1141, 1983

1024. Petrovich Z, Ohanian M, Cox JD: Clinical research on the treatment of locally advanced lung cancer. Cancer 42:1129–1134, 1978

1025. Carr DT, Childs DS Jr, Lee RE: Radiotherapy plus 5-FU compared to radiotherapy alone for inoperable and unresectable bronchogenic carcinoma. Cancer 29:375–380, 1972

1026. Choi CH, Carey RW: Small cell anaplastic carcinoma of the lung: Reappraisal of current management. Cancer 37:2651–2657, 1976

1027. Johnson BE, Ihde DC, Matthews MJ et al: Non-small cell lung cancer: Major cause of late mortality in patients with small cell lung cancer. Am J Med 80:1103–1110, 1986

1028. Baillie–Johnson H, Twentyman PR, Fox NE et al: Establishment and characterisation of cell lines from patients with lung cancer (predominantly small cell carcinoma). Cancer 52:495–504, 1985

1029. Klein JC, Zurcher C, Van Bekkum DW: Differential behavior of human bronchial carcinoma cells in culture. Cancer Res 47:3251–3258, 1987

1030. Bepler G, Jaques G, Neumann K, Aumuller G, Gropp C, Havemann K: Establishment, growth properties, and morphological characteristics of permanent human small cell lung cancer cell lines. J Cancer Res Clin Oncol 113:31–40, 1987

1031. Ruckdeschel JC, Oie HK, Gazdar AF: In vitro characterization of non-small cell lung cancer. Cancer Treat Res 28:49–59, 1986

1032. Kaiser LR, Kern DH, Campbell M, Mann PD, Holmes EC: In vitro assessment of antineoplastic therapy: New indication for thoracotomy? J Thorac Cardiovasc Surg 82:538–541, 1981

1033. Shorthouse AJ, Jones JM, Steel GG, Peckham MJ: Experimental combination and single-agent chemotherapy in human lung-tumor xenografts. Br J Cancer 46:35–44, 1982

1034. Ruckdeschel JC, Carney DN, Oie HK, Russell EK, Gazdar AF: In vitro chemosensitivity of human lung cancer cell lines. Cancer Treat Rep 71:697–704, 1987

1035. Douple EB, Cate CC, Curphey TJ et al: Evaluation of drug efficacy in vitro using human small cell carcinoma of the lung spheroids. Cancer 56:1918–1925, 1985

1036. Roed H, Vindelov LL, Spang–Thomsen M, Engelholm SA: Limitations and potentials of in vitro sensitivity testing of human small cell carcinoma of the lung. Cancer Treat Res 28:77–89, 1986

1037. Casero RA Jr, Go B, Theiss HW et al: Cytotoxic response of the relatively difluoro-methylornithine-resistant human lung tumor cell line (NCI-H157 to the polyamine analogue N1,N8-bis(ethylo)spermidine. Cancer Res 47:3964–3967, 1987

1038. Munker M, Munker R, Sazton RE, Koeffler HP: Effect of recombinant monokines, lymphokines, and other agents on clonal proliferation of human lung cancer cell lines. Cancer Res 47:4081–4085, 1987

1039. Bepler G, Carney DN, Nau MM, Gazdar AF, Minna JD: Additive and differential biological activity of alpha-interferon A, difluoromethylornithine, and their combinations on established human lung cancer cell lines. Cancer Res 46:3413–3419, 1986

1040. Teraskai T, Shimosato Y, Nakajima T et al: Reversible squamous cell characteristics induced by vitamin A deficiency in a small cell lung cancer cell line. Cancer Res 47:3533–3537, 1987

1041. Doyle A, Giangiulio D, Hussain A, Park H, Borges M: Retinoic acid changes variant small cell lung cancer (SCLC) to a classic morphology (abstract). Proc Am Soc Clin Oncol 6:A57, 1987

1042. Curt GA, Jolivet J, Carney DN et al: Determinants of the sensitivity of human small-cell lung cancer cell lines to methotrexate. J Clin Invest 76:1323–1329, 1985

1043. Twentyman RP, Fox NE, Wright KA, Bleehen NM: Derivation and preliminary characterisation of Adriamycin resistant lines of human lung cancer cells. Br J Cancer 53:529–537, 1986

1044. Zijlstra JG, de Vries EG, Mulder NH: Multifactorial drug resistance in an Adriamycin-resistant human small cell lung carcinoma cell line. Cancer Res 47:1780–1784, 1987

1045. Carney DN, Mitchell JB, Kinsella TJ: In vitro radiation and chemotherapy sensitivity of established cell lines of human small cell lung cancer and its large cell morphological variants. Cancer Res 43:2806–2811, 1983

1046. Fox NE, Twentyman PR: A comparison of clonogenic and radionuclide uptake assays for determining the radiation response of human small-cell lung cancer xenografts and cell lines. Br J Radiol 60:381–388, 1987

1047. Duchesne GM, Peakcock JH, Steel GG: The acute in vitro and in vivo radiosensitivity of human lung tumour lines. Radiother Oncol 7:353–361, 1986

1048. Von Hoff DD, Casper H, Bradley E et al: Association between human tumor colony-forming assay results and response of an individual patient's tumor to chemotherapy. Am J Med 70:1027, 1981

1049. Von Hoff DD, Forseth B, Warfel LE: Use of a radiometric system to screen for antineoplastic agents: Correlation with a human tumor cloning system. Cancer Res 45:4032, 1985

1050. Weisenthal LM, Morsden JA, Dill PL, Macaluso CK: A novel dye exclusion method for testing in vitro chemosensitivity of human tumors. Cancer Res 43:749, 1983

1051. Kanzawa F, Matsushima Y, Ishihara J et al: In vitro chemosensitivity patterns of carcinoma of the lung in human tumor clongenic assay. J Pharmacobiodyn 9:715–721, 1986

1052. Cole SPC: Rapid chemosensitivity testing of human lung tumour cells using the MTT assay. Cancer Chemother Pharmacol 17:259, 1986

1053. Carmichael J, DeGraff WG, Gazdar AF, Minna JD, Mitchell JB: Evaluation of a tetrazolium-based semiautomated colorimetric assay: Assessment of chemosensitivity testing. Cancer Res 47:936–942, 1987

1054. Carmichael J, DeGraff WG, Gazdar AF, Minna JD, Mitchell JB: Evaluation of a tetrazolium-based semiautomated colorimetric assay: Assessment of radiosensitivity. Cancer Res 47:943–946, 1987

1055. Carmichael J, Mitchell JB, DeGraff WG et al: Chemosensitivity testing of human lung cancer cell lines using the MTT assay. Br J Cancer (in press)

1056. Carney DN: Recent advances in the biology of small cell lung cancer. Chest 89 Suppl:253S–257S, 1986

1057. Gazdar AF: Advances in the biology of non-small cell lung cancer. Chest 89 Suppl:277S–283S, 1986

1058. Funa K, Gazdar AF, Minna JD, Linnoila RI: Paucity of beta 2-microglobulin expression on small cell lung cancer, bronchial carcinoids and certain other neuroendocrine tumors. Lab Invest 55:186–193, 1986

1059. Doyle A, Martin J, Gazdar A et al: Markedly decreased or absent expression of class I histocompatibility antigens in human small cell lung cancer. J Exp Med 161:1135–1151, 1985

1060. Bernal SD, Baylin SB, Shaper JH et al: Cytoskeleton-associated proteins of human lung cancer cells. Cancer Res 43:1798–1808, 1983

1061. Lehto VP, Stenman S, Miettinen M et al: Expression of a neural type of intermediate filament as a distinguishing feature between oat cell carcinoma and other lung cancers. Am J Pathol 110:113–118, 1983

1062. Broers JL, Carney DN, Klein RM et al: Intermediate filament proteins in classic and variant types of small cell lung carcinoma cell lines: a biochemical and immunochemical analysis using a panel of monoclonal and polyclonal antibodies. J Cell Sci 83:37–60, 1986

1063. Bunn Pa, Linnoila I, Minna JD et al: Small cell lung cancer, endocrine cells of the fetal bronchus, and other neuroendocrine cells express the Leu-7 antigenic determinant present on natural killer cells. Blood 65:764–768, 1985

1064. Cole SP, Mirski S, McGarry RC et al: Differential expression of the Leu-7 antigen on human lung tumor cells. Cancer Res 45:4285–4290, 1985

1065. Baylin SB, Gazdar AF, Minna JD, Shaper JH: A unique cell surface protein phenotype distinguishes human small cell from non-small cell lung cancer. Proc Natl Acad Sci USA 79:4650–4654, 1982

1066. Ball ED, Sorenson GD, Pettengill OS: Expression of myeloid and major histocompatibility antigens on small cell carcinoma of the lung cell lines analyzed by cytofluorography: modulation by gamma-interferon. Cancer Res 46:2335–2339, 1986

1067. Hellstrom I, Horn D, Linsley P et al: Monoclonal mouse antibodies raised against human lung carcinoma. Cancer Res 46:3917–3923, 1986

1068. Moss F, Bobrow LG, Sheppard MN et al: Expression of epithelial and neural antigens in small cell and non small cell lung carcinoma. J Pathol 149:103–111, 1986

1069. Roth KA, Barchas JD: Small cell carcinoma cell lines contain opioid peptides and receptors. Cancer 57:769–773, 1986

1070. Cerny T, Barnes DM, Hasleton P et al: Expression of epidermal growth factor receptor (EGF-R) in human lung tumours. Br J Cancer 54:265–269, 1986

1071. Sakiyama S, Nakamura Y, Yasuda S: Expression of epidermal growth factor receptor gene in cultured human lung cancer cells. Jpn J Cancer Res 77:965–969, 1986

1072. Knop RH, Carney DN, Chen CW et al: Levels of high energy phosphates in human lung cancer cell lines by 31^P nuclear magnetic resonance spectroscopy. Cancer Res 47:3357–3359, 1987

1073. Spitalnik SL, Spitalnik PF, Dubois C et al: Glycolipid antigen expression in human lung cancer. Cancer Res 46:4751–4755, 1986

1074. Ruff MR, Farrar WL, Pert CB: Interferon gamma and granulocyte–macrophage colony-stimulating factor inhibit growth and induce antigens characteristic of myeloid differentiation in small-cell lung cancer cell lines. Proc Natl Acad Sci USA 83:6613–6617, 1986

J. C. ROSENBERG

CHAPTER 23 *Neoplasms of the Mediastinum*

Mediastinal masses are asymptomatic in a little less than half the patients who are discovered to have them (Fig. 23-1).[1] Asymptomatic masses are usually detected when a chest roentgenogram is obtained for a reason unrelated to the mediastinal tumor. One can expect asymptomatic patients to harbor a benign lesion, because 90% of the lesions occurring in asymptomatic patients are benign.[1-3] The most common symptoms produced by mediastinal masses are listed in Table 23-1.

Some patients with benign tumors of the mediastinum are at risk of disability or death if the lesion's size or position interferes with cardiopulmonary function. Because of this hazard and the high incidence of malignant tumors in the mediastinum, a mass in this location cannot be "passively observed or treated by radiation without benefit of a specific diagnosis," as was occasionally the practice in the past.[4] The lesion must be diagnosed with precision and treated appropriately.

ANATOMICAL CONSIDERATIONS

The boundaries of the mediastinum are the diaphragm inferiorly, the parietal pleura laterally, the sternum anteriorly, the vertebral column and adjacent ribs posteriorly, and the thoracic outlet superiorly. The thoracic outlet is the area encompassed by the superior extent of the thoracic cage, that is, the level of the first thoracic vertebra and the first ribs.

Because of the constancy with which anatomical structures are located within specific areas of the mediastinum and the predilection of different lesions to occur within certain mediastinal areas, it is clinically relevant to divide the mediastinum into compartments. The superior mediastinum is the area between the thoracic outlet and a line drawn from the sternal angle of Louis (the junction of the manubrium and body of the sternum) to the fourth intervertebral disc. Since the mediastinum is trapezoidal in shape, the superior mediastinum is narrowed by the approximation of its lateral boundaries and cannot easily be subdivided further. However, the remainder of the mediastinum can be subdivided into anterior, middle, and posterior divisions.

The anterior mediastinum extends from the sternum to the pericardium and great vessels. The posterior mediastinum is bounded by the posterior rib cage and spinal column and extends anteriorly for a variable distance. Some authors define the anterior extent of the posterior mediastinum as the pericardium (Fig. 23-2C). Others set it at a line drawn along the anterior borders of the bodies of the vertebrae (Figs. 23-2A and 23-2B). In the latter case, the posterior mediastinum would consist of the costovertebral (or paravertebral) areas.

The middle mediastinum includes the section between the anterior and posterior compartments. It is also referred to as the hilar or visceral area since it contains the heart and great vessels.

Burkell and colleagues have suggested a different map of the mediastinum.[5] They speak of only three areas, the

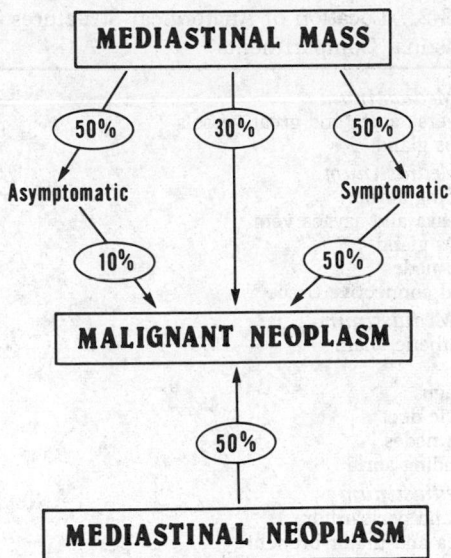

FIG. 23-1. Symptomatic mediastinal masses are often malignant neoplasms. Half of all new growths of the mediastinum are malignant.

anterosuperior, posterior, and the middle mediastinal divisions. They consider it impractical to designate the superior mediastinum as a distinct division of the mediastinum because many lesions that are found in the superior mediastinum are also found in the anterior mediastinum. Furthermore, superior mediastinal masses tend to extend down into the chest and also occupy the anterior mediastinum. Many posterior mediastinal lesions extend upwards, also occupying the superior mediastinum. Thus there is merit to their suggestion that the anterior and superior mediastinal compartments be combined into one division. Another way of looking at the mediastinum divided into three compartments is illustrated in Figure 23-2D.

TABLE 23-1. Mediastinal Masses: Signs and Symptoms

Nonspecific
- Chest discomfort—fullness, tightness, pain
- Anorexia
- Weight loss
- Malaise

Secondary to Compression or Displacement of Adjacent Mediastinal Structures
- Tracheo-bronchial compression—
  - cough, wheezing, stridor, dyspnea, recurrent respiratory infections
- Esophageal compression—dysphagia
- Superior vena cava syndrome
- Horner's syndrome
- Vocal cord paralysis—dysphonia
- Pulmonic stenosis—murmurs
- Cardiac tamponade or arrhythmias

Secondary to Endocrine Function
- Cushing's disease
- Gynecomastia
- Hypertension
- Hypoglycemia

Systemic Syndromes
- Thymoma*
  - Myasthenia gravis
  - Red cell aplasia
  - Hypogammaglobulinemia
  - Autoimmune diseases
- Carcinoid of thymus
  - Multiple endocrine abnormalities (type I)
  - Cushing's syndrome
- Neurofibroma
  - Osteoarthritis
- Lymphoma
  - Alcohol-induced pain
  - Fever
- Teratoma
  - Hypoglycemia—insulin-producing tumor

* See Table 23-4 for a complete list of systemic syndromes associated with thymomas.

FIG. 23-2. Various recommendations for dividing the mediastinum into compartments.

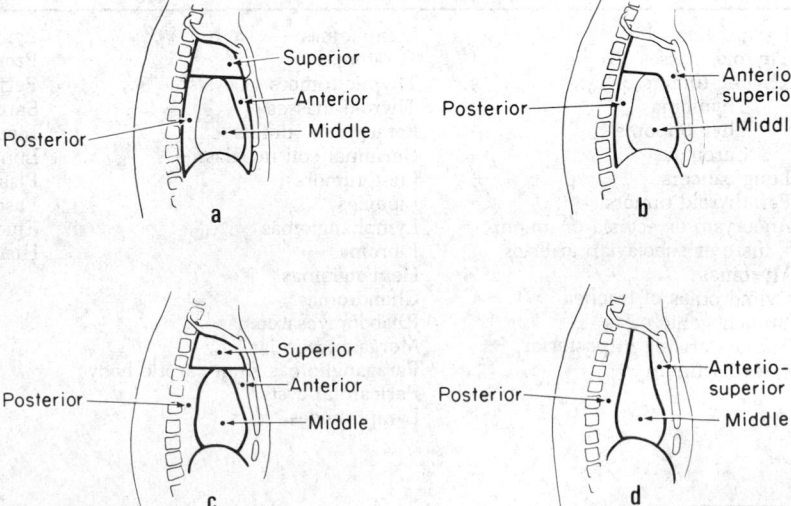

The anatomical structures normally found in the mediastinal compartments are listed in Table 23-2. Many of the lesions outlined in Table 23-3 can be derived from the list in Table 23-2. In addition to lesions arising from structures normally found in the mediastinum, abnormalities in the mediastinum may arise from adjacent anatomical areas, such as the abdomen, neck, lungs, and chest wall.

FREQUENCY OF MEDIASTINAL MASSES

Although lesions occur predominantly in one or another of the anatomic divisions of the mediastinum, there is an overlap in their distribution (Table 23-3). The most constant relationships are the thyroid masses, teratomas, and thymomas, which are located anteriorly and superiorly 90% of the time. Eighty percent of neurogenic tumors are located in the posterior mediastinum, and 50% of mediastinal lymphomas occur in the middle mediastinum.[6]

Mediastinal tumors and cysts in the adult are distributed throughout the mediastinal compartments in the following manner: 55% are in the anterior-superior compartment, 20% in the middle mediastinum, and 25% in the posterior mediastinum.[7] Some lesions cannot be localized because of their large size or indistinct margins. In children, the posterior mediastinum will contain 63% of the lesions; 26% occur in the anterior mediastinum, and 11% occur in the middle compartment.[8]

Tables 23-3 and 23-4 are fairly comprehensive lists of the lesions encountered in the mediastinum. Table 23-3 includes lesions arising outside the mediastinum that are located so close to it that they often extend into the mediastinum and may present as a primary mediastinal mass. In addition, physicians must be alert to the odd lesions that inevitably occur, such as an osteophyte of the spine protruding into the posterior mediastinum. Some spurious mediastinal masses that are on the surface of the patient appear on x-ray film to

lie within the mediastinum. A considerable number of "mediastinal masses" will eventually not be found within the mediastinum or will be lesions that secondarily involve the mediastinum, such as lung cancers.

Because primary tumors of the mediastinum are infrequent and not readily classified in a tabulation of malignancies, the best approximation of their incidence is to determine how often a major referral center with an interest in mediastinal masses encounters these lesions. Approximately 1 in every 3400 admissions to Duke University Medical Center was found to have a primary mediastinal tumor or cyst.[1] At the University of Wisconsin, 7 to 10 patients with different kinds of mediastinal lesions were seen each year.[5]

TABLE 23-2. Location of Anatomical Structures Within the Mediastinal Compartments

Superior Mediastinum
    Transverse aorta and great vessels
    Thymus gland
Anterior Mediastinum
    Ascending aorta
    Vena cava and azygos vein
    Thymus gland
    Lymph nodes
    Fat and connective tissue
Posterior Mediastinum
    Sympathetic chain
    Vagus
    Esophagus
    Thoracic duct
    Lymph nodes
    Descending aorta
Middle Mediastinum
    Heart and pericardium
    Trachea and major bronchi
    Pulmonary vessels
    Lymph nodes
    Fat and connective tissue

TABLE 23-3. Mediastinal Masses and Their Distribution

Superior	Anterior	Middle	Posterior
Lymphomas	Lymphomas	Lymphomas	Neurogenic tumors
Thyroid masses	Teratomas	Bronchogenic cysts	Lymphomas
Thymic tumors or cysts	Thymic tumors or cysts	Pericardial cysts	Bronchogenic cysts
Thymoma	Thyroid masses	Sarcoidosis	Enteric cysts
Thymolipoma	Parathyroid tumors	Lipomas	Xanthogranulomas
Carcinoid	Germinal cell neoplasms	Lung cancers	Esophageal masses and diverticula
Lung cancers	Lung tumors	Plasma cell myeloma	Lung cancers
Parathyroid tumors	Lipomas	Vascular tumors	Thyroid masses
Aneurysm or ectasia of innominate or subclavian arteries	Lymphangiomas	Epicardial fat pads	Hiatal hernias
Myxomas	Fibromas	Hiatal hernias	Paravertebral abscesses
Cylindromas of trachea	Hemangiomas		Fibrosarcomas
Bronchogenic cysts	Chondromas		Meningoceles
Tumors arising in posterior mediastinum	Rhabdomyosarcomas		Myxomas
	Morgagni hernias		Chondromas
	Paragangliomas from carotid body		Pheochromocytomas
	Pericardial cysts		Aneurysms of descending aorta
	Lymph nodes		Enlargement of azygous and hemiazygous veins
			Thoracic duct cysts
			Tumors of spinal column

TABLE 23-4. Classification of Mediastinal Tumors

Neurogenic
  Arising from peripheral nerves
    Neurofibroma
    Neurilemomma (Schwannoma)
    Neurosarcoma
  Arising from sympathetic ganglia
    Ganglioneuroma
    Ganglioneuroblastoma
    Neuroblastoma
  Arising from paraganglionic tissue
    Pheochromocytoma
    Chemodectoma (paraganglioma)

Thymic
  Thymoma
  Caarcinoid
  Thymolipoma

Lymphoma
  Hodgkin's disease
  Histiocytic lymphoma
  Undifferentiated

Germ Cell Tumors
  Seminoma
  Nonseminomatous tumors
  Pure embryonal cell
  Mixed embryonal cell
    with seminomatous elements
    with trophoblastic elements
    with teratoid elements
    with entodermal sinus elements
    (yolk sac tumors)
  Teratoma, benign

Aneurysms

Mesenchymal Tumors
  Fibroma and fibrosarcoma
  Lipoma and liposarcoma
  Myxoma
  Mesothelioma
  Leiomyoma and leiomyosarcoma
  Rhabdomyosarcoma
  Xanthogranuloma
  Mesenchymoma
  Hemangioma
  Hemangioendothelioma
  Hemangiopericytoma
  Lymphangioma
  Lymphangiomyoma
  Lymphangiopericytoma

Endocrine Tumors
  Thyroid
  Parathyroid

Cysts
  Pericardial
  Bronchogenic
  Enteric
  Thymic
  Thoracic duct
  Meningoceles

Hernias
  Hiatal
  Morgagni

Lymphadenopathy
  Inflammatory
  Granulomatous
  Sarcoid

Overall, the rate of malignancy of mediastinal masses is estimated at about 40%.[7] The relative incidence of tumors and cysts in a large combined group of patients is shown in Table 23-5.

In the Mayo Clinic series (1064 patients from 1929 to 1968), the incidence of malignant tumors in children was approximately the same as that encountered in adults (25%).[9] Most of the cancers in children were of neurogenic, teratomatous, or vascular origin. The types of benign lesions found in children also differed from those seen in adults. Neurogenic and teratomatous tumors and enterogenous cysts made up approximately 78% of the mediastinal masses seen in the pediatric age group. Vascular tumors and cystic hygromas occurred more frequently in infants and children than in adults. Only 1 of the 206 patients with thymoma in the Mayo Clinic series was younger than 20 years of age.[9] Pericardial cysts and intrathoracic goiters were also rare in children.

The data presented in Table 23-5 differ significantly from those presented in earlier publications on this subject. In a series of 2251 mediastinal tumors collected from the literature from 1946 to 1971, neurogenic tumors were most frequently found (38%), followed by thymoma and thymic cysts (13.5%). Currently, the incidences of both are about 20%. This change is thought to be the result of the recent, more assiduous search for thymomas in patients with myasthenia gravis and autoimmune disorders.[1,7] Another factor that may distort these statistics is the criteria used for including lym-

TABLE 23-5. Relative Frequency (%) of Primary Mediastinal Tumors and Cysts

Tumor or Cyst	Adults (n = 1950)	Children (n = 437)
Neurogenic tumors	21	40
Thymomas	19	0
Lymphomas	13	18
Germ cell neoplasms	11	11
Mesenchymal tumors	7	9
Endocrine tumors (thyroid, parathyroid, and carcinoid)	6	0
Primary carcinomas	3	4
Cysts (pericardial, bronchogenic, enteric, and others)	20	18

Silverman NA, Sabiston NC Jr: Mediastinal masses. Surg Clin North Am 60:757, 1980.

phomas in tabulations of mediastinal tumors. Lymphomas presenting as a mediastinal mass should be included, but not all lymphomas with mediastinal involvement qualify as primary mediastinal neoplasms. Primary mediastinal lymphomas do have some unique characteristics, but they are not sufficiently unique to merit separate consideration in this chapter.[10]

A recent review of the frequency of primary anterior mediastinal tumors in a combined series of 702 adults and 179 children resulted in the data shown in Table 23-6.

TABLE 23-6.   Relative Frequency (%) of Primary
Anterior Mediastinal Tumors

Tumors	Adults (n=702)	Children (n=179)
Thymic lesions (cysts, hyperplasia, and thymoma)	47	17
Germ cell neoplasms	15	24
Lymphomas	23	45
Endocrine tumors (thyroid and parathyroid)	16	0
Mesenchymal tumors	0	15

Mullen B, Richardson JD: Primary anterior mediastinal tumors in children and adults. Ann Thorac Surg 42:338, 1986.

Only 5 cases of thymoma in children are included in this study.[11]

DIAGNOSIS

IMAGING TECHNICS

Roentgenographic examinations constitute the most important diagnostic studies that can be performed to define the location and extent of a mediastinal mass. Chest roentgenograms in posteroanterior and lateral projections can identify most lesions and localize the bulk of the mass to one of the mediastinal compartments (Fig. 23-3). The shape, size, and density of the mass as it is seen on the chest roentgenogram do not differentiate whether it is benign or malignant. Most malignant primary lesions are located in the anterosuperior compartment of the mediastinum. The value of comparing current films with previously obtained chest roentgenograms cannot be overemphasized, because growth rates can be estimated and indistinct lesions more clearly defined.

Small lesions located in front of or behind the heart may be missed on a routine roentgenographic examination of the chest, especially in those patients with a large amount of fat. Suspected mediastinal masses or those that are ill-defined can be best delineated and localized by computed tomography (CT). Before the introduction of this valuable diagnostic tool in 1975, a long list of procedures were recommended in the diagnostic evaluation of mediastinal masses, such as penetrated views in various projections and coned views looking for bony projections and erosions of the spine, tomograms in various projections, barium contrast studies of the esophagus (still valuable in detecting a hiatal hernia presenting as a mediastinal mass), fluoroscopy, aortograms (Fig. 23-4 and 23-5), pulmonary arteriograms, venograms, azygograms, selective thymic venography, angiocardiography, pneumomediastinography, myelography (for posterior mediastinal masses accompanied by neurologic abnormalities), ultrasonography, echocardiography, and nuclide imaging procedures, such as thyroid, bone, and gallium scans.[12,13] The information obtained by performing these procedures can usually be derived from CT of the mediastinum.[7,14-18]

CT of the mediastinum offers two great advantages over conventional radiographic procedures. First is the ability to examine the mediastinum's cross-sectional anatomy. CT is better than lateral or oblique views for visualizing the mediastinum. Some mediastinal tumors may blend in with adjacent mediastinal structures in chest roentgenograms. CT can more precisely identify the margins between the tumor and adjacent anatomic structures, and anatomy heretofore not visible by noninvasive technics can be examined by the clinician (Fig. 23-6).

Widening of the mediastinum because of physiologic fat deposition or by dilation or ectasia of the great vessels can be readily detected by CT. Cystic areas and areas of calcification in the mediastinum can be precisely identified. The extent of involvement by a tumor or structures within the mediastinum can also be assessed by CT.

Magnetic resonance imaging (MRI), unlike CT, can define vascular structures without the use of contrast material. Several publications have appeared comparing CT with MRI without clearly defining the role of each.[19,20] MRI can define

FIG. 23-3. Posteroanterior (A), lateral (B), and oblique (C) view of an anterior mediastinal mass that was found to be an encapsulated thymoma on exploration of the mediastinum (see Fig. 23-6).

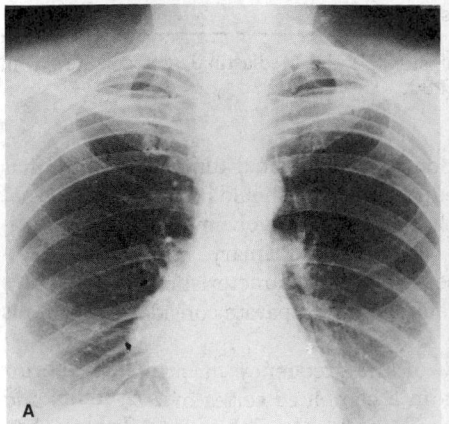
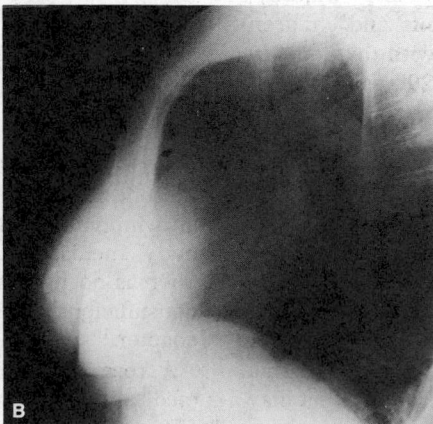
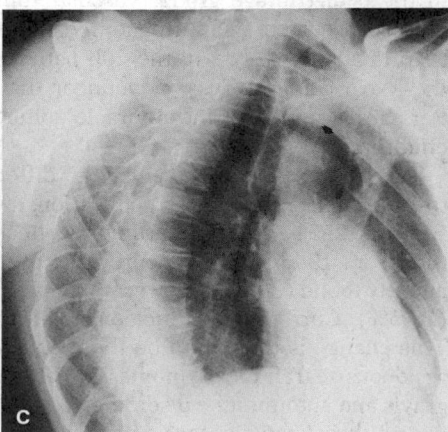

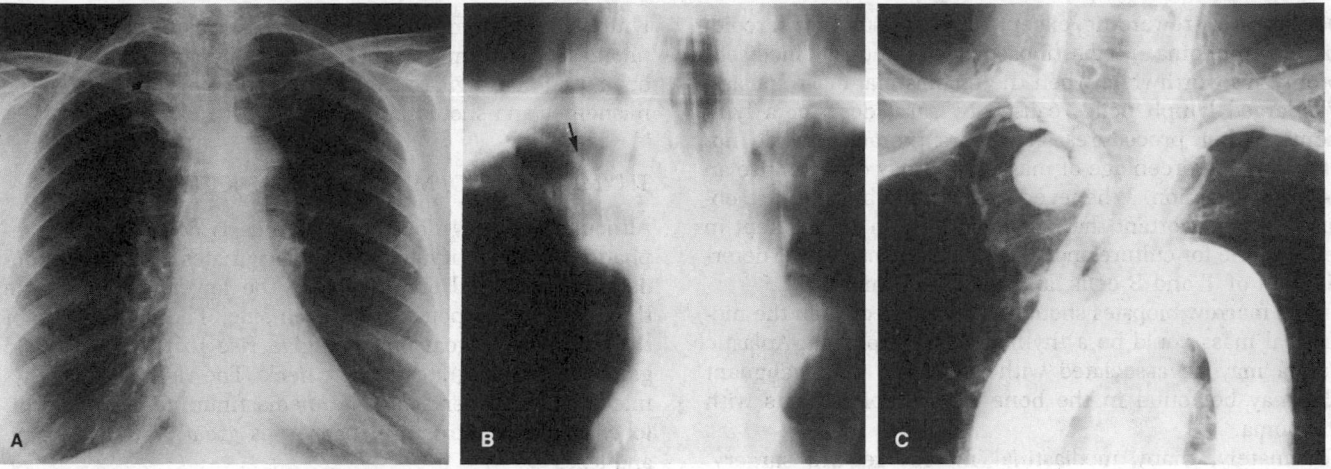

FIG. 23-4. Anterosuperior mediastinal mass seen on a plain film of the chest (**A**) and by tomography (**B**)was revealed to be a saccular aneurysm of the innominate artery when an arteriogram was obtained (**C**).

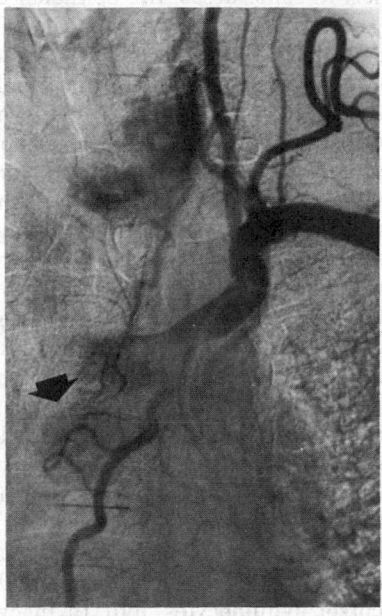

FIG. 23-5. Anteriograms delineate a parathyroid adenoma located within the thymus gland.

the mediastinal anatomy very well but has the disadvantage of requiring long scanning times, great expense, and limited availability.

If a thyroid scan is to be carried out to delineate a mass in the anterosuperior mediastinum, ^{131}I must be used rather than technetium pertechnetate, which will not identify mediastinal masses because of the high background of this nuclide in the vascular structures of the chest.[21] Iodine-131 will localize in the thyroid in most patients with mediastinal thyroid tissue. As many as 10% of mediastinal masses may be goiter, with as many as 25% in the posterior mediastinum.

ENDOSCOPY

Bronchoscopy and esophagoscopy should be performed whenever the radiographic abnormality could in any way be caused by a lung or esophageal tumor. The frequency of lung cancer requires that it be considered in patients with a smoking history who are 40 years of age or older.

BIOPSY PROCEDURES

If cervical or supraclavicular nodes are palpable, they should be biopsied. Scalene node biopsy in the absence of palpable

FIG. 23-6. Computed tomography of the patient with the thymoma depicted in Figure 23-3. The thymoma (*T*) is located immediately anterior to the base of the heart (*H*).

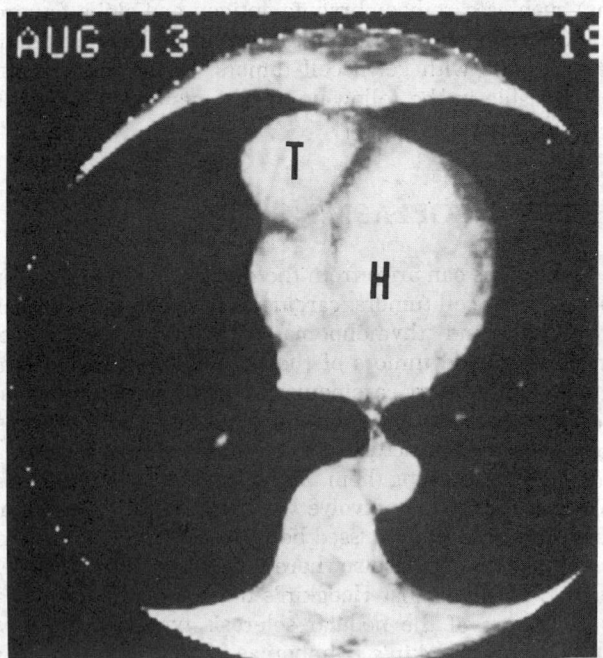

nodes is rarely rewarding, except when one suspects sarcoidosis or lymphoma. Mediastinoscopy and anterior mediastinotomy are worthwhile when the mediastinal mass consists of enlarged lymph nodes caused by sarcoidosis or a lymphoma. Other procedures short of a thoracotomy do not detect a high percentage of masses and may compromise an adequate resection. Whenever lymph node biopsies are obtained, it is important that portions of the node are kept in sterile saline for culture and sensitivity studies, for the determination of T and B cells, and for direct imprints.

Bone marrow biopsies should be considered when the mediastinal mass could be a thymoma or lymphoma. Aplastic anemia may be associated with thymoma, and malignant cells may be found in the bone marrow of patients with lymphoma.

Ultimately, many mediastinal masses require surgery. Thoracotomy will be required, using a median sternotomy or posterolateral incision. However, even under these circumstances, biopsy of a mass that cannot be completely removed occasionally leaves the pathologist confused if light microscopy alone is relied upon. Electron microscopy should be used in these instances.

If the patient with a mediastinal mass cannot tolerate a thoracotomy because of cardiopulmonary insufficiency, one of the limited biopsy procedures, an aspiration, or a needle biopsy of the mass may be attempted.[22] However, before this is done, be sure the structure being biopsied is not of vascular origin by using one or more of the imaging procedures.

HORMONAL ASSAYS AND TUMOR MARKERS

Hormonal assays and the determination of tumor markers may be of value in selected instances. Pheochromocytomas and some neurogenic tumors will be accompanied by elevated urinary catecholamine, homovanillic acid, or vanillyl mandelic acid levels. Germ cell tumors, teratomas, and some carcinomas will also elaborate glycoproteins (oncofetal antigens) such as carcinoembryonic antigen and alpha-fetoprotein. Chorionic gonadotrophin levels may be elevated in some patients with germ cell tumors. These markers are most valuable in the follow-up of patients and occasionally useful for diagnosis.

THYMIC NEOPLASMS

Several lesions can arise from the thymus: lymphomas, thymomas, germ cell tumors, carcinoids of the thymus, thymic carcinomas, and thymolipomas. Thymomas, germ cell tumors, carcinoid tumors of the thymus, mediastinal lymphomas, and primary carcinomas of the thymus may be confused with each other because of similarities in their gross and microscopic structure. Electron microscopy is of great value in differentiating them. Both Hodgkin's and non-Hodgkin's lymphomas may involve the thymus, but thymic lymphomas will not be discussed because they act the same as lymphomas that occur elsewhere (see Chap. 50). However, it should be noted that Hodgkin's disease of the thymus is almost always of the nodular sclerosis type and the most common non-Hodgkin's lymphomas of the thymus are the lymphoblastic lymphomas and the large-cell diffuse lymphomas. The term, "granulomatous thymoma," which has been used to designate Hodgkin's disease of the thymus, is a misnomer and should be discarded.[23]

THYMIC DEVELOPMENT AND FUNCTION

Although the fully developed thymus is considered a lymphatic organ, embryologically it originates from the endoderm as epithelial outgrowths of the lower portion of the third pharyngeal pouches on each side. The upper parts of the third pharyngeal pouches give rise to the parathyroid glands, which migrate into the neck. The right and left thymic anlagen descend into the mediastinum to become a bilobed glandular structure that varies greatly in both shape and size.[24-26]

The cords of epithelial cells that initially make up the thymus grow out into the surrounding mesenchyma. These cords subsequently constitute the medullary areas of the lobules of the thymus.[27] The epithelial cells in the cords eventually spread out to form a reticulum but never lose contact with each other. In some areas, the epithelial cells pile up and undergo keratinization and degeneration, forming distinctive structures known as Hassall's corpuscles. These structures are found in the medulla of the lobules.

As the epithelial cords proliferate and send out side branches into the mesenchyma, lymphocytes appear within the spaces between the epithelial cells of the cortex of the lobules. These lymphocytes are derived from hematopoietic stem cells that arise in the bone marrow and migrate to the thymus. The stem cells are concentrated in the periphery of the cortex of the thymic lobules. They give rise to the smaller lymphocytes, which are located in the deeper cortex of the lobule and fill the spaces between the epithelial cells. Medullary areas of the lobules in the mature thymus contain few lymphocytes and are largely epithelial in character. Germinal centers and lymphoid follicles are normally not found in the thymus.[26]

The process of lymphoblastic differentiation into mature thymocytes requires a humoral factor produced by the epithelial cells of the thymus. One preparation of this hormone (thymosine) is a polypeptide that can support the development of precursor lymphocytes into thymocytes.[28] This preparation and others, such as the thymic humoral factor of Trainin, are common to all mammals studied thus far.[29]

The differentiation of human lymphoblasts into thymocytes by the thymus takes place in fetal and early postnatal life. The thymocytes in the deeper cortex of the thymic lobules enter the circulation and populate all of the lymphatic tissue as thymus-derived lymphocytes (T lymphocytes). They have characteristic surface markers and specialized immunological functions, but are morphologically similar to the other major class of lymphocytes, the bone-marrow-derived lymphocytes (B lymphocytes).

Congenital absence of the thymus (DiGeorge syndrome) or its removal early in life results in a deficiency of cellular immune function. Thymectomy in the adult will also result in a decrease in immunological competence. However, because the half-life of thymus-derived lymphocytes in man is several years, the decrease in immunologic function due to the loss of T lymphocytes is gradual and less evident than when the thymus is removed at birth or shortly thereafter.

Although the mature thymus glands of individuals vary greatly with respect to size and shape, there is a relatively predictable pattern with respect to their size and the age of the patients. The thymus gland reaches a maximum size of 30 to 40 g in the adolescent, but its greatest size relative to the rest of the body is attained at about 4 years of age.[26] Following puberty, the thymus gradually involutes and the lymphoid component disappears. The parenchyma is largely replaced by fat. Hassell's corpuscles remain to identify the gland. The thymus never completely disappears.

A study of the morphology of the adult thymus by Bell and colleagues quantitated the variation in the dimensions and configuration of the thymus (Fig. 23-7).[24] The gland is generally situated beneath the upper part of the sternum. Its lower tip may end at any point between the first intercostal space and the costal cartilage of the seventh rib. In two thirds of the cases studied by Bell and colleagues, the caudal extremity of the thymus was between the third and fourth ribs. The thoracic portion of the thymus is usually thickest where it rests on pericardium. The cervical extent of the thymus is usually the least distinct of the gland's margins. The upper end of the thymus blends imperceptibly into the cervical fat and may extend up to the level of the sixth cervical vertebra.

THYMOMA

It is the epithelium of the thymus gland derived from the third pharyngeal pouches that may undergo neoplastic change to create a thymoma. Lymphocytic elements may be present and even dominate the histologic appearance of a

FIG. 23-7. The caudal tip of thymus gland was found between the third and fourth ribs in 66% of the 125 cadavers studied by Bell and colleagues.[24] Almost all of the glands terminated at some point above the xyphoid.

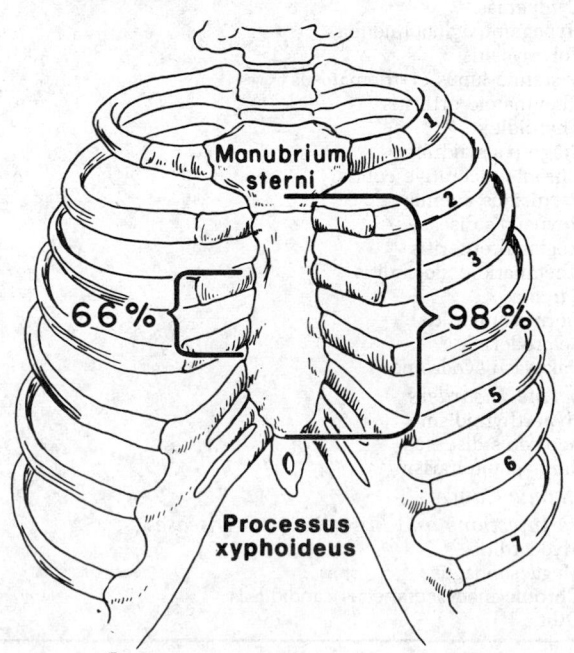

thymoma. Nevertheless, a neoplasm of the thymus is not considered to be a thymoma unless the epithelial component is the neoplastic element. The immunologic characteristics of the lymphocytic component of thymomas are similar to the phenotype of immature lymphocytes (thymocytes) found in the normal thymus, thus supporting the contention that thymomas are strictly tumors of thymic epithelium.[30]

Pathology

Thymomas have fibrous septae on cut section. Cystic areas are seen in 40% to 60% of specimens.[26] Several classifications of thymomas have been devised, based on the histopathology of these tumors. Rosai and Levine have reviewed this aspect of thymomas completely in their monograph.[26] The simplest classification designates three types, based on the predominant cell type comprising the tumor: lymphocytic, epithelial, and mixed (lymphoepithelial). A cell type is considered predominant by Bergh and colleagues if more than 80% of the tumor is made up of that cell.[31] By their standards, 23% of 43 thymomas studied were lymphocytic; 35% were lymphoepithelial; and 42% were epithelial.

The pathologists at the Mayo Clinic reviewed 197 thymomas and classified them into four types: lymphocytic (35% of tumors), epithelial (18%), mixed (25%), and spindle cell (22%).[9] Spindle cell thymomas are considered variants of epithelial thymomas.

Another variant of the epithelial thymoma is the pseudorosette type characterized by a predominant pattern of pseudorosette formation by the neoplastic epithelial cells.

The Mayo Clinic group found that patients with thymomas of mixed or predominantly epithelial cell types had lower survival rates than patients with spindle cell or predominantly lymphocytic cell types.[9] At the University of Michigan, epithelial thymomas also tended to be more extensive and pursue a more aggressive course.[32]

Most researchers do not find a correlation between the histopathology of a specific thymoma and its invasive potential.[26] Nor is there a correlation between the histopathology of a thymoma and the coexistence of associated systemic syndromes.[26] The malignancy of a thymoma is determined by its invasive characteristics rather than the microscopic appearance of the tumor. The number of mitotic figures seen is low in all thymomas, regardless of the invasiveness of the tumor.[26,31-37]

In general, thymomas are slow-growing tumors. Some have stayed the same size for as long as 15 years.[26] This has led to the designation of some thymomas as benign and others as malignant. A "benign" thymoma has been defined as a tumor that is well-encapsulated and does not invade adjacent mediastinal structures. Fifty percent to 65% of the thymomas fit this definition (Fig. 23-8). However, the distinction between a benign and a malignant thymoma is artificial and should be replaced by the designation encapsulated and invasive.[1] All thymomas are potentially invasive, and therefore they should all be considered malignant.

The surgeon is usually in the best position to determine whether a thymoma has infiltrated the surrounding tissue. Frozen-section analyses of dense fibrous attachments between the thymoma and surrounding tissue may be neces-

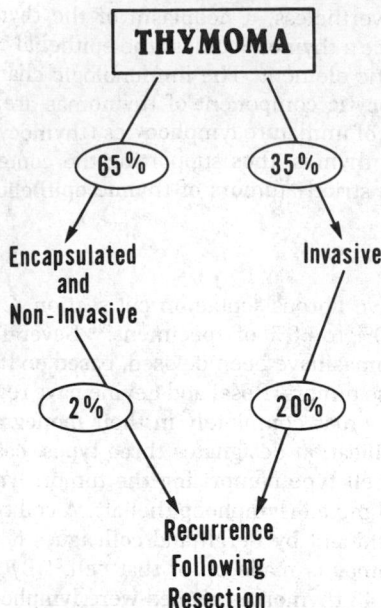

FIG. 23-8. Although figures vary from series to series, generally about two thirds of thymomas are "benign." The recurrence rate after removal of these tumors is low, in contrast to the higher recurrence rate after resection of invasive thymomas.

sary to be sure that the tumor is truly confined by its capsule. The capsule should be carefully examined for any discontinuity, which may represent an area of local invasion. The most common form of metastatic involvement is the occurrence of pleural or pericardial implants. They are thought to result from the shedding of tumor cells from the primary thymoma.

Staging of thymomas is based on the extent of invasiveness. The following staging system has been suggested by Bergh and colleagues:[31]

Stage I: Intact capsule or growth within the capsule
Stage II: Pericapsular growth into the mediastinal fat tissue
Stage III: Invasive growth into the surrounding organs, intrathoracic metastases or both

In the series from the University of Goteborg in Sweden, 40% of patients were stage I, 19% were stage II, and 41% were stage III. Thymomas over 500 g were all stage III tumors. Pleural metastases occurred in half of the patients with stage III thymomas. A more comprehensive staging system has been proposed, which subdivides the three stages based on additional pathologic findings at the time of surgery.[38] The drawback to these more detailed staging systems is the small number of patients available for analysis if they are classified into more than three groups.

Metastases to regional nodes or distant organs is uncommon. Only 30 instances of blood-borne metastases to extrathoracic sites were reported before 1976.[1] More have been reported since then. The organs involved were the liver, bone, colon, kidney, brain, and spleen. Epithelial thymomas gave rise to these metastases more often than other

tumors. Thymomas, although rare in children, appear to run a more malignant course in them than in adults.[39]

Clinical Findings

Fortuitous discovery of a thymoma when a chest roentgenogram is obtained for reasons unrelated to the tumor occurs in 30% to 40% of patients with this neoplasm. Patients are usually between 40 and 60 years of age. No more than 10% of thymomas are found in patients younger than 20 years of age.[36] There is very little difference in the frequency with which men and women are affected, although some series report a slightly increased incidence in women.

Vague, nonspecific symptoms may be present, such as cough, dyspnea, dysphagia, chest tightness, and chest pain. Chest pain may be a sign of an advanced malignant lesion. A superior vena cava syndrome may also result from an advanced lesion.

Thymoma-associated Systemic Syndromes

The systemic syndromes that may be associated with a thymoma are listed in Table 23-7, and the three most common will be discussed. The occurrence of these syndromes often leads to the discovery of a thymoma.

Because both the parathyroid and thymus glands are derived from the third pharyngeal pouches, the group at the Mayo Clinic thought it would be reasonable to compare the incidence of diseases associated with thymomas and parathyroid adenomas, the latter acting as a control to the former.[40] They reviewed 146 of their own patients with thymoma and

TABLE 23-7. Syndromes and Diseases Associated with Thymomas

Autoimmune or Immune Phenomena
    Myasthenia gravis
    Cytopenias
    Hypogammaglobulinemia
    Polymyositis
    Systemic lupus erythematosus
    Rheumatoid arthritis
    Thyroiditis
    Sjögren's syndrome
    Chronic ulcerative colitis
    Pernicious anemia
    Raynaud's disease
    Regional enteritis
    Rheumatic endocarditis
    Sarcoid
    Dermatomyositis
    Scleroderma
    Takayasu syndrome
Endocrine Disorders
    Hyperthyroidism
    Addison's disease
    Panhypopituitarism
Nonthymic Cancer
Severe Infections and Miscellaneous Diseases
    Myocarditis
    Megaesophagus
    Chronic macrocutaneous candidiasis
    Other

452 found in the literature with sufficient data to evaluate whether or not an associated disease occurred. The incidence of other diseases with thymomas was 71%, compared with a 12% incidence in 177 patients with parathyroid adenomas. The diseases associated with thymomas were classified into categories (Table 23-7).

In some patients more than one disease was associated with the thymoma, such as myasthenia gravis and thrombocytopenia. Almost 70% of the patients with thymoma and other diseases will have immunologic disorders. About 10% will have a malignancy and 5% will have an endocrine disorder. The remaining 15% will have a severe infection or another seemingly unrelated condition, such as megaesophagus. The most frequent association is between thymoma and myasthenia gravis. Some 40% to 50% of patients with syndromes associated with thymoma have myasthenia gravis. Some of the endocrine disorders, such as Cushing's syndrome, are concomitants of carcinoid tumor of the thymus, which may be mistakenly diagnosed as a thymoma.

MYASTHENIA GRAVIS. The pathophysiologic characteristic of myasthenia gravis is the rapid exhaustion of voluntary muscular contractions, with a slow return to a normal state. Repetitive stimulation of the motor nerve to a muscle in patients with myasthenia gravis results in a progressive decrement of muscle action potentials. Thus, the major symptoms of patients with this disease are weakness and fatigability. Another characteristic is that these symptoms are relieved by drugs that inhibit acetylcholinesterese, an enzyme located within the synaptic junction (the end plate) between the motor neuron and striated muscle. Because of these features of myasthenia gravis, the disease is considered an abnormality of neuromuscular transmission.[41]

It is widely accepted that myasthenia gravis is an autoimmune disease caused by antibodies directed against acetylcholine receptors in voluntary muscle. A myasthenic state can be produced in rabbits by immunizing them with a purified protein having the properties of acetylcholine receptors.[42] The effect of the immune response is to eliminate acetylcholine receptors and impair postsynaptic structure and functions. Patients with myasthenia gravis have 70% to 90% fewer acetylcholine receptors per neuromuscular junction than do normal people.[41] Because there is a decreased number of acetylcholine receptors present within the end plate of patients with myasthenia gravis, acetylcholine, which is responsible for neuromuscular transmission across the synaptic junction, is less effective in transmitting the signal from nerve to muscle.

An association between the thymus and myasthenia was first suspected when pathologic changes were found in the thymus gland of 75% to 85% of patients with this neuromuscular disease (Fig. 23-9). Germinal centers are not normally present in the thymus gland; yet 70% of patients with myasthenia gravis and thymic abnormalities demonstrate this form of "thymic lymphoid (follicular) hyperplasia."[43] It is characterized by germinal center proliferation in the medullary and cortical areas of the thymus, without necessarily increasing the gross appearance or weight of the thymus. Furthermore, 15% to 50% of patients with myasthenia will have gross or microscopic (occult) thymomas, depending

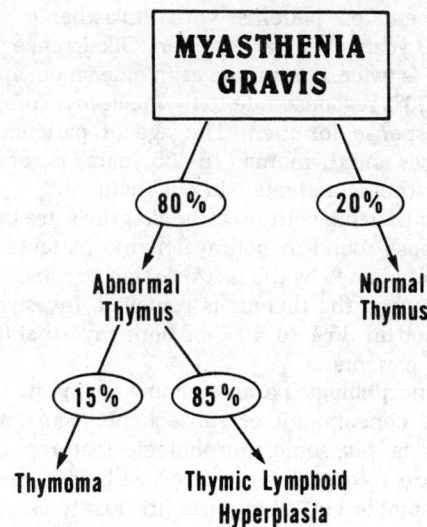

FIG. 23-9. Thymic abnormalities are frequent in patients with myasthenia. Both thymic lymphoid hyperplasia and thymoma may be present in the same patient.

upon the frequency with which patients with myasthenia gravis have thymectomy or have an autopsy to search for this lesion. Follicular hyperplasia of the nonneoplastic portions of the thymus may accompany a thymoma.

Thymectomy in patients with myasthenia gravis can be effective in producing a complete remission of the disease in 20% to 36% of patients. An additional 57% to 86% will be improved (Fig. 23-10).[41] The presence of a thymoma in a patient with myasthenia carries a poorer prognosis than for myasthenia patients without thymomas. Improvement in muscle strength following thymectomy can be anticipated in only 25% of patients with myasthenia and a thymoma. A 40% to 60% response rate may result when myasthenic patients have a thymectomy and do not have a thymoma.

FIG. 23-10. Response to thymectomy varies depending on age and sex of the patient and whether a thymoma is present.

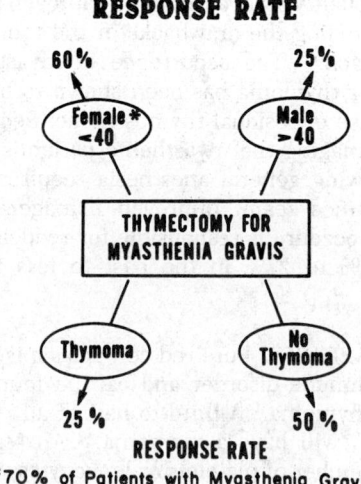

Seventy percent of patients with myasthenia gravis younger than 40 years of age are women. Occurrence of the disease in them is twice as common as in older men, and the women have a 60% response rate to thymectomy, compared with a 25% response for men. The age of patients with myasthenia gravis and thymoma (15–35 years) is generally older than myasthenic patients without thymoma.

Thymomas in patients with myasthenia gravis are usually smaller than those found in nonmyasthenic patients. This finding may be explained by the fact that they are discovered serendipitously when the thymus is removed. Invasive thymomas are found in 35% to 40% of both myasthenic and nonmyasthenic patients.

There is no morphologic parameter in a thymoma that is specific for the concomitant or subsequent occurrence of myasthenia gravis, but some morphologic features of thymomas are more frequently associated with myasthenia.[43] For example, spindle cell thymomas are rarely associated with myasthenia gravis. Another feature of thymomas and myasthenia gravis is the high frequency of lymphoid follicles with germinal centers in the thymic tissues surrounding the thymoma.[26]

The association of the thymus, thymomas, and myasthenia gravis remains an enigma despite all that has been learned in the past decade. There are data to suggest that myoid or muscle-like cells in the thymus and thymomas cross-react with antimuscle antibodies. These cells may be responsible for initiating the antibodies.[41] It has been suggested that a virally induced "thymitis" could trigger the process in which antigenic components within the thymus are recognized by the T lymphocytes and that these antigens cross-react with acetylcholine receptors.[41]

Myasthenic patients may show significant improvement after receiving immunosuppressive drugs, such as corticosteroids and azathioprine.[41,44] The salutory effect of thymectomy may also be explained by the immunosuppressive effect of extirpation of this gland.

Two important aspects of thymectomy for patients with thymomas and myasthenia gravis deserve mention. First, the entire thymus must be removed, along with the thymoma, and an aggressive surgical approach demands the wide resection of invaded structures if possible. Transcervical thymectomy may qualify as an acceptable approach to removing the thymus, avoiding the drawbacks of the more extensive thoracic approach.[45] The occurrence of myasthenia after thymectomy for thymoma has been shown to be related to recurrent disease of residual thymus tissue. Second, the intricacies of managing the myasthenic patient's respiratory problems following general anesthesia requires an experienced, well-trained team. Improved management of this phase of the procedure is responsible for reducing the mortality from 10% to 27% in the past to less than 6% at present.[41]

RED CELL APLASIA. Pure red cell aplasia is also considered an autoimmune disorder and can be found in 5% of patients with thymoma.[1] A third to half of all patients with red cell aplasia will have a thymoma.[46] An associated decrease in the number of platelets or leukocytes will be found in 30% of patients with red cell aplasia. This syndrome appears after the age of 40 in 96% of the patients who develop it. The diagnosis is based on examination of the bone marrow. Red cell precursors are absent, but platelet and leukocytic elements are normal. Thymectomy will result in a 25% to 30% remission of the disease.[46] The relationship between thymoma and red cell aplasia is not yet understood.

HYPOGAMMAGLOBULINEMIA. This abnormality is present in 5% to 10% of patients with thymoma.[40] Patients with hypogammaglobulinemia have a 10% incidence of thymoma. More than a third of those patients also have red cell hypoplasia. Combined humoral and cellular immunodeficiencies are present. Almost all patients are over the age of 40 years. Thymectomy has not proved beneficial in this condition.

Roentgenographic Features of Thymomas

Seventy-five percent of tumors are located in the anterior mediastinum and are the most frequent neoplasms found in this compartment (see Fig. 23-3). Approximately 15% occupy both the anterior and superior mediastinum, and 6% are primarily in the superior mediastinum. No more than 5% to 10% of thymomas occur in other locations, such as the neck and middle and posterior mediastinum. The lesion is characteristically located anterior to the junction of the great vessels, which may be displaced posteriorly by the tumor. Thymomas are round or oval, with smooth or lobulated margins. The mass may protrude to one or both sides of the mediastinum. Calcifications may be seen in as many as 20% of thymomas, either at the periphery of the tumor or throughout its substance.[26] Calcifications are best visualized by overpenetrated films, laminograms, or by CT (see Fig. 23-6).

CT allows precise definition of the extent of involvement and the nature of a tumor mass suspected of being a thymoma.[47] Among 19 patients with myasthenia gravis, CT was accurate in detecting 9 of the masses that were present but could not differentiate thymomas from nonthymomatous masses. Glands with thymic hyperplasia could not be differentiated from normal glands.[48] Cysts can be more easily differentiated from solid tumors by CT. By measuring the thickness of the thymic lobes, thymic hyperplasia and lymphoma can be diagnosed.[49] Pleural metastases are also more easily identified by CT than by conventional roentgenograms or laminograms of the chest.[47]

Treatment of Thymoma

SURGERY. The most effective therapy of a thymoma is its complete removal. When the thymoma is encapsulated and can be removed with the entire thymus, without disturbing the integrity of the capsule, virtually all patients will be cured of the tumor. As few as 2% will develop recurrences, which take the form of pleural, pericardial, or diaphragmatic implants or of a localized mediastinal tumor (Fig. 23-11).[37]

Poor prognostic determinants are invasiveness of the tumor and an associated syndrome such as myasthenia gravis.[34,50] Associated diseases are present in half of all patients who develop a recurrence following surgery. Fortu-

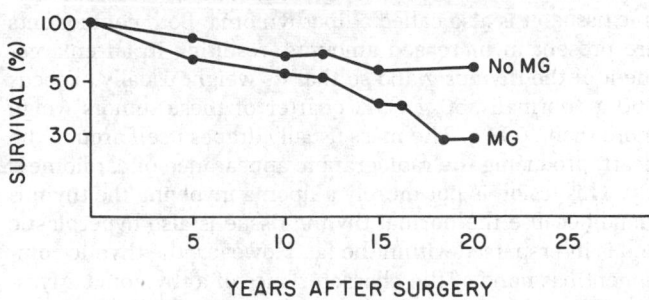

SURVIVAL FOLLOWING OPERATION
FOR ENCAPSULATED THYMOMA

FIG. 23-11. Bernatz found that patients with thymoma and myasthenia gravis had a poorer prognosis than did those without myasthenia gravis (*MG*). (Bernatz PE, Khonsari S, Harrison EG et al: Thymomas: Factors influencing prognosis. Surg Clin North Am 53:885, 1973)

nately, 65% of thymomas are well-encapsulated and not associated with myasthenia gravis. As expected of patients with a neuromuscular disorder, survival following resection of encapsulated thymomas is also poor when myasthenia gravis is present (Fig. 23-11). However, recent experiences have shown that patients with thymoma and myasthenia gravis do as well as those without myasthenia.[51]

Because of the propensity of thymomas to recur or develop local metastases when the integrity of the capsule is violated, biopsy of these tumors should be avoided. The tumor should be removed intact whenever possible. Biopsy should be reserved for the patient who is unable to tolerate a resection. Needle aspiration is another option for such patients.[22]

Thymectomy and resection of a thymoma is best carried out using a midline sternal-splitting incision. A bilateral submammary incision transecting the sternum may provide a more cosmetic result. However, the exposure this incision provides is not optimal, and it may be more difficult to deal with any invasive lesions encountered. The poor exposure provided by a cervical incision renders this approach unsatisfactory, although it may be used for smaller lesions. Standard right or left thoracotomies have been performed if the tumor appears to be present largely on one side or the other.

Resection of encapsulated noninvasive thymomas presents few problems to the surgeon because they are easily removed.[34] Invasive tumors, on the other hand, can be difficult and challenging. An aggressive surgical approach should be adopted because these tumors are slow-growing and remain localized in the chest for long periods. In order to obtain sufficient exposure to resect all of the tumor, the median sternotomy may have to be combined with a thoracotomy. Pericardium, phrenic nerve, pleura, diaphragm, and lung can be resected if these structures are involved. Lobectomy and pneumonectomy may be required, depending upon the specific circumstances and extent of involvement. Resection of the innominate vein and portions or all of the superior vena cava has been performed when these vessels are invaded.[52] A patch graft of autogenous vein or prosthetic material or a vascular graft of Teflon or Dacron can be used to bridge the resulting venous defect, with expectation of a

good functional result. When extensive involvement precludes complete resection, such as with invasion of the heart, great vessels, or trachea, as much tumor as can be safely resected should be removed to prevent cardiac tamponade or tracheal occlusion and asphyxiation. Resection should also be considered in the treatment of local recurrences and pleural and pericardial metastases.

RADIOTHERAPY. Thymomas are relatively radiosensitive. Radiation therapy constitutes excellent adjuvant therapy and is considered mandatory for all patients with invasive thymomas, whether or not a complete resection is performed.[53,54] The surgeon should therefore mark off the extent of the resected tumor and thymus with metallic radiopaque clips in order to facilitate treatment planning by the radiotherapist. Preoperative radiation therapy was used by several groups and was not helpful.[55] Investigative efforts are currently underway to determine if intraoperative radiation therapy may be of benefit.

There is some disagreement concerning the role of adjuvant radiotherapy for patients with encapsulated noninvasive thymomas. Because the recurrence rate is low (about 2%) and radiotherapy carries some morbidity, Rosai and Levine oppose the use of postoperative radiotherapy if these tumors are removed in toto.[26] At the other extreme is the view that no patient with thymoma can be considered to have been adequately treated unless he receives radiotherapy.[38] It is reasonable to adopt either course, depending upon the circumstances. If long-term follow-up is not possible or likely, and experienced radiotherapists are able to treat the area with minimal side effects, patients with noninvasive thymomas may be advised to undergo postoperative radiotherapy. On the other hand, easily followed patients with small, encapsulated tumors, which were removed with the entire thymus, can receive radiation if recurrences appear. Reresection should also be considered. In the absence of a prospective controlled randomized study, no definitive statement can be made concerning the role of adjuvant radiotherapy for Stage I thymomas.

Radiotherapy as adjuvant therapy, for the treatment of recurrences or to treat unresectable primary thymomas, usually consists of 3500 to 4500 rad given over 3 to 6 weeks. Dosages in excess of 4500 rad do not significantly increase response rates but do increase the risk of postirradiation complications if large fields are used. If the tumor is small, Penn and Hope-Stone recommend using two large anterior oblique wedge fields.[54] Field size in their experience was about 15 cm by 8 cm. More extensive lesions are treated with large parallel opposed fields, which can be supplemented with a wedge pair or an additional direct anterior field. Field sizes up to 20 cm by 15 cm are used. These techniques minimize exposure to the spinal cord.

In addition to irradiating the tumor, it is also often important to treat the entire thymus gland, which extends from the sixth cervical vertebra to the level of the fourth to seventh costal cartilage. Skeggs recommends a single anterior and two posterior oblique fields to provide satisfactory dose distribution.[56]

Marks and colleagues recommend a dose of 4000 rad to the tumor bed in 4 to 5 weeks if the invasive thymoma is completely removed. The last 1000 rad should be given with a pair of anterior oblique fields to reduce the total dose to the spinal cord. For unresectable or partially resectable disease, a dose of 4500 rad in 5 to 6 weeks is recommended. Shrinking fields should be used as the tumor responds. A split course of irradiation should be considered for large tumors in order to spare the spinal cord.[57] This approach has resulted in 100% local tumor control in 9 patients when used in conjunction with resection.

Pneumonitis is a frequent (40%) side effect of radiotherapy when large fields are used.[54] To minimize radiation damage to the lungs in patients with pleural implants, Ariaratnam and colleagues use a moving strip technique.[53] Mediastinitis, pericarditis, and myocarditis are additional infrequent complications of thymic radiation when unresectable or residual thymomas require large fields and high doses. However, if unresectable or residual tumor is carefully marked out at operation by the surgeon, it should be possible to treat a small tumor volume to a high dose without undue complications.

CHEMOTHERAPY. Corticosteroids have caused regression of some unresectable thymomas that do not respond to radiotherapy.[45] Chemotherapy for thymomas should be reserved for patients with advanced disease who respond neither to radiation nor steroids. Effective single drugs are cisplatin and doxorubicin.[58] Responses have also been reported with the use of alkylating agents.[45] Daugaard and colleagues reported complete responses, which lasted a median of 37 months, in four of nine patients treated with vincristine, cyclophosphamide, lomustine, and prednisone.[59] These are the best results in the largest series of patients treated with chemotherapy. The overall response rate was 56%. Partial remissions have been reported with combinations of cyclophosphamide, vincristine, prednisone, and procarbazine and with combinations of bleomycin, doxorubicin, cisplatin, and prednisone.[38,60,61]

RESULTS OF THERAPY. At the Mayo Clinic, the 10-year survival rate for noninvasive tumors was 65%, compared with 30% for invasive tumors.[50] The 5-year survival at the Memorial Hospital for encapsulated and invasive tumors was 83% and 54%, respectively.[36] Less than half of the patients with invasive thymomas who survived for 5 years were free of disease. Ten-year survival of patients with thymoma treated at the Massachusetts General Hospital are 57% overall; totally resected, 72%; encapsulated tumor without myasthenia gravis, 85%; and invasive tumor with myasthenia gravis, 8.7%. In France, patients with noninvasive thymomas had survival rates of 85% at 5 years and 80% at 10 years. Patients with invasive tumors had a survival rate of about 50% at 5 years and 35% at 10 years. In this series, associated autoimmune diseases had no influence on survival. All patients were treated with radiation postoperatively. Recurrences were found in 6% of patients with noninvasive tumors and in 36% of patients with invasive tumors. Slightly invasive, completely excised thymomas had the same rate of recurrence as largely invasive tumors in which only biopsy had been performed.[38]

THYMOLIPOMA

This tumor is a curious mixture of fat and hyperplastic thymic tissue. It is also called a lipothymoma. Both components are present in increased amounts, resulting in an enlargement of the thymus gland so that its weight usually exceeds 500 g (normally 50 g).[26] A quarter of these tumors weigh more than 2000 g. The mass usually drapes itself around the heart, producing the radiographic appearance of cardiomegaly. This lesion is not merely a lipoma involving the thymus gland because the normal thymic tissue is also hyperplastic and is interspersed within the fat. However, the thymic component has none of the characteristics of a thymoma. Myasthenia gravis has not occurred in association with this tumor. This is a rare, benign tumor that has never been reported to invade adjacent structures, to metastasize, or to recur following removal.

CARCINOID OF THE THYMUS

Until 1972, many carcinoid tumors of the thymus were not recognized as distinct lesions and were mistakenly labeled as variants of thymomas.[26,62-64] The fact that they have a similar morphology and similar biologic characteristics with respect to their malignant potential and that they respond to the same therapy probably accounts for the confusion between carcinoids and thymomas. However, significant morphological and biochemical differences exist between these two tumors, and they can be readily differentiated.

Thymic carcinoids develop from cells of neural crest origin, which differentiate into Kulchitsky cells. They can undergo malignant change to become carcinoid tumors. No more than 100 thymic carcinoids have been reported in the literature as of 1980.[64] Their gross appearance is similar to that of thymomas. The tumors may be encapsulated or invade adjacent structures. Invasiveness is seen in 50% of thymic carcinoids, compared with 35% of thymomas. Furthermore, thymomas rarely have extrathoracic metastases, but thymic carcinoids metastasize to bone, often forming blastic lesions, and other sites in up to 73% of patients with this tumor. Metastases may appear as long as 8 years after initial diagnosis.[64]

Fibrous compartmentalization and cystic changes seen in thymomas do not occur with thymic carcinoids. The two tumors may have similar appearances by light microscopy, but electron microscopy can accurately differentiate carcinoid tumors from thymomas. Carcinoids are characterized by numerous cytoplasmic neurosecretory granules, as are other foregut carcinoids. Thymomas will have desmosones, tonofilaments, and elongated cytoplasmic processes not seen in carcinoids. Carcinoids will also contain argyrophil cells that can be detected by appropriate staining techniques.

Thymic carcinoids have been classified among the "amine precursor uptake and decarboxylation" tumors (APUDomas), which are known to have the potential of elaborating peptides, amines, kinins, and prostaglandins. The only endocrine syndrome reported to be directly caused by thymic carcinoids is Cushing's syndrome. In these instances, the carcinoid produces elevated levels of ACTH. Patients with carcinoid syndrome caused by thymic carcinoids have not been reported, but other endocrine tumors have occurred with thymic carcinoids. Approximately one third to one half of thymic carcinoids have been associated with paraneoplastic syndromes. Although most of these have been Cushing's syndrome, patients with thymic carcinoids have been described with Type I multiple endocrine neoplasias (MEN I; Werner's syndrome; pituitary, parathyroid, and pancreatic islet cell tumors). In two thirds of these patients, the carcinoids have been malignant. Carcinoid tumors of the thymus have also been reported to coexist with medullary carcinomas of the thyroid (MEN II: Sipple's syndrome, medullary thyroid carcinoma, pheochromocytoma, and hyperparathyroidism). It has been postulated that the rare oat cell carcinomas of the thymus can arise from a carcinoid tumor of the thymus.[63,65]

Carcinoid tumors of the thymus are treated by wide excision of the thymus containing the tumor. The resection should include contiguous invaded structures that can be sacrificed or replaced. Postoperative radiation therapy has helped patients with persistent or recurrent tumor.

GERM CELL TUMORS

Much of the material covered in Chapter 35 on testicular tumors applies to this section as well since testicular and mediastinal germ cell tumors share many characteristics. All types of germinal tumors found in the testes have been reported in the mediastinum.[25] Approximately 10% of all mediastinal tumors are of germinal origin.

HISTOGENESIS

Extragonadal germ cell tumors are usually situated along the body midline in the cranium, the mediastinum, and the retroperitoneal and presacral areas. The histogenesis of these tumors is not clear. Those arising within the thymus presumably originate from germ cells that may have migrated into this gland during embryogenesis. Because the urogenital ridge extends from C6 to L4, its juxtaposition to the thymic anlage favors such a possibility. Alternatively, germ cell tumors may arise from a maldevelopment of a thymic anlage during embryogenesis or from potentially biphasic germ cells left within the thymus.

Germ cell tumors of the mediastinum are considered thymic neoplasms because they most likely arise within the gland. Many studies have demonstrated that they do not represent metastases from a primary gonadal site. Autopsies of patients with these tumors have enabled pathologists to examine multiple sections of the patient's gonads, and no evidence of testicular or ovarian involvement has been found in the vast majority of patients with mediastinal germ cell tumors.[26] Other autopsies of patients with germ cell tumors of the testes have shown that metastases solely to the anterior mediastinum do not occur.[66] If anterior mediastinal metastases are present from a testicular tumor, middle and posterior mediastinal nodes are also involved.[67]

INDICATIONS FOR TESTICULAR BIOPSY

Suggestions have been made to remove or biopsy the testes to exclude the possibility of an occult testicular primary tumor giving rise to mediastinal germ cell tumors. If the testes are abnormal on physical examination, these procedures are indicated. However, testes that appear normal on physical examination and on high-resolution ultrasonography need not be removed nor explored when a mediastinal germ cell tumor is present.[68] However, a testicular biopsy is indicated when lymphangiography or CT demonstrates involvement of pelvic or retroperitoneal lymph nodes or if an isolated retroperitoneal germ cell tumor is discovered.

CLASSIFICATIONS

Several classifications of germ cell tumors have been devised. Mediastinal germ cell tumors are often difficult to fit into any classification because they contain mixtures of various types. Rosai and Levine classify mediastinal germ cell tumors as germinomas (seminomas), adult teratomas, embryonal carcinomas, teratocarcinomas, choriocarcinomas, and yolk sac tumors (endodermal sinus tumors).[26] A simpler system of classification considers tumors as either pure seminomas or nonseminomatous carcinomas.[67] The latter may be pure embryonal carcinomas, pure teratocarcinomas, pure choriocarcinomas, pure entodermal sinus carcinomas, or mixtures of all these elements. Most often, the nonseminomatous tumors are of mixed composition, with or without seminomatous elements.

It is reasonable to classify mediastinal germ cell tumors into primary seminomas of the mediastinum and primary nonseminomatous germ cell tumors of the mediastinum. This division separates the tumors on the basis of their treatment and also by their prognosis. Seminomas have a better prognosis and are more responsive to therapy than the other pure and mixed malignant germ cell tumors of the mediastinum.

PRIMARY SEMINOMAS

Seminomas of the mediastinum make up half of all germ cell tumors of the mediastinum and occur in men 20 to 40 years of age. No more than 5% of these tumors occur in women.[69] They usually cause symptoms by impinging upon structures in the anterior mediastinum. Chest pain, cough, dyspnea, and superior vena caval obstruction are the most prominent symptoms. In a small percentage of patients, other germ cell elements are present in the malignancy in small amounts, resulting in elevated serum levels of alpha-fetoprotein or of the beta unit of human chorionic gonadotrophin (β-HCG). Radioimmunoassays may be required to detect these increases, because immunodiffusion techniques are not sufficiently sensitive. If the levels are very high, the pathologic diagnosis should be reevaluated and a diagnosis of a nonseminomatous tumor of the mixed type should be considered.

Most patients with mediastinal seminoma have extensive involvement of the great vessels when they are first seen. Only 20% of the tumors could be completely excised in the patients reported by the Memorial Hospital and the Mayo

Clinic.[67,70] The role of tumor reductive surgery (debulking) for mediastinal seminomas is questionable. If performed, it should be conservative and not add to the morbidity and mortality of the patient.

Because this tumor is extremely radiosensitive, local disease can usually be well-controlled. The excellent response of seminomas to radiation therapy is in marked contrast to the nonseminomatous germ cell tumors, which are relatively radioresistant. A recent review of the contribution of radiotherapy to the management of primary malignant mediastinal germ cell tumors revealed that the actuarial 5-year survival for seminomas was 100%, but it was only 8.8% for the remaining germ cell varieties.[71]

Megavoltage radiation therapy should be given to all patients. A shaped mediastinal field should be used with a midplane dose of up to 4500 rad over 5 to 6 weeks.[72] This dose is greater than that recommended for gonadal seminoma because it is the experience of some radiotherapists that lower doses may result in local recurrences.[72] A split course therapy with interruption after approximately 2000 to 3000 rad is a possible alternative. A more conservative dose of 3500 to 4000 rad is recommended by the Mayo Clinic group.[70]

It is important to emphasize that radiation therapy is the mainstay of curative therapy for primary mediastinal seminoma. Because the supraclavicular and infraclavicular low cervical lymph nodes can be easily included in the field of radiation, these areas should be treated as well. Prophylactic irradiation of the upper abdominal and para-aortic lymph nodes is recommended by some groups and not deemed necessary by others.

The combination of surgery and radiotherapy will result in a 58% to 82% 5-year survival rate.[72,73] Martini and colleagues reported that the local component of mediastinal seminomas could be controlled by resection and radiation in all patients with this tumor, regardless of the extent of mediastinal involvement.[67] Most patients in their series had disseminated disease, which caused their deaths. For this reason, they recommended early systemic chemotherapy even if there is no disease evident outside the mediastinum.

Metastases from the seminoma are commonly present. Involvement of bone, liver, spleen, tonsil, thyroid, skin, and the central nervous system has been reported. Factors that may predict the presence of distant metastases are age greater than 35 years, fever, superior vena caval obstruction, cervical and supraclavicular lymph node involvement, and hilar disease.[71]

A review of the management of primary mediastinal seminomas pointed out that combination chemotherapy with vinblastine, bleomycin, and cis-platinum (VBP) with or without doxorubicin can induce complete remissions (58%) and long-term disease-free survival.[73] Alkylating agents have also been recommended. A patient treated exclusively with chlorambucil and actinomycin D was free of disease 11 years after diagnosis. These observations and the results obtained in the treatment of testicular seminomas provide an encouraging outlook for patients with mediastinal seminoma.

NONSEMINOMATOUS PURE AND MIXED GERM CELL CARCINOMAS

Nonseminomatous tumors can be pure or mixed germ cell carcinomas. Mixed types contain seminomatous, embryonal, endodermal sinus, teratomatous, or trophoblastic elements. The latter subtype has the appearance and functional characteristics of a choriocarcinoma. Teratocarcinomas can be cystic or solid. All of these tumors occur most often in men. Of 20 patients with mixed germ-cell carcinomas of the mediastinum of various kinds treated at Memorial Sloan-Kettering Cancer Center from 1949 through 1971, 14 were men and 6 were women.[67] In many smaller series, all of the patients have been men. The majority of patients are between 15 and 35 years of age.

Pleuritic or substernal pain with dyspnea, cough, and hemoptysis are frequent presenting symptoms. Gynecomastia is present in 33% to 50% of men with choriocarcinoma. Patients with Kleinfelter's syndrome may be predisposed to the development of nonseminomatous extragonadal germ cell tumors and should be followed carefully.[74]

Elevated levels of β-HCG may be present in patients with choriocarcinoma and can be used to evaluate the efficacy of therapy and detect early recurrences and metastases. Elevated levels of β-HCG are present in 60% of patients with nonseminomatous germ cell tumors.[75] Serum levels of alpha-fetoprotein and carcinoembryonic antigen may also help in identifying some of these tumors preoperatively. If the tumors demonstrate a predominant pattern of endodermal sinus elements, serum alpha-fetoprotein levels are likely to be very high. Approximately 70% of patients with nonseminomatous germ cell tumors have elevated levels of alpha-fetoprotein.[75] These markers can also be used to follow the tumor's response to therapy and to detect recurrences.

Teratocarcinomas usually contain elements of embryonal cell carcinoma, but other malignant components, such as adenocarcinoma, squamous cell carcinoma, and sarcoma may be present.[76]

The mainstay of therapy for nonseminomatous germ cell tumors is intensive chemotherapy. VBP with or without doxorubicin resulted in complete remission in approximately 65% of patients with nonseminomatous germ cell tumors; choriocarcinomas showed the poorest response.[77] Patients with pure endodermal sinus tumors have poor prognoses also. The single most important prognostic indicator for mediastinal endodermal sinus tumors is whether they can be completely excised before or after chemotherapy.[78]

VBP is a toxic regimen, but attempts at lessening the drug dosages seem to reduce its efficacy.[79] A combination of vinblastine, actinomycin D, bleomycin, cis-platinum, and cyclophosphamide (VAB-3) has also been recommended.[80] There is some dissatisfaction with the results of these regimens, and several groups continue to search for better approaches to these tumors.[75,79,81] Some success has recently been achieved with VP-16, ifosfamide, and cisplatin as salvage therapy.[82] The benefit of radiation therapy for control of local and metastatic disease is questionable. Neither irradiation nor surgery can control the local disease for a significant length of time. Resection of the tumor after treatment with combination chemotherapy is recommended and may be beneficial.[75]

BENIGN (ADULT) TERATOMAS

Teratomas are neoplasms that originate in pluripotent cells, and are composed of a wide diversity of tissues foreign to the organ or anatomic site in which they arise. The tumors frequently occur in young adults, with equal incidence in both sexes. Approximately 20% of mediastinal teratomatous tumors are teratocarcinomas.[1] When they are malignant, they can contain any of the varieties of germ cell cancers. The subject of extragonadal teratomas has been comprehensively covered by Gonzalez-Crussi in the Armed Forces Institute of Pathology *Atlas of Tumor Pathology,* which contains a section on mediastinal teratomas.

In adults, the mediastinum is the second most frequent location of a teratoma, after the gonads. In children, the sacrococcygeal area is the most frequent site of teratomas, followed by the mediastinum. Teratomas are found almost exclusively in the anterosuperior mediastinum, at the junction of the heart and great vessels. Calcifications are present in 75% of the lesions. Occasionally, they occur in the pericardium or posterior mediastinum. The tumors contain representations of all three germ layers in a rather mature state. When the lesions are cystic and contain hair and teeth, they have been called dermoid cysts, but this is a misnomer because these tumors, like the ovarian dermoids, are not of ectodermal origin.

Most patients with teratomas are asymptomatic. Those with symptoms have them because of the size of the tumor and compression of adjacent structures. Tumors have reached 30 cm in diameter. Erosion into a bronchus is an uncommon complication, as is rupture into the pericardium. Insulin production by a teratoma may produce hypoglycemia.

Benign teratomas are easily excised after exposing them through a sternal-splitting or standard thoracotomy incision.

THYMIC CARCINOMA

The histogenesis of thymic carcinoma is indeterminate.[1] Wick and colleagues reviewed a large series of patients with this diagnosis and presented evidence suggesting that the tumors are more malignant variants of thymic epithelium, which differ from thymomas morphologically as well as biologically.[83] About half are highly undifferentiated. The others may have adenocarcinomatous, sarcomatous, or a squamous cell appearance. Some of the latter subtypes have the appearance of lymphoepitheliomas seen in the nasopharynx. This similarity in appearance has recently been shown to have a common cause—Epstein-Barr viral (EBV) penetration and replication in the epithelial elements of the thymus, which also occurs in the epithelial cells of the nasopharyngeal lymphoid tissue. A patient with a thymic carcinoma of the lymphoepithelioma type has recently been shown to have the serological profile of EBV, the presence of

EBV-associated nuclear antigens in the carcinoma cells, and a high level of viral genomes of EBV detected in the DNA. All of this indicates that EBV is involved in the genesis of some thymic carcinomas and some undifferentiated nasopharyngeal carcinomas.[84]

Because these cancers are most common in the anterosuperior compartment, they probably arise from thymic epithelium or embryonic nests within the thymus. These tumors should not be classified with thymomas and, like the lymphomas of the thymus, should be considered a separate entity with a poorer prognosis than the true thymomas.[81] Rarely, an oat cell tumor may also arise from the thymus.[65]

NEUROGENIC TUMORS

Neurogenic tumors vie with thymomas as the most common primary neoplasm of the mediastinum in adults and are the most common neoplasms in children (Table 23-5).[1-6,9,85,86]

HISTOGENESIS

Neural crest tissue gives rise to the nerve cells and the supporting elements (Schwann cells) that surround them. The sheath cells undergo neoplastic transformation to become neurilemmomas or schwannomas. Neurofibromas arise from the Schwann cells also but contain neuronal elements.

In the transformation of neural crest cells into neurones (ganglion cells), there is a certain progression. Sympathogonia develop from the embryonic neural crest and can be identified as the cells of origin of the tumor called a sympathogonioma. Sympathogonia become neuroblasts, the cells of origin of neuroblastomas. The neuroblast can either develop into a sympathicoblast or a pheochromocyte. The latter gives rise to pheochromocytomas (chromaffin positive or chemodectomas) and paragangliomas (chromaffin negative). Sympathicoblasts give rise to ganglioneuroblastomas.

Mature ganglion cells are derived from sympathicoblasts and can give rise to ganglioneuromas. Both malignant neuroblastomas and ganglioneuroblastomas can revert to the benign, more differentiated ganglioneuroma in 25% of instances.

NEURILEMMOMAS AND NEUROFIBROMAS

Neurilemmomas (Schwannomas) and neurofibromas can arise from the intercostal nerves or the sympathetic ganglia in the posterior mediastinum. The vagus and phrenic nerves are very rarely the sites of this neoplasm. Neurilemmomas and neurofibromas make up at least 65% of all neurogenic tumors, and about 66% to 75% will be found in the upper half of the chest. These tumors will also be found on the right side 65% to 75% of the time.

Differentiation between neurilemmomas and neurofibromas by the pathologist may be difficult at times. In most series neurilemmomas predominate over neurofibromas and are thus considered the most frequently encountered neurogenic tumor.[87] Ganglioneuromas may also have a histopathologic picture similar to the nerve sheath tumors.

From 25% to 40% of patients with nerve sheath tumors will have multiple neurofibromatosis (von Recklinghausen's disease). However, if a patient with von Recklinghausen's disease presents with a posterior mediastinal mass, it will more often be a meningocele than a posterior mediastinal neurofibroma.

Neurofibrosarcomas and malignant neurilemmomas constitute 10% to 20% of the tumors and are more frequently seen in patients with von Recklinghausen's disease. Radiation therapy and chemotherapy for those lesions are outlined in Chapters 39 and 46. These neoplasms carry a poor prognosis. Recurrences may occur even when the lesion is originally thought to be benign. Because malignant degeneration and recurrence can take place, patients operated upon for neurogenic tumors should be followed closely for many years.[87]

TUMORS OF NERVE CELLS

Neuroblastomas and ganglioneuroblastomas are poorly differentiated malignant tumors found predominantly in children (see Chap. 46). If present in the posterior mediastinum, their treatment is the same as for those encountered elsewhere in the body. These tumors are often unresectable.

The benign ganglioneuroma is easily excised at the time of thoracotomy.

Intrathoracic pheochromocytomas do not differ from those arising in the abdomen. Chemodectomas (paragangliomas) of the thorax may be locally invasive, involving the aorta, aortic branches, and the pulmonary artery. The capacity to synthesize catecholamines is the distinguishing feature of pheochromocytomas, but it is not unique to these neurogenic tumors. Any of the cells derived from the neural crest can develop this ability.

It may be possible to use this property of neurogenic tumors in the follow-up of patients with these tumors. The urinary metabolites of the catecholamines, vanillyl mandelic acid and homovanillic acid, can be used as tumor markers. Metanephrine and normetanephrine, the metabolites of epinephrine and norepinephrine, can be similarly used.

INTRASPINOUS INVOLVEMENT

One unique aspect of neurogenic tumors of the posterior mediastinum is the possibility that they may extend through an intervertebral foramen to assume a dumbbell shape.[85] Among 706 patients with mediastinal neurogenic tumors seen at the Mayo Clinic, 10% presented in this manner. Sixty percent of patients with dumbbell-shaped neurogenic tumors had symptoms of spinal cord compression. Roentgenologic studies demonstrating erosion or vertebral pedicles or enlargement of the intervertebral foramina adjacent to a mediastinal mass suggest the possibility of a dumbbell tumor. A myelogram can establish whether there is an intraspinous component of the posterior mediastinal neurogenic tumor. If such is the case, a one-stage combined intrathoracic and intraspinal approach can completely excise the tumor. The spinal component should be dealt with first to minimize bleeding into the spinal canal. If this occurs, the patient can become paraplegic.[87] If a dumbbell-shaped tumor is inadvertently found during a thoracotomy, a two-stage procedure can be effective. Dumbbell tumors carry the same 10% to 20% malignancy rate that other neurogenic tumors of the posterior mediastinum do.

MESENCHYMAL TUMORS

Most of the connective tissue tumors found in the soft tissues and discussed in Chapter 40 can also be found in the mediastinum. They constitute 6% to 7% of mediastinal neoplasms, and about half are malignant.[1] Benign tumors are permanently eradicated by surgical excision. Malignant mesenchymal tumors should be treated, as other soft tissue sarcomas are, with combined resection, radiation, and chemotherapy.

Seventy-five percent of mediastinal lipomas are located anteriorly and may present the same roentgenographic appearance as a pericardial cyst in the right cardiophrenic angle. Large lipomas extend into adjacent mediastinal compartments in an unpredictable manner. Liposarcomas, on the other hand, tend to occur in the posterior compartment where they may be confused with neurogenic tumors and the rare xanthogranulomas. Lipomatous tumors can be easily recognized by CT.

Mediastinal lymphangiomas can be difficult tumors to completely excise because they grow in a budding fashion and become densely adherent to the great vessels and other mediastinal structures. They are most often found in the anterior mediastinum.

Mesotheliomas may also present as mediastinal masses arising from parietal or pericardium. When they are localized, resection is curative. Diffuse invasive lesions have a poorer prognosis. Histologic criteria cannot differentiate benign from malignant lesions.

OTHER MEDIASTINAL TUMORS

There are a wide variety of lesions in this category, all of which are infrequently encountered, except for cysts. Cysts can now be readily diagnosed by CT and ultrasonography. Cysts are of congenital origin, have no neoplastic elements, and are pertinent only in the context of their differential diagnosis from other tumors of the mediastinum. Substernal goiters presenting in the anterosuperior mediastinum, like mediastinal cysts, make up a relatively large number of mediastinal masses and are of interest in differential diagnosis. Like cysts, they are readily managed by excision in order to eliminate the danger of sudden, life-threatening compressive complications, which can occur in asymptomatic and symptomatic patients.[88]

Mediastinal hemangiomas are rare lesions, which have been reported in 103 patients.[89] They can be found in either the anterosuperior or posterior mediastinum. Radical resection of these tumors to achieve total excision is not recommended, but they can be removed without undue blood loss. Local recurrences are possible, but they cause few problems and have shown no evidence of malignant degeneration.[89]

Inflammatory pseudotumors of the mediastinum are another group of rare lesions. They are not neoplastic, consist of chronic inflammatory fibrous tissue, and have an obscure cause. They can appear in either of the two major mediastinal compartments, anterosuperior or posterior, and are similar to those described in the lung.[90]

REFERENCES

1. Silverman NA, Sabiston DC Jr: Mediastinal masses. Surg Clin North Am 60:757, 1980
2. Oldham HN Jr: Mediastinal tumors and cysts. Ann Thorac Surg 11:246, 1971
3. Hammon JW Jr, Sabiston DC Jr: The mediastinum. In Ellis HE, Goldsmith HS (eds): Thoracic Surgery. Hagerstown, MD, Harper & Row, 1979
4. Lyons HA, Calvy GL, Sammons BP: The diagnosis and classification of mediastinal masses: 1. A study of 782 cases. Ann Intern Med 51:897, 1959
5. Burkell CC, Cross JM, Kent HP et al: Mass lesions of the mediastinum. Curr Prob Surg (Chicago), 1969
6. Herlitzka AJ, Gale JW: Tumors and cysts of the mediastinum, Arch Surg 76:697, 1958
7. Davis RD Jr, Oldham HN Jr, Sabiston DC Jr: Primary cysts and neoplasms of the mediastinum: Recent changes in clinical presentation, methods of diagnosis, management and results. Ann Thorac Surg 44:229, 1987
8. Grosfeld JL, Weinberger M, Kilman JW et al: Primary mediastinal neoplasms in infants and children. Ann Thorac Surg 12:179, 1971
9. Wychulis AR, Payne WS, Clagett OT et al: Surgical treatment of mediastinal tumors. J Thorac Cardiovasc Surg 62:379, 1971
10. Lichtenstein AK, Levine A, Taylor CR et al: Primary mediastinal lymphomas in adults. Am J Med 68:509, 1980
11. Mullen B, Richardson JD: Primary anterior mediastinal tumors in children and adults. Ann Thorac Surg 42:338, 1986
12. Strother CM, Schett JS, Crummy AB et al: Clinical application of computerized fluoroscopy: the extracranial carotid arteries. Radiology 136:781, 1980
13. Sone S, Higashihara T, Morimoto S et al: Normal anatomy of thymus and anterior mediastinum by pneumomediastinography. Am J Roentgenol 134:81, 1980
14. Pugatch RD, Foling LJ: Computed tomography of the thorax: A status report. Chest 80:618, 1981
15. Livesay JJ, Mink JH, Fee HJ et al: The use of computed tomography to evaluate suspected mediastinal tumors. Ann Thorac Surg 27:305, 1979
16. Miller GA, Heaston DK, Moore AV et al: CT differentiation of thoracic aneurysm from pulmonary masses adjacent to the mediastinum. J Comput Assist Tomogr 8:437, 1984
17. McLoud TC, Wittenberg J, Ferrucci JT: Computed tomography of the thorax and standard radiographic evaluation of the chest: A comparative study. J Comput Assist Tomogr 3:170, 1979
18. Goldwin RL, Heitzman ER, Proto AV: Computed tomography of the mediastinum: Normal anatomy and indications for the use of CT. Radiology 124:235, 1977
19. Webb WR, Gamou G, Stark DD et al: Evaluation of magnetic resonance sequences in imaging mediastinal tumors. Am J Radiol 143:525, 1984
20. vonShulthess GK, McMurdo K, Tscholakoff D et al: Mediastinal masses: MR imaging. Radiology 158:289, 1986
21. Irwin RS, Braman SS, Arvanitidis AN et al: Thyroid scanning in preoperative diagnosis of mediastinal goiter. Ann Intern Med 89:73, 1978
22. van Sonnenberg E, Lin AS, Deutsch AL et al: Percutaneous biopsy of difficult mediastinal hilar and pulmonary lesions by computed tomographic guidance and a modified coaxial technique. Radiology 148:300, 1983
23. Keller AR, Castleman B: Hodgkin's disease of the thymus gland. Cancer 33:1615, 1974
24. Bell RH, Knapp BI, Anson BJ et al: Form, size, blood supply and relations of the adult thymus. Bull Northwest Univ Med Sch 28:156, 1954
25. Sloan HE Jr: The thymus in myasthenia gravis. Surgery 13:154, 1943
26. Rosai J, Levine GD: Tumors of the thymus. Atlas of Tumor Pathology, Second Series, Fascicle 13. Washington DC, Armed Forces Institute of Pathology, 1976
27. Ham AW, Cormack DH: Histology, 8th ed. Philadelphia, JB Lippincott, 1979
28. Schulof RS, Goldstein AL: Thymosin and the endocrine thymus. Adv Intern Med 22:121, 1977
29. Trainin N: Thymic hormones and the immune response. Physiol Rev 54:272, 1974
30. Lauriola L, Maggiano N, Marino M et al: Human thymoma: Immunologic characteristics of the lymphocyte component. Cancer 48:1992, 1981
31. Bergh NP, Gatzinsky P, Larsson S et al: Tumors of the thymus and thymic region: I. Clinicopathological studies of thymomas. Ann Thorac Surg 25:91, 1978
32. LeGolvan DP, Abell MR: Thymomas. Cancer 39:2142, 1977
33. Gray GF, Gutowski WT: Thymoma: A clinicopathologic study of 54 cases. Am J Surg Pathol 3:235, 1979
34. Gerein AN, Srivastava SP, Burgess J: Thymoma: A ten-year review. Am J Surg 136:49, 1978
35. Salyer WR, Eggleston JC: Thymoma: A clinical and pathological study of 65 cases. Cancer 37:229, 1976
36. Batata MA, Martini N, Huvos AG et al: Thymomas: Clinicopathologic features, therapy, and prognosis. Cancer 34:389, 1974
37. Fechner RE: Recurrence of noninvasive thymomas. Cancer 23:1423, 1969
38. Verley JM, Hollmann KH: Thymoma: A comparative study of clinical stages, histologic features, and survival in 200 cases. Cancer 55:1074, 1985
39. Welch KJ, Tapper D, Vawter GP: Surgical treatment of thymic cysts and neoplasms in children. J Pediatr Surg 14:691, 1979
40. Souadjian JV, Enriquez P, Silverstein MN et al: The spectrum of diseases associated with thymoma. Arch Intern Med 134:374, 1974
41. Drachman DB: Myasthenia gravis. N Engl J Med 298:136, 186, 1978
42. Lindstron J: Autoimmune response to acetylcholine receptors in myasthenia gravis and its animal model. Adv Immunol 27:1, 1979
43. Alpert LI, Papatestas A, Kark A et al: Histologic reappraisal of thymus in myasthenia gravis. Arch Pathol 91:55, 1971
44. Shellito J, Khandekar JD, McKeever WP et al: Invasive thymoma responsive to oral corticosteroids. Cancer Treat Rep 62:1397, 1978
45. Papatestas AE, Pozner J, Genkins G et al: Prognosis in occult thymomas in myasthenia gravis following transcervical thymectomy. Arch Surg 122:1352, 1987
46. Zeok JV, Todd EP, Dillon M et al: The role of thymectomy in red cell aplasia. Ann Thorac Surg 28:257, 1979
47. Zerhouni EA, Scott WW, Baker RR et al: Invasive thymomas: Diagnosis and evaluation by computed tomography. J Comput Assist Tomogr 6:92, 1982
49. Baron RL, Lee JKT, Sagel SS et al: Computed tomography of the abnormal thymus. Radiology 142:127, 1982
50. Bernatz PE, Khonsari S, Harrison EG et al: Thymoma: Factors influencing prognosis. Surg Clin North Am 53:885, 1973
51. Wilkins EW, Castleman B: Thymoma: A continuing survey at the Massachusetts General Hospital. Ann Thorac Surg 28:252, 1979
52. Tanabe T, Kubo Y, Hashimoto M et al: Patch angioplasty of the superior vena caval obstruction (case reports with long follow-up results). J Cardiovasc Surg 20:519, 1979
53. Ariaratnam LS, Kalnicki S, Mincer F et al: The management of malignant thymoma with radiation therapy. Int J Radiat Oncol Biol Phys 5:77, 1979
54. Penn CRH, Hope-Stone HF: The role of radiotherapy in the management of malignant thymoma. Br J Surg 59:533, 1972
55. Sellors TH, Thackray AC, Thompson AD: Tumors of the thymus. Thorax 22:193, 1967
56. Skeggs DBL: Complications associated with the radiotherapy of thymic tumors. Proc R Soc Med 66:155, 1973
57. Marks RD, Wallace KM, Petit HS: Radiation therapy control of 9 patients with malignant thymoma. Cancer 41:117, 1978
58. Boston B: Chemotherapy of invasive thymoma. Cancer 38:49, 1976
59. Daugaard G, Hansen HH, Rorth M: Combination chemotherapy for malignant thymoma. Ann Intern Med 99:189, 1983
60. Evans WK, Thompson DM, Simpson WJ et al: Combination chemotherapy in invasive thymoma: Role of COPP. Cancer 46:1523, 1980
61. Chahinian AP, Bhardroj S, Meyer RJ et al: Treatment of invasive or metastatic thymoma: Report of eleven cases. Cancer 47:1752, 1981
62. Levine GD, Rosai J: Thymic hyperplasia and neoplasia: A review of current concepts. Hum Pathol 9:495, 1978
63. Salyer WR, Salyer DC, Eggleston JC: Carcinoid tumors of the thymus. Cancer 37:958, 1976
64. Wick MR, Carney JA, Bernaty PE et al: Primary mediastinal carcinoid tumors. Am J Surg Pathol 6:195, 1982
65. Wick MR, Scheithauer BW: Oat cell carcinoma of the thymus. Cancer 49:1652, 1982
66. Luna MA, Valenzuela-Tamariz J: Germ-cell tumors of the mediastinum, postmortem findings. Am J Clin Pathol 65:450, 1976
67. Martini N, Golbey RB, Hajdu SJ et al: Primary mediastinal germ cell tumors. Cancer 33:763, 1974
68. Kirschling RJ, Krols LK, Charboneau JW et al: High-resolution ultrasonographic and pathologic abnormalities of germ cell tumors in patients with clinically normal testes. Mayo Clin Proc 58:648, 1983
69. Polansky SM, Barwick KW, Ravin CE: Primary mediastinal seminoma. Am J Roentgenol 132:17, 1979
70. Hurt RD, Bruckman JE, Farrow GM et al: Primary mediastinal seminoma. Cancer 49:1658, 1982
71. Kersh CR, Eisert DR, Constable WC et al: Primary malignant mediastinal germ-cell tumors and the contribution of radiotherapy: A southeastern multi-institutional study. Am J Clin Oncol 10:302, 1987
72. Bush SE, Martinez A, Bagshaw MA: Primary mediastinal seminoma. Cancer 48:1877, 1981
73. Clamon GH: Management of primary mediastinal seminoma. Chest 83:263, 1983
74. Nichols CR, Heerema NA, Palmer C et al: Klingfelter's syndrome associated with mediastinal germ-cell neoplasms. J Clin Oncol 5:1290, 1987
75. Economou JS, Trump PL, Holmes EC et al: Management of primary germ cell tumors of the mediastinum. J Thorac Cardiovasc Surg 83:643, 1982
76. Fox RM, Woods RL, Tattersall MH et al: Undifferentiated carcinoma in young men. The atypical teratoma syndrome. Lancet 1:1316, 1979
77. Hainsworth JD, Einhorn LH, Williams SD et al: Advanced extragonadal germ-cell tumors: Successful treatment with combination chemotherapy. Ann Intern Med 97:7, 1982
78. Truong LD, Harris L, Mattioli C et al: Endodermal sinus tumor of the mediastinum. A report of seven cases and review of the literature. Cancer 58:730, 1986
79. Feun LG, Samson MK, Stephens RL: Vinblastine, bleomycin, cis-diamminedichlorplatinum in disseminated extragonadal germ cell tumors: A Southwest Oncology Group study. Cancer 45:2543, 1980
80. Vugrin D, Martini N, Whitmore WF et al: VAB-3 combination chemotherapy in primary mediastinal germ cell tumors. Cancer Treat Rep 66:1405, 1982

81. Vogelzang HJ, Raghaven D, Anderson RW et al: Mediastinal nonseminomatous germ cell tumors: The role of combined modality therapy. Ann Thorac Surg 33:333, 1982
82. Loehrer PJ Sr, Einhorn LH, Williams SD: VP-16 plus ifosfamide plus cisplatin as salvage therapy in refractory germ cell cancer. J Clin Oncol 4:528, 1986
83. Wick MR, Weiland LH, Scheithauer BW et al: Primary thymic carcinomas. Am J Surg Pathol 6:613, 1982
84. Leysraz S, Henle W, Chahinian AP et al: Association of Epstein-Barr virus with thymic carcinoma. N Engl J Med 312:1296, 1985
85. Akwari OE, Payne WS, Onofrio BM et al: Dumbbell neurogenic tumors of the mediastinum. Mayo Clin Proc 53:353, 1978
86. Gale AW, Jelihovsky T, Grant AF et al: Neurogenic tumors of the mediastinum. Ann Thorac Surg 17:434, 1974
87. Hajula A, Mattila S, Luosto R et al: Mediastinal neurogenic tumors. Early and late results of surgical treatment. Scand J Thorac Cardiovasc Surg 20:115, 1986
88. Katlic MR, Wang C, Grillo HC: Substernal goiter. Ann Thorac Surg 39:391, 1985
89. Cohen A, Sbaschnig RJ, Hochholzer L et al: Mediastinal hemangiomas. Ann Thorac Surg 43:656, 1987
90. Harpaz N, Gribety AR, Krellenstein DJ et al: Inflammatory pseudotumors of the thymus. Ann Thorac Surg 42:331, 1986

J. C. ROSENBERG

ALLEN S. LICHTER

LAWRENCE P. LEICHMAN

CHAPTER 24 *Cancer of the Esophagus*

Cancer of the esophagus was first recorded in China more than 2000 years ago when it was referred to as "Ye Ge," meaning dysphagia and belching.[1] Galen in the second century and Avenzoar (Ibn Zuhr), 1000 years later described the manifestations of what must have been a cancer of the esophagus. Avenzoar wrote about a condition "beginning with mild pain and difficulty in swallowing, and going on gradually to its complete prevention."[2] He treated these patients with silver sounds and nutritive enemas, palliative measures that were not improved upon for almost 750 years.

More aggressive attempts than those of Avenzoar at improving the outcome of a patient with malignant obstruction of the esophagus were undertaken in the middle of the 19th century. In 1849, Sédillot of Strasbourg performed the first gastrostomy for a patient suffering from severe dysphagia.[3] Unfortunately, the patient died less than 24 hours after the operation. At autopsy, an epithelial tumor of the esophagus was found. Bilroth, in 1871, wrote about resection of the esophagus for cancer after experimenting with animals, but it was Czerny, his co-worker in this project, who first attempted this surgery for a carcinoma of the cervical esophagus in 1877.[4]

The first successful resection of a thoracic esophageal malignancy was performed in 1913 in New York City by Franz Torek.[5] Like Czerny, he did not attempt to reconstruct the gastrointestinal tract but chose to allow the patient, a 67-year-old woman, to use an external rubber tube to connect a cervical esophagostomy to a gastrostomy tube while she ate. The patient survived for 13 years after this procedure. In 1920, Kirschner suggested that an esophagogastrostomy should be performed to reconstruct the esophagus after an esophagectomy.[6] It was not until 1932 that this was success-fully carried out by Ohsawa in Japan.[7] Reconstruction was first performed in the United States by Adams and Phemister in 1938.[8]

Because of the high mortality following resection of the esophagus during the third and fourth decades of the 20th century, radiation therapy was often chosen as a means of controlling the growth and spread of these malignancies. Radiation therapy using radium bougies and external radiation for esophageal carcinoma was introduced in the 1920s. Radium bougies were applied intermittently with disappointing results.[9] Deep seated lesions such as carcinomas of the esophagus were poorly handled by external radiation ($\sim$250 KeV) using orthovoltage therapy. Skin reactions and damage to structures close to the esophagus were frequent. In 1945, Nielsen reported on the use of radiation as primary treatment for esophageal cancer and introduced the use of a rotating chair to limit the side-effects of the roentgen beam.[10]

The most recent innovation in the treatment of carcinoma of the esophagus has been the use of multimodality therapy, employing combinations of chemotherapy, radiotherapy, and surgery. Preliminary studies have suggested that this approach may enhance the outlook of patients with this disease.

BENIGN NEOPLASMS OF THE ESOPHAGUS

Non-neoplastic tumors of the esophagus that may present as neoplasms comprise small islands of gastric heterotopia, cysts of various types (inclusion cysts, retention cysts

725

or duplication cysts), or granulomatous (fibrovascular) polyps.[11]

SQUAMOUS CELL PAPILLOMA

Benign neoplasms of epithelial origin are rare; the only type known is the squamous cell papilloma. Half the patients with squamous cell papillomas have multiple lesions, and most patients are asymptomatic. It is not known whether these lesions are precursors of squamous cell carcinoma. Occasionally, one may encounter difficulty in differentiating the squamous cell papilloma of the esophagus from a carcinoma or condylomata. Positive reactions to the human papillomavirus have been reported in these lesions. Treatment usually consists of endoscopic removal of the lesions.

BENIGN TUMORS OF MESODERMAL ORIGIN

The most common benign neoplasm of the esophagus is the leiomyoma, which accounts for 75% of all benign esophageal tumors.[12] The ratio of leiomyomas to leiomyosarcomas is 100:1. Leiomyomas are found in men two times more often than in women and are most often located in the lower third of the esophagus. Dysphagia is the most frequent presenting complaint, but half the patients with leiomyomas are asymptomatic. The treatment of choice is submucosal enucleation. Esophageal resection may be required for larger lesions. When resection is necessary, morbidity is increased; however, recurrences are rare.

Other benign nonepithelial neoplasms that occur in the esophagus are fibromyomas, lipomyomas, fibromas, lipomas, neurofibromas, giant cell tumors, osteochondromas, and granular cell myoblastomas.

SQUAMOUS CELL CARCINOMA OF THE ESOPHAGUS

PATHOLOGY

A list of malignant primary esophageal neoplasms based on the World Health Organization (WHO) classification is presented in Table 24-1.[11] More than 90% of malignant esophageal tumors are squamous cell carcinomas, arising from the squamous cell epithelium lining the lumen of the esophagus. The well-differentiated cancers have the characteristic features of keratin formation (epithelial pearls), intercellular bridges, and minimal pleomorphism. Poorly differentiated tumors do not contain keratin or demonstrate intercellular bridges, but they do have marked nuclear and cellular pleomorphism. The moderately differentiated tumors are intermediate between these two. The degree of differentiation has no prognostic value.

Spindle cell carcinoma, pseudosarcoma, carcinosarcoma, and verrucous carcinoma of the esophagus are pathologic variants of squamous cell carcinoma. They are discussed near the end of this chapter with other infrequent cancers of the esophagus.

TABLE 24-1. Malignant Esophageal Tumors

Epithelial Tumors
  Squamous cell carcinoma
    Well differentiated
    Moderately differentiated
    Poorly differentiated
  Variants of squamous cell carcinoma
    Spindle cell carcinoma
    Pseudosarcoma and carcinosarcoma
    Verrucous carcinoma
    In situ carcinoma
  Adenocarcinoma
    Adenoacanthoma
  Adenoid cystic carcinoma (cylindroma)
  Mucoepidermoid carcinoma
  Adenosquamous carcinoma
  Carcinoid
  Undifferentiated carcinoma
    Oat cell carcinoma
Nonepithelial Tumors
  Leiomyosarcoma
  Malignant melanoma
  Rhabdomyosarcoma
  Myoblastoma
  Choriocarcinoma

EPIDEMIOLOGIC AND ETIOLOGIC CONSIDERATIONS

The age-adjusted incidence of cancer of the esophagus in the United States is low. In 1984, it was 3.5 per 100,000 for all races (5.6 per 100,000 men and 1.9 per 100,000 women).[13] The age-adjusted mortality rate in the United States in 1984 was 5.7 per 100,000 men and 1.5 per 100,000 women.[13] These data vary significantly according to race. A statistically significant ($p < 0.05$) change of 0.6% has been observed in the average annual esophageal cancer mortality rate between 1975 and 1984. Esophageal cancer was responsible for approximately 8800 deaths in 1986, and during 1987, almost 9300 new cases were diagnosed. Cancer of the esophagus constitutes 1.5% of all cancers and 7% of all gastrointestinal carcinomas in the United States.[14]

The data from the United States are by no means representative of the incidence of this disease throughout the world or among different groups within a given country. Geographic variations in the incidence of squamous cell carcinoma of the esophagus are greater than for any other malignancy. Data obtained by WHO and published in 1977 show that mortality, standardized to the world population, was highest in China. Puerto Rico and Singapore were second and third (Fig. 24-1).[1]

There is also great variation in the geographic distribution of esophageal cancer in China. A 700-fold difference in mortality exists between the highest and lowest incidence areas. The highest rates in China were found in the north along the Taihang Mountain range. Honan Province is in this area. The age-adjusted mortality from esophageal cancer in Honan Province is 436 per 100,000 men and 22.5 per 100,000 women. In Yunan Province, on the southern border of China, the rates are 1.4 and 0.7 per 100,000, respectively. The Linxian county in Honan Province has the highest mortality rate from esophageal carcinoma (131.8 per

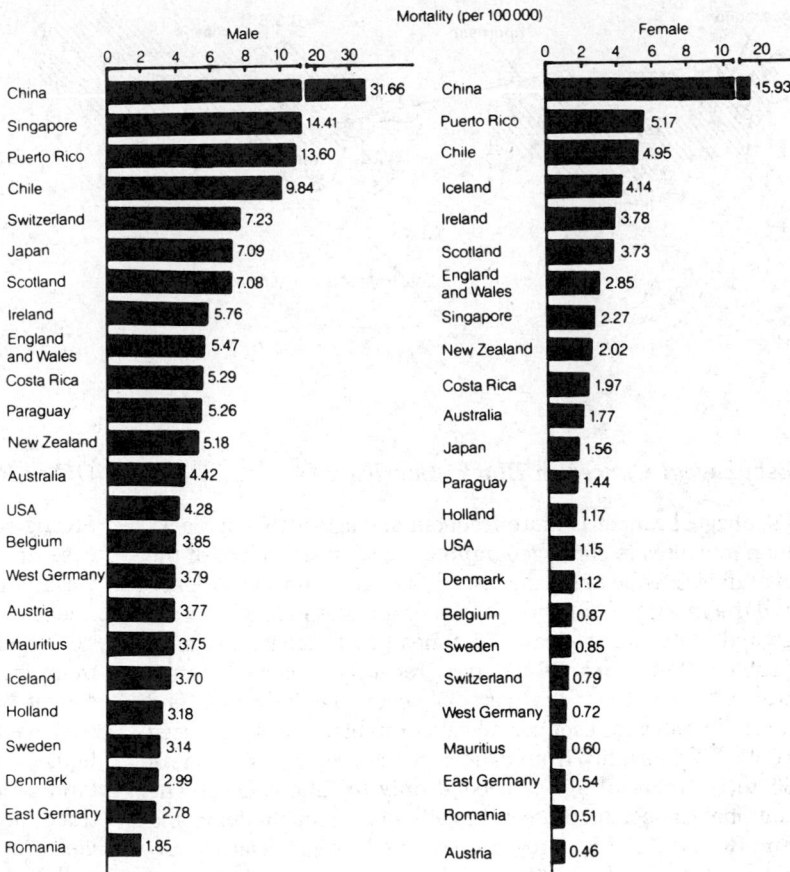

FIG. 24-1. Age-adjusted mortality for esophageal cancer as determined by the World Health Organization and published in 1977.[1]

100,000).[15] Chickens in Honan Province were also found to have esophageal cancer. When residents of Honan moved to the Hobei Province, both they and their chickens retained their high esophageal cancer rate. This observation led to the discovery of nitrosamines in food samples from areas of high incidence.[15] It is postulated that esophageal carcinoma is the end result of the combined effects of several etiologic factors.

Examples of variations in the geographic distribution of esophageal cancer can also be found in Africa, where the incidence has changed with time.[16] The incidence of esophageal cancer increased dramatically between 1940 and 1950 in the Transkei region of the Cape Province in South Africa. Before 1940, the disease was unknown, but the incidence is now 246 per 100,000 black men 35 to 64 years of age. In Nigeria (West Africa), the incidence is similar: 3 per 100,000.[17] The sex ratio (males:females) is also much higher among the black population of Cape Province than among the white people (9:1 for blacks and 4:1 for whites). Environmental factors seem to be responsible for these phenomena. Certain alcoholic drinks (kachosu, home-brewed from sugar and maize husks rather than the kafir beer made from sorghum), homegrown tobacco smoked in homemade pipes, and nutritional deficiencies may be responsible for the increased incidence. The etiologic relationships in the Transkei and in China are not clear.

Perhaps the area of the world with the highest incidence and most obscure etiologic relationships is in Iran and the Soviet Union around the Caspian Sea.[18] There is no significant alcohol or tobacco consumption among the Moslem population in this area. Dietary factors are most suspect. The Caspian littoral forms part of an "Asian esophageal cancer belt" which extends through northern China (Fig. 24-2). However, within this area there are striking variations in the frequency and sex incidence of esophageal carcinoma. The age-standardized incidence rates in Gorgan and Gonbad in the northeastern parts of the province of Mazandaran in Iran are approximately 108 per 100,000 men and 174 per 100,000 women.[18]

Cancer of the esophagus is common in France, Switzerland, Finland, Iceland, and Puerto Rico. The disease is less frequently seen in Norway, Britain, and Australia and among the white population of the United States. Alcohol consumption is thought to be a carcinogenic agent in the United States, Britain, France (Brittany), Sweden, and Japan. Tobacco consumption may be a factor in the United States, France, Britain, Sweden, India, and South Africa. Tobacco and excessive alcoholic intake are widely accepted as the major reason why squamous cell carcinoma of the esophagus is seen in many western countries. Each increases the risk of developing esophageal cancer, and, when combined, as is often the case, the risks are multiplied. The risk of developing esophageal cancer in smokers is increased ten-fold for beer drinkers and about 25-fold for whiskey drinkers compared with smoking matched nondrinkers.[19] Racial and genetic factors have been studied with inconclusive results.

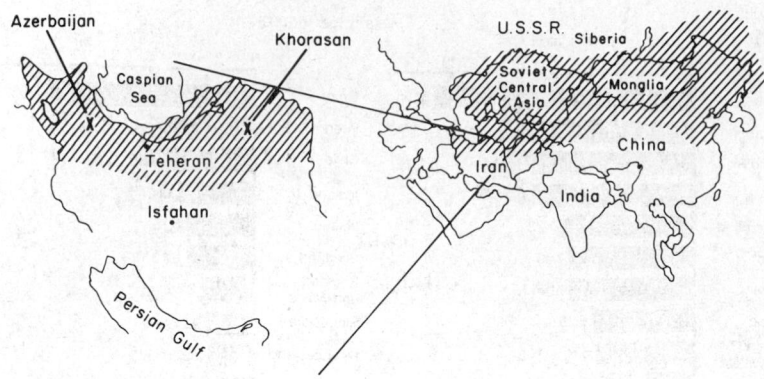

FIG. 24-2. An "esophageal cancer belt" extends across Asia from the southern shore of the Caspian Sea in Iran, through Soviet Central Asia and Mongolia, to Northern China. The incidence of cancer of the esophagus in the area around the Caspian Sea is higher than in any other area of the world. (Kmet J, Mahboudi E: Esophageal cancer in the Caspian littoral of Iran: Initial studies. Science 175:846, 1972)

Esophageal Cancer in Black Americans

Esophageal cancer is more frequent and aggressive in blacks than in whites in some geographic areas, independent of the overall incidence of the disease.[20] The fact that the incidence and the mortality of cancer of the esophagus in blacks in the United States are at least 3.5 times greater than in whites (Tables 24-2 and 24-3) has recently received much attention.[21-23] Over the past 25 years, the incidence and mortality rates for esophageal cancer in blacks has increased 105%.[20,23] Mortality from cancer of the esophagus in blacks 35 to 54 years of age is second only to lung cancer. The National Cancer Institute's Surveillance, Epidemiology, and End-Results (SEER) program reported 5-year relative survival rates (1974–1983) of 5.6% for white patients and 4.1% for black patients with esophageal cancer. The difference is statistically significant ($p<0.05$).[13]

It has been postulated that increased tobacco consumption among blacks or nutritional deficiencies may account for this increased risk. Alcohol potentiates the risk of developing esophageal cancer among smokers, and more black Americans smoke than white Americans (40% and 30%, respectively). More white Americans are former smokers than black Americans. However, nutritional surveys do not show that blacks are heavier drinkers than whites. The Health and Nutrition Survey carried out from 1971 to 1974, which included 20,749 persons, 20% of whom were black, showed that a smaller proportion of black men report heavy drinking than do white men of comparable age.[24]

In contrast to the higher incidence of squamous cell carcinoma of the esophagus in blacks than in whites is the higher incidence of adenocarcinomas of the esophagus in whites than in blacks. This relationship is discussed in the section on adenocarcinoma of the esophagus.

Other Risk Factors

Strong suspicions of nutritional factors involved in this disease are derived from the observation that there is a wide variation in the rates for men and women (from 5 : 1 to 1 : 1). Because the Plummer-Vinson syndrome is associated with a 10% incidence of esophageal or pharyngeal cancer and is more frequent in women, nutritional deficiencies have been sought as predisposing factors. No clear-cut relationships have been found. Heavy seasoning of foods and hot foods and liquids have been implicated, as have the use of betel nut, tannin-rich foods, contamination of food with silica particles, trace metal deficiencies and excesses, and vitamin deficiencies. Consideration has been given to poor oral hygiene, air pollution, radiation, exposure to asbestos, and previous gastric surgery as etiologic factors. These are speculations with little evidence to support them.

A recent review of dietary factors influencing esophageal cancer suggested that a high-risk diet depended on corn or wheat as staples, with marginal or deficient amounts of riboflavin, nicotinic acid, magnesium, and zinc.[25,26] Silica particles contaminating millet bran have also been implicated as an etiologic agent in areas with a high incidence of esophageal cancer.[27]

Predisposing Conditions

TYLOSIS. Attempts at correlating genetic factors with an increased incidence of esophageal cancer have failed to reveal a significant relationship, with the exception of patients with tylosis. In a classic article on this obscure condition, Howel-Evans described the occurrence of esophageal cancer in patients with this disease characterized by changes of the skin of the palms and soles (hyperkeratosis palmaris et plantaris) and papillomata of the esophagus. The syndrome is the

TABLE 24-2. Age-Adjusted Incidence of Cancer of the Esophagus, 1984*

	Race	Male	Female
Black	17.2	5.4	
White	4.6	1.5	

* 1986 Annual Cancer Statistics Review, incidence per 100,000; age-adjusted to the 1970 U.S. standard population.

TABLE 24-3. Age-Adjusted Mortality Rate for Cancer of the Esophagus, 1984*

	Race	Male	Female
Black	16.4	4.1	
White	4.7	1.3	

* 1986 Annual Cancer Statistics Review, incidence per 100,000; age-adjusted to the 1970 U.S. standard population.

result of an autosomal dominant gene. In some families, 95% of patients with tylosis will develop squamous cell carcinoma of the esophagus by the age of 65 years.[28]

ACHALASIA. Approximately 5% of patients with achalasia have developed squamous cell carcinomas of the esophagus. The cancers are located equally in the middle third and lower third of the esophagus.[29,30] Carcinomas occur after the achalasia has been present for 20 years or longer. In some instances, the cancer has been thought to be the cause of the achalasia.[31] Rarely, an adenocarcinoma may be found in the dilated esophagus.[32] Joske and Benedict suspected that the obstructive process somehow led to the squamous cell carcinoma, and literature continues to implicate retention esophagitis as a premalignant condition.[33,34] The esophagitis is thought to arise from stagnating retained food in the megaesophagus. The advent of fiberoptics for flexible endoscopy has promoted the use of esophagoscopy, which should generate increased reports of squamous cell cancer in patients with achalasia. The discovery of early lesions should improve survival rates.[35]

Treatment is the same as for any squamous cell carcinoma. Patients with this unusual association have as poor an outcome as do patients with esophageal cancer.[36]

ESOPHAGEAL DIVERTICULA. Isolated case reports constitute the basis of this uncommon association of conditions. As of 1976, 35 cases were collected from the literature. Two-thirds of the cancers occurred in pharyngoesophageal diverticula and the remainder at the epiphrenic level. Epithelial cysts of the esophagus do not develop cancers.[37] Of 1249 patients with a pharyngoesophageal diverticulum, 0.4% had an associated squamous cell carcinoma.[38] These cancers are treated as any other squamous cell carcinoma. In one series, diverticulectomy alone was curative in the absence of full-thickness penetration, nodal metastasis, or extension to the line of resection.[38]

LYE STRICTURE. Squamous cell carcinomas have occurred in esophageal strictures secondary to lye ingestion. The cancer occurs at the site of the stricture, which is frequently located at the level of the tracheal bifurcation.[39] The interval between the detection of the carcinoma and the ingestion of lye is between 30 and 45 years. The later in life that the lye is ingested, the shorter the interval before carcinoma develops.[40] The similarity of this lesion to squamous cell carcinomas occurring in chronic, draining sinus tracts and chronic skin ulcers suggests a common etiologic mechanism. These instances of carcinoma are less aggressive, have a slightly higher resectability rate, and may have a better prognosis than the usual forms of squamous cell carcinoma.

Resection of an extensively strictured esophagus not involved with cancer is a formidable procedure. Because the mortality may be higher than the risk of developing cancer in the esophagus, resection of the excluded esophagus is not advised, and a bypass procedure to relieve dysphagia may be the preferred procedure.

PLUMMER-VINSON   (PATERSON-KELLY)   SYNDROME. Sideropenic anemia, glossitis, and esophagitis are associated with a 10% incidence of pharyngeal or esophageal cancer, which is usually located in the upper esophagus. The syndrome and the cancers are more frequent in women than men. Nutritional deficiencies have been postulated as etiologic factors. The syndrome is seen less often now than when it was first described more than 65 years ago.[41] When strictures are present, dysplastic changes and in situ carcinoma can be found at the site of the narrowed esophagus.[42]

ANATOMIC CONSIDERATIONS OF CLINICAL SIGNIFICANCE

The esophagus begins at the level of C6, below the cricoid cartilage, where the cricopharyngeus muscle separates it from the pharynx. The length of the esophagus, from pharynx to stomach, is between 23 and 30 cm.

Endoscopists localize lesions in the esophagus by measuring the lesion's distance from the central incisor teeth. By this method of measurement, the esophagus begins 15 cm from the central incisors and terminates 38 to 45 cm distally, beneath the diaphragm. The thoracic inlet, the dividing line between the cervical and thoracic esophagus, is located 20 cm from the central incisors, at the level of T1 (Fig. 24-3).

The cervical esophagus is about 5 cm long. It extends down to the thoracic inlet, at the level of T1. The first 3 cm are located behind the larynx. This segment is the postcricoid portion of the cervical esophagus. Malignancies in this area present a special problem and are fully discussed in Chapter 21.

The thoracic esophagus begins at the thoracic inlet at the level of the clavicles and ends at T10. As the esophagus passes down the posterior mediastinum toward the left of the midline, it lies close behind the tracheal bifurcation and left main stem bronchus. This occurs at the level of T4 or T5, about 23 cm from the central incisors. The arch of the aorta passes in front of the left side of the esophagus at this level, producing a shallow depression that pulsates during endoscopy. These close anatomic relationships are demonstrated in Fig. 24-4. Because of the juxtaposition of these organs, malignant lesions can involve vital structures early in the

FIG. 24-3. Anatomic relationship and major subdivisions of the esophagus.

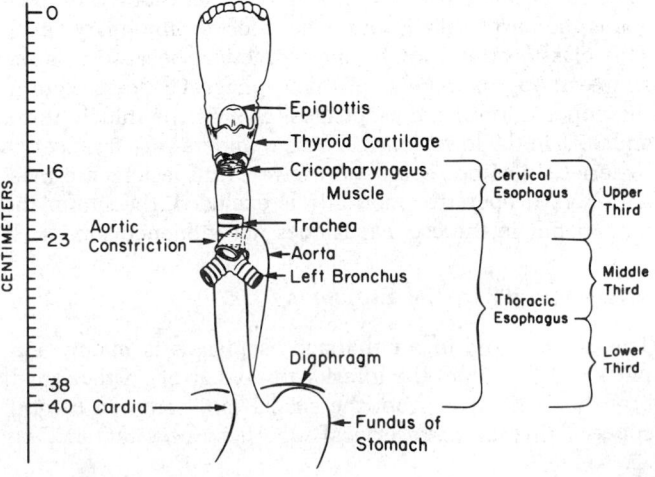

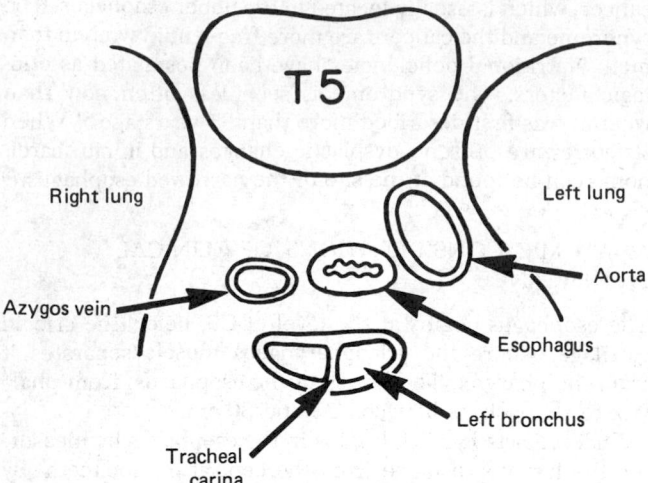

FIG. 24-4. Diagrammatic cross-sectional anatomy depicting the close relationship of the thoracic esophagus to the aorta, trachea, left mainstem bronchus, and azygos vein at the midthoracic (T4 and T5) level, 23 cm from the central incisors.

course of the disease. Tracheoesophageal fistulae are the most common problems encountered. These anatomic relationships contribute significantly to the higher operative mortality following resection of lesions at the midesophageal level.

The American Joint Committee for Cancer Staging and End-Results Reporting divides the esophagus into three principal regions: The cervical esophagus; the upper and midthoracic esophagus, extending from the thoracic inlet (18 cm from the upper incisor teeth) to a point 10 cm above the esophagogastric junction, usually located at T8 (31 cm from the upper incisor teeth); and the lower thoracic esophagus, which is the distal 10 cm of esophagus.[43] The Japanese Society for Esophageal Diseases has a similar system of dividing the esophagus into regions but further subdivides the upper and midthoracic esophagus and the lower esophagus each into two subdivisions.[44]

The esophagus can also be divided into thirds (Fig. 24-3). The cervical esophagus and upper thoracic esophagus are the upper third (above the aortic arch); the middle thoracic esophagus is the middle third (between the aortic arch and the inferior pulmonary vein); and the lower thoracic esophagus is the lower third (below the inferior pulmonary vein). This classification may be most practical because it is the simplest. Approximately 15% of esophageal cancers occur in the upper third of the esophagus, 50% in the middle third, and 35% in the lower third. These numbers vary from series to series. In some reports, the lower-third lesions are most common. If operative mortality is excluded, the site of the malignancy in the esophagus does not influence survival.[45]

Blood Supply to the Esophagus

The cervical and upper thoracic esophagus is mainly supplied by a branch of the inferior thyroid artery. Other small branches may arise from the subclavian, common carotid, superior thyroid, costocervical superficial cervical, and ver-

tebral arteries. The bronchial arteries and occasionally direct branches from the aorta supply the midesophagus, which is the most vascularized portion of the esophagus. Below the bifurcation of the trachea, the esophagus is supplied by arteries arising from the aorta.[46] The veins emanating from the thoracic esophagus drain directly into the azygos and hemiazygos systems and the intercostal veins, which are also tributaries of the azygos system.

Lymphatic Drainage of the Esophagus

A closely knit plexus of small lymphatic vessels in the mucosa merge with a less-dense network located in the submucosa.[47,48] Both of these plexuses communicate with five widely spaced lymphatic channels in the muscular layers of the esophagus, which, in turn, communicate with a network of cooperative lymphatics that extend throughout the esophagus (Fig. 24-5). Thus, lymphatic fluid can follow any one of a great number of pathways before emerging from the esophagus to drain into a lymph node. Because of the longitudinal course of the lymphatics and the interconnections between the mucosal, submucosal, and muscular lymphatics draining the esophagus, the pattern of flow to lymph nodes is unpredictable. Flow may be in the direction of adjacent lymph nodes or through the aforementioned network to more distant nodes. The pattern of lymphatics favors the flow of lymph in the direction of the long axis of the esophagus rather than in a circumferential direction.

Afferent lymphatics leaving the esophagus to drain into a lymph node tend to follow the arteries, which, as a rule, course longitudinally rather than radially. The lymphatics

FIG. 24-5. Lymphatics extend throughout the esophagus, draining the esophageal wall and passing to collections of lymph nodes that extend from the neck to the abdomen. Lymph node chains, which also may receive lymphatics from the esophagus, that are not illustrated are the cervical and supraclavicular lymph nodes.

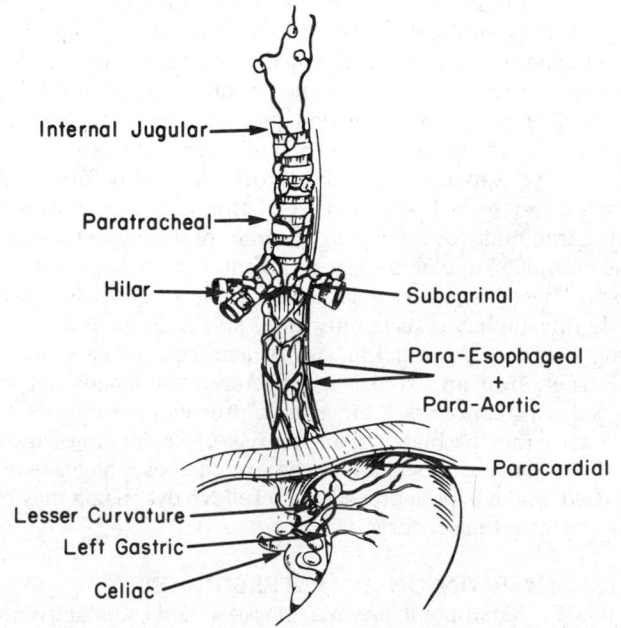

drain into the following lymph node chains: internal jugular, cervical, supraclavicular, paratracheal, hilar, subcarinal, paraesophageal, para-aortic, paracardial, lesser curvature, left gastric, and celiac (Fig. 24-5). Involvement of the paratracheal nodes on the right is more common than involvement of those on the left. The lowest right paratracheal lymph node is the azygos node. The posterior hilar lymph nodes are more frequently involved than the other hilar nodes. The paraesophageal and para-aortic group of lymph nodes are part of a chain of lymphatics extending from the inferior pulmonary vein to the diaphragm. Similarly, the celiac nodes are part of an extensive group of retroperitoneal lymph nodes.

Celiac node involvement occurs in 10% of the esophageal cancers located in the cervical and upper thoracic esophagus (up to the tracheal bifurcation). The middle third of the esophagus (up to the distal 10 cm of esophagus) may have celiac node involvement in 44% of patients.[49] The peculiar lymphatic drainage of the esophagus is responsible for the phenomenon of "skip areas" of involvement.[50] As much as 8 cm of normal esophagus may be interposed between the site of gross tumor and micrometastases within lymphatic vessels or the esophageal wall.

CLINICAL PRESENTATION

The patient with esophageal cancer will usually be a man between 55 and 65 years of age with a long-standing history of cigarette smoking and heavy alcohol intake. Dysphagia and weight loss are the initial symptoms of carcinoma of the esophagus in 90% of patients. Difficulty swallowing does not occur until the circumference of the esophagus is narrowed to a third or half of normal. Occasionally, the onset is sudden; most often symptoms have been present for 3 to 4 months. Pain on swallowing (odynophagia) is seen in about half the patients with cancer of the esophagus. When the pain radiates to the back, spinal column involvement should be suspected (Table 24-4). Regurgitation or vomiting and a discomfort in the throat, substernal area, or epigastrium may be additional symptoms. Aspiration pneumonia can be another presenting or concomitant feature of the disease. Advanced lesions may present with hematemesis, hemoptysis or melena, persistent cough caused by an esophagotracheobronchial fistula, dysphonia caused by involvement of the left recurrent laryngeal nerve with laryngeal paralysis, Horner's syndrome, or superior vena caval obstruction. Exsanguinating bleeding may occur if the cancer erodes into

TABLE 24-4. Signs and Symptoms Produced by Advanced Carcinoma of Esophagus

Pain radiating to the back on swallowing
Dysphonia (laryngeal paralysis)
Diaphragmatic paralysis (involvement of phrenic nerve)
Coughing when swallowing (tracheoesophageal fistula)
Superior vena cava syndrome
Palpable supraclavicular or cervical nodes
Malignant pleural effusion
Malignant ascites
Bone pain

the aorta. Other ominous findings are pleural effusion, palpable cervical or supraclavicular lymph nodes, and hepatomegaly. Hematuria can occur with renal involvement. Pain is prominent if there are metastases to the bones.

Occasionally a paraneoplastic syndrome is produced by an esophageal tumor. The most common is hypercalcemia unrelated to bone involvement.[51] Gonadotropin-producing and ACTH-producing tumors have been described but are rare.[52]

The gross appearance of an advanced carcinoma of the esophagus is best depicted by an esophagram. There are few lesions that can simulate the appearance of an esophageal carcinoma. Most confusion arises with lesions at the distal end of the esophagus. Adenocarcinoma of the esophagus or stomach, benign tumors, other malignant tumors, peptic strictures, and achalasia may have an appearance similar to squamous cell carcinoma radiographically and esophagoscopically.

DIAGNOSIS

Obtaining tissue for histopathologic confirmation of the diagnosis may not be easy when visualizing an esophageal tumor through an esophagoscope. Often, the submucosal extension of the tumor will push normal mucosa in front of it, and the biopsy forceps will not bite deeply enough to reach the malignant tissue. Brushings of the tumor will be diagnostic 90% of the time, compared with only 70% of the biopsies.[53,54] When both techniques are used and multiple biopsies (up to 7) obtained, a diagnosis can most often be established.[55] Exfoliative cytology also has diagnostic value.[56]

The Linxian County Hospital in the Honan Province of China developed the technique of abrasive cytology, using a catheter with a balloon covered by a cotton net to scrape loose esophageal mucosal cells. Cytologic examination has been 90% accurate in patients with very early cancer of the esophagus.[15] Dowlatshaki developed a similar technique using a brush passed through a nasogastric tube.[56]

EVALUATING THE PATIENT WITH ESOPHAGEAL CARCINOMA

Noninvasive Studies

The history and physical examination can provide important clues to the local extent and metastatic involvement of a cancer of the esophagus. The findings produced by advanced esophageal cancers were described above and are listed in Table 24-4.

The length of involvement of the esophagus by cancer, as determined by the esophagram, does not correlate well with resectability, cure, or the extent of involvement as determined by direct measurement of surgical or autopsy specimens.[45] The high frequency of metastases to the lungs, liver, adrenals, kidney, and bones has been used to justify computed tomography (CT) scans of the chest and upper abdomen, bone scans, and skeletal surveys.

Small esophageal carcinomas (<3.5 cm long) are not easily identified as malignant lesions by esophagrams.[57] Diagnostic accuracy approaches only 60% under these circumstances. A thickened posterior strip or band (wider than 4.5 cm) can be identified on the lateral chest x-ray film of patients with carcinoma of the esophagus. The thickened area is caused by periesophageal lymphatic involvement and can be seen as early as 6 months before the development of symptoms.[15,58]

Endosonography, also referred to as endoscopic ultrasonography, is valuable in diagnosing early lesions and contributes to the preoperative staging of esophageal carcinomas. Cancers of the esophagus appear as a hypoechoic mass or a mass containing heterogeneous echo spots. The length of the esophagus involved by the cancer, the infiltration by the cancer into adjacent organs, and the lymph node involvement can also be assessed by this technique.[59,60]

The results of several studies involving CT in esophageal cancer have recently been reviewed.[61,62] Those using preoperative CT, followed by surgical confirmation of stage, have shown that CT is best at assessing local extension of disease and at delineating liver or adrenal metastases. It is less accurate in assessing the degree of periesophageal lymph node involvement. In three different studies, CT underestimated the length of the esophageal lesion by 1 to 6 cm.[62-64] The current recommendation for staging purposes is to obtain both a barium esophagram and a CT scan to assess tumor length; the longer of the two measurements can be used. In addition to staging the tumor, CT has also proved helpful in radiation therapy planning and may be useful in assessing tumor response to both radiation and chemotherapy.[65]

Nuclear magnetic resonance imaging is used for precisely determining the extent of involvement of esophageal cancer. Experience with it thus far indicates that it has many of the same drawbacks as CT.[66]

Invasive Studies

Endoscopy, using the flexible esophagoscope, is best for evaluating esophageal cancers. Because of the high frequency of other malignancies within the upper and lower respiratory passageways, a careful examination of the mouth, pharynx, larynx, and tracheobronchial tree must be performed. Another compelling reason for performing laryngoscopy and bronchoscopy is the frequency of extension of midesophageal lesions into the tracheobronchial tree. Special attention should be given to the posterior wall of the left main stem bronchus and trachea where the esophagus crosses these structures. Narrowing in this area or infiltration of tumor, as evidenced by edema, prominent longitudinal folds, and bleeding upon contact are ominous findings.

Mediastinoscopy is used only if the patient is inoperable and a tissue diagnosis is required. Laparoscopy is helpful in identifying patients with malignant ascites, liver metastases, and extensive involvement of the stomach. All enlarged cervical or supraclavicular lymph nodes should be biopsied.

Biopsy of the celiac and lesser curvature lymph nodes is of great significance in planning therapy and providing prognostic data. Therefore, biopsy of these lymph nodes during laparotomy should be part of every therapeutic plan. Celiac node involvement occurs in 10% of patients with upper esophageal malignancies. With lower esophageal cancers, the incidence increases at least fivefold.[49]

STAGING

Because the esophagus is not an accessible organ, its clinical evaluation leaves a great deal to be desired. The use of invasive techniques, including biopsy procedures, is more appropriate. However, these techniques should be carried out before radiotherapy or chemotherapy is used if they are to be reliable. Because many esophageal cancers are being treated with preoperative radiation or chemotherapy, postsurgical evaluation may not accurately define the stage of the diagnosed cancer. The TNM staging system for the cervical and thoracic esophagus is outlined in Table 24-5. Stage grouping is given in Table 24-6.[43,67]

NATURAL HISTORY AND PATTERNS OF SPREAD

Esophageal cancers are characterized by extensive local growth and lymph node involvement before becoming widely disseminated. Follow-up of early asymptomatic patients with in situ carcinoma has demonstrated that it takes 3 to 4 years before advanced cancer develops.[68] Other studies of early superficial squamous cell carcinomas have resulted in estimates of 5 months for the doubling time of the longitudinal growth of these malignancies.[69] The unique lymphatic drainage of the esophagus and the long interval during which the tumor is asymptomatic account for the extensive involvement of lymph nodes and structures adjacent to the esophagus at the time of diagnosis. The poor prognosis of these patients is influenced by the proximity of the aorta and trachea and by the absence of a serosal covering.

The length of esophagus involved by the neoplasm is di-

TABLE 24-5.   TNM Staging for Esophageal Cancer

Primary Tumor (T)
TO   No demonstrable tumor
TIS   Carcinoma in situ
T1   Tumor involves 5 cm or less of esophageal length with no obstruction nor complete circumferential involvement nor extraesophageal spread.
T2   Tumor involves more than 5 cm of esophagus and produces obstruction with circumferential involvement of the esophagus but no extraesophageal spread.
T3   Tumor with extension outside the esophagus involving mediastinal structures.

Regional Lymph Nodes (N)
Cervical esophagus (cervical and supraclavicular lymph nodes)
N0   No nodal involvement
N1   Unilateral involvement (moveable)
N2   Bilateral involvement (moveable)
N3   Fixed nodes
Thoracic esophagus (nodes in the thorax, not those of the cervical, supraclavicular or abdominal areas)
N0   No nodal involvement
N1   Nodal involvement

Distant Metastases
M0   No metastases
M1   Distant metastases. Cancer of thoracic esophagus with cervical, supraclavicular, or abdominal lymph node involvement is classified as M1.

TABLE 24-6. Stage Grouping for Esophageal Cancer

Stage I

T1N0M0 Tumor that involves less than 5 cm of esophagus without obstruction and no circumferential, extraesophageal or nodal involvement and no metastases.

Stage II

T1N1M0
T1N2M0
T2N0M0
T2N1M0
T2N2M0

Cervical esophagus: No extraesophageal involvement with moveable regional lymph nodes but no metastases or a tumor more than 5 cm in size without lymph node involvement.

T2N0M0 Thoracic esophagus: Any tumor that is greater than 5 cm in length or produces obstruction or involves the entire circumference of the esophagus without extraesophageal spread.

Stage III

Any M1
Any T3

Any esophageal cancer with extraesophageal spread or distant metastases.
Cervical esophagus: fixed nodes (Any N3)
Thoracic esophagus: regional lymph node involvement (Any N1)

rectly correlated with the extent of involvement of adjacent structures and inversely related to curability. If the resected tumor (with no pretreatment) is 5 cm long or less, approximately 40% of the specimens demonstrate localized disease, 25% are locally advanced, and 35% have distant metastases or are unresectable. If the length exceeds 5 cm, as determined by pathologic examination, only 10% are localized, 15% are locally advanced, and 75% have distant metastases or exceed curative resection.[69-71]

Distant metastases do not usually dominate the initial clinical course of patients with esophageal cancer, but autopsies have shown that widespread distant metastases are almost always present at the time of death.[72,73] Esophageal carcinoma can spread to virtually any site, including lung, pleura, stomach, peritoneum, kidney, adrenal gland, brain, and bone; it is most likely present as subclinical metastatic tumor when the patient is first diagnosed.[74]

Autopsy studies have shown that disseminated tumor is frequently found in patients with disease that was thought to be limited to the local-regional area. In one review, 94% had residual cancer at postmortem.[75] Nine percent had local tumor only, and 85% had extensive disease, including residual local cancer. The most common sites of metastases were lymph nodes, lung, and liver, with the last two sites involved in approximately 50% of patients. Because the median survival of this group was only 4 months, the extensive disease found at autopsy cannot be ascribed to a prolonged interval between diagnosis and death. In a similar study of 113 autopsies, 73% had metastases.[76] In a third analysis, Bosch and his colleagues found that 32% had no residual local disease; however, more than half of these patients had died in the immediate postoperative period. Autopsies disclosed that 51% of their patients had nodal or visceral metastases.[77]

ASSOCIATED MALIGNANCIES AT OTHER SITES

Synchronous or metachronous malignant tumor of the aerodigestive tract occurs in 5% to 12% of patients with cancer of

the esophagus.[78-81] The oral cavity, pharynx, larynx, and lung are the most frequent sites. About half can be found in the head and neck areas, on the floor of the mouth, the tongue, tonsil, and larynx. Oral and pharyngeal cancers are most often associated with cancer of the esophagus, and laryngeal cancers are most often associated with cancer of the lung. Direct laryngoscopy, bronchoscopy, and esophagoscopy carried out in patients with head and neck cancer show that 5.5% of patients have synchronous lung or esophageal cancer, or both. Most of these patients (75%) are symptomatic.

At the Memorial Sloan-Kettering Cancer Center, 25% of patients with two primary cancers of the oral cavity, pharynx, larynx, or esophagus had synchronous cancers.[79] In 68%, the cancers appeared within 2 years of each other. The 60 patients with the multiple primary tumors came from a pool of 7000 patients seen during the same period for one of these malignancies.

TREATMENT

Despite all that surgeons have accomplished in recent years and the advances that have been made in radiation therapy and chemotherapy, the outlook for patients with squamous cell cancer of the esophagus remains poor. From 1974 to 1983, the average 5-year survival rate was 5%.[13]

Lack of progress in curing esophageal cancer has reinforced pessimism when considering the treatment of this disease. Many oncologists emphasize palliation rather than cure. Palliation is important because patients suffer greatly with malignant esophageal obstruction and tracheoesophageal fistulae. However, palliation and cure can be integrated into a management plan that can accomplish both objectives and compromise neither. The philosophy of this approach was most succinctly stated by Burdette, who advocated a plan of management for carcinoma of the esophagus "in which palliative measures were a part of the sequence leading to cure rather than a separate route of management."[82]

It is futile to attempt to determine which therapeutic approach is most likely to result in either cure or palliation because there are very few randomized comparisons of therapeutic approaches. Comparisons of reports from single institutions and historical data are not valid. Survival rates from both surgical and radiotherapy series can be markedly altered by reducing the denominator from which the survival percentage is determined.[83a,b] Surgical cure rates can be determined from the total number of patients evaluated, the number operated on, the number operated for attempted cure, the number successfully resected, or the number successfully resected who survive the immediate postoperative period. Similarly, radiation series can report survival based on various patient populations. The lack of standardized reporting continues to thwart an accurate assessment of 5-year survival rates, which range from 1% to 20%. These factors frustrate interpreting any report on therapy for carcinoma of the esophagus.

Although the three major modalities of therapy are discussed separately, the most important approach is combined modality therapy. Local eradication of squamous cell tumors will not suffice to improve the long-term survival of patients.

Effective chemotherapy in combination with surgery or radiation, or both, is the most promising approach to the treatment of esophageal malignancies.

Surgical Therapy

It must first be established whether the patient can withstand a thoracotomy and laparotomy. Advanced age is itself not a contraindication to surgical therapy. Inadequate cardiopulmonary function is the most frequent reason for declining to operate. Impaired cardiac and respiratory reserves frequently result from prolonged alcohol abuse and cigarette smoking, which are characteristic of patients with squamous carcinoma of the esophagus in the western hemisphere.

Because of the frequency of alcohol abuse, liver function tests are an important part of the preoperative assessment. Portal hypertension may also be severe enough to contraindicate an operation for esophageal cancer.

PREOPERATIVE PREPARATIONS. Debilitation from nutritional deficits should be corrected before considering surgery or any other therapy. Patients have fewer postoperative complications if they receive at least 5 days of preoperative nutritional support.[84] Protein and electrolyte derangements require immediate attention. Skin testing to determine whether the patient is anergic may be worthwhile. However, intense nutritional therapy with restoration of positive nitrogen balance may not suffice to correct anergy, and the ultimate benefits of nutritional supplementation have been questioned.[85,86] There is clear indication that prognosis can be related to the degree of weight loss. Patients with less than 10% weight loss do better than those with greater than 10% weight loss, but there is no evidence that correction of the weight loss improves prognosis.[87]

If the alimentary tract cannot be used, intravenous hyperalimentation should be employed. Gastrostomy should be avoided because the stomach is often used to replace or bypass the esophagus, but a feeding jejunostomy is acceptable. An excellent controlled randomized study has shown that the beneficial effects of enteral nutritional support are the same as by the venous parenteral route.[88]

Pulmonary function can be improved by eliminating cigarette smoking and by instituting chest physiotherapy and respiratory therapy in the form of intermittent positive-pressure breathing, incentive spirometry, bronchodilators, and antibiotics. Eliminating aspiration of oral secretions by placing a nasogastric tube above the malignant obstruction and attaching it to suction may be necessary for complete esophageal obstruction. Digitalization may be required, along with diuretics, to correct congestive heart failure.

Because the microbial flora of the esophagus of patients with cancer consist of many aerobic and anaerobic organisms, prophylactic antibiotics are used.[89] A third-generation cephalosporin or a combination of an aminoglycoside with clindamycin should be suitable.

These measures, vigorously applied, and equally effective postoperative care allow at least 50% of patients with cancer of the esophagus to undergo resection for either palliation or cure.

OPERATIVE CONSIDERATIONS. Patients who are operable should undergo a laparotomy to determine the extent of lymph node involvement and local (extraesophageal) spread. This information is vital in planning therapy. The surgeon should try to remove as much tumor as possible, leaving radiotherapy and chemotherapy the task of eliminating tumor that defies surgical removal. Radiopaque clips should be placed around the site of the tumor. This optimistic approach depends on the isolated case reports or the experience of surgeons who have struggled with the problem of esophageal cancer for many years. Wangensteen reported an 11-year cure for a patient with a cancer of the esophagus who had involvement of a lymph node on the greater curvature of the stomach.[4] Recent results reported by Ong and colleagues indicate that 10-year survival is possible even when a bronchoesophageal fistula is present from a lobar bronchus to the esophagus. Ong's patient had an esophagectomy and lobectomy.[90]

Ong cautions that if the main bronchus, trachea, or aorta is infiltrated by the malignancy, resection of these involved adjacent structures carries a high mortality and should not be performed. Patching the trachea or bronchus with pericardium is rarely successful. Most often the repair breaks down or infection causes the patched pericardium to slough.

Lymph node involvement following esophagectomy results in half of the 5-year survival rate of patients with negative regional lymph nodes. Even with positive regional lymph nodes, 10% to 15% of patients who have survived esophagectomy can be cured. However, 5-year survival rates may not be a valid basis for deciding whether a patient with esophageal cancer has been cured. After 5 years, as many as 78% of survivors may die of recurrences.[91]

Another cogent argument for proceeding with an esophageal resection whenever operable criteria are met is that this operation constitutes excellent palliation. Operative mortality for esophageal resection varies from 5% to 30%.[90] More recent reports have indicated that an operative mortality of less than 5% can be attained.[91]

ESOPHAGECTOMY. Because of the unusual lymphatic drainage of the esophagus, malignant cells can be found as far as 8 cm from the site of gross tumor with intervening skip areas free of tumor.[50] Lymph node involvement can also occur some distance from the site of the primary. The anatomic bases for these phenomena deserve emphasis because they support the generally accepted principle that the only adequate resection for a carcinoma of the thoracic esophagus is its complete removal. Esophagectomy should include a generous margin of the lesser curvature of the stomach, including the adjacent lymph node areas, and extend up to the cervical esophagus or the uppermost portion of the thoracic esophagus. The preferred method of reestablishing gastrointestinal continuity in most of these patients is an esophagogastrostomy. The mobilized stomach is brought up to the cervical esophagus or pharynx through a retrosternal tunnel or through the posterior mediastinum in the bed of the excised esophagus.

Watson's papers in the mid-1950s adequately documented the "case against segmental resection for esophageal carcinoma" and emphasized these principles.[50] Scanlon reported

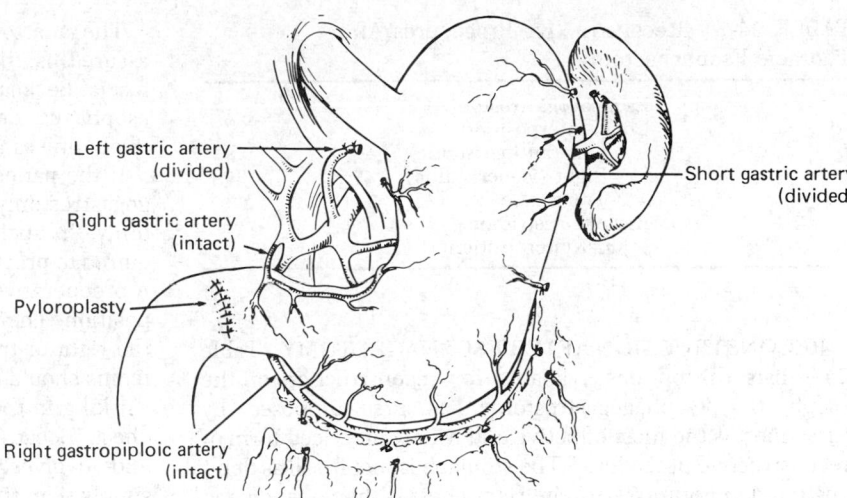

Left gastric artery
(divided)

Short gastric artery
(divided)

Right gastric artery
(intact)

Pyloroplasty

Right gastropiploic artery
(intact)

FIG. 24-6. Mobilization of the stomach for reconstruction of the esophagus involves division of the short gastric and left gastric arteries. The right gastric and gastroepiploic artery suffice to vascularize the stomach adequately. Since the vagus nerves are divided when the esophagus is resected, a pyloroplasty is required for adequate gastric drainage.

a 45% incidence of recurrence at the anastomotic site when a segmental resection of the esophagus was performed for carcinoma.[92] Wu and colleagues found cancerous tissue present at the margins in 14% of the resected specimens when they confined resection to 5 cm of esophagus above the cancer.[93] They advocate resection of the lower two-thirds of the esophagus for cancers of the lower third, and they perform an esophagogastrostomy in the chest above the level of the aortic arch. For midesophageal cancers, esophagogastrostomy is performed at the level of the dome of the pleural cavity. When the cancer extends above the level of the aortic arch, they perform an esophagogastrostomy in the neck. In one report, 43% of patients with cancer of the esophagus had cancer cells in the submucosa 5 cm above the tumor.[94] Thus, a resection that is less than a total thoracic esophagectomy will often be inadequate.

In addition to longitudinal resection of an esophageal cancer, a wide margin of surrounding normal tissues and as many as possible of the regional lymphatic channels, including the lymph nodes, should be removed. This is difficult in the upper thoracic esophagus because of the proximity of vital structures, including the aorta, the heart, the left main bronchus, and the inferior pulmonary veins. Skinner has advocated a radical en bloc resection of the esophagus, which was originally described by Logan.[95] This procedure aims to vacate the posterior mediastinum. It carried an 11% operative mortality and a complication rate of 52% in Skinner's hands. The difficulties encountered in performing an adequate resection of the upper esophagus provides a rationale for the use of radiotherapy or chemotherapy, or both, as adjuncts to local control of the tumor.

There are three approaches to esophageal resection: through a right thoracotomy, combined with a laparotomy; through a left thoracotomy, using a thoracoabdominal incision; and without thoracotomy, using separate abdominal and cervical incisions.

Esophagectomy through the right chest is the most widely accepted approach. During the same anesthetic, it is preceded by a laparotomy, during which the celiac and lesser curvature lymph nodes are biopsied and the stomach is mo-

bilized if it is to be used to replace the esophagus (Fig. 24-6).[96,97]

The esophagus can also be removed by blunt dissection through abdominal (transhiatal) and cervical incisions, thus avoiding thoractomy (Fig. 24-7). This operation was first described in England during the 1930s and was reintroduced by Kirk in 1974.[98] It has been used in the United States with acceptable results.[99-102] However, it does not allow for a wide resection of adjacent tissues and can be followed by disastrous complications.[103,104] It may be that esophagectomy without thoracotomy will suffice as a low-risk tumor reductive procedure, allowing radiotherapy and chemotherapy to eliminate the cancer that is left behind. It is most applicable for distal esophageal lesions and cervical esophageal lesions that can be mobilized adequately under direct vision.[105]

FIG. 24-7. The esophagus can be bluntly and blindly dissected free of surrounding structures through the esophageal hiatus and a cervical incision and thus removed.

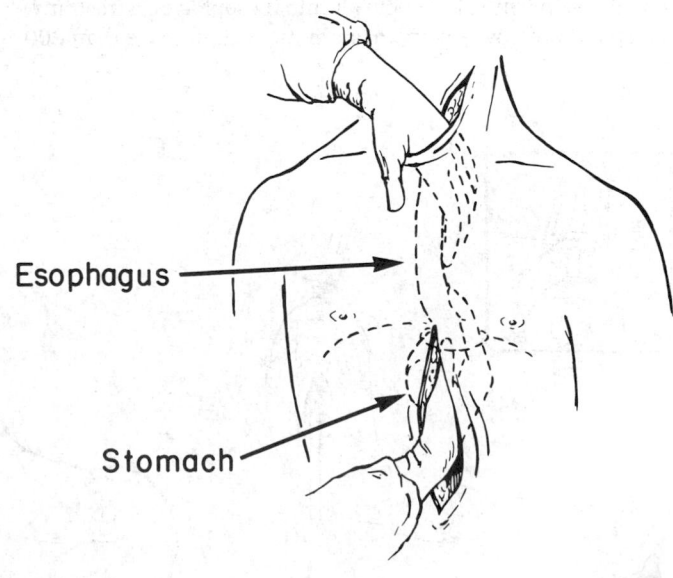

Esophagus

Stomach

TABLE 24-7.   Reconstructive Procedures After
Thoracic Esophagectomy

Esophagogastrostomy
Colon interposition
Left (antiperistaltic)
Right (isoperistaltic)
Transverse
Reverse gastric tube
Jejunal interposition

RECONSTRUCTION AFTER ESOPHAGECTOMY. Table
24-7 lists the options available for reconstruction of the
esophagus. Esophagogastrostomy, as first proposed by
Kirschner, is the most effective and widely practiced form of
reconstructive procedure.[6] The stomach is mobilized as demonstrated in Figure 24-6. The right chest is then opened and
the tumor removed. A right anterolateral thoracotomy has
been used by some surgeons rather than the right posterolateral thoracotomy demonstrated in the illustrations.[106] The
stomach is then brought up through the hiatus and anastomosed to the proximal esophagus (Figs. 24-8 and 24-9).
Alternatively, the stomach can be brought up to the neck
through the esophageal hiatus, or behind the sternum, and
anastomosed to the esophagus in the neck.[107]

Emphasis should be placed on the anastomosis between
the esophagus and stomach because its disruption is a major
cause of the morbidity and mortality following esophagogastrostomy. In addition to anastomotic disruption, strictures
can occur at the anastomotic site and gastroesophageal regurgitation can cause discomfort and disability resulting
from aspiration. Stapling devices can be used for this anastomosis with great success (Fig. 24-8).[108,109] An inkwell-type
anastomosis or fundoplication is performed if possible,
bringing the stomach around the esophagus, surrounding the
anastomosis with the stomach. This reinforces the anastomosis and diminishes the possibility of gastroesophageal reflux (Fig. 24-9).[110] Gastroesophageal reflux can be controlled by avoiding recumbency and by eating small meals.[111]
An innovative form of anastomosis developed by Shao and
associates in China is the intraluminal esophagogastrostomy,
which did not develop an anastomotic leak in more than 200
cases.[15]

The anastomosis should be free of tension. In order to
assure this, the stomach should be tacked to the prevertebral
fascia. Because a vagectomy is inevitable when removing the
esophagus, delayed gastric emptying can occur postoperatively unless a pyloroplasty is performed (Fig. 24-10).[112]

If the patient has had a previous gastrectomy, an esophagogastrostomy cannot be performed following esophagectomy. In such instances, a colon interposition will be required to provide a conduit to the stomach (Fig. 24-11).[113,114]
A preoperative barium enema is mandatory for a colon interposition. The left colon is best suited for this procedure, but
the right or transverse colon can also be used. Two surgical
teams should be used to limit operative time, with one team
working in the abdomen while the other team works in the
chest. Because this procedure requires three anastomoses
and involves the colon, which has a less adequate blood
supply than the stomach, the incidence of anastomotic leaks
is higher than after esophagogastrostomy.

Two other options exist for reconstruction of gastrointestinal continuity after a subtotal esophagectomy. A gastric
tube can be fashioned from the greater curvature of the
stomach (Fig. 24-12) or a jejunal loop can be used to bridge
the esophageal defect.[115,116] They have no advantages
over esophagogastrostomy and carry a higher rate of
complications.

Based on a review of several surgical series, the portion of
5-year survivors varies from 2% to 21%.[117] The average survival after the operation ranges from 7 to 28 months. Results
are generally better for smaller and more distally located
cancer.

The operative mortality with esophagogastrostomy ranges
from 4% to 30%.[117] Extremes of operative mortality for all
kinds of operations are 0.8% to 57%.[118] However, there appears to be a trend in recent years to lower operative mortality rates which should be less than 5%.[119] Cardiopulmonary
complications and anastomotic leaks lead the list of causes of
postoperative death.[120-123] Other complications are listed in
Table 24-8.

Radiation Therapy

Radiotherapy is rarely associated with acute mortality and,
when used by itself, frequently provides prompt relief of

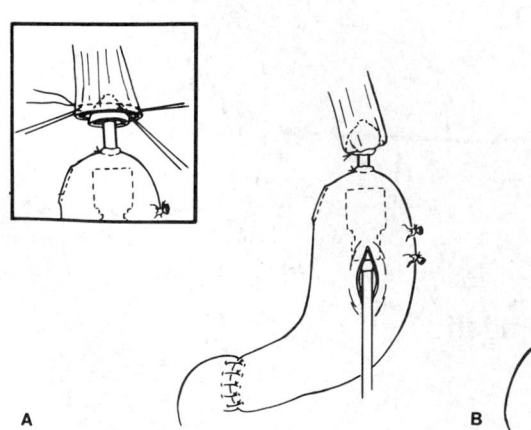

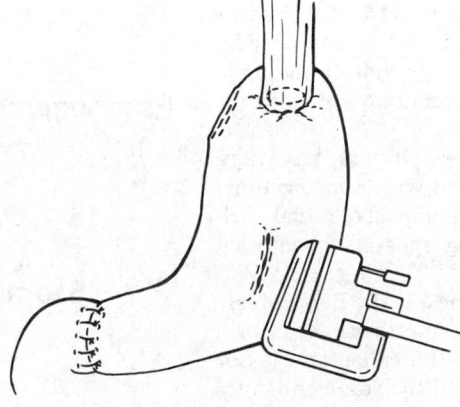

FIG. 24-8. **A.** Esophagogastrostomy is
performed using an end-to-end anastomosis stapler. The stapler may also
be inserted at the site of the pyloroplasty. The completed anastomosis is
shown in **B**. (Steichen FM, Ravitch
MM: Mechanical sutures in esophageal surgery. Ann Surg 191:373,
1980)

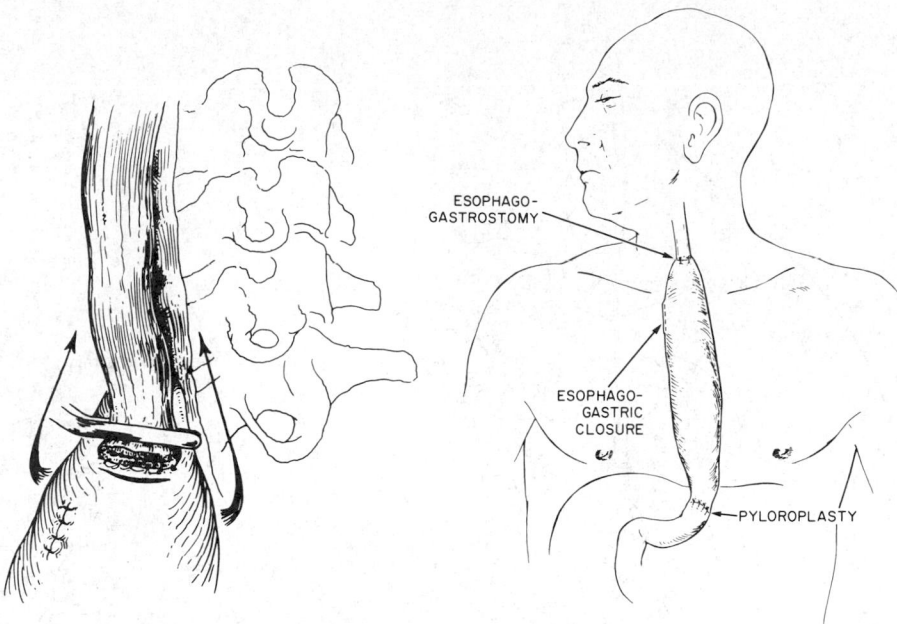

FIG. 24-9. A two-layered, end-to-side anastamosis is performed. After completion of the anastomosis, the stomach is wrapped around the esophagogastrostomy (*arrows*). **A.** The stomach also is sutured to the prevertebral fascia to prevent tension on the anastomosis. **B.** The finished operation.

FIG. 24-10. Barium contrast study following esophagogastrostomy.

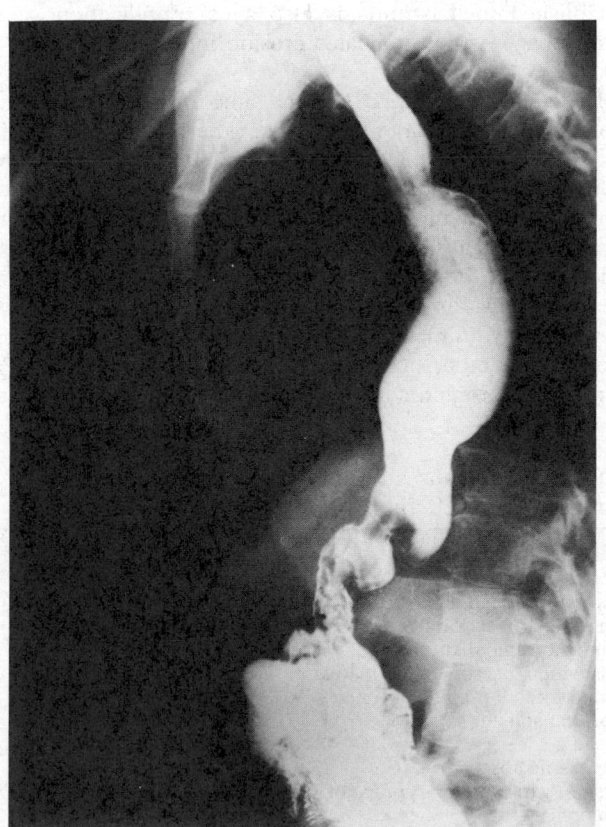

esophageal obstruction. However, definitive radiotherapy is a complex and demanding treatment, often requiring 6 to 8 weeks to complete. In a disease in which the median survival is measured in months, this is a substantial investment in time and resources for many of these patients. Furthermore, swallowing relief is only short-term in more than 50% of cases.

Radiotherapy alone is being used less frequently because newer techniques have been introduced that combine radiation with chemotherapy, with or without surgery. The radiotherapy is used to enhance local control and to control disease that may be difficult to resect, such as in mediastinal lymph nodes and periesophageal soft tissues.

PROGNOSTIC FACTORS AND PATIENT SELECTION. It is likely that radiotherapy alone will become confined to the elderly or infirm patient who is not a candidate for aggressive combined modality therapy, and radiation for palliation will be used in patients who present with metastatic disease. The optimal combined therapy for esophageal carcinoma has yet to be devised, but those in use are reviewed. Potential complications of surgery or chemotherapy still render many patients unsuitable for treatment with aggressive combined modality therapy, and radiotherapy alone will continue to play a role in the management of esophageal cancer.

A list of prognostic factors relevant to the radiotherapeutic treatment of esophageal cancer is presented in Table 24-9. In general, patients with small lesions (≤5 cm) are potentially curable with radiation, but those with lesions longer than 10 cm are rarely cured.[124] Although some institutions have not found tumor size to correlate with response, data from a large series of cases at The Princess Margaret Hospital indicate that response to radiation is 100% for lesions less than 5 cm, 66% for lesions 5 to 10 cm, and only 29% for tumors greater than 16 cm.[125,126] Circumferential lesions re-

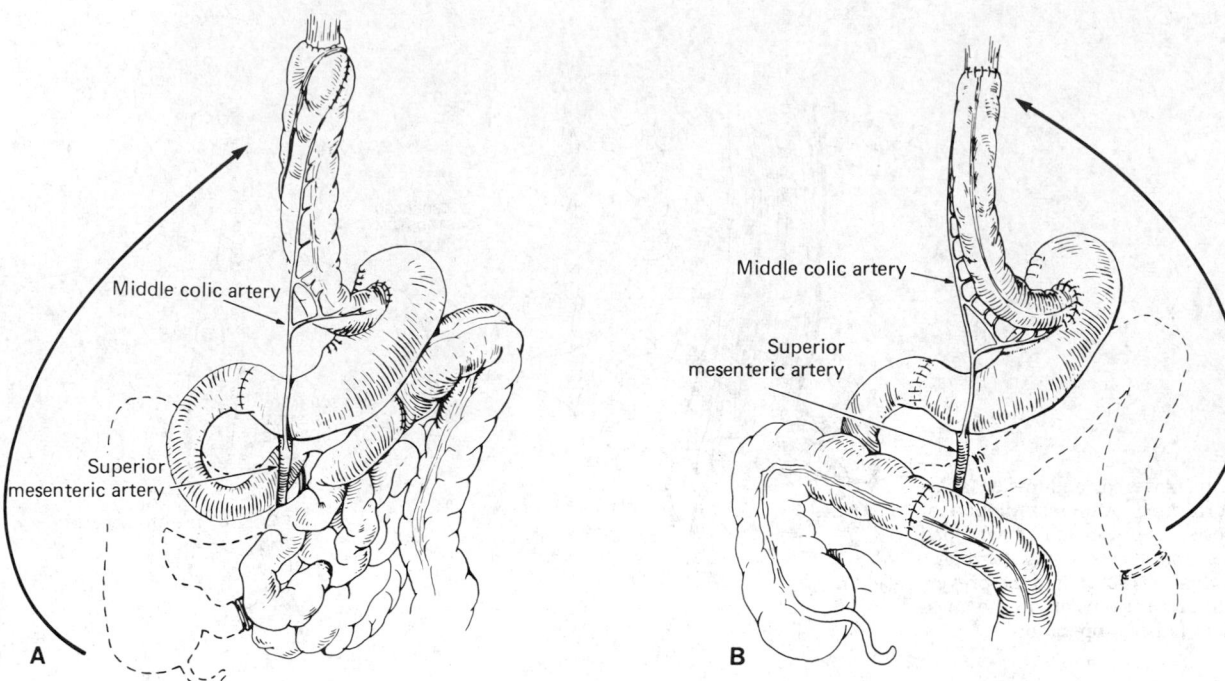

FIG. 24-11. Mobilization of the right colon to form an isoperistaltic conduit to the stomach (**A**) or the left colon to form an antiperistaltic esophageal substitute (**B**).

spond less well than do longitudinal tumors, probably a co-variable with size.[127] Women respond better than men; exo-phytic lesions respond better than ulcerative ones; older patients respond more frequently than younger patients; and upper-third lesions respond somewhat better than lesions in other areas of the esophagus.[124-128]

Several factors are relative contraindications to radiotherapy. Patients with a communication from the esophagus into the tracheobronchial tree have extremely short survivals and

FIG. 24-12. A gastric tube constructed from the greater curvature of the stomach can be used to reconstruct or bypass the esophagus. The gastric tube depicted here is isoperistaltic with the blood supply coming from the right gastroepiploic artery. A reverse gastric tube can be fashioned with the blood supply based at the fundus. (Postlethwait RW: Technique for isoperistaltic gastric tube for esophageal bypass. Ann Surg 189:673, 1979)

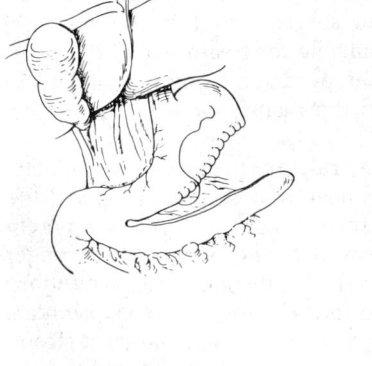 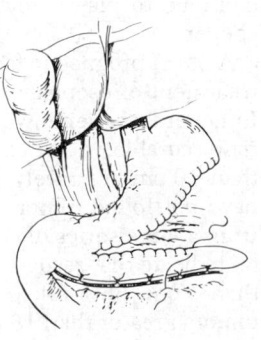

rarely benefit from radiation. Involvement of the trachea or bronchus without fistula often leads to fistulization as radiation shrinks the tumor, leaving behind a frank communication between the two structures that rarely will heal.[124] Established mediastinitis is also a contraindication, as is hemorrhage, which indicates erosion into a major vessel.

TECHNIQUE OF RADIATION. The intent of curative radiotherapeutic treatment is to treat the primary tumor, its potential microscopic extension, and the appropriate regional nodes to a cancericidal dose while respecting the tolerance of adjacent normal tissue. The radiotherapist must arrange the treatment fields and the patient's treatment position so that the setup can be reproduced accurately each treatment day for 6 to 7 weeks. Reproducibility is greatly facilitated by immobilization on the treatment table by a body cast or other customized molded support system. Patients with carcinoma of the esophagus often will be treated

TABLE 24-8.   Causes of Morbidity After Esophageal Resection

Anastomotic leak
Anastomotic stricture
Respiratory insufficiency
Congestive heart failure
Pulmonary embolism
Obstruction at esophageal hiatus
Wound infection or dehiscence
Ruptured spleen
Phlebitis
Subphrenic abscess
Torsion, gangrene or rupture of gastrointestinal replacement
Hemorrhage

TABLE 24-9. Prognostic Factors for Radiation Treatment of Esophageal Cancer

	Better	Worse
Female	Male
<5 cm length	>10 cm length
Less than circumferential	Circumferential
Upper one-third	Lower one-third
Older age	Younger age
Exophytic	Ulcerative

in the prone position to maximize the separation between the esophagus and spinal cord.[129-131] Many elderly patients find they cannot hold this treatment position long enough to accomplish simulation and subsequent treatment. In that case, patients are treated in the supine position. Arms are raised overhead to allow for access into the CT scanner in the treatment position.

Normal structures must be taken into account during esophageal irradiation to minimize complications. In esophageal carcinoma, the major dose-limiting structure is the spinal cord, which lies close to the esophagus. The radiation tolerance of the spinal cord is usually regarded as 4500 cGy, less than the dose required to eradicate the tumor. Therefore, some of the radiation treatment must be administered through oblique fields that avoid the spinal cord. These oblique fields, coupled with anterior or posterior fields, make up the commonly used three-field or four-field esophageal treatment plan (Fig. 24-13).[132]

The radiation therapy field is designed to encompass the gross and microscopic extensions of tumor, as well as regional lymph nodes. The radiographic extent of the tumor is covered with a 5-cm to 6-cm margin in the cephalad-caudad direction. Although esophageal cancer can spread more than 6 cm from the primary site in approximately 15% of cases, such patients are rarely cured with radiation therapy alone.[133] There is little evidence that radiation response or cure is associated with field size.[126] Pearson achieved the best results ever reported using a relatively limited field size.[134] Even when a 5- to 6-cm margin is taken around the tumor, field sizes will be 15 cm or longer, which is substantial (Fig. 24-14).

For treatment with radiation therapy alone, the field width is usually 7 to 8 cm, enough to cover the esophagus and nearby structures such as periesophageal lymph nodes. CT scans can detect significant amounts of periesophageal soft tissue extension that are difficult, if not impossible, to recognize on plain x-ray films taken with barium contrast.[62-65] CT scans display the location, size, and density of pulmonary tissue, which allows treatment to be performed with a correction built in for the increased radiation transmission that occurs through low-density lung tissue.[135]

CT scans can be used as a basis for radiotherapy treatment planning. The scan can be brought up on the treatment planning screen (Fig. 24-15A) and beams superimposed on this image. Dose calculations can be made, and the region of the esophagus and periesophageal soft tissues can be seen as encompassed within the high-dose volume (Fig. 24-15B). Furthermore, CT scans can be reformatted in the sagittal

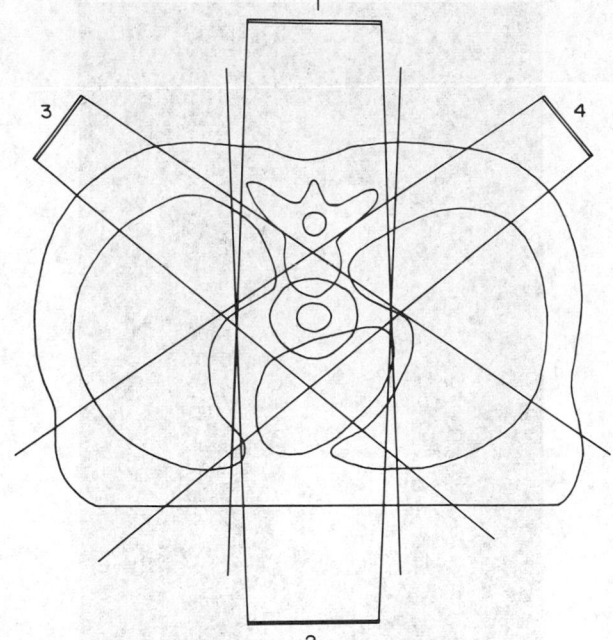

A

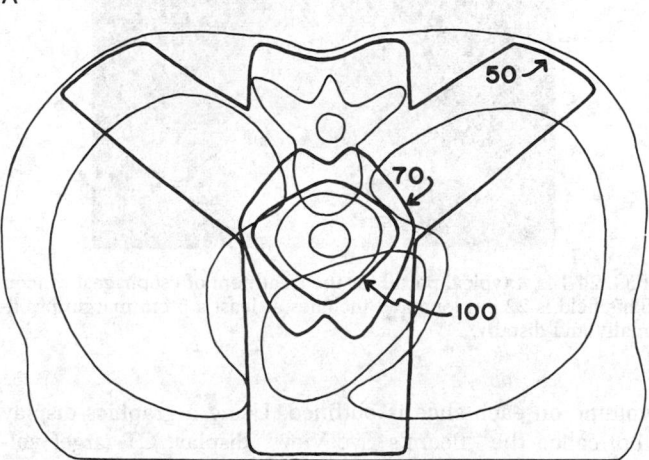

B

FIG. 24-13. **A.** The classic radiation field configuration for treatment of esophagus cancer. Two oblique fields are used matched to an anterior field, with or without a posterior field. This three- or four-field plan produces a high dose volume around the esophagus. The oblique fields spare the spinal cord so that dose to this structure can be kept below tolerance levels. **B.** Isodose curves for this treatment technique. The 100% volume encompasses the tumor while the spinal cord receives less than 70% of the dose.

plane. This allows a view of the region of the esophagus and the spinal cord throughout the treatment length. These displays are extremely valuable in planning treatment (Fig. 24-15C).

The CT scan can also verify the adequacy of the radiotherapy portals. First, the patient is simulated and films of each treatment port are taken using barium contrast (Fig. 24-14). The patient is then taken to the CT scanner, and CT slices throughout the esophageal tumor volume are obtained while the patient is positioned in a fashion to duplicate the treatment position. The CT scans are then viewed and the target

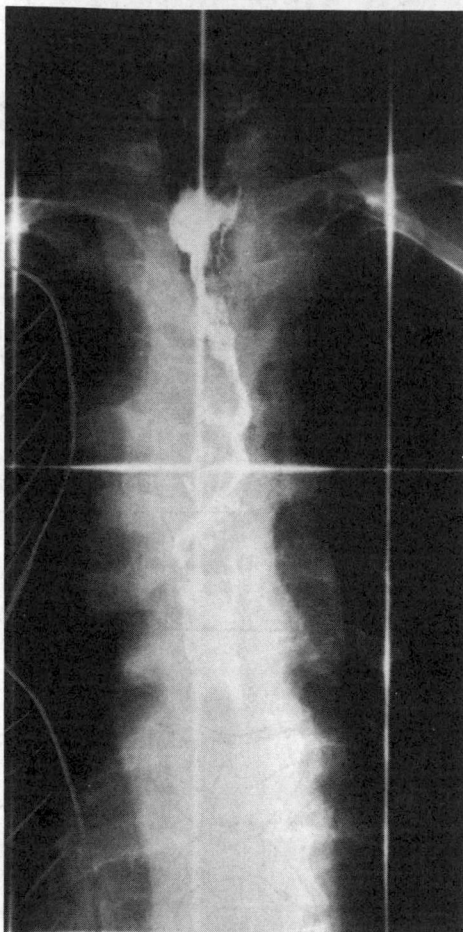

FIG. 24-14. A typical portal for the treatment of esophageal cancer. This field is 22 cm long and includes at least a 5 cm margin proximally and distally.

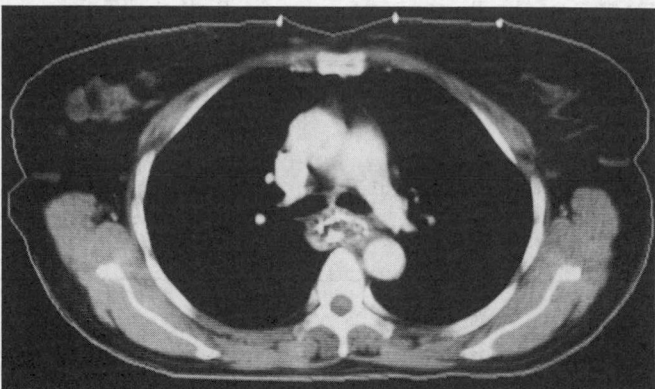

A

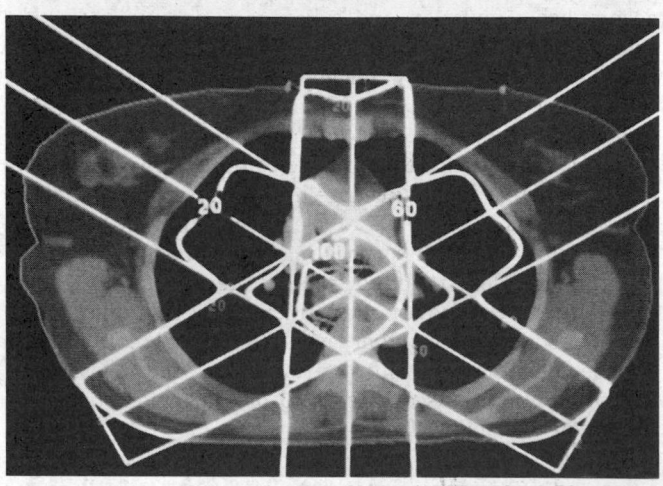

B

FIG. 24-15. **A.** CT scan of a patient with esophageal cancer. The patient is in the supine position on a flat couch that duplicates the treatment couch. The esophageal tumor with thickening of the esophageal wall can be clearly seen. **B.** Three-field plan (anterior and two posterior obliques) superimposed on the CT scan. The esophageal tumor is encompassed in the high dose zone, and the spinal cord is partially spared radiation with the oblique portals.

volume on each slice is outlined. Using a graphics display tool called the "Beam's Eye View" display, CT target volumes can be superimposed onto the simulator film.[136,137] It is then easy to determine whether the target volumes are adequately included in the radiation field and whether shielding blocks can be safely added to protect normal tissue (Fig. 24-16).[138]

The ability to see tumor and normal tissue anatomy on CT scans and the increasing use of combined modality therapy have refocused attention on regional lymph node treatment. Spread to regional nodes occurs in 40% to 70% of esophageal cancer patients, and sterilization of these areas is critical in the curative treatment of this disease. Many institutions now routinely include radiotherapy for supraclavicular nodes in their patients with upper esophageal lesions and for celiac nodes in their patients with middle and lower esophageal lesions.[138,140,141]

The dose of radiation varies from one institution to another and also depends on whether chemotherapy or surgery will be added to the treatment. Definitive doses of radiation range between 5000 cGy in 20 treatments over 4 weeks to 6600 cGy in 33 treatments over 7 weeks. In many instances, these doses are reduced when concurrent chemotherapy is

administered. No dose regimen has proved superior to any other, but, as combined modality therapy becomes more effective and systemic micrometastases are controlled, local control in the esophagus itself will take on increasing importance. In general, higher doses of radiation lead to higher local control rates.[142]

CLINICAL COURSE AFTER IRRADIATION. The squamous epithelium of the esophagus has approximately the same radiosensitivity as that of the oral mucosa.[143] Deepithelialization leads to clinical symptoms of esophagitis that begin 1 to 2 weeks after the start of treatment and can be severe in some patients. Tumor response usually begins during the second or third week. Improvement in swallowing and relief of tumor pain can make the discomfort of esophagitis more tolerable. Measures that reduce the symptoms of esophagitis include systemic analgesics and viscous lidocaine. The possibility of monilial esophagitis should always be considered, and antimonilial agents can benefit some patients. The radiation tolerance of the esophagus is usually

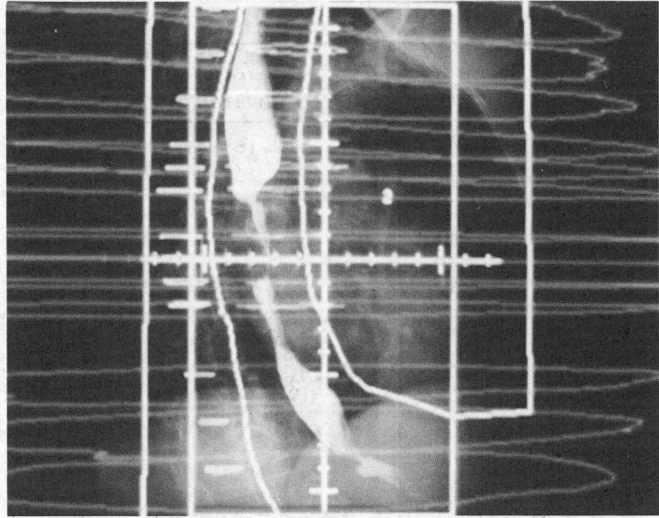

A

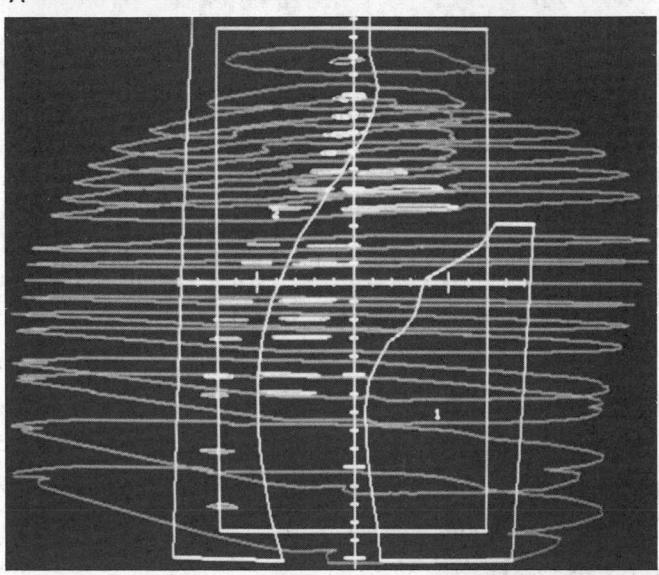

B

FIG. 24-16. **A**. Beam's eye view display for esophageal treatment. The CT target volumes and the spinal cord are superimposed on the simulator film with a barium esophagram. The shielding blocks treat the esophagus but can clearly be seen to encroach on the target volumes anteriorly. **B**. The blocks can be modified to better include the target volume. Here the spinal cord is protected by the posterior block, and the anterior block allows a generous margin around the target volume.

between 6000 and 6500 rad.[144] However, chemotherapeutic agents, especially doxorubicin, can dramatically increase the radiation sensitivity of the esophagus, and care must be exercised in the concurrent administration of drugs and radiation.[145]

RESULTS OF RADIATION THERAPY ALONE. Table 24-10 summarizes the result of radiation therapy alone and includes survival data for untreated patients. There is a suggestion that modern high-energy x-ray treatment produces an improvement compared with the natural history of the

disease. Between 60% and 80% of irradiated patients will have their dysphagia partially or completely relieved by irradiation (Fig. 24-17). This response is often rapid and in many patients occurs during treatment. In about one-third of treated patients, this restoration of swallowing will persist for the duration of their illness. This correlates reasonably well with the 15% to 30% complete tumor regression seen when radiation is used preoperatively in the treatment of esophageal cancer (Table 24-11).

COMPLICATIONS OF RADIATION THERAPY. Death or serious long-term morbidity caused by esophageal irradiation is uncommon. Occasionally, patients have been reported with radiation pneumonitis, pericarditis, myocarditis, or spinal cord damage. The most frequent complications from esophageal irradiation are stricture, fistula, and hemorrhage. Many of these complications are related to regrowth of the cancer itself. Although more than 50% of irradiated patients will develop stricture, many of these are due to persistent cancer.[125,126,150] Fistulas and hemorrhage following irradiation occur in 10% to 20% of cases and usually result from resolution of cancer that has invaded the neighboring trachea, bronchus, or aorta.[150,155,156] However, not all complications are tumor related, and benign esophageal stricture from radiation or infectious complications have been reported.[125]

INTRACAVITARY RADIATION. The concept of implanting radioactive sources within or around a tumor has a long history. The first cancer to be treated in this fashion was probably carcinoma of the cervix in which the cervical canal was a natural holder for the radium tube. In the early 1900s, Exner recognized that the lumen of the esophagus represented a natural opening for the introduction of radioactive material into the center of an esophageal cancer.[158] Since that time, several intraluminal applicators have been tried. In 1969, Rider reported on a series of patients treated with external radiation followed by an insertion of an intraluminal radium bougie.[159] These early results were encouraging, with a 37% 3-year survival. Since that time, a number of reports have appeared concerning intraluminal radiation, the most recent of which used remote after-loading sources to eliminate exposure of hospital staff.[160-165] The esophageal lesion suitable for such therapy is relatively small because the esophagus must be able to accept intubation and the dose distribution is about 1 to 1.5 cm. For these reasons, intraluminal therapy is being used in many cases after external-beam treatment has shrunk the primary tumor. The intraluminal treatment is then used as a boost dose, much as a radioactive implant of seeds is used in the head and neck or breast. Early reports of intraluminal therapy for rapid palliation of obstruction are encouraging.[165]

CONFORMATIONAL THERAPY. When the esophagus and periesophageal tissues are irradiated, a substantial amount of normal tissue is also irradiated. To reduce the dose to normal tissues, many radiotherapy centers have tried rotational therapy in which the treatment volume describes a tight circle around the target, with a rapid falloff in dose reaching the adjacent normal structures. However, the

TABLE 24-10.   Studies of Radiation Alone for Esophageal Cancer

Author	Reference	Dates	Patients Treated*	Dose (rad)	Median Survival (mo)	2-Year Survival	5-Year Survival
Roberts	146		975	Untreated	Not stated	20% (6 mo)	6% (1 yr)
Applequist	147	1965–74	50	5100–6800	12	12% (3 yr)	4%
Beatty	126	1969–75	146	4000–6000	9	20%	6%
Cedarquist	91	1945–69	388	4500–7000	8	11%	4%
Elkon	148	1968–73	50	5000–7000	11	28%	2%
Hussey	124	1945–75	69	5500–6500	10	16%	10%
Jobsen	149	1978–81	38	5500–6500	12	14%	4%
Lewinsky	130	1966–71	85	5000–6000	8	11%	4%
Lowe	150	1958–69	244	Not stated	5	7%	1%
Newaisky	151	1956–74	444	5000–5500	12	18%	9%
Pearson	134	1949–69	388	5000	12	28%	20%
Schuchmann	152	1950–78	77	4500	10	Not stated	0%
Van Andle	153	1970–78	115	6000–6600	Not stated	4%	1%
Van Houtte	154	1962–72	81	6000–7500	8	9%	3%
Wara	155	1950–73	103	5000–6000	7	8%	1%
Wei-Bo Yin	156	1968–69	1212	6000–7000	Not stated	11% (3 yr)	7%

* With curative doses; some data extracted from survival curves.

esophagus is rather difficult to treat in this fashion because the tissue that needs treatment is of different widths in different areas of the esophagus and because the esophagus has a curved shape.

Conformational therapy is a way around this dilemma. In this technique, the conventional radiation collimator is replaced by a device made up of 20 or 30 separate pairs of leaves. These leaves can independently be adjusted to any width, allowing the tumor to be treated with a shaped field that conforms to the tumor configuration. As the machine rotates around the patient, the leaves continuously change their position so that at every angle the treatment field is shaped to conform to the shape of the target volume. This creates a very tight dose distribution, which minimizes the dose to normal tissues.[166] In this manner, it may be possible to increase the dose of the esophagus while maintaining or diminishing the dose to the surrounding tissues.[127,166] Because increasing dose is usually related to increasing tumor

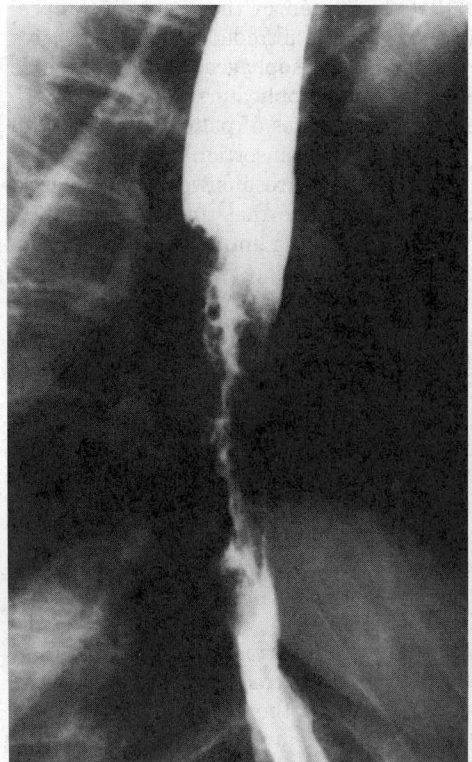
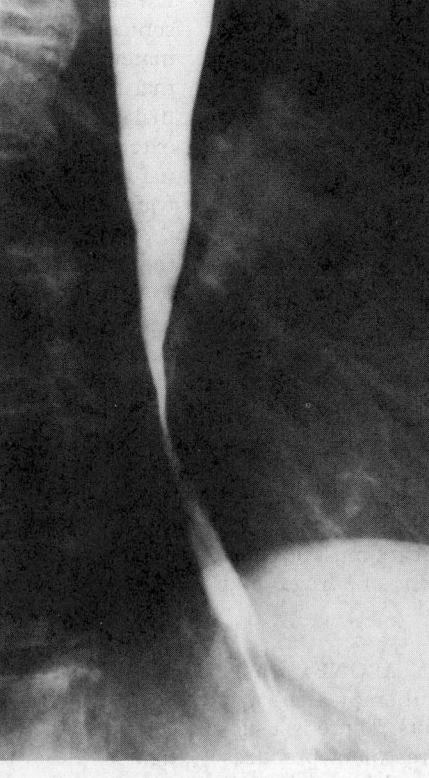

A   B

FIG. 24-17. **A.** Midesophageal lesion before treatment. **B.** Post-treatment esophagram. Swallowing was restored, and the surgical specimen was negative on pathologic examination.

TABLE 24-11. Ability of Radiation to Sterilize Esophageal Cancer

Reference		% Tumor-Free	Dose (rad) Specimen
	4000	21	213
	5000	23	
	4500	13	214
	4000	30	127
	3000	14	217

control, this therapy promises improved local control of esophageal cancer.

Chemotherapy

Autopsy studies of patients who died of locally controlled esophageal cancer indicate that treatment of the primary tumor and regional lymph nodes is insufficient.[72-77] The search for useful systemic therapies for squamous cell carcinoma of the esophagus has become an important goal because chemotherapy is no longer used solely as a treatment of last resort but has become a vital component of multimodality approaches.

Unfortunately, accurately assessing the effect of chemotherapy as part of initial treatment of esophageal lesions has posed special problems for clinical investigators. At best, measurement by CT of the chest, barium swallow, or endoscopy allows independent observers to declare a lesion improved. The classic partial response (50% reduction of the perpendicular diameters) as determined by barium swallow or endoscopy criteria is more likely to involve investigator bias than are measurements of pulmonary, soft tissue, and liver nodules. A clinically complete response demonstrated by x-ray film or endoscopy is far more elusive than a complete response confirmed by examination of the resected esophagus.[167,168] Despite their deficiencies, these diagnostic methods can determine partial responses with some reliability.

Data generated during the past decade have convincingly demonstrated that epidermoid tumors of the esophagus are relatively responsive to chemotherapy. Kelsen's review showed that nine adequately tested chemotherapeutic agents have modest but defined response rates for patients with measurable lesions.[169] Combinations of the active single agents have consistently yielded higher response rates than the single agents alone.[169]

Initial reports of clinical trials using single agents against epidermoid tumors of the esophagus concentrated on measurable lesions outside the esophagus itself. The modestly active agents, employed after esophagectomy or radiation therapy, produced responses lasting less than 3 months. Furthermore, palliation of symptoms was minimal. Occasionally, patients treated with chemotherapy who were not candidates for surgery or primary radiation experienced improvement of dysphagia, even if the distant measurable disease had not responded.[170,171]

It is no longer uncommon for investigators to report that chemotherapy given as first-line treatment before radiation or surgery improves dysphagia.[172,173] Subjective clinical improvement may or may not correlate with improvement in barium or endoscopy studies.[172,173] A complete response of the primary tumor to chemotherapy does not mean complete eradication of metastatic cancer of the esophagus.[174,175] Thus, current chemotherapy takes on some of the palliative properties of localized surgery and radiation.

SINGLE-AGENT CHEMOTHERAPY. Recent reviews outline the results of single-agent therapy for cancer of the esophagus, and Table 24-12 summarizes these data.[167,176,177] Most clinical trials of single agents enrolled patients whose disease was progressing after surgery or radiation. New Phase II chemotherapeutic agents are not commonly tested

TABLE 24-12. Standard Single Agents Against Squamous Cell Carcinoma of the Esophagus

Drug*	Dose	No. of Patients Treated		Response (%)		Dysphagia Relief	Reference
		1st Line	2nd Line	PR	CR		
Bleo	15 mg/m² 1V, twice weekly	15	0	3	1 (27)	?	178
Bleo	20 mg/m², IV, every day to 280 mg	0	14	0	0	?	179
Bleo	0.25 mg/kg, IV, every day to toxicity	0	4	0	0		180
Bleo	15 mg/m², IV, twice weekly × 4	?	?	1	1 (20)	40%	181
DDP	90 mg/m², every 3 weeks	0	10	2	2 (40)	?	182
DDP	2 mg/kg, every 4 weeks	17	0	1	0 (6)	35%	183
DDP	50 mg/m², IV, days 1 and 8, every 3 weeks	0	35	6	3 (26)	?	184
DDP	50 mg/m², IV, every 3 weeks	15	9	6	0 (25)	?	185
5-FU	500 mg/m², IV, every day × 5	0	23	4	0 (17)	?	186
5-FU	300 mg/m², continuous infusion every 6 weeks	11	0	0	11 (82)	100%	187
MMC3	0.05 mg/kg, IV, every day × 10	0	7	1	0 (14)	?	188
MMC	20 mg/m², IV, every 4 weeks × 2, then every 6 weeks	11	13	10	0 (42)	?	185
Dox	40 mg/m², IV, for 2 days	15	0	4	1 (33)	?	189
Dox	60 mg/m², IV, every 3 weeks	0	16	0	0	?	186
MTX	40 mg/m², IV, weekly	0	26	3	0 (12)	?	186
MTX	200 mg/m², IV, every 10 days × 2	44	0	20	1 (48)	73%	173

* Bleo = bleomycin; DDP = cisplatin; 5-FU = 5-fluorouracil; MMC = mitomycin C; Dox = doxorubicin; MTX = methotrexate.

against squamous cell tumors of the esophagus because the tumor is less common and less easy to measure than the classic signal tumors. Nevertheless, modest responses to bleomycin, mitomycin C, doxorubicin, 5-fluorouracil, and cisplatin were considered in designing combinations of chemotherapeutic agents used in initial treatments with surgery or radiation, or both. Investigational drugs, such as vindesine or mitoguazone (MGBG), were found to have modest but reproducible activity against advanced disease treated with other therapies.[190,191] A different picture might have emerged if intact, untreated primary tumors were studied

rather than advanced disseminated disease. Based on experience garnered from preoperative and preradiation chemotherapy regimens, single-agent therapy can produce responses in intact, untreated primary tumors in more than 50% of patients treated, and perhaps it is in this context that new and promising phase II agents should be tested.

COMBINATION CHEMOTHERAPY. Data reported for single-agent chemotherapy have been used to rationally combine agents. Table 24-13 is a partial listing of the combinations used to treat disseminated esophageal cancer. Most

TABLE 24-13. Combination Chemotherapy Trials for Disseminated Squamous Cell Carcinoma of the Esophagus

Chemotherapy*	No. of Patients	PR	CR	%	Median Survival†	Reference

DDP + Bleo
  DDP = 3 mg/kg day 1
  Bleo = 10 mg/m², IV, load day 3
      10 mg/m², 24-h infusion days 3–6
	18	2	1	17	4 mo	192

DDP + Bleo
  DDP = 20 mg/day × 8
  Bleo = 10 mg, infusion each day × 8
	17	1	3	24	?	193

DDP + Bleo + Vind
  DDP = 3 mg/kg, day 1
Bleo = 10 mg/m², IV, load day 3
      10 mg/m², 24-h infusion days 3–6
  Vind = 3 mg/m², IV, weekly
	24	8	0	33	4 mo	194

DDP + Bleo + Vind
  DDP = 50 mg/m², day 1
  Bleo = 15 mg/m² , day 1
  Vind = 3 mg/m² weekly
    Recycle every 3 weeks
	27	7	0	29	3.5 mo	195

DDP + Bleo + MTX
  DDP = 50 mg/m², day 3
  Bleo = 10 mg/m², IM, weekly
  MTX = 40 mg/m², IV, days 1 and 15
    Recycle every 3 weeks
	31	7	1	26	5 mo	196

DDP + Bleo + MTX
  DDP = 50 mg/m², day 4
  Bleo = 10 U, IM, weekly
  MTX = 40 mg/m², days 1 and 14
    Recycle every 3 weeks
	10	4	1	50	7.5 mo	197

DDP + Vind + MGBG
  DDP = 120 mg/m², day 1
  Vind = 3 mg/m², weekly
MGBG = 500 mg/m², days 1 and 14
    Recycle every 29 days × 1
	20	8	0	40	4.8 mo	198

DDP + Vind + MGBG
  DDP = 100 mg/m², day 2
  Vind = 1.6 mg/m², IV, days 1,2,3,4
  MGBG = 500 mg/m², IV, days 1 and 14
    Recycle every 29 days
	4	2	0	50	?	199

DDP + MGBG + MTX + Bleo
  DDP = 50 mg/m², day 4
  MGBG = 500 mg/m², days 1 and 14
  MTX = 40 mg/m², days 1 and 14
  Bleo = 10 U, IM, days 1 and 14
    Recycle every 21 days
	8	4	1	63	?	200

DDP + 5-FU + Dox
  DDP = 75 mg/m², day 1
  Dox = 30 mg/m², day 1
  5-FU = 600 mg/m², days 1 and 8
    Recycle every 29 days
	21	2	5	33	?	201

* DDP = cisplatin; Bleo = bleomycin; Vind = vindesine; MTX = methotrexate; MGBG = mitoquazone; 5-FU = 5-fluorouracil; Dox = doxorubicin.
† Median survival from time on study.

of the relatively successful regimens outlined in Table 24-13 have been used as first-line treatment for esophageal tumors in combination with radiation or surgery; because combined chemotherapy is used as primary therapy, its effect on survival becomes more important than its effect on tumor response. The signal contributions of Kelsen and colleagues at the Memorial Sloan-Kettering Cancer Center deserve special notation: they carefully defined partial and complete clinical responses, separated clinical and pathologic responses, and always kept sight of the ultimate aim of improving overall survival. They investigated the use of cisplatin and bleomycin infusion, basing their study on the work of Wittes and colleagues, which indicated that this combination had substantial activity in head and neck cancers.[202] Sixty-one patients were treated, producing a 15% complete and partial response rate, with a median duration of response of 6 months in patients with metastatic disease.[203]

After their initial studies had indicated activity for both bleomycin and doxorubicin, Kolaric and co-workers combined the two agents.[189] Of 16 patients, 3 had partial responses. Although the response rate observed was lower than that seen with doxorubicin alone, the 95% confidence limits overlap.

Using a combination of cisplatin, methotrexate, MGBG, and bleomycin, which had shown activity in head and neck cancers, Vogel and colleagues treated ten patients, nine of whom had metastatic disease.[200] Five patients had complete or partial responses, with remissions lasting 3.5 to 7 months.

Because their patients had different mechanisms of action and toxicities and appeared to lack cross-resistance, Kelsen and colleagues studied the three-drug combination of cisplatin, vindesine, and bleomycin (DVB).[204] Sixty-eight patients were treated. The response rate of patients with metastatic disease was 33%, and the median response for patients with extensive disease receiving chemotherapy alone was 7 months. Although DVB was fairly well tolerated, myelosuppression was dose-limiting. The median leukocyte nadir was 1700 cells/mm³. Other major toxicities were nephrotoxicity, nausea, vomiting, and a peripheral neuropathy.

Gisselbrecht and coworkers, treated 21 patients with advanced esophageal cancer, using a three-drug combination of 5-fluorouracil (5-FU), doxorubicin, and cisplatin.[201] Objective responses were seen in seven patients, including two complete remissions. The overall response rate was 33%. Cardiotoxicity was seen in one patient. Other toxicities included nausea, vomiting, myelosuppression, and occasional nephrotoxicity.

In the most recent studies, patients with poor Karnofsky performance status (*e.g.*, bedridden patients) have been excluded. Because responses are rare and toxicity is substantial in patients with severely impaired performance status, they should probably not receive aggressive therapy. For patients with a Karnofsky performance status of 50 or better, response rates between 15% and 80% have been reported, with response durations averaging 5 to 9 months. The complete response rate ranged from 0 to 20%. The lowest complete response rates were reported by investigators who restaged patients aggressively using endoscopy or surgery. Some patients have more durable remissions. However, for the smaller series, the 95% confidence limits are quite large.

Combined Modality Therapy

PREOPERATIVE RADIATION THERAPY. Several groups of radiation oncologists and surgeons have tested the hypothesis that for esophageal cancer treatment results improve by giving radiation therapy before resection (Table 24-14). The researchers hoped the two used together would cancel the disadvantages of each and reinforce their benefits. Radiation therapy carries a low mortality and morbidity and can, in higher doses, produce a marked regression in tumor bulk and sterilize microscopic disease in unresected areas (Table 24-11). It is possible to treat a wider area surrounding the esophageal cancer by radiation therapy than can be reasonably accomplished by surgery (Fig. 24-18). On the other hand, esophagectomy can treat a greater length of esophagus, contributing to local control of the tumor and providing a better chance of long-term palliation and possible cure. Reduction in tumor bulk from radiation can, in some cases, increase resectability rates and decrease operative mortality by making surgical procedures easier to perform. Preoperative radiation can prevent metastases and local recurrences that stem from clonogenic tumor cells being liberated by the surgical manipulations.

A variety of radiation dosages and schedules have been used (Table 24-14). In most studies, dosages of 3000 to 6000 cGy over 3 to 6 weeks have been employed. Surgery is undertaken 4 to 6 weeks after completion of the radiotherapy. Alternatively, some studies have used concentrated or large doses of radiation therapy consisting of 2000 to 3000 cGy over 7 to 10 days, with the operation taking place within a week. In most cases, difficulties encountered in operating in areas that received radiation did not increase morbidity and mortality. However, in some instances, the morbidity of preoperative radiation has been as high as either surgery or radiation therapy alone. Mortality rates have ranged from 4% to 33%.

Long-term survival from preoperative radiation correlates with the extent of tumor destruction seen in the operative specimen. For example, Morita found 44% 2-year and 28% 5-year survival rates when preoperative radiation showed extensive tumor destruction.[127] Survival rates were cut in half when this destructive effect was not seen histologically in the resected specimen. Sugimachi reports virtually identical findings.[217] However, Liu reported that long-term survival rates were unrelated to the degree of histologic destruction caused by preoperative radiation. In general, the disappearance of tumor is a significant goal in preoperative radiation, and most long-term survivors come from the groups whose tumor was nearly or completely eradicated by radiation. The fact that combined treatments of radiation plus chemotherapy increases this tumor-free rate is a possible explanation for the increased benefits of chemoradiation compared with radiation only before surgery.

The results of studies of preoperative radiation therapy must be interpreted with caution because many authors do not specify whether survival rates are based on the total number of patients examined, the total number of patients treated, the total number of patients taken to surgery, the total number of patients resected, or the total number of patients who survived the operation. If patients are omitted

TABLE 24–14. Studies of Preoperative Radiation Therapy for Esophageal Cancer

Author	Reference	Dates	Properative Dose (cGy)	No. Treated*	No. Operated on
Akakura	206	1963–68	5000–6000	117	117
Anderson	207	1977–81	3500	59	36
Doggett	208	1962–68	5000–6600	42	29
Gignoux	209	1976–81	3300	102	97
Groves	210	1964–71	2400	70	Not stated
Hussey	124	1944–75	3000–4000	56	41
Jobson	149	1978–81	4000	91	81
Huang	205	1977–82	4000	89	79
Kelsen	211	1965–76	2000–4500	76	66
Launois	212	1973–76	4000	67	62
Liu	213	1966–82	3000–7000	Not stated	74
Marks	214	1960–73	4500	332	137
Mortia	127	1971–80	3000–4000	130	Not stated
Nakayama	215	1959–79	2000–3000	Not stated	Not stated
Parker	216	1965–75	4500	75	75
Sugimachi	217	1972–83	2500–3000	Not stated	104
Van Andel	153	1970–77	4000	133	133

* Usually taken from larger series. Screening criteria often not specified.
† Distinction is often not made between curative and palliative resections.
‡ Many authors do not specify whether survival rates are calculated based on total number treated, number operated, or number surviving operation. Some data extracted from survival curves.

at each one of these branch points, thus reducing the denominator, long-term survival figures can be artificially inflated.

Two randomized studies involving preoperative radiation have been reported. Launois and colleagues studied 124 patients treated between 1973 and 1976.[212] In this trial, only middle-third or lower-third primary tumors were included. The two groups were similar in age, sex, tumor localization, and surgical approach. The resection rates for the two groups were similar, as was the operative mortality, which was substantial. Most disappointing were the median and long-term survival rates. When operative deaths were excluded from the analysis, the average survival was only 4.5 months for those receiving preoperative radiation and 8.2 months for those treated by surgery alone. There was no statistically significant difference for the two arms of the study or for the 5-year survival rates: 9.5% for combined treatment group and 11.5% for the patients treated by surgery alone. Although the preoperative radiation group had a higher operative mortality rate for patients with middle-third lesions, it was also not significant statistically.

A multi-institutional trial was performed by the European Organization for Research on Treatment of Cancer on 208 patients with resectable lesions.[209] The radiation regimen was 3300 cGy given in 10 fractions over 12 days. Resection was performed within 8 days. The control arm underwent surgery alone. The cure rate for resection alone was 57.5%. It was 49.5% in the group treated with preoperative radiation. There was no difference in resectability between the two treatment groups. The operative mortality was 24.7% for the group treated with preoperative radiation and 17.9% for the patients treated only with surgery. There was no difference in the 2-year survival or median survival for these groups.

Both studies used radiation doses that were relatively concentrated compared with the regimens used by others. In addition to the use of intense radiation, resection was undertaken 8 days after completion of radiation therapy, when the

inflammatory response to therapy was still present and before maximal shrinkage of the tumor took place. Despite these criticisms, the standard preoperative approach to esophageal carcinoma now frequently involves both radiation therapy and chemotherapy.

POSTOPERATIVE RADIATION THERAPY. When an exploratory thoracotomy or laparotomy reveals an unresectable advanced carcinoma of the thoracic esophagus, postoperative radiation therapy is often used to control the cancer. Radiation therapy under these circumstances should be considered palliative therapy. An unresectable lesion is unlikely to be cured by radiation therapy, although the possibility always exists.

The rationale for radiation therapy following curative resections of esophageal cancers is that irradiation will eradicate residual macroscopic or microscopic disease, which

FIG. 24-18. Portions of esophagus and adjacent tissues best treated by radiation and resection. (Adapted from Pearson JG: The present status and future potential of radiotherapy in the management of esophageal cancer. Cancer 39:882, 1977)

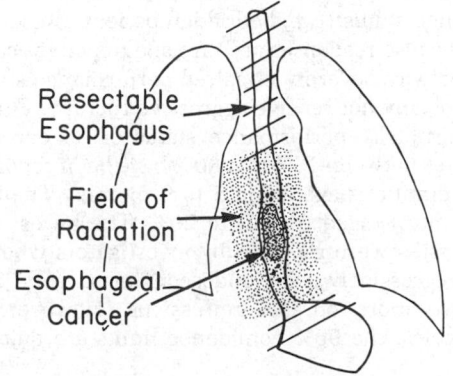

No. Resected	Operative Mortality (%)	Median Survival (mo)	2-Year Survival (%)*	5-Year Survival (%)*
96	21	11	32	25
19	6	7	19	Not stated
24	33	Not stated	12	5
75	25	Not stated	25	10
46	20	Not stated	11	Not stated
30	18	10	13	Not stated
69	20	18 (resected patients)	45	Not stated
79	4	Not stated	Not stated	Not stated
41	12	9	10	5
47	20	10	20	10
59	9	Not stated	70	60
101	18	25 (resected patients)	23	14
Not stated	Not stated		35	23
542	6	Not stated	Not stated	13
75	19	Not stated	15	10
104	6	Not stated	28	17
81	21	Not stated	Not stated	14

could be located within the unresected esophagus, at the margins of resection, or in regional lymphatics and lymph nodes that were not removed. Postoperative radiation may also be effective in controlling implantation or seeding of tumor cells, which may have occurred at the time of operation.

More effective radiation is possible postoperatively because the surgeon can demarcate the extent of the tumor with radiopaque clips at the time of operation, allowing the radiotherapist to direct the treatment accurately to the involved area. However, if the stomach or colon is brought up into the area formerly occupied by the esophagus, radiation therapy must be limited to 4500 to 5000 cGy to avoid radiation injury. Furthermore, the anatomy has been so distorted by these surgical procedures that it is difficult to delineate the volume that is at risk for tumor spread even with the aid of surgical clips and CT scans.

Of seven patients who underwent esophagectomy and postoperative radiation for the reasons enumerated above, Fraser and colleagues reported two 10-year survivors.[218] Both had cancer at the resected margins of the esophagus. Goodner reported 25 patients who had esophagectomy and esophagogastrostomy with postoperative irradiation.[219] Two patients survived for 5 years; the average survival was 9.9 months. At the Mayo Clinic, 14 patients with cancer of the upper thoracic esophagus were treated with postoperative radiation. Five of these patients were 3-year survivors.[220]

Hankins reported a doubling of median survival (7–13 months) for Stage III patients given postoperative irradiation.[221] Langer reported a 28% 2-year survival for nine patients treated with postoperative radiation.[222] Giuli and Gignoux found little effect if doses were less than 3000 cGy; at higher doses the rate of recurrence decreased.[223] In the only large-scale report concerning the use of irradiation after resection for cure, Stage I patients were excluded from this trial.[224] Treatment consisted of 6000 cGy to the mediastinum and neck. Patients with involved nodes at the time of surgery did not benefit, but patients with uninvolved nodes had an extraordinary survival rate (Table 24-15).

There is a paucity of data on the efficacy of postoperative radiation. The advantages of this approach over preoperative radiation are that an accurate anatomic staging of the disease is possible, surgery is not delayed, and it has no influence on operative mortality. On the other hand, esophageal reconstruction often requires lower doses of radiation. This combination of radiation and surgery is probably best used after low-dose preoperative radiation along with chemotherapy. Patients whose tumors are resectable but who have positive

TABLE 29-15. Survival After Postoperative Irradiation for Esophageal Carcinoma

Nodes	Mediastinal 1 Year	2 Years	5 Years
Negative (39)			
Radiation (20)	19/20 (95%)	17/18 (94.4%)	7/8 (87.5%)
No radiation (19)	10/19 (53%)	8/17 (47%)	3/11 (27%)
Positive (72)			
Radiation (32)	20/32 (63%)	11/30 (37%)	2/18 (11%)
No radiation (40)	21/40 (51%)	9/36 (24%)	4/22 (18%)
Overall Survival*			
Radiation		58%	35%
No radiation		30%	20%

* Not actuarial. Follow-up is 1 to 6 years.

or close tumor margins can have this area clipped and post-operative irradiation added through oblique portals.

PREOPERATIVE CHEMOTHERAPY. The rationale for using chemotherapy before and after surgery for squamous cell carcinoma of the esophagus has been described in the section on chemotherapy and is similar to that described for the use of preoperative radiation. Surgery following chemotherapy provides not only the potential of definitive treatment, but also an opportunity to assess pathologic responses to the chemotherapy program. Following resection of the esophageal cancer, chemotherapy can prevent recurrence and inhibit metastases.

Single-drug therapy with bleomycin, given daily or every other day to a total dose of 300 mg, followed by surgery resulted in a resectability rate of 47% and a 2-year survival of 21%.[225] Similar results were reported with this regimen from other centers in Japan.[226] Miller and colleagues used cisplatin as a single agent preoperatively and followed the resection with 4500 to 6000 cGy. More than half of these patients showed partial responses to cisplatin, but no patient had a complete response.[227]

Bleomycin was used as a continuous 3-day infusion after administration of cisplatin (Table 24-16).[192] Although approximately half the patients experienced subjective improvement in swallowing, only 14% were judged to have a partial response by barium swallow, and no patient had complete disappearance of all the cancer after esophagectomy. The median survival for those with local-regional cancer of the esophagus was 10 months.

After finding modest activity for the experimental vinca alkaloid, vindesine, Kelsen and his colleagues added it to bleomycin and cisplatin.[228] After the first 23 patients had been treated, two courses of chemotherapy were instituted before esophagectomy. Postoperative radiation was planned at 5000 cGy over 5 to 6 weeks for patients with T3 or N1 cancer found at operation. Nine percent of patients taken to resection were found to have no cancer in the resected esophagus. The median survival for the group was 16.2 months.

The report by Schlag and colleagues using the same regimen had similar results. Only one patient had a complete response. Fewer than half of the treated patients could be resected for cure.[229]

In the only prospectively randomized trial testing the efficacy of chemotherapy before surgery, 36 patients were randomly assigned to either immediate surgery or chemotherapy with cisplatin, vindesine, and bleomycin, using the dose and schedule recommended by Kelsen.[230] Although 8 (47%) of 17 patients treated before surgery responded to chemotherapy, no significant difference in resectability and survival was found between the two groups. Median survival was 9 months. When the eight patients responding to chemotherapy were compared with the cohort undergoing surgery without chemotherapy, a highly significant difference in median survival was detected.

After retesting an older drug, MGBG, with a new schedule, several investigators found modest activity against disseminated cancer of the esophagus.[231,232] Kelsen and colleagues hoped to be able to eliminate the bleomycin pulmonary toxicity by substituting MGBG.[198] The median duration of survival was greater than 2 years for all those having an operation after receiving MGBG, cisplatin, and vindesine.

After receiving preoperative vinblastine, cisplatin, and MGBG for 2 cycles scheduled 3 weeks apart, 9% of the patients treated had a pathologically confirmed complete response.[199] The median survival for the entire group of patients was 14 months.

Based on previous reports of the efficacy of 5-fluorouracil (5-FU) combined with cisplatin, Shields and colleagues used three courses of cisplatin and 5-FU before surgery for cancer of the esophagus.[233,234] Thirteen (76%) of 17 patients responded to the chemotherapy. No patient had a complete response. Postsurgical treatment consisted of three additional courses of chemotherapy. Those judged to have disease remaining after chemotherapy were offered radiation. Median survival reported for this group of patients is 17.3 months, with projected survival at 3 years of 36%.[234]

Carey and colleagues reported on 24 patients treated preoperatively with 5-FU and cisplatin.[235] Patients with tumor invading the mediastinum or with positive lymph nodes had postoperative radiation. Patients with complete clinical responses were offered four more courses of 5-FU and cisplatin. At the time of surgery 10 (43%) of 24 patients had no visible cancer; four patients who responded still had visible tumor. Only one patient was found pathologically to be free of cancer. Median survival for patients responding to the chemotherapy was projected at 20.4 months compared with 6.7 months for those patients who did not respond to the preoperative therapy.[234]

TABLE 24-16. Preoperative Chemotherapy

Combination*	Patients Operated on/ Patients on Study†	(%)	PR (%)	CR (%)‡	Median Survival§	Reference
DDP-Bleo	34/43	(79)	6 (14)	0	10.0 mo	192
DDP-Bleo-Vind	34/44	(77)	28 (63)	1 (2)	16.2 mo	194
DDP-Vind-MGBG	14/19	(74)	8 (42)	1 (5)	8.5 mo	198
DDP-Vind-MGBG	11/11	(100)	6 (55)	1 (9)	14.0 mo	199
DDP-5-FU	6/17	(35)	13 (76)	0	17.6 mo	233
DDP-5-FU	22/24	(92)	14 (58)	1 (4)		234

* For doses, see references listed. DDP = cisplatin; Bleo = bleomycin; Vind = vindesine; MGBG = mitoguazone; 5-FU = 5-fluorouracil.
† Patients operated on; all patients treated on study.
‡ Pathologic CR.
§ Median survival from time on study.

These experiences clearly indicate that combination chemotherapy can affect primary tumors in the esophagus (Table 24-16). Whether survival is enhanced by using chemotherapy before surgery awaits a randomized, controlled trial or more striking data than are available.

PREOPERATIVE CHEMORADIATION THERAPY. The earliest experiences with preoperative chemoradiation therapy used single agents. Fujimaki treated 76 patients with radiation and bleomycin before surgery.[225] Their results, as other reports from Japan, were encouraging.[226,236] Thirty percent of the 27 patients at risk for 3 or more years were still alive at the time of the report. A multi-institutional randomized trial from the Scandinavian countries involved 63 patients treated with preoperative radiation and 70 patients treated with preoperative radiation plus bleomycin. No significant differences in median survival or 2-year survival rates were observed.[207] Other studies of bleomycin combined with radiation have not been impressive either.[237]

Werner reviewed the results of a combination of methotrexate, leucovorin, and radiation.[238] Thirty-one percent of the resected patients had no tumor in the resected specimen. Operative mortality was 14%. The average survival reported for patients undergoing surgery was 2 years and 2 months. In a much smaller series from India, the results were similar.[173]

Beginning in 1976, Franklin and colleagues at Wayne State University (WSU) treated epidermoid tumors of the esophagus by using 5-FU and mitomycin C with radiation.[239] Franklin's study contained 30 patients judged to have resectable esophageal cancer.[240] The 23 patients (77%) who subsequently underwent surgery had preoperative barium swallows interpreted as "improved." Six patients (26%) who underwent esophagectomy did not have tumor in the resected esophagus. Four (13%) of these patients survived 5 or more years after their treatment ended. The median survival for the entire group treated was 12 months. Seven patients (30%) died after the operation. One of the patients who died in the postoperative period had no cancer in the resected esophagus.

Parker and colleagues reported on 34 patients treated with either one or two cycles of preoperative 5-FU and mitomycin C plus external-beam radiation of 3000 cGy over 3 weeks.[241] Thirty-four patients were treated in 3 years; 21 (62%) underwent surgery. Eleven had no cancer in the resected esophagus. Although the median survival for the group was not given, Parker clearly documented the problem of distant recurrence for patients rendered free of localized cancer by the preoperative treatment.

The WSU group attempted to decrease protocol mortality by eliminating the potential pulmonary complications of mitomycin C and, in its place, using cisplatin. Cisplatin was chosen as an alternative to mitomycin C because it had caused complete remissions in phase II trials.[184] Furthermore, there was a developing literature on cisplatin's radiation sensitizing properties.[242,243] Cisplatin is not initially toxic to the bone marrow, a property that allowed it to be combined with other chemotherapeutic agents, radiation, or surgery.

Leichman and colleagues reported on 21 patients treated with cisplatin and 5-FU.[233] Radiation and surgery were planned as in the 5-FU–mitomycin trial. Follow-up treatment was included only if cancer remained in the esophagus. Fifteen patients had esophageal resections; 7 (33%) patients were free of all cancer in the esophagus, but 2 of these patients had tumor within the celiac lymph nodes. The median survival for the entire group was 18 months. The median survival for those who could undergo resection was 24 months. Five patients (23%) survived for more than 3 years; three of these patients had no cancer in the resected esophagus and two had microscopic tumor in the resected esophagus.

Although these investigators believed that the patients who survived 3 years or more were cured, Leichman has reported that all these patients have died of recurrent esophageal cancer 3.5 to 5.5 years after treatment was completed. All patients who survived 2 or more years from the completion of surgery had documented distant recurrence of their cancer.

Several researchers reported data on 33 patients treated preoperatively with cisplatin, 5-FU, and radiation.[244,245] They compared the neoadjuvant patients with recent historical controls treated by surgery alone. Each group found a 2-year survival of more than 50% for those treated with neoadjuvant chemotherapy and radiation. Campbell reported no 2-year survivors for surgery alone, but Austin reported that 18% of those receiving surgery were alive at 2 years.

The Southwest Oncology Group (SWOG) and the Radiation Therapy Oncology Group (RTOG) treated patients with the WSU protocol.[175] The group was able to evaluate 106 patients; of this group, 71 (67%) underwent surgery. Eighteen (17%) of the patients (25% of those who underwent resection) were found to have no cancer in the resected esophagus. Operative mortality was 11%. Median survival for all patients who completed the protocol was 14 months. The median survival for those 18 without cancer in the resected esophagus was 32 months. When all patients are considered, 28% had 2-year survivals and 16% had 3-year survivals. In analyzing patterns of failure for patients treated on the SWOG and RTOG trials, Leichman found that 68% of the patients had distant recurrences, 20 had local (within the radiation field) and distant recurrences, and 12% had local recurrences only.[168]

Popp and colleagues used a combination of preoperative 5-FU, cisplatin, and vincristine sulfate with radiation.[246] They had utilized 5-FU mitomycin, and 5-FU–cisplatin on previous series of patients. Because of the small numbers of patients in each group, all patients treated by multimodality therapy are presented as a unit. Twenty-one percent of their combined modality group survived at least 30 months from treatment, compared with 4.8% of their patients treated with surgery alone. There were no long-term survivors who did not achieve a complete remission from preoperative chemoradiation. Their overall impression of multimodality therapy was that it was an improvement over previously used therapy.

Wolfe and co-workers used 5-FU, etopside, and radiation preoperatively.[247] At least 40% of the patients with squamous cell cancer of the esophagus resected had no tumor in the specimen. The 2-year survival for 17 patients completing the full course of treatment was 30%.

TABLE 24-17. Preoperative Chemoradiation

Drugs*	Radiation Dose (cGy)‡	Total No. of Patients	Patients Operated on	CR	Median Survival	Reference
5-FU-Mito C	3000	30	23 (77)	6 (20)	12 mo	218
5-FU-Mito C	3000	34	21 (62)	11 (32)		241
5-FU-DDP	3000	21	15 (71)	5 (24)	18 mo	232
5-FU-DDP or Mito C	3000	27	27 (100)	6 (24)		174
5-FU-DDP	3000	13	5 (38)	3 (23)		244
5-FU-DDP	3000	11	11 (100)	6 (55)	26 mo	245
5-FU-DDP	3000	106	71 (67)	18 (17)	14 mo	174
MTX with leucovorin	2000	58	58 (100)	18 (18)	26 mo	246

* 5-FU = 5-fluorouracil; Mito C = mitomycin C; DDP = cisplatin; MTX = methotrexate.
† Radiation given before surgery.

Clinical trials using chemotherapy and radiation before surgery for patients with untreated primary esophageal tumors can produce a partial response in at least half of the patients treated if the barium swallow and endoscopic improvement are used as indicators of response (Table 24-17). Fifteen percent to 30% of those treated will show a pathologically confirmed complete response upon review of the surgical specimen. Although it is true that radiation biologists have demonstrated that cisplatin and 5-FU enhance ionizing radiation, the degree of this sensitization has yet to be defined clinically.[52] Yet, Parker, Leichman, and Poplin have independently shown that distant recurrences are the rule, even for the patient with a pathologically proven complete response. No trial to date has shown a 5-year survival for even 20% of those treated. Moreover, toxicity and mortality from combining chemotherapy, radiation, and surgery have remained very troubling aspects of these trials.[249]

CHEMORADIATION THERAPY WITHOUT SURGERY. Surgery has been a very useful guidepost to instruct investigators as to the efficacy of chemotherapy alone or with radiation and may be indicated in clinical trials for this purpose. However, as a modality offering only local control for a disease that tends to disseminate early, surgery may be the modality most easily eliminated without sacrificing overall survival. Poplin's report on combined modality therapy found that the median survival for 113 patients entered on the SWOG trial was 12 months, and the median survival for the 71 patients undergoing surgery was only 2 months more.[175] Furthermore, because surgery and radiation therapy seem to have equal long-term results and their combination offers no apparent benefit, it seems worthwhile to attempt to treat esophageal cancer with chemoradiation without surgery to avoid the morbidity and mortality that occasionally follow esophagectomy.[85]

It must be stressed that in this discussion of therapy without surgery, we are referring to a combined modality approach that is designed as primary therapy for esophageal cancer. In the past, chemoradiation without surgery was considered only for patients who were unsuitable for operation because of advanced disease. The earlier literature reflects this latter approach and must be evaluated from this perspective.

As early as 1972, single-agent chemotherapy with irradiation was employed in a limited number of patients as primary treatment for esophageal carcinoma with encouraging results.[250] Kolaric evaluated the use of bleomycin, doxorubicin, and bleomycin–doxorubicin, in addition to radiation, in three sequential studies.[178,189,251] In each trial, a control group received chemotherapy alone. The number of patients in each arm was small (15–20 patients). In each study, the objective response rate to chemotherapy and radiation was superior to that seen with chemotherapy alone. Toxicity was, however, significant. The median duration of response for the radiation and chemotherapy group ranged from 5 to 9 months.

The results of a randomized trial involving bleomycin plus radiation or radiation alone were not encouraging.[252] Patients were given 5000 to 6000 cGy over 5 to 6 weeks; bleomycin was given at a dose of 15 units/day to a total dose of 210 mg. There was no improvement in swallowing function (objective regressions were not quantitated) or in survival for the bleomycin–radiation group compared with those receiving radiation alone.

A combination of methotrexate, bleomycin, 5-FU, and vincristine, followed by radiation, was used in a group of 26 patients.[253] After one to two cycles of chemotherapy, 55% had some degree of tumor shrinkage. After radiation, 66% had complete remissions; however, it was not clear how this evaluation was performed. There was one drug-related death. The median survival was 11 months.

Using cisplatin and bleomycin or cisplatin, vindesine, and bleomycin, Kelsen and co-workers treated 20 patients with local-regional tumor who either refused surgery or were poor surgical risks.[203,204] The response rates were similar to those seen in the larger group treated preoperatively (22% for cisplatin and bleomycin, 55% for cisplatin, vindesine, and bleomycin); radiation was well tolerated by most patients. Of the 20 patients, 5 were long-term survivors.

Abitbol and colleagues treated nine patients with radiation plus 5-FU, cisplatin, and methotrexate.[254] The median survival was 29 weeks.

Berenzweog and colleagues used a combination of cisplatin, methotrexate, bleomycin, and MGBG before radiation in 5 patients.[255] They were part of a larger group of 18 patients receiving this combination. The average survival of the whole group was 8 months.

The combination of vincristine, methotrexate, and cisplatin plus 5800 cGy did not appear to be an improvement over radiation alone. However, these studies were not carried out in a controlled fashion and can be compared only with historical controls.

Leichman and colleagues initiated a combined modality trial using criteria identical to those of the WSU studies in which surgery followed chemotherapy and radiation.[174] This group of patients received 5-FU, cisplatin, and radiation without intention to operate. Following the second course of 5-FU and cisplatin, mitomycin C and bleomycin were added. A second course of bleomycin was given 3 weeks after completion of the first cycle of mitomycin and bleomycin. Patients then received a follow-up radiation course of 2000 cGy over 2 weeks. Those with improvement in dysphagia were followed without further therapy.

The WSU group treated 20 patients on this protocol. The median lesion size was 7 cm; four patients were older than 80 years of age. Sixteen patients (80%) had an excellent clinical response as shown by subjective improvement in dysphagia and objective increase in body weight. Four patients who did not respond received esophagectomy without complication. The median survival for all patients treated had not been reached after 30 months. Pulmonary toxicity (presumably from bleomycin and radiation) necessitated steroids for 8 of the first 16 patients treated. The last 4 patients received cisplatin and 5-FU instead of bleomycin and radiation.

Lokich and co-workers reported the results of primary treatment of epidermoid tumors of the esophagus for 11 patients treated with 300 mg/m² of 5-FU continuously for 6 weeks.[187] All the patients treated reported symptomatic improvement. Nine (81.8%) of 11 had measurable improvement confirmed independently by barium swallow and endoscopy. These patients had further therapy with radiation and 5-FU. Two solid tumor trials have shown the superiority of this schedule for 5-FU compared with the bolus schedule.[256,257] Lokich's schedule may allow clinicians to take further advantage of Byfield's hypothesis that the best infusion schedule is the one that best potentiates the radiation sensitizing properties of 5-FU.[258] Lokich and colleagues have confirmed that low-dose continuous-infusion 5-FU without radiation is cytotoxic and can cause significant damage to the primary tumor without radiation.

Coia and colleagues treated 30 patients with squamous cell carcinoma of the esophagus with 5-FU, mitomycin C, and 6000 cGy of radiation over 6 to 7 weeks.[259] Some patients required breaks in their radiation therapy because of esophagitis, but no severe hematologic problems developed with this regimen. Complete responses based on clinical criteria were obtained in 84% of their patients. Two-year and 5-year actuarial survival rates were 47% and 32%, respectively.

Keane and colleagues from The Princess Margaret Hospital reported on 35 patients treated with 5-FU, mitomycin C, and radiation.[260] This group found significant improvement in both local disease-free survival and overall survival when compared with their own historical controls. The actuarial 2-year relapse-free rate was 47%, and the rate of local tumor control at 2 years was 54%, which was twice as long as their historical group.

John and co-workers treated 21 patients with inoperable cancer of the esophagus with infusion 5-FU, mitomycin C, and radiation followed by infusion 5-FU, cisplatin, and radiation.[261] Dysphagia was relieved within 7 to 14 days of starting therapy for 15 patients (71%), and the median survival for the entire group was 16 months. Six were alive 3 to 40 months after treatment.

Advani and colleagues, noting a paucity of data on the use of methotrexate in good-performance patients with squamous cell carcinoma of the esophagus, reported their experience with methotrexate as a single, first-line agent without leucovorin rescue.[173] Forty-eight percent of patients treated showed "good" responses by barium swallow criteria. When methotrexate was combined with cisplatin, response rates were increased to 76.2%. Twenty-nine of these 42 patients then received 6000 cGy of radiation. Twenty-three obtained further improvement in swallowing capability and esophagram changes. The median duration of response, however, was limited to 12 months, and a significant number of patients developed local-regional recurrences.

These reports indicate that little is lost in terms of survival if aggressive chemotherapy and radiation are used without surgical intervention in the primary treatment of epidermoid tumors of the esophagus. Nevertheless, the scientific rationale for combined radiation and chemotherapy needs refining. The definition of radiation sensitization should be clarified, because the chemotherapeutic agents once used as "sensitizers" for external-beam radiation possess cytotoxic properties against the primary tumor. Finally, a clearer understanding of why microscopic disseminated cancer is resistant to chemotherapy while gross esophageal mucosal tumors usually exhibit partial responses would be most helpful in designing regimens to overcome the differences in the sensitivities of the primary and metastatic cancers of the esophagus.

The past decade of clinical research in cancer of the esophagus has been the decade of emergence of chemotherapy as a primary modality in the therapeutic armamentarium. The clinical trials outlined have defined reproducible clinical and pathologic responses that radiation or surgery alone have not been able to produce in most series. The combined modality trials using chemotherapy with radiation or surgery, or both, have commonly reported median 2-year survivals between 25% and 30%, with median 3-year survivals between 12% and 25%. Unfortunately, there are only a few long-term survivors in each of these trials, and cure remains elusive.

Neither surgery alone nor radiation alone has been adequate. Nevertheless, it is incumbent on investigators to define a survival advantage for patients prospectively randomized to treatments of radiation with or without chemotherapy or surgery with or without chemotherapy. Without such proof, chemotherapy will join surgery and radiation as another toxic, inadequate therapy for primary cancer of the esophagus.

Treatment of Cervical Esophageal Carcinoma

Because of its intimate relationship to the larynx, cervical esophageal carcinomas present special kinds of problems. A recent review of 71 patients, seen from 1965 through 1980,

TABLE 24-18.   Reconstructive Procedures After Cervical
Esophagectomy

Pharyngogastrostomy
Reverse gastric tube
Skin tubes and skin grafts
    Wookey procedure
    Deltopectoral flap (Bakamjian)
    Others
Intestinal grafts with vascular anastomoses
    Jejunum
    Sigmoid
    Gastric antrum
Colonic interposition

revealed that extramural penetration was present in 77% of
the patients. Tracheal invasion was found in 35% and vocal
cord paralysis occurred in 24% of the patients.[262] These
findings carry a poor prognosis. Resection of a carcinoma of
the cervical esophagus usually requires removal of portions
of the pharynx, the entire larynx, the thyroid, and the proximal esophagus.[263] If cervical lymph nodes are involved and
the lesion is localized to that side, a unilateral radical neck
dissection may be included. This is a formidable procedure;
it leaves a large defect that is difficult to reconstruct and that
is followed by a high mortality and morbidity.[221] Table 24-18
outlines the techniques that can be used to reestablish pharyngoesophageal continuity.

The operation of choice is currently a pharyngogastrostomy.[263,264] The stomach is brought up through the posterior
mediastinum after it has been adequately mobilized. The
entire thoracic esophagus is bluntly dissected free of the
surrounding mediastinal structure and resected (Fig. 24-7).
Alternatively, a gastric tube may be constructed from the
greater curvature of the stomach to reestablish gastrointestinal continuity (Fig. 24-12). These extensive reconstructive
procedures further compromise the patient who has already
been stressed by the resection of the carcinoma. Harrison
has reported a 12% operative mortality for pharyngolaryngoesophagectomy with gastric anastomosis.[263] A review of
the mortality and morbidity of this operation was published
by Ong, who first described this operation in 1958.[265]

The surgical treatment of cervical esophageal malignancies carry a significant morbidity, leave the patient with a
great disability, and provide little hope for cure. Most recent
reports cite a 20% 2-year survival rate. However, if an
esophagogastrostomy is uncomplicated, significant palliation
is achieved, and the patient may swallow food and saliva
without difficulty.

Lesions in the cervical esophagus represent a particularly
vexing problem for the radiation therapist also. Generally,
these lesions are too low to allow good coverage with parallel, opposed lateral fields because irradiation would take
place through the patient's shoulders. Conversely, they are
often too high to allow treatment with posterior oblique
fields. However, it is possible to use anterior oblique fields,
often with wedges, to obtain satisfactory treatment. It must
be stressed that the proximity of dose-limiting structures
such as the spinal cord to the esophagus makes treatment of
this disease technically challenging in all patients.

Like squamous cell carcinomas in the thoracic esophagus,
multimodality therapy for these patients offers excellent
palliation, and the potential for cure exists when chemoradiation therapy is employed. Because of the disfigurement
and disability resulting from surgery, resection is best kept in
reserve as a salvage procedure.

ADENOCARCINOMA OF THE ESOPHAGUS

The literature on adenocarcinoma of the esophagus is difficult to summarize because so many authors include gastric
lesions that invade the esophagus. The rationale for doing so
is that the prognosis and treatment are the same. This may
be true for the advanced lesions, but, as diagnostic techniques such as esophagogastroscopy improve, early lesions
of the esophagus are found and a distinction can be made
between primary adenocarcinoma of the esophagus and
those that involve it by direct extension from the stomach.
Detection of the less-advanced lesion may be accompanied
by a better understanding of the factors responsible for the
emergence of these cancers and, hopefully, a better approach to their cure. Curative approaches also produce the
best palliation.

Until recently, many authorities doubted the existence of
primary adenocarcinoma of the esophagus because it was so
rare.[266] The Mayo Clinic reported 19 patients with this diagnosis who constituted 3.3% of the 1312 patients with cancer
of the esophagus or cardia seen from 1946 to 1963. Turnbull
and co-workers found an incidence of 2.3% among the 1918
patients with esophageal cancer seen from 1926 to 1968 at
the Memorial Hospital for Cancer in New York.[267] In a series
of 163 patients with esophageal cancer seen between 1975
and 1982, 6.7% had a primary adenocarcinoma of the esophagus.[268] This figure is close to the one reported from Denmark, in which 6.9% of the esophageal carcinomas were
found to be of the glandular type.[269]

HISTOGENESIS OF PRIMARY ADENOCARCINOMA

Three possible sources exist for the development of an adenocarcinoma of the esophagus: the superficial and deep
glands of the esophagus, persistence of embryonic remnants
of glandular epithelium in the esophagus, and metaplastic
glandular epithelium.

The superficial and deep glands of the esophagus are
mucus-secreting cells which are indistinguishable in appearance from the cardiac glands of the stomach. Secretions
from the superficial glands located within the mucosa enter
the lumen of the esophagus through ducts lined by a single
layer of mucus cells. The terminal portion of the ducts from
these glands is lined with squamous cells. The deep esophageal glands are thought to give rise to the mucoepidermoid
carcinomas occasionally found in the esophagus.[270]

Congenital persistence of columnar lining the esophagus
is possible because during early embryonic life the esophagus is a tube of stratified columnar cells that develops a
lumen and then becomes lined with ciliated columnar cells.
During the 14th week of embryonic life, squamous cells
appear in the middle third of the esophagus. They spread
craniad and caudad, gradually lining the entire lumen of the

esophagus by the 7th month of gestation. If this process is arrested during fetal life, segments of the esophagus could remain lined with glandular epithelium rather than squamous epithelium. Another possible explanation for small patches of fundic gastric mucosa in the esophagus is that they represent heterotopic deposits of displaced embryonic tissue, as are occasionally seen in a Meckel diverticulum.[270]

A columnar-lined esophagus resulting from glandular mucosa replacing the squamous cell mucosa occurs in some patients with reflux esophagitis (Barrett's esophagus). Although currently accepted, this explanation was not appreciated when Barrett first drew attention to the columnar-lined lower esophagus in 1950. He originally attributed the phenomenon to a congenitally short esophagus. He discarded the possibility that the shortened esophagus was acquired as a result of "reflux esophagitis," a term he coined. By 1957, he changed his views on the subject and postulated that the lower esophagus lined by columnar epithelium was most probably "the result of a failure of the embryonic lining of the gullet to achieve normal maturity," meaning that it was of congenital origin.[271]

As early as 1953, Allison and Johnstone pointed out the relationship between a hiatal hernia, reflux esophagitis, and the columnar-lined esophagus, but they did not understand that the reflux esophagitis was responsible for the appearance of the columnar epithelium. Indeed, it was thought that the "gastric mucosa" in the esophagus contributed to the esophagitis. One of the seven patients reported by Allison and Johnstone had an adenocarcinoma in the glandular ("gastric") lining of the esophagus.[272]

Barrett's explanation of the presence of a columnar-lined lower esophagus held sway for the next 20 years, and a columnar-lined esophagus is still commonly known as a "Barrett's esophagus."

Allison accumulated extensive experience with peptic esophagitis, recognizing that there was incompetence of the esophagogastric sphincter mechanism resulting in reflux. However, he focused on the anatomical abnormality rather than on the physiologic one, and he concentrated on repairing the hiatal hernia. He did not recognize that this did not correct the reflux. By 1970, he still considered the columnar-lined esophagus to be a failure of complete development but did recognize that it was inclined to malignant degeneration.[273] Others began to suspect as early as 1960 that reflux esophagitis could be responsible for the presence of the columnar epithelium. Adler's outstanding studies published in 1963 gave great credibility to this explanation—one that was subsequently substantiated and is now widely held.[274,275] It was also at this time that Nissen described his operation, the fundoplication, which effectively prevented reflux esophagitis and has become the standard operation for this condition.[276]

ADENOCARCINOMA IN BARRETT'S ESOPHAGUS

Etiologic and Pathologic Considerations

Barrett's esophagus is emphasized because 59% to 86% of adenocarcinomas of the esophagus arise in a Barrett's esophagus. It is thus possible that common factors are involved in the causation of both lesions.[277] The constituents of the refluxed material that are responsible for the conversion of the squamous epithelium to columnar epithelium are not known. It is difficult to reproduce the lesion in experimental animals.[278] Because it has been observed in 9 of 17 patients who had total gastrectomy with esophagojejunostomy, the alkaline small bowel contents have been suspected in its pathogenesis.[279]

Several explanations exist for the replacement of the squamous cell lining by the glandular epithelium. Epithelial cells from the stomach may grow up into an esophagus denuded of its mucosa. Submucosal esophageal glands or the cardiac glands in the lamina propria may proliferate and cover the denuded luminal surface of the esophagus. The squamous cell epithelium may undergo metaplasia under the influence of the esophagitis, which is the generally accepted explanation. However, there is a possibility that the columnar-lined esophagus can be of congenital origin. Ransom and colleagues considered the extended form of Barrett's esophagus (extending to 30 cm or more from the incisors) to be of congenital origin and to have a greater predilection for malignant degeneration. This group made up half of the 34 patients whom they studied.[280]

The microscopic changes that characterize a Barrett's esophagus have been carefully studied by both light and electron microscopy and by immunohistochemical techniques.[281-283] The mucosa can assume one of three forms, and there is usually a mixture of them in any given patient. There is a predilection of the gastric type of epithelium to be located distally. This type of tissue resembles the mucosa seen in the fundus of the stomach and contains parietal and chief cells. It has an atrophic appearance, and the functional status of the acid and pepsinogen secreting cells is unclear. Located proximally in the columnar-lined esophagus is intestinal-type epithelium, with villae lined by columnar and goblet cells. The changes in this type of mucosa closely resemble the process of "intestinalization" that is seen in the stomach of patients with atrophic gastritis. Unlike normal intestinal absorptive cells, the columnar cells of this specialized epithelium contain glycoprotein secretory granules, usually lack brush borders, and do not absorb lipids. Paneth and neuroendocrine cells can also be found in this tissue. The third type of epithelial cells seen in a Barrett's esophagus is cardiac-type glands, which tend to be found between the gastric-type and the proximal intestinal-type cells.

Barrett's esophagus has been found in 8% to 20% of patients who undergo esophagoscopy for evaluation of esophagitis. The frequency rises to 44% if a stricture complicates the esophagitis.[275] The percentage of patients with Barrett's esophagus who subsequently develop adenocarcinoma ranges from 0 to 46.5%.[277] Very little is known about the factors responsible for the malignant degeneration of this tissue. However, the finding of a progression of changes from dysplasia to in situ neoplasia to invasive malignancy is consistent with a metaplasic process that accounts for the presence of the columnar epithelium in the esophagus. The component of the Barrett's mucosa most often associated with the malignancy is the intestinal-type tissue, which is characterized by large numbers of goblet cells. Detailed studies of the adenocarcinomas in Barrett's esophagus reveal many cell types, including keratin-producing cells.[44] These investigations support the theory that adenocarcinoma, like the Barrett's esophagus itself, is an example of multidirectional differentiation.

Other important features of the adenocarcinoma are multiple foci of malignancy. There could be genetic components to both the occurrence of Barrett's esophagus and the adenocarcinoma arising from it because these lesions are rarely seen in blacks, but squamous cell carcinoma is far more common in blacks than in whites.[268,275,277] Because cigarette smoking and alcohol ingestion are thought to be related to the cause of squamous cell carcinoma, investigators have looked for this relationship in patients with adenocarcinoma in a Barrett's esophagus. Some reports suggest such a relationship; others do not.[277]

Clinical Features

Patients with adenocarcinoma that developed in a Barrett's esophagus are usually white men in the fifth and sixth decades of life with histories of esophagitis, hiatal hernias, and strictures who often smoke and may have a heavy alcohol intake (see Fig. 24-19). The higher frequency of cancer of all cell types of the esophagus in men is well established. Skinner and colleagues found that the male–female ratio among patients with Barrett's esophagus was 2:1. When adenocarcinoma complicated the columnar-lined esophagus, the ratio increased to 9:1.[285] Patients with reflux esophagitis caused by scleroderma and those with reflux caused by cardiomyotomy for achalasia may also be at risk. Peptic ulcer disease and extraesophageal tumors are other conditions frequently associated with Barrett's esophagus.

FIG. 24-19. Esophagram showing a deep ulcer (*arrow*) and a stricture of the distal esophagus in a patient with a columnar-lined esophagus and in situ adenocarcinoma.

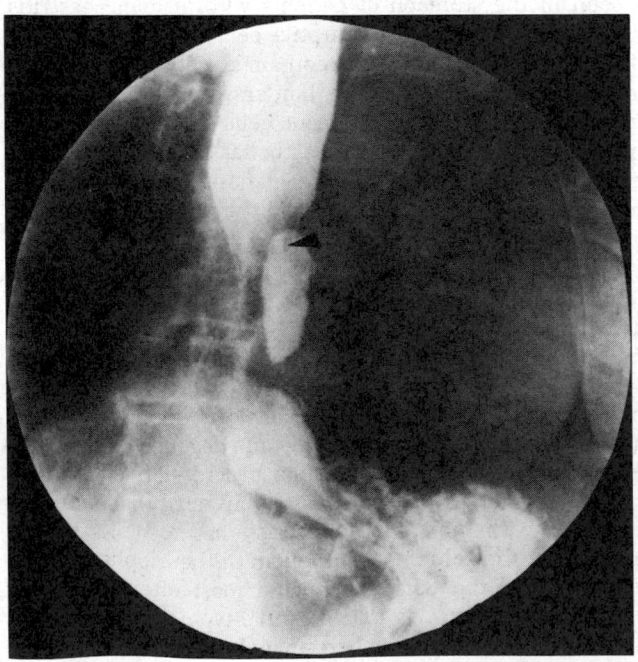

The absence of a history of Barrett's esophagus among patients found to have an adenocarcinoma in a columnar-lined esophagus is significant and underscores difficulty in recognizing the abnormally located epithelium in the esophagus. Its appearance on endoscopy is not strikingly different from that of squamous cell epithelium, and radiologic differentiation is unreliable. Pertechnetate scintigraphy has been recommended for the diagnosis of Barrett's esophagus, but this radionuclide will be concentrated by the columnar epithelium only if it is the gastric type.[286]

Barrett's mucosa may be granular with a salmon-pink color or have the velvety appearance of gastric mucosa. Biopsies must be taken to verify the diagnosis. Close surveillance of patients with reflux esophagitis and Barrett's esophagus may detect adenocarcinomas before they become extensive. Once adenocarcinomas cause symptoms, they are usually far advanced and have the same poor prognosis as squamous cell carcinomas.

Treatment

Patients with Barrett's esophagus who do not have dysplastic or neoplastic alterations in the columnar-lined esophagus may benefit from fundoplication, because some patients have experienced regression or stabilization of this process when the reflux of gastric contents was prevented.[285,287]

When patients show evidence of in situ or invasive malignancy in a Barrett's esophagus, esophagectomy followed by adjuvant chemotherapy of the type used for gastric adenocarcinoma is recommended.[277]

Dysplastic changes present within the Barrett's mucosa present a difficult therapeutic problem. It is difficult to recommend radical surgery under these circumstances, but evidence strongly indicates that dysplastic changes are the first stages of invasive carcinoma. This is especially true of "high-grade" dysplasia, which is considered a morphologic marker and precursor of adenocarcinoma.[275,288] Patients with this form of dysplasia are candidates for esophagectomy.[277,285]

The esophagectomy required is an extensive one, more extensive than can be performed using the Ivor Lewis approach. The columnar mucosa can extend quite high in the esophagus. By using an operation that places the esophagogastric or esophagocolic anastomosis in the neck, the sur-

TABLE 24-19. Staging of Adenocarcinoma Involving Barrett's Esophagus

Stage I
Carcinoma limited to the mucosa (including in situ carcinoma), not extending beyond the muscularis mucosa, with negative nodes
Stage II
Carcinoma limited to the esophageal wall but not extending to the adventitia, with negative nodes
Stage III
Any of the above with involved regional lymph nodes or full-thickness wall penetration of the tumor to the adventitia, without invasion of adjacent organs
Stage IV
Carcinoma invading adjacent organs or with distant metastases

geon can be more confident that all of the involved mucosa has been removed. A modification of the technique described by McKeown is recommended.[107]

The prognosis of patients with adenocarcinoma in a Barrett's esophagus depends on the pathologic stage of the tumor. The staging system proposed in Table 24-19 is similar to Duke's system of staging colon carcinoma and may more accurately predict the prognosis and progression than the TNM system. However, there have not been sufficient data available to prove this hypothesis.

PALLIATIVE THERAPY FOR CANCER OF THE ESOPHAGUS

RADIATION THERAPY

For patients not treated with a curative approach because of tumor extent, metastasis, or general medical condition, palliation of dysphagia and pain and the maintenance of a patent food passage are the goals of therapy. In some patients, this palliation is best achieved through surgery, but for many patients radiation continues to offer a reasonable expectation of symptom relief.[219] Dysphagia is relieved partially or completely in almost 80% of patients, resulting in stabilization or weight gain.[148,155,290] Simple anterior and posterior radiation fields can be used for the first 4000 cGy. If the patient is improving and tolerating treatment well, additional radiation may be administered through oblique or lateral fields that avoid the spinal cord. Fraction sizes are usually increased so that the overall time of treatment is kept to a minimum and the patient can spend the maximal time away from the hospital. Up to 5000 cGy have been delivered in 4 weeks of 250 cGy fractions.[126,134] In some cases, 400 cGy fractions have been used successfully.[291]

A significant percentage of patients whose symptoms are relieved by radiation will experience local tumor regrowth and a recurrence of their symptoms.[290] Pearson reported that 50% of irradiated patients will have a local recurrence, frequently within 6 months.[292] Beatty and colleagues studied 152 patients treated with "radical" radiation alone at The Princess Margaret Hospital.[126] Patients received at least 4000 cGy. Eighty-four percent of the patients had a shrinkage of their tumor. Only 28% (33% of responders) maintained their swallowing intact until death. Beatty also documented the high incidence of malignancy in esophageal strictures that were clinically judged to be benign. Of the 50 strictures that were diagnosed antemortem to be malignant, 24 were originally thought to be from "fibrosis," and 14 of these had an initial benign biopsy. Furthermore, autopsies on five patients who died with supposedly benign strictures revealed four who had tumor at the site of the stricture. These authors conclude that most benign strictures that do not resolve with dilation are related to persistent local tumor.

Wara and co-workers reported on a series of patients who received 5000 to 6000 cGy in 5.5 to 6.5 weeks.[155] The median survival was 7 months, whereas the median duration of palliation was only 3 months. Although 89% of patients had improvement in their dysphagia, most had recurrence of their symptoms.

TABLE 24-20. Palliative Procedures for Carcinoma of the Esophagus

Resect and reconstruct
   Intrathoracic
   Extrathoracic
      Presternal
      Retrosternal
Bypass
   Intrathoracic
   Extrathoracic
      Presternal
      Retrosternal
   Colon
   Stomach
Intraluminal intubation
Gastrostomy and cervical esophagogastrostomy with or without an external tube
Dilatation

These studies underscore the importance of proper identification of target volume and administration of an aggressive radiation dose even when palliation is the only goal. To deliver a low dose to an inadequate tumor volume may provide only temporary relief for a patient and may necessitate potentially hazardous surgery while the patient is in a reobstructed condition following radiation. In many respects, there is relatively little difference between the dose and field size that should be used for palliative or curative radiation. It may be worth taking an extra week or two to raise the radiation dose to a high level and taking an extra hour to plan the radiation with great care, even when the chances of cure are slim. Short-course, high-fraction radiotherapy should be reserved for patients whose life expectancy is extremely short because of metastatic disease or general physical condition.

SURGERY

The palliative operations available for patients with advanced carcinoma of the thoracic esophagus are outlined in Table 24-20 and have been reviewed by Orringer.[293]

A palliative esophagectomy should be performed only if the risk of morbidity and mortality are minimal and if at least a year of survival is reasonable. Patients who are not good candidates for palliative resection are those with the findings outlined in Table 24-21.

The rationale for esophageal resection to palliate esophageal cancer resides in the hope that the procedure can contribute to the patient's cure as well as palliation. If doubt

TABLE 24-21. Contraindications to Palliative Esophagectomy for Cancer of Thoracic Esophagus

Advanced inanition and debilitation
Inadequate cardiopulmonary function
Widespread (visceral) metastases
Malignant pleural effusion
Malignant ascites
Recurrent laryngeal, phrenic, or sympathetic nerve involvement
Superior vena cava obstruction
Tracheoesophageal fistula
Extension into the aortic wall or spinal column

exists about the removal of an esophageal lesion for cure, and the patient is judged to be a good surgical risk, the esophagus should be resected. The justification for this philosophy is twofold: occasionally, residual tumor may be successfully eliminated by radiotherapy and chemotherapy, and esophageal resection constitutes satisfactory palliative therapy. Payne said that "most efforts in the management of this condition [esophageal cancer] are palliative for most patients but not prejudicial to cure for the few.[294]

At the Mayo Clinic, more than 90% of patients undergoing resection had unobstructed swallowing throughout their subsequent survival.[294] Hankins and colleagues adapted a vigorous approach to palliation, a concept challenged by Orringer.[295,296]

The prognosis of patients with advanced esophageal cancer is so poor that the surgeon may question whether an undertaking of the magnitude of an esophageal resection is reasonable. When esophageal resection carries a prohibitive risk to the patient with concomitant cardiopulmonary disease or when resection cannot be performed because of technical reasons, a better palliative procedure is one that bypasses the malignant esophageal obstruction (Fig. 24-20).[297,298] Although this approach has had many advocates, more recent reports do not support bypass procedure as reasonable palliation because of the high mortality and morbidity that follow it, such as anastomotic leaks, mucocele formation, and infection in the excluded esophagus.[299-301] Orringer's patients with this operation had a postoperative mortality of 24%; 19% had anastomotic leaks, and 17% had

disruptions of the divided distal thoracic esophagus, a condition that frequently leads to an intra-abdominal abscess.[299] Major postoperative complications occurred in 59% of his patients. The average survival time of those leaving the hospital was 5.9 months. Blunt transhiatal esophagectomy has become his palliative procedure of choice. Gastric bypass of the esophagus is reserved for the occasional patient with a tracheoesophageal fistula who is capable of withstanding this operation.

INTRALUMINAL INTUBATION

Intubation of the esophagus with a prosthetic tube has been used for many years to allow patients with malignant esophageal obstruction to swallow. This procedure is successful for 4 to 6 months in 40% to 85% of patients.[117,302]

Patients who are candidates for this procedure are those who have such advanced malignant obstruction of the esophagus that no other therapy is possible. These are patients who are very debilitated and who have tracheoesophageal fistulae or invasion of the trachea, bronchus, or aorta. Patients who have malignant strictures after a course of chemoradiation and are not candidates for operative palliation may also benefit from intraluminal esophageal tubes. Another category of patients who have received endoesophageal tubes are those whose obstructing cancers are treated with laser vaporization.[303]

Two types of tubes are used: pulsion or push-through tubes, which depend entirely on being pushed blindly

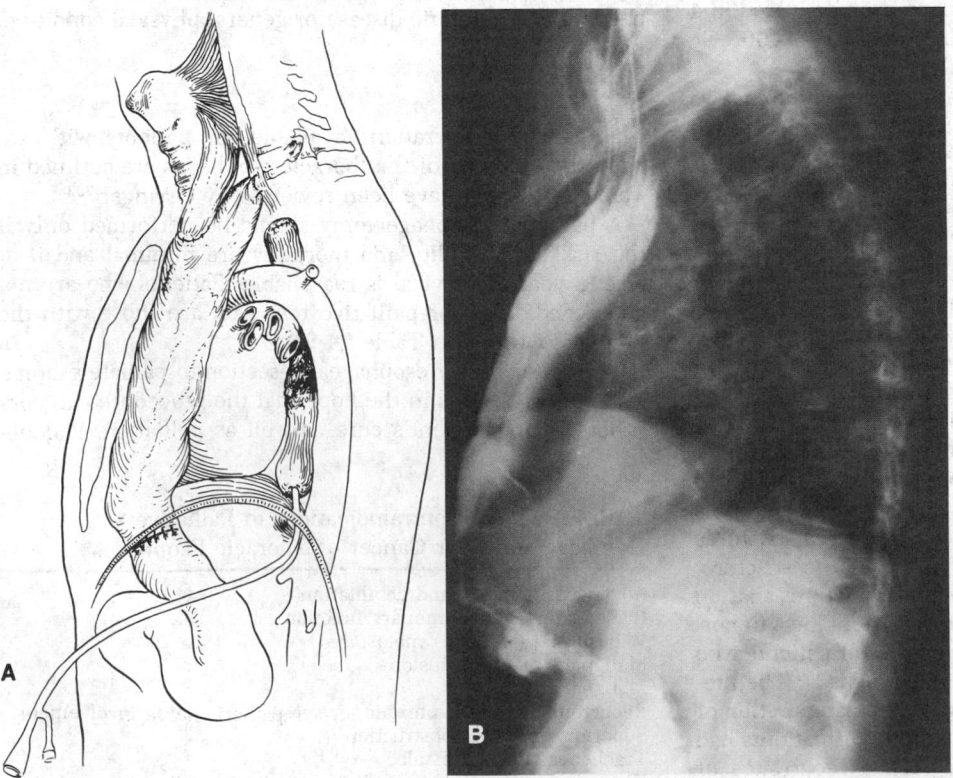

FIG. 24-20. **A**. The stomach is brought up behind the sternum and anastomosed to the esophagus. **B**. Radiographic appearance of a retrosternal gastric bypass.

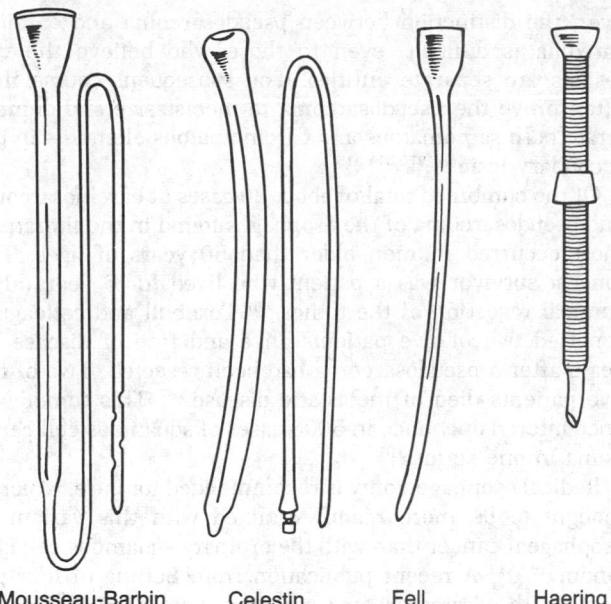

Mousseau-Barbin   Celestin   Fell   Haering

FIG. 24-21. Diagrammatic depiction of four commonly used intraluminal tubes.

through the area of obstruction, and traction tubes, which are pulled by a guide wire or string through the esophagus into the stomach. Pulsion tubes are usually limited to 10-cm segments and are best suited for middle-third and upper-third lesions. Traction tubes are best suited for middle-third or lower-third lesions. They are anchored to the stomach by a suture after being placed in proper position (Fig. 24-21). The use of introducers, such as the Nothingham introducer, and newer endoesophageal tubes, such as the Proctor-Livingston tube or Atkinson tube, has resulted in a preference for pulsion intubation over traction intubation and retrosternal gastric bypass for palliation of unresectable carcinoma of the esophagus.[304-306]

Endoesophageal tubes have several drawbacks as palliative procedures. A mortality of 10% to 40% accompanies placement of intraluminal tubes.[117,302] Perforation of the esophagus with mediastinitis may occur. Aspiration of gastric contents is frequent because the lower esophageal sphincter mechanism is blocked by the tube. Patients with this type of tube must be instructed to sleep with the head of the bed elevated. The tubes become dislodged and migrate in about 25% of patients; they also frequently become obstructed, and patients must be instructed to chew their food well or confine their diet to pureed foods.

Very often the malignant esophageal obstruction has to be dilated before an endoesophageal tube can pass through it.[307] Boyce has described his technique in detail.[308] The Eder-Peustow dilator is used for strictures that are very tight. When the lumen can take a 15-mm-dilator, Maloney bougies (tapered rubber tubes filled with mercury) are used. When a 15-mm dilator can be passed, the patient will no longer experience dysphagia. Dilatation with the mercury-filled bougies are continued daily or on alternate days for 1 week to 10 days, until the lumen of the esophagus will accept a 17-mm bougie. An endoesophageal tube can then be inserted and radiation given if indicated. Most patients (85%) can be maintained without a prosthesis by repeat dilatation. There was no increased incidence of perforation of the esophagus when radiation was combined with esophageal dilatation. During 5-years, 151 patients were treated by this technique with successful palliation in most of them.

Several precautions must be observed if dilatation of a malignant esophageal obstruction is to be used. The guide wire, as required with the Eder-Peustow dilator, should be passed under fluoroscopic control. Dilatation should not be carried out too rapidly. Physicians should never use more than three different-sized dilators during a single session. Patient discomfiture with this procedure is brief. Once the lumen is stretched to 17 mm, redilatation may be required no more than weekly or monthly. Intubation is necessary when dilatation cannot maintain a patent lumen for more than a day.

LASER THERAPY

Recently, endoscopic Nd:YAG and argon laser therapies have been used to reestablish esophageal continuity through malignant obstruction of the esophagus.[309-311] Fourteen patients were treated an average of five times to achieve luminal patency within a mean of 12 days.[309] Esophageal dilatation can be used after laser therapy. The mean survival was 14 weeks, but more than 75% of the patients could leave the hospital able to swallow. Nd:YAG laser equipment was used in this study, which employed an average of 4615 watt-seconds per treatment. Rather than using many treatments of lower energy to vaporize the tumor, some investigators advocate a single session of laser therapy to achieve luminal patency.[311] Complications of laser therapy are perforation of the esophagus, bleeding, and fistula formation. Occasionally, the lumen of the esophagus cannot be opened because of the distortion and twisting of the esophagus.

A tunable dye–argon laser system has been used in conjunction with the administration of sensitizing hematoporphyrin derivatives to destroy tumor tissue, using endoscopic techniques to deliver the light. This has been labeled photodynamic therapy and may be an additional modality of therapy available to patients with malignant obstruction of the esophagus.[310]

GASTROSTOMY AND CERVICAL ESOPHAGOSTOMY

The simplest palliative procedure is the creation of a gastrostomy to supply nutrition and a cervical esophagostomy to prevent aspiration of upper airway secretions or their passage into the tracheobronchial tree by a fistula to the esophagus. The cervical esophagostomy is of marginal benefit to the patient because there is a constant trickle of saliva through the esophagostomy that is difficult to collect. Personal hygiene and appearance are difficult to maintain. Eating or drinking is not possible with this form of palliation, unless a tube is fashioned to connect the cervical esophagostomy with the gastrostomy. Devices to accomplish this are not very effective.

OTHER CANCERS OF THE ESOPHAGUS

VARIANTS OF SQUAMOUS CELL CARCINOMAS OF THE ESOPHAGUS

Spindle Cell Carcinoma

This manifestation of squamous cell carcinoma is characterized histopathologically by spindle-shaped cells that resemble fibroblasts. It is a poorly differentiated squamous cell carcinoma that can be confused with a sarcoma. The spindle cells, however, have been studied by electron microscopy and have been shown to contain numerous tonofibrils and occasional well-developed desmosomes.[312] Desmosomes are characteristically found at the intercellular junction of epithelial cells. Tonofibrils radiate from them and contribute to the "stiffness" or cytoskeleton of this cell type. However, except for their large size and irregular shape, the spindle cells also resemble actively synthesizing fibroblasts and are closely associated with collagen fibrils. Battifora believes that the spindle cells originate from mesenchymal metaplasia of squamous cells and that collagen is produced by these metaplastic cells.[312] Similar tumors in the skin have shown a gradual transition of the spindle cells to typical squamous cells. This view has received support from others.[313]

Pseudosarcoma and Carcinosarcoma

Several observers argue that these two designations refer to the same lesion and should be referred to as polypoid carcinomas of the esophagus.[270,314,315] They both have the gross appearance of a polypoid lesion. Adenocarcinomas, inflammatory granulomas, smooth muscle tumors, and melanomas may also present as polypoid lesions.

In the case of pseudosarcomas or carcinosarcomas, the barium esophagram will usually reveal a large polypoid mass in the middle or lower third of the esophagus. The esophagus is usually distended at the site of the tumor, but the degree of esophageal obstruction is considerably less than one would expect from the size of the mass.

Histopathologically, they appear to be spindle cell carcinomas, which present a varying picture—from nests of squamous cells (which may or may not appear malignant) in a spindle cell stroma (referred to as pseudosarcoma) to an intimate mixture of carcinomatous- and sarcomatous-appearing cells growing together as a single tumor (carcinosarcoma). Although it is convincingly argued that these malignancies most likely arise from two different cell lines, carcinomatous and sarcomatous, that commingle, we regard them as highly undifferentiated squamous cell carcinomas of the spindle-cell type.[270]

Most carcinosarcomas do not invade very deeply into the underlying tissue. The carcinomatous elements are limited and may be found only at the base of the polypoid mass. Metastases from these tumors are usually sarcomatous in appearance.

According to authors who made a distinction between carcinosarcomas and pseudosarcomas, the latter differ from the former in that the seemingly sarcomatous tissue is considered nonmalignant because metastases do not occur. However, the distinction between pseudosarcoma and carcinosarcoma is difficult, even to those who believe the two lesions are separate entities. The subsequent course may often prove the pseudosarcoma to metastasize and demonstrate both sarcomatous and carcinomatous elements in the secondary lesions.[270,314,315]

Of the combined total of about 80 cases of carcinosarcoma and pseudosarcoma of the esophagus found in the literature, most occurred in men older than 50 years of ages. The longest survivor was a patient who lived for 6 years after surgical resection of the tumor.[270] Turnbull and colleagues reported two of five patients alive and free of disease 10 years after a pseudosarcoma had been resected. Two of the five patients died of metastatic disease.[267] This tumor was encountered only once in 5000 cases of squamous cell carcinoma in one series.[316]

Radical esophagectomy is recommended for cure, which is thought to be more readily attained with this variant of esophageal cancer than with the ordinary squamous cell carcinoma[317,318] A recent publication from Beijing of four patients with carcinosarcoma reported them all well 3 to 19 years after radical excision and esophagogastrostomy.[319]

Verrucous and Varicoid Carcinomas of the Esophagus

Verrucous and varicoid lesions are variants of fungating squamous cell carcinomas.[270,320] They may be confused with esophageal varices when an esophagram is obtained, which is their distinguishing feature. This lesion may also be confused with benign squamous cell papillomas of the esophagus.

ADENOID-CYSTIC CARCINOMA (CYLINDROMA)

Adenoid-optic carcinomas or cylindromas show histologic features that are identical with those found in the salivary glands, but they act more aggressively and have a poorer prognosis than do the relatively indolent salivary gland cylindromas.[270] Epstein and colleagues studied six cases of esophageal adenoid-cystic carcinomas and concluded that they were distinct morphologically and clinically from the adenoid-cystic carcinomas of salivary gland origin.[321] These tumors have the typical cystic or cribriform configuration of the tumor cells with some areas of solid or basaloid patterns. In the esophagus, the basaloid pattern predominates; the cells are more pleomorphic, and the overlying squamous mucosa contains focal areas of dysplasia and in situ carcinoma.

Based on a review of the 29 patients with this lesion who were reported in the literature before 1984, Epstein and colleagues found that 76% of the tumors occur in men during their sixth decade, in contrast to the salivary gland cylindromas, which predominate in women in the fourth and fifth decades of life.[321] The cancer's aggressive behavior is reflected in the 9-month median survival after diagnosis. It has been suggested that these lesions should be resected as is done for squamous cell carcinoma of the esophagus.[322] Recently, a combination of radiation therapy and cisplatin, cyclophosphamide, vincristine, and doxorubicin produced a complete response in a patient with metastases to the lung from an esophageal adenoid-cystic carcinoma. The 44 cases culled from the literature before 1986 confirmed the poor prognosis of these cancers, and further exploration of this combination chemotherapy has merit.[323]

MUCOEPIDERMOID CARCINOMA (ADENOCANTHOMA)

A mucoepidermoid carcinoma is an adenocarcinoma that contains squamous elements. The relative proportion of the two components varies both within and among these cancers. Ming suggests that when the tumor is a well-differentiated adenocarcinoma, some cells undergo squamous metaplasia and are surrounded by the unaffected glandular cells.[270] These lesions are typically referred to as adenocanthomas. They may arise from aberrant gastric epithelium; however, there are mucoepidermoid cancers of the esophagus that are thought to arise from the deep mucus glands of the esophagus. They are similar to those found in the salivary glands. In 1978, Woodard and colleagues collected only eight cases of this esophageal lesion, attesting to its rarity.[324]

Esophageal mucoepidermoid carcinomas are characterized by small groups of mucus cells scattered among large groups of squamous cells. These are very aggressive malignancies and are most often found at the lower end of the esophagus, although the tumor reported by Turnbull and co-workers was located in the upper thoracic esophagus.[267] Resection failed to cure this patient, and the poor prognosis was similar to that in patients with mucoepidermoid cancers arising from the bronchial glands.

CANCERS OF NEUROENDOCRINE ORIGIN

Primary Oat Cell Carcinoma

Various names are given to this cancer, which is similar in appearance and behavior to its counterpart in the lung. It is also referred to as a small cell carcinoma, a small cell undifferentiated carcinoma, or an apudoma (amine precursor uptake and decarboxylation tumor). A total of 88 cases of this lesion were recently collected from the literature.[325]

The tumors are thought to be of neuroectodermal origin because most investigators find them to be argyrophilic and on electron microscopy the cells contain neurosecretory granules.[326] Immunohistochemical studies have also revealed the presence of ACTH and calcitonin within some of the tumors that have been studied for their capacity to synthesize polypeptide hormones.[327] Evidence of Cushing's disease was not present in the patient found to have ACTH in the tumor. However, other patients have been reported with paraneoplastic syndromes, such as inappropriate antidiuretic hormone secretion and hypercalcemia.[328]

Because these tumors occasionally also have areas of squamous cell carcinoma within them, and even less often adenocarcinomatous elements, earlier authors had doubts about the origin of this malignancy. The accumulated evidence, however, leaves little doubt that it is of neuroectodermal origin.[329]

Like squamous cell carcinomas, most oat cell carcinomas are equally located in the middle and lower thirds of the esophagus. Men are more frequently affected than women (3:2) and the tumor is most common in the 50- to 70-year-old group.[325,328]

All of the patients with oat cell carcinoma of the esophagus have a very poor prognosis. All have died of disseminated disease. Overall survival is 4 to 5 months; the longest was 24 months.[325] Treatment has consisted of resection, radiation, and chemotherapy.[325,326,330] Combination chemotherapy used for patients with oat cell cancer of the lung has provided dramatic, albeit temporary, responses[330,331]

Carcinoid Tumors

Further evidence of the neuroendocrine basis of oat cell cancers is the rare carcinoid tumor, which is presumed to arise from the same cell type but which is a far less aggressive tumor. Resection of the esophagus is effective therapy.[332,333]

PRIMARY MALIGNANT MELANOMAS

Malignant melanomas are derived from neural crest tissue, as are apudomas and carcinoids. A review of the world literature revealed 110 patients with this infrequently encountered lesion of the esophagus.[334] The tumor is often polypoid and lymphatic and hematologic metastases are common, resulting in a 5-year survival rate of 4%. Resection is recommended and has resulted in a 10-year survival in one patient. Average survival, however, is only 13.4 months. Patients with secondary esophageal melanoma outnumber the patients with primary melanoma of the esophagus.

ESOPHAGEAL SARCOMAS

Leiomyosarcoma

This is the most common malignant nonepithelial tumor in the esophagus. Nonetheless, Choh and colleagues could find only 44 patients in the English literature with leiomyosarcoma of the esophagus.[335] Well-differentiated polypoid lesions respond best to surgical therapy. Radical excision may not be necessary in these extreme instances. Overall, the prognosis of patients with this rare cancer is poor, but resection has resulted in several 5-year survivors.

Rhabdomyosarcoma

These sarcomas, derived from striated muscle, are extremely rare. Resection can result in long-term survival.[336] Occasionally a granular cell myoblastoma may exhibit malignant characteristics.

CHORIOCARCINOMA

Three cases of choriocarcinoma of the esophagus were summarized in 1979.[337] The diagnosis was easily made by brush biopsy because the characteristic cytotrophoblastic and syncytotrophoblastic cells can be readily identified.

PRIMARY LYMPHOMA

Non-Hodgkin's and Hodgkin's lymphoma arising in the esophagus have been reported.[337-339] The radiographic appearance is characterized by a diffuse nodularity as a result of lymphomatous infiltration of the mucosa. This tumor is being seen increasingly in immunocompromised patients.[340]

METASTASES TO THE ESOPHAGUS

The esophagus is not a frequent site of metastatic disease. As indicated above, metastatic melanomas involve the esophagus more frequently than do primary melanomas. Lymphoma involving the esophagus as part of diffuse disseminated disease has also been reported. Direct extension from a tumor or its nodal involvement is responsible for 80% of the involvement of the esophagus by a malignancy arising in another organ.[341] Microscopic foci of tumor are seen at autopsy in 3% to 4% of patients dying of cancer and in 9% of women dying of breast cancer.[342,343] The relative frequency of involvement of the esophagus by metastatic breast cancer has resulted in recognition of the syndrome of postmastectomy dysphagia.[344,345] Fifty-eight cases of esophageal involvement in the course of breast cancer have been reported in the literature. Radiotherapy and chemotherapy may be beneficial in these instances.[345] Because the lesion often causes dysphagia by extrinsic compression, care must be taken during esophagoscopy that the esophagus is not perforated.[344] Biopsy by exploration of the neck or posterior mediastinum or by needle aspiration using CT can provide tissue for a definitive diagnosis. These lesions can mimic primary esophageal cancers. Other sites of cancer that have been reported to give rise to metastases to the esophagus are the kidneys, pancreas, cervix, and bladder.[343]

REFERENCES

1. Huang GJ, Wu YK: Carcinoma of the Esophagus and Gastric Cardia. New York, Springer-Verlag, 1984
2. Long ER: A History of Pathology. Baltimore, Williams & Wilkins, 1928
3. Wangensteen OH, Wangensteen SD: The Rise of Surgery: From Emperic Craft to Scientific Discipline. Minneapolis, University of Minnesota Press, 1978
4. Wangensteen OH: Cancer of the Esophagus and Stomach, 2nd ed. New York, American Cancer Society, 1956
5. Torek F: The first successful case of resection of the thoracic portion of the esophagus for carcinoma. Surg Gynecol Obstet 16:614, 1913
6. Kirschner H: Ein Neues Verfahren der Oesophagsplastik. Arch Klin Chir 114:606, 1920
7. Ohsawa T: The surgery of the esophagus. Arch Jpn Chir 10:605, 1933
8. Adams WE, Phemister DB: Carcinoma of the lower thoracic esophagus. Report of successful resection and esophagogastrostomy. J Thorac Surg 7:621, 1939
9. delRegato JA, Spjut HJ: Cancer: Diagnosis, Treatment and Prognosis, 5th ed. St. Louis, CV Mosby, 1977
10. Nielsen J: Clinical results with radiation therapy in cancer of the esophagus. Acta Radiol 26:361, 1945
11. Ota K, Shin LH: Histological typing of gastric and oesophageal tumors. Geneva, World Health Organization, 1977
12. Seremetic MG, Lyons WS, deGuzman VC et al: Leiomyomata of the esophagus: An Analysis of 838 cases. Cancer 38:2166, 1976
13. National Cancer Institutes: 1986 Annual Cancer Statistics Review. Division of Cancer Prevention and Control, NIH Publication No. 87-2889, Bethesda, MD, 1987
14. Cutler SJ, Devesa SS: Trends in cancer incidence and mortality in the USA. In Doll R, Vodopija I (eds): Host Environment Interactions in the Etiology of Cancer in Man. Lyon, France, World Health Organization International Agency for Research Cancer, 1973
15. Wu YK, Huang GJ, Shao LF et al: Progress in the study and surgical treatment of cancer of the esophagus in China, 1940–1980. J Thorac Cardiovasc Surg 84:325, 1982
16. Rose EF: A review of factors associated with cancer of the esophagus in Transkei. Prog Clin Biol Res 53:67–75, 1981
17. McGlashan ND: Oesophageal cancer and alcoholic spirits in central Africa. Gut 10:643, 1969
18. Kmet J, Mahboubi E: Esophageal cancer in the Caspian littoral of Iran: Initial studies. Science 175:846, 1972
19. Auerbach O, Stout AD, Hammond EC et al: Histologic changes in esophagus in relation to smoking habits. Arch Environ Health 11:4, 1965
20. Schoenberg BC, Bailar JC, Fraumeni JF: Certain mortality patterns of esophageal cancer in the United States, 1930–67. J Natl Cancer Inst 46:63, 1971
21. Potten LM, Morris LE, Blot WJ et al: Esophageal cancer among black men in Washington DC: I. Alcohol, tobacco and other risk factors. JNCI 67:777, 1981
22. Ziegler RG, Morris LE, Blot WJ et al: Esophageal cancer among black men in Washington DC: II. Role of nutrition. JNCI 67:1199, 1981
23. Rogers EL, Goldkind L, Goldkind SF: Increasing frequency of esophageal cancer among black male veterans. Cancer 49:610, 1982
24. Mettlin C: Nutritional habits of blacks and whites. Prev Med 9:601, 1980
25. vanRensburg SF: Epidemiologic and dietary evidence for a specific nutritional predisposition to esophageal cancer. JNCI 67:243, 1981
26. Munoz N, Crespi M, Grassi A et al: Precursor lesions of esophageal cancer in high-risk populations in Iran and China. Lancet 1:876, 1982
27. O'Neill C, Rani Q, Clarke G et al: Silica fragments from millet bran in mucosa surrounding oesophageal tumors in patients in northern China. Lancet 1:1202, 1982
28. Harper PS, Harper RMJ, Howel-Evans AW: Carcinoma of the oesophagus with tylosis. Q J Med 34:317, 1970
29. Lortat-Jacob JL, Richard CA, Fekete F et al: Cardiospasm and esophageal carcinoma: Report of 24 cases. Surgery 66:969, 1969
30. Just-Viera GO, Haight C: Achalasia and carcinoma of the esophagus. Surg Gynecol Obstet 128:1081, 1969
31. Rock LA, Latham PS, Hankins JR et al: Achalasia associated with squamous cell carcinoma of the esophagus: A case report. Am J Gastroenterol 80:526, 1985
32. Sigurgeirsson B, Johannson KB, Haroarson S et al: Acute thoracic inlet obstruction in achalasia with adenoid cystic and squamous cell carcinoma. Ann Thorac Surg 40:516, 1985
33. Joske RA, Benedict EB: The role of benign esophageal obstruction in the development of carcinoma of the esophagus. Gastroenterology 36:749, 1959
34. Hankins J Jr, McLaughlin JS: The association of carcinoma of the esophagus with achalasia. J Thorac Cardiovasc Surg 69:355, 1975
35. Lamb RK, Edwards CH, Pattison CW et al: Squamous carcinoma in situ of the esophagus in a patient with achalasia. Thorax 40:795, 1985
36. Wychulis AR, Woolam GL, Andersen HA et al: Achalasia and carcinoma of the esophagus. JAMA 215:1638, 1971
37. McGregor DH, Mills G, Boudet RA: Intramural squamous cell carcinoma of the esophagus. Cancer 37:1556, 1976
38. Huang B, Unni KK, Payne WS: Long-term survival following diverticulectomy for cancer in pharyngoesophageal (Zenker's) diverticulum. Ann Thorac Surg 38:207, 1984
39. Hopkins RA, Postlethwaite RW: Caustic burns and carcinoma of the esophagus. Ann Surg 194:146, 1981
40. Appelquist R, Salmo M: Lye corrosion carcinoma of the esophagus: A review of 63 cases. Cancer 45:2655, 1980
41. Ahlbom HE: Simple achlorhydric anaemia, Plummer-Vinson syndrome, and carcinoma of the mouth, pharynx and oesophagus in women: Observations at Radiumhemmet, Stockholm. Br Med J 2:331, 1936
42. Entwistle CC, Jacobs A: Histological findings in the Paterson-Kelly syndrome. J Clin Pathol 18:408, 1965
43. American Joint Committee for Cancer Staging and End-Results Reporting: Manual for Staging of Cancer. Chicago, American Joint Committee for Cancer Staging and End-Results Reporting, 1978
44. Japanese Society for Esophageal Diseases: Guidelines for the clinical and pathologic studies on carcinoma of the esophagus. Jpn J Surg 6:69, 1976
45. Younghusband JD, Aluwihare APR: Carcinoma of the oesophagus: Factors influencing survival. Br J Surg 57:442, 1970
46. Shapiro AL, Robillard GL: The esophageal arteries. Ann Surg 131:171, 1950
47. Haagenson CD, Feind CR, Herter FP et al: The Lymphatics in Cancer. Philadelphia, WB Saunders, 1972
48. Sarrazin R, Voilin C, Bade B et al: L'anatomie du drainage lymphatique de l'oesophage et so lymphologie sont encore mal connues. In Giuli R: Les Cancers de l'Oesophage en 1984: 135 Questions. Malonie SA, 1984
49. Guernsey JM, Knudsen DF: Abdominal exploration in the evaluation of patients with carcinoma of the thoracic esophagus. J Thorac Cardiovasc Surg 59:62, 1970
50. Watson WL, Goodner JT, Miller TP et al: Torek esophagectomy: The case against segmental resection for esophageal cancer. J Thorac Cardiovasc Surg 32:347, 1956
51. Stephens RL, Hansen HH, Muggia Fm: Hypercalcemia in epidermoid tumors of the head and neck and esophagus. Cancer 31:1487, 1973
52. Lohrenz FN, Custer GS: ACTH-producing metastases from carcinoma of the esophagus. Ann Intern Med 62:1017, 1965
53. Kobayashi S, Kasugai T: Brushing cytology for the diagnosis of gastric cancer involving the cardia of the lower esophagus. Acta Cytol 22:155, 1978
54. Winaiwer SJ, Sherlock P, Belladonna JA et al: Endoscopic brush cytology in esophageal cancer. JAMA 232:1358, 1975
55. Graham DY, Schwartz JT, Cain GD et al: Prospective evaluation of biopsy number in the diagnosis of esophageal and gastric carcinoma. Gastroenterology 81:228, 1982

56. Skinner DB, Dowlatshaki K, Delmeester TR: Potentially curable cancer of he esophagus. Cancer 50:2571, 1982

57. Moss AA, Koehler RE, Margulis AR: Initial accuracy of esophagograms in detection of small esophageal carcinoma. Am J Roentgenol 127:909, 1976

58. Putnam CE, Curtis AM, Westfried M et al: Thickening of the posterior tracheal strip: A sign of squamous cell carcinoma of the esophagus. Radiology 121:533, 1976

59. Murata Y, Muroi M, Yoshida M et al: Endoscopic ultrasonography in the diagnosis of esophageal carcinoma. Surg Endosc 1:11, 1986

60. Heyder N: Endoscopic ultrasonography of tumors of the esophagus and stomach. Surg Endosc 1:17, 1986

61. Halvorsen RA, Thompson W: Computed tomographic evaluation of esophageal carcinoma. Semin Oncol 11:1013, 1984

62. Moss AA, Schnyder P, Thoeni RF et al: Esophageal carcinoma: pre-therapy staging by computed tomography. AJR 136:1051, 1981

63. Lea JW, Prager RL, Bender H: The questionable role of computed tomography in preoperative staging of esophageal cancer. Ann Thorac Surg 38:479, 1984

64. Picus D, Balfe DM, Koehler R et al: Computed tomography in staging esophageal carcinoma. Radiology 146:433, 1983

65. Lichter AS, Fraass BA, van de Geijn J et al: An overview of clinical requirements and clinical utility of computed tomography based radiotherapy treatment planning. In Ling C, Rogers C, Morton R (eds): Computed Tomography in Radiation Therapy, p 1–22. New York, Raven Press, 1983

66. Quint LE, Glazer L, Orringer MB: Esophageal imaging by MR and CT: Study of normal anatomy and neoplasms. Radiology 156:727, 1985

67. Clinical staging system for carcinoma of the esophagus. CA 25:50, 1975

68. Guanrei Y, He H, Sunghong Q et al: Endoscopic diagnosis of 115 cases of early esophageal carcinoma. Endoscopy 14:157, 1982

69. Takagi I, Karasawa K: Growth of squamous cell esophageal carcinoma observed by serial esophagographies. J Surg Oncol 21:57, 1982

70. Merendino KA, Merk VJ: An analysis of 100 cases of squamous cell carcinoma: II. With special reference to its theoretical curability. Surg Gynec Obstet 94:110, 1952

71. Clayton ES: Carcinoma of the esophagus. Surg Gynecol Obstet 46:52, 1928

72. Mantravadi R, Lad T, Briele H et al: Carcinoma of the esophagus: Sites of failure. Int J Radiat Oncol Biol Phys 8:1897, 1982

73. Mandard AM, Chasle J, Marnay J et al: Autopsy findings in 111 cases of esophageal cancer. Cancer 48:329, 1981

74. Arbitol A, Straus M, Franklin G et al: Infusional chemotherapy and cyclic chemotherapy inoperable esophageal and gastric cardia carcinoma. Am J Clin Oncol 6:195, 1983

75. Anderson L, Lad T: Autopsy findings in squamous cell carcinoma of the esophagus. Cancer 50:1587, 1982

76. Attah E, Hadju S: Benign and malignant tumors of the esophagus at autopsy. J Thorac Cardiovasc Surg 55:396, 1980

77. Bosch A, Frias Z, Caldwell W et al: Autopsy findings in carcinoma of the esophagus. Acta Radiol Oncol 18:103, 1979

78. Cahan WG: Multiple primary cancers of the lung, esophagus and other sites. Cancer 40:1954, 1977

79. Goldstein HM, Zornoza J: Association of squamous cell carcinoma of the head and neck with cancer of the esophagus. Am J Roentgenol 131:791, 1978

80. Shibuya H, Tahogi M, Horiuchi J, et al: Carcinomas of the esophagus with synchronous or metachronous primary carcinoma in other organs. Acta Radiol Oncol 21:39, 1982

81. Shons AR, McQuarrie DG: Multiple primary epidermoid carcinomas of the upper aerodigestive tract. Arch Surg 120:1007, 1985

82. Burdette WJ: Palliative operation for carcinoma of cervical and thoracic esophagus. Ann Surg 173:714, 1971

83a. Earlam R, Cunha-Melo JR: Oesophageal squamous cell carcinoma: I. A critical review of surgery. Br J Surg 67:381, 1980

83b. Earlam R, Cunha-Melo JR: Oesophageal squamous cell carcinoma: II. A critical review of radiotherapy. Br J Surg 67:457, 1980

84. Daly JM, Massar E, Giacco G et al: Parenteral nutrition in esophageal cancer patients. Ann Surg 196:203, 1982

85. Haffejee AA, Angorn IB: Nutritional status and the nonspecific cellular and humoral immune response in esophageal carcinoma. Ann Surg 189:475, 1979

86. Brister SJ, Chin RCJ, Brown RA et al: Clinical impact of intravenous hyperalimentation on esophageal carcinoma: Is it worthwhile? Ann Thorac Surg 38:617, 1984

87. Pedersen H, Hansen HS, Cederquist C et al: The prognostic significance of weight loss and its integration in stagegrouping of oesophageal cancer. Acta Chir Scand 148:363, 1982

88. Burt ME, Gorschboth CM, Brennan MF: A controlled prospective randomized trial evaluating the metabolic effects of enteral and parenteral nutrition in the cancer patient. Cancer 49:1092, 1982

89. Finlay IG, Wright PA, Menzies T et al: Microbial flora in carcinoma of oesophagus. Thorax 37:181, 1982

90. Ong GB, Lam KH, Wong J et al: Factors influencing morbidity and mortality in esophageal carcinoma. J Thorac Cardiovasc Surg 76:745, 1978

91. Cedarquist C, Nielsen J, Berthelsen A et al: Cancer of the esophagus. II. Therapy and outcome. Acta Chir Scand 144:233, 1978

92. Scanlon EF, Morton DR, Walker JM et al: The case against segmental resection for esophageal carcinoma. Surg Gynecol Obstet 101:290, 1955

93. Wu Y, Chen P, Fang J et al: Surgical treatment of esophageal carcinoma. Am J Surg 139:805, 1980

94. Maillet P, Baulieux J, Boulez J et al: Carcinoma of the thoracic esophagus: Results of one-stage surgery (271 cases). Am J Surg 143:629, 1982

95. Skinner DB: En bloc resection for neoplasms of the esophagus and cardia. J Thorac Cardiovasc Surg 85:59, 1983

96. Lewis I: The surgical treatment of carcinoma of the esophagus. With special reference to a new operation for growths of the middle third. Br J Surg 34:18, 1946

97. Carey JS, Plested WG, Hughes RK: Esophagogastrectomy: Superiority of the combined abdominal-right thoracic approach (Lewis operation). Ann Thorac Surg 14:59, 1972

98. Kirk RM: Palliative resection of esophageal carcinoma without formal thoracotomy. Br J Surg 61:689, 1974

99. Orringer MB, Sloan H: Esophagectomy without thoracotomy. J Thorac Cardiovasc Surg 76:643, 1978

100. Szentpetery S, Wolfgang T, Lower R: Pull-through esophagectomy without thoracotomy for esophageal carcinoma. Ann Thorac Surg 27:399, 1979

101. Stewart JR, Starr MG, Sharp KW, et al: Transhiatal (blunt) esophagectomy for malignant and benign esophageal disease: Clinical experience and technique. Ann Thorac Surg 40:343, 1985

102. Hankins JR, Miller JE, Attar S et al: Transhiatal esophagectomy for carcinoma of the esophagus: Experience with 26 patients. Ann Thorac Surg 44:123, 1987

103. Postlethwait RW: Esophagectomy without thoracotomy. Ann Thorac Surg 27:395, 1979

104. Shakian DM, Neptune WB, Ellis FH et al: Transthoracic versus extrathoracic esophagectomy: Mortality, morbidity and long-term survival. Ann Thorac Surg 41:237, 1986

105. Steiger Z, Wilson RF: Comparison of the results of esophagectomy with and without a thoractomy. Surg Gynecol Obstet 153:653, 1981

106. Fisher RD, Brawley RK, Kieffer RF: Esophagectomy in the treatment of carcinoma of the distal two-thirds of the esophagus. Ann Thorac Surg 14:658, 1972

107. McKeown KC: Total three-stage oesophagectomy for cancer of the esophagus. Br J Surg 63:259, 1976

108. Steichen FM, Ravitch MM: Mechanical sutures in esophageal surgery. Ann Surg 191:373, 1980

109. Wong J: Stapled esophagogastric anastomosis in the apex of the right chest after subtotal esophagectomy for carcinoma. Surg Gynecol Obstet 164:569, 1987

110. Pearson FG, Henderson RD, Parrish RM: An operative technique for the control of reflux following esophagogastrostomy. J Thorac Cardiovasc Surg 58:668, 1969

111. Ward AS, Collis JL: Late results of oesophageal and oesophagogastric resection in the treatment of oesophageal cancer. Thorax 26:1, 1971

112. Cheung HC, Siu KF, Wong J: Is pyloroplasty necessary in esophageal replacement by stomach? A prospective, randomized controlled trial. Surgery 102:19, 1987

113. Wilkins EW, Burke JF: Colon esophageal bypass. Am J Surg 129:394, 1975

114. Postlethwait RW: Colonic interposition for esophageal substitution. Surg Gynecol Obstet 156:377, 1983

115. Postlethwait RW: Technique for isoperistaltic gastric tube for esophageal bypass. Ann Surg 189:673, 1979

116. Griffen WO, Daugherty ME, McGee EM et al: Unified approach to carcinoma of the esophagus. Am Surg 183:511, 1976

117. Cukingman RA, Carey JS: Carcinoma of the esophagus. Ann Thorac Surg 26:274, 1978

118. Mannell A: Carcinoma of the esophagus. Curr Probl Surg 19:554, 1982

119. Morstyn G, Thomas RJ, Mullerworth M et al: Improved survival in esophageal cancer in the period 1978 to 1983. J Clin Oncol 4:1062, 1986

120. Wilson SE, Stone R, Scully M et al: Modern management of anastomotic leak after esophagogastrectomy. Am J Surg 144:95, 1982

121. Isono K, Onoda S, Ishikawa T et al: Studies on the causes of deaths from esophageal carcinoma. Cancer 49:2173, 1982

122. Postlethwait RW: Complications and deaths after operation for esophageal carcinoma. J Thorac Cardiovasc Surg 85:827, 1983

123. Giuli R, Sancho-Garnier H: Diagnostic, therapeutic, and prognostic features of cancers of the esophagus: Results of the international prospective study conducted by the OESO group (790 patients). Surgery 99:614, 1986

124. Hussey DH, Barkley HT Jr, Bloedorn FG: Carcinoma of the esophagus. In Fletcher GH (ed): Textbook of Radiotherapy. pp 688–703. Philadelphia, Lea & Febiger, 1980

125. Levine MS, Langer J, Laufer I et al: Radiation therapy of esophageal carcinoma: Correlation of clinical and radiographic findings. Gastrointest Radiol 12:99, 1987

126. Beatty JD, DoBoer G, Rider WD: Carcinoma of the esophagus—pretreatment assessment, correlation of radiation treatment parameters with survival and identification and management of radiation treatment failure. Cancer 43:2254, 1979

127. Morita K, Takagi I, Watanabe M et al: Relationship between the radiologic features of esophageal cancer and the local control by radiation therapy. Cancer 55:2668, 1985

128. Hishikaw Y, Kamikonya N, Tanaka S et al: A multiple regression analysis for predicting local control of esophageal carcinoma treated by intracavitary irradiation. Radiat Med (Suppl 3)4:97, 1986

129. Smoron GL, O'Brien CA, Sullivan CA: Tumor localization and treatment technique for cancer of the esophagus. Radiology 111:735, 1974

130. Lewinsky BS, Annes GP, Mann SG et al: Carcinoma of the esophagus: An analysis of results and of treatment techniques. Radiol Clin North Am 44:192, 1975

131. Vijayakumar S, Muller-Runkel R: Irradiation of the thoracic esophagus: Prone versus supine treatment positions. Acta Radiol Oncol 25:187, 1986

132. Kagan AR, Wollin M, Rao AR et al: Treatment planning of esophagus, stomach, rectum and pancreas. Front Radiat Ther Oncol 21:236, 1987

133. Miller C: Carcinoma of the thoracic oesophagus and cardia. Br J Surg 49:507, 1962

134. Pearson JG: The present status and future potential of radiotherapy in the management of esophageal cancer. Cancer 39:882, 1977
135. McKenna WG, Yeakel K, Klink A et al: Is correction for lung density in radiotherapy treatment planning necessary? Int J Radiat Oncol Biol Phys 13:273, 1987
136. McShan DL, Fraass BA, Lichter AS: Treatment plan verification using portal images and beam's eye view treatment planning. Int J Radiat Biol Phys (in press)
137. Fraass BA, McShan DL, Weeks KJ: 3-D treatment planning: III. Complete beam's eye view planning capabilities. In Bruinvis IAD (ed): The Use of Computers in Radiation Therapy, pp 193–196. Amsterdam, Elsevier North-Holland, 1987
138. Bruso C, Perez-Tamayo C, McShan D et al: Results of beam's eye view treatment planning for esophageal carcinomas (abstr). Int J Radiat Oncol Biol Phys (Suppl 1) 13:195, 1987
139. Akiyama H, Tsurumaru M, Kawamara T et al: Principles of surgical treatment for carcinoma of the esophagus. Analysis of lymph node involvement. Ann Surg 194:438, 1981
140. Richmond J, Seydel HG, Bae Y et al: Comparison of three treatment strategies for esophageal cancer within a single institution. Int J Radiat Oncol Biol Phys 13:1617, 1987
141. Fisher SA, Brady LW: Carcinoma of the esophagus. In Perez CA, Brady LW (eds): Principles and Practice of Radiation Oncology, pp 700–722. Philadelphia, JB Lippincott, 1987
142. Fletcher DH: Clinical dose-response curves of human malignant epithelial tumors. Br J Radiol 46:1, 1973
143. Fajardo LF: Pathology of Radiation Injury, pp 50–53. New York, Masson, 1982
144. Seaman WB, Ackerman LV: The effect of radiation on the esophagus. Radiology 68:534, 1957
145. Phillips TL, Fu KK: Acute and late effects of multimodal therapy on normal tissues. Cancer 40:489, 1977
146. Roberts JG: Cancer of the oesophagus—How should tumor biology affect treatment? Br J Surg 78:791, 1980
147. Appelquist O, Silvo J, Rissanen P: The results of surgery and radiotherapy in the treatment of small carcinomas of the thoracic oesophagus. Ann Clin Res 11:184, 1979
148. Elkon D, Lee MS, Hendrickson FR: Carcinoma of the esophagus: Sites of recurrence and palliative benefits after definitive radiotherapy. Int J Radiat Oncol Biol Phys 4:615, 1978
149. Jobsen JJ, van Andel JG, Eijkenboom WMH et al: Carcinoma of the esophagus: Treatment results. Radiother Oncol 5:101, 1986
150. Lowe WC: Survival with carcinoma of the esophagus. Ann Intern Med 77:915, 1972
151. Newaishy GA, Read GA, Duncan W et al: Results of radical radiotherapy of squamous cell carcinoma of the esophagus. Clin Radiol 33:347, 1982
152. Schumann GF, Heydorn WH, Hall RV et al: Treatment of esophageal carcinoma. J Thorac Cardiovasc Surg 79:67, 1980
153. Van Andel JG, Dees J, Diskhuis CM et al: Carcinoma of the esophagus—results of treatment. Ann Surg 190:684, 1979
154. Van Houtte P: Radiotherapie du Cancer l'oesophage. Acta Gastroenterol Belg 40:121, 1977
155. Wara WM, Mauch PM, Thomas AN, Phillips TL: Palliation for carcinoma of the esophagus. Radiology 121:717, 1976
156. Yin W, Zhang LJ, Miao Y et al: The results of high-energy electron therapy in carcinoma of the oesophagus compared with telecobalt therapy. Clin Radiol 34:113, 1983
157. Robertson R, Coy P, Mokkhavesa S: The results of radical surgery compared with radical radiotherapy in the treatment of squamous carcinoma of the thoracic esophagus. J Thorac Cardiovasc Surg 53:430, 1967
158. Exner A: Veber die behandlung von oesophagus Karzinomen mit radiumstrahlen. Wien Klin Wochenschr 17:96, 1904
159. Rider W, Mendoza R: Some opinions on the treatment of cancer of the oesophagus. Am J Radiol 105:514, 1969
160. Moorthy CR, Nibhanupudy JR, Ashayeri E et al: Intraluminal radiation for esophageal cancer: A Howard University technique. J Natl Med Assoc 74:261, 1982
161. Bottrill DO, Plane JH, Newaishy GA: A proposed afterloading technique for irradiation of the esophagus. Br J Radiol 52:573, 1979
162. George FW: Radiation management in esophageal cancer. Am J Surg 139:795, 1980
163. Abe M, Kitagawa T: Treatment of esophageal cancer with high dose rate intracavitary irradiation. Tohoku J Exp Med 134:159, 1981
164. Hishikawa Y, Tanaka S, Miura T: Early esophageal carcinoma treated with intracavitary irradiation. Ther Radiol (Suppl 2)156:519, 1985
165. Rowland CG, Pagliero KM: Intracavitary irradiation in palliation of carcinoma of oesophagus and cardia. Lancet:981, 1985
166. Tate T, Brace JA, Morgan H, Skeggs DBL: Conformation therapy: A method of improving the tumour treatment volume ratio. Clin Radiol 37:267, 1986
167. Kelsen D, Bains M, Hilaris B et al: Combined-modality therapy of esophageal cancer. Semin Oncol 11:169, 1984
168. Leichman L, Steiger Z, Seydel HG et al: Combined preoperative chemotherapy and radiation therapy for cancer of the esophagus: The Wayne State University, Southwest Oncology Group and Radiation Therapy Oncology Group experience. Semin Oncol 11:178, 1984
169. Kelsen D: Chemotherapy of esophageal cancer. Semin Oncol 11:159, 1984
170. Folke S, Edsmyr F: Treatment of oesophagus carcinoma in Africa. Gann Monogr Cancer Res 19:187, 1976
171. Nabeya K: The use of bleomycin in the treatment of carcinoma of the esophagus. Gann Monogr Cancer Res 19:177, 1976
172. Resbeut M, Prise-Fleury E, Ben-Hassel M et al: Squamous cell carcinoma of the esophagus: Treatment by combined vincristine-methotrexate plus folinic acid rescue and cisplatin before radiotherapy. Cancer 56:1246, 1985
173. Advani SH, Saikia TK, Swaroop S: Anterior chemotherapy in esophageal cancer. Cancer 56:1502, 1985
174. Leichman L, Werskovic A, Leichman G et al: Non-operative therapy for squamous cell cancer of the esophagus. J Clin Oncol 5:365, 1987
175. Poplin E, Fleming T, Leichman L et al: Combined therapies for squamous cell cancer of the esophagus: A Southwest Oncology Group (SWOG 8037) Study. J Clin Oncol 5:633, 1987
176. Falkson G, Ckoetzer BJ, Terblanch AP: Oesophageal cancer—chemotherapy overview. S Afr Med J 71:21, 1987
177. Leichman L, Lokich JJ, Leichman CG: Esophageal and anal cancer. In Lokich JJ (ed): Cancer Chemotherapy by Infusion. Precept Press, 1987
178. Kolaric K, Moricic Z, Dujmovic I et al: Therapy of advanced esophageal cancer with bleomycin, irradiation and combination bleomycin and irradiation. Tumori 62:255, 1976
179. Ravry M, Moertel CG, Schutt AJ et al: Treatment of advanced squamous cell carcinoma of the gastrointestinal tract with bleomycin (NSC 125066). Cancer Chemother Rep 57:493, 1973
180. Yagoda A, Mukherji B, Young C et al: Bleomycin, an antitumor antibiotic: Clinical experience in 274 patients. Ann Intern Med 77:861, 1972
181. Bonnadonna G, de Lena M, Monfardini S et al: Clinical trial with bleomycin in lymphomas and solid tumors. Eur J Cancer Clin Oncol 8:205, 1972
182. Ravry M, Moore M: Phase II pilot study of cisplatinum (II) in advanced squamous cell esophageal cancer. Proc ASCO 21:353, 1980
183. Davis S, Shanmugathasa M, Kessler W: Cis-dichlorodiammine platinum (II) in the treatment of esophageal carcinoma. Cancer Treat Rep 64:709, 1980
184. Panettiere F, Leichman L, Tilchen E et al: Chemotherapy for advanced epidermoid carcinoma of the esophagus with single agent cisplatin: Final report on Southwest Oncology Group Study. Cancer Treat Rep 68:1023, 1984
185. Engstrom P, Lavin P, Lassen D: Phase II evaluation of mitomycin and cisplatin in advanced esophageal carcinoma. Cancer Treat Rep 67:713, 1983
186. Ezdinli E, Gelber R, Desai et al: Chemotherapy of advanced esophageal carcinoma: Eastern Cooperative Oncology Group experience. Cancer 46:2149, 1980
187. Lokich J, Shea M, Chaffey J: Sequential infusional 5-fluorouracil followed by concomitant radiation for tumors of the esophagus and the gastroesophageal junction. Cancer 60:275, 1987
188. Whitington R, Clos H: Clinical experience with mitomycin C. Cancer Chemother Rep 54:195, 1970
189. Kolaric K, Maricic Z, Roth A et al: Combination of bleomycin and adriamycin with and without radiation in the treatment of inoperable esophageal cancer. Cancer 45:2265, 1980
190. Bezwoda WR, Derman DP, Weaving A et al: Treatment of esophageal cancer with vindesine: An open trial. Cancer Treat Rep 68:783, 1984
191. Kelsen DR, Chapman R, Bains M: Phase II study of methyl-GAG in the present treatment of esophageal carcinoma. Cancer Treat Rep 66:1427, 1982
192. Coonley DJ, Bains M, Hilaris B et al: Cisplatin and bleomycin in the treatment of esophageal carcinoma: A final report. Cancer 54:2341, 1984
193. Bosset J, Hurteloup P, Bontemas P et al: A phase II trial of bleomycin and cisplatin in advanced oesophagus carcinoma (abstr). Proceedings of the 13th International Cancer Congress, 1982, p. 41.
194. Kelsen DP, Bains M, Hilaris B et al: Combination chemotherapy of esophageal carcinoma using cisplatin, vindesine and bleomycin. Cancer 49:1174, 1982
195. Dinwoodie WR, Bartolucci AA, Lyman GH et al: Phase II evaluation of cisplatin, bleomycin and vindesine in advanced squamous cell carcinoma of the esophagus: A Southeastern Study Group trial. Cancer Treat Rep 70:533, 1986
196. DeBasi P, Salvagno L, Endrizzi L et al: Cisplatin, bleomycin and methotrexate in the treatment of advanced oesophageal cancer. Eur J Cancer Clin Oncol 20:743, 1984
197. Vogl SE, Greenwald E, Kaplan BH: Effective chemotherapy for esophageal cancer with methotrexate, bleomycin, and cis-diamminedichloroplatinum II. Cancer 48:2555, 1981
198. Kelsen DP, Fein R, Coonley C et al: Cisplatin, vindesine and mitoguazone in the treatment of esophageal cancer. Cancer Treat Rep 70:255, 1986
199. Forastiere A, Gennis M, Orringer M et al: Cisplatin, vinblastine and mitoguazone chemotherapy for epidermoid and adenocarcinoma of the esophagus. J Clin Oncol 5:1143, 1987
200. Vogl SE, Camacho F, Berenzweig et al: Chemotherapy for esophageal cancer with mitoguazone, methotrexate, bleomycin and cisplatin. Cancer Treat Rep 69:21, 1985
201. Gisselbrecht C, Calvo F, Mignot L et al: Fluorouracil, adriamycin and cisplatin combination chemotherapy of advanced esophageal carcinoma. Cancer 52:974, 1983
202. Wittes R, Brescia F, Young CW: Combination chemotherapy with cis-diamminedichloroplatinum (II) and bleomycin in tumors of the head and neck. Oncology 32:202, 1975
203. Kelsen DP, Cvitkovic E, Bains M et al: Cis-diamminedichloroplatinum (II) and bleomycin in the treatment of esophageal carcinoma. Cancer Treat Rep 62:1041, 1978
204. Kelsen DP, Hilaris B, Coonley C et al: Cisplatin, vindesine and bleomycin combination chemotherapy of local-regional and advanced esophageal carcinoma. Am J Med 75:645, 1983
205. Huang GJ, Gu XZ, Wang LJ et al: Experience with combined preoperative irradiation and surgery for carcinoma of the esophagus. Gann Monogr Cancer Res 31:159, 1986
206. Akakura I, Nakamura Y, Kakegawa T et al: Surgery for carcinoma of the esophagus with preoperative irradiation. Chest 57:47, 1970

207. Andersen AP, Berdal P, Edsmyr F et al: Irradiation, chemotherapy and clinical study. Radiother Oncol 2:179, 1984

208. Doggett RLS, Guernsey JM, Bagshaw MA: Combined radiation and surgical treatment of carcinoma of the thoracic esophagus. Front Radiat Ther Oncol 5:147, 1970

209. Gignoux M, Roussel A, Paillot B et al: The value of preoperative radiotherapy in esophageal cancer: Results of a study of the EORTC. World J Surg 11:426, 1987

210. Groves LK, Rodriguez-Antunez A: Treatment of carcinoma of the esophagus and gastric cardia with concentrated preoperative irradiation followed by early operation. Ann Thorac Surg 15:333, 1973

211. Kelsen DP, Ahuja R, Hopfan S et al: Combined modality therapy of esophageal carcinoma. Cancer 48:31, 1981

212. Launois B, DeLaRue D, Campion JP et al: Preoperative radiotherapy for carcinoma of the esophagus. Surg Gynecol Obstet 153:690, 1981

213. Liu G, Huang Z, Rong T et al: Measures for improving therapeutic results of esophageal carcinoma in stage III: Preoperative radiotherapy. J Surg Oncol 32:248, 1986

214. Marks RD Jr, Scruggs HJ, Wallace KM: Preoperative radiation therapy for carcinoma of the esophagus. Cancer 38:84, 1976

215. Isono K, Onoda S, Ishikawa T et al: Studies on the causes of deaths from esophageal carcinoma. Cancer 49:2173, 1982

216. Parker EF, Gregorie HB, Prioleau WH Jr et al: Carcinoma of the esophagus — observations of 40 years. Ann Surg 195:618, 1982

217. Sugimachi K, Matsufuji H, Kai H et al: Preoperative irradiation for carcinoma of the esophagus. Surg Gynecol Obstet 162:174, 1986

218. Fraser RW, Wara WM, Thomas AN et al: Combined treatment methods for carcinoma of the esophagus. Radiology 128:461, 1978

219. Goodner JT: Surgical and radiation treatment of cancer of the thoracic esophagus. Am J Roentgenol Rad Ther Nucl Med 105:523, 1969

220. Gunnlaugsson GH, Wychulis AR, Roland et al: Analysis of the records of 1657 patients with carcinoma of the esophagus and cardia of the stomach. Surg Gynecol Obstet 130:997, 1970

221. Hankins JR, Cole FN, Ahar S et al: Carcinoma of the esophagus: Twelve years' experience with a philosophy for palliation. Ann Thorac Surg 33:464, 1982

222. Langer M, Choi NC, Orlow E et al: Radiation therapy alone or in combination with surgery in the treatment of carcinoma of the esophagus. Cancer 58:1208, 1986

223. Giuli R, Gignoux M: Treatment of carcinoma of the esophagus — retrospective study of 2400 patients. Ann Surg 192:44, 1980

224. Kasai M, Mori S, Watanabe T: Follow-up results after resection of thoracic esophageal carcinoma. World J Surg 2:543, 1980

225. Fujimaki M et al: Role of preoperative administration of bleomycin and radiation in the treatment of esophageal cancer. Jpn J Surg 5:48, 1975

226. Wada T, Matoumoto Y, Amano T: Chemotherapy of esophageal cancer with bleomycin. Prog Antimicrob Anticancer Chemother 2:696, 1970

227. Miller JJ, McIntyre B, Hatcher CR: Combined treatment approach in surgical management of carcinoma of the esophagus: A preliminary report. Ann Thorac Surg 40:289, 1985

228. Kelsen DP, Bains MS, Cvitkovic E et al: Vindesine in the treatment of esophageal carcinoma: A phase II study. Cancer Treat Rep 63:2019, 1979

229. Schlag P, Hermann R, Fritze D et al: Preoperative chemotherapy in localized cancer of the esophagus with cis-platinum, vindesine and bleomycin. Primary chemotherapy. In Cancer Medicine, pp 253–258. New York, Alan R Liss, 1985

230. Roth JA, Pass HI, Flanagan MM et al: Clinical trials with cisplatin, vindesine and bleomycin: Neoadjuvant chemotherapy for epidermoid carcinoma of the esophagus. In Levin B (ed): Gastrointestinal Cancer: Current Approaches to Diagnosis and Treatment. Austin, University of Texas Press, 1988

231. Falkson G: Methyl-GAG (NSC-32946) in the treatment of esophagus cancer. Cancer Chemother Rep 55:209, 1971

232. Kelsen DP, Yagoda A, Warrell R et al: Phase II trials of methyl-glyoxal bis [guanylhydrazone] (methyl-GAG). Am J Clin Oncol 5:221, 1982

233. Leichman L, Steiger Z, Seydel HG et al: Preoperative chemotherapy for patients with cancer of the esophagus: Potentially curative approach. J Clin Oncol 2:75, 1984

234. Shields TW, Rosen ST, Hellerstein SM et al: Multimodality approach to treatment of carcinoma of the esophagus. Arch Surg 119:558, 1984

235. Carey RW, Hilgenberg AD, Wilkens EW et al: Preoperative chemotherapy followed by surgery with possible postoperative radiotherapy in squamous cell carcinoma of the esophagus: Evaluation of the chemotherapy component. J Clin Oncol 4:697, 1986

236. Karasawa K, Okada Y, Akamire Y et al: The result of surgical treatment for esophageal cancer in combination with preoperative irradiation and bleomycin therapy (abstr). Nippon Gan Chiryo Gakkai Shi 12:209, 1975

237. Pedersen H, Hansen HS, Bertelsen S et al: Combined modality therapy for oesophageal squamous cell carcinoma. Acta Oncol 26:175, 1987

238. Werner ID: The multidisciplinary approach in the management of squamous carcinoma of the esophagus: The Groote Schmit Hospital experience. Front Gastrointest Res 5:130, 1979

239. Rosenberg JC, Franklin R, Steiger Z: Squamous cell carcinoma of the thoracic esophagus. Curr Probl Cancer 5:1–52, 1981

240. Franklin R, Steiger Z, Vaishanapayan G et al: Combined modality therapy for esophageal squamous cell carcinoma. Cancer 51:1062, 1983

241. Parker FP, Marks RD, Kratz JM et al: Chemoradiation therapy and resection for carcinoma of the esophagus: Short-term results. Ann Thorac Surg 40:121, 1985

242. Douple EB: Therapeutic potentiation in a mouse mammary tumor and an intracerebral rat brain tumor by combined treatment with cis-dichloroplatinum II and radiation. Hematol Oncol 7:585, 1977

243. Leipzig B, Wetmore SJ, Putzeys R et al: Cisplatin potentiation of radiotherapy. Arch Otolaryngol Head Neck Surg 11:114, 1985

244. Campbell WR, Taylor SA, Pierce GE et al: Therapeutic alternative in patients with esophageal cancer. Am J Surg 150:665, 1985

245. Austin JC, Postier RG, Elkins RC: Treatment of esophageal cancer: The continued need of surgical resection. Am J Surg 152:592, 1986

246. Popp MB, Hawley D, Reising J et al: Improved survival in squamous esophageal cancer. Arch Surg 121:1330, 1986

247. Wolfe WG, Burton GV, Seigler HF et al: Early results with combined modality therapy for carcinomas of the esophagus. Ann Surg 205:563, 1987

248. Vietti T, Eggerding F, Valeriote F: Combined effect of x-irradiation and 5-fluorouracil on survival of transplanted leukemic cells. J Natl Cancer Inst 47:865, 1971

249. Kelsen DP: Editorial: Multimodality therapy of esophageal carcinoma: Still an experimental approach. J Clin Oncol 5:530, 1987

250. Mathews CP: Results of combined chemo and radiotherapy in carcinoma oesophagus. Indian J Cancer 9:160, 1972

251. Kolaric K, Maricic Z, Roth A et al: Adriamycin alone and in combination with radiotherapy in the treatment of inoperable esophageal cancer. Tumori 63:485, 1977

252. Earle J, Gelbar R, Moertel C et al: A controlled evaluation of combined radiation and bleomycin therapy for squamous cell carcinoma of the esophagus. Int J Radiat Oncol Biol Phys 6:821, 1980

253. Marcial V, Velez-Garcia E, Clintron J et al: Radiotherapy preceded by multi-drug chemotherapy in carcinoma of the esophagus. Cancer Clin Trials 3:127, 1980

254. Abitbol A, Straus M, Franklin G et al: Infusional chemotherapy and cyclic radiation therapy in inoperable esophageal and gastric cardia carcinoma. Am J Clin Oncol 6:195, 1983

255. Berenzweig M, Vogl S, Camacho F et al: Esophageal squamous cancer chemotherapy with MGBG, methotrexate, bleomycin and dichlorodiammine platinum-MGBG-MBD. Pro Am Soc Clin Oncol 2:125, 1983

256. Seifert P, Baker LH, Reed ML et al: Comparison of continuously infused 5-fluorouracil with bolus injection in treatment of patients with colorectal adenocarcinoma. Cancer 36:123, 1975

257. Kish J, Ensley J, Weaver A et al: Superior response rates with 96-hour 5-fluorouracil infusional versus 5-FU bolus combined with cisplatinum (CACP) in a randomized trial for recurrent and advanced squamous head and neck cancer (HNC) (abstr). Proc Am Soc Clin Oncol 3:179, 1984

258. Byfield JE, Barone R, Mendelsohn J et al: Infusional 5-fluorouracil (5-Fu): Molecular and clinical scheduling implications. Proc Am Assoc Cancer Res 18:74, 1977

259. Coia LR, Engstrom PF, Paul A: Nonsurgical management of esophageal cancer. Report of a study of combined radiotherapy and chemotherapy. J Clin Oncol 5:1783, 1987

260. Kean TJ, Harwood AR, Tahany E et al: Radical radiation therapy with 5-fluorouracil infusion and mitomycin C for oesophageal squamous carcinoma. Radiother Oncol 4:205, 1985

261. John M, Flam M, Wittlinger P et al: Inoperable esophageal carcinoma: Results of aggressive synchronous radiotherapy and chemotherapy. Am J Clin Oncol 10:310, 1987

262. Collin CF, Spiro RH: Carcinoma of the cervical esophagus: Changing therapeutic trends. Am J Surg 148:460, 1984

263. Harrison DFN: Surgical repair in hypopharyngeal and cervical esophageal cancer: Analysis of 162 patients. Ann Otol Rhinol Laryngol 90:372, 1981

264. Ujiki GT, Pearl GJ, Poticha S et al: Mortality and morbidity of gastric pull-up for replacement of the pharyngoesophagus. Arch Surg 122:644, 1987

265. Lam KH, Wong J, Lim STK et al: Pharyngogastric anastomosis following pharyngolaryngoesophagectomy: Analysis of 157 cases. World J Surg 5:509, 1981

266. Raphael HA, Ellis HF, Dockerty MB: Primary adenocarcinoma of the esophagus: 18-year review and review of literature. Ann Surg 164:785, 1966

267. Turnbull AD, Rosen P, Goodner JT et al: Primary malignant tumors of the esophagus other than typical epidermoid carcinoma. Ann Thorac Surg 15:463, 1973

268. Steiger Z, Wilson RF, Leichman L et al: Primary adenocarcinoma of the esophagus. J Surg Oncol 36:68, 1987

269. Cedarquist C, Nielsen J, Berthelsen A et al: Adenocarcinoma of the esophagus. Acta Chir Scand 146:411, 1980

270. Ming SC: Tumors of the esophagus and stomach. In: Atlas of Tumor Pathology, 2nd series, fascile 7, Washington DC, Armed Forced Institute of Pathology

271. Barrett N: The lower esophagus lined by columnar epithelium. Surgery 41:881, 1957

272. Allison PR, Johnstone AS: The oesophagus lined with gastric mucous membrane. Thorax 8:87, 1953

273. Allison PR: Peptic oesophagitis and oesophageal stricture. Lancet 2:199, 1970

274. Adler RH: The lower esophagus lined by columnar epithelium: Its association with hiatal hernia, ulcer, stricture and tumor. J Thorac Cardiovasc Surg 45:13, 1963

275. Spechler SJ, Goyel RK: Barrett's esophagus. N Eng J Med 315:362, 1986

276. Nissen R: Eine einfache operation zur beinflussung der Refluxoesophagitis. Schweiz Med Wochenschr 86:590, 1956

277. Rosenberg JC, Budev H, Edwards RC et al: Analysis of adenocarcinoma in Barrett's esophagus utilizing a staging system. Cancer 55:1353, 1985

278. Bremner CG, Lynch VP, Ellis FH: Barrett's esophagus: Congenital of acquired? An experimental study of esophageal mucosal regeneration in the dog. Surgery 68:309, 1970

279. Hamilton SR, Yardley JG: Regeneration of cardiac type mucosa and acquisition of Barrett mucosa after esophagogastrostomy. Gastroenterology 72:669, 1977

280. Ranson JM, Patel GK, Clift SA et al: Extended and limited types of Barrett's esophagus in the adult. Ann Thorac Surg 33:19, 1982

281. Paull A, Trier JS, Dalton D et al: The histologic spectrum of Barrett's esophagus. N Engl J Med 295:576, 1976
282. Berenson MM, Herbst JJ, Freston JW: Enzyme and ultrastructural characteristics of esophageal columnar epithelium. Dig Dis Sci 19:895, 1974
283. Jass JR: Mucin histochemistry of the columnar epithelium of the oesophagus: A retrospective study. J Clin Pathol 34:866, 1981
284. Banner BF, Memoli VA, Warren WH et al: Carcinoma with multidirectional differentiation arising in Barrett's esophagus. Ultrastruct Pathol 4:205, 1983
285. Skinner DB, Walther BC, Riddell RH et al: Barrett's esophagus: Comparison of benign and malignant cases. Surgery 198:554, 1983
286. Mangla JC: Barrett's esophagus: An old entity rediscovered. J Clin Gastroenterol 3:347, 1981
287. Brand DL, Ylvisaker JT, Gelfand M et al: Regression of columnar esophageal (Barrett's) epithelium after anti-reflux surgery. N Engl J Med 302:844, 1980
288. Lee RG: Dysplasia in Barrett's esophagus: Clinicopathologic study of 6 patients. Am J Surg Pathol 9:845, 1985
289. Stoller JL, Brumwell ML: Palliation after operation and after radiotherapy for cancer of the esophagus. Can J Surg 27:491, 1984
290. Marcial VA, Tome JM, Ubinas J et al: The role of radiation therapy in esophageal cancer. Radiology 87:231, 1966
291. Schwade JG, Kinsella TJ, Kelly B et al: Clinical experience with intravenous misonidazole for carcinoma of the esophagus. Cancer Invest 2:91, 1984
292. Pearson JG: The value of radiotherapy in the management of esophageal cancer. Am J Roentgenol 105:500, 1969
293. Orringer MB: Palliative procedures for esophageal cancer. Surg Clin North Am 63:941, 1983
294. Payne WS: Palliation of esophageal carcinoma. Ann Thorac Surg 28:208, 1979
295. Hankins JR, Cole FN, Attar S et al: Carcinoma of the esophagus: Twelve years' experience with a philosophy for palliation. Ann Thorac Surg 33:464, 1982
296. Orringer MB: Esophageal carcinoma: What price palliation? Ann Thorac Surg 36:377, 1983
297. Orringer MB, Sloan H: Substernal gastric bypass of the excluded thoracic esophagus for palliation of esophageal carcinoma. J Thorac Cardiovasc Surg 70:836, 1975
298. Steiger Z, Nickel WD, Wilson RF et al: Improved surgical palliation of advanced carcinoma of the esophagus. Am J Surg 125:782, 1978
299. Orringer MB: Substernal gastric bypass of the excluded esophagus—Results of an ill-advised operation. Surgery 96:467, 1984
300. Olsen CO, Hopkins RA, Poltlethwait RW: Management of an infected mucocele occurring in a bypassed excluded esophageal segment. Ann Thorac Surg 40:73, 1985
301. Kamath MV, Ellison RG, Rubin JW et al: Esophageal mucocele: A complication of blind loop esophagus. Ann Thorac Surg 43:263, 1987
302. Angorn IB: Intubation in the treatment of carcinoma of the esophagus. World J Surg 5:535, 1981
303. Ghazi A, Nussbaum M: A new approach to the management of malignant esophageal obstruction and esophagorespiratory fistula. Ann Thorac Surg 41:531, 1986
304. Unruh HW, Pagliero KM: Pulsion intubation versus traction intubation for obstructing carcinoma of the esophagus. Ann Thorac Surg 40:337, 1985
305. Angorn IB, Haffegee AA: Pulsion intubation in v. retrosternal gastric bypass for palliation of unresectable carcinoma of the upper thoracic oesophagus. Br J Surg 70:335, 1983
306. Rose JDR, Smith PM: Fibre endoscopic insertion of palliative oesophageal tubes with the Nottingham introducer. J R Soc Med 76:266, 1983
307. Celestin LR, Campbell WB: A new and safe system for oesophageal dilatation. Lancet 1:74, 1981
308. Boyce HW: Medical management of esophageal obstruction and esophageal-pulmonary fistula. Cancer 50:2597, 1982
309. Fleischer D, Kessler F, Hage O: Endoscopic Nd:YAG laser therapy for carcinoma of the esophagus: A new form of palliative treatment. Gastroenterology 85:600, 1983
310. McCaughan JS, Williams TE, Bethel BH: Palliation of esophageal malignancy with photodynamic therapy. Ann Thorac Surg 40:113, 1985
311. Pietrafitta JJ, Dwyer RM: Endoscopic laser therapy of malignant esophageal obstruction. Arch Surg 121:395, 1986
312. Battifora H: Spindle cell carcinoma: Ultrastructural evidence of squamous origin and collagen production by the tumor cells. Cancer 37:2275, 1976
313. Agha FP, Keren DF: Spindle-cell squamous carcinoma of the esophagus: A tumor with biphasic morphology. AJR 145:541, 1985
314. Osamura RY, Shinamura K, Hata J et al: Polypoid carcinoma of the esophagus: A unifying term for "carcinosarcoma" and pseudosarcoma. Am J Surg Pathol 2:201, 1978
315. Matsusaka T, Watanabe H, Enjoji: Pseudosarcoma and carcinosarcoma of the esophagus. Cancer 37:1546, 1976
316. Fennell WM, Perold JI: Pseudosarcoma of the esophagus: A case report. S Afr Med J 52:37, 1977
317. Postlethwait RW, Wechsler AS, Shelburne JD. Pseudosarcoma of the esophagus. Ann Thorac Surg 19:198, 1975
318. DeMeester TR, Skinner DB: Polypoid sarcomas of the esophagus: A rare but potentially curable neoplasm. Ann Thorac Surg 20:405, 1975
319. Xu LT, Sun CF, Wu LH et al: Clinical and pathological characteristics of carcinosarcoma of the esophagus: Report of 4 cases. Ann Thorac Surg 37:197, 1978
320. Yates CW, LeVine MA, Jensen KM: Varicoid carcinoma of the esophagus. Radiology 122:605, 1977
321. Epstein JI, Sears VL, Tucker RS et al: Carcinoma of the esophagus with adenoid cystic differentiation. Cancer 53:1131, 1984
322. Pourzand A, Freant L, Levin R et al: Primary adenoid cystic carcinoma of the esophagus: Report of a case and review of the literature. J Thorac Cardiovasc Surg 69:785, 1975
323. Petersson SR: Adenoid cystic carcinoma of the esophagus: Complete response to combination chemotherapy. Cancer 57:1464, 1986
324. Woodard BA, Shelburne JD, Vollmer RT et al: Mucoepidermoid carcinoma of the esophagus: A case report. Hum Pathol 9:352, 1978
325. Sabnathan S, Graham GP, Salama FD: Primary oat cell carcinoma of the esophagus. Thorax 41:318, 1986
326. Imai T, Sannoke Y, Okano H: Oat cell carcinoma (APUDOMA) of the esophagus: A case report. Cancer 41:358, 1978
327. Johnson FE, Clawson MC, Bashiti HM et al: Small cell undifferentiated carcinoma of the esophagus. Cancer 53:1746, 1984
328. Doherty MA, McIntyre M, Arnott SJ: Oat cell carcinoma of the esophagus: A report of six British patients with a review of the literature. Int J Radiat Oncol Biol Phys 10:147, 1984
329. Reyes CV, Chejfec G, Jao W et al: Neuroendocrine tumors of the esophagus. Ultrastruct Pathol 1:367, 1980
330. Kelsen DP, Weston E, Kurty R et al: Small cell carcinoma of the esophagus: Treatment by chemotherapy alone. Cancer 45:1558, 1980
331. Rosenthal SN, Lemkin JA. Multiple small cell carcinomas of the esophagus. Cancer 51:1944, 1983
332. Rankin R, Nirodi NS, Browne MK: Carcinoid tumor of the esophagus: Report of a case. Scott Med J 25:245, 1980
333. Siegel A, Swartz A: Malignant carcinoid of oesophagus. Histopathology 10:761, 1986
334. Chalkiadokis G, Wihlm JM, Morand G et al: Primary malignant melanoma of the esophagus. Ann Thorac Surg 39:472, 1985
335. Choh JH, Khazei AH, Ihm JH: Leiomyosarcoma of the esophagus: Report of a case and review of the literature. J Surg Oncol 32:223, 1986
336. Wobbes T, Rinsma SG, Holla AT et al: Rhabpdomyosarcoma of the esophagus. Arch Chir Neerl 27:69, 1975
337. Trillo AA, Accettulo LM, Yecter TL: Choriocarcinoma of the esophagus: Histologic and cytologic findings. A case report. Acta Cytol 23:69, 1979
338. Matsuura H, Saito R, Nakajing S et al: Non-Hodgkin's lymphoma of the esophagus. Am J Gastroenterol 80:941, 1985
339. Agha FP, Schnitzer B: Esophageal involvement in lymphoma. Am J Gastroenterol 80:412, 1985
340. Gedgaudos-McClees RK, Maglinte DD: Lymphomatous esophageal nodules: The difficulty in radiological differential diagnosis. Am J Gastroenterol 80:529, 1985
341. Agha FP: Secondary neoplasms of the esophagus. Gastrointest Radiol 12:187, 1987
342. Marshall ME: Gastrointestinal metastasis from carcinoma of the breast. J Ky Med Assoc 81:154, 1973
343. Anderson MF, Harrell GS: Secondary esophageal tumors. Am J Radiol 135:1243, 1980
344. Laforet EG, Kondi ES: Postmastectomy dysphagia. Am J Surg 121:368, 1971
345. Boccardo F, Merlano M, Canobbio L et al: Esophageal involvement in breast cancer: Report of six cases Tumori 68:149, 1982

JOHN S. MACDONALD

GLENN STEELE, JR.

LEONARD L. GUNDERSON

CHAPTER 25 *Cancer of the Stomach*

Cancer of the stomach is the eighth most common cause of cancer deaths in the United States. In 1986 25,000 new cases occurred, and 14,000 deaths resulted from stomach cancer. Although gastric cancer still remains a major health problem in the United States, the death rate from this disease in males has decreased from approximately 22.8:100,000 in 1950 to 9:100,000 in the 1980s. The corresponding changes in women are from 12.3 to 4.3:100,000. This represents a 59% and 65% decrease in age-adjusted mortality due to stomach cancer in men and women, respectively. This decline is steepest in older persons and in whites.[1,2] The decreasing mortality is a result of the decreasing incidence of stomach cancer. There has been no adequate explanation for the decreasing incidence of gastric adenocarcinoma in the United States.

This unexplained decrease in a highly lethal malignancy has intrigued and stimulated epidemiologists. The decline in gastric cancer in the United States is particularly striking when considered in the context of the very high incidence rates of the disease in such countries as Japan (78:10,000) and Chile (70:100,000).[3] In the United States the approximate incidence of gastric cancer is 10:100,000. The fact that populations emigrating from high- to low-incidence countries experience a significant decrease in the occurrence of the disease clearly suggests that the cause of this cancer must be related to the environment.[3] The first-generation immigrants have a higher risk of stomach cancer than do natives of the host country. This finding suggests an etiological factor that may persist in the migrant population for some time[4,5]—perhaps a learned dietary practice that disappears as migrant groups are assimilated into the host culture. A variety of environmental factors have been associated with a high incidence of gastric cancer, including consumption of smoked foods, salted foods, and foods contaminated with aflatoxin.[6]

In the United States and Western Europe, stomach cancer is twice as frequent in the lower as in the highest socioeconomic groups. Increased stomach cancer rates have been associated with a number of occupations, including coal mining, farming (in Japan), and nickel refining (in the Soviet Union). Rubber workers and workers who process timber also have been reported to have an increased risk of stomach cancer. Whether these occupations are truly associated with an increased risk for gastric cancer or merely reflect the socioeconomic characteristics of the employees is not clear.[7] Stomach cancer also is more common in asbestos workers, and it is likely that this increase is due to exposure to asbestos fibers.[8]

Familial occurrence of gastric cancer is rare, and associations between gastric cancer and blood group A and intestinal metaplasia are discussed in subsequent sections of this chapter.[9,10] There appears to be no increased risk of gastric cancer in persons using alcohol or tobacco.

PATHOLOGY

Of the malignant neoplasms of the stomach, 95% are adenocarcinomas, and generally when the term gastric cancer is used, it refers to adenocarcinoma of the stomach. Although adenoacanthoma, squamous cell carcinoma, and carcinoid tumors do occur in the stomach, they each represent less than 1% of gastric malignancies.[11] Leiomyosarcomas of the stomach may account for 1% to 3% of malignant gastric tumors.[12,13] The stomach is the most common site for lymphoma of the gastrointestinal (GI) tract.[6] With the relative decrease in incidence of carcinoma of the stomach, lymphomas represent a larger proportion of malignancies diagnosed.[14] Pathologists and clinicians must be alert to the possibility that a gastric neoplasm represents lymphoma rather than carcinoma.

In evaluating the pathology of gastric cancer, several factors have important clinical significance. The gross appearance, site, and degree of local invasion of the tumor all bear on prognosis, as does the histology of the cancer. The macroscopic appearance of gastric cancer has been described according to several schemes.[11,15] Fifty years ago, the German pathologist Borrmann developed a classification scheme that divided gastric cancer into five types, according to macroscopic appearance.[15] Type 1 represented polypoid or fungating cancers, type 2 encompassed ulcerating lesions surrounded by elevated borders, type 3 represented ulcerating lesions infiltrating the gastric wall, type 4 tumors were diffusely infiltrating carcinomas, and type 5 were unclassifiable cancers. In the United States, a less formalized descriptive classification of gastric cancers generally is used.[11] This scheme divides the gross pathologic features of stomach cancer into four categories. Most lesions are ulcerative. The lesions may have the appearance of a benign gastric ulcer, or they may exhibit the findings classically attributed to malignant gastric ulcers, including a diameter greater than 2 cm and heaped-up borders, making the ulcer appear raised above the level of the surrounding stomach. Approximately 10% of gastric cancers can be classified grossly as polypoid. These lesions may be large without showing evidence of significant invasion or metastases. This may result from the fact that, histologically, these tumors are well differentiated. In the European literature, such well-differentiated types of stomach cancers have been classified as being of the intestinal type and have a better prognosis than tumors with diffuse anaplastic histopathology.[16] The third type of gross appearance of gastric cancer is the scirrhous pattern. Approximately 10% of cancers fall into this category. Scirrhous tumors result in thickening and rigidity of the gastric wall owing to diffuse infiltration with anaplastic cancer cells. These malignant cells produce a marked fibrous reaction in the gastric wall, leading to a stiffened stomach, giving the appearance of linitis plastica. Scirrhous carcinoma is almost invariably fatal. In a series of 504 patients with resectable gastric cancer reported by the Veterans Administration Surgical Oncology Group, the 5-year survival rate after gastric resection for patients with scirrhous carcinoma was 2%.[17] The fourth type of gastric cancer, the superficial variety, is uncommon in the United States. This tumor, found in fewer than 5% of surgical specimens, is characterized by sheet-like collections of cancer cells replacing the normal mucosa.

Gastric cancer does not arise from all sites in the stomach with equal frequency.[11,18] Most tumors develop in the antrum, or lower third of the stomach. Cancers are generally less common in the body of the stomach and least common in the cardia. However, recent information in the United States[19,20] suggests a slight increase in the incidence of cardioesophageal junction carcinomas and a decrease in the incidence of more distal lesions. These proximal lesions may invade the distal esophagous. Gastric cancers are more common in the lesser curvature than in the greater curvature of the stomach. Berkson, in reviewing the site of origin in 587 cases of gastric cancer, noted that the tumors arose in the lesser curvature in 18% of cases but from the greater curvature in only 3% of cases.[21] Multicentric involvement of the stomach has also been reported in patients with stomach cancer. Moertel reported that 2.2% of 1835 patients with gastric cancer showed gross evidence of having more than one primary gastric tumor.[11] If the stomachs of patients with gastric cancer are carefully examined histologically for the presence of multicentric tumor, in as many as 22% tumors will be found arising from several sites.[22] This phenomenon is more common in patients with gastric cancer following pernicious anemia.

Adenocarcinoma occurring in the stomach may be classified according to degree of histologic differentiation. Although not an independent prognostic variable, differentiation is important because prognosis is worse in the poorly differentiated lesions.[23] If Broder's classification is used, which grades tumor cells from 1 (well differentiated) to 4 (anaplastic), patients with unresectable stomach cancer and well-differentiated lesions (Grades 1 and 2) have a median survival of 7 months. Patients with Grade 3 or 4 tumor histology have a median survival of only 4 months. It should be emphasized that histologic grade of the tumor and the gross pathology are not independent variables. For example, linitis plastica is never seen with well-differentiated tumors, occurring only with the more undifferentiated cancer. Conversely, polypoid tumors are very likely to have well-differentiated histology.

ANATOMICAL RELATIONSHIPS OF THE STOMACH

From the oncologist's point of view, the important features of the stomach relate to the other viscera with which it comes in contact, its vascular supply, its lymphatic supply, and which surgical procedures may be performed on the stomach without endangering patient survival (Fig. 25-1).

Since the stomach begins at the gastroesophageal junction and ends at the pylorus, direct spread to the esophagus or the duodenum or so-called skip submucosal metastases must be taken into account when determining appropriate visual as well as microscopic margins in planning resections of tumors at the proximal or distal ends of the stomach. In addition, the stomach is in contact with the diaphragm, the anterior abdominal wall, the liver, the transverse colon and mesocolon, the spleen, the left adrenal, the left kidney, the pancreas, the splenic flexure of the colon, the greater omentum, and various loops of small intestine.

The blood supply to the stomach is derived from the celiac axis. The major vessels involved are the left gastric artery, the right gastric artery, and the gastroduodenal artery (all branches of the hepatic artery), the right and left gastroepiploic vessels, and the short gastric or vasa brevia (branches of the splenic artery). Other arteries of concern in terms of dissemination of gastric carcinoma or in terms of operative procedures on the stomach include the splenic, the hepatic,

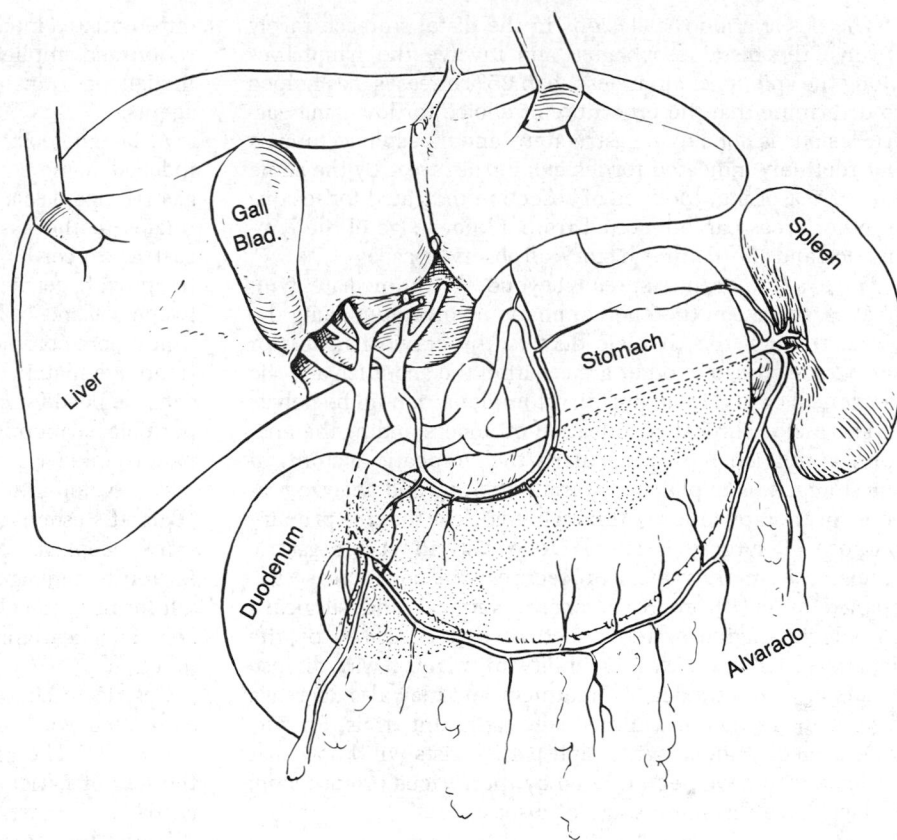

FIG. 25-1. Major anatomical relationships of the stomach, showing its blood supply, and the other organs most likely to be involved by primary malignant lesions in the stomach.

and the middle colic, any of which might be involved by an extensive tumor arising within the stomach or might be encountered during surgical procedures to remove these lesions.

In general, the venous drainage of the stomach parallels the arterial supply. The major additional vein is the coronary vein, which runs along the lesser curvature of the stomach and eventually drains into the portal vein.

The lymphatics of the stomach have been described in greater detail by Rouviere, and reference to his work is essential for anyone interested in the routes of potential spread of carcinoma of the stomach (Table 25-1).[18] Although there is a rich interconnecting lymphatic network within the stomach, the more important pathways with respect to gastric carcinoma are those that deal with the collecting trunk. Rouviere has divided these into three major systems: the region of the left gastric chain, the region of the splenic chain, and the region of the hepatic chain. The lymphatic pathways are complex and highly interconnected but, in general, follow the pathways of the major vascular supply to the stomach. It is clear from this that lymphatics can be involved along both the lesser and the greater curvatures of the stomach, extending to the hilum of the spleen on the left side and up the portal triad on the right side, across the surface of the pancreas, and down along the course of the duodenum inferiorly. The highly complex nature of the lymphatic pathways explains, to a certain extent, the problems with early and extensive spread of tumors from the stomach to other areas.

The gastric lymphatic pathways have been defined (see Table 25-1) to show that lesions in particular areas of the stomach generally follow a given direction, but this is not an invariable rule; if there is early blockage of the normal pathway, lymphatic drainage can then go in a different direction, thus causing even more extensive retrograde lymphatic blockage. The relatively rich lymphatic supply of the stomach makes accurate prediction of lymphatic spread of tumor more difficult, for example, than in colon or rectal cancer.

TABLE 25-1.   Lymphatic Drainage of the Stomach

The lymphatic networks
  The mucous network
  The submucous network
  The muscular network
  The subserous or subperitoneal network
The collecting trunks
  Left gastric chain
    Left gastropancreatic fold
    Lesser curvature nodes
    Parietal group
    Juxtacardiac nodes
  Splenic chain
    Suprapancreatic nodes
    Infrapancreatic nodes
    Afferent and efferent lymph vessels
  The hepatic chain
    Hepatic group
    Right gastroepiploic and infrapyloric group
    Right gastric group, suprapyloric nodes
    Pancreaticoduodenal group
    Afferent and efferent vessels

The observation that lesions in the distal stomach rarely involve the distal esophagus, and involve the lymphatics along the splenic chain in less than 25% of cases, has helped to determine that the procedure of choice for low-lying gastric lesions is not a total gastrectomy and that splenectomy is not routinely indicated for lesions in this area. By the same line of reasoning, the type of resection indicated for lesions in other areas can be plotted from a knowledge of the lymphatics and the natural history of observed cases.

Once a tumor has spread beyond the immediate lymphatics, there can then be lymphatic involvement along the aorta, through the thoracic duct to the cervical nodes, or retrograde spread to other areas within the abdomen and the peritoneal cavity, including direct implantation in the pelvis.

The major clinical ramification of understanding the anatomical relationships, particularly the lymphatic anatomy of the stomach, is to plan appropriate therapy and analyze reasons for therapy failure. Although it is clear that the primary purpose of surgery is simply to excise all visible gastric cancer (i.e., more radical procedures will not increase the chance of cure), more extensive surgical and surgical–pathologic staging systems such as that described by the Japanese will increase our ability to analyze why disease recurs after multimodality treatment and may also decrease discrepant results of multimodality adjuvant trials, for surgeons, medical oncologists, and pathologists will know that patients who have been treated by the various protocols do, in fact, have the same stage of disease.

NATURAL HISTORY

PREMALIGNANT LESIONS

The premalignant histology of the normal stomach may have an important influence on the occurrence of gastric cancer. For example, intestinal metaplasia of the stomach is more frequent in countries where the incidence of stomach cancer is high.[24-26] This lesion is defined as a replacement of stomach epithelium by intestinal epithelium containing goblet and paneth cells. In Japan, where gastric cancer causes 40% of all deaths from malignancy, intestinal metaplasia is found in 80% of stomachs resected for gastric cancer.[26,27] The type of stomach cancer associated with intestinal metaplasia is well differentiated.[28,29] In cases in which metaplasia is not observed, the tumor is poorly differentiated and frequently has a scirrhous carcinoma pattern.[27] The scirrhous histologic pattern is more common in Western countries, where intestinal metaplasia is less frequent than in Japan.

Experimental evidence suggests that the metaplastic change in intestinal metaplasia is a carcinogen-induced precursor lesion of gastric cancer.[28-30] In studies done in rats, Japanese workers have shown that nitro-N-nitrosoguanidines, known gastric carcinogens, first induce gastric intestinal metaplasia, which is followed by gastric cancer. Tumors did not occur in rats that did not develop intestinal metaplasia after carcinogen exposure. The relationship between a well-defined premalignant pathologic finding (intestinal metaplasia) induced by a known carcinogen and predisposition of the stomach to a specific type of adenocarcinoma (well-differentiated intestinal type) clearly deserves further exploration and implies that intestinal metaplasia is capable of malignant transformation when exposed to promoting agents.

Although most gastric cancers appear to be carcinogen induced, some conditions predispose to the development of gastric neoplasia. The firmest, most convincing evidence relates to the association between pernicious anemia and gastric cancer.[11,31] The incidence of gastric cancer in patients with pernicious anemia has been reported to be between 5% and 10%, and gastric cancer is estimated to be 20 times more common in patients with pernicious anemia than in an age-matched control population.[32] These results indicate the need for careful monitoring of patients with chronic pernicious anemia for the development of gastric malignancy. Likewise, patients with chronic reflux esophagitis may develop glandular metaplasia of the distal esophagus (Barrett's esophagus), which may progress to dysplasia and frank neoplasia. Malignancies developing in patients with Barrett's esophagus are discussed in more detail in Chapter 24; for now, the clinician should be aware that these esophageal adenocarcinomas may involve the cardioesophageal junction.

Gastric resection for benign peptic ulcer disease is also associated with an increased risk of subsequent stomach cancer.[33,34] The reason for this association is not clear, but the loss of parietal cell mass and the resulting decrease in gastric acid may favor the development of intestinal metaplasia of the stomach,[33] which may be a premalignant precursor to stomach cancer. The typical lag time between gastric resection and the manifestations of carcinoma is 15 to 40 years.[32] Giarelli and associates,[34] in an autopsy study of 480 patients who had undergone gastric resection for benign conditions, found a 6.5% incidence of gastric stump carcinomas. The long-term risk of developing gastric cancer was 2.45 times increased in persons who had undergone gastric resection before age 45.

The relationship between gastric polyps and gastric ulcers and malignancy has been debated in the literature for many years.[35-37] In general, it is agreed that polyps are rarely precursor lesions to gastric cancer.[36,38] There are three histologic types of gastric polyps: hyperplastic adenomatous polyps, hamartomatous adenomatous polyps, and villous adenomas. The hyperplastic adenomatous polyps are the most common type and appear to have no malignant potential. Hamartomatous adenomatous polyps are composed of normal gastric mucosal cells and are identical to the lesions seen in the Peutz-Jeghers syndrome. These polyps are the rarest form of gastric polyps and do not become malignant. The lesion that does appear to have malignant potential is the villous adenoma.[36,39,40] These polyps are ten times less common than hyperplastic polyps but are clearly premalignant, since foci of carcinoma are found in approximately 40%.

The experience at the Aichi Cancer Center in Japan confirms the importance of polyp histologic type in relationship to malignant potential.[40] On histologic examination of 198 consecutive cases of gastric polyps, 87.8% were found to be hyperplastic, and only 2% were villous adenomas. In 10 of 198 cases in which cancers of the stomach were present, villous adenomatous pathology was found in 9, and hyperplastic polyps in only 1. Thus, 69% of the villous adenomas but only 0.6% of the hyperplastic polyps were associated with malignancy.

There is controversy between U.S. and Japanese investigators concerning the association between gastric ulcer and malignancy.[11,35-37] The U.S. data can be shown to support the hypothesis that gastric cancer may commonly ulcerate but benign gastric ulcers rarely, if ever, become cancers. In the United States, carcinoma has been found in only 3% of resected gastric ulcers.[41] Conversely, in Japan, the experience at the Yokohama Cancer Hospital initially suggested a very high correlation between chronic gastric ulcer and cancer.[42] In the 1950s, 70% of the early cancers resected consisted of a deep chronic ulcer surrounded by a narrow cancerous lesion, suggesting a preexisting chronic ulcer with malignancy developing at its border. Interestingly, this pathologic entity has been identified progressively less frequently in Japan coincident with the introduction of fiberoptic gastroscopy. In 1974, only 10% of gastric cancers were associated with chronic gastric ulcers, whereas 75% of resected tumors consisted of a primary malignant tumor with ulceration. This finding may be explained in part by the fact that the frequency of chronic gastric ulcer also decreased in Japan by 50% during the period 1958 to 1974.[42]

In general, it appears that now, even in Japan, the risk of gastric cancer occurring in conjunction with gastric ulcer disease is small. This is borne out by the experience of Larson and associates in the United States.[43] These workers followed the course of 664 patients with clinically benign gastric ulcers less than 4 cm in diameter. All patients were treated medically. Only 21% of the patients experienced healing, and 40% eventually required surgery for persistent symptoms or acute problems, such as hemorrhage. The overall incidence of gastric cancer in this group after 5 to 10 years of follow-up was small. Malignancy was demonstrated in 60 (9%) of 664 cases.

Fiberoptic endoscopy now permits safe and rapid inspection and biopsy of gastric ulcers to rule out malignancy. It would seem prudent to follow carefully patients with apparently benign gastric ulcers and to consider prompt surgical intervention if healing does not occur rapidly. The clinician should understand, however, that the likelihood of finding malignancy at surgery is small.

Several conditions once thought to be associated with gastric cancer now appear to have at best a tenuous relationship with that entity. For example, a number of epidemiologic studies seem to have suggested that gastric cancer is more common in persons with blood group A than in those with blood group O.[9,11] More than 55 studies from around the world have supported this finding. However, the risk ratio for gastric cancer in persons with blood group A compared to those with blood group O is only a modest 1.2. In addition, several large studies from the Scandinavian countries have found no correlation between gastric cancer and blood group A.

For many years, a relationship between atrophic gastritis and gastric cancer has been postulated.[11,36] Atrophic gastritis is very commonly associated with gastric malignancy, but it does not follow that atrophic gastritis is a precursor to gastric carcinoma. In the older age group in which gastric cancer occurs, approximately 80% to 95% of individuals have some degree of atrophic gastritis. Thus a large percentage of older patients without stomach cancer have atrophic gastritis, making untenable the hypothesis that atrophic gastritis is a definite precursor of gastric cancer. It is possible that atrophic gastritis is a condition that is permissive for the development of gastric cancer, just as removing parietal cell mass by gastrectomy for benign disease may increase the risk of subsequent gastric carcinoma.[33,34]

PATTERN OF SPREAD

The choice of treatment for any given lesion of the stomach presupposes knowledge of the natural history of the disease and the more common routes of spread.[44] The TNM staging system, which is gaining increasing acceptance, should be used as a baseline to allow appropriate comparisons to be made among series reported from different institutions or at different times. Determination of disease stage requires careful definition by the surgeon and pathologist of local and regional spread during surgical staging.

Complete surgical resection in which all resection margins are rendered free of microscopic disease is possible in only 30% of patients. The tumor stage as determined at surgery will depend on the surgeon's experience and knowledge, and the thoroughness of the surgical and pathologic staging criteria. Nevertheless, multiple studies have confirmed the Charity Hospital series in which only 11% of 423 patients operated on were found to have lesions grossly limited to the stomach.[45,46] In an additional 11%, the only evidence of disease beyond the stomach was clinically positive nodes. Contiguous extension was found in 27% and distant metastatic disease in 31%. Although clinical assessment suggested that only 11% of patients had lymphatic metastases, histologic studies demonstrated nodal involvement in 52% of cases. When the gross surgical or autopsy findings are compared with the final diagnoses based on histologic examination, it is apparent that the surgeon's and the pathologist's gross observations are inadequate. There is a need to stress increased detail in the surgical–pathologic correlation.

The routes of spread of gastric carcinoma are similar to those for other GI lesions.[44] They include (1) direct spread within the involved stomach and into the adjacent esophagus or pylorus, or both; (2) spread to adjacent viscera; (3) spread through lymphatic chains; (4) spillage of tumor cells either from the serosal surface of the stomach or from the lumen at the time of an operative procedure; and (5) blood-borne metastases (Table 25-2).

Studies by Arhelger et al[47] and Coller et al[48] have demonstrated that although the size and location of the primary tumor have some bearing on the frequency and location of lymphatic metastases, these factors are not significantly predictive.

The pattern of distant organ involvement was recorded in the Charity Hospital experience with 348 autopsy cases, and this experience[46] is tabulated along with the reports of Clarke and co-workers,[49] Warren,[50] and Warwick[51] in Table 25-3. In all these studies the liver was the most frequent site of metastasis, being involved almost twice as frequently as the peritoneum or omentum, which are the next two in

TABLE 25-2.   Patterns of Spread of Gastric Cancer

Direct extension
    Lesser and greater omentum
    Liver and diaphragm
    Pancreas
    Spleen
    Biliary tract
    Transverse colon
Nodal metastases
    Local
    Distant
        Virchow's node
        Left axillary (Irish's) node
        Umbilical node
Vascular metastases
    Liver
    Pulmonary system
    Bone
    Brain
Peritoneal metastases
    Disseminated
    Pelvic
        Krukenburg tumor—ovary
        Blumer's rectal shelf

sequence. The distant organs most commonly involved were the lungs, followed by the adrenals. Histologic involvement of the spleen was relatively uncommon, accounting for less than 10% of the entire series, in contrast to the received opinion that the spleen is involved in a large proportion of the patients with gastric carcinoma.[11] The infrequent involvement of the spleen indicates that routine splenectomy is not necessary and, for lesions originating in the distal stomach without gross involvement of either the spleen or the lymph nodes adjacent to it, that splenectomy is valuable only because it facilitates a more complete lymph node dissection.

PATTERNS OF FAILURE

Although disseminated disease can be found in 75% of patients at autopsy (see Table 25-3), the importance of locoregional failure should not be underestimated. The magnitude of the problem has been demonstrated in clinical,[52]

autopsy,[53-55] and reoperation series.[56] McNeer and colleagues[53] have presented complete information on 92 patients autopsied after subtotal gastrectomies performed with curative intent. Some component of local failure was found in 74 (80%) patients, as follows: in 46 (50%), disease in the stomach wall or site or gastroenterostomy; in 14 (15%), tumor in the duodenum, in 5 cases associated with recurrence in the gastric remnant; and in 48 (52%), disease in the perigastric lymph nodes and stomach bed. Thomson and Robins[54] analyzed 28 cases with previous subtotal resection. In 5 (18%) cases disease recurred in the gastric stump alone, in 3 (11%) in the duodenal stump, in 13 (46%) in the gastric bed, and in 6 (21%) in the gastric bed and gastric stump. In a more recent autopsy analysis from the University of Washington, findings in 85 patients who died of gastric cancer were analyzed.[55] Of 16 who had undergone potentially curative resection, 15 (94%) had a locoregional component of failure. The liver was involved in 7 (44%), and peritoneal seeding was found in 8 (50%). Peritoneal seeding occurred in 7 of 10 patients with initial serosal involvement versus 1 of 6 with less extensive disease. Extra-abdominal spread occurred in 9 (69%) of 13 patients with primary lesions involving the gastroesophageal junction versus 35 (49%) of 72 patients with more distal lesions.

Gunderson and Sosin[56] approached the problem of defining sites of failure differently. These workers analyzed patterns of failure in a prospective study in which patients who had undergone gastric resection were subjected to periodic reoperation at the University of Minnesota. After the initial operative procedure, 109 patients underwent one or more reoperations. Since 2 had residual disease after the first procedure, 107 were evaluable for purposes of assessing sites of failure. All patients were treated by operation alone without preoperative or postoperative adjuvant therapy. The extent of the operative procedure was at the discretion of the surgeon, with a large group of patients undergoing a radical procedure, including splenectomy, omentectomy, and radical lymph node dissection in addition to some form of gastrectomy. Of the 107 evaluable patients, 86 (80%) had later evidence of cancer. Incidence and patterns of failure were analyzed in detail (Tables 25-4 and 25-5; Fig. 25-2). Distant

TABLE 25-3.   Metastasis at Autopsy or Operation

Site	Warwick[51] (n = 176)	DuPont et al[46] (n = 348)	Warren[50] (n = 67)	Clark et al[49] (n = 250)
Liver	38	54	34	40
Peritoneum	20	24	28	17
Omentum	13	21		
Lungs	12	22	9	19
Mesentery	9			
Pleura	8		4	
Pancreas	7	29	10	
Adrenals	5	15	3	12
Intestine	4		6	
Genitourinary		3		8
Spleen	2	13	1	
Gallbladder/biliary tract	2	4	6	
Bone	6	1	6	9
Central nervous system	1	0.2		2
No metastasis	23	11	24	22

TABLE 25-4. Patterns of Failure in Reoperation Series After Curative Resection*

Pattern of Failure†	Only Failure‡			Any Component‡		
	No.	%	(%)	No.	%	(%)
LF-RF	24	29.3	(22.9)	72	87.8	(68.6)
+ Localized PS (20 patients)	44	53.7	(41.2)			
PS	3	3.7	(2.9)	44	53.7	(41.9)
Localized				20	24.4	(19)
Diffuse				24	29.3	(22.9)
DM	5	6.1	(4.8)	24	29.3	(22.9)

* Gunderson LL, Sosin H: Adenocarcinoma of the stomach—areas of failure in a reoperation series, second or symptomatic looks. Clinicopathologic correlation and implications for adjuvant therapy. Int J Radiat Oncol Biol Phys 8:1–11, 1982.
† Of the 107 evaluable patients, 86 had failure, which was totally documented in 82. LF-RF = locoregional failure, PS = peritoneal spread, DM = distant metastases.
‡ Open figures represent number and percentage of the failure group of 82 patients, and figures in parentheses represent percentage of the 107 patients with complete follow-up.

metastases alone were uncommon but occurred as some component of failure in 29% of the failure group. Nearly half of the peritoneal failures were localized. Of those that had a diffuse component, nearly all also had a fairly massive local recurrence. Locoregional failure occurred as the only failure in 29% of the failure group (53% if localized peritoneal seeding was included) and as any component of failure in 88%. Locoregional failure was primarily limited to lymph nodes and organs and structures of the gastric bed, with a smaller but significant number of failures in the anastomosis, gastric remnant, or duodenal stump. Very few failures occurred in the abdominal incision or stab wounds. Distant metastases were primarily to the liver.

In the reoperative series, the extent of the initial operative procedure had little if any effect on either the incidence or type of subsequent failure (Tables 25-6 and 25-7). Lymph node failures were found in a fairly high percentage of patients who supposedly had undergone radical lymph node dissections. Table 25-8 lists sites of failure according to histopathologic stage of the primary tumor. Patterns of failure by stage were analyzed in detail in a recent series of 130 patients who underwent resection performed with curative intent at the Massachusetts General Hospital.[57] Locoregional failure occurred as any component of failure in 49 patients (38%) and as the sole failure in 21 (16% of 130 at risk and 24% of 88 with any disease progression). The incidence of

locoregional failure by stage was in excess of 35% for Stages B_2, B_3, C_2, and C_3 (see Table 25-8); the locations at highest risk for locoregional failure were the gastric bed (27 of 130 patients, 21%) and the anastomosis or stump (33 of 130 patients, 25%). Distant metastases occurred as any component of relapse in 52% (67 of 130 patients) and exceeded 50% for Stage B_2, B_3, C_2, and C_3 lesions. A majority of such failures were confined to the abdomen (61 of 67 patients, or 91%) with a liver component in 39 (30%) of 130 and peritoneal seeding in 30 (23%). A 20% or greater incidence of peritoneal seeding was found with only C_2 and C_3 lesions but if liver metastases were present, a 20% or greater incidence of peritoneal seeding was seen with all but Stage A lesions. The true incidences of gastric bed, nodal, and peritoneal failures may be higher, as this was not a reoperative or autopsy series (see comparative findings in Table 25-5).

All these data suggest that although systemic therapy is clearly important, the development of an effective therapy for regional disease as an adjuvant to surgery could potentially benefit at least 20% of patients.

CLINICAL PRESENTATION

Articles on cancer of the stomach stress the vague, nondiagnostic symptoms and the fact that patients are likely to be

TABLE 25-5. Patterns of Locoregional Failure in Clinical, Reoperative, and Autopsy Series

Site	Incidence—Any Component							
	MGH[57] (clinical) (N = 130)*		University of Minnesota[56] (reoperation) (N = 105)*		McNeer et al[53] (autopsy) (N = 92)*		Thomson and Robins[54] (autopsy) (N = 28)*	
	No.	%	No.	%	No.	%	No.	%
Gastric bed	27	(21)	58	(55)	48	(52)	19	(68)
Anastomosis or stumps	33	(25)	28	(27)	55	(60)	15	(54)
Abdominal or stab wounds	...	...	5	(5)	...	...	...	...
Lymph node(s)	11	(8)	45	(43)	48	(52)	...	...

*Number at risk.

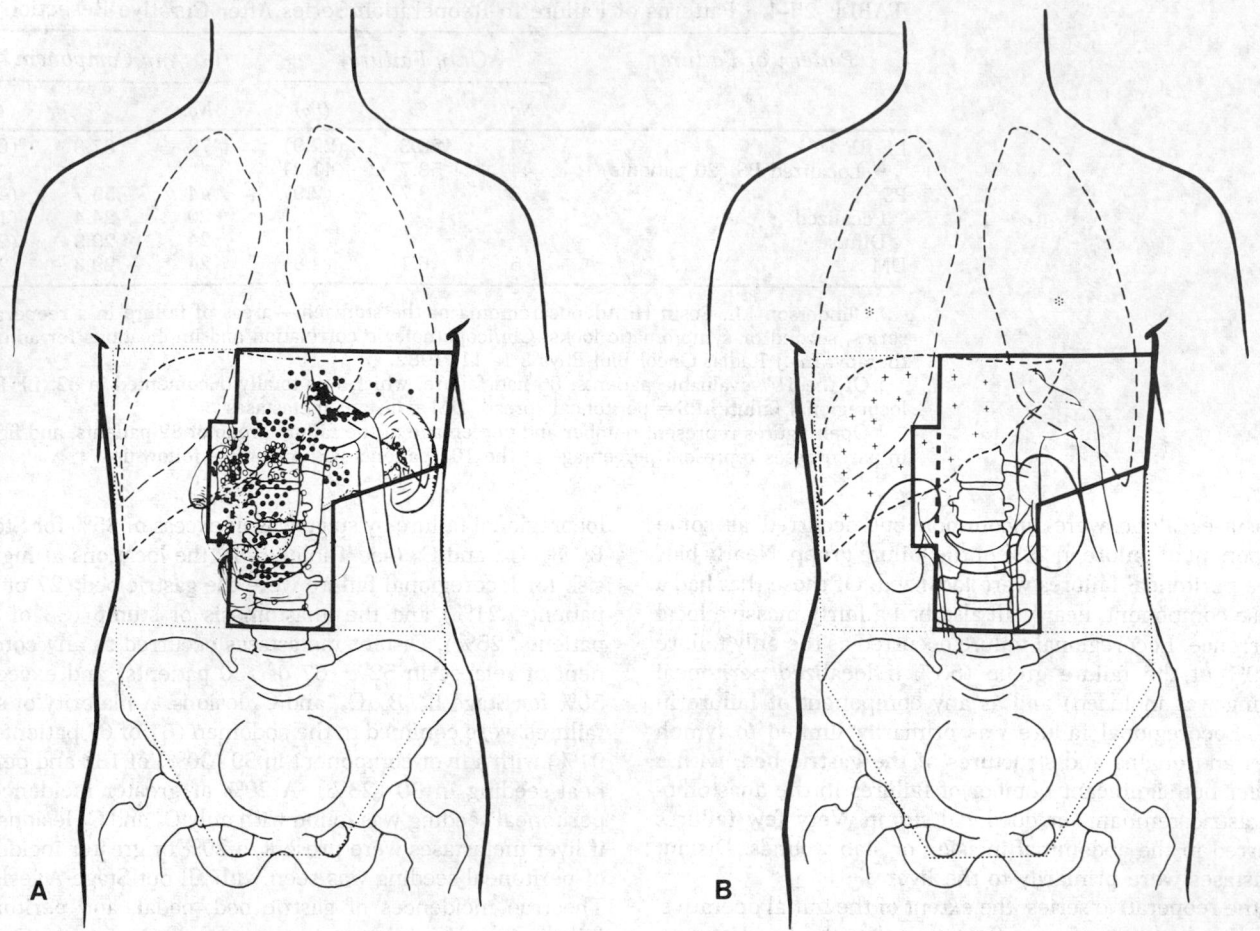

FIG. 25-2. Patterns of failure in the University of Minnesota reoperation series of 82 evaluable patients with evidence of gastric carcinoma after the initial operative procedure. Superimposed radiation portals: postsurgical gastric remnant, anastamoses, duodenal stump, gastric bed structures, and primary and secondary areas of lymph node drainage (*solid lines*), upper or total abdomen fields (*interrupted lines*), **A** • = local failures in surrounding organs or tissues; **B**, 0 = lymph node failures; * = lung metastasis; + = liver metastasis. Each marking indicates a single instance of such failure occurring alone or as any component except for lymph node failures where each major area of involvement is indicated.

unaware of their disease. Often patients present with a clinical picture that fails to trigger the proper diagnostic impressions in the physician's mind. Article after article stresses the "vague," "indefinite," "nonspecific" symptoms and then proceeds to list such things as epigastric uneasiness, mild anemia, fatigability, ulcer history, and weight loss. Clearly, none of these symptoms unequivocally indicates gastric cancer, and unless the clinician is alert to that possibility, the patient may be treated empirically for ulcer disease, not treated at all, or allowed to think there are no serious problems.[58-62]

Five different reviews covering the years 1950 to 1970 show essentially no change in the incidence of the key symptoms and show the vague, nonspecific nature of all of the findings in each individual study (Table 25-9).[49,58-61] The fact that the major presenting finding in some series could be a palpable mass in one third of the patients, ascites, or the less frequent findings of metastases to supraclavicular nodes

or jaundice suggests that extensive disease can exist before the patient seeks medical help.

One study compared the incidence of the various symptoms in resectable versus nonresectable cases and found very little difference.[63] The same study evaluated extent of weight loss, duration of symptoms, and location of the tumor in the stomach in relation to symptoms. There were no differences in any of these parameters except for the relatively higher incidence of dysphagia and regurgitation with lesions located in the proximal stomach. Specific symptoms may indicate complicating factors in individual cases. For example, a patient with dysphagia may have a cardioesophageal junction lesion with partial obstruction from involvement of the distal esophagus. Patients with persistent nausea and vomiting, indicating bowel obstruction, may have several syndromes associated with gastric cancer.[11] An antral carcinoma may produce obstruction and gastric dilation. Gastric cancer occasionally invades the transverse mesocolon directly, result-

TABLE 25-6. Extent of Gastrectomy and Node Dissection Versus Patterns of Failure, Reoperation Series

		Patterns of Failure*																
		LF-RF						PS						DM					
		Alone			Component			Alone			Component			Alone			Component		
Operative† Procedure	No. of Failure/ Total at Risk	No.	%	(%)	No.	%	(%)	No.	%	(%)	No.	%	(%)	No.	%	(%)	No.	%	(%)
Subtotal gastrectomy	53/72	16	30	(22)	45	85	(63)	3	6	(4)	27	51	(38)	4	8	(6)	17	32	(24)
Method 1	25/36	9	36	(25)	23	92	(64)	1	4	(3)	12	48	(33)	0			7	28	(19)
Method 2	15/17	3	20	(18)	11	73	(65)	1	7	(6)	8	53	(47)	3	20	(18)	5	33	(29)
Method 3	13/19	4	31	(21)	11	85	(58)	1	8	(5)	7	54	(37)	1	8	(5)	5	39	(26)
Total gastrectomy	27/33	7	26	(21)	25	93	(76)	0			17	63	(52)	1	4	(3)	6	22	(18)
Method 1	0																		
Method 2	14/15	3	21	(20)	13	93	(87)	0			9	64	(60)	0			4	29	(27)
Method 3	13/18	4	31	(22)	12	92	(67)	0			8	62	(44)	1	8	(6)	2	15	(11)
Total	80/105	23	29	(22)	70	88	(67)	3	4	(3)	44	55	(42)	5	6	(5)	23	29	(22)

*Of the 86 patients with failure, 80 were evaluable by all parameters. Open figures represent number and percentage of the failure group, and figures in parentheses represent percentage of patients with complete follow-up. LF-RF, local-regional failure; PS, peritoneal spread; DM, distant metastases.

†Method 1 (pre-1950), subtotal or total gastrectomy, greater omentectomy, regional node dissection; method 2 (1950–1954), method 1 plus splenectomy, total omentectomy, additional node dissection regarding splenic suprapancreatic and central celiac axis; method 3 (1954 on), methods 1 and 2 plus extension of node dissection to porta hepatis and pancreaticoduodenal (intent: total lymph node dissection of all primary node areas).

ing in transverse colon obstruction. Patients who develop peritoneal dissemination with gastric cancer may have distal bowel obstruction. A Blumer's shelf resulting from metastatic gastric carcinoma can cause rectal obstruction.

By the time physical signs of gastric cancer are present, the disease is incurable. The commonly found physical findings with stomach cancer are direct manifestations of the pattern of spread of this disease, as outlined in Table 25-2. Gastric adenocarcinoma disseminates by both lymphatic and hematogenous routes. The earliest sites of lymphatic metastases are the regional nodes and clearly cannot be detected by physical examination. However, three sites of nodal metastases are detectable by examination. Careful evaluation of the supraclavicular fossae is necessary in cases of suspected gastric cancer. The finding of a firm left supraclavicular (Virchow's) node may allow a tissue diagnosis without abdominal exploration. Two less common sites of metastases are worth noting. Patients with systemic symptoms consistent with stomach cancer should undergo careful digital examination of the periumbilical area and left axilla. Gastric

TABLE 25-7. Extent of Gastrectomy and Node Dissection Versus Type of LF-RF, Reoperation Series

| | | Any Component of LF-RF* | | | | | | | | | | | |
| | | Gastric Bed | | | Anastomosis or stumps | | | Abdomen or Stab Wound | | | Lymph Nodes | | |
Operative† Procedure	No. of Failure/ Total at Risk	No.	%	(%)	No.	%	(%)	No.	%	(%)	No.	%	(%)
Subtotal gastrectomy	53/72	36	68	(50)	18	34	(25)	3	6	(4)	29	55	(40)
Method 1	25/36	18	72	(50)	13	52	(36)	0			11	44	(31)
Method 2	15/17	9	60	(53)	4	27	(24)	1	7	(6)	9	60	(53)
Method 3	13/19	9	69	(47)	1	8	(5)	2	15	(11)	9	69	(47)
Total gastrectomy	27/33	20	74	(61)	8	30	(24)	2	7	(6)	15	56	(45)
Method 1	0												
Method 2	14/15	10	71	(67)	5	36	(33)	1	7	(7)	11	79	(73)
Method 3	13/18	10	77	(56)	3	23	(17)	1	8	(6)	4	31	(22)
Total	80/105‡	56	70	(53)	26	33	(25)	5	6	(5)	44	55	(42)

*Open figures represent number and percent of the failure group, and numbers in parentheses represent percent of patients with complete follow-up. LF-RF, local-regional failure; PS, peritoneal spread; DM, distant metastases.

†For operative procedure, see Table 25-6.

‡An additional 6 patients had failure, but only 80 of 86 were evaluable for operative method and pattern of failure.

TABLE 25-8. Incidence and Patterns of Failure by Stage After Resection with Curative Intent, MGH Single Institution Study*

Stage†	No. of Patients	Local Regional Failure				Distant Failure					
		Only		Total		Only		Total		Abdominal‡	
		No.	%	No.	%	No.	%	No.	%	No.	%
A	4	0	(6)	0	(0)	0	(0)	0	(0)	0	(0)
B_1	16	1	(6)	3	(19)	3	(19)	5	(31)	5	(31)
B_2	12	1	(8)	6	(50)	1	(8)	6	(50)	6	(50)
B_3	5	0	(0)	2	(40)	1	(20)	3	(60)	3	(60)
C_1	17	2	(12)	4	(24)	3	(18)	5	(29)	4	(24)
C_2	44	10	(23)	16	(36)	18	(41)	24	(55)	21	(48)
C_3	32	7	(22)	18	(56)	13	(41)	24	(67)	22	(61)
Total	130	21	(16)	49	(38)	39	(40)	67	(52)	61	(47)

*Modified from Landry J, Tepper JE, Wood WL et al: Patterns of failure following curative resection of gastric carcinoma: ASTRO Proceedings 1986. Int J Radiat Oncol Biol Phys 12(1):119, 1986.
†Gunderson Sosin modification of Astler Coller system (see Ref. 56).
‡Abdominal = liver and peritoneal seeding.

cancer has been reported to metastasize to both these areas.[11] Nodular metastases to the umbilical area and left axillary lymph node metastases (Irish's node) should be searched for assiduously, since their presence allows a simple tissue diagnosis to be made in the patient with gastric cancer. Umbilical metastases may not be in lymph nodes but rather may represent peritoneal dissemination.

The most common site of hematogenous metastases in stomach cancer is the liver. Firm, smooth, or nodular hepatomegaly may be apparent on physical examination as an indication of hepatic metastases. Patients with locally extensive stomach cancer may have a palpable epigastric mass that may be mistaken for the left lobe of an enlarged liver, when it actually represents the gastric tumor itself.

Rarely does the patient with gastric carcinoma present with significant bleeding. Although minor blood loss that may be detected as occult blood in the stool is common in gastric cancer, massive upper GI bleeding is uncommon. In fact, the patient with a gastric mass and upper GI hemorrhage is more likely to have gastric leiomyosarcoma than adenocarcinoma of the stomach.[6,11] Hemorrhage in the absence of a gastric mass suggests benign gastric ulcer.

Syndromes of remote effects of carcinoma are rare with stomach cancer. This disease, however, does represent the most common visceral malignancy associated with acanthosis nigricans.[11] This syndrome is characterized by hypertrophic pigmented skin lesions, particularly noted in the axilla. Glucose intolerance also may be present. The syndrome of thrombotic nonbacterial endocarditis has been associated with gastric cancer but is not specific and may be seen in any patient with advanced wasting from malignant disease.

STAGING

As more sophisticated combined modality approaches have been used in the treatment of gastric cancer, staging has become more important. In the past, an informal staging scheme was used by physicians treating this disease. Thus, the surgeon at the time of operation determined the stage of the cancer, and this stage determined which treatment option might be useful. Therapy was dictated by stage: (1) completely resectable, (2) locally unresectable or only par-

TABLE 25-9. Symptons of Gastric Carcinoma

Symptom	La Due et al[61] (n = 1,121)	Adashek et al[58] (n = 501)	Goldsmith et al[59] (n = 270)	Clarke et al[49] (n = 250)	Kelsey[60] (n = 245)
Weight loss	85	24	58	68	56
Pain	69	38	48	67	56
Vomiting	43	24	21	47	
Bowel symptoms	41		5		
Anorexia	30	4	21		
Dysphagia	20	13	17		9
Nausea	20		4	65	
Nausea and vomiting					38
Weakness	19	17			
Eructation	17				
Hematemesis	6	16	13	18	
Regurgitation	6				
Rapid satiation	5		2		
No symptoms	0.4			5	6

TABLE 25-10. TNM Classification*

Primary Tumor (T)

T_x Minimum requirements to assess the primary tumor cannot be met.

T_0 No evidence of primary tumor.

T_{is} Tumor limited to mucosa without penetration into the lamina propria.

T_1 Tumor limited to mucosa or mucosa and submucosa regardless of its extent (or location).

T_2 Tumor involves the mucosa and the submucosa (including the muscularis propria), and extends to or into the serosa but does not penetrate through the serosa.

T_3 Tumor penetrates through the serosa without invading contiguous structures.

T_{4a} Tumor penetrates through the serosa and involves immediately adjacent tissues, such as lesser omentum, perigastric fat, regional ligaments, greater omentum, transverse colon, spleen, esophagus, or duodenum by way of intraluminal extension.

T_{4b} Tumor penetrates through the serosa and involves the liver, diaphragm, pancreas, abdominal wall, adrenal glands, kidney, retroperitoneum, small intestine or esophagus, or duodenum by way of serosa.

Nodal Involvement (N)

N_x Minimum requirements to assess the regional nodes cannot be met.

N_0 No metastases to regional lymph nodes.

N_1 Involvement of perigastric lymph nodes within 3 cm of the primary tumor along the lesser or greater curvature.

N_2 Involvement of the regional lymph nodes more than 3 cm from the primary tumor, which are removed or removable at operation, including those located along the left gastric, splenic, celiac, and common hepatic arteries.

N_3 Involvement of other intra-abdominal lymph nodes, such as the para-aortic, hepatoduodenal, retropancreatic, and mesenteric nodes.

Distant Metastasis (M)

M_x Minimum requirements to assess the presence of distant metastasis cannot be met.

M_0 No (known) distant metastasis.

M_1 Distant metastasis present. Specify sites according to the following notations:

Peritoneal	PER
Pulmonary	PUL
Osseous	OSS
Hepatic	HEP
Brain	BRA
Lymph nodes (above diaphragm or nonabdominal)	LYM
Bone marrow	MAR
Pleura	PLE
Skin	SKI
Eye	EYE
Other	OTH

Stage Grouping

Stage 0	T_{is}, N_0, M_0
Stage I	T_1, N_0, M_0
Stage II	T_2, T_3, N_0, M_0
Stage III	T_1–T_3, N_1, N_2, M_0
	T_{4a}, N_0–N_2; M_0
Stage IV	T_1–T_3, N_3, M_0
	T_{4b}, any N, M_0
	Any T, any N, M_1

Tumor Grade (G)

G_1 Well differentiated

G_2 Moderately well differentiated

G_3–G_4 Poorly to very poorly differentiated.

Postgastrectomy Residual Tumor (R)

R_0 No residual tumor

R_1 Microscopic residual tumor

R_2 Macroscopic residual tumor

—Specify _____

Performance Status of Host (H)

	AJCC Performance	ECOG Scale	Karnofsky Scale (%)
H_0	Normal activity	0	90–100
H_1	Symptomatic but ambulatory, cares for self	1	70–80
H_2	Ambulatory more than 50% of time, occasionally needs assistance	2	50–60
H_3	Ambulatory 50% or less of time, nursing care needed	3	30–40
H_4	Bedridden, may need hospitalization	4	10–20

*Beahrs OH, Myers MH (eds): Manual for Staging of Cancer, p 67. Philadelphia, JB Lippincott, 1983.

tially resectable, indicating the use of radiation therapy, and (3) disseminated disease requiring chemotherapy.

More formal staging plans have been attempted during the last 50 years. In 1941, Coller and associates[48] reviewed 53 cases in detail in order to correlate lymphatic metastases and other features of primary lesions in the stomach. They divided the lymphatics into four zones, all four of which they recommended should be removed in all resectable cases. Their lymph node classification has served as the background for much that has been written about the staging of gastric cancer.

A suggestion for gross surgical classification of lesions of the stomach was advocated by Hoerr.[64,65] His original presentation and the subsequent reviews based on that classification have provided an additional means for studying the clinical significance of lesions in the stomach. This classification is based on the extent of invasion of the wall of the stomach and adjacent viscera, plus the extent of lymph node and distant involvement. Overall classification by this technique assists in determining whether a tumor is likely to be resectable and whether there is clear-cut evidence of distant spread. Another more recently proposed pathologic staging system is a modification of the Astler Coller system for stag-

TABLE 25-11. Five-Year Survival and Initial Stage of Gastric Cancer*

Extent of Disease	5-Year Survival (%)
Lymph nodes (−)	
Mucosa only	85
Mucosa and gastric wall	52
Through gastric wall	47
Lymph nodes (+)	
Extent of lymph node involvement	
Regional only	17
Other areas	5

*Data from Kennedy BJ: TNM classification for stomach cancer. Cancer 26:971, 1970.

ing colon cancer. This system, elaborated by Gunderson and Sosin,[56] gives the same type of information as the Hoerr[64,65] system and predicts failure rates after surgery.

The importance of the TNM classification (Table 25-10) has been established, and a review by Kennedy (Table 25-11) of 1241 patients demonstrated correlations between extent of disease (lymph node involvement, depth of penetration of the stomach by the lesion, presence of distant metastases) and survival.[66,67] More detailed clinicopathologic correlations have been provided by several large Japanese studies.[68,69] The system used by the Japanese as a basis for operative and adjuvant treatment staging should perhaps be considered for wider use in the United States in order to limit discrepancies in surgical staging. Such staging discrepancies may explain conflicting results in recently completed adjuvant multimodality treatment protocols.

Careful understanding of the patterns of dissemination as defined by staging systems may be helpful in dictating primary surgical therapy. Desmond[70] reviewed findings in 1363 cases and divided lymphatic drainage into seven different groups, with recommendations on appropriate surgical measures to be used for lesions involving any or all of these groups. The value of this approach will need to be comfirmed in prospective studies. However, it should be emphasized that, although the simple staging of disease into "resectable," "locally advanced," and "disseminated" still has some descriptive value, use of a formalized staging plan such as the TNM system allows much more accurate comparison of different treatment results.

PROGNOSIS

The prognosis for patients with gastric cancer depends on the extent of the disease and on treatment. Extension of disease, whether local or regional, adversely affects survival. Until recently, only patients who had undergone complete excision of localized cancer had any potential for long-term survival. Lymph node involvement is an adverse prognostic factor. However, most important is the extent of nodal metastases. Minimal lymphatic involvement adjacent to the tumor has little if any adverse prognostic effect. Extensive and distant nodal metastases are very poor prognostic factors.

Experience with 1497 cases at a single hospital provides the background for a number of different evaluations of survival based on various forms of operative treatment.[45,46] The 5-year survival rate for all patients observed 5 years or more in this study was 7.45%. The best 5-year survival figure in the entire study — 30.3% — was in the relatively small group of 149 patients with localized disease. Dupont and associates[46] reviewed survival data in 18,767 gastric cancer patients from 11 series and found disappointing results. The 5-year survival rate varied from 4.7% to 16.9%, but only 4 of 11 series reported 5-year survival rates greater than 10%.

A detailed statistical study of 11,817 patients at the Mayo Clinic by ReMine and co-workers[71] demonstrated relationships among survival, size of lesion, age of patient at operation, operative mortality, year of operation, pathologic stage of the disease, and other features. An additional prognostic factor noted in recent trials is location of the tumor. The more proximal or gastroesophageal junction tumors are more ominous, stage for stage, than are body or distal gastric adenocarcinomas.[72] Since tumors with an intestinal (or glandular) histologic pattern are known to be less aggressive than those with a less differentiated structure, and since proximal gastric cancers may be more frequently composed of poorly differentiated tumor cells than the distal lesions,[73] it is difficult to distinguish the prognostic importance of site versus histologic variability. Prognosis is more clearly related to resectability. Recent data from the combined chemotherapy and radiation therapy regional treatment for locally advanced gastric carcinoma of the Gastrointestinal Tumor Study Group[74] implied that surgical resection of bulk disease may be the most important criterion for better patient survival with combined modality treatment. Approximately 25% of patients with known cancer who underwent resection for bulk disease were long-term survivors after continued radiation therapy and chemotherapy. Patients with unresected bulk disease had no survival benefit. Naturally, it is impossible to determine if the benefit in patients who had most of their tumor removed surgically was due simply to biologic selection or if the surgery itself improved the effectiveness of subsequent combined modality therapy. The keys to significant improvements in survival in the future will be more reliable diagnostic tests allowing the diagnosis to be established at a time when the disease is still confined to the stomach, and the application of aggressive combined modality therapy for earlier disease. The effects of the various forms of therapy on prognosis in gastric cancer will be dealt with in detail in other sections of this chapter. In addition, more recent survival data obtained from the various nontreatment control arms of completed and ongoing multi-institutional combined modality adjuvant trials will provide more updated survival figures on patients who are well staged.

DIAGNOSIS

A sequence of diagnostic procedures for gastric cancer is outlined in Table 25-12. In the past, the keystone of diagnosis of stomach cancer was the barium upper GI series.[11,75,76] Although most patients with gastric cancer present with relatively advanced disease, which should be detected by the conventional upper GI series, recently reported studies indicate this is not the case. Current information suggests that the barium upper GI series is now most useful as a tool to direct the endoscopist to the area of the

TABLE 25-12. Sequence of Diagnostic Procedures in Suspected Gastric Cancer

1. Physical examination
   ? Lymph node metastasis → biopsy
   ? Hepatomegaly → biopsy
   ? Abdominal mass
2. Double contrast barium upper gastrointestinal series
3. Fiberoptic endoscopy with biopsy and cytology
4. Diagnostic/therapeutic laparotomy

stomach requiring careful examination and biopsy. A review of contemporary series that correlated roentgenographic findings with findings on endoscopic biopsy demonstrated that 9% to 40% of endoscopically positive lesions are not detected on previous barium studies.[76] These results suggest that, on the average, 10% of symptomatic carcinomas are missed in barium studies. An older study raised the question of faulty interpretation of abnormal findings on upper GI roentgenography.[75] This series reported data showing that 15% of malignant abnormalities may be misinterpreted as benign findings.

The diagnostic accuracy of barium roentgenography may be improved by the use of a double-contrast technique (Figs. 25-3 and 25-4).[76,77] This procedure makes use of high-density barium combined with an effervescent agent and glucagon administration to induce gastric atony. A double-contrast study allows careful evaluation of the proximal stomach, where malignant lesions are most likely to be missed by conventional barium studies. It should be emphasized that the vast majority of gastric ulcers should be examined endoscopically and biopsied. It is inappropriate to diagnose a gastric ulcer as benign solely on the basis of a barium study unless there is some compelling reason why upper GI endoscopy should not be performed.

With the advent of the flexible fiberoptic gastroscope, the preferred way to make a tissue diagnosis of gastric cancer has been by endoscopy to obtain material for either tissue biopsy or exfoliative cytology. Older studies reported wide variation in the success rate of endoscopic biopsy and cytology in gastric cancer.[11] In a review of several series, Bockus[78] reported positive cytologic findings in 37% to 97% of gastric cancer patients, with false-positive rates of 0.5% to 13%.[78] With improvement in both endoscopic technique and pathologic examination procedures, the success rate has improved. Winawer and colleagues[79,80] have pointed out several factors that bear on the likelihood of making a successful endoscopic tissue diagnosis. If the tumor mass is exophytic, endoscopy usually is successful in establishing a tissue diagnosis. In 24 (92%) of 26 such patients, Winawer et al obtained positive biopsy or cytologic brush pathology.[80] However, in 24 patients with infiltrative gastric cancer, the diagnosis was made in only 12 (50%). Other factors reducing the success of endoscopic biopsy are tumor diameter less than 3 cm, tumor location at the cardia or on the lesser curvature, and recurrent disease. In such unfavorable situations, lavage cytology may increase the accuracy of brush cytology or biopsy.[79] The use of endoscopic techniques in gastric cancer is described in greater detail in Chapter 20.

The recommended sequence for establishing a tissue diagnosis in the patient thought to have gastric cancer is the following: (1) careful physical examination for pathologic findings amenable to biopsy (nodal or liver involvement), (2) upper GI series with double contrast to establish the site of abnormality in the stomach, (3) endoscopy with biopsy and cytology, and (4) diagnostic/therapeutic laparotomy.

Other procedures that may be of ancillary use in cases of

FIG. 25-3. **A.** Normal appearance of the gastric antrum and body on double-contrast upper gastrointestinal study. **B.** Normal appearance of gastric fundus. (Laufer I: Double contrast radiology in the diagnosis of gastrointestinal cancer. Jerzy Glass GB [ed]: Progress in Gastroenterology, p 649. New York, Grune & Stratton, 1977)

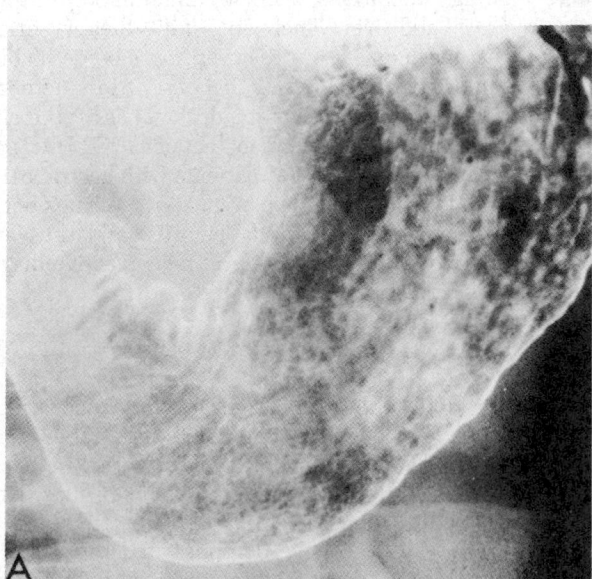

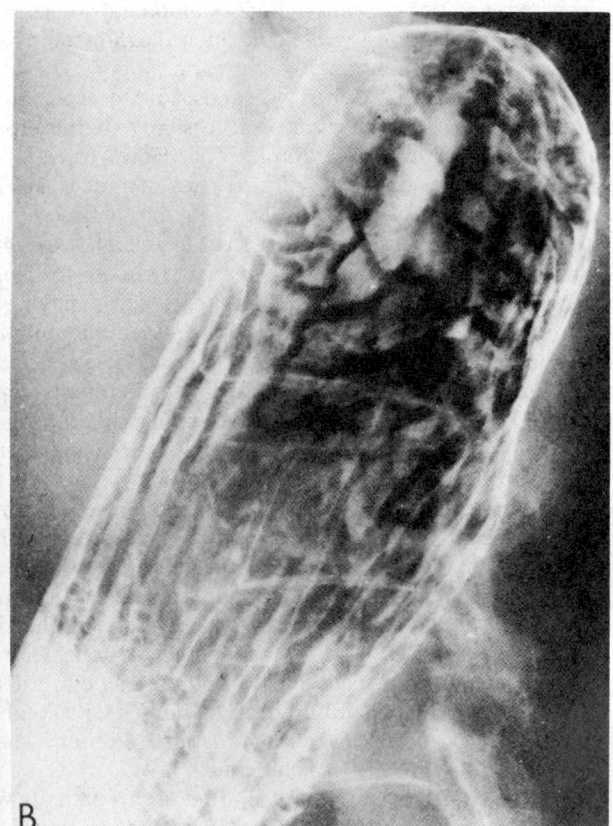

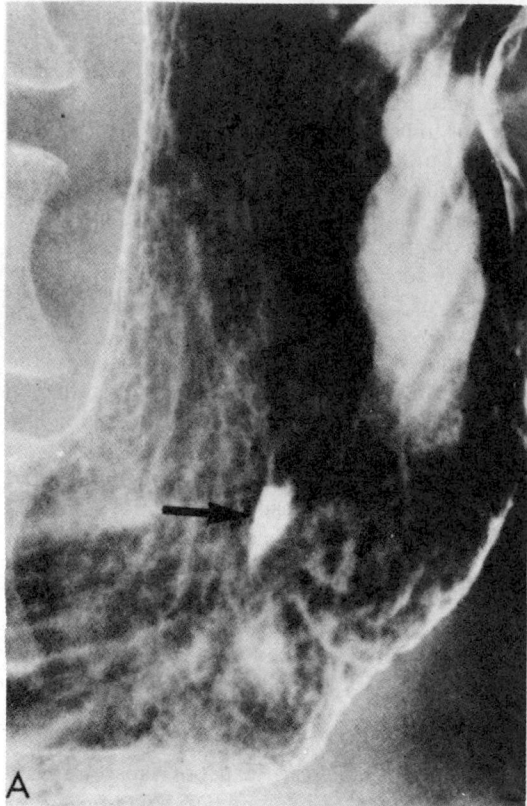

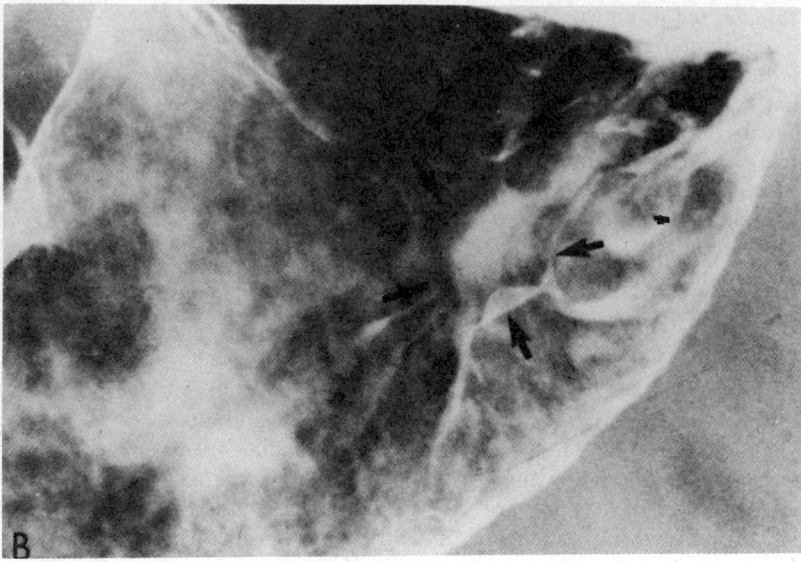

FIG. 25-4. **A**. Benign gastric ulcer on double-contrast UGI. The ulcer crater has smooth, sharply defined borders. **B**. Malignant gastric ulcer. Elevated irregular borders are present, and the ulcer crater is poorly circumscribed. (Laufer I: Double contrast radiology in the diagnosis of gastrointestinal cancer. In Jerzy Glass GB [ed]: Progress in Gastroenterology, p 652. New York, Grune & Stratton, 1977. By permission)

suspected gastric cancer include computed tomography (CT), ultrasonography (US), and identification of plasma tumor markers. In contrast to pancreatic cancer, CT and US are of little use in the primary diagnosis of stomach cancer, largely because the stomach is so accessible to barium roentgenographic studies and to endoscopy. However, both CT and US may be helpful in defining sites of metastases and extragastric extension.[81] This is particularly important in attempting to define surgical resectability. Complete obliteration of the lesser sac or involvement of the gastrohepatic tissues by direct extension of gastric carcinoma may be determined with CT or US. Tumors of the lesser curvature that encircle the left gastric and celiac vessels are also reasonably well defined by these techniques. This information is important for any surgeon attempting to circumscribe the gastric cancer, particularly in a patient known to have distant spread. For instance, in a patient with a biopsy-proven Virchow's node and CT evidence of extensive lesser sac tumor, palliative surgical attempts might not be appropriate prior to the use of chemotherapy or combined modality therapy to improve resectablity. The liver may also be evaluated with CT or US, along with radionuclide scanning, to elucidate suspected metastases. More disseminated peritoneal spread of gastric carcinoma is occasionally demonstrated by CT and US. Pelvic masses resulting from either the Krukenberg tumor or pelvic peritoneal dissemination (Blumer's shelf) may be detected by these techniques.

Plasma tumor markers are of limited use in patients with gastric cancer who have other manifestations of tumor.[82,83]

Levels of carcinoembryonic antigen (CEA) and some newer monoclonal antibody–defined, tumor-associated antigen epitopes, such as GI cancer antigen 19-9, are frequently elevated in the plasma of patients with gastric cancer. Elevations of these substances are not useful as screening diagnostic tests. Although these markers are increased in more than 50% of advanced gastric cancer cases, they are also increased in patients with other manifestations of tumor and in benign conditions, such as inflammation of the bowel, pancreas, and liver. Their only utility lies in serial evaluations that may correlate with other, more objectifiable evidence of tumor growth or tumor response. Alpha-fetoprotein (AFP), another oncofetal protein, does not assist the clinician in the early diagnosis of stomach cancer. AFP levels are increased in only 15% to 20% of patients with gastric carcinoma; they are also increased in patients with various benign diseases, including cirrhosis and hepatitis, and thus are associated with both false-negative and false-positive diagnoses of gastric cancer.

SCREENING

Because of the extent of the gastric cancer problem in some countries other than the United States, there has been interest in developing techniques of screening to detect early lesions. Screening methods have been most extensively developed in Japan.

The Japanese have demonstrated the value of mass surveys for gastric carcinoma in their population. They have detected early cancers through mass upper GI surveys using sophisticated endoscopic and radiologic techniques.[84] These techniques undoubtedly are useful in a cancer-prone population such as exists in Japan.

The ultimate aim of screening programs is to decrease the mortality from gastric cancer. The Japanese have succeeded in this endeavor. Operative attempts are highly successful when gastric cancer is limited to the mucosa, but the incidence of such early lesions is less than 5% in most U.S. series. In Japan, the incidence of lesions initially confined to the mucosa or submucosa was only 3.8% in the years 1955 to 1956, but, because of screening procedures, this figure had increased to 34.5% by 1966, with a corresponding survival rate of 90.9%.[85]

TREATMENT

Gastric cancer treatment uses three therapeutic modalities: surgery, radiation therapy, and chemotherapy. The choice of an individual treatment and the appropriate combination of treatments depends on the stage of disease. Patients with localized gastric cancer are candidates for surgery with curative intent with or without adjunctive chemotherapy or irradiation. Patients with unresectable, partially resectable, or disseminated cancer require treatment designed around chemotherapy with or without irradiation or palliative surgery. The treatment section of this chapter examines the therapeutic options in the management of the patient with gastric cancer in relation to the stage of disease with which the patient presents.

SURGICAL MANAGEMENT OF LOCALIZED GASTRIC CANCER

The most favorable gastric cancer is a fully resectable tumor confined to the stomach. The major treatment modality in such cases is surgery.

Surgical procedures for gastric cancer should be based on anatomical considerations, knowledge of the natural history of the disease, and specific surgical goals—curative or palliative—in a particular case. Increased demands for more detailed surgical–pathologic correlation, particularly in the setting of adjuvant multimodality treatment protocols, will increase the need for appropriate staging as exemplified by the extensive surgical staging procedures of the Japanese protocols. Because the stomach is not vital to a normal life span, the surgical procedure can involve anything up to and including a total gastrectomy (Fig. 25-5). Resection also can entail removal of the omentum, removal of the spleen, removal of the distal portion of the esophagus, removal of the proximal portion of the duodenum, and even simultaneous removal of a portion of the transverse colon. Although such an extensive procedure is not recommended as a routine, experience has indicated that any or all of these structures can be removed without jeopardizing the patient's long-term survival. Lesser resections of the stomach are anatomically, surgically, and oncologically possible, and the extent of the resection can be determined partly by the extent of the lesion and partly by knowledge of its usual pathways of extension.

For most of the 20th century the preferred treatment for gastric carcinoma has been some form of radical subtotal gastrectomy (Fig. 25-6). There have been significant swings in opinion toward and away from total gastrectomy as the

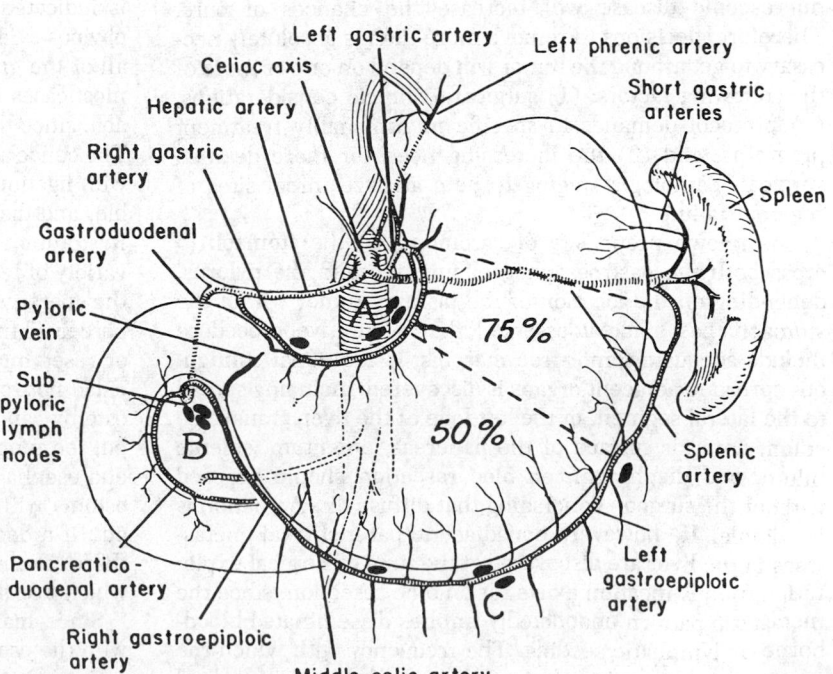

FIG. 25-5. Vascular supply and lymphatic drainage of the stomach in relation to the extent of gastrectomy commonly used in gastric cancer. Proximal resection margins for 50% and 75% subtotal gastrectomies are indicated. (Zollinger RM, Zollinger RM Jr: Atlas of Surgical Operations, 4th ed, plate XIX, no 1. New York, Macmillan, 1977. Copyright ©, 1975 by Macmillan Publishing Co., Inc.)

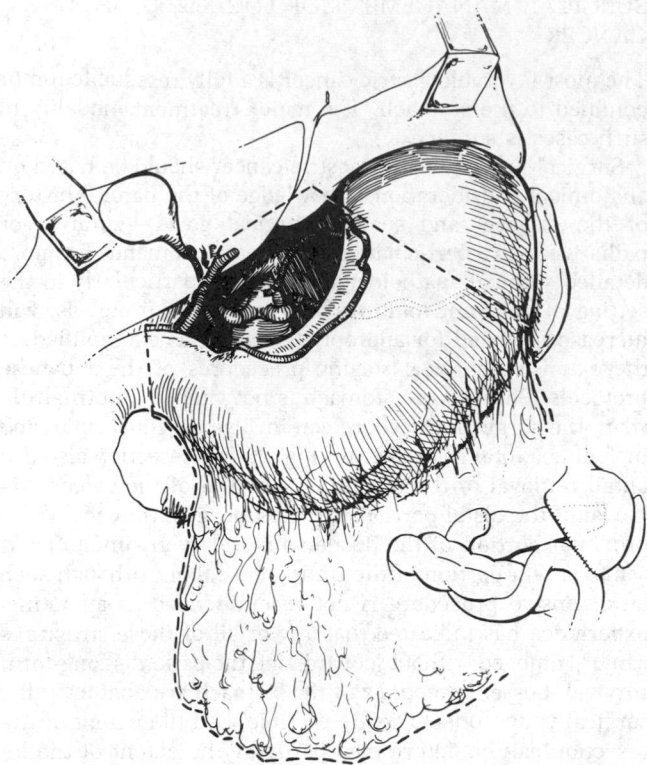

FIG. 25-6. Extent of resection margins of radical subtotal gastrectomy for distal gastric carcinoma. Inset shows appearance after anastomoses have been performed.

treatment of choice, and this has been coupled with various extensions of total gastrectomy that have been advocated from time to time.[86-92] At present, there is no evidence that surgery beyond that necessary to encompass all gross and microscopic disease will increase the chances of cure. Therefore, decisions to remove more than is absolutely necessary to get around the tumor will depend on one or more of the following factors: (1) surgical technical considerations, (2) protocol demands in specific multimodality treatment programs, and (3) the increasing need for more detailed surgical–pathologic staging to help analyze initial sites of regional failure.

The known propensity of carcinoma of the stomach to cross both the gastroesophagael junction and the pylorus, depending on the location of the primary tumor within the stomach, has made it essential that a curative procedure include adequate tumor-free margins. If additional contiguous spread to adjacent organs is discovered, including spread to the lateral segment of the left lobe of the liver, transverse colon, anterior surface of the pancreas, omentum, splenic hilum, and diaphragm, en bloc resection should proceed without the surgeon concluding that diffuse dissemination is inevitable. If, however, nonadjacent parenchymal metastases in the liver are discovered at the time of surgical exploration, no justification exists for en bloc resection, since the metastatic pattern undoubtedly implies disseminated bloodborne or lymphatic seeding. The frequency with which the transverse colon or its blood supply, or both, may be involved

makes it mandatory that the colon be appropriately prepared before any elective procedure on a patient suspected of having carcinoma of the stomach.

Almost every retrospective study on the surgical treatment of patients with gastric carcinoma has found that the morbidity and mortality are higher than expected, which emphasizes the importance of careful preoperative evaluation and patient preparation. In addition to all the standard studies that one should do before any major abdominal procedure, certain other considerations are of major importance in the patient with gastric cancer. Appropriate studies, beyond history and physical examination, should be completed to determine if there is any evidence of distant metastases. Chest roentgenography and physical examination for hepatic and splenic enlargement should be followed by scans of the liver or spleen if there is any suggestion of involvement of these organs. Since anemia and weight loss are common accompaniments of gastric cancer, appropriate blood cell counts, serum protein studies, and evaluations of liver function should be completed. Replacement of blood volume, red cell mass, and protein stores should be accomplished insofar as possible. Depending on the patient's preoperative cancer-related cachexia, hyperalimentation may be considered as a part of the preoperative preparation. However, parenteral or enteral alimentation should be reserved only for the patient who will be undergoing an appropriate palliative or curative surgical attempt. Under no circumstances should nutritional support be considered if no appropriate palliative or curative therapy is contemplated.

The major procedures used for curative attempts in gastric cancer are total gastrectomy and some modification of a radical subtotal gastrectomy. A brief outline of the operative and postoperative problems associated with each of these procedures follows.

A total gastrectomy should entail removal of the entire stomach, as much of the adjacent duodenum or esophagus as is indicated by the location of the primary tumor and by obvious evidence of its spread into the organ in question, and all of the greater omentum. The spleen may be removed in most cases if the lesion is in the proximal half of the stomach, since this results in the most complete node dissection. The celiac axis should be dissected as completely as possible, with ligation of the major vessels at as high a level as possible, and dissection of the hepatic artery as far as possible. Restoration of GI continuity can be achieved by any one of a variety of techniques, depending on the patient's response to the operative procedure, the length of the operation, and the perceived importance of providing a substitute gastric pouch or reservoir at the time of the initial procedure. If it is decided not to make a pouch, an end-to-end esophagoduodenostomy can be fashioned in some cases, or, if this appears to put too much tension on the anastomosis, either an end-to-end esophagojejunostomy or an end-to-side esophagojejunostomy with or without a Roux-en-Y loop should be carried out. If a decision is made at the outset to fashion a pouch, there are a number of pouches which can be utilized, some of which are illustrated in Figure 25-7.

Since many of these procedures involve an anastomosis with the esophagus, a major problem is leak. Leak is a serious postoperative complication and can be avoided by pre-

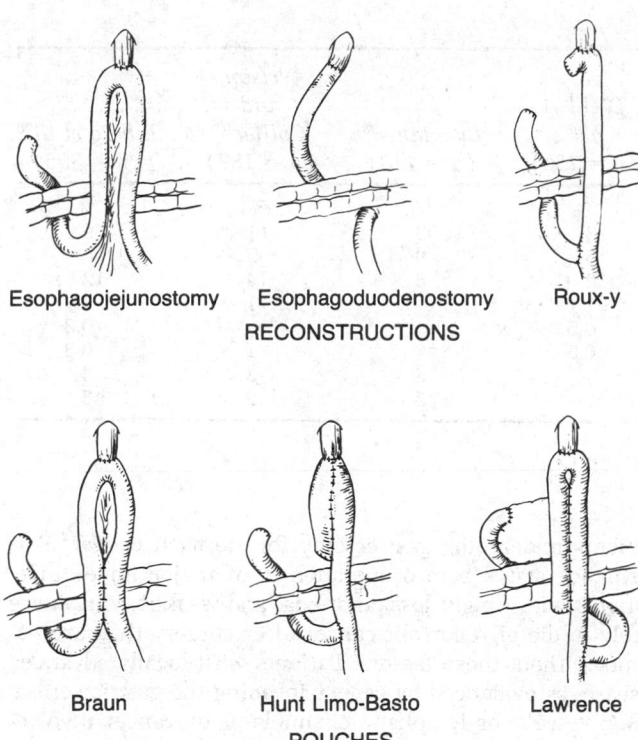

Esophagojejunostomy   Esophagoduodenostomy   Roux-y

RECONSTRUCTIONS

Braun   Hunt Limo-Basto   Lawrence

POUCHES

FIG. 25-7. Major variations in types of reconstructions possible after total gastrectomy. Examples of gastric reservoir pouches that can be used to increase the capacity of the substitute stomach after a total gastrectomy.

serving a rim of proximal stomach if the gross and microscopic examination of margins confirms that the tumor has been completely resected. Additional techniques for decreasing the probability of a leak have to do with good surgical technique, regardless of whether hand-sewn anastomoses or automatic stapling devices are used for reconstructing GI continuity. If a gastric cancer involves a sufficient portion of the stomach to require a total gastrectomy, that is the procedure of choice. It must be emphasized, however, that the extent of operation is determined by the surgical goal: resection of all of the tumor. Increasing the amount of stomach or adjacent tissue removed when excising a small tumor has not demonstrated superior curative potential compared to a resection that simply encompasses the tumor.[45] If frozen section examination of surgical margins has shown microscopic clearance but permanent histologic evaluation contradicts the earlier results, the surgeon should not reoperate to obtain microscopically clear disease. There is no evidence that such a reoperation will increase the curative potential in such a setting, and the morbidity and mortality of a second procedure will not be justified.

The preferred treatment for gastric carcinoma, particularly for a lesion located in the distal half of the stomach, is a subtotal resection of the stomach that adequately removes the tumor (see Fig. 25-6). This often includes removal of 80% to 85% of the stomach, the omentum, the first portion of the duodenum, and node-bearing tissue of the hepaticoduodenal pedicle, the gastrohepatic omentum, and the gastrocolic omentum. The spleen should be removed only if

there is direct evidence of spread to the spleen or to the splenic nodes, or if the lesion is encroaching on the proximal half of the stomach. For cancers involving the proximal stomach or cardioesophageal junction, a variant of the radical subtotal gastrectomy, the proximal subtotal gastrectomy, should be performed.[6] This procedure may require an abdominal or thoracoabdominal surgical approach.

Many individual investigators have attempted to determine whether one or another type of surgical procedure gives the best curative result. Almost all of these experiences are retrospective or, at best, prospective nonrandomized studies. The evaluation of survival figures in such trials is biased, and conclusions concerning a best surgical approach will reflect mainly the contribution of biologic selection. Thus, such trials as reported from the Charity Hospital indicating that radical subtotal gastrectomy gives the best survival results (Fig. 25-8)[45] should be cautiously interpreted. No randomized trials have shown that one or another type of surgical resection will increase the cure rate as long as all the gastric cancer is removed. Design of surgery should be based on techniques that allow safe removal of all tumor, meet the specific demands of combined modality treatment or surgical staging protocols, palliate the patient's symptoms (bleeding, obstruction), and produce the least surgical mortality and morbidity (Table 25-13).[93-98]

Since there is often involvement of the transverse colon or its blood supply, and since this involvement does not contraindicate resection, adequate mechanical and antibiotic preparation of the large bowel should be performed preoperatively in every patient undergoing an elective procedure for removal of stomach cancer. Additional adjacent organs may be involved by contiguous extension of the tumor, not neces-

FIG. 25-8. Survival, computed by the life-table method, after various procedures for adenocarcinoma of the stomach. (Dupont JB, Cohn I: Gastric adenocarcinoma. Curr Probl Cancer 4:25, 1980)

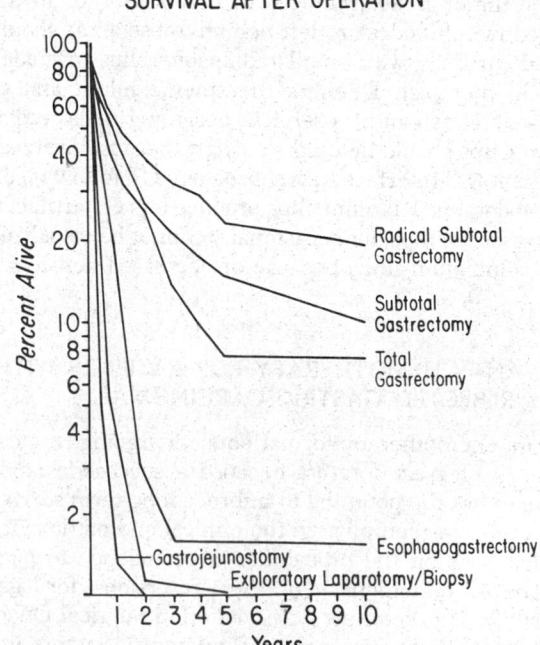

SURVIVAL AFTER OPERATION

TABLE 25-13. Postoperative Complications

Complication	CHNO* (n = 130)	Adashek et al[58] (n = 369)	Ekbom and Gleysteen[94] (n = 144)	Diehl et al[95] (n = 150)	Lygidakis[96] (n = 118)	Nelson and Collier[97] (n = 187)	Inberg et al[98] (n = 305)
	%	%	%	%	%	%	%
Pulmonary	55	11		3	3	11	9
Infectious	22		3	5	9	5	9
Anastomotic	21	9	18	3	8	14	12
Cardiac	10	6		1		1	3
Renal	8	1		0.5			0.3
Bleeding	5	4	4	0.5		1	0.3
Pulmonary embolus	4	1		1	3	3	4
Miscellaneous	5	1	6		3	2	3

* Charity Hospital of Louisiana at New Orleans.

sarily implying disseminated blood-borne or lymphatic metastases. En bloc resection of these structures should be part of the curative or palliative approach, and appropriate preoperative preparation, according to results of noninvasive staging procedures, should be individualized. Only in the case of complete obliteration of the lesser sac, as defined by CT or US, should the symptomatic gastric cancer be considered inoperable or unresectable prior to a laparotomy.

A specific point of surgical concern is the finding of disease in the lateral segment of the left lobe of the liver. If disease in this location is thought to represent contiguous extension, it is reasonable to remove the segment of the involved liver during the gastric resection. Attention must be paid to the aberrant arterial anatomy in a minority of patients whose left hepatic blood flow occurs from the left gastric artery. If this is not noted at the time of surgery, the lateral and medial segments of the left lobe may necrose, resulting in abscess formation, a long postoperative convalescence, and often multiple reoperations.

If the tumor is not removed in its entirety, or if known involved lymph nodes are left behind, these areas should be marked carefully with small radiopaque clips to guide the radiation therapist. Defining the splenic hilum and porta hepatis by clips can be useful in designing nodal radiation portals. Clips should be used sparingly, because overzealous placement will interfere with subsequent CT follow-up of the upper abdomen. Titanium clips produce less CT artifact than small vascular clips but occasionally cannot be visualized on lateral simulation films because of decreased density.

ADJUVANT CHEMOTHERAPY FOR PATIENTS WITH FULLY RESECTED GASTRIC CARCINOMA

Adjuvant chemotherapy for patients undergoing surgical resection is of great interest because a successful adjuvant treatment has the potential to improve long-term survival. It is important to reemphasize the clinical and pathologic factors that bear on the probability of recurrence in patients who have undergone curative resection for gastric cancer.[17,93] The Veterans Administration Surgical Oncology Group (VASOG)[93] has examined prognostic factors in 503

patients undergoing gastrectomy for stomach cancer. Performance status before operation is of major importance: patients with weight loss, anorexia, and weakness are more likely to die of recurrent cancer after surgery than are patients without these factors. Patients with locally advanced disease, as evidenced by cancer invading the gastric serosa, blood vessels, or lymphatic channels or by cancer involvement of perigastric lymph nodes, have a poor prognosis. Patients with extensive evidence of such local invasion have a less than 20% probability of being cured by gastric resection. A proximal location of the primary tumor in the stomach, necessitating a total gastrectomy, is an adverse prognostic factor. In the Veterans Administration studies,[93] only 15% of patients requiring proximal or total gastrectomies for resectable gastric cancer survived 5 years, as opposed to approximately 30% of those who had distal gastrectomies. The pathologic characteristics of the primary tumor are important in predicting survival. Only 2% of patients with linitis plastica survived 5 years after resection.

Most well-designed adjuvant chemotherapy studies that have been reported have failed to show significant benefit for treatment with chemotherapy. Table 25-14 describes a series of studies in which a large number of patients were evaluated.[72,99-104] In an adjuvant therapy study it is exceedingly important that a prospectively randomized design be used. Only in this way can one be assured of balancing prognostic factors between treatment and control groups. All of the studies detailed in Table 25-14 were prospectively randomized controlled trials of chemotherapy versus surgery alone. In the United States, VASOG was a pioneer in performing these studies. The data from this group have shown that single-agent chemotherapy with thiotepa or fluorodeoxyuridine (FUdR) fails to influence disease-free survival at 5 years after resection.[99,100] In the thiotepa study, treatment with chemotherapy appeared to influence survival adversely; however, the difference was not significant.[99]

Because of the high incidence of gastric cancer in Japan, there has been great interest in the surgical adjuvant therapy of the disease in that country. Table 25-14 describes a recent randomized controlled trial in which 223 patients were entered. Patients treated with adjuvant chemotherapy had a better disease-free survival rate than those treated with sur-

TABLE 25-14. Surgical Adjuvant Chemotherapy of Gastric Cancer

Group	No. of Patients	Treatment	Randomized Untreated Controls	Survival Benefit for Treated Group	Reference
VASOG	73	Thiotepa vs. control	Yes	No	99
	276	FudR vs. control	Yes	5-Year Survival: _Treated_ 25.5% _Control_ 33.7% No	100
	134	5-FU + methyl-CCNU vs. control	Yes	5-Year Survival: _Treated_ 23.9% _Control_ 21.3% No	101
GITSG	142	5-FU + methyl-CCNU vs. control	Yes	4-Year Survival: _Treated_ 37.8% _Control_ 38.9% Survival (4-year median follow-up): _Treated_ 59% _Control_ 44% (p < 0.03)	72
ECOG	160	5-FU + methyl-CCNU vs. control	Yes	Survival (4-year median follow-up): _Treated_ 44% _Control_ 47% (p = 0.68)	102
SWOG	180	FAM vs. control	Yes	See text	103
MAOP	300	FAM vs. control	Yes	See text	
International gastric adjuvant study NCCTG	120	5-FU + doxorubicin vs. control	Yes	Survival (4-year median follow-up): _Treated_ 52% _Control_ 51% (p = 0.49)	103a
Cancer Institute of Toyko	73	Mitomycin C + Ara-C + 5-FU vs.	Yes	68% 5-yr survival	104
	76	Mitomycin-C + Ftorafur Ara-C vs.		63% 5-yr survival	
	74	Control		51% 5-yr survival	

VASOG = Veterans Administration Surgical Oncology Group; GITSG = Gastrointestinal Tumor Study Group; ECOG = Eastern Cooperative Oncology Group; SWOG = Southwest Oncology Group; HAOP = Mid-Atlantic Oncology Program; NCCTG = North Central Cancer Treatment Group. 5-FU = 5-fluorouracil; FudR = fluorodeoxyuridine.

gery alone. This result is at odds with results of other studies, and it is important to be aware that the biology of gastric cancer, the stage at diagnosis, and the natural history of this disease may differ between the United States and Japan. Thus, the benefits of Japanese treatment strategies must be confirmed in U.S. studies before treatments are adopted for noninvestigational use.

Both the Gastrointestinal Tumor Study Group (GITSG)[72] and the Eastern Cooperative Oncology Group (ECOG)[102] have reported adjuvant chemotherapy studies using 5-fluorouracil (5-FU) + methyl-CCNU. Both of these studies were prospectively controlled randomized clinical trials initiated in the mid-1970s when 5-FU + methyl-CCNU was thought to produce objective remission in approximately 40% of patients with advanced gastric cancer. The current analysis of these two studies reveals differing results. The GITSG program showed statistical benefit for treatment, the ECOG study did not. The VASOG also performed a Phase III study of 5-FU + methyl-CCNU as adjuvant therapy for gastric cancer and found no benefit with such treatment.[101] It is not clear why the GITSG trial demonstrated benefit and the ECOG and VASOG studies did not.

Table 25-14 also shows that two randomized comparisons of 5-FU, doxorubicin (Adriamycin), and mitomycin C (FAM), an active treatment in advanced gastric cancer, have been performed. The Middle Atlantic Oncology Group (MAOP) study has 300 patients enrolled and evaluable. The Southwest Oncology Group (SWOG) study has 180 patients enrolled. An interim report of the SWOG trial showed no significant differences in relapse rate and survival between patients receiving postoperative FAM and those receiving no additional therapy.[103] This study is ongoing and will require more time for data accrual. The value of adjuvant therapy for gastric cancer is unproved at present, and such treatment cannot be recommended as a routine in patients who have undergone surgical resection.

The adjuvant therapy studies that have been completed have demonstrated the need to have a surgery-only control group. It may be noted from the 5-FU + methyl-CCNU studies that the surgery-only groups have disease-free survival rates of 39% to 47%. If the 20% survivals of "historical controls" in these studies were compared with survival in the treatment arms, all three would be considered to demonstrate improved survival.

MEDICAL MANAGEMENT OF PATIENTS WITH GASTRIC RESECTION

Patients with stomach cancer have all had major disruptions of the GI tract. Patients who have undergone significant gastric resection may have special metabolic problems. The syndromes associated with gastric resection have been reviewed by Lawrence.[105] The most common complication of total gastric resection is the dumping syndrome. This symptom complex results from lack of antral function and includes epigastric fullness, hyperperistalsis, borborygmi, cramps, and occasionally nausea, vomiting, and diarrhea. Other subjective postprandial complaints include diaphoresis, tachycardia, weakness, and dizziness. The mechanisms of the dumping syndrome are due to major fluid shift out of the intravascular space and into the bowel after the sudden dumping of hypertonic foodstuffs into the small bowel in gastrectomized patients.

High-carbohydrate meals, which are most likely to be hyperosmolar, increase symptoms. Many of the symptoms of the dumping syndrome may be produced by the release of serotonin, and antiserotonin agents occasionally may ameliorate the syndrome. Symptomatic therapy for the patient with the dumping syndrome centers on decreasing the osmotic load presented to the small bowel. Small, frequent feedings of low-carbohydrate, high-protein meals usually will improve symptoms. A high fat content in the diet is useful because the high caloric value of fat makes it easier to provide the patient with adequate calories.

All patients who have undergone gastric resection eventually become deficient in vitamin B_{12}, since the stomach produces the intrinsic factor necessary for distal ileal absorption of this vitamin. Because of liver storage of vitamin B_{12}, megaloblastic anemia may not occur for up to 4 years after gastric resection. The administration of 100 μg of this vitamin every month will prevent deficiency.

Less commonly, patients who have undergone a gastrectomy may manifest malabsorption from the afferent or blind loop syndrome.[105] A blind loop of bowel is one that allows ingress of bowel contents but not adequate egress. Bacterial overgrowth may occur, with bacterial metabolism of bile acids resulting in malabsorption. Antibiotic therapy may be helpful in this situation.

All patients with gastric cancer who are undergoing active treatment by surgery, radiation therapy, or chemotherapy and who are manifesting significant malnutrition (>10% weight loss, albumin < 2.5 g/100 ml) should be considered for nutritional support. It makes no sense to support nutritionally a patient with advanced gastric cancer who has failed to respond to appropriate therapy. However, if poor nutritional status itself prevents the optimal application of a potentially useful treatment, nutritional support should be provided. Either parenteral or enteral hypernutrition may be used; both are described in Chapter 59, section 1.

TREATMENT OF LOCALLY UNRESECTABLE OR LOCALLY RECURRENT GASTRIC CANCER

Patients with stomach cancer frequently have advanced local tumors that are either unresectable or only partially resectable. Patients with completely resected gastric cancer may also have a tumor recur in the gastric bed and require management of locally advanced stomach carcinoma. The major issues facing clinicians dealing with locally advanced or recurrent gastric tumors are (1) what is the role of surgery in these patients, (2) how does one coordinate surgery with radiation therapy and cytotoxic chemotherapy in the management of these patients?

Because surgical resection is the curative treatment for gastric carcinoma, the disease should be considered operable and potentially resectable until proved otherwise. The patient whose stomach is involved with extensive local tumor on roentgenographic examination, one with evidence of widespread metastatic involvement, or one with ascites on the basis of peritoneal carcinomatosis should be considered to have an inoperable cancer. The presence of a Virchow's node or other evidence of lymphatic dissemination does not make the cancer inoperable, although it is likely to be incurable with present methods of therapy. The gastric lesion should not be considered unresectable until operation proves it so. As long as the stomach is mobile or the stomach and the organs to which it has become adherent can be removed without compromising the patient's survival, every attempt should be made to resect the primary lesion regardless of its size and the other organs involved. Leaving behind a mass lesion in the stomach is an open invitation to bleeding, perforation, or further obstruction and greatly diminishes the likelihood of success with adjuvant therapy.[106] Not only can removal of the primary tumor reduce the bulk and thereby improve the chances for chemotherapy, it also diminishes the likelihood of the other complications just named. Thus, whenever possible, a lesion in the stomach should be removed, even if this is done for purposes of palliation. Both the surgeon and the patient or the patient's family should be aware of the difference between an attempted curative procedure and a palliative one; nevertheless, a vigorous attempt at palliation is justified.

Many investigators have proved the inefficacy of various bypass procedures if the tumor cannot be removed. The surgeon should be wary of being pressured to "do something" surgically in patients with obstructing unresectable gastric cancer. A recent review of the Charity Hospital experience in New Orleans has concluded correctly that palliative bypass procedures do not increase survival and probably do not increase the quality of life.[45,46,66] The physiologic mechanism of inadequate relief of obstruction is not understood, but results are unsatisfactory regardless of the surgical techniques utilized to bypass unresectable gastric carcinomas.

Although as previously described, palliative gastrectomy is reasonable, a total gastrectomy should not be undertaken as a palliative procedure. The palliation achieved with a total gastrectomy is not good, and the mortality and morbidity of the procedure are too high to justify its use as a palliative procedure.

RADIATION THERAPY

Radiation therapy, usually in conjunction with chemotherapy, plays a major role in patients with locally advanced or recurrent stomach cancer. The effective use of radiation in patients with gastric cancer depends on defining in which clinical situation this modality will be most useful and on developing plans of treatment with tolerable morbidity. This section addresses considerations in planning and executing the radiotherapeutic management of gastric cancer, then reviews the results of existing studies.

The patterns of locoregional failures in the University of Minnesota reoperative group[56] were in a distribution suitable for inclusion within a shaped radiation portal (see Fig. 25-2), which should be modified according to the initial extent of the disease. In Figures 25-9 and 25-10, these portals are superimposed on the limiting organs of tolerance. With accurate field definition, aided by clip placement in the splenic hilum and porta hepatis, one half to two thirds of the left kidney could be spared in many patients, and inclusion of the porta hepatis and retroduodenal areas would include only a minor portion of the right kidney.

Dose-limiting organs and structures in the upper abdomen (stomach, small intestine, liver, kidneys, and spinal cord) are numerous. Because of the posterior extent of the gastric fundus, it is impractical to use lateral portals routinely for a portion of treatment, as is done with tumors of the head of

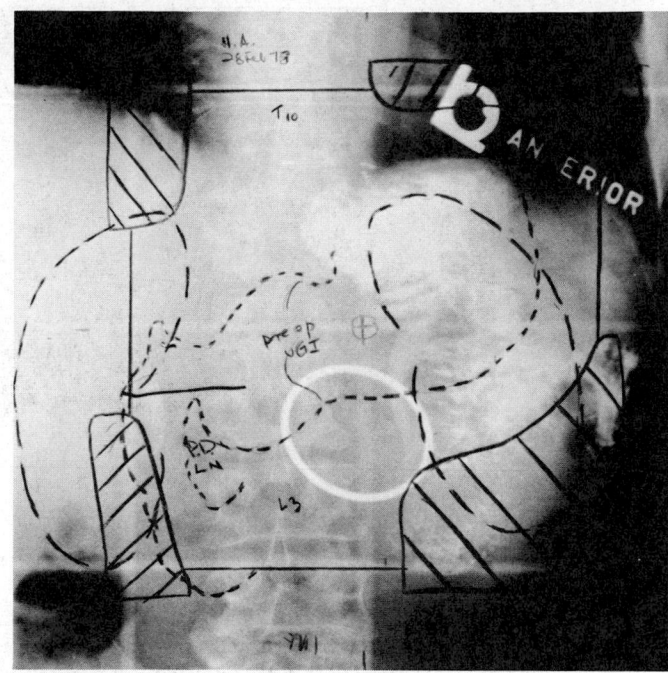

FIG. 21-10. Portals for radiation showing inclusion of the gastric bed plus 70% of the left kidney but excluding 75% or more of the right kidney.

FIG. 25-9. Potential radiation portals are superimposed on organs and structures of tolerance (gastric remnant, duodenal stump, jejunum, liver, kidneys, spinal cord, and spinal and pelvic marrow).

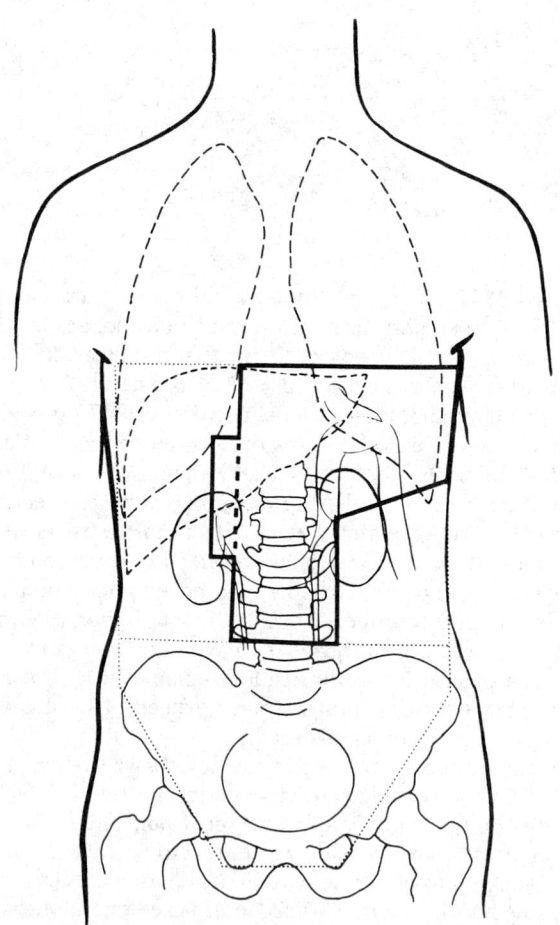

the pancreas, in order to spare the spinal cord or kidney. Since parallel opposed portals are the most practical field arrangement for delivering most tumor and nodal radiation, one must limit either the volume of normal tissue included or the upper dose level. Multiple-field techniques should be considered when this would improve long-term normal tissue tolerance. (For example, with unresectable lesions at the level of the esophagogastric junction, if moderate lateral extension is noted on CT, lateral fields can be useful in decreasing the volume of heart within the radiation field.)

The exact tolerance of kidneys, when portions of both are included in the radiation field, is somewhat uncertain. When both kidneys are to be included in their entirety, Luxton and Kunkler[107] prefer to limit the dose to the upper third of each kidney to 1700 rad but believe their experience suggests that a dose of 2300 rad delivered over 5 weeks to the whole of both kidneys may be acceptable. When portions of both kidneys are to be included in the radiation field, the preference is to exclude two thirds to three fourths of one kidney.[108,109] For proximal gastric lesions, at least one half of the left kidney usually lies within the radiation portal (see Fig. 25-11), and the right kidney must be appropriately spared. For distal lesions with narrow or positive duodenal margins, a similar amount of right kidney often is included (Fig. 25-11), and then every effort must be made to spare enough left kidney. When this approach is followed, problems with radiation nephritis have not been encountered.[109,110] In a series reported from the Massachusetts General Hospital,[110] renal tolerance was evaluated in a group of 86 patients with upper abdominal malignancies who received irradiation with curative intent. At least 50% of the unilateral kidney received 300 rad or more, and all patients survived 1 year or

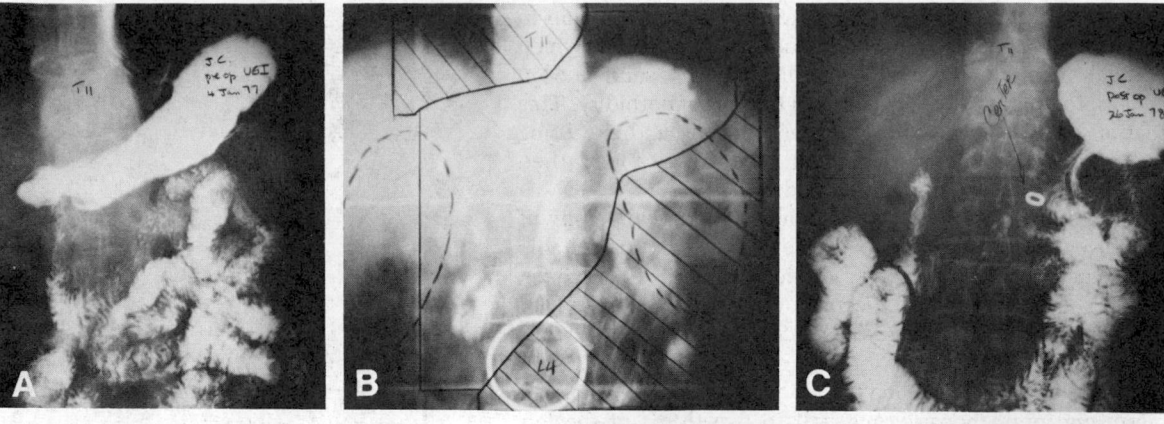

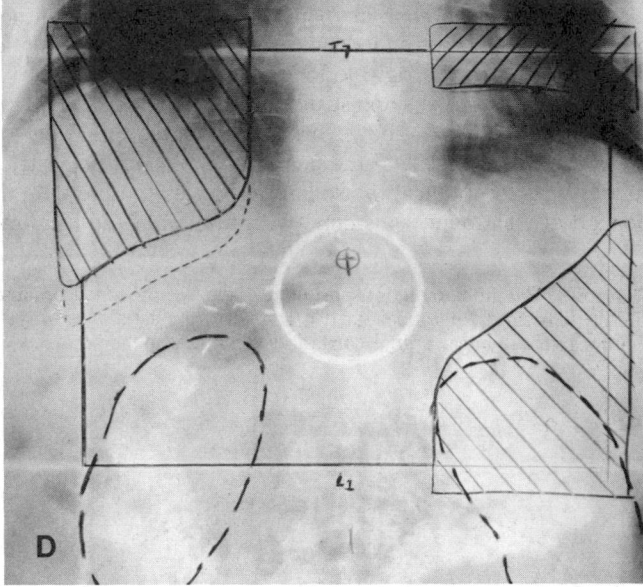

FIG. 25-11. Patient J.C. (**A–C**) had a subtotal gastrectomy with gastrojejunostomy for adenocarcinoma of the stomach and was referred to MGH for postoperative radiation. The initial intent was inclusion of the duodenal stump, a portion of the duodenal loop, the tumor bed and nodal areas, yet sparing 75 + % of the left kidney with blocks (*cross-hatched areas*). **A.** Position of the duodenum in the preoperative UGI. **B, C.** Good visualization of both the duodenal stump and gastric pouch in both the radiation planning film (**B**) and the postoperative diagnostic UGI (**C**).

Patient A.X. had an unresectable carcinoma of the stomach. (**D**) The lesion's extent was marked with clips at exploratory laparotomy. Since the radiation therapy portal included nearly 50% of the right kidney, cerrobend blocking was used to exclude the left kidney. Other blocks (*cross-hatched areas*) were used to exclude portions of liver and heart. Additional liver blocking was added after 3500 rad. (Parts **A–C** from Gunderson L: Part IX. In Alimentary Tract Radiology, p 606. St. Louis, C V Mosby, 1979)

longer. No patient developed acute or chronic renal failure. Of 73 patients who were normotensive before irradiation, 2 became hypertensive (easily controlled with medication in one; malignant hypertension required nephrectomy in the second).

The most commonly used dose schedules of 4000 to 5000 rad delivered over 4 to 5 weeks as continuous irradiation for various upper abdominal malignancies have been tolerated by the stomach and small intestine, with a complication rate ranging from 0 to 8.3% in recent series.[111,112] Roswit and co-workers[113] summarized the older Walter Reed Hospital testicular data, which showed a higher incidence of gastric and intestinal complications. This may have resulted from the following factors: lower voltage radiation (maximum 1 MeV), short fractionation schedules (4500 to 5400 rad delivered over 3 to 4 weeks), and treatment of one field per day. Duodenal and distal gastric tolerance were evaluated in a series of 36 patients treated with curative intent at Mayo Clinic with irradiation ± 5-FU for locally advanced biliary duct cancer.[114] Multiple-field techniques and 180-rad fraction size were used in most patients, and specialized irradiation supplements were used in 18 (transcatheter iridium in 10, IORT electrons in 8). Two (11%) of 19 patients who received 5500 rad or less by external beam ± iridium to a portion of duodenum or distal stomach developed duodenal ulcers or upper GI bleeding. When that dose was exceeded, the incidence increased to 33% (2 of 6 patients).

In the upper abdomen, daily single doses of 170 to 180 rad are better tolerated than doses of 200 rad or more. Weekly weights should be followed closely. When doses of 170 to 180 rad are used, about half of patients require pretreatment antiemetics. Most patients with intact stomachs, however, have some degree of anorexia and need encouragement to eat adequate amounts. Patients who have undergone partial or subtotal gastrectomies seem to tolerate upper abdominal irradiation better than those who have not undergone resection. Use of oral hyperalimentation should be encouraged, and if weight loss during treatment exceeds 10%, hyperalimentation should be considered.

With proximal gastric lesions or lesions at the esophagogastric junction, inclusion of a major portion of the left hemidiaphragm is indicated when the lesion extends through the entire alimentary wall. In these circumstances, cerrobend blocking to decrease cardiac irradiation can be important, since doxorubicin is a frequently used chemotherapeutic agent in this malignancy.

Method of Radiation

Differences of opinion may exist on the preferred way to combine surgery and irradiation for gastric carcinoma. Preoperative, intraoperative, and postoperative radiation therapy have been used to some degree in the past, mainly in Japan.[115-119] The main problem with using intraoperative radiation as the sole method of radiation, as is done in Japan, is that the pathologic extent of disease is not known and radiation portals cannot be individualized. A possible advantage is that dose-limiting tissues, such as the small intestine, colon, and liver, can be retracted outside the radiation field. Such retraction, however, might result in margin failures, since a significant number of locoregional failures in the Minnesota reoperative series involved those organs. A preferred method may be to combine external beam and intraoperative irradiation.

The direct controversy of preoperative versus postoperative radiation therapy versus a combination thereof is probably of greatest interest, since intraoperative irradiation is not feasible in most institutions. Theoretical considerations in this regard are discussed in Chapter 15. Since 30% to 50% of gastric lesions are technically unresectable, some preoperative irradiation to alter implantability or to shrink disease would be attractive. Because the routine diagnostic techniques often reveal only the "tip of the iceberg" regarding extent of disease, CT should be performed to define extragastric disease extent, and peritoneoscopy or minilaparotomy could be considered to rule out peritoneal seeding or minimal disease on the surface of the liver. If moderate-dose preoperative irradiation (4500–5000 rad) were used in an attempt to shrink disease to improve resectability, risks of anastomotic leaks probably would increase unless resections were wide and at least one of the limbs of the anastomosis was not irradiated.

With postoperative irradiation, field setup (portals) and dose could be individualized to some degree with potential portals according to extent of disease, as follows:

1. Negative lymph nodes, extension beyond mucosa but confined to gastric wall. Small field irradiation to the anastomotic area, including duodenal stump if it was a distal lesion. If only a small number of lymph nodes were sectioned, consider inclusion of primary lymph nodes.
2. Negative lymph nodes, extension beyond gastric wall. Moderate field radiation therapy to cover the stomach bed structures with or without nodal areas. Entire left hemidiaphragm should be considered for inclusion, especially in proximal lesions.
3. Positive lymph nodes, confined to gastric wall. Cover both the primary and secondary nodal drainage areas. Do not need to include the entire left hemidiaphragm, and therefore treat less lung and heart.
4. Positive lymph nodes, extension beyond gastric wall. Cover entire gastric bed plus primary and secondary lymph node drainage areas (major solid line field as shown in Figs. 25-2 and 25-9).

The nodal areas considered at risk for primary spread include the gastric and gastroepiploic nodes (usually resected), and the entire celiac axis, including porta hepatis, subpyloric, gastroduodenal, splenic suprapancreatic, and retropancreaticoduodenal nodes (paraesophageal nodes if the tumor is proximal). Secondary chains at risk include the superior mesenteric and para-aortic nodes.

The usual dose aim is 4500 to 5000 rad in 5 to 6 weeks delivered in 170 to 180 rad fractions to the initial field. A boost field can be safely carried to 5000 rad and occasionally is brought to 5500 rad for unresected or residual disease. Some European and Scandinavian centers use upper dose levels of 6000 rad in 6 to 9 weeks for unresected or residual disease, but these centers have provided only minimal information on long-term tolerance. Parallel opposed fields usually are necessary for the initial large field to the tumor or tumor bed and lymph node areas. Doses greater than 4500 to 5000 rad are discouraged with treatment energies of 4 MeV or less unless multiple-field techniques can be used for a portion of the treatment. If residual or unresected disease is marked with clips, that possibility exists. On rare occasions, the dose for residual disease in lymph nodes or tumor bed may be boosted to 6000 rad if clips are placed and an upper GI study is done to define the relationship of residual disease to the gastric pouch and small intestine.

Results

RADIATION WITH OR WITHOUT CHEMOTHERAPY. Radiation alone has been shown to have curative potential in a small percentage of patients with resected but residual[115] or with unresectable but localized disease.[119,120] Its greatest benefit has been when used in combination with chemotherapy, as noted for some time in studies from the Mayo Clinic[109,121] and a number of foreign centers.[116-120]

Adjuvant radiation alone or in combination with chemotherapy would be attractive for high-risk subgroups of patients with resected gastric carcinoma. Local failure after curative resection is common. Although some cures have been obtained with irradiation alone,[119,120] indicating that gastric cancer is radiosensitive, this is not a viable single-modality approach because the bulk of disease and the limited tolerance of the stomach and surrounding organs prevent a suitable therapeutic ratio between cure and complications. The preferred use of radiation as an aid to local regional control would be in combination with operative removal of all gross disease in the primary area and lymph nodes, with radiation usually in combination with chemotherapy being used to treat microscopic or subclinical residual disease.

RADIATION AND SURGERY. Available literature supports the concept that adenocarcinoma of the stomach is a radioresponsive lesion.[115-120] Wieland and Hymmen[120] used 6000 rad when feasible (150 to 200 rad daily) with 11% (9 of 82) 3-year and 7% (5 of 72) 5-year survivals. Takahashi[119] compared historical controls with patients with inoperable disease or patients who had undergone palliative procedures and received postoperative irradiation (no mention of chemotherapy). The average survival for the group treated by radiation therapy was longer by 9 to 10 months, with 74% survival (32 of 43 patients) at 1 year and 28% survival (12 of 43 patients) at 2.5 years. In a preoperative series, Hoshi[118] found histologic changes of tumor necrosis in 28% of patients with doses less than 2000 rad, in 74% with doses of 2000 rad, and in 88% with higher doses. Asakawa and associates[116,117] found a greater than 50% decrease in the size of tumor in 60% and total regression in 10% of 40 patients treated with radiation alone or in combination with chemotherapy prior to surgery.

CONVENTIONAL RADIATION AND CHEMOTHERAPY. Most reports on combined treatment deal with results in the patient with unresectable cancer and show suggestive improvement for irradiation plus 5-FU over that achieved with either irradiation alone or 5-FU alone.[121-123] In the Mayo Clinic series,[121] a randomized double-blind study of patients with unresectable disease, 5-FU was used during the first 3 days of radiation (3500–4000 rad at 900–1200 rad/week). For the combined therapy versus radiation therapy groups, mean survival was 12 versus 5.9 months, and 5-year survival rate was 12% (3 of 25 patients) versus 0% (0 of 23). Asakawa and co-workers[116,117] reported treatment results in 54 patients, of whom 42 received some 5-FU. At the 2-year interval, 3 of 33 patients treated without surgical resection and 4 of 8 treated with partial resection were alive (6000 rad over 6 to 9 weeks was the aim).

In a recent report of the randomized GITSG study (protocol 8274), including 90 patients with unresectable or residual disease,[74] the combination of radiation therapy plus 5-FU followed by maintenance 5-FU plus methyl-CCNU was statistically superior to 5-FU plus methyl-CCNU alone with regard to long-term survival, with a plateau of 20% reached after 3 years of follow-up (p < 0.05). The short-term advantage to 5-FU plus methyl-CCNU (median survival, 70 versus 36 weeks) was believed due to early tumor-related and toxicity deaths with the 5-FU–radiation therapy combination during the first 26 weeks of treatment. Irradiated patients received 5000 rad in 8 weeks in split-course fashion (2500 rad in 3 weeks, followed by 2 weeks' rest, followed by an additional 2500 rad in 3 weeks; 500 mg/m² of 5-FU was given on days 1, 2, and 3 of each radiation therapy sequence, followed by 5-FU plus methyl-CCNU maintenance chemotherapy). Patients with residual disease after resection had better long-term survival rates than those whose cancers were never resected.

In a series of 46 patients with localized gastric cancer treated with radiation alone (6 patients) or in combination with chemotherapy at the Massachusetts General Hospital,[109] toxicity-related deaths were not encountered. The numbers of patients by disease category were as follows: recurrent disease, 4; medically inoperable, 4; surgically unresectable, 9; resected but residual, 15; and resected but high risk for local recurrence, 14. Patients treated with radiation therapy plus chemotherapy followed two sequences: radiation therapy plus 3 days of 5-FU followed by maintenance 5-FU or combined drugs (26 patients); and single course of 5-FU plus *bis*-chloroethylnitrosourea (BCNU) or FAM, followed by radiation therapy and maintenance combination chemotherapy (14 patients). Radiation with 10 or 25 MeV photons was delivered to tightly contoured portals, sparing as much bone marrow and bowel as possible and delivering 4500 to 5200 rad in 25 to 29 fractions over 5 to 6 weeks. Only 4 patients (9%) had poor tolerance, and 2 of those completed radiation therapy. Hematologic parameters delayed the radiation therapy or chemotherapy course in 11 patients. The difference in treatment-related toxicity in the GITSG versus Massachusetts General Hospital series may in part be due to the use of tightly contoured portals in the latter series, an aspect of technique more difficult to coordinate in a multi-institution study.

Although patterns of failure and lack of positive chemotherapy trials help justify the incorporation of radiation therapy into future adjuvant trials, data from pilot trials are minimal. In the initial publication from the Massachusetts General Hospital,[109] 14 of the 46 patients had curative resection but were at high risk for locoregional failure and received postoperative irradiation + 5-FU. Local progression as any component of failure was subsequently documented in 2 (14%), and the 4-year actuarial survival rate was 46%. In a randomized trial from the Mayo Clinic,[124] 62 patients with involved nodes were randomized to no further treatment or postoperative irradiation (3750 rad over 4–5 weeks) plus 5-FU (15 mg/kg IV bolus on days 1–3). The 5-year survival rate in patients assigned to receive additional treatment was 23%, versus 4% in those treated by surgery alone (p < 0.05). However, 10 patients who refused additional treatment had a 5-year survival rate of 30%, compared to the 23% rate in patients given additional treatment. Local failure was documented as a component of initial progression in 39% of treated patients versus 55% of those treated with surgery alone. In view of the high rate of nonacceptance to assigned treatment, end results are difficult to interpret but suggest a decrease in local failure. It would be reasonable to evaluate further the combination of external radiation + 5-FU in subsequent randomized trials (alone or in combination with more aggressive chemotherapy).

RADIATION AND FAM. Combinations of FAM and radiation have been used in pilot studies for unresectable gastric or pancreatic cancer (MGH, Middle Atlantic Oncology Program [MAOP]), as well as in resected but high-risk (MGH) or resected but residual gastric cancer (MGH, SWOG). In the SWOG pilot study,[125] 12 patients were treated with concomitant FAM and radiation. The MGH trial used a sequential FAM plus irradiation plus FAM regimen (1 cycle of FAM, radiation therapy of 4500 to 5000 rad delivered over 5 to 5½ weeks in 180-rad fractions, FAM for 5 cycles).[109] Although some patients with pancreatic cancer have been treated at Massachusetts General Hospital, the major focus has been on gastric cancer, with 24 gastric patients having completed treatment as of a September 1985 report.[126] In a MAOP trial of 42 patients reported by Schein and colleagues[127] (gastric cancer, 21 patients; pancreatic cancer, 21 patients), FAM was used before and after a course of split-course radiation combined with 5-FU (4500 rad over 7 weeks: 2250 rad per sequence plus 5-FU, 350 mg/m², on days 1, 2, and 3 of each X-irradiation sequence). Both the MGH and MAOP trials used 1 cycle of FAM before radiation and 5 to 6 cycles afterward, with radiation instituted in week 7 in the MGH pilot and in week 10 in the MAOP pilot (5-FU was added to the X-irradiation course in the MAOP pilot but not at MGH). In the MGH and MAOP trials, GI tolerance was acceptable

TABLE 25-15. Component of Failure After Radiation and Chemotherapy*†

Treatment Group	No. of Failures/ Total Group‡	Local			Liver			Peritoneal			Lung		
		No.	%	(%)	No.	%	(%)	No.	%	(%)	No.	%	(%)
Curative	8/14	2	25	(14)	5	63	(36)	2	25	(14)	2	25	(14)
Residual microscopic	8/8	1	13	(13)	3	38	(38)	2	25	(25)	1	13	(13)
Gross	6/7	1	17	(14)	1	17	(14)	2	33	(29)	4	67	(58)
Unresectable	9/9	6	67	(67)	3	33	(33)	2	22	(22)	4	44	(44)

*Modified from Gunderson LL, Hoskins B, Cohen AM et al: Combined modality treatment of gastric cancer. Int J Radiat Oncol Biol Phys 9:965–975, 1983.

†Open figures represent number and percentage of failure group, and numbers in parentheses represent percentage of total evaluable patients.

‡An additional 8 patients were treated in this series (medically inoperable, 4; recurrent, 4), and 6 of the 16 local failures occurred in these 8 patients.

(mild to moderate nausea and vomiting), with myelosuppression representing the dose-limiting toxicity. In the larger MAOP trial, the median white blood cell nadir was $2.3 \times 10^3/mm^3$ (range, $0.2–6.6 \times 10^3/mm^3$) and the platelet nadir was $84 \ 10^3/mm^3$ (range, $20–288 \times 10^3/mm^3$). Median survival was 13+ months (range, 1+ to 15 months) for gastric patients in the MAOP trial and 19 months at MGH. In the MGH analysis, 2-year actuarial survival was 41%. While these trials indicate that such treatment combinations can be used with acceptable toxicity, randomized trials will be needed to determine whether the therapeutic effect of such combined treatment is better than that achieved with either irradiation plus 5-FU or multiple drug chemotherapy alone.

PATTERNS OF FAILURE. Sites of failure were analyzed in the group of 46 patients treated with combined radiation and chemotherapy for gastric cancer at MGH (Table 25-15). Disease progression was identified in 70 sites in 37 patients. Most sites were intra-abdominal (47 of 70 sites, or 67.2%; 32 of 46 patients, or 70%), with frequent liver metastases and peritoneal seeding (21 of 46 patients, or 46%, had either or both, 17 with a single component, 4 with both). A component of local or regional failure was noted in 16 patients (23% of sites and 35% of total patient group). Such failures were outside the irradiation field in 1 patient and possibly at the margin of the failed in 1 additional patient. Three failures were associated with peritoneal seeding. Pleural or pulmonary failure was noted in approximately 18% of sites or 28% of the total patient group.

In Table 25-15, the four major causes of failure are analyzed by treatment group. Although tissue confirmation of failure was available in 18 of the 37 patients, confirmation of failure sites by reoperation or autopsy was available in only 7. Interestingly, only 4 (14%) of 29 patients with curative resection or resection but residual disease had any evidence of failure within the radiation field, as opposed to 6 (66%) of 9 with unresectable disease. In 2 of the 4 patients in the former group, such failure probably was due to the use of a posterior cord block during irradiation, which was not used by the senior author of the MGH series and is thought not to be necessary at the dose levels in that series (4500 rad in 25

fractions to the large field, 5000 rad to the boost field). Of the 24 patients treated with FAM plus irradiation at MGH, 20 died with disease.[126] Local control was maintained in 16. Distant metastases were found in all 20 patients.

RADIATION (MULTIPLE DAILY FRACTIONS) PLUS CHEMOTHERAPY. In view of major local and systemic problems with gastric cancer identified in various series, a pilot study was instituted at the Mayo Clinic in an attempt to optimize the use of combination chemotherapy and irradiation.[128] The intent was to sequence combined drug regimens before and after radiation therapy and to use two fractions a day of irradiation with or without 5-FU. This was an attempt to shorten intervals from operative intervention to the institution of combined drug chemotherapy and between chemotherapy regimens, and to improve the radiation response of patients with poorly differentiated lesions (a majority of patients with gastric cancer) on the basis of less repopulation between radiation fractions. Such a schema contrasts markedly with the use of split-course irradiation regimens, which may be inappropriate with poorly differentiated lesions.

Eighteen patients with unresectable or residual regional gastric cancer without evident distant metastases were treated with an intensive combined modality regimen to determine patient tolerability (16 of 18 received irradiation and 12 had some maintenance chemotherapy).

1. Induction chemotherapy: 5-FU, 350 mg/m² IV on days 1 through 5, plus doxorubicin, 50 mg/m² IV on day 1.
2. Radiation therapy: beginning on day 21, 4500 rad given in two 165-rad fractions daily, plus 5-FU, 500 mg/m² IV on days 28 through 30.
3. Maintenance chemotherapy: beginning 4 weeks from the end of radiation therapy, 5-FU, 225 mg/m² IV on days 1 through 5 every 5 weeks; doxorubicin, 30 mg/m² IV on day 1 every 5 weeks; methyl-CCNU, 80 mg/m² PO on day 1 every 10 weeks.

Six of 7 patients treated with the combined regimen experienced prolonged anorexia and nausea during radiation therapy and for several weeks thereafter, requiring a delay in instituting maintenance chemotherapy in 5 of 6 patients.

Three of 6 patients also experienced leukopenia (white blood cell count ≤ 2500), one of whom was unable to receive maintenance chemotherapy because of prolonged leukopenia. Increasing the rest interval after induction chemotherapy by 1 week and decreasing the radiation dose per fraction to 150 rad did not reduce the severe nutritional effects in 2 of 3 patients thus treated. Nine additional patients have received either hyperfactionated radiation without 5-FU (6 patients) or single daily doses of radiation plus 5-FU (3 patients) with improved tolerance. At the last evaluation, disease in 11 patients had progressed (time to progression in weeks: median, 19; range, 4–49). All 13 patients evaluable for patterns of progression developed distant metastases. Only 2 of 11 who received radiation therapy also had initial local progression.

INTRAOPERATIVE RADIATION. Most information on the use of intraoperative radiation therapy (IORT) for the treatment of gastric cancer is based on data reported by Abe and Takahashi from Japan.[129] Abe has been treating gastric carcinoma with a relatively constant technique of IORT alone after gastrectomy (no external beam irradiation). A pentagonal treatment field, designed to cover the tumor bed and major nodal sites, receives 2800 to 4000 rad in a single fraction (measured at the 100% isodose line) with high-energy electrons.

Although formal randomization has not been performed, patients are selected for IORT on the basis of the day they are admitted to the hospital. In a prospective study, 110 patients were treated by surgery alone and 84 patients by surgery plus IORT.

Abe's results are shown in Table 25-16. Five-year survival is very similar in both treatment groups for Stage I disease, but there is a suggestion of a survival advantage for both Stage II (77.6% versus 54.5%) and Stage III (44.6% versus 36.8%) for the IORT group. The most impressive difference, however, is seen in patients with Stage IV disease who had direct local extension posteriorly or residual disease without distant metastases. In this subset, there were no survivors among 18 patients treated with operation alone, compared to a 19.5% 5-year survival rate among 27 patients treated with surgery plus IORT. This percentage is similar to the incidence of locoregional failure occurring as the only failure in the University of Minnesota reoperative series (29% of failure group, or 23% of total group at risk) and indicates that radiation therapy may add to survival in a subset of patients who are at high risk for local failure. There has been a small

(less than 40 patients) randomized IORT study in resected gastric cancer performed at the National Cancer Institute. Neither disease-free nor overall survival was improved by IORT.

Recommendations for Nonprotocol Radiation plus Chemotherapy

The major role of radiation therapy today in the treatment of gastric cancer is in the management of locally unresectable, partially resectable, or recurrent disease. The recommended nonprotocol therapy is the radiation plus 5-FU plus methyl-CCNU regimen previously outlined in this chapter, or continuous radiation plus 5-FU, possibly followed by FAM (4500–5000 rad in 180-rad fractions over 5–5½ weeks with a 500 mg/m^2 IV 5-FU push for 2 consecutive days in weeks 1 and/or 5, depending on blood cell counts and GI tolerance). With the 5-FU + methyl-CCNU program, the drugs are given in the following schedule: 5-FU, 325 mg/m^2 on days 1 through 5, 375 mg/m^2 on days 36 through 40; methyl-CCNU, 150 mg/m^2 on day 1. The schedule is repeated every 9 to 10 weeks, depending on tolerance, and is not initiated until radiation therapy has been completed and radiation-associated acute toxicities have cleared. Methyl-CCNU is currently not available for other than investigational use. Also, caution should be exercised in using methyl-CCNU in patients who may be long-term survivors. Boice and colleagues[130] have demonstrated that methyl-CCNU increases the incidence of acute leukemia (relative risk: 12.4) in patients with GI cancer who had received this drug as adjuvant therapy. It should be emphasized that there are no combined modality regimens that are dramatically successful, and there is continued need for active investigation in the use of combined radiation plus chemotherapy.

TREATMENT OF PATIENTS WITH DISSEMINATED CANCER

The major treatment modality currently available for metastatic gastric cancer is chemotherapy. The chemotherapy of advanced gastric cancer has aroused considerable interest[106,131–133] because several studies have documented response rates of 40% to 50% with combination chemotherapy. Whether currently available therapies result in improved survival for treated patients is not clear.

In evaluating the reported results of chemotherapy in advanced gastric cancer, several prognostic factors are important. Available data suggest that patients who have a good performance status, who are only minimally symptomatic, and who have evaluable disease confined to the abdomen are more likely to respond to chemotherapy than are patients with either widely disseminated metastatic disease or poor performance status.[106] Therefore, it becomes important in evaluating the results of chemotherapy studies that data on performance status and sites of metastatic disease be analyzed carefully. Clearly, any chemotherapy regimen used in totally asymptomatic patients with limited disease would appear to be more effective than a treatment program used in significantly symptomatic patients with widely disseminated cancer.

TABLE 25-16.   Gastric Cancer — Surgery and IORT, Japan

| | 5-Year Survival | | | |
| | Surgery | | Surgery + IORT | |
	No.	%	No.	%
Stage I	43	93	20	88.1
Stage II	11	54.5	18	77.6
Stage III	38	36.8	19	44.6
Stage IV (no distant metastases)	18	0	27	19.5

In evaluating the results of chemotherapy trials in gastric cancer, the following criteria for response are used. A complete response consists in the disappearance of all objective evidence of cancer. A partial response is defined as a greater than 50% decrease in the products of the two largest perpendicular diameters of clearly measurable metastatic lesions. An alternative, stricter interpretation of partial response requires a greater than 50% decrease in all metastatic lesions. A minimal response is defined as a less than 50% but greater than 25% decrease in measurable metastatic lesions. In general, lesion diameters may be measured physically or from radiographs. Radionuclide scans of the liver may be used if perfusion defects are clearly measurable and greater than 3 cm in diameter.[132] Similarly, large abnormalities on CT or US occasionally may serve as measurable disease. However, further clinical correlation with the changes in CT or US tumor images after chemotherapy is necessary. When response to chemotherapy is referred to in this chapter, only partial and complete responses are meant. Minimal responses will not be considered as objective disease regression.

Study design is another factor that must be evaluated carefully when assessing results of chemotherapy trials in patients with stomach cancer. Study design is particularly important when claims of improved survival with a particular regimen are made. The only proper way to demonstrate improved survival with a chemotherapy regimen is to evaluate that treatment program prospectively in a Phase III trial. In advanced gastric carcinoma, a disease in which complete remissions secondary to chemotherapy are exceedingly rare, it is difficult to sustain the claim that chemotherapy improves survival in partially responding patients. It may be entirely possible that response to a chemotherapy program does not result in prolongation of survival, but rather that the patients who will have the longest survival if untreated are the ones most likely to respond to chemotherapy. Thus response to chemotherapy may merely be another indication of good prognosis, as are other factors such as good performance status, relatively minimal disease, and well-differen-

tiated histology.[106] With the above caveats firmly established, this section reviews the results of single-agent chemotherapy and combination chemotherapy of gastric cancer.

Single-Agent Chemotherapy

The use of systemic chemotherapy for disseminated gastric cancer has depended on documentation of antitumor activity of various single agents against this disease. Table 25-17 reviews objective response rates reported for single agents in patients with stomach cancer.[106,131,134-148] Many other agents have been reported anecdotally in the literature, but Table 25-17 reports studies in which 18 or more patients were evaluated.

The fluorinated pyrimidine 5-fluorouracil (5-FU), which has been tested in almost 400 patients, is the most completely evaluated single agent.[134] The dosage schedule most frequently used is the loading course method in which the drug is administered IV for 4 to 5 days, followed by half-doses every other day until toxicity is produced. Various maintenance schedules have been used; the most common are weekly IV doses or repeated loading courses at monthly intervals. The objective partial response rate with 5-FU is a disappointing 21%. Complete responses are exceedingly rare, and the median duration of 5-FU response can be expected to range from 3 months to 6 months.

The antibiotic mitomycin C, first developed in Japan, has been evaluated in gastric cancer. The original reports of Japanese clinical trials suggested an overall objective response rate of 35%.[134] The initial experience in the United States was considerably less impressive, however. Administration of mitomycin C on a daily schedule was found to produce significant delayed myelosuppression and a cumulative, persistent bone marrow injury.[149] In addition, inadvertent extravasation during IV administration resulted in a severe inflammatory reaction, with potential skin slough. Drug-related deaths occurred in 11% of the patients, and the objective response rate was only 18%. More recent experi-

TABLE 25-17. Single-Agent Chemotherapy in Advanced Gastric Cancer

Drug	No. of Responses/ No. of Patients	% Response	Reference
5-Fluorouracil	84/392	21	134
Mitomycin C	63/211	30	134
Adriamycin	17/68	25	135–137
Hydroxyurea	6/31	19	138
BCNU	6/33	18	131
Chlorambucil	3/18	17	139
Mechlorethane	3/23	13	140
Methyl-CCNU	3/37	8	106
Cisplatin	8/36	22	141,142
Triazinate	4/26	15	143
Methotrexate	3/28	11	143
Razoxane	0/19	0	143
4'-Epidoxorubicin	8/22	36	144
Carboplatin (CBDCA)	0/22	0	145
Bisantrene	1/26	4	146
m-AMSA	0/125	0	147
Ftorafur	5/19	27	148

TABLE 25-18.   Combination Chemotherapy in Advanced Gastric Cancer

Drug Combination	No. of Responses/ No. of Patients	% Responses	Median Duration of Survival (Months)	Reference
Adriamycin + mitomycin C	13/46	29	3.5	151
5-FU + methyl-CCNU	12/30	40 (20% CR, 20% PR)	5.0	106
	6/44	14	3.0	151
	5/54	9	4.5	152
	6/29	21	4.5	153
	12/49	24	4.5	137
	1/18	6	5.5	154
Total	42/224	19		
5-FU+mitomycin C	6/43	14	6.0	152
	17/53	32	4.0	137
Total	23/96	24		
5-FU + Adriamycin	3/11	27	7.0	155
	1/19	5	6.0	156
Total	4/30	13		
5-FU + BCNU	14/34	41	7.7	131
	5/28	18	3.0	157
	2/18	11	4.0	158
Total	21/80	26		
Triazinate + mitomycin C	8/28	29	5.5	159
5-FU + high-dose folinic acid	13/27	48 (4% CR, 44% PR)	11 *	160
FAM	6/11	55	16.5*	161
(5-FU + Adriamycin + mitomycin C)	26/62	42	12.5*	132
	20/45	44	11.5*	163
	6/27	22	5.5	164
	28/81	35	17.0*	165
	7/33	21	5.5	166
	4/22	18	6.2	167
	25/83	30	5.8	168
	3/12	25	6.8	154
	3/18	17	6.2	156
	18/46	39	6.4	151
	5/13	38	7.2	155
Total	151/453	33		

(continued)

ence has shown an overall response rate for mitomycin C in gastric cancer of 15% to 30%.[134] There has been renewed interest in the use of this drug with the demonstration that single treatments of 10 mg/m² to 20 mg/m², at 6- to 8-week intervals, result in manageable hematologic toxicity while retaining therapeutic activity.[150]

The anthracycline antibiotic doxorubicin (Adriamycin) is a drug with a wide range of antitumor activity in human solid tumors that has recently been evaluated in gastric cancer. Early trials reported a response rate of 36% with doxorubicin.[135] More recently, the GITSG[138] and the ECOG have performed Phase II trials testing the efficacy of doxorubicin.[137] Both of these studies confirm the activity of this drug. Doxorubicin was administered at 60 mg/m² every 3 to 4 weeks, and objective responses were demonstrated in 4 of 17 cases (24%) and 8 of 37 cases (22%).[136,137] The median duration of response to doxorubicin was 4 months. These studies have demonstrated that doxorubicin is at least as active as the fluorinated pyrimidines and indicated a need to test this drug in combination chemotherapy regimens. Another anthracycline, 4'-epidoxorubicin,[144] which may cause fewer or less severe cardiac toxic effects than doxorubicin, has been evaluated in Phase II trials in stomach cancer. One small study reported 8 (36%) of 22 patients achieving a partial response.[144] This result will require confirmation.

The chloroethylnitrosoureas BCNU and methyl-CCNU represent another class of single agents evaluated in advanced gastric cancer patients.[106,131] BCNU produced objective partial remissions in 6 (18%) of 33 patients treated, with a 4-month duration of response. The methylated chloroethylnitrosourea, methyl-CCNU, also has been tested by ECOG and produced responses in 3 (8%) of 37 patients.[106] Median survival of patients receiving this drug was less than 15 weeks. Other single agents that have been reported to have minimal activity (<20%) in gastric cancer include hydroxyurea, carboplatin, bisantrene, and the alkylating agents mechlorethamine and chlorambucil (see Table 25-17).

Cisplatin[141,142] is reported to produce response in 22% of patients and its role in combination chemotherapy regimens will be discussed later in this chapter. Triazinate is of interest because it is a folate antagonist that has demonstrated modest activity (15% partial response) in heavily pretreated

TABLE 25-18. *(continued)*

Drug Combination	No. of Responses/ No. of Patients	% Responses	Median Duration of Survival (Months)	Reference
FAMtx (5-FU + Adriamycin + methotrexate)	22/62	35 (15% CR, 20% PR)	6.0	169
	59/100	59 (12% CR, 47% PR)	9.0	170
Total	81/162	50		
FAMe (5-FU + Adriamycin + methyl-CCNU)	7/15	47	6.0	136
	3/10	30	8.5	154
	4/16	25	7.1	156
	11/39	29	5.5	151
Total	25/80	31		
FAP (5-FU + Adriamycin + cisplatin)	10/35	29	5.5	171
	8/16	50	10.5	172
	13/26	50 (11% CR, 39% PR)	9.0	173
	5/16	31	13.0	174
Total	36/93	39		
5-FU + mitomycin C + cytosine arabinoside	3/18	17	3.2	136
5-FU + Adriamycin + BCNU	18/35	51	12 *	175
	4/17	24	5.5	157
	40/94	43	8.2	176
Total	62/146	42		
FAM + triazinate	4/22	18	NA	177
FAM + BCNU	9/41	22	6	178
FAM + methyl-CCNU	2/18	11	6.2	179
	12/31	39	7.1	180
Total	14/49	29		

CR = complete response, PR = partial response.
* Survival duration in responders only.

patients with gastric cancer (see Table 25-17).[143] The response rate may be significantly higher in previously untreated patients. Triazinate may be useful in investigational combination therapy programs because it has single-agent activity and also may synergize with fluorinated pyrimidines. Although some single agents do have activity in stomach cancer, it should be emphasized that all the single agents have the shared liability of low response rates and short duration of response (3–5 months); also, complete responses to single agents are very rare. Therefore, single-agent chemotherapy for gastric cancer is of minimal practical benefit to the patient. For this reason, the polychemotherapy of stomach cancer is being pursued with increasing intensity.

Combination Chemotherapy

There have been numerous attempts to develop effective combination chemotherapy regimens using both single-agents known to be active and agents that have not been evaluated for single-agent activity. Table 25-18 reviews the published results of 16 combination chemotherapeutic regimens tested in patients with gastric cancer.

Two of the most extensively evaluated regimens in the United States have used 5-FU in combination with either BCNU or methyl-BCNU.[106,131] In a study reported by Kovach et al,[131] the combination of 5-FU and BCNU was compared with each drug alone in a randomized Phase III trial. All drugs were given IV in the following doses: 5-FU alone, 13.5 mg/kg/day for 5 days; BCNU alone, 50 mg/m²/day for 5 days; 5-FU + BCNU, 10 mg/kg/day and 40 mg/m²/day, respectively, for 5 days. Objective responses to therapy were 29% for 5-FU alone, 17% for BCNU alone, and 41% for 5-FU + BCNU. Median survival for patients treated with the combination was 7 months and was not significantly different from that seen with the single agents alone. However, there was a significant improvement in survival at 18 months for the patients treated with 5-FU + BCNU. At that point, 25% of the group receiving combination chemotherapy were alive, compared to fewer than 10% of those receiving either single agent.

The ECOG conducted a controlled randomized trial in advanced gastric cancer comparing the combination of 5-FU + methyl-CCNU with methyl-CCNU used alone.[106] The dosages in the combination were as follows: 5-FU, 300 mg/m²/day IV for 5 days with methyl-CCNU, 175 mg/m² given orally on the first day; this regimen was repeated at 7-week intervals. The dosage of methyl-CCNU alone was 200 mg/m² given in a single oral dose and repeated at 7-week intervals. The combination produced a 40% response rate and definitely was superior to methyl-CCNU alone, which produced an 8% response (p < 0.05).[106] A significant survival benefit was reported for the patients treated with 5-FU + methyl-CCNU in this trial. The median survival of patients treated with the combination was 20 weeks, whereas patients treated with methyl-CCNU lived a median of 13 weeks. The differences in survival may reflect the inferior response rate produced by methyl-CCNU (8%). Also, this modest improvement in survival may be secondary to the relatively high order of complete response in the patients treated with 5-FU plus methyl-CCNU (see Table 25-18).

An ECOG study reported in 1979 also brings into question the high response rate originally reported for 5-FU + methyl-CCNU.[137] This study compared 5-FU + methyl-CCNU, 5-FU + mitomycin C, and doxorubicin used as a single agent. The 5-FU + methyl-CCNU was used in a dosage schedule identical to that which had earlier produced a 40% response.[106] That response rate was not confirmed in the more recent study. Twelve (24%) of 49 patients receiving 5-FU + methyl-CCNU responded in this study, compared to 17 (32%) of 53 responding to 5-FU + mitomycin C. The patients in all arms of this study were similar as to sites of disease, extent of disease, and performance status. The survival curves for all arms were identical, with a median survival of 17 weeks. Finally, an ECOG study published in 1984 showed only a 14% response rate in 44 patients with advanced gastric cancer treated with 5-FU + methyl-CCNU.[151] The median survival for patients in this study was only 8 months.

The regimen of 5-FU + doxorubicin + methyl-CCNU has been shown to be active in gastric cancer.[136,154] This treatment produced an average response of 31% (see Table 25-18) and is well tolerated. Levi and associates[175] reported a 52% response in 35 patients treated with 5-FU + doxorubicin + BCNU. Two other studies performed with this combination reported response rates of 24% and 43%.[157,176] The overall experience with 5-FU + Adriamycin + BCNU has yielded a response rate of 42% (62 of 146 patients). The combination of 5-FU + Adriamycin + cisplatin has been evaluated in advanced gastric cancer.[171-174] Two studies report response rates of 31%[174] and 29%[171]; two other studies report response rates of 50%. The clinical trial reported by Moertel et al[173] is of particular interest since 11% of patients had complete responses. This treatment program is currently undergoing confirmation in a Phase III trial.

Triazinate in combination chemotherapy may have a role in the treatment of patients with advanced stomach cancer. A recent Phase III trial performed by the GITSG[162] has shown that the combination of 5-FU + Adriamycin + triazinate (FAT) produces significantly prolonged median survival (29 weeks) when compared to that produced by FAM (24 weeks). The respective year survival rates are 28% for FAT and 15% for FAM.

The combination of 5-FU + doxorubicin (Adriamycin) + mitomycin C (FAM) has been tested in 520 patients in 12 separate clinical trials with a cumulative response rate of 33% (173 of 520 patients). A large Phase II evaluation of FAM in 62 patients[132] reported an overall response rate of 42%. There was significant response in patients with major metastatic liver disease and large abdominal masses. Response was correlated with palliation of symptoms, and responding patients had marked improvement in performance status. In this Phase II trial responding patients survived a median of 13 months, compared to 3 months for nonresponding patients; however, there were no complete responses. FAM was well tolerated, with the only significant toxic effect being moderate myelosuppression.

The activity of the FAM regimen has been confirmed in both Phase II and Phase III trials.[161,168] Bitran and coworkers[161] in a small study found that 6 (55%) of 11 patients responded to FAM. In an ECOG Phase III study published in 1984,[151] 18 (39%) of 46 patients treated with FAM responded. This result is consistent with the order of response seen with FAM in Phase II studies. In a Phase III trial, the SWOG compared two dose schedules of FAM. The drugs given in the simultaneous schedule developed at Georgetown[132] were superior to the same drugs given sequentially. With the simultaneous schedule, 8 (40%) of 20 patients responded. With the sequential schedule, the response rate was 11% (4 of 26 patients). Differences in survival between these two treatment regimens were not significant. Of interest, the substitution of the furanyl derivative of 5-FU, Ftorafur, which may have less myelosuppressive toxicity than the other fluorinated pyrimidines, decreased the activity of FAM. Woolley and associates[181] reported responses in 3 (20%) of 15 patients with advanced gastric cancer treated with the regimen. The toxicity seen with the Ftorafur-substituted FAM regimen was significant and qualitatively different, since the Ftorafur caused major transient cerebellar dysfunction.

The North Central Cancer Therapy Group (NCCTG)[155] has reported results of a Phase III trial comparing 5-FU, 5-FU + doxorubicin, and the FAM regimen. Patients with both gastric and pancreatic cancer were included in the study. In gastric cancer, median survivals were between 6 and 7 months for all regimens. However, in the small number of patients with measurable cancer, FAM produced a superior response rate. Five (38%) of 13 patients treated with FAM had objective tumor regression, whereas the response rates for 5-FU + doxorubicin and 5-FU alone were 27% and 18%, respectively. It is not surprising that median survival was not improved with any of these regimens because fewer than 50% of patients responded.

Although partial response will not improve median survival, this outcome does result in palliation of symptoms. Combination chemotherapy produces partial response more frequently than single-agent treatment. Although FAM produces a consistent, if modest, response rate with tolerable toxic effects, FAM is far from ideal therapy. The major problem with FAM is that this regimen only rarely produces complete responses. In an analysis of 302 patients treated with FAM, only 7 (2%) had complete regression of disease.[182] It is clear that without a high rate of complete remission, no chemotherapy program will produce prolonged survival in patients with any form of advanced cancer.

Presently there has been interest in chemotherapy regimens utilizing biochemical modulation of antimetabolites in the treatment of gastric cancer. Machover et al[160] used 5-FU + folinic acid to treat 27 patients with advanced gastric cancer. Reduced folates stabilize the fluorodioxyuridylate (Fdump) thymidylate synthetase enzyme complex and thereby increase the effective cytotoxicity of 5-FU. Thirteen (48%) of 27 patients responded to 5-FU + folinic acid. One patient evidenced complete response. The value of fluorinated pyrimidine plus folinic acid in gastric cancer therapy must be confirmed in subsequent clinical trials. Another biochemical modulation of potential interest in stomach cancer is the use of methotrexate-"directed" 5-FU. Table 25-18 reports two studies[169,170] in which methotrexate, 5-FU, and Adriamycin produced responses in 81 (50%) of 162 patients. This response rate is particularly impressive, since 27% of patients had complete responses. These protocols used high-dose methotrexate (1.5 g/m²) with folinic acid rescue and were associated with considerable methotrexate-related toxicity, including treatment-related deaths. The results of these two European studies are of interest and will require confirmation.

The most important observation about the combination chemotherapy of advanced gastric cancer is the high order of activity evidenced by several regimens in this disease.[106,131,169,170,177] Response rates of 40% to 50% are distinctly uncommon in advanced GI adenocarcinomas, and the apparent responsiveness of gastric cancer has encouraged active investigation of polychemotherapy. In reviewing Table 25-18, however, it is apparent that not all studies with FAM, FAP, FAMe, or 5-FU + methyl-CCNU report response rates of 40% to 50%. Clinical oncologists must evaluate clinical trial design carefully for similarity of response criteria, prognostic factors, and other factors relating to patient selection to ensure that differences in response to the same regimens are not artifactual. It is hoped that confirmation of active combination chemotherapy regimens in advanced disease will translate into effective treatment for earlier stages of disease.

Recommendations

The first option in the treatment of any eligible patient with advanced gastric cancer should be entrance into a clinical trial. If this is not feasible, one could consider the use of a combination chemotherapy regimen such as FAM or FAP, because this approach may increase the probability of attaining partial remission and palliation of symptoms.

FUTURE CONSIDERATIONS

A major effort toward early diagnosis of gastric cancer is a necessity in countries with a high incidence of this disease. This chapter has described the success the Japanese have had with such an approach.[84] However, in the United States, where stomach cancer is not a major public health problem and, if anything, has been decreasing in incidence, massive screening programs for early diagnosis would hardly be cost-effective. Therefore, the future direction in gastric cancer management that the American clinician will deal with will concern attempts to improve therapy of this disease.

SURGERY

Complete surgical resection of the tumor remains the major curative therapy modality in patients with stomach cancer. There has also been interest in reoperation for attempted curative resection of recurrent disease in gastric cancer patients. The curative benefit of planned reoperations for gastric carcinoma was minimal in the University of Minnesota series—four conversions to disease-free status, but three operative deaths.[56] There is no justification for reoperation unless it has specific palliative intent. However, in future aggressive regional treatment protocols, reoperation may be indicated. At present, there is no indication that conventional treatment should include reoperation aimed at cure.

CHEMOTHERAPY PLUS RADIATION

In view of the patterns of treatment failure in gastric cancer, it appears that innovative combinations of chemotherapy plus radiation therapy versus polychemotherapy alone may be necessary to alter both short- and long-term survival in resectable as well as unresectable disease. Even after so-called curative resection, locoregional failure is a significant problem, as noted in both the University of Minnesota reoperative series[52] and autopsy series.[52,54] This knowledge must be tempered, however, by the fact that distant failures (distant metastases plus peritoneal spread occur more commonly than with colorectal cancer and the natural history is much shorter, perhaps because of the much higher incidence of poorly differentiated gastric lesions. Early tumor-related deaths in the GITSG study (protocol 8274) may be related to the fact that combined drug chemotherapy was not instituted until at least day 71 after onset of treatment, which may have been 4 to 6 weeks after operative resection or exploration (overall time after diagnosis, 13–17 weeks or more). If one saves the best chemotherapy for 3 to 4 months from the time of diagnosis in such a disease, the systemic component, if present, may then be beyond control.

In view of the major systemic failure problem with gastric cancers, there is a need to optimize the use of combination chemotherapy and irradiation. This may involve idealized sequencing of combined drug regimens before or concomitantly with irradiation in a manner that will result in acceptable toxicity, yet shorten intervals from operative intervention to the institution of combined drug chemotherapy, and the time between chemotherapy courses. The problem with systemic failures, however, was not alleviated in pilot programs at the MGH and the Mayo Clinic that used combined drug chemotherapy before and after either conventional radiation therapy (MGH: 5-FU + BCNU, or FAM) or radiation therapy given in two fractions per day (Mayo: FA + XRT + FAMe).

Since chemotherapy has not been shown to have definite

curative potential for advanced disease, the only patients with curable disease may be those without occult dissemination at initiation of treatment. Therefore, an alternate treatment approach is to provide the most effective locoregional treatment "up front" (x-irradiation, one or two daily fractions ± 5-FU, combined with resection whenever this can be accomplished before or after irradiation), followed by the most effective systemic treatment, such as FAM, FAP, or perhaps 5-FU + folinic acid if initial promising results are confirmed with this biochemical modulation. Other more recent approaches to chemotherapy with fluorinated pyrimidines may be useful in gastric cancer combined modality programs. Lokich et al[183] have demonstrated in a Phase III study in patients with advanced colon cancer that continuous IV infusion of 5-FU at 300 mg/m²/day is superior to bolus IV administration of the drug. The response rate in the infusion patients was 31%, versus 8% in patients treated with bolus 5-FU. Continuous low-dose infusion of 5-FU through a central catheter has minimal toxicity (mainly hand/foot syndrome) and is not associated with myelosuppression or GI toxicity. Such low-dose continuous fluorinated pyrimidine therapy may have a role in combination with radiation therapy in patients with stomach cancer.

Since liver metastases and peritoneal seeding are common both after resection and in patients with unresectable or residual disease treated with radiation therapy plus chemotherapy, such failures could possibly be prevented or delayed by extending external beam radiation portals to include the entire upper abdomen or total abdomen for a portion of treatment, or by treating the peritoneal surfaces with intraperitoneal radiocolloids or chemotherapy (of less potential value in lesions at or extending to the esophagogastric junction or beyond, since failures in the lung are also common). An external beam upper abdomen portal has an advantage over a total abdomen beam in that it would not significantly increase the amount of bone marrow included in the irradiation field, yet it potentially alters both liver failures (distant metastases) and upper abdomen peritoneal disease. In the Minnesota reoperative series,[52] peritoneal seeding was localized in 20 of 44 patients and, on the basis of serial reoperations in several other patients, was seen to progress from upper abdominal involvement to diffuse abdominal involvement. In a Japanese gastric cancer series by Nakajima and co-workers,[184] of 96 patients who had peritoneal seeding, 29 (30%) had implants only in the upper abdomen (above the transverse colon mesentery). In that series, the finding of positive peritoneal cytology was an independent negative prognostic factor with regard to survival, and peritoneal cytology might be used to make decisions on upper versus total abdomen prophylaxis. With either approach, the risks of radiation-induced hepatitis or nephritis may be increased, and tolerance problems should be worked out with residual or unresected disease before being considered in an adjuvant setting.

RADIATION TECHNIQUES AND DOSE MODIFIERS

The limited tolerance of the stomach and surrounding organs and tissues prevents a major increase in dose levels above 5000 to 5500 rad. With residual, unresectable, or re-

current disease, the most likely gains will come from combined radiation therapy and chemotherapy (chemotherapy plus radiation therapy plus chemotherapy), dose modifiers (sensitizers, protectors, hyperthermia), or, in selected cases, dose localization and increased doses with external beam or intraoperative irradiation.

For patients found to have locally unresectable cancers at initial exploration, it would be worthwhile to obtain a baseline CT study, deliver 4500 to 5000 rad, and restage the patient 3 to 4 weeks later. If the patient is without evidence of metastases and the lesion has shrunk or is stable on repeat CT, it would be justifiable to consider operative exploration and resection with an intraoperative or postoperative boost dose of irradiation. This sequence may in fact be preferable to the alternative of resecting lesions found to have disease adherence or fixation at the initial exploration, since this usually results in cutting through tumor and may produce an increased incidence of peritoneal or hematogenous failure.

The Japanese experience of achieving some long-term cures after partial resection with the addition of a single large dose of intraoperative radiation supports continued use of intraoperative irradiation alone or in combination with fractionated external beam irradiation or chemotherapy in Japan and other countries. In the latter circumstance, a dose of 1000 to 2000 rad could be delivered as a boost to the tumor bed and primary nodal areas after resection, or to areas of residual disease plus primary nodal sites after subtotal resection. Postoperative radiation therapy would then be used to deliver 4500 to 5000 rad to the areas at risk, based on both operative findings and pathologic reconstruction.

SUMMARY

Gastric malignancies present us with many challenges. Innovative combined modality approaches will be needed if survival is to be improved and toxic effects of treatment are to be acceptable. Careful and detailed intraoperative staging is imperative if seminal clinical trials are to be designed that will provide the information necessary for developing appropriate treatment strategies for this disease. Such strategies may include combinations of external beam and intraoperative irradiation plus resection for the local component, and systemic or intraperitoneal chemotherapy or wide-field irradiation, or a combination of these three, for therapy of intraabdominal or systemic disease. The role of biological response modifiers (cytokines, adoptive immunotherapy, and differentiating agents) in gastric cancer needs to be defined. The possibilities for clinical research in stomach cancer therapy are manifold.

REFERENCES

1. Silverberg E, Lubera J: Cancer Statistics. CA 36:9–25, 1986
2. Devesa SS, Silverman DT: Cancer incidence and mortality trends in the United States 1935–1974. JNCI 60:545–561, 1978
3. Dunham LJ, Bailar JC III: World maps of cancer mortality rates and frequency ratios. JNCI 41:155–203, 1968
4. Staszewski J: Migrant studies in alimentary tract cancer. Recent Results Cancer Res 39:85–97, 1971

5. Haenszel W, Kurihara M, Segi M et al: Stomach cancer among Japanese in Hawaii. JNCI 49:969–988, 1972
6. Moertel CG: The stomach. In Holland JF, Frei E III (eds): Cancer Medicine, pp 1760–1774. Philadelphia, Lea & Febiger, 1982
7. Haas JF, Schottenfeld D: Epidemiology of gastric cancer. In Lipkin M, Good RA (eds): Gastrointestinal Tract Cancer. Sloan-Kettering Cancer Series. New York, Plenum Medical, 1978
8. Selikoff IJ: Cancer risk of asbestos exposure. In Hiatt HH, Watson JD, Winsten JA (eds): Origins of Human Cancer, Book C, pp 1765–1784. New York, Cold Spring Harbor Laboratory, 1977
9. Aird I, Benthall HH, Roberts JAF: A relationship between cancer of the stomach and the ABO blood groups. Br Med J 1:799–801, 1953
10. Imai T, Kubo T, Watanabe H: Chronic gastritis in Japanese with reference to high incidence of gastric carcinoma. JNCI 47:179–195, 1971
11. Moertel CG: The stomach. In Holland JH, Frei E III (eds): Cancer Medicine, pp 1527–1541. Philadelphia, Lea & Febiger, 1973
12. Pack GT: Unusual tumors of the stomach. Ann NY Acad Sci 114:985, 1964
13. Phillips JC, Linsay JW, Kendall JA: Gastric leiomyosarcoma: Roentgenologic and clinical findings. Am J Dig Dis 15:239, 1970
14. Macon WL: Gastric lymphoma vs adenocarcinoma. A diagnostic problem. Arch Surg 114:305–306, 1979
15. Piper SW (ed): Stomach Cancer, p 41. Geneva, UICC Technical Report Series, 1978
16. Morson BC: Carcinoma arising from areas of intestinal metaplasia in the gastric mucosa. Br J Cancer 9:377, 1955
17. Higgins GA, Serlin O, Amadeo JH et al: Gastric cancer factors in survival. Surg Gastrointest 10:393, 1976
18. Rouviere H: Anatomy of the Human Lymphatic System, pp 183–187. Ann Arbor, Edwards Bros, 1938
19. Cady B, Choed DS: Changing patterns of gastric cancer. In Nieburgs HE (ed.): Third International Symposium on Detection and Prevention of Cancer, pp 2041–2049. New York, Decker, 1980
20. O'Brien MJ, Bunakoff R, Robbins EA et al: Early gastric cancer: Clinicopathologic study. Am J Med 78:195–202, 1985
21. Berkson J: Statistical smmary. In ReMine JH, Priestley JT, Berkson J (eds): Cancer of the Stomach, p 207. Philadelphia, WB Saunders, 1964
22. Collins WT, Gall EA: Gastric carcinoma, multicentric lesion. Cancer 5:62, 1952
23. Moertel CG, Reitemeier RJ: Advanced Gastrointestinal Cancer: Clinical Management and Chemotherapy, pp 3–21. New York, Harper & Row, 1969
24. Correa P: IAP Maude Abbott Lecture. Geographic pathology of cancer in Colombia. Int Pathol 11:16, 1970.
25. Correa P, Cuello C, Duque E: Carcinoma and intestinal metaplasia of the stomach in Colombian migrants. J Natl Cancer Inst 44:297, 1970
26. Piper DW (ed): Stomach Cancer, p 16. Geneva, UICC Technical Report Series, 1978
27. Kawachi T, Sugimura T: Abnormal differentiation of stomach epithelium: Intestinalization as the possible beginning of neoplastic change. In Ebert J, Okada T (eds): Mechanisms of Cell Change. New York, John Wiley & Sons, 1979
28. Piper DW (ed): Stomach Cancer, p 27. Geneva, UICC Technical Report Series, 1978
29. Matsukura N, Kawachi T, Sasajima K et al: Induction of intestinal metaplasia in the stomach of rats by N-methyl-N'-nitro-N-nitrosoguanadine. J Natl Cancer Inst 61:141, 1978
30. Sasajima K, Kawachi T, Matsukura N et al: Intestinal metaplasia and adenocarcinoma induced in the stomach of rats by N-propyl-N'-nitro-N-nitrosoguanidine. J Cancer Res Clin Oncol 94:201, 1979
31. Hofman NR: The relationship between pernicious anemia and cancer of the stomach. Geriatrics 25:90, 1970
32. Hitchcock CR, Schneiner SL. Early diagnosis of gastric cancer. Surg Gynecol Obstet 113:655, 1961
33. Lygidakis NJ: Gastric stump cancer after surgery for gastroduodenal ulcer. Ann R Coll Surg Engl 63:203–205, 1981
34. Giarelli L, Melato M, Stauta G et al: Gastric resection a cause of high frequency of gastric carcinoma. Cancer 52:1113–1116, 1983
35. Kuru M: On cancers developed upon ulcerative lesions of the stomach: A study of the regeneration of the mucous membrane of the stomach with special reference to its malignant transformation. Gann 44:47, 1953
36. Ming SC: Histogenesis and premalignant lesions. JAMA 228:886, 1974
37. Oota K: On the nature of the ulcerative changes in early carcinoma of the stomach. Gann Monogr 3:141, 1968
38. Tomaslo J: Gastric polyps. Histologic types and their relationship to gastric carcinoma. Cancer 27:1346, 1971
39. Ming SC, Goldman H: Gastric polyps: A histogenetic classification and its relation to carcinoma. Cancer 18:721, 1965
40. Piper DW (ed): Stomach Cancer, p 30. Geneva, UICC Technical Report Series, 1978
41. Thunold S, Wetteland P: Ulcer-carcinoma of the stomach in a 10-year biopsy series. A follow-up study of 19 patients. Arch Pathol Microbiol Scand 56:155, 1962
42. Piper DW (ed): Stomach Cancer, p 31. Geneva, UICC Technical Report Series, 1978
43. Larson NE, Cain JC, Bartholomew LG: Prognosis of the medically treated small gastric ulcer; comparison of follow-up data in two series. N Engl J Med 164:119, 1961
44. Cohn I Jr: The meaning of lymph node metastases and their treatment: Cancer of the stomach, pancreas, and small bowel. In Weiss L, Gilbert HA, Ballon SG (eds): Lymphatic System Metastases, p 262. Boston, GK Hall, 1980
45. Dupont JB Jr, Cohn I Jr: Gastric adenocarcinoma. Curr Probl Cancer 4:25, 1980
46. Dupont JB Jr, Lee JR, Burton GR et al: Adenocarcinoma of the stomach: Review of 1497 cases. Cancer 41:941, 1978
47. Arhelger SW, Lober PH, Wangensteen OH: Dissection of the hepatic pedicle and retropancreaticoduodenal areas for cancer of the stomach. Surgery 38:675, 1955
48. Coller FA, Kay EB, McIntyre RS: Regional lymphatic metastases of carcinoma of the stomach. Arch Surg 43:748, 1941
49. Clarke JS, Cruze K, El Farra S et al: The natural history and results of surgical therapy for carcinoma of the stomach: An analysis of 250 cases. Am J Surg 102:143, 1961
50. Warren S: Studies on tumor metastasis: IV. Metastases of cancer of the stomach. N Engl J Med 209:825, 1933
51. Warwick M: Analysis of one hundred and seventy-six cases of carcinoma of the stomach submitted to autopsy. Ann Surg 88:216, 1928
52. Papachristou DN, Fortner JG: Local recurrence of gastric adenocarcinomas after gastrectomy. J Surg Oncol 18:47–53, 1981
53. McNeer G, Vandenberg H, Donn FY et al: A critical evaluation of subtotal gastrectomy for the cure of cancer of the stomach. Ann Surg 134:2, 1951
54. Thomson FB, Robins RE: Local recurrence following subtotal resection for gastric carcinoma. Surg Gynecol Obstet 95:351, 1952
55. Wisbeck WA, Becker EM, Russell AH: Adenocarcinoma of the stomach: Autopsy observations with therapeutic implications for the radiation oncologist. Radiother Oncol 7:13–18, 1986
56. Gunderson LL, Sosin H: Adenocarcinoma of the stomach—areas of failure in a reoperation series (second or symptomatic looks): Clinicopathologic correlation and implications for adjuvant therapy. Int J Radiat Oncol Biol Phys 8:1–11, 1982
57. Landry J, Tepper JE, Wood WL et al: Patterns of failure following curative resection of gastric carcinoma: ASTRO Proceedings 1986. Int J Radiat Oncol Biol Phys vol 12(1):119, 1986
58. Adashek K, Sanger J, Longmire WP Jr: Cancer of the stomach. Review of consecutive ten-year intervals. Ann Surg 189:6, 1979
59. Goldsmith HS, Ghosh BC: Carcinoma of the stomach. Am J Surg 120:317, 1970
60. Kelsey JR Jr: Cancer of the Stomach: A Clinical Guide for Diagnosis and Treatment. Springfield, Ill, Charles C Thomas, 1967
61. LaDue JS, Murison PJ, McNeer G et al: Symptomatology and diagnosis of gastric cancer. Arch Surg 60:305, 1950
62. Shahon DB, Hdorowitz S, Kelly WD: Cancer of the stomach: An analysis of 1,152 cases. Surgery 39:204, 1956
63. McNeer G, Pack GT: Malignant tumors of the stomach. In Pack GT, Ariel IM (eds): Treatment of Cancer and Allied Diseases, vol 5, pp 111–268. New York, Paul B Hoeber, 1962
64. Hoerr SO: Prognosis for carcinoma of the stomach. Surg Gynecol Obstet 137:205, 1973
65. Hoerr SO, Hodgman RW: Carcinoma of the stomach: An interpretive review. Am J Surg 107:620, 1964
66. Beahrs OH, Myers MH (eds): Manual for Staging of Cancer, p 67. Philadelphia, JB Lippincott, 1983
67. Kennedy BJ: TNM classification for stomach cancer. Cancer 26:971, 1970
68. Japanese Research Society for Gastric Cancer: The general rules for the gastric cancer study in surgery. Jpn J Surg 3:61, 1973
69. Okajima K: Surgical treatment of gastric cancer with special reference to lymph node removal. Acta Med Okayama 31:3269, 1977
70. Desmond AM: Radical surgery in treatment of carcinoma of the stomach. Proc R Soc Med 69:867, 1976
71. ReMine WH, Priestley JT, Berkson J: Cancer of the Stomach. Philadelphia, WB Saunders, 1964
72. Gastrointestinal Tumor Study Group: Controlled trial of adjuvant chemotherapy following curative resection for gastric cancer. Cancer 49:1116–1122, 1982
73. Antoniolli DA, Goldman H: Changes in the location and type of gastric adenocarcinoma. CA 50:775–781, 1982
74. Gastrointestinal Tumor Study Group: A comparison of combination chemotherapy and combined modality therapy for locally advanced gastric carcinoma. Cancer 49:1771–1777, 1982
75. Cooley RN: The diagnostic accuracy of upper gastrointestinal radiologic studies. Am J Med Sci 242:628, 1961
76. Laufer I: Double contrast radiology in the diagnosis of gastrointestinal cancer. In Glass J (ed): Progress in Gastroenterology, pp 643–669. New York, Grune & Stratton, 1977
77. Laufer I: A simple method for routine double contrast study of the upper gastrointestinal tract. Radiology 117:513, 1975
78. Bockus HL: Gastroenterology, 2nd ed, vol I, pp 743–801. Philadelphia, WB Saunders, 1963
79. Winawer SJ, Melamed M, Sherlock P: Potential of endoscopy, biopsy, and cytology in the diagnosis and management of patients with cancer. Clin Gastroenterol 5:575, 1976
80. Winawer SJ, Sherlock P, Hajdu SI: The role of upper gastrointestinal endoscopy in patients with cancer. Cancer 37:440, 1976
81. Wittenberg J: Computed tomography of the body. N Engl J Med 309:1224–1230, 1983
82. Nathanson L: Remote effects of cancer in the host. In Horton J, Hill L (eds): Clinical Oncology, pp 49–85. Philadelphia, WB Saunders, 1977

83. Schein PS: Tumor markers. In Beeson P, McDermott W, Wyngaarden J (eds): Textbook of Medicine, pp 1411–1413. Philadelphia, WB Saunders, 1979

84. Kaneko E, Nakamura T, Umeda N et al: Outcome of gastric carcinoma detected by gastric mass survey in Japan. Gut 18:6–26, 1977

85. Prolla JC, Kobayashi S, Kirsner JB: Gastric cancer: Some recent improvements in diagnosis based upon the Japanese experience. Arch Intern Med 124:238, 1969

86. Longmire WP Jr: Total gastrectomy for carcinoma of the stomach. Surg Gynecol Obstet 84:21, 1947

87. Miwa K: Advances in treatment of stomach carcinoma in Japan. In Hirayama T (ed): Epidemiology of Stomach Cancer: Key Questions and Answers, pp 105–110. Tokyo, WHO, 1977

88. Pack GT, McNeer G: Total gastrectomy for cancer. A collective review of the literature and an original report of twenty cases. Int Abstr Surg 77:265, 1943

89. Paulino F. Roselli A: Carcinoma of the stomach, with special reference to total gastrectomy. Curr Probl Surg, pp 1–72, Dec 1973

90. Ransom HK: Cancer of the stomach. Surg Gynecol Obstet 96:275, 1953

91. Rush BF Jr, Brown MW, Ravitch MM: Total gastrectomy: An evaluation of its use in the treatment of gastric cancer. Cancer 13:643, 1960

92. Lumpkin WM, Crow RL Jr, Hernandez CM et al: Carcinoma of the stomach: Review of 1,035 cases. Ann Surg 159:919, 1964

93. Serlin O, Keehn RJ, Higgins GA et al: Factors related to survival following resection for gastric carcinoma. Cancer 40:1318, 1977

94. Ekbom GA, Gleysteen JJ: Gastric malignancy: Resection for palliation. Surgery 88:476, 1980

95. Diehl JT, Hermann RE, Cooperman AM, Hoerr SO: Gastric carcinoma. A ten-year review. Ann Surg 198:9, 1983

96. Lygidakis NJ: Total gastrectomy for gastric carcinoma: A retrospective study of different procedures and assessment of a new technique of gastric reconstruction. Br J Surg 68:649, 1981

97. Nelson PG, Collier N: Carcinoma of the stomach: The need for a new approach. Aust NZJ Surg 52:358, 1982

98. Inberg MV, Heinonen R, Lauren P et al: Total and proximal gastrectomy in the treatment of gastric carcinoma: A series of 305 cases. World J Surg 5:249, 1981

99. Dixon WJ, Longmire WP, Holden WD: Use of triethylenethiophosphoramide as an adjuvant to the surgical treatment of gastric and colorectal carcinoma: Ten year follow-up. Ann Surg 173:16, 1971

100. Serlin O, Wolkoff JS, Amadeo JM et al: Use of 5-fluorodeoxyuridine (FudR) as an adjuvant to the surgical management of carcinoma of the stomach. Cancer 24:223, 1969

101. Higgins GA, Amadeo JH, Smith DE et al: Efficacy of prolonged intermittent therapy with combined 5-FU and methyl-CCNU following resection for gastric carcinoma. Cancer 52:1105, 1983

102. Engstrom P, Lavin P: Post-operative adjuvant therapy for gastric cancer patients. Proc Am Soc Clin Oncol 2:114, 1983

103. Galiano R, McCracken JD, Chen T: Adjuvant chemotherapy with 5-fluorouracil, adriamycin, and mitomycin (FAM) in gastric cancer. Proc Am Soc Clin Oncol 2:114, 1983

103a. Krook JE, O'Connell MJ, Wieand HS et al: Adjuvant therapy of gastric cancer with doxorubicin and 5-fluorouracil. Proc Am Soc Clin Oncol 7:93, 1988

104. Nakajima T, Takahashi T, Takagi K: Comparison of 5-FU with Ftorafur in adjuvant chemotherapies with combined inductive and maintenance therapies for gastric cancer. J Clin Oncol 2:1366–1371, 1984

105. Lawrence W: Nutritional consequences of surgical resection of gastrointestinal tract for cancer. Cancer Res 37:2379, 1977

106. Moertel CG, Mittelman JA, Bakermeier RF et al: Sequential and combination chemotherapy of advanced gastric cancer. Cancer 38:678, 1976

107. Luxton RW, Kunkler PB: Radiation nephritis. Acta Radiol 2:169, 1964

108. Goffinet DR, Glatstein E, Zuks Z, Kaplan HS: Abdominal irradiation in non-Hodgkin's lymphoma. Cancer 37:2797, 1976

109. Gunderson LL, Hoskins B, Cohen A et al: Combined modality treatment of gastric cancer. Proc ASTR Int J Radiol Oncol 5:118, 1979

110. Willett C, Tepper JE, Orlow EL et al: Renal complications secondary to treatment of upper abdominal malignancies. ASTRO Proceedings, 1985

111. Goldstein HM, Rogers LF, Fletcher GH, Dodd GD: Radiological manifestations of radiation-induced injury to the normal upper gastrointestinal tract. Radiology 117:135, 1975

112. Nordman E, Kauppinen C: The value of megavolt therapy in carcinoma of the stomach. Strahlentherapie 144:635, 1972

113. Roswit B, Malsky SJ, Reid CB: Radiation tolerance of the gastrointestinal tract. Radiat Ther Oncol 6:160–181, 1972

114. Buskirk SJ, Gunderson LL, Nagorney DM et al: Analysis of failure following curative radiation of extrahepatic bile duct cancers. Int J Radiat Oncol Biol Phys 12:120, 1986

115. Abe M, Yabumoto E, Takahashi M, Adachi H, Yoshi M, Mori K: Intra-operative radiotherapy of gastric cancer. Cancer 45:40, 1980

116. Asakawa H, Otawa K, Watarai J: High energy x-ray therapy for stomach carcinoma, second report: The evaluation of radiotherapy for the early and the inoperable stomach carcinoma. Nippon Acta Radiol 31:505, 1971 (English tables and extended summary)

117. Asakawa H, Takeda T: High energy x-ray therapy of gastric carcinoma. J Jpn Soc Cancer Ther 8:362, 1973

118. Hoshi H: Histologic study on the effect of preoperative irradiation on gastric cancer. Tohoku J Exp Med 96:293, 1968

119. Takahashi T: Studies on preoperative and postoperative telecolbalt therapy in gastric cancer. Nippon Acta Radiol 24:129, 1964 [English tables and abstract]

120. Wieland C, Hymmen U: Megavoltage therapy for malignant gastric tumors (abstr). Strahlentherapie 140:20, 1970

121. Childs DS, Moertel CG, Holbrook MA et al: Treatment of unresectable adenocarcinomas of the stomach with a combination of 5-fluorouracil and radiation. AJR 102:541, 1968

122. Falkson G, Falkson HC: Fluorouracil and radiotherapy in gastrointestinal cancer. Lancet 2:1252, 1969

123. Lagunova IG, Cybulskij BA, Kornev II et al: Ausseinander folgende Strahlentherapie mit einem 25-meV Betatron and Chemotherapie mit Fluoruracil zur Behandlung von Kranken mit fortgeschrittenem Krebs des oberen Magenabschnittes (abstr). Radiobiol Radiother (Berl) 13:307, 1978

124. Moertel CG, Childs DS, O'Fallon JR et al: Combined 5-fluorouracil and radiation therapy as a surgical adjuvant for poor prognosis gastric carcinoma. J Clin Oncol 2:1249, 1984

125. Haas L, Vaikevicius V, Bukowski R et al: Southwest Oncology Group (SWOG) pilot study of radiotherapy (R) + 5-fluorouracil (F) + adriamycin (A) + mitomycin C (M) in patients with minimal residual gastric cancer (abstr). Proc Am Soc Clin Oncol 21:342, 1980

126. Lingos T, Tepper JE, Gunderson LL et al: Adjuvant FAM–Rad–FAM after resection of high risk gastric carcinoma. Int J Radiat Oncol Biol Phys 11:110, 1985

127. Schein PS, Smith FP, Dritschilo A et al: Phase I-II trial of combined modality FAM plus split-course radiation (FAM-RT-FAM) for locally advanced gastric and pancreatic cancer: A Mid-Atlantic Oncology Program study. Abstr Am Soc Clin Oncol 1983:126, 1983

128. O'Connell MJ, Gunderson LL, Moertel CG et al: A pilot study to determine clinical tolerability of intensive combined modality therapy for locally unresectable gastric cancer. Int J Radiat Oncol Biol Phys 11:1827, 1985

129. Abe M, Takahashi M: Intraoperative radiotherapy: The Japanese experience. Int J Radiat Oncol Biol Phys 5:863–868, 1981

130. Boice JD, Greene MH, Killen JY et al: Leukemia and preleukemia after adjuvant treatment of gastrointestinal cancer with Semustine (methyl-CCNU). N Engl J Med 309:1079–1084, 1983

131. Kovach JS, Moertel CG, Schutt AJ: A controlled study of combined 1, 3-bis-2-chloroethyl-l-nitrosourea and 5-flurouracil therapy for advanced gastric and pancreatic cancer. Cancer 33:563, 1974

132. Macdonald JS, Schein PS, Woolley PV et al: 5-Fluorouracil, mitomycin-C, and adriamycin (FAM): A new combination chemotherapy program for advanced gastric carcinoma. Ann Intern Med 93:533, 1980

133. Schein PS, Smith FP, Woolley PV et al: Current management of advanced and locally unresectable gastric carcinoma. Cancer 50:2590–2596, 1982

134. Comis RL, Carter SK: Integration of chemotherapy into combined modality treatment of solid tumors: III. Gastric cancer. Cancer Treat Rev 1:221, 1974

135. Moertel CG: Chemotherapy of gastrointestinal cancer. Clin Gastroenterol 5:777, 1976

136. Gastrointestinal Tumor Study Group: Phase II–III chemotherapy studies in advanced gastric cancer. Cancer Treat Rep 63:1871, 1979

137. Moertel CG, Lavin PT: Phase II–III chemotherapy studies in advanced gastric cancer. Cancer Treat Rep 63:1863, 1979

138. Livingston RB, Carter SK: Single Agents in Cancer Chemotherapy. New York, IFI/Plenum, 1970

139. Moore G, Bross I, Ausman R et al: Effects of chlorambucil (NSC 3088) in 374 patients with advanced cancer. Cancer Chemother Rep 52:661, 1968

140. Hurley JD, Ellison EH, Carey LL: Treatment of advanced cancer of the gastrointestinal tract with antitumor agents. Gastroenterology 41:557, 1961

141. Lacave A, Izarzugaza I, Aparicio L et al: Phase II clinical trial of cisdichlorodiamminoeplatinum in gastric cancer. Am J Clin Oncol 6:35–38, 1983

142. Beer M, Cocconi G, Ceci G et al: A phase II study of cisplatin in advanced gastric cancer. Eur J Cancer Clin Oncol 19:717–720, 1983

143. Bruckner HW, Lokich JJ, Stablein DM: Studies of Baker's antifol, methotrexate, and Razoxane in advanced gastric cancer: A gastrointestinal tumor study group report. Cancer Treat Rep 66:1713–1717, 1982

144. Cazap E, Bruno M, Levy D et al: Phase II trial of 4'-epi-doxorubicin (4'-epi-dx) in advanced gastric cancer. Proc Am Soc Clin Pathol 5:91, 1986

145. Kelsen D, Sternberg C, Einzig A et al: Phase II study of carboplatin (CBDCA) in advanced upper gastrointestinal tract malignancy. Proc Am Soc Clin Oncol 3:141, 1984

146. Panettiere F, Jones S, Oishi N et al: Bisantrene hydrochloride in gastric adenocarcinoma: A Southwest Oncology Group study. Med Pediatr Oncol 14:78–80, 1986

147. The Southeastern Cancer Study Group: m-AMSA treatment of advanced colorectal, pancreatic, and gastric carcinoma. Proc Am Soc Clin Oncol 22:454, 1981

148. Bjerkeset T, Fjosne H: Comparison of oral ftorafur and intravenous 5-fluorouracil in patients with advanced cancer of the stomach, colon or rectum. Oncology 43:212–215, 1986

149. Jones R: Mitomycin-C: A preliminary report of studies of human pharmacology and initial therapeutic trial. Cancer Chemother Rep 2:3, 1959

150. Baker IH, Caoili EM, Izbick VK: A comparative study of mitomycin-C and profiromycin. Proc Am Soc Clin Oncol 15:182, 1974

151. Douglass H, Lavin P, Goudsmit A et al: An Eastern Cooperative Oncology Group evaluation of combinations of methyl-CCNU, mitomycin-C, Adriamycin, and 5-fluorouracil in advanced measurable gastric cancer (Est 2277). J Clin Oncol 2:1372–1381, 1984

152. Buroker T, Kim P, Grappe C et al: 5-FU infusion with mitomycin-C versus 5-FU infusion with methyl-CCNU in the treatment of advanced upper gastrointestinal cancer. Cancer 44:1215–1221, 1979

153. The Southwest Oncology Group: Randomized prospective trial comparing 5-fluorouracil (NSC-19893) to 5-fluorouracil and methyl-CCNU (NSC-95441) in advanced gastrointestinal cancer. Cancer Treat Rep 60:733–737, 1976

154. The Gastrointestinal Tumor Study Group: A comparative clinical assessment of combination chemotherapy in the management of advanced gastric carcinoma. Cancer 49:1362–1366, 1982

155. Cullinan S, Moertel C, Fleming T et al: A comparison of three chemotherapeutic regimens in the treatment of advanced pancreatic and gastric carcinoma. JAMA 253:2061–2067, 1985

156. The Gastrointestinal Tumor Study Group: randomized study of combination chemotherapy in unresectable gastric cancer. Cancer 53:13–17, 1984

157. Jamieson G, Gill P: A prospective trial of 5-FU and BCNU in the treatment of advanced gastric cancer. Aust NZ J Surg 5:16–19, 1981

158. Schnitizler G, Queisser W, Heim M et al: Phase III study of 5-FU and carmustine versus 5-FU, carmustine and doxorubicin in advanced gastric cancer. Cancer Treat Rep 70:477–479, 1986

159. O'Connell M, Schutt A, Moertel C et al: Phase II clinical trial of triazinate in combination with mitomycin-C for patients with advanced gastric cancer. Proc Am Soc Clin Oncol 5:82, 1986

160. Machover D, Goldschmidt E, Chollet P et al: Treatment of advanced colorectal and gastric adenocarcinomas with 5-fluorouracil and high dose folinic acid. J Clin Oncol 4:685–696, 1986

161. Bitran JD, Desser RK, Kozloff MF et al: Treatment of metastatic pancreatic and gastric adenocarcinomas with 5-fluorouracil, Adriamycin, and mitomycin-C (FAM). Cancer Treat Rep 63:2049, 1979

162. Bruckner HW, Stablein DM (for the Gastrointestinal Tumor Study Group): A randomized study of 5-FU, methyl-CCNU, cis-platinum, or triazinate for treatment of advanced gastric cancer. Proc Am Soc Clin Oncol 5:90, 1986

163. Benetta G, Fraschini P, Labianca R et al: The value of FAM polychemotherapy in advanced gastric cancer. Proc Am Soc Clin Oncol 1:103, 1982

164. The Southwest Oncology Group: 5-Fluorouracil, Adriamycin, and mitomycin-C ± vincristine (FAM vs V-FAM) compared to chlorozotocin, mAMSA and dihydroxyanthracenedione with unimpressive differences. Proc Am Soc Clin Oncol 2:122, 1983

165. Cummingham D, Soukop M, McArdle C et al: Advanced gastric cancer: Experience in Scotland using 5-fluorouracil, Adriamycin, and mitomycin-C. Br J Surg 71:673–676, 1984

166. Haim N, Cohen Y, Honigman J et al: Treatment of advanced gastric carcinoma with 5-fluorouracil, Adriamycin, and mitomycin-C (FAM). Cancer Chemother Pharmacol 8:277–280, 1982

167. Haim N, Epelbaum R, Cohen Y et al: Further studies on the treatment of advanced gastric cancer by 5-fluorouracil, Adriamycin, and mitomycin-C (modified FAM). Cancer 54:1999–2002, 1984

168. Panettiere F, Haas C, McDonald B et al: Drug combinations in the treatment of gastric adenocarcinoma. J Clin Oncol 2:420–424, 1984

169. Wils J, Bleiberg H, Dalesio O et al: An EORTC Gastrointestinal Group evaluation of the combination of sequential methotrexate and 5-fluorouracil, combined with Adriamycin in advanced measurable gastric cancer. J Clin Oncol 4:1799–1803, 1986

170. Klein H, Wickramanayake P, Farrokh G: 5-FU, adriamycin, and methotrexate: A combination protocol (FAMTX) for treatment of metastasized stomach cancer. Proc Am Soc Clin Oncol 5:84, 1986

171. Cazap E, Gisselbrecht C, Smith F et al: Phase II trials of 5-FU, doxorubicin, and cisplatin in advanced, measurable adenocarcinoma of the lung and stomach. Cancer Treat Rep 70:781–783, 1986

172. Wagener D, Burghouts J, van Dam F et al: A Phase II trial of 5-fluorouracil, Adriamycin, and cisplatin (FAP) in advanced gastric cancer. Proc Am Soc Clin Oncol 115, 1983

173. Moertel C, Rubin J, O'Connel M et al: A phase II study of combined 5-fluorouracil, doxorubicin, and cisplatin in the treatment of advanced upper gastrointestinal adenocarcinomas. J Clin Oncol 4:1053–1057, 1986

174. Robinson E, Haim N, Eppelbaum R et al: Phase II trials in the treatment of advanced gastric cancer. Proc Am Soc Clin Oncol 4:77, 1985

175. Levi J, Dalley D, Aroney R: Improved combination chemotherapy in advanced gastric cancer. Br Med J 2:1471–1473, 1979

176. Levi J, Fox R, Tattersall M et al: Analysis of a prospectively randomized comparison of doxorubicin versus 5-fluorouracil, doxorubicin, and BCNU in advanced gastric cancer: Implications for future studies. J Clin Oncol 4:1348–1355, 1986

177. Ahlgren J, Smith F, Harvey J et al: A phase II study of FAM plus triazinate for advanced measurable gastric carcinoma. Proc Am Soc Clin Oncol 3:145, 1984

178. De Lisi V, Cocconi G, Tonato M et al: Randomized comparison of 5-FU alone or combined with carmustine, doxorubicin, and mitomycin (BAFMi) in the treatment of advanced gastric cancer. Cancer Treat Rep 70:481–485, 1986

179. Bunn P, Nugent J, Ihde D et al: 5-Fluorouracil, methyl-CCNU, Adriamycin, and mitomycin C in the treatment of advanced gastric cancer. Cancer Treat Rep 62:1287–1293, 1978

180. Karlin D, Stroehlein J, Bennetts R et al: Phase I–II study of the combination of 5-FU, doxorubicin, mitomycin, and semustine (FAMMe) in the treatment of adenocarcinoma of the stomach, gastroesophageal junction, and pancreas. Cancer Treat Rep 66:1613–1617, 1982

181. Woolley PV, Macdonald JS, Smythe I et al: A phase II trial of Ftorafur, Adriamycin, and mitomycin-C (FAM II) in advanced gastric adenocarcinoma. Cancer 44:1211, 1979

182. Macdonald JS, Gohmann J: Chemotherapy of gastric cancer. Semin Oncol 15(suppl 4):42–49, 1988

183. Lokich J, Ahlgren J, Gullo J, Mid-Atlantic Oncology Program: A randomized trial of standard bolus 5-FU vs. protracted infusional 5-FU in advanced colon cancer. Proc Am Soc Clin Oncol 6:81, 1987

184. Nakajima T, Harashima S, Hirata M et al: Prognostic and therapeutic values of peritoneal cytology in gastric cancer. Acta Cytol 22:225–229, 1978

MURRAY F. BRENNAN

TIMOTHY KINSELLA

MICHAEL FRIEDMAN

CHAPTER 26 *Cancer of the Pancreas*

Pancreatic cancer is the fourth largest cancer killer in adults in the United States. The incidence of new cases of the disease and the death rate each year remain very close. In 1988, approximately 27,000 new cases will be seen in the United States, and 24,500 deaths will eventually result. The incidence is exceeded only by lung, colon and rectum, prostate, and breast cancer(s).

EPIDEMIOLOGIC CONSIDERATIONS

Because most patients with pancreatic cancer die of the disease, mortality data can be a good indicator of incidence provided that diagnostic accuracy is high.[1] Diagnostic accuracy can be checked by comparing the number of cases histologically confirmed at operation, biopsy, or autopsy with the number of cases diagnosed. For cancer of the pancreas, this varies from 75% to 95%.[1]

Cancer of the pancreas is increasing, and age-specific death rates increase with age (Fig. 26-1). The median age of presentation in national surveys is 69.2 years for men and 69.5 years for women from 1973 through 1977.[2] The overall male–female ratio of patients suspected of having peripancreatic cancer, presenting to Memorial Sloan-Kettering Cancer Center from October 1983 to October 1986, was 1.2:1. This differs from the male–female ratio of 1.7:1.0 for pancreatic cancer deaths in other series.[3] The male–female ratio differs according to age and has been previously reported for pancreatic cancer deaths varying from 2:1 for patients younger than age 40 to 1:1 for patients older than age 80. Our present data suggest that the male–female ratios for age at presentation younger than 40 are 3:1, 1.8:1 for 41 to 50 years; 1.2:1 for 51 to 80 years; and 1.1:1 for patients older than 80. The overall persistent male preponderance is completely reversed, however, in the Native Indian population in New Mexico (Fig. 26-2).[4]

The incidence of pancreatic cancer in several predominantly Spanish populations varies from 3.0 per 100,000 women in Puerto Rico to 11.7 per 100,000 Spanish men in New Mexico (Table 26-1). These racial differences are emphasized by the incidence in black men in Los Angeles (9.5 per 100,000) compared with the rate in Chinese men in the same city of 2.0 per 100,000 (Fig. 26-3). Intermediate rates are seen for the United States white population, the Spanish population, and the Japanese population.

The incidence in countries of origin and in first-generation and second-generation immigrants has been examined (Fig. 26-4). The rate in the first generation rapidly increases to the rate of U.S. whites. This is not solely due to smoking, although it may account for the effect in Japanese and Chinese populations.[5]

The influence of birthplace has been examined in Israel, and the incidence of carcinoma of the pancreas varies from 10.4 per 100,000 men born in Europe or America to 5.6 per

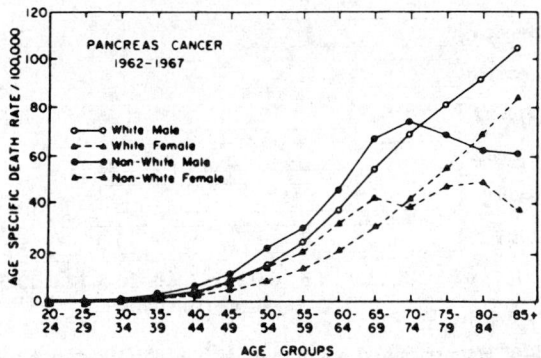

FIG. 26-1. Increasing U.S. age-specific mortality rates for cancer of the pancreas, by race and sex. (Levin DL, Connelly RR: Cancer of the pancreas. Available epidemiologic information and its implications. Cancer 31:1231–1236, 1973)

TABLE 26-1. Incidence of Pancreatic Cancer in Selected Areas by Sex

Location	Men*	Women*
New Mexico		
Spanish	11.7	9.2
Other white	10.1	6.6
American Indian	5.2	10.4
Cuba	4.9	3.2
Puerto Rico	4.9	3.0
Los Angeles		
Spanish	7.5	5.0
Other white	8.1	5.0
Cali, Colombia	5.0	3.2
Spain		
Navarra	4.0	2.6
Zaragoza	4.9	1.8

World Health Organization: Cancer Incidence in Five Continents, vol IV. IARC Sci Publ 42, 1982.
*Per 100,000 population.

100,000 men born in Israel. In non-Jewish residents, the incidence is 3.3 per 100,000 (Fig. 26-5).

Similar wide variations can be demonstrated in male incidence at various sites within different countries. For example, incidences vary from 11.0 per 100,000 in Ontario, Canada, to 3.7 in the Northwestern Territory of Canada. Countries with a high incidence are illustrated in Figure 26-6. There has been a progressive international increase in the incidence of pancreatic cancer. In England and Wales, from 1911 to 1971, the mortality from cancer of the pancreas in both men and women has increased at least fivefold.[6]

ETIOLOGY

Several environmental factors have been associated with an increased risk of pancreatic carcinoma, although the exact cause remains unclear. Pancreatic carcinoma, like several other common malignancies, appears to be more prevalent among persons in lower socioeconomic groups.[7] Close scrutiny of the available epidemiologic studies shows that pancreatic carcinoma has less of a demographic association with

social class than do other common malignancies such as breast and lung carcinoma.[3,7]

Several dietary factors have been implicated. At least one study showed a positive correlation between coffee consumption and pancreatic carcinoma.[8] In this case-control study, patients with carcinoma of the pancreas were found to have a history of greater coffee consumption than the control group of patients with benign gastrointestinal disorders. Because the control group contained patients with peptic ulcer disease and had an overall average coffee intake below the level of consumption for the general population, it is difficult to confirm whether patients with cancer of the pancreas actually consumed more coffee than would be considered average. There have been at least two other studies that have not confirmed the association of coffee intake and pancreatic carcinoma.[9,10]

One study suggested an association between alcohol consumption and an increased risk of carcinoma of the pancreas.[11] In this study of Finnish men with a history of alcohol abuse, an excess of pancreatic carcinoma was found, compared with the overall Finnish male population. At least three other studies have shown little or no correlation between alcohol consumption and pancreatic carcinoma.[12-14]

FIG. 26-2. Male-to-female ratio for varying populations with pancreatic cancer. Note the major difference in the American Indian population in New Mexico. (World Health Organization: Cancer Incidence in Five Continents, vol IV. IARC Sci Publ 42, 1982)

FIG. 26-3. Incidence of pancreatic cancer. Influence of race in a single geographic area: Los Angeles. (World Health Organization: Cancer Incidence in Five Continents, vol IV. IARC Sci Publ 42, 1982)

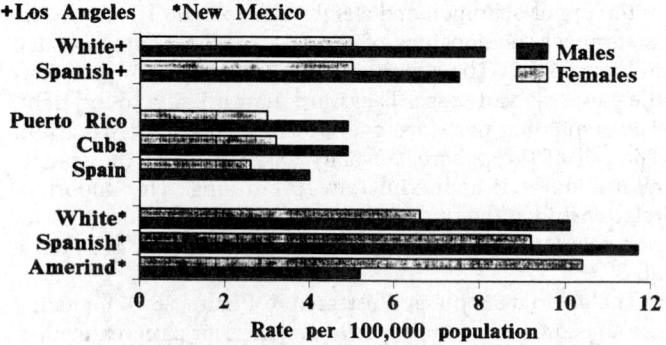

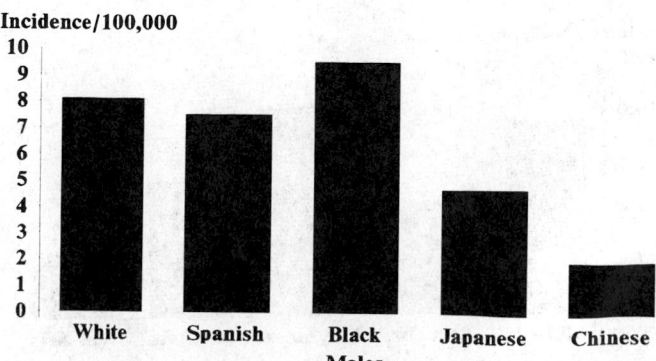

MALES

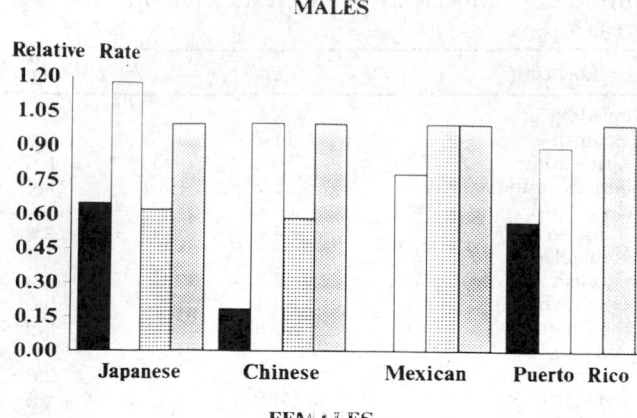

FEMALES

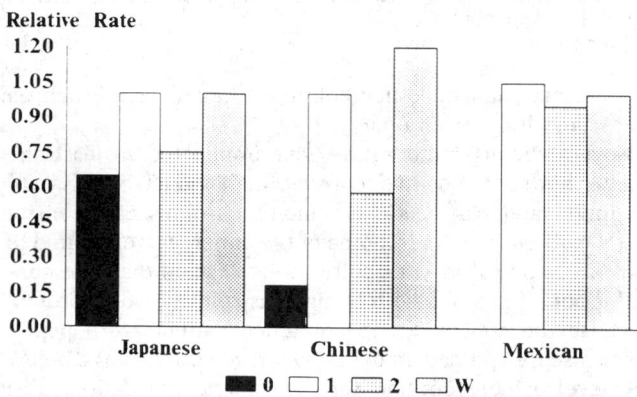

FIG. 26-4. Rates of pancreatic cancer in countries of origin and in first and second generation migrants relative to rates in white Americans. 0, country of origin; 1, first generation; 2, second generation; W, United States whites. (Thomas DB, Karagas MR: Cancer in first and second generation Americans. Cancer Res 47:5771, 1987)

Cigarette smoking has also been associated with an increased risk of pancreatic carcinoma.[1,15,16] In heavy cigarette smokers (at least two packs daily), a study from Veterans Administration hospitals showed almost twice the rate of pancreatic carcinoma compared with nonsmokers.[17] Cigarette smoke contains carcinogens, including the nitrosoamines that have induced pancreatic malignancies in laboratory animals.[18,19]

FIG. 26-5. Incidence of pancreatic cancer in Israel: effect of birthplace. Eur, Europe; Amer, North America; Afr, Africa. (World Health Organization: Cancer Incidence in Five Continents, vol IV. IARC Sci Publ 42, 1982)

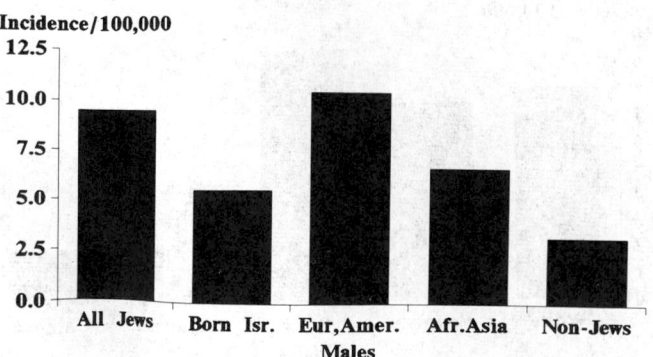

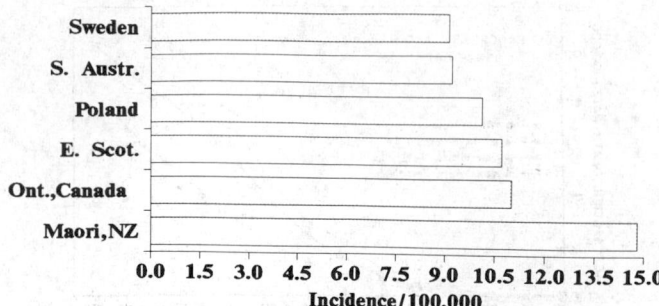

FIG. 26-6. Countries and population with a high incidence of pancreatic cancer. (World Health Organization: Cancer Incidence in Five Continents, vol IV. IARC Sci Publ 42, 1982)

An increased incidence of pancreatic carcinoma is present in patients with chronic pancreatitis.[20,21] Calcifications associated with chronic pancreatitis have been found in 3% of patients with documented pancreatic carcinoma.[22,23] However, there appears to be no association between biliary calcifications and carcinoma of the pancreas.[24] Epidemiologic studies of patients have also shown that almost 15% have a history of diabetes mellitus, which appears to be higher than expected.[25,26] However, in more than half of the patients with diabetes and pancreatic carcinoma, the onset of clinical diabetes preceded the diagnosis of pancreatic carcinoma by no longer than 3 months.[24,26] This suggests that the carcinoma may cause pancreatic endocrine insufficiency. Diabetes mellitus, presenting many months to years before the development of pancreatic carcinomas, would be better evidence for an etiologic correlation, but this type of temporal relationship is not commonly found.[25]

Long-term exposures to solvents and petroleum compounds appear to increase the risk of pancreatic carcinoma.[24] A prospective study of workers exposed to benzidine and beta-naphthylamine showed a higher incidence.[27] The nitrosoamines are recognized as potent pancreatic carcinogens in hamsters.[28] Azaserine has also been shown to produce pancreatic tumors in rats.[29] Exposure for 10 years or longer to these industrial chemicals may increase the risk of pancreatic carcinoma by a factor of five.[24]

ANATOMICAL CONSIDERATIONS

The pancreas lies transversely in the posterior peritoneum of the upper abdomen and weighs approximately 100 g. The anatomical relationships of the pancreas are demonstrated in Figure 26-7. The superior part of the duodenum overlaps the pancreas and passes backward, upward, and to the right. The remaining parts are overlapped by the pancreas itself. The tail of the pancreas usually extends out to the splenic hilum, and it is approximately 15 cm long. The important relationship to the transverse mesocolon and the deep posterior relationship of the pancreas are illustrated in Figure 26-8.

The arterial supply is illustrated in Figure 26-9, including the anastomoses of the superior and inferior pancreaticoduo-

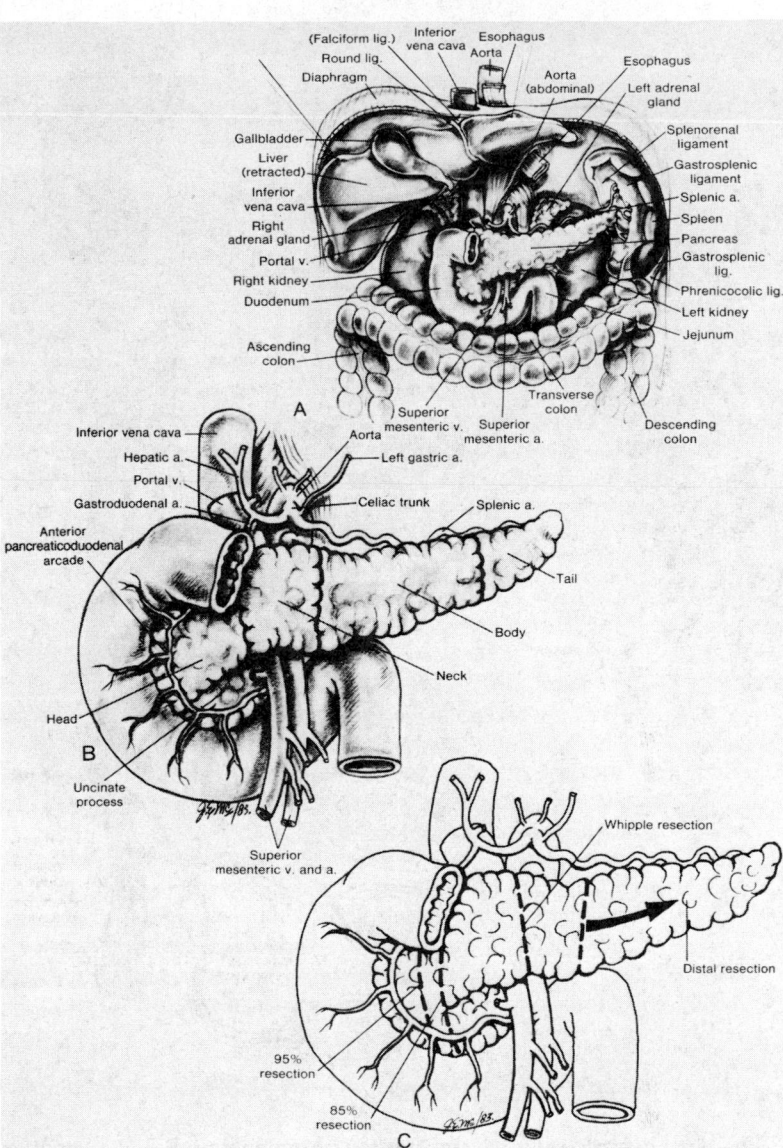

FIG. 26-7. Anatomical relationships of the pancreas. (Gray SW, Skandalakis JE, McCluskey DA: Atlas of Surgical Anatomy for General Surgeons. Baltimore, Williams & Wilkins, 1985)

denal arteries. The important venous drainage is illustrated in Figure 26-10. The surgically important lymphatic drainage is in intimate relationship with the surface and borders of the pancreas and indirectly with the celiac, preaortic, and superior mesenteric groups. Because of the diffuse, surrounding lymphatic drainage, it is thought that tumors in the pancreas can drain virtually to any of the surrounding nodal-bearing areas.

The diameter of the pancreatic duct varies: within the head, it is 3 to 4.8 mm; within the body, 2 to 3.5 mm; and within the tail, 0.9 to 2.4 mm.[30] Two milliliters to 3 ml of contrast material can fill the main pancreatic duct, and 7 to 10 ml can fill the smaller ducts.[31] The pancreatic duct variations have been widely described (Fig. 26-11). From the standard, both ducts open into the duodenum, with communication between the accessory and the main duct, to a blind accessory duct, an independent accessory duct, or missing accessory duct.

The extent of the uncinate process is variable: It can extend from just behind the vessels to the left of the superior mesenteric artery and is an important feature of transection during surgery. Failure to remove this portion of the uncinate process completely in a pancreatoduodenectomy can result in troublesome intraoperative and postoperative bleeding.

The most important anatomical abnormalities that influence pancreatic resection are those of vascular supply. There are usually variations in the hepatic artery, the most common abnormality being the right hepatic artery, arising from the superior mesenteric artery. The course is variable and usually proceeds behind the common duct and the portal vein. This can occur in as many as 25% of patients. The accessory left hepatic artery is rarely a problem because it tends to rise from the common hepatic or left gastric artery and passes in the left omentum. However, on rare occasions it may arise from the superior mesenteric or from the gastroduodenal artery. In 2% to 4% of patients the common hepatic artery arises from the superior mesenteric and occasionally passes through the head of the pancreas, which can be a major problem during resection.[32]

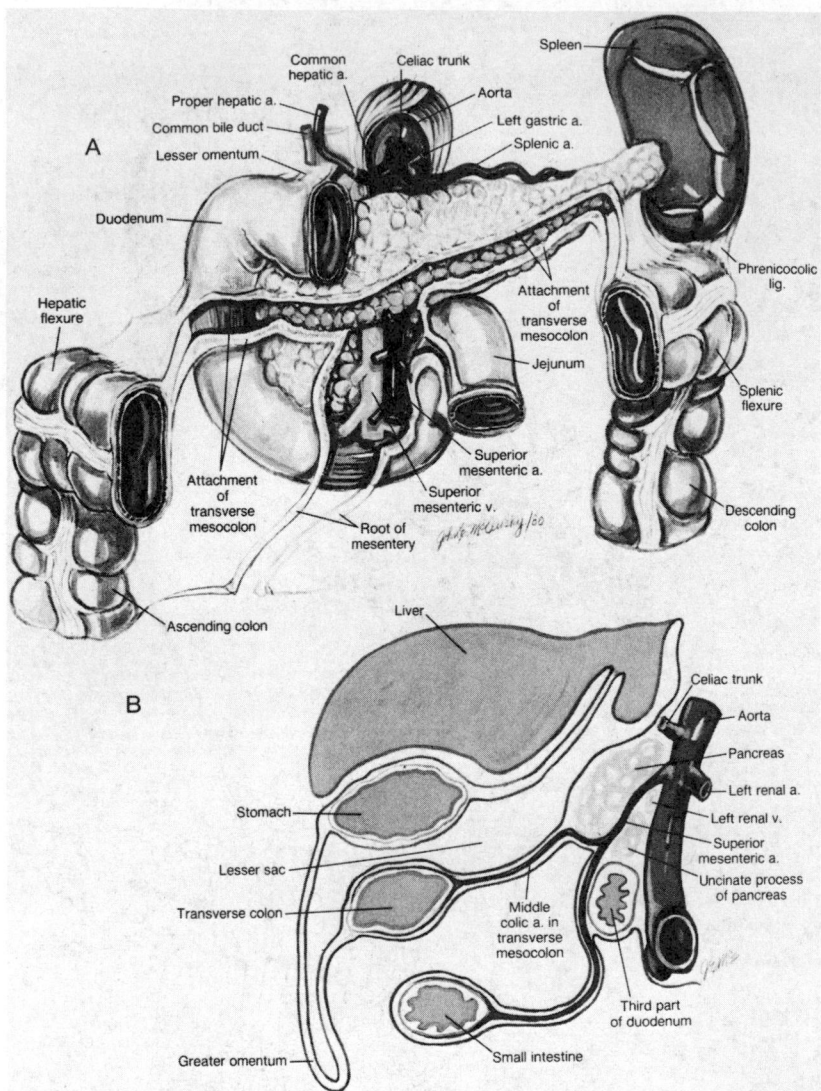

FIG. 26-8. Important relationship to the transverse mesocolon and the deep posterior relationship to the pancreas. (Gray SW, Skandalakis JE, McCluskey DA: Atlas of Surgical Anatomy for General Surgeons. Baltimore, Williams & Wilkins, 1985)

The portal vein rarely lies anterior to the duodenum. Biliary tract abnormalities usually accompany this vascular abnormality. The portal vein may communicate with the superior vena cava, and rarely, a pulmonary vein joins the portal vein. Congenital strictures in the portal vein can occur, and the preduodenal portal vein is often associated with other abnormalities of the pancreas, including malrotation.

PATHOLOGIC CLASSIFICATION

Pancreatic cancers arise from both the exocrine and endocrine parenchyma of the gland.[33,34] Approximately 95% occur within the exocrine portion of the pancreas and may arise from ductal epithelium, acinar cells, connective tissue, or lymphatic deposits. Only 2% of tumors of the exocrine pancreas are benign.[35] The less common tumors of the endocrine pancreas arise from islet of Langerhans cells, and most are benign. An overview of the classification of benign and malignant tumors of the pancreas is presented in Table 26-2. Tumors of endocrine origin are covered in Chapter 39.

The most common pancreatic cancer is a ductal adenocarcinoma, which accounts for about 80% of all pancreatic cancers.[36] In a recent analysis of patients presenting to the Memorial Sloan-Kettering Cancer Center, 79% of 575 admitted during 46 months with peripancreatic cancer had adenocarcinoma of the pancreas. Less common ductal cancers include squamous cell carcinomas, giant cell carcinomas, and carcinosarcomas. Carcinomas of the pancreas usually arise in the proximal gland, which includes the head, neck, and uncinate process.[37] Carcinomas arise in the distal gland less commonly, with 20% of all carcinomas occurring in the body and 5% to 10% occurring in the tail. Grossly, carcinomas appear hard and gritty and often are whitish. Microscopic changes of acute and, more commonly, chronic pancreatitis often surround a pancreatic carcinoma and can make the diagnosis difficult, especially when small amounts of tissue are obtained with a percutaneous biopsy.

Because most pancreatic tumors are ductal in origin, pancreatic ductal obstruction is a common finding. Cancers in the pancreatic head often produce obstruction of both the pancreatic and common bile ducts. Invasion of adjacent duodenum, with ulceration and partial or complete duodenal obstruction, occurs in as many as 25% of pancreatic head

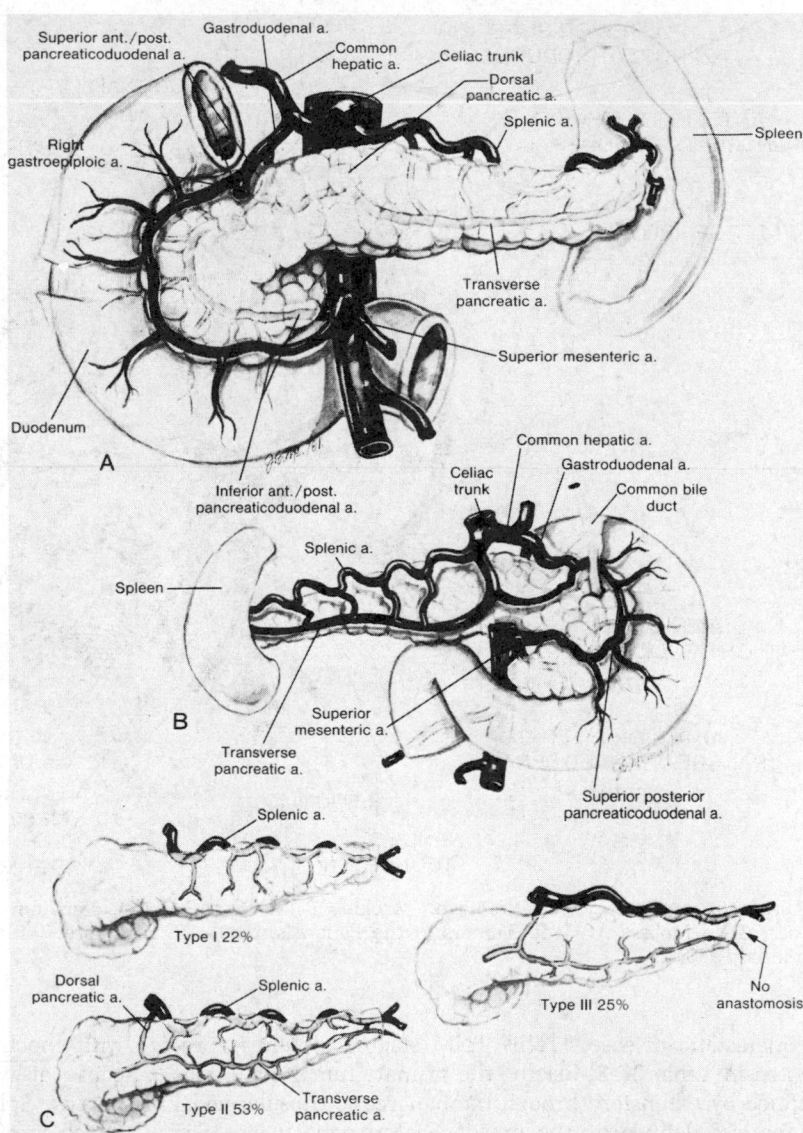

FIG. 26-9. Arterial drainage. (Gray SW, Skandalakis JE, McCluskey DA: Atlas of Surgical Anatomy for General Surgeons. Baltimore, Williams & Wilkins, 1985)

cancers.[37] Obstruction of the portal or superior mesenteric vein can result from local invasion of tumors of the proximal pancreas. Tumors of the distal gland are often larger at diagnosis (5–10 cm) than proximal gland tumors.[33,34] These distal tumors of the pancreatic body and tail can cause obstruction of the splenic vein.

A characteristic pathologic feature of pancreatic adenocarcinomas is the early development of subclinical metastases.[24,37] Fewer than 20% of patients have disease macroscopically confined to the pancreas at diagnosis; 40% of patients present with locally advanced disease, including involvement of regional lymph nodes and adjacent pancreatic tissue, and more than 40% have identifiable visceral metastases at presentation, usually involving the liver.[24] Peritoneal implants occur in 35% of patients at presentation. The natural history of pancreatic carcinomas is highlighted by widespread metastases to other abdominal viscera and extra-abdominal spread to lung, bone, and brain.

Cystic neoplasms of the pancreas are rare tumors that have characteristic pathologic features.[33,34] These tumors are usually large, filled with mucinous secretions, and may be multilocular. Microscopically, the cysts are lined with columnar epithelium alone (cystadenomas) or with a mixture of columnar epithelium and atypical malignant epithelial cells (cystadenocarcinomas). These carcinomas are usually localized, and approximately 50% of patients can be cured with surgery alone. Other rare (<1%) tumors of the nonendopancreas include acinar cell carcinomas, pancreatic sarcomas, and lymphomas. Islet cell tumors are covered in Chapter 39.

CLINICAL FEATURES

STAGING

In 1981, the American Joint Committee for Cancer Staging and End Results Reporting published a staging system for pancreatic carcinoma based on the extent of the primary tumor, the status of regional lymph nodes, and the presence

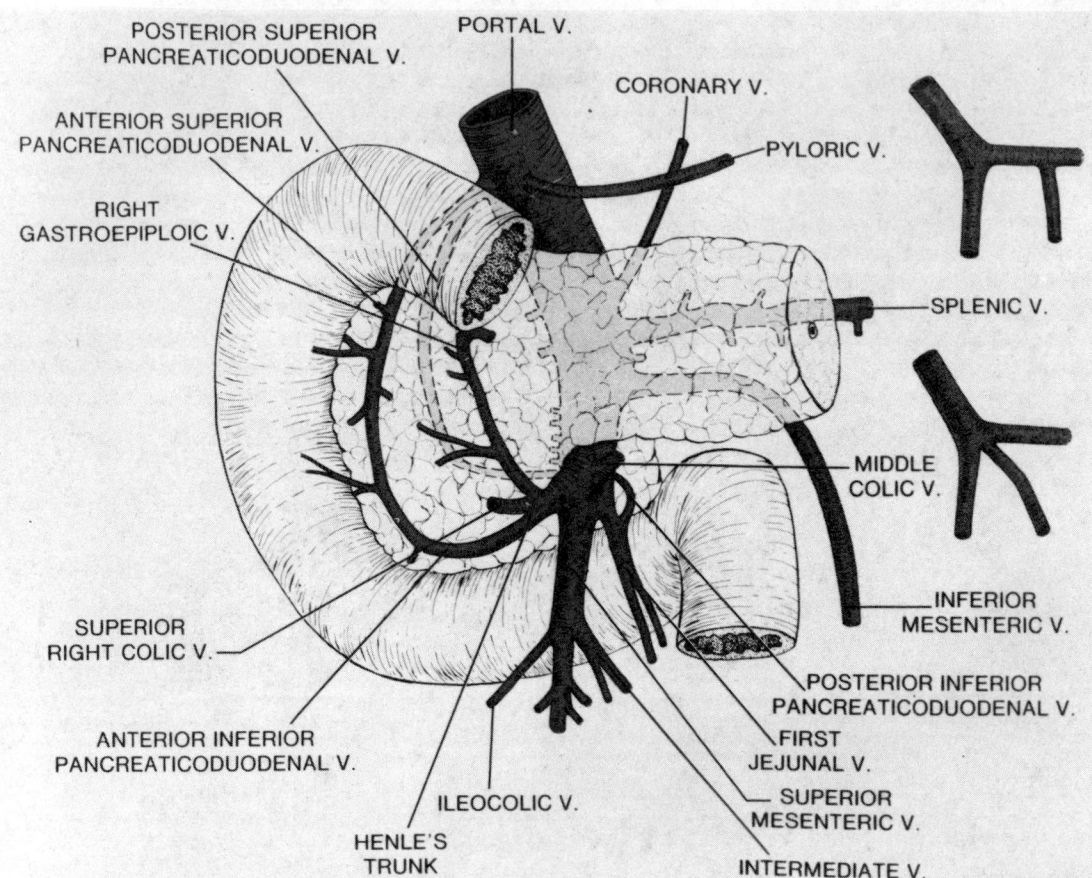

FIG. 26-10. Important venous drainage. (Mackie CR, Moossa AR: Surgical anatomy of the pancreas. In Moossa AR [ed]: Tumors of the Pancreas, pp 1–19. Baltimore, Williams & Wilkins, 1980)

of metastatic disease.[38] This TNM staging system is presented in Table 26-3. Briefly, the primary tumor status was defined by extension through the pancreatic capsule; nodal status was defined by the presence of regional pancreatic lymph node involvement; and metastatic disease status was defined by the presence of distal lymph node, peritoneal, or visceral metastatic disease. The surgical staging system based on the TNM system was defined as follows: Stage I disease is localized within the pancreatic capsule and amenable to surgical resection; Stage II disease is locally advanced with invasion of duodenum or peripancreatic soft tissues and not surgically resectable; Stage III disease has regional lymph node involvement; and Stage IV disease has distant metastases. The staging system used at Memorial Sloan-Kettering Cancer Center is illustrated in Table 26-4.[39]

SIGNS AND SYMPTOMS

Cancer of the pancreas is a highly malignant disease. The majority of patients present with disease advanced beyond the scope of potentially curative treatment. The hallmarks of pancreatic carcinoma are pain and clinical wasting. Tumors in the head of the pancreas often cause biliary obstruction. Patients also develop signs and symptoms of gastric outlet and duodenal obstruction because of local tumor invasion,

with mechanical obstruction and motility problems, the cause of which is probably infiltration of the splanchnic nerves. Splanchnic nerve invasion results in severe pain, which is often difficult to eradicate by medication. Carcinoma of the body and tail rarely produces gastric obstruction because of local infiltration and is often asymptomatic until well advanced. Even in the absence of mechanical obstruction of the stomach and duodenum, marked loss of appetite is a common symptom. A typical patient with pancreatic carcinoma has lost more than 10% of his body weight at diagnosis, and wasting is progressive. Distant metastases, particularly to liver, occur early in the course of the disease.

The initial symptoms are nonspecific and insidious at onset. The typical patient reports a gradual onset of anorexia, nausea, upper abdominal to midabdominal pain, and weight loss. Because of the nonspecific nature of these symptoms, early diagnosis of pancreatic cancer is difficult and requires a high index of suspicion on the part of the physician initially involved in the patient's care. A delay in diagnosis of several months from the initiation of symptoms is common. In a report from the Cancer of the Pancreas Task Force, fewer than 33% of patients experienced symptoms for 2 months or less before diagnosis.[38] Delays in diagnoses are reported in other large reviews.[37,40]

Pain is the most common symptom in patients with pan-

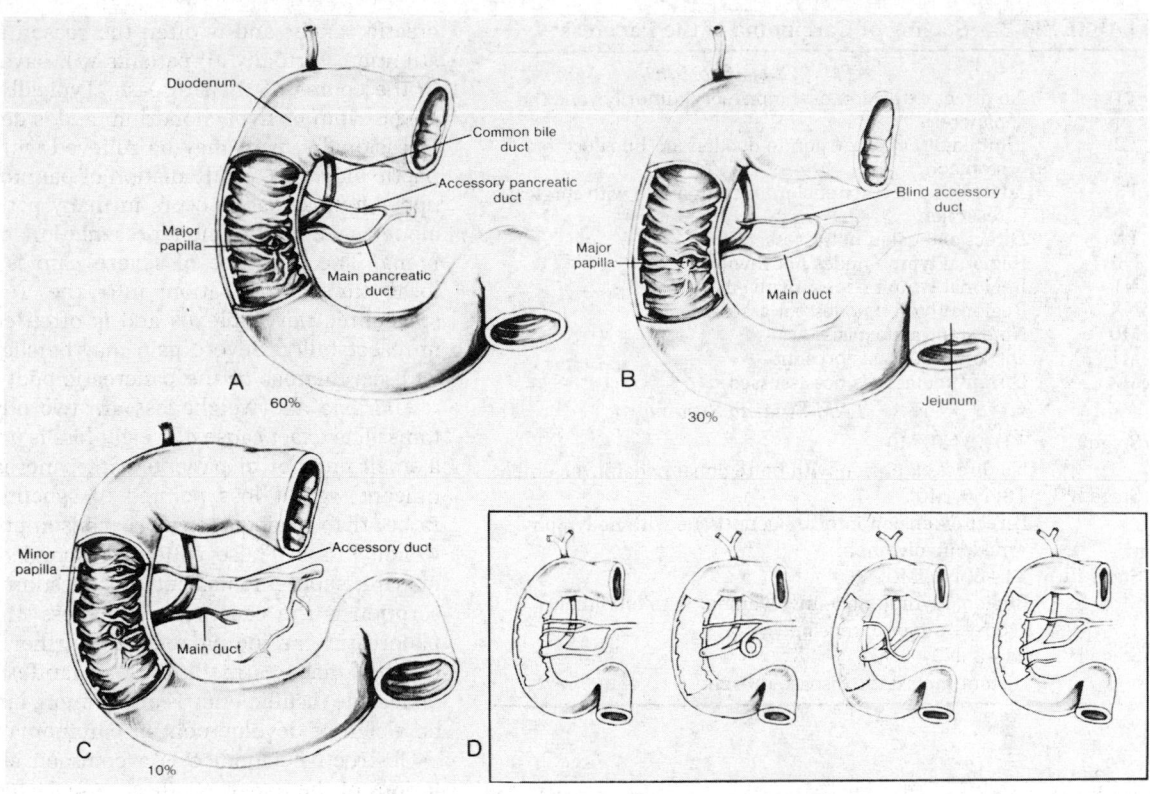

FIG. 26-11. Pancreatic duct variations. (Gray SW, Skandalakis JE, McCluskey DA: Atlas of Surgical Anatomy for General Surgeons. Baltimore, Williams & Wilkins, 1985)

TABLE 26-2.   Histogenetic Classification of Pancreatic Neoplasms

Origin	Benign	Malignant
Duct Cell	Polyp	Duct cell carcinoma
	Papilloma	Giant cell carcinoma
	Adenoma	Adenosquamous carcinoma
	Cystadenoma	Microglandular adenocarcinoma
	Oncocytoma	Mucinous carcinoma
	Benign papillary cystic neoplasm	Cystadenocarcinoma
		Papillary cystic carcinoma
Acinar Cell	Acinar cell adenoma	Acinar cell carcinoma
	Acinar cell cystadenoma	Acinar cell cystadenocarcinoma
Connective Tissue	Lipoma	Malignant fibrous histiocytoma
	Leiomyoma	Fibrosarcoma
	Benign peripheral nerve tumor	Liposarcoma
	Hemangioma	Leiomyosarcoma
	Lymphangioma	Malignant peripheral nerve tumor
		Rhabdomyosarcoma
		Hemangiosarcoma
		Lymphangiosarcoma
		Hemangiopericytoma
		Malignant lymphoma
		Plasmacytoma
Islet Cell	Insulinoma	Malignant insulinoma
	Glucagonoma	Malignant glucagonoma
	Gastrinoma	Malignant gastrinoma
	Adenoma, functionally inactive	Islet cell carcinoma, functionally inactive
		Islet cell carcinoma carcinoid type
Uncertain	Fibroadenoma	Pancreaticoblastoma

Modified from Cubilla AL, Fitzgerald PJ: Tumors of the exocrine pancreas. Washington DC, Armed Forces Institute of Pathology, 1984, and from Legg MA: Pathology of the pancreas. In: Brooks JR (ed): Surgery of the Pancreas, pp 41–77. Philadelphia, WB Saunders, 1983.

TABLE 26-3.   Staging of Carcinoma of the Pancreas

TNM Classification

T1	No direct extension of the primary tumor beyond the pancreas
T2	Limited direct extension to duodenum, bile duct, or stomach
T3	Advanced direct extension, incompatible with surgical resection
TX	Direct extension not assessed
N0	Regional lymph nodes not involved
N1	Regional lymph nodes involved
NX	Regional lymph nodes not assessed
M0	No distant metastasis
M1	Distant metastasis present
MX	Distant metastasis not assessed

TNM Staging System

Stage I	T1–2, N0, M0
	No direct extension with no regional nodal involvement
Stage II	T3, N0, M0
	Direct extension into adjacent tissue with no lymph node involvement
Stage III	T1–3, N1, M0
	Regional lymph node involvement with or without direct tumor extension
Stage IV	T1–3, N0–1, M1
	Distant metastatic disease present

creatic cancer and is often the reason for seeking medical attention. Virtually all patients will have pain at some point in the course of their disease. Typically, the pain is in the epigastrium or hypochondrium and is described as gnawing. Occasionally, pain may be relieved with meals, mimicking peptic ulcer disease. Radiation of pain to the low thoracic or upper lumbar back occurs in many patients, but back pain alone is an uncommon presentation of pancreatic carcinoma. The presence of severe pain is often indicative of local tumor infiltration into the retroperitoneum and splanchnic nerve plexus and is often considered a sign of unresectability. Severe pain may be slightly more common with carcinomas of the pancreatic body and tail.[37]

Anorexia and weight loss are two other common symptoms. The exact cause of weight loss is unknown. A report on a small number of patients with pancreatic cancer and significant weight loss pointed to subclinical malabsorption, rather than inadequate caloric consumption, as the source of weight loss.[41] These patients responded to oral pancreatic enzyme supplements, but the question of whether malabsorption is the cause of weight loss in most patients with pancreatic carcinoma requires further study. The sudden onset of diabetes mellitus as a manifestation of pancreatic endocrine insufficiency is uncommon, but is often thought to be a sign of development of carcinoma of the pancreas.[42]

Obstructive jaundice is a common sign, particularly for lesions of the pancreatic head. Associated symptoms of dark

---

TABLE 26-4.   Postsurgical Staging for Cancer of the Pancreatic Region

Primary Tumor: T

T1	2 cm or less in diameter
T2	2 to 6 cm in diameter
T3	Over 6 cm in diameter
T4	Direct extension to contiguous structures
TX	Unknown or unrecorded

Nodes: N

N0   None
N1   Anterior, posterior, superior, inferior pancreatic nodes
   a) Microscopic focus in one node
   b) Solitary, macroscopic
   c) Multiple nodes (microscopic or macroscopic)
N2   Porta hepatic, common hepatic, celiac, proximal superior mesenteric lymph nodes
   a) Microscopic focus in one node
   b) Solitary, macroscopic
   c) Multiple nodes (microscopic or macroscopic)
N3   Periaortic, distal superior mesenteric, or other abdominal lymph nodes
NX   Unknown or unrecorded

Metastases Beyond Regional Nodes: M

M0   None
M1   Liver only
M2   Other Intra-abdominal metastases
   a) Without liver
   b) With liver
M3   Multiple peritoneal implants or malignant ascites
M4   Extra-abdominal metastases
MX   Unknown or unrecorded

Clinical (cTNM) and Pathologic (pTNM) Staging

Stage I	T1–4,	N0,	M0
Stage II	T1–4,	N1–2,	M0
Stage III	T1–4,	N0–3,	M1–4

urine, light stools, and pruritus may proceed the clinical detection of jaundice. Totally painless jaundice is not common in pancreatic carcinoma and occurs more often in ampullary carcinoma or a primary bile duct carcinoma.[43] Although the gallbladder is commonly distended at exploration, fewer than 33% of patients will have a palpable gallbladder at presentation (Courvoisier's sign).[43] Splenomegaly, another uncommon physical finding, usually occurs with tumors of the distal gland involving splenic vein obstruction. Early spread of tumor to the liver and peritoneum may occur in 15% to 25% of patients and presents with the signs of a palpable liver or abdominal distension with ascites.[37]

Patients may have a higher risk of depression at diagnosis, compared with other abdominal tumors. One study reported depression in 67% of 46 patients with pancreatic carcinoma, compared with less than 10% of 64 patients with colon carcinoma.[44] Considering the delay in diagnosis of several months in most patients, a reactive depression may be expected. Patients with pancreatic carcinoma may have a higher frequency of venous thrombosis and migratory thrombophlebitis (Trousseau's sign).[45] Thrombophlebitis appears more commonly in patients with tumors of the distal pancreas, but there is no clear correlation between the development of thrombophlebitis with an underlying pancreatic carcinoma in an otherwise healthy patient.[43]

DIAGNOSIS

The algorithm for the diagnosis of adenocarcinoma of the pancreas is outlined in Figure 26-12. Once a suspicion of pancreatic cancer has been raised—because of nonspecific upper abdominal symptoms, weight loss, or jaundice—then clinical confirmation is required. This is usually obtained by physical examination to confirm jaundice, ascites, palpable mass, or metastatic disease. Chemical confirmation of the jaundice can be obtained by serum indices. Radiologic tests can also evaluate the extent of the disease. Radiologic confirmation requires ultrasonography to demonstrate a mass in the pancreas, dilated extrahepatic biliary ducts, or metastatic disease in the liver.

Computed tomography (CT) is the mainstay of both diagnostic confirmation and the evaluation of the extent of disease (Fig. 26-13). CT can demonstrate the mass in the pancreas, metastatic disease in the liver and the periaortic and retropancreatic lymph nodes, and ascites. Enormous masses arising from the pancreas suggest diagnoses such as lymphoma or sarcoma (Fig. 26-14). Clear identification of cystic changes, with or without calcification, suggests the possibility of cystadenoma or cystadenocarcinoma. Masses in young people suggest the possibility of pancreaticoblastoma.

Endoscopic retrograde cholangiopancreatography (ERCP) is a valuable tool in the diagnosis, or in the localization of the tumor to the ampulla or the demonstration of obstructed stenotic or sclerosed ducts (Fig. 26-15), all highly suggestive of adenocarcinoma. Conversely, the presence of a lesion on CT scans with a subsequently normal pancreatic duct (Figs. 26-13 and 26-14) may suggest an islet cell neoplasm or exclude pancreatic adenocarcinoma. Care must be taken, however, not to misinterpret a normal duct as an islet cell

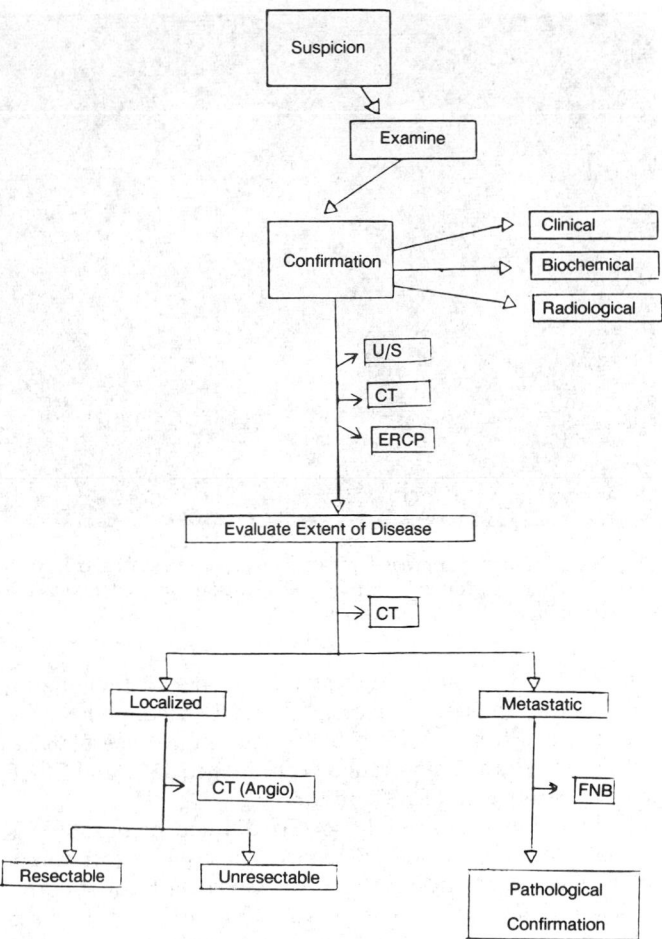

FIG. 26-12. Algorithm: diagnosis of pancreatic adenocarcinoma.

FIG. 26-13. Obvious mass on CT scan, shown to have normal pancreatic duct and benign minimal enlargement by operation and long-term follow-up.

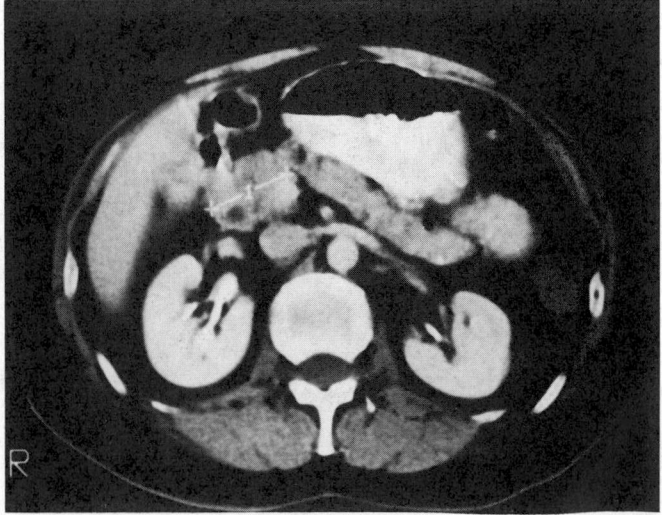

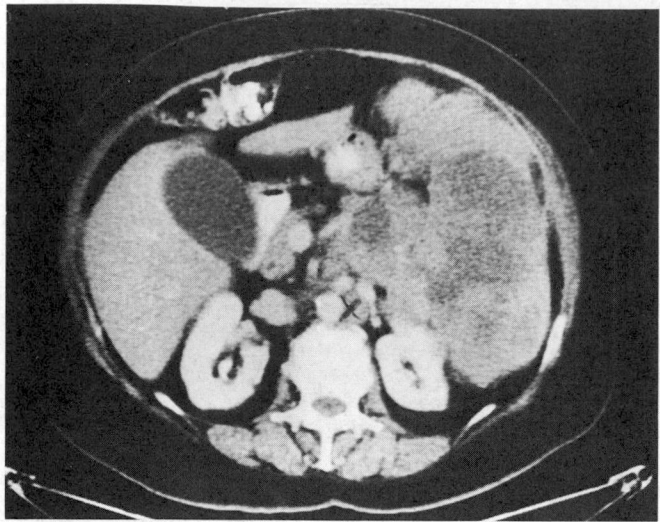

FIG. 26-14. Large pancreatic mass shown subsequently to have a normal pancreatic duct by ERCP. The patient proved to have a primary pancreatic lymphoma.

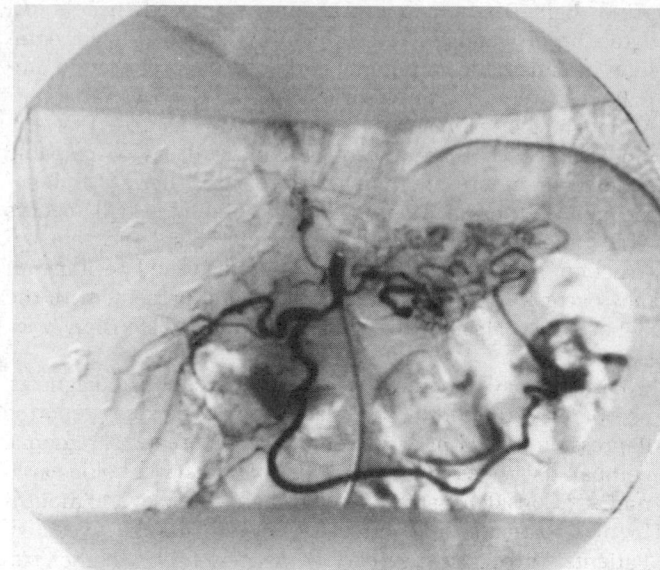

FIG. 26-16. Arteriogram demonstrating encasement of the common hepatic and splenic arteries, indicating unresectability.

tumor when the pancreatic lesion is an adenocarcinoma involving the uncinate process. CT results had positive response rates from 63% to 100%, with an average of 65%. Ultrasound has a similar range, from 23% to 95%, and ERCP had a positive rate of 53% to 96%.[40]

If the tumor appears to be localized, then the next step is to evaluate for resectability. Again CT plays a central role in determination of the involvement, particularly of superior mesenteric and celiac axis vessels (Fig. 26-13).[40] If these vessels are not involved and a reasonable assessment can be made about obstruction of the portal vein on the basis of CT, then resection can be considered. If the tumor is clearly unresectable, or if metastatic disease is identified, based on the CT scan, we proceed to pathologic confirmation. However, if there is concern about resectability and if there are compelling reasons not to explore the patient, then we use angiography (Fig. 26-16).

Angiography is used to determine the presence of abnormal vasculature, such as a right hepatic artery arising from the superior mesenteric artery, and to determine unresectability based on encasement of the superior mesenteric or, rarely, hepatic or celiac axis arteries (Fig. 26-17). The abnormal vasculature does not warrant the uniform use of angiography before surgery. This vessel can usually be detected in the porta hepatis at the time of resection and often runs behind the pancreas, rather than directly through it. Conversely, the complete encasement of the superior mesenteric or celiac arteries is an absolute contraindication to resection.

If the tumor is deemed unresectable or metastatic disease is identified, then histopathologic confirmation should be

FIG. 26-17. Encasement of an abnormal right hepatic artery arising from the superior mesenteric artery.

FIG. 26-15. ERCP of patient with a localized mass in the head and body of the pancreas, confirmed as an unresectable adenocarcinoma.

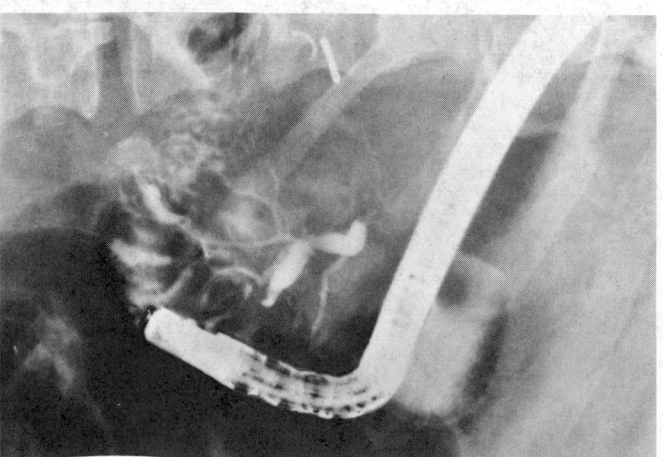

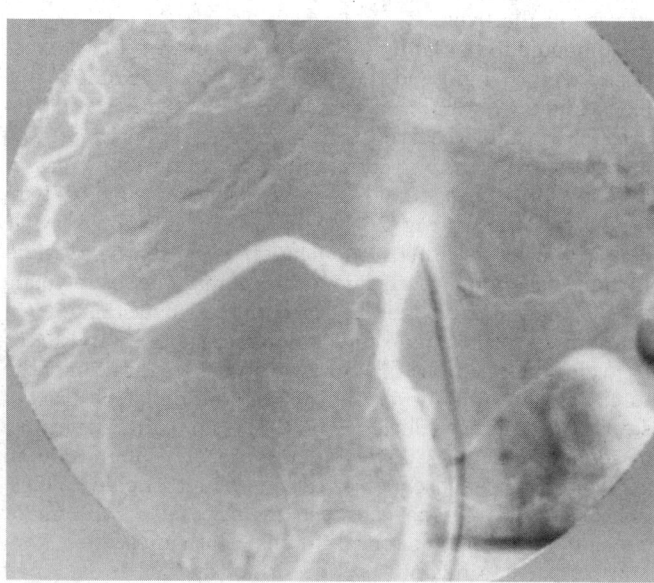

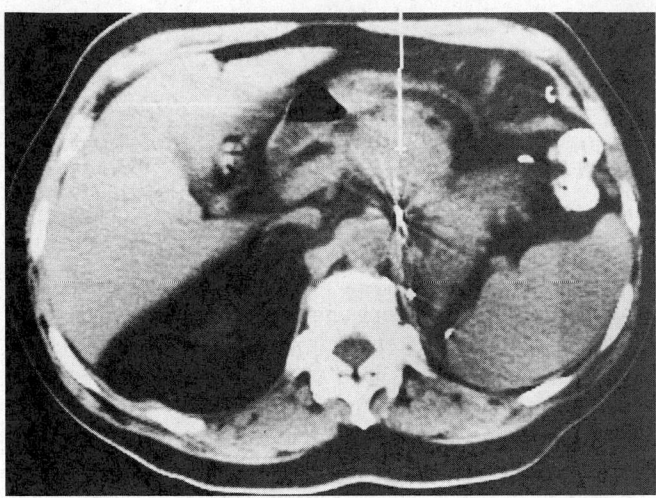

FIG. 26-18. Histopathologic confirmation obtained by "skinny" needle biopsy of the pancreas.

obtained, either by direct fine-needle biopsy of the pancreas (Fig. 26-18) or percutaneous biopsy of a liver metastasis.

Upper gastrointestinal (GI) contrast studies, which are rarely of value, are much less valuable than CT. This test is also redundant because most patients will have endoscopy as part of the ERCP. Magnetic resonance imaging (MRI) is only now undergoing serious evaluation in the pancreatic area. MRI may eventually displace CT, but for the present CT is the procedure of choice.

A new modality is endoscopic ultrasound. It is used mainly for staging gastric and esophageal cancer and can demonstrate local invasion by pancreatic neoplasms into the portal vein (Fig. 26-19).

Percutaneous transhepatic cholangiograms (PTHC) are indicated on limited occasions. They are primarily used if there is concern about a distal common bile duct lesion and

the proximal extent of such a tumor is unclear. By use of ultrasound and CT, it is usually possible to determine the dilation of the extrahepatic biliary ducts and the proximal extent of any stenotic lesion of the common bile duct. It is appropriate at the time of ERCP, if the common bile duct can be entered, to place a stent or a nasobiliary catheter before considering further surgical intervention.

SEROLOGIC MARKERS

Serologic markers of pancreatic cancer are of interest for a variety of reasons. If sufficiently sensitive and specific, markers aid in the differential diagnosis of patients with abdominal or retroperitoneal disease. Markers can also identify a prognostically more favorable population of patients with resectable, curable disease. For postoperative and advanced pancreatic cancer patients with poorly measurable tumor, a convenient, reproducible, and accurate serologic test can assist in clinical follow-up.

The summarized results of four potential markers are shown in Table 26-5. One of the first markers to be investigated systematically was the carcinoembryonic antigen (CEA). CEA is a high-molecular-weight glycoprotein and the normal product of fetal gut tissue. This widely available test identifies about half of the pancreatic cancer patients and can discriminate malignant from benign pancreatic disease in over 90% of cases. However, CEA is not an efficient marker for either diagnosis or follow-up because it is elevated in many benign states, such as ulcerative colitis or biliary disease, and in many malignancies, such as colon or lung cancer.[53-56]

The CA 125 antigen is a well-recognized marker for epithelial ovarian neoplasms and has been screened in GI malignancies as well.[57-59] This large glycoprotein is identified by a murine monoclonal antibody raised against a human ovarian cell line.[60] In pancreatic cancer patients, CA 125 is detected less than 50% of the time. As a single test, CA 125

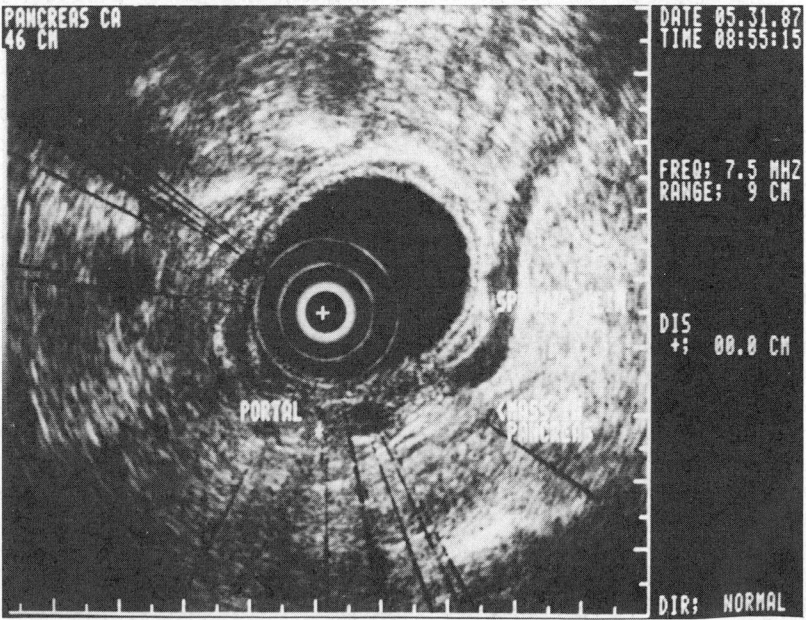

FIG. 26-19. Tissue to be removed. All of the finely shaded area, including distal stomach, duodenum, head of pancreas, gallbladder, and common bile duct, will be resected.

TABLE 26-5.   Selected Tumor Markers in Pancreatic Cancer

Marker	Reference	Serum Level	Pancreatic Cancer	Pancreatitis	Normal Levels
CEA	46–49	2.5–50 ng/ml	114/231 (49%)	10/188 (5%)	0/34
CA 125	48–50	35 U/ml	55/132 (42%)	15/75 (20%)	0/38
CA 19-9	46–48, 50, 51	37 U/ml	255/319 (80%)	18/233 (8%)	1/72
DU-PAN-2	52	300 U/ml	31/33 (94%)		0/126

is not clinically satisfactory for pancreatic cancer and is probably more useful for ovarian cancer.

The tumor-associated carbohydrate antigen, CA 19-9, is detectable by a murine monoclonal antibody raised against a human colorectal adenocarcinoma cell line.[61] This mucin-like molecule is a sialated Lewis antigen, which has been associated more often with pancreatic than with other intra-abdominal malignancies.[62] The findings of five representative studies are summarized in Table 26-5. With this monoclonal antibody, approximately 80% of pancreatic cancer patients are correctly detected, compared with 8% of patients with pancreatitis and 1% of normal subjects incorrectly identified. Steinberg found CA 19-9 was statistically more specific than CEA (86.5% versus 48.4%) but only slightly more sensitive (92.5% versus 87.3%).[46] Data from Piantino demonstrated an identical superiority for CA 19-9.[47] Tempero suggests that CA 19-9 may provide a useful clinical marker for detecting pancreatic cancer progression in patients with recurrent or advanced disease.[63]

More recently, a murine monoclonal antibody directed against a pancreatic adenocarcinoma glycoprotein has been evaluated. The DU-PAN-2 antigen appears to be an oncofetal surface antigen that is quite specific for identifying and following pancreatic cancer.[52] DU-PAN-2 may be elevated in those with biliary cirrhosis, gastric cancer, and biliary cancer but seems to be sensitive and specific for pancreatic cancer and deserves further evaluation.

With the enthusiasm for and increasing sophistication of monoclonal antibody production, it is likely that new markers will be forthcoming. The simultaneous use of several species (e.g., CA 19-9 and CA 125) may yield even more satisfactory discrimination between diseases and clinical results.[64,65]

SURGICAL TREATMENT

PREOPERATIVE BILIARY DECOMPRESSION FOR OBSTRUCTIVE JAUNDICE

Preoperative biliary drainage before surgery has been practiced for a number of years. Dr. Alan O. Whipple's early experience with a pancreaticoduodenectomy was preceded by relief of obstruction by bypass.[66] Retrospective studies suggested that preliminary decompression by cholecystectomy resulted in a decrease in operative mortality from 50% to 8%![67]

Percutaneous transhepatic biliary drainage (PTBD) resulted in a striking reduction in operative mortality to 8.2%, compared with 28% in historical controls.[68] Several other retrospective studies using historical controls and other trials, including concurrent nonrandomized controls and no controls, suggested benefit.[69-72] The combined results of these studies suggested an operative mortality of 13.7% among patients undergoing preoperative PTBD, compared with 26% among patients undergoing surgery without it (Table 26-6). Two of the five trials suggested a significant reduction in mortality and in morbidity. The apparent improvement associated with PTBD in these studies may be explained further by other factors, such as the exclusion of high-risk patients from subsequent operations or the use of PTBD as the definitive form of palliation. In fact, 98 (40%) of 246 of patients undergoing PTBD did not proceed to subsequent laparotomy.

More recent prospective randomized trials have challenged the value of PTBD. In 1982 the first prospective evaluation in a single-arm trial of 37 patients, 35 of whom had malignant obstruction, resulted in drainage-related morbidity of 54% and drainage-related mortality of 13.5%.[73] Postoperative mortality was 24%. In two well-controlled randomized trials, 127 patients, 94% of whom had malignant disease, showed no benefit in either morbidity or mortality by PTBD.[74,75] Overall mortality was 14% with or without preliminary drainage (Table 26-6). In-hospital mortality was 23% among patients drained and 16% among those not drained. In one of the trials, there was a 19% mortality among 31 patients not drained and 32% mortality among 34 patients drained, including five deaths before any operation and two additional deaths resulting from complications of drainage procedure. Five patients required early surgery for bile peritonitis.[75]

In all these trials, there have been many complications related to PTBD. A prospective controlled trial has been completed that showed no benefit in operative mortality and showed a prolongation of hospital stay with the drainage procedure for patients with both benign and malignant biliary obstruction.[76] Overall, no objective benefit other than decrease in bilirubin has been shown to result from preoperative drainage. The high complication rate with the percutaneous procedure has obscured any potential benefit from the biliary decompression.

The alternative is endoscopically placed biliary drainage, which has theoretical appeal in providing similar drainage with less risk of complication. In a comprehensive series of 595 cases collected from six centers in Japan and Europe, a 97.5% success rate has been claimed.[77] This is far in excess of any success rate that most North American centers have been able to provide. Complication rates are small (4%). The principal complication is cholangitis. Mortality is less than 2%. Current trials examine benefits of preoperative

TABLE 26-6.   Postoperative Mortality in Obstructive Jaundice*: Results of Preoperative Drainage Studies

Author	Year	Method	Mortality	
			Drainage	No Drainage
Retrospective				
Whipple[66]	1983	Cholecystostomy	8% (2/25)	50% (16/32)
Nakayama[68]	1978	PTBD†	8% (4/49)	28% (36/148)
Dooley[72]	1979	PTBD	24% (5/21)	Not reported
Denning[69]	1981	PTBD	18% (4/22)	27% (7/26)
Norlander[20]	1982	PTBD	18% (8/44)	33% (14/42)
Gundry[71]	1984	PTBD	4% (1/25)	20% (5/25)‡
Total			14% (22/161)	26% (62/241)
Prospective, Nonrandom				
McPherson[73]	1982	PTBD	24% (8/33)	Not reported
Prospective, Random				
Hatfield[74]	1982	PTBD	5% (1/22)	8% (2/25)
McPherson[75]	1984	PTBD	22% (6/27)	19% (6/31)
Total			14% (7/49)	14% (8/56)

*Data presented for malignant causes only unless otherwise noted.
†PTBD = percutaneous transhepatic biliary drainage.
‡Twenty-eight percent were benign.

nasobiliary drainage in alleviating the risks and complications of postoperative patients. In centers where the overall operative mortality is less than 5%, it is unlikely that any benefit in mortality can be shown by such studies without large numbers of patients. In a randomized trial comparing endoscopic and percutaneous stent insertion in 75 patients with malignant obstructive jaundice, the endoscopic route had a greater success rate in relieving jaundice and was associated with a significantly lower complication rate and 30-day mortality.[78] Proponents of the percutaneous route have challenged this study based on a too high percutaneous complication rate.[79]

RESECTION

Surgical resection remains the only possible chance for cure and allows confirmation of the histologic and site-specific subtypes. Candidates for resection can be carefully chosen by preoperative testing.

Incision and Evaluation

The bilateral subcostal incision with the extensive use of an upper-hand retractor to gain complete and adequate access to the upper abdomen is preferred. Rarely, an upper midline extension (Mercedes-Benz) is required.

Primary contraindications to resection are liver metastasis or extrapancreatic serosal implantation. It is important to examine the inferior surface of the mesocolon to be sure there is no tumor extending through the base. For many, this is an indication of unresectability. In essence, as resectability is evaluated, part of the dissection for the subsequent resection is completed. In most patients, evidence of obvious nodal involvement with cancer in the portal area precludes subsequent resection. If an ampullary or islet cell lesion is suspected, positive nodes are an absolute contraindication to further dissection.

Once it is clear that the tumor, duodenum, and the head of the pancreas are mobile, the histopathologic diagnosis is obtained, if it has not been obtained preoperatively. This is done by a single pass of a transduodenal tru-cut needle, holding the pancreas and tumor with the fingers and thumb of the left hand. Although difficulty may be encountered in obtaining a histologic diagnosis, most physicians have reported a very low false-negative rate, and a diagnosis was readily obtained.[37,80]

On rare occasions a decision has to be made to proceed with a pancreatic resection when no histologic diagnosis of carcinoma can be obtained. Some authors advocate this approach, but, whenever possible, a clear histologic diagnosis should be obtained. Conversely, repetitive transduodenal or open biopsies should be discouraged. Difficulties are encountered with persistent attempts at aggressive biopsy with no subsequent progression to resection than if the surgeon proceeds with conventional resection because of the very high likelihood that a pancreatic or periampullary carcinoma exists. Provided that this issue has been discussed preoperatively with the patient, the procedure can be continued.

If tumor invades or adheres to the celiac axis or origin of the common hepatic artery, it is a contraindication for further resection, and the procedure should be terminated. Once the hepatic vessels are free, the suprapancreatic portal vein is dissected just medial to the curve of the hepatic artery. This can be easily identified between common duct and hepatic artery, and its freedom from any local tumor invasion should be established. This exposure is limited, and the vein will be more easily demonstrated from the inferior approach.

The relationship of the tumor to the portal vein is then established inferiorly through the lesser sac. Gross and encompassing involvement and difficulty in obtaining dissection between vein and pancreas are limits to resection. Minimal adherence to the vein, however, does not prevent resection and can be dealt with by resection of the vein. The surgeon should assess whether the superior mesenteric artery is involved. It is rare that involvement of the origin of the superior mesenteric artery will exist without virtually complete encasement of the portal vein, often with obvious venous collaterals and varices. Once it has been established that the superior mesenteric artery is free and that the portal vein is free or only minimally involved, the decision to proceed is made.

Pancreaticoduodenectomy

The tissue to be resected includes the distal stomach, the gallbladder, the common bile duct, the head of the pancreas with the contained tumor, all four parts of the duodenum, and the first part of the small intestine (Fig. 26-20). The topography of the tumor in its relation to these tissues is illustrated in Figure 26-21. The common duct is commonly dilated and there may be some dilatation of the pancreatic duct. This may not be appreciated. Preoperative assessment can determine the degree of expected dilatation of the common hepatic duct, and the failure to find what was assessed preoperatively raises the question of an erroneous diagnosis.

The order in which dissection proceeds is a matter of personal preference. The continued mobilization of the third and fourth parts of the duodenum, at the ligament of Treitz, and the first part of the jejunum, early in the procedure rather than following the gastric dissection, is often appropriate. It may be easier to divide the stomach earlier in the procedure to gain access to the pancreas. Procedures reserving the pylorus can, on rare occasions, be done for very small lesions involving the ampulla.

FIG. 26-20. All tissues are now removed and the reconstruction can begin.

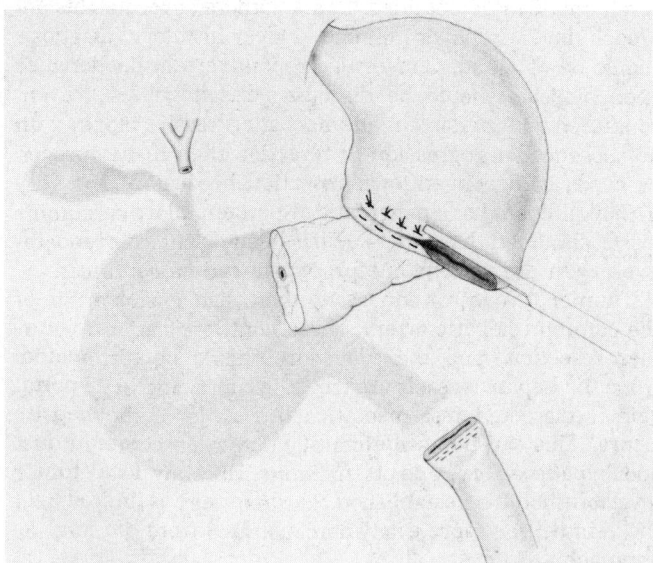

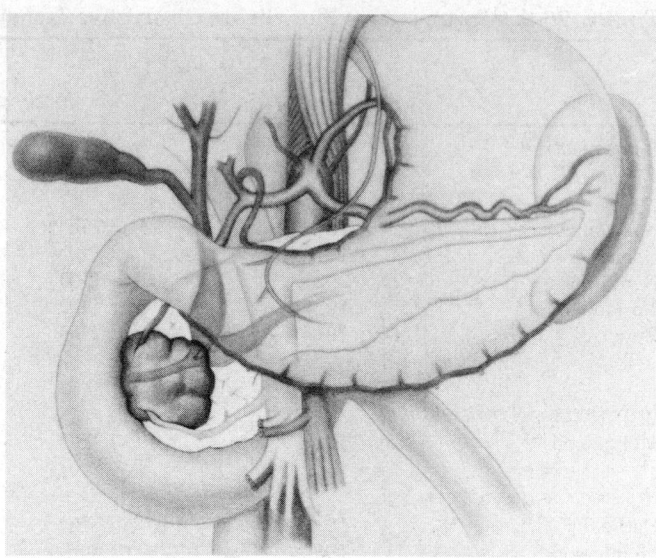

FIG. 26-21. Topography of the tumor, demonstrating both the dilatation of the common bile duct and pancreatic duct and the tissues that need to be exposed and resected.

Once the pancreas has been divided, then the final dissection of the porta hepatis is continued. The cholecystectomy is performed, and, when the duct enters low on the common duct, surgery can be done conventionally from fundus to duct such that the gallbladder will come with the specimen. If the entrance of the cystic duct is quite high on the common duct or into the right hepatic duct, then cholecystectomy is done in conventional fashion as an isolated procedure, ligating duct and artery and removing the gallbladder, discontinuous with the specimen.

Careful and diligent attention is then paid to the uncinate process. Many surgeons do not remove the uncinate process completely, but it is important to do so because it can be a worrisome site of subsequent bleeding. In uncinate process tumors, unresectability may be encountered quite late in the procedure. If that is suspected by the early assessment, then the uncinate process should be dissected before the small bowel is divided. If invasion of the portal vein is encountered, isolation above and below can be obtained and the vein transected if necessary. Conversely, a lateral sidebiting, vascular clamp can be placed along the pancreatic vein and a small portion of the vein taken. If the vein is taken, mobilization of the small intestine can easily make up several centimeters such that end-to-end approximation with vascular 4-0 sutures can be achieved. This allows the specimen to be removed, and the tissue remaining (see Fig. 26-20) is now ready for reconstruction.

Reconstruction

Choledochojejunostomy is performed first because it is the deepest anastomosis. A small longitudinal incision is made with a cautery over the serosa of the small bowel, and the serosa is gently teased from the mucosa to allow a greater entry site for mucosa than for serosa. The horizontal running everting mattress suture of 3-0 or 4-0 prolene is then used to

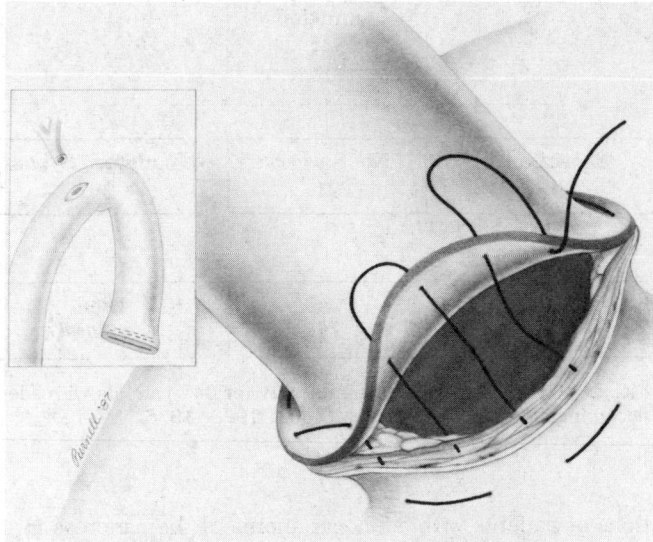

FIG. 26-22. The choledochojejunostomy is performed by a running, everting, nonabsorbable, monofilament suture.

settle the back wall and the anterior separate line suture (Fig. 26-22). This gives a comfortable, easy-to-place anastomosis that can slide down to approximate the tissues under direct vision. By taking a larger bite on the serosal site and a small bite on the mucosal site, a satisfactory mucosa-to-mucosa anastomosis can be obtained.

The pancreaticojejunostomy is performed next. A similar incision in the small intestine is made along the jejunal wall, and horizontal nonabsorbable mattress sutures are placed to attach the pancreas to the small bowel. A direct duct to the mucosal anastomosis is then performed with three interrupted 4-0 or 5-0 prolene sutures, bringing the duct directly to mucosa. A similar row of horizontal mattress sutures is then encompassed to place the remainder of the pancreas into the small intestine (Fig. 26-23). Once this has been completed the standard gastrojejunostomy is performed, usually with one absorbable and one nonabsorbable layer of sutures. The completed anastomoses appear as in Figure

FIG. 26-23. The choledochojejunostomy is complete and the pancreaticojejunostomy is begun. The posterior layer of horizontal mattress sutures fixes the pancreas to the jejunum and two or three interrupted 5-0 nonabsorbable prolene complete a mucosa-to-mucosa anastomosis of the pancreatic duct to the jejunum.

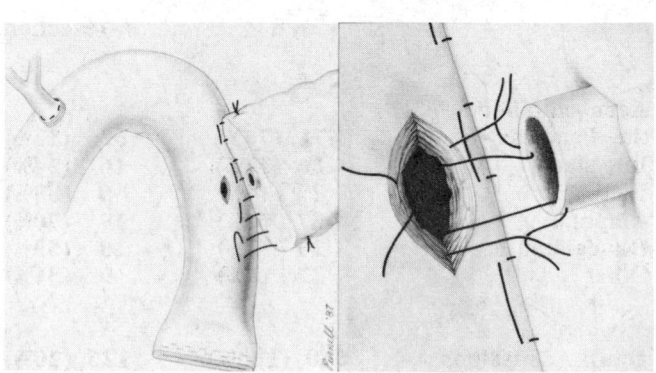

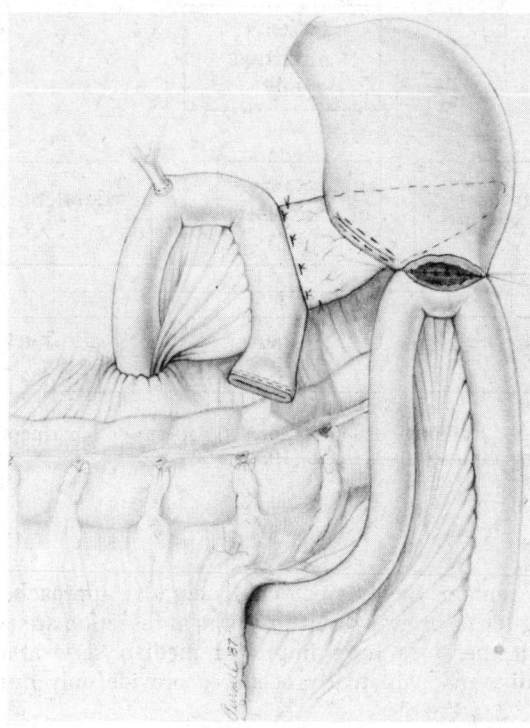

FIG. 26-24. The completed reconstruction, showing the pancreaticojejunostomy, the choledochojejunostomy, and gastrojejunostomy being performed. The pancreatic and jejunal anastomosis is usually done retrocholic and the gastrojejunostomy can be either retrocholic, as shown here, or anticholic.

26-24, although on occasion the gastrojejunostomy will be retrocolic. We prefer to use two Reliavac drains, one in the right upper quadrant and one from the left side of the pancreaticojejunostomy. The wound is closed in standard fashion with a running mass closure with nonabsorbable #1 suture material.

Extended Resections

Extended pancreatic resections have been proposed to include resection of the portal vein, superior mesenteric artery, and celiac axis and an extended nodal dissection.[81] This "regional pancreatectomy" has undergone considerable evolution and refinement and has an improved operative morbidity and mortality.

Current approaches to pancreatic resection for adenocarcinoma have evolved from major arterial resection, but they have encompassed more extensive nodal dissection, liberal use of portal vein resection, and primary reanastomosis, if necessary.

The debate about total pancreatectomy as a preferred procedure over more limited resections continues. As operative morbidity from leakage from pancreaticojejunostomy has decreased, arguments for total pancreatectomy have become less forceful. Because the results in long-term survival do not clearly depend on the type of pancreatic resection, most experienced surgeons rely on the procedure that most easily and adequately removes the primary cancer.

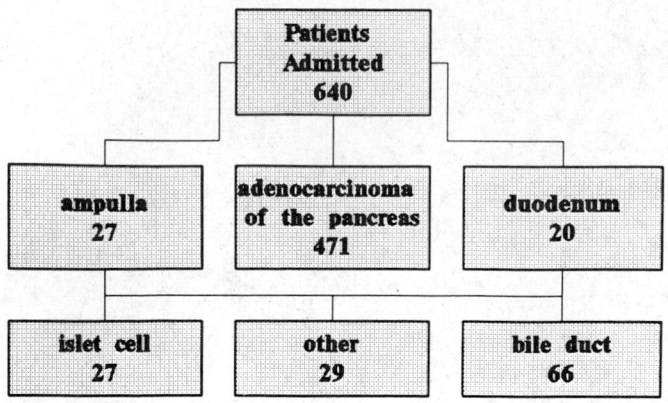

FIG. 26-25. Definitive diagnoses for 640 patients with peripancreatic cancer admitted to MSKCC, 1983–1987.

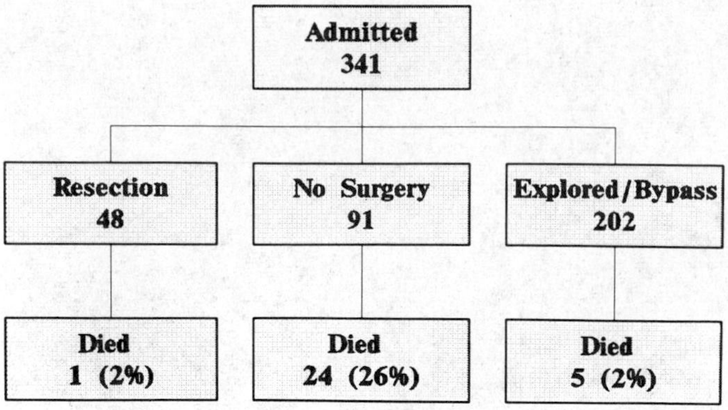

```
            Admitted
              341
   ┌────────────┼────────────┐
Resection   No Surgery   Explored/Bypass
   48           91            202
   │            │             │
 Died         Died          Died
 1 (2%)      24 (26%)       5 (2%)
```

FIG. 26-27. In-hospital 30-day mortality for 341 patients with adenocarcinoma of the pancreas, MSKCC, 1983–1986.

Results

Surgery remains the only potentially curative approach, and the long-term survival results of surgical resection are poor. Adjuvant therapies have improved median survival only minimally, and palliative procedures provide only limited benefit.

The number of patients who present with suspected adenocarcinoma of the pancreas is clearly greater than the actual incidence. From 1983 through 1987, the Memorial Sloan-Kettering Cancer Center (MSKCC) admitted 640 adult patients suspected of having peripancreatic carcinoma. Of these, 471 (73%) had adenocarcinoma of the pancreas. The remainder had bile duct cancer (10%), islet cell cancer (4%), or ampullary or duodenal cancer (7%) (Fig. 26-25). Of 442 patients suspected of having a peripancreatic carcinoma admitted to the same institution between 1983 and 1986, 341 (77%) had adenocarcinoma of the pancreas. The age range for these patients was 31 to 90 years (Fig. 26-26).

OPERABILITY. Of 341 patients, 250 (73%) underwent exploration and 48 (19%) were resected (Fig. 26-27). Comparable figures for the resectability rate of other peripancreatic tumors are shown in Figure 26-28.

The majority of these patients require a pancreaticoduodenectomy or total pancreatectomy. In 63 successive resec-

tions of patients with adenocarcinoma of the pancreas in 4 years, there were only five distal pancreatic resections (8% of those resected). Operations lasted for an average of 6.4 hours (range, 2.2–14.5 hours), and the median intraoperative blood replacement was 1000 ml (0–6500 ml).

The results of resection, bypass, and pancreatic implantation have been previously reported from MSKCC.[82] Until 1980, operative and in-hospital mortality was between 16% and 20% for resection, biopsy, or bypass (Tables 26-7, 26-8, and 26-9). This was similar to the operative mortalities of 15% to 25% reported before 1982 (Table 26-8). In a recent report on 50 cases of adenocarcinoma, patients operated on between 1969 and 1980 were compared with those operated on between 1981 and 1986.[100] The operative mortality rate fell from 24% in the first period to 2% in the second, remarkably similar to the operative mortality of 18% until 1980 at MSKCC and of 2% between 1983 and 1986, with similar numbers of patients (Fig. 26-27). Age has not been a barrier to resection. Patients who are older than 70 years of age have no greater operative mortality and similar survival compared with younger patients (Fig. 26-29).

SURVIVAL. Operative morbidity and mortality have been markedly decreased. Long-term survival, however, is little changed (Table 26-8). The MSKCC experience is shown in Figure 26-30. The influence of brachytherapy on survival

FIG. 26-26. Age range of 341 patients with adenocarcinoma of the pancreas, MSKCC, 1983–1986.

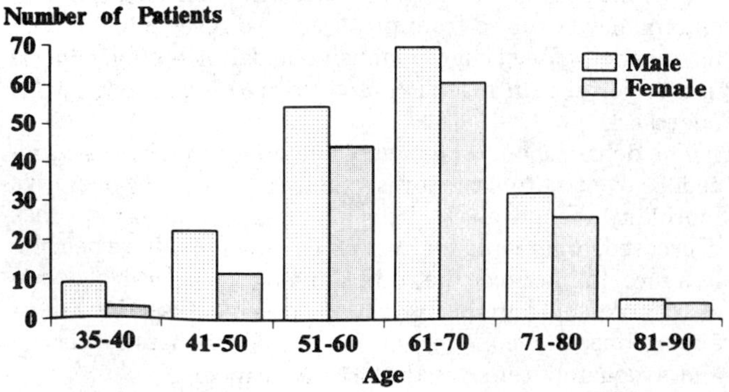

FIG. 26-28. Resectability rates of peripancreatic tumors, MSKCC, 1983–1987.

	n		# resections	
Adenocarcinoma of the Pancreas	471	(74%)	63	(13%)
Bile duct	66	(10%)	16	(24%)
Islet cell	27	(4%)	9	(33%)
Ampulla	27	(4%)	19	(70%)
Duodenum	20	(3%)	10	(50%)
Other	29	(4%)	9	(31%)
Total Admissions	640	(100%)	126	(20%)

TABLE 26-7.   In-Hospital and Long-Term Survival by Procedure

Procedure	No. of Patients	Mortality (%) 30-day	Mortality (%) In-Hospital	Median Surviva (mo)
Biopsy	80	15	16	4
Biopsy, alone	48	19	20	3
Biopsy, previous bypass	32	9	9	6
Bypass	76	12	14	4
Implant	33	0	3	8
All resection for cure	39	18	23	18
Conventional resection*	16	19	19	14
Resection	19	16	16	17

Morrow M, Hilaris B, Brennan MF: Comparison of conventional surgical resection, radioactive implantation, and bypass procedures for exocrine carcinoma of the pancreas, 1975–1980. Ann Surg 199:1–5, 1984.
*Figures exclude cystadenocarcinoma.

was shown to be a median of 8 months, with no in-hospital mortality (Table 26-7). Current experience is similar, with small improvement in those receiving brachytherapy (Fig. 26-31). Hospital stay was not affected by brachytherapy treatment (Table 26-10).

BYPASS PROCEDURES

Between 1970 and 1979, 34% of 46,888 patients in England and Wales had operations for pancreatic cancer, and 95% of these were biliary bypasses for relief of jaundice. Only 5% of the 34% underwent resection; between 1970 and 1979, fewer than 800 pancreatic resections were performed in all of England and Wales, despite their very high incidence of pancreatic cancer.[6] The hospital mortality for pancreatic by-

pass was 20%, compared with 14% mortality for resection in the same series.

Because more than 80% of the patients with carcinoma of the pancreas present with obstructive jaundice and resection is possible in only 25%, palliative bypass has received considerable attention.[98–100] In a collected series of more than 8000 patients with unresectable carcinoma of the pancreas, Sarr and Cameron showed that patients undergoing biliary bypass had a lower operative mortality rate (19%) than did patients subjected to diagnostic laparotomy only (26%).[101] The overall survival was longer (5.4 months) in the patients having bypass than for those patients subject to diagnostic laparotomy (3.5 months). For the 341 patients with adenocarcinoma of the pancreas admitted from 1983 through 1986, the operations performed are illustrated in Figures 26-32 and 26-33.

TABLE 26-8.   Results of Pancreatic Resection for Cure of Exocrine Cancer

Author	Year	Years of Treatment	No. of Patients	No. per Year	Operative Mortality (%)	Mean Survival (mo)
Bowden[83]	1958	26	51	2	31	9
Portland Surg. Coop.[84]	1967	10	27	2	22	22
Crile[85]	1970	Selected	28		NS*	6
Feduska[86]	1971	11	16	1	44	7
Wilson[87]	1974	16	13	1	23	10
Brooks[88]	1975	10	16	1	13	23
Shapiro[89]	1975	Selected	24		8	11
Nakase[90]	1975	25	430	17	22 / 10 b + t / 5 total	12 (head)
Tepper[91]	1976	10	31	3	16	11
Knight[92]	1978	10	16	1	14	16
Moosa[93]	1979	7	52	7	8	23
Longmire[94]	1980	21	50	2	NS	16†
Edis[95]	1980	25	162	6	16	10†
Fortner[96]	1981	9	36	4	15	NS
Herter[97]	1982	39	82	2	19	9
All patients			1034	4‡	18‡	12‡
Memorial Sloan-Kettering Cancer Center	1982	6	39	7	18%	18

Modified from Morrow M, Hilaris B, Brennan MF: Comparison of conventional surgical resection, radioactive implantation, and bypass procedures for exocrine carcinoma of the pancreas, 1975–1980. Ann Surg 199:1–5, 1984.
*NS = not stated; b + t = body and tail of pancreas.
†These figures are medians.
‡These figures are averages.

TABLE 26-9.   Bypass Procedures

Author	Year	No. of Patients	Mortality (%)	Mean Survival (mo)
Bowden[83]	1958	114	57	5
Portland Coop.[84]	1967	248	18	5.4
Crile[85]	1970	28		8
Feduska[86]	1971	60	33	6
Wilson[87]	1974	80	14	6
Brooks[88]	1975	35	15	5.8
Shapiro[89]	1975	24	4	8
Nakase[90]	1975	1791	21	5 head
				3 b + t*
				3 total
Knight[92]	1978	155	22	7
Moosa[93]	1979	31	6	6
Longmire[94]	1980	103		6
Van Heerden[98]	1980	151	6	6†
Brooks[99]	1980	51	24	7
Herter[97]	1982	152	17	6
All patients		3023	18‡	6‡
Memorial Sloan-Kettering Cancer Center	1982	76	12	4

Modified from Morrow M, Hilaris B, Brennan MF: Comparison of conventional surgical resection, radioactive implantation, and bypass procedures for exocrine caracinoma of the pancreas, 1975–1980. Ann Surg 199:1–5, 1984.
*b + t = body and tail of pancreas.
†This is a median figure.
‡These figures are averages.

The question of the preferred biliary diversion—gallbladder to intestine or common bile duct to intestine—has been addressed.[101] The debate centers on the ease of doing cholecystojejunostomy versus the slower decline in bilirubin than in choledochal drainage. Other objections to the cholecystojejunostomy are that the cystic duct will become obstructed by the primary neoplasm and that the cystic duct must enter the common bile duct well above the malignant distal obstruction at the time of initial bypass.[102–104] Conversely, the choledochojejunal anastomosis is technically more difficult and requires greater exposure but has been favored by many.

There have been questions about the merits in terms of survival.[101] In a collected series of over 900 patients, the operative mortality was identical in patients undergoing biliary drainage through the common duct (20%) to those undergoing cholecystojejunostomy (16%). In addition, survival in more than 1600 patients was similar after biliary decompression using the common bile duct (6.5 months) to the gallbladder (5.3 months). These comparisons, although not addressing stage or extent of disease, suggest that either method is equally acceptable.

The problem of recurrent jaundice is poorly addressed. At worst, less than 5% to 10% of patients with obstructive jaundice in which the cholecystojejunostomy was used as the decompression route have recurrent jaundice, which can be resolved with an endoscopic procedure. The particular methods of diversion include not only simple cholecystojejunostomy with a loop but also other procedures such as Roux-en-Y cystojejunostomy, cholecystoduodenostomy, choledochoduodenostomy, and choledochojejunostomy by a loop or by the Roux-en-Y method. These have been looked at

FIG. 26-29. Age range of 48 patients resected for adenocarcinoma of the pancreas, MSKCC, 1983–1986.

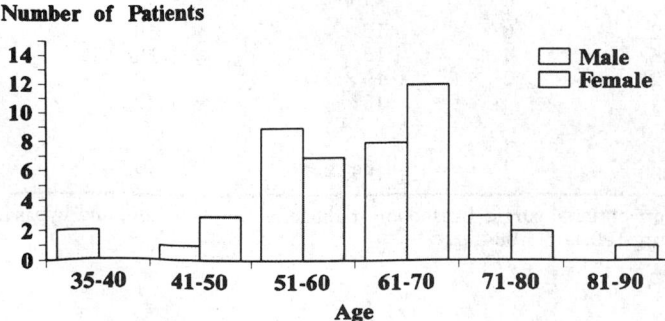

FIG. 26-30. Survival for adenocarcinoma of the pancreas, MSKCC, 1983–1987.

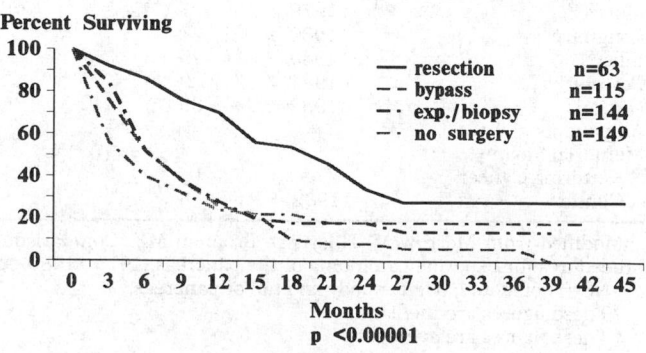

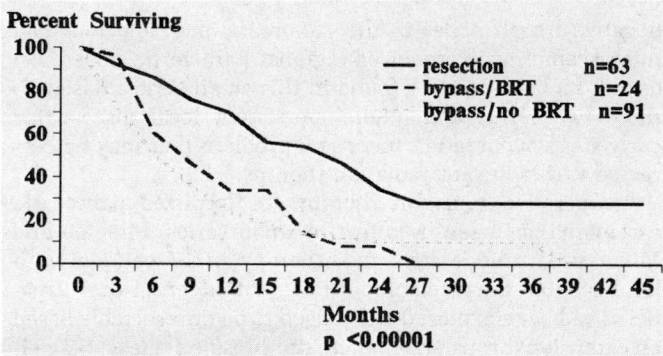

FIG. 26-31. Influence of brachytherapy on survival for adenocarcinoma of the pancreas, MSKCC, 1983–1987.

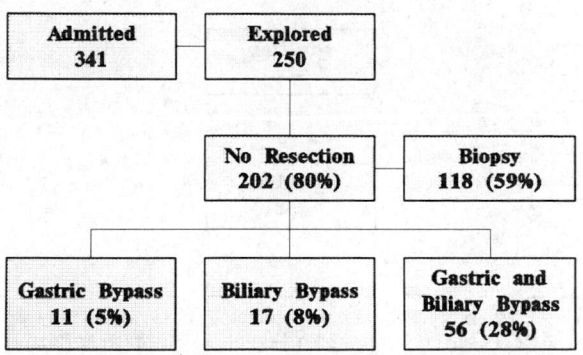

FIG. 26-32. Types of operations performed on 341 patients with adenocarcinoma of the pancreas, MSKCC, 1983–1986.

in terms of survival, and they do not seem to show any significant benefit. A review of 1114 patients shows all methods to give a range of survival between 4.8 and 7.8 months, with considerable overlap.[101]

Gastric Bypass for Obstructive Jaundice

Complete duodenal obstruction is an unusual presenting symptom of pancreatic cancer but is often a component of the disease. Many patients will have some abnormality of the duodenal outlet, detected either by endoscopy or by upper GI radiologic studies. Approximately 30% of patients will present with nausea and vomiting, some of which is associated with duodenal obstruction.[37,105] There has been considerable debate whether gastroenterostomy should be performed in all patients or only when apparently imminent obstruction is present. The objection to routine gastroenterostomy is based on the fact that most patients will not require it, that it increases morbidity due to increased operative time and additional anastomoses, and that some extrapolations have suggested increased mortality. The possibility of subsequent stomal ulceration or some contribution of the gastroenterostomy to functional gastric emptying delay has also been raised.

Reoperations for subsequent duodenal obstruction in patients who had not had previous gastroenterostomy appear to be quite high, ranging from 2% to 50% (Table 26-11). Sarr and Cameron suggest that 13% of patients not undergoing gastroenterostomy at the time of the initial operation subsequently required gastroenterostomy for development of duodenal obstruction.[101] One review reported that almost 50% of

patients who did not have a gastric duodenal bypass initially and survived for 6 months or more were likely to develop duodenal obstruction and needed reoperation.[106] Others suggested a mortality of 10% to 20%.[107,112]

In a collected series of more than 500 patients, there was an average survival of 5.8 months for patients with gastroenterostomy and an average of 6.6 months for those not undergoing gastroenterostomy.[101] Similar figures for operative mortality are suggested in a review of 648 patients: 17% operative mortality with gastroenterostomy and 18% mortality without gastroenterostomy. We believe that gastroenterostomy should be routinely employed unless there is some circumstance specifically arguing against it.

RADIATION THERAPY

ADJUVANT RADIATION THERAPY FOR RESECTABLE DISEASE

Radiation therapy in combination with surgical resection has been used in an attempt to improve local disease control and survival. The pattern of failure after surgical resection by pancreaticoduodenectomy was analyzed for 31 patients from the Massachusetts General Hospital, in which survival (median, 10.5 months) and operative mortality (16%) were equivalent to other surgical series at that time (1963–1973).[91] Of 26 postoperative survivors, 22 patients died of recurrent (persistent) pancreatic carcinoma, 13 cases of which were confirmed by reexploration for suspected recurrence or by autopsy. When the clinical and pathologic findings were combined, 13 patients (50%) were believed to

TABLE 26-10. Hospital Stay for Patients with Pancreatic Adenocarcinoma*

Factors	Resection	Explored Biopsy	Explored Bypass	Explored Brachytherapy	No Operation
Number of patients	48	118	84	19	279
Median	26	17	19	18	14
Range	8–62	2–131	2–84	10–72	1–176
Estimated median survival (mo)	18	4	4	9	3
Hospital stay survival	5%	14%	16%	6%	16%

*Figures for Memorial Sloan-Kettering Cancer Center from October 15, 1983, to October 15, 1986.

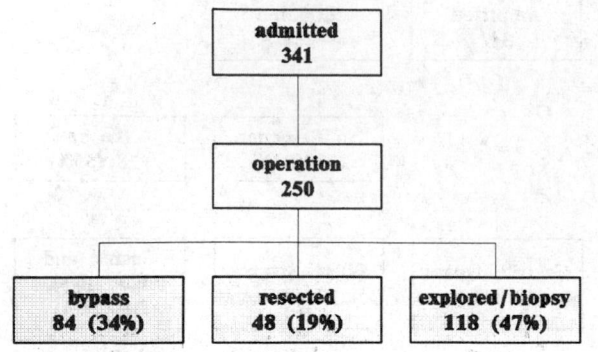

FIG. 26-33. Adenocarcinoma of the pancreas, Memorial Sloan-Kettering Cancer Center, 1983–1986.

have locoregional recurrence within the surgical bed. Only 4 (15%) of 26 patients demonstrated distant metastases without evidence of local failure.

The problem of persistent locoregional disease following surgical resection of Stage I disease was highlighted in a recent autopsy series from Japan.[127] Of eight patients with T1 and T2 tumors, six had microscopic metastases in grossly negative lymph nodes in the pancreatic bed, and four had microscopic involvement of regional para-aortic nodes. No distant metastases were found in this small series. Based on these two series and others, persistent local disease for early-stage pancreatic cancer is a problem that may be corrected with adjuvant radiation therapy.[82]

Preoperative radiation therapy for localized pancreatic carcinoma has been used in two small series. Pilepich and Miller used preoperative radiotherapy in 17 patients with localized, but unresectable, lesions.[128] Sixteen of the 17 patients had been explored and judged to be unresectable based on extension through the pancreatic capsule (at least Stage II disease). The primary tumor was less than 5 cm in 4 patients and 5 cm or larger in the remaining 13 patients. These patients then received conventionally fractionated 200 cGy/ fraction) radiation therapy of 40 to 50 Gy in 4 to 5 weeks. Eleven of the 17 patients were reexplored, with 6 patients undergoing resection of tumors of the pancreatic head. Two patients remained disease-free at 5 years. The second series involved 7 patients with tumor of the pancreatic head or periampullary area who received a pancreaticoduodenectomy procedure and 45 Gy of radiation delivered preoperatively (5 patients) or postoperatively (2 patients).[129] Two

TABLE 26-11.   Incidence of Duodenal Obstruction Requiring Gastroenterostomy (GE) After Initial Laparotomy or Biliary Bypass, 1965–1980

Author	Total	% Undergoing GE at Initial Celiotomy	% Requiring GE in Future	Operative Mortality of Subsequent GE
Glantz[107]	93	26	10*	40
Richards[108]	106	20	34	10
Webster[109]	74	4	26†	14
Pipes[110]	28	8	28‡	
Hertzberg[111]	169	3		
Collure[112]	79	37	20§	
Stuart[113]	48	0	20	
Elmslie[104]	27	20	23	
Douglass[114]	64	8	17	
Vijayanagar[115]	50	30	23	
Mendoza[116]	32	54	14	
Monge[117]	23	12	27	
Buckwalter[118]	296	69	6	
Winegarner[119]	112	29	6	
Williams[120]	135	10	8	
McDevitt[121]	13	46	15	
Howard[37]	81	15	2	
Brooks[88]	60		9	
Glassman[122]	20		20	
Blievernicht[103]	93	45	38	15
Linn[123]	43		16‖	
du Plessis[124]	4		50	
Reed[125]	56		11	
Forrest[126]	159	31	13	
Mean			13	16
Total	1865			

Sarr MG, Cameron JL: Surgical management of unresectable carcinoma of the pancreas. Surgery 91:123–133, 1982.

*Eleven additional patients died with duodenal obstruction.
†Six additional patients had symptoms of duodenal obstruction at death.
‡One additional patient died with duodenal obstruction.
§Two additional patients died with duodenal obstruction.
‖Only 25% of these patients had abnormal UGI series findings originally.

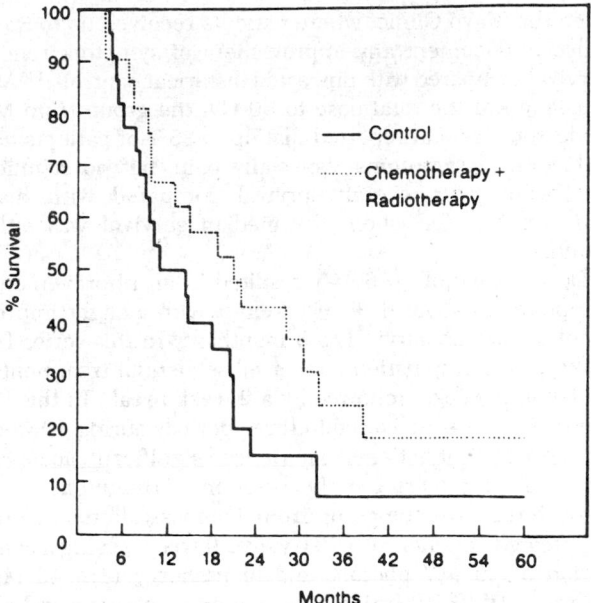

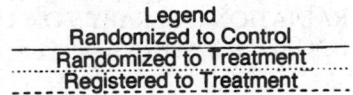

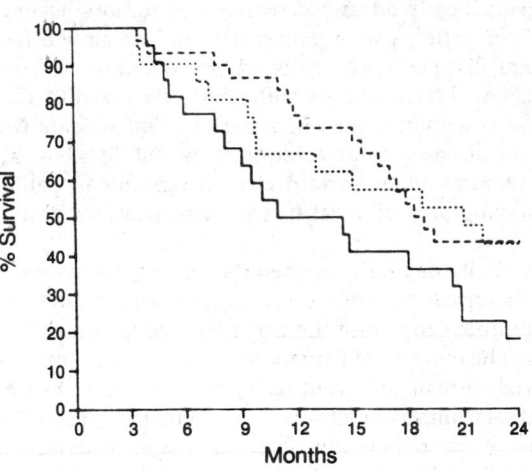

FIG. 26-34. GITSG: comparison of survival in treated with control group. Survival was greater in treated as compared with control groups throughout follow-up period (adjusted p = 0.03) (Kalser MH, Ellenberg SS: Pancreatic cancer: Adjuvant combined radiation and chemotherapy following curative resection. Arch Surg 120:901, 1985)

FIG. 26-35. GITSG: probability of survival by treatment. (Gastrointestinal Tumor Study Group [GITSG]: Further evidence of effective adjuvant combined radiation and chemotherapy following curative resection of pancreatic cancer. Cancer 59:2006–2010, 1987)

patients survived for 5 years, and there were no clinically detected local recurrences.

More recently, two groups have performed randomized prospective trials of postoperative radiation therapy in patients with resected carcinoma of the pancreas. In a study at the National Cancer Institute, 32 patients with locally confined pancreatic carcinoma underwent total or regional pancreatectomy and were randomly allocated to receive either intraoperative radiotherapy (IORT) as adjuvant treatment or conventional treatment.[130] The IORT group of 16 patients received 20 Gy, using 9 to 12 MeV electrons to the tumor bed and regional nodal basins immediately after resection. The surgical and radiotherapeutic details of IORT are described elsewhere.[131,132] The control group of 16 patients received surgery alone for Stage I disease and external-beam radiation therapy (50 Gy in 5–6 weeks) postoperatively for Stage II and Stage III disease. More than 90% of patients on both arms of this study were Stages II and III.

Operative mortality was high (9 of 32 patients) but was similar in both IORT and control groups, as was the incidence of complications in the postoperative period. When operative deaths were excluded from analysis, the disease-free survival was increased in the IORT patients (20 months) compared with the control group (12 months, p = 0.1), but overall survival was similar. Local disease control was significantly improved in the IORT group. Although the number of patients on this trial was modest, it appears that IORT can improve local disease control in locally advanced disease following pancreatectomy with acceptable morbidity.

The Gastrointestinal Tumor Study Group (GITSG) reported on a prospective randomized trial comparing surgery

(usually a Whipple procedure) to postoperative adjuvant therapy with external-beam irradiation (40 Gy in 6 weeks) and 5-fluorouracil (500 mg/m² × 3 days, repeated monthly for 2 years).[133] Forty-three patients were randomized to surgery alone (22 patients) or postoperative adjuvant therapy (21 patients), with an equal distribution of patients with Stages I, II, and III disease. There was a significant improvement in median survival (21 months versus 11 months, p = 0.05) and 2-year survival (43% versus 18%, p = 0.05) in patients receiving postoperative combined modality therapy (Fig. 26-34). Median disease-free survival, however, was 9 months and 11 months in the control and treated groups, respectively, and the overall death rates were 86% and 71%, respectively. Subsequently, the GITSG entered an additional 30 patients with similar clinical and pathologic features into the postoperative combined modality treatment arm.[134] In this study (Fig. 26-35), results similar to the treated arm were obtained. However, the survival curves are carried to 60 months in the earlier study (see Fig. 26-34), whereas in the latter study results are only given for 24 months.

Although these reports from the National Cancer Institute and the GITSG support the use of postoperative adjuvant treatment, the routine use of external-beam irradiation with or without 5-fluorouracil (5-FU) cannot be recommended. Without studies of alternative therapies, postoperative radiation therapy with 5-FU appears to be the adjuvant therapy most likely to prolong survival, but the use of this therapy, given the limited survival prolongation, requires individualization. A series of resected pancreatic carcinoma shows considerable variation in the median survival of 10 to 23 months, with the upper limit similar to the results of the adjuvant therapy trials.[82,93–95,97]

RADIATION THERAPY FOR UNRESECTABLE LOCAL DISEASE

Radiation therapy continues to be a primary treatment for patients with locally advanced, resectable tumors. Overall, up to 50% of patients with pancreatic carcinoma will have locoregional disease at the time of presentation, but only 10% to 15% will have tumors sufficiently localized to allow for surgical resection. Thus, in a majority of patients with locoregional disease, curative surgery is not feasible, and radiation therapy under certain circumstances can palliate signs and symptoms of local disease and possibly prolong survival.

In 1922, Richards first described the use of external-beam radiation therapy for pancreatic carcinoma and reported excellent pain relief in two of the three treated patients.[135] All patients had histologic confirmation of adenocarcinoma, and one survived without recurrent pain for 27 months. A three-field treatment approach similar to the currently used field arrangements for pancreatic carcinoma was described by Richards. In the 1920s and 1930s, there were anecdotal case reports of effective palliation of pain in patients with pancreatic carcinoma by using external orthovoltage radiation.[136,137] Unfortunately, the limited tissue penetration of the available low-energy orthovoltage beams and the proximity of radiosensitive normal structures did not allow for delivery of homogeneously distributed, high doses of fractionated orthovoltage radiation, which we now recognize as being necessary for even a palliative tumor response.

The use of brachytherapy radiation for pancreatic carcinoma was initially described by Upcott in 1912, when he placed radium capsules in a cholecystostomy following resection of an ampullary carcinoma.[138] In 1934, Handley used multiple radium tubes to implant a patient with an unresectable pancreatic carcinoma.[137] The tubes contained up to 35 mg of radium and were removed through the operative wound 15 to 50 hours after implantation. Three of the seven patients treated in this fashion survived for more than 1 year. In the late 1930s, Pack and McNeer used a permanent radium implant in three patients with unresectable pancreatic carcinoma, one of whom survived pain-free for 16 months.[139]

In the 1950s and 1960s, the development of the betatron and the linear accelerator, which were capable of generating megavoltage x-rays, allowed the delivery of high doses of radiation to deep-seated tumors, such as pancreatic carcinoma, with relative sparing of adjacent normal tissues. Phillips from Memorial Hospital, reported the first series of megavoltage irradiation in unresectable pancreatic carcinoma and recorded the effective palliation of symptoms, particularly pain, in 25% of the patients treated to doses of 4400 to 5000 roentgens delivered during 4 weeks.[140] Shortly thereafter, Miller and Fuller from M.D. Anderson Hospital, reported an improvement in symptom palliation and in normal tissue tolerance, compared with orthovoltage radiation, in a series of patients with pancreatic carcinoma.[141]

A dose-response relationship for unresectable pancreatic carcinoma to megavoltage radiation therapy, at least in the palliation of symptoms, is suggested in a comparison of several radiation therapy series. Additionally, there may be a dose-response relationship for overall survival. Early reports from the Mayo Clinic, where patients received up to 35 Gy, failed to document any improvement of symptom relief or survival compared with untreated historical controls.[142] With escalation of the total dose to 50 Gy, the group from M.D. Anderson Hospital reported that up to 33% of patients had a reduction of symptoms, especially pain, but no significant improvement in overall survival compared with historical controls, for whom the median survival was only 6 months.[141]

Dose escalation to 60 Gy resulted in an improvement in symptoms in about 67% of patients, with a slight improvement in median survival to 8 months.[143] In this series from Duke University, patients received sequential treatments of 20 Gy in 2 weeks, followed by a 2-week break. In this regimen, 60 Gy was delivered in three periods during 10 weeks, and only 10% of patients experienced significant, acute radiation effects requiring early cessation of treatment.

More recently, the group from Thomas Jefferson University treated patients with 70 Gy over 9 weeks, using a combination of 45 MV photons and high-energy (15–40 MeV) electrons.[144,145] With this combination of photons and electrons, effective palliation was noted in 50% to 70% of patients, depending on the type and severity of symptoms. Thirty-six of 40 patients completed treatment, and there were only two cases of significant late radiation injury to bowel. A median survival of 10 months was observed, which is similar to some surgical series of resectable pancreatic carcinoma.[24,94]

Although it is difficult to compare retrospective treatment series because of varying and often unknown patient selection factors, as the total dose of external-beam radiation was increased from 35 to 70 Gy a trend of an increased tumor response, as measured by palliation of signs and symptoms and by increased overall survival, was evident. However, it is important to point out that even with doses as high as 70 Gy, local tumor control was achieved clinically in only 50% of patients.[144,145] Unfortunately, many patients who initially respond favorably to the external-beam irradiation of unresectable pancreatic carcinoma will later show evidence of tumor regrowth and the return of local signs and symptoms before death. Even with high-dose external-beam irradiation of 70 Gy, only a rare patient will be a long-term survivor of 5 years or more.[143,144] Because of these poor treatment results, experimental irradiation techniques have been used either alone or in combination with conventional external-beam photon irradiation in an attempt to improve local control and influence overall survival.

EXTERNAL-BEAM PHOTON IRRADIATION FOR UNRESECTABLE DISEASE

Selection of optimal treatment for a patient with a locally advanced unresectable pancreatic carcinoma poses a major problem to the radiation oncologist. Considerations in determining the radiation therapy technique include the extent of local tumor, the volume of normal tissues included within the radiation fields, and the baseline medical and nutritional status of the patient. Although the role of external-beam radiation therapy must be determined on an individual basis, certain guidelines should be followed.

Patients presenting with widespread metastatic disease are clearly not candidates for high-dose external-beam radiation. If local symptoms of pain and intestinal obstruction are the predominant symptoms in a patient presenting with metastasis, then lower doses of radiation (50 Gy) may be used in an attempt to provide temporary palliation. For the unresectable patient presenting with biliary obstruction and clinical jaundice, surgical bypass or endoscopic or percutaneous transhepatic biliary drainage is preferable to palliative external-beam radiation therapy. For a patient with no clinical evidence of visceral metastasis but with significant weight loss (> 10–15% of body weight) and locally advanced unresectable disease, high-dose external-beam irradiation again is not warranted because this type of radiation is typically

complicated by acute symptoms of nausea, vomiting, anorexia, and diarrhea.[146] In the nutritionally depleted patient, the acute radiation symptoms are often severe enough to abort a planned course of high-dose radiation therapy. Even in selected patient series, at least 10% do not complete the planned course of high-dose radiation therapy.[143,144]

Patients with unresectable pancreatic carcinoma found suitable for aggressive external-beam radiation therapy should have locally advanced disease without evidence of dissemination and should demonstrate adequate nutritional status. In this patient group, the intent of external-beam radiation is to deliver a dose of at least 60 Gy to gross disease and 45 to 50 Gy to microscopic disease. The local tumor volume is determined by CT scanning with oral contrast

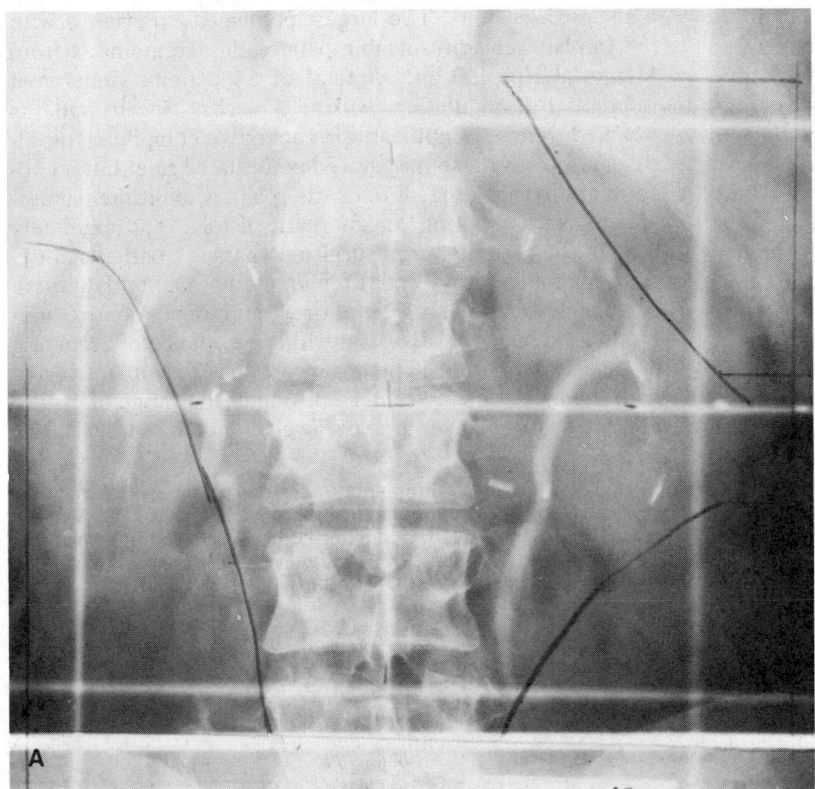

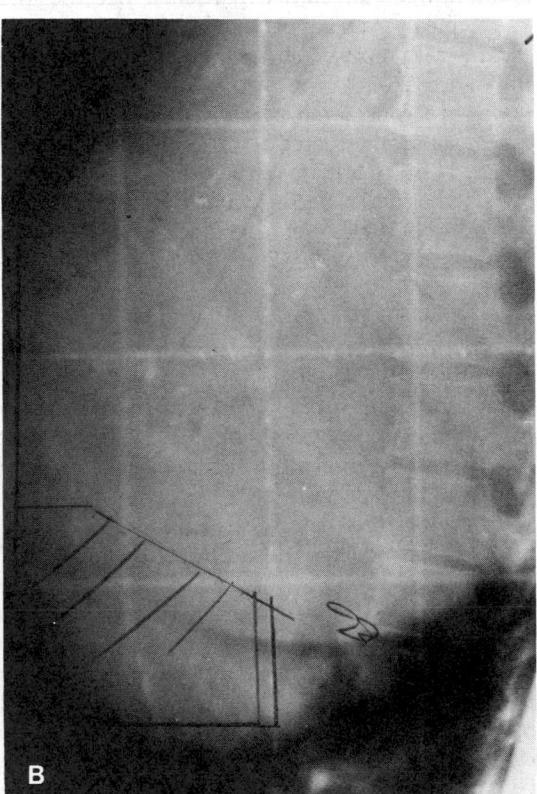

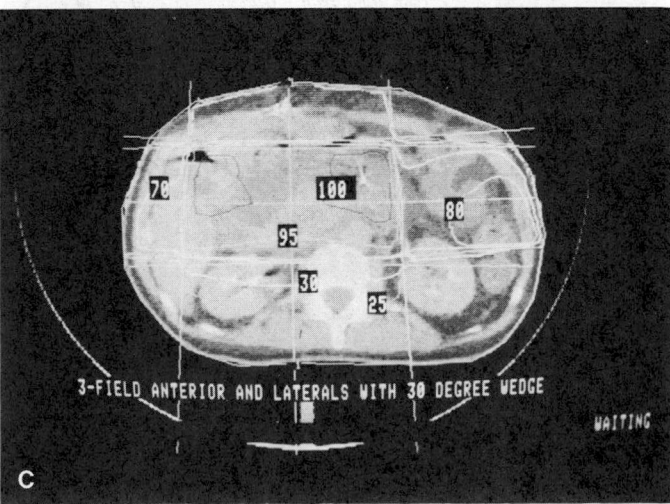

FIG. 26-36. Radiation therapy treatment for carcinoma of the pancreas. **A.** Anterior field including blocks to protect the kidneys. **B.** Lateral field including blocks. **C.** Transverse computer-generated scan with percentages of composite dose distribution from the anterior and lateral wedged fields.

material, by surgical clips placed at the time of exploration, and, if possible, by operative consultation with the radiation therapist or by a review of the surgical and pathology reports. The role of MRI scanning in defining the tumor volume for radiation therapy of unresectable pancreatic carcinoma has not been clearly defined at this time.

A major concern in radiation treatment planning for this patient group is the amount of normal tissues included within the high-dose volume. Organs that limit upper abdominal irradiation include stomach, small bowel, large bowel, liver, kidney, and spinal cord. Although the tolerance of each of these organs is reasonably well defined, when using conventionally fractionated irradiation (1.8–2.0 Gy daily), factors such as previous surgical procedures or the use of concomitant chemotherapy may lower the threshhold for acute and late radiation injury, particularly to the intestine.[146]

A typical external-beam radiation treatment plan for a patient with unresectable pancreatic carcinoma is illustrated in Figure 26-36. The primary tumor and regional lymph nodes are considered part of the initial treatment volume, which is usually treated at 1.8-Gy to 2.0-Gy daily fractions to a dose of 45 to 50 Gy. At the time of simulation, an intravenous pyelogram is performed to visualize the kidneys on both the anteroposterior and lateral radiation fields. Oral contrast material is used to visualize the stomach and proximal small bowel. Typically, a three-field plan, with an anterior field and two wedged lateral fields, usually results in the best dose distribution to cover the initial tumor volume and maximally spare normal tissues. Customized cerrobend blocks are used if appropriate to further protect normal tissue. Additionally, CT scanning in the radiation treatment position often is helpful to best direct the radiation dose distribution to the initial tumor volume.

Following treatment of the initial tumor volume by 45 to 50 Gy, a second simulation is done to plan an increase of the radiation dose to the primary gross disease by an additional 20 to 25 Gy. Although the "boost" field volume often requires a similar three-field or simple anteroposterior/posteroanterior field arrangement, rotational fields may be used for tumor volumes of 5 cm or smaller. Although some series have advocated the use of split-course radiotherapy (20 Gy over 2 weeks, followed by a 2-week break, with a total of 60 Gy administered over 10 weeks), other series have treated continuously to 60 to 70 Gy over 7 to 8 weeks. Although the rationale for split-course external-beam irradiation includes minimizing the acute effects of radiation, increasing the ability to integrate external-beam radiation therapy and chemotherapy, and providing the opportunity to reevaluate patients during treatment breaks for the development of metastasis, protraction of the radiation dose may reduce the radiobiologic effect. At present, there does not appear to be any significant advantage of split-course treatment over continuous fractionation with respect to relief of symptoms, local control, or overall survival.

SPECIALIZED METHODS OF RADIATION THERAPY

Because local control is achieved in fewer than 50% of patients with unresectable pancreatic carcinoma, experimental methods of radiation have been used, often in conjunction with external-beam therapy, to deliver higher effective tumor doses. These specialized experimental techniques include the use of interstitial implants, IORT, high linear energy transfer (high LET) or fast-neutron therapy, and charged-particle irradiation.

Interstitial Therapy

Interstitial irradiation involves implantation of radioactive sources into the pancreatic parenchyma (Fig. 26-37). The use of interstitial implants is attractive in theory because of the rapid falloff in dose from a radioactive source and because of the low dose rate delivered (< 1 Gy per hour), which can result in a greater biologic effectiveness.

The most commonly used isotope for pancreatic implants is iodine-125 (^{125}I). The largest published experience with ^{125}I implants in unresectable pancreatic carcinoma is from Memorial Hospital.[82,147] A total of 33 patients underwent interstitial implantation with ^{125}I seeds. Seven patients (21%) developed significant postoperative complications, although four of these may have been related to either a concomitant bypass procedure or the result of multiple pancreatic biopsies creating a pancreatic fistula. Approximately 67% of the patients had a surgical bypass, 11 patients at the time of implantation and 11 patients before implantation. The median survival for the entire group was 8 months, with the longest survivor alive and without evidence of recurring disease at 33 months. The dose from the ^{125}I implant varied with the extent of the tumor but was in the range of 160 to 200 Gy delivered over 1 year. Twelve patients in this series

FIG. 26-37. Interstitial implantation of the pancreas with radioactive sources for brachytherapy. (Shipley WU, Nardi GL, Cohen AM et al: Iodine-125 implant and external beam irradiation in patients with localized pancreatic carcinoma. A comparative study to surgical resection. Cancer 45:709–714, 1980)

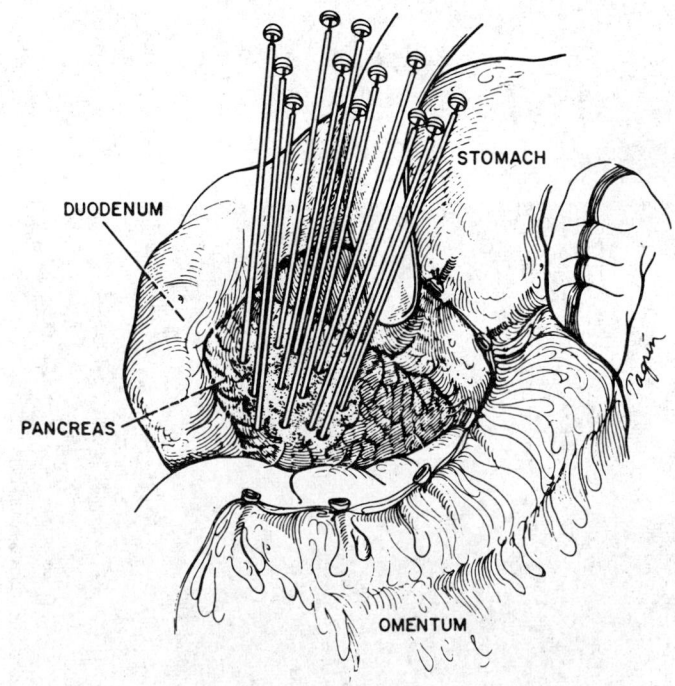

also received external-beam photon irradiation using conventional fractionation to a dose of 30 to 40 Gy.

There was no significant difference in overall survival in this series of 33 implanted patients (median, 8 months) compared with a separate group of 39 patients (median, 18 months) who underwent resection at Memorial Hospital during the same period (Table 26-8).[82] The recent experience with resection shows a highly significant improvement in survival between resection and no resection, with or without brachytherapy (Fig. 26-32).[148] Nine of 33 patients receiving the ^{125}I implant had documented liver metastasis at the time of implantation, and the other 24 patients had locally advanced unresectable disease. The 30-day mortality for this group was 0, compared with 18% for the surgically resected patients. Although showing improved survival, this does not demonstrate statistical significance for brachytherapy over bypass alone, but follow-up is short. Theoretically, significant complications can result from this therapy, but in the MSKCC experience hospital stay was not different for those patients receiving or not receiving brachytherapy (Table 26-10).

There are two other series using ^{125}I implants and external-beam irradiation for unresectable pancreatic carcinoma. At the Massachusetts General Hospital, Shipley and coworkers treated 12 patients with locally advanced pancreatic carcinoma with a combination of ^{125}I implantation (calculated dose of 160 Gy) and external-beam irradiation (45 Gy in 5 weeks), encompassing both the primary tumor and regional lymph nodes.[149] The median survival in this series was 11 months, with 30 months for the longest surviving patient. Clinical local tumor control was achieved in 9 of the 12 patients. Pancreatic fistulas developed in 2 patients, and both responded to conservative management. The group at Thomas Jefferson University also combined the ^{125}I implant with postoperative external-beam irradiation.[145] In this series, 18 patients received a ^{125}I implant (120 Gy) and external-beam radiation therapy (60 Gy); they had a median survival of 12 months, and only 1 patient was thought to have failed locally. Treatment complications included abscess formation in 3 patients, duodenal ulceration with perforation in 1 patient, and pancreatitis in 1 patient.

Intraoperative Radiotherapy

IORT involves the use of large single doses of radiation delivered directly to an exposed tumor and potential areas of regional spread at the time of surgical exploration. High-energy electrons have been used most frequently in Japan and in the United States. IORT has been used alone in patients with locally advanced unresectable pancreatic carcinoma with little obvious therapeutic gain.

In pilot studies from Howard University, the median survival of patients with unresectable pancreatic carcinoma treated with IORT was only 6 months, although 10 of the 19 treated patients had liver metastases documented at surgery and certainly represented a poor prognostic group.[150] The largest experience with IORT alone is from Kyoto University in Japan, where 108 patients were treated.[151] This study noted pain relief in patients receiving an IORT dose of greater than 20 Gy, although there was no documentation of

the extent or duration of pain relief. The median survival was 6 months, and most patients died of progressive disease within 12 months. Ulceration and hemorrhage of the duodenum included within the IORT field occurred in 25% of the patients, but there were no treatment-related deaths. The investigators concluded that the IORT dose should be limited to less than 30 Gy if a significant segment of duodenum needs to be included within the IORT field. In a more recent study from two other Japanese centers, 33 patients received an IORT dose of 20 to 40 Gy, which gave prompt pain relief (within 1 week) in 50% of patients. There was a suggestion of an improved survival in IORT patients (median, 6 months) compared with patients treated with only surgical bypass (median, 2.5 months).[152]

A combination of intraoperative electron-beam irradiation and external-beam photon irradiation has been used in patients with unresectable pancreatic carcinoma at three major medical centers within the United States. A total of 63 patients with locally advanced disease were treated at the Massachusetts General Hospital between 1978 and 1985 on a single-arm pilot study.[153,154] All patients received preoperative external-beam radiation of 10 Gy delivered in five fractions during the week before exploration. At exploration, the patients received introperative electron-beam radiation of 15 to 20 Gy, with most receiving 20 Gy. Misonidazole, a hypoxic cell sensitizer, was given at a dose of 3.5 g/m² immediately before IORT in 41 of 63 patients. A surgical bypass of the bile duct or duodenum was performed as indicated. Postoperatively, the patients received an additional 39.6 Gy of external-beam radiation over 5 weeks. The median survival of the group was 14 months, with a 16.5-month median survival in patients receiving IORT without misonidazole and a 12-month median survival in patients receiving IORT with misonidazole. Approximately 60% of patients were alive at 1 year, and 25% were alive at 2 years. As determined clinically by follow-up CT scans, about 67% of patients had local control at 1 year, but only 40% continued to have local control at 2 years. The longest survival in the series was 52 months.

At the Mayo Clinic, a total of 44 patients with primary unresectable pancreatic carcinoma have been treated with a combination of IORT to 20 Gy and external-beam radiation therapy of 45 to 50 Gy, using conventional fractionation.[155] Some patients also received 5-FU given intravenously for three consecutive days at 500 mg/m² during weeks 1 and 5 of the external-beam irradiation. Median survival was in the range of 12 months, with only 10% of patients alive at 2 years. There was no significant difference in survival based on tumor size of less than or greater than 6 cm. Local tumor progression with the external-beam or IORT fields was uncommon and occurred in only 3 of 42 (7%) evaluable patients. Most patients died of metastatic disease. The most common postoperative problem was a periodic delay in gastric emptying. There were no major problems with duodenal hemorrhage.

At the National Cancer Institute there has been a randomized trial of IORT in patients with unresectable carcinoma of the pancreas.[130] In this study, 32 patients with unresectable Stage III disease or with limited Stage IV disease (liver and peritoneal metastases detected at exploration) were entered into a prospectively randomized trial. The patients in the treatment group received surgical biliary and gastric bypass followed by intraoperative radiation therapy to the primary tumor of 25 Gy using 18 to 22 MeV electrons. These patients then received postoperative external-beam radiation therapy of 50 Gy over 6 to 7 weeks. The control group received the biliary and gastric bypass and postoperative external beam radiation of 60 Gy delivered in split courses of 20 Gy over 2 weeks, with cycles separated by a 2-week break. Both the experimental and control groups received 5-FU begun concomitant with external-beam irradiation at 500 mg/m² for 3 days, repeated every 4 weeks for a year. In this study, in which a majority of patients had Stage IV disease, the median survival for both the IORT and control patients was 8 months. All patients on the control arm died within 18 months, and patients on the IORT arm died within 24 months. Time to local disease progression was longer in the IORT arm, but more than 50% of patients were judged to fail locally. Four patients had complete autopsies. Radiation-related changes were seen, with widespread necrosis and little or no viable tumor identified in two patients.[156] Although the treatment-related complication rates were similar for both the IORT and control groups, three patients receiving IORT developed severe, but not fatal, late duodenal hemorrhage.

Based on the published experience with IORT alone or with the combination of IORT and external-beam irradiation, there does not appear to be any major improvement in overall survival in patients with locally advanced unresectable pancreatic carcinoma. Although the initial experience on the contribution of misonidazole as a radiation sensitizer was positive, further follow-up at Massachusetts General Hospital and from the study at the National Cancer Institute suggests that there is no benefit from the addition of the sensitizer to IORT.[130,153,154] Some of these series suggest a decrease in local failure, but the development of widespread metastatic disease during or shortly after treatment continues to be the major problem.

High Linear Energy Transfer Radiation

The use of high LET radiation can theoretically improve tumor response because its ability to kill cells has little dependence on oxygen concentration. With photon irradiation, which is low linear energy radiation, cell kill can vary by a factor of 2.5 to 3.0, depending on the tissue concentration of oxygen. Fast-neutron irradiation is a type of high LET commonly used in the United States, although it is available only at a limited number of centers.

At the Fermi Laboratory in Illinois, 31 patients with unresectable pancreatic carcinoma received two or three treatments with fast neutrons weekly for up to 7 weeks.[157] These patients received approximately 1950 neutron cGy in 13 fractions, which is estimated to be biologically equivalent to 60 Gy of photon irradiation delivered in conventional fractionation. The median survival in this group was 9 months, with 25 of 31 patients showing clinical evidence of local failure. Additionally, almost 33% of the patients had severe late toxicity, with two treatment-related deaths from GI hemorrhage. At the Mid-Atlantic Neutron Therapy Facility outside Washington, D.C., 19 patients received 1750 neutron cGy in 24 fractions over 6 weeks.[158] Although local control was achieved in approximately 50% of the patients, median survival was only 6 months. There was an unacceptably high rate of late radiation complications, with seven patients experiencing significant GI injuries and one patient developing a transverse myelitis. At the M.D. Anderson Hospital, combined neutron and photon irradiation has been used in 13 patients, who received two neutron and three photon treatments weekly for up to 10 weeks.[159] Although acute and late radiation effects were minimal, median survival was 8 months.

Charged-Particle Irradiation

Both helium ions and negative pi mesons have been used to treat locally advanced pancreatic carcinoma. In contrast to photons or neutrons, for which the beam energy is attenuated continuously in tissue, the dose distribution of charged particles is characterized by a discrete stopping region called the Bragg peak, which is dependent on the initial beam energy. A relatively homogeneous dose distribution can be obtained for a tumor volume using beam modulators. These charged particles are biologically more effective than photons, with factors of relative biological effectiveness of 1.2 for helium ions and 1.5 for negative pi mesons, compared with 1.0 for photons. At the University of California at Berkeley, 34 patients with unresectable pancreatic carcinoma were treated with helium ions, receiving the equivalent of 50 to 60 Gy of photon irradiation over 8 weeks.[160] The median survival in this group was only 9 months, and 24 of the 34 patients had persistent local disease. Additionally, 4 patients developed late GI hemorrhage several months after treatment. At Los Alamos Laboratory, 10 patients received negative pi meson irradiation comparable to 45 to 55 Gy of photon irradiation; they had a survival of only 5 months.[161]

COMPLICATIONS OF TREATMENT

Many physicians have argued against pancreatic resection for adenocarcinoma of the pancreas because of operative mortality in the range of 20% to 30%. The operative mortality in our hands is less than 5%, similar to other reported series. Estimated median operative blood loss in the 48 resections performed at MSKCC for adenocarcinoma of the pancreas from 1983 to 1986 was 2200 ml, with a median replacement of 10,000 ml (0–6500 ml). Mortality is usually associated with a leak of the pancreaticojejunal anastomosis, with the second most common complication being postoperative hemorrhage. The high frequency of leakage from pancreaticojejunostomy has been used as an argument in favor of performing total pancreatectomy. We believe that these complications are small and uncommon, and with operative mortality less than 5%, they should not be used as an argument against resection.

One early postsurgical complication is delayed gastric emptying, which is usually self-limiting and requires agents such as Reglan. If drainage is adequate, pancreaticojejunal leaks and biliary leaks can usually be treated conservatively. On rare occasions, reexploration for such anastomotic difficulties is justified. Later technical complications include stenosis at the choledochojejunal anastomosis. Stenoses are often associated with the development of cholangitis and with progressive deterioration in liver function. The symptoms are intermittent fever and chills, accompanied by mildly elevated liver function test findings. Diagnosis can be confirmed by ultrasound or CT scanning, which can demonstrate a dilated duct and the presence of intraductal stones. If sufficient doubt exists, then transhepatic percutaneous cholangiography can clearly demonstrate the problem. This can be remedied by re-resection of the anastamosis, performed after all the biliary stones have been removed.

Metabolic complications include diabetes mellitus and pancreatic exocrine insufficiency. The development of insulin-dependent diabetes mellitus depends on the amount of normal pancreas left, and various tests of pancreatic reserve are being explored.[162] For most patients who do not have diabetes preoperatively and who require resection only of the head of the pancreas, no supplemental insulin is needed after the procedure.

Unless there was extensive antecedent pancreatitis or chronic obstruction and glandular obstruction, pancreatic insufficiency is usually mild. If there is significant diarrhea or fat malabsorption, then the addition of pancreatic enzyme supplementation before each meal is of significant benefit. Other complications are usually indicators of recurrent disease. Most commonly, the recurrence of pain, jaundice from obstruction or intrahepatic metastases, and the development of ascites are harbingers of relatively imminent demise and require only symptomatic or palliative treatment.

Complications of intraoperative radiation therapy can be significant, with pancreatic leak, the development of pancreatic ascites, and, occasionally, prolonged delays in return to normal GI function. Despite this, we were not able to demonstrate prolonged hospital stays because of brachytherapy (Table 26-10). In all of these situations, nutritional deficits are common, and perioperative use of nutritional support by the parenteral or enteral route is to be encouraged.

CHEMOTHERAPY

The overwhelming majority of pancreatic adenocarcinoma patients have unresectable, incurable disease. These patients have a predictably short survival, averaging only 14 weeks, and fewer than 10% are alive 1 year after diagnosis.[163] Moreover, they have severe, debilitating symptoms that require palliation. The typical patient has evidence of a poor performance status, malabsorption, weight loss, abdominal pain, bowel dysmotility, hepatic synthetic and detoxification derangement, obstructive jaundice, and effusions. Because of this constellation of symptoms, most patients cannot tolerate intensive chemotherapy. There are pharmacokinetic and pharmacodynamic reasons for intolerance of vigorous treatment, including hypoalbuminemia, ascites, anemia, and hepatic dysfunction. For these fragile patients, surviving so short a time, there is a thin therapeutic index and little opportunity for therapy to exert antitumor effects.

In addition to host disability and risk factors, the tumor itself has a virulently expressed biology. Arising within the retroperitoneum and involving deep abdominal structures, this cancer is usually detected in an advanced stage. These sites of original and metastatic disease have the two-fold effect of rarely providing easily measurable disease for judging objective antitumor effects and of presenting a complex picture of physiological derangement.

Pancreatic cancer cells are relatively resistant to conventional chemotherapy, but the reasons for this resistance have not been clearly defined. There has been no systemic evaluation of pancreatic adenocarcinoma cells to screen for the presence of the multiple-drug-resistant phenotype (mdr-1 gene or P-glycoprotein gene).[164,165] Nor has there been a full elucidation of possible intracellular mechanisms of biochemical resistance to nitrosoureas or fluoropyrimidines. A more thorough understanding of the cellular biology of this tumor is needed.

The general pessimism that accompanies chemotherapy for those with advanced disease is well founded but poorly understood. With more than 20,000 deaths in the United States each year, there are too few pancreatic cancer patients being treated in a formal research protocol manner and an insufficient effort to correlate laboratory insights with clinical outcome.

SINGLE-AGENT CHEMOTHERAPY

For more than three decades, efforts have been made to identify effective systemic agents.[163,166,167] Because pancreatic cancer is rarely a locoregional problem, systemic therapy has been the major clinical thrust. Unfortunately, many flaws have consistently characterized chemotherapy studies. Despite the number of new cases diagnosed each year, relatively small series of patients have usually been assembled and reported. Attempts to use objective response rate as a measure of effect have been confounded by interobserver variation or inaccuracy, and attempts to replicate clinical findings have often been frustrating. Differences in the mix of prognostic features of study populations seem to have more often accounted for a "therapeutic advance" than the new treatment itself. Comparisons of the survival of responders and nonresponders have inappropriately been used as prima facie evidence of the identification of new, effective treatments. These study design and analysis difficulties have limited the value of some clinical research efforts and should be considered in the design of future trials.

A therapy can be considered effective if it results in an appreciable number of complete tumor regressions; if it shifts the overall survival for a treated population, including both responders and nonresponders; or if it results in long-term survival for even a minority of patients, affecting the tail on the survival curve. By these criteria, there has been no satisfactory agent yet identified for patients with pancreatic adenocarcinoma.[167,168]

Table 26-12 provides an overview of many of the single agents that have been used in patients with advanced and metastatic pancreatic cancer. These data are a compilation of series reported to NCI Cancer Therapy Evaluation Program Information System (CTEP-IS) or found in the medical literature.[178] The objective response rates are displayed with 95% confidence intervals. The drugs most commonly used

TABLE 26-12.   Single-Agent Chemotherapy in Pancreatic Cancer

Drug	Author	Number of Patients	Response Rate ± 95% CI*
Commonly Used			
5-Fluorouracil	Carter[166]		
	Moertel[169]	251	26 ± 3%
Mitomycin C	Crooke[170]	53	21 ± 6%
Streptozotocin	Carter[166]	27	11 ± 6%
Doxorubicin	GITSG[171]		
	Carter[166]		
	Crooke[170]	28	7 ± 5%
Semustine (methyl-CCNU)	Moertel[169]	91	4 ± 2%
Nitrosoureas			
Carmustine (BCNU)	Moertel[169]	31	0
Lomustine (CCNU)	Carter[166]	19	16 ± 8%
Chlorozotocin	Moertel[169]		
	GITSG[172]	53	6 ± 3%
Intercalators			
Amsacrine	Inamasu[173]		
	Omura[174]		
	Sternberg[175]	109	0
Mitoxantrone (DHAD)	Bedikian[176]	14	0
4′DMDR	Mittleman[177]		
	CTEP-IS[178]	58	10 ± 7%
Epirubicin	Hochster[179]		
	Wils[180]	50	22 ± 6%
Esorubicin	Blayney[181]	16	0
Mitoxantrone	DeSimone[182]		
	CTEP-IS[178]	48	0
Aclacinomycin	CTEP-IS[178]	9	22 ± 14%
Alkylator			
Melphalan	Horton[183]		
	Smith[184]	58	5 ± 3%
Ifosfamide	Gad-El-Mawla[185]		
	Einhorn[186]		
	Bernard[187]	83	26 ± 5%
Miscellaneous			
AZQ	DeSimone[188]	17	0
BTGDR	GITSG[189]		
	CTEP-IS[178]	32	6 ± 4%
Cisplatin	CTEP-IS[178]	15	0
Dactinomycin	GITSG[171]	28	4 ± 4%
Dianhydrogalanul	CTEP-IS[178]	44	5 ± 3%
Etoposide	CTEP-IS[178]		
	Horton[183]	38	0
Hexamethylmelamine	CTEP-IS[178]	54	7 ± 3%
L-Asparaginase	Lessner[190]	10	0
Maytansine	GITSG[172]	33	0
Methotrexate	GITSG[171]	25	4 ± 4%
Metoprine	Sternberg[191]	27	0
MGBG	Inamasu[192]		
	Ravry[193]	66	6 ± 3%
Razoxane (ICRF159)	GITSG[189]	24	8 ± 6%
Tamoxifen	Crowson[194]	14	0
Vindesine	Smith[195]	15	7 ± 7%

*95% confidence interval for responses.

are 5-FU, mitomycin C, streptozotocin, doxorubicin, and methyl-CCNU. Of these agents, only 5-FU has been reported to have a minimum 95%-confidence-boundary response rate of greater than 20%. Whether administered in a bolus intravenous loading or by weekly schedule, there is not convincing evidence that any particular 5-FU regimen is supe-

rior.[196,197] As with other enteric adenocarcinomas, the response rates reported for 5-FU range from 0 to more than 50%.[198] Given the pharmacology of 5-FU, there is evidence that oral 5-FU is unpredictably and inconsistently absorbed and should never be used.[197]

Mitomycin C has become a very popular agent in combination therapy of pancreatic cancer patients. Because of delayed hematologic suppression, it has been used in an intermittent schedule of bolus dosing every 6 to 8 weeks. The chronic toxicities of cumulative marrow depletion, nephrotoxicity, and hemolytic-uremic syndrome are not commonly seen because pancreatic cancer patients rarely benefit sufficiently or live long enough to receive large total doses.[166,170]

The nitrosoureas have also been investigated. Streptozotocin has been the particular focus of study because it is toxic to both pancreatic islet and ductular epithelial cells.[199] Because the drug has relatively little bone marrow toxicity, it can be conveniently combined with other agents in combination programs. However, it does induce nausea, vomiting, anorexia, and renal tubular toxicity, which many patients find intolerable.[168,200,201] Other nitrosoureas, such as BCNU, CCNU, methyl-CCNU, and chlorozotocin, have also been screened, but they benefitted very few patients as single agents.[166,202]

The other interesting compounds are the anthracyclines. Doxorubicin has been evaluated in a small population of patients as a single agent.[203] Although the response rate is low, it has been incorporated in some combination programs.[170]

In recent years, many drugs have been used as first-line therapies. The attempt to study the best possible patient population is thought to aid the identification of potentially effective therapies. Anthracycline analogues, including epirubicin, 4'demethoxydoxorubicin (4'DMDR), and aclacinomycin A, have resulted in objective responses.[177-180] However, it is not clear whether they are superior to doxorubicin in terms of efficacy or toxicity. Responses have also been noted with the alkylators, melphalan and ifosfamide, but further evaluation is necessary.[183-187] There is no single agent of dramatic efficacy.

COMBINATION CHEMOTHERAPY

Attempts to improve on the unsatisfactory state of single-agent chemotherapy for pancreatic adenocarcinoma have led investigators to explore drug combinations. Clinical investigators recognized the variability and imprecision of small Phase II studies and began to perform larger, randomized studies to define activity more reliably. Table 26-13 summarizes selected randomized two-drug studies, based on 5-FU, which provided the therapeutic rationale for the subsequent three-drug combinations. Response rates for these two-drug regimens, including BCNU, streptozotocin, methyl-CCNU, and mitomycin C, are clustered between 5% and 33%, with 95% confidence limits of ± 3% to 9%. The median survival time for the entire treated population varies between 9 and 26 weeks. No two-drug combination provides satisfactory palliation or survival benefits.[169,208]

Some biologic similarities between gastric and pancreatic cancer have been noted, and similar therapeutic regimens have been applied. The most widely employed three-drug regimens derived from work begun at Georgetown University in the early 1970s. Patients with enteric adenocarcinoma were treated with, and responded to, combinations of 5-FU, mitomycin C, and either Adriamycin or streptozotocin, administered in a cyclic weekly program. In 1978, the SMF program was described.[209] All agents were administered by bolus or short-infusion IV injection: streptozotocin (1 gm/m²) and 5-FU (600 mg/m²) on days 1, 8, 29, and 36; mitomycin C (10 mg/m²) on day 1 of each 8-week treatment cycle. Of 23 patients treated with SMF, there were 10 (43%) objective responses, and there was an overall median survival of 24 weeks. Other investigators found a similar efficacy for the SMF program.[210,211]

In 1980, Smith and colleagues described their results with the FAM program: 5-FU (600 mg/m²) on day 1, 8, 29, 36; Adriamycin (30 mg/m²) on day 1 and 29; mitomycin C (10 mg/m²) on day 1, repeated every 8 weeks. An objective response rate of 37% in 27 patients was described.[212] Both SMF and FAM demonstrated increased survival times for responding patients compared with nonresponding patients; the toxicity proved tolerable, and some patients enjoyed meaningful palliation. However, these initial studies consisted of small numbers of patients, and the results of other Phase II attempts to confirm these FAM and SMF data were not entirely consistent. Response rates of as low as 13% were reported.[195,214-216] Table 26-14 lists some of the more popular three- or four-drug combinations tested. Where replica-

TABLE 26-13. Selected Two-Drug Combination Chemotherapy in Randomized Trials for Pancreatic Cancer

Author	Treatment	Number	Objective Response Rate (±95% CI)*	Median Survival (weeks)
Kovach[204]	5-FU + BCNU†	30	10 (33 ± 9%)	24
	5-FU	31	5 (16 ± 7%)	26
	BCNU	21	0 (0%)	22
Moertel[205]	5-FU + streptozotocin	42	5 (12 ± 5%)	13
	Streptozotocin + cyclophosphamide	51	6 (12 ± 5%)	9
Moertel[206]	5-FU + spironolactone	89		18
	5-FU + streptozotocin ± spironolactone	87		16
Buroker[207]	5-FU + mitomycin C	45	10 (22 ± 6%)	19
	5-FU + methyl-CCNU	43	2 (5 ± 3%)	17

*95% confidence interval.
†5-FU = 5-fluorouracil; BCNU = carmustine; methyl-CCNU = semustine.

TABLE 26-14.   Selected Combination Chemotherapy in Pancreatic Cancer

References	Common Regimen Designations	Range of Response Rates	Range of Median Survival (weeks)
195, 198, 212, 213	FAM*	13–40%	12–24
195, 209, 211, 214, 215	SMF	14–43%	13–24
216	FAC	21%	16
217	FAM-chlorozotocin	13%	25
218	FAM-streptozotocin	18–48%	18–22
219	FAMMe	22%	

*FAM = 5-fluorouracil, doxorubicin, mitomycin C; SMF = streptozotocin, mitomycin C, 5-fluorouracil; FAMMe = 5-fluorouracil, doxorubicin, mitomycin C, semustine; FAC = 5-fluorouracil, doxorubicin, cisplatin.

tion has been performed, the range of responses is given. With variable response rates and minimal impact on overall survival, no combination therapy demonstrates apparent superiority.

To define more precisely the efficacy of the competing FAM and SMF programs and to compare FAM with simpler, less-toxic regimens, three important randomized trials have been performed (Table 26-15). The Gastrointestinal Tumor Study Group (GITSG) compared several chemotherapy programs, including FAM and two SMF programs, in 1976. The FAM and SMF I regimens were modeled to conform exactly to the Georgetown University protocols, whereas SMF II was a modification, employing a 5-day loading course for 5-FU.[209,212,220] A total of 92 previously untreated patients were studied, 34 of whom had a performance status 0 or 1. The response rates were indistinguishable, and median survival very nearly so. The investigators concluded that SMF I "ranked first" among the regimens tested, but neither FAM nor SMF could be recommended for routine use.[220]

In 1986, Oster and colleagues described 184 patients treated with either FAM or SMF (as used by GITSG and Georgetown).[221] More than 70% of patients had a performance status 0 or 1 and had undergone a prior celiotomy. Objective responses were slightly more frequent for FAM (1 complete response and 8 partial responses in 90 patients) compared with SMF (3 partial responses in 94 patients), but there were no statistically significant differences in response or survival (medians, 18.3 for FAM versus 26.4 weeks for SMF). Reasonable levels of toxicity were produced, with 50% of FAM and 39% of SMF groups having severe or life-threatening toxicity. These investigators also concluded that neither regimen was truly satisfactory.

The third important study was reported by the North Central Cancer Treatment Group (NCCTG).[222] This was a Phase II comparison of 5-FU (500 mg/m^2 per day × 5, repeated at 4 weeks × 2, then at 5 weeks); 5-FU (400 mg/m^2 daily × 4) plus doxorubicin (40 mg/m^2 every 4 weeks × 2, then every 5 weeks); and FAM. A total of 144 cases were evaluated for survival, and 33 with measurable disease were evaluated for objective response. There was a nonsignificant greater number of responses for 5-FU and 5-FU plus doxorubicin than for FAM. The median survival times were clustered at 17 to 23 weeks. Although somewhat more marrow toxicity resulted with FAM, about 30% of the 5-FU and 5-FU plus doxorubicin groups had leukopenia (2000/mm^3). Considering toxicity, cost, and survival, the authors concluded that neither drug combination was superior to 5-FU.[222]

Based on all the available data, it is difficult to recommend any particular combination program for patients outside a clinical trial setting. Simple attempts to combine the minimally effective agents in an empirical manner produce combinations of two to four drugs that more often yield toxicity rather than efficacy.[218,219,223-225] Trivial differences may exist between regimens, but the vast majority of patients are not benefitted.

CHEMOTHERAPY TRIALS

For patients with incurable disease, there is an ongoing effort to identify effective systematic chemotherapy drugs and

TABLE 26-15.   Selected Combination Chemotherapy in Pancreatic Cancer: FAM and SMF Comparisons

Author	Treatment	Number	Objective Response Rate (±95% CI)*	Median Survival (weeks)
GITSG[220]	FAM†	90	9 (14% ± 4%)	18.3
	SMF	94	3 (4% ± 2%)	26.4
Oster[221]	FAM	29	4 (14% ± 6%)	11.6
	SMF I	28	4 (14% ± 7%)	17.7
Cullinan[222]	5-FU	50	3/10 (30% ± 15%)	23
	5-FU + doxorubicin	44	3/10 (30% ± 15%)	23
	FAM	50	1/13 (8% ± 7%)	17

*95% confidence interval.
†FAM = 5-fluorouracil (5-FU), doxorubicin, mitomycin C; SMF = streptozotocin, mitomycin C, 5-fluorouracil.

biologicals. Formal disease-oriented Phase II screening efforts, sponsored by pharmaceutical companies or by the National Cancer Institute, are the focus of most clinical efforts. Additionally, there is a randomized trial being conducted by the NCCTG, which seeks to confirm the efficacy of a combination chemotherapy program described by Mallinson et al in 1980.[226] These authors randomized 40 patients either to supportive care only (no chemotherapy) or to a regimen consisting of 5-FU (270 mg/m² daily for 5 days), cyclophosphamide (160 mg/m² on day 1 and 5), methotrexate (11 mg/m² on day 1 and 4) and vincristine (0.7 mg/m² on day 2 and 5), followed in 5 weeks with 5-FU (350 mg/m²) plus mitomycin C (3.5 mg/m²), both daily for 5 days. The median survival of the control group was 9 weeks, compared with 44 weeks for those treated with chemotherapy (p = 0.0006). The toxicity was acceptable, and the treatment appeared to demonstrate substantial benefit. To assess this treatment, the NCCTG plans to randomize approximately 200 patients to one of three treatments: 5-FU (500 mg/m² daily for 5 days every 5 weeks); the Mallinson regimen; or 5-FU (300 mg/m², daily for 5 days, plus doxorubicin (40 mg/m² on day 1) plus cisplatin (60 mg/m², daily) repeated every 5 weeks.[216] This study should complete accrual in 1988 and should provide definitive confirmation or refutation of this therapy.

Studies based on laboratory information have produced Phase III trials comparing combinations of cisplatin, Ara-C, and caffeine to the more conventional SMF regimen.[227]

NEW DIRECTIONS

Several new themes in pancreatic adenocarcinoma clinical research are likely to develop in the near future. Formal clinical trials investigating biologic response modifiers (BRM) are anticipated. There are few data on the use of interferons in pancreatic cancer, and small studies with recombinant gamma-interferon and other products have neither been promising nor definitive.[228,229] There has been relatively little clinical exploration of interleukins, with or without activated lymphocytes, in these patients.[230,231]

There has been more, albeit incomplete, data on therapeutic monoclonal antibodies. Experience with the 17-1A antibody has been the best described. This is a murine-derived IgG2a monoclonal antibody generated against a human colorectal adenocarcinoma cell line. It binds to human enteric cancers in vitro and inhibits adenocarcinoma xenografts in athymic nude mice.[232-234] Preliminary studies in man demonstrated that 17-1A was tolerable, but antimouse antibodies were detected circulating in those treated.[235] Phase II studies in pancreatic cancer patients have used both 17-1A alone and 17-1A absorbed on autologous peripheral mononuclear white cells that are reinfused.[236,237]

Sindelar reported objective responses in 4 of 25 pancreatic cancer patients treated with 17-1A, but these benefits were brief, ranging from 6 to 40 weeks, with a median overall survival of 12 weeks.[236] Further analyses of these data suggest no significant objective response.[238] Patients have also been treated with 17-1A plus FAM chemotherapy.[239] Clinical responses have been noted, but the inclusion of conventional chemotherapy complicated the interpretation of the data. There are other monoclonal antibodies, such as DU-PAN-1 through DU-PAN-5 and ACI, that may prove to be of clinical relevance for pancreatic cancer patients.[240,241] This is a promising area of clinical investigation which is now only beginning to be explored.[66]

RELATIVE THERAPEUTIC EFFECTIVENESS

It is very difficult to evaluate cost effectiveness in the treatment of pancreatic adenocarcinoma. Length of hospital stay has been used as an indication of the effectiveness of treatment. Table 26-10 outlines the length of stay at the Memorial Sloan-Kettering Cancer Center in New York. It is clear that length of stay varies by only a small degree for patients undergoing major resection, those undergoing bypass procedures, with or without radiation therapy, or those being admitted and not undergoing surgery. Basing the length of subsequent survival on the length of stay, if the average survival for a bypass procedure is 4 months, the length of stay as a percentage of life expectancy is 14%. Conversely, if we do the same for resections, then the length of stay is 5% of mean estimated survival rates. This does not take into account perioperative or in-hospital mortality, and because mortality was greater in patients with advanced disease and shorter life expectancy, this only exaggerates these effects. In similar fashion, if conventional radiation therapy is delivered over 6 weeks for unresectable disease, patients will be in active daily treatment for 25% of their life expectancy. A clear indication of the costs or charges accrued by such a treatment has yet to be produced.

PAIN RELIEF

Epigastric pain is the most common symptom in patients with pancreatic carcinoma and often is the reason for seeking medical attention. Increase in the severity of epigastric pain, associated with radiation to the back or diffuse radiation in the abdomen, occurs in most patients during the course of their disease. Severe pain is the most incapacitating symptom of pancreatic cancer. In a study of pain prevalence in patients with lung, prostate, uterine, cervical, or pancreatic cancer that has recently been completed, 60% of patients with pancreatic cancer reported "moderate to bad" pain in the past week.[242] Patients (86%) were interviewed within 6 months of diagnosis and tended to be those who had survived after surgery. Daily "moderate to bad" pain occurred in 38% of these patients.

The cause of severe pain is believed to result from tumor infiltration into the retroperitoneum and splanchnic nerve plexus.[243] Treatment to palliate pain includes medical management with narcotic analgesics, surgical neurotomy, chemical neurolysis, and radiation therapy. Three treatment approaches are discussed here, and a discussion of the judicious use of narcotic analgesics in cancer patients is presented in Chapter 59. Medical management alone often is not successful in relieving pain in patients with pancreatic carcinoma.

Three types of surgical neurotomy have been used to ease pain in patients with pancreatic carcinoma, including a neurotomy of the preganglionic sympathetic plexus, a neurotomy of the celiac and superior mesenteric ganglions, and a neurotomy of the postganglionic plexus of the celiac ganglion.[244-246] Considerable expertise is required to perform these procedures, particularly in the patient with locally advanced or locally recurrent pancreatic carcinoma. Unfortunately, most patients will experience only partial and temporary pain relief following neurotomy, presumably resulting from inadequate surgical denervation or subsequent tumor infiltration of other nerve roots in the retroperitoneum.

Chemical neurolysis, using either an intraoperative or percutaneous approach, is used more often today than surgical neurotomy to relieve pain in patients with pancreatic carcinoma. The percutaneous injection of 50 ml of 50% alcohol after a diagnostic injection of pontocaine was described by Bridenbaugh and colleagues in 1964.[247] The efficacy of neurolytic block of the celiac plexus approaches 90%.[248,249] Needle verification by radiographic techniques, particularly CT scanning, appears to reduce morbidity and improve efficiency.[250,251] Serious complications of a percutaneous nerve block are rare (<1%) and result from inadvertent injection into the peritoneal cavity (causing peritonitis) or into the subarachnoid space (causing paralysis). Transient hypotension as a result of splanchnic pooling following injection occurs more commonly and responds to supportive care.

Chemical neurolysis may be more easily performed intraoperatively.[243] At laparotomy, both sides of the celiac axis are directly injected with 50% alcohol or 6% phenol. No increased morbidity or mortality, compared with laparotomy and surgical bypass alone, is reported by the University of Michigan.[243] Approximately 90% of their patients had effective and, occasionally, permanent pain relief.

External-beam radiation therapy is often effective in reducing pain associated with pancreatic carcinoma. Based on a comparison of retrospective series, doses of > 50 Gy (usually > 60 Gy) are required.[143-145] Between 50% and 70% of patients will experience significant pain relief. Japanese investigators have used large, single doses of intraoperative electron-beam radiation.[151,152] Doses of 20 to 40 Gy delivered to unresectable pancreatic carcinoma results in effective and often prompt (within 1–2 weeks) pain relief in as many as 50% of patients. However, intraoperative radiation therapy remains an experimental approach available only in a limited number of medical centers within the United States.

REFERENCES

1. Levin DL, Connelly RR: Cancer of the pancreas: Available epidemiologic information and its implications. Cancer 31:1231, 1973
2. Pollack ES: The epidemiology of cancer and the delivery of medical care services. Public Health Rep 99:476, 1984
3. Buncher CR: Epidemiology of pancreatic cancer. In Moosa AR (ed): Tumors of the Pancreas, p 415. Baltimore, Williams & Wilkins, 1980
4. World Health Organization: Cancer Incidence in Five Continents, vol IV. IARC Sci Publ 42, 1982
5. Thomas DB, Karagas MR: Cancer in first and second generation Americans. Cancer Res 47:5771, 1987
6. Allen-Mersh TG, Earlam RJ: Pancreatic cancer in England and Wales: Surgeons look at epidemiology. Ann R Coll Surg Engl 68:154, 1986
7. Hoover R, Mason T, McKay F et al: Geographic patterns of cancer mortality in the United States. In Fraumeni JF (ed): Persons at High Risk of Cancer. An Approach to Cancer Etiology and Control, pp 343–360. New York, Academic Press, 1975
8. MacMahon B, Yen S, Trichopoulos D, et al: Coffee and cancer of the pancreas. N Engl J Med 304:630, 1981
9. Feinstein A, Horowitz R, Spitzer W et al: Coffee and pancreatic cancer: The problems of etiologic science and epidemiologic case-control research. JAMA 246:957, 1981
10. Wynder E, Hall N, Polansky M: Epidemiology of coffee and pancreatic cancer. Cancer Res 43:3900, 1983
11. Hakulinen T, Lehtimaki L, Lehtonen M et al: Cancer morbidity among two male cohorts with increased alcohol consumption in Finland. J Natl Cancer Inst 52:1711, 1974
12. Wynder E, Mabuchi K, Maruchi N et al: A case control study of cancer of the pancreas. Cancer 31:641, 1973
13. Wynder E, Mabuchi K, Maruchi N et al: Epidemiology of cancer of the pancreas. J Natl Cancer Inst 50:645, 1973
14. Monson R, Lyon J: Proportional mortality among alcoholics. Cancer 36:1077, 1975
15. Wynder E: An epidemiologic evaluation of the causes of cancer of the pancreas. Cancer Res 35:2228, 1975
16. Krain L: The rising incidence of carcinoma of the pancreas. An epidemiologic appraisal. Am J Gastroenterol 54:500, 1970
17. Kahn H: The Dorn study of smoking and mortality among U.S. veterans: Report on eight and one-half years of observation. Natl Cancer Inst Monogr 19:1, 1966
18. Pour P, Wilson R: Experimental tumors of the pancreas. In Moosa A (ed): Tumors of the Pancreas, p 37. Baltimore, Williams & Wilkins, 1980
19. Sindelar W, Kurman C: Nitrosamine-induced pancreatic carcinogenesis in outbred and inbred Syrian hamsters. Carcinogenesis 3:1021, 1982
20. Bartholomew L, Gross J: Carcinoma of the pancreas associated with chronic relapsing pancreatitis. Gastroenterology 35:473, 1958
21. Lundh G, Nordenstam H: Pancreas calcification and pancreas cancer. A discussion of two cases. Acta Chir Scand 136:493, 1970
22. Robin A, Scott J, Rosenfeld D: The occurrence of carcinoma of the pancreas in chronic pancreatitis. Radiology 94:289, 1970
23. Mainz D, Webster P: Pancreatic carcinoma. A review of etiologic considerations. Am J Dig Dis 19:459, 1974
24. Brooks J: Cancer of the pancreas. In Brooks JR (ed): Surgery of the Pancreas, p 263. Philadelphia, WB Saunders, 1983
25. Sasaki A, Kamado K, Horiuchi N: A changing pattern of causes of death in Japanese diabetics. Observations over fifteen years. J Chronic Dis 312:433, 1978
26. Karmody A, Kyle J: The association between carcinoma of the pancreas and diabetes mellitus. Br J Surg 56:362, 1969
27. Mancuso T, El-Attar A: Cohort study of workers exposed to betanaphythylamine and benzidine. J Occup Med 9:277, 1967
28. Pour P, Althoff J, Kruger F et al: The effect of N-Nitrosobis (2-oxopropyl)almine after oral administration to hamsters. Cancer Lett 2:323, 1977
29. Longnecker D, Curphey T: Adenocarcinoma of the pancreas in azaserine-treated rats. Cancer Res 35:2249, 1975
30. Skandalakis JE, Gray SW, Rower JS et al: Anatomical complication of pancreatic surgery. Contemp Surg 15:17, 1979
31. Kasugai T, Kuno N, Kobayashi S: Endoscopic pancreatocholangiography. Gastroenterology 63:217, 1972
32. Michels NA: The hepatic, cystic and retroduodenal arteries and their relations in the biliary ducts. Ann Surg 133:503, 1951
33. Cubilla AL, Fitzgerald PJ: Surgical pathology of tumors of the exocrine pancreas. In Moosa AR (ed): Tumors of the Pancreas, pp 159–193. Baltimore, Williams & Wilkins, 1980
34. Cello JP: Carcinoma of the pancreas. In Sleisenger MH, Fordtran JS (eds): Gastrointestinal Disease: Pathophysiology, Diagnosis, Management, 3rd ed, pp 1514–1527. Philadelphia, WB Saunders, 1983
35. Cubilla AL, Fitzgerald PJ: Tumors of the Exocrine Pancreas. Washington DC, Armed Forces Institute of Pathology, 1984
36. Legg MA: Pathology of the pancreas. In Brooks JR (ed): Surgery of the Pancreas, pp 41–77. Philadelphia, WB Saunders, 1983
37. Howard JM, Jordan GL: Cancer of the pancreas. Curr Probl Cancer 2:1, 1977
38. Cancer of the Pancreas Task Force: Staging of cancer of the pancreas. Cancer 47:1631, 1981
39. Fortner JG: Regional pancreatectomy for cancer of the pancreatic ampulla with other related sites: Tumor staging and results. Ann Surg 199:418, 1984
40. Gudjonsson B, Livestone EM, Spiro HM: Cancer of the pancreas. Diagnostic accuracy and survival statistics. Cancer 42:2494, 1978
41. Perez MM, Newcomer AD, Moertel CG et al: Assessment of weight loss, food intake, fat metabolism, malabsorption, and treatment of pancreatic insufficiency in pancreatic cancer. Cancer 52:346, 1983
42. Go VLW, Taylor WF, DiMagno EP: Efforts at early diagnosis of pancreatic cancer: The Mayo Clinic experience. Cancer 47:1698, 1981
43. Moertel CG: Exocrine pancreas. In Holland JF, Frei E (eds): Cancer Medicine, 2nd ed, pp 1792–1804. Philadelphia, Lea & Febiger, 1982
44. Fras I, Litin EM, Pearson JS: Comparison of psychiatric symptoms in carcinoma of the pancreas with those in some other intra-abdominal neoplasms. Am J Psychiatry 123:1553, 1967

45. Sack GH, Levin J, Bell WR: Trousseau's syndrome and other manifestations of chronic disseminated coagulapathy in patients with neoplasms: Clinical, pathophysiologic, and therapeutic features. Medicine 56:1, 1977
46. Steinberg WM, Gelfand R, Anderson KK et al: Comparison of the sensitivity and specificity of the CA 19-9 and carcinoembryonic antigen assays in detecting cancer of the pancreas. Gastroenterology 90:343, 1986
47. Piantino P, Andriulli A, Gindro T et al: CA 19-9 assay in differential diagnosis of pancreatic carcinoma from inflammatory pancreatic diseases. Am J Gastroenterol 81:436, 1986
48. Haglund C, Roberts PJ, Kuusela P et al: Gastrointestinal cancer associated antigen CA 19-9 in histological specimens of pancreatic tumors and pancreatitis. Br J Cancer 53:189, 1986
49. Haglund C: Tumour marker antigen CA 12-5 in pancreatic cancer: A comparison with CA 19-9 and CEA. Br J Cancer 54:897, 1986
50. Pasquali C, Sperti C, D'Andrea AA et al: Evaluation of carbohydrate antigens 19-9 and 12-5 in patients with pancreatic cancer. Pancreas 2:34, 1987
51. Sakahara H, Endo K, Nakajima K et al: Serum CA 19-9 concentrations and computed tomography findings in patients with pancreatic carcinoma. Cancer 57:1324, 1986
52. Mahvi DM, Meyers WC, Bast RC et al: Therapeutic efficacy as defined by a seriodiagnostic test utilizing a monoclonal antibody in carcinoma of the pancreas. Ann Surg 202:440, 1985
53. Moosa AR, Levin B: The diagnosis of "early" pancreatic cancer: The University of Chicago experience. Cancer 47:1688, 1981
54. Moosa AR, Mackie CR, Gelder FB et al: The value of tumor markers in the diagnosis and management of nonendocrine tumors of the pancreas. In Moosa AR (ed): Tumors of the Pancreas, pp 355–380. Baltimore, Williams & Wilkins, 1980
55. Holyoke ED, Evans JT, Mittleman A: Biochemical Markers for Cancer, pp 61–80. New York, Marcel Dekker, 1982
56. Cooper MJ, Mackie CR, Skinner DB et al: A reappraisal of the value of carcinoembryonic antigen in the management of patients with various neoplasms. Br J Surg 66:120, 1979
57. Van Nagell Jr: Tumor markers in ovarian cancer. Clin Obstet Gynecol 10:197, 1983
58. Pentti K, Keinonen KT, Koiwla T et al: Tumor associated antigen CA 12-5 in patients with ovarian cancer. Br J Obstet Gynaecol 92:528, 1985
59. Bast RC, Klug TL, St John E et al: A radioimmunoassay using a monoclonal antibody to monitor the course of epithelial ovarian cancer. N Engl J Med 309:883, 1983
60. Bast RC, Feeney M, Lazarus H et al: Reactivity of a monoclonal antibody with human ovarian carcinoma. J Clin Invest 68:1331, 1981
61. Koprowski H, Steplewski Z, Mitchell K et al: Colorectal carcinoma antigens detected by hybridoma antibodies. Somatic Cell Mul Genet 5:957, 1979
62. Ritts RE, Del Villano BC, Go VLM et al: Initial clinical evaluation of an immunoradiometric assay for CA 19-9 using the NCI serum bank. Int J Cancer 33:339, 1984
63. Tempero M, Uchida E, Takasaki H et al: Serial CA 19-9 levels and tumor response in pancreatic cancer (abstr). Proc Am Soc Clin Oncol 6:81, 1987
64. Benini L, Cavallini G, Zordan D et al: Prospective clinical evaluation of the diagnostic accuracy of monoclonal (CA 19-9, CA 50, CA 12-5) and polyclonal (CEA, TPA) antigens in respect to pancreatic cancer. Dig Dis Sci (66S) 31:254, 1986
65. Schlom J, Weeks MO: Potential clinical utility of monoclonal antibodies in the management of human carcinomas. In DeVita VT Jr, Hellman S, Rosenberg SA (eds): Important Advances in Oncology 1985, p 170. Philadelphia, JB Lippincott, 1985
66. Whipple AO, Parsons WB, Mullins CR: Treatment of carcinoma of the ampulla of Vater. Ann Surg 102:763, 1935
67. Maki T, Sato T, Kakizaki G: Pancreatoduodenectomy for periampullary carcinomas: Appraisal of a two-stage procedure. Arch Surg 92:825, 1966
68. Nakayama T, Ikeda A, Okuda K; Percutaneous transhepatic drainage of the biliary tract: Technique and results in 104 cases. Gastroenterology 74:554, 1978
69. Denning DA, Ellison EC, Carey LC: Preoperative percutaneous transhepatic biliary decompression lowers operative morbidity in patients with obstructive jaundice. Am J Surg 141:61, 1981
70. Norlander A, Kalin B, Sundblad R: Effect of percutaneous transhepatic drainage upon liver function and postoperative mortality. Surg Gynecol Obstet 155:161, 1982
71. Gundry SR, Strodel WE, Knol JA et al: Efficacy of preoperative biliary tract decompression in patients with obstructive jaundice. Arch Surg 119:703, 1984
72. Dooley JS, Dick R, Olney J et al: Non-surgical treatment of biliary obstruction. Lancet 2:1043, 1979
73. McPherson GAD, Benjamin IS, Habib NA et al: Percutaneous transhepatic drainage in obstructive jaundice: Advantages and problems. Br J Surg 62:261, 1982
74. Hatfield ARW, Tobias R, Terblanche J et al: Preoperative external biliary drainage in obstructive jaundice: A prospective controlled clinical trial. Lancet 2:896, 1982
75. McPherson GAD, Benjamin IS, Hodgson HJF et al: Preoperative percutaneous biliary drainage: The best results of a controlled trial. Br J Surg 71:371, 1984
76. Pitt HA, Cameron JL, Postier RG et al: Factors affecting mortality in biliary tract surgery. Am J Surg 141:66, 1981
77. Hagenmuller F, Classen M: Therapeutic endoscopic and percutaneous procedures for biliary disorders. Prog Liver Dis 7:299, 1982
78. Speer AG, Cotton PB, Russell RC et al: Randomised trial of endoscopic versus percutaneous stent insertion in malignant obstructive jaundice. Lancet 2:57, 1987
79. Bornman PC, Terblanche J, Harries-Jones EP et al: Endoscopic versus percutaneous stents for malignant jaundice. Lancet 2:689, 1987
80. Isaacson R, Weiland LH, McIlrath DC: Biopsy of the pancreas. Arch Surg 109:227, 1974
81. Fortner JG: Regional resection of the pancreas: A new surgical approach. Surgery 73:307, 1973
82. Morrow M, Hilaris B, Brennan MF: Comparison of conventional surgical resection, radioactive implantation, and bypass procedures for exocrine carcinoma of the pancreas, 1975–1980. Ann Surg 199:1, 1984
83. Bowden L, McNeer G, Pack G: Carcinoma of the head of pancreas—Five-year survival in four patients. Am J Surg 109:578, 1965
84. Portland Surgical Society Cooperative Study: A ten-year experience with carcinoma of the pancreas. Arch Surg 94:322, 1967
85. Crile G: The advantages of bypass operations over radical pancreaticoduodenectomy in the treatment of pancreatic carcinoma. Surg Gynecol Obstet 130:1049, 1970
86. Feduska N, Dent T, Lindenauer S: Results of palliative operations for carcinoma of the pancreas. Arch Surg 103:330, 1971
87. Wilson S, Block G: Periampullary carcinoma. Arch Surg 108:539, 1974
88. Brooks J, Culebras J: Cancer of the pancreas—palliative operation, Whipple procedure, or total pancreatectomy? Am J Surg 131:516, 1976
89. Shapiro T: Adenocarcinoma of the pancreas: A statistical analysis of biliary bypass vs. Whipple resection in good risk patients. Ann Surg 182:715, 1975
90. Nakase A, Matsumoto Y, Uchida K et al: Surgical treatment of cancer of the pancreas and the periampullary region: Cumulative results in 57 institutions in Japan. Ann Surg 185:52, 1977
91. Tepper J, Nardi G, Suit H: Carcinoma of the pancreas: Review of MGH experience from 1963 to 1973. Cancer 37:1519, 1976
92. Knight R, Scarborough J, Goss J: Adenocarcinoma of the pancreas—A ten-year experience. Arch Surg 113:1401, 1978
93. Moosa A, Lewis M, Mackie C: Surgical treatment of pancreatic cancer. Mayo Clin Proc 54:468, 1979
94. Longmire W, Transero L: The Whipple procedure and other standard operative approaches to pancreatic cancer. Cancer 47:1706, 1981
95. Edis A, Kiernan P, Taylor W: Attempted curative resection of ductal carcinoma of the pancreas. Review of Mayo Clinic experience: 1951–1975. Mayo Clin Proc 55:531, 1980
96. Fortner J: Surgical principles for pancreatic cancer: Regional total and subtotal pancreatectomy. Cancer 47:1712, 1981
97. Herter F, Cooperman A, Ahlborn T et al: Surgical experience with pancreatic and periampullary cancer. Ann Surg 195:274, 1982
98. Van Heerden J, Heath P, Alden C: Biliary bypass for ductal adenocarcinoma of the pancreas: Mayo Clinic experience, 1970–1975. Mayo Clin Proc 55:537, 1980
99. Brooks DC, Osteen R, Gray E et al: Evaluation of palliative procedures of pancreatic cancer. Am J Surg 141:430, 1981
100. Crist DW, Sitzmann JV, Cameron JL: Improved hospital morbidity, mortality, and survival after the Whipple procedure. Ann Surg 206:358, 1987
101. Sarr MG, Cameron JL: Surgical management of unresectable carcinoma of the pancreas. Surgery 91:123, 1982
102. Bufkin WJ, Smith PE, Krementz FT: Evaluation of palliative operations for carcinoma of the pancreas. Arch Surg 94:240, 1967
103. Blievernicht SW, Neifeld JP, Terz JJ et al: The role of prophylactic gastrojejunostomy for unresectable periampullary carcinoma. Surg Gynecol Obstet 151:794, 1980
104. Elmslie RG, Slovatinek AH: Surgical objectives in unresected cancer of the head of the pancreas. Br J Surg 59:500, 1972
105. Hart PF, Gillett DJ: Non-functioning palliative gastroenterostomy. Aust NZ J Surg 41:354, 1972
106. Gudjonsson B: Cancer of the pancreas: 50 years of surgery. Cancer 60:2284, 1987
107. Glantz G, Ozeran RS: Role of gastroenterostomy in management of pancreatic carcinoma. Am J Surg 32:670, 1966
108. Richards AB, Chir M, Sosin H: Cancer of the pancreas: The value of radical and palliative surgery. Ann Surg 177:325, 1973
109. Webster DJT: Carcinoma of the pancreas and periampullary region: A clinical study in a district general hospital. Br J Surg 62:130, 1975
110. Pipes KE, Pareira MD: Duodenal obstruction appearing after palliative biliary diversion for pancreatic carcinoma. Surgery 44:636, 1958
111. Hertzberg J: Pancreatico-duodenal resection and bypass-operation in patients with carcinoma of the head of pancreas, ampulla, and distal end of the common duct. Acta Chir Scand 140:523, 1974
112. Collure DWD, Burns GP, Schenk WG Jr: Clinical, pathological, and therapeutic aspects of carcinoma of the pancreas. Am J Surg 128:683, 1974
113. Stuart M, Keo T, Hermann RE et al: Palliation of malignant obstruction of the common bile duct by side to side choledochoduodenostomy. Am J Surg 121:505, 1971
114. Douglass HO, Holyoke ED: Pancreatic cancer: Initial treatment as the determinant of survival. JAMA 229:793, 1974
115. Vijayanagar R, Tobins SH: Evaluation of palliative operations for carcinoma of the head of the pancreas: A ten-year study. Mt Sinai J Med (NY) 37:115, 1970
116. Mendoza CB, Easley GW: Bypass procedure for palliation in obstructive jaundice. W Va Med J 70:27, 1974
117. Monge JJ: Survival of patients with small carcinomas of the head of the pancreas: Biliary intestinal bypass vs pancreaticoduodenectomy. Ann Surg 166:908, 1967
118. Buckwalter JA, Lawton RL, Tidrick RT: Bypass operations for neoplastic biliary tract obstruction. Am J Surg 109:100, 1965
119. Winegarner FG, Haguea WH, Elliott DW: Tissue diagnosis and surgical management of malignant jaundice. Am J Surg 111:5, 1966
120. Williams RD, Elliott DW, Zollinger RM: Surgery for malignant jaundice. Arch Surg 80:992, 1960

121. McDevitt JB: Parenchymatous carcinoma of the head of the pancreas. J Ir Med Assoc 62:390, 1969
122. Glassman WS, Johnston PW: Palliative surgery in carcinoma of the pancreas. Geriatrics 10:456, 1955
123. Linn BS, Goldstein HS: Judgement in palliation of pancreatic carcinoma: With an assist by the computer. South Med J 62:116, 1969
124. du Plessis DJ: The palliative operation for obstructive jaundice due to carcinoma of the pancreas. S Afr J Surg 8:11, 1970
125. Reed K, Vose PC, Jarstfer BS: Pancreatic cancer: 30-year review (1947–77). Am J Surg 138:929, 1979
126. Forrest JF, Longmire WP Jr: Carcinoma of the pancreas and periampullary region: A study of 279 patients. Ann Surg 189:129, 1979
127. Nagai H, Kuroda A, Morioka Y: Lymphatic and local spread of T_1 and T_2 pancreatic cancer. Ann Surg 204:65–71, 1986
128. Pilepich MV, Miller HH: Pre-operative irradiation in carcinoma of the pancreas. Cancer 46:1945, 1980
129. Kopelson G: Curative surgery for adenocarcinoma of the pancreas/ampulla of Vater: The role of adjuvant pre- or post-operative radiation therapy. Int J Radiat Oncol Biol Phys 9:911, 1983
130. Sindelar WF, Kinsella TJ: Randomized trial of intraoperative radiotherapy in resected carcinoma of the pancreas. Int J Radiat Oncol Biol Phys (Suppl 1)12:148, 1986
131. Fraass BA, Miller RW, Kinsella TJ et al: Intraoperative radiation therapy at the National Cancer Institute: Technical innovations and dosimetry. Int J Radiat Oncol Biol Phys 11:1299, 1985
132. Sindelar WF, Hoekstra HJ, Kinsella TJ: Surgical approaches and techniques in intraoperative radiotherapy for intra-abdominal, retroperitoneal, and pelvic neoplasms. Surgery (in press)
133. Gastrointestinal Tumor Study Group: Pancreatic cancer: Adjuvant combined radiation and chemotherapy following curative resection. Arch Surg 120:899, 1985
134. Gastrointestinal Tumor Study Group: Further evidence of effective adjuvant combined radiation and chemotherapy following curative resection of pancreatic cancer. Cancer 59:2006, 1987
135. Richards GE: Possibilities of roentgen-ray treatment in cancer of the pancreas. Am J Roentgenol 9:150, 1922
136. Merritt EA, Rathbone RR: The diagnosis and roentgen treatment of carcinoma of the head of the pancreas. Radiology 26:459, 1936
137. Handley WS: Pancreatic cancer and its treatment by implanted radium. Ann Surg 100:215, 1934
138. Upcott H: Tumors of the ampulla of Vater. With a report of two cases. Ann Surg 56:710, 1912
139. Pack GT, McNeer G: Radiation treatment of pancreatic cancer. Am J Roentgenol Rad Ther Nucl Med 40:708, 1938
140. Phillips R: Principles and results of palliative radiotherapy in nonresectable cancer. Med Clin North Am 40:807, 1956
141. Miller TR, Fuller LM: Radiation therapy of carcinoma of the pancreas. Report on 91 cases. Am J Roentgenol Rad Ther Nucl Med 80:787, 1958
142. Billingsley JS, Bartholomew LG, Childs DS: A study of radiation therapy in carcinoma of the pancreas. Proc Staff Meet Mayo Clin 33:426, 1958
143. Haslam JB, Cavanaugh PJ, Stroup SL: Radiation therapy in the treatment of irresectable adenocarcinoma of the pancreas. Cancer 32:1341, 1973
144. Dobelbower RR, Borgelt BB, Strubler KA et al: Precision radiotherapy for cancer of the pancreas: Technique and results. Int J Radiat Oncol Biol Phys 6:1127, 1980
145. Whittington R, Dobelbower RR, Mohiuddin M et al: Radiotherapy of unresectable pancreatic carcinoma: A six-year experience with 104 patients. Int J Radiat Oncol Biol Phys 7:1639, 1981
146. Kinsella TJ, Sindelar WF, Bloomer WD: Radiation enteritis: Pathophysiology, clinical manifestations and management. In Nyhus LM, Nelson RL (eds): Surgery of the Small Intestine, pp 193–203. Norwalk, CT, Appleton-Century-Crofts, 1987
147. Hilaris B, Moorthy C, Kim J: Radiotherapeutic management of pancreatic cancer at Memorial Sloan-Kettering Cancer Center. In Conn I (ed): Pancreatic Cancer: New Directions in Therapeutic Management, pp 251–262. New York, Masson, 1980
148. Brennan MF, Hilaris B: Unpublished data
149. Shipley WU, Nardi GL, Cohen AM et al: Iodine-125 implant and external beam irradiation in patients with localized pancreatic carcinoma. A comparative study of surgical resection. Cancer 45:709, 1980
150. Goldson AL, Ashaveri E, Espinoza MC et al: Single high-dose intraoperative electrons for advanced stage pancreatic cancer: Phase I pilot study. Int J Radiat Oncol Biol Phys 7:869, 1981
151. Abe M, Takahashi M: Intraoperative radiotherapy: The Japanese experience. Int J Radiat Oncol Biol Phys 7:863, 1981
152. Nishamura A, Nakano M, Otsu H et al: Intraoperative radiotherapy for advanced carcinoma of the pancreas. Cancer 54:2375, 1984
153. Shipley WU, Wood WC, Tepper JE et al: Intraoperative electron beam irradiation for patients with unresectable pancreatic carcinoma. Ann Surg 200:289, 1984
154. Tepper JE, Shipley WU, Warshaw AL et al: The role of Misonidazole combined with intraoperative radiation therapy in the treatment of pancreatic carcinoma. J Clin Oncol 5:579, 1987
155. Gunderson LL, Martin JK, Kvols LT et al: Intraoperative and external beam irradiation ± 5-FU for locally advanced pancreatic cancer. Int J Radiat Oncol Biol Phys 13:319, 1987
156. Sindelar WF, Hoekstra H, Rstrepo C et al: Pathological tissue changes following intraoperative radiotherapy. Am J Clin Oncol 9:504, 1986

157. Kaul R, Cohen L, Hendrickson F et al: Pancreatic carcinoma: Results with fast neutron therapy. Int J Radiat Oncol Biol Phys 7:173, 1981
158. Smith FP, Schein PS, Macdonald JS et al: Fast neutron irradiation for locally advanced pancreatic cancer. Int J Radiat Oncol Biol Phys 7:1527, 1981
159. Al-Abdulla ASM, Hussey DH, Olson MH et al: Experience with fast neutron therapy for unresectable carcinoma of the pancreas. Int J Radiat Oncol Biol Phys 7:165, 1981
160. Castro JR, Quivey JM, Lyman JT et al: Current status of clinical particle radiotherapy at Lawrence Berkeley Laboratory. Cancer 46:633, 1980
161. Kligerman MM, Sala JM, Smith AR et al: Tissue reaction and tumor response with negative pi mesons. J Can Assoc Radiol 31:13, 1980
162. Bajorunas D, Horowitz DG, Dresler C et al: Amino acid kinetics under glucagon replacement in pancreatectomized patients (in preparation)
163. Moertel CG, Reitemeier RJ: Advanced Gastrointestinal Cancer: Clinical Management and Chemotherapy. New York, Harper & Row, 1969
164. Pastan I, Gottesman M: Multiple drug resistance in human cancer. N Engl J Med 316:1388, 1987
165. Myers C, Cowan K, Sinha B et al: The phenomenon of pleotropic drug resistance. In: DeVita VT Jr, Hellman S, Rosenberg SA (eds): Important Advances in Oncology 1987, pp 27–37. Philadelphia, JB Lippincott, 1987
166. Carter SK: The integration of chemotherapy into a combined modality approach for cancer treatment: VI. Pancreatic adenocarcinoma. Cancer Treat Rev 3:193, 1975
167. O'Connell MJ: Current status of chemotherapy for advanced pancreatic and gastric cancer. J Clin Oncol 3:1032, 1985
168. Schein PS: The role of chemotherapy in the management of gastric and pancreatic carcinoma. Semin Oncol 12:49, 1985
169. Moertel CG: Chemotherapy of gastrointestinal cancer. Clin Gastroenterol 5:777, 1976
170. Crooke ST, Bradner WT: Mitomycin C: A review. Cancer Treat Rev 3:121, 1976
171. Gastrointestinal Tumor Study Group: Randomized phase II clinical trial of adriamycin, methotrexate, and actinomycin D in advanced measurable pancreatic carcinoma. Cancer 42:19, 1978
172. Gastrointestinal Tumor Study Group: Phase II trials of maytansine, low-dose chlorozotocin, and high-dose chlorozotocin as single agents against advanced measurable adenocarcinoma of the pancreas. Cancer Treat Rep 69:417, 1985
173. Inamasu M, Oishi N, Chen T et al: Phase II trial of amsacrine in pancreatic carcinoma: A Southwest Oncology Group study. Cancer Treat Rep 68:1411, 1984
174. Omura GA, Bartolucci AA, Lessner HE et al: Phase II evaluation of amsacrine in colorectal, gastric, and pancreatic carcinomas: A Southeastern Cancer Study Group trial. Cancer Treat Rep 68:929, 1984
175. Sternberg CN, Magill GB, Sordillo PP et al: Phase II evaluation of m-AMSA (4'-(9-acridinylamino)-methane-sulfon-m-anisidide) in patients with adenocarcinoma of the pancreas. Am J Clin Oncol (CCT) 6:459, 1983
176. Bedikian AY, Stroehlein J, Korinek J et al: Phase II evaluation of dihydroxyanthracenedione (DHAD, NSC 301739) in patients with upper gastrointestinal tumors. A preliminary report. Am J Clin Oncol 6:473, 1983
177. Mittelman A, Magill GB, Raymond V et al: Phase II trial of Idarubicin in patients with pancreatic cancer. Cancer Treat Rep 712:657, 1987
178. National Cancer Institute: Cancer Therapy Evaluation Program Information System (CTEP-IS), 1987
179. Hochster H, Green MD, Speyer JL et al: Activity of epirubicin in pancreatic cancer. Cancer Treat Rep 70:299, 1986
180. Wils J, Bleiberg H, Blijham G et al: Phase II study of epirubicin in advanced adenocarcinoma of the pancreas. Eur J Cancer Clin Oncol 21:191, 1985
181. Blayney DW, Goldberg DA, Leong LA et al: Phase II trial of esorubicin in advanced pancreatic adenocarcinoma. Cancer Treat Rep 70:683, 1986
182. DeSimone PA, Gams R, Bartolucci A: Weekly mitoxantrone in the treatment of advanced pancreatic carcinoma: A Southeastern Cancer Study Group trial. Cancer Treat Rep 80:929, 1986
183. Horton J, Gelber R, Engstrom P et al: Trials of single agent and combination chemotherapy for advanced cancer of the pancreas. Cancer Treat Rep 65:65, 1981
184. Smith DB, Kenny JB, Scarffe JH et al: Phase II evaluation of melphalan in adenocarcinoma of the pancreas. Cancer Treat Rep 69:917, 1985
185. Gad-El-Mawla N: Ifosfamide in advanced pancreatic cancer. Cancer Chemother Pharmacol 18:555, 1986
186. Einhorn LH, Loehrer PJ: Ifosfamide chemotherapy for pancreatic carcinoma. Cancer Chemother Pharmacol 18:551, 1986
187. Bernard S, Noble S, Wilcosky T et al: A phase II study of ifosfamide (IFOS) plus N-acetyl cysteine (NAC) in metastatic measurable pancreatic adenocarcinoma (pc) (abstr). Proc Am Soc Clin Oncol 5:328, 1986
188. DeSimone P, Kramer B, Omura GA et al: Phase II evaluation of diaziquone in gastric and pancreatic cancers: A Southeastern Cancer Study Group trial. Am J Clin Oncol (CCT) 9:401, 1986
189. Gastrointestinal Tumor Study Group: Phase II trials of hexamethylmelamine, dianhydrogalactitol, razoxane, and beta-2'-deoxythioguanosine as single agents against advanced measurable tumors of the pancreas. Cancer Treat Rep 69:713, 1985
190. Lessner HE, Valenstein S, Kaplan R et al: Phase II study L-asparaginase in the treatment of pancreatic carcinoma. Cancer Treat Rep 64:1359, 1980
191. Sternberg CN, Magill GB, Sordillo PP et al: Phase II evaluation of metoprine in advanced pancreatic adenocarcinoma. Cancer Treat Rep 68:1053, 1984
192. Inamasu MS, Oishi N, Chen TT et al: Phase II study of mitoguazone in pancreatic cancer: A Southwest Oncology Group study. Cancer Treat Rep 70:531, 1986
193. Ravry MJR, Omura GA, Hill GJ et al: Phase II evaluation of mitoguazone in cancers of

the esophagus, stomach, and pancreas: A Southeastern Cancer Study Group trial. Cancer Treat Rep 70:533, 1986

194. Crowson MC, Dorrell A, Rolfe EB et al: A phase II study to evaluate tamoxifen in pancreatic adenocarcinoma. Eur J Surg Oncol 12:335, 1986

195. Smith FP, Stablein DM, Schein PS: Phase II combination chemotherapy trials in advanced measurable pancreatic cancer (abstr). Proc Am Soc Clin Oncol 3:150, 1984

196. Lokich J, Chawla PL, Brooks J et al: Chemotherapy in pancreatic carcinoma: 5-fluorouracil (5-FU) and 1,3, bis-(2 chlorethyl)-1-nitrosourea (BCNU). Ann Surg 179:450, 1974

197. Stolinsky DC, Pugh RP, Bateman JR: 5-fluorouracil (NSC-19383) therapy for pancreatic carcinoma: Comparison of oral and intravenous routes. Cancer Chemother Rep 59:1031, 1975

198. Mater MW, Theologides A, Cooper MR et al: Fluorouracil (F) + adriamycin (A) + mitomycin (M) (FAM) versus fluorouracil (F) + streptozotocin (S) + mitomycin (M) (FSM) in advanced pancreatic cancer (abstr). Proc Am Soc Clin Oncol 1:90, 1982

199. Schein PS, O'Connell MJ, Blom J et al: Clinical antitumor activity and toxicity of streptozotocin (NSC-85998). Cancer 34:993, 1974

200. Stolinsky DC, Sadoff L, Braunwald J et al: Streptozotocin in the treatment of cancer. Cancer 30:61, 1972

201. DuPriest RW, Huntington MC, Massey WH et al: Streptozotocin therapy in 22 patients. Cancer 25:358, 1975

202. Moertel CG, Doublass HO, Hanlet J et al: Phase II study of methyl-CCNU in the treatment of advanced pancreatic carcinoma. Cancer Treat Rep 60:1659, 1976

203. Schein PS, Lavin PT, Moertel CG et al: Randomized phase II clinical trial of adriamycin in advanced measurable pancreatic carcinoma: A Gastrointestinal Tumor Study Group report. Cancer 42:19, 1978

204. Kovach JS, Moertel CG, Schutt AJ et al: A controlled study of combined 1,3-bis-(2-chlorethyl)-1-nitrosorea and 5-fluorouracil therapy for advanced gastric and pancreatic cancer. Cancer 33:563, 1974

205. Moertel CG, Douglass HO Jr, Hanley J et al: Treatment of advanced adenocarcinoma of the pancreas with combinations of streptozotocin plus 5-fluorouracil and streptozotocin plus cyclophosphamide. Cancer 40:605, 1977

206. Moertel CG, Engstrom P, Lavin PT et al: Chemotherapy of gastric and pancreatic carcinoma. Surgery 85:509, 1979

207. Buroker T, Kim PN, Groppe C et al: 5-FU infusion with mitomycin C vs 5-FU infusion with methyl CCNU in the treatment of advanced upper gastrointestinal cancer. Cancer 44:1215, 1979

208. Stephens RL, Hoogstraten B, Haas C et al: Pancreatic cancer treated with carmustine, fluorouracil and spironolactone. A randomized study. Arch Intern Med 138:115, 1978

209. Wiggans RG, Wooley PV, MacDonald JS et al: Phase II trial of streptozotocin, mitomycin-C and 5-fluorouracil (SMF) in the treatment of advanced pancreatic cancer. Cancer 41:387, 1978

210. Aberhalden RT, Bukowski RM, Groppe CW et al: Streptozotocin (STZ) and 5-fluorouracil (5-FU) with and without mitomycin-C (Mito) in the treatment of pancreatic adenocarcinoma (abstr). Proc Am Soc Clin Oncol 18:301, 1977

211. Bukowski RM, Abderhalden RI, Hewlett JS et al: Phase II trial of streptogotocin, mitomycin-C, and 5-fluorouracil in adenocarcinoma of the pancreas. Cancer Clin Triasl 3:321, 1980

212. Smith FP, Hoth DF, Levin B et al: 5-fluorouracil in adenocarcinoma of the pancreas. Cancer Clin Trials 3:321, 1980

213. Bitran JD, Desser RK, Kozloff MF et al: Treatment of metastatic pancreatic and gastric adenocarcinoma with 5-fluorouracil, adriamycin, and mitomycin-C (FAM). Cancer Treat Rep 63:2049, 1979

214. Bukowski RM: Randomized comparison of 5-FU and mitomycin-C (MF) versis 5-FU, mitomycin-C and streptozotocin (SMF) in pancreatic adenocarcinoma. A Southwest Oncology Group study (abstr). Proc Am Soc Clin Oncol 22:543, 1981

215. Bukowski RM, Balcerzak ST, O'Bryan RM et al: Randomized trial of 5-fluorouracil and mitomycin-C with or without streptozotocin for advanced pancreatic cancer. A Southwest Oncology Group study. Cancer 52:1577, 1983

216. Moertel CG, Rubin J, O'Connell MJ et al: A phase II trial of combined 5-fluorouracil, doxorubicin and cisplatin in the treatment of advanced upper gastrointestinal adenocarcinoma. J Clin Oncol 4:1053, 1986

217. Smith FP, Rustgi VK, Schertz G et al: Phase II study of 5-FU, doxorubicin, and mitomycin (FAM) and chlorozotocin in advanced measurable pancratic cancer. Cancer Treat Rep 66:2095, 1982

218. Bukowski RM, Schacter LP, Groppe CT et al: Phase II trial of 5-fluorouracil, adriamycin, mitomycin-C and streptozotocin (FAM-S) in pancreatic cancer. Cancer 50:197, 1982

219. Karlin DA, Stroehlein JR, Bennetts RW et al: Phase I-II study of the combination of 5-FU, doxorubicin, mitomycin, and semustine (FAMMe) in the treatment of adenocarcinoma of the stomach, gastroesophageal junction, and pancreas. Cancer Treat Rep 66:1613, 1982

220. Gastrointestinal Tumor Study Group: Phase II studies of drug combination in advanced pancreatic carcinoma: Fluorouracil plus doxorubicin plus mitomycin-C plus fluorouracil. J Clin Oncol 4:1794, 1986

221. Oster MW, Gray R, Panasci L et al: Chemotherapy for advanced pancreatic cancer: A comparison of 5-fluorouracil, adriamycin, and mitomycin-C (FAM) with 5-fluorouracil, streptozotocin and mitomycin-C (FSM). Cancer 57:29, 1986

222. Cullinan SA, Moertel CG, Fleming TR et al: A comparison of chemotherapeutic regimens in the treatment of advanced pancreatic and gastric carcinoma. JAMA 253:2061, 1985

223. Bukowski RM, Inamasu M, Taylor S et al: Randomized trials of combination chemotherapy vs. a Phase II drug in metastatic adenocarcinoma of the pancreas. A Southwest Oncology Group Study (abstr). Proc Am Soc Clin Oncol 4:80, 1985

224. Magill GB, Jakubowski AA, Sternberg CN et al: Phase II trial of MIFA IV chemotherapy for advanced adenocarcinoma of the pancreas (abstr). Proc Am Soc Clin Oncol 6:88, 1987

225. Bukowski RM: Characteristics of long-term survivors receiving chemotherapy for pancreatic adenocarcinoma in Southwest Oncology Group studies (abstr). Proc Am Soc Clin Oncol 3:149, 1984

226. Mallinson CN, Rake MO, Cocking JB et al: Chemotherapy in pancreatic cancer: Results of a controlled, prospective, randomized, multicenter trial. Br Med J 281:1589, 1980

227. Kyriazis AP, Kyriazis AA, Yagoda AA: Enhanced therapeutic effect of cis-diamminodichloroplatinum against nude mouse grown human pancreatic adenocarcinoma when combined with I-B-D-arabionfuranosylcytosine and caffeine. Cancer Res 45:6083, 1985

228. Roh JK, Wooley PV, Reich SD et al: Phase II evaluation of recombinant interferon gamma (IF) in advanced pancreatic and gastric adenocarcinoma (abstr). Proc Am Soc Clin Oncol 5:85, 1986

229. Chachoua A, Green M, Muggia FM: Immune modulating therapy in gastrointestinal cancer. Am J Gastroenterol 81:623, 1986

230. Rosenberg SA, Lotze MT, Muul LM et al: A progress report on the treatment of 157 patients with advanced cancer using lymphokine-activated killer cells and interleukin-2 or high-dose interleukin-2 alone. N Engl J Med 316:889, 1987

231. West WH, Tauer KW, Yannelli JR et al: Constant-infusion recombinant interleukin-2 in adoptive immunotherapy of advanced cancer. N Engl J Med 316:898, 1987

232. Herlyn M, Steplewski Z, Herlyn D et al: Colorectal carcinoma-specific antigen: Detection by means of monoclonal antibodies. Proc Natl Acad Sci USA 76:1438, 1979

233. Herlyn DM, Steplewski Z, Herlyn MF et al: Inhibition of growth of colorectal carcinoma in nude mice by monoclonal antibody. Cancer Res 44:717, 1980

234. Herlyn DM, Koprowski H: IgG2a monoclonal antibodies inhibit human tumor growth through interaction with effector cells. Proc Natl Acad Sci USA 79:4761, 1982

235. Sears HF, Herlyn D, Steplewski Z et al: Effects of monoclonal antibody immunotherapy on patients with gastrointestinal adenocarcinoma. J Biol Response Mod 3:138, 1984

236. Sindelar WF, Maher MM, Herlyn D et al: Trial of therapy with monoclonal antibody 17-1A in pancreatic carcinoma: Preliminary results. Hybridoma 5:125, 1986

237. Tempero MA, Pour PM, Uchida E et al: Monoclonal antibody C017-1A and leukopheresis in immunotherapy of pancreatic cancer. Hybridoma 5:133, 1986

238. Glenn J, Steinberg WM, Kurtzman SH et al: Evaluation of the utility of a radioimmunoassay for serum CA 19-9 levels in patients before and after treatment of carcinoma of the pancreas. J Clin Oncol 6:462, 1988

239. Paul AR, Engstrom PD, Weiner LM et al: Treatment of advanced measurable evaluable pancreatic carcinoma with 17-1A murine monoclonal antibody alone or in combination with 5-fluorouracil, adriamycin and mitomycin (FAM). Hybridoma 5:171, 1986

240. Metzgar RS, Gaillard MT, Levine SJ et al: Antigens of human pancreatic adenocarcinoma cells defined by murine monoclonal antibodies. Cancer Res 42:601, 1982

241. Parsa I: Identification of human acinar cell carcinoma by monoclonal antibody and in vitro differentiation. Cancer Lett 15:115, 1982

242. Greenwald HP, Bonica JJ, Bergner M: The prevalence of pain in four cancers. Cancer 60:2563, 1987

243. Flanigan D, Kraft R: Continuing experience with palliative chemical splanchniectomy. Arch Surg 113:509, 1978

244. de Takats G, Walter L, Lasner J: Splanchnic nerve section for pancreatic pain. Ann Surg 131:44, 1949

245. Grimson K, Hesser F, Kitchin W: Early clinical results of transabdominal celiac and superior mesenteric ganglionectomy, vagotomy, or transthoracic splanchnioectomy in patients with chronic abdominal visceral pain. Surgery 22:230, 1947

246. Yoshioka H, Wakabavashi T: Therapeutic neurotomy on head of pancreas for relief of pain due to chronic pancreatitis. Arch Surg 76:546, 1958

247. Bridenbaugh L, Moore D, Campbell D: Management of upper abdominal cancer pain: Treatment with celiac plexus block with alcohol. JAMA 190:99, 1964

248. Jones J: Coeliac plexus block with alcohol for relief of upper abdominal pain due to cancer. Ann Coll Surg Engl 59:46, 1977

249. Thompson G, Moore D, Bridenbaugh L: Abdominal pain and alcohol celiac plexus nerve block. Anesth Analg 56:1, 1977

250. Hanowell S, Kennedy S, MacNamara T et al: Celiac plexus block. Diagnostic and therapeutic applications in abdominal pain. South Med J 73:1330, 1980

251. Buy JN, Moss A, Singler R: CT guided celiac plexus and splanchnic nerve neurolysis. J Comput Assist Tomogr 6:315, 1982

HAROLD J. WANEBO

GEOFFREY FALKSON

STANLEY E. ORDER

CHAPTER 27 *Cancer of the Hepatobiliary System*

Hepatobiliary cancer is relatively uncommon in the United States. In 1987, approximately 14,000 new cases were reported.[1] Worldwide, however, primary hepatocellular carcinoma may be the most common fatal cancer, having an estimated annual incidence between 300,000 and 1.2 million and a fatality ratio of 0.92.[2] In the United States primary cancers of the liver and biliary passages are considered collectively for incidence. It is estimated that gallbladder cancer is the most common, accounting for 4000 to 6000 deaths each year, followed by 4000 hepatocellular cancer deaths and a slightly smaller number of bile duct cancer deaths. In recent years, our understanding of the cause and distribution of hepatobiliary cancer has improved markedly, and newer technologics have become available for diagnosis and management. Therapeutic advances have been made through experimental approaches that combine the efforts of the radiation oncologist, the surgeon, and the medical oncologist.[3-6]

HEPATOCELLULAR CARCINOMA

EPIDEMIOLOGY

Primary hepatocellular carcinoma (HCC) or malignant hepatoma is one of the most common malignancies in the world, and it is estimated to be responsible for up to 1,250,000 deaths every year.[2,7,8] It occurs infrequently in the United States and North America, with fewer than 10,000 new patients annually, accounting for less than 2% of all malignancies.[1,7-9] The age-standardized annual incidence is 2.9 per 100,000 men and 1.2 per 100,000 women. A similar low incidence is found in Britain, Canada, Australia, and South America. In portions of Africa and Asia, HCC is the most common malignant tumor.[10-12] The incidence ranges from 34 per 100,000 men in Singapore of Chinese descent to 65 per 100,000 men in Zimbabwe to more than 100 per 100,000 men in Mozambique and Taiwan.[13] The incidence of HCC is so high in parts of China that population screening is advocated.[14] Worldwide, the disease occurs predominately in men over 30 years of age.[14,15] Five times more men have HCC than women in high-incidence regions, whereas in low-incidence areas the ratio is 2 : 1.[7] The fibrolamellar variant of HCC occurs in a younger population (mean, 23–26 years), occurs equally in both sexes, and has a relatively longer survival period (Table 27-1).[16-19]

Chinese immigrants to Singapore or low-risk areas, such as the United States, retain their high-risk rates for HCC, but this is not the case with black migrants. Blacks in South Africa have a higher incidence (28 per 100,000) than American blacks (8 per 100,000), in whom the rate is slightly higher than in American whites (2.4 per 100,000).[7,20] There is a close relationship between the distribution of hepatitis B virus (HBV) infections and HCC, and the carrier rate for HBV is high among native born and migrant Chinese and black Africans but low for blacks outside Africa and for whites in South Africa, Europe, and North America.[11,21,22-34]

TABLE 27-1. Incidence of Heptocellular Carcinoma

Country	Incidence	Reference
North America Britain, Canada, Australia and South America	10,000 cases per year	1-4, 7-9
	No figures cited	2, 4, 7
Mozambique and Taiwan	100 per 100,000	10, 11, 13
Singapore	34.2 per 100,000 Chinese men	14
Zimbabwe	65 per 100,000 men	14
South Africa	28 per 100,000 black men	7, 20
United States	8 per 100,000 black men	20
United States	2.4 per 100,000 white men	20

ETIOLOGY

There are many risk factors related to HCC, including malnutrition, dietary carcinogens, parasitic infections, cirrhosis from various causes (Tables 27-2 and 27-3), caval outflow obstruction, and hormone ingestion.[36-59] Although some of these factors may have a role in the disease, it appears that HBV plays a major role in the pathogenesis of most HCC.[23-34,50-54,60]

Although the association of HCC in West Africa with viral hepatitis was reported by Paget in 1956, it was not until the identification of HBV (Australian antigen) by Blumberg in 1967 and a marker for hepatitis A that the role of hepatitis could be defined.[7,25,27] Studies of the etiologic relationship between HBV and HCC were advanced by the demonstration of a human tumor cell line that has HBV DNA integrated into the cellular genome, which replicates HBsAg.[35] Integration of HBV DNA has been demonstrated both in hepatoma cell lines and in tumor samples from HCC patients.[24,34,35] The cirrhosis seen in HCC patients is usually the macronodular or postnecrotic type, which is caused by chronic HBV infection.[2,15,21,22] Prospective data from Taiwan strongly suggest a direct role for HBV in HCC.[26] Beasley's 4-year study of 3500 HBV carriers and 19,250 controls established a relative risk of 234, with HCC occurring in 40 carriers and 1 control subject.[28]

PATHOLOGY

About 90% of primary carcinomas of the liver are HCC, the remaining are cholangiocarcinomas (about 7%) and less common tumors such as hepatoblastomas, angiosarcomas, and sarcomas (Table 27-4).[60-73] The gross appearance varies from a single, large, dominant nodule or mass, which may be well-circumscribed or infiltrating, to a multicentric tumor. The tumor itself is characteristically soft, a factor that may lead to rupture and intraperitoneal hemorrhage. There may be areas of necrosis or hemorrhage, especially in large tumors. Intermediate forms of the large nodular tumor are often seen. Multicentric tumors frequently are found in cirrhotic livers, and in some cases, it may be difficult to distinguish neoplastic from regenerative nodules.[63-65] In livers with multiple small nodules, it is difficult to distinguish be-

TABLE 27-2. Risk Factors for Hepatocellular Carcinoma

Risk Factor	Observation	Reference
Chronic hepatic injury	Associated with HCC in North and South America in 22% to 60% of HCC patients	1, 7, 13, 14
Cirrhosis	Associated with HCC in Asia and Africa in 60% to 90% of HCC patients	7, 10-12, 23, 26, 37, 38, 51
Chronic hepatitis B infection	Increases the chance of developing HCC; persistent viral infection found in sera from 20% to 90% of HCC patients worldwide	7, 25, 34, 41, 42, 52
Aflatoxin	Implicated in etiology of HCC in Africa and Asia	7, 39, 41, 42
Alcoholism	Implicated in etiology of HCC, but association between alcoholism and HCC is less strong than between chronic alcohol intake and cancer of the mouth, larynx, and esophagus; possible promoter for hepatitis B virus	7, 29, 43, 44
Chronic hepatic outflow obstruction (CHOO)	Associated with HCC in 20% of South African cases and well documented in Japan; 61.6% of CHOO cases studied by Simson had HCC	45-49
Male sex	Most HCC occurs in men; suggested hormonal involvement	50, 53-59

TABLE 27-3.   Clinical Features of Hepatocellular Carcinoma in High- and Low-Incidence Areas

Variables	High Incidence	Low Incidence
Geographic location	Asia, Africa	North America, Europe
Race	Asians, blacks	Mostly whites
Median age	Asians, 40–50 yr	50–60 yr
	Blacks, 20–30 yr	
Duration of symptoms	Usually short, especially in young blacks	Can be indolent
Abdominal pain or discomfort	70–90%	50–70%
Anorexia and weight loss	Common	Common
Hemorrhage secondary to ruptured tumor	10–20%	<10%
Cirrhosis	60–80%	60–80%
Cirrhosis evolving to hepatocellular carcinoma	50% or more	5–10%
Type of cirrhosis	Mostly macronodular	Mostly micronodular
Etiology of cirrhosis	HBV probably most important	Often alcohol and HBV
Hepatocellular carcinoma associated with hepatitis B virus	80% or more	30–50%
Hepatitis B antigen	70–90%	15–40%
Possible exposure to aflatoxin	High	Most unlikely
AFP > 400 ng/ml (radioimmunoassay)	70–85%	30–65%

tween a multicentric HCC or intrahepatic metastatic spread.[67] A high frequency of portal vein invasion may be responsible for retrograde tumor spread and multiple intrahepatic metastases.[65] Okuda and colleagues have drawn attention to an important encapsulated HCC.[66] This tumor is common in Japan but is less frequently seen in other areas.[63] Sclerotic tumors are uncommon and may be mistaken for carcinoma on gross examination.

Peters recognized six different histologic patterns of HCC: microtrabecular, macrotrabecular, acinar, pseudoglandular, cobblestone, and pelioid types.[63,67] Cytologically, HCC may range from a well-differentiated tumor that is difficult to distinguish from normal hepatocytes to a poorly differentiated neoplasm. Cells may be uniform or markedly pleomorphic or may form giant cells. Cell cytoplasm may be clear, containing large amounts of glycogen, or have large lipid-containing vacuoles. Hyland bodies and Mallory bodies may be present. The trabecular hepatic portal canaliculi are reproduced in well-differentiated tumors, and exaggerations of these histologic features are responsible for most of the microscopic subtypes. Well-differentiated carcinomas may secrete bile and formed bile plugs may be recognized in the canaliculi. Canaliculi lined by two or three hepatocytes may assume the appearance of rosettes, similar to those seen in non-neoplastic livers in chronic acute hepatitis—the pseudoglandular pattern.

Some have suggested that histologic classification of HCC should be simplified into two subtypes: trabecular or undifferentiated tumors. The macrotrabecular, microtrabecular, acinar, pseudoglandular, and adenomatous carcinomas are all considered trabecular. Other histologic variants of trabecular tumors are the carcinoid-like tumors and highly vascu-

TABLE 27-4.   Classification of Hepatic Tumors

Epithelial		Mesenchymal		Others
Benign	Malignant	Benign	Malignant	
Focal nodular hyperplasia	Hepatoblastoma	Hemangioma	Mixed	Cysts
Adenoma	Hepatocellular carcinoma	Hemangioendothelioma (types I and II)	Mesenchyumal tumors	Metastasis
Bile duct adenoma	Cholangiocellular carcinoma	Mesenchymal hamartoma	Rhabdomyosarcoma	
Bile duct cystadenoma		Peliosis hepatitis	Undifferentiated sarcoma	
Adrenal rest			Angiosarcoma	
Nodular hyperplasia			Malignant histiosarcoma	
			Neuroblastoma	
			Germ cell tumor	
			Endodermal sinus tumor	
			Lymphoma	
			Leiomyosarcoma	
			Malignant tumor of bile duct origin, carcinomas, rhabdomyosarcoma	

Data from Rao BN, Green AA: Hepatic tumors in children and adolescents. In Wanebo HJ (ed): Hepatic and biliary cancer, pp 187–218. New York, Marcel Dekker, 1987.

larized types resembling peliosis hepatitis, called "peleoid" by Peters.[63,68]

Two histologic subsets of HCC can be classified separately because of their clinical and prognostic features. Fibrolamellar carcinoma occurs in younger patients of either sex and is associated with better resectability rates and survival than is the usual form of HCC.[67,69-72] Distinctive features include the marked fibrosis, which is arranged in a lamellar fashion around the neoplastic hepatocytes. These tumors have also been called "polygonal cell type" with fibrous stroma by Berman, Libbey, and Foster.[71] The more favorable prognosis of these patients, compared with those with other forms of HCC, has been disputed by Christopherson and his co-workers.[72]

Sclerosing HCCs (cholangiocarcinoma, carcinoma of bile duct) are adenocarcinomas that have a ductular arrangement.[73] They may secrete mucus but not bile. On gross examination they present as a solitary white mass containing more fibrous stoma than does HCC. It is histologically indistinguishable from the cholangiocarcinomas that arise in extrahepatic bile ducts. Sclerosing HCC is associated with hypercalcemia.[73]

Related Liver Tumors

Benign liver tumors include adenoma, focal nodular hyperplasia (FNH), hemangioma, and mesenchymal hamartoma.[61,62] In Christopherson's Liver Registry, FNH was the most common, diagnosed in 106 of the 201 cases. The median age was 31 years, compared with 30 years in the 83 patients with adenomas. Hemoperitoneum occurred in 9%, and 83% had a history of birth control pill use for an average of 71 months. FNH is usually described as having a large central scar from which radiates wide fibrous bands, somewhat resembling macronodular cirrhosis.

Of the patients with liver cell adenomas, 83% used oral contraceptives for an average of 80 months. In most cases, there was a single tumor, ranging in diameter from 1 to 22 cm. Adenomas were composed exclusively of hepatocytes, tended to be circumscribed, and were usually described as encapsulated.

Other malignant tumors include angiosarcoma of the liver which is related to ingestion or exposure to Thorotrast, an organic arsenical vinyl chloride, androgenic anabolic steroids, birth control pills, and diethylstilbestrol for prostatic cancer.[62] Patients usually die from liver destruction, even though at the time of diagnoses only a small number (12%) have distant metastases. The disease is multicentric and widespread throughout the liver, and there have been no survivors.

The ethnically global mixture of the American population and the infrequent incidence of HCC in North America limit the study of hepatoma. There is a diversity of underlying disease, including macronodular cirrhosis, primarily in Chinese men; diffuse cirrhosis, primarily in whites; and nodular and diffuse cirrhosis in patients with nonresectable HCC. The disease may be alpha-fetoprotein (AFP) positive or negative. This variable mixture must be analyzed in toto to develop realistic prognoses and therapeutic approaches.

Pathophysiologic Classification

HCC can be described morphologically by histologic characteristics, but a pathophysiologic classification that deals with underlying disease, as observed by CT scan and analyzed by biochemical markers, may be of more value in guiding chemical decisions than is the histologic description. One exception is the fibrolamellar form of HCC, which appears to be associated with prolonged survival.[66,67]

Underlying Disease

CHRONIC ACTIVE HEPATITIS. Patients with chronic active hepatitis present difficult management problems because most major cytotoxic agents adversely affect chronic active hepatitis and the damaged liver. The regenerative capacity of the normal liver decreases with relapsing viral infection. In addition, these patients are often managed with prednisone, Imuran, and other immunosuppressive agents that further complicate management. Even with reduced dosages of chemotherapy, a reactivation of hepatitis and further injury of tissue may occur.[74]

DIFFUSE CIRRHOSIS. Diffuse cirrhosis, common in the United States, is often associated with a loss of regenerative capacity in the normal liver. Experience suggests that if the liver involved by HCC is also small and cirrhotic, it is unlikely that it will be able to regenerate in response to tumor resection.[75] Depending on the degree of cirrhosis, sequelae such as modest liver failure and ascites may occur, and, in more marked circumstances, esophageal varices caused by portal hypertension and jaundice may occur. Each of these factors makes therapy more difficult and increases the complication rate, regardless of the treatment modality used.[76] A milder form of diffuse cirrhosis is one in which the regenerative capacity of the normal liver is suggested by increased liver size as detected by physical examination or CT scans. The expansion of the normal liver, in addition to the presence of the tumor, suggests to the oncologist a potential for liver regeneration after treatment of the tumor.

MACRONODULAR CIRRHOSIS. Macronodular cirrhosis is particularly prominent in Asians, in contrast to the more diffuse cirrhosis seen in North Americans. Hepatitis B has been commonly associated with macronodular cirrhosis.[77] The distinctive large and nodular liver is also associated with a poor regenerative capacity, as is the case with diffuse cirrhosis, and it severely limits the ability to resect. However, AFP screening has permitted identification of a large series of patients in China with early HCC. The majority of these patients underwent curative wedge resections of these early lesions.[77] Although this result has not been duplicated for diffuse cirrhosis, there are methods for converting nonresectable HCC to a resectable state through cytoreduction by means of isotopic labeled antibody therapy.[78] Furthermore, HCC that occurs in conjunction with macronodular cirrhosis is usually hypervascular, which enhances certain treatment methods, particularly radiolabeled antibodies.[78]

TUMOR MARKERS. AFP is the major tumor marker associated with HCC and is elevated in over 70% of patients with disease.[79-82] Correlations between tumor differentiation and the levels of AFP have been demonstrated.[69] Patients with high levels of the marker protein have short survival times and poorly differentiated carcinomas. Moderately differentiated tumors are associated with intermediate levels of AFP and intermediate survival times. Patients with low AFP levels fall into two groups. One group consists of long-term survivors with extremely well-differentiated tumors, and the second group with anaplastic carcinomas have ultrashort survival times.[69] Other series have shown that high AFP levels are associated with better survival rates than normal AFP levels, but these data may reflect a particular patient mix.[33]

Carcinoembryonic antigen (CEA) is elevated in more than 70% of patients with HCC, but it lacks specificity. There is no correlation between CEA and AFP concentrations: the CEA may rise when the AFP decreases. Alkaline phosphatase is invariably elevated, but it also lacks specificity.[83]

Other tumor markers have been found in patients with HCC, especially in low-incidence areas and usually in patients without HBV and without elevated AFP. Increased levels of chorionic gonadotropin, of chorionic somatotropin, and of calcitonin have been reported.[84,85] Elevated neurotensin levels have been found in patients with fibrolamellar carcinoma.[86]

In China, 70% to 75% of patients with HCC have positive AFP titers. Between 90% and 95% have either hepatitis B antigen or antibody. However, 25% to 30% of the patients with HCC are AFP negative.[87,88] These patients have not attracted general attention in Chinese medical practice.

In the randomized prospective study carried out through the Radiation Oncology Study Group (RTOG) in the eastern United States, 63% of the patients were AFP positive and 37% were AFP negative. Ten percent of the patients have HBV antigen, according to a study by DiBisceglie and coworkers.[25a] Twenty-one percent of 63 patients had positive anti-HBV antibody titers. This contrasts with no HBV-antigen positivity (p < 0.004) and 10% anti-HBV antibody positive titers (p = 0.08) in 98 consecutive cancer patients. In the western United States, however, the higher incidence of patients of Asian background leads to a higher incidence of AFP positivity, HBS antigenicity, and antibody levels. Finally, based on the original Phase I–II study with radiolabeled antibody, tumors that do not elevate AFP seem to grow slower than AFP-producing tumors.

CLINICAL PRESENTATION

Most patients complain of right upper quadrant pain or distention and weight loss. The pain is usually dull or aching, but it can be acute and frequently radiates to the right shoulder. Fatigue and loss of appetite are common, and unexplained fever may occur. Patients may present with hepatic decompensation and have ascites, variceal bleeding, jaundice, or encephalopathy.

The findings of firm nodular hepatomegaly and an arterial bruit, combined with a hepatic rub, strongly suggest HCC in an advanced stage. Earlier stages may have hepatomegaly

only or have no specific findings. Among 569 patients referred to a hospital in South Africa as possible HCC cases based on hepatomegaly, more than 60% were confirmed to have HCC, 11% had cirrhosis only, 7.5% had tuberculosis, and 5% had amoebiasis.[81] Only 3.5% had metastatic cancer to the liver.

In high-risk patients having chronic HVB or cirrhosis, ultrasound and AFP monitoring may lead to earlier diagnoses. Metastases occur commonly in HCC, accounting for the variable modes of presentation. Lung metastases are found in approximately 20% of patients, and pulmonary or chest wall symptoms may be the first symptom. Occasionally, metastases to bone or other uncommon sites may draw attention to the disease. Although the liver disease dominates the clinical picture, more than half of the patients will have extrahepatic spread during the clinical course of the disease. Other modes of presentation include an acute abdomen from a spontaneous rupture of the tumor (more common in Asia), acute Budd-Chiari syndrome due to extension of the tumor into the inferior vena cava, and portal hypertension due to invasion of the portal venous system.[89,90] There are rare modes of presentation that receive undue attention, including endocrine and paraneoplastic complications. Erythrocytosis is the most common. Hypoglycemia occurs in the late stages of the disease but is very seldom the reason for suspecting HCC. Hypercalcemia, hyperthyroidism, and carcinoid syndrome are also described. Hypertrophic pulmonary osteoarthropathy is common in South African patients with HCC but is seldom symptomatic.[81]

METASTATIC DISEASE

HCC can invade the diaphragm and adjacent organs like the stomach, which may be related to the propensity for membranous obstruction of the inferior vena cava in patients with HCC.[90] HCC may also invade the portal vein and, less frequently, the hepatic veins. Bile duct obstruction and early jaundice can result, even in the setting of limited tumor burden.[91] Perineural metastases and intraperitoneal rupture of the hepatic tumor and hemorrhage can also occur.

Metastatic disease is present in a minority of patients at operation, but at the time of autopsy more than 50% of the patients have metastases. These occur most commonly in regional nodes, lung, bone, adrenal gland, and brain. Series by Simson, Peters, and Anthony show a distribution of metastases similar in African and non-African studies.[63,64,68] Approximately 40% of all patients have tumor in regional nodes. Other metastatic sites are very rare, with less than 10% involving bone, adrenal gland, heart, and central nervous system. Sternal metastases may be a specific type of spread in patients with membranous obstruction of the inferior vena cava.[90] Direct venous spread is an important factor in HCC. Invasion of the portal and hepatic vein is common, and tumor frequently involves the inferior vena cava. The gallbladder is invaded directly in approximately 6% of the cases, and the tumor obstructs large bile ducts in the porta hepatis or in the larger ducts within the liver.[91] The subsequent jaundice in these patients can falsely suggest a terminal status usually seen in patients with HCC who are jaundiced. Spontaneous hemoperitoneum caused by rupture, evident in 25% of Anthony's series, and hemorrhage from esophageal varices, evident in 19% of the same series, are serious complications of HCC.[68]

DIAGNOSIS

In areas of the world where HCC is common, chronic HBV infection, chronic membranous obstruction of the inferior vena cava, chronic hepatic outflow obstruction (CHOO), and male sex are factors that should draw attention to the possibility of developing HCC. These clear associations also apply to low-incidence areas of the world. HCC is insidious. If clinical signs and symptoms directly referable to HCC have developed, the prognosis is usually only a few months.

Tumor Markers

The presence of AFP in the serum of patients with HCC has led to its use as a screening method in high-risk populations. This has been effective in China, in patients with chronic hepatitis in Japan, and among Alaskan Eskimos, and it may have value in selected patients with HBV-positive hepatitis.[79,82,92-97] Elevated AFP, unfortunately, is not specific for the diagnosis of HCC, and histologic confirmation is essential. In a series of black South African patients suspected to have HCC and who had elevated levels of serum AFP, several nonhepatic malignancies of the gallbladder and the extrahepatic bile ducts and pancreas were demonstrated.[81]

Elevation of AFP levels is a well-recognized feature of metastatic liver cancer, endodermally derived tumors, and islet cell tumors.[80] Unlike germ cell tumors, in which the elevation of AFP may be related to the amount of tumor present, the levels vary in patients with HCC. The heterogeneity of AFP expression may relate to the cause of HCC, although in classic HCC, elevated AFP levels should raise concern about the diagnosis of HCC. Although AFP occurs in fetal blood in levels reaching 500 to 700 ng/ml, it decreases rapidly after birth.[92] Within the first year, infants achieve normal adult values of less than 10 ng/ml. The frequency of AFP elevation in HCC varies from 30% to 90%.[79-93] Although a normal AFP does not exclude HCC, very high values strongly suggest HCC.

A general diagnostic approach is outlined in Figure 27-1. The finding of an upper abdominal mass in a high-risk patient, who is HBV positive or who lives in an indigenous area for HCC, should prompt an AFP test, followed rapidly by an ultrasound and CT scan. If disease is extensive, a fine-needle biopsy may suffice. If liver resection is considered, an exploration with operative biopsy is preferred.

Radiologic Studies

Plain films of the chest and abdomen may provide some information.[98] An unusual hump or elevation of the diaphragm may correspond to an invasive liver tumor, pending exclusion of a primary nerve palsy or eventration. Abdominal films may show hepatomegaly and, occasionally, calcification is seen in primary hepatic tumors. An upper gastrointestinal (GI) series may show gross displacement of the stomach in patients with advanced disease. Some patients may present with hemothorax and corresponding ascites, along with metastases to the lung detected as large "cannonball lesions" or the rarer micronodule shadows.

Radionuclide-labeled colloids, in particular ^{99m}Tc-labeled sulfur colloid, are sensitive in evaluating space-occupying liver lesions. In a large Singapore study, ^{99}Tc-sulfur colloid detected HCC in 94% of the patients, ^{198}Au-colloid detected lesions in 81%, and gallium in 89%.[99] Gallium was more useful in distinguishing primary HCC from secondary lesions or abscesses. Most of the difficulties arose from background effects of a highly cirrhotic liver; here gallium may be more useful and provide better quality scanning, with improved specificity and sensitivity. A technetium scan would appear to be the preferred initial diagnostic examination, but gallium may be more useful if metastases are suspected.[100]

Ultrasound is a very versatile and inexpensive early diagnostic test. It is noninvasive, nontoxic, and rapidly used. It may be of equal or greater sensitivity than radionuclide scanning. Lesions less than 3 cm can be detected by ultrasound; for the small tumors, ultrasound is considered by some to be the most sensitive of imaging techniques, in which cases it is hypoechoic.[101] It also can guide an aspiration needle. Intraoperative ultrasound is useful in the detection of deep-seated small tumors.[102]

CT can detect and delineate the extent of hepatic tumors. The presence of isodense tumors or small lesions may lead to false-negative results, and occasionally false-positive results are also given. Magnetic resonance imaging (MRI) has been shown comparable to CT scanning and in some cases may be preferable. The degree of contrast between the

FIG. 27-1. Evaluation of hepatocellular cancer. A general guideline to the diagnostic workup of the patient at risk for hepatocellular carcinoma. An arteriogram is generally done if resection is planned. A biopsy could be done at that time, unless the patient is considered unresectable, at which time a percutaneous biopsy could be done. *Paraneoplastic syndrome may elevate or depress calcium or glucose. **Must indicate safety of biopsy or be corrected.

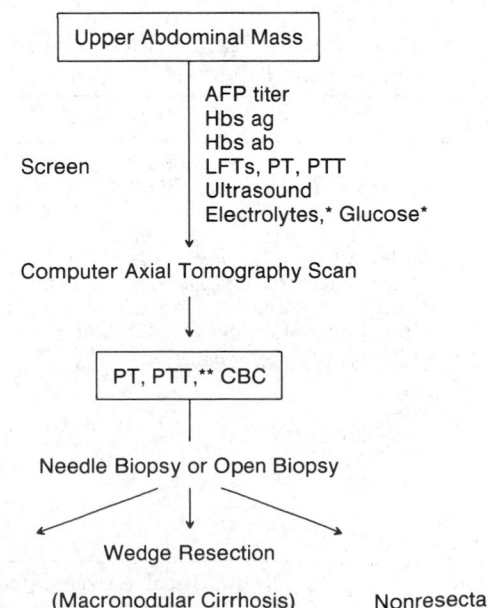

tumor and normal liver is better with MRI and distinguishes among HCC and angioma, cysts, and cirrhosis.

Comparisons of these methods suggest that scintography with technetium may be a good first choice, although if adequate ultrasound is available it is considered preferable by many. CT and technetium scanning are probably similar in sensitivity, but the CT scan better defines the anatomy of the disease and also shows the extrahepatic extent of tumor. Ultrasound in skilled hands is useful in distinguishing cysts and possible vascular lesions, as well as for detecting small HCC not visualized by the CT scan.[101]

Diagnosis by needle biopsy is frequently possible.[102] Caution is required because of the potential for hemorrhage from a hypervascular HCC or a misdiagnosed hemangioma. Peritoneoscopic visualization with biopsy is recommended by some.[103] This would allow direct assessment of the liver during the biopsy and minimize the potential for hemorrhage. In patients who are candidates for resection, a needle biopsy is not recommended in view of the risk for hemorrhage and tumor-cell contamination. Such patients are better explored and resected if curative surgery is undertaken.

Patients who are considered candidates for surgery (*i.e.*, localized lesion limited to one lobe or segment without extrahepatic spread) should have hepatic angiography.[104,105] This provides information about the tumor extent and an arterial and venous system road map essential for planned resection. These tumors are usually hypervascular, and, in some cases, the angiogram may demonstrate lesions in both lobes of the liver not detected by noninvasive techniques.[103-105] A late-phase angiogram can demonstrate the portal vein and its major branches, and a direct inferior vena cavogram may be useful in determining the metastasic or direct invasion. Angiography provides data for resection and for other surgical approaches, such as hepatic artery infusion therapy.

Although staging is essential to the primary management of all major cancers, an accepted system is not currently in use for HCC. One suggested system was based on risk factors in Ugandan patients (Table 27-5).[106] This system categorizes patients according to the presence or absence of ascites, weight loss, portal hypertension, or jaundice, and it further subdivides categories by the anatomical extent of tumor. In the Ugandan patients, the survival ranged from greater than 3 months in those with no ascites, weight loss <10%, no portal hypertension, and normal bilirubin to less than 2 months in those with all these factors present. Prognostic factors in advanced HCC are discussed in the section on chemotherapy.[107]

SURGERY

The preoperative assessment by the clinical and radiologic techniques described should provide the major determination of resectability.[103-105,108,109] During the laparotomy, the final decisions are made, based on the extent of tumor, the involvement of major vascular structures, lymph node metastases, or extrahepatic spread. Extension to the diaphragm or to the lateral parities under the rib cage requires a more extensive resection to insure adequate margins. In general, extension into the suprahepatic portion of the inferior vena cava or extension into the porta hepatis with involvement of the ducts or vessels on the contralateral major lobe precludes conventional resection.

In a jaundiced patient, a percutaneous cholangiogram or endoscopic cholangiopancreatiography (ERCP) may reveal a bile duct extension with contralateral hepatic duct involvement or common bile duct involvement, probably precluding resection except by very experienced surgeons or for patients selected for transplant surgery. Cirrhosis is also a major risk factor governing the extent of resection. Extensive cirrhosis, especially that associated with portal hypertension, precludes resection in most patients, except for very small tumors. Intraoperative ultrasound can determine the presence of small intrahepatic tumors, especially the presence of multicentric tumors, and can influence the plan for resection.

TABLE 27-5. Revised Staging Criteria for Hepatocellular Carcinoma in African Patients

Stage	Cancer Presentation
I	No ascites, weight loss or portal hypertension Serum bilirubin less than 2 mg/dl
II	Ascites and/or moderate weight loss (<25% of body weight), no portal hypertension Serum bilirubin less than 2 mg/dl
III	Severe weight loss (>25% body weight) Portal hypertension Serum bilirubin greater than 2 mg/dl

Anatomic Extent of Involvement

A One lobe only
B Two lobes
C Metastatic disease

Cirrhosis

(+) = present
(−) = absent
(?) = uncertain

Primack A, Vogel CL, Kyalwazi et al: A staging system for hepatocellular carcinoma: Prognostic factors in Ugandan patients. Cancer 35:1357–1364, 1975.

FIG. 27-2. The liver in transparency to show the branching and relative position of the parts of the portal and hepatic veins. (Goldsmith NA, Woodburne RT: The surgical anatomy pertaining to liver resection. Surg Gynecol Obstet 105:310, 1957. By permission of Surgery, Gynecology & Obstetrics)

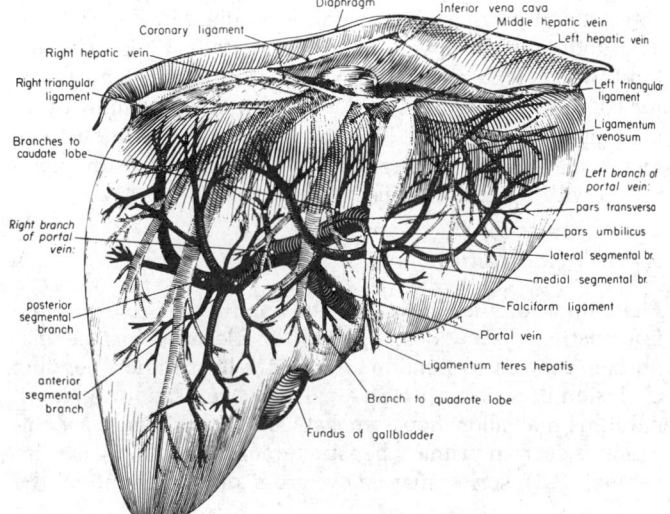

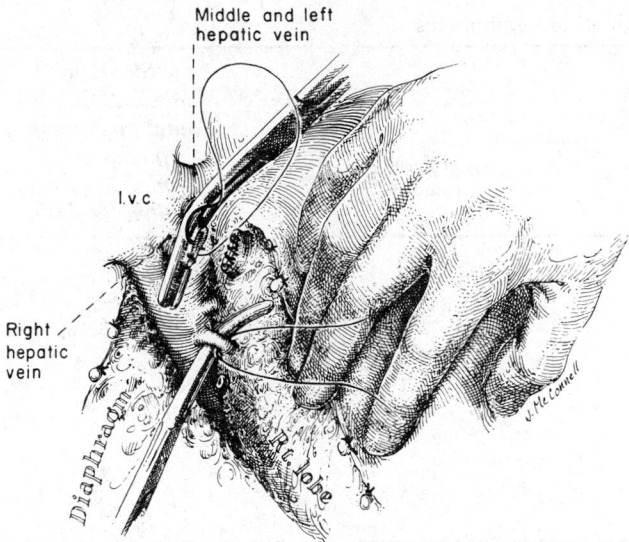

FIG. 27-3. Division of the right hepatic vein. With the right lobe of the liver retracted anteriorly and to the left, the vein is divided between Pott's clamps and oversewn with vascular sutures. Several smaller hepatic veins must be ligated as they enter the retrohepatic vena cava more inferiorly. (Starzl TE, Bell RH, Beart RW, et al: Hepatic trisegmentectomy and other liver resections. Surg Gynecol Obstet 141:429, 1974. By permission of Surgery, Gynecology & Obstetrics)

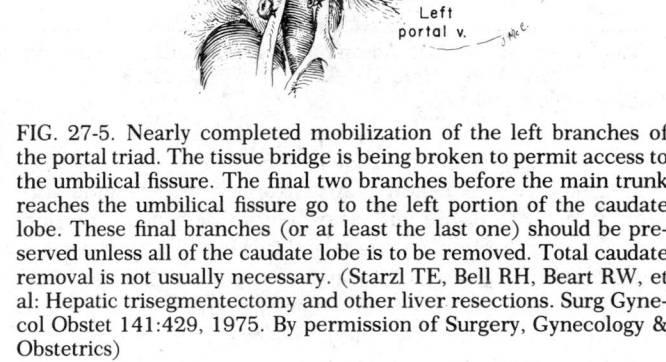

FIG. 27-5. Nearly completed mobilization of the left branches of the portal triad. The tissue bridge is being broken to permit access to the umbilical fissure. The final two branches before the main trunk reaches the umbilical fissure go to the left portion of the caudate lobe. These final branches (or at least the last one) should be preserved unless all of the caudate lobe is to be removed. Total caudate removal is not usually necessary. (Starzl TE, Bell RH, Beart RW, et al: Hepatic trisegmentectomy and other liver resections. Surg Gynecol Obstet 141:429, 1975. By permission of Surgery, Gynecology & Obstetrics)

FIG. 27-4. Devascularization of the true right lobe. The cystic artery and cystic duct are ligated and divided to aid in the dissection. Of the structures of the portal triad, the bifurcation of the duct is almost always the most superior, that of the portal vein is intermediate, and that of the hepatic artery is most inferior. The lateral suture closure of the portal vein is at the site of detachment of the right portal branch. The tissue bridge conceals the umbilical fissure, behind which a finger can be inserted. The bridge is present in about half the patients. (Starzl TE, Bell RH, Beart RW, et al: Hepatic trisegmentectomy and other liver resections. Surg Gynecol Obstet 141:429, 1975. By permission of Surgery, Gynecology & Obstetrics)

FIG. 27-6. Liver transection nearly completed along the exact line of color change demarcated by viable and cyanotic liver tissue. Intersegmental veins are left attached to the lateral segment if possible. The last major structure to be encountered is the middle hepatic vein. (Starzl TE, Bell RH, Beart RW, et al: Hepatic trisegmentectomy and other liver resections. Surg Gynecol Obstet 141:429, 1975. By permission of Surgery, Gynecology & Obstetrics)

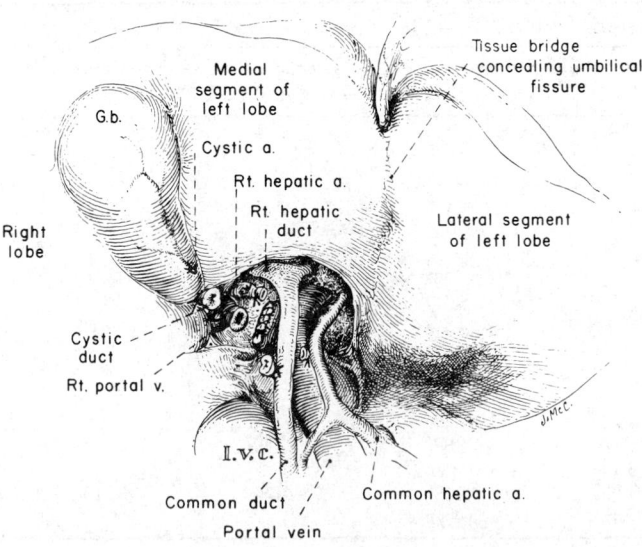

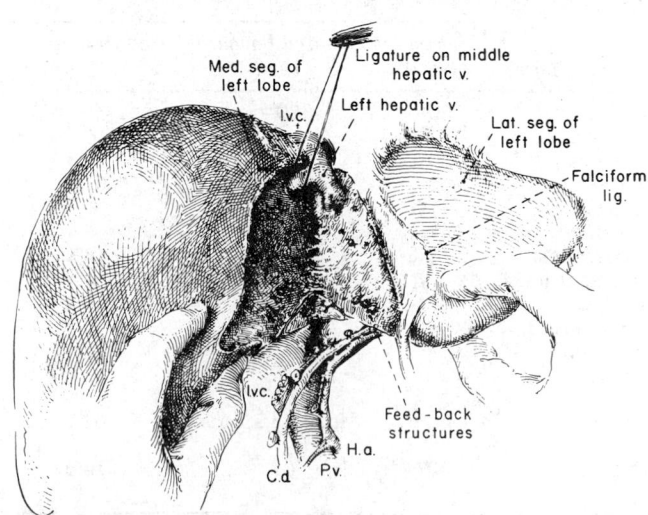

TABLE 27-6. Summary of Resection Experience with Primary Hepatic Malignancies

Resection Data	Clinical Cancers			Small or "Minute" Cancers Found by Screening in High-Risk Groups Requiring Limited Resections
	Western Experience	Eastern Experience	Japan National Study	
Total patients	~2000	4983	5496	147
No. of resections	482	969	1186	110
Resectability rate (range)	20–25%	19% (7–46%)	21.5%	73% (54–76%)
With cirrhosis, mean (range)	17% (0–43%)	68% (40–90%)	~80%	90%
Hospital mortality after resection	15%	18%		0–5%
Overall survival				
1 year	81%	48%	55%	73%
3 years	46%	24%	30%	66%
5 years	30%	14.5%		33–70%

Data from Nagorney DM, Adson MA: Major hepatic resections for hepatoma in the west. In Wanebo HJ (ed): Hepatic and biliary cancer, pp 167–185. New York, Marcel Dekker, 1987; Okuda K, Liver Cancer Study Group of Japan: Primary liver cancers in Japan. Cancer 45:2663–2669, 1980.

The operative exposure is important.[105,109–112] Some surgeons are comfortable with the bilateral subcostal incision with anterior traction on the costal border by a rigid retractor. Others may make liberal use of thoracoabdominal incisions, which afford improved exposure and may be necessary in patients having large lesions that involve the proximal portion of the inferior vena cava in the superior portion of the liver. This incision may also be necessary in patients in whom proximal control of the vena cava is required.

Anatomical Considerations

The liver substance is arranged segmentally. The classic descriptions of Goldsmith and Woodburne divide the liver into two major lobes, with the division line on a plane from the bed of the gallbladder to the inferior vena cava (Fig. 27-2).[113] Couinaud categorized eight hepatic subsegments.[114] The subsegments, based on the portobiliary drainage, have been more commonly used by European than North American surgeons, perhaps because of their greater familiarity with Couinaud's work.[115]

The classic approach consists of hilar dissection, with vascular control and subsequent resection of major portobiliary segments using various methods of dissection to maximize hemostasis (Figs. 27-3 through 27-6).[3,105,110,116,117] Refinements of the finger fracture technique include disruption by the sucker tip or the ultrasonic dissector. Numerous methods of disrupting the liver substance are available that permit identification of the thread-like portal triad structures and

TABLE 27-7. Resection of Hepatocellular Carcinoma: Results of Selected Series

Author (Year)	Western Series						
	Adson (1986)	Lim and Bongard (1984)	Sorenson et al (1979)	Fortner et al (1981)	Bengmark et al (1982)	Iwatshi et al (1983)	Thompson et al (1983)
Total study population	230	86					
% cirrhosis	50%	43%					
No resections	62	22	31	42	21	43	35
Resectability rate	27%	26%					
% resections with cirrhosis	3%	43%	16%		0%	12%	20%
Hospital mortality after resections		39%	26%	17%	14%	9%	20%
Survival							
1 year				85%		78%	
2 year	53%	Median 18.7 mo	62%	50% (3 yr)	38% (2 yr)	60%	
5 years	30%		16%	37%	20% (4 yr)	46%	31%

larger segmental vessels and ducts, which can be ligated, clipped, or in some cases, electrocoagulated. Larger vessels are easily identified within the liver substance and are formally ligated and bisected. Control of the hepatic veins is controversial and depends primarily on the experience of the individual surgeon rather than on any accepted surgical anatomical study. Although the right and left hepatic veins may be easily exposed in some patients, more commonly they are buried within the liver substance. Because of its position superior and posterior in the liver, the early exposure of this vein can be treacherous, and many prefer to expose and ligate it near the completion of the resection.[124] Many approaches have been described in the literature.[105,108-117]

The basic principles of safe hepatic resection require adequate exposure and complete mobilization of the liver, with division of ligamentous attachments (*i.e.*, the triangular ligament superiorly and the attachments of the right lobe posteriorly and laterally for right hepatic resections) and exposure of the superior hepatic cava. Isolation of the suprahepatic cava and vascular control with a looped umbilical tape may provide an additional safety measure for control of the suprahepatic cava in the event of a mishap. Although rarely necessary, use of a large-bore cardiac venous shunt, placed by means of the right atrium into the inferior vena cava using a large-bore shunt for very high-risk lesions, is possible.

Hilar dissection and vascular isolation of the major branches of hepatic artery and portal vein, encircling these with a vascular loop or an umbilical tape or ligating these structures directly, will markedly reduce the bleeding of both portal veins and arterial inflow to the segments. Some surgeons espouse total inflow occlusion by clamping the porta hepatis with a vascular clamp.[118] Occlusion times up to 1 hour have been reported, and blood loss and operative time have been markedly reduced from conventional approaches. If feasible, the numerous retrohepatic veins should be exposed and ligated. This may not be possible in all patients because of the extensive encircling of the cava by the liver. The same can be said for the hepatic veins, which may be located deep in liver. In some cases, however, the veins may be easily seen, mobilized, and ligated during the dissection.

Blood loss may be moderate or profound, depending on the extent of the resection and the presence of underlying cirrhosis or coagulopathy; it is imperative to minimize blood loss by all mechanical methods. Autotransfusions may be useful, although there are concerns about the potential for spreading cells unwittingly shed during the operative procedure. Adequate replacement with fresh-frozen plasma and platelets, if necessary, early in the dissection, especially in cirrhotic patients, may help reduce blood loss.

Lateral sublobar segmental resections (*i.e.*, tumors less than 5 cm in the lateral portion of the liver) may not require routine hilar vascular control. In contrast, even small tumors in the proximity of the hepatic vein on the posterior dome (segments 7 and 8) may preclude a safe resection for most surgeons. Intraoperative ultrasound can locate small nonpalpable HCC and major portal inflow to the subsegment, which allows for a more limited resection in cirrhotic patients.

After completion of the resection, the liver surface is irrigated copiously, small open ducts or vessels are ligated as necessary, and the open liver substance is covered with omentum. Most surgeons make use of a closed drainage system to provide egress of blood and bile during the immediate postoperative period. Antibiotics and adequate replacement of fluids and clotting factors are prerequisites to good clinical outcome.

Resectability

Twenty-five percent of patients with primary HCC seen at major centers have potentially resectable lesions (Tables 27-6 and 27-7).[119-128] Approximately 10% to 12% are actually resected.

Most surgeons consider severe cirrhosis to be a contraindication to major resection.[124-128] This is suggested from studies demonstrating retrospectively that cirrhosis and HCC

TABLE 27-7. Resection of Hepatocellular Carcinoma: Results of Selected Series *(continued)*

			Eastern Series				
Honjo and Mizusoto (1974)	Lin (1976)	Okuda et al (1980)	Wu et al (1980)	Lee et al (1982)	Okamato et al (1984)	Nagasue et al (1986)	Nagoa et al (1987)
76	382	2411	748	935	266		
40%		83%			90%		
21	181	213	181	165	103	94	98
26%	31%	9%	24%	18%	46%		
48%	21%	71%	70%	85%		86%	75%
9%	12%	28%	9%	20%	13%	7.6%	19%
	35%	33%	56%	45%	65%	55%	73%
23% (3 yr)	20% (3 yr)	20% (3 yr)	29% (3 yr)	20% (3 yr)	27%		42%
14%	19%	12%	16%	18%	13%	3.5%	25%

coexisted in 81% of patients examined at autopsy, in only 35% of patients examined at laparotomy, and in only 21% of patients with resectable tumors.[124] Most experienced surgeons have recognized that the greater the extent of the liver resection, the more dangerous is the procedure in patients with cirrhosis.[123,126] This recognition has led to mass screenings of patients at risk for HCC, many of whom have cirrhosis, with the hope of finding small resectable tumors. Kanematsu and colleagues have explored the risk and the value of limited hepatic resection for smaller encapsulated hepatomas from cirrhotic livers.[129] They found operative mortality rates of 1% to 15% for limited resections in patients with severe hepatic impairment and for major resections in cirrhotic patients with better hepatic reserve.[129]

Patient selection remains a problem for cirrhotics. Lee and co-workers found that bromosulfaphthalein excretion greater than 10% at 45 minutes or serum albumin less than 3 g/dl contraindicated major resection.[130] Tobe observed that major resection was generally contraindicated in patients who were Child's C class and who had impaired clearance of indocyanine green.[131] Schemes to define liver reserve in cirrhotics and to determine safe hepatic resection limits have been offered by several clinicians.[131-133]

Table 27-6 presents an overview of the eastern and western experience.[119-135] In the western series fewer than 20% of patients have cirrhosis, and the overall resectability is about 20% to 25%, with a 15% operative mortality rate. The 5-year cure rate is approximately 30%. In the eastern series, the percentage of cirrhosis ranged between 40% and 90%. The overall resectability rate ranged from 7% to 46%. The overall hospital mortality after resection ranged from 9% to 33%; Okuda in Japan reports 28% and Okamoto reports 13%.[133,135] Among cirrhotics in the Japanese overview, the overall mortality was approximately 30%, but in other series it was less: 20% in Honjo and Mizsumoto's series and 12% in the Wu series.[123,127a] The 5-year survival rate in those resected ranged from 11% to 19%.

An update of the Japanese experience reviewed survival rates and the impact of cirrhosis in HCC patients undergoing surgery between 1980 and 1981.[135a] Cirrhosis had a significant, adverse impact on survival after resection (Fig. 27-7). In a review of the medical and surgical experience at the Chiba University Hospital, Okuda and Tobe reported HCC was resected in 64 (19.8%) of 324 patients, with an operative death rate of 9.9%; multiple resections were performed in 6 patients.[135a] The extent of resection in 71 patients included partial resection for 48, segmentectomies for 8, and lobectomy or trisegmentectomy in 15. The relationship of mortality to the extent of resection was 15% to 27% in the group having major resections and was only 5% (3 of 56) in those patients undergoing partial resections or segmentectomies. The operative mortality according to Child's class was 4% (47 cases) with Child A, 7% (18 cases) with Child B, and 50% (6 cases) with Child C.[135] This series also used intraoperative ultrasonography to detect nonpalpable or unrecognizable tumors smaller than 5 cm, of particular importance in cirrhotics.

The relationships of tumor size, AFP levels, and the diagnostic measures of ultrasound, CT, and angiography in this well-studied group of patients is shown in Table 27-8, and

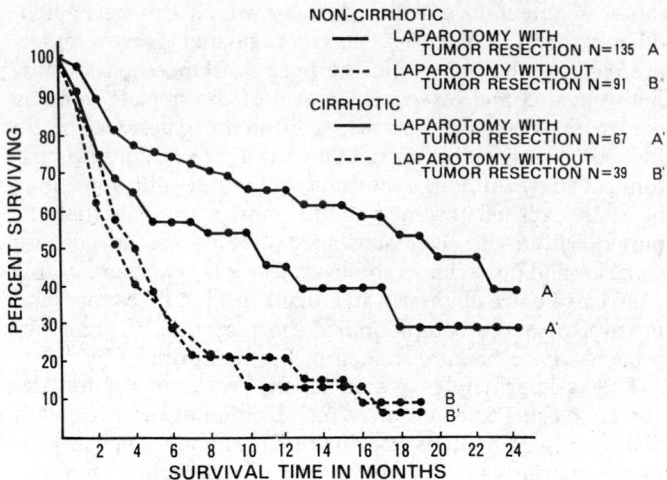

FIG. 27-7. Survival curves for the laparotomized cases in the latest National Study (1980–1981): (A) 135 noncirrhotic cases with resection; (B) 91 noncirrhotic cases without resection; (A') 67 cirrhotic cases with resection; (B') 39 cirrhotic cases without resection. There are significant differences between A and A', between A and B, and between A' and B', but not between B and B'.

the surgical survival data relevant to Child's class and extent of resection are shown in Table 27-9. The survival rate at 3 years in this series was 80% for patients with small tumors (≥2 cm), compared with 20% for those with tumors larger than 5 cm. High rates of resectability and survival have been reported for other Japanese and Chinese series for small HCC lesions diagnosed at an early stage.[135a-135c] In patients with tumors larger than 5 cm, approximately half died from tumor recurrence and the remaining from hepatic failure. This selective series emphasizes the need for concentrated experience with the disease.

Pediatric Liver Tumors

HEPATOBLASTOMA. Hepatoblastoma is a distinctive tumor of the liver in infants and children, with the male-female ratio of 1.5:2.1.[136-141] It is usually diagnosed in the first 2 to 3 years of life and is rarely seen in children older than age 6. It may be associated with congenital anomalies, such as tetralogy of Fallot, persistent ductus arteriosis, or extrahepatic biliary atresia. The most common presentation is as an asymptomatic abdominal mass found by the parent or during a routine physical examination. Jaundice is rare. Abdominal roentgenographic examination usually shows a mass density in the upper abdomen, and liver scan usually shows decreased isotope uptake. About 67% of the tumors arise in the right lobe. The serum levels of AFP are elevated in 80% to 90% of all patients. Microscopically, hepatoblastoma is classified into the more common pure epithelial type and a mixed epithelial mesenchymal type.[136-142]

HCC is also seen in the pediatric population, but it is less frequent than hepatoblastoma, occurs in older children (median, 10–12 years), and has a male-female ratio of about 8:1. At the time of diagnosis most patients are symptomatic, with weight loss, abdominal pain, jaundice, and anemia, and serum AFP levels are elevated in 30% to 80%. Although it is

TABLE 27-8.   Accuracy of Various Diagnostic Modalities for Hepatocellular Carcinoma (Chiba University Hospital Experience)

Size of Tumor (cm)	No. of Patients	Alpha-Fetoprotein Levels (ng/ml)			Diagnosis Made by (%)		
		<20	20–499	>500	Ultrasound	CT	Angiography
<2	12	5	7		75	92	67
<3	19	10	7	2	93	93	80
<5	23	5	13	5	100	94	95
<5.1	17	3	4	10	100	100	100
Total	71	23	31	17	94	95	89

From Okuda K, Ryu M, Tobe T: Surgical management of hepatoma. The Japanese experience. In Wanebo HJ (ed): Hepatic and biliary cancer, pp 219–238. New York, Marcel Dekker, 1987.

similar in its histologic pattern and clinical presentation to the adult form, the incidence of cirrhosis is only 5% in the children compared with about 75% in the adults.[136] In a review of pediatric hepatic tumors from St. Jude's Children's Research Hospital by Rao and Green, 29 of 76 hepatic tumors were hepatoblastomas, 18 were HCC, 8 were sarcomas, 1 was neuroblastoma, 7 were hemangiomas or hemangioendotheliomas, 3 were visceral larval migrans, 2 were hepatic abscesses, and 8 were other miscellaneous non-neoplastic tumors (Table 27-10).[136]

Of 29 hepatoblastomas, 7 had associated congenital abnormalities (a major CNS defect in 4), and 10 were resectable by hepatic lobectomy.[136] Eight of ten patients survived 3 to 18 years after resection, and two patients developed intrahepatic recurrences resistant to chemotherapy and died after 17 and 31 months, respectively. Among the 18 patients with HCC, all but 2 had asymptomatic masses. Five had congenital abnormalities, and only three had complete tumor resection of their tumors. Two of these were alive 5 and 17 years after surgery, and one died with local tumor recurrence. Of the eight primary liver sarcomas, six were malignant mesenchymoma and two were intrahepatic rhabdomyosarcoma. Five patients were resected, and three were long-term survivors with adjuvant chemotherapy. Two patients not given adjuvant therapy developed metastases and died.[136]

Transplantation

PRIMARY LIVER CANCER. In view of the limited resectability rate of 15% to 30% in most of the series, the potential for retrieval by total hepatectomy and transplantation has intrigued and challenged surgeons for years. The largest experience has been reported by Starzl and his group, although other surgeons have participated.[142-146] In the Starzl experience, a total of 55 patients received orthotopic liver transplants who had primary hepatic malignancies. There were 32 women and 23 men, with ages between 2 and 68 years (Table 27-11). Malignancies included HCC in 38 patients (69%), of which 7 were the fibrolamellar variant; bile duct carcinoma (Klatskin's tumor) in 8 (14.5%); epithelioid hemangioendothelial sarcoma in 3 (5.5%); and cholangiocarcinoma in 2 (3.6%). Four additional tumors included hepatoblastoma, hemangiosarcoma, unclassified sarcoma, and adenocarcinoma from an unknown primary. Of 40 patients, 76% were thought to have unresectable lesions and received liver transplants as the primary method of therapy. In the first 20 of these the immune suppression regimen included azathioprine, prednisone, and antilymphocyte globulin; the other 19 were immunosuppressed with cyclosporin and prednisone.

Thirteen patients received transplants for non-neoplastic

TABLE 27-9.   Hepatic Resection for Primary Liver Cancer: Relationship of Surgical Procedure, Child's Classification, and Operative Mortality (Chiba University Hospital Experience)

Child's Classification	No. of Cases	Extent of Resection		
		Partial	1 Segment	2–3 Segments
A	47	28	7	12
	(2)* (4.3%)	(1)†		(1)
B	18	16		2
	(2) (11.1%)			(2)
C	6	4	1	1
	(3) (50%)	(1)	(1)	(1)
Total	71	48	8	15
	(7) (9.9%)	(2) (4.1%)	(1) (12.5%)	(4) (26.7%)

Okuda K, Ryu M, Tobe T: Surgical management of hepatoma. The Japanese Experience. In Wanebo HJ (ed): Hepatic and Biliary Cancer, pp 219–238. New York, Marcel Dekker, 1987.
*Number in parentheses are operative deaths.
†Due to variceal bleeding.

TABLE 27-10.   Therapy for Primary Malignant Liver Tumors (St. Jude Children's Research Hospital Experience)

Disease	Total	Resected	AWD*	DOD	DWD	NED
Hepatoblastoma	29	10	1	14	3	11
Hepatocellular carcinoma	18	3	2	14	0	2
Sarcoma	8	5	0	5	0	3
Neuroblastoma	1	1				1

Rao BN, Green AA: Hepatic tumors in children and adolescents. In Wanebo HJ (ed): Hepatic and biliary cancer, pp 187–218. New York, Marcel Dekker, 1987.

*AWD = alive with disease; DOD = died of disease; DWD = died without disease; NED = no evidence of disease.

end-stage liver disease and were found to have coincidental primary liver malignancy. Hepatocellular carcinoma was found in 12 and hepatoblastoma in 1. Twelve of 13 patients are alive and free of disease from 10 months to more than 15 years. Among those operated for clinical HCC, the recurrence rate was 50%. All the HCCs recurred within 1 year (mean, 6 months; range, 4–12 months), but patients with the fibrolamellar type had recurrences after 1 year (mean,

20 months). There was a continued decline in survival because of recurrent malignancy. Of the 42 patients with unresectable malignancy, only 10 (24%) were alive and only 6 (14%) were free of tumor from 4 months to 9 years. In contrast, among the 13 patients who had liver replacements for non-neoplastic liver disease and were found to have incidental HCC, none had recurrence and 12 are living 10 months to 15 years after treatment. Thus, it appears that

TABLE 27-11.   Liver Transplantation in Patients with Unresectable Liver Cancer (Starzl Group)

Histology	Method of Immune Suppression*	No. of Patients	Months Until Recurrence, (%)	Time of Survival (Mean)	No. of Survivors, (%)
HCC	Az/ALG	8	5 (63)	2–13 mo / 4 mo	0
	Cy/P	8	4 (50)	4–12 mo / 6 mo	3 (38)
HCC fibrolamellar variant	Az/ALG	1	1 (10)	13 mo	0
	Cy/P	6	3 (50)	13–30 mo	4 (66)
Bile duct	Az/ALG	3	2 (66)	21–42 mo	0
(Klatskin) cholangiocarcinoma	Cy/P	2	2	6–10 mo	0
		1	1	15 mo	0
Sarcoma	Az/ALG	2	1 (50)		1 (50)
	Cy/P	2	1 (50)		1 (50)

TOTAL: Az/ALG, group (20) of 14 survivors:
 6 postoperative deaths
 9 (64%) died of recurrence
 4 died NED; infection, 2, 2, 3, 6 mo
 1 survival—9 yr

Cy/P group (22) of 21 survivors:
 1 postoperative death
 9 (41%) alive 4–48 mo (mean 23 mo)
 4 died NED; infection, 1, 2, 2, 13 mo
 8 DOD

Data from Esquirel CO, Iwatsuki S, Gordon RD et al: Transplantation for primary liver cancer. In Wanebo HJ (ed): Hepatic and biliary cancer, pp 477–486. New York, Marcel Dekker, 1987.

*Immunosuppression regimen: Az/ALG = azathioprine + antilymphocyte globulin; Cy/P = cyclosporine + prednisone.

Liver Transplantation in Patients with Incidental Primary Liver Cancer

Histology	No. of Patients	Months Until Recurrence	No. of Survivors
HCC	11	0	10 (10 mo–15 yr), 1 Postoperative death
Hepatoblastoma	1	0	1

HCC per se is not an absolute contraindication to total resection and transplantation. The extent of tumor in HCC appears to be the main determining factor, emphasizing the need for effective drug treatment.

CHEMOTHERAPY

Despite the poor prognosis of patients with inoperable HCC, there is sufficient prognostic diversity to confuse the analysis of the outcome of therapeutic trials, if known prognostic factors are not taken into account. Important factors of the natural history of the disease, such as sex, age, performance status, cirrhosis, race, and country of origin, should be considered in predicting survival in therapeutic trials. In many cases, these factors are more significant than the treatment used. Unique data are available in the analysis of 432 patients with advanced HCC prospectively studied by ECOG, in which eligibility and availability were standardized for all patients. Furthermore, the 301 North American patients and the 131 South African patients received similar treatment at the same time.[147]

Factors that had the most significant adverse effect on survival were impaired performance status, male sex, older age, and the presence of jaundice and reduced appetite. Cirrhosis by itself was associated with poorer survival but, viewed relative to sex and age, lost its statistical significance. Country of origin, but not race, was significant; North American patients had a longer survival. The importance can be seen in the following example: For patients with a good performance status, a South African man older than 45 years of age, with jaundice and reduced appetite, has a 5% probability of surviving 6 months, but a North American woman younger than 45 years of age, without jaundice or loss of appetite, has a 68% chance of surviving 6 months. The median survival time of the 432 ECOG patients was 14 weeks. Patients with a performance status of 4, with renal insufficiency or with any evidence of encephalopathy, were not entered into the study. The overall median survival time of all patients with advanced HCC was therefore even shorter.

In a French study, prognostic factors for 127 untreated patients were analyzed.[148] The median survival time was 73 days; four of these untreated patients survived longer than 1 year. A survival time longer than 60 days was seen in only 1 of 25 patients with evidence of encephalopathy. Predictive of very poor prognosis were encephalopathy, alcohol consumption, and elevated AFP, BUN, and bilirubin levels. The authors conclude that the natural history of patients with HCC in France shows no difference from those in Asia or Africa. Malaysian patients had a survival time between that of North American and South African patients.[160]

Although HBV infection has not been shown to have prognostic significance, a growing body of evidence suggests that North American and European patients without cirrhosis have a better prognosis than do patients in the high-incidence areas for cirrhosis of Africa and most of Asia.[33] In Pretoria, Simson's postmortem studies highlight the importance of membranous occlusion of the hepatic veins and demonstrate the paradoxical finding that survival is poorer for patients without cirrhosis than for those patients with cirrhosis.[90] It is important, therefore, to have ongoing Phase

II trials in different parts of the world, in which standard eligibility criteria are used to compensate for known and unknown factors.

In evaluating clinical trials of HCC, certain rules must be observed: histologic confirmation of the diagnosis, proper stratification by important prognostic variables, and inclusion of all patients in the study for response and survival data. Early deaths should not be excluded.

Unfortunately, most of the literature on the treatment of HCC consists of uncontrolled trials with selected patients that do not take into account any of the above factors. Although important information can be gained from these trials, the results must be interpreted both in the light of selection factors, purposeful or not, and of exclusion factors.

Determination of Tumor Response

The criteria for objective response are as follows: *Complete response* is the absence of any clinically detectable tumor mass (*i.e.*, normal physical examination, liver chemistries, appropriate radiographic studies, and normal AFP if elevated before therapy); and a *partial response* is a reduction by at least 50% of the product of the largest perpendicular diameters of the most clearly measurable lesions, with no increase in any other indicator lesion, and the absence of new areas of malignant disease. If hepatomegaly is the primary indicator, there must be a reduction by at least 30% of the sum of liver measurements below each costal margin at the midclavicular line and xyphoid process. For complete and partial responses, there can be no significant deterioration in weight or performance status.

Survival time is the best objective measure of the effects of treatment in patients with HCC, but it is important to include patients who do not complete the prescribed program.

Single Agents

In controlled studies, no alkylating agent has been found to be of value in the treatment of patients with primary liver cancer. Response rates with these drugs are less than 10%, and median survival times are comparable to those achieved with placebos.[148-150] Various antimetabolites have been tested, and none have proved useful as single agents in the treatment of patients with HCC.[151-160,171] Data on single-agent results for 5-fluorouracil and dichloromethotrexate are given in Table 27-12. None of the plant alkaloids have been shown to be of value, nor has diaminodichloroplatinum (DDP).[161-168]

Various antibiotics and related substances have been tested, but none have been shown to be of definite value in controlled studies.[11,160,164,169-187] Data from the longer series of patients treated with doxorubicin, idarubicin, epirubicin, esorubicin, mitoxantrone, and neocarzinostatin are shown in Table 27-12.

Other diverse agents have been tested, including hormones, and biological response modifiers, but none have proved to be of clinical value.[162,170,188-201]

TABLE 27-12.   Liver Cancer: Single-Agent Studies with ≥10 Patients

Agent	No. of Patients	No. of Responses	Mean Survival (mo)	Author, Year	Reference
5-Fluorouracil					
IV	19	2		Brennan, 1964	154
	16	0	2	Gailani, 1972	150
	10	1	5	Davis, 1974	153
Oral	9	0	2	Link, 1977	158
	12	6		Kennedy, 1977	159
	45	0	2	Falkson, 1978	172
Doxorubicin	13	2	3	Ihde, 1977	174
	41	7		Vogel, 1977	173
	44	14	3	Johnson, 1978	177
	74	22		Olweny, 1980	176
	31	8	4	Melia, 1983	164
	12	0	3	Barbare, 1984	179
	52	6	4	Chlebowski, 1984	175
	45	11	3	Choi, 1984	180
	63	6	3	Falkson, 1978–1984	170, 171
	109	1	4	Sciarrino, 1985	178
Idarubicin	15	0		Cheng, 1985	183
Epirubicin	18	3	3	Hochster, 1985	181
	17	0	4	Shiu, 1986	182
Esorubicin	35	3	3	Perry, 1987	167
Mitoxantrone	19	2	3	Falkson, 1984	185
	33	3	>4	Davis, 1986	184
	34	0	<3	Falkson, 1987	187
Neocarzinostatin	28	2	3	Falkson, 1980	169
	30	7	2	Falkson, 1984	170
m-AMSA	35	1	3	Falkson, 1981	189
	23	3	5	Bukowski, 1982	190
	16	0		Cheng, 1983	191
	20	1		Amrein, 1984	192
	24	0	3	Falkson, 1984	170
CDDP	13	1		Melia, 1981	166
	20	1	2	Ravry, 1986	168
	35	2	<3	Falkson, 1987	187
VP-16	25	3	<3	Cavalli, 1981	163
	24	3	2	Melia, 1983	164
DCMTX	17	1		Vogel, 1972	151

TABLE 27-13.   Liver Cancer: Combination Chemotherapy in Series with ≥10 Patients

Agent	No. of Patients	No. of Responses	Mean Survival (mo)	Author, Year	Reference
5-FU + Ara C	22	1	2	Gailani, 1972	156
5-FU + BCNU	14	1		McIntire, 1976	202
5-FU PO + MeCCNU	44	2	<3	Falkson, 1978	172
5-FU PO + MeCCNU	20	4	4	Joishy, 1982	160
5-FU IV + MeCCNU	55	7	<3	Falkson, 1984	171
5-FU + MMC	13	5	2	Umsawasdi, 1978	203
5-FU + STZ	33	4	<3	Falkson, 1978	172
5-FU + STZ	49	4	<3	Falkson, 1984	171
5-FU + MTX, CYT, VCR	10	0	5	Cochrane, 1977	206
5-FU + MTX, CYT, VCR	19	0	1	Choi, 1984	180
DOX + 5-FU	38	5	3	Baker, 1977	207
DOX + DCMTX	12	1		Olweny, 1980	176
DOX + PRED	17	6	4	Oon, 1980	208
DOX + 5-FU, PRED, VCR	17	5	4	Oon, 1980	208
DOX + MeCCNU	21	3	3	Chlebowski, 1981	209
DOX + 5-FU, VM-26	36	16		Bezwoda, 1982	210
DOX + STZ	23	2	3	Morstyn, 1983	211
DOX + 5-FU, MeCCNU	38	8	3	Falkson, 1984	171
DOX + BLEO	49	8	2	Ravry, 1984	212
DOX + 5-FU, MMC	40	5	2	Al-Idrissi, 1985	213

*5-FU = 5-fluorouracil;   Ara   C = cytarabine;   BCNU = carmustine;   MeCCNU = methyl-lomustine;   MMC = mitomycin-c;   ST2 = streptozotocin;   CYT = cyclophosphamide;   VCR = vincristine;   DOX = doxorubicin;   PRED = prednisone;   VM-26 = teniposide;   BLEO = bleomycin.

TABLE 27-14.   Liver Cancer: Chemotherapy Overview by Agent Class

Agent	Response	Reference
Alkylating Agents		
Cyclophosphamide, triethyleneglycol diglycidylether, alanine mustard, DL-serine bis (2-chloropropyl) carbamate ester, chlorethylcyclohexylnitrosourea, chloroethyl-methyl-cyclohexyl-nitrosourea	Response rates are less than 10% and median survival time is comparable to that achieved with placebo	149, 150
Antimetabolites		
Methotrexate Dichloromethotrexate 6-Mercaptopurine Hydroxyurea Cytosine-arabinoside 5-Fluorouracil	Various antimetabolites have been tested; none have proved of value as single agents	151–159, 196
Plant Alkaloids		
Vinblastine SPG 827 (podophyllin derivative) VP-16-213 (etoposide)	Vinblastine and SPG 827 of no therapeutic value; variable response for etoposide ranging from median survival of 22 weeks in one trial to no survival advantage in other trials;	161–165
Antibiotics and Related Substances		
Mitomycin-C Actinomycin-D Carzinophyllin Chromomycin-A_3 Neocarzinostatin	No value shown for mitomycin-C, actinomycin-D, carzinophyllin or chromomycin-A_3; neocarzinostatin showed response in 2/25 patients and median survival time of 11 weeks in one clinical trial	169–170
Doxorubicin		
Doxorubicin 4'-Epidoxorubicin Oral demethoxydaunorubicin Mitoxantrone Menogaril	For doxorubicin, clinical trials report response rates of 17%, 15%, 11%; for all patients in all trials median survival is less than 4 months; other analogues have been equally ineffective	171–186
Other Agents		
Dehydroemitine, Procarbazine, cobalt proporphyrin complex, Butyryloxyethylglyoxal Dithiosemicarbazone, [4'-(9-Acridinlyamino)-methanesulphon-m-anisidide] (m-AMSA) Acivin Alpha-interferon Gamma-interferon Beta-interferon	No therapeutic responses for all agents; minimal response rates for m-AMSA	166, 168, 170, 187–195
Cis-diamino-dichloroplatinum (DDP)	DDP shows little or no effect	166, 168, 187
Hormone Treatment		
Magesterol acetate Tamoxifen Cyproterone acetate Buserelin	No beneficial results for these agents, although the anti-androgen cyproterone acetate shows some promise in HCC patients with cirrhosis; the gonadotrophic agonist, Buserelin, is in clinical trials but is not yet evaluable	197–101
Combination Chemotherapies and Chemotherapy/Radiotherapy Combinations		
Vincristine (VCR) + methotrexate (MTX) + 6-mercaptopurine (6MP) + prednisone (Pred); BCNU + cytosine-arabinoside; 5-FU + thiotepa; 5-FU + mitomycin C (MMC); 5-FU + cyclophosphamide (CTX) + MTX + VCR; 5-FU + ara-C; 5-FU + MeCCNU; 5-FU + streptozotocin; Doxorubicin (ADM) + 5-FU; ADM + 5-FU + Pred + VCR; ADM + MeCCNU; ADM + 5-FU + VM26; ADM + STZ; ADM + bleomycin; ADM + 5-FU + MMC; radiotherapy (RT) + 5-FU + CTX + MTX + VCR; RT + intra-arterial 5-FU + ADM; RT + MTX or MMC + 5-FU + ADM.	No response or limited response in combination chemotherapies with high toxicity in 5-FU studies; chemoradiotherapies show no survival differences with combined chemotherapies	156, 171–172, 176, 180, 202–203, 206–213

Combination Chemotherapy

With few exceptions, it has been shown that nothing is gained by adding cytostatics that do not have single-agent activity to a drug combination regimen. This procedure leads to increased toxicity, necessitating a decrease in the amount of the therapeutically active agents that can be given at the same time. Various small series of uncontrolled trials of drug combinations in patients with primary liver cancer are reported in the literature, in which patient selection was ignored and the results can be explained by variations in the natural history of the disease.

None of the combination treatments have given results superior to single agents in clinical trials.[11,157,180,202-213] The response and the survival for larger series of patients treated with 5-fluorouracil (5-FU) or doxorubicin combinations are given in Table 27-13. An overview of the response to chemotherapy by agent class is shown in Table 27-14.

Chemoradiation Therapy

Combination treatment with chemotherapy and radiotherapy has been tried in various smaller series. Procarbazine and radiotherapy were randomly compared to other treatments and placebo and not found to be effective; nor was radiotherapy combined with 5-FU, cyclophosphamide (CTX), methotrexate (MTX), and vincristine (VCR).[11,206] Early trials of radiotherapy and intra-arterial (IA) 5-FU and doxorubicin (ADM) did give promising results, as did radiotherapy with MTX or mitomycin C in addition to 5-FU and ADM.[214-216] In a larger trial, no survival improvement was reported for patients given radiotherapy only or given radiotherapy with mitomycin C, ADM, and 5-FU given intra-arterially or intravenously.[215,225]

Status of Chemotherapy

Until better response rates can be documented for single agents or there is sufficient rationale for combination chemotherapy in patients with HCC, physicians cannot justify treating small groups of patients with combination of poorly active agents. The recommended approach is to have well-designed Phase II trials of new agents. The expanding knowledge about HCC as a disease may promote better clinical trials. Even in Phase II trials, patient discriminants such as age, sex, performance status, and country of origin are important. It may also be important to stratify patient categories according to type of HCC: normal and cirrhotic or pre-cirrhotic patterns; encapsulated hepatocellular carcinomas (common in Japan), excluding the status of hepatitis B viral infection, and fibrosing varieties of expanding types of HCC, including fibrolamellar HCC. Although no cytostatic has shown reproducible response rates of 20% or more in patients with HCC, at least agents with occasional activity can be selected over others that are totally inactive.

Hepatic Artery Infusion

Although careful postmortem examination shows that metastases occur in the vast majority of patients with HCC, liver disease dominates the clinical picture in most of the patients, and only 25% of patients have extrahepatic metastases at the time of diagnosis. This has motivated attempts at regional chemotherapy. Results of treatment by hepatic artery infusion appear better than they are because of selection factors. In 1968, optimism was justified because early results seemed promising.[218] In 1970, continuous intra-arterial MTX was shown to be superior to intra-arterial 5-FU.[219] The median survival time of these selected patients was 375 days for the group treated intra-arterially with MTX, 118 days for 5-FU, and 55 days for the control group. The controls were patients who met the selection criteria for intraoperative placement of the catheter in the hepatic artery. Despite this survival difference, this form of treatment was not regarded as practical or advisable. No other controlled studies comparing intra-arterial to systemic chemotherapy or to no treatment have been done despite numerous publications on intra-arterial fluorinated pyrimidines and on intra-arterial doxorubicin in patients with HCC.[153,157,220-225]

No evidence from any of these studies supports the contention that intra-arterial treatment prolongs survival, nor is there evidence of a change in prognosis after intra-arterial HN_2, dichloromethotrexate, mitomycin C, or cisplatin.[226,227] Optimistic claims have been made and 50% response rates have been quoted for these therapies.[228-231] These series consist of selected patients with good pathologic discriminants. Most of the studies of intra-arterial chemotherapy require that the patients have adequate enough performance status to tolerate a laparotomy for placing the catheter, no distal metastases, and adequate liver function. With these preconditions, the median survival time should be good because these known prognostic factors give a 50% chance of surviving 1 year. The total number of patients with HCC seen was also not given.

Although adequate pharmacologic rationale for intra-arterial treatment is available, the clinical case remains to be proved. Intra-arterial chemotherapy is only indicated in a clinical trial setting if it is compared with systemic treatment and if *all* patients, including postoperative and early deaths, entered on the study are included in the denominator. These results of intra-arterial cytostatics in HCC are similar to those for patients with liver metastases from colon cancer. Local tumor shrinkage does occur, but considerable toxicity and morbidity and even mortality are associated with this approach, even in selected patients with good prognostic features.

In a randomized study comparing intra-arterial cytostatics and hepatic artery ligation with hepatic artery ligation and partial vein infusion with symptomatic treatment, no difference in survival between treated and untreated patients was observed.[232] Hepatic artery ligation was performed in a large series of patients with HCC in Mozambique before 1978, with disastrous results in this African population with advanced disease.[233] More recent experience has been more optimistic, with both simple ligation of the hepatic artery and selective arterial ligation to the specific lobe where the tumor is located and with total hepatic dearterialization.[176,231,232]

Hepatic arterial occlusion has been used with MTX, 5-FU, doxorubicin, and mitomycin C.[176,232,234-240] Causes of death included hepatic failure and hepatorenal syndrome. Various refinements in techniques, such as intermittent occlusion of the hepatic artery, selective transcatheter embolization, and introduction of Gelfoam or Ivalon particles have been introduced.[241-243]

Particles to which doxorubicin, mitomycin C, or a combination of mitomycin C, fluorodeoxyuridine (FudR), and doxorubicin have been added have been tried.[242,243] Neocarzinostatin suspended in a lipid lymphographic agent and injected into the arterial system has been tried in Japan.[245] Definite tumor necrosis can be produced by injecting ethiodol or lipiodol with doxorubicin, with or without nimustine hydrochloride (ACNU).[246,247] Intra-arterial BCNU has been given with starch microspheres.[248] In Japan, where resection is more often possible because of the nature of the disease, intra-arterial embolization and chemotherapy are being used as neoadjuvant therapy.[249-251]

Intra-arterial therapy by continuous infusion or by microspheres, with or without hepatic arterial occlusion, has many enthusiastic followers. In the absence of controlled clinical trials in which all patients entered on the study are evaluated, there can be no real assessment of its value.

A problem has already arisen in that intra-arterial doxorubicin is considered to be effective treatment. In a study on 64 patients with nonresectable HCC treated with intra-arterial epirubicin, tumor size was evaluated only in 53 patients, 8 of whom had objective improvement. The reported response rate was 15.1% but should have been 12.5%. The median survival time of 205 days was compared with the historic survival time obtained with intra-arterial doxorubicin. It was concluded that the epirubicin was more effective than doxorubicin in the intra-arterial treatment of nonresectable HCC.[252] As with systemic treatment, the results of the different intra-arterial treatments can be interpreted only in terms of the HCC subtype and the patient's prognostic factors.[253]

RADIATION

Evaluation for Radiotherapy

The distinctions between diffuse or nodular patterns of HCC are important for any review of the role of CT in hepatocellular cancer. A widely dispersed, nonmarginated, diffuse tumor is not only nonresectable, but also unlikely to have sufficient tumor remission to be resectable.[254] In contrast, nonresectable massive nodular disease with clear margins on CT scans can be converted to a resectable state by new techniques.[254,255] Similarly, multifocal, nodular, clearly demarcated patterns of HCC can be converted to a resectable state by new treatment modalities that include external radiation, sensitizing drugs, and radiolabeled antiferritin.[254]

In the past, a partial response of HCC was defined to be at least a 30% reduction in the sum of liver measurements below each costal margin at the midclavicular lines and the xyphoid process.[256] The dorsal to ventral dimension could not be obtained accurately by clinical measurement. CT scans in 8-mm sections now allow total reconstruction of the entire liver volume. Pixels may then be examined to determine density. Standardization of the pixels before scanning each patient provides uniform analysis and a more accurate comparison of results. When all pixels from the entire CT series are analyzed, a bimodal pattern of density is established for tumor and for normal tissue (Fig. 27-8). This more

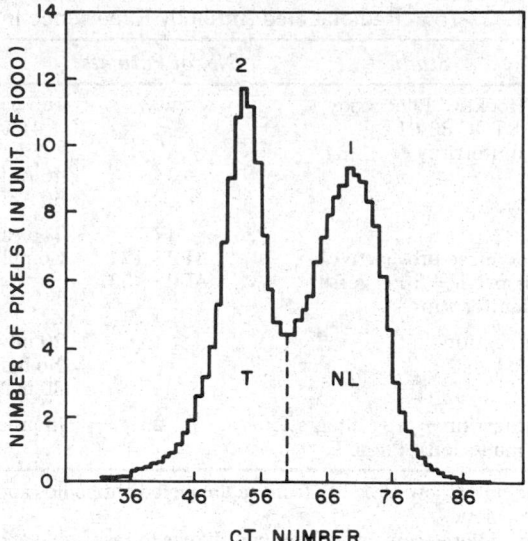

FIG. 27-8. When all of the pixels from the entire computerized axial tomographic series are analyzed, a bimodal pattern of density is established for tumor and another for normal tissue. This more accurate method to determine tumor volumetrics was originally designed from the dosimetry of radiolabeled antibody which requires tumor volumetrics. (Yang N-C, Leichner PK, Fishman EK et al: CT volumetrics of primary liver cancers. J Comput Assist Tomogr 10:621–628, 1986. Used with permission of Raven Press)

FIG. 27-9. Hepatocellular cancer with chronic active hepatitis. Note that with modest tumor reduction there is a greater normal liver reduction. The top line indicates the total liver volume, the intermediate line indicates normal liver volume, and the bottom line indicates the tumor volume. The reduced normal liver tolerance when chronic active hepatitis is an underlying disease is characteristic. See new methods of evaluation for tumor volumetrics and normal liver volumetrics. Compare normal liver volumetrics to Figure 27-10.

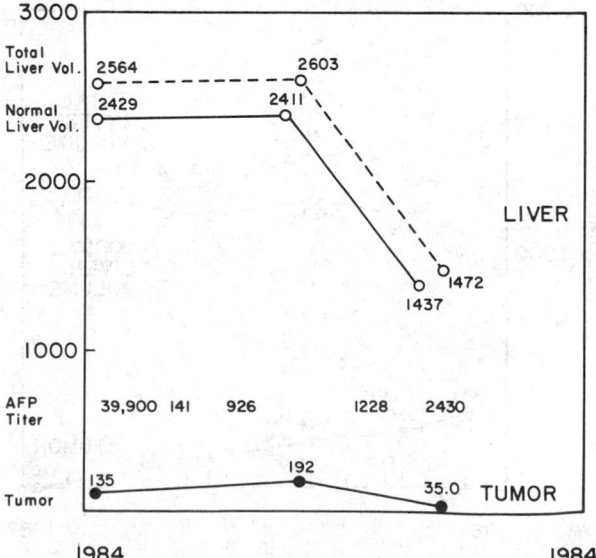

TABLE 27-15. Radiolabeled Antibody Experience in Hepatoma*

Study	No. of Patients	Results
Johns Hopkins' Pilot Study And RTOG 83-01 ^{131}I-antiferritin	263	105 patients reported 41% PR 7% CR 46 AFP+: 5 months median survival 59 AFP−: 10.5 month median survival
RTOG 83-19 Randomized prospective† Adriamycin + 5-FU versus ^{131}I-antiferritin	177 AFP+ 124 AFP− 53	Too early to evaluate Completion expected 1.5 years
[90]Y-antiferritin* Phase I	15	20 mCi Yttrium No hematologic toxicity† 30 mCi grade 3
[90]Y-antiferritin + drug integration and monoclonal Phase I	25	In progress

*The only known toxicity from radiolabeled antibodies applied to hepatocellular cancer has been hematopoietic.
†Ten patients converted from two studies to resectable and NED.

accurate method was originally designed for the dosimetry of radiolabeled antibody, which requires tumor volumetrics.[257]

The pragmatic application of tumor volumetrics for progression and remission analysis has become a valuable tool in determining patient response to therapy (Fig. 27-9).[258] Tumors of varying sizes cannot be quantitatively analyzed in terms of percentage of remission. If two tumors weighing 500 g and 2500 g regressed by 30%, the reduction would be 150 g and 750 g, respectively. From the viewpoint of applied cytotoxic therapy, more quantitative analyses offer better and more accurate appreciation of a given modality than does percent reduction. As use of the computer program becomes more pervasive in the major medical centers, a

clearer understanding of the cytoreductive power of agents used to treat HCC will emerge.[257,258]

External Radiation

Radiation doses greater than 3000 rad within 3 weeks have caused radiation hepatitis.[259] In the treatment of metastatic lesions, 2100 rad was successful in achieving partial remission. This dose was later integrated with Adriamycin and 5-FU in the treatment of metastatic liver disease.[260-262] This same combination was then used as an induction therapy for a multimodality treatment program and achieved a 15% partial remission rate during the treatment course.[75] A variety of other radiation sources, including yttrium-90 microspheres and [131]ethiodol, have been proposed, but without meaningful dosimetry.[263-265]

FIG. 27-10. A 22-year-old woman, AFP negative, with no underlying pathology and with recurrent nonresectable nodular hepatocellular cancer. Volumetrics demonstrate total liver volume, normal liver volume, and tumor volume following radiolabeled antibody treatment.

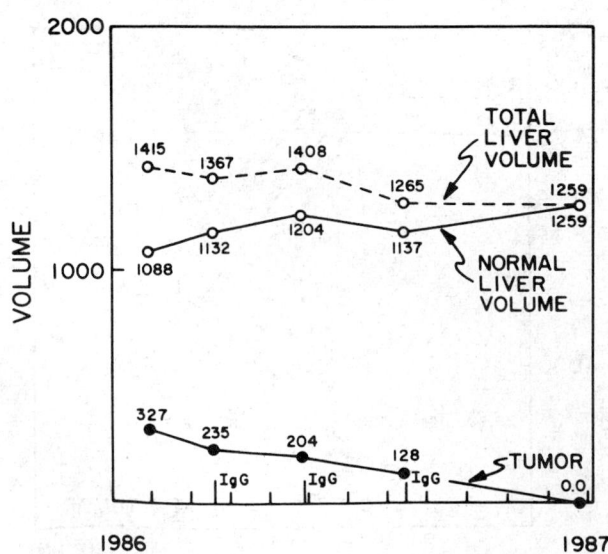

FIG. 27-11. An 83-year-old man with nodular massive nonresectable AFP negative hepatocellular cancer treated with multiple courses of ^{131}I-antiferritin radiolabeled antibodies.

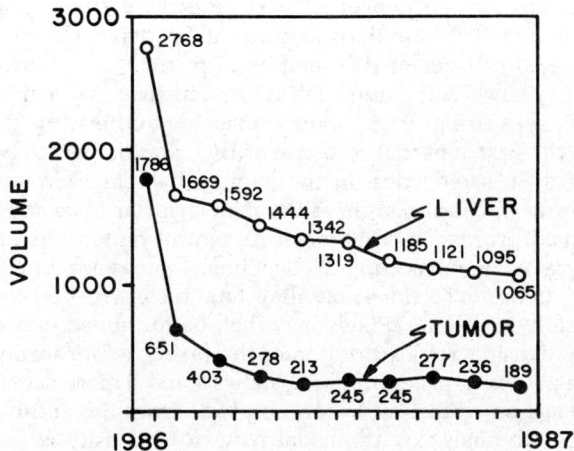

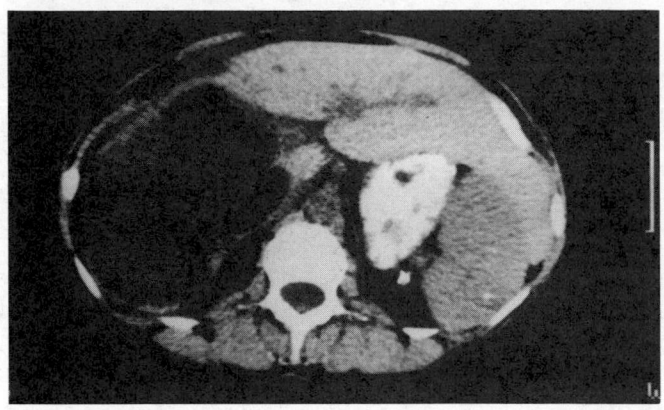

A

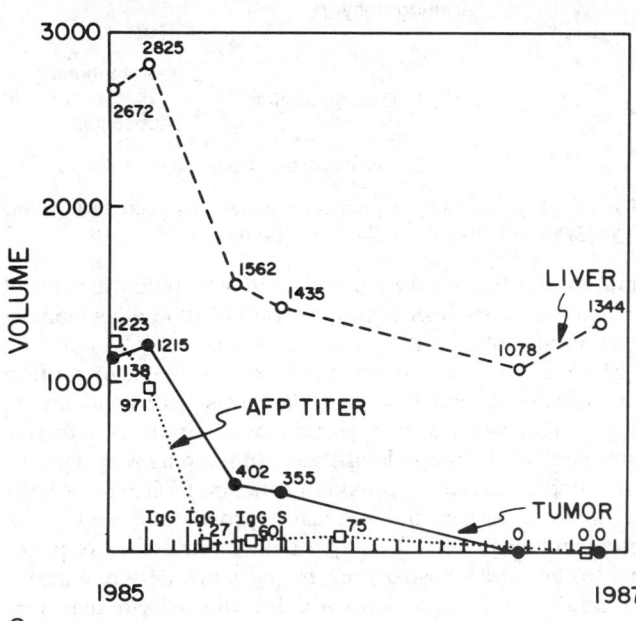

C

1985   1987

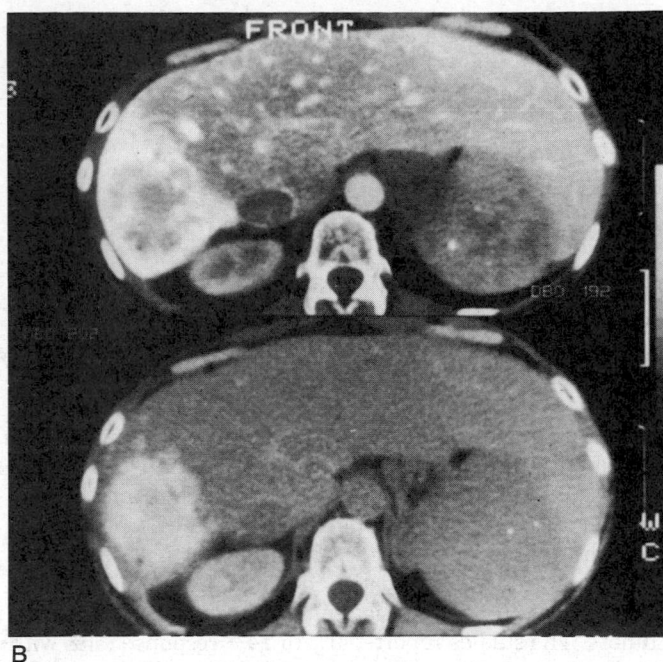

B

FIG. 27-12. **A.** A 56-year-old woman with nodular massive nonresectable AFP positive hepatocellular cancer with presenting computed tomogram. Bracket at right represents 5 cm. **B.** After treatment, the arteriographic computed tomographic arterial and venous phase before resection. Bracket at right represents 5 cm. **C.** Total liver, tumor volumetrics, and AFP titer of this patient converted from nonresectable to resectable. The patient remains disease-free. (Sitzman JV, Order SE, Klein JL et al: Conversion by new treatment modalities of nonresectable to resectable hepatocellular cancer. J Clin Oncol 5:1566–1578, 1987. Reproduced with permission of Grune & Stratton)

Radioactive Antibodies

HCC was known to produce ferritin.[266] This protein, normally associated with iron storage, is in the apoferritin form (*i.e.*, lacking iron) and is produced ubiquitously by a variety of malignancies.[266,267] The finding that selective tumor deposition of ^{131}I-antiferritin occurred due to increased tumor vascular permeability was described both in experimental models and in clinical investigation.[268–272] Tumor saturation, the dose of ^{131}I-antiferritin that binds accessible tumor ferritin, and the tumor effective half-life of 3 to 4 days led to the development of this new agent.[75] Two intravenous infusions led to a median dose of 1100 to 1200 rad and were later integrated with 15 mg of Adriamycin and 500 mg of 5-fluorouracil, which acted as potential sensitizers.[75] The newest laboratory information indicates that Adriamycin shifts the tumor cells into G2 and early M, both positions in the cell cycle in which increased radiosensitivity has been reported.[269]

The initial experience in 105 patients indicated an advantageous response in AFP-negative patients, who had a me-

dian survival of 10.5 months, and no significant difference from conventional therapy in AFP-positive patients, who had a median survival of 5 months.[75] The conversion from nonresectable to resectable disease in patients with nodular massive or nodular multifocal HCC has offered new treatment possibilities (Table 27-15; Figs. 27-10, 27-11, and 27-12).[254] The modification in China of the ^{131}I-antiferritin therapy by intra-arterial infusion was also followed by partial wedge resections in patients with macronodular HCC.[75] In both limited series of patients, an elevated serum AFP level was not a distinguishing factor because conversion to a resectable state occurred in patients with and without elevated AFP levels.[254,273]

Currently under investigation is the use of ^{90}Y, which is a more powerful beta-emitting isotope than [131]I (0.3 MeV versus 0.9 MeV).[271,272,274] Yttrium-90 has demonstrated remissions of metastatic lesions and primary HCC.[272,274]

The influence of radiolabeled antibody treatment on complete remissions, conversions to resectability, and remissions of metastasis indicate that more should be expected from further clinical research with them. Iodine-131-anti-

AFP has been reported by some investigators to have therapeutic activity, but others have not been able to document significant tumor deposition.[275,276] It would be reasonable to expect that Adriamycin, cis-platinum, and 5-FU may act as sensitizing agents for radiolabeled antibodies.[277,277a,278]

INTRAHEPATIC BILIARY CANCER

Intrahepatic biliary cancer occurs less frequently than extrahepatic Klatskin's tumor, and it represents about 0.5% of primary liver tumors in the United States. In contrast to extrahepatic bile duct cancer, this tumor has an associated significant neovasculature, produces CEA, and may be treated with ^{131}I-anti-CEA to achieve a partial remission. In 37 patients, a 25.9% partial remission and 7.4% complete remission rates were achieved.[279] These results took 8 years to accumulate, indicating the rarity of the disorder. It was also observed that elevated AFP levels do not distinguish hepatoma from intrahepatic cholangiocarcinoma because there are AFP-positive patients with intrahepatic biliary tumors. The studies reported 9% to 14% response rates with 14-day to 4-month median survivals. Overall, the median survival was 6.5 months, and the 33% of patients who responded to therapy demonstrated a median survival of 15.2 months.[279]

BILIARY TRACT CANCER

Primary malignancies of the biliary tract were first described by Fardel in 1890 with a subsequent description by Courvoisier in the last decade of the 19th century.[280,281] Baudoin performed the first biliary enteric bypass of a biliary malignancy in 1896, and in 1903 Mayo reported the first successful resection.[282,283]

The autopsy frequency of bile duct carcinoma is approximately 0.01 to 0.46%, and carcinoma is found in approximately 1 of every 200 operations involving the biliary tree.[284,285]

DIAGNOSIS

The clinical presentation of the patient with cancer of the bile duct is usually painless jaundice. Fatigue, pruritus, fever, and nonspecific abdominal pain are frequent accompanying findings.[286,287] Laboratory findings are often nonspecific. Hemoglobin, leukocyte counts, and serum electrolyte values are usually unaltered. Liver function tests reflect obstructive jaundice in more than 80% of cases.[286-288] A variety of diagnostic measures are available, and an orderly sequence is noted (Fig. 27-13).

Ultrasound is the simplest noninvasive test that can suggest extrahepatic biliary obstruction by confirming the presence of dilatation of intrahepatic biliary ducts.[289]

Cholangiography is the next consideration, and the options include endoscopic retrograde cholangiography (ERCP), percutaneous transhepatic cholangiography (PTC), or intraoperative cholangiography. Careful preoperative cholangiography is helpful in assessing the resectability of tumors and in planning the operative approach. Intraoperative cholangi-

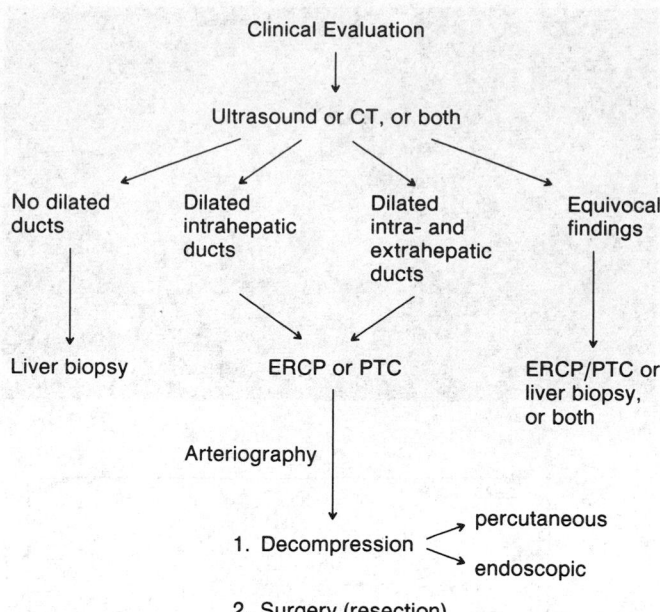

FIG. 27-13. Evaluation of jaundiced patient suspected of having cholangiocarcinoma or bile duct carcinoma.

ography assists the surgeon in the finer technical aspects of the operation, such as documentation of tube placement or location of multicentric tumors or stones.

ERCP is an effective preoperative tool that can confirm ductal anatomy and histologic diagnosis with concomitant biopsy. This procedure is particularly helpful in detecting carcinoma of the ampulla of Vater. In patients with obstructive jaundice caused by proximal cancers, PTC is most helpful. In these tumors the surgical approach and question of resectability can be settled by the ductal architecture proximal to the tumor obstruction. In the University of Virginia series, all 16 PTC in patients with bile duct carcinomas were interpreted as abnormal, and 15 (94%) were diagnosed as consistent with "malignancy." Although three patients (18%) had complications, none were fatal.[286] Elias and colleagues conducted a prospective randomized comparison of ERCP and PTC in jaundiced patients and concluded that both techniques had similar diagnostic accuracy.[291] PTC can also provide effective decompression of the biliary system and normalization of liver function test findings. PTC requires that any clotting abnormalities be corrected before the procedure.

Arteriography is not routinely used in the preoperative workup of obstructive jaundice but may be used for diagnosis in more difficult or confusing cases and in those cases in which resection is contemplated. The findings of neovascu-

TABLE 27-16A. Bile Duct Cancer (The UCLA Experience)

Laboratory Finding	Mean	% Abnormal
Alkaline phosphatase (U)	582	94
Total bilirubin (mg/dl)	17.4	84
SGOT (IU)	96	55
SGPT (IU)	121	50
Creatinine (mg/dl)	1.1	10
Albumin (g/dl)	3.3	52

TABLE 27-16B.   Bile Duct Cancer (The UCLA Experience)

Test	1954–1978		1979–1983	
	No. Performed	Accuracy (%)	No. Performed	Accuracy (%)
Ultrasound	9	56	35	91
CT scan	0		19	95
Transhepatic cholangiogram	13	100	33	100
Transjugular cholangiogram	12	100	0	
ERCP	7	43	12	92

larity, major arterial encasement, or occlusion can lead to evaluation of nonresectability, particularly in tumors located in or near the hilum.[287] Late-phase arteriography allows visualization of the portal system and its relation to the neoplasm. Percutaneous transhepatic portography with direct cannulation of the portal system can also be done to evaluate tumor invasion.[292] The sensitivity of diagnostic measures is shown in Table 27-16, A and B.

Voyles and co-workers reported their experience with cholangiography and arteriography (with late-phase portography) in evaluation of the resectability of tumors of the proximal biliary tree.[293] All 37 patients in the study received PTC, and 20 received arteriography. Of the tumors, 32% were judged unresectable by cholangiography; 54% were judged unresectable by cholangiography and arteriography; and 65% were judged unresectable by cholangiography, arteriography, and "clinical considerations." Only 7 patients (18.9%) underwent resection. This represented 38.5% of those predicted to be unresectable and 8.3% of the patients whose tumors were predicted to be unresectable. The authors concluded that cholangiography with arteriography can predict resectability with a high degree of certainty and perhaps present laparotomy if cytological diagnosis can be confirmed by transcutaneous biopsy.

Although CT was not evaluated in the study, it can evaluate the hepatic parenchyma for other space-occupying lesions or metastases. In addition, CT allows a more precise evaluation of the head of the pancreas, which is important because carcinoma in this location is a common lesion.[287,294] Percutaneous needle aspiration for cytodiagnosis may also be done and may obviate laparotomy in those patients judged to be unresectable by preoperative studies. A fine needle can be advanced into the tumor under ultrasound or CT guidance. Evander and colleagues reported a 53% correct diagnosis in biliary tract and pancreatic carcinoma.[295] There were no false positives and no complications. This technique should probably not be performed in patients planned for resection because there is potential for tumor growth along the needle tract.[296]

Selected radiologic procedures in the patient with obstructive jaundice should allow a 90% to 95% accurate diagnosis of the malignancy of the biliary tract. Ultrasound is the first choice, and, if intrahepatic biliary dilatation is observed, PTC or fine-needle aspiration for cytodiagnosis can effectively be used for tissue evaluation and hepatic decompression. In some centers, ERCP has proved most useful in diagnosis of malignancy in the distal biliary tree. ERCP, CT, and arteriography can be used for evaluation of more confusing or difficult cases.

MANAGEMENT

Percutaneous Transhepatic Catheter

PTC drainage procedures can be effective diagnostic tools. In addition, PTC can provide internal or external drainage with biliary decompression of partial or complete obstructions. With proper hygiene and attention to catheter care, a patient can maintain a biliary catheter and provide decompression for many months.[287]

Resection of hilar tumors is often impossible. An alternative approach in such cases is to provide satisfactory drainage of bile through the occluding tumor.[308-311] In the past, this was accomplished by dilatation of the tumor and insertion of the proximal limb of a T tube through the tumor into the proximal duct so that the distal limb provided drainage into the common bile duct. Two additional techniques have been described and are probably superior to simple T tubes. Terblanche and colleagues suggested the use of the U tube for palliation of bile duct tumors.[311] The U tube is a Silastic tube passed into the distal common duct through the tumor and out the hepatic parencyhma proximally through the affected right or left hepatic duct. Each end of the tube is brought out through the abdominal wall. This apparatus can provide both internal and external drainage. An advantage of this tube is that it can be changed percutaneously as necessary.

Cameron and co-workers suggested stenting bile duct tumors and benign strictures with Silastic tubing introduced transhepatically into the common bile duct.[308-310] In addition to providing satisfactory splinting of the obstruction, only one tube remains external, and it can be easily changed over a guide wire. The rationale for employing stents is that primary bile duct carcinomas often do not metastasize to distant sites and the tumors may remain small for extended periods. Because the primary causes of death are the sequelae of obstructive jaundice, significant palliation may be achieved by biliary decompression, with prolongation of life and relief of the aggravating symptoms of obstructive jaundice. Stenting in particular is applicable for proximal bile duct cancers that are not resectable.[308-310]

In some cases, the bile ducts may be satisfactorily drained by hepaticojejunostomy using the approach to the left duct described by Blumgart or by intrahepatic cholangiojejunostomy.[312-316] For lesions in the common duct, resection should be employed.[317-322] The proximity of the hepatic artery and portal vein to these lesions, however, frequently limits the extent or possibility of resection because of direct invasion. If the lesion in the mid-duct is unresectable, palliation can be achieved by insertion of a stent or by performing a biliary enteric anastomosis. A Roux-en-Y jejunal anastomosis to the duct proximal to the tumor is the preferred approach.[308,309] For lesions of the distal duct that are resectable, pancreaticoduodenectomy is the preferred treatment.[317-322] For distal lesions that are not resectable, a bypass procedure, either cholecystojejunostomy or choledochojejunostomy, is preferable.

Preoperative decompression is a matter of debate. In 1978, Nakayama and co-workers suggested that a period of preoperative biliary decompression might improve liver function and the nutritional status, thereby decreasing morbidity and mortality of surgery for obstructive jaundice.[297] Although this view was held by many surgeons, Norlander and colleagues reported no significant difference in postoperative mortality patients with obstructive jaundice caused by benign or malignant processes.[298] Results continue to be mixed.[299] A recent report by Denning strongly suggests that preoperative decompression does lower surgical morbidity, but not mortality, for surgery for malignancies in the biliary tract.[300] MacPherson and co-workers reported a prospective randomized trial in Great Britain that entered 65 patients with obstructive jaundice.[301] Of these, 31 patients underwent exploration and were compared with 34 who received drainage for a mean duration of 18 days before exploration. Hospitalization was prolonged for the drainage group (40 versus 24 days). The mortality rate was 19% (6 of 31) for the laparotomy group and 32% (11 of 34) for the drainage group. The authors concluded that preoperative percutaneous biliary drainage fails to improve the mortality rate in patients treated surgically for obstructive jaundice.[301] More recently, Pitt and colleagues reported a prospective randomized trial that agrees with these results.[302]

Surgery

Traditional treatment for carcinoma of the bile duct has been surgical (Table 27-16C). The long-term results of surgery and other therapies have been exceedingly poor. Treatment has been palliative in most cases, although some patients with lesions detected early had fully resectable disease. Fortunately, today most patients operated on for bile

duct cancer have the site of obstruction delineated preoperatively by PTC or ERCP, which optimizes treatment planning.

An important step in the intraoperative management of the patient suspected of having a bile duct tumor is a biopsy to establish the diagnosis. It is sometimes difficult to obtain biopsy specimens, particularly when the tumor is located in a relatively inaccessible area. Intraoperative choledoctoscopy permits direct visualization and biopsy of tumors and may aid in evaluating the extent of the tumor.[303]

The surgical approach to primary bile duct tumors depends on several factors, including the anatomical site of the tumor and the age and general condition of the patient. A localized intrahepatic cholangiocarcinoma can be resected in the patient in good general condition, ordinarily by lobectomy. A more difficult problem is presented by the tumor located at the ductal confluence (Klatskin's tumor), which may involve both right and left hepatic ducts and the common hepatic duct.[304] The preferred treatment is excision of the tumor and the involved ductal system, establishing enteric bile drainage by a Roux-en-Y hepaticojejunostomy. In a small number of cases, the tumor may involve only one hepatic duct, and the affected duct and its lobe can be removed by hepatic lobectomy, sparing the contralateral lobe. Biliary-enteric continuity is reestablished by a Roux-en-Y hepaticojejunostomy or hepaticocholedochostomy.[305-307]

PROGNOSIS

The overall results of treatment of primary biliary tract cancer have been poor. The strategic location of these tumors precludes excision in most cases.

In 1979, Akwari and Kelly reported 30 patients with cancers in the hilium.[305] Of 4 resected, 3 (75%) were alive at 1 year; 26% of 26 patients having drainage and none of the 8 who had laparotomies alone were alive at 1 year. In 1980, Evander and colleagues reported on 80 patients, of whom 27 (34%) were resected.[323] In that group there were 9 bile duct resections, 15 bile duct plus hepatic lobe resections, 2 pancreaticoduodenectomies with total pancreatectomy, and 1 local excision. The postoperative mortality was 11% after resection and 30% if the tumor was nonresectable. The median survival was 20 months after radical resection, 7.5 months after palliative resections, and 2.5 months for patients with unresectable tumors.[323]

In the UCLA series of 146 patients, the overall morbidity rate during the most recent 5 years was 67% and the overall mortality was 11%.[324] Complications were primarily wound

TABLE 27-16C. Bile Duct Cancer (The UCLA Experience)

Procedure	1954–1978		1979–1983	
	No.	%	No.	%
Resection	50	53	13	27
Palliation	45	47	33	73
PTD	0		5	10
Laparotomy, biopsy	23	24	8	11
Biliary-enteric bypass	21	22	23	50
Pancreatoduodenectomy	15	16	4	9
Cholangioscopy			25	54

Pitt H, Roslyn JJ, Tompkins R: Surgical resection of bile duct cancer. The UCLA Experience. In Wanebo HJ (ed): Hepatic and Biliary Cancer, pp 339–355. New York, Marcel Dekker, 1987.

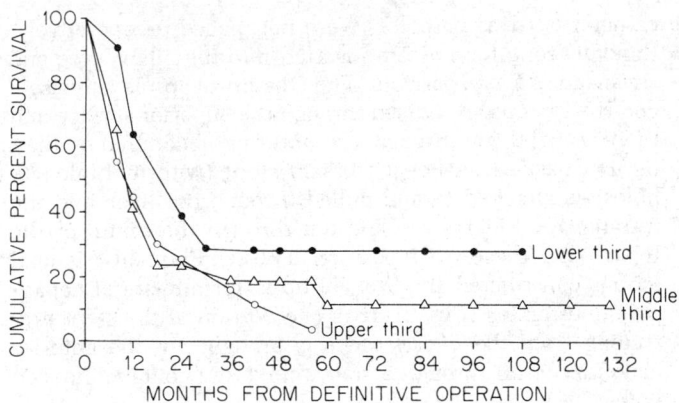

FIG. 27-14. Postoperative survival curves of 96 patients treated from 1954 to 1978 according to location of lesion within biliary system. Forty-seven were upper third, 24 were middle third and 18 were lower third. Six had diffuse lesions. (Tompkins RH, Thomas D, Longmire WP: Prognostic factors in bile duct carcinoma. Ann Surg 194:447–457, 1981)

and intra-abdominal infections. The mortality after resection was 13% in 63 patients, compared with 10% in 33 patients who underwent palliative procedures. The mortality after laparotomy alone, with or without chloecystectomy, was 2%, and it was 11% for choledochotomy with T tube or U tube insertion. For patients undergoing radical pancreatic resection or biliary enteric bypass, it was about 10%. The survival in this group was determined by the location, extent, and histology of the tumor and the operative procedure performed (Figs. 27-14 and 27-15).

Cumulative survival at 5 years was 8%. The rates were best for lower-third lesions (28%), which were commonly treated by Whipple procedure. For the upper-third lesions the 1- and 2-year survivals were 45% and 25%, respectively, but there were no 5-year survivors (Figs. 27-14 and 27-15). The total series of long-term survivors included one patient with a middle-third lesion who was alive at 11 years and another patient with a lower-third tumor who was alive with no recurrence at 9 years. There was no significant difference in mortality between biliary enteric anastomosis (9%) and intubation (7%). Survival was also related to microscopic pathology. Five-year survival was 31% in patients with papillary lesions, 20% in those with sclerosing cholangiocarcinomas, 8% in those with well-differentiated tumors, and 0 in patients with poorly differentiated bile duct cancers. Before 1979, 22 of 47 patients underwent resection of proximal lesions, and there were no 5-year survivors. Operative mortality was 23% in the resected patients and 19% for the entire group of 47 patients. Since 1979, only 7 (18%) of 40 patients with upper-third lesions have undergone resection with no mortality; the in-hospital mortality was 7.5% for the whole group. Thus, there has been a shift from resection to palliative bypass for proximal lesions.

In a report by Blumgart's group, there were 94 patients with proximal lesions, of whom 19% underwent a resection.[307,325] Six had local resection with no mortality, and 12 had major resections with two 30-day mortalities and one delayed death. Of the 17 surgical survivors, 7 were alive and well at 2 years, with one surviving more than 70 months. The mean survival of this group was 36 months. Ten died of disease between 6 and 30 months (mean survival, 15.5 months), and two patients died of other causes at 7 and 9 months.[325] Of 57 treated by biliary enteric or intubational bypass, 19 died, primarily from infection. Previous surgery or biliary drainage appeared to complicate matters and increase morbidity and mortality rates. Of 24 patients previously manipulated, the mortality was 33%, compared with 18% in 22 patients palliated without previous interference. The long-term survival rate was not given.[325]

The Hopkins' approach has been to correct metabolic and septic problems by vitamin K administration and IV antibiotics. If a patient does not respond within 24 hours, percutaneous transhepatic cholangiographic decompression of the biliary tree is carried out with insertion of multiholed ring catheters, which are placed in a dilated hepatic duct and advanced through the tumor-constricted site into the duodenum.[308–310] If the catheter cannot be passed through the tumor at first attempt, external drainage for 2 to 3 days may reduce edema and allow a successful passage through the stricture in the duodenum. The side holes in the tube allow internal decompression. Decompressing the biliary tree reduces the need for urgent surgical intervention and may decrease operative morbidity and mortality. The ring catheter also assists in identifying the bile ducts during surgery. In the case of a Klatskin's tumor obstructing both the left and right hepatic ducts, it may be necessary to insert ring catheters into each side of the biliary tree. Biliary ring catheters were required in 6 of the 27 patients in the Hopkins' series, and preoperative internal drainage was maintained for a mean period of 7 days.[309] All patients received penicillin or ampicillin, gentamicin, and clindamycin or flagyl before surgery.

The surgical technique is shown in (Figs. 27-16 and 27-17). Preoperative insertion of the ring catheters allows easy identification of the ducts above the bifurcation. After the entire extrahepatic biliary tree has been removed, transhepatic stents are placed in both the right and left hepatic ducts. These stents can be placed by attaching them to their previously placed ring catheters and withdrawn by the ring

FIG. 27-15. Postoperative survival curves of 96 patients treated from 1954 to 1978 according to type of operation performed. Results of pancreatic duodenectomy (Whipple procedure, 15 patients) for middle and lower third lesions were significantly better than biliary anterior bypass (21 patients) or intubation (45 patients). (Tompkins RH, Thomas D, Longmire WP: Prognostic factors in bile duct carcinoma. Ann Surg 194:447–457, 1981)

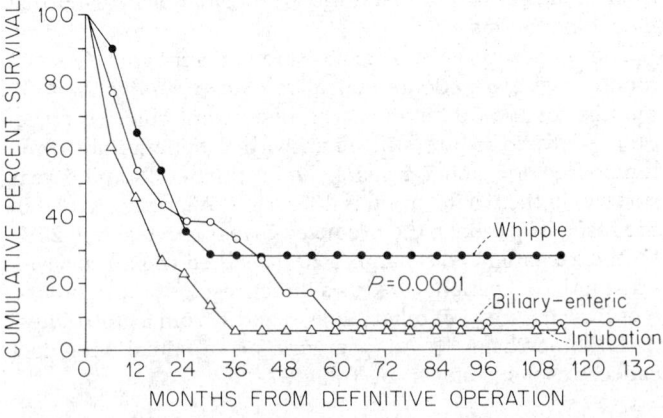

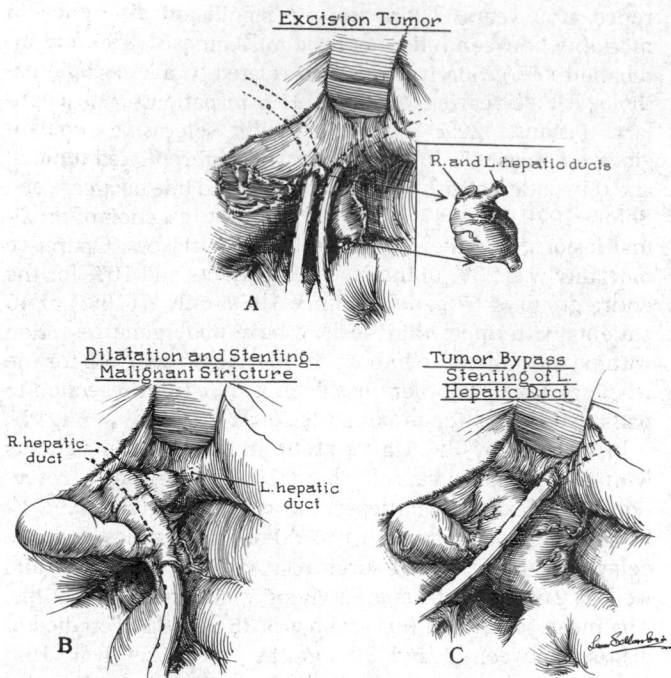

FIG. 27-16. Malignant biliary strictures can be resected (**A**), dilated from below (**B**), or bypassed by entubating the left hepatic duct above the tumor (**C**). A hepaticojejunostomy is then constructed over the stent. (Cameron JL, Gayler BW, Zuidema GD: The use of silastic transhepatic stents in benign malignant biliary strictures. Ann Surg 188:552–561, 1978)

FIG. 27-17. Procedure for replacing transhepatic biliary stents under fluoroscopic control. A stylet is threaded through the old silastic stent into the Roux-en-Y loop. The old stent is then removed, leaving the stylet in place, and the new stent is easily threaded back into place over the stylet. (Broe PJ, Cameron JL: Management of proximal biliary tract tumors. In Maclean LD (ed): Advances in Surgery, vol 15. Chicago, Year Book, 1981)

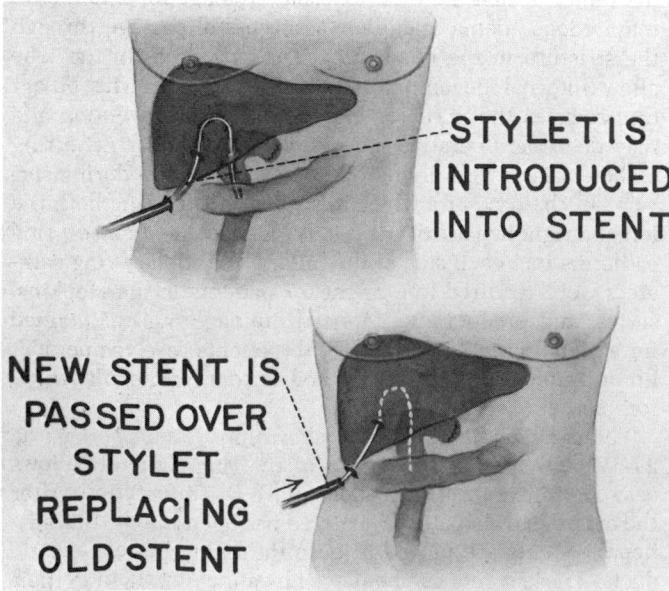

STYLET IS INTRODUCED INTO STENT

NEW STENT IS PASSED OVER STYLET REPLACING OLD STENT

catheters. If ring catheters were not placed preoperatively, Randall-Stone forceps are inserted into the biliary tree and advanced as far as possible. The Glisson's capsule is incised, and the forceps are passed through the superior surface and then brought out through the anterior abdominal wall. A 6-mm Silastic transhepatic biliary stent (with multiple site holes) is attached to and pulled through the liver into the intrahepatic biliary tree and out through the hilum of the liver. When these are in position, a 60-cm Roux-en-Y jejunal loop is constructed and brought up to form bilateral hepaticojejunostomies (Fig. 27-16). The portion of the stent protruding from the liver surface is brought out the anterior abdominal wall through a stab wound and contains no side holes.

The stents are left in place permanently and are irrigated by the patient. They are replaced every 3 months as an outpatient procedure, using the guide wire technique (Fig. 27-17). If the tumor is resectable, that is the best option; if not, the tumor can be dilated and one or more intrahepatic ducts intubated with stents. It is advisable to place stents in both ducts if the lesion is not resected to reduce the risk of infection in the undrained duct. After palliative tumor dilatation and intubation, a Roux-en-Y jejunal loop is constructed and a hepaticojejunostomy performed. If it is not possible to dilate the stricture, the tumor is bypassed by inserting the stent into the left hepatic duct, proximal to the lesion. A hepaticojejunostomy is then fashioned over the distal end of the biliary stent.

In the Hopkins' series of 27 patients treated for proximal bile duct cancer, there was one postoperative death from sepsis secondary to cholangitis developing in an undrained left duct after an effort at dilatation and stent insertion in the right hepatic duct.[309] Thirteen patients had previous cholecystectomies or common duct explorations; 93% were jaundiced and had preoperative PTC placement of ring catheters as described. All gross tumor was removed in 10 of 13 patients in whom resection was attempted. Palliative dilatation and stenting was carried out in the remaining 14 patients. Hepaticojejunostomies were done in 25 patients and hepaticoduodenostomy in 1 patient.

Postoperative irradiation of the tumor bed was given to 20 patients, of whom 9 received a full course of 5000 rad and 5 received less than 3000 rad. Six patients who had undergone curative resection received 5000 rad externally and 2500 rad delivered by local radium-192 seeds placed in the Silastic stents for 24 to 48 hours (Fig. 27-18). All had a reduction of their jaundice, with a restoration to normal or near-normal liver function tests.

The mean survival for 26 surgical survivors was 22 months, with 6 patients still alive. Mean survival was 30 months for the 10 patients who underwent curative resection. Of these, 5 are still alive, with 2 patients alive and tumor-free at 5 and 7.5 years. The estimated 2- and 5-year survival in the whole group is 40% and 15%, respectively. In the resected patients, the predicted 5-year survival was 25%. Of the 26 patients discharged, 20 have died (mean survival, 15 months); 8 patients died as a direct result of their tumors, 5 of liver failure, 4 of biliary sepsis, and 1 from a gastrointestinal hemorrhage.[309] An overview of proximal bile duct cancer results is shown in Table 27-17.

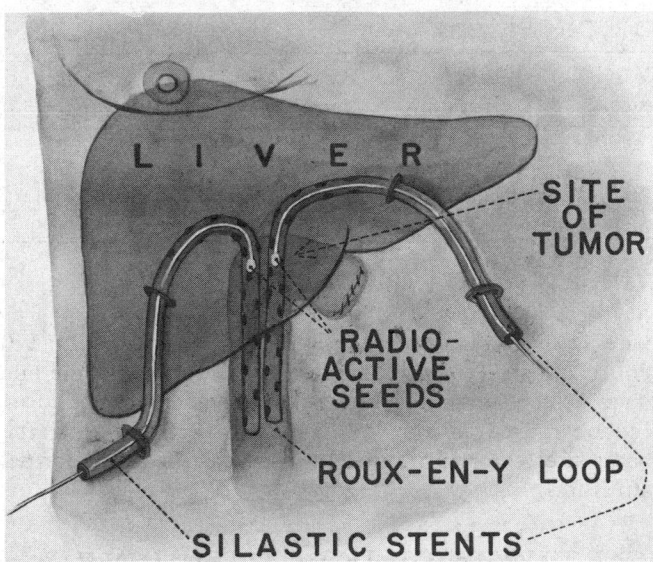

FIG. 27-18. The silastic transhepatic stents can be used as conduits for lowering radioactive ¹⁹²Ir seeds to the site of the tumor. These seeds are left in place for 24 to 48 hours and then removed. (Broe PJ, Cameron JL: Management of proximal biliary tract tumors. In Maclean LD (ed): Advances in Surgery, vol 15. Chicago, Year Book, 1981)

RESECTION OF MIDDLE AND DISTAL DUCT CANCERS. Cancer of the middle portion of the common bile duct is refractory to curative therapy. These tumors are within a few millimeters of the hepatic artery and portal vein. Of the 12 patients seen at the Lahey Clinic between 1965 and 1978, 4 were resected, and none survived beyond 2 years.[317-321]

Their most extensive experience has been with distal bile duct cancers. Between 1939 and 1978, the Lahey Clinic had experience with 282 patients with primary cancer of the bile duct, all but 6 of which were adenocarcinomas.[342-345] Of 173 patients treated between 1939 and 1965, most died of cancer 5 to 26 weeks after surgery, and only 25 survived more than 1 year.[319] Of 109 patients seen between 1965 and 1978, the median survival was 11 months. Of 41 patients with distal lesions resected by Whipple procedures (pyloris preserving), there were 10 (24%) postoperative deaths, and 8 (26%) of 31 survived free of disease beyond 5 years.[321]

Herter and colleagues also reported on pyloris-preserving Whipple procedures with pancreatic enteric anastomoses in 48 patients, of whom 33 had periampullary area neoplasms and 15 had pancreatitis without any postoperative deaths. Ten patients with distal bile duct cancers were alive 1 to 42 months after surgery (mean follow-up, 9 months).[322] A composite of experience with distal bile duct cancer is shown in Table 27-18.

Radiation Therapy

Although radiotherapy has a long history of use in treating patients with extrahepatic bile duct cancer, most of the published experiences have been anecdotal and retrospective and describe a variety of doses, fields, and delivery techniques.

Kopelson and co-workers reported on eight patients, of whom two were resected and six had palliative radiation only.[326] Doses ranged from 3800 to 7225 cGy in 25 to 29 treatments, using anterior and posterior fields. Obstructive jaundice was relieved. Palliation was achieved in seven of eight patients, with a mean survival of 7.4 months. In a Cleveland Clinic series of 79 bile duct cancer patients treated from 1958 to 1977, 16 were radiated postoperatively.[327] Intubation or bypass was done in 14; one was resected and one was biopsied only. The tumor was at the bifurcation in ten patients, in the common hepatic duct in four, and in the common bile duct in two. Cobalt irradiation of 2400 to 5000 rad was given. The proximal duct cancer patients survived an average of 1.7 years, and one patient was alive and tumor-free at 6 years. Nonirradiated patients survived an average of 6 months.

In a report by Wheeler, radiation was given to 9 of 21 patients with hepatic duct lesions in whom a T tube or U tube internal drain had been inserted.[328] Four patients received external radiation (4000–4500 rad), four had a radium wire passed through a T tube or U tube, delivering a dose of 4000 rad in 2 days, and one was treated by external and internal radiation. Actuarial survival appeared enhanced in those treated with radiation compared to patients treated with drainage only.[328] Fletcher and colleagues used internal radiation with iridium-192 wire to treat eight patients with proximal bile duct lesions.[329] A radiation dose of 4000 to 4800 rad at 0.5 cm from the wire was delivered over 48 hours. The median survival was 11 months, with two patients alive at 22

TABLE 27-17.   Survival Data in Patients Undergoing Surgery for Proximal Biliary Tumors

Procedure	No. of Patients	Postoperative Deaths (%)	Mean survival (mo)
Laparotomy and biopsy	41	5 (12)	5.6 ± 4.2
Palliative Y- or T-tube stenting	251	44 (17)	9.9 ± 5.3
Intrahepatic cholangiojejunostomy	68	11 (16)	11.0 ± 7.6
Palliative transhepatic stenting	35	3 (9)	18.6 ± 15.3
Tumor resection	88	11 (12)	22.2 ± 16.7
Total	483	74 (15)	

Data from Cameron JL, Sanfey H: Surgical management of proximal cholangiocarcinomas. In Wanebo HJ (ed): Hepatic and Biliary Cancer, pp. 395–415, New York, Marcel Dekker, 1987.

TABLE 27-18.   Survival After Surgical Resection of Distal Bile Duct Cancer

Author	Institution	Series	Reference	No. of Patients	Whipple Operation	Postoperative Mortality (%)	5-Year Survival (%)
Braasch	Lahey Clinic	1939–1965	319	62	27	26	30
		1965–1978	317	14	14	21	18
Herter	Cleveland Clinic	1940–1978	322	21	10	Not reported	33
Pitt	UCLA	1954–1983	324	22	15	13	30

and 23 months. An update of the experience to 18 patients continues to show a similar trend.

In the Johns Hopkins' experience with proximal bile duct cancers, 20 of 27 patients had postoperative radiation. Nine patients received 5000 rad externally and six patients received iridium-192 wire irradiation (2500 rad) and 5000 rad externally after tumor resection. The mean survival rate of the entire group was 18 months, with 11 patients remaining alive with the tumor controlled.[330] Between 1974 and 1981, Hashikawa treated 25 patients with hepatic duct lesions.[331] Most had percutaneous transhepatic drainage before irradiation, three had T tubes placed, and three had no surgical procedures. Survival appeared to be longer in patients treated with doses greater than 4000 rad. One of the 25 patients has survived disease-free for more than 6.5 years.

Intraoperative radiation has also been applied to bile duct cancers, primarily in Japan. Todoroki treated 25 patients with unresectable advanced cancer of the bile duct, using a single dose of 3000 rad with 11 to 20 MeV electrons.[332] Treatment was well-tolerated and palliation was effective, with recanalization of the obstructed ducts documented in all cases. Median survival was 13 months. Abe and Takahashi reviewed results of intraoperative therapy in Japan. A total of 59 patients with biliary cancer were treated in 12 institutions. Single doses of 2500 to 4000 rad were administered. Recanalization of the bile duct was demonstrated radiographically in 90% of the patients. Analysis of autopsied patients suggested that a single dose of 3500 rad was potentially curative.[333]

RADIOTHERAPEUTIC CONSIDERATIONS. A recent analysis of radiation for bile duct cancer by Pilepich suggested that radiation may have a potentially curative role in patients with local regional disease.[234] Because of slow growth, low propensity to metastasize, and small tumor bulk, the volume of normal tissues in irradiation treatment fields is generally small. External radiation doses of 6000 rad in 6 weeks, and preferably 7000 rad in 7 to 8 weeks, are suggested for consistent control of gross tumor. A dose of 4500 to 5000 rad is considered adequate for irradiation of microscopic disease.

The delivery of full tumoricidal doses of external-beam radiation is feasible for proximal bile duct lesions but difficult for distal duct cancers because of potential damage to the duodenum and stomach. In these cases, the best approach may be a combination of external-beam radiation of 5000 to 6000 rad and internal brachiotherapy as a boost. Internal radiation alone cannot be expected to provide adequate dosage to gross tumor unless the lesion is small and superficial. This is due to a rapid falloff of dosage around the wire. Delivery of adequate dosage for distances of 1.0 to 2.0 cm requires very high exposures at the surface of the bile ducts, which can produce scarring and stenosis of the ducts. Intraoperative radiation is another way of providing the boost after external irradiation while sparing some normal structures.

CARCINOMA OF THE GALLBLADDER

Carcinoma of the gallbladder is the fifth most common malignancy of the GI tract in the United States, after cancers of the colon, pancreas, stomach, and esophagus.[335] It occurs in about 1% of patients undergoing cholecystectomy for gallstones. It carries a grave prognosis, with most large series reporting 5-year survival rates of less than 5%. The disease is advanced and unresectable in most patients. A patient in whom the carcinoma was an incidental finding at the time of routine cholecystectomy may be cured by cholecystectomy alone. These are primarily patients with carcinoma in situ or with small cancers showing limited invasion of the gallbladder wall.[335–343] About 75% of the patients are women whose median age is in the seventh decade and in whom the diagnosis is made only on surgical exploration. More than 75% have associated cholelithiasis.[335,343]

PATHOLOGY

Cancer of the gallbladder usually presents as a locally extensive tumor.[335,337,343] The entire gallbladder may be involved, appearing thickened, contracted, and plastered into the liver, and it may be filled with purulent material, mucus, or stones.[343–345] Occasionally, extensive areas of hemorrhage and necrosis are present, even leading to perforation.[345] Frequently, one or more gallstones are present in the specimen, and about 85% of the cases have associated cholelithiasis. Carcinoma is most often present in the fundus and may present as a mucosal plaque, a polypoid or papillary excrescence, or discrete thickening of the wall, sometimes with an attached gallstone.[335,344,345] Papillary tumors are shaggy, friable lesions projecting into the lumina, and they may extend to and obstruct the cystic duct. A thickened gallbladder wall may exhibit diffuse calcification, a result of long-standing inflammation. A calcified or "porcelain gallbladder" is demonstrable radiographically and has about a 15% to 20% chance of containing cancer.[346,347] The series by Polk and colleagues included 22 cases of gallbladder cancer in approximately 100 porcelain gallbladders.[347]

Histologic types include adenocarcinoma in about 85% of patients and pure squamous cancers or mixed carcinomas with glandular and squamous elements in 10%.[345] About 5%

of the cases have neither squamous nor glandular differentiation and by light microscopy are found to be true sarcomas.

The adenocarcinomatous glands vary in size and may blend into the surrounding stoma and may be unrecognized. Occasionally, such cases are overlooked in the routine cholecystectomy but will be manifested subsequently by metastases; the occult cancer will be found frequently on reexamination of the original specimen.[345] Intramucosal lesions should be examined by multiple sections to determine the presence of invasion, which is frequently difficult if the tumor has grown into a Rokitansky-Aschoff sinus. Among the adenocarcinomas, 15% are predominantly papillary and about 9% are mucinous. The mucinous tumors contain large pools of mucin, with clusters of freely floating tumor cells, and such cases often have peritoneal implants and obstruction of the extrahepatic bile ducts.[344,345] Distant metastases are infrequent.[344]

Some adenocarcinomas may be poorly differentiated or anaplastic and are difficult to separate from sarcomas. Spindle-cell malignancies of the gallbladder are carcinomas, not sarcomas.[345,348,349] The distinction between carcinomas and rhabdomyosarcomas in children is important because of chemotherapeutic implications. Tumors with squamous components are observed commonly in North Americans, constituting almost 35% of gallbladder cancers in this population.[350] Mixed lesions with both glandular and squamous elements may occur. These have been called adenoacanthomas, but a better label may be adenosquamous carcinomas.[343-345]

Clear cell carcinomas of the gallbladder have been described by Albores-Saavedra and are historically identical to small cell undifferentiated cancers found in other sites.[351] Of 19 cases, all metastasized, and 9 patients were dead within 1 year.[351] Well-differentiated neuroendocrine tumors, such as carcinoids, have also been incidental findings at cholecystectomy.[345]

METASTATIC DISEASE

Modes of spread of carcinoma of the gallbladder have been examined in surgical cases and autopsy material. In a review by Fahim and co-workers, about 25% of 151 patients had nodal metastases at the time of surgery.[352] Most of the involved nodes were in the drainage of the cystic duct and the common hepatic and bile ducts. Vascular invasion was noticed in 14% and nerve invasion occurred in 24%. None of the patients had intraperitoneal tumor spread, but invasion of adjacent organs was common. Thirty-four percent had spread to the liver, and in 84% of these the involvement was restricted to the gallbladder bed. Satellite nodules surrounded the main hepatic extension in 8% and multiple distant nodules occurred in the right hepatic lobe in 8%.

At autopsy, carcinoma of the gallbladder involves the liver (90%) and bile ducts (60%) and extends to regional nodes in about 70% of the cases.[353] Over 60% had para-aortic nodal metastases and 33% had supraclavicular nodal disease. Approximately 33% had extension to the stomach, duodenum, pancreas, and peritoneum. The lung was involved in about 33%.[353] Most of the long-term survivors have had tumors that were unsuspected clinically at the time of surgery. In

Piehler and Crichlow's review, survival was 14.9% among 15 patients whose tumors were detected by the pathologist after cholecystectomy and only 2.9% among 70 patients whose lesions were discovered by the surgeon and were resected completely.[335]

CLINICAL FEATURES

Common symptoms as noted in a representative series included pain (79%), nausea and vomiting (53%), weight loss (42%), jaundice (34%), anorexia (27%), abdominal distention (24%), pruritus (15%), and melena (3%). Most patients had multiple symptoms (Table 27-19A).[360] The major clinical findings included tenderness or a mass in the right upper quadrant or epigastrium in more than half the patients, hepatomegaly and jaundice in one third, and cachexia, fever, and ascites in about 10% to 15%. The duration of symptoms was variable, ranging from 1 month in 33% of the patients to 2 to 6 months in 50%, and 6 to 12 months in the remaining patients (Table 27-19).

Preoperative testing was distinctly inaccurate in most cases. The preoperative diagnosis based on both clinical and laboratory findings in one series was a benign process in 60% and a malignant process in 40% of the cases.[337] Acute or chronic cholecystitis and cholelithiasis were the most common of the preoperative benign diagnoses, considered in more than 60% of the patients; pancreatic cancer and biliary tract cancer were considered to be the most likely malignant diagnoses.[337] Liver function studies and radiologic tests failed to pinpoint the diagnosis in most cases. Percutaneous transhepatic cholangiography, although useful for showing obstruction and suggesting a possible cause, did not distinguish primary gallbladder cancer from other lesions in this region. Of the patients in the University of Virginia series, 75% had cholelithiasis, findings that are similar to those of most series.[337]

The diagnostic problems resulting in delayed diagnosis of gallbladder cancer have been confirmed by other studies. The University of Minnesota series listed a high percentage of abnormal oral or intravenous cholangiography, but other test findings, such as upper GI series, were abnormal in less than 50% of cases (Table 27-19B).[338] The Charity Hospital series reported by Hamrick and colleagues concluded that none of the preoperative tests were diagnostic.[354] Hyperbilirubinemia occurred in 44% of their patients, and anemia, leukocytosis, and hypoalbuminemia were frequent abnormalities, as were hepatic enzyme elevations in patients with more advanced disease. In most of their patients, the gallbladder was not visualized by oral cholecystogram, and intravenous cholangiography added no new information. The upper GI series was abnormal in 33% of the patients, and in half of these cases, there was gastric outlet obstruction. External duodenal compression was observed in about 33% of the cases. Percutaneous transhepatic cholangiograms helped to visualize the site of obstruction, but they were not diagnostic.

Although few of these patients had ultrasonography, it might be helpful in some patients to document a thickened wall or identify adenomata.[355-357] In addition, CT scans may assist in the earlier identification of a neoplastic process in the gallbladder fossa.

TABLE 27-19A. Symptoms in Patients with Carcinoma of the Gallbladder (University of Virginia Series, 1981)

Symptom*	% Patients	Duration
Pain	79	<1 month, 30%
Nausea and vomiting	53	2–6 months, 50%
Weight loss	42	7–12 months, 20%
Jaundice	34	
Anorexia	27	
Abdominal distention	24	
Pruritus	15	
Melena	3	

Wanebo HJ, Costle WN, Fechner RE: Is carcinoma of the gallbladder a curable lesion? Ann Surg 195:624–631, 1982.
*Multiple symptoms in most patients.

SURGERY

Because of the variety of clinical presentations, ranging from occult malignancy to advanced diseases, surgical management has been quite varied in most series. In the University of Virginia series of 100 gallbladder cancer patients, surgical approaches consisted of cholecystectomy alone or with common duct drainage in 40 patients, cholecystectomy and partial liver resection in 8 patients, exploration with bypass or biopsy only in 44 patients, and autopsy only in 8 patients.[337] The median survival after cholecystectomy was 6 months, with two long-term survivals of 11 and 24 years. In many cases, the carcinoma was diagnosed postoperatively by the pathologist. The median survival after resection of the gallbladder and associated liver bed was 14 months, with one of seven long-term survivors (14%). Among 44 patients having miscellaneous procedures, the median survival time was 2 months with no long-term survivors.[337]

The impact of occult gallbladder cancer and the role of histopathologic stage has been addressed by many authors. In a Mayo Clinic report by Appleman, 21 of 166 patients who underwent definitive gallbladder surgery survived 5 years or longer.[340] None of the 21 involved adjacent structures, but 10 invaded the muscle of the gallbladder wall. Frank and Spjut described 16 patients whose tumors were first detected by the pathologist.[341] The cancer invaded the muscularis propria in 12 patients, the serosa in 3 patients, and the adjacent liver in 1 patient. The 5-year survival for the group was only 13%.[341]

Bergdahl reviewed 32 patients with clinically occult

TABLE 27-19B. Diagnostic Procedures Used in Primary Gallbladder Cancer*

Procedure	% Abnormal Tests
Oral cholecystogram, 42/47	89
Intravenous cholecystogram, 6/7	86
Upper gastrointestinal series, 24/53	45
Selective hepatic arteriogram, 1/3	33
Abdominal film, 7/109	6

Morrow CE, Sutherland DE, Florack G et al: Primary gallbladder carcinoma: Significance of suberosal lesions and results of aggressive surgical treatment and adjuvant chemotherapy. Surgery 94:709–714, 1983.
*University of Minnesota series, 1983.

cancer whose gallbladders were removed for clinically benign disease. Among the 21 patients whose tumors involved all layers of the gallbladder, the longest survival was 2.5 years.[339] Among the 11 patients with tumors confined to the mucosa or submucosa, 7 were alive after 5 years.

Nevin and colleagues attempted to reconcile the prognostic heterogeneity of gallbladder cancer by formulating a staging system based on depth of invasion and spread of disease.[336] Five stages were delineated: Stage 1 (intramucosal); Stage 2 (mucosa and muscularis); Stage 3 (involvement of all three layers); Stage 4 (involvement of all three layers and cystic lymph nodes); and Stage 5 (involvement of liver by direct extension or metastases to distant organs). Of 17 patients with Stage 1 or Stage 2 disease, all survived. Of 23 patients with Stage 3, 2 survived 5 years, and of 5 with Stage 4 there was one 5-year survival. None of the 21 Stage 5 patients survived beyond 1 year.

In a similar study from the University of Virginia, microscopic staging failed to identify a favorable subgroup of patients.[337] Among 46 stageable patients, only two had Stage I and four had Stage II disease. Only 2 of these survived 5 years, and 1 had a carcinoid of the gallbladder. If the latter patient is excluded, there was a survival rate of 20% for lesions confined to the muscularis. This is not different from other studies with similarly staged patients.[337–339,357] The greatest number of cases was in the Stage III group, of whom only 3 of 21 survived 2 years and only 1 survived beyond 5 years. None of the Stage IV patients survived, and only 1 of 13 Stage V patients survived (a patient with extension to the liver). The disease was limited to the gallbladder in only 25% of the patients.

In most cases, extension was into the liver or metastasis to the common duct nodes, the ducts themselves, the pancreas, or the duodenum (Fig. 27-19). In some of the patients, the gallbladder and liver were not available for the definitive study that would have allowed those patients to be included in the staging system. Liver metastases alone occurred in 19 patients, and secondary GI tract carcinomas accompanied the primary disease in 13 patients.

Somewhat similar results occurred in the University of Minnesota series. Of 11 patients with invasive cancer of the muscular wall that did not extend through the serosa, 1 (20%) of 5 patients survived after cholecystectomy alone, and 4 of 6 survived after more radical resection: cholecystectomy and lymphadenectomy (with three hepatic wedge re-

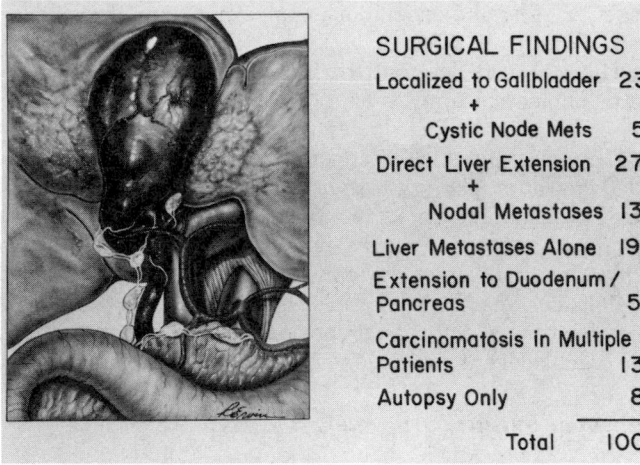

SURGICAL FINDINGS

Localized to Gallbladder	23
+	
Cystic Node Mets	5
Direct Liver Extension	27
+	
Nodal Metastases	13
Liver Metastases Alone	19
Extension to Duodenum / Pancreas	5
Carcinomatosis in Multiple Patients	13
Autopsy Only	8
Total	100

FIG. 27-19. Locoregional extent of disease in the University of Virginia series is enumerated above. Primary sites of extension are liver nodes, with occasional patients having extension to duodenum and pancreas.

sections and one pancreatic duodenectomy).[338] The three patients treated by cholecystectomy alone died of recurrent cancer at 18, 48, and 60 months, respectively. The overall survival rate in 11 patients with cancer confined to the wall was 46% (5 of 11). Of the 13 patients with cystic node metastases (Stage IV), 9 had cholecystectomy alone, 3 had lymphadenectomy, and 1 had pancreaticoduodenectomy. The cumulative survival was only 37% at 6 months, and all patients were dead within 18 months. Of 14 patients with advanced disease treated by aggressive surgery (lymphadenectomy in 6, hepatic wedge resection in 6, and right hepatic lobectomy in 2), the mean survival time was only 3 months.

The surgical results of four microstaged Western series are shown in Table 27-20 and emphasize the need to standardize the staging and reporting for surgical outcome. It would appear from the surgical series that the patient most likely to benefit from a cholecystectomy alone would be one with intramucosal disease only, but a composite resection (cholecystectomy with removal of the gallbladder bed by hepatic wedge resection and lymphadenectomy) would be required for those with invasive cancer confined to the wall (muscular coat or subserosal).

Among the Stage IV and V patients in the Minnesota series were 38 patients who were treated with either chemotherapy (35 patients) or radiation (3 patients) and who had a mean survival time of 4.5 months, compared with 3 months for the group of 14 patients receiving surgery only (p = 0.0001).[338] Although this series was not randomized, it suggests a rationale for pursuing adjuvant therapy in these patients.

The treatment is probably valid for early gallbladder cancer in which disease is limited to the gallbladder. In a report by Adson of 112 patients, 16 had carcinoma extending just beyond the gallbladder or regional nodes, which was theoretically resectable.[358] Of these, 12 had cholecystectomy, all but 1 died within 15 months. Four patients had a cholecystectomy plus wedge resection of the liver and lymphadectomy; all remained free of disease, but 3 died without cancer (3.5, 6, and 14 years), and 1 is alive at 9 years. This suggests the need for a more aggressive approach in the Stage III patients.

In the Scandinavian series by Bergdahl, 32 of 120 patients had a cholecystectomy performed for benign disease, whereupon cancer was found by the pathologist.[339] The survival was poor (longest, 2.5 years) in the 21 patients with cancer involving all layers of the wall, but it was 64% in the 11 patients with mucosal or submucosal cancers. Of the group having cholecystectomies, only 5 died of recurrence, suggesting the need for radical cholecystectomy (wedge resection of the liver and lymph node dissection). It also suggested a rationale for adjuvant therapy in patients with disease involving the entire wall.

In a review of 2567 patients with gallbladder cancer from

TABLE 27-20.   Five-Year Survival After Resection of Gallbladder Cancer in Staged Series

		Surviving/Total				
Stage	Extent of Invasion	Nevin (336)	Wanebo (337)	Morrow (338)	Bergdahl (339)	Composite Survival
I	Mucosa	6/10	1/2	NS/4* 2/26 (8%)	6/11 (64%)	(Stage 1-II) 18/33 (55%)
II	Muscularis	5/7 [13/40 (33%)]	0/3	NS/4 7/8 (88%) at 3 yr		(Stage 1-III) 27/106 (26%)
III	Subserosal	2/23	1/21	NS/3 5/8 (63%) at 5 yr	0/21 (0)	
IV	Cystic LN+	1/5	0/6	0/13	NS	1/24 (4.2%)
Va	Extension to liver or adjacent organ (resectable)	0/21	1/3	0/14	NS/88 = 0? (presumed, not stated)	1/123 (8%)
Vb	Regionally advanced or metastatic (unresectable)			0/74		
Total series	(microstaged)	14/66 (21%)	3/46 (65%) 3/100 total series	5/112 (4.5%)	6/120 (5%) (calculated, not stated)	28/398 (7%)

Data from Wanebo HJ: Carcinoma of the gallbladder. In Wanebo HJ (ed): Hepatic and biliary cancer, pp 431–445. New York, Marcel Dekker, 1987.

*NS = not stated.

Japan, Tashiro and colleagues found 467 patients (20.6%) who were treated by radical resection.[359] Those with Stages I and II lesions had good survival times, but those with more extensive disease did poorly. As in the Western series, most patients (59%) had associated gallstones, and only a small percentage (1.6%) were diagnosed preoperatively. These authors recommend that patients with cancer extending through the wall should have an extended cholecystectomy, a right hepatic lobectomy, and pancreaticoduodenectomy.[359]

A surprisingly high survival rate was obtained in the 467 patients who had radical resections of various types. The 5-year survival by stage ranged from 97% to 58% for Stages I and II to 25% to 20% for Stages III and IV. Even Stage V had an 11% survival rate. These Japanese survival rates are quite superior to any of the American or European series. The reasons for these differences are not clear, but possible racial, cultural (nutritional), and pathobiologic differences should be studied. It is unlikely that the extent of surgery or basic treatment differences would explain these survival results. An international symposium to compare differences may be of value.

Most of the series from the United States and Europe are in agreement that a more extended cholecystectomy (including the gallbladder bed and a regional node dissection) should be done. Although there are reported 5-year survivors after hepatic lobectomy, most investigators believe that formal lobectomies or other organ resections are probably not indicated and that a wedge resection or subsegmental resection should suffice.[360-363]

Related Epithelial Abnormalities

Other epithelial abnormalities should be pointed out in addition to carcinoma. Benign tumors, such as papillomas, adenomas, lipomas, and hemangiomas, may occur.[364-367] Noncarcinomatous malignancies may also occur, such as melanoma, carcinosarcoma, and malignant mixed tumors.[345] For the most part, the epithelial abnormalities are generally related to chronic cholecystitis and are probably precursor lesions to cancer. The relationship of cholecystitis to epithelial abnormalities has been examined by Albores-Saavedra and colleagues.[366] In a report from Mexico, 13.5% of patients with cholecystitis had atypical hyperplasia, and 3.5% had what was thought to be carcinoma in situ.[366] Carcinoma in situ is very common in surgical cases of gallbladder cancer, suggesting that this epithelial abnormality is probably a precursor of invasive cancer. Removal of this level of disease should result in improved survival. The presence of polyps is also a consideration for surgery.

A series reported by Kozuka and colleagues of 1605 cholecystectomies included 11 benign adenomas (all <12 mm), 9 adenomas with malignant change (all >12 mm), and 79 patients with invasive cancer (most >30 mm).[367] Of the 79 patients, 15 had adenomatous residues. The average ages were 50 years in the adenoma group, 58 years in the patients with in situ cancer, and 64 years in the invasive cancer patients. Some of the long-term survivors of cholecystectomy alone may be patients with relatively benign lesions such as adenomas or in situ cancers. It also suggests a ratio-

nale for early and expeditious cholecystectomy in older patients with cholelithiasis.

There is evidence that the retained diseased gallbladder after cholecystostomy is at increased risk for the development of cancer. In the University of Virginia series, 8 of 100 patients presented with cancer developing in retained gallbladders after cholecystostomy.[368] These patients had all been observed for a median of 8 years before developing the symptoms that led to the diagnosis of the gallbladder cancer. Physicians can reasonably consider patients with a diseased gallbladder retained after cholecystostomy to be at increased risk for cancer and should consider expeditious removal of the gallbladder if the patient is fit medically.

Optimal Surgical Approach

The optimal surgical approach has not been defined from any published clinical trial data. Considering the infrequency of the cancer, it is unlikely that the answer will be available soon, but recommendations can be made on the basis of some of the findings of the larger clinical series, in particular the studies performed at the Mayo Clinic.[352] This group described a major route of spread of gallbladder cancer, which appears to be locoregional rather than distant. Direct extension to the liver is common, with frequent spread to cystic, common duct, and peripancreatic nodes. Further direct extension along the nodal pathways may also involve the pancreas and duodenum. Similar findings have been reported from several of the recent larger series.[337,338,343] Liver metastasis or direct liver extension occurs in about 30% to 40% of the cases.

A logical surgical approach is total removal of the organ and the gallbladder bed, with a wedge of 3 to 4 cm of underlying liver, and a node dissection of the draining lymphatics. A right hepatic lobectomy is probably unnecessary. The lymph node dissection should include the nodal drainage of the entire bile duct, including the superior and inferior peripancreatic nodes, the common duct nodes, nodes in the porta hepatis (the common hepatic duct), and periportal vein and perihepatic artery nodes.

Biopsies should be taken from strategic areas of the resection site to ensure that the margins are clear. If all margins are clear, the nodes are negative, and the lesions seem confined to the gallbladder only, then the physician may observe the patient, obtaining frequent CT scans. If the nodes are positive, the margins are positive, or the disease extends into the liver, then postoperative radiation and chemotherapy are indicated.

The surgeon should be suspicious of gallbladder cancer in the high-risk patient who is older, has stones, has a very thick-walled gallbladder, or has a calcified gallbladder that is not completely compatible with the expected findings of chronic cholecystitis. If cancer is suspected, a small biopsy should be obtained before the dissection of the gallbladder. This prevents the unnecessary spillage of tumor cells that invariably occurs if a cholecystectomy is done and the carcinomatous communication between gallbladder and liver is disrupted. Tumor spillage may account for the frequent rapid dissemination of this disease in many patients after cholecystectomy. If a cancer is recognized early, then the operative procedures outlined could be carried out at that time or delayed if the patient and family are not prepared for a more extended resection. If there are questions about the diagnosis (infection and inflammation versus tumor), a fine-needle aspiration of the gallbladder fluid for cytology and bacteriology could be done to assess drainage or malignancy.

In the event that a cholecystectomy was done for a clinically occult lesion, the physician should consider reexploration with resection of the gallbladder bed and lymph node dissection. In the medically high-risk patient, observation only should be considered for cancer limited to mucosa or submucosa, and radiation plus chemotherapy should be given for lesions invading beyond these layers.

RADIATION

The pattern of failure after resection clearly points to the limitation of surgical procedures for most patients.[326,369] Local recurrence is a common cause of death in patients who relapse after cholecystectomy.[326] In Kopelson's review, local recurrence was present or was a cause of death in 86% of 110 patients who died within 5 years after simple cholecystectomy.[326]

Radiation data for gallbladder cancer are sparse. Hanna and Rider reviewed data on 51 patients treated at the Princess Margaret Hospital in Toronto.[370] Radiation doses ranged from an average of 2600 rad in those treated for palliation to 4000 rad in 4 weeks in those treated with curative intent.[370] Two-thirds of the patients had disease confined to the right upper quadrant. Although all the patients eventually died of disease, survival was stated to be significantly longer for those who received postoperative radiotherapy than for those who had surgery only.[393] Similar impressions of the survival benefit of irradiation were recorded by other researchers, but patient numbers were very small.[326,334,371] In a retrospective review by Vaittinen, the median survival was 29 months with surgery alone and 63 months for patients who were irradiated postoperatively.[343] These data may reflect case selection bias, and more data on external-beam therapy are needed to evaluate the role of irradiation for these tumors.

Several preliminary reports on the use of intraoperative radiotherapy indicate that this technique may play a part in the palliative and curative management of biliary tract malignancies.[372]

Effective radiation for gallbladder carcinoma depends on the volume of the treatment fields necessary to encompass the tumor, the residual tumor burden, and the total dose and fractionation. The relationship between tumor bulk and tumor control is well established. A dose of 4500 to 5000 rad, using conventional 175 to 200 rad/day fractionation, is required to eradicate microscopic disease but will not control gross tumor.

The ideal candidates for adjuvant, postoperative radiotherapy are patients who have had resection of all gross disease and are at high risk of harboring microscopic, residual tumor. A dose of 4500 to 5000 rad in approximately 5 weeks delivered to the gallbladder bed and regional lymphatics is likely to provide permanent local-regional control and, in a subset of patients, cure. For patients who have gross residual disease after resection or who had unresectable disease, consistent locoregional control will require higher doses, in the range of 7000 rad in 7 to 8 weeks. Such doses cannot be delivered safely to intra-abdominal sites unless the treated volume is small and removed from vulnerable structures, such as small bowel, or unless such procedures as a radioactive implant or intraoperative radiotherapy are used in conjunction with external-beam radiotherapy.

Combined radiotherapy and chemotherapy have a potential for improving locoregional control. 5-FU has been used as a radiation potentiator in the treatment of other GI malignancies and appears to have improved locoregional control with radiotherapy in several trials.[373] Similar trials should be conducted in patients with carcinoma of the gallbladder, particularly in those with gross residual tumor after surgery.

CHEMOTHERAPY

Single-Agent Chemotherapy

The infrequent occurrence of biliary cancer has limited the evaluation of its response to chemotherapeutic agents (Table 27-21).[374] Because many reports have included data on hepatic and pancreatic cancer under hepatobiliary malignan-

TABLE 27-21.   Chemotherapeutic Responses of Biliary Cancer

Drugs	Response (%)	References
5-Fluorouracil	4/17 (24)	Haskell (1980) [375]
	3/23 (13)	Davis et al (1980) [376]
Mitomycin C	7/15 (42)	Crooke and Bradner (1976) [377]
	0/10 (0)	Von Eyben et al (1980) [378]
BCNU	2/2 (100)	Haskell (1980) [375]
Adriamycin	1 (anecdotal)	Adolphson and Carpenter (1981) [379]
Neocarzinostatin	Anecdotal response	Bodey et al (1981) [380]
m-AMSA	2/23 (9)	Bukowski et al (1983) [381]
FAM	4/14 (31)	Harvey et al (1984) [382]
Ftorafur, Adriamycin, and BCNU	3/7 (43)	Hall et al (1979) [383]
Adriamycin and bleomycin	1/5	Ravey and Hester (1979) [384]
5-FU and mitomycin C via hepatic artery	9/13 (69)	Misra et al (1977) [385]

Andrews W, Smith F: Chemotherapy for cholangiocarcinoma and gallbladder cancer. In Wanebo HJ (ed): Hepatic and biliary cancer, pp 453–457. New York, Marcel Dekker, 1987.

cies, information on chemotherapy for these tumors lags behind that of the more common GI malignancies.

Several drugs beneficial in other upper GI malignancies have apparent single-agent activity in biliary cancer. In all of these single-agent trials, however, durations of response have been very short, on the order of weeks. This paucity of single-agent therapy needs to be remedied before combination chemotherapy or combined modality therapy for biliary cancer can be developed. The most commonly reported drug has been 5-FU. Haskell reported responses in 4 of 17 patients (24%).[375] Davis and co-workers reported three responses in 23 patients (13%).[376] Mitomycin C was effective in 7 of 15 patients (42%) in a study by Crooke and Bradner, but Von Eyben and colleagues noted no responses in 10 patients given mitomycin C.[377,378] Anecdotal reports of responses to BCNU, Adriamycin, and neocarzinostatin have also been published.[379-380]

Bukowski and colleagues reported on 23 cases of gallbladder carcinoma and cholangiocarcinoma treated with m-AMSA.[381] Doses of 60 to 120 mg/m^2, given IV at 4-week intervals, produced partial responses in 1 of 12 patients with gallbladder cancer and 1 of 11 patients with cholangiocarcinoma.

Combination Chemotherapy

Several combination chemotherapy regimens have been studied in biliary tract carcinomas. One used the FAM protocol developed for gastric carcinomas. This consisted of treatment in 8-week cycles, giving 5-FU at a dose of 600 mg/m^2 on days 1, 8, 29, and 36; Adriamycin at 30 mg/m^2 on days 1 and 29; and mitomycin C at 10 mg/m^2 only on day 1 of each cycle. Harvey and co-workers reported on 17 consecutive patients with metastatic disease treated with FAM, of whom 14 had objectively measurable disease.[382] Partial responses were noted in 4 patients (31%), with a median duration of 8.5 months and a median survival of 11.5 months. Seven patients had disease stabilization for a median of 6.7 months (range, 3–18 months) and a median survival of 8.4 months. Progressive disease was seen during the first cycle of FAM in 4 patients, with this group surviving from 2 to 5 months.

Hall and colleagues evaluated a combination chemotherapy (FAB) using 4 mg/m^2 of Ftorafur given IV on days 1 and 22 and 2 mg/m^2 on days 4 and 26; 60 mg/m^2 of Adriamycin given IV on day 1 and 45 mg/m^2 on day 22; and 150 mg/m^2 of BCNU given IV on day 1. This regimen was given on a 6- to 8-week cycle in a mixed population of seven patients with gallbladder and bile duct cancer.[383] They reported three responders (43%), with two complete responses. Responders had an 11-month median survival. Ravey and Hester used a combination of 60 mg/m^2 of Adriamycin given IV every 3 weeks, combined with 10 U/m^2 of bleomycin every 2 weeks. They reported one partial remission among five patients.[384]

Mirsa and co-workers reported the use of chemotherapy given directly into the hepatic artery.[385] This seemed to be more effective than intravenous therapy. By delivering 5-FU plus mitomycin C directly into the hepatic artery in patients with gallbladder carcinoma metastatic to the liver, they noted 9 responses in 13 treated patients (69%).[385]

Adjuvant chemotherapy was explored in a nonrandomized trial using 5-FU with and without other drugs as adjuvant therapy in 13 patients with gallbladder cancer.[386] Treated patients had a median survival of 20 weeks, compared with 8 weeks for untreated patients. Of these, 1 treated patient with gross disease remaining after surgery was alive at 6 years.

The paucity of chemotherapy and combined modality data in the treatment of biliary cancer and cancer of the gallbladder delineates the need for clinical trials to address these issues.[373,387] Intergroup studies are probably needed to provide adequate patient numbers.

REFERENCES

1. Silverberg E: Cancer statistics 1987. CA 38:5–22, 1988
2. Cook GG, Moosa B: Hepatocellular carcinoma: One of the world's most common malignancies. Am J Med 233:705–708, 1985
3. Cady B, MacDonald JS, Sunderson LL: Cancer of the hepatobiliary system. In DeVita VT Jr, Hellman S, Rosenberg SA (eds): Cancer: Principles and Practice of Oncology, 2nd ed, pp 741–770. Philadelphia, JB Lippincott, 1985
4. Knop R, Berg CD, Ihde D: Primary liver cancer in the adult. In Moossa AR, Robson MC, Schimpff SC (eds): Comprehensive Textbook of Oncology, pp 1087–1096, Baltimore, Williams & Wilkins, 1986
5. Herfarth C, Schlag P, Hohenberger P (eds): Therapeutic Strategies in Primary and Metastatic Liver Cancer, Berlin, Springer-Verlag, 1986.
6. Wanebo HJ (ed): Hepatic and Biliary Cancer. New York, Marcel Dekker, 1987

EPIDEMIOLOGY

7. Linsell A: Primary liver cancer: Epidemiology and etiology. In Wanebo HJ (ed): Hepatic and Biliary Cancer, pp 3–15. New York, Marcel Dekker, 1987
8. Chlebowski R, Tong M, Weissman J et al: Hepatocellular carcinoma–diagnostic and prognostic features in North American patients. Cancer 53:2701–2706, 1984
9. Lopez-Corella E, Ridaura-Sanz C, Albores-Saavedra J: Primary carcinoma of the liver in Mexican adults. Cancer 22:678–684, 1968
10. Sung J, Wang T, Yu J: Clinical study of primary carcinoma of the liver inTaiwan. Am J Dig Dis 12:1036–1049, 1967
11. Geddes EW, Falkson G: Malignant hepatoma in the Bantu. Cancer (Suppl 6) 25:1271–1278, 1970
12. Okuda K, Liver Cancer Study Group of Japan: Primary liver cancers in Japan. Cancer 45:2663–2669
13. Falk H: Liver. In Schottenfeld J, Fraumeni J (eds): Cancer Epidemiology and Prevention, pp 668–682. Philadelphia, WB Saunders, 1982
14. Tang Z-Y, Yank B-I: Early detection of subclinical hepatocellular carcinoma. In Tang Z-Y (ed): Subclinical Hepatocellular Carcinoma, pp 12–21. Berlin, Springer-Verlag, 1985
15. Cook GG, Mozaffari P, Van Rensberg S: Cancer of the liver. Br Med Bull 40:342–345, 1984
16. Berman M, Libbey P, Foster J: Hepatocellular carcinoma: Polygonal cell type with fibrous stroma—an atypical variant with a favorable prognosis. Cancer 46:1448–1455, 1980
17. Craig J, Peters R, Edmondson H et al: Fibrolamellar carcinoma of the liver: A tumor of adolescents and young adults with distinctive clinicopathologic features. Cancer 46:372–379, 1980
18. Lack E, Neave C, Vawter G: Hepatocellular carcinoma—Review of 32 cases in childhood and adolescence. Cancer 52:1510–1515, 1983
19. Ihde D, Matthews M, Makuch R et al: Prognostic factors in patients with hepatocellular carcinoma receiving systemic chemotherapy—Identification of two groups of patients with prospects for prolonged survival. Am J Med 78:399–406, 1985
20. Dunham LJ, Bailar JC III: World maps of cancer mortality rates and frequency ratios. JNCI 41:155–203, 1968
21. Omato M, Ashcavaii M, Liew CT et al: HCC in USA; etiologic consideration. Localization of hepatitis B antigen. Gastroenterology 76:279–287, 1979
22. Trichopolous D, Tabor E, Goetz RJ et al: Hepatitis B and primary hepatocellular carcinoma in European population. Lancet 2:1217–1219, 1978
23. Liver Cancer Study Group of Japan: Primary liver cancer in Japan. Cancer 54:1747–1755, 1984
24. Lin D, Liaw Y, Chu C et al: Hepatocellular carcinoma in noncirrhotic patients—A laparoscopic study of 92 cases in Taiwan. Cancer 54:1466–1468, 1984
25. DiBisceglie AM, Hoofnagle JH: Hepatitis B virus infection and hepatocellular carcinoma: Etiologic relationships and clinical implications. In Updates: Cancer: Principles and Practice of Oncology, vol 10, pp 1–10. Philadelphia, JB Lippincott, 1987
25a. DiBisceglie AM, Sjogren M, Klein J et al: Role of hepatitis B virus infection in hepatocellular carcinoma in the United States. Presented at International Sympo-

sium on Molecular Probes: Technology Medical Applications, Florence, Italy, April 11-13, 1988

26. Lai C, Lam K, Wong K et al: Clinical features of hepatocellular carcinoma: Review of 211 patients in Hong Kong. Cancer 47:2746-2755, 1981

27. Hall AJ, Winter PD, Wright R: Mortality of hepatitis B positive blood donors in England and Wales. Lancet 1:91-93, 1985

28. Beasley RP, Linn CC, Hwang LY et al: Hepatocellular carcinoma and hepatitis B virus: A prospective study of 22,707 men in Taiwan. Lancet 2:1129-1132, 1981

29. Bassendine MF, Della Seta L, Salmeron J et al: Incidence of hepatitis B virus infection in alcoholic liver disease, HBsAg negative chronic active liver disease and primary liver cell cancer in Britain. Liver 3:65-70, 1983

30. Yeh FS, Mo CC, Luo S et al: A serological case control study of primary hepatocellular carcinoma in Los Angeles. Cancer Res 43:6077-6079, 1983

31. Lohija G, Pirkle H, Hoefs J et al: Hepatocellular carcinoma in young mentally retarded HBsAg carriers without cirrhosis. Hepatology 5:824-826, 1985

32. Van den Heever A, Pretorius FJ, Falkson G et al: Hepatitis B surface antigen and primary liver cancer. S Afr Med J 54:359-361, 1978

33. Falkson G, Bohmer RH, Adam M et al: Hepatitis-B as a prognostic discriminant in patients with primary liver cancer. Cancer 57:812-815, 1986

34. Wen Y: Hepatitis B virus and hepatocellular carcinoma—cellular and molecular aspects. In Tang Z-Y (ed): Subclinical Hepatocellular Carcinoma, pp 218-231. Berlin, Springer-Verlag, 1985

35. MacNab GM, Alexander JJ, Lecatsas G et al: Hepatitis B surface antigen produced by a human hepatoma cell line. Br J Cancer 34:509-515, 1976

36. Smalley SR, Moertel CG, Hilton JF et al: Hepatoma in the noncirrhotic liver (in press)

37. Hislop W, Masterson N, Bouchier I et al: Cirrhosis and primary liver cell carcinoma in Tayside—A five year study. Scott-Med J 27:29-36, 1982

38. Fisher RL, Schauer PS, Sherlock S: Primary liver cancer in the presence or absence of hepatitis B-antigen. Cancer 38:901-905, 1976

39. Linsell CA, Peers FG: Aflatoxin and liver cell cancer. Trans R Soc Trop Med Hyg 71:471-473, 1977

40. Yaobin W, Lizun L, Benfa Y et al: Relationship between geographical distribution of liver cancer and climate—aflatoxin B_1 in China. Sci Sin [B] 26:1166-1175, 1983

41. Troillais P: Evidence that hepatitis B virus has a role in liver cell carcinoma in alcoholic liver disease. N Engl J Med 306:1384-1387, 1982

42. Kew MC, Roussow E, Paterson A et al: Hepatitis B virus status of black women with hepatocellular carcinoma. Gastroenterology 84:693-696, 1983

43. McSween RNM: Alcohol and cancer. Br Med Bull 38:31-33, 1982

44. Nakanuma J, Ohta G: Morphology of cirrhosis and occurrence of hepatocellular carcinoma in alcoholics with and without HBsAg and in nonalcoholic HBsAg positive patients. A comparative study. Liver 3:231-237, 1983

45. Simson IW: Budd Chiari syndrome and veno-occlusive disease in contemporary issues in surgical pathology. In Peters RL and Craig JR (eds): Liver Pathology, pp 299-314. Edinburgh, Churchill Livingstone, 1986

46. Simson IW: Membranous obstruction of the inferior vena cava and hepatocellular carcinoma in South Africa. Gastroenterology 82:171-178, 1982

47. Rector WG, Xu Y, Goldstein L et al: Membranous obstruction of the inferior vena cava in the United States. Medicine 64:134-143, 1985

48. Simson IW: The causes and consequences of chronic hepatic venous outflow obstruction. S Afr Med J 72:11-14, 1987

49. Nakamura S, Takezawa Y: Obstruction of the inferior vena cava in the hepatic portion and hepatocellular carcinoma. Tohoku J Exp Med 138:119-120, 1982

50. Johnson PJ, Krasner N, Portman B et al: Hepatocellular carcinoma in Great Britain: Influence of age, sex, HBsAg status and etiology of underlying cirrhosis. Gut 19:1022-1026, 1978

51. Melia WM, Wilkinson ML, Portman BC et al: Hepatocellular carcinoma in the non-cirrhotic liver: A comparison with that complicating cirrhosis. Q J Med (211)53:391-400, 1984

52. Cobden I, Bassendine MF, James OFW: Hepatocellular carcinoma in North East England: Importance of hepatitis B infection and extropical military service. Q J Med (233)60:855-863, 1986

53. Schonland MM, Millward-Sadler GH, Wright DH et al: Hepatocellular carcinoma. In Wright R, Millward-Sadler GH, Alberti KGMM et al (eds): Liver and Biliary Disease, 2nd ed, pp 1138-1184. London, Balliere Tindall, 1985

54. Iqbal MJ, Wilkinson ML, Forbes A et al: Preponderance of serum and intrahepatic 5-alpha-dihydrotestosterone in males with hepatocellular carcinoma despite low circulating androgen levels. J Hepatol 3:304-309, 1986

55. Iqbal MJ, Wilkinson ML, Johnson PJ et al: Sex steroid receptor proteins in foetal adult and malignant human liver tissue. Br J Cancer (Suppl 6)48:791-796, 1983

56. Wilkinson ML, Iqbal MJ, Williams R: Characterisation of high affinity binding sites of androgens in primary hepatocellular carcinoma. Clin Chim Acta 152:105-113, 1985

57. Nagasue N, Ito A, Yukaga H et al: Androgen receptors in hepatocellular carcinoma and surrounding parenchyma. Gastroenterology 89:643-647, 1985

58. Ohnishi S, Murakami T, Moriyama T et al: Androgen and estrogen receptors in hepatocellular carcinoma and in the surrounding non-cancerous liver tissue. Hepatology 6:440-443, 1986

59. Nagasue N, Yukaya H, Chang Y-C et al: Active uptake of testosterone by androgen receptors of hepatocellular carcinoma in humans. Cancer 57:2162-2167, 1986

60. Edmondson HA, Steiner PE: Primary carcinoma of the liver: An autopsy study of 100 cases among 48,900 necropsies. Cancer 7:462-502, 1954

61. Christopherson WM, Mays ET, Barrows GH: Liver tumors in young women: A clinical pathologic study of 201 cases in the Louisville registry. In Fenoglio CM, Wolff M (eds): Progress in Surgical Pathology, vol II, pp 187-205. New York, Masson Publishing USA, 1980

62. Christopherson WM, Mays ET: Risk factors, pathology and pathogenesis of selected benign and malignant liver neoplasms. In Wanebo HJ (ed): Hepatic and Biliary Cancer, pp 17-43. New York, Marcel Dekker, 1987

PATHOLOGY

63. Peters RL: Pathology of hepatocellular carcinoma. In Okuda K, Peters RL (eds): Hepatocellular Carcinoma, pp 107-168. New York, John Wiley & Sons, 1976

64. Simson IW: Personal communication, 1987

65. Steiner PE: Cancer of the liver and cirrhosis in Trans-Saharan Africa and the United States of America. Cancer 13:1085-1166, 1960

66. Okuda K, Musha H, Nakajima Y et al: Clinicopathologic features of encapsulated hepatocellular carcinoma. A study of 26 cases. Cancer 40:1240-1245, 1977

67. Nakashima T, Sakamoto K: A study of hepatocellular carcinoma among Japanese from the point of veiw of morpho-developmental pathology—gross anatomical types classified in its relation to capsule formation. Kurume Med J 24:S43-62, 1977

68. Anthony PP: Primary carcinoma of the liver: A study of 282 cases in Ugandan Africans. J Pathol 110:37-48, 1973

69. Matsumoto Y, Suzuki T, Asada I et al: Clinical classification of hepatoma in Japan according to serial changes in serum alpha-fetoprotein levels. Cancer 49:354-360, 1982

70. Craig JR, Peters RL, Edmondson HA et al: Fibrolamellar carcinoma of the liver. A tumor of adolescents and young adults with distinctive clinico-pathologic features. Cancer 46:372-379, 1980

71. Berman MM, Libbey NP, Foster JH: Hepatocellular carcinoma. Polygonal cell type with fibrous stroma—an atypical variant with a favorable prognosis. Cancer 46:1448-1455, 1980

72. Christopherson WM, Mays ET, Barrows GH: Liver tumors in young women: A clinical pathologic study of 201 cases in the Louisville registry. In Fenoglio CM, Wolff M (eds): Progress in Surgical Pathology, vol II, pp 187-205. New York, Masson Publishing USA, 1980

73. Omata M, Peters RL, Tatter D: Sclerosing hepatic carcinoma: Relationship to hypercalcemia. Liver 1:33-49, 1981

74. Rizzo PA, Young RC: Infections in the cancer patient. In DeVita VT Jr, Hellman S, Rosenberg SA (eds): Cancer: Principles and Practice of Oncology, 2nd ed. p 1963, Philadelphia, JB Lippincott, 1985

75. Order SE, Stillwagon GB, Klein JL et al: Iodine 131 antiferritin, a new treatment modality in hepatoma: A Radiation Therapy Oncology Group study. J Clin Oncol 3:1573, 1985

76. Tommasini M, Colombo M, Sangiovanni A et al: Intrahepatic doxorubicin in unresectable hepatocellular carcinoma: The unfavorable role of cirrhosis. Am J Clin Oncol 9:8, 1986

77. Tang Z-Y, Yu Y, Linz Zhou Y et al: Small hepatocellular carcinoma: Clinical analysis of 30 cases. Chin Med J [Engl] 92:455, 1979

78. Rostock RA, Klein JL, Leichner PK et al: Distribution of physiologic factors that affect 131-I antiferritin tumor localization in experimental hepatoma. Int J Radiat Oncol Biol Phys 10:1135, 1984

79. Okuda K, Kotoda K, Obata H et al: Clinical observations during a relatively early stage of hepatocellular carcinoma with special reference to serum alpha-fetoprotein levels. Gastroenterology 69:226-234, 1975

80. McIntyre KR, Waldmann TA, Moertel CG et al: Serum alpha-fetoprotein in patients with neoplasms of the gastrointestinal tract. Cancer Res 35:991-996, 1975

81. Geddes EW, Falkson G: Differential diagnosis of primary malignant hepatoma in 569 Bantu mineworkers. Cancer (Suppl)31:1216-1221, 1973

82. Waldmann TA, McIntire KR: The use of radioimmunoassay for alpha-fetoprotein in the diagnosis of malignancy. Cancer 34:1510-15, 1974

83. Melia WM, Johnson PJ, Carter S et al: Plasma carcinoembryonic antigen in the diagnosis and management of patients with hepatocellular carcinoma. Cancer 48:1004-1008, 1981

84. Nakagawara A, Ikeda K, Tsuneyoshi M et al: Hepatoblastoma producing both alphafetoprotein and human chorionic gonadotropin. Clinicopathologic analysis of four cases and a review of the literature. Cancer 56:1636-1642, 1985

85. Conte N, Ceccettin PM, Manente P et al: Calcitonin in hepatoma and cirrhosis. Acta Endocrinol (Copenh) 106:109-111, 1984

86. Collier NA, Weinbren K, Bloom SR et al: Neurotensin secretion by fibrolamellar carcinoma of the liver. Lancet 1:538-540, 1984

87. Anderson JR, Cain KC, Gelber RD et al: Analysis and interpretation of the comparison of survival by treatment outcome variables in cancer clinical trials. Cancer Treat Rep (Suppl 10)69:1139-1144, 1985

88. Falkson G: Personal communication

89. Ong GB, Taw JL: Spontaneous rupture of hepatocellular carcinoma. Br Med J 4:146-149, 1972

90. Simson IW: Membranous obstruction of the inferior vena cava and hepatocellular carcinoma in South Africa. Gastroenterology 82:171-178, 1982

91. van Sonnenberg E, Ferrucci JT: Bile duct obstruction in hepatocellular carcinoma (hepatoma)—clinical and cholangiographic characteristics. Report of 6 cases and review of the literature. Radiology 130:7-13, 1979

92. Alpert E: Human alpha-fetoprotein (AFP): Developmental biology and clinical significance. In Popper H, Schaffner E (eds): Progress in Liver Diseases, vol V, pp 337–349. New York, Grune and Stratton, 1976
93. McIntire KR, Vogel CL, Primack A: Effect of surgical and chemotherapeutic treatment on alpha-fetoprotein levels in patients with hepatocellular carcinoma. Cancer 37:677–683, 1976
94. The Co-ordinating Group for the Research of Liver Cancer, People's Republic of China: Application of serum alpha-fetoprotein assay in mass survey of primary carcinoma of liver. Am J Clin Med 241:241–245, 1974
95. Heyward WL, Bender TR, Lanier AP et al: Serological markers of heptatitis B virus and alpha-fetoprotein levels preceding primary hepatocellular carcinoma in Alaskan eskimos. Lancet 2:889–891, 1982
96. Dodd RY, Vyas GN, Dienstag VL et al: HbsAg as a risk factor for hepatocellular carcinoma among Americans In Viral Hepatitis and Liver Disease, p 638. Orlando, Grune & Stratton, 1984
97. Lotze MT, Wanebo HJ: Current and future research directions in management of hepatic cancer. In Wanebo HJ (ed): Hepatic and Biliary Cancer, pp 501–534. New York, Marcel Dekker, 1987
98. Teates CD: Radiological techniques in the diagnoses and treatment of liver tumors. In Wanebo HJ (ed): Hepatic and Biliary Cancer, pp 57–95. New York, Marcel Dekker, 1987
99. Oon CJ, Yo SL, Chio LF et al: The evaluation of tumour marker proteins in the diagnosis of primary hepatocellular carcinoma. Ann Acad Med Singapore, (Suppl 2) 9:228–233, 1980
100. Ihde DC, Sherlock P, Winawer SJ et al: Clinical manifestations of hepatoma: A review of 6 years' experience at a cancer hospital. Am J Med 56:83, 1974
101. Ohto M et al: Detection of minute hepatocellular carcinoma for early diagnosis of real-time ultrasonography (abstr). Gastroenterology 79:1117, 1980
102. Ohto M, Karasawa E, Tsuchiya et al: Ultrasonically guided percutaneous contrast medicine injection and aspiration biopsy using a real time puncture transducer. Radiology 136:171–176, 1980
103. Cheng W-KE, Lightdale CJ: Primary liver cancer: Diagnosis and laboratory findings. In Wanebo HJ (ed): Hepatic and Biliary Cancer, pp 45–55. New York, Marcel Dekker, 1987
104. Fortner JG, Kim DK, McSweeney J et al: Tumors of the liver as demonstrated by angiography, scan and laparotomy. Surg Gynecol Obstet 141:409–411, 1975
105. Fortner JG: Current management of tumors of the liver. Surg Clin North Am 57:465–472, 1977
106. Primack A, Vogel CL, Kyalwazi SK et al: A staging system for hepatocellular carcinoma: Prognostic factors in Ugandan patients. Cancer 35:1357–1364, 1975
107. Falkson G, Moertel CG, Lavin P et al: Chemotherapy studies in primary liver cancer. Cancer 42:2149–2156, 1978
108. Adson NA, Beart RW: Elective hepatic resections. Surg Clin North Am 57:339, 1977
109. Adson MA: Diagnosis and surgical treatment of primary and secondary solid hepatic tumors in the adult. Surg Clin North Am 61:181–196, 1981
110. Adson MA: Hepatic resections: Technical considerations—One surgeons view. In Wanebo HJ (ed): Hepatic and Biliary Cancer, pp 487–499. New York, Marcel Dekker, 1987
111. Fortner JG, Maclean BA, Kim DK et al: The seventies' evolution in liver surgery for cancer. Cancer 47:2162–2166, 1981
112. Tobe T: Hepatectomy in patients—cirrhotic liver: Clinical and basic observations. In Nyhus LM (ed): Surgery Annual, pp 177–202. Norwalk, Appleton, 1984
113. Goldsmith NA, Woodburne RT: The surgical anatomy pertaining to liver resection. Surg Gynecol Obstet 105:310, 1957
114. LeFoie CC: Etudes anatomiques et chirurgicales. Paris, Masson, 1957
115. Bismuth H: Surgical anatomy and anatomical surgery of the liver. World J Surg 6:3–9, 1982
116. Starzl TE, Bell RH, Beart RW et al: Hepatic trisegmentectomy and other liver resections. Surg Gynecol Obstet 141:429, 1975
117. Foster JH, Berman MM: Solid liver tumors. Major Probl Clin Surg 22:1, 1977
118. Huguet C, Gallot D, Offenstadt G: Normothermine complete hepatic vascular exclusion for extensive resection of the liver. N Engl J Med 294:51, 1976
119. Nagorney DM, Adson MA: Major hepatic resections for hepatoma in the west. In Wanebo HJ (ed): Hepatic and Biliary Cancer, pp 167–185. New York, Marcel Dekker, 1987
120. Inouye AA, Whelan TJ Jr: Primary liver cancer: A review of 205 cases in Hawaii. Am J Surg 138:53, 1979
121. Harrison NW, Dhru D, Primack A et al: The surgical management of primary hepatocellular carcinoma in Uganda. Br J Surg 60:565, 1973
122. Lee NW, Wong J, Ong GB: The surgical management of primary carcinoma of the liver. World J Surg 6:66, 1984
123. Wu M, Chen H, Zhang X et al: Primary hepatic carcinoma resection over 18 years. Chin Med J [Engl] 93:723, 1980
124. Lin T-Y: Recent advances in technique of hepatic lobectomy and results of surgical treatment for primary carcinoma of the liver. Prog Liver Dis 4:668, 1976
125. Okuda K: Liver Cancer Study Group of Japan: Primary liver cancers in Japan. Cancer 45:2663, 1980
126. Tobe T: Current status of surgical therapy for primary liver cancer in Japan. Jpn J Surg 13:86, 1983
126a. Nagasue N, Yukaya H, Ogawa Y et al: Clinical experience with 118 hepatic resections for hepatocellular carcinoma. Surgery 99:694–701, 1986
126b. Nagao T, Inoue S, Goto S et al: Hepatic resection for hepatocellular carcinoma. Clinical features and long-term prognosis. Ann Surg 205:33–40, 1987
127. Okuda K, Musha H, Nakajima Y et al: Clinicopathologic features of encapsulated hepatocellular carcinoma. A study of 26 cases. Cancer 40:1240, 1977
127a. Honjo I, Mitzumoto R: Primary carcinoma of the liver. Am J Surg 128:31, 1974
128. Balasegram M, Joishy SK: Hepatic resection. The logical approach to surgical management of major trauma to the liver. Am J Surg (Suppl 5)142:580–583, 1981
129. Kanematsu T, Takenatio K, Matsumata T et al: Limited hepatic resection effective for selected cirrhotic pts with primary liver cancer. Ann Surg 199:51, 1984
130. Lee Y-T N: Primary carcinoma of the liver: Diagnosis, prognosis, and management. J Surg Oncol 22:17, 1983
131. Tobe T: Hepatectomy in patients with cirrhotic livers: Clinical and basic observations. Surg Annu 16:177 1984
132. Gill RA, Goodman MW, Golfus GE et al: Aminopyrine breath test predicts surgical risk for patients with liver disease. Ann Surg 198:701, 1983
133. Okamoto E, Kyo A, Yamanaka N et al: Prediction of the safe limits of hepatectomy by combined volumetric and functional measurements in patients with impaired hepatic function. Surgery 95:586, 1984
134. Tsuzuki T, Ogata Y, Iida S et al: Hepatic resection in 125 patients. Arch Surg 119:1025, 1984
135. Okuda K, Ryu M, Tobe T: Surgical management of hepatoma. The Japanese experience. In Wanebo HJ (ed): Hepatic and Biliary Cancer, pp 219–238. New York, Marcel Dekker, 1987
135a. Chen D, Sung J, Shev J et al: Serum AFP in early stage of human hepatocellular carcinoma. Gastroenterology 86:1404, 1984
135b. Shinagawa T, Ohto M, Kimura K et al: Diagnosis and clinical features of small hepatocellular carcinoma with emphasis on the utility of real-time ultrasonography. A study in 51 patients. Gastroenterology 86:495, 1984
135c. Ebara M, Ohto M, Shingawa T et al: Natural history of minute HCC smaller than 3 cm complicating cirrhosis. A study in 22 patients. Gastroenterology 90:289, 1986
136. Rao BN, Green AA: Hepatic tumors in children and adolescents. In Wanebo HJ (ed): Hepatic and Biliary Cancer, pp 187–218. New York, Marcel Dekker, 1987
137. Weinberg AG, Finegold MJ: Primary hepatic tumors of childhood. Hum Pathol 14:512–537, 1983
138. Edmondson HA: Differential diagnosis of tumors and tumor-like lesions of the liver in infancy and childhood. Am J Dis Child 91:168, 1956
139. Ishak KG: Primary hepatic tumors in childhood. In Popper H, Schafner R (eds): Progress in Liver Disease, Vol 5, pp 636–667. New York, Grune & Stratton, 1976
140. Lack EE, Neave C, Vawter GF: Hepatoblastoma: A clinical and pathological study of 54 cases. Am J Surg Pathol 6:693–702, 1982
141. Gonzales-Crussi F, Upton MP, Maurer HS: Hepatoblastoma: Attempt at characterization of histologic subtypes. Am J Surg Pathol (Suppl 7)6:599–612, 1982
142. Esquivel CO, Iwatsuki S, Gordon RD et al: Transplantation for primary liver cancer. Wanebo HJ (ed): Hepatic and Biliary Cancer, pp 477–486. New York, Marcel Dekker, 1987
143. Starzl TE, Putnam CW: Experiences in Hepatic Transplantation. Philadelphia, WB Saunders, 1969
144. Calne RY: Liver transplantation. In Calne RY (ed): The Cambridge and King's College Hospital Experience, pp 306–311. London, Grune & Stratton, 1983
145. Iwatsuki S, Gordon RD, Shaw BW Jr et al: Role of liver transplantation in cancer therapy. Ann Surg (Suppl 4)202:401–407, 1985
146. Starzl TE, Iwatsuki S, Shaw BW Jr et al: Treatment of fibrolamellar hepatoma with partial or total hepatectomy and transplantation of the liver. Surg Gynecol Obstet 162:145–148, 1986
147. Falkson G, Cnaan A: Prognostic factors in hepatocellular cancer (in press)
148. Attali P, Prod'Homme S, Pelletier G et al: Prognostic factors in patients with hepatocellular carcinoma. Attempts for the selection of patients with prolonged survival. Cancer 59:2108–2111, 1987
149. Falkson G, Snyman HJ: Experience with chemotherapy of cancer at the University of Pretoria. Acta Union Internationale Contre le Cancer (Suppl 1–2)20:439–446, 1964
150. South African Primary Liver Cancer Research Group: Malignant hepatoma—controlled therapeutic trials. S Afr Med J 41:309–314, 1967
151. Vogel C, Adamson R, DeVita V et al: Preliminary clinical trials of dichloromethotrexate (NSC-29630) in hepatocellular carcinoma. Cancer Chemother Rep 56:249–258, 1972
152. Tester W, Donhower R, Eddy J et al: Evaluation of weekly escalating doses of dichloromethotrexate in patients with hepatocellular carcinoma and other solid tumors. Cancer Chemother Pharmacol 8:305–310, 1982
153. Davis H, Ramirez G, Ansfield F: Adenocarcinomas of stomach, pancreas, liver and biliary tracts: Survival of 328 patients treated with fluoropyrimidine therapy. Cancer 33:193–197, 1974
154. Brennan M, Talley R et al: Critical analysis of 594 cancer patients treated with 5-fluorouracil. In Plattner A (ed): Proceedings of the International Symposium on Chemotherapy of Cancer, pp 118–149. New York, Elsevier North-Holland, 1964
155. Ramierz G, Ansfield F, Curreri A: Hepatoma: Long-term survival with disseminated tumor treated with 5-fluorouracil. Am J Surg 120:400–403, 1970
156. Gailani S, Holland JF, Falkson G et al: Comparison of treatment of metastatic gastrointestinal cancer with 5-fluorouracil (5-FU) to a combination of 5-FU with cytosine arabinoside. Cancer 29:1308–1313, 1972
157. Al-Sarraf M, Go T, Kithier K et al: Primary liver cancer. A review of the clinical features, blood groups, serum enzymes, therapy, and survival of 65 cases. Cancer 33:574–582, 1974
158. Link J, Bateman J, Paroly W et al: 5-Fluorouracil in hepatocellular carcinoma—Report of twenty-one cases. Cancer 39:1936–1939, 1977

159. Kennedy P, Lahane D, Smith F et al: Oral fluorouracil therapy of hepatoma. Cancer 39:1930–1935, 1977
160. Joishy SK, Bennett JM, Balasegaram M et al: Clinical and chemotherapeutic study of hepatocellular carcinoma in Malaysia—A comparison with African and American patients. Cancer 50:1065–1069, 1982
161. Damrongsak C, Viranuvatti V, Chearanai O et al: Vinblastine in the treatment of carcinoma of the liver. J Med Assoc Thai 56:370–372, 1973
162. Falkson G: The treatment of liver cell cancer. In Cameron HM, Linsell DA, Warwick GP (eds): Liver Cell Cancer, pp 81–92. Amsterdam, Elsevier Scientific Publishing, 1976
163. Cavalli F, Rozencweig M, Renard J et al: Phase II study of oral VP-16-213 in hepatocellular carcinoma. Eur J Cancer Clin Oncol (Suppl 10)17:1079–1082, 1981
164. Melia WM, Johnson PJ, Williams R: Induction of remission in hepatocellular carcinoma: A comparison of VP-16 with adriamycin. Cancer 51:206–210, 1983
165. Domingo GO, Lingao AL, Lao JY et al: Therapeutic activity and efficiency of etoposide in hepatocellular carcinoma. Phil J Intern Med 20:106–112, 1982
166. Melia WM, Westaby D, Williams R: Iamminodichloride platinum (cisplatinum) in the treatment of hepatocellular carcinoma. Clin Oncol 7:275–280, 1981
167. Perry DJ, Van Ecco DA, Mick R: A Phase II study of deoxydoxorubicin in patients with advanced liver cancer. Cancer Treat Rep 71:1117–1118, 1987
168. Ravery MJR, Omura GA, Bartolucci AA et al: Phase II evaluation of cisplatin in advanced hepatocellular carcinoma and cholangiosarcoma: A Southwestern Cancer Study Group trial. Cancer Treat Rep (Suppl 2)70:311–312, 1986
169. Falkson G, Von Hoff D, Klaassen D et al: A phase II study of neocarzinostatin (NSC 157365) in malignant hepatoma. An Eastern Cooperative Oncology Group pilot study. Cancer Chemother Pharamcol 4:33–36, 1980
170. Falkson G, MacIntyre J, Coetzer B et al: Phase II-III trial of neocarzinostatin versus m-AMSA adriamycin in hepatocellular carcinoma. J Clin Oncol (Suppl 6)2:581–584, 1984
171. Falkson G, Coetzer BJ, Terblance APS: Phase II trial of mitoxantrone in patients with primary liver cancer. Cancer Treat Rep (Suppl 10)68:1311–1312, 1984
172. Falkson G, Moertel C, Lavin P et al: Chemotherapy studies in primary liver cancer a prospective randomized clinical trial. Cancer 42:2149–56, 1978
173. Vogel CL, Bayley AC, Rocker RJ et al: A phase II study of adriamycin (NSC 123127) in patients with hepatocellular carcinoma from Zambia and the United States. Cancer 39:1923–1929, 1977
174. Ihde D, Kane R, Cohen M et al: Adriamycin therapy in American patients with hepatocellular carcinoma. Cancer Treat Rep 61:1385–1387, 1977
175. Chlebowski R, Brzechwa-Adjunkiewicz A, Cowden A et al: Doxorubicin (75 mg/m²) for hepatocellular carcinoma: Clinical and pharmacokinetic results. Cancer Treat Rep 68:487–491, 1984
176. Olweny CL, Katongole-Mbidde E, Bahendeka S et al: Further experience in treating patients with hepatocellular carcinoma in Uganda. Cancer 46:2717–2722, 1980
177. Johnson P, Thomas H, Williams R et al: Induction of remission in HCC with doxorubicin. Lancet 1:1006–1009, 1978
178. Sciarrino E, Simonetti R, LeMoli S et al: Adriamycin treatment for hepatocellular carcinoma—Experience with 109 patients. Cancer 56:2751–2755, 1985
179. Barbare J, Ballet F, Petit J et al: Carcinoma hepatocellulaire sur cirrhose: Traitment par la doxorbucine. Essaie phase II. Bull Cancer (Paris) 71:442–445, 1984
180. Choi T, Lee N, Wong J: Chemotherapy for advanced hepatocellular carcinoma. Adriamycin versus quadruple chemotherapy. Cancer 53:401–405, 1984
181. Hochster HS, Green MD, Speyer S et al: 4'-Epidoxorubicin (epirubicin): Activity in hepatocellular carcinoma. J Clin Oncol (Suppl 3)3:1535–1540, 1985
182. Shiu W, Mok S, Tsao S et al: Phase II trial of epirubicin in hepatoma. Cancer Treat Rep 70:1035–1036, 1986
183. Cheng E, Chun H, Schiff C et al: Phase II trial of oral 4'demethoxydaunorubicin (DMDR) in patients (pts) with primary liver carcinoma (PLC) (abstr). Proc Am Soc Clin Oncol 4:88, 1985
184. Davis RB, Van Ecco DA, Leone LA et al: Phase II trial of mitoxantrone in advanced primary liver cancer: A cancer and leukemia group B study. Cancer Treat Rep 70:1125–1126, 1986
185. Falkson G, Coetzer BJ, Terblanche APS. Phase II trial of mitoxantrone in patients with primary liver cancer. Cancer Treat Rep (Suppl 10)68:1311–1312, 1984
186. Falkson G, Coetzer B: Phase II studies of mitoxantrone in patients with liver cancer. Invest New Drugs 3:187–189, 1985
187. Falkson G, Ryan LM, Johnson LA et al: Randomized phase II study of mitoxantrone and cis-platinum in patients with HCC. An ECOG study. Cancer 60:2141–2145, 1987
188. Falkson G: Therapeutic approaches to hepatoma. Cancer Treat Rev 2:73–76, 1975
189. Falkson G, Coetzer B, Klaassen DJ: A phase II study of m-AMSA in patients with primary liver cancer. Cancer Chemother Pharmacol 6:127–129, 1981
190. Bukowski RM, Legha S, Saiki J et al: Phase II trial of m-AMSA in hepatocellular carcinoma. A Southwest Oncology Group study. Cancer Treat Rep 66:1651–1652, 1982
191. Cheng E, Lightdale C, Young C et al: Phase II trial of (m-AMSA) 4'-9-(acridinlyamino)-methanesulfon-m-anisidide in primary liver cancer. Am J Clin Oncol 6:211–213, 1983
192. Amrein P, Richards F, Coleman M et al: Phase II trial of amsacrine in patients with hepatoma: A Cancer and Leukemia Group study. Cancer Treat Rep 68:923–924, 1984
193. Nair PV, Tong MJ, Kemp F et al: Clinical, serological and immunological effects of human leukocyte interferon in HBsAg positive hepatocellular carcinoma. Cancer 56:1018–1022, 1985
194. Sachs E, Bisceglie AM, Dusheiko GM et al: Treatment of hepatocellular carcinoma with recombinant leukocyte interferon. A pilot study. Br J Cancer 52:105–109, 1985
195. Forbes A, Johnson PJ, Williams R: Recombinant human gamma interferon in primary hepatocellular carcinoma. J R Soc Med 78:826–829, 1985
196. Falkson G: Chemoterapie van primere lewerkarsinoom. Spekulum 3:5–11, 1954
197. Gillman T, Hathorn M, Lamont NME: Alloxan as a possible therapeutic agent for primary carcinoma of the liver. Lancet 2:687–688, 1957
198. Friedman MA, Demanes DJ, Hoffman PG Jr: Hepatomas: Hormone receptors and therapy. Am J Med 73:362–366, 1982
199. Paliard R, Clement G, Saez S et al: Traitment du carcinome hepatocellulaire par le tamoxifene. Gastroenterol Clin Biol 8:680–681, 1984
200. Trinchet J-C, Roudil F, Vayasse J et al: Effects d'une association tamoxifene—norethisterone chez 16 malades de carcinome hepatocellulaire. Gastroenterol Clin Biol 9:455, 1985
201. Forbes A, Wilkinson ML, Iqbal MJ et al: Possible role of antiandrogens in treatment of hepatocellular carcinoma. Gut 27:A596, 1986
202. McIntyre K, Vogel C, Primack A et al: Effect of surgical and chemotherapeutic treatment on alpha fetoprotein levels in patients with hepatocellular carcinoma. Cancer 37:677–683, 1976
203. Umsawasdi T, Chainuvati T, Viranuvatti V: Combination chemotherapy of hepatocellular carcinoma (HC) with 5-fluorouracil (5-FU) and mitomycin-C (MMC) (abstr). Proc Am Assoc Cancer Res 19:193, 1978
204. Lee Y-TM: Systemic and regional treatment of primary carcinoma of the liver. Cancer Treat Rev 4:195–212, 1977
205. Falkson G: The management of tumors of the liver and biliary tract. In Carter SK, Glatstein E, Livingston RB (eds): Principles of Cancer Treatment, pp 426–433. New York, McGraw-Hill, 1982
206. Cochrane A, Muray-Lyon I, Brinkly D et al: Quadruple chemotherapy versus radiotherapy in treatment of primary hepatocellular carcinoma. Cancer 40:609–614, 1977
207. Baker LH, Saiki JH, Jones SE et al: Adriamycin and 5-fluorouracil in the treatment of advanced hepatoma. A Southwest Oncology Group study. Cancer Treat Rep 61:1595–1597, 1977
208. Oon CJ, Chua EJ, Foong WC et al: Adriamycin in the treatment of resectable and intersectible primary hepatocellular carcinoma. Ann Acad Med Singapore 9:256–259, 1980
209. Chlebowski R, Chan K, Tong M et al: Adriamycin and methyl-CCNU. Combination therapy in hepatocellular carcinoma: Clinical and pharmacokinetic aspects. Cancer 48:1088–1095, 1981
210. Bezwoda W, Derman D: Treatment of advanced malignant hepatoma with adriamycin or AMSA in combination with VM-26 plus 5-FU (abstr). Proc Am Soc Clin Oncol 1:91, 1982
211. Morstyn G, Ihde D, Eddy J et al: Combination chemotherapy of hepatocellular carcinoma with doxorubicin and streptozotocin. Am J Clin Oncol 6:547–551, 1983
212. Ravery MJR, Omura GA, Bartolucci AA: Phase II evaluation of epidoxorubicin plus bleomycin in hepatocellular carcinoma. A Southeastern Cancer Group trial. Cancer Treat Rep 68:1517–1518, 1984
213. Al-Idrissi H, Ibrahim E, Satir A et al: Primary hepatocellular carcinoma in the Eastern Province of Saudi Arabia: Treatment with combination chemotherapy using 5-fluorouracil, Adriamycin and mitomycin-C. Hepatogastroenterology 32:8–10, 1985
214. Friedman MA, Volberding P, Cassidy M et al: Therapy for hepatocellular cancer with intrahepatic arterial adriamycin and 5-fluorouracil combined with whole-liver irradiation: A Northern California Oncology Group study. Cancer Treat Rep 63:1885–1888, 1979
215. South African Primary Liver Cancer Research Group. Malignant hepatoma—Controlled therapeutic trials. S Afr Med J 41:309–314, 1967
216. Volberding P, Friedman M, Phillips T: Hepatoma treated with intraarterial (IA) polychemotherapy plus whole liver radiation (abstr). Proc Am Soc Clin Oncol 21:418, 1980
217. Okuda K, Peters RL, Simson IW: Gross anatomic features of hepatocellular carcinoma from three disparate geographic areas. Proposal of new classification. Cancer 54:2165–2173, 1984
218. Falkson G, Geddes EW: Infusion of liver tumours. Br Med J 4:454, 1968
219. Lange M, Falkson G, Geddes E: Intra-arterial chemotherapy in the treatment of primary liver cancer. S Afr J Surg (Suppl 4)12:245, 1974
220. Watkins E, Khazei A, Nahara K: Surgical basis for arterial infusion chemotherapy of disseminated carcinomas of the liver. Surg Gynecol Obstet 130:581–605, 1970
221. Cady B, Oberfield R: Arterial infusion chemotherapy of hepatoma. Surg Gynecol Obstet 138:381–4, 1974
222. Sullivan RD: Systematic and arterial infusion chemotherapy for metastatic liver cancer. Int J Radiat Oncol Biol Phys 1:973–976, 1976
223. Pettavel J, Morgenthaler F: Protracted arterial chemotherapy of liver tumors: An experience of 107 cases over a 12-year period. Prog Clin Cancer 7:217–233, 1978
224. Urist M, Balch C: Intra-arterial chemotherapy for hepatoma using adriamycin administered via an implantable infusion pump (abstr). Proc Am Soc Clin Oncol 3:148, 1984
225. Friedman MA, Volberding PA, Cassidy MJ: Therapy of hepatocellular cancer with combined intra hepatic arterial chemotherapy and whole liver irradiation. Ann Acad Med Singapore 9:260–268, 1980
226. Chearanai O, Plengvanit U, Tuchinda S et al: Treatment of advanced primary liver

carcinoma using intermittent intraarterial nitrogen mustard. Southeast Asian J Trop Med Public Health 5:96–104, 1974

227. Cheng E, Watson R, Fortner J et al: Regional intraarterial infusion of cisplatin in primary liver cancer: A phase II trial (abstr). Proc Am Soc Clin Oncol 22:179, 1982

228. Misra N, Jaiswal M, Singh R et al: Intrahepatic arterial infusion of the combination of mitomycin-C and 5-fluorouracil in treatment of primary and metastatic liver carcinoma. Cancer 39:1425–1429, 1977

229. Shildt R, Baker L, Stuckey W: Hepatic artery infusion (HAI) with 5-FUDR (F), Adriamycin (A) and streptozotocin (St) in unresectable hepatoma. A Southwest Oncology Group study (abstr). Proc Am Soc Clin Oncol 3:150, 1984

230. Douglass H: Prolongation of survival with periodic percutaneous multidrug arterial infusions in patients with primary and metastatic hepatic gastrointestinal carcinoma to liver (abstr). Proc Am Soc Clin Oncol 21:416, 1980

231. Patt Y, Charnsangavej C, Saski M: Hepatic arterial infusion of floxuridine, adriamycin, and mitomycin C for primary liver neoplasms. Dev Oncol 26:125–140, 1984

232. Lai EC, Choi TK, Tong SW et al: Treatment of unresectable hepatocellular carcinoma: Results of a randomized controlled trial. World J Surg 10:501–509, 1986

233. Coccia-Portugal MA: Personal communication

234. Almersjo O, Bengmark S, Rudenstam C et al: Evaluation of hepatic dearterialization in primary and secondary cancer of the liver. Am J Surg 124:5–9, 1972

235. Balasegaram M: Complete hepatic dearterialization for primary carcinoma of the liver—Report of twenty-four patients. Am J Surg 124:340–345, 1972

236. Fortner J, Mulcare R, Solis A et al: Treatment of primary and secondary liver cancer by hepatic artery ligation and infusion chemotherapy. Ann Surg 178:162–172, 1973

237. Al-Jurf A, Jochimsen P, Shirazi S et al: Hepatic artery ligation and chemotherapeutic infusion in the treatment of hepatic malignancy. J Surg Oncol 27:119–123, 1984

238. Almersjo O, Bengmark S, Hafstrom L et al: Results of liver dearterialization combined with regional infusion of 5-fluorouracil for liver cancer. Acta Chir Scand 142:131–138, 1976

239. Takagi H, Morimoto R, Yasue M et al: Ligation and catheterization of the hepatic artery for palliative treatment of malignant hepatic tumors. J Surg Oncol 23:219–222, 1983

240. Nagasue N, Inokuchi K, Kobayashi M et al: Hepatic dearterialization for nonresectable primary and secondary tumors of the liver. Cancer 38:2593–2603, 1978

241. El-Domeiri A, Mojab K: Intermittent occlusion of the hepatic artery and infusion chemotherapy for carcinoma of the liver. Am J Surg 135:771–775, 1978

242. Yamada R, Sato M, Kawabata M et al: Hepatic artery embolization in 120 patients with unresectable hepatoma. Radiology 148:397–401, 1983

243. Charnsangavej C, Chuang V, Wallace S et al: Work in progress: Transcatheter management of primary carcinoma of the liver. Radiology 147:51–55, 1983

244. Kinami Y, Miyazaki I: The supersuperselective and the selective one shot methods for treating inoperable cancer of the liver. Cancer 41:1720–1727, 1978

245. Konno K, Maeda H, Iwai K et al: Effect of arterial administration of high-molecular-weight anticancer agents SMANCS with lipid lymphographic agent on hepatoma: A preliminary report. Eur J Cancer Clin Oncol 19:1053–1065, 1983

246. Tashiro S, Maeda H: Clinical evaluation of artyerial administration of SMANCS in oily contrast medium for liver cancer. Jpn J Med 2479–80, 1985

247. Kanematsu T, Inokuchi K, Sugimachi K et al: Selective effects of lipiodolized antitumor agents. J Surg Oncol 25:218–226, 1984

248. Dakhil S, Ensminger W, Cho K et al: Improved regional selectivity of hepatic arterial BCNU with degradable microspheres. Cancer 50:631–635, 1982

249. Nakamura H, Tanaka T, Hori S et al: Transcatheter embolization of hepatocellular carcinoma: Assessment of efficacy in cases of resection following emoblization. Radiology 147:401–405, 1983

250. Okamura J, Monden M, Kambayashi J et al: Experience of the multidisciplinary treatment of hepatocellular carcinoma. Follow-up studies on chemoembolization with surgical excision. Excerpta Med Int Cong Ser 629:400–417, 1984

251. Sakurai M, Okamura J, Kuroda C: Transcatheter chemo-embolization effective for treating hepatocellular carcinoma—A histopathologic study. Cancer 54:387–392, 1984

252. Epirubicin Study Group for Hepatocellular Carcinoma: Intra-arterial administration of epirubicin in the treatment of nonresectable hepatocellular carcinoma. Cancer Chemother Pharmacol 19:183–189, 1987

253. Ihde DC, Matthews MJ, Makuch RW et al: Prognostic factors in patients with hepatocellular carcinoma receiving systemic chemotherapy. Am J Med 78:399, 1985

254. Sitzmann JV, Order SE, Klein JL et al: Conversion by new treatment modalities of nonresectable to resectable hepatocellular cancer. J Clin Oncol 5:1566, 1987

255. Liu TF: Distribution of malignancies in China. Proceedings of the First International Radiation Therapy Congress, Shanghai, 1986

256. Falkson G, Lavin P, Moertel CG et al: Chemotherapy studies in primary liver cancer: A prospective randomized clinical trial. Cancer 42:2149, 1978

256a. Yang N-C, Leichner PK, Fishman EK et al: CT volumetrics of primary liver cancers. J Comput Assist Tomogr 10:621–628, 1986

257. Leichner PK, Klein JL, Siegelman SS et al: Dosimetry of 131-I labeled antiferritin in hepatoma: Specific activities in the tumor and liver. Cancer Treat Rep 66:647, 1983

258. Ettinger DS, Leichner PK, Siegelman SS et al: Computed tomography assisted volumetric analysis of primary liver tumors as a measure of response to therapy. Am J Clin Oncol 8:413, 1985

259. Kaplan HS, Bagshaw MA: Radiation hepatitis possible prevention by combined isotopic and external radiation therapy. Radiology 91:12, 1968

260. Sherman DM, Weichselbaum R, Order SE et al: Palliation of hepatic metastasis. Cancer 41:2013, 1978

261. Friedman MA, Volberding PA, Cassidy MJ et al: Therapy in hepatocellular cancer with intrahepatic arterial Adriamycin and 5-fluorouracil combined with whole liver irradiation. A Northern California Group study. Cancer Treat Rep 63:1885, 1979

262. Friedman MA: Primary hepatocellular cancer—present results and future prospects. Int J Radiat Oncol Biol Phys 9:1841, 1983

263. Grady ED, Nolan TR, Crumbley AJ et al: Internal radiation therapy of liver cancer. J Med Assoc Ga 66:625, 1977

264. Ohishi H, Uchida M, Yoshimura H et al: Hepatocellular carcinoma detected by iodized oil: Use of anticancer agents. Radiology 154:25, 1985

265. Park CH, Suh JH, Yoo HS et al: Evaluation of intrahepatic I-131 Ethiodol on a patient with hepatocellular cancer. Clin Nucl Med 11:514, 1986

266. Richter GW: Comparison of ferritin from neoplastic and nonneoplastic human cells. Nature 207:616, 1965

267. Lenhard RE, Order SE, Spunberg JJ et al: Isotopic immunoglobulin: A new systemic therapy for advanced Hodgkin's disease. J Clin Oncol 3:1296, 1985

268. Rostock RA, Klein JL, Leichner PK et al: Selective tumor localization in experimental hepatoma by radiolabeled antiferritin antibody. Int J Radiat Oncol Biol Phys 9:1345, 1983

269. Rostock RA, Klein JL, Kopher KA et al: Variables affecting the tumor localization of 131-I antiferritin in experimental hepatoma. Am J Clin Oncol 6:9, 1984

270. Rostock RA, Kopher KA, Bauer TW et al: Factors that affect antiferritin localization in four rat hepatoma models. In Freeman AI (ed): Cancer Drug Delivery, vol 2, p 139. New York, Mary Ann Liebert, 1985

271. Leichner PK, Yang NC, Frenkel TL et al: Dosimetry and treatment planning for ^{90}Y-labeled antiferritin in hepatoma. Int J Radiat Oncol Biol Phys 14:2775, 1988

272. Williams J: Personal communication, 1987

273. Tang ZY, Liu KD, Guo YD et al: Tumor imaging and targeting therapy for hepatocellular carcinoma: Preliminary results of experimental and clinical studies: Chung Hua I Hsueh Tsa Chih 99:855, 1986

274. Order SE, Klein JL, Leichner PK et al: 90-Yttrium antiferritin: A new therapeutic radiolabeled antibody. Int J Radiat Oncol Biol Phys 12:277, 1986

275. Kusumoto Y, Nakata K, Muro T et al: Serotherapy of AFP producing tumors with the purified antibody to AFP. Oncoder Bio-Med 4:95, 1983

276. Koji T, Ishi N, Munehisa T et al: Localization of radioiodinated antibody to alpha fetoprotein in hepatoma transplanted in rats and a case report of alpha fetoprotein antibody treatment of a hepatoma patient. Cancer Res 40:3013, 1980

277. Matsumoto Y, Suzuki T, Asada I et al: Clinical classification of hepatoma in Japan according to serial changes in serum alpha fetoprotein levels. Cancer 49:354, 1982

277a. Fu KK, Lam KN, Rayner PA: The influence of time sequence of Cisplatin administration and continuous low dose rate irradiation (CLDRI) on their combined effects on a murine squamous cell carcinoma. J Radiat Oncol Biol Phys 11:2119, 1985

278. Johnson PJ, Williams R: Serum alpha fetoprotein estimations and doubling time in hepatocellular carcinoma. Influence of therapy and possible value in early detection. JNCI 64:1329, 1980

279. Stillwagon GB, Order SE, Klein JL et al: Multi-modality treatment of primary nonresectable intrahepatic cholangiocarcinoma with 131-I anti-CEA—A Radiation Therapy Oncology Group study 13:687, 1987

280. Fardel D: Malignant neoplasms of the extrahepatic biliary ducts. Ann Surg 76:205, 1922

281. Courvoisier LG: Casuistisch-Statistische Beitrage zur Pathologie und Chirurgie der Gallenwege. Leipzig, Vogel, 1890

282. Baudoin CE: Surgery of the upper abdomen: II. Surgery of the Gallbladder, Liver, Pancreas and Spleen, vol 24, p 409. Philadelphia, Blakiston, 1913

283. Mayo WJ: Malignant disease of the common bile duct. In Mayo WJ, Mayo CH (eds): Collection of Papers Published Previous to 1909, p 401. Philadelphia, Saunders, 1912

284. Sako K, Seitzinger GL, Garside E: Carcinoma of the extrahepatic bile ducts: Review of the literature and report of six cases. Surgery 41:416, 1957

285. Neibling HH, Dockerty MB, Waugh JM: Carcinoma of the extrahepatic bile ducts. Surg Gynecol Obstet 89:429, 1949

286. Gibby DG, Hanks JB, Wanebo HJ et al: Bile duct carcinoma: Diagnosis and treatment. Ann Surg 202:139, 1985

287. Jones RS, Hanks J: Overview of Cancer of Bile Duct. In Wanebo HJ (ed): Hepatic and Biliary Cancer, pp 329–338. New York, Marcel Dekker, 1987

288. Faintuck J and Levin B: Diagnosis of Bile Duct Cancer. In Wanebo HJ (ed): Hepatic and Biliary Cancer, pp 299–338. New York, Marcel Dekker, 1982

289. McKay AJ, Duncan JG, Lau P et al: The role of gray scale ultrasonography in the investigation of jaundice. Br J Surg 66:162, 1979

290. Broughton NS, Evensen A, Osnes M: Endoscopic retrograde cholangiography in primary biliary tract carcinoma. Clin Radiol 29:647, 1978

291. Elias E, Hamlyn AN, Jain S et al: A randomized trial of percutaneous transhepatic cholangiography with the Chiba needle versus ERCP for bile duct visualization in jaundice. Gastroenterology 71:439, 1976

292. Hoevels J, Ihse I: Percutaneous transhepatic portography in bile duct carcinoma. Correlation with percutaneous transhepatic cholangiography and angiography. ROFO 131:140, 1979

293. Voyles CR, Bowley NJ, Allison DJ et al: Carcinoma of the proximal extrahepatic biliary tree: Radiologic assessment and therapeutic alternatives. Ann Surg 197:188, 1983

294. Goldberg HI, Filly RA, Korobkin M et al: Capability of CT body scanning and ultrasonography to demonstrate the status of the biliary ductal system in patients with jaundice. Radiology 129:713, 1978

295. Evander A, Ihse I, Lunderquist A et al: Percutaneous cytodiagnosis of carcinoma of the pancreas and bile duct. Ann Surg 188:90, 1978
296. Cutherell L, Wanebo HJ, Tegtmeyer CJ: Catheter tract seeding after percutaneous biliary drainage for pancreatic cancer. Cancer 57:2057–2060, 1986
297. Nakayama T, Ikeda A, Okuda K et al: Percutaneous transhepatic drainage of the biliary tract. Technique and results in 104 cases. Gastroenterology 74:554, 1978
298. Norlander A, Kalin B, Sunblad R: Effect of percutaneous transhepatic drainage upon liver function and post-operative mortality. Surg Gynecol Obstet 155:161, 1982
299. Ferrucci JV, Mueller PR: Interventional radiology of the biliary tract. Gastroenterology 82:974, 1982
300. Denning DA, Ellison EC, Carey LC: Pre-operative percutaneous transhepatic biliary decompression lowers operative morbidity in patients with obstructive jaundice. Am J Surg 141:61, 1981
301. MacPherson GAD, Benjamin IS, Hodgson HJF et al: Pre-operative percutaneous transphepatic biliary drainage: The results of a controlled trial. Br J Surg 71:371, 1984
302. Pitt HA, Gomes AS, Lois JF et al: Does pre-operative percutaneous biliary drainage reduce operative risk or increase hospital cost? Ann Surg 201:545, 1985
303. Tompkins RK, Johnson J, Storm FK et al: Operative encoscopy in the management of biliary tract neoplasms. Am Surg 132:174, 1976
304. Klatskin G: Adenocarcinoma of the hepatic duct with distinctive clinical and pathological features. Am J Med 38:241, 1965
305. Akwari OE, Kelly KA: Surgical treatment of adenocarcinoma. Location: Junction of the right, left and common biliary ducts. Arch Surg 114:22, 1979
306. Tompkins RK, Thomas D, Wile A et al: Prognostic factors in bile duct carcinoma. Analysis of 96 cases. Ann Surg 4:447–457, 1981
307. Beazley RM, Hadjis NS, Benjamin IS et al: Clinicopathological aspects of high bile duct cancer. Experience with resection and bypass surgical treatments. Ann Surg 199:623–636, 1984
308. Cameron JL, Gayler BW, Zuidema GD: The use of silastic transhepatic stents in benign and malignant biliary strictures. Ann Surg 188:552, 1978
309. Cameron JL, Sanfey H: Surgical management of proximal cholangiocarcinomas. In Wanebo HJ (ed): Hepatic and Biliary Cancer, pp 395–416. New York, Marcel Dekker, 1987
310. Broe PJ, Cameron JL: The management of proximal biliary tract tumors. Adv Surg 15:47–91, 1981
311. Terblanche J, Saunders SJ, Louw JH: Prolonged palliation in carcinoma of the main hepatic duct junction. Surgery 71:720, 1972
312. Blumgart LH, Kelley CJ: Hepaticojejunostomy in benign and malignant high bile duct strictures: Approaches to the left hepatic ducts. Br J Surg 71:257–261, 1984
313. Longmire WP Jr, Sanford MD: Intrahepatic cholangiojejunostomy with partial hepatectomy for biliary obstruction. Surgery 24:264, 1948
314. Longmire WP Jr, Lippman HN: Intrahepatic cholangiojejunostomy: An operation for biliary obstruction. Surg Clin North Am 36:849, 1956
315. Smith R: Hepaticojejunostomy with transhepatic intubation. A technique for very high strictures of the hepatic ducts. Br J Surg 51:186, 1964
316. Bismuth H, Corlette MB: Intrahepatic cholangioenteric anastimosis in carcinoma of the hilus of the liver. Surg Gynecol Obstet 140:170–178, 1975
317. Alexander F, Rossi RL, O'Bryan M et al: Biliary carcinoma: A review of 109 cases. Am J Surg 147:503–509, 1984
318. Braasch JW: Surgical resection of cancer of the mid-duct and distal common bile duct in hepatic and biliary cancer. In Wanebo HJ (ed): Hepatic and Biliary Cancer, pp 357–373. New York, Marcel Dekker, 1987
319. Braasch JW, Warren KW, Kune GA: Malignant neoplasms of the bile ducts. Surg Clin North Am 47:627–638, 1967
320. Braasch JW: Carcinoma of the bile duct. Surg Clin North Am 53:1217–1227, 1973
321. Braasch JW, Jin G, Rossi RL: Pancreatoduodenectomy with preservation of the pylorus. World J Surg 8:900–905, 1984
322. Herter FP, Cooperman AM, Ahlborn TN et al: Surgical experience with pancreatic and periampullary cancer. Ann Surg 195:274–281, 1982
323. Evander A, Fredlund P, Hoevels J et al: Evaluation of aggressive surgery in carcinoma of the extrahepatic bile ducts. Ann Surg 191:23, 1980
324. Pitt HA, Roslyn JJ, Tompkins RK: Surgical resection of bile duct cancer: The UCLA experience. In Wanebo HJ (ed): Hepatic and Biliary Cancer, pp 339–355. New York, Marcel Dekker, 1987
325. Blumgart LH, Hadjis NS: Proximal bile duct cancer: Curative resection or palliative bypass. In Wanebo HJ (ed): Hepatic and Biliary Cancer, pp 375–394. New York, Marcel Dekker, 1987
326. Kopelson G, Harisiadis L, Tretter P et al: The role of radiation therapy in cancer of the extra-hepatic biliary system: An analysis of thirteen patients and a review of the literature of the effectiveness of surgery, chemotherapy and radiotherapy. Int J Radiat Oncol Biol Phys 2:883–894, 1977
327. Lees CD, Zapolanski A, Cooperman AM et al: Carcinoma of the bile ducts. Surg Gynecol Obstet 151:193–198, 1980
328. Wheeler PG, Dawson JL, Nunnerley H et al: Newer techniques in the diagnosis and treatment of proximal bile duct carcinoma—an analysis of 41 consecutive patients. Q J Med 199:247–258, 1981
329. Fletcher MS, Brinkley D, Dawson JL et al: Treatment of hilar carcinoma by bile drainage combined with internal radiotherapy using 192-iridium wire. Br J Surg 70:733–735, 1983
330. Cameron JL, Broe P, Zuidema GD: Proximal bile duct tumors. Surgical management with silastic transhepatic biliary stents. Ann Surg 196:412–419, 1982
331. Hashikawa Y, Shimada T, Miura T et al: Radiation therapy of carcinoma of the extrahepatic bile ducts. Radiology 146:787–789, 1983
332. Todoroki T, Iwasaki Y, Okamura T et al: Intraoperative radiotherapy for advanced carcinoma of the biliary system. Cancer 46:2179–2184, 1980
333. Abe M, Takahashi M: Intraoperative radiotherapy: The Japanese experience. Int J Radiat Oncol Biol Phys 7:863–868, 1981
334. Pilepich MV: Radiation for carcinoma of the extrahepatic bile duct and Radiotherapy in carcinoma of gallbladder. In Wanebo HJ (ed): Hepatic and Biliary Cancer, pp 417–427, 447–452. New York, Marcel Dekker, 1987
335. Piehler JM, Crichlow RW: Primary carcinoma of the gallbladder. Surg Gynecol Obstet 147:929–942, 1978
336. Nevin JE, Moran TJ, Kay S et al: Carcinoma of the gallbladder. Cancer 37:141–148, 1976
337. Wanebo HJ, Castle WN, Fechner RE: Is carcinoma of the gallbladder a curable lesion? Ann Surg 195:624–631, 1982
338. Morrow CE, Sutherland DE, Florack G et al: Primary gallbladder carcinoma: Significance of suberosal lesions and results of aggressive surgical treatment and adjuvant chemotherapy. Surgery 94:709–714, 1983
339. Bergdahl L: Gallbladder carcinoma first diagnosed at microscopic examination of gallbladders removed for presumed benign disease. Ann Surg 191:19–22, 1980
340. Appleman RM, Morlock CG, Dahlin DC et al: Long-term survival in carcinoma of the gallbladder. Surg Gynecol Obstet 17:459–464, 1963
341. Frank SA, Spjut HJ: Inapparent carcinoma of the gallbladder. Am Surg 33:367–372, 1967
342. Jones CJ: Carcinoma of the gallbladder. A clinical and pathological analysis of fifty cases. Ann Surg 132:110–120, 1950
343. Vaittinen E: Carcinoma of the gallbladder: A study of 390 cases diagnosed in Finland 1953–1967. Ann Chir Gynaecol [Suppl] 168:7–81, 1970
344. Edmonsdon HA: Tumors of the Gallbladder and Extrahepatic Bile Ducts, Section VII, Fascicle 26. Washington DC, Armed Forces Institute of Pathology, 1967
345. Frierson HF, Fechner RE: Pathology of malignant neoplasms of the gallbladder and extrahepatic bile ducts. In Wanebo HJ (ed): Hepatic and Biliary Cancer, pp 281–297. New York, Marcel Dekker, 1987
346. Berk RN, Armbuster TG, Saltzstein SL: Carcinoma in the porcelain gallbladder. Radiology 106:29–31, 1973
347. Polk HC Jr: Carcinoma and the calcified gall bladder. Gastroenterology 50:582–585, 1966
348. Alpers CE, Smuckler EA: Pleomorphic carcinoma of the gallbladder. Case report and ultrastructural study. Ultrastruct Pathol 6:29–38, 1984
349. Appleman HD, Coopersmith N: Pleomorphic spindle-cell carcinoma of the gallbladder. Relation to sarcoma of the gallbladder. Cancer 25:535–541, 1970
350. Black WC, Key CR, Carmany TB et al: Carcinoma of the gallbladder in a population of Southwestern American Indians. Cancer 39:1269–1279, 1977
351. Albores-Saavedra J, Soriano J, Larraza-Hernandez O et al: Oak cell carcinoma of the gallbladder. Hum Pathol 15:639–646, 1984
352. Fahim RB, McDonald JR, Richards JC et al: Carcinoma of the gallbladder: A study of its modes of spread. Ann Surg 156:114–124, 1962
353. Ohlsson EG, Aronsen KF: Carcinoma of the gallbladder. A study of 181 cases. Acta Chir Scand 140:475–480, 1974
354. Hamrick RE Jr, Liner FJ, Hastings PR et al: Primary carcinoma of the gallbladder. Ann Surg 195:270–273, 1982
355. Detweiler DG, Biddinger P, Staab EV et al: The appearance of adenomyomatosis with the newer imaging modalities: A case with pathologic correlation. J Ultrasound Med 1:295–298, 1982
356. Lampman LE, Meijer JG, Stroucken AA: Sonographic detection of early gallbladder cancer. Diagn Imag Clin Med 53:99–103, 1984
357. Sato T, Koyama K, Yamauchi H et al: Early carcinoma of the gallbladder. Gastroenterol Jpn 16:459–464, 1981
358. Adson MA: Carcinoma of the gallbladder. In Moody F (ed): Advances in Diagnosis and Treatment of Biliary Tract Disease, Ch 12. New York, Masson, 1983
359. Tashiro S, Konno T, Mochinaga M et al: Treatment of carcinoma of the gallbladder in Japan. Jpn J Surg 12:98–104, 1982
360. Pack GT, Miller TR, Brasfield RD: Total right hepatic lobectomy for cancer of the gallbladder: Report of three cases. Ann Surg 142:6–16, 1955
361. Brasfield RD: Right hepatic lobectomy for carcinoma of the gallbladder: A five-year cure. Ann Surg 153:563–566, 1961
362. Pemberton LB, Diffenbaugh WF, Strohl EL: The surgical significance of carcinoma of the gallbladder. Am J Surg 122:381–383, 1971
363. Burdette WJ: Carcinoma of the gallbladder. Ann Surg 145:832, 1957
364. Shepard VD, Walters W, Dockerty MD: Benign neoplasms of the gallbladder. Arch Surg 45:1, 1942
365. Arbab A, Brasfield R: Benign tumors of the gallbladder. Surgery 61:535–540, 1967
366. Albores-Saavedra J, Alcantra-Vazquez A, Cruz-Ortiz H et al: The precursor lesions of invasive gallbladder carcinoma: Hyperplasia, atypical hyperplasia and carcinoma in situ. Cancer 45:919–927, 1980
367. Kozuka S, Tsubone N, Yasui A et al: Relation of adenoma to carcinoma in the gallbladder. Cancer 50:2226–2234, 1982
368. Castle WN, Wanebo HJ, Fechner RE: Carcinoma of the gallbladder and cholecystectomy. Arch Surg 117:946–948, 1982
369. Nagashima H, Watanabe A, Hayashi S et al: Primary carcinoma of the gallbladder and the extrahepatic bile duct. Gastroenterology 17:246–253, 1982
370. Hanna SS, Rider WD: Carcinoma of the gallbladder or extrahepatic bile ducts: The role of radiotherapy. Can Med Assoc J 118:59–61, 1978

371. Treadwell TA, Harding WJ: Primary carcinoma of the gallbladder. The role of adjunctive therapy in its treatment. Am J Surg: 703–706, 1976
372. Abe M, Takahashi M: Intraoperative radiotherapy: The Japanese experience. Int J Radiat Oncol Biol Phys 7:863–868, 1981
373. Schein DS, Stablein DM, Novah JW et al: A comparison of combination chemotherapy and combined modality therapy for locally adrenal gastric cancer. Cancer 49:1771–1777, 1982
374. Andrews W, Smith F: Chemotherapy for cholangiocarcinoma and gallbladder cancer. In Wanebo HJ (ed): Hepatic and Biliary Cancer, pp 453–457. New York, Marcel Dekker, 1987
375. Haskell CM: Cancer of the liver. In Haskell CM (ed): Cancer Treatment, pp 319–357. Philadelphia, WB Saunders, 1980
376. Davis HL Jr, Ramirez G, Ansfield FJ: Adenocarcinoma of stomach, pancreas, liver, and biliary tracts: Survival of 328 patients treated with fluoropyrimidine therapy. Cancer 33:193–197, 1974
377. Crooke ST, Bradner WT: Mitomycin-C: A review. Cancer Treat Rev 3:121–139, 1976
378. Von Eyben F, Hellekant C, Mattson M et al: Mitomycin-C in advanced gallbladder carcinoma. Acta Radiol [Diagn] (Stockh) 19:81–84, 1980
379. Adolphson CC, Carpenter JT Jr: Response to doxorubicin and mitomycin in cholangiocarcinoma: A case report. Cancer Treat Rep 66:209–210, 1982
380. Bodey GP, Bedikian AY, Valdivieso M et al: Chemotherapeutic management of hepatobiliary and pancreatic cancer. In Stroehlein JR, Romsdahl MM (eds): Gastrointestinal Cancer, pp 279–292. New York, Raven Press, 1981
381. Bukowski RM, Leichman LP, Rivkin SE: Phase II trial of m-AMSA in gallbladder and cholangiocarcinoma: A Southwest Oncology Group study. Eur J Cancer Clin Oncol 6:721–723, 1983
382. Harvey JH, Smith FP, Schein PS: 5-Fluorouracil, mitomycin, and doxorubicin (FAM) in carcinoma of the biliary tract. J Clin Oncol (Suppl 11)2:1245–1248, 1984
383. Hall SH, Benjamin RS, Murphy WK et al: Adriamycin, BCNU, Ftorafur chemotherapy of pancreatic and biliary tract cancer. Cancer 44:2008–2013, 1974
384. Ravey M Jr, Hester M: Phase II study of adriamycin plus bleomycin for the treatment of hepatocellular and biliary tract carcinoma. Proc Am Soc Clin Oncol 20:415, 1979
385. Misra NC, Jaiswal MSD, Singh RV et al: Intrahepatic arterial infusion of combination of mytomycin-C and 5-fluorouracil in treatment of primary and metastatic liver carcinoma. Cancer 39:1425–1429, 1977
386. Oswalt CE, Cruz AB: Effectiveness of chemotherapy in addition to surgery in treating carcinoma of the gallbladder. Rev Surg 34:436–438, 1977
387. Pilepich MV, Lambert PM: Radiotherapy of carcinomas of the extrahepatic biliary system. Radiology 127:767–770, 1978
388. Wanebo HJ: Carcinoma of the gallbladder. In Wanebo HJ (ed): Hepatic and Biliary Cancer, pp 431–445. New York, Marcel Dekker, 1987

WILLIAM F. SINDELAR

CHAPTER 28 *Cancer of the Small Intestine*

Neoplasms are uncommon in the duodenum and small intestine. The small bowel accounts for more than 75% of the length and more than 90% of the mucosal absorptive surface of the entire gastrointestinal (GI) tract; however, fewer than 5% of all GI neoplasms arise in the small intestine.[1,2] Cancers of the duodenum and small intestine constitute about 1% of all gastrointestinal tract malignancies.[3–5]

The diagnosis of neoplasms of the duodenum or small intestine can be difficult to establish because symptoms may be vague and nonspecific.[6,7] Metastatic disease is frequently present at the time of diagnosis of malignant tumors, and the prognosis is not favorable for small bowel cancers.[7,8] Surgical resection can cure some patients with small intestinal malignancies.[7–10] However, radiotherapy, chemotherapy, and other treatment modalities have been of little benefit in managing malignant diseases of the small intestine.[7,8,11–15]

HISTORY

Neoplasms occurring in the small intestine were first recognized in 1655.[16] The first clinically reported small bowel tumor was a duodenal carcinoma described in 1746.[17] Wesner discovered a leiomyosarcoma of the small intestine in 1883.[18] The first successful surgical resection of a small intestinal tumor was reported by Fleiner in 1885.[19]

Early reviews of small intestinal neoplasms were compiled by Heurtaux in 1899 and by King in 1917.[20,21] Modern reviews have examined benign or malignant tumors of the duodenum and small intestine.[1,3,4,6–10,14–16,22–32]

EPIDEMIOLOGY

Duodenal and small intestinal tumors have been reported in patients whose ages range from 1 year to 84 years, with a mean age of 59 years.[1,7,8,23] The average age at presentation of patients with benign neoplasms is 62 years, whereas patients with intestinal malignancies present at a mean age of 57 years.[33] The annual incidence of clinically diagnosed small bowel neoplasms in the United States is approximately 1200 cases.[5,34] The age-adjusted incidence in the United States for clinically diagnosed small intestinal neoplasms in the white population is 1.2 per 100,000 for men and 0.8 per 100,000 for women.[34] The incidence per 100,000 blacks is 1.6 for men and 0.7 for women.[34] The incidence and distribution of small intestinal tumors appears to be uniform worldwide.[5,8]

The autopsy incidence of small intestinal tumors is 0.2%, but the operative incidence of neoplasms of the small bowel is less than 0.01%.[35] Most benign tumors are asymptomatic and clinically innocent, but most malignancies become symptomatic and require surgical intervention.[8,36–39] Clinical series of symptomatic patients have revealed symmetric distribution of benign and malignant small intestinal tumors.[7–10,24,33–43] Table 28-1 summarizes the distribution of benign and malignant neoplasms of the duodenum and small intestine in various clinical series.[7–10,24,33,36–43]

Duodenal and small intestinal neoplasms are associated with certain inherited disorders of the GI tract, including familial polyposis, Gardner's syndrome, Peutz–Jeghers syndrome, Crohn's disease, celiac disease, and neurofibromatosis.

875

TABLE 28-1. Benign and Malignant Neoplasms of the Duodenum and Small Intestine

Author	Year	Number of Neoplasms		
		Benign	Malignant	Total
Darling et al[24]	1959	46	86	132
Krouse et al[36]	1961	24	12	36
Botsford et al[33]	1962	71	44	115
Skandalakis et al[9]	1962	340	257	597
Sawyer et al[37]	1963	23	27	50
Schmutzer et al[38]	1964	59	41	100
Ebert et al[10]	1965	48	29	77
Ostermiller et al[39]	1966	77	122	199
Spratt[40]	1966	11	19	30
Freund et al[41]	1978	37	79	116
Miles et al[42]	1979	11	31	42
Herbsman et al[8]	1980	20	54	74
Mittal et al[7]	1980	15	39	54
Giuliani et al[43]	1985	5	43	48
TOTAL		787 (47%)	883 (53%)	1670

ETIOLOGY

There have been no factors identified as having a definite role in the etiology of duodenal and small intestinal neoplasms. Because of the rarity of small bowel tumors compared with neoplasms occurring in the large bowel, stomach, or esophagus, there have been proposals that local factors in the small intestine may function in the prevention of neoplasia or in the deactivation of possible carcinogens.

The lack of acid in the small intestinal lumen has been suggested to be protective against tumorigenesis.[8,9] Neoplasms frequently are encountered in areas of GI tract acidity, such as the stomach and colon. Nitrosamines, which are potent experimental GI carcinogens, are formed only in acid environments.[44]

The rapid peristalsis of the small bowel has been suggested to protect against neoplasia in the duodenum and small bowel, possibly by minimizing the time of mucosal exposure to carcinogenic agents.[45] It has been proposed that the liquid small bowel content may be less abrasive or irritating to the mucosa than are particulates in the esophagus, chyme in the stomach, or fecal matter in the colon.[46]

Benzopyrene hydroxylase is present in large amounts in the mucosa of the small intestine and may detoxify carcinogens.[8,47] A large concentration of secretory immunoglobulin in the small intestine has been considered protective against the development of tumors, possibly by neutralizing oncogenic viruses.[28]

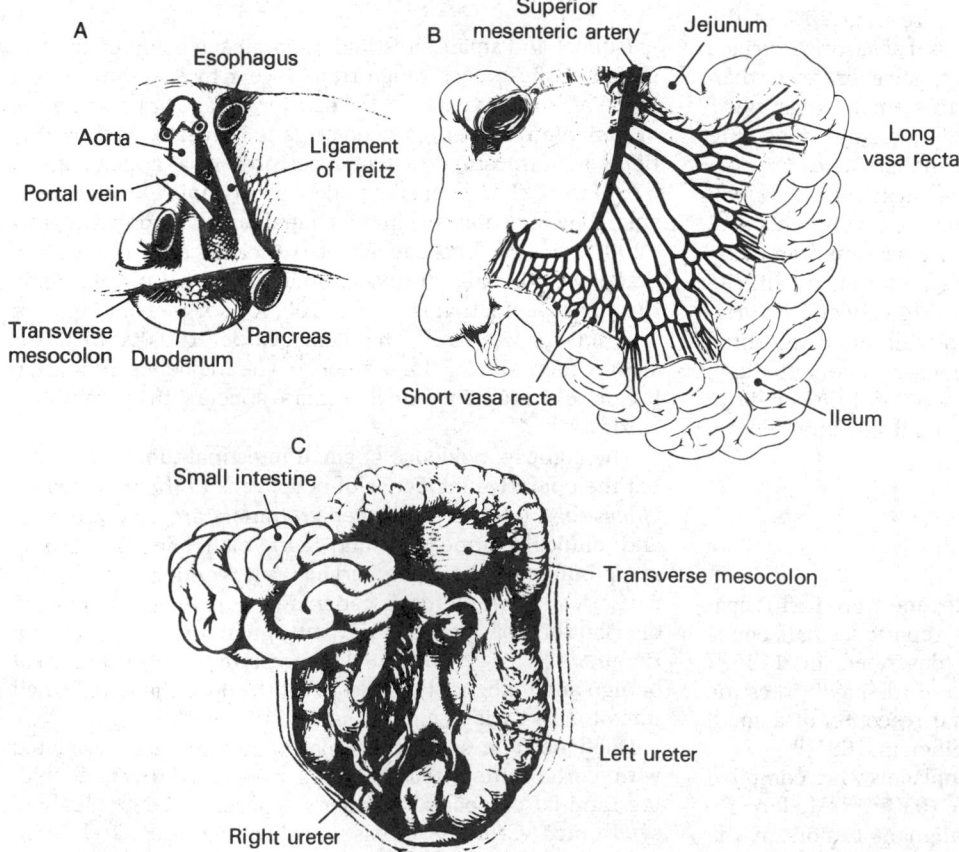

FIG. 28-1. Anatomy of the small intestine. **A.** Relationships of the duodenum. **B.** Vascular supply of the small intestine. **C.** Mesentery of the small intestine. (Adapted from Healey JE: A Synopsis of Clinical Anatomy, p 179. Philadelphia, WB Saunders, 1969)

The relative absence of bacteria in the duodenum and small intestine, compared with the esophagus or colon, may protect against neoplastic transformation resulting from bacterially produced carcinogens.[28]

ANATOMY

ANATOMIC RELATIONSHIPS

The small bowel is more than 600 cm long, extending from the gastric pyloric ring to the colonic ileocecal valve. The small bowel comprises the duodenum, jejunum, and ileum (Fig. 28-1).

The duodenum extends horizontally to the right from the pyloric ring as an intraperitoneal structure and then turns caudally to become retroperitoneal, surrounding the head of the pancreas and receiving openings from the biliary and pancreatic ducts. The duodenum then extends horizontally to the left, passing dorsally to the superior mesenteric vessels before turning superiorly and emerging as an intraperitoneal segment at the ligament of Treitz. The duodenum derives its arterial supply from the gastroduodenal branches of both the celiac axis and superior mesenteric artery. Duodenal venous drainage is into the portal system. Figure 28-2 illustrates the vascular anatomy in the region of the duodenum. Duodenal lymphatics drain behind the head of the pancreas into the pancreaticoduodenal group and into the celiac nodes.

The jejunum begins at the ligament of Treitz, situated to the left of the second lumbar vertebra, and extends caudally from the free border of the mesentery. The arterial supply is derived from branches of the superior mesenteric artery. Venous drainage is through mesenteric tributaries that terminate in the portal vein through the superior mesenteric vein. Lymphatic drainage flows through the mesentery, with nodes located within the mesenteric leaflets.

The ileum is located distal to and is continuous with the jejunum, with an indistinct division between the distal jejunum and proximal ileum. Arterial branches supply the ileum from the ileocolic artery, which arises as a branch of the superior mesenteric artery. Venous drainage into the portal system is through the superior mesenteric vein. Numerous lymph nodes occur along lymphatic channels that pass through the mesentery.

The mesentery attaches obliquely to the dorsal abdominal wall in a line extending from the left of the second lumbar vertebra to the right iliac fossa. The free mesenteric border fans out to allow convolutions within the abdominal cavity of the small intestine, which attaches to the edge of the mesentery. The small intestinal arterial supply, venous drainage, and lymphatic channels are supported within the mesentery. Blood vessels anastomose freely in the mesentery through arcades that supply the intestine through segmental branches.

MICROSCOPIC ANATOMY

The small intestine is a tubular organ containing an inner mucosal layer, a middle muscular layer composed of an inner circular and outer longitudinal array of smooth muscle, and an outer serosal layer of peritoneum and connective tissue.

The lining of the small intestine is arranged into circular folds, the valvulae conniventes, which increase the surface area of the mucosa. Valvulae are prominent in the duodenum, well developed in the jejunum, and poorly developed in the ileum. Mucosal villi are formed by epithelial foldings and provide a large absorptive surface area. The lining epithelium comprises columnar epithelial cells, goblet cells, and enterochromaffin cells.

The submucosa contains supportive connective tissue and carries the intestinal blood supply in both longitudinal and circular directions through a submucosal plexus. The submucosa contains considerable amounts of connective tissue throughout the small intestine, with increasing concentrations distally in the bowel.

The muscular portion of the small intestinal wall is formed of smooth muscle with small amounts of connective tissue, as well as blood vessels and lymphatics. The inner, circular muscular layer is thick. The thin, outer muscular layer is longitudinally oriented. The myenteric nerve plexus is con-

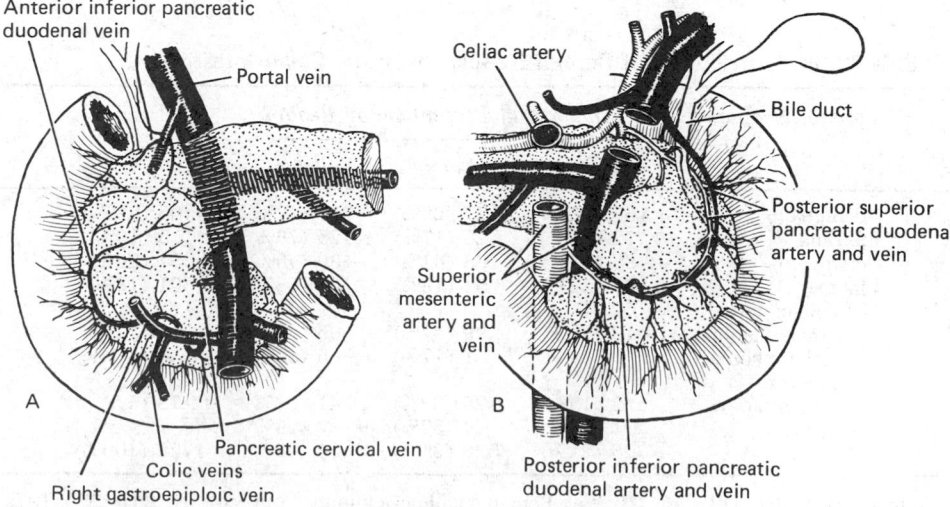

FIG. 28-2. Anatomy of the duodenum. **A.** Anterior view with pancreatic and duodenal vessels. **B.** Posterior view with posterior vascular arcades. (Edwards EA, Malone PD, MacArthur JD: Operative Anatomy of Abdomen and Pelvis, p 127. Philadelphia, Lea & Febiger, 1975)

TABLE 28-2.   Classification of Neoplasms of the Duodenum and Small Intestine

Tissue of Origin	Benign	Malignant
Epithelium	Adenoma	Adenocarcinoma
Connective tissue	Fibroma	Fibrosarcoma
Smooth muscle	Leiomyoma	Leiomyosarcoma
Fat	Lipoma	Liposarcoma
Vascular tissue	Hemangioma	Angiosarcoma
	Lymphangioma	
Lymphoid tissue	Pseudolymphoma	Lymphoma
Nerve	Neurofibroma	Neurofibrosarcoma
	Neurilemmoma	Malignant schwannoma
Argentaffin	—	Carcinoid

tained in the connective tissue that separates the circular and longitudinal muscular layers.

The serosa is composed of epithelium that forms a peritoneal surface over a subserosa of loose connective tissue. The serosa covers the intestinal tube, except at the point of mesenteric attachment, where the intestinal serosa is continuous with the peritoneal epithelium of the mesentery.

PATHOLOGY

Benign or malignant intestinal neoplasms can arise from any portion of the duodenum, jejunum, or ileum.[48,49] Small intestinal tumors are classified in Table 28-2.

The most frequently encountered benign tumors of the small intestine are adenomas, leiomyomas, and lipomas.[48–51] Fibromas and neurofibromas are uncommon small bowel neoplasms.[50–52] Intestinal neurofibromas are sometimes seen in patients with neurofibromatosis. Vascular tumors, such as hemangiomas and lymphangiomas, are unusual. Hamartomas of the small intestine are associated with the Peutz–Jeghers syndrome. Lymphoid hyperplasia in the small intestine can lead to the formation of polypoid masses, and small intestinal pseudolymphoma can occur.[5,53,54] The distribution of benign neoplasms in the duodenum, jejunum, and ileum is given in Table 28-3.[29]

Adenocarcinomas make up about half of the malignancies involving the small intestine, and carcinoid tumors account for about 35% of malignant lesions.[3,8] Leiomyosarcomas are among the most common of the small intestine sarcomas which develop in the small intestine, and angiosarcomas and liposarcomas are seen rarely.[50] Neurofibrosarcomas occur in the small bowel and occasionally are associated with neurofibromatosis. Although secondary lymphomatous involvement of the small bowel regularly is seen in disseminated lymphomas, malignant lymphomas occur rarely as primary tumors. The distribution of malignant neoplasms in the duodenum, jejunum, and ileum is given in Table 28-4.[28,30,54]

CLINICAL FEATURES

SYMPTOMS

Benign small bowel tumors may remain occult and cause no symptoms, being found incidentally at autopsy.[24,33] The lack of symptoms may be due to the distensibility of the small intestine and the low viscosity of bowel fluid, which allow the passage of small bowel content in spite of partial occlusion of the intestinal lumen.[8] Approximately half of all patients with benign small bowel tumors eventually become symptomatic, usually presenting with abdominal pain.[2,24] The pain may be related to partial or complete intestinal obstruction, which is present in more than 50% of symptomatic cases. Intussusception is often the cause of intestinal obstruction, with the tumor acting as a lead point. Benign small bowel neoplasm is the most frequent cause of adult intussusception.[24] Intestinal obstruction often is chronic and intermittent, probably because of the distensibility of the small bowel, allowing the passage of bowel content around lesions of substantial size.[1,2,8,13–15] The symptoms produced by a proximal obstruction in the duodenum or jejunum usually are unrelenting nausea and vomiting with cramping epigastric pain. Distal obstructing lesions in the ileum typically result in intermittent vomiting, abdominal distension, and cramping periumbilical pain.

Hemorrhage may occur from benign tumors resulting from mucosal involvement by the neoplastic process, which becomes manifest in approximately 25% of symptomatic

TABLE 28-3.   Distribution of Benign Neoplasms in the Small Intestine

Type of Neoplasm	Number and Percentage by Region			Total
	Duodenum	Jejunum	Ileum	
Adenoma	167 (33%)	127 (25%)	211 (42%)	505 (29%)
Fibroma	12 (7%)	28 (17%)	125 (76%)	165 (10%)
Leiomyoma	86 (19%)	188 (41%)	180 (40%)	454 (26%)
Lipoma	72 (24%)	54 (18%)	175 (58%)	301 (18%)
Hemangioma and lymphangioma	18 (8%)	99 (47%)	95 (45%)	212 (12%)
Pseudolymphoma	0	1 (17%)	5 (83%)	6 (<1%)
Neurofibroma and neurilemmoma	12 (15%)	25 (32%)	41 (53%)	78 (5%)
Hamartoma	1 (14%)	4 (57%)	2 (29%)	7 (<1%)
TOTAL	368 (21%)	526 (31%)	834 (48%)	1728 (100%)

Wilson JM, Melvin DB, Gray GF et al: Benign small bowel tumor. Ann Surg 181:247–250, 1975.

TABLE 28-4. Distribution of Malignant Neoplasms in the Small Intestine

Type of Neoplasm	Number and Percentage by Region			Total
	Duodenum	Jejunum	Ileum	
Adenocarcinoma	427 (40%)	408 (38%)	241 (22%)	1076 (46%)
Sarcoma	46 (10%)	162 (36%)	239 (54%)	447 (19%)
Lymphoma	4 (16%)	9 (36%)	12 (48%)	25 (1%)
Carcinoid	48 (6%)	78 (10%)	682 (84%)	808 (34%)
TOTAL	525 (22%)	660 (28%)	1171 (50%)	2356 (100%)

Loehr WH, Mujahed Z, Zahn FD, et al: Primary lymphoma of the gastrointestinal tract: A review of 100 cases. Ann Surg 170:232–238, 1969; Wilson JM, Melvin DB, Gray GF, et al: Primary malignancies of the small bowel: A report of 96 cases and review of the literature. Ann Surg 180:175–179, 1974; Barclay THC, Schapira DV: Malignant tumors of the small intestine. Cancer 51:878–881, 1983.

patients.[9,10,38] Hemorrhage is usually slow and chronic, resulting in anemia, weakness, and debilitation.[39] Severe intestinal bleeding sufficient to warrant surgical intervention is unusual in benign small bowel tumors.[24]

Malignant tumors of the small intestine produce symptoms in more than 75% of patients.[7–9,14,15,21,24–28,50,51] Pain is the most common presenting symptom, occurring in more than 65% of cases of malignant small bowel tumors.[8,14,24,37,51] The pain may occur intermittently as cramps or as diffuse, dull aches that may radiate through the abdomen or to the back. Weight loss occurs in more than half of the patients.[28,37,51] The most profound weight loss occurs in intestinal lymphomas. Symptoms of partial intestinal obstruction develop in approximately 35% of patients with malignant lesions.[8,15] Obstruction is usually due to malignant invasion of the intestinal wall, unlike benign intestinal tumors that frequently result in intussusception.

Hemorrhage may occur with small bowel malignancies.[10,39] Bleeding is often chronic and occult, leading to anemia. Rarely, massive hemorrhage may be the presenting complaint. Approximately 10% of patients with malignant small bowel tumors present with an acute abdomen resulting from bowel perforation and peritonitis.[24] Frequently the symptoms resulting from small intestinal malignancies may be vague and nonspecific, leading to difficulties in diagnosis.[52,54] Diarrhea or steatorrhea may occur, particularly with lymphomas involving the duodenum or jejunum.[53] Carcinoids can produce the carcinoid syndrome, characterized by cutaneous flushing, cyanosis, chronic diarrhea, and intermittent respiratory distress.[55,56] The carcinoid syndrome is manifest only in the presence of metastatic disease.

SIGNS

The clinical examination in patients with benign small intestinal tumors may be unrewarding, with many patients presenting with no abnormal findings.[57] Benign tumors are not palpable unless they are very large. If palpable, benign neoplasms typically are freely moveable.[5,10] Distension and visible peristaltic waves may be present in intestinal obstruction. Intussusception may cause the appearance of a tender, palpable mass, and melanotic stool may be present. Benign tumors may cause intestinal bleeding, which produces anemia and stools positive for gross or occult blood.

Malignancies of the small intestine often present without specific clinical findings but with indications of intestinal dysfunction or obstruction. Signs of weight loss are common as presenting findings, and cachexia may be present if the disease is advanced.[33] An abdominal mass is palpable in approximately 25% of cases.[4,8,33] Intestinal obstruction develops in about 25% of patients, with abdominal distension a frequent finding.[57,58] Gross or occult blood may be present in the stool if there has been hemorrhage from the tumor, and anemia frequently is present. Clinical jaundice is seen routinely with duodenal malignancies. Peritonitis can occur with tumors that have perforated the intestinal wall. Steatorrhea and malabsorption can be present with small intestinal malignancies, especially with lymphomas, in which villous atrophy of the intestinal mucosa occurs.[54,58–61] Peripheral lymphadenopathy may be present in disseminated lymphomas. Hypertension and cutaneous hyperemia may be present as a consequence of advanced carcinoid tumor.

DIAGNOSIS

GENERAL CONSIDERATIONS

The diagnosis of benign or malignant small intestinal tumors is difficult before surgical exploration because clinical symptoms and signs may be nonspecific and because diagnostic efforts may not confirm neoplasms. A correct preoperative diagnosis can be expected in less than half of the symptomatic patients.[39,50]

LABORATORY STUDIES

Laboratory studies rarely reveal specific abnormalities in patients with small intestinal neoplasms. A hypochromic, microcytic anemia may result from chronic blood loss from tumor ulceration. Elevations of bilirubin and hepatic enzymes routinely result from duodenal neoplasms that obstruct the bile duct. Hyperamylasemia can evolve following obstruction of the pancreatic duct by duodenal tumors. Tumor markers, such as carcinoembryonic antigen, are rarely elevated in small intestinal tumors unless metastatic disease is present in the liver. Carcinoid tumors frequently cause elevated levels of 5-hydroxyindoleacetic acid in the urine.

RADIOLOGIC STUDIES

Roentgenographic examinations are useful in the diagnosis of small intestinal neoplasms. Abdominal films are generally nonspecific in asymptomatic patients. If intestinal obstruction is present, air–fluid levels and intestinal dilatation can be observed. In bulky intestinal tumors, a mass may be visible on routine abdominal roentgenography.

Contrast radiography is the most valuable roentgenographic modality for diagnosing small intestinal tumors. Upper GI series with small bowel follow-through have been successful in demonstrating tumors of the small intestine, particularly in obstructing malignant lesions, for which the diagnostic accuracy can be as high as 50%.[27] The GI series can sometimes distinguish among various types of small bowel lesions.[8] Intraluminal masses typically represent benign intestinal lesions such as polyps or leiomyomas. Intramural masses that thicken the intestinal wall but cause little or no mucosal changes suggest mural sarcomas or malignant lymphomas. Ulcerative mucosal lesions generally result from carcinomas. GI series may demonstrate intussusception. Through the administration of glucagon or anticholinergic agents, hypotonic duodenography may improve the visualization of the duodenum and small bowel by arresting intestinal motility at the time of contrast roentgenography.[62] Selective intubation of the small intestine may be possible using Miller-Abbott or Cantor tubes, allowing detailed study of isolated intestinal segments through the direct instillation of contrast material and air. The distal ileum usually is poorly visualized in upper GI contrast studies, but it may be demonstrated through barium enemas in which contrast material from the colon is refluxed into the distal small intestine.

Angiography may be of benefit in the diagnosis and localization of small intestinal neoplasms. A tumor blush may be present on angiogram in vascular neoplasms such as carcinoids or hemangiomas. Displacement of normal bowel vascular architecture can occur with hypovascular tumors such as carcinomas. Vascular malformations of the small intestine are often demonstrated angiographically by the appearance of abnormal concentrations of blood vessels or arteriovenous shunting. Actively bleeding intestinal neoplasms may be localized by angiographic examination.

Chest roentgenography should be performed in the evaluation of patients for small intestinal tumors to examine for possible metastatic tumor deposits. Lung tomography should be performed to evaluate any questionable pulmonary metastatic lesions.[63]

Computed tomographic (CT) body scans have improved roentgenographic sensitivity and accuracy over conventional x-rays in diagnosing intra-abdominal neoplasms. However, body scans are rarely helpful in the detection of small intestinal tumors. The presence of fluid and gas within the small bowel can obscure masses within the intestinal wall or obscure projections into the bowel lumen. CT scans may benefit the definition of large tumors extending beyond the intestinal wall and may assist in the demonstration of advanced metastatic disease by resolving hepatic metastases or by revealing mesenteric lymphadenopathy or peritoneal tumor implants.

Magnetic resonance imaging (MRI) demonstrates neoplasms of the small intestine as intra-abdominal masses with signal intensities varying from the characteristics and configuration of normal bowel. Metastatic deposits may be detected by MRI in the mesentery, retroperitoneum, or liver.

Diagnostic ultrasonography is useful in evaluating intra-abdominal masses, particularly in distinguishing solid from cystic lesions. Ultrasonography has little role, however, in the diagnosis of small intestinal neoplasms because the fluid content of the bowel assumes a sonic density similar to the density of the intestinal wall and of intestinal tumors, obscuring the ultrasonic detection of small bowel masses. The presence of gas in the small bowel blocks the ultrasonic transmission and thereby eliminates the possibility of detection of masses in regions of gaseous bowel distension. Large tumors extending outside the intestine can be visualized, and ultrasound can reveal disseminated disease, particularly liver metastases.

RADIOISOTOPIC SCANS

Radionuclide scans have little role in diagnosing small bowel neoplasms because intestinal tumors rarely take up imaging agents selectively. Nonspecific intestinal incorporation of imaging material may obscure the visualization of bowel tumors in gallium scans. However, radioisotopic scans may be of benefit in detecting small bowel neoplasms that have metastasized. Liver scans show metastatic foci as hepatic filling defects, and bone scans demonstrate radionuclide uptake by osseous metastases.

ENDOSCOPIC EXAMINATIONS

Endoscopy can be used to examine the duodenum. Using flexible fiberscopes, the entire duodenum and portions of the proximal jejunum can be visualized. Direct biopsies or cytologic samples can be obtained. Periampullary lesions can be evaluated directly by endoscopic cannulation of the biliary and pancreatic ducts through the papilla of Vater and by directly injecting contrast material for roentgenographic visualization. The distal ileum occasionally can be examined by fiberoptic colonoscopy by passing the endoscope through the ileocecal valve and viewing the ileum retrograde. Experimental endoscopes capable of visualizing the entire small intestine are being developed.

TREATMENT

Therapy depends on the histologic type of small intestinal tumor and upon the malignant potential of the neoplasm. General principles can be followed in treating tumors of the duodenum and small intestine.

Surgery is the indicated treatment for virtually all symptomatic tumors of the small intestine. Benign tumors can be removed by local excision. Small tumors, particularly pedunculated neoplasms, can be removed adequately by enterotomy and simple excision of the lesion. Large sessile tumors may require segmental resection of the involved portion of intestine, with reestablishment of bowel continuity by end-to-end intestinal anastomosis. Malignant tumors require extensive surgical excision, which includes segmental resection of the involved bowel with wide margins around the neoplasm, including the mesentery with the vascular and lymphatic pedicle. Lesions in the jejunum and ileum are amenable to radical segmental resection. However, anatomic difficulties are encountered in attempts to radically extirpate tumors in the duodenum because of the retroperitoneal location of the duodenum and its proximity to the pancreas, biliary system, portal venous system, and stomach. Duodenotomy and local excision of benign tumors are possible. Segmental resection can be performed only in the distal free portion of the duodenum. Adequate resection of malignant duodenal lesions in the proximal portion or in the C-loop usually requires pancreaticoduodenectomy (Whipple's operation).

For nonresectable small intestinal tumors, surgical palliation is indicated if intestinal obstruction is present. Usually an obstruction is palliated through bypass, anastomosing unobstructed intestine proximal to the lesion to bowel located distal to the site of obstruction.

Radiation therapy has little role in the treatment of primary small intestinal neoplasms, although it sometimes palliates advanced disseminated disease by relieving pain in areas of metastatic deposits, such as the liver or bone. Chemotherapy has little impact on primary small intestinal neoplasms and is used only for the treatment of metastatic bowel malignancies. Adjuvant radiotherapy and chemotherapy are controversial treatment modalities in small bowel tumors and are subjects of current clinical investigations.

BENIGN NEOPLASMS

ADENOMAS

Adenomas are benign proliferations of epithelium arising from the mucosa or glandular elements. They comprise approximately 30% of all benign small intestinal neoplasms.[8,27,37,64,65] Adenomas can occur as adenomatous polyps, villous adenomas, and Brunner's gland adenomas.

Adenomatous polyps are found throughout the small intestine. They are located commonly in the ileum and in the duodenum but are also found in the jejunum.[8,23,24,27,51] Adenomatous polyps are usually solitary, but multiple polyps may occur within the small bowel. Rarely, the entire GI tract is involved in a polyposis syndrome.[23,37,66] Adenomatous polyps typically are pedunculated, but sessile polyps sometimes can be found. Adenomatous polyps often are asymptomatic and are identified incidentally at autopsy.[24,33] Symptomatic polyps usually present with intermittent intestinal obstruction caused by intussusception, with the polyp acting as the lead point.[2,13-15] Polyps frequently produce chronic, slow intestinal hemorrhage, leading to anemia.[10] Rarely, small intestinal adenomatous polyps result in profuse bleeding.[39]

Indications for the treatment of small intestinal adenomatous polyps include obstruction and hemorrhage. Pedunculated polyps may be excised at the base of the stalk by ente-

rotomy. Some duodenal polyps may be removed endoscopically. For sessile polyps, complete excision of the base is required. Segmental intestinal resection may be necessary to prevent luminal narrowing after the removal of large polyps. Intussuscepted bowel segments must be reduced in all cases of intestinal obstruction, and segmental resection should be performed on any portion of the intestine suspected of vascular compromise. If no ischemic or damaged bowel results after intussusception reduction, simple enterotomy and polyp excision are sufficient treatment.

Villous adenomas are sessile polyps that form exuberant fronds.[67-69] They occur rarely in the small bowel. They are found most often in the duodenum but occasionally occur in the jejunum and ileum.[70,71] Most villous adenomas are smaller than 5 cm in diameter, but some may attain large sizes before becoming symptomatic.[72-74] Malignant degeneration has been reported in almost half of the villous adenomas exceeding 5 cm.[74,75] Malignancy is rare in small villous adenomas. Typical symptoms produced by villous adenomas are intestinal bleeding and intermittent cramping pain.[76] Bouts of intermittent partial intestinal obstruction develop in approximately 35% of patients.[74] Intestinal hemorrhage is seen in about half of the symptomatic patients and is usually associated with malignant degeneration.[74] Bleeding is usually occult or mild; however, massive bleeding from villous adenomas has been reported.[66] Villous adenomas in the small intestine are not heavily secretory and do not produce diarrhea and electrolyte loss as can villous adenomas located in the colon.[8] The diagnosis of intestinal villous adenomas can be established by contrast radiography in approximately 75% of cases.[71,77,78] Villous adenomas characteristically produce filling defects with striated patterns on roentgenographs, indicating where the contrast material infiltrates among the villous fronds.

The treatment of villous adenomas of the small intestine is surgical excision. Lesions should be removed because of the possibility of hemorrhage and malignant transformation. Although some small duodenal lesions may be amenable to endoscopic resection, the majority of villous adenomas require laparotomy for removal. Small lesions can be excised locally through enterotomy, but large lesions may require segmental bowel resection. For villous adenomas with evidence of malignant transformation, resection with wide margins of bowel and mesentery should be performed.

Adenomas of Brunner's glands are rare, pedunculated, solitary neoplasms found in the duodenum, which arise from the submucosal Brunner's glands that produce alkaline duodenal mucus.[26,79-81] Usually Brunner's gland adenomas are less than 1 cm in diameter. Malignant transformation has not been recognized, but adenomas of Brunner's glands can cause duodenal obstructive and hemorrhagic symptoms.[79] Clinically, they may mimic peptic ulcer disease, with epigastric pain, vomiting, and bleeding.[8] The diagnosis of Brunner's gland adenoma may be made by contrast roentgenography, which may show a duodenal polypoid lesion. Endoscopy and biopsy may establish the diagnosis. Symptomatic Brunner's gland adenomas should be surgically excised. Large tumors that are not amenable to local excision should be bypassed by gastroenterostomy, rather than performing a potentially hazardous pancreaticoduodenectomy for a benign neoplasm with no recognized potential for malignant transformation.

BENIGN TUMORS OF CONNECTIVE TISSUE

Benign tumors involving the small intestine can arise from connective tissues and include fibromas, lipomas, and tumors of vascular tissues.

Fibromas are rare benign neoplasms of connective tissue that typically are located within the intestinal wall.[82] Usually fibromas are smaller than 2 cm in diameter, although large tumors have been reported.[83] Fibromas can be pedunculated lesions, but most are sessile.[82,83] Most are asymptomatic and are discovered incidentally. Occasionally, intestinal fibromas can cause symptoms, including hemorrhage from mucosal ulceration and intestinal obstruction, chiefly intussusception. Symptomatic fibromas should be treated by surgical excision. Simple local excision suffices for small tumors, but large lesions may require segmental bowel resection.

Lipomas are neoplasms of mature adipose tissue that can be found throughout the GI tract as well-circumscribed tumors within the intestinal submucosa. More than 50% of all GI lipomas are found in the small intestine, accounting for approximately 20% of all benign small bowel neoplasms.[82] The incidence of lipomas increases distally in the small intestine, with 60% of lipomatous lesions in the ileum, 20% in the jejunum, and 20% in the duodenum.[24,29,84] Lipomas are usually solitary but can occur as multiple lesions. Their frequency increases with advancing age, and they are slightly more common in men than in women.[8] Lipomas of the small intestine remain asymptomatic in at least 35% of cases, being discovered incidentally.[83] Symptomatic lipomas usually cause cramping pain and intestinal obstruction, with intussusception occurring frequently.[29] Hemorrhage from intestinal lipomas is not common. The diagnosis of intestinal lipoma occasionally can be made on the basis of a GI series detecting the presence of a small bowel filling defect. Lipomas frequently occur at the ileocecal valve, where a filling defect may be demonstrated during a barium enema that refluxes into the small bowel. The treatment of symptomatic intestinal lipomas is surgical excision. Local excision is sufficient for small lesions, but for large or obstructing tumors, segmental intestinal resection is recommended.

Benign tumors of vascular tissue can occur in the duodenum and small intestine. Vascular neoplasms are considered to represent proliferative developmental malformations of vascular or lymphatic channels.[82,85]

Intestinal *hemangiomas* are rare benign tumors arising from a proliferation of vascular channels within the submucosal vascular plexus.[86-89] They account for approximately 10% of all benign tumors in the small bowel.[23,83] Hemangiomas are polypoid lesions that usually extend intraluminally. Large tumors may become annular, causing bowel constriction and mucosal ulceration.[86] Approximately 40% of intestinal hemangiomas are solitary. Single hemangiomas can be small and isolated or can involve long segments of the bowel.[82,86] Multiple lesions occur in 60% of patients with intestinal hemangiomas, with lesions found throughout the GI tract.[82,84,87,88] Hemangiomas are slightly more common in the jejunum than in the ileum, and they are unusual in the duodenum.[82,89] Hemangiomas appear grossly as congested small submucosal nodules. Multiple hemangiomas occurring in the GI tract are commonly designated as multiple phlebectasia. Although most cases of GI multiple phlebectasia are sporadic, a hereditary form exists, called the Osler–Weber–Rendu syndrome, in which telangiectatic lesions involve long segments of the small intestine.[85]

Most patients with intestinal hemangiomas develop clinical manifestations, especially diffuse intestinal bleeding.[8,82,87-90] Rarely, vague abdominal pain, intestinal obstructive symptoms, or intussusception characterize the clinical presentation. The diagnosis of intestinal hemangioma is difficult but should be suspected if hemangiomatous lesions are present in the skin or are detected on endoscopic examination of the esophagus, stomach, or colorectum. Hemangiomas of the small intestine may be revealed on contrast roentgenographic studies. Occasionally, they may be thrombosed and calcified, a condition that may be apparent on abdominal x-ray film.[91] Visceral angiography can detect arteriovenous malformations in hemangiomas and is often successful in confirming and locating intestinal hemangiomas when active hemorrhage is present.[92]

The treatment of symptomatic hemangiomas of the small intestine is surgical excision. Generally, the entire involved segment of bowel must be removed to ensure complete extirpation of the abnormal blood vessels giving rise to the tumor. Obstructing lesions should be removed by segmental bowel resection. Most instances of surgical intervention are for intestinal hemorrhage. Unless preoperative angiography can localize the point of hemorrhage, operative identification of the site of bleeding can be challenging. If a single lesion is present in the intestine, it may be identified by palpation or by inspection for fullness in the bowel wall. However, when multiple hemangiomas are present, localization of the bleeding can be difficult. Transillumination of the intestinal wall for hemorrhagic lesions, examination for engorgement of mesenteric vessels in the region of bleeding, division of the intestine and examination for bleeding in the lumen to determine whether hemorrhage is proximal or distal to the point of division, and multiple enterotomies to examine possible bleeding sources have been used to operatively localize bleeding hemangiomas in the small intestine.[86-89,92] Even if the bleeding site can be identified and resected, the patient may suffer future hemorrhage from unresected lesions if multiple phlebectasia is present.[8,87-90,93]

Lymphangiomas of the small intestine are rare tumors that arise from masses of dilated lymphatic vessels within the submucosa.[82,94] Lymphangiomas occur throughout the GI tract, usually as solitary intramural lesions, but occasionally as multiple lymphangiomas.[95] Most intestinal lymphangiomas are asymptomatic and are discovered incidentally. Rarely, lymphangiomas produce intussusception and intestinal obstruction. Symptomatic lymphangiomas should be treated by segmental resection of the involved bowel segment.

BENIGN TUMORS OF SMOOTH MUSCLE

Leiomyomas of the small intestine are benign neoplasms of smooth muscle. They are relatively common small bowel tumors, comprising about 25% of all benign intestinal tumors.[9,29,96] Leiomyomas are found throughout the small intestine, occurring equally in the jejunum and ileum and less commonly in the duodenum.[9,29,82] The benign tumors can occur in patients of any age, but the frequency increases with advancing age.[23,81,96] They typically occur with equal frequency in males and females.[9,23,96]

Leiomyomas grow as intramural masses that expand the intestinal wall. Tumor growth usually causes compression of the lumen and subserosal bulging.[29] A characteristic growth feature of leiomyomas involves central ulceration, probably from the compression of feeding blood vessels and resultant necrosis. The tumors typically are well-circumscribed but lack a true capsule. Leiomyomas frequently erode the overlying bowel mucosa. Leiomyomas produce clinical symptoms in more than 70% of patients.[9,23,29,82] Cramping, intermittent abdominal pain is a presenting symptom in at least 65% of patients.[29] Chronic intestinal obstructive symptoms are present in about 30% of cases.[29] Intussusception develops in about 15% of patients.[9,29] A palpable mass is present in up to 25% of patients with symptomatic leiomyomas.[9] Intestinal bleeding is a common clinical feature, often intermittent and frequently manifested as melena. Hematemesis can occur with lesions in the duodenum. Massive hemorrhage from intestinal leiomyomas is rare.[82] Patients with leiomyomas of the small bowel usually complain of fatigue, and many patients experience weight loss. The diagnosis of small intestinal leiomyoma sometimes can be established clinically. Detection of occult blood in the stool is possible in more than 50% of the symptomatic patients, and anemia usually is present.[8,16,23] Contrast radiography may identify an intestinal neoplasm, and ulcerations in the bowel mucosa sometimes are present at the site of the lesion. Leiomyomas of the small intestine should be treated surgically. Lesions should be removed by segmental bowel resection with margins of surrounding normal tissue.

OTHER BENIGN TUMORS OF THE SMALL INTESTINE

A variety of benign neoplasms can occur within the small intestine, including pseudolymphomas, neurogenic tumors, and hamartomas.

Pseudolymphoma of the small intestine presents as hyperplasia of lymphoid tissue in the bowel wall, which can occur with infectious stimuli such as viral illnesses or bacterial enteritis. Lymphoid hyperplasia has been reported with hypoglobulinemia, and lymphoid polyposis has been noted occasionally to precede the development of lymphoma or leukemia.[97,98] Enlarged lymphoid aggregates may cause abdominal pain or symptoms of intestinal obstruction. Usually, the enlarged lymphoid tissue collections are located in the ileum, but significant hypertrophy of lymphoid patches can occur in the jejunum. The duodenum rarely develops pseudolymphoma. Contrast radiologic studies may demonstrate enlarged lymphoid aggregates. Pseudolymphoma is a benign condition that resolves after treatment or removal of the infectious stimulus.

Benign tumors of neuroectodermal origin occur with low frequency in the small intestine, accounting for about 5% of all benign small bowel neoplasms.[23,29] *Neurofibromas* are composed of nerve elements and appear in the small intestine as nonencapsulated, intramural tumors. They can occur at any age as single, isolated lesions or as multiple neoplasms. Intestinal neurofibromas are found in von Recklinghausen's disease.[23,99–101] Neurofibromas usually occur in the ileum, but they also have been reported in the jejunum and duodenum.

Neurofibromas can remain asymptomatic, but an estimated 70% of patients eventually develop symptoms.[101] Pain occurs as the presenting symptom in approximately 40% of patients, and intestinal bleeding develops in 35%.[29] Intermittent intestinal obstruction can occur, often from intussusception.[82] The diagnosis of neurofibroma of the small intestine should be suspected in patients with the clinical manifestations of neurofibromatosis, including cutaneous neurofibromas, axillary freckling, and patchy skin pigmentation. The stool is usually positive for occult blood. Abdominal x-ray films may show signs of intestinal obstruction, and contrast roentgenography may demonstrate small bowel filling defects. Symptomatic intestinal neurofibromas are treated by surgical excision. Segmental intestinal resections are often necessary for bleeding lesions or obstruction. Small pedunculated tumors can be removed by local excision.

Neurilemmomas are benign tumors of nerve sheaths that are rare in the small intestine.[102] The tumors are small, encapsulated lesions that can occur in all areas of the small intestine, causing pain, hemorrhage, and intestinal obstruction. Symptomatic neurilemmomas should be excised.

Hamartomas are polyps containing myoepithelial elements and are formed from developmental overgrown portions of the bowel wall.[5,8,51] Hamartomatous polyps can cause pain, intussusception, intestinal obstruction, or bleeding. Occasionally, hamartomas may remain asymptomatic. Small intestinal hamartomatous polyps can occur as manifestations of various clinical syndromes. Multiple hamartomas have been identified in adenomatosis of the entire GI tract. A well-recognized clinical entity associated with multiple small intestinal hamartomas is the Peutz–Jeghers syndrome.[103–105] The disease is a hereditary condition carried as a simple mendelian dominant trait characterized by multiple polyps of the small intestine, circumoral pigmentation, and perianal mucosal melanosis. Polyps in the Peutz–Jeghers syndrome are hamartomatous. The polyps are concentrated in the jejunum but also occur in the ileum, duodenum, stomach, and occasionally the colon.

Most cases of Peutz–Jeghers polyps can be managed conservatively. However, symptomatic polyps may require surgical exploration and excision. Because polyps are multiple, it can be a difficult problem to distinguish the area of intestine that is responsible for clinical symptoms. Preoperative localization of obstructed intestinal segments or areas of bleeding by roentgenographic studies may be helpful. Frequently, patients with symptomatic Peutz–Jeghers intestinal polyps require multiple operations for recurrent obstruction or GI hemorrhage. Simple excision of symptomatic polyps is sufficient. If polyp removal compromises the bowel wall, lumen size, or vascular supply, segmental bowel resection must be performed. Although GI malignancies have been reported in the presence of the Peutz–Jeghers syndrome, malignant transformation of the hamartomatous polyps is unlikely.[2,105–107]

MALIGNANT NEOPLASMS

ADENOCARCINOMA

General Considerations

Adenocarcinomas are the most common small intestinal malignancies, accounting for approximately 50% of all cancers of the small bowel.[3,24,27,28,41,42,108-114] Adenocarcinomas increase in frequency with advancing age, with a peak incidence after age 70.[29] Small intestinal adenocarcinomas are slightly more frequent in males than females.

The distribution of adenocarcinomas tends to be greatest proximally in the duodenum, with reduced frequency in the jejunum, and with the lowest incidence distally in the ileum.[8,15,24,30,37,38,108-114] The duodenum is the site of approximately 40% of small bowel carcinomas, the jejunum 35%, and the ileum 25%. Considering the average length of the duodenum as 10% of the length of either the jejunum or the ileum, the frequency of occurrence of small bowel carcinomas in relation to intestinal length is lowest in the ileum, higher in the jejunum by a factor of approximately twofold, and highest in the duodenum by a factor of 20-fold. In the duodenum, approximately 65% of carcinomas occur in the periampullary region, 20% occur proximal to the ampulla, and 15% occur distal to the ampulla.[82] Carcinomas of the jejunum tend to develop proximally, with 70% of jejunal cancers located within 100 cm of the ligament of Treitz.[82] Ileal carcinomas are chiefly distal, with 70% of ileal cancers located within 100 cm of the ileocecal valve.[82]

Adenocarcinomas of the small intestine are derived from the glandular epithelium. Carcinomas tend to grow through the intestinal mucosa to form ulcerative lesions and tend to infiltrate the bowel wall and penetrate through the serosa. Adenocarcinomas can metastasize through lymphatics to the regional lymph nodes, locally to the peritoneal cavity and serosal surfaces, and hematogenously to the liver, lungs, bone, and other sites.

Clinical Features

The clinical manifestations of carcinoma of the small intestine depend upon the size and location of the neoplasm. They include abdominal pain, nausea and vomiting, weakness, weight loss, anemia, GI hemorrhage, bowel obstruction, or intestinal perforation.[5,8,35]

Duodenal carcinomas produce jaundice in more than half of the patients.[82] Periampullary lesions result in biliary obstruction in more than 75% of cases.[8,115] Hemorrhage is common with duodenal carcinomas, resulting in anemia and the presence of occult blood in the stool in more than 75% of patients.[34] Pain, usually epigastric, is often present, with a burning quality that often mimics an ulcer diathesis.[8] Obstruction is unusual in duodenal carcinomas. A palpable mass is present in 25% of cases and usually represents a dilated gall bladder rather than a neoplastic mass.[8]

Carcinomas of the jejunum produce complaints of vague, cramping abdominal pain, weight loss, and weakness. Hemorrhage is common and is usually chronic. Intestinal obstruction occurs in approximately 25% of patients.[28] A mass is palpable in about 30% of cases.[8,82]

Ileal carcinomas present clinically as cramping pain, chiefly in the lower abdomen. Weakness and weight loss are common. Chronic hemorrhage frequently occurs in carcinomas of the ileum. Obstructive symptoms can develop in 35% of patients. Tumors usually occur distally in the ileum and frequently grow circumferentially around the bowel. Approximately 35% of patients present with a palpable abdominal mass.[8,82] Some association between Crohn's disease and ileal carcinomas has been reported.[116-118]

Diagnosis

Duodenal carcinomas can be diagnosed by upper GI series, which may demonstrate filling defects, mucosal ulcerations, or visceral displacement suggestive of neoplasm (Fig. 28-3). In cases of jaundice, transhepatic cholangiography may reveal a malignant obstruction in the ampullary area. CT of the abdomen may reveal a duodenal or peripancreatic mass. Diagnostic ultrasonography can demonstrate a duodenal mass or confirm biliary obstruction and dilatation. Endoscopy allows duodenal carcinomas to be visualized and directly biopsied. Endoscopic retrograde cholangiopancreatography, with endoscopic cannulation of the pancreatic and biliary ducts for the injection of radiographic contrast material, can help in differentiating obstructive jaundice caused by neoplasm from jaundice resulting from biliary lithiasis or inflammatory pancreatic masses. Occasionally, duodenal carcinomas can be diagnosed from cytologic specimens obtained from the duodenum by intubation and aspiration or by endoscopic brushings.[8] Percutaneous needle aspiration has routinely enabled the diagnosis of malignancies in the region of the duodenum and head of pancreas.[119,120]

Carcinomas of the jejunum can be diagnosed by contrast radiography. GI series with small bowel follow-through can demonstrate filling defects, intramural lesions, mucosal abnormalities, or intestinal displacement suggestive of neoplasm. Arteriography can delineate jejunal neoplasms suspected of hemorrhage. CT body scans of the small intestine resolve poorly owing to shadow artifacts caused by intraluminal air and fluid. However, body scans can visualize large tumors and enlarged regional metastatic lymph nodes or metastatic disease in the liver. Ultrasonography resolution of jejunal cancers is limited by the inability of sound waves to pass through intestinal gas. Metastatic deposits, particularly in the liver, can be detected by ultrasonic examination. Endoscopy is not routinely possible beyond the ligament of Treitz and is not helpful in diagnosing carcinoma of the jejunum.

Carcinomas of the ileum generally can be diagnosed roentgenographically. GI series can show filling defects, ulcerations, or bowel loop displacements. Barium enemas with reflux of contrast material through the ileocecal valve into the terminal ileum can identify distal ileal lesions. Arteriography can detect carcinomas presenting with intestinal bleeding. Carcinomas occurring in the distal ileum and ileocecal valve areas occasionally can be visualized endoscopically by using colonoscopy and retrograde examination through the ileocecal valve. Usually, body scans and diagnostic ultrasonography are not helpful in diagnosing tumors of

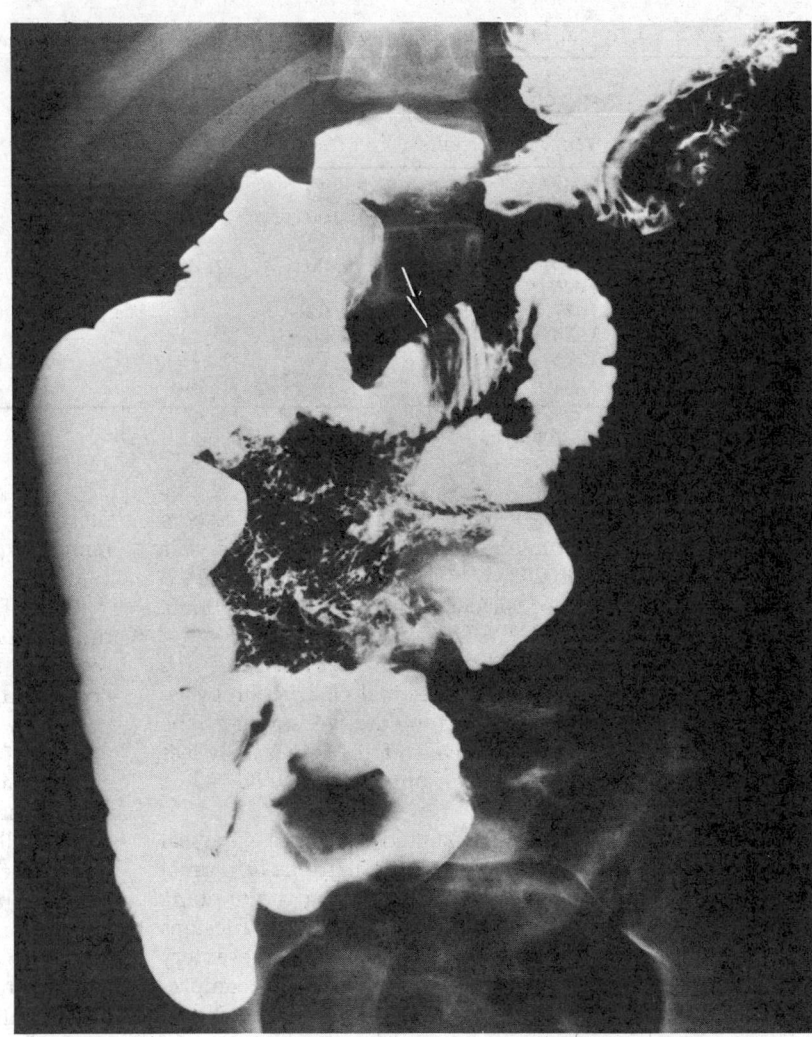

FIG. 28-3. Adenocarcinoma of the duodenum. A filling defect (*arrow*) is present in the duodenum proximal to the ligament of Treitz.

the ileum, except in detecting metastatic deposits in lymph nodes or in the liver.

Treatment and Prognosis

SURGERY. Carcinomas of the small intestine are treated by surgical resection, which should be radical to ensure complete excision of the tumor and the surrounding tissue. The resection should include the segment of bowel containing the tumor, the lymphovascular mesenteric pedicle, and the regional draining lymph nodes. In advanced nonresectable or metastatic disease, local resection or bypass of the tumor may be necessary to palliate obstructive symptoms.

Localized duodenal carcinomas should be treated by radical resection. Although segmental resections are sometimes possible for tumors occurring proximally or distally in the duodenum away from the pancreas, most duodenal carcinomas require extirpation of the entire duodenum and the head of the pancreas. Duodenal carcinomas are usually treated by pancreaticoduodenal resection, which includes duodenectomy, antrectomy, resection of the head of the pancreas, and resection of the distal common bile duct.[121-123]

GI tract reconstruction after pancreaticoduodenectomy requires pancreaticojejunostomy, choledochojejunostomy, and gastrojejunostomy.[121-123] Radical resection for duodenal carcinomas has resulted in 5-year survival rates in most series averaging 20%.[43,114,115,123-129] Table 28-5 summarizes the clinical results for patients surgically treated for carcinoma of the duodenum.[43,114,115,125-129]

Patients with metastatic duodenal cancers or with malignant duodenal lesions not amenable to radical surgical resection should undergo palliative surgical bypass to correct or prevent biliary and gastric obstruction.[129,130] Survival after palliative treatment for duodenal cancers is usually short, averaging 4 months.[129] The survival in patients with untreated duodenal carcinomas is typically less than 3 months from diagnosis.[82]

Carcinoma occurring in the jejunum should be treated by radical surgical resection that includes the segment of intestine containing the neoplasm, wide margins of normal bowel around the tumor, and resection of the mesentery supporting the involved intestine, including all draining lymph nodes down to the mesenteric root. Tumor involvement of mesenteric blood vessels may limit radical resection if the sacrifice of most of the small intestine or its blood supply is not

TABLE 28-5. Clinical Series of Carcinoma of the Duodenum

Author	Year	Number of Patients	Resection Rate (%)	Operative Mortality (%)	Mean Survival (months)*	5-Year Survival* (%)
Spinazzola et al[125]	1963	12	50	0	16	0
Mongé et al[126]	1964	25	100	24	10	37
Cortese et al[127]	1972	32	44	29	46	30
Warren et al[128]	1975	39	100	21	31	23
Shulka et al[115]	1976	8	50	25	9	0
Nakase et al[129]	1977	50	62	16	19	8
Ouriel et al[114]	1984	34	56	11	28	29
Giuliani et al[43]	1985	13	77	40	36	17
TOTAL		213	69	20	24	22

* Survival of resected group.

feasible. The overall prognosis for resected jejunal cancers is not favorable, with tumor recurrence likely. The 5-year survival rate is less than 20%.[8,14,25,28,106-114,131,132] Table 28-6 summarizes the results of various surgical series of patients with jejunal carcinomas.[3,15,24,27,28,43,114]

Palliative segmental bowel resection or bypass may be necessary to relieve or prevent intestinal obstruction by jejunal carcinomas too extensive for curative surgery. The survival of patients given palliative treatment is usually less than 6 months, and the survival of untreated patients is less than 4 months.[8,82]

Adenocarcinomas of the ileum should be treated by radical resection of the involved intestine, wide margins of normal surrounding tissue, and mesentery containing the draining lymph nodes. Frequently, radical resections for ileal lesions require right colectomy because resection of the mesentery containing the lymph nodes that drain the ileum compromises the blood supply to the right colon. Tumor extension into the root of the mesentery may not permit wide excision. For patients with carcinomas of the ileum who can undergo surgical resection, 5-year survival rates average 20%.[8,14,28,43,109-114] Results of patients treated surgically for carcinoma of the ileum are given in Table 28-7.[3,15,24,27,28,43,114]

Palliative segmental intestinal resection or bypass may be required to relieve or to prevent obstruction in patients with carcinoma of the ileum that are metastatic or which are too extensive to cure by resection. The survival following palliative treatment of cancers of the ileum usually is less than 6 months.[8,82] The survival of untreated patients with carcinoma of the ileum is typically less than 4 months.[8,82]

RADIATION THERAPY. Carcinomas of the small intestine may be treated with radiation therapy if curative surgical resection is not possible. Radiotherapy has been reported occasionally to produce remissions and to prolong survival in patients with advanced disease. Palliative radiotherapy may decrease pain and relieve obstructive symptoms.[5,8,133] Many carcinomas are radioresistant, and the overall results of the role of radiation therapy in promoting survival in patients with small intestinal cancers are discouraging.[8] Radiotherapy to the intestinal tract is poorly tolerated, resulting in malaise, nausea, vomiting, and enteritis. Often, radiation toxicity prevents the delivery of sufficient tumoricidal dosage. A combination of radiation therapy and surgery may benefit situations in which the surgical resection is likely to leave behind microscopic residual tumor that can be sterilized subsequently by radiotherapy. The use of intraoperative radiation therapy may prove useful when, at the time of surgery, a single large dose of radiation can be given to the tumor or resected tumor bed and to areas at risk for residual tumor contamination and possible recurrence.[134-136] Normal tissues not at risk for tumor contamination may be moved operatively from the radiation beam path or may be shielded to prevent exposure to radiosensitive normal tissues.[134-139]

CHEMOTHERAPY. Chemotherapy may be used in the treatment of disseminated small intestinal carcinomas or in

TABLE 28-6. Clinical Series of Carcinoma of the Jejunum

Author	Year	Number of Patients	Resection Rate (%)	5-Year Survival (Resected Group) (%)
Darling et al[24]	1959	16	44	14
Rochlin et al[3]	1961	9	67	17
McPeak[15]	1967	17	100	6
Silberman et al[27]	1974	5	80	50
Wilson et al[28]	1974	16	88	21
Ouriel et al[114]	1984	21	76	50
Giuliani et al[43]	1985	16	81	38
TOTAL		100	77	27

TABLE 28-7.   Clinical Series of Carcinoma of the Ileum

Author	Year	Number of Patients	Resection Rate (%)	5-Year Survival (Resected Group) (%)
Darling et al[24]	1959	4	75	0
Rochlin et al[3]	1961	4	75	33
McPeak[15]	1967	3	100	0
Silberman et al[27]	1974	4	75	33
Wilson et al[28]	1974	13	85	0
Ouriel et al[114]	1984	10	70	14
Giuliani et at[43]	1985	19	68	38
TOTAL		57	75	19

the treatment of small bowel cancers that are not amenable to curative surgical resection. Chemotherapy occasionally has been useful in advanced intestinal cancers, resulting in tumor regressions and improved survival in some patients.[13-15,26,28,132] The usual chemotherapeutic agents used in carcinomas of the small intestine are 5-fluorouracil and the nitrosoureas. Combination chemotherapy regimens have improved response rates in various GI cancers compared with single agents.[140,141] The roles of chemotherapy following surgical resection and in combination with radiotherapy in the treatment of small intestinal malignancies are under investigation.

SARCOMA

General Considerations

Sarcomas are malignant tumors that arise in tissues derived from embryonic mesoderm. Sarcomas can develop in all organs and may occur as neoplasms of the small intestine. The many types of sarcomas originate in connective tissue, muscle, fat, vascular tissue, neural elements, and other tissues. Despite a broad spectrum of histogenesis, all sarcomas have similar clinical behaviors and can be considered as a single class of malignant neoplasms for the purposes of diagnosis and management.

Sarcomas account for approximately 20% of all malignant small bowel tumors.[9,17,24,28,38,39,108] Sarcomas of the small intestine have been reported at all ages, with a general increase in frequency with advancing age and with most tumors presenting after the age of 50.[8] The frequency of small bowel sarcomas is approximately equal in men and women. Sarcomas may develop in all regions of the small intestine, but they are least common in the duodenum, which harbors approximately 10% of small intestinal sarcomas.[9,24,28,36] The jejunum is the site of about 35% of intestinal sarcomas, and the ileum is the site of 55% of the sarcomas of the small intestine.[9,24,28,36]

Small intestinal sarcomas usually develop in intramural locations and grow predominantly toward serosal surfaces, so that the tumors often extend outside the bowel wall where they may invade surrounding structures. The growth of intramural sarcomas toward intestinal mucosa can take place, producing ulceration. Intestinal sarcomas frequently develop into neoplasms of large size, with more than 75% being larger than 5 cm in diameter.[108] Because of their large sizes,

sarcomas frequently outgrow their vascular supplies and develop ischemic central necrosis.

Sarcomas of the small intestine typically spread by direct extension into tissues that surround the bowel, such as mesentery, abdominal wall, retroperitoneum, and adjacent intestine or other viscera. Intestinal sarcomas disseminate chiefly by the hematogenous route, with the most frequent sites of metastases being the lungs and liver.[9,24,28,38,39] Lymphatic metastases are unusual in sarcomas.[8,82]

Histologic Types

Fibrosarcomas are derived from malignant connective tissue elements. Fibrosarcomas occurring in the small intestine are rare, accounting for less than 10% of small intestinal sarcomas.[24] Fibrosarcomas have been reported in both men and women, chiefly in persons over the age of 50. Fibrosarcomas are reported most frequently in the ileum, with moderate distribution in the jejunum and rare occurrence in the duodenum. The average 5-year survival is 35%.[82]

Leiomyosarcomas arise from malignant smooth muscle elements. Leiomyosarcomas are the most common small intestinal sarcomas, comprising more than 75% of GI sarcomas and accounting for approximately 15% of all malignant small bowel tumors.[8,9,16,38,39] Leiomyosarcomas have been reported at all ages, with a general increase in frequency with advancing age.[8] There is a slight male predominance over females in incidence in most series.[8,9,38,39] Intestinal leiomyosarcomas occur most often in the ileum, with a moderate incidence in the jejunum and least often in the duodenum. Leiomyosarcomas usually grow in an intramural location with serosal extension, and the neoplasms often become large masses that invade outside the intestine. The tumors often develop necrotic centers, which can lead to fistula or abscess formation. Leiomyosarcomas often exhibit protracted, slow growth, with approximately 50% of patients surviving 5 years or longer after diagnosis.[8,108]

Liposarcomas are malignant neoplasms derived from lipoblasts. Liposarcomas are found frequently in the retroperitoneum and abdominal wall but are quite rare as tumors arising within the small bowel. Intestinal liposarcomas typically occur in the serosa and develop into masses that result in extrinsic compression and intestinal obstruction, often growing slowly and achieving large sizes before causing clinical symptoms.[8] Intestinal liposarcomas are found chiefly in the ileum but can occur in the jejunum. Liposarcomas are extremely rare in the duodenum.

Angiosarcomas develop from vascular elements and are rare in the small intestine.[82] Angiosarcomas typically are aggressive, rapidly growing lesions with a poor clinical prognosis. They have been reported in all areas of the small intestine in both men and women. The lesions are intramural, with mucosal extension and ulceration. Angiosarcomas are highly vascular, often presenting with GI hemorrhage.

Neural sarcomas can occur in the small intestine and are derived from neural elements. Intestinal neural sarcomas include *neurofibrosarcomas* and *malignant schwannomas*. Neurofibrosarcomas are malignant tumors arising from neural elements and occur only rarely in the small intestine. Neurofibrosarcomas tend to be aggressive neoplasms that exhibit rapid growth and early dissemination.[82] The tumors develop intramurally and extend toward both the serosa and mucosa. Neurofibrosarcomas occur in all regions of the small bowel and develop equally in men and women. There is an increased incidence of intestinal neurofibrosarcomas in patients with von Recklinghausen's disease.[82]

Malignant schwannomas are sarcomas derived from nerve sheath cells. Schwannomas of the intestinal tract are rare.[82] Schwannomas generally develop in the intestinal wall and extend in subserosal directions, although mucosal invasion and ulceration can occur. Schwannomas are found most often in the ileum, less in the jejunum, and least in the duodenum. Most schwannomas grow slowly, and patient survivals of over 2 years are common even with metastatic disease.

Clinical Features

Patients with sarcomas of the small intestine often complain of cramping abdominal pain that is intermittent. Occasionally, the pain may be a steady discomfort or feeling of fullness. Pain is a feature at clinical presentation in more than 65% of patients.[4,16,24,28,108] Weight loss is seen in 30% of patients. Nausea and vomiting, although typically intermittent, are part of the clinical presentation in approximately 40% of cases.[24,28] An abdominal mass is palpable in more than 50% of patients at the time of presentation.[8,9,28] GI hemorrhage develops in about 50% of patients with sarcomas of the small intestine, usually with leiomyosarcomas.[8,9,24,28] Bleeding is usually chronic, resulting in melena and anemia. Hematemesis is occasionally present with tumors of the proximal intestine, and profuse hemorrhage can occur in some cases.[8] Intestinal obstruction develops in approximately 20% of patients from direct tumor occlusion of the bowel lumen, from intestinal kinking around a tumor mass, or from intussusception.[9,28,39]

Diagnosis

The diagnosis of sarcoma of the small intestine frequently depends on surgical exploration. However, intestinal sarcoma is suggested by the presence of an abdominal mass on radiographs. If extensive necrosis is present, a fluid level may be visible within the mass. Radiographic contrast studies can show intestinal filling defects, ulcerative lesions, or displacement of bowel loops. A barium enema can show colonic displacement by a large abdominal mass, and the reflux of contrast through the ileocecal valve can demonstrate neoplasms in the distal small bowel. Arteriography can show a mass or tumor blush.

CT can delineate the extent of an abdominal mass and identify areas where the tumor has invaded surrounding structures. Ultrasonography can show cystic or necrotic areas within a tumor mass. Metastatic disease in the liver, peritoneum, or retroperitoneum may be revealed by body scans or ultrasonography. Radionuclide liver scans can show hepatic metastatic disease, and gallium scintigraphy occasionally reveals the extent of a primary intestinal tumor or metastatic deposits, particularly if areas of necrosis are present within the neoplasm.

Endoscopy can provide a diagnosis of sarcoma located proximally in the intestine located within the reach of the fiberoptic gastroduodenoscope or distally within the viewing distance of the colonoscope passed retrograde through the ileocecal valve. Because many sarcomas grow subserosally and spare the mucosa, endoscopic biopsies may be negative for tumor unless mucosal invasion has taken place.

Treatment and Prognosis

SURGERY. Surgical excision should be performed whenever possible in sarcomas of the small intestine. Resection should include the intestinal segment giving rise to the tumor, along with surrounding normal tissues in areas of potential tumor spread. In addition, wide resection for intestinal sarcoma may require sacrifice of portions of tissues adjacent to the intestine, such as liver, retroperitoneum, or abdominal wall. Because lymphatic metastases are unusual in sarcomas, extensive dissections of the nodal drainage beds usually are not performed. Five-year survivals as high as 50% have been reported following resection.[8,108]

In nonresectable tumors, palliative segmental bowel excision or bypass of the tumor should be performed to relieve or prevent obstruction. Nearly all patients treated palliatively for unresected tumors succumb to their disease within 12 months of diagnosis.[108]

Pulmonary metastases should be treated by thoracotomy and wedge excision if all metastatic disease is removable from the lung and if no extrapulmonary dissemination is present. In many sarcomas, salvage rates as high as 25% are seen following aggressive surgical excision of pulmonary metastatic disease.[142-144]

If isolated hepatic metastases are present, surgical excision of the metastatic deposits should be considered. Hepatic metastases should be removed by wedge excision or by hepatic lobectomy if the deposits can be approached and extirpated with reasonable morbidity. Although the overall survival of patients with hepatic metastases is poor, some patients may derive long-term benefit from the surgical excision of metastatic deposits within the liver.[145] Patients with solitary hepatic metastases are likely to have longer survival after resection than patients with multiple or bilobar metastases.

RADIATION THERAPY. Radiotherapy may be of benefit in the palliation of patients with nonresectable intestinal sarcomas.[8,24,146] Sarcomas may respond to high-dose radiation, occasionally with long-term survivals resulting even in the presence of gross residual tumor.[147]

Radiation therapy should be considered as an adjunct following surgical resection of intestinal sarcoma, particularly if extraintestinal tissue invasion by microscopic residual disease remaining at the surgical margin is possible. Surgical resection combined with radiation therapy has achieved satisfactory disease control in some intra-abdominal sarcomas, even when incompletely resected.[148,149]

CHEMOTHERAPY. Chemotherapy can be of benefit in the palliation of advanced sarcomas.[150,151] Doxorubicin has broad activity against sarcomas. In metastatic sarcoma, objective response rates in excess of 65% have been reported using combination chemotherapy including doxorubicin, cyclophosphamide, vincristine, and imidazole carboxamide.

Adjuvant chemotherapy following surgical resection of sarcomas has been suggested to reduce the chance of local recurrence and of disease dissemination.[148,149] Adjuvant chemotherapy following surgery or given in combination with radiation therapy is being evaluated for possible benefit in the treatment of various sarcomas.

LYMPHOMA

Lymphoid elements are found throughout the small intestine, and the small bowel can become involved in lymphoid malignancies. Lymphoma can originate in the small bowel as a primary neoplasm, or the small intestine can become involved secondarily as a manifestation of systemic lymphoid malignancy.

Primary lymphoma of the small intestine typically is localized to a single segment of bowel, although multiple separate lesions may be present in up to 20% of cases.[152] All anatomic regions of the small intestine may develop lymphoma. The frequency of lymphoma is lowest in the duodenum, moderate in the jejunum, and highest in the ileum, a pattern consistent with the relative increase in the concentration of lymphatic tissue from the lymphatic-poor duodenum through the jejunum to the lymphatic-rich ileum.[152,153] Primary GI lymphoma constitutes approximately 5% of all lymphoid malignancies and accounts for about 1% of small bowel neoplasms.[8,53,152,153] There appears to be an epidemiologic association between intestinal lymphoma and chronic celiac disease, with chronic immunodeficiency diseases, and with ethnic origins from the Middle East.[154-157] Intestinal lymphomas occur in increased frequency below the age of 10, in low incidence between ages 10 and 50, and in dramatically increased incidence above 50 years of age.[158,159] Intestinal lymphoma shows a slight male predominance, with the male:female incidence ratio being approximately 1.5:1. In areas of the Middle East, the incidence of intestinal lymphoma is high, men and women are affected equally, and the disease tends to be manifested before the age of 30.[155]

Intestinal lymphoma arises in the lymphoid tissue of the submucosa. The tumor expands the bowel wall, invades and ulcerates the mucosa, and penetrates the intestinal wall into the serosa. The histologic architecture of the neoplasm can be nodular, with aggregations of lymphoid cells, or diffuse, with a uniform infiltration of malignant lymphoid elements. Involvement of the mesentery and regional lymph nodes in areas of small bowel lymphoma is common. Bowel involvement may be limited or may extend for considerable distances. Most intestinal lymphomas are large in size, with 70% of the lesions exceeding 5 cm in diameter.[108]

Lymphomas of the small intestine manifest clinical signs and symptoms attributable to the presence of a mass that may be ulcerated or obstructing.[159] Cramping abdominal pain is common and often associated with nausea and vomiting. Frequently, lymphoma causes partial intermittent intestinal obstruction. Complete obstruction can occur but is unusual. GI hemorrhage is frequent and usually chronic, leading to anemia. Rarely, massive intestinal bleeding can occur with acute ulceration of the tumor. Fever may be present, usually indicating systemic lymphoma. Occasionally, intestinal lymphomas cause perforation, with the clinical presentation of an acute abdomen. A palpable abdominal mass frequently is present. Diffuse lymphadenopathy or organomegaly suggests advanced systemic disease. Ascites can be present if there is extensive intra-abdominal or retroperitoneal lymphoma. The ascites may represent a malignant effusion or may be a chylous accumulation of intestinal lymph resulting from lymphomatous disruption of mesenteric and retroperitoneal lymphatic channels.

In many instances, the diagnosis of intestinal lymphoma can be made roentgenographically. GI contrast studies may show infiltration of the bowel wall with ulceration or thickening of the mucosa. Segmental intestinal constriction may be present. Displacement of bowel loops can occur with extensive bulky disease. A barium enema can show colonic displacement by large tumors or reveal abnormalities in the distal ileum by retrograde filling of the small intestine. Lymphangiography can determine lymphomatous involvement of intra-abdominal and retroperitoneal nodes. CT and MRI body scans can delineate large masses.

The treatment of lymphoma isolated to the small intestine should be surgical and should involve wide resection of the involved bowel segment, the surrounding tissues, and the regional mesenteric lymph nodes. Extensive disease or intestinal lymphoma presenting together with systemic disease may require palliative resection or bypass to relieve or prevent intestinal obstruction or hemorrhage. Many series report 5-year survival rates of patients with resected intestinal lymphoma averaging 40%.[108,153,159] Patients with nonresectable disease have an overall 5-year survival of 25%.[8] Radiotherapy is of benefit in the palliation of extensive, nonresectable intestinal lymphomas, and chemotherapy is indicated for the treatment of intestinal lymphoma patients unable to undergo curative resections.[8,159,160] Chemotherapy is universally administered for disseminated lymphoma. Chemotherapeutic agents with activity against malignant lymphomas include methotrexate, vincristine, cyclophosphamide, and 6-mercaptopurine.[159]

There is considerable debate over the possible roles of adjuvant radiation therapy and adjuvant chemotherapy following complete surgical excision of lymphoma isolated to the small intestine. Many centers advocate systemic treatment whenever lymphomatous involvement of the GI tract is diagnosed.[12] Although resection of isolated lymphoma of the small bowel can be curative in some patients, studies currently are being performed to evaluate whether adjuvant radiotherapy and chemotherapy after surgery can result in prolonged patient survival.[159]

CARCINOID

Carcinoids are malignant neoplasms that arise from argentaffin cells.[161] Carcinoids represent unusual tumors that can develop throughout the GI tract, in the respiratory tract, and in the gonads.[162,163] The appendix and the small intestine are the sites most frequently affected by carcinoid tumors. Carcinoids account for more than 30% of all small intestinal malignancies, and they typically occur in the intestine as small submucosal nodules.[164,165] Carcinoids are usually solitary, although multiple tumors can be seen in approximately 30% of cases.[166] Carcinoids are rarely located in the duodenum, are infrequent in the jejunum, and are most frequently located in the ileum.[163-168]

Small intestinal carcinoids typically exhibit a slow growth rate. As many as 70% of lesions may remain clinically asymptomatic and are discovered incidentally at autopsy or at laparotomy performed for reasons unrelated to small intestinal neoplasms.[39,163,164] When carcinoids of the small intestine produce symptoms, the clinical features can be vague and nonspecific. Abdominal pain is the chief symptom, although nausea and vomiting may be prominent features of the clinical presentation.[167,168] Intestinal obstruction may occur from fibrosis around the neoplasm or from intussusception. Occasionally, an abdominal mass is palpable. By the time patients present with clinical symptoms, metastatic disease has developed in as many as 90%.[164,169] Despite the high incidence of disseminated disease at the time of diagnosis, the overall 5-year survival rate of patients with carcinoid of the small intestine averages over 20%.[163]

The carcinoid syndrome is an infrequently occurring but well recognized clinical constellation of symptoms that develops in fewer than 10% of patients with carcinoid tumors of the small bowel.[167,170] Because of their derivation from argentaffin cells, which can produce various kinins, carcinoid tumors produce 5-hydroxytryptamine (serotonin) in large amounts, along with histamine, catecholamines, and kinins that are released into the circulation to produce vasoactive manifestations.[163,170,171] The clinical features of the carcinoid syndrome include cutaneous flushing, episodic watery diarrhea, and paroxysmal dyspnea or asthma. The carcinoid syndrome is clinically manifested only with advanced cases of carcinoid tumor when liver metastases are present. Circulating 5-hydroxytryptamine is metabolized and excreted in the urine as 5-hydroxyindoleacetic acid, which serves as a chemical marker for the carcinoid syndrome.

The diagnosis of carcinoid tumor of the small intestine can be difficult to establish before surgical exploration. Contrast roentgenography may reveal small bowel filling defects, obstructing lesions, or mural thickening. Carcinoids in the ileum occasionally can be demonstrated retrograde by a barium enema that is refluxed through the ileocecal valve. Arteriography often reveals a tumor blush because carcinoids typically are highly vascular. Urinary excretion of 5-hydroxyindoleacetic acid may be elevated particularly in patients with advanced disease.

The treatment of carcinoid tumor of the small intestine depends upon the extent of the disease. Curative surgical removal is possible for localized tumors. Carcinoids of the jejunum should be treated by wide segmental bowel resection. Carcinoids in the ileum should be segmentally resected and may require right hemicolectomy if the blood supply to the right colon is compromised by resection of the tumor. Duodenal carcinoids often require pancreaticoduodenectomy. The surgical treatment of advanced cases of carcinoid is indicated if the patient can clinically tolerate surgical intervention, because reducing primary tumor bulk and metastatic deposits can prolong survival.[25,163,172] The treatment of advanced cases demonstrating the carcinoid syndrome should consist of the pharmacological management of the symptoms of flushing, diarrhea, and dyspnea with antiserotonin and antibradykinin agents.[173,174] Although radiation therapy is of limited benefit in carcinoids, palliative liver irradiation has been successful in improving symptoms in some patients with extensive hepatic metastatic disease.[163,175] Chemotherapy has been of limited success. Streptozotocin has shown some efficacy against carcinoid tumors.[176] Intra-arterial chemotherapy for hepatic metastatic disease has palliative benefit in some patients.[177]

METASTATIC TUMORS

Nonintestinal malignancies may metastasize to the small bowel, involving the intestine by direct invasion or by spread to the bowel wall through peritoneal seeding, lymphatic spread, or hematogenous dissemination.

The small intestine may be involved by tumors that originate outside the bowel and invade the intestine secondarily. The duodenum can be involved by tumor extension from cancers of the colon, stomach, pancreas, biliary system, or kidney.[178-181] Metastatic tumors involving retroperitoneal lymph nodes may enlarge, spread, and invade intestine.[182] The jejunum can be invaded directly by malignancies of the colon, stomach, pancreas, kidney, or retroperitoneum.[8,183] The ileum may be affected by cancers arising in the colon or pelvis.[8,183]

Direct tumor extension into the small intestine produces clinical symptoms and signs of intestinal obstruction or of hemorrhage if the tumor ulcerates. The diagnosis of small bowel involvement by direct neoplastic extension may be made by radiologic contrast studies, which can demonstrate compression, displacement, or ulceration of the intestine. However, the diagnosis of a primary extraintestinal tumor must be established to distinguish secondary intestinal involvement from tumors arising primarily within the small bowel. GI series may demonstrate gastric or pancreatic malignancies. Barium enemas can show colonic tumors, and pyelography can reveal renal neoplasms. Lymphangiography localizes malignant retroperitoneal lymphadenopathy. CT or

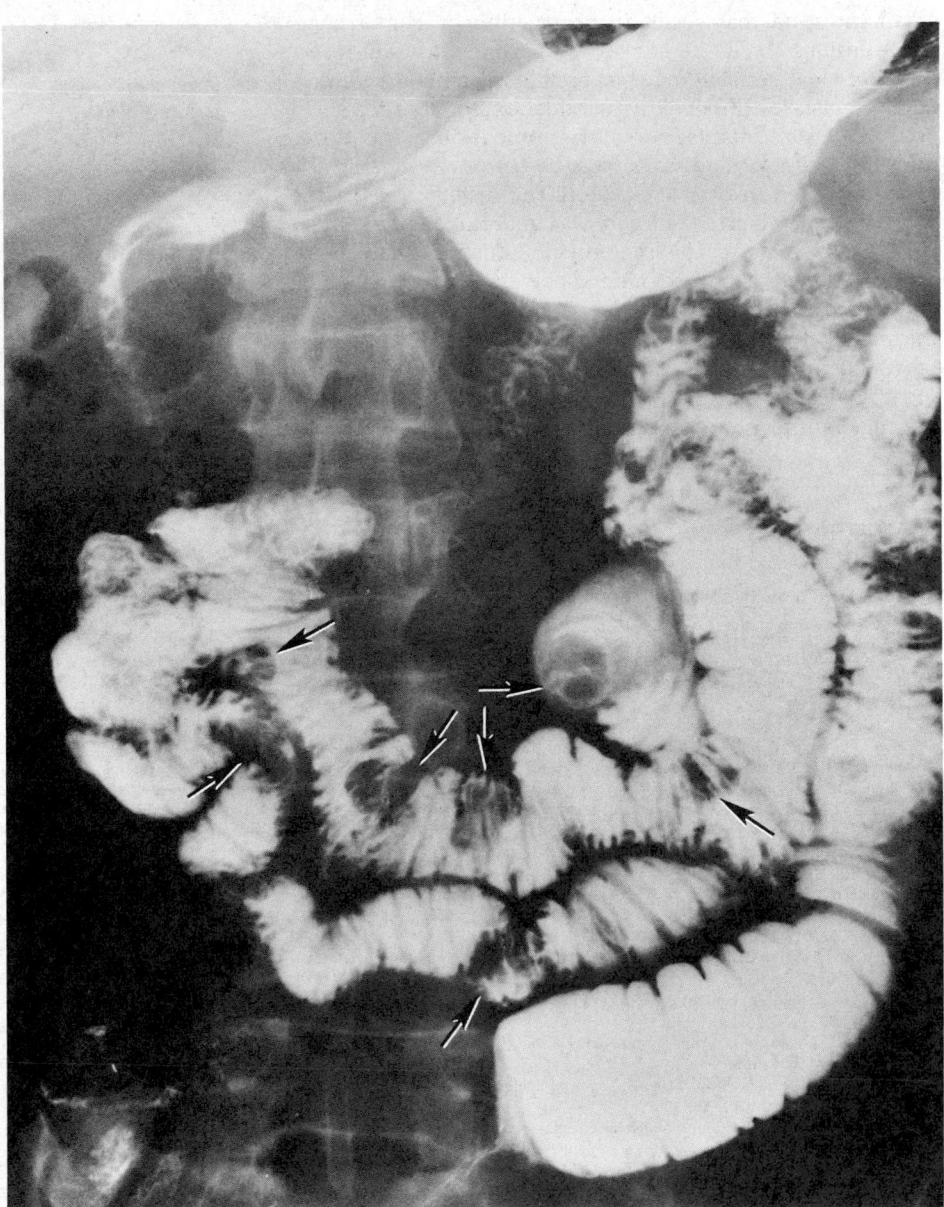

FIG. 28-4. Metastatic melanoma in the small intestine. Multiple filling defects (*arrows*) are present in the small bowel.

MRI body scans can demonstrate intra-abdominal tumor masses and indicate areas of small bowel invasion.

The treatment of tumors invading the small bowel should include surgical excision of the primary tumor, including the segment of bowel invaded. Resection may be quite extensive to include all areas at risk for tumor extension.[181,183,184]

The small intestine may be the site of metastatic deposits from malignancies arising outside the small bowel that involve the intestine by hematogenous, lymphatic, or transperitoneal spread.[185,186] Although the incidence of metastatic involvement of the small bowel is low, tumors that give rise to small intestinal metastases include carcinoma of the cervix, malignant melanoma, carcinoma of the lung, carcinoma of the esophagus, and carcinoma of the ovary.[181,182,185–189] Small intestinal metastatic deposits typically develop in the submucosa and produce intramural lesions. Metastases to

the small intestine may form expansile segments within the bowel wall that lead to obstruction, ulcerated mucosal lesions that produce intestinal hemorrhage, or submucosal polypoid masses that result in intussusception. The most common presenting clinical complaint of patients with metastatic lesions to the small bowel is partial intestinal obstruction.[185] Chronic intestinal hemorrhage may be present, resulting in anemia and possibly intermittent melena.[185,186]

The diagnosis of metastatic involvement of the small intestine may be difficult. Roentgenographic contrast studies may reveal masses or filling defects in the small intestine (Fig. 28-4); however, in approximately 50% of cases of small bowel metastases no radiographic abnormalities can be demonstrated.[8]

Surgical resection should be used to treat metastases to the small intestine that result in obstruction or hemorrhage. Large lesions should be excised by segmental bowel resection, but local excision may be possible in small or pedunculated metastases. Frequently, surgical exploration for small bowel metastatic disease reveals multiple lesions. If multiple metastases are present, care must be taken intraoperatively to identify and to treat adequately the lesions causing the symptoms for which the surgery was undertaken. If a solitary small bowel metastasis is the only demonstrable site of disseminated malignancy, segmental bowel resection should be performed, because there is a small chance that resection of the metastatic deposit will be curative.[186] In resections of metastatic melanoma, the mesenteric lymph nodes draining the involved intestinal segment should be removed because the regional nodes frequently contain tumor.[186]

REFERENCES

1. Braasch JW, Denbo HF: Tumors of the small intestine. Surg Clin North Am 44:791–809, 1964
2. Schier J: Diagnostic and therapeutic aspects of tumors of the small bowel. Int Surg 57:789–792, 1972
3. Rochlin DB, Longmire WP: Primary tumors of the small intestine. Surgery 50:586–592, 1961
4. Good CA: Tumors of the small intestine. Am J Roentgenol 89:685–705, 1963
5. Moertel CG: Small intestine. In Holland JF, Frei E (eds): Cancer Medicine, 2nd ed, pp 1808–1818. Philadelphia, Lea & Febiger, 1982
6. Croom RD, Newsome JF: Tumors of the small intestine. Am Surg 41:160–167, 1975
7. Mittal VK, Bodzin JH: Primary malignant tumors of the small bowel. Am J Surg 140:396–399, 1980
8. Herbsman H, Wetstein L, Rosen Y et al: Tumors of the small intestine. Curr Probl Surg 17:121–184, 1980
9. Skandalakis JE, Gray SW, Shepard D et al: Smooth Muscle Tumors of the Alimentary Tract. Leiomyomas and Leiomyosarcomas—A Review of 2525 Cases, pp 1–468. Springfield, Charles C Thomas, 1962
10. Ebert PA, Zuidema GD: Primary tumors of the small intestine. Arch Surg 91:452–455, 1965
11. Sternlieb P, Mills M, Bellamy J: Hodgkin's disease of the small bowel. Am J Med 31:304–309, 1961
12. Weaver DK, Batsakis JG: Primary lymphomas of the small intestine. Am J Gastroenterol 42:620–625, 1964
13. Rochlin DB, Smart CR, Silva A: Chemotherapy of malignancies of the gastrointestinal tract. Am J Surg 109:43–46, 1965
14. Dorman JE, Floyd CE, Cohn I: Malignant neoplasms of the small bowel. Am J Surg 113:131–136, 1967
15. McPeak CJ: Malignant tumors of the small intestine. Am J Surg 114:402–411, 1967
16. Sarr GF, Dockerty MB: Leiomyomas and leiomyosarcomas of the small intestine. Cancer 8:101–111, 1955
17. Hamberger GE: Propempticum Auspicale quo Dissertationem Solemnen: Indicit et de Ruptura Intestini Duodeni Disserit, pp 1–8. Jena, Litteris Ritterianis, 1746
18. Wesner F: Beiträge zur Casuistik der Geschwülste: I. Ueber ein Telangiectatisches Myom des Duodenum von Ungewöhnlicher grösse. Virchows Arch [Pathol Anat] 93:377–386, 1883
19. Fleiner W: Zwei Fälle von Darmgeschwülsten mit Invagination. Virchows Arch [Pathol Anat] 101:484–523, 1885
20. Heurtaux A: Nôte sur les temeurs bénignes de l'intestin. Arch Prov Chir 8:701–712, 1899
21. King EL: Benign tumors of the intestines with special reference to fibroma. Surg Gynecol Obstet 25:54–71, 1917
22. Shallow TA, Eger SA, Carty JB: Primary malignant disease of the small intestine. Am J Surg 69:372–383, 1945
23. River L, Silverstein J, Tope JW: Benign neoplasms of the small intestine. A critical comprehensive review with reports of 20 new cases. Int Abstr Surg 102:1–38, 1956
24. Darling RC, Welch CE: Tumors of the small intestine. N Engl J Med 260:397–408, 1959
25. Brookes VS, Waterhouse JAH, Powell DJ: Malignant lesions of the small intestine: A ten-year survey. Br J Surg 55:405–410, 1968
26. Reyes L, Talley RW: Primary malignant tumors of the small intestine. Am J Gastroenterol 54:30–43, 1970
27. Silberman H, Crichlow RW, Caplan HS: Neoplasms of the small bowel. Ann Surg 180:157–161, 1974
28. Wilson JM, Melvin DB, Gray GF et al: Primary malignancies of the small bowel: A report of 96 cases and review of the literature. Ann Surg 180:175–179, 1974
29. Wilson JM, Melvin DB, Gray G et al: Benign small bowel tumor. Ann Surg 181:247–250, 1975
30. Barclay THC, Schapira DV: Malignant tumors of the small intestine. Cancer 51:878–881, 1983
31. Johnson AM, Harman PK, Hanks JB: Primary small bowel malignancies. Am J Surg 51:31–36, 1985
32. Ciccarelli O, Welch JP, Kent GG: Primary malignant tumors of the small bowel. The Hartford Hospital experience, 1969–1983. Am J Surg 153:350–354, 1987
33. Botsford TW, Crowe P, Crocker DW: Tumors of the small intestine: A review of experience with 115 cases including a report of a rare case of malignant hemangioendothelioma. Am J Surg 103:358–365, 1962
34. Cutler SJ, Young JL: Third National Cancer Survey: Incidence data. Natl Cancer Inst Monogr 41:1–454, 1975
35. Spiro HM: Clinical Gastroenterology, 3rd ed, pp 643–666. New York, Macmillan, 1983
36. Krouse JM, Eyerly RC, Babcock JR: Tumors of the small bowel. Am J Surg 101:121–127, 1961
37. Sawyer RB, Sawyer KC, Sawyer KC et al: Benign and malignant tumors of the small intestine. Am Surg 29:268–272, 1963
38. Schmutzer KJ, Holleran WM, Regan JF: Tumors of the small bowel. Am J Surg 108:270–276, 1964
39. Ostermiller W, Joergenson EJ, Weibel L: A clinical review of tumors of the small bowel. Am J Surg 111:403–409, 1966
40. Spratt JS: Prevalence of neoplastic and pseudoneoplastic lesions of the small intestine. Geriatrics 21:231–238, 1966
41. Freund H, Lavi A, Pfeffermann R et al: Primary neoplasms of the small bowel. Am J Surg 135:757–759, 1978
42. Miles RM, Crawford D, Duras S: The small bowel tumor problem: An assessment based on a 20-year experience with 116 cases. Ann Surg 189:732–740, 1979
43. Giuliani A, Caporale A, Teneriello F et al: Primary tumors of the small intestine. Int Surg 70:331–334, 1985
44. Schmahl D: Carcinogenic substances and carcinogens: Their clinical significance. In Herfarth C, Schlag P (eds): Gastric Cancer, pp 15–18. New York, Springer-Verlag, 1979
45. Wattenberg LW: Carcinogen-detoxifying mechanisms in the gastrointestinal tract. Gastroenterology 51:932–935, 1966
46. Lowenfels AB: Why are small bowel tumors so rare? Lancet 1:24–25, 1973
47. Wattenberg LW: Studies of polycyclic hydrocarbon hydroxylases of the intestine possibly related to cancer: Effect of diet on benzopyrene hydroxylase activity. Cancer 28:99–102, 1971
48. Barnett WO: Benign tumors of the duodenum. Am Pract 13:625–632, 1962
49. Stassa G, Klingensmith WC: Primary tumors of the duodenal bulb. Am J Roentgenol 107:105–110, 1969
50. Everson TC: Carcinoma of the small intestine. In Everson TC, Cole WH (eds): Cancer of the Digestive Tract. Clinical Management, pp 75–85. New York, Appleton–Century–Crofts, 1969
51. Lowe WC: Neoplasms of the Gastrointestinal Tract, pp 125–144. Flushing, Medical Examination Publishing, 1972
52. Hancock RJ: An 11-year review of primary tumours of the small bowel including the duodenum. Can Med Assoc J 103:1177–1179, 1970
53. Loehr WJ, Mujahed Z, Zahn FD et al: Primary lymphoma of the gastrointestinal tract: A review of 100 cases. Ann Surg 170:232–238, 1969
54. Haghighi P, Nasr K: Primary upper small intestine lymphoma (so-called Mediterranean lymphoma). Pathol Annu 8:231–255, 1973
55. Cassidy M: Abdominal carcinomatosis associated with vasomotor disturbances. Proc R Soc Med 27:220–221, 1934
56. Thorson A, Biörck G, Björkman G, Waldenström J: Malignant carcinoid of the small intestine with metastases to the liver, valvular disease of the right side of the heart (pulmonary stenosis and tricuspid regurgitation without septal defects), peripheral vasomotor symptoms, bronchoconstriction, and an unusual type of cyanosis: A clinical and pathologic syndrome. Am Heart J 47:795–817, 1954
57. Montgomery GE, Liechty RD: Malignant small-bowel tumors. J Iowa Med Soc 56:249–251, 1966
58. Lee FD: Nature of the mucosal changes associated with malignant neoplasms in the small intestine. Gut 7:361–367, 1966
59. Brzechwa-Ajdukiewicz A, McCarthy CF, Austad W et al: Carcinoma, villous atrophy, and steatorrhea. Gut 7:572–577, 1966
60. Jinich H, Rojas E, Webb JA et al: Lymphoma presenting as malabsorption. Gastroenterology 54:421–425, 1968
61. Brunt PW, Sircus W, Maclean N: Neoplasia and the coeliac syndrome in adults. Lancet 1:180–184, 1969
62. Chernish SM, Miller RE, Rosenak BD et al: Hypotonic duodenography with the use of glucagon. Gastroenterology 63:392–398, 1972
63. Sindelar WF, Bagley DH, Felix EL et al: Lung tomography in cancer patients: Full-lung tomography in screening for pulmonary metastases. JAMA 240:2060–2063, 1978
64. Morson BC, Dawson IMP: Gastrointestinal Pathology, pp 352–377. London, Blackwell Scientific Publications, 1972
65. Muto T, Bussey HJR, Morson BC: The evolution of cancer of the colon and rectum. Cancer 376:2251–2270, 1975
66. Ravitch MM: Polypoid adenomatosis of the entire gastro-intestinal tract. Ann Surg 128:283–298, 1948

67. Perry EC: Papilloma of the duodenum. Trans Pathol Soc London 44:84–85, 1893
68. Wechselmann L: Polyp und Carcinom in Magen-darmkanal. Beitr Klin Chir 70:855–904, 1910
69. Joyeux R: Tumeur adenomato-villeuse du duodenum. J Chir (Paris) 66:437–448, 1950
70. Steinberg LS, Sheiber W: Villous adenomas of the small intestine. Surgery 71:423–428, 1972
71. Kutin ND, Ranson JHC, Gouge TH et al: Villous tumors of the duodenum. Ann Surg 181:164–168, 1975
72. Golden R: Non-malignant tumors of the duodenum: Report of two cases. Am J Roentgenol 20:405–413, 1928
73. Hoffman BP, Grayzel DM: Benign tumors of the duodenum. Am J Surg 70:394–400, 1945
74. Shulten MF, Dyasu R, Beal JM: Villous adenoma of the duodenum: A case report and review of the literature. Am J Surg 132:90–96, 1976
75. Bremer EH, Battaile WG, Bulle PH: Villous tumors of the upper gastrointestinal tract: Clinical review and report of a case. Am J Gastroenterol 50:135–143, 1968
76. Meltzer AD, Ostrum BJ, Isard HJ: Villous tumors of the stomach and duodenum. Radiology 87:511–513, 1966
77. Waters CA: The roentgenologic diagnosis of papilloma of the duodenum. Am J Roentgenol 24:544–557, 1930
78. Ring EJ, Ferrucci JT, Eaton SB et al: Villous adenomas of the duodenum. Radiology 104:45–48, 1972
79. Silverman L, Waugh JM, Huizenga KA et al: Large adenomatous polyp of Brunner's glands. Am J Clin Pathol 36:438–443, 1961
80. Deutschberger O, Tchertkoff V, Daino J et al: Benign duodenal polyp: Review of the literature and report of a giant adenomatous polyp of the duodenal bulb. Am J Gastroenterol 38:75–84, 1962
81. de Silva S, Chandrasoma P: Giant duodenal hamartoma consisting mainly of Brunner's glands. Am J Surg 133:240–243, 1977
82. Wood DA: Atlas of Tumor Pathology. Tumors of the Intestines, section VI, fascicle 22, pp 19–120. Washington, Armed Forces Institute of Pathology, 1967
83. Rankin FW, Newell CE: Benign tumors of the small intestine. Report of twenty-four cases. Surg Gynecol Obstet 57:501–507, 1933
84. Smith FR, Mayo CW: Submucous lipomas of the small intestine. Am J Surg 80:922–928, 1950
85. Gentry RW, Dockerty MB, Clagett OT: Vascular malformations and vascular tumors of the gastrointestinal tract. Int Abstr Surg 88:281–323, 1949
86. Moore RM, Schmeisser HC: Benign tumors of the small intestine. South Med J 27:386–393, 1934
87. Sivula A: Intestinal haemangioma: Observation on two cases treated surgically. Acta Chir Scand 131:485–491, 1966
88. Bilton JL, Riahi M: Hemangioma of the small intestine. Am J Gastroenterol 48:120–124, 1967
89. Hyun BH, Palumbo VN, Null RH: Hemangioma of the small intestine with gastrointestinal bleeding. JAMA 208:1903–1905, 1969
90. Brown AJ: Vascular tumors of the intestine. Surg Gynecol Obstet 39:191–199, 1924
91. Nys A, Buyssens N: Diffuse cavernous hemangiomatosis of the small intestine. Gastroenterology 45:663–666, 1963
92. Alfidi RJ, Esselstyn CD, Tarar R et al: Recognition and angio-surgical detection of arteriovenous malformations of the bowel. Ann Surg 174:573–582, 1971
93. Calem WS, Jimenez FA: Vascular malformations of the intestine. Their role as a source of hemorrhage. Arch Surg 86:571–579, 1963
94. Arnett NL, Friedman PS: Lymphangioma of the colon: Roentgen aspects. A case report. Radiology 67:882–885, 1956
95. Puppel ID, Morris LE: Lymphangioma of the jejunum. Arch Pathol 38:410–412, 1944
96. Golden T, Stout AP: Smooth muscle tumors of the gastrointestinal tract and retroperitoneal tissues. Surg Gynecol Obstet 73:784–810, 1941
97. Hermans PE: Nodular lymphoid hyperplasia of the small intestine and hypogammaglobulinemia: Theoretical and practical considerations. Fed Proc 26:1066–1611, 1967
98. Shaw EB, Hennigar GR: Intestinal lymphoid polyposis. Am J Clin Pathol 61:417–422, 1974
99. Shaw RC: Von Recklinghausen's disease of the small intestine associated with skin lesions. Am J Surg 80:360–363, 1950
100. Brasfield RD, Das Gupta TK: Von Recklinghausen's disease: A clinicopathological study. Ann Surg 175:86–104, 1972
101. Hochberg FH, DaSilva AB, Galdabini J et al: Gastrointestinal involvement in von Recklinghausen's neurofibromatosis. Neurology (Minneap) 24:1144–1151, 1974
102. Cedermark J: Neurinomas of the gastrointestinal tract. J Int Coll Surg 12:5–11, 1949
103. Jeghers H, McKusick VA, Katz KH: Generalized intestinal polyposis and melanin spots of the oral mucosa, lips and digits: A syndrome of diagnostic significance. N Engl J Med 241:993–1005, 1949
104. Dormandy TL: Gastrointestinal polyposis with mucocutaneous pigmentation (Peutz-Jeghers syndrome). N Engl J Med 256:1093–1102, 1141–1146, 1186–1190, 1957
105. Reid JD: Duodenal carcinoma in the Peutz-Jeghers syndrome: Report of a case. Cancer 18:970–977, 1965
106. Williams JP, Knudsen A: Peutz-Jeghers syndrome with metastasizing duodenal carcinoma. Gut 6:179–184, 1965
107. Humphries AL, Shepherd MH, Peters HF: Peutz-Jeghers syndrome with colonic adenocarcinoma and ovarian tumor. JAMA 197:296–298, 1966
108. Pagtalunan RJG, Mayo CW, Dockerty MB: Primary malignant tumors of the small intestine. Am J Surg 108:13–18, 1964
109. Goel IP, Didolkar MS, Elias EG: Primary malignant tumors of the small intestine. Surg Gynecol Obstet 143:717–719, 1976
110. Rich JD: Malignant tumors of the intestine: A review of 37 cases. Am Surg 43:445–454, 1977
111. Sager GF: Primary malignant tumors of the small intestine. A twenty-two-year experience with thirty patients. Am J Surg 135:601–603, 1978
112. Coutsoftides T, Shibata HR: Primary malignant tumors of the small intestine. Dis Colon Rectum 22:24–26, 1979
113. Williamson RC, Welch CE, Malt RA: Adenocarcinoma and lymphoma of the small intestine: Distribution and etiologic associations. Ann Surg 197:172–178, 1983
114. Ouriel K, Adams JT: Adenocarcinoma of the small intestine. Am J Surg 147:66–71, 1984
115. Shukla SK, Elias EG: Primary neoplasms of the duodenum. Surg Gynecol Obstet 142:858–860, 1976
116. Morowitz DA, Block GE, Kirsner JB: Adenocarcinoma of the ileum complicating chronic regional enteritis. Gastroenterology 55:397–402, 1968
117. Tyers GFO, Steiger E, Dudrick SJ: Adenocarcinoma of the small intestine and other malignant tumors complicating regional enteritis: Case report and review of the literature. Ann Surg 169:510–518, 1969
118. Frank JD, Shorey BA: Adenocarcinoma of the small bowel as a complication of Crohn's disease. Gut 14:120–124, 1973
119. Smith EH, Bartrum RJ, Chang YC et al: Percutaneous aspiration biopsy of the pancreas under ultrasonic guidance. N Engl J Med 292:825–828, 1975
120. Goldman ML, Naib ZM, Galambos JT et al: Preoperative diagnosis of pancreatic carcinoma by percutaneous aspiration biopsy. Am J Dig Dis 22:1076–1082, 1977
121. Howard JM: Pancreatico-duodenectomy: Forty-one consecutive Whipple resections without an operative mortality. Ann Surg 168:692–640, 1968
122. Gilsdorf RB, Spanos P: Factors influencing morbidity and mortality in pancreaticoduodenectomy. Ann Surg 177:332–337, 1973
123. Howard JM, Jordan GL: Cancer of the pancreas. Curr Probl Cancer 2:1–52, 1977
124. Brunschwig A, Tiholiz IC: Surgical treatment of malignant tumors of the duodenum exclusive of those arising from the papilla of Vater. Surg Clin North Am 26:163–175, 1946
125. Spinazzola AJ, Gillesby WJ: Primary malignant neoplasms of the duodenum: Report of twelve cases. Am Surg 29:405–412, 1963
126. Mongé JJ, Judd ES, Gage RP: Radical pancreatoduodenectomy: A 22-year experience with the complications, mortality rate, and survival rate. Ann Surg 160:711–722, 1964
127. Cortese AF, Cornell GN: Carcinoma of the duodenum. Cancer 29:1010–1015, 1972
128. Warren KW, Choe DS, Plaza J et al: Results of radical resection for periampullary cancer. Ann Surg 181:534–540, 1975
129. Nakase A, Matsumoto Y, Uchida K et al: Surgical treatment of cancer of the pancreas and the periampullary region: Cumulative results in 57 institutions in Japan. Ann Surg 185:52–57, 1977
130. Coutsoftides T, MacDonald J, Shibata HR: Carcinoma of the pancreas and periampullary region: A 41-year experience. Ann Surg 186:730–733, 1977
131. Vuori JVA: Primary malignant tumors of the small intestine. Analysis of cases diagnosed in Finland, 1953–1962. Acta Chir Scand 137:555–561, 1971
132. Morgan DF, Busuttil RW: Primary adenocarcinoma of the small intestine. Am J Surg 134:331–333, 1977
133. Cavanaugh PJ: Considerations appropriate to a clinical trial of definitive radiation therapy in adenocarcinoma of the pancreas. J Surg Oncol 7:135–137, 1975
134. Abe M, Takahashi M, Yabumoto E et al: Techniques, indications and results of intraoperative radiotherapy of advanced cancers. Radiology 116:693–702, 1975
135. Abe M, Takahashi M, Yabumoto E et al: Clinical experiences with intraoperative radiotherapy of locally advanced cancers. Cancer 45:40–48, 1980
136. Gunderson LL, Tepper JE, Biggs PJ et al: Intraoperative±external beam irradiation. Curr Probl Cancer 7:1–69, 1983
137. Sindelar WF, Kinsella T, Tepper J et al: Experimental and clinical studies with intraoperative radiotherapy. Surg Gynecol Obstet 157:205–219, 1983
138. Kinsella TJ, Glatstein E, Sindelar WF: Intraoperative radiotherapy. Hosp Pract 20:125–127, 130–131, 137–138, 140–141, 1985
139. Kinsella TJ, Sindelar WF, Tepper JE et al: Intraoperative radiotherapy. In Withers HR, Peters LJ (eds): Innovation in Radiation Oncology, pp 143–153. New York, Springer-Verlag, 1988
140. Bunn PA, Nugent JL, Ihde DC et al: 5-Fluorouracil, methyl-CCNU, adriamycin, and mitomycin-C in the treatment of advanced gastric cancer. Cancer Treat Rep 62:1287–1293, 1978
141. Higgins GA: Chemotherapy in advanced gastric cancer. In Herfarth C, Schlag P (eds): Gastric Cancer, pp 361–366. New York, Springer-Verlag, 1979
142. Thomford NR, Woolner LB, Clagett OT: The surgical treatment of metastatic tumors in the lungs. J Thorac Cardiovasc Surg 49:357–363, 1965
143. Ochsner A, Rush V: Treatment of pulmonary metastatic disease. Surg Clin North Am 46:1469–1473, 1966
144. Fallon RH, Roper CL: Operative treatment of metastatic pulmonary cancer. Ann Surg 166:263–265, 1967
145. Foster JH, Berman MH: Solid Liver Tumors, pp 209–234. Philadelphia, WB Saunders, 1977
146. McNeer GP, Cantin J, Chu F et al: Effectiveness of radiation therapy in the management of sarcoma of the soft somatic tissues. Cancer 22:391–397, 1968

147. Suit HD, Russell WO, Martin RG: Management of patients with sarcoma of soft tissue in an extremity. Cancer 31:1247–1255, 1973
148. Rosenberg SA, Kent H, Costa J et al: Prospective randomized evaluation of the role of limb-sparing surgery, radiation therapy, and adjuvant chemoimmunotherapy in the treatment of adult soft-tissue sarcomas. Surgery 84:62–69,1978
149. Rosenberg SA, Sindelar WF: Surgery and adjuvant radiation-chemoimmunotherapy in soft tissue sarcomas: Result of treatment at the National Cancer Institute. In van Oosterom AT, Muggia FM, Cleton FJ (eds): Therapeutic Progress in Ovarian Cancer, Testicular Cancer and the Sarcomas, pp 397–412. Boston, Martinus Nijhoff, 1980
150. Jacobs EM: Combination chemotherapy of metastatic testicular germinal cell tumors and soft part sarcomas. Cancer 25:324–332, 1970
151. Gottlieb JA: Combination chemotherapy for metastatic sarcoma. Cancer Chemother Rep 58:265–270, 1974
152. Rosenberg SA, Diamond HD, Jaslowitz B et al: Lymphosarcoma: A review of 1269 cases. Medicine (Baltimore) 40:31–84, 1961
153. Naqvi MS, Burrows L, Kark AE: Lymphoma of the gastrointestinal tract: Prognostic guides based on 162 cases. Ann Surg 170:221–231, 1969
154. Eidelman S, Parkins RA, Rubin CE: Abdominal lymphoma presenting as malabsorption: A clinico-pathologic study of nine cases in Israel and a review of the literature. Medicine (Baltimore) 45:111–137, 1966
155. Harris OD, Cooke WT, Thompson H et al: Malignancy in adult coeliac disease and idiopathic steatorrhoea. Am J Med 42:899–912, 1967
156. Whitehead R: Primary lymphadenopathy complicating idiopathic steatorrhoea. Gut 9:569–575, 1968
157. Dutz W, Asvadi S, Sadri S et al: Intestinal lymphoma and sprue: A systematic approach. Gut 12:804–810, 1971
158. Mestel AL: Lymphosarcoma of the small intestine in infancy and childhood. Ann Surg 149:87–94, 1959
159. McGovern VT: Lymphomas of the gastrointestinal tract. In Yardley JH, Morson BC, Abell MR (eds): The Gastrointestinal Tract, pp 184–205. Baltimore, Williams & Wilkins, 1977
160. Treadwell TA, White RR: Primary tumors of the small bowel. Am J Surg 130:749–755, 1975
161. Pearse AGE: The APUD cell concept and its implications in pathology. Pathol Annu 9:27–41, 1974
162. Ritchie AC: Carcinoid tumors. Am J Med Sci 232:311–328, 1956
163. Marks C: Carcinoid Tumors. A Clinicopathologic Study, pp 1–154. Boston, GK Hall, 1979
164. Moertel CG, Sauer WG, Dockerty MB et al: Life history of the carcinoid tumor of the small intestine. Cancer 14:901–912, 1961
165. Horsley BL, Baker RR: Fibroplastic response to intestinal carcinoid. Am Surg 36:676–680, 1970
166. Cunningham PJ, Norman J, Cleveland BR: Malignant carcinoid associated with thoraco-abdominal aneurysm and analysis of thirty-one cases of gastrointestinal carcinoid tumors. Ann Surg 176:613–619, 1972
167. Ostermiller WE, Joergenson EJ: Carcinoid tumors of the small bowel. Arch Surg 93:616–619, 1966
168. Sterling JA, Jayasanker MR, Galvez M: Carcinoids of the gastrointestinal tract. Am J Gastroenterol 47:373–378, 1967
169. Dockerty MB: Carcinoids of the gastrointestinal tract. Am J Clin Pathol 25:794–796, 1955
170. Diffenbaugh WG, Anderson RE: Carcinoid (argentaffin) tumors of the gastrointestinal tract. Arch Surg 73:21–37, 1956
171. Sjoerdsma A, Weissbach H, Udenfriend S: A clinical, physiologic and biochemical study of patients with malignant carcinoid (argentaffinoma). Am J Med 20:520–532, 1956
172. Chandler JJ, Foster JH: Malignant carcinoid syndrome treated by resection of hepatic metastases. Am J Surg 109:221–222, 1965
173. Melmon KL, Sjoerdsma A, Oates JA et al: Treatment of malabsorption and diarrhea of the carcinoid syndrome with methysergide. Gastroenterology 48:18–24, 1965
174. Tilson MD: Carcinoid syndrome. Surg Clin North Am 54:409–423, 1974
175. Herbsman H, Hassan A, Gardner B et al: Treatment of hepatic metastases with a combination of hepatic artery infusion chemotherapy and external radiotherapy. Surg Gynecol Obstet 147:13–17, 1978
176. Schein P, Kahn R, Gorden P et al: Streptozotocin for malignant insulinomas and carcinoid tumor. Report of eight cases and review of the literature. Arch Intern Med 132:555–561, 1973
177. Sparks FC, Mosher MB, Hallauer WC et al: Hepatic artery ligation and postoperative chemotherapy for hepatic metastases: Clinical and pathological results. Cancer 35:1074–1082, 1975
178. Grinnell RS: Lymphatic metastases of carcinoma of the colon and rectum. Ann Surg 131:494–506, 1950
179. Lawson LJ, Holt LP, Rooke HWP: Recurrent duodenal haemorrhage from renal carcinoma. Br J Urol 38:133–137, 1966
180. Treitel H, Meyers MA, Maza V: Changes in the duodenal loop secondary to carcinoma of the hepatic flexure of the colon. Br J Radiol 43:209–213, 1970
181. Veen HF, Oscarson JEA, Malt RA: Alien cancers of the duodenum. Surg Gynecol Obstet 143:39–42, 1976
182. Ngan H: Involvement of the duodenum by metastases from tumours of the genital tract. Br J Radiol 43:701–705, 1970
183. Van Prohaska J, Govostis MC, Wasick M: Multiple organ resection for advanced carcinoma of the colon and rectum. Surg Gynecol Obstet 97:177–182, 1953
184. Ellis H, Morgan MN, Wastell C: "Curative" surgery in carcinoma of the colon involving duodenum: A report of 6 cases. Br J Surg 59:932–935, 1972
185. de Castro CA, Dockerty MB, Mays CW: Metastatic tumors of the small intestines. Surg Gynecol Obstet 105:159–165, 1957
186. Das Gupta TK, Brasfield RD: Metastatic melanoma of the gastrointestinal tract. Arch Surg 88:969–973, 1964
187. Farmer RG, Hawk WA: Metastatic tumors of the small bowel. Gastroenterology 47:496–504, 1964
188. Beckly DE: Alimentary tract metastases from malignant melanoma. Clin Radiol 25:385–389, 1974
189. McNeill PM, Wagman LD, Neifeld JP: Small bowel metastases from primary carcinoma of the lung. Cancer 59:1486–1489, 1987

ALFRED M. COHEN

BRENDA SHANK

MICHAEL A. FRIEDMAN

CHAPTER 29 *Colorectal Cancer*

Adenocarcinoma of the large bowel affects approximately one person in 20 in the United States and in most Westernized countries. With more than 140,000 new cases diagnosed in the Unites States each year, representing 15% of all cancers, this disease constitutes a major public health problem. However, when diagnosed in its early stages, this common malignancy is highly curable by surgical treatment, with minimal morbidity and mortality. Because of the high potential cure rate, defining populations at risk and screening asymptomatic patients are important considerations. The presence of a number of "biomarkers" associated with colorectal cancer, such as adenomatous polyps and abnormal mucosal cell proliferation, will allow clinicians to test the efficacy of a number of preventive strategies in the next decade.[1]

This chapter reviews recent advances in the multidisciplinary treatment of primary colorectal cancer. Incremental benefits, risks, and toxic effects of these combined modality approaches are defined, and recent developments in chemotherapeutic protocols for metastatic disease are examined. Much of the discussion will consider *colon* cancer separately from *rectal* cancer. Although certain features of their biology and natural history are similar, patterns of tumor recurrence, surgical treatment, and adjuvant treatment programs are so disparate as to warrant the distinction. Treatment of patients with potentially curable cancers will be discussed separately from treatment of patients with unresectable, recurrent, or metastatic disease.

Figure 29-1 provides an overview of the end results of treatment of patients with colorectal adenocarcinoma. It demonstrates the need for improved earlier diagnosis and control of micrometastatic disease. Figure 29-2 suggests that

efforts in these directions have reduced the overall death rate from this cancer. The 5-year relative survival rate from colon cancer increased from 41% in the 1950s to 54% in the 1980s; that for rectal cancer increased from 40% to 51.5% in the same period.[2]

ANATOMY

GROSS ANATOMY OF THE LARGE BOWEL

The large bowel is divided into the colon and rectum. However, for treatment purposes, it is also important to consider the large bowel in terms of free intraperitoneal location versus extraperitoneal location. Treatment failure of intraperitoneal tumors is more likely to be expressed as peritoneal seeding, whereas treatment failure of extraperitoneal tumors manifests as local recurrence. Extraperitoneal sites of tumor include the pelvis and the abdominal retroperitoneum.

The cecum, transverse colon, and sigmoid loop are mobile structures that lie free in the peritoneal cavity and are completely covered with serosa (visceral peritoneum). The dorsal or posterior aspect of the ascending and descending colon, and both flexures frequently lack serosa. Tumor spread from these segments may involve the retroperitoneal soft tissues, kidney, ureter, and pancreas. Although the rectum is frequently considered to be extraperitoneal, the anterior surface of the upper rectum is covered with serosa and is therefore intraperitoneal. Patterns of recurrence of high rectal cancer may depend on whether the location of the tumor is anterior or posterior.

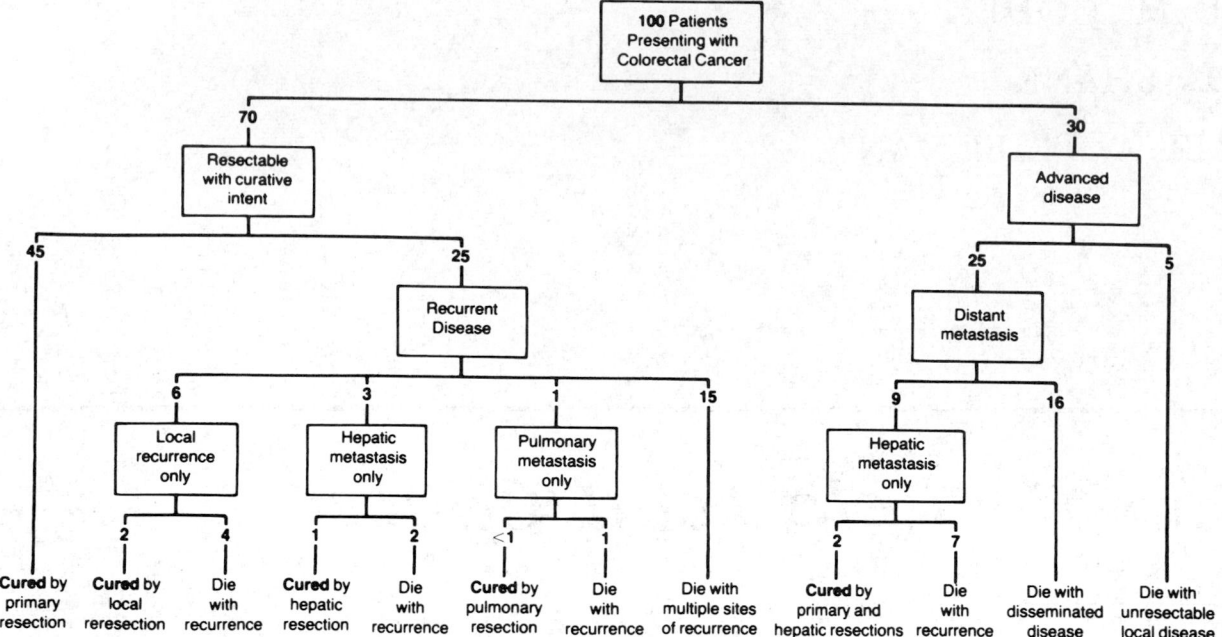

FIG. 29-1. Patterns of failure in 100 patients presenting with large bowel cancer. (August DA, Ottow RT, Sugarbaker PH: Clinical perspectives on human colorectal cancer metastases. Cancer Metastasis Rev 3:303–324, 1984)

RECTUM

The rectum in the adult is about 15 cm long; for treatment purposes it is divided into 5-cm segments. However, actual rectal length and division into surgical segments reflect several patient features, such as height, body habitus, pelvic width (gynecoid versus android), and curve of the sacral hollow, within which the rectum resides. The backward displacement of the rectum onto the sacrum is important in fecal continence, to be discussed later.

Frequently the lowermost location of a rectal cancer is defined in terms of distance from the anus. It should be stated whether the determination is made with a rigid or flexible endoscope, and whether the reference point is the anal verge (the lowermost portion of the anal canal) or the dentate line. Once the rectum is surgically mobilized from the sacral hollow, a posteriorly based tumor easily palpable on digital rectal examination may be well out of the pelvis.

About 1 to 2 cm above the dendate line is the posteriorly

palpable muscular anorectal ring, or puborectalis sling. The dentate line is well defined visually, and the distance above this demarcation as determined with a rigid proctoscope is the most reliable way of defining the lowest extent of a rectal cancer (Fig. 29.3).

The rectal diameter, particularly 5 to 12 cm from the anal verge, is two to three times the diameter of the sigmoid and left colon, which allows the rectum to serve as a reservoir. Although rectal resection with anastomosis establishes intestinal continuity, the reservoir function of the rectum is abolished. This may lead to urgency and frequency in defecation, which usually improves with time and with dilation of the neorectum.

NORMAL HISTOLOGY

The histology of the large bowel directly reflects its functions of water absorption and mucus secretion. Water is absorbed primarily in the proximal half, with storage in the distal bowel. Mucus facilitates evacuation of the partially desiccated feces. The bowel wall consists of mucosa, lamina propria, muscularis mucosa, submucosa, muscularis propria, and, when present, visceral peritoneum (serosa). A layer of fat (subserosa) is present between the muscularis propria and the serosa. The serosa wraps around the colon to envelop the vascular/lymphatic structures and form the mesentery. This explains why tumors that grow completely through the muscularis are not necessarily "transmural" (see section on Surgical-Pathologic Staging, below).

The inside of the colon is relatively smooth, lacking the plicae of the small intestine. Only large folds (haustrations) are present. Microscopically, the entire thickness of the mucosa is composed of rather straight glands between which are

FIG. 29-2. Improvement in 5-year relative survival rates from colorectal cancer (white men and women).[2]

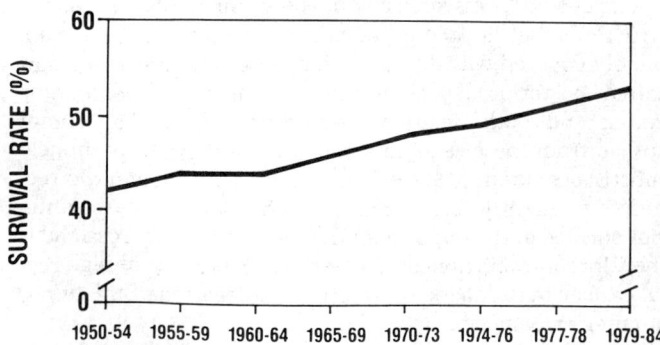

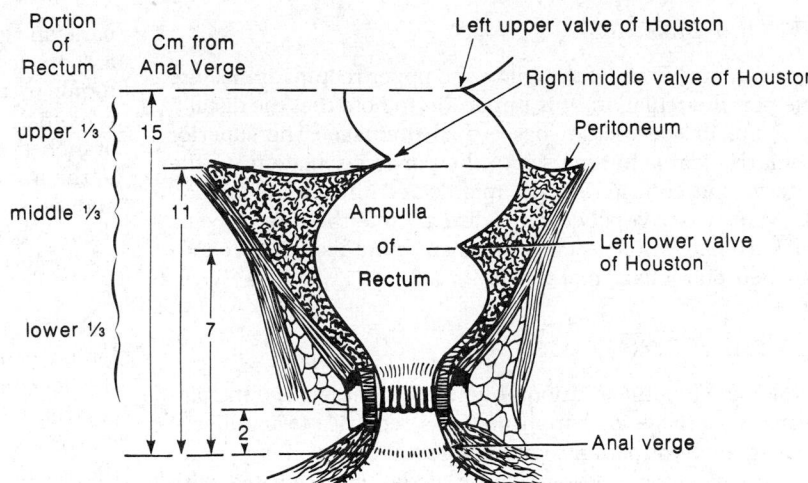

FIG. 29-3. Division of the rectum into upper, middle, and lower thirds. (Goligher JC [ed]: Surgical anatomy. In Surgery of the Anus, Rectum and Colon, 3rd ed. London, Baillière Tindal, 1975) Diseases of the Colon and Anal Rectum. Philadelphia, WB Saunders, 1959)

the crypts of Lieberkühn. Goblet cells are interspersed with tall columnar cells. Mitoses are present primarily in the base of the crypts, and new cells move up the glands with continuous exfoliation into the bowel lumen.

ARTERIAL SUPPLY TO THE LARGE BOWEL

Although standard surgical treatment of large bowel cancer includes resection of the potentially involved node-bearing mesentery, the extent of mesenteric resection frequently depends on arterial supply (Fig. 29-4).

The cecum and the ascending and transverse colon are nourished by branches from the superior mesenteric artery. The ileocolic artery is quite constant, feeding the distal ileum as well as the proximal colon. When a right colectomy is performed, at least 15 cm of ileum is included to ensure adequate blood supply to the distal small bowel. The right colic artery is quite variable: it may be a branch of the superior mesenteric artery or a subdivision of the ileocolic artery. It is usually diminutive, which precludes a cecectomy and necessitates a full right hemicolectomy, even for early lesions in the cecum. The middle colic artery routinely divides proximally into a left and right branch.

The descending colon, the sigmoid, and the upper rectum are supplied by branches of the inferior mesenteric artery. Approximately 4 cm below the origin of the inferior mesenteric artery is the takeoff of the left colic artery. This ascending branch connects via the marginal artery of Drummond with the left branch of the middle colic artery. If there is significant stenosis of the origin of the superior mesenteric artery, the left colic artery may provide the major blood supply to the transverse and right colon, as well as to the entire small bowel. Pulses in the superior mesenteric artery and middle colic artery should always be felt before dividing the inferior mesenteric or left colic artery to prevent this potentially catastrophic complication. The collateral blood supply to the left colon from the middle colic artery must also be examined whenever the inferior mesenteric artery is ligated, as the marginal arterial arcade may be incomplete.

The upper rectum receives its blood supply from the superior hemorrhoidal artery, the continuation of the inferior mesenteric artery. The diminutive middle hemorrhoidal and

the inferior hemorrhoidal arteries are branches of the internal iliac artery. In addition, blood is supplied to the anus and lower rectum via pudendal branches of the internal iliac artery. The blood supply to the distal 5 cm of rectum comprises a rich network of multiple small branches, which allows surgical clearance of all perirectal tissue down to the level of the levator muscles without producing an ischemic rectal remnant.

FIG. 29-4. Anatomical segments and vascular supply to the colon and rectum. (Jones T, Shepard WC: A Manual of Surgical Anatomy. Philadelphia, WB Saunders, 1945)

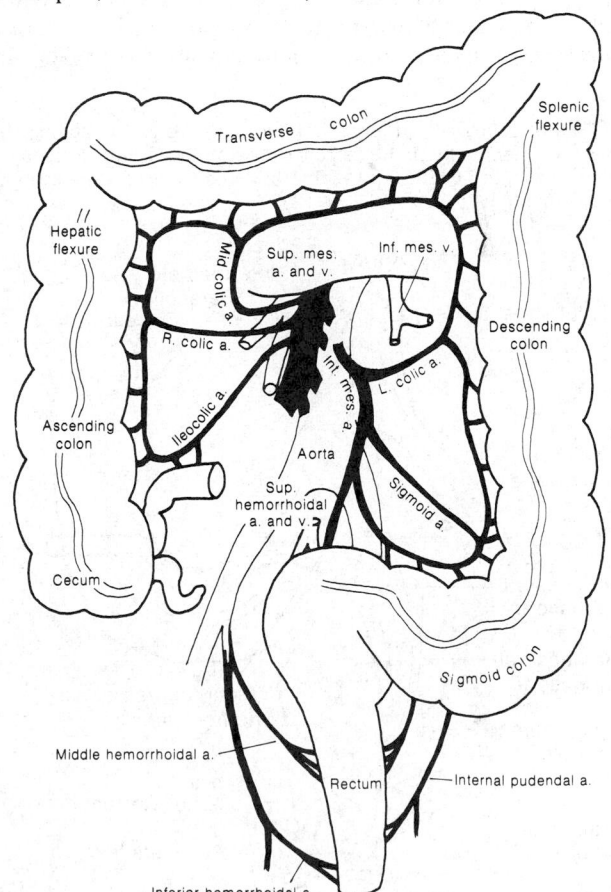

VENOUS DRAINAGE

The venous system of the colon and upper rectum drains into the portal circulation. It is important to note that the distal 5 to 7 cm of the rectum has a dual drainage. The superior hemorrhoidal vein drains into the portal circulation via the inferior mesenteric vein; the middle and inferior hemorrhoidal veins pass via pelvic veins directly into the inferior vena cava. Hence, distal rectal cancers are more likely to produce isolated pulmonary metastases.

LYMPHATIC DRAINAGE

Understanding the location of lymphatic vessels and the patterns of drainage to lymph nodes is requisite to intelligent management of patients with colorectal cancer. Surgical resection of tumor-bearing lymph nodes is associated with cure, albeit in a minority of patients. Hence, surgical lymphadenectomy should be considered a therapeutic procedure as well as a staging procedure.

The intramural lymphatics of the large bowel begin as a plexus beneath the lamina propria, superficial to the muscularis mucosa. This anatomical relationship explains the absence of lymph node metastases associated with in situ tumors. The lymphatics pass into the submucosa, where they follow blood capillaries. Efferent lymphatic vessels proceed radially outward through the circular and longitudinal muscle layers to communicate with an intramuscular and subserosal lymphatic plexus (Fig. 29-5).

Some lymphatics drain into subserosal epicolic lymph nodes. The majority of extramural lymphatics enter the mesentery and converge toward the major arterial trunks. The paracolic groups of lymph nodes along the marginal vascular arcades are the most numerous and are important sites of tumor metastases. The intermediate nodal groups are more proximal, involving the bifurcation of major arterial branches. Central or principal nodes are present contiguous to the inferior mesenteric and superior mesenteric arteries, and ultimately the entire para-aortic chain. Table 29-1 lists the numbers of lymph nodes in surgically cleared specimens; the largest number of nodes are in the paracolic group.[3]

RIGHT COLON. The cecal paracolic area is rich with lymph nodes. The dominant intermediate nodes are along the ileocolic artery. Medial to the ileocolic artery is the avascular space of Treves. Lateral to this space, the lymphatics all pass centrally and proximally, without any connection to the nodes of the small intestine. Anterior to the superior mesenteric vein, a continuous series of nodes follows the ileocolic artery, extending to the superior mesenteric artery. Some lymphatics pass up the superior mesenteric vein, which accounts for the portal lymph node metastases from right colon cancer.

TRANSVERSE COLON. The hepatic flexure and proximal two thirds of the transverse colon drain into the middle colic intermediate lymph nodes. The midcolic lymphatics pass directly into the superior mesenteric nodes. There are occasional connections from the transverse paracolic lymphatics to the omental and splenic hilar nodes.

SPLENIC FLEXURE AND DESCENDING COLON. The lymphatics of the splenic flexure and upper descending

FIG. 29-5. Lymphatic drainage of the large bowel, including the colon wall. (Villemin F, Huard P, Montague M: Recherches Anatomiques Sur les Lymphatiques du Rectum, et De l'Anus. Rev Surg Chir 63:39–80, 1925, and Cole PP: The intramural spread of rectal carcinoma. Br Med J 1:431–433, 1913)

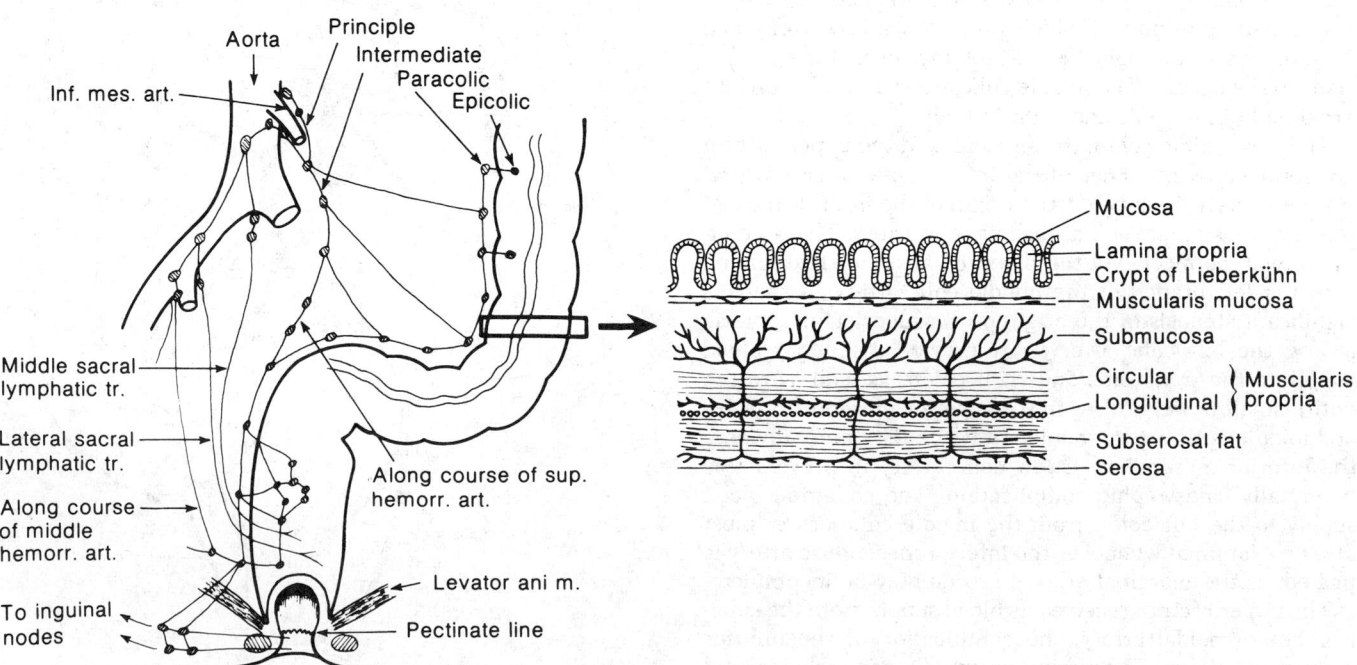

TABLE 29-1.   Lymph Nodes in Various Nodal Groups

Regional Lymphatic Chain	Average No. of Nodes		
	Paracolic	Intermediate	Central
Ileocolic	19.0	6.7	3.3
Right colic	7.3	2.3	1.5
Middle colic	16.2	3.7	2.5
Left colic	19.5	4.6	1.3

Data modified from Slanetz CA Jr, Herter FP: The large intestine. In Haagensen CD, Feind CR, Harter FP et al (eds): The Lymphatics in Cancer, pp 489–564. Philadelphia, WB Saunders, 1972.

colon follow the course of the marginal vascular arcade and the left colic artery to reach the inferior mesenteric artery.

SIGMOID AND RECTOSIGMOID.   The paracolic nodes in this area are numerous. Some intramural lymphatics bypass these nodes, passing directly to intermediate or central nodes, which explains the occasional finding of a skip metastasis. Approximately 20% of patients have predominantly paracolic and central lymph nodes, with few intermediate nodes. Even in this group, only an average of 4.3 lymph nodes can be obtained from along the inferior mesenteric artery proximal to the origin of the left colic artery.

RECTUM.   The major portion of the lymphatic drainage of the rectum passes along the superior hemorrhoidal arterial trunk toward the inferior mesenteric artery. Only a few lymphatics pass along the inferior mesenteric vein. The pararectal nodes above the level of the middle rectal valve drain exclusively along the superior hemorrhoidal lymphatic chain. Below this level (approximately 7–8 cm above the anal verge), some lymphatics pass to the lateral rectal pedicle. These lymphatics are associated with nodes along the middle hemorrhoidal artery, obturator fossa, hypogastric, and common iliac arteries. In addition, extensive lymphatics are present in women contiguous with the rectovaginal septum, and in men along Denonvilliers' fascia.[4,5] The entire extraperitoneal soft tissue (mesorectum) is permeated with lymphatics.

NORMAL PHYSIOLOGY

The function of the large bowel is to absorb water from the small bowel contents and to act as a reservoir for fecal material. The right colon is primarily responsible for the solidification of ileal contents by the absorption of water. The left colon and the rectum are fecal storage sites. Mucus secretion by colonic goblet cells facilitates passage of the more solidified stool.

Two muscular mechanisms are involved in maintaining fecal continence. The internal and external sphincter muscles control the anal canal lumen. The puborectalis sling system elevates the distal rectum when intra-abdominal pressure increases, leading to kinking at the anorectal angle and enhanced continence, despite sneezing or coughing.

This is the "flap-valve" theory of continence.[6] The intrarectal balloon proctogram defines the anorectal angle at rest and with straining.[7,8] Anorectal manometry and electromyography can be used to study subtle functional differences.[9]

Sphincter-saving treatment of rectal cancer may result in impaired function. Frequency and urgency occur when the normal rectal reservoir is replaced with the less capacious proximal colon. Poor control of gas and fecal soilage, particularly with coughing, may lead to considerable embarrassment. Besides impairing motor function of the sphincter systems, surgery can cause sensory changes. Normal innervation is sensitive enough to distinguish gas, liquid, and solid feces, resulting in controlled differential release of these substances.

EPIDEMIOLOGY

Worldwide, the incidence rates of colorectal cancer vary widely, from 3.4 cases per 100,000 population in Nigeria to 35.8 cases per 100,000 population in Connecticut.[10] In addition to North America, both Australia and New Zealand, as well as portions of northern and western Europe, have a relatively high incidence of the disease.[11,12] In the United States, the Northeast has had a particularly high mortality from bowel cancer, with a marked clustering of cases in more densely populated areas. These trends are gradually becoming less apparent but still exist.[11] Also, American immigrants from Germany, Ireland, Czechoslovakia, and Greece have a higher incidence of disease than immigrants from other nations.[13,14]

The age-specific incidence of disease in the United States appears to rise steadily from the second to the ninth decade. Men have proportionately more rectal cancer than women, but both sexes are relatively equally represented.[15]

In the United States two religious groups have a diminished risk of large bowel cancer. Seventh-Day Adventists and Mormons have a standardized mortality ratio of 0.52 to 0.81 for bowel cancer at all sites, compared to geographic cohorts of other religions. Both groups refrain from using alcohol and tobacco and practice some form of dietary moderation.[16–19] The reasons for the 20% to 50% risk reduction are not clear; these populations continue to be the subjects of careful scrutiny.

Colorectal cancer is a dynamically changing disease entity.[11] There has been a progressive trend toward disease of the more proximal colon and away from disease of the rectosigmoid bowel.[10,20–22] Less than 60% of cases are currently diagnosable with only rigid proctosigmoidoscopy.

ETIOLOGY

It has long been postulated that colorectal cancer is caused or promoted by environmental factors, and especially by dietary factors that affect the enteric milieu.[23,24] It is suspected that carcinogens are present and identifiable in feces.[25,26] Although it is not possible to identify a specific cause of colon cancer, epidemiologic studies of nutritional habits and migration patterns are revealing. Both national and international studies point to a clear association of colorectal cancer with certain diets (such as those rich in animal fats and meat and poor in fiber) and certain high-risk populations.[11,14,27,28]

Japanese in their native country have a low incidence of colorectal cancer, approximately 6 to 8 cases per 100,000 population.[10] However, first-generation Japanese emigrants to Hawaii have a 2.5-fold greater rate of large bowel cancer, similar to that of caucasians living in Hawaii.[29,30] Exposure to the typical American diet, rich in cholesterol and fat and low in fiber, appears to affect the risk even in first-generation immigrants.[31] Moreover, since 1945, the incidence of colorectal cancer has increased in Japan, perhaps related to a more American-style diet there.[32] Immigrants to Puerto Rico, Europe, Israel, Australia, and Poland assume the risk of these host countries.[33-38] Studies that relate cultural, dietary, and genetic factors with colorectal cancer incidence offer important insights into disease etiology and identify the test populations for intervention efforts. A variety of possibilities are being considered in order to identify the causative factors more precisely. Currently at least six etiologic hypotheses are being tested preclinically, epidemiologically, or with clinical intervention, as described below.

1. FECAPENTAENES. These potent mutagenic compounds, found in human feces and thought to be produced by gut microflora, were active in the Ames *Salmonella* assay[39] and mammalian cell systems.[40] Moreover, there is a correlation between the level of stool fecapentaenes and tumor incidence in select high- and low-risk populations in South Africa.[41] Bruce[42] and Correa et al[43] have suggested a positive association between fecapentaene levels and the incidence of colonic polyps. Intraluminal levels of fecapentaenes can be lowered by fiber, vitamin C, and vitamin E intake.[44,45]

2. 3-KETOSTEROIDS. These are potential tumor promoters or initiators, presumed to be derived from metabolic products of cholesterol. They induce genetic damage in cell cultures and rodent bowel.[46,47] At least two have been identified in human feces, and they may be present in higher concentrations in persons at higher risk for colon cancer.[48-50]

3. PYROLYSIS PRODUCTS. Compounds such as benzo [a] pyrene, which result from the broiling or frying of meat at high temperatures, have proved carcinogenic in rodents[51,52] and are suspected of contributing to gastric and esophageal cancers.[24]

4. NORMAL BILE ACIDS. Directly related to the intake of fat, bile acids such as deoxycholic and cholic acid are thought to induce gut lumen proliferation.[53,54] Populations that consume more fat have more bile acid secretion and an associated increased incidence of colonic cancer. Removing the gallbladder results in high levels of bile acids in the cecum, ascending colon, and stool[55,56] and may be associated with a greater frequency of right-sided colon cancer.[57] It is the free, not total, bile acid concentration that is most critical.[58,59]

5. INSUFFICIENT DIETARY CALCIUM. Calcium salts appear to modulate the damage described above by reducing the concentration of free bile acids by forming insoluble bile salt complexes.[58] At least one cohort study found that individuals with colon cancer tend to have a lower intake of calcium.[60]

6. FECAL PH. Alkaline environments support higher concentrations of free bile acids and other potential carcinogens.[61,62] In such an environment, bile acids are more soluble and carcinogens more damaging in animal model systems.[62,63] Epidemiologic studies from South Africa and the United States reveal a higher incidence of colon cancer in subjects with a higher stool *p*H.[60,64,65]

PRIMARY PREVENTION

Despite the inability to precisely identify the factor or factors responsible for colon cancer, a variety of dietary interventions have been considered and are being tested. Painter and Burkitt, observing dietary patterns in different African groups, postulated that those who ingested large volumes of fiber and consequently had high stool bulk had a lower incidence of many types of bowel disease, including colorectal cancer.[66,67] They suggested that high bulk stools promote faster colonic transit time, and thus intraluminal carcinogens have less opportunity to be formed or to interact with the epithelium at risk. However, this explanation is incomplete, since in some normal individuals fiber can slow fecal transit time. In addition to simple dilution, fiber may directly bind carcinogens, may favorably change the fecal *p*H, or may participate in other complex interactions.[68-70] Case–control and population studies in Scandinavia, Israel, and the United States support the contention that increased dietary fiber is of value.[25,71,72] Of the many types of fiber, cellulose and bran fiber may be more effective in reducing carcinogenesis than other fiber types.[73-75]

Limitation of total dietary fat and cholesterol has been proposed.[24] Studies of immigrant populations to Hawaii, populations in Nebraska,[14] and Seventh-Day Adventists[76] confirm that increased fat and cholesterol ingestion can be associated with increased risk of colorectal cancer. The use of *oral calcium* to potentially counteract bile acid effects has been suggested.[77] The use of *antioxidants* is also being evaluated. Vitamin C, tocopherol, and selenium are micronutrients that have many diverse biochemical effects but which also serve to protect gut epithelium from fecapentaene and other carcinogen (oxidative) damage.[78-80] However, simple dietary supplementation with these agents has not proved to be of dramatic benefit.[81,82]

With the identification of a number of phenotypic "intermediate biomarkers" associated with colorectal cancer, clinical prevention trials may generate useful insights without having to wait decades for the end results.[1]

SECONDARY PREVENTION. It is possible, in part, to identify patients at high risk for developing colorectal cancer. So-called secondary prevention strategies in these patients may include removal of precancerous lesions (neoplastic polyps), or excising the entire end-organ at risk. Management of patients with precancerous diseases will be discussed in a later section.

CLINICAL RISK FACTORS FOR COLORECTAL CANCER (TABLE 29-2)

GENETIC

FAMILIAL POLYPOSIS SYNDROMES. Several heritable syndromes are associated with adenomatous polyposis and a high risk of large bowel cancer.[83] The most important of these is the familial adenomatosis syndrome. Numerically, few colon cancer patients have this condition, since its incidence in the United States is between 1:6850 and 1:8300.[84] However, without intervention, virtually all affected individuals will develop colorectal cancer. The disease is inherited as an autosomal dominant trait, with greater than 90% penetrance. Affected persons develop pancolonic adenomatous polyposis. The polyps are not present at birth, but by late adolescence more than 1000 may be visualized. If the polyposis is untreated, the risk of cancer rises progressively with age so that by 40 years, nearly 80% of affected persons will have at least one adenocarcinoma. New mutations may arise in 20% to 30% of these cases of polyposis, and a careful evaluation of family members is necessary.[85-88]

Gardner's syndrome, also inherited as an autosomal dominant trait, occurs with half the frequency of familial adenomatosis syndrome. The entire large and small bowel may be affected by adenoma.[83] Other mesenchymal abnormalities that may coexist include desmoid tumors of the mesentery and abdominal wall, lipomas, sebaceous cysts, osteomas, and fibromas. Because the full clinical spectrum may not be expressed in a given patient, an evaluation of family members is warranted.[89,90] Related to this clinical entity may be the Oldfield syndrome of multiple sebaceous cysts associated with polyposis and adenocarcinoma.[91] It is likely that all of these syndromes are variations of the same genetic defect. Familial adenomatous polyposis is the generic appellation most recently selected to identify these groups. Less common is the Turcot syndrome, probably an autosomal recessive condition, which is associated with malignant central nervous system tumors in addition to bowel polyposis.[92]

Bodmer and co-workers have putatively identified one locus for the familial adenomatous polyposis gene on chromosome 5 near the fq21–22 bands.[93] Such molecular landmarks would permit screening in utero or before the development of signs or symptoms of disease. Moreover, the same researchers have identified a chromosome 5 allele loss in sporadic, noninherited colon cancer. Such molecular probes offer unprecedented opportunities for improved understanding of disease biology, diagnosis, prevention, and therapy.

HEREDITABLE SYNDROMES NOT PARTICULARLY ASSOCIATED WITH COLON CANCER. Both the Peutz-Jeghers syndrome and generalized juvenile polyposis are characterized by hamartomatous polyps of the bowel. The patient with Peutz-Jeghers syndrome has multiple tumors, usually clustered more in the small bowel (duodenum) than in the large intestine, and mucocutaneous pigmented lesions.[94] There is a small chance (2%–3%) of malignant degeneration.[95] The juvenile polyposis syndrome also is characterized by multiple hamartomas of the entire bowel. The chance of malignancy is considered to be quite small.[95,96]

FAMILIAL CANCER SYNDROMES. Certain families appear to have a high frequency of colon cancer without adenomatous polyposis of the bowel. A clinical condition described by Lynch and Lynch is inherited as an autosomal dominant trait with greater than 90% penetrance.[97] It has several unusual clinical features, including the development of multiple colon cancers at a relatively early age in several generations. The majority of these cancers are located in the proximal colon. A more generalized condition, also inherited as an autosomal dominant trait, has been described by Lynch et al and Law et al for some families with multiple colonic and extracolonic adenocarcinomas (familial adenocarcinomatosis).[97-99] This syndrome is characterized by the relatively early onset of colon, endometrial, breast, or gastric adenocarcinomas.[98]

For the majority of colorectal cancer patients, those with so-called sporadic disease, there is also evidence of an increased incidence in family members. Macklin has demonstrated that the relatives of individuals with sporadic colon cancer have a twofold to threefold greater chance of developing large bowel cancer than the general population.[100] The clustering of colon and rectal cancer in those with a positive family history but without an excess number of polyps has not been characterized as a specific genetic disorder.[83] Rather, environmental and dietary factors may be of greater importance—or, more likely, the etiology lies in a subtle interplay of heredity and environmental factors.[101] Burt et al analyzed a large family with multiple colon cancer cases but without a precisely definable pattern of inheritance and noted adenomatous polyps in 21% of 191 family members but in only 9% of 132 controls.[102] They proposed that this excess of polyps and colon cancer was the result of an unspecified autosomal dominant gene for susceptibility rather than chance occurrence. This group of patients is also the subject of investigation as to genotypic changes.[103]

INFLAMMATORY BOWEL DISEASE

There is a well-recognized increased risk (up to 30-fold) of colonic cancer in patients with inflammatory bowel disease. For patients with ulcerative colitis the incidence of malignancy increases with the extent of bowel involvement, age at onset, severity, and duration of the disease.[104-107] Patients who have had pancolitis for 30 years have a greater than 35% chance of developing bowel cancer.[108-111] At even

TABLE 29-2. Clinical Risk Factors for Colorectal Cancer

Genetic
    Familial adenomatous polyposis syndrome
    Gardner, Oldfield, or Turcot syndrome
    Peutz-Jegher syndrome
Familial
    Familial colorectal cancer syndrome
    Hereditary adenocarcinomatosis syndrome
    Family history of colorectal cancer
Preexisting disease
    Inflammatory bowel disease
    Colorectal cancer
    Pelvic cancer post irradiation
    Neoplastic colorectal polyps
General
    All men and women over age 40

greater risk are those in whom severe pancolitis began in childhood. Other atypical aspects of malignancy include multifocal disease (10%–20% of cases) and proximal colon primary sites (40%–50%).[106,112,113]

GRANULOMATOUS COLITIS

Crohn's disease also carries an increased risk of large as well as small bowel cancer.[114] Although granulomatous colitis is not as frequently associated with cancer as is ulcerative colitis, bowel adenocarcinomas with atypical presentations at younger ages are often noted.[113,115,116] Tumors usually arise in affected portions of the bowel, but they may also be metachronous and may occur in sites of prior surgery.[117]

PREVIOUS MALIGNANT DISEASE

Patients who have undergone treatment for a large bowel adenocarcinoma are at greater risk for developing a second colorectal tumor. There is at least a threefold greater likelihood that a second primary bowel cancer will develop either coincident with the index lesion or at a later time.[118-120] The implications for the follow-up of patients after definitive resection are obvious: regular reevaluation is required. Clustering of breast, ovarian, and colon cancer in the same patients has also been demonstrated. The aggregation of multiple adenocarcinomas is similar to the pattern described for familial adenocarcinoma syndrome.[121]

Irradiation of the pelvis also seems to enhance the risk of developing sigmoid cancer. Patients who have undergone radiation therapy for cervical, endometrial, or bladder cancer may be at enhanced risk of developing large bowel cancer, possibly related to irradiation-induced carcinogenesis.[122,123]

PRIOR NONCANCER SURGERY

Patients who have undergone cholecystectomy or ureterosigmoidostomy have a higher incidence of large bowel cancer. It is postulated that the high concentration of inciting or promoting compounds in the secretions accounts for the increased risk of neoplasia.[124-126]

POLYPS

Neoplastic and inflammatory polyps occur in the large bowel. Adenomatous polyps may be tubular or villous. The tubular adenomas are four times more common than the villous adenomas and are usually smaller. In general, large polyps are more likely to contain a malignant focus than the smaller ones; nearly half of polyps larger than 2 cm in diameter will contain malignancy.

Approximately 25% of patients with one tubular polyp will have others. Tubular adenomas are relatively more evenly distributed throughout the large bowel, while villous tumors are more frequently found in the rectum.[127] Villous adenomas are reported to have eight to ten times the probability of cancer than tubular polyps.[127-130]

Predictably, the larger the number of these adenomas, the greater the chance that cancer will develop.[131] Although it is not necessary to have a polyp prior to or coincident with a cancer, this sequence occurs five times more frequently than cancer alone.[10]

GENERAL POPULATION

By far the largest population at risk for colorectal cancer are men and women over the age of 40. Although colorectal cancer is sometimes found in children, the incidence of disease increases steadily up to the eighth decade.[132,133]

DIAGNOSIS

Colorectal cancer may be diagnosed when a patient presents with symptoms or as the result of a screening program. Except for patients with obstructing or perforating cancers, the duration of symptoms does not correlate with prognosis.[134-136] However, since early colorectal cancer produces no symptoms, and since many of the symptoms of colorectal cancer are nonspecific, aggressive efforts at detection through screening programs are essential.

We cannot adequately stress the vagueness of abdominal symptoms in colorectal cancer. Twelve percent of otherwise healthy patients without colorectal cancer complain of a change in bowel habits in the recent past, and 11% report abdominal pain.[137] Even rectal bleeding has a very low predictive value in the diagnosis of colorectal cancer.[138] Screening strategies will be discussed in subsequent sections.

EVALUATION OF THE SYMPTOMATIC PATIENT

COLON CANCER. Symptoms of colon cancer—intermittent abdominal pain, nausea, or vomiting—are secondary to bleeding, obstruction, or perforation. A palpable mass is common with right colon cancer. Bleeding may be acute and most commonly appears as red blood mixed with stool. Dark blood is most commonly secondary to diverticular bleeding. Occasionally, melena may be associated with a right colon cancer. Chronic blood loss with iron deficiency anemia can occur. Such patients may present with weakness and high output congestive heart failure. Lesser degrees of bleeding may be detected as part of a fecal occult blood test (discussed below under screening). Rectal bleeding associated with warfarin use should be investigated to rule out a colon cancer.

Malignant obstruction of the large bowel is most commonly associated with cancer of the sigmoid. If the ileocecal valve is competent, such obstructions manifest as acute abdominal illness. If the ileocecal valve is incompetent, the illness is more insidious, with increasing constipation and abdominal distention noted over many days. The major differential diagnosis in such cases includes cancer and diverticulitis. A limited barium enema examination may yield only suggestive data, and even fiberoptic endoscopy may not be diagnostic if associated edema precludes reaching the cancer with the endoscope. Cytology of a brush biopsy specimen obtained through the fiberoptic endoscope may be diagnostic.

TABLE 29-3. Qualitative Analysis of Screening Options for Colorectal Cancer

Technique	Sensitivity for Cancer	Sensitivity for Polyps	Cost	Patient Discomfort
Digital rectal examination	+	$\frac{1}{2}$+	$\frac{1}{2}$+	+
Fecal occult blood	++	+	$\frac{1}{2}$+	$\frac{1}{2}$+
Rigid sigmoidoscopy	++	++	++	++
Flexible sigmoidoscopy (60–65 cm)	+++	+++	++	+
Single column barium enema	++	+	++	++
Air contrast barium enema	+++	+++	++	+++
Colonoscopy	++++	++++	++++	+++

The perforation of colon cancer may be acute or chronic. The clinical picture of acute perforation may be identical to that of appendicitis or diverticulitis, with pain, fever, and a palpable mass. In the presence of obstruction, there may be a perforation either through the tumor or through proximal nontumorous colon (cecum). The distinction is important from a prognostic viewpoint. Chronic perforation with fistula formation into the bladder from sigmoid colon cancer is similar to diverticulitis. Gross pneumaturia may occur, or the patient may present only with recurrent urinary tract infections. The continued presence of multiple enteric organisms despite repeated treatment mandates diagnostic studies. Bladder cytologies, cystoscopy, brushings, and biopsies may not lead to the correct diagnosis. Fiberoptic endoscopy of the colon is the most valuable diagnostic procedure.

RECTAL CANCER. Rectal and rectosigmoid cancer is much more likely to be symptomatic prior to diagnosis. Gross red blood (mixed or covering stool, or by itself) is frequent. Hemorrhoidal bleeding should always be a diagnosis of exclusion. All patients with rectal bleeding should be evaluated. If the blood is minimal and bright red in appearance, is located only on the toilet paper, and is associated with normal-colored stool, a sigmoidoscopy (preferably fiberoptic sigmoidoscopy with a 60- to 65-cm instrument) may suffice. All other patients should undergo sigmoidoscopy and barium enema examination, or colonoscopy. Since a rectal cancer may be missed on barium enema examination, proctosigmoidoscopy complements the radiologic study.

With compromise of the rectal reservoir by tumor, a change in bowel activity may occur. Unexplained constipation or reduction in stool caliber should lead to evaluation. Obstructing rectal cancers frequently cause diarrhea rather than constipation. Rigid sigmoidoscopy and barium enema examination or colonoscopy are the appropriate studies.

In cases of locally advanced rectal cancer with circumferential growth and extensive transmural penetration, urgency and inadequate emptying lead to tenesmus. This is usually a grave sign. Some degree of tenesmus may occur with less extensive distal rectal cancer as part of the normal rectal reflex. Urinary symptoms may occur with compression of the bladder, invasion of the prostate, or destruction of the high sacral nerve roots. Buttock or perineal pain from posterior extension also is a grave sign.

METASTATIC DISEASE. Synchronous liver metastases occur in 5% to 10% of patients and occasionally are the presenting manifestation of colorectal cancer. The patient may complain of pain in the right upper quadrant, right hypochondrium, right posterior chest, or right shoulder. The pain may be a continuous ache, or it may be experienced as an acute episode related to hemorrhage or necrosis of a metastasis. Hepatomegaly may be detected on routine physical examination of an otherwise asymptomatic patient. It is important to evaluate the gastrointestinal (GI) tract in such patients, even if the fecal occult blood test is negative, before proceeding with a premature liver biopsy.

SCREENING

The early detection of colorectal cancer is potentially associated with a dramatic reduction in disease-related mortality. The relatively slow growth of most colorectal cancers and the high diagnostic sensitivity of colonoscopy and air contrast barium enema examination justify aggressive screening strategies. In addition, some screening approaches may detect not only early cancers, but benign neoplastic polyps as well. Endoscopic removal of such polyps may, to some extent, prevent subsequent colorectal cancer. Screening strategies must take into account the risk of the population being screened, the segments of the large bowel at greatest risk, the cost-effectiveness of screening, the availability of various technologies, and patient compliance.[139]

A qualitative assessment of the various screening options is outlined in Table 29-3. The reader should keep in mind that there has been a proximal shift in the location of many colorectal cancers, leading to a considerable increase in right colon cancers, particularly in women.[140-142] Predictive values for the various screening methods have not been included in Table 29-3, since they are prevalence dependent. For example, the predictive value of a positive fecal occult blood test in an otherwise healthy 40-year-old person will be much lower than in a 65-year-old person with a strong family history of colorectal cancer. The incidence of colorectal cancer in the 65-year-old population is 10 times as great as in the 40-year-old population.

HIGH-RISK FACTORS

FAMILY HISTORY. In persons with a family history of colorectal cancer, screening should begin at age 35 to 40 years with a yearly fecal occult blood test and probably some type of endoscopic surveillance.[143] Flexible sigmoidoscopy (with the 60- to 65-cm instrument) every 3 to 5 years should be considered, with full colonoscopy if an adenomatous polyp is identified.[144] Autosomal dominant cancer families require frequent invasive screening with colonoscopy or sigmoidoscopy combined with air contrast barium enema examinations every 3 to 5 years beginning at age 40.[139]

FAMILIAL ADENOMATOUS POLYPOSIS. Once the diagnosis of familial adenomatous polyposis is made, many patients will undergo either a total colectomy with ileorectal anastomosis, or total proctocolectomy with ileostomy or ileal pouch–anal anastomosis. Those with retained rectum should undergo rigid proctoscopy with fulguration of polyps every 6 months for the rest of their lives.

PERSONAL HISTORY OF CANCER OR POLYP. Endoscopic surveillance of the entire remaining bowel is appropriate every 1 to 3 years.[145] An air contrast barium enema examination combined with limited endoscopy is also reasonable. The National Polyp Study is prospectively gathering data on the frequency and type of follow-up appropriate for these patients.[146] Preliminary data indicate that patients with multiple polyps, particularly villous lesions, are at a greater risk for subsequent polyp formation.

ULCERATIVE COLITIS. Patients with a history of extensive ulcerative colitis (except patients with isolated ulcerative proctitis) present for at least 10 years and not treated by proctocolectomy, require colonoscopic surveillance every 1 to 2 years. Any worrisome area is biopsied, and multiple blind biopsies of "normal" mucosa are performed to detect dysplasia.[147,148] A recent review questions the efficacy of endoscopic screening in this population.[149]

SCREENING STRATEGIES FOR THE GENERAL POPULATION

DIGITAL RECTAL EXAMINATION. The digital rectal examination is a traditional part of the annual physical examination. In addition to low rectal cancers, anal and prostatic cancers may also be detected; and a stool specimen is obtained for occult blood determination. The sensitivity of the digital rectal examination has decreased with the more proximal shift in the location of colorectal cancer. Although it is difficult to demonstrate a reduction in cancer mortality from periodic rectal digital examinations, the procedure should remain part of any regular physical examination.[150]

RIGID SIGMOIDOSCOPY. Rigid sigmoidoscopy is comparatively inexpensive, but its usefulness is restricted by the length of bowel that can be examined and by patients' unwillingness to undergo the procedure. In a series of 26,000 patients over the age of 45 studied at the Strang Clinic, asymptomatic cancer was detected in 58 patients.[151] The cure rate in these patients was 90%. Gilbertsen et al studied 18,000 patients with serial sigmoidoscopies and polypectomies.[152] Although the variable length of follow-up makes accurate analysis difficult, their data indicate a substantial reduction in the incidence of subsequent rectal cancer in patients from whom premalignant polyps were removed.

FLEXIBLE SIGMOIDOSCOPY. Flexible proctosigmoidoscopes are available in 25 to 35 cm lengths and 60 to 65 cm lengths. The light source is provided by fiberoptic technology. Viewing may use fiberoptics or direct videoendoscopic technology. The shorter scopes are relatively easy to learn to use, more comfortable for the patient, and more applicable for screening programs using nonphysician personnel.[153,154] The longer flexible sigmoidoscopes reach on the average 45 cm proximal to the anus (the junction of the descending colon and sigmoid) and allow detection of approximately two thirds of colorectal cancers and polyps.[144,154-160] Any patient found to have a neoplastic polyp on screening endoscopy should be considered at high risk and should undergo complete examination of the remaining colon and more intense surveillance.

BARIUM ENEMA AND COLONOSCOPY. Because most studies compare these two procedures, a joint discussion follows. The standard barium enema examination is unsatisfactory for the detection of early cancers or polyps, missing one third of early cancers in a study by Gilbertsen et al.[152] Colonoscopy is the most accurate way of diagnosing early colorectal cancers and allows resection of premalignant polyps at the same time. However, the air contrast barium enema examination may be almost as accurate, except for diminutive polyps, and has the advantage of routine visualization of the ascending colon, not possible in 5% to 10% of colonoscopies.[161-164] Endoscopy is not completely accurate: polyps may not be visualized because of blind corners and mucosal folds, and the cecum may not be reached in every case.[165] The prospective data from the National Polyp Study will more clearly define the efficacy of these two modalities.

TABLE 29-4. Screening Programs for Colorectal Cancer Using Fecal Occult Blood Tests

Study	No. of Patients	Compliance	Positive Tests (%)	No. of Cancers Detected	Predictive Value (%)
Gilbertsen et al[152]	23,000	72	2.3	54	11.3
Winawer et al[177]	13,127	74	2.5	59	17.7
Winchester et al[184]	54,101	26	4.4	29	4.7
Sontag et al[185]	13,522	22	4.6	14	10.3
Cummings et al[178]	58,934	20	2.3	17	6.4
Hardcastle et al[176]	10,253	39	2.4	17	13.7

EXFOLIATIVE CYTOLOGY. Lavage-induced exfoliative cytology and brush biopsies can be used as an adjunct to endoscopic examination. Lavage cytology does not appear to improve the diagnostic yield, although brush techniques may be helpful.[166]

FECAL CARCINOEMBRYONIC ANTIGEN. This approach is at the earliest stages of investigation.[167] The concept of detecting shed tumor antigens in the feces needs to be explored in additional studies.

FECAL OCCULT BLOOD TESTING. Guaiac-impregnated paper slide tests for fecal occult blood have been available for 20 years. The relatively low cost and the potential for patient testing at home have generated considerable interest in this approach. All guaiac tests measure hemoglobin indirectly by the determination of its peroxidase activity. Two other approaches are being studied. The HemoQuant test, a quantitative assay for fecal hemoglobin, is based on the conversion of heme to fluorescent porphyrins.[168,169] The test is more costly and requires more complicated testing support. Data are not yet available comparing this test with existing guaiac-based systems in a large screening program. An immunochemical approach to the detection of human fecal hemoglobin is possible, which would obviate false positive test results associated with dietary hemoglobin and ingestion of peroxidase-containing foods.[170,171]

In considering the overall impact of fecal occult blood screening programs, a number of features must be stressed. False positive tests are extremely expensive and at best inconvenient for the patient. Patients with positive test results undergo extensive diagnostic testing, which may include sigmoidoscopy, barium enema, colonoscopy, and upper GI endoscopy.[172] Patients with false negative results may be inappropriately reassured, and may disregard subsequent symptoms.

All guaiac-based fecal occult blood tests are unreliable to some degree. Ahlquist and Beart[173] reported positive Hemoccult test results with as little as 0.04 mg hemoglobin per gram of stool (normal, <2 mg/g) and negative results with as much as 42.5 mg/g. Fecal occult blood testing as a screening technique assumes that colorectal cancers (many of which are ulcerated) are associated with detectable intraluminal blood loss. However, some colorectal cancers bleed intermittently, and others not at all. In several studies of patients with known colorectal cancer, 20% to 30% of patients had negative fecal occult blood tests.[174-176] Less than one third of patients with polyps have stools positive for occult blood.[176]

Several factors affect the accuracy of fecal occult blood tests.[169,178,179] The initial studies by Greegor suggested that dietary restriction was important in order to minimize peroxidase from red meat, fresh fruit, and raw vegetables. Macrae and associates did not find this to be very important, as long as the slides were not dehydrated.[180] This issue has yet to be completely resolved. The number of stool specimens tested will influence the reliability of the technique.[181] Separate specimens taken on three consecutive days is the usual recommendation. Slide hydration before testing reactivates the fecal peroxidase activity. Although this maneuver decreases the false negative rate, it dramatically increases the false positive rate.[177] Certain medications, including iron, cimetidine, antacids, and particularly large amounts of ascorbic acid, may interfere with the peroxidase reaction, leading to an increased false negative rate.[182]

Evaluation of the Positive Fecal Occult Blood Test. Because the predictive value of a positive test is less than 20%, the few dollars spent for the fecal occult blood test leads to a great expenditure of funds to identify patients with true positive results.[172] Although a complete colonoscopy is probably the most direct way to exclude cancer and polyps, an air contrast barium enema examination may be the most cost-effective approach to the evaluation of the patient with a positive test result.[183] Rigid or flexible sigmoidoscopy should complement the barium study.

Screening Programs. Data from selected large series are presented in Table 29-4.[152,176-178,184,185] Approximately 2.5% of tested patients are Hemoccult (or Hemoccult II) positive, with compliance rates ranging from 20% to 97%.

Three large-scale prospective population-based programs are attempting to demonstrate a reduction in colorectal cancer mortality with fecal occult blood test-screening, and to define compliance and cost issues associated with this test. These studies are taking place at the University of Minnesota; New York; Nottingham, England; and Goteborg, Sweden.[176,184]

SCREENING RECOMMENDATIONS FOR THE GENERAL POPULATION. We recommend yearly fecal occult blood tests and sigmoidoscopy every 3 to 5 years beginning at age 40. We would encourage the greater use of flexible sigmoidoscopy as part of a screening strategy.

PATHOLOGY

GROSS APPEARANCE

Tumor configuration may be divided into fungating (exophytic), ulcerating, stenosing, or constricting (annular, circumferential). Approximately two thirds of all tumors are ulcerating and one third are fungating.[186] These configurations do not represent different kinds of tumors but different phases of an orderly progression. Most malignant bowel tumors start out as a small polypoid lesions. These lesions may grow into the lumen, or into the bowel wall itself. As they grow laterally or circumferentially, they are termed *infiltrating.* Right-sided cancers, usually fungating in nature, tend to grow more into the lumen and extend along one wall, especially in the capacious cecum. Left-sided cancers tend to grow more into the bowel wall and circumferentially, having a typical "napkin ring" configuration on barium enema examination. These cancers are thought to start as sessile masses that gradually span the circumference over a 1- to 2-year period. Growth along circumferential lymphatics may account for much of this behavior. As tumors grow into the bowel, they eventually interfere with the blood supply, occasionally leading to necrosis, ulceration, and perforation.[187,188]

HISTOLOGIC TYPES

The major histologic type of large bowel cancer is adenocarcinoma, which accounts for 90% to 95% of all large bowel tumors.[189,190] It is the only histologic type further classified by grade. Adenocarcinoma consists of columnar or cuboidal epithelium with varying degrees of loss of the normal differentiation pattern.

A number of histologic types of large bowel cancer have been identified. The World Health Organization (WHO) has developed a classification of both benign and malignant tumors.[191] The classification of malignant tumors is given in Table 29-5. Descriptions of most of these pathologic types may be found in the Armed Forces Institute of Pathology Series[192]; illustrations of each may be found in that series and in the WHO series.[191]

Mucinous or "colloid" adenocarcinoma represents approximately 10% of large bowel tumors.[193] These adenocarcinomas are defined by large amounts of *extracellular* mucin retained within the tumor. A separate WHO classification is the rare (4% of mucinous carcinomas) *signet-ring cell* carcinoma, which contains intracellular mucin, which pushes the nucleus to one side. Some signet-ring tumors appear to form a linitis plastica type of tumor by spreading intramurally, usually not involving the mucosa.[194] Other rare variants of epithelial tumors include squamous cell carcinomas, of which about 40 cases have been reported in the literature.[195] Another rare variant is the adenosquamous carcinoma, sometimes called adenoacanthoma. This tumor has elements of both adenocarcinoma and squamous carcinoma and usually manifests as an ulcerated tumor. About 50 cases have been reported in the literature.[190]

Finally, there are the undifferentiated carcinomas, which contain no glandular structures or other features such as mucus secretions. Other designations for undifferentiated carcinoma include carcinoma simplex, medullary carcinoma, and trabecular carcinoma. Gibbs has emphasized that undifferentiated carcinomas are not necessarily anaplastic.[196] He describes undifferentiated carcinoma as a malignant epithelial neoplasm that does not differentiate into formed tubules, but exhibits little nuclear pleomorphism and few bizarre mitoses.

TABLE 29-5.   World Health Organization Classification of Malignant Primary Tumors of the Large Intestine

Epithelial tumors
   Adenocarcinoma
   Mucinous adenocarcinoma
   Signet-ring cell adenocarcinoma
   Squamous cell carcinoma
   Adenosquamous carcinoma
   Undifferentiated carcinoma
   Unclassified carcinoma
Carcinoid tumors
   Argentaffin
   Nonargentaffin
   Composite
Nonepithelial tumors
   Leiomyosarcoma
   Others
Hematopoietic and lymphoid neoplasms
Unclassified

About 4% to 17% of carcinoids may appear in the rectum, and 2% to 7% may appear in the colon.[197-199] These small, firm, polypoid nodules are covered by an intact mucosa and rarely produce the carcinoid syndrome. The nonepithelial tumors include a variety of sarcomas, all rare; leiomyosarcomas appear to predominate. In one report of intestinal leiomyosarcoma, 4 of 41 cases were in the rectum and none were in the colon.[199] Primary malignant lymphomas that occur in the colon and rectum are usually of a diffuse histiocytic (large cell) type.[190]

DEGREE OF DIFFERENTIATION

Broders was a pioneer in classifying the adenocarcinomas by their degree of differentiation.[200] He designated four grades, based on the percentage of differentiated tumor cells. "Well differentiated" in Broders' system meant well-formed glands, resembling an adenoma. Broders included the mucinous carcinomas in his system. Dukes considered mucinous carcinomas separately.[201] Because of their poor prognosis, others group them with the most undifferentiated tumors.

Dukes' grading system considered the arrangement of cells rather than the percentage of differentiated cells. Dukes' initial approach evolved into a three-grade system, now most widely used. Grade 1 is the most differentiated, with well-formed tubules and the least nuclear polymorphism and fewest mitoses. Grade 3 is the least differentiated, having only occasional glandular structures, pleomorphic cells, and a high incidence of mitoses. Grade 2 is intermediate between Grades 1 and 3.[189,202]

Jass and colleagues use seven parameters in their grading criteria: histologic type, overall differentiation, nuclear polarity, tubule configuration, pattern of growth, lymphocytic infiltration, and amount of fibrosis.[203] It is clear that not everybody agrees on the grading criteria, but most agree on the use of a three-grade system, similar to that described in this section.

SPREAD OF COLORECTAL CANCER

Much of what we know about the local and distant spread of colorectal cancer is due to the meticulous and elegant studies of Cuthbert Dukes, a pathologist at St. Mark's Hospital in London, who did extensive studies on the local invasion of rectal cancer and on lymphatic involvement by this disease. In 1930, Dukes and his colleague Gordon-Watson described the spread of rectal cancer,[187] which Dukes amplified in later papers.[188,201,204]

LOCAL INVASION. After the initial mucosal growth, there are several directions in which a tumor may progress, but usually it protrudes first into the lumen. Dukes found that subsequent lateral invasion was greater in the transverse rather than the longitudinal direction, leading to circumferential growth.[201,205] Black and Waugh found that the same growth pattern occurred in colon cancer.[206]

In addition to intramural and circumferential spread, the growth of rectal cancer proceeds cephalad and caudad (longitudinally). Dukes described the growth as more extensive in the submucosa.[201] However, Miles in 1920 concluded that submucosal intramural spread was comparatively trivial.[207] In a 1966 study of curative resections, Grinnell found no retrograde submucosal spread in 67 of 76 cases.[208]

As the tumor traverses the muscularis mucosa and infiltrates the submucosa, it is termed *invasive*. As it reaches the muscle and blood supply becomes inadequate, ulceration may occur. As the tumor penetrates the rectal wall and extrarectal tissues, it directly invades neighboring structures.[204] Dukes and Bussey defined various degrees of local spread: slight local spread denotes invasion only of the extrarectal tissues; moderate spread refers to tumor well established in the mesentery; and extensive spread refers to deeply invasive carcinoma, possibly extending into neighboring organs.[204] They also found that the extent of spread increases with the grade of the tumor.

One of the more interesting ways of looking at histologic sections is with whole mounts of the cross-section of the bowel.[209,210] This histologic procedure allows one to define the invasion profile of lateral transmural penetration. This has not been used extensively yet, but it may prove to be of great use in future studies.

An additional pattern of local spread is perineural invasion, or spread along the perineural spaces, which may reach as far as 10 cm from the primary tumor.[211] Perineural invasion increases with the degree of local extension. In one study, no patient with Dukes' A tumors had perineural invasion, whereas 24% of those with Dukes' B and 69% with Dukes' C tumors did have perineural invasion, as did 23% of patients with Broders Grade 2 lesions and 58% with Grade 3 lesions.[212] Too few patients had Broders Grade 1 or 4 lesions to evaluate.

LYMPHATIC EXTENSION. In 1930 Dukes concluded, incorrectly, that lymph node metastases occurred only after local tumor spread into the perirectal tissues.[187] The exceptions were generally high-grade tumors. More recent studies have demonstrated a 10% to 20% incidence of nodal metastases from rectal cancer limited to the bowel wall.[213-225]

In 1935 Gabriel et al described the orderly and predictable course of spread of lymphatic disease in rectal cancer.[226] First, disease metastasizes to the perirectal nodes at the level of the primary tumor or immediately above it. Then the chain accompanying the superior hemorrhoidal vessels is involved. Very rarely are there discontinuous or skip metastases.[226-229] The pericolic lymph nodes along the mesenteric border of the pelvis usually are not involved by these rectal tumors unless there is extensive tumor with lymphatic blockage. Gabriel et al pointed out that in late stages of the disease, when the hemorrhoidal lymphatics are blocked, there is lateral or downward spread.[226] Grinnell also noted such retrograde flow in 34 (3.7%) of 913 cases of colon and rectum tumors.[230]

In colon carcinoma, the normal lymphatic flow is through the lymphatic channels along the major arteries, with three echelons of lymph nodes: pericolic, intermediate, and principal lymph nodes. If tumors lie between two major vascular pedicles, lymphatic flow may drain in either or both directions, as shown in Figure 29-6. If the central lymph nodes

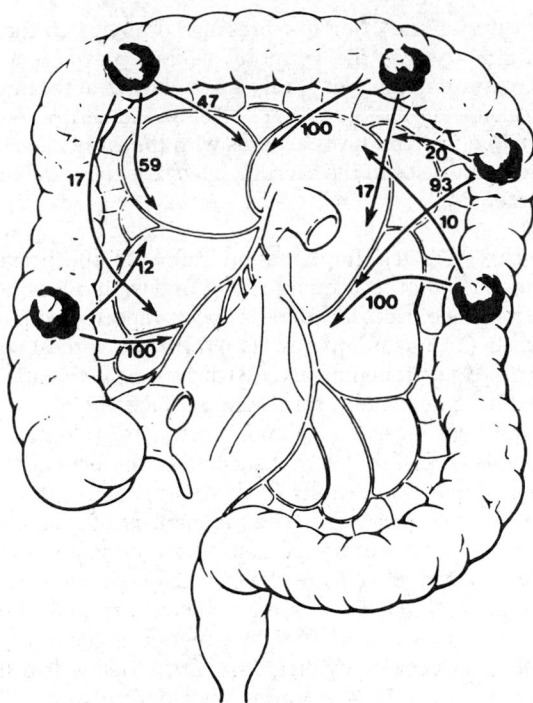

FIG. 29-6. For tumors that lie between two pedicles, lymphatic flow may drain in either or both directions. From a study of cleared specimens, it was possible to determine the preferential route by the location of lymphatic metastases. The numbers above signify the percentage of metastasizing carcinomas in the above locations that have demonstrated positive nodes along a given vascular route. For example, tumors lying between the ileocolic and right colic arcades metastasize along the ileocolic pedicle in 100% and along the right colin in 12%. (Hertzer FP, Slanetz CA: Patterns and significance of lymphatic spread from cancer of the colon and rectum. In Weiss L, Gilbert HA, Ballon SC (eds): Lymphatic System Metastasis. Boston, GK Hall, 1980)

are blocked by tumor, lymphatic flow can become retrograde along the marginal arcades, both proximally and distally.[231]

The risk of lymph node metastases increases with increasing tumor grade.[204] Dukes found that 30% of low-grade tumors were associated with positive lymph nodes, compared to 81% of high-grade tumors. The number of lymph nodes involved also increased with grade: an average of 3.2 nodes were involved for low-grade tumors and 6.8 for high-grade tumors.

HEMATOGENOUS SPREAD. The liver is the primary site of hematogenous metastases, followed by the lung. In approximately 40% of autopsy studies the liver is the only site involved.[232-234] Involvement of other sites in the absence of liver or lung involvement is rare.

The major venous drainage of the lower rectum is by a dual system: drainage from the superior hemorrhoidal veins enters the portal system to the liver, drainage from the middle and inferior hemorrhoidal veins eventually reaches the vena cava to get to the lungs. Bone metastases in the sacrum and the vertebral bodies may occur through the vertebral venous plexus, as originally described by Batson.[235] In 1977 Vider et al proposed that this system represented another mechanism of metastatic spread.[236] The portal mesenteric and caval systems offer low-pressure drainage to the liver and lungs, whereas the vertebral venous plexus is a high-pressure system that may only open during defecation, allowing metastases to go to the skeleton and central nervous system. Such a hypothesis accords with the early appearance of bone metastases in the sacrum, coccyx, pelvis, and lumbar vertebrae.

IMPLANTATION. Implantation refers to the release of tumor cells from the primary tumor and their deposition on another surface. Implantation has been reported with tumor cells shed (1) intraluminally, (2) from the serosal surface through the peritoneum, and (3) by surgical manipulation and resulting deposition on wound surfaces.[237]

Intraluminal spread of tumor occurs by release of the tumor cells from the mucosal surface of the primary tumor and their deposition distally in the bowel, either in fistulas, abscesses, or hemorrhoids. The mechanism of such implantation is considered to be the deposition of viable cells onto the raw surface of a fistula or an ulcerated or surgically treated hemorrhoid. There are a number of reports of tumor growth in hemorrhoids.[238-240] McGrew et al found that the percentage of positive cytologic smears varied with distance from the tumor in 50 specimens studied. Smears were positive in 42% at the proximal ends of resected specimens (average length, 21 cm) and in 65% at the distal ends (average length, 10 cm).[241]

Transcoelomic spread accounts for intraperitoneal seeding and carcinomatosis seen, even in the absence of nodal or hematogenous spread.

Other forms of implantation may be related to surgery. The incidence of disease recurrence at suture lines is about 10%.[242,243] At least half of these recurrences might be explained by implantation of cells from the stump.[242]

Tumor can also be implanted into the abdominal surgical scar,[244-246] into the perineal scar after an abdominoperineal resection,[247-249] or even into the mucocutaneous margin of a colostomy.[242,250] Pomeranz and Garlock performed studies to ascertain how easily cells might be dislodged from the serosal surface during surgery.[246] They looked at cells obtained by gently rubbing the serosal surface with a slide or cotton tip. Tumor cells were found in 2 of 20 cases. Boreham tried such studies in 52 patients and could not easily dislodge cells from the serosa.[245] However, in 4 of 16 samples, sections through areas of serosal puckering or ulceration opposite the growth revealed malignant cells on the peritoneal surface.

A concern is that surgical manipulation could also release cells into the venous circulation. Cole et al found malignant cells in the veins when isotonic saline was perfused from the artery to the vein when the vein and artery had been tied off before any colonic manipulation.[243] Fisher and Turnbull found tumor cells in the mesenteric veins in 32% of 25 consecutive bowel resections.[251]

STAGING AND PROGNOSTIC FEATURES

The staging of colorectal carcinoma has been complicated by the fact that it has evolved over half a century, and various authors have developed systems that use the same descrip-

tors to represent different stages. Even one common and simple staging system, the Dukes classification for cancer of the rectum, has been misinterpreted by various authors.[252] This is perhaps not surprising, since the definitions changed even in Dukes' personal series of publications.[187,201] Because of these discrepancies in coding for the same stages, comparison of clinical studies reported in the literature is often impossible.

The ultimate value of any staging system lies not only in treatment planning but in comparing results of different studies and predicting recurrence patterns and survival.[253] Many pathologic features of colorectal carcinoma influence predictions of recurrence and survival. Independent pathologic variables include the depth of penetration through the bowel wall, whether lymph nodes are involved, and the number of involved lymph nodes. Nonindependent features that have been incorporated into a few staging systems include extent of local invasion,[214,254] level of lymph node involvement,[226] blood vessel invasion, lymphatic invasion, histologic grade,[255] and carcinoembryonic antigen (CEA) level.[256,257]

SURGICAL–PATHOLOGIC STAGING

This section describes various pathologic staging systems. Operative findings of liver metastases, peritoneal seeding, and adherence to or invasion of contiguous organs must be combined with the histologic findings.

Dukes' Classification and Its Modifications

The first practical staging system was Dukes' classification,[201] which classified rectal tumors from A to C, with stage A indicating penetration into but not through the bowel wall, stage B representing penetration through the bowel wall, and stage C representing involvement of lymph nodes, regardless of the extent of bowel wall penetration. This system, developed from an earlier clinical grouping by Lockhart-Mummery,[258] had the virtue of being simple and predictive of prognosis. However, it has since been modified by many authors, including Dukes,[226] to reflect finer levels of penetration and nodal metastases, and has been extended to include the colon as well as the rectum.

The most important of the staging systems that utilize the A, B, C terminology are shown in Figure 29-7. Kirklin and colleagues split Dukes' stage A into a new A (mucosa only) and B1 (into but not through the muscularis propria), and changed Dukes' stage B to B2.[259] The Astler–Coller staging system[213] allowed separation of wall penetration and nodal status.

A recent analysis of clinical trials in the National Surgical Adjuvant Breast and Bowel Project (NSABP) compared the prognostic abilities of various modifications of the original Dukes classification.[260] In Dukes' stage C the level of positive node involvement, defined as either less than 2 cm or 2 cm or more beyond the bowel wall, was not very predictive of ultimate survival. Researchers analyzing the clinical trial results found that depth of penetration and the number of positive nodes were significant predictors of survival, and the number of positive nodes was the strongest factor in this

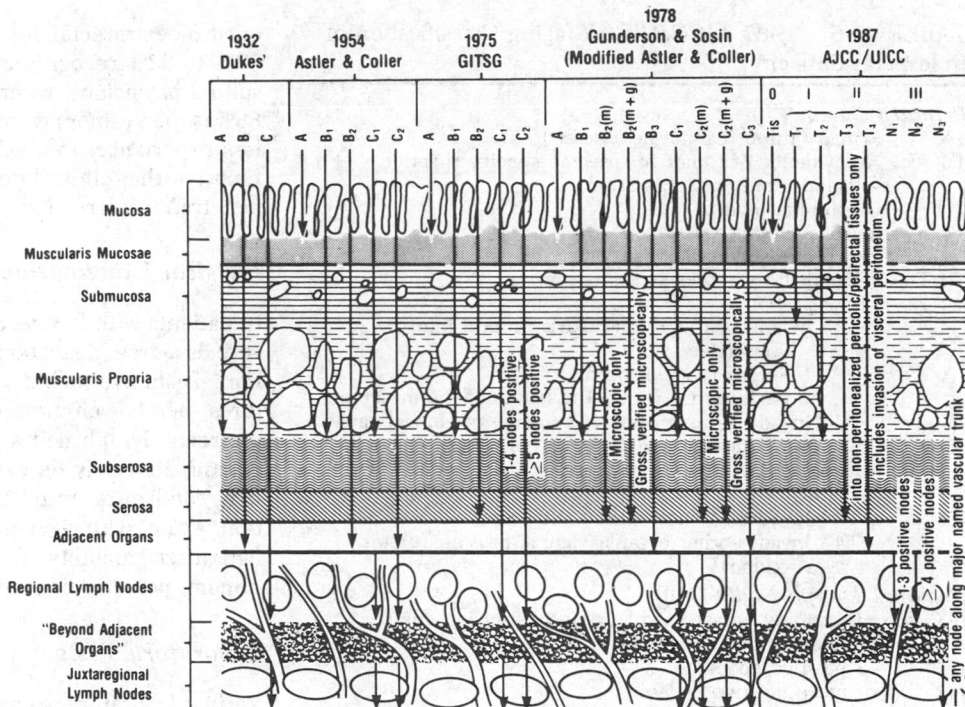

FIG. 29-7. Schematic comparison of the various pathological staging systems.

analysis. The number of positive nodes was also independently prognostic in the multivariate analysis from the Large Bowel Cancer Project in London.[261] Until now, the number of positive nodes has been included only in the Gastrointestinal Tumor Study Group (GITSG) classification.[262] The data suggest that any classification or staging system devised in the future should certainly consider the number of positive nodes as a predictive discriminant.

The TNM Classification

Both the American Joint Committee on Cancer (AJCC)[263] and the International Union Against Cancer (UICC)[264] have proposed staging systems utilizing the TNM classification. There was not, however, total agreement between the staging systems, and neither system specifically considered the number of positive nodes. In studies which looked at the prognostic ability of pathologic TNM staging,[265-267] survival was identical or even reversed for Stages II and III.

A revised, 1987 joint AJCC/UICC TNM staging system unified the two systems. The revised system is simpler and considers the important prognostic factor, the number of positive nodes.[268-270] Free mesothelial penetration is also considered.[271] We strongly recommend the universal use of the new TNM system for reporting end results. Table 29-6 defines the three most widely used systems: Dukes, Astler–Coller, and the 1987 TNM.

CLINICAL STAGING SYSTEMS

Pretreatment Evaluation

Because all three systems described above involve postsurgical pathologic staging, they cannot be used for making treatment decisions, and they are not applicable when sphincter-conserving procedures are used, such as fulguration, local excision, or contact radiation therapy. Therefore, clinical staging systems have been considered. Abrams tried to correlate the size of the tumor, the presence or absence of ulceration, and the degree of differentiation with the final Dukes' stage.[272] Ulceration was the principal feature, with 63% of nonulcerated cancers classified as Dukes' A, compared with only 28% of ulcerated lesions. Another clinical staging system, devised by a group from the Princess Margaret Hospital in Toronto,[273] was based on several prognostic variables: the presence or absence of metastases, whether the rectal tumor was fixed or mobile, whether it was annular, and whether the clinical symptoms of weight loss, anorexia, weakness, and anemia were present. These variables were grouped into four clinical classes. In Class I none of the variables were present; Class II was characterized by annular rectal tumor or the systemic symptoms; Class III denoted a fixed rectal tumor; and in Class IV metastases were present. Patient survival correlated well with breakdown into these classes and with breakdown by Dukes' stages, but the correlation between clinical classes and Dukes' stages was not good. Recently, univariate and multivariate analyses of prognostic features were done on 824 rectal cancer patients in the Medical Research Council's preoperative radiation therapy trial in the United Kingdom.[274,275] Mobility of the tumor was the most important preoperative assessment related to curative resection.

An Australian Clinicopathological Staging System combines features of both a pathologic staging system and a clinical system, based on local tumor characteristics alone.[276,277]

York Mason has also suggested the use of a clinical staging system based on mobility of the primary tumor. Clinical

TABLE 29-6. 1987 AJCC/UICC Staging Classification of
Colorectal Cancer*

Primary Tumor (T)
TX   Primary tumor cannot be assessed
T0   No evidence of tumor in resected specimen (prior
—polypectomy or fulguration)
Tis   Carcinoma in situ
T1   Invades submucosa
T2   Invades into muscularis propria
T3/T4   Depends on whether serosa is present
Serosa present:
     T3   Invades through muscularis propria into
          Subserosa
          Serosa (but not through)
          Pericolic fat within the leaves of the mesentery
     T4   Invades through serosa into free peritoneal cavity,
          —or through serosa into a contiguous organ
No serosa (distal two thirds rectum, posterior left of right
—colon)
     T3   Invades through muscularis propria
     T4   Invades other organs (vagina, prostate, ureter,
          —kidney)

Regional Lymph Nodes (N)
NX   Nodes cannot be assessed (*e.g.*, local excision only)
N0   No regional node metastases
N1   1–3 positive nodes
N2   4 or more positive nodes
(N3   central nodes positive)

Distant Metastases (M)
MX   Presence of distant metastases cannot be assessed
M0   No distant metastases
M1   Distant metastases present

Dukes' staging system correlated with TNM
Dukes' A = T1N0M0
           T2N0M0
Dukes' B = T3N0M0
           T4N0M0
Dukes' C = T(any)N1M0, T(any)N2M0
Dukes' D = T(any)N(any)M1

Modified Astler–Coller (MAC) system correlated with TNM
MAC A = T1N0M0
MAC B1 = T2N0M0
MAC B2 = T3N0M0, T4N0M0
MAC B3 = T4N0M0
MAC C1 = T2N1M0, T2N2M0
MAC C2 = T3N1M0, T3N2M0
         T4N1M0, T4N2M0
MAC C3 = T4N1M0, T4N2M0

Note: In all pathologic staging systems, particularly those applied to rectal cancer, the abbreviations (m) and (g) may be used: (m) denotes microscopic transmural penetration; (g) or (m + g) denotes transmural penetration visible on gross inspection and confirmed microscopically.

* Modified from American Joint Committee on Cancer: Manual for Staging of Cancer, 3rd ed. Philadelphia, JB Lippincott, 1987; and Union Internationale Contre le Cancer: TNM Classification of Malignant Tumors, 4th ed. Geneva, UICC, 1987; by permission.

Stage I represents a freely mobile tumor; Stage II, a mobile tumor; Stage III, tethered mobility; and Stage IV, fixed tumor.[278] Clinical Stages I and II should comprise cases in which local curative excision may be possible. Nicholls et al tested the accuracy of the digital examination by comparing it with the final pathologic stage.[279] They assessed the morphology, number of quadrants involved, fixation, and pres-

ence of extrarectal involvement. In 70 tumors, there was 67% to 83% recognition of the final pathology by the consulting physicians, whereas the correlation was less (44%–68%) when tumors were assessed by the registrars, who had less experience. In a subsequent publication, Nicholls et al reported that clinical determination of the local extent and penetration correlated positively with survival.[280]

Physical Examination

In patients with low rectal cancer, digital examination often reveals a great deal about the primary tumor size, configuration, friability, mobility, involvement of contiguous structures, percent circumference, and possibly involvement of perirectal lymph nodes. With rigid endoscopy, the physical examination may be extended to higher rectal tumors and may confirm or amplify the results of the digital examination. Again, with rigid endoscopy one may assess tumor configuration, mobility (using the endoscope to move the tumor), percent circumference, and size.

Laboratory Tests

Various laboratory tests such as standard liver function tests, 5'-nucleotidase, and γ-glutamyl transpeptidase (GGTP) may be useful in suggesting liver metastases. However, the results are not specific, and a liver imaging study is necessary, and sometimes even a biopsy, to verify metastases. Although it was hoped that the CEA level would be useful for staging, Moertel et al reported that whereas CEA levels usually increase with increasing stage of colorectal cancer, a large proportion of patients with tumors of all stages have no increase in CEA levels.[257]

Imaging Studies

Many imaging modalities have been used to rule out distant metastases in patients preoperatively. Chest radiography is performed to rule out lung metastases and to assess the patient's ability to tolerate surgery. Intravenous pyelography (IVP) has usually been done to look for ureteral deviation or hydronephrosis. However, computed tomography (CT) is making IVP obsolete.[281,282]

PRIMARY TUMOR AND NODES. Imaging studies for staging of the primary tumor must be capable of revealing the extent of penetration through the bowel wall. A barium enema or air contrast barium enema study is inadequate for this purpose, since either study offers only intraluminal images. Several authors report that intrarectal ultrasound (US) is extremely sensitive, as good as or better than CT for assessing extent of bowel wall penetration.[283-286] For example, Hildebrandt and Feifel compared the rectal US findings with pathologic findings in 25 patients.[283] The findings on digital examination correlated with pathologic findings in 15 of 17 patients and overestimated disease in 2 patients. Sonography correlated with the pathologic assessment in 23 of 25 patients; the other 2 were overstaged. These authors proposed a US staging category, uTNM. Nyberg et al have suggested a potential application for intraluminal US in assessing colon tumors as well.[287] In an in vitro study, they compared US examinations of colon specimens with the histopathology and found a good correlation. It has even been suggested that US may be useful in detecting metastases in lymph nodes. In a study by Rifkin and Marks,[285] CT demonstrated only 2 of 7 positive lymph nodes, with no false positives, whereas sonography demonstrated 6 of 7 positive nodes, with 2 false positives. The positive nodes were 0.5 to 1.0 cm in size. The single positive case not detectable with US had normal-sized nodes with only microscopic invasion. Neither CT nor US could detect such nodal disease.

Mayes and Zornoza reviewed 80 CT examinations done for colon and rectal carcinoma and concluded that CT was useful in assessing pelvic masses, para-aortic nodes, adrenals, and liver.[288] Nicholls et al[279] found that CT correctly demonstrated extensive local spread in rectal carcinoma in 89% of patients but was no better than the digital examination in cases of lesser spread or lymph node involvement.

Several investigators have indicated that CT staging is quite accurate,[282,289-292] with one study offering a CT staging system.[289] Staging was based on bowel wall thickness and penetration into surrounding fat, any positive lymph nodes, or distant disease in the liver. Other authors have indicated that CT staging is not accurate, primarily because of inability to assess the depth of invasion accurately from CT scans, or to detect positive lymph nodes.[293-299] Grabbe et al[294] indicated that CT staging was better than the clinical staging system of York Mason, but the problem of assessing slight perirectal spread and tumor in lymph nodes made CT staging inaccurate. On the other hand, Netri et al[296] indicated that CT staging was less accurate than the rectal examination in assessing extraparietal invasion but had a 77% accuracy for detecting positive lymph nodes.

Magnetic resonance (MR) imaging has been compared with CT in several studies[300-302]; the two modalities have been found to be roughly equivalent in demonstrating positive lymph nodes. CT affords better spatial resolution but MR imaging affords better contrast resolution.[301] Butch et al thought that CT and MR imaging were equally effective in staging but that neither modality could demonstrate the extent of bowel wall infiltration or tumor spread to normal-sized perirectal nodes.[302]

Other methods of assessing lymph node involvement include lymphangiography and lymphoscintigraphy. The lymphangiogram "inconstantly" demonstrated nodes associated with internal iliac vessels.[303] Ege and Cummings found pelvic lymphoscintigraphy feasible,[304] but Reasbeck et al found it of no use.[305] Some of the newer radiolabeled monoclonal antibodies may be of use in the future in assessing the presence of tumor in lymph nodes, as well as distant disease.[306,307]

LIVER. Radionuclide scintigraphy, once the prominent method for imaging the liver, has a low spatial resolution and does not demonstrate metastases less than 2 cm in size.[308-310] Although US is of low cost and widely available, it is less accurate than CT for imaging of hepatic disease.[296] The best modality for detecting small metastases at this time is CT.[311,312] MR imaging has generally proved not as useful as CT,[313] although in one study in which two very specific MR

techniques were used,[314] MR imaging was better than conventional CT and comparable to CT enhanced with ethiodized oral emulsion-13.

STAGING OF ADVANCED DISEASE

As newer, more aggressive approaches are adopted for metastatic disease, particularly to the liver, a classification of the extent of metastatic disease becomes more pressing. There have been attempts to define classifications[312,314] based on extent of hepatic replacement, symptoms, extrahepatic disease, resectability, or liver function test results, but the definitive system has not yet evolved. An International Staging System has been proposed that is simple and logical.[314] It has four stages: O = curatively resected; I = <25% hepatic replacement (HR) with no extrahepatic disease (E) or symptoms attributable to liver metastases (S); II = 25% to 75% HR with no E and no S; III = >75% HR with no E and no S, or any HR with E and/or S. If this system is adopted, its utility will only be determined by prospective analyses of its predictive value.

ADDITIONAL PROGNOSTIC VARIABLES

Although operative findings and pathologic stage are the major determinants of prognosis, many clinical and pathologic features may be prognostic for ultimate survival. Many of these factors are interrelated and merely reflections of the same overall characteristic of the cancer. Very few multivariate analyses have been performed.[253,271]

Clinical Features

AGE. Ever since Hoerner in 1958 reported the poor prognosis for colorectal cancer in the very young,[315] numerous articles have supported this conclusion in patients less than 40 years old. Various explanations have been offered, including delay in diagnosis of the disease and the large number of mucoid adenocarcinomas in this group. Dukes and Bussey suggested that the much higher rate of lymphatic metastases in patients less than 40 years old was due to a delay in receiving treatment or to more rapid progression of the disease in young patients; they favored the latter explanation.[204] Their data indicated that the average age (62 years) of patients with low-grade malignancies was considerably higher than those with high-grade malignancies (55 years).[204] Recio and Bussey[316] found that 53% of tumors in young patients were high grade, versus only 20% of tumors in the older age groups where colorectal carcinoma is more common. They also noted an increased number of mucoid tumors in younger patients. Many other authors have supported these findings.[317-319] Adolescent patients less than 20 years old have presented with high-stage, mucin-producing, high-grade tumors and have had a poor survival as a result.[320]

When stage-adjusted survival has been analyzed, in almost all reports there is no difference in relative prognosis for the younger age group.[320-324] In one study, only Dukes' Stage C patients less than 30 years old had a worse outcome than older patients.[325]

GENDER. Women do better than men in terms of survival from colorectal cancer, just as they often survive better with other malignancies.[326,327] In the randomized preoperative radiation therapy study for rectal cancer at Memorial Sloan-Kettering Cancer Center,[328] the only variable besides stage that was predictive of prolonged survival was female gender. Four large analyses showed an improved survival for females.[329-332] However, other studies have not shown a difference in prognosis by gender.[323,325,333,334] Since women generally live longer than men, studies should address the causes of death to ascertain whether the improved long-term survival merely reflects fewer non-cancer-related deaths. Koch analyzed relative survival, independent of deaths from other causes, and still found a higher survival rate for women.[335]

SYMPTOMS. Beahrs and Sanfelippo[336] reported that symptomatic colorectal cancer patients had a 5-year survival rate of 49%, compared with 71% for asymptomatic patients. It is logical to assume that patients in whom colorectal cancer is detected by a screening technique such as fecal occult blood testing or sigmoidoscopy might be treated at an earlier stage and therefore might have a greater chance for cure. Several reports note high survival rates in patients in whom colorectal cancer was detected by screening. In these studies, the number of patients with positive lymph nodes has been small and the survival rates high.

DURATION OF SYMPTOMS. It appears that patients with symptoms lasting longer than 6 months have an increased 5-year survival rate. This improved survival may reflect the slow growth rate of tumors in these patients. In a study of 1084 patients reported by Copeland and colleagues, the 5-year disease-free survival rate for patients with symptoms of 6 months' duration or less was 31%, compared to 37% for patients who had had symptoms longer than 6 months.[337] In a study of 161 patients, Pescatori et al found that patients with symptoms for more than 6 months had a significantly higher rate of radical operations, a lower postoperative mortality, and a higher 5-year survival rate — 43%, versus only 32% for patients with symptoms of less than 6 months' duration.[338] Pescatori et al found no correlation between the duration of symptoms and pathologic stage.[338] In a recent multivariate analysis, there was no effect of duration of symptoms on survival when stage was controlled.[332]

OBSTRUCTION OR PERFORATION. Obstruction and perforation appear to reduce survival.[223,332,339-348] One reason for the poor prognosis in this group of patients is the high operative mortality.[349] In one study, after resection performed with curative intent, patients whose lesions had obstructed or invaded other organs had the same 5-year survival rate as the curative resection group as a whole.[349] However, patients with perforating lesions had only half this life expectancy. A study of 2524 patients in the Large Bowel Cancer Project in the United Kingdom confirmed that obstruction was an important contributor to mortality during the initial in-patient period.[334] Obstruction was the only symptom that had an independent effect in the multivariate analysis of 709 patients in Sydney.[332]

A Danish study compared outcome in 219 patients who had obstruction and perforation and 732 patients who did not have these complications.[323] The 5-year survival rate was 23% for patients with either or both of these complications and 35% for patients without them. In the NSABP clinical trial, data from 1021 patients were analyzed.[347] The presence of bowel obstruction strongly influenced the prognostic outcome. Of interest, bowel obstruction in the right colon was associated with a significantly diminished disease-free survival, whereas obstruction in the left colon was not associated with a similar diminution in survival. Obstruction and circumferential growth were separate prognostic factors; neither one completely explained the effects of the other. The relative risk for patients with tumors that were both obstructing and encircling compared to patients with tumors that were neither obstructing nor encircling was 3.27. The GITSG used multivariate analysis to examine prognostic features in 572 patients.[348] Obstruction was an important indicator of prognosis, completely independent of Dukes' stage. Bowel perforation was important as a prognostic feature only for disease-free survival. In light of the findings of the NSABP study, it is of interest that the GITSG found no differences in the relative failure risks for obstruction in different sites in the bowel. A study reported from Massachusetts General Hospital indicated that both local failure and intra-abdominal metastatic failure were increased in patients with obstruction or perforation, compared with a control group of patients without these symptoms.[223] In regard to perforating cancers, one should distinguish between perforation through the tumor and perforation proximal to an obstructing cancer.

HEMORRHAGE OR RECTAL BLEEDING. Hemorrhage or rectal bleeding has been associated with an improved prognosis, perhaps because it is related to a surface erosion that can manifest early and lead to early intervention, and not a symptom reflective of tumor penetration.[350] In the GITSG experience, the presence of melena or rectal bleeding marginally prolonged survival ($p = 0.08$) even after the effects of Dukes' stage were accounted for.[348] In another study, symptomatic or asymptomatic anemia had no effect on prognosis.[337] In the analysis of the Sydney Hospital experience, patients with rectal bleeding had a significantly longer survival on univariate analysis; however, the significance of bleeding disappeared on multivariate analysis.[332]

LOCATION OF THE PRIMARY TUMOR. It has generally been found that the 5-year survival rate is less for patients with cancer of the rectosigmoid and rectum than for patients with cancer elsewhere in the colon.[329,330,333,337,347,351] In regard to colon primaries, some authors suggest a worse prognosis for patients with lesions in the right colon.[329,347] Others find no difference[323,331]; still others report a worse prognosis for patients with disease in the left colon.[338] For rectal disease, a decreased survival has been noted for patients with lesions below the peritoneal reflection, compared with patients with lesions above the peritoneal reflection.[352] These data are supported by the Medical Research Council's preoperative radiation therapy trial for rectal cancer.[275]

PRIMARY TUMOR SIZE. Colorectal cancer is unusual in that the majority of studies report no adverse relationship of tumor size to survival.[202,219,221,224,329,330,332,353,354] A few studies have shown improved survival with smaller tumors.[217] A recent study found that colon tumors 6 to 10 cm in size were associated with an improved survival, compared to lesions larger than 11 cm.[225] The relationship of size to survival did not hold for rectal tumors.[224] Of interest, some studies have shown increased tumor penetration through the bowel wall with larger tumors,[221,355] but not an increase in lymph node metastases.[221] The GITSG analysis of 572 colon patients in a randomized chemoimmunotherapy trial found that although tumor size was unimportant when analyzed as a single factor, when the effects of other factors were adjusted for, increasing size had a negative effect on survival and disease-free survival.[348]

PRIMARY TUMOR CONFIGURATION. As early as 1939 Grinnell reported that survival was higher in patients with tumors projecting into the lumen (83%) than in patients whose tumors were either intermediate (45% survival) or infiltrating (38%).[228] The reasons for such differences in survival include the lower frequency of penetration of the bowel wall by exophytic tumors compared with ulcerating tumors (24% versus 39%),[355] less frequent nodal metastases with exophytic tumors than with ulcerating lesions,[355-357] and fewer hematogenous metastases (23% versus 31%).[185] Overall, exophytic tumors are more frequently limited to the bowel wall (46%) than are ulcerating tumors (24%).[355] One recent study that has looked at exophytic versus nonexophytic tumors is the GITSG colon adjuvant study.[348] This study found that the presence of an exophytic lesion had a significantly beneficial effect on survival.

BLOOD TRANSFUSION. Several authors have suggested that perioperative blood transfusions have a negative effect on disease-free interval in patients with colorectal or colonic cancer.[358,359] Other prognostic variables were not considered in these studies. Foster et al did consider other variables and claimed a worse survival for patients with colonic cancers, regardless of stage, receiving perioperative transfusions but no adverse effects of transfusion for rectal cancers.[360] After adjusting for stage, age, and gender by Cox regression analysis, Nathanson et al found that blood transfusions were not detrimental.[361] Weiden and associates, in a retrospective multivariate analysis of 171 patients with colorectal cancer, found no relationship between perioperative blood transfusion and survival or disease recurrence.[362] Corman and associates also were unable to show an adverse effect after a multivariate analysis.[333] However, when they considered the number of units transfused, both as a single variable and in the multivariate analysis, this feature had a very strong prognostic value for colorectal cancer, and in particular for colon cancer (p = 0.005). It was not prognostic when patients with rectal cancer were analyzed separately, but there were only 74 patients in this group. In addition to perioperative blood transfusion, other surgical complications such as fever and sepsis may play a role.[365]

TABLE 29-7.   Percent Survival as a Function of Histologic Tumor Grade

Study	(No. of Patients)	% Survival by Grade:			
		1	2	3	4
Broders[200]	Rectum (598)	56	38	25	15
Grinnell[228]	Colon/rectum (204)	66	48	25	*
Sunderland[378]	Rectum/sigmoid (210)	75	76	58	*
Dukes and Bussey[204]	Rectum (2097)	77	61	29	*
Copeland et al[337]	Colon/rectum (654)	58	42	21	*
Rao et al[219]	Rectum/sigmoid (107)	59	38	11	*
Riboli et al[366]	Colon/rectum (90)	65	33	25	*
Minsky et al[373]	Colon (158)	100	80	56	*
Minsky et al[373]	Rectum (82)	86	71	55	*

* No Grade 4 in system employed.

Pathologic Features

ADJACENT ORGAN INVOLVEMENT. Adjacent organs are involved in about 10% of colorectal cancer cases. Spratt and Spjut found that removal of a contiguous pathologically invaded organ did not alter 5- and 10-year survival rates.[329] To address this issue, Gunderson and Sosin devised a modification of the Astler–Coller staging system which added B3 and C3 stages, denoting adjacent organ involvement for node-negative or node-positive disease, respectively.[214] Several studies have analyzed both locoregional recurrence and 5-year survival rates by this modified Astler–Coller staging system.[227,363,364] The additional B3 and C3 staging predicted increased local recurrence, as well as decreased 5-year survival. Nathanson et al, in a multivariate analysis of prognostic factors, indicated that the second most important factor was involvement of adjacent organs, which increased the relative risk of dying of colorectal cancer to 2.6.[361] Minsky and colleagues analyzed patients with colon or rectal cancer according to whether they had stage B3 or C3 disease clinically or verified microscopically.[224,225] Patients with Stage B3 colon cancer verified pathologically had a 27% 5-year actuarial survival rate, significantly lower than the 88% survival in patients with B3 disease who were thought to have only clinical adjacent organ involvement.[225]

DEGREE OF DIFFERENTIATION. Dukes and others pointed out a correlation of grade with lymph nodal and distant metastases found at operation.[188,204,215] Disease grade has also been correlated with the likelihood of venous spread,[184,204] the risk of lymphatic penetration,[184] extent of local spread,[204] average number of lymphatic metastases,[355] and increasing wall penetration.[355] In another study, grade was not associated with the extent of local invasion.[366]

Univariate analysis has shown a definite relationship between survival and histologic grade in both colon and rectal cancer (Table 29-7). The relationship was significant in node-negative patients,[366] but too few patients with positive nodes were available to assess the influence of grade in this group. In several recent multivariate analyses, grade was independently prognostic of survival.[261,275,331,332,348,367]

The trend of the data indicates that grade should be consid-

TABLE 29-8.   Scoring System for Prognostic Model Based on Grade- and Stage-Related Parameters*

Parameter	Score
Lymphocytic infiltration	
Marked	0
Moderate	3
Little or none	6
No. of Nodes involved	
0	0
—1–4	4
—≥5	8
Spread through bowel wall	
None	0
Slight to moderate	3
Extensive	6

* Grinnell RS: The grading and prognosis of carcinoma of the colon and rectum. Ann Surg 109:500–533, 1939.

Range of possible total scores: 0–20. A set of five prognostic categories (I to V) based on the model was highly predictive of survival. Scores of 0 are assigned to category I, scores of 1 to 6 to category II, scores of 7 to 11 to category III, scores of 12 to 16 to category IV, and scores of 17 to 20 to category V.

ered an independent prognostic factor; however, several problems are associated with its use, including the nonuniformity of grading systems, the designation of the majority of tumors as "intermediate" in grade, variability of grade in different parts of the tumor,[369] and concern as to pathologists' agreement on grading of the same tumor. The question of the adequacy of biopsies has been addressed.[228,281,370] Agreement between the grade of a resected rectal cancer specimen and the grade of the original biopsy specimen obtained at proctosigmoidoscopy varied from 56% to 78%. It was worse for poorly differentiated tumors, 38% to 52%, and somewhat better for moderately well differentiated tumors, 64%.[281,370] The proctosigmoidoscopy biopsy specimen was usually assigned a lower grade than the surgical specimen.[228] Complete agreement among three pathologists with respect to multiple biopsy specimens obtained under anesthesia and the resected specimens was only 44%.[281]

An interesting study from St. Mark's Hospital and St. Bartholomew's Hospital in London has addressed the problem of subjectivity in grading by defining the parameters of grading and then determining those most predictive of survival with a multivariate analysis.[203] The best-fitting parsimonious model comprised the grading variables of lymphocytic infiltration, tubular configuration, and pattern of growth (expanding versus infiltrating). A four-grade system was devised that proved to be reproducible and predictive of survival. The investigators took this one step further, allowing grade-related parameters to compete with stage-related parameters in an overall model of pathologic prognostic categories. The best model consisted of the number of affected lymph nodes, the presence of lymphocytic infiltration, and the extent of spread through the bowel wall (Table 29-8).[234] A set of five prognostic categories based on the model was highly predictive of survival.

COLLOID   CARCINOMA   (MUCINOUS   CARCINOMA).   Colloid or mucinous adenocarcinomas have a poor prognosis and frequently are grouped with high-grade carci-

nomas since their prognosis is quite similar. The percentage of regional or synchronous distant metastases is higher than in noncolloid carcinomas; Trimpi and Bacon reported a 70% incidence of regional or distant metastases.[371] Sundblad and Paz reported 43% Stage C or D carcinomas in patients with colloid carcinomas, compared with only 15% for patients with noncolloid carcinomas.[372] Cohen et al reported an 83% frequency of positive nodes and an increased incidence of gross transmural penetration in patients with colloid carcinomas, findings similar to those in patients with poorly differentiated adenocarcinomas.[355] Minsky et al noted that local recurrence and abdominal failure were higher.[373]

Many authors have reported a poorer survival rate in patients with colloid carcinomas—less than half in some series.[374,375] Symonds and Vickery reported a 34% survival in all patients with colloid colorectal carcinomas, compared to 53% for patients with other adenocarcinomas. The survival rate for patients with colloid rectal carcinoma was only 18%,[376] versus 49% for those with noncolloid rectal carcinoma. Others have found less dramatic differences.[373,377]

Signet-ring cell carcinoma is rarely cured. All four cases reported by Symonds and Vickery were fatal within 1 year of diagnosis.[376]

BLOOD VESSEL INVASION. It would be logical to assume that blood vessel invasion might signify dissemination to distant organs. However, as pointed out by Dukes, emboli within a vein may not mean dissemination but only spread along a path of least resistance.[188] Furthermore, failure to find emboli within a vein does not preclude earlier dissemination. Brown and Warren reported increased blood vessel invasion with higher grade of disease, increased bowel wall penetration, and increased visceral metastases.[232] The frequency of visceral metastases was reduced in the absence of blood vessel invasion: only 1 of 70 patients without blood vessel invasion had visceral metastases.[232] In a 1983 study, Knudsen et al found that liver metastases were three times as frequent in patients with venous invasion than in patients without it.[212] All seven patients with synchronous metastases studied by Madison and associates had blood vessel invasion, whereas only 31% of those patients without metastases had this finding.[368] Dukes and Bussey noted an increase in blood vessel invasion with both increasing grade and increasing local spread,[204] and verified an earlier study showing an increase in blood vessel invasion with positive lymph nodes.[188]

Blood vessel invasion is detected in 17% to 50% of cases.[202,211,221,251,368,378–380] This feature may predict decreased survival.[329,337,348,378,379,381–384] However, because blood vessel invasion is related to many other factors, whether it is an independent variable remains unclear. Blood vessel invasion is associated with a poor prognosis in Dukes' B and C patients, independent of lymph node status[378,381,382] and of Dukes' stage.[378,382] In the colon, a survival difference has been reported only for patients with Stage C2 disease.[383] In the rectum and sigmoid, a survival difference has been noted only for patients with Dukes' C disease.[378]

In multivariate analyses, vascular invasion was not an independent variable in one study,[384] but it was in five other large studies.[212,261,275,332,367]

LYMPHATIC VESSEL INVASION. Grinnell was one of the first to look at lymphatic vessel invasion.[233] Spratt and Spjut noted decreased survival at 5 and 10 years when lymphatic vessel invasion was present.[329] From their data it appears that once lymphatic vessel invasion was present, neither venous invasion nor perineural invasion decreased the survival rate much further. Khankanian et al grouped lymphatic vessel invasion with blood vessel invasion and designated the combined entity "vascular invasion."[385] They studied this phenomenon within the bowel wall only and noted no difference in disease-free interval with vascular invasion. Analysis of the GITSG data indicated that lymphatic invasion was "potentially harmful" (p = 0.08 in their analysis).[348] A recent multivariate study of rectal and rectosigmoid cancer considered stage, blood vessel invasion, and lymphatic vessel invasion.[384] Lymphatic vessel invasion was an independent prognostic feature (p = 0.04).

PERINEURAL INVASION. The classic study of perineural invasion was reported by Seefeld and Bargen,[211] who noted that malignant spread by growth along perineural spaces occurred as far as 10 cm from the primary tumor. The incidence of perineural invasion was 30% in 100 cases, increasing with grade and Dukes' stage. Patients with perineural invasion had more local recurrences in the scar or anastomotic site than those free of perineural invasion (81% versus 30%). The 5-year survival rate was also lower in the former group (7% versus 35%). Spratt and Spjut confirmed this survival difference.[329] One multivariate analysis included nerve invasion and found it to be an independent prognostic variable.[212]

IMMUNE RESPONSE TO THE PRIMARY TUMOR. Crude indicators of patients' general immune response have been analyzed for prognostic usefulness. Two studies of peripheral blood lymphocyte counts are contradictory. Kim and associates noted that when the peripheral blood lymphocyte count was less than $1000/mm^3$, survival was 30%, compared to about 60% survival in patients with higher counts.[386] Corman et al, in a multivariate analysis, found no difference in survival by preoperative lymphocyte counts.[333] In a study of lymphocyte subsets, T-lymphocytes were depressed in 57% of preoperative and postoperative patients with colorectal carcinoma; B-lymphocyte counts were normal.[387] The impact of T-cell depression on prognosis was not evaluated.

A recent Southwestern Oncology Group (SWOG) study that analyzed humoral immunity reported no survival difference as a function of serum IgM concentration but prolonged survival with higher levels of IgA and IgG.[388] Baseler and associates noted that circulating IgA immune complexes were increased in patients with various carcinomas compared with healthy subjects or patients undergoing surgery for benign disease.[389] The highest levels of circulating IgA immune complexes were found in patients with colon carcinoma.

Considerable interest has been expressed in the prognostic value of local inflammatory reactions at the primary tumor site. Spratt and Spjut noted a decrease in survival with a lack of inflammatory response around the tumor periphery.[329]

Murray et al reported an increased 5-year survival rate for patients with Dukes' B and C colon cancer when local inflammation was present (89% versus 46%).[390] Local inflammation has been found in approximately 50% to 75% of tumors.[202,390] Jass et al demonstrated that lymphocytic infiltration was the most important factor in their grading model (Cox regression analysis) and was also important in their "best" model with grade- and stage-related parameters.[203] Carlon et al similarly noted that lymphocytic infiltration around the primary and the pattern of growth were the most significant prognostic features.[391] Svennevig and associates reported a higher number of mononuclear cells in both the peritumoral stroma and within the tumor parenchyma from those patients cured by surgery.[392]

REACTIVE LYMPH NODES. Multiple investigators have shown that an apparent immunologic response in regional lymph nodes correlates with improved survival.[390,393-395] In sigmoid colon cancer, Patt and associates noted that sinus histiocytosis and paracortical immunoblastic activity individually correlated with an increased survival.[393] When both features were present, survival was even better. There was no benefit from increased germinal center activity in this study. Murray et al also reported an increased survival with sinus histiocytosis of the draining lymph nodes, and an even greater increase in survival when this feature was present with a local inflammatory reaction to the primary.[390] Pihl and colleagues observed that paracortical lymph node hyperplasia occupying more than 15% of the lymph node section was favorably associated with survival.[395]

CARCINOEMBRYONIC ANTIGEN AND OTHER BIOMARKERS. The value of the preoperative CEA level as an independent prognostic indicator is unclear. The preoperative CEA level does reflect tumor burden.[396-398] Many authors have reported that an increased level (5 ng/ml) indicates an increased risk of recurrence,[398-405] but others have not found it to be a good prognostic variable.[406-409] Steele et al reported that an increased CEA level was prognostic for colon cancer but not for rectal cancer.[410] Recently, a group from the Mayo Clinic reported that the CEA level was strongly associated with survival, but within stages, it was only independently prognostic for Dukes' C patients with four or more positive lymph nodes.[257]

The CEA level not only correlates with the extent of the tumor burden, it also correlates highly with venous invasion.[411] Tabuchi et al looked at peripheral as well as portal vein CEA levels immediately after laparotomy. In peripheral blood, increased CEA levels correlated only with venous invasion. In portal venous blood, CEA elevation correlated with venous invasion, tumor size, lymphatic invasion, Dukes' stage, and depth of invasion.[411]

De Mello et al looked at a large number of factors as potential prognostic variables.[331] They found that the CEA level was prognostic as a single variable, but not if age, stage, and sex were included in the model. Similarly, the possible tumor markers of γ-glutamyl transpeptidase and pseudouridine were found to be prognostic only as single variables. Phosphohexoseisomerase and three acute phase reactant proteins (APRP), α_1-antichymotrypsin, C-reactive protein, and α_1-acid glycoprotein, were found to be prognostic. When α_1-antichymotrypsin was included in the model, the other markers were no longer significant, although phosphohexoseisomerase was of borderline significance. Ward et al in 1977 found other APRP to be prognostic.[412] Durdey and colleagues demonstrated that APRP combined with CEA level were most useful in determining fixed versus mobile tumors, and whether tumors were fixed because of inflammation or invasion.[413] By using the criteria of increased APRP and CEA (>45 ng/ml) levels, Williams and co-workers were able to identify 10 of 11 tumors with extensive or moderate malignant spread, 4 of 5 with inflammatory spread, and 21 of 23 with no spread.[281] These were not very good criteria for determining minimal malignant spread, but for moderate and extensive spread, the sensitivity, specificity, and accuracy were 91%, 96%, and 94%, respectively. Others have found that preresection APRP levels are of no value in predicting who will develop metastases, or the site of metastases.[414]

CELL CYCLE PARAMETERS AND PLOIDY. In 100 patients, Meyer and Prioleau found no relationship between the fraction of cells in S-phase and histologic grade or other clinicopathologic features, such as age, sex, site of tumor, size, Dukes' stage, number of positive lymph nodes, presence of adenomas, or even relapse-free survival.[415] The question of alteration of prognosis was also considered by Blijham et al who noted an increased rate of recurrences with a high percentage of S-phase cells in Dukes' C colorectal cancer.[416] On the other hand, Bleiberg et al found no correlation between the mean labeling index and age, sex, tumor localization, Dukes' classification, or disease-free survival at 5 years.[417]

Some authors have found a relationship between aneuploidy and Dukes' stage[418-420]; others have not.[421-423] No significant relationship of aneuploidy to grade has been established.[416,421] Ota et al looked at primary colorectal cancer specimens for labeling index, flow cytometry parameters, and primer-available DNA-dependent polymerase index (PDPI), all of which bore no relation to Dukes' stage, tumor location, tumor size, or frequency of nodal metastases.[423]

Flow cytometry parameters may bear a relation to recurrence or survival. Streffer et al reported a high incidence of local recurrence in patients with rectal carcinoma who had a high ratio of S-phase cells.[424] For rectal carcinoma, the incidence of either lymph node metastases or distant metastases increased with an increased percentage of S-phase cells in the tumor. For tumors with more than 19.7% cells in S-phase, the incidence of lymph node or distant metastases was 82%. For tumors with less than 19.7% cells in S-phase, the incidence of positive lymph nodes or distant metastases was only 14%.

Several authors have found an increase in survival with diploid tumors and a worse survival with aneuploid tumors.[419,424-427] Scott et al found significantly better survival in patients with diploid tumors than in patients with aneuploid or tetraploid tumors.[427] Local recurrence was twice as common in patients with nondiploid tumors as in patients with diploid tumors. Using a Cox multivariate analysis that included multiple clinical and pathologic factors, Scott et al found that DNA ploidy and the operative assessment of tumor spread were the most important prognostic variables. Nondiploid tumors also were associated with an increased incidence of vascular invasion, tumor fibrosis, and high Dukes' stage. In a series of 33 patients with at least a 3-year follow-up, Melamed and associates were unable to document a poorer prognosis for patients with aneuploid tumors when ploidy was corrected for stage.[428] The potential for cell cycle analysis and its use in prognosis is only beginning to be realized.

SUMMARY OF STAGING AND PROGNOSTIC VARIABLES

Although the presence of hematogenous or nodal metastases are major determinants of curability, recent analyses utilize multivariate regression models to provide sophisticated outcome projections. These data have been applied toward unifying end-results reporting.[428d,428e]

ADDITIONAL TUMOR BIOLOGIC FEATURES

Oncogenes

The *ras* and *myc* oncogenes have been implicated in colorectal carcinoma. Der et al initially reported that carcinoma of the colon was associated with the activated oncogene (c-Ki-ras-2-gene).[429] Elevated expression of the *ras* oncogene family was also found in premalignant and malignant tumors of the colorectum by Spandidos and Kerr.[430] The *ras* oncogene protein product (p21) was detected by Gallick et al in 9 of 17 colon cancers.[431] However, in 4 of 5 patients with distant metastases this protein product was not elevated, suggesting that *ras* oncogene activation is an early phenomenon in carcinogenesis. Thor and associates demonstrated a correlation of p21 expression with the depth of invasion.[432] Overall, the protein was found to be increased in 22 of 47 malignant colon carcinomas but not in benign colon conditions or normal colon. Recently, two groups (the State University of New York at Stony Brook, and the University of Leiden with Johns Hopkins University) have detected specific mutations to the *ras* oncogene from the normal counterpart in about 40% of colon cancers.[433-435] These mutations were often present in villous adenomas as well, indicating strongly that *ras* oncogene activation is a relatively early event.

The c-*myc* oncogene has also been found in polyps and colon cancer.[436,437] In one study of 15 patients, tumors and adjacent normal tissues were examined for expression of c-*myc*.[437] The authors found no gene amplification or rearrangement of c-*myc*. However, the c-*myc* mRNA transcripts were elevated in 12 of 15 tumors and the protein product, p62 c-*myc*, was elevated in 8 of 15 tumors. In both cases the transcript elevation and protein product elevation were greatest in the well-differentiated tumors and lowest in the poorly differentiated tumors. Since there was no gene amplification, it was proposed that the increased transcripts were due to enhanced transcription or to an increase in mRNA stability.

Growth Factors and Receptors

Tumor growth is a function of the fraction of cells actively in cycle (growth fraction), the cell cycle time, and the amount of cell loss. Primary colon cancers have been radiologically observed to double in size in 138 to 1155 days.[438] Doubling times of human colon carcinoma in cell culture are from 16 to 36 hours. These rates of growth are exceedingly rapid compared with the observed doubling times of such cancers in situ, probably reflecting both a low growth fraction and a large cell loss to desquamation or necrosis.

Colorectal cancer cells have been found to secrete transforming growth factors (TGF) and tumor inhibitory factors (TIF).[439,440] Gastrin receptors have been found in cultured cells.[441,442] Androgen receptors at low levels have been detected.[443] Alford and colleagues studied hormone receptors in 23 primary tumors and found estrogen receptors in 30% and glucocorticoid receptors in 23%; in six patients, there were receptors for the three hormones estrogen, progesterone, and dihydrotesterone.[444] In that study, at least 70% of the tumors had at least one positive receptor. McClendon et al also found estrogen-binding activity in 5 of 21 human colon carcinomas.[445] Additional data have substantiated the presence of multiple hormone receptors.[446]

Ornithine Decarboxylase

The enzyme ornithine decarboxylase (ODC) has been implicated in both tumor promotion and proliferation by increasing polyamine synthesis.[447] It is the rate-limiting enzyme that is essential for mucosal proliferation in the colon.[448] A group at Johns Hopkins has shown that ODC activity increases from normal mucosa, through normal-appearing mucosa in patients with familial polyposis, to nondysplastic polyps in such patients, to dysplastic polyps.[448] Porter and associates found ODC levels eight times greater in cancer specimens than in normal adjacent mucosa; adenomatous polyps were intermediate, although there was a considerable overlap.[449]

Immunology and Markers

A large group of biologically interesting antigens has been detected in association with colorectal cancer cells. The CEA level was discussed earlier as a preoperative prognostic factor. Monoclonal antibody technology will allow identification of multiple additional antigens in the coming years. An overview of various antigens follows.

CARCINOEMBRYONIC ANTIGEN. CEA was referred to as an "Oncofetal protein" after Gold and Freeman isolated it in 1965 from human adult colon cancer and fetal colon epithelium using adsorption and tolerance techniques.[450] It is a heavily glycosylated, single chain peptide of 200,000 daltons molecular weight. Electron microscopic immunochemical techniques demonstrate the protein in normal colonic columnar and goblet cells.[451] Monoclonal antibody technology has indicated a large number of epitopes.[452,453] Studies with these epitopes are under way with the hope of improving the specificity of this antigen in the detection and treatment of colorectal cancer.

BLOOD GROUP ANTIGENS. Multiple investigators have confirmed the lack of expression of normal blood group ABH antigens in the distal colon and rectal mucosa and the presence of such antigens on cancers in these locations.[454-457] A recent report suggests that ABH antigens appear in neoplastic (adenomatous) polyps but not in hyperplastic polyps.[458] Many of the tumor-associated antigens detected with monoclonal antibodies are modified blood group glycolipids.[459] The modified Lewis antigens represent another group of oncofetal antigens[460-462]; variations in their expression are currently of great interest.

CA 19-9. Of the large number of antigens defined on colorectal cancers (albeit not exclusively), one of the most widely studied has been the carbohydrate cell surface antigen, designated 19-9, which was identified by Koprowski and associates.[463] This antigen is a sialylated lacto-N-fucopentose that is related to the Lewis blood group substance.[464] CA 19-9 is released into the blood of cancer-bearing patients and is detected with the CA 19-9 assay system. The antigen recognized by this antibody appears to be a class 3 differentiation antigen.[465]

ADDITIONAL MONOCLONAL ANTIBODY-DEFINED ANTIGENS. Koprowski's group defined another antigen identified with monoclonal antibody 17-1A.[466,467] This system has been of particular interest because immunologic inhibition of growth can result with infusion of this antibody. Johnson, Schlom, and associates defined a high molecular weight glycoprotein (referred to as TAG-72) using monoclonal antibody B72.3.[468] Although this antigen is present in 85% of colorectal cancers, there is considerable heterogeneity in its expression in the primary tumor, lymph nodes, and distant metastases.[469]

HUMAN CHORIONIC GONADOTROPIN. Human chorionic gonadotropin (hCG) has been found in approximately 50% of colorectal carcinomas, although increased serum levels are found considerably less often.[470,471] In an immunohistochemical study of 50 colorectal carcinomas, 20 adenomas, 8 ulcerative colitis specimens, and 10 normal mucosa specimens, Campo et al found hCG-producing cells in 52% of the carcinomas but in none of the normal mucosa or benign lesions.[471] They suggest that hCG may be a marker of prognostic significance: hCG was detected in the primary tumor in 15 of 19 patients with lymph node or hepatic metastases, but in only 9 of 23 patients without metastases.

TREATMENT OF PRECANCEROUS COLORECTAL DISEASE

NEOPLASTIC POLYPS (ADENOMAS)

Histologically, neoplastic polyps are tubular, villous, or a combination of both. Villous tumors have a higher propensity to be associated with cancer in the polyp. In addition, patients with multiple villous polyps are more likely to develop additional polyps following removal of the initial lesions. Since the finding of a polypoid mass on endoscopy or barium enema examination does not connote benignity, such lesions should be removed except in the most infirm patients. Almost all pedunculated polyps can be removed by endoscopic snare polpectomy. Sessile lesions can frequently be removed piecemeal, but with an increased risk of perforation. Several sessions may be necessary. Large villous lesions in the cecum and ascending colon may require colectomy.

Data accruing from the National Polyp Study will define more precisely the appropriate follow-up strategies for patients with polyps. Current data from several sources allow us to endorse the follow-up algorithms in Figures 29-8 and 29-9 as general guidelines.[472-475]

The large villous adenoma of the rectum can pose a difficult management problem. Transanal local excision at the level of the submucosa allows complete histologic examination. Some 75% of soft, nonulcerated tumors will prove benign on subsequent examination, 15% will contain superficial cancer, and 10% will contain invasive cancer.[476] Random biopsies of grossly benign-appearing lesions are unreliable and make subsequent surgical excision more difficult.[477] Electrocoagulation with cautery, piecemeal snare excision, and neodymium/yttrium-aluminum-garnet (Nd-YAG) laser ablation have all been used, but preclude complete histologic assessment. Very large tumors can be excised and the mucosa closed by muscle plication and mucosal advancement.[478,479] Low anterior resection, coloanal procedures, and abdominoperineal resection all play a role in the management of extensive benign rectal polyps.

FAMILIAL ADENOMATOUS POLYPOSIS

There is continued controversy as to the appropriate surgical management of patients with familial adenomatous polyposis. Because almost all untreated patients develop colorectal cancer by age 40, prophylactic surgery is warranted. Total abdominal colectomy with ileorectal anastomosis is usually the procedure of choice if the rectum is relatively free of polyps. Bowel function is acceptable, and bladder and sexual function are preserved. The rectal stump must be examined frequently (as often as every 6 months) for signs of cancer. Polyps must be regularly removed or fulgurated. Cancer has been reported to develop in the retained rectal stump in 5% to 60% of patients. The results from the major centers are summarized in Table 29-9. Unquestionably, there is increased risk with increased duration of follow-up. The risk is considerably less if the rectum is not involved by the polyposis (20% of polyposis patients).[480] In patients not willing to risk developing cancer in the retained rectum, or in patients with a carpet of polyps in the rectum, total proctocolectomy is appropriate. In most younger patients, restorative proctocolectomy with a distal mucosal proctectomy and an ileal pouch–anal anastomosis will enhance the quality of life.[485] Multiple aspects of the management of these patients are described in a recent monograph.[486]

ULCERATIVE COLITIS

As described in the section on screening, many patients with ulcerative colitis can be followed endoscopically, with selective surgery performed in those who develop high-grade dys-

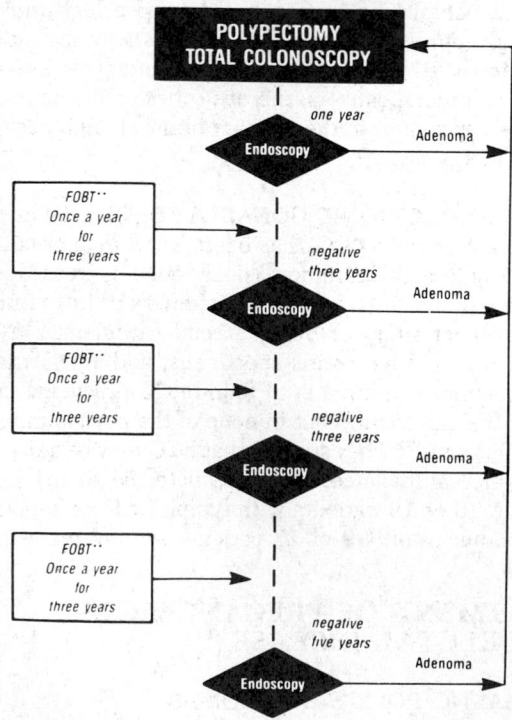

FIG. 29-8. Management of the minimal-risk patient with colorectal adenomas, defined as the patient with a solitary adenoma less than 2 cm, pedunculated, if sessile then having tubular histology, with only mild or moderate dysplasia.[472]

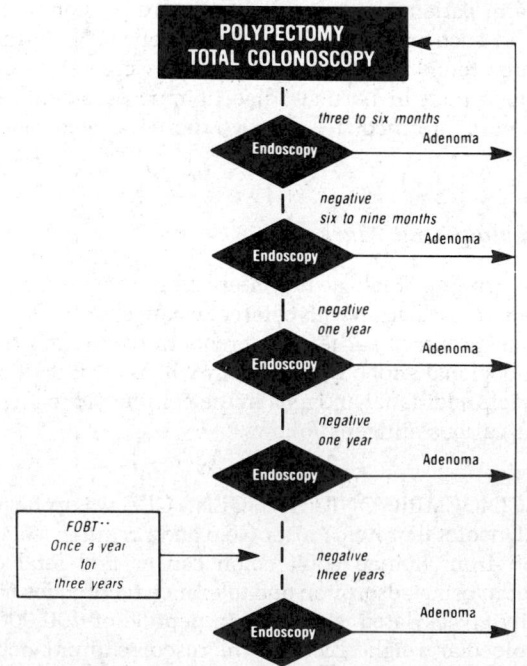

FIG. 29-9. Management of the high-risk patient with colorectal adenomas, defined as multiple adenomas, ≥2 cm, sessile, villous, or tubulovillous, with severe dysplasia, carcinoma in situ, or invasive cancer.[472]

TABLE 29-9. Risk of Rectal Cancer After Abdominal Colectomy for Polyposis

Center	No. of Patients	Subsequent Rectal Cancer
St. Marks Hosp.[481]	174	13% (at 25 yr)
Mayo Clinic[482]	178	59% (at 23 yr)
Memorial Hospital[483]	27	10%
Cleveland Clinic[484]	133	7.5%

plasia or cancer.[487-491] Restorative total proctocolectomy with distal submucosal proctectomy and ileal pouch–anal anastomosis should be considered in the younger patient undergoing elective surgery.[492,493]

TREATMENT OF POTENTIALLY CURABLE COLORECTAL CANCER

The remainder of this chapter describes multimodality treatment strategies for colorectal cancer, cure rates, and patterns of recurrence. Treatment strategies and end results are presented separately for four major disease groups: (1) resectable colon cancer (including cancer of the rectosigmoid), (2) resectable rectal cancers, (3) potentially curable but primarily surgically unresectable colorectal cancers, and (4) recurrent or metastatic disease.

PRETREATMENT EVALUATION

The following are general guidelines for the pretreatment evaluation of potentially curable colorectal disease:

History: In addition to the personal medical history, the family history of colorectal cancer, polyps, and other cancers should be obtained.

Physical Examination: Check for hepatomegaly, ascites, and lymphadenopathy. If rectal cancer is present, determine its distance from the anal verge and dentate line, distance from levators, configuration, mobility, involvement of contiguous organs or the pelvis, and involvement of pararectal nodes. In women, rule out synchronous ovarian pathology and breast cancer.

Laboratory Data: Blood count, CEA, liver chemistries.

GI: Full colonoscopy or proctosigmoidoscopy and air contrast barium enema (in the absence of obstruction or perforation).

Imaging: A preoperative chest radiograph is appropriate. Rectal cancer patients should undergo CT of the abdomen and pelvis, particularly if preoperative radiation therapy is planned. If available, intrarectal US may be helpful. Colon cancer patients need a perioperative CT or US study of their liver as a baseline. This study need not be performed preoperatively if liver chemistries are normal and hepatomegaly is not present.

Surgical: Examination under anesthesia and cystoscopy may be helpful in selected cancer cases.

TREATMENT OF RESECTABLE COLON CANCER, AND END RESULTS

Treatment strategies for potentially curable colon and intraperitoneal rectal cancer remain primarily surgical. However, preliminary data indicate that postoperative chemotherapy may improve the disease-free survival rate in patients who have undergone potentially curative surgery. Results from recent adjuvant systemic and regional portal vein chemotherapy studies supporting this statement will be presented. The rationale for adjuvant radiation in selected patients will be discussed.

GENERAL SURGICAL PRINCIPLES

The morbidity of elective colon surgery is directly related to mechanical and oral antibiotic bowel preparation, the use of perioperative systemic antibiotics, and the skill of the surgical and anesthesia team.

Extent of Bowel Resection

Except for the occasional minimally invasive polypoid cancer, which can frequently be cured by endoscopic polypectomy, en bloc surgical resection is the primary treatment approach in patients with colon cancer. Fortunately, almost all of these cancers can be treated without a permanent or even temporary colostomy. This should be explained to the patient and family at an early point in the consultation, since concern about a colostomy frequently supersedes all other considerations of the patient.

Surgical treatment of colon cancer requires excision of an adequate amount of normal colon proximal and distal to the tumor, adequate lateral margins if the tumor is adherent to a contiguous structure, and removal of the regional lymph nodes. Pathologic studies indicate that tumor rarely spreads more than 1.2 cm longitudinally beyond the area of gross involvement, and a 5-cm margin is more than adequate.[206] However, removal of intermediate and more central (principal) lymph nodes requires ligation and division of multiple main vascular trunks. Hence, the extent of the colonic resection for potentially curable colon cancer is determined by the biology of local tumor growth and by the associated lymphadenectomy.

Extent of Lymph Node Dissection

Patients with colon cancer metastatic to regional lymph nodes may still be cured with surgery. Hence, lymphadenectomy is not only necessary for staging, it is also therapeutic. The paracolic and intermediate lymph nodes are routinely resected, but it is not clear to what extent removal of more central or principal lymph nodes is therapeutic. Enker, Laffer, and Block described excellent results in the treatment of colon cancer which they believed were due in part to an extensive lymphadenectomy.[494] However, Grinnell reported that all 17 patients with carcinoma of the descending colon, sigmoid, or rectum and positive nodes around the origin of the inferior mesenteric artery died of cancer.[495]

Adequate regional lymph node dissection is therefore part of effective therapy for colon cancer. Small segmental resections with removal of only the paracolic lymph nodes are suitable only in the presence of liver metastases or peritoneal seeding, or in medically poor-risk patients. Relevant intermediate nodes should be routinely removed. The extent of resection of central nodes will depend on the patient's age, body habitus, overall medical condition, and the operative findings.

"No Touch" Technique

The discovery of large numbers of tumor cells within the portal vein associated with intraoperative manipulation of the tumor led to the suggestion that the lymphovascular pedicle be ligated prior to mobilization of the primary tumor.[496-498] Current concepts of tumor biology suggest that in the large majority of patients with subsequent liver metastases, micrometastases are already established before the primary tumor is resected. Thus, intraoperative vascular dissemination may play only a small role in the metastatic process. From a practical surgical viewpoint, it can be very difficult and potentially dangerous to isolate vascular structures prematurely. A randomized prospective trial of the "no touch" technique is underway in the Netherlands.[499] Preliminary results suggest a small benefit with preliminary vascular ligation only in the subset of patients with sigmoid colon cancer and histologic evidence of venous invasion. A complete analysis of mature data will be of interest in resolving this controversial issue.

Prevention of Intraluminal Spread

There appears to be little doubt that tumor cells are exfoliated into the intestinal lumen. It is likely that some of these cells are alive and capable of implanting on exposed cut surfaces of the bowel.[237,500] Isolated suture line recurrences are very rare after right colectomy, occurring more often after left-sided colectomies and in rectal operations. The greater longitudinal bowel margins with right-sided colon cancers, and the presence of active digestive enzymes and cytotoxic bile, may explain some of this discrepancy. Stapled anastomoses do not seem to be any more susceptible to tumor implantation than those that are hand-sewn. Precautions to minimize the implantation of cancer cells have been advised[501-503]; those that have shown efficacy in animal studies include isolation of the tumor with ligatures proximal and distal, irrigation of the lumen, Formalin or electrocautery treatment of bowel edges, and use of iodized suture material. No randomized clinical trial has ever tested these hypotheses.

Prophylactic Oophorectomy

Since 2% to 8% of women with colorectal cancer will have synchronous ovarian metastases,[504-506] and 1% to 7% of those who undergo potentially curative resections will develop subsequent ovarian metastases, prophylactic oophorectomy appears to be useful in the overall management of such patients. In addition, such an approach would reduce or eliminate the risk of primary ovarian cancer, which is approximately 1% for women over age 40, and is perhaps higher in colorectal cancer patients.[507] Extensive ovarian metastases are almost always part of widespread recurrent tumor, but it remains unclear as to whether prophylactic removal of grossly normal ovaries containing micrometastatic colonic cancer will actually increase the cure rate.

The mechanism of spread to ovaries remains unclear. It does not appear to be by peritoneal seeding, but more likely by lymphatic or hematogenous pathways. Most authors report that node-positive patients are at greater risk.[505,507,508] However, others are unable to show a predominance of ovarian metastases in node-positive patients.[509,510] Premenopausal women are at greater risk.[504,507] Whether this is related to the presence of steroid receptors in colon cancer cells is unknown.[444]

When nonrandomized patient groups that underwent prophylactic oophorectomy have been compared with appropriate matched controls, no survival benefit has been demonstrated.[505,511] It is likely that a 5% survival benefit is the maximum to be gained from prophylactic oophorectomy.

We recommend that women with colorectal cancer be asked preoperatively for permission to perform a bilateral oophorectomy. If the ovaries are grossly abnormal they should be removed. A hysterectomy is not required in the treatment of ovarian metastases. If a premenopausal woman is considering childbirth, prophylactic oophorectomy is not warranted. However, in the large majority of perimenopausal and postmenopausal women with potentially curable colorectal cancer, consideration should be given to removal of grossly normal ovaries.

SITE-SPECIFIC SURGERY

General guidelines for appropriate operative resection for colon cancers involving the major locations follow. The exact anastomotic technique (e.g., hand-sewn versus stapled anastomoses, use of different suture materials, one or two layers) is not important for the purposes of this chapter; in general, all of these issues are a function of the surgeon's preference.[512]

CECUM/ASCENDING COLON. Tumors in the cecum or ascending colon are treated by right hemicolectomy. The ileocolic and right colic arteries are divided, and usually the right branch of the middle colic (Fig. 29-10). The right ureter, spermatic or ovarian veins, inferior vena cava, superior mesenteric vein, and duodenum are at risk during this procedure. In the obese patient, overly aggressive lymphadenectomy along the superior mesenteric artery can cause catastrophic damage to the superior mesenteric vein, which lies adjacent.

HEPATIC FLEXURE. An extended right hemicolectomy is necessary for tumors in the hepatic flexure. This procedure is identical to that for cancer in the ascending colon, except that the middle colic artery is resected at its origin (Fig. 29-11). The splenic flexure may be mobilized to facilitate anastomosis as well as subsequent endoscopy.

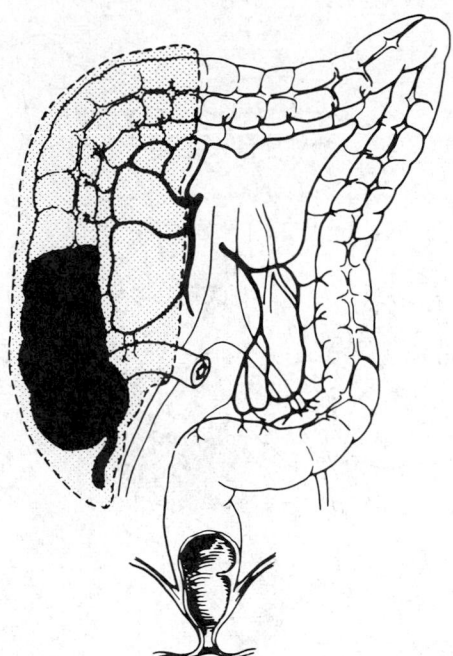

FIG. 29-10. Surgical resection for a cecal or ascending colon cancer.

TRANSVERSE COLON. Lesions of the middle and left transverse colon usually require resection of all colon proximal to the descending colon (Fig. 29-12). The right colon is removed for technical surgical reasons, and not to enhance cancer treatment. A more limited transverse colectomy is also acceptable, particularly with a lengthy ascending colon.

SPLENIC FLEXURE. As described for transverse colon lesions, an extensive resection of all proximal colon gener-

FIG. 29-11. Surgical resection for a cancer at the hepatic flexure.

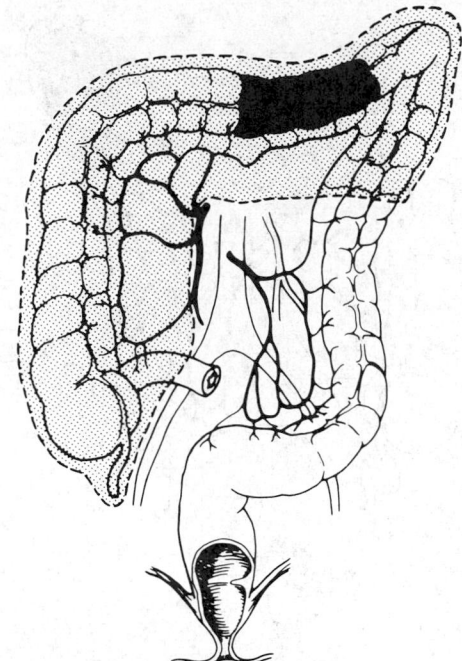

FIG. 29-12. Preferable surgical resection for cancer for the transverse colon. A segmental resection may be appropriate in poor-risk patients.

ally is preferred. The inferior mesenteric artery is preserved but cleared of contiguous nodes (Fig. 29-13). It is also acceptable to preserve the right branch of the middle colic artery and all proximal colon, with the mid-transverse colon anastomosed to the mid-descending colon (Fig. 29-14). Care must always be taken to avoid an unnecessary splenectomy, which may adversely affect survival.[513]

FIG. 29-13. Preferred extensive resection for cancer at the splenic flexure.

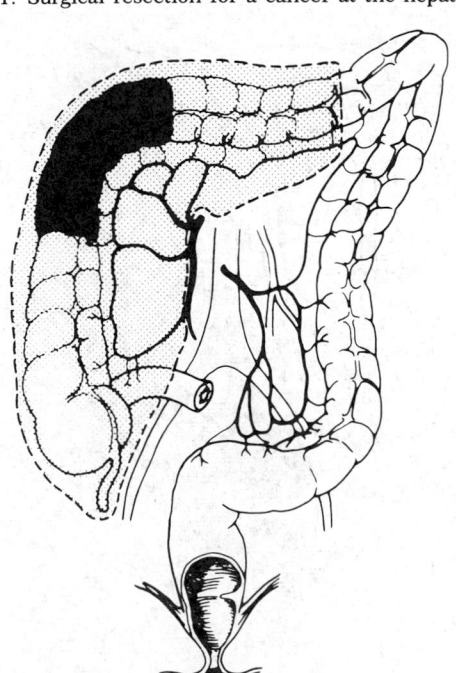

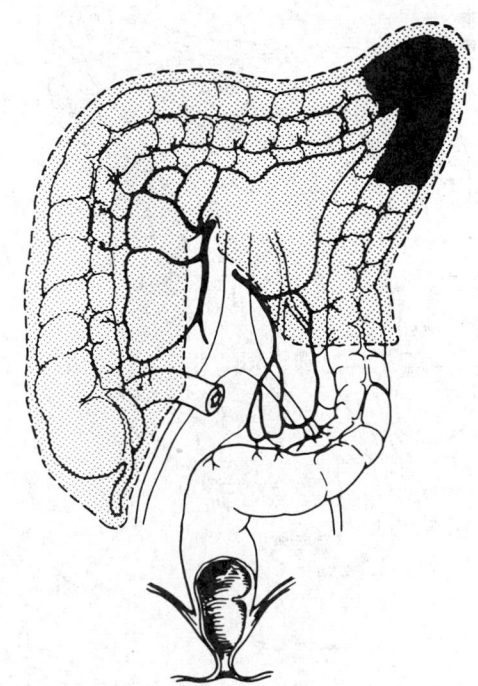

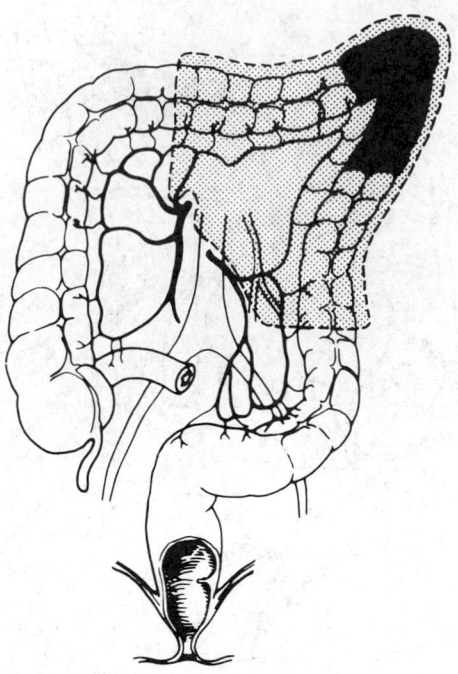

FIG. 29-14. A more limited resection for cancer of the splenic flexure in poor risk patients.

DESCENDING COLON. A left hemicolectomy with high ligation of the inferior mesenteric artery and vein is necessary for cancers of the descending colon. The transverse colon is brought to the distal sigmoid colon at the level of the pelvic brim (Fig. 29-15). The ureters, spermatic or ovarian veins, spleen, and pancreas are all at risk.

FIG. 29-15. Surgical resection for a descending colon cancer.

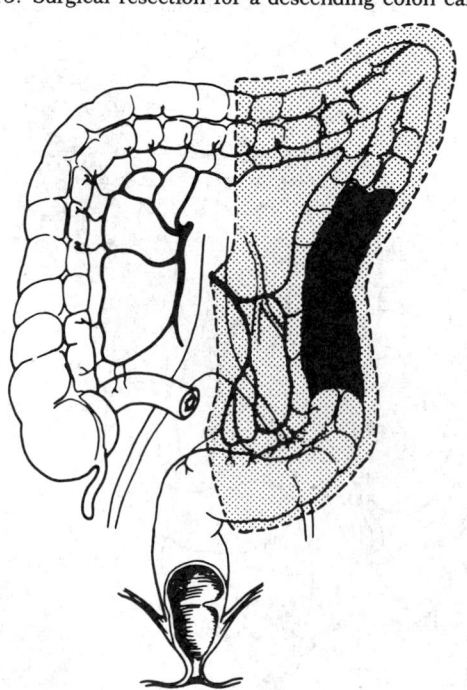

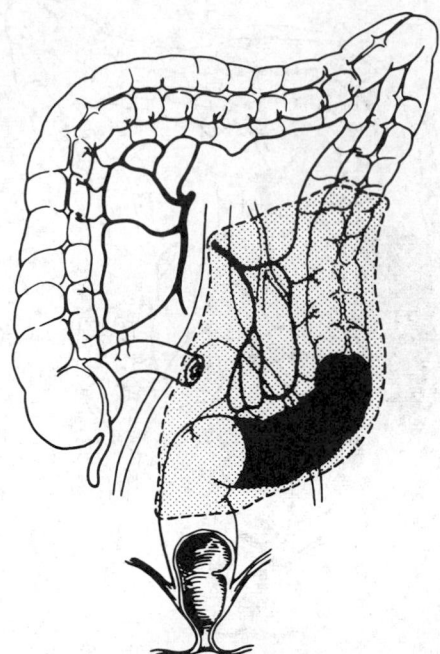

FIG. 29-16. Preferred surgical procedure for cancer of the mid and proximal sigmoid colon. In poor-risk patients, the inferior mesenteric artery and the left colic artery may be preserved.

SIGMOID COLON. Tumors in the sigmoid colon may be resected by wide sigmoid resection, with the superior hemorrhoidal artery ligated just distal to the origin of the left colic artery; or by a complete left hemicolectomy (Fig. 29-16). Both ureters must be identified and the presacral space entered.

FIG. 29-17. Surgical resection for cancer of the rectosigmoid.

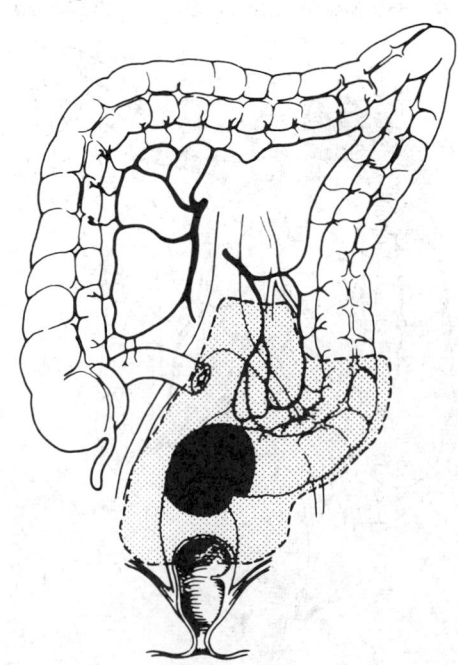

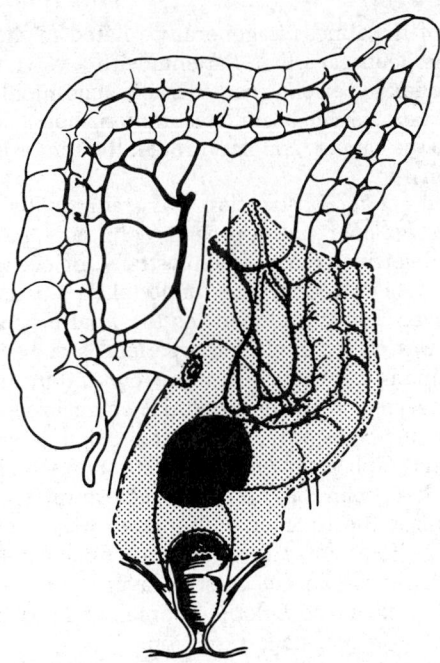

FIG. 29-18. A more radical surgical resection for cancer of the rectosigmoid.

RECTOSIGMOID (INTRAPERITONEAL RECTUM). Tumors of the distal sigmoid and intraperitoneal rectum are treated by "anterior" resection. Both ureters must be identified. The rectum is mobilized from the presacral space. The pelvic peritoneum is incised completely. The anterior prerectal plane along the prostate or vagina is opened. The lateral attachments of the rectum may be preserved. The middle sacral vessels are ligated. The proximal vessels may be ligated just distal to the left colic artery origin (Fig. 29-17) or at the level of the origin of the inferior mesenteric artery (Fig. 29-18). The higher ligation may be necessary to allow mobilization of the splenic flexure and adequate length of the proximal bowel to allow a tension-free anastomosis.

TREATMENT RESULTS

Many variables affect the curability of colorectal cancer. Multivariate analysis indicates that the surgical–pathologic stage is the most important. This section examines expected end results after surgery for potentially curable colon cancer as a function of stage. The impact of the many other prognostic variables on outcome was discussed earlier in the chapter. The management of patients with unresectable primary cancer or synchronous hematogenous metastases is discussed later.

Data appear to suggest that the 5-year survival rates after surgical resection have improved somewhat in recent years. Although such results may indicate the widespread application of appropriate surgical techniques in resecting these cancers, the use of perioperative CT may increase our ability to detect early liver metastases, and therefore to define more accurately the patient population selected for potentially curative surgery. However, whether one looks at a very large

TABLE 29-10. Five-Year Survival Rates in Node-Negative Colon Cancer

Study	Stage	Survival (%)
Willet et al[363]	T1N0M0	97
	T2N0M0	90
	T3N0M0	78
	T4N0M0	63
Eisenberg et al[325]	Dukes' A	82
	Dukes' B	73
GITSG[560,561]	T3N0M0	80

experience of a single surgeon (such as that of E. S. R. Hughes in Australia)[327] or the multicenter experience of the United Kingdom Large Bowel Cancer Project,[261] it appears that the majority of patients with colon cancer resectable at the time of laparotomy are cured by surgical extirpation.

CURE RATES FOR NODE-NEGATIVE PATIENTS. The 5-year survival rate for patients with tumors involving the mucosa or submucosa is in excess of 90%. Muscle wall invasion decreases the 5-year survival rate slightly, to 80%. Transmural penetration is still associated with cure in the majority of patients, with survival in the 60% to 80% range. Data from selected series are listed in Table 29-10.

CURE RATES FOR NODE-POSITIVE PATIENTS. The overall 5-year cure rate for patients with regional lymph node metastases is approximately one third. However, recent data are consistent with a relatively good prognosis in patients with four or fewer lymph nodes involved. The end results reported by the GITSG indicate a survival of 56% in patients with one to four positive nodes. Results from the National Surgical Adjuvant Breast and Bowel Project (NSABP)[514] and the United Kingdom Large Bowel Cancer Project[261] support this distinction. Data from selected series are listed in Table 29-11.

PATTERNS OF RECURRENCE. We will examine local (direct extension), regional (lymphatic/nodal), and peritoneal seeding recurrence patterns.

The major risk of recurrence in patients with colon cancer remains disseminated disease. The liver is involved in as many as two thirds of patients who die of colon cancer.[363] Ovarian metastases develop in up to 7% of women with colon cancer and are a symptomatic problem in approximately half of those patients.

The risk of locoregional failure varies with the pathologic

TABLE 29-11. Five-Year Survival Rates in Node-Positive Colon Cancer

Study	Stage	Survival (%)
Willet et al[363]	T2N1M0	74
	T3N1M0	48
	T4N1M0	38
Eisenberg et al[325]	Dukes' C	40
GITSG[560,561]	Dukes' C (1–4 nodes)	56
	Dukes' C (>4 nodes)	26

stage of the primary tumor. In addition, posterior penetration in a portion of the colon devoid of serosa may increase the local recurrence rate. In an autopsy series reported from the University of Florida, the local recurrence rate (in patients who died of cancer) was 27% in those with T3N0M0 disease, 21% in those with T2N1M0 disease, and 52% in those with T3N1M0 disease.[515] A similar analysis from the University of Washington identified a 27% recurrence rate in patients with transmural tumor, but 69% if the tumor adhered to or invaded adjacent structures.[516] However, only 19% of the 53 patients autopsied had isolated locoregional recurrences. The rate of disease recurrence in retroperitoneal lymph nodes was 64% in that report, and included some patients with negative nodes in the originally resected specimen.

Recurrence patterns have been analyzed in a group of 533 patients with colon cancer treated at the Massachusetts General Hospital.[363,364] The overall locoregional failure rate was 19%, with only 6% isolated local failures. However, two thirds of the patients with disease recurrence at any site had some component of locoregional failure. The local recurrences correlated with gross transmural penetration of the primary, and particularly with adherence to or invasion of surrounding organs. The local failure rate approached 50% in patients with five or more positive lymph nodes. These findings are supported by a report from the Peter Bent Brigham Hospital, in which patients with sigmoid colon cancer had an overall regional recurrence rate of 18%.[217] However, this represented a two-thirds failure rate in patients with disease recurrence at any site. In half of these patients, failure was expressed as isolated regional recurrence.

In a clinical analysis of node-positive patients at Memorial Hospital, local recurrence was documented in only 6% of 148 patients, representing only 13% of those patients with overall tumor recurrence (Enker WE: Personal communication, 1988).

The incidence of peritoneal seeding has not been well documented. In the autopsy series reported from the University of Washington, treatment failure manifested as peritoneal seeding was identified in 36% of patients who died of colon cancer. Of note, peritoneal seeding occurred in the absence of locoregional recurrence in 58% of those cases.[516] The Massachusetts General Hospital autopsy series has yielded comparable data, a 32% failure rate by peritoneal seeding.[515a]

SPECIFIC MANAGEMENT PROBLEMS IN COLON CANCER

SYNCHRONOUS CANCERS. Synchronous colorectal cancers occur in 3% to 5% of patients.[517,518] In addition, approximately one third of cancer-bearing patients will have associated benign neoplastic polyps. These data suggest that preoperative clearance of the remaining colon is required, either by air contrast barium enema examination or, preferably, by colonoscopy.[519]

OBSTRUCTING CANCERS. Circumferential cancers of the colon may manifest as large bowel obstruction. The acuteness of the illness is generally related to the competence of the ileocecal valve. Patients with a valve that does not allow reflux experience considerable abdominal pain and distention. Perforation is not uncommon, but it is usually proximal to the cancer, and not through the tumor itself (see next section).

Left-sided colonic obstruction was traditionally managed by a three-stage operative approach.[345] Initially, patients underwent a diverting transverse colostomy, or occasionally a cecostomy. The second stage, undertaken 10 to 14 days later, involved tumor resection. As the final procedure, the colostomy was closed. Unless the patient is quite ill, a two-stage Hartmann procedure is more commonly used. The tumor is resected, with the proximal colon brought to the skin as an end-colostomy. The distal colon is sutured or stapled closed. The second operation reestablishes intestinal continuity. If a preliminary diverting colostomy is chosen, it is important at the time of initial surgery to examine the cecum for perforation and the liver for metastases.

Intraoperative whole gut colonic lavage may be used to mechanically clear the colon proximal to an obstruction. This may allow a one-stage resection.

The patient with an obstructing cancer of the ascending or transverse colon can usually be treated with a single-stage resection (Fig. 29-12). An ileal–colon anastomosis is performed, which even in the absence of bowel preparation usually heals without complication. Perioperative systemic antibiotics are essential.

PERFORATING CANCERS. Perforation of the colon can occur proximal to an obstructing cancer. Recognition of this catastrophe and the timely performance of radical surgical resection, peritoneal cavity irrigation, drainage, and antibiotic administration have lessened the morbidity and mortality. Chronic perforations into a contiguous organ with or without fistula formation will be discussed subsequently. Acute free perforations into the peritoneal cavity leading to generalized peritonitis or localized abscess formation can be catastrophic. The differential diagnosis primarily includes appendicitis, diverticulitis, or perforated gastroduodenal ulcer.

CONTIGUOUS ORGAN INVOLVEMENT. Direct involvement of adjacent organs occurs in approximately 10% of patients. Extended surgery in such patients is associated with cure rates of 20% to 50%.[346,520,521] The tumor-bearing colon may be adherent due to inflammatory adhesions, or may be attached by direct penetration of tumor. Penetration into an adjacent hollow organ such as bladder or small bowel may lead to a fistula. Almost one half of clinically adherent or invaded viscera are attached by inflammatory adhesions only.[521] All such attachments should be presumed to be due to direct tumor penetration and should not be divided and biopsied. If such attachments are inadvertently torn, the survival (albeit by retrospective analysis) is half that associated with direct multivisceral resection.[521,522]

CANCER IN POLYPS. Cancer is present in approximately 5% of adenomatous polyps.[523] Cancers invasive to the level of the muscularis mucosa do not have access to the lym-

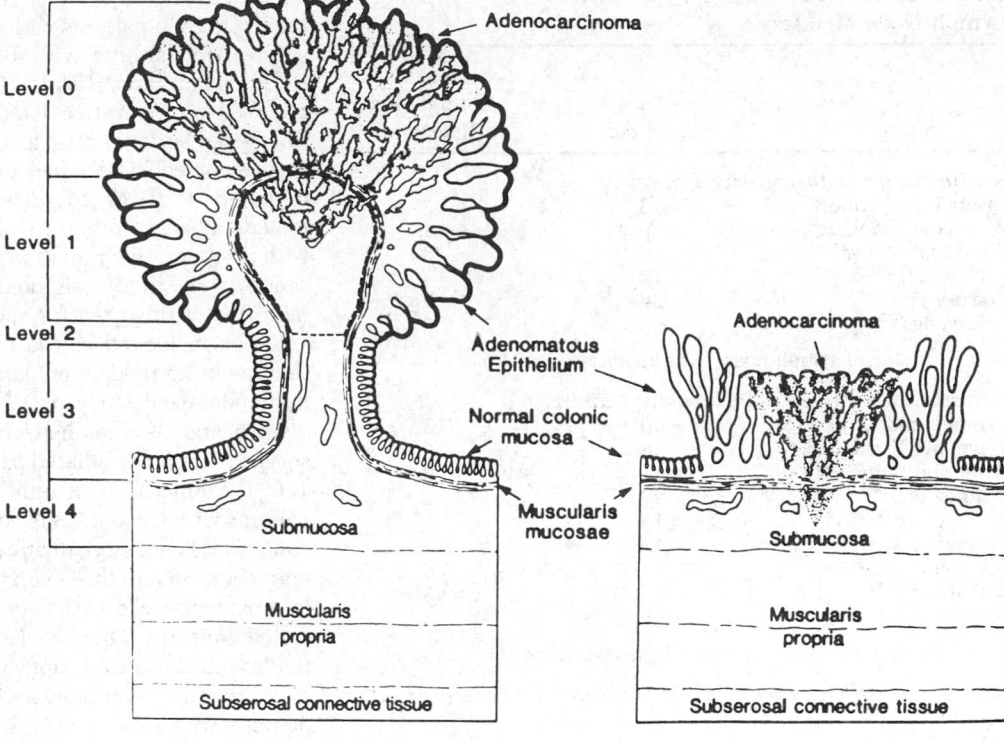

FIG. 29-19. Levels of invasion in a pedunculated adenoma (*left*) and a sessile adenoma (*right*). The stippled areas represent zones of carcinoma. Note that any invasion below the muscularis mucosae in a sessile lesion represents Level 4 invasion (submucosa). In contrast, invasive carcinoma in a pedunculated adenoma must traverse a considerable distance before it reaches the submucosa of the underlying bowel wall. However, any cancer that penetrates the muscularis mucosae is at risk for dissemination. (Haggitt RC, Glotzbach RE, Soffer EE, et al: Prognostic factors in colorectal carcinomas arising in adenomas: Implications for lesions removed by endoscopic polypectomy. Gastroenterology 89:328–336, 1985)

phatic pathways and can be cured by endoscopic or surgical polypectomy. This section considers the treatment of cancer invasive at least through the muscularis mucosa in an otherwise benign adenomatous or villous polyp. The extent of invasion must be considered, and whether the polyp is pedunculated or sessile. After endoscopic polypectomy of such lesions, one must address the risk of residual localized or nodal cancer versus the risk of definitive colectomy. Decision analysis theory can be applied for more elegant help with this troublesome problem.[524]

Figure 29-19 defines the various levels of invasion and helps in conceptualizing the problem. In addition to the level of invasion, histopathologic features to be taken into account include the degree of differentiation (grade), the presence of lymphatic or blood vessel invasion, and the adequacy of endoscopic resection (margin). Patients at high risk for local residual or nodal metastatic cancer have polyps containing one or several of the following features: poorly differentiated cancer, lymphatic vessel invasion, tumor invasive to level 3 or 4, or a positive or close polypectomy margin.[525–528]

The major issue is the risk of lymph node metastases. Colacchio and colleagues have documented what they feel is an unacceptable risk associated with conservative (nonresective) management of most of these patients.[529] The overall risk of nodal metastases is reported by these authors to be 10%. Nivatongs looked only at patients who subsequently underwent surgical resection and defined subsets based on polyp configuration and gross extent of invasion. His data and review of the literature provide the most realistic appraisal of the risk of lymph node metastases (Table 29-12). Since approximately half of patients with lymph node me-

tastases die of cancer, the incremental survival benefit from surgery for cancer limited to the head of a polyp is only 1.5%.

In summary, polypectomy alone can cure almost all patients with a moderately or well-differentiated cancer limited to the head of a pedunculated adenomatous polyp, with clear margins on the stalk, and no histopathologic evidence of lymphatic vessel invasion. The polypectomy site should be examined endoscopically in 4 to 6 months to confirm the absence of mucosal recurrence.

Not all polyps can be removed endoscopically. Large sessile lesions, particularly of the thin-walled ascending colon, pose a major therapeutic challenge. Large villous tumors have a high likelihood (up to 40%) of containing carcinoma in the polyp. Hence, limited biopsies are subject to extensive sampling error false negatives. If endoscopic removal is attempted, piecemeal removal with the snare cautery over several sessions is required. Such patients should be observed as inpatients for 1 to 2 days to rule out a perforation. Large benign sessile adenomas may require surgical resection as the least morbid approach to removal.

ADJUVANT THERAPIES FOR COLON CANCER

Adjuvant Radiation Therapy

Adjuvant radiation therapy for colon carcinoma has been approached with two different philosophies, which we will consider separately: (1) localized irradiation to the tumor bed and potentially positive nodal sites, and (2) whole abdominal irradiation.

TABLE 29-12.   Cancer in Polyps: Risk of
Lymph Node Metastases

Study	No. Resected	No. of Lymph Node Metastases
Sessile Polyps with Invasive Cancer		
Grinnell and Lane[531]	13	3
Waye and Frankel[532]	9	1
Wolff and Shinya[523]	5	2
Locke et al[533]	12	4
Kodaira et al[534]	34	2
Nivatvongs[530]	25	3
% of lymph nodes with metastases = 15%		
Pedunculated Polyps with Invasive Cancer		
Grinnell and Lane[531]	39	3
Waye and Frankel[532]	8	0
Wolff and Shinya[523]	11	0
Shatney et al[535]	23	1
Locke et al[533]	15	1
Coutsoftides et al[536]	13	0
Colacchio et al[529]	24	6
Kodaira et al[534]	64	3
Nivatvongs[530]	16	3
% of lymph nodes with metastases = 8%		
Pedunculated Polyps with Invasive Cancer Limited to Head of Polyp		
Grinnell and Lane[531]	28	0
Shatney et al[535]	14	0
Nivatvongs[530]	12	0
Colacchio et al[529]	11	2
% of lymph nodes with metastases = 3%		

Nivatongs S: Management of polyps containing invasive carcinoma. In Codner IJ, Fry RD, Roe JP (eds): Colon, Rectal, and Anal Surgery 1985, pp 183–188. St. Louis, CV Mosby, 1985.

Adjuvant radiation therapy for colon carcinoma is associated with special problems of toxicity because of the large amount of small bowel that may lie in the treatment field. Radiologic imaging with contrast materials can be used to determine the location and mobility of small bowel while planning the treatment. A good shift of the small bowel can be achieved by placing the patient in the lateral decubitus position, allowing the target area to be treated with a minimum of bowel present.[537] Other techniques to reduce radiation toxicity will be discussed later.

Locoregional Adjuvant Irradiation

Several nonrandomized reports indicate that locoregional adjuvant irradiation improves local control of cancer of the cecum, a site at high risk for local recurrence. Doses of 4000 to 6000 cGy plus boost treatment have been used on primary and nodal drainage sites.[538–541] Shehata et al used postoperative radiation therapy on 40 patients and found that after a median follow-up of 4 years, 21 of the 31 living patients had had no recurrences. There were four local failures, one being an isolated local recurrence.[540]

In a study of 80 patients with Stages B2(g) to C3 colon tumors at various sites, Duttenhaver and associates gave 4500 cGy to the tumor bed, occasionally with a 540-cGy boost to the nodal areas.[542] Radiation therapy decreased local recurrences in patients with B3 and C2 disease and improved survival in patients with B3, C2, and C3 disease. At the Princess Margaret Hospital in Toronto, 82 patients who had received postoperative irradiation had a 67% local recurrence-free survival rate at 5 years.[541] Patients in whom disease recurred locally had primarily Stage B2 (3 of 18 patients) or C (9 of 24) disease. Duttenhaver et al did not include adjacent organ involvement in their analysis. Even with postoperative radiation therapy, 8 of the 25 local recurrences were in the sigmoid colon, which emphasizes the high risk of this area for recurrent disease.

Kopelson looked at the effect of postoperative radiation therapy in sigmoid colon cancer after curative resection in a nonrandomized study of 17 patients with Stages B2 to C3 disease and 39 matched controls.[543] The 5-year actuarial survival rate for irradiated patients with B2 or B3 disease was 100%, compared with only 64% in the control group. For patients with C2 and C3 lesions, the survival difference from controls was not statistically significant. At 3 years there was one recurrence in the seven irradiated patients with B2 or B3 lesions, compared with four recurrences in the 17 nonirradiated controls. There were no recurrences in the five patients with C2 or C3 lesions who received postoperative radiation therapy, compared with three recurrences in eight patients with similar stages of disease who did not receive such treatment. The Radiation Therapy Oncology Group (RTOG) and Eastern Cooperative Oncology Group (ECOG) are cooperating in a randomized study to compare the effects of "sandwich" radiation therapy versus postoperative radiation therapy alone. Patients are randomly assigned to receive preoperative low-dose radiation therapy for tumors in fixed portions of the large bowel and rectum. After surgery, patients with Stage B2, B3, or C tumors receive radiation therapy.[544] The ECOG also has a study in progress involving adjuvant large-field radiation therapy with low dose per fraction irradiation to the tumor bed, draining nodes, and liver for C1 and C2 colon tumors that have been completely excised.

Whole Abdomen Adjuvant Irradiation

Whole abdominal radiation therapy for patients with colon carcinoma has been explored by several investigators. In a series of papers from the Albert Einstein Medical Center, Turner, Ghossein, and their colleagues have described results in patients who received approximately 2100 cGy to the whole abdomen by a moving strip technique.[545–547] The right lobe of the liver received a dose of 1500 cGy. Seventeen of 31 patients were alive after a minimum follow-up of 1 year (mean follow-up, 2 years).[546] In five patients disease recurred locally with or without distant metastases; eight had distant metastases only. One patient died of radiation enteritis. Other studies of whole abdominal radiation therapy suggest a benefit.[548,549]

The Princess Margaret Hospital is conducting a randomized trial in patients with completely resected B2 and C colon carcinoma. Patients are randomly assigned to surgery alone, or 2200 cGy delivered over 4½ weeks to the whole abdomen.[549]

Abdominal Irradiation and Chemotherapy

Intraperitoneal 5-fluorouracil (5-FU) combined with local–regional radiation therapy may enhance local, peritoneal cavity, and hepatic control.[544] The SWOG has completed a Phase I–II trial of concomitant bolus 5-FU and whole abdominal irradiation, with modest toxicity.[550] The same group has recently activated a program of concomitant continuous infusion of 5-FU with whole abdominal irradiation.

Adjuvant Systemic Therapy for Colon Cancer

As the natural history of colon cancer has been better defined, patient populations at increased risk for overall recurrence after surgery have been identified. Systemic chemotherapy has been administered after primary resection for those with poor prognoses. The first generation of adjuvant trials was initiated in the late 1950s and is summarized in Table 29-13.[351,551-554] These were studies of heterogeneous patient groups, often including patients with colonic and rectal primaries, patients who had undergone curative and palliative resections, and all Dukes' stages. Only thiotepa and the fluoropyrimidines, 5-FU and floxuridine (FUDR), were available, and were usually employed with suboptimal intensity.

Despite these flaws in study design and conduct, relatively large patient cohorts were accrued and studied, establishing the clinical and scientific basis for subsequent adjuvant efforts. The trials listed in Table 29-13 are conventionally considered "negative studies," since dramatic benefits were not elicited. However, the third and fourth Veterans Administration Surgical Oncology Group (VASOG)[553] and the Central Oncology Group (COG)[554] studies demonstrated a 5% to 10% benefit in 5-year survival. For Dukes' C colon cancer, a significant disease-free survival benefit was noted (p = 0.026): 40% of adjuvantly treated patients had recurrences at 5 years, versus 52% of patients not given systemic adjuvant treatment.[554] Moreover, an overall analysis of the fluoropyrimidine trials indicates a relatively consistent therapeutic effect, confirmed by statistical pooling methodology.[555,556] Given the available drugs, existing pharmacologic understanding, size of patient groups studied, and dose intensity of therapy offered, it is not surprising that a major therapeutic impact was not observed. Rather, it is interesting that benefits were noted for any of the trials.

The second generation of studies focused on combinations of agents and included both chemotherapy and immunotherapy. Table 29-14 describes six major trials initiated in the 1970s.[557-561] Five of the six studies employed a surgery-only control group (the exception was the ECOG 2276 study). Five utilized a combination of 5-FU + methyl-CCNU, with (MOF) or without (MF) vincristine. Combination chemotherapy — MF or MOF — was presumed to be more active than 5-FU alone in advanced disease. The empirical application of nonspecific immunotherapy with bacillus Calmette-Gúerin (BCG), BCG-MER (BCG with methanol extraction residue of BCG), or levamisole was studied. More than 4000 patients were evaluated; a trend favoring chemotherapy was noted in several studies, but statistically significant benefit was detected only in the NSABP C01 and the North Central Cancer Treatment Group (NCCTG) 78-48-52 studies.

In the NSABP C01 study, conducted from 1977 to 1983, 1116 patients were randomly assigned to observation, chemotherapy, or immunotherapy. There was a statistically significant superiority in both disease-free survival (p = 0.05) and overall survival (p = 0.04) for the MOF chemotherapy group compared to the control group. A patient not receiving adjuvant chemotherapy had a 1.34 greater likelihood of dying than his counterpart who did, a 5% to 8% survival improvement at the interim analysis.[559] Patients with right-sided colonic tumors appeared to derive the most salutary benefits. BCG treatment had no discernible impact on overall survival.

Based on preliminary data reported by Verhaegen et al,[562] the NCCTG assigned 408 patients to receive either the presumed immunomodulatory agent levamisole, 5-FU + levamisole, or observation only (see Table 29-14). With a median follow-up of 56 months, the levamisole and 5-FU + levamisole regimens improved disease-free survival (p = 0.02 to 0.04), especially for patients with Dukes' C lesions. Toxic effects were generally mild and reversible. These beneficial effects formed the rationale for the large intergroup study (INT 0035) described in Table 29-15.

Several preliminary conclusions were drawn from these second-generation studies. The benefits of adjuvant therapy were confidently observed only in large-scale clinical trials. No single therapeutic program could be recommended for all patients, but several attractive options existed. Another lesson learned was that methyl-CCNU had unexpected chronic bone marrow toxicity; acute nonlymphocytic leukemia was noted in 14 of 2067 adjuvantly treated patients. The excess risk to those receiving large doses of methyl-CCNU as an adjuvant was estimated to be 2.3:1000 persons per year. The promising leads developed in the second-generation trials are being pursued in the currently active group studies (see Table 29-15).

The NSABP in protocol C03 plans to utilize MOF as its standard control regimen. However, the total amount of therapy is decreased to 46 weeks (five cycles) to attempt to reduce the chance of nitrosourea-associated leukemia. A program of 5-FU biochemical modulation by folinic acid (leucovorin) will be compared to MOF (see Chemotherapy for Metastatic Colorectal Disease). Of interest will also be the results of a National Cancer Institute of Canada (NCIC) adjuvant study of 5-FU + folinic acid, initiated in 1987. This

TABLE 29-13. First-Generation Randomized Trials of Adjuvant Therapy for Large Bowel Cancer*

Study	Study Period	Treatment Regimen	Treatment Duration	Total Accrual
Dixon et al,[551]	1957–60	Thiotepa	2 days	695
Dwight et al,[351]	1957–61	Thiotepa	2 days	1064
Dwight et al,[552]	1961–64	FUDR	7 wk	548
Higgins et al,[553]	1965–69	5-FU	6 wk	308
	1969–73	5-FU	18 mo	518
Grage and Moss,[554]	1971–76	5-FU	12 mo	233

*All studies had a surgery-only control group.
FUDR = floxuridine; 5-FU = 5-fluorouracil.

TABLE 29-14.   Second-Generation Colon Cancer Adjuvant Trials

Study	Total Accrual	Chemotherapy	Immunotherapy	Chemoimmunotherapy	Results
VASOG 5[557]	654	5-FU, 9 mg/kg on d 1, + methyl-CCNU, 120 mg/m² on d 1, every 7 wk for 12 cycles			MF results in survival benefit for Dukes' C1
GITSG 6175[558]	621	5-FU, 325 mg/m² on d 1–5, 375 mg/m² on d 36–40, + methyl-CCNU, 130 mg/m² on d 1, every 10 wk for 7 cycles	BCG-MER, 1 mg intradermally (ID) on d 1 and 0.5 mg ID once weekly at wk 1, 5, 10, 15, 20, 25, 40, 55, 70	MF + BCG-MER	Apparent overall improved survival compared to historical controls
ECOG 2276 —(unpublished)	866	5-FU + methyl-CCNU, same as GITSG 6175, for 8 cycles or 5-FU, 450 mg/m²/d × 5 d, every 5 wk for 15 cycles			
NSABP C01[559]	1166	MF, same as in GITSG 6175 protocol, + VCR, 1 mg/m² on d 1 every 10 wk for 8 cycles	BCG, 6 × 10⁸ organisms by scarification weekly for 12 wk, then every other week for 33 wk		MOF results in 67% 5-year survival, vs. 58% for control
SWOG 7510[560]	626	5-FU, 400 mg/m² on d 1, 8, 15, + methyl-CCNU, 175 mg/m² on d 1, every 8 wk for 7 cycles		MF + BCG (6 × 10⁸ organisms PO) every other wk for 26 wk	Superior disease-free survival benefit for MF ± BCG
NCCTG 78-48-52[561]	398		Levamisole, 150 mg on d 1, 2, 3 every 3 wk	Levamisole + 5-FU, 450 mg/m², weekly for 52 wk	5-FU ± levamisole results in superior disease-free survival

MF = methyl-CCNU + 5-FU; VCR = vincristine; BCG = bacillus Calmette-Guérin; MER = methanol extraction residue of BCG; VASOC = Veterans Administration Surgical Oncology Group; GITSG = Gastrointestinal Tumor Study Group; ECOG = Eastern Cooperative Oncology Group; NSABP = National Surgical Adjuvant Breast and Bowel Project; SW = Southwest Oncology Group; NCCTG = North Central Cancer Treatment Group.

TABLE 29-15.   Currently Active Cooperative Group Trials of Adjuvant Systemic Therapy for Colon Cancer

Study	Projected Accrual	Treatment/Arm	Comments
INT 0035	300	Control 5-FU + levamisole	Dukes' B
	900	Control Levamisole 5-FU + levamisole	Dukes' C (Study duplicates and attempts to confirm NCCTG 78-48-52)
NSABP C03	855	MOF 5-FU + folinic acid	Similar to NSABP C01, but only 5 —courses Similar to regimen of Petrelli et al[817]
NCIC C03	400	Control 5-FU + folinic acid MOF	Similar to regimen of Ehrlichman et al[825]; high-dose FA
NCCTG 87-46-51	450	Control 5-FU + folinic acid. γ-interferon	Low-dose FA

INT = Intergroup; NSABP = National Surgical Adjuvant Breast and Bowel Project; NCIC = National Cancer Institute of Canada; NCCTG = North Central Cancer Treatment Group.

study has a surgery-alone control arm. The intergroup study (INT 0035) is attempting to confirm the NCCTG levamisole ± 5-FU experience. Begun in 1985, NCCTG, SWOG, and ECOG plan to accrue 1200 Dukes' B and C patients by late 1987.

There has never before been so much documentation to support the contention that adjuvant systemic therapy is of value for Dukes' B and C colon cancer patients. It is not possible to specify precisely which regimen is optimal for each patient subgroup at this time. Nonetheless, the current generation of national trials presents an ideal opportunity to confirm the magnitude and character of the impact of adjuvant therapy, and patients and physicians should be encouraged to participate. However, it is important to note that four of five major trials continue to use a surgery only control.

Adjuvant Portal Vein Chemotherapy

The rationale for adjuvant perioperative infusion of chemotherapy into the portal vein is based on the observation that, at the time of surgery, tumor cells embolize the portal venous system, seeding the liver.[337,563] Fisher and Turnbull in 1955 demonstrated tumor cells in the portal circulation in 32% of patients at the time of colonic carcinoma resection.[251] Moreover, there is considerable clinical and autopsy evidence that the liver may be the most frequent, and sometimes the only, site of metastasis.[337,563] Although established metastases are fed primarily by the hepatic artery, micrometastases are likely to still be dependent on the portal venous blood.

In 1975 Taylor et al began a randomized study of intraportal 5-FU, 700 mg/m^2/d, with heparin, infused continuously for 7 days immediately postoperatively for patients with Dukes' A, B, and C lesions. Approximately 250 patients were studied; by 1985, with a greater than 50-month median follow-up, 80 deaths had occurred. Patients with Dukes' B colon cancer appeared to have a substantial survival benefit (p = 0.002) with intraportal venous 5-FU.[564] This preliminary study stimulated several randomized trials of generally similar design.

The Australia and New Zealand Trial evaluated 372 patients with colon cancer randomly allocated to observation alone or immediate postoperative chemotherapy with 5-FU, 600 mg/m^2/d for 7 days given intravenously or intraportally. Compared to the other two groups, portal vein 5-FU infusion resulted in a highly significant superior disease-free and overall survival in Dukes' C patients.[565] These data are not fully mature and require further follow-up in order to determine the magnitude and duration of benefits.

A second study of similar design was conducted by the Swiss Group for Clinical Cancer Research (SAKK).[566] From 1981 to 1986, 378 evaluable patients who had undergone resection for Dukes' A, B, or C lesions were allocated to a control or a chemotherapy group; the chemotherapy group received immediate postoperative intraportal 5-FU, 500 mg/m^2/d, with 5,000 units of heparin, given by continuous infusion for 7 days. On the first day of therapy, a 10 mg/m^2 bolus of mitomycin C was also administered. After a median follow-up of 24 months, recurrences were detected in 43 of 187 control patients, compared with 34 of 191 infused patients

TABLE 29-16. Currently Active U.S. Studies of Adjuvant Portal Vein Chemotherapy

Study	Projected Accrual	Treatment/Arm
NCCTG 69-46-04	220	Control
		5-FU, 500 mg/m^2/d $\times$ 7 d, + heparin
NSABP C02	1334	Control
		5-FU, 600 mg/m^2/d $\times$ 7 d, + heparin

(p < 0.05). Too few deaths have occurred to establish a significant observable difference in survival, and a longer follow-up period is required before definitive conclusions can be drawn.

In the United States there are currently two active Phase III trials evaluating perioperative portal venous chemotherapy. Described in Table 29-16, these two studies should provide considerable information. Of special importance is the NSABP C02 study, since, with 1,334 patients, it will be the largest single trial of portal venous chemotherapy. It is anticipated that both studies will complete accrual by 1988 and that preliminary survival data will be available 1 to 3 years thereafter.

Use of a chemotherapy program such as that described by Taylor et al[564] in the immediate postoperative recovery period is attractive because of its convenience, modest toxicity, and relative lack of added expense. The clinical results reported to date are promising, but the impact of adjuvant portal venous chemotherapy on overall survival is not yet sufficiently clear that this therapy can be routinely recommended at this time. If ongoing trials confirm efficacy, subsequent programs will have to integrate systemic and portal venous chemotherapy.

Summary of Adjuvant Treatment for Colon Cancer

Less than 1% of all patients with colorectal cancer are entered into randomized trials. In order to help define further benefits of adjuvant treatment, patient participation in randomized trials is strongly encouraged. Preliminary data suggest a potential survival benefit with adjuvant chemotherapy. Pending maturation of recently initiated studies, high-risk patients should be considered for treatment. Adjuvant irradiation may also play a role in highly selected patients.

TREATMENT OF RESECTABLE RECTAL CANCER, AND END RESULTS

In the patient's mind, the treatment of rectal cancer is frequently associated with a colostomy. In some patients such concern may lead to a delay in seeking medical care. Fortunately, at most only one third of patients with rectal cancer require a permanent colostomy. For most patients, the primary treatment modality is radical surgical resection. As described in this section, the results of these primarily surgical approaches can be improved with adjuvant therapy, and several techniques can be utilized to maximize both local and overall cure rates of resectable colon cancers.

TABLE 29-17.   Treatment of Cancers of the Extraperitoneal Rectum (<11 cm from Anal Verge)*

Abdominoperineal resection
Low anterior resection
  End-to-end versus side-to-end
  Sutures versus staples
Abdominosacral resection
Coloanal resection
  Endoanal versus pull-through
  Staples versus sutures
Localized procedures
  Local excision
  Fulguration
  Endocavitary radiation/brachytherapy

*Exclusive of adjuvant therapies.

SITE-SPECIFIC TREATMENT OPTIONS

For surgical resections, the rectum is generally considered in three distinct sections in relation to the anal verge: the upper third, middle third, and lower third. These sections roughly correlate with 5-cm intervals. Treatment options for cancers of the lower two thirds of the rectum (extraperitoneal rectum) are outlined in Table 29-17.

UPPER THIRD. Treatment of cancers in the distal sigmoid or intra-abdominal rectum (rectosigmoid), cure rates, and patterns of recurrent cancer are similar to those of the more proximal colon. Tumors in the upper third of the rectum have their lowermost edge 11 to 12 cm from the anal verge. Extirpation is primarily surgical, by anterior or low anterior resection. In an anterior resection of the rectosigmoid, the rectum is mobilized from the sacral hollow. However, with a low anterior resection, the lateral rectal attachments (middle hemorrhoidal arteries) are divided. Bowel continuity is always restorable, either end to end or side to end. Single- or double-layer sutures or staples are suitable.

MIDDLE THIRD. Cancers in the middle third of the rectum are quite problematic to treat, because abdominoperineal resection with permanent colostomy does *not* yield superior results to those achieved with sphincter-saving surgical treatment.[567] Hence, every effort should be made to restore intestinal continuity in patients with cancers 6 to 11 cm from the anal verge. Overall surgical success depends not only on surgical expertise but also on patient body habitus, pelvic width, and the presence of associated colonic disease such as diverticulosis.

LOWER THIRD. Almost all cancers in the lower 5 cm of the rectum require an abdominoperineal resection. The abdominosacral resection or stapled low anterior resection may be feasible with early tumors if small margins are accepted. The restorative proctectomy with a coloanal anastomosis can be used in selected patients. Local procedures may also be appropriate for selected patients with low rectal cancers (see below).

EXTENT OF SURGERY ISSUES

Prior to describing the essential features of the various approaches outlined in Table 29-17, we will address a number of issues relevant to radical extirpative surgery.

DISTAL MUCOSAL MARGIN. One of the pivotal aspects of sphincter-saving surgery for patients with distal rectal cancers is the requirement to obtain an "adequate distal margin." A 5-cm distal margin is traditionally cited in surgical texts. The data do not support this rule. Distal spread may be via submucosal direct extension or intramural lymphatics. The spread may be continuous or discontinuous (satellites). Histologic examination of the bowel wall distal to the gross tumor reveals a predominance of tumors without any distal spread, and only 2.5% with spread greater than 2 cm.[567] The few patients with extensive distal spread usually have poorly differentiated, node-positive rectal cancers that disseminate rapidly.[568] A recent report from Copenhagen confirmed that a margin of 1.5 cm is adequate for potentially curable tumors.[569] There is no correlation between the risk of suture line or local recurrence and the extent of distal margin in excess of 2 cm.[570,571]

Measured operative surgical margins always exceed pathologically measured margins, because of shrinkage of the specimen. Because of the potential for miscalculation during the operative procedure, we recommend a surgical margin of 3 cm. If the transanal intraluminal circular stapler is used, margins of 2 cm plus the additional distal "donut" specimen are adequate. Exceptions are bulky, poorly differentiated or anaplastic carcinomas, which may require a longer distal margin to maximize local control. It is unacceptable to intraoperatively surgically transect a rectal cancer in a desperate attempt to avoid a permanent colostomy.

EXTENT OF PROXIMAL LYMPH NODE DISSECTION. In patients with rectal cancer the mesorectum should be removed to the level of the aortic bifurcation. This will include all nodes just distal to the origin of the left colic artery, but not the periaortic nodes or those along the inferior mesenteric artery. A nonrandomized comparison of "high ligation" of the inferior mesenteric artery and resection distal to the left colic artery, reported by the St. Mark's Hospital group, did not elicit any survival benefit for the higher lymphadenectomy group.[572] The results in patients from whom pathologically positive nodes along the inferior mesenteric artery were surgically removed justify limiting routine resection to below the left colic origin: Hojo et al had only one 5-year survivor,[573] and Grinnell none.[574] However, technically it is frequently necessary to divide the inferior mesenteric artery and vein in order to mobilize an adequate length of proximal colon to reach the rectal or anal remnant in sphincter-saving surgical procedures.

EXTENT OF PELVIC (DISTAL AND LATERAL) DISSECTION. Although the studies reviewed above justify a more limited mucosal distal margin than was recommended in the past, the extent of surgical excision of distal lymphatics or lymph nodes has not been discussed. These structures reside within the mesorectum. In a report by Williams and colleagues, only 3 of 50 patients who underwent abdominoperineal resection had positive lymph nodes caudad to the tumor within the mesorectum;[568] these cases were poorly differentiated cancers. Heald et al have strongly advocated complete excision of the mesorectum for distal rectal cancers, reporting an astonishing local recurrence rate of only 3.7% with such an approach.[575,576]

The appropriate extent of the lateral dissection for rectal cancer remains controversial. A formal pelvic lymphadenectomy is feasible in young slender patients. Not only does the procedure remove iliac and obturator lymph nodes, it may remove pararectal tissue more effectively. An adequate lateral dissection is crucial to effective local control.[576a] Such surgery may be associated with greater blood loss, a greater overall complication rate, more bladder dysfunction, and uniform erectile impotence in males.

Interest in formal pelvic lymph node dissection has been limited to a number of centers: Memorial Sloan–Kettering Cancer Center, the University of Chicago, St. Mark's Hospital, and the National Cancer Center Hospital in Tokyo. Elegant studies by Hojo et al have defined the incidence of metastasis to the various nodal groups.[573] These data were presented earlier in this chapter. An approximate 10% improvement in 5-year survival has been reported by a number of authors from these centers.[577-580] The survival benefit was most notable in patients who underwent a sphincter-saving procedure.[581] In a nonrandomized comparative report from St. Mark's Hospital, no survival advantage could be demonstrated with extended abdominopelvic nodal dissection.[582]

In summary, although a limited (2–3 cm) distal mucosal margin is adequate, local cure of rectal cancer requires maximum extirpation of mesorectal and lateral pararectal tissues. The role of formal pelvic lymphadenectomy is not defined.

RADICAL TREATMENT OPTIONS

ABDOMINOPERINEAL RESECTION. Abdominoperineal resection can be performed as a synchronous transabdominal/perineal procedure with two operative teams, or sequentially. Surgery is greatly facilitated by placing the patient in the modified lithotomy position with a single skin preparation and draping.

The abdomen is explored for nodal metastases, other primary cancers, and liver metastases. The superior hemorrhoidal vessels are ligated just caudad to the origin of the left colic artery (Fig. 29-20). If extensive nodal disease is present, higher arterial ligation may be appropriate (Fig. 29-21). The mid-sacral vessels are ligated. The rectum is mobilized from the sacral hollow beneath Waldeyer's fascia. The rectosacral fascia is incised to mobilize the rectum to beyond the coccyx. The peritoneum at the base of the bladder or posterior vagina is incised, and the rectum separated from the prostate or posterior vagina. If there is any suggestion of involvement of the rectovaginal septum, a hysterectomy with posterior vaginectomy will facilitate adequate tumor clearance. The "lateral ligaments" are divided, and the anus with pelvic floor muscles is excised.

An end sigmoid colostomy is brought out through the rectus sheath to minimize subsequent hernia. If postopera-

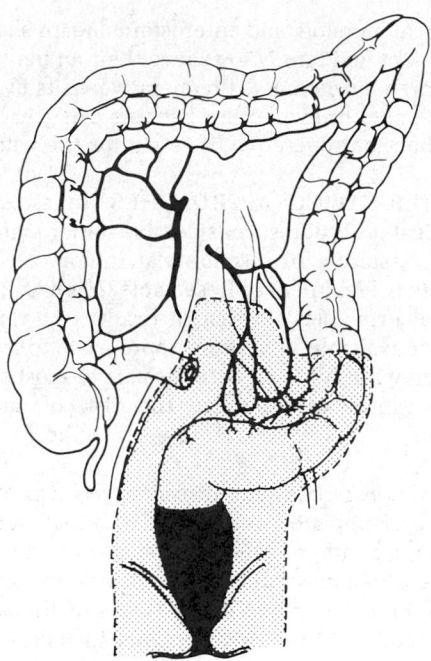

FIG. 29-20. Preferred extent of surgery in an abdominoperineal resection.

tive radiation therapy is a possibility, clips should be placed around the tumor area to facilitate delivering the boost dose. Efforts to exclude the small bowel from the radiation field using the uterus, omentum, peritoneum, or absorbable mesh should be considered. The perineum was traditionally left open to heal by granulation, but in most patients the pelvic fat and skin can be closed primarily, with greatly improved recovery.

FIG. 29-21. Extended proximal lymphadenectomy in selected patients having abdominoperineal resection.

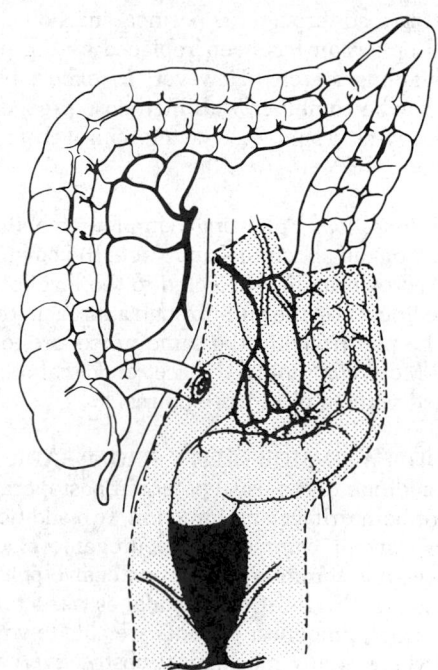

The surgical, nursing, and enterostomal team should work with the patient and family to relieve their anxiety concerning colostomy management. Preoperative visits by specially trained personnel or even other patients can greatly reduce concerns about postoperative life-style for the colostomate.

SPHINCTER-SAVING APPROACHES. In all sphincter-saving surgical procedures, considerable tumor manipulation is required, resulting in intraluminal tumor cell shedding (see section on Treatment of Resectable Colon Cancer: General Surgical Principles). Although results of a randomized study are not available, it appears appropriate to irrigate the distal rectum with saline or water as part of most sphincter-saving procedures to minimize the risk of suture line recurrences.

Low Anterior Resection. If a transanal reconstruction with a stapler is contemplated, the patient is draped in the modified lithotomy position. The initial stages of the operation with complete mobilization of the rectum to the level of the levators are identical to the initial stages of the abdominoperineal resection. Restorative options include end-to-end and side-to-end anastomoses constructed with sutures or staples. The most widely used approach utilizes the intraluminal circular stapler placed via a transanal approach. This approach allows the creation of very low anastomoses in the pelvis,[583] but the leak rate may be slightly higher.[584] Temporary protective transverse colostomy is no longer a routine adjunct with low anterior resection.

Abdominosacral Resection. An operation pioneered by D'Allaines in the 1940s has been modified by a number of surgeons to allow direct anastomosis through a perineal incision.[585,586] The rectum is mobilized to the pelvic floor, as in the operations described above. A second incision is made just above the anus, the coccyx is removed, and the pelvis is entered through the posterior fascia. An end-to-end anastomosis is performed through the perineal incision. To a great extent, this operation has been replaced by the use of the transanal stapling system. However, in expert hands, the operation may be combined with high-dose preoperative radiation therapy as a sphincter-saving approach to very low rectal cancers.[587,588]

Coloanal Resection. Following complete mobilization of the rectum from an abdominal approach, the bowel continuity is restored by bringing the colon to the level of the anus and dentate line. With the pull-through approach, the anastomosis can be performed at the same procedure, or delayed 10 days.[580] More commonly, a direct endoanal anastomosis is performed with staples[590] or sutures.[591]

MORBIDITY AND MORTALITY FROM RADICAL SURGERY. In addition to the usual potential postoperative complications of hemorrhage and infection, two additional areas of concern warrant comment. A neurogenic bladder with inability to void is common after an extensive pelvic dissection. Catheter drainage of the bladder is used for 7 to 10 days, after which time most patients are able to void spontaneously. If there is any mechanical obstructive component

from urethral stricture or prostate enlargement, transurethral surgery may be required before voiding is possible. Bethanechol chloride may be useful in improving bladder emptying. Intermittent or continuous catheterization for months may be necessary in some patients.

Sexual dysfunction, particularly in males, is the rule. Retrograde ejaculation despite normal orgasm is the most common complaint. Erectile impotency is very common after abdominoperineal resection.

The mortality from radical surgery for rectal cancer is 2% to 6%, with no difference between abdominoperineal resection or sphincter-saving procedures.[592-594]

LOCAL TREATMENT OPTIONS FOR RECTAL CANCER

PATIENT SELECTION. Local treatment alone for rectal cancer was first applied to patients with medical contraindications to radical surgery. Severe cardiopulmonary disease may preclude extensive surgery because of high surgical mortality. Patient blindness has always been a concern if a colostomy is required, which makes subsequent self-care difficult. However, a small subset of patients with early rectal cancers may be treated preferentially by one of a number of more limited approaches. Exophytic, small (<3 cm), well-differentiated tumors, clinically limited to the submucosa, are ideal for a limited approach. However, tumors invasive into the muscle wall have also been treated in limited fashion, with good results. Improved clinical staging systems, combined with careful histologic and biologic analyses of various phenotypic markers, may enable us to define appropriate subsets of rectal cancer patients for these treatment strategies.[280] A detailed analysis of these considerations is outside the scope of this book, but the various approaches will be described to familiarize the reader with these therapeutic options. The results are presented in subsequent sections.

TRANSANAL LOCAL EXCISION. A transanal local excision is the most straightforward approach to removing rectal cancers. The deep plane of dissection can be submucosal or full-thickness, generally the latter. Adequate dilation of the anus and the use of special retractors, fiberoptic light, and traction sutures facilitate the procedure. Primary closure of the defect minimizes subsequent scarring, which is important in follow-up of these patients.

POSTERIOR PROCTOTOMY. For lesions too large or too proximal for transanal local excision, two other surgical approaches are available—the posterior proctotomy (Kraske procedure) and transsphincteric excision. In the posterior proctotomy, a perineal incision is made just above the anus, the coccyx is removed, and the fascia divided. The rectum is mobilized and a wide local excision is performed, or even a sleeve resection.[595]

TRANSSPHINCTERIC PROCEDURE. Also known as the Bevan or York Mason procedure, the transsphincteric approach is identical to the posterior proctotomy, except that the entire anal sphincter is divided posteriorly in the midline. As long as each portion of the sphincter mechanism is identified and marked, the anus can be reconstructed at the completion of the operation with minimal risk of functional impairment.[596]

FULGURATION. Fulguration or cauterization has been used as an alternative to abdominoperineal resection by Madden, Crile, Turnbull and others.[597,598] The procedure is done in multiple stages under general or regional anesthesia. Tumor is charred, then scraped with a curette. This approach is not without risk, primarily a delayed hemorrhage (in 10%–20% of cases) from the slough of the scar at 7 to 10 days.

ENDOCAVITARY IRRADIATION. Radiation has been used as a single modality approach to early rectal cancer with curative intent. External beam x-rays alone have been used,[599] but most investigators have used intracavitary irradiation, either alone or combined with temporary isotope implants.[600] The anus is dilated and a 4-cm proctoscope is introduced. A low-energy x-ray unit is placed through the scope almost against the tumor. Generally, 50-kV x-rays, in doses of 3000 cGy per treatment, are given using this "contact" approach. Three or four such sessions are required. Bulky tumors may require additional irradiation with iridium implants or external beam therapy to reach the deeper pararectal tissues.

OTHER LOCAL OPTIONS. Multiple other local treatment strategies have been used. Cryosurgery and Nd-YAG laser ablation may play a role in future years.

Treatment Results in Rectal Cancer

This section presents the end results after surgery for rectal cancer. Overall, cure rates for cancers in the lowermost third of the rectum are less than those for cancers in the upper two thirds.[601,602] In the discussion of patterns of recurrence, pelvic failure will be explored in detail.

CURE RATES FOR NODE-NEGATIVE RECTAL CANCER. Three fourths of patients with node-negative rectal cancer will be cured by radical surgical resection.[261,592] The 5-year survival figures from several major centers are listed in Table 29-18.

CURE RATES FOR NODE-POSITIVE RECTAL CANCER. Only a minority of patients whose rectal cancers have spread to regional lymph nodes are cured by surgery.

TABLE 29-18. Cure Rates in Node-Negative Rectal Cancer

Study	Stage	5-Year Survival (%)
Wilson and Beahrs[594]	Dukes' A, B	79
Eisenberg et al[325]	Dukes' A	88
McDermott et al[136]	Dukes' A	93
Eisenberg et al[325]	Dukes' B	79
McDermott et al[136]	Dukes' B	71

TABLE 29-19. Cure Rates in Node-Positive Rectal Cancer

Study	Stage	5-Year Survival (%)
Wilson and Beahrs[594]	Dukes' C	41
Eisenberg et al[325]	Dukes' C	29
McDermott et al[136]	Dukes' C	41

About one third of such patients achieve a 5-year disease-free survival (Table 29-19).

RESULTS WITH LOCAL TREATMENT OPTIONS. In analyzing the long-term results achieved with the various limited treatment options, it is important to appreciate that case selection favors excellent results.[602b] When in situ cancers were excluded, a local control rate of 82% was obtained in a total of 378 patients with invasive cancer treated by local excision.[602c–602g] In the most recent report from St. Marks Hospital, treatment failed locally in 4 of 39 patients.[602h] Hager and associates from Erlangen reported that 3 of 36 patients with T_1 cancers and 3 of 18 with T_2 cancers had local recurrences.[602i] The largest series has been reported from the Mayo Clinic, with a local failure rate of 27% (38 of 141 patients).[603]

Local failure after *fulguration* occurs in 10% to 50%.[602d,602e,604] Multiple sessions (average of 3.5) may be required to maximize local control.[602d,604] A subset of patients with recurrence are cured by subsequent radical surgery.[602d,602e,604–606]

Papillon and colleagues in Lyon, France, pioneered the treatment of selected patients with rectal cancers using *endocavitary irradiation*. Exophytic superficial cancers exclusive of poorly differentiated or colloid histology and less than 4.5 cm in diameter were treated. If the tumor was felt to invade muscle, interstitial iridium-192 was added. In 245 patients, the 5-year disease-free survival rate was 76%. The local failure rate was only 5.3%.[602g] Sischy and associates have reported equally good results.[607] The local failure rate in 94 patients treated with endocavitary irradiation alone was 5%.

Five-year survival rates with local treatment options vary from 50% to 90%, with many deaths secondary to medical illnesses and unrelated to cancer. In selected patients, a 10% cancer-related 5-year mortality can be expected with local excision, fulguration, or primary irradiation.

PATTERNS OF RECURRENCE AFTER RADICAL SURGERY. Despite radical surgery, local–regional failure occurs in 20% to 50% of patients with transmural or node-positive rectal cancers. Pelvic recurrence can be secondary to suture line tumor, retained lymph nodes, intralymphatic tumor, or shed tumor cells. The incidence of treatment failure in the pelvis is directly related to the extent of transmural penetration (microscopic versus gross) and the additive risks of lymph node metastases. Pelvic failure rates as a function of various pathologic parameters are listed in Tables 29-20 and 29-21.

Failure patterns determined at autopsy provide the most accurate insight into the relative risks of local and distant recurrence. In the series reported from the Massachusetts

TABLE 29-20. Pelvic Recurrence Rates After Surgery for Node-Negative Rectal Cancer

Study	Stage	Locoregional Recurrence
McDermott et al[610]	Dukes' B	15
Phillips et al[609]	Dukes' B	15
Pilipshen et al[608]	Dukes' B	30
Pilipshen et al[608]	T2N0M0	14
Pilipshen et al[608]	T3N0M0	30
Rich et al[221]	T3(m)N0M0*	17
Rich et al[221]	T3(g)N0M0*	25
Rich et al[221]	T4N0M0	53

*(m) denotes microscopic transmural extension; (g) denotes gross transmural extension.

General Hospital, isolated pelvic recurrences were documented in 25% of patients, but a total of 75% of cancer-related deaths were associated with tumor in the pelvis. These data suggest that improved local control through multimodality treatment of the primary cancer not only will dramatically reduce cancer-related morbidity, but also may improve survival, particularly in node-negative patients.

SPECIFIC MANAGEMENT PROBLEMS IN RECTAL CANCER

OBSTRUCTION. Subtotal obstruction from rectal cancers may manifest as increasing constipation or frank obstipation, more commonly as diarrhea and tenesmus. If dietary management with a minimal residue regimen is not effective in allowing an elective operation (perhaps including preoperative irradiation), a preliminary colostomy should be considered.

CONTIGUOUS ORGAN INVOLVEMENT. In patients with rectal cancer, contiguous organ involvement usually entails direct invasion of the prostate and base of the bladder in men, and of the vagina in women. In women who have previously undergone a hysterectomy, a cancer of the upper third of the rectum may invade the base of the bladder. Management issues are discussed in a later section on unresectable, recurrent cancer—locally advanced rectal cancer.

TABLE 29-21. Pelvic Recurrence Rates After Surgery for Node-Positive Rectal Cancer

Study	Stage	Locoregional Recurrence (%)
McDermott et al[610]	Dukes' C	32
Phillips et al[609]	Dukes' C	21
Pilipshen et al[608]	Dukes' C	39
Pilipshen et al[608]	T2 N1 M0	22
Pilipshen et al[608]	T3 N1 M0	49
Rich et al[221]	T3(m)N1M0*	28
Rich et al[221]	T3(g)N1M0*	52
Rich et al[221]	T4N1M0	67

*(m) denotes microscopic transmural extension; (g) denotes gross transmural extension.

ADJUVANT THERAPIES FOR RECTAL CANCER

Limited Local Surgery and Adjuvant Irradiation

As described previously, limited local treatment strategies such as local excision, fulguration, and intracavitary irradiation may be selected as palliative approaches, and, with appropriate case selection, as curative approaches. It is reasonable to postulate that locoregional failure secondary to microscopic residual primary tumor or pelvic lymph node metastases may be reduced with adjuvant radiation. Relatively little data are available in this regard, and none of it is randomized.

Some investigators have used supplementary radiation therapy in a subset of patients who were treated with electrocoagulation.[598,606,611–613] Wittoesch and Jackman reported a 47% 5-year survival rate in their poor-risk patients, of whom 62% had received some form of adjuvant irradiation.[614] Preoperative irradiation to about 2000 cGy was used in a local excision series at Memorial Hospital, in which many patients had undergone reexcision for recurrent disease.[615] The 5-year survival rate was 83%, similar to the 84% survival rate reported by that institution for primary local excisions without irradiation, with only 6% dead of disease during the 5-year interval.[616]

Rich et al described 17 patients with adenocarcinoma in the lower two thirds of the rectum who underwent a local procedure to remove gross tumor, either a local excision (in 16 patients) or fulguration (1), and who received adjuvant irradiation. There was only one local failure (6%) despite positive margins in 11 of the 17 patients.[617]

Radical Surgery and Adjuvant Irradiation

The multimodality management of patients with rectal cancer is directed toward maximizing local control, as well as increasing overall survival. The following discussion addresses the complex issues of radiation dose, sequencing, and toxicity prior to analyzing the end results of adjuvant radiation therapy.

Until recently, analyses of adjuvant irradiation for rectal carcinoma were nonrandomized, retrospective studies that compared results in patients who had received adjuvant radiation therapy as a complement to a radical surgical procedure with results in historical or, at best, concurrent controls. In the discussion of adjuvant radiation therapy, we will distinguish nonrandomized from randomized studies.

DOSE CONSIDERATIONS. If one looks at the series of preoperative radiation therapy studies done in the past, there appears to be a trend toward increasing local control as the preoperative dose of radiation therapy increased.[618] In a recent preoperative radiation therapy study, the local control rate was 67% with 4000 cGy, increasing to 91% with 5000 cGy.[619] A study of patients with gross residual cancer demonstrated a local control rate of 67% with doses between 5000 and 5499 cGy, increasing to 89% with doses above 6000 cGy.[620] In the randomized GITSG postoperative radiation therapy study, the local control rate was 76% without pelvic irradiation in the control group but increased only to 80% in the radiation therapy alone group, which had received only 4400 to 4800 cGy.[262] It seems apparent that doses of 5000 cGy or higher are needed to control microscopic disease.

SEQUENCING CONSIDERATIONS. *Preoperative Radiation.* The rationale for using preoperative radiation therapy is (1) to increase resectability, (2) to abrogate potential seeding of tumor during surgery, and (3) to destroy microscopic foci of tumor that may lie beyond the surgical margins or in lymph nodes outside the operative field.[621]

The potential advantages of delivering radiation therapy preoperatively are several. (1) The radiation is delivered under well-vascularized and well-oxygenated conditions, so that the cells are maximally radiosensitive. (2) One can avoid implantation of viable cells, either locally or through vascular channels, as the tumor is manipulated during surgery. (3) The radiation is delivered with a freely mobile small bowel (*i.e.*, without any adhesions resulting from a surgical procedure), so that any given portion of the small bowel lies within the radiation fields only part of the time during irradiation. (4) If there is a question regarding fixation, preoperative irradiation increases the chance of resectability. A decrease in the number of positive nodes has also been noted after preoperative radiation therapy,[622-624] but the ultimate effect of such a downstaging on survival is unclear.

Postoperative Radiation. A major reason for choosing postoperative irradiation is that the stage and extent of disease are known, and one may select the patients most likely to benefit from adjuvant therapy on the basis of these prognostic features. Other advantages include the following: (1) The extent of disease is determined at surgery, so that the radiation therapy field, including boost fields, may be more carefully defined. (2) Sphincter-preserving procedures can be done without (unfounded?) fear of healing of irradiated tissue. (3) Surgery is not delayed. (4) Patients with distant metastases found at surgery may be excluded from the treatment program or may be placed on a combined radiation-chemotherapy regimen. Potential disadvantages include the loss of the advantages that preoperative radiation therapy offers: (1) after surgery tumor cells may be in a hypoxic state because vascularity is compromised, and therefore the cells may be less radiosensitive; (2) the small bowel may be fixed within the radiation fields; and (3) the potential advantage of preventing seeding of viable cells at surgery cannot exist.

"Sandwich" Radiation Therapy. This technique entails a combination of preoperative radiation therapy, usually with relatively small doses (500–2000 cGy), and postoperative radiation therapy, to a high total dose only in high stage cases. The technique may offer the advantages of both preoperative and postoperative radiation therapy.

TECHNIQUES TO MINIMIZE TOXICITY. At the doses necessary to control microscopic disease before or after surgery for rectal carcinoma, the major organ of concern for tolerance is the small bowel.[625] If a large portion of the small bowel receives more than 5000 cGy, the risk of treatment-associated complications increases. These complications include obstruction, perforation, and fistula. The risk of complications may also be increased with other patient-related factors, such as hypertension or diabetes,[626] or a history of multiple surgical procedures in the abdomen. Many techniques have been developed to prevent such toxic effects (Table 29-22). These may be divided into surgical and radiation therapy techniques.

Surgical techniques include pelvic reconstruction to exclude small bowel from the pelvis.[537] An omental transposition flap[627] or retroverted uterus may be used, or an absorbable synthetic polyglycolic mesh pelvic sling.[628-631] Insertion of a tissue expander has also been described.[632]

During radiation therapy planning, small bowel radiographs with contrast material in the small bowel to determine its location and mobility are essential.[537,633-635] The severity of acute GI effects has been correlated with the small bowel volume included in the radiotherapy fields.[635] There was no diarrhea when the average volume of small bowel included in the fields was 58 cm³, whereas when this volume was increased to 485 cm³, unresponsive diarrhea developed. Late GI effects correlated with prior pelvic surgery and with the volume of small bowel that received more than 4500 cGy.

A three- or four-field technique with careful blocking is used for the large pelvic portion of treatment, with AP/PA and two lateral fields, to a dose of 4600 to 5000 cGy. After this, a carefully planned boost dose (1000–1500 cGy) is given to the tumor bed area, guided by the location of the original tumor as defined by various imaging methods and by clips placed at surgery. The boost field may be planned most effectively in this era with the aid of CT (Fig. 29-22).

During treatment of the prone patient, the bladder may be distended, which will push small bowel superiorly out of the pelvic fields.[537] External compression with the patient in the

---

TABLE 29-22. Techniques to Minimize Toxic Effects in Small Bowel with Pelvic Radiation Therapy

Surgical Techniques:
  Pelvic reconstruction to exclude small bowel from pelvis:
    Reperitonealize pelvic floor
    Retrovert the uterus
    Construct omental sling
    Use temporary prosthesis
  Place clips to delineate high-risk areas
  Perform temporary colostomy
Radiation Therapy Techniques:
  During planning:
    Small bowel radiographs during simulation
    Liberal use of other diagnostic tools such as US, CT, or MR imaging to delineate tumor–small bowel relationship
    Place patient prone
    Use multiple fields for pelvic treatment, with judicious blocking
    Use carefully planned boost fields
  During treatment:
    Bladder distention (with patient prone)
    Use external compression
    Use "false tabletop"
    Use small doses per fraction (180 cGy) or hyperfractionation (b.i.d.)
    Diet regulation
    Potential: use of radioprotectors

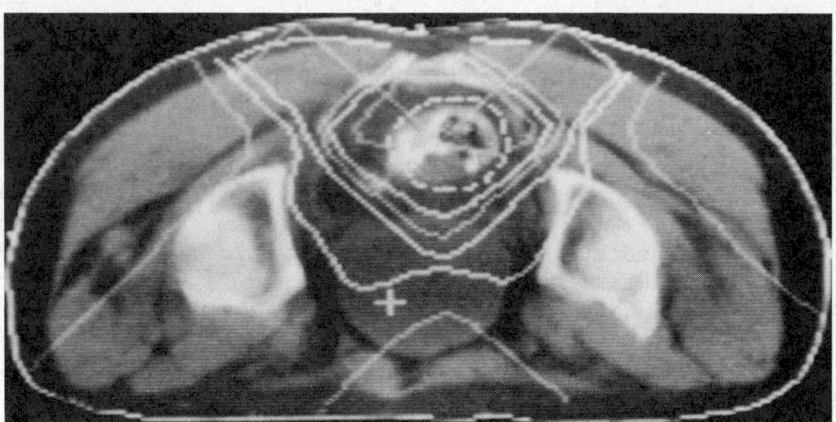

FIG. 29-22. Planning "boost" treatment for a rectal primary in an inoperable patient utilizing a computerized tomography treatment planning system. Dashed inner line = biological target volume. Other lines are isodoses from two wedged posterior oblique fields.

prone position has also been used. Gallagher et al demonstrated a reduction of small bowel within the fields when they combined the prone position, bladder distention, and external compression, in comparison with the supine position.[635]

It has been suggested that the use of special diets during a course of radiation therapy may be an advantage in preventing acute radiation effects.[636] Diets have included (1) a powdered elemental diet, (2) a lactose-restricted diet, and (3) a combination low-fat, low-residue, low-lactose diet. The elemental diet was of value in animal studies,[637] and preliminary results suggest benefit in clinical trials.[638] A lactose-restricted diet has not been shown to be of value in patients undergoing whole pelvis irradiation.[639] A randomized trial with a low-fat, low-residue, low-lactose diet is in progress at Memorial Sloan–Kettering Cancer Center for gynecologic patients receiving pelvic radiation therapy; the trial has been expanded to patients with other carcinomas receiving pelvic radiation therapy.[640]

Some pharmaceutical agents may possibly protect the small bowel while not jeopardizing the radiation effect on the tumor. The radioprotector, WR-2721, has been studied in mice.[641,642] A Phase II trial was initiated in April 1987 by the RTOG in which WR-2721 was administered before protracted fractionated radiation therapy for carcinoma of the rectum, cervix, or bladder. Other analogues may prove to be of more use in the future. A study in mice has shown that prostaglandin E_2 protected against acute toxicity, as measured by jejunal cell survival, when given 1 hour before radiation therapy.[643] At present, the best protection against toxic effects in the small bowel is careful coordination from the outset by the surgeon and radiation therapist.

Results of Preoperative Radiation Therapy

NONRANDOMIZED STUDIES. Seminal studies from Memorial Hospital[644,645] suggested a survival benefit at doses approximating 1500 to 2000 cGy. A variety of radiation techniques were used (radon seeds, orthovoltage, etc.) The overall 5-year survival rate was 55% in irradiated patients versus 45% in those treated by surgery alone. In subsequent studies doses have ranged from 2000 to 6000 cGy. In all of these studies, the local recurrence rates have been low (5%–15%),[587,646–651] considerably lower than in patients treated with surgery alone at the same institution.[647,649,650] The results with high-dose preoperative therapy are summarized in Table 29-23.

High-dose preoperative radiation therapy has also allowed downstaging of disease in some cases. In most series, the percentage of patients with positive lymph nodes is reduced from 30% to 40% without radiation therapy to a level of 20% to 25%.[647–649] In a few studies, no microscopic tumor was

TABLE 29-23. Nonrandomized Studies of High-Dose Preoperative Radiation Therapy

Study	Date	Dose (cGy)	Local Recurrence S	RT	Survival S		RT
Jewish Hospital of St. Louis and Mallinckrodt Institute of Radiology	1982	2000 or 4500	14%	2000 cGy } 8% 4500 cGy } 4%	. . .		. . .
University of Florida	1985	3000–4500	29%	8%	41%	5-yr NED	71%
Baystate Medical Center	1985	4000–4500	15%	6%	48%	5-yr adjusted overall	74%
					52%	Adjusted NED	79%
Thomas Jefferson Hospital	1987	4000–5000	All: 14%		. . .	4-yr all	66%
			Low lesions:	11%	41%	Low lesions (Memorial Hosp. comparison)	72%

S = surgery; RT = radiation therapy.

TABLE 29-24. Randomized Studies of Preoperative Radiation Therapy

Study	Date	Dose (cGy)	No. of Patients S	No. of Patients RT	LR S	LR RT	5-Year Survival S	5-Year Survival RT
Princess Margaret Hosp., Toronto[655]	1977	500	56	55	. . .	. . .	35% Overall	35%
							17% Stage C	35%
Medical Research Council[274,655a]	1982	500	275	277	57%	55%	38% Overall	42%
	1984	2000		272		53%		40%
Memorial Hosp.[328]	1974	2000	414	376	23%† Stage C	13%†	65% Overall	67%
					From autopsy:			
VASOG I[622,657]	1975	2000–2500	353	347	36% All	29%	32% Overall	40%
					40% APR	29%*	28% APR	41%
							32% Stage C	54%
Stockholm Rectal Group, Stockholm[656]	1987	2500	274	271	20 (p < .01)	8%	. . .	. . .
VASOG II[658]	1986	3150	180	181	. . .	. . .	50% APR	50%
Mainz[663,664]	1977, 1984	3450	106	64	20%	12.5%	64% (p < .05)	80%
EORTC[654,665]	1985, 1987	3450	166	152	35% (p = 0.002)	15%	60% (p = .08)	70%

LR = local recurrence; S = surgery alone; RT = adjuvant preoperative radiation therapy; APR = abdominoperineal resection.
*Statistically significant.
†Unpublished data (Shank et al).

found in 3% to 17% of the operative specimens.[651–653] A recent study stressed the safety and ability of preoperative radiation therapy to complement sphincter-saving procedures in low rectal cancer.[587] Complications have tended to be minimal, similar to the complications of surgery alone, although an increase in wound sepsis in one series was reported.[647] Friedmann et al noted an increase in bowel obstruction and organ injury during surgery to 5% with radiation therapy, compared with 1% without.[649]

RANDOMIZED STUDIES. Many randomized studies have used relatively low doses of preoperative irradiation, ranging from 500 cGy to 3450 cGy. Although large numbers of patients were treated in several of these studies, the lower doses produced little benefit in local recurrence rates. The major preoperative studies are summarized in Table 29-24.[654–665] The most impressive results are reported by the European Organization for Research on Treatment of Cancer (EORTC).[654] At 5 years, the actuarial local control rate was 85% in the group treated with preoperative radiation therapy group (3450 cGy in 230 cGy per day fractions) compared with 65% for the surgery-alone group (p = 0.001). Similar data have been reported by the group in Mainz, Federal Republic of Germany,[664] and the Stockholm Rectal Cancer Study Group.[656]

In the studies with doses less than 3000 cGy, there has been no improvement in overall survival. An exception is the VASOG I study in which patients who received preoperative irradiation (2500 cGy) before abdominoperineal resection had a 41% 5-year survival rate, compared with a 28% survival rate for those treated by surgery alone. Of the studies utilizing doses higher than 3000 cGy, the EORTC and the Mainz group report a difference in disease-free survival with preoperative irradiation.[664,665] A small study from Yale randomizing patients to 4500 cGY noted an improved 5-year survival, from 25% to 41%. Two studies from the Soviet Union have shown statistically significant increases in sur-

vival, but it is not clear whether they were truly randomized.[659,660]

In terms of complications with low-dose radiation therapy, the most complete observations have been done in the Medical Research Council study.[661] In this study, the complications were essentially identical between the two radiation therapy groups and the surgery-alone group, except for a significant decrease in anastomotic leaks in the radiation therapy groups compared with the surgery-alone group. In addition, there were no increases in long-term complications.[661] In the VASOG II study, most complications were similar in the two groups, except for an increase in moderate to severe complications, especially perineal infections, in the group treated with preoperative radiation therapy.[658]

SUMMARY OF PREOPERATIVE IRRADIATION. Adjuvant preoperative irradiation in sufficiently high doses likely improves the local control rate and may increase survival. To confirm these conclusions, the United Kingdom Medical Research Council (MRC) has begun trial II, randomizing patients with "tethered" cancers to receive 4,000 cGY preoperatively.

Results of Postoperative Radiation Therapy

NONRANDOMIZED STUDIES. The largest nonrandomized studies (Table 29-25) have been reported from the M. D. Anderson Hospital[666] and from the Massachusetts General Hospital.[662] In both studies, high doses were delivered to the pelvis (4000–5000 cGy at M. D. Anderson Hospital and 4500 cGy at Massachusetts General Hospital), with additional boost doses to high-risk areas in some cases. The results show a reduction in the local recurrence rate for patients with B2 and C2 lesions (the stages for which sufficient patients were available to draw valid comparisons with historical controls). In the Massachusetts General Hospital series, 5-year survival was higher with radiation therapy. The

TABLE 29-25.   Nonrandomized Studies of Postoperative Radiation Therapy

Study	Year	Dose (cGy)	Total No. of Patients		Local Recurrence			5-Year Actuarial Survival	
			S	RT	Stage	S	RT	S	RT
M.D. Anderson Hosp.[666] (Follow-up range, 24–138 mo)	1987	4000–5000 to pelvis, + 600–1000 boost	?	105	B2	13%	4%	. . .	65%
					B3	26%	31%	. . .	48%
					C2	30%	18%	. . .	48%
					C3	49%	1/5		3/5
Mass. General Hosp.[662] (Median follow-up, 56 mo)	1987	4500 to pelvis, ± ≥540 boost	142	165 (79)*	B2	23%	9%	. . . (47%)	71% (76%)†
					B3	53%	0/7	. . . (27%)	67% (69%)
					C2	47%	21%	. . . (27%)	39% (34%)
					C3	4/6	53%	. . . (0/6)	17% (13%)
Thomas Jefferson Univ. Hosp.[668] (Follow-up range, 2–9 yr)	1985	4500 to pelvis	88	26	B2	26%	11%	34%	32%
					C1				
					C2				

S = surgery only; RT = adjuvant postoperative radiation therapy.
*Surgery done at the same institution
†( ) = NED survival; patients dying of intercurrent disease were excluded from analysis at time of death.

M. D. Anderson Hospital report does not include historical surgery-only controls in the survival analysis. The incidence of small bowel obstruction requiring surgery was higher at M. D. Anderson Hospital (13%) than at Massachusetts General Hospital (6%). However, the former group used larger parallel opposed anteroposterior pelvic fields for most of their patients, whereas the group at Massachusetts General Hospital used a four-field technique for the pelvic portion of the radiation therapy. A report from Thomas Jefferson University Hospital also suggests an advantage for postoperative radiation therapy (4500 cGy) in preventing local recurrences, but not in improving overall survival.[668]

RANDOMIZED STUDIES. Three major randomized studies of postoperative radiation therapy have included a surgery-only arm for comparison: a GITSG study, an NSABP study, and a study from multiple institutions in Denmark (Table 29-26).[262,669–671] In all three studies a slightly lower dose of radiation was used than in the nonrandomized stud-

TABLE 29-26.   Randomized Studies of Postoperative Radiation Therapy for Rectal Carcinoma

Study	Year	Dose (cGy)	No. of Patients		Stage	Local Recurrence		Survival		
			S	RT		S	RT	S		RT
								At 5 yr:		
GITSG[262,669]	1985, 1986	4000–4800	58	50	B2–C:	24%	20%	43%		52%
								At 5 yr:		
NSABP[670]	1987	4600–4700 ≥ perineal boost	184	184	B2–C:	25%	16%	43%	Overall	41%
								30%	DFS	34%
								At 2 yr:		
Denmark[671]	1986	5000 (split course: 3000 →2 wk 2000)	250	244	B:	12%	12%	67%	LRF	82%
					C:	25%	21%			
					If > 4500 cGy delivered:					
					B:		9%			
					C:		16%			

S = surgery only; RT = adjuvant postoperative radiation therapy; DFS = disease-free survival; LRF = local recurrence free.

ies, and there were frequently many protocol violations with respect to the actual dose of radiation delivered. Nevertheless, all of the studies show some advantage for postoperative radiation therapy in terms of decreasing local recurrences. No survival difference has been seen at 5 years in any of these studies, although the study from Denmark is not yet mature.

These studies have shown disparate results in terms of complications. In the GITSG trial there was an 18% rate of severe or life-threatening toxicity(4% life-threatening) due to enteritis.[672] This was not a function of radiation dose. However, in the combined therapy arm, there was a 61% incidence of severe, life-threatening, or fatal toxic effects. In contrast, in the NSABP study, no severe complications were associated with radiation therapy. The Denmark study indicated a higher rate of severe complications in the radiation therapy group, 21%, versus only 8% in the surgery-only group.

SUMMARY OF POSTOPERATIVE IRRADIATION. A decreased local recurrence rate in nonrandomized studies of postoperative radiation therapy for rectal carcinoma has been confirmed in randomized studies. However, this has not yet been translated into any increase in overall 5-year survival. The studies are still maturing, and one must bear in mind that the doses of radiation used were somewhat lower than in the nonrandomized studies, or were given as a split course, as in the Denmark study.

A Swedish trial is comparing moderate dose/high fraction (2500–500 rad/day) preoperatively versus postoperative treatment of B2/C patients with >5000–200 rad/day.[667]

"Sandwich" Radiation Therapy

In nonrandomized studies, many authors have explored the use of combined preoperative and postoperative radiation therapy, or "sandwich" radiation therapy (Table 29-27). Preoperative doses have varied from 500 cGy as a single fraction[668,673] to as high as 2000 cGy.[674] In all trials, the preoperative portion of radiation therapy has been well tolerated. Mohiuddin et al reported the Thomas Jefferson University results in Stage B2 to C rectal cancer, comparing (1) combined preoperative and postoperative radiation therapy, (2) the preoperative portion of treatment only, (3) surgery alone, and (4) surgery plus postoperative radiation therapy (4500 cGy).[668] Local control was improved in the groups that had received high total doses of radiation therapy, namely the sandwich radiation therapy group and the postoperative radiation therapy group. Distant metastases were fewer in the patients who received 500 cGy preoperatively, either alone or with postoperative treatment, than in the surgery-alone group (24%, 13%, and 57% rate of distant metastases for the respective groups). The only significantly improved 5-year survival rate was in the group given sandwich radiation therapy — 78%, compared with only 34% in the surgery-alone group.

In a study from the Massachusetts General Hospital,[673] in which patients were selected to receive postoperative irradiation based on pathologic criteria (C, B2(m+g), B2(m) with poor margins), the 4-year survival rate was 79% in the sandwich arm, similar to the results reported from Thomas Jefferson University. In a study reported by Brenner et al[674] in which 2000 cGy was given preoperatively and 2600 cGy postoperatively, there were no local recurrences in 26 patients with Dukes' B and C lesions after a follow-up of 14 to 42 months. In another nonrandomized study, reported by Shank et al,[675] about equal numbers of patients were assigned to receive either 1500 cGy in five fractions preoperatively or sandwich radiation therapy, consisting of 1500 cGy preoperatively and 4140 cGy postoperatively. There was only one local recurrence, in the group given preoperative radiation therapy only.

The RTOG and the ECOG have joined in a randomized study of patients with rectal lesions less than 12 cm from the anal verge. Patients were randomly assigned to receive 500 cGy preoperative radiation therapy or no preoperative radiation therapy. All patients with B2 to C disease received 4500 rad postoperatively. Results of this study are not yet available.

TABLE 29-27.   Results of "Sandwich" Radiation Therapy for Rectal Cancer: Nonrandomized Studies

Study	Date	No. of Patients			Dose (cGy)		Local Recurrence			% Survival		
		S	P	C	Preop.	Postop.	S	P	C	S	P	C
										At 5 years		
Thomas Jefferson Univ. Hosp.[668]	1985	88	29	31	500	4500	26%	34%	7%	34	52	78
										At 4 years:		
Mass. General Hosp.[673]	1983	...	16	15	500	4500–5000 (6000–6500 for gross disease)	...	13%	29%	...	93	79
										At 3 years:		
Memorial Hosp.[675]	1987	...	24	23	1500	4140	...	4%	0%	...	92	82

S = surgery only; P = preoperative radiation therapy only; C = combined preoperative and postoperative radiation therapy.

Radical Surgery and Adjuvant Chemotherapy or Chemotherapy–Radiation Therapy Combinations for Rectal Cancer

The local anatomy and natural history of rectal adenocarcinoma require clinical attention to issues of both regional and systemic control of tumor. Three recently completed randomized studies are of particular relevance. As summarized in Table 29-28, these studies evaluated postoperative pelvic radiation therapy; two had surgery-only control groups and two had combined radiation therapy and chemotherapy arms.[262,669,670,676]

The GITSG[262,669] Study 7175, initiated in 1975, allocated patients with completely resected Dukes' B2 and C lesions to one of four treatment groups: (1) surgical control; (2) methyl-CCNU (130 mg/m² on day 1) and 5-FU (325 mg/m² on days 1–5, and 375 mg/m² on days 36–40), repeated every 10 weeks for 18 months; (3) radiation therapy, 4000 to 4800 cGy to the pelvis; or (4) radiation therapy, 4000 to 4400 cGy, plus 5-FU and methyl-CCNU as in (2). Although initially projected to accrue more than 500 patients, this trial was terminated after the entry of only 227 patients because of observed outcome differences between the regimens. At an 80-month median follow-up time, the control population had a 55% recurrence rate as compared to a 33% rate for the combination radiation therapy plus chemotherapy group ($p < 0.009$). There were 14 local recurrences in the 32 control patients and 5 local recurrences in the 46 patients treated by combination therapy. A subsequent analysis at 94 months' median follow-up showed an even larger margin of benefit for the combination therapy. In addition to a disease-free survival advantage, combination chemotherapy–radiation therapy was associated with a statistically significant overall survival benefit ($p = 0.005$). There was an approximate 20 percentage point superiority in survival at 6 years for the 96 patients at risk.[669] Although these data support an aggressive multimodality approach to patients with rectal cancer, the morbidity of combined radiation therapy plus 5-FU and methyl-CCNU must be considered.[672] Severe or life-threatening acute toxic effects occurred in 18% of patients in the radiation therapy arm and in 61% of those in the combined radiation therapy–chemotherapy arm. Three late deaths occurred, two from enteritis in the combined treatment group and one from nonlymphocytic leukemia in a chemotherapy-alone patient.

The second major trial of adjuvant therapy for rectal cancer was initiated by the NCCTG (study 79-47-51) in 1979.[676] A total of 200 patients with Dukes' B2 and C rectal cancer were randomly assigned to either postoperative radiation therapy only (4500 cGy with a 500-cGy boost) or to an integrated program of methyl-CCNU (130 mg/m² on day 1) plus 5-FU (350 mg/m²/d on days 1–5; 400 mg/m²/d on days 36–40), radiation therapy beginning on day 64, followed by one additional cycle of methyl-CCNU + 5-FU (sandwich therapy). The radiation therapy dose was 4500 to 5000 cGy. At a median follow-up time of 29 months, there were 38 recurrences in the group treated with radiation therapy alone, compared with only 23 recurrences in those treated with combination therapy. The disease-free survival doubled in patients who underwent sphincter-saving surgery followed by the combination treatment, compared with postoperative radiation therapy alone. The local failure rate in the combination treatment group was 11%, versus 20% in those treated with postoperative irradiation only. The overall disease-free survival was superior with combined treatment ($p = 0.001$). The time interval to tumor recurrence was statistically superior for the combination therapy group ($p = 0.025$). Overall survival differences could not be reported since the data were not sufficiently mature.

The largest study was performed by NSABP (R01) and required a decade (1977–1987) to complete accrual.[670] A total of 528 patients with Dukes' B2 and C lesions were randomized to (1) postoperative observation; (2) postoperative pelvic radiation therapy, 4700 cGy with a boost to 5300 cGy maximum; or (3) MOF chemotherapy (methyl-CCNU, vincristine, 5-FU) as utilized in the NSABP C01 study. After a 54-month mean follow-up time, there was a statistically significant disease-free survival advantage for MOF chemotherapy ($p = 0.05$) and an overall survival improvement for selected subsets of patients receiving MOF (particularly males and those less than 65 years old). Patients given only postoperative irradiation had no statistically demonstrable

TABLE 29-28.   Recently Completed U.S. Trials of Adjuvant Therapy for Rectal Cancer

Study	Total Accrual	Treatment* (Arms)	Results
GITSG 7175[669]	227	Control MF Pelvic RT RT + 5-FU, then MF	RT + CT resulted in 59% 5-year survival versus 43% in controls ($p < 0.01$)
NCCTG 79-47-51[676]	200	Pelvic RT Sandwich MF + RT + MF	RT + MF resulted in 55% 5-year survival versus 49% for RT alone
NSABP R01[670]	551	Control Pelvic RT MOF	MOF resulted in 52% 5-year survival versus 42% in controls

MF = methyl-CCNU + 5-FU; MOF = methyl-CCNU + vincristine (Oncovin) + 5-FU.
*All patients underwent complete surgical resection.

improvement in overall or relapse-free survival. There was, however, a reduction in the locoregional recurrence rate from 25% without radiation therapy to 16% with radiation therapy. Despite the 80 weeks of MOF chemotherapy, no leukemias had yet been observed; other toxic effects were predictable and tolerated.[670]

In contrast to the above studies, the EORTC was unable to show a benefit with combined treatment.[677] This study of preoperative adjuvant therapies compared irradiation (3450 cGy in 230-cGy fractions) with the same radiation regimen combined with only an intravenous bolus of 5-FU (375 mg/m²) on the first four days of irradiation. In the 247 patients followed up, overall survival was better with radiation therapy only. However, the incidence of liver metastases was reduced (p = 0.07) in the combined radiation therapy + 5-FU group.

As an integrated experience, the three recent U. S. studies summarized in Table 29-28 indicate that meaningful survival benefits can be achieved with programs utilizing postoperative chemotherapy. These data are supported by two earlier trials of adjuvant single-agent 5-FU in colorectal cancer patients; the results in the rectal cancer patients were reported separately. Survival benefits with intensive 5-FU regimens have been reported by Grage et al[554] for the Central Oncology Group and by Higgins et al for the VA group.[553]

Although radiation therapy alone has had little apparent impact on survival, the combination of radiation therapy and chemotherapy may offer the greatest survival advantage.[556] Several issues remain unclear: the exact choice of chemotherapy agent(s) that will provide the most benefit at the least toxicity, the duration of chemotherapy, the scheduling and dosage of radiation therapy, and the integration of all three modalities (surgery, radiation therapy, and chemotherapy). In an attempt to address some of the therapeutic issues, new studies have been initiated.

Currently, two large cooperative group randomized efforts are ongoing in the United States (Table 29-29). The NCCTG Study 864751 is using a 2 × 2 factorial statistical design and attempting to quantify the relative benefits of continuous infusion versus bolus 5-FU, as well as the value of including methyl-CCNU in the chemotherapy regimen. All patients receive pelvic radiation therapy and concomitant 5-FU in the sandwich sequence of chemotherapy–radiation–

chemotherapy. Half the patients receive MF chemotherapy as in the previous NCCTG trial (79-4751), the other half receive 5-FU, 500 mg/m² on days 1 to 5 and days 36 to 40 before radiation therapy, and 450 mg/m² on days 1 to 5 and days 36 to 40 1 month after the completion of radiation therapy. During the irradiation interval patients receive either standard 5-FU, 500 mg/m² on days 1 to 3 and days 36 to 39 as an IV bolus, or 225 mg/m²/d as a continuous IV infusion for 5 weeks. The planned pelvic radiation therapy dose is 4500 cGy, with a boost to a total of 5400 to 5900 cGy.

The recently activated NSABP R02 study is also summarized in Table 29-29. This protocol compares the standard NSABP MOF chemotherapy regimen with a 5-FU + folinic acid program and is complementary to NSABP Study C03 for patients with colon cancer. Half the patients will receive radiation therapy in conjunction with chemotherapy. Because of preliminary evidence of qualitative therapy interactions in specific subgroups, women will receive 5-FU + folinic acid, with or without radiation therapy; men will be randomly assigned to the four therapy options. The chemotherapy doses are identical to those used in NSABP Study C03.

These two active studies address some of the most demanding questions in the treatment of rectal cancer. Programs entailing pelvic irradiation and 5-FU + methyl-CCNU have demonstrated both benefits and toxicities. The new NSABP and NCCTG studies will help redefine the therapeutic ratio, and in addition will evaluate promising new ways of using 5-FU, by infusion or with folinic acid modulation.

Summary of Adjuvant Treatment for Rectal Cancer

Until a complete analysis of the above studies becomes available, some form of adjuvant therapy is recommended for most patients with T3 or T4 and/or N1 rectal cancer. Whenever possible, participation in a formal clinical trial is to be encouraged. However, for those not entering a clinical study, the choice of adjuvant therapy is contingent on many medical, psychological, and financial factors, which must be considered by the patient and physician. For many patients the use of high-dose preoperative or postoperative radiation therapy with postoperative 5-FU chemotherapy is entirely reasonable and justifiable.

TABLE 29-29. Currently Active U.S. Trials of Adjuvant Therapy for Rectal Cancer

Study	Total Accrual	Treatment (Arms)
NCCTG 86-47-51	450	MF/RT + 5-FU/MF (5-FU infusion) MF/RT + 5-FU/MF (5-FU bolus) 5-FU/RT + 5-FU/5-FU (5-FU infusion) 5-FU/RT + 5-FU/5-FU (5-FU bolus)
NSABP R02	800	Men ⎡ MOF MOF + RT 5-FU/FA 5-FU/FA + RT ⎤ Women

FA = folinic acid; MF = methyl-CCNU + 5-FU.

MANAGEMENT OF UNRESECTABLE, RECURRENT, AND METASTATIC DISEASE

TREATMENT OF INITIALLY ADVANCED COLON CANCER

Synchronous Metastatic Cancer

Approximately 10% to 15% of patients with primary colon cancers will present with synchronous metastatic cancer. The treatment of patients with synchronous liver metastases is discussed under Treatment of Recurrent and Metastatic Cancer. The operative finding of peritoneal seeding or extensive unresectable intra-abdominal nodal metastases beyond the central nodal drainage should not deter surgical resection. An extended surgical lymphadenectomy in selected younger patients may be curative in a small subset despite gross involvement of high nodes, albeit probably at most 10% to 15%.

Locally Unresectable Colon Cancer

Such tumors may be unresectable for cure, whether or not distant metastases are present. Extensive direct extension into the retroperitoneum, pelvic side wall, or duodenum or pancreas may be found. In the presence of concomitant metastatic disease, a bypass enteroenterostomy is usually appropriate. In the absence of distant disease, an aggressive local surgical approach to these "unresectable" tumors should be taken in otherwise healthy patients.

TREATMENT OF INITIALLY ADVANCED RECTAL CANCER

Synchronous Metastatic Cancer

Synchronous metastatic cancer, particularly to the liver, is not a contraindication to resection of the rectal primary. Maximum surgical effort should be made to avoid a permanent colostomy if the surgery is considered palliative. However, a palliative abdominoperineal resection is appropriate in the presence of minimal distant disease, in order to prevent or treat bleeding, obstruction, or diarrhea. However, if massive liver metastases are present, palliation may be achieved with dietary restriction, radiation therapy, fulguration, or laser therapy. A diverting colostomy alone is to be avoided if at all possible.

Locally Advanced and Unresectable Rectal Cancer

Such cancers are adherent to or directly invade contiguous organs or structures. Many are *curable* with radical surgery and high-dose radiation therapy. Anterior exenteration in women with vaginal involvement is appropriate. The rectal tumor is resected in continuity with a hysterectomy and a posterior vaginectomy. Anterior extension of rectal cancer into the prostate or base of the bladder in men, or into the bladder in women who have had a hysterectomy, is surgically curable in one third of cases by pelvic exenteration.[678-680] Posterior extension into bone can be surgically treated by including the sacrum in the rectal resection.[681]

In the absence of distant disease, locally advanced rectal cancer that invades contiguous organs or pelvic structures is best treated locally with a combination of surgery and radiation therapy.[681]

PREOPERATIVE IRRADIATION. For unresectable or marginally resectable rectal cancer, the goal of preoperative irradiation is to increase the likelihood of pathologically negative margins at surgery. Such an approach would potentially lead to an increased local control rate as well as (one hopes) survival. The problem in evaluating any series involving preoperative irradiation is the use of variable subjective criteria for resectability. The doses needed to increase resectability must be high, 4500 cGy or above.

The results of preoperative radiation therapy in lesions that were considered marginally resectable or unresectable are shown in Table 29-30. Resectability and the complete resection rate are seen to be highly variable, as are the local failure rate and the survival rate.[619,652,682-685] The data in Table 29-30 suggest that if a sufficiently high dose of preoperative irradiation is given, a large percentage of tumors may become resectable, and many patients in this group may have a long survival. However, since the local failure rate remains high, with survival of only 25% to 50% of patients on average, better local and systemic control is needed. As a result, there have been attempts to add intraoperative therapy in the form of radioactive implants or electron beam irradiation to these preoperative irradiation regimens for enhanced local control, or to provide chemotherapy concurrently with radiation therapy for better systemic control.

Several studies of combined chemotherapy and irradiation have included small numbers of patients with advanced rectal carcinoma.[686-689] The definition of advanced disease has varied from study to study, but in general the tumors have been circumferential, fixed or partially mobile, large (≥ 4 cm), involving adjacent structures, and/or deeply ulcerated. Chemotherapy has consisted of 5-FU alone[686,689] or combined 5-FU and mitomycin C.[686-688] After the combined treatment, 71% to 98% of the patients underwent surgical resection. In two of the studies[686,687] no tumor was found in 13% to 20% of the operative specimens. Local failure rates varied from 7% to 22%, and the rate of distant metastases from 23% to 39%. Overall survival rates varied from 59% to 86%, with disease-free survival rates of 48% to 64%. The data of Taylor et al did not suggest any additive benefit to the 5-FU.[689] Because the follow-up time in these studies has been relatively short and no randomized studies have been done, it is difficult to ascertain whether the addition of chemotherapy will affect the long-term survival in patients with marginally resectable or unresectable disease.

INTRAOPERATIVE IRRADIATION. Intraoperative radiation therapy may be defined as the use of some form of irradiation during a surgical procedure. Low-energy photon beams, electron beams, and interstitial radioactive implants have been used.[690] The value of intraoperative radiation therapy is that the field of a boost dose may be reduced by directly visualizing the target volume. In addition, one may minimize the dose received by normal tissues by physically moving normal tissues out of the way of an external beam or

TABLE 29-30. Preoperative Radiation Therapy for Marginally Resectable or Unresectable Rectal Cancer

Study	No. of Patients	Dose (cGy)	Follow-up	Resectability (%)*	Complete Resection (%)*	Local Failure (%)†	Survival (%)*
Netherlands Cancer Inst.[682]	21	3500 (marginally resectable)	$2\frac{1}{2}$–$6\frac{1}{2}$ yr	95	95	15	48
	38	6400 (unresectable)	$\frac{1}{2}$–$2\frac{1}{2}$ yr	0	0	. . .	18
Univ. of Oregon[652]	58	5000	≥4 yr	41	24	. . .	9
Univ. Hosp. of Bergen[683]	24	3150	4 mo to $3\frac{1}{2}$ yr	67	46	6	33
Tufts–New Engl. Med. Ctr.[684]	44	4500–5000‡	>3 yr	75	59	36	41
Mass. Genl. Hosp.[685]	25	4000–5200	2–6 yr	80	64	43	28
Univ. of Virginia[619]	60	4000–6000	>$3\frac{1}{2}$ yr (mean)	. . .	87	12	45
Thomas Jefferson Univ. Hosp.[588]	45	4500 (partially fixed)	≥3 yr	100	. . .	2	79
	19	5500 (totally fixed)	≥3 yr	84	. . .	29	52
	12	6500 (unresectable)	≥3 yr	58	. . .	43	24

* Original number of patients used as a denominator.
† Local failure as a percentage of patients resected.
‡ Two patients received higher doses (5400 and 6000 cGy).

by using rapid dose decrements at the periphery of the target volume with radioactive implants. As a result, a better therapeutic ratio may ensue. In this situation one may use a relatively high boost dose given in minutes as intraoperative beam therapy, or a relatively high localized dose given over a few days by means of an interstitial implant.

Pilot studies combining external irradiation and intraoperative electron beam therapy have been done by Gunderson et al at both Massachusetts General Hospital and the Mayo Clinic on patients with residual, unresectable, or recurrent disease of the colon or rectum.[691-693] At both institutions, preoperative external radiation therapy was given in doses of 4500 to 5000 cGy, with electron beam boosts of 1000 to 1500 cGy, usually with 6- to 18-MeV electrons. In both studies, the local recurrence rate has been low (6%–15%), and the survival rate without evidence of disease has been about 60%. In an analysis of unresectable rectal carcinoma cases at the Massachusetts General Hospital, Tepper et al reported a 92% actuarial local control rate at 3 years in patients with completely resected disease.[694] In patients with residual disease the actuarial local control rate at 3 years was 67%. Survival overall was 60% at 3 years, with 70% actuarial survival for those with completely resected disease and 30% for those with gross residual tumor. In an update from the Mayo Clinic, the disease-free survival rate was 53% after a follow-up of 10 to 64 months.[693] In an RTOG Phase I/II study of intraoperative radiation therapy for unresectable or recurrent carcinoma of the rectum, no toxic effects have been observed other than minor bladder problems. The RTOG is now planning to proceed with Phase III trials.[695]

Interstitial implants have been used for advanced and recurrent carcinoma of the colon and rectum.[696-698] A study reported from the University of Southern California involved locally extensive carcinoma of the anorectum.[697] Forty patients were treated, although only 32 had adenocarcinomas of the rectum. A preoperative radiation dose of 4000 to 5000 cGy was given to the pelvis, followed by insertion of an iridium-192 afterloading implant, either once to a dose of 3500 to 4000 cGy (in four patients treated early in the program) or twice to a dose of 1500 to 2000 cGy for each implant, spaced 2 to 3 weeks apart (for the remainder of the patients). With a 3-year average follow-up, the local recurrence rate was 30%.

In summary, combined preoperative external radiation therapy and intraoperative irradiation techniques may improve local control and survival rates in some patients. Complications with intraoperative electron beam therapy have been relatively few (ureteral obstruction, healing problems, or infectious complications), while complications with interstitial implants have been relatively serious, although it is reported that when implants are fractionated (i.e., two separate implantations), complications are fewer.[697]

POSTOPERATIVE IRRADIATION. Wang and Schulz reported a few "cures" in patients treated with postoperative radiation therapy who had residual disease after surgery for initially advanced lesions.[699] In a series of papers from the Albert Einstein College of Medicine, the disease-free survival rate was about 67% after an average follow-up of about 3 years in patients with advanced rectal and rectosigmoid cancer treated postoperatively with 4600 cGy to the pelvis followed by a 1000 to 2000 cGy boost to areas of residual disease.[545,547,700] Allee et al differentiated between patients with gross residual and microscopic residual disease.[620] Those with gross residual disease had a local failure rate of 52% and an actuarial 3-year survival rate of only 6%, whereas those with microscopic residual disease had a local failure rate of 26% and an actuarial 3-year survival rate of 59%. These patients were treated with relatively high doses, initially to 4500 cGy, to pelvic fields, followed by a boost to 6000 to 7000 cGy if small bowel could be excluded.

Patients with advanced or residual local disease who have not received any preoperative or intraoperative irradiation should be considered for high-dose postoperative irradiation, although no randomized studies have been done to show a survival benefit in these patients.

FOLLOW-UP AFTER POTENTIALLY CURATIVE TREATMENT

PURPOSES OF REGULAR FOLLOW-UP

The detection of asymptomatic recurrence, discussed below, is only one facet of patient follow-up. Maximizing the quality of life by management of treatment-related problems is extremely important in patients with colorectal disease.

Management of Treatment-Related Problems

DISTURBANCES IN BOWEL FUNCTION. Dietary modifications and medications may be necessary for control of bowel function, in the short or long term. Severe diarrhea secondary to loss of the ileocecal valve and bile salt intolerance can occur after a right-sided colectomy. Many patients are chronically constipated before colorectal surgery and may need to continue increased intake of dietary roughage and the use of stool softeners. After sphincter-saving rectal surgery, fecal urgency and frequency may be ameliorated with stool bulking agents.

SMALL BOWEL OBSTRUCTION. This late-occurring problem, related to surgical scarring or radiation enteritis, necessitates surgery in 5% of patients.

COLOSTOMY-ASSOCIATED PROBLEMS. The need for continued advice about colostomy management, irrigation techniques, prevention of skin irritation, and so forth may necessitate consultation with an enterostomal therapist.

DISTURBANCES IN SEXUAL FUNCTION. Surgery or pelvic irradiation in females may lead to menopause and vaginal dryness with dyspareunia. Male impotence due to both psychological and organic factors may require intervention. Implants can improve erectile impotence. Retrograde ejaculation is the rule after pelvic surgery in males.

Detection of New Primary Colorectal Cancers

Since approximately 5% of patients will develop a metachronous large bowel cancer, the detection of new primary colorectal cancers is one of the more important aspects of follow-up. If colonoscopy was not performed preoperatively, it should be performed 4 to 6 months after surgery.

Detection of Other Primary Cancers

Patients who have had primary colorectal cancer may be at high risk for the development of other cancers, particularly of the female breast, ovary, and cervix. Coordinated screening for these potentially curable cancers is important.

DETECTION OF RECURRENT COLORECTAL CANCER

A subset of patients with recurrent colorectal cancer can be cured[702]; hence, a nihilistic approach to follow-up is not appropriate. Local failure in the pelvis and limited distant metastases to the liver or lung may be curable if detected at an asymptomatic stage.

Follow-up strategies directed toward the detection of recurrent cancer in asymptomatic patients will vary, based on the risks of such recurrence and the likelihood that such detection would lead to early intervention. The availability of multiple expensive tests has led to some uncertainty as to appropriate follow-up strategies. A recent prospective study from the National Institutes of Health provides common-sense guidelines for the follow-up of high-risk patients.[703] Interval history and physical examination were combined with serial abdominal CT, chest radiography, lung tomography, liver–spleen radionuclide scintigraphy, intravenous pyelography, bone scans, and barium studies. CEA levels were monitored monthly for 3 years, then every 3 months for an additional 2 years. Serial CEA testing combined with regular physician visits was the most useful approach to the detection of recurrent colorectal cancer. The controversial issue of CEA determinations is addressed below.[704,705]

General guidelines for the follow-up of patients after potentially curative treatment for colorectal cancer are outlined in Table 29-31. A more detailed discussion of various tests follows.

Blood Tests in the Detection of Recurrent Cancer

CARCINOEMBRYONIC ANTIGEN. Studies from a number of groups have confirmed that serial CEA assays do detect recurrent colorectal cancer in asymptomatic patients.[706-713] In approximately two thirds of patients with recurrent disease, an increased CEA level will be the first indicator of the tumor. The pattern of recurrence influences the likelihood of CEA elevation: 25% to 50% of patients with local or regional recurrences and 95% of those with liver metastases have increased CEA levels.[714] Primary anaplastic tumors that do not stain positively with immunohistochemical stains for CEA frequently are not associated with an elevated CEA level despite the presence of metastatic disease.[715]

The sensitivity and specificity of the CEA assay will depend to a great degree on the definition of an "elevated" CEA level. Minimal transient CEA elevations are common after surgery, and can be influenced not only by smoking history, chronic bronchitis, hepatitis, and colitis, but also simple factors such as the time of day the blood sample was drawn. A diurnal variation in CEA levels in normal people has been documented.[714,716] Minton and associates have developed a nomogram to identify pathologic elevations for an individual patient that may still fall within the normal range for large populations.[708] The rate of CEA elevation (the slope) may be a more accurate indicator, with a more rapid rise suggestive of liver metastases.[717] Denstman and colleagues have looked at decision matrices for various CEA levels, as well as rate of CEA elevation. Receiver-operating characteristic curve analysis has been used to define 6.0 ng/ml as the ideal upper limit of normal.[718] However, despite this analysis, Denstman et al point out that with this value the data indicate only a sensitivity of 62% and specificity of 83%.

In using the CEA test, it is important to consider the prognostic group (pathologic stage) and the interval between

TABLE 29-31. General Guidelines for Follow-up of Patients After Potentially Curative Surgery

Procedure/Test	Frequency	Comment
History/examination	Every 3–4 mo for 3 yr, then every 6 mo for 2 yr	Detects ⅓ of recurrences
Fecal occult blood	Same	
Sigmoidoscopy	Same	Only if anastomosis in pelvis
Colonoscopy	Preoperatively or 4–6 mo postoperatively, then every 6–36 mo	Every 3 yr once free of polyps
Chest x-ray	Yearly	
CEA	Every 2–4 mo	
Liver chemistries		
Chest CT		
Abdominal CT	As indicated by findings on history, examination, or elevated CEA levels	
Pelvic CT		
Liver–spleen scan		
Liver US		
IVP		
Bone scan		

tests. Even if we accept a 95% sensitivity and 95% specificity, the predictive value will vary greatly based on the likely prevalence of recurrent cancer.[718] If an early node-negative cancer patient undergoes CEA testing monthly, the prevalence of interval disease may only be 1%. The predictive value of a positive test will be only 16%, with a 99.9% predictive value for a negative CEA test. At the other extreme, if a multiple node-positive patient undergoes CEA testing every 4 months, a tumor recurrence prevalence of 20% may be estimated. Under these circumstances, a positive CEA test will have a predictive value of 82.6% and a negative test will have a predictive value of 98.7%.[719]

Considering the speculative benefit of early detection of asymptomatic recurrent colorectal cancer, a number of oncologists have suggested that CEA assays should not be performed at all outside of clinical trials. By contrast, a group at Ohio State University recommends testing every 4 to 6 weeks to maximize the efficacy of second-look surgery.[720] The IUCC Workshop on the Immunodiagnosis of Cancer recommended that CEA assays be performed every 6 to 12 weeks.[721]

LIVER FUNCTION TESTS. Because the CEA level is elevated in 95% of patients with liver metastases, the CEA assay may be the most sensitive "liver function test" for the diagnosis of this condition. The following is limited to the various biochemical tests normally performed when liver disease is suspected. Unfortunately, published reports do not focus on the detection of early or minimal metastatic disease, but include in the analyses patients with gross metastatic cancer.

Lind and Singer, using Bayesian analysis, analyzed the predictive value of bilirubin, alkaline phosphatase (AP), lactic dehydrogenase (LDH), and SGOT values in the diagnosis of liver metastases.[722] Interested readers are encouraged to study this report. The accuracy of such tests is the highest when the prevalence of liver metastases is low. With a prevalence of 5% (in the range for screening purposes), accura-

cies are as follows: AP, 76%; SGOT, 86%; bilirubin, 90%; and LDH, 71%.

A prospective analysis of both single and multiple blood chemistries in the detection of liver metastases was reported by Kemeny, Sugarbaker, and colleagues.[311] CEA and γ-glutamyl transpeptidase (GGTP) were the most sensitive, while SGOT and 5'-nucleotidase were the most specific. The sensitivity of the CEA assay as a single test was 86%, the specificity was 60%, and the accuracy was 79%. Combinations of liver chemistries with and without CEA assay yielded accuracies only in the range of 60%. Tartter et al also found the combination of CEA and AP to be the most useful screening test for liver metastases.[723] With CEA values above 10 ng/ml and AP values above 135 IU/ml, the combination had a sensitivity of 88%, with a false negative rate of only 2%. In another prospective study of liver metastases, Kemeny et al looked at the subset of patients with resectable (minimal) liver metastases. Only 40% had an elevated AP level, and only 30% an elevated LDH level.[724]

ADDITIONAL BLOOD TESTS. Podolsky and associates reported results with galactosyl transferase isoenzyme II (GT II) in patients with colorectal cancer. The isoenzyme was elevated in 75% of patients with metastatic cancer; in three patients, increased levels preceded clinical recurrence by 3 to 7 months.[725]

The cancer-associated carbohydrate antigen 19-9 (CA 19-9), detected by monoclonal antibody, is present in the serum of patients with a diversity of cancers. Reports from a number of authors indicate that it is not as useful as the CEA assay.[726-728]

Diagnostic Imaging in the Detection of Recurrent Cancer

Chest radiographs are useful for the early detection of asymptomatic *lung metastases*. Before a major liver resection is undertaken, lung tomography or chest CT is appropriate.

For the detection of recurrent disease in the *pelvis and abdomen*, CT is the imaging modality of choice after a complete physical examination. It remains unclear whether magnetic resonance (MR) imaging will be superior to CT in this anatomical area or even complementary.

A variety of imaging techniques are available for the detection of *liver metastases*. The sensitivity of the modality is important, but specificity must also be considered because hepatic cysts and hemangiomas are common. The type of patient being studied is important in the selection of an imaging technique. For patients with symptomatic hepatomegaly, radionuclide scintigraphy of the liver allows excellent visualization of multifocal metastases.

The evaluation of patients with one or a few space-occupying lesions less than 3 cm in diameter is a more difficult problem. Kemeny and associates, reporting on 60 patients, noted that CT correctly demonstrated the size and location of the lesions in only 43%.[724] In 40% of patients lesions found at surgery were not visualized on CT. In a similar study reported by Sugarbaker's group, CT, radionuclide scintigraphy, and US all were unreliable for lesions less than 3 cm in diameter.[311,729] Overall, CT had the highest accuracy at 84%.

Gunven and colleagues in Tokyo studied CT and US preoperatively.[730] For lesions under 1 cm, CT was the most accurate, but still detected less than 50% of the lesions. Even with 1- to 2-cm lesions, the sensitivity of CT was only 50%, and that of US was only 40%.

The three-dimensional imaging capabilities of MR imaging have yet to be fully explored in characterizing liver metastases. Stark and associates found MR imaging to be superior to CT, and MR displayed definitive diagnostic features in small hemangiomas.[731] At present, MR imaging should not supplant CT in the search for minimal intra-abdominal and hepatic metastatic cancer.

TREATMENT OF RECURRENT AND METASTATIC CANCER

SPECIFIC MANAGEMENT PROBLEMS

Liver Metastases

Surgical excision of liver metastases is discussed in depth in Chapter 62, Section 3. It is important to stress that surgical resection of liver metastases is the only curative option and should be considered in most patients in otherwise good general health and lacking evidence of any tumor outside the liver. Overall, surgical resection is associated with a 25% to 30% 5-year disease-free survival rate. Results are better if the primary was node negative. Wedge resection with a 2-cm margin is adequate, unless size or location requires anatomical lobectomy. Although the presence of a single metastatic focus is ideal for treatment purposes, excision of as many as four lesions is associated with cure, particularly if the lesions are all greater than 4 cm or are unilobar.

Since hamartomas, bile duct cysts, hemangiomas, and granulomas are common in the liver, every attempt should be made to biopsy suspicious liver nodules found during surgery for the primary tumor. If an incisional biopsy is not feasible, flexible needle aspiration may be used to obtain material for cytological analysis.[732] A limited wedge resection of a single liver metastasis is reasonable at the time of surgery for the primary. More extensive resections should be delayed 4 to 6 weeks after surgery for the primary, particularly if a preoperative CT scan is not available.

Lung Metastases

Lung metastases are usually associated with widespread metastatic disease. However, isolated lung metastases may occur, and if they are single, resection should be considered. Lung metastases occur most commonly with cancers of the distal 5 cm of the rectum because of the dual venous drainage. In highly selected patients with isolated single lung lesions, resection results in a 20% 5-year survival rate.[733]

Local Failure in Rectal Cancer

Local or regional failure may occur after treatment of the primary cancer by local measures, sphincter-saving surgery, or abdominoperineal resection. Because recurrent pelvic cancer is frequently symptomatic and difficult to eradicate when it occurs, efforts should be directed toward maximizing the local cure at the time of the original treatment. Unexplained perineal or buttock pain that develops a few months to a few years after treatment of rectal cancer should be considered to indicate recurrence until proven otherwise. Most apparently localized pelvic recurrences are associated with more extensive diffuse pelvic cancer, which makes cure difficult. Some 25% to 50% of patients with rectal cancer have isolated locoregional recurrences, so aggressive treatment may lead to cure. Since management differs greatly, depending on the initial surgical treatment, the following discussion is organized according to the original approach to the primary tumor. In addition, aggressive multimodality locoregional treatment options are more limited in patients in whom disease recurs despite full-dose adjuvant radiation therapy.

RECURRENCE AFTER LIMITED LOCAL TREATMENT. After treatment of rectal cancer by local excision, intracavitary radiation, or fulguration, some patients with limited local recurrences can be cured by radical surgery, perhaps combined with radiation therapy. Selected patients with very superficial recurrences can be given additional local treatment prior to radical extirpative surgery, particularly if their medical condition would render radical surgery excessively risky. Although the data are scant, low anterior resection or abdominoperineal resection can often be performed (in the absence of distant disease), with 25% to 50% salvage rates.

RECURRENCE AFTER RADICAL SURGERY. Although isolated resectable local recurrences occur, most patients with pelvic failure have diffuse locoregional recurrences. In addition, many of these patients will also have distant metastatic disease. Patients with asymptomatic or minimally symptomatic pelvic recurrences and tumor outside the pelvis are usually treated with systemic chemotherapy. Regional chemotherapy of the pelvis is an experimental approach, with an encouraging initial report on the use of 5-FU and mitomycin C given by internal iliac artery infusion.[734] Results may be enhanced with hyperthermia.[735]

Irradiation is the most useful palliative technique in patients with symptomatic pelvic recurrence. Although 80% to 90% of patients will obtain initial pain relief, long-term symptom-free survival is uncommon with external beam irradiation alone.[736,737] If disease recurs in the pelvis despite adjuvant high-dose irradiation, additional palliative irradiation is frequently not feasible. In patients with uncontrolled pelvic pain despite irradiation, symptomatic relief must be sought with pain control measures, not cancer treatment.

Localized pelvic recurrences should be resected if feasible. These include instances of limited presacral tumor, vaginal apex masses, and isolated suture line and perineal recurrences. The useful surgical procedures include wide local excision, abdominoperineal resection, resection of pelvic tumors with en bloc partial sacrectomy, and total pelvic exenteration. Resection may be combined with external beam irradiation, intraoperative brachytherapy with iodine-125, intraoperative electron beam or photon radiation, or after-loading isotope catheter systems.

Surgical resection of highly selected patients with pelvic recurrence can be curative.[738] Exenteration can result in a 20% to 30% 5-year survival rate.[739] Posterior fixation to the lower sacrum may necessitate en bloc excision. As long as the S3 nerve roots are left intact, bladder function will be acceptable. Composite resection has been reported by Wanebo and associates, with 6 of 24 patients surviving 4 years.[740]

Patients with localized pelvic recurrences without prior irradiation have been treated at the Massachusetts General Hospital and Mayo Clinic with an aggressive multimodality approach. Patients undergo high-dose external beam irradiation and radical surgical resection with an intraoperative electron beam boost. In the Massachusetts General Hospital series of 22 patients, an actuarial local control rate of 56% was obtained at 4 years in the subset of patients with tumors amenable to complete resection.[690] Thirty-six patients have been treated at the Mayo Clinic, with only a 17% local failure rate after a short median follow-up.[741] Intraoperative brachytherapy has yielded comparable results at Memorial Hospital.[698]

SUTURE LINE RECURRENCE AFTER LOW ANTERIOR RESECTION. Limited suture line recurrence in a patient with metastatic cancer may not require treatment. Radiation therapy may be useful for more advanced disease, and to control bleeding. Prophylactic colostomy should be avoided if at all possible, with partial obstruction managed by diet restriction and stool softeners. The Nd-YAG laser may play a role in keeping the lumen patent. In patients without distant metastases, long-term disease-free survival can be achieved with abdominoperineal resection, although cures are infrequent.[742-744]

PERINEAL RECURRENCE AFTER ABDOMINOPERINEAL RESECTION. It is important to distinguish between pelvic and perineal recurrences after abdominoperineal resection.[745] Isolated perineal recurrences can be palliated by wide local excision, but the disease is rarely cured.[746,747]

Treatment Initiated on the Basis of CEA Assay

The definition of an elevated CEA level and the evaluation of patients with elevated levels were discussed earlier. After transient CEA elevations, associated benign disorders, and laboratory error have been ruled out, asymptomatic patients will fall into one of three groups: they will have a new primary cancer; they will have a recurrent colorectal cancer, which can be ascertained by a more complete history, physical examination, or a panoply of tests and scans; or they will have an entirely negative evaluation. This section discusses the management of the latter group.

Options in managing asymptomatic patients with elevated CEA levels and negative evaluations include (1) continued observation and repeat examinations and tests, (2) chemotherapy, and (3) surgical exploration (second-look surgery).

CHEMOTHERAPY. Because of the relative inefficacy of systemic chemotherapy, it is difficult to use this modality in asymptomatic patients without some way to monitor response to treatment. In a randomized trial of 5-FU and methyl-CCNU, a survival benefit could not be demonstrated in patients receiving early cytotoxic therapy rather than continued observation.[748]

SURGERY. In analyzing data on the usefulness of CEA-directed second-look surgery, a number of issues are important (Table 29-32).

The frequency with which CEA assays should be performed was discussed earlier in the section on Detection of Recurrent Colorectal Cancer. However, if second-look surgery is shown to be efficacious, it is likely that CEA assays will need to be done every 1 to 2 months to maximize this benefit. The Ohio State University group has strongly endorsed monthly CEA assays, followed by early reoperation if necessary (see below).[749] Currently, a prospective randomized trial is underway at the Memorial Sloan–Kettering Cancer Center comparing CEA assays performed monthly versus every 4 months.

Sites Most Amenable to Curative Resection. In the various studies of CEA-directed second-look operations, the term curative resection is used. This term is loosely applied to tumors amenable to complete surgical resection. It is unlikely that resection of para-aortic nodes, omental tumor, or other peritoneal nodules is truly curative. However, selected liver or lung metastases and some locally recurrent cancer may be resected for cure in a subset of patients.

Negative Exploration. Most groups have documented tumor recurrence in over 90% of patients selected for second-look surgery. At Ohio State University, tumor was confirmed in 139 of 146 surgical explorations.[720,749,750] The Memorial Hospital group found recurrence in 33 of 37 patients explored.[751] Staab and associates reported tumor confirmation in 29 of 32 patients.[752] However, most of the patients in whom surgical exploration is negative will likely develop clinical signs of recurrent cancer in the future.

Surgical Resections. There has been great variability in the reports of second-look operations in regard to the frequency of potentially curative resections. In a series of four reports from the Ohio State University group, a total of 146 patients underwent surgical exploration; 58% subsequently underwent resection with curative intent.[708,720,749,750] This high re-

TABLE 29-32.   CEA-Initiated Second-Look Surgery Issues

Is overall survival, as well as symptom-free survival, prolonged compared to that achieved with regular interval history and physical examination?

Optimum CEA assay frequency

Optimum definition of abnormal CEA

Optimum timing of second-look surgery in patients with elevated CEA levels and negative evaluation for recurrent cancer

Value of adjuvant chemotherapy after second-look surgery

Cost–benefit analysis

---

sectability rate was ascribed to a policy of frequent CEA determinations (every 4–6 weeks), and early operation with CEA values less than 10 ng/ml. At Memorial Hospital, 43% of patients had resectable tumors.[751] However, Steele et al at Harvard University could resect only 27%,[753] Wilking et al at Roswell Park Memorial Cancer Institute only 15%,[754] and Staab et al in the Federal Republic of Germany only 12%.[752]

Cures. Despite considerable variability in long-term survival data, some patients who undergo second-look operations based on CEA assay results will have tumor resected and will be alive and free of cancer at 5 years. Most reports refer to actuarial 5-year survival rates. However, in a recent publication from the Ohio State University group, the 5-year survival rate in the 45 patients who underwent curative resection and were at risk for 5 years was 31%.[720]

Cost. The cost of CEA follow-up programs is considerable. When the expenses of the assays, additional laboratory tests and scans, and exploratory surgery are tabulated, such programs cost $25,000 per patient found to have resectable cancer.[755] If 25% of such patients are actually cured, then the true cost is $100,000 per patient cured.

Overall Impact on Survival. August, Ottow, and Sugarbaker have analyzed colorectal cancer from the perspective of the potential for surgical cure of recurrent cancer.[702] They estimate that 15% of patients have isolated local recurrence, with a cure rate of 20%. This results in a 3% incremental survival. Approximately 25% of patients appear to have isolated hepatic metastases, with one fourth of these appropriate for resection. With a 30% cure rate following liver resection, the overall incremental survival will be an additional 2%. Hence, it is likely that surgery, either based on clinical criteria or on a CEA blood test, can improve overall survival only by 5% (3% + 2%) of the entire patient population undergoing potentially curative resection of colorectal cancer.

Current Studies. The National Institutes of Health and the Medical Research Council are sponsoring a large cooperative trial in the United Kingdom to answer the following question: Does monthly CEA monitoring, added to quarterly routine histories and physical examinations, actually reduce the morbidity and mortality of colorectal cancer?[756] Following resection of B2 or C colon or rectal cancer, patients undergo monthly CEA assays. The results of the tests are unknown to the patient and the physician. If recurrence is detected because of symptoms or physical examination, appropriate treatment is instituted. If the patient remains asymptomatic but has a rising CEA level (> 10 ng/ml), the patient is randomized. In the standard follow-up arm, again the physician and patient are not notified. In the intensive follow-up arm, the physician is notified, additional tests and scans are obtained, and second-look surgery is performed, if appropriate, based on the complete evaluation.

At this time, no groups are studying the issue of the optimum timing of second-look surgery in asymptomatic patients with a negative evaluation. Since most patients have no benefit from these explorations, a strategy of delayed surgery until tumor is detectable on a radiograph, scan, or examination or until symptoms develop may maximize symptom-free survival for the entire group.

One approach to focusing second-look surgery despite normal routine radiographs and scans is the use of isotope-labeled monoclonal antibodies to define recurrent tumor, both with external scanning and with intraoperative gamma detection. Iodine-131, iodine-125, and indium-111 isotopes with CEA antibody and monoclonal B72.3 have been studied.[757-760] The exact usefulness of these techniques is not yet known.

CHEMOTHERAPY FOR METASTATIC COLORECTAL CANCER

Single-Agent Chemotherapy

The fluoropyrimidines remain the most widely employed single chemotherapeutic agents for patients with colorectal cancer. Since the introduction of 5-FU in 1957,[761] tens of thousands of patients have been treated, and objective response rates of 8% to 85% have been reported.[701,762] The reasons for the wide range of response rates include various patient selection factors, such as performance status and co-morbid conditions; disease factors, such as sites of metastases and prior therapy; and treatment-related factors. A particularly important treatment-related variable seems to be the intensity of 5-FU administration. Moertel found a 9% response rate for 5-FU therapy that induced no leukopenia, compared with a 30% response rate for 5-FU therapy that reduced the white blood cell count to 4500 to 1500 cells/mm³.[763] The Central Oncology Group compared four programs with different schedules, routes, and intensities of 5-FU.[764] They found that IV 5-FU, 12 mg/kg/d for 5 days, followed by 6 mg/kg every other day for 11 days, followed by 15 mg/kg/wk resulted in a superior response rate (35%) and response duration (p < 0.001). Associated with this benefit was a higher incidence of drug toxicity, with 18% of patients experiencing severe or life-threatening leukopenia. This loading course schedule of 5-FU did not, however, result in a significantly longer survival. It has been asserted that an objective response rate of about 20% is generally achievable with the fluoropyrimidines.[701,763] Overall, 5-FU does not demonstrably affect survival for all patients treated; it is associated with a median survival of 6 or 8 months. However, for the minority of patients who do evidence an objective response, the median survival may be in the 12- to 18-month range.[762] If 5-FU is administered with proper vigor, most patients experience mucositis, diarrhea, or leukopenia as dose-limiting effects of therapy.[762,765] Even after three decades of use, no single schedule or dose scheme has yet been shown to be ideal, but administration with proper intensity (to the point of definite but acceptable toxic effects) is appropriate.

Attempts to improve upon the therapeutic benefit of 5-FU have included modifications of route and schedule. Administering 5-FU by the oral rather than parenteral route has been abandoned because of erratic GI absorption and poor response rates.[765-768] However, the use of prolonged or nearly continuous IV infusions of 5-FU has gained in popularity. The advantages of ambulatory infusion 5-FU given over

TABLE 29-33. Hepatic Intra-arterial Floxuridine Therapy for Liver Metastases in Colorectal Cancer

Study	Mode	No. of Patients	Dose (mg/kg/d × 14 d q 28 d)	Objective Response Rate (%)
Kemeny et al, 1986[783]	IV	49	0.125	20
	IA	45	0.3	50
Hohn et al, 1987[784]	IV	46	0.075	10
	IA	67	0.20	37

IV = intravenous; IA = intra-arterial.

several days to months include the ability to deliver a relatively higher dose per unit time and the lack of myelotoxicity.[769-771] In order for continuous IV infusion to be practical and economically feasible, dependable and affordable infusion devices had to be developed. The current pump technology makes these devices easily available. Lokich et al[772] have demonstrated that for 5-FU the major toxic effect of 300 mg/m²/d given by continuous IV infusion for weeks to months is mucositis; an additional 5% to 25% of patients experience a hand-foot syndrome of painful erythroderma.[773] The relative lack of hematologic toxicity makes this regimen attractive for combinations with myelotoxic drugs. Response rates ranging from 25% to 50% have been reported,[774-779] and some comparative studies suggest that infusion is more efficacious than bolus therapy.[770] Prospective randomized trials comparing conventional with continuous infusion 5-FU are ongoing.[772,780] Because of the added expense and bother of this mode of therapy, it is hoped that substantial clinical advantages will be demonstrated.[781] Preliminary data indicate a 29% response rate with continuous IV infusion of 5-FU, compared to a 9% response rate with bolus administration.

Another special mode of administration of a fluoropyrimidine is hepatic intra-arterial (IA) therapy for those with liver metastases. Because of the favorable pharmacodynamics of fluorodeoxyuridine (FUDR), there is high hepatic extraction and drug concentration with relatively little systemic exposure. Moreover, preliminary Phase II studies with continuous intrahepatic arterial infusion of FUDR at 0.2 to 0.4 mg/kg/d for 14 days out of 28 have reported 80% objective response rates.[781,782] In order to confirm these findings, two randomized studies have been completed comparing IV with IA FUDR (Table 29-33). Although two to three times higher response rates can be obtained with IA therapy, the impact on disease-free and overall survival is unclear.[783,784]

Historically, the next most important family of compounds for colorectal cancer patients has been the nitrosoureas. Response rates of 10% to 15% have been reported for BCNU, CCNU, chlorozotocin, and methyl-CCNU.[701,785,786] Because of the convenience of oral administration and of single-agent activity equivalent to that of 5-FU demonstrated in one randomized trial, methyl-CCNU has probably been the most frequently employed.[785] There are, however, no firm data to support the contention of superiority for any particular nitrosourea.[787] The chloroethyl nitrosoureas have characteristic delayed and cumulative toxic effects on bone marrow, which often limits the ability to administer therapy for prolonged periods. In addition, patients receiving methyl-CCNU are at greater risk for myelodysplasia, preleukemia, and acute nonlymphatic leukemia. For 2067 patients retrospectively evaluated, the relative risk of such a hematologic syndrome was estimated to be 12.4 times greater than in those treated with other forms of chemotherapy. The chance of a leukemic syndrome was greater for those receiving higher total doses and living for a longer time. Obviously, patients receiving large total doses of methyl-CCNU as part of an adjuvant program are at the greatest risk.[788] Mitomycin C has produced the same general quantitative and qualitative responses as the nitrosoureas.[765,787,789] Since both mitomycin C and methyl-CCNU have potential for substantial chronic hematologic and renal toxicity and yield median response durations of approximately 3 months, there is little to recommend one agent over the other.

Unfortunately, although dozens of new drugs are being screened there is no convincing evidence of meaningful efficacy for any of them. Table 29-34 lists the other agents, which have produced a total response rate of 4% in almost 4000 patients studied.

The modest responsiveness of colon adenocarcinoma to currently available chemotherapy has been the subject of intense basic science investigation. Adenocarcinoma of cer-

TABLE 29-34. Single Chemotherapeutic Agents Examined in Phase II Studies

Acivicin	Ftorafur
Aclacinomycin A	F3TDR
Alanosine	Hexamethylmelamine
Aminothiadiazole	Ifosfamide
AMSA	Indicine-n-oxide
Anguidine	Maytansine
5-Azacytidine	Methyl-CCNU
B-TGDR	MGBG
Bisantrene	Mitoxantrone
Bleomycin	PALA
Chlorozotocin	PCNU
Cisplatin	Piperazinedione
Cyclocytidine	Razoxane
3-Deazauridine	Rubidazone
4-Deoxydoxorubicin	Streptonigrin
Dianhydrogalactidol	Streptozotocin
Diaziquone	Teniposide
Dibromodulcitol	TMCA
Dichloromethotrexate	Triazinate
Diglycoaldehyde	Tubercidin
4-DMDR	Vindesine
DON	Yoshi-864
Doxorubicin	Zinostatin
Etoposide	

tain other organs (breast, ovary, stomach) is initially responsive to a wide variety of alkylating and anthracycline agents, so histopathology is not an adequate explanation. One possible explanation for the poor response of colon adenocarcinoma to chemotherapy may lie in the observation of high expression of the *mdr* 1 gene in colon cancer cells de novo. This gene encodes a drug transport protein that modulates the access of cytotoxics to the interior of the cell. Other mechanisms of drug resistance, both acquired and arising de novo, are being explored.[790] Colon carcinoma cells also evidence other aspects of the pleotropic drug resistance phenomenon,[791] and characterization of the p170 glycoprotein, glutathione transferase and other biochemical marker activity is being pursued.

Combination Chemotherapy

Because of the limited number of chemotherapeutic options available, most attempts to improve systemic treatment have consisted of empirically adding drugs to 5-FU.[701,787] One such popular regimen is based on the addition of methyl-CCNU to 5-FU. Enthusiasm for this combination arose from a small randomized comparison of methyl-CCNU + Oncovin + 5-FU (MOF) versus 5-FU in metastatic bowel cancer patients at the Mayo Clinic. As initially reported, the objective response rate for MOF was twice that for 5-FU (43% versus 19%), but no significant survival advantage was observed.[792] Subsequent attempts to confirm this superiority have not been uniformly successful, and response rates for MOF or MF type regimens have ranged from 4% to 40%.[787,793-799] This observed heterogeneity should not be surprising, since the reported response rate for 5-FU alone varies tenfold. Perhaps MF combinations result in higher response rates than 5-FU alone, but most of the responses are partial and last less than 6 months. Nonetheless, the initial activity of MOF or MF combinations has influenced the design of adjuvant trials in both colon and rectum cancer for more than a decade.

Simple attempts to substitute or add another alkylating-type agent such as mitomycin C, for the nitrosourea have not generally resulted in clinically meaningful differences.[800,801] There have been attempts to combine multiple alkylating-type agents, such as 5-FU + methyl-CCNU + mitomycin C or MOF + streptozotocin. Randomized trials with appropriate control groups have failed to demonstrate a significant survival superiority for any such combination despite considerable increases in response rates.[799,802]

Loehrer and colleagues combined bolus IV 5-FU, 15 mg/kg/wk, with cisplatin, 60 mg/m² every 3 weeks, and noted a 32% response rate in 38 patients.[803] They presumed that this combination represents a special synergy, since at this dose cisplatin alone is nearly inactive in colon cancer.[804] This combination has been evaluated not only with bolus 5-FU[803,805] but also with infusion 5-FU, resulting in 21 responses in 30 patients.[806] As was noted for methyl-CCNU + 5-FU combinations, provocative preliminary results require confirmation in larger series. At least one trial comparing bolus 5-FU with 5-FU + cisplatin (as utilized by Loehrer[803]) has shown equivalent response and survival results.[807] Bolus

TABLE 29-35. Selected Randomized Trials of Chemotherapy for Patients with Metastatic Large Bowel Cancer

Study	Treatment/Arms (mg/m²)
GITSG	5-FU, 500/d × 5 d q 4 wk FA, 500/wk, + 5-FU, 600/wk FA, 25/wk, + 5-FU, 600/wk
NCOG	5-FU, 440/d × 5 d, then 550/wk FA, 200/d × 5 d, + 5-FU, 400/d × 5 d q 28 d MTX, 50/6 h × 5 followed in 24 h by 5-FU, 500, and FA 10/6 h × 8 (rescue)
NCCTG	5-FU, 500/d × 5 d FA, 20/d × 5 d, + 5-FU, 425/d × 5 d FA, 200/d × 5 d, + 5-FU, 370/d × 5 d MTX, 200, followed in 7 h by 5-FU, 1000, and FA 15/6 h × 8 (rescue) MTX, 40, followed in 24 h by 5-FU, 700 5-FU, 300/d × 5 d, + CDDP, 20/d × 5 d
ECOG	5-FU, 500/d × 5 d, then 600/wk 5-FU, 500/d × 5 d, + CDDP, 20/d × 5 d 5-FU, 300/d by continuous infusion 5-FU, 300/d by continuous infusion, + CDDP, 20/d × 5 d

FA = folinic acid; CDDP = cisplatin.

and infusion 5-FU + cisplatin combinations are being evaluated in large-scale randomized trials (Table 29-35), with the appropriate comparison to 5-FU alone.

Fluorouracil Modulation

Another scientific theme currently being explored is the attempt to increase the effectiveness of the 5-FU. Efforts to biochemically modulate fluoropyrimidine cytotoxicity have recognized the crucial and complex interactions of fluoropyrimidine and folate molecular species. These studies have concentrated on altering folate metabolism with either methotrexate (MTX) or folinic acid (FA, leucovorin). The sequential use of MTX followed by 5-FU results in enhanced cell kill in various cell culture and animal tumor model systems.[808-810] This effect is assumed to result from MTX inhibition of purine metabolism causing more PRPP production or increasing dTMP synthetase binding, resulting in more 5-FU effect on RNA.[809,810] Many MTX dosages (ranging from 200-800 mg/m²), intervals (1-24 hours before 5-FU), and schedules (bolus to infusion, weekly to monthly) have been reported. Mucositis and leukopenia have been the most notable toxic effects. Responses have been observed in untreated patients as well as patients who have failed 5-FU regimens, but currently there is no single regimen of proven superior therapeutic index.[806,811-816] Moreover, there is no convincing evidence that MTX/5-FU is better than 5-FU alone.[817]

Another and potentially more promising avenue of research is the modulation of 5-FU by folinic acid. Considerable preclinical evidence indicates that intracellular reduced folate cofactor enhances cytotoxicity by stabilizing the covalent ternary complex of thymidylate synthetase and

FdUMP.[818-820] Folinic acid effectively provides the pool of required reduced folates and is clinically available. Numerous Phase II studies have been performed with varying doses of folinic acid (25 to 250 mg/m² per course) and 5-FU (150–200 mg/m² per course). Response rates of 10% to 60% have been noted both in those with and without prior 5-FU exposure.[821-824] At least three randomized studies have suggested superiority for 5-FU + FA combinations. Ehrlichman and colleagues[825] concluded that the combination of FA in a dosage of 200 mg/m²/d for 5 days and 5-FU in a dosage of 370 mg/m²/d for 5 days every 28 days produces more objective responses than the single-agent schedule of 5-FU, 370 mg/m²/d for 5 days. Doroshow et al, using the same 5-FU dose with 500 mg/m² FA, demonstrated similar benefits.[826] Petrelli et al[817] suggested that weekly FA, 500 mg/m², plus 5-FU, 600 mg/m², produced a higher response rate than 5-FU, 450 mg/m²/d for 5 days, followed by 200 mg/m² every other day for 6 days. The toxicity of FA-modulated 5-FU therapy is noteworthy. When administered weekly, the combination results in relatively mild leukopenia in approximately 10% of patients. The dose-limiting toxic effects are enteritis and diarrhea, which can be life-threatening. In contrast, daily administration of the combination for 5 days produce oral mucositis in approximately 33% of all patients. In addition to these medical side-effects, the cost of administering high doses of folinic acid can exceed several thousand dollars for a treatment course.

In order to resolve the unanswered questions concerning efficacy and therapeutic index of 5-FU–modulating combination chemotherapy schedules, several major randomized trials have been initiated (see Table 29-35). With so many variables in dose intensity, schedule, and frequency of administration, it would be impossible to test all possible permutations. Nonetheless, those regimens which in Phase II testing appear to be the most promising candidates are being directly compared with 5-FU alone. The implications for adjuvant programs are obvious, since more active regimens could translate into greater therapeutic impact on Dukes' B and C patients. There are already two ongoing adjuvant studies of 5-FU + FA, the NSABP C03 and NCIC C02 studies.

Chemotherapy for Patients Not Benefiting from 5-FU Therapy

The majority of patients who receive 5-FU as a single agent will not benefit, and many are candidates for subsequent systemic therapy. Outside of a formal research program, the options available for such patients are limited. Occasional responses to nitrosoureas have been observed in those not benefiting from 5-FU. Moertel et al noted a 10% response rate in 112 patients treated with a chlorethyl nitrosourea as second-line therapy.[792] Likewise, two-drug combinations containing methyl-CCNU have proved to be effective in less than 10% of patients.[797] Some patients have been reported to respond to 5-FU + FA or 5-FU + MTX as subsequent therapy,[821,823,824] and to high-dose alkylators with autologous bone marrow support, but lasting benefits are not observed. However, in no situation have better response rates to such programs been demonstrated in those who failed prior 5-FU therapy than in previously untreated patients.

INNOVATIVE THERAPIES FOR COLORECTAL CANCER

BIOLOGICAL RESPONSE MODIFIERS

There has been a dramatic expansion in the understanding and synthesis of biological response modifiers. Historically, nonspecific immunostimulants such as BCG or MER-BCG were widely studied. Several adjuvant protocols tested BCG alone or in conjunction with conventional chemotherapy.[670,827,828] Hoover and colleagues have combined BCG with an autologous tumor cell vaccine.[829] None of these studies has demonstrated that a BCG product increases overall survival. Another nonspecific immunostimulant is the phenyl midazothiazole, levamisole. As described in the section on Adjuvant Therapies for Colon Cancer, levamisole, either alone or with 5-FU, appears to increase disease-free time.[561]

More intensive activity has centered on testing of the interferons (IFN) (Table 29-36).[830-845] At least three studies of an α-IFN preparation in patients with advanced colon cancer patients have been reported. A total of 45 patients were treated with various doses or schedules (up to 50 × 10⁶ U/d for 5 days every 14–21 days), but no objective responses were noted.[830-832] α-IFN has been combined with 5-FU in Phase II studies and responses have been observed.[833,834] It is not yet known whether IFN adds to 5-FU efficacy in any way. Multiple other IFN species are being evaluated.[835-838]

Interleukin-2, either alone or with specific activated killer lymphocytes, is being tested, and some responses have been noted.[839,840]

Monoclonal antibodies directed against colon cancer are also being investigated.[841,842] The 17-1A antibody has been the most widely tested, and objective responses have been noted.[843,845] Although preliminary data do not permit any

TABLE 29-36.   Selected Biological Response Modifiers

Class	Biological Response Modifier	Reference
Interferon (IFN)	Leukocyte IFN Lymphoblastoid IFN	830, 838
	RIFN-α₂	
	RIFN leukocyte A RIFN-β RIFN-γ	
	RIFN-γ + 5-FU RIFN-α + 5-FU	
Interleukins (IL)	IL-2 + LAK cells	839
	IL-2	839
	IL-2	840
Monoclonal antibodies	17-1A	841, 843
	44 × 14	845
	B 72.3	842
Autologous tumor vaccine	Antigen + BCG	844

From the Cancer Therapy Evaluation Program Information System.

definite conclusion of activity, the potential for this approach seems bright.[846]

BONE MARROW TRANSPLANTATIONS

Based on the responses noted in leukemias and lymphomas with very high dose chemotherapy accompanied by autologous bone marrow reconstitution, colon cancer patients have recently been treated with similar regimens. Leff et al treated 20 patients with IV bolus L-PAM at 180 mg/m² plus bone marrow transfusion and observed three complete and six partial responses.[847] In a similar program the same workers obtained 9 responses in 19 patients.[848] Responses have also been seen with combinations of very high dose alkylating agents, such as cyclophosphamide + cisplatin + BCNU.[829] Unfortunately, despite the impressive objective response rates, the duration of regression has been only 1 to 3 months and the toxicity is truly formidable. Attempts to evaluate high-dose chemotherapy and bone marrow reconstitution are continuing, and methods of integrating this approach with conventional therapies are being explored.

MISCELLANEOUS COLORECTAL TUMORS

CARCINOID TUMORS

Most alimentary tract carcinoids occur in the ileum and the appendix. The rectum is the next most common site, with occasional tumors in the colon.[849] Almost all rectal carcinoids present as asymptomatic submucosal nodules less than 2 cm in size. In contrast to other sites, hematogenous and lymph node metastases are rare (<15%).[850] Malignant potential is seen almost exclusively in patients with tumors larger than 2 cm.[851] Transanal local excision suffices for tumors less than 2 cm, with radical surgery reserved only for larger tumors and those with histologic evidence of invasion of the muscularis propria.[852]

SARCOMA

Almost all smooth muscle tumors in the bowel occur in the stomach and small bowel. A few cases of rectal leiomyosarcoma have been reported.[853-855] The tumors may be small and asymptomatic, or greater than 10 cm with typical rectal cancer symptomatology. The smaller, submucosal tumors arise from the muscularis mucosa. Most are low grade, and almost all are curable by local excision. Tumors arising in the muscularis propria are frequently high grade. Local recurrence is common with limited surgical approaches.[853,855] With high-grade tumors, metastases to liver and lung occur in almost all patients despite radical surgery.[854,855]

LYMPHOMA

Primary rectal lymphoma is rare; it can be cured by surgery and postoperative irradiation.[856]

This Chapter was critically reviewed and edited by Ms. Millicent Cranor, whose efforts are gratefully recognized.

REFERENCES

1. Lipkin M: Biomarkers of increased susceptibility to gastrointestinal cancer. Gastroenterology 92:1083-1086, 1987
2. National Institutes of Health: Annual Cancer Statistics Review, Including Cancer Trends; 1950-1985. NIH publication No. 88-2789, Bethesda, Md, February 1988
3. Slanetz CA Jr, Herter FP: The large intestine. In Lymphatics in Cancer pp 489-564. Haagensen CD, Feind CR, Herter FP et al (eds): Philadelphia, WB Saunders, 1972
4. Enquist IF, Block IR: Rectal cancer in females: Selection of proper operation based upon anatomic studies of rectal lymphatics. Prog Clin Cancer 2:73-85, 1966
5. Reinhold P: Contribution a l'Etude des Facteurs de Recidives Postoperatoire du Cancer Rectal. These, Paris, 1924
6. Bartolo DCC, Row AM, Locke-Edmunds JC et al: Flap-valve theory of anorectal continence. Br J Surg 73:1012-1014, 1986
7. Preston DM, Lennard-Jones JE, Thomas BM: The balloon proctogram. Br J Surg 71:29-32, 1984
8. Lahr CJ, Rothenberger DA, Jensen LL et al: Balloon topography. Dis Colon Rectum 29:1-5, 1986
9. Read NW, Bartolo DCC, Read MG: Differences in anal function in patients with incontinence to solids and in patients with incontinence to liquids. Br J Surg 71:39-42, 1984
10. Schottenfeld D, Winawer SJ: Large intestine. In Schottenfeld D, Fraumeni JF Jr (eds): Cancer: Epidemiology and Prevention, pp 703-709. Philadelphia, WB Saunders, 1982
11. Ziegler RG, Devesa SS, Fraumeni JF Jr: Epidemiology pattern of colorectal cancer. In Devita VT Jr, Hellman S, Rosenberg SA (eds): Important Advances in Oncology 1986, pp 209-232. Philadelphia, JB Lippincott, 1986
12. Waterhouse J, Muir C, Correa P et al: Cancer Incidence in Five Continents, Vol III. Lyon, International Agency for Research on Cancer, 1976
13. Blot WJ, Fraumeni JF, Stone BJ et al: Geographic patterns of large bowel cancer in the United States. JNCI 57:1225-1231, 1976
14. Pickle LW, Greene MH, Ziegler RG et al: Colorectal cancer in rural Nebraska. Cancer RES 44:363-369, 1984
15. Burdette WJ (ed): Carcinoma of the Colon and Antecedent Epithelium. Springfield, Ill, Charles C Thomas, 1970
16. Phillips RL, Kuzma JW, Lotz TM: Cancer mortality among comparable members versus non-members of the Seventh Day Adventist Church. In Cairns J, Lyon JL, Skolnick M (eds): Cancer Incidence in Defined Populations, pp 83-102. Banbury Report No. 4, Cold Spring Harbor, New York, Cold Spring Harbor Laboratory, 1980
17. Phillips RL, Garfinkel L, Kuzma JW et al: Mortality among California Seventh-Day Adventists for selected cancer sites. JNCI 65:1097-1107, 1980
18. Enstrom JE: Health and dietary practices and cancer mortality among California Mormons. In Cairns J, Lyon JL, Skolnick M (eds): Cancer Incidence in Defined Populations, pp 69-90. Banbury Report No. 4, Cold Spring Harbor, New York, Cold Spring Harbor Laboratory, 1980
19. Lyon JL, Sorenson AW: Colon cancer in a low-risk population. Am J Clin Nutr 31:227-230, 1978
20. Cady B, Persson AV, Monson DO et al: Changing patterns of colorectal cancer. Cancer 33:433-436, 1974
21. Axtell LM, Chiazze L: Changing relative frequency of cancers of the colon and rectum in the United States. Cancer 19:750-754, 1966
22. Rhodes JB, Holmes FF, Clarke GM: Changing distribution of primary cancers in the large bowel. JAMA 235:1641-1643, 1977
23. Bruce WR, Dion PW: Studies relating to a fecal mutagen. Am J Clin Nutr 33:2511-2512, 1980
24. Weisburger JH, Wynder EL: Etiology of colorectal cancer with emphasis on mechanism of action and prevention. In Devita VT, Hellman S, Rosenberg SA (eds): Important Advances in Oncology 1987, pp 197-221. Philadelphia, JB Lippincott, 1987
25. Modan B: Dietary role in cancer etiology. Cancer 40:1887-1891, 1977
26. Willett NC, MacMahon B: Diet and cancer—an overview. N Engl J Med 310:697-703, 1984
27. Palmer S, Bakshi K: Diet, nutrition, and cancer: I. Interim dietary guidelines. JNCI 70:1151-1170, 1983
28. Jain M, Cook GM, Davis FG et al: A case-control study of diet and colorectal cancer. Int J Cancer 26:757-768, 1980
29. Haenszel WM, Kurihara M: Studies of Japanese immigrants: I. Mortality from cancer and other diseases among Japanese in the United States. JNCI 40:43-47, 1968
30. Correa P, Haenszel W: The epidemiology of large-bowel cancer. Adv Cancer Res 26:1-141, 1978
31. Armstrong B, Doll R: Environmental factors and cancer incidence and mortality in different countries with special reference to dietary practices. Int J Cancer 15:617-631, 1975
32. Lee JAH: Recent trends of large bowel cancer in Japan compared to United States and England and Wales. Int J Epidemiol 5:187-194, 1976
33. Waterhouse J, Shanmugaratnam K, Mair C et al: (eds): Cancer Incidence in Five Continents, Vol IV. IARC Scientific Publication No. 42, Lyon, International Agency for Research on Cancer, 1982
34. Waterhouse J, Carrea P, Muir et al (eds): Cancer Incidence in Five Continents, Vol III. IARC Scientific Publication No. 15, Lyon, International Agency for Research on Cancer, 1976

35. McMichael AJ, McCall MG, Hartshorne JM et al: Patterns of gastrointestinal cancer in European migrants to Australia: The role of dietary change. Int J Cancer 25:431–437, 1980

36. Monk M, Warshauer ME: Stomach and colon cancer mortality among Puerto Ricans in New York City and Puerto Rico. J Chronic Dis 28:349–358, 1975

37. Martinez I, Torres R, Frias Z et al: Factors associated with adenocarcinoma of the large bowel in Puerto Rico. In Birch JM (ed): Advances in Medical Oncology Research and Education, Vol 3, pp 45–52. New York, Pergamon Press, 1979

38. Zhang YQ, MacLennan R, Berry G: Mortality of Chinese in New South Wales, 1969–1978. Int J Epidemiol 13:188–192, 1984

39. Ames BN, McCann J, Yamasaki E: Methods for detecting carcinogens and mutagens with the *Salmonella* mammalian microsome test. Mutat Res 31:347–364, 1975

40. Curren RD, Putman DL, Yang LL et al: Genotoxicity of fecapentaene-12 in bacterial and mammalian cell assay systems. Carcinogenesis 8:349–353, 1987

41. Ehrich M, Aswell JE, Van Tassell RL et al: Mutagens in the feces of three South African populations at different levels of risk for colon cancer. Mutat Res 64:231–240, 1979

42. Bruce WR: Recent hypotheses for the origin of colon cancer. Cancer Res 47:4237–4242, 1987

43. Correa P, Paschal J, Pizzolato P et al: Fecal mutagens and colorectal polyps: Preliminary report of an autopsy study. In Bruce WR, Correa P, Lipkin M et al (eds): Gastrointentinal Cancer: Endogenous Factors, pp. 119–123. Cold Spring Harbor, New York, Cold Spring Harbor Laboratory, 1981

44. Dion PW, Bright-See EB, Smith CC et al: The effect of dietary ascorbic acid and α-tocopherol on fecal mutagenicity. Mutat Res 102:27–37, 1982

45. Reddy BS, Sharma C, Simi B et al: Metabolic epidemiology of colon cancer: Effect of dietary fiber on fecal mutagens and bile acids in healthy subjects. Cancer Res 47:644–648, 1987

46. Susuki K, Bruce WR, Baptista J et al: Characterization of cytotoxic steroids in human feces and their putative role in the etiology of human colon cancer. Cancer Lett 33:307–317, 1986

47. Smith LL: Carcinogenic cholesterol products. In Cholesterol Autoxidation, pp 432–446. New York, Plenum Press, 1981

48. Lipkin M, Reddy BS, Weisburger J et al: Non-degradation of fecal cholesterol in subjects at high risk for cancer of the large intestine. J Clin Invest 67:304–307, 1981

49. Bird RP, Bruce WR: Toxicity of dietary components to colonic mucosa in vivo. Proc Am Assoc Cancer Res 24:89, 1983

50. Bird RP: Effect of dietary components on the pathobiology of colonic epithelium: Possible relationship with colon tumorigenesis. Lipids 21:289–291, 1986

51. Sugimura T: Carcinogenicity of mutagenic heterocyclic amines formed during the cooking process. Mutat Res 150:33–42, 1985

52. Tanaka T, Barnes WS, Weisburger JH et al: Multipotential carcinogenicity of the fried food mutagen 2-amino-3-methylimidazo[4,b-f]quinoline (IQ) in rats. Jpn J Cancer Res (Gann) 76:570–576, 1985

53. Suzuki K, Bruce WR: Increase by deoxycholic acid of the colonic nuclear damage induced by known carcinogens in C57B1/6J mice. JNCI 76:1129–1132, 1986

54. Hill MJ, Drasar BS, Williams RED et al: Faecal bile-acid and clostridia in patients with cancer of the large bowel. Lancet 1:535–539, 1975

55. Linos DA, Beard CM, O'Fallon et al: Cholecystectomy and carcinoma of the colon. Lancet 2:379–381, 1981

56. Vernick LF, Kuller LH: Cholecystectomy and right-sided colon cancer; An epidemiological study. Lancet 2:381–383, 1981

57. Vernick LJ, Kuller LH, Lohsoonthorn P et al: Relationship between cholecystectomy and ascending colon cancer. Cancer 45:392–395, 1980

58. Bird RP, Medline A, Furrer et al: Toxicity of orally administerd fat to the colonic epithelium of mice. Carcinogenesis 6:1063–1066, 1985

59. Caderni G, Stuart E, Bruce WR: Dietary factors affecting the proliferation of epithelial cells in the colon of the mouse. Gastroenterology 92:1336, 1987

60. Garland C, Shekelle RB, Barrett-Connor E et al: Dietary vitamin D and calcium and risk of colorectal cancer: A 19-year prospective study in men. Lancet 1:307–309, 1985

61. Thornton JR: High colonic pH promotes colorectal cancer. Lancet 1:1081–1082, 1981

62. Van Dokkum W, de Boer BCJ, van Faassen A et al: Diet, faecal pH and colorectal cancer. Br J Cancer 48:109–110, 1983

63. Samelson SL, Nelson RL, Nyhus LM: Protective role of faecal pH in experimental colon carcinogenesis. JR Soc Med 78:230–233, 1984

64. Walker ARP, Walker AJ: Faecal pH, dietary fibre intake, and proneness to colon cancer in four South African populations. Br J Cancer 53:489–495, 1986

65. Pietroiusti A, Guliano M, Vita S et al: Faecal pH and cancer of the large bowel. Gastroenterology 84:1273, 1983

66. Painter NS, Burkitt DP: Diverticular disease of the colon: A deficiency disease of Western civilization. Br Med J 12:450–454, 1971

67. Burkitt DP, Walker ARP, Painter NS: Dietary fiber and disease. JAMA 229:1063–1074, 1974

68. Doll R, Peto R: The causes of cancer: Quantitative estimates of avoidable risks of cancer in the United States today. JNCI 66:1193–1308, 1981

69. Reddy BS: Dietary fiber and colon carcinogenesis: A critical review. In Vahouny GV, Kritchevsky D (eds): Dietary Fiber in Health and Disease, pp 265–285. New York, Plenum Press, 1982

70. Kritchevsky D: Diet, nutrition and cancer. Cancer 58:1830–1836, 1986

71. Jensen OM, Mosbech J, Salaspuro M et al: A comparative study of the diagnostic basis for cancer of the colon and cancer of the rectum in Denmark and Finland. Int J Epidemiol 3:183–186, 1974

72. Modan B, Barell V, Lubin F et al: Low fiber intake as an etiologic factor in cancer of the colon. JNCI 55:15–18, 1975

73. Greenwald P, Lanza E: Role of dietary fiber in the prev of cancer. In DeVita VT Jr, Hellman S, Rosenberg SA (eds): Important Advances in Oncology 1986, pp 37–54. Philadelphia, JB Lippincott, 1986

74. Glauert HP, Bennick MR, Sander CH: Enhanced 1,2-dimethylhydrazine-induced colon carcinogenesis in mice by dietary agar. Food Cosmet Toxicol 19:281–286, 1981

75. Freeman HJ, Spiller GA, Kim YS: A double blind study of the effect of purified cellulose dietary fiber on 1,2-dimethylhydrazine-induced rat colonic neoplasia. Cancer Res 38:2912–2917, 1978

76. Reddy BS, Ekelund G, Bohe M et al: Metabolic epidemiology of colon cancer: Dietary pattern and fectal sterol concentrations of three populations. Nutr Cancer 5:a34–40, 1978

77. Lipkin M, Newmark H: Effect of added dietary calcium on colonic epithelial cell proliferation in subjects at high risk for familial colon cancer. N Engl J Med 313:1381–1384, 1985

78. Clark LC: The epidemiology of selenium and cancer. Fed Proc 44:2584–2589, 1985

79. Shamberger RJ: Nutrition and Cancer. New York, Plenum Press, 1984

80. Banner WP, DeCosse JJ, Tan QH et al: Selective distribution of selenium in colon parallels its antitumor activity. Carcinogenesis 5:1543–1546, 1984

81. Bussey HJ, DeCosse JJ, Deschner EE: A randomized trial of ascorbic acid in polyposis coli. Cancer 50:1434–1439, 1982

82. McKeown-Eyssen GE, Bright-See E: Dietary prevention of recurrences of adenomatous polyps in the colon and rectum. In: UICC Cancer Congress, Budapest, 1986. Geneva, International Union Against Cancer, 1986

83. McKusick VA: Genetics and large-bowel cancer. Am J Dig Dis 19:954–957, 1974

84. Lipkin M, Sherlock P, DeCosse JJ: Risk factors and preventative measures in the control of cancer of the large intestine. Curr Probl Cancer 4:1057, 1980

85. Bussey HJR: Gastrointestinal polyposis. Gut 11:970–978, 1970

86. Bussey AJR: Familial Polyposis Coli. Baltimore, Johns Hopkins University Press, 1975

87. Erbe RW: Inherited gastrointestinal polyposis syndromes. N Engl J Med 294:1101–1104, 1976

88. DeCosse JJ, Adaurs MB, Condon RF: Familial polyposis. Cancer 39:267–273, 1977

89. Kelly PB, McKinnon DA: Familial multiple polyposis of the colon: Review and description of a large kindred. McGill Med J 30:67–85, 1961

90. Gardner EJ: Follow-up study of a family group exhibiting dominant inheritance for a syndrome including intestinal polyps, osteomas, fibromas and epidermal cysts. Am J Hum Genet 14:376–390, 1962

91. Oldfield MC: The association of familial polyposis of the colon with multiple sebaceous cysts. Br J Surg 41:534–541, 1954

92. Turcot J, Despres JP, St. Pierre F: Malignant tumors of the central nervous system associated with familial polyposis of the colon: Report of two cases. Dis Colon Rectum 2:465–68, 1959

93. Bodmer WF, Bailey CJ, Bodmer J et al: Localization of the gene for familial adenomatous polyposis on chromosome 5. Nature 328:2–4, 1987

94. Jeghers H, McKusick VA, Katz KH: Generalized intestinal polyposis and melanin spots of the oral mucosa, lips and digits. N Engl J Med 241:993–1005, 1949

95. Reid JD: Intestinal carcinoma in the Peutz-Jeghers syndrome. JAMA 229:833–834, 1974

96. Kussin SZ, Lipkin M, Winawer SJ: Inherited colon cancer: Clinical implications. Am J Gastroenterol 72:443–457, 1979

97. Lynch HT, Lynch PM: Heredity and gastrointestinal tract cancer. In Lipkin M, Good RA (eds): Gastrointestinal Tract Cancer. New York, Plenum Press, 1978

98. Lynch HT, Albano WA, Lynch JF et al: Recognition of the cancer family syndrome. Gastroenterology 84:672–673, 1983

99. Law JP, Herberman RB, Oldham RL: Familial occurrence of colon, uterine and of lymphoproliferative malignancies: Clinical description. Cancer 39:1224–1228, 1977

100. Macklin MT: Inheritance of cancer of the stomach and large intestine in man. JNCI 24L:551–557, 1960

101. Sherlock P: Heredity versus environment in colorectal cancer. In Winawer S, Schottenfeld D, Sherlock P (eds): Colorectal Cancer: Prevention, Epidemiology and Screening, pp 65–66. New York, Raven Press, 1980

102. Burt RW, Bishop DT, Cannon LA et al: Dominant inheritance of adenomatous colonic polyps and colorectal cancer. N Engl J Med 12:1540–1544, 1985

103. Mulvihill JJ: Clinical ecogenetics: Cancer in families. N Engl J Med 312:1569–1570, 1985

104. Edwards FC, Truelove SC: The course and prognosis of ulcerative colitis. Gut 5:1–22, 1964

105. Morson BC: Cancer and ulcerative colitis. Gut 7:425–426, 1966

106. Mir-Modjlessi SH, Farmer RG, Easley KA et al: Colorectal and extracolonic malignancy in ulcerative colitis. Cancer 58:1569–74, 1986

107. MacDougall PM: The cancer risk in ulcerative colitis. Lancet 2:655–658, 1966

108. Ohman U: Colorectal carcinoma in patients with ulcerative colitis. Am J Surg 144:344–349, 1982

109. Kewenter J, Ahlman H, Hulten L: Cancer risk in extensive ulcerative colitis. Ann Surg 188:824–828, 1978

110. Katzka I, Body RS, Morris E et al: Assessment of colorectal cancer risk in patients with ulcerative colitis. Experience from a private practice. Gastroenterology 85:22–29, 1983

111. Prior P, Gyde SN, Macartney JC et al: Cancer morbidity in ulcerative colitis. Gut 23:490–497, 1982

112. Devroede GJ, Taylor WF, Sauer WG: Cancer risk and life expectancy of children with ulcerative colitis. N Engl J Med 285:17–21, 1971

113. Kirsner JB, Shorter RG: Inflammatory bowel disease of the large bowel and anal canal. In Kirsner JB, Shorter RG (eds); Diseases of the Colon, Rectum and Anal Canal, chap 17. Baltimore, Williams & Wilkins, 1987

114. Hamilton SR: Colorectal carcinoma in patients with Crohn's disease. Gastroenterology 89:398–407, 1985

115. Heaton K: Crohn's disease and ulcerative colitis. In Trowell H, Burkitt D, Heaton K et al (eds): Dietary Fibre, Fibre-Depleted Foods and Disease, pp 205–216. New York, Academic Press, 1985

116. Greenstein AJ, Sachar DB, Smith H et al: Patterns of neoplasia in Crohn's disease and ulcerative colitis. Cancer 46:403–407, 1980

117. Weedon DD, Shorter RG, Ilstrup DM et al: Crohn's disease and cancer. N Engl J Med 289:1099–1104, 1973

118. Morson BC: Genesis of colorectal cancer. Clin Gastroenterol 5(3): 505–525, 1976

119. Heald RJ, Bussey HJR: Clinical experience at St. Mark's Hospital with multiple synchronous cancers of the colon and rectum. Dis Colon Rectum 18:6, 1975

120. Schottenfeld D, Berg JW, Vitsky B: Incidence of multiple primary cancers: II. Index cancers arising in the stomach and lower digestive system. JNCI 43:77–86, 1969

121. Burbank F: Patterns in cancer mortality in the United States: 1950–1967. Natl Cancer Inst Monogr 33, 1971

122. MacMahon CE, Rowe JW: Rectal reaction following radiation therapy of cervical carcinoma: Particular reference to subsequent occurrence of rectal carcinoma. Ann Surg 173:264–269, 1971

123. Castro EB, Rosen PP, Quan SH; Carcinoma of large intestine in patients irradiated for carcinoma of cervix and uterus. Cancer 31:45–52, 1973

124. McMichael AJ, Potter JD: Host factors in carcinogenesis: Certain bile-acid metabolic profiles that selectively increase the risk of proximal colon cancer. JNCI 75:185–191, 1985

125. Lowenfels AB, Domellof L, Lindstrom CG et al: Cholelithiasis, cholecystectomy, and cancer: A case–control study in Sweden. Gastroenterology 83:672–676, 1982

126. Bristol JB, Williamson RCN: Ureterosigmoidostomy and colon carcinogenesis. Science 214:351, 1981

127. Appel MF, Spjut HJ, Estroda RG: The significance of villous component in colonic polyps. Am J Surg 134:770–771, 1977

128. Morson BC: Evolution of cancer of the colon and rectum. Cancer 34:845–849, 1974

129. Lipkin M: Phase 1 and phase 2 proliferative lesions of colonic epithelial cells in diseases leading to colonic cancer. Cancer 34:878–888, 1974

130. Muto T, Bussey HJR, Morson BC: The evolution of cancer of the colon and rectum. Cancer 36:2251–2270, 1975

131. Ekelund GR: Cancer risk with single and multiple adenomas, synchronous and metachronous tumors. In Winawer SJ, Schottenfeld D, Sherlock P (eds): Progress in Cancer Research and Therapy, Vol 13, Colorectal Cancer: Prevention, Epidemiology and Screening, pp 151–155. New York, Raven Press, 1980

132. Sherlock P, Lipkin M, Winawer SJ: The prevention of colon cancer. Am J Med 68:917–931, 1980

133. Winawer SJ, Miller DG, Sherlock P: Risk and screening for colorectal cancer. Adv Intern Med 30: 471–496, 1984

134. Devlin HB, Plant JA, Morris D: The significance of symptoms of carcinoma of the rectum. Surg Gynecol Obstet 137:399–402, 1973

135. Irvin TT, Greaney MG: Duration of symptoms and prognosis of carcinoma of the colon and rectum. Surg Gynecol Obstet 144:883–886, 1977

136. McDermott FT, Hughes ESR, Paihl E et al: Prognosis in relation to symptom duration in colon cancer. Br J Surg 68:846–849, 1981

137. Farrands PA, Hardcastle JD: Colorectal cancer by self completion questionnaire. Gut 25:4445–4447, 1984

138. Chapuis PH, Goulston KJ, Dent OF et al: Predictive value of rectal bleeding in screening for rectal and sigmoid polyps. Br Med J Clin Res 290:1546–1548, 1985

139. Eddy DM, Nugent FW, Eddy JF et al: Screening for colorectal cancer in a high-risk population: Results of a mathematical model. Gastroenterology 92:682–692, 1987

140. Snyder DN, Heston JF, Meigs JW et al: Changes in site distribution of colorectal carcinoma in Connecticut, 1940–1973. Dig Dis 22:791–797, 1977

141. Stewart RJ, Stewart AW, Turnbull PRG et al: Sex differences in subsite incidence of large bowel cancer. Dis Colon Rectum 26:658–660, 1983

142. Butcher D, Hassanein K, Dudgeon M et al: Female gender as a major determinant of changing subsite distribution of colorectal cancer with age. Cancer 56:714–716, 1985

143. Rozen P, Fireman Z, Figer A et al: Family history of colorectal cancer as a marker of potential malignancy within a screening program. Cancer 60:248–254, 1987

144. Gryska PV, Cohen AM: Screening asymptomatic patients at high risk for colon cancer with full colonoscopy. Dis Colon Rectum 30:18–20, 1987

145. Nava H, Pagana TJ: Postoperative surveillance of colorectal carcinoma. Cancer 49:1043–1047, 1982

146. Winawer SJ, Ritchie M, Diaz B et al: The National Polyp Study: Aims and Organization. In Rozen P, Winawer SJ (eds): Frontiers of Gastrointestinal Research, Vol 10, Secondary Prevention of Colorectal Cancer: An International Perspective, pp 216–225. Basel, Karger, 1986

147. Morson BC: Use of dysplasia as an indicator of risk for malignancy in patients with ulcerative colitis. In Winawer SJ, Schottenfeld D, Sherlock P (eds): Colorectal Cancer: Prevention, Epidemiology and Screening, pp 347–354. New York, Raven Press, 1980

148. Dobbins WO, Stock M, Ginsberg AL: Early detection and prevention of carcinoma of the colon in patients with ulcerative colitis. Cancer 40:25–48, 1977

149. Collins RH, Geldman M, Fordtran JS: Colon cancer, dysplasia, and surveillance in patients with ulcerative colitis. N Engl J Med 316:1654–1658, 1987

150. Dales LG, Friedman GD, Collen MF: Evaluating periodic multiphase health check-ups: A controlled trial. J Chronic Dis 32:385–404, 1979

151. Hertz RE, Deddish MR, Day E: Value of periodic examination in detecting cancer of the rectum and colon. Postgrad Med 27:290, 1960

152. Gilbertsen VA, Williams SE, Schuman L et al: Colonoscopy in the detection of carcinoma of the intestine. Surg Gynecol Obstet 149:877–878, 1979

153. Winawer SJ, Cummins R, Baldwin NP et al: A new flexible sigmoidoscope for the generalist. Gastrointest Endosc 28:233–236, 1982

154. Dubow RA, Katon RM, Benner KG et al: Short (36 cm) versus long (60 cm) flexible sigmoidoscopy: A comparison of findings and tolerance in asymptomatic patients screened for colorectal neoplasia. Gastrointest Endosc 31:305–308, 1985

155. Wilking N, Petrelli NJ, Herrera L et al: A comparison of the 25 cm rigid proctosigmoidoscope with the 65 cm flexible endoscope in the screening of patients for colorectal carcinoma. Cancer 57:669–671, 1986

156. Winnon G, Beri G, Parnish J: Superiority of the flexible to the rigid sigmoidoscope in routine proctosigmoidoscopy. N Engl J Med 302:1011–1012, 1980

157. Marks G, Boggs HW, Castro AF et al: Sigmoidoscopic examinations with rigid and flexible fiberoptic sigmoidoscopes in the surgeon's office: A comparative prospective study of effectiveness in 1,012 cases. Dis Colon Rectum 22:162–168, 1979

158. Lipshutz GR, Katon RM, McCool MF et al: Flexible sigmoidoscopy as a screening procedure for neoplasia of the colon. Surg Gynecol Obstet 148:19–22, 1979

159. Marks G, Gathright JB, Boggs W et al: Guidelines for use of the flexible sigmoidoscope in the management of the surgical patient. Dis Colon Rectum 25:187–190, 1982

160. Wherry DC: Screening for colorectal neoplasia in asymptomatic patients using flexible fiberoptic sigmoidoscopy. Dis Colon Rectum 24:521–522, 1981

161. Rex DK, Rehman GA, Coppas JC et al: Sensitivity of double contrast barium study for left colon polyps. Radiology 158:69–72, 1986

162. Fork FT, Lindstrom C, Ekelund GR: Reliability of double contrast examination of the large bowel in polyp detection: A prospective clinical study. Gastrointest Radiol 8:163–172, 1983

163. Ott DJ, Albin OS, Gelfand GW et al: Predictive value of a diagnosis of colonic polyp on the double contrast barium enema. Gastrointest Radiol 8:75–80, 1983

164. Thoeni RF, Petras A: Double contrast barium enema and endoscopy in the detection of polypoid lesions in the cecum and ascending colon. Radiology 144:257–260, 1982

165. Miller RE, Lehman G; Polypoid colonic lesions undetected by endoscopy. Radiology 129:295–297, 1978

166. Winawer SJ, Leidner SD, Hajdu SI, et al: Colonoscopic biopsy and cytology in the diagnosis of colon cancer. Cancer 42:2849–2853, 1978

167. Shimano T, Okuda H, Mondes T et al: Usefulness of carcinoembryonic antigen measurement in feces of patients with colorectal cancer. Dis Colon Rectum 30:607–10, 1987

168. Ahlquist DA, McGill DB, Schwartz S et al: Hemoquant, a new quantitative assay for fecal hemoglobin. Ann Intern Med 101:297–302, 1984

169. Ahlquist DA, McGill DB, Schwartz S et al: Fecal blood levels in health and disease. N Engl J Med 312:22–1428, 1985

170. Songster CL, Barrows GH, Jarrett DD: Immunochemical detection of fecal blood— the fecal smear pinch disc test. A new non-invasive screening test for colorectal cancer. Cancer 45:1099–1102, 1980

171. Saito H, Tsuchida S, Nakaji S et al: An immunological test for fecal occult blood by counter immunoelectrophoresis. Cancer 56:1549–1552, 1985

172. Barry MJ, Mulley AG, Richter JM: Effect of workup strategy of the cost-effectiveness of fecal occult blood screening for colorectal cancer. Gastroenterology 93:301–310, 1987

173. Ahlquist DA, Beart RW Jr: Use of fecal occult blood test in the detection of colorectal neoplasia. Curr Probl Gen Surg 2:200–210, 1985

174. Winawer SJ, Fleisher M: Sensitivity and specificity of the fecal occult blood test for colorectal neoplasia. Gastroenterology 82:986–991, 1982

175. Griffith CDM, Turner DJ, Saunders JH: False-negative results of hemoccult test in colorectal cancer. Br J Med 283:472, 1981

176. Hardcastle JD, Armitage NC, Chamberlin J et al: Fecal occult blood screening for colorectal cancer in the general population. Cancer 58:397–403, 1986

177. Winawer SJ, Andrews M, Flehinger B et al: Progress report on controlled trial of fecal occult blood testing for the detection of colorectal neoplasia. Cancer 45:2959–2964, 1980

178. Cummings KM, Michalek AJ, Tidings J et al: Results of a public screening program for colorectal cancer. NY State Med 86:68–72, 1986

179. Simon JB: Occult blood screening for colorectal carcinoma: A critical review. Gastroenterology 88:820–837, 1985

180. Macrae FA, St. John DJ, Couligiore P et al: Optimal dietary conditions for hemoccult testing. Gastroenterology 82:889–903, 1982

181. Gnauck R, Macrae FA, Fleisher M: How to perform the occult blood test. CA 34:134–147, 1984

182. Jaffe RM, Kasten B, Young DS et al: False negative stool occult blood test caused by the ingestion of ascorbic acid. Ann Intern Med 83:824–826, 1975

183. Feczko PJ, Halpert RD: Reassessing the role of radiology and hemoccult screening. AJR 146:697–701, 1986
184. Winchester DP, Shull JH, Scanlon EF et al: A mass screening program for colorectal cancer using chemical testing for occult blood in the stool. Cancer 45:2955–2958, 1980
185. Sontag SJ, Durczak C, Aranha GV et al: Fecal occult blood screening for colorectal cancer in a Veteran's Administration hospital. Am J Surg 145:89–93, 1983
186. Jackman RJ, Beahrs OH: Tumors of the Large Bowel. Philadelphia, WB Saunders, 1969
187. Gordon-Watson C, Dukes C: The radium problem: III. The treatment of carcinoma of the rectum with radium. With an introduction on the spread of cancer of the rectum. Br J Surg 17:643–669, 1930
188. Dukes CE: Cancer of the rectum: An analysis of 1000 cases. J Pathol Bacteriol 50:527–539, 1940
189. Hermanek P: Evolution and pathology of rectal cancer. World J Surg 6:502–509, 1982
190. Spjut HJ: Pathology of neoplasms. In Spratt JS (ed): Neoplasms of the Colon, Rectum, and Anus: Mucosal and Epithelial. Philadelphia, WB Saunders, 1984
191. Morson BC, Sobin LH: Histological typing of intestinal tumours. Technical report No. 15, Geneva, World Health Organization, 1976
192. Wood DA: Tumors of the intestines. In: Atlas of Tumor Pathology, Section VI, Fascicle 22. Washington, DC, Armed Forces Institute of Pathology, 1967
193. Bonello JC, Sternberg SS, Quan SHQ: The significance of the signet-cell variety of adenocarcinoma of the rectum. Dis Colon Rectum 23:180–183, 1980
194. Mathews JL, Coyle D Jr, Little WP: Primary linitis plastica of the rectum: Report of a case. Dis Colon Rectum 25:488–490, 1982
195. Cooper HS: Carcinoma of the colon and rectum. In Norris HT (ed): Pathology of the Colon, Small Intestine, and Anus. New York, Churchill Livingstone, 1983
196. Gibbs NM: Undifferentiated carcinoma of the large intestine. Histopathology 1:77–84, 1977
197. MacDonald RA: A study of 356 carcinoids of the gastrointestinal tract: Report of four new cases of the carcinoid syndrome. Am J Med 21:867–878, 1956
198. Orloff MJ: Carcinoid tumors of the rectum. Cancer 28:175–180, 1971
199. Evans HL: Smooth muscle tumors of the gastrointestinal tract: A study of 56 cases followed for a minimum of 10 years. Cancer 56:2242–2250, 1985
200. Broders AC: The grading of carcinoma. Minn Med 8:726–730, 1925
201. Dukes CE: The classification of cancer of the rectum. J Pathol 35:323–332, 1932
202. Qizilbash AH: Pathologic studies in colorectal cancer: A guide to the surgical pathology examination of colorectal specimens and review of features of prognostic significance. Pathol Annu 17(part 1):1–46, 1982
203. Jass JR, Atkin WS, Cuzick I et al: The grading of rectal cancer: Historical perspectives and a multivariate analysis of 447 cases. Histopathology 10:437–459, 1986
204. Dukes CE, Bussey HJR: The spread of rectal cancer and its effect on prognosis. Br J Cancer 12:309–320, 1958
205. Cole PP: The intramural spread of rectal carcinoma. Br Med J 1:431–433, 1913
206. Black WA, Waugh JM: The intramural extension of carcinoma of the descending colon, sigmoid, and rectosigmoid: A pathologic study. Surg Gynecol Obstet 87:457–464, 1948
207. Miles WE: Discussion on the surgical treatment of cancer of the rectum. Br Med J 2:730–742, 1920
208. Grinnell RS: Lymphatic block with atypical and retrograde lymphatic metastasis and spread in carcinoma of the colon and rectum. Ann Surg 163:272–280, 1966
209. Montessori GA, Donald JC, Invasion profile of colorectal carcinoma. Dis Colon Rectum 21:26–28, 1978
210. Templeton A: The value of whole mount sections in determining adequacy of surgical margins and in staging carcinoma of the colorectum. Presented at the 24th annual meeting of the American Society of Therapeutic Radiology and Oncology, Oct 28, 1982
211. Seefeld PH, Bargen JA: The spread of carcinoma of the rectum: Invasion of lymphatics, veins and nerves. Ann Surg 118:76–90, 1943
212. Knudsen JB, Nilsson T, Sprechler M et al: Venous and nerve invasion as prognostic factors in postoperative survival of patients with resectable cancer of the rectum. Dis Colon Rectum 26:613–617, 1983
213. Astler VB, Coller FA: The prognostic significance of direct extension of carcinoma of the colon and rectum. Ann Surg 139:846–851, 1954
214. Gunderson LL, Sosin H: Areas of failure found at reoperation (second or symptomatic look) following "curative surgery" for adenocarcinoma of the rectum: Clinicopathologic correlation and implications for adjuvant therapy. Cancer 34:1278–1292, 1974
215. Gilbert SG: Symptomatic local tumor failure following abdomino-perineal resection. Int J Radiat Oncol Biol Phys 4:801–807, 1978
216. Cass AW, Million RR, Pfaff WW: Patterns of recurrence following surgery alone for adenocarcinoma of the colon and rectum. Cancer 37:2861–2865, 1976
217. Olson RM, Perencevich NP, Malcolm AW et al: Patterns of recurrence following curative resection of adenocarcinoma of the colon and rectum. Cancer 45:2969–2974, 1980
218. Malcolm AW, Perencevich NP, Olson RM et al: Analysis of recurrence patterns following curative resection for carcinoma of the colon and rectum. Surg Gynecol Obstet 152:131–136, 1981
219. Rao AR, Kagan AR, Chan PM et al: Patterns of recurrence following curative resection alone for adenocarcinoma of the rectum and sigmoid colon. Cancer 48:1492–1495, 1981
220. Mendenhall WM, Million RR, Pfaff WW: Patterns of recurrence in adenocarcinoma of the rectum and rectosigmoid treated with surgery alone: Implications in treatment planning with adjuvant radiation therapy. Int J Radiat Oncol Biol Phys 9:977–985, 1983
221. Rich T, Gunderson LL, Lew R et al: Patterns of recurrence of rectal cancer after potentially curative surgery. Cancer 52:1317–1329, 1983
222. Pilipshen SJ, Heilweil M, Quan SHQ et al: Patterns of pelvic recurrence following definitive resections of rectal cancer. Cancer 53:1354–1362, 1984
223. Willett C, Tepper JE, Cohen A et al: Obstructive and perforative colonic carcinoma: Patterns of failure. J Clin Oncol 3:379–384, 1985
224. Minsky BD, Mies C, Recht A et al: Resectable adenocarcinoma of the rectosigmoid and rectum: 1. Patterns of failure and survival. Cancer (in press)
225. Minsky BD, Mies C, Rich TA et al: Potentially curative surgery of colon cancer: 1. Patterns of failure and survival. J Clin Oncol 6:106–118, 1988
226. Gabriel WB, Dukes C, Bussey HJR: Lymphatic spread in cancer of the rectum. Br J Surg 23:395–413, 1935
227. Wood WQ, Wilkie DPD: Carcinoma of the rectum: An anatomico-pathologic study. Edinburgh Med J 40:321–331, 1933
228. Grinnell RS: The grading and prognosis of carcinoma of the colon and rectum. Ann Surg 109:500–503, 1939
229. Villemin F, Huard P, Montague M: Récherches anatomiques sur les lymphatiques du rectum et de l'anus. Rev Chir 63:39–80, 1925
230. Grinnell RS: Lymphatic block with atypical and retrograde lymphatic metastasis and spread in carcinoma of the colon and rectum. Ann Surg 108:621–642, 1938
231. Herter FP, Slanetz CA: Patterns and significance of lymphatic spread from cancer of the colan and rectum. In Weiss L, Gilbert HA, Ballon SC (eds); Lymphatic System Metastasis. Boston, GK Hall, 1980
232. Brown CE, Warren S: Visceral metastases from rectal carcinoma. Surg Gynecol Obstet 66:611–621, 1938
233. Grinnell RS: The lymphatic and venous spread of carcinoma of the rectum. Ann Surg 116:200–215, 1942
234. Weiss L, Grundmann E, Torhorst J et al: Haematogenous metastatic patterns in colonic carcinoma: An analysis of 1541 necropsies. J Pathol 150:195–203, 1986
235. Batson OV: The function of the vertebral veins and their role in the spread of metastases. Ann Surg 112:138–149, 1940
236. Vider M, Maruyama Y, Narvaez R: Significance of the vertebral venous (Batson's) plexus in metastatic spread in colorectal carcinoma. Cancer 40:67–71, 1977
237. Umpleby HC, Williamson RCN: Anastomotic recurrence in large bowel cancer. Br J Surg 74:873–878, 1987
238. Beahrs OH, Phillips JW, Dockerty MB: Implantation of tumor cells as a factor in recurrence of carcinoma of the rectosigmoid: Report of four cases with implantation at dentate line. Cancer 8:831–838, 1955
239. LeQuesne LP, Thompson AD: Implantation recurrence of carcinoma of rectum and colon. N Engl J Med 258:578–582, 1958
240. Boreham P: Implantation metastases from cancer of the large bowel. Br J Surg 46:103–108, 1958
241. McGrew EA, Laws JF, Cole WH: Free malignant cells in relation to recurrence of carcinoma of the colon. JAMA 154:1251–1254, 1954
242. Goligher JC, Dukes CE, Bussey HJR: Local recurrences after sphincter-saving excisions for carcinoma of the rectum and rectosigmoid. Br J Surg 39:199–211, 1951
243. Cole WH, Packard D, Southwick HW: Carcinoma of the colon with special reference to prevention of recurrence. JAMA 155:1549–1553, 1954
244. Lawrie H: Letter: Cancer contagion and inoculation. Br Med J 1:198–199, 1906
245. Ryall C; Cancer infection and cancer recurrence: A danger to avoid in cancer operations. Lancet 2:1311–1316, 1907
246. Pomeranz AA, Garlock JH: Postoperative recurrence of cancer of colon due to desquamated malignant cells. JAMA 158:1434–1436, 1955
247. Moossa AR, Ree PC, Marks JE et al: Factors influencing local recurrence after abdominoperineal resection for cancer of the rectum and rectosigmoid. Br J Surg 62:727–730, 1975
248. Walz BJ, Green MR, Lindstron BJ et al: Anatomical prognostic factors after abdominooperineal resection. Int J Radiat Oncol Biol Phys 7:477–484, 1981
249. Thomas PRM, Stablein DM, Kinzie JJ et al: Perineal effects of postoperative treatment for adenocarcinoma of the rectum. Int J Radiat Oncol Biol Phys 12:167–171, 1986
250. Mayo WJ: Grafting and traumatic dissemination of carcinoma in the course of operations for malignant disease. JAMA 60:512–513, 1913
251. Fisher ER, Turnbull RB Jr: The cytologic demonstration and significance of tumor cells in the mesenteric venous blood in patients with colorectal carcinoma. Surg Gynecol Obstet 100:102–108, 1955
252. Goligher JC: The Dukes' A, B and C categorization of the extent of spread of carcinomas of the rectum. Surg Gynecol Obstet 143:793–794, 1976
253. Wiggers T, Arends JW, Volovics A: Regression analysis of prognostic factors in colorectal cancer after curative resections. Dis Colon Rectum 31:33–41, 1988
254. Wood CB, Gillis CR, Hole D et al: Local tumour invasion as a prognostic factor in colorectal cancer. Br J Surg 68:326–328, 1981
255. Davis NC, Evans EB, Cohen JR et al: Staging of colorectal cancer: The Australian Clinico-Pathological Staging (ACPS) System compared with the Dukes' system. Dis Colon Rectum 27:707–713, 1984
256. Midiri G, Amanti C, Consorti F et al: Usefulness of preoperative CEA levels in the assessment of colorectal cancer patient stage. J Surg Oncol 22:257–260, 1983

257. Moertel CG, OFallon JR, Go VL et al: The preoperative carcinoembryonic antigen test in the diagnosis, staging, and prognosis of colorectal cancer. Cancer 58:603–610, 1986

258. Lockhart-Mummery JP: Two hundred cases of cancer of the rectum treated by perineal excision. Br J Surg 14:110–124, 1927

259. Kirklin JW, Dockerty MB, Waugh JM: The role of the peritoneal reflection in the prognosis of carcinoma of the rectum and sigmoid colon. Surg Gynecol Obstet 88:326–331, 1949

260. Wolmark N, Fisher B, Wieand HS: The prognostic value of the modifications of the Dukes' C class of colorectal cancer. Ann Surg 203:115–122, 1986

261. Phillips RKS, Hittinger R, Blesovsky L et al: Large bowel cancer: Surgical pathology and its relationship to survival. Br J Surg 71:604–610, 1984

262. Gastrointestinal Tumor Study Group: Prolongation of the disease-free interval in surgically treated rectal carcinoma. N Engl J Med 312:1465–1472, 1985

263. American Joint Committee on Cancer: Manual for Staging of Cancer, 2nd ed. Philadelphia, JB Lippincott, 1983

264. Harmer MH (ed): TNM Classification of Malignant Tumours, pp 69–76. Geneva, International Union Against Cancer [Union Internationale Contre le Cancer], 1978

265. Chapuis PH, Dent OF, Newland RC et al: An evaluation of the American Joint Committee (pTNM) staging method for cancer of the colon and rectum. Dis Colon Rectum 29:6–10, 1986

266. Enderlin F, Gloor F: Colorectal cancer: The relationship of staging to survival. A cancer registry study of 800 cases in St. Gallen-Appenzell. Soz Praventivmed 31:85–88, 1986

267. Hermanek P: Problems of pTNM classification of carcinoma of the stomach, colorectum and anal margin. Pathol Res Pract 181:296–300, 1986

268. American Joint Committee on Cancer: Manual for Staging of Cancer, 3rd ed. Philadelphia, JB Lippincott, 1987

269. Hermanek P, Sobin LH (eds): TNM Classification of Malignant Tumours (International Union Against Cancer), 4th ed. Berlin, Springer-Verlag, 1987

270. Nathanson SD, Schultz L, Tilley B et al: Carcinoma of the colon and rectum: A comparison of staging classifications. Am Surg 52:428–433, 1986

271. Newland RC, Chapuis PH, Smyth EJ: The prognostic value of substaging colorectal carcinoma: A prognostic study of 1117 cases with standardized pathology. Cancer 60:852–857, 1987

272. Abrams JS: Clinical staging of rectal cancer. Am J Surg 139:539–543, 1980

273. Zorzitto M, Germanson T, Cummings B et al: A method of clinical prognostic staging for patients with rectal cancer. Dis Colon Rectum 25:759–765, 1982

274. Duncan W, Smith AN, Freedman LF et al: Clinico-pathological features of prognostic significance in operable rectal cancer in 17 centres in the U.K. Br J Cancer 50:435–442, 1984

275. Freedman LS, Macaskill P, Smith AN: Multivariate analysis of prognostic factors for operable rectal cancer. Lancet 2:733–736, 1984

276. Davis NC, Newland RC: The reporting of colorectal cancer: The Australian clinico-pathological staging system. Aust NZ J Surg 52:395–397, 1982

277. Davis NC, Evans EB, Cohen JR et al: Clinicopathological staging of colorectal cancer: Has the time arrived? Br J Surg 72 (suppl):S47–S52, 1985

278. York Mason A: Rectal cancer: The spectrum of selective surgery. Proc R Soc Med 69:237–244, 1976

279. Nicholls RJ, York Mason A, Borson BC et al: The clinical staging of rectal cancer. Br J Surg 69:404–409, 1982

280. Nicholls RJ, Galloway DJ, Mason AY et al: Clinical local staging of rectal cancer. Br J Surg 72 (suppl):S51–S52, 1985

281. Williams NS, Durdey P, Quirke P et al: Pre-operative staging of rectal neoplasm and its impact on clinical management. Br J Surg 72:868–874, 1985

282. Clark J, Bankoff M, Carter B et al: The use of computerized tomography scan in the staging and follow-up study of carcinoma of the rectum. Surg Gynecol Obstet 159:335–342, 1984

283. Hildebrandt U, Feifel G: Preoperative staging of rectal cancer by intrarectal ultrasound. Dis Colon Rectum 28:42–46, 1985

284. Romano G, de Rosa P, Vallone G et al: Intrarectal ultrasound and computed tomography in the pre- and postoperative assessment of patients with rectal cancer. Br J Surg [Suppl]:S117–S119, 1985

285. Rifkin MD, Marks GJ: Transrectal US as an adjunct in the diagnosis of rectal and extrarectal tumors. Radiology 157:499–502, 1985

286. Beynon J, Mortensen NJ, Foy DM et al: Endorectal sonography: Laboratory and clinical experience in Bristol. Int J Colorect Dis 1:212–215, 1986

287. Nyberg DA, Kimmey MB, Wang K et al: Sonographic staging of colon neoplasms: Accuracy in determining depth of spread (abst). Radiology 154: 1986

288. Mayes GB, Zornoza J: Computed tomography of colon carcinoma. AJR 135:43–46, 1980

289. Thoeni RF, Moss AA, Schnyder P, Margulis AR: Detection and staging of primary rectal and rectosigmoid cancer by computed tomography. Radiology 141:135–138, 1981

290. Hamlin DJ, Burgener FA, Sischy B: New technique to stage early rectal carcinoma by computed tomography. Radiology 141:539–540, 1981

291. Zaunbauer W, Haertel M, Fuchs WA: Computed tomography in carcinoma of the rectum. Gastrointest Radiol 6:79–84, 1981

292. van Waes PFGM, Koehler PR, Feldberg MAM: Management of rectal carcinoma: Impact of computed tomography. AJR 140:1137–1142, 1983

293. Dixon AK, Fry IK, Morson BC et al: Pre-operative computed tomography of carcinoma of the rectum. Br J Radiol 54:655–659, 1981

294. Grabbe E, Lierse W, Winkler R: The perirectal fascia: Morphology and use in staging of rectal carcinoma. Radiology 149:241–246, 1983

295. Adalsteinsson B, Glimelius B, Graffman S et al: Computed tomography in staging of rectal carcinoma. Acta Radiol Diagn 26:45–55, 1985

296. Netri G, Coco C, Valentine V et al: Clinical staging of rectal cancer: Results of a prospective continuing study. Ital J Surg Sci 15:169–174, 1985

297. Freeny PC, Marks WM, Ryan JA, Bolen JW: Colorectal carcinoma evaluation with CT: Preoperative staging and detection of postoperative recurrence. Radiology 158:347–353, 1986

298. Thompson WM, Halvorsen RA, Foster WL Jr et al: Preoperative and postoperative CT staging of rectosigmoid carcinoma. AJR 146:703–710, 1986

299. Shank B, Dershaw D, Caravelli J et al: A prospective, blinded trial of CT staging for rectal carcinoma (unpublished data)

300. Lee JKT, Heiken JP, Ling D et al: Magnetic resonance imaging of abdominal and pelvic lymphadenopathy. Radiology 153:181–188, 1984

301. Dooms GC, Hricak H, Crooks LE, Higgins CB: Magnetic resonance imaging of the lymph nodes: Comparison with CT. Radiology 153:719–728, 1984

302. Butch RJ, Stark DD, Wittenberg J et al: Staging rectal cancer by MR and CT. AJR 146:1155–1160, 1986

303. Fuchs WA: Normal anatomy. In Fuchs WA, Davidson JW, Fisher HW (eds): Lymphography in Cancer. Recent Results Cancer Res 23: 42–86, 1969

304. Ege GN, Cummings BJ: Interstitial radiocolloid ilio-pelvic lymphoscintigraphy: Technique, anatomy and clinical application. Int J Radiat Oncol Biol Phys 6:1483–1490, 1980

305. Reasbeck PG, Manktelow A, McArthur AM et al: An evaluation of pelvic lymphoscintigraphy in the staging of colorectal carcinoma. Br J Surg 71:936–940, 1984

306. Moldofsky PJ, Powe J, Mulhern CB Jr et al: Metastatic colon carcinoma detected with radiolabeled $F(ab')_2$ monoclonal antibody fragments. Radiology 149:549–555, 1983

307. Mach J–P, Chatal J–F, Lumbroso J–D et al: Tumor localization in patients by radiolabeled monoclonal antibodies against colon carcinoma. Cancer Res 43:5593–5600, 1983

308. Alderson PO, Adams DF, McNeil BJ et al: Computed tomography, ultrasound, and scintigraphy of the liver in patients with colon or breast carcinoma: A prospective comparison. Radiology 149:225–230, 1983

309. Zeman RK, Paushter DM, Schiebler ML et al: Hepatic imaging: Current status. Radiol Clin North Am 23:473–487, 1985

310. Thompson WM: Imaging strategies for tumors of the gastrointestinal system. CA 37:165–185, 1987

311. Kemeny NM, Sugarbaker PH, Smith TJ et al: A prospective analysis of laboratory tests and imaging studies to detect hepatic lesions. Ann Surg 195:163–167, 1982

312. Gennari L, Doci R, Bozzetti F et al: Surgical treatment of hepatic metastases from colorectal cancer. Ann Surg 203:49–54, 1986

313. Reinig JW, Dwyer AJ, Miller DL et al: Liver metastasis detection: Comparative sensitivities of MR imaging and CT scanning. Radiology 162:43–47, 1987

314. van de Velde CJH: The staging of hepatic metastases arising from colorectal cancer. Recent Results Cancer Res 100:85–90, 1984

315. Hoerner MT: Carcinoma of the colon and rectum in persons under twenty years of age. Am J Surg 96:47–53, 1958

316. Recio P, Bussey HJR: The pathology and prognosis of carcinoma of the rectum in the young. Proc R Soc Lond 58:789–790, 1965

317. Mayo CW, Pagtalunan JG: Malignancy of the colon and rectum in patients under 30 years of age. Surgery 53:711–718, 1963

318. Coffey RJ, Cardenas F: Cancer of the bowel in the young adult. Dis Colon Rectum 7:491–492, 1964

319. van Langenberg AV, Ong GB: Carcinoma of large bowel in the young. Br Med J 3:374–376, 1972

320. Odone V, Chang L, Caces J et al: The natural history of colorectal carcinoma in adolescents. Cancer 49:1716–1720, 1982

321. Safford KL, Spebar MJ, Rosenthal D: Review of colorectal cancer in patients under age 40 years. Am J Surg 142:767–769, 1981

322. Simstein NL, Kovalcik PJ, Cross GH: Colorectal carcinoma in patients less than 40 years old. Dis Colon Rectum 2:169–171, 1978

323. Bülow S: Colorectal cancer in patients less than 40 years of age in Denmark, 1943–1967. Dis Colon Rectum 23:327–336, 1980

324. Umpleby HC, Williamson RCN: Carcinoma of the large bowel in the first four decades. Br J Surg 71:272–277, 1984

325. Eisenberg B, DeCosse JJ, Harford F et al: Carcinoma of the colon and rectum: The natural history reviewed in 1704 patients. Cancer 49:1131–1134, 1982

326. Welch CE, Burke JF: Carcinoma of the colon and rectum. N Engl J Med 266:211–219, 1962

327. McDermott FT, Hughes ESR, Pihl E et al: Comparative results of surgical management of single carcinomas of the colon and rectum: A series of 1939 patients managed by one surgeon. Br J Surg 68:850–855, 1981

328. Stearns MW, Deddish MR, Quan SHQ et al: Preoperative reontgen therapy for cancer of the rectum and rectosigmoid. Surg Gynecol Obstet 138:584–586, 1974

329. Spratt JS Jr, Spjut HJ: Prevalence and prognosis of individual clinical and pathologic variables associated with colorectal carcinoma. Cancer 20:1976–1985, 1967

330. Godwin JD, Brown CC: Some prognostic factors in survival of patients with cancer of the colon and rectum. J Chronic Dis 28:441–454, 1975

331. deMello J, Struthers L, Turner R et al: Multivariate analysis as aides to diagnosis and assessment of prognosis in gastrointestinal cancer. Br J Cancer 48:341–348, 1983

332. Chapuis PH, Dent OF, Fisher R et al: A multivariate analysis of clinical and pathological variables in prognosis after resection of large bowel cancer. Br J Surg 72:698–702, 1985

333. Corman J, Arnoux R, Peloquin A et al: Blood transfusions and survival after colectomy for colorectal cancer. Can J Surg 29:325–329, 1986

334. Fielding LP, Phillips RKS, Fry JS et al: Prediction of outcome after curative resection for large bowel cancer. Lancet 2:904–907, 1986

335. Koch M, McPherson TA, Egedahl RD: Effect of sex and reproductive history on the survival of patients with colorectal cancer. J Chronic Dis 35:69–72, 1982

336. Beahrs OH, Sanfelippo PM: Factors in the prognosis of colon and rectal cancer. Cancer 28:213–217, 1971

337. Copeland EM, Miller LD, Jones RS: Prognostic factors in carcinoma of the colon and rectum. Am J Surg 116:875–881, 1968

338. Pescatori M, Maria G, Beltrani B et al: Site, emergency, and duration of symptoms in the prognosis of colorectal cancer. Dis Colon Rectum 25:33–40, 1982

339. Ulin AW, Ehrlich EW: Current views related to management of large bowel obstruction caused by carcinoma of the colon. Am J Surg 104:463–467, 1962

340. Chang WYM, Burnett WE: Complete colonic obstruction due to adenocarcinoma. Surg Gynecol Obstet 114:353–356, 1962

341. Miller LD, Boruchow IB, Fitts WT: An analysis of 284 patients with perforative carcinoma of the colon. Surg Gynecol Obstet 123:1212–1218, 1966

342. Floyd CE, Cohn I: Obstruction in cancer of the colon. Ann Surg 165:721–731, 1967

343. Crowder VH, Cohn I: Perforation in cancer of the colon and rectum. Dis Colon Rectum 10:415–420, 1967

344. Glenn F, McSherry CK: Obstruction and perforation in colorectal cancer. Ann Surg 173:983–992, 1971

345. Welch JP, Donaldson GA: Management of severe obstruction of the large bowel due to malignant disease. Am J Surg 127:492–499, 1974

346. Welch JP, Donaldson GA: Perforative carcinoma of colon and rectum. Ann Surg 180:734–740, 1974

347. Wolmark N, Wieand HS, Rockette HE et al: The prognostic significance of tumor location and bowel obstruction in Dukes B and C colorectal cancer: Findings from the NSABP clinical trials. Ann Surg 198:743–752, 1983

348. Steinberg SM, Barkin JS, Kaplan RS et al: Prognostic indicators of colon tumors: The Gastrointestinal Tumor Study Group experience. Cancer 57:1866–1870, 1986

349. Kelley WE Jr, Brown PW, Lawrence W Jr et al: Penetrating, obstructing, and perforating carcinomas of the colon and rectum. Arch Surg 116:381–384, 1981

350. Thomas WH, Larson, RA, Wright HK et al: An analysis of patients with carcinoma of the right colon. Surg Gynecol Obstet 127:313–318, 1968

351. Dwight RW, Higgins GA, Keehn RJ: Factors influencing survival after resection in cancer of the colon and rectum. Am J Surg 117:512–522, 1969

352. Gilchrist RK, David VC: A consideration of pathological factors influencing five year survival in radical resection of the large bowel and rectum for carcinoma. Ann Surg 126:421–438, 1947

353. Osnes S: Carcinoma of the colon and rectum: A study of 353 cases with special reference to prognosis. Acta Chir Scand 110:378–388, 1956

354. McSherry CK, Cornell GN, Glen F: Carcinoma of the colon and rectum. Ann Surg 169:502–512, 1969

355. Cohen AM, Wood WC, Gunderson LL et al: Pathological studies in rectal cancer. Cancer 45:2965–2968, 1980

356. Wolmark N, Fisher ER, Wieand HS et al: The relationship of depth of penetration and tumor size to the number of positive nodes in Dukes C colorectal cancer. Cancer 53:2707–2712, 1984

357. Coller FA, Kay EB, MacIntyre RS: Regional lymphatic metastasis in carcinoma of the colon. Ann Surg 114:56–63, 1941

358. Burrows L, Tartter P: Effect of blood transfusions on colonic malignancy recurrence rate. Lancet 2:662, 1982

359. Agarwal M, Blumberg N: Colon cancer patients transfused perioperatively have an increased incidence of recurrence (abst) Transfusion 23:421, 1983

360. Foster RS Jr, Costanza MC, Foster JC: Adverse relationship between blood transfusions and survival after colectomy for colon cancer. Cancer 55:1195–1201, 1985

361. Nathanson SD, Tilley BC, Schultz L et al: Perioperative allogeneic blood transfusions: Survival in patients with resected carcinomas of the colon and rectum. Arch Surg 120:734–738, 1985

362. Weiden PL, Bean MA, Schultz P: Perioperative blood transfusion does not increase the risk of colorectal cancer. Cancer 60:870–874, 1987

363. Willett CG, Tepper JE, Cohen AM et al: Failure patterns following curative resection of colonic carcinoma. Ann Surg 200:685–690, 1984

364. Willett C, Tepper JE, Cohen AM et al: Local failure following curative resection of colonic adenocarcinoma. Int J Radiat Oncol Biol Phys 10:645–651, 1984

365. Fucini C, Bandettini L, Dlia M et al: Are postoperative fever and/or septic complications prognostic factors in colorectal cancer resected for cure? Dis Colon Rectum 28:94–95, 1985

366. Riboli EB, Secco GB, Lapertosa G et al: Colorectal cancer: Relationship of histologic grading to disease prognosis. Tumori 69:581–584, 1983

367. Godwin JD II: Carcinoid tumors: An analysis of 2837 cases. Cancer 36:560–569, 1975

368. Madison MS, Dockerty MB, Waugh JM: Venous invasion in carcinoma of the rectum as evidenced by venous radiography. Surg Gynecol Obstet 99:170–178, 1954

369. Qualheim RE, Gall EA: Is histopathologic grading of colon carcinoma a valid procedure? Arch Pathol 56:466–472, 1953

370. Thomas GDH, Dixon MF, Smeeton NC et al: Observer variation in the histological grading of rectal carcinoma. J Clin Pathol [Suppl] 36:385–391, 1983

371. Trimpi HD, Bacon HE: Mucoid carcinoma of the rectum. Cancer 4:597–609, 1951

372. Sundblad AS, Paz RA: Mucinous carcinomas of the colon and rectum and their relation to polyps. Cancer 50:2504–2509, 1982

373. Minsky BD, Mies C, Rich TA et al: Colloid carcinoma of the colon and rectum. Cancer 60:3103–3112, 1987

374. DeMascarel A, Coindre JM, DeMascarel I et al: The prognostic significance of specific histologic features of carcinoma of the colon and rectum. Surg Gynecol Obstet 153:511–514, 1981

375. Walton WW, Hagihara PF, Griffen WO: Colorectal adenocarcinoma in patients less than 40 years old. Dis Colon Rectum 19:529–534, 1976

376. Symonds DA, Vickery AL Jr: Mucinous carcinoma of the colon and rectum. Cancer 37:1891–1900, 1976

377. Umpleby HC, Ranson DL, Williamson HC: Peculiarities of mucinous colorectal carcinoma. Br J Surg 72:715–718, 1985

378. Sunderland DA: The significance of vein invasion by cancer of the rectum and sigmoid: A microscopic study of 210 cases. Cancer 2:429–437, 1949

379. Grinnell RS: Lymphatic metastases of carcinoma of the colon and rectum. Ann Surg 131:494–506, 1950

380. Burns FJ, Pfaff J Jr: Vascular invasion in carcinoma of the colon and rectum. Am J Surg 92:704–709, 1956

381. Swinton NW: Cancer of the colon and rectum: A statistical study of 608 patients. Surg Clin North Am 39:745–753, 1959

382. Talbot IC, Ritchie S, Leighton MH et al: Spread of rectal cancer within veins: Histologic features and clinical significance. Am J Surg 141:15–17, 1981

383. Minsky BD, Mies C, Rich TA et al: Potentially curative surgery of colon cancer: 2. The influence of blood vessel invasion. J Clin Oncol 6:119–127, 1988

384. Minsky BD, Mies C, Recht A et al: Resectable adenocarcinoma of the rectosigmoid and rectum: 2. The influence of blood vessel invasion. Cancer 61:1408–1416, 1988

385. Khankanian N, Mavligit GM, Russell WO et al: Prognostic significance of vascular invasion in colorectal cancer of Dukes' B class. Cancer 39:1195–1200, 1977

386. Kim US, Papatestas AE, Aufses AH Jr: Prognostic significance of peripheral lymphocytic counts and carcinoembryonic antigens in colorectal carcinoma. J Surg Oncol 8:257–262, 1976

387. Shafir M, Bekesi JG, Papatestas A et al: Preoperative and postoperative immunological evaluation of patients with colorectal cancer. Cancer 46:700–705, 1980

388. Panettiere FJ, Chen TT: Prognostic significance of serum immunoglobulin levels in colorectal adenocarcinoma: Data from a SWOG study. Proc Am Soc Clin Oncol 6:73, 1987

389. Baseler MW, Maxim PE, Veltri RW: Circulating IgA immune complexes in head and neck cancer, nasopharyngeal carcinoma, lung cancer, and colon cancer. Cancer 59:1727–1731, 1987

390. Murray D, Hreno A, Dutton J et al: Prognosis in colon cancer: A pathologic reassessment. Arch Surg 110:908–913, 1975

391. Carlon CA, Fabris G, Arslan-Pagnini C et al: Prognostic correlations of operable carcinoma of the rectum. Dis Colon Rectum 28:47–50, 1985

392. Svennevig JL, Lunde OC, Holter J et al: Lymphoid infiltration and prognosis in colorectal carcinoma. Br J Cancer 49:375–377, 1984

393. Patt DJ, Byrnes RK, Vardiman JW et al: Mesocolic lymph node histology is an important prognostic indicator for patients with carcinoma of the sigmoid colon: An immunomorphologic study. Cancer 35:1388–1397, 1975

394. Tsakraklides V, Wanebo HJ, Sternberg SS et al: Prognostic evaluation of regional lymph node morphology in colorectal cancer. Am J Surg 129:174–180, 1975

395. Pihl E, Malahy MA, Khankanian N et al: Immunomorphological features of prognostic significance in Dukes' class B colorectal carcinoma. Cancer Res 37:4145–4149, 1977

396. LoGerfo P, Herter FP: Carcinoembryonic antigen and prognosis in patients with colon cancer. Ann Surg 181:81–84, 1975

397. Herrera MA, Chu TM, Holyoke ED: Carcinoembryonic antigen (CEA) as a prognostic and monitoring test in clinically complete resection of colorectal carcinoma. Ann Surg 183:5–9, 1976

398. Wanebo HJ, Rao B, Pinsky CM et al: Pre-operative carcinoembryonic antigen level as a prognostic indicator in colorectal cancer. N Eng J Med 299:448–451, 1978

399. Band PR, Beck IT, Dinner PJ et al: Two year follow-up study of patients with known serum concentrations of carcinoembryonic antigen. Can Med Assoc J 117:657–659, 1977

400. Evans JT, Mittleman A, Chu M et al: Pre- and post-operative uses of CEA. Cancer 42:1419–1421, 1978

401. Kohler JP, Simonowitz D, Paloyan D: Pre-operative CEA level: A prognostic test in patients with colorectal carcinoma. Am Surg 46:449–452, 1980

402. Staab HJ, Anderer FA, Brummendorf T et al: Prognostic value of pre-operative serum CEA level compared to clinical staging: I. Colorectal carcinoma. Br J Cancer 44:652–662, 1981

403. Szymendera J, Nowacki MP, Szalowski AW et al: Predictive value of plasma CEA levels: Preoperative prognosis and postoperative monitoring of patients with colorectal carcinoma. Dis Colon Rectum 25:46–52, 1982

404. Onetto M, Paganuzzi M, Secco GB et al: Preoperative carcinoembryonic antigen and prognosis in patients with colorectal cancer. Biomed Pharmacother 39:392–395, 1985

405. Aabo K, Pedersen H, Kjaer M: Carcinoembryonic antigen (CEA) and alkaline phos

phatase in progressive colorectal cancer with special reference to patient survival. Eur J Cancer Clin Oncol 22:211–217, 1986

406. Goslin R, Steele G, MacIntyre J et al: The use of pre-operative plasma CEA levels for the stratification of patients after curative resection of colorectal cancer. Ann Surg 192:747–751, 1980

407. Chapuis PH, Newland RC, Payne JE et al: Preoperative carcinoembryonic antigen level and prognosis in colorectal cancer. Med J Aust 2:140–143, 1980

408. Blake KE, Dalbow MH, Concannon JP et al: Clinical significance of preoperative plasma carcinoembryonic antigen (CEA) level in patients with carcinoma of the large bowel. Dis Colon Rectum 25:24–32, 1982

409. Lewi H, Blumgart LH, Carter DC et al: Pre-operative carcinoembryonic antigen and survival in patients with colorectal cancer. Br J Surg 71:206—208, 1984

410. Steele G Jr, Ellenberg S, Ramming K et al: CEA monitoring among patients in multi-institutional adjuvant G.I. therapy protocols. Ann Surg 196:162–169, 1982

411. Tabuchi Y, Deguchi H, Imanishi K et al: Comparison of carcinoembryonic antigen levels between portal and peripheral blood in patients with colorectal cancer: Correlation with histopathologic variables. Cancer 59:1283–1288, 1987

412. Ward AM, Cooper EH, Turner R et al: Acute-phase reactant protein profiles: An aid to monitoring large bowel cancer by CEA and serum enzymes. Br J Cancer 35:170–178, 1977

413. Durdey P, Williams NS, Brown DA: Serum carcinoembryonic antigen and acute phase reactant proteins in the pre-operative detection of fixation of colorectal tumours. Br J Surg 71:881–884, 1984

414. Walker C, Grace BN: Acute-phase reactant proteins and carcinoembryonic antigen in cancer of the colon and rectum. Cancer 52:150–154, 1983

415. Meyer JS, Prioleau PG: S-phase fractions of colorectal carcinomas related to pathological and clinical features. Cancer 48:1221–1228, 1981

416. Blijham G, Schutte B, Reynders M et al: Flow cytometric (FCM) determination of ploidy level and life cycle analysis on 297 paraffin embedded colorectal carcinoma specimens. Proc Am Soc Clin Oncol 4:22, 1985

417. Bleiberg H, Buyse M, van den Heule B et al: Cell cycle parameters and prognosis of colorectal cancer. Eur J Cancer Clin Oncol 20:391–396, 1984

418. Mauro F, Teodori L, Schumann J, Gohde W: Flow cytometry as a tool for the prognostic assessment of human neoplasia. Int J Radiat Oncol Biol Phys 12:625–636, 1986

419. Wolley RC, Schreiber K, Koss LG et al: DNA distribution in human colon carcinomas and its relationship to clinical behavior. JNCI 69:15–22, 1982

420. Tribukait B, Hammarberg C, Rubio C: Ploidy and proliferation patterns in colorectal adenocarcinomas related to Dukes' classification and to histopathological differentiation. Acta Pathol Microbiol Immunol Scand [A] 91:89–95, 1983

421. Hiddemann W, von Bassewitz DB, Kleinemeier H–J et al: DNA stemline heterogeneity in colorectal cancer, Cancer 58:258–263, 1986

422. Frankfurt OS, Slocum HK, Rustum Ym et al: Flow cytometric analysis of DNA aneuploidy in primary and metastatic human solid tumors. Cytometry 5:71–80, 1984

423. Ota D, Johnston D, Drewinko B: Colorectal carcinoma (CA) cell kinetics: Need for new therapeutic strategies. Proc Am Soc Clin Oncol 6:13, 1987

424. Streffer C, van Beuningen D, Gross E et al: Predictive assays for the therapy of rectum carcinoma. Radiother Oncol 5:303–310, 1986

425. Armitage NC, Robins RA, Evans DF et al: Tumour cell DNA content in colorectal cancer and its relationship to survival. Br J Surg 72:828–830, 1985

426. Kokal W, Sheibani K, Terz J et al: Tumor DNA content in the prognosis of colorectal carcinoma JAMA 255:3123–3127, 1986

427. Scott NA, Rainwater LM, Wieand HS et al: The relative prognostic value of flow cytometric DNA analysis and conventional clinicopathologic criteria in patients with operable rectal carcinoma. Dis Colon Rectum 30:513–520, 1987

428. Melamed MR, Enker WE, Banner P et al: Flow cytometry of colorectal carcinoma with three-year followup. Dis Colon Rectum 29:184–186, 1986

428a. Chapuis PH, Dent OF, Fisher R et al: A multivariate analysis of clinical and pathological variables in prognosis after resection of large bowel cancer. Br J Surg 72:698–702, 1985

428b. Fielding LP, Phillips RK, Frey JS et al: The prediction of outcome after curative resection for large bowel cancer. Lancet 2:904–907, 1986

428c. Jass JR, Love SB, Northover JM: A new prognostic classification of rectal cancer. Lancet 1:1303–1306, 1987

428d. Fielding LP: Clinical-pathologic staging of large-bowel cancer: A report of the ASCRS committee. Dis Colon Rectum 31:204–209, 1988

428e. Williams NS, Jass JR, Hardcastle JD: Clinicopathological assessment and staging of colorectal cancer. Br J Surg 75:649–652, 1988

429. Der CJ, Cooper GM: Altered gene products are associated with activation of cellular ras genes in human lung and colon carcinomas. Cell 32:201–208, 1983

430. Spandidos DA, Kerr IB: Elevated expression of the human ras oncogene family in premalignant and malignant tumours of the colorectum. Br J Cancer 49:681–688, 1984

431. Gallick GE, Kurzrock R, Kloetzer WS et al: Expression of p21ras in fresh primary and metastatic human colorectal tumors. Proc Natl Acad Sci USA 82:1795–1799, 1985

432. Thar A, Hand PH, Wunderlich D et al: Monoclonal antibodies define differential ras gene expression in malignant and benign colonic diseases. Nature 311:562–565, 1984

433. Marx JL: Research news: ras oncogene activated in human colon cancers. Science 237:603, 1987

434. Bos JL, Fearon ER, Hamilton SR et al: Prevalence of ras gene mutations in human colorectal cancers. Nature 327:293–297, 1987

435. Forrester K, Almoguera C, Han K et al: Detection of high incidence of K-ras ongogenes during human colon tumorigenesis. Nature 327:298–303, 1987

436. Stewart DJ, Evan G, Watson JV, Sikora K: Detection of the c-myc oncogene product in colonic polyps and carcinomas. Br J Cancer 53:1–6, 1986

437. Sikora K, Chan S, Evan G et al: c-myc oncogene expression in colorectal cancer. Cancer 59:1289–1295, 1987

438. Welin S, Youker J, Spratt JS Jr et al: The rates and patterns of growth of 375 tumors of the large intestine and rectum observed serially by double contrast enema study (Malmo technique). AJR 90:673–687, 1963

439. Hanauske AR, Buchok J, Scheithauer W, Von Hoff DD: Human colon cancer cell lines secrete alpha TGF-like activity. BR J Cancer 55:57–59, 1987

440. Coffey RJ Jr, Shipley GD, Moses HL: Production of transforming growth factors by human colon cancer lines. Cancer Res 46:1164–1169, 1986

441. Beauchamp RD, Townsend CM Jr, Singh P et al: Proglumide, a gastrin receptor antagonist, inhibits growth of colon cancer and enhances survival in mice. Ann Surg 202:303–309, 1985

442. Singh P, Walker JP, Townsend CM Jr et al: Role of gastrin and gastrin receptors on the growth of a transplantable mouse colon carcinoma (MC-26) in BALB/c mice. Cancer Res 46:1612–1616, 1986

443. Stebbings WS, Farthing MJ, Vinson GP et al: Androgen receptors in rectal and colonic cancer. Dis Colon Rectum 29:95–98, 1986

444. Alford TC, Do HM, Geelhoed GW et al: Steroid hormone receptors in human colon cancers. Cancer 43:980–984, 1979

445. McClendon JE, Appleby D, Claudon DB et al: Colonic neoplasms: Tissue estrogen receptor and carcinoembryonic antigen. Arch Surg 112:240–241, 1977

446. Geelhoed GW, Crandall A, Lippman ME: Biologic implications of steroid hormone receptors in cancers of the colon. South Med J 78:252–254, 1985

447. Tempero M: Bile acids, ornithine decarboxylase, and cell proliferation in colon cancer: A review. Dig Dis 4:49–56, 1986

448. Luk GD, Baylin SB: Ornithine decarboxylase as a biologic marker in familial polyposis. N Engl J Med 311:80–83, 1984

449. Porter CW, Herrera-Ornelas L, Pera P et al: Polyamine biosynthetic activity in normal and neoplastic human colorectal tissues. Cancer 60:1275–1281, 1987

450. Gold P, Freeman SO: Specific carcinoembryonic antigens of the human digestive system. J Exp Med 122:467–481, 1965

451. Ahnen DJ, Nakane PK, Brown WR: Ultrastructural localization of carcinoembryonic antigen in normal intestine and colon cancer. Cancer 49:2077–2090, 1982

452. Primus FJ, Kuhns WJ, Goldenberg DM; Immunological heterogeneity of carcinoembryonic antigen: Immunohistochemical detection of carcinoembryonic determinants in colonic tumors with monoclonal antibodies. Cancer Res 43:693–701, 1983

453. Herlyn M, Blaszczyk M, Sears HF et al: Detection of carcinoembryonic antigen and related antigens in sera of patients with gastrointentinal tumors using monoclonal antibodies in double-determinant radioimmunoassays. Hybridoma 2:329–339, 1983

454. Wiley EL, Murphy P, Mendelson G, Eggleston JC: Distribution of blood group substances in normal human colon. Am J Clin Pathol 76:806–809, 1981

455. Ernst C, Thurin J, Atkinson B: Monoclonal antibody localization of A and B iso-antigens in normal and malignant fixed human tissues. Am J Pathol 117:451–461, 1984

456. Schoentag R, Primus FJ, Kuhns W: ABH and Lewis blood group expression in colorectal carcinoma. Cancer Res 47:1695–1700, 1987

457. Compton C, Wyatt R, Konugres A et al: Immunohistochemical studies of blood group substance H in colorectal tumors using a monoclonal antibody. Cancer 59:118–127, 1987

458. Itzkowitz SH, Yuan M, Ferrell LD et al: Cancer-associated alterations of blood group antigen expression in human colorectal polyps. Cancer Res 46:5976–5984, 1986

459. Hakomori S: Blood group glycolipid antigens and their modifications as human cancer antigens. Am J Clin Pathol 82:635–648, 1984

460. Abe K, Hakomori S, Ohshiba S: Differential expression of difucosyl type II chain (Eey) defined by monoclonal antibody AH6 in different locations of colonic epithelia, various histological types of colonic polyps and adenocarcinomas. Cancer Res 46:2639–2644, 1986

461. Sakamoto J, Furukawa K, Cordon-Cardo C et al: Expression of Lewis A, Lewis B, X, Y blood group antigens in human colonic tumors and normal tissue in human tumor-derived cell lines. Cancer Res 46:1553–1561, 1986

462. Itzkowitz SH, Yuan M, Fukushi Y et al: Lewis X- and sialylated Lewis X-related antigen expression in human malignant and non-malignant colonic tissues. Cancer Res 46:2627–2632, 1986

463. Koprowski H, Steplewski Z, Mitchell K et al: Colorectal carcinoma antigens detected by hybridoma antibodies. Somatic Cell Mol Genet 5:957–972, 1979

464. Magnani JL, Nilsson B, Brockhaus M et al: A monoclonal antibody–defined antigen associated with gastrointestinal cancer is a ganglioside containing sialylated lacto-N-fucopentose. J Biol Chem 257:14365–14369, 1982

465. Atkinson BF, Ernst CS, Herlyn M et al: Gastrointentinal cancer-associated antigen in immunoperoxidase assay. Cancer Res 42:4820–4823, 1982

466. Herlyn D, Herlyn M, Steplewski Z, Koprowski H: Monoclonal antibodies in cell mediated cytotoxicity against human melanoma and colorectal carcinoma. Eur J Immunol 9:657–659, 1979

467. Herlyn D, Steplewski Z, Herlyn M, Koprowski H: Inhibition of growth of colorectal carcinoma in nude mice by monoclonal antibody. Cancer Res 40:717–721, 1980

468. Johnson VG, Schlom J, Patterson AJ et al: Analysis of a human tumor associated glycoprotein (TAG-72) identified by monoclonal antibody B72-3. Cancer Res 46:850-857, 1986

469. Lottich SC, Szpak CA, Johnston WW et al: Phenotypic heterogeneity of a tumor-associated antigen in adenocarcinomas of the colon and their metastases as demonstrated by monoclonal antibody B72.3. Cancer Invest 4:387-395, 1986

470. Skinner JM, Whitehead R: Tumor-associated antigens in polyps and carcinoma of the large bowel. Cancer 47:1241-1245, 1981

471. Campo E, Palacin A, Benasco C et al: Human chorionic gonadotropin in colorectal carcinoma. Cancer 49:1611-1616, 1987

472. Lambert R, Sobin LH, Waye JD et al: The management of patients with colorectal adenomas. CA 34:167-176, 1984

473. Wegener M, Borsch G, Schmidt G: Colorectal adenomas: Distribution, incidence of malignant transformation, and rate of recurrence. Dis Colon Rectum 29:383-387, 1986

474. Neugut AI, Johnsen CM, Forde KA et al: Recurrence rates for colorectal polyps. Cancer 55:1586-1589, 1985

475. Nava H, Carlsson G, Petrelli NJ et al: Followup colonoscopy in patients with colorectal adenomatous polyps. Dis Colon Rectum 30:465-468, 1987

476. Nivatvongs S, Nicholson JD, Rothenberger DA et al: Villous adenomas of the rectum: The accuracy of clinical assessment. Surgery 87:549-551, 1980

477. Taylor EW, Thompson H, Oates GD et al: Limitations of biopsy in reoperative assessment of villous papilloma. Dis Colon Rectum 24:259-262, 1981

478. Groff W, Rubin RJ, Salvati EP et al: A method of management of a circumferential villous tumor of the rectum. Dis Colon Rectum 24:151-154, 1981

479. Pello MJ: Transanal excision of large sessile villous adenomas using an endorectal traction flap. Surg Gynecol Obstet 164:281-279, 1987

480. Bess MA, Adson MA, Elveback LR, Moertel CG: Rectal cancer following colectomy for polyposis. Arch Surg 115:460-467, 1980

481. Bussey HJR, Eyers AA, Ritchie SM et al: The rectum in adenomatous polyposis: The St. Mark's policy. Br J Surg 72:S29-S35, 1985

482. Moertel CG, Hill JR, Adson MA: Management of multiple polyposis of the large bowel. Cancer 28:160-164, 1971

483. Harvey JC, Quan SHQ, Stearns MW: Management of familial polyposis with preservation of the rectum. Surgery 84:476-482, 1978

484. Sarre RG, Jagelman DG, Beck GJ et al: Colectomy with ileorectal anastomosis for familial adenomatous polyposis: The risk of rectal cancer. Surgery 101:20-26, 1986

485. Heimann TM, Gelernt I, Salky B et al: Familial polyposis coli: Results of mucosal proctectomy with ileoanal anastomosis. Dis Colon Rectum 30:424-427, 1987

486. Herrera-Irbelas L (ed): Familial polyposis coli. Semin Surg Oncol 3:66-139, 1987

487. Kewenter J, Hulten L, Ahren C: The occurrence of severe epithelial dysplasia and its bearing on treatment of longstanding ulcerative colitis. Ann Surg 195:209-213, 1982

488. Nugent FW, Haggitt RC, Colcher H et al: Malignant potential of chronic ulcerative colitis. Gastroenterology 76:1-5, 1979

489. Lennard-Jones JE, Morson BC, Ritchie JK et al: Cancer and colitis—assessment of the individual risk by clinical and histological criteria. Gastroenterology 73:1280-1289, 1977

490. Lennard-Jones JE; Cancer risk in ulcerative colitis—surveillance or surgery? Br J Surg 72(suppl):S84-S86, 1985

491. Rosenstock E, Farmer RG, Petras R et al: Surveillance for colonic carcinoma in ulcerative colitis. Gastroenterology 89:1342-1346, 1985

492. Wong WD, Rothenberger DA, Goldberg SA: Ileoanal pouch procedures. Curr Probl Surg 22:1-78, 1985

493. Taylor BA, Dozois RR: The J ileal pouch-anal anastomosis. World J Surg 11:727-734, 1987

494. Enker WE, Laffer UT, Block GE: Enhanced survival of patients with colon and rectal cancer is based upon wide anatomic resection. Ann Surg 190:350-360, 1979

495. Grinnell RS: Results of ligation of inferior mesenteric artery at the aorta in resections of carcinoma of the descending and sigmoid colon and rectum. Surg Gynecol Obstet 120:1031-1036, 1965

496. Ault GW: A technique for cancer isolation and extended dissection for cancer of the distal colon and rectum. Surg Gynecol Obstet 106:467-477, 1958

497. Cole WH, Roberts SS, Strehl FW: Modern concepts of cancer of the colon and rectum. Cancer 19:1347-1358, 1966

498. Turnbull RB Jr, Kyle K, Watson FR, Spratt J: Cancer of the colon: The influence of the no-touch isolation technique on survival rates. Ann Surg 166:420-427, 1967

499. Wiggers T, Jeekel J, Arends JW et al: The no-touch isolation technique in colon cancer: A prospective controlled multi-center trial. Proc Am Soc Clin Oncol 5:269, 1986

500. Cohn I Jr, Gonzalez EA Jr, Atik M: Spillage and recurrence of colonic carcinoma. Surg Forum 12:153-155, 1961

501. Cohn I Jr, Floyd CE, Atik M: Control of tumor implantation during operations on the colon. Ann Surg 157:825-838, 1963

502. Cohn I Jr, Corley RG, Floyd CE: Iodized suture for control of tumor implantation in a colon anastomosis. Surg Gynecol Obstet 116:366-370, 1963

503. Douglass HO Jr, LeVeen HH: Tumor recurrence in colon anastomoses: Prevention by coagulation and fixation with formalin. Ann Surg 173:201-205, 1971

504. MacKeigan JM, Ferguson JA: Prophylactic oophorectomy in colorectal cancer in premenopausal patients. Dis Colon Rectum 22:401-405, 1979

505. Cutait R, Lesser ML, Enker WE: Prophylactic oophorectomy in surgery for large bowel cancer. Dis Colon Rectum 26:6-11, 1983

506. Graffner HOL, Alm POA, Oscarson JEA: Prophylactic oophorectomy in colorectal carcinoma. Am J Surg 146:233-235, 1983

507. O'Brien PH, Newton BB, Metcalf JS et al: Oophorectomy in women with carcinoma of the colon and rectum. Surg Gynecol Obstet 153:827-830, 1981

508. Blamey S, McDermott F, Pihl E et al: Ovarian involvement in adenocarcinoma of the colon and rectum. Surg Gynecol Obstet 153:42-44, 1981

509. Herrerra LO, Ledesma E, Natarajan N et al: Metachronous ovarian metastases from adenocarcinoma of the colon and rectum. Surg Gynecol Obstet 154:531-534, 1982

510. Morrow M, Enker WE: Late ovarian metastases in carcinoma of the colon and rectum. Arch Surg 119:1385-1388, 1984

511. Ballantyne GH, Raigel MM, Wolff BG et al: Oophorectomy in colon cancer: Impact on survival. Ann Surg 202:209-214, 1985

512. Wolmark N, Gordon PH, Fisher B et al: A comparison of stapled and hand-sewn anastomoses in patients undergoing resection of Duke's B and C colorectal cancer: An analysis of disease-free survival and survival from the NSABP prospective trials. Dis Colon Rectum 29:344-350, 1986

513. Davis CJ, Ilstrup DM, Pemberton JH: Influence of splenectomy on survival rate of patients with colorectal cancer. Am J Surg 155:173-179, 1988

514. Wolmark N, Fisher B, Wieand HS: The prognostic value of modifications of the Duke's C class of colorectal cancer: An analysis of the NSABP clinical trials. Ann Surg 203:115-122, 1986

515. Cass AW, Million RR, Pfaff WW: Patterns of recurrence following surgery alone for adenocarcinoma of the colon and rectum. Cancer 37:2861-2865, 1976

515a. Welch JP, Donaldson GA: The clinical correlation of an autopsy study of recurrent colorectal cancer. Ann Surg 189:496-502, 1979

516. Russell AH, Pelton J, Reheis CE et al: Adenocarcinoma of the colon: An autopsy study with implications for new therapeutic strategies. Cancer 56:1446-1451, 1985

517. Enker WE, Dragacevic S: Multiple carcinomas of the large bowel. Ann Surg 187:8-11, 1978

518. Langevin JM, Nivatvongs S: The true incidence of synchronous cancer of the large bowel. Am J Surg 147:330-333, 1984

519. Isler JJm Brown PC, Lewis FG et al: The role of preoperative colonoscopy in colorectal cancer. Dis Colon Rectum 30:435-439, 1987

520. Kelly WE Jr, Brown PW, Lawrence W, Tertz JJ: Penetrating, obstructing, and perforating carcinomas of the colon and rectum. Arch Surg 116:381-384, 1985

521. Gall FP, Tonak J, Altendorf A: Multivisceral resections in colorectal cancer. Dis Colon Rectum 30:337-341, 1987

522. Hunter JA, Ryan JA Jr, Schultz P: En bloc resection of colon cancer adherent to other organs. Am J Surg 154:67-71, 1987

523. Wolff WI, Shinya H: Definitive treatment of "malignant" polyps of the colon. Ann Surg 182:516-524, 1975

524. Wilcox GM, Beck JR: Early invasive cancer in adenomatous colonic polyps: Valuation of the therapeutic options by decision analysis. Gastroenterology 92:1159-1168, 1987

525. Cranley JP, Petras RE, Carey WD et al: When is endoscopic polypectomy adequate therapy for colonic polyps containing invasive carcinoma? Gastroenterology 91:419-427, 1987

526. Wilcox JM, Anderson PB, Colaccio TA: Early invasive carcinoma in colonic polyps: A review of the literature with emphasis on the assessment of the risk of metastasis. Cancer 57:160-171, 1986

527. Haggitt RC, Glotzbach RE, Soffer EE et al: Prognostic factors in colorectal carcinomas arising in adenomas: Implications for lesions removed by endoscopic polypectomy. Gastroenterology 89:328-336, 1985

528. Bartnik W, Butruk E, Orlowska J: A conservative approach to adenomas containing invasive carcinoma removed colonoscopically. Dis Colon Rectum 28:673-675, 1985

529. Colaccio TA, Forde KA, Scantlebury VP: Endoscopic polypectomy: Inadequate treatment for invasive colorectal carcinoma. Ann Surg 194:704-707, 1981

530. Nivatvongs S: Management of polyps containing invasive carcinoma. In Codner IJ, Fry RD, Roe JP (eds): Colon, Rectal, and Anal Surgery 1985, pp 183-188. St Louis, CV Mosby, 1985

531. Grinnell RS, Lane N: Benign and malignant adenomatous polyps and papillary adenomas of the colon and rectum: An analysis of 1,856 tumors in 1,335 patients. Int Abstr Surg 106:519, 1958

532. Waye JD, Frankel A: Treatment of early colon cancer. Gastroenterology 66:796, 1974

533. Locke MR, Cairns DW, Ritchie JK, Lockhart-Mummery HE: The treatment of early colorectal cancer by local excision. Br J Surg 65:346-349, 1978

534. Kodaira S, Teramoto T, Oro S et al: Lymph node metastases from carcinomas developing in pedunculated and semi-pedunculated colorectal adenomas. Aust NZ J Surg 51:429-433, 1981

535. Shatney CH, Lober PH, Gilbertsen VA, Sosin H: The treatment of pedunculated adenomatous colorectal polyps with focal cancer. Surg Gynecol Obstet 139:845-850, 1974

536. Coutsoftides T, Lavery I, Benjamin SP, Sivak MV Jr: Malignant polyps of the colon and rectum: A clinical pathological study. Dis Colon Rectum 22:82-86, 1979

537. Gunderson LL, Russell AH, Llewellyn HJ et al: Treatment planning for colorectal cancer: Radiation and surgical techniques and value of small-bowel films. Int J Radiat Oncol Biol Phys 11:1379-1393, 1985

538. Kopelson G: Adjuvant postoperative radiation therapy for colorectal carcinoma

above the peritoneal reflection: II. Antimesenteric wall ascending and descending colon and cecum. Cancer 52:633–636, 1983

539. Loeffler RK: Postoperative radiation therapy for adenocarcinoma of the cecum using two fractions/day. Int J Radiat Oncol Biol Phys 10:1881–1883, 1984

540. Shehata WM, Meyer RL, Jazy FK et al: Regional adjuvant irradiation for adenocarcinoma of the cecum. Int J Radiat Oncol Biol Phys 13:843–846, 1987

541. Wong CS, Harwood AR, Cummings BJ et al: Postoperative local abdominal irradiation for cancer of the colon above the peritoneal reflection. Int J Radiat Oncol Biol Phys 11:2067–2071, 1985

542. Duttenhaver JR, Hoskins RB, Gunderson LL et al: Adjuvant postoperative radiation therapy in the management of adenocarcinoma of the colon. Cancer 57:955–963, 1986

543. Kopelson G: Adjuvant postoperative radiation therapy for colorectal carcinoma above the peritoneal reflection: I. Sigmoid colon. Cancer 51:1593–1598, 1983

544. Richards F II, Atkins JN, Scarantino C et al: Phase I study of intraperitoneal 5-fluorouracil (IP-5FU) with local radiation therapy (RT) as adjuvant therapy in stage B3 and C1, 2, 3 colon cancer (abst). Proc Am Soc Clin Oncol 5:80, 1986

545. Turner SS, Vieira EF, Ager PJ et al: Elective postoperative radiotherapy for locally advanced colorectal cancer: A preliminary report. Cancer 140:105–108, 1977

546. Ghossein NA, Ager PJ, Ragins H et al: The treatment of locally advanced carcinoma of the colon and rectum by a surgical procedure and radiotherapy postoperatively. Surg Gynecol Obstet 148:917–920, 1979

547. Ghossein NA, Samala EC, Alpert S et al: Elective postoperative radiotherapy after incomplete resection of colorectal cancer. Dis Colon Rectum 24:252–256, 1981

548. Meek AG, Lam WC, Order SE: Carcinoma of the colon: Irradiation by delayed split whole-abdominal technique. Radiology 148:845–849, 1983

549. Wong CS, Harwood AR, Cummings BJ et al: Total abdominal irradiation for cancer of the colon. Radiother Oncol 2:209–214, 1984

550. Fabian CJ, Reddy E, Jewell et al: Phase I–II pilot of whole abdominal radiation and concomitant 5-FU as an adjuvant in colon cancer. A Southwest Oncology Group Study (unpublished manuscript)

551. Dixon WJ, Longmire WP Jr, Holden WD: Use of triethylenethiophosphomamide as adjuvant to the surgical treatment of gastric and colorectal cancer: Ten year follow-up. Ann Surg 173:26–39, 1971

552. Dwight RW, Humphrey EW, Higgins GA et al: FUDR as an adjuvant to surgery in cancer of the large bowel. J Surg Oncol 5:243–249, 1973

553. Higgins GA, Lee LE, Dwight RW et al: The case for adjuvant 5-fluorouracil in colorectal cancer. Cancer Clin Trials 1:35–41, 1978

554. Grage TB, Moss SE: Adjuvant chemotherapy in cancer of the colon and rectum: Demonstration of effectiveness of prolonged 5-FU chemotherapy in a prospectively controlled randomized trial. Surg Clin North Am 61:1321–1329, 1981

555. Buysce ME, Zeleniuch-Jacquotte A, Chalmers TC: Adjuvant therapy of colorectal cancer: Why we still don't know (unpublished manuscript)

556. Macdonald JS: Adjuvant therapy of gastrointestinal cancer. In Salmon SE (ed): Adjuvant Therapy of Cancer V, pp 479–496. New York, Grune & Stratton, 1987

557. Higgins GA, Amadeo JH, McElhinney J et al: Efficacy of prolonged intermittent therapy with combined 5-fluorouracil and me-CCNU following resection for carcinoma of the large bowel. Cancer 53:1–8, 1984

558. Gastrointestinal Tumor Study Group: Adjuvant therapy of colon cancer: Results of a prospectively randomized trial. N Engl J Med 310:737–743, 1984

559. Wolmark N, Fisher B, Rockette H: Adjuvant therapy in carcinoma of the colon: Five year results of NSABP protocol C-01. In Salmon SE (ed): Adjuvant Therapy of Cancer V, pp 531–536. New York, Grune & Stratton, 1987

560. Panettiere FJ, Chen TT: The SWOG large bowel study benefits from therapy (abst). Proc Am Soc Clin Oncol 4:76, 1985

561. Laurie J, Moertel C, Flemming T et al: Surgical adjuvant therapy of poor prognosis colorectal cancer with levamisole alone or combined levamisole and 5-fluorouracil: A North Central Cancer Treatment Group and Mayo Clinic Study (abst). Proc Am Soc Clin Oncol 5:81, 1986

562. Verhaegen H, DeCree J, DeCock W et al: Levamisole therapy in patients with colorectal cancer. In Terry WD, Rosenberg SA (eds): Immunotherapy of Human Cancer, pp 225–230. New York, Excerpta Medica, 1982

563. Pestana C, Reitemeyer RJ, Moertel CG et al: The natural history of carcinoma of the colon and rectum. Am J Surg 108:826–829, 1964

564. Taylor I, Machin D, Mullee M et al: A randomized controlled trial of adjuvant portal vein cytotoxic perfusion in colorectal cancer. Br J Surg 72:359–362, 1985

565. Gray BN, deZwart J, Fisher R et al: The Australia and New Zealand Trial of Adjuvant Chemotherapy in Colon Cancer. In Salmon SE (ed): Adjuvant Therapy of Cancer V, pp 537–554. New York, Grune & Stratton, 1987

566. Metzger U, Mermillod B, Aeberhard P et al: Intraportal chemotherapy in colorectal carcinoma as an adjuvant modality. World J Surg 11:452–458, 1987

567. Williams NS: The rationale for preservation of the anal sphincter in patients with low rectal cancer. Br J Surg 71:575–518, 1984

568. Williams NS, Dixon MF, Johnston D: Reappraisal of the 5 centimetre rule of distal excision for carcinoma of the rectum: A study of distal intramural spread and of patients' survival. Br J Surg 70:150–154, 1983

569. Madsen PM, Christiansen J: Distal intramural spread of rectal carcinomas. Dis Colon Rectum 29:279–282, 1986

570. Hojo K: Anastomotic recurrence after sphincter-saving resection for rectal cancer: Length of distal clearance of the bowel. Dis Colon Rectum 29:11–14, 1986

571. Pollett WG, Nicholls RJ: The relationship between the extent of distal clearance and survival and local recurrence rates after curative anterior resection for carcinoma of the rectum. Ann Surg 198:159–163, 1984

572. Pezim ME, Nicholls RJ: Survival after high or low ligation of the inferior mesenteric artery during curative surgery for rectal cancer. Ann Surg 200:729–733, 1984

573. Hojo K, Koyama Y, Moriya Y: Lymphatic spread and its prognostic value in patients with rectal cancer. Am J Surg 144:350–354, 1982

574. Grinnell RS: Results of ligation of inferior mesenteric artery at the aorta in resections of carcinoma of the descending and sigmoid colon and rectum. Surg Gynecol Obstet 120:1031–1036, 1965

575. Heald RJ, Husband EM, Ryall RDH: The meso-rectum in rectal cancer surgery: The clue to pelvic recurrence? Br J Surg 69:613–616, 1982

576. Heald RJ, Ryall RDH: Recurrence and survival after total meso-rectal excision for rectal cancer. Lancet 1:1479–1482, 1986

576a. Quirke P, Durdey P, Dixon MF et al: Local recurrence of rectal adenocarcinoma due to inadequate surgical resection. Histopathological study of lateral tumor spread and surgical excision. Lancet 1:996–999, 1986

577. Deddish MR: Surgical procedures for carcinoma of the left colon and rectum with five year end results following abdomino-pelvic dissection of lymph nodes. Am J Surg 99:188–191, 1960

578. Enker WE, Laffer UT, Block GE: Enhanced survival of patients with colon and rectal cancer is based upon wide anatomic resection. Ann Surg 190:350–360, 1979

579. Hojo K, Koyama Y: The effectiveness of wide anatomical resection and radical lymphadenectomy for patients with rectal cancer. Jpn J Surg 12:111–116, 1982

580. Koyama Y, Moriya Y, Hojo K: Effects of extended systemic lymphadenectomy for adenocarcinoma of the rectum: Significant improvement of survival rate and decrease of local recurrence. Jpn J Clin Oncol 14:623–632, 1984

581. Enker E, Heilweil ML, Hertz REL et al: En bloc pelvic lymphadenopathy and sphincter preservation in the surgical management of rectal cancer. Ann Surg 203:426–433, 1986

582. Glass RE, Ritchie JK, Thompson HR et al: The results of surgical treatment of cancer of the rectum by radical resection and extended abdomino-iliac lymphadenectomy. Br J Surg 72:599–601, 1985

583. Beart RW Jr, Kelly KA: Randomized prospective evaluation of the EEA stapler for colorectal anastomoses. Am J Surg 141:143–147, 1981

584. McGinn FP, Gartell PC, Clifford PC et al: Staples or sutures for low colorectal anastomoses: A prospective randomized trial. Br J Surg 72:603–605, 1985

585. Donaldson GA, Rodkey GV, Behringer GE: Resection of the rectum with anal preservation. Surg Gynecol Obstet 123:571–580, 1966

586. Localio SA, Eng K, Coppa GF: Abdominosacral resection for mid-rectal cancer. Ann Surg 198:320–324, 1983

587. Higgins GA, Humphrey EW, Dwight RW et al: Preoperative radiation and surgery for cancer of the rectum: Veterans Administration Surgical Oncology Group trial II. Cancer 58:352–359, 1986

588. Mohiuddin M, Yelovich RM, Komarnicky LT et al: Preoperative radiation and surgery in unfavorable cancers of the rectum (abst). Proc Am Soc Clin Oncol 6:97, 1987

589. Cutait DE, Cutait R, Ioshimoto M et al: Abdominoperineal endoanal pull-through resection: A comparative study between immediate and delayed colorectal anastomosis. Dis Colon Rectum 28:294–299, 1985

590. Enker WE, Stearns MW Jr, Janov AJ: Peranal coloanal anastomosis following low anterior resection for rectal carcinoma. Dis Colon Rectum 28:576–581, 1985

591. Parks AG, Percy JP: Resection and sutured colo-anal anastomosis for rectal carcinoma. Br J Surg 69:301–304, 1982

592. Welch JP, Donaldson GA: Recent experience in the management of cancer of the colon and rectum. Am J Surg 127:258–266, 1974

593. McDermott FT, Hughes ESR, Pihl EA et al: Changing survival prospects in rectal carcinoma: A series of 1,306 patients managed by one surgeon. Dis Colon Rectum 29:798–803, 1986

594. Slanetz CA Jr, Herter FP, Grinnell RS: Anterior resection versus abdominoperineal resection for cancer of the rectum and rectosigmoid. Am J Surg 123:110–117, 1972

595. Hargrove WC III, Gertner MH, Fitts WT Jr: The Kraske operation for carcinoma of the rectum. Surg Gynecol Obstet 148:931–933, 1979

596. Bevan AD: Carcinoma of the rectum: Treatment by local excision. Dis Colon Rectum 29:906–910, 1986

597. Madden JL, Kandalaft SI: Electrocoagulation as a primary curative method in the treatment of carcinoma of the rectum. Surg Gynecol Obstet 157:164–179, 1983

598. Crile G, Turnbull RB: Role of electrocoagulation in the treatment of carcinoma of the rectum. Surg Gynecol Obstet 135:391–396, 1972

599. Cummings BJ Jr, Rider WD, Harwood AR et al: Radical external beam radiation therapy for adenocarcinoma of the rectum. Dis Colon Rectum 26:30–36, 1983

600. Papillon J: New prospects in the conservative treatment of rectal cancer. Dis Colon Rectum 27:695–700, 1984

601. Lockhart-Mummery HE, Ritchie JK et al: The results of surgical treatment for carcinoma of the rectum at St. Marks Hospital from 1948 to 1972. Br J Surg 63:673–677, 1976

602. Whittaker M, Goligher JC: The prognosis after surgical treatment for carcinoma of the rectum. Br J Surg 63:384–388, 1976

602a. Wilson SM, Beahrs OH: A curative treatment of carcinoma of the sigmoid, recto-sigmoid and rectum. Ann Surg 183:556–565, 1976

602b. Accarpio G, Scopinaro G, Claudiani F et al: Experience with local rectal excision in light of two recent preoperative diagnostic methods. Dis Colon Rectum 30:296–298, 1987

602c. Allgower M, Durig M, Hochstetter A et al: The parasacral sphincter-splitting approach to the rectum. World J Surg 6:539–548, 1982

602d. Killingback MJ: Indications for local excision of rectal cancer. Br J Surg 2S:54–56, 1985

602e. Wilson E: Local treatment of cancer of the rectum. Dis Colon Rectum 16:194–199, 1973

602f. Mason AY: Transsphincteric approach to rectal lesions. Surg Ann 9:171–194, 1977

602g. Grigg M, McDermott FT, Pihl EA et al: Curative local excision in the treatment of carcinoma of the rectum. Dis Colon Rectum 27:81–83, 1984

602h. Whiteway J, Nicholls RJ, Morson BC: The role of surgical local excision in the treatment of rectal cancer. Br J Surg 72:694–697, 1985

602i. Hager T, Gall FP, Hermanek P: Local excision of cancer of the rectum. Dis Colon Rectum 26:149–151, 1983

603. Biggers OR, Beart RW Jr, Ilstrup DM: Local excision of rectal cancer. Dis Colon Rectum 29:374–377, 1986

604. Salvati EP, Rubin RJ: Electrocoagulation as primary therapy for rectal carcinoma. Am J Surg 132:583–586, 1976

605. Wanebo HJ, Quan SHQ: Failures of electrocoagulation of primary carcinoma of the rectum. Surg Gynecol Obstet 138:174–176, 1974

606. Eisenstat TE, Duke ST, Rubin RJ et al: Five year survival in patients with carcinoma of the rectum treated by electrocoagulation. Am J Surg 143:127–131, 1982

607. Sischy B, Granez MJ, Hinson EJ: Endocavitary irradiation for adenocarcinoma of the rectum. Cancer 34:333–339, 1984

608. Pilipshen SJ, Heilweil M, Quan SHQ et al: Patterns of pelvic recurrence following definitive resections of rectal cancer. Cancer 53:1354–1362, 1984

609. Phillips RKS, Hittinger R, Blesovsky L et al: Local recurrence following curative surgery for large bowel cancer. Br J Surg 71:17–20, 1984

610. McDermott FT, Hughes ESR, Pihl E et al: Local recurrence after potentially curative resection for rectal cancer in a series of 1,008 patients. Br J Surg 72:34–37, 1985

611. Jackman RJ: Conservative management of selected patients with carcinoma of the rectum. Dis Colon Rectum 4:429–434, 1961

612. Culp CE: Conservative management of certain selected cancers of the lower rectum: In Controversies in Surgery, pp 407–414. Philadelphia, WB Saunders, 1976

613. Gingold BS, Mitty WF Jr, Tadros M: Importance of patient selection in local treatment of carcinoma of the rectum. Am J Surg 145:293–296, 1983

614. Wittoesch JH, Jackman RS: Results of conservative management of cancer of the rectum in poor risk patients. Surg Gynecol Obstet 107:618, 1958

615. Deddish MR: Local excision. Surg Clin North Am 54:877–880, 1974

616. Stearns MW Jr, Sternberg SS, DeCosse JJ: Treatment alternatives: Localized rectal cancer. Cancer 54:2691–2694, 1984

617. Rich TA, Weiss DR, Mies C et al: Sphincter preservation in patients with low rectal cancer treated with radiation therapy with or without local excision or fulguration. Radiology 156:527–531, 1985

618. Enker WE, Kemeny N, Shank B et al: Defining the needs for adjuvant therapy of rectal and colonic cancer. Surg Clin North Am 61:1295–1310, 1981

619. Fortier GA, Krochak RJ, Kim JA et al: Dose response to preoperative irradiation in rectal cancer: Implications for local control and complications associated with sphincter sparing surgery and abdominal resection. Int J Radiat Oncol Biol Phys 12:1559–1563, 1986

620. Allee PE, Gunderson LL, Munzenrider JE: Postoperative radiation therapy for residual colorectal carcinoma (abst). Int J Radiat Oncol Biol Phys 7:1208, 1981

621. Powers WE, Tolmach LJ: Preoperative radiation therapy: Biological basis and experimental investigation. Nature 201:172–204, 1964

622. Higgins GA Jr, Conn JH, Jordan PH et al: Preoperative radiotherapy for colorectal cancer. Ann Surg 181:624–631, 1975

623. Boulis Wassif S, Langenhorst BL, Hop WCJ: The contribution of preoperative radiotherapy in the management of borderline operability rectal cancer. In: Jones SE, Salmon SE (eds): Adjuvant Therapy of Cancer II, pp 613–620. New York, Grune & Stratton, 1979

624. Kligerman MM, Urdanetta N, Knowlton A et al: Preoperative irradiation of rectosigmoid carcinoma including its regional lymph nodes. Am J Roentgenol Radium Ther Nucl Med 114:498–503, 1972

625. Kinsella TJ, Bloomer WD: Tolerance of the intestine to radiation therapy. Surg Gynecol Obstet 151:273–284, 1980

626. Maruyama Y, Van Nagell JR Jr, Utley J et al: Radiation and small bowel complications in cervical cancer. Radiology 112:699–703, 1974

627. Russ JE, Smoron GL, Gagnon JD: Omental transposition flap in colorectal carcinoma: Adjunctive use in prevention and treatment of radiation complications. Int J Radiat Oncol Biol Phys 10:55–62, 1984

628. Sugarbaker PH: Pelvic displacement prosthesis to prevent small bowel damage with pelvic irradiation. Surg Gynecol Obstet 157:269–271, 1983

629. Devereux DF, Kavanah MT, Feldman MI et al: Small bowel exclusion from the pelvis by a polyglycolic acid mesh sling. Surg Oncol 26:107–112, 1984

630. Kavanah MT, Feldman MI, Devereux DF et al: New surgical approach to minimize radiation-associated small bowel injury in patients with pelvic malignancies requiring surgery and high-dose irradiation: A preliminary report. Cancer 56:1300–1304, 1985

631. Devereux DF, Chandler JJ, Eisenstat T et al: Efficacy of an absorbable mesh in keeping the small bowel out of the human pelvis following surgery. Dis Colon Rectum 31:17–21, 1988

632. Dische S, Dowdell JW: A method to reduce radiation injury to intestine—a preliminary report. Radiother Oncol 1:277–279, 1984

633. Green N, Iba G, Smith WR: Measures to minimize small intestine injury in the irradiated pelvis. Cancer 35:1633–1640, 1975

634. Green N: The avoidance of small intestine injury in gynecologic cancer. Int J Rad Oncol Biol Phys 9:1385–1390, 1983

635. Gallagher MJ, Brereton HD, Rostock RA et al: A prospective study of treatment techniques to minimize the volume of pelvic small bowel with reduction of acute and late effects associated with pelvic irradiation. Int J Rad Oncol Biol Phys 12:1565–1573, 1986

636. Pezner R, Archambeau JO: Critical evaluation of the role of nutritional support for radiation therapy patients. Cancer 55:263–267, 1985

637. McArdle AH, Wittnich C, Duguid W, Freeman CR: The use of an elemental diet as prophylaxis in radiation enteropathy. [Works-in-Progress]. Am Soc Ther Radiol Mtg., September, 1981

638. McArdle AH, Reid EC, Laplante HP et al: Prophylaxis against radiation injury: The use of elemental diet prior and during radiotherapy for invasive bladder cancer and in early postoperative feeding following radical cystectomy and ileal conduit. Arch Surg 121:879–885, 1986

639. Stryker JA, Bartholomew M: Failure of lactose-restricted diets to prevent radiation-induced diarrhea in patients undergoing whole pelvic irradiation. Int J Radiat Oncol Biol Phys 12:789–792, 1986

640. Shike M: Personal communication, 1987

641. Ito H, Meistrich ML, Barkley HT Jr et al: Protection of acute and late radiation damage of the gastrointestinal tract by WR-2721. Int J Radiat Oncol Biol Phys 12:211–219, 1986

642. Travis EL, Thames HD Jr, Tucker SL et al: Protection of mouse jejunal crypt cells by WR-2721 after small doses of radiation. Int J Radiat Oncol Biol Phys 12:807–814, 1986

643. Hanson WR, Thomas C: 16,16-dimethyl prostaglandin E$_2$ increases survival of murine intestinal stem cells when given before photon radiation. Radiat Res 96:393–398, 1983

644. Stearns MW Jr, Deddish MR, Quan SH et al: Preoperative roentgen therapy for cancer of the rectum. Surg Gynecol Obstet 109:285–289, 1959

645. Quan SHQ, Deddish MR, Stearns MW: The effect of preoperative roentgen therapy upon the 10- and 5-year results of the surgical treatment of cancer of the rectum. Surg Gynecol Obstet 111:507–508, 1960

646. Gary-Bobo J, Pujol H, Solassol CI et al: L'irradiation préoperatoire du cancer rectal: résultats a 5 ans de 116 cas. Bull Cancer [Paris] 66:491–496, 1979

647. Glimelius B, Graffman S, Pahlman et al: Preoperative irradiation with high-dose fractionation in adenocarcinoma of the rectum and rectosigmoid. Acta Radiol Oncol 21:373–379, 1982

648. Mendenhall WM, Million RR, Bland KI et al: Preoperative radiation therapy for clinically resectable adenocarcinoma of the rectum. Ann Surg 202:215–222, 1985

649. Friedmann P, Garb JL, Park WC et al: Survival following moderate-dose preoperative radiation therapy for carcinoma of the rectum. Cancer 55:967–973, 1985

650. Roe JP, Kodner IH, Walz B et al: Preoperative radiation therapy for rectal carcinoma. Dis Colon Rectum 25:471–473, 1982

651. Papillon J: The future of external beam irradiation as initial treatment of rectal cancer. Br J Surg 74:449–454, 1987

652. Stevens KR Jr, Fletcher WS, Allen CV: A review of the value of radiation therapy for adenocarcinoma of the rectum and sigmoid. Front Gastrointest Res 5:93–101, 1979

653. Sischy B: The place of radiotherapy in the management of rectal adenocarcinoma. Cancer 50:2631–2637, 1982

654. Gerard A, Berrod J-L, Pene F et al: Interim analysis of a phase III study on preoperative radiation therapy in resectable rectal carcinoma: Trial of the Gastrointestinal Tract Cancer Cooperative Group of the European Organization for Research on Treatment of Cancer (EORTC). Cancer 55:2373–2379, 1985

655. Rider WD, Palmer JA, Mahoney LJ et al: Preoperative irradiation in operable cancer of the rectum: Report of the Toronto Trial. Can J Surg 20:335–338, 1977

655a. Duncan W: Adjuvant radiotherapy in rectal cancer: The MRC trials. Br J Surg 72 (suppl):S59–S62, 1985

656. Stockholm Rectal Cancer Study Group: Short-term preoperative radiotherapy for adenocarcinoma of the rectum. Am J Clin Oncol 10:369–375, 1987

657. Roswit B, Higgins GA Jr, Keehn R: Preoperative irradiation for carcinoma of the rectum and rectosigmoid colon: Report of a national Veterans Administration randomized study. Cancer 35:1597–1602, 1975

658. Higgins GA, Humphrey EW, Dwight RW et al: Preoperative radiation and surgery for cancer of the rectum: Veterans Administration Surgical Oncology Group trial II. Cancer 58:352–359, 1986

659. Dedkov IP, Zibina MA: Intensive preoperative gammatherapy in combined treatment of cancer of the rectum. Am J Proctol 27:43–47, 1976

660. Simbirtseva LP, Sneshko LI, Smirnov NM: Results of intensive combined therapy for carcinoma of the rectum. Vopr Oncol 21:7–12, 1975

661. Duncan W, Smith AN, Freedman LS et al: A trial of preoperative radiotherapy in the management of operable rectal cancer: First report of an MRC working party. Br J Surg 69:513–519, 1982

662. Tepper JE, Cohen AM, Wood WC et al: Postoperative radiation therapy of rectal cancer. Int J Radiat Oncol Biol Phys 13:5–10, 1987

663. Bruckner R, Kempf P, Kutzner J, Brunner H: Preliminary results of preoperative radiotherapy in carcinoma of the rectum. Dtsch Med Wochenschr 102:195–198, 1977

664. Kutzner J, Bruckner R, Kempf P: Präoperative Strahlentherapie beim Rektum Karzinomen. Strahlenther 160:236–238, 1984

665. Gerard A: Personal communication, 1988

666. Vigliotti A, Rich TA, Romsdahl MM et al: Postoperative adjuvant radiotherapy for

adenocarcinoma of the rectum and rectosigmoid. Int J Radiat Oncol Biol Phys 13:999–1006, 1987

667. Pahlman L, Glimelius B, Graffman S: Pre- versus postoperative radiotherapy in rectal carcinoma: An interim report from a randomized multicentre trial. Br J Surg 72:961–966, 1985

668. Mohiuddin M, Derdel J, Marks G et al: Results of adjuvant radiation therapy in cancer of the rectum: Thomas Jefferson University Hospital experience. Cancer 55:350–353, 1985

669. Douglass HO, Moertel CG, Mayer RJ et al: Survival after postoperative combination treatment of rectal cancer. N Engl J Med 315:1294–1295, 1986

670. Fisher B, Wolmark N, Rockette HE et al: Adjuvant chemotherapy or postoperative radiation for rectal cancer: Five year results of NSABP R01. In Salmon SE (ed): Adjuvant Therapy of Cancer V, pp 547–554. New York, Grune & Stratton, 1987

671. Balslev I, Pedersen M, Teglbjaerg PS et al: Postoperative radiotherapy in Dukes' B and C carcinoma of the rectum and rectosigmoid: A randomized multicenter study. Cancer 58:22–28, 1986

672. Thomas PRM, Lindblad AS, Stablein DM et al: Toxicity associated with adjuvant postoperative therapy for adenocarcinoma of the rectum. Cancer 57:1130–1134, 1986

673. Gunderson LL, Dosoretz DE, Hedberg SE et al: Low-dose preoperative irradiation, surgery, and elective postoperative radiation therapy for resectable rectum and rectosigmoid carcinoma. Cancer 52:446–451, 1983

674. Brenner S, Lanter BH, Seligman BR: Adjuvant therapy in treatment of rectal carcinoma (abst). Int J Radiat Oncol Biol Phys 6:1378, 1980

675. Shank B, Enker W, Santana J et al: Local control with pre-operative radiotherapy alone versus "sandwich" radiotherapy for rectal carcinoma. Int J Radiat Oncol Biol Phys 13:111–115, 1987

676. Krook J, Moertel C, Wieand H et al: Radiation vs. sequential chemotherapy–radiation–chemotherapy: A study of the North Central Cancer Treatment Group, Duke University and the Mayo Clinic. Proc Am Soc Clin Oncol 5:82, 1986

677. Boulis-Wassif S, Gerard A, Loygue J et al: Final results of a randomized trial on the treatment of rectal cancer with preoperative radiotherapy alone or in combination with 5-fluorouracil, followed by radical surgery. Cancer 53:1811–1818, 1984

678. Boey J, Wong J, Ong GB: Pelvic exenteration for locally advanced colorectal carcinoma. Ann Surg 195:513–518, 1982

679. Ledesma EJ, Bruno S, Mittelman A: Total pelvic exenteration in colorectal disease. Ann Surg 194:701–703, 1981

680. Bricker EM, Kraybill WG, Lopez MJ et al: The current role of ultraradical surgery in the treatment of pelvic cancer. Curr Probl Surg 23:871–953, 1986

681. Sugarbaker PH: Partial sacrectomy for en bloc excision of rectal cancer with posterior fixation. Dis Colon Rectum 25:708–711, 1982

682. Tierie AH: Radiotherapy in marginal resectable and non-resectable rectum cancer. Radiol Clin 47:222–227, 1978

683. Bjerkeset T, Dahl O: Irradiation and surgery for primarily inoperable rectal and adenocarcinoma. Dis Colon Rectum 23:298–303, 1980

684. Emami B, Pilepich M, Willett C et al: Effect of preoperative irradiation on resectability of colorectal carcinomas. Int J Radiat Oncol Biol Phys 8:1295–1299, 1982

685. Dosoretz DE, Gunderson LL, Hedberg S et al: Preoperative irradiation for unresectable rectal and rectosigmoid carcinomas. Cancer 52:814–818, 1983

686. Schnetzer G, Brickner T, Stone W et al: Adjuvant preoperative chemotherapy and radiation therapy in moderately advanced adenocarcinoma of rectum (abst). Proc Am Soc Clin Oncol 3:133, 1984

687. Haghbin M, Sischy B, Hinson J: Adjuvant preoperative irradiation and chemotherapy for primary large rectal carcinoma: nine-year follow-up (abst). Proc Am Soc Clin Oncol 5:80, 1986

688. Sedlacek S, Pearlman N: Locally advanced adenocarcinoma of the rectum (ACR): Concurrent preoperative chemotherapy (CT) and radiation therapy (RT) (abst). Proc Am Soc Clin Oncol 6:93, 1987

689. Taylor RE, Karr GR, Arnott SJ: External beam radiotherapy for rectal adenocarcinoma. Br J Surg 74:455–459, 1987

690. Cohen AM: Intraoperative radiation therapy for colorectal cancer. Probl Gen Surg 4:76–82, 1987

691. Gunderson LL, Cohen AC, Dosoretz DD et al: Residual, unresectable, or recurrent colorectal cancer: External beam irradiation and intraoperative electron beam boost ± resection. Int J Radiat Oncol Biol Phys 9:1597–1606, 1983

692. Gunderson LL, Martin JK Jr, Earle JD et al: Intraoperative and external beam irradiation with or without resection: Mayo pilot experience. Mayo Clin Proc 59:691–699, 1984

693. Gunderson LL, Martin JK, Beart RW et al: Intraoperative and external beam irradiation ± 5-FU for locally advanced colorectal cancer. Ann Surg (in press)

694. Tepper JE, Cohen AM, Wood WC et al: Intraoperative electron beam radiotherapy in the treatment of unresectable rectal cancer. Arch Surg 121:421–423, 1986

695. Calkins AR: Personal communication, 1987

696. Syed AMN, Puthawala A, Neblett D et al: Primary treatment of carcinoma of the lower rectum and anal canal by a combination of external irradiation and interstitial implant. Radiology 128:199–203, 1978

697. Puthawala AA, Syed AMN, Gates C et al: Definitive treatment of extensive anorectal carcinoma by external and interstitial irradiation. Cancer 50:1746–1750, 1982

698. Fourquet A, Enker WE, Shank B et al: The value of interstitial radiation in advanced and recurrent colorectal cancer. Endocr Hypertherm Oncol 1:113–117, 1985

699. Wang CC, Schulz MD: The role of radiation therapy in the management of carcinoma of the sigmoid, rectosigmoid and rectum. Radiology 79:1–5, 1962

700. Ghossein NA, Ager PJ, Ragins H et al: The treatment of locally advanced carcinoma of the colon and rectum by a surgical procedure and radiotherapy postoperatively. Surg Gynecol Obstet 148:917–920, 1979

701. Carter SK: Large bowel cancer: The current status of treatment. JNCI 56:3–10, 1976

702. August DA, Ottow RT, Sugarbaker PH: Clinical perspective of human colorectal cancer metastasis. Cancer Metastasis Rev 3:303–324, 1984

703. Sugarbaker PH, Gianola FJ, Dwyer A et al: A simplified plan for follow-up of patients with colon and rectal cancer supported by prospective studies of laboratory and radiologic test results. Surgery 102:79–87, 1987

704. Fletcher RH: Carcinoembryonic antigen. Ann Intern Med 104:66–73, 1986

705. Northover J: Carcinoembryonic antigen and recurrent colorectal cancer. Gut 27:117–122, 1986

706. Beart RW, Metzger PP, O'Connor MJ et al: Postoperative screening of patients with carcinoma of the colon. Dis Colon Rectum 24:585–589, 1981

707. Boey J, Cheung HC, Lai CK et al: A prospective evaluation of serum carcinoembryonic antigen levels in the management of colorectal carcinoma. World J Surg 8:279–286, 1984

708. Minton JP, James KK, Hurtubise PE et al: The use of serial carcinoembryonic antigen determinations to predict recurrence of carcinoma of the colon and the time for a second-look operation. Surg Gynecol Obstet 147:208–210, 1978

709. Smith AN, Gordon A, Browning GCP et al: Postoperative monitoring of CEA in the prediction of surgical outcome in colorectal cancer. J R Coll Surg Edinb 30:294–298, 1985

710. Sorokin JJ, Sugarbaker PH, Zamcheck N et al: Serial carcinoembryonic antigen assays: Use in detection of cancer recurrence. JAMA 228:49–53, 1974

711. Wanebo HJ: Are carcinoembryonic antigen levels of value in the curative management of colorectal cancer? Surgery 89:290–295, 1981

712. Sugarbaker PH, Zamcheck N, Moore FD: Assessment of serial carcinoembryonic antigen assays in postoperative detection of recurrent colorectal cancer. Cancer 38:2310–2315, 1976

713. Wedell J, Eisen PM, Luu TH et al: A retrospective study of serial CEA determinations in the early detection of recurrent colorectal cancer. Dis Colon Rectum 24:618–621, 1981

714. Moertel CG, Schutt AJ, Go LW: Carcinoembryonic antigen test for recurrent colorectal cancer. JAMA 239:1065–1066, 1978

715. Midiri G, Amanti C, Benedetti M et al: CEA tissue staining in colorectal cancer patients. Cancer 55:2624–2629, 1985

716. Focan C: Circadian CEA variability: When to sample. J Clin Oncol 3:607, 1985

717. Staab HJ, Anderer FA, Hornung A et al: Doubling time of circulating CEA and its relation to survival of patients with recurrent colorectal cancer. Br J Cancer 46:773–781, 1982

718. Denstman F, Rosen L, Khubchandani IT et al: Comparing predictive decision rules in postoperative CEA monitoring. Cancer 58:2089–2095, 1986

719. Vecchio TJ: Predictive value of a single diagnostic test in unselected populations. N Engl J Med 274:1171–1173, 1966

720. Martin EW Jr, Minton JP, Carey LC: CEA-directed second-look surgery in the asymptomatic patient after primary resection of colorectal cancer. Ann Surg 202:310–317, 1985

721. Neville AM: International Union Against Cancer Workshop on Immunodiagnosis. Cancer Res 46:3744–3746, 1986

722. Lind SE, Singer DE: Diagnosing liver metastases: A Bayesian analysis. J Clin Oncol 4:379–388, 1986

723. Tartter PI, Slater G, Gelernt I et al: Screening for liver metastases from colorectal cancer with carcinoembryonic antigen and alkaline phosphatase. Ann Surg 193:357–360, 1981

724. Kemeny NM, Ganteaume L, Goldberg DA et al: Preoperative staging with computerized axial tomography and biochemical laboratory tests in patients with hepatic metastases. Ann Surg 303:169–172, 1986

725. Podolsky DK, Weiser MM, Isselbacher KJ et al: A cancer-associated galactosyltransferase isoenzyme. N Engl J Med 299:703–705, 1978

726. Putzki H, Student A, Jablonski M et al: Comparison of the tumor marker CEA, TPA, and CA 19-9 in colorectal carcinoma. Cancer 59:223–226, 1987

727. Szymendera JJ, Nowacki MP, Kozlowicz-Gudzinska I et al: The value of serum levels of carcinoembryonic antigen, CEA, and gastrointestinal cancer antigen, GICA or CA 19-9, for preoperative staging and postoperative monitoring of patients with colorectal carcinoma. Dis Col Rectum 28:895–899, 1985

728. Novis BH, Gluck E, Thomas P et al: Serial levels of CA 19-9 and CEA in colonic cancer. J Clin Oncol 4:987–993, 1986

729. Smith TJ, Kemeny NM, Sugarbaker PH et al: A prospective study of hepatic imaging in the detection of metastatic disease. Ann Surg 195:486–491, 1982

730. Gunven P, Makuchi MM, Takayasu K et al: Preoperative imaging of liver metastases: Comparison of angiography, CT scan, and ultrasonography. Ann Surg 202:573–579, 1985

731. Stark DD, Felder RC, Wittenberg et al: Magnetic resonance imaging of cavernous hemangioma of the liver: Tissue specific characterization. Am J Radiol 145:213–222, 1985

732. Cohen AM: Needle biopsy technique to confirm suspected liver metastases at laparotomy. Surg Gynecol Obstet (in press)

733. McCormack PM, Attiyeh FF: Resected pulmonary metastases from colorectal cancer. Dis Colon Rectum 22:553–556, 1979

734. Patt YZ, Peters RE, Chuang VP et al: Palliation of pelvic recurrence of colorectal

cancer with intra-arterial 5-fluorouracil and mitomycin. Cancer 56:2175–2180, 1985

735. Estes NC, Morphis JG, Hornback NB, Jewell WR: Intraarterial chemotherapy and hyperthermia for pain control in patients with recurrent rectal cancer. Am J Surg 152:597–601, 1986

736. Dobrowsky W, Schmid AP: Radiotherapy of presacral recurrence following radical surgery for rectal carcinoma. Dis Colon Rectum 28:917–919, 1985

737. Pacini P, Cionini L, Pirtoll L et al: Symptomatic recurrence of carcinoma of the rectum and sigmoid: The influence of radiotherapy on the quality of life. Dis Colon Rectum 29:865–868, 1986

738. Benotti PN, Bothe A, Eyre RC et al: Management of recurrent pelvic tumor. Arch Surg 122:457–460, 1987

739. Pearlman NW, Donohue RE, Stiegmann GV et al: Pelvic and sacropelvic exenteration for locally advanced or recurrent anorectal cancer. Arch Surg 122:537–541, 1987

740. Wanebo HJ, Gaker DL, Whitehill R et al: Pelvic recurrence of rectal cancer: Options for curative resection. Presented at the 98th annual meeting of the Southern Surgical Association, Palm Beach, Fla, November–December, 1986

741. Beart RW Jr, Martin JK Jr, Gunderson LL: Management of recurrent rectal cancer. Mayo Clin Proc 61:448–450, 1986

742. Sannella NA: Abdominoperineal resection following anterior resection. Cancer 38:378–381, 1976

743. Vassilopoulos PP, Yoon JM, Ledesma EJ et al: Treatment of recurrence of adenocarcinoma of the colon and rectum at the anastomotic site. Surg Gynecol Obstet 152:777–780, 1981

744. Pihl E, Hughes ESR, McDermott FT et al: Recurrence of carcinoma of the colon and rectum at the anastomotic suture line. Surg Gynecol Obstet 153:495–496, 1981

745. Stearns MW Jr: Diagnosis and management of recurrent pelvic malignancy following combined abdominoperineal resection. Dis Colon Rectum 23:359–361, 1980

746. Polk HC Jr, Spratt JS Jr: The results of treatment of perineal recurrence of cancer of the rectum. Cancer 43:952–955, 1979

747. Wilking N, Herrera L, Petrelli NJ, Mittelman A: Pelvic and perineal recurrences after abdominoperineal resection for adenocarcinoma of the rectum. Am J Surg 150:561–563, 1985

748. Hine KR, Dykes PW: Prospective randomized trial of early cytotoxic therapy for recurrent colorectal carcinoma detected by serum CEA. Gut 25:682–688, 1984

749. Martin EW Jr, Cooperman M, King G et al: A retrospective and prospective study of serial CEA determinations in the early detection of recurrent colorectal cancer. Am J Surg 137:167–169, 1979

750. Martin EW Jr, Cooperman M, Carey LC, Minton JP: Sixty second-look procedures indicated primarily by rise in serial carcinoembryonic antigen. J Surg Res 28:389–394, 1980

751. Attiyeh FF, Stearns MW: Second-look laparotomy based on CEA elevations in colorectal cancer. Cancer 47:2119–2125, 1981

752. Staab HJ, Anderer FA, Stumpf E et al: Eighty-four second look operations based on sequential carcinoembryonic antigen determinations and clinical investigations in patients with recurrent gastrointestinal cancer. Am J Surg 179:198–204, 1985

753. Steele G Jr, Zamcheck N, Mayer R et al: Results of CEA-initiated second-look surgery for recurrent colorectal cancer. Am J Surg 139:544–548, 1980

754. Wilking N, Petrelli NJ, Derrera L et al: Abdominal exploration for suspected recurrent carcinoma of the colon and rectum based upon elevated carcinoembryonic antigen alone or in combination with other methods. Surg Gynecol Obstet 162:465–468, 1986

755. Sandler RS, Freund DA, Herbst CA et al: Cost effectiveness of postoperative carcinoembryonic antigen monitoring in colorectal cancer. Cancer 53:193–198, 1984

756. Northover J, Slack WW: A randomized controlled trial of CEA-prompted second look surgery in recurrent colorectal cancer: A preliminary report. Dis Colon Rectum 27:576, 1984

757. Beatty JD, Duda RB, Williams LE et al: Preoperative imaging of colorectal carcinoma with indium 111-labelled anticarcinoembryonic antigen monoclonal antibody. Cancer Res 46:6494–6502, 1986

758. Martin DT, Hinkel GH, Tuttle S et al: Intraoperative radio immunodetection of colorectal tumor with a hand-held radiation detector. Am J Surg 150:671–674, 1985

759. Lyden MJ, Thompson CH, Liechtenstein M et al: Visualization of metastases from colon carcinoma using an iodine 131-radio-labeled monoclonal antibody. Cancer 57:1135–1139, 1986

760. Begent RHJ, Keep PA, Searle F et al: Radioimmunolocalization and selection for surgery in recurrent colorectal cancer. Br J Surg 73:64–67, 1986

761. Heidelberger C, Chandhari NK, Dannenberg P et al: Fluorinated pyrimidines: A new class of tumor inhibitory compounds. Nature 179:665–666, 1957

762. Moertel CG, Reitemeyer RJ: Advanced Gastrointestinal Cancer: Clinical Management and Chemotherapy. New York, Harper & Row, 1969

763. Moertel CG: Large bowel. In Holland JF, Frei E (eds): Cancer Medicine, pp 1497–1626. Philadelphia, Lea & Febiger, 1973

764. Ansfield F, Klotz J, Nealor T et al: A phase III study comparing the clinical utility of four regimens of 5-fluorouracil. Cancer 39:34–40, 1977

765. Moertel CG: Clinical management of advanced gastrointestinal cancer. Cancer 36:675, 1975

766. Christophidis N, Vajda FJE, Lucas I et al: Fluorouracil therapy in patients with carcinoma of the large bowel: A pharmacokinetic comparison of various rates and routes of administration. Clin Pharmacokinet 3:330–336, 1978

767. Bateman J, Irwin L, Pugh R et al: Comparison of intravenous and oral administration of 5-fluorouracil for colorectal carcinoma. Proc Am Assoc Cancer Res 16:242, 1975

768. Hahn RG, Moertel CG, Shutt AJ et al: A double-blind comparison of intensive course 5-FU by oral vs. intravenous route in the treatment of colon carcinoma. Cancer 35:1031–1036, 1975

769. Lokich J, Bothe A, Fine N et al: Phase I study of protracted venous infusion of 5-fluorouracil. Cancer 48:2565–2568, 1981

770. Seifert P, Baker LH, Reed MD et al: Comparison of continuously infused 5-fluorouracil with bolus injection in treatment of patients with colorectal adenocarcinoma. Cancer 36:123–128, 1975

771. Caballero GA, Ausman RK, Quebbeman EJ: Long-term, ambulatory, continuous intravenous infusion of 5-fluorouracil for treatment of advanced adenocarcinoma. Cancer Treat Rep 69:13–15, 1985

772. Lokich J, Gillings D, Gallo J et al: Bolus versus infusion 5-fluorouracil (5-FU): A randomized clinical trial in advanced measurable colorectal cancer. Proc Am Soc Clin Oncol 5:83, 1986

773. Lokich JJ, Moor C: Chemotherapy associated palmar-plantar erythrodysesthesia syndrome. Ann Intern Med 101:798–800, 1984

774. Quebbeman E, Ausman R, Hansen R et al: Long-term ambulatory treatment of metastatic colorectal adenocarcinoma by continuous intravenous infusion of 5-fluorouracil. J Surg Oncol 30:60–65, 1985

775. Wade JL, Herbst S, Greenburg A: Prolonged venous infusion (PVI) of 5-fluorouracil (5-FU) for metastatic colon cancer. Proc Am Soc Clin Oncol 5:88, 1986

776. Benedetto P, Davila E, Solomon J: Chronic continuous systemic infusion of 5-fluorouracil (CCI-5-FU) in the treatment of metastatic colorectal carcinoma (CCA). Proc Am Soc Clin Oncol 3:142, 1984

777. Hansen E, Quebbeman R, Ausman R et al: Continuous 5-fluorouracil (5-FU) infusion in colorectal cancer: Update of the MCW experience. Proc Am Soc Clin Oncol 6:80, 1987

778. Belt RJ, Davidner ML, Myron MC et al: Continuous low dose 5-fluorouracil (5-FU) for adenocarcinoma: Confirmation of activity. Proc Am Soc Clin Oncol 4:90, 1985

779. Leichman L, Seichman CG, Kinzie J et al: Long term low dose 5-fluorouracil (5-FU) in advanced measurable colon cancer: No correlation between toxicity and efficacy. Proc Am Soc Clin Oncol 4:86, 1985

780. NCIC Ongoing Clinical Trial, initiated 1986

781. Lokich J: Optimal schedule for 5-fluorouracil chemotherapy: Intermittent bolus or continuous infusion? Am J Clin Oncol 8:445–448, 1985

782. Niederhuber JE, Ensminger W, Gyves J et al: Regional chemotherapy of colorectal cancer metastatic to the liver. Cancer 53:1336–1343, 1984

783. Kemeny N, Reichman B, Oderman P et al: Update of randomized study of intrahepatic (H) vs systemic (S) infusion of fluorodeoxyuridine (FUdR) in patients with liver metastases from colorectal carcinoma (CR). Proc Am Soc Clin Oncol 5:86, 1986

784. Hohn D, Stagg R, Friedman M et al: The NCOG randomized trial of intravenous (IV) vs. hepatic arterial (IA) FUDR for colorectal cancer metastatic to the liver. Proc Am Soc Clin Oncol 6:85, 1987

785. Moertel CG: Therapy of advanced gastrointestinal cancer with the nitrosoureas. Cancer Chemother Rep 3/4:27, 1973

786. Macdonald JS, Neefe J: Chemotherapy in the management of gastrointestinal cancer. Abdom Surg 21:126–131, 1979

787. Moertel CG: Chemotherapy of gastrointestinal cancer. N Engl J Med 299:1049–1052, 1978

788. Boice JD, Greene MH, Killen JY et al: Leukemia and pre-leukemia after adjuvant treatment of gastrointestinal cancer with semustine (methyl-CCNU). N Engl J Med 309:1079–1083, 1983

789. Wasserman TH, Comis RL, Goldsmith M et al: Tabular analysis of clinical chemotherapy of solid tumors. Cancer Chemother Rep 6:399, 1975

790. Pastan I, Gottesman M: Multiple-drug resistance in human cancer. N Engl J Med 316:1388–1393, 1987

791. Myers C, Cowan K, Sinha B et al: The phenomenon of pleiotropic drug resistance. In DeVita VT, Hellman S, Rosenberg SA (eds): Important Advances in Oncology 1987, pp 27–37. Philadelphia, JB Lippincott, 1987

792. Moertel CG, Schutt AJ, Hahn RG et al: Therapy of advanced colorectal cancer with a combination of 5-fluorouracil, methyl 3-cis-(2-chlorethyl)-1-nitrosourea and vincristine. JNCI 54:69, 1975

793. Posey L, Morgan LR: Methyl CCNU versus methyl CCNU and 5-fluorouracil in carcinoma of the large bowel. Cancer Treat Rep 61:1453–1458, 1977

794. Baker LH, Talley RW, Matter R et al: Phase III comparison of the treatment of advanced gastrointestinal cancer with bolus weekly 5-FU vs. methyl-CCNU plus bolus weekly 5-FU: A Southwest Oncology Group study. Cancer 38:1–7, 1976

795. Falkson G, Falkson HC: Fluorouracil, methyl-CCNU, and vincristine in cancer of the colon. Cancer 38:1468–1470, 1976

796. Macdonald JS, Kisner DF, Smythe T et al: 5-Fluorouracil (5-FU), methyl-CCNU and vincristine in the treatment of advanced colorectal cancer: Phase II study utilizing weekly 5FU. Cancer Treat Rep 60:1597, 1976

797. Kemeny N, Yagoda A, Braun D et al: Randomized study of 2 different schedules of methyl CCNU, 5-FU, and vincristine for metastatic colorectal carcinoma. Cancer 43:78–82, 1979

798. Engstrom P, MacIntyre J, Douglass H Jr et al: Combination chemotherapy of advanced bowel cancer. Proc AACR-ASCO 19:384, 1978

799. Kemeny N, Yagoda A, Braun J: Metastatic colorectal carcinoma: A prospective trial of methyl CCNU, 5-fluorouracil (5FU) and vincristine (MOF) versus MOF plus streptozotocin (MOF-Strep). Cancer 51:20–25, 1983

800. Buroker T, Kim PN, Groppe C et al: 5FU infusion with mitomycin C vs. 5FU infusion with methyl CCNU in the treatment of advanced colon cancer. Cancer 42:1228–1233, 1978

801. Ramming KP, Tesler AS, Haskell CM: Gastrointestinal tract neoplasms. In Haskell CM (ed): Cancer Treatment, pp 300–301. Philadelphia, WB Saunders, 1980

802. Richards FD, Case LD, White DR et al: Combination chemotherapy (5-fluorouracil, methyl-CCNU, mitomycin C) versus 5-fluorouracil alone for advanced previously untreated colorectal carcinoma: A phase III study of the Piedmont Oncology Association. J Clin Oncol 4:565–570, 1986

803. Loehrer PJ, Einhorn LH, Williams JD et al: Cisplatin plus 5-FU for the treatment of adenocarcinoma of the colon. Cancer Treat Rep 69:1359–1363, 1985

804. Kovach JS, Moertel CG, Shutt AS et al: Phase II study of cis-diamminedichloroplatin (NSC-119875) in advanced carcinoma of the large bowel. Cancer Chemother Rep 57:357–358, 1973

805. O'Connell MJ, Moertel CG, Kvols LK et al: Clinical trial of cisplatin and intensive 5-fluorouracil for the treatment of advanced colo-rectal cancer. Am J Clin Oncol 9:192–195, 1986

806. Cantrell J, Hart R, Taylor R et al: A Phase II trial of continuous infusion (CI) 5-FU and weekly low dose cis-platin (DDP) in colorectal carcinoma. Proc Am Soc Clin Oncol 5:84, 1986

807. Loehrer PJ, Turner S, Kubilis P et al: A prospective randomized study of 5-fluorouracil (5FU) alone or with cisplatin (P) in the treatment of metastatic colorectal cancer: A Hoosier Oncology Group trial. Proc Am Soc Clin Oncol 6:297, 1987

808. Bertino JR, Sawicki WL, Lindquist A et al: Schedule dependent autitumor effects of methotrexate and 5-fluorouracil. Cancer Rev 37:327–328, 1977

809. Cadman E, Heimer R, Davis L: Enhanced 5-fluorouracil nucleotide formation after methotrexate adminstration: Explanation for drug synergism. Science 205:1135–1137, 1979

810. Benz C, Cadman E: Modulation of 5-fluorouracil metabolism and cytotoxicity by antimetabolite pretreatment in human colorectal adenocarcinoma HCT-8. Cancer Rev 41:994–999, 1981

811. Mehrotra S, Rosenthal CJ, Gardner B: Biochemical modulation of antineoplastic response in colorectal carcinoma: 5-fluorouracil (F), high dose methotrexate (M) with calcium leukovorin (L) rescue (FML) in two sequences of administration. Proc Am Soc Clin Oncol 1:95, 1982

812. Kemeny N, Michaelson R: Phase II trial of low dose methotrexate and sequential 5-fluorouracil in the treatment of metastatic colorectal carcinoma. Proc Am Soc Clin Oncol 1:95, 1982

813. Mahajan SL, Ajan JA, Kanoj A et al: Comparison of two schedules of sequential high-dose methotrexate (MTX) and 5-fluorouracil (5-FU) for metastatic colorectal carcinoma. Proc Am Soc Clin Oncol 2:122, 1983

814. Rangineni RR, Ajani JA, Bedikian AY et al: Sequential conventional dose methotrexate (MTX) and 5-fluorouracil (5-FU) in the primary therapy of metastatic colorectal carcinoma. Proc Am Soc Clin Oncol 2:125, 1983

815. Hansen R, Ritch P, Anderson T: Sequential methotrexate (MTX), 5-fluorouracil (5-FU), and leukovorin (LCV) in colorectal cancer. Proc Am Soc Clin Oncol 2:117, 1983

816. Drapkin R, McAloon E, Lyman G: Sequential methotrexate (MTX) and 5-fluorouracil in advanced measurable colorectal cancer. Proc Am Soc Clin Oncol 2:118, 1983

817. Petrelli N, Herrera L, Stulc J et al: A phase III study of 5FU versus 5FU + methotrexate versus 5FU + high-dose leucovorin in metastatic colorectal adenocarcinoma. Proc Am Soc Clin Oncol 6:286, 1987

818. Ullman B, Lee M, Martin DW et al: Cytotoxicity of 5-fluoro-2'-deoxyuridine: Requirement for reduced folate cofactors and antagonism of methotrexate. Proc Natl Acad Sci USA 75:980–983, 1978

819. Evans RM, Laskin JD, Hakala MT: Effect of excess folates and deoxyinosine on the activity and site of action of 5-fluorouracil. Cancer Res 41:3283–3295, 1981

820. Houghton JA, Maroda SJ Jr, Philips JO et al: Biochemical determinants of responsiveness to 5-fluorouracil and its derivatives in xenografts of human colorectal adenocarcinomas in mice. Cancer Res 41:144–149, 1981

821. Machover D, Schwarzenberg L, Goldschmidt E et al: Treatment of advanced colorectal and gastric adenocarcinomas with 5-FU combined with high-dose folinic acid: A pilot study. Cancer Treat Rep 66:1803–1807, 1982

822. Greene H, Desai A, Levick S et al: Combined 5-fluorouracil infusion and high dose folinic acid in the treatment of metastatic gastrointestinal cancer. Proc Am Soc Clin Oncol 5:89, 1986

823. Lopez AR, Van Tilburg A, Bradley T et al: Treatment of advanced malignancy with 5-fluorouracil combined with folinic acid. Proc Am Assoc Cancer Res 25:178, 1984

824. Schmoll HJ, LeBlanc S: Sequential high dose folinic acid and 5-fluorouracil in advanced colorectal cancer with measurable, progressive disease. Proc Am Soc Clin Oncol 4:94, 1985

825. Ehrlichman C, Fine S, Wong A et al: A comparison of 5-fluorouracil and folinic acid versus 5FU in metastatic colorectal cancer. Proc Am Soc Clin Oncol 5:82, 1986

826. Doroshow JH, Bertrand M, Multhauf P et al: Prospective randomized trial comparing 5FU versus 5FU and high dose folinic acid (hdfa) for treatment of advanced colorectal cancer. Proc Am Soc Clin Oncol 6:374, 1987

827. Mavligit GM, Burgess MA, Seibert GB et al: Adjuvant immunotherapy and chemoimmunotherapy in colorectal cancer of the Dukes C classification. Cancer 36:2421–2427, 1975

828. Higgins GA, Donaldson R, Rogers L et al: Efficacy of MER immunotherapy when added to a regimen of 5-fluorouracil and methyl-CCNU following resection for carcinoma of large bowel. Cancer 54:193–198, 1984

829. Antman K, Eder JP, Schryber et al: Fifty-eight solid tumor patients treated with a high dose combination alkylating agent preparative regimen with autologous bone marrow support: The DFCI/BIH experience (abst). Proc Am Soc Clin Oncol 5:40, 1986

830. Silgals RM, Ahern JD, Neefe JR et al: A phase II trial of high dose intravenous interferon alpha 2 in advanced colorectal cancer. Cancer 54:2257–2261, 1984

831. Figlin RA, Callaghan N, Sarna G: Phase II trial of interferon administered daily in adenocarcinoma of the colon/rectum. Cancer Treat Rep 67:493–494, 1983

832. Niederle N, Kurschel E, Schmidt CG: Biologic effect of recombinant leukocyte 2 interferon in metastatic colorectal carcinomas. Dtsch Med Wochenschr 109:779–782, 1984

833. Wrigley PFM, Slevin ML, Clark P et al: Alpha-2 interferon in combination with 5-fluorouracil for advanced colorectal carcinoma. Proc Am Soc Clin Oncol 3:14, 1984

834. Kreuser ED, Porzsolt F, Digel W et al: Interferon alpha-2C in combination with 5-fluorouracil for refractory colorectal carcinoma (abst 611). Presented at the Fifth NCI–EORTC Symposium on New Drugs and Cancer Therapy, Amsterdam, 1986

835. Lillis PK, Brown T, Beougher K et al: Phase II trial of recombinant beta interferon (beta-seron) in advanced colorectal cancer. Proc Am Soc Clin Oncol 6:A336, 1987

836. O'Connell MJ, Moertel CG, Shutt AJ et al: Phase II clinical trial of human recombinant gamma interferon (RIFN-gamma) in patients (Pts) with advanced colorectal cancer. Proc Assoc Cancer Res 27:181, 1986

837. Rios A, Levin B, Ajani J et al: Combination of recombinant human interferon gamma (RIFN gamma) and 5-fluorouracil in the treatment of patients with advanced colorectal carcinoma (CRC). Proc Am Soc Clin Oncol 6:A328, 1987

838. Crown SE, Mintzer D, Cunningham-Rundles S et al: High-dose human lymphoblastoid interferon in metastatic colorectal cancer: Clinical results and modification of biological responses. Cancer Treat Rep 71:39–45, 1987

839. Rosenberg SA, Lotze MT, Muul LM et al: A progress report on the treatment of 157 patients with advanced cancer using lymphokine-activated killer cells and interleukin-2 alone. N Engl J Med 316:889–897, 1987

840. West WH, Tauer KW, Yannelli JR et al: Constant-infusion recombinant interleukin-2 in adoptive immunotherapy of advanced cancer. N Engl J Med 316:898–905, 1987

841. Sears H, Herlyn D, Steplewski Z, Koprowski H: Effects of monoclonal antibody immunotherapy on patients with gastrointestinal adenocarcinoma. J Biol Res Mod 3:138–150, 1984

842. Gallagher WJ, Burk MW: Monoclonal antibody ricin A chain conjugates (immunotoxins): Potential therapeutic agents for human colon carcinoma. J Surg Res 40:159–166, 1986

843. Douillard JY, LeMevel B, Curtet et al: Immunotherapy of gastrointestinal cancer with monoclonal antibodies. Med Oncol Tumor Pharmacother 3:141–146, 1986

844. Hoover HC Jr, Surdyke M, Dangel RB et al: Prospectively randomized trial of adjuvant active specific immunotherapy for human colorectal cancer. Cancer 55:1236–1243, 1985

845. Mellstedt H, Frodin JE, Christensson B et al: Application of monoclonal antibodies (Mab 17-1A) in the treatment of colo-rectal carcinomas. In Carrano RA, Douillard JY (eds): Monoclonal Antibodies in Clinical Oncology. New York, Marcel Dekker, 1988

846. Schlom J, Weeks MO: Potential clinical utility of monoclonal antibodies in the management of human carcinomas. In DeVita VT, Hellman S, Rosenberg SA (eds): Important Advances in Oncology, 1985, pp 170–192. Philadelphia, JB Lippincott, 1985

847. Leff RS, Thompson JM, Johnson DB et al: Phase II trial of high-dose melphalan and autologous bone marrow transplantation for metastatic colon carcinoma. J Clin Oncol 4(11):1586–1591, 1986

848. Leff RS, Johnson DB, Daly MB et al: High response rate with minimal toxicity in the treatment of metastatic colon carcinoma with high dose melphalan and autologous bone marrow transplantation (ABMT). (abst). Proc Soc Clin Oncol 5:88, 1986

849. Orloff MJ: Carcinoid tumors of the rectum. Cancer 28:175–180, 1971

850. Naunheim KS, Zeitels J, Kaplan EL et al: Rectal carcinoid tumors: Treatment and prognosis. Surgery 94:670–675, 1983

851. Quan SHQ, Bader G, Berg JW: Carcinoid tumors of the rectum. Dis Colon Rectum 7:197–206, 1964

852. Morgan JG, Marks C, Hearn D: Carcinoid tumors of the gastrointestinal tract. Ann Surg 180:720–727, 1974

853. Khalifa AA, Bong WL, Rao VK et al: Leiomyosarcoma of the rectum: Report of a case and review of the literature. Dis Colon Rectum 29:427–432, 1986

854. Walsh TH, Mann CV: Smooth muscle neoplasms of the rectum and anal canal. Br J Surg 71:597–599, 1984

855. Evans HL: Smooth muscle tumors of the gastrointestinal tract. Cancer 56:2242–2250, 1985

856. Devine RM, Beart RW Jr, Wolff BG: Malignant lymphoma of the rectum. Dis Colon Rectum 29:821–824, 1986

BRENDA SHANK

ALFRED M. COHEN

DAVID KELSEN

CHAPTER 30 *Cancer of the Anal Region*

The treatment of epidermoid cancer of the anal region has undergone a major change over the past decade. From radical surgery only—abdominoperineal resection—treatment has evolved to entail radiation therapy, either alone or combined with chemotherapy, with sphincter-sparing surgery.[1-3] This combined modality approach is now regarded as the model for successful combined modality therapy of cancer.

EPIDEMIOLOGY AND ETIOLOGY

INCIDENCE, AGE, AND SEX

In the United States, cancer of the anal region accounts for 1% to 2% of all large bowel cancers[4-6] and 3.9% of all anorectal carcinomas.[7] The figures are similar in the United Kingdom, where cancer of the anal region constitutes 3% to 3.5% of all anorectal tumors.[8,9] Most of these tumors are epidermoid carcinoma (Table 30-1).[10]

Epidermoid carcinoma of the anal region most commonly occurs between age 30 years and the late 80s, with the preponderance of cases occurring in persons aged 58 to 64 years.[4,5,7,11-13] McConnell correlated the site with age and found that 80% of *anal canal* carcinomas occurred in people over the age of 60, whereas more than 50% of the *anal margin* carcinomas occurred in people younger than 60 years old.[9] However, Stearns et al reported no age differences for patients with carcinomas in these two sites.[7]

In the United States, anal carcinoma occurs more frequently in females than in males (Table 30-2).[4,5,7,10,14] This is generally true for anal *canal* cancers in the Western world.[8,9,15-18] Anal *margin* cancers, however, are more frequent in males. In contrast, Kapur et al noted a strong male preponderance for anal cancer in New Delhi, India.[19]

Several recent studies have implicated male homosexuality in anal canal carcinoma, presumably from anal intercourse.[10,13,20-24] A case-control study reported by Daling et al compared potential risk factors in 148 patients with anal cancer and 166 controls with colon cancer.[24] A history of anal-receptive intercourse in men (but not in women) was strongly associated with anal cancer (relative risk [RR] = 33.1).

In a study by Peters and Mack of 970 Los Angeles County residents, the incidence of anal carcinoma was 6.1 times greater in single men than in married men (p < 0.001).[10] The increased incidence was limited to squamous and transitional cell carcinomas in the anus and did not apply to adenocarcinoma; single women were not at an increased risk. In the age group less than 35 years old, anal carcinoma was more common in men, the reverse of the sex ratio for patients over 35 years old, where again there was a substantial female predominance. Peters and Mack regarded these findings as consistent with the hypothesis that anal sexual activity is related to anal cancer. They also noted an increase in the incidence of anal carcinoma in 1980–1981 to twice that expected for men less than 45 years old (18 cases versus 8.3 expected). An increased incidence was not seen in women of any age or in men more than 45 years old. The investigators

965

TABLE 30-1.   Anal Carcinoma: Distribution of Histologic Types in 970 Patients*

Type	% of Patients
Squamous cell carcinoma	63
Transitional (cloacogenic) carcinoma	23
Adenocarcinoma	7
Paget's disease	2
Basal cell carcinoma	2
Melanoma	2

* Modified from Peters RK, Mack TM: Patterns of anal carcinoma by gender and marital status in Los Angeles County. Br J Cancer 48:629–636, 1983.

could not rule out the possibility that the increased incidence in young single men may have been related to acquired immune deficiency syndrome (AIDS), which was also occurring in the same population. Mechanisms postulated were physical irritation of the anal canal, genital carcinogens (*e.g.*, lubricants), or the transmission of oncogenic viruses by sexual contact.

VIRUSES AND OTHER INFECTIOUS AGENTS

There appears to be a relationship between papillomaviruses and the development of genital warts (condylomata acuminata), which can convert to squamous cell carcinomas after a long latent period of 5 to 40 years.[25] Anal canal carcinoma has been associated with condylomata[26-29] in the general population and in male homosexuals.[30] In the case-control study reported by Daling et al,[24] squamous cell carcinoma (but not transitional cell carcinoma) was strongly associated with a history of genital warts (RR = 26.9 in males and 32.5 in females). Nine (64%) of 14 patients with tumors positive for human papillomavirus by in situ hybridization techniques had a history of warts.

In women without a history of genital warts, anal cancer was associated with seropositivity for herpes simplex virus type 2 (RR = 4.1) and *Chlamydia trachomatis* (RR = 2.3). In men without a history of warts, there was an association with gonorrhea (RR = 17.2).

OTHER ASSOCIATED CONDITIONS

Anal canal carcinomas, in particular mucinous adenocarcinomas, have been associated with anal fistulas[4,31-34] and

TABLE 30-2.   Anal Carcinoma: Geographic Variability in Male:Female Ratios

Geographic Area	Male:Female Ratio		
	All	Anal Canal	Anal Margin
United States[4,5,7,10,14]	1:2	3:7	2:1
United Kingdom[8,9,15-17]	1:1	3:4	3–4:1
France[18]	. . .	1:3	. . .
India (New Delhi)[19]	3:1	. . .	. . .

Ellipses indicate data not reported or not subdivided by location.

other benign conditions such as lymphogranuloma venereum[35,36] and leukoplakia.[16] Brennan and Stewart reported the relationship with condylomata acuminata and fistulas as well as fissures, abscesses, and hemorrhoids.[37] In one study, 41% of anal canal carcinomas were preceded by benign anorectal disease for at least 5 years.[38] There is a sexual difference in susceptibility to development of anogenital malignancies in the presence of condylomata: in a study reported by Chuang et al that spanned 28 years, 41 of 500 women with condylomata acuminata developed anogenital malignancies, while only one of 246 men developed anogenital malignancies.[39]

Prior radiation therapy may play a role in the development of anal carcinoma,[16,40,41] as may immunosuppression. Immunosuppressed renal transplant patients have a 100-fold increase in anogenital tumors compared with the rest of the population.[42] Many of these patients have a history of condylomata acuminata (29%) or herpes genitalis. In the case-control study reported by Daling et al, current cigarette smoking was a major risk factor in both sexes (RR = 7.7 in women and 9.4 in men).[24] This substantiates the report by Daniell, who noted that 54% of 13 women with anal cancer were current smokers, in comparison to only 26% of 202 age-matched patients with colon cancer.[43]

Several general conclusions with regard to etiology can be made. Anal canal carcinoma appears to be related to immunosuppression and correlates highly with preexisting condylomata acuminata, which are probably caused by viruses. There is a clear-cut relationship with male homosexuality, which may relate both to the presence of other viral diseases in these individuals and to immunosuppression. The relationship between anal cancer and AIDS is unclear,[44] but numerous and diverse gastrointestinal tract disorders are associated with AIDS, and an increase in anal cancer incidence has been seen recently in the AIDS-prone population in Los Angeles County.

ANIMAL STUDIES

Animal studies offer some clues to the genesis of anal tumors. In mice, anal carcinomas may be induced by chemical carcinogens.[45,46] In a study by Kingsnorth et al, the induction of anal squamous cell carcinomas was promoted by epidermal growth factor (EGF).[46] The frequency of anal squamous cell carcinomas induced by dimethylhydrazine (DMH) alone was only 10%, whereas in mice treated with both DMH and EGF, the frequency was 33% (p < 0.05). Kingsnorth et al postulated that this potentiation was a result of EGF-stimulated squamous cell hyperplasia, with the EGF thus acting as a co-carcinogen. It is of particular interest that EGF did not promote the development of DMH-induced tumors in the rest of the colon, which occur at a high rate (approximately 75%) with DMH alone.

ANATOMIC CONSIDERATIONS

Squamous cell cancer of the anus can occur in the anal canal proper, the lowermost rectum, or the perianal skin.[47,48] Important gross anatomic landmarks associated with these lo-

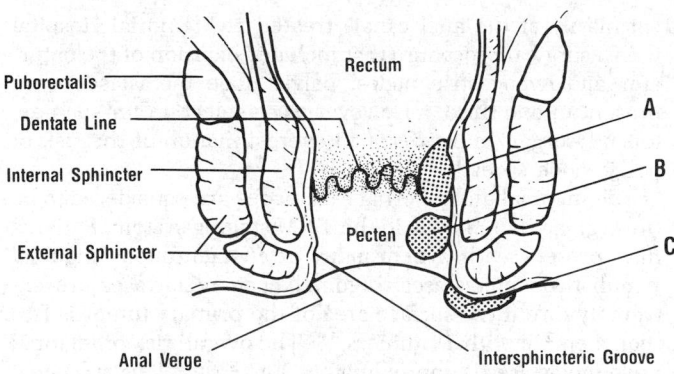

FIG. 30-1. Gross anatomy of the anal canal. A tumor in location *A* is always considered anal *canal* cancer; in location *C* it is anal *margin* cancer; in location *B* it is anal canal *or* margin, depending on institutional preference.

cations are illustrated in Figure 30-1. Each level is associated with histologically distinct epithelium.

The lowermost region lies caudad to the anal verge and is covered with keratinized stratified squamous epithelium. Pigmentation and hair follicles are present. Anal cancers are defined distally as those that are within 5 cm of the anal verge, and are referred to as *perianal* or *anal margin* cancers. Extending proximally from the anal verge to the pectinate or dentate line is the hairless stratified squamous epithelium of the anal canal. The rectal columns (columns of Morgagni) extend for 1.0 to 1.5 cm proximal to the level of the anorectal ring. Proximal to the ring the mucosa is columnar. The mucosa over the rectal columns is cuboidal, giving rise to the transitional cell or cloacogenic anal cancers. Squamous epithelium can extend proximally to the pectinate line, which explains the finding of squamous cell cancers in the distal rectum proper. The anal crypts are located in the distal columns of Morgagni. From microscopic glandular components within these crypts the rare mucoepidermoid cancers arise.

The definition of the proximal extent of tumors referred to as *anal margin* varies. The St. Marks Hospital, London, Memorial Hospital, New York (part of Memorial Sloan-Kettering Cancer Center), and Melbourne, Australia, groups consider all tumors below the dentate line as anal margin.[49–51] All tumors involving the dentate line are then considered *anal canal* cancers. The Mayo Clinic and other groups define anal margin tumors as those below the anal verge.[52] Figure 30-1 shows the various potential tumor sites within the anal region.

The *intersphincteric groove* is easily palpable on rectal examination. It represents the potential plane between the internal and external sphincter mechanism. The external sphincter surrounds the internal sphincter circumferentially and extends more caudad than the internal sphincter. Hence, the most superficial muscle beneath the anal verge is the superficial *external sphincter*. This is an important anatomic consideration when local excision is attempted. The superficial external and internal sphincter muscles can be resected without loss of continence in most patients. The entire sphincter mechanism caudad to the puborectalis sling can be resected over a partial circumference with acceptable continence (compared to a permanent colostomy).

The anal region is extremely well vascularized and has an extensive lymphatic system (Fig. 30-2). The lymphatics drain into the inguinal nodes, the lateral pelvic nodes, and the mesorectal nodes.[7] Tumors below the anal verge drain primarily into the inguinal nodal system. The distal 5 cm of rectum and the anal canal to the anal verge drain into the inguinal nodes, as well as along the middle hemorrhoidal vessels to the pelvic side walls, and into the inferior mesenteric system. Lymph node metastases are the rule with advanced anal cancer.

PATHOLOGY

HISTOLOGY

Many different histologic cell types may occur in the anal area.[53] In addition to the more common types (see Table 30-1), other rare histologic entities can arise, such as small cell carcinomas similar to oat cell carcinoma of the lung,[54] lymphoma, basal cell carcinoma, and Paget's disease.[55] Melanomas constitute 1% to 2% of all anal cancers, and anal melanoma constitutes only 1.6% of all melanomas.[56] The importance of anal melanoma lies in its poor prognosis, with a 5-year survival rate of only 8% to 12%[57,58]; survival is associated with tumors less than 2 mm in diameter.[57]

Some pathologists divide anal canal tumors into those that exhibit keratinization and those that do not,[49] and further subdivide nonkeratinizing tumors into basosquamous, basaloid, and cloacogenic carcinomas. Other investigators have found no difference in clinical outcome with such subdivisions and believe that all histologic varieties are subsets of squamous cell carcinoma.[59,60]

FIG. 30-2. Lymphatic drainage of the anus. Drainage is through three pathways: (1) inferiorly, from the *margin* and *canal*, across the perineum to the superficial inguinal lymph nodes; (2) from the upper canal and just superior to the dentate line, along the inferior and middle hemorrhoidal vessels to the hypogastric nodes; and (3) superiorly, from the rectum, along the superior hemorrhoidal vessels to the inferior mesenteric nodes.

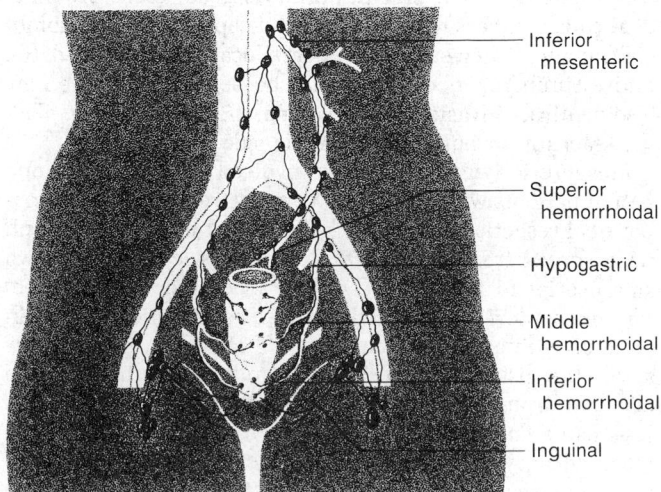

PRECANCEROUS CHANGES

Precancerous changes seen histologically in the anal canal, such as intraepidermal carcinoma of the Bowenoid type,[51] have been studied by a number of investigators. Fenger and Nielsen studied the incidence of precancerous changes in the anal canal epithelium.[61,62] Of 306 specimens, obtained at minor surgery, that included at least 1 cm of the anal transition zone (ATZ), seven (2.3%) showed squamous cell dysplasia, although the dysplasia was severe in only one. With an average follow-up of 27 months, no case of dysplasia had progressed to carcinoma. In a group of 139 patients who underwent abdominoperineal resections (most with carcinomas of the rectum, but some with anal canal tumors), 15 (10.8%) had dysplasia that was thought to be precancerous or to represent carcinoma in situ. Of the 16 patients with squamous cell carcinoma of the anal canal, severe dysplasia or carcinoma in situ was seen in 13 (81%). Fenger and Nielsen concluded that most anal canal tumors arising in the ATZ are preceded by multicentric areas of dysplasia.

Flow cytometric analysis of normal epithelium along the ATZ and, in smaller groups of patients, of anal canal tumors has been performed in fresh specimens by Fenger and Bichel.[63] A normal diploid population was seen in normal squamous epithelium in the ATZ, along with a small hyperdiploid peak, the relevance of which was unclear. Three patients with squamous cell carcinoma of the anal canal had a high proliferative index but near-diploid peaks. In contrast, Goldman et al found that most anal tumors had an aneuploid pattern.[64] Additional studies in larger numbers of patients are needed to clarify these findings.

NATURAL HISTORY

Squamous cell cancer of the anus and its variants spread by direct extension into contiguous soft tissues, with early dissemination via the lymphatics. Hematogenous spread is less common. The basaloid or cloacogenic subtypes have less biologic relevance than tumor location in a consideration of the natural history of anal cancer.[65,66]

Anal margin cancers invade local tissues and cause clinically apparent local ulceration and spread. More proximal anal canal cancers frequently spread cephalad in the submucosal plane. When such cancers are locally far advanced, the entire sphincter mechanism may be penetrated; there may also be direct invasion of the vagina, urethra, prostate, bladder, sacrum, or bone of the pelvic side walls.

Mesenteric lymph nodes are involved in one third to one half of patients with anal *canal* cancers treated by abdominoperineal resection,[6,16,51,59,67,68] The risk of mesenteric lymph node spread from anal *margin* cancers is less clear. In two small series of patients treated by abdominoperineal resection, mesenteric lymph node spread was identical to that in patients with anal canal cancers.[51,67] However, in two other series the risk was almost nil.[6,69] In addition, because the cure rate from local excision alone with anal margin cancers less than 5 cm in diameter is 90%,[50] it appears that spread to mesenteric lymph nodes is infrequent, except in cases of massive disease. In a series of 45 patients with anal cancer (primarily of the anal canal) treated at Memorial Hospital with a surgical procedure that included excision of the obturator and hypogastric nodes, pelvic node metastases were present in one third.[59] However, case selection for such extensive surgery must result in overestimation of the risk of pelvic node spread.

The inguinal and external iliac nodes are considered to be the regional lymphatics in the TNM staging system. Patients may present with synchronous or metachronous inguinal lymph node metastases. Inguinal node metastases are extremely rare if the surface area of the primary tumor is less than 4 cm² or with T1 tumors.[5,67] The overall risk of inguinal node metastases is approximately 30%.[59,67,70] This was equal to the incidence of pelvic node metastases in the Memorial Hospital series.[7] If inguinal nodes originally negative on physical examination are destined to become clinically positive, they usually do so within 18 months of treatment of the primary tumor.[67]

Hematogenous metastases occur in a minority of patients. Because of the dual venous drainage of the area, metastases occur equally to the liver and lung.[71]

Despite radical surgery, almost all recurrences of disease after surgery alone represent locoregional treatment failure. Most cancer-related deaths are secondary to uncontrolled pelvic and perineal disease.[52,54,68,72,73]

DIAGNOSIS

Because the initial symptoms of anal cancer are similar to those of common benign conditions, patient-related delay in diagnosis is very frequent. Because anal cancer is rare and examination may be painful and difficult if spasm is present, physician-related delay also occurs. Almost one third of the patients at Memorial Hospital with squamous cell cancer of the anorectum were thought to have had benign disease until a biopsy proved otherwise.[59] More than half of the patients in the Mayo Clinic study had associated benign anal pathology such as fistula-in-ano, fissure, or hemorrhoids.[52]

Bleeding, pain, and a sensation of a mass are the most common symptoms. Pruritus is less frequent, except in patients with perianal cancer.[52] Physical examination should include digital anorectal examination, anoscopy and proctoscopy, and palpation of the inguinal lymph nodes. Associated Bowen's or Paget's disease of the perianal skin increases the index of suspicion for anal carcinoma. The differential diagnosis of bleeding, pain, and/or a mass sensation includes thrombosed hemorrhoids, fissures, fistula, perianal or crypt abscess, benign anal papilloma, and adenocarcinoma of the rectum. Patients with severe pain and spasm may be treated empirically with analgesics, stool softeners, warm baths, and topical ointments for 1 to 2 weeks. Persistent symptoms may require examination under sedation or general anesthesia to avoid missing the diagnosis of cancer or an inadequately treated infection.

An incisional biopsy is necessary to confirm the diagnosis. Excision should not be attempted, except for superficial lesions detected very early. In general, suspicious inguinal lymph nodes should be biopsied to distinguish inflammatory from metastatic lymphadenopathy. Formal groin dissection should be avoided. Needle aspiration of the groin nodes for cytology may be attempted first. If the results are negative, surgical biopsy should follow. In addition to physical examination and surgical staging of a suspicious inguinal node site, an extent-of-disease staging includes chest radiography, liver function tests, and computed tomography of the abdomen and pelvis.

STAGING

An early attempt at staging was made at the Mayo Clinic in 1962.[5] This staging was similar to the Dukes' staging of rectal cancer, with Stage A representing invasion into sphincter muscle, Stage B, invasion through the sphincter muscle, and Stage C, lymph node involvement. They also graded the tumors by Broders' system. This simple system was found to be prognostic for 5-year survival. Because the sphincter muscle is thick, Stage B was later subclassified further and Stage D was added, representing unresectable regional tumor or distant metastases.[54] This classification was found to be prognostic for local and distant recurrence and for survival. Both of these classifications developed at the Mayo Clinic were pathologic classifications and applicable solely to anal canal carcinomas.

A similar surgical-pathologic staging classification was developed at the Roswell Park Memorial Institute[74] for application to the perianal area as well as the anal canal. A Stage O was introduced for carcinoma in situ, and perirectal and inguinal nodes were subclassified. That system was found to be prognostic, but the major decrements in survival came from sphincter muscle or inguinal node involvement. Involvement of perirectal nodes only was not particularly detrimental to survival compared with sphincter muscle involvement.[74]

The International Union Against Cancer (UICC) established a dual staging system with a clinical staging and a pathologic staging post-surgery,[75] to be used only for carcinoma in the anal region. Separate classifications were developed for the anal canal and for the anal margin, the anal margin staging system being analogous to that for other skin tumors. There were criticisms[76]; suggestions were incorporated into an illustrated guide of the UICC staging system.[77] A 1987 edition of the UICC staging system has now been published.[78] The American Joint Committee on Cancer (AJCC) adopted the same staging system for anal carcinoma.[79] This unified AJCC/UICC system (Table 30-3) takes into account the fact that anal canal carcinoma is increasingly treated by nonsurgical methods, such as radiation therapy alone or multimodality therapy.

Regardless of treatment, this standard clinical TNM staging system should be used to facilitate comparison of results. T staging is by size and invasion into other organs or tissues. The N classification for the anal canal subdivides the regional nodes, recognizing the poor prognosis of inguinal node involvement. Anal margin tumors are staged as for skin cancers, the T staging being almost the same as for the anal canal (see Table 30-3). Grading is also stipulated, with Grade 1 representing well-differentiated disease; Grade 2, moderately differentiated disease; Grade 3, poorly differen-

tiated disease; and Grade 4, undifferentiated disease. Other variations of a TNM system have been used.[18,80]

In devising a staging system it is important to ascertain which clinical features are the most prognostic. Many studies have shown that survival correlates with size of the anal lesion (see section on Prognostic Factors). In one study survival correlated with the 1978 UICC clinical staging (circumferential invasion or invasion of adjacent organs) and with grade.[64] However, size, which may be more objectively assessed, also correlates with circumferential invasion. Therefore, any staging system should logically be based on tumor size and invasion into adjacent organs, and should also consider grade, as does the new AJCC/UICC system. We recommend that this system be used routinely so that results between institutions may be compared.

TABLE 30-3. AJCC/UICC Staging for Anal Canal and Anal Margin Cancer*

Primary tumor (T)
TX Primary tumor cannot be assessed
T0 No evidence of primary tumor
Tis Carcinoma in situ
T1 ≤2 cm in greatest dimension
T2 >2 cm but ≤5 cm in greatest dimension
T3 >5 cm in greatest dimension
Anal canal:
T4 Any size, invading adjacent organ(s): vagina, urethra, bladder
Anal margin:
T4 Invading deep extradermal structures: skeletal muscle, bone

Regional Lymph Node Involvement (N)
NX Regional lymph nodes cannot be assessed
N0 No regional lymph node involvement
Anal canal:
N1 Metastasis to perirectal lymph nodes
N2 Metastasis to unilateral internal iliac and/or unilateral inguinal lymph nodes
N3 Metastasis to perirectal and inguinal lymph nodes and/or bilateral internal iliac and/or bilateral inguinal lymph nodes
Anal margin:
N1 Ipsilateral inguinal lymph node metastasis

Distant Metastasis (M)
MX Distant metastasis cannot be assessed
M0 No distant metastasis
M1 Distant metastasis

Stage Grouping

Stage 0	Tis	N0	M0
Stage I	T1	N0	M0
Stage II	T2	N0	M0
	T3	N0	M0

Anal canal:

Stage IIIA	T4	N0	M0
	T1–3	N1	M0
Stage IIIB	T4	N1	M0
	Any T	N2, 3	M0

Anal margin:

Stage III	T4	N0	M0
	Any T	N1	M0

Both:

Stage IV	Any T	Any N	M1

* Postsurgical histopathologic staging is the same, except determined by the pathologic examination (pT and pN).

PROGNOSTIC FACTORS

STAGE

Clinical stage (as measured by 1978 UICC T stage) has been correlated with prognostic outcome. Goldman and co-workers retrospectively analyzed findings in a group of 43 patients from Sweden with anal canal cancers.[64] Clinical stage was highly statistically correlated with outcome: patients with T1 and T2 cancers had a greater than 80% 5-year survival rate, while those with T3 and T4 disease had survival rates in the range of 0 to <20%; however, very few patients had T3 or T4 disease. This relationship is probably not an independent relationship, as T stage is related to size.

Metastasis to inguinal lymph nodes is also an indicator of a poor prognosis.[66,81] However, Greenall and co-workers found a 55% 5-year survival rate despite the presence of inguinal lymph node metastases, if lymphadenectomy could be performed.[81] It is not yet clear how the use of multimodality therapy will alter the historically poor prognosis associated with positive inguinal nodes. Treatment failure carries a poor prognosis, as might be expected. In one series patients in whom disease recurred despite treatment with chemotherapy and radiation, or radiation alone, had a median survival of 7 to 14 months.

SIZE

Tumor size (related to T stage) is of prognostic importance. A number of investigators have found that patients with lesions less than 2 cm in diameter have a markedly better prognosis than those with larger lesions.[54,67] Dillard et al found a 75% 5-year survival rate in a group of 12 patients with tumors less than 8 cm²; only 47% of patients with tumors larger than 8 cm² survived.[67] Boman et al reported that of a total of 108 patients with anal canal tumors, 13 had small (<2 cm in diameter), superficially invasive lesions.[54] All were treated with local excision, and although one later required abdominoperineal resection, all were cured. Kuehn et al[82] reported no survivors with tumors >6 cm in diameter; and even with aggressive therapy, Wanebo et al found very poor survival in patients with lesions more than 10 cm in diameter.[83] Salmon et al also found that size was significantly related to survival in a study in which radiation therapy alone was the primary treatment.[66] In another radiation therapy series, size (≤4 cm or >4 cm in diameter) was prognostic for 5-year survival but not for tumor control.[84]

OTHER PROGNOSTIC FEATURES

Histologic cell type for squamous cancers of the anal canal (epidermoid versus cloacogenic) has not been found to be of major prognostic relevance. The cloacogenic carcinomas have been considered to have a slightly better prognosis in some series[66,85]; however, in 243 patients with resectable anal canal tumors, Papillon and Montbarbon found a worse prognosis for patients with nonkeratinizing and basaloid carcinoma than for patients with keratinizing lesions.[84] Small cell carcinomas of the anus, like extrapulmonary small cell cancers in other parts of the body, appear to have a worse prognosis, with a high propensity for systemic dissemination.[54]

Asymptomatic patients do better than symptomatic patients, but this may be directly related to the size of the tumor.[86] *Location* may be of slight prognostic importance, with anal margin tumors having a better outcome than those in the anal canal. On the other hand, Paradis et al found no difference in survival rates between patients with tumors within the anal canal and those with tumors in the perianal region.[74] No difference in survival according to *sex* was observed by Papillon and Montbarbon.[84]

Goldman et al looked at *DNA content,* (i.e., whether tumors were diploid or greater than diploid) and found no correlation of survival with this factor.[64]

TREATMENT

ANAL MARGIN

Local Surgery

Superficial perianal skin carcinomas outside the anal verge may be treated with wide local excision with good results. A skin graft can be placed if the surgical defect is large. Rarely are formal skin flaps necessary or desirable. A split-thickness skin graft will shrink with time, leaving a relatively small defect that will not interfere with the detection of local recurrence. Primary abdominoperineal resection is almost never indicated as the initial treatment of these lesions. As with squamous cell cancer elsewhere on the integument, the cure rate after local excision for superficial tumors exceeds 80%.[49,50,52,70,87] Local failure rates are higher if the anal margin includes cancers in the anal canal distal to (not involving) the dentate line.[50] In the Memorial Hospital experience disease recurred locally in nine of 31 patients treated with local excision for such anal margin cancers.[50] Eight of these cases were amenable to a second local excision. In four patients, disease recurred in the inguinal nodes. There were only three cancer-related deaths in the 31 patients initially treated by local excision, and only one patient ultimately required abdominoperineal resection.

Deeply infiltrative anal margin lesions have been treated with abdominoperineal resection.[50,67] Although most patients are cured, the small number of reported cases of disease defined as anal margin cancers precludes detailed analysis of end results and patterns of failure.

External Irradiation

Epidermoid carcinoma of the anal margin tends to be early or only moderately advanced at the time of diagnosis,[88,89] with lymph nodes only rarely involved (0–15%),[88,90] usually in larger tumors (≥5 cm in diameter).[91] Although these early cancers of the anal margin are very successfully treated by local excision, radiation therapy should be considered in some patients. Papillon suggested that radiation therapy should be used in patients with anal margin carcinoma that is considered unresectable, or in patients who have extensive or recurrent lesions[80]; in addition, patients who are medically inoperable may have radiation therapy to this area.

Although some early studies of anal margin irradiation were done with interstitial radium needle implants,[80,88] the high incidence of radionecrosis and the relatively poor geometry indicate that external-beam radiation therapy is the radiation modality of choice.[80] Although photons are most frequently used for such treatments, electron-beam therapy may also be successfully utilized for early perineal epidermoid carcinomas.[92] Results in perineal anal canal lesions, stage for stage, are similar to results in anal canal lesions[89,93]; more extensive lesions therefore require more aggressive therapy. Although some authors have recommended abdominoperineal resections for extensive lesions,[89] from reported results radiation therapy appears to be an excellent alternative that yields a good cure rate with sphincter preservation.

Most studies group together patients with anal margin and anal canal carcinomas. Recently two groups reported on the results in anal margin carcinomas alone.[91,94] Neither study was a pure radiation therapy study, as chemotherapy with mitomycin C and 5-FU was given concurrently with radiation therapy in a large proportion of the patients. The study from the Centre Leon Berard used direct perineal fields and cobalt-60 as the source to deliver a surface dose of 4000 cGy in ten fractions. In a few patients with residual disease, iridium-192 implants were also used.[94] In the study from Princess Margaret Hospital, external-beam radiation therapy was used in most of the patients, who received a dose of 5000 cGy in 4 weeks, or in 8 weeks as a split course.[91] In both studies, local control was similar (80%–85%). In the Centre Leon Berard study, the 5-year disease-free survival rate was 50%, and only half of the deaths were secondary to cancer.[94] Treatment failed locally in five of 35 patients, but two patients were salvaged. Lymph node failures tended to occur later and were fatal in three patients. In the Princess Margaret Hospital study, local control was achieved in all 13 patients with a primary lesion less than 5 cm in diameter but in only two of five patients with a primary lesion larger than 10 cm.[91] Four patients had positive lymph nodes in this study, and disease in two was controlled by treatment. The investigators noted that local necrosis developed in three of 11 patients treated with radiation therapy alone.

In a study of both perianal and anal canal tumors, five patients with perianal tumors without nodal involvement were treated with radiation therapy (4000–6000 cGy) plus bleomycin; two of these patients with advanced disease (T4NO) also underwent abdominoperineal resection after chemotherapy and radiation therapy.[95] All five patients were alive and disease-free on follow-up of 16 to 84 months.

ANAL CANAL

Local Disease

LOCAL EXCISION. In a small series reported from the Cleveland Clinic, none of ten patients treated initially by local excision experienced recurrence of the disease.[96] Included were cancers of the anal margin and anal canal that extended less than one-half the circumference; cancers involving the dentate line were excluded. Internal or full-thickness sphincter excision with skin-graft coverage resulted in acceptable continence. In a review from the Connecticut Cancer Registry reported by Kuehn et al, 26 patients with anal cancer including distal anal canal cancers were treated by local excision, and 76% were cured.[47]

The Mayo Clinic experience[54] with anal cancers between the dentate line and the anal verge includes 19 patients treated by local excision. Treatment failed locally in one of 12 superficial tumors, which was subsequently cured with abdominoperineal resection. Seven patients with underlying sphincter muscle invasion refused radical surgery and were treated by wide local excision, some with adjuvant irradiation. Disease recurred locally in three.[54] In a group of five patients (four with T1 disease) treated at the Lahey Clinic by local excision, none had disease recurrence.[12] Of 144 patients treated at Memorial Hospital for anal canal cancers (dentate line involvement), only 11 were suitable candidates for local excision. The 5-year survival rate was only 45%, and the majority had local recurrence.[97] Less than 10% of the 91 anal canal tumors treated at St. Mark's Hospital with curative intent (dentate line involvement) were amenable to local excision; of these, 75% were cured.[70] Klotz et al compiled reports of anal canal "basaloid" cancers, 33 of which had been treated by local excision.[11] Most of the tumors had been found incidentally in hemorrhoidectomy specimens. The 5-year cure rate was 60%. Local excision should be considered only for small (T1) tumors with no evidence of nodal involvement, and in patients who can be followed up closely.

Locoregional Disease

MULTIMODALITY THERAPY. *Diagnostic Surgery.* Because integrated multimodality therapy not only improves overall survival but also allows radical surgery to be avoided in the majority of patients, the scope of initial diagnostic surgery should be limited to maximize the final functional result.

For anal margin cancers distal to the anal verge, a punch or surgical incisional biopsy performed in the office will suffice. For patients with considerable spasm and pain, examination and incisional biopsy under general anesthesia is appropriate. If a decision is made to proceed with local excision only (small anal margin or T1 anal canal lesion), the bowel is prepared and elective surgery is done.

Grossly positive inguinal lymph nodes are studied initially by needle aspiration cytology; open biopsy is performed if the result is benign. Minimally suspicious nodes warrant an excisional biopsy of one or two lymph nodes, with great care to avoid a hematoma or lymphatic leak. A superficial groin dissection is not necessary or useful as part of the initial treatment strategy, will delay definitive chemotherapy and radiation treatment, and may increase the risk of leg edema following combined treatment.

Combined Chemotherapy and Irradiation. In the past 10 to 15 years, increasing evidence amassed from single-arm Phase II studies has indicated that initial chemotherapy plus radiation therapy yields a very high rate of tumor regression

TABLE 30-4. Epidermoid Anal Canal Carcinoma: Treatment Plans and Results, by Institution

Treatment and Results	Wayne State University, Detroit	Memorial Hospital, New York	Highland Hospital, Rochester, NY	Princess Margaret Hospital, Toronto	Fresno Community Hospital, Fresno, CA
5-FU	1000 mg/m² × 4 d × 2 cycles	750 mg/m² × 5 d	1000 mg/m² × 4 d × 2 cycles from d 2	1000 mg/m² × 4 d	1000 mg/m² × 4 d × 2 cycles
Mitomycin C	15 mg/m², d 1	15 mg/m², d 1	10 mg/m², d 2	10 mg/m², d 1	10–15 mg/m², on d 1, × 2 cycles
RT	30 Gy/15 fx from d 1	30 Gy/15 fx starting d 6–9	50–57.5 Gy/25–32 fx from d 1 with boost	50 Gy/20 fx from d 1†	41–50 Gy/23–28 fx from d 1 with boost
Surgery	APR or LE 4–6 wk after RT	APR or LE 2–4 wk after RT	APR in 4 patients; no surgery in others; ¹⁹²Ir implant for residual disease	None	None
Maintenance Chemotherapy	None	For gross or microscopic residual disease*	None	None	None, but additional chemotherapy for residual disease
Total cases	45	44	33	30	30
Primary cases	45	44	33	30	27
Measurable response to chemotherapy and RT:					
CR	38	26	30	28	26
PR	7	. . .	3	2	4
No. having surgery	45	44	4	2‡	22
No. with sphincter preservation	27	20	29	30	30
No. with histologically neg. specimens	38	26	4	0	21
No. continuously NED	34	32	24	24§	27
5-Year Actuarial Survival	. . .	78%	. . .	72%	. . .
Median follow-up, mo (range)	50 (18–124)	39 (1–89)	51 (12–108)	25 (8–50)	? (9–76)

5-FU = 5-fluorouracil, RT = radiation therapy, CR = complete response, PR = partial response, APR = abdominoperineal resection, LE = local excision, fx = fraction(s), d = day, NED = no evidence of disease.
*Most patients did not receive maintenance chemotherapy.[106]
†Continuous radiation therapy in 16 patients and split course in 14.
‡Surgery for known residual disease only.
§One half of patients with local failure were salvaged with local resection.

(including a high complete remission rate) and that further surgery, if needed, can be limited to an excisional biopsy of residual scar. Thus, for many patients with relatively large anal epidermoid tumors, a colostomy can be avoided with an excellent survival expectation.

Table 30-4 summarizes the results of therapy in a number of large series.[98-103] Because anal canal tumors are rare, there are no prospective controlled randomized trials comparing chemotherapy plus irradiation with irradiation alone or surgery alone. However, because the combined approach yields comparable or superior results with modest morbidity and a high rate of sphincter preservation, a prospective controlled study does not seem to be required to accept multimodality therapy as conventional treatment for the majority of patients with anal canal disease. One retrospective study that compared multimodality therapy with surgery or radiation therapy alone suggested a higher cure rate with multimodality therapy in patients with higher stage disease (sphincter muscle and/or perirectal node involvement).[104]

All of the larger series have followed a chemotherapy protocol similar to that pioneered by Nigro and co-workers[105]: 5-FU given by continuous 24-hour infusion for 4 to 5 days, plus a single bolus dose of mitomycin C. Combined therapy has been given concurrently or sequentially. In the concurrent regimen, radiation therapy and chemotherapy are initiated on the same day. In the sequential regimen, chemotherapy is given before radiation therapy. In addition to differences in timing of administration, the dose of radiation therapy has also varied (see Table 30-4). Furthermore, in centers such as Wayne State University and the Memorial Sloan-Kettering Cancer Center, chemotherapy plus radiation therapy has been given prior to a planned surgical procedure—initially abdominoperineal resection, later local excision. At Highland Hospital in Rochester, New York, and the Princess Margaret Hospital, radiation therapy to higher total doses was definitive treatment; surgery was not part of the treatment plan. Despite these differences between trials, there is little evidence from these four studies, all of which were conducted on relatively small groups of patients, that one schedule or dose level is markedly superior to another. Response and survival rates are similar, although fewer patients may require an abdominoperineal resection after concurrent chemotherapy and radiation therapy to higher doses.

Some investigators have found that any patient with a positive biopsy result after completion of the initial treatment was certain to have recurrence of disease. All seven patients at Wayne State University with positive biopsy findings at that point had recurrent disease, despite salvage abdominoperineal resection performed in six patients.[98] However, this is not the experience of others.[99,106]

Combined therapy can be given in a community setting,[107] but because this approach involves careful interdigitation of several disciplines, it should be initiated only if there is a sufficient patient load to make such interactions workable (e.g., more than ten patients per year). Results in 30 patients with anal canal tumors treated at a community hospital[102,103] in California (see Table 30-4) were similar to results achieved at the larger centers, with no patient experiencing more than group II toxicity on a modified scale.[108]

The best chemotherapy–radiation therapy regimen and the most appropriate radiation dose to use for patients with anal canal tumors limited to the primary site have not yet been defined. Distant recurrence is not the major problem in these patients. Local recurrence is more common, especially if the radiation dose is low (3000 cGy). 5-FU probably acts as a radiosensitizer,[109] while mitomycin is probably not synergistic.[110] Byfield and co-workers treated 11 patients with a 120-hour infusion of 5-FU at 25 mg/kg/24 h and concurrent irradiation, and omitted mitomycin.[111] Radiation therapy was given in 4-day cycles (1000 cGy/cycle) separated by at least 9 days, to a total dose of 3000 to 4750 cGy. All patients had complete clinical regressions; only one had active disease histologically. There was only one local recurrence.

The chemotherapy regimen of mitomycin C and 5-FU is quite active against anal canal tumors, with major response rates in the 50% to 60% range when used in chemotherapy alone trials. However, some patients do not respond or have less than a complete remission with this combination. It may be possible to identify subsets of patients at greater risk for failure who would be candidates for aggressive investigational chemotherapy–radiation therapy regimens.

RADICAL SURGERY. Before the widespread use of multimodality therapy, more than 90% of patients with potentially curable anal canal cancers required abdominoperineal resection. A wide perineal dissection in association with a posterior vaginectomy in women was recommended.[14,68] Despite initial enthusiasm from the group at Memorial Hospital in regard to vaginectomy, a more recent analysis discounted its routine application.[7] Lateral pelvic lymphadenectomy was initially advocated by the same group on the basis of a 24% incidence of pathologically positive nodes.[59] Subsequent analysis could not define any therapeutic benefit for this extended abdominoperineal resection.[7] The overall cure rate with abdominoperineal resection is approximately 50%.[112]

The Mayo Clinic experience initially reported in 1976 by Beahrs and Wilson[52] has been updated by Boman et al.[54] Disease recurred in 40% of the 114 patients, with subsequent treatment resulting in a 71% 5-year survival rate. At the Ellis Fischel State Cancer Hospital in Columbia, Missouri, the 5-year survival rate in 46 patients was 58%.[67] The M. D. Anderson Hospital group reported a 62% 5-year survival rate in 109 patients treated with only abdominoperineal resection.[90] One sixth of the cases were anal margin cancers. The most recent Memorial Hospital update includes 103 patients treated by radical surgery, with a 55% 5-year survival rate.[97] All of these tumors involved the dentate line. The 5-year survival in patients with tumors larger than 5 cm was only 40%. At St. Mark's Hospital, the 5-year survival rate in 83 patients with anal cancers involving the dentate line treated by radical surgery was 48%.[70]

Treatment failure despite radical surgery is both locoregional and distant. In the Mayo Clinic experience, 84% of initial sites of failure included local and regional disease.[54] The majority of cancer-related deaths are secondary to uncontrolled locoregional tumor. One third to one half of patients with locally advanced anal cancers treated by abdominoperineal resection at the major centers known for their expertise in this disease still had local recurrence in the pelvis or perineum.[54,68,70,90,97]

Today, with the success of combined modality therapy, an abdominoperineal resection should be reserved for salvage of the few patients in whom multimodality treatment fails.

INTERSTITIAL RADIATION THERAPY. Interstitial radiation therapy was originally used because of the limitations of orthovoltage irradiation. It had the potential of curing only early lesions that were unlikely to spread to the lymph nodes. Radium needles have been used primarily, although interstitial implants with ^{192}Ir have also been used. Radium needles were used for several years at the Christie Hospital in Manchester, England,[88,93] and are still used there for early anal lesions. In a recent update from that institution, radium needles were the exclusive treatment modality in 74 patients, 43 with anal canal lesions and 31 with anal margin lesions.[93] The minimum follow-up period was 5 years. Of the 68 evaluable patients, 33 (49%) were disease-free at 5-year follow-up or at death and were considered to have been cured. Of the 35 locoregional failures, 7 were salvaged by a surgical procedure. Local control was achieved in 64% of tumors less than 5 cm in diameter but in only 23% of tumors 5 cm or larger. The investigators recommend only local excision or an implant for tumors less than 5 cm in diameter with clinically negative nodes, and close follow-up and surgical resection for any recurrence.

Radium implantation has also been used extensively by Papillon,[80] but he has abandoned this technique because of painful local reactions and inability to achieve nodal control because of the small target volume.[84] Early studies with radium needles yielded a severe necrosis rate of about 25%.[88,113,114] Utilizing ^{192}Ir to a dose of 6000 cGy, Keiling and co-workers observed no local failures in 12 patients but a 16% local necrosis rate, although all healed with conservative treatment.[115] In two patients disease recurred in regional lymph nodes, again emphasizing the lack of control outside the very small target volume.

Combined multimodality techniques are yielding better

local control, sphincter preservation, and survival rates and should be considered for locoregional anal canal disease.

EXTERNAL IRRADIATION. External irradiation may be used with fields designed to cover the pelvic and inguinal node areas, which are at risk in anal canal cancer. In the modern megavoltage era, there is less morbidity from external irradiation than there was in the orthovoltage era. Computed tomography (CT) may aid in the planning of treatment. For example, boost doses, whether given by external irradiation or by interstitial implant, may be better designed with the use of CT. A study reported from Duke University Medical Center found excellent definition of tumor extent (local spread, lymph node involvement, and distant metastases) with CT of the pelvis, and CT was also useful for follow-up for potential recurrence.[116]

The results of major studies using external irradiation alone are given in Table 30-5. Local control overall ranges from 60% to 80%, while overall survival ranges from 50% to 80%. Two French studies, from the Institut Curie[108] and the Institut Gustave Roussy,[117] show that 5-year survival is related to the extent of the primary tumor as determined from either tumor size or the 1978 UICC T staging. A study from San Francisco found that survival is better in tumors less than 5 cm in diameter with negative nodes.[13,118] Of interest, in an update of the Institut Curie external irradiation data, the investigators expressed the belief that multimodality therapy is now the best approach for curative therapy.[119] Investigators at the Princess Margaret Hospital, who compared multimodality therapy with external irradiation, also concluded that multimodality therapy affords better local control and therefore a better colostomy-free survival.[100] In a study from Russia, in which the length of follow-up is unclear, similar results were obtained for 5-year survivals by T stage.[120]

In all of the studies listed in Table 30-5, the rate of complications requiring surgery remains around 5% to 15%, probably reflecting the high doses (6000–7000 cGy) that must be delivered to the primary site to control this disease when radiation therapy is the sole treatment modality. The addition of bleomycin to external irradiation in ten patients has not offered any added benefit in terms of decreased recurrence.[121]

COMBINED INTERSTITIAL AND EXTERNAL IRRADIATION. Several studies on small numbers of patients have been done with external irradiation combined with implants (^{137}Cs, ^{192}Ir, radium needles).[90,92,122,123] Good local control was achieved, but there was still a relatively high rate of complications requiring surgery or leading to death. Delouche et al reporting on 22 patients followed up for 5 to 13 years, noted a 32% rate of moderate to severe complications with 3000 to 4000 cGy external radiation therapy and 3500 to 4000 cGy ^{192}Ir implant.[122] However, a 78% local control rate was achieved, with an overall survival of 45%.

The most extensive series is that from the Centre Leon Berard in which 222 patients were treated over a 15-year period with external radiation therapy (^{60}Co) to a dose of 3000 to 4200 cGy across the target volume, followed by an ^{192}Ir implant 2 months later to a dose of 1500 to 2000 cGy.[84] The investigators reported only a 3% rate of serious complications, 65% 5-year disease-free survival, and 79% locoregional control. Combined brachytherapy and external irradiation may also be useful in very extensive lesions,[124,125] described below in the section on Locally Advanced and Recurrent Cancer.

In summary, combined interstitial and external radiation therapy may yield high local control rates but a significant complication rate. However, a 5-year disease-free survival rate of 65%, as reported by Papillon,[84] is excellent and compares favorably with results in surgically treated patients.

Locally Advanced and Recurrent Cancer

Recurrent *anal margin* cancer, after local excision, may require only further local excision for salvage. In a study from Memorial Sloan-Kettering Cancer Center, 16 patients in whom disease recurred underwent additional surgical procedures; of these, 12 were alive at 5 years and only two had died of disease.[81] One patient was unavailable for follow-up. Eleven of the 12 patients with local failure underwent local excision only for salvage. More advanced primary or recur-

TABLE 30-5.   Anal Canal Carcinoma: Treatment with External Radiation Therapy Alone

Study	No. of Patients	Primary Site Dose (cGy)	Follow-up (Yr)	Complications Requiring Surgery	5-Year Survival		Local Control
Institut Curie[108]	158	6500–7000	3–14	8%	T ≤ 4 cm:	70%	
					>4 cm T≤ 6 cm:	57%	
					T > 6 cm:	33%	
					All:	51%	67%
					UICC 1978 stage		
Inst. Gustave Roussy[117]	64	6000–6500	2–13	14%	T1, T2:	72%	91%
					T3, T4:	35%	T3: 76%
							T4: 4/6
					All:	50%	81%
St Francis Hosp. et al[13,118]	39[13]	6500	0.5–8.5	13%	All:	79%	80%
	35[118]	4525–7550		6%	N0, <5 cm:	92%	77%
Princess Margaret Hosp.[100]	25	4500–6000	5–25	12%	All:	72%	60%

rent anal margin lesions may be salvaged by external radiation therapy.[80]

Patients with recurrent *anal canal* cancer after surgery should be considered for multimodality therapy (described in section on Multimodality Therapy for locoregional disease of the anal canal). Locoregional failures after initial multimodality therapy have been successfully treated with abdominoperineal resection[2] or with additional radiation and chemotherapy.[103]

Multimodality therapy for locally advanced primary anal canal tumors may yield good palliation and, in some cases, even cure. In a study reported from the University of Virginia, major regressions were observed in six of seven patients, three of whom were treated with chemotherapy alone and three with chemotherapy plus irradiation.[58] An abdominoperineal resection was performed on all patients, and all had delayed wound healing. Three of the seven patients remained disease-free for 24 to 26 months and four died, two of cancer and two of other causes. Another form of multimodality therapy, mitomycin C and 5-FU with external irradiation and interstitial ^{192}Ir implant, has been tried in 29 patients with advanced local disease.[126] With a follow-up of 5 to 54 months, 25 of 29 patients were alive and disease-free, only two of these having required radical salvage surgery with loss of sphincter function.

Brachytherapy combined with external irradiation has been used for advanced disease.[124,125] In a study from the University of California,[125] among 40 patients with anorectal cancer, eight had squamous cell or cloacogenic carcinoma and received combined external and interstitial ^{192}Ir irradiation. With a 2 to 6 year follow-up, there was a 10% rate of complications requiring surgery or leading to death. Although one cannot separate out the patients with epidermoid carcinomas in this study, there was a 70% local control rate and a 3-year disease-free survival rate of 60% in the entire group of 40 patients.

Inguinal Node Involvement

The initial experience from Memorial Hospital suggested that patients with grossly positive inguinal lymph nodes *synchronous* with the primary tumor were incurable.[127] A subsequent report indicated that two of 13 patients survived 5 years after abdominoperineal resection followed 6 weeks later by inguinal lymphadenectomy.[72] Other studies have confirmed a small cure rate for surgical treatment of patients with synchronous unilateral inguinal nodes.[52,67] Current recommendations are for limited surgical sampling, combined chemotherapy and radiation therapy with boost doses to the involved groin, and surgical salvage for isolated inguinal recurrence.

The development of unilateral *metachronous* inguinal lymph nodes does not carry such an ominous prognosis. After therapeutic groin dissection, the 5-7 year survival rate as reported from Memorial Hospital and St. Mark's Hospital exceeded 50%,[69,81] but it was nil in a small series reported from the Mayo Clinic.[52] Current strategies in patients with metachronous isolated inguinal node metastases after multimodality therapy include a formal groin dissection followed

by chemotherapy. The use of radiation under these circumstances would depend on prior dose and fields.

Metastatic Disease

Because of its rarity and because many patients with anal canal tumors have locoregional disease that has been successfully treated by surgery alone, radiation therapy alone, or multimodality therapy, data on the use of chemotherapy as a single modality in the treatment of advanced disease are scanty. A number of anecdotal reports are available, however. Single-agent trials of Adriamycin and of cisplatin have been reported by several investigators. Fisher et al reported response to both Adriamycin as a single agent and cisplatin at a dosage of 2 mg/kg in an elderly man with advanced disease.[128] Salem et al studied cisplatin as a single agent in three patients: one achieved complete remission and the other two had partial regressions.[129] Earlier trials with 5-FU and vinblastine in small groups of patients were ineffective. Bleomycin and vincristine were used by Livingston et al in a single patient and a partial regression was observed.[130] Combination chemotherapy with cisplatin plus 5-FU has now been reported in two patients, again with major objective responses, one of which was a complete remission.[131]

One of the larger series of patients with advanced anal canal tumors treated with chemotherapy as primary management has been reported by Wilkin et al.[132] They treated a group of 15 patients with advanced disease with a non-cisplatin-containing combination of bleomycin, vincristine and high-dose methotrexate, with leucovorin rescue (BOM). Major objective regressions were seen in three (25%) of 12 patients with measurable disease, but the duration of response ranged from only 1 to 5 months. Toxicity was severe in one third of the patients, and four patients probably died as a result of toxicity. Wilkin et al concluded that although one fourth of the patients had responses, these were of short duration and associated with severe toxicity.

Magill et al treated a group of 19 patients (11 of whom had had prior chemotherapy) with a combination of cisplatin, bleomycin, and a vinca alkaloid (either vinblastine or vindesine). Six of 15 evaluable patients responded.[133]

In summary, anal canal tumors are sensitive to several chemotherapeutic agents, including cisplatin and mitomycin–5-FU. The optimal regimen remains to be defined. Complete remissions are possible, but relapse of distant metastases has always been seen.

FOLLOW-UP

Patients with squamous cell cancer of the anus require careful follow-up. Those with local or regional recurrence can be treated curatively, and those with systemic disease are eligible for effective chemotherapy. Follow-up should include interval history, physical examination, and liver function tests every 2 to 3 months for the first 3 years, then semiannually for another several years. The detection of local and inguinal node recurrence requires follow-up by the same physicians in order to differentiate post-treatment scar and inflammatory lymphadenitis from progressive recurrent tumor. Regular chest radiography and abdominal or pelvic CT at least yearly for the first 3 years is appropriate.

Management of patients with residual or recurrent local disease, as well as those with metachronous regional lymph nodes, was discussed earlier. The most recent report from the Memorial Hospital group documents the efficacy of surgical treatment of such patients.[81] Additional chemotherapy as definitive treatment or as a surgical adjuvant will likely improve these results further.[103]

ANORECTAL MELANOMA

Anorectal melanomas are rarely diagnosed at a curable stage, and most patients die within a year of diagnosis from systemic metastases. Fortunately, such tumors are rare, accounting for approximately 1% of anal cancers. Ultraradical surgery involving an abdominoperineal resection with inguinal and pelvic lymphadenectomy was the recommended approach for many years.[134] The end results with such approaches are poor, and current recommendations encourage a sphincter-saving local treatment if at all feasible.

Clinical and Pathologic Features

The diagnosis of anorectal melanoma is frequently delayed because the tumor is located deep within the anal canal and because symptoms are typically nonspecific "hemorrhoidal" complaints. Anal burning, pruritus, and minor intermittent blood on the toilet paper are usual. A mass, frequently nonpigmented, is seen at the dentate line, consistent with a thrombosed internal hemorrhoid. With progression, a prolapsing mass with increasing hemorrhage occurs, perhaps with palpable inguinal adenopathy. However, primary tumor progression is almost always cephalad. Although the majority of anal melanomas are pigmented on microscopic examination, only a small minority are grossly melanotic.[135] Asymptomatic anal melanoma is diagnosed as an incidental finding in hemorrhoidectomy specimens.

Patterns of Spread

Extensive proximal submucosal spread into the rectum occurs. Lymph node metastases are found in the mesorectal nodes in 50% of patients treated by radical surgery, and in the inguinal nodes in 20%.[134-136] Hematogenous metastases occur early and widely, primarily to the liver and lungs.

Treatment and End Results

The Memorial Hospital,[58,136-138] St. Mark's Hospital,[139] and Mayo Clinic[140] groups report the largest experience with these tumors, in addition to a composite experience from Israel.[141] In the initial reports from Memorial Hospital, abdominoperineal resection, alone or combined with pelvic and inguinal lymphadenectomy, was recommended for all patients without distant disease, but there were only three 5-year survivors of 50 patients so treated. In a smaller experience at St. Mark's Hospital, there were no 5-year survivors. In the few patients treated by wide local excision (2-cm margins), all patients died of distant disease without local recurrence. The Mayo Clinic experience with abdominoper-

ineal resection is equally grim. In a report from Israel, only two of 30 patients survived 5 years, both after local excision.

A more recent analysis of the Memorial Hospital experience includes some patients treated by local measures, such as local excision, fulguration, and cryosurgery.[58] The end results as a function of tumor thickness provided the greatest insight into the far-advanced nature of these cancers when treatment is undertaken. All three patients with melanomas less than 2.0 mm thick were cured with abdominoperineal resection. No patient with a tumor thicker than 2.0 mm survived longer than 5 years, and 85% were dead in 2 years. Hence, it appears that only patients with "incidentally diagnosed" melanomas, usually as part of a hemorrhoidectomy specimen, are likely to be cured by surgery. Although the long-term survivors at Memorial Hospital were treated with radical surgery, that does not preclude cure with a more limited approach.[142] More advanced lesions may be treated by local excision combined with external-beam radiation therapy, at doses of at least 400 cGy per fraction.[143]

Summary

Patients with incidental anal melanomas less than 2 mm thick detected in hemorrhoidectomy specimens should undergo wide local excision. If the location of the tumor is unknown (multiple unmarked specimens sent to pathology), the patient may either be observed closely for signs of local recurrence or may undergo abdominoperineal resection.

Intermediate tumors, those more than 2 mm thick but not overly bulky, may be palliated with a local procedure — wide local excision, fulguration, laser vaporization, or cryosurgery. External-beam or implant radiation therapy may play an adjuvant role.

Despite the incurability of bulky anal melanoma, if the lesion cannot be controlled with a local approach, abdominoperineal resection or radiation therapy may still be necessary to palliate symptoms of bleeding, tenesmus, or obstruction.

Patients with systemic disease should be considered for chemotherapy and immunotherapy regimens appropriate for skin melanoma.

FUTURE DIRECTIONS

PREVENTION AND EARLY DETECTION. Prevention of epidermoid carcinoma of the anal canal will require better knowledge of etiologic factors. Meanwhile, because accumulating evidence implicates papillomaviruses as causative factors, and because the incidence of anal cancer appears to be increasing in the male homosexual community, it would be wise to direct further epidemiologic and virologic studies along these lines. Increasing use of measures for "safe sex" initiated to stem the spread of AIDS may also affect the incidence of anal cancer. Early detection could result from increased awareness in high-risk individuals; both male homosexuals and immunosuppressed renal transplant patients should be educated about anal cancer. Basic studies, such as the search for tumor markers or flow cytometric analyses for possible premalignant or diagnostic changes, may aid in detection as well as follow-up. Animal studies, such as those with epidermal growth factor, may offer insights into etiology and potentially lead to means of prevention.

THERAPY. Multimodality therapy has made great inroads in the sphincter-saving cure of anal cancer. Studies are now addressing issues such as the following: (1) decreasing thrombocytopenia during treatment by omitting mitomycin C from the regimen; (2) optimizing the treatment of patients with positive inguinal lymph nodes by limiting surgical excision to clinically grossly positive nodes and relying increasingly on high-dose nodal irradiation in combination with chemotherapy; (3) investigating more aggressive multimodality regimens for advanced local disease (*i.e.*, chemotherapy plus external-beam irradiation plus radioactive implants); and (4) exploring new aggressive chemotherapy regimens for patients with metastatic disease.

REFERENCES

1. Cummings BJ: The place of radiation therapy in the treatment of carcinoma of the anal canal. Cancer Treat Rev 9:125–147, 1982
2. Shank B: Treatment of anal canal carcinoma. Cancer 55:2156–2162, 1985
3. Papillon J: The responsibility of radiologists in the preservation of breast and rectum in cancer treatment. Clin Radiol 37:303–309, 1986
4. Grinnell RS: An analysis of forty-nine cases of squamous cell carcinoma of the anus. Surg Gynecol Obstet 98:29–39, 1954
5. Richards JC, Beahrs OH, Woolner LB: Squamous cell carcinoma of the anus, anal canal, and rectum in 109 patients. Surg Gynecol Obstet 114:475–482, 1962
6. Sawyers JL, Herrington JL Jr, Main FB: Surgical considerations in the treatment of epidermoid carcinoma of the anus. Ann Surg 157:817–824, 1963
7. Stearns MW Jr, Urmacher C, Sternberg SS et al: Cancer of the anal canal. Curr Probl Cancer 4:1–44, 1980
8. Morson BC, Volkstadt H: Malignant melanoma of the anal canal. J Clin Pathol 16:126–132, 1963
9. McConnell EM: Squamous cell carcinoma of the anus: A review of 96 cases. Br J Surg 57:89–92, 1970
10. Peters RK, Mack TM: Patterns of anal carcinoma by gender and marital status in Los Angeles County. Br J Cancer 48:629–636, 1983
11. Klotz RG, Pamukcoglu T, Souilliard DH: Transitional cloacogenic carcinoma of the anal canal. Cancer 20:1727–1745, 1967
12. Corman ML, Haggitt RC: Carcinoma of the anal canal. Surg Gynecol Obstet 145:674–676, 1977
13. Cantril ST, Green JP, Schall GL et al: Primary radiation therapy in the treatment of anal carcinoma. Int J Radiat Oncol Biol Phys 9:1271–1278, 1983
14. Welch JP, Malt RA: Appraisal of treatment of carcinoma of the anus and anal canal. Surg Gynecol Obstet 145:837–841, 1977
15. Gabriel WB: Discussion on squamous cell carcinoma of the anus and anal canal. Proc R Soc Med 53:403–409, 1960
16. Wolfe HRI, Bussey HJR: Squamous cell carcinoma of the anus. Br J Surg 55:295–301, 1968
17. Morson BC, Pang LSC: Pathology of anal cancer. Proc R Soc Med 61:623–624, 1968
18. Rousseau J, Mathieu G, Fenton J et al: La télécobaltothérapie des cancers du canal anal. J Radiol Electrol Med Nucl 54:622–626, 1973
19. Kapur BML, Dhawan IK, Singhal KK: Epidermoid carcinoma of the anorectum: Review of 13 cases. Dis Colon Rectum 20:252–254, 1977
20. Cooper HS, Patchefsky AS, Marks G: Cloacogenic carcinoma of the anorectum in homosexual men: An observation of four cases. Dis Colon Rectum 22:557–558, 1979
21. Li FP, Osborn D, Cronin CM: Anorectal squamous carcinoma in two homosexual men. Lancet 2:391, 1982
22. Austin DF: Etiologic clues from descriptive epidemiology: Squamous carcinoma of the rectum or anus. Natl Cancer Inst Monogr 62:89–90, 1982
23. Daling JR, Weiss NS, Klopfenstein LL et al: Correlates of homosexual behavior and the incidence of anal cancer. JAMA 247:1988–1990, 1982
24. Daling JR, Weiss NS, Hislop G et al: Sexual practices, sexually transmitted diseases, and the incidence of anal cancer. N Engl J Med 317:973–977, 1987
25. zur Hausen H: Human papillomaviruses and their possible role in squamous cell carcinomas. Curr Top Microbiol Immunol 78:1–30, 1977
26. Siegel A: Malignant transformation of condyloma acuminatum: Review of the literature and case report. Am J Surg 103:613–617, 1962
27. Friedberg MJ, Serlin O: Condyloma acuminatum: Its association with malignancy. Dis Colon Rectum 6:352–355, 1963
28. Oriel JD, Whimster IW: Carcinoma in situ associated with virus-containing anal warts. Br J Dermatol 84:71–73, 1971
29. Prasad ML, Abcarian H: Malignant potential of perianal condyloma acuminatum. Dis Colon Rectum 23:191–197, 1980
30. Croxson T, Chabon AB, Rorat E et al: Intraepithelial carcinoma of the anus in homosexual men. Dis Colon Rectum 27:325–330, 1984
31. McAnally AK, Dockerty MB: Carcinoma developing in chronic draining cutaneous sinuses and fistulas. Surg Gynecol Obstet 88:87–96, 1949
32. Winkelman J, Grosfeld J, Bigelow B: Colloid carcinoma of anal-gland origin: Report of a case and review of the literature. Am J Clin Pathol 42:395–401, 1964
33. Bretlau P: Carcinoma arising in anal fistula. Acta Chir Scand 133:496–500, 1967
34. Chaos A, Garrido H, Fernandez-Villoria JM: Carcinoma associated with fistula in ano. Int Surg 58:497–499, 1973
35. Binkley GE, Derrick WA: The association of squamous cancer with anal manifestations of lymphogranuloma venereum. Am J Dig Dis 12:46–47, 1945
36. Rainey R: The association of lymphogranuloma inguinale and cancer. Surgery 35:221–235, 1954
37. Brennan JT, Stewart CF: Epidermoid carcinoma of the anus. Ann Surg 176:787–790, 1972
38. Buckwalter JA, Jurayj MN: Relationship of chronic anorectal disease to carcinoma. Arch Surg 75:352–361, 1957
39. Chuang TY, Perry HO, Kurland LT et al: Condyloma acuminatum in Rochester, Minnesota, 1950–1978: II. Anaplasias and unfavorable outcomes. Arch Dermatol 120:476–483, 1984
40. Cabrera A, Tsukada Y, Pickren JW et al: Development of lower genital carcinomas in patients with anal carcinoma: A more than casual relationship. Cancer 19:470–480, 1966
41. Goligher JC: Surgery of the Anus, Rectum and Colon, 3rd ed, p 815. London, Bailere, Tindell and Cassell Ltd, 1975
42. Penn I: Cancers of the anogenital region in renal transplant recipients: Analysis of 65 cases. Cancer 58:611–616, 1986
43. Daniell HW: Re: causes of anal carcinoma. JAMA 254:358, 1985
44. Cone LA, Woodard DR, Potts BE et al: An update on the acquired immunodeficiency syndrome (AIDS): Associated disorders of the alimentary tract. Dis Colon Rectum 29:60–64, 1986
45. Kawaura A, Kumagai H, Shibata M et al: Tumors of the anal region induced in mice painted with methyloxymethanol acetate. Gann 72:886–890, 1981
46. Kingsnorth AN, Abu-Khalaf M, Ross JS et al: Potentiation of 1,2-dimethylhydrazine-induced anal carcinoma by epidermal growth factor in mice. Surgery 97:696–700, 1985
47. Kuehn PG, Beckett R, Eisenberg H et al: Epidermoid carcinoma of the perianal skin and anal canal. N Engl J Med 270:614–617, 1964
48. Adam YG, Efron G: Current concepts and controversies concerning the etiology, pathogenesis, diagnosis and treatment of malignant tumors of the anus. Surgery 101:253–266, 1987
49. Morson BC: The pathology and results of treatment of squamous cell carcinoma of the anal canal and anal margin. Proc R Soc Med 53:414–420, 1960
50. Greenall MJ, Quan SHQ, Stearns MW et al: Epidermoid cancer of the anal margin. Am J Surg 149:95–101, 1985
51. Hardy KJ, Hughes ESR, Cuthbertson AM: Squamous cell carcinoma of the anal canal and anal margin. Aust NZ J Surg 38:301–305, 1969
52. Beahrs OH, Wilson SM: Carcinoma of the anus. Ann Surg 184:422–428, 1976
53. Wood DA: Tumors of the intestines. In: Atlas of Tumor Pathology, pp 200–223. Washington, DC, Armed Forces Institute of Pathology, 1967
54. Boman BM, Moertel CG, O Connell MJ et al: Carcinoma of the anal canal: A clinical and pathologic study of 188 cases. Cancer 54:114–125, 1984
55. Ordonez NG, Awalt H, Mackay B: Mammary and extramammary Paget's disease: An immunocytochemical and ultrastructural study. Cancer 59:1173–1183, 1987
56. Remigio PA, Der BK, Forsberg RT: Anorectal melanoma: Report of two cases. Dis Colon Rectum 19:350–356, 1976
57. Quinn D, Selah C: Malignant melanoma of the anus in a Negro: Report of a case and review of the literature. Dis Colon Rectum 20:627–631, 1977
58. Wanebo HJ, Woodruff JM, Farr GH et al: Anorectal melanoma. Cancer 47:1891–1900, 1981
59. Stearns MW, Quan SH: Epidermoid carcinoma of the anorectum. Surg Gynecol Obstet 191:953–957, 1970
60. Dougherty B, Evans H: Carcinoma of the anal canal: A study of 79 cases. Am J Clin Pathol 83:159–164, 1985
61. Fenger C, Nielsen VT: Precancerous changes in the anal canal epithelium in resection specimens. Acta Pathol Microbiol Immunol Scand [A] 94:63–69, 1986
62. Fenger C, Nielsen VT: Dysplastic changes in the anal canal epithelium in minor surgical specimens. Acta Pathol Microbiol Immunol Scand [A] 89:463–465, 1981
63. Fenger C, Bichel P: Flow cytometric DNA analysis of anal canal epithelium and ano-rectal tumours. Acta Pathol Microbiol Scand [A] 89:351–355, 1981
64. Goldman S, Auer G, Erhardt K et al: Prognostic significance of clinical stage, histologic grade, and nuclear DNA content in squamous-cell carcinoma of the anus. Dis Colon Rectum 30:444–448, 1987
65. Singh R, Nime F, Mittelman A: Malignant epithelial tumors of the anal canal. Cancer 48:411–415, 1981
66. Salmon RJ, Zafrani B, Habib A et al: Prognosis of cloacogenic and squamous cancers of the anal canal. Dis Colon Rectum 29:336–340, 1986
67. Dillard BM, Spratt JS Jr, Ackerman LV et al: Epidermoid cancer of anal margin and canal. Arch Surg 86:772–777, 1963
68. Clark J, Petrelli N, Herrera L et al: Epidermoid carcinoma of the anal canal. Cancer 57:400–406, 1986
69. Wolfe HRI: The management of metastatic inguinal adenitis in epidermoid cancer of the anus. Proc R Soc Med 61:626–629, 1961
70. Hardcastle JD, Bussey HJR: Results of surgical treatment of squamous cell carcinoma of the anal canal and anal margin seen at St. Mark's Hospital 1928–66. Proc R Soc Med 61:629–630, 1968
71. Kuehn PG, Beckett R, Eisenberg H et al: Hematogenous metastases from epidermoid carcinoma of the anal canal. Am J Surg 109:445–449, 1965

72. Greenall MJ, Quan SHQ, DeCosse J: Epidermoid cancer of the anus. Br J Surg 72:S97–S103, 1985
73. Pyper PC, Parks TG: The results of surgery for epidermoid carcinoma of the anus. Br J Surg 72:712–714, 1985
74. Paradis P, Douglass HO Jr, Holyoke ED: The clinical implications of a staging system for carcinoma of the anus. Surg Gynecol Obstet 141:411–416, 1975
75. Harmer MH (ed.): TNM Classification of Malignant Tumors, 3rd ed, pp 77–81. Geneva, International Union Against Cancer (Union Internationale Contre le Cancer), 1978
76. Hermanek P: Problems of pTNM classification of carcinoma of the stomach, colorectum and anal margin. Pathol Res Pract 181:296–300, 1986
77. Spiessl B, Hermanek P, Scheibe O et al (ed): TNM-Atlas: Illustrated Guide to the TNM/pTNM Classification of Malignant Tumours, 2nd ed, pp 114–123. New York, Springer-Verlag, 1982
78. Hermanek P, Sobin LH (eds): TNM Classification of Malignant Tumours, 4th ed, pp 50–52, 83–88. New York, Springer-Verlag, 1987
79. American Joint Committee on Cancer: Manual for Staging of Cancer, 3rd ed. Philadelphia, JB Lippincott Co, 1987
80. Papillon J: Rectal and Anal Cancers, pp 124–125. New York, Springer-Verlag, 1982
81. Greenall M, Magill G, Quan S et al: Recurrent epidermoid cancer of the anus. Cancer 57:1437–1441, 1986
82. Kuehn PG, Eisenberg H, Reed JF: Epidermoid carcinoma of the perianal skin and anal canal. Cancer 22:932–938, 1968
83. Wanebo H, Futrell W, Constable W: Multimodality approach to surgical management of locally advanced epidermoid carcinoma of the anorectum. Cancer 47:2817–2826, 1981
84. Papillon J, Montbarbon JF: Epidermoid carcinoma of the anal canal: A series of 276 cases. Dis Colon Rectum 30:324–333, 1987
85. Serota AI, Weil M, Williams RA et al: Anal cloacogenic carcinoma. Arch Surg 116:456–459, 1981
86. Grodsky L: Unsuspected anal cancer discovered after minor anorectal surgery. Dis Colon Rectum 10:471–478, 1967
87. Turell R: Epidermoid squamous cell cancer of the perianus and anal canal. Surg Clin North Am 42:1235–1241, 1962
88. Dalby JF, Pointon RS: The treatment of anal carcinoma by interstitial irradiation. AJR 85:515–520, 1961
89. Schraut WH, Wang C-H, Dawson PJ et al: Depth of invasion, location, and size of cancer of the anus dictate operative treatment. Cancer 51:1291–1296, 1983
90. Frost DB, Richards PC, Montague ED et al: Epidermoid cancer of the anorectum. Cancer 53:1285–1293, 1984
91. Cummings BJ, Keane TJ, Hawkins NV et al: Treatment of perianal carcinoma by radiation (RT) or radiation plus chemotherapy (RTCT) (abstr). Int J Radiat Oncol Biol Phys 12:170, 1986
92. Hintz BL, Charyulu KKN, Sudarsanam A: Anal carcinoma: Basic concepts and management. J Surg Oncol 10:141–150, 1978
93. James RD, Pointon RS, Martin S: Local radiotherapy in the management of squamous carcinoma of the anus. Br J Surg 72:282–285, 1985
94. Papillon J, Renard L, Pipard G: Le cancer de la marge de l'anus: Experience du Centre Leon Berard. J Eur Radiother 6:29–34, 1985
95. Glimelius B, Påhlman L: Recurrent epidermoid cancer of the anus. Cancer 57:1437–1441, 1986
96. Al-Jurf AS, Turnbull RB, Fazio VW: Local treatment of squamous cell carcinoma of the anus. Surg Gynecol Obstet 148:576–578, 1979
97. Greenall MJ, Quan SHQ, Urmacher C et al: Treatment of epidermoid carcinoma of the anal canal. Surg Gynecol Obstet 161:509–517, 1985
98. Leichman L, Nigro N, Vaitkevicius VK et al: Cancer of the anal canal: Model for preoperative adjuvant combined modality therapy. Am J Med 78:211–216, 1985
99. Enker WE, Heilweil M, Janov AJ et al: Improved survival in epidermoid carcinoma of the anus in association with pre-operative multi-disciplinary therapy. Arch Surg 121:1386–1390, 1986
100. Cummings B, Keane T, Thomas G et al: Results and toxicity of the treatment of anal canal carcinoma by radiation therapy or radiation therapy and chemotherapy. Cancer 54:2062–2068, 1984
101. Sischy B: The use of radiation therapy combined with chemotherapy in the management of squamous cell carcinoma of the anus and marginally resectable adenocarcinoma of the rectum. Int J Radiat Oncol Biol Phys 11:1587–1593, 1985
102. John MJ, Flam M, Lovalvo L et al: Feasibility of non-surgical definitive management of anal canal carcinoma. Int J Radiat Oncol Biol Phys 13:299–303, 1987
103. Flam MS, John M, Mowry P et al: Definitive combined modality therapy of carcinoma of the anus: A report of 30 cases including results of salvage therapy in patients with residual disease. Dis Colon Rectum 30:495–502, 1987
104. Ajlouni M, Mahrt D, Milad MP: Review of recent experience in the treatment of carcinoma of the anal canal. Am J Clin Oncol 73:687–691, 1984
105. Nigro ND, Vaitkevicius VK, Considine B Jr: Combined therapy for cancer of the anal canal: A preliminary report. Dis Colon Rectum 17:354–356, 1974
106. Michaelson RA, Magill GB, Quan SHQ et al: Pre-operative chemotherapy and radiation therapy in the management of anal epidermoid carcinoma. Cancer 51:390–395, 1983
107. Nigro ND: Multi-disciplinary management of cancer of the anus. World J Surg 11:446–451, 1987
108. Salmon RJ, Fenton J, Asselain B et al: Treatment of epidermoid anal canal cancer. Am J Surg 147:43–48, 1984
109. Byfield JE, Calabro-Jones P, Klisak I et al: Pharmacologic requirements for obtaining sensitization of human tumor cells in vitro to combined 5-fluorouracil or ftorafur and x rays. Int J Radiat Oncol Biol Phys 8:1923–1933, 1982
110. Rockwell S: Cytotoxicities of mitomycin C and X rays to aerobic and hypoxic cells in vitro. Int J Radiat Oncol Biol Phys 8:1035–1039, 1982
111. Byfield JE, Barone RM, Sharp TR et al: Conservative management without alkylating agents of squamous cell anal cancer using cyclical 5-FU alone and X-ray therapy. Cancer Treat Rep 67:709–712, 1985
112. Golden GT, Horsley JS III: Surgical management of epidermoid carcinoma of the anus. Am J Surg 131:275–280, 1976
113. Bond WH: Proc R Soc Med 53:411–414, 1960
114. Devois A, Decker R: La curiepuncture du cancer de l'anus. Arch Fr Mal Appar Dig Mal Nutr 49(suppl):54–67, 1960
115. Keiling R, Grunewald JM, Achille E: Radiothérapie des cancers malpighiens de l'anus: La curiethérapie interstitielle à l'iridium 192 des epitheliomas du canal anal. J Radiol Electrol Med Nucl 54:634–635, 1973
116. Cohan RH, Silverman PM, Thompson WM et al: Computed tomography of epithelial neoplasms of the anal canal. AJR 145:569–573, 1985
117. Eschwege F, Lasser P, Chavy A et al: Squamous cell carcinoma of the anal canal: Treatment by external beam irradiation. Radiother Oncol 3:145–150, 1985
118. Doggett SW, Green JP, Cantril ST: Efficacy of radiation alone for limited squamous cell carcinoma of the anal canal. Int J Radiat Oncol Biol Phys 12(suppl):170–171, 1986
119. Fenton J, Cutuli B, Rousseau J et al: Anal canal carcinoma: Survival and sphincter preservation after radiotherapy (195 cases) (abstr). Presented at the fifth annual meeting of the European Society of Radiologic Therapy and Oncology, 1986
120. Chruscov MM, Semakina EP, Raifel BA: Die Strahlentherapie des rektalen Epidermoidkarzinoms. Radiobiol Radiother (Berlin) 19:683–689, 1978
121. Glimelius B, Påhlman L: Radiation therapy of anal epidermoid carcinoma. Int J Radiat Oncol Biol Phys 13:305–312, 1987
122. Delouche G, Bachelot F, Cohen M et al: La radiothérapie des cancers malpighiens de l'anus. J Radiol Electrol Med Nucl 54:642–646, 1973
123. Ager P, Samala E, Bosworth J et al: The conservative management of anorectal cancer by radiotherapy. Am J Surg 137:228–230, 1979
124. Martinez A, Edmundson GK, Cox RS et al: Combination of external beam irradiation and multiple-site perineal applicator (MUPIT) for treatment of locally advanced or recurrent prostatic, anorectal, and gynecologic malignancies. Int J Radiat Oncol Biol Phys 11:391–398, 1985
125. Puthawala AA, Syed N, Gates TC et al: Definitive treatment of extensive anorectal carcinoma by external and interstitial irradiation. Cancer 50:1746–1750, 1982
126. Pipard G, Peytremann R, Marti MC: Conservative multidisciplinary treatment of locally advanced epidermoid and cloacogenic cancer of the anal canal (abst). Proc Am Soc Clin Oncol 5:268, 1986
127. Stearns MW Jr: Epidermoid carcinoma of the anal region. Surg Gynecol Obstet 106:92–96, 1958
128. Fisher W, Herbst K, Sims J et al: Metastatic cloacogenic carcinoma of the anus: Sequential responses to Adriamycin and cis-dichlorodiamineplatinum (II). Cancer Treat Rep 62:91–97, 1978
129. Salem P, Habboubi N, Naanasissie E et al: Effectiveness of cisplatin in the treatment of anal squamous cell carcinoma. Cancer Treat Rep 69:891–893, 1985
130. Livingston R, Bodey G, Gottlieb J et al: Kinetic scheduling of vincristine and bleomycin in patients with lung cancer and other malignant tumors. Cancer Chemother Rep 57:219–224, 1973
131. Khatr R, Frenay M, Bourry J et al: Cisplatin plus 5-fluorouracil in the treatment of metastatic anal squamous cell carinoma: A report of two cases. Cancer Treat Rep 70:1345–1346, 1986
132. Wilkin N, Petrelli N, Herrera L et al: Phase II study of combination of bleomycin, vincristine and high-dose methotrexate (BOM) with leucovorin rescue in advanced squamous cell carcinoma of the anal canal. Cancer Chemother Pharmacol 15:300–302, 1985
133. Magill GB: Personal communication, 1987
134. Pack GT, Martins FG: Treatment of anorectal malignant melanoma. Dis Colon Rectum 3:15–24, 1960
135. Morson BC, Volkstadt H: Malignant melanoma of the anal canal. J Clin Pathol 16:126–132, 1963
136. Quan SH, Deddish MR: Noncutaneous melanoma. CA 16:111–114, 1966
137. Quan SHQ, White JE, Deddish MR: Malignant melanoma of the anorectum. Dis Colon Rectum 2:275–283, 1959
138. Pack GT, Oropeza R: A comparative study of melanoma and epidermoid carcinoma of the anal canal: A review of 20 melanomas and 29 epidermoid carcinomas. Dis Colon Rectum 10:161–176, 1967
139. Ward MW, Romano G, Nicholls RJ. The surgical treatment of anorectal malignant melanoma. Br J Surg 73:68–69, 1986
140. Chiu YS, Unni KK, Beart RW: Malignant melanoma of the anorectum. Dis Colon Rectum 23:122–124, 1980
141. Siegel B, Cohen D, Jacob ET: Surgical treatment of anorectal melanomas. Am J Surg 146:336–338, 1983
142. Garnick M, Lokich JJ: Primary malignant melanoma of the rectum: Rationale for conservative surgical management. J Surg Oncol 10:529–531, 1978
143. Harwood AR, Cummings BJ: Radiotherapy for mucosal melanomas. Int J Radiat Oncol Biol Phys 8:1121–1126, 1982

W. MARSTON LINEHAN

WILLIAM U. SHIPLEY

DAN L. LONGO

CHAPTER 31 *Cancer of the Kidney
and Ureter*

RENAL CELL CARCINOMA

Each year in the United States there are approximately 18,000 cases of renal cell carcinoma, resulting in more than 9,000 deaths. This tumor accounts for approximately 3% of adult malignancies and occurs in a male–female ratio of 2:1. It is more common among urban than rural residents. Although most cases of renal cell carcinoma occur in persons aged 50 to 70 years, it has been observed in children as young as 6 months of age. Between 1975 and 1984 there was a modest increase in the incidence of renal cell carcinoma, about 2% per year.[1-7]

Renal cell carcinoma was first described by Konig in 1826. As early as 1855 Robin concluded that the renal tubular epithelium was the most probable tissue of origin of the cancer, an observation that was confirmed by Waldeyer in 1867. In 1883 Grawitz, noting that the fatty content of the cancer cells was similar to that of adrenal cells, concluded that the tumors arose from adrenal rests within the kidney and introduced the term "stroma lipomatodes aberrata renis" for these clear cell tumors. The term "hypernephroid tumors" was introduced in 1894 by Birch-Hirschfeld. Since then the conceptually incorrect term "hypernephroma" has frequently been applied to renal tumors.[8-11]

Rarely, renal cell carcinoma occurs in a familial form. There is an increased incidence of renal cell carcinoma with von Hippel–Lindau syndrome: up to 35% of patients with von Hippel–Lindau syndrome will develop renal cell carcinoma. In both familial syndromes the renal cancer is often bilateral and tends to occur in a younger age group.[12-15] An increased incidence of renal cell carcinoma has also been observed in patients with autosomal dominant polycystic kidney disease.[16]

ETIOLOGY

A number of environmental, hormonal, cellular, and genetic factors have been studied as possible causal factors in the development of renal cell carcinoma. Cigarette smoking is a definite risk factor for the development of kidney cancer. It has been estimated that 30% of renal cell carcinomas in men and 24% in women may be directly due to smoking.[17-19] Obesity is associated with an increased risk of development of renal cell carcinoma, particularly in women.[18-20] Analgesic abuse, which is known to be associated with renal pelvis cancer, is also associated with an increased incidence of kidney cancer. The increased risk for the development of renal cell carcinoma is observed primarily in patients who abuse phenacetin-containing analgesics and develop analgesic nephropathy.[18,21]

A number of environmental and occupational factors have been associated with the development of kidney cancer. There is an increased incidence of renal cell carcinoma among leather tanners, shoe workers, and workers exposed to asbestos.[22,23] Exposure to cadmium is associated with an increased incidence of kidney cancer, particularly in men who smoke.[24] Patients exposed to thorotrast, a 2.5% solution of thorium dioxide used in the 1920s as a contrast medium for renal and hepatic visualization, have an increased incidence of kidney cancer. Thorium dioxide is a radioactive agent that produces α-rays, β-rays, and γ-rays; it is thought that chronic exposure to radiation emitted by this agent is responsible for the development of renal cancer.[25] An association between gasoline exposure and kidney cancer has been observed in animal studies. Although there is an increased incidence of renal cell carcinoma reported with exposure to petroleum, tar, and pitch products, studies of oil refinery workers and petroleum products distribution workers do not identify a definite relationship between gasoline exposure and renal cancer. There may be an increased risk of kidney cancer in older workers or in workers exposed to gasoline for prolonged periods of time.[26,27]

There is an increased incidence of renal cell carcinoma in patients who develop acquired cystic disease while on long-term hemodialysis.[28-31] Acquired cystic disease is a recently described phenomenon in which patients on long-term dialysis for renal failure develop cysts in their native kidneys. Renal cell carcinoma has been found in association with the papillary hyperplasia observed in the cyst epithelium of these kidneys. It is estimated that 35% to 47% of patients on long-term dialysis will develop acquired cystic disease, and about 5.8% of the patients with acquired cystic disease will develop renal cell cancer. Although most of these cancers are clinically insignificant and are found incidentally in autopsy or after bilateral nephrectomy, some will have an aggressive course.[28-30]

A hormonal etiology for renal cell carcinoma was suggested in 1947 based on a series of animal studies by Matthews and co-workers, who reported the induction of kidney tumors in male Syrian golden hamsters by prolonged administration of estrogen.[32,33] In a subsequent study published in 1952, Kirkman and Bacon reported treatment with estrogen of 100 male hamsters for 250 days; 97 developed renal tumors.[34] Bloom et al demonstrated that cortisone plus medroxyprogesterone acetate (Provera) could inhibit the growth of estrogen-induced, transplantable renal tumors, and that an estrogen antagonist could inhibit the growth of these tumors in the hamster.[35,36] The current role of hormonal therapy in the management of patients with metastatic renal cell carcinoma will be discussed.

GROWTH FACTORS

The role of tumor-produced growth factors in the initiation or progression of genitourinary malignancies is currently under study. In many patients with renal cell carcinoma there is evidence of tumor-produced factors that have systemic effects. Pyrexia, cachexia, abnormal liver function, increased alkaline phosphatase levels, hypercalcemia, polycythemia, neuromyopathy, and amyloidosis have all been reported in association with renal cell carcinoma.[37] Humoral hypercalcemia of malignancy, frequently observed in patients with renal cell carcinoma, is thought to be caused by a tumor-produced, systemically active bone-resorbing factor. Some studies suggest that this tumor-produced factor is parathyroid hormone (PTH)-like, others suggest that it is more transforming growth factor (TGF)-like.[38] A PTH-related protein that has been implicated in malignant hypercalcemia has been cloned from a human lung cancer cell line and expressed in mammalian cells.[39] Whether or not this PTH-

like factor induces paracrine or endocrine effects such as bone resorption or hypercalcemia of malignancy in patients with renal cell carcinoma is currently under study.

It has been suggested that the bone-resorbing factor produced by human tumors may have TGF-like bioactivity. Derynck et al[40] have shown that renal cell carcinoma and renal cell carcinoma cell lines have increased expression of TGF-α, TGF-β, and epidermal growth factor (EGF) receptor.[40,41] Gomella and co-workers found greater expression of TGF-α and TGF-β in renal cell carcinoma than in normal renal tissue from the same patient.[42] TGF-α is known to bind to the EGF receptor and can induce reversible transformation of nontransformed cell lines.[43,44] TGF-β has been shown to inhibit both the growth of lymphokine-mediated stimulation of peripheral blood lymphocytes[45] and the lytic activity of lymphokine-activated killer cells.[46,47] These and other studies suggest the possibility that tumor-produced growth factors could have a number of roles in renal cell carcinoma. TGF-α, for example, could have an autocrine role in either initiation or progression of renal cell carcinoma by stimulation through the EGF-receptor and induction of unregulated cell growth. Bone resorption induced by TGF-α[48] or a PTH-like factor could release TGF-β from the bone (one of the largest reservoirs of TGF-β in the body), which could inhibit the host's immune response to the tumor.[45-47] It is hoped that an understanding of the role of soluble factors involved in regulation of growth of renal cell carcinoma will lead to new strategies for treatment of this disease. Studies of peptides that block growth factor receptor activation, antibodies that block growth factor receptors, and other agents that affect growth factor production and action are in progress.

MOLECULAR GENETICS

In the past ten years much information on the genetics of renal cell carcinoma has become available. In 1979 Cohen and co-workers described a pedigree with familial renal cell carcinoma in which the pattern of inheritance was consistent with an autosomal dominant gene.[49] Of particular interest was the association of renal cell carcinoma with a karyotypic abnormality, a balanced reciprocal translocation between the short arm of chromosome 3 and the long arm of chromosome 8. This abnormality was present in constitutional tissue and, therefore, presumably in tumor tissue of affected family members. All members of the family who developed renal cell carcinoma had a 3;8 translocation; no family member without a 3;8 translocation developed renal cell carcinoma. It has since been shown that in this kindred the cellular oncogene c-myc is translocated from chromosome 8 to chromosome 3 and the cellular oncogene c-raf is translocated from chromosome 3 to chromosome 8.[50] A second pedigree with renal cell carcinoma was described in 1982 by Pathak and co-workers.[51] In the propositus, the major karyotypic abnormality was a chromosome 3 to chromosome 11 translocation. This pedigree differed from the one described by Cohen et al. in that the karyotypic abnormality was limited to the tumor. Recently, chromosomal analysis performed on tumor cells from a patient with von Hippel–Lindau disease revealed a proximal deletion in the short arm of chromosome 3 in the 3p14 region.[52]

The studies of chromosomal abnormalities in familial renal cell carcinoma focused attention on the possible role of alterations in the short arm of chromosome 3 in the genesis of nonfamilial renal cell carcinoma. Chromosomal analysis by Yoshida et al,[53,54] Szucs et al,[55] and Carroll et al[56] suggested that a structural change in chromosome 3 is linked to sporadic as well as hereditary renal cell carcinoma. This information led to the use of restriction length fragment polymorphism (RFLP) analysis of chromosome 3 in constitutional and tumor tissue in patients with sporadic renal cell carcinoma.[57] The technique of RFLP analysis for detection of DNA sequence deletions in tumors, described by Cavanee et al in 1983, is more sensitive than karyotype analysis for detecting DNA sequence deletions.[58] RFLP analysis has been used to detect DNA sequence deletions in a number of human tumors, including Wilms' tumor,[59-62] retinoblastoma,[63] bladder cancer,[64] small cell lung carcinoma,[65] and colorectal carcinoma.[66] The use of RFLP analysis to define the somatic mechanisms involved in tumor development relies on the variability of DNA recognition sequences of bacterial restriction endonucleases.[63,67] Study of these RFLPs permits comparison of normal and tumor tissue for the presence or absence of DNA sequences. For example, the RFLP obtained with a particular probe for chromosome 3, pH3H2 (DNF15S2), detects a polymorphic locus at the 3p21 region.[68]

Zbar and co-workers performed RFLP analysis on normal and tumor tissue from 18 patients with renal cell carcinoma using three recombinant probes that have been mapped to the short arm of chromosome 3.[57] These investigators found evidence for a DNA sequence deletion (see Fig. 31-1) in 11 of 11 evaluable patients with renal cell carcinoma. The frequency of loss of 3p sequences in renal cell carcinoma is greater than that observed at other chromosomal loci in bladder carcinoma (42%), Wilms' tumor (55%), and colorectal carcinoma (20%) and suggests that loss of heterozygosity in this region is a nonrandom alteration and that a functioning gene located on 3p may be involved in the origin or evolution of renal cell carcinoma.[57,64,66]

Many of the biologic and genetic alterations in renal cell carcinoma are similar to those in retinoblastoma. Both neoplasms exist in hereditary and sporadic forms, and the hereditary form is associated with an earlier age at onset than is the sporadic form. The conceptual basis that seems to fit the current genetic data on retinoblastoma is consistent with the current molecular genetic data on renal cell carcinoma. The two-mutation theory of Knudson postulates that at least two mutations are necessary for the development of cancer (Fig. 31-2).[69,70] The data generated by chromosomal and RFLP analysis of renal cell carcinoma suggest that a somatic mutation is a chromosomal event that may involve the loss of the wild-type allele of a particular gene. In Wilms' tumor, which is associated with a DNA sequence deletion in the 13p region of chromosome 11, the introduction of a normal human chromosome 11 suppresses the tumorigenicity of Wilms' tumor cell lines.[71] Analogously, the introduction of a normal chromosome 3 back into a renal cell carcinoma cell line may be used to assess its effect on tumorigenesis.

FIG. 31-1. Chromosome 3 showing the area of interstitial deletion in renal cell carcinoma at 3p14-21 locus. * denotes the site of the c-erb a-2 oncogene; ** the c-raf-1 locus.

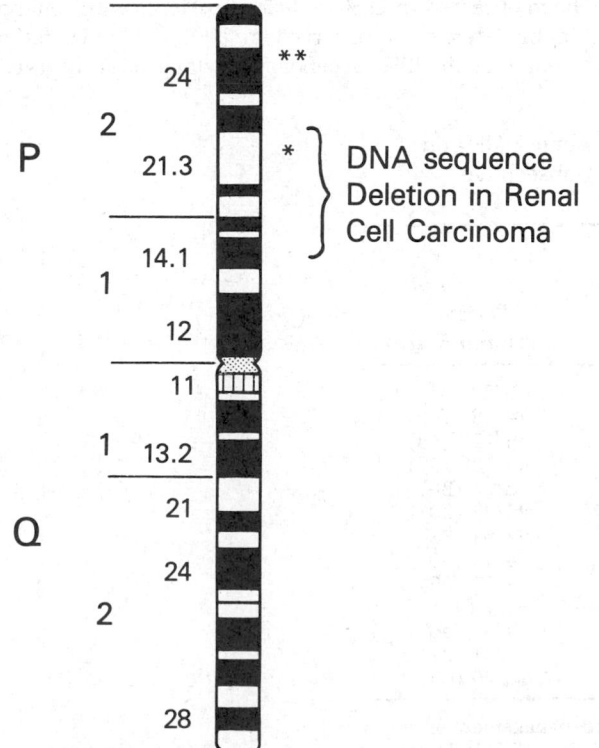

FIG. 31-2. Knudsen's hypothesis[69,70] as applied to renal cell carcinoma would suggest that RFLP analysis uncovers a DNA sequence deletion in allele A with a coexistent mutation at the same locus on allele A. In this region could be a gene that codes for a protein that regulates or suppresses growth factor or oncogene expression. (Comings, 1973).

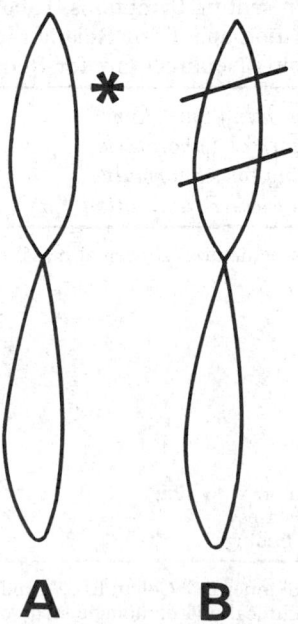

PATHOLOGY

For a number of years it was thought that renal cell carcinoma originated in adrenal rests within the kidney; immuno-histologic and ultrastructural analysis has now established that the proximal renal tubular epithelium is the true tissue of origin.[1,72] Renal cell tumors tend to be round, but may vary widely in size. The average diameter is approximately 7 cm; however, renal tumors can often grow to fill the entire retroperitoneum. Previously, renal lesions 2 cm or less in diameter were considered to be renal adenomas, while lesions 2 cm or more in diameter were considered to be carcinomas. The distinction between benign and malignant tumors is no longer made on the basis of size but on the basis of classic histologic criteria.[72,73] Although renal cell carcinoma tends to arise in the cortex of the kidney, it can originate in the interior of the kidney. There is often a pseudo-capsule formed around the tumor by compression of surrounding tissue. Hemorrhage and necrosis may be present, and frequently large areas of sclerosis and fibrosis are found within the tumor. Calcification and single or multiple fluid-filled cysts may be seen within the tumor. Sporadic renal cell carcinoma appears in either kidney with equal frequency; it is most often solitary and unilateral.

Renal cell carcinoma can occur in three different cellular types: clear cell, granular cell, and spindle or sarcomatoid variant. Clear cell carcinomas contain lightly staining cells with vacuolated cytoplasm containing cholesterol-like substances, neutral lipids, phospholipids, and glycogen.[1,74] Granular cell carcinomas contain cells that have a ground-glass–appearing, eosinophilic-staining cytoplasm with abundant mitochondria. The large nuclei of granular cells stain darker than the nuclei of clear cells. In sarcomatoid renal cell carcinoma there are spindle type cells which may resemble fibroblasts, rhabdomyoblasts, lipoblasts, or pleomorphic mesenchymal cells.[1,74-76] Few tumors are purely clear or granular cell type; most are mixtures of clear and granular cells. Depending on the series, 1% to 6% of renal cell carcinomas are sarcomatoid variant.[77,78]

Some studies suggest that there is slightly better prognosis with clear cell variant than with granular or mixed renal cell carcinomas.[79] The sarcomatoid variant is associated with a significantly poorer prognosis than are carcinomas of the clear, granular, or mixed cell type.[78,80-82] Sella and co-workers recently reported a median survival of only 6.6 months in 44 patients with sarcomatoid-type renal cell carcinoma, versus a 19.0-month median survival in 814 patients with nonsarcomatous renal cell carcinoma.[82] Although infrequently used in renal cell carcinoma, tumor grading may correlate with survival, particularly in patients with non-metastatic cancer.[79,80,83]

CLINICAL PRESENTATION

Renal cell carcinoma may remain clinically occult for most of its course. The classic presentation of pain, hematuria, and flank mass occurs in only about 19% of patients and often is indicative of advanced disease.[1] A tumor in the kidney can progress unnoticed to a large size in the retroperitoneum until a metastasis appears. Approximately 30% of patients with renal cell carcinoma present with metastatic disease, 25% with locally advanced renal cell carcinoma, and 45% with localized disease (Table 31-1).[7,84] Some 75% of patients with metastatic renal cell carcinoma have metastases to the lung, 36% to soft tissues, 20% to bone, 18% to liver, 8% to cutaneous sites, and 8% to the central nervous system.[85]

A considerable number of patients with renal cell carcinoma develop systemic symptoms of this disease.[86-89] Hypochromic anemia, due to either hematuria or hemolysis, has been observed in 29% to 88% of patients with renal cell carcinoma. Pyrexia is observed in 20%; cachexia, fatigue, and weight loss in 33%. Secondary amyloidosis is observed in

TABLE 31-1. Presenting Symptoms, Laboratory Abnormality, or Abnormality on Physical Examination and Their Relation to Survival Rate in 309 Consecutive Patients Undergoing Nephrectomy for Renal Cell Carcinoma*

Presenting Symptom, Abnormal Laboratory Finding, or Abnormality on Physical Examination	No. of Patients (% of total) (n = 309)	No. (%) of Patients Surviving 5 Years
Classic triad (gross hematuria, abnormal mass, pain)	29 (9)	9/29 (31)
Hematuria	183 (59)	74/183 (40)
Pain	127 (41)	56/127 (44)
Abdominal mass	139 (45)	49/139 (35)
Fever	21 (7)	8/21 (38)
Weight loss	85 (28)	29/85 (39)
Anemia	64 (21)	24/64 (38)
Erythrocytosis	10 (3)	4/10 (40)
Hypercalcemia	11 (3)	4/11 (35)
Acute varicocele	7 (2)	3/7 (43)
Tumor calcification on x-ray film	39 (13)	18/39 (46)
Symptoms of metastases	31 (10)	1/31 (3)
Cancer, incidental finding	20 (7)	13/20 (65)

* Modified from Skinner DG, Colvin RB, Vermillion CD et al: Diagnosis and management of renal cell carcinoma: A clinical and pathologic study of 309 cases. Cancer 28:1165–1177, 1971.

3% to 5%.[37] Nonmetastatic hepatic dysfunction, initially described by Stauffer in 1961, is a reversible syndrome associated with renal carcinoma that tends to occur in association with fever, fatigue, and weight loss and resolves when the primary tumor is removed. Nonmetastatic hepatic dysfunction, which is usually associated with poor long-term prognosis, occurs in up to 7% of patients with renal cell carcinoma. Abnormal hepatic function is observed in up to 40%.[81,90-92]

Renin levels are often elevated in patients with renal cell carcinoma, but tend to return to normal after the kidney is removed. Whether the tumor itself produces renin or whether it induces renin production by compression of adjacent tissue is unclear. Immunocytochemical studies suggest that renal cell carcinoma may produce renin, which, however, may be biologically inactive.[89,93,94] Plasma fibrinogen levels are elevated in patients with renal cell carcinoma and may correlate with tumor stage, disease activity, and response to therapy.[95] Acquired dysfibrinogenemia has also been reported in association with renal cell carcinoma and can be a sensitive plasma marker for the disease and for tumor progression.[96]

RADIOGRAPHIC EVALUATION

It is often difficult to determine whether a space-occupying renal mass lesion is benign or malignant. In a series of 940 asymptomatic space-occupying renal mass lesions reported by Lang, 515 (55%) were benign renal cysts, and only 52 (5.5%) were malignant neoplasms (Table 31-2).[97] A number of diagnostic modalities are used to evaluate and stage renal mass lesions (Fig. 31-3), including excretory urography, computed tomography (CT), arteriography, venography, ultrasound, and magnetic resonance imaging (MRI). Excretory urography is commonly used in the initial evaluation of renal mass lesions, but because it is neither sensitive nor specific in renal cell carcinoma, a small to medium-sized tumor may be present when the excretory urogram appears normal. Excretory urography does provide important information

TABLE 31-2. Underlying Pathologic Conditions in 940 Asymptomatic Space-Occupying Lesions of the Kidney*

Type of Lesion	No. of Lesions	% of Total No. of Lesions
Cystic lesions		58
Benign cysts	515	
Benign hemorrhagic cysts	4	
Hydronephrosis	8	
Cystic dysplastic kidney	3	
Polycystic kidney	17	
Malignant neoplasms		5.5
Hypernephromas	21	
Other malignant neoplasms	31	
Benign neoplasms	40	4.2
Inflammatory lesions (pyelonephritis, abscess)	213	23
Intrarenal hematoma	7	0.7
Pseudotumors	81	8.6

* Modified from Lang EK: Diagnosis of renal and parenchymal tumors. In Skinner DG, deKernion JB (eds): Genitourinary Cancer, p 42. Philadelphia, WB Saunders, 1978.

about the location and function of the contralateral kidney, and this is particularly useful when surgery is being considered.

Ultrasound examination provides excellent staging and diagnostic information and can provide accurate anatomic detail of extrarenal extension of tumor, adrenal involvement, involvement of lymph nodes, and infiltration of adjacent viscera.[1,98-100] It can also aid in the detection and delineation of renal vein or inferior vena caval involvement. Ultrasound examination is frequently used in the evaluation of renal cystic lesions that are detected on excretory urography or CT. If a cystic renal mass lesion appears potentially malignant on excretory urography, ultrasound, or CT, further evaluation by percutaneous cyst puncture under ultrasound or CT guidance may be performed. This procedure has two components: evaluation of cyst fluid and radiographic examination of the interior of the cyst. Cyst fluid aspirate is assessed for color, turbidity, and the presence of blood; and fat, protein, lactic acid dehydrogenase (LDH), and glucose content is measured. If the cyst is benign, there is typically a clear, straw-colored fluid that is low in fat, protein, and LDH content. When a cystic or necrotic tumor is aspirated, the fluid may be bloody and may have a high fat, protein, or LDH content. After the fluid is removed, the cyst is filled with contrast medium and air and imaged radiographically. A benign cyst should appear as a homogeneous sphere with a regular border; a tumor may show up as a nodule or mass protruding into the cyst.[98] The combination of ultrasound and cyst puncture enables the clinician to make the correct diagnosis in a very high percentage of suspicious renal mass lesions.[1]

Renal arteriography (see Figs. 31-4B, 31-4C) has historically been a standard part of the evaluation of patients with a suspicious renal mass. In a renal cell carcinoma the arteriogram will often show neovascularity, arteriovenous fistulas, pooling of contrast medium, and accentuation of capsular vessels. Epinephrine may be used as an aid in the diagnosis of an equivocal renal mass lesion. When epinephrine is infused into a normal kidney during arteriography the renal vessels constrict; the vessels in a renal cell carcinoma do not constrict owing to lack of musculature in the tumor vessels.[1] A renal arteriogram is particularly useful in evaluating an indeterminant small renal mass lesion and as an aid to the surgeon in defining the vasculature during the surgical removal of a large tumor.[101,102] Although renal arteriography can be performed with minimal risk, false aneurysms, arterial emboli, hemorrhage, and decreased renal function secondary to contrast agent injection have been reported.[1] Digital subtraction arteriography can define the tumor vasculature without the morbidity associated with standard arteriography and adequately demonstrates the main renal arterial anatomy in more than 80% of cases. The combination of CT and digital subtraction angiography yields satisfactory diagnostic and anatomic detail in most cases of renal cell carcinoma.[103]

CT is a useful imaging technique for renal cell carcinoma (see Fig. 31-5A).[5,100,101,104-109] In a study in which CT results were correlated with pathologic findings in 111 patients, perirenal extension was correctly identified in 79% of cases, lymph node involvement in 87%, renal vein involvement in

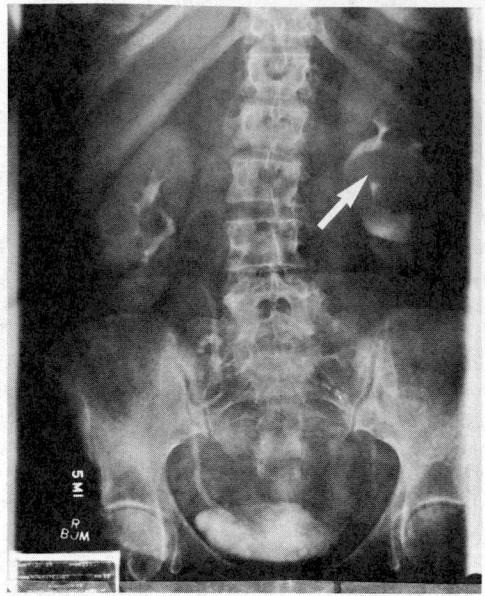

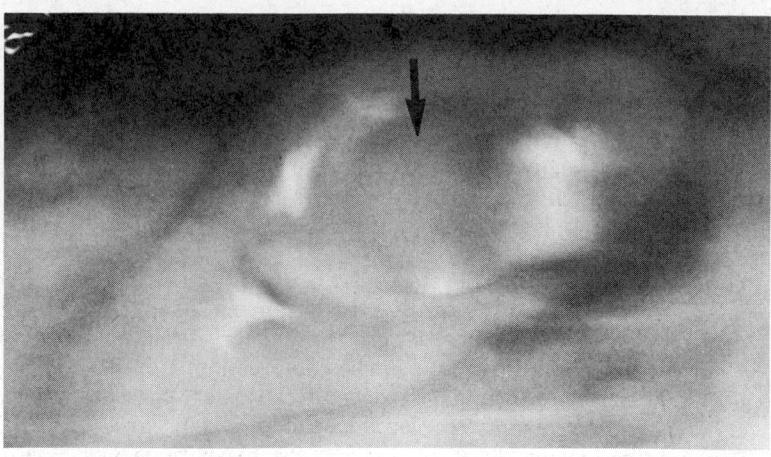

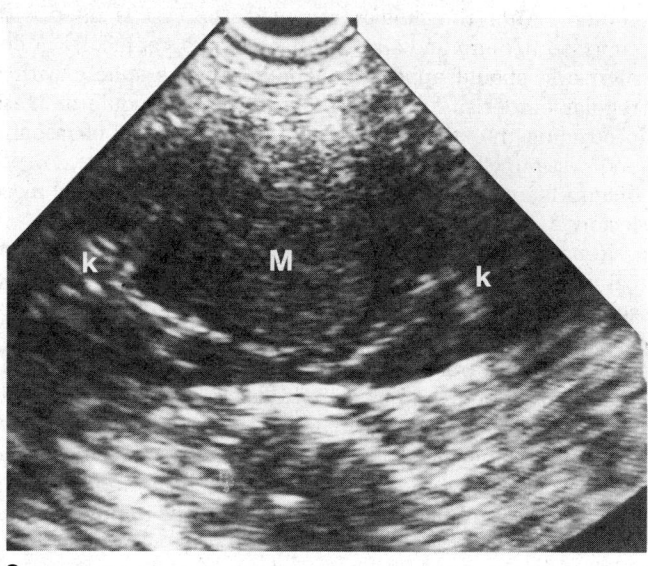

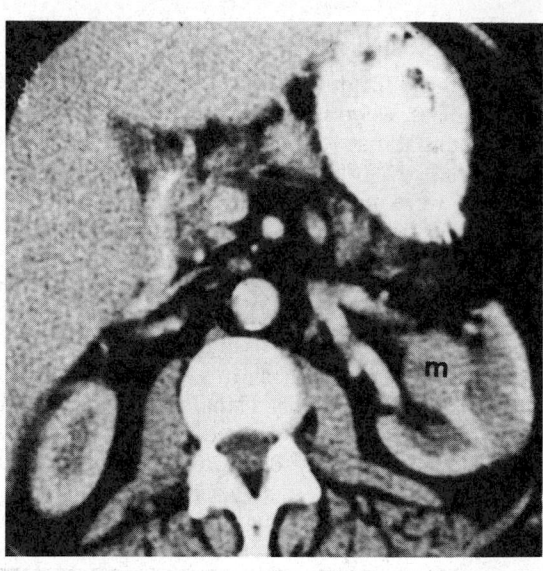

FIG. 31-3. Renal cell carcinoma involving the renal pelvis. **A.** Intravenous urogram demonstrates displacement of renal collecting system by a large mass (*arrow*). The appearance could be mistaken for a parapelvic cyst. **B.** Linear tomogram demonstrates the pelvic filling defect more precisely (*arrow*). **C.** Sagittal ultrasound through the left kidney demonstrates normal renal parenchymal (*k*) and a solid mass near the renal pelvis (*M*). **D.** Bolus enhanced CT scan demonstrates enhancing mass (*m*) near the renal pelvis.

91%, and local advancement into adjacent viscera in 96%.[106] Although arteriography and CT are equivalent in depicting renal vein involvement, CT is better for demonstrating local nodal involvement.[104] The use of contrast agent enhancement has greatly increased the sensitivity of CT for abnormal renal mass lesions.[107,108] Contrast-enhanced CT allows the clinician to detect very small changes in the density of a renal lesion that might indicate the presence of an early neoplastic lesion. In a comparison study, dynamic CT was superior to standard CT arteriography, ultrasonography, and radionuclide scanning. Dynamic CT correctly demonstrated tumor involvement of the kidney, involvement of the renal fascia, or extension into adjacent organs in all of the 22 patients studied.[100]

Inferior venacavography is performed when there is a large renal tumor or when there is uncertainty about tumor involvement of the vena cava. Ultrasound, CT, and MRI (Fig. 31-6) can provide information about tumor involvement of the vena cava; however, the inferior venacavogram is the most reliable means of accurately determining the precise

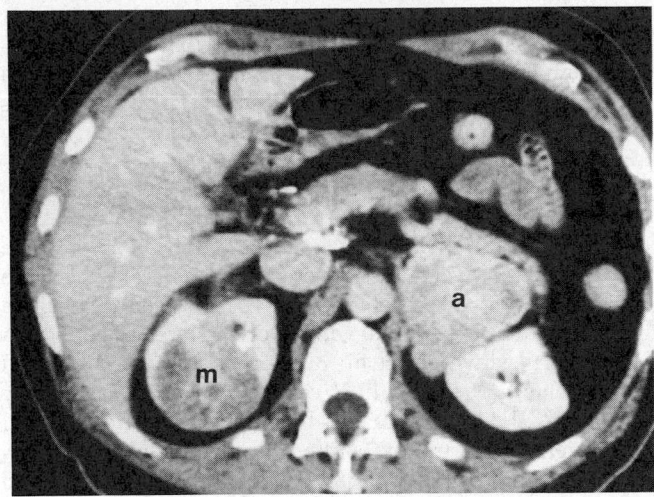

A

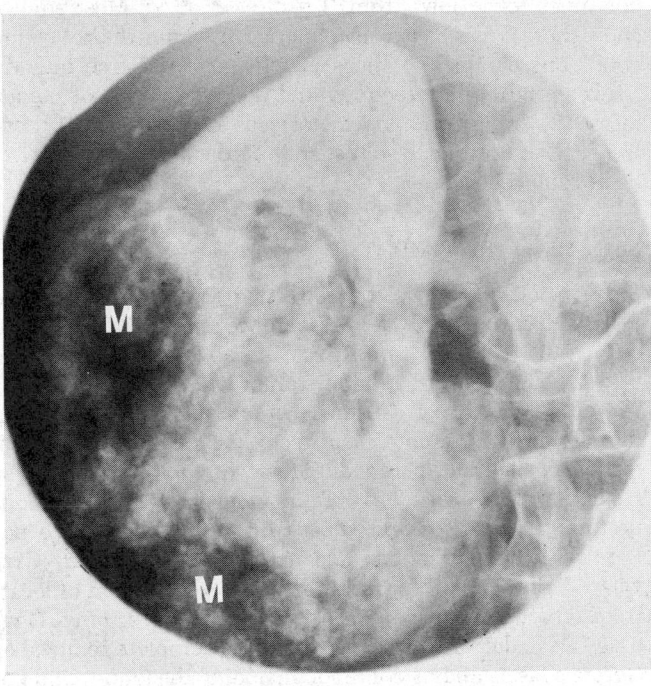

C

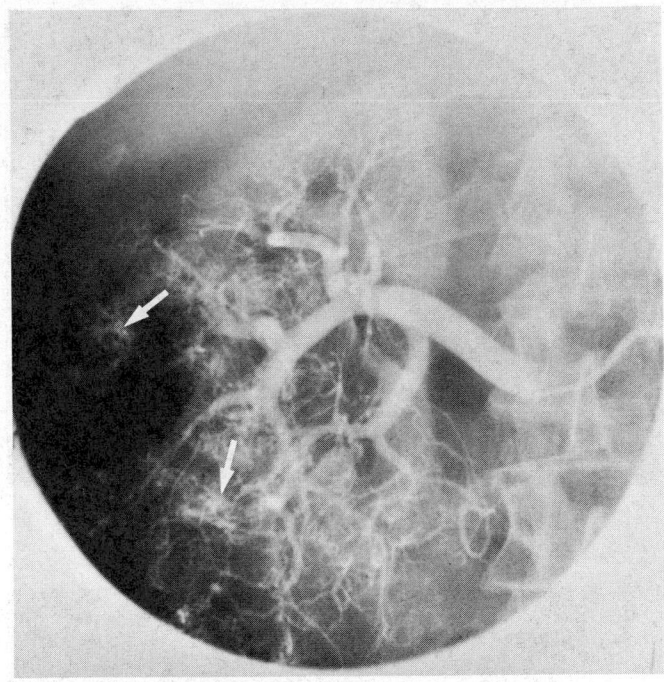

B

FIG. 31-4. Angiographic appearance of a renal cell carcinoma. **A.** CT demonstrates a right renal carcinoma (*m*) with a large contralateral adrenal metastasis (*a*). **B.** Early phase of arteriogram demonstrates vascular changes indicative of a malignancy with puddling and tortuosity (*arrows*). **C.** Late phase of the arteriogram demonstrates that the tumor (*M*) is relatively avascular despite its early appearance.

extent of vena caval involvement by tumor. This information is important to the surgeon in planning the vascular aspect of the operative procedure.

MRI is very useful for staging renal cell carcinoma.[110] MRI can produce a unique three-dimensional picture of the tumor which, in the case of a large tumor, may be an invaluable aid to the surgeon in planning the operative approach.

There is no single imaging technique that is best for all patients with renal cell carcinoma. Depending on the size of the primary tumor and the extent of extrarenal disease, excretory urography, CT, ultrasound, arteriography, venography, and MRI each can provide unique information in an individual case. Because CT, MRI, and ultrasound are outpatient procedures and are less invasive than arteriography,

arteriography is now less frequently used. Multiple imaging modalities are often used to provide the most complete information, particularly when surgical removal of a large tumor is being considered.

STAGING AND PROGNOSIS

The staging system (Fig. 31-7) currently in use by most physicians in the United States is the Robson modification of the system of Flocks and Kadesky (Table 31-3).[111] In the Robson classification, Stage I renal cell carcinoma is confined to the kidney, Stage II carcinoma extends through the renal capsule but is confined to Gerota's fascia, and Stage III carcinoma involves the renal vein or inferior vena cava (III-

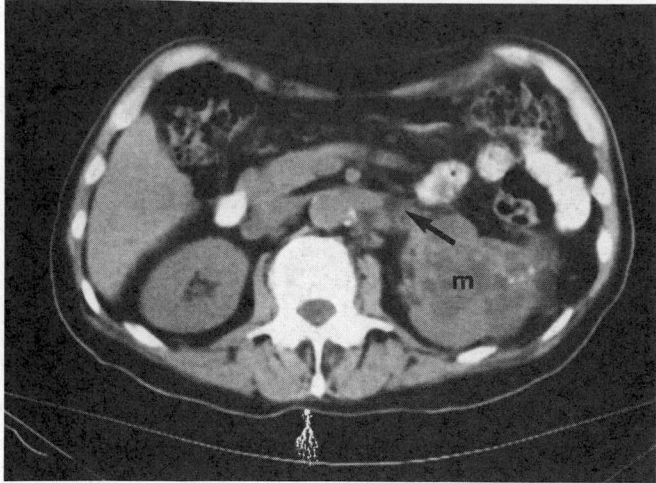

A

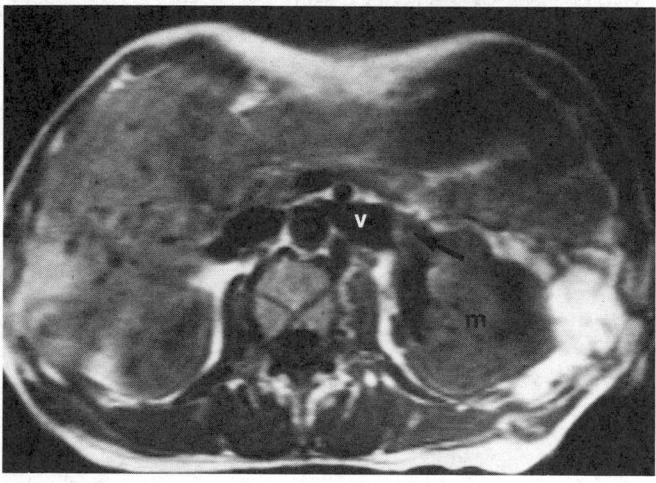

B

FIG. 31-5. Renal vein invasion by a renal carcinoma as shown by CT and MRI. **A.** Nonenhanced CT shows large left renal mass with calcification (*m*) invading the left renal vein (*arrow*). **B.** T1-weighted MRI demonstrates tumor (*m*) and vascular invasion (*arrow*). Flowing blood (*v*) in the left renal vein is black on this scan.

A) or the local hilar lymph nodes (III-B). In Stage IV renal cell carcinoma the tumor has spread to local, adjacent organs (other than the adrenal gland) or to distant sites. The Robson staging system is uncomplicated and widely used. A disadvantage of this system is that it combines stages that may have significantly different survival prognoses. In this classification system renal vein or inferior vena caval involvement (III-A) is the same stage as local lymph node metastasis (III-B). Although patients with Stage III-B renal cell carcinoma have a greatly decreased survival,[112,113] the prognosis for patients with Stage III-A renal cell carcinoma is not particularly different from that for patients with Stage I or Stage II renal cell carcinoma.

The TNM classification provides a more accurate method for classifying extent of tumor involvement. In the TNM classification, T1 denotes a small tumor confined to the kid-

ney, T2 denotes a large tumor that deforms the kidney or collecting system but is still confined to the kidney, T3 denotes tumor with perinephric or hilar extension, and T4 denotes tumor that has extended to neighboring organs (Table 31-4). N+ indicates local nodal involvement, and in M+ disease there are metastases.

The 5-year survival initially reported by Robson and co-workers in 1969 was 66% for Stage I renal cell carcinoma, 64% for Stage II, 42% for Stage III, and only 11% for Stage IV.[111] These survival statistics remained essentially the same for a number of years (Table 31-5).[79,90] However, it has since been noted that while renal vein involvement does not have a markedly negative effect on prognosis, the 5-year survival for patients with Stage III-B renal cell carcinoma is only 18%.[7,79,80,90,114] Recent studies have reported better survival for patients with tumor confined to the kidney: approximately 95% 5-year survival for T1 renal cell carcinoma and 92% 5-year survival for Stage T2 disease.[80,106] The 5-year survival for patients with metastatic renal cell carcinoma continues to be low, from 0 to 20%.[7,80,85,115] Most studies show increased survival in patients in whom the following conditions obtain: (1) there is a long disease-free interval between initial nephrectomy and the appearance of metastases, (2) only pulmonary metastases are present, (3) there is a good performance status, and (4) the primary tumor has been removed.[85]

SURGICAL TREATMENT

Surgery is the only known effective therapy for localized renal cell carcinoma. The first nephrectomy was performed by Erastus B. Walcott in Milwaukee on June 4, 1861, on a 58-year-old man with a kidney tumor who died 15 days after surgery.[116] Professor Gustave Simon, after completing a number of experimental nephrectomies on dogs, undertook the first deliberate, planned and successful nephrectomy in Heidelberg on August 2, 1869, in a patient with a persistent ureteral fistula. The first successful nephrectomy in a patient with kidney cancer was performed in 1883 by Grawitz.[116] The standard procedure today for treatment of localized renal cell carcinoma is radical nephrectomy (Fig. 31-8).[117] Radical nephrectomy includes complete removal of Gerota's fascia and its contents, including the kidney and the adrenal gland, and provides a better surgical margin than simple removal of the kidney.

There are a number of different surgical approaches to removal of a kidney cancer. Common approaches are the anterior transperitoneal approach, the flank approach, and the thoracoabdominal approach. The choice of surgical approach depends on the location and size of the tumor and the body habitus of the patient. The type of incision is chosen to ensure that the tumor may safely be removed. A flank incision, with or without removal of a portion of the 10th or 11th rib, is often used for small tumors without venous involvement. A subcostal transabdominal incision may be used when there is a large tumor in the middle or lower aspect of the kidney or when vascular involvement is anticipated and access to the major vessels is essential. A thoracoabdominal incision is often required when there is a large middle or upper pole tumor. In a thoracoabdominal incision a rib is

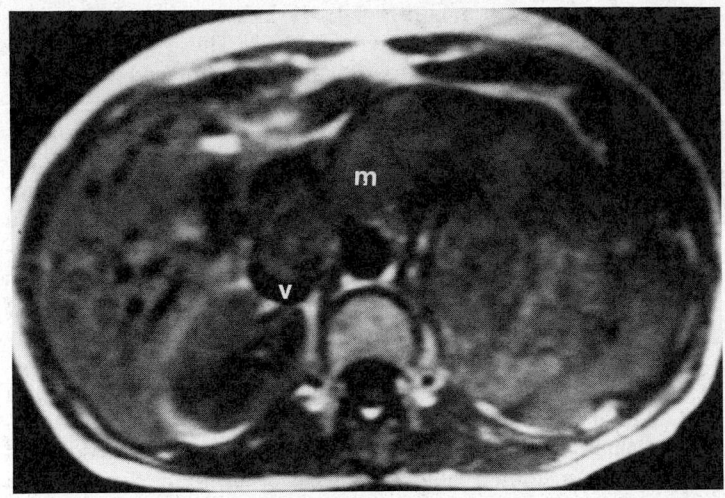

A

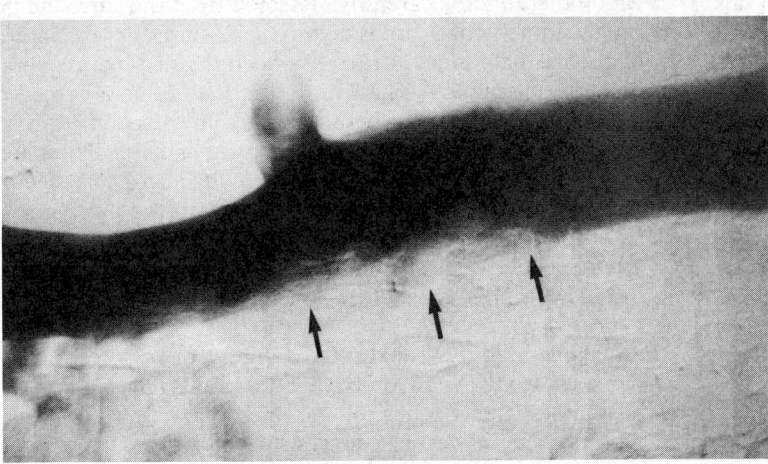

C

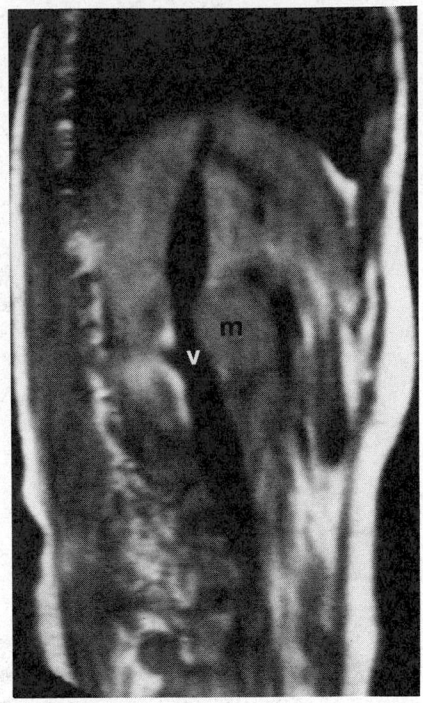

B

FIG. 31-6. Invasion of IVC by renal carcinoma demonstrated by MRI and venography. **A**. Axial T1-weighted image demonstrates a large left renal carcinoma with extension into the left renal vein (*m*) with protrusion into the IVC (*v*). **B**. Sagittal T1-weighted image shows the relation of the tumor thrombus (*m*) to the IVC (*v*) in the lateral projection. **C**. An AP image of the interior cavagram demonstrates tumor in the medial aspect of the inferior vena cava.

removed, the thoracic cavity is opened, and the diaphragm is incised. The incision is then carried down transabdominally to allow maximal exposure of the upper abdominal region and the great vessels. In removal of a right-sided tumor, the hepatic flexure of the colon is mobilized toward the midline away from the kidney and duodenum. The duodenum is also dissected up anteriorly and medially to the great vessels, and the renal artery and vein are identified. The renal vessels are divided and ligated early in the surgical procedure to decrease the vascularity of the tumor so that it may be removed with a minimum of blood loss. Following ligation of the vessels, Gerota's fascia is incised away from the posterior abdominal wall, diaphragm, and liver (pancreas and spleen on a left-sided tumor) (see Fig. 31-9). Once Gerota's fascia and its contents have been dissected away from the surrounding structures and the vasculature has been ligated with nonabsorbable suture, the specimen can be lifted out of the retroperitoneum. When there is tumor in the renal vein, the renal vein can be ligated distal to the tumor thrombus. If there is tumor extension into the vena cava, the vena cava may need to be partially resected. If the tumor has grown into the side wall of the vena cava or if the vena caval involvement is too extensive for a simple partial wall resection, a portion of the vena cava itself may be resected. When

the tumor is in the right kidney, the adjacent vena cava can often be resected safely. If, however, the tumor in the left kidney and the adjacent vena cava are resected, vascular reconstruction of the right renal vein may be needed to establish adequate venous drainage.[114,118,119] If the suprahepatic caval extension of a renal tumor thrombus extends up to the right atrium, cardiopulmonary bypass may be required for tumor removal.[119,120]

Regional lymphadenectomy is often performed at the time of radical nephrectomy, although its role in prolonging survival has not been demonstrated. In a regional lymphadenectomy, ipsilateral nodal tissue from the diaphragm to the bifurcation of the aorta as well as nodal tissue in the interaortocaval region at the hilum of the kidney is removed. Proponents of regional lymphadenectomy point out that 5-year survival in patients with N+ renal cell carcinoma is greatly decreased, and there is no known effective therapy for metastatic renal cell carcinoma. If local nodes were the first site of metastasis, resection of microscopic disease might be of benefit. Long-term survival in patients with N+ disease who underwent lymphadenectomy has been reported. The ultimate role of regional lymphadenectomy remains to be determined in further randomized trials.[79,111–113,121–123]

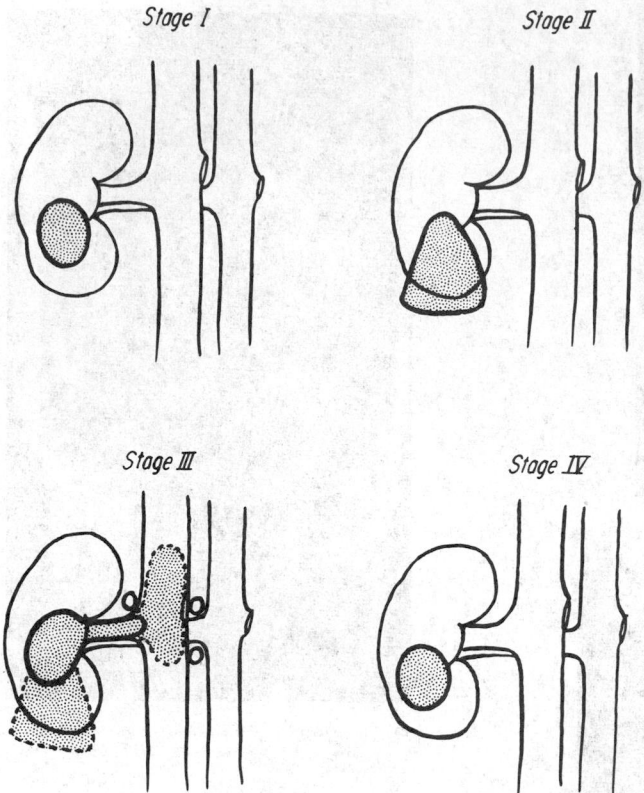

FIG. 31-7. Staging system for renal adenocarcinoma. (Modified from Skinner DG, Vermillion CD, Colvin RB: The surgical management of renal cell carcinoma. J Urol 107:705–716, 1972)

BILATERAL RENAL CELL CARCINOMA OR TUMORS IN SOLITARY KIDNEYS

The treatment of patients who present with either bilateral renal cell carcinoma or renal cell carcinoma in a solitary kidney is challenging. Patients with tumor in a solitary kidney may be treated by either partial nephrectomy or nephrectomy followed by dialysis and/or transplantation.[124-127] A 5-year survival of 60% in patients with bilateral renal cell carcinoma or tumor in a solitary kidney treated by partial nephrectomy has been reported.[128] Some surgeons advocate surgical enucleation of a tumor in a patient with a solitary kidney. In one series patients with either bilateral renal cell

TABLE 31-3. Comparison of the Two Classification Systems for Staging of Renal Cell Carcinoma*

	TNM (1978)	Robson
Small tumor, no enlargement of kidney	T1	A
Large tumor, cortex not broken	T2	A
Perinephric or hilar extension	T3	B
Extension to neighboring organs	T4	D
Nodal invasion	N+	C
Renal vein involved	V1	C
Vena cava involved	V2	C
Distant metastases	M+	D

* Selli C, Hinshaw WM, Woodard BH, Paulson DF: Stratification of risk factors in renal cell carcinoma. Cancer 52:899, 1983.

carcinoma or tumor in a solitary kidney treated with enucleation had a 90% 3-year survival. There was excellent renal function in all patients; none required dialysis.[129] Others advocate caution in using surgical enucleation and favor partial nephrectomy instead. Marshall and co-workers evaluated standard nephrectomy specimens that were enucleated ex vivo and found positive margins, satellite tumor nodules, and occult metastatic disease in lymph nodes in a number of cases that were not appreciated fully in the operating room.[130] Most surgeons favor resection of a narrow rim of normal tissue around the tumor in the kidney instead of simple enucleation.[131] Extracorporeal partial nephrectomy plus autotransplantation is a technique that allows the surgeon to accurately remove large tumors in the center of a solitary kidney.[128] This ex vivo procedure entails radical excision of the kidney and division of the ureter. The kidney is then placed on a table and is intermittently perfused with a chilled solution to enhance viability. Under optical magnification the tumor is carefully dissected from the surrounding renal parenchyma. Care is taken to preserve the vasculature of the normal kidney, which has been defined by preoperative arteriography. A small rim of normal tissue is removed along with the tumor to provide a tumor-free margin of resection. After the kidney has been surgically reconstructed it is autotransplanted back into the iliac space. Vascular anastomosis of the renal artery and vein to the iliac vessels and ureteroureterostomy are performed. If multiple tumors are encountered in which small tumors are distributed throughout the parenchyma, autotransplantation is not indicated.[124]

Although familial renal cell carcinoma or renal cell carcinoma associated with von Hippel–Lindau syndrome is often bilateral, sporadic renal cell carcinoma is only rarely bilateral.[132] Bilateral (synchronous or asynchronous) renal cell carcinoma has been reported to occur in 1.8% to 3.8% of cases.[117] Patients with synchronous bilateral renal cell carcinoma have a better prognosis than patients with asynchronous disease. Zincke and co-workers reported a 78% 5-year survival for patients seen initially with bilateral renal cell carcinoma versus only a 38% 5-year survival for patients whose metastases in the contralateral kidney appeared after the primary had been removed.[132]

RADIATION THERAPY AS AN ADJUVANT TO NEPHRECTOMY

The cure rates for patients with high pathologic stage renal cell carcinoma (N+, M+) treated by nephrectomy are only fair and have improved little in the last two decades. However, because patients with renal cell carcinoma can have variable and protracted courses, the benefit in survival from any adjunctive therapy to nephrectomy is difficult to demonstrate. Currently no data clearly indicate that radical nephrectomy plus lymph node dissection provides enhanced cure rate over treatment by nephrectomy alone.[115] In addition, studies looking at the possible benefit of adjuvant irradiation combined with nephrectomy are few and inconclusive (Table 31-6). Reports of benefit with radiation therapy come from only one nonrandomized trial.[133] Two randomized studies found no benefit from postoperative irradia-

TABLE 31-4. TNM Classification—Kidney

Primary Tumor (T)
TX Minimum requirements cannot be met
T0 No evidence of primary tumor
T1 Small tumor, minimal renal and calyceal distortion or deformity. Circumscribed neovasculature surrounded by normal parenchyma
T2 Large tumor with deformity or enlargement of kidney or collecting system
T3a Tumor involving perinephric tissues
T3b Tumor involving renal vein
T3c Tumor involving renal vein and infradiaphragmatic vena cava
Note: Under T3, tumor may extend into perinephric tissues, into renal vein, and into vena cava as shown on cavography. In these instances, the T classification may be shown as T3a, b, and c, or some appropriate combination, depending on extension, e.g., T3a,b is tumor in perinephric fat and extending into renal vein.
T4a Tumor invasion of neighboring structures (e.g., muscle, bowel)
T4b Tumor involving supradiaphragmatic vena cava

Nodal Involvement (N)
The regional lymph nodes are the para-aortic and paracaval nodes. The juxtaregional lymph nodes are the pelvic nodes and the mediastinal nodes.
NX Minimum requirements cannot be met
N0 No evidence of involvement of regional nodes
N1 Single, homolateral regional nodal involvement
N2 Involvement of multiple regional or contralateral or bilateral nodes
N3 Fixed regional nodes (assessable only at surgical exploration)
N4 Involvement of juxtaregional nodes
Note: If lymphography is source of staging, add "1" between "N" and designator number; if histologic proof is provided "+" if positive, and "−" if negative. Thus N1+ indicates multiple positive nodes seen on lymphography and proved at operation by biopsy.

Distant Metastasis (M)
MX Not assessed
M0 No (known) distant metastasis
M1 Distant metastasis present
Specify
Specify sites according to the following notations

Pulmonary—PUL   Bone Marrow—MAR
Osseous—OSS   Pleura—PLE
Hepatic—HEP   Skin—SKI
Brain—BRA   Eye—EYE
Lymph Nodes—LYM Other—OTH

Note: Add "+" to the abbreviated notation to indicate that the pathology (p) is proved.

TABLE 31-5. Summary of Published Survival Rates in Renal Cell Carcinoma

Study, Year	Length of Survival (yr)	Survival (%) by Stage			
		I	II	III	IV
Robson et al, 1969[111]	5	66	64	42	11
	10	60	67	38	0
Skinner et al, 1971[79]	5	65	47	51	8
	10	56	20	37	7
Boxer et al, 1979[81]	5	56	100	50	8
	10	20	66	25	0
McNichols et al, 1981[83]	5	67	51	34	14
	10	56	28	20	3
Cherrie et al, 1982[114]	5	. . .	. . .	0–53	0
	10	. . .	. . .	. . .	. . .
Selli et al, 1983[80]	5	93	63	80	13
	10	. . .	. . .	. . .	. . .
Bassil et al, 1985[115]	5	91–100	. . .	. . .	18
	10	. . .	. . .	. . .	. . .
Golimbu et al, 1986[7]	5	88	67	40	2
	10	66	35	15	. . .

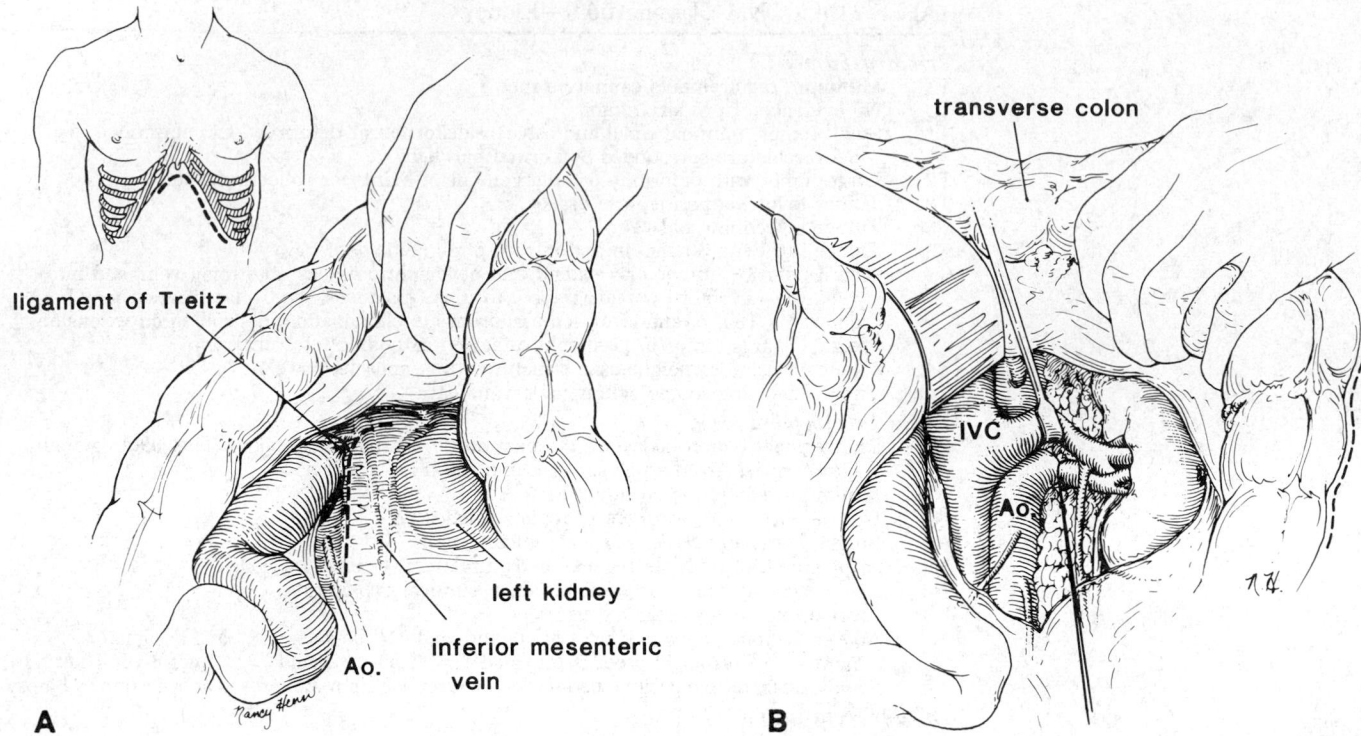

FIG. 31-8. Area of dissection for lymph node dissection for radical nephroureterectomy should be from the superior mesenteric artery to the level of the inferior mesenteric artery with the anatomic structures identified. The dotted line to the right of the descending colon indicates a line of incision on the left pericolic gutter that should extend superiorly to include division of the splenocolic attachments. (Paulson DF, Perez CA, Anderson T: Cancer of the kidney and ureter. In DeVita VT Jr, Hellman S, Rosenberg SA (eds): Cancer: Principles and Practice of Oncology, 2nd ed, p 898. Philadelphia, JB Lippincott, 1985)

FIG. 31-9. The left colon can be reflected from the anterior surface of Gerota's fascia with exposure of the renal artery before ligation and division. (Paulson DF, Perez CA, Anderson T: Cancer of the kidney and ureter. In DeVita VT Jr, Hellman S, Rosenberg SA (eds): Cancer: Principles and Practice of Oncology, 2nd ed, p 900. Philadelphia, JB Lippincott, 1985)

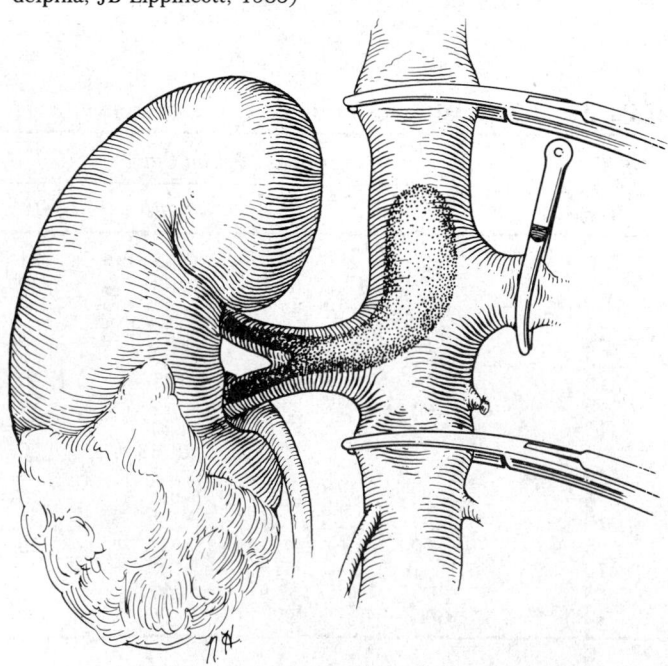

tion.[134,135] However, any possible benefit from radiation therapy in the latter two studies was likely compromised by either the radiation technique or the radiation dose. Four fatal liver complications occurred after postoperative irradiation of up to 5500 cGy in the 1973 study reported by Finney.[134] In a study in Denmark, reported in 1987, a high complication rate was noted.[135] In this series the dose per fraction was 250 cGy, for a total dose of 5000 cGy delivered over approximately 4 weeks. Because of complications (44% severe, 19% fatal), mainly gastrointestinal, this trial was stopped.[135]

Two studies of preoperative radiation therapy given before partial nephrectomy have been reported. The first, reported by van der Werf-Messing,[136] found no benefit with a dose of 3000 cGy given prior to nephrectomy. However, 37% of the patients had tumors of low pathologic stage and thus would have been unlikely to benefit from the adjuvant treatment. Likewise, in the Phase III trial reported from Finland of 3600 cGy given preoperatively, 70% of patients had tumors of low pathologic stage (pT1 and pT2). Thus, to date there are no wholly satisfactory analyses of the efficacy of well-tolerated modern megavoltage preoperative or postoperative radiation therapy as an adjunct to radical nephrectomy in patients judged to be at high risk for locoregional failure—those with high pathologic stage tumors.

Present information indicates that patients with pathologic stage T1 or T2 tumors without lymph node metastases are not good candidates for adjunctive therapy as they are likely

TABLE 31-6.   Renal Cell Carcinoma: Treatment Results with and Without Adjuvant Radiation Therapy

Study, Year	No. of Patients	Local Treatment	5-Year Survival (%)	Local Recurrences (%)	Comments
Peeling et al, 1969[294]	96	Nephrectomy	52	. . .	Not randomized; ? RT
	68	Nephrectomy + RT	25	. . .	dose
Rafla, 1970[133]	96	Nephrectomy	37	25	Not randomized; ? RT
	94	Nephrectomy + RT	56	7	dose
Finney, 1973[134]	49	Nephrectomy	44	. . .	Randomized; RT dose
	51	Nephrectomy + RT	36	. . .	to 5500 cGY
van der Werf-Messing, 1973[136]	85	Nephrectomy	50	. . .	Randomized; 37% of
	89	RT (3000 cGy) + nephrectomy	45	. . .	patients had small tumors (pT1–2)
Juusela et al, 1977[295]	44	Nephrectomy	63	. . .	Randomized; 70% of
	38	RT (3600 cGy) + nephrectomy	47		patients had small tumors (pT1–2)
Kjaer et al, 1987[296]	33	Nephrectomy	62	3	Randomized; RT
	32	Nephrectomy + RT (5000 cGy; 20 fractions)	38	0	group with high complication rate—44% serious, 19% lethal

RT = radiation therapy.

to have an 80% or greater 5- to 10-year survival after radical nephrectomy alone.[113,115] Candidates for possible postoperative adjunctive radiation therapy include those with pathologic evidence of deep invasion of Gerota's fascia, adjacent organs, or regional lymph nodes and who have no known metastatic disease. Such patients are probably best treated by daily fractions of 180 to 200 cGy with 10- to 25-MV beams from linear accelerators to fields that include the renal fossa and tumor bed as well as the para-aortic and paracaval lymph nodes, to a total dose of 4500 cGy in 5 weeks. The usual parallel-opposed anterior-posterior isocentric fields are secondarily shaped with individual corner blocks. For right-sided tumors there is often a need for field reduction at the 3600 to 4600 cGy level to include only the tumor bed and the retroperitoneal lymph node regions, so that not more than 30% of the liver parenchyma receives a high dose. A postnephrectomy, preirradiation CT scan is very useful as a baseline for subsequent comparison. Unless there is clear evidence of wound contamination by tumor spill at the time of nephrectomy, usually no effort is made to include the entire surgical incision in the treatment fields.

METASTATIC RENAL CELL CARCINOMA

NEPHRECTOMY AND RESECTION OF METASTASES

Adjuvant or palliative nephrectomy is not infrequently performed in patients with metastatic renal cell carcinoma, particularly those with pain, hemorrhage, malaise, hypercalcemia, erythrocytosis, or hypertension. Removal of the primary tumor may alleviate some or all of these abnormalities.[137,138] Although there are isolated reports of regression of metastatic renal cell carcinoma following removal of the primary tumor, only four (0.8%) of 474 patients in nine series who underwent nephrectomy experienced "regression" of metastatic foci.[139] DeKernion and co-workers reported results in 26 patients with metastatic renal cell carcinoma who underwent palliative or adjuvant nephrectomy

and found no increase in survival, compared with survival in the entire group of 79 patients with metastatic renal cell carcinoma.[140] Middleton reported on 141 patients with metastatic renal cell carcinomas; 33 underwent adjuvant nephrectomy, however, none of the 141 patients survived more than 24 months.[141] Adjuvant nephrectomy is not recommended for the purpose of inducing spontaneous regression; rather, it is performed to decrease symptoms or to decrease tumor burden in preparation for subsequent therapy in carefully controlled environments.

Of the approximately 30% of patients with renal cell carcinoma who present with metastases, only 1.5% to 3.5% have solitary metastasis.[141–143] Patients with a solitary metastasis synchronous with a primary lesion have decreased survival when compared with patients who develop metastasis after the primary tumor is removed.[133,140,142] Surgical resection is appropriate in selected patients with metastatic renal cell carcinoma. In one study, 59 patients with renal cell carcinoma who underwent surgical resection for a solitary metastasis had a 45% 3-year survival and a 34% 5-year survival.[141] O'Dea et al reported on patients who presented with primary tumor in place and a solitary metastasis. Of the patients who underwent nephrectomy and who later developed metastasis, 23% lived more than 5 years after removal of the metastatic lesions. Three of the 26 patients were alive 58, 94, and 245 months after resection of the metastatic lesion.[142] Nephrectomy and resection of metastases will render few cures but will frequently produce some long-term survivors.

ANGIOINFARCTION

Angioinfarction of the kidney is used both with and without nephrectomy in the treatment of metastatic renal cell carcinoma. A number of techniques have been developed to occlude the renal artery for this purpose. Short-term embolization can be accomplished with alcohol, autologous blood clot, or gelatin sponge pads (Gelfoam). Other inert substances such as Silastic spheres, stainless steel pellets, or Gianturco steel coils are also used to embolize the renal artery.[144] Most patients develop a postinfarction syndrome consisting of pain, fever, and gastrointestinal complaints almost immediately after infarction.[137] Transcatheter arterial occlusion may decrease vascularity prior to nephrectomy in patients with large, locally advanced renal cell carcinoma or may lessen tumor bleeding, pain, or other systemic symptoms in patients with unresectable tumors.[144] Angioinfarction has not been demonstrated to be an effective method for inducing regression in patients with metastatic renal cell carcinoma. In a study by Swanson et al of patients with metastatic renal cell carcinoma who underwent angioinfarction followed by nephrectomy, a small number experienced complete or partial response of the metastatic disease to this therapy; however, there was no difference in survival between these patients (n = 100) and the patients who were treated with nephrectomy alone (n = 43).[145]

ROLE OF RADIATION THERAPY

The major sites of hematogenous metastases from renal cell carcinoma are bone, lung, and brain. Treatment in virtually all instances is noncurative, and thus the role of radiation therapy, neurosurgery, orthopedic surgery, or thoracic surgery in the local management of these metastases is nearly always palliative. However, patients presenting with an initially solitary metastatic lesion have a 30% to 40% chance of surviving for 5 years. Thus, in these patients it is important to ensure as durable a palliative response as possible. In patients presenting with a solitary metastasis to the lung, spine, or brain, initial or de novo surgery should be considered, usually followed by postoperative irradiation. For a solitary metastasis to the spine, vertebral body resection by the anterior approach has proved satisfactory in carefully selected patients.[146,147] External-beam radiation therapy, the usual initial palliative approach for patients with symptomatic metastases, has been reported to yield a subjective or objective response in one half to two thirds of patients.[148-150] In a selected and carefully reviewed subset of patients irradiated for metastatic renal carcinoma, subjective improvement was noted in 16 of 19 analyzed patients, whereas objective evidence of regression, usually radiographic, was documented in only 13 of 26 treated patients. The external-beam radiation doses were most commonly in the range of 4000 cGy.[148] Doses the equivalent of at least 5000 cGy in 5½ weeks are necessary to achieve a durable palliative response.[149] To deliver such high doses, multiple-field techniques are often necessary. Palliation of large renal bed recurrences by external-beam irradiation has been unsatisfactory. Some relief of pain has been achieved in about 50% of the patients, but it is usually of very short duration.[150]

SYSTEMIC THERAPY

The treatment of patients with metastatic renal cell carcinoma has been one of the most frustrating endeavors of medical oncology. A huge number of chemotherapeutic agents, hormones, and combinations have been tested, but none has yielded reproducible therapeutic effects. The his-

tory of the therapy of metastatic renal cell carcinoma is dotted with positive pilot studies that fail to remain positive when tested in another institution or in another group of patients. Recently it has been found that renal tubular epithelium, the tissue of origin of renal cell carcinoma, constitutively expresses the multidrug resistance gene, mdr, which encodes a transport protein called p170.[151] Whether this gene is responsible for the de novo drug resistance seen in nearly all renal cell carcinomas has not been examined.

In contrast to the results with chemotherapeutic agents and hormones, several biologic approaches to renal cell carcinoma have produced response rates so encouraging that many oncologists feel justified in offering biologic agents as primary treatment. When response rates in patients with metastatic disease approach 30%, it is probably reasonable to begin to apply the therapy in the adjuvant setting to patients with locally advanced disease with a high probability of relapse after surgery. Such studies are being planned for at least two biological therapies.

CHEMOTHERAPY

The conventional treatment for metastatic renal cell carcinoma is vinblastine, 0.2 or 0.3 mg/kg/wk. Hrushesky and Murphy found that the response rate among 39 patients receiving weekly doses of vinblastine of 0.2 mg/kg was 31%, but the response rate among 96 patients receiving less vinblastine was only 15%.[152] Responders have markedly prolonged survival. Dose-related variables and dose intensity have not been carefully evaluated prospectively in renal cell carcinoma. Most workers administer lower doses because of concern about toxic effects, and most agree that the response rate is closer to 15% than 30%.

Efforts to improve the response rate to vinblastine by adding other agents have been largely unsuccessful.[32] Usually the agents added to vinblastine are not active in renal cell carcinoma as single agents (a violation of one of the cardinal rules for building a more effective combination regimen), and often the dose of vinblastine is lowered or the frequency of administration decreased because of toxic effects produced by the less effective agents in the combination. A recent report of a 30% response rate to vinblastine (4 mg/m²), bleomycin (30 mg), and methotrexate (500 mg/m² with leucovorin rescue) may represent a possible exception to this bleak picture.[153] However, it must be remembered that other initial reports of high response rates with combination therapy have uniformly failed to be confirmed.

An innovative approach to the use of chemotherapy in the treatment of metastatic renal cell carcinoma has been taken by Hrushesky and his colleagues.[154] Using programmable Medtronic pumps for automatic drug delivery, they found that the maximum tolerated dose of fluorodeoxyuridine (FUDR) infusions was more than twice that of conventional infusions if the FUDR infusion rate was sinusoidal, with the peak centered around 6 PM. Among 18 evaluable patients, five achieved partial responses and one a complete response. This small study suggests that a clever treatment design takes into account circadian influences on the therapeutic ratio and may allow augmentation of dose intensity to a clinically significant degree.

A complete response to neocarzinostatin has been reported, but the denominator is unknown.[155] A series of patients with primarily pulmonary disease were treated with chemotherapy infusions into the bronchial arteries.[156] Five of 12 patients were said to have responded, but the results are not evaluable because of extreme heterogeneity in agent, dose, and timing of administration.

CHEMOTHERAPY FOR LOCALLY ADVANCED RENAL CELL CARCINOMA

There are very few studies of adjuvant chemotherapy in renal cell cancer, and those few are not prospective and randomized.[157] However, one small study reported that the adjuvant use of bleomycin and lomustine (CCNU) was associated with fewer relapses and longer survival than in historical controls.[158] The intra-arterial administration of chemotherapeutic agents has been tried as a means of controlling locally advanced disease in single-arm studies that are difficult to interpret. Although tumors resected after intra-arterial chemotherapy with 5-FU[159] or mitomycin C in liposomes[160] are commonly found to be necrotic, it is not clear that this method prevents local or distant recurrences. This field of inquiry has been hampered by the paucity of active chemotherapeutic agents. It is hoped that the development of new approaches will allow a more careful assessment of the impact of treatment on locally advanced disease.

HORMONAL THERAPY

The possibility that hormonal therapy might be useful in renal cell cancer was briefly addressed earlier. Because prolonged estrogen administration induces renal tumors in male Syrian golden hamsters, it was reasoned that human renal cell cancer might be responsive to hormonal manipulation. Experimental studies showed that renal tumors in animals could be modulated by hormonal influences, and the findings were extrapolated to men on the basis of the more frequent occurrence of the tumor in men than in women. Human renal cancer was not evaluated for the presence of hormone receptors, but it was felt that there was little other effective therapy to offer and that the toxic effects of hormonal manipulation were less than those of experimental chemotherapy. Patients received progestogens (chiefly medroxyprogesterone acetate), testosterone, or antiestrogens, alone, in combination, or together with corticosteroids, chemotherapy, or immunotherapy.[32] Objective response rates in the compiled data range from 5% to 9%, with nearly all responses being partial and short-lived and affecting mainly pulmonary metastatic disease. In fact, one analysis suggested that as stricter response criteria are applied, the response rate to hormonal manipulation falls to less than 2%.[152] One study from Japan attempted to evaluate the role of medroxyprogesterone acetate given after definitive surgery in patients with Stages I to III disease.[161] Although a difference that was not statistically significant was seen between the treated and control groups, the study was not prospective and randomized, and it is not clear that both groups underwent similar surgical-pathologic staging. Recent work has documented the presence of receptors for some sex steroids on some human renal cell carcinomas, but efforts to correlate the presence of progesterone receptors, estrogen receptors, and androgen receptors with response have usually been fruitless.[162] Careful study of bona fide human cell lines of renal cell carcinoma is in the initial stages, but it appears that sex steroid hormones exert little trophic effect on human renal cell carcinoma. Any effect of hormonal manipulation could be due more to immune stimulation by the progestogen than to direct effects on the tumor. Although the side-effects of hormonal therapy are not life-threatening, they can be unpleasant. The recent development of biologic treatments with measurable response rates has relegated hormonal therapy to the third line of treatment approaches for metastatic renal cell carcinoma.

BIOLOGIC THERAPY

Several exciting developments in biologic therapy have altered substantially the prospects for the treatment of renal cell carcinoma. The development by Rosenberg and colleagues at the Surgery Branch of the National Cancer Institute (NCI) of adoptive cellular therapy with lymphokine-activated (LAK) cells plus interleukin-2 (IL-2) has changed our view of this resistant disease.[163,164] These investigators have obtained objective response rates of over 30%, and 10% of patients with metastatic disease achieve complete remissions that appear to have affected survival. Other biologic agents such as interferon, tumor necrosis factor, and monoclonal antibodies are being tested that may be effective alone or may have additive therapeutic effect when administered in combination with IL-2–based immunotherapy. Various interferons have been tested and have been found to be effective in 15% to 20% of patients, most of whom had had disease progression on chemotherapy.[165-167] A pilot study of cimetidine plus coumarin, two biologic response modifiers whose immune effects are not well characterized, has also demonstrated objective responses.[168] Active specific and nonspecific approaches have been explored, and monoclonal antibodies are just beginning to be characterized.

The new approach to the treatment of patients with metastatic renal cell carcinoma with adoptive immunotherapy developed by Rosenberg et al involves two elements, IL-2 and LAK cells. This therapy begins with 4 to 5 days of intravenous IL-2 every 8 hours. Patients are then given a 2-day rest, and those scheduled to receive LAK cells undergo four or five daily leukophoreses to harvest lymphocytes. The lymphocytes are cultured in medium containing IL-2 to generate LAK cells, which are then reinfused along with intravenous IL-2. Patients who receive intravenous IL-2 alone receive a second cycle of IL-2 beginning approximately 1 week after the last dose of IL-2 given in the first cycle. (Further details on the basic and clinical aspects of this therapy are given in Chapter 17, Principles and Applications of Biologic Therapy.) Because there were no responses in nine patients with metastatic renal cell carcinoma with the primary tumor in place who were treated in the Surgery Branch of the NCI with either IL-2 or IL-2 plus LAK cells, most patients who present with a kidney tumor in place undergo nephrectomy before receiving adoptive immunotherapy. The nephrectomy decreases the tumor bulk and provides tissue for possible subsequent use for therapy with tumor-infiltrating lymphocytes (discussed below). It is important that immunotherapy in patients with metastatic renal cell carcinoma not be instituted until the patient has fully recovered from surgery and renal function is normal. One of the toxic effects of IL-2 therapy involves the development of renal insufficiency. Although the renal insufficiency resolves quickly after IL-2 is withdrawn, patients with one kidney who have recently had surgery must be evaluated and monitored carefully.

Currently, 124 patients with metastatic renal cell carcinoma have been treated in the Surgery Branch of the NCI. Most of the patients underwent nephrectomy prior to treatment, and many had had chemotherapy, radiation, hormone, or other therapies previously. Seventy-two evaluable patients with metastatic renal cell carcinoma received IL-2 plus LAK cell therapy, 52 received IL-2 alone. Some received lower-dose IL-2 (30,000 U/kg every 8 hours), most received higher-dose IL-2 (100,000 U/kg every 8 hours).

Of the 72 evaluable patients who received LAK cells plus IL-2, 8 had complete responses and 17 had partial responses, for a 35% complete or partial response rate. Of the 52 evaluable patients who received IL-2 alone, 4 had complete responses and 7 had partial responses. Durations of responses to the two different regimens are given in Table 31-7. There were responses at a number of different sites, including lung, liver, soft tissue, subcutaneous tissue, and bone (Figs. 31-10, 31-11, 31-12, 31-13, 31-14).

A randomized trial is currently under way at the NCI comparing response to therapy with IL-2 plus LAK cells to IL-2 alone. Currently 48 patients with advanced renal cell carcinoma have been randomized to receive IL-2 plus LAK cells and 48 to receive IL-2 alone. Among the 46 evaluable patients who have received IL-2 plus LAK cells, 7 have achieved a complete response and 8 have had partial responses. Among the 42 evaluable patients who received IL-2 alone, so far 3 patients have achieved a complete response and 7 have achieved a partial response. (Inevaluable patients are those who for some reason did not receive IL-2; also, two patients in the LAK/IL-2 group, one with a complete response and one with no response, did not receive LAK cells. [Rosenberg SA et al: Submitted for publication].)

Other groups have also reported responses in metastatic renal cell carcinoma with adoptive immunotherapy with IL-2 plus LAK cells.[165] The NCI IL-2/LAK Extramural Working Group reported two complete and three partial responses in 32 evaluable patients treated with IL-2 plus LAK cells, for a

16% response rate.[169] The difference in response rate seems to be accounted for by the greater tumor burden present in the patients treated at the extramural centers. In the extramural trial there were more patients with bulky abdominal disease than in the NCI series, and 9 of 35 patients treated had not undergone nephrectomy before receiving adoptive immunotherapy. It has been reported that patients with renal cell cancer may have defects in their immune systems that correct with the excision of the primary tumor.[170] It seems likely that overcoming the immunosuppressive effects of factors produced by solid tumors would be easier at lower tumor burdens. Perhaps these further arguments support performing nephrectomy in the setting of metastatic disease. The success in treating metastatic disease has stimulated interest in performing adoptive cellular therapy with LAK cells plus IL-2 in a surgical adjuvant setting. A prospective randomized study in patients with N+ or T4A renal cell carcinoma is currently being conducted by Linehan, Rosenberg, and their colleagues.

Other recent *in vivo* and *in vitro* preclinical studies suggest that major improvements in adoptive immunotherapy are likely to occur. In an attempt to identify more potent cells for use in adoptive transfer, Rosenberg et al have performed murine studies in which lymphocytes grown from the tumor, tumor-infiltrating lymphocytes (TIL), have proved much more potent than LAK cells in mediating regression of established metastases.[171] It has been demonstrated recently that TIL from a number of human tumors, including renal cell carcinoma, can be isolated and expanded.[172-175] Based on these studies and on clinical experience demonstrating that selected patients who have recently undergone nephrectomy can safely undergo adoptive immunotherapy with IL-2 or IL-2 plus LAK cells, a clinical trial has been initiated in which the primary kidney tumor or accessible metastatic tissue is resected, the lymphocytes from the tumor are expanded in media containing IL-2, and the TIL cells plus intravenous IL-2 and cyclophosphamide are administered back into the patient.[176] A pilot trial has demonstrated that this therapeutic strategy is practical and that in carefully selected patients with renal cell carcinoma, IL-2 plus TIL cell therapy can safely be administered. Currently, after the renal tumor is removed, the enzyme-dispersed cells (containing tumor cells and lymphocytes) are cryopreserved and stored. After the patient has fully recovered from surgery and renal function is normal, the cells are thawed and the TIL cells are expanded for therapy.

The potential for improved outcome by combining adop-

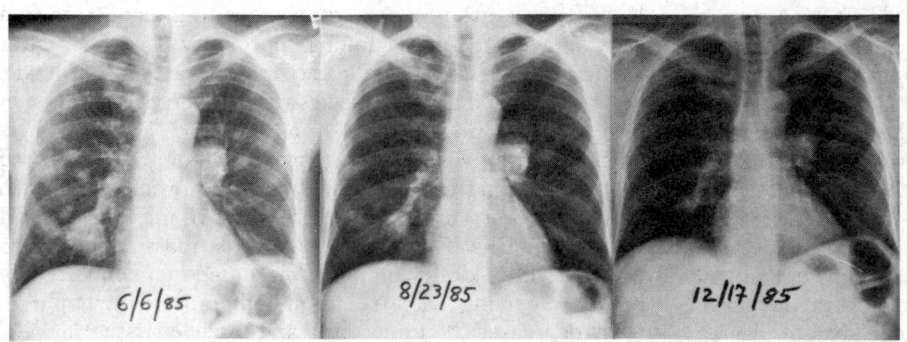

FIG. 31-10. Chest radiographs of multiple pulmonary nodules in a patient with metastatic renal cell cancer before (*left panel*) and after (*middle and right panels*) treatment with IL-2 and LAK cells. All of the nodules underwent a marked regression; most resolved completely.

TABLE 31-7. Results of Immunotherapy for Renal Cell Carcinoma, Surgery Branch, National Cancer Institute

Total Evaluable Patients	LAK Cells + IL-2		IL-2	
	No. of Patients	Response Duration (mo)	No. of Patients	Response Duration (mo)
	72		52	
No. with CR	8	20+, 17+, 15, 13+, 13, 11, 9, 6	4	24+, 18+, 17+, 15+
No. with PR	17	26+, 17+, 13, 11, 10+, 10+, 10, 9, 7, 7, 6, 6, 6, 6, 3, 1, 1	7	17+, 17+, 15+, 11+, 11, 9+, 5+
Total no. of CR + PR	25	(35%)	11	(21%)

tive cellular therapy with chemotherapy has been demonstrated in other animal experiments. Salup, Back, and Wiltrout found, in a murine renal cell carcinoma model, that neither LAK cells plus IL-2 nor single-agent doxorubicin were very effective therapy in advanced stage renal cancer. However, when doxorubicin and LAK cells plus IL-2 were combined and administered both systemically and intraperitoneally, 80% of animals with locally advanced and metastatic disease were cured of renal cell carcinoma.[177] A clinical trial applying the principles learned from these experiments is under way. Among the effects demonstrated for doxorubicin is that on the trafficking of adoptively transferred cells. When doxorubicin is administered with the cells, nearly twice as many cells home to a tumor-bearing kidney than to a normal kidney. Another drug, flavone-8-acetic acid (FAA), has been demonstrated to be a potent inducer of interferon. When used together with IL-2 in a

FIG. 31-11. Lung tomograms of a patient with metastatic renal cell carcinoma with a right hilar mass, before treatment with IL-2 and LAK cells (*lower panels*) and afterward (*upper panels*). The tumor regresses almost completely.

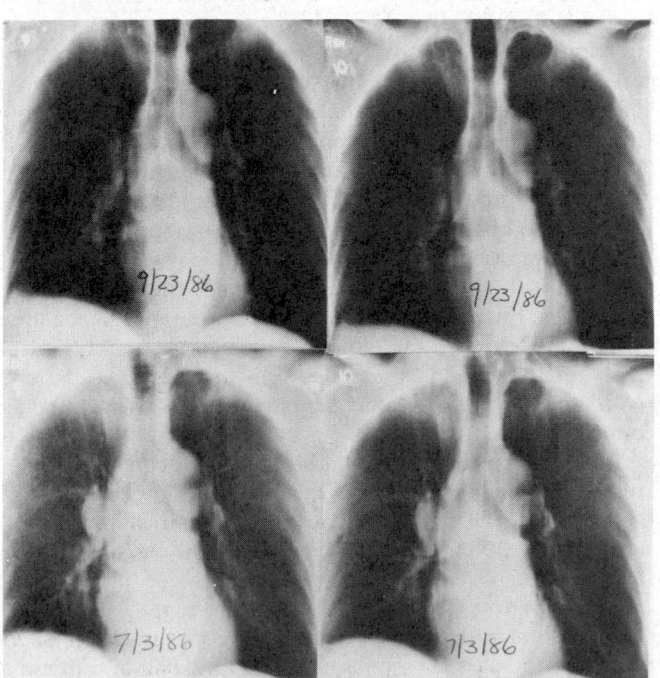

murine model, FAA cured 80% or more of animals with advanced renal cell carcinoma.[178] Thus, the exploration of combined modality therapy may improve on the advances made to date.

Interferon is perhaps the most extensively evaluated biologic agent in renal cell cancer treatment.[167,168] A large number of patients have been treated with purified and recombinant interferon-α, interferon-β, and interferon-γ; the results of such studies are summarized in Table 31-8.[179-198] The data suggest that the best response rates occur when interferon is administered daily at close to the maximum tolerated dose, rather than intermittently at high doses. The response rate for daily doses of interferon-α between 10 and 20 megaunits/m² is around 25%, and about 5% of the responses are complete. Responses last a median of 8 months. It would be expected that interferon might act additively or synergistically with certain other biologic agents like LAK cells plus IL-2, IL-2, other interferons, tumor necrosis factor, and other cytokines. Interferon should also potentiate the effects of antitumor monoclonal antibodies. A number of clinical trials employing combinations of biologic agents are under way. Substantial preclinical data support the use of interferon in combination with chemotherapeutic agents.[199] Clinical trials of interferon plus vinblastine[200-202] and interferon plus BCNU[203] have not shown dramatic enhancement or antitumor responses. A study conducted at the Mayo Clinic appears to show nearly a doubling of the response rate in patients with renal cell carcinoma treated with interferon (20 megaunits/m² three times weekly) with the addition of aspirin (2 tablets orally four times a day) to the therapeutic regimen.[204] Ten (34%) of 29 patients achieved objective responses lasting a median of over 10 months. This observation is being tested in a prospective randomized study by the North Central Oncology Group. The mechanism by which aspirin enhances the antitumor effects of interferon is unknown but could relate to the inhibition of lipoxygenase or the induction by aspirin of a protein that blocks phospholipase C, which is involved in cell proliferation through phosphoinositol turnover. Certainly the single-agent activity of interferon-α is at least comparable to that of the best chemotherapeutic agents. Interferon may form a building block for a combined modality regimen that includes chemotherapeutic agents and LAK cells plus IL-2. The M. D. Anderson group has suggested that tumors that progress after an interferon-induced partial or complete remission may be more

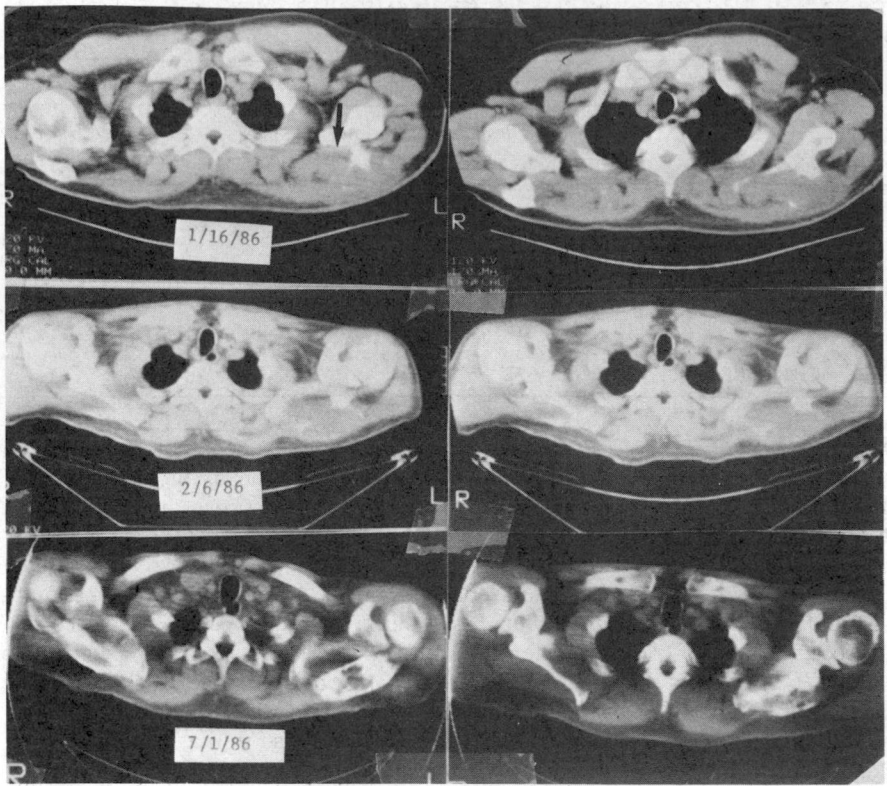

FIG. 31-12. CT scan of a patient with renal cell carcinoma with a metastasis in the scapula before treatment with IL-2 and LAK cells (*upper panels*) and afterward (*middle and lower panels*). All tumors regressed completely.

FIG. 31-13. Radiograph of the pelvis of a patient with metastatic renal cell carcinoma who had a large osseous metastasis before treatment with IL-2 and LAK cells (*upper panel*) and afterward (*lower panel*). The osseous lesion regressed completely and the bone recalcified.

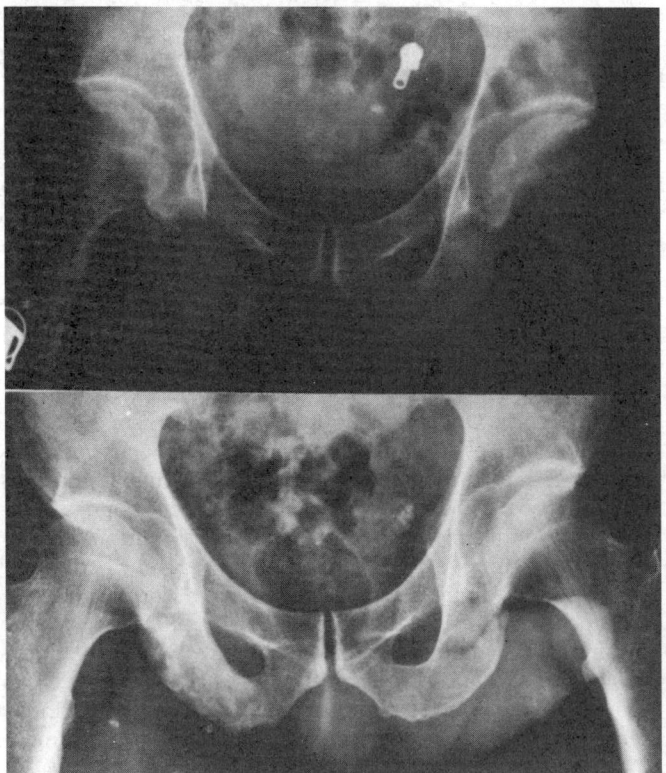

responsive to subsequent treatment with chemotherapeutic agents.[205] Sequential therapy also needs to be evaluated.

Ribonucleic acid (RNA) has been used in the treatment of patients with renal cell carcinoma, in the form of synthetic double-stranded polymer, polyinosinic-polycytidylic acid (poly IC), which induces interferon,[206] and in the form of xenogeneic immune RNA, RNA extracted from the lymphoid cells of animals immunized with human renal cell carcinoma cells.[207,208] Poly IC did not produce responses at the maximum tolerated dose.[206] The incubation of patient lymphocytes with immune RNA extracted from the lymphocytes of guinea pigs that had been immunized with the patient's tumor results in the development of tumor-specific cellular immunity by a mechanism that is not yet established. When such cells were reinfused into the patient, most patients had measurable changes in immune function, and complete or partial responses were obtained in 6 (22%) of 27 patients.[207] Patients with pulmonary metastases were the most likely to respond to this form of passive immunotherapy. Xenogeneic immune RNA from the lymphoid cells of sheep immunized with renal cancer has also been given directly to patients with renal carcinoma, but has not been shown to produce tumor regression.[208]

Active nonspecific immunotherapy has recently produced responses in a pilot study of 42 patients with metastatic renal cell cancer.[168] The use of two orally administered agents, coumarin (100 mg/d) and cimetidine (300 mg/four times a day), produced complete responses in three patients and partial responses in 11 (overall response rate, 33%). Response durations are not yet available for complete responders, but the partial responses lasted a median of 5 months. All the responses occurred in patients who had undergone

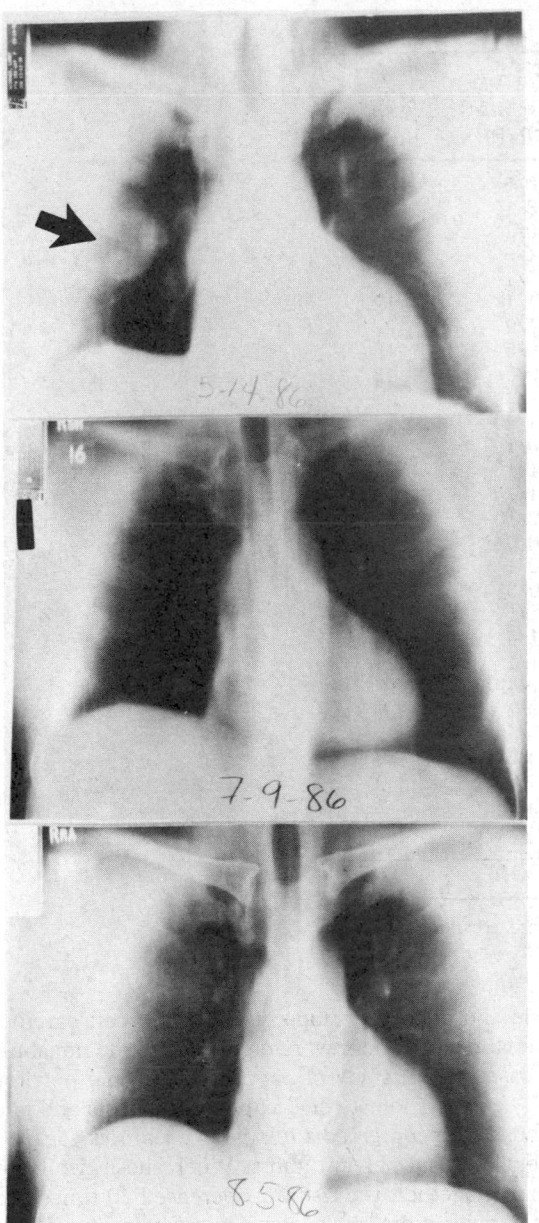

FIG. 31-14. Lung tomograms of a patient with renal cell carcinoma who had a large pulmonary metastasis before IL-2 treatment (*upper panel*) and afterward (*middle and lower panels*). The pulmonary nodule regressed completely.

when administered in the adjuvant setting. BCG has been given as a component of a multimodality treatment program that included combination chemotherapy and hormonal manipulation, but the response rate was not higher than that obtained with interferon or vinblastine as single agents.[210] In another study of vincristine, doxorubicin, medroxyprogesterone, and BCG, patients whose primary tumors were resected had a higher probability of responding than those in whom the primary tumor was left in place.[211] Thymosin fraction V appears to have no antitumor effects in renal cancer,[212] but an acid mucopolysaccharide called catrix-s, extracted from bovine tracheal cartilage, produced a dramatic complete remission in one of two patients with renal cell carcinoma who were treated with it.[213]

A variety of approaches to inducing tumor-specific immunity have been taken. Treatment with autologous cells modified by dimethyldioctadecyl ammonium bromide,[214] or with autologous cells irradiated and given with adjuvants like *Corynebacterium parvum* with[215] and without[216] cyclophosphamide to eliminate suppressor cells, is associated with response rates of 10% to 20%.[217] Antigens have been extracted from tumors, polymerized, and administered together with immune stimulants like BCG,[218,219] and attenuated vaccinia virus[220] has been given in an effort to elicit a tumor-specific immune response. Such approaches have been minimally effective at eliciting appropriate immune responses, and antitumor responses in vivo have been rare. However, the success that has been demonstrated in colorectal cancer using an autologous tumor vaccine plus BCG, and the availability of recombinant molecules such as IL-2 that may be superior at boosting cell-mediated immunity, make this approach to treatment worthy of further exploration.

An early attempt at using an immunologic approach to the treatment of renal cell cancer was reported in 1971. Horn and Horn infused plasma from a patient previously cured of renal cell carcinoma into a family member who had diffusely metastatic renal cell carcinoma, and produced a complete remission that lasted almost 2 years.[221] The patient relapsed with metastases to the cerebrum, a site that might be considered a sanctuary from the effects of antibodies. Investigators have been slow to apply the field of serotherapy to renal cell carcinoma. Only very recently have efforts been made to characterize the cell surface of renal cell cancers and the polyclonal and monoclonal antibodies that recognize the cell surface antigens.[222,223] Antibodies directed against renal cell cancer are expected to be useful adjuncts to therapy with interferons and LAK cells plus IL-2.

CARCINOMA OF THE RENAL PELVIS

Carcinoma of the renal pelvis is a relatively rare tumor that accounts for 5% of all renal tumors. It occurs more frequently in men than in women (2–3:1). Upper urinary tract carcinoma is a multifocal process; patients with cancer at one site in the upper urinary tract are at greater risk of developing tumors elsewhere. The probability of multifocal occurrence is greater in patients with larger lesions and in those with carcinoma in situ. A patient with one upper tract urothelial tumor has a 30% to 50% chance of developing a bladder tumor as well. Some 2% to 4% of patients with an

nephrectomy (14 of 31, or 45%). Although cimetidine has been thought to modulate suppressor cells, the effects of coumarin on the immune system are unclear. These results need to be confirmed and extended. In contrast, the use of bacillus Calmette-Guérin (BCG) has not been associated with convincing therapeutic results in patients with metastatic disease. Pulmonary lesions may regress, but it is not known if such responses prolong survival. In one study of BCG given in the adjuvant setting after nephrectomy, survival did not appear to be improved.[209] However, if BCG and its related nonspecific immunostimulants are to be successfully applied to the treatment of cancer, one would expect their greatest effect to be seen in locally advanced disease

TABLE 31-8.   Response Rate of Renal Cell Carcinoma to Various Interferons

Interferon Type and Source	Dose (megaunits/m²), Route, and Schedule	No. of Evaluable Patients	No. of Responses (CR/PR)	Response Rate (%)
HuIFN(Le)[179,180]	3 IM daily	19	0/5	26
	3 IM daily	50	3/10	26
HuIFN(Le)[181]	6 IM daily × 3 d, for 4 wk	4	0/1	25
HuIFN(Le)[182]	3 IM daily × 5 d, for 12 wk	43	1/6	16
HuIFN(Le)[183]	1 IM daily × 28 d	14	0/1	7
	10 IM daily × 28 d	16	1/1	12.5
HuIFN(Le)[184]	3 IM daily	11	1/2	27
HuIFN(Ly)[185]	5 IM 3 times a wk × 24 wk	33	0/5	15
HuIFN(Ly)[186]	3 IM on d 1, 5 on d 2, 10 on d 3, 20 on d 4–10	39	0/5	13
HuIFN(Ly)[187]	3 IM daily	18	1/2	17
HuIFN(Ly)[188]	3 IM 3 times a wk × 6 wk	21	0/1	5
HuIFN(Ly)[189]	5 IM daily	73	1/16	23
αA	3–36 IM daily	45	1/7	18
rIFN-α2	6–10 IM daily	108	2/13	14
rIFN-α2[190]	2 SC 3 times a wk,	10	0/0	0
	30 IV daily × 5 d, for 2–3 wk	10	0/1	10
rIFN-α2[191]	2 IM daily	15	0/0	0
	20 IM daily	41	1/11	29
rIFN-α2[192]	3–36 IM daily × 5 d × 14 wk	19	1/4	26
rIFN-α2[193]	10 IM daily × 3 mo	8	1/1	25
rIFN-α2[194]	2 SC 3 times a wk,	51	1/4	10
	30 IV daily × 5 d, for 3 wk	46	1/2	7
rIFN-α2[195]	3–36 IM daily × 10 wk	22	0/5	23
rIFN-β[196]	150 IV twice a wk × 4 wk	15	0/2	13
rIFN-γ[197]	Up to 75 IV twice a week	13	0/0	0
rIFN-γ[198]	Varying doses IM	14	0/1	7
	Varying doses IV	16	0/1	6
Total		747	16/107	16.5

IM = intramuscular,   SC = subcutaneous,   IV = intravenous,   CR = complete   response,   PR = partial response.

upper tract urothelial tumor develop bilateral renal pelvic tumors. If a patient has both a renal pelvic tumor and a ureteral tumor at the same time, there is a 75% chance that a bladder tumor will develop. Alternatively, a patient with a bladder tumor initially has a 2% to 3% chance of developing an upper tract tumor.[224-228]

ETIOLOGY

In 1965 Hultengren et al first identified a connection between epithelial tumors of the renal pelvis and abuse of compound analgesics.[229,230] Since then a number of other reports from Sweden,[231,232] Australia,[233-235] the Netherlands,[236] Denmark,[237] Italy,[238] and Germany[239] have demonstrated an association between analgesic abuse and renal pelvic tumors. Most of the patients ingested a significant amount (5 kg) of compound analgesics, usually containing phenacetin, phenazone, and caffeine.[228,234] Typically, upper genitourinary (GU) tract tumors occur in patients in whom prolonged and heavy analgesic ingestion is followed by renal papillary necrosis.[234] Although the precise mechanism is not completely understood, studies have suggested a possible etiologic role of orthoaminophenols, the major phenacetin metabolites, in the development of renal pelvic tumors.[228] In a study of 192 patients with chronic pyelonephritis, 104 had pyelonephritis secondary to analgesic abuse. Of the 104 an-

algesic abusers, 8 developed transitional cell carcinoma of the renal pelvis. There were no tumors in the nonabusers.[231] In a case-control study of patients with renal pelvic transitional cell carcinoma, renal papillary necrosis and phenacetin abuse both conferred a relatively equal risk for the development of renal pelvic tumors. When these two conditions occurred together, the risk was increased 20 times over that for nonconsumers of analgesics without renal papillary necrosis.[235]

There is also an association between cancer of the renal pelvis and Danubian endemic familial nephropathy (Balkan nephropathy). Balkan nephropathy is a slowly progressive inflammation of the interstitium of the kidney that ultimately results in renal failure. This disorder, which is prevalent in the Balkan countries (Yugoslavia, Rumania, Bulgaria, and Greece), is associated with multifocal, slow-growing, superficial, low-grade tumors of the renal pelvis.[228] The cause of Balkan nephropathy is unclear; however, a number of potential etiologic agents such as fungal toxins, viruses, silicates, and heavy metals have been studied.[224]

An association has been observed between renal pelvic tumors and urban residence as well as occupation in the aniline dye, textile, plastics, and rubber industries.[228,240] There is a significant increase in risk for upper genitourinary tract urothelial cancer in smokers; the risk is highest among the heaviest smokers.[228] Chronic inflammation and irritation are associated with the development of renal pelvic tumors, particularly in patients who have upper urinary tract stones.

There are in-depth studies of the molecular genetics of transitional cell carcinoma. DNA sequence deletions have been detected by RFLP analysis at the *c-H-ras* locus in 42% of patients with bladder carcinoma, suggesting the possibility of a recessive or activated oncogene at this site.[64] There are reports of nine kindreds exhibiting a familial pattern in the development of transitional cell carcinoma of the urinary tract.[241,242] Of the affected family members, 22% had upper tract tumors, 59% had bladder cancer, and 18% had both upper and lower tract tumors.[241] One member of another cancer-prone family (Li-Fraumeni syndrome) developed bilateral upper tract urothelial carcinoma. A molecular defect, an activated *c-raf*-1 gene, has been isolated from noncancerous cells from members of a family with Li-Fraumeni syndrome; however, material from affected family members with bladder or upper tract transitional cell carcinoma has not yet been analyzed.[243] Studies of the molecular and cellular aspects of urothelial transformation should provide further insight into the etiology and mechanisms of progression and metastasis of this disease.

PATHOLOGY

Transitional cell carcinoma accounts for 90% of the tumors of the renal pelvis and can be in situ, papillary, or planar. Squamous cell carcinoma, which is usually associated with chronic inflammation or infection of the renal pelvis, accounts for 7% of renal pelvic tumors. Squamous cell cancer of the renal pelvis is often deeply invasive and is associated with a worse prognosis than is transitional cell carcinoma. Adenocarcinoma of the renal pelvis has been reported in few patients and occurs in association with inflammation, infection, or calculi.[224,228,240,244]

DIAGNOSTIC AND STAGING TECHNIQUES

The differential diagnosis of renal pelvic carcinoma is given in Table 31-9. Hematuria is the initial presenting symptom in the majority of patients. Gross hematuria is present in 62% to 75%, microscopic hematuria in 10%. The triad of flank mass, pain, and hematuria is encountered frequently, in 20% or less, and often is associated with advanced disease.[228,240,245-248]

Excretory urography is frequently used to evaluate patients with renal pelvic tumors and will often reveal a filling defect in the collecting system. There may also be either a hydronephrotic or a nonfunctional kidney due to obstruction by a blood clot or mass.[224,227] Retrograde pyelography (in which contrast medium is injected into the ureter through an endoscope) accurately delineates upper tract filling defects. If there is uncertainty about the nature of a renal pelvic lesion, CT performed before and after administration of intravenous contrast material will differentiate a tumor from another radiolucent mass such as a stone. Angiography is not often used in the diagnostic evaluation of a suspected renal pelvic tumor. However, a renal mass lesion that lacks the characteristic neovascularity of a renal cell carcinoma may

TABLE 31-9.   Differential Diagnosis of Cancer of the Renal Pelvis*

Intrinsic Lesions
  Calculus
  Blood clot
  Cholesteatoma
  Malakoplakia
  Inflammatory lesions of urothelium (pyelitis cystica, etc.)
  Benign ureteropelvic junction obstruction
  Benign (connective tissue) tumors of renal pelvis
  Renal cell carcinoma
  Suburothelial hemorrhage
Extrinsic Lesions
  Vascular impressions
  Parapelvic cyst

* Modified from Fraly EE: Cancer of the renal pelvis. In Skinner DG, de Kernion JB (eds): Genitourinary Cancer, p 141. Philadelphia, WB Saunders, 1978.

be the first indication of a renal pelvic tumor invading the renal parenchyma.[249-251]

Urine cytology is useful in evaluating a renal pelvis mass, and endoscopically obtained barbotage specimens allow an accurate diagnosis to be made in about 80% of cases.[252,253] Tissue can also be obtained by introducing a biopsy brush into the ureter and removing a specimen for cytologic or histologic examination. Brush biopsy increases diagnostic accuracy to between 80% and 90%. Endoscopic ureteroscopy and percutaneous nephroscopy are recently developed clinical techniques that have improved the diagnosis of upper tract tumors. With currently available flexible endoscopic instruments, the renal pelvis can be inspected visually in almost 90% of patients.[240,246,254,255]

STAGE AND GRADE

The most significant prognostic factors for survival of patients with renal pelvic carcinoma are stage and grade of tumor.[246,256] Renal pelvic cancer is divided into four stages. Stage I is papillary carcinoma without evidence of invasion, Stage II denotes tumor that is superficially invasive but limited to the lamina propria, Stage III denotes involvement of the muscularis, Stage III denotes involvement of the muscularis, and stage IV denotes extent to adjacent structures or metastatic disease (Table 31-10). Renal pelvic tumors are graded from I to III. The 5-year survival for patients with

TABLE 31-10.   Renal Pelvic Cancer*

Stage I	Papillary or planar (nonpapillary) carcinoma with no evidence of invasion.
Stage II	Papillary or planar carcinoma. Superficially invasive but with invasion limited to the lamina propria.
Stage III	Papillary or planar carcinoma, extending to the level of the muscularis (may extend beyond the muscularis in intrarenal portions of the renal pelvis if confined to the kidney.)
Stage IV	Papillary or planar carcinoma extending to the adventitial surface and either involving adjuvant structures or metastatic or both.

* Modified from Bennington JL, Beckwith JB: Armed Forces Institute of Pathology, 2nd ed, Fasc 12, 1975.

Grade I transitional cell carcinoma of the renal pelvis approaches 100%; for Grade II, it is 60% to 70%; and for Grade III, it is 5%. Invasion of the renal hilum occurs in 95% of patients who ultimately develop metastases.[246,256,257]

TREATMENT

Carcinoma of the renal pelvis may be treated with a radical nephrectomy that includes removal of Gerota's fascia and its contents, total removal of the ipsilateral ureter, and removal of a cuff of bladder.[224,228,246,248,258-260] Simple intrafascial nephrectomy is associated with a decreased 5-year survival rate compared to that for radical nephrectomy, particularly in patients with Stage III or IV tumors.[259] When transitional cell carcinoma of the renal pelvis invades the renal vein or vena cava, an extensive surgical procedure including thrombus extraction and/or partial vena cava resection may be required.[224,228,240,246,248,258-262]

A more conservative surgical excision is advocated by some who note that renal pelvic carcinoma can be bilateral and that survival of patients with low-stage, low-grade renal pelvic carcinoma treated with a conservative surgical procedure is approximately the same as in patients treated with more radical surgery.[263-265] The incidence of low-grade, low-stage renal pelvic carcinoma is approximately 8% and that of bilateral disease is 2%. There is also often a long latent period prior to recurrence.[240,247,260] In most studies reporting a low recurrence rate after local excision, the follow-up period is short. When even low-stage, low-grade tumors were resected from the renal pelvis, a 29% to 30% incidence of recurrence in the ipsilateral ureter was found during a 10-year follow-up.[240] Although the availability of new techniques such as intraoperative nephroscopy and brush cytology have made staging much more accurate, intraoperative pyeloscopy is not without risk. In a recent series of 18 patients with renal pelvic carcinoma who underwent intraoperative pyeloscopy for evaluation and staging, two experienced disease recurrence in the renal fossa.[266] Currently, most clinicians consider that local, partial excision is most appropriate for patients with a solitary kidney, with bilateral renal pelvic carcinoma, or with renal insufficiency. New treatment strategies involving percutaneous resection of renal pelvic tumors followed by either laser irradiation or supplemental intracavitary therapy with mitomycin C or BCG are currently being evaluated.[255]

FOLLOW-UP

Conscientious follow-up after surgery for renal pelvic carcinoma is essential. Urinalysis, urine cytology, and cystourethroscopy are performed every 3 months for 2 to 3 years, then less frequently. For patients who undergo a conservative upper tract procedure, periodic retrograde pyelography is also performed.[240]

URETERAL CARCINOMA

Ureteral carcinoma is an uncommon neoplasm that accounts for only 1% of all malignancies of the upper GU tract. Ureteral carcinoma was first described by the French pathologist

TABLE 31-11. Classification of Tumors of the Ureter*

Primary Tumors
Epithelial
  Malignant
    Transitional cell carcinoma (71%)
    Transitional cell carcinoma with differentiation (20%)
      Squamous differentiation
      Glandular differentiation
      Mixed
    Squamous cell carcinoma (pure) (8%)
    Adenocarcinoma (1%)
    Undifferentiated carcinoma (1%)
  Benign
    Papilloma
Mesodermal
  Malignant
    Leiomyosarcoma
  Benign
    Fibroepithelial polyp
    Leiomyoma
    Neurilemmoma
    Angioma
Secondary Tumors (All Malignant)
Drop metastases
Metastases via blood or lymph
Direct extension

* Modified from Bennington JL, Beckwith JB: Armed Forces Institute of Pathology, 2nd ed, Fasc 12, 1975.

Rayer in 1841; the first ureteral carcinoma to be removed by nephroureterectomy was reported by Vorphl in 1905. Ureteral carcinoma tends to occur in the older age groups, predominantly in the sixth, seventh, and eighth decades of life. The male–female ratio is 2:1. The most common site for the occurrence of a ureteral tumor is in the lower third of the ureter, with a lesser incidence higher up.[267-272]

HISTOLOGY AND ETIOLOGY

Ninety percent of malignant tumors of the ureter are transitional cell carcinomas; 20% have squamous or glandular differentiation. Eight percent of the tumors are pure squamous cell carcinomas and 1% are adenocarcinomas (Table 31-11). Tumors of the ureter share embryologic, morphologic, and etiologic characteristics with renal pelvic tumors. As with renal pelvic tumors, there is an increased incidence of ureteral carcinoma associated with Balkan nephropathy, prolonged exposure to phenacetin, or prolonged exposure to environmental agents such as aniline dyes.[273]

CLINICAL PRESENTATION

Hematuria is the most common presenting symptom and is present in 75% of patients with ureteral carcinoma. The hematuria is usually painless; however, colicky pain due to obstruction by clot or by tumor occurs in up to 35%. Urinary frequency or dysuria, present in only 10% of patients with renal pelvic carcinoma, occurs in up to 50% of patients with ureteral carcinoma.[269,273]

Ureteral carcinoma is divided into five stages (Table 31-12). Stage 0 ureteral carcinoma is confined to the mucosa of the ureter; Stage A disease involves the lamina propria. In Stage B the tumor involves the muscularis of the ureter; in Stage C the tumor extends through the muscularis to the

TABLE 31-12.   Staging of Ureteral Carcinoma

Stage 0	Limited to mucosa
Stage A	Lamina propria invasion
Stage B	Confined to muscularis
Stage C	Invasion through muscularis with involvement of adjacent structures or metastases
Stage D	Metastatic

adventitia. Stage D is metastatic disease. Although up to 100% of Grade I tumors and 85% of Grade II tumors may be noninvasive, only 30% of Grade III and 8% of Grade IV tumors are noninvasive.[273]

DIAGNOSIS

Excretory urography is an initial part of the evaluation of a suspected ureteral mass lesion. On excretory urography the upper tract above the tumor may be completely normal or there may be hydronephrosis or complete nonfunction. Retrograde pyelography is performed to delineate accurately the precise location of the ureteral lesion.[273,274] Urine is collected for cytologic examination, and brush biopsy may be performed to obtain tissue for histologic examination. The availability of flexible endoscopy has greatly improved the surgeon's ability to visualize and biopsy ureteral lesions.[255] Abdominal CT also provides useful staging information, particularly with regard to extension of the tumor outside the ureter.

TREATMENT

Carcinoma of the ureter is treated by either nephroureterectomy (Fig. 31-15) or partial ureterectomy.[227,268,269,275] The advantage of a partial ureterectomy is that the more conservative procedure preserves the kidney. However, mapping studies of the urothelium have demonstrated that carcinoma of the upper urinary tract is a multifocal disease. There is often atypia and carcinoma in situ in multiple areas of the urothelium, particularly in high-grade, high-stage carcinomas. Ureteral carcinoma treated by partial ureterectomy or by nephrectomy plus partial ureterectomy is associated with a 12% to 40% recurrence rate.[269,275] Those who advocate more conservative management of ureteral carcinoma note that recent studies demonstrate that in low-stage, low-grade carcinomas, distal ureterectomy with reimplantation of the distal ureter is associated with excellent survival,[227,264] and that survival is more dependent on grade and stage of disease (Table 31-13) than on the type of operation performed.[247,276] In a study reported by Babain and Johnson there was a 100% 5-year survival rate in patients with Stage 0 or A distal ureteral carcinoma who were treated with distal ureterectomy plus reimplantation.[227] Currently, distal ureterectomy plus reimplantation is recommended for patients with low-stage, low-grade disease that occurs in the distal third of the ureter. Nephroureterectomy is recommended for patients with high-grade or high-stage tumor and for those with disease at a location other than the distal third of the ureter.

The surgical procedure of radical nephrectomy plus ureterectomy entails removal of the kidney and the entire con-

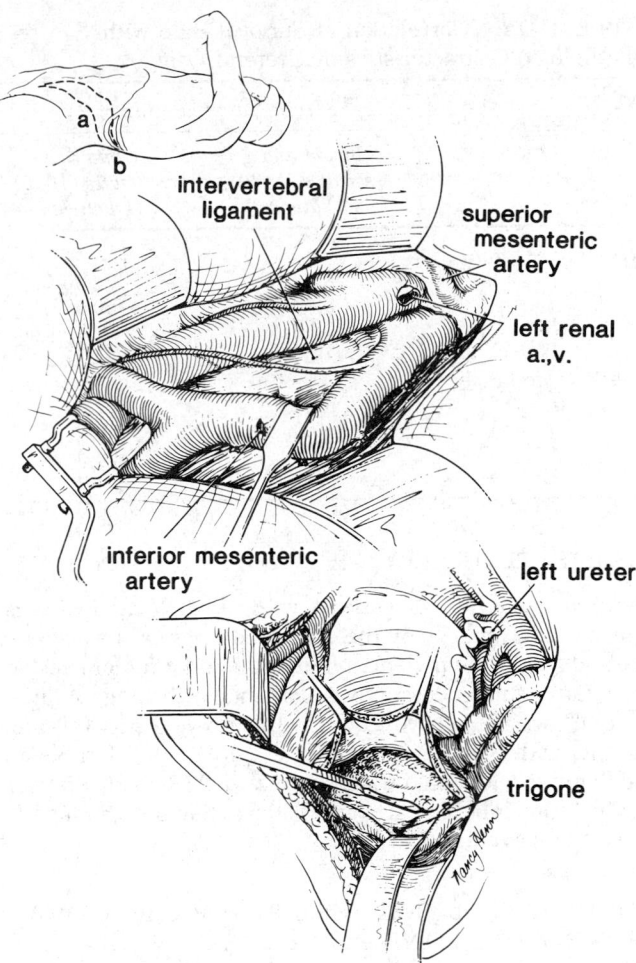

FIG. 31-15. The patient for a nephroureterectomy with lymph node dissection should be placed in a modified flank position and an incision made either through line a or line b. The area of dissection is as indicated in the middle panel, being divested from the superior mesenteric artery to the bifurcation. The ureter is removed by opening the bladder, circumscribing the orifice, and sharply dissecting the ureter from the surrounding detrusor muscle. The defect in the bladder is then closed appropriately. (Paulson DF, Perez CA, Anderson T: Cancer of the kidney and ureter. In DeVita VT Jr, Hellman S, Rosenberg SA (eds): Cancer: Principles and Practice of Oncology, 2nd ed, p 907. Philadelphia, JB Lippincott, 1985)

tents of Gerota's fascia, the ureter, and a cuff of bladder including the ureteral orifice and intramural ureter. Regional lymph nodes may be removed, particularly if there is indication of involvement. This surgical procedure may be performed using one or two incisions, depending on the patient's body habitus and the surgeon's preference. When partial ureterectomy is performed, urinary tract continuity is reestablished with either ureteroureterostomy or ureteroneocystostomy.

New strategies involving endoscopic fulguration and laser photocoagulation have been developed for treatment of patients with ureteral carcinoma. Carcinoma in situ of the distal ureter has been treated with endoscopic fulguration, with encouraging preliminary results.[277] These new therapeutic strategies will be important in the future evaluation of the role of radical versus local surgery for treatment of this disease.

TABLE 31-13. Correlation of Survival Rate with Pathologic Characteristics of Ureteral Cancer

	5-Year Survival Rate (%)	
	Bloom and Associates (1970) (54 Patients)	Batata and Associates (1975) (41 Patients)
Histologic Grade		
I	83.0	78.0
II	52.0	50.0
III	18.0	0
IV	12.0	0
Pathologic Stage		
0,A	62.0	91.0
B	50.0	43.0
C	33.3	23.0
D	0	0

RESULTS OF THERAPY

The 5-year survival of patients with ureteral carcinoma is determined primarily by the grade and stage of the disease. Sex and age of the patient and multiplicity of tumor sites do not greatly influence survival. Patients with Stage A or 0 ureteral carcinoma have a 90% to 100% 5-year survival rate. Patients with Stage B disease have a 45% to 85% survival, and patients with Stage C disease have a 25% to 30% 5-year survival rate. The 5-year survival for patients with Stage D disease is currently 0 to 5%.

ADJUVANT RADIATION THERAPY FOR CARCINOMA OF THE RENAL PELVIS AND URETER

There would seem to be no role for adjuvant therapy for low-stage upper tract transitional cell tumors; most series report less than 20% of the patients failing treatment or dying within 5 years after surgical resection.[270,245] Moreover, the results of surgical resection for patients with high-stage tumors—those with pathologic evidence of periurethral, peripelvic, or perirenal extension, or those with regional lymph node metastases—are also poor; less than 30% of the patients are cured by surgery alone.[278-280] Autopsy studies indicate that lymph node involvement occurs in 37% to 82% of patients with pelvic tumors.[245,281] In patients with ureteral tumors, lymph node involvement occurs in 22% to 41% of cases.[271] Local recurrence rate has been reported to be higher after surgical resection for invasive pelvic tumors (43%) than for invasive tumors of the ureter (14%).[269,244] A recent retrospective review of patients with poor-risk (high-stage or high-grade) transitional cell carcinoma of the renal pelvis and ureter found that patients treated with postoperative irradiation of 4000 to 5000 cGy had a lower incidence of local recurrence (1% versus 46%) and a higher 5-year survival (27% versus 17%) than patients treated with surgery alone.[280] Also, 45% of the patients in the poor prognosis group developed distant metastases.

A study of the best available information suggests that postoperative radiation therapy following radical surgical resection should be considered only for patients with locally advanced disease—those with pathologically confirmed periureteral, perirenal, or peripelvic extension of tumor, or those with proven regional lymph node metastases. Some centers are embarking on Phase I or II studies or pilot studies combining such local radiation therapy with adjuvant cisplatin-based chemotherapy regimens.[282] The dose of radiation therapy if no adjuvant chemotherapy is given would be in the range of 4500 cGy delivered in 180-cGy fractions over 5 weeks to the tumor bed, and to the regional lymph nodes with a boost to the tumor bed of up to 5000 cGy. However, if adjuvant chemotherapy is given, these doses should be decreased by 10% to 15%.

CHEMOTHERAPY FOR CARCINOMAS OF THE RENAL PELVIS AND URETER

Carcinomas arising in the ureters and renal pelvis are mainly transitional cell carcinomas,[227] can be multiple (either metachronously or synchronously),[283] occur with increased frequency in Balkan nephropathy (a toxic nephropathy indigenous to the Danube basin),[284] and give rise to metastases in about 40% of patients.[227] The histology, biology, and natural history make it senseless for the medical oncologist to consider transitional cell carcinomas of the ureter and renal pelvis as pathologic entities distinct from transitional cell carcinoma of the bladder. There are certainly distinctive features to the surgical management of ureteral and renal pelvis tumors based on anatomic differences; however, the patterns of local recurrence and systemic spread and response to treatment are very similar to histologically identical tumors arising in the bladder.[285]

In light of the frequent epithelial atypia in a normal-appearing ureter adjacent to primary tumors and the high incidence of local recurrence (up to 64%) and subsequent development of bladder tumors (21%),[286] it is surprising that adjuvant chemotherapy has been reported only anecdotally.[287] Topical thiotepa has been employed, but it is not possible to discern whether it exerts beneficial effects. A systematic study of postoperative or preoperative chemotherapy or immunotherapy is indicated.

The treatment of metastatic disease is the treatment for metastatic bladder cancer. At the moment, the most active regimen is M-VAC, a four-drug regimen consisting of methotrexate, vincristine, doxorubicin, and cisplatin, developed by Yagoda and colleagues at Memorial Sloan-Kettering Cancer Center.[288] M-VAC produces objective responses (complete and partial) in 69% of patients with metastatic transitional cell carcinoma of bladder, ureter, and renal pelvis.[288] The use of cyclophosphamide, doxorubicin, and cisplatin in varying doses, routes (intravenous, intra-arterial), and schedules has produced a similar response rate.[289] Both regimens are being tested in neoadjuvant trials. The administration of doxorubicin followed by cyclophosphamide 12 hours later allowed nearly 100% of the projected doses of the two drugs to be given, with a 57% overall response rate and a 23% complete response rate.[290] The capacity of WR-2721 to enhance the antitumor effects of cisplatin in patients with melanoma[291] makes it important to test its use in transitional cell tumors, which are also highly responsive to cisplatin-containing regimens. The apparent superiority of BCG over thiotepa in superficial bladder cancer[292] has suggested that immunotherapy approaches may also be useful. In addition to the active nonspecific approaches (BCG, interferon) and passive nonspecific approaches, there is a burgeoning preclinical literature on monoclonal antibodies that alone or conjugated to a drug or toxin or used in combination with other treatment modalities may prove useful in treating transitional cell tumors.[293] The reader is referred to Chapter 32 for a more complete discussion of treatment options and the direction of current treatment approaches.

REFERENCES

1. DeKernion JB: Renal tumors. In Walsh PC, Gittes RF, Perlmutter AD et al (eds): Campbell's Urology, 5th ed, pp 1294–1342. Philadelphia, WB Saunders, 1986
2. Goodman MT, Morgenstern H, Wynder EL: A case-control study of factors affecting the development of renal cell carcinoma. Am J Epidemiol 124:926–941, 1986
3. Lack EE, Cassady R, Sallan SE: Renal cell carcinoma in childhood and adolescence: A clinical and pathological study of 17 cases. J Urol 133:822–828, 1985
4. Lieber MM, Tomera FM, Taylor WF et al: Renal adenocarcinoma in young adults: Survival and variables affecting prognosis. J Urol 125:164–168, 1981
5. Castellanos RD, Aron BS, Evans AT: Renal adenocarcinoma in children: Incidence, therapy and prognosis. J Urol 111:534–537, 1974
6. National Institutes of Health: 1986 Annual Cancer Statistics Review. NIH publication No. 87–2789, Washington, DC, 1986
7. Golimbu M, Joshi P, Sperber A et al: Renal cell carcinoma: Survival and prognostic factors. Urology 27:291–301, 1986
8. Carson WJ: Tumors of the kidney: Histologic study. In: Transactions of the Section on Urology, American Medical Association, 1928
9. Glenn JF: Renal tumors. In Harrison JH, Gittes RF, Perlmutter AD et al (eds): Campbell's Urology, 4th ed, pp 967–1009. Philadelphia, WB Saunders, 1979
10. Grawitz P: Die sogenannten Lipome der Niere. Virchows Arch Pathol Anat 93:39–63, 1883
11. Doderlein A, Birch-Hirschfeld FV: Embryonale Drusengeschwulst der Nierengegend im Kindesalter. Sex Organe 3:88–99, 1984
12. Outzen HC, Maguire HC Jr: The etiology of renal-cell carcinoma. Semin Oncol 10:378–384, 1983
13. Lauritsen JG: Lindau's disease: A study of one family through six generations. Acta Chir Scand 139:482–486, 1973
14. Green JS, Bowmer MI, Johnson GJ: Von-Hippel-Lindau disease in a Newfoundland kindred. Can Med Assoc J 134:133–146, 1986
15. Malek RS, Omess PJ, Benson RC Jr et al: Renal cell carcinoma in von Hippel–Lindau syndrome. Am J Med 82:236–238, 1987
16. Gregoire JR, Torres VE, Holley KE et al: Renal epithelial hyperplastic and neoplastic proliferation in autosomal dominant polycystic kidney disease. Am J Kidney Dis 9:27–38, 1987
17. Kantor AF: Current concepts in the epidemiology and etiology of primary renal cell carcinoma. J Urol 117:415–417, 1977
18. McLaughlin JK, Mandel JS, Blot WJ et al: A population-based case-control study of renal cell carcinoma. J Natl Cancer Inst 72:275–284, 1984
19. Yu MC, Mack TM, Hanisch R et al: Cigarette smoking, obesity, diuretic use, and coffee consumption as risk factors for renal cell carcinoma. J Natl Cancer Inst 77:351–356, 1986
20. Whittemore AS, Paffenbarger RS Jr, Anderson K et al: Early precursors of urogenital cancers in former college men. J Urol 132:1256–1261, 1984
21. Lornoy W, Becaus I, de Vleeschouwer M et al: Renal cell carcinoma, a new complication of analgesic nephropathy. Lancet 1:1271–1272, 1986
22. Malker HR, Malker BK, McLaughlin JK et al: Kidney cancer among leather workers. Lancet 1:56, 1984
23. Maclure M: Asbestos and renal adenocarcinoma: A case-control study. Environ Res 42:353–361, 1987
24. DeKernion JB, Smith RB: The kidney and adrenal glands. In Paulson DF (ed): Genitourinary Surgery, pp 1–153. New York, Churchill-Livingstone, 1984
25. Kauzlaric D, Barmeir E, Luscieti P et al: Renal carcinoma after retrograde pyelography with thorotrast. AJR 148:897–898, 1987
26. Enterline PE, Viren J: Epidemiologic evidence for an association between gasoline and kidney cancer. Environ Health Perspect 62:303–312, 1985
27. McLaughlin JK, Blot WJ, Mehl ES et al: Petroleum-related employment and renal cell cancer. J Occup Med 27:672–674, 1985
28. Grantham JJ, Levine E: Acquired cystic disease: Replacing one kidney disease with another. Kid Int 28:99–105, 1985
29. Hughson MD, Buchwald D, Fox M: Renal neoplasia and acquired cystic kidney disease in patients receiving long-term dialysis. Arch Pathol Lab Med 110:592–601, 1986
30. MacDougall ML, Welling LW, Wiegmann TB: Renal adenocarcinoma and acquired cystic disease in chronic hemodialysis patients. Am J Kidney Dis 9:166–171, 1987
31. Bretan PN, Busch MP, Hricak H et al: Development of acquired renal cysts and renal cell carcinoma: Case reports and review of the literature. Cancer 57:1871–1879, 1986
32. Harris DT: Hormonal therapy and chemotherapy of renal-cell carcinoma. Semin Oncol 10:422–430, 1983
33. Matthews VS, Kirkman H, Bacon RL: Kidney damage in the golden hamster following chronic administration of diethylstilbestrol and sesame oil. Proc Soc Exp Biol Med 66:195–196, 1947
34. Kirkman H, Bacon RL: Estrogen-induced tumors of the kidney: I. Incidence of renal tumors in intact and gonadectomized male golden hamsters treated with diethylstilbestrol. J Natl Cancer Inst 13:745–755, 1952
35. Bloom HJG, Dukes CE, Mitchley BCV: Hormone-dependent tumours of the kidney: I. The oestrogen-induced renal tumour of the syrian hamster. Hormone treatment and possible relationship to carcinoma of the kidney in man. Br J Cancer 17:611–646, 1963
36. Bloom HJG, Roe FJC, Mitchley BCV: Sex hormones and renal neoplasia: Inhibition of tumor in hamster kidney by an estrogen antagonist, an agent of possible therapeutic value in man. Cancer 20:2118–2124, 1967
37. Chisholm GD: Nephrogenic ridge tumors and their syndromes. Ann NY Acad Sci 230:403–423, 1974
38. Strewler GJ, Williams RD, Nissenson RA: Human renal carcinoma cells produce hypercalcemia in the nude mouse and a novel protein recognized by parathyroid hormone receptors. J Clin Invest 71:769–774, 1983
39. Suva LJ, Winslow GA, Wettenhall EH et al: A parathyroid hormone-related protein implicated in malignant hypercalcemia: Cloning and expression. Science 237:893–895, 1987
40. Derynck R, Goeddel DV, Ullrich A et al: Synthesis of messenger RNAs for transforming growth factors alpha and beta and the epidermal growth factor receptor by human tumors. Cancer Res 47:707–712, 1987
41. Derynck R, Roberts AB, Winkler ME et al: Human transforming growth factor-alpha: Precursor structure and expression in E. coli. Cell 38:287–297, 1984
42. Gomella LG, Sargent EF, Wade TP et al: Expression of transforming growth factor alpha in normal adult kidney and enhanced expression of transforming growth factor alpha and beta in renal cell carcinoma (submitted for publication)
43. Rosenthal A, Lindquist PB, Bringman TS et al: Expression in rat fibroblasts of a human transforming growth factor-alpha cDNA results in transformation. Cell 46:301–309, 1986
44. Coffey RJ Jr, Derynck R, Wilcox JN et al: Production and autoinduction of transforming growth factor-alpha in human keratinocytes. Nature 328:817–820, 1987
45. Kehrl JH, Wakefield LM, Roberts AB et al: Production of transforming growth factor beta by human T lymphocytes and its potential role in the regulation of T cell growth. J Exp Med 163:1037–1050, 1986
46. Mule JJ, Schwarz SL, Roberts AB et al: Transforming growth factor-beta inhibits the in vitro generation of lymphokine-activated killer cells and cytotoxic T cells (unpublished manuscript)
47. Kasid A, Director EP, Bell GI: Effects of TGF-beta on human lymphokine activated killer cell precursors: Autocrine inhibition of cellular proliferation and differentiation to immune killer cells (unpublished manuscript)
48. Ibbotson KJ, Harrod J, Gowen M et al: Human recombinant transforming growth factor alpha stimulates bone resorption and inhibits formation in vitro. Proc Natl Acad Sci USA 87:2228–2232, 1986
49. Cohen AJ, Li FP, Berg S et al: Hereditary renal-cell carcinoma associated with a chromosomal translocation. N Engl J Med 301:592–595, 1979
50. Drabkin HA, Bradley C, Hart I et al: Translocation of c-myc in the hereditary renal cell carcinoma associated with a t(3:8) (p14.2;q24.13) chromosomal translocation. Proc Natl Acad Sci USA 82:6980–6984, 1985
51. Pathak S, Strong LC, Ferrell RE et al: Familial renal cell carcinoma with a 3;11 chromosome translocation limited to tumor cells. Science 217:939–941, 1982
52. King CR, Schimke RN, Arthur T et al: Proximal 3p deletion in renal cell carcinoma cells from a patient with von Hippel–Lindau disease. Cancer Genet Cytogenet 27:345–348, 1987
53. Yoshida HA, Ohyashiki K, Ochi H et al: Cytogenetic studies of tumor tissue from patients with nonfamilial renal cell carcinoma. Cancer Res 46:2139–2147, 1986
54. Yoshida HA, Ohyashiki K, Ochi H et al: Rearrangement of chromosome 3 in renal cell carcinoma. Cancer Genet Cytogenet 19:351–354, 1986
55. Szucs S, Muller-Brechlin R, DeRiese W et al: Deletion 3p: The only chromosome loss in a primary renal cell carcinoma. Cancer Genet Cytogenet 26:369–373, 1987
56. Carroll PR, Murty VVS, Reuter V et al: Abnormalities at chromosome region 3p 12-14 characterize clear cell renal carcinoma. Cancer Genet Cytogenet 26:253–259, 1987
57. Zbar B, Brauch H, Talmadge C et al: Loss of alleles of loci on the short arm of chromosome 3 in renal cell carcinoma. Nature 327:721–727, 1987
58. Cavenee WK, Dryja TP, Phillips RA et al: Expression of recessive alleles by chromosomal mechanisms in retinoblastoma. Nature 305:779–784, 1983
59. Koufos A, Hansen MFM, Lampkin BC et al: Loss of alleles at loci on human chromosome 11 during genesis of Wilms' tumour. Nature 309:170–172, 1984
60. Orkin SH, Goldman DS, Sallan SE: Development of homozygosity for chromosome 11p markers in Wilms' tumour. Nature 309:172–174, 1984
61. Reeve AE, Hiusiaux PJ, Gardner RJM et al: Loss of a Harvey ras allele in sporadic Wilms' tumour. Nature 309:174–176, 1984

62. Fearon ER, Vogelstein B, Feinberg AP: Somatic deletion and duplication of genes on chromosome 11 in Wilms' tumours. Nature 309:175–177, 1984

63. Cavenee WK, Murphree AL, Shull MM et al: Prediction of familial predisposition to retinoblastoma. N Engl J Med 314:1201–1207, 1986

64. Fearon ER, Feinberg AP, Hamilton SH et al: Loss of genes on the short arm of chromosome 11 in bladder cancer. Nature 318:377–380, 1985

65. Brauch H, Johnson B, Hovis J et al: Molecular analysis of the short arm of chromosome 3 in small-cell and non-small-cell carcinoma of the lung. N Engl J Med 317:1109–1113, 1987

66. Solomon E, Voss R, Hall V et al: Chromosome 5 allele loss in human colorectal carcinomas. Nature 328:616–619, 1987

67. White R, Leppert M, Bishop T et al: Construction of linkage maps with DNA markers for human chromosomes. Nature 313:101–105, 1985

68. Carritt B, Welch HM, Parry-Jones NJ: Sequences homologous to the human D1S1 locus present on human chromosome 3. Am J Hum Genet 38:428–436, 1986

69. Knudson AG Jr: Genetics of human cancer. Annu Rev Genet 20:231–251, 1986

70. Moolgavkar SH, Knudson AG Jr: Mutation and cancer: A model for human carcinogenesis. J Natl Cancer Inst 66:1037–1051, 1981

71. Weissman BE, Saxon PJ, Pasquale SR et al: Introduction of a normal human chromosome 11 into a Wilms' tumor cell line controls its tumorigenic expression. Science 236:175–180, 1987

72. Tannenbaum M: Ultrastructural pathology of human renal cell tumors. Pathol Annu 6:249–277, 1971

73. Fisher ER, Horvat B: Comparative ultrastructural study of so-called renal adenoma and carcinoma. J Urol 108:382–386, 1972

74. Mostofi FK, Davis CJ Jr: Pathology of urologic cancer. In Javadpour N (ed): Principles and Management of Urologic Cancer, 2nd ed, pp 54–126. Baltimore, Williams & Wilkins, 1983

75. Thoenes W, Storkel ST, Rumpelt HJ: Histopathology and classification of renal cell tumors (adenomas, oncocytomas and carcinomas): The basic cytological and histopathologoical elements and their use for diagnostics. Pathol Res Pract 181:125–143, 1986

76. Bonsib SM, Fischer J, Plattner S et al: Sarcomatoid renal tumors: Clinicopathologic correlation of three cases. Cancer 59:527–532, 1987

77. Bertoni F, Ferri C, Bacchini BP et al: Sarcomatoid carcinoma of the kidney. J Urol 137:25–28, 1987

78. Ro JY, Ayala AG, Sella A et al: Sarcomatoid renal cell carcinoma: Clinicopathologic. A study of 42 cases. Cancer 59:519–526, 1987

79. Skinner DG, Colvin RB, Vermillion CD et al: Diagnosis and management of renal carcinoma: A clinical and pathologic study of 309 cases. Cancer 28:1165–1177, 1971

80. Selli C, Hinshaw WM, Woodard BH et al: Stratification of risk factors in renal cell carcinoma. Cancer 52:899–903, 1983

81. Boxer RJ, Waisman J, Lieber MM et al: Renal carcinoma: Computer analysis of 96 patients treated by nephrectomy. J Urol 122:598–601, 1979

82. Sella A, Logothetis CJ, Ro JY et al: Sarcomatoid renal cell carcinoma: A treatable entity. Cancer 60:1313–1318, 1987

83. McNichols DW, Segura JW, DeWeerd JH: Renal cell carcinoma: Long-term survival and late recurrence. J Urol 126:17–23, 1981

84. Silverberg E: Cancer statistics. CA 31:13–28, 1981

85. Maldazys JD, deKernion JB: Prognostic factors in metastatic renal carcinoma. J Urol 136:376–379, 1986

86. Samaan NA: Paraneoplastic syndromes associated with renal carcinoma: A pilot study. J Clin Oncol 6:862, 1987

87. Pinals RS, Krane SM: Medical aspects of renal carcinoma. Postgrad Med J 38:507–519, 1962

88. Cherukuri SV, Johenning PW, Ram MD: Systemic effects of hypernephroma. Urology 10:93–97, 1977

89. Sufrin G, Mirand EA, Moore RH et al: Hormones in renal cancer. J Urol 117:433–438, 1977

90. Utz DW, Warren MM, Gregg JA et al: Reversible hepatic dysfunction associated with hypernephroma. Mayo Clin Proc 45:161, 1970

91. Boxer RJ, Waisman J, Lieber MM et al: Non-metastatic hepatic dysfunction associated with renal carcinoma. J Urol 119:468–471, 1978

92. Hanash KA, Utz DC, Khalil L et al: Syndrome of reversible hepatic dysfunction associated with hypernephroma: An experimental study. Invest Urol 8:399–404, 1971

93. Lindop GB, Fleming S: Renin in renal cell carcinoma: An immunocytochemical study using an antibody to pure human renin. J Clin Pathol 37:27–31, 1984

94. Lindop GB, Leckie B, Winearls CG: Malignant hypertension due to renin-secreting renal cell carcinoma: An ultrastructural and immunocytochemical study. Histopathology 10:1077–1088, 1986

95. Sufrin G, Mink I, Moore FR et al: Coagulation factors in renal adenocarcinoma. J Urol 119:727–730, 1978

96. Dawson NA, Barr CF, Alving BM: Acquired dysfibrinogenemia: Paraneoplastic syndrome in renal cell carcinoma. Am J Med 78:682–686, 1985

97. Lang EK: Asymptomatic space-occupying lesions of the kidney: A programmed sequential approach and its impact on quality and cost of health care. South Med J 70:277–285, 1977

98. Frohmuller HGW, Grups JW, Heller V: Comparative value of ultrasonography, computerized tomography, angiography and excretory urography in the staging of renal cell carcinoma. J Urol 138:482–484, 1987

99. Juul N, Torp-Pedersen S, Gronvall S et al: Ultrasonically guided fine needle aspiration biopsy of renal masses. J Urol 133:579–581, 1985

100. Lang EK: Comparison of dynamic and conventional computed tomography, angiography, and ultrasonography in the staging of renal cell carcinoma. Cancer 54:2205–2214, 1984

101. Karp W, Ekelund L, Olafsson G et al: Computed tomography, angiography and ultrasound in staging of renal carcinoma. Acta Radiol 22:625–632, 1981

102. Mauro MA, Wadsworth DE, Stanley RJ et al: Renal cell carcinoma: Angiography in the CT era. AJR 139:1135–1138, 1982

103. Zabbo A, Novick AC, Risius B et al: Digital subtraction angiography for evaluating patients with renal carcinoma. J Urol 134:252–255, 1985

104. Richie JP, Garnick MC, Seltzer S et al: Computerized tomography scan for diagnosis and staging of renal cell carcinoma. J Urol 129:1114–1116, 1983

105. Stephenson TF, Tyengar S, Rashid HA: Comparison of computerized tomography and excretory urography in detection and evaluation of renal masses. J Urol 131:11–13, 1984

106. Jashke W, Kaick GV, Peter S et al: Accuracy of computed tomography in staging of kidney tumors. Acta Radiol (Stockh) 23:593–598, 1982

107. Kothari K, Segal AJ, Spitzer RM et al: Preoperative radiographic evaluation of hypernephroma. J Comput Assist Tomogr 5:702–704, 1981

108. Yokoyama M, Watanabe K, Inatsuki S et al: Computerized tomography of the kidney: Tissue-plasma ratio of contrast enhancement with bolus injection and renal function. J Urol 127:721–723, 1982

109. Lang EK: Angio-computed tomography and dynamic computed tomography in staging of renal cell carcinoma. Radiology 151:149–155, 1984

110. Karstaedt N, McCullough DL, Wolfman NT et al: Magnetic resonance imaging of the renal mass. J Urol 136:566–570, 1986

111. Robson CJ, Churchill BM, Anderson W: The results of radical nephrectomy for renal cell carcinoma. J Urol 101:297–301, 1969

112. Peters PC, Brown GL: The role of lymphadenectomy in the management of renal cell carcinoma. Urol Clin North Am 7:705–709, 1980

113. Siminovitch JMP, Montie JE, Straffon RA: Prognostic indicators in renal adenocarcinoma. J Urol 130:20–23, 1983

114. Cherrie RJ, Goldman DG, Lindner A et al: Prognostic implications of vena caval extension of renal cell carcinoma. J Urol 128:910–912, 1982

115. Bassil B, Dosoretz DE, Prout GR Jr: Validation of the tumor, nodes and metastasis classification of renal cell carcinoma. J Urol 134:450–454, 1985

116. Gilbert JB: Diagnosis and treatment of malignant renal tumors. J Urol 39:223–237, 1938

117. McDonald MW: Current therapy for renal cell carcinoma. J Urol 127:211–217, 1982

118. Kearney GP, Waters WB, Klein LA et al: Results of inferior vena cava resection for renal cell carcinoma. J Urol 125:769–773, 1981

119. Sogani PC, Herr HW, Bains MS et al: Renal cell carcinoma extending into the inferior vena cava. J Urol 130:660–663, 1983

120. Marshall FF, Reitz BA, Diamond DA: A new technique for management of renal cell carcinoma involving the right atrium: Hypothermia and cardiac arrest. J Urol 131:103–107, 1984

121. deKernion JB, Berry D: The diagnosis and treatment of renal cell carcinoma. Cancer 45:1947–1956, 1980

122. deKernion JB: Lymphadenectomy for renal cell carcinoma. Urol Clin North Am 7:697–703, 1980

123. Marshall FF, Powell KC: Lymphadenectomy for renal cell carcinoma: Anatomical and therapeutic considerations. J Urol 128:677–681, 1982

124. Zincke H, Engen DE, Henning KM et al: Treatment of renal cell carcinoma by in situ partial nephrectomy and extracorporeal operation with autotransplantation. Mayo Clin Proc 60:651–662, 1985

125. Mandel J, Kjellstrand CM: Long-term results of dialysis and transplantation in patients with end-stage renal failure from hypernephroma. Nephron 44:111–114, 1986

126. Smith RB, deKernion JB, Ehrlich RM et al: Bilateral renal cell carcinoma and renal cell carcinoma in the solitary kidney. J Urol 132:450–454, 1984

127. Jacobs SC, Berg SI, Lawson RK: Synchronous bilateral renal cell carcinoma: Total surgical excision. Cancer 46:2341–2345, 1980

128. Topley M, Novick AC, Montie JE: Long-term results following partial nephrectomy for localized renal adenocarcinoma. J Urol 131:1050–1052, 1984

129. Novick AC, Zincke H, Neves RJ et al: Surgical enucleation for renal cell carcinoma. J Urol 135:235–238, 1986

130. Marshall FF, Taxy JB, Fishman EK et al: The feasibility of surgical enucleation for renal cell carcinoma. J Urol 135:231–234, 1986

131. deKernion JB, Mukamel E: Selection of initial therapy for renal cell carcinoma. Cancer 60:539–546, 1987

132. Zincke H, Swanson SK: Bilateral renal cell carcinoma: Influence of synchronous and asynchronous occurrence on patient survival. J Urol 128:913–915, 1982

133. Rafla S: Renal cell carcinoma: Natural history and results of treatment. Cancer 25:26–40, 1970

134. Finney R: Radiotherapy in the treatment of hypernephroma: A clinical trial. Br J Urol 45:258–269, 1973

135. Kjaer M, Frederiksen PL, Engelholm SA: Postoperative radiotherapy in stage II and III renal adenocarcinoma: A randomized trial by the Copenhagen renal cancer study group. Int J Radiat Oncol Biol Phys 13:665–672, 1987

136. van der Werf-Messing B: Carcinoma of the kidney. Cancer 32:1056–1062, 1973

137. deKernion JB: Treatment of advanced renal cell carcinoma: Traditional methods and innovative approaches. J Urol 130:2–7, 1983

138. Freed SZ: Nephrectomy for renal cell carcinoma with metastases. Urology 9:613–615, 1977

139. Montie JE, Stewart BH, Straffon RA et al: The role of adjunctive nephrectomy in patients with metastatic renal cell carcinoma. J Urol 117:272–275, 1977
140. deKernion JB, Ramming KP, Smith RB: The natural history of metastatic renal cell carcinoma: A computer analysis. J Urol 120:148–151, 1978
141. Middleton RG: Surgery for metastatic renal cell carcinoma. J Urol 97:973–977, 1967
142. O'Dea MJ, Zincke H, Utz DC et al: The treatment of renal cell carcinoma with solitary metastasis. J Urol 120:540–542, 1978
143. Tolia BM, Whitmore WF Jr: Solitary metastasis from renal cell carcinoma. J Urol 114:836–838, 1975
144. Swanson DA, Wallace S, Johnson DE: The role of embolization and nephrectomy in the treatment of metastatic renal carcinoma. Urol Clin North Am 7:719–730, 1980
145. Swanson DA, Johnson DE, von Eschenbach AC et al: Angioinfarction plus nephrectomy for metastatic renal cell carcinoma: An update. J Urol 130:449-452, 1983
146. Sundaresan N, Galicich JH, Baines MS et al: Vertebral body resection in the treatment of cancer involving the spine. Cancer 53:1393–1396, 1984
147. Sundaresan N, Scher H, Whitmore WF Jr: Spinal cord compression in kidney cancer (abstr). Proceedings of the American Society of Clinical Oncology, March 1986, p 267
148. Fossa SD, Kjolseth I, Lund G: Radiotherapy of metastasis from renal cancer. Eur Urol 8:340–342, 1982
149. Onufrey V, Mohiuddin M: Radiation therapy in the treatment of metastatic renal cell carcinoma. Int J Radiat Oncol Biol Phys 11:2007–2009, 1985
150. Halperin EC, Harisiadis L: The role of radiation therapy in the management of metastatic renal cell carcinoma. Cancer 51:614–617, 1983
151. Fojo AT, Ueda K, Slamon DJ et al: Expression of a multidrug-resistance gene in human tumors and tissues. Proc Natl Acad Sci USA 84:265, 1987
152. Hrushesky WJ, Murphy GP: Current status of the therapy of advanced renal carcinoma. J Surg Oncol 9:277, 1977
153. Bell DR, Aroney RS, Fisher RJ et al: High-dose methotrexate with leucovorin resue, vinblastine, and bleomycin with or without tamoxifen in metastatic renal cell carcinoma. Cancer Treat Rep 68:587, 1984
154. Hrushesky WJM, Roemeling R, Rabatin J et al: Continuous FUDR infusion is effective in progressive renal cell cancer. Proc Am Soc Clin Oncol 6:108, 1987
155. Satake I, Tari K, Yamamoto M et al: Neocarzinostatin-induced complete regression of metastatic renal cell carcinoma. J Urol 133:87, 1985
156. Kakizoe T, Matsumoto K, Nishio Y et al: Chemotherapy by bronchial arterial infusion for pulmonary metastases of renal cell carcinoma. J Urol 131:1053, 1984
157. Poster DS, Pinna K, Bruno S et al: Current status of chemotherapy, hormonal therapy, and immunotherapy in the treatment of renal cell carcinoma. Am J Clin Oncol 5:53, 1982
158. Miller CF: Adjuvant chemotherapy of renal cell carcinoma using a combination of bleomycin and lomustine. Proc Am Soc Clin Oncol 21:C-171, 1980
159. Leiter E, Edelman S, Brendler H: Continuous preoperative intraarterial perfusion of renal tumors with chemotherapeutic agents. J Urol 95:169, 1966
160. Kato T, Nemoto R, Mori H et al: Transcatheter arterial chemoembolization of renal cell carcinoma with microencapsulated mitomycin C. J Urol 125:19, 1981
161. Satomi Y, Takai S, Kondo I et al: Postoperative prophylactic use of progesterone in renal cell carcinoma. J Urol 127:919, 1982
162. Ronchi E, Pizzocaro G, Miodini P et al: Steroid hormone receptors in normal and malignant human renal tissue: Relationship with progestin therapy. J Steroid Biochem 21:329, 1984
163. Rosenberg SA, Lotze MT, Muul LM et al: Observations on the systemic administration of autologous lymphokine-activated killer cells and recombinant interleukin-2 to patients with metastatic cancer. N Engl J Med 313:1485, 1985
164. Rosenberg SA, Lotze MT, Muul LM et al: A progress report on the treatment of 157 patients with advanced cancer using lymphokine-activated killer cells and interleukin-2 or high dose interleukin-2 alone. N Engl J Med 316:889, 1987
165. West WH, Tauer KW, Yannelli JR et al: Constant infusion recombinant interleukin-2 in adoptive immunotherapy of advanced cancer. N Engl J Med 316:898–905, 1987
166. Krown SE: Interferon treatment of renal cell carcinoma: Current status and future prospects. Cancer 59:647, 1987
167. Goldstein D, Laszlo J: Interferon therapy in cancer: From imaginon to interferon. Cancer Res 46:4315, 1986
168. Marshall ME, Mendelsohn L, Butler K et al: Treatment of metastatic renal cell carcinoma with coumarin (1,2-benzopyrone) and cimetidine: A pilot study. J Clin Oncol 6:682, 1987
169. Fisher RI, Coltman CA, Doroshow JH et al: Phase II clinical trial of interleukin-2 plus lymphokine activated killer cells in metastatic renal cancer. Proc Am Soc Clin Oncol 6:244, 1987
170. Krishnan EC, Mebust WK, Weigel JW et al: Culture of peripheral monocytes in vitro in patients with renal cell carcinoma: A possible prognostic indicator. J Urol 130:597, 1983
171. Rosenberg SA, Spiess P, Lafreniere R: A new approach to the adoptive immunotherapy of cancer with tumor-infiltrating lymphocytes. Science 233:1318, 1986
172. Belldegrun A, Linehan WM, Robertson CN et al: Isolation and characterization of lymphocytes infiltrating human renal cell cancer: Possible application for therapeutic adoptive immunotherapy. Surg Forum 37:671, 1986
173. Belldegrun A, Muul LM, Rosenberg SA: Interleukin-2 expanded tumor infiltrating lymphocytes in human renal cell cancer: Isolation, characterization and antitumor activity. Cancer Res 48:206–214, 1988
174. Topalian SL, Muul LM, Solomon D et al: Expansion of human tumor infiltrating lymphocytes for use in immunotherapy trials. J Immunol Methods 102:127–141, 1987
175. Muul LM, Spiess PJ, Director EP et al: Identification of specific cytolytic immune responses against autologous tumor in humans bearing malignant melanoma. J Immunol 138:989–995, 1987
176. Topalian SL, Solomon D, Avis FP et al: Immunotherapy of patients with advanced cancer using tumor infiltrating lymphocytes and recombinant interleukin-2: A pilot study. J Clin Oncol 6:839–853, 1988
177. Salup RR, Back TC, Wiltrout RH: Successful treatment of advanced murine renal cell cancer by bicompartmental adoptive chemoimmunotherapy. J Immunol 138:641, 1987
178. Wiltrout RH, Boyd MR, Back TT et al: Flavone-8-acetic acid augments systemic natural killer cell activity and synergizes with interleukin-2 for treatment of murine renal cancer. J Immunol 140:3261–3265, 1988
179. Quesada JR, Swanson DA, Trindade A et al: Renal cell carcinoma: Antitumor effects of leukocyte interferon. Cancer Res 43:940, 1983
180. Quesada JR, Swanson DA, Gutterman JU: Phase II study of interferon alpha in metastatic renal-cell carcinoma: A progress report. J Clin Oncol 3:1086, 1985
181. Medenica R, Slack N: Clinical results of leukocyte interferon-induced tumor regression in resistant human metastatic cancer resistant to chemotherapy and/or radiotherapy—pulse therapy schedule. Cancer Drug Deliv 2:53, 1985
182. deKernion JB, Sarna G, Figlin R et al: The treatment of renal cell carcinoma with human leukocyte alpha-interferon. J Urol 130:1063, 1983
183. Kirkwood JM, Harris JE, Vera P et al: A randomized study of low and high doses of leukocyte alpha interferon in metastatic renal cell carcinoma: The American Cancer Society collaborative trial. Cancer Res 45:863, 1985
184. Edsmyr F, Eposti PL, Andersson L et al: Interferon therapy in disseminated renal cell carcinoma. Radiother Oncol 4:21, 1985
185. Neidhart JA, Gagen MM, Yound D et al: Interferon-alpha therapy of renal cancer. Cancer Res 44:4140, 1984
186. Trump DL, Elson PJ, Borden EC et al: High-dose lymphoblastoid interferon in advanced renal cell carcinoma: An Eastern Cooperative Oncology Group study. Cancer Treat Rep 71:165, 1987
187. Marumo K, Murai M, Hayakawa M et al: Human lymphoblastoid interferon therapy for advanced renal cell carcinoma. Urology 24:567, 1984
188. Vugrin D, Hood L, Taylor W et al: Phase II study of human lymphoblastoid interferon in patients with advanced renal carcinoma. Cancer Treat Rep 69:817, 1985
189. Umeda T, Niijima T: Phase II study of alpha interferon on renal cell carcinoma: Summary of three collaborative trials. Cancer 58:1231, 1986
190. Kempf RA, Grunberg SM, Daniels JR et al: Recombinant interferon alpha-2 (Intron A) in a phase II study of renal cell carcinoma. J Biol Response Mod 5:27, 1986
191. Quesada JR, Rios A, Swanson D et al: Antitumor activity of recombinant-derived interferon alpha in metastatic renal cell carcinoma. J Clin Oncol 3:1522, 1985
192. Sarna G, Figlin R, deKernion J: Interferon in renal cell carcinoma: The UCLA experience. Cancer 59:610, 1987
193. Kuzmits R, Kokoschka EM, Micksche M et al: Phase II results with recombinant interferons: Renal cell carcinoma and malignant melanoma. Oncology 42 (suppl):26, 1985
194. Muss HB, Costanzi JJ, Leavitt R et al: Recombinant alpha interferon in renal cell carcinoma: A randomized trial of two routes of administration. J Clin Oncol 5:286, 1987
195. Buzaid AC, Robertone A, Kisals C et al: Phase II study of interferon alpha-2a, recombinant (Roferon-A) in metastatic renal cell carcinoma. J Clin Oncol 5:1083, 1987
196. Rinehart J, Malspeis L, Young D, Neidhart J: Phase I/II trial of human recombinant beta-interferon serine in patients with renal cell carcinoma. Cancer Res 46:5364, 1986
197. Rinehart J, Malspeis L, Young D et al: Phase I/II trial of human recombinant interferon gamma in renal cell carcinoma. J Biol Response Mod 5:300, 1986
198. Quesada JR, Kurzrock R, Sherwin SA et al: Phase II studies of recombinant human interferon gamma in metastatic renal cell carcinoma. J Biol Response Mod 6:20, 1987
199. Trotta PP: Preclinical biology of alpha interferons. Semin Oncol 13 (suppl 2):3, 1986
200. Figlin RA, deKernion JB, Maldazys J et al: Treatment of renal cell carcinoma with alpha (human leukocyte) interferon and vinblastine in combination: A phase I-II trial. Cancer Treat Rep 69:263, 1985
201. Fossa SD, DeGaris ST, Heier MS et al: Recombinant interferon alpha-2a with or without vinblastine in metastatic renal cell carcinoma. Cancer 57:1700, 1986
202. Schnornagel J, Verwey J, tenBokkel Huinink W et al: Phase II study of recombinant interferon alpha-2 and vinblastine in advanced renal carcinoma. Proc Am Soc Clin Oncol 6:106, 1987
203. Creagan ET, Kovach JS, Long HJ et al: Phase I study of recombinant leukocyte A human interferon combined with BCNU in selected patients with advanced cancer. J Clin Oncol 4:408, 1986
204. Creagan ET, Kovach JS, O'Connell MJ et al: Improved response of renal cell carcinoma to alpha interferon by the addition of aspirin. Cancer (in press)
205. Dexeus FH, Logothetis CJ, Quesada J et al: Potential increase in efficacy of chemotherapy after treatment of patients with metastatic renal cell carcinoma with interferon. Proc Am Soc Clin Oncol 6:100, 1987
206. Droller MJ: Immunotherapy of metastatic renal cell carcinoma with polyinosinic-polysytidylic acid. J Urol 137:202, 1987
207. deKernion JB, Ramming KP: The therapy of renal adenocarcinoma with immune RNA. Invest Urol 17:378, 1980
208. Richie JP, Steele GD Jr, Wilson RE et al: Current treatment of metastatic renal cell carcinoma with xenogeneic immune ribonucleic acid. J Urol 131:236, 1984
209. Morales A, Wilson JL, Pater JL Loeb M: Cytoreductive surgery and systemic bacillus

Calmette-Guerin therapy in metastatic renal cancer: A phase II trial. J Urol 127:230, 1982

210. Stanisic TH: Renal cell carcinoma (hypernephroma). Ariz Med 37:164, 1980

211. Ishmael DR, Burpo LJ, Bottomley RH: Combined therapy of advanced hypernephroma with medroxyprogesterone, BCG, Adriamycin, and vincristine. Proc Am Soc Clin Oncol 19:407, 1978

212. Dimitrov NV, Arnols D, Munson J et al: Phase II study of thymosin fraction 5 in the treatment of metastatic renal cell carcinoma. Cancer Treat Rep 69:137, 1985

213. Romano CF, Lipton A, Harvey HA et al: A phase II study of catrix-s in solid tumors. J Biol Response Mod 4:585, 1985

214. Prager MD, Baechtel FS, Peters PC et al: Specific immunotherapy of human metastatic renal cell carcinoma. Proc Am Assoc Cancer Res 22:163, 1981

215. Sahasrabudhe DM, deKernion JB, Pontes JE et al: Specific immunotherapy with suppressor function inhibition for metastatic renal cell carcinoma. J Biol Response Mod 5:581, 1986

216. McCune CS, Patterson WB, Henshaw EC: Active specific immunotherapy with tumor cells and Corynebacterium parvum. Cancer 43:1619, 1979

217. McCune CS: Immunologic therapies of kidney carcinoma. Semin Oncol 10:431, 1983

218. Tallberg T, Tykka H, Mahlberg K et al: Active specific immunotherapy with supportive measures in the treatment of palliatively nephrectomized, renal adenocarcinoma patients: A thirteen-year follow-up study. Eur Urol 11:233, 1985

219. Neidhart JA, Murphy SG, Hennick LA et al: Active specific immunotherapy of stage IV renal carcinoma with aggregated tumor antigen adjuvant. Cancer 46:1128, 1980

220. Arakawa S Jr, Hamami G, Umezu K et al: Clinical trial of attenuated vaccinia virus AS strain in the treatment of advanced adenocarcinoma: Report on two cases. J Cancer Res Clin Oncol 113:95, 1987

221. Horn L, Horn JL: An immunological approach to the therapy of cancer? Lancet 2:466, 1971

222. Yoshida SO, Imam A, Olson CA et al: Proximal renal tubule surface membrane antigens identified in primary and metastatic renal cell carcinoma. Arch Pathol Lab Med 110:825, 1986

223. Iizumi Y, Yazaki T, Kanoh S et al: Fluorescence study of renal cell carcinoma with antibodies to renal tubular antigens, intermediated filaments, and lectins. Urol Int 41:57, 1986

224. Fraley EE: Cancer of the renal pelvis. In Skinner DG, deKernion JB (eds): Genitourinary Cancer, pp 134–149. Philadelphia, WB Saunders, 1978

225. Mahadevia PA, Larwa GL, Koss LG: Mapping of urothelium in carcinomas of the renal pelvis and ureter: A report of nine cases. Cancer 51:890–897, 1983

226. McCarron JP Jr, Chasko SB, Gray GF Jr: Systemic mapping of nephroureterectomy specimens removed for urothelial cancer: Pathological findings and clinical correlations. J Urol 128:243–246, 1982

227. Babaian RJ, Johnson DE: Primary carcinoma of the ureter. J Urol 123:357–359, 1980

228. Droller MJ: Transitional cell cancer: Upper tracts and bladder. In Walsh PC, Gittes RE, Perlmutter AD et al (eds): Campbell's Urology, pp 1343–1440. Philadelphia, WB Saunders, 1986

229. Hultengren N, Lagergren C, Ljungqvist A: Carcinoma of the renal pelvis in renal papillary necrosis. Acta Chir Scand 130:314–320, 1965

230. Palvio DHB, Andersen JC, Falk E: Transitional cell tumors of the renal pelvis and ureter associated with capillarosclerosis indicating analgesic abuse. Cancer 59:972–976, 1987

231. Bengtsson U, Angervall L, Ekman H et al: Transitional cell tumors of the renal pelvis in analgesic abusers. Scand J Urol Nephrol 2:145–150, 1968

232. Bengtsson U, Johansson S, Angervall L: Malignancies of the urinary tract and their relation to analgesic abuse. Kidney Int 13:107–113, 1978

233. Adam WR, Dawborn JK, Price CG et al: Anaplastic transitional-cell carcinoma of the renal pelvis in association with analgesic abuse. Med J Aust 1:1108–1109, 1970

234. Mahony JF, Storey BG, Ibanez RC et al: Analgesic abuse, renal parenchymal disease and carcinoma of the kidney or ureter. Aust NZ J Med 7:463–469, 1977

235. McCredie M, Stewart JH, Carter JJ et al: Phenacetin and papillary necrosis: Independent risk factors for renal pelvic cancer. Kidney Int 30:81–84, 1986

236. Gaakeer HA, De Ruiter HJ: Carcinoma of the renal pelvis following the abuse of phenacetin–containing analgesic drugs. Br J Urol 51:188–192, 1979

237. Hoybye G, Nielsen OE: Renal pelvic carcinoma in phenacetin abusers. Scand J Urol Nephrol 5:190–192, 1971

238. Campo B, Zanitzer L, Torelli T et al: Renal cell carcinoma and transitional cell carcinomas of the pelvis and bladder in a patient affected by chronic renal failure due to abuse of phenacetin. Tumori 72:215–217, 1986

239. Rathert P, Melchior H, Lutzeyer W: Phenacetin: A carcinogen for the urinary tract. J Urol 113:653–657, 1975

240. Clayman RV, Lange PH, Fraley EE: Cancer of the upper urinary tract. In Javadpour N (ed): Principles and Management of Urologic Cancer, pp 544–559. Baltimore, Williams & Wilkins, 1983

241. Orphali SLJ, Shols GW, Hagewood J et al: Familial transitional cell carcinoma of renal pelvis and upper ureter. Urology 27:394–396, 1986

242. Frischer Z, Waltzer WC, Gonder MJ: Bilateral transitional cell carcinoma of the renal pelvis in the cancer family syndrome. J Urol 134:1197–1198, 1985

243. Cahng EH, Pirollo KF, Zou ZQ et al: Oncogenes in radioresistant, noncancerous skin fibroblasts from a cancer-prone family. Science 237:1036–1041, 1987

244. Blacher EJ, Johnson DE, Abdul-Karim FW et al: Squamous cell carcinoma of the renal pelvis. Urology 25:124–126, 1985

245. Johansson S, Angervall L, Bengtsson U et al: A clinicopathologic and prognostic study of epithelial tumors of the renal pelvis. Cancer 37:1376–1383, 1976

246. Grabstald H, Whitmore WF, Melamed MR: Renal pelvic tumors. JAMA 218:845–854, 1971

247. Murphy DM, Zincke H, Furlow WL: Management of high grade transitional cell cancer of the upper urinary tract. J Urol 125:25–29, 1981

248. Wagle DG, Moore RH, Murphy GP: Primary carcinoma of the renal pelvis. Cancer 33:1642–1648, 1974

249. Lang EK: The arteriographic diagnosis of primary and secondary tumors of the ureter or ureter and renal pelvis. Radiology 93:799–805, 1969

250. Pontes JE, Christensen LC, Pierce JM Jr: Angiographic aspects of tumors of renal pelvis and ureter. Urology 7:334–336, 1976

251. Gatewood OMB, Goldman SM, Marshall FF et al: Computerized tomography in the diagnosis of transitional cell carcinoma of the kidney. J Urol 127:876–887, 1982

252. Cullen TH, Pophom RR, Vos HJ: Urine cytology and primary carcinoma of the renal pelvis and ureter. Aust NZ J Surg 41:230–236, 1972

253. Highman WJ: Transitional carcinoma of the upper urinary tract: A histological and cytopathological study. J Clin Pathol 39:297–305, 1986

254. Smith AD, Orihuela E, Crowley AR: Percutaneous management of renal pelvic tumors: A treatment option in selected cases. J Urol 137:852–856, 1987

255. Bagley DH, Huffman JL, Lyon ES: Flexible ureteropyeloscopy: Diagnosis and treatment in the upper urinary tract. J Urol 138:280–285, 1987

256. Davis BW, Hough AJ, Gardner WA: Renal pelvic carcinoma: Morphological correlates of metastatic behavior. J Urol 137:857–861, 1987

257. Tumors of the renal pelvis and ureter. In Bennington JL, Beckwith JB (eds): Tumors of the Kidney, Renal Pelvis, and Ureter, pp 243–310. Washington, DC, Armed Forces Institute of Pathology, 1975

258. Cummings KB: Nephroureterectomy: Rationale in the management of transitional cell carcinoma of the upper urinary tract. Urol Clin North Am 7:569–578, 1980

259. Johansson S, Wahlqvist L: A prognostic study of urothelial renal pelvic tumors. Cancer 43:2525–2531, 1979

260. Johnson DE, deBerardinis M, Ayala AG: Transitional cell carcinoma of the renal pelvis: Radical or conservative surgical treatment? South Med J 67:1183–1186, 1974

261. Geiger J, Fong O, Fay R: Transitional cell carcinoma of renal pelvis with invasion of renal vein and thrombosis of subhepatic inferior vena cava. Urology 28:52–54, 1986

262. Jitsukawa S, Nakamura K, Nakayama M et al: Transitional cell carcinoma of kidney extending into renal vein and inferior vena cava. Urology 25:310–312, 1985

263. Gittes RF: Management of transitional cell carcinoma of the upper tract: Case for conservative local excision. Urol Clin North Am 7:559–568, 1980

264. Bazeed MA, Scherge T, Becht E et al: Local excision of urothelial cancer of the upper urinary tract. Eur Urol 12:89–95, 1986

265. Wallace DMA, Wallace DM, Whitfield HN et al: The late results of conservative surgery for upper tract urothelial carcinomas. Br J Urol 53:537–541, 1981

266. Tomera KM, Leary FJ, Zincke H: Pyeloscopy in urothelial tumors. J Urol 127:1088–1089, 1982

267. McIntyre D, Pyrah LN, Raper FP: Primary ureteric neoplasms with a report of forty cases. Br J Urol 37:160–191, 1965

268. Foord AG, Ferrier PA: Primary carcinoma of the ureter with report of seven cases. JAMA 112:596–601, 1939

269. Abeshouse BS: Primary benign and malignant tumors of the ureter: A review of the literature and report of one benign and twelve malignant tumors. Am J Surg 91:237–271, 1956

270. Heney NM, Nocks BN, Daly JJ et al: Prognostic factors in carcinoma of the ureter. J Urol 125:632–636, 1981

271. Hawtrey CE: Fifty-two cases of primary ureteral carcinoma: A clinical-pathologic study. J Urol 105:188–193, 1971

272. Batata MA, Whitmore WF Jr, Hilaris BS et al: Primary carcinoma of the ureter: A prognostic study. Cancer 35:1626–1632, 1975

273. Richie JP: Management of ureteral tumors. In Skinner DG, deKernion JB (eds): Genitourinary Cancer, pp 150–165. Philadelphia, WB Saunders, 1978

274. Bergman H, Friedenberg RM, Sayegh V: New roentgenologic signs of carcinoma of the ureter. Am Roentgen Ray Soc 86:707–717, 1961

275. Strong DW, Pearse HD: Recurrent urothelial tumors following surgery for transitional cell carcinoma of the upper urinary tract. Cancer 38:2178–2183, 1976

276. Bloom NA, Vidone RA, Lytton B: Primary carcinoma of the ureter: A report of 102 new cases. J Urol 103:590–598, 1970

277. Herr HW, Whitmore WF Jr: Ureteral carcinoma in situ after successful intravesical therapy for superficial bladder tumors: Incidence, possible pathogenesis and management. J Urol 138:292–294, 1987

278. Heney NM, Nocks BN, Daly JJ et al: Prognostic factors in carcinoma of the ureter. J Urol 125:632–636, 1981

279. Johannson A, Angerval L, Benstsson U et al: A clinicopathologic and prognostic study of epithelial tumors of the renal pelvis. Cancer 37:1376–1381, 1976

280. Brookland RK, Richter MP: Postoperative irradiation of transitional cell carcinoma of the renal pelvis and ureter. J Urol 133:952–955, 1985

281. Saitoh H, Hida N, Nakamura K et al: Distant metastases urothelial tumors of the renal pelvis and ureter. Tokai J Exp Clin Med 7:355–361, 1982

282. Shipley WU: Radiation therapy in the management of patients with genitourinary malignancies. In Wang CC (ed): Clinical Radiation Oncology: Indications, Techniques, and Results. Boston, PSG, 1987

283. Maruf NJ, Godec CJ, Kahn A et al: Synchronous tumors in both ureters and left renal pelvis. Urology 21:305, 1983

284. Hall P, Dammin G: Balkan nephropathy. Nephron 22:281, 1968

285. Trindade A, Samuels ML, Logothetis CJ: Chemotherapy of carcinoma of renal pelvis: Preliminary report. Urology 18:54, 1981

286. Nocks BN, Heney NM, Daly JJ et al: Transitional cell carcinoma of renal pelvis. Urology 19:472, 1982

287. DeKock MLS, Breytenbach IH: Local excision and topical thiotepa in the treatment of transitional cell carcinoma of the renal pelvis: A case report. J Urol 135:566, 1986

288. Sternberg C, Scher H: Current status of chemotherapy for urothelial tract tumors. Oncology 1:41, 1987

289. Logothetis CJ, Samuels ML, Selig DE et al: Combined intravenous and intraarterial cyclophosphamide, doxorubicin, and cis-platin (CISCA) in the management of select patients with invasive urothelial tumors. Cancer Treat Rep 69:33, 1985

290. Hrushesky WJM, Roemeling RV, Wood PA et al: High-dose intensive systemic therapy of metastatic bladder cancer. J Clin Oncol 5:450, 1987

291. Glover D, Glick JH, Weiler C et al: WR-2721 and high-dose cisplatin: An active combination in the treatment of metastatic melanoma. J Clin Oncol 5:574, 1987

292. Pinsky CM, Camacho FJ, Kerr D et al: Intravesical administration of bacillus Calmette-Guerin in patients with recurrent superficial carcinoma of the urinary bladder: Report of a prospective, randomized trial. Cancer Treat Rep 69:47, 1985

293. Bander NH: Monoclonal antibodies in the diagnosis and treatment of bladder cancer. In Yagoda A (ed): Bladder Cancer: Future Directions for Treatment, p 75. New York, John Wiley & Sons, 1986

294. Peeling WB, Mantell BS, Shepheard BGF: Post-operative irradiation in the treatment of renal cell carcinoma. Br J Urol 41:23–31, 1969

295. Juusela H, Malmio K, Alfthan D et al: Preoperative irradiation in the treatment of renal adenocarcinoma. Scand J Urol Nephrol 11:277–281, 1977

296. Kjaer M, Frederiksen PL, Engelholm SA: Postoperative radiotherapy in stage II and III renal adenocarcinoma. A randomized trial by the Copenhagen Renal Cancer Study Group. Int J Radiat Oncol Biol Phy 13:665–772, 1987

JEROME P. RICHIE

WILLIAM U. SHIPLEY

ALAN YAGODA

CHAPTER 32 *Cancer of the Bladder*

Carcinoma of the urinary bladder accounts for approximately 2% of all malignant tumors. The American Cancer Society has estimated that there will be 46,400 new cases of bladder cancer in 1988, with an estimated 10,400 deaths.[1] Although the disease is localized at the time of initial diagnosis in 90% of patients, as many as 80% will subsequently develop recurrent tumors. Close follow-up is mandatory because of both the potential for recurrence and the potential change in the biologic behavior of recurrent tumors. Indeed, patients with recurrent superficial bladder tumors give a glimpse of the process of carcinogenesis in vivo, with polychronotopism and subsequent invasion of the muscle wall and metastases.

Traditionally, management of the patient with carcinoma of the bladder has been the responsibility of the urologic surgeon. Currently, however, proper management requires the concerted effort of a team approach, with involvement from the radiotherapist and medical oncologist as well as the urologist. The increased incidence of bladder cancer and the rising mortality from bladder cancer underscore the need for effective combination treatment programs for all stages of disease in order to reduce recurrences and improve survival rates.

EPIDEMIOLOGY

The incidence of carcinoma of the bladder is higher in industrialized countries than in underdeveloped regions such as Asia and Africa. Bladder cancer is more prevalent in urban than in rural areas, giving credence to the effects of industrial carcinogens on the development of bladder cancer. The

incidence of bladder cancer increases with age, with a peak incidence in the seventh decade of life. The male to female ratio is $3:1$.

The association of occupational factors with the development of bladder malignancies was first suggested by Rehn[2] in 1895, who observed an increased risk of bladder cancer in aniline dye workers. Subsequent studies over the next 50 years have identified benzidine, 1 naphthylamine, and 2 naphthylamine as the primary agents. The average latency between exposure and development of bladder cancer is between 16 and 22 years. Other occupational categories associated with bladder cancer have been the dye, rubber, leather, paint, and organic chemical industries.

A consistent relationship has been demonstrated between cigarette smoking and bladder cancer. The rate of development of bladder cancer is about twice as high in smokers as in nonsmokers.[3] Winder and Goldsmith[4] reported a consistent relationship between the amount and duration of smoking and the incidence of bladder cancer in both men and women. The disparity in habits of cigarette smoking may account for the male to female ratio in bladder cancer of $3:1$, which seems to be decreasing as more women have smoked for longer periods of time. A Canadian study[5] showed that the risk ratio of bladder cancer in men who smoked 10 cigarettes a day, between 10 and 20, and more than 20 cigarettes a day was 1.0, 3.8, and 5.1 respectively. The relationship of artificial sweeteners to bladder cancer was highlighted by the Food and Drug Administration. Some pioneering work by Hicks and associates[6] has shown that both cyclamate and saccharine function as potent promoting agents in the rat model in which a single subthreshold initiating dose of methyl-nitrosourea (MNU) is followed by oral

1008

saccharine or cyclamates. These promoters increase the rate of tumors from 2% to 50% and telescope the time of induction from 2 years to 8 weeks. These findings were explained by the subthreshold dose of MNU serving as an initiator, with cyclamate or saccharine serving as a promoter. Although epidemiologic studies have suggested that artificial sweeteners are only weak human carcinogens,[7] these studies would be expected to show only an increased risk of 30% or more. Although the studies did not reach statistical significance, in the small group of nonsmoking females who represent the lowest risk the relative risk ratio for development of bladder cancers with cyclamates was 2.9.

A close relationship exists between bilharziasis and squamous cell carcinoma of the bladder. A recent review has focused on the presence of urinary nitrite in association with squamous cell carcinoma secondary to bilharziasis. Urinary tract infection associated with urinary nitrites and the production of nitrosourea may act as a proximate carcinogen for the production of squamous cell cancer of the bladder.[8]

PATHOLOGY

Ninety percent of urothelial bladder tumors are of the transitional cell variety. These tumors are usually papillary and often multicentric, reflecting the field change phenomena so often observed in transitional cell malignancies. Squamous cell carcinoma accounts for 6% to 8% of bladder tumors, and 2% are adenocarcinomas, usually arising in the dome of the bladder from the urachus. Tumors in association with exstrophy of the bladder are often adenocarcinomas.

Tumors are graded by the degree of cellular atypia and nuclear abnormalities as well as the number of mitotic figures. Broder's classification segregates tumors on a scale of I to IV, based on the degree of anaplasia. Some pathologists prefer to use a three grade system because the behaviors of grades III and IV are so similar that combining these two into a single grade seems justified.[9]

Mostofi and the World Health Organization (WHO) have called attention to the importance of recognizing and recording the growth pattern of bladder cancer (papillary or infiltrating, or both, or nonpapillary and noninfiltrating). Papillary tumors seem to have pushing borders that do not invade the muscularis on a broad front and therefore have a relatively better prognosis. Nonpapillary lesions, however, tend to invade on a broader front and hence have a more ominous prognosis.[10] A major problem in treating patients with bladder cancer has been in distinguishing the benign "papilloma" from malignant epithelial tumors. For many years, the variable nature of the benign-appearing papilloma has caused most pathologists to classify this lesion as a low grade carcinoma. Based on studies by Lerman et al and Koss,[11,12] it would appear that sufficient data exist to justify the separation of papilloma from carcinoma. The WHO has defined a papilloma as a papillary tumor with a delicate fibrovascular core covered by normal transitional cell epithelium that is less than six layers thick.[10] These benign transitional cell lesions have a recurrence rate of up to 50%; hence, semiannual surveillance is required for patients with this diagnosis.

Carcinoma in situ is defined as diffuse presence of highly anaplastic malignant cells within the confines of the urothelial lining. This term is used to designate a flat intraurothelial cancer with crowding of the larger nuclei and numerous mitoses. The lamina propria reveals no specific abnormalities. A lesion may appear cystoscopically as normal bladder mucosa or as a red velvety area related to vascular proliferation and dilatation. Carcinoma in situ, in association with overt bladder tumors, signifies a field change and indicates the need for more aggressive therapy.

CLINICAL PRESENTATION

There are no pathognomonic signs or symptoms of bladder cancer. Hematuria, with or without irritative symptoms, occurs in 75% of patients with bladder cancer. Vesical irritability alone is the persisting symptom in 30% of patients and often signifies the presence of carcinoma in situ. Advanced cases may present with rectal obstruction, pelvic pain, or lower extremity edema secondary to lymphatic or venous occlusion. Urinary cytology or flow cytometry may lead to a presumptive diagnosis of bladder cancer, especially in patients with higher grade lesions. Many patients will have an excretory urogram, which often suggests an intraluminal filling defect in the bladder.[13] The diagnosis of bladder cancer is confirmed by cystoscopic examination and transurethral biopsy of the suspected area. At the time of biopsy, bimanual examination is conducted to ascertain the extent of tumor and the presence or absence of fixation to adjacent pelvic structures. The biopsy should be adequate to determine the presence or absence of muscle invasion. Random biopsies at sites adjacent to and distant from the tumor should be evaluated for carcinoma in situ. A cold cup or punch biopsy forceps is useful for obtaining tissue without cautery artifact.

STAGING

Bladder carcinoma that has invaded the muscular wall or deeper is a potentially lethal disease, often metastasizing before major urinary symptoms appear in the patient. Once a diagnosis has been ascertained by biopsy, a chest roentgenogram, radionuclide bone scan, and liver and renal function studies should be performed. The first site of failure in patients with invasive bladder cancer is usually in the bones or the lungs; therefore these areas should be evaluated carefully.[14] Computed tomography scans or magnetic resonance imaging have gained increasing popularity as an adjunct to staging. Ultrasonography of the bladder has been evaluated but has yet to be very helpful in delineating the extent of local involvement.

Modern-day staging began with the observations of Jewett and Strong[15] in 1946, in a study that related the depth of penetration of the bladder wall to the incidence of local extension in metastases. This staging system was modified by Marshall into an O, A, B, C, D system that was based on the bimanual examination under anesthesia and the histologic evaluation of the tumor resected transurethrally.[16] The Jewett, Strong, Marshall staging system and its counterpart in the UICC and the American Joint Committee tumor,

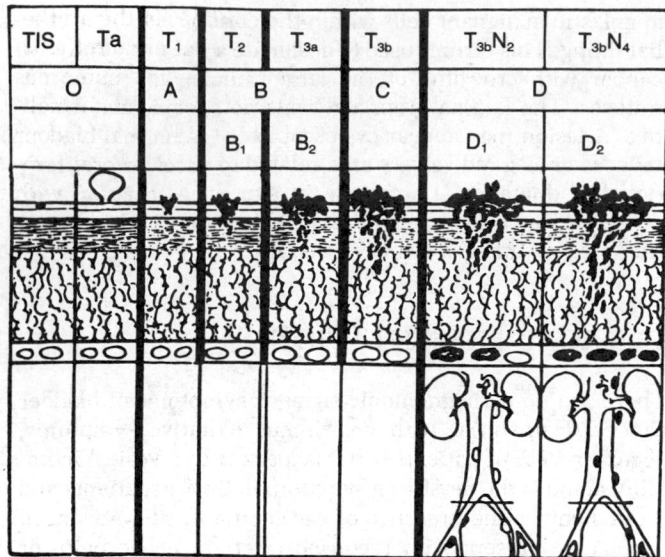

TIS	Ta	T₁	T₂	T₃ₐ	T₃ᵦ	T₃ᵦN₂	T₃ᵦN₄
O	A	B		C		D	
			B₁	B₂		D₁	D₂

FIG. 32-1. Comparison of TNM system and Jewett, Marshall, Strong (O, A, B, C, D) system for staging of transitional cell carcinoma of the bladder. (Prout GR Jr: Bladder carcinoma. In Pilch YH [ed]: Surgical Oncology, p 683. New York, McGraw-Hill, 1984)

nodes, and metastases (TNM) system are illustrated in Figure 32-1.[18] The stage O lesion indicated tumor that is limited to the mucosa, which includes both a visible papillary carcinoma (T$_a$) and carcinoma in situ (TIS). Clinical stage T1 (A) lesions have invaded into the lamina propria but not beyond. Clinical T2–T4 (B,C) are tumors that invade at least into muscle. Clinical T2 (B1) tumors infiltrate muscle but have no palpable mass or induration on bimanual examination after transurethral resection. A stage T3 (B2-C) tumor infiltrates muscle and has a palpable mass or induration present on bimanual examination after transurethral resection. (T3A or B2 tumors do not have evidence of invading beyond the bladder muscle; stage T3B or C tumors have invasion documented into perivesical fat.) The clinical T4 tumors are those that extend into neighboring structures (T4A invasion into vagina, uterus, or prostate with histologic confirmation; T4B tumors are fixed to the bony pelvis or abdominal wall or invade rectum). The staging criteria for lymph nodal involvement are based on the surgical and pathologic staging of the lymph nodes. In the absence of any histologic confirmation of nodal metastasis, the disease is staged as Nx. Patients with biopsy-proven metastatic lymph nodes limited to

the pelvis have either stage D$_1$ or N$_{1-3}$. N$_1$ is involvement of a single homolateral node; N$_2$ is involvement of contralateral or multiple pelvic lymph nodes; N$_3$ is involvement of fixed pelvic lymph node(s). Patients with involvement of lymph nodes outside the pelvis are classified either D$_2$ or N$_4$. Among the muscle-invading tumors the prognostic difference between clinical stage T2 (B1) and clinical T3 (B2-C) is significant in some series,[15,16,40–42,54,56,59] but in others no difference was noted.[17,39,57]

One difficulty with clinical staging systems is that they are only as good as the techniques available to assess the extent of disease. Many American urologists continue to use the Jewett, Strong, Marshall system of classification, but there is a growing trend in the United States to join international colleagues in using the TNM system. The National Surgical Adjuvant Group and the Memorial Sloan-Kettering Cancer Center have documented an error rate as high as 50% between clinical and pathologic stages for patients with muscle-invading tumors.[54,64] Skinner and associates,[19] in a review of 130 patients, found that clinical and pathologic stages were concordant in 53% of patients with Stage T1 tumors, in only 13% of patients with clinical Stage T2 tumors, and in 50% of patients with Stage T3 tumors. The overall rate of agreement was only 36%, with 41% of patients understaged and 23% overstaged. Refinements in the clinical staging system with more emphasis on histopathologic information of the biopsy such as degree of invasion, grade of tumor, configuration of tumor, and the presence or absence of carcinoma in situ are in order. It is hoped that many of these factors can be consistently shown independently to influence prognosis following treatment for patients with muscle-invading tumors. The TNM pathologic staging criteria by microscopic evaluation of the tumor in the radical cystectomy specimen are quite accurate for predicting prognosis (Table 32-1). A refined clinical staging system that would correlate well with the TNM pathologic staging will be quite useful if and when such refinements can be developed and tested prospectively.

TREATMENT

PHILOSOPHIC CONSIDERATIONS

Treatment of the patient with bladder carcinoma should be selected so as to prevent death from the malignancy and to do so with as little treatment-related morbidity as possible. In

TABLE 32-1. Therapeutic Results for Radical Cystectomy for Invasive Bladder Cancer (Patients Grouped by Pathologic Stage)

Series (Year)	No. of Patients	5-Year Survival Rate (%) for Pathologic Stage				
		P0/P1/Pcis	P2	P3a	P3b	P4 or N+
Bowles and Cordonier,[4] 1963	50		63	50	20	0
Jewett, King, Shelley,[45] 1964	61		50	16	12	
Pearse, Reed, Hodges,[46] 1978	52		50	16	12	
Mathur, Krahn, Ramsey,[47] 1981	58	71	88	57	40	29
Skinner, Lieskovsky,[48] 1984	197	75	64	44		36
Skinner, Lieskovsky,[49] 1988	189	83	83	69	29	27

patients with superficial tumors, recurrences are likely and increase with the size and the multiplicity of the tumor and the association of carcinoma in situ. Treatment directed toward recurrent superficial bladder tumors is mainly for patient convenience and the reduction of the need for resection; fewer than 25% of these patients will progress to invasive disease. In patients with muscle-invading tumors, surgical extirpation remains as the gold standard for long-term tumor-survival. However, innovative approaches for patients with muscle-invading tumors that incorporate more extensive transurethral surgery with chemotherapy or radiation therapy, or both, and selective bladder preservation are now being studied in careful prospective protocols.[119,120]

SUPERFICIAL BLADDER CANCER

Stage O (in situ) tumors are frequently treated with transurethral resections or fulguration. Many of these lesions are papillary and can be controlled locally with conservative therapy in more than 80% of the cases. However, some lesions are more infiltrating and less differentiated, and recurrences in more than 50% of the patients have been reported. It is important for the urologist to remove the base of the lesion with an adequate margin.

Intravesical Chemotherapy

Postoperative intravesical chemotherapy has been used to reduce recurrence rates. Agents such as doxorubicin have been used in a cyclic fashion, beginning on the day of surgery, with good success.[20] Randomized trials have been undertaken specifically to destroy existing tumors or tumor implants that could occur during local resection or fulguration, and to prevent recurrence of resected primary tumors or development of new cancers.[21,22] Ideally, agents for intravesical administration should be poorly absorbed through the bladder mucosa, thereby preventing systemic toxicity and exposing local lesions to a high drug concentration.

Thiotepa, which has been studied extensively in the carcinogen-induced FANFT murine bladder cancer model, has little effect on normal murine urothelium, destroys established cancers, inhibits tumor reimplantation, and retards development of new lesions.[21,22] The usual dose is 30 to 60 mg/30 to 60 ml given intravesically for 1 to 2 hours weekly for 4 weeks and thereafter monthly. When given to patients with established tumors, approximately 30% achieve complete and 30% achieve partial remissions. In a randomized trial using 90 mg for 30 minutes given immediately after complete resection of all tumors versus no therapy, tumor recurrence (or implants) decreased by 40%.[23] In a study in patients with no visible tumor, 66% of the thiotepa group versus 40% of the control group remained tumor free at 1 year.[24] Because of its low molecular weight, 189, thiotepa is absorbed and myelosuppression can be seen in 18% to 40% of cases; pancytopenia is uncommon.[25]

Mitomycin-C in doses of 20 to 60 mg/20 to 40 ml weekly for eight doses produces complete response in approximately half and partial response in one third of the cases.[26] Higher response rates are noted with doses greater than 40 mg/40 ml. The drug seems to be as effective as thiotepa as

primary therapy and can induce complete remission in patients failing thiotepa therapy. Myelosuppression is rare because the molecular weight, 334, is too large for absorption through the bladder mucosa. Bladder irritation and genital and palmar rashes secondary to direct contact with the drug have been described.[21] Doxorubicin, epodyl, and tenoposide (VM-26) have been used extensively in Europe and Japan. In two randomized studies, doxorubicin, given three times per week in doses of 20 mg to 30 mg, 50 mg, and 60 mg, produced responses in 31% to 56%, 69% to 72%, and 59% to 74% of cases, respectively.[27] Other studies have described complete remission with negative cytologic and endoscopic findings in two thirds of the cases.[21] However, bladder irritation is frequent, 27% to 44%, and severe when given immediately after fulguration. Of note, cisplatin, intravesically as well as intravenously, is ineffective and can induce severe hypersensitivity reactions.[28]

Bacillus Calmette-Guerin (BCG) in doses of 120 mg/50 ml of normal saline intravesically with weekly intradermal administration for 6 weeks has also proved extremely effective. Prospective randomized trials by Lamm et al[29] and Pinsky et al[30] have shown a 50% prophylaxis versus untreated cases. In a study of 86 cases, half of whom served as controls, the number of recurrent tumors was reduced, and the disease-free interval, including negative cytology, and the time to progression locally and to cystectomy (BCG 3 of 43 cases versus control 15 of 43 cases) was significantly (p = 0.001) prolonged.[31] Conversion to a negative cytology was frequently observed (p = 0.05).[32] A few patients who after achieving complete remission eventually required surgery for recurrent, abnormal cytology showed new tumors only in the renal pelvis, ureter, or urethra; areas that had direct contact with BCG remained free of disease. Present data suggest that intradermal administration can be omitted.[32]

Lamm[32] reported his experience in patients with superficial bladder cancer receiving intravesical BCG (Pasteur) strain (120 mg/50 ml saline weekly for 6 weeks). A highly significant reduction recurrence rate was noted: 20% versus 52% in controls. Brosman[33] reported 35 patients treated with TICE strain of BCG for carcinoma in situ. By 24 weeks, all 27 patients who tolerated BCG were rendered tumor free and placed on maintenance regimen. Six patients did not receive full treatment; thus, 31 of 33 patients (94%) were rendered free of disease.

CARCINOMA IN SITU

Management of carcinoma in situ may present specific problems in patients with transitional cell carcinoma. Carcinoma in situ is noninvasive but has a high potential for subsequent invasion. Carcinoma in situ is multifocal and diffuse and reflects the potential for the entire urothelial surface to undergo exposure to potential carcinogens.

If the lesion involves only a small portion of the bladder (<5 cm), is reasonably well delineated, does not involve the prostatic urethra, vesical neck, or either ureteral orifice, and there is no evidence of positive cytologic findings from the upper urinary tract, thorough electrofulguration of the involved areas is indicated followed by a course of intravesical thiotepa or doxorubicin for 6 months. Another alternative is

BCG weekly for 6 to 12 weeks. The patient should be followed post-treatment with cystoscopic and urinary cytologic studies at 2- to 3-month intervals for the first year, at 4-month intervals for the second year, and at 6-month intervals thereafter. If the lesion does not respond, if cytologic findings do not convert to negative, and if the irritative bladder symptoms remain after treatment, cystoprostatectomy with urinary diversion is recommended. In patients who have diffuse lesions, involvement of the prostatic urethra, or severe irritative bladder symptomatology, radical cystectomy is warranted.

Involvement of the prostatic urethra with carcinoma in situ should prompt in-continuity urethrectomy.

The initiation of aggressive treatment of carcinoma in situ is prompted by the previous experience of Utz and co-workers.[34] In their initial series in which carcinoma in situ was treated primarily by transurethral electroresection and fulguration, subsequent invasion developed in 73% of patients, with 57% of these patients dying of their disease in 5 years. The more aggressive approach of cystectomy after diagnosis of carcinoma in situ demonstrated no deaths in 15 subsequent patients. Three of these patients had microinvasion with more than 80% of the bladder replaced by in situ cancer at the time of pathologic examination.

In a more recent series, however, Utz and co-workers[35] have identified a subset of patients with positive cytologic findings in whom carcinoma in situ has been found without associated irritative symptoms or overt bladder tumors. These patients seem to represent an earlier state along the road to invasion and metastases, and some have been followed for longer than 10 years without progression. Thus, management of the patient with carcinoma in situ should be individualized, with more conservative treatment such as intravesical chemotherapy used for those patients at lower risk of progression.

INVASIVE DISEASE

PARTIAL CYSTECTOMY

The role of segmental resection in the management of transitional cell carcinoma of the bladder remains controversial. However, this operative option presents an attractive alternative for carefully selected patients. Selection of patients for partial cystectomy is complicated by the tendency of the entire vesical urothelium to be unstable in the presence of an isolated and well-defined lesion, and because of the probability of undetected microinvasion and carcinoma in situ in remote areas of the bladder. The additional problem of wound seeding at the time of partial cystectomy must not be underemphasized.

A series of specific criteria must be established in order to select the appropriate patient for surgery. The tumor should be invasive. The tumor should be less than 6 cm to 8 cm in size to permit resection with sufficient tumor-free margins for acceptable functional bladder capacity. The lesion should be solitary and primary and, ideally, located in the upper part of the bladder or on the posterior wall. Invasion of the vesical

neck or the prostate is a contraindication. Transitional cell carcinomas have a better response to partial cystectomy than do squamous cell carcinomas owing to the tendency of the latter to extend intramurally via lymphatics and venous plexus of the bladder wall. The appearance of carcinoma in situ adjacent or distant to the lesion itself indicates urothelial instability and is a contraindication to partial cystectomy.

Before partial cystectomy, preoperative radiotherapy in the form of a minimum dose of 1000 to 2000 rad should be established to devitalize the tumor cells and prevent wound seeding. Before opening the bladder, the bladder should be irrigated with sterile water. When laterality of the lesion can be established, a unilateral pelvic node dissection should be established in continuity.

The necessity for rigid patient selection makes segmental resection appropriate for only 5% of patients with bladder cancer. Five-year survival rates in patients with Stage O, A, or B bladder cancer carefully selected for treatment by partial cystectomy range from 65% to 81%.[36,37]

RADICAL CYSTECTOMY: TREATMENT RESULTS

For most patients whose tumor demonstrates invasion of the muscle wall, more aggressive treatment is clearly indicated. Once the urothelial malignancy has penetrated into the muscularis, radical cystoprostatectomy in men or anterior exenteration in women has been the treatment of choice. This operation satisfies the treatment of field changes that are common in urothelial malignancy and results in reasonable potential for cure if the cancer is still confined within the bladder wall. Unfortunately, many tumors have progressed beyond the point of curability by means of local therapy with radical cystectomy alone. Failures in patients managed by radical cystectomy are usually due to distant metastases, with fewer than 10% of patients failing locally.

Prognosis in patients with carcinoma of the bladder who have undergone cystectomy has traditionally been reported on the basis of 5-year survival rates. Originally, this was based on observed survival data, with all patients followed at least 5 years. Beginning in the 1970s, however, actuarial survival rates using statistical correlation such as Kaplan Meyer curves have been used to present projected 5-year survival rates (Table 32-1). This technique allows the incorporation of patients followed for less than 5 years but considered at risk for the interval over which they have been followed. One problem with reports of survival is that most 5-year survivals have been based on pathologic stage (Table 32-1), which may be at some variance from the clinical stage (Table 32-2).

Up until the 1950s, survival rates had little meaning since the operative mortality varied from 25% to 60%. In 1966, Glantz[50] reported a mortality rate of 20% in patients who underwent total cystectomy in the 1950s and early 1960s. Whitmore and Marshall[51] reported a mortality rate of 14% in radical cystectomies done between 1945 and 1955. Richie and associates[17] reported a 15% overall operative mortality from 1955 to 1971 but a 2% operative mortality in the most recent 50 patients done in the early 1970s. Johnson and Lamy[52] reported a 3.3% mortality rate in 214 radical cystec-

TABLE 32-2. Therapeutic Results for Radiation Therapy and Radical Cystectomy for Invasion Bladder Cancer

Series and Year	No. of Patients	Clinical Stage	Total Dose (cGY)	Maintained Local Control (%)	5-Year Survival Rate (%)
Radiation Therapy					
Miller and Johnson,[38] 1973	263	T2,T3	5800–6500	56	22
Shipley et al,[40] 1985	37	T2,T3	6400–6840	49	39
Timmer et al,[41] 1985	76	T2,T3	6000–6500	41	38
Quilty and Duncan,[42] 1986	333	T3	5000–5750	24	26
Blandy,[43] 1988	138	T2,T3	6000	40	
Preoperative Radiation and Surgery			*Preoperative XRT*		
Boileau and Johnson et al,[39] 1980	112	T2,T3	5000	90	50
Batata et al,[117] (1981)	133	T3,T4	2000	88	35
van der Werf-Messing et al,[58] 1982	183	T3	4000	100	52
National Bladder Cancer Group[59]	175	T2–T4	4000	92	52

tomies done from 1969 to 1975. More recently, Skinner[53] reported a less than 1% operative mortality in 128 radical cystectomies from 1971 to 1977.

With the improvement in postoperative mortality rate, survival data have become more meaningful (see Table 32-1). Before 1975, most survival rates were broken down into patients with superficial (O,A and B1; T-O,TA, T1) and deep (B2, C or T3A, T3B) pathologically staged lesions. Whitmore and associates[54] reported a 63% 5-year survival rate for superficial tumors by pathologic stage and a 20% 5-year survival rate for deep lesions by pathologic stage in 137 patients who underwent radical cystectomy alone from 1949 to 1958. With preoperative radiation therapy of 4500 rad and improved surgical techniques, 5-year survival rates for 119 patients operated on from 1959 to 1966 were 58% for the superficial group and 48% for the deep group. Eighty-six patients who received a short course (2000 rad) to the bladder and true pelvis and then radical cystectomy from 1966 to 1970 had a 5-year survival rate of 56% for the superficial lesions and 58% for the deep lesions. Although this series suggests improvement in survival rate related to preoperative radiation, an equally plausible alternative explanation relates to improved survival rates from improved techniques of surgical approach, anesthetic management, and patient monitoring.

In an effort to improve patient survival, various combinations of radiation therapy along with radical cystectomy have been advocated. Randomized trials of radiation therapy prior to radical cystectomy have shown a trend in improvement in survival but not one that is statistically significant when compared with surgery alone.[62,64] Nonrandomized concurrent studies have not shown any survival advantage to preoperative radiation therapy versus current surgical cystectomy.[48,55] At present, one has the clear impression that for patients with tumors that minimally invade muscle (clinical and pathologic stage T2 or B$_1$), there seems to be no benefit from radiation therapy in addition to immediate radical cystectomy. Such opinion is supported by the fact that the 5-year survival rates with radical cystectomy alone for patients with pathologic stage T1 or T2 are 80% or more in recent series (see Table 32-1).

FULL-DOSE RADIATION THERAPY: TREATMENT RESULTS

External Beam Irradiation

Full-dose radiation therapy as definitive treatment has yielded 5-year survival rates of 22% to 39% for patients presenting with clinical stage T2 and T3 (B1, B2-C) tumors (see Table 32-1).[38,40-43] The major clinical problem in such patients is that permanent eradication of the cancer in the bladder occurs in only 30% to 50% of the patients (see Table 32-2) compared to more than 85% in patients treated by cystectomy following preoperative radiation therapy.[39,58,59,117] However, patients who do have an excellent response to radiation therapy have an excellent survival probability. In the retrospective review from the Massachusetts General Hospital, the survival of patients with clinical stage T2 and T3 tumors from their bladder cancer was 79% in patients who had local control of their cancer compared to only 11% for patients who developed a local recurrence.[40] In these retrospective series, several clinically useful observations can be made: fewer than half of the treated patients will have a complete response to conventional external beam radiation therapy, and only one third to two fifths of the whole group will have permanent control of their local bladder tumor; radical cystectomy may be deferred in the completely responding patients, most of whom will not require this operation; patients needing salvage cystectomy have been, during the most recent decade, better able to tolerate that operation, perhaps because of improvements in surgery, radiation therapy, and perioperative care; and, finally, the radiation response rate has not changed over the past two decades, and thus expecting further progress with conventional radiation therapy alone and prompt salvage cystectomy seems unrealistic. Salvage cystectomy still carries significant risks, with mortality rates from 2% to 19%.[41,52]

Tumor-related prognostic factors that contribute to an improved treatment outcome by full-dose radiation therapy in patients with muscle-invading tumors include the clinical stage of the tumor, the accomplishment of a visibly complete transurethral resection of the tumor, the histologic characteristic of a papillary tumor surface, and the absence of

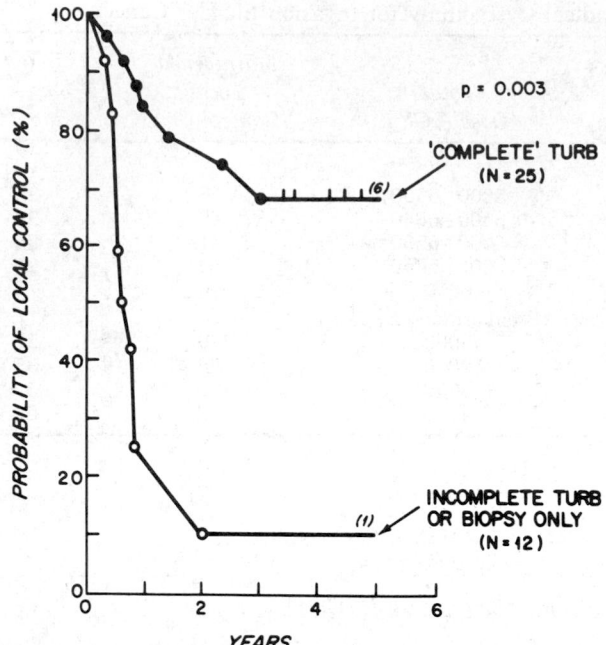

FIG. 32-2. Probability of local control by full-dose radiation therapy in patients with Stages T2 and T3 bladder cancer in whom a "visibly complete" transurethral resection of the bladder tumor (TURB) was possible, and in patients in whom only an incomplete resection or biopsy was done. The numbers in parentheses indicate the number of patients followed up more than 5 years. (Shipley WV, Prout GE Jr, Kaufman SD et al: Full-dose irradiation for patients with invasive bladder carcinoma: Clinical and histological factors prognostic of improved survival. Cancer 60:511, 1987)

ureteral obstruction by tumor. In patients with clinical stage T2 and T3 tumors, the local control rate at 5 years in 25 patients in whom the urologist judged that a visibly complete transurethral resection had been accomplished was 68% versus 10% for those patients who had undergone a biopsy only or incomplete resection (p = 0.003).[40] The 5-year survival rate from bladder cancer in the group who underwent a complete resection was 54% versus 17% in the group who did not (Figure 32-2). There are almost certainly some inaccuracies in the endoscopic estimate of the extent of tumor debulking. Nevertheless, this is a favorable prognostic factor and very likely correlates both with initial tumor size and with the number of remaining tumor cells that must be inactivated by irradiation.

Many reports have documented that papillary tumors are of less malignant potential than are solid tumors.[60-63] Muscle invading papillary tumors are more effectively treated by radiation therapy than are solid tumors.[40,62,64,65] For tumors of the same clinical stage, radiation therapy has led to both better local tumor control and patient survival in those tumors of papillary histology, as compared to the solid tumors for patients treated with external beam radiation therapy[40] and by combined external beam and interstitial radiation therapy.[65]

Intraoperative Radiation Therapy

The ability to deliver selectively more radiation therapy directly to the tumor and less to the uninvolved portion of the

bladder can be provided in appropriate patients by open surgery. Brachytherapy using radium-226 (^{226}Ra) needle implantation has been used with great success over the past 25 years by van der Werf-Messing and colleagues at the Rotterdam Radiotherapy Institute for patients with solitary tumors of less than 5 cm in greatest diameter. Intraoperatively, the radium needles are inserted into and immediately adjacent to the tumor at the time of open cystotomy. Recently, however, the radioactive source has been changed to cesium-137 (^{137}Cs).[66] Sutures that are attached to the needles are brought out through a separate track from the incision and are used to remove the needles in 3 to 6 days, or following the delivery of 3,250 to 6,500 cGy of radiation. Problems of wound seeding by tumor resulting from the open cystotomy have been solved by the use of preoperative radiation therapy with doses of 1,050 cGy over 3 elapsed days in 3 fractions. The largest number of patients (328) who have been treated by this approach have had clinical stage T2 tumors, although not all of these patients have had proof of muscle invasion. Seventy-seven percent have remained free of recurrence of tumor in their bladder for at least 5 years (Table 32-3), for an overall survival of 56%.[66] For patients with clinical stage T2 tumors a similarly high 5-year local tumor control rate as well as survival rate is seen by groups from Amsterdam and Creteil.[67,68]

Intraoperative radiation therapy by electron beam has been used with similar success in Japan.[69] The treatment was also done at the time of open cystotomy but without tumor resection or fulguration. The electron beam dose of 2,500 to 3,000 cGy by 3.5 to 7.5 MeV electrons was delivered via cylinders of 4, 5, or 6 cm in internal diameter. Three thousand to 4,000 cGy of external beam irradiation was given postoperatively to the whole bladder in 15 to 20 treatments. In 28 patients treated for stage T2 tumors there was freedom from local recurrence in 82%, with an overall 62% 5-year survival rate.

RECENT MODIFICATIONS IN TREATMENT TECHNIQUES

Surgical Techniques

POTENCY PRESERVING TECHNIQUE FOR RADICAL CYSTECTOMY. Before the early 1980s, virtually all patients who had undergone radical cystectomy were impotent postoperatively. Following the pioneering work by Walsh and associates of delineation of the anatomy of Santorini's plexus[70] and the description of the anatomic relationships between the nerves supplying the corpora cavernosum and the apex of the prostate,[71] anatomical approaches have been described for radical prostatectomy and radical cystectomy that can preserve potency in a high percentage of patients. Radical cystectomy proceeds in standard fashion, including bilateral pelvic lymph node dissection and division of the lateral pedicles to the prostate. A plane is developed between the bladder and rectum by incising the peritoneum and using gentle blunt dissection to free the rectum from the prostate at Denonvilliers' fascia. Dissection is stopped before encountering lateral pedicles of the bladder near the pelvic fascia. Attention is then turned to the dorsal-venous complex and plexus of Santorini as for radical retropubic prostatec-

TABLE 32-3. Intraoperative Radiation Therapy: Clinical Stage T2 Bladder Cancer

Series	No. of Patients	Treatment	5-Year Local Control (%)	5-Year Survival (%)
van der Werf-Messing et al[66]	328	XRT, [226]Ra	77	56
Batterman et al[67]	85	XRT, [226]RA	74	55
Mazeron et al[68]	24	Resection, ^{192}Ir, XRT	92	58
Matsumoto et al[69]	28	IORT, XRT	82	62

XRT, external Beam irradiation; [226]Ra, brachytherapy by radium needles; ^{192}Ir, brachytherapy by after-loading iridium in catheters; IORT, single dose electron beam irradiation.

tomy. Isolation of the dorsal-venous complex is achieved and the membranous urethra transected with division of the lateral pelvic fascia and pedicles to the prostate. The seminal vesicles are then dissected away from the neurovascular bundle on each side and the remainder of the lateral bladder pedicles ligated.

Using these principles, radical removal of bladder cancer can be performed with preservation of the neurovascular bundles and therefore preservation of potency. Indeed, approximately two thirds of the patients who were potent preoperatively will recover potency from 3 months to 1 year after radical cystectomy using this modified technique.

URINARY DIVERSION. The standard method of urinary diversion following cystectomy in 1988 remains the ileal conduit. However, newer techniques have been described to include continent forms of urinary diversion such as the Kock pouch, Camey procedure, or ileocecal segment. These techniques involve innovative use of bowel segments either brought to the skin or sutured to the urethra, allowing the patient to void in a normal fashion or be catheterized intermittently rather than wearing an external collecting device. The Kock pouch involves use of a long segment of ileum and creation of an internal pouch with antirefluxing intussuscepted nipple connected to both ureters and a second nipple to preserve continence. The pouch is usually brought to the abdominal wall but may, on rare occasions, be placed down to the urethra.[72] The Camey procedure involves use of a long segment of ileum hooked to the end of the urethra in an end-to-side anastomotic fashion.[73] Each ureter is implanted into one end of the upper portion of the U using an antirefluxing ureteroileal anastomosis. The patients void normally during the daytime but have problems with nocturnal enuresis. The ileocecal segment can be used with the ileocecal valve as an antireflux mechanism and the cecum brought to the skin for intermittent catheterization or a cecoileal segment anastomosed directly to the urethra for normal voiding.[74,75] All of these techniques are somewhat experimental and should be used only in selected patients. Urinary diversion continues to evolve through a variety of new techniques, all of which will require long-term follow-up to be certain that complications not yet suspected do not arise.

NORMAL TISSUE-SPARING TECHNIQUES WITH IRRADIATION. Over the past decade improvements in the use of higher energy megavoltage irradiation (XRT) primarily from linear accelerator beams have been used for full-dose or definitive treatment of patients with bladder cancer. These have been well tolerated by the pelvic soft tissues and likely represent a clinically significant reduction in late radiation sequelae in the pelvic tissues without compromising bladder and bowel function. The four-field box technique has become the accepted method of treating the bladder tumor volume and the pelvic lymph nodes.[38] These fields are based inferiorly 1.0 cm below the lower border of the obturator foramena so as to include adequate urethral tissue distally. (The fields may have to be even lower in women with cystoceles.) The width is 1 to 1.5 cm lateral to the bony pelvis at its widest point to cover adequately the external iliac lymph nodal tissues. For conventional radiation fractionation, daily doses (5 sessions per week) in the 180 to 200 cGy range were judged to offer an optimal therapeutic index. For instance, when 180 cGy per fraction doses were used with full-dose radiation therapy, only 4 of 35 patients developed severe frequency or hematuria, or both, either causing incontinence or requiring surgery.[40] In a series in which high radiation doses per fraction (240–275 cGy) were delivered to the whole bladder and to some surrounding nodal tissues in patients with T3 tumors to total doses of 4,750 to 5,500 cGy, the incidence of severe bladder damage was 45% in patients who lived 3 years or more after treatment.[76]

The technique of administering the boost to the tumor volume depends on the equipment available and the size of the patient. The goal is to exclude as much uninvolved normal tissue as possible from the region that receives the total dose (6,000–7,000 cGy in 7–8 weeks). Ideally the technique should limit the total dose to less than 6,000 cGy to the uninvolved section of the bladder and the posterior half of the rectosigmoid, and to less than 4,500 to 5,000 cGy to the anus and the head and neck regions of the femorae. The information allowing the boost dose to be only to the bladder tumor volume and not the whole bladder requires close coordination between the urologist and radiation oncologist. A diagram of the bladder tumor, the extent of transurethral resection, the bimanual examination, and the selected mucosal biopsies are all helpful in planning the cone-down boost field to the tumor volume. The boost can be optimally given with treatment beams of 10 MV x-rays or greater by paired lateral fields that maximally exclude the rectum. However, if the beam of a 4 or 6 MV accelerator is to be used, the 120 degree arc rotation is usually the most desirable boost technique (Fig. 32-3).

CHEMOTHERAPY FOR ADVANCED DISEASE

Transitional cell carcinoma of the urothelium (renal pelvis, ureter, urinary bladder, urethra, and prostatic ducts) is a chemotherapeutically responsive tumor, evidenced by com-

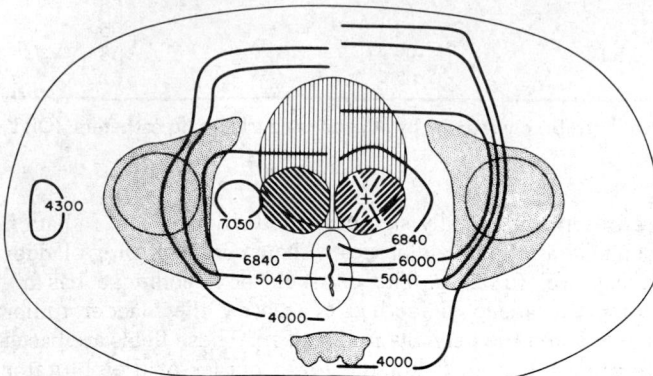

10 MV X-RAYS

7 cm LATERAL BOOST

4 MV X-RAYS

6 cm 120° ARC BOOST

FIG. 32-3. A comparison for full-dose radiation therapy (XRT) of invasive T2–T3 bladder tumor by 10 MV x-rays or 4 MV x-rays. The XRT dose to the whole pelvis is 5040 cGy; the XRT boost dose to the bladder tumor volume is 1800 cGy.

plete and partial remissions observed in 45% to 70% of selected cases with some combination regimens.[77,78] Single agents can produce objective tumor regression in 10% to 30% of cases; only with multidrug regimens have a significant number of complete remissions been reported. Of cardinal importance, such combinations still need to be proved in prospective randomized Phase III studies against active single agents such as cisplatin or methotrexate.

The major problem in evaluating therapy in this tumor is patient selection bias owing to different patient populations, sites of metastases being evaluated, extent of prior therapies, and response criteria.[79-81] The last-mentioned problem has

come under scrutiny in a Consensus Development Conference on Guidelines for Clinical Research in Bladder Cancer.[80,81]

Single Agents

The most active single agents are cisplatin and methotrexate (Table 32-4).[77,78] Cisplatin has been evaluated in more than 320 cases, generally in a dose of 70 mg/m² IV every 3 to 4 weeks. Response is observed within 3 to 6 weeks and persists for 3 to 5 months; complete remission is uncommon. No evidence exists to suggest that higher cisplatin doses will induce a better or a more prolonged response. In randomized Phase III studies, cisplatin singly has produced response in 17% to 20% of cases.[82-84] Although some data suggest that cisplatin may be more effective against soft tissue metastases than against primary intravesical disease,[84] two studies[85,86] using cisplatin alone neoadjuvantly described significant efficacy. Methotrexate produces remission in 30% of cases.[77,78] The optimum dose is still unknown, but the schedule most frequently used is 40 mg/m² IV weekly. Tumor regression occurs within 2 to 4 weeks and persists for 3 to 4 months. Complete remission is infrequent. No randomized trial has evaluated high- versus low-dose methotrexate, but in 57 cases culled from the literature giving high dose with citrovorum favor rescue, the response rate was 45% (95% confidence intervals, 32–50%).

Doxorubicin and the vinca alkaloids have also shown moderate antitumor activity. Doxorubicin, 45, 60, and 75 mg/m² IV every 3 weeks, produces response in 17% of cases. Complete remission for 17 to 48 months has been reported; most responses are partial and persist a median of 3 months. A possible dose response relationship has been suggested. Vin-

TABLE 32-4.   Single-Agent Trials in Previously Treated and Untreated Patients with Advanced Urothelial Tract Tumors[77,78]

Drugs	No. of Patients	% Complete and Partial Remission
Amsacrine (AMSA)	61	12 (4–20)*
Bisantrene	13	0 (0–23)
Bleomycin	79	5 (0–10)
Carboplatin	80	11 (7–15)
Cisplatin	**320**	**30 (25–35)**
Cyclophosphamide	26	7 (0–17)
10-Deazaaminopterin	15	20 (0–40)
Diaziquone (AZQ)	16	0 (0–17)
Doxorubicin	**248**	**17 (12–23)**
Etoposide (VP-16-213)	47	2 (0–4)
5-Fluorouracil	105	15 (18–22)
Gallium nitrate	26	27 (11–48)
Hexamethylmelamine	24	13 (0–31)
Methotrexate	**236**	**29 (23–35)**
(high dose)	57	45 (32–50)
Mitomycin-C	42	13 (3–23)
Mitoxantrone	28	0 (0–10)
Neocarcinostatin	19	5 (0–19)
PALA	18	0 (0–16)
Teniposide (VM-26)	64	11 (3–19)
(intravesical)	148	13 (8–18)
Vinblastine	**38**	**16 (4–28)**
Vincristine	42	14 (3–25)

* Numbers in parentheses indicate range of 95% confidence intervals.

blastine sulfate and vincristine in limited trials were observed to induce remission in 16% and 14% of cases, respectively.[77,78] Both agents are now being used only in combination regimens.

Few trials have investigated lymphokines or immunologic agents. Interferon exhibited significant antiproliferative activity against five human bladder lines,[87] and interleukin-2 has induced tumor regression of T2–T4 primary bladder lesions with intralesional administration.[88] Of note, three of six patients were observed to have had complete tumor regression, and two additional patients obtained a partial remission.[88] Both agents have not yet been investigated in a systematic disease-site trial for bladder cancer.

Combination Regimens

Cisplatin has been combined with various drugs; the most common are doxorubicin and cyclophosphamide. In most Phase II studies, significantly higher response rates have been observed only with cisplatin and doxorubicin combinations, with or without cyclophosphamide (Table 32-5).[77,78] However, randomized Phase III trials have generally been unable to find a statistically significant prolongation in survival for such combinations compared to a single drug therapy.[82,84,89] Many Phase II studies of cisplatin plus doxorubicin have noted an increased number of complete responses, with some patients living 2 to 8 years. In a trial by the Eastern Cooperative Oncology Group,[84] 33% of 45 patients responded to cisplatin, adriamycin, and cyclophosphamide

(CAP) combination compared to 17% of 48 patients given cisplatin alone. However, in another Phase III randomized trial in 46 cases, response rates were similar, 20% and 16%, respectively.[77,78] This CAP combination has also been given intra-arterially to patients with advanced local disease.[78] In contrast, the doxorubicin non-cisplatin non-methotrexate-containing regimen and the methotrexate non-cisplatin-containing regimen have generally shown no enhanced antitumor activity greater than that which could be achieved with doxorubicin or with methotrexate alone.[78]

The most efficacious new regimens combine cisplatin and methotrexate.[77,78,90,91] The European Organization for Research on Treatment of Cancer (EORTC)[90] has had the most experience, using a schedule of cisplatin, 70 mg/m² administered on day 1, and methotrexate, 40 mg/m² administered on days 8 and 15, IV, every 3 weeks. In 43 evaluable cases, 23% achieved complete and 23% partial remissions (95% confidence intervals, 31–61%).[90] Median remission duration was 54 and 24 weeks, respectively; survival had not been reached at 26 months for those achieving complete remission compared to 9 months for partial responders and stable disease cases. Toxicity was significant, with more than 50% having severe mucositis, resulting in 83% of cases never receiving the protocol as planned. Other investigators have used this two-drug combination in various schedules and dosages and have reported a significant response rate in the primary bladder lesion as well as in metastatic sites.[77,78] In a randomized trial[83] comparing the two-drug combination against cisplatin alone, the response rate was 45% in 49

TABLE 32-5. Combination Agent Trials in Previously Treated and Untreated Patients with Advanced Urothelial Tract Tumors[77,78]

Drugs	No. of Patients	% Complete and Partial Remission
Cisplatin	**320**	**30 (25–35)**
+Cyclophosphamide	113	25 (17–33)
+Doxorubicin +	142	51 (43–59)
cyclophosphamide	351	46 (41–51)
5-fluorouracil	44	44 (29–59)
5-fluorouracil + teniposide	12	58 (29–82)
+Teniposide (VM-26)	41	51 (36–67)
+Vinca + bleomycin	18	50 (24–76)
Cistaplatin + Dichloromethotrexate	49	47 (33–61)
Cisplatin + Methotrexate +	**160**	**46 (38–54)**
cyclophosphamide + doxorubicin	13	38 (17–67)
vinblastine (CMV)	**50**	**56 (42–70)**
vinblastine + doxorubicin (M-VAC)	**83**	**67 (55–76)**
Doxorubicin	**248**	**17 (12–23)**
+Cyclophosphamide +	56	23 (12–34)
5-fluorouracil	58	19 (9–29)
bleomycin	23	35 (15–55)
+5-Fluorouracil +	103	39 (29–48)
teniposide + mitomycin-C	29	48 (30–66)
+Teniposide (VM-26)	27	19 (8–36)
+Bleomycin	7	0 (0–96)
Methotrexate	**236**	**29 (23–35)**
+Cyclophosphamide + doxorubicin +	38	39 (27–52)
bleomycin + vinicristine +		
mitomycin-C	22	32 (13–58)
+Mitomycin-C	16	31 (9–54)
+Vinblastine	47	40 (22–55)

* Numbers in parentheses indicate range of 95% confidence limits.

cases (95% confidence intervals, 31–59%) compared with 33% in 51 cases (95% confidence intervals, 20–46%), respectively. In more than 160 patients given this two-drug combination, the response rate was 46% (95% confidence limits, 38–54%), with a 14% (95% confidence intervals, 9–19%) complete remission rate.[77,78] At this time, the cisplatin, methotrexate, vinblastine (CMV) and the methotrexate, vinblastine, Adriamycin (doxorubicin), cisplatin (M-VAC) regimens have not been evaluated against cisplatin plus methotrexate, and these three- and four-drug regimens may be no more active than the two-drug combination. Dichloromethotrexate, a drug excreted by way of the biliary system, thereby avoiding additive toxicity with cisplatin, in a weekly dosage schedule of 300 to 400 mg/m² was combined with cisplatin 50 to 70 mg/m² on days 1, 28, and thereafter every 6 weeks.[92] Remission rates were similar to those achieved with methotrexate and cisplatin combinations. This antifol analogue is potentially a useful agent in such combinations because of its mode of excretion, and future trials are planned.

Harker et al[93] using the CMV regimen (Table 32-6) achieved a 28% complete (95% confidence intervals, 16–41%) and 28% partial remission rate in 50 adequately treated patients: overall response rate was 56% ± 14%. Dose modifications were made for myelosuppression, changes in creatinine clearance, nausea and vomiting, and age. Approximately 31% of cases required a dose modification. Six patients (12%) experienced nadir sepsis, and 2 (4%) died secondary to chemotherapy. Median duration of complete remission was 9 months, with 6 patients in remission for 6 to 35 months. Median survival for complete remission was 44 weeks compared to 29 weeks for partial remission and 25 weeks for nonresponders. Four additional patients who had significant tumor regression with CMV plus irradiation had all disease surgically removed (CR_s). In 17 patients who still had an intact bladder, 11 had complete tumor regression: 6 given CMV alone and 5 given CMV plus irradiation.[94] Of these 11 patients, 10 clinical complete responses ($_cCR$) and 1 pathologic complete response ($_pCR$), 5 had no evidence of disease for 4 to 41 months.

Using the M-VAC regimen (Table 32-7), Sternberg et al[95] reported complete remission in 37% (95% confidence inter-

TABLE 32-6.   CMV Regimen* [93]

Drugs†	Days		
	1	2	8¶
Cisplatin‡		100	
Vinblastine	40		40
Methotrexate§	4		4

* All doses in mg/m² with cycles repeated on day 22.
† Patients > 70 years old receive 80% of all doses; if vomiting persists to day 8, no drug is given.
‡ For each cycle adjust cisplatin to 100% for Ccr > 60 ml/min; 50% of dose for Ccr 50–60 ml/min; none for Ccr < 50 ml/min.
§ No drug for a decrease on day 8 of > 30 ml/min compared to day 1 or Ccr < 50 ml/min or Cr > 1.8 mg/dl.
¶ Major dose modifications for both drugs depending on myelosuppression.

TABLE 32-7.   M-VAC Regimen* [95]

Drugs	Days			
	1	2	15	22‡
Methotrexate	30		30	30
Vinblastine		3†	3	3
Doxorubicin		30		
Cisplatin		70		

* All doses are in mg/m² and cycles are repeated every 28–32 days (see text).
† For patients having prior pelvic irradiation equivalent to > 2500 rad in 5 days, reduce the dose of doxorubicin 15 mg/m².
‡ No doses given when the WBC < 2500 cells/mm³, platelets > 100,000 cells/mm³, or mucositis present.

vals, 21–41%). Of 92 patients entered, 83 were adequately treated and had transitional cell carcinoma: 19 with $N_{3-4} M_o$ and 64 with M + disease. $_cCR$ was achieved in 13%, $_pCR$ in 12%, and CR_s in 12%. Median survival for the whole CR group has not yet been reached and will exceed 30 months: median survival for $_cCR$ and $_pCR$ will exceed 28 and 33 months, respectively; median survival has been reached for CR_s at 27 months. Considering only the N + cases, 53% achieved complete remission versus 33% for the M + cases. Liver and bone metastases were not as responsive as nodal, soft tissue, and pulmonary lesions. Patients who achieved a partial or minor remission survived a median of 11 months and nonresponders only 7 months. There were no 2-year survivors for partial or minor responders and nonresponders, whereas 71% of complete responders survived 2 years and 55% were projected to survive 3 years. Brain metastases have been noted in 18% of responders beginning 6 to 42 months after remission, half of whom never experienced systemic relapse. Nontransitional cell histologies (two cases) and carcinoma in situ lesions did not respond. Toxicity was moderately severe, with nadir sepsis in 20% of cases and 4% having a drug-related death. Renal toxicity greater than + 1 was noted in 31% and mucositis in 41%. Of note, in 25 patients who underwent surgical restaging, 24% were clinically understaged, confirming the inaccuracy of $_cCR$ status.

Although preliminary data from other M-VAC trials have found similar efficacy,[96-98] others have described significantly less responsiveness and considerably more toxicity.[99-101] In one study,[99] only three patients (15%) achieved complete remission and four (20%) had a partial response; two complete responders are alive without evidence of disease for 2 to 3.5 years. These data suggest that M-VAC may be beneficial only for low volume metastatic disease. In other trials, 1 of 12 (8%)[100] and 10 of 23 (43%)[101] patients responded. M-VAC is now being evaluated in two randomized series against methotrexate and cisplatin, each used singly; results of these Phase III studies should define more clearly the role for this regimen.

Adjuvant Neoadjuvant

Increasing efficacy of combination regimens in treatment of patients with advanced disease has led to many pilot Phase II trials employing chemotherapy adjuvantly and neoadjuvantly. Since clinically staged high-grade, high-stage (T_{3B-4}) bladder lesions are frequently (40–60%) found at radical cystectomy to have lymph node involvement ($_pN+$) and such metastases denote a poor prognosis (17%, 2-year survival, and less than 7%, 5-year survival) because of eventual tumor dissemination,[102] the rationale for systemic therapy is obvious. Additionally, if primary bladder lesions can be significantly downstaged, further therapy with irradiation or other modalities may permit surgical resection or even bladder preservation.[107–110,119,120]

While nonrandomized Phase II trials[85,86] have described significant clinical (pretherapy T versus post-therapy T stage) and, in some series, pathologic (P < T) downstaging with chemotherapy and radiation therapy, used singly or together, these positive results still need prospective randomized Phase III trials to confirm such efficacy. Many cooperative groups recently have undertaken such prospective studies; until results become available, investigators in this area need not feel compelled to institute adjuvant or neoadjuvant therapies because published randomized neoadjuvant and adjuvant studies,[103–105] generally with less than 50 cases in each arm, have yet to demonstrate benefit with chemotherapy.

These pilot trials, however, have delineated future difficulties in interpreting results from neoadjuvant therapy, suggesting that disease-free survival with or without bladder preservation at designated intervals may be the only appropriate end-point. Generally, significant clinical downstaging can be observed cystoscopically in 50% to 70% of cases,[85,106–110] cystoscopically in 60%, and pathologically in 30% to 40%.[106,111–115] The more noninvasive diagnostic T procedures used (CT and MRI scan, transrectal or abdominal sonography, urine cytology and flow cytometry, and transurethral resection with biopsy) in one series[106] decreased the clinical T remission rate to 24%. Using T staging by cystoscopic examination alone leads to significant clinical understaging (T < P), whereas noninvasive procedures can also be confusing and lead to clinical overstaging (T > P).[106] Most regimens seem to be ineffective against mixed histologies (transitional cell carcinoma plus squamous cell carcinoma or adenocarcinoma) and carcinoma in situ. Definitions of response and time to clinical and pathologic restaging vary, thereby leading to confusion in the interpretation of results. In some series, disappearance of a T_{3-4} lesion with persistence of carcinoma in situ has been interpreted as a complete response; in others, response is downgraded to a partial remission—yet both may be correct and simply represent different response criteria. Additionally, small lesions, T_2, may have been completely removed after an aggressive surgical transurethral resection, thereby rendering the patient disease-free (T_0) at the next cystoscopy[106,109–110]; chemotherapy, in this instance, actually was administered adjuvantly rather than neoadjuvantly since response may have been secondary to surgery alone. Aggressive surgical transurethral resection of tumor may explain the favorable reports of neoadjuvant chemotherapy for T_2 lesions. However, so-called radical transurethral resection of 5 to 7 cm lesions described by Hall et al[109,110] prior to initiating chemotherapy may be an important factor in increasing survival and in maintaining bladder preservation. Of 60 patients subjected to radical transurethral resection followed by 2 g IV of methotrexate every 3 weeks for 8 doses, 57% were tumor-free at 3 years, 12% experienced a recurrent T_{1-2} lesion, 12% had progressive disease and died, and 20% still had muscle invasive tumors. The 1-, 2-, and 3-year survival rates were 81%, 60%, and 52%, respectively, a rate believed to be similar to that of historical controls with irradiation and surgery alone; however, bladder preservation was possible. Preliminary results using cisplatin plus methotrexate suggested even better control (11 of 14 patients tumor-free), and this combination is now being evaluated in a prospective trial.[110] Thus, the benefit of complete endoscopic resection at the onset of treatment for removal of tumor bulk is difficult to ignore, and randomized phase III studies will need to stratify such patients, based on surgical resection, before randomization.

Adjuvant trials, which define more precisely tumor stage prior to chemotherapy, should require fewer patient entries because there is less need to compensate for the 30% to 50% error in clinical staging. Patient selection can be minimized but still may be a major factor in the interpretation of results, as illustrated in one series in which 475 patients were considered for therapy, 220 were entered onto the study, 180 completed radiation and radical cystectomy, and only 83 were able to be randomized to cisplatin versus no therapy. Of note, of the 43 patients randomized to cisplatin, only 9 received the planned 8 doses.[103] It is not surprising that there was no major improvement in the disease-free survival for the cisplatin-treated group.

The roles for combined cisplatin and radiation therapy for selected patients in whom medical indications precluded radical cystectomy[98,107,115] and for a sandwich technique of chemotherapy and radiation therapy are also under investigation, with interesting preliminary results.

The National Bladder Cancer Group treated patients with muscle-invading bladder cancer (clinical stages T2–T4) who were *not* candidates for cystectomy. The initial complete response rate was high (77%), however, among the 57 patients who had gross residual disease and who were evaluated cystoscopically, 23% of the completely responding tumors have recurred to date, mostly in patients with large tumors.[115] The actuarial 4-year survival rate for the entire group, whether or not they completed the planned treatment, is 35% and is significantly better for patients with clinical stage T2 tumors (64%) than those with clinical stage T3 or T4 cancers (Fig. 32-4). Jakse and colleagues[116] from Innsbruck report a similar experience in 44 patients, with a complete response rate of 75% and with local relapse in only 15% of the completely responding group. The actuarial 5-year survival for all patients in this series is 46% and is 66% for the completely responding patients. Currently, many institutions and multidisciplinary groups are using combinations of chemotherapy and radiation therapy,[119,120] both together and alone, as "upfront" or neoadjuvant treatment in patients with invasive bladder carcinoma to evaluate the possibility of selecting for treatment with bladder preservation only patients who have a complete response to this regimen following chemotherapy and 4000 cGy of irradiation, and thus who have a high probability of having had, without cystectomy, the local cure of their bladder cancer. The complete responding patients undergo consolidation with irradia-

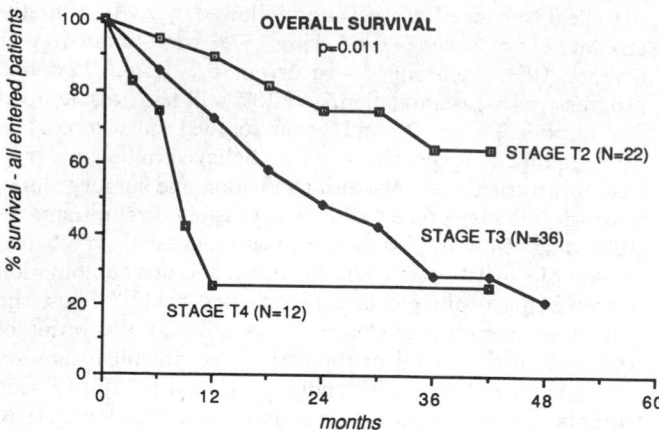

FIG. 32-4. Actuarial survival by clinical stage for all 70 patients entered on the National Bladder Cancer Group protocol of cisplatin and full-dose radiation therapy.[115]

tion to 6000 to 6500 cGy plus cisplatin. The patients whose tumors do not respond completely to chemotherapy plus 4000 cGy are recommended to undergo immediate cystectomy.

In the final analysis, however, we must await the data from investigative prospectively randomized trials before accepting adjuvant or neadjuvant treatment modalities.

FUTURE CONSIDERATIONS

Improvement in survival rates must rely on earlier detection and development of new therapeutic strategies to combat unrecognized micrometastases. Flow cytomery holds promise as an automated technique to identify changes in DNA/RNA ratio and, when further refined, may serve an important screening function. Identification of oncogenes related to cellular transformation should open exciting new pathways for diagnosis and treatment. Although surgical extirpation has been the mainstay of treatment, therapy combining local–regional control with systemic control, with agents such as cisplatin in combination with other chemotherapeutic agents, may help to reduce the overall mortality from distant metastases and result in improved long-term disease-free survival rate. Phase III trials randomized with or without adjuvant cisplatin-and-methotrexate-containing regimens are underway to evaluate this hopeful possibility. Innovative selective bladder-sparing approaches await confirmation of efficacy by prospective multi-institutional trials.

REFERENCES

1. Silverberg E: Cancer Statistics, 1988. CA 38:14, 1988
2. Rehn L: Blasen Geschwulste Bei Fuchsin—Arbeitern. Arch Klin Chir 50:588, 1895
3. Clayson DB: Epidemiology of Bladder Cancer. In Cooper EH, Williams RE, (eds): The Biology and Clinical Management of Bladder Cancer p, 65. Oxford, England, Blackwell Scientific Publications, 1975
4. Winder EL, Goldsmith R: The Epidemiology of Bladder Cancer: The Second Look. Cancer 40:1246, 1977
5. Miller AB: Bladder Cancer—Epidemiology. In Wilkinson PM (ed): Advances in Medical Oncology, Research and Education; Vol XI, Clinical Cancer—Principal Sites II, p 201. Elmsford, New York, Pergamon Press, 1979
6. Hicks RM, Chowaniec J: Experimental induction, histology and ultrastructure of hyperplasia and neoplasia in the urinary bladder epithelium. International Review Experimental Pathology 18:199, 1978
7. Morrison AS, Buring JE: Artificial sweeteners in cancer of the lower urinary tract. N Eng J Med 302:537, 1980
8. El-Asar AA, et al: Study of the etiological factor of bilharzial bladder cancer in Egypt: Five-urinary nitrite in a rural population. Tumori 66:409, 1980
9. Collan Y, Makinen J, Heikkenen A: Histologic grading of transitional cell tumors of the bladder: Value of histologic grading (WHO) in prognosis. Eur Urol 5:311, 1979
10. Mostofi FK: Pathology in staging of bladder cancer. In Wilkinson PM (ed): Advances in Medical Oncology Research and Education, Vol XI, Clinical Cancer—Principal Site II, p 213. Elmsford, New York, Pergamon Press, 1979
11. Lerman RI, Hutter RVP, Whitmore WF Jr: Papilloma of the urinary bladder. Cancer 25:333, 1970
12. Koss LG: Mapping of the urinary bladder: Its impact on the concepts of bladder cancer. Hum Pathol 10:533, 1979
13. DeFelippo N, Fortunato R, Mellins HZ, et al: Intravenous urogram: Important adjunct for the diagnosis of bladder tumors. Br J Urol 56:502, 1984
14. Prout GR Jr, Griffin PP, Shipley WU: Bladder carcinoma as a systemic disease. Cancer 43:2532, 1979
15. Jewett HJ, Strong GH: Infiltrating carcinoma of the bladder: Relation of depth of penetration of the bladder wall to incidence of local extension in metastases. J Urol 55:366, 1946
16. Marshall VF: The relation of the preoperative estimate to the pathologic demonstration of the extent of vesical neoplasms. J Urol 68:714, 1952
17. Richie JP, Skinner DG, Kaufman JJ: Radical cystectomy for carcinoma of the bladder: 16 years of experience. J Urol 113:186, 1975
18. American Joint Committee for Cancer Staging, Beahrs OH, Myers MH (eds): Manual for Staging of Cancer, 2nd ed, p 171. Philadelphia, JB Lippincott, 1983
19. Skinner DG, Tift JP, Kaufman JJ: High-dose, short-course preoperative radiation therapy and immediate single stage radical cystectomy with pelvic node dissection in the management of bladder cancer. J Urol 127:671, 1982
20. Garnick MB, Schade D, Israel M, et al: Intravesical doxorubicin for prophylaxis in the management of recurrent superficial bladder carcinoma. J Urol 131:43, 1984
21. Soloway MS: Surgery and intravesical chemotherapy in the management of superficial bladder cancer. Semin Urol 1:23, 1983
22. Soloway MS, Murphy WM: Experimental chemotherapy of bladder cancer systemic and intravesical. Semin Oncol 6:168, 1979
23. Burnand KG, Boyd PJR, Mayo ME, et al: Single dose intravesical thiotepa as an adjuvant to cystodiathermy in the treatment of transitional cell bladder carcinoma. Br J Urol 50:237, 1978
24. Koontz WW Jr, Prout GR Jr, Smith W, et al: The use of intravesical thio-tepa in the management of non-invasive carcinoma of the bladder. J Urol 125:307, 1981
25. Hollister D, Coleman M: Hematologic effects of intravesicular thiotepa therapy for bladder cancer. JAMA 244:2065, 1980
26. Bracken RB, Johnson DE, von Eschenbach AC, et al: Role of intravesical mitomycin-C in management of superficial bladder tumors. Urology 16:11, 1980
27. Niijima T: Intravesical therapy with adriamycin and new trends in the diagnostics and therapy of superficial urinary bladder tumors. In Montedison Laekermedol AB (ed): Diagnostics and Treatment of Superficial Urinary Bladder Tumours, p 37. Stockholm, WHO Collaborating Centre for Research and Treatment of Urinary Bladder Cancer, 1979
28. Blumenreich MS, Needles B, Yagoda A, et al: Intravesical cisplatin for superficial bladder tumors. Cancer 50:863, 1982
29. Lamm DL, Thor DE, Winters WD, et al: BCG immunotherapy of bladder cancer: Inhibition of tumor recurrence and associated immune response. Cancer 48:82, 1981
30. Pinsky C, Camacho F, Kerr D, et al: Treatment of superficial bladder cancer with intravesical BCG. Proc Am Soc Clin Oncol (abstract C-223). 2:57, 1983
31. Herr HW: Carcinoma in situ of the bladder. Semin Urol 1:15–22, 1983
32. Lamm DL: Bacillus Calmette-Guerin immunotherapy for bladder cancer. J Urol 134:40, 1985
33. Brosman SA: The use of Bacillus Calmette-Guerin in the therapy of bladder carcinoma in situ. J Urol 134:36, 1985
34. Utz DC, Hanash KA, Farrow GM: The plight of the patient with carcinoma in situ of the bladder. J Urol 103:160, 1970
35. Utz DC, Farrow GM, Rife CC, et al: Carcinoma in situ of the bladder. Cancer 45:1842, 1980
36. Marshall VF, Holden J, Ma KT, et al: Survival of patients with bladder carcinoma treated by simple segmental resection. Cancer 9:568, 1956
37. Masina F: Segmental resection for tumors of the urinary bladder: Ten-year follow-up. Br J Surg 52:279, 1965
38. Miller LS, Johnson DE: Megavoltage radiation for bladder carcinoma: Alone, post-operative, or pre-operative, p 771. Seventh National Cancer Conference Proceedings, 1973
39. Boileau MA, Johnson ED, Chan RC, et al: Bladder carcinoma: Results with preoperative radiation therapy and radical cystectomy. Urology 16: 569–576, 1980
40. Shipley WU, Rose MA, Perrone TL, et al: Full-dose irradiation for patients with invasive bladder carcinoma: Clinical and histological factors prognostic of improved survival. J Urol 134:679–683, 1985
41. Timmer PR, Hartlief HA, Hooijkaas JA: Bladder cancer: Pattern of recurrence in 142 patients. Int J Radiat Oncol Biol Phys 11:899–905, 1985
42. Quilty PM, Duncan W: Primary radical radiotherapy for T3 transitional cell cancer of

the bladder: An analysis of survival and control. Int J Radiat Oncol Biol Phys 12:853–860, 1986

43. Blandy JP, Jenkins BJ, Fowler CG, et al: Radical radiotherapy and salvage cystectomy for T2 and T3 cancer of the bladder. In Smith PM, Pavone-Macaluso MM (eds): The Treatment of Advanced Bladder Cancer. New York, AR Liss (in press)

44. Bowles WT, Cordonnier JJ: Total cystectomy for carcinoma of the bladder. J Urol 90:731, 1963

45. Jewett HJ, King LR, Shelley WM: A study of 365 cases of infiltrating bladder cancer: Relation of certain pathological characteristics to prognosis after extirpation. J Urol 92:668, 1964

46. Pearse HD, Reed RR, Hodges CV: Radical cystectomy for bladder cancer. J Urol 119:216, 1978

47. Mathur VK, Krahn HP, Ramsey EW: Total cystectomy for bladder cancer. J Urol 125:784, 1981

48. Skinner DG, Lieskovsky G: Contemporary cystectomy with pelvic node dissection compared to preoperative radiation therapy plus cystectomy in management of invasive bladder cancer. J Urol 131:1069, 1984

49. Skinner DG, Lieskovsky G: Management of invasive and high-grade bladder cancer. In Skinner DG, Lieskovsky G (eds): Diagnosis and Management of Genitourinary Cancer pp 295–312. Philadelphia, WB Saunders, 1988

50. Glantz GN: Cystectomy and urinary diversion. J Urol 96:714, 1966

51. Whitmore WF Jr, Marshall VF: Radical total cystectomy for cancer of the bladder: 230 consecutive cases five years later. J Urol 87:853, 1962

52. Johnson DE, Lamy SM: Complications of a single stage radical cystectomy and ileal conduit diversion: review of 214 cases. J Urol 117:171, 1977

53. Skinner DG: Current perspectives in the management of high-grade invasive bladder cancer. Cancer 45:1866–1874, 1980

54. Whitmore WF Jr, Batata MA, Ghoneim MA, et al: Radical cystectomy with or without prior radiation in the treatment of bladder cancer. J Urol 118:184, 1977

55. Montie JE, Straffon RA, Stewart BH: Radical cystectomy without radiation therapy for carcinoma of the bladder. J Urol 131:477, 1984

56. Goffinet DR, Schneider NJ, Glatstein EJ, et al: Bladder cancer: Results of radiation therapy in 384 patients. Radiology 117:149, 1975

57. Blandy JP, England HR, Evans SJW, et al: T3 bladder cancer—the case for salvage cystectomy. Br J Urol 52:506, 1980

58. van der Werf-Messing B: Carcinoma of the urinary bladder T3 NX MO treated by preoperative radiation followed by simple cystectomy. Int J Radiat Oncol Biol Phys 8:1849–1855, 1982

59. Shipley WU, Coombs LJ, Prout GR Jr: Preoperative irradiation and radical cystectomy for invasive cancer—patterns of failure and prognostic factors associated with patient survival and disease progression. J Urol 135:222A, 1986

60. Jewett HJ, King LR, Shelley WJ: A study of 365 cases of infiltration bladder cancer: Relation of certain pathologic characteristics to prognosis after extirpation. J Urol 92:668, 1964

61. Soto EA, Friedell GH, Tiltman AJ: Bladder cancer as seen in giant histologic sections. Cancer 39:447, 1977

62. Slack NH, Prout GR Jr: The heterogeneity of invasive bladder carcinoma and different responses to treatment. J Urol 123:644, 1980

63. Heney NM, Proppe K, Prout GR Jr, et al: Invasive bladder cancer: Tumor configuration, lymphatic invasion and survival. J Urol 130:895, 1983

64. Prout GR Jr: Radiation therapy and cystectomy. Urol 23(Suppl 4):104, 1984

65. van der Werf-Messing B, Menon RS, Hop WCJ: Carcinoma of the urinary bladder category T2, T3, Nx, MO, treated by interstitial radium implant. In Smith PH, Pavone-Macaluso MM (eds): The Treatment of Advanced Bladder Cancer. New York, AR Liss, (in press)

66. van der Werf-Messing B, Menon RS, Hop WL: Cancer of the urinary bladder T2, T3 (NXMO) treated by interstitial radium implant: Second report. Int J Radiat Oncol Biol Phys 7:481–485, 1983

67. Battermann JJ, Tierie AH: Results of implantation for T1 and T2 bladder tumors. Radiother Oncol 5:85–90, 1986

68. Mazeron JJ, Marinello G, Pierquin B, et al: Treatment of bladder tumors by iridium-192 implantation: The Creteil technique. Radiother Oncol 4:111–119, 1985

69. Matsumoto L, Kakizoe T, Mikuriya S, et al: Clinical evaluation of intraoperative radiotherapy for carcinoma of the urinary bladder. Cancer 47:509–513, 1981

70. Reiner WG, Walsh PC: An anatomical approach to the surgical management of the dorsal vein and Santorini's plexus during radical retropubic surgery. J Urol 121:998, 1978

71. Walsh PC, Donker PJ: Impotence following radical prostatectomy: Insight into etiology and prevention. J Urol 128:492, 1982

72. Kock NG, Nilson AE, Nilsson LO, et al: Urinary diversion via a continent ileal reservoir: Clinical results in 12 patients. J Urol 128:469, 1982

73. Lilien OM, Camey M: 25-year experience with replacement of the human bladder (Camey procedure). J Urol 132:886, 1984

74. Rowland RG, Mitchell ME, Bihrle R, et al: Indiana continent urinary reservoir. J Urol 137:1136, 1987

75. Thuroff JW, Alken P, Riedmiller H, et al: The Mainz pouch (mixed augmentation ileum and cecum) for bladder augmentation and continent diversion. J Urol 136:17, 1986

76. Duncan W, Williams JR, et al: An analysis of the radiation related morbidity observed in a randomized trial of neutron therapy for bladder cancer. Int J Radiat Oncol Biol Phys 12:2085–2092, 1986

77. Yagoda A: Chemotherapy of urothelial tract tumors. Cancer 60:1879, 1987

78. Yagoda A: Chemotherapy for advanced bladder cancer. In Yagoda A (ed): Bladder Cancer: Future Directions for Treatment, p 87. New York, John Wiley & Sons, 1986

79. Yagoda A: Future implications of phase II chemotherapy trials in 95 patients with measurable advanced bladder cancer. Cancer Res 37:2775–2780, 1977

80. Yagoda A: Progress in treatment of advanced urothelial tract cancer tumors. J Clin Oncol 3:1448, 1985

81. Van Oosterom AT, Akaza H, Hall R, et al: Response criteria phase II/phase III invasive bladder cancer. In Denis L, Niijima A, Prout GR Jr, et al (eds): Developments in Bladder Cancer, p 301. New York, Alan R Liss, 1986

82. Soloway MS, Einstein A, Corder MP, et al: A comparison of cisplatin and the combination of cisplatin and cyclophosphamide in advanced urothelial cancer. Cancer 52:767, 1983

83. Hillcoat BL, Raghavan D: A randomized comparison of cisplatin (C) versus cisplatinum and methotrexate (C + M) in advanced bladder cancer. Proc Am Soc Clin Oncol 5(Abstr 426):110, 1986

84. Khandekar JD, Elson PJ, DeWys WD, et al: Comparative activity and toxicity of cis-diamminedichloroplatinum (DDP) and a combination of doxorubicin, cyclophosphamide, and DDP in disseminated transitional cell carcinoma of the urinary tract. J Clin Oncol 3:539, 1985

85. Ragahavan D, Pearson B, Duval P, et al: Initial intravenous cisplatin therapy: Improved management for invasive high risk bladder cancer. J Urol 133:399, 1985

86. Fagg SL, Dawson-Edwards P, Hughes MA, et al: Cis-diamminedichloroplatinum (DDP) as initial treatment of invasive bladder cancer. Br J Urol 56:296, 1984

87. Borden EC, Groveman DS, Nasu T, et al: Antiproliferative activities of interferons against human bladder carcinoma cell lines in vitro. Int J Cancer 34:359, 1984

88. Pizza G, Severni G, Menniti D, et al: Tumor regression after intralesional injection of interleukin 2 (IL-2) in bladder cancer: preliminary report. Int J Cancer 34:359, 1984

89. Al-Sarraf M, Frank J, Smith J Jr, et al: Phase II trial of cyclophosphamide, doxorubicin and cisplatin (CAP) versus amsacrine in patients with transitional cell carcinoma of the urinary bladder: A southwest oncology group study. Cancer Treat Rep 69:189, 1985

90. Stoter G, Splinter TAW, Child JA, et al: Combination chemotherapy with cisplatin and methotrexate in advanced transitional cell cancer of the bladder. J Urol 137:663, 1987

91. Carmichael J, Cornbleet MA, MacDougall RH, et al: Cis-platin and methotrexate in treatment of transitional cell carcinoma of the urinary tract. Br J Urol 57:299, 1985

92. Natale RB, Wheeler RH, Ensminger W, et al: Cisplatin and dichloromethotrexate (DCM): A pharmacologically rational combination with high activity. Proc Am Assoc Cancer Res 24:166(Abstr. 659), 1983

93. Harker WG, Meyers FJ, Freiha FS, et al: Cisplatin, methotrexate and vinblastine (CMV): An effective chemotherapy regimen for metastatic transitional cell carcinoma of the urinary tract. A Northern California oncology group study. J Clin Oncol 134:1118, 1985

94. Meyers FJ, Palmer JM, Freiha FS, et al: The fate of the bladder in patients with metastatic bladder cancer treated with cisplatin, methotrexate, and vinblastine: A Northern California Oncology group study. J Urol 134:118, 1985

95. Sternberg CN, Yagoda A, Scher HI, et al: M-VAC (methotrexate, vinblastine, adriamycin, and cisplatin) for advanced transitional cell carcinoma of the urothelium. J Urol 139:461, 1988

96. Hasun R, Pont J, Marberger M, et al: M-VAC for recurrent urothelial tumor after radical surgery. 10th International Symposium on the Chemotherapy of Bladder Cancer, Abstr 149. Vienna, Austria, February 18–21, 1987

97. Chong C, Logothetis CJ, Dexus FH, et al: M-VAC as salvage chemotherapy in transitional cell carcinoma (TCC) of the urothelium previously treated with cisplatin combination chemotherapy. Proc Am Assoc Cancer Res 28(Abstr 810):204, 1987

98. Srougi M: Estrategia de tratamento do cander de bexiga. J Brasil Urol (in press)

99. Tannock I: Chemotherapy with M-VAC at the Princess Margaret Hospital (Abstr 9). Acta Urol Ital 1(Suppl 1):7, 1987

100. Droz JP, Lupera H, Gliosen M, et al: Phase I trial of methotrexate (M), vinblastine (V), adriamycin (A), and cisplatin (C) (M-VAC regimen) in advanced stage bladder cancer (Abstr 11). Acta Urol Ital 1(Suppl 1):8, 1987

101. de La Pena J, Martinez-Peneiro JM, Cisneros J, et al: M-VAC chemotherapy in disseminated bladder cancer (Abstr 10). Acta Urol Ital 1(Suppl 1):7, 1987

102. Smith JA, Whitmore WF: Regional lymph node metastases from bladder cancer. J Urol 126:591, 1981

103. Einstein A, Coombs J, Pearse H, et al: Cisplatin (CP) adjuvant therapy following pre-operative radiotherapy plus radical cystectomy (RT + RCy) for invasive bladder carcinoma: A randomized trial of the National Bladder Cancer group (NBCP). Am Urol Assoc 133(Abstr 433):222, 1985

104. de La Pena J, Martinez-Pineiro JM, Leon JJ, et al: Cisplatinum plus cystectomy vs. cystectomy alone in invasive bladder cancer: Preliminary results of a randomized multicentre study (Abstr 19). Acta Urol Ital 1(Suppl 1):10, 1987

105. Daniels JR, Skinner DG, Lieskovsky G: Chemotherapy of carcinoma of the bladder. In Skinner DG, Lieskovsky G: Diagnosis and Management of Genitourinary Cancer, pp 313–322. Philadelphia, WB Saunders, 1988

106. Scher HI, Yagoda A, Herr H, et al: Neoadjuvant M-VAC (methotrexate, vinblastine, adriamycin, and cisplatin): The effect on the primary bladder lesion. J Urol (in press)

107. Shipley WU, Coombs LJ, Einstein AB, et al: Cisplatin and full dose irradiation for patients with invasive bladder cancer: A preliminary report of tolerance and local response. J Urol 132:899, 1984

108. Jaske G, Frommhold H, Nedden DZ: Combined radiation and chemotherapy for

locally advanced transitional cell carcinoma of the urinary bladder. Cancer 52:767, 1983

109. Hall RR, Newling DWW, Ramsden PD, et al: Treatment of invasive bladder cancer by local resection and high dose methotrexate. Br J Urol 56:668, 1984

110. Hall RR: Transurethral resection and systemic chemotherapy as primary treatment for T₃ bladder cancer. In Yagoda A (ed): Bladder Cancer: Future Directions for Treatment, p 111. New York, John Wiley & Sons, 1986

111. Scher HI, Yagoda A, Herr H, et al: Neoadjuvant M-VAC (methotrexate, vinblastine, adriamycin and cisplatin) for extravesical urinary tract tumors. J Urol (in press)

112. Simon SD, Srougi M: Systemic M-VAC chemotherapy for primary treatment of locally invasive transitional cell carcinoma of the bladder (TCCB): A pilot study. Pro Am Soc Clin Oncol 5(Abstr 432):11, 1987

113. Bukowski RM, Montie JE, Lee M, et al: Neoadjuvant M-VAC with intraarterial (i.a.) cisplatin in locally advanced transitional cell carcinoma of the bladder. J Urol 137(Abstr 211):156A, 1987

114. Sabri SE, Zincke H, Keating JP, et al: Neoadjuvant chemotherapy (M-VAC) prior to cystectomy for high stage (T2-4NxMo) bladder cancer: Do local pathological findings suggest a potential for bladder salvage. J Urol 137(Abstr 212):156A, 1987

115. Shipley WU, Prout GR Jr, Einstein AB Jr, et al: Treatment of invasive bladder cancer by cisplatin and radiation in patients unsuited for surgery. JAMA 258:931–935, 1987

116. Jakse G, Frommhold H, Nedden DZ: Combined radiation and chemotherapy for locally advanced transitional cell carcinoma of the urinary bladder. Cancer 55:1659–1664, 1985

117. Batata MA, Chu FCH, Hilaris BS, et al: Preoperative whole pelvis versus through pelvis irradiation and cystectomy for bladder cancer. Int J Radiat Oncol Biol Phys 7:1349–1355, 1981

118. Bloom HCG, Hendry WR, Wallace DM, et al: Treatment of T3 Bladder Cancer: A controlled trial of preoperative radiotherapy and radical cystectomy versus radical radiotherapy, 2nd report and review. Br J Urol 54:136, 1982

119. Prout GR Jr, Kaufman SD, Shipley WU, et al: Combined therapy in the treatment of patients with muscle-invading bladder cancer: A preliminary report of a bladder-sparing effort. J Urol 139:268A, 1988

120. Wajsman Z, Klimberg IW, Parsons JJ, et al: Bladder sparing treatment for muscle invasive transitional cell carcinoma: Cystemic chemotherapy followed by radiation therapy with adjunctive cysplatin. J Urol 139:268A, 1988

CARLOS A. PEREZ
WILLIAM R. FAIR
DANIEL C. IHDE

CHAPTER 33 *Carcinoma of the Prostate*

Adenocarcinoma of the prostate is a common tumor in man. In 1987 it was estimated that in the United States 90,000 new cases were clinically diagnosed and 26,000 patients died of the disease.[1]

The prostatic cell is the target for many hormonal and chemical substances that control the gland's proliferative rate and biologic behavior[2]; this influence stems from organs as close as the testicle or the adrenal cortex and as far away as the pituitary and the hypothalamus.[3] Recently tissue- and tumor-specific antigens and associated antigens have been identified in several animal tumor systems.[4,5]

The role of the prostate in causing bladder outlet obstruction was first defined by Ferri of Naples in 1530.[6] The earliest anatomical illustration depicting the prostate was published in the Tabulae Anatomicae by Vesalius in 1538. The first known reference to a prostatic tumor causing obstruction of the bladder neck was by Riolan in 1649,[7] but the earliest specific reference to carcinoma of the prostate was made by Baillie in 1794.[8]

In 1786 John Hunter, the great English anatomist, demonstrated that removing the testicles from young male animals prevented the growth of the prostate; in a mature animal orchiectomy was followed by prostatic atrophy.[9] Some 150 years later Huggins and Hodge demonstrated that regression of carcinoma of the prostate could be induced by endocrine manipulation.

EPIDEMIOLOGY AND GENETICS

The annual incidence of prostatic cancer in the United States is approximately 58 per 100,000 white men and 95 per 100,000 black men. Although some reports indicate that the incidence of prostatic cancer is rising,[10] the overall incidence from 1940 to 1980 remained unchanged. The 5-year survival rate in white men increased to 63% for those diagnosed between 1970 and 1973, compared with 50% for those diagnosed a decade earlier. For blacks, the 5-year survival rate for those diagnosed between 1970 and 1973 was 55%, a 20% increase over the survival rate for those diagnosed in the period 1960 to 1963.[11]

There is a 40-fold difference in incidence of prostatic cancer between U.S. blacks, who have one of the highest rates in the world, and residents of Japan, who have one of the lowest rates.[12] Breslow and co-workers found significant differences between the low rate of latent carcinoma in Chinese populations from Hong Kong and Singapore compared with the high rate in men in Sweden, the Federal Republic of Germany, and blacks from Jamaica; an intermediate frequency was found for Israelis and black Ugandans.[13] The prevalence of small latent carcinomas was about 12% in all areas studied, and they occurred at a constant frequency in all age groups. Support for the concept that these differences may be related to environmental factors stems from the observation that persons emigrating from low-risk countries to the United States have rates of clinical disease intermediate between those of their country of origin and the United States.[14,15]

No particular influence of urban or rural residence on the subsequent development of prostatic cancer has been demonstrated; this is inconsistent with the hypothesis that environmental factors may play a major role in causing the disease.[10,16-20] The prostate is one of the major cancer sites in man for which an association with smoking has not been demonstrated.[21] An intensive study of the incidence of prostatic cancer in Japanese men found no relationship between residence in the Hiroshima and Nagasaki areas at the time of the atomic bomb explosions and the subsequent development of prostatic carcinoma.[22] A familial association has been reported in several studies.[17,18,23,24]

Steele and co-workers identified an increased number of sexual partners and a higher occurrence of venereal disease in a patient group compared with controls, suggesting a possible viral-venereal relationship to prostatic cancer.[24] Although there is little agreement in the literature as to the possible roles of coital frequency or numbers of sexual partners, some studies confirm a higher frequency of previous venereal disease in patients with prostatic cancer.[25,26] The role of circumcision in the development of prostatic cancer was studied by Wynder et al[18] and Rotkin[27]; no significant correlations were found. Despite long debate, the role of hormones in the etiology of carcinoma of the prostate is obscure, for the following reasons: (1) prostatic cancer does not develop in eunuchs; (2) many cases of metastatic disease of the prostate appear to be hormonally dependent; and (3) latent prostatic cancer is lower than expected in cirrhotic men who have elevated blood levels of endogenous estrogens.[28,29] Despite the decrease in latent carcinoma of the prostate in patients with cirrhosis, when worldwide mortality rates for patients with cirrhosis are correlated with the rate of prostatic cancer, the presence or absence of cirrhosis appears entirely unrelated to death from prostatic cancer.[30]

Prostatic cancer and benign prostatic hyperplasia are often found concurrently in older men. Greenwald and co-workers observed 838 patients with benign prostatic hyperplasia and 802 age-matched controls for an average of 10 years and found no difference in the prevalence of prostatic cancer between the two groups[31] Armenian et al,[32] in a study of 296 patients with benign prostatic hyperplasia diagnosed either histologically or clinically and 299 age-matched controls followed up for 7 to 27 years, found the incidence of prostatic cancer to be 3.7 times higher in men with benign prostatic hyperplasia than in the controls. This issue is still unsettled.

ANATOMICAL CONSIDERATIONS

The prostate gland is a solid organ that surrounds the urethra between the base of the bladder and the urogenital diaphragm. It has a walnut-shaped, somewhat pyramidal configuration and is situated just distal to the bladder neck, its apex resting against the urogenital diaphragm (Fig. 33-1). The normal prostate has a consistency similar to that of the tip of the nose, carcinoma characteristically having a firmer consistency.[33] The normal prostate weighs about 20 g. The lateral margins of the prostate are delineated usually against the levator ani muscles forming the lateral prostatic sulci. Often there is a midline furrow that demarcates the left and right lobes of the prostate. These anatomical structures may be lost when there is extensive involvement of the gland by tumor or periprostatic extension. The prostate consists of fibrous acinar, glandular, muscular, and vascular elements.

Anteriorly the prostate is attached to the pubic symphysis by the puboprostatic ligaments; posteriorly it is separated from the rectum by Denonvilliers' fascia. In the fetus the

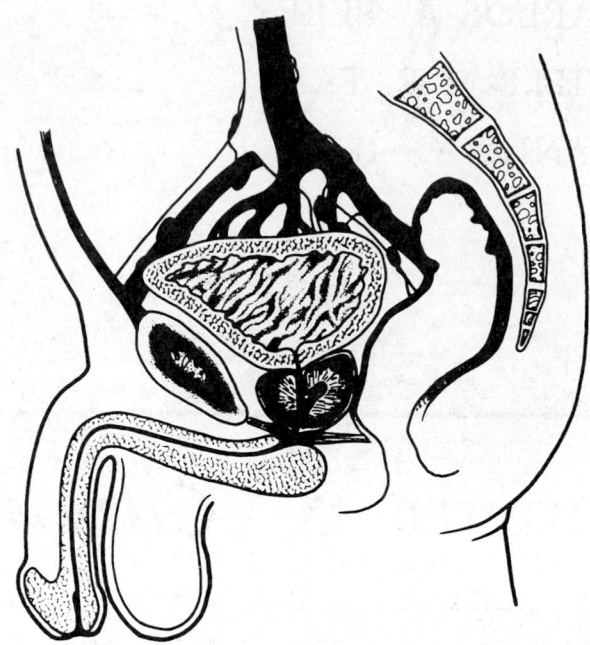

FIG. 33-1. Anatomy of male urogenital system (sagittal section).

peritoneum of the pelvic floor extends down as a continuation of the pouch of Douglas behind the prostate gland. In later life the two layers are fused, with a potential space between them. Denonvilliers' fascia is attached above to the peritoneum and below to the urogenital diaphragm; it limits the posterior extension of prostatic carcinoma into the rectum. Attached to the posterior superior aspect of the prostate are the seminal vesicles and the vas deferens, which pierce the gland to enter the urethra at the verumontanum.

Classically the prostate has been described as consisting of five lobes: anterior, posterior, median, and two lateral lobes. The posterior lobe extends across the entire posterior surface of the gland and is the portion of the gland felt by the examining rectal finger. McNeal, in an elegant study of the morphological anatomy of the prostate, defined four basic anatomical areas[34]:

1. The peripheral zone, constituting 70% of the glandular prostate. Almost all carcinomas of the prostate arise in this gland.
2. The central zone, constituting 25% of the glandular prostate. The central zone is markedly different histologically from the peripheral zone.
3. The preprostatic region, the urethral segment proximal to the verumontanum. The preprostatic region is the exclusive site of benign prostatic hyperplasia.
4. The anterior fibromuscular stroma, which forms the anterior surface of the prostate.

The prostatic acini are lined with a columnar epithelium with two cell layers (basal and principal cells); the peripheral ducts are lined by a single layer of glandular epithelium that merges with the transitional epithelium of the central prostatic ducts and urethra.

NATURAL HISTORY AND ROUTES OF SPREAD

More than 95% of prostatic carcinomas arise in the glandular epithelium of the peripheral glands of the prostate,[35-37] in contrast to benign prostatic hyperplasia, which originates from the central or periurethral portions of the gland. These observations led McNeal to conclude that "evidence from volume distribution data suggests that there are not two types of prostatic carcinoma with different biologic potential, but a single species having slow growth rate with a logarithmic growth curve. The development of carcinoma in the gland follows predictable patterns, including early involvement of the capsule and perineural spaces. The later course of tumor growth is characterized by a loss of differentiation and the ability to penetrate the capsule and periurethral stroma."[35]

Breslow et al demonstrated that carcinoma is more common in the apex (caudal portion) of the prostate; 64% of 350 carcinomas were detected in a section taken 5 mm from the distal end of the prostate.[13] Thus, unless the urethra is transected distal to the prostate, the likelihood of leaving prostatic cancer behind is extremely high; this is a further argument against the common practice of leaving a "button" of distal prostate to facilitate the urethrovesical anastomosis.[35,38-40]

An increased incidence of Stage A lesions has been found in older patients.[41-44] As stated by Whitmore, "although it is reasonable to assume that the stage A prostatic lesion is the source of all clinically evident prostatic cancers, it is also apparent that most stage A tumors never become clinically manifest."[41] The clinical incidence of Stage A tumors is about half of that predicted by autopsy studies, strongly suggesting that these lesions do not become clinically manifest within the lifetime of the host.

The tumor may form one or more nodules involving one or more lobes; in 77% of pathologic specimens of radical prostatectomies resected by Jewett, multiple tumor foci were found throughout the gland.[45] Because of the peripheral location of the lesions, tumor later extends into and through the capsule of the gland, and invades periprostatic tissues. It may extend into the seminal vesicles, and later involve the bladder neck or the rectum. Tumor invasion of the perineural spaces and the lymphatics as well as the blood vessels explains the tendency of the tumor to produce lymphatic or distant metastases.

LYMPH NODE METASTASES

Depending on the extent of the tumor and the degree of differentiation, the tumor may metastasize to the regional lymphatics. Flocks et al in a study of 411 patients were among the first to correlate the size of the gland and the probability of lymphatic metastases.[46] Table 33-1 shows the relationship of clinical stage and degree of differentiation of the tumor with the frequency of nodal metastases.[47]

McLaughlin et al found that multiple lymph nodes were frequently affected in patients with well-differentiated tumors, not only those with poorly differentiated tumors.[48] The lymph nodes most commonly involved were the obturator and hypogastric, followed by the external iliac group.

The earliest lymph nodes to be involved are those in the periprostatic and obturator area (Fig. 33-2). The tumor subsequently involves the external iliac and hypogastric lymph nodes, and later the common iliac and periaortic nodes. Approximately 7% of patients have involvement of the presacral and presciatic lymph nodes (including promontorial and middle hemorrhoidal group) without evidence of metastases to the external iliac or hypogastric lymph nodes.[49]

Pistenma et al reported findings in 93 patients in whom lymphangiography and pelvic and retroperitoneal lymph node dissections were carried out.[50] Table 33-2 lists the frequency of lymph node involvement by anatomical site in these 93 patients.

Prout et al reported similar findings in 92 patients with various stages of prostatic carcinoma who underwent pelvic lymphadenectomy.[51] More patients with extracapsular extension had pelvic nodal metastases. Solitary lymph node metastases were noted in 11 of 32 patients with positive nodes. Bilateral pelvic lymph node involvement was present in 14 of 24 patients with more than one metastatic lymph node.

Prognosis is closely related to the presence or absence of lymph node metastases (Fig. 33-3).[51] Prout et al found that

TABLE 33-1. Frequency of Pelvic Node Metastasis by Histologic Grade and Clinical Stage*

| | Grade | | | |
| | Well Differentiated | Moderately Differentiated | Poorly Differentiated | |
Stage	No./Total (%)	No./Total (%)	No./Total (%)	Total (%)
A1	0/28	0/12	0/1	0/41
A2	0/7	5/19 (26)	3/7 (43)	8/33 (24)
B1	2/53 (4)	13/94 (14)	3/9 (33)	18/156 (12)
B2	5/27 (18)	29/106 (27)	9/21 (43)	43/154 (28)
C	5/10 (50)	18/44 (41)	13/14 (93)	36/68 (53)
Total	12/125 (10)	65/275 (24)	28/52 (54)	105/452 (23)

*Middleton RG: Value of and indications for staging pelvic lymph node dissection. Presented at the NIH Consensus Development Conference, Management of Clinically Localized Prostate Cancer, Bethesda, MD, June 15–17, 1987.

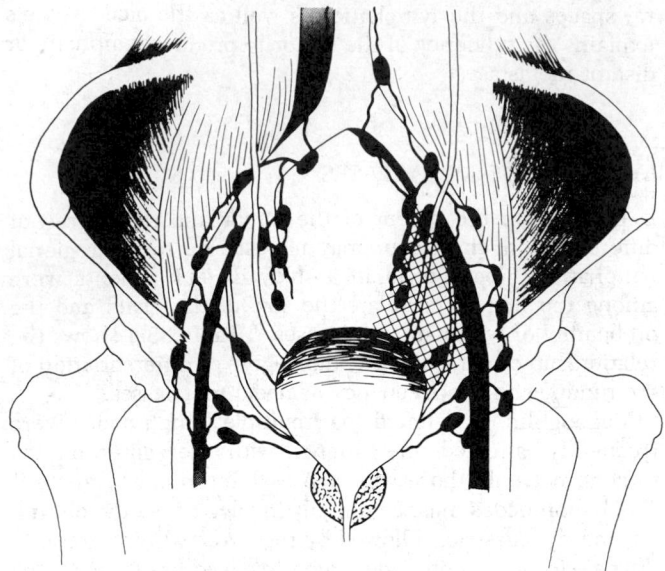

FIG. 33-2. Anatomy of prostate and lymphatic drainage. Shaded area depicts boundaries of limited staging lymphadenectomy.

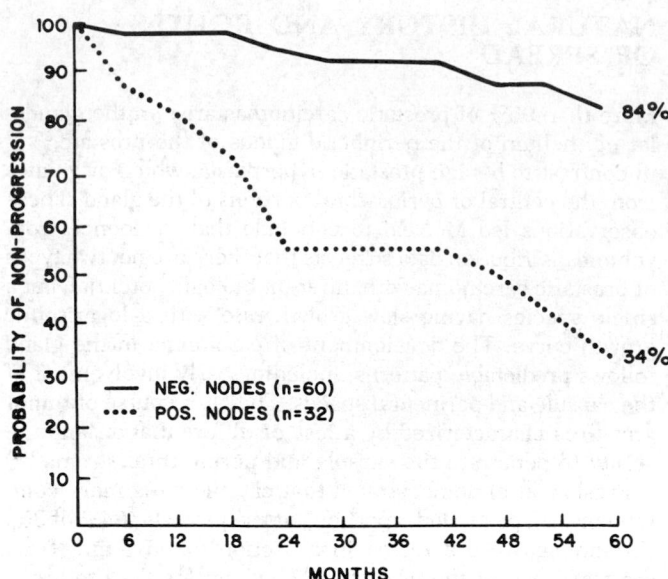

FIG. 33-3. Probability of survival without progression of clinical prostatic adenocarcinoma related to presence of pelvic lymph node metastases. (Prout GR et al: Nodal involvement as a prognostic indicator in patients with prostatic carcinoma. J Urol 124:226–231, 1980)

the presence of a single nodal metastasis was not an unfavorable prognostic sign: only 2 (18%) of 11 patients experienced tumor progression, in comparison to 16 (76%) of 21 with multiple lymph node involvement.

DISTANT METASTASES

Distant metastases usually occur to the skeleton, liver, and lungs, and less frequently to the brain or other sites. It is generally accepted that prostatic carcinoma metastasizes preferentially to the bones of the pelvis and the spine by way of the vertebral veins, a concept popularized by Batson.[52] However, Dodds et al found that the distribution of skeletal metastases is comparable in patients with prostatic or other primary tumors,[53] thus not confirming Batson's hypothesis. The preponderance of metastases to the axial skeleton and proximate long bones may be a function of regional arterial blood flow and not of any specific venous drainage.

PATHOLOGY

The most common tumor arising in the prostate is adenocarcinoma, which originates from the peripheral acinar glands. Adenocarcinomas are classified by some pathologists as well, moderately, and poorly differentiated, according to cellular characteristics, nuclear content, number of nuclei, pleomorphism, invasion of the stroma, and so forth.

Mostofi has used the following criteria for defining the various histological grades.[54] Well-differentiated tumors form glands that may be large, intermediate, or small, and have a papillary configuration. Of the moderately differentiated tumors, only 50% to 75% form glands, and there may be a cribriform, less papillary pattern. In poorly differentiated tumors, cells are arranged in rows, columns, or sheets; 25% or less of the tumors will form glands. Poorly differentiated tumors carry a much worse prognosis than the better

TABLE 33-2.   Frequency of Lymph Node Involvement by Tumor in Adenocarcinoma of the Prostate (93 Patients)*

Lymph Node Group	No. of Patients Undergoing Biopsy	No. (%) with Tumor	% Opacified†
Para-aortic	74	13 (18)	93
Common iliac	76	13 (17)	95
External iliac	74	16 (22)	94
Internal iliac	63	15 (24)	87
Obturator	51	16 (31)	94

*Pistenma DA, Bagshaw MA, Freiha FS: Extended-field radiation therapy for prostatic adenocarcinoma: Status report of a limited prospective trial. In Johnson DE, Samuels ML (eds): Cancer of the Genitourinary Tract, pp 229–247. New York, Raven Press, 1979.
†Refers to histologic evidence of retained contrast material within the lymph node specimen.

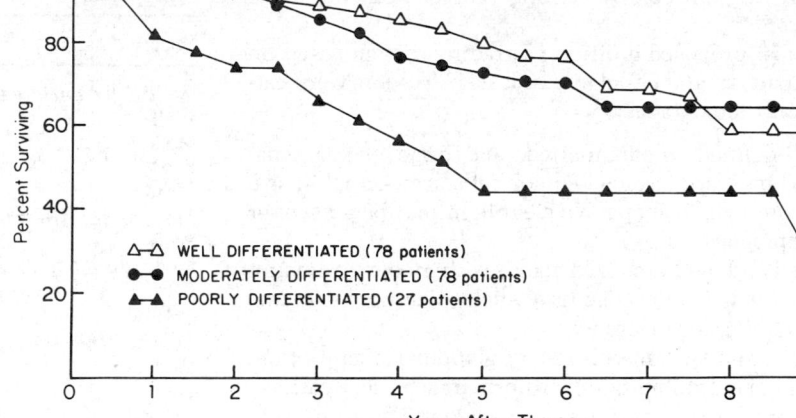

FIG. 33-4. Tumor-free survival according to histologic degree of differentiation of the tumor in patients with carcinoma of the prostate treated at Washington University from 1967 to 1983. **A**. Stage B. **B**. Stage C. (Perez CA et al: Definitive radiation therapy in carcinoma of the prostate localized to the pelvis: Experience at the Mallinckrodt Institute of Radiology. Natl Cancer Inst Monogr [in press])

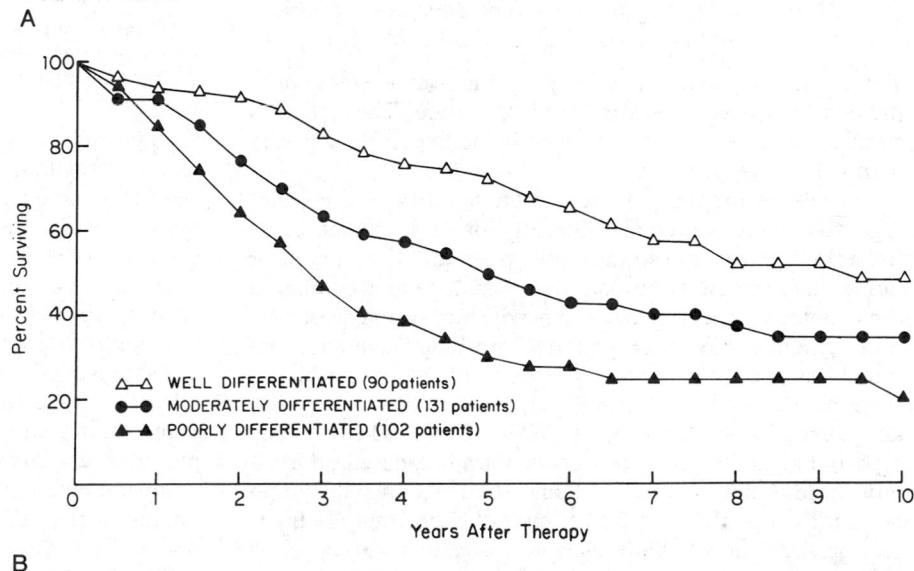

differentiated lesions (Fig. 33-4). The poorer prognosis is closely related to the tendency of such tumors to metastasize to regional lymph nodes and distant sites (Fig. 33-5).[55]

Gleason and associates proposed a prognostic classification system based on the clinical stage and the degree of differentiation of primary and secondary patterns of the tumor.[56] Patients with tumors with a Gleason score of less than 5 have relatively early stage disease and well-differentiated lesions, with excellent prognosis. Patients with scores of 6 through 10 usually have Stage B or C tumors, with moderate differentiation and an intermediate prognosis. Scores higher than 10 in general correspond to anaplastic lesions and are associated with a poor prognosis. As Gleason pointed out, the degree of histologic differentiation of prostatic adenocarcinoma is the simplest, strongest, and most readily available measure of the biologic malignancy of this tumor.[57]

Paulson and the Uro-Oncology Research Group[58] and Kramer et al[59] have concluded that the Gleason grade of prostatic carcinoma as determined from needle biopsy specimens is an accurate predictor of pelvic lymph node metas-

FIG. 33-5. Anatomical sites of failure in patients with carcinoma of the prostate according to pathologic degree of tumor differentiation (1967–1983). (Perez CA et al: Definitive radiation therapy in carcinoma of the prostate localized to the pelvis: Experience at the Mallinckrodt Institute of Radiology. Natl Cancer Inst Monogr [in press])

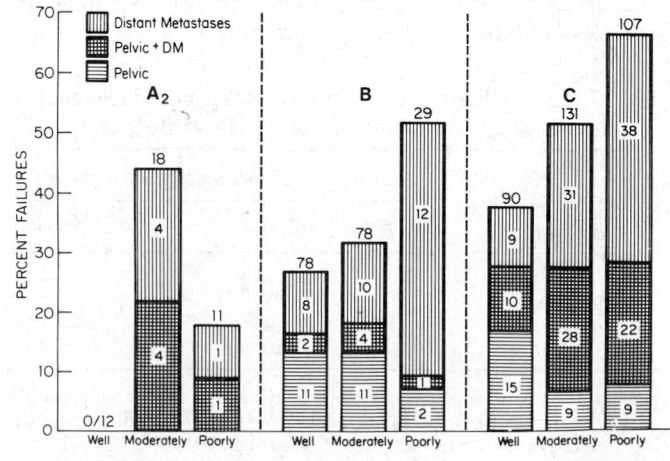

tases. Others not using the Gleason grading system have not found a particularly strong correlation of these parameters.[51,60]

Gaeta et al proposed a different grading system based on glandular pattern and cellular anaplasia.[61] Tumors were categorized into four grades:

1. Well-defined, medium-sized, and large glands separated by scant stroma. Tumor cells are normal in size and uniform in shape. No clear light may be present or conspicuous.
2. Small and medium-sized glands with moderate amount of stroma. Tumor cells have slight pleomorphism and the nuclei are prominent.
3. More small ascini with loss of glandular organization, the glands exhibiting a cribriform or scirrhous pattern. The nuclei are vesicular with acidophilic nuclei.
4. Absence of gland formation. The cells are quite pleomorphic and show significant mitotic activity.

The tumor is graded according to the worse component present in at least one third of the specimen. The system is simple, reproducible, and has been found to correlate closely with cancer death rates.

One of the problems in accurately identifying the histologic subtype or degree of differentiation of the tumor arises from the vagaries of the needle biopsies and the amount of tissue that is submitted for analysis. Catalona et al compared the histologic appearance of the needle biopsy and prostatectomy specimens from 66 patients with Stage B disease and found that the tumor was undergraded in the needle biopsy specimens in 22 cases (33%), overgraded in five cases (8%), and correctly classified in 39 (59%) (Table 33-3).[62] They reported a good correlation between grading based on prostatic needle biopsy specimens and the frequency of lymph node metastases (Table 33-4), even though multiple bilateral prostatic needle biopsies were associated with appreciable errors in tumor grading.

Brawn reported on 54 patients with prostatic carcinoma who underwent two transurethral resections of the prostate separated by 3 to 11 years.[63] He observed significant dedifferentiation of the tumors, going into higher grades, in 19 (73%) of 26 initially Grade 1 tumors, 9 (75%) of 12 Grade 2 tumors, and 7 (88%) of 8 Grade 3 tumors. Even the tumors that did not change grade between the two examinations were less differentiated at the time of the second transure-

TABLE 33-3. Errors in Tumor Grading on Needle Biopsy Specimens of Adenocarcinoma of the Prostate*

Grade on Needle Biopsy	Grade on Prostatectomy Specimen			
	Well	Moderate	Poor	Totals
Well	21	17	2	40
Moderate	3	11	3	17
Poor	0	2	7	9
Total	24	30	12	66

*Catalona WJ, Stein AJ, Fair WR: Grading errors in prostatic needle biopsies: Relation to the accuracy of tumor grade in predicting pelvic lymph node metastases. J Urol 127:919–922, 1982.
Well, poor, and moderate refer to degree of tumor differentiation.

TABLE 33-4. Grading Errors in Prostatic Needle Biopsies: Relation to Lymph Node Metastases*

Specimen	Positive Nodes/Total	%
Well differentiated on needle biopsy, 40 cases		
Well	0/21	0
Moderate	1/17	6
Poor	0/2	0
Total	1/40	3
Moderately differentiated on needle biopsy, 17 cases		
Well	1/3	33
Moderate	4/11	36
Poor	1/3	33
Total	6/17	35
Poorly differentiated on needle biopsy, 9 cases		
Moderate	0/2	0
Poor	5/7	71
Total	5/9	56

*Catalona WJ, Stein AJ, Fair WR: Grading errors in prostatic needle biopsies: Relation to the accuracy of tumor grade in predicting pelvic lymph node metastases. J Urol 127:919–922, 1982.

thral prostatic resection when compared with the first one. A direct correlation between dedifferentiation and metastases was noted: no Grade 1 lesions in the second analysis showed evidence of metastases, whereas 4 (19%) of 21 Grade 2 lesions, 10 (55%) of 18 Grade 3 lesions, and 28 (80%) of 35 Grade 4 lesions showed evidence of metastases at the time.

Periurethral duct carcinoma has been described as a separate clinicopathologic entity.[64-69] Histologic sections show a transitional cell type of carcinoma in most instances, while in others a mixture of glandular and transitional cells is noted. Clusters of large anaplastic tumor cells often fill the periurethral prostatic ducts and spread into the prostatic stroma. A high number of mitoses is seen.[70] This tumor does not invade the perineural spaces as commonly as adenocarcinoma of the prostate for localized tumors.

Some authors believe periurethral duct carcinomas are relatively benign,[71] yet most reports indicate aggressive behavior, with invasion of the prostatic stroma and the bladder neck and metastases to the lymph nodes, bone, and lung. In most series the majority of patients died of the tumor within 4 years.[68,72]

The treatment of choice is radical cystoprostatectomy.[73] Kopelson et al reported a good prognosis in patients with early stage disease; however, in patients with Stage C disease the 5-year survival rate was only 34.5%.[69] It is important to recognize this tumor, since it is not hormonally responsive but is moderately sensitive to radiation therapy. Kopelson et al reported a 76% local tumor control and a 58% 5-year survival rate in patients treated with irradiation, in contrast to 14% local tumor control and 24% 5-year survival rate in patients not receiving this treatment.

Another rare type of epithelial tumor in the prostate is the *adenoid cystic carcinoma* (representing less than 0.01% of all tumors of the prostate). Its histologic appearance is similar to that of the salivary gland counterpart, with a cribriform pattern and cystic structures associated with gland formation.

Endometrioid tumors occasionally arise from the verumontanum. These tumors may have an exophytic configuration in the prostatic urethra or may infiltrate the adjacent tissues. Endometrial glands and cells with numerous mitotic figures may be seen. Melicow and Pachter postulated that this tumor originates in müllerian duct tissue of the prostatic utricle.[74]

Carcinosarcoma of the prostate represents 0.1% of prostatic neoplasias. As in the endometrial counterpart, there is a mixed pattern of adenocarcinoma invading the stroma and sarcomatous elements. Smooth or striated muscle, fibroblasts, or other mesenchymal malignant cells may be identified.

Sarcomas constitute about 0.1% of all primary neoplasias of the prostate gland[70] and may be characterized histologically as leiomyosarcoma, rhabdomyosarcoma, or fibrosarcoma. These tumors have the propensity to develop early lymphatic and vascular invasion with widespread regional lymphatic and distant metastases.

Primary *malignant lymphomas* of the prostate are rare. The tumors may be of the lymphocytic, histiocytic, or mixed cell type.[75] These tumors behave similarly to extranodal malignant lymphomas in other sites and should be treated accordingly.

CLINICAL FEATURES

SYMPTOMS

Patients with localized prostatic carcinoma frequently are asymptomatic and the diagnosis is suspected during a routine rectal examination. Patients with Stage A disease may have symptoms of bladder outlet obstruction and rectal findings compatible with benign prostatic hyperplasia. Larger tumors may produce symptoms of urethral obstruction with resulting frequency, nocturia, hesitancy, and narrow stream. Occasional patients have severe irritative bladder symptoms in the absence of clinical evidence of infection. Isolated hematuria or hematospermia is rare.

In advanced disease the majority of patients present with symptoms of bony metastases manifested by back pain or stiffness; occasionally the disease is erroneously treated as degenerative arthritis. Pathologic fractures are occasionally seen, with lytic metastases in the subtrochanteric areas of the femur.

SCREENING STUDIES

Mass screening for prostate cancer is somewhat difficult, because rectal examination still remains the most effective means of detecting early carcinoma of the prostate, other tests not being particularly sensitive or specific for this malignancy.[76,77] The efficacy of a screening test is a function of three factors: (1) the sensitivity of the test, (*i.e.*, the proportion of true positive tests), (2) the specificity of the test (*i.e.*, the proportion of true negative tests), and (3) the prevalence of prostatic carcinoma in the population being screened. Digital rectal examination has about 80% sensitivity and 50% specificity. Radioimmunoassays for prostatic acid phosphatase (PAP) have a sensitivity of only 10% and a specificity of 90% for tumors.

Recently, clinical application of prostate-specific antigen (PSA) has come under investigation. This antigen, initially identified and purified by Wang et al in 1979 from prostatic tissue,[78] is a protein with a molecular weight of 33,000 in about 7% carbohydrate. PSA is detected not only in prostatic tissue (normal, benign hyperplasia, malignant tumors) and seminal fluid but also in the sera of patients with prostatic cancer. PSA is localized within the cytoplasm ductal epithelial cells and in secretory materials in ductal lamina.[79,80] Seamonds et al reported a specificity of PSA assay of 95% in 40 patients with newly diagnosed carcinomas of the prostate and 97.1% in 35 patients with recurrent tumors.[81] The corresponding values for PAP were 24 of 40 (60%) and 23 of 35 (65.7%), respectively. The overall sensitivity of PSA was 96% compared with 62.7% for PAP. The specificity of PSA and PAP assays is comparable in their experience (96.8% and 98.9%, respectively). Seamonds et al believe that the PSA assay is more sensitive for monitoring therapy, since the PSA titer usually rises before the PAP level and always precedes clinical signs of relapse. Although there may be some false positive tests, since PSA titers may be elevated more frequently than PAP levels in selected patients with benign prostatic hypertrophy or prostatitis, Seamonds et al postulate that these patients may fall into a high-risk population that may have early undetected carcinoma of the prostate or precancerous conditions, and they recommend close follow-up. The PSA titer used at our institution is 0.4 to 4 ng/ml. Elevated titers have been found to be associated with a greater probability of lymph node metastases or distant dissemination.

Recently Stamey et al reported a comparison of PSA and PAP as measured by radioimmunoassay in 2200 serum samples from 699 patients, 378 known to have prostatic carcinoma.[82] The PSA titer was elevated in 122 of 127 patients with newly diagnosed and treated prostatic carcinoma. The antigen titer increased with advancing clinical stage and was proportional to estimated volume of the tumor. On the other hand, the PAP concentration was elevated in only 57 of the patients with cancer and correlated less closely with tumor volume. However, the PSA titer was increased in 86% and the PAP concentration in 14% of the patients with benign prostatic hyperplasia. After radical prostatectomy for cancer, PSA titers routinely fell to undetectable ranges with a half-life of 2.2 days. PAP concentration, if initially elevated, fell to normal levels within 24 hours but always remained detectable. PSA but not PAP appeared to be useful in detecting residual and early recurrence of tumor and in monitoring response to radiation therapy. Stamey et al concluded that the PSA titer is more sensitive than the PAP level in the detection of prostatic carcinoma and probably will be more useful in monitoring response and recurrence after therapy. However, a caveat is that both PSA and PAP levels may be elevated in benign prostatic hyperplasia.

DIAGNOSTIC STUDIES

Rectal examination of the prostate is critical. The examination is best performed with a well-lubricated glove and with the patient standing, bent over at the waist with his elbows resting comfortably on a firm surface. The examiner notes

TABLE 33-5.   Results of Screening Tests for Prostate Cancer*

Test	No. of Patients	Sensitivity	Specificity	Predictive Value Positive Test	Predictive Value Negative Test	Efficiency
Rectal examination	300	0.69	0.89	67	91	85
Acid phosphatase—enzyme	300	0.56	0.94	72	88	84
Acid phosphatase—RIA	100	0.20	0.85	29	78	70
Acid phosphatase—CIEP	100	0.20	0.95	56	80	78
Urine cytology before massage	202	0.17	0.98	67	80	79
Prostatic secretion cytology after massage	211	0.29	0.98	78	82	81
Urine cytology after massage	209	0.22	0.98	71	81	80
Aspiration cytology	200	0.55	0.91	65	88	83
Lactic dehydrogenase V/I ratio	132	0.47	0.82	44	83	73
Leukocyte adherence inhibition	113	0.50	0.79	43	83	72

*Guinan P, Bush I, Ray V et al: The accuracy of the rectal examination in the diagnosis of prostate carcinoma. N Engl J Med 303:499–503, 1980.

the size of the gland, its overall consistency, and the presence of any firm areas. A typical neoplastic nodule of prostatic carcinoma is extremely firm, often not elevated above the surface of the gland, but surrounded by compressible prostatic tissue. The examiner should determine whether or not the lateral sulcus is involved by the tumor and also the degree of spread superiorly. In most patients the seminal vesicles cannot be palpated as discrete structures, and the finding of a firm area extending above the prostate suggests involvement of the seminal vesicles by malignancy. After palpating the prostate the physician should always examine the posterior aspect of the rectum as well. Not all areas of induration felt on prostatic examination represent carcinoma. Other causes of induration are prostatic calculi, infections, granulomatous prostatitis, prostatic infarction, and firm nodules of benign prostatic hyperplasia. Approximately 50% of prostatic nodules found on rectal examination are confirmed to be malignant on biopsy.[83-85]

In a study by Guinan and associates,[86] the digital rectal examination had the highest overall efficacy of ten screening tests for prostatic cancer (Table 33-5).

Although the rectal examination remains the keystone for early detection, the actual diagnosis of carcinoma of the prostate can be made only with histologic or cytologic evaluation. Needle biopsy is the standard method of diagnosing this tumor in the United States. Closed needle biopsy of the prostate can be performed via either the perineal or the

transrectal route. The transperineal route minimizes the risk of infection because the needle is not placed through the rectum. Proponents of the transrectal route (Fig. 33-6) believe that this approach allows the surgeon to guide the point of the biopsy needle into the suspect area more accurately.

Currently there is little enthusiasm for routine transurethral biopsy of the prostate. Although by definition, this is the only method of diagnosing Stage A cancer of the prostate, it is of no value in determining the nature of a solitary nodule felt on rectal examination and may miss even larger tumors that have not extended to the periurethral area.

In Europe and especially Scandinavia, aspiration biopsy has been utilized for many years with impressive results; it is a relatively simple procedure and permits the physician to make the diagnosis in an outpatient procedure with a minimum of expense and patient morbidity. The most commonly used instrument is the needle described by Franzen et al,[87] which is guided by the rectal examining finger to the nodule; an aspirate is obtained directly from the suspect area. No anesthesia is required. With sufficient experience in obtaining a specimen and interpreting the cytology, the results of cytologic aspiration compare favorably with histologic results in material obtained by needle biopsy. With adequate examiner skills, unsatisfactory cell samples resulting from faulty biopsy technique are found in fewer than 1% of all specimens.[88,89] False negative diagnoses range from less than 5% to 30%. False positive diagnoses are relatively rare,

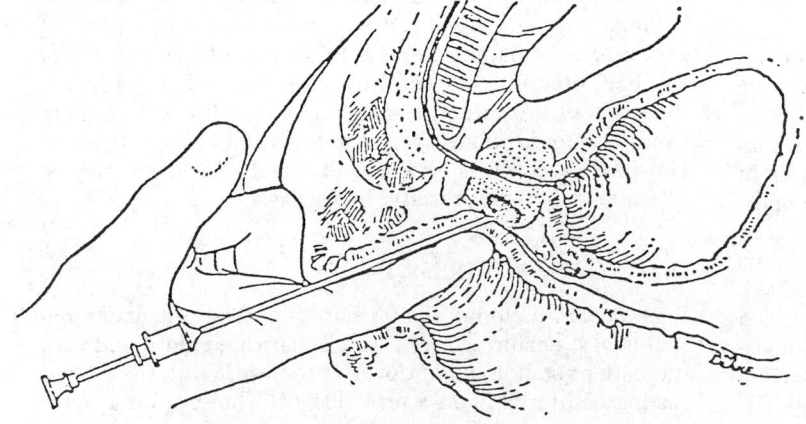

FIG. 33-6.   Transrectal needle biopsy of the prostate.

TABLE 33-6. Transrectal Aspiration Biopsy for Clinical Staging and Cytologic Grade in Carcinoma of the Prostate*

Cytologic Grade	No. of Patients	Stage (%)		
		B	C	D
High	131	62 (47.3)	56 (42.8)	13 (9.9)
Moderate	265	65 (24.5)	172 (64.9)	28 (10.6)
Poor	73	7 (9.6)	42 (57.5)	24 (32.9)
Total	469	134 (28.6)	270 (57.5)	65 (13.9)

*Esposti PL: Cytologic malignancy grading of prostatic carcinoma by transrectal aspiration biopsy. Scand J Urol Nephrol 5:199–209, 1971.

but granulomatous prostatitis or aspiration of cells from the seminal vesicle can confuse the cytopathologist.

Esposti found a significant correlation between the cytologic grade of the specimen and the clinical stage of disease (Table 33-6).[90]

STANDARD WORKUP

The standard tests currently required in the evaluation of patients with prostatic carcinoma are listed below.

Standard Workup for Prostatic Carcinoma

    Physical examination
    Rectal examination
    Serum acid phosphatase
    Serum alkaline phosphatase
    Prostate-specific antigen (PSA)
    Chest radiograph
    Radioisotope bone scan
    Needle biopsy (or TURP)

Other Tests as Indicated

    Pelvic CT
    Ultrasonography
    Bipedal lymphangiography
    Pelvic lymphadenectomy
    Radiographic bone survey

The value of serum acid phosphatase in the detection or staging of prostatic cancer is limited.[91-93] Neither radioimmunoassay nor conventional enzymatic methods are accurate enough to use as routine screening tests for the detection of carcinoma of the prostate.[92,93] In patients with surgical Stage D disease the acid phosphatase level may be in the normal range.[94] There is little evidence to warrant the routine use of bone marrow acid phosphatase assays in staging carcinoma of the prostate.[95]

In a large-scale study conducted by the Uro-Oncology Research Group (UROG), 509 men with newly diagnosed prostatic adenocarcinoma were assigned a preliminary clinical stage based on the results of physical examination, routine bone survey, and serum phosphatase levels.[96] Patients underwent, in sequence, a radioisotope bone scan, lymphangiography, and a staging pelvic lymph node dissection before being assigned a final clinical stage. Technetium-99 medronate bone scanning demonstrated bony metastases in ap-

proximately 25% of all patients judged free of disease from a routine bone survey, the incidence being related to the stage of the disease (Table 33-7). Lund et al[97] and Merrick et al[98] have stressed the value of bone scanning in the staging of patients with clinically localized carcinoma of the prostate in whom radiation therapy or a surgical procedure is planned. Abnormalities in the bone scan coupled with elevation of either the PAP level or PSA titer are strongly suggestive of clinically inapparent metastatic disease. Merrick et al noted that repeated follow-up bone scans may be of value in detecting post-treatment metastases, since patients with normal bone scans will live longer than those with abnormal scans.[98] However, from a clinical standpoint, this procedure in follow-up is of questionable value since treatment of symptomatic bone metastases may not be justifiable. Of course, bone scans will be of substantial diagnostic help in patients with bone pain and normal radiographs. Roentgenograms may sometimes be necessary to better evaluate areas of increased uptake on the radioisotope bone scan, but routine radiographic bone surveys are of little value and add unnecessary expense to the evaluation of the patient, even though occasionally a lesion seen on radiographs may not appear on the bone scan.[99]

Lymphangiography has shown an overall accuracy of 75% in several studies.[100,101] Pistenma et al described a true negative rate of 88% (52/59) but a true positive rate of only 50% (15/30).[101] The lymphangiogram cannot demonstrate microscopic metastases, or lymph nodes that are totally replaced by metastatic tumor. On bipedal lymphangiography the internal iliac and obturator nodes, frequently involved in early nodal tumor extension, do not opacify. This accounts

TABLE 33-7. Adenocarcinoma of the Prostate: Incidence of Positive Bone Scans as a Function of Preliminary Clinical Stage*

Preliminary Stage	No. of Patients	Bone Scan Positive, No. (%)
IA	31	3 (10)
IB	51	4 (8)
II	101	20 (20)
III	79	19 (24)
IVA	94	33 (35)
IVC	69	65 (94)

*Paulson DF, Uro-Oncology Research Group: The impact of current staging procedures in assessing disease extent of prostatic adenocarcinoma. J Urol 121:300–302, 1979.

TABLE 33-8.   Adenocarcinoma of the Prostate: Impact of Radioisotope Bone Scan and Staging Pelvic Node Dissection on Change in Assigned Clinical Stage*

Preliminary Stage	No. of Patients (N = 452)	Final Stage												
		IA No.	(%)	IB No.	(%)	II No.	(%)	III No.	(%)	IVA No.	(%)	IVB No.	(%)	IVC No.	(%)
IA	70	67	(95)	1										2	
IB	41	1		22	(53)	4	(54)	1		1		10	(24)	2	(5)
II	83	1		1		45		5	(57)	6		17	(20)	8	(10)
III	73	0		0		0		42		4	(26)	12	(16)	15	(20)
IVA	82	3		1		1		6		22		14	(16)	35	(42)
IVC	103	0		0		0		0		0		0		103	

*Paulson DF, Uro-Oncology Research Group: The impact of current staging procedures in assessing disease extent of prostatic adenocarcinoma. J Urol 121:300–302, 1979.

for the relatively high incidence — 22% to 40% — of false negative results with routine lymphangiography.[60,96,100,102]

Computed tomography (CT) also has problems in detecting positive pelvic lymph nodes in patients with cancer of the prostate. CT does not accurately demonstrate intranodal metastasis unless the nodes are enlarged more than 2 cm.[103] Large lymph nodes in a patient with prostatic cancer do not necessarily indicate metastatic tumor in the nodes, because they may be enlarged for other reasons (e.g., hyperplasia). In a study by Golimbu et al, the accuracy of CT was only 70% for assessing the lymph node status and 47% for determining the tumor extent.[104]

In the UROG study, almost 50% of patients with Stages IB, II, and III disease were shifted to a more advanced disease category as a result of radioisotope bone scans and lymph node biopsy. The impact was greatest in those patients originally thought to have disease confined to the prostate (Table 33-8.)[96] Failure to determine the presence of bone or nodal extension with these studies would have resulted in inappropriate treatment selection.

Several reports have described the technique of transrectal ultrasound (US) as well as the anatomy of the prostate and preliminary US findings in benign hyperplasia or carcinoma of the prostate.[105,106] In a study of 443 men who underwent transrectal endosonography of the prostate, Rifkin found 130 pathologically proven cancers and 313 cases of benign prostatic disease.[105] Cancers were hyperechoic in 69% of cases and had poorly defined margins, whereas benign lesions were hyperechoic in only 46% of cases and tended to be more accurately measured because of their sharper borders. However, Rifkin concluded that there are no specific characteristics on transrectal US that differentiate among many cases of benign prostatic disease and malignancy, and therefore biopsy is always required.[105] Rectal US may assist in determining the location of the areas to be biopsied, and a needle inserted through the perineum or the rectum can be guided to the suspect nodule by means of US.

Chodak et al, in a prospective randomized study of transrectal US in 216 men, reported a sensitivity of 86% but a specificity of only 41%.[107] Tumors less than 1 cm in diameter were the most difficult to detect. To date, the use of transrectal US remains a controversial issue: in our experience at the Memorial Sloan-Kettering Cancer Center, only 5% of patients with positive findings on transrectal US will have carcinoma confirmed on subsequent biopsy.[108] Further evaluation of this procedure will be required before more definite conclusions can be made regarding its usefulness in the early detection of carcinoma of the prostate.

STAGING AND PROGNOSIS

LYMPHADENECTOMY

Because of increased morbidity associated with pelvic lymph node dissection extending from the common iliac artery superiorly to the genitofemoral nerve laterally and the obturator fossa medially, a number of surgeons recommend a more limited dissection.[109,110] The incidence of identified nodal spread by clinical stage is similar whether the dissection is limited or more extensive. The limited dissection outlined by Paulson et al is the procedure of choice (see Fig. 33-2).[58] Dissection is begun at the bifurcation of the common iliac vessels and carried down the medial inferior margin of the external iliac artery to the pelvic floor, medially across the pelvic floor to the inferior border of the prostate, and then superiorly along the hypogastric vessels back to the bifurcation of the common iliacs. The tissue surrounding the obturator nerve should be included in the specimen. The obturator artery and vein may be sacrificed if necessary. The UROG failed to find a single case of positive periaortic nodes among 54 patients with negative pelvic nodes,[111] confirming similar observations by Flocks et al[46] and Arduino and Glucksman.[112]

Is a staging pelvic lymphadenectomy of prognostic value in patients with prostatic cancer? The answer is clearly yes. Whitmore et al found that 40% of patients with positive lymph nodes after a pelvic lymph node dissection and ^{125}I prostate implantation had recurrent disease within 24 months.[113] Furthermore, more than 75% of the patients with positive pelvic nodes had evidence of distant metastases within 60 months after treatment. Cline and co-workers, in a series of patients treated with pelvic lymph node dissection and radical perineal prostatectomy, found that 50% of patients with positive lymph nodes had recurrent disease within 24 months after treatment.[114]

Is pelvic lymph node dissection of value in planning radiation therapy? The rationale is that if the nodes are negative, irradiation should be confined to the prostate, whereas if the nodes are positive, irradiation should be extended to pelvic and/or periaortic lymph nodes. Freiha et al have questioned whether radiation therapy can sterilize metastatic pelvic lymph nodes.[115] Paulson studied 90 patients with surgical Stage D1 carcinoma.[116] The mean time to failure was 23 months in a group of patients who received extended field radiation therapy (inverted T field extending from the diaphragm to the prostate with lateral extension to the pelvic side walls, with a total of 7000 cGy delivered to the prostate and 5000 cGy to the periaortic and pelvic nodes). The mean relapse-free survival period was 12 months in patients receiving delayed hormonal treatment (p = 0.02). Although radiation therapy might delay the onset of recurrent or metastatic disease, it may have little impact on prolonging overall survival in these patients.

Is pelvic node dissection curative? Controversy still exists over the curative value of pelvic lymph node dissection. Barzell et al[117] in a study of patients treated with interstitial radiation and pelvic node dissection, reported that when the total tumor volume in the lymph nodes was less than 3 cc there was some therapeutic benefit from the lymph node dissection. However, a more recent study at the same institution[118] and one by Kramer et al[119] do not confirm these findings and provide convincing evidence that in most patients, staging lymphadenectomy is not a curative procedure. In the series reported by Kramer et al, of 11 patients with Stage D1 carcinoma of the prostate who were treated with radical perineal prostatectomy plus pelvic lymph node dissection, 50% had recurrent disease within 18.3 months. In 33 other patients with Stage D1 disease who were treated

with either radiation therapy or delayed hormonal therapy, the time to 50% patient failure was 19.2 months. The same authors found no notable difference between the mean time to treatment failure in 17 patients with one positive node and in 10 patients with multiple positive nodes. It appears that either surgery or radiation therapy is rarely curative in the presence of positive lymph nodes. Hence, staging lymph node dissection should be considered only if the physician has predetermined that if positive nodes are found, no attempt at curative therapy will be made.

DIGITAL EXAMINATION

Experienced digital examination of the prostate yields relatively accurate information about tumor volume. Byar and Mostofi noted that 85% of the nodules in 208 patients treated with radical prostatectomy were multifocal or extensive[2]; 17% of the patients with Stage A2 and B tumors had extracapsular tumor extension in the specimen. Jewett reported that after radical prostatectomy, 25% of patients with Stage A and B disease had seminal vesicle involvement in the operative findings.[85]

CLINICAL STAGING SYSTEMS

The American Joint Committee schema for staging carcinoma of prostate is shown in Table 33-9 and Figure

TABLE 33-9.   TNM Classification—Prostate*

Primary Tumor (T)

TX   Minimum requirement to assess the primary tumor cannot be met.
T0   No tumor present
    T1a   No palpable tumor; on histologic sections no more than three high-power fields of carcinoma found
    T1b   No palpable tumor; histologic sections revealing more than three high-power fields of prostatic carcinoma
    T2a   Palpable nodule less than 1.5 cm in diameter with compressible, normal-feeling tissue on at least three sides
    T2b   Palpable nodule more than 1.5 cm in diameter or nodule or induration in both lobes
T3   Palpable tumor extending into or beyond the prostatic capsule
    T3a   Palpable tumor extending into the periprostatic tissues, or involving one seminal vesicle
    T3b   Palpable tumor extending into the periprostatic tissues, involving one or both seminal vesicles; tumor size more than 6 cm in diameter
T4   Tumor fixed or involving neighboring structures

Nodal Involvement (N)

The regional nodes are those within the true pelvis; all others are distant nodes. Histologic examination is required for stages N0 through N3, except for subset "c."
NX   Minimum requirements to assess the regional nodes cannot be met.
N0   No involvement of regional lymph nodes
N1   Involvement of a single homolateral regional lymph node
N2   Involvement of contralateral, bilateral, or multiple regional lymph nodes
N3   A fixed mass present on the pelvic wall with a free space between this and the tumor

Distant Metastasis (M)

MX   Minimum requirements to assess the presence of distant metastasis cannot be met
M0   No (known) distant metastasis
M1   Distant metastasis present
        Specify_____
Specify sites according to the following notations:

Distant lymph nodes	LYM	Pleura	PLE
Pulmonary	PUL	Skin	SKI
Osseous	OSS	Eye	EYE
Hepatic	HEP	Other	OTH
Brain	BRA		

*Beahrs OH, Myers MH (eds): Manual for Staging Cancer, American Joint Committee on Cancer. Philadelphia, JB Lippincott, 1983.

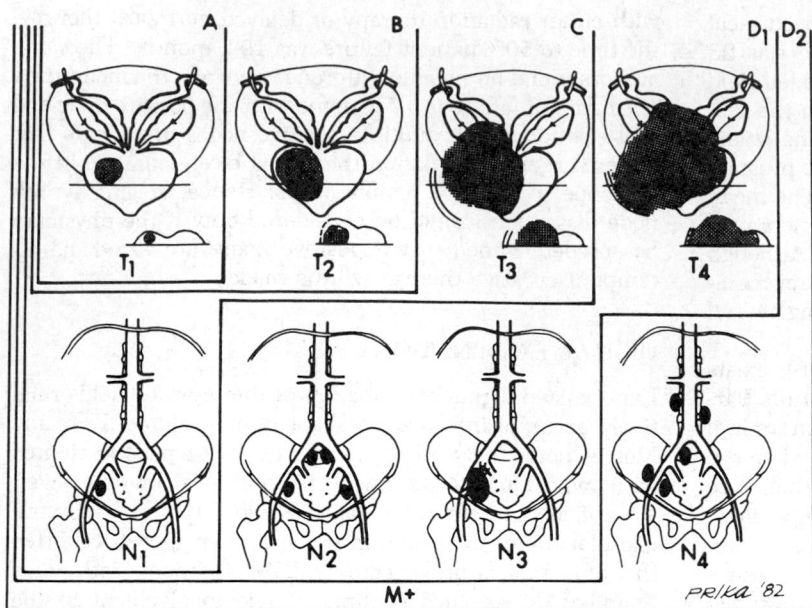

FIG. 33-7. Anatomic staging for carcinoma of the prostate. Stage groupings follow the T categories and are incorporated into the American Urologic System of Stage A1, B1, C1, D1, and D2. The AJC and UICC do not stage group. Regional nodes are N1 = T3 and D1 and juxtaregional nodes are considered metastatic; therefore, T4–N1 equivalence, same as D2. The AJC and UICC classification systems are identical. The American (Jewett-Marshall) system utilizes A, B, C, D designations that are translated to correspond to TNM categories. Modified from AJC. (Frank IN et al: Urologic and male genital cancers. In Rubin P [ed]: Clinical Oncology. American Cancer Society, 1983)

33-7.[120,121] Other systems such as the American Urological Society system are used to express the clinical extent of this tumor (Table 33-10). *Stage A1* lesions are well-differentiated local adenocarcinomas that are not clinically apparent but are found incidentally during transurethral prostatic resection or needle biopsy of the prostate.[122] *Stage A2* tumors also are not clinically apparent, but they have a more diffuse pattern or larger volume, frequently with multifocal involvement of the prostate, and are not well differentiated histologically.

McMillen and Wettlaufer[123] repeated transurethral resection 3 months after the first procedure in 27 patients with an initial diagnosis of Stage A adenocarcinoma of the prostate; 7 (26%) of the 27 patients were found to have substantial residual tumor at the time of repeat resection and were reclassified as having Stage A2 disease. Parfitt et al in similar studies found that only 7% to 9% of patients originally diagnosed as having focal carcinoma of the prostate had more extensive disease on repeat transurethral resection or radical prostatectomy.[124]

Golimbu and Morales analyzed findings in 24 patients with clinical Stage A2 tumors and concluded that such tumors are more aggressive biologically than Stage B1 lesions.[125] Re-

view of several papers in the literature disclosed a 24% incidence of lymph node metastases in this group of patients. Bauer and associates analyzed the 10-year survival of 24 patients with clinically unsuspected prostatic carcinoma (Stages A1 and A2) and noted that 50% of those with moderately and poorly differentiated lesions (Stage A2) died of the disease.[126] Furthermore, if the lesion was diffusely infiltrating the gland, the deaths from or with cancer rose to 80%. Similar findings have been reported by Heaney et al,[127] Barnes et al,[128] and DeVere White et al.[129]

Stage B represents palpable tumor confined within the capsule of the prostate gland. It has been divided into B1, in which the nodule involves a single lobe and is less than 1.5 cm in diameter, and B2, in which there is more extensive intraglandular palpable tumor.

Stage C denotes lesions with extracapsular extension. These lesions have been subclassified as C1, when there is involvement of the periprostatic tissues, and C2, when the tumor involves the seminal vesicles. Neglia et al also include in the C2 subgroup tumors that extend into the bladder neck, rectum, or pelvic wall.[130]

Stage D tumors can be subclassified as D1 when there is metastatic disease to the regional lymph nodes or when, as

TABLE 33-10.   Preliminary Stage Classification—Prostate

AUS Stage	Stage	AJC-UICC Classification	Local Lesion	Prostatic Acid Phosphatase	Bone Metastases By Bone Roentgenogram
A1—focal	IA	T0NxM0	Not palpable, focal	Not elevated	No
A2—diffuse	IB	T0NxM0	Not palpable, diffuse	Not elevated	No
B	II	T1T2NxM0	Confined to prostate	Not elevated	No
C	III	T3NxM0	Local extension	Not elevated	No
D1	IVA	TanyNxM0	Any	Elevated	No
D1	IVB	*TanyN1–4M0	Any	Any	No
D2	IVC	TanyNanyM1	Any	Any	Yes

*IVB patients cannot be assigned a stage classification until after node dissection as this category is reserved for patients with lymph node extension.

used by Perez et al,[131] there is extensive involvement of the bladder, rectum, or pelvic tissues extending to the pelvic wall (by clinical examination). Stage D2 denotes clinically evident metastatic carcinoma when the patient is first seen, as evidenced by abnormal radionuclide bone scans, liver and spleen scans, skeletal radiographs, or surgically proved extrapelvic soft tissue or lymph node metastases.

In general, 10% of newly diagnosed cases of prostatic adenocarcinoma belong to Stage A, 15% to 20% to Stage B, 40% to stage C, and the remaining to Stage D. The proportion of patients with Stage D2 lesions has decreased from about 40% 20 years ago to 25% at the present time, a reflection of professional and public education that has increased the awareness of the disease.

It should be kept in mind that the accuracy of clinical staging is not optimal. In 175 prostatectomy specimens thought to be clinical Stage I or II, Byar and Mostofi reported definite histologic evidence of seminal vesicle involvement in 37 (21%).[2] Furthermore, the presence of metastatic lymph nodes in the pelvis, which significantly alters the prognosis, frequently correlates with clinical stage as well as with histologic differentiation of the tumor.

PROGNOSTIC FACTORS

There is a striking correlation between clinical stage, degree of differentiation of the tumor, and biologic behavior and prognosis. Secondary prognostic factors, which are closely dependent on the former, include (1) extent (size) of the tumor within each clinical stage, (2) plasma acid phosphatase levels, (3) regional lymph node involvement by tumor, (4) findings on radionuclide bone scan, and (5) response to therapy.

McNeal noted that 80% of the tumors less than 10 mm in diameter were focal, whereas 78% of those larger than 10 mm were diffuse, and 84% of the latter had penetrated and spread outside the capsule.[35] This work was confirmed by Scott et al.[132] Byar and Mostofi have shown that the depth of penetration of the tumor in the capsule before there is periprostatic involvement has prognostic implications.[2]

Of the diagnostic tests used to determine tumor extent, the plasma acid phosphatase levels have been shown to correlate closely with tumor dissemination and prognosis,[93,94] with elevations over 25% of maximum normal values carrying a poorer prognosis.

Oesterling et al reported on 275 patients with clinically localized carcinoma of the prostate treated surgically.[133] They noted that the serum prostatic acid phosphatase and Gleason degree of tumor differentiation correlated very well with prognostic factors such as capsular penetration, seminal vesical involvement, and lymph node involvement (Fig. 33-8).

Hilaris et al[100] noted very few distant metastases in patients with Stage T1 and T2 disease and negative pelvic lymph nodes; of those with T3–T4 disease and negative nodes, about 50% have distant metastases after 5 years. Patients with positive lymph nodes, regardless of the initial stage of the primary tumor, have a 75% to 80% rate of distant metastases during the same period of observation.

The location of the metastatic lymph nodes has great prog-

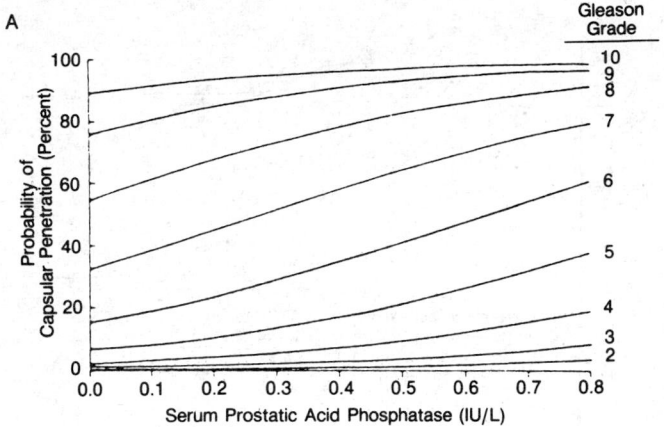

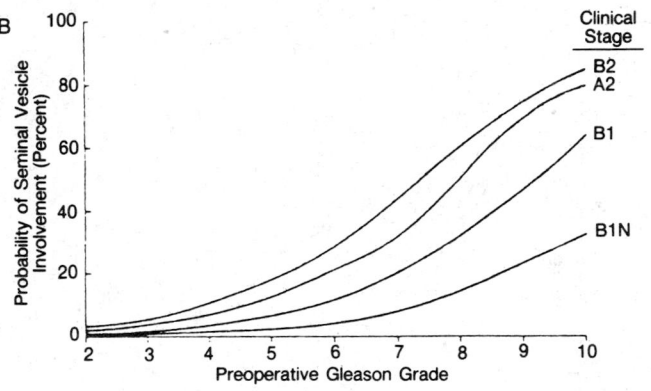

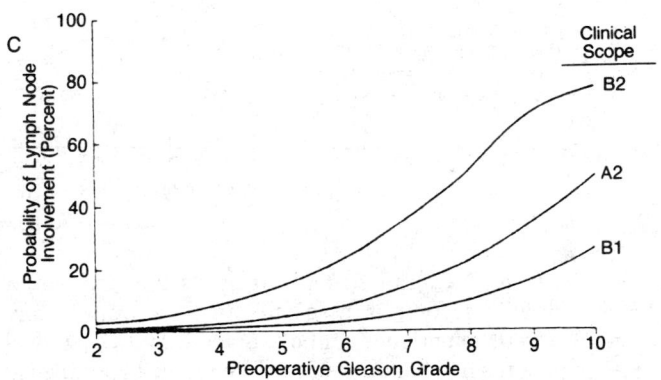

FIG. 33-8. **A.** Probability of capsular penetration as a function of serum prostatic acid phosphatase level and preoperative Gleason grade. **B.** Probability of seminal vesicle involvement as a function of preoperative Gleason grade and clinical stage. There is no curve for A1 disease because no patient in this series with that clinical stage cancer had seminal vesicle involvement. **C.** Probability of lymph node involvement as a function of preoperative Gleason grade and clinical stage. There are no curves for A1 and B1N disease because no patient with either of these clinical stages had positive lymph nodes. (Oesterling JE et al: Correlation of clinical stage, serum prostatic acid phosphatase and preoperative Gleason grade with final pathological stage in 175 patients with clinically localized adenocarcinoma of the prostate. J Urol 138:92–98, 1982)

nostic importance. Bagshaw et al reported that the disease-free survival rate in patients with negative lymph nodes was 86%, in those with positive pelvic lymph nodes it was 71%, while in those with positive periaortic lymph nodes it was only 30%.[134]

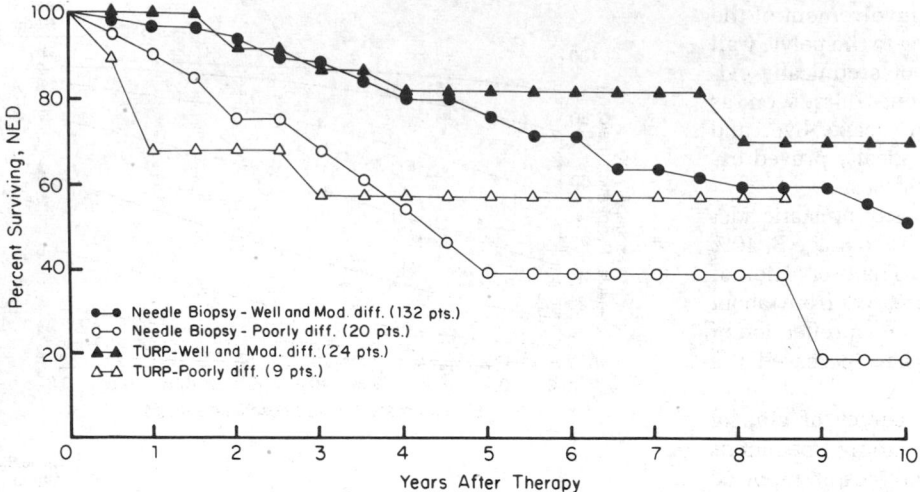

A

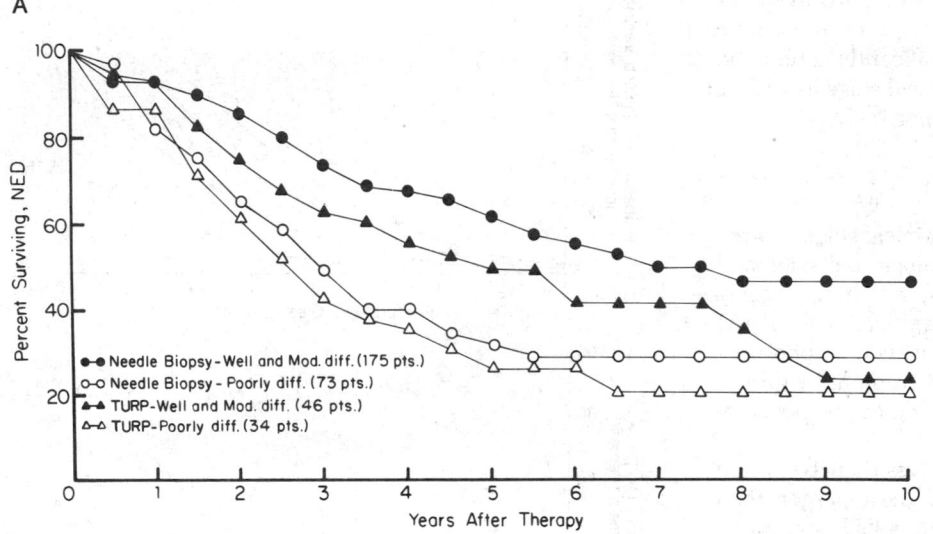

B

FIG. 33-9. NED survival of patients with carcinoma of the prostate correlated with method of diagnosis (needle biopsy or transurethral prostatic resection) and histologic grade. **A.** Stage B. **B.** Stage C. (Perez CA et al: Definitive radiation therapy in carcinoma of the prostate localized to the pelvis: Experience at the Mallinckrodt Institute of Radiology. Natl Cancer Inst Monogr [in press])

A report by McGowan strongly suggests that the use of transurethral resection is associated with a worse prognosis.[135] In our experience, in both Stage B and C, survival rates in patients in whom this procedure has been performed are comparable to survival rates in those with disease diagnosed by needle biopsy, if the patients are grouped according to tumor differentiation (Fig. 33-9). It is likely that the bulk of tumor, which presumably will be greater in patients requiring transurethral resection of the prostate because of urethral obstruction, and the lesser differentiation may account for the worse prognosis. Similar conclusions were reached by Kuban et al[136] but not by Hanks et al.[137] These observations need to be further investigated.

Hormonal Receptors

In 75% to 80% of cases, tumors of the prostate respond to hormonal therapy. Huggins et al in 1939 and subsequently others demonstrated experimentally the dependency of prostatic enlargement on circulating androgens.[138] Animal studies have confirmed the correlation between prostatic tumor growth and hormonal stimulation by androgens, and be-

tween tumor depression and androgen deprivation or estrogen administration. Huggins and Hodges in 1941 reported historical observations on the treatment of carcinoma of the prostate with hormonal manipulation.[139]

There are some technical difficulties to the characterization of hormonal receptors in human prostatic tissues,[140] which are related to the following factors:

1. The composition of the prostate, with intermixed epithelial and stromal cells; 17β-estradiol receptors are present in both epithelial and stromal tissues from normal, benign prostatic hyperplasic, and adenocarcinoma prostatic specimens.
2. Cellular heterogeneity in prostatic carcinoma.
3. Contamination of tissue with serum testosterone-estradiol binding globulin.
4. High endogenous content of dihydroxytestosterone in human prostate, with near saturation of receptor protein.
5. High content of proteolytic enzymes, difficult to homogenize, which leads to receptor inactivation.

6. The presence of a protein in cytosol of human prostate that binds with high affinity to methyltrienolone (R1881), but has the features of a progesterone receptor.

Nevertheless, Ekman et al in a study of 23 patients reported a significant correlation between the presence of steroid receptors and response to hormonal therapy.[141] Fifteen (83%) of 18 patients with "positive" receptors experienced clinical tumor regression, in contrast to only one response (20%) in 5 patients with "negative" receptors.

TREATMENT

At present, several therapeutic options are available:

1. Observation (in patients with Stage A1 disease), although Walsh[142] believes radical prostatectomy is justified in selected cases.
2. Radical prostatectomy, including the nerve-sparing operation (limited to selected patients with Stage A2 or B disease).
3. Interstitial irradiation combined with staging lymphadenectomy (for selected patients with Stage A2 or B disease).
4. External irradiation (for patients with Stage A2, B, C, or D1 disease).
5. Hormonal manipulation (for various stages).
6. Chemotherapy.

Patients with Stage A1 disease found incidentally on transurethral resection require no treatment because the disease has many years of natural evolution before it becomes a clinical problem.[143] Byar et al reported on 148 patients with Stage A focal carcinoma treated conservatively or not at all.[144] Only 6.8% of these patients experienced disease progression. A literature review disclosed a death rate of only 1.9% in 262 patients with stage A1 cancer.

Barnes and Ninan demonstrated comparable survival for patients with Stage A and B lesions treated with either radical prostatectomy or endocrine therapy.[145] On the other hand, the survivals reported by Thompson[146] from the Mayo Clinic in patients treated with transurethral resection before 1940 are well below those reported with more aggressive therapy. Hanash et al reviewed findings in 200 patients with histologically proven carcinoma of the prostate treated with only transurethral resection between 1934 and 1942 (probably the same population studied by Thompson).[44] Patients were not clinically staged. In those with clinically latent (occult) tumors, the 5-year survival rate was about 50%; the 10-year survival rate for all histologic grades was 30%. This was similar to the expected survival for a comparable normal population. In contrast, patients with clinically manifest tumors had a 5-year survival rate of 20% for those with Grade 1, 2 or 3 disease and less than 5% for those with Grade 4 disease. The 10-year survival rate was below 10% for all grades, significantly below the expected normal survival rate (about 40%). Patients with Stage A2 or B tumors may be treated with a radical prostatectomy, external irradiation, or interstitial ^{125}I implants combined with a staging pelvic lymphadenectomy.

Today many urologists agree that patients with Stage C tumors may be treated with definitive external irradiation, or in some instances palliatively with hormonal manipulation. Patients with distant metastases should be initially treated with hormonal therapy or chemotherapy; irradiation may be useful in controlling local or metastatic tumor growth.

RADICAL PROSTATECTOMY

Radical prostatectomy, initially described by Young in 1905,[147] was popularized by Jewett.[45] Radical prostatectomy is a therapeutic option only when the tumor is confined to the prostate; it has no role in the management of extracapsular disease or in the presence of positive lymph nodes. Freiha reviewed specimens obtained at autopsy or during radical prostatectomy in more than 300 patients and concluded that the largest optimal volume amenable to cure by radical prostatectomy is 1 to 4 cc (1.4-cm nodule), if capsular penetration is considered a proved prognostic sign.[148]

Radical prostatectomy should not be performed for at least 6 to 8 weeks after transurethral resection or open prostatectomy, to minimize technical difficulties. The obliteration of tissue planes during open surgery or a particularly aggressive transurethral resection may make radical prostatectomy difficult to perform, and other therapeutic modalities may have to be considered.

The anatomical location of the prostate makes successful removal of the organ technically difficult and has led to the development of several approaches for radical prostatovesiculectomy, whether by a retropubic or a perineal approach.[149-151] The procedure consists of radical in-continuity removal of the prostate and its investing capsule, together with the seminal vesicles, the ampulla, and the vas deferens (Fig. 33-10). The prostate should be completely removed by excision of the urethra at the prostatomembranous junction; no residual "button" of prostatic tissue should be left at the apex. The fascia extending between the bladder and seminal vesicles should be removed with the specimen despite the potential danger of damage to the posterior bladder wall and ureters. These two fascia layers do provide an area for containment of local tumor growth.

The vascular supply to the prostate arises from the inferior vesical artery, and both veins and arteries course together with their fascia at the vesicoprostatic junction in a posterior lateral direction. The vascular supply of the seminal vesicles also arises from the inferior vesical plexus and is routinely controlled during division and ligation of the vascular pedicles of the prostate.

Arterial bleeding during a radical prostatectomy will often cease spontaneously; however, bleeding from branches of the internal pudendal artery adjacent to the prostate may be difficult to control as these vessels retract into the fat surrounding the rectum. Venous bleeding usually causes the major blood loss during the performance of radical prostatectomy, particularly when the dorsal vein of the penis is divided as it courses under the symphysis pubis. At this point, the vein courses over the anterior surface of the prostate and forms free anastomoses with the veins from Santorini's

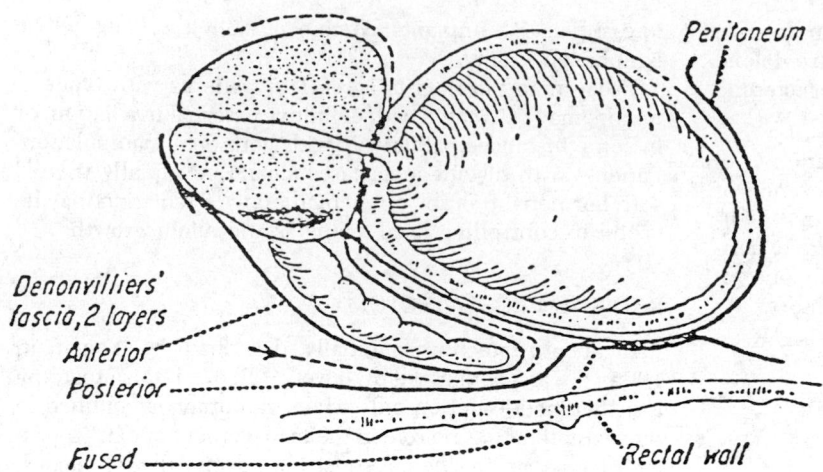

FIG. 33-10. Limits of dissection for radical prostatectomy.

plexus. Any laceration of these friable structures can lead to considerable blood loss that is often difficult to control.

The retropubic approach to radical prostatectomy is preferred by many surgeons. As a rule, urologic oncologists are more familiar with the pelvic anatomy than with the perineal approach. The retropubic prostatectomy also allows the simultaneous performance of a bilateral pelvic lymph node dissection. The use of nerve-sparing techniques to avoid impotence following radical prostatectomy[152] has led to renewed enthusiasm among surgeons for the retropubic approach.

The disadvantages of the retropubic approach to the prostate are the vascularity of the field and the difficulty in establishing a direct vesicourethral anastomosis beneath the pubis, particularly in obese patients. Removal of the pubic symphysis has been advocated. This does not decrease stability of the pelvis postsurgically, but may enhance the degree of postoperative incontinence. Additionally, a nerve-sparing prostatectomy may be more difficult to perform from the perineal approach. The primary contraindications to a surgical procedure are ankylosis of the hips and previous prostatic surgery, which may fix the prostate and bladder in the pelvis and make reconstruction of the vesicourethral junction difficult.

Perineal prostatoseminovesiculectomy has the advantage of providing a relatively avascular field for dissection, good exposure for reconstruction of the vesicourethral anastomosis, and postoperative drainage. The procedure is well tolerated by elderly patients, in whom an intra-abdominal approach may compromise pulmonary function. The principal disadvantage is that it does not afford simultaneous exposure of the pelvic lymphatic drainage and thus a second operative procedure is required.

NERVE-SPARING RADICAL RETROPUBIC PROSTATECTOMY

The successful performance of a nerve-sparing radical prostatectomy is based on attention to important recent observations concerning the prostatic and pelvic anatomy. The first of these, which described the anatomy of the dorsal vein complex and Santorini's plexus, led to modifications in the surgical procedure that reduced blood loss and improved surgical exposure, thereby facilitating the ease of identification and preservation of the nerves.[153] The second observation delineated the location of the autonomic nerves that innervate the corpora cavernosa and modified the operative approach to avoid damaging these structures, thereby retaining potency in many patients.[154] Additionally, improved visualization of the anatomy of the urethrovesical function has led to improvements in the technique of performing the anastomosis between the urethra and the bladder neck, with a resulting decrease in the frequency of postoperative incontinence.[155,156]

The improvement in the rate of impotence and incontinence associated with radical surgery for carcinoma of the prostate has led to a renewed enthusiasm for total prostatectomy to control localized prostatic cancer. The details of the operative technique should be familiar to all urologic oncologists.

The operation is best performed under regional anesthesia. An epidural anesthetic has the advantage of allowing excellent anesthetic control during the surgery, and the resulting peripheral vasodilation appears to greatly reduce blood loss during pelvic surgery. The epidural catheter also allows additional anesthetic agents to be administered in the immediate postoperative period and obviates the need for injectable narcotic medication in many patients.

Before the prostatectomy is begun, a bilateral pelvic lymph node dissection is performed. In the presence of metastatic disease in the lymph nodes, there are no data to support the position that total prostatectomy is a curative procedure, and our policy is not to proceed with the prostatectomy if positive nodes are found.

If the frozen section samples of the lymph nodes are negative for metastatic cancer, the operative procedure is carried out as described by Walsh.[157] After the endopelvic fascia has been incised bilaterally and the puboprostatic ligaments cut to allow the prostate to drop dorsally, the dorsal vein complex is ligated and divided. This maneuver allows direct visualization of the urethroprostatic junction. The neurovascular bundles run parallel and in close proximity to the prostatic capsule and the lateral walls of the proximal urethra.

An important step at this juncture is to spread the tips of

the dissecting scissors just adjacent to the lateral walls of the urethroprostatic junction. This maneuver separates the neurovascular bundles laterally from the urethra and allows passage of a right angle clamp under the urethra. This in turn makes possible the division of the urethra under direct vision and enables the surgeon to cut only the urethra and avoid transecting the neurovascular bundles at the apex of the prostate. Once the urethra is transected, the prostate is separated from the rectum in the midline. This maneuver is facilitated by upward traction on the cut end of the Foley catheter, the balloon of which is still inflated in the bladder. The surgeon can now visualize the relationship of the neurovascular bundles to the tumor and decide whether they must be excised or can be safely preserved. If the decision is made to excise the neurovascular bundle on the side of the tumor, the neurovascular bundle on the contralateral side can usually be preserved. With wide excision of the neurovascular bundle, it is now possible to obtain wider soft tissue margins than were previously attainable with standard radical prostatectomy.[158] The specific operative steps in the surgical procedure have been detailed elsewhere.[159,160]

If a bilateral nerve-sparing technique is appropriate, the lateral pelvic fascia is then divided between fine silk ligatures close to the prostatic capsule. Proceeding in a cephalad direction will bring the seminal vesicles into view, and these structures are excised in their entirety with the prostate.

The bladder neck is then transected at its junction with the prostatic urethra. In performing this maneuver it is important to define a plane between the prostate and the bladder that will allow a relatively small bladder neck opening when the junction between the prostate and bladder is cut.

To ensure coaptation of the bladder mucosa to the proximal urethra, the bladder mucosa is exteriorized by a series of 0000 chromic catgut sutures everting the mucosa over the cut bladder neck. The anastomosis between the bladder and urethra is also done under direct vision using five or six 00 chromic catgut sutures. A Foley catheter is left in place for 3 weeks before removal.

PRESERVATION OF SEXUAL FUNCTION. Walsh recently described the results in 320 men who had undergone a nerve-sparing prostatectomy and were followed up for 1 year or longer.[158] Of the 320 men, 259 were potent preoperatively and had sexual partners. Postoperatively, 192 (74%) were potent.

Potency, which was defined as the ability to achieve an erection sufficient for vaginal penetration and orgasm, returned gradually over the first 2 years following surgery. Potency correlated with both the age of the patient and the stage of the disease (Table 33-11). Thus, potency returned in 93% of patients with Stage A1 disease, 72% with Stage A2 disease, 92% with Stage B1N disease, 72% with Stage B1 disease, and 56% with Stage B2 disease. Of note, in those patients in whom it was necessary to sacrifice the neurovascular bundle on one side, 69% were potent postoperatively.[161]

Of concern has been the possibility that preservation of the neurovascular bundle might compromise the adequacy of the surgical margins obtained. In a recent analysis of 414 patients treated by Walsh and colleagues (Table 33-12), 10% of patients had disease in the surgical margin, a frequency similar to that reported with the older techniques of radical prostatectomy.[158]

IRRADIATION

Interstitial Irradiation

Starting with Pasteau in 1911,[162] radium was used in the treatment of patients with prostatic carcinoma, either by implanting needles through a perineal route or by inserting special applicators through the rectum or the prostatic urethra.[163-166] Bumpus[167] and Nitch[168] utilized rectal, urethral, or external applicators or interstitial implantation into the prostate gland through a suprapubic cystostomy; Caulk[169] combined brachytherapy with supplemental external x-ray therapy. Flocks[170] used interstitial injection of radioactive

TABLE 33-11. Influence of Age and Clinical Stage on Postoperative Potency in 320 Men Followed for at Least 1 Year

Clinical Stage	Age (years)					Total
	30–39	40–49	50–59	60–69	70–75	
A1		100% (2/2)	90% (9/10)	100% (3/3)		93% (14/15)
A2			90% (9/10)	57% (4/7)	0% (0/1)	72% (13/18)
B1N	100% (2/2)	80% (4/5)	97% (30/31)	92% (11/12)	0% (0/1)	92% (47/51)
B1		79% (11/14)	82% (42/51)	65% (39/60)	20% (1/5)	72% (93/130)
B2		67% (2/3)	68% (15/22)	40% (8/20)		56% (25/45)
Total	100% (2/2)	79% (19/24)	85% (105/124)	64% (65/102)	14% (1/7)	74% (192/259)

Walsh PC: Preservation of sexual function in the surgical treatment of prostatic cancer—an anatomic surgical approach. In DeVita VT Jr, Hellman S, Rosenberg SA (eds): Important Advances in Oncology 1988, p 165. Philadelphia, JB Lippincott, 1988.

TABLE 33-12. Pathologic Findings in 414 Consecutive Radical Prostatectomies (in %)

Clinical Stage	No. of Patients	Pathologic Findings (%)				
		Organ Confined	Capsular Penetration	Seminal Vesicle Involvement	Positive Surgical Margin	Positive Lymph Nodes
A1	16	94	6	0	0	0
A2	40	83	17	15	15	10
B1N	78	82	18	3	3	0
B1	196	65	35	10	9	3
B2	84	29	71	31	19	23
Total	414	64	36	13	10	7

Walsh PC: Preservation of sexual function in the surgical treatment of prostatic cancer—an anatomic surgical approach. In DeVita VT Jr, Hellman S, Rosenberg SA (eds): Important Advances in Oncology 1988, p 167. Philadelphia, JB Lippincott, 1988.

colloidal gold into the prostate gland. A local control of over 50% was achieved, with few complications.

In the early 1970s Whitmore et al popularized the retropubic implantation of ^{125}I for clinical Stage A2, B, and selected C cases.[171] A limited staging lymphadenectomy is always performed, and in general, only patients with negative lymph nodes are treated with radioactive implants. The prostate is freed from the endopelvic fascia and the puboprostatic ligament is partially sectioned for better exposure; metallic stylettes are placed in the prostate gland, about 1 cm apart, and not too close to the rectum or the bladder neck (Fig. 33-11A). [125]I seeds, usually 0.4 to 0.5 mCi strength, are inserted at various intervals. In general, an adequate seed implant will deliver 7000 to 8000 cGy to the tumor, with higher doses to the central portion of the gland. The rectum and bladder receive 5000 to 6000 cGy (Fig. 33-11B). Patients who have undergone a complete transurethral prostatic resection have insufficient tissue left to support the ^{125}I seeds.

Charyulu et al[172] and Syed et al[173] described a peritoneal approach with afterloading techniques for implantation of radon or ^{125}I seeds or removable ^{192}Ir implants.

Carlton et al have used radioactive gold ([198]Au) grains combined with external irradiation in the treatment of carcinoma of the prostate.[174] After staging pelvic lymphadenectomy, gold grains are implanted into the prostate gland through a suprapubic incision to deliver 3000 to 3500 cGy, followed by external pelvic irradiation to the pelvis (approximately 4000 cGy).

External Irradiation

With the advent of megavoltage equipment, irradiation has been increasingly used for the treatment of prostatic carcinoma.[175,176] A variety of techniques have been used, varying from parallel anterioposterior (AP) ports with a perineal appositional field, to lateral ports (box technique), or rotational fields to supplement the dose to the prostate. At present, it is not known whether pelvic and periaortic lymph node irradiation may improve survival.[177,178] In patients with obstructive lower urinary tract symptoms who have undergone transurethral resection, 4 weeks should elapse before radiation therapy is initiated, in order to decrease sequelae (urinary incontinence, urethral strictures).

Hormonal manipulation concurrent with irradiation has not been shown to improve survival or tumor control.[131,166,179] Therefore, it is strongly recommended that hormonal therapy be withheld until there is evidence of tumor progression after initial therapy.

PORTALS, BEAM ENERGY, AND TUMOR DOSES. If it is decided to treat the pelvic lymph nodes, as is customarily done at Washington University, the field size for Stage A2 and B lesions is 15 × 15 cm at the patient surface (16.5 cm at isocenter). For Stages C and D1 tumors, the field size is increased to 15 × 18 cm at the patient surface (16.5 × 20.5 cm at isocenter) to cover the common iliac lymph nodes (Fig. 33-12A)

The reduced field for treatment of the prostatic volume can be about 7 × 9 cm to 10 × 12 cm, depending on the size of the gland and periprostatic extensions (Fig. 33-12B). Pilepich et al have issued practical guidelines on the size of the gland as determined by CT in 100 patients and have recommended specific landmarks for use in determining field sizes.[180]

The periaortic lymph nodes can be treated through a separate periaortic port placed above the pelvic fields, in which case an appropriate gap should be calculated. If large-field linear accelerator beams are available, it is more convenient to use a single port that includes both the pelvic and periaortic lymph nodes.

The use of high-energy photon beams (above 10 MV) will simplify the technique and decrease morbidity. Up to 5000 cGy total dose can be delivered through AP and PA ports; the additional dose is administered through rotational ports. Although anterior arc rotation has been employed, a better distribution is obtained with bilateral 120-degree arc rotations that skip the midline anteriorly and posteriorly (Fig. 33-13). With lower energy photon beams (4–10 MV), lateral ports are necessary to deliver part of the dose (box technique) (Fig. 33-14). Posterior oblique fields are occasionally used for the same purpose.

The usual dose of irradiation is 4500 to 5000 cGy to the pelvic and periaortic lymph nodes (when the latter are to be irradiated), with a boost to the prostate. The minimal total tumor dose to the prostate in Stage A2 or B tumor is 6500 cGy, and for Stage C, 7000 cGy. For Stage D1 lesions,

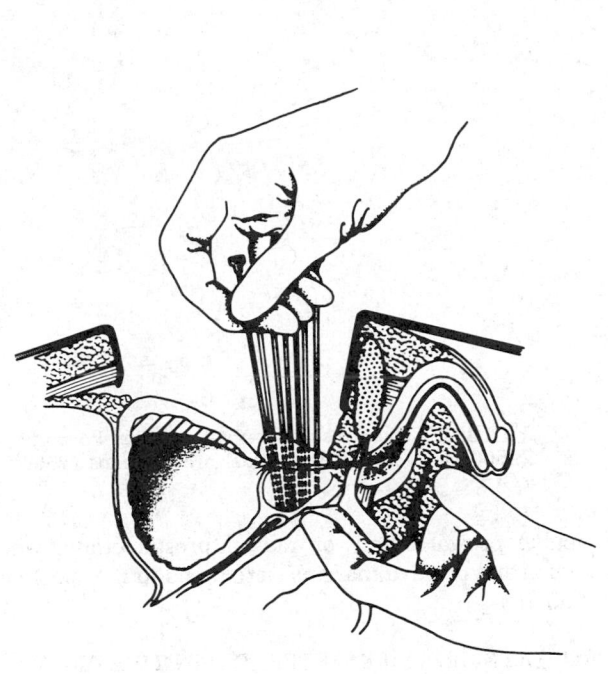

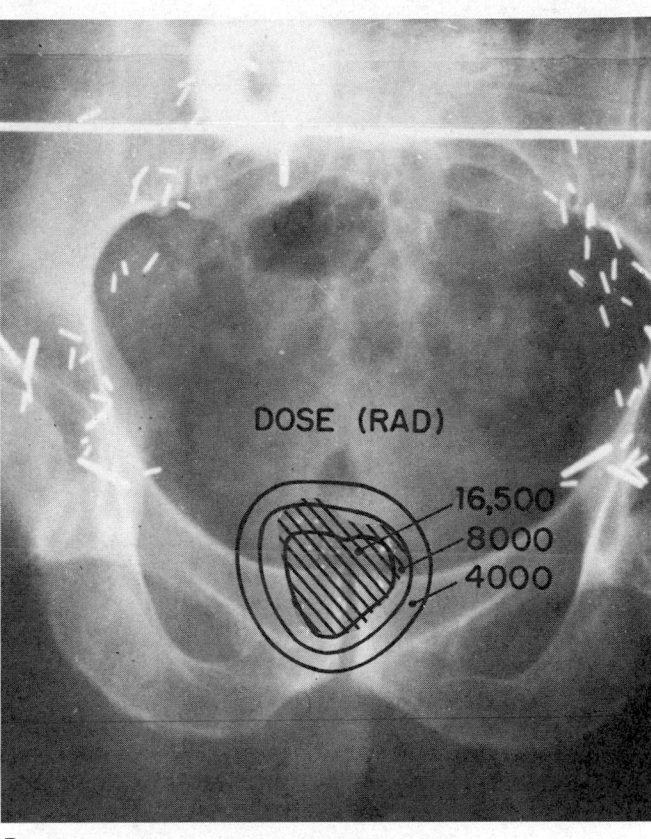

DOSE (RAD)

16,500
8000
4000

A

B

FIG. 33-11. **A**. Suprapubic interstitial implantation in the prostate. **B**. Anteroposterior radiograph of pelvis showing iridium-192 seed implant in the prostate and isodose curves.

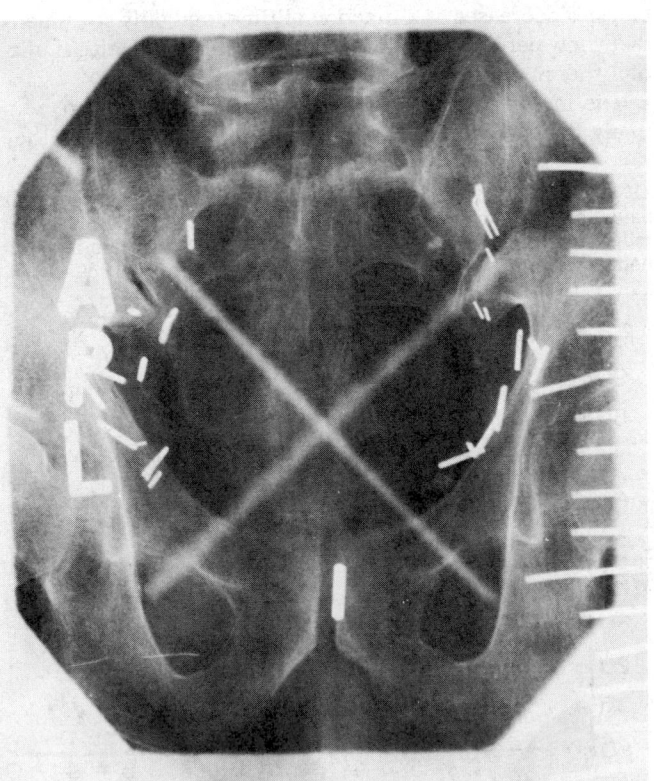

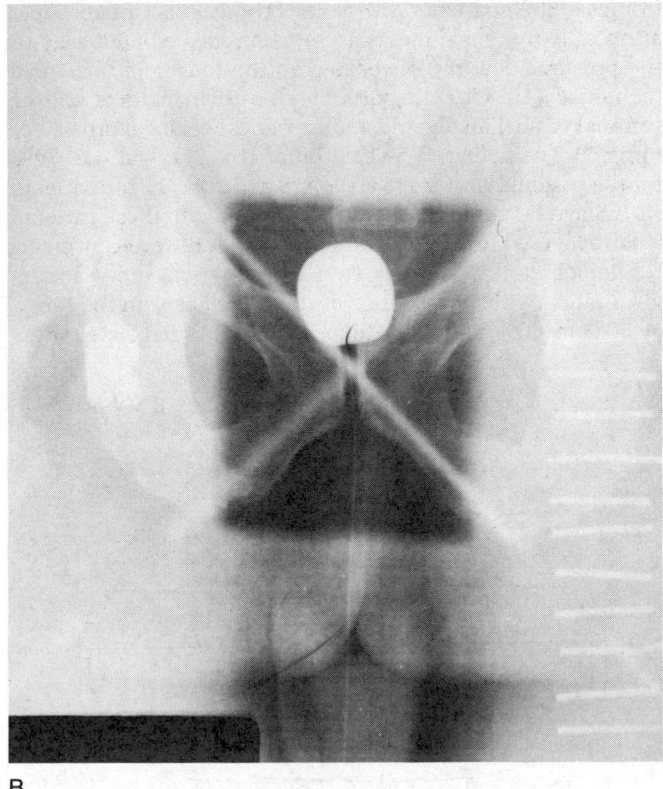

A

B

FIG. 33-12. **A**, **B**. Ports for pelvic lymph nodes and prostate boost.

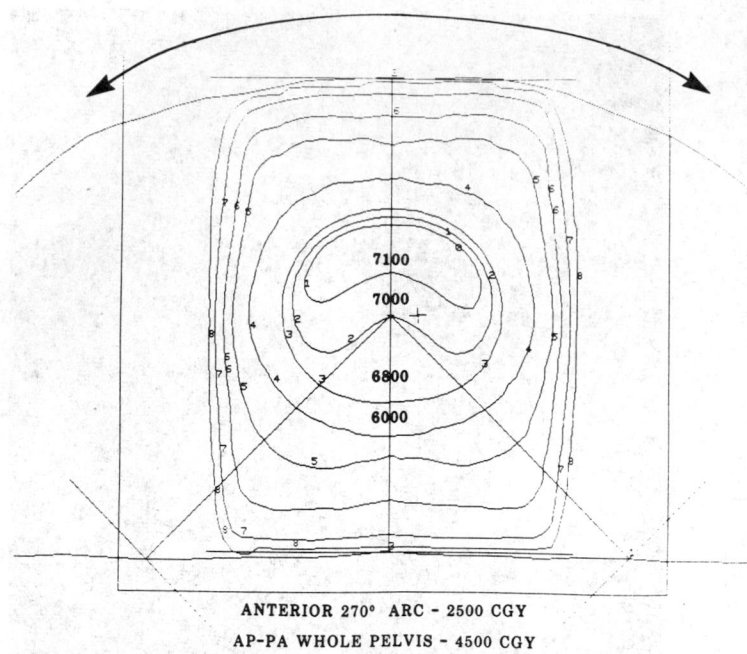

ANTERIOR 270° ARC - 2500 CGY

AP-PA WHOLE PELVIS - 4500 CGY

FIG. 33-13. Dose distribution with AP and PA ports (4500 cGy) and bilateral 120° arc rotations (2500 cGy).

because this treatment is palliative, the minimal tumor dose can be held at 6500 cGy to decrease morbidity.

Most institutions treat with daily fractions of 180 to 200 cGy, five fractions per week.

Irradiation After Prostatectomy

Lang reported treatment results in 30 patients with Stage C lesions and 26 patients with Stage D1a lesions (microscopic areas of lymph node metastases) who received 6000 cGy to the prostatic bed in 6½ weeks with the four-field isocentric technique (10 × 10 cm ports) for positive margins and/or seminal vesical involvement after radical perineal prostatectomy.[181] The actuarial 5-year tumor-free survival was 72% for the patients with Stage C tumors and 70% for the patients with Stage D1 tumors. Therapy was limited to those patients who recovered fully from the operation and were continent.

Pilepich et al[182] and Ray et al[183] also reported 5-year survival rates (without evidence of tumor relapse) in the range of 50% to 60% in small groups of patients irradiated after

suprapubic prostatectomy or radical prostatectomy when carcinoma and positive margins were found in the specimen (Fig. 33-15).

PROSTATE BIOPSIES AFTER DEFINITIVE IRRADIATION. Numerous reports describe the microscopic disappearance of tumor, fibrosis, obliteration of glandular structure, and occasionally calcifications in the prostate after definitive radiation therapy.[184-188] The number of positive biopsies decreases as a function of time, and only specimens that show persistent tumor more than 18 months after radiation therapy may have clinical import.

It is important to determine whether biopsies were routinely done regardless of clinical findings or whether they

FIG. 33-15. Disease-free survival (actuarial life-table method) for patients with carcinoma of the prostate treated with postoperative radiotherapy. (Pilepich MV et al: Postoperative irradiation in carcinoma of the prostate. Int J Radiat Oncol Biol Phys 10:1869–1873, 1984)

FIG. 33-14. Dose distribution with box technique, 6-MV photons.

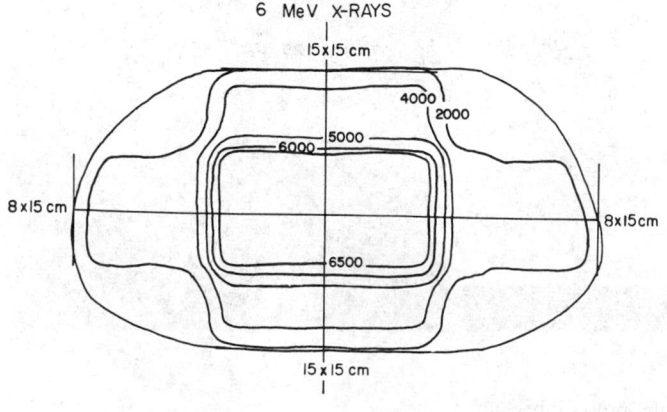

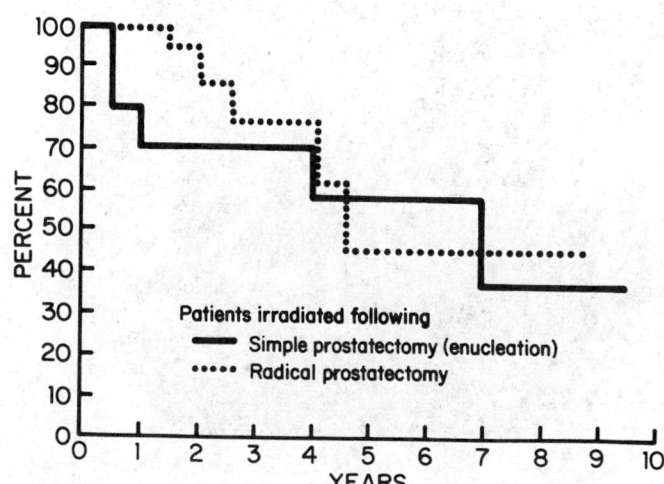

were indicated because of clinical suspicion of tumor progression. In a report by Freiha and Bagshaw on biopsies performed in 64 of 146 patients 2 or more years after completion of irradiation, only 29% of the prostates normal on digital rectal examination contained cancer, in contrast to 85% of those that seemed abnormal.[115]

Cox and Kline recently reported on 46 consecutive patients, many of whom underwent serial transperineal needle biopsies of the prostate following definitive radiation therapy (7000 cGy in 30 to 37 fractions); a decreased incidence of positive specimens was noted, with 19% showing persistent tumor after 24 months and 15% after 42 months.[184] Perez et al recorded the time at which complete tumor regression took place after definitive radiation therapy in patients with Stage B or C carcinoma of the prostate.[55] Figure 33-16 superimposes Perez's clinical findings on the pathologic observations of Cox and Kline. There is a similar pattern of clinical and histologic tumor regression, with about 20% of the cases showing persistent tumor by either method. Therefore, careful periodic digital examination is adequate for evaluating the effects of irradiation on local control of prostatic carcinoma, and biopsies are required only when the gland remains persistently indurated after 18 months or there is evidence of tumor regrowth.

Another important issue discussed in many of the reports is the import of positive biopsy specimens. In general, if the biopsies are done routinely, there is no significant correlation between the positive needle biopsy findings and the clinical course of the patients.[55,184-188] However, Freiha et al[115] and Carlton et al[189] noted that residual viable prostatic carcinoma in needle biopsy specimens more than 2 years after external irradiation is associated with a high rate of local recurrence and distant metastases.

Scardino reported on 475 patients with clinical Stage A2, B, or C1 prostatic carcinoma treated with radioactive gold seed implantation and external beam irradiation.[190] In 124 patients, one or more needle biopsies of the prostate were performed 6 to 36 months after completion of the radiation therapy. Biopsy results were consistently negative in 81 (65%) of the 124 patients and were positive for cancer on one or more occasions in 43 (35%). The rate of local recurrence was 14% in patients with negative biopsy results and

47% in those with positive biopsy results. Distant metastases were noted in 30% of those with negative biopsies and in 51% of those with positive biopsies.

Palliative Irradiation

Patients with massive pelvic extensions of prostatic carcinoma or with lymph node involvement may complain of pelvic pain or hematuria, or may develop urethral obstruction or leg edema due to lymphatic obstruction. Radiation therapy in the range of 5000 cGy may be quite efficacious in the treatment of these symptoms. Carlton et al reported relief of bladder neck obstruction in 20 (50%) of 40 patients treated palliatively, improvement of hydronephrosis in 8 (73%) of 11 patients, and disappearance of intractable hematuria in 7 (100%) of 7 patients who had either failed to respond to estrogen therapy or had been treated with hormones after irradiation.[189]

Kraus et al reported satisfactory results in the palliative treatment of locally advanced prostatic cancer with doses ranging from 2250 to 6600 cGy; most patients received between 4000 and 5000 cGy.[191] Disappearance of gross hematuria was noted in 13 (100%) of 13 patients, and a definitive decrease in the size and induration of the gland was observed in 19 (82%) of 23 patients. Marked improvement in rectal symptoms (pain, constipation, tenesmus) was reported in 5 (100%) of 5 patients after irradiation, and severe rectal bleeding due to tumor invasion was controlled in one patient. Symptoms of lower urinary tract obstruction showed improvement after irradiation in 14 patients; 4 of 5 patients treated for urethral obstruction had a favorable response. Severe edema of the lower extremities improved in 3 patients, and perineal and inguinal pain was relieved in 3 patients.

Increasing urinary difficulty may develop in patients with partial urethral obstruction because of swelling during the initial phase of irradiation. An indwelling catheter may avert a complete blockage, but this should not be used for more than 2 or 3 weeks because of irritation and the danger of superimposed infection. A transurethral resection may be performed occasionally if the obstruction does not improve during the initial course of irradiation.

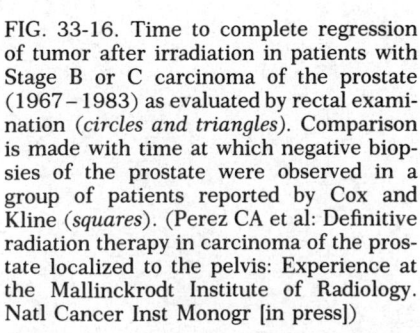

FIG. 33-16. Time to complete regression of tumor after irradiation in patients with Stage B or C carcinoma of the prostate (1967–1983) as evaluated by rectal examination (circles and triangles). Comparison is made with time at which negative biopsies of the prostate were observed in a group of patients reported by Cox and Kline (squares). (Perez CA et al: Definitive radiation therapy in carcinoma of the prostate localized to the pelvis: Experience at the Mallinckrodt Institute of Radiology. Natl Cancer Inst Monogr [in press])

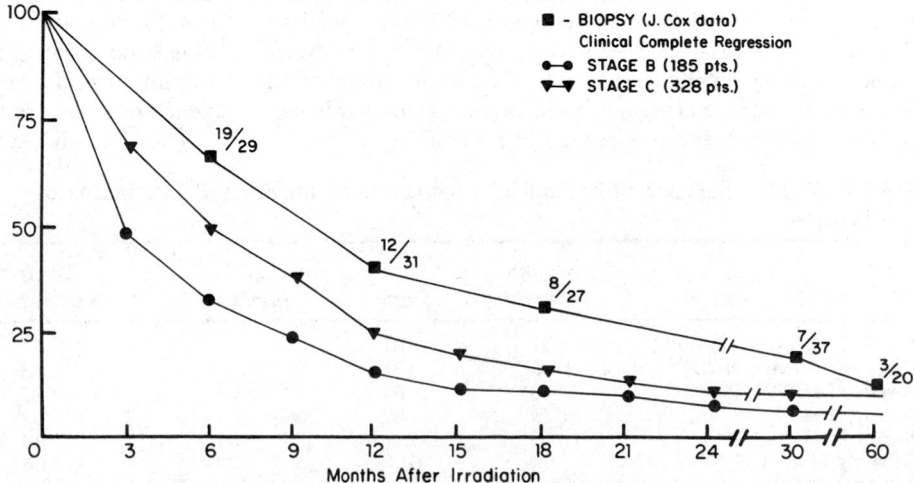

Radiation therapy is also used in the treatment of *distant metastases* from prostatic carcinoma. Marked symptomatic relief is noted in over 80% of the patients treated with doses of 3000 to 3500 cGy in 2 to 3 weeks. Large ports to include the entire bone, such as in the extremities of the pelvis, must be used. Also, portals encompassing the entire thoracic or lumbar spine, as the case may be, will decrease the need for retreatment. Brain metastases may be successfully treated with doses in the range of 3000 to 3500 cGy delivered over 2 or 3 weeks to the entire cranial contents (75% of the patients have multiple lesions).

When practically all the bones of the body are involved by tumor, several investigators have advocated systemic administration of radioactive phosphorus (^{32}P) after priming with testosterone[192-194] or parathormone.[195,196] Testosterone cyprionate, 100 mg, is given intramuscularly each day for 7 to 15 days. After the first 5 or 6 days, ^{32}P (sodium phosphate) administration is begun, either orally or intravenously (1.5 mCi for 6–7 days). Others advocate administration of a single dose of 5 to 7 mCi. Edland reported good to excellent relief of pain in 86% of 42 patients treated.[197]

Pinck and Alexander treated 32 patients with parathormone prior to ^{32}P administration and noted acute pain relief in 22 (69%) and extended (1 year or longer) pain relief in 14 (44%).[198] In these patients, the usual acute gastrointestinal symptoms secondary to irradiation may appear, and there is a certain degree of bone marrow depression.

Straffon et al reported the use of yttrium-90 hypophysectomy in the palliative treatment of patients with painful widespread bony metastases.[199] About half of 13 patients had good response, including 7 that had not responded to orchiectomy or estrogen therapy.

Prophylactic Breast Irradiation Before Hormonal Therapy

Gynecomastia is a common and unwanted side-effect of estrogen therapy that may cause pain, discomfort, and embarrassment. The prevention of gynecomastia and related symptoms has been reported in approximately 80% of patients treated with irradiation in the range of 1000 cGy delivered as a single dose through small appositional ports with superficial x-rays.[200-202] We employ tangential ports with a cobalt-60 or 4-MV photons and deliver a 1200 cGy midplane dose to each breast in three fractions. The entire breast glandular tissue must be irradiated before orchiectomy or the initiation of estrogen therapy, because once glandular hyperplasia is initiated, the process is not reversible.

RESULTS OF THERAPY

SURVIVAL

Radical Prostatectomy

Table 33-13 gives the 10- and 15-year survival rates after radical prostatectomy for Stage B carcinoma of the prostate.[85,203-207] The major difficulties in accurately assessing the impact of treatment on disease that is presumably localized to the prostate are as follows.

1. Patients treated in the past, included to allow an adequate follow-up period, were not staged by modern techniques, such as radioisotope bone scanning, CT, and sensitive tumor biomarkers.
2. None of the studies included bilateral pelvic lymphadenectomy to determine the presence of lymph node metastases at the time of surgery.
3. In many older series, patients with Stage A and B disease were grouped together. Some patients received empirical hormonal therapy in addition to surgery, making it impossible to assess the effect of surgery alone.

In 1970 Jewett described the results of prostatectomy in 111 consecutive patients with tumors less than 1.5 cm in diameter.[205] Ten-year tumor-free survival was 41%. Overall tumor-free survival was 27%. Of the 38 patients who died with disease, 17 had microscopic invasion of the seminal vesicles at the time of prostatectomy; in the remaining 21 the disease was histologically limited to the prostate. In Jewett's series, of 79 patients with Stage B2 disease, 18% survived 15 years, 50% had invasion of the seminal vesicles, and only 5% lived without evidence of tumor for 15 years.

In 1987 Lepor et al updated the results of radical perineal prostatectomy performed at Johns Hopkins University between 1951 and 1963.[208] Seventy patients with clinical Stage I disease, 57 of whom were followed up, had a 5-year survival rate of 83%, a 10-year survival rate of 63%, and a 15-year survival rate of 52%. Survival in these patients was virtually identical to the projected life expectancy of age-matched men in the general population. These results are similar to those reported by Bagshaw in 491 patients with clinical Stage A2 and B carcinoma of the prostate treated with radiation therapy alone, 60% of whom survived 15 years.[209] Gibbons reported that 46 (84%) of 55 patients followed up for a minimum of 15 years were alive or had died without evidence of tumor recurrence.[210]

The Veterans Administration Cooperative Urological Re-

TABLE 33-13.   Survival After Radical Prostatectomy for Stage B Carcinoma of the Prostate

Study, Year	No. of Patients	Stage	10-Year Survival (%)	15-Year Survival (%)
Walsh and Jewett, 1980[203]	57	B1	. . .	51
Culp and Meyer, 1973[204]	86	B1	. . .	33
Jewett, 1970[205]	103	B1	50	27
Jewett, 1956[84]	79	B2		33
Berlin et al, 1968[206]	116	Localized	57	39
Gibbons et al, 1984[207]	54	B1/B2	74	55

search Group reported a randomized trial of radical prostatectomy plus placebo (37 patients) versus placebo alone (29 patients) in patients with Stage A and B tumors.[211] Nine of the placebo-treated patients and seven of the prostatectomy patients were omitted from analysis for various reasons. The results were comparable at a median 7.7-year follow-up of all survivors. Madsen et al noted that six patients in the prostatectomy group had Gleason scores of 8 to 10, in contrast to none in the placebo group. Of the patients treated with radical prostatectomy plus placebo, 45% were alive at 8.5 years, compared to 62% of those treated with placebo alone. The differences were not statistically significant. Also, there was no significant difference in the rate of progression of Stage B prostatic carcinoma after either therapy, only two patients dying with tumor.[212]

Long-term results with the nerve-sparing radical prostatectomy are awaited with high expectation. Unfortunately, patients have not been followed up for a long enough time, and survival results are not yet available.

Direct randomized comparison of radiation therapy versus radical prostatectomy for early prostatic carcinoma was reported by Paulson et al in 97 patients with clinical Stage A2 or B disease.[213] Fifty-six patients received radiation therapy and 41 were treated with radical prostatectomy. The authors did not specify the stratification criteria used or why, in a randomized study, 59 patients were assigned to radiation and 47 to radical prostatectomy. Also, 7 patients in the radiation treatment group and 9 patients in the surgical group did not receive the prescribed treatment. The actuarial disease-free survival was 85% for the surgical patients and 60% for the radiation therapy group. Most treatment failures occurred because of metastases to bone (as evidenced by a positive bone scan) or other distant sites. This certainly should not have been the direct effect of the local irradiation and may be related to the initial distribution of the patients in the two study groups. Furthermore, serious reservations regarding the statistical processing of the data have been raised.[214]

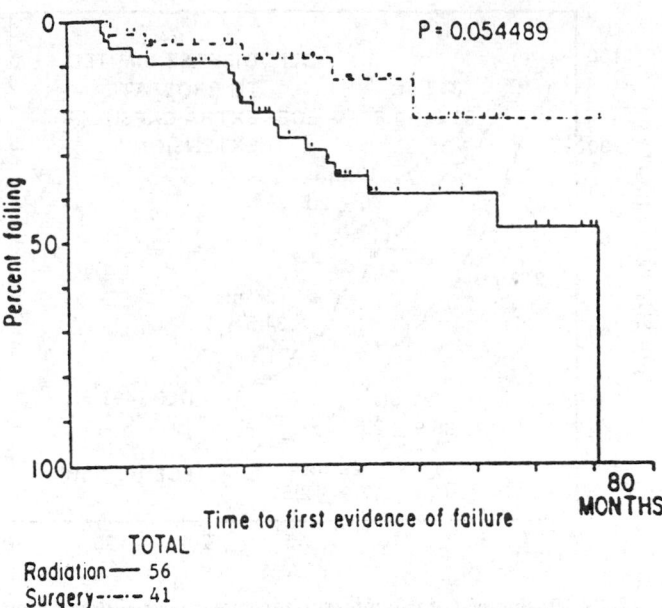

FIG. 33-17. Disease-free survival after additional 20 months of follow-up. (Paulson DF: Randomized series of surgery versus radiation therapy. Presented at the NIH Consensus Development Conference, Management of Clinically Localized Prostate Cancer, Bethesda, MD, June 15–17, 1987).

In 1987 Paulson updated the results in these patients and again noted better survival in the prostatectomy patients (Fig. 33-17).[215] However, the results obtained with radiation therapy in this series are inferior to those reported by other authors.[216] Figure 33-18 illustrates a comparison of survival in patients with similar surgical stage treated with radiation therapy alone by Bagshaw.[209] Therefore, a properly designed prospective clinical trial to compare these two modalities is warranted.

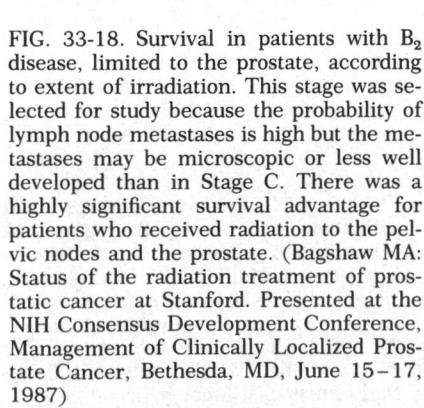

FIG. 33-18. Survival in patients with B₂ disease, limited to the prostate, according to extent of irradiation. This stage was selected for study because the probability of lymph node metastases is high but the metastases may be microscopic or less well developed than in Stage C. There was a highly significant survival advantage for patients who received radiation to the pelvic nodes and the prostate. (Bagshaw MA: Status of the radiation treatment of prostatic cancer at Stanford. Presented at the NIH Consensus Development Conference, Management of Clinically Localized Prostate Cancer, Bethesda, MD, June 15–17, 1987)

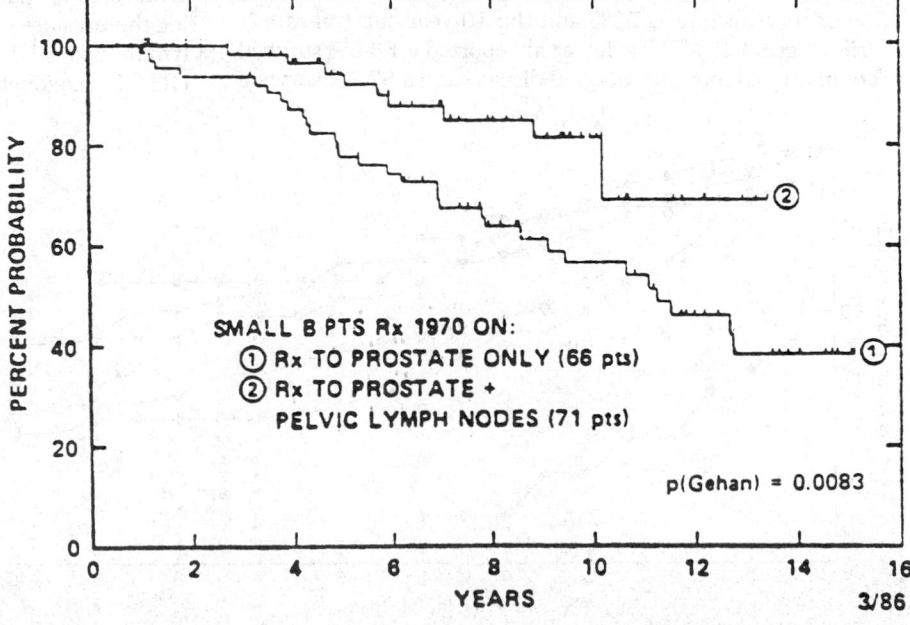

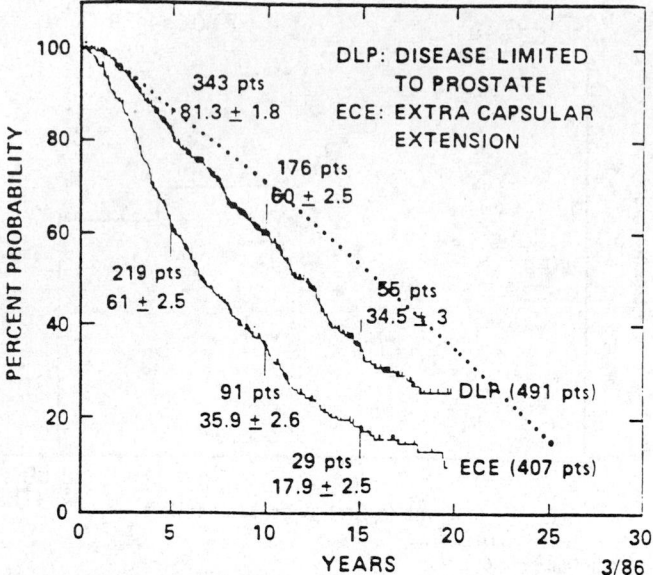

FIG. 33-19. Survival of patients with prostate cancer after radiation therapy, Stanford University. Each upward tick indicates the length of survival for each survivor and that the patient was alive at the time of the last follow-up notation. A downward step indicates the death of one or more patients. The curves are uncorrected, and deaths due to all causes are counted. The expected survival of an age-adjusted cohort of American men is plotted as a separate curve. Percentage survival ±SD at 5-year intervals is annotated to 15 years. (Bagshaw MA: Status of the radiation treatment of prostatic cancer. Presented at the NIH Consensus Development Conference, Management of Clinically Localized Prostate Cancer, Bethesda, MD, June 15–17, 1987)

Irradiation

The largest experience with the use of external irradiation in the treatment of prostatic carcinoma localized to the pelvis has been reported by Stanford University. Their results indicate that at 5 years the disease-free survival rate for patients with tumors localized to the prostate is about 75%, and at 10 years it is 60%. In patients with extracapsular extension the 5-year survival rate is 50% and the 10-year survival rate is 30% (Fig. 33-19).[209] Taylor et al reported a 58.8% survival rate in 36 patients with Stage B disease and a 57.7% survival

rate in 221 patients with Stage C disease with a minimum follow-up of 2 to 3 years.[217] Perez et al recently reported results in 577 patients with various stages of prostatic carcinoma who were followed up for a minimum of 3 years after therapy (median follow-up, 6.5 years).[55] The actuarial disease-free 5-year survival rate was 78% for patients with Stages A2 and B disease, 60% for those with Stage C disease, and 15% for those with Stage D1 disease (Fig. 33-20). The 10-year tumor-free survival rate was 60% for patients with Stages A2 and B disease and 40% for those with Stage C disease (Table 33-14). The local failure rate was about 12% ($5/41$) in patients with Stage A2 tumors and 17% ($31/185$) in those with Stage B tumors; no particular difference was noted with doses ranging from 6000 to 7000 cGy. A significantly higher failure rate was noted in patients with Stage C disease treated with doses below 7000 cGy than in those treated with higher doses (Fig. 33-21). Approximately half of the pelvic failures were also associated with distant metastases. The overall rate of distant metastases was 20% in Stage B, 40% in Stage C, and 65% in Stage D1. Others have reported similar results.[130,135,218–221]

Hanks et al reported the results of definitive radiation therapy (6000–7000 cGy) in 619 patients treated throughout the United States and reported in the Patterns of Care Study.[222] The 5-year survival rate was 75% for Stage A, 85% for Stage B, and 58% for Stage C. The 10-year survival rate was 50% for Stage A2, 61% for Stage B, and 38% for Stage C. These figures are comparable to those reported by single institutions. Furthermore, Hanks et al noted a greater probability of in-field recurrences in patients treated with less than 6500 cGy for Stage T3 or T4 tumors. The complication rate was 6.9% in 174 patients treated with doses above 7000 cGy and 3.5% in those treated with doses below this level (p = 0.03).

McGowan reported that patients with Stage B2 and C tumors in whom the pelvic lymph nodes were treated had a better survival than those who underwent irradiation to the prostate only.[135] By contrast, Neglia et al noted similar survival rates for patients treated either with fields encompassing the prostate only or with larger ports including the pelvic lymph nodes.[130] The Radiation Therapy Oncology Group (RTOG) conducted two randomized studies assessing the

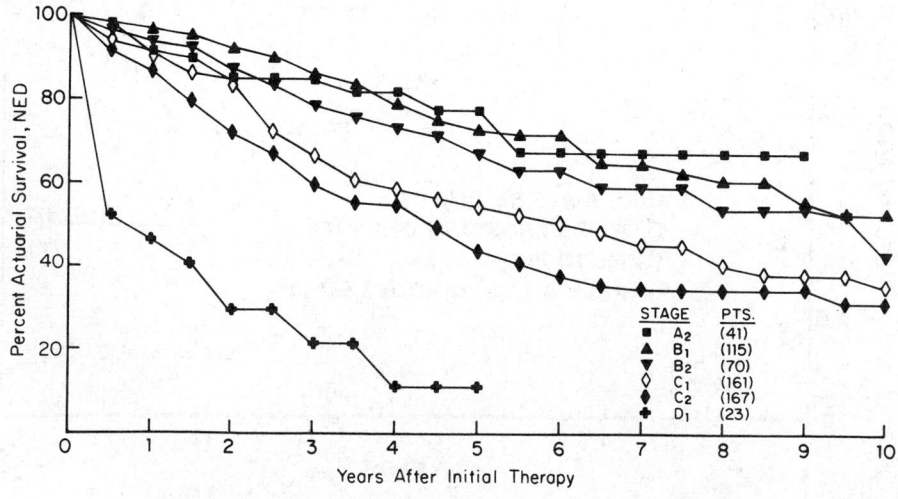

FIG. 33-20. NED survival by stage for 577 patients with carcinoma of the prostate localized to the pelvis treated with definitive irradiation at Mallinckrodt Institute of Radiology (1967–1983). (Perez CA et al: Definitive radiation therapy in carcinoma of the prostate localized to the pelvis: Experience at Mallinckrodt Institute of Radiology. Natl Cancer Inst Monogr [in press])

TABLE 33-14. Carcinoma of the Prostate, 1967–1983: 10-Year Survival

Clinical Stage	No. of Patients at Risk	10-Year Direct Survival		Death — ICD	Adjusted Survival (%)
		No.	(%)		
A2	3	2	(66.7)	1	100
B1	30	21	(70)	2	75
B2	16	10	(62.5)	4	83.3
C1	76	30	(39.5)	16	50
C2	61	20	(32.8)	10	39.2
D1	12	2	(16.7)	2	20

value of irradiation to the pelvic nodes in Stage B disease or the periaortic nodes in Stage C disease.[223,224] Preliminary data reported by Asbell et al[225] and Pilepich et al[177,178] show similar survival, whether or not the pelvic lymph nodes are electively irradiated, in Stage A2 or B tumors. Elective irradiation of the periaortic lymph nodes in patients with Stage C disease or with Stage A2–B disease and positive pelvic nodes failed to improve survival. However, a slightly higher survival rate has been reported by Pistenma et al for patients with positive nodes when the pelvic and periaortic lymph nodes were irradiated.[50]

Hilaris et al[100,226] and Sogani et al[227] reported 5-year survival rates of 80% or higher for patients with T1 and T2 tumors and 55% to 60% for those with T3 tumors treated with ^{125}I implants and staging lymph node dissection. The local failure rate was approximately 15%. Local recurrence was 10% or less with doses over 15,000 cGy and 30% or greater with lower doses.

FIG. 33-21. Correlation of pelvic recurrences and dose of irradiation for patients with Stage B carcinoma of the prostate (1967–1983). (Perez CA et al: Definitive radiation therapy in carcinoma of the prostate localized to the pelvis: Experience at Mallinckrodt Institute of Radiology. Natl Cancer Inst Monogr [in press])

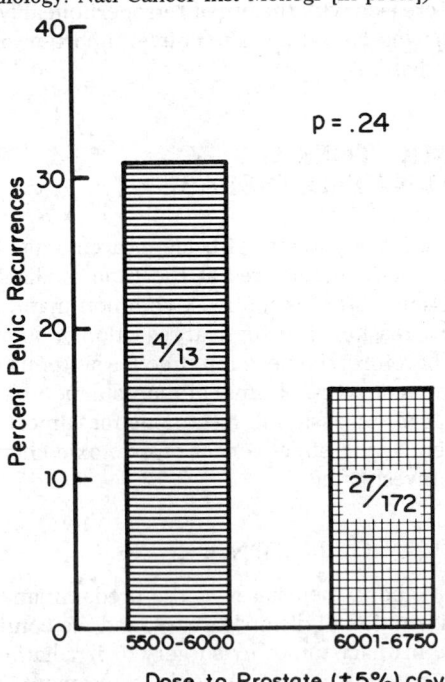

Carlton et al reported results in 542 patients treated with [198]Au grains and external irradiation, with a minimum follow-up of 1 year.[174,189] The survival rates are comparable to those reported after radical prostatectomy or other radiation therapy techniques. Approximately 65% of the patients with Stage A, B, or C1 disease had negative biopsies 1 year or longer after therapy. Exact patterns of failure were not reported.

Batata et al reported on 28 patients who had positive nodes at the time of interstitial therapy and pelvic lymphadenectomy and who then received irradiation to the whole pelvis alone or to the pelvis and the periaortic lymph nodes; they were compared with a group of 24 patients not given external irradiation. The determinate 5-year survival rate was 54% in both groups; the tumor-free 5-year survival rate was 15% (⅔₁₃) with and 21% (5/24) without external irradiation.[228] Similar results were reported by Prout et al, who compared results in 16 patients given external irradiation and 16 patients who received no additional therapy after ^{125}I implantation in the prostate.[51] Nodal external irradiation is probably not effective because 75% to 80% of these patients develop distant metastases and few survive more than 5 years.

TREATMENT SEQUELAE

Surgery

The major objection to the routine use of radical prostatectomy to control localized prostatic carcinoma has been the nearly 100% rate of impotence. However, after the nerve-sparing radical retropubic prostatectomy described by Walsh, 83% of his patients retained potency,[152] whereas Catalona et al observed preservation of potency in only 22 (52%) of 42 sexually potent patients treated with this procedure.[229] From 3% to 7% of the patients will experience urinary incontinence of varying degrees; in a small percentage it can be permanent and disabling.

Other complications of radical prostatectomy include excessive blood loss and fistula formation between the bladder and rectum due to injury to the rectum when the prostate is freed off this structure. The ureters may be damaged if the surgeon dissects within layers of the trigone while attempting to define a cleavage plane between the bladder and seminal vesicles. Fortunately, injuries to the surrounding structures are relatively rare. They occur most commonly in patients who have had previous prostatic surgery or pelvic irradiation.

Thrombophlebitis may occur in a small percentage of patients following bilateral pelvic lymphadenectomy. The incidence does not appear to be appreciably reduced by the routine use of preoperative minidose heparin.[230] Modification of the limits of the node dissection may minimize this problem.

Irradiation

Acute side-effects of irradiation include diarrhea, abdominal cramping, rectal discomfort, and occasionally rectal bleeding, which may be related to a transient enteroproctitis. Patients with hemorrhoids may experience discomfort earlier than other patients, and aggressive symptomatic treatment should be instituted promptly. The symptoms can be controlled with the administration of diphenoxylate hydrochloride with atropine sulfate (Lomotil), opium preparations such as paregoric, Imodium, and emollients such as kaolin and pectin. The local symptoms of proctitis and rectal discomfort can be relieved by administration of small enemas with cod liver oil, and suppositories containing bismuth, benzyl benzoate, zinc oxide, or Peruvian balsam (Anusol, Wyanoids, Medicone, etc.). Some of the suppositories may contain cortisone. Other preparations that can be quite effective are small enemas with hydrocortisone (Proctofoam, Cortifoam). An adequate diet with low residue and no grease or spices usually helps to decrease gastrointestinal symptoms.

Genitourinary symptoms are secondary to cystourethritis and are characterized by dysuria, frequency, and nocturia. The urine is usually clear, although occasionally it may show microscopic or even gross hematuria. Preparations such as mandelamine and antispasmodics, phenazopyridine HCl (Pyridium), or a smooth muscle antispasmodic such as flavoxate HCl (Urispas, Cistopaz) can be effective in relieving symptoms. An adequate fluid intake is extremely important (at least 2000–2500 ml daily). Superimposed infections of the urinary tract may occur and should be diagnosed with appropriate urine culture studies, including tests of sensitivity to sulfonamides and antibiotics. Therapy should be promptly instituted.

Erythema and dry or moist desquamation may develop in the perineum or intergluteal fold. Good skin hygiene and topical application of Vaseline, Aquaphor, or lanolin should suffice. However, if more severe reactions develop, use of zinc oxide ointment or Desitin and intensive skin care are necessary.

More severe late sequelae of treatment include persistent proctitis or proctosigmoiditis, with an occasional patient requiring a colostomy. This complication was noted in 1% of 577 patients. The incidence of rectal ulcers is 2% to 3%, and that of persistent proctitis is about 6%.[55]

Hazra and Giri noted a 43% incidence of proctitis, with 2% of the patients requiring colostomy, in a group of 32 patients with localized prostatic carcinoma treated with 5000 cGy to the pelvic lymph nodes and 1000 cGy to the prostate and adjacent tissues with conventional fractionation, and an additional 800 cGy single-dose exposure to the pelvic girdle.[231] This is not usual and customary therapy.

Chronic cystitis is observed in less than 5% of the patients; with doses of more than 7500 cGy to the bladder hemor-

rhagic cystitis may occasionally develop, requiring a cystectomy (less than 1% of the patients). Urethral stricture has been reported in approximately 5% of patients,[128,232,233] most frequently in patients who underwent transurethral prostatic resection before or during radiation therapy.

A complete tabulation of the reported incidence of severe intestinal or urinary complications was published by Dewit et al.[234]

One of the most vexing sequelae of irradiation is sexual impotence, which has been reported in about 40% of initially potent patients treated with external radiation therapy, but in only 15% of those treated with interstitial ^{125}I. Age may be a factor in this difference, since implants tend to be used in younger patients and external beam irradiation in older patients. Possible causes of sexual impotence include decreased testosterone and dihydroxytestosterone levels, fibrosis or decreased external glandular secretions, pudendal or sympathetic nerve injury, and anxiety or depression.

Serial determinations of plasma dihydroxytestosterone and testosterone levels in patients treated with external irradiation showed no notable changes in hormone levels.[235]

Combined Surgery and Irradiation

The combination of a surgical procedure and definitive radiation therapy is associated with a higher complication rate. Pilepich et al described no excessive edema of the lower extremities in 236 patients treated with definitive radiation therapy alone, in contrast to 15.5% ($^{18}/_{116}$) of patients who had undergone limited pelvic lymph node dissection and 66% ($^{4}/_{6}$) of patients who had undergone extended lymphadenectomy.[236]

Pistenma et al reported a high frequency of small bowel complications in patients in whom a transperitoneal periaortic lymph node dissection was performed and 5500 cGy was delivered through AP and PA ports.[50] The frequency was greatly decreased with the use of retroperitoneal lymph node dissections and lateral ports to deliver a portion of the periaortic irradiation.

SYSTEMIC THERAPY FOR DISSEMINATED DISEASE

Up to one third of patients with adenocarcinoma of the prostate have distant metastases at the time of diagnosis, and distant dissemination is the most common manifestation of disease progression after surgical resection or definitive irradiation. Therefore, the need for effective systemic therapy of this cancer is obvious. Hormonal manipulation has been the standard form of systemic treatment for almost 50 years. More recently, the effectiveness of cytotoxic chemotherapy has been investigated.

EVALUATION OF RESPONSE

Osteoblastic bone metastases as the predominant and often sole manifestation of distant disease, and the continued control of the primary tumor by surgery or irradiation in many men with systemic cancer, make the assessment of response to chemotherapy in prostatic carcinoma especially difficult. Because of this, response in therapeutic trials reported in the literature has been determined by variable and often subjective methods. The need for reproducible and standardized response definitions in prostatic cancer is emphasized by the observation that the "objective" response to cisplatin in one chemotherapy trial ranged from 4% to 23%, depending on which of several published systems of response determination was employed.[237] Methods frequently employed to monitor tumor response are listed in Table 33-15.

Since most patients receiving systemic therapy will have bone metastases, reliable response assessment with radionuclide bone scintigraphy and bone radiography would be of great value. Improvement on serial bone scans and radiographs provides specific evidence of tumor response and is associated with improved survival,[97,238] but radiographic resolution of osteoblastic lesions is rare, scan improvement often lags behind other evidence of response, and the detection of scintigraphic changes requires careful attention to technical details of scanning. Findings on both examinations often worsen with tumor progression, but worsening on either, especially radiography, can also occur with osteoblastic activity associated with bone healing in responding patients[239] and cannot be relied on as the sole evidence of disease progression.

Some investigators do not find primary tumor assessment to be helpful,[240] but the National Prostatic Cancer Project (NPCP) found that regression of the primary tumor correlates with favorable response at 12 weeks of therapy and with normalization of acid phosphatase levels.[241,242] Recent experience suggests that rectal US improves the ability to detect changes in the primary tumor volume during therapy.[243,244]

Substantial declines in elevated values of serum acid phosphatase, which are present in most men with disseminated prostatic cancer, correlate with improved survival on both hormonal therapy[245] and chemotherapy,[246] pain relief, and reduction in size of the primary tumor.[242] Furthermore, elevated values normalize significantly more often in patients with stable disease than in those with progressive disease by NPCP criteria.[247] Radioimmunoassays for acid phosphatase appear no more useful than enzymatic assays for monitoring

TABLE 33-15. Methods for Monitoring of Tumor Response in Patients with Metastatic Prostatic Cancer Given Systemic Therapy

---

Assessment of primary prostatic tumor:
  Physical examination
  Ultrasound examination
Radionuclide bone scans and bone radiographs
Measurement of serum acid phosphatase levels
Determination of serum specific prostatic antigen
Nonspecific indicators of disease status:
  Performance status
  Bone pain
  Weight
  Hemoglobin level
Measurable or evaluable tumor masses:
  Physical examination
  Chest radiographs and/or other radiographs or radionuclide
    studies
  Computed tomography

---

tumor status on systemic treatment.[248] Because of fluctuation in results of repeated measurements of acid phosphatase,[249] reliance should be placed only on confirmed, substantial (twofold or greater) changes in values that persist for at least a month, preferably longer.[248,249] Recent studies of a newly characterized prostate-specific antigen indicate that this test could prove useful in evaluating tumor response.[250]

Until recently, the nonspecific indicators of performance status, bone pain, weight, and hemoglobin level have been the most commonly utilized end points for the evaluation of response in metastatic prostate cancer. Although these parameters frequently worsen with tumor progression and improve with response, especially response to hormonal therapy, 23% to 63% of improvements can occur in patients who experience tumor progression within 12 weeks of initiation of therapy.[241]

Sites of clearly measurable or evaluable masses in metastatic prostatic cancer are infrequently documented with routine tests. Pulmonary metastases are found in 10% to 20% of patients, liver metastases in 10% to 15%, and peripheral lymph node metastases in 10%,[246,251-253] but these patients probably have a worse prognosis than men without such measurable lesions.[246,254] Abnormally enlarged pelvic and abdominal lymph nodes can be detected in 30% to 35% of patients with bone metastases if CT is performed.[252] Objective responses in these more "measurable" sites are associated with improved survival[237,246,251,255] and in one series with improvement in a mean of 4.6 other objective and subjective indicators of response.[252]

Currently, the most widely used response criteria are those of the NPCP, which require normalization of acid phosphatase level, improvement in some evaluable tumor lesion if present, and no new tumor lesions or symptomatic deterioration for 12 weeks in order to declare a partial response.[256] If only the last two criteria plus the failure of any evaluable lesion to worsen are observed, the patient is declared to have stable disease. These criteria may fail to identify some objective tumor regressions. More importantly, studies that utilize NPCP response criteria often report results in terms of "objective response rate," which includes both partial response and stable disease categories.

When NPCP criteria are applied, survival and response duration are similar for patients with partial response or stable disease on both hormonal therapy and chemotherapy.[256] This is also true when other response criteria emphasizing measurable disease are utilized.[255] Criteria that emphasize disease stability are clearly inadequate to document antitumor activity in nonrandomized Phase II trials. A simple, reproducible, universally applicable system for unequivocally and objectively demonstrating tumor response in prostatic cancer remains elusive. This enhances the importance of survival as a measure of therapeutic efficacy in this disease. Response criteria and prognostic factors in prostatic cancer have been reviewed.[257]

HORMONAL THERAPY OF PROSTATIC CARCINOMA

Multiple types of hormonal therapy have been employed since 1941 when Huggins and colleagues demonstrated

TABLE 33-16. Effect of Endocrine Therapy on Hormonal Levels in Prostatic Cancer Patients*

| Therapy | Testosterone Levels | | | Luteinizing Hormone Levels | Estradiol Levels |
	First Week	Long-term	Duration		
Orchiectomy	Castrate	Castrate	Indefinite	Increased	Decreased
Estrogens	Decreased	Castrate	Reversible	Decreased	Increased
LHRH Agonists	Increased	Castrate	Reversible	Increased, then decreased	Decreased
Progestational agents	Decreased	May rebound	Reversible	Decreased	Unknown
Pure antiandrogens	Increased	Increased	Reversible	Increased	Increased
Inhibitors of steroid synthesis	Castrate	Unknown	Reversible	Increased	Decreased

*Modified from Grayhack JT, Keeler TC, Kozlowski JM: Carcinoma of the prostate: Hormonal therapy. Cancer 60:589-601, 1987.

tumor regression and diminution of serum acid phosphatase levels after orchiectomy or estrogen administration in patients with prostatic cancer.[139,258] All protocols seek to reduce androgenic stimulation of the carcinoma by one or more of four mechanisms: ablation of androgen-producing tissue, suppression of pituitary gonadotropin release, inhibition of androgen synthesis, or interference with androgen action in target tissues.[259] Changes in hormone levels induced by, and side-effects of various types of endocrine treatments are summarized in Tables 33-16 and 33-17.

Orchiectomy removes the source of 95% of circulating testosterone and is followed by a prompt, long-lasting decline in serum testosterone levels. Elevated levels of this hormone are not routinely observed with tumor recurrence after orchiectomy.[260] Adrenalectomy reduces extratesticular sources of androgen production in castrated patients, but is now infrequently performed.

The principal action of estrogens in prostatic cancer is thought to be suppression of pituitary gonadotropin release with consequent reduced stimulus for testicular testosterone synthesis, although direct interference with hormonal synthesis or a direct effect on the prostatic cancer cell may also be contributory.[259,260] The nonsteroidal estrogen diethylstilbestrol (DES) suppresses serum testosterone to castrate levels in a dosage of 3 mg/day, while higher dosages have no additional effect.[261] Testosterone is not uniformly suppressed by a 1 mg/day dosage, which nonetheless appears to have similar antitumor effects. Progestational agents suppress gonadotropin release[262] and may also directly interfere

with hormonal synthesis or, in some cases, act as antiandrogens in target tissues.[259,260] With prolonged use of progestins, however, suppressed testosterone levels may rise in some patients.[259] The newly introduced leutinizing hormone-releasing hormone (LHRH) agonists such as leuprolide and buserelin induce an initial rise in gonadotropin levels followed by a sharp decline associated with castrate levels of testosterone within 2 to 3 weeks.[263] Hypophysectomy eliminates gonadotropin and adrenocorticotropic hormone stimulation of testicular and adrenal androgen secretion.

Androgen production in the adrenal gland and the testicle may be inhibited at several points in the synthetic pathway. Aminoglutethimide, which is administered with a glucocorticoid, inhibits the synthesis of all adrenal steroids and leads to further reduction of serum testosterone in castrate patients that may correlate with tumor regression.[264,265] Ketoconazole, an antifungal agent, impairs steroid synthesis, including testicular and adrenal androgens, and can often be administered without supplemental glucocorticoids.[266] Spironolactone, which also has some direct antiandrogenic effects, inhibits male sex hormone production further down the synthetic pathway,[267] and estrogens and progestational agents exert such effects even more distally.[260]

Cyproterone acetate is the most potent of the progestational antiandrogens, which are thought to act by inhibiting formation of the dihydrotestosterone-receptor complex in prostatic nuclei.[259,260] Flutamide is a nonsteroidal antiandrogen that does not suppress gonadotropin or testosterone levels but does have estrogenic side-effects.[268] In contrast to

TABLE 33-17. Morbidity of Endocrine Therapy in Prostatic Cancer Patients*

Effect	Orchiectomy	Estrogens	LHRH Agonists	Antiandrogens
Cardiovascular	−	+†	−	−
Tumor flare	−	−	++	−
Gastrointestinal distress	−	+	−	+
Impotence	++	++	+++	−
Gynecomastia	−	+++	−	++
Hot flashes	+	±	+	−

*Modified from Grayhack JT, Keeler TC, Kozlowski JM: Carcinoma of the prostate: Hormonal therapy. Cancer 60:589-601, 1987.
†Dose dependent.

other forms of hormonal manipulation, it infrequently induces impotence.[259,268] Tamoxifen is a nonsteroidal antiestrogen that has been studied in prostatic cancer because of some evidence of estrogen receptors in neoplastic cells, but it appears to have minimal or no antitumor effects.[269]

Orchiectomy, DES, or LHRH agonists (especially leuprolide) are the most common initial hormonal treatments for metastatic prostate cancer in the United States. When NPCP objective response criteria are applied to patients with disseminated cancer, 37% to 46% of patients have complete or partial responses to any of these maneuvers, and in an additional 39% to 48% the disease stabilizes for 12 weeks or more.[270–272] Pain and impaired ambulatory status improve in 40% to 70% of cases.[271,272] In a large randomized study by the Veterans Administration Cooperative Urologic Research Group (VACURG), DES in a dosage of 5 mg/day, orchiectomy, or the combination was markedly superior to placebo after 6 months in terms of pain relief, improved ambulation, and reduction in primary tumor size, soft tissue metastases, and ureteral dilation. All hormonal therapies delayed the development of distant metastases compared with placebo,[273] and none of the three treatments was superior to another by any parameter.

In contrast to breast cancer, objective response with a second endocrine manipulation is only infrequently observed (5%–15% of cases) in carcinoma of the prostate after termination of response to initial hormonal therapy. Subjective improvement of short duration, however, is not uncommon. DES or orchiectomy,[274] adrenalectomy,[275] hypophysectomy,[276] high-dose DES-diphosphate,[277] progestins,[262] LHRH agonists,[278] aminoglutethimide,[265,279] ketoconazole,[266] antiandrogens,[259] and antiestrogens[280] have been employed in this setting. For most patients their value is undefined. In an early randomized study,[281] DES was not superior to a placebo in orchiectomized patients with progressive tumor.

There is no doubt of the palliative efficacy, both subjective and objective, of hormonal therapy in prostatic cancer, and survival beyond 10 years can occur in up to 10% of patients with bony metastases on such treatment.[282] The influential study of Nesbit and Baum,[274] published in 1950, compared the survival of men given hormonal treatment with survival in a control group treated from 1925 to 1940, before the introduction of endocrine therapy (and of antibiotics), and concluded that orchiectomy, DES, or the combination improved survival in locally advanced or metastatic tumor. A more recent study employing multivariate analysis, however, found that improvement in survival after 1940 in prostatic cancer patients could potentially be explained by a trend toward lower mortality which was occurring from 1937 to 1944 independently of treatment.[283]

The principal prospectively collected data addressing the impact of hormonal therapy on survival was generated by the VACURG in a series of randomized trials. In men with Stage A cancer who did not receive any locoregional therapy, hormone treatment had no impact on survival,[284] and DES in a dosage of 5 mg/day given as an adjuvant after radical prostatectomy to men with Stages A and B disease significantly shortened survival.[285] Adjuvant therapy with DES in patients treated with prostatic or pelvic irradiation confers no survival advantage in randomized studies.[130] Therefore, hormonal treatment should not be administered to any patient with localized or locally advanced cancer unless it is the most feasible method of relieving tumor-related symptoms.

The first large VACURG study randomized patients with locally advanced or metastatic cancer to receive DES (5 mg/day), orchiectomy, both treatments simultaneously, or placebo. In patients with Stage III (locally advanced) disease, estrogen-containing treatments actually shortened survival because of the increased risk of death from cardiovascular causes, while patients with Stage IV disease (distant metastases or elevated serum acid phosphatase levels) had a similar survival rate regardless of treatment.[273] Since changes in treatment were allowed in this study for patients with worsening symptoms, and since almost half the patients with Stage IV disease who were initially given placebo received some form of active treatment within the first year, this trial actually evaluated the merits of immediate hormonal treatment versus withholding such therapy until symptoms worsen.[273] The results imply that hormonal treatment can be withheld in symptomatic patients without compromising survival, provided that therapy is later given when needed. This concept has recently been questioned on theoretical grounds, but no conclusive data that mandate immediate therapy in asymptomatic patients have been forthcoming.[259]

In the second VACURG study in advanced disease, placebo was compared with DES in dosages of 5, 1, or 0.2 mg/day. Excessive cardiovascular deaths in patients with Stage III disease were again noted with the 5-mg dose of DES, but with the 1-mg dose cardiovascular deaths were no greater than with placebo. The 1- and 5-mg doses of DES were similar in retarding progression from Stage III to IV and in reducing overall cancer deaths.[286] Despite the ability of DES to retard development of metastases in Stage III disease, initial therapy with placebo yielded better survival than DES 5 mg/day in Stage III disease and was no worse than the 1-mg dose regimen,[287] once again confirming that withholding hormonal treatment in less advanced disease is not deleterious provided that it is administered when metastases develop. Later analysis of this randomized trial[288] revealed that survival is modestly but significantly better with DES, 1 or 5 mg/day, than with DES, 0.2 mg/day, or placebo in men less than 75 years old (those with the least cardiovascular risk from estrogens) with Stage IV or high-grade tumor, the subgroup most in need of effective anticancer therapy. Recent mature results of this study are said to demonstrate superior survival with DES, 1 mg/day, as initial therapy for men with Stages III and IV disease combined. Nonetheless, proof that hormonal therapy prolongs survival in metastatic prostatic cancer cannot be considered to be established.

A few large trials have compared different forms of hormonal manipulation as initial systemic therapy for prostate cancer. Recent studies have shown that LHRH agonists produce antitumor effects and survival rates similar to those seen with DES and orchiectomy.[272,289] The initial increase in levels of circulating androgens induced by LHRH agonists is not of clinical import in most patients, but in less than 10% worsening pain or urinary symptoms can occur.[272] Some investigators do not advise use of LHRH agonists as sole treatment in patients with impending neurologic compromise.[290] In a European trial in men with locally advanced and metastatic disease, DES, 3 mg/day, and the progestational antiandrogen cyproterone acetate were both superior to medroxyprogesterone acetate in terms of time to tumor progression and survival. Antitumor effects of the former two agents were not significantly different.[291] When a lower dose of medroxyprogesterone acetate was compared with DES, 1 mg/day, in a VACURG study, the progestational agent was again inferior to DES in retardation of tumor progression, though not in overall survival.[292] Some of these randomized trials have established that the 3 mg/day dosage of DES, which currently is often utilized, is associated with more frequent fluid retention and cardiovascular toxicity than the LHRH agonist[272] or antiandrogen[293] to which DES was compared.

Recently the concept of "total blockade" of the effects of both testicular and adrenal androgen production has aroused renewed interest because of the availability of pharmacologic means of achieving this effect with an LHRH agonist and an antiandrogen. Whether adrenal androgens contribute to the growth of prostatic cancer, either supplementary to the testicular hormonal source or after castration, is controversial, but elevated levels of dihydrotestosterone, the active metabolite of testosterone, have been demonstrated in prostatic cancer tissue after orchiectomy.[290,294] The lowest concentration of androgen that is capable of stimulating prostatic cancer growth is unknown, however.[290]

Early promising results with the combination of an LHRH agonist or orchiectomy and an antiandrogen as initial treatment for Stage D2 prostate cancer were obtained by Labrie and colleagues. Recently published data in 131 such patients indicate complete or partial response rates by NPCP criteria of 61%, disease stability in another 34%, actuarial 2-year freedom from tumor progression of 61%, and actuarial 2-year survival of 89%.[295] These results, if reproducible, appear superior to those achieved with previous forms of endocrine therapy. Preliminary results of a randomized study of leuprolide alone versus leuprolide plus flutamide in more than 600 patients with Stage D2 cancer indicate improvement in time to tumor progression with the combination regimen, but the magnitude of this difference is quite modest, with an increase from 13.8 to 16.5 months at the median point. The frequency of improvement in pain and serum acid phosphatase levels after 12 weeks of therapy also favors the two-drug regimen, but there is no significant difference in overall response to therapy or survival with the addition of flutamide to leuprolide, compared to results with leuprolide alone.[296]

Orchiectomy, an LHRH agonist (currently leuprolide in the U.S.), or DES in a dosage of 1 mg/day is presently the recommended standard therapy when hormonal therapy is required in prostatic cancer. Orchiectomy is preferred in men with cardiovascular disease or those who do not wish to take daily medication. LHRH agonists avert some of the psychological effects of orchiectomy, but leuprolide requires daily parenteral administration. Currently there is no proof that any form of hormonal therapy is superior to orchiectomy,[259,290] and initial therapy can be selected based on patient preference, consideration of side-effects, and expense.

The presence of elevated levels of nuclear androgen receptor proteins in prostatic tumor specimens is associated with improved response and survival on initial hormonal manipulation in most[297,298] but not all[299] studies. Heterogeneity of receptor content among tumor cells, sampling problems with small tissue specimens, and technical complexities of current assay systems limit widespread application of these tests. After patients fail initial treatment, a receptor assay would have major clinical utility if it could identify the small minority of patients with a high likelihood of response to a second endocrine therapy.

CYTOTOXIC CHEMOTHERAPY

In addition to major difficulties in objectively documenting tumor response, there are several other reasons for the modest utilization of chemotherapeutic agents in this disease. Prostatic cancer is a disease of older men, many of whom will die of intercurrent illness rather than of the tumor. Even in men with osseous metastases, the course of the disease varies markedly, making survival a poor criterion of treatment efficacy except in prospective randomized clinical trials. Customarily employed endocrine therapies are relatively nontoxic compared with chemotherapy. Finally, and perhaps most important, there are major limitations to the effectiveness of currently available drugs. The present status of chemotherapy in this tumor has been the subject of several reviews.[300-302]

Table 33-18 summarizes results of single-agent chemotherapy in hormone-resistant metastatic prostate cancer. Only drugs administered to at least 40 patients in Phase II or randomized NPCP trials that report "objective" response rates are included.[300] Although response criteria are variable, no chemotherapeutic agent has reproducibly yielded even a 20% complete plus partial remission rate in this setting. Despite its failure to produce tumor regression in all reported studies, doxorubicin had a superior response rate and was associated with better survival (after adjustment for prognostic factors) in a randomized comparison with 5-fluorouracil.[246] Estramustine phosphate, a nitrogen mustard covalently bound to estradiol, produces a high response rate in patients who have not had previous hormone therapy.[303] However, castrate levels of testosterone result from administration of the drug,[304] and the therapeutic contribution of the alkylating moiety is uncertain. As shown in Table 33-18, objective antitumor effects are minimal in men failing hormonal manipulation.

The initial prospective randomized trials of the NPCP compared single-agent cytotoxic chemotherapy in men with Stage D cancer who had failed endocrine treatment with "standard therapy," which included continued administration of other hormonal treatments and palliative irradiation. Of those who had not had major previous irradiation, 41% and 36% of men given cyclophosphamide and 5-fluorouracil, respectively, had *not* developed tumor progression after 12 weeks of treatment, compared with 19% given standard therapy. The difference in freedom from progressive disease between the cyclophosphamide and standard therapy treatment groups was statistically significant[305] and provided an impetus for further evaluation of chemotherapy in prostatic cancer. There was no significant difference in survival

TABLE 33-18.   Single-Agent Chemotherapy in Hormone-Resistant Metastatic Prostatic Cancer*

Drug	No. of Evaluable Patients	CR + PR (%)	Stable Disease (%)
Doxorubicin	88	15	20
Cyclophosphamide	119†	6	34
Cisplatin	117	20	7
	92†	2	27
Estramustine phosphate	86	17	20
	163	3	25
5-Fluorouracil	14	29	21
	33†	12	42
Hydroxyurea	30	50	13
	28†	7	7
Prednimustine	23	0	0
	62†	0	13
Dacarbazine	55†	4	24
Methotrexate	58†	5	36
Amsacrine	40	0	25

*Modified from Eisenberger MA, Simon R, O'Dwyer PJ et al: A reevaluation of nonhormonal cytotoxic chemotherapy in the treatment of prostatic carcinoma. J Clin Oncol 3:827–841, 1985.
†NPCP trial.
CR = complete response, PR = partial response.

among the treatment arms, however.[300] In men who had had prior irradiation, the less myelosuppressive agents estramustine phosphate and streptozocin were compared with standard therapy. There were no significant differences in response rates or survival.[300,306] No other randomized trials of cytotoxic chemotherapy versus further endocrine management or supportive care in hormone-resistant prostate cancer have been reported to date.

Given the very modest efficacy of the available individual drugs, it is perhaps not surprising that randomized trials have failed to demonstrate any superiority of combination chemotherapy to single agent treatment (Table 33-19). In these studies, the intensity of drug administration was less

than in some Phase II studies that were able to demonstrate objective response rates over 20% in good-prognosis patients who were extensively evaluated to document sites of measurable or evaluable tumor.[251,255] A two-drug combination that included doxorubicin produced a significantly higher response rate than hydroxyurea alone, although the survival rate was unaffected.[307]

Cytotoxic chemotherapy has also been administered to prostatic cancer patients without prior hormonal therapy, either in addition to or instead of an endocrine manipulation. The NPCP reported two prospective randomized trials in men with newly diagnosed Stage D2 disease who had not received prior systemic therapy; control patients received

TABLE 33-19.   Randomized Trials of Combination Chemotherapy Versus Single-Agent Chemotherapy in Prostatic Cancer*

Study, Treatment	No. of Evaluable Patients	CR + PR	Stable Disease	Median Survival
Smalley et al[308]				
5-FU	32	2	5	34 wk
CTX + DXR + 5-FU	39	2	4	25 wk
Chlebowski et al[309]				
CTX	15	0	8	7.2 mo
CTX + DXR + 5-FU	12	0	6	8.9 mo
Muss et al[310]				
CTX	17	0	9	8 mo
CTX + MTX + 5-FU	15	1	7	5 mo
Herr[311]				
CCNU	20	0	6	24 wk
CTX + MTX + 5-FU	20	3	4	26 wk
Stephens et al[307]				
HU	69	1/24†	9	28 wk
CTX + DXR	68	6/19†	18	27 wk

*Modified from Eisenberger MA, Simon R, O'Dwyer PJ et al: A reevaluation of nonhormonal cytotoxic chemotherapy in the treatment of prostatic carcinoma. J Clin Oncol 3:827–841, 1985.
†Patients with measurable disease only.
5-FU = 5-fluorouracil, CTX = cyclophosphamide, DXR = doxorubicin, MTX = methotrexate, CCNU = lomustine, HU = hydroxyurea, CR = complete response, PR = partial response.

DES or orchiectomy. DES plus cyclophosphamide or estramustine phosphate plus cyclophosphamide were compared with standard therapy in the first study; DES plus cyclophosphamide plus 5-fluorouracil and estramustine phosphate were evaluated in the second study. There were no significant differences in response rate, time to tumor progression, or survival rate among treatment groups in either study.[259,260] Other studies have also confirmed that estramustine is not superior to DES as initial hormonal therapy in terms of time to tumor progression[303] or survival rate.[303,312]

Combination chemotherapy followed by hormone manipulation only after tumor progression has been given as initial treatment for good-risk patients presenting with distant metastases. Although the anticipated high response to subsequent endocrine treatment did occur, the response rate to chemotherapy alone was not remarkably higher than in the authors' experience with similar chemotherapy given after development of hormone resistance.[313]

Because male hormones are trophic for the malignant tissue in most prostatic cancer patients, an enhanced sensitivity to chemotherapy after stimulation of tumor growth by androgen administration has been postulated. Both early[314] and more recent[315,316] experience, however, suggests that even in men who have failed standard hormone treatment, androgens can produce subjective, objective, and possibly fatal tumor stimulation. A recent randomized study in hormone-refractory patients showed no benefit to "androgen priming" prior to administration of combination chemotherapy.[316]

Tumor regressions with cytotoxic chemotherapy do occur in patients with prostatic cancer resistant to hormonal therapy. Chemotherapy may be modestly better than continued hormone manipulation in delaying further tumor progression in this setting. Its impact is still marginal, however, and no drugs or regimens can be recommended as "standard treatment." Research to identify more drugs with greater antitumor activity is needed.

REFERENCES

1. American Cancer Society 1987 Cancer Facts & Figures. New York, American Cancer Society, 1986
2. Byar DP, Mostofi FK, Veterans Administration Cooperative Urological Research Group: Carcinoma of the prostate: Prognostic evaluation of certain pathologic features in 208 radical prostatectomies examined by the step-section technique. Cancer 30:5–13, 1972
3. Catalona WJ, Chretien P, Trahan EE: Abnormalities of cell-mediated immunocompetence in genitourinary cancer. J Urol 111:229–237, 1974
4. Wang MC, Papsidero LD, Valenzuela LA et al: Prostate antigen: A new potential marker for prostatic cancer. Prostate 2:89–96, 1981
5. Coffey DS, Isaacs JT: Requirements for an idealized animal model of prostatic cancer. In Murphy GP (ed): Models for Prostate Cancer pp 379–391. New York, Alan R Liss, 1980
6. Ferri A: Decaruncla Cusive callo quae cervici vesicae innascitur. Naples, 1553
7. Riolan J: Encheiridium Anatomicum et Pathologicum. Lugd Batav, 1649
8. Baillie M: The morbid anatomy of the human body. London, Longmans, 1794
9. Hunter J: Treatise on the Venereal Disease. London, 1788
10. Winkelstein W Jr, Ernster FL: Epidemiology and etiology of prostatic cancer. In Murphy GP (ed): Prostatic Cancer, pp 1–18. Littleton, Mass, PSG Publishing, 1979
11. Rotkin ID: Distribution and risk of prostatic cancer. In: Cancer Epidemiology in the USA and USSR, pp 111–123. NIH publication AD-2044, Washington, DC, US Government Printing Office, 1980
12. Doll R: Geographic variation in cancer incidence: A clue to causation. World J Surg 2:595–602, 1978
13. Breslow N, Chan CW, Dhom G et al: Latent carcinoma of prostate at autopsy in seven areas. Int J Cancer 20:680–688, 1977
14. Staszewski J, Haenszel W: Cancer mortality among the Polish-born in the U.S. JNCI 35:291–297, 1965
15. Haenszel W, Kurihara M: Studies of Japanese migrants: I. Mortality from cancer and other disease among Japanese in the United States. JNCI 40:43–68, 1968
16. Malcolm D: Potential carcinogenic effect of cadmium in animals and man. Ann Occup Hyg 15:33–36, 1972
17. Krain LS: Epidemiologic variables in prostatic cancer. Geriatrics 2:93–97, 1973
18. Wynder EL, Mabushi K, Whitmore WJ Jr: Epidemiology of cancer of the prostate. Cancer 18:344–360, 1971
19. Haenszel WM, Marcus SC, Zimmerer EG: Cancer morbidity in urban and rural Iowa. Public Health Service monograph 37, Bethesda, Md, US Department of Health, Education and Welfare, 1957
20. Akazaki K, Stemmermann GN: Comparative study of latent carcinoma of the prostate among Japanese in Japan and Hawaii. JNCI 50:1137–1144, 1973
21. Hammond EC: Tobacco in persons at high risk of cancer. In Fraumani JF (ed): Persons at High Risk of Cancer: An Approach to Epidemiology and Control, pp 131–138. New York, Academic Press, 1975
22. Bean MA, Yatani R, Liu PI et al: Prostatic carcinoma at autopsy in Hiroshima and Nagasaki Japanese. Cancer 32:498–506, 1973
23. Woolf CM: An investigation of the familial aspects of carcinoma of the prostate. Cancer 13:739–744, 1960
24. Steele R, Lees REM, Kraus AS et al: Sexual factors in the epidemiology of cancer of the prostate. J Chronic Dis 24:29–37, 1971
25. Krain LS: Some epidemiologic variables in prostatic carcinoma in California. Prev Med 3:154–159, 1974
26. Schumman LM, Mandel J, Blackard C et al: Epidemiologic study of prostatic cancer: Preliminary report. Cancer Treat Rep 61:181–186, 1977
27. Rotkin ID: Studies in the epidemiology of prostatic cancer: Expanded sampling. Cancer Treat Rep 61:173–179, 1977
28. Glantz GM: Cirrhosis and carcinoma of the prostate gland. J Urol 91:291–293, 1964
29. Robson MC: Cirrhosis and prostatic neoplasms. Geriatrics 21:150–154, 1966
30. Rotkin ID: Epidemiology clues to increase risk of prostatic cancer. In Spring-Mills E, Hafez ESE (eds): Male Accessory Sex Glands: Biology and Pathology, pp 289–309. New York, Elsevier/North-Holland, 1980
31. Greenwald PKV, Polan AK et al: Cancer of the prostate among men with benign prostatic hyperplasia. JNCI 53:335–340, 1974
32. Armenian HK, Lilienfeld AM, Diamond EL et al: Relationship between benign prostatic hyperplasia and cancer of the prostate. Lancet 2:115–117, 1974
33. Catalona WJ: Prostate Cancer. Orlando, Fla, Grune & Stratton, 1984
34. McNeal JE: Zonal anatomy of the prostate. Prostate 2:35–49, 1981
35. McNeal JE: Origin and development of carcinoma in the prostate. Cancer 23:24–34, 1969
36. McNeal JE: Morphogenesis of prostatic carcinoma. Cancer 18:1659–1666, 1965
37. McNeal JE: Regional morphology and pathology of the prostate. Am J Clin Pathol 49:347–356, 1968
38. Franks LM: Benign nodular hyperplasia of the prostate: A review. Ann R Coll Surg Engl 14:92–106, 1954
39. McNeal JE: Anatomy of the prostate: An historical survey of divergent views. Prostate 1:3–13, 1980
40. Blennerhassett JB, Vickery AL: Carcinoma of the prostate gland: An anatomical study of tumor location. Cancer 19:980–984, 1966
41. Whitmore WF Jr: The natural history of prostatic cancer. Cancer 32:1104–1112, 1973
42. Halpert B, Sheehan EE, Schmalhorst WR et al: Carcinoma of the prostate: A survey of 5,000 autopsies. Cancer 16:737–742, 1963
43. Halpert B, Schmalhorst WR: Carcinoma of the prostate in patients 70 to 79 years old. Cancer 19:695–698, 1966
44. Hanash KA, Utz DC, Cook EN et al: Carcinoma of the prostate: A 15-year follow up. J Urol 107:450–453, 1972
45. Jewett HJ: Radical perineal prostatectomy for palpable, clinically localized, non-obstructive cancer: Experience at the Johns Hopkins Hospital 1909–1963. J Urol 124:492–494, 1980
46. Flocks RH, Culp D, Porto R: Lymphatic spread from prostatic cancer. J Urol 81:194–196, 1959
47. Middleton RG: Value of and indications for staging pelvic lymph node dissection. Presented at the NIH Consensus Development Conference, Management of Clinically Localized Prostate Cancer, Bethesda, Md, June 15–17, 1987
48. McLaughlin AP, Saltzstein SL, McCullough DL et al: Prostatic carcinoma: Incidence and location of unsuspected lymphatic metastases. J Urol 115:89–94, 1976
49. Golimbu M, Morales P, Al-Askari S et al: Extended pelvic lymphadenectomy for prostatic cancer. J Urol 121:617–619, 1979
50. Pistenma DA, Bagshaw MA, Freiha FS: Extended-field radiation therapy for prostatic adenocarcinoma: Status report of a limited prospective trial. In Johnson DE, Samuels ML (eds): Cancer of the Genitourinary Tract, pp 229–247. New York, Raven Press, 1979
51. Prout GR Jr, Heaney JA, Griffin P et al: Nodal involvement as a prognostic indicator in patients with prostatic carcinoma. J Urol 124:226–231, 1980
52. Batson OV: The role of the vertebral veins in metastatic processes. Ann Intern Med 16:38–45, 1942

53. Dodds PR, Caride VJ, Lytton B: The role of vertebral veins in the dissemination of prostatic carcinoma. J Urol 126:753–755, 1981

54. Mostofi FK: Grading of prostatic carcinoma. Cancer Chemother Rep 59:111–117, 1975

55. Perez CA, Pilepich MV, Garcia D et al: Definitive radiation therapy in carcinoma of the prostate localized to the pelvis: Experience at the Mallinckrodt Institute of Radiology. Natl Cancer Inst Monogr (in press)

56. Gleason DF, Mellinger GT, Veterans Administration Cooperative Urological Research Group: Prediction of prognosis for prostatic adenocarcinoma by combined histological grading and clinical staging. J Urol 111:58–64, 1974

57. Gleason DF, Veterans Administration Cooperative Urological Research Group: Histologic grading and clinical staging of prostatic carcinoma. In Tannenbaum M (ed): Urologic Pathology: The Prostate, pp 171–198. Philadelphia, Lea & Febiger, 1977

58. Paulson DF, Uro-Oncology Research Group: The impact of current staging procedures in assessing disease extent of prostatic adenocarcinoma. J Urol 121:300–302, 1979

59. Kramer SA, Spahr J, Brendler CB et al: Experience with Gleason's histopathologic grading in prostatic cancer. J Urol 124:223–224, 1980

60. Freiha FS, Pistenma DA, Bagshaw MA: Pelvic lymphadenectomy for staging prostatic carcinoma: Is it always necessary? J Urol 122:176–177, 1979

61. Gaeta JF, Asirwatham JE, Miller G et al: Histologic grading of primary prostatic cancer: A new approach to an old problem. J Urol 123:689–693, 1980

62. Catalona WJ, Stein AJ, Fair WR: Grading errors in prostatic needle biopsies: Relation to the accuracy of tumor grade in predicting pelvic lymph node metastases. J Urol 127:919–922, 1982

63. Brawn N: The dedifferentation of prostate carcinoma. Cancer 52:246–251, 1983

64. Albert PS, Mallouh C, Nagamatsu GR: Transitional-cell carcinoma of the prostate. Urology 2:128–130, 1973

65. Bates RH Jr: Transitional cell carcinoma of the prostate. J Urol 101:206–207, 1969

66. Dube VE, Farrow GM, Greene LF: Prostatic adenocarcinoma of ductal origin. Cancer 32:402–409, 1973

67. Greene LF, O'Dea MJ, Dockery MD: Primary transitional cell carcinoma of the prostate. J Urol 116:761–763, 1976

68. Johnson DE, Hogan JM, Ayala AG: Transitional-cell carcinoma of the prostate: A clinical morphological study. Cancer 29:287–293, 1972

69. Kopelson G, Harisiadis L, Romas NA et al: Periurethral prostatic duct carcinoma: Clinical features and treatment results. Cancer 42:2894–2902, 1978

70. Tannenbaum, M: Histology of the prostate gland. In Tannenbaum M (ed): Urologic Pathology: The Prostate, pp 312–315. Philadelphia, Lea & Febiger, 1977

71. Bates HR: Transitional cell carcinoma of the prostate. J Urol 101:206–207, 1969

72. Greene LF, Mulcahy JJ, Warren MM et al: Primary transitional cell carcinoma of the prostate. J Urol 110:235–237, 1973

73. Wolfe JHN, Lloyd-Davis RW: The management of transitional cell carcinoma in the prostate. Br J Urol 53:253–257, 1981

74. Melicow MM, Pachter MR: Endometrial carcinoma of prostatic utricle (uterus masculinua). Cancer 20:1715–1722, 1967

75. Mostofi FK, Price EB Jr: Malignant tumors of the prostate. In: Atlas of Tumor Pathology: Tumors of the Male Genital System, 2nd series, fascicle 8, p 253. Washington, DC, Armed Forces Institute of Pathology, 1973

76. Galen RS, Gambino SR: Beyond Normality: The Predictive Value and Efficiency of Medical Diagnosis. New York, John Wiley & Sons, 1978

77. Watson RA, Tang DB: The predictive value of prostatic acid phosphatase as a screening test for prostatic cancer. N Engl J Med 303:497–499, 1980

78. Wang MC, Valenzuela LA, Murphy GP et al: Purification of a human prostatic specific antigen. Invest Urol 17:159–163, 1979

79. Papsidero LD, Kuriyama M, Wang MC et al: Prostate antigen: A marker for human prostate epithelial cells. JNCI 66:37–42, 1981

80. Papsidero LD, Wang MC, Valenzuela LA et al: A prostate antigen in sera of prostatic cancer patients. Cancer Res 40:2428–2432, 1980

81. Seamonds B, Yang N, Anderson K et al: Evaluation of prostate-specific antigen and prostatic acid phosphatase as prostate cancer markers. Urology 28:472–479, 1986

82. Stamey TA, Yang N, Hay AR et al: Prostate-specific antigen as a serum marker for adenocarcinoma of the prostate. N Engl J Med 317:909–916, 1987

83. Emmett JL, Barber KW Jr, Jackman RJ: Transrectal biopsy to detect prostatic carcinoma: A review and report of cases. J Urol 87:460–474, 1962

84. Jewett HJ: Significance of a palpable prostatic nodule. JAMA 160:838–839, 1956

85. Jewett HJ: The present status of radical prostatectomy for stages A and B prostatic cancer. Urol Clin North Am 2:105–124, 1975

86. Guinan P, Bush I, Ray V et al: The accuracy of the rectal examination in the diagnosis of prostatic carcinoma. N Engl J Med 303:499–503, 1980

87. Franzen S, Giertz G, Zajicek J; Cytological diagnosis of prostatic tumor by transrectal aspiration biopsy: A preliminary report. Br J Urol 32:193–196, 1960

88. Andersson L, Jonsson G, Brunk U: Puncture biopsy of the prostate in the diagnosis of prostatic cancer. Scand J Urol Nephrol 1:227–234, 1967

89. Willems JS, Lowhage T: Transrectal fine needle aspiration biopsy for cytologic diagnosis in grading of prostatic carcinoma. Prostate 2:381–395, 1981

90. Esposti PL: Cytologic malignancy grading of prostatic carcinoma by transrectal aspiration biopsy. Scand J Urol Nephrol 5:199–209, 1971

91. Foti AG, Cooper JF, Herschman H et al: Detection of prostatic cancer by solid phase radio-immunoassay of serum prostatic acid phosphatase. N Engl J Med 297:1357–1361, 1977

92. Fair WR, Heston WDW, Kadmon D et al: Prostatic cancer, acid phosphatase, creatinine kinase-BB and race: A prospective study. J Urol 128:735–738, 1982

93. Yam LT: Clinical significance of the human acid phosphatase: A review. Am J Med 56:604–616, 1974

94. Whitesel JA, Donohue RE, Mani JH et al: Acid phosphatase-its influence on pelvic lymph node dissection (abstr 236). Presented at the annual meeting of the American Urologic Association, Kansas City, MO, May 1982

95. Belleville WD, Mahan DE, Sepulveda RA et al: Bone marrow acid phosphatase by radio-immuno assay: Three years of experience. J Urol 125:809–811, 1981

96. Paulson DF, Uro-Oncology Research Group: The impact of current staging procedures in assessing disease extent of prostatic adenocarcinoma. J Urol 121:300–302, 1979

97. Lund F, Smith PH, Suciu S, EORTC Urological Group: Do bone scans predict prognosis in prostatic cancer? A report of the EORTC protocol 3762. Br J Urol 56:58–63, 1984

98. Merrick MV, Ding CL, Chisholm GD et al: Prognostic significance of alkaline and acid phosphatase and skeletal scintigraphy in carcinoma of the prostate. Br J Urol 57:715–720, 1985

99. Murphy GP, Natarajan N, Pontes JE et al: The national survey of prostate cancer in the United States by the American College of Surgeons. J Urol 127:928–934, 1982

100. Hilaris BS, Whitmore WF, Batata MA et al: Behavioral patterns of prostate adenocarcinoma following an I-125 implant and pelvic node dissection. Int J Radiat Oncol Biol Phys 2:631–637, 1977

101. Pistenma DA, Bagshaw MA, Freiha FS: Extended-field radiation therapy for prostate adenocarcinoma: Status report of a limited prospective trial. In Johnson DE, Samuels ML (eds): Cancer of the Genitourinary Tract, pp 229–247. New York, Raven Press, 1979

102. Ray GR, Pistenma DA, Castellino RA et al: Operative staging of apparently localized adenocarcinoma of the prostate: Results in 50 unselected patients. I. Experimental design and preliminary results. Cancer 38:73–83, 1976

103. Gore RM, Moss AA: Value of computed tomography in interstitial ^{125}I brachytherapy of prostatic carcinoma. Radiology 146:453–458, 1983

104. Golimbu M, Morales P, Al-Askari S et al: CAT scanning in staging of prostatic cancer. Urology 18:305–308, 1981

105. Rifkin MD: Endorectal sonography of the prostate: Clinical implications. AJR 148:1137–1142, 1987

106. Lee F, Gray JM, McLeary RD et al: Prostatic evaluation of transrectal sonography: Criteria for diagnosis of early carcinoma. Radiology 158:91–95, 1986

107. Chodak GW, Wald V, Parmer E et al: Comparison of digital examination and transrectal ultrasonography for the diagnosis of prostate cancer. J Urol 135:951–954, 1986

108. Stone NN, Sogani PC, Rosenberg SM et al: Screening of ambulatory patients for prostate cancer by transrectal ultrasonography (unpublished manuscript)

109. Fisher H, Herr H, Sogani P et al: Modified pelvic lymph node dissection in patients undergoing I-125 implantation for carcinoma of the prostate (abstr). Presented at a conference on Prostate and Bladder Cancer, San Francisco, Oct 9–10, 1981

110. Paulson DF: The prognostic role of lymphadenectomy in adenocarcinoma of the prostate. Urol Clin North Am 7:615–622, 1980

111. Paulson DF, Perez CA, Anderson T: Genitourinary malignancies in cancer. In DeVita VT, Hellman S, Rosenberg SA (eds): Cancer: Principles and Practice of Oncology, ed 1, pp 732–785. Philadelphia, JB Lippincott, 1982

112. Arduino LJ, Glucksman MA: Lymph node metastases in early carcinoma of the prostate. J Urol 8:91–93, 1962

113. Whitmore WF Jr, Batata MA, Hilaris BS: Prostate irradiation: Iodine-125 implementation. In Johnson DE, Samuels ML (eds): Cancer of the Genitourinary Tract. New York, Raven Press, 1979

114. Cline WA, Kramer SA, Farnham R et al: Impact of pelvic lymphadenectomy in patients with prostatic adenocarcinoma. Urology 17:129–131, 1981

115. Freiha FS, Bagshaw MA: Carcinoma of the prostate: Results of post-irradiation biopsy. Prostate 5:19–25, 1984

116. Paulson DF, Cline WA, Hinshaw W, Uro-Oncology Research Group: Extended field radiation therapy vs delayed hormonal therapy in node positive prostatic adenocarcinoma. J Urol 127:935–937, 1982

117. Barzell W, Bean MA, Hilaris BS et al: Prostatic adenocarcinoma: Relationship of grade and local extent to pattern of metastases. J Urol 118:278–282, 1977

118. Grossman HB, Batata M, Hilaris D et al: I-125 implantation for carcinoma of prostate: Further follow-up of first 100 cases. Urology 20:591–598, 1982

119. Kramer SA, Cline WA Jr, Farnham R et al: Prognosis of patients with stage D-1 prostatic adenocarcinoma. J Urol 125:817–819, 1981

120. American Joint Committee on Cancer: Manual for Staging of Cancer. Beahrs OH, Myers MH (eds): Philadelphia, JB Lippincott, 1983

121. Rubin P (ed): Clinical Oncology. New York, American Cancer Society, 1983

122. Sheldon CA, Williams RD, Fraley EE: Incidental carcinoma of the prostate: A review of the literature and critical appraisal of classification. J Urol 124:626–631, 1980

123. McMillen SM, Wettlaufer JN: The role of repeat transurethral biopsy in stage A carcinoma of the prostate. J Urol 116:759–760, 1976

124. Parfitt HE, Smith JA, Gliedman JB et al: Accuracy of staging in A1 carcinoma of the prostate. Cancer 51:2346–2350, 1983

125. Golimbu M, Morales P: Stage A2 prostatic carcinoma: Should staging system be reclassified? Urology 13:592–596, 1979

126. Bauer WC, McGavran MH, Carlin MR: Unsuspected carcinoma of the prostate in

suprapubic prostatectomy specimens: A clinico-pathological study of 55 consecutive cases. Cancer 13:370–378, 1960

127. Heaney JA, Chang HC, Daly JJ et al: Prognosis of clinically undiagnosed prostatic carcinoma and the influence of endocrine therapy. J Urol 118:283–287, 1977

128. Barnes R, Hirst A, Rosenquist R: Early carcinoma of the prostate: Comparison of stages A and B. J Urol 115:404–405, 1976

129. DeVere White R, Paulson DF, Glenn JF: The clinical spectrum of prostate cancer. J Urol 117:323–327, 1977

130. Neglia WJ, Hussey DH, Johnson DE: Megavoltage radiation therapy for carcinoma of the prostate. Int J Radiat Oncol Biol Phys 2:873–882, 1977

131. Perez CA, Walz BJ, Zivnuska FR et al: Irradiation of carcinoma of the prostate localized to the pelvis: Analysis of tumor response and prognosis. Int J Radiat Oncol Biol Phys 6:555–563, 1980

132. Scott R Jr, Mutchnik DL, Laskowski TZ et al: Carcinoma of the prostate in elderly men: Incidence, growth characteristics and clinical significance. J Urol 101:602–607, 1969

133. Oesterling JE, Brendler CB, Epstein JI et al: Correlation of clinical stage, serum prostatic acid phosphatase and preoperative Gleason grade with final pathological stage in 175 patients with clinically localized adenocarcinoma of the prostate. J Urol 138:92–98, 1987

134. Bagshaw MA, Pistenma DA, Ray GR et al: Evaluation of extended-field radiotherapy for prostatic neoplasm: 1976 progress report. Cancer Treat Rep 61:297–306, 1977

135. McGowan DG: The value of extended field radiation therapy in carcinoma of the prostate. Int J Radiat Oncol Biol Phys 7:1333–1339, 1981

136. Kuban DA, El-Mahdi AM, Schellhammer PF: The effect of TURP on prognosis in prostatic carcinoma. Int J Radiat Oncol Biol Phys 13:1653–1659, 1987

137. Hanks GE: Optimizing the radiation treatment and outcome of prostate cancer. Int J Radiat Oncol Biol Phys 11:1235–1246, 1985

138. Huggins C, Masino MH, Eichelberger L et al: Quantitative studies of prostatic secretion. Characteristics of the normal secretion: The influence of thyroid suprarenal and testis extirpation and androgen substitution on the prostatic output. J Exp Med 70:543–556, 1939

139. Huggins C, Hodges CV: Studies on prostatic cancer: I. The effect of castration of estrogen and of androgen injection on serum phosphatases in metastatic carcinoma of the prostate. Cancer Research 1:293–297, 1941

140. Murphy GP, Sandberg AA (eds): Progress in Clinical and Biological Research, Vol 23, Prostate Cancer and Hormone Receptors. New York, Alan R Liss, 1979

141. Ekman P, Snochowski M, Zetterberg A et al: Steroid receptor content in human prostatic carcinoma and response to endocrine therapy. Cancer 44:1173–1181, 1979

142. Walsh PC: Radical prostatectomy with preservation of sexual function. Presented at the NIH Consensus Development Conference, Management of Clinically Localized Prostate Cancer, Bethesda, Md, June 15–17, 1987

143. Stamey TA: Cancer of the prostate: An analysis of some important contributions and dilemmas. Monogr Urol 67–94, 1982

144. Byar DP, Veterans Administration Cooperative Urological Research Group: Survival of patients with incidentally found microscopic cancer of the prostate: Results of a clinical trial of conservative treatment. J Urol 108:908–913, 1972

145. Barnes RW, Ninan CA: Carcinoma of the prostate: Biopsy and conservative therapy. J Urol 108:897–900, 1972

146. Thompson GJ: Transurethral resection of malignant lesions of the prostate gland. JAMA 120:1105–1109, 1942

147. Young YH: Early diagnosis and radical cure of carcinoma of the prostate: Being a study of 40 cases and presentations of radical operation. Bull Johns Hopkins Hosp 16:315–321, 1905

148. Freiha FS: Selection criteria for radical prostatectomy based on morphometric studies. Presented at the NIH Consensus Development Conference, Management of Clinically Localized Prostate Cancer, Bethesda, Md, June 15–17, 1987

149. Hutch JA: A new theory of anatomy of the internal urinary sphincter and the physiology of micturition: IV. the urinary sphincteric mechanism. J Urol 97:705–712, 1967

150. Vickery AL Jr, Kerr WS Jr: Carcinoma of the prostate treated by radical prostatectomy: A clinical pathological survey of 187 cases followed for five years and 148 cases followed for ten years. Cancer 16:1598–1608, 1983

151. Weyrauch HM: Surgery of the Prostate. Philadelphia, WB Saunders, 1959

152. Walsh PC: Radical prostatectomy with preservation of sexual function. Urologist Letter Club, March 24, 1983

153. Reiner WG, Walsh PC: An anatomical approach to the surgical management of a dorsal vein and Santorini's plexus during radical retropubic surgery. J Urol 121:198–200, 1979

154. Walsh PC, Donker PJ: Impotence following radical prostatectomy: Insight into etiology and prevention. J Urol 128:492–497, 1982

155. Fowler JE Jr, Clayton M, Roohallah S et al: Early experience with Walsh technique of radical retropubic prostatectomy. Urology 29:242–246, 1987

156. O'Donnell PD, Finan B: Urinary continence following nerve sparing radical prostatectomy. J Urol 137:225A, 1987

157. Walsh PC: Radical retropubic prostatectomy with preservation of sexual function: Evolution of a surgical procedure. AUA Update Series, vol 5, lesson 5, American Urological Association, 1985

158. Walsh PC: Preservation of sexual function and the surgical treatment of prostatic cancer: An anatomic surgical approach. In DeVita VT Jr, Hellman S, Rosenberg SA (eds): Important Advances in Oncology 1988. Philadelphia, JB Lippincott, 1988

159. Walsh PC: Radical retropubic prostatectomy and cystoprostatectomy: Surgical technique for preservation of sexual function. Film produced by Aegis Productions, distributed by Norwich Eaton Pharmaceuticals, 1984

160. Walsh PC: Radical retropubic prostatectomy. In Walsh PC, Gittes RF, Perlmutter AD et al (eds): Campbell's Textbook of Urology, 5th ed, vol 3, pp 2754–2775. Philadelphia, WB Saunders, 1986

161. Walsh PC, Epstein JI, Lowe FC: Potency following radical prostatectomy with wide unilateral excision of the neurovascular bundle. J Urol 138:823–827, 1987

162. Pasteau O: Traitement du cancer de la prostate par le radium. Rev Mal Nutr 1911, p 363

163. Young YH: Use of radium in cancer of the prostate and bladder. JAMA 68:1174–1177, 1917

164. Manon G: D'un moyen simple et facile d'applique le radium dans le cancer de la prostate. J Urol (Paris) 7:335, 1918

165. Deming CL: Results of 100 cases of cancer of the prostate and seminal vesicles treated with radium. Surg Gynecol Obstet 34:99–118, 1922

166. Barringer BS: Radium in the treatment of prostatic carcinoma. Ann Surg 80:881–884, 1924

167. Bumpus HC Jr: Radium in cancer of the prostate: Report of 217 cases. JAMA 78:1374–1376, 1922

168. Nitch CAR: The conservative treatment of carcinoma of the prostate. Br J Urol 8:329–336, 1936

169. Caulk JR: Carcinoma of the prostate. J Urol 37:832–839, 1937

170. Flocks RH: Interstitial irradiation therapy with a solution of Au198 as part of combination therapy for prostatic carcinoma. J Nucl Med 5:691–705, 1964

171. Whitmore WF Jr, Hilaris B, Grabstald H: Retropubic implantation of Iodine 125 in the treatment of prostatic cancer. J Urol 108:918–920,1972

172. Charyulu K, Block N, Sudarsanam A: Preoperative extended field radiation with I-125 seed implant in prostatic cancer: A preliminary report of a randomized study. Int J Radiat Oncol Biol Phys 5:1957–1961, 1979

173. Syed AMN, Puthwala AA, Tansey LA et al: Management of prostate carcinoma: Combination of pelvic lymphadenectomy, temporary IR-192 implantation and external irradiation. Radiology 19:829–833, 1983

174. Carlton CE Jr, Hudgins PT, Guerriero WG et al: Radiotherapy in the management of stage C carcinoma of the prostate. Trans Am Assoc Genitourinary Surg 67:70–74, 1975

175. Cosgrove MD, George FW III, Terry R: The effects of treatment on the local lesion of carcinoma of the prostate. J Urol 109:861–865, 1973

176. DelRegato JA: Long term curative results of radiotherapy of patients with inoperable prostatic carcinoma. Radiology 131:291–297, 1979

177. Pilepich MV, Krall JM, Sause WT et al: Prognostic factors in carcinoma of the prostate: Analysis of RTOG Study 75-06. Int J Radiat Oncol Biol Phys 13:339–349, 1987

178. Pilepich MV, Asbell SO, Krall JM et al: Correlation of radiotherapeutic parameters and treatment related morbidity: Analysis of RTOG Study 77-06. Int J Radiat Oncol Biol Phys 13:1007–1012, 1987

179. van der Werf-Messing D, Sourek-Zikova V, Blonk DI: Localized advanced carcinoma of the prostate: Radiation therapy vs hormonal therapy. Int J Radiat Oncol Biol Phys 1:1043–1048, 1976

180. Pilepich MV, Prasad SC, Perez CA: Computed tomography in definitive radiotherapy of prostatic carcinoma: Part 2. Definition of target volume. Int J Radiat Oncol Biol Phys 8:235–240, 1982

181. Lang PH: Adjuvant postoperative radiation therapy following radical prostatectomy. Presented at the NIH Consensus Development Conference, Management of Clinically Localized Prostate Cancer, Bethesda, Md, June 15–17, 1987

182. Pilepich MV, Walz BJ, Baglan RJ: Postoperative irradiation in carcinoma of the prostate. Int J Radiat Oncol Biol Phys 10:1869–1873, 1984

183. Ray GR, Cassady JR, Bagshaw MA: External beam megavoltage radiation treatment of post-radical prostatectomy residual or recurrent tumor: Preliminary results. J Urol 114:98–101, 1975

184. Cox JD, Kline RW: Do prostate biopsies 12 months or more after external irradiation for adenocarcinoma stage III, predict long-term survival? Int J Radiat Oncol Biol Phys 9:299–303, 1983

185. Leach GE, Cooper JF, Kagan AR et al: Radiotherapy for prostatic carcinoma: Postirradiation prostatic biopsy and recurrent patterns with long term followup. J Urol 128:505–509, 1982

186. Kiesling VJ, McAninch JW, Goebel JL et al: External beam radiotherapy for adenocarcinoma of the prostate: A clinical followup. J Urol 124:851–854, 1980

187. Kagan AR, Gordon J, Cooper JF et al: A clinical appraisal of post-irradiation biopsy in prostatic cancer. Cancer 39:637–641, 1977

188. van der Werf-Messing B: Prostatic cancer treated at the Rotterdam Radiotherapy Institute. Strahlentherapie 154:537–541, 1978

189. Carlton CE Jr, Dawoud F, Hudgins P et al: Irradiation treatment of carcinoma of the prostate: A preliminary report based on 8 years of experience. J Urol 108:924–927, 1972

190. Scardino PT: Local control of prostate cancer with radiation therapy: Frequency and significance of positive postirradiation prostatic biopsy results. Presented at the NIH Consensus Development Conference, Management of Clinically Localized Prostate Cancer, Bethesda, Md, June 15–17, 1987

191. Kraus PA, Lytton B, Weiss RM et al: Radiation therapy for local palliative treatment of prostatic cancer. J Urol 108:612–614, 1972

192. Joshi DP, Seery WH, Goldberg LG et al: Evaluation of phosphorus 32 for intractable pain secondary to prostatic carcinoma metastases. JAMA 193:621–623, 1965

193. Kaplan E, Fels IG, Kotlowski BR et al: Therapy of carcinoma of the prostate metastatic to bone with P32 labeled condensed phosphate. J Nucl Med 1:1, 1960

194. Smart JG: The use of P32 in the treatment of severe pain from bone metastases of carcinoma of the prostate. Br J Urol 37:139–147, 1965

195. Tong ECK, Finkelstein P: The treatment of prostatic bone metastases with parathormone and radioactive phosphorus. J Urol 109:71–75, 1973

196. Rubenfeld S: Treatment of bone metastases from carcinoma of the prostate with parathyroid hormone and radioactive phosphorus. Urology 1:268–269, 1973

197. Edland RW: Testosterone potentiated radiophosphorus therapy of osseous metastases in prostatic cancer. AJR 120:678–683, 1974

198. Pinck BD, Alexander S: Parathormone potentiated radiophosphorus therapy in prostatic carcinoma. Urology 1:201–204, 1972

199. Straffon RA, Kiser WS, Robitaille M et al: Yttrium hypophysectomy in the management of metastatic carcinoma of the prostate gland in 13 patients. J Urol 99:102–105, 1968

200. Larsson L-G, Sundbom C-M: Roentgen irradiation of the male breast. Acta Radiol Ther Phys Biol 58:253–256, 1962

201. Corvalan JG, Gill WM, Egleston TA et al: Irradiation of the male breast to prevent hormone produced gynecomastia. Am J Roentgenol Radiat Ther Nucl Med 106:839–840, 1969

202. Rodriguez-Antunez A, Cook SA, Jelden GL et al: Management of primary and metastatic carcinoma of the prostate by the radiotherapist. AJR 118:876–880, 1973

203. Walsh PC, Jewett HJ: Radical surgery for prostatic cancer. Cancer 45:1906–1908, 1980

204. Culp OS, Meyer JJ: Radical prostatectomy in the treatment of prostatic cancer. Cancer 32:1113–1118, 1973

205. Jewett HJ: The case for radical perineal prostatectomy. J Urol 103:195–199, 1970

206. Berlin BB, Cornwell PM, Connelly RR et al: Radical perineal prostatectomy for carcinoma of the prostate survival in 143 cases treated from 1935-1958. J Urol 99:97–101, 1968

207. Gibbons RP, Korrea RJ, Brannen GE et al: Total prostatectomy for localized prostatic cancer. J Urol 131:73–76, 1984

208. Lepor H, Kimball AW, Walsh PC: Cause-specific survival analysis following radical prostatectomy: The Johns Hopkins Experience. Presented at the NIH Consensus Development Conference, Management of Clinically Localized Prostate Cancer, Bethesda, Md, June 15–17, 1987

209. Bagshaw MA: Status of the radiation treatment of prostatic cancer at Stanford. Presented at the NIH Consensus Development Conference, Management of Clinically Localized Prostate Cancer, Bethesda, Md, June 15–17, 1987

210. Gibbons RP: Total prostatectomy for localized prostatic cancer: Long-term surgical results and current morbidity. The Virginia Mason Clinic experience. Presented at the NIH Consensus Development Conference, Management of Clinically Localized Prostate Cancer, Bethesda, Md, June 15–17, 1987

211. Byar DP, Corle DK: VACURG randomized trial of radical prostatectomy for stages I and II prostate cancer. Urology 17(suppl):7–11, 1981

212. Madsen PO, Corle DK, Byar DP: Radical prostatectomy for carcinoma of the prostate: Stages I and II. In Rost A, Fielder U (eds): Proceedings, International Symposium on the Treatment of Carcinoma of the Prostate, p 46. Berlin, Berlin Urologische Klinik, Klinikum Steglitz, Freie Universität, 1980

213. Paulson DF, Lin GH, Hinshaw W, Stephani S, Uro-Oncology Research Group: Radical surgery versus radiotherapy for adenocarcinoma of the prostate. J Urol 128:502–504, 1982

214. Hanks GE: National practice results of external beam radiation for prostate cancer. Presented at the NIH Consensus Development Conference, Management of Clinically Localized Prostate Cancer, Bethesda, Md, June 15–17, 1987

215. Paulson DF: Randomized series of surgery versus radiation therapy. Presented at the NIH Consensus Development Conference, Management of Clinically Localized Prostate Cancer, Bethesda, Md, June 15–17, 1987

216. Pilepich MV, Bagshaw MA, Asbell SO et al: Definitive radiotherapy in resectable (stage A2 and B) carcinoma of the prostate: Results of a nationwide overview. Int J Radiat Oncol Biol Phys 13:659–663, 1987

217. Taylor WJ, Richardson RG, Hafermann MD: Radiation therapy for localized prostate cancer. Cancer 43:1123–1127, 1979

218. Gibbons RP, Mason JT, Correa RJ Jr et al: Carcinoma of the prostate: Local control with external beam radiation therapy. J Urol 121:310–312, 1979

219. Hussey DH, Chan R, Delclos L et al: Radiotherapy for carcinoma of the prostate. Cancer Bull 30:131–134, 1978

220. Harisiadis L, Veenema RJ, Senyszyn JJ et al: Carcinoma of the prostate: Treatment with external radiotherapy. Cancer 41:2131–2152, 1978

221. Lipsett JA, Cosgrove MD, Green N et al: Factors influencing prognosis in the radiotherapeutic management of carcinoma of the prostate. Int J Radiat Oncol Biol Phys 1:1049–1058, 1976

222. Hanks GE, Leibel SA, Krall JM et al: Patterns of care studies: Dose-response observations for local control of adenocarcinoma of the prostate. Int J Radiat Oncol Biol Phys 11:153–157, 1985

223. Radiation Therapy Oncology Group: Protocol 75-06 randomized radiation therapy for adenocarcinoma of the prostate, stage C or stage B, with positive pelvic nodes. Philadelphia, Radiation Therapy Oncology Group, 1975

224. Radiation Therapy Oncology Group: Protocol 77-06 randomized radiation therapy for adenocarcinoma of the prostate, stage B or A2. Philadelphia, Radiation Therapy Oncology Group, 1977

225. Asbell SO, Krall JM, Pilepich MV et al: Elective pelvic irradiation in stage A$_2$, B carcinoma of the prostate: Analysis of RTOG 77-06. Int J Radiat Oncol Biol Phys (in press)

226. Hilaris BS, Whitmore WF, Batata MA et al: ^{125}I implantation of the prostate: Dose-response considerations. Front Radiat Ther Oncol 12:82–90, 1978

227. Sogani PC, DeCosse JJ Jr, Montie J et al: Carcinoma of the prostate: Treatment with pelvic lymphadenectomy and 125 iodine implants. Clin Bull 9:24–31, 1979

228. Batata MA, Hilaris BS, Chu FCH et al: Radiation therapy in adenocarcinoma of the prostate with pelvic lymph node involvement on lymphadenectomy. Int J Radiat Oncol Biol Phys 6:149–153, 1980

229. Catalona WJ, Dresner SM: Nerve-sparing radical prostatectomy: Extraprostatic tumor extension and preservation of erectile function. J Urol 134:1149–1151, 1985

230. Hindsley JP Jr, Sanfelippo CJ, Fowler JE Jr et al: Mini dose heparin therapy in pelvic lymphadenectomy and ^{125}I implantation for localized prostatic cancer. Urology 15:272–274, 1980

231. Hazra TA, Giri S: Prophylactic pelvic girdle irradiation in the treatment of prostatic carcinoma. Int J Radiat Oncol Biol Phys 7:817–819, 1981

232. Pilepich MV, Perez CA, Walz BJ et al: Complications of definitive radiotherapy for carcinoma of the prostate. Int J Radiat Oncol Biol Phys 7:1341–1348, 1981

233. Ray GR, Cassady R, Bagshaw MA: Definitive radiation therapy of carcinoma of the prostate: A report on 15 years of experience. Radiology 106:407–418, 1973

234. Dewit L, Ang KK, van der Schueren E: Acute side effects and late complications after radiotherapy of localized carcinoma of the prostate. Cancer Treat Rev 10:79–89, 1983

235. Perez CA: Carcinoma of the prostate, a vexing biological and clinical enigma. Int J Radiat Oncol Biol Phys 9:1427–1438, 1983

236. Pilepich MV, Pajak T, George FW et al: Preliminary report on phase III RTOG studies on extended-field irradiation in carcinoma of the prostate. Am J Clin Oncol 6:485–491, 1983

237. Yagoda A, Watson RC, Natale RB et al: A critical analysis of response criteria in patients with prostatic cancer treated with cis-diamminedichloride platinum: II. Cancer 44:1553–1562, 1979

238. Pollen JJ, Gerber K, Ashburn WL et al: Nuclear bone imaging in metastatic cancer of the prostate. Cancer 47:2585–2594, 1981

239. Levenson RM, Sauerbrunn BJL, Bates HR et al: Comparative value of bone scintigraphy and radiography in monitoring tumor response in systemically treated prostatic carcinoma. Radiology 146:513–518, 1983

240. Paulson DF, Berry WR, Cox EB et al: Treatment of metastatic endocrine-unresponsive carcinoma of the prostate gland with multiagent chemotherapy: Indicators of response to therapy. JNCI 63:615–622, 1979

241. Schmidt JD, Johnson DE, Scott WW et al: Chemotherapy of advanced prostatic cancer: Evaluation of response parameters. Urology 7:602–610, 1976

242. Johnson DE, Scott WW, Gibbons RP et al: Clinical significance of serum acid phosphatase levels in advanced prostatic carcinoma. Urology 8:123–126, 1976

243. Fujino A, Scardino PT: Transrectal ultrasonography for prostate cancer: II. The response of the prostate to definitive radiotherapy. Cancer 57:935–940, 1986

244. Kojima M, Watanabe H, Ohe H et al: Kinetic evaluation of the effect of LHRH analog on prostatic cancer using transrectal ultrasonography. Prostate 10:11–17, 1987

245. Byar DP: VACURG studies on prostatic cancer and its treatment. In Tannenbaum M (ed): Urologic Pathology: The Prostate, pp 241–267. Philadelphia, Lea & Febiger, 1977

246. DeWys WD, Begg CB, Brodovsky H et al: A comparative clinical trial of Adriamycin and 5-fluorouracil in advanced prostatic cancer: Prognostic factors and response. Prostate 4:1–11, 1983

247. Slack NH, Mittelman A, Brady MF et al: The importance of the stable category for chemotherapy treated patients with advancing and relapsing prostate cancer. Cancer 46:2393–2402, 1980

248. Zweig MH, Ihde DC: Assessment of serum radioimmune and enzymatic prostatic acid phosphatase and radioimmune creatine kinase BB for monitoring response to therapy in metastatic prostate cancer. Cancer Res 45:3945–3950, 1985

249. Brenckman WD, Lastinger LB, Sedor F: Unpredictable fluctuations in serum acid phosphatase activity in prostatic cancer. JAMA 245:2501–2504, 1981

250. Killian CS, Yang N, Emrich LJ et al: Prognostic importance of prostate specific antigen for monitoring patients with stages B2 to D1 prostate cancer. Cancer Res 45:886–891, 1985

251. Logothetis CJ, Samuels MJ, von Eschenbach AC et al: Doxorubicin, mitomycin-C, and 5-fluorouracil (DMF) in the treatment of metastatic hormonal refractory adenocarcinoma of the prostate, with a note on the staging of metastatic prostate cancer. J Clin Oncol 1:368–379, 1983

252. Winkler CF, Dunnick NR, Eddy J et al: Computed tomography of the abdomen and pelvis: Documentation of tumor response and progression in disseminated prostate cancer. Med Pediatr Oncol 4:20–25, 1986

253. Torti FM, Aston D, Lum BL et al: Weekly doxorubicin in endocrine-refractory carcinoma of the prostate. J Clin Oncol 1:477–482, 1983

254. Berry WR, Laszlo J, Cox E et al: Prognostic factors in metastatic and hormonally unresponsive carcinoma of the prostate. Cancer 44:763–775, 1979

255. Ihde DC, Bunn PA, Cohen MH et al: Effective treatment of hormonally-unresponsive metastatic carcinoma of the prostate with Adriamycin and cyclophosphamide: Methods of documenting tumor response and progression. Cancer 45:1300–1310, 1980

256. Slack NH, Brady MF, Murphy GP et al: A reexamination of the stable category for evaluating response in patients with advanced prostate cancer. Cancer 54:564–574, 1984

257. Torti FM: Response criteria in urologic malignancies: Recent results. Cancer Res 85:50–57, 1983

258. Huggins C, Stevens RE, Hodges CV: Studies on prostatic cancer: II. The effects of castration on advanced carcinoma of the prostate gland. Arch Surg 43:209–223, 1941

259. Grayhack JT, Keeler TC, Kozlowski JM: Carcinoma of the prostate: Hormonal therapy. Cancer 60:589–601, 1987

260. Menon M, Walsh PC: Hormonal therapy for prostatic cancer. In Murphy GP (ed): Prostatic Cancer, pp 175–200. Littleton, Ma, PSG Publishing, 1979

261. Shearer RJ, Hendry WF, Sommerville IF et al: Plasma testosterone: An accurate monitor of hormone treatment of prostatic cancer. Br J Urol 45:668–677, 1973

262. Geller J, Albert J, Yen SSC: Treatment of advanced cancer of prostate with megestrol acetate. Urology 12:537–541, 1978

263. Warren B, Worgul TJ, Drago J et al: Effect of very high dose D-leucine-6-gonadotropin-releasing hormone proethylamide on the hypothalamic-pituitary testicular axis in patients with prostatic cancer. J Clin Invest 71:1842–1853, 1983

264. Worgul TJ, Santen RJ, Samojlik E et al: Clinical and biochemical effect of aminoglutethimide in the treatment of advanced prostatic carcinoma. J Urol 129:51–55, 1983

265. Ahmann FR, Crawford ED, Kreis W et al: Adrenal steroid levels in castrated men with prostatic carcinoma treated with aminoglutethimide plus hydrocortisone. Cancer Res 47:4736–4739, 1987

266. Tapazoglou E, Subramanian MG, Al-Sarraf M et al: High-dose ketoconazole therapy in patients with metastatic prostate cancer. Am J Clin Oncol 9:369–375, 1986

267. Walsh PC, Siiteri PK: Suppression of plasma androgens by spironolactone in castrated men with carcinoma of the prostate. J Urol 114:254–256, 1975

268. Sogani PC, Vagaiwala MR, Whitmore WF: Experience with flutamide in patients with advanced prostatic cancer without prior endocrine therapy. Cancer 54:744–750, 1984

269. Torti FM, Lum BL, Lo R et al: Tamoxifen in advanced prostatic carcinoma: A dose escalation study. Cancer 54:739–743, 1984

270. Murphy GP, Huben RP, Priore R: Results of another trial of chemotherapy with and without hormones in patients with newly diagnosed metastatic prostatic cancer. Urology 28:36–40, 1986

271. Murphy GP, Beckley S, Brady MR et al: Treatment of newly diagnosed metastatic prostate cancer patients with chemotherapy agents in combination with hormones versus hormones alone. Cancer 51:1264–1272, 1983

272. Leuprolide Study Group: Leuprolide versus diethylstilbestrol for metastatic prostatic cancer. N Engl J Med 311:1281–1286, 1984

273. Blackard CE, Byar DP, Jordan WP: Orchiectomy for advanced prostatic carcinoma: A reevaluation. Urology 1:553–560, 1973

274. Nesbit RM, Baum WC: Endocrine control of prostatic carcinoma: Clinical and statistical survey of 1,818 cases. JAMA 143:1317–1320, 1950

275. Bhanalaph T, Varkarakis MJ, Murphy GP: Current status of bilateral adrenalectomy for advanced prostatic carcinoma. Ann Surg 179:17–23, 1974

276. Silverberg GD: Hypophysectomy in the treatment of disseminated prostatic carcinoma. Cancer 39:1727–1731, 1977

277. Citrin DL, Kies MS, Wallemark C-B et al: A phase II study of high dose estrogens (diethylstilbestrol diphosphate) in prostate cancer. Cancer 56:457–460, 1985

278. Eisenberger MA, O'Dwyer PJ, Friedman MA: Gonadotropin hormone-releasing hormone analogues: A new therapeutic approach for prostatic cancer. J Clin Oncol 4:414–424, 1986

279. Drago JR, Santen RJ, Liptonk A et al: Clinical effect of aminoglutethimide, medical adrenalectomy, in treatment of 43 patients with advanced prostatic cancer. Cancer 53:1447–1450, 1984

280. Glick JH, Wein A, Padavic K et al: Phase II trial of tamoxifen in metastatic carcinoma of the prostate. Cancer 49:1367–1372, 1982

281. Brendler H, Prout G: A cooperative group study of prostatic cancer: Stilbestrol versus placebo in advanced progressive disease. Cancer Chemother Rep 16:323–328, 1962

282. Reiner WG, Scott WW, Eggleston JC et al: Long-term survival after hormonal therapy for stage D prostatic cancer. J Urol 122:183–184, 1979

283. Lepor H, Ross A, Walsh PC: The influence of hormonal therapy on survival of men with advanced prostatic cancer. J Urol 128:335–340, 1982

284. Byar DP: Survival of patients with incidentally found microscopic cancer of the prostate: Results of a clinical trial of conservative treatment. J Urol 108:908–913, 1972

285. Arduino LJ, Bailar JC, Becker LE et al: Carcinoma of the prostate: Treatment comparisons. J Urol 98:516–522, 1967

286. Byar DP: The Veterans Administration Cooperative Urologic Research Group's studies of cancer of the prostate. Cancer 32:1126–1130, 1973

287. Bailar JC, Byar DP: Estrogen treatment for cancer of the prostate: Early results with 3 doses of diethylstilbestrol and placebo. Cancer 26:257–261, 1970

288. Byar DP, Green SB: The choice of treatment for cancer patients based on covariate information. Bull Cancer 67:477–490, 1980

289. Parmer H, Edwards L, Phillips RH et al: Orchiectomy versus long-acting D-trp-6-LHRH in advanced prostatic cancer. Br J Urol 59:249–254, 1987

290. Smith JA: New methods of endocrine management of prostatic cancer. J Urol 137:1–10, 1987

291. Pavone-Macaluso M, de Voogt HJ, Viggiano G et al: Comparison of diethylstilbestrol, cyproterone acetate, and medroxyprogesterone acetate in the treatment of advanced prostatic cancer: Final analysis of a randomized phase III trial of the EORTC urological group. J Urol 136:624–631, 1986

292. Byar DP: Hormone therapy: Results of the VACURG studies. In: Management of Clinically Localized Prostate Cancer: NIH Consensus Development Conference, pp 117–119. Bethesda, MD, National Cancer Institute, 1987

293. de Voogt HJ, Smith PH, Pavone-Macaluso M et al: Cardiovascular side effects of diethylstilbestrol, cyproterone acetate, medroxyprogesterone acetate, and estramustine phosphate used for the treatment of advanced prostatic cancer: Results from EORTC trials 30761 and 30762. J Urol 135:303–307, 1986

294. Geller J: Rationale for blockade of adrenal as well as testicular androgens in the treatment of advanced prostate cancer. Semin Oncol 12(suppl 1):28–35, 1985

295. Labrie F, Dupont A, Giguere M et al: Advantages of the combination therapy in previously untreated and treated patients with advanced prostate cancer. J Steroid Biochem 25:877–883, 1986

296. Crawford ED, McLeod D, Dorr A et al: A comparison of leuprolide with flutamide and leuprolide in previously untreated patients with clinical stage D2 cancer of the prostate. J Urol 137:256A, 1987

297. Trachtenberg J, Walsh PC: Correlation of prostatic nuclear androgen receptor content with duration of response and survival following hormonal therapy in advanced prostatic cancer. J Urol 127:466–471, 1982

298. Benson RC, Gorman PA, O'Brien PC et al: Relationship between androgen receptor binding activity in human prostate cancer and clinical response to endocrine therapy. Cancer 59:1599–1606, 1987

299. Gorelic LS, Lamm DL, Ramzy I et al: Androgen receptors in biopsy specimens of prostate adenocarcinoma: Heterogeneity of distribution and relation to prognostic significance of receptor measurements for survival of advanced cancer patients. Cancer 60:211–219, 1987

300. Eisenberger MA, Simon R, O'Dwyer PJ et al: A reevaluation of nonhormonal cytotoxic chemotherapy in the treatment of prostatic carcinoma. J Clin Oncol 3:827–841, 1985

301. Tannock IF: Is there evidence that chemotherapy is of benefit to patients with carcinoma of the prostate? J Clin Oncol 3:1013–1021, 1985

302. Torti FM: Prostatic cancer chemotherapy: Recent results. Cancer Res 85:58–69, 1983

303. Smith PH, Suciu S, Robinson RG et al: A comparison of the effect of diethylstilbestrol with low dose estramustine phosphate in the treatment of advanced prostate cancer: Final analysis of a phase III trial of the EORTC. J Urol 136:619–623, 1986

304. Nickel CJ, Morales A: Estramustine phosphate versus stilbestrol as primary treatment for metastatic cancer of the prostate. Can J Surg 26:434–438, 1983

305. Scott WW, Johnson DE, Schmidt JE et al: Chemotherapy of advanced prostatic carcinoma with cyclophosphamide or 5-fluorouracil: Results of first national randomized study. J Urol 114:909–911, 1975

306. Murphy GP, Gibbons RP, Johnson DE et al: A comparison of estramustine phosphate and streptozotocin in patients with advanced prostatic carcinoma who have had extensive irradiation. J Urol 118:288–291, 1977

307. Stephens RL, Vaughn C, Lane M et al: Adriamycin and cyclophosphamide versus hydroxyurea in advanced prostatic cancer: A randomized Southwest Oncology Group study. Cancer 53:406–410, 1984

308. Smalley RV, Bartolucci AA, Hemstreet G et al: A phase II evaluation of a 3-drug combination of cyclophosphamide, doxorubicin, and 5-fluorouracil in patients with advanced bladder carcinoma or stage D prostatic carcinoma. J Urol 125:191–195, 1981

309. Chlebowski RT, Hestorff R, Sardoff L et al: Cyclophosphamide versus the combination of Adriamycin, 5-fluorouracil, and cyclophosphamide in the treatment of metastatic prostate cancer: A randomized trial. Cancer 42:2546–2552, 1978

310. Muss HB, Howard V, Richards F et al: Cyclophosphamide versus cyclophosphamide, methotrexate, and 5-fluorouracil in advanced prostatic cancer: A randomized trial. Cancer 47:1949–1953, 1981

311. Herr HW: Cyclophosphamide, methotrexate, and 5-fluorouracil combination chemotherapy versus chlorethyl-cyclohexyl-nitrosourea in the treatment of metastatic prostatic cancer. J Urol 127:4620–4625, 1982

312. Benson RC, Gill GM: Estramustine phosphate compared with diethylstilbestrol: A randomized, double-blind, crossover trial for stage D prostate cancer. Am J Clin Oncol 9:341–351, 1986

313. Seifter EJ, Bunn PA, Cohen MH et al: A trial of combination chemotherapy followed by hormonal therapy for previously untreated metastatic carcinoma of the prostate. J Clin Oncol 4:1365–1373, 1986

314. Fowler JE, Whitmore WF: Considerations for the use of testosterone with systemic chemotherapy in prostatic cancer. Cancer 49:1373–1377, 1982

315. Suarez AJ, Lamm DL, Radwin HM et al: Androgen priming and cytotoxic chemotherapy in advanced prostatic cancer. Cancer Chemother Pharmacol 8:261–265, 1982

316. Manni A, Santen RJ, Boucher AE et al: Androgen priming and response to chemotherapy in advanced prostatic cancer. J Urol 136:1242–1256, 1986

WILLIAM R. FAIR

CARLOS A. PEREZ

TOM ANDERSON

CHAPTER 34 *Cancer of the Urethra and Penis*

Malignant lesions of the urethra and penis are uncommon tumors. This fact has contributed somewhat to the controversy regarding their treatment, in that no single institution has sufficient patients to define the natural history and proper therapy. Treatment has often been empiric and published reports anecdotal.

Squamous cell carcinoma is the most common cancer in the penis and urethra. The pattern of spread is primarily a reflection of the area of the organ affected. Likewise, the treatment approach, and in large measure the overall prognosis, is directly related to the region of the urethra or penis involved.

CARCINOMA OF THE MALE URETHRA

Carcinoma of the male urethra is extremely rare, with only approximately 600 cases reported in the world literature.[1] Such carcinomas have been reported in boys as young as 13 years and in men as old as 91, although most patients are over 50 years of age with a peak incidence at 58 years.[2] Significant etiologic factors have not been identified, but chronic inflammation is thought to play a role in the initiation of the disease on the basis of the observation that many patients give a history of prior venereal disease, urethritis, or urethral stricture. The incidence of urethral stricture in men with carcinoma of the male urethra is reported to range from 24% to 76%, with the most frequent site also being the most frequent site of malignancy.[3-6] No racial predisposition has been recorded.

As in bladder cancer, a high percentage of males with carcinoma of the urethra give a history of smoking or occupational exposure to known carcinogens. However, no epidemiologic studies have unequivocally linked these factors to the development of urethral carcinoma.

SYMPTOMS

The lesion is often insidious at onset, with the symptoms being attributed primarily to benign stricture disease rather than to malignancy. Urethral stricture or bleeding in a patient without a history of trauma or venereal disease, or the onset of a perineal abscess or fistula in an elderly man, should suggest the possibility of urethral carcinoma. Because of the nonspecific nature of the symptoms, the interval between the initiation of symptoms and the diagnosis is as long as 15 years with an average of 5 months.[7] The most common presenting symptoms are listed in Table 34-1; most reflect local involvement by the lesion.

PATHOLOGY

Tumors of the male urethra may be categorized according to the histology of the cells lining the anatomic region of origin (Fig. 34-1). The transitional epithelium of the prostatic urethra gives rise to transitional cell malignancy that is histologically and clinically distinct from the adenocarcinoma commonly associated with prostatic malignancy. Benign lesions of condyloma acuminatum, benign papillomas, and urethral caruncles are found within the distal penile urethra and

1059

TABLE 34-1. Presenting Symptoms of Carcinoma of the Male Urethra in 47 Cases

Symptoms	Number	(%)
Palpable urethral mass	34	(72)
Obstructive symptoms (with or without retention)	32	(65)
Pain	12	(26)
Urethral fistula/periurethral abscess	10	(21)
Hematuria	10	(21)
Palpable inguinal mass	9	(19)

TABLE 34-2. Staging System for Carcinoma of the Male Urethra

Stage	Criteria
O	Confined to mucosa only (in situ)
A	Into but not beyond lamina propria
B	Into but not beyond substance of corpus spongiosum or into but not beyond prostate
C	Direct extension into tissues beyond corpus spongiosum (corpora cavernosa, muscle, fat, fascia, skin, direct skeletal involvement), or beyond prostatic capsule
D_1	Regional metastasis including inguinal and/or pelvic lymph nodes (with any primary tumor)
D_2	Distant metastasis (with any primary tumor)

Modified from Ray B, Canto AR, Whitmore W: Experience with primary carcinoma of the male urethra. J Urol 117:591–594, 1977.

EVALUATION AND STAGING

The diagnosis is made by transurethral or needle biopsy. The extent of local involvement can be determined by careful inspection and palpation of the external genitalia and perineum at the time of cystourethroscopy and by bimanual examination with the patient under anesthesia. Cytologic studies of voided urine may be helpful for the diagnosis in some patients.[1] A CT scan or MRI is helpful in evaluating the pelvic and para-aortic nodes. A lymphangiogram may be of value in selected cases but is not required routinely.

The most common staging system currently is that proposed by Ray and associates (Table 34-2). A system proposed by the American Joint Committee (AJC) based on the extent of the primary tumor and the presence or absence of regional lymph node involvement or distant metastases is given in Table 34-3.

meatus. In published reports, 59% of tumors occurred in the bulbomembranous urethra, 34% in the penile urethra, and 7% in the prostatic urethra. Histologically, 78% of male urethral carcinomas were squamous cell carcinoma, 15% transitional carcinoma, 6% adenocarcinoma, and 1% undifferentiated carcinoma.

Male urethral carcinoma tends to spread by direct extension to adjacent structures and usually involves the vascular spaces of the corpus spongiosum and the periurethral tissues. Carcinoma of the bulbomembranous urethra often extends to the urogenital diaphragm, prostate, perineum, and scrotal skin. Hematogenous spread is uncommon except in advanced disease. Metastasis occurs by lymphatic embolization to regional lymph nodes. The lymphatics from the anterior urethra drain into the superficial and deep inguinal nodes and occasionally to the external iliac nodes, whereas the lymphatics from the posterior urethra drain into the external iliac, obturator, and hypogastric nodes. Tumors of the anterior urethra generally metastasize to the inguinal nodes and tumors of the posterior metastasize to pelvic nodes; however, there are some exceptions.[8]

FIG. 34-1. Anatomy and pathology of urethral carcinoma.

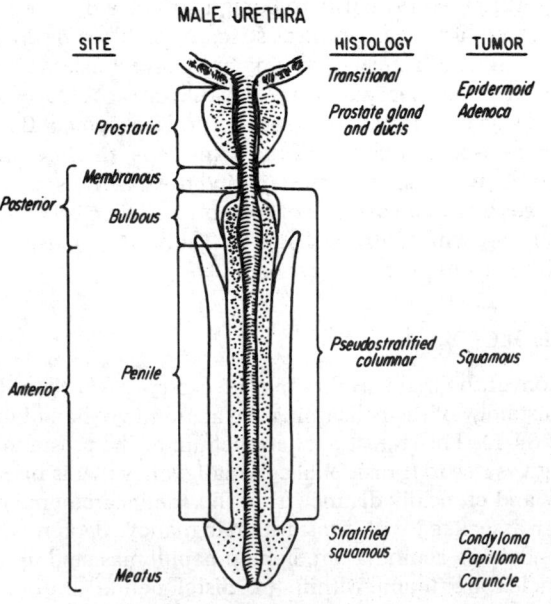

TABLE 34-3. Staging System for Urethral Cancer (American Joint Committee)

T – Primary Tumor (Male)
Tx   Primary tumor cannot be assessed
T0   No evidence of primary tumor
Tis   Carcinoma in situ
Ta   Noninvasive papillary, polypoid, or verrucous carcinoma
T1   Tumor invades subepithelial connective tissue
T2   Tumor invades corpus spongiosum or prostate or periurethral muscle
T3   Tumor invades corpus cavernosum or beyond prostatic capsule or bladder neck
T4   Tumor invades other adjacent organs
N – Regional Lymph Nodes
Nx   Regional lymph nodes cannot be assessed
N0   No regional lymph node metastasis
N1   Metastasis in a single lymph node, 2 cm or less in greatest dimension
N2   Metastasis in a single lymph node, more than 2 cm but no more than 5 cm in greatest dimension, or multiple lymph nodes, none more than 5 cm in greatest dimension
N3   Metastasis in a lymph node(s) more than 5 cm in greatest dimension
M – Distant Metastasis
Mx   Presence of distant metastasis cannot be assessed
M0   No distant metastasis
M1   Distant metastasis

TREATMENT

General Philosophy

The primary mode of therapy for carcinoma of the male urethra is surgical excision of the lesion. The extent of surgery depends on the location and stage of the tumor. In general, anterior urethral carcinoma seems more amenable to surgical control than does posterior urethral carcinoma; perhaps as a consequence, the prognosis for patients with lesions originating in the anterior urethra is better than that of those with tumors situated posteriorly.

A comparison of the results of surgical excision and radiation therapy is difficult because of the low incidence of the disease. As with surgery, the results of radiation therapy are very much dependent on the site of the tumor, with anterior urethral lesions responding better than posterior ones.[2]

Modern combinations of chemotherapy are capable of producing meaningful objective regression of regionally advanced or metastatic urothelial carcinomas. The MVAC regimen (methotrexate, vinblastine, doxorubicin, and cisplatin) has produced significant tumor regression in a majority of patients with transitional cell carcinoma of the urinary tract.[9-11] Of note is that tumors of nontransitional histology appear to be resistant to this combination. The MVAC regimen causes significant myelosuppression, and the potential for nephrotoxicity and cardiotoxicity necessitate careful attention to detail in drug administration. However, on the basis of the response to MVAC chemotherapy in bladder and upper tract urothelial tumors, investigation into its use in transitional cell carcinoma of the urethra is warranted.

Untreated patients with carcinoma of the urethra can anticipate a median survival of 3 months, with a range of 1 week to 15 months. Only 16% of these patients will survive more than 5 years.[12]

Carcinoma of the Distal Urethra

Carcinoma of the penile urethra may be treated by transurethral resection, local excision, partial amputation, or radical amputation with or without emasculation. For superficial, papillary, or in situ tumor, transurethral resection may be sufficient. For tumor infiltrating the corpus and localized to the distal half of the penis, a partial amputation with a 2-cm margin proximal to any visible or palpable lesion is the generally accepted treatment. If the infiltrating tumor is located in the proximal penile urethra or involves the entire penile urethra, radical amputation should be done. Emasculation is indicated only when the scrotal skin is involved.

Unlike the situation in carcinoma of the penis, clinically palpable adenopathy in the groin of patients with urethral carcinoma usually represents metastases and is not often the result of reactive inflammation. Ilioinguinal node dissection is indicated only if the inguinal nodes are palpable; there is no evidence of benefit from prophylactic groin dissection. After excision of the primary tumor, the patient should be followed with careful examination of the inguinal areas for evidence of lymphadenopathy, and a groin dissection should be done on the finding of metastatic disease.[1,3,5,7,13] In general, the survival rates correlate with the location and type of lesion and overall are poor (Table 34-4).

Carcinoma of the Bulbomembranous Urethra

Early lesions of the bulbomembranous urethra have been treated successfully by transurethral resection or by resection of the involved urethral segment with end-to-end anastomosis, but cases appropriate for such limited resection are rare.[13,14] Poor survival figures have been recorded with all forms of treatment; however, it appears that radical excision offers the best opportunity for long-term disease control with the lowest incidence of local recurrence. Unfortunately, most patients with bulbomembranous urethral carcinoma present with locally advanced disease.

In-continuity resection of the pubic rami has been suggested as a means of improving local control,[15] but the small number of patients thus treated prevents definitive conclusions. Patients with carcinoma of the posterior urethra should have simultaneous deep pelvic node dissection to determine the presence of nodal metastatic disease. There is no evidence that cure can be effected in patients with gross pelvic disease by either surgical excision or radiation therapy alone.

Carcinoma of the Prostatic Urethra

Carcinoma arising from the prostatic urethra is rare. There are no characteristic symptoms of this lesion, and the serum acid phosphatase concentration is not elevated. Superficial lesions of the prostatic urethra have been managed successfully by transurethral resection in some patients;[1] however, such tumors are uncommon. In the majority of instances, the tumor involves the bulk of the prostate with variable exten-

TABLE 34-4.   Five-Year Survival in Carcinoma of Male Urethra

Histologic Type	No. of Cases (%)			
	Penile	Bulbomembranous	Prostatic	Total
Squamous	12/27 (44)	4/40 (10)	0/1 (0)	
Transitional	1/3 (33)	0/4 (0)	4/13 (31)	
Adenocarcinoma	–	1/4 (25)	–	
Undifferentiated	–	0/1 (0)	–	
Total	13/30 (43)	5/49 (10)	4/14 (29)	

Modified from Ray B, Canto AR, Whitmore WF: Experience with primary carcinoma of the male urethra. J Urol 117:591–594, 1977.

sion to the bulbomembranous urethra or the bladder neck and trigone. In this situation, radical prostatectomy alone may not provide a tumor-free margin, and anterior exenteration is the treatment of choice. As with other carcinomas in the posterior urethra, the overall 5-year survival rates for invasive prostatic urethral carcinoma are poor.[5]

The results of radiation therapy for carcinoma of the male urethra are difficult to evaluate because the incidence of the tumor is so low and few cases have been treated. In lesions of the distal urethra, the response to either penectomy or radiation therapy is similar.[16] Aggressive external radiation to the prostate (6000–7000 cGy) in combination with transurethral resection has produced an occasional long-term survivor.

CARCINOMA OF THE FEMALE URETHRA

Carcinoma of the urethra is unusual among genitourinary tract neoplasms in occurring more often in females than in males. The tumors most commonly present in older, postmenopausal women, with 75% of patients being over 50 years of age. The disease is more prevalent in whites than in other races.

ETIOLOGY

The etiology of urethral carcinoma in females has not been established, although a causal relation is reported between chronic irritation and malignancy. Proliferative lesions such as caruncles, papillomas, adenomas, and polyps have been reported to be associated with subsequent malignancy. Leukoplakia of the urethra should be considered a premalignant lesion and treated accordingly.

SYMPTOMS

The tumor usually presents as a papillary growth and later becomes a soft, fungating mass that bleeds easily. Ulcerative lesions may produce a foul-smelling discharge. Spread from the primary lesion is by local extension and infiltration with subsequent involvement of the bladder neck and vulva. It may be difficult on initial physical examination to differentiate malignant tumors of the urethra from those of the vulva.

The lymphatic drainage of the various segments of the female urethra is poorly defined. However, it is generally accepted that the lymphatics of the distal urethra drain into the inguinal region, whereas the drainage from the more proximal urethra is to the obturator and iliac nodes. Between 25% and 50% of patients will have inguinal node involvement at the time of initial diagnosis[2,17–19]; an additional 15% of patients will develop tumorous nodes during follow-up. As with urethral carcinoma in males, inguinal lymphadenopathy usually indicates malignant involvement.

PATHOLOGY

Stratified squamous epithelium lines the distal two thirds of the female urethra, whereas transitional epithelium lines the proximal one third (Fig. 34-2). Tumor histology is a reflec-

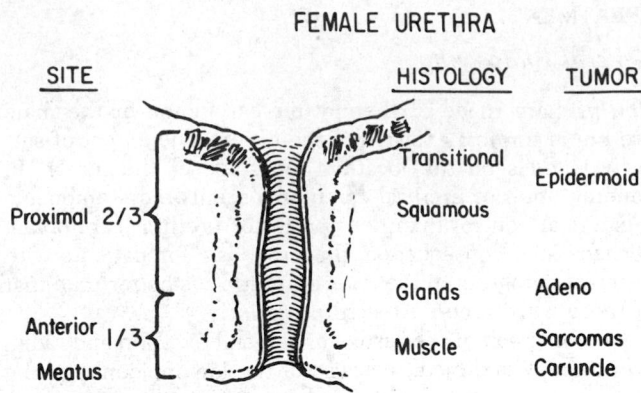

FIG. 34-2. Anatomy and pathology of the female urethra.

tion of the site, with the predominant tumor being squamous cell carcinoma, usually presenting in the proximal two thirds. In general, carcinomas of the anterior urethra are low grade, whereas carcinomas of the proximal or entire urethra are of higher grade. However, histologic characteristics do not significantly affect the prognosis; thus, for practical purposes, transitional cell carcinoma, squamous cell carcinoma, and adenocarcinoma are treated in a similar fashion, although for metastatic transitional cell carcinoma, combination chemotherapy may be considered.[9,10]

TREATMENT

The most significant prognostic factor is the anatomical location of the tumor. For example, meatal tumors, when diagnosed early, are associated with an excellent 5-year survival rate.[20,21] The treatment is based primarily on the tumor stage at the time of presentation. Local excision is often sufficient in selected patients with carcinoma of the distal urethra, as the incidence of lymph node metastasis with distal urethral carcinoma is low.

For tumors involving the proximal urethra or with extension beyond the urethra into the adjacent structures, more extensive surgical resection is necessary, including total urethrectomy, cystectomy with pelvic node dissection, and, in cases of palpable inguinal lymph nodes, inguinal lymphadectomy. Removal of the vulva and vagina have also been advocated as part of an anterior exenteration.[13,22]

Bracken and co-workers reported on 81 cases of carcinoma of the female urethra,[21] with the overall 5-year survival rate of the entire group being 32%. There is a high incidence of local recurrence for all forms of single-modality therapy ranging from 46% to 64%, suggesting the need to explore combination treatment.

Radiation Therapy

In carcinoma of the urethral meatus, irradiation can control the tumor and preserve the function of the urethra. Meatal carcinomas are usually treated with interstitial implants; large tumors that extend into the labia, vagina, or urinary bladder require the addition of external beam therapy. The combination of surgery and brachytherapy irradiation[23] or external beam irradiation[15] has been advocated to improve the results in advanced urethral tumors.

RADIATION THERAPY TECHNIQUES. Declois[24] thoroughly described the techniques for interstitial irradiation of the female urethra. Single- or double-plane or a volume implant is performed, depending on the volume of tumor to be treated. With the advent of ^{192}Ir, after-loading implants utilizing this material have largely replaced radium or [60]Co. Pierquin et al[25] described the use of "directional gutters" through which ^{192}Ir pins are inserted. Should the tumor involve the inferior aspect of the urethral meatus, care must be exercised to encompass this part of the lesion adequately, sometimes utilizing "crossing" needles. In this case, it is advisable to use a vaginal cylinder that will extend the periphery of the implant into the labia minora.

Radiographs are obtained to verify the insertion of the sources, and computer calculation displays the dose distributions in multiple planes. An estimated dose of 6000 to 7000 cGy is given, depending on tumor extent.

For larger tumors involving the labia, vagina, or the base of the urinary bladder, an implant technique alone will be inadequate to control the disease. For these patients, a combination of external beam radiotherapy with an interstitial implant is recommended.

Tumors involving the posterior urethra should be treated in a manner similar to those of the urinary bladder.[26]

RESULTS. Small meatal tumors show 5-year cure rates in the range of 70% to 90%.[20,26-28] Neoplasms involving the proximal urethra or the entire urethra are more difficult to treat, and the overall control rate for these tumors is only 20% to 30%. In some studies, the combination of preoperative radiotherapy and radical cystourethrectomy appeared to increase the survival rate in patients with advanced disease.[29,30]

SEQUELAE. Urethral strictures will develop in some patients, necessitating dilatation. More severe complications are necrosis secondary to overdosage and, occasionally, fistula, primarily vesicovaginal or urethrovaginal.[21,26] In the case of advanced neoplasms, fistula formation is unavoidable because of tumor erosion of the organ and subsequent tumor necrosis.[30] Other less common complications include osteomyelitis of the symphysis pubis, radiation cystitis and urinary incontinence or stress incontinence, radiation enteritis, and small-bowel obstruction. Johnson and O'Connell[29] encountered a 42% complication rate in patients treated by radiotherapy, whereas in the series by Prempree et al,[28] two of ten patients treated definitively by means of radiotherapy developed strictures. Bracken et al[21] reported a complication rate of 45% among their patients who were treated with radiation, whereas Taggart et al[26] encountered severe complications in 5 of 37 patients.

CANCER OF THE PENIS

INCIDENCE

Carcinoma of the penis represents 2% to 5% of all urogenital cancers.[31] Although rare in North America, tumors of the penis are a significant clinical problem in populations where circumcision is not a common practice and proper hygiene is lacking. Indeed, in some populations, squamous cell carcinoma of the penis accounts for 10% to 12% of all malignancies in males. Although malignant penile lesions have been found in young men, most patients are more than 50 years of age.

ETIOLOGY

The occurrence of penile carcinoma correlates strongly with the presence of a foreskin and the irritative effects of smegma combined with the products of poor hygiene within the preputial sac. Carcinoma is rare among men who were circumcised in the neonatal period,[32] but circumcision performed at puberty or in adulthood does not have the same

TABLE 34-5. Malignant Lesions of the Penis

Lesions	Characteristics	Treatment
Squamous carcinoma	Mass of foreskin or glans; phimosis often	Partial penectomy ± lymph node dissection; local excision or radiation therapy in appropriate, localized lesions
Malignant melanoma	Mass of foreskin or glans; phimosis often	Excision with wide margins; partial/total penectomy may be required. Lymph node dissection
Basal cell carcinoma	Extremely rare. Rolled, well-defined edges	Local excision with adequate margins.
Carcinoma in situ	Red or scaly plaque, no deep invasion	Local excision
Mesenchymal tumors	From stromal/connective tissue of penis. Approximately 50% are malignant. Sarcomas (Kaposi's and fibrosarcoma) most common malignant lesions	Partial/total penectomy
Metastatic tumors	Usually from genitourinary tract	Local control only
Leukemic or lymphomatous infiltrate	Rare	Treatment of systemic disorder

TABLE 34-6.   Premalignant Lesions of the Penis

Lesion	Characteristics	Treatment
Leukoplakia	White plaque	Local excision
Erythroplasia of Queyrat	Raised, red, velvet lesion; cellular disorientation with multiple mitoses; identical to carcinoma in situ of skin; 10%–20% may develop areas of squamous cell carcinoma. May be painful	Local excision; topical 5-fluorouracil; radiation
Bowen's disease	Red plaque	Local excision
Balanitis xerotica obliterans	Scaly, atrophic with fissure or ulceration; meatus often involved	Local excision; topical steroids (?)
Buschke–Lowenstein tumor	Large verrucous lesion, histologically benign; may undergo malignant degeneration	Local excision with negative margins. Topical therapy doubtful; radiation therapy has limited effectiveness

protective potential as does neonatal circumcision.[33–35] Although the annual age-adjusted incidence of carcinoma of the penis for males in the United States is only 1.0 per 100,000, the incidence in uncircumcised males is approximately 1 in 600.[36] Smegma, the product of bacterial action or desquamated epithelial cells, has been identified as carcinogenic in animal systems, although the specific component responsible for malignant degeneration in human males has not been identified.

Conflicting reports both support and deny the association of penile carcinoma with the presence of cervical carcinoma in sexual partners as well as a possible relation to herpetic infection.[37,38] No persistent etiologic relation has been documented between carcinoma of the penis and the venereal diseases of syphilis, granuloma inguinale, and chancroid.

SYMPTOMS

The most common presenting clinical manifestation of penile cancer is a mass or a persistent sore or ulcer of the glans or foreskin.[31,39] Most penile carcinomas are painless, and there may be significant ulceration and bleeding without

TABLE 34-7.   Minimal Diagnostic Criteria for Carcinoma of the Penis

T = primary tumor
    Clinical examination
    Incisional/excisional biopsy
N = Regional lymph nodes
    Clinical examination
    CT/MRI
    Intravenous urography (optional)
    Lymphangiography (optional)
    Superficial femoral node biopsy (optional but recommended)
M = Distant Metastases
    Clinical examination
    Chest radiography
    CT/MRI
    Biochemical determinations (liver function, calcium)
    Liver scan, bone scan (optional)

patient concern. Less commonly, the initial symptoms are related to inguinal lymphadenopathy.

It has been estimated that more than one-half of patients will delay more than a year in seeking treatment after the appearance of the lesion.[12,35,39–41]

PATHOLOGY

Penile carcinoma is most often squamous cell in origin, although a variety of other malignancies may also involve the penis (Table 34-5). In addition, a number of premalignant lesions have been identified (Table 34-6).

STAGING

The initial diagnosis must be made by incisional or, preferably, excisional biopsy. Careful physical examination to determine the extent of local invasion and the status of the inguinal lymph nodes is essential to proper staging. A CT scan or MRI to evaluate the pelvic or abdominal lymph nodes or both is also required. A lymphangiogram appears to be optional (Table 34-7).

Table 34-8 shows the Jackson staging system for penile carcinoma.[42] Although widely used, this system suffers to the extent that inguinal nodal involvement is not subcategorized; all patients with tumorous nodes are grouped together.[43] The tumor–node–metastasis (TNM) classification, outlined in

TABLE 34-8.   Jackson Classification for Penile Cancer

Stage	Criteria
I	Tumor confined to glans or prepuce
II	Invasion into shaft or corpora; no nodal or distant metastases
III	Tumor confined to penis; inguinal metastases that are operable
IV	Tumor involves adjacent structures; inoperable and/or distant metastases

TABLE 34-9. TNM Classification of Squamous Carcinoma of Penis*

T		N		M	
TX	Minimum requirements cannot be met	NX	Minimum requirements cannot be met	MX	Minimum requirements cannot be met
T0	No evidence of primary tumor	N0	No evidence of involvement of regional lymph nodes	M0	No evidence of distant metastases
TIS	Carcinoma *in situ* (Bowen's disease, erythroplasia of Queyrat)			M1	Distant metastases present
T1	Tumor not more than 1 cm in largest dimension and clearly superficial	N1	Involvement of a single regional node	M1a	Evidence of occult metastases based on biochemical and/or other tests
T2	Tumor 1 cm in any dimension and clearly superficial	N2	Involvement of single bilateral inguinal nodes or multiple unilateral nodes	M1b	Single metastasis in a single organ site
T3	Tumor of any size invading underlying tissues	N3	Fixation of regional nodes or ulceration of skin over involved regional nodes	M1c	Multiple metastases in a single site
T4	Tumor invading adjacent structures, that is, corpus, urethra, symphysis, perineum	N4	Involvement of juxtaregional lymph nodes	M1d	Metastases in multiple organ sites

* Minimal requirements for tumor (*T*) include clinical examination with biopsy; for nodes (*N*) clinical examination, lymphography, or urography; for distant metastasis (*M*) clinical examination, chest x-ray film, lymphography or metastatic bone studies. The regional nodes are those of the superficial inguinal region. Juxtaregional nodes are those of the external iliac chain below the bifurcation of the common iliac artery and those of the hypogastric region.

Table 34-9, is an attempt to quantify more precisely the nodal and metastatic disease.

TREATMENT PRINCIPLES

Adequate therapy of patients with penile cancer implies an accurate assessment of the extent of the disease with particular reference to the status of the regional lymph nodes. Surgery, in the form of partial or total penectomy with or without inguinal and pelvic lymph node dissection is the most commonly accepted treatment. Radiation therapy as external irradiation, penile brachytherapy, or both, also have been given in an attempt to lessen the functional sacrifice associated with ablation of the primary tumor.

Paramount in any treatment philosophy is a consideration of the lymphatic drainage of the penis as a prelude to rational therapeutic planning (Fig. 34-3). The skin of the penis and the lymphatics of the prepuce drain primarily into the superficial inguinal nodes. As a result of a freely anastomosing system and crossover at the base of the penis, bilateral drainage occurs.[44] The glans is likewise drained by the superficial inguinal nodes, but, along with those of the corpora, the glans lymphatics also empty into the deep inguinal and iliac nodes. The superficial nodes are located in the deep portion of Camper's fascia superficial to the deep fascia of the thigh, the fascia lata. Subsequently, the superficial lymphatics drain into the deep inguinal lymphatics surrounding the femoral vessels and thence to the external iliac, common iliac, and periaortic lymphatic channels. Tumor invasion of the corpora cavernosa or the posterior urethra also is consistent with involvement of the deep pelvic lymphatic structures of the internal iliac and obturator regions.

Surgical Treatment

Two areas of surgical concern in disease management are the selection of the appropriate treatment for the primary lesion and the role of surgery in the evaluation and therapy of nodal disease.

TREATMENT OF PRIMARY LESION. Adequate control of the primary tumor must be accomplished for a cure to be expected. Surgical therapy involves removal of the lesion with adequate margins to minimize the risk of local recur-

FIG. 34-3. Lymphatic drainage of penis.

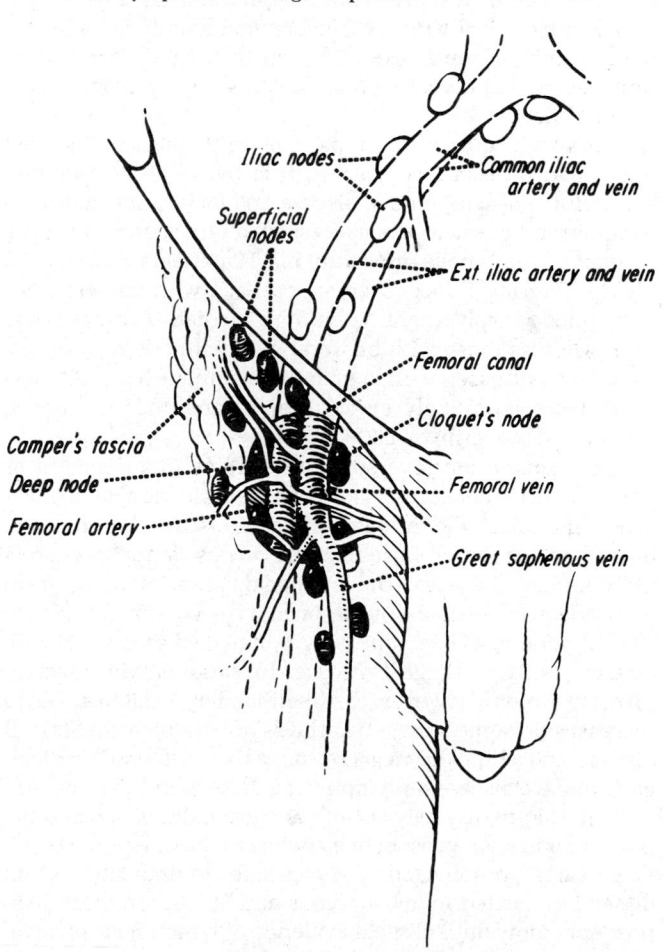

rence. Small tumors that are limited to the prepuce are treated by circumcision alone. Lesions that on physical examination involve only the skin, not the underlying structures, may be controllable by excisional biopsy. Penectomy, either partial or total, is indicated for lesions that, because of their size, invasiveness, or location on the shaft, are not amenable to more conservative treatment. Partial penectomy requires that a 2-cm margin of grossly normal shaft be available proximal to the primary lesion. For lesions that approach the base of the shaft or that are extensive, total penectomy should be accomplished with excision of both corpora and creation of a perineal urethrostomy.[45]

MANAGEMENT OF REGIONAL LYMPH NODES. Several important facts should be kept in mind concerning the role of regional lymphadectomy in patients with penile cancer. First, between 35% and 60% of patients with squamous cell penile cancer will present with palpable inguinal lymph nodes.[46,47] Second, the incidence of false-positive lymph nodes on clinical examination averages 40%, with various series reporting figures between 13% and 82%,[12,43,45] because of the well-known association of inflammatory inguinal lymphadenopathy with ulcerated or infected penile lesions. Clinical assessment of the lymph nodes thus should be delayed until after a 4- to 6-week course of antibiotic therapy, especially in patients with obviously infected or inflamed penile lesions. Third, approximately 20% of patients with clinically tumor-free inguinal lymph nodes in fact have lymphatic metastases.[45,46] Fourth, lymph node dissection can be curative in some patients with tumor-bearing inguinal nodes.

Overall, 40% to 50% of patients with positive inguinal nodes can be rendered disease free by surgical resection. The volume of lymph node disease and its location appear to be important predictors of success. In a recent analysis of the results of lymph node dissection in 119 patients at Memorial Sloan-Kettering Cancer Center, patients with unilateral inguinal-node involvement had a 56% median 5-year survival rate, whereas those with bilateral inguinal-node metastases, extranodal disease, or iliac node involvement had a 9% survival. Cure is unlikely by surgical means once the pelvic lymph nodes are involved.[44]

The primary controversy in the surgical management of penile cancer concerns lymph node dissection in the absence of clinically identifiable inguinal disease. Whereas the overall incidence of false-negative nodes is approximately 20%, in Stage I disease, the late nodal extension to the groin after adequate excision of the primary occurs in only 5% to 11% of patients, Thus, routine lymph node dissection is difficult to justify in Stage I disease. In patients with invasive primary tumors, however, the likelihood of nodal metastases increases; in some series, two-thirds of patients with Stage II disease and clinically negative nodes were found histologically to have disease on lymph node dissection.[48] The significant morbidity that may accompany groin dissection and the lack of controlled prospective studies to document the benefit of early "prophylactic" versus late "therapeutic" groin dissection has led many surgeons and centers to delay lymphadenectomy until clinical evidence of lymph node involvement exists.[37,47]

Ekstrom and Edsmyr identified a 50% disease control rate in patients who had node dissection delayed until adenopathy was evident.[49] Frew et al[50] could identify no cancer deaths in patients in whom lymph node excision was deferred until clinical node disease was present. Beggs and Spratt reported no significant adverse effect on survival in patients with delayed groin dissection; the 1% mortality rate from lymphadenectomy was essentially the same as the percentage of patients who died from cancer as a result of therapeutic delay.[47] More recently, others have reported a significant decrease in 5-year survival rates in patients with therapeutic as opposed to prophylactic groin dissection[48,51] and have suggested that delayed surgery is inappropriate.

Cabanas[52] has described a technique of "sentinel node" biopsy followed by a formal node dissection if metastatic disease is found. The sentinel lymph node is found radiographically, on the anteroposterior view, at the junction of the femoral head and the ascending pubic ramus. Anatomically, the sentinel node is part of the lymphatic system around the superficial epigastric vein located medial to and above the superficial epigastric–saphenous junction. In Cabanas' series, inguinel–femoral–iliac node involvement was not demonstrated in the absence of a positive sentinel node biopsy. However, subsequently, Perinetti et al[53] reported a case of a patient with a negative sentinel-node biopsy who had unresectable bilateral groin disease 3 months later.

It thus seems appropriate that patients with noninvasive tumor and clinically negative nodes (Stage I) be followed carefully and groin dissection considered only if lymphadenopathy occurs. In patients with Stage II disease, the sentinel node biopsy is appealing as a means of increasing diagnostic and prognostic accuracy without significant morbidity, although proponents of both prophylactic and therapeutic groin dissection exist. In patients with clinically positive nodes (Stage II), initial bilateral dissection should be performed because of the high incidence (60%) of bilateral inguinal node involvement.[49] Unilateral node dissection in patients managed by delayed lymphadenectomy is reasonable because the incidence of contralateral involvement in these patients is less than 10%.[12] Controversy also exists over the benefit obtained by pelvic node dissection in the presence of pelvic nodal metastatic disease. Although positive pelvic nodes appear to be an indicator of incurable disease, some authors report a 20% to 29% cure rate with surgery in these patients. Whether this apparent long-term survival reflects a beneficial impact of surgery or represents a subset of patients with apparently indolent disease is undetermined.[52]

Technical Aspects of Lymphadenectomy. The operation is performed essentially as described by Whitmore and Vagaiwala.[54] The patient is placed in the supine position with the thighs slightly flexed, abducted, and externally rotated with support under the knees. The incision for the bilateral pelvic node dissection, which may be performed before (usually) or after the inguinal dissection, is a midline incision from the umbilicus to the pubis. The dissection limits are defined by the genitofemoral nerve laterally, the bladder medially, the bifurcation of the common iliac artery superiorly, and the fascia covering the obturator internus and levator ani mus-

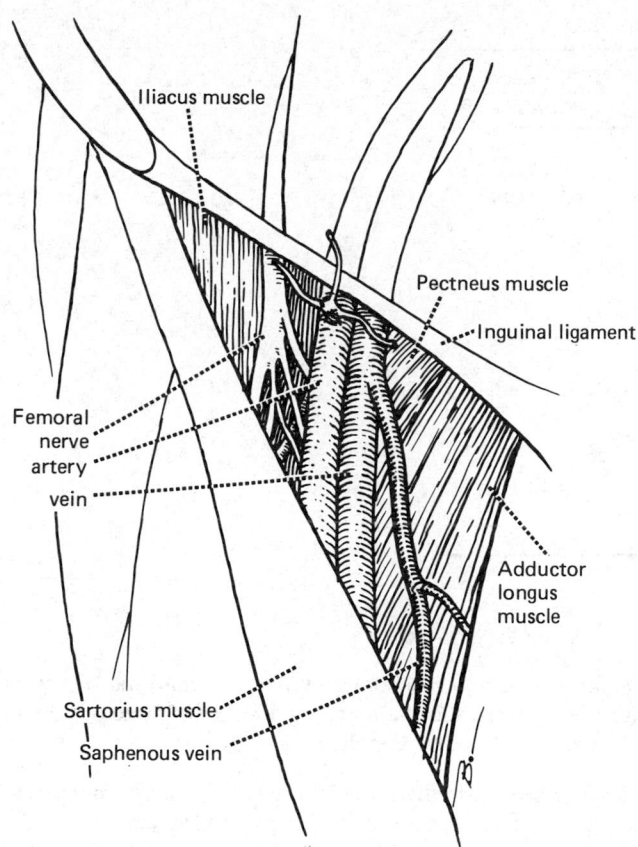

FIG. 34-4. Anatomical limits of deep groin dissection.

Labels on figure: Iliacus muscle; Pectneus muscle; Inguinal ligament; Femoral nerve; artery; vein; Adductor longus muscle; Sartorius muscle; Saphenous vein

cles inferiorly (Fig. 34-4). Cloquet's node can usually be removed through the pelvic incision as the vessels are cleaned as they enter the femoral canal. The inguinal incision is planned to provide adequate margins surrounding lymph nodes containing obvious tumor and simultaneously to remove the area of skin at greatest risk of devitalization and necrosis. An elliptical incision is made over the inguinal ligament from the anterosuperior iliac spine toward, but lateral to, the pubic tubercle. The borders of the ellipse parallel the inguinal ligament and extend 4 to 6 cm in a vertical diameter at the widest point. The incision is bevelled outward from the skin down so as to describe a pyramidal wedge of tissue, truncated by the skin surface. Because penile cancers appear to involve the inguinal lymph nodes by tumor embolization rather than through permeation of lymphatic channels, wide, thin skin flaps and a thorough dissection, such as is required for malignant melanoma, are not indicated. The surgeon's goal should be to remove completely the nodes in the superficial and deep inguinal areas; this can be done without widely undermining the skin flaps.

Complications. The most common complication is skin flap necrosis. Particular attention to operative detail, especially with regard to skin flap thickness, infection control, protection of femoral vessels by sartorius transfer, appropriate drainage, and postoperative immobilization appears to lessen this most disturbing complication. Other problems include lymphedema (19%–45%), wound infection (10%), and, rarely, hemorrhage, hernia, or death. The presence of persistent lymphedema can be a particular problem. Meticulous ligation of lymphatic channels during the dissection by cautery, metal clips, or fine ligatures appears to reduce the likelihood of severe, persistent lymphedema. The use of preoperatively fitted compression stockings, elevation, and immobilization also appears to be important in reducing the incidence of this problem.

Radiation Therapy

As with surgery, radiation therapy has been used in treatment of both the primary lesion and nodal disease.

RADIATION OF THE PRIMARY LESION. The principal advantage of irradiation in treating the primary lesion is preservation of the penis. Irradiation alone will control the tumor in a significant number of patients, thus avoiding anatomic and functional deficits that may produce devastating psychological effects. In addition, if radiation therapy fails, a surgical procedure may control the recurrent disease if it is not too extensive and metastases are not present.

Before initiation of radiotherapy for carcinoma of the penis, routine circumcision must be performed. This procedure will minimize the radiotherapy-associated morbidity, swelling and irritation of the skin, moist desquamation, and secondary infection.[55]

RADIATION THERAPY. A wide variation of techniques, doses, and fractionation schemes have been employed.[56–60] Implants, molds, contact therapy, orthovoltage therapy, and megavoltage therapy are used. The most commonly employed techniques are as follows.

Low-energy orthovoltage (60–150 kVp) has been used for the treatment of relatively superficial invasive carcinoma or for carcinoma in situ (including the erythroplasia of Queyrat). The lesion is treated with a margin of 1 to 2 cm beyond visible or palpable tumor. Doses in the range of 6000 cGy in 5 to 6 weeks will produce local control in most instances.

Megavoltage irradiation is necessary for infiltrating tumors with thickness greater than 0.5 cm. It also is required for the inguinal lymph nodes. When the tumor in the lymph nodes is infiltrating the skin, bolus therapy should be used to avoid skin-sparing effect. For the treatment of the primary lesion, the entire penis should be included in the irradiated volume. This can be done with appositional portals using special positioning devices. The doses of irradiation should be 6500 to 7000 cGy, in five-weekly fractions, for 5 to 7 weeks, depending on the volume treated.

External beam radiotherapy requires specially designed accessories to achieve adequate bolus over the organ and homogeneous dose distribution. The device usually consists of a plastic box with a central opening that can be fitted over the organ; the space between the skin and the box must be filled with tissue-equivalent material. This box can then be treated with a parallel opposed megavoltage beam.

Although external beam radiotherapy has become a prevalent modality in the treatment of the primary lesion in carci-

TABLE 34-10. Control of Primary Lesion with Radiotherapy

Author	No. of Patients	Treatment Method	Dosage	Local Control (%)
Engelstad[58]	72	Mold, teleradium	3500–3700 R 500–700 R/day	50
Jackson[42]	39	Mold (most cases), external beam (some cases)	?	49
Murrell & Williams[59]	108	External beam	3000–6700 cGy 200 cGy/day	52
Kelley et al.	10	External beam (electrons)	5100–5400 cGy 300 cGy/day	100
Haile & Delclos	20	Mold, implant, external beam	?	90
Pointon[61]	32	External beam	5250–5500 cGy in 16 Rx/22 days	84
Salverria	41	Iridium mold	6000 cGy/several days	84

noma of the penis, molds are still used. The mold is usually built as a box with a central opening, and radioactive sources should be sufficiently long to prevent underdosage at the tip of the penis. A dose of 6500 cGy at the surface and approximately 6000 cGy at the center of the organ is delivered over 6 to 7 days.

Control rates of the primary lesions with radiation therapy achieved by several authors are summarized in Table 34-10.

RADIATION OF REGIONAL LYMPHATICS. Irradiation of the involved regional lymph nodes in patients with carcinoma of the penis may result in permanent control and cure of a substantial percentage of patients.[60]

In cases in which irradiation is used to treat lymph nodes, both inguinal and pelvic nodes as far as the common iliac bifurcation should be irradiated with paralleled anteroposterior and posteroanterior portals. Because of the anterior position of the lymph nodes, an unequal loading favoring the anterior portals can be used. For elective treatment (without clinical evidence of metastatic tumor), doses of approximately 5000 cGy in 5 weeks are adequate. In those patients with palpable lymph nodes, doses on the order of 7000 to 8000 cGy over 7 to 8 weeks (180–200 cGy per day) are indicated.

Special skin care must be instituted to prevent moist epidermitis and serious discomfort. The prevention of infection is critical to the satisfactory completion of the radiation therapy.

PALLIATION. Good palliative effects can be achieved in patients with extensive, advanced, infiltrating, or ulcerated tumors. A direct appositional port may be adequate, and doses in the range of 4000 to 6000 cGy may cause temporary tumor regression with decreased pain and bleeding and healing of neoplastic ulceration.

POSTOPERATIVE IRRADIATION. In those patients with incomplete tumor resections or positive margins of resection, postoperative radiation using doses of 5000 to 6000 cGy over 6 weeks may be beneficial.

SEQUELAE. Irradiation of the penis produces moist desquamation of the skin and swelling of the subcutaneous tissue of the shaft. Albeit uncomfortable, this is a reversible reaction that subsides within a few weeks. Telangiectasia is a common late consequence of radiation therapy and is usually asymptomatic (Fig. 34-5).

Ulceration, necrosis of the glans, or necrosis of the skin of the shaft area are rare. Lymphedema of the legs has been reported following inguinal and pelvic radiotherapy, but the role of radiotherapy in the development of this complication remains controversial; the majority of the patients with this symptom have disease in the lymphatics that may be responsible for lymphatic blockage.

In the reported series, meatal–urethral strictures occur with a frequency ranging from 0 to 40%.[7,14-17] This incidence compares favorably with the incidence of urethral stricture following penectomy. Most of the strictures after radiotherapy are at the meatus.

Chemotherapy

Primarily because of the rarity of penile cancer in those countries that have the most experience in doing controlled clinical trials, optimal chemotherapy for this lesion has not yet been defined. Bleomycin is the most active drug tested to date, with rates of objective response ranging from 21% to 60%.[62,63] Methotrexate in doses necessitating leucovorin rescue has produced objective responses in 61% of patients,[62] including an occasional complete remission.[64] Cisplatin has produced responses in 21% of patients.[62]

As yet, no meaningful combination regimens have been tested. The drugs with demonstrable activity could be judiciously combined. However, current chemotherapy must be considered primarily palliative.

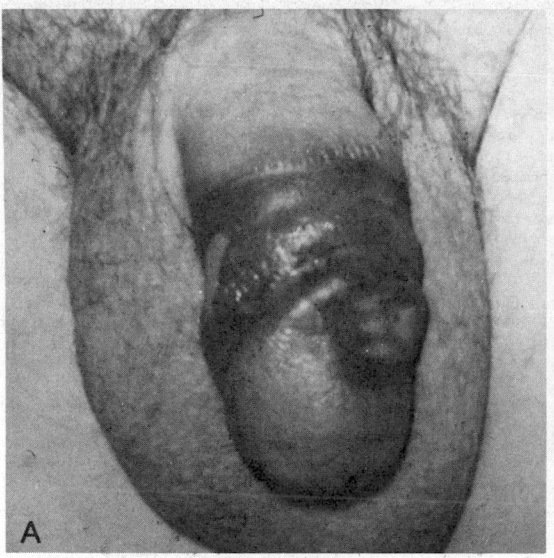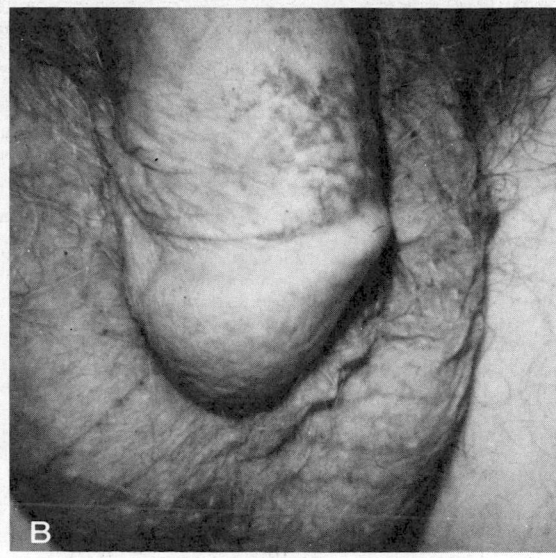

FIG. 34-5. Squamous-cell carcinoma of balanopreputial region with extension into glans (Stage I). Patient was treated with 120 kVp x-rays, 0.3 mm³ HVL, receiving 6000 cGY skin dose in 5 weeks. **A.** Before treatment. **B.** Same patient 4 years later; no evidence of disease. Telangiectasia is present. (Reproduced with permission from Pilepich MV: Carcinoma of the penis and male urethra. In Perez CA, Brady LW [eds]: Principles and Practice of Radiation Oncology, pp 912–918. Philadelphia, JB Lippincott, 1987)

REFERENCES

1. Fair WR, Yang CR: Urethral carcinoma in males. In Resnick M, Kursh E (eds): Current Therapy in Surgery. Toronto, BC Decker, 1987
2. Grabstald H: Tumors of the urethra in men and women. Cancer 32:1236–1255, 1973
3. Kaplan GW, Bulkey GJ, Grayhack JT: Carcinoma of the male urethra. J Urol 96:365–371, 1967
4. King LR: Carcinoma of the urethra in male patients. J Urol 92:555–559, 1964
5. Ray B, Canto AK, Whitmore WF Jr: Experience with primary carcinoma of the male urethra. J Urol 117:591–594, 1977
6. Zaslow J, Priestly JT: Primary carcinoma of the male urethra. J Urol 58:207–211, 1947
7. Mandler JT, Pool TL: Primary carcinoma of the male urethra. J Urol 96:67–72, 1966
8. Yang CR, Fair WR, Whitmore WF Jr: Urethral carcinoma in males (submitted for publication)
9. Sternberg CN, Yagoda A, Scher HI, et al: Preliminary results of M-VAC (methotrexate, vinblastine, Adriamycin and cisplatin) for transitional cell carcinoma of the urothelium. J Urol 33:403–407, 1985
10. Scher HI, Yagoda A, Herr HW, et al: Neoadjuvant M-VAC (methotrexate, vinblastine, Adriamycin and cisplatin) for extravesical urinary tract tumors. J Urol (in press)
11. Scher HI, Yagoda A, Herr HW, et al: Neoadjuvant M-VAC (methotrexate, vinblastine, Adriamycin and cisplatin): Effect on the primary bladder lesion (submitted for publication)
12. Paulson DF, Perez CA, Anderson T: Cancer of the urethra and penis, In Devita VT Jr, Hellman S, Rosenberg SA (eds): Principles and Practice of Oncology, vol 1, pp 965–977. Philadelphia, JB Lippincott, 1985
13. Pointon RCS, Poole-Wilson DS: Primary carcinoma of the urethra. Br J Urol 40:682–685, 1968
14. Lower WE, Hausfeld KF: Primary carcinoma of the male urethra: Report of 10 cases. J Urol 58:192–206, 1947
15. Klein FA, Whitmore WF Jr, Herr HW, et al: Inferior pubic rami resection with en bloc radical excision for invasive proximal urethral carcinoma. Cancer 51:1238–1242, 1983
16. Raghavaiah NV: Radiotherapy in the treatment of carcinoma of the male urethra. Cancer 41:1313–1316, 1978
17. Desai S, Libertino JA, Zinman L: Primary carcinoma of the female urethra. J Urol 110:693–695, 1973
18. Staubitz WJ, Carden LM, Oberkircher OJ, et al: Management of urethral carcinoma in the female. J Urol 73:1045–1053, 1955
19. Ritter DW: Primary malignancy of the female urethra. West J Surg Obstet Gynecol 51:420–429, 1953
20. Antoniades J: Radiation therapy in carcinoma of the female urethra. Cancer 24:70–76, 1969
21. Bracken RB, Johnson DE, Miller LS, et al: Primary carcinoma of the female urethra. J Urol 116:188–192, 1976
22. Grabstald H, Hilaris B, Henschike U, Whitmore WF Jr: Cancer of the female urethra. JAMA 197:835–837, 1966
23. Hopkins SC, Vider M, Nag SK, et al: Carcinoma of the female urethra: Reassessment of the modes of therapy. J Urol 129:958–961, 1983
24. Declois L: Carcinoma of the female urethra: Interstitial irradiation in genitourinary tumors, In Johnson DE, Boileau MA (eds): Fundamental Principles and Surgical Techniques, pp 275–286. New York, Grune & Stratton, 1982
25. Pierquin B, Chassange D, Cox JD: Toward consistent local control of certain malignant tumors: Endoradiotherapy with iridium 192. Radiology 99:661–667, 1971
26. Taggart CG, Castro JR, Rutledge FN: Carcinoma of the female urethra. Am J Roentgenol 114:145–151, 1972
27. Prempree T, Amoremarn R, Patanaphan V: Radiation therapy in primary carcinoma of the female urethra. Cancer 54:729–733, 1984
28. Prempree T, Wizenberg MJ, Scott RM: Radiation treatment of primary carcinoma of the female urethra. Cancer 42:1177–1184, 1978
29. Johnson DE, O'Connell JR: Primary carcinoma of the female urethra. Urology 21:42–45, 1983
30. Antoniades J, Pilepich MV: Carcinoma of the female urethra, In Perez CA, Brady LW (eds): Principles and Practice of Radiation Oncology, pp 863–866. Philadelphia, JB Lippincott, 1987
31. Hanash K, Furlow W, Utz D, et al: Carcinoma of the penis: A clinicopathologic study. J Urol 104:291–297, 1970
32. Jackson SM: The treatment of carcinoma of the penis. Br J Surg 53:33–35, 1966
33. Kuruvilla JT, Garlic RH, Mamnen KE: Results of surgical treatment of carcinoma of the penis. Aust NZ J Urol 41:157–159, 1971
34. Schellhammer PF, Spaulding JP: Carcinoma of the penis, In Paulson DF (ed): Genitourinary Surgery, p 629. New York, Churchill Livingstone, 1983
35. Thomas JA, Small CS: Carcinoma of the penis in southern India. J Urol 160:520–524, 1963
36. Paymaster JC, Gangadharin P: Cancer of the penis in India. J Urol 97:110–113, 1967
37. Gursel EO, Georgountzod C, Uson AC, et al: Penile cancer. Urology 1:569–578, 1973
38. Schrek L, Lenowitz H: Etiologic factors in carcinoma of the penis. Cancer Res 7:180–184, 1947
39. Hardner GJ, Bhanalaph T, Murphy GP, et al: Carcinoma of the penis: Analysis of therapy in 100 consecutive cases. J Urol 108:428–430, 1972
40. Buddington WT, Kickham CJ, Smithy WE: An assessment of malignant disease of the penis. J Urol 89:442–446, 1963
41. Dean AL: Epithelioma of the penis. J Urol 33:252–254, 1935
42. Jackson SM: The treatment of carcinoma of the penis. Br J Surg 53:33–35, 1966
43. Srinivas V, Morse MJ, Herr HW, et al: Penile cancer: Relation of extent of nodal metastasis to survival. J Urol 137:880–882, 1987
44. Skinner DG, Leadbetter WR, Kelley SP: The surgical management of squamous cell carcinoma of the penis. J Urol 107:273–277, 1972
45. Persky L, deKernion JB: Carcinoma of the penis. CA 36:258–272, 1986
46. deKernion JB, Tynberg P, Persky L, et al: Carcinoma of the penis. Cancer 32:1256–1262, 1973

47. Beggs JH, Spratt JS Jr: Epidermoid carcinoma of the penis. J Urol 91:166–172, 1964
48. McDougal WS, Kirchner FK Jr, Edwards RH, et al: Treatment of carcinoma of the penis: The case for primary lymphadenectomy. J Urol 136:38–41, 1986
49. Ekstrom T, Edsmyr F: Cancer of the penis: A clinical study of 29 cases. Acta Chir Scand 115:25–45, 1958
50. Frew ID, Jefferies JD, Swinney J: Carcinoma of the penis. Br J Urol 39:398–401, 1967
51. Johnson DE, Lo RK: Management of regional lymph nodes in penile carcinoma: Five-year results following therapeutic groin dissections. Urology 24:308–311, 1984
52. Cabanas RM: An approach for the treatment of penile carcinoma. Cancer 39:456–466, 1977
53. Perinetti EP, Crane DD, Catalona WJ: Unreliability of sentinel lymph node biopsy for staging penile carcinoma. J Urol 124:734–735, 1980
54. Whitmore WF Jr, Vagaiwala MR: A technique of ilioinguinal lymph-node dissection of carcinoma of the penis. Surg Gynecol Obstet 159:573–578, 1984
55. Pilepich MV: Carcinoma of the penis and male urethra, In Perez CA, Brady LW (eds): Principles and Practice of Radiation Oncology, pp 912–918. Philadelphia, JB Lippincott, 1987
56. Almgard LE, Edsmyr F: Radiotherapy in treatment of patients with carcinoma of the penis. Scand J Urol Nephrol 7:1–5, 1973
57. Engelstad RB: Treatment of cancer of the penis at the Norwegian Radium Hospital. Radiology 60:801–806, 1948
58. Murrell DS, Williams JL: Radiotherapy in the treatment of carcinoma of the penis. Br J Urol 37:211–222, 1965
59. Newaisy GA, Deeley TG: Radiotherapy in the treatment of carcinoma of the penis. Br J Urol 41:519–521, 1968
60. Pointon RCS: External beam therapy. Proc R Soc Med 68:779–781, 1975
61. Narayana AS, Olney LE, Loening SA, et al: Carcinoma of the penis: Analysis of 219 cases. CA 49:2185–2191, 1982
62. Ahmed T, Sklaroff R, Yagoda A: Sequential trials of methotrexate, cisplatin, bleomycin. J Urol 132:465–468, 1984
63. Kyalwazi SK, Bhana D, Harrison NW: Carcinoma of the penis and bleomycin chemotherapy in Uganda. Br J Urol 46:689–696, 1974
64. Garnick MB, Szkarin AT, Ceele GD Jr: Metastatic carcinoma of the penis: Complete remission after high dose methotrexate chemotherapy. J Urol 122:265–266, 1979

LAWRENCE H. EINHORN

E. DAVID CRAWFORD

WILLIAM U. SHIPLEY

PATRICK J. LOEHRER

STEPHEN D. WILLIAMS

CHAPTER 35 *Cancer of the Testes*

Although testicular cancer is a relatively uncommon disease, accounting for only 1% of all male malignancy,[1] it is important for several reasons. Because testis cancer is the most common carcinoma in the 15- to 35-year-old age group, it has the potential for reducing productive years of life in this young patient population. Moreover, testicular cancer is one of the few neoplasms associated with accurate serum markers: human chorionic gonadotropin (hCG) and alpha-fetoprotein (AFP). Also, whereas in most disseminated cancers, if a complete remission is not attained with chemotherapy, the patient ultimately dies of the disease, in testicular cancer, it is possible to resect residual disease surgically, changing a partial remission (PR) to a surgical complete remission (CR) and curing the patient. Finally, testicular cancer has become a model for a curable neoplasm.[2]

ANATOMY AND HISTOLOGY OF THE TESTIS

The normal testis measures about $4 \times 3 \times 2.5$ cm. The testes acquire various tunics or coverings during their descent from the area of the genital ridge in the retroperitoneum through the inguinal canal into the scrotum. These tunics are the tunica vaginalis, the internal spermatic fascia, the cremasteric fascia, the external spermatic fascia, and the scrotum, which consists of skin and the dartos tunic. The testicular tubules themselves have a dense fascial covering called the tunica albuginea, which posteriorly is invaginated into the body of the testis to form the mediastinum testis. This mediastinum sends fibrous septae into the testis, thus separating it into several hundred lobules. The upper pole of the testis has a vestigial structure, the appendix testis. Posteriorly, the adnexal structures associated with the testis are the epididymis, the vas deferens, and the spermatic cord.

Histologically, each lobule of the testis contains convoluted seminiferous tubules, which are freely anastomotic. An estimated 250 to 400 lobular ducts converge at the mediastinum testis, where they connect with 12 to 20 efferent ducts that drain into the globus major of the epididymis.[3] The testicular seminiferous tubule is surrounded by a basement membrane of connective and elastic tissue. The basement membrane encloses the seminiferous cells, which are of two types: the supporting, or Sertoli, cells and the spermatogenic cells, called spermatogonia. The stroma between the seminiferous tubules is connective tissue in which the interstitial (Leydig) cells are located.

The blood supply to the testes is derived from their site of origin at the genital ridges. The arteries to the testes are the internal spermatic arteries arising from the aorta just below the renal arteries. They course through the spermatic cords directly to the testes, where they anastomose with the vas deferential arteries, which are branches of the hypogastric artery. The venous return from the testis begins as a pampiniform plexus of the spermatic cord. At the internal ring, this plexus joins to form the common spermatic vein. The right spermatic vein enters the vena cava anteriorly, usually several centimeters below the right renal vein. The left spermatic vein empties directly into the left renal vein, usually at a right angle. The lymphatics of the testis pass up the cord to the lumbar lymph nodes, the distribution of which is discussed in a separate section of this chapter.

The appendages of the testis and epididymis are embryologic remnants. The appendix testis is a remnant of the müllerian duct, whereas the remaining appendages (epididymis, superior and inferior vas aberrans, and paradidymis) arise from the mesonephric (wolffian) duct and are attached to the globus major, the upper and lower epididymis, and the junction of the epididymis and vas deferens, respectively. The appendage most commonly present is the appendix testis, found in 90% of autopsies. The appendix epididymis is present in one-third of patients, and the remaining appendages are found in only 1% to 3% of patients.

ETIOLOGY OF TESTICULAR TUMORS

The etiology of germinal cell tumors is unknown. There is an increased frequency in patients with abnormal testicular development and descent.[4,5] For example, in atrophic cryptorchid (undescended) testes, tumors are much more frequent even after orchiopexy. Gilber and Hamilton report that 12% of all testicular neoplasms arise in cryptorchid testes, and the chance of a tumor developing in an undescended testis is more than 40 times greater than in a normally descended scrotal testis.[6]

HISTOLOGY

The classification of malignant tumors for practical clinical purposes in this country is based on the classification of Dixon and Moore as reported in the Armed Forces Institute of Pathology fascicles (Table 35-1).[7] Ninety-six percent of

TABLE 35-1. Pathologic Classification of Testicular Neoplasms

Primary Neoplasms
    Germinal neoplasms (may demonstrate any one or more of the following components):
      1. Seminoma
        a. Classic (typical)
        b. Anaplastic
        c. Spermatocytic
      2. Embryonal carcinoma
      3. Teratoma
        a. Mature
        b. Immature
      4. Chloriocarcinoma
      5. Yolk sac tumor (endodermal sinus tumor; embryonal adenocarcinoma of the prepubertal testis)
    Nongerminal neoplasms
      1. Specialized gonadal stromal neoplasms
        a. Leydig cell tumors
        b. Other gonadal stromal tumors
      2. Gonadoblastomas*
      3. Miscellaneous neoplasms
        a. Adenocarcinoma of the rete testis
        b. Neoplasms of mesenchymal origin
        c. Adrenal rest "tumors"
        d. Adenomatoid tumor
Secondary neoplasms
    Reticuloendothelial neoplasms
    Metastatic carcinomas

* Gonadoblastomas show both germ-cell and gonadal stromal elements and, strictly speaking, should not be considered nongerminal. They are included under this heading for convenience, as they differ clinically from germ-cell tumors.

all primary tumors are malignant and arise from germinal cells. They are either seminomas or nonseminomatous tumors.

There have been at least six major attempts since 1940 to classify germinal tumors along clinically meaningful lines. Beginning with the work of Freedman and Moore in 1946,[8] Dixon and Moore in 1952,[7] and Mostofi and Price in 1973,[9] this nomenclature is now incorporated in a classification proposed by the World Health Organization International Reference Center.[10] In Table 35-2, it can be noted that the British refer to all nonseminomatous germ-cell tumors as "malignant teratomas" of one type or another. American pathologists prefer the term "embryonal carcinoma" to signify a tumor that appears as the most undifferentiated form of teratoma. Despite these differences in language, the classifications are easily correlated (Table 35-2).

CLASSIC SEMINOMA

Classic seminoma usually presents in the fourth or fifth decade of life and accounts for about 40% of testicular tumors. The most common presenting symptom is gradual, painless testicular enlargement. The tumor is homogeneous on cut section and tan to pink with areas of infarct-like granular necrosis. Microscopically, it forms sheets of uniform cells segregated into compartments by slender fibrous septae containing a lymphocytic infiltrate that may vary in density. The nuclei are large, central, and hyperchromatic; the cytoplasm is clear or granular; and the cell borders are well defined. Occasional giant cells may occur in seminoma in the form of a Langerhans' giant cell and also a multinucleated giant cell, which may resemble that of a syncytiotrophoblast. Of course, when the seminoma is combined with other teratomatous or embryonal elements, it is not considered a pure or classic seminoma.

Whether anaplastic seminoma is truly intrinsically distinct from typical seminoma is doubted seriously. Consequently, a panel of pathologists at a 1980 international symposium on testicular cancer suggested the deletion of this term from the literature.[11] Until recently, the histologic diagnosis of anaplastic seminoma was made on the basis of the following microscopic features: (1) a large number of mitotic figures (an average count exceeding five per high-power field); (2) tumor cell anaplasia; and (3) a low-power impression of a solid neoplasm that does not appear as well nested and organized as the classic counterpart. In one report, 55% of a series of primary "anaplastic seminomas" contained multinucleated giant cells with positive histochemical staging for intracytoplasmic hCG, yet the clinical behavior of these tumors of low clinical stage was favorable when patients were treated with radiotherapy in the conventional manner.[12,13]

Approximately 10% of seminomas will be associated with an elevated serum hCG concentration. An elevated AFP concentration is never seen in pure seminoma.

SPERMATOCYTIC SEMINOMA

Spermatocytic seminoma accounts for about 7% of all seminomas and carries a good prognosis. It occurs in older patients, with an average age of 65 years. It is slow growing and

TABLE 35-2.   Comparison of Classifications of Testicular Germ-Cell Tumors*

Dixon and Moore	Mostofi and Price	WHO	British Testicular Tumour Panel
	Tumors of one histologic type	Tumors of one histologic type	
Seminoma	Seminoma (typical) Spermatocytic seminoma Anaplastic seminoma†	Seminoma Spermatocytic seminoma	Seminoma Spermatocytic seminoma
Embryonal carcinoma	Embryonal carcinoma Polyembryoma Adult	Embryonal carcinoma Polyembryoma	Malignant teratoma, undifferentiated (MTU)
Teratoma, adult	Teratoma Mature Immature With malignant change‡	Teratoma Mature Immature With malignant transformation	Teratoma, differentiated
	Embryonal carcinoma juvenile	Yolk sac tumor (embryonal carcinoma, juvenile type; endodermal sinus tumor)	Yolk sac tumor
Choriocarcinoma	Choriocarcinoma	Choriocarcinoma	
	Tumors of more than one histologic type	Tumors of more than one histologic type	
Teratoma with embryonal carcinoma ("teratocarcinoma")	Embryonal carcinoma with teratoma ("teratocarcinoma") Specify types	Embryonal carcinoma with teratoma ("teratocarcinoma")	Malignant teratoma, intermediate (MTI)
		Choriocarcinoma and any other types (specify)	Malignant teratoma trophoblastic (MTT)
	Specify types	Other combinations (specify)	"Combined tumor" when seminoma present

* Excluding intratubular germ-cell neoplasia.
† This term has been discarded in a more recent formulation.
‡ Refers to malignant areas independent of seminoma, embryonal carcinoma, or choriocarcinoma.

rarely metastasizes. The cut surface is pale gray, soft, and friable with a gelatinous or mucoid appearance. The tumor cells form solid sheets with poor segregation by fibrous septae, in contrast to its classic counterpart, which is well segregated by septae. A marked variation in the size of the tumor cells is a classical confirming histologic feature. Cells range from giant cells (50–100 μm) to many small cells (6–8 μm). There is no lymphocytic infiltration or granuloma formation, as would be seen in the classic seminoma.

EMBRYONAL CARCINOMA

Embryonal carcinoma is a highly malignant tumor with a cellular structure that is anaplastic with embryoid features such as immature tubular, papillary, or reticular appearance. The adult type has a variable histologic pattern. The polyembryonic type contains embryonal bodies that resemble those in its ovarian counterpart. Infantile embryonal carcinoma usually occurs as endodermal sinus (yolk sac) tumors. It varies in its size grossly, and cut surfaces show a varied appearance, with hemorrhagic necrosis often interspersed among yellow or gray bulging soft tissue. Its microscopic appearance is of characteristic primitive epithelial cells that are distinctly malignant in appearance. There is great variation in their size and arrangement, including some with very large pleomorphic nuclei and without distinct cell borders and others that are small with obvious borders. Mitotic figures and multinucleation are common. Acinar and papillary

structures are noted frequently. The stroma is variable; it may be loose or quite thick and fibrous. Some tumors contain trophoblastic cells. These tumors generally are more aggressive and have a high metastatic potential compared with seminoma. Embryonal cells can secrete hCG, AFP, or both.

TERATOCARCINOMA

"Teratocarcinoma" describes a germinal tumor with elements of histologically mature teratoma. Behaviorally, it lies somewhere between the mature teratoma and the highly anaplastic and malignant embryonal carcinoma. On cut surface, it has a mixture of solid and cystic spaces, the solid spaces often containing hemorrhagic or necrotic material. Histologically, there is a mixture of frankly malignant tissue, as in embryonal carcinoma, and fully differentiated cartilage, muscle, or epithelial tissue. Trophoblastic cells may also be found. The British would classify this as malignant teratoma, intermediate.

ADULT (MATURE) TERATOMA

Adult teratoma has elements of one or more of the three germinal layers showing evidence of complete histologic maturity. It is necessary to sample such a tumor thoroughly to exclude undifferentiated foci. Although this type is the least aggressive of the nonseminomatous tumors, it can metastasize in the adult and so cannot be regarded as biologically benign. In fact, only 75% of patients with mature teratoma survived when treated with orchiectomy alone; the remaining 25% died of metastatic disease. Therefore, appropriate pathologic staging is indicated in adults. However, this is not the case in children, particularly newborn infants and those under the age of 2. When an adult teratoma has cellular and active stroma with mitotic figures, it is referred to as immature teratoma.

YOLK SAC TUMOR

Yolk sac (endodermal sinus) tumor presents more commonly in infants and young children but also can present in its histologically distinct form in adults. It is an aggressive tumor in the adult, with early hematogenous dissemination. It is especially virulent when it presents as a primary in the mediastinum. In contrast, its clinical behavior is considerably less aggressive in infants and young children.[14,15] Pure yolk sac tumors routinely are associated with an elevated AFP and a normal hCG.

CHORIOCARCINOMA

Choriocarcinoma is the most aggressive of the nonseminomatous tumors and is rare in its pure form. More frequently, it is seen mixed with other germ cell elements such as embryonal carcinoma and teratocarcinoma. It is recognized grossly by focal hemorrhages on the cut surface. The microscopic diagnosis requires definition of syncytiotrophoblastic cells, which are giant cells with multiple hyperchromatic nuclei and abundant eosinophilic cytoplasm, in relation to cytotrophoblasts, which are sheets of cells with single nuclei, abundant clear cytoplasms, and well-defined borders. HCG has long been used as a diagnostic marker of trophoblastic neoplasia. Beta subunits of hCG (β-hCG) have been identified, and accurate radioimmunoassays have been developed. Monitoring of this diagnostic marker now forms an indispensable part of the management and follow-up of patients with germ-cell tumors of the testis.[16]

BENIGN TUMORS

Tumors of stromal cell origin represent about 3% to 4% of primary testicular tumors. They are grouped as tumors of the specialized gonadal stroma and are called interstitial (Leydig) cell tumors, Sertoli cell tumors, granulosa cell tumors, androblastomas, testicular tubular adenomas, and so on.[17] Histologically, they have the appearance of the supporting tissues of the gonads of either sex and therefore may resemble Sertoli cells, granulosa cells, or theca cells. They constitute almost 20% of childhood testicular tumors.[18] Their behavior usually is benign; no more than 10% are reported to have malignant potential.[19,20] Gynecomastia occurs in about 15% of adults having interstitial cell tumors and in about one-third of adults with Sertoli cell tumors.[20] Management is accomplished with orchiectomy alone and clinical staging with CT scan and lymphangiography. Routine lymphadenectomy is not considered necessary if these studies are negative.

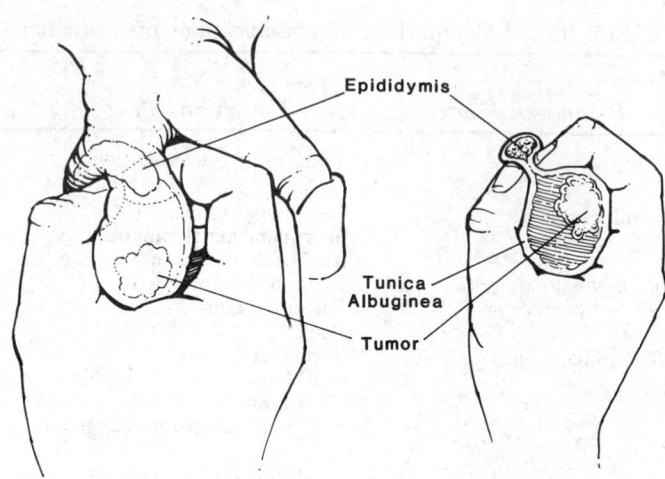

FIG. 35-1. Male scrotal examination. (Einhorn LH, Donohue JP, Peckham MJ, et al: Cancer of the testis. In DeVita VT Jr, Hellman S, Rosenberg SA [ed]: Cancer: Principles and Practice of Oncology, 2nd ed, p 985. Philadelphia, JB Lippincott, 1985)

SIGNS AND SYMPTOMS

The usual presentation of a testicular cancer is a painless enlargement of one gonad with the patient seeking medical evaluation of a lump, swelling, or hardness of the testis. In our experience, approximately 40% of patients also complain of a dull ache or heavy sensation in the scrotum, inguinal area, or lower abdomen. Acute onset of pain is rare unless the patient has concomitant epididymitis or develops bleeding within the testis, as expansion of the tunica albuginea produces pain.

Physical examination of the testis is performed by carefully palpating the organ between the thumb and first two fingers. The normal testis is homogeneous in consistency and freely movable (Fig. 35-1). Any nodular, hard, or fixed area discovered within the substance must be considered neoplastic until proved otherwise. The contralateral testis provides a comparative model for the examiner.

Simple palpation of a testis mass may give some clue as to its pathology. For example, seminomas tend to expand through the entire testicular substance, whereas teratomas and embryonal cell tumors tend to produce discrete nodular masses within the substance of the testis. Evaluation of the epididymis and cord structure is recommended.

DIFFERENTIAL DIAGNOSIS

The differential diagnosis of a testicular mass includes torsion, epididymitis, and tumor. Ancillary studies, including ultrasonography, are helpful in establishing a diagnosis, but suspicion is raised by the physical examination alone. In a retrospective review of our testicular cancer population, 55% of patients were initially treated for presumed epididymitis, resulting in a delay of definitive therapy from several weeks to 9 months or longer.

LABORATORY INVESTIGATION

Along with the blood cell count and urinalysis, the basic laboratory studies for patients suspected of having testicular tumors are specified radiologic studies and measurement of serum markers. HCG and AFP have become the ultimate tumor markers, and their use is routine in all stages of germ-cell tumors. In disseminated nonseminomatous germ-cell tumors, approximately 40% of all patients will have an elevated AFP and 75% an elevated hCG, and 85% will have one or both markers elevated. A marker that fails to return to normal or rises after a chemotherapy-induced CR almost invariably implies persistent or recurrent disease. The half-life of hCG is 18 to 24 hours and that of AFP, 5 days. Marked elevations of AFP may take several months to normalize after a curative treatment, either surgery (retroperitoneal lymphadenectomy; RPLND) or chemotherapy.

Occasionally, elevated hCG or AFP levels are found in the absence of active germ-cell tumors. The most obvious cause of such a result is a laboratory error. No patient should be treated as having a relapse purely on the basis of a single elevation of hCG. Although there is a sense of urgency to treat patients immediately with chemotherapy for a post-RPLND or first-line chemotherapy relapse, in reality, there is no necessity for prompt institution of chemotherapy as long as there is no obvious hematogenous spread (normal chest radiograph) or extensive nodal disease (on physical examination, abdominal CT, or both). For example, if a patient achieves a CR with cisplatin combination chemotherapy and subsequently has an hCG of 18 mIU/ml (normal less than 1.50-mIU/ml) while all other studies are normal, the worst error an oncologist can make is to start salvage chemotherapy; in reality, there may not be a relapse at all. Initially, we would repeat the hCG assay with another laboratory if appropriate. We also would query the patient about recent marijuana abuse, as this can cause gynecomastia and modest elevations of hCG. Finally, some patients will have cisplatin-induced atrophy in the remaining normal testis, with resultant low serum testosterone levels. The pituitary gland, by normal feedback mechanisms, will secrete large quantities of luteinizing hormone (LH) to stimulate the Leydig cells of the testis to secrete more testosterone. The beta subunit of hCG is not supposed to have cross-reactivity with LH; however, there is always some degree of interference even in the best radioimmunoassays. A simple test in this clinical situation is to give a patient a single injection of 300 mg of depotestosterone and repeat the hCG assay in 2 weeks. If hCG has been suppressed, the cause of the apparent elevation is cross-reactivity of the assay with LH.

Only rarely is a false-positive AFP elevation observed. This marker can be elevated in other tumors, especially hepatoma. Also, regenerating hepatitis or cirrhotic nodules can cause a false-positive elevation of AFP, but this is usually obvious clinically.

Markers are also of value in seminoma. HCG is elevated in only 10% of seminoma; however, 50% of patients Stage III seminomas will have elevated hCG. Moreover, AFP is never elevated in pure seminoma, so if an orchiectomy reveals pure seminoma, but the AFP is elevated, the patient should be managed as having nonseminomatous disease.[13]

Lactic dehydrogenase (LDH) is a nonspecific marker akin to the erythrocyte sedimentation rate in Hodgkin's disease. Most patients with bulky metastases of germ-cell tumor will have an elevated LDH.

A potential new marker has recently been described for metastatic seminoma. Kuzmits and colleagues measured serum neuron-specific enolase (NSE) in 11 patients with metastatic seminoma, and eight had elevated levels.[21] Only 3 of 11 had elevated hCG, and all 11 had normal AFP levels. The NSE levels fell to normal with cisplatin combination chemotherapy. These authors also documented the localization of NSE in seminoma cells immunohistochemically. NSE assays may be of particular value in bulky Stage II–III seminoma with persistent radiographic abnormalities after cisplatin-based chemotherapy in helping to determine the need for subsequent laparotomy or radiotherapy.

RADIOGRAPHIC STUDIES AND STAGING

In nonseminomatous disease, Stage I (or A) refers to tumor confined to the testis; this implies tumor-free lymph nodes and a clear chest. Stage II (or B) indicates metastatic disease in the node-bearing area of the periaortic or vena caval zone but with no demonstrable metastases above the diaphragm or in visceral organs. Stage III (C) designates clinical or radiographic evidence of metastases above the diaphragm or in other viscera. Stages IIA (B_1) and IIB (B_2) refer to microscopic (IIA with fewer than five positive nodes) and grossly positive nodes or more than 5 positive nodes, respectively.

Radiographic studies are designed to rule out Stage III disease (pulmonary metastases) and retroperitoneal nodal metastases (Stage II disease). Useful in this regard are chest CT, which we consider essential before embarking on lymphadenectomy. Of less value are lymphangiography and intravenous urography. The possible error in pedal lymphangiography is roughly 25% false negative and 5% to 10% false positive.[22] With such overall inaccuracy, lymphangiography is no longer needed for staging purposes in our view. We have been impressed with the value of CT as a staging mechanism for the retroperitoneal space. Gross nodal metastases usually are detected by this method, although microscopic metastases are not, and our overall accuracy rate with CT is 70% to 80%.[23,24] Independent clinical studies in the United States reveal at least a 20% understaging rate when combining all diagnostic tests such as CT scan and serum markers.[22-24]

SEMINOMA

Seminoma is the most common histologic subtype of testis tumors in adults, accounting for about 60% of all germ-cell tumors. Its treatment is one of the most gratifying endeavors in all of oncologic clinical practice: with the advent of multidrug chemotherapy that allows the cure of men with disseminated disease, the overall cure rate for all stages is now at or above 90% in most treatment centers. Because these tumors occur in a young population, and because surgical resection, external-beam radiation, and multidrug chemotherapy are

TABLE 35-3. Staging of Seminoma

Stage I	Tumor confined to the testis
Stage II	Nodal metastases (usually based on radiologic studies) but limited to the infradiaphragmatic lymphatics
	A. Minimal retroperitoneal disease
	B. Bulky metastases
Stage III	Tumor involving lymphatics above the diaphragm
Stage IV	Extranodal metastases

all effective (either alone or in combinations) in treating patients with metastatic deposits, consideration of cure *with* maintenance of fertility *and* avoidance of potential harmful sequelae is very important.

Seminoma is exquisitely sensitive to radiation and usually presents at an early stage. Postorchiectomy external-beam radiation therapy to the retroperitoneal lymph nodes achieves very high cure rates for patients with low-stage tumors. The optimum treatment of patients presenting with distant metastases is chemotherapy initially. The role, if any, of consolidation surgery or radiotherapy in clinical scenarios in which there are persistent radiographic abnormalities remains controversial. Likewise, the optimal treatment of bulky Stage II disease is uncertain.

After radical orchiectomy (see below) that reveals seminoma, the clinical evaluation for possible extragonadal metastatic disease should always include postorchiectomy serum radioimmunoassays for hCG and AFP, tomography, a retroperitoneal CT scan, and a bipedal lymphangiogram if the retroperitoneal CT scan is negative. Because the AFP concentration is never elevated with pure seminoma and the serum hCG rarely is, these markers contribute nothing to the clinical staging of patients with seminoma (Table 35-3). The absolute incidence of occult retroperitoneal lymph node metastases in Stage I seminoma (CT and lymphangiograms are normal) is not known because for the last three decades, patients have been treated by regional radiation after noninvasive staging. The accepted incidence of occult metastases is 10% to 25% [22,25,26]

Recently, several specific histopathologic characteristics of the primary tumor have been evaluated with regard to their influence on metastatic spread in men with pure seminoma.[27,28] Unfortunately, no significant predictors have been identified, although because all patients evaluated had retroperitoneal irradiation, the false-negative rate of noninvasive staging has not truly been tested. In preliminary data from the Massachusetts General Hospital, no difference has been found in the incidence of either vascular invasion or invasion of the epididymis or spermatic cord in patients clinically staged as I compared with those in Stage II.

POSTORCHIECTOMY RADIATION TECHNIQUE (STAGES I AND IIA)

The retroperitoneal lymph nodal groups usually included in the radiation treatment fields are the ipsilateral external iliac, the bilateral common iliac, the paracaval, and the para-aortic nodes superiorly including coverage of the cisterna cyli. Lymphangiographic study of the retroperitoneal lymph nodes is very useful in the design of the treatment fields at

the time of simulation. An excretory urogram or an abdominal CT scan must be carefully evaluated prior to or at the time of simulation with the patient in the treatment position to assure the exact localization of the kidneys with respect to the treatment fields. When such care is taken to localize the kidneys properly, the risk of radiation-induced damage is essentially eliminated.

The exact definition of the fields depends on the unique characteristics of the individual patients and the type of megavoltage equipment available. The boundaries of the fields usually are *superiorly* to the origin of the thoracic duct or to include the entire anterior surface of the T11 vertebral body; *inferiorly* to the internal inguinal ring and the inguinal excision; and *laterally* to include the ipsilateral renal hilum, usually more generously on the left than on the right. The contralateral para-aortic or paracaval and common iliac lymph node groups are contoured with individually cut Cerrobend blocking and treated with 4 to 12 MeV linear accelerator beams.

These fields should be expanded to include additional areas in the following not-uncommon situations. First, in patients who have a history of herniorrhapy or orchiopexy, which may predispose to atypical lymphatic drainage, the inferior portion of the field should be extended to include the contralateral inguinal region. Second, in patients with histo-

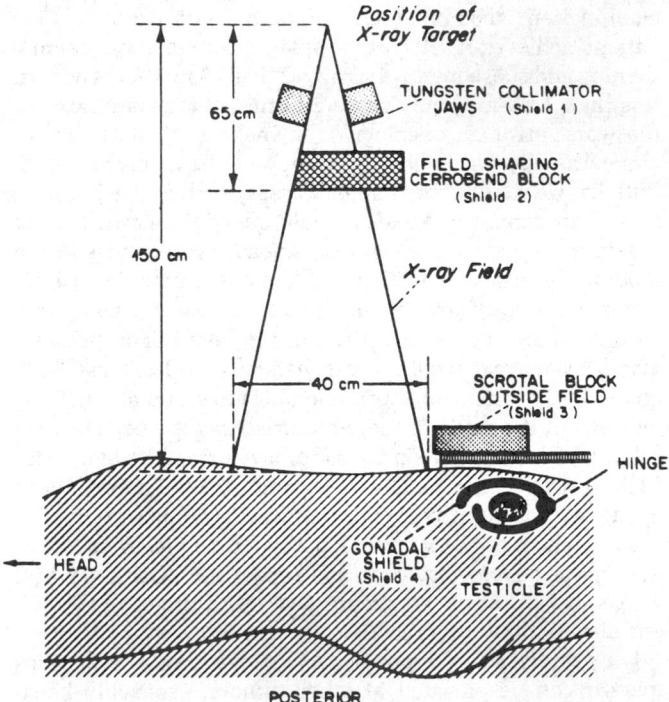

FIG. 35-2. A schematic sagittal diagram of the treatment set-up and shielding for the treatment of a patient with a testicular seminoma following radical orchiectomy. Patient is supine and the contralateral testis is shown diagrammatically. Field size is 40 cm in the longitudinal direction, and the treatment distance from source to skin is 150 cm. Four shielding devices are illustrated: the collimator jaws of the linear accelerator, cerrobend field shaping blocks, a lead scrotal block, and a gonadal shield whose front or cephalad wall separates the testicle from the horizontal internal scatter. (Kubo HD, Shipley WU: Int J Radiat Oncol Biol Phys 8:1741–1745, 1982)

logic evidence of epididymal or spermatic cord invasion, the field should be enlarged to include the ipsilateral hypogastric lymph nodes as potential site of metastases.

Recent improvements in shielding the contralateral testis include using three additional shields outside the primary beam. A system that has proved convenient, effective, and useful at the Massachusetts General Hospital is shown in Figure 35-2 and includes a 10-cm lead shield immediately above the contralateral testis; an extension of Cerrobend block for an additional 5 cm below the inferior border of the field at the level of the blocking tray; and a more comprehensive gonadal shielding, preventing the majority of internally scattered photons from hitting the remaining testis. This combination has lowered the dose received by the contralateral testis to approximately 0.1% of the treatment dose.[29]

The fields are treated with conventional fractionations (150 cGy per day, five sessions per week) using 10-MeV linear accelerator beam. Both the anterior and the posterior fields are treated each day. If the patient has had a huge primary tumor invading part of the scrotum but not requiring a hemiscrotectomy, or if the tumor has been removed through a scrotal incision, the ipsilateral hemiscrotum is treated by a 12 to 15 MeV electron-beam field that is matched to the lower border of the photon field. The ipsilateral hemiscrotum is held to the involved side with a soft clamp while the patient places and holds his remaining testis high in the inguinal canal and under a 2-cm-thick lead cup. With this technique, the contralateral testis can usually be moved more than 4 cm from the electron beam edge and has been consistently found to receive 3% or less of the given electron dose by scatter.

TREATMENT RESULTS: STAGE I

The results from many major centers in clinical Stage I seminoma treated with postorchiectomy radiation therapy are all outstanding (for examples, see Table 35-4). The 3- to 5-year disease-free survival rates are very near the absolute cure rates in patients with testicular seminoma in that there are very few late relapses with death in these series. Now, with the advent of chemotherapy effective against disseminated disease, we would anticipate being able to cure nearly all of these few patients who will relapse with distant disease.

The outstanding 3- to 5-year survival rates (all above 95%)

TABLE 35-4.   Results of Postorchiectomy Radiation Therapy in Stage I Seminoma

Treatment Center	Total Patients	5-Year Survival (%)
Walter Reed Army Hosp.[30]	284	97
Royal Marsden Hosp.[31]	232	98
M.D. Anderson Hosp.[28]	161	95
Stanford Univ. Hosp.[32]	71	100
Massachusetts General Hosp.[33]	135	98
U.S Patterns of Care Study[34]	229	98
Cross Cancer Institute[35]	139	98
Total	1151	98

TABLE 35-5.   Results of Postorchiectomy Radiation Therapy in Stage II Seminoma

Treatment Center	Total Patients	5-Year Survival (%)
Walter Reed Army Hosp.[30]	34	76
Royal Marsden Hosp.[36]	63	79
M.D. Anderson Hosp.[39]	48	88
Ontario Cancer Institute[37]	86	74
Massachusetts General Hosp.[33]	25	92
Cross Cancer Institute[35]	32	70
Total	288	79

seem not to be influenced by whether the reporting institution did or did not use prophylactic mediastinal irradiation. In the absence of any data to support its usefulness,[36,37] prophylactic mediastinal irradiation has been discontinued by most treatment centers for at least 5 years. Moreover, supradiaphragmatic irradiation will certainly compromise a patient's ability to receive and tolerate multidrug chemotherapy should it be necessary.[38] Thus, this practice seems further contraindicated.

Patients treated with postorchiectomy radiation therapy for Stage I seminoma have only a 2% probability of developing metastatic disease, a 2% incidence of a second testis tumor, and a less than 0.5% incidence of leukemia.[28,31,33] The incidence of second tumors has been no higher than the age-standardized national incidence rates.[31]

TREATMENT RESULTS: STAGE II

Postorchiectomy radiation therapy for patients with Stage II seminoma has been reported to yield a 70% to 88% survival rate (Table 35-5). The "correct" management of these patients has become increasingly controversial over the last 5 years with the demonstrated effectiveness of multidrug chemotherapy against advanced or disseminated seminoma. Several not completely satisfactory staging systems for the size of the metastatic deposits in retroperitoneal lymph nodes exist. However, it is clear from all series that those patients with bulky retroperitoneal metastases (Stage IIB) have had, with radiation alone before the cisplatin and chemotherapy era, survival or cure rates in the 60% range, compared with rates above 90% in those with minimal disease (Stage IIA), which statistically is not significantly lower than for Stage I. Patterns of failure following radiation for Stage IIB seminoma by wide-field or extended-field radiation therapy alone in the 1960s and 1970s suggest, in most[33,36,39] (Tables 35-6 and 35-7), but not all,[40] series, that 30% or more of the patients so treated will develop metastatic disease outside the treated volume. In contrast, those patients with Stage IIA disease have a very low incidence of distant metastases whether or not they are given prophylactic mediastinal irradiation.[37,39]

Observations 15 to 20 years ago in patients with testicular seminoma suggested that those with anaplastic tumor histology or an elevated urinary gonadotropin titer did uniquely poorly. However, recent reviews by several large institutions, including the Walter Reed Army Hospital[41] and the

TABLE 35-6.   Results of Treatment in Stage II Seminoma: Royal Marsden Hospital 1962–1979

Stage	Size of Retroperitoneal Node Metastases (cm)	No. of Patients	Total Relapsing (%)	Died of Seminoma	Died of Intercurrent Disease
IIA	<2	31	3 (9.7)	2	5
IIB	<5	11	2 (18)	1 0	
IIC	>5	21	tap(38)	6	3
Total		63	13 (21)	9 (14%)	8 (13%)

Memorial Sloan-Kettering Cancer Center,[42] documented that patients with Stages I and IIA disease and anaplastic histology have, when treated with conventional radiation therapy, as high an overall success rate as do patients with well-differentiated seminoma. Also, in recent reviews, all patients with Stage I or Stage IIA disease who had an elevated serum hCG by radioimmunoassay have remained in complete remission after conventional radiation therapy.[43,44] Thus, patients with Stages I and IIA pure seminoma with elevated serum hCG, as well as those with anaplastic seminoma, should be treated by radiation therapy with doses that are usual for the patient's clinical stage.

TREATMENT OF ADVANCED SEMINOMA

Radiation therapy was the treatment of choice for Stage IIB, III, or IV seminoma before the advent of cisplatin combination chemotherapy. The cure rate for Stage IIB was about 60%, and the cure rate for Stages III and IV ranged from 20% to 60%.[33,36,45] Extended radiation therapy to both infradiaphragmatic and supradiaphragmatic fields often precludes the administration of effective doses of chemotherapy to control any later failure.[38]

Alkylating agents were used against metastatic seminoma in the 1970s. However, beginning in 1974, the combination of cisplatin, vinblastine, and bleomycin (PVB) was instituted as first-line chemotherapy in disseminated testicular seminoma at Indiana University. Seminoma was judged at least as chemosensitive as any other germ-cell type to cisplatin-based chemotherapy, and even as a single agent, cisplatin has produced excellent results. For example, Oliver at the Institute of Urology in London utilized cisplatin 50 mg/m² on days one and two every 3 weeks for four courses and achieved a CR in 13 of 14 patients.[46] The response rates are high whether cisplatin-based chemotherapy is given as the first treatment with no prior radiation (Table 35-8) or as salvage treatment for relapse after initial radiation (Table 35-9). Although most authors have not reported separately the maintained CR rate with and without prior radiation therapy, it seems clear that extensive prior radiation is a significant negative influence on both the chemotherapy tolerance and the CR rate. The Southeastern Cancer Study Group has recently published the largest experience in the treatment of patients with advanced seminoma with and without prior radiation therapy.[38] In their series, 43 of 62 patients treated by PVB with or without VP-16 or doxorubicin have achieved and maintained CR. However, in 13 of these 43 patients the response was "consolidated" by surgery, radiation therapy, or both to the site of original tumor bulk. There were six drug-related fatalities and 12 patients dying of progressive disease, 11 of whom were never disease-free.

In patients treated with cisplatin-containing chemotherapy regimens, one difficulty has been that 50% or more will not have a radiographic CR. The need for further treatment versus observation in these patients is still unclear. Surgical resection following such chemotherapy is difficult because of the severe fibrotic reaction frequently noted in the retroperitoneum. Friedman and associates reported two perioperative deaths in three patients who underwent surgery to remove residual disease.[48] In a recent Memorial Sloan-Kettering Cancer Center review of patients with bulky Stage II or Stage III seminoma, residual viable tumor was found only when the residual mass was 3 cm or greater radiologically and clear rather than desmoplastic.[49]

In summary, advanced seminoma is a rare disease and one that is chemosensitive and has a cure potential with chemotherapy competitive with that seen in nonseminomatous germ-cell tumors: 93 of 111 (84%) patients achieved a continuous disease-free status with cisplatin combination chemotherapy. A reasonable approach, shared by many

TABLE 35-7.   Sites of Initial Relapse After Radiotherapy for Stage II Seminoma: Royal Marsden Hospital, 1962–1979

Stage	Size of Retroperitoneal Node Metastases (cm)	No. of Patients	Lung± Mediastinum	Cervical	Scrotum or Groin Nodes*	Liver	Extradural	Multiple Sites
IIA	2	31	1	0	2	0	0	0
IIB	2–4.9	11	0	0	1	0	1	0
IIC	5–9.9	9	2	0	0	1	0	0
IID	10	12	1	2	0	0	0	2
Total		63	4	2	3	1	1	2

* Two of three patients who had scrotal interference prior to orchiectomy and who did not receive scrotal and groin-node irradiation suffered relapses.

TABLE 35-8.   Results of Postorchiectomy Initial Chemotherapy in Stages IIB, III, and IV Seminoma

Treatment Center	Chemotherapy	No. of Patients	Maintained CR*
London Inst. Urology[46]	Cisplatin	10	9
M.D. Anderson Hosp.[39]	Cisplatin ± cyclophosphamide	10	8
University of Munich[47]	VIP	6	5
Southeastern Cancer Study Group[38]	PVB ± doxorubicin or PVP-16B	27	21
Norwegian Random Hosp.[51]	PVB or PVP-16B	39	33
National Cancer Inst., Milan[52]	PVB or PVP-16B	19	17
Total		111	93(84%)

* Includes some patients receiving postchemotherapy surgery or radiation to remove residual disease.

treatment centers, is to use multidrug cisplatin-based chemotherapy initially and to use no further treatment in the patients with a radiographic CR. In those with residual masses, either careful close observation or consolidation by radiation therapy or surgery is appropriate.[50,51] Possibly the recent identification of two potentially useful serum markers for seminoma, placental alkaline phosphatase[52] and neuron-specific enolase[21] will aid in the difficult decision concerning appropriate management of patients with persistent radiographic abnormalities.

ORCHIECTOMY

Removal of the testis through an inguinal approach is the definitive procedure for both pathologic diagnosis and local control of the primary tumor. The inguinal approach is preferred as it permits early control of both the vascular and lymphatic supply of the testis as well as the en bloc removal of the paratesticular fascial layers. Scrotal orchiectomy and biopsy are to be condemned and have been associated with a 24% incidence of local recurrence or spread to inguinal lymph node areas.[53] Although (β-hCG and AFP) are sensitive markers germ-cell tumors, 30% of patients with nonseminomatous germ-cell tumor and 92% of those with seminomas will have normal marker levels. Therefore, a decision against surgical exploration of a testicular mass should not be based on negative results of tumor markers.

The management of the patient who has undergone a scrotal orchiectomy is predicated on whether a testicular biopsy was performed prior to the orchiectomy. If the operating surgeon recognized the presence of a tumor and did not biopsy the testis, then the inguinal portion of the spermatic cord can be removed through a metachronous inguinal incision or at the time of an RPLND. If a biopsy was performed and a nonseminomatous germ-cell tumor identified, a hemiscrotectomy should be done; an inguinal lymphadenectomy is performed only in the unusual case where palpable nodes are identified. In patients who have a seminoma, the groin and lateral scrotum should be included within the irradiated field.

The surgical procedure for orchiectomy is as follows. The patient is placed supine on the operative table, and adequate anesthesia is attained. The inguinal area is prepared and draped, and an incision is made 2 cm superior and parallel to the inguinal ligament. The incision is carried through the subcutaneous tissue, and the several large veins encountered are identified and ligated. The aponeurosis of the external oblique and the external inguinal ring are identified, and an incision is made in the external fascia. Care is taken to dissect bluntly the underlying medial muscle and nerve from the fascia. The medial and inferior aspects of the spermatic cord are dissected free from the external fascia, exposing the pubic tubercle. At this point, a Penrose drain is placed around the spermatic cord at the level of the pubic tubercle. After the cremasteric vessels have been divided, the drain is doubled around the spermatic cord and clamped securely 1 inch from the internal ring. By both blunt and sharp dissection, the testis is delivered from the scrotum to the operative field. With large tumors, it is often necessary to extend the incision down to the upper aspects of the scrotum.

If a tumor appears obvious, then the surgeon should proceed with division of the spermatic cord at the internal ring. If the existence of a neoplasm is questionable, a frozen section may be performed by isolating the testis away from the operative field, covering the incision, and performing the biopsy with the testis encircled by towels or sponges. In order

TABLE 35-9.   Results of Chemotherapy After Orchiectomy and Radiation Therapy for Disseminated Relapse of Seminoma Salvage (Chemotherapy)

Treatment Center	Chemotherapy	No. of Patients	Maintained CR*
London Inst. Urology[46]	Cisplatin, etoposide	4	4
University of Munich[47]	VIP	7	5
Southeastern Cancer Study Group[38]	PVB ± doxorubicin or PVP-16B	33	20
Norwegian Radium Hosp.[50]	PVB or PVP-16	15	9
National Cancer Institute, Milan[51]	PVB or PVP-16B	13	6
Total		72	44(61%)

* Includes some patients receiving postchemotherapy surgery for residual disease.

to remove the testis, the structures of the spermatic cord should be identified and divided. It is necessary to identify and ligate the vas separately from the spermatic vessels. The cord stump is placed in the retroperitoneum so that the distal aspects of the cord can be removed without difficulty in the event a RPLND is performed.

RADICAL RETROPERITONEAL LYMPH NODE DISSECTION

Retroperitoneal lymphadenectomy remains the mainstay of surgical therapy for nonseminomatous germ-cell tumors. In patients with low-volume disease, including Stages I, IIA, and IIB, RPLND permits accurate staging, minimizes the risk of retroperitoneal recurrence, and cures a substantial number of patients without chemotherapy. Controversies surrounding management by observation for clinical Stage I disease as well as the role of primary and adjuvant chemotherapy for early Stage II are discussed elsewhere in this chapter. RPLND is also performed to remove residual disease after chemotherapy and to define further therapy in this subset of patients.

HISTORICAL PERSPECTIVES

Jamieson and Dobson in 1910 described the lymphatic drainage of the testis, establishing the primary echelon of drainage for right-sided tumors to the interaortocaval, preaortic, and precaval nodes and for left-sided tumors to the left periaortic and preaortic nodes.[54] There exists some crossover, especially from right to left, of these lymphatics. Their anatomical study was the basis for lymph node dissection in the management of these tumors. The first site of metastases is the retroperitoneal lymph nodes in nearly 90% of patients who have nonseminomatous tumors; in only 7% to 15% of patients will the site of first metastasis be outside the surgical margins of the lymph node dissection.

The first successful retroperitoneal lymph node dissection was reported by Cuneo and Marcille.[55] Other investigators soon described performing lymph node dissections in an attempt to cure testicular tumors.[56,57] The classic report by Lewis in 1948 was the first to establish RPLND as a primary therapy for nonseminomatous germ-cell tumors.[58] He reported a 46% 5-year survival rate among 28 patients who were treated with combined retroperitoneal lymphadenectomy and radiation after orchiectomy.

Various surgical approaches have been advocated for the removal of the retroperitoneal lymph nodes. Cooper and associates were among the first to popularize the transthoracic approach[59] based on Sweet's gastroesophageal procedures. The transabdominal approach was popularized by Staubitz, Whitmore, and others.[60,61] Donohue and his co-workers later modified this dissection by including an extended bilateral suprahilar removal using a transabdominal midline incision with mobilization of the pancreas and surrounding structures.[62] In addition, Donohue's group depicted the distribution of retroperitoneal lymph node metastases in patients who had Stages IIA, IIB, and IIC disease.[62] This significant, meticulously performed study provides the ratio-

nale for tailoring the surgical procedure to the amount of disease present. Furthermore, it serves as a rationale for modifying RPLND in order to preserve ejaculatory function in patients with clinical Stage I disease.

There is minimal morbidity and virtually no mortality associated with RPLND.[62,63] The principal long-term complication remains loss of ejaculation. However, recent reports by Lange and colleagues reveal that fertility can be preserved in selected patients undergoing radical retroperitoneal dissection,[64] and this subject will be discussed later in this chapter.

Radiologic tests to detect lymph node metastases, including magnetic resonance imaging (MRI), CT scanning, and lymphangiography, have false-positive and false-negative rates that range from 15% to 25%.[65] Therefore, RPLND is the most accurate way to detect retroperitoneal metastases. Moreover, it is therapeutic in the majority of patients with Stages I through IIB disease, being associated with a recurrence rate of less than 2% in the retroperitoneum.[66]

Adequate preoperative preparation of the patient undergoing an RPLND is imperative. Vigorous preoperative overnight hydration with 5% dextrose in 0.45% saline at a rate of 150 ml per hour is instituted; in combination with intravenous mannitol at the time of dissection of the renal hilum, this fluid reduces the risk of arterial thrombosis and renal ischemia. Broad-spectrum antimicrobials are administered preoperatively. General anesthesia is routine. Occasionally, in patients with residual disease after chemotherapy, sodium nitroprusside-induced hypotension is employed to reduce blood loss when resecting bulky retroperitoneal disease associated with a dense desmoplastic reaction around the vessels and other retroperitoneal structures. Central venous lines and arterial lines are helpful in monitoring hemodynamic status in patients judged to be at high risk for bleeding or other complications.

SURGICAL PROCEDURE: THORACOABDOMINAL LYMPH NODE DISSECTION

Patient position for thoracoabdominal RPLND is of paramount importance. The patient is placed on the ipsilateral side of the operating table with the break located just above the iliac crest (Fig. 35-3). The ipsilateral shoulder is positioned 30° off the horizontal, and the arm is extended across the chest and placed on a Mayo stand or a Kraus armrest. The hips are nearly flat. Once the incision is made, this position results in an uncoiling phenomenon similar to that observed when opening an empty paper towel roll.

The incision is made over an appropriately selected rib so that the medial aspect of the incision lies halfway between the xiphoid process and the umbilicus. The lateral extent of the incision is the posterior axillary line. The costochondral junction is crossed, and a gentle curve like that of a hockey stick is made so that the incision becomes either a left paramedian or a midline. In general, the thoracic and abdominal limbs of the incision should be of equal length.

With the electrocautery device, the subcutaneous tissues and latissimus dorsi muscle are divided. The distal two-thirds of the selected rib is identified and resected. At this point, the surgeon can proceed either in an extraperitoneal or in-

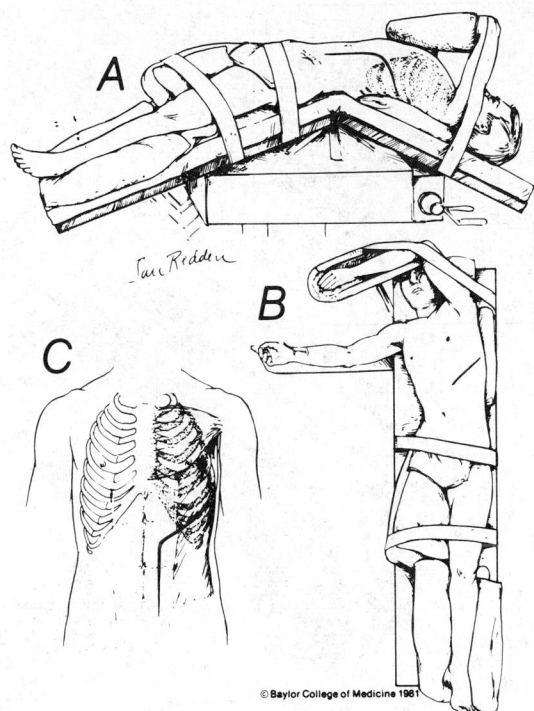

FIG. 35-3. Position and incision for left thoracoabdominal retroperitoneal lymphadenectomy. **A.** The soft tissue of the flank is placed directly over the break in the table, with the contralateral leg triangulated and the ipsilateral leg straight. The table is maximally hyperextended. **B.** The right arm rests on an arm board; the left arm is elevated on a well-padded Kraus support. **C.** The incision begins over the rib at the left posterior axillary line, is directed toward a point midway between the xiphoid and the umbilicus, and then turns over the abdomen to become a paramedian incision. (Scardino PT: Thoracoabdominal retroperitoneal lymphadenectomy for testicular cancer. In Crawford ED, Borden TA [eds]: Genitourinary Cancer Surgery. Philadelphia, Lea & Febiger, 1982)

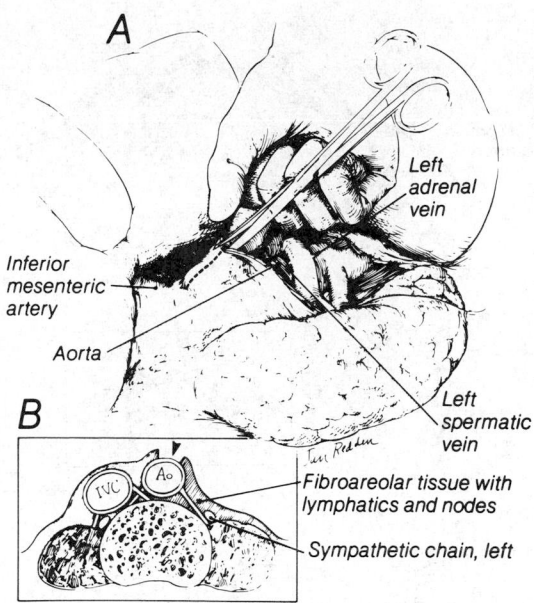

FIG. 35-4. **A.** The left renal vein is mobilized by dividing the adrenal and spermatic veins. The plane between the aorta and the retroperitoneal tissue to be dissected can be established bluntly as illustrated. **B.** The dissection is viewed in cross-section to illustrate the tissue to be dissected from the great vessels. (Scardino PT: Thoracoabdominal retroperitoneal lymphadenectomy for testicular cancer. In Crawford ED, Borden TA [eds]: Genitourinary Cancer Surgery. Philadelphia, Lea & Febiger, 1982)

traperitoneal fashion after division of the costochondral junction. In general, an extraperitoneal approach is indicated in patients who have not had chemotherapy or who have small amounts of retroperitoneal disease. In patients undergoing RPLND after chemotherapy, it is difficult to proceed extraretroperitoneally, and the peritoneum should be opened to expose the retroperitoneal structures.

With both sharp and blunt dissection, the diaphragm and peritoneum are dissected from the posterior sheath medially to the linea alba. Once the peritoneal envelope is retracted, a plane must be developed between the Gerota's fascia and the posterior peritoneum. After the peritoneal envelope is freed from the retroperitoneal structures, a Finochietto retractor is placed in the wound in such a fashion as to allow the costochondral margins to protrude through its open blades. For a left-sided dissection, the left renal vein represents the center of the anatomic dissection. Located immediately above the left renal vein is the superior mesenteric artery; laterally is the kidney, posteriorly and laterally is the left renal artery, posteriorly are the aorta and right renal artery, inferiorly are the aorta and inferior mesenteric artery, and medially is the inferior vena cava.

The initial dissection proceeds along the root of the supe-

rior mesenteric artery. This artery is an important landmark, and great care must be observed so that the vessel is not injured. There are numerous lymphatics that circumscribe the superior mesenteric artery, and these must be clipped and divided carefully. The dissection is carried laterally to the crus of the left hemidiaphragm and then continued medially and superiorly to the adrenal gland (Fig. 35-4).

Once this is accomplished, the dissection is carried over to the inferior vena cava, further delineating the upper limits of the dissection. The areolar tissues surrounding the left renal vein are divided and ligaclipped. The dissection then proceeds to the superior aspect of this vein, where the adrenal vein is identified and ligated. As the dissection is carried posteriorly, the lumbar vein will be encountered and should be identified and ligated, as it can be the source of troublesome bleeding (Fig. 35-5). In general, with anterior and superior traction, the aorta and root of the left renal artery are identified. A plane is located and developed between the adventitia of the aorta and the anteriorly located areolar and nodal tissues. Dissection is carried inferiorly on the aorta, identifying the inferior mesenteric artery. This artery may be divided; however, in older patients and in patients in whom ejaculatory function is to be preserved, this artery is not divided.

Both the renal artery and renal vein can now be dissected from proximal to distal or from the hilum to the root. Bivalving Gerota's fascia provides safe access to the renal hilar area and easy identification of aberrant renal arteries and veins (Fig. 35-5). Prior to dissection of the renal vessels, administration of 12.5 g of mannitol intravenously is recom-

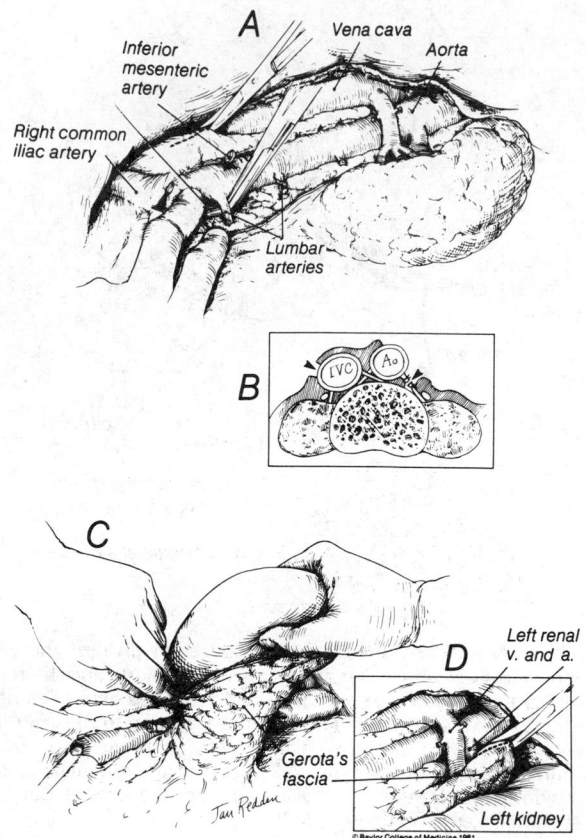

FIG. 35-5. **A**. The lateral border of the dissection is the lateral aspect of the inferior vena cava. Hemoclips must be applied along this margin. The lumbar arteries are identified, ligated, and divided. **B**. Cross-sectional view. **C**. Gerota's fascia is divided over the lateral border of the kidney and split into an anterior and posterior bundle. **D**. The ring of perirenal fat can be divided at the renal hilum while the renal vessels are directly visible. (Scardino PT: Thoracoabdominal retroperitoneal lymphadenectomy for testicular cancer. In Crawford ED, Borden TA [eds]: Genitourinary Cancer Surgery. Philadelphia, Lea & Febiger, 1982)

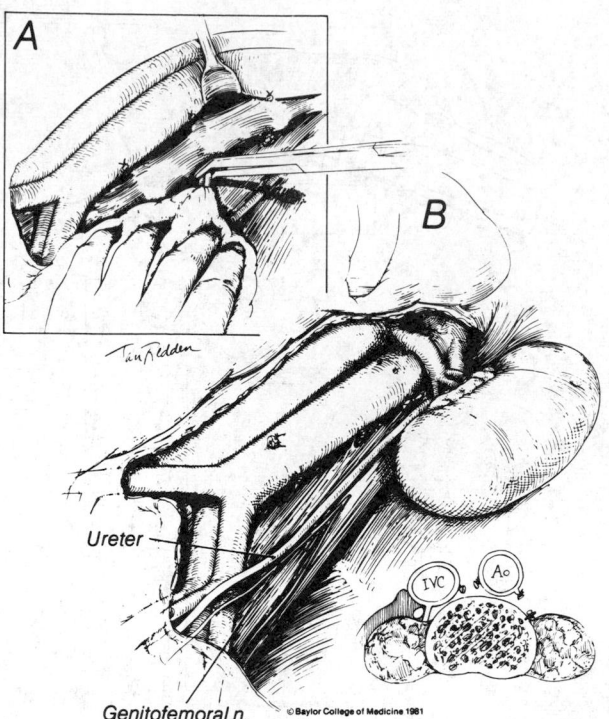

FIG. 35-6. **A**. Clips are applied to the vessels along the left aortic groove in the area of the sympathetic chain. **B**. The completed dissection is illustrated both as an overview and as a cross-section. The left common iliac artery and vein are dissected to a point just beyond their bifurcation. (Scardino PT: Thoracoabdominal retroperitoneal lymphadenectomy for testicular cancer. In Crawford ED, Borden TA [eds]: Genitourinary Cancer Surgery. Philadelphia, Lea & Febiger, 1982)

mended. In patients requiring extensive dissection after chemotherapy, intravenous mannitol is again administered 20 minutes after vessel manipulation.

With both blunt and sharp dissection, Gerota's fascia is freed from the anterior and posterior surface of the kidney. This maneuver allows for the removal of node-bearing hilar tissue en bloc with the surgical specimen. We routinely remove the adrenal gland with the specimen.

Once this tissue is freed, attention is directed to the inferior margins of the great vessels. Areolar and nodal tissues are divided in and around the aorta and vena cava, and the lumbar arteries and veins are isolated and divided. A right-angle clamp is passed around each vessel prior to ligation with 4-0 silk suture. The left renal vein is retracted to expose the origin of the right renal artery. The areolar tissue cephalad to the right renal artery is mobilized, clipped, and divided. Dissection continues behind the vena cava, exposing the prevertebral ligaments. On the ipsilateral side, the dissection should be carried down to the great vessels to just below the bifurcation of the external and internal common iliac arteries. Dissection on the ipsilateral side includes all

tissue lateral to the aorta and medial to the ureter (Fig. 35-6).

In patients who have lymph node involvement clinically judged as IIB or IIC, a similar margin is obtained on the contralateral side. Modification of the lymph node dissection to preserve ejaculatory function can be performed by preserving the sympathetic supply roots and postganglionic fibers (Fig. 35-7). All remnants of the spermatic cord are removed with the surgical specimen by tracing the testicular vessels to the internal ring, palpating the ligature on the stump, and dissecting the vas from the vessels. The margins of the dissection have now been outlined, and attention is directed to removing the remaining retroperitoneal node tissue.

Modification of the operation is necessary in patients who have residual disease after chemotherapy, as it is frequently impossible to remove all tumor en bloc, because the normal anatomic cleavage plane between the nodal tissue and the great vessels may be obliterated. Sharp dissection with a No. 10 knife blade on a scalpel may be necessary for removal of tumor, as may ligation and resection of the inferior vena cava. Rarely, aortic resection with graft placement is required. Nephrectomy and bowel resection may be performed in order to remove all gross tumor. Cytoreductive surgical procedures of this nature may require 12 to 15 hours of operating time and should be performed only by surgeons

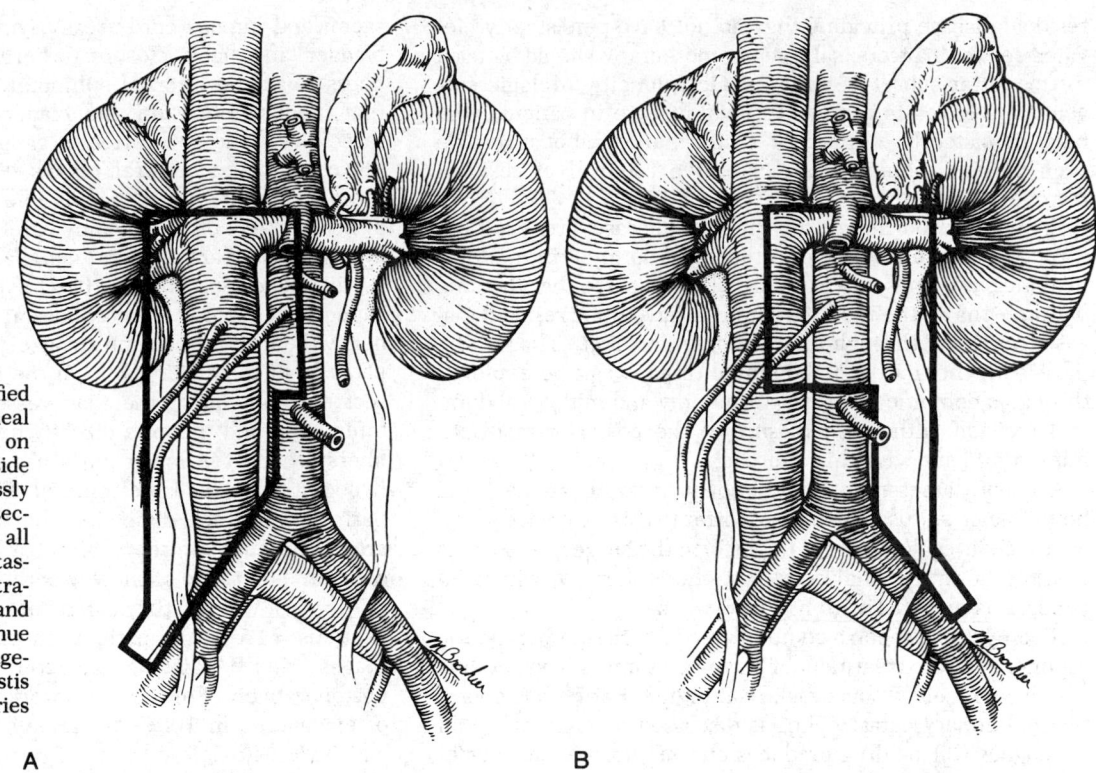

FIG. 35-7. Limits of modified nerve sparing retroperitoneal lymph node dissection on right side (**A**) and left side (**B**) for patients with grossly negative nodes. The dissection is designed to remove all nodes likely to contain metastases yet preserve the contralateral sympathetic chain and hypogastric plexus. (Donohue JP: Options in the management of low stage testis cancer. AUA Update Series 6:27, 1987)

A   B

well versed in retroperitoneal anatomy and surgery. After properly administered and effective chemotherapy, this operation is indicated in patients with partial resolution of retroperitoneal or thoracic disease as demonstrated on CT scan or other radiographic studies. Patients who have persistently elevated serum markers are, in general, not candidates for this surgical procedure. In patients who have both abdominal and thoracic disease, we have modified the incision to include a median sternotomy coupled with a midline abdominal incision. A complete bilateral dissection, including the suprahilar areas, is indicated in all postchemotherapeutic node dissections.

As Donohue has pointed out, the "heterogenicity of the tissue in the retroperitoneum makes it visually impossible to distinguish between necrotic changes, teratoma, and carcinoma" (cited by Einhorn and associates).[67] The surgeon must be cognizant of the existence of the lymph nodes in the retrocrural space, especially in patients with lower abdominal lymphadenopathy. CT scans may demonstrate lymph node enlargement in this area.[68]

RADIATION THERAPY FOR PATIENTS WITH NONSEMINOMATOUS GERM-CELL TUMORS

Because of the very high success rate with first-line chemotherapy, the quite satisfactory response rates with second-line chemotherapeutic regimens, and the excellent results using surgical resection of residual disease, many clinicians do not appreciate the marked sensitivity of embryonal carcinoma and teratocarcinoma to local radiation—about that of

non-Hodgkin's lymphoma. The best of the documentation of the efficacy of external-beam radiation with conventional fractionation in doses of 4500 to 5000 cGy comes from the Royal Marsden Hospital experience. In that series, only 2 of 84 patients with clinical Stage I disease developed a retroperitoneal recurrence, 1 each in 44 patients with primary teratocarcinoma and 40 patients with primary embryonal carcinoma. In patients with clinical Stage II tumors with metastases that were 2 cm or smaller by lymphangiography, radiation therapy sterilized these deposits in 93%. However, radiation was effective in permanently sterilizing the retroperitoneum in only 31% of the patients with bulky retroperitoneal metastases.[69] Radiation in nonseminomatous germ-cell tumors is reserved for those patients with incompletely responding (radiographically) metastases that are not amenable to postchemotherapy surgical resection, such as metastases in the central mediastinum, the bone, and the brain when there is clinical or pathologic evidence of persistent carcinoma. Doses with conventional fractionation are used in this setting, usually approximately 3600 cGy over 4 weeks. In sites in which the heart and central nervous system can be completely excluded, boosts to higher doses should be considered.

SURGICAL RESECTION OF RESIDUAL DISEASE

The incidence of demonstrable residual disease in the retroperitoneum, chest, or both after combination chemotherapy is between 30% and 60%.[53,63,70] Patients who achieve a PR to chemotherapy are considered candidates for resection of the residual disease providing they do not have persistently elevated serum markers; salvage chemotherapy should be used in this latter subset of patients. Occasionally, urologic surgeons are asked to remove residual disease in patients who have persistently elevated or rising markers, but rarely do such patients benefit from extensive removal of residual retroperitoneal or chest disease.

Patients harboring retroperitoneal disease are explored through either a midline or a thoracoabdominal intraperitoneal incision. Those with unilateral disease in either the lung parenchyma or the mediastinum can have their residual disease removed through thoracotomy incision. Those who have both thoracic and abdominal disease can be explored through a combined median sternotomy and midline abdominal incision, although exposure of the posterior mediastinum is difficult with this approach.

Adequate assessment of pulmonary, cardiovascular, and hematologic status is mandatory prior to this extensive surgical procedure. We attempt to perform the surgery as soon as possible after the final course of chemotherapy, which, in general, is anywhere from 4 to 6 weeks.

Bleomycin has been a component of the chemotherapeutic regimens for the treatment of germ-cell tumors, and patients who have received this drug are at high risk for a postoperative pulmonary catastrophe, as discussed by Goldinger and colleagues.[71] This drug produces chronic fibrotic changes in the lung leading to restrictive pulmonary disease and impaired carbon monoxide diffusion. These changes are subtle and require pulmonary function testing to be appreciated. Patients who are overhydrated during surgery and who have a fixed pulmonary arterial resistance can develop interstitial edema, enhancing the diffusion defect caused by bleomycin. Elevated FiO_2 concentrations can lead to destruction of Type I and Type II pneumocytes, producing an adult respiratory distress syndrome (ARDS). In order to avert this complication, the patient should be maintained at a relative hypovolemic state, being carefully monitored by a Swan-Ganz catheter to assess central and pulmonary pressures. In addition, there should be judicious use of crystalloids in fluid replacement. Colloids are preferable. Inspired FiO_2 concentration should not exceed 25% both intraoperatively and postoperatively.

FERTILITY ISSUES AFTER RPLND

The majority of patients undergoing a bilateral radical RPLND will be rendered infertile by virtue of the development of retrograde ejaculation or ejaculatory failure. This complication has surfaced as an important issue that often determines the type of therapy for a patient. There are several reasons for the contemporary interest in this complication, including the fact that the majority of patients with germ-cell tumors can expect to be cured of their cancer.

The neuroanatomy of ejaculation is not completely understood. The efferent impulses are mediated by sympathetic fibers from the thoracolumbar outflow at T12 to L3 and travel by the paravertebral ganglia and hypogastric neuroplexus.[72] Efferent impulses that mediate ejaculation are carried by autonomic and somatic nerves originating in the

sacral and lumbar cord areas. Sympathetic fibers augment bladder and neck closure, whereas the parasympathetic fibers relax the internal sphincter. The sympathetic fibers that mediate emission and bladder neck closure traverse three paths: the paravertebral ganglia, the aortomesenteric plexus, and the ureteral plexus. Preservation of many of these sympathetic paths is possible by modifying the extent of node dissection and also by carefully dissecting the tissue overlying the paravertebral ganglia.

Lange and associates at the University of Minnesota have supported changing from a bilateral to a unilateral dissection below the inferior mesenteric artery in order to preserve the pathway of these nerves.[72] On the ipsilateral side, they dissect only on top of the iliac vessels and avoid the aortic bifurcation and the area directly below it. The sympathetic fibers around the lower aorta are thus preserved, and the hypogastric plexus is not injured. Those authors continue to perform a bilateral dissection above the inferior mesenteric artery. Because the thoracolumbar sympathetic ganglia are deep on either side of the vertebral column under the edges of the great vessels, they can be preserved. With these modifications, 51% of the patients in the Minnesota series with Stages I and IIA disease had return of ejaculatory function postoperatively. Fossa and co-workers have reported return of ejaculation in 100% of patients with right-sided tumors and 56% with left-sided tumors with a limited dissection above the inferior mesenteric artery.[73]

The majority of patients with testicular cancer can expect to achieve a long-term disease-free status. Because this population is sexually active and frequently concerned about fathering children, both the short-term and the long-term effects of treatment on their reproductive system is of concern. Lange and co-workers stated that 25% of patients with testis cancer are permanently infertile before any therapy is instituted, 35% are temporarily infertile, and 40% are fertile.[64] Therefore, approximately 75% of the patients are at risk for loss of fertility from either lymph node dissection, chemotherapy, or both. The exact reasons for the impaired fertility at the time of diagnosis remain poorly understood. Berthelsen and Skakkeback evaluated 218 patients with testicular cancer and found 9% had a history of cryptochidism.[74] When the contralateral testes were biopsied, irreversible changes were noted in 24%, and carcinoma in situ was found in 5%. Fifteen percent had lowered serum testosterone, and LH was elevated in 12%.

CHEMOTHERAPY FOR DISSEMINATED TESTIS CANCER

HISTORICAL PERSPECTIVES: PRE-CISPLATIN ERA

Even in the 1950s and 1960s, disseminated testicular cancer was considered a chemosensitive tumor, with a respectable 50% objective response rate and a modest 5% to 10% cure rate with dactinomycin-based chemotherapy.[75,76] During the 1960s, several other single agents such as mithramycin, vinblastine, and bleomycin demonstrated similar activity.[77-79] These early chemotherapy studies achieved a 10% to 20% CR rate, and approximately half of these patients relapsed,

TABLE 35-10.   VAB-VI Chemotherapy Regimen

Drug	Dose	Day
Vinblastine	4 mg/m^2	
Cyclophosphamide	600 mg/m^2	1
Dactinomycin	1 mg/m^2	1
Bleomycin	30 units by IV push	1
	20 units/m^2 by continuous IV infusion	1–3
Cisplatin	120 mg/m^2	4

usually within 1 year. With modern cisplatin combination chemotherapy, patients achieving a CR have only a 10% relapse rate owing to the more effective induction therapy and the availability of tumor markers and CT scans to define CR more accurately.

Combination chemotherapy with vinblastine plus bleomycin was first described by Samuels and colleagues at M.D. Anderson Hospital and Tumor Institute.[80] In 1973, these authors switched from intermittent therapy to continuous infusion bleomycin in combination with vinblastine.[81]

The discovery of cisplatin was a major advance in the field of medical oncology. Cisplatin is one of a group of coordination compounds of platinum identified by Rosenberg, Van Camp, and Krigas that strongly inhibits bacterial replication.[82] Cisplatin as a single agent had significant activity in refractory advanced testicular cancer.[83] Indeed, it is the single most active agent in the treatment of testicular cancer and has become an integral part of combination chemotherapy programs for disseminated disease.

VAB PROGRAMS: MEMORIAL SLOAN-KETTERING CANCER CENTER

The Memorial group evaluated combination chemotherapy with vinblastine plus actinomycin D (dactinomycin) plus bleomycin (VAB-1) from June 1972 to April 1974.[84] This regimen was utilized in 71 evaluable patients and produced 14% CR and 22% PR rates. From June 1974 to January 1976, cisplatin administered every 3 to 4 months plus continuous-infusion bleomycin was added to the VAB regimen (VAB-II).[85] There was a 50% CR rate in 50 evaluable patients, and 12 (24%) remained alive and disease-free.[84] Slight modifications were made in the protocol from July 1975 through September 1976, creating VAB-III. Forty-four per cent of these 80 patients were disease free with follow-up 17 to 31 months.[86] In September 1976, another slight modification resulted in VAB-IV, with 50% of 48 patients disease free with shorter follow-up than for VAB-III.[86]

Between January 1979 and November 1982, 166 patients were treated with VAB-VI. This regimen represented a major departure from the prior VAB programs in that cisplatin (120 mg/m^2) was given monthly for three courses (Table 35-10). Therapy was repeated every 4 weeks for three courses. Bleomycin was not given on the third cycle. The complete response rate was 78%, with 67% of patients disease free with chemotherapy alone and 11% after chemotherapy plus resection of viable residual carcinoma.[87] The overall relapse rate was 12% and was greater in tumors of extragonadal origin (21%) than for testis primary (11%).

The Memorial group has recently completed a randomized prospective study comparing VAB-VI with the two-drug regimen of cisplatin plus VP-16 in good-risk disseminated testicular cancer.[88] The therapeutic results were identical, but there was a highly statistically significant reduction in toxicity with the two-drug regimen.

PVB STUDIES AT INDIANA UNIVERSITY

In August 1974, we began studies at Indiana University in disseminated testicular cancer with the already-established two-drug regimen of vinblastine plus bleomycin and adding to this the then-experimental drug, cisplatin.[89] The original regimen is depicted in Table 35-11. The cisplatin was dissolved in 50 ml of normal saline and given at a rate of 1 mg/min. Saline hydration at a rate of 100 ml/hour was given continuously during all 5 days of cisplatin administration. Mannitol diuresis was not employed and has never been felt to be necessary in any of our subsequent studies. In this trial, 33 of 47 patients (70%) achieved a CR, and an additional five patients (11%) were rendered disease free by post-PVB resection of teratoma or carcinoma. Thirty patients (64%) survived 5 years and 28 (60%) 10 years.

Today, after four courses of PVB, if the markers are normal and there are persistent radiographic abnormalities, we resect residual disease 4 to 6 weeks after the final cisplatin chemotherapy if anatomically feasible. Surgery consists of RPLND, lateral thoracotomy, median sternotomy with wedge resection of bilateral pulmonary metastases, or a combined thoracoabdominal procedure.[93] If carcinoma is found in the completely resected specimen and the markers remain normal, two postoperative courses of the original induction regimen (fifth and sixth courses of cisplatin combination chemotherapy) are given. This strategy will result in a 67% long-term disease-free survival rate in such patients.[90] Similar results have been obtained with post-VAB-VI resection at Memorial.[87]

The principal serious toxicity of the original PVB protocol was related to the high-dose (0.4 mg/kg) vinblastine. Myalgias, constipation, neuropathy, and paralytic ileus all were troublesome, but severe granulocytopenia and potential

TABLE 35-11.   Original PVB Regimen

Cisplatin	20 mg/m^2 every 3 weeks × 4
Vinblastine	0.2 mg/kg day 1 and 2 every 3 weeks × 4
Bleomycin	30 units IV push weekly × 12

Maintenance vinblastine 0.3 mg/kg monthly × 21 months

TABLE 35-12. Three Treatment Arms of PVB Study No. 2

Cisplatin 20 mg/m² × 5 every 3 weeks × 4
Vinblastine 0.4 mg/kg
Bleomycin 30 units IV weekly × 12

Cisplatin 20 mg/m² × 5 every 3 weeks × 4
Vinblastine 0.3 mg/kg
Bleomycin 30 units weekly × 12

Cisplatin 20 mg/m² × 5 every 3 weeks × 4
Vinblastine 0.2 mg/kg every 3 weeks × 4
Doxorubicin 50 mg/m² every 3 weeks × 4
Bleomycin 30 units weekly × 12

sepsis was the most worrisome toxicity. Therefore, in 1976, we started a randomized prospective trial comparing our original PVB with the same regimen but with a 25% reduction in the vinblastine dosage (to 0.3 mg/kg). A third arm adding doxorubicin to PVB with vinblastine at 0.2 mg/kg was also studied (Table 35-12). Once again, maintenance vinblastine was employed for a total of 2 years.

Seventy-eight patients were entered on this study. The 25% reduction in the vinblastine dosage resulted in the expected decrease in hematologic and neuromuscular toxicity. There was no significant difference in the efficacy of the three induction arms (Table 35-13).[91] Fifty-eight patients (73%) are currently alive and disease free for 9+ years.

On the basis of the results of this study, we abandoned our original PVB regimen in 1978 in favor of the equally effective but less toxic regimen involving the reduced dosage of vinblastine. A similar but larger study was conducted by the EORTC in 214 patients randomized to vinblastine 0.4 or 0.3 mg/kg in combination with cisplatin and bleomycin.[92] This study also showed no benefit for the higher dose of vinblastine: the CR rates were 68% for the regimen using vinblastine at 0.4 mg/kg versus 71% with 0.3 mg/kg. There was no significant difference in the disease-free or overall survival rates, but there was a significant increase in both hematologic (p = 0.01) and nonhematologic toxicity with the higher dose of vinblastine.

We began a third-generation study in 1978 in conjunction with the Southeastern Cancer Study Group. This study randomized patients achieving CR or disease-free status after resection of teratoma to maintenance vinblastine, as in our first two studies, versus no maintenance therapy (just four courses of PVB over 12 weeks). This study confirmed the fact that optimal cure rates were achieved with induction PVB and that maintenance vinblastine was unnecessary.[93] One hundred forty-seven patients from Indiana University entered this study, and 117 (80%) are alive and disease free

with a minimum follow-up of 5 years. The Memorial group has also evaluated maintenance therapy (vinblastine plus dactinomycin) with VAB-VI and likewise found no value.[87]

The results of these three PVB studies are depicted in Table 35-14. Overall, with follow-up of 6 to 13 years, 201 of 272 (74%) patients with disseminated testicular cancer are alive and presumably cured of their disease. Similar results with PVB have been published by numerous other investigators and cooperative groups around the world.

PVB VERSUS CISPLATIN PLUS VP-16 PLUS BLEOMYCIN (PVP-16B)

Etoposide (VP-16) is an epipodophyllotoxin derivative with definite single-agent activity in refractory testicular cancer.[94] In preclinical systems, there is marked synergy with VP-16 plus cisplatin.[95] In 1978, we began our initial salvage chemotherapy studies with cisplatin plus VP-16 in patients who were not cured with PVB or similar induction therapy (vide infra). VP-16, unlike vinblastine, is essentially devoid of neuromuscular toxicity.

The three-drug combination of cisplatin, VP-16, and bleomycin was initially used as first-line induction chemotherapy at the Royal Marsden Hospital.[96] Thirty-seven of 43 patients (86%) achieved disease free status.

From 1981 through 1984, the Southeastern Cancer Study Group conducted a randomized prospective study comparing PVB and PVP-16B as initial induction chemotherapy (Table 35-15).[97] Once again, no maintenance therapy was given in either arm, and if the markers were normal postchemotherapy but there was persistent radiographic abnormalities, appropriate surgery was done. If carcinoma was found, two more courses of the original induction regimen were given.

A total of 244 patients from 24 institutions entered this trial. Of 121 patients treated with PVB, 74 (61%) had a CR, and another 15 (13%) became disease free after resection of teratoma (10 patients) or carcinoma (5 patients). Among the 123 patients given PVP-16B, 74 (60%) had a CR, and 28 (23%) became free of disease after resection of teratoma (22 patients) or carcinoma (6 patients). Thus, 74% became disease free after treatment with PVB and 83% after PVP-16B. Nine patients on PVB and six receiving PVP-16B subsequently had recurrences. The 2-year survival rate was approximately 80% in both arms, with a slight but not statistically significant survival advantage for PVP-16B. However, in the subgroup of advanced disseminated disease, there was a clear survival advantage for this combination (p = 0.02).

Granulocytopenic toxicity, including granulocytopenic fever, was similar in the two arms. Severe thrombocytopenia

TABLE 35-13. Results of PVB Study No. 2

	PVB (0.4 mg/kg) (n = 26)	PVB (0.3 mg/kg) (n = 27)	PVB + Doxorubicin (n = 25)
NED*	23 (88%)	21 (78%)	20 (80%)
Relapses	5 (19%)	2 (10%)	3 (15%)
Currently NED	20 (77%)	19 (70%)	18 (72%)

* No evidence of disease.

TABLE 35-14. Summary of PVB Studies at Indiana University

Study No.	Time	No. of Patients	CR (%)	NED with Surgery (%)	Currently NED (%)
1	1974–76	47	33 (70)	5 (11)	27 (57)
2	1976–78	78	53 (68)	13 (17)	57 (73)
3	1978–81	147	92 (63)	31 (21)	117 (80)

was more common with PVP-16B, as 14% had a platelet count below 50,000/mm³ at some time during treatment compared with 5% of the patients given PVB. However, hemorrhage was seen in two patients given PVB but in none given PVP-16B. There was a major reduction in neuromuscular toxicity, as manifested by paresthesia, abdominal cramps and ileus, and myalgias. This was significant not only statistically but also clinically (Table 35-16). On the basis of this study, which demonstrated a reduction in morbidity and equivalent, if not superior, survival, we now utilize PVP-16B as first-line therapy for disseminated testicular cancer.

EXTRAGONADAL GERM-CELL TUMORS

Primary extragonadal germ-cell tumors may arise in midline structures such as the mediastinum and retroperitoneum or in the pineal gland, prostate, stomach, or thymus. During early embryogenesis, germinal epithelium arises in the yolk sac and undergoes a midline migration (from the sixth cervical vertebra to the second sacral vertebra) down the dorsal mesentery of the hindgut to the urogenital ridge and eventually forms aggregrates of testicular tissue in the scrotum. During the migration, germinal epithelium may be sequestered along the route and ultimately undergo malignant transformation.

Patients with presumed primary retroperitoneal germ-cell tumors must have a careful search for an occult testicular primary. This is critically important, because the testis is a relative sanctuary site from the effects of chemotherapy, and a missed small primary there will not necessarily be eradicated with chemotherapy.[98] Patients with a normal testis on palpation should have bilateral testicular ultrasound performed. If physical examination or ultrasound is abnormal, an orchiectomy should be performed, usually after completion of chemotherapy. Also, a primary retroperitoneal germ-cell tumor should be a midline mass: if the abdominal CT scan reveals predominantly right- or left-sided adenopathy, this is compatible with an occult primary site of origin in the ipsilateral testis, and strong consideration should be given to removal of the suspected testis.

TABLE 35-15. Treatment Arms of Southeastern Cancer Study Group Comparison of PVB and PVP-16B

Cisplatin 20 mg/m² × 5 every 3 weeks × 4
Vinblastine 0.15 mg/kg days 1 and 2 every 3 weeks × 4
Bleomycin 30 units weekly × 12

Cisplatin 20 mg/m² × 5 every 3 weeks × 4
VP-16 100 mg/m² × 5 every 3 weeks × 4
Bleomycin 30 units weekly × 12

The treatment philosophy for a primary retroperitoneal germ-cell tumor should parallel that for the testicular tumors in general, and the prognosis for cure is similar to that of testicular primaries with similar amounts of disease and marker elevation.

There is a paucity of literature guidelines for the management of suprasellar germ-cell tumors (pinealomas). Most of these are seminoma, but anatomical location often precludes accurate histologic diagnosis. An area of significant controversy is whether cranial irradiation alone is adequate or whether the entire neuroaxis should be radiated. The incidence of positive spinal-fluid cytology ranges from 6% to 55% in various series, and about 35% of patients relapse in the spine. However, the routine use of craniospinal radiotherapy makes the subsequent delivery of myelosuppressive chemotherapy very difficult should the patient relapse. The Harvard Joint Center for Radiotherapy recently detailed their results in 25 suprasellar germ-cell tumors.[99] Nineteen of the patients (76%) are continuously disease free, and most of these received radiation to the entire neuroaxis.

Primary mediastinal germ-cell tumors are fascinating biologic entities and therapeutically challenging disorders. The curve rate with cisplatin combination chemotherapy for nonseminomatous tumors is well below 50% and that for endodermal sinus (yolk sac) tumors below 25%. However, primary mediastinal seminomas have an extremely high cure rate with either radiotherapy or chemotherapy. There are a variety of known, suspected, and unknown reasons for the poor prognosis of primary mediastinal nonseminomatous tumors. One obvious reason is the initial presence of teratoma, which is often unresectable after chemotherapy because of anatomical constraints that do not exist in the retroperitoneum. However, even when a CR is achieved with resection of just necrotic fibrous tissue after cisplatin combination chemotherapy, there is a higher than expected relapse rate.

Primary mediastinal nonseminomatous germ-cell tumors have recently been associated with hematologic disorders and Klinefelter's syndrome. Nichols and coworkers described three patients with such tumors and hematologic malignancy (two cases of megakaryocytic leukemia and one myelodysplastic syndrome). These authors reviewed the case records of 688 patients with germ-cell tumors treated at Indiana University and the Dana Farber Cancer Institute.[100] Thirty-four (4.9%) of these tumors arose in the mediastinum, and three of these patients had hematologic malignancies. By contrast, there were no hematologic malignancies in the 654 patients with primary testicular or retroperitoneal germ-cell tumors. Subsequent to this report, we have seen six additional cases of hematologic malignancies associated with primary mediastinal germ-cell tumors.

TABLE 35-16. Neuromuscular Toxicity (% of Patients)

	PVB (N = 114)		PVP-16B (N = 110)
Paresthesias		p = 0.0003	
None	62		77
Mild	27		19
Moderate	11		4
Abdominal Cramps		p = 0.0008	
None	80		95
Mild	12		3
Moderate	8		2
Myalgias		p = 0.00002	
None	81		99
Mild	5		1
Moderate	14		0

The Indiana group has also prospectively performed chromosomal studies on 22 consecutive patients with mediastinal germ-cell tumors.[101] Five (22%) had karyotypic or pathologic evidence of Klinefelter's syndrome. All five had tumors with nonseminomatous histology and were relatively young (median age 15).

Extragonadal germ-cell tumors must always be considered in the diagnosis of "carcinoma, primary unknown," especially in young patients with mediastinal or retroperitoneal masses. Assays for hCG and AFP should be performed. The investigators at Vanderbilt accumulated data on 119 patients with poorly differentiated carcinoma, primary unknown.[102] Reviewing pathologists found features suggestive of germinal neoplasm in only six cases, and only two of these achieved CR with cisplatin combination chemotherapy. Overall, 27 of 96 patients (28%) who received at least one course of chemotherapy attained a CR and an additional 42 (44%) a PR. Sixteen patients (17%) are currently without evidence of disease 16 to 133 months (median 65 months) after completion of chemotherapy. Only three of the 27 achieving a CR were hCG or AFP positive. This article points out that neither light microscopy nor marker elevation can differentiate curable and incurable patients.

The results of PVB in extragonadal germ-cell tumors at Indiana and Vanderbilt have been published.[103] Eighteen of 32 (56%) patients had no evidence of disease for 1 to 5+ years at the time of publication. Identical chemotherapy was employed by the Southeastern Cancer Study Group with similar results.[104] VAB-VI gave similar results at Memorial Sloan-Kettering Cancer Center.[105] All eight patients with extragonadal seminomas achieved a CR compared with 6 of 11 whose tumors had nonseminomatous elements. Twelve of nineteen (63%) were continuously disease free at the time of publication. Investigators at M.D. Anderson used a complicated five-drug regimen and, again, achieved similar results, with 16 of 19 patients with seminomas and 12 of 30 with nonseminomatous tumors without evidence of disease.[106]

CENTRAL NERVOUS SYSTEM METASTASES

Metastasis in the central nervous system (CNS) is an uncommon initial presentation, occurring in less than 5% of all patients with Stage III disease. Most of these patients have concomitant advanced pulmonary metastases with testicular-tumor histology mainly of choriocarcinoma or yolk sac elements. The presence of CNS metastases does not preclude cure, and such patients should be treated aggressively.

At M.D. Anderson Hospital and Tumor Institute, 12 patients with disseminated testicular cancer and CNS metastases were treated from 1977 to 1979 with chemotherapy plus whole-brain radiotherapy.[107] Although none of the six patients with multiple CNS metastases were cured, four of the six with single CNS metastases were disease free at 13+ to 41+ months.

A unique approach for CNS metastases has been advocated by investigators at Charing Cross Hospital in London, England.[108] Ten patients with germ-cell tumors and CNS metastases were treated from 1977 to 1984 with no CNS irradiation. A complicated chemotherapy regimen (POMB/ACE or EP/OMB) was employed in conjunction with high-dose (1 g/m²) methotrexate and intrathecal methotrexate. Eight patients were disease free at 3+ to 54+ months.

At Indiana University, five patients presented with CNS metastases, and four are without evidence of disease at 2+ to 8+ years with cisplatin combination chemotherapy plus simultaneous cranial irradiation (5000 rad in 5 weeks). In addition, five patients had the termination of a chemotherapy CR with the development of CNS metastases, and three of these are disease free 2+ to 8+ years. We have not seen any acute or delayed neuropsychological sequelae from this combined-modality approach.[109]

Our current recommendation at Indiana University for CNS metastases at the time of diagnosis is to initiate full-dose cisplatin combination chemotherapy plus 5000 rad of whole-brain irradiation in 5 weeks with both modalities starting on day 1. If a patient with a chemotherapy CR relapses with only CNS metastases, we employ identical CNS irradiation plus two courses of cisplatin combination chemotherapy, because we feel that a CNS relapse can herald a systemic relapse, similar to meningeal relapse of childhood acute lymphoblastic leukemia.

THE TESTIS AS A SANCTUARY SITE

Testicular relapse can terminate a CR in childhood acute lymphoblastic leukemia in the absence of marrow or meningeal relapse, implying that the testis is a sanctuary site. In germ-cell tumors, the testis is affected by chemotherapy, with resultant testicular atrophy and impaired spermatogenesis. Nevertheless, the primary tumor in the testis is not always eradicated by systemic chemotherapy. Greist and coworkers described 20 patients with occult testicular primaries who underwent a delayed orchiectomy after cisplatin combination chemotherapy.[110] These patients were initially believed to have a primary retroperitoneal germ-cell tumor but subsequently were found to have a testicular primary upon careful palpation or bilateral testicular ultrasound demonstrating a characteristic hypoechogenic mass. Three of these patients had embryonal cell carcinoma in the testis after cisplatin chemotherapy, and an additional six had teratoma. None of the 20 patients had persistent carcinoma in the original areas of bulky retroperitoneal disease. Similar results have been reported by others.[111,112]

An orchiectomy therefore must be performed initially or after chemotherapy in any patient with a known or suspected testicular primary, as it is erroneous to assume that the chemotherapy will eradicate the primary. If carcinoma is found in the orchiectomy specimen, we recommend two postoperative courses of cisplatin combination induction chemotherapy, as we do if carcinoma is found in the retroperitoneum or chest after chemotherapy. However, this view is controversial,[111] and there is not enough information to permit a firm recommendation based on hard data.

SALVAGE CHEMOTHERAPY

First-line cisplatin combination chemotherapy will cure 70% of patients with disseminated germ-cell tumors. By definition, then, 30% become candidates for salvage chemotherapy.

It is our philosophy to resect residual disease after a maximum of four courses of induction therapy if the serum markers are normal and if it is anatomically feasible to extirpate the persistent disease. We traditionally do not give more than four courses of induction therapy even if there is continued serologic and radiographic regression. Most patients with persistently elevated markers at this time demonstrate a plateau in their marker decline, allowing the physician to realize that a fifth or sixth course will be incapable of normalizing the markers. Furthermore, by continuing the same "ineffective" induction regimen beyond four courses, there is a risk that the disease will worsen, thereby depriving the patient of the opportunity to enroll on a potentially curative cisplatin salvage regimen. A patient who progresses *during* cisplatin combination chemotherapy is not a candidate for a cisplatin salvage chemotherapy regimen, whereas a patient progressing while no longer receiving cisplatin is still potentially curable with agents to which his tumor has not been exposed.

The marker results of a hypothetical patient of this type are shown in Table 35-17. This patient had his maximal marker regression with his first course of chemotherapy. He still had a greater than 1 log reduction with his second course; however, he subsequently had a clear plateau in his hCG decline. It should be obvious that giving a fifth and sixth course of the identical induction regimen would never normalize his hCG. Instead, because of continuation of a noncurative regimen, he eventually develops marker-evidenced

TABLE 35-17. Hypothetical Example of Disease Progression During Cisplatin Combination Chemotherapy (see text for discussion)

Chemotherapy Course	hCG
1	100,000
2	5000
3	450
4	300
5	240
6	220
7	2000

progression and is no longer a candidate for a cisplatin-based salvage regimen, as his disease has progressed during cisplatin chemotherapy.

If a patient has a PR with anatomically unresectable disease but has normal serum markers, he is observed monthly (on no therapy) until he develops serologic or radiographic evidence of progressive disease. This practice is followed because some patients with an "unresectable PR" have no remaining tumor; that is, they have persistent necrotic fibrous tissue with or without teratoma. Some of these patients will become radiographically free of disease with the passage of time as their necrotic fibrous deposits spontaneously dissipate.

The two-drug combination of cisplatin and VP-16 is highly synergistic in preclinical systems.[113] Single-agent VP-16 is an active, albeit noncurative, drug in refractory testicular cancer. We first began PVP-16 salvage chemotherapy in 1978 and documented a 30% cure rate.[114] These results have subsequently been confirmed by other single institutions as well as by the Southeastern Cancer Study Group.[115] This represented the first curative salvage regimen for an adult solid tumor.

Another active drug in refractory testicular cancer is ifosfamide, with a 22% single-agent response rate after PVB and PVP-16.[116] We have evaluated cisplatin plus ifosfamide in refractory testicular cancer.[117] Perhaps the most impressive results are with this therapy as a third-line or later regimen in patients previously given PVB or PVP-16 combinations: 16 of 54 patients (30%) achieved disease-free status, and 10 (18%) are 18+ months continuously disease free, including seven who are 2+ years free of disease with this third-line regimen.[118] Our current first-line regimen is PVP-16B. Therefore, our present initial salvage regimen is cisplatin plus vinblastine plus ifosfamide (Table 35-18). The uroprotector mesna, in a dosage of 120 mg/m² by intravenous push, is given just prior to starting ifosfamide and then by continuous infusion 1200 mg/m² per day for all 5 days of each ifosfamide course.

The second course of salvage chemotherapy always begins

TABLE 35-18. Initial Salvage Chemotherapy at Indiana University

Cisplatin 20 mg/m² × 5
Vinblastine 0.22 mg/kg on day 1
Ifosfamide 1.2 g/m² × 5
Drugs are given every 3 weeks for four courses.

on day 22, regardless of the blood count. We try to give courses three and four on time also, and if we do delay therapy, we never delay by more than 7 days. If, on day 5 of a course of salvage chemotherapy, there is no obvious hematologic recovery, we delete the fifth day of ifosfamide. We do not ever lower drug dosages based on nadir blood counts or day-of-treatment counts. However, if granulocytopenic fever or thrombocytopenic bleeding occurs, we reduce subsequent ifosfamide and vinblastine 25%. We never reduce cisplatin dosages. If the serum creatinine exceeds 2 mg/dl, we reduce ifosfamide (alone) 25%, and if hematuria (more than 10 erythrocytes per high-power field) is found, during daily urinalysis, we hold ifosfamide that particular day and resume regular dose after hematuria clears.

We are now evaluating high-dose chemotherapy with autologous bone-marrow transplantation in patients who are otherwise incurable (progression during cisplatin or prior PVB, VP-16, and ifosfamide). Results with this approach in the past have been disappointing, with virtually no 1+-year remissions. However, most preparative regimens used chemotherapy regimens without cisplatin (e.g., cyclophosphamide, VP-16, BCNU). Carboplatin (CBDCA) is as active as cisplatin, with myelosuppression as its dose-limiting toxicity, making it ideal for high-dose therapy with bone-marrow transplantation in refractory testicular cancer. Furthermore, in preclinical systems, the drug is highly synergistic with VP-16. We are currently evaluating very high-dose CBDCA plus VP-16 with marrow transplantation in this setting, with very encouraging (albeit early) results.

MANAGEMENT OF POOR-PROGNOSIS TESTICULAR CANCER

The first important issue is determining which patients with germ-cell tumors have advanced disease and would be candidates for more aggressive (and therefore, by definition, more toxic) chemotherapy. No author disputes the fact that patients with advanced disease have a relatively poor prognosis with standard-dose cisplatin plus vinblastine (or VP-16) plus bleomycin; however, not all authors agree on the criteria for

TABLE 35-19.   Indiana University Staging System for Disseminated Testicular Cancer

Minimal Extent
1. Elevated markers only
2. Cervical nodes (±nonpalpable retroperitoneal nodes)
3. Unresectable nonpalpable retroperitoneal disease
4. Fewer than five pulmonary metastases per lung field AND largest <2 cm (±nonpalpable retroperitoneal nodes)

Moderate Extent
1. Palpable abdominal mass only (no supradiaphragmatic disease)
2. Moderate pulmonary metastases: 5–10 metastases per lung field and largest <3 cm OR solitary pulmonary metastasis of any size >2 cm (±nonpalpable retroperitoneal disease)

Advanced Extent
1. Advanced pulmonary metastases: primary mediastinal nonseminomatous germ-cell tumor OR >10 pulmonary metastases per lung field, OR multiple pulmonary metastases with largest >3 cm (±nonpalpable retroperitoneal disease)
2. Palpable abdominal mass plus supradiaphragmatic disease
3. Liver, bone, or CNS metastases

TABLE 35-20.   Therapeutic Results in Advanced Testicular Cancer According to Indiana Staging System, 1978–1983*

Minimal	Moderate	Advanced
102/103 (99%)	50/55 (91%)	43/81 (53%)

* Numerator is all patients who became disease free with PVB or PVP-16B with or without surgery for residual disease.

advanced disease. Tumor volume, variously defined, is important prognostically in all series. Serum markers, especially hCG, are independently important in most, but not all, series.[119]

At Indiana University, we have developed a staging system that places patients with disseminated germ-cell tumors into three separate categories: minimal, moderate, or advanced disease (Table 35-19).[119] Table 35-20 demonstrates the therapeutic outcome of these patients. It should be noted that our "moderate disease" category included patients who did extremely well with standard chemotherapy, with 50 of 55 (91%) achieving disease-free status. These patients would have been classified as having advanced disease in many other staging systems and would have been inappropriately subjected to a newer, more aggressive chemotherapy regimen instead of standard chemotherapy.

A recent British study from six medical centers treating patients from 1976 to 1982 also identified three separate prognostic categories with 3-year survival rates of 91%, 72%, and 47% and overall a 75% 3-year survival rate.[120] Therapeutic results improved with the passage of time, presumably because of greater familiarity of cisplatin combination chemotherapy regimens and surgical resection of residual disease (Table 35-21). If the 1981–1982 regimen had been a newer, more aggressive regimen, the authors might have erroneously believed a therapeutic advance had been made when comparing the results with those of the 1976–1978 regimens. This table demonstrates the hazard of historical control analysis in documenting superiority of a new regimen. The improved results with time were seen in both advanced and less advanced disease.

A similar demonstration of the importance of experience with chemotherapy was also observed in patients with disseminated germ-cell tumors treated at Indiana University (Table 35-22). As discussed in detail earlier, our original regimen (1976–1976) consisted of cisplatin plus vinblastine plus bleomycin (PVB). Our second study demonstrated that we could achieve identical therapeutic results with less hematologic and neuromuscular toxicity by reducing the vin-

TABLE 35-21.   Improvement of Outcome in Advanced Disease with Time (Multicenter British Study)

Year(s)	No. of Patients	3-Year Survival Rate (%)
1976–78	110	68
1979	102	72
1980	101	81
1981–82	145	89

TABLE 35-22. Comparison of Results of Sequential PVB Studies at Indiana University

Study No. (Year)	No. of Patients	No. with CR (%)	NED with Surgery (%)	Now NED (%)
1 (1974–76)	47	33 (70)	5 (11)	27 (57)
2 (1976–78)	78	51 (65)	13 (17)	57 (73)
3 (1978–81)	147	92 (63)	31 (21)	117 (80)

blastine dosage from 0.4 to 0.3 mg/kg, and our third study documented that optimal cure rates could be achieved with 12 weeks (four courses of PVB) and that maintenance vinblastine was unnecessary. In these studies, our cure rate increased from 57% to 80% with the identical chemotherapy regimens except for the reduction in the vinblastine dosage and the elimination of maintenance vinblastine. Unfortunately, many descriptions of "new improved" regimens compare the results in a small number of patients with brief follow-up with our original regimen despite the fact that their new, more aggressive regimens were all given in the 1980s. Such claims of superiority obviously must be viewed with caution, if not skepticism.

Cisplatin plus VP-16 plus bleomycin has been recently utilized as initial chemotherapy in both Europe and the United States. Peckham and associates treated 43 patients, with 37 (86%) becoming disease-free. Cisplatin was given in a dosage of 20 mg/m² five times a week, bleomycin at 30 mg weekly, and VP-16 at 120 mg/m² on one through three days. Fourteen of these patients had advanced disease, and 12 (86%) were continuously disease free at the time of the publication.[96]

From 1981 to 1984, the Southeastern Cancer Study Group randomized patients with disseminated germ-cell tumors to 12 weeks of PVB or 12 weeks of PVP-16B.[97] The cisplatin and bleomycin in both regimens were the same (20 mg/m² five times weekly every 3 weeks for four courses and 30 units weekly for 12 weeks); the vinblastine dosage was 0.15 mg/kg on days one and two and the VP-16 dosage was 100 mg/m² five times a week every 3 weeks for four courses. In the subgroup of patients with advanced disease, 48% are continuously disease-free with PVP-16B and 33% with PVB, and there is a statistically significant survival advantage (p = 0.02) for the PVP-16B arm in these patients with advanced disseminated disease (Table 35-23).

Pizzocaro and colleagues recently published their results with PVP-16B in advanced germ-cell cancer.[121] The cisplatin dosage was 20 mg/m² for five consecutive days, the VP-16 dosage was 100 mg/m² for three consecutive days, and the

bleomycin dosage 30 units weekly. Forty patients were treated from August 1981 through November 1983. Any patient with a larger than 10-cm abdominal mass, a larger than 5-cm pulmonary nodule, metastases outside the nodes and lung (e.g., liver, bone, CNS), a serum AFP exceeding 1000 ng/ml, or a serum hCG exceeding 50,000 mIU/ml was eligible. All but three patients (92%) achieved disease-free status, and with a median follow-up of 24 months (range 13–40 months), 34 (85%) remain free of disease.

An innovative aggressive regimen for advanced testicular cancer was devised by Ozols and colleagues at the U.S. National Cancer Institute (NCI). This pilot regimen tested double-dose cisplatin (40 mg/m² five times weekly) combined with vinblastine, VP-16, and bleomycin (PVeBV). Starting in May 1981, the NCI performed a randomized study comparing the new regimen with standard PVB. Of 30 patients, 26 (87%) achieved a CR with PVeBV, and 21 of the 30 (70%) are continuously free of disease. There were two deaths secondary to bleomycin and one death from recurrent embryonal carcinoma (malignant teratoma, undifferentiated), and two patients had recurrent teratoma (teratoma, differentiated). In this randomized study, 10 of 16 (62%) achieved a CR on standard dose PVB; however, only 5 of 16 (31%) are continuously free of disease (one death from bleomycin pulmonary fibrosis; two patients with recurrent teratoma). Although there is a trend favoring PVeBV, after 4 years, the only parameter that has achieved statistical significance is the number of patients who are alive and without recurrent embryonal carcinoma or teratoma (p = 0.027).

High-dose cisplatin plus high-dose VP-16 in 22 poor-prognosis patients was reported by Daugaard and Rørth.[122] Their criteria for advanced disease included greater than 10-cm abdominal nodes, liver metastases, greater than 5-cm supradiaphragmatic metastases, multiple pulmonary metastases with at least one larger than 5 cm, extragonadal primary tumor with elevated marker(s), or hCG greater than 100,000 mIU/ml. Drug dosages were cisplatin 40 mg/m² five times weekly, plus VP-16 200 mg/m² five times weekly, plus bleomycin 15 mg/m² weekly, with courses repeated every 3 weeks. Nineteen patients (86%) achieved a CR, and 17 (77%) had no evidence of disease with a median follow-up of 11 months (range 1⁺–19⁺ months). However, toxicity was severe, with five drug-related deaths and 20 of 22 patients having at least one episode of granulocytopenic fever and 15 having two to five episodes of granulocytopenic fever, including four cases of documented bacteria.

A present national intergroup study of two cisplatin doses (20mg/m² × 5 versus 40 mg/m² × 5) in combination with VP-16 and bleomycin in advanced disseminated germ cell tumors (Table 35-24) will clarify the role of high-dose cisplatin in this patient population.

TABLE 35-23. Randomized Southeastern Cooperative Group Comparison of PVB and PVP-16B: Number (%) of Patients Achieving CR

Initial Extent of Disease	PVB	PVP-16B
Minimal	52/54 (96)	54/56 (97)
Moderate	22/26 (85)	23/30 (77)
Advanced	12/36 (33)	17/35 (48)
Total	116	121

TABLE 35-24.   Protocol for Randomized High-Dose Cisplatin Trial in Advanced Disease

Cisplatin Dose*	Other Drugs (Both Arms)
20 mg/m² OR 40 mg/m²	VP-16 100 mg/m² × 5 q 3 weeks × 4 Bleomycin 30 units weekly × 12

* Dose given five times weekly every 3 weeks for four courses.

The principal reason for chemotherapy failure and subsequent death from disseminated testicular cancer is bulky advanced diseases, but it must be remembered that another cause of treatment failure is moderate-size or bulky teratoma that persists after chemotherapy and is unresectable.[123] Alternatively, teratoma may be associated with non-germ-cell elements that are as chemoresistant as is teratoma.[124] More aggressive chemotherapy will not solve either of these latter two problems.

SURVEILLANCE VERSUS RPLND FOR CLINICAL STAGE I DISEASE

Retroperitoneal lymph dissection remains the only modality that can prove that clinical Stage I nonseminomatous germ-cell tumor is in fact pathologic Stage I. (Even in the most experienced of hands, clinical understaging of the disease occurs in approximately 25% of patients and overstaging in 20%). Nevertheless, approximately 70% of patients undergoing RPLND will receive no definitive therapeutic benefit from the operation. Additionally, 10% to 13% of patients undergoing the procedure will nevertheless experience relapse, usually outside of the operative field. Moreover, in the past, loss of ejaculation and sterility occurred in most patients who underwent RPLND. Because of these drawbacks of surgery, and in view of the development of sensitive tumor markers and effective chemotherapeutic agents, postorchiectomy observation or surveillance is appealing. As previously discussed, the overall survival rate for patients with pathologic Stage I disease who undergo a RPLND should approach 100%, so the standard by which surveillance programs must be judged is formidable.

The results of several large surveillance programs throughout the world consistently show a disease progression rate of approximately 30%,[72] and unfortunately, there have been several deaths in these programs, although, as expected, the majority of patients do well. Recent reports suggest that, even with monitoring, 80% of relapses are of a more advanced stage,[65,72] compared to those patients undergoing RPLND who tend to relapse in the chest with a lower volume of disease.

As more experience is generated, it becomes clear that patient selection for surveillance protocols requires individualization. A meticulous work-up should be performed and interpreted by a multidisciplinary team consisting of urologists, medical oncologists, radiologists, and pathologists experienced in evaluating these patients and tests. As a minimum for consideration of entry into an observation protocol,

the patient should have undergone a radical inguinal orchiectomy with negative surgical margins. Postorchiectomy, the tumor markers β-hCG, AFP, and LDH should fall to normal within their expected metabolic half-lives. Both CT scan of the abdomen and chest or whole-lung tomograms should show no suspicious nodes or evidence of pulmonary parenchymal metastases. Finally, a lymphangiogram should be unequivocally negative.

If all these criteria are met, known prognostic factors are analyzed. Patients who have an embryonal carcinoma are felt to be at high risk of relapse, as are patients having vascular, lymphatic, or cord invasion by tumor. Finally, a judgment must be made about the reliability of the patient in returning for rigorous follow-up examination. Because, in effect, surveillance is a form of treatment, the physician also maintains a degree of responsibility for ensuring the follow-up. It should be emphasized to the patient that surveillance is an as yet-unproven method of therapy, whereas RPLND has been performed in many large centers with few complications and no deaths. The principal criticism is the ejaculatory dysfunction that occurs, but with the modifications in the operation recently described by Lange and others, this argument no longer seems important. Thus, patients with a grossly normal retroperitoneum can be offered a modified nerve-sparing lymphadenectomy, which will maintain antegrade ejaculation and subsequent fertility in approximately 90% of cases. In our experience, once these matters are discussed with the patient, the majority opt for surgical staging and therapy by RPLND.

Regardless of the initial form of therapy, careful follow-up during the perioperative period is mandatory. Physical examination, chest radiography, and serum marker assays are performed monthly during the first year, every 2 months during the second year, and every 6 months thereafter. Patients who elect surveillance should have a CT scan approximately every 2 to 3 months for the first 2 years.

LATE CONSEQUENCES OF CISPLATIN COMBINATION CHEMOTHERAPY

Approximately 80% of patients with disseminated cancer are cured with initial cisplatin combination chemotherapy or salvage chemotherapy. At Indiana University, we recently reviewed 207 patients with a minimum follow-up of 5+ years.[125] The overwhelming majority of these patients have returned to a productive life with few, if any, long-term toxicities other than sterility and Raynaud's phenomenon. In our experience, only rarely is the Raynaud's condition of sufficient severity to impair health.

FERTILITY

Drasga and associates have evaluated with serial semen analyses 69 patients with disseminated germ-cell tumors who did not undergo an RPLND.[126] Before any chemotherapy was administered, 77% of patients were severely oligospermic and 17% azoospermic. After four courses of PVB, 96% were azoospermic. However, 2 years after initiation of chemotherapy, 50% had recovered a normal sperm count and motility, and approximately half of the patients who had attempted to impregnate their wives had been successful, with the infants having no congenital abnormalities. Fossa and colleagues at the Norwegian Radium Hospital in Oslo reported similar results,[127] with 50% to 60% of patients having active spermatogenesis 1 to 3 years after PVB. In contrast, Nijman and associates recently reported that 2 years after PVB, only 28% of patients had greater than 60,000,000 spermatozoa/ml; however, unlike the previous two studies, these patients all received maintenance cisplatin for 12 months.[128]

RAYNAUD'S PHENOMENON

Vogelzang and colleagues were among the first to observe the relation of Raynaud's phenomenon to testicular cancer chemotherapy.[129] In their series, 22 of 60 men (37%) treated with vinblastine plus bleomycin with or without cisplatin developed Raynaud's. Digital ischemia occurred in 21% of patients treated with vinblastine plus bleomycin and in 41% treated with PVB. This complication began a median of 10 months after chemotherapy was instituted (range 2–28 months). Other authors have reported on Raynaud's phenomenon with vinblastine plus bleomycin.[130]

VASCULAR COMPLICATIONS

The incidence of Raynaud's phenomenon with distal arteriolar narrowing raises the specter of generalized vascular disease with acute myocardial infarction secondary to coronary artery disease, deep venous thrombosis, and cerebrovascular

accident. Bleomycin and vinca alkaloids such as vinblastine have been anecdotally associated with myocardial ischemia.[131,132] In 1979, Edwards and associates reported two patients in their 20s treated with PVB for eight courses who died of far-advanced testicular cancer and at autopsy had clinically unsuspected severe arteriosclerosis of the coronary arteries.

Two recent reports have increased concern about vascular complications of cisplatin combination chemotherapy. Samuels and colleagues described five patients with both acute and long-term vascular toxicity,[134] and three of these patients had no evidence of cancer at autopsy (Table 35-25). These cases were culled from 65 patients treated at the University of Minnesota from 1978 to 1982. However, one of these patients came from the University of Chicago, and the denominator at that institution is unknown. Thus, the frequency of these problems cannot be determined at present.

These five cases are not proof of PVB-based toxicity. Patient 1 may have had clostridial sepsis as the causative agent of rectal infarction. Patient 3 had sepsis and hypotension during high-dose ara-C and a questionable myocardial infarction. Patient 4 received doxorubicin, a known cardiotoxic drug, as well as other agents. Finally, in patient 5, Koch's postulates were not fulfilled, as rechallenge with five more courses of PVB produced no immediate further problems.

Doll and associates described four additional cases of vascular complications after cisplatin combination chemotherapy in 23 patients treated from 1983 to 1985 (Table 35-26).[135] None of these patients had known risk factors

TABLE 35-25. Vascular Complications Associated with Cisplatin Combination Chemotherapy[134]

Age	Vascular Event	Timing Postchemotherapy (mo)	Comments
23	Rectal infarction	Course 4 PVB	Rectal pain and bleeding with blood cultures positive for Clostridia
24	Myocardial infarction	18	Obese; sudden death with 75% occlusion left anterior descending coronary artery
33	Myocardial infarction	6	PVB, then cisplatin+ VP-16, then high-dose ara-C; developed sepsis, hypotension, and questionable MI.
42	Myocardial infarction	46	Prior radiotherapy to abdomen + cyclophosphamide, bleomycin, and doxorubicin; subsequent PVB
58	Cerebrovascular accident	Course 1 PVB	CVA resolved; received 5 further cycles of PVB without problems. Subsequent cyclophosphamide + dactinomycin + methotrexate with worsening left hemiparesis and subsequent death

TABLE 35-26.   Vascular Complications Associated with Cisplatin Combination Chemotherapy

Age	Vascular Event	Timing Postchemotherapy (mo)	Comments
21	Cerebrovascular accident	7	Double-dose cisplatin + VP-16 + bleomycin; developed headaches, slurred speech, and right hemiparesis with normal head CT, MR, and cerebral arteriogram
24	Myocardial infarction	18	No risk factors
25	Cerebrovascular accident	course 3	No risk factors
27	Myocardial infarction	course 2	Double-dose cisplatin + VP-16 + bleomycin; PVB 5 years previously; patient completed 3 additional courses without further problems

such as prior mediastinal radiotherapy, family history of cardiac disease, heavy smoking, hypertension, diabetes, or hyperlipedemia.

There are several plausible explanations for vascular toxicity, including the previously mentioned Raynaud's phenomenon progressing to generalized vascular disease. Also, bleomycin can cause endothelial changes cumulatively in capillaries and arterioles.[136] Cisplatin-induced hypomagnesemia can cause ventricular irritability and coronary artery spasm. High levels of circulating von Willebrand's factor antigen have been associated with Raynaud's, may be a marker for endothelial damage,[137] and may lead to thrombosis.[138]

There are several conclusions and statements that can be made:

1. The incidence of vascular complications is low (less than 5%).
2. Vascular complications are various.
3. Some patients with complications can be retreated with the same chemotherapy without apparent problems.
4. It is not possible to know whether these vascular complications are secondary to treatment or to the disease process (*e.g.*, tumor emboli, deep venous thrombosis in association with large pelvic mass). If treatment is implicated, which drug or drug combination is the culprit remains unknown.

The recently completed adjuvant intergroup Stage I–II study provides a unique forum to address these important concerns. Questionnaires concerning deep venous thrombosis, pulmonary embolus, myocardial infarction, and cerebrovascular accident have been sent to several hundred patients. It will be of great interest to see if there is an increase in vascular complication in patients who received cisplatin combination chemotherapy versus those patients who were cured with surgery alone.

BLEOMYCIN-RELATED COMPLICATIONS

Barneveld and colleagues evaluated 93 patients treated with PVB, of whom eight had clinical evidence of bleomycin pneumonitis.[139] One of these patients died from bleomycin toxicity; the other seven were fully recovered with a minimum follow-up of 2 years. Chest films normalized at a median of 9 months (range 6–13 months), and all symptoms abated in 4 to 5 months.

A different bleomycin-related complication relates to radiographic abnormalities that can simulate metastatic pulmonary nodules.[140,141] Subclinical bleomycin pulmonary fibrosis can produce a coalescence of fibrous tissue that on chest roentgenography or, especially, CT has the appearance of metastatic nodules. If such nodules are seen after chemotherapy in areas different from those of the original pulmonary metastases, they are assumed to be secondary to bleomycin, and it is not necessary to biopsy these areas by fine-needle aspiration or thoracotomy.

LEUKEMIA

Testicular cancer patients are immunologically intact and receive short-duration chemotherapy, and there is no appreciable risk of secondary leukemia. However, if alkylating agents are used long term, secondary leukemia can be a late consequence of curative therapy.[142] The Memorial Sloan-Kettering Cancer Center group retrospectively evaluated patients treated from 1950 through 1979 and found four cases of acute myeloblastic leukemia and one of chronic myelomonocytic leukemia, with a relative risk estimate of 13.7 in the total patient population and 50.1 in the group receiving chemotherapy. Two of these patients were treated with VAB-III (2 years of chlorambucil), two with radiotherapy alone, and one with radiotherapy plus 18 months of chemotherapy.

TABLE 35-27. Characteristics of Late Relapses at Walter Reed Army Medical Center[143]

Patient	Timing of Relapse (mo)	Initial Chemotherapy	Comments
1	45	VAB-III	Large abdominal mass ? CR; late relapse in abdomen with elevated AFP
2	54	VAB-III	Large abdominal mass with abdominal recurrence
3	76	Adjuvant dactinomycin	CR with PVB for 65+ months
4	87	Mithramycin	Initial pulmonary metastases, recurred in lungs
5	56	PVB	Recurred with solitary pulmonary metastases
6	51	Adjuvant VAB-III	Pelvic recurrence of teratocarcinoma with elevated AFP
7	86	VAB-III	Late abdominal and pelvic recurrence with elevated AFP

LATE RELAPSES

Perhaps the most ominous late consequence is a relapse. In our experience at Indiana University, we see occasional late (more than 2 years) relapses after chemotherapy. The usual scenario is a patient presenting with bulky teratocarcinoma who has normalization of markers with chemotherapy and undergoes an RPLND with resection of large-volume teratoma. Theoretically, microscopic teratoma may have been left behind; it can be biologically inert, grow slowly as teratoma, or, possibly, transform as teratocarcinoma with the preponderant mass consisting of mature and immature teratoma with small components of embryonal cell carcinoma. Such patients relapse in the original area of bulk teratoma, frequently with elevated AFP concentrations. Our present recommendations for patients with postchemotherapy resection of teratoma that is larger than 5 cm is to obtain abdominal CT scans every 3 to 4 months for 2 years and then one or two times per year for an additional 2 to 3 years.

The Walter Reed group has reported seven patients with late relapse (45–87 months after chemotherapy).[143] These patients are detailed in Table 35-27.

Another issue of "late relapse" is a second primary germ-cell tumor, which will occur in 1% to 3% of all cured patients. Instruction in testicular self-examination as well as physician palpation of the testis is part of our routine follow-up in all patients.

ADJUVANT CHEMOTHERAPY

The criteria for successful application of adjuvant chemotherapy are (1) poor prognosis for cure with primary therapy alone, and (2) evidence that the proposed adjuvant therapy is effective in metastatic disease. However, in nonseminomatous germ-cell tumors, there is a third consideration, namely, whether similar cure rates can be achieved by using

chemotherapy when a patient relapses after an RPLND; adjuvant chemotherapy may be unnecessary.

A national intergroup study has been recently completed in patients with pathologic Stage II nonseminomatous germ-cell tumors. Patient entry was from 1979 to 1987, and there were 197 evaluable patients.[144] Median time on study is in excess of 4 years. Patients were randomized to two postoperative courses of cisplatin combination chemotherapy versus observation, which consisted of history and physical examination, and hCG and AFP assays, and posteroanterior and lateral chest films monthly the first postoperative year, every 2 months during the second year, and subsequently every 6 months. Ninety-seven patients entered the adjuvant arm, and only one patient has relapsed. This patient subsequently died of metastatic testicular cancer. Forty-eight of 98 patients on the observation arm have relapsed. However, with this close follow-up, relapse was detected in a favorable setting: only three of these patients have died from recurrent testicular cancer, and the remaining 95 remain disease free. There was no independent risk factor for relapse that would mandate adjuvant chemotherapy in any subtype (e.g., marker-negative patients, vascular invasion). Two courses of cisplatin-based adjuvant chemotherapy will almost always prevent relapse. However, when surgery, follow-up, and chemotherapy are optimal, either approach produces excellent cure rates.

NEW STUDIES

In addition to the studies already mentioned in this chapter, there are other important studies that are still awaiting final analysis (Table 35-28). In the Memorial study, the results with the two-drug regimen of cisplatin and VP-16 produced therapeutic results equivalent to those of the five-drug regimen of VAB-VI with considerably less treatment-related morbidity. In the Southeastern Cancer Study Group protocol,

TABLE 35-28. New Studies

Institution	Patient Population	Study Design
Memorial Sloan-Kettering	Favorable prognosis	VAB-VI versus PVP-16
Southeastern Cancer Study Group	Minimal and moderate disseminated disease	PVP-16B × 4 courses versus PVP-16B × 3 courses
EORTC	Favorable prognosis	PVP-16B versus PVP-16
ECOG	Advanced disseminated disease	PVP-16B versus cisplatin + VP-16 + ifosfamide

approximately 200 patients were randomized, and at present, it appears that three courses of PVP-16B over 9 weeks gives results identical to those of four courses over 12 weeks. The EORTC study is still too early for any conclusions, and the ECOG study has just recently begun patient accrual.

REFERENCES

1. Drain LS: Testicular cancer in California from 1942–1969: The California Tumor Registry experience. Oncology 27:45–51, 1973
2. Einhorn LH: Testicular cancer: A model for a curable neoplasm. Cancer Res 41:3275–3280, 1981
3. Strecker JF, Floyd JW III: The testis. In Devine CJ, Stecker JF (eds): Urology in Practice, pp 73–79. Boston, Little, Brown, 1978
4. Hausfeld KF, Schrandt D: Malignancy of testis following atrophy: Report of three cases. J Urol 94:69–72, 1965
5. Herr HW, Silber I, Martin DC: Management of inguinal lymph nodes in patients with testicular tumors following orchiopexy, inguinal, or scrotal operation. J Urol 110:223–224, 1973
6. Gilbert JB, Hamilton JB: Incidence and nature of tumors in ectopic testes. Surg Gynecol Obstet 71:731–743, 1940
7. Dixon FJ, Moore RA (eds): Atlas of Tumor Pathology, Fascicle 31B, section 8, p 32. Washington, DC, Armed Forces Institute of Pathology, 1952
8. Friedman NB, Moore RA: Tumors of the testis: A report on 922 cases. Milit Surgeon 99:573–593, 1946
9. Mostofi FK, Price EB (eds): Tumors of the Male Genital System Atlas of Tumor Pathology, Second Series, Fascicle 8, p 7. Washington, DC, Armed Forces Institute of Pathology, 1973
10. Mostofi FK, Sobin LH: Histological Typing of Testis Tumors. International Histological Classification of Tumors, No. 16. Geneva, World Health Organization, 1977
11. Rosai J, Heyderman E, Kurman RJ, Mostofi FK, Nochomovitz LE, Scully RA: Report of the Pathology Review Committee. International Symposium on Human Testis Cancer, Mouse Teratocarcinoma and Oncofetal Proteins. Minneapolis, 1980
12. Rosen SW, Weintraub BD, Vaitukaitis JL et al: Placental proteins and their subunits as tumor markers. Ann Intern Med 82:71–83, 1975
13. Lange PH, Nochomovitz LE, Rosai J, et al: Serum alpha-fetoprotein and human chorionic gonadotropin in patients with seminoma. J Urol 124:472–478, 1980
14. Drago JR, Nelson RP, Palmer JM: Childhood embryonal carcinoma of the testis. Urology 12:499–503, 1978
15. Duckett J: Panel on testis tumors, American Cancer Society. Atlanta, October, 1980
16. Lange PH, Fraley EE: Serum alpha-fetoprotein and human chorionic gonadotropin in the treatment of patients with testicular tumors. Urol Clin North Am 4:393–406, 1977
17. Mostofi FK, Theiss EA, Ashley DJB: Tumors of specialized gonadal stroma in human male patients: Androblastoma, Sertoli cell tumor, granulosa-theca cell tumor of the testis, and gonadal stromal tumor. Cancer 12:944–957, 1959
18. Holtz F, Abell MR: Testicular neoplasms in infants and children I: Tumors of non-germ cell origin. Cancer 16:982–986, 1963
19. Silverberg SG, Thompson JW, Higashi G, Baskin AM: Malignant interstitial cell tumor of the testis: Case report and review. J Urol 96:356–363, 1966
20. Hopkins GB: Interstitial cell tumor of the testis: Case report and review of the literature. J Urol 103:449–451, 1970
21. Kuzmits R, Schernthaner G, Krisch K: Serum neuron-specific enolase: A marker for response to therapy in seminoma. Cancer 60:1017–1021, 1987
22. Barzell W, Whitmore WF: Neoplasms of the testis. In Harrison JH, Gittes RF, Perlmutter AD et al (eds): Campbell's Urology, 4th Ed, p 1141. Philadelphia, WB Saunders, 1979
23. Richie JP, Garnick MB, Finberg H: Computerized tomography: How accurate for abdominal staging of testis tumors? J Urol 127:715–717, 1982
24. Rowland RG, Weisman D, Williams S, Einhorn L, Donohue, JP: Accuracy of preoperative staging in Stage A and B non-seminomatous germ cell testis tumors. J Urol 127:718–720, 1982
25. Maier JG, Sulak MH, Mittemeyer BT: Seminoma of the testis: Analysis of treatment success and failure. 102:596–602, 1968
26. Heiken JP, Balfe DM, McClennan BL: Testicular tumors: Oncologic imaging and diagnosis. Int J Radiat Oncol Biol Phys 10:275–287, 1984
27. Hoeltl W, Kosak D, Pont J et al: Testicular cancer: Prognostic implications of vascular invasion. J Urol 137:683–685, 1987
28. Zagars GK, Babaian RJ: Stage I testicular seminoma: Rationale for post-orchiectomy radiation therapy. Int J Radiat Oncol Biol Phys 13:155–162, 1987
29. Kubo HD, Shipley WU: Reduction of the scatter dose to the testicle outside the radiation treatment fields. Int J Radiat Oncol Biol Phys 8:1741–1745, 1982
30. Maier JG, Sulak MH: Radiation therapy in malignant testis tumors seminoma. Cancer 32:1212–1216, 1973
31. Hamilton C, Horwich A, Peckham MJ et al: Radiotherapy for Stage I seminoma testis: Results of treatment and complications. Radiat Ther Oncol 6:115–120, 1986
32. Earle JD, Bagshaw MA, Kaplan HS: Supervoltage radiation therapy of testicular tumors. Am J Roentgenol 117:653–661, 1973
33. Dosoretz DE, Shipley WU, Blitzer PH et al: Megavoltage irradiation for pure testicular seminoma: Results and patterns of failure. Cancer 48:2184–2190, 1981
34. Hanks GE, Herring DF, Kramer S: Patterns of care outcome studies: Results of the National Practice in Seminoma of the Testis. Int J Radiat Oncol Biol Phys 7:1413–1417, 1981
35. Willan BD, McGowan DG: Seminoma of the testis: A 22 year experience with radiation therapy. Int J Radiat Oncol Biol Phys 11:1769–1775, 1985
36. Peckham MJ: Testicular tumors: Investigation and staging. In The Management of Testicular Tumors, pp 89–101. London, Edwin Arnold, 1981
37. Thomas GM, Rider WD, Dembo AJ et al: Seminoma of the testis: Results of treatment and patterns of failure after radiation therapy. Int J Radiat Oncol Biol Phys 8:165–174, 1982
38. Loehrer PJ, Birch R, Williams SD et al: Chemotherapy of metastatic seminoma: The Southeastern Cancer Study Group experience. J Clin Oncol 5:1212–1220, 1987
39. Zagars GK, Babian RJ: The role of radiation therapy in Stage II testicular seminoma. Int J Radiat Oncol Biol Phys 13:163–170, 1987
40. Smalley SR, Evans RG, Richardson RL et al: Radiotherapy as initial treatment for bulky Stage II seminoma. J Clin Oncol 3:1333–1338, 1985
41. Percarpio B, Clements JC, McLeod DG et al: Anaplastic seminoma: An analysis of 77 patients. Cancer 43:2510–2513, 1979
42. Cockburn AG, Vugrin D, Batata M et al: Poorly differentiated (anaplastic) seminoma of the testis. Cancer 53:1991–1994, 1984
43. Mauch P, Weichselbaum R, Botnick L: The significance of positive chorionic gonadotropins in apparently pure seminoma of the testis. Int J Radiat Oncol Biol Phys 5:887–889, 1979
44. Mirimanoff RO, Shipley WU, Dosoretz DE et al: Pure seminoma of the testis: The results of radiation therapy in patients with elevated human chorionic gonadotropin titers. J Urol 134:1124–1126, 1985
45. Quivey JM, Fu KK, Herzog KA et al: Malignant tumors of the testis: Analysis of treatment results and sites and causes of failure. Cancer 39:1247–1253, 1977
46. Oliver RTD: Surveillance for Stage I seminoma in single agent cisplatinum for metastatic seminoma (abstr). Proc Am Soc Clin Oncol 3:162, 1984
47. Clemm C, Hartenstein R, Willich N et al: Vinblastine–ifosfamide–cisplatinum treatment of bulky seminoma. Cancer 58:2203–2207, 1986
48. Friedman EL, Garnick MB, Stomper PC et al: Therapeutic guidelines and results in advanced seminoma. J Clin Oncol 3:1325–1332, 1985
49. Motzer R, Bosl G, Heelan R et al: Residual mass: An indication for surgery in patients with advanced seminoma following systemic chemotherapy. J Clin Oncol 5:1064–1070, 1987
50. Fossa S, Borge L, Aass N et al: The treatment of advanced metastatic seminoma: Experience in 55 cases. J Clin Oncol 5:1071–1077, 1987
51. Pizzocaro G, Salvioni R, Piva L et al: Cisplatin combination chemotherapy in advanced seminoma. Cancer 58:1625–1629, 1986
52. Horwich A, Tucker DF, Peckham MJ: Placenta alkaline phosphatase as a tumor marker in seminoma using the H17E2 monoclonal antibody assay. Br J Cancer 51:625–629, 1985
53. Crawford ED, Scardino PT: Testicular carcinoma: An overview. In Crawford ED, Borden TA (eds): Genitourinary Cancer Surgery, pp 249–261. Philadelphia, Lea & Febiger, 1982
54. Jamieson JK, Dobson JF: The lymphatics of the testicle. Lancet 1:493–495, 1910
55. Cuneo B, Marcille M: Topographie des ganglions iliopelviens. Bull Soc Anat [Paris], 6s(III):653, 1901
56. Howard RJ: Malignant disease of the testis. Practitioner 79:794–810, 1907
57. Hinman F: The operative treatment of tumor of the testicle. JAMA 63:2009–2015, 1914
58. Lewis LG: Radioresistant testis tumors: Results in 133 cases—Five-year followup. J Urol 69:841–844, 1953
59. Cooper JF, Leadbetter WF, Chute R: The thoracoabdominal approach for retroperitoneal gland dissection: Its application to testis tumors. Surg Gynecol Obstet 90:486–496, 1950
60. Staubitz WJ, Early KS, Magoss IV, Murphy GP: Surgical management of testis tumors. J Urol 111:205–209, 1974
61. Whitmore WF: Surgical treatment of adult germinal testis tumors. Semin Oncol 6:55–68, 1979
62. Donohue JP, Zachary JM, Maynard BR: Distribution of nodal metastases in non-seminomatous testis cancer. J Urol 128:315–320, 1982
63. Donohue JP: Surgical management of testicular cancer. In LH Einhorn (ed): Testicular Tumors: Management and Treatment, pp 29–46. New York, Masson Publishing, 1980
64. Lange P, Narayan P, Fraley E: Fertility issues following therapy for testicular cancer. Semin Urol 4:264, 1985
65. Rowland RG, Weisman D, Williams S et al: Accuracy of preoperative staging in Stage A and B non-seminomatous germ cell testis tumors. J Urol 127:718–720, 1982
66. Pizzocaro G, Musumeci R: The relative value of lymphangiography (LAG) and computed tomography (CT) in diagnosing small retroperitoneal metastases. In S Khoury (ed): Testicular Cancer, p 261. New York, 1985
67. Einhorn LH, Donohue JP, Peckham MJ et al: Cancer of the testes. In DeVita VT, Hellman S, Rosenberg SA (eds): Cancer: Principles and Practice of Oncology, pp 979–1011. Philadelphia, JB Lippincott, 1985

68. Crawford ED, Mettler FA, Duncan PR: Retrocrural lymphadenopathy in testicular cancer. J Urol 131:343–345, 1984

69. Tyrell CJ, Peckham MJ: The response of lymph node metastases of testicular teratoma to radiation therapy. Br J Urol 48:363–370, 1976

70. Skinner DG: Surgical management of germ cell tumors of the testis. In DG Skinner (ed): Urological Cancer, pp 301–304 Grune & Stratton, 1983

71. Goldinger PL, Scheweizer O: The hazards of anesthesia and surgery in bleomycin-treated patients. Semin Oncol 6:121–124, 1979

72. Lange PH, Narayan P, Vogelzang NJ et al: Return of fertility after treatment for non-seminomatous testicular cancer: Changing concepts. J Urol 129:1131–1135, 1983

73. Fossa SD, Klepp O, Molne K et al: Testicular function after unilateral orchiectomy for cancer and before further treatment. Int J Androl 5:179–184, 1982

74. Berthelsen JG, Skakkeback NE: Gonadal function in men with testis cancer. Fertil Steril 39:68–75, 1983

75. Li MC, Whitmore WF, Golbey R et al: Effects of combined drug therapy on metastatic cancer of the testis. JAMA 174:145–153, 1960

76. MacKenzie AR: Chemotherapy of metastatic testis cancer: Results in 154 patients. Cancer 19:1369–1376, 1966

77. Kennedy BJ: Mithramycin therapy in advanced testicular neoplasms. Cancer 26:755–766, 1970

78. Blum RH, Carter S, Agre K: A clinical review of bleomycin: A new anti-neoplastic agent. Cancer 31:903–914, 1973

79. Samuels ML, Howe CD: Vinblastine in the management of testicular cancer. Cancer 25:1009–1017, 1970

80. Samuels ML, Johnson DE, Holoye PY: Continuous intravenous bleomycin therapy with vinblastine in Stage III testicular neoplasia. Cancer Chemother Rep 59:563–570, 1975

81. Samuels ML, Lanzotti VJ, Holoye PY et al: Combination chemotherapy in germinal cell tumors. Cancer Treat Rev 3:185–204, 1976

82. Rosenberg B, VanCamp L, Krigas T: Inhibition of cell division in E. coli by electrolysis products from a platinum electrode. Nature 205:678–699, 1965

83. Higby DJ, Wallace HJ, Albert DJ et al: Diamminedichloroplatinum: A Phase I study showing responses in testicular and other tumors. Cancer 33:1219–1225, 1974

84. Wittes RE, Yagoda A, Silvay O et al: Chemotherapy of germ cell tumors of the testis. Cancer 37:637–645, 1976

85. Cheng E, Cvitkovic E, Wittes RE et al: Germ cell tumor: VAB II in metastatic testicular cancer. Cancer 42:2162–2168, 1978

86. Cvitkovic E, Wittes R, Golbey R et al: Primary combination chemotherapy for metastatic or unresectable germ cell tumors (abstract). Proc Am Assoc Cancer Res 19:174, 1978

87. Bosl GJ, Gluckman R, Geller NL et al: VAB-6: An effective chemotherapy regimen for patients with germ cell tumors. J Clin Oncol 4:1493–1499, 1986

88. Bosl GJ, Geller NL, Cirrincione CC et al: Multivariate analysis of prognostic variables in patients with metastatic testicular cancer. Cancer Res 43:3403–3407, 1983

89. Einhorn LH, Donohue JP: Cis-diamminedichloroplatinum, vinblastine, and bleomycin combination chemotherapy in disseminated testicular cancer. Ann Intern Med 87:293–298, 1977

90. Nichols C, Gupta S, Loehrer P et al: Outcome in patients with residual germ cell cancer after post-chemotherapy surgery (abstr). Proc Am Soc Clin Oncol 6:100, 1987

91. Einhorn LH, Williams SD: Chemotherapy of disseminated testicular cancer. Cancer 46:1339–1344, 1980

92. Stoter G, Sleyfer DT, Bokkel Huinink WW et al: High-dose versus low-dose vinblastine in cisplatin–vinblastine–bleomycin combination chemotherapy of non-seminomatous testicular cancer: A randomized study of the EORTC Genitouurinary Tract Cancer Cooperative Group. J Clin Oncol 4:1199–1206, 1986

93. Einhorn LH, Williams SD, Troner M et al: The role of maintenance therapy in disseminated testicular cancer. N Engl J Med 305:727–731, 1981

94. Fitzharris BM, Kaye SB, Saverymuttu S et al: VP-16-213 as single agent in advanced testicular tumors. Eur J Cancer 16:1193–1197, 1980

95. Schabel FM Jr, Trader MW, Laster WR Jr et al: Cis-dichlorodiammineplatinum: Combination chemotherapy and cross-resistance studies with tumors of mice. Cancer Treat Rep 63:1459–1473, 1979

96. Peckham MJ, Barrett A, Liew KH et al: The treatment of metastatic germ cell testicular tumors with bleomycin, etoposide, and cisplatin (BEP). Br J Cancer 47:613–619, 1983

97. Williams SD, Birch R, Einhorn LH et al: Treatment of disseminated germ-cell tumors with cisplatin, bleomycin, and either vinblastine and etoposide. N Engl J Med 316:1435–1440, 1987

98. Greist A, Einhorn LH, Williams SD et al: Pathologic findings at orchiectomy following chemotherapy for disseminated testicular cancer. J Clin Oncol 2:1025–1027, 1984

99. Rich TA, Cassady JR, Strand RD et al: Radiotherapy for pineal and suprasellar germ cell tumors. Cancer 55:932–940, 1985

100. Nichols CR, Hoffman R, Einhorn LH, et al: Hematologic malignancies associated with primary mediastinal germ cell tumors. Ann Intern Med 102:603–609, 1985

101. Nichols CR, Heerema NA, Palmer C et al: Klinefelter's syndrome associated with mediastinal germ cell neoplasms. J Clin Oncol 5:1290–1294, 1987

102. Hainsworth JD, Wright EP, Gray GF, Greco FA: Poorly differentiated carcinoma of unknown primary: Correlation of light microscopic findings with response to cisplatin-based combination chemotherapy. J Clin Oncol 5:1275–1280, 1987

103. Hainsworth JD, Einhorn LH, Williams SD et al: Advanced extragonadal germ cell tumors. Ann Intern Med 97:7–11, 1982

104. Vugrin D, Einhorn LH, Williams SD et al: A multi-institutional experience in extragonadal germ cell tumors: An SECSG study (abstr). Proc Am Assoc Cancer Res 26:172, 1985

105. Israel A, Bosl GJ, Golbey RB et al: The results of chemotherapy for extragonadal germ-cell tumors in the cisplatin era: The MSKCC experience (1975–1982). J Clin Oncol 3:1073–1078, 1985

106. Logothetis CJ, Samuels ML, Selig DE et al: Chemotherapy of extragonadal germ cell tumors. J Clin Oncol 3:316–325, 1985

107. Logothetis CJ, Samuels ML, Trindode A: The management of brain metastases in germ cell tumors. Cancer 49:1278–1281, 1982

108. Rustin GJS, Newlands ES, Bagshawe KD et al: Successful management of metastatic and primary germ cell tumors in the brain. Cancer 57:2108–2113, 1986

109. Lester SG, Morphis JG, Hornback NB et al: Brain metastases and testicular tumors: Need for aggressive treatment. J Clin Oncol 2:1397–1403, 1984

110. Greist A, Einhorn LH, Williams SD et al: Pathologic findings at orchiectomy following chemotherapy for disseminated testicular cancer. J Clin Oncol 2:1025–1027, 1984

111. Chong C, Logothetis CJ, von Eschenbach A et al: Orchiectomy in advanced germ cell carcinoma following intensive chemotherapy: A comparison of systemic to testicular response. J Urol 136:1221–1223, 1986

112. Fowler JE Jr, Whitmore WF Jr: Intratesticular germ cell tumors: Observations on the effect of chemotherapy J Urol 126:412–415, 1981

113. Schabel FM Jr, Trader MW, Laster WR Jr et al: Cis-dichlorodiammineplatinum: Combination chemotherapy and cross-resistance studies with tumors of mice. Cancer Treat Rep 63:1459–1573, 1979

114. Williams SD, Einhorn LH, Greco FA et al: VP-16-213 salvage therapy for refractory germinal neoplasms. Cancer 46:2154–2158, 1980

115. Hainsworth JD, Williams SD, Einhorn LH et al: Successful treatment of resistant germinal neoplasms with VP-16 and cisplatin: Results of a Southeastern Cancer Study Group trial. J Clin Oncol 3:666–671, 1985

116. Wheeler BM, Loehrer PJ, Williams SD, Einhorn LH: Ifosfamide in refractory germ cell tumors. J Clin Oncol 4:28–34, 1986

117. Loehrer PJ, Einhorn LH, Williams SD: Salvage therapy for refractory germ cell tumors with VP-16 + ifosfamide + cisplatin. J Clin Oncol 4:528–536, 1986

118. Lauer RL, Roth B, Loehrer PJ et al: Cisplatin + ifosfamide + either VP-16 or vinblastine as third-line therapy for metastatic testicular cancer (abstr). Proc Am Soc Clin Oncol 6:99, 1987

119. Birch R, Williams SD, Cone A et al: Prognostic factors for favorable outcome in disseminated germ cell tumors. J Clin Oncol 4:400–407, 1986

120. Peckham MJ, Oliver RTD, Bagshawe KD et al: Prognostic factors in advanced non-seminomatous germ-cell testicular tumors: Results of a multicentre study. Lancet 1:8–11, 1985

121. Pizzocaro G, Piva L, Salvioni R et al: Cisplatin, etoposide, bleomycin as first-line therapy and early resection of residual tumor in far-advanced germinal testis cancer. Cancer 56:2411–2415, 1985

122. Daugaard G, Rorth M: High-dose cisplatin and VP-16 with bleomycin in the management of advanced metastatic germ cell tumors. Eur J Cancer Clin Oncol 22:477–485, 1986

123. Loehrer PJ, Sledge GW, Einhorn LH: Heterogeneity among germ-cell tumors of the testis. Semin Oncol 12:304–316, 1985

124. Ulbright TM, Loehrer PJ, Roth LM et al: The development of non-germ cell malignancies within germ cell tumors. Cancer 54:1824–1833, 1984

125. Greist A, Roth B, Einhorn LH et al: Cisplatin-combination chemotherapy for disseminated germ cell tumors: Long-term followup (abstr). Proc Am Soc Clin Oncol 4:98, 1985

126. Drasga RE, Einhorn LH, Williams SD et al: Fertility after chemotherapy for testicular cancer. J Clin Oncol 1:179–183, 1983

127. Fossa SD, Ous S, Abyholm T et al: Post-treatment fertility in patients with testicular cancer. Br J Urol 57:210–214, 1985

128. Nijman JM, Koops HS, Kremer J et al: Gonadal function after surgery and chemotherapy in men with Stages II and III non-seminomatous testicular tumors. J Clin Oncol 5:651–656, 1987

129. Vogelzang NJ, Bosl GJ, Johnson K et al: Raynaud's phenomenon: A common toxicity after combination chemotherapy for testicular cancer. Ann Intern Med 95:288–292, 1981

130. Teutsch C, Lipton A, Harvey HA: Raynaud's phenomenon as a side effect of chemotherapy with vinblastine plus bleomycin for testicular cancer. Cancer Treat Rep 61:925–926, 1977

131. Subar M, Muggia FM: Apparent myocardial ischemia associated with vinblastine administration. Cancer Treat Rep 70:690–691, 1986

132. Vogelzang NJ, Freming DH, Kennedy BJ: Coronary artery disease after treatment with bleomycin and vinblastine. Cancer Treat Rep 64:1159–1160, 1980

133. Edwards GS, Lane M, Smith FE: Long-term treatment with PVB: Possible association with severe coronary artery disease. Cancer Treat Rep 63:551–552, 1979

134. Samuels BL, Vogelzang NJ, Kennedy BJ: Severe vascular toxicity associated with vinblastine, bleomycin, and cisplatin chemotherapy. Cancer Chemother Pharmacol 19:253–256, 1987

135. Doll DC, List AF, Greco FA et al: Acute vascular ischemic events after cisplatin-based combination chemotherapy for germ cell tumors of the testis. Ann Intern Med 105:48–51, 1986

136. Burkhardt A, Haltje WJ, Gebbens JO et al: Vascular lesions following perfusion with bleomycin: Electron microscopic observations. Virchows Arch [Pathol Anat] 372:227–236, 1976

137. Kahaleh MD, Osborn I, LeRoy EC: Increased Factor VIII antigen in scleroderma and Raynaud's phenomenon. Ann Intern Med 94:842–845, 1981

138. Pui CH, Chesney CM, Weed J et al: Altered von Willebrand factor molecule in children with thrombus following asparaginase–prednisone–vincristine therapy for leukemia. J Clin Oncol 3:1266–1271, 1985

139. Barneveld PW, Sleijfer DT, van der Mark TW et al: Natural course of bleomycin induced pneumonitis. Am Rev Resp Dis 135:48–51, 1987

140. Nachman JB, Baum ES, White H et al: Bleomycin-induced pulmonary fibrosis mimicking recurrent metastatic disease in a patient with testicular cancer. Cancer 47:236–239, 1981

141. McCrea ES, Diaconis JN, Wade JC et al: Bleomycin toxicity simulating metastatic nodules to the lungs. Cancer 48:1096–1100, 1981

142. Redman JR, Vugrin D, Arlin ZA et al: Leukemia following treatment of germ cell tumors in men. J Clin Oncol 2:1080–1087, 1984

143. Terebelo HR, Taylor HG, Brown A et al: Late relapse of testicular cancer. J Clin Oncol 1:566–571, 1983

144. Williams SD, Stablein DM, Einhorn LH et al: Pathologic Stage II testis cancer: Immediate adjuvant chemotherapy versus observation with treatment relapse: A report from the Testicular Cancer Intergroup Study. N Engl J Med 317:1433–1438, 1987

WILLIAM J. HOSKINS

CARLOS PEREZ

ROBERT C. YOUNG

CHAPTER 36 *Gynecologic Tumors*

Gynecologic cancer represents 14.9% of all cancers in women and accounts for 10% of all cancer deaths.[1] Table 36-1 lists the estimated number of new cases and deaths of the female genital cancers for 1987. For the physician called on to diagnose and treat patients with female genital cancer, it is important to have a thorough understanding of the pathophysiology of the disease as well as an understanding of the various therapeutic options available. In this chapter we present current information on all of the female genital cancers except ovarian cancer, which is covered separately in Chapter 37. Epidemiology, natural history, and routes of spread are presented as well as the essential pathologic characteristics necessary for planning therapy. Major emphasis is placed on methods of diagnosis and current therapeutic options.

CARCINOMA OF THE VULVA

Carcinoma of the vulva accounts for approximately 3% of all female genital cancers.[1] Squamous cancer accounts for 90% of these cancers. Other cell types encountered are malignant melanoma, basal cell carcinoma, and adenocarcinoma of the Bartholin's and Skene's glands. Occasionally, primary vulvar sarcoma and verrucous carcinoma are seen. Paget's disease, which is discussed under the section on preinvasive cancer, may be associated with invasive adenocarcinoma of the sweat glands.

Usually vulvar cancers tend to develop slowly and spread by direct continuity to adjacent tissues or via the lymphatics to the inguinal lymph nodes. Treatment is most often surgical and results in physical disfigurement and sexual dysfunction.[2] Ongoing clinical protocols in this disease are evaluat-

ing alternative methods of therapy that researchers hope will allow modifications of treatment so as to reduce disfigurement and improve survival.

EPIDEMIOLOGY

The median age for patients with carcinoma in situ of the vulva is 44[3-9] and for those with microinvasive carcinoma it is 58.[8,10,11] Patients with frankly invasive carcinoma have a median age of 61.[12-14] Some authors have suggested that carcinoma in situ and microinvasive carcinoma are being seen more frequently and are occurring in younger women, but there are too few large series to document that impression. There does not appear to have been any change in the age incidence of invasive cancer.

Japaze et al[6] reported no increased incidence of vulvar cancer in any ethnic group, but Mack and Casagrande[15] reported an incidence in women of the lowest socioeconomic class that was three times the incidence in women of the highest socioeconomic class. Medical illnesses associated with vulvar cancer are hypertension, cardiovascular disease, obesity, and diabetes.[5,11,16-18] A variety of sexually transmitted diseases have been found in association with vulvar carcinoma including granulomatous venereal disease, syphilis, herpes hominis type II, and condylomata acuminata.[9,19] An increased incidence of anogenital carcinoma, especially cervical cancer, has been reported in patients with vulvar cancer.[20,21]

NATURAL HISTORY AND PATTERNS OF SPREAD

The association of carcinoma in situ, microinvasive carcinoma, and invasive vulvar carcinoma indicates that there is a

TABLE 36-1. Estimated New Cases and Deaths from Female Genital Cancer in 1988

Site	Estimated New Cases	Estimated Deaths
Corpus	34,000	3,000
Ovary	19,000	12,000
Cervix	12,900	7,000
Other	4,800	1,100
Total	70,700	23,100

Adapted from Silverberg E, Lubera J: Cancer statistics, 1988. CA 38:5, 1988.

continuum from preinvasive to invasive disease. There seems little doubt, however, that this process is much slower in the vulva than in the vagina or cervix, with almost two decades separating the peak incidence of vulvar carcinoma in situ and invasive carcinoma. Some authors have suggested that the multifocal carcinoma in situ of women in their 30s or 40s may not be as likely to progress to invasive cancer as the localized carcinoma in situ of the older woman. Although this may be true, there is no definite proof of this theory, and certainly one should not delay therapy in young women on this basis.

Plentl and Friedman[22] reported that primary vulvar lesions are most common in the labia and next most common on the clitoris. Labial lesions occurred three times more frequently on the labia majora as on the labia minora. These same authors pointed out the predictable spread of metastatic lesions to the inguinal lymph nodes followed by spread to the pelvic nodes. With the possible exception of vulvar melanoma, it is unusual for vulvar cancer to spread via the bloodstream.

The embryologic derivation of the lymphatics of the vulvar skin is similar to that of the abdominal skin,[22] and it is logical that primary drainage would be to the superficial and deep inguinal lymph nodes. Direct drainage to the pelvic lymph nodes occurs infrequently. The labia minora are characterized by a fine network of lymphatics that extend to the folds between the labia minora and labia majora. At these folds the lymphatic vessels become more coarse and extend cephalad. The lymphatics of the labia majora are more coarse than those of the labia minora and run laterally to the crural fold where they turn cephalad. Both of these lymphatic channels drain to the inguinal nodes. The clitoral vessels drain into the connecting trunks of the labia minora. All of these channels eventually drain into the superficial inguinal nodes that lie beneath Camper's fascia and anterior to the cribriform fascia. Connecting lymphatics lead to the deep inguinal nodes that surround the femoral vessels and drain into the iliac nodal system. Although it appears that clitoral lymphatics also drain directly into the pelvic lymphatics,[22] metastases to pelvic nodes without inguinal involvement are rare. Way[23] found involvement of the pelvic lymph nodes in the absence of inguinal lymph nodes in only 3% of his cases.

The overall incidence of positive lymph nodes (both inguinal and pelvic) in vulvar cancer was found to be 46% in a literature review of more than 1,100 patients by Plentl and Friedman.[22] Since the incidence of pelvic node metastases is

5% to 10%, one can expect inguinal node metastases to occur in 35% to 40% of cases. These same authors reported a 62% incidence of metastases in clinically palpable lymph nodes and a 35% incidence of metastases in nonpalpable lymph nodes. The incidence of positive lymph nodes increases with the size of the lesion, with the depth of invasion, and by location, with midline lesions having a higher incidence of bilateral positive lymph nodes.

PATHOLOGY

Intraepithelial neoplasia of the vulva exhibits a variety of gross and microscopic patterns. Grossly, the lesions may be flat and raised (maculopapular) or verrucous. They may be brown (hyperpigmented), red (erythroplastic) or white (leukoplakia). The various gross and microscopic patterns led to these lesions being termed Bowen's disease, erythroplasia of Queyrat, carcinoma simplex, and Paget's disease.[24] In order to standardize nomenclature, the International Society for the Study of Vulvar Disease published a classification in 1976 that is widely accepted throughout the world.[26] A summary of that classification is shown in Table 36-2. In this classification system only two types of true intraepithelial neoplasia are accepted: carcinoma in situ and Paget's disease. Histologically, carcinoma in situ is characterized by disordered orientation and maturation of the epithelial cells that extend the full thickness of the epithelium. Giant cells, multinucleated cells, dyskeratosis, parakeratosis, and increased density of cells are seen as well as abnormal nuclear morphology with irregular nuclear borders and clumped chromatin.[26] Paget's disease is characterized microscopically by the Paget's cells, which are large and round or oval with pale, vacuolated cytoplasm. These cells appear singly and in nests surrounded by small hyperchromatic basaloid cells. Helwig and Graham[27] reported that one third of their cases of Paget's disease of the vulva were associated with underlying adenocarcinomas of an adnexal structure. Associated carcinomas of the breast[28] and of Bartholin's gland[29] and squamous carcinoma of the cervix[30] have been reported.

Invasive squamous cancer is the most common vulvar malignancy and accounts for more than 90% of all cases. Grossly, the lesions will be ulcerated and endophytic in one third of cases and exophytic in the remainder.[26] Histologically, squamous cancers are usually well differentiated with whorls and nests of keratin. Gosling et al[31] and Way[32] have reported that 5% to 10% of these cancers will be anaplastic.

TABLE 36-2. International Society for the Study of Vulvar Disease: Classification of Vulvar Diseases*

A.	Hyperplastic dystrophy
	1. Without atypia
	2. With atypia
B.	Lichen sclerosis
C.	Mixed dystrophy
	1. Without atypia
	2. With atypia
D.	Paget's disease of the vulva
E.	Carcinoma in situ

* Abbreviated classification.

Squamous cancers that are less than 2 cm in diameter and invade less than 5 mm are often termed microinvasive carcinoma.[33,34] The actual metastatic potential and the proper management of such patients are currently being evaluated. Two varieties of squamous cancer that occur rarely are adenoid squamous cancer described by Lasser et al[35] and verrucous carcinoma.[36] Verrucous carcinoma resembles extensive condylomata acuminata and is very well differentiated. It invades locally but rarely metastasizes.[37]

Melanoma accounts for 2% to 9% of vulvar cancers.[26] Two varieties of melanoma are described: the nodular melanoma and the superficial spreading melanoma.[26] Depth of invasion is directly related to the incidence of nodal metastases and survival.[38] Although a common finding in other parts of the body, basal cell carcinomas of the vulva occur infrequently.[39] Sarcomas may rarely arise in the vulvar connective tissue and, although leiomyosarcoma is the most common, neurofibrosarcomas, rhabdomyosarcomas, fibrosarcomas, and angiosarcomas have been reported.[40] Adenocarcinomas may occasionally arise from the periurethral Skene's glands, but most adenocarcinomas are either of the Bartholin's gland or from vulvar adnexal structures associated with Paget's disease.

Bartholin's carcinomas can be squamous if they originate near the orifice of the duct, papillary if they arise from the transitional epithelium of the duct, and adenocarcinoma if they arise from the gland itself. The adenoid cystic variety of Bartholin's gland carcinoma is similar to the adenoid cystic tumor of the salivary gland and tends to invade locally with metastases occurring late, if at all.[26]

CLINICAL PRESENTATION AND STAGING

The most common complaint of the patient with vulvar cancer is of a growth or mass of the vulva.[18] Pruritus vulvae, bleeding, and pain are also seen, and up to 20% of patients will be asymptomatic.[16,41] Although both physician and patient delay have been attributed to delays in diagnosis, better education appears to have had an influence since most recent series report smaller lesions and there is a growing body of literature on microinvasive cancer.

The best method of diagnosis of vulvar cancer is a high index of suspicion and early biopsy. Either a wedge biopsy with a knife or a circular biopsy with a Keye's dermal punch under local infiltration anesthesia will provide an excellent specimen and early diagnosis. The Keye's punch is especially good since hemostasis can usually be obtained with silver nitrate application without need for suture. Colposcopy will often be of use in defining the limits of the lesion, but it is too time-consuming to be significantly useful as a screening procedure. Toluidine blue staining of the vulva has been advocated as a method of identifying areas for biopsy but has a 20% false positive rate.

If invasive carcinoma is found on biopsy, the patient should undergo a metastatic evaluation. The vagina and cervix should be carefully inspected and a Papanicolaou smear of the cervix obtained. A careful bimanual examination, cystoscopy, proctoscopy, barium enema, intravenous pyelogram, chest radiograph, and biochemical profile are required. Computed tomography or nuclear magnetic

resonance imaging (MRI) of the pelvis may be helpful in evaluating retroperitoneal nodal areas. Since most of these patients will be elderly, a thorough medical evaluation is often indicated before treatment.

The International Federation of Gynecology and Obstetrics classification for vulvar cancer is based on the tumor, nodes, and metastases (TNM) classifications with descriptive phraseology. Both the TNM classifications and the descriptions for each stage are listed in Table 36-3. For malignant melanoma, either the Clark[42] or Breslow[43] classifications of depth of invasion should also be provided. Bartholin's gland carcinomas are staged by the International Federation of Gynecology and Obstetrics (FIGO) system and

TABLE 36-3. Carcinoma of the Vulva: FIGO Method of Staging (TNM Classification)

T	Primary tumor
T1	Tumor confined to the vulva—2 cm or less in larger diameter
T2	Tumor confined to the vulva—more than 2 cm in diameter
T3	Tumor of any size with adjacent spread to the urethra or vagina or perineum or anus
T4	Tumor of any size infiltrating the bladder mucosa or the rectal mucosa or both, including the upper part of the urethral mucosa, or fixed to the bone
N	Regional lymph nodes
N0	No nodes palpable
N1	Nodes palpable in either groin, not enlarged, mobile (not clinically suspicious of neoplasm)
N2	Nodes palpable in either one or both groins, enlarged, firm and mobile (clinically suspicious of neoplasm)
N3	Fixed or ulcerated nodes
M	Distant Metastases
M10	No clinical metastases
M1a	Palpable deep pelvic lymph nodes
M1b	Other distant metastases

Definitions of the different clinical stages in carcinoma of the vulva (FIGO)

Stage I	
T1 N0 M0	Tumor confined to the vulva—2 cm or less in the larger diameter. Nodes are not palpable, or are palpable in either groin, not enlarged, mobile (not clinically suspicious of neoplasm)
Stage II	
T2 N0 M0	Tumor confined to the vulva—more than 2 cm in diameter. Nodes are not palpable, or are palpable in either groin, not enlarged, mobile (not clinically suspicious of neoplasm)
Stage III	
T3 N0 M0	Tumor of any size with adjacent spread to the
T3 N1 M0	lower urethra or the vagina, perineum, or anus,
T3 N2 M0	or nodes palpable in either one or both groins,
T1 N2 M0	enlarged, firm and mobile, not fixed (but
T2 N2 M0	clinically suspicious of neoplasm)
Stage IV	
T4 N0 M0	Tumor of any size infiltrating the bladder mucosa
T4 N1 M0	or the rectal mucosa or both, including the
T4 N2 M0	upper part of the urethral mucosa, or fixed to
T1 N3 M0	the bone or other distant metastases. Fixed or
T2 N3 M0	ulcerated nodes in either one or both groins
T3 N3 M0	
T4 N3 M0	

All other conditions containing M1 or M1b

metastatic tumors are not staged. It must be realized that the above staging system does not include a subdivision for microinvasive vulvar cancer. It is thus important to describe accurately the depth of invasion for Stage I tumors. For future prognostic evaluation, the presence or absence of lymphovascular invasion should also be noted.

TREATMENT

Historically, vulvar carcinoma has been considered to be effectively managed only by radical surgery with little place for radiation therapy, chemotherapy, or conservative surgery. The slow growth of the disease with its orderly progression of metastases to regional lymph nodes lends itself to en bloc surgical resection, and survival rates of 80% to 85% for patients with negative lymph nodes and 40% to 50% for those with positive inguinal nodes have been consistently reported. Table 36-3A shows 5-year survival rates in patients with carcinoma of the vulva. Unfortunately, the operation of radical vulvectomy and inguinal or inguinal and pelvic node dissection results in significant disruption of normal anatomy and is complicated by wound breakdown, lymphedema, and sexual dysfunction. Because of the above, several innovative approaches are being evaluated to decrease the short- and long-term morbidity of treatment of this disease. It is quite possible that the next decade will see rapid changes in the therapy of vulvar cancer.

STAGE 0

In the 1960s, Collins et al[44] advocated radical vulvectomy for carcinoma in situ of the vulva, pointing out that 4 of their 41 patients had unsuspected invasive cancer in the final specimen. Boutselis[4] reported survival rates approaching 100% with simple vulvectomy, and Rutledge and Sinclair[45] described the skinning vulvectomy that removed the skin of the vulva but preserved the fat, muscular, and glandular structures. When covered with a split-thickness skin graft from the thigh or buttocks, better cosmesis was obtained. Forney et al[7] used this procedure in 8 patients and noted only 1 recurrence. In 1983, Barnhill et al[46] described the rhomboid flap technique for vulvar reconstruction following wide local excision of carcinoma in situ.

Current management of carcinoma in situ of the vulva is wide local excision using either primary closure, skin flaps, or skin graft for restoration of normal anatomy. Many authors[7,9,47,48] have reported successful control of the disease with recurrence rates of 9% to 12%. Given the improved function and cosmesis with wide local excision, there is little doubt that optimal management consists of this method of therapy and close follow-up. Most patients, even if they re-

TABLE 36-3A. Survival Rates for Carcinoma of the Vulva

Stage	Five-Year Survival Rate (%)
Stage I	70
Stage II	50
Stage III	30
Stage IV	10

quire repeat excisions for recurrence, can be managed by wide local excision providing they adhere to a schedule of frequent follow-up examinations. Other methods of treating carcinoma in situ of the vulva include topical 5-fluorouracil, cryosurgery, dinitrochlorobenzene-induced hypersensitivity, and laser vaporization. Of these methods, only laser vaporization has proved significantly useful, and none provide a pathologic specimen for histologic review.

Paget's disease of the vulva extends subepithelially and requires wide excision in order to achieve free margins. Frozen section of the margins in the operating room may assist the surgeon in ensuring complete removal. Although some authorities recommend simple vulvectomy, this lesion, like carcinoma in situ, can usually be managed by less radical excision so that sexual function is maintained. A slightly deeper excision to remove the epidermis and corium down to the level of the underlying fat is indicated to ensure removal of the adnexal skin structures. Breen et al[49] reported a 12.4% recurrence rate after surgical excision, many of these patients having undergone simple vulvectomy initially. Some authors[50] have reported success with topical chemotherapy for recurrent Paget's disease, but such treatment should not be used as primary therapy because of the possibility of missing an underlying adenocarcinoma. If an invasive adenocarcinoma is found, the patient should be managed according to the extent of the invasive disease.

STAGE I

Stage I vulvar cancer encompasses all tumors that show any invasion (of any depth) as long as the tumor is less than 2 cm in diameter, does not involve the anus, vagina, or urethra, and there are no palpably enlarged lymph nodes. There is a growing body of literature, however, that indicates that certain early lesions should be separated into a category called microinvasive vulvar carcinoma. Wharton et al[33] in 1974 described a series of patients with vulvar cancers that were less than 2 cm in diameter and exhibited less than 5 mm of stromal invasion. They performed lymphadenectomies in 10 of 25 such patients and found no positive lymph nodes. Parker et al,[34] using the same definition of microinvasion, found inguinal metastases in 3 of 37 patients. Since those reports, several authors have reported small series of patients with an average incidence of inguinal node metastases of 5% to 10%.[8,11,51,52] Factors that may influence the incidence of nodal metastases are invasion greater than 2 mm,[52] anaplastic tumors,[11,34,52] confluency of invading foci,[11] and lymphovascular invasion.[34]

At present, there is no consensus as to how patients with microinvasive carcinoma should be managed. Nor is there clear-cut evidence in the literature that enables us to establish firm guidelines. DiSaia et al[53] have recommended an operative procedure in which the superficial inguinal lymph nodes are removed and sent for frozen section. If positive nodes are found, bilateral complete groin dissections and radical vulvectomy are performed; but if the nodes are negative, wide local excision of the primary cancer is performed and the procedure terminated. This therapeutic option appears to offer the best treatment plan to date, based on the meager information available. However, no large prospective trial of this method of therapy has been conducted to date. The Gynecologic Oncology Group (GOG) is currently evaluating prospectively all patients with tumor diameter of less than 2 cm and tumor invasion of less than 5 mm. In this protocol, patients are being managed by modified radical hemivulvectomy and ipsilateral node dissection. Perhaps a large number of patients, followed prospectively, will allow us to set reasonable treatment guidelines.

All other Stage I carcinomas of the vulva (those with invasion greater than 5 mm) should be managed by radical vulvectomy and bilateral inguinal lymphadenectomy. The therapeutic options for these patients are the same as those for Stage II carcinoma discussed below.

STAGES II AND III

Stage II vulvar carcinoma is a cancer that is greater than 2 cm in diameter, does not involve the anus, vagina, or urethra, and in which there are no palpable suspicious inguinal lymph nodes. The treatment of Stage II carcinoma of the vulva is radical vulvectomy and bilateral inguinal lymphadenectomy. There are three basic surgical approaches. The so-called butterfly incision removes the skin over the mons from the level of the iliac crest, the vulva, and a wedge of skin over the inguinal dissection. An alternative to this is to mobilize a skin flap over the inguinal dissection without excision of this skin. Finally, some authors have advocated separate groin incisions for the inguinal dissections coupled with a radical excision of the vulva. The incidence of local recurrence is similar in each type, and the choice of incision is primarily a matter of preference. Although some authors still recommend routine performance of pelvic lymphadenectomy as part of this operation,[54] most surgeons who perform pelvic lymphadenectomy do so only if the inguinal lymph nodes are positive. Green[16] found no patients with pelvic nodal metastases in patients with negative inguinal nodes. Recently, the GOG completed a randomized trial of pelvic irradiation or pelvic lymphadenectomy in patients with positive inguinal nodes and demonstrated statistically significant improved survival and no increased morbidity in the group receiving pelvic irradiation.[55] They have since begun a randomized trial of pelvic and inguinal irradiation versus inguinal lymphadenectomy in patients with Stages I and II vulvar cancer.

STAGES III AND IV CARCINOMA OF THE VULVA

Stage III vulvar carcinoma is a tumor of any size with spread to the urethra, vagina, or anus, or with clinically suspicious nodes in the inguinal area. In these patients, radical vulvectomy often requires removal of a portion of the distal urethra or vagina and may require excision of a portion of the anus. Exenteration is rarely required. Based on the GOG study cited earlier, these patients should undergo postoperative pelvic irradiation if the inguinal lymph nodes contain cancer.

Stage IV vulvar cancer involves the upper one third of the urethra or involves the bladder or rectum. Patients will also be considered Stage IV if they have fixed inguinal lymph nodes, fixation of tumor to bone, or distant metastases. Treatment of tumors involving the bladder or upper urethra

is best managed by the addition of anterior exenteration to the radical vulvectomy and inguinal node dissections. Posterior exenteration is used when the lesion involves the rectum. When the tumor is fixed to bone or there are distant metastases, treatment is usually palliative and consists of combinations of irradiation and chemotherapy.

MALIGNANT MELANOMA OF THE VULVA

Chung et al[38] found no lymph node metastases in patients with Clark's level I or II malignant melanoma. Positive lymph nodes were present in deeper levels. Current recommendations for treatment are radical vulvectomy and bilateral inguinal node dissection for levels of invasion greater than Clark's level II and wide local excision for Clark's level I and II. Some authorities recommend wide local excision and ipsilateral inguinal node dissection for all cases of vulvar melanoma. The GOG is prospectively evaluating wide local excision and inguinal lymphadenectomy for all cases of vulvar melanoma.

BARTHOLIN'S GLAND CARCINOMA

Bartholin's gland carcinoma is managed by radical vulvectomy and bilateral inguinal node dissection. Resection of the local tumor must be extensive because of its deep location. Although some authors recommend pelvic node dissection in all Bartholin's gland carcinoma, current evidence would suggest that pelvic irradiation may be an acceptable treatment option. Adenoid cystic carcinoma of the Bartholin's gland usually requires only wide local excision because lymph node metastases are rare.

OTHER VULVAR TUMORS

Basal cell carcinoma and verrucous carcinoma are managed by wide local excision. Lymph node dissection is not indicated in these patients. Metastatic tumors of the vulva should usually be excised, if possible, to control local symptoms. Further treatment will depend on the site of the primary cancer. All soft tissue sarcomas should be locally excised, if possible. After excision, treatment should include combinations of systemic chemotherapy and local and regional irradiation.

SURGICAL TREATMENT OF VULVAR CARCINOMA

Radical vulvectomy was first described in 1912 by Basset.[56] The classical operation as practiced until the mid-1960s included both bilateral inguinal and pelvic lymph node dissection. In the middle to late 1960s, many surgeons began to perform pelvic lymph node dissections only if the inguinal lymph nodes contained metastatic cancer. The validity of this approach has been clearly documented by several authors who have shown that pelvic node metastases rarely occur in patients with negative inguinal lymph nodes.[57-59] Additionally, the literature indicates that survival in patients with positive pelvic lymph nodes is very poor.

For many years, most surgeons utilized some form of en bloc dissection of the vulva and inguinal lymph nodes with

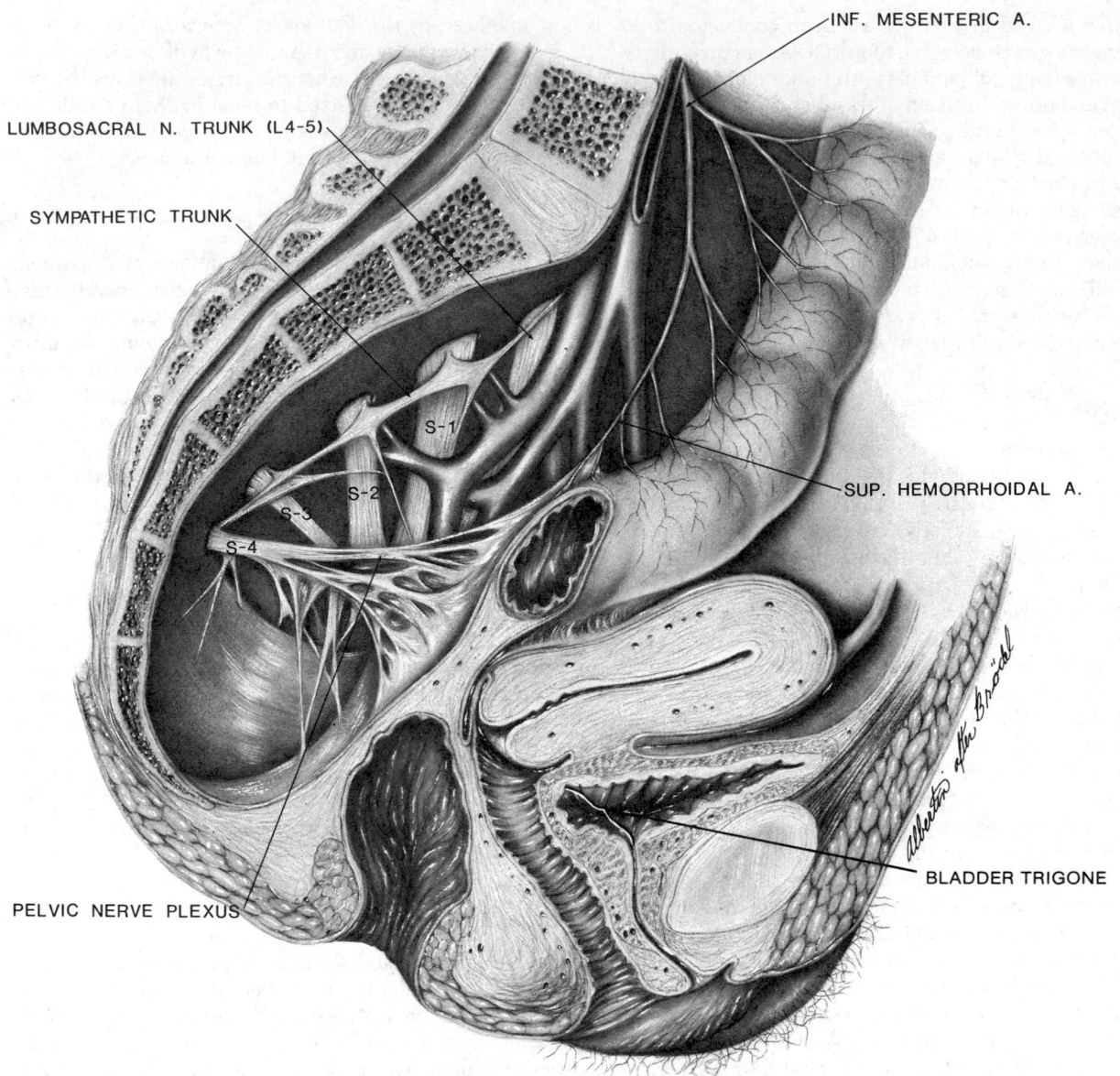

FIG. 36-1**A**. Sagittal view of female pelvis, including relationships of pelvic viscera, vasculature, and nerve plexuses. (*Figure continues on facing page.*)

the overlying skin as illustrated in Figure 36-1C. In recent years, many surgeons have used separate inguinal incisions without removal of the skin overlying the nodal areas. When combined with a radical vulvectomy, this procedure leaves a "bridge" of skin between the vulvectomy and the inguinal incision. Hacker et al[60] reviewed 100 cases and reported no recurrence of tumor in this skin bridge; they found a 14% incidence of wound breakdown compared to more than 40% wound breakdown in patients managed by a classical type of en bloc dissection. Figure 36-1D illustrates the lines of incision for a radical vulvectomy with separate inguinal incisions.

The necessity of performing a bilateral inguinal lymph node dissection in all patients was first questioned by Morris in 1977.[61] A review of Way's total experience indicates that only 5% of patients with negative ipsilateral inguinal lymph nodes had contralateral nodal involvement.[62] Recent prospective series by the GOG also indicate a low incidence of contralateral positive lymph nodes in patients with negative ipsilateral nodes.[63]

Iversen et al[64] have recommended hemivulvectomy and ipsilateral inguinal dissection for lesions of less than 1 cm with no vascular invasion and the GOG is currently evaluating hemivulvectomy for lesions of less than 2 cm with invasion of less than 5 mm. Figure 36-1E illustrates this procedure. Although there is currently no consensus about the necessary radicality of the approach to vulvar cancer, it is apparent that many investigators are questioning the uniform practice of the classical radical vulvectomy and bilateral inguinal node dissection. Further investigations into the results of less radical approaches are necessary before definite recommendations can be made.

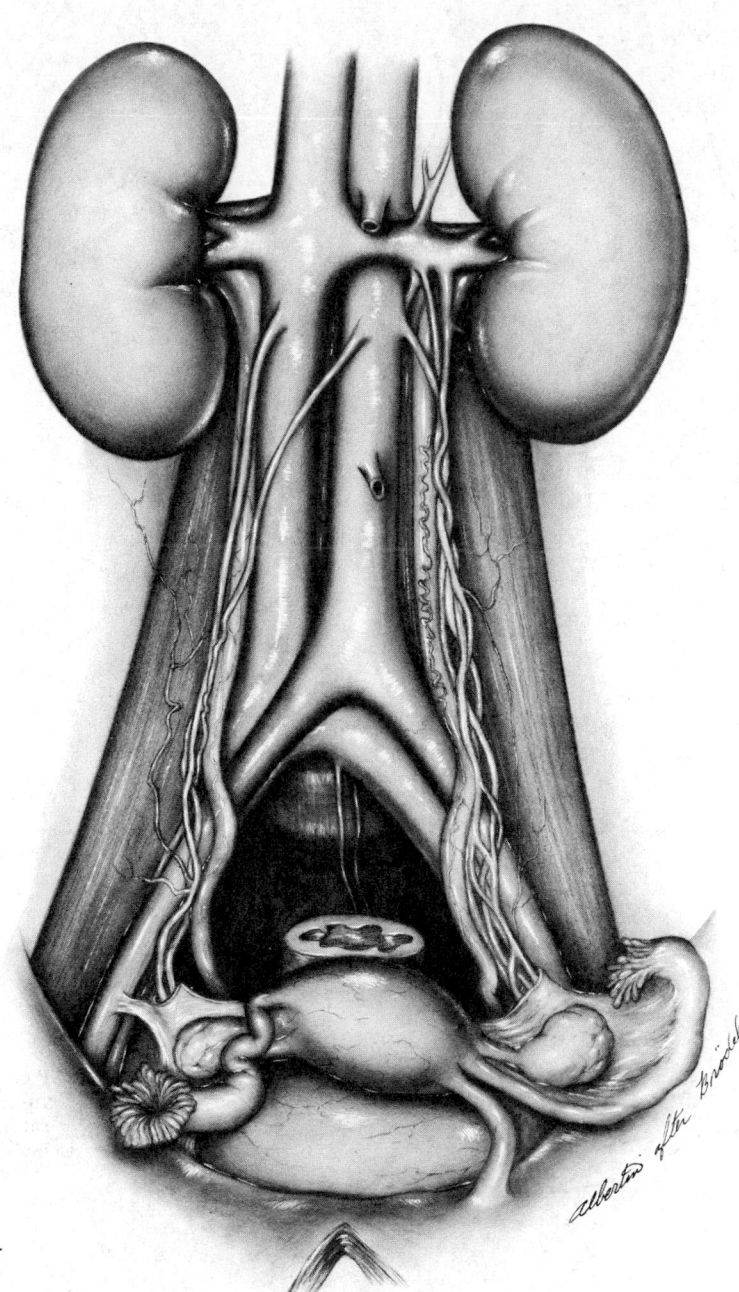

FIG. 36-1**B**. Abdominal and pelvic anatomy of the female reproductive tract. (*Figure continues on next page.*)

The major surgical complication associated with radical vulvectomy is wound breakdown with rates of 30% to 80% depending on the definition used. The use of perioperative antibiotics, separate inguinal incisions, and careful attention to a lack of tension on the wound edges will help minimize this complication. The formation of lymphocysts and chronic lymphedema can be minimized by use of suction drains but still remains a significant problem in patients who undergo surgical therapy of vulvar carcinoma. Catastrophic hemorrhage from the denuded femoral vessels is a rare complication if the sartorius muscle is transposed to cover the inguinal dissection. Introital stenosis can be minimized by use of skin flaps and avoidance of excessive tension at the time of closure of the surgical incision.

Despite better patient and physician education, one occa-sionally sees patients with vulvar cancers that involve the rectum or bladder. In such cases, anterior or posterior exenteration must be combined with radical vulvectomy and inguinal node dissection. It is possible that continued development of radiation therapy techniques will make possible combined therapy that can spare these organs.

RADIATION THERAPY IN VULVAR CANCER

The role of radiotherapy in the management of carcinoma of the vulva remains a controversial issue, primarily because of the lack of data on the results of treatment with modern techniques. The traditional belief that vulvar tissues cannot tolerate therapeutic doses of radiation has limited the role of

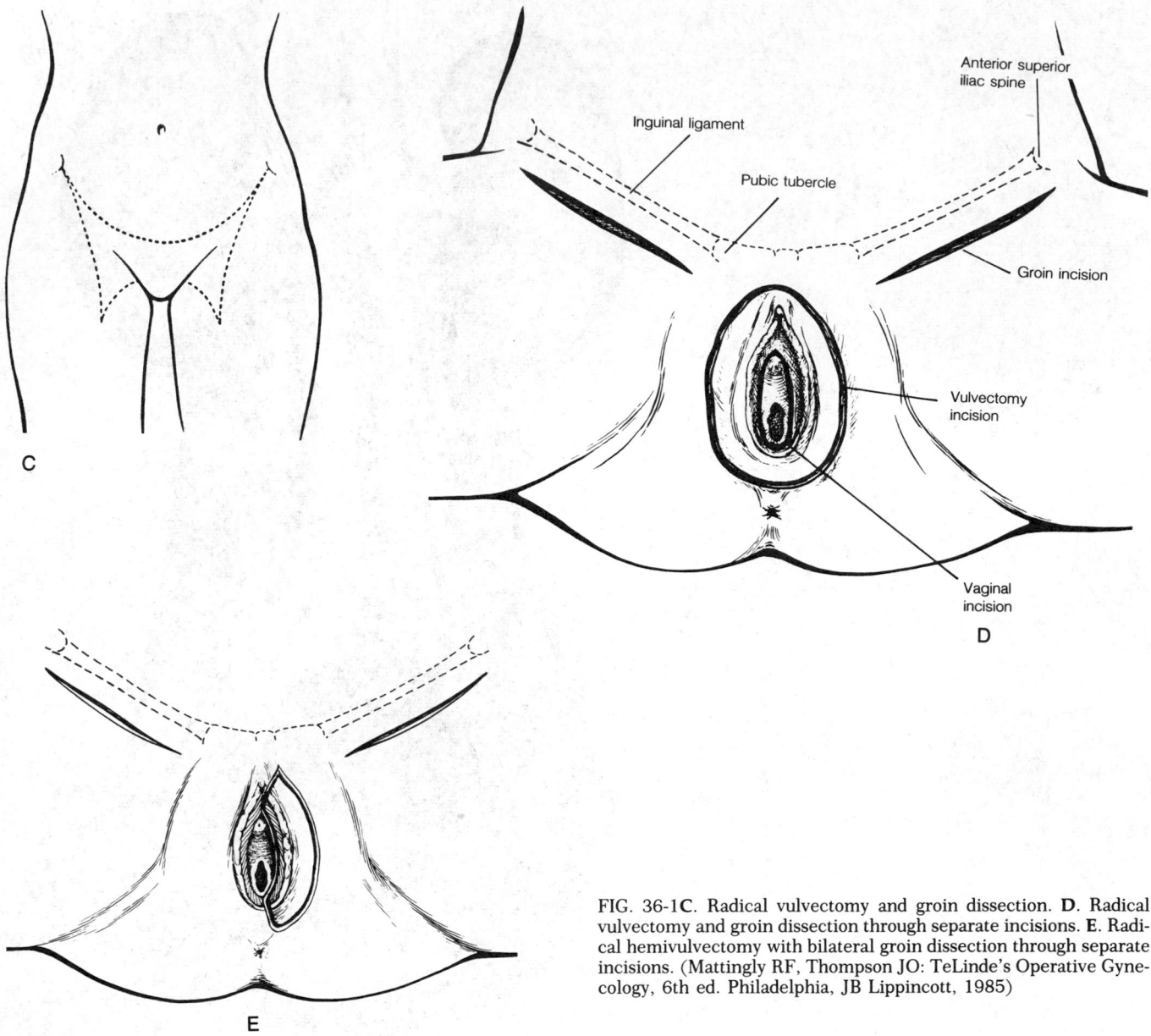

FIG. 36-1C. Radical vulvectomy and groin dissection. **D**. Radical vulvectomy and groin dissection through separate incisions. **E**. Radical hemivulvectomy with bilateral groin dissection through separate incisions. (Mattingly RF, Thompson JO: TeLinde's Operative Gynecology, 6th ed. Philadelphia, JB Lippincott, 1985)

radiotherapy to palliation or for treatment of patients who are not amenable to surgical resection.

Radiation Therapy Techniques for the Primary Site (Vulva)

In patients who are not candidates for surgical resection, the primary tumor site needs to be irradiated to the customary tumoricidal dose of approximately 7000 cGy in 35 to 40 treatments. Very small lesions may be controlled with somewhat lower doses (6000–6500 cGy). It is important to use a daily fraction size of 180 cGy or less. Usually, parallel opposed AP-PA portals are used, preferentially loaded anteriorly (or using a high energy single anterior beam), that cover the vulva and the regional lymphatics. An electron beam or

low energy photon beam supplement aimed directly at the vulva is needed at the end of the course to bring doses to full tumoricidal level. An implant may also be considered as a means of providing a boost to the primary tumor site. Use of appropriate bolus material over the areas of the skin (vulva) at risk for tumor involvement is essential. Interruption of the course is often necessary in the third or fourth week of treatment to prevent severe moist desquamation and maceration of tissues.

Radiation Therapy Techniques for the Regional Lymphatics

In patients with no clinical indications of regional lymphatic involvement, the inguinal lymph nodes are treated electively (prophylactically) to a dose of 5000 cGy (180–200 cGy per day). Depending on the available equipment, either an anteroposterior beam or a differentially loaded parallel opposed beam or an electron beam (for part of the treatment) can be used. Care should be taken to deliver adequate doses not only to the superficial inguinal nodes but also to the femoral nodes and the first echelon of deep pelvic nodes (Figs. 36-1 and 36-2).

In patients with findings indicative of regional lymph node involvement, the doses to the involved lymph nodes need to be in the range of 6500 to 7000 cGy, depending on the size of the involved nodes. In patients with evidence of involvement of the inguinal lymph nodes, the pelvis should be treated with prophylactic irradiation of 4500 to 5000 cGy. In patients with evidence of spread to the pelvic nodes, these fields may be boosted to 5500 to 6000 cGy (Fig. 36-3). Because some of the patients with involved pelvic lymph nodes remain curable, irradiation of the lower para-aortic chain in the presence of pelvic lymph node involvement might be appropriate.

Postoperative Radiotherapy

Radiotherapy is used increasingly in combination with surgery. In patients who have undergone a resection of the primary lesion and are considered at high risk for recurrence because of inadequate resection margins, postoperative irradiation is well indicated and should consist of at least 4500 cGy, preferably 5000 cGy, (175–200 cGy per day). If the resection margins are clearly involved or there is known

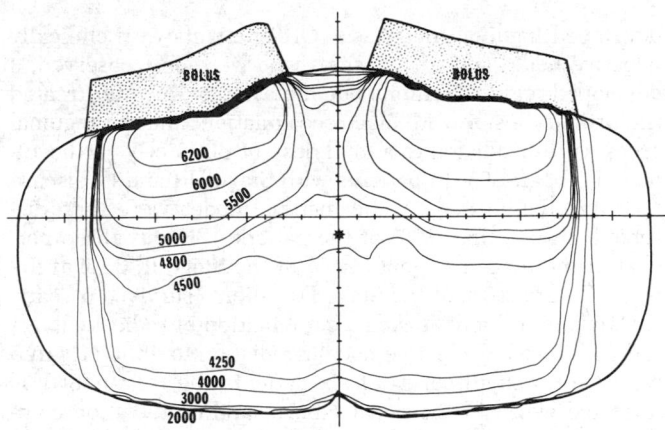

FIG. 36-3. Representative treatment plans for irradiation of regional lymphatics. Parallel opposed 18 MV photon beams are preferentially loaded anteriorly (2700 cGy anteriorly, 1800 cGy posteriorly), and a bolus is added over the inguinal areas to improve dose distribution in subcutaneous tissues in that area. A boost of 1500 cGy using 16 MeV electrons (without bolus) is added to the groin. (Pilepich MV: Carcinoma of the vulva. In Perez CA, Brady LW [eds]: Principles and Practice of Radiation Oncology, pp 1036–1043. Philadelphia, JB Lippincott, 1987)

gross residual tumor, higher doses of irradiation (6000–7000 cGy) are required.

Preoperative Radiotherapy

Patients with advanced primary lesions involving surrounding structures that are either of questionable resectability or are clearly unresectable can be treated with preoperative intent. By delivering moderately high doses of 4500 to 5500 cGy preoperatively, one can expect an increase in the resectability rate and also avoid mutilating procedures such as exenteration.

Irradiation of Recurrent Lesions

Recurrences following surgical resection remain potentially curable and need to be treated aggressively in the manner described above, with doses in the range of 6500 to 7000 cGy, and daily fractions of 180 cGy.

RESULTS OF RADIATION THERAPY IN VULVAR CANCER

There have been numerous attempts to combine radiotherapy and surgery in order to improve the therapeutic results.[65-72] Frankendal et al[65] reported on 55 patients of whom 22 had palpable lymph nodes considered tumerous; in 19 of these there was histologic confirmation of nodal involvement. Primary lesions were either electrocoagulated, resected, or irradiated. The regional nodes were dissected if clinically involved. Clinically negative nodes were observed without treatment unless the primary tumor was quite large or poorly differentiated. In such a situation, the groins were irradiated to a dose of 3000 to 6000 cGy in 15 to 55 days. Of the 12 patients who were irradiated prophylactically to the inguinal areas because of unfavorable primary lesions, none

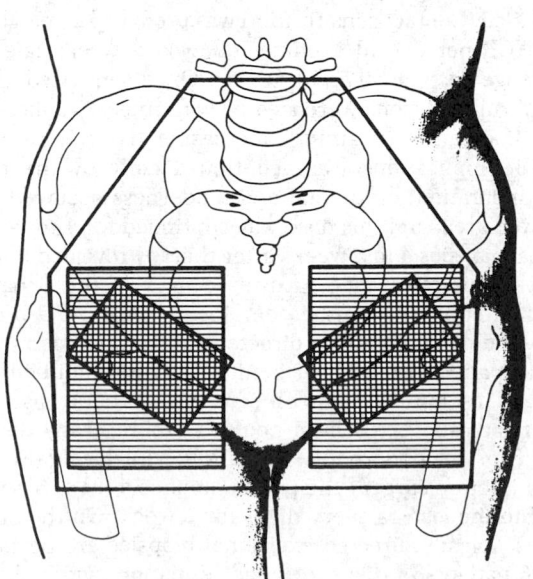

FIG. 36-2. Set-up for patients with positive inguinal lymph nodes. The entire pelvis is treated to a dose of 4500 to 5000 cGy. This is followed by a boost to the inguinal-femoral areas and distal iliac chain to bring the total dose to that area to 5500 to 6000 cGy and a final boost to the positive inguinal lymph nodes consisting of 500 to 1000 cGy, bringing the total dose to that area to approximately 6500 cGy (calculated at 3–4 cm). (Pilepich MV: Carcinoma of the vulva. In Perez CA, Brady LW [eds]: Principles and Practice of Radiation Oncology, pp 1036–1043. Philadelphia, JB Lippincott, 1987)

developed inguinal metastasis. Of 7 patients with clinically negative nodes and early lesions who were only observed, 3 developed regional lymph node metastases. Kucera[71] treated the primary lesion with electrocoagulation, and the inguinal areas were irradiated to a total dose of 6000 cGy (orthovoltage or cobalt-60). In patients with Stages III and IV disease (positive lymph nodes), the inguinal nodes were then dissected (in less than 20% of the patients). Eighty-three percent of the Stage I patients, 69% of the Stage II, 58% of the Stage III, and 10% of the Stage IV patients survived 5 years.

Daly and Million[69] tested a combination of radical vulvectomy followed by elective nodal irradiation to 4500 cGy in 5 weeks. In a small series of six patients the treatment was tolerated well with no nodal failures and no radiation complications. No delay in healing of the surgical site was recorded. Homesley et al[55] reported on 114 patients with invasive carcinoma of the vulva and positive inguinal nodes randomized (after radical vulvectomy and bilateral groin lymphadenectomy) to receive postoperative radiation therapy to the pelvic and groin lymph nodes (4500–5000 cGy in 5–6 weeks). The irradiated patients had a recurrence rate of 32.3% and a 68% 2-year survival rate in contrast to a recurrence rate of 45.5% and a 2-year survival rate of 54% in the nonirradiated group. The incidence of recurrence at the primary site was similar in both groups (8.5% in the irradiated and 9.1% in the pelvic lymph node dissection groups). Surgical morbidity and late side effects of irradiation and surgery were similar in both groups.

The rationale for a combination of radiotherapy and conservative surgery in advanced tumors that would ordinarily require exenteration has been discussed by Boronow.[68] In a series of nine cases, only one local recurrence was observed. The incidence of operative morbidity was minimal, and five patients remained disease-free for a period ranging from 11 months to 4.5 years. This experience has recently been updated,[67] indicating a 75% to 80% 5-year salvage probability in advanced primary and recurrent cancer. Hacker et al[70] treated eight patients with locally advanced vulvar cancer, who would ordinarily require an exenteration, with 4400 to 5400 cGy prior to resection (vulvectomy). Significant tumor regression was observed in seven and there was no viable tumor in the surgical specimen in four patients. Five of eight patients (62.5%) remained alive without evidence of disease from 15 months to 10 years.

Pao et al[74] reported the results on 40 patients with histologically confirmed primary or recurrent vulvar carcinoma treated with radiation therapy for locoregional disease at Washington University Medical Center. Nineteen of the patients with primary tumors received postoperative radiotherapy (5000 cGy in 6 weeks) after wide local excision or simple vulvectomy (9 patients) or radical vulvectomy (10 patients). Fifteen of the 19 exhibited local tumor control. Five patients with Stage III or IV disease were managed with radiotherapy alone. Four had a complete response with two currently with no evidence of disease (NED). Two patients who received preoperative radiotherapy with local excision are also currently free of disease. The 4-year NED survival rate for the study population is 100%, 28%, 50%, 0% and 10% for Stages I, II, III, IV and recurrent tumors, respectively. The poor results obtained in Stage II tumors are prob-

ably due to selection because 4 of 7 patients developed distant metastases. Two of 14 patients treated for recurrent disease remain NED after local excision of their tumors and irradiation. No dose response for subclinical disease could be found between 4500 and 7000 cGy. Treatment morbidity was acceptable with 2 patients developing severe long-term complications requiring surgical intervention.

The wide range of techniques, doses, and fractionation patterns makes it difficult to evaluate accurately the side effects of radiotherapy using modern techniques and treatment schemes. When dealing with a tumor at the skin or mucosal surface, which requires that the peak dose be at the surface, it is to be expected that all patients will have a significant acute (cutaneous and mucosal) irritation. Of more concern, however, is the incidence of late sequelae, some of which can be attributed to the fractionation schemes. Schulz et al,[75] for example, reported a very high incidence in patients who were treated with 500 cGy fractions. The complication rate has been consistently low in patients who were treated with the conventional 200 cGy per day or similar fractionation schemes. Prospective, large scale, multidimensional studies are needed to define the optimal indications for radiotherapy in vulvar carcinoma and its efficacy using modern techniques.

CHEMOTHERAPY OF CARCINOMA OF THE VULVA

Topical chemotherapy has been used for treatment of selected patients with vulvar or vaginal intraepithelial neoplasia. Topical 5-fluorouracil (5-FU) has been the most commonly used agent.[76] Often, three 7-day courses of 5% 5-FU cream are given 2 weeks apart. A study of 27 patients treated in this manner demonstrated that although 3 patients required retreatment at 3, 9, and 11 months, all 25 evaluable patients were free of disease for 3+ to 40+ months after treatment.[77]

Foster and Woodruff[73] treated six patients with histologically documented atypical vulvar dystrophy with topical dinitrochlorobenzene (DNCB) after surgery and topical 5-FU had failed. Contact sensitization was produced using 2000 μg of DNCB per 0.1 ml acetone followed 2 weeks later by a challenge dose of 50 μg of DNCB. Once sensitized, the patients' vulvar lesions were treated with topical application of DNCB cream containing increasing concentrations of DNCB. Applications were continued daily by the patient until induration, erythema, and tenderness occurred in the involved area, and this dose was continued for 1 to 2 weeks. Repeat biopsies 4 to 6 weeks after therapy revealed improvement or disappearance of disease in 5 of the 6 patients. Stillman et al[78] have used combined topical 5-FU pretreatment and colposcopically directed surgical excision to manage 16 patients with lower genital tract intraepithelial neoplasia. This approach was based on the authors' observation that neoplastic epithelium could be more easily dissected away from the underlying stroma following local 5-FU application. Before surgery the patient applies 4 ml of 5% topical 5-FU to the lesions every night for 1 week. On the 8th day, colposcopically directed excisional biopsies are performed. All 16 patients in this series had remission, and, although 2 have required retreatment, no patient has had a recurrence of severe dysplasia.

Levin et al[79] have used preoperative chemotherapy (mitomycin C and 5-FU) followed by pelvic irradiation prior to surgery for advanced carcinoma of the vulva. On day 1, mitomycin C (10 mg/m²) is given intravenously followed 30 minutes later by a 24-hour infusion of 5-FU (1000 mg/m²). 5-FU is repeated for 3 additional days at a similar dose and schedule followed by 10 days of equal fractions of radiation therapy. Courses of chemotherapy and radiation therapy last 2 weeks. Once adequate response was achieved (usually 1–2 cycles), surgery was performed. The researchers observed marked local tumor shrinkage in six patients that allowed more definitive surgery following the chemotherapy.

FUTURE CONSIDERATIONS IN CARCINOMA OF THE VULVA

Future studies in vulvar cancer should be directed toward defining microinvasive carcinoma and continuing the search for methods to reduce the radicality of the surgical therapy. Further investigations of plastic surgical reconstruction of the vulva should be directed at restoring normal anatomy and function, especially for the young patient.[80,81]

If the ongoing GOG study shows inguinal and pelvic irradiation to be as good as or better than bilateral inguinal node dissection, attention should next be turned to combining local excision with vulvar irradiation in an attempt to improve functional and cosmetic results.

From our limited experience as well as the reports in the literature, it is possible that radiation therapy may play a significant role in the management of patients with carcinoma of the vulva:

1. Radical vulvectomy could, in selected patients (those with tumors less than 2 cm and clinically negative nodes), be replaced by a wide local excision of the tumor to be followed by irradiation of the vulvar region as well as elective irradiation of the regional lymphatics in patients with clinically negative inguinal-femoral lymph nodes (5000 cGy). The margins of the primary tumor specimen should be microscopically negative (no residual tumor).

2. In patients with lesions smaller than 2 cm and clinically positive regional lymph nodes, the primary tumor could be removed by wide local excision, a superficial inguinal lymph node dissection carried out, and post-operative irradiation delivered (5000 cGy to the primary tumor area and 6000 cGy to the inguinal-femoral and pelvic lymph nodes).

3. Patients on whom a radical vulvectomy is carried out when the surgical margins at the primary site are negative and the regional lymph nodes have no evidence of metastatic tumor should not require postoperative radiation therapy. However, in patients with positive lymph nodes, postoperative irradiation has been shown to improve the probability of tumor control and survival. Frankendal et al[65] reported on 19 of 55 patients on whom there was histologic evidence of lymph node metastases and who received postoperative radiation

therapy (3000–6000 cGy in 15–55 days). Of 12 patients given elective irradiation because of unfavorable primary tumors, none developed inguinal lymph node recurrences. Seven patients who were observed developed regional lymph node metastases.

4. In patients with advanced inoperable carcinoma of the vulva, radiation therapy combined with chemotherapy (cisplatin and 5-FU) is beginning to be used with encouraging preliminary results.[82] Continued research into combinations of chemotherapy and irradiation may make even large tumors curable.

None of these approaches to therapy of vulvar cancer have been widely used, and careful, prospective trials of patients treated by these methods are necessary. The prospect of irradiation playing a major role in the management of carcinoma of the vulva is very promising.

CARCINOMA OF THE VAGINA

Carcinoma of the vagina is defined as a primary carcinoma arising in the vagina that does not involve the cervix or vulva. As a primary carcinoma, it is not a common cancer and accounts for about 2% of all gynecologic cancers.[83–85] The most common carcinomas of the vagina are actually tumors that involve the vagina by direct extension or are metastases from other genital areas, particularly the cervix. The vagina is also frequently involved by tumors of the rectum. With the exception of diethylstilbestrol (DES)-related clear cell carcinomas, primary carcinomas of the vagina are squamous cell cancers. Primary sarcomas occur but are rare.

EPIDEMIOLOGY

The median age for patients with carcinoma in situ of the vagina is the early fifth decade,[86–88] whereas the median age for patients with invasive cancer is the mid-sixth decade.[83–85,89] One percent to 3% of patients who develop squamous carcinoma of the vagina will have had squamous neoplasia of the cervix.[87] Hummer et al[88] reported that carcinoma in situ of the vagina followed carcinoma in situ of the cervix within up to 17 years, but that one third of the cases were diagnosed within 2 years. Prior radiation therapy may be a predisposing factor in primary vaginal carcinoma.[83,89,90] Pride et al[89] noted that 9 of 43 patients (20.9%) with invasive cancer of the vagina had a history of radiation therapy. The interval from previous irradiation to development of the primary squamous cancer was 7 to 20 years. Other authors[83,90] have noted intervals from 10 to 15 years.

In 1971 Herbst et al[91] related an increase in the number of clear cell carcinomas of the vagina to maternal ingestion of DES during pregnancy. The youngest DES exposed patient to develop clear cell adenocarcinoma was 7 years old and the peak incidence occurred at age 19.[92,93] The actual risk of an exposed female developing clear cell adenocarcinoma is 0.14 to 1.4 per 1,000 through age 24.[92] A plateau of cases was reached in the mid-1970s with a gradual decline in the number of cases each year since that time. It is not known whether these women will be at risk for the development of other cancers of the genital tract as they become older.

Primary sarcomas of the vagina account for about 2% of all vaginal cancer.[94,95] Leiomyosarcoma is the most frequent, but reticulum cell and stromal sarcomas have been reported. Age at diagnosis is in the fifth and sixth decades.[94] Sarcoma botryoides, although rare, is the most common tumor of the genital tract in female children.[96] The mean age for the appearance of these tumors is between 2 and 3 years.

Malignant melanomas occur in the vagina infrequently as a primary neoplasm. As in other parts of the genital tract, they spread locally by direct extension as well as by lymphatics and via the bloodstream.[97,98]

NATURAL HISTORY AND PATTERNS OF SPREAD

The location of primary vaginal carcinoma was evaluated in an extensive literature review of more than 1,200 cases by Plentl and Friedman.[85] They found that 26.9% occurred on the anterior wall, 57.2% on the posterior wall, and 15.9% on the lateral walls. Of 743 cases reviewed for axial location, they found that 50.7% occurred in the upper third of the vagina, 18.8% in the middle third, and 30.4% in the lower third. Clear cell adenocarcinomas of the vagina associated with maternal DES ingestion occur more commonly on the anterior vagina and are more frequently seen in the upper third of the vaginal canal.

Vaginal carcinomas spread to adjacent structures by direct extension or via lymphatics. By convention, tumors that involve the cervix or vulva are considered as primary in those sites because they are more common. The proximity of the urethra, bladder, and rectum results in early involvement of those structures and has a major effect on treatment planning. When spreading laterally, the tumor may invade the paracolpial, parametrial, and pararectal tissues, with extension to the pelvic side walls.

The lymphatic drainage of the vagina begins with the fine capillary meshwork in the mucosa and submucosa.[85] Both of these systems flow into collecting trunks near the lateral aspect of the vagina. The ventral portion of the vagina drains primarily to lateral pelvic lymph nodes while the posterior portion drains into the rectal and para-aortic lymph nodes. There is significant overlap in these patterns of drainage. The upper third of the vagina drains primarily like the cervix, whereas the middle third tends to spread both into the pelvic nodes and into the inferior gluteal nodes in the area of the ischial spine. The lower third of the vagina drains laterally, posteriorly, and to the femoral nodes.

In addition to the above distribution of lymphatics, there is a rich interconnection between the lymphatics of the vagina and those of the bladder and rectum. In their review of the literature, Plentl and Friedman[85] reported an overall positive node rate of 20.8% for vaginal carcinoma. These results were obtained both from surgical series and autopsy reports. Patients with clear cell carcinoma have distant spread (supraclavicular nodes or lungs) more frequently than would be expected for a similar group of patients with squamous cell carcinoma of the vagina or cervix.[93]

Pathology

Squamous carcinomas of the vagina may appear grossly as either ulcerated and endophytic tumors or they may be exo-phytic and protrude into the vaginal canal. Microscopically, they are epidermoid carcinomas with pleomorphic squamous cells that display a lack of organization and loss of cellular cohesion.[99] The lesions may exhibit patterns of dysplasia, carcinoma in situ, and invasion. Premalignant lesions may be multifocal.

Most clear cell adenocarcinomas of the vagina are polyploid or nodular with a reddish color. Some, however, are flat with a granular surface. Microscopically, three histologic patterns have been described: a tubulocystic pattern, a solid pattern, and a papillary pattern.[100]

Leiomyosarcoma of the vagina has a similar gross and microscopic appearance to leiomyosarcoma of other sites. Tavassoli and Norris[101] reviewed smooth muscle tumors of the vagina and concluded that tumors with moderate to marked atypia and greater than 5 mitoses per 10 high power fields should be considered leiomyosarcomas. The sarcoma botyroides of infancy is characterized by friable polypoid growths that appear like a bunch of grapes. Microscopically, these tumors comprise poorly differentiated spindle cells and a myxoid stroma and tend to grow around blood vessels.[99]

CLINICAL PRESENTATION, DIAGNOSIS, AND STAGING

Preinvasive lesions of the vagina are asymptomatic, and diagnosis is usually made during the evaluation of an abnormal Pap smear. Examination of the vagina by colposcopy should be conducted in all patients with abnormal cytology, even if there is a lesion of the cervix that appears to explain the cytology. Although not totally painless, vaginal biopsies do not usually require local anesthesia. A skin hook used to tent up the vaginal mucosa and stabilize it is often helpful in obtaining an adequate biopsy.

Abnormal vaginal bleeding is the most common symptom of invasive vaginal carcinoma.[94,102] The bleeding is often postmenopausal because that is the most common age group to develop the disease, but may also be postcoital or, in younger patients, intermenstrual. Vaginal discharge is also common. Pain or symptoms referable to the bladder or rectum usually occur with more advanced disease.[103] Brady[104] has reported that the average duration of symptoms before diagnosis is up to 7.4 months.

Detection of invasive vaginal carcinoma is made by inspection, palpation, and biopsy. In performing a speculum examination, it is important to either rotate the speculum or remove it slowly so as to visualize the entire vagina. Lesions arising on the posterior vaginal wall are particularly likely to be missed because they can be obscured by the posterior blade of the speculum. Any lesions noted during examination should be biopsied. Wharton et al[102] published data from M.D. Anderson Hospital that showed that 67.5% of patients seen at that institution had lesions larger than 2 cm when initial diagnosis was made.

The staging workup of the patient with vaginal cancer includes careful inspection of the vagina and cervix with biopsies as needed and a careful bimanual examination. Chest radiograph, biochemical profile, intravenous pyelogram, barium enema, cystoscopy, and proctoscopy are necessary. CT, MRI, and lymphangiography may be helpful in

TABLE 36-4. International Federation of Gynecology and Obstetrics Classification for Carcinoma of the Vagina

Stage 0	Carcinoma in situ: intraepithelial carcinoma
Stage I	Carcinoma limited to the vaginal wall
Stage II	Carcinoma has invaded the subvaginal tissue but has not extended to the pelvic wall
Stage III	Carcinoma has extended to the pelvic wall
Stage IV	Carcinoma has extended beyond the true pelvis or has involved the mucosa of the bladder or rectum. Bullous edema as such does not permit a case to be alloted to Stage IV
Stage IVA	Spread of the growth to adjacent organs
Stage IVB	Spread to distant organs

certain situations. The FIGO classification of vaginal carcinoma is listed in Table 36-4.

TREATMENT OF VAGINAL CANCER

The anatomical position of the vagina, lying between the urethra and bladder anteriorly and the rectum posteriorly, has been the predominant factor in treatment planning. The vaginal tube is thin walled, and the thickness of the vesicovaginal and rectovaginal septa is usually measured in millimeters.

Surgical extirpation of carcinoma of the vagina is often not feasible because the proximity of the bladder and rectum requires exenterative procedures to achieve adequate surgical margins. Therefore, with the exception of clear cell adenocarcinoma of the vagina occurring in young women and localized to the upper third of the vaginal canal, the primary treatment of vaginal carcinoma, especially squamous cell carcinoma, has been radiotherapy. Chau[105] pointed out the complexity of management of these patients and the need for careful radiotherapeutic techniques, which has resulted in survival similar to that for carcinoma of the uterine cervix. Perez et al[106] suggested that a correlation can be drawn between the doses of irradiation given to various tumor stages and the probability of local tumor control.

Carcinoma in situ

A wide range of therapeutic options are available for carcinoma in situ of the vagina and the choice of the correct option depends on the location of the lesion, the size of the lesion, and whether it is a single focus or multiple foci. Local excision is ideal therapy for patients with either single lesions or several lesions located in a single portion of the vagina, especially patients who develop recurrence in the vaginal cuff following hysterectomy. Total vaginectomy, on the other hand, is a difficult procedure and requires split thickness grafts for repair. Multiple lesions may often be treated in stages, with multiple excisions and primary closure. Cryotherapy has limited usefulness in the treatment of vaginal carcinoma in situ as it usually must be performed under anesthesia, requires multiple applications, and can easily damage the urethra, bladder, or rectum because of the difficulty in controlling the depth of the freeze. CO_2 laser has become very popular recently and has the advantage of being able to be tailored to rather exact depth and extent of dis-

ease. Further studies with long-term follow-up are needed to define the extent of its usefulness in this disease. Woodruff et al[107] reported the use of topical 5-FU in preinvasive vaginal carcinoma and noted complete eradication of lesions in 8 of 9 patients. Townsend[108] recommends 5 g of 5-FU cream instilled in the vagina every night for 5 days. He repeats these courses of therapy every 6 to 12 weeks until eradication of the lesion is documented. Contamination of the vulva must be prevented because 5-FU cream can produce an intense chemical reaction on the vulva. Radiation therapy of carcinoma in situ is rarely indicated; however, in selected cases in which the patient is a poor operative risk, irradiation of the vagina has been reported to afford excellent cure rates using intracavitary and interstitial sources alone.[109,110] Radiation therapy may also be considered in cases in which extensive surgical resection is necessary because of multifocal involvement of the entire vagina.

Stage I

Stage I lesions of the vagina that are located in the upper one third of the vagina can be managed by either radical hysterectomy, partial vaginectomy and pelvic lymphadenectomy, or standard radiotherapy. Some authors[110-113] have recommended a surgical approach in most of these cases. Lesions of the middle or lower vagina, unless they are very superficial and do not lie in the rectovaginal or vesicovaginal septa, often require either anterior or posterior exenteration for primary surgical therapy. Frick et al[111] have considered low and middle vaginal posterior lesions similar to rectal carcinoma and thus justified posterior exenteration as a logical choice of therapy. Although there is little doubt that individualization of therapy may often be best for any given patient, the difficulties encountered in surgical therapy of vaginal carcinoma because of the proximity of the bladder and rectum have resulted in most of these cancers being managed by irradiation. Irradiation appears to allow considerably more flexibility than does surgery, and good functional results are obtained with adequate radiation therapy. Surgical procedures may be reserved for the treatment of irradiation failures.

Brown et al[109] and Perez and Camel[110] have reported excellent tumor control and survival in patients with Stage I vaginal carcinoma. These authors have cautioned against an overly aggressive therapy in these early lesions because of the possibility of producing mucosal injury and interference with sexual function. Most patients with Stage I superficial tumors can be treated adequately with intracavitary and interstitial sources alone. If the carcinoma is less than 0.5 cm thick, intracavitary irradiation with a vaginal cylinder to deliver 8000 cGy to the mucosa will yield excellent results (over 90% tumor control). If the lesion is thicker or localized to one of the walls of the vagina, the addition of an interstitial single plane implant will deliver an adequate dose of irradiation to the tumor, limiting the exposure to the uninvolved normal tissues.

In patients with more extensive Stage I lesions, external irradiation should be administered to treat the paravaginal tissues and the regional lymph nodes, in addition to intracavitary and interstitial therapy.

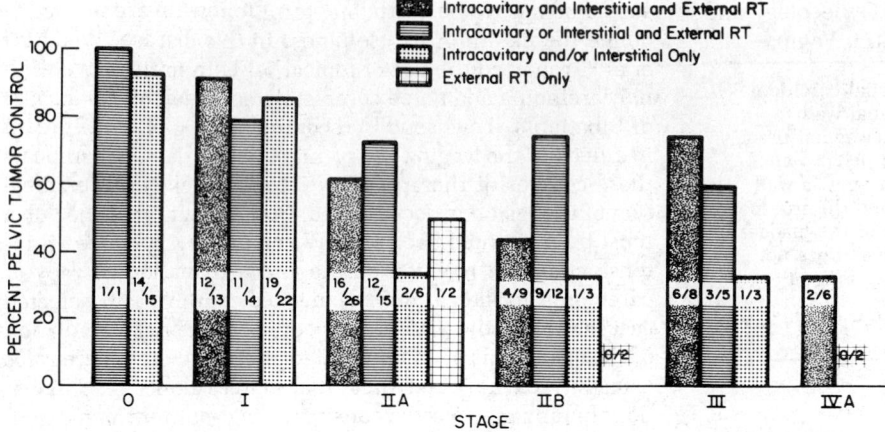

FIG. 36-4. Tumor control in the vagina and the pelvis (MIR 1950–1984) as a function of the type of treatment used and the anatomical stage of the disease. In patients with tumor beyond Stage I there is a critical need for the addition of external beam irradiation in order to improve tumor control. (Perez CA, Camel HM, Galakatos AE, et al: Definitive irradiation in carcinoma of the vagina. Long-term evaluation. Personal communication, 1987)

Stage II

Patients with Stage II carcinoma of the vagina require a more comprehensive approach that should include external beam irradiation and brachytherapy. Better survival has been observed by Perez et al[106] in Stage II carcinomas with the addition of external irradiation in comparison to brachytherapy alone (Fig. 36-4). They reported 65% survival with brachytherapy plus external irradiation and 40% survival with brachytherapy alone. In general, doses of 2000 cGy to the whole pelvis are delivered followed by a supplemental dose (3000 cGy) to the parametria with a midline shielding block. This is combined with interstitial and intracavitary therapy to deliver a minimum of 6500 to 7000 cGy to the base of the tumor and 5000 cGy to the pelvic lymph nodes.

Stages III and IV

In the more advanced lesions (Stages III and IVA) the results with irradiation have been less than satisfactory, with only 25% to 30% pelvic tumor control and survival. Therefore, higher irradiation doses with a greater contribution from the external irradiation are used. Table 36-5 summarizes the results in 165 patients with carcinoma of the vagina treated at the Mallinckrodt Institute of Radiology, Washington University School of Medicine Center.[106] Several authors have suggested a combination of irradiation and surgery in an effort to improve therapeutic results.

TECHNIQUES OF RADIATION IN VAGINAL CARCINOMA

The pelvic portals should encompass the entire vagina down to the introitus and the pelvic lymph nodes to the upper portion of the common iliac chain. Portals of 15 × 15 cm or 15 × 18 cm are usually adequate. In lesions of the lower two thirds of the vagina, it is necessary to electively include the inguinal lymph nodes in the irradiated field even when no palpable lymph nodes are present.

Intracavitary therapy is carried out with varying diameter vaginal cylinders, such as the Burnett, Bloedorn, or Delclos applicators. The largest possible diameter should be used to improve the ratio of mucosa/tumor dose (Fig. 36-5).[114,115] A new afterloading vaginal applicator retaining the characteristics of the Bloedorn applicator has recently been designed at Washington University Medical Center by Perez et al.[116] Interstitial therapy with ^{137}Cs, ^{226}Ra needles or afterloading ^{192}Ir needles have been employed. Single plane, double plane, or volume implants should be planned depending on the extent and thickness of the tumor.

When the lesion is in the upper third, it is the authors' practice to treat the upper vagina with the same intracavitary arrangement as in carcinoma of the uterine cervix, including an intrauterine tandem and vaginal colpostats. The middle and distal vagina are treated with a vaginal cylinder. For smaller lesions (carcinoma in situ and Stage I), a dose of 6000 cGy at 0.5 cm under the mucosa is adequate. For larger lesions, doses in the range of 7000 to 8000 cGy are neces-

TABLE 36-5. Carcinoma of the Vagina, Mallinckrodt Institute of Radiology: Anatomical Sites of Failure

Stage	No. of Patients	Local/Parametrial Only	Local/Parametrial + Distant Metastases	Distant Metastases Only	Dead of Intercurrent Disease
0	16	1 (6.3%)	0	0	6 (37.5%)
I	50	4 (8%)	3 (6%)	5 (10%)	20 (40%)
IIA	49	10 (20.4%)	9 (18.4%)	6 (12.2%)	15 (30.6%)
IIB	26	5 (19.2%)	7 (26.9%)	5 (19.2%)	6 (23.1%)
III	16	0	6 (37.5%)	4 (25%)	1 (6.3%)
IVA	8	2 (25%)	4 (50%)	0	1 (12.5%)

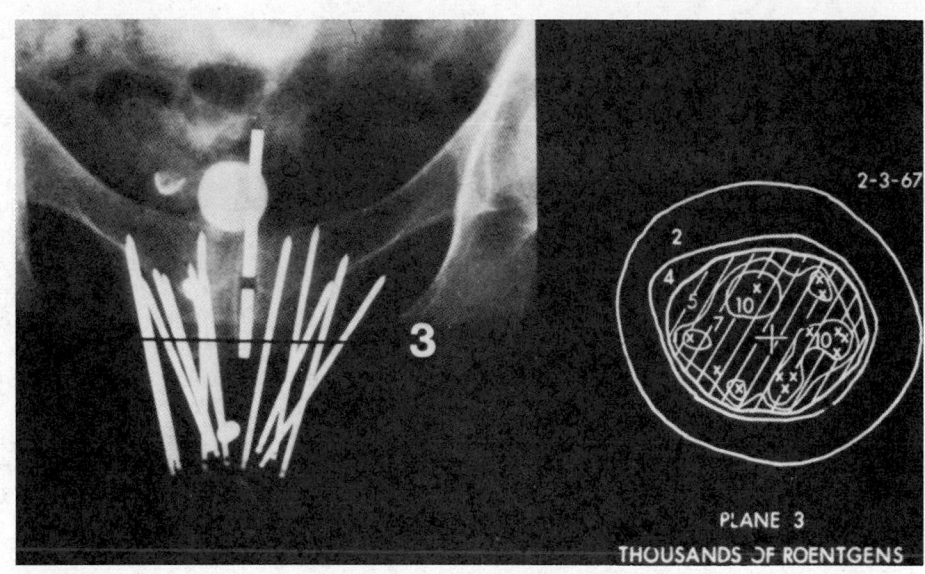

FIG. 36-5. **A.** Example of an intracavitary and double plane interstitial implant used to treat an extensive carcinoma of the vagina. This was combined with external beam 22 MV photon irradiation (4000 cGy whole pelvis and additional 2000 cGy parametrial dose). **B.** Distribution of radioactive sources and minimal tumor doses around primary tumor. **C.** Dose profile for patients with advanced vaginal carcinoma, using a combination of whole pelvic (WP) and parametrial external irradiation (SF), and intracavitary and double plane interstitial implant. (Perez CA, Korma A, Sharma S: Dosimetric considerations in irradiation of carcinoma of the vagina. Int J Radiat Oncol Biol Phys 2:639, 1977)

A

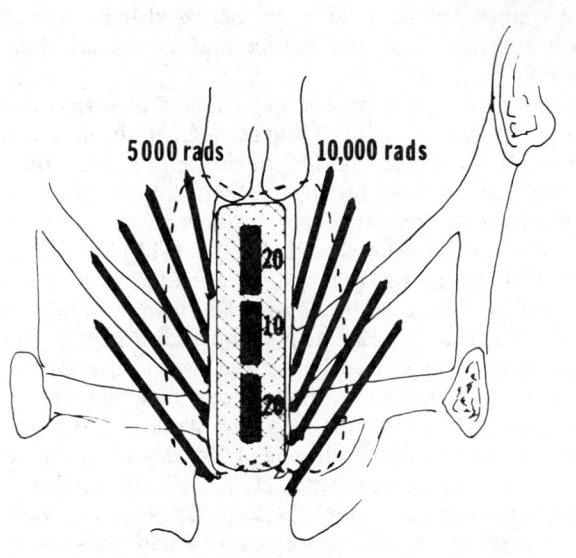

B

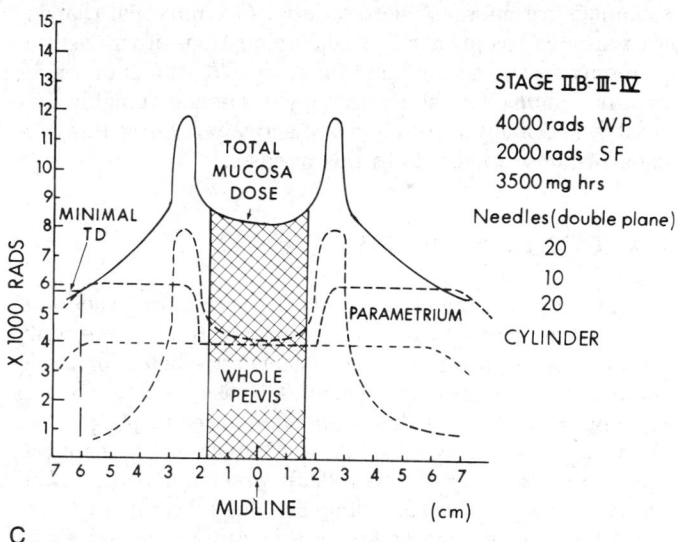

C

sary. In general, the vaginal mucosa receives an estimated 9000 to 10,000 cGy, which usually is well tolerated. The pelvic lymph nodes usually receive 5000 to 6000 cGy with whole pelvis and split fields.

TREATMENT OF CLEAR CELL CARCINOMA OF THE VAGINA

Stage I lesions of the cervix or vagina can be treated with either surgery or radiation therapy.[93,117] All other stages should be treated with radiation therapy.

Surgery for Stage I clear cell carcinoma may have the advantage of ovarian preservation and better vaginal function following skin graft although Wharton et al[117] have advocated intracavitary or transvaginal irradiation for the treatment of small tumors. They describe excellent tumor control with a functional vagina and preservation of ovarian function.

A radical hysterectomy and vaginectomy with radical lymph node dissection are necessary for vaginal clear cell carcinoma. Para-aortic nodes should be sampled before the procedure to determine whether there is lymphatic disease beyond the pelvis.

Fletcher[118] reported the results in 19 young women treated with irradiation alone (2 treated with irradiation combined with surgery), 15 of them followed for more than 2 years. Eighteen of the patients are surviving, 17 of them tumor free. One patient with an extensive lesion has a vaginal recurrence, and 1 patient died of a pulmonary embolus after removal of radium needles.

TREATMENT OF NONEPITHELIAL TUMORS OF THE VAGINA

The treatment of embryonal rhabdomyosarcoma of the vagina has undergone significant change in the past few years.

Combined treatment with chemotherapy, irradiation, and surgery has allowed many children to be treated without performing pelvic exenteration.[119,120] Survival rates of 46% to 63% have been reported using such combinations of therapy.[120,121] Sordillo et al[122] and Kinsella and Glatstein[123] have reported on the use of combinations of chemotherapy or radiation sensitizer and irradiation in adult soft tissue sarcomas. These same principles may be applicable to adult sarcomas of the vagina.

The results of surgical or irradiation therapy or both for vaginal melanoma are poor. Morrow and DiSaia[124] reported only 21% survival following radical surgery. These authors reported an 80% recurrence rate in cases managed by excisions with or without irradiation. Further studies of these patients are needed to determine optimal methods of therapy.

CHEMOTHERAPY OF VAGINAL CARCINOMA

Chemotherapy for squamous carcinoma of the vagina is no different from that outlined later in this chapter for cervical squamous carcinoma. The treatment of embryonal rhabdomyosarcoma has primarily used combinations of vincristine, actinomycin D, and cyclophosphamide. Treatment of malignant melanoma with chemotherapy has not been highly successful, and many institutions are actively investigating biologic response modifiers in this disease.

CARCINOMA OF THE CERVIX

Carcinoma of the uterine cervix is the third most frequent of the female genital cancers.[1] Although there were only 12,900 cases of invasive cervical cancer predicted for 1988, this does not include more than 50,000 cases of carcinoma in situ and several times that number of cases of preinvasive dysplasias of the cervix.[1] Of all the female genital cancers, only cervical cancer can be reliably prevented by use of an effective, inexpensive screening technique that allows detection of precancerous conditions that can be treated effectively so as to prevent the development of invasive cancer. Thus, the vast majority of deaths due to cervical cancer each year can be said to be preventable if women avail themselves of routine screening with cervical cytology.

EPIDEMIOLOGY

The peak age incidence for carcinoma of the cervix is between 48 and 55 years with the mean age 53.8 years and the median age 51.5 years.[125,126] This compares to a peak age incidence between the ages of 25 and 40 for carcinoma in situ.[126] Barber[127] reviewed data from the state of Connecticut and the Third National Cancer Survey and found that only 9% of women with invasive cancer were under age 35 whereas 53% of women with carcinoma in situ were under age 35.

Cervical cancer is more frequent in women of low socioeconomic status, women who begin sexual intercourse at a young age, women with a larger number of sexual partners, women who become pregnant at a young age, multiparous women, and prostitutes.[127-131] In contrast, carcinoma of the cervix is infrequent in nulliparous women, in those with inactive sexual lives, such as nuns, and in women married to one husband without children.[127,131,132] Cancer of the cervix is infrequent in Jewish and Moslem women, and circumcision of Jewish and Moslem men has been postulated as a cause.[133] Abou-Daoud[134] questioned the role of circumcision as a protective factor when he found an equal incidence of cervical cancer in Lebanese Moslems and Christians. Ackerman and del Regato[135] postulated genetic factors as a cause of the low incidence of cervical cancer in Jewish women. Kessler[136] has shown that the risk of cervical cancer may be increased in the wives of men who have been previously married to women who developed cervical cancer.

Chemical irritants have not been demonstrated to increase the incidence of cervical carcinoma in women, although cervical carcinoma has been induced in animals by direct application of chemical carcinogens.[137] Hormonal compounds in the form of oral contraceptives cannot be linked to an increased incidence of cervical cancer, but use of DES by pregnant women has resulted in an increased incidence of clear cell carcinoma of the cervix and vagina in their offspring.[138-140]

Recently, major attention has been directed toward the possibility of infectious agents being etiologic in the development of cervical cancer. The identification of herpes virus type 2 (HSV-2) and the finding of higher antibody titers against the virus in cervical cancer patients than in controls are suggestive of a cause and effect relationship.[141,142] Hollinshead et al[143] reported that the sera of 88% of patients with invasive cervical cancer contained antibodies to herpes virus tumor-associated antigens as compared to 11% of the sera of controls. Several authors have demonstrated that HSV-2 viruses can transform animal cells[144] or human embryonic cells[145] into malignant cells, and Wentz et al[146] produced in situ and invasive carcinoma of the cervix and vagina of mice inoculated with inactivated HSV-2. Finally, Notter et al[147] were able to demonstrate HSV-2 tumor-associated antigens in biopsies of cervical cancer using a peroxidase-antiperoxidase stain.

Meisels and Fortin[148] first demonstrated the high frequency of human papillomavirus (HPV) infection in 1976 and noted its association with dysplasias of the cervix. Kurman et al[149] studied 322 cases of cervical dysplasia and carcinoma in situ for the presence of papilloma antigen and found these proteins in over 20% of cases. Current studies would indicate that almost 50% of intraepithelial neoplasia will show evidence of HPV infection,[150,151] and viral particles have been demonstrated in invasive cervical cancer.[151] HPV types 6 and 11 are common in non-neoplastic condylomata acuminata, and HPV types 16 and 18 (and less often types 31, and 33–35) are common in cervical intraepithelial neoplasia and invasive cervical cancer. Several authors have recently found HPV infections of the penis in sexual partners of women with cervical intraepithelial neoplasia.[152,153] Krebs and Schneider[154] examined 127 male partners of women with cervical intraepithelial neoplasia and found 83 men (65%) with penile HPV lesions of which 3 had penile dysplasia.

Although definitive answers as to the exact mechanism for

the development of cervical cancer are not available, considerable insight has been obtained during the past few years. High-risk populations can be identified, and it would appear that viral infection may play an important role in the development of the disease process.

NATURAL HISTORY AND PATTERNS OF SPREAD

Squamous cell carcinoma usually arises from the squamocolumnar junction of the cervix and is preceded by cervical dysplasia and carcinoma in situ.[155,156] Petersen[154a] reported 127 patients with untreated carcinoma in situ of the cervix and described invasive carcinoma in 30% of cases by the 10th year. Clemmesen and Poulsen[157] reported a progression rate of 40% from carcinoma in situ to invasive cancer, whereas Kottmeier[157a] reported that of 31 patients with carcinoma in situ 71% developed invasive cancer within 12 years and 80% within 30 years. Although most authorities agree that dysplasias and carcinoma in situ do proceed to invasive cancer, there is less agreement on the time scale of this progression. The Walton report[158] described intervals of 1 to 20 years.

Invasive carcinoma occurs when the malignant epithelial cells break through the basement membrane and enter the stroma. Continued growth results in a visible lesion that involves progressively more of the cervical tissue. Cervical cancer spreads by direct extension into the paracervical tissue, the vagina, or the endometrium. Continued local growth will involve the pelvic side walls laterally, the bladder anteriorly, or the rectum posteriorly. Metastases occur primarily by means of the lymphatics, although blood-borne metastases do occur.

The cervix has a rich lymphatic network. Microscopic lymphatics lie beneath the squamous mucosa and surround the endocervical glands.[159] In the outer third of the cervix the lymphatics turn cephalad. In these lateral channels the cervical lymphatics are joined by vaginal lymphatics. Plentl and Friedman[159] comment on the interconnection of all of the lymphatics from the various levels of the cervix with those of the uterus and upper vagina. The lateral collecting trunks are relatively large and leave the cervix with the uterine artery and veins. The upper branches of these collecting lymphatics drain into the interiliac lymph nodes, whereas the middle branches drain into the obturator and deep hypogastric lymph nodes. The lower branches drain into the inferior gluteal and sacral lymph nodes and then into the lower aortic nodes. The interiliac, obturator, and hypogastric nodes drain into the common iliac and aortic lymph nodes.

In a review of 31 reports (more than 6,000 patients), Plentl and Friedman[159] found that the average incidence of positive lymph nodes was 15.4% in Stage I and 28.6% in Stage II. A recent series from Memorial Sloan-Kettering Cancer Center evaluated 431 patients and reported 15% positive lymph nodes in Stage IB and 22% in Stage IIA cervical cancer.[160] Table 36-6 shows the distribution of para-aortic nodal metastases reported by several authors.[161-169] As can be seen, the incidence of positive para-aortic nodes is 6% in Stage IB, 12% in Stage IIA, 19% in Stage IIB, and 29% in Stage IIIB.

Spread by hematogenous dissemination is relatively unusual in early stages of cervical cancer but increases with more advanced stages. Carlson et al[170] reported distant metastases in 4.7% of patients with Stage IB and 9.2% in Stage IIA. In Stage IIB through Stage IV the average incidence of distant metastases was 20.4%, ranging from 16.2% in Stage IIB to 24% of Stage IV.

PATHOLOGIC CHARACTERISTICS

Gross Characteristics

In situ and microinvasive cervical cancers are, in general, diagnosed by exfoliative cytology and colposcopy and do not present with gross abnormalities. The term "occult" carcinoma refers to an invasive cancer that is not clinically apparent and usually is the result of an endophytic carcinoma that develops high in the endocervix. Visible lesions are usually divided into endophytic and exophytic lesions. A variant of the endophytic type of tumor extends into and expands the endocervix so that the diameter of the corpus and cervix appear to be equal, resembling a barrel. These so-called barrel-shaped carcinomas are usually described as having transverse diameters of 6 cm or more and present special treatment problems.[171] Just as endophytic tumors can have a misleading appearance and be more extensive than they appear at first examination, exophytic tumors may appear more extensive than they actually are when examined more

TABLE 36-6. Metastases to Para-Aortic Lymph Nodes in Carcinoma of the Cervix

	Stage					
	IB	*IIA*	*IIB*	*IIIA*	*IIIB*	*IV*
Sudarsanam et al[161]	11/53 (7%)	3/31 (14%)	4/22 (18%)	2/3 (66%)	3/16 (19%)	0/3 (0)
Nelson et al[162]		5/31 (16%)			13/28 (46%)	
Piver et al[163]			6/46 (13%)		18/49 (36%)	4/7 (57%)
Wharton et al[164]	0/21 (0)	0/10 (0)	10/47 (21%)		14/42 (33%)	
Lagasse et al[165]	8/143 (5%)	4/22 (18%)	19/58 (33%)	0/3 (0)	19/61 (31%)	1/4 (25%)
Buchsbaum[166]	0/23 (0)	1/12 (7%)			7/20 (35%)	1/2 (50%)
Averette et al[167]	3/40 (8%)	1/12 (7%)	2/9 (22%)		2/20 (10%)	1/2 (50%)
Welander et al[168]			8/41 (20%)	2/6 (33%)	8/32 (25%)	4/12 (33%)
Berman et al[169]	8/158 (5%)	3/25 (12%)	40/240 (17%)	1/3 (33%)	44/177 (25%)	3/17 (18%)
Total	30/438 (6%)	13/109 (12%)	94/494 (19%)	5/15 (33%)	128/445 (29%)	14/47 (30%)

carefully. Often an exophytic tumor appears to fill the upper vagina and be connected to the cervix by a relatively small stalk with only moderate invasion into, or enlargement of, the cervix.

Microscopic Characteristics

Preinvasive cervical carcinoma is usually described by one of two different classifications, both of which are common usage. The first system divides lesions into dysplasias (mild, moderate, and severe) and carcinoma in situ. The second system uses three divisions of the term cervical intraepithelial neoplasia (CIN-1, CIN-2, and CIN-3). This precursor stage of cervical carcinoma begins with minimal morphologic changes (CIN-1 or mild dysplasia) and progresses to the point that the entire epithelium from the basement membrane to the surface is composed of malignant cells (CIN-3 or carcinoma in situ).

The vast majority of invasive carcinomas of the cervix are squamous cell carcinomas. Although many authors state that these carcinomas represent 90% or more of all cervical cancer, Regan and Ng[172] have pointed out that when rigid histologic criteria are used, only 75% to 80% are of the squamous cell type. Regan and Ng[172] have proposed that squamous carcinomas be classified as large-cell nonkeratinizing, large-cell keratinizing, and small-cell nonkeratinizing. They reported survival by cell type of 68.3% with large-cell nonkeratinizing carcinomas, 41.7% with large-cell keratinizing carcinomas, and 20% with small-cell nonkeratinizing carcinomas. Other authors have used different types of histologic grading. Wentz[173] divided these cancers into well-differentiated, moderately differentiated, and poorly differentiated carcinomas and reported differences in survival by grade. Many other terms have been used including high grade and low grade, anaplastic, and grades 1 through 4. This lack of uniformity has often made comparison of results difficult and often prohibits rational clinical protocol development that might be based on differentiation of the carcinomas.

Adenocarcinomas of the cervix arise from the endocervical columnar cells.[174] They account for 10% to 15% of cervical carcinomas,[172,174] although some authors have recently reported incidences of 16% to 34%.[175,176] This relative increase in incidence has been postulated to be due to improved detection and treatment of squamous cancers during their relatively prolonged preinvasive stage.[176] Histologically, endocervical adenocarcinoma is composed of glands formed of malignant columnar cells with enlarged, bizarre nuclei and increased mitoses. As these adenocarcinomas become less differentiated, they may lose their glandular appearance and become more solid.

Adenosquamous carcinomas of the cervix represent 2% to 5% of all cervical carcinomas[172,177] and are a mixture of malignant adenocarcinoma and malignant squamous cell carcinoma. These tumors are poorly differentiated and associated with decreased survival.[172,178] Clear cell carcinoma[178,179] glassy cell carcinoma,[180] adenoid cystic carcinoma[181] and mucoepidermoid carcinoma[182] are seen infrequently, but in general behave as poorly differentiated carcinomas. Also reported rarely as primary carcinomas arising in the cervix are malignant melanoma,[183] carcinoid,[184] sarcomas,[185] malignant lymphoma and Hodgkin's disease,[186,187] and verrucous carcinoma.[188] The last carcinoma mentioned, verrucous carcinoma, is a very well-differentiated squamous cell carcinoma that invades locally but rarely metastasizes.

CLINICAL MANIFESTATIONS

Preinvasive cervical carcinoma is detected by the Papanicolaou smear at the time of routine periodic examination and is not associated with symptoms. Any symptoms the patient might have, such as vaginal discharge, represent coexisting problems. Early invasive carcinoma can produce a vaginal discharge or vaginal bleeding (the most common type of vaginal bleeding being postcoital spotting). As the tumor of the cervix becomes more extensive, a serosanguinous or prurulent discharge is more pronounced and bleeding may become intermenstrual and more copious in quantity.

Pain is a late symptom in cervical carcinomas as are symptoms relative to the urinary tract or rectum. Dull aching pain low in the pelvis may be associated with chronic inflammation, tumor necrosis, or a combination of these factors. Low back pain or leg pain may be due to compression of lumbosacral nerves, direct involvement of lumbosacral nerve roots, pressure from a large tumor mass, or, on occasion, ureteral obstruction. Urinary frequency or urgency, hematuria, rectal tenesmus, and rectal bleeding result from direct invasion of the bladder or rectum from advanced disease.

DIAGNOSIS, CLINICAL EVALUATION, AND STAGING

Diagnosis

The purpose of periodic cytologic screening by means of the Papanicolaou smear is to prevent invasive cervical cancer. Although microinvasive and early invasive cervical cancers will be detected and this early detection is valuable in decreasing the death rate from cervical cancer, the ideal is to detect all cervical abnormalities in the premalignant stage and thus prevent invasive cervical cancer.

Papanicolaou smears are performed at the time of routine pelvic examination, and there appears to be little doubt that this technique has resulted in a decline in the mortality from cervical cancer.[189,190] The frequency with which this routine screening examination should be performed, however, is the subject of considerable debate. In 1976, the task force appointed by the Conference of Deputy Ministers of Health of Canada was reported (The Walton Report).[158] They identified two major categories of risk. The "low risk" group is made up of women who have never had a period of sexual activity during their lives, who have had a hysterectomy for nonmalignant disease, or who have reached the age of 60 after regular participation in a screening program never having had an abnormal cytologic smear. The "at risk" group is made up of women who have reached the age of 18, who are sexually active, and who do not otherwise fall into the low risk group. Within the "at risk" group is a "high risk" subgroup made up of women who have had an early onset of sexual activity with multiple partners. Largely as a result of this report, the American Cancer Society recommended that asymptomatic women 20 years of age and older and those under 20 years of age who are sexually active have cytologic screening for 2 consecutive years and at least one screening every 3 years until age 65. They further recommended that women at high risk of developing cervical carcinoma because of early age at first coitus, multiple sexual partners, and multiparity should have a yearly cytologic screening. A complete gynecologic examination should be performed when the vaginal smears are obtained.[191] The American College of Obstetricians and Gynecologists refused to accept this recommendation, however, and still recommends that cervical cytologic screening take place at the time of an annual gynecologic examination.[192]

To date, there is no clear and unified recommendation concerning periodic screening of women by cervical cytology in the United States. Although the distribution of women into risk groups seems reasonable, that distribution in practice is quite difficult. To effectively establish risk categories, one must have a detailed and reliable sexual history, and even then there is the question of whether the woman's risk status is also influenced by the sexual history of her partner (which may be even more difficult to determine accurately). Also unanswered is whether the value of annual screening is influenced by the bimanual examination and the breast examination and whether that annual examination by the gynecologist is the only periodic health screening that the woman receives.

If the cytologic smear reveals dysplastic or malignant cells, the patient should be evaluated by colposcopy and biopsy. Atypical smears due to inflammation should be managed by treating the inflammation and repeating the Papanicolaou smear. Persistent atypical smears that do not clear with treatment of infection require colposcopic evaluation and biopsy.

Colposcopy is the recommended method of evaluating an abnormal Papanicolaou smear. Using a bright light with a green filter to enhance vascular patterns and 10 to 15 power magnification, abnormal areas can be visualized and identified for biopsy with considerable accuracy. Most obstetrics and gynecology programs in the United States provide a thorough experience in this technique, and colposcopes are a relatively inexpensive piece of office equipment. Colposcopy is designed to allow properly directed biopsies; it is not a substitute for cervical biopsy and endocervical curettage. When colposcopy is inadequate in the patient with dysplastic or malignant cells on a Papanicolaou smear, cervical conization is mandatory.

Cervical conization is the removal of a cone shaped portion of tissue from the cervix that includes most or all of the transformation zone. This procedure is indicated in any patient who has dysplastic or malignant cells on cervical cytology, inadequate colposcopy, and no grossly visible lesion on the cervix. It is also indicated in patients with microinvasive cancer and in patients where the depth of invasion cannot be determined by biopsy. A cone biopsy should not be performed on a patient with a visible lesion of the cervix unless a cervical biopsy of the area fails to make the diagnosis of invasive cancer.

As mentioned above, any grossly visible cervical lesion should be biopsied. The performance of a Papanicolaou smear or colposcopy, or both, does not substitute for cervical biopsy. The inflammation that accompanies many cervical carcinomas can be misleading on both colposcopic examination and on the Papanicolaou smear, resulting in false negative evaluation.

Clinical Evaluation

The standard clinical evaluation for patients with cervical carcinoma includes examination by inspection and palpation (under anesthesia, if necessary), biochemical profile to include evaluation of liver and renal functions, chest radiograph, cytoscopy, proctosigmoidoscopy, and intravenous pyelography. In patients with advanced stage or in all patients over age 40, a barium enema should be obtained. CT scan can be helpful in evaluating retroperitoneal lymph nodes or in treatment planning of bulky lesions for irradiation. The reliability of this method of evaluation of lymph nodes has been reported in nonsurgically staged patients[193] and is currently under investigation in patients who are undergoing surgical staging by the GOG. Lymphangiograms have been used in the nonsurgical evaluation of cervical cancer and may be helpful when clearly positive. Piver and Chung[194] reported 98% accuracy by biopsy or laparotomy in patients with a positive lymphangiogram but a 20% false negative rate in those studies reported as negative. MRI is being evaluated and may prove to be helpful. Other symptoms may also require evaluation with appropriate studies.

Clinical Staging of Cervical Carcinoma

The staging of cervical carcinoma is a clinical staging classification that consists of physical examination (inspection, palpation, and biopsy), laboratory studies, and roentgenographic evaluation as outlined above. Surgical staging, if performed, does not alter the official stage of the patient for the purpose of reporting treatment results. Whenever possible, cervical cancer should be staged as part of a multidisciplinary effort involving the gynecologist, radiation therapist, and medical oncologist. The staging examination can usually be performed adequately in the outpatient setting, but if there is significant question about the adequacy of the examination or the examination is perceived not to be adequate, examination under anesthesia should be performed.

In 1985 the Oncology Committee of the FIGO made changes in the FIGO classification of cervical carcinoma. Although these changes will not officially be published until the 20th annual report in 1988, FIGO allowed publication of the changes in early 1987.[195] The new FIGO classification is listed in Table 36-7. As can be seen, the changes in the staging system are limited to Stage I. Stage IA, which in the 19th report published in 1985 was described as "microinvasive carcinoma (early stromal invasion)," is now divided into two categories. Stage IA$_1$ is defined as "preclinical carcinomas of the cervix, that is, those diagnosed only by microscopy," and should be limited to the very earliest forms of microinvasion, including cases in which invasion can be seen but the area of invasion is too small for measurement. Stage IA$_2$ are "lesions detected microscopically that can be mea-

TABLE 36-7. Staging of Invasive Carcinoma of the Uterine Cervix Adopted in 1987 by the International Federation of Gynecology and Obstetrics (FIGO)

Stage 0	Carcinoma in situ, intraepithelial carcinoma Cases of Stage 0 should not be included in any therapeutic statistics for invasive carcinoma
Stage I	The carcinoma is strictly confined to the cervix (extension to the corpus should be disregarded)
Stage IA1	Preclinical carcinomas of the cervix, that is, those diagnosed only by microscopy
Stage IA2	Lesions detected microscopically that can be measured. The upper limit of the measurement should not show a depth of invasion of more than 5 mm taken from the base of the epithelium, either surface or glandular, from which it originates, and a second dimension, the horizontal spread, must not exceed 7 mm. Larger lesions should be staged as IB
Stage IB	Lesions of greater dimensions than Stage IA2 whether seen clinically or not. Preformed space involvement should not alter the staging but should be specifically recorded so as to determine whether it should affect treatment decisions in the future
Stage II	The carcinoma extends beyond the cervix, but has not extended on to the pelvic wall. The carcinoma involves the vagina but not the lower third
Stage IIA	No obvious parametrial involvement
Stage IIB	Obvious parametrial involvement
Stage III	The carcinoma has extended to the pelvic wall. On rectal examination there is no cancer-free space between the tumor and the pelvic wall The tumor involves the lower third of the vagina All cases with a hydronephrosis or nonfunctioning kidney should be included, unless they are known to be due to other cause
Stage IIIA	Extension on to the pelvic wall
Stage IIIB	Extension on to the pelvic wall and hydronephrosis or nonfunctioning kidney
Stage IV	The carcinoma has extended beyond the true pelvis or has clinically involved the mucosa of the bladder or rectum. A bullous edema as such does not permit a case to be allotted to Stage IV
Stage IVA	Spread of the growth to adjacent organs
Stage IVB	Spread to distant organs

sured." The upper limit of the measurement should not show a depth of invasion of more than 5 mm taken from the base of the epithelium (either surface or glandular) from which it originates, and a second dimension, the horizontal spread, should not exceed 7 mm. Larger lesions should be staged as IB. Stage IB is now defined as "lesions of greater dimensions than Stage IA$_2$ whether seen clinically or not." Performed space involvement should not alter the staging but should be specifically recorded to determine whether it might affect treatment decisions in the future. The remainder of the staging classification is unchanged.

The impact of these changes on the staging system is not clear at this time since most authorities in the United States use "less than 3 mm of invasion without lymphovascular invasion" as the definition of Stage IA cervical carcinoma. It appears doubtful at this time that clinical practice patterns will be changed by this new classification, and its effect on reporting of results cannot be defined.

Surgical Staging of Cervical Carcinoma

In the early 1970s, Averette et al[167,196] and Nelson et al[162] introduced the concept of pretreatment surgical staging of cervical carcinoma. Averette et al[167] reported a high lack of correlation between clinical staging and the results of surgical exploration with reported errors of 26% in Stage IB, 45% in Stage IIA, 60% in Stage IIB, 66% in Stage IIIA, and 95% in Stage IIIB. Both authors demonstrated the relatively high frequency of para-aortic nodal metastases in cervical carcinoma, particularly in more advanced stages. Table 36-6 summarizes the results of several reports of positive para-aortic lymph nodes in cervical cancer.

Wharton et al[164] and Piver and Barlow[163] reported on the treatment of patients with positive para-aortic nodes with extended field radiotherapy. Wharton et al[164] gave 5500 cGy to the para-aortic area and noted a 27% serious complication rate with a 13% treatment related mortality rate. Piver and Barlow[163] used 6000 cGy and noted a similar high complication rate. Berman et al[197] reported fewer intestinal complications using a retroperitonial approach to the para-aortic lymph nodes, and Welander et al,[168] using a transperitoneal approach to the para-aortic lymph nodes, reported that a 4400 cGy dose to the para-aortics was not associated with a high complication rate.

Survival in patients with positive para-aortic lymph nodes has been addressed by several authors and is summarized in Table 36-8. The average disease-free survival is approximately 18%. Welander et al[168] pointed out that because the maximum tolerated para-aortic irradiation appears to be in the range of 4400 to 4500 cGy, it is unlikely that patients with more than microscopic disease will be cured by extended field irradiation. They also pointed out that because many patients with positive para-aortic lymph nodes have bulky local disease, control of para-aortic disease may not benefit survival because of inability to control the local disease. Also, spread to para-aortic lymph nodes may be a sign only of systemic disease. Buchsbaum[166] reported that 34.8% of patients with positive para-aortic lymph nodes had metastatic cancer in the scalene lymph nodes, and Welander et al[168] found that 54.8% of patients with positive para-aortic lymph nodes developed distant metastases as compared to 25% of a similar group of patients with negative para-aortic lymph nodes.

The place of pretreatment surgical staging in cervical carcinoma of the cervix remains unclear. Several large institutions across the United States routinely perform such procedures as prospective protocols and the GOG has used pretreatment laparotomy as an integral part of many of their advanced cervix protocols. Certainly the operation has a place in a research setting. Whether data being accumulated

TABLE 36-8. Survival in Cervical Carcinoma Patients with Positive Para-Aortic Lymph Nodes

Author	Year Published	Survival (%)	Duration of Survival Analysis (yr)
Wharton et al[164]	1977	14.2	2
Piver and Barlow[163]	1977	12.5	
Nelson et al[162]	1977	13	4
Buchsbaum[166]	1979	18.8	2
Welander et al[168]	1981	25.8	2+
Berman et al[169]	1984	25	3
Mean		18.2	

in these studies will show enough survival benefit to recommend the procedure routinely remains to be elucidated.

PROGNOSTIC FACTORS IN CERVICAL CANCER

Prognosis in cervical cancer is worse with advancing stage of disease, which in general represents increasing tumor bulk or increasing extent of tumor involvement of adjacent or distant organs. In early stage disease, however, survival appears to be influenced by multiple factors. The accurate identification of these risk factors has been addressed by several authors. Patients with Stages IB and IIA carcinoma treated by radical hysterectomy and pelvic lymphadenectomy have survival rates of 82% to 92% when there are no metastases to pelvic lymph nodes, compared to survival rates of 45% to 61% in patients with positive lymph nodes (Table 36-9). The incidence of positive lymph nodes in these patients has, in turn, been related to tumor diameter greater than 4 cm,[194,198,208] lymphovascular invasion,[198,208,209] deep invasion into the cervical stroma,[198,210,211] and histologic grade.[198,211] At least two of these authors also looked at recurrence in patients who had negative lymph nodes.[198,211] Fuller et al[198] found that after stratifying for nodal metastases, size of the primary tumor, depth of invasion into the cervix, and histologic grade were associated with an increased incidence of recurrence. They also noted an increased incidence of recurrence in patients who had adenocarcinoma as compared to squamous histology, even though patients with adenocarcinoma did not have an increased incidence of positive lymph nodes. Burke et al[211] found adenomatous cell type and lymphovascular invasion to place patients with negative lymph nodes at increased risk. Figge and Tamimi[212] noted an increased recurrence rate in patients with adenocarcinoma, but in their series this was only in association with lymphovascular space involvement and positive lymph nodes. Several authors have reported increased recurrence rates and decreased survival as the number of metastatic lymph nodes or the number of metastases in lymph node groups increase.[194,199,213]

In patients managed by radiotherapy, several authors have reported lower survival and an increased incidence of pelvic recurrences in patients with anemia.[214,215] Jenkin and Stryker[216] found more pelvic recurrences and complications in patients with hypertension, whereas Van Herik[217] found decreased survival when patients had oral temperatures over 100° F. Although some patients with elevated temperatures had pelvic infection, over half of them had no specific etiologic factor for the temperature elevation.

Prempree et al[218] reported an increased incidence of poorly differentiated tumors and decreased survival in patients with cervical cancer who were younger than 35 years of age. Other authors, however, have not found age at onset of the disease to affect survival.[219,220]

TREATMENT OF CERVICAL CARCINOMA

General Principles of Management

The primary method of therapy for preinvasive (Stage 0) and microinvasive (Stages IA$_1$ and IA$_2$) carcinoma of the cervix is surgery. Only rarely is there a place for radiation therapy in the management of such early disease. Stages IB and IIA carcinoma of the cervix can be managed equally effectively by either radical surgery or irradiation therapy.[221] There is no purpose in comparing the efficacy of these two treatment modalities because there has been, and should be, definite selection of patients in that some patients are better managed surgically whereas others will benefit most from primary therapy with irradiation. The optimum approach is that all patients be treated in institutions that have personnel

TABLE 36-9. Influence of Positive Pelvic Lymph Nodes on Survival in Stages IB and IIA Carcinoma of the Cervix

	Percent Survival	
	Positive Lymph Nodes	Negative Lymph Nodes
Piver and Chung (1975)[194]	45	82
Fuller et al (1987)[198]	50	85
Burghardt et al (1987)[199]	60.9	88.1
Martimbeau et al (1982)[200]	53	92
Mean	52.2	86.8

and equipment suitable for either type of therapy and that selection of therapy be a joint decision among the surgeon, the radiation oncologist, and the patient. Only in this setting will the very best results be obtained for all patients.

Patients with Stage IIB through Stage IVA are usually managed by radiotherapy. Although the rare patient with IVA carcinoma of the cervix may be a candidate for primary pelvic exenteration, such patients are usually managed by radiotherapy. Patients with IVB cervical carcinoma are usually managed by combinations of chemotherapy and irradiation. Recently, there have been reports of Phases I and II trials of concomitant chemotherapy and irradiation in patients with locally advanced disease. Although this is an intriguing concept, its usefulness is uncertain as yet.

Selected types of cervical carcinoma may be managed by combinations of surgery and irradiation. Those specific areas will be discussed later in this chapter.

Stage 0 (Carcinoma in situ)

Although the standard therapy for cervical intraepithelial neoplasia (CIN), grade 3 (severe dysplasia and carcinoma in situ) is conization of the cervix, selected patients can be managed by outpatient therapy using either cryotherapy or laser ablation. For these patients to be candidates for such therapy, their lesions should be entirely visible by colposcopy, the squamocolumnar junction must be visible, the endocervical curettage must be negative, and the colposcopically directed biopsy must be at least as severe as the cytologic smear. Some authorities also require that the lesion occupy no more than one quadrant of the cervix and there be no gland involvement. To be a candidate for outpatient therapy, the patient must be reliable and agree to long-term follow-up. Townsend et al[222] reviewed cases of invasive carcinoma following outpatient therapy and found that in most cases in which invasive cancer developed, there had been obvious deviation from above criteria. Similar findings were reported by Sevin et al.[223]

In the past, abdominal or vaginal hysterectomy has been considered the treatment of choice for CIN-3. Based on the evidence now available in the literature, this is no longer justified. In an extensive review of the literature, Coppleson[224] found that only 18 of 5,442 women (0.3%) treated for carcinoma in situ by conization of the cervix subsequently developed overt invasive cancer. This compared to 38 of 8,995 women (0.4%) who developed invasive carcinoma of the vagina after hysterectomy for carcinoma in situ. Based on these results, routine hysterectomy for CIN-3 cannot be recommended. Patients who do not desire further childbearing and have intraepithelial neoplasia that involves the margins of the cone biopsy may be treated by hysterectomy. Hysterectomy can also be indicated in patients with other gynecologic disorders that require removal of the uterus. It is the rare patient desirous of further childbearing who will ever require hysterectomy for preinvasive cancer.

Stage IA Carcinoma of the Cervix

In the 1987 classification of cervical carcinoma by FIGO, microinvasive carcinoma is divided into IA_1 and IA_2 (see Table 36-7). Stage IA_1 (microinvasive carcinoma that is so small it cannot be measured) should be treated by abdominal or vaginal hysterectomy in the healthy patient who is not desirous of further childbearing. Women who desire preservation of fertility or who are poor surgical risks can be managed by conization and followed closely, providing the cone margins are free of disease.

The proper management of Stage IA_2 is less clear. Averette et al[225] found no cases with positive lymph nodes if invasion was less than 1 mm without lymphovascular invasion but reported a 3.5% incidence of positive nodes in the literature if invasion extended to 5 mm. Simon et al[226] found no metastases to lymph nodes in 43 patients with invasion less than 3 mm and 3.9% positive lymph nodes in 26 patients with invasion of 3.1 to 5 mm. These same authors reviewed the literature and reported 8% nodal metastases in patients with invasion of 3 to 5 mm. In addition to depth of invasion, several authors have reported an increased incidence of nodal metastases if there was lymphovascular space invasion.[227,228] Based on these results, most authorities in the United States recommend abdominal or vaginal hysterectomy for Stage IA cervical cancer if invasion is less than 3 mm and there is no lymphovascular space involvement. Cervical carcinoma with invasion of more than 3 mm or in which there is lymphovascular invasion is managed in the same way as Stage IB. The influence of volume of invasive cancer as a criteria for planning therapy has been recommended by Burghardt.[227,232] Because such measurements are now part of the new FIGO classification, further data may be available in the future.

Patients with Stage IA may also be treated with intracavitary irradiation. In 32 patients with microinvasive carcinoma treated at Washington University, 18 of whom received intracavitary therapy alone, no local or regional failures occurred, and the corrected 5-year survival (for intercurrent disease) was 100%.

Hamberger et al[229] reported on 151 patients with Stage IA or IB lesions less than 1 cm in diameter treated with intracavitary therapy alone. No failures were noted in 41 patients with Stage IA, and only 4 failures in 93 (4%) were seen in patients with small volume Stage IB carcinoma. However, of 17 patients with more advanced Stage IB lesions, 3 patients (18%) treated with intracavitary therapy alone had regional failures.

Stages IB and IIA Carcinoma of the Cervix

Stages IB and IIA cervical carcinoma can be managed equally effectively by either radical hysterectomy and pelvic lymphadenectomy or full pelvic irradiation.[221] Surgical therapy is preferred by some because ovarian function is preserved in young women, the vagina is usually more pliable than when irradiation is used, overall treatment time is shorter, and long-term radiation complications in pelvic tissues are avoided. Other reasons for selection of surgery are concomitant inflammatory gastrointestinal disease, pelvic inflammatory disease, presence of an adnexal mass, and pregnancy. Radiation therapy has the advantages that it avoids major intraoperative and postoperative surgical complications, the patient can receive most of the therapy as an outpatient, and

TABLE 36-10. Survival Rates for Stages I and II Carcinoma of the Cervix Treated by Radical Hysterectomy and Pelvic Lymphadenectomy

Author	Stage	No. of Patients	Survivors*	Survival (%)
Blaikley et al[201]	IB	98	64	65.5
	IB and IIA	161	96	50.8
Brunschwig and Barber[202]	IB (A)	173	141	81.5
	IB and IIA			
	(B)†	308	231	76.0
Christensen et al[203]	IB	168	137	82.7
	IB and IIA	219	168	77.0
Ketcham et al[204]	IB	28	Actuarial	86.0
	IB and IIA	42		87.0
Liu and Meigs[205]	IB	116	91	78.4
	IB and IIA	165	119	72.1
Masterson[206]	IB	120	105	87.5
	IB and IIA	150	124	82.5
Park et al[207]	IB	126	Actuarial	91.0
Average	IB			81.9
	IB and IIA			74.2

Modified from Hoskins WJ, Ford JH Jr, Lutz MH, et al: Radical hysterectomy and pelvic lymphadenectomy for the management of early invasive carcinoma of the cervix. Gynecol Oncol 4:278, 1976.
* Patients dead of intercurrent disease were included with survivors when data were available.
† Surgical and pathologic classification.

it is suitable for virtually any patient. Several authors[207,230,231] have reported noncontrolled studies that demonstrate that both methods are equally effective therapy for Stages IB and IIA cervical cancer. Newton[233] and Roddick and Greenlow[234] have reported similar survival and complication rates in Stages IB and IIA cervical cancer when patients were prospectively randomized to either radiation therapy or radical hysterectomy. The results of a literature review that compared the two modalities were reported by Hoskins et al[221] and are presented in Tables 36-10 and 36-11.

Volterrani and Lombari[242] reported a 5-year survival rate of 82.6% in 23 patients with occult Stage IB carcinoma of the cervix treated with intracavitary radium only (^{226}Ra application using a derivation from the Paris method to deliver 7500 mgh). However, in Stage IB the 5-year survival rate was only 65.8%, in Stage II 50%, and in Stage III 29.8%. The results are substantially inferior to those obtained with a combination of intracavitary and external irradiation. It is obvious that intracavitary therapy alone is grossly inadequate to effectively irradiate the larger primary tumors, including the

TABLE 36-11. Five-Year Survival Rates of Patients with Stages I and II Carcinoma of the Cervix Treated by Radiotherapy

Author	Stage	No. of Patients	Survivors*	Survival (%)
Blaikley et al[201]	I	183	123	67.2
	I and II	551	296	53.7
Dickson[235]	IB	348	249	71.6
	IB and IIA	983	598	60.0
Fletcher[236]	IB	549	Actuarial	91.5
	IB and IIA	973		83.5
Kline et al[237]	IB	45	37	81.4
	IB and IIA	64	47	70.5
Kottmeier[238]	IB	611	547	89.5
	IB and IIA	1576	1244	78.9
Muirhead and Green[239]	I	194	152	78.0
	I and II	306	208	68.0
Perez et al[240]	IB	312	Actuarial	87.0
	IIA	98	NED	73.0
Wall et al[241]	I	101	87	86.4
	I and II	208	153	73.5
Average	I			83.5
	I and II			75.6

Modified from Hoskins WJ, Ford JH Jr, Lutz MH, et al: Radical hysterectomy and pelvic lymphadenectomy for the management of early invasive carcinoma of the cervix. Gynecol Oncol 4:278, 1976.
* Patients dead of intercurrent disease were included with survivors when data were available.

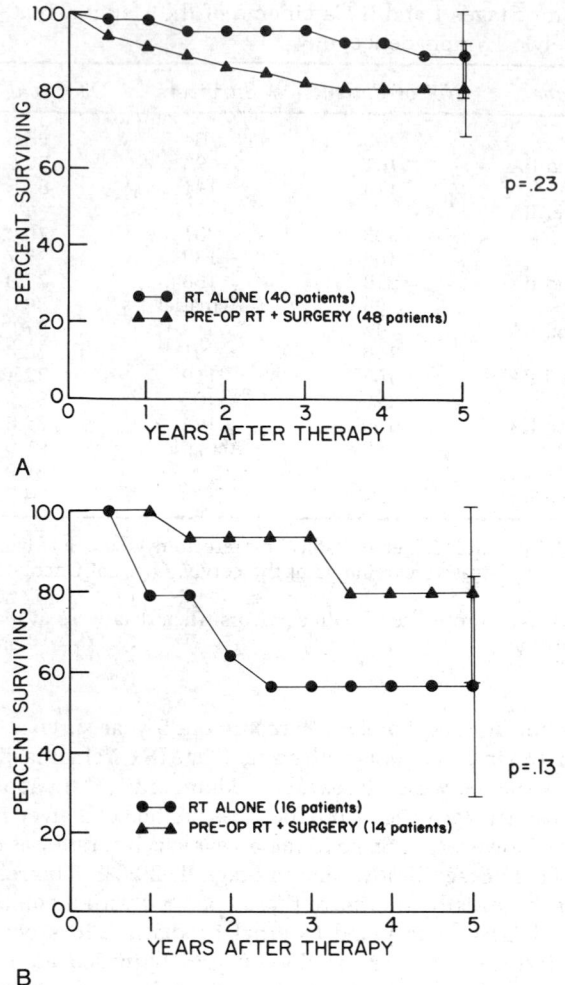

FIG. 36-6. A, B. NED actuarial survival in patients with Stage IB (**A**) or IIA (**B**) carcinoma of the uterine cervix treated with either irradiation alone (*solid circles*) or a combination of low dose preoperative irradiation and surgery (*solid triangles*). Randomized study, 1966–1979. Difference in survival is not statistically significant. (Perez CA, Camel HM, Kao MS, et al: Randomized study of preoperative radiation and surgery or irradiation alone in the treatment of stage IB and IIA carcinoma of the uterine cervix: Final report. Gynecol Oncol 27:129, 1987)

barrel-shaped lesions as well as any parametrial extension. Unfortunately, the authors did not report the exact location of the failures.

Van Nagell et al,[243] after radical hysterectomy or irradiation for Stage IB disease, found that the recurrence rate was 5% for tumors less than 2 cm in diameter treated with either modality. In lesions 2 to 5 cm in diameter, the failure rate was 24% for surgery but only 11% for radiation. Kielbinska et al,[244] in a long-term follow-up of 792 women treated by irradiation and 789 women treated with hysterectomy and irradiation for Stage I cervical carcinoma, found no difference in survival, general health, incidence of recurrent carcinoma, or appearances of second primary malignancies. Perez et al[245] have recently reported a randomized trial of preoperative irradiation and radical hysterectomy versus ir-

radiation alone in Stage IB and Stage IIA cervical cancer (Fig. 36-6).

Bulky endocervical carcinoma (barrel-shaped cervix) has been reported to have a higher incidence of central recurrence, pelvic and para-aortic node metastases, and distant metastases.[246] Because of the difficulty of obtaining central control of these large lesions, higher doses of irradiation to the central pelvis or a surgical procedure to remove the uterus or both have been advocated.[247] Currently, the GOG is evaluating the benefit of postirradiation hysterectomy in such patients in a prospective, randomized trial.

The use of irradiation for patients with positive lymph nodes following radical hysterectomy is controversial. In a panel report summarizing the experience at several institutions in the United States, Morrow[248] reported no consistent practice and no evidence of benefit from such therapy. Recently, investigators from the Memorial Sloan-Kettering Cancer Center reported improved survival in patients with nodal metastases at radical hysterectomy when they were treated postoperatively with a combination of whole pelvis irradiation and chemotherapy.[249]

Stages IIB, III, and IV Carcinoma of the Cervix

The treatment of cervical cancer more advanced than Stage IIA is irradiation. Isolated cases of Stage IVA cervical cancer with involvement of the bladder or rectum without pelvic sidewall involvement can be treated by primary pelvic exenteration, but the better choice of therapy, even in these patients, is primary irradiation.

In Stage IIB the 5-year survival rate is 60% to 65% and practically all patients are treated with irradiation alone. Occasionally a conservative hysterectomy is performed after high-dose preoperative irradiation in patients with a barrel-shaped cervix and limited medial parametrial infiltration that regresses completely 4 to 6 weeks after completion of irradiation.

In Stage IIIB, the 5-year survival rates range from 25% to 48%. This may be related to the socioeconomic status of the patients, extent of the disease, technique of irradiation, and dose delivered to the parametrium. Johns[250] reported better pelvic tumor control and survival and fewer complications in a group of 65 patients with Stages IIB and III cervical carcinoma treated with 23 MV photons in comparison with 61 patients treated with ^{60}Co external irradiation and intracavitary insertions (Fig. 36-7).

Interstitial parametrial implants have been used to supplement standard external and intracavitary techniques. Prempree[251] reported a 96% local tumor control rate and a 61% 5-year disease-free survival rate in 23 patients with an intact uterus and Stage IIIB carcinoma of the cervix treated with a combination of external irradiation and intracavitary and interstitial implants to the parametrium. Likewise, he described a 23% local failure rate and a 69% 5-year survival rate in 26 patients with similar stage carcinoma of the cervix treated in the same manner but on whom the uterine cavity could not be probed or was absent.

Aristizabel et al[252] described the treatment of 21 patients with locally advanced invasive carcinoma of the uterine cervix treated with transperineal interstitial implants using a

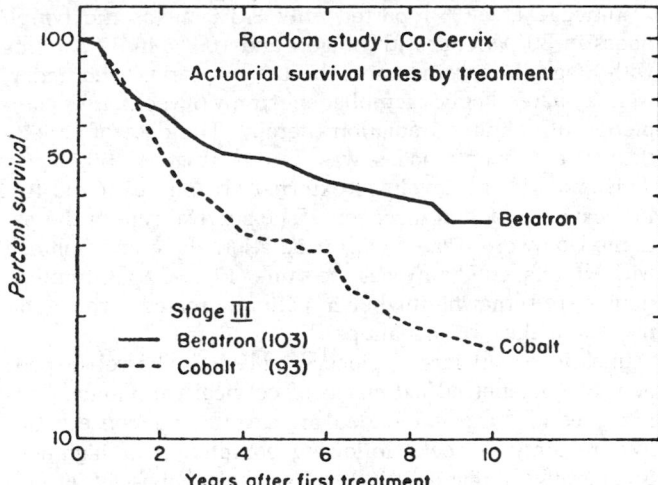

FIG. 36-7. Survival curves for patients with Stage III carcinoma of the uterine cervix on a randomized treatment study with either betatron or cobalt-60 external beams in addition to intracavitary insertion (unpublished data). (Johns HE: Optimization of energy and equipment. In Kramer S, Suntharalingam N, Zinniger GF [eds]: High Energy Photons and Electronics: Clinical Applications in Cancer Management, p 333. New York, John Wiley and Sons, 1976)

Maruyama and Muir[254] have used Californium-252 (^{252}Cf) neutron brachytherapy in conjunction with fractionated external irradiation to treat carcinoma of the uterine cervix. They reported on 41 patients with Stage IB treated with 4000 to 5000 cGy to the whole pelvis followed by 500 to 1500 cGy boost dose to the lateral pelvic wall. Cs neutron-252 therapy was usually delivered in a single intracavitary insertion in about 8 hours. Nearly total tumor clearance was achieved in more than 90% of the patients by the completion of therapy, only a small group exhibiting a slow clearance pattern.

When brachytherapy procedures cannot be performed because of medical reasons or unusual anatomical configuration of the pelvis or the tumor (*i.e.*, extensive lesion and inability to identify the cervical canal), higher doses of external irradiation alone may be used. Castro et al[255] reported results in 118 patients with invasive cervical carcinoma treated with 5000 to 6000 cGy to the whole pelvis (four-field box technique) and additional doses to residual tumor with reduced AP-PA portals to complete 7000 cGy tumor dose. With doses below 5000 cGy, no pelvic tumor control was obtained in 32 patients, but disease control and survival were significantly enhanced with higher doses. Complications increased with higher doses.

specially designed plastic template. With a mean follow-up of 26 months, local tumor control was reported in 18 of the patients (85%). Seven patients (33%) developed grade 2 or 3 complications, which included vesicovaginal (1 patient), rectovaginal (1 patient), or both fistulae (1 patient). Three patients developed severe radiation proctitis or cystitis, or both (one each).

Martinez et al,[253] using a special applicator consisting of two acrylic cylinders, a template with an array of holes that serve as guides to localize the trocars, and a cover plate, treated 37 patients with advanced or recurrent carcinoma of the cervix and 26 with vaginal-urethral tumors. They reported six local failures in the patients with cervical lesions and five in the group with vaginal-urethral tumors. The overall complication rate was 5.1%.

Combinations of Irradiation and Surgery in Carcinoma of the Cervix

The results of several series are similar to those obtained with irradiation alone. Perez et al[245] reported on a prospectively randomized study of 118 selected patients with Stages IB and IIA carcinoma of the uterine cervix. All patients were followed for a minimum of 5 years or until death. Patients were randomly assigned to be treated with irradiation alone (as described previously) or with irradiation and surgery (2000 cGy to the whole pelvis and one intracavitary insertion for 5000–6000 mgh followed by a radical hysterectomy with pelvic lymphadenectomy 26 weeks later). The tumor-free actuarial 5-year survival rate for 40 Stage IB patients treated with irradiation alone was 80% and for 48 patients treated with preoperative irradiation and surgery was 82%

TABLE 36-12. Carcinoma of the Uterine Cervix, Stages IB and IIA: Percentage of Metastatic Pelvic Lymph Nodes and Dose of Irradiation Delivered to Lymph Nodes

Author	Stage IB		Stage IIA		Estimated Dose (cGy) to Nodes
	Surgery Alone	Preoperative XRT	Surgery Alone	Preoperative XRT	
Christensen[203]	29/167 (17.4%)		27/104 (26%)		0
Morley[257]	18/143 (12.6%)				0
Morton[258]	9/38 (23.7%)	4/32 (12.5%)			1800
Sweeney and Douglas[259]		5/39 (13%)		9/54 (17%)	3500
Rampone[260]		81/137 (15%)			2000
Decker[261]		5/38 (13.2%)		11/45 (24.4%)	4000
Quigley[262]		13/136 (9.6%)			1800
Parker[263]	15/95 (16%)	6/73 (8%)	7/16 (44%)	20/71 (28%)	Not stated
Gray[264]	5/44 (11.4%)	3/58 (5.2%)	6/17 (35.3%)	Inc. with I	4500
Perez[265]		2/43 (4.6%)		2/24 (8.3%)	3000–4000
Perez[265]	0/32 (0)				4001–5000
Rutledge[266]		1/30 (3.3%)		4/39 (10.3%)	5000

Modified from Perez CA, Breaux S, Askin F, et al: Irradiation alone or in combination with surgery in Stage IB and IIA carcinoma of the uterine cervix. A non-randomized comparison. Cancer 43:1062, 1979.

(p = 0.23). In 16 patients with Stage IIA, actuarial tumor-free survival was 56% with irradiation alone and 79% in 14 patients treated with irradiation and surgery (p = 0.13). In the patients with Stage IB treated with irradiation alone, the pelvic failure rate was 2.5% and distant metastases 7.5%. In the preoperative irradiation-surgery group, the pelvic failure rate was 12.5% and distant metastases 4.2%. In Stage IIA, patients receiving radiotherapy alone had a pelvic failure rate of 6.3%, combined pelvic recurrence with distant metastases of 18.8%, and distant metastases alone of 12.5%. The incidence of grade 2 to 3 complications in the patients receiving radiation therapy alone was 13.8% (two vesicovaginal fistulae, one rectovaginal fistula, and one rectal stricture). In the patients treated with preoperative irradiation and surgery, 11% developed grade 2 to 3 complications (one rectal stricture, one severe proctitis, one small bowel obstruction, and three ureteral strictures).

Einhorn et al[256] in a nonrandomized study reported better survival in 49 patients with Stage IB using a combination of surgery and irradiation (100% at 5 years) in comparison with 64 patients treated with irradiation alone (81% at 5 years). No difference was observed in 25 patients with Stage IIA treated with combined therapy and 40 treated with irradiation alone (about 75% 5-year survival rate). Patients with metastatic lymph nodes have survival rates that are approximately 50% of those with negative nodes.

The dose of irradiation delivered to the lymph nodes, the time of the operation, and the pathologic examination of the specimens are critical in determining the presence of postirradiation residual tumor (Table 36-12). Rampone et al[260] reported a 15% incidence of metastatic lymph nodes in a group of 537 patients with Stage IB treated with two preoperative intracavitary insertions (total of 6000 mgh), which delivered 1500 cGy to the pelvic lymph nodes. All patients with positive nodes in the operative specimen were given postoperative external radiation to the pelvis. The 5-year survival rate was 92.9% for 456 patients with negative nodes in contrast to 52% in 81 patients with positive nodes.

Rutledge et al[266] reported only 3.3% metastatic lymph nodes in 30 patients with Stage I and 10.3% in 39 patients with Stage IIA carcinoma of the uterine cervix who underwent a bilateral pelvic lymphadenectomy 6 weeks after completion of definitive radiation therapy. The dose of irradiation to the lymph nodes was in the range of 5000 cGy delivered with megavoltage external photon beam and two intracavitary radium insertions. The survival rate in the patients who were treated with irradiation alone or combined with lymphadenectomy was the same (Fig. 36-8). Complications were somewhat higher in patients treated with combinations of the two modalities.

In patients with large endocervical lesions (barrel-shaped) or with endometrial extension of cervical carcinoma, Durrance et al[267] recommended an extrafascial conservative hysterectomy 6 weeks following completion of high-dose preoperative radiation (2000 cGy whole pelvis, 3000 cGy split fields, and one intracavitary insertion of 6000 mgh). Perez et al[268] reported that in patients with primary carcinoma of the uterine cervix who have endometrial stromal invasion of tumor only in the curettings, the addition of a hysterectomy did not improve the survival since most of the patients failed because of distant dissemination. Stage IVB cancer is managed by combinations of irradiation and chemotherapy.

RADIATION THERAPY TECHNIQUES

The application of radium therapy in the treatment of carcinoma of the cervix was first presented in 1913 at the Congress at Halle. Despite a slower regression after irradiation, reflecting cellular kinetics and slow growth, no difference in tumor control or survival has been observed in adenocarcinomas when compared with epidermoid carcinoma.[268,269] Because of the predilection for endocervical involvement in adenocarcinoma, a combination of irradiation and conservative hysterectomy has been advocated.[231,271]

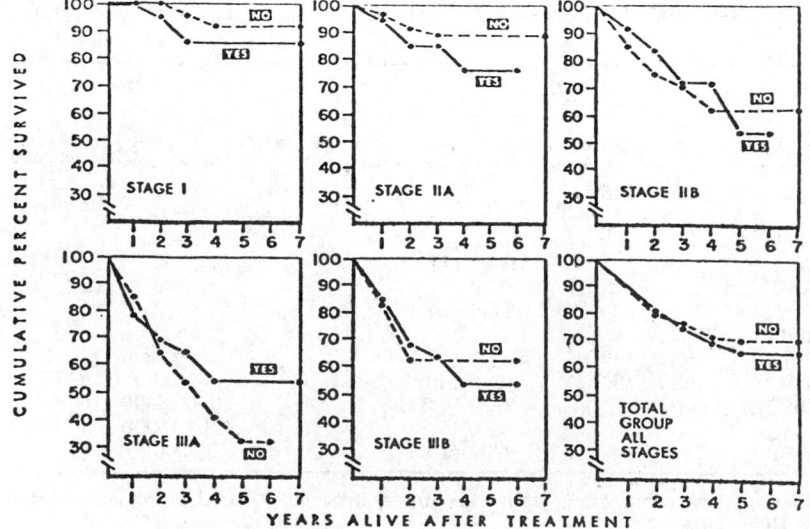

FIG. 36-8. Survival curves of patients treated for squamous cell carcinoma of the cervix, Stages I, IIA, IIB, IIIA, IIIB, and all stages combined. Patients who had lymphadenectomy after definitive irradiation to their treatment are represented by solid line curves. The broken line curves are for patients who had radiation treatment only. (Rutledge FM, Fletcher GM, Macdonald EJ: Pelvic lymphadenectomy as an adjunct to radiation therapy in treatment for cancer of the cervix. Am J Roentgenol Radium Ther Nucl Med 106:831, 1969)

External Irradiation

External irradiation is used to treat the whole pelvis and the parametria including the common iliac lymph nodes, whereas the central disease (cervix, vagina, and medial parametria) is primarily irradiated with intracavitary sources. External pelvic irradiation is delivered before intracavitary insertions in patients with the following:

1. Bulky cervical lesions, to improve the geometry of the intracavitary application
2. Exophytic easily bleeding tumors
3. Tumors with necrosis or infection.

Volume

In the treatment of invasive carcinoma of the uterine cervix, it is critical to deliver adequate doses of irradiation to the pelvic lymph nodes. For Stage IB carcinoma, 15 × 15 cm portals (at the surface of the patient) are sufficient. For patients with IIA-B, III, and IVA carcinoma, somewhat larger portals, 18 × 15 cm, are required to cover all of the common iliac nodes in addition to the cephalad half of the vagina (Fig. 36-9). A 2 cm margin lateral to the bony pelvis is sufficient. If there is no vaginal extension, the lower margin of the port is at the inferior border of the obturator foramen. When there is vaginal involvement, the entire length of this organ should be treated down to the introitus.

If metastatic periaortic lymph nodes are suspected or confirmed, the retroperitoneal tissues need to be irradiated either through a separate portal or with a field that includes both the periaortic nodes and the pelvic tissues (anterior and posterior, occasionally lateral portals).

FIG. 36-9. Simulation AP film of pelvis showing volume treated with external irradiation that includes uterus, upper vagina, parametria, and pelvic lymph nodes.

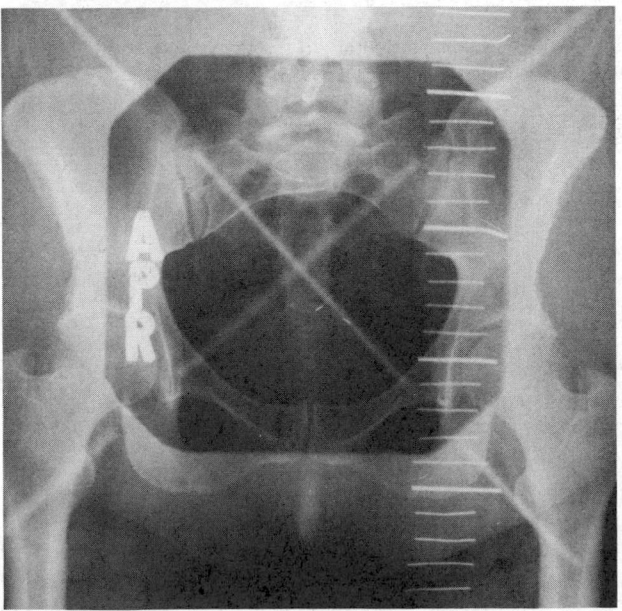

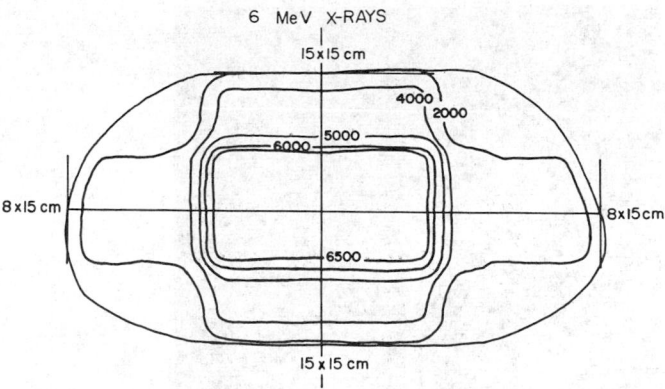

FIG. 36-10. Example of "box technique" with anterior/posterior and lateral portals used for the treatment of pelvic tumors.

Beam Energies

Because of the thickness of the pelvis, high-energy beams are especially suited for this treatment. They decrease the dose of radiation delivered to the peripheral normal tissues and provide a more homogeneous dose distribution in the central pelvis. With lower-energy megavoltage beams (^{60}Co, 4–6 MV photons), higher maximum doses must be given and there is a need to use more complex portal arrangements (three fields or pelvic box technique) to minimize the dose to the bladder and the rectum while delivering an adequate dose in the cervix and the parametria (Fig. 36-10).

Brachytherapy

Brachytherapy can be delivered with intracavitary techniques using applicators consisting of an intrauterine tandem and vaginal colpostats or, when necessary, with vaginal cylinders. Also, intersitital implants with needles in limited tumor volumes are helpful in specific clinical situations (i.e., localized residual tumor).

The intracavitary therapy, with its rapid dose fall-off as a function of distance, yields a high dose to the uterus and paracervical tissues, but as the only modality it is inadequate to treat the pelvic lymph nodes (Fig. 36-11). Several isotopes are available, such as ^{226}Ra and ^{60}Co, although currently ^{137}Cs is the most popular. Various applicators are used for intracavitary therapy, most at present being afterloading. Afterloading applicators allow a better application because the operators are not concerned with radiation exposure; also, the technique can be exploited to achieve more optimal dose distribution with replacement or removal of sources in the tandem or the vaginal ovoids at different times. Radiographs of the application can be obtained using dummy sources; the active sources will be inserted only after the films have been reviewed and the position of the applicators is believed to be satisfactory.

In general, the first intracavitary insertion is scheduled after 1000 to 2000 cGy of external irradiation if an adequate geometry exists in the pelvis. Otherwise, 2000 to 4000 cGy are delivered before the first application to decrease the size of the lesion and improve the relationship of the applicators

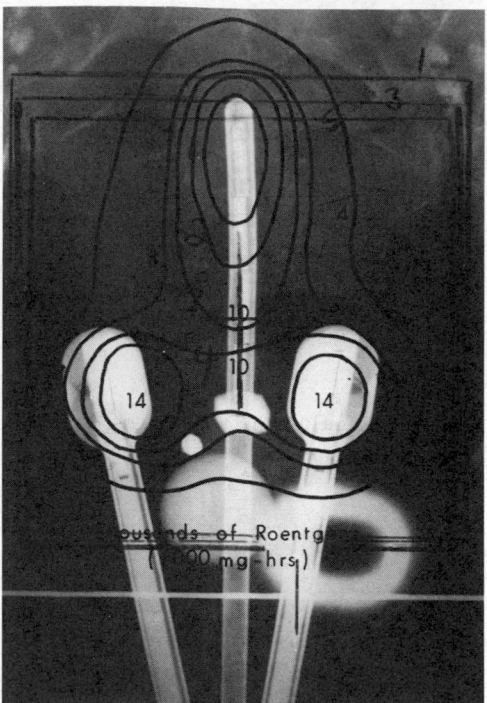

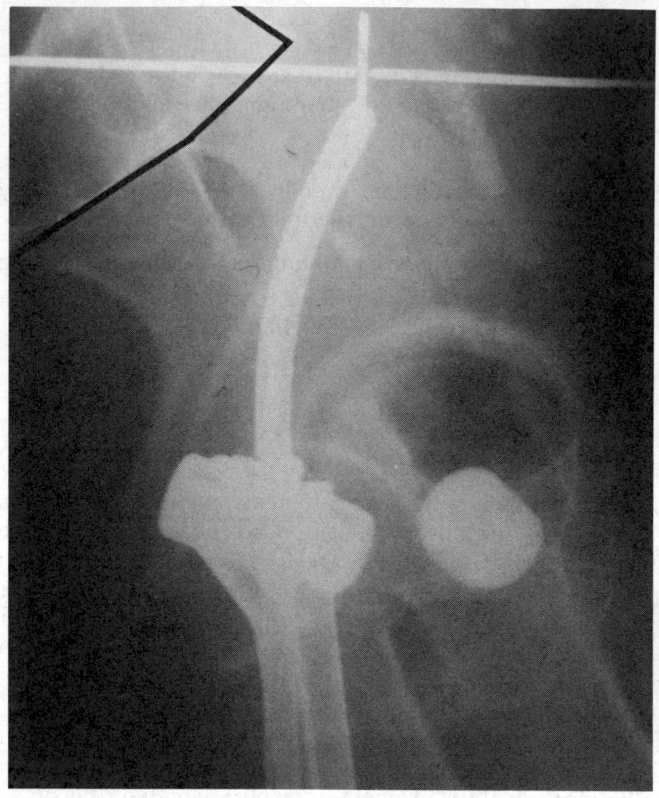

FIG. 36-11. AP (**A**) and lateral (**B**) radiographs of the pelvis showing an intracavitary application with interuterine tandem and vaginal colpostats. Isodose dose curves on a coronal plane are superimposed on AP port.

to the cervix and vagina. The second application is performed 1 to 3 weeks after the first insertion.

Doses of Irradiation

Optimal dose for invasive carcinoma of the cervix is delivered with a combination of whole pelvis, intracavitary, and, at times, interstitial therapy. Some institutions use lower doses of whole pelvis, external irradiation (1000 cGy for Stage IB and 2000 cGy for Stages IIA–B, III, and IVA) in addition to parametrial doses to complete 5000 cGy in Stages IB and IIA–B and 6000 cGy for more advanced stages. An assortment of step wedges designed in accordance with the isodose curves of the intracavitary applications or a 3 cm wide rectangular 5 half value lead block are used to shield the midline. This is combined with two intracavitary insertions that deliver 7000 to 8000 mgh (6500–7200 cGy to point A).

This technique affords a high central dose to the cervix, paracervical tissues, and parametria and a moderate homogeneous dose to the external iliac lymph nodes without exceeding the bladder and rectal tolerance doses (Fig. 36-12). Other institutions prefer higher doses of whole pelvic external irradiation (usually 4000 cGy) with an additional parametrial dose to complete 5000 cGy in patients with Stages IB and IIA and 6000 cGy for patients with IIB, III, or IVA tumors. This is usually combined with one or two intracavitary insertions for approximately 5000 to 6000 mgh (4500–5500 cGy to point A). When residual tumor is palpated at the

completion of the prescribed course of therapy, an additional 1000 cGy through a small 8 × 12 cm field to one parametrium or 12 × 12 cm to both parametria may be used to deliver an additional 1000 cGy. The midline block is left in place.

FIG. 36-12. Isodose distribution in the pelvis with combined external and intracavitary irradiation showing doses to be delivered to the cervix and parametria without exceeding irradiation of bladder and rectum.

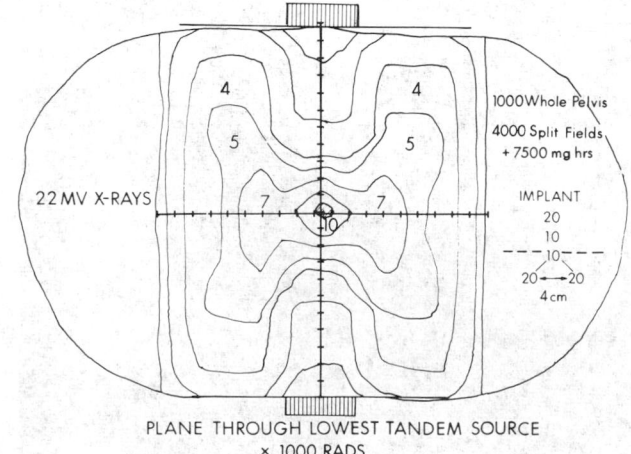

Techniques for Combination of Irradiation and Surgery

PREOPERATINE IRRADIATION. At some institutions the combination of preoperative irradiation and a hysterectomy has been used to treat patients with Stages IB and IIA.[272,273] Sometimes an intracavitary insertion alone is used (5000–6000 mgh) before radical hysterectomy with pelvic lymphadenectomy. At some institutions this brachytherapy is combined with external irradiation (2000 cGy to the whole pelvis in which case a radical hysterectomy and pelvic lymphadenectomy is performed). In other patients 2000 cGy to the whole pelvis plus 3000 cGy to the parametria and an intracavitary insertion (5000–6000 cGy to point A) are delivered, to be followed 4 to 6 weeks later by a conservative extrafascial hysterectomy.[272,273] The rationale for the use of an operation in addition to irradiation has been the alleged inability of irradiation to eradicate completely the tumor at bulky primary sites or in the pelvic lymph nodes[274,275] and the belief of some gynecologists that a more functional vagina in sexually active patients will be left after the surgical procedure.[276]

POSTOPERATIVE IRRADIATION. When metastatic pelvic lymph nodes or positive surgical margins are found after a hysterectomy, postoperative irradiation is delivered. If only intracavitary therapy was given preoperatively, 2000 cGy whole pelvis and 3000 cGy to the parametrial are administered, shielding the midline. If some external therapy is delivered preoperatively, an additional parametrial dose to complete 5500 cGy should be given again, shielding the midline with an appropriate block.

In patients not irradiated preoperatively on whom postoperative irradiation is indicated because of positive (central) surgical margins, we administer a combination of external irradiation (2000 cGy whole pelvis and 3000 cGy to the parametria with a small midline block) combined with an intracavitary insertion for 6000 cGy to the vaginal mucosa (1800 mgh) with two colpostats. In patients with metastatic pelvic lymph nodes external irradiation alone (5000 cGy to the midplane of the pelvis) has been administered.

In patients receiving postoperative irradiation, extreme care should be exercised in designing treatment techniques that include intracavitary insertions; because of the surgical extirpation of the uterus, the bladder and the rectosigmoid may be closer to the radioactive sources than in the patient with an intact uterus.[277] Furthermore, vascular supply may be affected by the surgical procedure and adhesions can prevent mobilization of the small bowel loops that occasionally may be fixed in the pelvis, which increases the risk of complications.

Hyperbaric Oxygen, Hypoxic Sensitizer, and Hyperthermia Combined with Irradiation

Several reports have been published on clinical trials evaluating the efficacy of hyperbaric oxygen (HBO)[278] combined with irradiation in the treatment of a variety of human tumors, one of them carcinoma of the uterine cervix. Watson and co-workers,[279] in a randomized clinical trial involving 320 patients (Stages III and IVA) treated at four institutions, reported a 5-year survival rate of 33% in the oxygen-treated group in contrast to 27% in the control patient group treated in air (p = 0.08). The greatest improvement in survival was observed in women below the age of 55, in whom the 5-year survival rate for those treated with oxygen was 50% in contrast to 30% for the control group treated in air. The local recurrence rate was 33% in the 161 patients treated with oxygen and 53% in 159 patients treated in air. The difference is statistically significant (p = 0.001). The morbidity in the patients treated with oxygen was greater (20 severe and 13 moderate) than in those treated in air (6 severe and 8 moderate). The difference was particularly striking in the bowel (13 versus 2 severe complications, respectively).

On the other hand, an extensive trial of carcinoma of the cervix reported by Fletcher et al[280] in 233 patients with Stages IIB, III, and IV randomized to be treated with conventional irradiation in air or with hyperbaric oxygen demonstrated no significant benefit in survival or tumor control (20 of 109 patients treated with oxygen failing in the pelvis in contrast to 29 of 124 treated in air). Further, the morbidity was greater (26 complications) in patients treated with hyperbaric oxygen compared with the control group (15 complications). A smaller series reported by Glassburn and colleagues[281] showed no benefit in survival but increased morbidity with hyperbaric oxygen in carcinoma of the cervix. It is possible that hyperbaric oxygen administered with fewer high-dose fractions may be more efficacious than when combined with conventional dose and fractionation schemes.[282] The trials reported have not shown an increased incidence of distant metastasis, which has been reported in a clinical study and in some animal experiments.[283]

Thomas and co-workers[284] described a Phase I study of metronidazole carried out on 80 patients with various stages of carcinoma of the uterine cervix. The authors suggested that a daily dose of 1.3 g/m² was well-tolerated but no tumor response data were reported; Phase III clinical trials were recommended.

Dische[285] reported preliminary observations on the use of misonidazole in the treatment of advanced carcinoma of the cervix in 10 patients. The morbidity of this therapy is similar to that observed with irradiation alone, except for some misonidazole neurotoxicity. All 10 patients had more than 50% tumor regression, results believed to be very promising. A randomized study was recently carried out by the Radiation Therapy Oncology Group to evaluate the sensitizing effects of misonidazole in Stages III and IVA carcinoma of the cervix (daily dose of 400 mg/m² for a total of 12 g/m²) treated with conventional fractionation. Preliminary results show no significant differences in survival, tumor control, or morbidity. The GOG has developed a protocol to compare misonidazole or hydroxyurea in combination with definitive irradiation in patients with Stages IIB, III, or IV carcinoma of the uterine cervix.

Because of technological limitations to deliver adequate heat to large parts of the body such as the pelvis, the evaluation of hyperthermia in the treatment of carcinoma of the uterine cervix has been sparse. Hornback and co-workers[286] recently reported on a nonrandomized study stating that the combination of microwave hyperthermia and irradiation

TABLE 36-13. Carcinoma of the Uterine Cervix, MIR 1959–1977, Irradiation Alone: Type of Grade III Severe Treatment Sequelae

| | \multicolumn{7}{c}{Stage} |
	IA	IB	IIA	IIB	IIIA	IIIB	IVA
Total no. of patients treated	26	277	86	215	10	183	14
Number of complications (%)	1 (3.8)	22 (7.9)	7 (8.1)	32 (14.9)		13 (7.1)	2 (14.3)
Intestinal							
Rectovaginal fistula		2		5			
Sigmoid perforation		1		3			
Small bowel perforation			1				
Proctitis		2		2		2	
Rectal ulcer			3				
Sigmoid stricture		3	1	3		1	
Small bowel obstruction		1		4		4	
Other GI	1	1		2			
Urinary							
Cystitis		1					
Bladder ulcer		2		1			
Vesicovaginal fistula		3		2		3	1
Ureteral stricture		4	2	4		2	
Other GU							1
Other							
Pulmonary embolus						1	
Pelvic hemorrhage				1			
Pelvic abscess		1		1			
Arteriosclerosis				2			
Other		1		2			

Perez CA, Breaux S, Madoc-Jones H, et al: Radiation therapy alone in treatment of carcinoma of the uterine cervix: II. Analysis of complications. Cancer 54:235, 1984.

TABLE 36-14. Carcinoma of the Uterine Cervix, MIR 1966–1979, Stages IB and IIA: Major Complications of Treatment

| | \multicolumn{4}{c}{Stage IB} | \multicolumn{4}{c}{Stage IIA} |
| | \multicolumn{2}{c}{Radiation Therapy Alone (40 Patients)} | \multicolumn{2}{c}{Preoperative Radiation Therapy + Surgery (48 Patients)} | \multicolumn{2}{c}{Radiation Therapy Alone (16 Patients)} | \multicolumn{2}{c}{Preoperative Radiation Therapy + Surgery (14 patients)} |
	Grade 2	Grade 3	Grade 2	Grade 3	Grade 2	Grade 3	Grade 2	Grade 3
Rectovaginal fistula		1 (2.5%)						
Vesicovaginal fistula		2 (5%)						
Ureteral stricture		1 (2.5%)		1 (2.1%)				2 (14.3%)
Wound infection			1 (2.1%)					
Subcutaneous fibrosis	1 (2.5%)							
Vault necrosis	1 (2.5%)		1 (2.1%)		1 (6.3%)		1 (7.1%)	
Pelvic infection		1 (2.5%)						
Vaginal stenosis	6 (15%)		1 (2.1%)		2 (12.5%)			
Thrombophlebitis			2 (4.2%)					
Pelvic arteriosclerosis	1 (2.5%)							
Proctitis								1 (7.1%)
Rectal stricture						1 (6.3%)		1 (7.1%)
Acute pelvic cellulitis							1 (7.1%)	
Small bowel stricture								1 (7.1%)
Lymphocyst							1 (7.1%)	

Perez CA, Camel HM, Kao MS, et al: Randomized study of preoperative radiation and surgery or irradiation alone in the treatment of Stage IB and IIA carcinoma of the uterine cervix: Final report. Gynecol Oncol 27:129, 1987.

(433 mgh) resulted in improved tumor control in a group of 79 patients with Stage IIIB (72% local tumor control) in comparison with previously irradiated controls (35% and 53% tumor control). However, 5-year survival rates were similar in all groups (22–30%).

COMPLICATIONS OF IRRADIATION

Major complications of radiation therapy for Stages I and IIA carcinoma of the cervix range from 3% to 5% and for Stages IIB and III, between 10% and 15%. The most frequent major complications for the various stages are listed in Tables 36-13 and 36-14. Perez et al,[287] Kottmeier,[288] Pourquier et al,[289] and others have demonstrated a greater incidence of complications with higher doses of irradiation. Higher doses of external irradiation to the whole pelvis have also been associated with a greater number of complications (Fig. 36-13)[287] Injury to the gastrointestinal tract usually appears within the first 2 years after radiotherapy, whereas complications of the urinary tract are seen more frequently 3 to 4 years after treatment.[290] When preoperative radiation is combined with surgery, the complication rate tends to be somewhat higher (5–10%), particularly because of injury to the ureter or the bladder (ureteral stricture or uretero-vaginal or vesicovaginal fistula).

The dose and techniques of irradiation and the type of surgical procedures performed are important in determining the morbidity of combined therapy. Nelson et al[272] reported an incidence of severe complications of 17.5% in a group of 80 patients treated with radiation and radical hysterectomy in contrast to 7.4% major complications in a group of 95 patients treated with high-dose preoperative radiation and a conservative extrafascial hysterectomy.

The pretherapy staging laparotomy is fraught with a significant number of complications, particularly if irradiation is given (over 5000–5500 cGy) when metastatic para-aortic lymph nodes are found. The usual operative complications may be noted, such as pneumonia, thrombophlebitis, cardio-

vascular accident, hepatitis, or evisceration. Late complications include those of combined surgery and irradiation in the abdomen and pelvis, such as small bowel obstruction, stricture and fibrosis of the intestine or rectosigmoid, and rectovaginal or vesicovaginal fistula. With improving anesthesia, surgical techniques, and antibiotic therapy, the mortality for radical hysterectomy with pelvic lymphadenectomy has decreased to 1% or less.[221] Other complications include ureterovaginal fistula, the incidence of which has decreased to less than 3%.

The incidence of complications has been listed between 5% and 20%, depending on the extent of the periaortic lymph node dissection, the transperitoneal or retroperitoneal approach for the operation, and the dose of irradiation given.[291,292] Tewfik et al[293] reported 27.8% complications in a group of 23 patients mostly with Stage IIIB carcinoma of the cervix treated with laparotomy and pelvic/periaortic nodal irradiation. Komaki et al[292] observed 3 small bowel obstructions in 22 patients (14%) receiving 5000 to 5500 cGy to the periaortic areas for histologically proven nodal metastases from carcinoma of the cervix or endometrium. In contrast, Potish et al[294] described only 2 patients with small bowel obstructions and 3 with large bowel complications in 81 patients (6%) with cervical carcinoma treated with radiotherapy alone (including periaortic lymph nodes) and not undergoing a surgical exploration. The risk of para-aortic nodal irradiation, when indicated, must be evaluated with respect to survival. Several authors[292,293,295] have reported survival rates of 30% to 40%, but, as previously noted in Table 36-9, other authors have reported lower survival rates.[292,293,295]

SURGICAL TECHNIQUES FOR CARCINOMA OF THE CERVIX

From the first hysterectomy for cervical cancer in 1878 by Freund[296] until the description of total pelvic exenteration by Brunschwig in 1948,[297] surgical treatment has played a vital role in the management of cervical cancer. In the following sections, the major surgical procedures are discussed briefly. No attempt has been made to describe the procedures in detail or to show drawings of the operations more suitable to a surgical text. The interested reader is referred to *Telinde's Operative Gynecology*.[298]

Cervical Conization

Conization of the cervix may be either diagnostic or therapeutic. It is indicated for the diagnostic evaluation of patients with cervical intraepithelial neoplasia or microinvasive carcinoma and is the standard therapeutic option for patients with CIN-3. Complications associated with cervical conization are hemorrhage, cervical stenosis, and uterine perforation.

Total Extrafascial Abdominal Hysterectomy

Total abdominal hysterectomy for the treatment of cervical carcinoma includes the removal of the uterus and the cervix.

FIG. 36-13. Major treatment sequelae (grades 2 and 3), radiation only, carcinoma of the uterine cervix. MIR, 1959–1977. (Perez CA, Breaux S, Mudoc-Jones H, et al: Radiation therapy alone in treatment of carcinoma of the uterine cervix. II. Analysis of complications. Cancer 54:235, 1984)

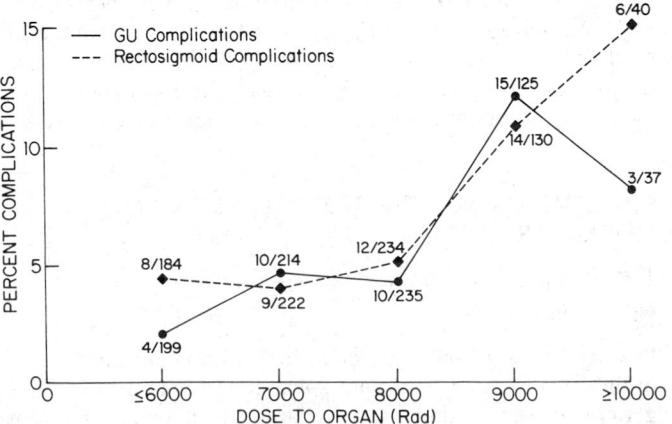

The plane of excision lies just outside the pubocervical fascia and does not require unroofing of the ureters as they pass through the cardinal ligaments. A small vaginal cuff can easily be excised. Hysterectomy is indicated in selected cases for CIN-3 and for microinvasive cervical carcinoma when invasion is less than 3 mm and there is no lymphovascular invasion. Extrafascial hysterectomy is also used by some authorities after irradiation for barrel-shaped Stages IA and IB cervical carcinoma and after irradiation in early stage disease if the endometrium is involved.

Modified Radical Hysterectomy

In the modified radical hysterectomy, the ureter is unroofed from its canal, but the lateral attachments with their blood supply are preserved. Parametrial and paracervical tissue medial to the ureter is removed and a larger vaginal cuff is taken. Some authorities have recommended this operation for carcinoma in situ or microinvasive carcinoma of the cervix, but it is rarely used today.

Radical Abdominal Hysterectomy with Bilateral Pelvic Lymphadenectomy

In the radical hysterectomy, the ureters are dissected completely free from their tunnels through the paracervical tissues and the bladder is dissected free of the upper one third of the vagina. The uterosacral ligaments are severed near their point of origin posteriorly and the cardinal ligaments are severed at the lateral pelvic sidewall. This allows complete removal of the parametrial, paracervical, and upper paravaginal tissues as well as removal of the upper one fourth to one third of the vagina. The lymphadenectomy begins at the middle of the common iliac vessels and consists of removal of the distal one half of the common iliac and complete removal of the external iliac, hypogastric, obturator, and presacral lymph nodes. Many surgeons combine this operation with a selective para-aortic lymphadenectomy and begin the pelvic dissection at the bifurcation of the aorta.[221]

Average blood loss from radical hysterectomy and pelvic lymphadenectomy for cervical cancer is 1,500 to 1,800 ml, and most patients will require blood transfusions.[176,221] Aside from minor postoperative infections, the most common complication is neurogenic bladder dysfunction, and Webb and Symmonds[299] have reported poor bladder sensation in 31.5% of patients who required catheter drainage more than 14 days after surgery. Urinary tract fistulae are the most common serious complications of radical hysterectomy, but most modern series report the incidence to be less than 2%.[176,221,300] Pelvic lymphocysts and pelvic abscess are infrequent problems resulting from the use of closed suction drainage of the pelvis by most surgeons.

Radical hysterectomy is used for Stages IB and IIA cervical carcinoma. Its advantages and disadvantages have been cited previously. In the hands of well-trained, experienced surgeons it has an acceptable complication rate that is similar to that for full pelvic irradiation. Symmonds[300] has pointed out that the complications of radical hysterectomy are more often amenable to correction than the late complications of irradiation.

Selective Para-Aortic Lymphadenectomy

Selective para-aortic lymphadenectomy or para-aortic lymph node biopsy is an integral part of the management of patients with cervical carcinoma. Its use in pretreatment surgical staging has already been discussed. Many surgeons perform this procedure prior to radical hysterectomy, believing that if these lymph nodes contain metastatic cancer, the patient is better treated by extended field irradiation. Enlarged or suspicious lymph nodes seen on CT scan or lymphangiography can sometimes be sampled by fine needle aspiration guided by CT scan or fluoroscopy. If this sampling procedure is inadequate, para-aortic node biopsy is indicated.

Pelvic Exenteration

The use of pelvic exenteration for recurrent cervical cancer after irradiation therapy was introduced at Memorial Sloan-Kettering Cancer Center by Brunschwig in 1948.[297] In 1960 Brunschwig and Daniel[301] reported on 592 exenterations with a 5-year survival rate of 17% and an operative mortality of 23%. In 1987, Lawhead et al[302] reviewed the Memorial Sloan-Kettering Cancer Center experience with pelvic exenteration for the years 1972 through 1981 and reported an operative mortality of 9.8% and a 5-year survival rate of 23%. As of December 1981, 1,129 pelvic exenterations had been performed on the Gynecology Service at Memorial Sloan-Kettering Cancer Center.

Total pelvic exenteration consists of removal of the bladder, urethra, uterus, cervix, vagina, and rectum along with all lateral supporting tissues. Most surgeons differentiate between supralevator exenterations which stop at the floor of the pelvis and infralevator exenterations which excise part or all of the pelvic floor and include removal of the vulva. Posterior exenteration allows preservation of the urinary tract and anterior exenteration preserves the rectum. The urinary conduit can be constructed from the ileum, sigmoid, or transverse colon. On occasion, in a supralevator exenteration, the continuity of the large intestine can be maintained by low rectal anastomosis.

In recent years, improved radiation therapy equipment, improved training of radiotherapists, and better techniques for administration of irradiation have made central recurrence alone an unusual finding in cervical carcinoma. Between 1948 and 1971, 1,064 exenterations were performed at Memorial Sloan-Kettering Cancer Center, an average of 46.3 per year. From 1972 until 1981, 65 exenterations were performed, an average of 6.5 per year. Similar experiences have been found at most centers that treat cervical cancer.

SURGICAL OR IRRADIATION TREATMENT OF SPECIAL PROBLEMS

Palliation of Locally Advanced Carcinoma of the Cervix

Irradiation can be quite effective for palliation of pelvic pain or bleeding or in patients with advanced tumors in whom the general condition does not warrant a prolonged course of external irradiation with conventional fractionation. If vaginal bleeding is the main concern, a single intracavitary insertion with tandem and colpostats for about 6000 mgh (5500 cGy to point A) will suffice. If previous irradiation was delivered, lower intracavitary doses should be prescribed (4500–5000 mgh).

Several high dose fractionation schedules have been used, and Meoz et al[303] described satisfactory palliation with single doses of 1000 cGy combined with misonidazole, delivered every 3 to 6 weeks for a total 3000 cGy. Complications in the long-term survivors were relatively high (15%). The Radiation Therapy Oncology Group is conducting a Phase I/II trial using multiple (twice daily) fractions of 370 cGy each to deliver 740 cGy on two consecutive days, repeating every 3 to 6 weeks for a total of 4400 cGy.

Treatment of Recurrent Carcinoma of the Cervix

AFTER DEFINITIVE IRRADIATION. The irradiation of previously irradiated patients must be undertaken with extreme caution. It is very important to analyze the techniques used in the initial treatment (beam energy, volume, doses delivered with external or intracavitary irradiation) and the period of time between the two treatments. In general, we give external irradiation to limited volumes (4000–4500 cGy, 180 cGy total dose per fraction preferentially using lateral portals). Occasionally, intracavitary or interstitial irradiation can be used to treat relatively circumscribed recurrences.

Puthawala et al[304] treated 14 patients with interstitial implants who had received definitive radiotherapy at the time of initial treatment for carcinoma of the uterine cervix that recurred in the pelvis. Seven of them exhibited tumor control (50%). Palliation of symptoms after reirradiation was obtained in about 80% of the patients. The authors described no postoperative mortality. Severe complications occurred in 15% of the patients (soft tissue necrosis and one instance each of rectovaginal fistula, vesicovaginal fistula, enterovaginal fistula, and rectal stricture).

Prasavinichai et al[305] noted a 17.6% 5-year survival rate in 51 patients with recurrent tumors limited to the pelvis, treated with irradiation alone, pelvic exenteration (10 patients), or combination of exploratory laparatomy, debulking, and irradiation (10 patients). Prempree et al[306] treated 8 patients with late invasive cervical carcinoma recurrent after primary irradiation. Three survived tumor free more than 5 years after retreatment.

AFTER PREVIOUS SURGERY. It is easier to treat surgical recurrences with irradiation. We believe that a combination of external irradiation (2000–4000 cGy total dose) depending on volume of tumor and an additional parametrial dose with midline shielding for a total of 5000 to 6000 cGy is needed. In addition, an intracavitary insertion that may cover the vaginal vault or the entire vagina depending on tumor volume should be delivered. The total mucosal dose from the external and intracavitary therapy can approach 12,000 cGy without a high risk. It is extremely useful to combine these techniques with interstitial irradiation to boost the dose to

the vaginal vault or the parametrium or paravaginal tissues when the volume of disease requires it. Doses in the range of 2000 to 3000 cGy are administered with single, double, or volume implants, depending on the extent of the tumor.

Friedman and Pearlman[307] reported a 42% tumor-free survival rate in 38 patients treated with irradiation after primary surgical therapy (7 were irradiated electively for close or positive margins, lymphatic permeation, or pelvic lymph node involvement). Six of the 7 patients were tumor free for 2 to 5 years. Of 14 patients with limited central recurrence, 8 were tumor free from 3.5 to 9 years. The worst results were noted with persistent or recurrent peripheral pelvic tumor (3 of 11 patients survived tumor free more than 5 years) or with massive pelvic recurrences (in 6 patients only palliation was achieved). Evans et al[308] reported on 114 patients found to have unresectable recurrent carcinoma of the cervix after primary irradiation or surgical treatment. Seventy patients were treated with irradiation (external, interstitial, or combination). Ten percent of the patients lived 15 months or longer and 5% survived 5 or more years (Fig. 36-14). Satisfactory palliation was observed in a large proportion of the patients.

FIG. 36-14. Survival of 70 patients in nonrandomized study with recurrent carcinoma of the uterine cervix treated with radiation therapy (external, brachytherapy, or a combination). (Evans SR Jr, Hilaris BS, Borber HRK: External vs. interstitial irradiation in unresectable recurrent cancer of the cervix. Cancer 28:1284, 1971)

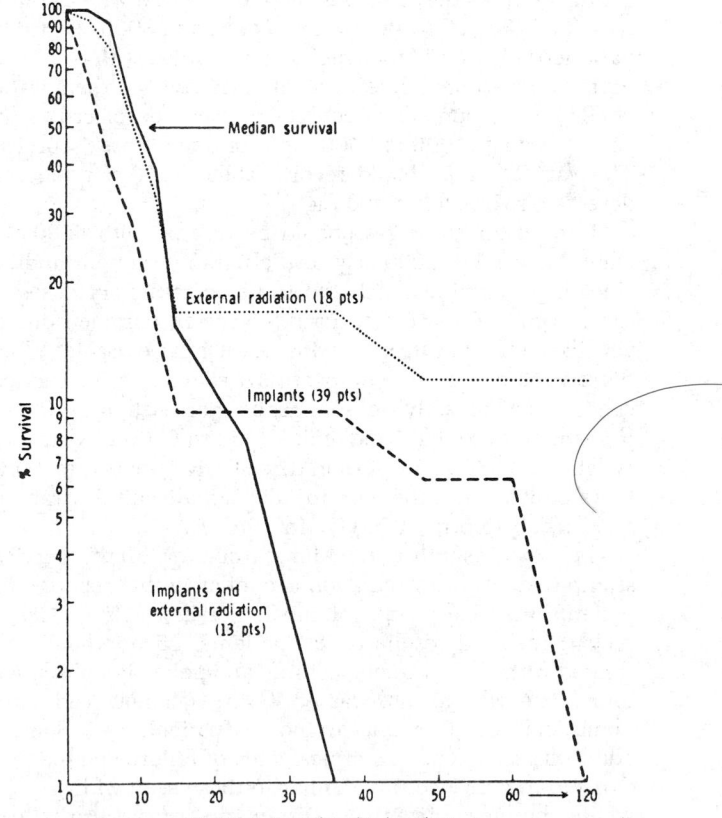

Carcinoma of the Cervical Stump

Subtotal hysterectomy, a relatively popular procedure for benign conditions of the uterus in past years, is performed rarely today. These patients are, of course, at risk to develop carcinoma of the uterine cervix. It is important to divide patients with carcinoma of the cervical stump into the following groups: *true,* when the first symptom occurs 3 or more years after subtotal hysterectomy, or *coincidental,* when the symptoms are noticed before the third postoperative year.[309] Moss et al[310] recommend two elapsed years after hysterectomy as the time for the classification of these lesions. This distribution is important because the prognosis for carcinoma of the true stump is significantly better than for coincidental lesions, which probably means that carcinoma was present at the time the hysterectomy was performed. The natural history and patterns of spread of carcinoma of the cervical stump are similar to those for the cervix in the intact uterus. The diagnostic workup, clinical staging, and basic principles of therapy are the same. When surgery is performed for Stage I tumors, it is somewhat more difficult because of the previous surgical procedures and the presence of adhesions in the pelvis.

When irradiation is administered, the lack of a uterine cavity into which to insert a tandem containing three or more sources makes intracavitary therapy more difficult. Whenever possible, sources should be inserted in the remaining cervical canal. Occasionally, transvaginal irradiation may be used to boost the dose delivered to central disease in the stump. It is important to deliver more whole pelvis irradiation.

In general, patients with Stage I are treated with a combination of 2000 cGy to the whole pelvis and 3000 cGy to the parametria with midline shielding combined with two intracavitary insertions. The dose of intracavitary therapy depends on the number of sources that can be placed in the cervical canal (1000 to 3000 mgh for one to three sources). The vaginal vault should receive about 7000 cGy mucosal dose (approximately 2000 mgh).

More advanced stages should be treated with 4000 cGy whole pelvis and 2000 cGy to the parametria with midline shielding, combined with the same intracavitary doses. If there is bulky disease present in the cervix, parametrium, or vagina, interstitial therapy with needles is advisable. When there is no opportunity to insert any sources in the cervical canal, the whole pelvis dose must be increased to 6000 cGy. In using intravaginal irradiation, 3000 to 5000 cGy air dose is delivered in 2 to 4 weeks in three to five weekly fractions. Moss et al[310] limit the dose to the vaginal vault for transvaginal irradiation to 3000 cGy in 10 days.

The 5-year survival rate for carcinoma of the cervical stump treated with irradiation is similar to that reported for patients with carcinoma of the intact uterus.[309,311] Creadnick[312] reported results on 83 patients, 25 of whom were treated with radical trachelectomy and pelvic lymphadenectomy. The salvage rate was 85.7% in squamous cell carcinoma and 50% in adenocarcinoma (patients with Stages I and II disease). The anatomical sites of failure and the incidence of recurrences are similar to those seen with cases in whom the uterus in intact. Distant metastasis also follows the same distribution.

Because of the proximity of the bladder, rectum, and small intestine to the intracavitary sources and the often higher doses of whole pelvis external beam irradiation given, complications are somewhat more frequent than in the carcinoma of the cervix with intact uterus. Wimbush and Fletcher[311] reported 5 fistulas, 6 cases of severe proctosigmoiditis, and 12 cases of vault necrosis in 238 patients treated with definitive radiotherapy.

Carcinoma of the Cervix During Pregnancy

Preinvasive and invasive cervical carcinoma that occurs during pregnancy requires the combined expertise of the gynecologic oncologist, maternal-fetal medicine specialist, and on occasion, the radiation oncologist. An abnormal Papanicolaou smear in the pregnant patient should be evaluated by colposcopy and biopsy.[313] Although an endocervical curettage should not be performed, the physiologic eversion of the cervix in pregnancy usually allows easy visualization of the squamocolumnar junction. Biopsy of the cervix requires a well-equipped treatment room because of the likelihood of profuse bleeding. Although conization of the cervix should be performed in patients with biopsies or Papanicolaou smears suspicious for invasion, less severe lesions can usually be followed by colposcopy and Papanicolaou smears with biopsy as necessary until the postpartem period. Several authors have reported the use of cervical conization in pregnancy with small to significant increases in morbidity and pregnancy wastage.[314,315]

When invasive cancer of the cervix is encountered, it is imperative that the patient be evaluated by the oncologist and the specialist in maternal-fetal medicine. The patient must be informed of all therapeutic options and their possible effects on both her fetus and her. In 1988, a tertiary level intensive care nursery can reliably obtain survival rates of about 80% for fetuses delivered at 28 weeks of gestation (1000-g fetus).[316] For patients less than 24 weeks gestation the pregnancy should be disregarded, whereas patients who are 28 weeks pregnant or more should have delivery of the fetus by cesarean section. Between 24 and 28 weeks, the patient and her physician must weigh the advantages and disadvantages of all courses of action because even though fetal survival rates at 28 weeks' gestation may be excellent, there is significant morbidity associated with the small birth weight infant.

The actual treatment of the cancer depends on the stage of disease and the usual considerations for selecting therapy. Radical hysterectomy can be performed either with the fetus in situ or in the case of a viable fetus immediately after delivery by cesarean section. If radiation is to be used, the patient will usually abort during the course of whole pelvis irradiation. If this does not occur, the uterus must be evacuated before insertion of intracavitary irradiation.[317,318] Survival has been reported to be similar in pregnant and nonpregnant patients matched by stage of disease regardless of the gestational age of the pregnancy.[317,319] Common practice is to avoid vaginal delivery in pregnancy because of the fear that delivery through a cervix involved with carcinoma will result in more rapid spread of the disease. However, Creasman et al[317] were not able to document decreased survival in

Stage I patients who had vaginal delivery before definitive treatment.

CHEMOTHERAPY OF CARCINOMA OF THE CERVIX

Because effective initial therapy with surgery and irradiation is available for most patients with cervical carcinoma, chemotherapy has been studied less completely.[320,321] Nevertheless, there are circumstances in which chemotherapy would play an important role, if effective regimens were identified. Groups of patients who are candidates for chemotherapy include those with advanced (Stages III and IV) disease, patients who have recurrent disease after surgery and radiation therapy, and patients who present with pelvic and periaortic nodal metastasis and therefore have a low potential for cure with standard treatment modalities.

In addition, chemotherapy could play a role as a radiation sensitizer, enhancing conventional irradiation. Finally, the location of cervical carcinoma and the regional localization in the pelvis have provided a rationale for the study of regional perfusion of the chemotherapy using intra-arterial infusion.

Factors that complicate the effective use of chemotherapy in cervical carcinoma include decreased pelvic vascular perfusion, limited bone marrow reserve, and poor renal function related to ureteral obstruction from tumor or fibrosis.

Single-Agent Chemotherapy

Table 36-15 lists the single agents that have some activity in cervical carcinoma. These data can be used only to suggest activity because, for the most part, they represent collected information from the literature in which variable criteria for response were used. Significant activity in well-designed studies with adequate patient numbers has been documented only for 5-FU and cisplatin,[322,323] although activity for dibromoducitol,[324] dianhydrogalactitol,[325] ifosfamide[325] and the platinum derivatives CHIP,[326] and carboplatin[327] has recently been documented.

Cisplatin remains the single agent with the best-documented activity.[323] The GOG evaluated 497 patients on three separate dose schedules: 50 mg/m² every 3 weeks; 100 mg/m² every 3 weeks; or 20 mg/m² × 5 every 21 days. Responses were seen in 20%, 31%, and 25%, with complete responses in 10%, 13%, and 9%, respectively. The median duration of response was 4 months and the median survival 6.5 months. Significant nephrotoxicity and myelosuppression were seen with all regimens. Although there was a statistically significant difference in response rates favoring the high dose schedule, there were no differences in complete response rates or survival.

Combination Chemotherapy

Because there are several classes of cytotoxic agents with different mechanisms of action that have activity in carcinoma of the cervix, a number of combinations have been used. None of these combinations has been definitely shown to be more effective than single agents. Recently, however, several studies show 10% to 29% complete remission rates, suggesting some enhancement of effect. Table 36-16 lists combination chemotherapy studies in which reasonable numbers of evaluable patients have been studied, and the response rates appear to exceed those of single agents. However, the majority of the studies have not compared combination chemotherapy regimens to standard single agents, and the toxicity of these combinations is substantial. Although some of these combinations produce higher response rates, none has been definitely shown to be superior to single agent cisplatin in either duration of response or survival, particularly in patients who have recurrent disease after primary therapy.

Intra-arterial Chemotherapy

Intra-arterial infusions of chemotherapeutic agents in cervical carcinoma have been of considerable theoretical interest for some years based on the distinct arterial supply to the

TABLE 36-15. Single-Agent Chemotherapy in Cervical Cancer

Drugs	Responders/Total Treated	Overall Response (%)
Alkylating Agents		
Cyclophosphamide	31/228	14
Chlorambucil	11/44	25
Dibromodulcitol	4/15	27
Dianhydrogalactitol	7/36	17
Ifosfamide	10/30	30
Antimetabolites		
5-Fluorouracil	68/348	20
Methotrexate	12/77	16
Mitotic Inhibiters		
Vincristine	10/44	23
Antitumor Antibiotics		
Doxorubicin (Adriamycin)	8/78	10
Bleomycin	17/172	10
Other Agents		
Cisplatin	21/52	40
CHIP	7/36	21
Carboplatin	11/39	28
Piprazinedione	5/38	13

TABLE 36-16.   Combination Chemotherapy in Cervical Carcinoma

Regimen	Evaluable Patients	Number of Responses (%)	Complete Responses (%)
Doxorubicin (Adriamycin) and methotrexate	59	39 (66)	13 (22)
	24	7 (28)	0 (0)
Doxorubicin and methyl-CCNU	13	14 (45)	9 (29)
Doxorubicin and cisplatin	19	6 (31)	2 (10)
Mitomycin C and bleomycin	33	12 (36)	5 (15)
Mitomycin C, vincristine and bleomycin	91	46 (51)	14 (15)
Mitomycin C, vincristine, bleomycin and cisplatin	14	6 (43)	4 (29)
Cisplatin, bleomycin and velban	33	22 (66)	6 (18)
Cisplatin, bleomycin, vincristine and methotrexate	15	10 (66)	3 (20)

tumor-bearing area. Unfortunately, the responses have been limited and the toxicity significant. Morrow et al[328] and Swenerton et al[329] each studied 20 patients using bleomycin or a combination of bleomycin and mitomycin-C and vincristine. Morrow et al[328] observed only 2 of 26 objective regressions; Swenerton et al[329] reported 3 of 20. The approach continues to be evaluated, using injections of either single drugs or combinations into the internal iliac arteries, and some studies report a reduction in complications related to the procedure and some responses.[330-333] However, randomized comparisons will be required to establish the benefits, if any, of intra-arterial chemotherapy infusions.

Chemotherapy as a Radiosensitizer

Continued interest in the use of chemotherapeutic agents as radiation sensitizers has been stimulated by the initial positive results with hydroxyurea. Piver et al[334] studied 130 patients with Stages IIB–IIIB cervical carcinoma in a prospective double-blind randomized study in which patients received split-course radiation therapy with or without hydroxyurea. In clinical Stage IIB patients, a significant improvement in 2-year survival was achieved for the group receiving hydroxyurea (74%) in comparison to the control group treated with radiotherapy and a placebo (43.5%). In clinically staged IIIB patients, 52% of those receiving hydroxyurea were alive at 2 years compared with 33% of those receiving a placebo with radiation (p = 0.22). Increased toxicity was noted in the hydroxyurea arm.[335,336]

Hreshchyshyn et al[337] and Piver[338] compared hydroxyurea or placebo combined with irradiation in Stages IIIB and IV cervical cancer. In 104 evaluable patients randomized to two treatment regimens, the complete response rate was 68% for the hydroxyurea-treated group and 48% for the placebo group (p < 0.05).[337] Duration of progression-free intervals and survival were also significantly better in the patients receiving hydroxyurea. Hematologic toxicity was more common and more severe in those patients receiving hydroxyurea. However, the results are less secure because the patients were not all surgically staged and substantial numbers of randomized patients were inevaluable. With effective radiotherapy alone, Fletcher[339] and Perez et al[340] demonstrated survival and tumor control similar to those observed with the addition of hydroxyurea in the two series described. Nevertheless, the two studies do suggest a potential role for

radiation sensitizers in cervical carcinoma. Recently, cisplatin has been used as a radiation sensitizer in cervix carcinoma. Studies by Choo et al[341] randomized 45 Stage I and II patients to receive either radiation alone or radiation therapy with cisplatin 25 mg/m² intravenously weekly. Significantly higher complete response rates were noted in the radiotherapy and chemotherapy group (55%) compared with radiation alone (20%), but no differences in local recurrence rates or survival were reported. Two other studies have demonstrated that weekly low-dose cisplatin with irradiation is feasible and not associated with significant increases in toxicity but may be associated with a modest improvement in disease-free survival (54% versus 45%).[342,342a]

FUTURE DIRECTIONS

Conservative therapy (less than hysterectomy) is well established for Stage 0 (CIN-3) of the cervix. Prospective studies may show that conization of the cervix with negative margins and close follow-up may be sufficient for some patients with microinvasive cervical cancer. For patients with Stages IB and IIA cervical cancer, identifications of high risk subgroups may allow early use of adjunctive therapy with further improvements in survival. Combination therapy using irradiation and chemotherapy may be able to improve survival in advanced disease. Most important, every effort should be expended to develop chemotherapeutic agents effective in the therapy of squamous cell and adenocarcinoma of the cervix. All patients with advanced and recurrent cervical cancer should be considered for entry in clinical trials.

CARCINOMA OF THE ENDOMETRIUM

Carcinoma of the endometrium is the most common of the female genital cancers. It is estimated that there will be 34,000 new cases in 1988, which represents 48% of all female genital cancers and 6.9% of all malignancies occurring in women.[1] Although carcinoma of the endometrium accounts for 48% of all new cases of female genital cancer, it will cause only 13% of all gynecologic cancer deaths.[1] The low death rate in this disease is primarily due to early diagnosis. Approximately 78% of all uterine cancer is diagnosed while it is still confined to the uterus.[1]

EPIDEMIOLOGY

The largest number of cases of endometrial cancer occurs between the ages of 55 and 60, although 75% to 80% of cases occur after menopause and a significant number of cases are reported in each decade after age 50. The median age is 61.1 years.[343] Obesity,[344-346] nulliparity,[346,347] late menopause,[343] polycystic ovarian disease,[343,348] estrogen secreting tumors of the ovary,[348,349] and exogenous estrogen[350,351] are associated with an increased incidence of endometrial cancer. Nachtigall et al[352] and Gambrel[353] have shown that when progesterone is given with exogenous estrogen, there is no increased risk of endometrial cancer. Medical disorders associated with the development of endometrial cancer include diabetes, hypertension, arthritis, and hypothyroidism. Of these, hypertension and diabetes mellitus are most frequently observed.[343,354,355]

Carcinoma of the endometrium has been observed more frequently in Jewish women and is rare among Japanese women.[355] Sommers et al[356] have reported an increased susceptibility to endometrial cancer in some families, but in general the familial association does not appear to be strong.[357]

NATURAL HISTORY, ROUTES OF SPREAD, AND CLINICAL MANIFESTATIONS

The association of hyperplasia of the endometrium with endometrial carcinoma is well documented.[358] Cystic and adenomatous hyperplasias may be physiologic when they occur in an anovulatory hormonal environment before menopause but must be of more concern in a postmenopausal woman. Atypical adenomatous hyperplasia is a cause of concern in any woman, regardless of menstrual status.

Carcinoma of the endometrium may spread along the uterine cavity to the cervix, penetrate the uterine wall, or spread through the fallopian tubes. The carcinoma can spread by local extension to the ovary, broad ligament, vagina, or other pelvic organs. Malignant cells may spread by way of the lymphatics or less frequently through the bloodstream. The endometrial lymphatics begin beneath the glandular lining cells of the endometrium and drain into lymphatic vessels in the myometrium. Myometrial lymphatics, in turn, drain into the subserosal network which coalesces into larger channels before exiting the uterus. Lymph flow from the fundus travels toward the adnexa and infundibulopelvic ligaments, whereas flow from the lower and middle thirds tends to spread in the base of the broad ligament toward the lateral pelvic sidewall.[359] There are four drainage channels from the uterus according to Plentl and Friedman[359]: (1) from the fundus with the ovarian vessels, (2) in the folds of the broad ligament, (3) along the mesosalpinx and fallopian tubes, and (4) along the round ligaments to the femoral nodes.

In a review of the literature, Plentl and Friedman[359] found nodal metastases in 202 of 1,978 cases (10%) undergoing lymphadenectomy at the time of surgical therapy for endometrial carcinoma. In autopsy series, these same authors reported an incidence of 65%. Creasman et al,[360] reporting on a pilot study of the GOG in which patients with Stage I adenocarcinoma had selective pelvic and para-aortic lymph node sampling, reported an incidence of positive pelvic lymph nodes of 11.4% and of aortic nodes of 5.7%.

Metastases or extension of endometrial cancer to the fallopian tubes or the ovaries has been reported to occur in 5% to 10% of patients.[361] Cervical involvement has been found to occur with the same frequency.[362] Extension to the vagina occurs in about 7% of cases.[359] Metastases to the peritoneal cavity and the omentum are occasionally seen. Creasman et al[363] reported a recurrence rate of 34% in patients wtih positive peritoneal cytology as compared to a 10% recurrence rate in patients with negative peritoneal cytology. However, other authors have not confirmed this high recurrence rate.[364]

Almost all women with endometrial cancer report abnormal vaginal bleeding. Since 70% to 75% of women who develop the disease are postmenopausal, this symptom should be easily identified. The character of the abnormal bleeding varies from a serosanguinous discharge to frank bleeding. Pyometria and hematometria may be seen in patients with stenosis of the cervical canal. The finding of a pyometria in a postmenstrual woman should be considered highly suggestive of endometrial cancer. Pain is usually a symptom of advanced disease.

PATHOLOGY

Grossly, endometrial carcinoma is a polypoid growth that arises most often in the fundus of the uterus. The tumor may be small and focal or diffusely involve the uterine cavity. The diffuse lesions often show extensive hemorrhage and necrosis. The posterior wall is more likely to be involved than the anterior wall.

Histologically, most endometrial carcinomas are adenocarcinomas.[365] There is no evidence that adenoacanthoma behaves differently from pure adenocarcinoma. Recently several pathologists have begun using the term "adenocarcinoma with squamous metaplasia" to describe an adenocanthoma. Adenosquamous carcinoma of the endometrium contains malignant adenocarcinoma and malignant squamous carcinoma. Ng et al[366] and Silverberg[367] have described these lesions in detail, and both have reported a worse prognosis for them compared to pure adenocarcinomas. Both Silverberg et al[367] and Salazar et al[368] have related prognosis in these tumors to the differentiation of the adenocarcinoma portion of the tumor.

Infrequently seen carcinomas of the endometrium include clear cell carcinoma,[369] secretory carcinoma,[370] and squamous carcinoma.[371] Recently attention has been directed toward the papillary variety of endometrial carcinoma. Two varieties are recognized: an endometrioid papillary carcinoma and a serous papillary carcinoma. Although both have been reported to behave as poorly differentiated tumors, the serous papillary variety appears to carry the worse prognosis.[372,373]

The histologic grading of endometrial carcinoma is divided by FIGO into well differentiated (Grade 1), moderately differentiated (Grade 2), and poorly differentiated (Grade 3). In a GOG pilot study of 222 patients, Boronow et al[374] found the distribution of cases to be 42% Grade 1, 40% Grade 2, and 18% Grade 3. These authors were able to correlate increasing grade with an increased frequency of nodal metastases.

DIAGNOSIS, CLINICAL EVALUATION, AND STAGING

The diagnosis of endometrial carcinoma is made on the basis of a fractional dilation and curettage. The endocervical curettage should be performed before sounding or dilating the cervix to prevent contamination of the cervical sample by endometrial tissue that may be dislodged by the sound or dilator. If there is a visible lesion or a suspicious area on the cervix, biopsies should be obtained. If the diagnosis was made by office biopsy, a separate endocervical curettage should be obtained. Some authorities recommend that a formal dilatation and curettage be performed if carcinoma is diagnosed on office biopsy to be sure that the worst lesion is sampled. The Papanicolaou smear is not a reliable method of detecting endometrial cancer, even though occasionally malignant endometrial cells may be found in the Papanicolaou smears of asymptomatic patients with endometrial cancer. In such cases, a dilatation and curettage is indicated.

Patients diagnosed as having endometrial carcinoma should undergo a thorough history and physical examination, a careful pelvic examination, a chest radiograph, an intravenous pyelogram, a barium enema, cystoscopy, and proctosigmoidoscopy. Laboratory studies should include a complete blood count and biochemical profile to include renal and liver function tests. Other diagnostic studies such as CT, MRI, and lymphangiography may occasionally be helpful. Additional tests should be performed if warranted by symptoms.

The FIGO staging classification is listed in Table 36-17. As with other gynecologic cancers, staging should be performed jointly by the gynecologic oncologist, radiation oncologist, and medical oncologist. Stage I tumors are subclassified according to the grade of the tumor.

TABLE 36-17. FIGO Classification of Endometrial Carcinoma

Stage I	The carcinoma is confined to the corpus
Stage Ia	The length of the uterine cavity is 8 cm or less
Stage Ib	The length of the uterine cavity is 8 cm or more
	Stage I cases should be subgrouped with regard to the histologic type of the adenocarcinoma as follows:
	G1 — Highly differentiated carcinoma
	G2 — Differentiated adenocarcinomas with partly solid areas
	G3 — Predominantly solid or entirely undifferentiated carcinomas
Stage II	The carcinoma involves the corpus and the cervix
Stage III	The carcinoma extends outside the corpus, but not outside the true pelvis (it may involve the vaginal wall or the parametrium but not the bladder or rectum)
Stage IV	The carcinoma involves the bladder or rectum or extends outside the pelvis

PROGNOSTIC FACTORS IN CARCINOMA OF THE ENDOMETRIUM

Age at time of diagnosis of endometrial carcinoma has long been known to be a prognostic factor. Frick et al[354] reported improved survival in patients under age 59 with Stage I disease even after correcting for deaths from intercurrent disease. Other authors[375a,376] have reported similar findings. Jones[376] attributed the improved survival to an increased incidence of less extensive, better differentiated lesions in younger women. Stage at diagnosis is directly related to survival. Creasman and Weed[343] reviewed three large series and reported average survivals of 79% for Stage I, 50% for Stage II, 27% for Stage III, and 9% for Stage IV. Cervical involvement has been associated with a worse prognosis in most series. Surwit et al[377] reviewed 117 patients with histologic involvement of the cervix. Overall survival for the entire group was 58%. However, when divided into those with stromal invasion and those with only involvement of endocervical glands, the survival rates were 47% and 74%, respectively. Uterine size in Stage I disease appears to be a less reliable indicator of prognosis. Lutz et al[378] state that uterine size does not always reflect actual tumor volume because of the association of benign uterine disease such as leiomyomata. Creasman et al,[360] however, noted an increased incidence of both pelvic and para-aortic lymph node metastases in stage IB as compared to Stage IA.

Perhaps the most significant prognostic factors for planning therapy in patients with early disease are histologic grade, depth of myometrial penetration, and lymph node metastases. Lewis et al[375] in 1970 reported an 11.2% incidence of nodal metastases in Stage I endometrial cancer, and in a literature review Morrow et al[360] reported that 10.6% of 369 patients with Stage I and 36.5% of 85 patients with Stage II disease had positive lymph nodes. Creasman et al[360] and Boronow et al,[375] reporting on a GOG pilot study, found that the incidence of both pelvic and para-aortic nodal metastases was related to increasing histologic grade, increasing depth of myometrial invasion, and, to a lesser extent, uterine size. DiSaia et al[379] evaluated recurrence and survival in that same group of patients and found those risk factors to be related to both increased rates of recurrence and decreased survival. Plentl and Friedman,[359] in an extensive review of the literature, found decreased survival in endometrial cancer to be directly related to both histologic grade and depth of tumor penetration of the myometrium. These same authors found that vaginal recurrence was also directly related to histologic grade. They reported 4.3% vaginal recurrence with Grade 1 tumors, 9.2% with Grade 2, and 24.4% with Grade 3.

TREATMENT OF CARCINOMA OF THE ENDOMETRIUM

Although the numbers of deaths from endometrial carcinoma are low in relation to cervical carcinoma and ovarian carcinoma, this is due to the large percentage of patients diagnosed in Stage I rather than the survival rates per stage. In a literature review, Morrow et al[380] reported survival rates of 76% for Stage I, 51% for Stage II, 26% for State III, and 9% for Stage IV. Boronow[381] found that survival in endometrial cancer was very similar to cervical cancer when corrected for stage distribution. In other series, the 5-year survival rate of surgery alone or combined with preoperative or postoperative radiation therapy has varied from 80% to 95%.[382-385]

The therapeutic approach for endometrial cancer is determined by FIGO stage, histologic type and grade, depth of myometrial penetration, and the medical condition of the patient.[386,387] Hysterectomy is the central feature of the management of most cases. The place of radiation therapy is in the adjunctive therapy of high-risk early-stage disease, in the management of advanced disease, and for those patients with early disease who are medically unsuitable for hysterectomy.[388,389]

Stages IA and IB Carcinoma of the Endometrium

Patients with Stages IA and IB endometrial carcinoma whose tumor is grade 1 can be managed by total abdominal hysterectomy and bilateral salpingo-oophorectomy. Removal of pelvic or para-aortic lymph nodes is not indicated as the incidence of nodal metastases is less than 5%.[360,374] If pathologic analysis of the uterus reveals invasion of greater than 50%, whole pelvic irradiation should be added even though the major effect of this irradiation may be to decrease the incidence of central recurrence rather than improve survival.[379,390] DiSaia et al[379] found that only 4% of grade 1 patients had deep myometrial invasion. Whether postoperative vaginal irradiation should be added in grade 1 patients with minimal myometrial invasion is controversial. The incidence of vaginal metastases is reported to be less than 5%[359,391] in grade 1 carcinomas.

Patients with histologic grade 2 or grade 3 carcinomas have a 15% and 39% incidence, respectively, of deep myometrial invasion.[374] The incidence of metastases to pelvic lymph nodes is 10% for grade 2 and 36% for grade 3, and aortic lymph nodes are involved in 4% of grade 2 tumors and 28% of grade 3 tumors.[360] Because of these factors, preoperative whole pelvis irradiation is used at Memorial Sloan-Kettering Cancer Center and para-aortic nodal sampling is performed at the time of hysterectomy. Vaginal irradiation is added postoperatively.

In preoperative insertions (^{137}Cs) for Stage I tumors, Perez at Washington University has used 3500 to 4000 mgh in the endometrial cavity. A surface dose of 6000 to 6500 cGy is also delivered to the surface of the vaginal fornices (1800–2000 mgh). Surgery is usually scheduled 3 days to 1 week after removal of the brachytherapy insertion to ensure that the true pathologic extent of the tumor can be adequately evaluated histologically. Although a higher degree of tumor sterilization is observed when surgery is performed 4 to 6 weeks after the brachytherapy placement, the pathologic features that can be helpful in determining whether further treatment is necessary, such as depth of myometrial invasion, are more difficult to evaluate.[392-394] Preoperative brachytherapy has the disadvantage that inadequate radiation dose is delivered to the pelvic lymph nodes. If tumor extension greater than 50% thickness of the myometrium or tumor extension beyond the uterus is demonstrated

at the time of surgery, external beam irradiation should be added postoperatively.

In patients treated after total abdominal hysterectomy and bilateral salpingo-oophorectomy, the irradiation fields are the same as those used for preoperative irradiation. Whole pelvis fields are used for this boost, using a midline shield at some point during the treatment course as determined by calculating the bladder and rectal doses from the intracavitary insertion. Usually, 2000 cGy are delivered to the whole pelvis and 3000 cGy to the parametria with a midline block. If the patient has residual tumor left in the pelvis, a boost to the area of residual tumor is indicated. The indications for postoperative radiation therapy are deep myometrial invasion, transection of tumor, unsuspected advanced stage (ovary/tube/node involvement), and unsuspected poorly differentiated tumors.

Creasman and Weed[343] have recommended initial total abdominal hysterectomy with selective pelvic and para-aortic lymph node sampling in all Stage IA and IB grade 2 and 3 patients. These authors would then add postoperative pelvic or vaginal irradiation based on findings at surgery.

Stage II Carcinoma of the Endometrium

In Stage II endometrial carcinoma, the cancer has involved the cervix (corpus et collum). There appears to be little doubt that survival is significantly lower in these patients.[359,367,377,395] Surwit et al[377] reported survival rates of 74% if only the endocervical glands were involved. Homesley et al[345] in a review from Memorial Sloan-Kettering Cancer Center reported survival rates of 61% if cervical involvement was occult and 48% if there was gross involvement of the cervix. Recently, however, Larson et al[396] from M.D. Anderson Hospital divided patients into three groups: gross cervical involvement, occult stromal invasion, and no evidence of stromal invasion. They reported survival rates of 70%, 65%, and 67% in each group respectively and concluded that there is no prognostic significance in the extent of cervical involvement.

Most authorities use a combination of whole pelvis irradiation and a single intracavitary application of cesium followed by total abdominal hysterectomy and bilateral salpingo-oophorectomy for Stage II carcinoma of the endometrium.[396,397] At Washington University, based on previous experience recently reported by Grigsby et al,[398] patients with Stage II endometrial carcinoma who have only microscopic involvement of the endocervix are treated with a preoperative intracavitary insertion followed by an extrafascial hysterectomy and bilateral salpingo-oophorectomy. In general, the dose delivered is 3500 to 4000 mgh to the body of the uterus and 6000 cGy to the vaginal vault (1800 to 2000 mgh) with 2 cm colpostats. If there is gross or multiple quadrant microscopic involvement of the exocervix, in addition to the intracavitary insertion, the patient receives external irradiation (2000 cGy whole pelvis and 3000 cGy additional dose to the parametria with midline shield) followed by an extrafascial hysterectomy approximately 4 weeks later. For the inoperable patient, or in the case in which surgery is refused, radiation alone is used. At Memorial Sloan-Kettering Cancer Center, whole pelvis irradiation followed in 3 to 4 weeks by modified radical hysterectomy with para-aortic nodal sampling is used for Stage II endometrial carcinoma.

Although some series have reported the use of radical hysterectomy and bilateral pelvic lymphadenectomy in these patients, Rutledge[399] has pointed out that therapy with irradiation followed by hysterectomy has greater usefulness for most patients and the cure rate is comparable.

Stages III and IV Carcinoma of the Endometrium

Most patients with advanced endometrial cancer will not be candidates for operation. Because the distribution of tumor within the pelvis may vary, no single technique is applicable to all patients. External beam therapy is the mainstay of treatment; whole pelvis irradiation is given for 2000 to 4000 cGy, with an additional boost to the parametria given with midline shield to complete 5000 to 6000 cGy in 5 to 7 weeks. The central dose is supplemented with at least two brachytherapy applications for approximately 8000 mgh. Afterloading Simon-Heyman capsules and the Fletcher-Suit applicators lend themselves best to the differential loading necessary to achieve the best possible dose distribution. If lower third vaginal extension is present, volume interstitial implantation with brachytherapy sources is indicated.

Endometrial carcinoma that is Stage III based on involvement of the upper vagina may be managed by preoperative whole pelvis and intracavitary irradiation and total abdominal or modified radical hysterectomy and a wide vaginal cuff.

RESULTS OF TREATMENT USING RADIATION THERAPY IN CARCINOMA OF THE ENDOMETRIUM

Statistically valid data are not available to support the impact of adjuvant radiotherapy on survival. However, in a randomized study, Graham[400] reported better 5-year survival rates with combination therapy as opposed to hysterectomy alone, although the differences between the preoperative and postoperative irradiation groups were not statistically significant. Nolan et al[384] in a nonrandomized study also demonstrated improved survival with combined therapy in patients with Stage I in high risk groups (large uterus or less differentiated lesions).

Nevertheless, there has been a significantly decreased incidence of vaginal recurrences in patients treated with irradiation (1–3%) in contrast to those treated with hysterectomy alone (15%). A review of 304 patients treated at the Mallinckrodt Institute of Radiology, using preoperative intracavitary therapy alone in 199 patients, in addition to 43 patients on whom additional external irradiation was given (usually 2000–3000 cGy whole pelvis), demonstrated an overall pelvic recurrence rate of 4% for grade 1, 3% for grade 2, and 9% for grade 3 lesions.[401] Survival is shown in Figure 36-15. Table 36-18 shows 5-year survival figures for patients with Stage I disease, as reported in the literature.

Several authors have reported a greater incidence of vaginal pelvic recurrences and distant metastases in patients with poorly differentiated (grade 3 tumors) or in those with advanced stage. However, radiation therapy has been shown to decrease the incidence of pelvic recurrences. Bedwinek et al[407] reported a 71% overall 5-year disease-free survival,

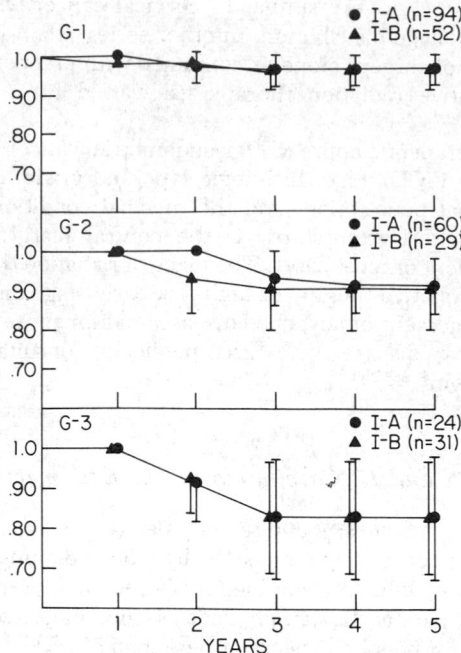

FIG. 36-15. Disease-free survival by grade and stage. (Stokes S, Bedwinek JM, Kao M-S, et al: Treatment of Stage I adenocarcinoma of the endometrium by hysterectomy and adjuvant irradiation: A retrospective analysis of 304 patients. Int J Radiat Oncol Biol Phys 12:339, 1986)

9.6% incidence of pelvic recurrences, and 15.6% distant failures in 83 patients with Stage I grade 3 endometrial carcinoma treated with either intracavitary irradiation alone or combined with pelvic external radiotherapy.

Uterine size in Stage I has been found to correlate with prognosis only if the enlargement is related to tumor infiltration in the myometrium (Table 36-19). Wade et al[415] and Javert[416] noted that often benign conditions such as myomata and adenomyosis may contribute to uterine enlargement and have no significant impact on prognosis. Stokes et al[401] observed similar survival rates in Stages IA and IB patients regardless of the tumor differentiation. Myometrial invasion decreases the 5-year survival rate from 85% to 90% when it is absent to 60% to 79% when involvement is more

TABLE 36-18. Stage I Endometrial Carcinoma Survival at 5 Years

Author	No. of Patients	% Survival at 5 Years
Bleiler et al[402]	282	64 crude
Wharam et al[403]	269	81 NED
Graham[400]	123	74 crude
Malkasian et al[404]	409	82 actuarial
Underwood et al[385]	220	91 actuarial
Frick et al[354]	239	78 crude
Salazar et al[405]	307	84 actuarial
Brady et al[406]	99	88 crude
Stokes et al[401]	304	

Modified from Glassburn JR, Brady LW: Carcinoma of the endometrium. In Perez CA, Brady LW (eds): Principles and Practice of Radiation Oncology, pp 966–987. Philadelphia, JB Lippincott, 1987.

TABLE 36-19.   Five-Year Survival Rates Correlated with Depth of Myometrial Invasion

	No Invasion		Superficial Invasion		Deep Invasion	
	No. of Patients	5-Year Survival Rate (%)	No. of Patients	5-Year Survival Rate (%)	No. of Patients	5-Year Survival Rate (%)
Author						
Anderson[408]	12	100	22	86	7	42
Gusberg[409]	245	67	96	70	94	34
Climie[335]	56	87	20	80	23	56
Austin[336]	133	91	239	95	163	81
Cheon[410]	181	81	91	77	73	42
Nilson[411]			205	89	131	76
Lewis[375]	16	93	41	88	22	54
Ng[412]	129	88	48	72	22	27
Sall[413]			75	92	16	75
Nahhas[414]	75	85	33	82	28	56
Frick[354]	63	79	101	77	42	45
Total patients	910		971		621	
Total survivors	736		827		376	
Average 5-year survival rate		80		85		50

Adapted from Jones HW III: Treatment of adenocarcinoma of the endometrium. Obstet Gynecol Surv 30:147, 1975.

than half way through the myometrium (Fig. 36-16).[376,379] Similar results are correlated with the degree of differentiation of the tumor (Table 36-20).

A few reports have compared the effectiveness of external irradiation or intracavitary radium without conclusive results. Sala and del Regato[422] compared the survival after 4000 cGy external irradiation to the pelvis (70 patients) or a radium implant for 6000 cGy (48 patients). The 3-year survival rate was 87% and 77%, respectively. No vaginal recurrences were noted in either group. The survival rate was similar whether residual tumor was present in the surgical specimen or not. Similar findings were reported by Silverberg and DeGeorgi[423] in 76 patients treated with preoperative irradiation and hysterectomy. Weigensberg[424] in a randomized study involving small groups of patients in two community hospitals observed a 5-year actuarial disease-free survival rate of 75% in 53 patients treated with intracavitary irradiation and hysterectomy and of 48% in 38 patients treated with external beam irradiation. Patients treated with intracavitary radium received 5400 cGy and with external beam irradiation, 4000 cGy. Only 2 of the intracavitary therapy patients had pelvic recurrences in contrast to 9 in the external beam group. Uterine size and degree of tumor differentiation were similar in both groups. Aalders et al[390] in a randomized trial, and Bedwinek et al[407] in a nonrandomized retrospective review, reported similar survival rates with intracavitary therapy alone or combined with external irradiation. However, pelvic recurrences can be decreased with external irradiation in patients with less differentiated tumors from about 20% to 5%.

In 19 patients with Stage II endometrial carcinoma treated by an intracavitary insertion and external beam radiation to the whole pelvis, a 63% 5-year survival rate was obtained.[425] A report by Grigsby et al[398] from the Mallinkrodt Institute of Radiology disclosed 8 pelvic recurrences in 79 patients (10%) with stage II endometrial carcinoma treated by a combination of preoperative or postoperative intracavitary insertion and external irradiation. Eleven patients with microscopic endocervical involvement treated only with a preoperative intracavitary insertion had no pelvic or vaginal recurrence. In a small group of 26 patients with Stage II endometrial carcinoma treated with irradiation alone, the overall incidence of pelvic failure was 34.6%, in contrast to only 8.9% in those treated with a combination of irradiation and surgery. The survival and NED survival rates are illustrated in Figure 36-17.

It is known that gross involvement of the cervix carries a

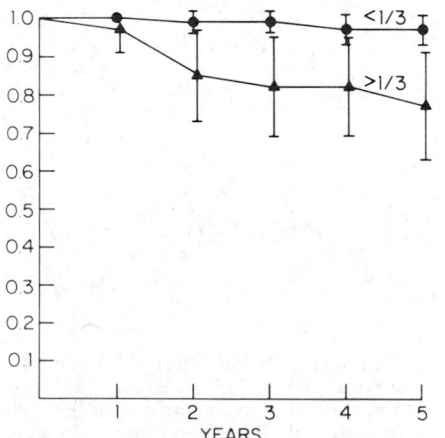

FIG. 36-16. NED survival by depth of myometrial invasion (quick or postoperative radiotherapy) for endometrial carcinoma patients. (Stokes S, Bedwinek JM, Kao M-S, et al: Treatment of Stage I adenocarcinoma of the endometrium by hysterectomy and adjuvant irradiation: A retrospective analysis of 304 patients. Int J Radiat Oncol Biol Phys 12:339, 1986)

TABLE 36-20. Relationship Between Tumor Differentiation and 5-Year Survival Rates in Patients with Endometrial Carcinoma

Author	Grade I		Grade II		Grade III	
	No. of Patients	5-Year Survival Rate (%)	No. of Patients	5-Year Survival Rate (%)	No. of Patients	5-Year Survival Rate (%)
Webb[417]	32	84	155	52	37	30
Lindgren[418]	120	88	153	82	56	80
Gusberg[409]	204	62	85	53	65	32
Boutselis[419]	81	75	42	64	49	14
Anderson[408]	14	100	51	82	26	65
Climie[335]	56	93	24	75	18	44
Dobbie[420]	147	81	74	78	45	73
Roman[421]	47	87	105	78	113	51
Wade[415]	65	84	150	78	50	42
Austin[336]	126	96	239	96	163	75
Cheon[410]	196	81	72	78	77	44
Ng[412]	91	86	101	75	62	37
Nahhas[414]	106	84	57	75	35	48
Beiler[402]	54	83	130	65	67	40
Frick[354]	218	79	76	54	54	30
Total patients	1558		1515		917	
Total survivors	1267		1124		462	
Average 5-year survival rate		81		74		50

Adapted from Jones HW III: Treatment of adenocarcinoma of the endometrium. Obstet Gynecol Surv 30:147, 1975.

worse prognosis than microscopic involvement. Noteably, Grigsby et al[398] reported lower survival in patients with ectocervical tumor invasion, even if it was microscopic only. Patterns of failure reported by various authors in patients with Stage II endometrial carcinoma are summarized in Table 36-21.

Unfortunately the results of treatment for Stage III disease are poor. A 25% 5-year survival is to be expected with aggressive therapy, with somewhat better results being obtained in patients who had ovarian involvement only (Table 36-22). Patients with Stage IV disease are rarely cured, and most authors report 5% of the patients alive at 5 years.

SURGERY FOR CARCINOMA OF THE ENDOMETRIUM

The usual surgical procedure for adenocarcinoma of the endometrium is abdominal hysterectomy and bilateral salpingo-oophorectomy. On occasion, some authorities will recommend modified radical hysterectomy or radical hysterectomy for Stage II disease. The techniques for these procedures are identical to those described under the section on cervical cancer and need not be repeated here. Most surgeons do not recommend that the cervix be sutured closed before abdominal hysterectomy for endometrial carcinoma although this was common practice in the past. Nei-

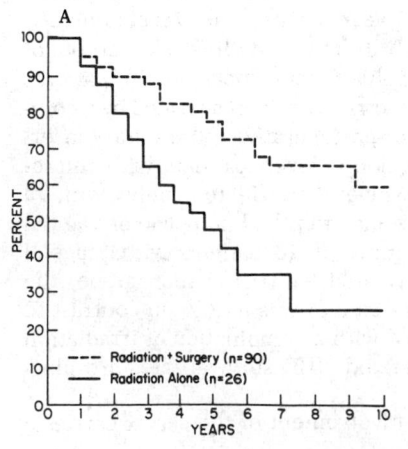
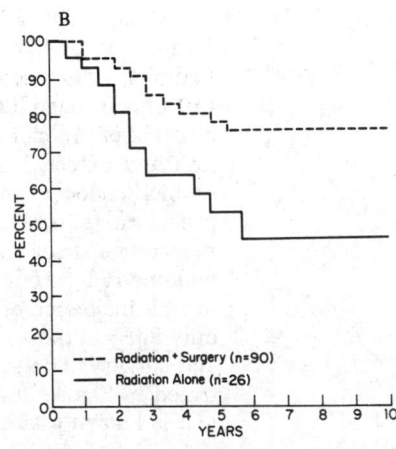

FIG. 36-17. Overall survival (A) and disease-free survival (B) in 116 patients with Stage II carcinoma of the endometrium. MIR, 1960–1981. (Grigsby PW, Perez CA, Camel HM, et al: Stage II carcinoma of the endometrium: Results of therapy and prognostic factors. Int J Radiat Oncol Biol Phys 11:1915, 1985)

TABLE 36-21.   Carcinoma of the Endometrium: Treatment Outcome of Stage II Disease

Investigator	No. of Patients	Survival (%)	Vagina	Pelvis	Vagina + Pelvis	Pelvis + DM	DM
					No. of Recurrences (%)		
Stage II—Radiation Therapy and Surgery							
Gagnon et al[426]	20	44.8*		1 (5)			2 (10)
Onsrud et al[427]	44†	85			1 (2.3)		4 (9.1)
	40‡	85	2 (5)	2 (5)	3 (7.5)		4 (10)
Salazar et al[405]	20			1 (5)			3 (15)
Spanos et al[428]	61				12 (19.7)§		Not reported
Total‖	124		2 (1.6)	4 (3.2)	4 (3.2)	0	13 (10.5)
				Total pelvis 8%		Total DM 10.5%	
Stage II—Radiation Therapy Alone							
Landgren et al[429]	38	65**		3 (7.9)		4 (10.5)	9 (23.7)
Salazar et al[405]	8			3 (37.5)			2 (25)
Spanos et al[428]	21				4 (19)††		Not reported
Total‖	46			6 (13)		4 (8.7)	11 (23.9)
				Total pelvis 21.7%		Total DM 32.6%	

Perez CA, Bedwinek JM, Breaux SR: Patterns of failure after treatment of gynecological tumors. Cancer Treat Symp 2-217, 1983.
* Five years.
† Radium only.
‡ Radium + external.
§ Value = combined total or recurrences in pelvis, vagina and pelvis, and pelvis + DM in study by Spanos et al.
‖ Excluding Spanos et al.
** Actuarial, 5 years.
†† Value = combined total of recurrences in pelvis and pelvis + DM in study by Spanos et al.

ther do most surgeons tie the fimbriated ends of the fallopian tubes upon opening the abdomen, although most do recommend placing clamps across the cornual region to occlude the fallopian tubes and provide traction during the procedure. Pelvic exenteration has been used for central recurrence after irradiation, but the utility of this procedure in endometrial carcinoma is limited.[437]

TECHNIQUES OF IRRADIATION FOR CARCINOMA OF THE ENDOMETRIUM

Combinations of Irradiation and Surgery

A variety of techniques have been used combining irradiation and surgery in the treatment of Stage I endometrial cancer, including external beam, brachytherapy, or combinations of

TABLE 36-22.   Stage III Endometrial Carcinoma: Survival Rates at 5 Years

Author	No. of Patients	Survival at 5 Years (%)
Antoniades et al[430]	37	25
Rutledge and Ehrlich[431]		21
Buchler et al[357]	32	22
Kottmeier[432]	136	30
Homesley et al[433]	23	4
Boronow[434]	49	18
Geisler and Gibbs[435]	19	5.3
Ng and Reagan[412]	14	13.6
Danoff et al[436]	17	11.7

Danoff BF, McDay J, Louka M, et al: Stage III endometrial carcinoma: Analysis of patterns of failure and therapeutic implications. Int J Radiat Oncol Biol Phys 6:1491, 1980.

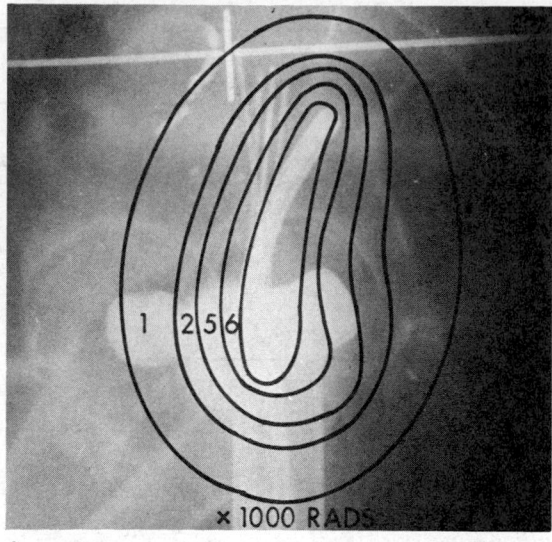

A

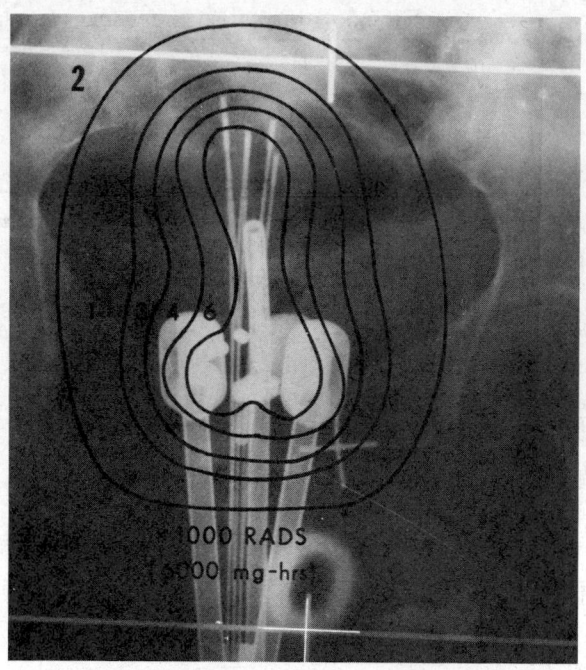

B

FIG. 36-18. Frontal (**A**) and lateral (**B**) radiographs of intracavitary insertion in patient with carcinoma of the endometrium showing Heyman-Simon afterloading capsule in the uterine fundus, tandem in the lower uterine segment, and ovoids in the vaginal vault. (Perez CA, DiSaia PJ, Knapp RC: Gynecologic tumors. In DeVita VT Jr, Hellman S, Rosenberg SA [eds]: Cancer: Principles and Practice of Oncology, 2nd ed, pp 1013–1081. Philadelphia, JB Lippincott, 1985)

both. Irradiation has been administered preoperatively or postoperatively or as a combination of both.

Preoperative irradiation has several aims: to decrease the opportunity of viable tumor cells seeded in the operative field to develop into a local recurrence, to render the tumor cells nonviable and decrease the possibility of distant dissemination of the tumor, and to irradiate the areas of frequent nodal involvement that are not removed at the time of surgery. The techniques of external beam irradiation, volume to be treated, and portals used are similar to those used in the treatment of carcinoma of the uterine cervix.

For the intracavitary insertions, in addition to afterloading tandem and vaginal ovoids, it is common practice to pack the uterine cavity with Heyman or afterloading Heyman-Simon capsules (Fig. 36-18). This technique allows the placement of sources in the body of the uterus around the tumor and, at the same time, some pressure can be exerted on the uterine wall, it is hoped with some reduction in its thickness. These two effects may result in higher doses of irradiation delivered to the serosa of the uterus and immediately adjacent paracervical tissues. The lower segment of the uterus and the endocervical canal can be treated with capsules or with a tandem. The vaginal vault is always irradiated with vaginal colpostats. If there is tumor extension into the vagina, the entire length of this organ should be treated with a cylinder or special applicator (*i.e.*, Burnett, Bloedorn, Delclos) to include the suburethral regions and introitus because of the propensity of advanced endometrial adenocarcinoma to metastasize to this site through submucosal venous and lymphatic plexuses.

Radiation Therapy Alone

Medically inoperable patients with Stage I or II disease in a significant percentage of cases can be cured with a combination of external beam therapy and brachytherapy. Usually two intracavitary insertions are carried out, 2 weeks apart, to deliver 4500 to 5000 mgh to the uterine cavity and an additional 3000 mgh to the vaginal vault. This is combined with external beam therapy for an additional 2000 to 4000 cGy to the whole pelvis, and subsequent boosting of the lateral pelvic dose to a total of 5000 cGy with a midline pelvic shield to protect the bladder and bowel. Survival rates of 74% to 78% at 5 years have been reported.[389,438]

COMPLICATIONS OF THERAPY

Surgical or combined treatment by surgery and adjuvant irradiation in endometrial carcinoma is well tolerated. Major complications, as reported by Stokes et al,[439] with a preoperative implant and hysterectomy, were noted in 1% of 199 patients. However, if the intracavitary insertion was given postoperatively, 12% of the patients (3 of 26) had significant complications. When external irradiation was given—the dose to the whole pelvis combined with an intracavitary insertion—the complication rate was 2% (5 in 264 patients) but increased to 18% (7 in 40 patients) when the whole pelvis dose exceeded 3000 cGy. A total of 8 major gastrointestinal and 4 urinary complications were noted in 304 patients, the most frequent being bowel obstruction, ureterovaginal fistula, uretheral stricture, hemorrhagic cystitis, and rectal ulcer.

CHEMOTHERAPY OF CARCINOMA OF THE ENDOMETRIUM

Hormonal Therapy

The most commonly used systemic treatment in recurrent endometrial carcinoma has been synthetic progestational agents. The response rates range from 30% to 37%.[440] Responses are associated with prolonged survival; median survival for patients responding to progesterone therapy has been 23 to 29 months compared to 6 months for patients without an objective response.[440] Response to hormonal therapy is related to the histologic grade of the tumor, and well-differentiated tumors respond more frequently than do those with poorly differentiated histologies. Other factors that influence response to hormonal therapy include disease-free interval, age, and presence of areas of squamous metaplasia within the tumor. Responses are more likely in vaginal or lung metastases and lymph nodes and less likely in pelvic recurrences.

The progesterone receptor content of endometrial tumors correlates well with subsequent response to progesterone therapy.[441,442,443] Even though well-differentiated tumors tend to have the highest progesterone receptor positivity, the receptor positivity appears to be a better correlate than grade.

In studies on 114 endometrial adenocarcinomas, the mean progesterone-binding capacity was inversely related to tumor grade.[441] Although more data are needed to firmly establish the value of progesterone receptor (PR) analysis, it is noteworthy that this study reported that 88% (30 of 34) of progesterone-responsive lesions were PR(+) and 94% (34 of 36) of unresponsive lesions were PR(−).

Systemic hormonal therapy with progestogens has been well established as first-line systemic therapy for patients with recurrent or disseminated disease. The most commonly used progestogens have been hydroxyprogesterone (Delalutin) or medroxyprogesterone (Depo-Provera, 400 mg intramuscularly weekly). Oral megastrol acetate (Megase), 160 mg/day, produces similar results. These progestogens should be continued indefinitely until recurrence or distant metastases develop.

Studies using alternative endocrine therapy for advanced endometrial cancer, including the antiestrogen tamoxifen[444,445] and the synthetic 17-ethinyl testosterone derivative danazol, have suggested some activity. Data from several studies with tamoxifen[446-449] suggest an overall response rate of approximately 39% with well-differentiated tumors being more likely to respond. Recently, attempts have been made to enhance the activity of hormonal therapy by sequential therapy with tamoxifen that induces progesterone receptors.[450] Although an increase in progesterone receptors was documented, the overall response rate was 33%, not significantly different from progesterone alone. However, further studies to study the modulation of progesterone receptors in endometrial cancer are warranted.

The use of progestogen therapy as prophylaxis in early-stage endometrial carcinoma remains controversial. In one large adjuvant trial, Stage I patients received either adjuvant Depo-Provera or a placebo.[451] Despite unbalanced stratification with regard to prognostic factors and frequent unevaluability, there was no difference in 5-year survival rates. Another study of 35 Stage IA and Stage IB patients treated with surgery with or without subsequent treatment with 6-methyl-17-hydroxyprogesterone reported no benefit.[452] Despite this, several investigators have advocated the use of prophylactic progestational agents in high risk patients.[453-457] However, the worth, if any, of adjuvant progesterone therapy in early-stage endometrial carcinoma must be considered unproven. Two ongoing trials, one in Australia[440] and one in Italy[458] that include only high risk patients, suggest some beneficial effect, but further follow-up is needed in this important subgroup of patients.

Single-Agent Chemotherapy

Nonhormonal chemotherapy has been studied to a limited degree. Table 36-23 lists the single agents that appear to have some activity in advanced endometrial cancer.[459-462] These data can be used only to suggest activity because of the small numbers of patients studied and the variability of prognostic factors. Of these agents, only doxorubicin, hexamethylmelamine, and cisplatin appear to have clearly established

TABLE 36-23. Single Agent Chemotherapy in Endometrial Carcinoma

Drugs	Patients Responding/Total Treated	Response Rate (%)
Alkylating agents		
Cyclophosphamide	7/33	21
Nitrogen mustard	3/11	27
Antimetabolites		
5-Fluorouracil	10/43	23
Antitumor Antibiotics		
Doxorubicin (Adriamycin)	33/92	36
Bleomycin	3/8	37
Miscellaneous Agents		
Hexamethylmelamine	6/29	30
Cisplatin	11/26	42
Cisplatin	4/13	31

activity[463,464] with response rates in the 30% to 40% range.

Of all the single agents, doxorubicin has been most extensively evaluated and appears to be the standard single agent to which new agents or combinations should be compared. Thigpen et al[465] treated 43 patients with advanced or recurrent disease using 60 mg/m² intravenous doxorubicin every 3 weeks. They reported a 37% response rate (16 of 43), and 26% (11 of 43) had clinical complete regression of disease. Median survival was 14 months for patients achieving a complete response, 6.8 months for those with a partial regression, and 3.5 months for patients with progressive disease. Age, time to first recurrence, histologic grade of primary site of metastasis, and previous therapy had no effect on probability of response. Toxicity was similar to other studies in which doxorubicin was used as a single agent.

Conflicting reports on the activity of cisplatin in this disease may relate to its low activity (1 of 25, 4%) when used as second-line treatment[460] and its reasonable response rate (46%) when used at higher doses (100 mg/m²) in patients who had not been previously treated with chemotherapy.[461]

Combination Therapy

Combination chemotherapy for advanced endometrial carcinoma has not been studied extensively. The relatively few studies that have been published generally include small patient numbers.[463,464] Recent studies employing doxorubicin and cisplatin[466,467] report higher response rates (30–90%) but with only a few patients treated. Comparison of this two-drug regimen with doxorubicin alone[468] demonstrates a 45% response rate for the combination compared to 20% for the single agent. Cisplatin, doxorubicin (Adriamycin), and cyclophosphamide (PAC) demonstrated a 45% overall response rate in 209 patients at a cost of moderate to severe toxicity.[469] Another study of the three-drug regimen CAP, including cisplatin 50 mg/m², cyclophosphamide 500 mg/m², and doxorubicin 50 mg/m² intravenously every 4 weeks, produced a 58% response rate, including 28% complete remissions in 18 patients with advanced disease.[470] Both the AP and CAP combinations appear to have some enhanced activity and should be compared to doxorubicin alone in larger trials. Other studies have added combination chemotherapy and progestogens, but the independent contribution of the drugs and the hormone cannot be assessed in these single-arm studies.[471–474]

The combination of megestrol, cyclophosphamide, and doxorubicin with or without 5-FU was given to 126 patients in a cooperative group study.[475] The response rate (22%) and the median survival (27 weeks) were the same in both arms and represent only a marginal improvement over the 19% response rate achieved by the same group with doxorubicin alone.

Whether the use of combinations of hormones with single agent chemotherapy or combinations enhances the antitumor effect substantially remains unresolved and should be subjected to well-controlled clinical trials.

FUTURE DIRECTIONS

Major efforts should be made to better define the relative risk groups in early-stage endometrial cancer. The GOG has closed its surgical staging protocol in which more than 1,000 cases of patients have undergone rigidly controlled surgical staging. When these data are available, a great deal of information will be gleaned from careful analysis of those cases. Prospective studies should then be undertaken to improve therapeutic results in high risk groups.

It is imperative that chemotherapeutic agents useful in endometrial cancer be developed. Not only will this provide hope for recurrent disease, but also it will allow the development of useful neoadjuvant regimens. At this time, all patients with advanced and recurrent disease should be considered candidates for investigational protocols.

UTERINE SARCOMAS

Uterine sarcomas account for 1% to 6% of all cancers of the corpus uteri.[476–484] These variations in reported incidence depend on the criteria used to classify these cancers as well as the nature of the series on which the reports are based. Table 36-24 lists a classification of uterine sarcomas. It is based on Kempson's[479] simplification of the classification by Ober.[479a] For practical purposes, however, there are three main histologic types of uterine sarcomas that are of clinical significance: (1) malignant mixed mullerian tumors, (2) leiomyosarcomas, and (3) stromal sarcomas. Although there is no FIGO staging classification for uterine sarcomas, most authors utilize a modification of the FIGO classification for endometrial carcinoma. This classification is listed in Table 36-25. As has been pointed out by Lewis et al,[476] this classification is a surgical classification based on the findings at initial surgical treatment of the sarcoma.

TABLE 36-24.   Classification of Uterine Sarcomas

I.   Pure sarcomas
   A.   Pure homologous
      1.   Leiomyosarcoma
      2.   Stromal sarcoma
      3.   Angiosarcoma
      4.   Fibrosarcoma
   B.   Pure heterologous
      1.   Rhabdomyosarcoma
      2.   Chondrosarcoma
      3.   Osteogenic sarcoma
      4.   Liposarcoma
II.   Mixed sarcomas
   A.   Mixed homologous
   B.   Mixed heterologous
   C.   Mixed homologous and heterologous
III.   Malignant mixed mullerian tumors
   A.   Malignant mixed mullerian tumor, homologous type; carcinoma plus one or more of the homologous sarcomas listed under IA above
   B.   Malignant mixed mullerian tumor, heterologous type; carcinoma plus one or more of the heterologous sarcomas listed under IB; homologous sarcoma(s) may also be present
IV.   Sarcoma, unclassified
V.   Malignant lymphoma

TABLE 36-25.   Staging Classification of Uterine Sarcomas

Stage I	Sarcoma is confined to the corpus
Stage II	Sarcoma is confined to the corpus and cervix
Stage III	Sarcoma has spread outside the uterus but is confined to the true pelvis
Stage IV	Sarcoma has spread outside the true pelvis

MALIGNANT MIXED MULLERIAN TUMORS

Malignant mixed mullerian tumors or mesodermal mixed tumors are composed of two types of cells: an adenocarcinoma of the endometrium and a sarcomatous element. They are termed homologous if the sarcomatous element is from a cell type found in the uterus and referred to as heterologous if the sarcomatous element is from cell types not found in the uterus (rhabdomyosarcoma, chondrosarcoma, osteosarcoma, or liposarcoma). The reported peak age incidence for malignant mixed mullerian tumors is between 55 and 65 years.[476,477] Vaginal bleeding is the most common presenting symptom.[480,481] Prior irradiation is reported in 5% to 30% of patients.[480,481] Diagnosis is made by dilatation and curettage. Spread of disease is usually by local extension in the pelvis, to lymph nodes, and to the lungs similar to endometrial adenocarcinoma, although these tumors are more aggressive than most endometrial adenocarcinomas. Major et al[482] reported at 15.5% incidence of positive lymph nodes in 174 cases of malignant mixed mullerian tumors and correlated these metastases with depth of myometrial penetration, lymphovascular invasion, and cervical involvement.

The primary treatment for malignant mixed mullerian tumors is surgical removal of the uterus, fallopian tubes, and ovaries. Adjunctive radiotherapy has been reported to decrease the incidence of local recurrence but not to enhance survival.[477]

Perez et al[483] reported on a group of 54 patients with mixed mesodermal sarcomas of the uterus who received combined radiation therapy and surgery as their treatment. In Stage I disease, a preoperative uterine packing for 6000 mgh was recommended. Treatment for patients with Stage II disease consisted of an intracavitary insertion for 5000 to 6000 mgh, combined with external beam whole pelvis irradiation for 2000 cGy and a 3000 cGy boost to the parametrium with a midline shield. They found that local failures were decreased, as compared with other series in which surgery alone was the only local treatment.[484] This increase in local control with radiation has been confirmed by others, and there is a tendency in the combined radiation and surgery group toward improved survival.[485-487] However, numbers in most series are quite small, the reports are unrandomized, and it is quite difficult to make a definite statement about treatment efficacy.

Belgrad et al,[487] in reviewing patients treated at four institutions, also found improved 2-year survival rates in patients treated by combined radiation and surgery for both endometrial stromal sarcomas and mixed mesodermal sarcomas. In the mixed mesodermal category, 35% survived 2 years with combined modality therapy, whereas 20% survived with surgery only. Salazar et al[488] found that in patients who received local radiotherapy as part of their program of management, local failures decreased but survival was not changed.

In a GOG randomized trial of chemotherapy in advanced uterine sarcomas, responses to Adriamycin alone or Adriamycin plus DTIC were noted in 10% to 23% of patients.[489] This same group was unable to demonstrate a statistically significant survival advantage with the adjunctive use of Adriamycin in early (Stages I and II) disease.[490]

Prognosis of malignant mixed mullerian tumors is directly related to the extent of disease at the time of diagnosis. Kempson and Bari[479] reported that all of their patients with disease extending into the outer half of the myometrium died. Piver and Lurain[491] reviewed 610 cases and reported an overall survival rate of 21%. Most reports in their review indicated survival rates of 15% to 30%.

LEIOMYOSARCOMA

Leiomyosarcomas are tumors of the smooth muscle and arise in the myometrium. The exact dividing line between cellular leiomyomata and leiomyosarcoma is not clear. Taylor and Norris[492] found that tumors of less than 10 mitoses per 10 high power fields did not recur or metastasize and called these tumors cellular leiomyomata. Kempson and Bari[479] reported death from tumor or metastases in all of their patients if the tumors had 5 to 9 mitoses per 10 high power fields. Silverberg[493] reported death or metastases in one-half of his patients if the tumor had 5 to 9 mitoses per 10 high power fields. Other factors that seem to influence prognosis are cellular atypia, vascular invasion, and infiltrating tumor margins.[493] It thus appears clear that most, if not all, tumors with less than 5 mitoses per high power field are benign, all with greater than 10 mitoses per 10 high power fields are malignant, and those with 5 to 9 mitoses per 10 high power fields are of uncertain malignant potential. Piver and Lurain[491] in a literature review of 265 cases reported 99% survival for 0 to 4 mitoses per 10 high power fields, 30% survival for 5 to 9 mitoses per 10 high power fields, and 16% survival for tumors with 7 to 10 mitoses per 10 high power fields.

The median age for patients who develop leiomyosarcoma is between 43 and 56 years.[494,495] The presenting symptoms are abnormal vaginal bleeding, an enlarging pelvic mass, and pain or pressure in the pelvis. Dilatation and curettage will result in a correct diagnosis in fewer than one third of cases.[496] Spread of disease is by direct extension to other pelvic viscera, through the lymphatics, and by invasion of blood vessels and hematogenous spread, especially to the lung. Treatment consists of removal of the uterus and adnexa. Adjuvant radiotherapy has not been found to be of benefit in patients with leiomyosarcoma.[447,448] Adjuvant chemotherapy with Adriamycin in Stages I and II disease was evaluated by the GOG.[490] The recurrence rate was 40% in patients receiving Adriamycin and 57% in the no therapy group. The difference was not significant. Responses of 25% and 30% were seen in advanced disease by the GOG using Adriamycin alone versus Adriamycin and DTIC.[489] Prognosis for uterine leiomyosarcoma varies from essentially nil in advanced disease to 20% to 30% for disease confined to the uterus at initial diagnosis.[478]

ENDOMETRIAL STROMAL SARCOMA

Two varieties of this tumor are recognized: endometrial stromal sarcoma and endolymphatic stromal myosis. A third type of this tumor is referred to as stromal nodule, but this is a universally benign tumor. Stromal sarcomas arise from the endometrial stroma, and the distinction between stromal sarcoma and endolymphatic stromal myosis is on the basis of mitotic count. Tumors with 10 or more mitoses per 10 high power fields are stromal sarcomas, and those with fewer mitoses are endolymphatic stromal myosis.[476,492]

Stromal tumors are seen most frequently between the ages of 45 and 50 years, and the most common symptoms are vaginal bleeding and an enlarged, boggy uterus. Diagnosis is made by dilatation and curettage or as an unexpected finding at hysterectomy for leiomyomata. Endolymphatic stromal myosis spreads by direct extension and via the lymphatics. It has extended beyond the uterus by the time of diagnosis in 40% of cases, although two thirds of cases will have the disease confined to the pelvis.[491] Recurrence rates of 50% are reported, but spread outside of the pelvis is not usually seen.[497] Endometrial stromal sarcomas are highly malignant neoplasias with tumor-free survival rates of 0 to 33% being reported.[479,490,498] Distant metastases are more frequent in this group of patients.

The treatment of endolymphatic stromal myosis and endometrial stromal sarcoma is removal of the uterus and adnexa. More radical local resection has been recommended for endolymphatic stromal myosis, but no large series supports this recommendation. Adjunctive irradiation for stromal sarcoma is probably effective in obtaining local control and preventing pelvic recurrences, and Belgrad et al[487] have reported modest improvements in survival. In their report, the 2-year survival rate in patients with endometrial stromal sarcoma treated by radiation therapy and surgery was 57% while in those treated by surgery alone it was 37%.

Norris and Taylor[498] reported a beneficial effect of irradiation on residual disease with endolymphatic stromal myosis, and Koss et al[499] recommended pelvic irradiation for recurrences as well as postsurgical residual disease. There are very few data on chemotherapy for stromal sarcomas, although Baggish and Woodruff[500] have reported responses with high-dose progestins.

CONCLUSIONS AND FUTURE DIRECTIONS

Surgery remains the treatment of choice for all sarcomas arising from the uterus. A total abdominal hysterectomy and bilateral salpingo-oophorectomy are the preferred treatment, although there are advocates of a more radical surgical approach for endolymphatic stromal myosis. In general, lymph node dissections or lymph node sampling, although adding information with regard to prognosis, have not improved survival. Although local failures are unfortunately quite common, the vast majority of patients will fail because of hematogenous dissemination of their tumor. The role of radiation therapy in the treatment of uterine sarcomas remains controversial, with no clear evidence at present that its use, either preoperatively or postoperatively, improves survival. In patients with Stages III and IV disease who are not operative candidates, some palliation and control of local symptoms can be achieved by the judicious use of both external beam therapy and brachytherapy placements.

Since the major pattern of failure is that of disseminated tumor, either alone or in combination with local failure, an effective systemic means of therapy must be devised if a significant improvement in survival is to be obtained. Because of the rarity of sarcomas arising from the uterus, multi-institutional studies are necessary to evaluate new treatment approaches.

CARCINOMA OF THE FALLOPIAN TUBE

Of all the organs of the female genital tract, the fallopian tube gives rise to the smallest number of primary malignant tumors. Such tumors comprise between 0.5% and 1.1% of all gynecologic malignancies.[501-504] Because of its anatomical location in association with the uterus and ovary (the two most common sites of gynecologic cancers), rigid criteria have been recommended to label a tumor as being a primary cancer of the fallopian tube.[503,504] To be considered a primary carcinoma of the fallopian tube, the tumor must be located grossly within the fallopian tube, the uterus and ovary must either not contain carcinoma or, if they contain carcinoma, it must be clearly different from the fallopian tube carcinoma, and the tubal carcinoma must involve the tubal mucosa with transition from benign to malignant epithelium (except in the case of sarcomas arising from nonmucosal structures). By far the most common malignant tumors involving the fallopian tube are metastatic from other genital organs.[505]

EPIDEMIOLOGY

Benedet and White[506] reviewed eight reports of fallopian tube carcinomas reported between 1961 and 1979 (393 cases) and found a mean age incidence of 55 years. They stated that although the disease had been reported to occur between 18 and 87 years, the vast majority of cases occurred between the ages of 40 and 65. The most commonly associated conditions are infertility and chronic salpingitis. However, the common association of infertility and salpingitis and the high frequency in which salpingitis is found, compared to the rarity of fallopian tube carcinoma, renders chronic infection as an etiologic factor unlikely. Some authors have also found an increased incidence of tuberculous salpingitis in association with tubal carcinoma, but again no definite etiologic link has been proved.

PATHOLOGY

The most common malignant tumors of the fallopian tube are adenocarcinomas. Grossly, adenocarcinoma of the fallopian tube presents as a swollen, dilated fallopian tube that, when opened, is filled with papillary and solid tumor. Areas of degeneration with hemorrhage and necrosis are commonly seen.[504] The fimbriated end of the tube is closed in approximately one half of cases, and, prior to opening the tube, it is difficult to differentiate tubal carcinoma from a hydrosalpinx or tubo-ovarian abscess.[507] Microscopically, alveolar, papillary, and medullary patterns of tumor growth have been described with abrupt transitions from normal to neoplastic epithelium.[508] Mixtures of the above patterns are common. Grading of fallopian tube carcinomas has not been proved to be of prognostic significance by some authors,[509] but this may be due to the relatively small numbers in most series. Hu et al[503] did relate survival to histologic grade and found that grade was important in those cases in which the serosa was not involved but that after involvement of the serosa, metastases developed irrespective of grade.

Pure sarcomas of the fallopian tube such as leiomyosarcoma and chondrosarcomas have been reported but are exceedingly rare.[510] Mixed mesodermal tumors of the fallopian tube contain mixtures of adenocarcinoma and sarcoma and are either homologous, when they contain sarcomas of tubal elements such as smooth muscle, or heterologous, when they contain tissues not found in the tube such as cartilage or bone.[511]

Other rare tumors that may be seen in the fallopian tube are lymphomas,[512] hydatidiform moles,[513] and choriocarcinoma.[512] The last two types are probably associated with tubal pregnancies. A primary adenosquamous carcinoma has recently been reported.[514]

PATTERNS OF SPREAD, CLINICAL MANIFESTATION, AND STAGING

Malignant tumors of the fallopian tube spread by exfoliation of clonogenic cells into the lumen of the fallopian tube that then migrate into the pelvic and abdominal cavity, or in the case of tumors that penetrate the serosa, shed cells directly into the pelvic and abdominal cavity. Although a large percentage of tubal carcinomas exhibit occlusion of the fimbriated end of the tube, one must assume that the potential for transtubal migration may have existed earlier in the course of the disease. Following entry of cells into the abdominal cavity, spread is similar to that of ovarian carcinoma. Fallopian tube cancer also spreads by contiguous invasion of adjacent structures and via the lymphatics. Hematogenous spread appears to occur less frequently. Commonly involved organs are the pelvic peritoneum, broad ligament, omentum, diaphragm, and surfaces of the intestines.[501,515] Plentl and Friedman[515] described the lymphatics of the fallopian tube. Efferent lymphatics travel in the mesosalpinx to join efferent channels from the ovary and uterus and follow the ovarian vessels to para-aortic lymph nodes. Lymphatics also course within the broad ligament to the iliac lymph nodes and superior gluteal lymph nodes. Metastatic disease to pelvic and para-aortic nodes is most common, although inguinal node metastases are occasionally seen.[515]

Bilateral tubal involvement was reported in one half of their cases by Novak and Woodruff.[516] Benedet and White[506] in their review of more than 400 cases from the literature reported the incidence of tumors to be roughly equal in the right and left fallopian tubes and found bilaterality in 21%. Whether bilaterality is due to multicentric involvement of paired organs or due to metastases is not clear.

Frick[517] has stated that the diagnosis of fallopian tube cancer is made preoperatively in only 5% of cases. The most common symptoms are abnormal vaginal bleeding and abdominal pain. Benedet and White[506] reviewed 8 series of cases and found that of 203 patients, 101 (50%) reported abnormal vaginal bleeding or discharge, 62 (30%) described abdominal pain, and in 25 (12%) a mass was the presenting symptom. Pain may be intermittent and colicky or dull and aching in nature and probably results from tubal distension similar to that seen with a tubal pregnancy. On rare occasions, an asymptomatic patient may present with adenocarcinoma cells on a Papanicolaou smear.[504] The symptoms complex of hydrops tubae profluens consists of the triad of a profuse vaginal discharge, abdominal pain, and an adnexal mass. This triad is said to be pathognomonic for tubal carcinoma but is uncommon in most series.

Staging of carcinoma of the fallopian tube is determined at surgical exploration, as in ovarian carcinoma. The preoperative diagnostic evaluation is also the same as for ovarian carcinoma since most patients undergoing surgery will do so with the diagnosis of a pelvic mass. Only rarely will fallopian tube cancer be high on the list of differential diagnoses. There is no FIGO staging classification for fallopian tube carcinoma. Dodson et al[518] in 1970 modified the staging for ovarian carcinoma and adapted it to tubal carcinoma by substituting fallopian tube for ovary, and vice versa. Shiller and Silverberg[519] in 1971 developed a different system that is more like the Dukes' classification for colon cancer. Benedet and White[506] modified the staging system reported by Erez et al[520] in 1967 and reported survival in 142 patients staged by their "modified Erez" classification. They found 5-year survival rates of 60% in Stage I, 30% in Stage II, 16% in Stage III, and 19% in Stage IV. Table 36-26 lists and compares the three staging systems mentioned above.

TREATMENT OF CARCINOMA OF THE FALLOPIAN TUBE

General Principles

Because of the relative rarity of fallopian tube carcinoma and because its histology and patterns of spread are so similar to carcinoma of the ovary, most authors have recommended treatment plans of surgery, radiation therapy, and chemotherapy similar to carcinoma of the ovary.

Surgery

The recommended surgical approach for tubal carcinoma is total abdominal hysterectomy, bilateral salpingo-oophorectomy, omentectomy, and resection of as much gross disease as possible. If the disease is limited to the pelvis or if all gross disease is resectable, a full surgical staging operation to include multiple peritoneal biopsies, diaphragmatic biopsy, and sampling of the pelvic and para-aortic nodes is required. Because of the potential early exfoliation of malignant cells via the tubal lumen, no recommendation for conservative surgery in the young patient can be made. This same potential for early dissemination of malignant cells has led most authorities to recommend that all patients with tubal cancer be treated adjunctively with either irradiation or chemother-

TABLE 36-26.   Three Suggested Classifications for Fallopian Tube Carcinoma

Stage		FIGO Type*	Dukes' Type†	Modified Erez‡
0			Carcinoma in situ	
I		Growth limited to tube	Tumor extends into submucosa or muscularis, not serosa	Tumor limited to the tube (mucosa or muscularis)
	IA	One tube, no ascites		
	IB	Both tubes, no ascites		
	IC	One or both tubes with ascites with malignant cells		
II		Growth limited to the true pelvis	Tumor extends to serosa	
	IIA	Extension to uterus or ovary		Tumor has extended through the serosa but not to contiguous organs
	IIB	Extension to other pelvic tissues		Tumor directly invading surrounding organs in pelvis or abdomen or metastases to pelvic organs
III		Growth involving one or both ovaries with intraperitoneal metastases	Tumor extends to ovary or endometrium	True metastatic lesions outside the pelvis but confined to the abdomen
IV		Growth involving one or both tubes with distant metastases outside the peritoneal cavity	Tumor extends beyond reproductive organs	Metastatic disease outside the abdomen

* Modified from Dodson MG, Ford JH Jr, Averette HE: Clinical aspects of fallopian tube carcinoma. Obstet Gynecol 36:935, 1970.
† Modified from Shiller HM, Silverberg SG: Staging and prognosis in primary carcinoma of the fallopian tube. Cancer 28:389, 1971.
‡ Modified from Benedet JL, White GW: Malignant tumors of fallopian tube. In Coppleson M (ed): Gynecologic Oncology: Fundamental Principles and Clinical Practice, pp 621–629. New York, Churchill Livingstone, 1981.

apy. McMurray et al[521] suggested that all patients with disease greater than Stage I be treated with aggressive postoperative therapy. They state that in their series of 30 patients, 50% of failures were in the upper abdomen and 44% failed in extraperitoneal sites. As with ovarian cancer, there does not seem to be any place for radical hysterectomy, complete lymphadenectomy, or pelvic exenteration in this disease.

Radiation Therapy for Carcinoma of the Fallopian Tube

Postoperative radiotherapy in patients with fallopian tube carcinoma has been recommended by some investigators and questioned by others.[502,509,522,523] Radiotherapy techniques currently used include 5000 cGy whole pelvis external beam irradiation for the more aggressive Stages I and II tumors. For Stage III disease, whole pelvic and abdominal radiation is required. Techniques resemble those used for ovarian tumors.[524] Instillation of radioactive colloidal gold ([198]Au) and chromic phosphate (^{32}P) has been recommended in cases in which no macroscopic disease is present in the peritoneal cavity.

Several studies have suggested benefits from postoperative radiotherapy. In 1957 Engstrom[525] reported significant improvement in his cases of fallopian tube carcinoma treated with postoperative radium and deep external beam radiation (patients treated with postoperative radiotherapy showed a 38% 5-year survival rate versus a 15% 5-year survival rate in patients treated with surgery only). Greene and Scully[526] reported an average survival of 2 years with postoperative radiation and no survivors 1 year after surgery without radiotherapy.

Boutselis and Thompson[522] reported an increased 5-year survival rate in 7 of 8 patients treated with postoperative

radiotherapy. Phelps and Chapman[527] reported good results for patients with Stages I and II disease treated with megavoltage irradiation. Nine patients with Stage I or II disease received 2500 to 5000 cGy to the pelvis or abdomen. Six also received intraperitoneal radioactive colloidal gold or phosphate. Eight of the 9 patients were alive at the time of publication of the study, with 6 patients being 5-year survivors. Six patients with Stage III disease were treated with postoperative radiotherapy; none survived. In a study of 34 patients, Amendola et al[528] reported 1 of 4 patients alive 5 years after therapy consisting of less than 3000 to 5000 cGy. However, 5 of 14 patients who received more than 5000 cGy were alive and disease free.

McMurray et al[521] reported on 30 patients with adenocarcinoma of the fallopian tube treated at Washington University. Nine had Stage I disease, 11 had Stage II, 7 had Stage III, and 3 had Stage IV. Primary surgical treatment consisted of total abdominal hysterectomy and bilateral salpingo-oophor-

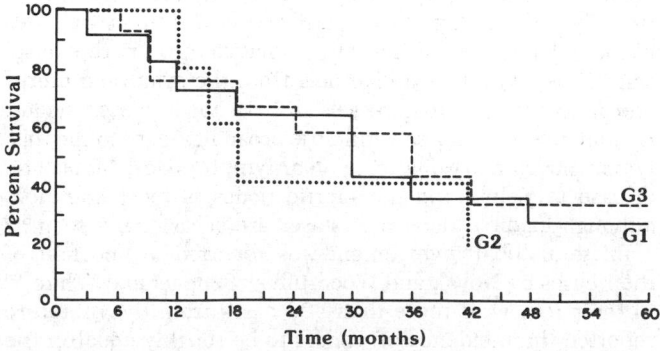

FIG. 36-19. Grade versus survival in fallopian tube carcinoma according to histologic differentiation, Washington University, 1950–1981.

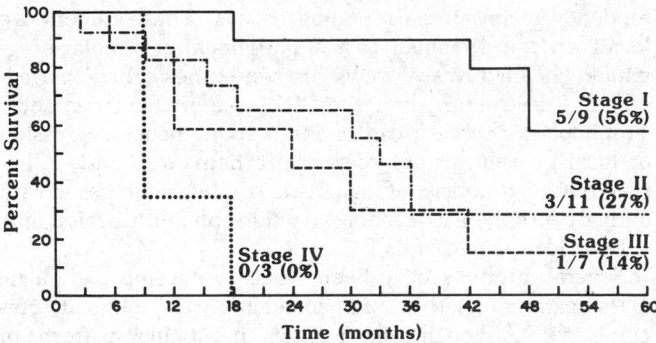

FIG. 36-20. Stage versus survival in fallopian tube carcinoma according to surgical stage, Washington University, 1950–1981.

PATTERNS OF FAILURE

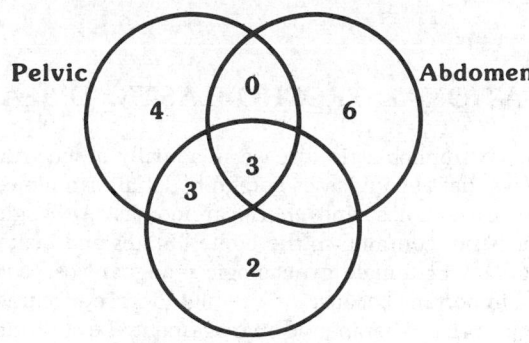

FIG. 36-21. Site of recurrence in fallopian tube carcinoma, Washington University, 1950–1981.

ectomy in 70% of patients; 23% had more extensive surgery than this, whereas 13% had incomplete extirpation of the female genitalia. Three patients with Stage I tumors were treated with surgery alone, and the remainder received postoperative radiation, chemotherapy, or both. Survival was unrelated to grade (Fig. 36-19), but highly dependent upon stage. Disease-free survival at 3 years was 86% for Stage I, 27% for Stage II, 29% for Stage III, and 0% for Stage IV (Fig. 36-20). Four of 5 patients treated after surgery with a combination of cisplatin, doxorubicin, and cyclophosphamide survived at least 3 years. Patterns of initial treatment failure showed 56% with a component of pelvic failure, 50% with a component of upper abdominal failure, and 44% with extraperitoneal metastases as a component of failure (Fig. 36-21). The results according to method of treatment (Table 36-27) suggest that aggressive postoperative adjuvant therapy targeted at upper abdominal and distant sites for metastases in all lesions beyond Stage I will improve survival and tumor control.

Chemotherapy of Carcinoma of the Fallopian Tube

Because it is a rare tumor, data on the chemosensitivity of tubal carcinoma must be obtained from individual case reports and small series. There are anecdotal reports of responses to triple drug therapy with cyclophosphamide, dactinomycin, and 5-FU[529] and to cyclophosphamide, doxorubicin, and progestogens.[530] Adjuvant chlorambucil has

been used with pelvic irradiation with some long-term survivors.[531] Raju et al[523] reported experience with 22 cases of tubal carcinoma collected from 1955 to 1980. Six patients had been treated with chemotherapy, and only 1 showed an objective regression following treatment with cisplatin (100 mg/m² every 4 weeks).

A recent experience with chemotherapy for recurrent disease documented complete responses in one of six patients treated with oral alkylating agents and two of three patients treated with intravenous cisplatin.[532] Recently, the CAP (cyclophosphamide, Adriamycin, and cisplatin) regimen has been used in nine patients. Four complete remissions were seen; three of the four were without evidence of disease at 18 to 56 months.[532] This small study suggests significant activity for this combination, and it should be further investigated.

Because of the paucity of specific data about the chemosensitivity of this tumor and because its histology and pattern of spread resemble that of epithelial ovarian tumors, it has been common practice to treat these rare carcinomas with chemotherapeutic regimens active in epithelial ovarian cancer. However, a recent review of 30 patients[521] suggests that although the tumors behave similarly to ovarian cancer, they present at earlier stages and there is an increased frequency of failure due to distant metastases. Both these obser-

TABLE 36-27. Survival According to Treatment and Stage (Treatment of Patients Surviving 3 Years or More)

Stage	S	S + RT	S + CT	S + PAC	S + CT + RT	Total
I	3/3	1/2	3/3*		1/1	8/9
II		2/5	0/2	3/3†	0/1	5/11
III			0/3	1/2	1/2*	2/7
IV			0/1		0/2	0/3

Jacob AJ, Perez CA, et al: Carcinoma of the fallopian tube: Management and sites of failure. Cancer 58:2070, 1986.
* Two patients received RT.
† One patient alive with disease.
S, surgery; RT, radiotherapy; CT, chemotherapy; PAC, cisplatin, Adriamycin (doxorubicin), and Cytoxan (cyclophosphamide).

vations coupled with the generally poor prognosis suggest a potential role for adjuvant chemotherapy after surgery.

GESTATIONAL TROPHOBLASTIC DISEASE

Gestational trophoblastic disease is actually a spectrum of neoplasias that encompasses benign hydatidiform moles, locally invasive moles, and choriocarcinomas. Although the disorder is not common in the United States and makes up less than 1% of female gynecologic malignancies, it is extremely important because of the high degree of curability with appropriate therapeutic management. Because of the rarity of the disease, most patients should be treated at trophoblastic disease centers where sufficient expertise exists to deal with the complex and life-threatening nature of this disorder. Because of adherence to these principles, death from this disease is now rare, and in 1983 there were only 24 deaths reported in the United States from choriocarcinoma.[533]

EPIDEMIOLOGY

Although rare in the United States, the disease is much more common in other areas of the world, particularly in Asia and in South America, where incidences as high as 1:120 pregnancies have been reported. Although the precise explanation for this increase is unknown, many investigators have suggested nutritional or dietary factors. Studies in Philippine populations[534] revealed a lower incidence in the meat-eating, wealthy populations than in the poorer populations whose diets were heavily based on fish and rice and whose incidence of molar pregnancy was as high as 1 in 200. This contrasts to the incidence of approximately 1 in 1,200 pregnancies in the United States. In most series, increasing age, particularly above the age of 40, increases the risk. This is true in all countries but is most dramatic in countries in which a high baseline risk is already existent. Studies in Singapore demonstrate a 12-fold increase in risk for women above the age of 45.[535] Although risk increases with pregnancies over age 40, there appears to be no increasing risk with advancing parity. Furthermore, the patient's age or the parity does not affect the outcome of a molar pregnancy.

CLASSIFICATION AND PATHOLOGY

Approximately half of all trophoblastic tumors develop after a molar pregnancy, but they can develop after an abortion, an ectopic pregnancy, or after an apparently normal term pregnancy. If the disease occurs after a molar pregnancy, the tumor can be either a hydatidiform mole or a choriocarcinoma. However, if the disease develops in any of the other settings, virtually all the tumors are choriocarcinoma. Generally, the trophoblastic neoplasias can be classified morphologically as hydatidiform mole, invasive mole, and choriocarcinoma.

Hydatidiform moles have clusters of hydropic villi, absence of fetal vessels, and trophoblastic hyperplasia. Invasive moles have similar histologic findings but display a greater tendency to invade surrounding tissues. These tumors are locally invasive in about 15% of patients after a molar pregnancy. Locally invasive moles are sometimes called chorioadenoma destruens when they follow a molar pregnancy. Trophoblastic disease can undergo spontaneous regression or local invasion or can metastasize hematogenously. Choriocarcinomas consist of anaplastic trophoblastic tissue with both cytotrophoblastic and syncytiotrophoblastic elements and no identifiable villi.

Several attempts have been made to develop pathologic classifications that would correlate wtih clinical outcome.[536,537] Although classifications that include patterns of growth, extent of stromal invasion, nuclear grade, and lymphocytic infiltration have broadly correlated, the management and outcome generally have been based on staging and clinical definition of low, moderate, and high risk patients.

TUMOR MARKERS (HUMAN CHORIONIC GONADOTROPIN [HCG])

A major reason for the successful management of this tumor has been the availability of this marker substance that is invariably present with the disease. All types of trophoblastic disease produce hCG, and the quantity produced is proportional to the volume of the disease.[538] As a result, one can use hCG titers as an accurate monitor of disease response to therapy. Both diagnosis and management depend on careful radioimmunoassay of this substance. Pregnancy tests or biological assays have no place in the management of the disease. hCG consists of an alpha and beta chain. Because the alpha chain is cross-reactive with leutinizing hormone (LH), it has been the source of some confusion in diagnosis and subsequent management. As a result, a specific assay for the beta subunit was developed[539] and will selectively assay hCG in the presence of normal LH. Use of this specific radioimmunoassay is required for monitoring all patients with trophoblastic disease. Generally, after evacuation of a molar pregnancy, the elevated hCG titers disappear in 8 to 10 weeks, although in about 25% of patients clearance may be delayed as long as 14 to 16 weeks.[540]

CLINICAL EVALUATION AND STAGING

Generally, molar pregnancies are associated with first trimester bleeding, ectopic pregnancies, or threatened abortions. Often, the uterus is large for the estimated length of the gestation and the hCG titers are elevated in excess of a normal pregnancy. Fetal heart sounds are absent and obviously fetal parts are not palpable. Early toxemia of pregnancy may be present. Expulsion of grape-like villi will often provide the diagnosis of hydatidiform mole although vaginal bleeding is the most common presenting finding with invasive mole or choriocarcinoma. Occasionally patients will present with metastatic disease as their first manifestation of the illness.

Ultrasound evaluation is increasingly used to diagnose molar pregnancies, and the characteristic findings can be diagnostic. These techniques may also define extrauterine extension but are not always diagnostic.[541] Amniography also produces a typical moth-eaten appearance that is also characteristic. Neither amniography or angiography is frequently used because of the current sophistication of ultrasonography. The diagnosis is generally based on the clinical findings, hCG titer, ultrasound, and pathological confirmation. Patients with molar pregnancy should be evaluated further with chest radiographs, careful pelvic examinations, and weekly serial monitoring of the hCG titers. Patients who have evidence of persistent disease and those found to have choriocarcinoma should have chest radiographs and brain and liver scans to define the extent of metastatic spread.

Distant metastases are noted in about 5% of those patients who have molar pregnancies. Choriocarcinoma spreads hematogenously, and the common metastatic sites are lungs (80%), vagina (30%), pelvis (20%), liver (10%), brain (10%), bowel, kidney and spleen (5%).[542]

Unfortunately, no uniform staging classification has received widespread adoption. Many investigators classify patients according to whether disease is metastatic or nonmetastatic and then, among those with metastatic disease, further divide patients into those with low risk and high risk.[543] Several staging schemes have been used, including those of Bagshawe,[543] the Dutch Working Group for trophoblastic tumors,[544] and the New England Trophoblastic Disease Center.[543] Comparisons of all three staging classifications generally documented similar degrees of specificity and prognostic value.[544] The last two classifications are easier to apply because they are based on data readily available and do not require information about the husband's blood group, lymphocytic infiltration of the tumor, or the patient's immune status. Unfortunately, none of these retrospective comparisons identify a particular staging classification as superior. Nevertheless, the staging classification used by the New England Trophoblastic Disease Center is straightforward and useful as outlined in Table 36-28. Patients are divided into high risk and low risk molar pregnancies, patients with disease confined to the corpus of the uterus (Stage I), patients wtih local pelvic spread (Stage II), and patients with more advanced disease (Stages III and IV). Patients believed to have low risk molar pregnancies include those with hCG titers less than 100,000 IU/ml, small uterine size, ovarian enlargement less than 6 cm, and no other poor-prognosis metabolic or epidemiologic factors.[545] Patients at high risk include those with hCG titers greater than 100,000 IU/ml, uterine size greater than normal for date of gestation, enlarged ovaries, and any of the poor-prognosis metabolic or epidemiologic factors, including maternal age over 40, toxemia, coagulopathy, trophoblastic tumor with or without embolization, and hyperthyroidism.

TABLE 36-28. Staging of Gestational Trophoblastic Neoplasms

Stage 0	Molar pregnancy
	A. Low risk
	B. High risk
Stage I	Confined to uterine corpus
Stage II	Metastases to pelvis and vagina
Stage III	Metastasis to lung
Stage IV	Distant metastases

Goldstein DP, Berkowitz RS: The management of gestational trophoblastic neoplasms. Curr Prob Obstet Gynecol 4:1, 1980.

The majority of patients with Stage I disease (75%) have classical invasive mole, and the remaining 25% have locally invasive choriocarcinoma. Stages 0 to 3 all have good prognoses when treated with currently available therapies. Stage IV patients include those with poor prognostic findings. All have choriocarcinoma and include those with initial hCG titers of greater than 100,000 IU/ml, persistence of disease longer than 4 months after initial therapy, and those with brain or liver metastasis.

TREATMENT

Patients with hydatidiform mole require evacuation of the uterus by suction curettage and oxytocin. After evacuation, patients generally have a dilatation and curettage. In 80% of patients, no further therapy will be needed. Subsequent follow-up requires weekly hCG assay until the titer returns to normal.

The mainstay of treatment for the other gestational trophoblastic neoplasias is chemotherapy. Before chemotherapy, only 40% of patients could be cured with hysterectomy alone even when the disease appeared localized. In the presence of any evidence of metastatic spread, fewer than 10% of those patients survived despite aggressive surgery and irradiation. The classical reports of Li and colleagues[546] of the activity of methotrexate in the 1950s and the subsequent documentation of the curative capacity of chemotherapy by Hertz et al[547] represent milestones in cancer treatment and ushered in the era of modern chemotherapy.

Chemotherapy is now commonly used to manage patients with gestational trophoblastic neoplasia. Patients with hydatidiform mole receive chemotherapy if there is a persistent plateau in the weekly β-hCG level, a rise in the β-hCG titer, or the development of metastases. Patients with invasive mole or choriocarcinoma or those who present with metastatic disease require immediate chemotherapy.

Generally, patients requiring chemotherapy are divided into good risk patients who can be cured with single-agent chemotherapy and poor risk patients who generally require initial combination chemotherapy for best results. Poor-risk features include Stage IV disease, cerebral or hepatic metastases, β-hCG levels of greater than 100,000 IU/ml, previous unsuccessful treatment, persistence of symptoms for greater than 4 months, or disease after a full-term pregnancy. Using these criteria, treatment selection can be based on risk factors and stage.

Treatment of Low Risk Patients (Stages I and II and Low Risk Metastatic Disease)

Historically, single-agent chemotherapy is most commonly used for these patients. Intramuscular methotrexate (Mtx) or actinomycin D (Act D) have been the standard single-agent therapies with Mtx given intramuscularly 0.4 mg/kg/day × 5 days every 2 weeks or Act D 10 to 12 μg/kg/day × 5 days every 2 weeks. Although this therapy is extremely effective for low risk trophoblastic disease, both regimens have significant toxicity, and more recently moderate dose Mtx with leucovorin rescue has achieved similar results wtih less toxicity. The New England Trophoblastic Disease Center has recently summarized its 10-year experience with this regimen.[548] One hundred eighty-five patients were treated. Complete remissions were achieved in 88% of patients, including 90% of the 163 patients with nonmetastatic disease and 68% of those with low risk metastatic disease. In 82% of these patients, complete remission was achieved with a single course of methotrexate and leucovorin. The regimen includes Mtx 1 mg/kg intramuscularly every other day for 4 doses, followed by leucovorin intramuscularly 0.1 mg/kg 24 hours after each Mtx dose.

After the initial course of chemotherapy, the response to therapy is monitored by β-hCG regression curves.[549] One log or greater fall in hCG titer over the subsequent 18 days allows the physician to withhold further therapy. If the βhCG titer does not fall to this degree, reaches a plateau, or begins rising, a second course of therapy is administered. Therapy continues until the βhCG titer has normalized for 3 weeks. Patients are subsequently monitored at monthly intervals for 1 year. If βhCG titers remain normal for a year, pregnancy may be allowed.

Toxicity was modest. Granulocytopenia occurred in 6% of patients and thrombocytopenia in less than 2%. There was no alopecia, and nausea and vomiting were rare. Although 14% of patients developed enzyme evidence of hepatic toxicity, this resolved within 2 weeks of completing therapy. All of the patients in this series, who failed initial induction therapy with Mtx-leucovorin, achieved a complete remission with subsequent combination chemotherapy. On the basis of this extensive experience, this regimen appears to be the treatment of choice for low risk gestational trophoblastic disease.

Treatment of High Risk Patients

All high risk patients should receive initial combination chemotherapy. The most common regimen used contains methotrexate 0.3 mg/kg intramuscularly, actinomycin D 10 μg/kg intravenously, and chlorambucil 10 mg orally daily × 5 days with courses repeated as required until 3 successive weeks of normal β-hCG levels are achieved.[550] Other effective regimens include the CHAMOCA regimen of Bagshawe,[551,552] MAC,[553,554] or PVB (cisplatin, vinblastine, bleomycin).[554] Using these regimens, complete responses are generally achieved in approximately 80% of patients, although generally lower responses (60–70%) are seen in patients with hepatic or cerebral metastases.[555]

Salvage chemotherapy for patients failing initial induction therapy for high risk disease has generally employed six to seven drug combinations.[556,557] Although many of these early trials achieved some salvage, small numbers of patients were included. One salvage regimen using high-dose cisplatin, vincristine, and methotrexate with leucovorin achieved durable complete remissions in 35% of previous failures.[558] With the identification of VP-16[497,559] and cisplatin[560] as active agents in a salvage setting, several investigators have used these drugs in new regimens.

PVB, after failure of conventional triple therapy, achieved a complete remission in 50% of patients, although only 20% (2 of 11) had a sustained complete remission. More recently, high dose Mtx (1 g/m²) with leucovorin rescue, VP-16, and

bleomycin were used in 9 patients failing initial therapy with the modified Bagshawe regimen. Eight of the 9 (89%) achieved a sustained remission for more than 2 years. Bone marrow toxicity was universal and substantial.[498]

Patients with brain or liver metastasis are generally treated with local irradiation to the sites. Patients with proven brain metastasis or elevations of cerebrospinal fluid hCG are treated with 3000 cGy whole brain irradiation. Surgery is rarely required. Patients with hepatic metastasis are often treated with 2500 cGy before the start of chemotherapy to reduce the risk of intrahepatic hemorrhage during chemotherapy.

Long-Term Complications of Chemotherapy

Several studies of the long-term consequences of successful therapy for this disease have been published, and as yet there is no evidence of increased risk of maternal complications or fetal abnormalities associated with these treatments.[562,563]

POSTIRRADIATION GYNECOLOGIC MALIGNANCIES

Several reports have been published on the incidence of malignant tumors of the endometrium or other pelvic organs in patients treated with irradiation for benign or malignant pelvic conditions. Smith and Doll[564] reported an increased incidence of leukemia (7 deaths observed against 2.3 expected) and cancers of the heavily irradiated sites (59 observed versus 40.1 expected) 5 years or more after irradiation to the pelvis for benign metropathia haemorrhagica. The mean dose of radiation to the bone marrow was estimated to correlate with the projected excess rate of leukemia, which is about 1.1 case/woman/cGy/year. However, other authors such as Hutchinson[565] have not observed this increased incidence (3 cases observed versus 16 expected). Dickson[566] reported 2 deaths from leukemia whereas only 1.1 were expected. Wagoner[507] observed no excess of leukemia among 7,835 women treated with radium and roentgen rays for primary uterine cancer. Arneson and Schellhas[568] and Spratt and Hoag[569] observed no significant increase of malignancy in patients treated with irradiation for carcinoma of the uterine cervix.

Lee et al[570] reviewed 1,150 patients treated with irradiation for carcinoma of the uterine cervix at Washington University. Table 36-29 shows the observed and expected incidence of malignancy in several series. Thus, the current data fail to support the suggestion that irradiation may increase the incidence of malignancy in patients irradiated for gynecologic cancer.

Wagoner[567] also studied 1,803 patients treated for benign gynecologic disorders with radium and observed 10 deaths from leukemia against 3.6 expected; in a similar series in Connecticut, 9 cases of leukemia were seen against 2.8 expected. A decreased death rate from carcinoma of the breast has been observed by Smith and Doll[564] and others[571,572] with an artificial inducement of menopause. In the patients treated for carcinoma of the cervix at Washington University, a similar lower mortality from breast cancer was noted. It is possible that the castration induced by irradiation in younger women may influence the subsequent development

TABLE 36-29. Incidence of Postirradiation Gynecologic Malignancy

	Average Age (yr)	No. of Patients	No. 2 NDI	Human Years Observed	CA per Human Year	Rate per 100,000
Lee et al[570]	52	1053	49	6244	0.00785	785
Arneson and Schellhas[567]	49	874	36	6142	0.00586	586
Spratt and Hoag[569]	54	1853	36	6264	0.00574	574

Lee JY, Perez CA, Ettinger N, et al: The risk of second primaries subject to irradiation for cervix cancer. Int J Radiat Oncol Biol Phys 8:207, 1982.

of carcinoma of the breast. Villasanta and Rubel[573] reported 15 cases of pelvic malignancy in 174 patients irradiated for benign uterine bleeding in contrast to only 3 malignant tumors in 147 nonrandomized control patients who were not irradiated. Most of the tumors developed in the endometrium or the ovary. The dose of irradiation was relatively small (2000–2400 mgh). In contradistinction, the same authors observed only 19 patients developing a second pelvic malignancy in 569 women with malignant tumors of the gynecologic tract treated wtih doses of irradiation above 5000 cGy and followed for 4 years or longer. Dickson[566] pointed out that the incidence for malignancy after irradiation for benign uterine bleeding was significantly less in patients treated with external irradiation than in those treated with intracavitary radium. As reported by Thomas et al[574] most postirradiation malignancies of the uterus are adenocarcinomas of the endometrium, followed by mixed mullerian tumors and sarcomas of the uterine cervix. The prognosis of these patients after treatment was similar to that of patients who had not had irradiation.[574]

The principles of management for these patients are similar to those patients who receive no previous irradiation. Most authors agree that the primary treatment of these patients is surgical. There is some controversy whether preoperative or postoperative irradiation should be delivered. However, the number of patients is small, and no definite conclusions can be drawn.

REFERENCES

1. Silverberg E, Lubera J: Cancer statistics, 1988. CA 38:5, 1988
2. Anderson BL, Hacker NF: Psychosexual adjustment after vulvar surgery. Obstet Gynecol 62:457, 1983
3. Collins CG, Roman-Lopez JJ, Lee FYL: Intraepithelial carcinoma of the vulva. Am J Obstet Gynecol 108:1187, 1987
4. Boutselis JG: Intraepithelial carcinoma of the vulva. Am J Obstet Gynecol 113:733, 1972
5. Franklin EW, Rutledge FD: Epidemiology of epidermoid carcinoma of the vulva. Obstet Gynecol 39:165, 1972
6. Japaze H, Garcia-Buneul R, Woodruff JD: Primary vulvar neoplasia. Obstet Gynecol 49:404, 1977
7. Forney JP, Morrow CP, Townsend DE, et al: Management of carcinoma in situ of the vulva. Am J Obstet Gynecol 127:801, 1977
8. Kunschner A, Kanbour AI, David B: Early vulvar carcinoma. Am J Obstet Gynecol 132:599, 1978
9. Friedrich EG, Wilkinson EJ, Fu YS: Carcinoma in situ of the vulva: A continuing challenge. Am J Obstet Gynecol 136:880, 1980
10. Parker RT, Duncan I, Rampone J, et al: Operative management of early invasive epidermoid carcinoma of the vulva. Am J Obstet Gynecol 123:349, 1975
11. Magrina JF, Webb MJ, Gaffey TA, et al: Stage I squamous cell cancer of the vulva. Am J Obstet Gynecol 134:453, 1975
12. Podratz KC, Symmonds RE, Taylor WF, et al: Carcinoma of the vulva: Analysis of treatment and survival. Obstet Gynecol 61:63, 1983
13. Rutledge F, Smith JP, Franklin EW: Carcinoma of the vulva. Am J Obstet Gynecol 106:1117, 1970
14. Hacker NF, Leuchter RS, Berek JS, et al: Radical vulvectomy and bilateral inguinal lymphadenectomy through separate groin incisions. Obstet Gynecol 58:574, 1981
15. Mack T, Casagrande JT: Epidemiology of gynecologic cancer: II. Endometrium, ovary, vagina, vulva. In Coppleson M (ed): Gynecologic Oncology: Fundamental Principles and Clinical Practice, pp 28–30. New York, Churchill Livingstone, 1981
16. Green TH: Carcinoma of the vulva: A reassessment. Obstet Gynecol 52:462, 1978
17. Collins CC, Lee FYL, Ramon Lopez JJ: Invasive carcinoma of the vulva with lymph node metastases. Am J Obstet Gynecol 109:446, 1971
18. Morley GW: Infiltrative carcinoma of the vulva: Results of surgical treatment. Am J Obstet Gynecol 124:874, 1976
19. Josey WE, Nahmais AJ, Naib ZM: Viruses and cancer of the lower genital tract. Cancer 38:526, 1976
20. Deligdisch L, Szulman AE: Multiple and multifocal carcinoma in female genital organs and breast. Gynecol Oncol 3:181, 1975
21. Stern BD, Kaplan L: Multicentric foci of carcinoma arising in structures of cloacal origin. Am J Obstet Gynecol 104:255, 1969
22. Plentl AA, Friedman EA: Lymphatic System of the Female Genitalia: The Morphologic Basis of Oncologic Diagnosis and Therapy, pp 15–50. Philadelphia, WB Saunders, 1971
23. Way S: Carcinoma of the vulva. In Meigs JV, Sturgis SH (eds): Progress in Gynecology, vol 3. New York, Grune & Stratton, 1957
24. Kaufman RH, Gardner HL: Intraepithelial carcinoma of the vulva. Clin Obstet Gynecol 8:1035, 1965
25. International Society for the Study of Vulvar Disease. New nomenclature for vulvar disease: I. Obstet Gynecol 47:122, 1976
26. Friedrich EG Jr, Wilkinson EJ: The vulva. In Blaustein A (ed): Pathology of the Female Genital Tract, pp 13–58. New York, Springer-Verlag, 1977
27. Helwig EB, Graham JH: Anogenital (extramammary) Paget's disease. Cancer 16:387, 1963
28. Friedrich EG Jr, Wilkinson EJ, Steingraeber PH, et al: Paget's disease of the vulva and carcinoma of the breast. Obstet Gynecol 46:130, 1975
29. Tchang F, Okagaki T, Richart R: Adenocarcinoma of Bartholin's gland associated with Paget's disease of vulvar area. Cancer 31:221, 1973
30. Woodruff JD, Richardson EH: Malignant vulvar Paget's disease. Obstet Gynecol 10:10, 1957
31. Gosling JRG, Abell MR, Drolette BM, et al: Infiltrative squamous cell carcinoma of the vulva. Cancer 14:330, 1961
32. Way S: Carcinoma of the vulva. Am J Obstet Gynecol 79:692, 1960
33. Wharton JT, Gallagher S, Rutledge FN: Microinvasive carcinoma of the vulva. Am J Obstet Gynecol 118:159, 1974
34. Parker RT, Duncan I, Rampone J, et al: Operative management of early invasive epidermoid carcinoma of the vulva. Am J Obstet Gynecol 123:349, 1975
35. Lasser A, Cornorg JT, Morris JM: Adenoid squamous carcinoma of the vulva. Cancer 33:224, 1974
36. Gallousis S: Verrucous carcinoma. Obstet Gynecol 40:502, 1972
37. Lucas WE, Bernischke K, Lebherz TB: Verrucous carcinoma of the female genital tract. Am J Obstet Gynecol 119:435, 1974
38. Chung AF, Woodruff JM, Lewis JL Jr: Malignant melanoma of the vulva. Obstet Gynecol 45:638, 1975
39. Breen JL, Neubecker RD, Greenwald E, et al: Basal cell carcinomas of the vulva. Obstet Gynecol 46:122, 1975
40. Tavassoli FA, Norris HJ: Smooth muscle tumors of the vulva. Obstet Gynecol 53:213, 1979
41. Buscema J, Woodruff JD, Parmley TH, et al: Carcinoma in situ of the vulva. Obstet Gynecol 55:225, 1980
42. Clark WH Jr: A classification of malignant melanoma in man correlated with histogenesis and biologic behavior. In Montagna W, Hu F (eds): Advances in Biology of Skin and Pigmentary System, pp 621–647. London, Pergamon Press, 1967
43. Breslow A: Thickness, cross-sectional areas and depth of invasion in the prognosis of cutaneous melanoma. Ann Surg 172:902, 1970
44. Collins CG, Ramon-Lopez JJ, Lee FYL: Intraepithelial carcinoma of the vulva. Am J Obstet Gynecol 18:1187, 1970
45. Rutledge FN, Sinclair M: Treatment of intraepithelial carcinoma of the vulva by skin excision and graft. Am J Obstet Gynecol 102:806, 1986

46. Barnhill DR, Hoskins WJ, Metz P: Use of the rhomboid flap after partial vulvectomy. Obstet Gynecol 62:444, 1983
47. Woodruff JD, Julian C, Puray T, et al: The contemporary challenge of carcinoma in situ of the vulva. Am J Obstet Gynecol 115:677, 1973
48. Dean RE, Taylor ES, Weisbrod DM, et al: The treatment of premalignant and malignant lesions of the vulva. Am J Obstet Gynecol 119:59, 1974
49. Breen JL, Smith CI, Gregori CA: Extramammary Paget's disease. Clin Obstet Gynecol 21:1107, 1978
50. Watring WG, Roberts JA, Lagasse LD, et al: Treatment of recurrent Paget's disease of the vulva with topical bleomycin. Cancer 41:10, 1978
51. DiPaola GR, Gomez-Rueda N, Arrighi L: Relevance of microinvasion in carcinoma of the vulva. Obstet Gynecol 45:647, 1975
52. Kneale BLG, Elliott PM, McDonald IA: Microinvasive carcinoma of the vulva: Clinical features and management. In Coppleson M (ed): Gynecologic Oncology: Fundamental Principles and Clinical Practice, pp 320–328. New York, Churchill Livingstone, 1981
53. DiSaia PJ, Creasman WT, Rich WM: An alternate approach to early cancer of the vulva. Am J Obstet Gynecol 133:825, 1979
54. Krupp PJ: Invasive tumors of vulva: clinical features and management. In Coppleson M (ed): Gynecologic Oncology: Fundamental Principles and Clinical Practice, pp 329–338. New York, Churchill Livingstone, 1981
55. Homesley HD, Bundy BN, Sedlis A, et al: Radiation therapy versus pelvic node resection for carcinoma of the vulva with positive groin nodes. Obstet Gynecol 68:733, 1986
56. Basset A: Traitement chirurgical operatoire de l'epithelioma primitf du clitoris. Rev Chir 46:546, 1912
57. Krupp PJ, Bohm JW: Lymph node metastases in invasive squamous cell cancer of the vulva. Am J Obstet Gynecol 130:943, 1978
58. Hacker NF, Berek JS, Lagasse LD: Management of regional lymph nodes and their prognostic influence in vulvar cancer. Obstet Gynecol 61:408, 1983
59. Podratz KC, Symmonds RE, Taylor WF, et al: Carcinoma of the vulva: Analysis of treatment and survival. Obstet Gynecol 61:63, 1983
60. Hacker NF, Leuchter RS, Berek JS, et al: Radical vulvectomy and bilateral inguinal lymphadenectomy through separate groin incisions. Obstet Gynecol 58:574, 1981
61. Morris JM: A formula for selective lymphadenectomy: Its application to cancer of the vulva. Obstet Gynecol 50:152, 1977
62. Mattingley RF, Thompson JD: Surgical conditions of the vulva. In Mattingley RF, Thompson JD (eds): Telinde's Operative Gynecology, p 720. Philadelphia, JB Lippincott, 1985
63. Sedlis A, Marshall R, Homesley H, et al: Positive groin lymph nodes in vulvar cancer with superficial penetration. Gynecol Oncol 17:259, 1984
64. Iversen T, Abeler D, Aalders J: Individualized treatment of Stage I carcinoma of the vulva. Obstet Gynecol 57:158, 1976
65. Frankendal B, Larsson LG, Westing P: Carcinoma of the vulva. Acta Radiol [Ther] (Stockh) 12:165, 1973
66. Acosta AA, Given FT, Frazier AB, et al: Preoperative radiation therapy in the management of squamous cell carcinoma of the vulva: Preliminary report. Am J Obstet Gynecol 132:198, 1978
67. Boronow RC: Combined therapy or an alternative to exenteration for locally advanced vulvovaginal cancer. Cancer 49:1085, 1982
68. Boronow RC: Therapeutic alternative to primary exenteration for advanced vulvo-vaginal cancer. Gynecol Oncol 1:233, 1973
69. Daly JW, Million RR: Radical vulvectomy combined with elective node irradiation to TxNO squamous carcinoma of the vulva. Cancer 34:161, 1974
70. Hacker NF, Berek JS, Juillard GJF, et al: Preoperative radiation therapy for locally advanced vulvar cancer. Cancer 54:2056, 1984
71. Kucera H: Die Behandlung des Vulvakzinoms an der I. Universitats-Frauenklinik Wien (386 Falle). Strahlentherapie 156:598, 1980
72. Simonsen E, Nordberg UB, Johnson JE, et al: Radiation therapy and surgery in the treatment of regional lymph nodes in squamous cell carcinoma of the vulva. Acta Radiol Oncol 23:433, 1984
73. Foster DC, Woodruff JD: The use of dinitrochlorobenzene in the treatment of vulvar carcinoma in situ. Gynecol Oncol 11:330, 1981
74. Pao WM, Perez CA, Kuske RR, et al: Radiation therapy and conservation surgery for primary and recurrent carcinoma of the vulva: Report of 40 patients and a review of the literature. Int J Radiat Oncol Biol Phys (in press)
75. Schulz U, Callies R, Kruger KG: Effizienz der postoperativen electronentherapie des lekalisierten vulvarkarzinoms. Strahtertherapie 156:326, 1980
76. Stillman FH, Sedlis A, Boyce JG: A review of lower genital intraepithelial neoplasia and the use of topical 5-fluorouracil. Obstet Gynecol Surf 40:190, 1985
77. Calgar H, Hertzog AW, Hreschyshyn MM: Topical 5-fluorouracil treatment of vaginal intraepithelial neoplasia. Obstet Gynecol 5:580, 1981
78. Stillman FH, Boyce JG, Macasaet MA, et al: 5-Fluorouracil/chemosurgery for intra-epithelial neoplasia of the lower genital tract. Obstet Gynecol 58:356, 1981
79. Levin W, Rad FF, Goldberg G, et al: The use of concomitant chemotherapy and radiotherapy prior to surgery in advanced stage carcinoma of the vulva. Gynecol Oncol 25:20, 1986
80. Hoskins WJ, Burke TW, Weiser EB, et al: The use of rotation flaps in vulvar surgery. Contemp Ob/Gyn 28:159, 1986
81. Julian CG, Callison J, Woodruff JD: Plastic management of extensive vulvar defects. Obstet Gynecol 38:193, 1971
82. Lovett RD, Kuske RR, Perez CA, et al: Preliminary evaluation of toxicity and tumor response to radiotherapy with cis-platinum and 5-fluorouracil for advanced or recurrent gynecologic malignancies. Presented at the 29th Annual Meeting of American Society for Therapeutic Radiology and Oncology, October 1987
83. Rutledge F: Cancer of the vagina. Am J Obstet Gynecol 97:635, 1967
84. Herbst AL, Green TH Jr, Ulfelder H: Primary carcinoma of the vagina. Am J Obstet Gynecol 106:210, 1970
85. Plentl AA, Friedman EA: Lymphatic System of the Female Genitalia: The Morphologic Basis of Oncologic Diagnosis and Therapy, pp 51–74. Philadelphia, WB Saunders, 1971
86. Gallup DG, Morley GW: Carcinoma in situ of the vagina. Obstet Gynecol 46:334, 1975
87. Graham JB, Meigs JV: Recurrence of tumor after total hysterectomy for carcinoma in situ. Am J Obstet Gynecol 64:1159, 1952
88. Hummer WK, Massey E, Decker DG, et al: Primary invasive squamous carcinoma of the vagina. Obstet Gynecol 53:218, 1959
89. Pride GL, Schultz AE, Chuprevich TW, et al: Primary invasive squamous carcinoma of the vagina. Obstet Gynecol 53:218, 1979
90. Novak ER, Woodruff JD: Postirradiation malignancies of the pelvic organs. Am J Obstet Gynecol 77:667, 1959
91. Herbst AL, Ulfelder H, Poskanzer DC: Adenocarcinoma of the vagina: Association of maternal stilbestrol therapy with tumor appearance in young women. N Engl J Med 11:284, 1971
92. Herbst AL, Cole P, Colton T, et al: Age-incidence and risk of diethylstilbestrol-related clear cell adenocarcinoma of the vagina and cervix. Am J Obstet Gynecol 128:48, 1977
93. Herbst AL, Robboy SJ, Scully RE, et al: Clear cell adenocarcinoma of the vagina in girls: Analysis of 170 registry cases. Am J Obstet Gynecol 119:713, 1974
94. Park RC, Parmley TH: Vaginal cancer. In McGowan L (ed): Gynecologic Oncology, pp 174–184. New York, Appleton-Century-Crofts, 1978
95. Perez C, Arneson AN, Galakatos A, et al: Malignant tumors of the vagina. Cancer 31:36, 1973
96. Smith J: Malignant gynecologic tumors in children. Am J Obstet Gynecol 116:201, 1973
97. Norris HJ, Taylor HB: Melanomas of the vagina. Am J Clin Pathol 46:420, 1966
98. Ragiri MV, Tobon H: Primary malignant melanoma of the vagina and vulva. Obstet Gynecol 43:658, 1974
99. Blaustein A: Diseases of the vagina. In Blaustein A (ed): Pathology of the Female Genital Tract, pp 59–86. New York, Springer-Verlag, 1977
100. Scully RE, Robboy SJ, Welch WR: Pathology and pathogenesis of diethylstilbestrol-related disorders of the female genital tract. In Herbst AL (ed): Intrauterine Exposure to Diethylstilbestrol in the Human. Chicago, The American College of Obstetricians and Gynecologists, 1978
101. Tavassoli FA, Norris HJ: Smooth muscle tumors of the vagina. Obstet Gynecol 53:689, 1979
102. Wharton JT, Fletcher GH, Declos L: Invasive tumors of vagina: Clinical features and management. In Coppleson M (ed): Gynecologic Oncology: Fundamental Principles and Clinical Practice, pp 345–359. New York, Churchill Livingstone, 1981
103. Livingstone RC: Primary carcinoma of the vagina. Springfield, IL, Charles C Thomas, 1950
104. Brady LW: Radiation therapy for carcinoma of the vagina. In McGowan L (ed): Gynecologic Oncology, pp 185–190. New York, Appleton-Century-Crofts, 1978
105. Chau PM: Radiotherapeutic management of malignant tumors of the vagina. Am J Roentgenol Radium Ther Nucl Med 89:502, 1963
106. Perez CA, Camel HM, Galakatos AE, et al: Definitive irradiation in carcinoma of the vagina. Long-term evaluation (personal communication)
107. Woodruff JD, Parmley TH, Julian CG: Topical 5-flourouracil in the treatment of vaginal carcinoma in situ. Gynecol Oncol 3:124, 1975
108. Townsend DE: Intraepithelial neoplasia of the vagina. In Coppleson M (ed): Gynecologic Oncology: Fundamental Principles and Clinical Practice, pp 339–344. New York, Churchill Livingstone, 1981
109. Brown GR, Fletcher GH, Rutledge FN: Irradiation of 'in situ' and invasive squamous cell carcinomas of the vagina. Cancer 28:1278, 1971
110. Perez CA, Camel HM: Longterm followup in radiation therapy of carcinoma of the vagina. Cancer 49:1308, 1982
111. Frick HC, Jacox HW, Taylor HC Jr: Primary carcinoma of the vagina. Am J Obstet Gynecol 101:695, 1968
112. Herbst AL, Green TH, Ulfelder H: Primary carcinoma of the vagina. Am J Obstet Gynecol 106:210, 1970
113. Underwood PB, Smith RT: Carcinoma of the vagina. JAMA 217:46, 1971
114. Perez CA, Korba A, Sharma S: Dosimetric considerations in irradiation of carcinoma of the vagina. Int J Radiat Oncol Biol Phys 2:639, 1977
115. Perez CA, DiSaia PJ, Knapp RC: Gynecologic tumors. In DeVita VT Jr, Hellman S, Rosenberg SA (eds): Cancer: Principles and Practice of Oncology, 2nd ed, pp 1013–1081. Philadelphia, JB Lippincott, 1985
116. Perez CA, Grigsby DW, Slessinger E: A new afterloading vaginal applicator (personal communication) 1987
117. Wharton JT, Rutledge FN, Gallagher HS, et al: Treatment of clear cell adenocarcinoma in young females. Obstet Gynecol 45:365, 1975
118. Fletcher GH (ed): Textbook of Radiotherapy, 3rd ed, pp 821–824. Philadelphia, Lea & Febiger, 1980
119. Piver MS, Barlow JJ, Wang JJ, et al: Combined radical surgery, radiation therapy and

chemotherapy in infants with vulvo-vaginal embryonal rhabdomyosarcoma. Obstet Gynecol 42:522, 1973

120. Grosfeld JL, Smith JP, Clatworthy JR: Pelvic rhabdomyosarcoma in infants and children. J Urol 107:673, 1973

121. Ghavimi F, Exelby PR, D'Angio GJ, et al: Combination therapy of urogenital embryonal rhabdomyosarcoma in children. Cancer 32:1178, 1973

122. Sordillo P, Magill GB, Shauer PK, et al: Preliminary trial of combination therapy with Adriamycin and radiation therapy in sarcomas and other malignant tumors. J Surg Oncol 21:23, 1982

123. Kinsella TJ, Glatstein E: Clinical experience with intravenous radiosensitizers in unresectable sarcoma. Cancer 59:908, 1987

124. Morrow CP, DiSaia PJ: Malignant melanoma of the female genitalia: A clinical analysis. Obstet Gynecol Surv 31:233, 1976

125. Barber HRK: Incidence, prevalence and median survival rates of gynecologic cancer. In van Nagell JR Jr, Barber HRK (eds): Modern Concepts of Gynecologic Oncology, pp 1–19. Boston, John Wright PSG Inc, 1982

126. Cramer D, Cutler SJ: Incidence and histopathology of malignancies of the female genital organs in the United States. Am J Obstet Gynecol 118:443, 1974

127. Barber HRK: Cervical Cancer. In McGowan L (ed): Gynecologic Oncology, pp 206–216. New York, Appleton-Century-Crofts, 1975

128. Christopherson WM, Parker JE: Relation of cervical cancer to early marriage and childbearing. N Engl J Med 273:235, 1965

129. Keighley E: Carcinoma of the cervix among prostitutes in a women's prison. Br J Vener Dis 44:254, 1968

130. Rotkin ID: Adolescent coitus and cervical cancer associations of related events with increased risk. Cancer Res 27:603, 1967

131. Rotkin ID: Sexual characteristics of a cervical cancer population. Am J Public Health 57:815, 1967

132. Taylor RS, Carroll BE, Lloyd JW: Mortality among women in 3 Catholic religious orders with special references to cancer. Cancer 12:1207, 1959

133. Terris M, Wilson F, Nelson JH Jr: Relation of circumcision to cancer of the cervix. Am J Obstet Gynecol 117:1056, 1973

134. Abou-Daoud KT: Epidemiology of cancers of the cervix in Lebanese Christians and Moslems. Cancer 20:1706, 1967

135. Ackerman LV, del Regato JA (eds): Cancer. Diagnosis, Treatment and Prognosis. St. Louis, CV Mosby, 1977

136. Kessler I: Human cervical cancer as a venereal disease. Cancer Res 36:783, 1976

137. Joneja MG, Coulson DB: Histopathology and cytogenetics of tumors induced by application of 7,12-dimethyl-benz (a) centhracene (DMBA) in mouse cervix. Eur J Cancer 9:367, 1973

138. Herbst AL, Cole P, Norusis MJ, et al: Epidemiologic aspects and factors related to survival in 384 registry cases of clear cell adenocarcinoma of the vagina and cervix. Am J Obstet Gynecol 135:876, 1979

139. Boyce JG, Lu T, Nelson JH Jr: Cervical carcinoma and oral contraceptives. Gynecol Obstet Invest 40:139, 1972

140. Drill VA: Oral contraceptives: Relation to mammary cancer, benign breast lesions and cervical cancer. Am Rev Pharmacol 15:367, 1975

141. Melnick JL, Adams E, Rawls WE: The causative role of herpes virus 2 in cervical cancer. Cancer 34:1375, 1974

142. Nahmias AJ, Naib ZM, Josey WE, et al: Prospective studies of the association of genital herpes simplex infection and cervical anaplasia. Cancer Res 33:1491, 1973

143. Hollinshead AC, Chretien PB, O'bong L, et al: In vivo and in vitro measurements of the relationship of human squamous carcinoma to herpes simplex virus tumor-associated antigen. Cancer Res 36:821, 1976

144. Rapp F, Duff R: Oncogenic conversion of normal cells by inactivated herpes simplex virus. Cancer 34:1353, 1974

145. Darai G, Munk K: Human embryonic lung cells abortively infected with herpes hominus Type 2 show properties of cell transformation. Nature New Biol 241:268, 1973

146. Wentz WB, Reagan JW, Heggie AD: Cervical carcinogenesis with herpes simplex virus, Type 2. Obstet Gynecol 46:117, 1975

147. Notter MFD, Docherty JJ, Martel R, et al: Detection of herpes simplex virus tumor associated antigen in uterine cervical tissue: Five case studies. Gynecol Oncol 6:574, 1978

148. Meisels A, Fortin R: Condylomatous lesions of the cervix and vagina I. Cytologic patterns. Acta Cytol 20:505, 1976

149. Kurman RJ, Jenson AB, Lancaster WD: Papillomavirus infections of the cervix: Relationship to intraepithelial neoplasia based on the presence of specific viral structural proteins. Am J Surg Pathol 7:39, 1983

150. Reid R, Crum CP, Herschman BR, et al: Genital warts and cervical cancer. III Subclinical papillomaviral infection and cervical neoplasia are linked by a spectrum of continuous morphologic and biologic change. Cancer 53:943, 1984

151. Crum CP, Levine RU: Human papillomavirus infection and cervical neoplasia: New perspectives. Int J Gynecol Pathol 3:376, 1984

152. Durst M, Gissman L, Ikenberg H, et al: A papillomavirus DNA from a cervical cancer and its prevalence in cancer biopsies from different geographical regions. Proc Natl Acad Sci USA 80:3812, 1983

153. Levine RU, Crum CP, Herman E, et al: Cervical papillomavirus infection and intraepithelial neoplasia: A study of male sexual partners. Obstet Gynecol 64:16, 1984

154. Krebs HB, Schneider V: Human Papillomavirus-associated lesions of the penis: colposcopy, cytology and histology. Obstet Gynecol 70:299, 1987

154a. Petersen O: Spontaneous course of cervical pre-cancerous conditions. Am J Obstet Gynecol 72:1063, 1956

155. Richart RM: Natural history of cervical intraepithelial neoplasia. Clin Obstet Gynecol 110:748, 1967

156. Reagan JW, Wentz WB: Genesis of carcinoma of the uterine cervix. Clin Obstet Gynecol 10:883, 1967

157. Clemmesen J, Poulsen H: Report of the Ministry of the Interior. Document 3, Copenhagen, 1971

157a. Kottmeier HL: Evolution et traitment des epitheliomas. Rev Fr Gynec Obstet 56:821, 1961

158. Walton Report: Cervical cancer screening program, epidemiological and natural history of cancer of the cervix. Can Med Assoc J 114:1003, 1976

159. Plentl AA, Friedman EA: Lymphatic system of the female genitalia: The morphologic basis of oncologic diagnosis and therapy, pp 75–115. Philadelphia, WB Saunders, 1971

160. Fuller AF, Elliott N, Kosloff C, et al: Lymph node metastases from carcinoma of the cervix, Stages IB and IIA: Implications for progress and treatment. Gynecol Oncol 13:165, 1982

161. Sudarsanam A, Komanduri C, Belinson J, et al: Influence of exploratory celiotomy on the management of carcinoma of the cervix. A preliminary report. Cancer 41:1049, 1978

162. Nelson JH Jr, Macasaet MN, Lu T, et al: The incidence and significance of para-aortic lymph node metastases in late invasive carcinoma of the cervix. Amer J Obstet Gynecol 118:749, 1974

163. Piver MS, Barlow JJ: High dose irradiation to biopsy confirmed aortic node metastases from carcinoma of the cervix. Cancer 39:1243, 1977

164. Wharton JT, Jones HW III, Day TG, et al: Preirradiation celiotomy and extended field irradiation for invasive carcinoma of the cervix. Obstet Gynecol 49:333, 1977

165. Lagasse LD, Creasnan WT, Singleton HM, et al: Results and complications of operative staging in cervical cancer: Experience of the Gynecologic Oncology Group. Gynecol Oncol 9:90, 1980

166. Buschbaum HJ: Extrapelvic lymph node metastases in cervical carcinoma. Am J Obstet Gynecol 133:814, 1979

167. Averette HE, Ford JH Jr, Dudan RC, et al: Staging of cervical cancer. Clin Obstet Gynecol 18:215, 1975

168. Welander CE, Pierce VK, Nori D, et al: Pretreatment laparatomy in carcinoma of the cervix. Gynecol Oncol 12:336, 1981

169. Berman ML, Keys H, Creasman W, et al: Survival and patterns of recurrence in cervical cancer metastatic to periaortic lymph nodes: A Gynecologic Group Study. Gynecol Oncol 19:8, 1984

170. Carlson V, Delclos L, Fletcher GH: Distant metastases in squamous-cell carcinoma of the uterine cervix. Radiology 88:961, 1987

171. Rutledge FN, Warton JT, Fletcher GH: Clinical studies with adjunctive surgery and irradiation therapy in the treatment of carcinoma of the cervix. Cancer 38:596, 1976

172. Regan JW, Ng ABP: The cellular manifestations of uterine carcinomas. In Norris HJ, Hertig AT, Abell MR (eds): The Uterus. International Academy of Pathology, Monographs in Pathology. Baltimore, Williams & Wilkins, 1973

173. Wentz WB: Histological grade and survival in cervical cancer with respect to cell type. Cancer 18:412, 1961

174. Abell MR, Gosling JRG: Gland cell carcinoma (adenocarcinoma) of the uterine cervix. Am J Obstet Gynecol 83:729, 1962

175. Davis JR, Moon LB: Increased incidence of adenocarcinoma of uterine cervix. Obstet Gynecol 45:79, 1975

176. Artman LE, Hoskins WJ, Bibro MC, et al: Radical hysterectomy and pelvic lymphadenectomy for stage IB carcinoma of the cervix: 21 years experience. Gynecol Oncol 28:8, 1987

177. Dougherty CM, Cottin N: Mixed squamous cell and adenocarcinoma of the cervix: Combined adenosquamous and mucoepidermoid types. Cancer 17:1132, 1964

178. Noller KL, Decker DG, Dockerty MD, et al: Mesonephric (clear cell) carcinoma of the vagina and cervix. Obstet Gynecol 43:640, 1974

179. Hart WR, Norris HJ: Mesonephric adenocarcinoma of the cervix. Cancer 29:106, 1972

180. Ulbright TM, Gersell DJ: Glassey cell carcinoma of the uterine cervix. A light and electron microscopic study of five cases. Cancer 51:2255, 1983

181. Hoskins WJ, Ng APB, Averette HE, et al: Cylindroma of the cervix uteri: Report of six cases and review of the literature. Gynecol Oncol 7:371, 1979

182. Dougherty CM, Cotten N: Mixed squamous cell and adenocarcinoma of the cervix: Combined, adenosquamous and mucoepidermoid types. Cancer 17:1132, 1964

183. Abell MR: Primary melanoblastoma of the uterine cervix. Am J Clin Pathol 36:248, 1961

184. Warner TFCS: Carcinoid tumor of the uterine cervix. J Clin Pathol 31:990, 1978

185. Abell MR, Ramirez JA: Sarcomas and carcinosarcomas of the uterine cervix. Cancer 31:1176, 1973

186. Charlton I, Karnei RF, King FM, et al: Primary malignant reticuloendothelial disease involving the vagina, cervix and corpus uteri. Obstet Gynecol 44:735, 1974

187. Retikas DG: Hodgkin's sarcoma of the cervix. Report of a case. Am J Obstet Gynecol 80:1104, 1960

188. Jennings RH, Barclay DI: Verrucous carcinoma of the cervix. Cancer 30:430, 1972

189. Breslow L: Cytology and the decline in uterine cervix mortality in California. In Clark RL, Cumley RW, McCoy JE, et al (eds): Oncology 1970. Proceedings of the

Tenth International Cancer Congress, vol IV. Diagnosis and Management of Cancer: Specific sites. Chicago, Year Book, 1971

190. Fidler HK, Boyes DA, Worth AJ: Cervical cancer detection in British Columbia. J Obstet Gynecol Br Comm 75:392, 1968

191. American Cancer Society: ACS report on the cancer-related health check-up. Cancer 30:194, 1980

192. The American College of Obstetricians and Gynecologists Statement of Policy. Periodic cancer screening for women. American College of Obstetricians and Gynecologists, June 1980

193. Walsh JW, Amendola MA, Konerding KF, et al: Computed tomographic detection of pelvic and inguinal lymph node metastases from primary and recurrent pelvic malignant disease. Radiology 137:157, 1980

194. Piver MS, Chung WS: Prognostic significance of cervical lesion size and pelvic node metastases in cervical carcinoma. Obstet Gynecol 46:507, 1975

195. Changes in definitions of clinical staging for carcinoma of the cervix and ovary: International Federation of Gynecology and Obstetrics. Am J Obstet Gynecol 156:263, 1987

196. Averette HE, Dudan RC, Ford JH: Exploratory celiotomy for surgical staging in cervical cancer. Am J Obstet Gynecol 113:1090, 1972

197. Berman ML, Lagasse LD, Watring WG, et al: The operative evaluation of patients with cervical carcinoma by an extraperitoneal approach. Obstet Gynecol 50:658, 1977

198. Fuller AF, Elliott N, Kosloff C, et al: Determinants of increased risk for recurrence in patients undergoing radical hysterectomy for stage IB and IIA carcinoma of the cervix. Gynecol Oncol (in press)

199. Burghardt E, Pickel H, Haas J, et al: Prognostic factors and operative treatment of stages IB to IIB cervical cancer. Am J Obstet Gynecol 156:988, 1987

200. Martimbeau PW, Kjorstad KE, Jenson T: Stage IB carcinoma of the cervix, the Norwegian Radium Hospital. II Results when pelvic nodes are involved. Obstet Gynecol 60:215, 1982

201. Blaikley JB, Lederman M, Pollard W: Carcinoma of the cervix at Chelsea Hospital for Women, 1935–1965. Five-year and 10-year results of treatment. J Obstet Gynecol Brit Commonw 76:729, 1969

202. Brunschwig A, Barber HRK: Surgical treatment of carcinoma of the cervix. Obstet Gynecol 27:21, 1966

203. Christensen A, Lange P, Neilsen E: Surgery and radiotherapy for invasive cancer of the cervix: Surgical treatment. Acta Obstet Gynecol 43:59, 1964

204. Ketcham AS, Hoye RC, Taylor PT: Radical hysterectomy and lymphadenectomy for carcinoma of the uterine cervix. Cancer 28:1272, 1971

205. Liu W, Meigs JV: Radical hysterectomy and pelvic lymphadenectomy: A review of 473 cases including 244 for primary invasive carcinoma of the cervix. Am J Obstet Gynecol 69:1, 1955

206. Masterson JG: The role of surgery in the treatment of early carcinoma of the cervix. Clin Obstet Gynecol 10:922, 1967

207. Park RC, Patow WE, Rogers RR, et al: Treatment for stage I carcinoma of the cervix. Obstet Gynecol 41:117, 1973

208. Chung CK, Nahlas WA, Stryker JA, et al: Analysis of factors contributing to treatment failures in stages IB and IIA carcinoma of the cervix. Am J Obstet Gynecol 138:550, 1980

209. van Nagell JR, Donaldson ES, Wood EG, et al: The significance of vascular invasion and lymphocytic infiltration in invasive cervical cancer. Cancer 41:228, 1978

210. Boyce J, Fruckter RC, Nicastri A, et al: Prognostic factors in stage I carcinoma of the cervix. Gynecol Oncol 12:154, 1981

211. Burke TW, Hoskins WJ, Heller PB, et al: Prognostic factors associated with radical hysterectomy failures. Gynecol Oncol 26:153, 1987

212. Figge DC, Tamimi HK: Patterns of recurrence of carcinoma following radical hysterectomy. Am J Obstet Gynecol 140:213, 1981

213. Fuller AF, Elliott N, Kosloff C, et al: Lymph node metastases from carcinoma of the cervix, stages IB and IIA. Implications for prognosis and treatment. Gynecol Oncol 13:165, 1982

214. Bush RS, Jenkin RDT, Alet WEC, et al: Definitive evidence for hypoxic cells influencing cure in cancer therapy. Br J Cancer 37:302, 1978

215. Vigario G, Kurohara SS, George FW III: Association of hemoglobin levels before and during radiotherapy with prognosis in uterine cervix cancer. Radiology 106:649, 1973

216. Jenkin RDT, Stryker JA: The influence of the blood pressure on survival in cancer of the cervix. Br J Radiol 41:913, 1968

217. Van Herik M: Fever as a complication of radiation therapy for carcinoma of the cervix. Am J Roentgenol Radium Ther Nuc Med 43:104, 1965

218. Prempree T, Patanaphan V, Sewchanel W, et al: The influence of patient's age and tumor grade on the prognosis of carcinoma of the cervix. Cancer 51:1764, 1983

219. Berkowitz RS, Ehrmann RL, Lavizzo-Mourey R, et al: Invasive cervical carcinoma in young women. Gynecol Oncol 8:311, 1979

220. Kyriakos M, Kempson RL, Perez CA: Carcinoma of the cervix in young women. Obstet Gynecol 8:311, 1979

221. Hoskins WJ, Ford JH Jr, Lutz MH, et al: Radical hysterectomy and pelvic lymphadenectomy for the management of early invasive carcinoma of the cervix. Gynecol Oncol 4:278, 1976

222. Townsend DE, Richart RM, Marks E, et al: Invasive carcinoma following outpatient evaluation and therapy for cervical disease. Obstet Gynecol 57:145, 1971

223. Sevin B, Ford JH, Girtanner RD, et al: Invasive cancer of the cervix after cryosurgery. Pitfalls of conservative management. Obstet Gynecol 53:465, 1979

224. Coppleson M: Cervical intraepithelial neoplasia: Clinical features and management. In Coppleson M (ed): Gynecologic Oncology: Fundamental Principles and Clinical Practice, pp 451–464. New York, Churchill Livingstone, 1981

225. Averette HE, Nelson JH, Ng ABP, et al: Diagnosis and management of microinvasive (stage IA) carcinoma of the uterine cervix. Cancer 38:414, 1976

226. Simon NL, Gore H, Shingleton HM, et al: Study of superficially invasive carcinoma of the cervix. Obstet Gynecol 69:19, 1986

227. Burghardt E: Microinvasive carcinoma. Obstet Gynecol Surv 34:836, 1979

228. van Nagell JR, Greenwell N, Powell DF, et al: Microinvasive cancer of the cervix. Am J Obstet Gynecol 145:981, 1983

229. Hamberger AD, Fletcher GH, Wharton JT: Results of treatment of early stage I carcinoma of the uterine cervix with intracavitary radium alone. Cancer 41:980, 1978

230. Pilleron JP, Durand JC, Lenoble JC: Carcinoma of the uterine cervix stages I and II, treated by radiation therapy and extensive surgery (1,000 cases). Cancer 29:593, 1972

231. Sall S, Pineda AA, Cananoq A, et al: Surgical treatment of stages IB and IIA invasive carcinoma of the cervix by radical abdominal hysterectomy. Am J Obstet Gynecol 135:442, 1979

232. Burghardt E: Early Histological Diagnosis of Cervical Cancer. Philadelphia, WB Saunders, 1973

233. Newton M: Radical hysterectomy or radiotherapy for stage I cervical cancer. Am J Obstet Gynecol 123:535, 1975

234. Roddick JW Jr, Greenlow RH: Treatment of cervical cancer. Am J Obstet Gynecol 19:754, 1971

235. Dickson RJ: Late results of radium treatment of carcinoma of the cervix. Clin Radiol 23:528, 1972

236. Fletcher GH: Cancer of the uterine cervix. Janeway Lecture. Am J Roentgenol Radium Ther Nucl Med 111:225, 1971

237. Kline JC, Schultz AE, Vermund H: High dose radiotherapy for carcinoma of the cervix. Method and results. Am J Obstet Gynecol 104:479, 1969

238. Kottmeier HL (ed): Annual Report on the Results of Treatment in Carcinoma of the Uterus, Vagina and Ovary, vol 15. Stockholm, International Federation of Gynecology and Obstetrics, 1973

239. Muirhead W, Green LS: Carcinoma of the cervix. Five-year results sequelae of treatment. Am J Obstet Gynecol 101:744, 1968

240. Perez CA, Camel HM, Kuske RR, et al: Radiation therapy alone in the treatment of carcinoma of the uterine cervix: A 20-year experience. Gynecol Oncol 23:127, 1986

241. Wall JA, Collins VP, Hudgins PT: Carcinoma of the cervix. Review of clinical experience during a 20-year period. Am J Obstet Gynecol 96:57, 1966

242. Volterrani F, Lombardi F: Long term results of radium therapy in cervical cancer. Int J Radiat Oncol Biol Phys 6:565, 1980

243. van Nagell JR, Rayburn W, Donaldson ES: Therapeutic implications of patterns of recurrence in cancer of the uterine cervix. Cancer 44:2354, 1979

244. Kielbinska S, Ludwika T, Fraczek O: Studies of mortality and health status in women cured of cancer of the cervix uteri: Comparison of long-term results of radiotherapy and combined surgery and radiotherapy. Cancer 32:245, 1973

245. Perez CA, Camel HM, Kao MS, et al: Randomized study of preoperative radiation and surgery or irradiation alone in the treatment of stage IB and IIA carcinoma of the uterine cervix. Final report. Gynecol Oncol 27:129, 1987

246. Lu T, Macasaet M, Nelson JH Jr: The barrel shape cervix. Am J Obstet Gynecol 124:596, 1976

247. O'Guinn AG, Fletcher GH, Wharton JT: Guidelines for conservative hysterectomy after irradiation. Gynecol Oncol 9:68, 1980

248. Morrow CP: Panel report: Is pelvic radiation beneficial in the postoperative management of stage IB squamous cell carcinoma of the cervix with pelvic node metastases managed by radical hysterectomy and pelvic lymphadenectomy? Gynecol Oncol 10:105, 1980

249. Wertheim MS, Hakes TB, Doghestani AN, et al: A pilot study of adjuvant therapy in patients with cervical cancer at high risk of recurrence after radical hysterectomy and pelvic lymphadenectomy. J Clin Oncol 3:912, 1985

250. Johns HE: Optimization of energy and equipment. In Kramer S, Suntharalingam N, Zinniger GF (eds): High Energy Photons and Electrons: Clinical Applications in Cancer Management, p 333. New York, John Wiley & Sons, 1976

251. Prempree T: Parametrial implant in stage IIIB cancer of the cervix. III. A five-year study. Cancer 52:748, 1983

252. Aristazabel SA, Surwit EA, Hevezi JM, et al: Treatment of advanced cancer of the cervix with transperineal interstitial irradiation. Int J Radiat Oncol Biol Phys 9:1013, 1983

253. Martinez A, Edmundson GK, Cox RS, et al: Combination of external beam irradiation and multiple-site perineal applicator (Mupit) for treatment of locally advanced or recurrent prostatic, anorectal, and gynecologic malignancies. Int J Radiat Oncol Biol Phys 11:391, 1985

254. Maruyuma Y, Muir W: Human cervical cancer clearance after ^{252}Cf neutron brachytherapy versus conventional photon brachytherapy. Am J Clin Oncol 7:347, 1984

255. Castro JR, Issa P, Fletcher GH: Carcinoma of the cervix treated by external irradiation alone. Radiology 95:163, 1970

256. Einhorn N, Bygdeman M, Sjoberg B: Combined radiation and surgical treatment for carcinoma of the uterine cervix. Cancer 45:720, 1980

257. Morley GW, Seski JC: Radical pelvic surgery versus radiation therapy for stage I carcinoma of the cervix (exclusive of microinvasion). Am J Obstet Gynecol 1126:785, 1976

258. Morton DG, Lagasse LD, Moore JG: Pelvic lymphadenectomy following radiation in cervical carcinoma. Am J Obstet Gynecol 88:932, 1964
259. Sweeney WJ III, Douglas RG: Treatment of carcinoma of the cervix with combined radiation and extensive surgery. Am J Obstet Gynecol 84:981, 1962
260. Rampone JF, Klem V, Kolstad P: Combined treatment of stage IB carcinoma of the cervix. Obstet Gynecol 41:163, 1973
261. Decker DG, Aaro LA, Hunt AB, et al: Sequential radiation and operation in carcinoma of the uterine cervix. Am J Obstet Gynecol 92:35, 1965
262. Quigley MM, Knab DR, McMahan ER: Carcinoma of the cervix. A third treatment. Obstet Gynecol 45:650, 1975
263. Parker RT, Wilbanks GD, Yowell RK: Radical hysterectomy with and without preoperative radiotherapy for cervical cancer. Am J Obstet Gynecol 99:993, 1967
264. Gray MJ, Gusberg SB, Guttman R: Pelvic lymph node dissection following radiotherapy. Am J Obstet Gynecol 76:629, 1958
265. Perez CA, Camel HM, Kao MS, et al: Randomized study of preoperative radiation and surgery or irradiation alone in the treatment of stage IB and IIA carcinoma of the uterine cervix. Preliminary analysis of failures and complications. Cancer 45:2759, 1980
266. Rutledge FN, Fletcher GH, Macdonald EJ: Pelvic lymphadenectomy as an adjunct to radiation therapy in treatment for cancer of the cervix. Am J Roentgenol Radium Ther Nucl Med 93:607, 1965
267. Durrance FY, Fletcher GH, Rutledge FN: Analysis of central recurrent disease in stage I and II squamous cell carcinomas of the cervix on intact uterus. Am J Roentgenol Radium Ther Nucl Med 106:831, 1969
268. Perez CA, Breaux S, Askin F, et al: Irradiation alone or in combination with surgery in stage IB and IIA carcinoma of the uterine cervix. A non-randomized comparison. Cancer 43:1062, 1979
269. Cuccia AA, Blodorn FG: Treatment of primary adenocarcinoma of the cervix. Am J Roentgenol Radium Ther Nucl Med 99:371, 1967
270. Rutledge FN, Galakatos AE, Wharton JT, et al: Adenocarcinoma of the uterine cervix. Am J Obstet Gynecol 122:236, 1975
271. Nelson AJ, Fletcher GH, Wharton T: Indications for adjunctive conservative extrafascial hysterectomy in selected cases of carcinoma of the uterine cervix. Am J Roentgenol Radium Ther Nucl Med 123:91, 1975
273. Perez CA, Kao M-S: Radiation therapy alone or combined with surgery in the treatment of barrel-shaped carcinoma of the uterine cervix (stages IB, IIA, IIB). Int J Radiat Oncol Biol Phys 11:1903, 1985
274. Leveuf J, Godord H: Le'exerese chirugicale des ganglions pelviens complement de la curtherapie des cancers du col de 'uterus. J Chir 43:177, 1934
275. Taussig FJ: Iliac lymphadenectomy with irradiation in the treatment of cancer of the cervix. Am J Obstet Gynecol 28:650, 1934
276. Abitol NM, Davenport JH: Sexual dysfunction after therapy for cervical carcinoma. Am J Obstet Gynecol 119:181, 1974
277. Perez CA: Carcinoma of the uterine cervix. In Perez CA, Brady LW (eds): Principles and Practice of Radiation Oncology, pp 919. Philadelphia, JB Lippincott, 1987
278. Fowler JF: Radiobiological considerations from the hyperbaric oxygen trials. A personal view. Br J Radiol 51:68, 1978
279. Watson ER, Halnan KE, Dische C, et al: Hyperbaric oxygen and radiotherapy: A Medical Research Council trial in carcinoma of the cervix. Br J Radiol 51:879, 1978
280. Fletcher GH, Lindberg RD, Caderao JB, et al: Hyperbaric oxygen as a radiotherapeutic adjuvant in advanced carcinoma of the uterine cervix. Preliminary results of a randomized trial. Cancer 39:617, 1977
281. Glassburn JR, Damsker JI, Brady LW, et al: Hyperbaric oxygen and radiation in the treatment of advanced cervical carcinoma. In Fifth International Hyperbaric Congress Proceedings, II, p 813, Simon Fraser University
282. Dische S: Hyperbaric oxygen: The Medical Research Council trials and their clinical significance. Br J Radiol 51:888, 1979
283. Johnson RJR, Walton RF: Sequential study on the effect of the addition of hyperbaric oxygen on the 5-year survival rates of carcinoma of the cervix treated with conventional fractional irradiations. Am J Roentgenol Radium Ther Nucl Med 120:111, 1974
284. Thomas GM, Rauth AM, Bush RS, et al: A toxicity study of daily dose metronidazole with pelvic irradiation. Cancer Clin Trials 3:223, 1980
285. Dische S: Misonidazole in the clinic at Mount Vernon. Cancer Clin Trials 3:175, 1980
286. Hornback HB, Shupe RE, Shidnia H, et al: Advanced stage IIIB cancer of the cervix treatment by hyperthermia and radiation. Gynecol Oncol 23:160, 1986
287. Perez CA, Breaux S, Madoc-Jones H, et al: Radiation therapy alone in treatment of carcinoma of the uterine cervix. II. Analysis of complications. Cancer 54:235, 1984
288. Kottmeier HL: Complications following radiation therapy in carcinoma of the cervix and their treatment. Am J Obstet Gynecol 88:854, 1964
289. Pourquier H, Dubois JB, Deland R: Cancer of the uterine cervix. Dosimetric guidelines for prevention of late rectal and rectosigmoid complications as a result of radiotherapeutic treatment. Int J Radiat Oncol Biol Phys 8:1887, 1982
290. Strockbine MJ, Hancock JE, Fletcher GH: Complications in 831 patients with squamous cell carcinoma of the intact uterine cervix treated with 3000 cGy or more whole pelvis irradiation. Am J Roentgenol Radium Ther Nucl Med 108:293, 1970
291. Piver MS, Vongtama V, Barlow JJ: Para-aortic lymph node irradiation for carcinoma of the uterine cervix using split-course technique. Gynecol Oncol 3:168, 1975
292. Komaki R, Mattingly RF, Hoffman RG, et al: Irradiation of para-aortic lymph node metastases from carcinoma of the cervix or endometrium. Radiology 147:245, 1983
293. Twefik HH, Buschbaum HJ, Latourette HB, et al: Para-aortic lymph node irradiation in carcinoma of the cervix after exploratory laparotomy and biopsy-proven positive aortic nodes. Int J Radiat Biol Phys 8:13, 1982
294. Potish R, Adcock L, Jones T, et al: The morbidity and utility of periaortic radiotherapy in cervical carcinoma. Gynecol Oncol 15:1, 1983
295. Rotman M, John M: Para-aortic irradiation in cervical carcinoma. Int J Radiat Oncol Biol Phys 5:2139, 1979
296. Freund AW: Zu meiner methods des totalen uterus-exstripation. Zentralbl Gynak 2:265, 1878
297. Brunschwig A: Complete excision of pelvic viscera for advanced carcinoma: A one-step abdominoperineal operation with end colostomy and bilateral ureteral implantation into the colon above the colostomy. Cancer 1:177, 1948
298. Mattingly RF, Thompson JD (eds): Telinde's Operative Gynecology, 6th ed. Philadelphia, JB Lippincott, 1985
299. Webb MJ, Symmonds RE: Wertheim hysterectomy: A reappraisal. Obstet Gynecol 54:140, 1979
300. Symmonds RE: Morbidity and complications of radical hysterectomy with pelvic lymph node dissection. Am J Obstet Gynecol 94:663, 1966
301. Brunschwig A, Daniel WW: Pelvic exenteration operations. Ann Surg 151:571, 1960
302. Lawhead RA, Clark DGC, Smith DH, et al: Pelvic exenteration for recurrent or persistent gynecologic malignancies: A ten-year review of the Memorial Sloan-Kettering Cancer Center experience (1972–1981). Gynecol Oncol (in press)
303. Meoz RT, Spanos WJ, Doss L, et al: Misonidazole combined with large-fraction pelvic irradiation in the treatment of patients with advanced pelvic malignancies. Preliminary report of an ongoing RTOG phase I–II study. Am J Clin Oncol 6:417, 1983
304. Puthawala AA, Syed AM, Fleming PA, et al: Re-irradiation with interstitial implant for recurrent pelvic malignancies. Cancer 50:2810, 1982
305. Prasavinichai S, Glassburn JR, Brady LW: Treatment of recurrent carcinoma of the cervix. Int J Radiat Oncol Biol Phys 4:957, 1978
306. Prempree T, Kwon T, VillaSanta U, et al: Management of late second or late recurrent squamous cell carcinoma of the cervix uteri after successful initial radiation treatment. Int J Radiat Oncol Biol Phys 5:2053, 1979
307. Friedman M, Pearlman AW: Carcinoma of the cervix; radiation salvage of surgical failures. Radiology 84:801, 1965
308. Evans SR Jr, Hilaris BS, Barber HRK: External vs. interstitial irradiation in unresectable recurrent cancer of the cervix. Cancer 28:1284, 1971
309. Sala JM, deLeon AD: Treatment of carcinoma of the cervical stump. Radiology 81:300, 1963
310. Moss WT, Brand WN, Battifor H (eds): Radiation Oncology. Rational, Technique, Results, p 408. St. Louis, CV Mosby, 1973
311. Wimbush PR, Fletcher GH: Radiation therapy of carcinoma of the cervical stump. Radiology 93:655, 1969
312. Creadnick RN: Carcinoma of the cervical stump. Am J Obstet Gynecol 75:5465, 1958
313. DePetrillo AD, Townsend DE, Morrow CP, et al: Colposcopic evaluation of the abnormal Papanicoloau test in pregnancy. Am J Obstet Gynecol 121:441, 1975
314. Averette HE, Nasser N, Yankow SL, et al: Cervical conization in pregnancy. Analysis of 180 operations. Am J Obstet Gynecol 106:543, 1970
315. Miluta JH, Enterline HT, Braun TE Jr: Carcinoma in situ of the cervix and pregnancy associated with pregnancy. JAMA 204:763, 1968
316. Boyle MH, Torrance GW, Sinclair JC, et al: Economic evaluation of neonatal intensive care of very low-birth-weight infants. N Engl J Med 308:1330, 1983
317. Creasman WT, Rutledge FN, Fletcher GH: Carcinoma of the cervix associated with pregnancy. Obstet Gynecol 36:495, 1970
318. Sablinska R, Tarlowska L, Stelmachar J: Invasive carcinoma of the cervix associated with pregnancy: Correlation between age advancement of cancer and gestation, and result of treatment. Gynecol Oncol 5:383, 1979
319. Kinch RAH: Factors affecting the prognosis of carcinoma of the cervix in pregnancy. Am J Obstet Gynecol 82:45, 1961
320. Bonomi PD, Yordan EL: Chemotherapy of cervical carcinoma. In Deppe G (ed): Chemotherapy of Gynecologic Cancer, p 103. New York, Alan R Liss, 1984
321. Wasserman TH, Carter SKL: The integration of chemotherapy into combined modality treatment of solid tumors: VIII. Cervical cancer. Cancer Treat Rep 4:25, 1977
322. Malkasian GD, Decker DG, Jorgensen EP: Chemotherapy of carcinoma of the cervix. Gynecol Oncol 5:109, 1976
323. Thigpen T, Shingleton H, Homsley H, et al: Cis-platinum in treatment of advanced or recurrent squamous cell carcinoma of the cervix: A phase II study of the Gynecologic Oncology Group. Cancer 48:899, 1981
324. Lira-Puerta V, Tenovio F, Wernz J, et al: Phase II study of cisplatin or dibromoducitol for carcinoma of the cervix. Proc Am Soc Clin Oncol 1:111, 1982
325. Stehman FB, Blom J, Blessing J, et al: Phase II trial of galactitol 1,2:5,6-dianhydro (NSC 132313) in the treatment of advanced gynecologic malignancies: a Gynecologic Oncology Group study. Gynecol Oncol 15:381, 1983
326. McGuire WP, Blessing JA, Hatch K, et al: A Phase II study of CHIP in advanced squamous cell carcinoma of the cervix (a Gynecologic Oncology Group study). Invest New Drugs 4:181, 1986
327. Arseneau J, Blessing JS, Stehman FB, et al: A Phase II study of carboplatin in advanced squamous cell carcinoma of the cervix (a Gynecologic Oncology Group study). Invest New Drugs 4:187, 1986
328. Morrow CP, DiSaia PJ, Mangan CF, et al: Continuous pelvic arterial infusion with bleomycin for squamous carcinoma of the cervix recurrent after irradiation therapy. Cancer Treat Rep 61:1403, 1977

329. Swenerton KD, Evers JA, White GW, et al: Intermittent pelvic infusion with vincristine, bleomycin and mytomycin C for advanced recurrent carcinoma of the cervix. Cancer Treat Rep 63:1379, 1979

330. Ohta A: Basic and clinical studies on the simultaneous combination treatment of cervical cancer (especially advanced cases) with a carcino-static agent and radiation. J Tokyo Med Coll 36:529, 1978

331. Oku T, Iwaskaki M, Tojo S: Study on surgical chemotherapy for advanced cancer of the uterine cervix — Particularly on the problem of clinical effect and drug concentration. Acta Obstet Gynaecol Jpn 31:1833, 1979

332. Kavanagh JJ, Rutledge F, Wharton JT, et al: Palliation of advanced recurrent pelvic malignancies by selective intra-arterial combination chemotherapy. Proc Am Soc Clin Oncol 1:109, 1982

333. Carlson JA, Freedman RS, Wallace S, et al: Intraarterial cis-platinum in the management of squamous cell carcinoma of the uterine cervix. Gynecol Oncol 12:92, 1981

334. Piver MS, Varlow JJ, Vongtama V, et al: Hydroxyurea and radiation therapy in advanced cervical cancer. Am J Obstet Gynecol 120:969, 1974

335. Climie ARW, Rachmaninoff N: A ten-year experience with endometrial carcinoma. Surg Gynecol Obstet 120:73, 1965

336. Austin JH, MacMahon B: Indicators of prognosis in carcinoma of the corpus uteri. Surg Gynecol Obstet 128:1247, 1969

337. Hreshchyshyn MM, Aron BS, Boronow RC, et al: Hydroxyurea or placebo combined with radiation to treat stages IIIB and IV cervical cancer confined to the pelvis. Int J Radiat Oncol Biol Phys 5:317, 1979

338. Piver MS, Barlow JJ, Vongtama V, et al: Hydroxyurea as a radiation sensitizer in women with carcinoma of the uterine cervix. Am J Obstet Gynecol 129:379, 1977

339. Fletcher GH: Cancer of the uterine cervix. Janeway Lecture. Am J Roentgenol Radium Ther Nucl Med 111:225, 1971

340. Perez CA, Breaux S, Madoc-Jones H, et al: Radiation therapy alone in the treatment of carcinoma of the uterine cervix: I. Analysis of tumor recurrence. Cancer 51:1393, 1983

341. Choo YC, Choy TK, Wong LC: Potentiation of radiotherapy by cis-dichlorodiammine platinum (II) in advanced cervical carcinoma. Gynecol Oncol 23:94, 1986

342. Twiggs LB, Potish RA, McIntyre S, et al: Concurrent weekly cis-platinum and radiotherapy in advanced cervical cancer: a preliminary dose escalating toxicity study. Gynecol Oncol 24:143, 1986

342a. Potish RA, Twiggs LB, Adcock LL, et al: Effect of cis-platinum on tolerance to radiation therapy in advanced cervical cancer. Am J Clin Oncol 9:387, 1986

343. Creasman WT, Weed JC Jr: Carcinoma of the endometrium (FIGO Stages I and II): Clinical features and management. In Coppleson M (ed): Gynecologic Oncology: Fundamental Principles and Clinical Practice, pp 562–574. New York, Churchill Livingstone, 1985

344. Damon A: Host factors in cancer of the breast and uterine cervix and corpus. J Natl Cancer Inst 24:485, 1960

345. Wynder EL, Escher GC, Montel N: An epidemiological investigation of cancer of the endometrium. Cancer 19:489, 1966

346. MacMahon B: Risk factors for endometrial cancer. Gynecol Oncol 2:122, 1974

347. Masubuchi K, Nemoto H: Epidemiologic studies on uterine cancer at Cancer Institute Hospital, Tokyo, Japan. Cancer 30:208, 1972

348. McDonald TW, Malkasian GD, Gaffney TA: Endometrial cancer associated with feminizing ovarian tumor and polycystic ovarian disease. Obstet Gynecol 49:654, 1977

349. Gusberg SB, Kardon P: Proliferative endometrial response to theca-granulosa cell tumors. Am J Obstet Gynecol 3:633, 1971

350. Smith DC, Prentice R, Thompson DJ, et al: Association of exogenous estrogen and endometrial carcinoma. N Engl J Med 293:1164, 1975

351. Amtunes CMF, Stolley PD, Rosensheim NB, et al: Endometrial cancer and estrogen use (Report of a large case-control study). N Engl J Med 300:9, 1979

352. Nachtigall LE, Nachtigall RH, Nachtigall RD, et al: Estrogen replacement therapy II: A prospective study in the relationship to carcinoma and cardiovascular metabolic problems. Obstet Gynecol 54:74, 1979

353. Gambrel DR Jr: Role of hormones in the etiology and prevention of endometrial and breast cancer. Acta Obstet Gynecol Scand [Suppl] 106:337, 1982

354. Frick HC, Munnell EW, Richart RM, et al: Carcinoma of the endometrium. Am J Obstet Gynecol 115:663, 1973

355. Moss WT: Common peculiarities of patients with adenocarcinoma of the endometrium, with special reference to obesity, body build, diabetes and hypertension. Am J Roentgenol Radium Ther Nucl Med 58:203, 1947

356. Sommers SC, Hertig AT, Beugloff H: Genesis of endometrial carcinoma. 11 cases 19 to 35 years old. Cancer 2:957, 1949

357. Buchler DA, Peckham BM, Carr WF: Treatment and results of endometrial carcinoma from 1956–1974. In Gray LA Sr (ed): Endometrial Carcinoma and Its Treatment: The Role of Irradiation, Extent of Surgery, and Approach to Chemotherapy, pp 146–150. Springfield, IL, Charles C Thomas, 1977

358. Gore H, Hertig AT: Premalignant lesions of the endometrium. Clin Obstet Gynecol 5:1148, 1962

359. Plentl AA, Friedman EA: Lymphatic system of the female genitalia: The morphologic basis of oncologic diagnosis and therapy, pp 116–152. Philadelphia, WB Saunders, 1971

360. Creasman WT, Boronow RC, Morrow CP, et al: Adenocarcinoma of the endometrium: Its metastatic lymph node potential. Gynecol Oncol 4:239, 1976

361. Berman ML, Ballon SC, Lagasse LD, et al: Prognosis and treatment of endometrial cancer. Am J Obstet Gynecol 136:679, 1980

362. Tak WK: Carcinoma of the endometrium, with cervical involvement (Stage II). Cancer 43:2504, 1979

363. Creasman WT, DiSaia PJ, Blessing J, et al: Prognostic significance of peritoneal cytology in patients with endometrial cancer and preliminary data concerning therapy and intraperitoneal pharmaceuticals. Am J Obstet Gynecol 141:931, 1981

364. Kennedy AW, Peterson FL, Becker SN, et al: Experience with pelvic washings in Stage I and II endometrial carcinoma. Gynecol Oncol 28:50, 1987

365. Reagan JW, Fu YS: Pathology of endometrial carcinoma. In Coppleson M (ed): Gynecologic Oncology: Fundamental Principles and Clinical Practice, pp 546–561. New York, Churchill Livingstone, 1981

366. Ng ABP, Reagan JW, Storaasli JP, et al: Mixed adenosquamous carcinoma of the endometrium. Am J Clin Pathol 59:765, 1973

367. Silverberg SG, Bolin MG, DeGiorgio LS: Adenoacanthoma and mixed adenosquamous carcinoma of the endometrium. A clinico-pathologic study. Cancer 30:1307, 1972

368. Salazar VM, DePapp EW, Bonifiglio TA, et al: Adenosquamous carcinoma of the endometrium: An entity with an inherent poor prognosis? Cancer 40:119, 1977

369. Kurman RJ, Scully RE: Clear cell carcinoma of the endometrium: an analysis of 21 cases. Cancer 37:872, 1976

370. Hertig AT, Gore H: Tumors of the female sex organs: Part 2. Tumors of the vulva, vagina and uterus. In Atlas of Tumor Pathology, Series 1, Fascicle 33. Washington, DC, Armed Forces Institute of Pathology, 1960

371. Fluhman CF: Squamous epithelium in benign and malignant conditions. Surg Gynecol Obstet 46:309, 1928

372. Hendrickson M, Ross J, Eifel P, et al: Uterine papillary serous carcinoma: A highly malignant form of endometrial adenocarcinoma. Am J Surg Pathol 6:93, 1982

373. Ramirez-Gonzalez CE, Adams K, Mangual-Vazquez TY, et al: Papillary Adenocarcinoma in the Endometrium. Obstet Gynecol 70:212, 1987

374. Boronow RC, Morrow CP, Creasman WT, et al: Surgical staging in endometrial cancer: Clinical-pathologic findings of a prospective study. Obstet Gynecol 63:825, 1984

375. Lewis BW, Stallworthy JA, Cowdell R: Adenocarcinoma of the body of the uterus. J Obstet Gynecol Br Commonw 77:343, 1970

376. Jones HW: Treatment of adenocarcinoma of the endometrium. Obstet Gynecol Surv 30:147, 1975

377. Surwit EA, Fowler WC Jr, Rogoff EE, et al: Stage II carcinoma of the endometrium. Int J Radiat Oncol Biol Phys 5:323, 1979

378. Lutz MH, Underwood PB, Kreutner A, et al: Endometrial carcinoma: A new method of classification of therapeutic and prognostic significance. Gynecol Oncol 6:83, 1978

379. DiSaia PJ, Creasman WT, Boronow RC, et al: Risk factors and recurrent patterns in Stage I endometrial cancer. Am J Obstet Gynecol 151:1009, 1985

380. Morrow CP, DiSaia PJ, Townsend DE: Current management of endometrial carcinoma. Obstet Gynecol 42:399, 1973

381. Boronow RC: Endometrial cancer: Not a benign disease. Obstet Gynecol 47:630, 1976

382. Arneson A: Clinical results and histologic changes following the radiation treatment of cancer of the corpus uteri. Am J Roentgenol Radium Ther Med 36:461, 1936

383. Kempson RL, Pokorny GE: Adenocarcinoma of the endometrium in women 40 years of age and younger. Cancer 21:650, 1968

384. Nolan JF, Dorough ME, Anson JH: The value of preoperative radiation therapy in Stage I carcinoma of the uterine corpus. Am J Obstet Gynecol 98:663, 1967

385. Underwood PB, Lutz MH, Kreutner A, et al: Carcinoma of the endometrium: Radiation followed immediately by operation. Am J Obstet Gynecol 128:86, 1977

386. Gusberg SB, Chen SY, Cohen CJ: Endometrial cancer: Factors influencing the choice of treatment. Gynecol Oncol 2:308, 1974

387. Malkasian GD Jr: Carcinoma of the endometrium: Effect of stage and grade on survival. Cancer 41:996, 1978

388. Kottmeier HL: Individualization of therapy in carcinoma of the corpus. In Cancer of the Uterus and Ovary. MD Anderson Hospital, pp 102–108. Chicago, Year Book, 1969

389. Landgren RD, Fletcher GH, Deldos L, et al: Irradiation of endometrial cancer in patients with medical contraindication to surgery or with unresectable lesions. Am J Roentgenol Radium Ther Nucl Med 126:148, 1976

390. Aalders H, Abler Z, Kolstad P, et al: Postoperative external irradiation and prognostic parameters in stage I endometrial carcinoma. Clinical and histopathologic study of 540 patients. Obstet Gynecol 56:419, 1980

391. Wharam MO, Phillips TL, Bagshaw MA: The role of radiation therapy in clinical stage I carcinoma of the endometrium. Int J Radiat Oncol Biol Phys 1:1081, 1976

393. Landgren RC, Fletcher GH, Delclos L, et al: Irradiation of endometrial cancer in patients with medical contraindications to surgery or with unresectable lesions. Am J Roentgenol Rad Ther Nucl Med 126:148, 1976

394. Strickland PL: Carcinoma corpus uteri: A radical intracavitary treatment. Br J Radiol 16:112, 1965

395. Homesley HD, Boronow RC, Lewis JL: Stage II Endometrial Adenocarcinoma: Memorial Hospital for Cancer, 1949–1965. Obstet Gynecol 49:604, 1977

396. Larson DM, Copeland LJ, Gallager HS, et al: Nature of cervical involvement in endometrial carcinoma. Cancer 59:959, 1987

397. Kinsella TJ, Bloomer WD, Lavin PT, et al: Stage II endometrial carcinoma: Ten-year followup of combined radiation and surgical treatment. Gynecol Oncol 10:290, 1980

398. Grigsby PW, Perez CA, Camel HM, et al: Stage II carcinoma of the endometrium:

Results of therapy and prognostic factors. Int J Radiat Oncol Biol Phys 11:1915, 1985

399. Rutledge F: The role of radical hysterectomy in adenocarcinoma of the endometrium. Gynecol Oncol 2:331, 1974

400. Graham H: The value of preoperative or postoperative treatment by radium for carcinoma of the uterine body. Surg Gynecol Obstet 1323:855, 1971

401. Stokes S, Bedwinek JM, Kao M-S, et al: Treatment of stage I adenocarcinoma of the endometrium by hysterectomy and adjuvant irradiation: A retrospective analysis of 304 patients. Int J Radiat Oncol Biol Phys 12:339, 1986

402. Beiler DD, Schmitz DA, O'Rourke TL: Carcinoma of the endometrium: Radiation and surgery versus surgery alone. Radiology 102:159, 1972

403. Wharam MO, Phillips TL, Bagshaw MA: The role of radiation therapy in clinical stage I carcinoma of the endometrium. Int J Radiat Oncol Biol Phys 1:1081, 1976

404. Malkasian GD Jr, McDonald TW, Pratt JH: Carcinoma of the endometrium. Mayo Clinic Experience. Mayo Clinic Proc 51:175, 1977

405. Salazar OM, Feldstein ML, DePapp EW, et al: Endometrial carcinoma: Analysis of failures with special emphasis on the use of initial preoperative external pelvic radiation. Int J Radiat Oncol Biol Phys 2:1101, 1977

406. Brady LW, Lewis GC, Antoniades J, et al: Evolution of therapeutic techniques. Gynecol Oncol 2:253, 1974

407. Bedwinek JM, Galakatos A, Camel HM, et al: Stage I, grade III adenocarcinoma of the endometrium treated with surgery and irradiation: Sites of failure and correlation of failure rate with irradiation technique. Cancer 54:40, 1984

408. Anderson JC, Meltzer HD, Scarborough JE, et al: Adenocarcinoma of the endometrium. Cancer 18:955, 1965

409. Gusberg SB, Yannopoulos D: Therapeutic decisions in corpus cancer. Am J Obstet Gynecol 120:73, 1964

410. Cheon HK: Prognosis of endometrial carcinoma. Obstet Gynecol 34:680, 1969

411. Nilson PA, Koller O: Carcinoma of the endometrium in Norway 1957–1960 with special reference to treatment results. Am J Obstet Gynecol 105:1099, 1969

412. Ng ABP, Reagan JW: Incidence and prognosis of endometrial carcinoma by histologic grade and extent. Obstet Gynecol 35:437, 1970

413. Sall S, Sonneblick B, Stone ML: Factors affecting survival of patients with endometrial adenocarcinoma. Am J Obstet Gynecol 107:116, 1970

414. Nahhas WA: Prognostic factors in endometrial carcinoma (personal communication, 1971)

415. Wade E, Kohorn EI, Morris JM: Adenocarcinoma of the endometrium. Evaluation of preoperative irradiation and factors influencing prognosis. Am J Obstet Gynecol 99:869, 1967

416. Javert CT: The spread of benign and malignant endometrium in the lymphatic system with a note on coexisting vascular involvement. Am J Obstet Gynecol 64:780, 1952

417. Webb GA, Margolis AJ, Traut HF: Adenocarcinoma of the endometrium: An evaluation of factors influencing prognosis and an outline of a plan of therapy based on these factors. West J Surg Obstet Gynecol 63:407, 1955

418. Lindgren L: The prognosis of carcinoma of the endometrium in its different stages treated by surgery combined with postoperative radiotherapy. Acta Obstet Gynecol Scand 36:426, 1957

419. Boutselis JG, Bair JR, Nichols V, et al: Carcinoma of the uterine corpus: A study of 269 cases, 1947–1959. Am J Obstet Gynecol 85:994, 1963

420. Dobbie BMW, Taylor CW, Waterhouse JAH: A study of carcinoma of the endometrium. J Obstet Gynaecol Br Commonw 72:659, 1965

421. Roman R, Beck R, Latour J: Correlation of histologic grading with 5-year survival rates in endometrial carcinoma. Am J Obstet Gynecol 97:117, 1967

422. Sala JM, del Regato JA: The treatment of carcinoma of the endometrium. Radiology 79:12, 1969

423. Silverberg SG, DeGiorgi LS: Histopathologic analysis of preoperative radiation therapy in endometrial carcinoma. Am J Obstet Gynecol 119:698, 1974

424. Weigensberg IJ: Preoperative radiation therapy in endometrial carcinoma: Preliminary report of a clinical trial. Am J Roentgenol Radium Ther Nucl Med 127:391, 1976

425. Greenberg SB, Glassburn JR, Antoniades J, et al: Management of carcinoma of the uterus stage II. Cancer Clin Trials 4:183, 1981

426. Gagnon JD, Moss WT, Gabourel LS, et al: External irradiation in the management of stage II endometrial carcinoma. A logical approach. Cancer 44:1247, 1979

427. Onsrud M, Aalders J, Abeler V, et al: Endometrial carcinoma with cervical involvement (stage II): Prognostic factors and value of combined radiological-surgical treatment. Gynecol Oncol 13:76, 1982

428. Spanos WJ, Fletcher GH, Wharton JT, et al: Patterns of pelvic recurrence in endometrial carcinoma. Gynecol Oncol 6:495, 1978

429. Landgren RC, Fletcher GH, Delclos L, et al: Irradiation of endometrial cancer in patients with medical contraindication to surgery or with unresectable lesions. Am J Roentgenol Radium Ther Nucl Med 126:148, 1976

430. Antoniades J, Brady LW, Lewis GC: The management of stage III carcinoma of the endometrium. Cancer 38:1838, 1967

431. Rutledge F, Ehrlich C: Adenocarcinoma of the endometrium. In Gray LA Sr (ed): Endometrial Carcinoma and Its Treatment: The Role of Irradiation, Extent of Surgery, and Approach to Chemotherapy, pp 128–137. Springfield, IL, Charles C Thomas, 1977

432. Kottmeier HL: Endometrial carcinoma and its treatment: Recent experience of the Radiumhemmet, Stockholm. In Gray LA Sr (ed): Endometrium Carcinoma and Its Treatment: The Role of Irradiation, Extent of Surgery and Approach to Chemotherapy, pp 118–126. Springfield, IL, Charles C Thomas, 1977

433. Homesley HD, Lewis JL Jr: Treatment of endometrial adenocarcinoma at Memorial Hospital, New York, 1884–1976. In Gray LA Sr (ed): Endometrial Carcinoma and Its Treatment: The Role of Irradiation, Extent of Surgery and Approach to Chemotherapy, pp 99–17. Springfield, IL, Charles C Thomas, 1977

434. Boronow RC: Endometrial cancers: Staging, pretreatment evaluation and factors in outcome. In Gray LA Sr (ed): Endometrial Carcinoma and Its Treatment: The Role of Irradiation, Extent of Surgery and Approach to Chemotherapy, pp 38–57. Springfield, IL, Charles C Thomas, 1977

435. Geisler HE, Gibbs CP: Invasive carcinoma of the endometrium. A 5 to 16 year followup of 183 patients. Am J Obstet Gynecol 102:516, 1968

436. Danoff BF, McDay J, Louka M, et al: Stage III endometrial carcinoma: Analysis of patterns of failure and therapeutic implications. Int J Radiat Oncol Biol Phys 6:1491, 1980

437. Barber HRK, Brunschwig A: Treatment and results of recurrent cancer of the corpus uteri in patients receiving anterior and posterior pelvic exenteration (1947–1963). Cancer 22:949, 1968

438. Stander RW: Vaginal metastases following treatment of endometrial carcinoma. Am J Obstet Gynecol 71:776, 1956

439. Stokes S, Bedwinek J, Breaux S, et al: Treatment of stage I adenocarcinoma of the endometrium by hysterectomy and adjuvant irradiation: Analysis of complications. Obstet Gynecol 65:86, 1985

440. Kneale BLG: Adjunctive and therapeutic progestins in endometrial cancer. Clin Obstet Gynecol 13:789, 1986

441. Ehrlich CE, Young PCM, Cleary RE: Cytoplasmic progesterone and estradiol receptors in normal, hyperplastic and carcinomatous endometria: Therapeutic implications. Am J Obstet Gynecol 141:539, 1981

442. Podratz KC, O'Brien PC, Malkasian GD Jr: Effects of progestational agents in treatment of endometrial carcinoma. Obstet Gynecol 66:106, 1985

443. Quinn MA, Cauchi M, Fortuna D: Endometrial carcinoma: Steroid receptors and response to medroxyprogesterone acetate. Gynecol Oncol 21:314, 1985

444. Swenerton KD: Treatment of advanced endometrial adenocarcinoma with tamoxifen. Cancer Treat Rep 64:805, 1980

445. Bonte J: Recente aanwinsten in de behandeling van endometriaal adenocarcinoma. Tijdschm. Voor Geneeskind 37:1377, 1981

446. Rendina GM, Donadio C, Saccucci P, et al: La nostra esperienza sulla terapia endocriva del carcinoma endometriale in fase avanzata (studio comparativo SW 269 casi). G Ital Oncol 3:153, 1983

447. Rendina GM, Donadio C, Fabri M, et al: Tamoxifen and medroxyprogesterone therapy for advanced endometrial carcinoma. Eur J Obstet Gynecol Reprod Biol 17:285, 1984

448. Slavik M, Petty WM, Blessing JA, et al: Phase II clinical study of tamoxifen in advanced endometrial adenocarcinoma. A Gynecology Oncology Group Study. Cancer Treat Rep 68:809, 1984

449. Hald I, Salimschick M, Mouridsen HT: Tamoxifen treatment of advanced endometrial carcinoma a phase II study. Eur J Gynecol Oncol 4:83, 1983

450. Carlson JA, Allegra JC, Day TG, et al: Tamoxifen and endometrial carcinoma: Alterations in estrogen and progesterone receptors in untreated patients and combination hormonal therapy in advanced neoplasia. Am J Obstet Gynecol 149:149, 1984

451. Lewis GC Jr, Slack NH, Mortel R, et al: Adjuvant progestogen therapy in the primary definitive treatment of endometrial cancer. Gynecol Oncol 2:368, 1974

452. Malkasian GD Jr, Decker DG: Adjuvant progesterone therapy for stage I carcinoma. Int J Gynecol Obstet 16:48, 1978

453. Beck RP: Experience in treating two hundred and eighty-eight patients with endometrial carcinoma from 1968 to 1972. Am J Obstet Gynecol 133:260, 1979

454. Gusberg SB: Current concepts in cancer: The changing nature of endometrial cancer. N Engl J Med 302:729, 1980

455. Kucera VH, Gerstner G, Michalica W, et al: Hormonprophylaxe bel der strahlenbehandlung des korpuskarzinomas mit hochdosierten gestagenen. Wien Med Wochenschr 129:395, 1979

456. Fournier D, Kubli F, Bauer M, et al: Hochdosierte gestagenlaznzeittherapie biem korpuskarizon, einflub aut uberlebenzeit. Geburtsh Frauenheilk 41:266, 1981

457. Bochman YV, Chepik OF, Volkova AT, et al: Can primary endometrial carcinoma stage I be cured without surgery and radiation therapy? Vopr Onkol 28:42, 1982

458. De Palo G, Spatti GB, Luciani L: Pilot study with adjuvant hormone therapy in FIGO Stage I endometrial carcinoma with myometrial invasion. Tumori 69:65, 1983

459. Lagasse L, Thigpen T, Morrison F: Phase II trial of piperazinedione in treatment of advanced endometrial carcinoma, uterine sarcoma, and vulvar carcinoma. Proc Am Assoc Cancer Res 20:388, 1970

460. Thigpen T, Blessing J, DiSaia P, et al: Phase II trial of cisplatinum in the management of advanced or recurrent endometrial carcinoma. Proc Am Soc Clin Oncol 22:469, 1981

461. Seski JC, Edwards CL, Herson J, et al: Cisplatin chemotherapy for disseminated endometrial cancer. Obstet Gynecol 59:225, 1982

462. Seski JC, Edwards CL, Copeland LG, et al: Hexamethylmelamine chemotherapy for disseminated endometrial cancer. Obstet Gynecol 58:361, 1981

463. Depe G, Malviya VK, Zbella E: Non-hormonal chemotherapy in endometrial cancer—a review. Wien Klin Wochenschr 96:747, 1984

464. Cohen CJ: Cytotoxic chemotherapy for patients with endometrial carcinoma. Clin Obstet Gynecol 13:811, 1986

465. Thigpen JT, Buschbaum HJ, Mangan C, et al: Phase II trial of adriamycin in the treatment of advanced or recurrent endometrial carcinoma. A Gynecologic Oncology Group Study. Cancer Treat Rep 63:21, 1979

466. Pasmantier MW, Coleman M, Silver RT, et al: Treatment of advanced endometrial carcinoma with doxorubicin and cisplatin: Effects on both untreated and previously treated patients. Cancer Treat Rep 69:539, 1985

467. Seltzer V, Vogl SE, Kaplan BH: Adriamycin and cisdiaminedichloroplatinum in the treatment of endometrial adenocarcinoma. Gynecol Oncol 19:308, 1984

468. Chauvergne J, Granger C, Mage PH, et al: Chimiotherapie palliative des cancers de l'endometre. Rev Fr Gynecol Obstet 81:547, 1986

469. Turbow MM, Thornton J, Ballon S, et al: Chemotherapy of advanced endometrial carcinoma with platinum, adriamycin, and cyclophosphamide. Proc Am Soc Clin Oncol 1:108, 1982

470. Hancock KC, Freedman RS, Edwards CL, et al: Use of cisplatin, doxorubicin, and cyclophosphamide to treat advanced and recurrent adenocarcinoma of the endometrium. Cancer Treat Rep 70:789, 1986

471. Bruckner HW, Deppe G: Combination chemotherapy of advanced endometrial adenocarcinoma with adriamycin, cyclophosphamide, 5-fluorouracil and medroxyprogesterone acetate. Obstet Gynecol 50:415, 1977

472. Cohen CJ, Deppe G, Bruckner HW: Treatment of advanced adenocarcinoma of the endometrium with melphalan, 5-fluorouracil and medroxyprogesterone acetate. A preliminary study. Obstet Gynecol 50:415, 1977

473. Lovecchio JL, Averette HE, Lichtinger M, et al: Treatment of advanced or recurrent endometrial adenocarcinoma with cyclophosphamide, doxorubicin, cis-platinum and megestrol-acetate. Obstet Gynecol 63:557, 1984

474. Piver MS, Lele SB, Patsner B, et al: Melphalan, 5-fluorouracil, and medroxyprogesterone acetate in metastatic endometrial carcinoma. Obstet Gynecol 67:261, 1986

475. Horton J, Elson P, Jordan P, et al: Combination chemotherapy for advanced endometrial cancer: An evaluation of three regimens. Cancer 49:2441, 1982

476. Lewis JL Jr, Berchuck A, Rubin SC, et al: Uterine Sarcomas in Shu MH, Brennan M (eds): Surgical Management of Soft Tissue Sarcoma. Philadelphia, Lea & Febiger (in press)

477. DiSaia PJ, Castro JR, Rutledge FN: Mixed mesodermal sarcoma of the uterus. Am J Roentgenol Rad Ther Nucl Med 117:632, 1973

478. Berchuck A, Rubin SC, Hoskins WJ, et al: Treatment of uterine leiomyosarcoma. Obstet Gynecol (in press)

479. Kempson RL, Bari W: Uterine sarcomas: Classification, diagnosis and prognosis. Hum Pathol 1:331, 1970

479a. Ober WB: Uterine sarcomas. Histogenesis and taxonomy. Ann NY Acad Sci 75:568, 1959

480. Norris HJ, Roth E, Taylor HB: Mesenchymal tumors of the uterus. II. A clinical and pathological study of 31 mixed mesodermal tumors. Obstet Gynecol 28:57, 1966

481. Salazar OM, Bonfiglio TA, Patten SF, et al: Uterine sarcomas. Natural history, treatment and prognosis. Cancer 42:1152, 1978

482. Major F, Silverberg S, Morrow P, et al: A preliminary analysis of prognostic factors in uterine sarcomas. A Gynecologic Oncology Group Study. Gynecol Oncol 26:411, 1987

483. Perez CA, Askin F, Baglan RJ, et al: Effect of irradiation on mixed mullerian tumors of the uterus. Cancer 43:1274, 1979

484. Edwards CL: Undifferentiated tumors. In Cancer of the Uterus and Ovary, pp 84–94. Chicago, Year Book, 1969

485. DiSaia PJ, Castro JR, Rutledge FN: Mixed mesodermal sarcoma of the uterus. Am J Roentgenol Radium Ther Nucl Med 117:632, 1973

486. Vongtama V, Karlen JR, Piver SM, et al: Treatment, results and prognostic factors in stage I and II sarcomas of the corpus uteri. Am J Roentgenol 126:139, 1976

487. Belgrad R, Elbadaw N, Rubin P: Uterine sarcoma. Radiology 114:181, 1975

488. Salazar OM, Bonfiglio TA, Patten SF, et al: Uterine sarcomas. Analysis of failures with special emphasis on the use of adjuvant radiation therapy. Cancer 42:1161, 1978

489. Omura GA, Major FJ, Blessing JA, et al: A randomized study of Adriamycin with and without Dimethyltriazenomidazole Carboxamide in advanced uterine sarcomas. Cancer 52:626, 1983

490. Omura GA, Blessing JA, Lifshitz S, et al: A randomized trial of adjacent Adriamycin in uterine sarcomas: A Gynecologic Oncology Group study. J Clin Oncol 3:1240, 1985

491. Piver MS, Lurain JR: Uterine sarcomas: Clinical features and management. In Coppleson M (ed): Gynecologic Oncology: Fundamental Principles and Clinical Practice, pp 608–618. New York, Churchill Livingstone, 1981

492. Taylor HB, Norris HJ: Mesenchymal tumors of the uterus. IV. Diagnosis and Prognosis of leiomyosarcomas. Arch Pathol 82:40, 1966

493. Silverberg SC: Leiomyosarcoma of the uterus: A clinicopathologic study. Obstet Gynecol 38:613, 1971

494. Bartsich EG, Bowe ET, Moore JG: Leiomyosarcoma of the uterus: A 50 year review of 42 cases. Obstet Gynecol 32:101, 1968

495. Christopherson WM, Williamson EO, Gray LA: Leiomyosarcoma of the uterus. Cancer 29:1512, 1972

496. Giarratano RC, Slate TA: Sarcoma of the uterus. Obstet Gynecol 38:472, 1971

497. Newlands ES: New chemotherapeutic agents in the management of gestational trophoblastic disease. Semin Oncol 9:239, 1982

497a. Hart WR, Yoonessi M: Endometrial stromatosis of the uterus. Obstet Gynecol 49:393, 1977

498. Wong LC, Choo YC, Ma HK: Etoposide, methotrexate, and bleomycin in drug-resistant gestational trophoblastic disease. Gynecol Oncol 24:51, 1986

498a. Norris HJ, Taylor HB: Mesenchymal tumors of the uterus. I. A clinical and pathologic study of 53 endometrial stromal tumors. Cancer 19:755, 1966

499. Koss LG, Spiro RH, Brunschwig A: Endometrial stromal sarcoma. Surg Gynecol Obstet 121:531, 1965

500. Baggish MS, Woodruff JD: Uterine stromatosis: Clinicopathologic features and hormone dependency. Obstet Gynecol 40:487, 1972

501. Sedlis A: Primary carcinoma of the fallopian tube. Obstet Gynecol 16:209, 1961

502. Roberts JA, Lifshitz S: Primary adenocarcinoma of the fallopian tube. Gynecol Oncol 13:301, 1982

503. Hu CY, Taymor ML, Hertig AT: Primary carcinoma of the fallopian tube. Am J Obstet Gynecol 59:58, 1950

504. Green TH, Scully RE: Tumors of the fallopian tube. Clin Obstet Gynecol 5:886, 1962

505. Woodruff JD, Julian CG: Multiple malignancy in the upper genital canal. Am J Obstet Gynecol 103:810, 1969

506. Benedet JL, White GW: Malignant tumors of fallopian tube. In Coppleson M (ed): Gynecologic Oncology: Fundamental Principles and Clinical Practice, pp 621–629. New York, Churchill Livingstone, 1981

507. Woodruff JD, Pauerstein CJ: The Fallopian Tube. Baltimore, Williams & Wilkins, 1969

508. Wheeler JE, Mastroianni L Jr: Pathology of the fallopian tube. In Blaustein A (ed): Pathology of the Female Genital Tract, pp 359–362. New York, Springer-Verlag, 1977

509. Hanton EM, Malkasian GD Jr, Dahlin DC, et al: Primary carcinoma of the fallopian tube. Am J Obstet Gynecol 94:832, 1966

510. Scheffey LC, Lang WR, Nugent FB: Clinical and pathologic aspects of primary sarcoma of the uterine tube. Am J Obstet Gynecol 52:904, 1941

511. Wu JP, Tanner WS, Fardal PM: Malignant mixed Mullerian tumor of the uterine tube. Obstet Gynecol 41:707, 1973

512. Hertig AT, Gore H: Tumors of the female sex organs: Part 3. Tumors of the ovary and fallopian tube. In Atlas of Tumor Pathology Series 1, fasc 33. Washington, DC, Armed Forces Institute of Pathology, 1961

513. Patton GWJ, Goldstein DP: Gestational choriocarcinoma of the tube and ovary. Surg Gynecol Obstet 137:608, 1973

514. Weiss PD, MacDougall MK, Regan JW, et al: Primary adenosquamous carcinoma of the fallopian tube. Obstet Gynecol 55:885, 1980

515. Plentl AA, Friedman EA: Lymphatic system of the female genitalia: The morphologic basis of oncologic diagnosis and therapy, pp 153–157. Philadelphia, WB Saunders, 1971

516. Novak ER, Woodruff JD: Novak's Gynecologic and Obstetric Pathology. Philadelphia, WB Saunders, 1971

517. Frick MC: Cancer of the fallopian tube. In Gusberg SG, Frick MC (eds): Corscaden's Gynecological Cancer. Baltimore, Williams & Wilkins, 1978

518. Dodson MG, Ford JH Jr, Averette HE: Clinical aspects of fallopian tube carcinoma. Obstet Gynecol 36:935, 1970

519. Shiller HM, Silverberg SG: Staging and prognosis in primary carcinoma of the fallopian tube. Cancer 28:389, 1971

520. Erez S, Kaplan AL, Wall JA: Clinical staging of the uterine tube. Obstet Gynecol 30:547, 1967

521. McMurray EH, Jacob AJ, Perez CA, et al: Carcinoma of the fallopian tube: Management and sites of failure. Cancer 58:2070, 1986

522. Boutselis JG, Thompson JN: Clinical aspects of primary carcinoma of the fallopian tube. Am J Obstet Gynecol 111:98, 1971

523. Raju KS, Barker GH, Wiltshaw E: Primary carcinoma of the fallopian tube: Report of 22 cases. Br J Obstet Gynaecol 88:1124, 1981

524. Pauerstein CJ: The Fallopian Tube: A Reappraisal. Philadelphia, Lea & Febiger, 1974

525. Engstrom L: Primary carcinoma of the fallopian tube. Acta Obstet Gynecol Scand 36:289, 1957

526. Greene TH Jr, Scully RE: Tumors of the fallopian tube. Clin Obstet Gynecol 5:886, 1962

527. Phelps MH, Chapman EK: Role of radiotherapy in treatment of primary carcinoma of the uterine tube. Obstet Gynecol 43:669, 1974

528. Amendola BE, LaRouere J, Amendola MA, et al: Adenocarcinoma of the fallopian tube. Surg Gynecol Obstet 158:223, 1983

529. Henderson SR, Harper RC, Salazar OM, et al: Primary carcinoma of the fallopian tube. Difficulties of diagnosis and treatment. Gynecol Oncol 5:168, 1977

530. Guthrie D, Cohen S: Carcinoma of the fallopian tube treated with a combination of surgery and cytotoxic chemotherapy. Br J Obstet Gynaecol 88:1051, 1981

531. Griffiths CT: Ovary and the fallopian tube. In Holland JF, Frei E III (eds): Cancer Medicine, p 1718. Philadelphia, Lea & Febiger, 1972

532. Jacobs AJ, McMurray EH, Parham J, et al: Treatment of carcinoma of the fallopian tube using cisplatin, doxorubicin, and cyclophosphamide. Am J Clin Oncol 9:436, 1986

533. U.S. Public Health Service, National Vital Statistics Division Vital Statistics of the United States, Annual 1930–1983, Washington, U.S. Government Printing Office, 1934–1985

534. Acosta-Sison H: Statistical study of chorionephithelioma in the Phillipine General Hospital. Am J Obstet Gynecol 58:125, 1949

535. Teoh ES, Dawood MY, Ratnam SS: Epidemiology of hydatidiform mole in Singapore. Am J Obstet Gynecol 110:53, 1947

536. Hertig AT, Sheldon WH: Hydatidiform mole—A pathologicoclinical correlation of 200 cases. Am J Obstet Gynecol 53:1, 1947

537. Deligdisch L, Driscoll SG, Goldstein DP: Gestational trophoblastic neoplasms: Morphologic correlates of therapeutic response. Am J Obstet Gynecol 130:801, 1978
538. Goldstein DP: Endocrine assay in chorionic tumors. Clin Obstet Gynecol 18:41, 1978
539. Vaitukaitis JL, Braunstein GD, Ross GT: A radioimmunoassay which specifically measures human chorionic gonadotropin in the presence of human luteinizing hormone. Am J Obstet Gynecol 38:453, 1976
540. Goldstein DP: Chorionic gonadotropin. Cancer 38:453, 1976
541. Woo JSK, Ngan HYS, Ma HK: Non-resolution of pelvic sonographic abnormality after chemotherapy for persistent trophoblastic disease — A word of caution. Eur J Obstet Gynecol Reprod Biol 22:153, 1983
542. Goldstein DP, Berkowitz RS: The management of gestational trophoblastic neoplasms. Curr Prob Obstet Gynecol 4:1, 1980
543. Bagshawe DK: Risk and prognostic factors in trophoblastic neoplasia. Cancer 38:1373, 1976
544. Dijkema HE, Aalders JG, DeBruijn HWA, et al: Risk factors in gestational trophoblastic disease, and consequences for primary treatment. Eur J Obstet Gynecol Reprod Biol 22:145, 1986
545. Goldstein DP, Berkowitz RS, Cohen SM: The current management of molar pregnancy. Curr Prob Obstet Gynecol 3:1, 1978
546. Li MC, Hertz R, Spence DB: Effect of methotrexate therapy upon choriocarcinoma and chorioadenoma. Proc Soc Exp Biol Med 93:361, 1956
547. Hertz R, Lewis JL Jr, Lipsett MB: Five years experience with the chemotherapy of metastatic choriocarcinoma and related trophoblastic disease. Gynecol Oncol 23:111, 1976
548. Berkowitz RS, Goldstein DP, Bernstein MR: Ten years experience with methotrexate and folinic acid as primary therapy for gestational trophoblastic disease. Gynecol Oncol 23:111, 1986
549. Berkowitz RS, Goldstein DP: Methotrexate with citrovorum factor rescue for non-metastatic gestational neoplasms. Obstet Gynecol 54:725, 1979
550. Surwit EA, Hammond CB: Treatment of metastatic trophoblastic disease with poor prognosis. Obstet Gynecol 53:207, 1979
551. Bagshawe KD: Treatment of trophoblastic tumors. Ann Acad Med 5:273, 1976
552. Weed JC, Barnard DE, Currie JL, et al: Chemotherapy with the modified Bagshawe protocol for poor prognosis metastatic trophoblastic disease. Obstet Gynecol 59:377, 1982
553. Berkowitz RS, Goldstein D, Bernstein M: Modified triple chemotherapy in the management of high risk metastatic gestational trophoblastic tumors. Gynecol Oncol 19:173, 1984
554. Hansen LA, Clayton BD: Treatment of gestational trophoblastic tumors. Drug Intell Clin Pharm 18:569, 1984
555. Ballon SC, Berman ML, Lagasse LD, et al: The unique aspects of gestational trophoblastic disease. Obstet Gynecol Surv 32:405, 1977
556. Bagshawe KD: Treatment of trophoblastic tumors. Ann Acad Med 5:273, 1976
557. Surwit EA, Suciu TN, Schmidt HJ, et al: A new combination chemotherapy for resistant trophoblastic disease. Gynecol Oncol 8:110, 1979
558. Newlands ES, Bagshawe KD: Activity of high dose cis-platinum (NCI 119875) in combination with vincristine and methotrexate in drug resistant gestational choriocarcinoma. A report of 17 cases. Br J Cancer 40:943, 1979
559. Newlands ES, Bagshawe KD: The role of BP16-213 (Etoposide) in gestational choriocarcinoma. Cancer Chemother Pharmacol 7:211, 1982
560. Amiel JL, Droz JP, Tursz T: Placental tumors resistant to usual chemotherapy: Treatment using cis-diaminedichloroplatinum. Two cases. Nouv Presse Med 7:1933, 1978
561. Gordan AN, Lavanagh JJ, Gershenson DM, et al: Cisplatin, vinblastine, and bleomycin combination therapy in resistant gestational trophoblastic disease. Cancer 58:1407, 1986
562. Ross GT: Congenital anomalies among children born to mothers receiving chemotherapy for gestational trophoblastic neoplasms. Cancer 37:1043, 1976
563. Kuten A, Cohen Y, Thatcher M, et al: Pregnancy and delivery after successful treatment of epidural metastatic choriocarcinoma. Gynecol Oncol 6:464, 1978
564. Smith PG, Doll R: Late effects of X irradiation in patients treated for metropathia haemorrhagica. Br J Radiol 49:224, 1976
565. Hutchinson GB: Leukemia in patients with cancer of the cervix uteri treated with radiation. A report covering the first five years of an international study. J Natl Cancer Inst 40:9591, 1968
566. Dickson RJ: The late results of radium treatment for benign uterine haemorrhage. Br J Radiol 42:582, 1969
567. Wagoner JK: Leukemia and other malignancies following radiation therapy for gynecological disorders. Boice, Fraumeni (eds): Radiation Carcinogenesis: Epidemiology and Biological Significance, pp 153–159. New York, Raven Press, 1984
568. Arneson AN, Schellhas HF: Multiple primary cancers in patients treated for carcinoma of the cervix. Am J Obstet Gynecol 106:1155, 1970
569. Spratt JS, Hoag MG: Incidence of multiple primary cancers per man years of follow-up: Twenty-year review from Ellis Fischel State Cancer Hospital. Ann Surg 164:775, 1966
570. Lee JY, Perez CA, Ettinger N, et al: The risk of second primaries subsequent to irradiation for cervix cancer. Int J Radiat Oncol Biol Phys 8:207, 1982
571. Wagoner JK: Presented at the 1969 meeting of the American Public Health Association
572. Feinleib M: Breast cancer and artificial menopause: A cohort study. J Natl Cancer Inst 41:315, 1968
573. Villasanta U, Rubel H: Radium treatment of benign uterine bleeding. Long-term follow-up. Obstet Gynecol 33:813, 1969
574. Thomas WO Jr, Harris HH, Enden JA: Postirradiation malignant neoplasms of the uterine fundus. Am J Obstet Gynecol 104:209, 1969

ROBERT C. YOUNG

ZVI FUKS

WILLIAM J. HOSKINS

CHAPTER 37 *Cancer of the Ovary*

Ovarian cancer is the fourth most frequent cause of cancer death in women and the leading cause of gynecologic cancer death in the United States. More women die of ovarian cancer yearly than from cervical and endometrial carcinoma combined. Incidence and mortality estimates for 1986 indicate that 19,000 new cases are diagnosed yearly and 11,600 women die.[1] A steady increase in the age-adjusted ovarian cancer death rates has been observed over the past 25 years, with similar increases in other industrialized nations as well.[2] Approximately 1 woman in 70 will develop the disease, and about 1% of all female deaths are due to ovarian cancer.

EPIDEMIOLOGY

The highest ovarian cancer rates are reported from highly industrialized countries, with age-adjusted mortality rates that range from 3.02:100,000 in Italy to 7.04:100,000 in the United States and 11.02:100,000 in Denmark. The notable exception is Japan, where rates of death from ovarian cancer are 1.69:100,000, among the lowest in the world. Studies of migrant populations suggest significant environmental influences. Japanese migrants to Hawaii and their first-generation offspring in the United States have an incidence significantly higher than women in Japan but lower that that in the indigenous white population of the United States.[3,4]

In the United States, the common epithelial ovarian neoplasms are most frequent in adult white populations. They are rarely seen before menarche but tend to increase significantly thereafter, with peak incidence in the 40- to 70-year-old group. In contrast, germ-cell ovarian tumors are seen primarily in children and young women and are more frequent in nonwhite populations.

Several epidemiologic studies suggest that disordered endocrine function may contribute to the development of ovarian cancer. For example, a higher incidence of epithelial tumors is seen in women with lower mean number of pregnancies, in those never pregnant, and in those with a history of infertility.[5-7] No clear-cut association between ovarian cancer and the administration of synthetic estrogens has been established,[8] but oral contraceptives appear to reduce the risk.[9] Also, cancer of the ovary and cancer of the breast appear to share some etiologic factors. For example, women with breast cancer have twice the expected risk of ovarian carcinoma, and women with ovarian cancer have a threefold to fourfold increase in the frequency of subsequent breast cancer.

No association with viral infections has been identified. Paradoxically, a lower-than-expected frequency of mumps and other viral exanthems is reported for women with ovarian cancer.[10]

Familial and genetic associations have been reported but are rare. Ovarian cancer has been reported in multiple members of the same or succeeding generations.[11] Several unusual genetic disorders seem to predispose to ovarian neoplasms, although the tumors are usually benign and stromal in origin. Females with Peutz–Jeghers syndrome (mucocutaneous pigmentation and intestinal polyps) have a 5% to 14% chance of developing ovarian tumors, and women with inherited basal-cell nevus syndrome develop benign fibromas or, rarely, other tumors. Patients with gonadal dysgenesis (46XY genotype or mosaic) are prone to gonadoblastomas, but, interestingly, patients with Turner's syndrome (45X0) and undeveloped gonads have no such tendency. An

1162

increased frequency of ovarian thecomas has been described in patients on long-term anticonvulsant therapy and is believed to be related to variations in the ability to metabolize these drugs.[12]

Although epidemiologic evidence strongly suggests environmental causes, few, if any, associations have been firmly established. There is no good evidence that either diagnostic or therapeutic irradiation increases the frequency of this malignancy. Likewise, there is no established association with known chemical carcinogens. Ovarian cancer has not been seen among women with industrial exposure to dyes, tars, or anthracene-containing compounds.[13] However, exposure to asbestos or talc is associated with an increased risk of ovarian carcinoma in humans. Studies indicate a higher-than-expected frequency of ovarian and peritoneal neoplasms in asbestos workers. Passage of such materials through the bowel wall or retrograde through the female reproductive tract has been described and could explain how such agents arrive at the ovarian epithelium.[14,15]

PATHOGENESIS AND BEHAVIOR

Epithelial carcinomas account for 80% to 90% of ovarian malignancies; the remaining ovarian tumors arise from the germ or stromal cells. Epithelial tumors arise from the serosal mesothelial layer of the gonads. In the embryo, the ovary develops from the genital ridge of thickened coelomic epithelium. The germ cells originate in the primitive streak and migrate to the gonad, where they proliferate to form the bulk of the cortex. The mesenchyma of the medulla gives rise to the ovarian stroma. All three of these cell types (coelomic epithelial cells, germ cells, and stromal cells) can give rise to malignant neoplasms.[16] Because the coelomic epithelium has the multipotential capability to differentiate into endometroid, mucinous, or serous epithelium, the common epithelial tumors of the ovary have these characteristic cell types.[17]

Epithelial tumors disseminate primarily by surface shedding, lymphatic spread, or, rarely, metastasizing hematogenously. Most of the errors committed by surgeons in the operative management of this disease can be directly related to a lack of understanding of the patterns of spread. Figure 37–1 illustrates the typical spread of the disease. Commonly, these tumors spread by continuity and intraperitoneal dissemination.[18] Spread to the opposite ovary occurs in 6% to 13% of patients with otherwise Stage IA disease,[19,20] and transperitoneal tumor implantation or lymphatic spread to the uterus and fallopian tubes occurs in approximately 5% of patients otherwise thought to be Stage IA (see below for discussion of staging system).[19] However, with more advanced stages of disease, the uterus is involved in 25%,[18] sometimes with demonstrable retrograde lymphatic tumor emboli. Direct spread may also involve the peritoneal surfaces of the bladder, the rectosigmoid, or the pelvic peritoneum.

The most common type of extraovarian spread is transperitoneal dissemination of cells shed from gross or microscopic excrescences on the surface of the primary tumor. The presence of malignant cells in the peritoneal cavity in

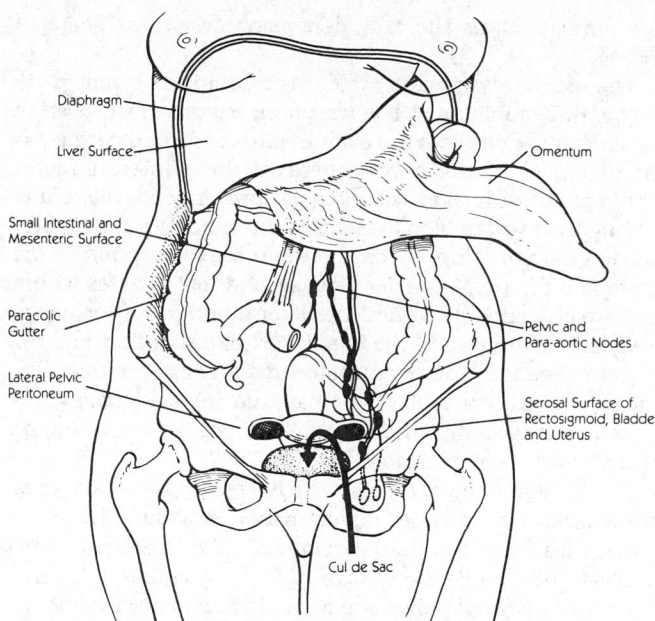

FIG. 37-1. Spread of disease in ovarian cancer.

spite of an apparently intact capsule indicates that some cancers exfoliate cells even before there is disruption of the capsule.[21] The exfoliated clonogenic cells attach to the peritoneal surfaces and form micrometastases, which continue to exfoliate clonogenic cells. These free-floating cells are removed from the peritoneal cavity through lymphatic channels located in the diaphragm.[22,23] Clearance does not take place evenly over the whole diaphragmatic surface, being more extensive on the right side overlying the liver[24] because respiratory movements create a flow of peritoneal fluid along the abdominal gutters that ultimately flows predominantly to the right hemidiaphragm.[25] Drainage then occurs into the submesothelial lymphatic capillaries of the diaphragm, which intercommunicate with the pleural surface and subsequently with the anterior mediastinal lymph nodes.[22,26,27] This pathway quantitatively accounts for 80% of the peritoneal clearance. Peritoneoscopic studies have shown that a significant fraction of patients otherwise thought to have Stage I or Stage II disease have involvement of the undersurface of the diaphragm,[28-30] and this fact accounts for the failure to cure some patients with "Stage I–II" disease. Partial or complete obstruction of the diaphragmatic lymphatics by tumor cells allows implantation on the omentum and at various other sites on the serosal surface of the peritoneum. It also causes accumulation of carcinomatous ascites.[31] The force of gravity in the upright patient leads to early implantation in the cul-de-sac and along the surface of the rectum.

Autopsy studies have demonstrated virtual 100% involvement of the omenta of patients dying of ovarian carcinoma. Occult omental metastases have been found in 3% to 11% of untreated patients who were thought to have Stage I or II disease at initial surgical exploration.[30,32] Steinberg and associates[33] reported that 22% of 55 grossly negative omenta had histologically proven tumor. In one-half of these patients, the omentum was the only demonstrable site of Stage III disease.

The ovarian lymphatic system is also an important pathway of dissemination.[34] The lymphatic vessels of the ovarian parenchyma drain into the ovarian hilus to form the subovarian plexus. From this plexus, there are three different routes of lymphatic drainage. The main pathway ascends bilaterally among the ovarian blood vessels and terminates in the para-aortic group of lymph nodes between the bifurcation of the aorta and the renal arteries. The second route passes within the broad ligaments toward the lateral and posterior pelvic wall and terminates in the uppermost external iliac and hypogastric nodes. The third route runs along the round ligaments and into the external iliac and inguinal nodes, accounting for the uncommon instances of ovarian carcinoma spread to the inguinal nodes.

Use of lymphangiography in early and advanced stages of the disease demonstrates dissemination in about 15% of patients with Stage I ovarian carcinoma, 17% in Stage II, 31% in Stage III, and 64% in Stage IV.[35-37] At autopsy, the frequency of involved pelvic and aortic lymph nodes is approximately equal, with 80% of patients showing metastases.[38] Burghardt and associates[39] performed complete pelvic and para-aortic lymphadenectomies in 48 patients with untreated ovarian cancer and found that 14% had positive lymph nodes in Stages I and II and 63% in Stages III and IV. Pelvic nodes were involved more frequently than para-aortic nodes, which were never involved unless pelvic nodes were involved. Preliminary data from a Gynecologic Oncology Group (GOG) surgical staging study indicate that in patients with disease in Stage I, Stage II, or optimal Stage III (defined in this study as less than 3 cm of abdominal disease prior to debulking), the incidence of positive pelvic lymph nodes is 11% and the incidence of positive para-aortic lymph nodes is 8%[40].

Although peritoneum, omentum, bowel surfaces, and retroperitoneal lymph nodes are the most frequent sites of spread, other organs are also at risk for metastasis. Among the distant organs that may be involved are (in order of decreasing frequency) liver, lung, pleura, kidney, bone, adrenal gland, bladder, and spleen.[18] Recent studies of recurrence after negative second-look laparotomy have found disease outside the abdominal cavity in as many as 50% of patients.[41,42]

PATHOLOGY

Several comprehensive reviews of the pathology of ovarian cancer have been published that provide detailed descriptions for each of the individual tumor types.[43-47] The World Health Organization (WHO) and the International Federation of Gynecology and Obstetrics (FIGO) have adopted a unified classification of the common epithelial tumors, the sex cord–stromal tumors, and the germ-cell tumors (Table 37–1). The vast majority (85%–90%) of malignant ovarian tumors seen in the United States are of the epithelial type, and their approximate overall frequency is as follows: serous cystadenocarcinoma, 42%; mucinous cystadenocarcinoma, 12%; endometrioid carcinoma, 15%; undifferentiated carci-

37-1. World Health Organization Classification of Malignant Ovarian Tumors

Common Epithelial Tumors
Malignant serous tumors
    Adenocarcinoma, papillary adenocarcinoma, papillary cystadenocarcinoma
    Surface papillary carcinoma
    Malignant adenofibroma, cystadenofibroma
Malignant mucinous tumors
    Adenocarcinoma, cystadenocarcinoma
    Malignant adenofibroma, cystadenofibroma
Malignant endometroid tumors
    Carcinoma
        Adenocarcinoma
        Adenoacanthoma
        Malignant adenofibroma, cystadenofibroma
    Endometroid stromal sarcomas
    Mesodermal (müllerian) mixed tumors: homologous and heterologous
Clear-cell (mesonephroid) tumors, malignant
    Carcinoma and adenocarcinoma
Brenner tumors, malignant
Mixed epithelial tumors, malignant
Undifferentiated carcinoma
Unclassified
Sex Cord–Stromal Tumors
Granulosa–stromal cell tumors
    Granulosa-cell tumor
    Tumors in the thecoma–fibroma group
    Fibroma
    Unclassified
Androblastomas: Sertoli–Leydig cell tumors
    Well-differentiated
        Tubular androblastoma, Sertoli cell tumor (tubular adenoma of Pick)
        Tubular androblastoma with lipid storage, Sertoli cell tumor with lipid storage (folliculome lipidique of Lecene)
        Sertoli–Leydig cell tumor (tubular adenoma with Leydig cells)
    Leydig cell tumor, hilus cell tumor
        Of intermediate differentiation
        Poorly differentiated (sarcomatoid)
        With heterologous elements
Gynandroblastoma
Unclassified
Lipid (Lipoid) Cell Tumors
Germ-Cell Tumors
    Dysgerminoma
    Endodermal sinus tumor
    Embryonal carcinoma
    Polyembryoma
    Choriocarcinoma
    Teratomas
        Immature
        Mature dermoid cyst with malignant transformation
        Monodermal and highly specialized
            Struma ovarii
            Carcinoid
            Struma ovarii and carcinoid
            Others
    Mixed forms
Gonadoblastoma
    Pure
    Mixed with dysgerminoma or other form of germ cell tumor

Modified from Serov SF, Scully RE, Solvin LH: International Histological Classification of Tumors, No. 9. Histological Typing of Ovarian Tumors. Geneva, World Health Organization, 1973.

noma, 17%; and clear-cell carcinoma, 6%. The remaining 8% of primary tumors are the sex cord–stromal and germ-cell tumors.

EPITHELIAL OVARIAN CARCINOMA

Tumors of Low Malignant Potential (Borderline Tumors)

Epithelial tumors are generally classified as benign, malignant (invasive), or carcinomas of low malignant potential (tumors of borderline malignancy). The latter group has neoplastic epithelial cells, cellular clusters detached from sites of origin, increased mitotic activity, and nuclear abnormalities. However, they lack obvious invasion of the supporting stroma. The incidence of these borderline epithelial tumors is variable but may approach 15% of all epithelial tumors.

These tumors clearly possess a different natural history; they grow and metastasize slowly. Five-year survival rates for patients with serous and mucinous low-malignant-potential epithelial tumors range from 74% to 98%.[48] In another study, the 5- and 10-year survival rates of patients with low-malignant-potential tumors were 93% and 91%, respectively, compared with 34% and 29% for patients with invasive epithelial carcinomas.[49] It is therefore important to identify patients with tumors of low malignant potential and to distinguish them from the patients with invasive ovarian carcinoma when planning treatment or analyzing results and survival.

The optimal treatment for borderline tumors is unclear. In early-stage (I and II) disease, surgical resection alone usually produces excellent results. However, in the more advanced stages, some investigators advocate therapeutic approaches similar to those used for more invasive tumors, for despite the fact that these tumors grow more slowly, approximately 10% to 15% of patients will die of their disease within the first 5 to 10 years.

Histology: Importance of Type and Grade

For the invasive epithelial carcinomas, an independent correlation of survival with histologic type has not been found consistently.[50-54] The current consensus is that there is limited prognostic significance to the histologic type of these cancers independent of clinical stage, extent of residual disease, and histologic grade.

In contrast to histologic type, the degree of cellular differentiation of epithelial cancers (histologic grade) is an important independent predictor of response to treatment and survival.[55-58] For example, studies from the Mayo Clinic of Stage II serous cystadenocarcinoma demonstrate an 80% survival for patients with Broder's Grade 1 tumors, 47% for Grade 2, and 10% for Grade 3 and 4 tumors.[56] Day and colleagues have made similar observations using the pattern system of grading.[57] In Stages I and II serous carcinoma of the ovary, patients with Grade 1 tumors had a 78% 7-year survival rate compared with 35% for Grade 2 and 0 for Grade 3. Although initial studies emphasized the effect of grade on prognosis in early-stage disease, subsequent studies suggest

it is important even in more advanced disease. Using grading systems based on cytologic detail (Broder's) or the pattern-grading classification based on the degree to which the tumor forms papillary structures or glands rather than solid sheets, several investigators have shown survival significance to grading systems for patients with advanced disease treated with chemotherapy.[58,59]

A study by Dembo and Bush suggests a more complex interaction of grade and histologic type.[60] In patients with serous tumors, the effect of grade was highly significant, whereas grade was not of prognostic significance in patients with mucinous, endometrioid, or clear-cell tumors. When the two variables of grade and histologic type were combined, it was possible to show significant survival differences between patients with "favorable" pathologies (serous well-differentiated and mucinous, endometrioid, and clear-cell types of all grades), in whom the 5-year survival rate was 59%, and patients with "unfavorable" pathologies (serous, moderately, and poorly differentiated and the unclassified type), in whom the 5-year survival rate was 19%.

Histologic grading of ovarian tumors has not been accepted enthusiastically by pathologists, primarily because no standardized and easily reproducible objective classification exists. Nevertheless, in spite of the different classifications used, virtually every published study thus far indicates an important survival impact of tumor grade, and grading is now a requirement in every carefully designed clinical study.

STROMAL AND GERM-CELL TUMORS

Stromal Tumors

Fewer than 10% of all ovarian tumors are of stromal origin. These include tumors containing granulosa, theca, Sertoli, Leydig, and collagen-producing stromal cells or their embryonic precursors.[47,61] Only the granulosa-cell tumor, of the many stromal tumors listed in Table 37–1, is seen with significant frequency. This tumor is composed of granulosa cells with or without an admixture of theca cells and may contain folliculoid structures known as Call–Exner bodies. These tumors can be associated with feminizing effects and precocious puberty secondary to tumor-related estrogen secretion. Presenting signs and symptoms are similar to those of epithelial ovarian tumors with the exception of those related to hyperestrogenism. These tumors tend to be discovered at earlier stages and to have a more indolent course than the epithelial tumors. Late recurrences sometimes can be treated effectively with repeated cytoreductive surgery. There is no convincing evidence that the tumor is particularly responsive to radiation therapy or chemotherapy, but responses to alkylating agents and Adriamycin (doxorubicin) have been described. Recently, 6 of 11 patients treated with a combination of cisplatin, vinblastine, and bleomycin (PVB) achieved pathologically documented complete remission (CR),[62] but follow-up is short and toxicity significant.

Sertoli–Leydig cell tumors are characterized by differentiation toward testicular structures. These contain various mixtures of Sertoli and Leydig cells and tissues similar to those of the fetal testis.

Gonadal stromal tumors occasionally contain granulosa-cell elements combined with tubules and Leydig cells characteristic of the arrhenoblastoma. Such tumors are called gynandroblastomas.

Germ-Cell Tumors

Although germ-cell tumors constitute less than 5% of all ovarian malignancies, they are important because they occur in young women, display a vastly different natural history than epithelial tumors, and require different treatment. Nearly all of these patients can be cured using combination chemotherapy and limited surgery. Irradiation is now used only for the dysgerminomas.

Of these tumors, dysgerminoma, endodermal sinus tumor, and embryonal carcinoma are most often encountered. The dysgerminomas comprise less than 2% of all ovarian malignancies, are cytologically similar to seminoma of the testis, and display a very similar natural history. These tumors are frequently (90%) unilateral and tend to be localized, with secondary spread by way of the lymphatics to the para-aortic nodes. The tumor is highly radiosensitive, and primary management is with surgery and radiation. Five-year survival rates with effective conventional therapy approach 80% to 90%.

The terms "endodermal sinus tumor" and "embryonal carcinoma" have, in the past, often been used interchangeably to describe highly malignant germ-cell tumors of the ovary. However, there is now convincing evidence that the two disorders are different.[61] Embryonal carcinoma, with patterns typical of embryonal carcinoma of the testis and associated with elevations of serum human chorionic gonadotropin (hCG) or alpha-fetoprotein (α-FP), is rarely seen in the ovary. Endodermal sinus tumors are more common and are similar morphologically to the infantile orchioblastoma. The endodermal sinus tumor, also called yolk sac tumor, is characterized by reticular patterns, papillary formations known as Schiller–Duval bodies, and both intracellular and extracellular hyaline droplets. This tumor is derived from extraembryonic rather than embryonic tissues. Both tumors are highly aggressive, metastasize hematogenously, and are poorly controlled even with radical surgery and irradiation. Chemotherapy is highly effective however and will be discussed in a later section.

DIAGNOSIS AND STAGING

There are no specific symptoms or signs of ovarian cancer, particularly in early stages, and as a result, when symptoms and signs appear, they are usually manifestations of advanced disease. Early on, ovarian cancer is often asymptomatic; symptoms of nausea, dyspepsia, and vague lower abdominal discomfort are frequently ignored by the patient or the doctor. Seventy-five percent of patients will have spread beyond the ovary at diagnosis, and 60% will have spread beyond the pelvis.[63,64] Sall and Stone[65] found that 37% of patients had abdominal discomfort or pain, 35% had abdominal swelling or masses, and 15% experienced vaginal bleeding. Gastrointestinal symptoms were present in 10% and urinary tract symptoms in 1.5% In two other large series, the presenting symptoms were pain (57%), abdominal distention (51%), and vaginal bleeding (25%).[66,67]

Because the ovary lies in the rather spacious pelvic cavity and is suspended loosely by the ovarian and infundibulopelvic ligaments, a mass may become quite large without producing symptoms of either pain or pressure. When pain does occur, it is probably caused by stretching of the supporting ligaments and may be both nonspecific and intermittent. Discomfort from compression of the bladder or rectum is also nonspecific. It is therefore essential that all women, particularly perimenopausal or postmenopausal women, with pelvic or abdominal symptoms have a thorough physical and pelvic examination with careful evaluation of the adnexal area. All too often, women are subjected to several weeks or months of expensive diagnostic radiographic studies when a pelvic examination in the office would have revealed the large pelvic mass that was finally discovered on computed tomography (CT) scan or magnetic resonance imaging (MRI). Of even more concern is the delay in diagnosis that results from trying various symptomatic therapies without having performed a pelvic examination.

Palpation of an adnexal mass in a premenarchal or postmenopausal female is one indication for exploratory laparotomy. Functional ovarian cysts should not occur in these age groups, and a palpable mass usually indicates neoplastic growth. The incidence of malignancy in such patients is difficult to determine, but the high mortality rate of ovarian cancer that has spread beyond the ovary mandates early surgical exploration. Barber and Graber[68] have pointed out that the normal ovary during the reproductive years is approximately $3.5 \times 2.0 \times 1.5$ cm but that in the postmenopausal patient it should be $2.0 \times 1.0 \times 0.5$ cm or less. As a result, palpation of an ovary in a postmenopausal woman indicates ovarian enlargement, and surgical exploration should be considered. However, Flynt and Gallup[69] performed exploratory laparotomy on 11 patients with a palpable postmenopausal ovary and found only one malignancy: a colon carcinoma. A larger series of patients is needed to clarify whether all such patients should undergo surgical exploration.

Ovarian enlargement in a woman during the reproductive years is more often benign. Most of these enlargements are attributable to either follicular or corpus luteum cysts (functional cysts), and the vast majority will regress in one to three menstrual cycles. Such patients should be followed by repeat pelvic examination at 4- to 6-week intervals. Some gynecologists recommend oral contraceptives to increase the speed of spontaneous resolution by preventing stimulation of the ovary by pituitary hormones. Table 37-2 outlines the suggested management of patients with an adnexal mass. Although still in the reproductive age group, patients who are over age 40 are at greater risk for ovarian cancer. Fortunately, retention of reproductive function is usually of less concern in these patients.

Conventional Papanicolaou smears offer little diagnostically because they are rarely positive and then only in advanced disease. However, any patient with adenocarcinoma cells on a Pap smear and a negative evaluation of the vulva, vagina, cervix, and endometrium should be considered to have carcinoma of the ovary, fallopian tubes, or other intra-

TABLE 37-2.   Management of the Patient with an
Adnexal Mass

Observe and Repeat Examination in 4–6 Weeks	Surgical Exploration
Reproductive age	Premenarchal
	Post-menopausal
Less than 8 cm	Greater than 8 cm
Decreasing size	Increase in size or persistence through 2–3 menstrual cycles
Cystic and smooth	Solid and irregular
Mobile	Fixed
Unilateral	Bilateral
Asymptomatic	Pain or other symptoms of acute intra-abdominal process
No ascites	Ascites

TABLE 37-3.   Evaluation of Patients with Suspected
Ovarian Carcinoma

Careful history and physical examination to include breast and
  pelvic examination and Papanicolaou smear
Complete blood count, biochemical profile, and CA-125 assay
Chest radiograph
Intravenous urogram
Cystoscopy
Proctoscopy
Barium enema
CT, MRI, or ultrasound*
Upper-gastrointestinal series with small-bowel follow-through in
  patients with upper gastrointestinal symptoms or symptoms of
  partial bowel obstruction

* As indicated by clinical evaluation.

abdominal organs. If a metastatic evaluation is negative, the patient should be considered for surgical exploration.

Some investigators have attempted mass screening of asymptomatic patients by peritoneal lavage with culdocentesis,[70-72] but poor patient acceptance and low positive yield make this an ineffective method of diagnosing ovarian cancer. Moreover, Rubin and associates[73] have recently shown that peritoneal washings were negative in more than 50% of patients with gross intraperitoneal disease at second-look surgical exploration.

Laparoscopy as a diagnostic tool for ovarian carcinoma should, in general, be discouraged. Although it may occasionally be useful in differentiating uterine leiomyomata or endometriosis from ovarian cancer, such cases are infrequent. Laparoscopic biopsy or needle aspiration of an unruptured ovarian mass should not be performed because malignant cells may be spilled into the peritoneal cavity.

Ultrasound is a safe, noninvasive procedure that may be used to define intra-abdominal disease. Solid elements and prominent papillary projections with involvement of adjacent viscera suggest a malignant neoplasm. Ultrasound can also be used to distinguish ascites from a large ovarian cyst. A mass separate from the uterus associated with internal echoes of normal sensitivity suggests ovarian cancer. Ultrasound can also be used to guide direct percutaneous needle aspiration of suspected metastasis or aspiration biopsies of aortic nodes.[74,75]

Lymphangiography is useful in the evaluation of patients with ovarian carcinoma[35-37,76] and detects nodal involvement in 30%. In those positive, 32% had disease in the pelvic nodes only, and in 46%, there was diffuse retroperitoneal involvement of both pelvic and para-aortic nodes.[19] Lymphangiography is accurate when the aortic lymph nodes are enlarged by tumor and the radiologist has sufficient expertise. In one study of 33 patients with positive preoperative lymphangiograms, histologic confirmation was obtained in 100%. In 63 patients with negative preoperative lymphangiograms, the lymphographic–histologic correlation was 87.3%. Eight of these 63 patients (12.7%) had microscopic nodal involvement at surgery. The overall accuracy of bipedal lymphangiography in this study thus was 91.7%.[37]

CT adds useful diagnostic and staging information to that obtained by ultrasound, lymphangiography, and surgery. CT may clearly delineate liver and pulmonary nodules, abdominal and pelvic masses, and retroperitoneal nodal involvement. However, it is costly and still cannot reliably detect masses smaller than 2 cm in diameter. The technique has been particularly useful in ovarian carcinoma when bowel ileus makes an ultrasonogram difficult to interpret.[77] CT has also been used to detect subcutaneous metastases in patients with ovarian cancer.[78]

Preoperative evaluation of a patient with suspected ovarian cancer is outlined in Table 37-3. The extent of such an evaluation requires that the physician use clinical judgment: a young woman with a persistent unilateral cystic mass may require only basic biochemical evaluation and an intravenous urogram, whereas a postmenopausal woman with a large, irregular mass should undergo a more extensive evaluation.

TUMOR MARKERS

Tumor markers that can detect early ovarian cancer would be valuable because most disease currently is diagnosed only when it is already advanced. Whereas markers have often been helpful in monitoring the rare germ-cell malignancies, they have not been very helpful thus far in detecting early epithelial ovarian malignancies.

The serial measurement of α-FP has facilitated the postsurgical evaluation of therapy for patients with endodermal sinus tumors.[79] After surgical resection, serum α-FP levels progressively decline and, with recurrence, become elevated prior to clinically palpable disease. Assays for α-FP are also helpful in diagnosing an endodermal sinus tumor in a woman with a rapidly enlarging, solid ovarian mass. Human chorionic gonadotropin or its beta subunit has been a valuable tumor marker in the postsurgical evaluation of patients with ovarian choriocarcinoma and embryonal carcinoma or in evaluating germ-cell tumors with choriocarcinomatous elements.[80]

Carcinoembryonic antigen (CEA) is elevated in approximately 58% of patients with Stage III epithelial ovarian cancer.[81] The frequency of elevated CEA levels increases progressively with advancing stage and bulk of tumor. However, because serum CEA levels have also been elevated in patients with cirrhosis, chronic pulmonary disease, inflammatory bowel disease, or a history of heavy cigarette smoking, CEA is of limited diagnostic use in ovarian cancer. Nevertheless, in patients who do have elevated CEA levels before therapy, serial measurements may be valuable in monitoring subclinical disease.

Numerous investigators have attempted to isolate tumor-specific antigens that could be used for both serologic diagnosis and monitoring of patients during therapy.[82-85] Of all of these, the monoclonal antibody OC-125 directed against the antigen CA-125 common to most nonmucinous epithelial ovarian tumors appears to be the most useful.[86] The OC-125 antibody recognizes multiple antigen determinants on a high-molecular-weight (> 500,000 daltons) glycoprotein. These determinants are found in coelomic epithelium during embryonic development and can be detected on fetal tissues, müllerian duct remnants, amnion, and amnionic fluid. The antigen is not found in normal ovarian tissue but is found in nonmucinous epithelial ovarian carcinomas. Eighty-two percent of ovarian cancer patients react positively, and rising or falling titers correlate with disease in 93% of patients. Approximately 25% of patients with nongynecologic malignancies, 5% of patients with benign disease, and 1% of apparently healthy persons have elevated antigen levels (> 35 units of CA-125 per ml of serum).

Recently, several studies have explored CA-125 use in the detection of ovarian carcinoma. Zurawski and colleagues[87] studied 915 nonhospitalized Roman Catholic nuns, in whom CA-125 levels ranged from 0 to 574 U/ml. Thirty-six women (3.9%) had CA-125 levels greater than 35 U/ml, and 7 had levels greater than 65 U/ml. Of the latter 7 women, 5 were found to have benign or malignant neoplasms, including one colon carcinoma, one uterine leiomyoma, one endometrioma, one fibroadenoma of the breast, and one sclerosing adenosis of the breast. None of the 36 patients with levels of greater than 35 U/ml was found to have an ovarian cancer. Einhorn and associates[88] measured CA-125 levels in 100 women undergoing diagnostic laparotomy for a palpable adnexal mass. Levels were greater than 35 U/ml in 11 of 18 patients (61%) with some form of ovarian cancer and were greater than 65 U/ml in 9 of these 11 patients. Malkasian and co-workers[89] studied 64 women with benign ovarian lesions and found 13 of 31 (42%) with endometriosis to have levels greater than 35 U/ml. Other authors[90] have also found elevated levels in patients with endometriosis or hepatitis,[91] during menses in women with and without endometriosis,[92,93] and in patients with pelvic inflammatory diseases or pregnancy.[94]

From these studies, it is clear that CA-125 is not at present specific enough to be an accurate diagnostic test for ovarian cancer. There are insufficient data to determine its sensitivity in an asymptomatic population. Continued evaluation of the test in patients at high risk because of either the presence of an adnexal mass or a family history of ovarian carcinoma is warranted.

On the other hand, a persistent elevation of CA-125 in patients with a history of ovarian cancer has invariably been associated with the finding of residual disease at second-look surgery. Unfortunately, the level may fall into the normal range even though disease remains. Bast and coworkers per-

formed second-look surgery on 15 women whose OC-125 levels had fallen into the normal range, and in 11 of the women residual disease was detected.[86]

The elevation of CA-125 levels may antedate the appearance of detectable disease or recurrence. Levels are often elevated 2 to 7 months before clinical detection of recurrent disease, and, in one unusual patient, elevated levels of CA-125 were present up to a year before the initial diagnosis of ovarian cancer. Unfortunately, the large amount of circulating antigen in most patients prevents the monoclonal antibody from being used effectively in its present form for either imaging or therapeutic purposes.

TREATMENT METHODS

SURGERY

Initial Surgical Staging

Unlike most gynecologic cancers, in which clinical evaluation is used to stage the diseases, ovarian cancer is staged surgically. The FIGO classification was revised in 1985, and although the official report has not been published, FIGO allowed publication of the changes in early 1987[95] (Table 37-4).

Major changes have been made in Stages I, II, and III. In Stages I and II, the former subdivisions "Ai and Aii" and "Bi and Bii" that identified tumor rupture or surface spread have been made part of subdivision C. It is required that malignant cells be identified in either washings or ascites to assign a patient to Stages IC or IIC; the presence of ascites alone without malignant cells is insufficient. In Stage III, subdivisions A, B, and C designate the size of the tumor found at surgical exploration. Inguinal node metastases are included in Stage IIIC. Of particular importance, this staging classification is based on the findings on opening the abdomen and *not* following surgical debulking: (i.e. a patient with disease larger than 2 cm confined to the omentum who has cytoreduction such that no residual tumor is apparent still has Stage IIIC disease). It is essential for the surgeon to define clearly the amount of disease found upon opening the abdomen.

Although only a few patients with ovarian cancer can be managed by surgery alone, the success of subsequent therapy is in large part determined by the accuracy and comprehensiveness of the initial surgical procedure. Proper selection of appropriate adjunctive therapy requires accurate assessment of the extent of residual disease at the conclusion of the initial operation, and the chance of achieving a complete pathologic response (negative second-look operation) is directly related to residual disease volume.

For best results, the surgeon must have a thorough understanding of the pathogenesis of the disease, be thorough in both preoperative preparation and postoperative care, and be appropriately aggressive intraoperatively. Most surgeons prefer a vertical midline incision for patients with suspected ovarian cancer because it provides excellent access to the pelvis and can be extended as far as proves necessary into the upper abdomen. Moreover, patients with apparent early-

TABLE 37-4. FIGO Stage Grouping for Primary
Carcinoma of the Ovary (1987)

Stage I	Growth limited to the ovaries	
	IA	Growth limited to one ovary; no ascites. No tumor on the external surface, capsule intact
	IB	Growth limited to both ovaries; no ascites. No tumor on the external surfaces; capsules intact
	IC*	Tumor either Stage IA or IB but with tumor on the surface of one or both ovaries, or with capsule ruptured, or with ascites present containing malignant cells, or with positive peritoneal washings
Stage II	Growth involving one or both ovaries with pelvic extension	
	IIA	Growth involving one or both ovaries with pelvic extension
	IIB	Extension and/or metastases to the uterus and/or tubes
	IIC*	Tumor either Stage IIA or IIB but with tumor on the surface of one or both ovaries, or with capsule(s) ruptured, or with ascites present containing malignant cells, or with positive peritoneal washings
Stage III	Tumor involving one or both ovaries with peritoneal implants outside the pelvis and/or positive retroperitoneal or inguinal nodes. Superficial liver metastases equal Stage III. Tumor is limited to the true pelvis but with histologically verified malignant extension to small bowel or omentum	
	IIIA	Tumor grossly limited to the true pelvis with negative nodes but with histologically confirmed microscopic seeding of abdominal peritoneal surfaces
	IIIB	Tumor of one or both ovaries with histologically confirmed implants of abdominal peritoneal surfaces, none exceeding 2 cm in diameter. Nodes negative
	IIIC	Abdominal implants greater than 2 cm in diameter and/or positive retroperitoneal or inguinal nodes
Stage IV	Growth involving one or both ovaries with distant metastasis. If pleural effusion is present, there must be positive cytologic test results to allot a case to Stage IV. Parenchymal liver metastasis equals Stage IV.	

* To evaluate the impact on prognosis of the different criteria for alloting cases to Stage IC or IIC, it would be of value to know if rupture of the capsule was (1) spontaneous or (2) caused by the surgeon, and if the source of malignant cells detected was (1) peritoneal washings or (2) ascites.

stage disease may require different therapy than those found to have microscopic metastases to the upper abdomen, and proper evaluation of the upper abdomen is rarely possible through a lower-abdominal incision. When gross disease is present in the upper abdomen, proper resection requires adequate exposure. Unfortunately, it is still common to see patients who have had two or more operations for ovarian cancer yet no abdominal scar that extends above the umbilicus.

In a young patient with a nonsuspicious pelvic mass, a low transverse incision may be quite appropriate but must be large enough to remove the mass without danger of rupture. It is never appropriate to aspirate an ovarian mass to reduce its size to fit the incision. In instances in which carcinoma is found and a Pfannenstiel's incision has been used, the incision should be converted to a true transverse incision by dividing the rectus muscles and a second, upper-abdominal midline, incision made to explore the upper abdomen adequately. The patient should be made aware of this possibility preoperatively.

Initial exploration of the abdomen must be thorough and methodical. Figure 37-2 illustrates the essentials. The presence, amount, and character of any ascitic fluid should be noted and the fluid submitted in toto for cytology study. In the absence of ascitic fluid, washings should be obtained from the pelvis, each abdominal gutter, and each subdiaphragmatic surface.

If a unilateral mass is found, the surgeon must decide whether simply to remove it or to remove the tube and ovary. Generally, a cystectomy would be indicated only in a young (less than age 40) patient. If cystectomy is to be performed, the abdomen should be protected by the use of laparotomy tapes from spillage secondary to inadvertent rupture. If frozen-section study indicates a malignant neoplasm, a full metastatic search is mandated. In a patient not concerned about future childbearing, a total abdominal hysterectomy and bilateral salpingo-oophorectomy are indicated. Unilateral salpingo-oophorectomy is indicated only in the young patient desirous of further childbearing in whom careful inspection reveals no evidence of disease other than in one ovary. If careful and methodical inspection of the entire abdomen is negative, biopsies, as outlined in Table 37-5, are performed. In general, it is best to establish a set sequence for inspecting the abdomen and obtaining biopsies so that nothing will be omitted; Table 37-5 outlines the recommended exploration and biopsy procedure. It is not unreasonable to maintain the written protocol in the operating room to ensure accuracy.

Cytoreductive Surgery

Cytoreductive surgery is an integral part of initial patient management and demands substantial skill and judgment. Technically difficult cytoreductive surgery requires not only detailed knowledge of gynecologic surgery but also readiness for complicated abdominal and urologic surgery. Formal residency programs in obstetrics and gynecology and in general surgery do not usually provide the depth of knowledge and experience necessary for the surgical management of ovarian cancer. Whenever possible, therefore, patients with ovarian cancer should be referred to individuals with special training in surgical or gynecologic oncology.

The surgeon faces a formidable task when ovarian carcinoma has spread throughout the abdomen and pelvis. Often, the tumor fills the pelvis, and there is little room for examination of vital structures such as the iliac vessels and ureter. All peritoneal surfaces may be involved, including the lateral pelvic sidewalls, the bladder peritoneum, and the serosa of the rectosigmoid. The optimal approach to the pelvis is via the retroperitoneum. By opening the peritoneum lateral to the iliac vessels (and, if necessary, the colon), the surgeon gains access to the pararectal and paravesical spaces, allowing identification of the major blood vessels, ureter, and

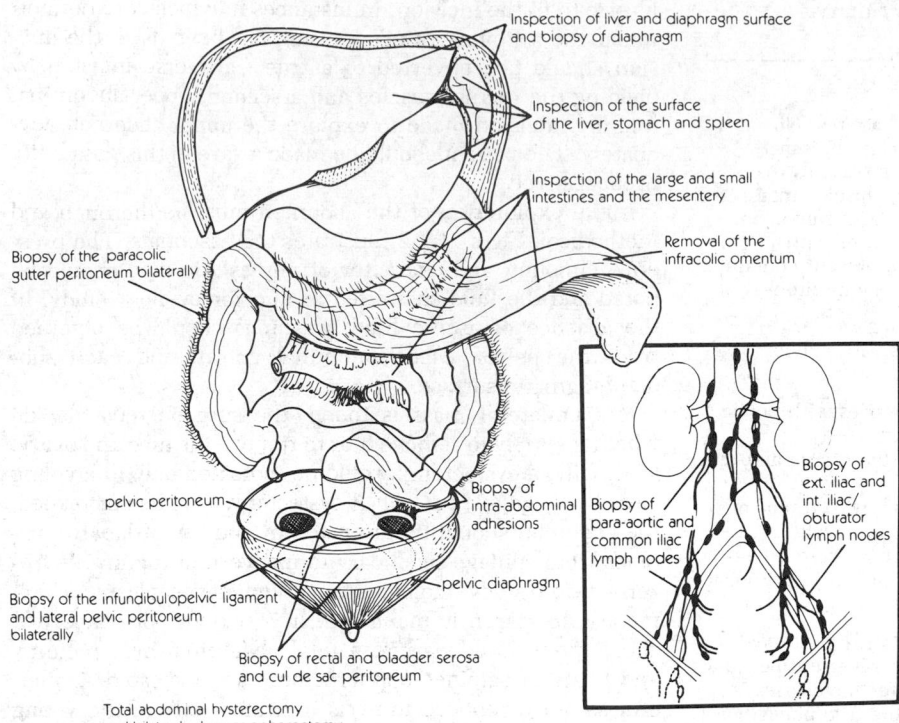

Inspection of liver and diaphragm surface
and biopsy of diaphragm

Inspection of the surface
of the liver, stomach and spleen

Inspection of the large and small
intestines and the mesentery

Removal of the
infracolic omentum

Biopsy of the paracolic
gutter peritoneum bilaterally

Biopsy of
ext. iliac and
int. iliac/
obturator
lymph nodes

Biopsy of
para-aortic and
common iliac
lymph nodes

Biopsy of
intra-abdominal
adhesions

pelvic peritoneum

pelvic diaphragm

Biopsy of the infundibulopelvic ligament
and lateral pelvic peritoneum
bilaterally

Biopsy of rectal and bladder serosa
and cul de sac peritoneum

Total abdominal hysterectomy
and bilateral salpengoophorectomy

FIG. 37-2. Staging laparotomy for the patient with ovarian cancer. (Hoskins WJ: The role of cytoreductive surgery in ovarian cancer. PPO Update 1(2), February 1987)

infundibulopelvic ligament. Ligation of this ligament and of the round ligament allows the surgeon to mobilize the pelvic viscera and tumor masses. The ureter can be dissected free of the medial flap of peritoneum, and the uterine artery can be identified and ligated. If the tumor is large or has extended into the obturator foramen, the obturator nerve should be identified and preserved. With the ureter, obturator nerve, and major blood vessels identified and the uterine artery and infundibulopelvic ligament ligated, the surgeon can remove the uterus, adnexa, and pelvic tumor. In some cases, the tumor will peel away from the peritoneum, whereas in other cases the peritoneum must be removed with the tumor. On occasion, it is necessary to remove a portion of the bladder or rectosigmoid colon. Primary reanastomosis of the rectum is usually feasible, although on occasion a colostomy will be necessary. In some patients, pelvic involvement of the cecum or terminal ileum necessitates resection of these structures with reconstruction of intestinal continuity by ileoascending or ileotransverse colostomy. Although the ureter can usually be separated from the pelvic tumor, resection and reimplantation into the bladder may be necessary to achieve complete cytoreduction.

Resection of disease in the abdominal cavity should be as complete as possible. If disease involves the infracolic omentum, it can be removed below the transverse colon. If disease involves the supracolic omentum, it should be detached from the transverse colon and resected along the greater curvature of the stomach, as shown in Figure 37-3. Particular attention should be given to carrying the dissection up toward the spleen in order to remove all gross tumor. On occasion, it is necessary to remove the spleen. Tumor implants in the paracolic gutters and on the surface of the intestine can usually be separated from the underlying structures, although it is sometimes necessary to resect portions of the intestine. Disease on the liver surface and undersurface of the diaphragm can often be partially debulked, and venous oozing can usually be controlled with pressure from a laparotomy pack.

The surgeon must often make difficult decisions as to how extensive the resection of gross tumor should be in relation to possible benefit. There is probably little benefit in leaving a patient with a colostomy or resecting large segments of small intestine if bulk disease cannot be removed from other sites. On the other hand, such resection may be quite feasible in order to leave the patient with minimal residual disease.

Impact of Primary Cytoreductive Surgery

In 1968, Munnel[96] reported improved survival in Stages III and IV ovarian carcinoma if omentectomy was performed. He further demonstrated improved survival in patients undergoing definitive operation rather than "partial removal" or "laparotomy and biopsy." A year later, Delcos and Quinlan[97] reported that patients with "nonpalpable" disease survived longer than patients with "palpable" ovarian cancer when treated with radiotherapy. For nonpalpable disease, the 4-year survival rates for Stages II and III were 72% and 25%, respectively, and for palpable disease, the rates were 33% and 9%, respectively.

In the mid-1970s, Griffiths[98] used chemotherapy after cytoreductive surgery and compared the survival of patients grouped by the amount of residual disease. He demonstrated

TABLE 37-5.   Operative Procedure for Proper Surgical Staging of the Patient with Ovarian Cancer

Step 1.   If ascites is present, remove as much as possible for cytology. If no ascites is present, obtain cell washings from the pelvis, both abdominal gutters, and both subdiaphragmatic areas.

Step 2.   Determine whether the mass is malignant; if malignant, perform appropriate pelvic procedure (total abdominal hysterectomy and bilateral salpingo-oophorectomy unless patient desires further childbearing and there is no evidence of spread beyond the ovary).

Step 3.   Carefully examine pelvic peritoneum; if lesions are present, remove as much as possible and biopsy any lesion that cannot be removed. If no lesions are seen, sample at a minimum the peritoneum of the lateral pelvic sidewalls, the bladder, the rectosigmoid, and the cul-de-sac.

Step 4.   Examine the paracolic gutters, and remove any lesions seen. If no lesions are seen, obtain a 1 × 3-cm strip of peritoneum on either side.

Step 5.   Examine the omentum, and remove any that contains visible tumor (including the supracolic omentum if involved by tumor). If no lesions are seen, remove the infracolic omentum.

Step 6.   Examine and palpate both diaphragms and the surface of the spleen and liver. If lesions are present, remove as much as possible; biopsy if they cannot be removed. If no lesions are seen, a strip of peritoneum 1 × 2 cm should be carefully excised from the right hemidiaphragm. (Note: only peritoneum is needed, and care should be taken not to create a pneumothorax.)

Step 7.   Beginning at either the rectum or cecum, carefully inspect the entire large colon and remove and/or biopsy any suspicious lesion of the intestine or mesentery.*

Step 8.   Beginning at either the ileocecal valve or ligament of Treitz, carefully inspect the entire small bowel and mesentery, removing and/or biopsing any lesions.*

Step 9.   If, after all of the above procedures, no gross disease larger than 1 or 2 cm is left, the pelvic and para-aortic lymph nodes should be sampled.

* If resection of intestine is necessary to cytoreduce the tumor optimally or to relieve obstruction, this should be performed.

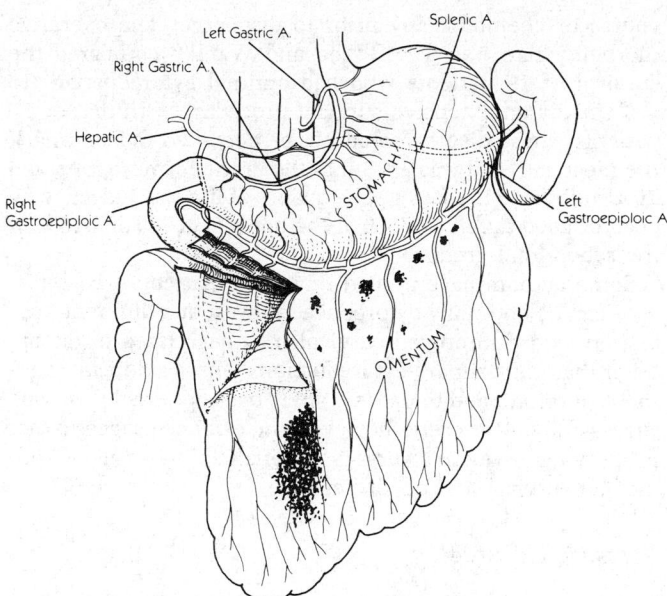

FIG. 37-3. Omentectomy in patients with metastatic ovarian cancer. (Hoskins WJ: The role of cytoreductive surgery in ovarian cancer. PPO Update 1(2), February 1987)

regimens, showed a significant difference in both the progression-free interval and the survival rate for patients with no residual disease compared with those with residual masses as large as 1 cm. Fuks and associates[104] described two radiotherapy series in which the median survival was 24 months for "small residual" or "no residual" disease compared with 6 to 11 months for "large residual" disease. Dembo[105] reported a 43% 5-year survival rate in Stage III with less than 2 cm of residual disease in patients treated with whole-abdominal irradiation compared with an 18% 5-year survival rate for patients with greater than 2 cm of disease.

To evaluate the operative morbidity and quality of life of primary cytoreductive surgery. Chen and co-workers[106] reviewed 60 patients who underwent optimal primary cytoreductive surgery. They reported a mean operating time of 3.6 hours, a mean blood loss of 1644 ml, and a mean hospital stay of 16 days, with most patients receiving their first

that the duration of survival was directly related to the amount of residual disease after initial cytoreductive surgery: patients with no residual disease had a mean survival of 39 months compared with 29 months for those with residual disease of no more than 0.5 cm and 18 months for those with residual disease of 0.6 cm to 1.5 cm. Patients with larger volumes of disease had a mean survival of 11 months, and none of these suboptimally cytoreduced patients survived beyond 26 months.

Table 37-6 summarizes four reports in which the median length of survival is reported based on primary cytoreductive surgery to less than, or greater than, 2 cm of residual disease. Most of these patients received postoperative multidrug chemotherapy. The mean survival was 29.4 months in the optimally cytoreduced group and 13.4 months in the group in whom cytoreductive surgery was suboptimal. A recent study of the GOG,[103] which compared two cisplatin-based

TABLE 37-6.   Effect of Volume of Residual Disease on Survival in Patients with Stage III Epithelial Ovarian Carcinoma Given Postcytoreduction Chemotherapy

| | Survival (mo) | | |
	< 2 cm	> 2 cm	Reference
	44.5	15.9	99
	25+	13.5	100
	30+	18	101
	18*	6*	102
Mean	29.4	13.4	

* 0.5–1.5 cm.

course of chemotherapy prior to discharge. The operative morbidity rate was 5%. Blythe and Wahl[107] compared the survival of 19 patients who had optimal cytoreduction (to <2 cm) by an extensive surgical procedure with that of 17 patients whose disease could not be debulked (suboptimal); the mean survival was 14.3 months in the former group and 10.2 months in the latter. The quality of life was judged to be good or good to fair in 75% of the optimal group and 18% of the suboptimal group.

Some authors have argued that these patients whose disease can be optimally cytoreduced represent a different population whose improved survival may be related to factors other than the primary cytoreduction. This is a difficult argument to refute, and to date no study has addressed this issue successfully. At present, however, the evidence suggests that primary cytoreductive surgery is beneficial in terms of both median survival and quality of life.

Postsurgical Staging

If the proper careful staging procedure was performed at initial surgery, then little additional evaluation is ordinarily required postoperatively. However, if the upper abdomen was not properly evaluated during the initial operation, postoperative reevaluation by either laparotomy or laparoscopy may be necessary even before other treatment is begun. Unfortunately, understaging as a result of inadequate initial surgery is common: several laparoscopy studies have documented unappreciated intra-abdominal spread in 30% to 40% of patients with early (FIGO Stages I and II) disease explored through lower-abdominal incisions.[28,29] Piver and co-workers found diaphragmatic metastases in 11% and aortic lymph node metastases in 13% of patients otherwise felt to have Stage I disease.[30]

The use of laparoscopy in patients with ovarian carcinoma is of value both for initial staging and as a means of surveillance to assess therapeutic response.[28,29] In the U.S. National Cancer Institute (NCI) experience, laparoscopy documented involved sites that had gone undetected during conventional radiologic and isotopic procedures in 42% of patients.[108] In addition, this technique provided the only evidence of disease in 38%. Twenty percent to 30% of patients referred with presumed Stage I or II disease were reclassified as having Stage III disease on the basis of diaphragmatic metastases detected at laparoscopy.

Laparoscopy was found to be safe and feasible even in patients who had had prior laparotomies.[108] In 6% of patients, technical problems occurred that precluded complete evaluation. Of 159 procedures performed, there were few serious complications; only 2.5% of the patients required medical therapy to manage a complication. Complications included pneumothorax (one case), bleeding necessitating transfusion (one), wound infection (one), and hypotension (two). Other complications not requiring therapy were pneumomediastinum and subcutaneous or mesenteric emphysema. There were no deaths or viscus perforations, and no patient required surgical exploration because of a complication.

Other institutions have had similar experiences. Berek, Griffiths, and Leventhal reviewed 112 laparoscopies performed in 57 patients without clinical evidence of disease.[109] In 80 (71%) of the procedures, the entire peritoneal cavity was examined; visibility was totally inadequate in only 16 procedures. Similar complications occurred in this series, but none was serious.

Second-Look Surgical Reassessment

The term "second-look surgical reassessment" should be restricted to a systematic surgical reexploration of patients who have completed a planned course of treatment after initial surgical staging and cytoreductive surgery. Such patients should be clinically without evidence of disease by physical examination and routine diagnostic studies such as chest film, liver function tests, CA-125 assay, intravenous urogram, barium enema, and CT scan. The fact that approximately 50% of patients so evaluated will be found to have residual disease illustrates the difficulty of nonsurgical evaluation in this disease.

Wangenstein and associates introduced the concept of second-look surgery,[110] and a series of studies from the M.D. Anderson Hospital and Tumor Institute defined its application to ovarian cancer.[111-113] The technique of second-look reassessment requires considerable care because most patients with negative second-look operations do not receive further therapy. The abdomen should be entered through a generous midline incision extending from the symphysis pubis to at least 6 cm above the umbilicus. If no disease is found or if upper-abdominal disease is to be cytoreduced, the incision will probably need to be extended further toward the xyphoid. All adhesions in the abdomen and pelvis should be lysed, and portions of these adhesions should be submitted for pathologic analysis. A thorough examination of the abdomen and pelvis is then done. In general, the same procedures are followed as for the primary staging of ovarian cancer (see Table 37-5). Washings of the pelvis, paracolic gutters, and subdiaphragmatic areas are essential. If no gross disease is found, pelvic and para-aortic lymph nodes should be biopsied. Usually, a second-look operation results in 20 to 40 pathologic specimens. Residual disease should be resected whenever possible, and any disease that cannot be resected should be noted in the operative report.

Table 37-7 summarizes the effect of initial residual disease on the outcome of second-look surgical reassessment in epithelial ovarian cancer. The likelihood of a complete pathologic response (negative second-look reassessment) is 82% if no apparent residual disease remained after the initial surgery, 53% if minimal residual disease remained, and 23% if only suboptimal resection was possible.

The timing of second-look surgical reassessment has varied since the concept was introduced. Patients treated with single alkylating agents were usually treated for 12 to 18 months, and Smith and associates[113] indicated that patients given at least 10 courses of melphalan had a better survival rate than those who had shorter courses of therapy prior to the second look. With the introduction of multidrug regimens, toxicity was greater and 10 to 12 months of such chemotherapy was difficult to administer without significant dose reduction or prolongation of chemotherapy intervals. Greco and Berek and their co-workers[114,115] have used sec-

TABLE 37-7. Effect of Residual Disease at End of Initial Cytoreductive Operation on Presence of Disease at Second-Look Surgical Reassessment

| | Percentage with Negative Second Look | | | |
	No Residual	Optimal Residual	Suboptimal Residual	Reference
	67	61	14	41
	76	50	28	118
	–	40	11	119
	75	–	25	120
	95	36	20	121
	82	44	33	122
	–	49	13	123
	79	45	22	124
	100	100	40	125
Mean	82	53	23	

ond-look laparotomy after six courses of therapy. In a prospective randomized trial under way at Memorial Sloan-Kettering Cancer Center, five courses of cyclophosphamide, Adriamycin, and cisplatin (CAP) are being compared with 10 courses of the same regimen. It is too early to provide final results, but a preliminary review[116] has indicated no difference in the frequency of negative second-look surgical reassessment in the two arms. Although the optimal timing for second-look surgery has not been established, the use of multiagent chemotherapy has decreased the interval from the onset of chemotherapy to the surgical reassessment.

Unfortunately, Rubin and co-workers[42] reported that shorter courses of cisplatin-based chemotherapy produce a higher complete response rate but a higher recurrence rate after negative second-look surgical reassessment. They suggest that the longer intervals of therapy with earlier regimens allowed a longer time for patients whose tumors had developed drug resistance to have recurrences and thus not have second-look surgery.

Second-look surgical reassessment has recently been reviewed by Rubin and Lewis,[117] and the results are summarized in Table 37-8. The chance of a patient having a negative second-look surgical reassessment is directly related to the stage of disease, the grade of tumor, and the amount of residual disease at the conclusion of the initial cytoreductive operation. Of 1255 patients included in the 16 reports reviewed by Rubin and Lewis, 53.9% had residual disease detected at second-look surgery.

Persistent disease at second-look reassessment has been described in the pelvis, on the surfaces of the intestine, on the diaphragm, in the omentum, and retroperitoneal lymph nodes.[120,122,126,127] Both Berek and colleagues[119] and Creasman and associates[128] have reported retroperitoneal lymph node spread as the sole positive finding at second-look surgery.

Second-look surgical reassessment is a significantly invasive procedure that involves the expense and discomfort of a major abdominal operation and disrupts the patient's normal activities. Nevertheless, published reports have documented acceptable morbidity. In the excellent review by Rubin and Lewis, there were no deaths in 682 operations, and the over-

all morbidity rate (including minor complications) was 19%. Most of these complications were infections involving the incision, the urinary tract, or the lungs.

Recurrent ovarian carcinoma after negative second-look surgery occurred in 15% to 20% of all cases in the many references previously cited. However, in certain groups of patients, the recurrence rate is much higher. Barnhill and co-workers[41] and Rubin et al[42] have reported recurrence rates of approximately 50% in patients with Stages III and IV, Grade 2 and 3 tumors after treatment with cisplatin-based chemotherapy. It is possible that patients in these high-risk categories should receive additional therapy after negative second-look surgical reassessment.

Several authors have questioned the value of second-look surgery because of the poor survival of patients with positive findings and the high recurrence rates of patients with negative ones. However, new second-line experimental therapeutic options are available and should encourage further use of the second-look reevaluation technique. In areas in which such second-line therapeutic options are not available, the patient should be referred to centers where investigational treatment is being used.

TABLE 37-8. Results (as %) of Second-Look Surgery in Ovarian Carcinoma (Collected Series)*

	Negative
Stage	
I	80
II	68
III	35
Grade	
1	61
2	50
3	41
Residual disease after cytoreductive operation	
None	77
"Optimal"	45
"Suboptimal"	25

* Adapted from Rubin and Lewis.[117]

Other techniques for monitoring the response to therapy short of second-look laparotomy can be used under some circumstances. For example, the NCI group has utilized peritoneoscopy.[108] In 66 restaging peritoneoscopies, residual disease was found in 33 patients; peritoneoscopic findings provided the only evidence of disease in 24 patients (36%). These patients were spared an unnecessary second-look laparotomy, whereas those patients with negative results on peritoneoscopy underwent laparotomy. Residual ovarian cancer was found in 55%, mainly in the pelvis and mesentery. Therefore, a negative peritoneoscopy must be followed by laparotomy before a patient with ovarian cancer can be considered disease free. However, in patients undergoing therapy, laparoscopy proved a useful tool for monitoring subclinical disease.

Secondary Cytoreductive Surgery

Although the worth of primary cytoreductive surgery is clear, the value of secondary cytoreduction is controversial. The recent availability of cisplatin analogues, intraperitoneal chemotherapy, and a new generation of biologic response modifiers has expanded our second-line treatment capabilities, and because these agents are most effective against minimal residual disease, secondary cytoreduction may be important.

Table 37-9 summarizes the frequency with which secondary cytoreduction can be accomplished. Berek and co-workers[129] performed secondary cytoreduction on 32 patients and found that in 12 (38%), residual disease could be reduced to optimal (less than 1.5 cm). Median survival for that group was 20 months compared with 5 months for the 20 patients whose disease could not be optimally cytoreduced. Factors that were associated with a greater likelihood of optimal secondary cytoreduction were previous optimal primary cytoreduction, less than 1000 ml of ascites, tumor size less than 5 cm at second operation, and interval from primary to secondary surgery of greater than 12 months. Age, tumor grade, type of subsequent chemotherapy, and the presence or absence of bowel obstruction did not influence survival following secondary cytoreductive surgery.

Griffiths and associates[130] compared the incidence of successful cytoreduction and survival in patients undergoing primary versus secondary operations. Although effective cytoreduction was equally possible in both types of patients,

survival was significantly less in those undergoing secondary cytoreduction. Wiltshaw et al[131] showed that partial responders to chemotherapy had improved survival if they underwent secondary cytoreductive surgery. Copeland and co-workers[132] evaluated nine patients who had undergone secondary cytoreduction and concluded that such surgery could contribute to long term survival. Several other groups also have reported successful secondary cytoreduction.[113,133–135]

Although the role of secondary cytoreduction surgery remains controversial, the increased availability of second-line therapy may increase the importance of such surgical procedures.

RADIATION THERAPY

Historical Considerations

The first report of radiation therapy for ovarian carcinoma was published in 1912 by Eymer,[136] who described long-term remissions in eight patients treated with low-dose whole-abdominal irradiation. The low-energy radiation beams available with the early orthovoltage machines had poor penetration and produced high skin doses and significant skin toxicity, which prevented the delivery of high-dose radiation to peritoneal tumors. Therefore, although radiation was shown to have significant palliative effects, its curative value was justifiably questioned.

The introduction of megavoltage radiotherapy in the early 1950s allowed more penetrating and skin-sparing radiation and made possible the application of large and shaped fields carried to high doses. However, the extreme radiation sensitivities of some of the normal abdominal contents have limited the use of radiotherapy as a curative modality in many patients, especially those with advanced disease. Nonetheless, when appropriate precautions are taken, radiotherapy does represent an effective curative modality for certain patients with ovarian carcinoma.

Tumoricidal Radiation Doses

The shape and distribution of the radiation fields as well as the dose and fractionation schemes employed in the treatment of ovarian carcinoma represent a compromise between the need to employ tumoricidal doses to eradicate tumor deposits and the desire to avoid injury to normal tissues included in the treatment fields. Although the tumoricidal dose levels for ovarian tumors have not been determined with great accuracy, there is ample evidence that radiation can permanently eradicate tumor deposits in patients with residual ovarian cancer. Fuks and Bagshaw[137] reported an actuarial 5-year disease-free survival rate of 46% in 16 Stage IIB patients with residual pelvic disease treated with 5000 to 6000 cGy. Schray and associates[138] treated 26 patients with small residual tumors (less than 2 cm in diameter) with similar radiation doses. Only four relapsed in the pelvis compared with 9 of 20 (45%) who had larger residual tumors. Dembo[139,140] treated patients with Stage I, II, or IIIA tumors with 4500 cGy to the pelvis and 2250 cGy to the upper abdomen. The 5-year survival rate in 50 patients with small

TABLE 37-9. Frequency of Successful Secondary Cytoreductive Operations in Patients with Advanced or Recurrent Epithelial Ovarian Cancer

	No. of Patients	Patients Optimally Cytoreduced (%)	Reference	
		32	12 (37.5)	129
	13	11 (84.6)	130	
	29	13 (44.7)	133	
	26	15 (57.7)	134	
	69	29 (42.0)	113	
	38	9 (24.0)	135	
Total	207	89 (43.0%)		

or no residual tumors was 78% compared with 19% in 26 patients with larger residua. These data suggest that tumoricidal doses are tumor size dependent. For large tumors, this dose probably exceeds 5000 to 6000 cGy, whereas for small (< 2 cm) tumors it is probably 4500 to 5000 cGy, and for microscopic tumor deposits, the existing data suggest that the tumoricidal dose levels may be even lower. The Princess Margaret Group randomized patients with no residual tumors after surgery to receive either 4500 cGy to the pelvis or the same dose to the pelvis and 2250 cGy to the upper abdomen.[140-142] The 5-year survival rate for the patients receiving abdominopelvic radiotherapy was 78% compared with 51% in the patients treated to the pelvis only, the survival difference resulting from a 30% higher control rate of occult upper-abdominal metastases in the group that received abdominopelvic radiation. These data suggest that the 2250 cGy given was tumoricidal to microscopic upper-abdominal tumor deposits. These observations are supported by data of Delclos and Smith,[143] who showed that patients with Stage II disease treated with 5000 cGy to the pelvis and 2600 to 2800 cGy to the upper abdomen by the moving-strip technique had an improved survival rate at 5 years (57%) compared with the patients treated to the pelvis only (17%). Similarly, Perez et al[144,145] report a 5-year survival rate of 57% in patients with Stage II disease treated with a similar technique to the whole abdomen and of 16% in patients receiving pelvic irradiation only. It is therefore generally accepted that a dose of 2500 to 3000 cGy given in daily fractions of 150 to 200 cGy is probably tumoricidal for microscopic ovarian carcinoma.

Design of Treatment Fields, Total Dose, and Fractionation

In carcinoma of the ovary, the entire peritoneal cavity is at risk. However, the doses that would be required to eradicate large tumors in the upper abdomen cannot be administered because of the limited tolerance of some abdominal organs, such as the liver, kidneys, spinal cord, stomach, and intestines. Therefore, restrictions of the dose and special shielding for vital viscera are necessary to ensure that normal-tissue tolerance is not exceeded.

Two radiotherapy techniques have been employed routinely in patients with ovarian carcinoma: the open-field technique[146] and the moving-strip technique.[147,148] The open field employs irradiation through two large fixed portals (anterior and posterior) shaped to encompass the entire peritoneal cavity (Fig. 37-7). In some patients with Stage I or Stage II disease, radiation portals have been restricted to the lower half of the peritoneal cavity. However, in view of the frequent involvement of the retroperitoneal para-aortic group of lymph nodes in early-stage ovarian carcinoma, Hanks and Bagshaw[146] suggested that treatment should include the para-aortic region. Further, because many of these patients also have metastatic deposits on the undersurface of the diaphragms,[28] Glatstein and colleagues[149] suggested further modifications to encompass, in addition to the para-aortic region, large portions of the diaphragms (Fig. 37-4).

Using the open-field techniques, radiation is delivered at a rate of 800 to 1000 cGy per week. The total dose to the lower

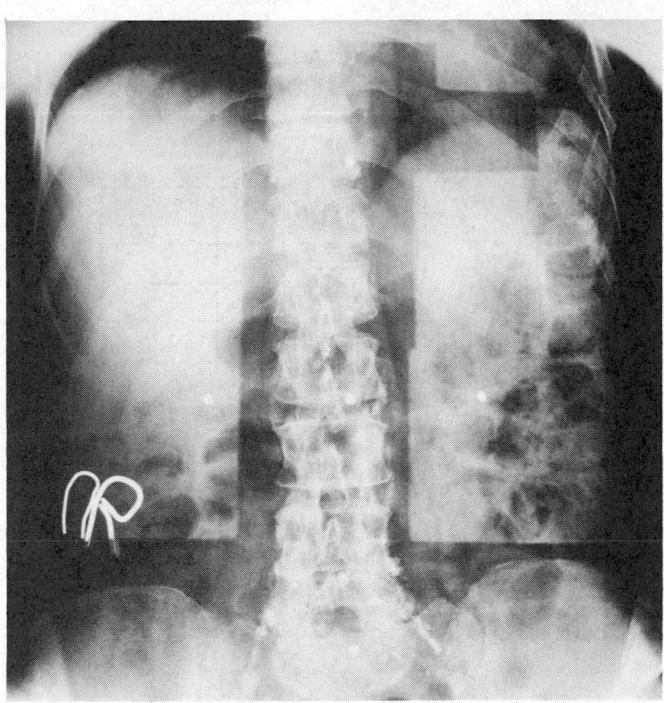

FIG. 37-4. Simulator portal film (Fuks Z, Bagshaw MA: The rationale for curative radiotherapy for ovarian carcinoma. Int J Radiat Oncol Biol Phys 1:21–32, 1975) demonstrating the anterior-posterior T-shaped field designed for the treatment of the para-aortic lymph nodes, the medial two thirds of the diaphragms, and the subpleural diaphragmatic lymph nodes. The technique, which is a four-field technique, also involves two opposed cross-table lateral fields. Its posterior margin is placed at the midplane of the lumbar vertebral bodies, providing protection to both kidneys from radiation damage. Its anterior margin is placed at the anterior periperitoneal fat line to encompass the total peritoneal cavity and the diaphragms. (Glatstein E, Fuks Z, Bagshaw MA: Diaphragmatic treatment in ovarian carcinoma: A new radiotherapeutic technique. Int J Radiat Oncol Biol Phys 2:357–362, 1977)

abdomen usually is 5500 cGy delivered in 27 fractions over 37 days. When calculated by the Ellis nominal standard dose (NSD) method,[150,151] the total dose to the pelvis is 1646 rets, and the corresponding tumor dose fractionation (TDF) value[152] is 89. When treating the upper abdomen, the dose usually is 4000 cGy delivered in 20 fractions over 33 days (1325 rets; TDF value 64), but shielding provided to the kidneys and liver (including the right hemidiaphragm) to protect these organs from radiation damage limits the effective dose to the underlying organs to approximately 2000 cGy.

A further modification of the open-field technique has recently been suggested by Martinez and associates[153,154] (Fig. 37-5). This modification involves a special field design and dose fractionation scheme designed to improve the tolerance of the open-field technique. Briefly, treatment is delivered by a series of anteroposterior–posteroanterior opposed fields. Beginning with radiation to the true pelvis, the field extends from the lower borders of the obturator foramina up to the level of L5. Five fractions of 180 cGy each are given in 1 week. The field is then opened to include the entire ab-

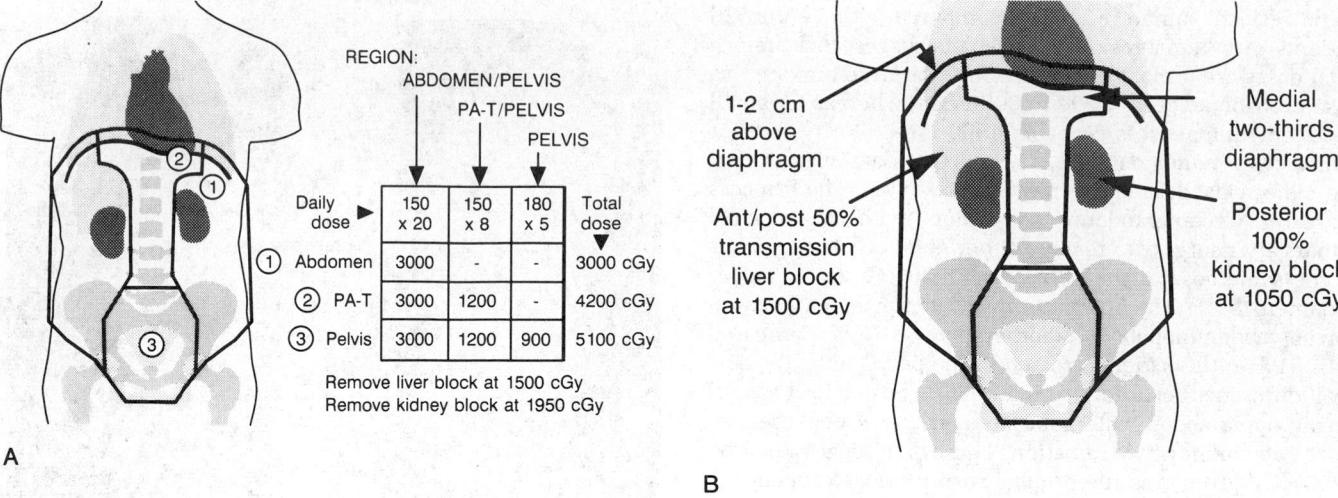

FIG. 37-5. Martinez technique and dose schedule. Field boundaries and blocks for treatment of gynecologic malignancies by whole-abdomen irradiation with diaphragmatic, para-aortic, and pelvic boost. PA'N, para-aortic nodes; DIAPH, diaphragm. (Martinez A, Schray MF, Howes AE, et al: Postoperative radiation therapy for epithelial ovarian cancer: The curative role based on a 24-year experience. J Clin Oncol 3:901–922, 1985)

dominal and pelvic peritoneum, extending up to 1 cm above the diaphragms. Twenty fractions of 150 cGy each are given to this volume in 4 weeks. A full-thickness posterior block is introduced after 1000 cGy to shield the kidneys, and a 50% transmission block is introduced anteriorly and posteriorly to shield the liver after 1500 cGy. The third and last field is a continuous pelvic, para-aortic, and partial diaphragmatic T-shaped field. Eight fractions of 150 cGy each are given in 10 days. In summary, the whole peritoneal cavity receives 3000 cGy in 20 fractions in 4 weeks, the pelvis receives 5100 cGy in 33 fractions in 6 to 7 weeks, and the para-aortic region, together with the medial part of the diaphragm, receives 4200 cGy in 28 fractions in 5 to 6 weeks. The total dose to the liver is 2250 cGy and to the kidneys 2000 cGy in 20 fractions in 4 weeks. This technique appears to be well tolerated.[154,155]

The moving-strip technique[147] involves the division of the peritoneal cavity into equal horizontal segments (strips) (Fig. 37-6). Treatment begins with irradiation to the lowest segments of the pelvis. At each radiotherapy session, a fixed number of adjacent segments are treated simultaneously. On consecutive days, the irradiated volume is moved cephalad from one segment to the adjacent segment in an orderly fashion until the entire abdomen has been treated. The dose to each point in the abdominal cavity usually is 3000 cGy delivered in 10 fractions over 12 days (1313 rets; TDF value 62). The kidneys and liver are usually shielded by partial-thickness lead blocks designed to allow the delivery of 50% of this dose. An additional dose of 2000 cGy in 10 fractions over 12 days usually is delivered to the pelvis by an open-field technique to increase the pelvic dose. When calculated by the NSD method, the total dose to the pelvis is 1713 rets (TDF value 95).

The moving-strip technique was designed to decrease the morbidity of whole-abdominal irradiation observed with the open-field technique.[143,147] However, when the NSD doses and the TDF values for the two techniques are compared, they prove similar. The NSD doses and the TDF values provide an estimate of normal tissue tolerance for fractionated radiation programs, and identical values imply biologically equivalent programs.[150-152] Indeed, studies comparing the open-field and moving-strip techniques[139,156] have shown that the rates of acute morbidity, chronic complications, and survival are similar.

FIG. 37-6. Total abdominal irradiation approach using the moving strip technique. Volume covered with the megavoltage moving strip technique. Kidneys are shielded from the posterior beam by two half-value layers of lead. The liver is shielded from the anterior beam by two half-value layers of lead. To compensate for the lower dose at both ends of the irradiated volume, treatment is started one strip below the lower margin of the pelvic field and completed one strip above the diaphragm.

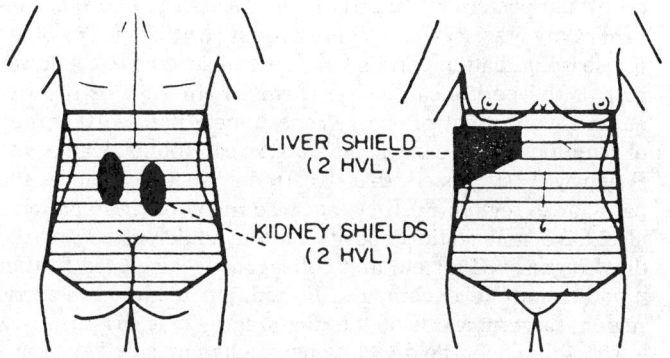

Acute Morbidity and Long-term Complications

The most common complication of radiation therapy for ovarian carcinoma is radiation-induced enteritis.[35,52,156] Its incidence and severity are directly related to the radiation dose. Acute morbidity, including diarrhea, nausea, vomiting, and weight loss, was seen in 78% of 167 patients treated with high-dose radiotherapy (4500 to 6000 cGy) to the lower abdomen.[157] In most of the patients, the gastrointestinal symptoms subsided within a few weeks after completion of treatment, although in 29% of the patients, diarrhea with or without gastrointestinal bleeding persisted for months to years. In 24 of the 167 patients (14%), severe bowel stenosis and bleeding developed, necessitating surgical intervention. Similar rates of acute and chronic radiation-induced enteritis have been reported by other investigators using the moving-strip technique.[158,159] Although still within acceptable limits, these rates of morbidity and complications are regarded as very high, despite the fact that they result from a treatment that is considered potentially curative for a malignant disease.

Some reduction in the peripheral blood counts almost always accompanies radiation.[35] Counts usually return to normal shortly after cessation of the treatment, but there is evidence that the activity of irradiated bone marrow remains impaired to a certain degree for extended periods.[160]

Radiation-induced hepatitis and nephritis are well-known hazards of doses exceeding 2500 cGy.[161,162] When careful port design and shielding are not performed, these syndromes are not uncommon in patients treated for ovarian carcinoma.[52,147,163] More recently, however, symptoms of hepatitis and nephritis have not been as common because of careful application of appropriate shielding of the liver and kidneys.

Preoperative Radiation

Preoperative radiation has been used sporadically.[164] Kottmeier reported a 40% (34/86) 3-year survival rate with preoperative radiation and total hysterectomy with bilateral salpingo-oophorectomy.[165] However, further information on these patients is not available. Kjorstad and co-workers[166] studied 145 patients with Stage III disease, 96 of whom had unresectable disease at initial surgery. Following a dose of 3000 cGy in 4 weeks to the whole abdomen, resection of the primary tumor, uterus, and omentum was possible in 38%. However, the operative mortality rate was 9% and the 5-year survival rate only 16%. The authors concluded that they achieved only a small increase in the salvage rate. Preoperative irradiation has not been popular for several reasons. One is the lack of histologic confirmation of malignancy without a laparotomy. Furthermore, after irradiation, the full extent of the disease is not known. Finally, there may be technical difficulties in carrying out surgery in the wake of high doses of preoperative irradiation.

Radioisotopes

The intraperitoneal instillation of radioactive colloidal gold (^{196}Au) or phosphorus (^{32}p) to irradiate the peritoneal cavity was popular in the past.[167,168] Colloidal ^{196}Au is no longer available for therapy. The colloidal particles increase isotope uptake by the mesothelial peritoneal cells and lymph nodes and decrease systemic radioisotope elution. Radioactive phosphorus (chromic phosphate) has a half-life of 14.2 days and emits only beta particles (1.7 MeV maximum energy). The range of beta particles in tissue is only 3 to 5 mm; thus, radioisotopes such as ^{32}p may sterilize microscopic peritoneal implants, but they are inadequate to treat large masses because of the short range of the beta particle. Also, because of adhesions or loculation, poor distribution in the peritoneal cavity may occur. This can be defined by injecting dilute Hypaque or by instilling technetium into the peritoneal cavity and scanning the patient before the therapeutic isotope is administered.

After radioisotope therapy, surgical management may be more difficult because of reactive fibrosis, although with ^{32}p, this problem has been infrequent. The usual dose of intraperitoneal radiophosphorus (as chromic phosphate) is 20 to 25 mCi diluted with sterile saline (1000–1500 ml) and properly distributed throughout the entire peritoneal cavity. If the average peritoneal surface is estimated at 30,000 cm^2, the dose of radiation delivered to the peritoneum is 6000 cGy and the dose delivered to the omentum is 7000 cGy.[168] Various methods for the administration of isotopes and verification of adequate distribution in the peritoneal cavity have been published.

The most common complication of intraperitoneal colloidal radioisotopes is small-bowel obstruction and stenosis. Pezner and co-workers[169] reviewing 104 patients treated intraperitoneally with radioisotopes, found that 11 required surgery for adhesions or fibrosis of the small intestine with severe chronic diarrhea; 1 patient with partial small-bowel obstruction was treated conservatively. In the patients receiving radioactive colloidal gold, only 1 of 45 (2.2%) developed small-bowel complications, in contrast to 12 of 50 (24%) treated with this technique in addition to pelvic external radiotherapy (about 4000 cGy in 4 weeks with ^{60}Co or 2-MeV photons). The frequency of small-bowel complications appears to be lower with ^{32}P than with ^{196}Au. Complications tend to be slightly more common in patients who have uneven distribution of the radioactive material in the peritoneal cavity.

CHEMOTHERAPY

Single Agents

Chemotherapy has ordinarily been used as the initial treatment in patients with advanced disease (FIGO Stages III and IV) and, in the past, for patients who were not considered appropriate candidates for radiation therapy.[170] Recently, with the discovery of more active agents, chemotherapy has become the most common form of therapy for patients with advanced disease.

Alkylating agents have been used more extensively than any other class of chemotherapeutic drugs. Melphalan, chlorambucil, cyclophosphamide, and thiotepa have produced similar objective response rates (33%–65%).[53] The median survival of treated patients is approximately 10 to 14 months; the median survival of those responding to chemotherapy is 17 to 20 months, and that for those not responding, 6 to 13 months. The 5-year survival rate of patients treated with alkylating agents ranges from 0 to 9% (mean 7%). The 5-year survival rate of the largest single series of patients treated with melphalan was 9%; approximately 20% of the responders in that series were alive at 5 years, with some patients alive and free of disease for periods in excess of 10 years. Second-look studies indicate that patients with no residual tumor at that time have a 5-year survival rate of 60% to 80% without further therapy.[171,172] It is therefore clear that some women with advanced ovarian cancer can be cured with single alkylating-agent therapy alone, although the number is small (5%–10%).

In addition to the alkylating agents, three other drugs—hexamethylmelamine,[173,174] Adriamycin, and cisplatin—have been fairly extensively studied and have response rates in the 20% to 35% range.[175] Cisplatin is one of the most active agents in ovarian cancer; overall response rates of 25% to 40% have been reported in single-agent trials.[176] In a randomized trial of cisplatin versus cyclophosphamide, a longer duration of response (18 versus 8 months) and significantly better survival (19 versus 12 months; p = 0.009) was seen with cisplatin.[177] Toxicities include nausea and vomiting, ototoxicity, peripheral neuropathy, nephrotoxicity, and bone-marrow suppression. Techniques are now available using hydration and chloruresis that markedly reduce the nephrotoxicity of the agent.[178-180] However, bone-marrow toxicity, peripheral neuropathy, and ototoxicity remain significant problems.

Several studies have demonstrated a clinically important dose–response relation with cisplatin.[181,182] Recently, Levin and Hryniuk[183] demonstrated a relation between dose intensity and outcome in 33 chemotherapy trials in ovarian cancer. The overall response rate and median survival correlated with the dose intensity (measured as mg/m² per week) for combinations of drugs, particularly those containing cisplatin. When analyzed as single drugs, the dose intensity relation was seen primarily for cisplatin. Because of the importance of dose intensity in cisplatin therapy, studies of high-dose (40 mg/m² daily for 5 days) cisplatin have been performed, demonstrating 32% response rates in refractory cases.[178]

Adriamycin is an active first-line agent in advanced ovarian cancer: collected experience indicates a response rate of approximately 30%.[175] Unfortunately, several studies indicate that the drug has very little activity when used as a second- or third-line agent, with only 3 of 56 patients (5%) responding to the drug after failing initial chemotherapy.[184,185]

One study of hexamethylmelamine in 54 previously untreated patients documented an overall response rate of 32%.[186] The drug was given orally continuously in this study, and there was significant gastrointestinal, hematologic, and neurologic toxicity. Recent studies suggest reduced toxicity with intermittent 14-day per month schedules. A recent update of information on hexamethylmelamine indicates definite single-agent activity.[187]

The cisplatin derivatives carboplatin (CBDCA) and CHIP have been studied extensively in ovarian cancer, and both have significant activity.[188-190] Carboplatin (400 mg/m²) appears to be roughly equivalent to 100 mg/m² of cisplatin.[188] The toxicity of carboplatin is primarily bone-marrow suppression with little or no nephrotoxicity, ototoxicity, or peripheral neuropathy. Preliminary evidence suggests that carboplatin has less cumulative toxicity than CHIP. Other single agents that appear to have some activity in advanced ovarian cancer after adequate testing include ifosfamide,[189-191] AZQ,[190] VP-16 (etoposide),[192,193] Peptichemio,[194] and low-dose mitomycin C.[195] Table 37-10 summarizes the activity of potentially important single agents in ovarian cancer.

Hormone Therapy

Although the ovary is the principal source of estrogen in women, the extent to which hormones regulate the ovarian epithelium is unclear. With the demonstration of the presence of both estrogen and progesterone receptors in approximately half of all ovarian carcinomas,[196-198] hormone treatment of the disease has been actively investigated. Initial reports of activity for megestrol (Megase),[199] medroxyprogesterone (MPA),[200,201] and tamoxifen[202,203] have been followed by larger studies with less-impressive results. One recent trial of MPA in 41 patients resulted in one partial response,[204] and two recent trials of tamoxifen have demonstrated no responses in 22[205] and 23[206] patients.

One recent study attempted to induce progesterone receptors by sequencing estradiol with MPA. Sixty-five patients were treated in two different dose schedules, and the overall response rate was 14%.[207] Although the toxicity of these agents is low, the activity appears to be extremely modest.

In Vitro Clonogenic Assays in Ovarian Cancer

For many years, attempts have been made to define the activity of potentially useful chemotherapeutic agents using a variety of in vitro screening techniques. These have not been particularly successful. An in vitro tumor colony assay that evaluates clonogenic potential after exposure to chemotherapy has been used in a variety of tumors and has received considerable study in ovarian carcinoma.[208] Unfortunately, subsequent larger studies with ovarian cancer, as well as other solid tumors, have highlighted serious shortcomings of the human tumor clonogenic assay.[209] The technical limitations of the assay include difficulty in preparation of single-cell suspensions, lack of optimum growth conditions for specific tumor types, and persistence of nonclonogenic clumps of tumor cells. In addition, it is unclear whether the assay is predictive for a specific drug or merely identifies those patients whose tumors are more generally responsive to chemotherapy. These technical limitations, coupled with the absence of sufficient numbers of active drugs for relapsed ovarian cancer patients and the short duration of response in relapsed patients, make the assay an experimental tool, not a clinically proven means for selection of chemotherapy.

Combination Chemotherapy

Combination chemotherapy in advanced ovarian cancer has been extensively studied over the past decade. From these

TABLE 37-10. Single Agents Active in Advanced Ovarian Adenocarcinoma

Drugs	No. of Patients	Percent Response (% CR)
Alkylating agents		
Melphalan	494	47 (20)
Chlorambucil	280	50
Thiotepa	144	65
Cyclophosphamide	126	49
Mechlorethamine	81	35
Ifosfamide	61	78
AZQ	26	15
Antimetabolites		
5-Fluorouracil	81	32 (18–20)
	21	33
Methotrexate	16	25
	23	13
Antitumor antibiotics		
Doxorubicin (Adriamycin)	18	28
	33	36
Mitomycin C	43	23
Plant Alkaloids		
Vinblastine	16	13
VP-16	22	32
Miscellaneous		
Hexamethylmelamine	53	41
Cisplatin	34	27
Carboplatin	22	50 (17)
Dianhydrogalacticol	39	15
Peptichemio	47	24 (14)

studies, important prognostic factors such as stage, histologic grade, and extent of residual disease have been well defined; the majority of trials now either stratify for important prognostic factors or at least analyze trials by these factors.[175] Nevertheless, response rates have varied from 20% to 90%, with CR rates ranging from 10% to 65% depending on the types of patients included and the criteria used for assessing response. The great variation in patient selection, prognostic factors, and response criteria makes it difficult, if not impossible, to compare many of these studies. Furthermore, in many of the studies, the differences in patient characteristics may have a more important influence on survival than the therapies being reported. In general, the recently published studies can be divided into three major groups: those comparing single agents with combinations, salvage chemotherapy studies on patients who have failed previous therapy, and studies on previously untreated patients.

SINGLE AGENTS VERSUS COMBINATION CHEMOTHERAPY. The first study to demonstrate significantly improved survival with any combination in a prospective comparison with a standard alkylating agent was published in 1978.[210] Eighty previously untreated patients were randomized to receive either melphalan in conventional doses, or Hexa-CAF (hexamethylmelamine, cyclophosphamide, methotrexate, and 5-fluorouracil [5-FU]). Treatment with the four-drug combination achieved a significantly higher overall response rate (75% versus 54%; p < 0.05), more complete remissions (33% versus 16%; p = 0.06), and significantly longer median survival (29 months versus 17 months; p < 0.02). However, Hexa-CAF was most effective in patients with small amounts of residual disease, in whom a

higher overall response rate was achieved than in patients with extensive residual disease (84% versus 53%; p < 0.05). Important stratification factors, such as the extent of residual disease and histologic grade, as well as age, stage, and histologic type, were well balanced in the two groups. Careful definition of CR using peritoneoscopy or second-look laparotomy was utilized. Patients achieving CR, documented by restaging, had a long survival: 60% of these women were alive more than 4 years later. The toxicity of the combination was greater than that of the single agent, primarily because of greater hematologic toxicity, along with nausea, vomiting, and alopecia.

Dutch investigators confirmed the activity of the Hexa-CAF combination in previously untreated patients (overall response rate 57% with 30% CR)[211] but also demonstrated that in previously treated patients, Hexa-CAF has a much lower overall response rate (3 of 13 with no CR) and increased toxicity. Their study emphasizes the marked reduction of activity of any regimen used as second-line therapy in advanced ovarian cancer and, in addition, illustrates the futility of beginning therapy with an alkylating agent, then later attempting to salvage relapsing patients with more aggressive combination chemotherapy.

Subsequently, a series of randomized trials comparing single-agent chemotherapy (generally alkylating agents) with combination chemotherapy have been published. Generally, these trials either show improved response rates, improved disease-free or overall survival, or all three (Table 37-11).[212-218] In addition to the Hexa-CAF study, two other prospective randomized trials have demonstrated better survival. The first was a multi-institutional Swedish study. Trope and co-workers compared melphalan plus Adriamycin

TABLE 37-11.   Combination Chemotherapy Versus Single Agents in Advanced Previously Untreated Ovarian Carcinoma

Regimen*	Results	Reference
Clinical Trials Demonstrating Increased CR Rates and/or Disease-Free Survival		
CHAD vs. LPAM	38% CR vs. 21% CR: progression-free survival increased for CHAD	212
CHF vs. LPAM	85% RR vs. 57% RR; 50% CR vs. 17% CR	213
AC vs. C	Improved progression-free survival with AC in patients with minimal residual disease	214
PAC vs. CLB	RR: 68% vs. 26%, p = 0.0004 PCR: 26% vs. 15%	215
Clinical Trials Demonstrating Improved Survival		
Hexa-CAF vs. LPAM	75% RR vs. 43%; 33% CR vs. 16%; median survival, 29 mo. vs. 17 mo.	210
A + LPAM vs. LPAM	67% RR vs. 40%; 23+ mo. vs. 8.1 mo. for duration of response; median survival, 17 mo. vs. 11 mo.	217
CP vs. C	2-year disease-free interval: 52% vs. 10%; 2-year survival: 62% vs. 19%	218

*CHAD = cyclophosphamide, hexamethylmelamine, Adriamycin, cisplatin; LPAM = melphalan; CHF = cyclophosphamide, hexamethylmelamine, 5-fluorouracil; AC = Adriamycin, cyclophosphamide; C = cyclophosphamide; PAC = cisplatin, Adriamycin, cyclophosphamide; CLB = chlorambucil; Hexa-CAF = hexamethylmelamine, cyclophosphamide, methotrexate, 5-fluorouracil; CP = cyclophosphamide, cisplatin.

with melphalan alone in 142 patients with bulky Stage III or Stage IV disease.[217] The combination was superior to the single agent in overall response rate (63% versus 40%; p < 0.01), duration of response (23+ months versus 8.1 months; p < 0.001), and overall median survival (16.8+ months versus 10.7 months; p < 0.03). The second study was a Mayo Clinic trial[218] of 41 patients and showed a 2-year survival rate of 52% for cyclophosphamide and cisplatin compared with 19% for cyclophosphamide alone. The projected median survivals were 40 months and 16 months, respectively.

These trials provide substantial evidence for the increased effectiveness of combinations compared with single agents in this disease. Other studies have not shown such benefit,[216,219,220] but patient compliance and substantial dose modifications may have played a significant role in the results of these negative studies. One recent example is a large cooperative trial in Australia and New Zealand that compared oral chlorambucil with cisplatin at relapse with the combination of chlorambucil and cisplatin.[215] Response rates (53% versus 51%) and median survival (16 versus 17 months) were similar. However, only 57% of patients on combination chemotherapy had any significant myelosuppression, and even fewer (25%) did on the sequential treatment, yet the authors demonstrated that myelosuppression had an important favorable effect on survival. The relatively poor survival for both arms of the trial (similar to that achieved with single alkylating agents alone) and the authors' demonstrated positive effect of myelosuppression on subsequent survival illustrate the problem with this and similar trials. One is likely to demonstrate equivalence of single agents and combinations if the trial is designed with insufficient dose intensity of the drugs used in combination.

Several recent trials have also utilized maintenance alkylating agent therapy for several years.[215,221] These trials have failed to show a benefit for such maintenance and have reported leukemias in long-term survivors. In light of the dangers of long-term alkylating agent therapy[222,223] and in the absence of demonstrated benefit, this approach should be abandoned.

Several general conclusions emerge from these prospective randomized trials. Combination chemotherapy continues to provide higher overall response rates and higher CR rates than single agents, although in some studies survival time is not altered significantly. Nevertheless, long-term disease-free survivors, although uncommon, are more frequent with combinations, particularly when the dose intensity is adequate. Several newer combinations may be more effective than those originally used in the prospective comparisons with single alkylating agents.

At present, it would appear that the best chance for achieving a complete remission in advanced ovarian carcinoma exists when the initial therapy is an effective combination used in full therapeutic doses.

COMBINATION CHEMOTHERAPY AFTER ALKYLATING AGENT FAILURE. Many investigators have used combination chemotherapy after the tumor has failed to respond to initial single-agent therapy. Details of these regimens are presented in the original publications, in recent reviews,[224-227] and in Table 37-12. Unfortunately, none of these trials really established any regimen as particularly successful in managing chemotherapy failures. In spite of the high overall response reported for many of these combinations, the number of patients in the studies is small, and the majority of the responses are partial and of short duration (4-6 months). Moreover, the toxicity, when reported, appears to be substantial. Very few of these patients, regardless of the regimen, are alive at 1 year.

Two recent studies suggest some activity for VP-16 and

TABLE 37-12. Combination Chemotherapy After Alkylating Agent Failure

Regimen*	No. of Patients	CR + Pr (%)	Survival of Responders (mo)	Reference
ADR/CDDP	20	42	NS	228
	43	36	7	229
	20	25	7.2	230
ADR/CDDP/5-FU	103	48	12	231
CTX/HEX/ADR/CDDP	35	49	NS	232
	21	49	15	233
HEX/ADR/CDDP	27	41	7.5	234
	21	19	5.3	230
CTX/MTX/CF ± VCR	55	30	7.5	235
HEX/CDDP	38	55	10.8	236
	10	20	NS	237
VP-16/CDDP	10	50	NS	238
	25	40	NS	239

* ADR = Adriamycin; CDDP = cisplatin; 5-FU = 5-fluorouracil; HEX = hexamethylmelamine; CTX = cyclophosphamide; VCR = vincristine; MTX = methotrexate; CF = citrovorum factor; NS = not stated.

cisplatin regimens, although only a small number of patients were treated.[238,239] With the currently available drugs and regimens, combination chemotherapy used after the initial treatment fails is not likely to improve the cure rate in this disease but can, at present, be thought of as a way to identify interesting regimens for primary therapy of the untreated patient.

COMBINATION CHEMOTHERAPY AS INITIAL TREATMENT. Many studies have now been published of combination chemotherapy as the initial treatment in advanced disease. These studies have either been single-arm studies or randomized trials in which two or more combinations have been compared. A summary of a representative group of the single-arm trials is shown in Table 37-13. Most of these

TABLE 37-13. Combination Chemotherapy in Advanced Ovarian Carcinoma

Regimen	Schedule	No. of Evaluable Patients	Complete and Partial Remissions (%)	No. of Clinical CR (%)	No. of Pathologic CR (%)
PAC[240]		56	44/56 (79)	23/56 (41)	10/56 (18)
Cisplatin	20 mg/m² IV day × 5 q 4 wk				
Adriamycin	50 mg/m² IV day 1 q 4 wk				
Cyclophosphamide	750 mg/m² IV day 1 q 4 wk				
A-C (Dana Farber)[241]		41	35/41 (83)	20/41 (48)	12/41 (29)
Cyclophosphamide	500 mg/m² IV				
Adriamycin	40 mg/m²				
Hexa-CAF (NCI)[210]		40	30/40 (75)		13/40 (33)
Hexamethylmelamine	150 mg/m² PO qd × 14				
Cyclophosphamide	150 mg/m² PO qd × 14				
Methotrexate	40 mg/m² IV days 1,8				
5-Fluorouracil	600 mg/m² IV days 1,8				
CHAD[114]		46	45/46 (98)	35/46 (76)	14/46 (30)
Cyclophosphamide	600 mg/m² IV day 1				
Hexamethylmelamine	200 mg/m² PO days 8–22				
Adriamycin	25 mg/m² IV day 1				
Cisplatin	50 mg/m² IV day 1				
CHEX-UP[171]		62	43/62 (69)	29/62 (47)	12/62 (19)
Cyclophosphamide	150 mg/m² PO days 2–8 and 2–16				
Hexamethylmelamine	150 mg/m² PO days 2–8 and 9–16				
5-Fluorouracil	600 mg/m² IV days 1 and 8				
Cisplatin	30 mg/m² IV days 1 and 8				
CHAP-5[244]		84	66/84 (79)	Not Stated	25/84 (30)
Cyclophosphamide	100 mg/m² PO days 15–29				
Hexamethylmelamine	150 mg/m² PO days 15–29				
Adriamycin	35 mg/m² IV day 1				
Cisplatin	20 mg/m² IV days 1–5				
PC[243]		52	Not Stated	Not Stated	12/52 (23)
Cisplatin	20 mg/m² IV days 1–5				
Cyclophosphamide	600 mg/m² IV day 4				

studies now contain sufficient information about prognostic factors, response duration, and survival to allow realistic comparisons with currently established combination chemotherapy regimens or single agents.

Several groups have reported results of two-, three-, and four-drug combinations in nonrandomized studies in previously untreated Stage III and Stage IV disease. Most of these trials have used combinations of cisplatin, Adriamycin, cyclophosphamide, hexamethylmelamine, methotrexate, or 5-FU.[114,171,210,240–245] The overall response rates have been 60% to 80%, with clinical CR in approximately 40% to 50% of patients. Approximately half of those clinically free of disease actually have residual disease at second-look laparotomy. As a result, about 25% to 30% of all patients treated with combination chemotherapy will be free of disease at restaging, and it is this subset of patients who experience long-term disease-free survival. At present, there does not seem to be a striking difference between combinations, although the addition of cisplatin appears beneficial. Randomized trials between platinum-containing combinations have generally demonstrated equivalent results in terms of survival (see Table 37-14).

Recently, several well-designed trials have been performed of various combination regimens in an attempt to define the relative contributions of individual drugs as well as the combinations themselves. Several of the more significant studies are summarized in Table 37-14.

Dutch investigators compared CHAP-5 (cyclophosphamide, hexamethylmelamine, Adriamycin, and cisplatin) with Hexa-CAF and demonstrated a statistically greater response rate (79% versus 50%) and CR rate (30% versus 17%) as well as an improved disease-free survival (19.5 versus 6.8 months) and improved overall survival (30.7 versus 19.6 months) for the CHAP-5 combination.[244] The GOG compared Adriamycin and cyclophosphamide (AC) with cisplatin, Adriamycin, and cyclophosphamide (PAC) in 227 patients with measurable disease.[246] The CR rate was 51% for CAP and 26% for AC (p < 0.0001). The progression-free interval (13 versus 7.7 months) and overall survival (19.7 versus 15.7 months) were also statistically better with the cisplatin-containing combination.

These trials provide substantial evidence of the importance of platinum in any ovarian cancer regimen. Indeed, it is not clear whether the addition of other agents to regimens that include full-dose intensities of cyclophosphamide and cisplatin is necessary or beneficial. The Netherlands Cancer Institute recently completed a large trial comparing CHAP-5 with cyclophosphamide and cisplatin (CP). The overall response rate (78% versus 76%) and the pathologically documented CR rate (34% versus 37%) were similar for the two regimens.[246] A study from the Mayo Clinic compared CP with hexamethylmelamine, cyclophosphamide, Adriamycin, and cisplatin (HCAP) in 181 patients.[247] At a median follow-up of 30 months, the regimens produced identical survivals (24.6 months). A similar experience was seen in the preliminary analysis of a GOG trial comparing CAP with CP.[248] In this trial, the numbers of negative second looks (39% versus 38%) were similar, as were the times to disease progression and survival for the two arms.

Two studies comparing CP with CAP have come to somewhat different conclusions. A study by Conte et al[249] compared CP and PAC in 125 patients, including some with localized as well as those with advanced disease. The objective response rates were similar for the two groups (54% versus 56%), but the PAC regimen induced a higher percentage of CRs (41% versus 20%) in patients with measurable disease and there were more surgically documented CRs (62% versus 40%). However, progression-free interval and survival were not statistically different. The second trial[250] compared CP and PAC in 154 patients with advanced disease. The CR rate favored PAC (24% versus 11%), and at 3 years' follow-up there was a better survival rate in the PAC-treated group (48% versus 20%).

On the basis of the available data, there is very little evidence that any combination regimen produces better results than the two-drug CP regimen used in full therapeutic doses.

Late Complications of Chemotherapy

As therapy for advanced ovarian cancer improves, a variety of late complications are being observed that are related either to the treatment or to the altered natural history of the disease. Late relapses with unusual lesions such as bone metastases or central nervous system involvement have now

TABLE 37-14.   Randomized Comparisons of Combination Chemotherapy in Advanced Ovarian Adenocarcinoma

Study	Results	Reference
CHAP-5 vs. Hexa-CAF	79% RR vs. 50%; 30% CR vs. 17%; median survival, 31 mo. vs. 20 mo.	244
PAC vs. AC	51% CR vs. 26% in patients with measurable disease. Response duration (15 mo. vs. 19 mo.), progression-free interval (13 mo. vs. 7 mo.), and overall survival (20 mo. vs. 16 mo.) all statistically significant	245
CHAP-5 vs. CP	78% RR vs. 76%. PCR 34% vs. 37% and no differences in survival	246
HCAP vs. CP	Survival at 30 months equivalent for the two regimens (24.6 mo.)	247
PAC vs. PC	41% clinical CR vs. 20% CR; in those patients going to second-look, significant increase in PCR for PAC (62% vs. 40%, p < 0.05). No difference in overall survival	249
PAC vs. CP	CR 24% vs. 11% (p < 0.05); at 3 yrs more PAC survivors (48% vs. 20%)	250

been reported.[251] Acute leukemia as a late complication of therapy has been reported in several studies. A published survey of 70 institutions with 5455 patients revealed 13 patients who developed leukemia, representing a 21-fold increase in risk.[222] Risks were highest in patients who had chemotherapy in excess of 2 years, and approximately two-thirds of the patients with leukemia had received radiation as well. Often, a long period of pancytopenia preceded frank leukemic transformation. Two-thirds of the leukemic patients who died had no evidence of ovarian cancer at autopsy. Similar results have been published in an analysis of 1399 women in five randomized trials in which the cumulative risk of acute nonlymphocytic leukemia was 9.6% at 7 years.[223] Nevertheless, it is important to emphasize that the overall risk of acute leukemia is small (0.3%).[222] However, techniques for minimizing the risk, such as cyclic intermittent chemotherapy rather than continuous daily treatment, avoidance of combined radiation–chemotherapy treatments, no maintenance alkylating-agent therapy, and better techniques for defining the CRs so that therapy can be discontinued, will undoubtedly be helpful.

Experimental Approaches

IMMUNOTHERAPY. Immunotherapy has been investigated in only a few studies, although a good theoretical basis for immunotherapy exists, including (1) the existence of tumor-associated antigens in ovarian cancer; (2) circulating lymphocytes that are reactive to the patient's tumor cells; (3) defects in B-cell function in patients with advanced ovarian cancer, although T-cell function appears intact; and (4) animal models of ovarian cancer that demonstrate enhanced tumor killing with chemotherapy and either nonspecific immunotherapy or specific antibodies generated against ovarian tumor cells.[252,253] Most studies have used nonspecific immunotherapy with chemotherapy. However, trials with intraperitoneal *Corynebacterium parvum*[255,256] interferon,[254] and melphalan–levamisole[257] have been reported.

Nonspecific immunotherapy in conjunction with chemotherapy has shown activity in two randomized studies in ovarian carcinoma,[258,259] and, although the independent contribution of immunotherapy to the therapeutic result is not completely clear, these studies are provocative. Further prospective studies with careful stratification of known prognostic factors will be required to define the role, if any, of this modality in advanced ovarian cancer.

Recently, studies have been done utilizing intraperitoneal IL-2 with or without lymphokine-activated killer (LAK) cells.[253,260] Some reduction in the systemic toxicity of this therapy is achieved when the biologicals are administered intraperitoneally, and objective regressions in ovarian cancer patients have been seen.[260] Unfortunately, at present, the therapy is associated with abdominal pseudocyst formation, which limits its effectiveness.

Several murine monoclonal antibodies have been generated against ovarian cancer specifically or are cross-reactive with ovarian cancer cell lines. Because for the most part these murine antibodies lack intrinsic cytotoxicity, they have been coupled to toxic moieties such as radioisotopes, chemotherapeutic agents, or natural toxins such as ricin or *Pseudomonas* exotoxin.[261,262] Preliminary results in cell lines in vitro and in a nude mouse model of human ovarian cancer[256] are encouraging, and these and other monoclonal antibodies are now entering clinical trial.[253]

DRUG RESISTANCE. The effectiveness of drug therapy in this disease is limited by the development of drug resistance. This resistance not only is drug–specific but also is frequently associated with a broad cross-resistance to structurally dissimilar drugs. Such pleiotropic resistance may be the result of presence of the *MDR*-1 gene with its protein product, the P-170 glycoprotein,[263,264] which enables the drug-resistant tumor to limit accumulation of structurally unrelated agents.[265-268] This cross-resistance is most frequently seen with natural products such as the vinca alkaloids, Adriamycin, and VP-16. Although this mechanism appears to be important in certain other tumors, it does not seem to be the primary mechanism of broad cross-resistance in ovarian cancer. Other mechanisms of resistance include the elevation of intracellular glutathione (GSH)[269] and increased DNA repair.[270]

Potential approaches to overcoming these mechanisms of drug resistance are now being explored. Certain calcium-channel blockers can overcome resistance associated with decreased drug accumulation. For example, verapamil reverses Adriamycin resistance in ovarian carcinoma cell lines[271] by blocking drug efflux. A pilot clinical trial has been completed;[272] levels of verapamil adequate for clinical effect could not be reached without unacceptable cardiac toxicity. Other calcium-channel blockers are now under study.

GSH is a tripeptide thiol found ubiquitously in human cells. Drug resistance in ovarian cancer cells is associated with a marked increase in intracellular GSH.[273,274] Buthionine sulfoximine (BSO), a synthetic amino acid analogue, inhibits the synthesis of GSH and markedly reduces intracellular GSH in vitro and in vivo.[277,278] This change is associated with a restoration of drug sensitivity in cell lines and a prolongation of survival in the in vivo nude mouse model of ovarian cancer. BSO has recently been approved for clinical trials in the salvage therapy of ovarian cancer.

It has also been demonstrated that drug resistance in ovarian cancer is associated with increased DNA repair after both chemotherapeutic or radiotherapeutic injury.[277] Aphidicolin, a potent inhibitor of α and β polymerase, can block this DNA repair and thus partially restore drug sensitivity in these resistant cell lines.[270] This approach may be applicable clinically.

These studies, taken as a whole, indicate that drug resistance in ovarian cancer is an interaction of multiple factors and that a single explanation of drug resistance is not likely. Nevertheless, there are now clinical trials under way to test a variety of ways in which resistance can be overcome.

RESULTS OF TREATMENT

Historically, the treatment of ovarian cancer has been discussed in the context of FIGO stage; that is, separating early disease (FIGO Stage I and Stage II) from advanced disease (FIGO Stage III and Stage IV). However, recent analyses of long-term survival results from several major institutions indicate that other patient- and tumor-related characteristics are extremely important. In addition to FIGO stage, the most important prognostic variables are tumor residuum, grade, histologic subtype, and the age of the patient at diagnosis.[49,60,154,278-281] A multivariate analysis of these variables in 430 ovarian carcinoma patients demonstrates that residual disease and tumor grade are the most important (p < 0.001) followed by stage (p = 0.002), age (p = 0.004), and histologic type (p = 0.058).[60] Thus, it appears that tumor residuum and stage are independent variables and that tumor residuum is significantly more powerful in predicting the therapeutic outcome than is the FIGO stage. This finding is now reflected in the change in the FIGO stage classification for advanced disease, as discussed earlier in this chapter.

That the amount of tumor remaining after initial surgery affects the final results of treatment has been known for years.[60,98,278] It is now common to describe three prognostically distinct subgroups based on early disease (Stages I and II) and the presence or absence of large postsurgical residual disease (usually > 2 cm). Patients with small amounts of residual disease stand a good chance of disease eradication by postoperative therapy and have the highest probability of long-term survival. For these reasons, it seems justified to discuss the treatment of three groups of patients separately: (1) those with early (FIGO Stages I and II) cancer and microscopic or no residual disease; (2) those with advanced disease but minimal residua (< 2 cm) after initial surgery; and (3) those more-frequent patients with bulky residual tumor and advanced (Stage III or IV) disease.

EARLY OVARIAN CANCER (FIGO STAGES I AND II) WITH MICROSCOPIC OR NO RESIDUAL DISEASE

The surgical management of Stage I ovarian cancer is influenced by the histologic type and grade of the tumor as well as by the reproductive desires of the patient. Although certain types of epithelial ovarian cancer are more likely than others to present at an early stage, there is probably little difference in either survival or recommended surgical management of these carcinomas when matched for stage and grade. Scully[43,47] summarized three series in which cancer was confined to a single ovary and reported a 78% survival rate with conservative surgical treatment and a 79% rate with radical therapy. Munnell[20] reported a 75% survival rate in two similar groups of patients, and Webb et al[283] reported 90% survival in patients with Stage I tumors with intact capsules and 57% survival when the tumor had penetrated the capsule or ruptured.

From these studies, it would appear that patients with epithelial cancer confined to one ovary with an otherwise-negative comprehensive surgical exploration can be managed by unilateral salpingo-oophorectomy and no further therapy providing the tumor is Grade 1 or 2 and the patient wants to have children. In patients who undergo conservative (unilateral salpingo-oophorectomy) therapy, the opposite ovary should be biopsied. In patients with Grade 3 tumors or those who do not desire to have children, a total abdominal hysterectomy and bilateral salpingo-oophorectomy should be performed.

A series of studies have attempted to define whether well-staged patients with IA and IB, well- or moderately well-differentiated tumors require further therapy. Dembo and associates[59] studied a group of 54 patients with Stage IA disease who were randomized between observation or pelvic radiotherapy after initial surgery. There were nine relapses among 30 patients with moderately or poorly differentiated tumors compared with none among 24 patients with well-differentiated tumors regardless of whether pelvic radiation was given. Similarly, the GOG[284,285] reported only one relapse among 56 patients with Stage IA–IB well- or moderately differentiated tumors randomized to receive either melphalan or no treatment postoperatively. On the basis of these observations, it has been suggested that patients with well-differentiated Stage I tumors who are without positive peritoneal cytology, densely adherent tumors, or cyst rupture do not require postoperative therapy.[142,284,285]

For patients with Stage II disease or with Stage I disease with incomplete surgical staging or poor prognostic findings, more aggressive management is required. Stage II epithelial ovarian carcinoma requires total abdominal hysterectomy, bilateral salpingo-oophorectomy, and a full staging operation in all cases. Particular care must be exercised to ensure that the carcinoma has not spread to the upper abdomen. Every effort should be made to remove all visible tumor in the pelvis utilizing techniques involving retroperitoneal approaches if necessary. If microscopic or small macroscopic residual disease remains, then adjuvant therapy is generally employed, and the management is similar to that used for patients with advanced stages and small residua.

The GOG, in an early trial, studied patients with Stage IA and IB epithelial ovarian cancer (staged in a conventional manner) and compared no additional therapy, pelvic irradiation, or intermittent oral melphalan.[284] Forty-nine percent of patients were not evaluable, and the three treatment arms were not well balanced for prognostic variables. The frequency of relapse was greatest after pelvic irradiation: 7 of 23 (30%) compared with observation (5 of 29; 17%) and intermittent oral melphalan (2 of 34; 6%), although there were no significant differences in overall survival. In subsequent trials that required careful surgical staging prior to entry, the Ovarian Cancer Study Group–GOG studied two groups of patients with early disease. The first, which was mentioned earlier, studied patients with good-prognosis Stage I disease; the second included patients with IC, IIA,B,C, and poor-prognosis Stage I disease and compared melphalan with intraperitoneal ^{32}p. Follow-up on this study is not complete, but the 5-year disease-free survival rate of both treatment approaches is good ($\cong$ 80%).[285] A replacement trial has been initiated in the same patient population comparing intraperitoneal ^{32}p with three courses of cyclophosphamide–cisplatin. Because radiocolloids are transported to the diaphragm and concentrated there,[167,286] this treatment technique delivers high-dose radiation to the diaphragm, perhaps explaining the improved survival rate observed in patients receiving intraperitoneal radioactive colloids.

PATIENTS WITH POOR-PROGNOSIS STAGE I AND STAGES II–IV WITH LITTLE OR NO RESIDUAL DISEASE POSTOPERATIVELY

Patients in this category include most of those with poor-prognosis Stage I or II disease and 20% to 30% of those with Stage III disease who are left without gross tumor after initial

surgery. Current evidence indicates that these patients require postoperative therapy, although it is not clear what
form of therapy is optimal.

One approach has been to use postoperative irradiation,
with doses of 4500 to 5000 cGy given to the pelvis and 2250
to 3000 cGy to the upper abdomen. Previous studies indicate
that whole-abdominal radiation is necessary. Bush[287] showed
that 4500 cGy given to the pelvis reduced the number of
pelvic recurrences in Stage I disease, but the overall risk of
relapse did not decrease, as most of the irradiated patients
relapsed in the upper abdomen. Similarly, Schray and associates[138] reported that 14 of 19 Stage I and II patients treated
with high-dose lower-abdominal irradiation relapsed in the
upper abdomen. Irradiation of the upper abdomen will decrease the risk of relapse there and improve survival. The
Princess Margaret Group studied patients with Stage IB, II, or
IIIA ovarian carcinoma who were randomized to receive pelvic radiation, pelvic radiation plus oral chlorambucil for 2
years, or pelvic and upper-abdominal radiation.[140,141] In 8 of
31 patients treated with radiation to the pelvis only, upper-
abdominal relapses without concomitant pelvic relapses
were observed, compared with none in patients receiving
whole-abdominal irradiation.[141] The 5-year survival rate for
patients with whole-abdominal irradiation was 78% compared with 51% in the patients receiving pelvic radiation
with or without chlorambucil.[287] Similarly, Delclos and
Smith[143] reported that only 17% of 18 Stage II patients irradiated to the pelvis alone survived at 5 years compared with
49% of 71 patients treated with whole-abdominal irradiation.
From these data, it is generally accepted that whole-abdominal radiotherapy is the optimal technique for this group of
patients.

Chemotherapy has also been used in this group of patients,
and the data suggest that results are similar to those observed
with external-beam radiotherapy. The M.D. Anderson group
studied patients with Stages I–IIIA and small amounts of
residual disease, comparing single-agent melphalan with
total-abdominal irradiation by moving strip in a slightly different dose and schedule than that used by the Princess
Margaret group.[288,289] The 2- and 5-year survival rates for the
groups were 86.5% and 71.5% for radiation and 90% and
78% for melphalan. Furthermore, now with 10 years' follow-up, there are still no differences in survival rates in the
two groups.[290] The M.D. Anderson group concluded that
chemotherapy is as effective as irradiation, has fewer serious
side-effects, and is less expensive.

In contrast, the Radiumhemmet Group randomized patients with Stage I or Stage IIA seropapillary ovarian carcinoma to adjuvant postsurgical treatment with either lower-
abdominal radiation, single alkylating-agent chemotherapy,
or radiotherapy followed by chemotherapy.[291] The lowest
5-year survival rate was observed in patients treated with
chemotherapy alone (68%) compared with 88% in the radiation alone group and 91% in the combined radiation–
chemotherapy group.

Many of these early studies did not require comprehensive
surgical staging before therapy. When systematic restaging
is performed prospectively in such patients, 31% are found
to have a more advanced stage, and 77% actually have Stage
III disease.[282] Thus, it is clear that a significant reason why
local treatment fails in many patients with apparently local-

ized disease is that they have unsuspected extrapelvic metastases that are not being treated by surgery or pelvic
irradiation.

Although both radiation and chemotherapy are effective
against small (< 2 cm) ovarian tumors, resulting in high
rates of clinical and pathologic CR, the cure rates for patients with residual tumor after initial surgery have been less
favorable than those in patients with no residual tumor.[142,154]
Whole-abdominal irradiation has frequently been employed
in such patients with doses of 5000 to 6000 cGy to the lower
abdomen and 3000 to 4000 cGy to the upper abdomen.
Using radiotherapy, Dembo[142] reported a 58% 5-year survival rate in 36 patients with Stage II disease and a 43% rate
in 55 patients with Stage III disease left with small residual
tumors after initial surgery. Martinez et al[154] reported a 54%
5-year survival rate in 42 similar patients with Stage II or III
disease.

Combination chemotherapy has been used in similar
groups of patients. The initial response rates are high, and
the pathologically confirmed complete remission rates are
about 56% (Table 37-15). These patients generally experience long survival. The M.D. Anderson Group reported 34%
4-year survival rate in 83 patients treated with a variety of
single-agent chemotherapies (melphalan, 5-FU, Adriamycin, cisplatin, hexamethylmelamine) and 51% in 66 patients
treated with various combinations (HAC, HMM-CYT, MEL-
DDP).[293,294] Lambert and Berry[177] reported a 35% 4-year
survival rate in 42 patients treated with high-dose cyclophosphamide or high-dose cisplatin, and Belinson and associates[293] reported a 53% survival rate in 21 patients treated
with CAP. These survival rates are generally similar to those
observed with total-abdominal radiation.

The frequency of surgically confirmed CRs is approximately half the clinical CR rate but is heavily dependent on
the volume of disease at initial therapy. The effect of extent
of residual disease on the frequency of a pathologic CR is
shown in Table 37-15.

Generally, patients who have negative second-look laparotomies after combination chemotherapy experience long
survival, although this varies from institution to institution.[295] Greco et al[296,297] reported a 74% 4-year disease-free
survival rate in patients with negative second-look operations postchemotherapy. The NCI experience is similar:
among patients treated with CHEX-UP, 63% of the patients
with pathologically documented CR are alive without relapse

TABLE 37-15. Effect of Residual Disease on Pathologic
Complete Remission Rate

Chemotherapy	Surgically Confirmed Complete Remissions (%)	
	<3 cm Residua	>3 cm Residua
Hexa-CAF[210]	8/8 (100)	5/32 (16)
CHEX-UP[242]	5/14 (36)	5/37 (14)
H-CAP[247]	18/21 (86)	3/29 (11)
A-C[241]	11/12 (92)	1/24 (4)
PAC[240]	5/17 (30)	5/39 (13)
PAC/Hexa-CAF[292]	6/22 (27)	1/17 (6)
Total	53/94 (56)	20/178 (11)

at 5 years.[242] In contrast, studies from Memorial Hospital on survival of patients with negative second-look operations project a 65% relapse rate by 48 months.[298] In a 7-year follow-up of patients treated with PAC, only three of eight were alive without recurrence 7 to 8 years after treatment.[240] It is not clear why there are significant differences from institution to institution in the survival of patients with negative second-look operations postchemotherapy.

PATIENTS WITH STAGES II–IV AND BULKY RESIDUAL DISEASE

Unfortunately, most patients with Stage III disease and some with Stage II disease are left with extensive residual disease after initial surgery. These patients respond poorly to conventional therapies of all types, and the major challenge for the future lies in the development of successful management approaches for this large group of women.

In recent years, the mainstay of therapy for this group has been systemic chemotherapy; however, some patients with unique presentations may be appropriately treated with radiation. It is worthwhile to separate patients with gross abdominal tumor from those with only retroperitoneal lymph node metastases, because the latter group may have a different prognosis when given appropriate irradiation. Hintz and colleagues noted that patients with retroperitoneal lymph nodes as the only site of extrapelvic disease have a survival rate of about 55% at 5 years, in contrast to 10% for patients with peritoneal spread.[299]

In contrast, the prognosis of patients with gross abdominal tumors exceeding 2 cm in diameter has been poor with whole-abdominal irradiation. Even when aggressive radiotherapeutic approaches were used, with radiation to the whole peritoneal cavity at maximal tolerable doses, the 5-year survival rates were only 9% to 12%.[96,301,302] Further, the tolerance of treatment in these patients generally has been extremely poor. Additional treatment with single alkylating-agent chemotherapy, given either before or after radiotherapy,[300,303–306] usually failed to improve survival and was even less well tolerated. Therefore, it has been generally accepted that postoperative whole-abdominal irradiation given as the primary modality with curative intent is not indicated for patients with large (> 2 cm) abdominal tumors unless effective cytoreductive surgery can be performed before radiotherapy, leaving the peritoneal cavity either without gross disease or with little (< 2 cm) residual disease.

The lack of satisfactory cure rates with either radiation or combination chemotherapy in patients with bulky disease, and the frequent inability to cytoreduce the tumors at the initial laparotomy, have led to the introduction of combined-modality therapy. Combination chemotherapy is highly effective in debulking such tumors, resulting in 80% to 90% significant clinical responses. If second-look surgery is performed, the residual tumors are often small, and their complete or nearly complete resection can frequently be achieved. The elimination of this minimal residual disease after induction therapy has been under intensive study.[307]

Fuks et al[308] gave 38 patients initial induction therapy using 3 to 14 courses of the CHAD combination for tumor mass reduction and a second laparotomy for resection of residual tumors, followed by a consolidation phase with curative doses of whole-abdominal irradiation. The initial clinical response (CR and partial response) to CHAD was 91%. After second-look surgery, 76% of patients were without residual disease. Whole-abdominal irradiation using the Martinez technique was then given. The actuarial 5-year survival and disease-free survival rates for the whole group were 27% and 17%, respectively. These survival data are similar to those of patients treated with CHAP-5 combination chemotherapy without subsequent whole-abdominal irradiation,[246,309] suggesting that the consolidation radiotherapy had little if any effect on the survival probability already achieved by chemotherapy.

This observation is consistent with other recent reports. Hacker et al[292] treated 30 patients with a variety of combination-chemotherapy protocols, followed by a second surgical tumor reduction and whole-abdominal radiotherapy. Only 4 of 16 patients with completely resected tumors during the second laparotomy survived 22 to 41 months after radiotherapy. Hainsworth and associates,[297] using a similar approach after H-CHAP or H-FAP combination chemotherapy, found that 14 of 17 patients relapsed between 2 and 20 months after completion of radiotherapy. Coltart et al[310] reported 30% 3-year survival rate in 10 Stage III patients treated with cisplatin–cyclophosphamide chemotherapy, second debulking surgery, and whole-abdominal radiation. Not only was survival poor, but also the authors reported poor tolerance to radiation, including early discontinuation of the radiation in

TABLE 37-16. Survival for ≥2 Years After Salvage Abdominal Irradiation Following Positive Second-Look Surgery

	Residual Disease			
Microscopic	*< 1 cm*	*> 1 cm*		*Reference*
1/4	0/3	0/1		311
3/11	0/5	0/1		297
2/10	0/4	0/2		312
4/16	2/6	0/18		292
0/1	0/6	0/1		313
2/9	0/7	0/6		314
0/4		0/4		315
Total 12/55 (22%)	2/31 (7%)	0/33 (0%)		

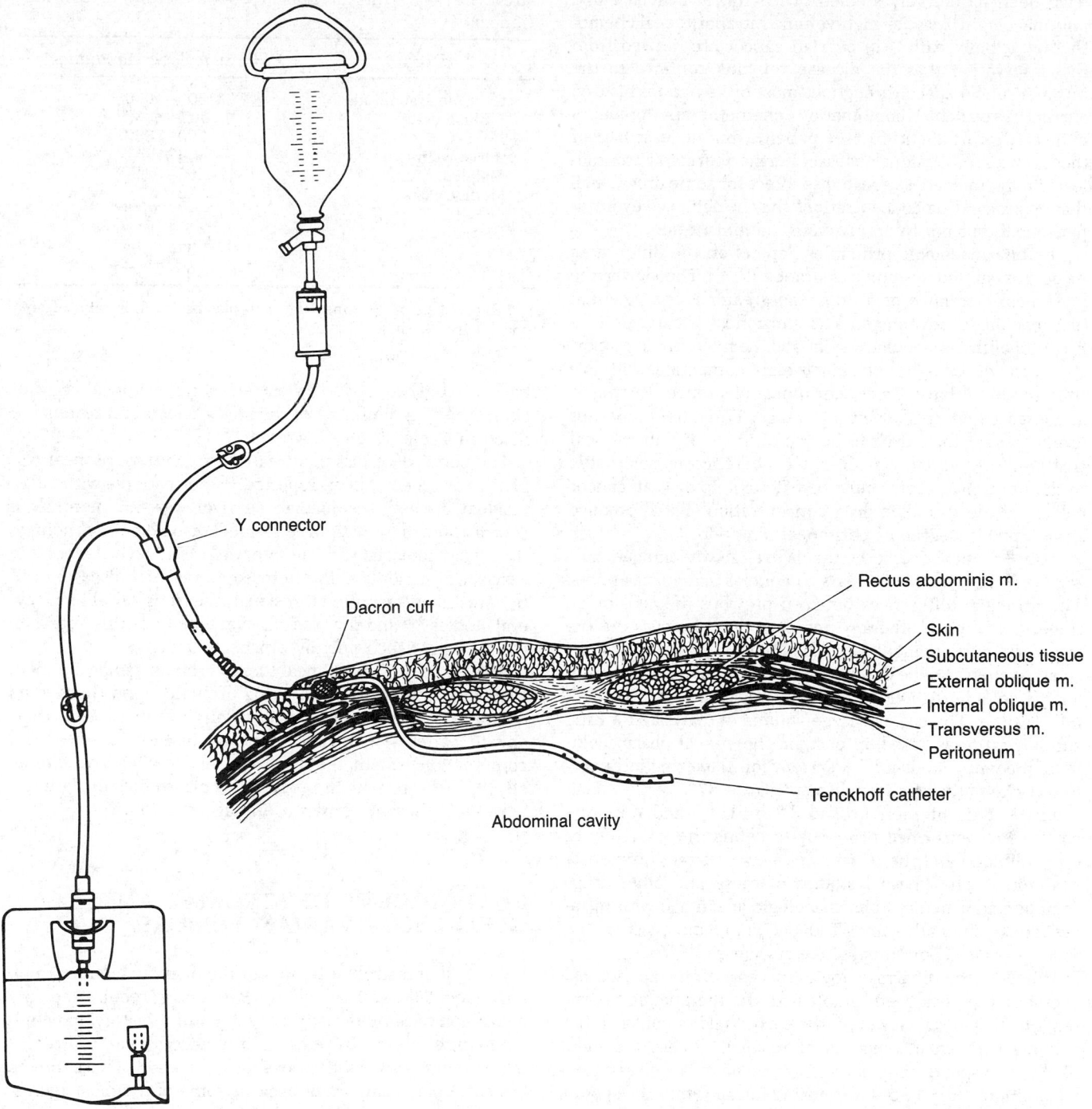

Y connector

Dacron cuff

Rectus abdominis m.

Skin
Subcutaneous tissue
External oblique m.
Internal oblique m.
Transversus m.
Peritoneum

Tenckhoff catheter

Abdominal cavity

FIG. 37-7. Tenckhoff dialysis catheter system for the delivery of intraperitoneal chemotherapy in ovarian cancer.

30% to 53% of patients because of marrow toxicity and radiation enteritis necessitating surgery in 27% to 63% of the patients. Indeed, the probability of achieving a long (> 2-year) disease-free survival using postchemotherapy total-abdominal irradiation is low in general and a function of the extent of residual disease (Table 37-16). Other attempts to control small amounts of residual disease remaining after

initial induction chemotherapy have included intraperitoneal radioisotopes (primarily ^{32}p) or chemotherapy.

Intraperitoneal Chemotherapy

Techniques for delivering chemotherapy to the patient with small amounts of peritoneally dispersed residual disease have been extensively studied. The clinical rationale and pharmacologic basis for high-volume intraperitoneal chemotherapy ("belly bath") in ovarian cancer are derived from the observation that the disease remains confined to the intraperitoneal space throughout most of its natural history; currently available combination chemotherapy produces clinical CRs in about 40% of patients, but at least half of these have some residual disease. Furthermore, in vitro studies demonstrate a dose–response effect for some drugs, such that cytotoxic drug concentrations may be achieved by intraperitoneal, but not by intravenous, administration.

The pharmacologic principles depend on the differences in peritoneal and systemic clearance.[317-319] The slower the peritoneal clearance of a drug, the greater is the potential pharmacologic advantage. The peritoneal clearance is a function of the molecular weight and the hydrophilic properties of the drug: high-molecular-weight compounds with low lipid solubility have a slow peritoneal clearance, leading to an increased pharmacologic advantage. Two other properties are necessary for a drug to be useful in the intraperitoneal treatment of ovarian cancer: the concentrations achievable in the peritoneal cavity must be cytotoxic to ovarian cancer cells, and the cytotoxic drug concentration should produce an acceptable degree of peritoneal irritation.

Intraperitoneal chemotherapy is not a new technique, having been used for many years to control malignant ascites. The principal differences between previous methods of intraperitoneal chemotherapy and current techniques are the use of a semipermanent Tenckhoff dialysis catheter or Port-a-cath system and the delivery of the antineoplastic agents in a large volume (2 liters of dialysate) instead of in 50 to 100 ml of saline. The use of a large volume of dialysate for drug administration is based, in part, on theoretical pharmacokinetic modeling studies.[317] A system for delivering intraperitoneal chemotherapy is shown in Figure 37-7.

Initial trials of methotrexate,[320] 5-FU,[321] and Adriamycin[322] were performed primarily to define the feasibility of the technique and the pharmacokinetics of the intraperitoneal route. The Phase I studies of these and other drugs documented a marked pharmacologic advantage with intraperitoneal chemotherapy (Table 37-17), and most of the Phase I trials reported objective responses.[319,320]

Although the pharmacologic success of intraperitoneal chemotherapy has been established, the therapeutic benefit remains less clear. However, the early trials established that patients with small amounts of residual disease are most likely to respond and that responses of bulky disease are uncommon.[331,332] Two studies using intraperitoneal cisplatin

TABLE 37-17. Intraperitoneal Chemotherapy in Ovarian Cancer

Drug	Pharmacologic Advantage*
Cytosine arabinoside	300–1000[323]
5-Fluorouracil	111–898[321]
	550–7852[324]
Adriamycin	474[322]
Melphalan	63–93[325]
Methotrexate	18–36[320]
	7–303[326]
Cisplatin	21[327]
	47–72[328]
	50–100[329]

* Ratio of peak peritoneal level to plasma level or ratio of area under curve (AUC).

have established it as the current intraperitoneal drug of choice.[333,334] A summary of the study design and results are listed in Table 37-18.

The survival of patients treated with intraperitoneal cisplatin has recently been reported.[335] For patients with bulky residual disease, the median survival was 6.5 months. In contrast, for those with little residual disease before therapy, the 2-year actuarial survival rate was 74%. Nevertheless, the survival of patients with microscopic residual disease, positive washings, or minimal residual disease is variable in several studies,[246] and the true survival benefit of this approach will be established only by prospective trials.

At present, intraperitoneal therapy remains experimental. Cisplatin appears to be the drug of choice, and there is no evidence of substantial activity of any intraperitoneal therapy in patients with bulky residual disease. Studies with combination chemotherapy administered intraperitoneally[332,336,337] are now in progress, as are studies using intraperitoneal therapy as part of initial induction.

MANAGEMENT OF STROMAL AND GERM-CELL OVARIAN TUMORS

Germ-cell and stromal tumors of the ovary, which make up only about 5% to 10% of all ovarian tumors, require separate discussion because of their unusual natural history and clinical manifestations. In addition, it is necessary to utilize different therapies for the various tumor types.[338] These tumors are particularly important because some of the most aggres-

TABLE 37-18. Intraperitoneal Cisplatin in Small Volume Residual Disease Ovarian Cancer After Induction Chemotherapy

	Mt Sinai[334]	Netherlands Cancer Institute[333]
No. of patients	23	21
Cisplatin dose	50 mg/m² in 2 liters every 3 wk	60–150 mg/m² in 2 liters every 2–3 wk
No. of cycles	6	6–10
Sodium thiosulfate	Not used	If toxicity developed in previous cycle
Catheter	Temporary in 75% of patients	Tenckhoff
Results	6/19 (32%) negative laparotomy	7/21 (33%) negative laparatomy

sive ones are now curable with combination chemotherapy and conservative surgery.

These tumors can be separated into three groups:

1. Those with ovarian stromal components, such as the granulosa-cell and Sertoli–Leydig cell tumors;
2. Those derived from germ-cell elements, such as malignant teratoma, embryonal carcinoma, endodermal sinus tumor, and dysgerminoma; and
3. Choriocarcinoma.

OVARIAN STROMAL TUMORS

Ovarian stromal tumors account for approximately 1% to 3% of all ovarian tumors, generally have an indolent natural history, and sometimes recur many years after initial therapy. They are sometimes associated with precocious feminization, and their association with unopposed estrogen secretion and an increased incidence of concomitant endometrial carcinoma (7.8%) has been well documented.[339] In a review of 51 patients, 43% of the tumors were theca-cell tumors, 24% were pure granulosa-cell tumors, and 33% were mixed granulosa–theca-cell tumors.[340] None of the patients with thecomas died as a result of their disease; deaths occurred only in patients having the granulosa cell-containing tumors with metastases.

Stromal tumors can be managed by unilateral salpingo-oophorectomy in young patients and rarely required adjunctive therapy. The incidence of bilaterality is very low. There are too few reported cases of Stage II stromal tumors to make definitive recommendations, but the lack of proven adjunctive therapy does not permit recommending conservative surgery in such patients. Factors such as tumor size, degree of differentiation, histologic patterns, and tumor spillage are of prognostic importance. Because of their protracted natural history, it is difficult to document the value of postoperative radiation. However, in tumors that are not completely resected, a dose of 5000 to 6000 cGy to the pelvis has been advocated. Such treatment of 37 patients at M.D. Anderson Hospital resulted in a 5-year survival rate of 75% for Stage I and 50% to 60% for Stages II and III.[338]

The role of chemotherapy in treating the granulosa–theca cell tumors has been poorly defined because so few patients have been studied. There are anecdotal reports of responses to alkylating agents[338,341] and Adriamycin.[342]

Experience with nine patients with Sertoli–Leydig cell tumors has been reported from the M.D. Anderson Hospital, five seen for initial therapy, and four with recurrent tumor. Two patients with recurrent lesions had a complete response after administration of a combination of vincristine, dactinomycin, and cyclophosphamide.[338] There is a report of partial regressions using CAP in two patients.[343] The largest recent study described 11 patients with granulosa-cell tumors who were treated with PVB.[62] Six of the 11 had surgically confirmed CRs. Substantial drug toxicity was seen, but this combination merits further study in stromal tumors in light of the paucity of activity with other regimens and with radiation therapy.

Recurrent stromal tumors are treated by resection and postoperative irradiation, if the residual tumor can be en-

compassed by external irradiation, or with chemotherapy, if the disease is extensive.

OVARIAN GERM-CELL TUMORS

Ovarian germ-cell tumors are rare, accounting for about 2% to 3% of all ovarian cancers. These tumors may have a mixed histologic pattern, and treatment should be designed to deal with the most malignant component. Historically, embryonal carcinoma, endodermal sinus tumors, and malignant teratomas had an extremely poor prognosis with surgery alone, and long-term survival was achieved only in a small percentage of patients even with Stage I disease.[344] For example, the Ovarian Tumor Registry of the American Gynecological Society reported in 1977 that 31 of 34 patients with endodermal sinus tumor were dead of disease after surgery alone; the three survivors, all with Stage IA disease, were living 2.5, 9, and 12 years after surgery.[345] Gallion and co-workers have reviewed the published literature on 150 cases of pure endodermal sinus tumors.[346] Before the use of chemotherapy, the overall 2-year survival rate of patients with Stage I disease was 27%, which did not differ from that of patients presenting with more advanced disease. Surgery alone was ineffective, producing only a 16% 2-year survival rate. Even total abdominal hysterectomy and bilateral salpingo-oophorectomy for Stage IA disease in one study produced only a 13% 2-year survival rate. Pelvic or total-abdominal radiation added little to these 2-year survival figures.

Improved cure rates for these tumors have followed the observation that germ-cell tumors are highly curable with combination chemotherapy. Surgery can now be more limited.

For germ-cell tumors confined to one ovary, unilateral salpingo-oophorectomy is the operation of choice for the young patient. For tumors that have spread to pelvic structures other than the opposite ovary, fallopian tube, or uterus, complete tumor removal without total abdominal hysterectomy or removal of the uninvolved adnexa is indicated. These patients can usually be cured with adjunctive chemotherapy and retain reproductive function.

Endodermal Sinus Tumors

Endodermal sinus tumors are unusual and aggressive tumors of germ-cell origin that reproduce the extraembryonic structures of the early embryo. The tumor is rarely bilateral. Before the use of combination chemotherapy, the tumor was almost invariably fatal.

The consensus at present is that all patients, regardless of stage, should receive chemotherapy. The earliest effective regimen reported was the VAC (vincristine, actinomycin D, cyclophosphamide) program. Two studies have summarized the results with VAC in a variety of more aggressive germ-cell tumors. Cangir and co-workers described 21 patients (8 with malignant teratomas, 6 with endodermal sinus tumors, 6 with mixed germ-cell tumors, and 1 with Sertoli–Leydig tumor),[347] 14 of whom showed no evidence of malignancy at a second-look operation after chemotherapy. These authors concluded that maximal surgical removal followed by adjuvant VAC was appropriate and that irradiation had no role in the initial management of these patients. Slayton and colleagues have recently summarized the experience of the GOG with VAC in aggressive germ-cell tumors.[348] Seventy-six patients were treated with VAC postoperatively, including 54 who were believed disease free after surgery, and 39 of these 54 (72%) remain disease free. The best results were seen in patients with immature (Grades II and III) teratoma, where 19 of 20 remained disease free. Results were not nearly as good in patients with significant residual disease after surgery; in this group, only 7 of 22 were disease free after VAC chemotherapy.

Although the largest experience has been with the VAC combination, recent reports indicate that PVB is at least as good as and may be better than VAC. Collected experience from published series[349-351] shows 53 of 61 (87%) of PVB-treated patients alive without evidence of disease. Recently, platinum, VP-16, and bleomycin (PVP-16B) has been used by the Royal Marsden group in nine patients (six with Stages III and IV disease), eight of whom are disease free at 6 to 62[+] months.[350] Although no randomized trials exist comparing VAC with PVB or P-VP-16B, it is likely that the last two regimens will become the therapy of choice for endodermal sinus tumors.

Malignant Teratoma

Malignant teratoma of the ovary is a rare, lethal germ-cell tumor. More than half of the patients present before the age of 20. The tumor is rarely bilateral. Prognosis seems to be related to the histologic grade of the tumor, according to the M.D. Anderson experience with 25 patients.[352]

Before the use of combination chemotherapy, patients were managed with aggressive surgery followed by irradiation or single-agent chemotherapy. Of eight patients managed in this manner, none survived, although all different grades of tumor were represented. In contrast, using the VAC combination without irradiation, 10 of 12 patients are surviving at a median of 43 months. A combination-chemotherapy approach with VAC or one of the other regimens mentioned in the previous section is now the therapy of choice for these tumors. Of all the germ-cell tumors, the Grade II and III immature teratomas appear to respond best to VAC.

Dysgerminoma

Dysgerminomas constitute only about 2% of all ovarian malignancies, and they are unique among the germ-cell tumors because of the high cure rate and sensitivity to radiation. They are the only ovarian germ-cell malignancy that occurs bilaterally with significant frequency (10% to 15%). Although these tumors are the counterpart of testicular seminoma in males, they are rarer. The tumor metastasizes to the regional lymph nodes in about 20% of the patients and can be cured with limited surgical procedures and low-dose radiation therapy.

Any other malignant germ-cell tumor components should be identified because they influence the prognosis. Asadourian and Taylor reported an admixture of germinal elements in 12 of 117 patients with dysgerminoma reviewed at the Armed Forces Institute of Pathology.[353] Several studies indicate that extension through the capsule of the tumor, extraovarian spread, large tumor size, or bilateral lesions are poor prognostic findings.[354,355]

At initial surgery, the contralateral ovary should be carefully examined. If there is any question of involvement, it should be bivalved, and wedge biopsies should be obtained for frozen section. If the tumor is localized to one ovary, a unilateral salpingo-oophorectomy should be performed. Also, the pelvic and periaortic nodes should be evaluated carefully by palpation; biopsies should be taken of any suspicious areas. If the tumor is localized inside the capsule of one ovary, no postoperative irradiation is indicated. Otherwise, a dose of 2000 to 2500 cGy should be delivered to the midplane of the hemipelvis on the side of the lesion, in addition to the pelvic and periaortic nodes.[355,356] If there is bilateral disease, bilateral salpingo-oophorectomy should be carried out and irradiation given to the pelvis and iliac and para-aortic nodes. If grossly metastatic nodes are present, a boost of 500 to 1000 cGy should be delivered with reduced fields. High-energy linear accelerator beams should be used to decrease the scatter dose to the contralateral ovary.

The group from the M.D. Anderson Hospital has reported results on 36 patients with pure dysgerminoma.[356] Sixty-one percent of the patients were in Stage I, and 34% had advanced disease (FIGO Stages III and IV). In 5 patients with Stage IA disease treated only with unilateral salpingo-oophorectomy, no recurrences were noted. All patients are alive 3 to 20 years after initial treatment, and 3 of these patients have had children. Management of the other patients was generally with aggressive debulking surgery followed by total-abdominal irradiation. Lymphangiography was used to assess disease in the para-aortic nodes. The overall survival for their group of patients was 86%. Similar results have been reported from the Radiumhemmet Institute.[355] Of 56 patients treated with radiation therapy, the overall 5-year survival rate was 75%, with 36% of the patients developing recurrences. The extent of the tumor was a critical factor in determining survival and recurrences. In 40 patients treated initially at the Radiumhemmet, 13 recurrences were noted, and of these patients 8 survived for 5 years or more after the beginning of therapy. Asadourian and Taylor reported recurrences or metastases in 23 of 105 patients (24%); additional therapy resulted in the cure of 10 of these patients.[353] These authors also observed a 96% 5-year actuarial survival rate in 78 patients with tumor localized to one or both ovaries, in contrast to 63% in 17 patients with extraovarian extension. There were 18 pregnancies after treatment in 10 patients. Fifteen of the babies were normal, 1 was malformed, and there were two abortions, one therapeutic and 1 spontaneous.

Recurrent tumors, when extensive or with distant metastasis, have been treated with combination chemotherapy.[357] In light of the activity of PVB in the testicular counterpart of this tumor, seminoma, the ovarian tumor has recently been treated with PVB. The Royal Marsden group treated seven patients with Stage III or IV dysgerminoma, four of whom had not responded to radiation, with PVB.[350] All seven had a CR, and six have been free of disease for more than 1 year.

Choriocarcinoma

This tumor is extremely rare (less than 1% of ovarian tumors). Chemotherapy, as in trophoblastic lesions, has been the treatment of choice.[358] The prognosis, however, is extremely poor. Rutledge reported a few patients responding to a combination of methotrexate, dactinomycin, and cyclophosphamide (MAC).[338] Recently, Fanning et al[359] reported the successful treatment of a patient with Stage III mixed germ-cell tumor with pure choriocarcinoma in the para-aortic nodes. The patient was treated with alternating sequences of VAC and PVB and at 30 months is free of disease. The authors state that this is the first reported long-term survival of a patient with pure choriocarcinoma metastases.

TREATMENT OF OVARIAN CARCINOMA ASSOCIATED WITH PREGNANCY

Although unusual, ovarian carcinoma does occur during pregnancy.[360] Palpation of an adnexal mass during the first trimester without other evidence of malignancy should be managed by close follow-up with pelvic examinations and, if necessary, ultrasound. A persistent corpus luteum cyst will usually resolve spontaneously, and surgical exploration for an asymptomatic mass is best carried out during the second trimester. Although most adnexal masses in pregnancy will be benign, a persistent mass should be removed. Creasman et al[361] reported on 17 patients with ovarian carcinoma managed at M.D. Anderson Hospital who were either pregnant or within 6 months of delivery at the time of diagnosis. One-third of the tumors were diagnosed at delivery.

Unless there is spread outside the ovary, unilateral salpingo-oophorectomy and a full staging operation are the treatments of choice. If the carcinoma has spread beyond the ovary, a full staging and debulking operation should be performed, although hysterectomy with sacrifice of the fetus should be undertaken only if necessary to debulk the tumor properly. Postoperative chemotherapy should be administered as indicated by the stage, cell type, and grade of the tumor, because most chemotherapeutic agents useful in ovarian cancer can be administered during pregnancy without known adverse effects on the fetus.

REFERENCES

1. Cancer Facts and Figures 1986. New York, American Cancer Society, 1986
2. Doll R, Muir C, Waterhouse J (eds): International Union Against Cancer: Cancer Incidence in Five Continents, vol 2. Berlin, Springer-Verlag, 1970
3. Buell P, Dunn JE: Cancer mortality among Japanese Issei and Nisei of California. Cancer 18:656–664, 1965
4. Haenszel W, Kurihara M: Studies of Japanese migrants: I. Mortality from cancer and other disease among Japanese in the United States. J Natl Cancer Inst 40:43–48, 1968
5. Joly DJ, Lilienfield AM, Diamond EL et al: An epidemiologic study of the relationship of reproductive experience to cancer of the ovary. Am J Epidemiol 99:190–209, 1974
6. Beral V, Fraser P, Chilvers C: Does pregnancy protect against ovarian cancer? Lancet 2:1083–1086, 1978
7. Lingeman CH: Etiology of cancer of the human ovary: A review. J Natl Cancer Inst 53:1603–1618, 1974
8. Hoover R, Gray LA, Fraumeni JF: Stilbestrol and the risk of ovarian cancer. Lancet 2:533–534, 1977
9. The Cancer and Steroid Hormone Study of the Centers for Disease Control and The National Institute of Child Health and Development: The reduction in risk of ovarian cancer associated with oral contraceptive use. N Engl J Med 316:650–655, 1987
10. West BO: Epidemiologic study of malignancies of the ovaries. Cancer 19:1001–1007, 1966
11. Fraumeni JF, Grundy GW, Creagan ET: Six families prone to ovarian cancer. Cancer 36:364–369, 1975
12. Schweisguth O, Gerard–Marchant R, Plainfosse B et al: Bilateral nonfunctioning thecoma of the ovary in epileptic children under anticonvulsant therapy. Acta Paediatr Scand 60:6–10, 1971
13. Hueper WC, Conway WD: Chemical Carcinogenesis and Cancers. Springfield, IL, Charles C Thomas, 1964
14. Longo DL, Young RC: Cosmetic talc and ovarian carcinoma. Lancet 2:349–351, 1979
15. Cramer DW, Welch WR, Scully RE, Wojciechowski CA: Ovarian cancer and talc. Cancer 50:372–376, 1982
16. Scully RE: Tumors of the Ovary and Maldeveloped Gonads. Armed Forces Institute of Pathology, Second Series, Fascicle 16. Washington, DC, Armed Forces Institute of Pathology, 1979
17. Janovski NA, Paramandandhan, TL: Tumors and tumor-like conditions of the ovaries, fallopian tubes and ligaments of the uterus. In Friedman EA (ed): Major Problems in Obstetrics and Gynecology, vol 4, p 12. Philadelphia, WB Saunders, 1973
18. Plentl AA, Friedman EA: Lymphatic System of the Female Genitalia: The Morphologic Basis of Oncologic Diagnosis and Therapy, pp 168–180. Philadelphia, WB Saunders, 1973
19. Fuks Z: Patterns of spread of ovarian carcinoma: Relation to therapeutic strategies. Adv Biosci 26:39–51, 1980
20. Munnell EW: Is conservative therapy ever justified in Stage I (Ia) cancer of the ovary? Am J Obstet Gynecol 103:641–650, 1969
21. Keettel WC, Pixley E: Diagnostic value of peritoneal washings. Clin Obstet Gynecol 1:592, 1958
22. Joffey JM, Courtice FC: Lymphatics, Lymph and Lymphoid Complexes, pp 295–305. New York, Academic Press, 1970
23. Feldman GB, Knapp RC: Lymphatic drainage of the peritoneal cavity and its significance in ovarian cancer. Am J Obstet Gynecol 119:991–994, 1974
24. Meyers MA: The spread and localization of acute intraperitoneal effusions. Radiology 95:547–554, 1970
25. Dyre JC: Intraperitoneal pressure in the human. Surg Gynecol Obstet 87:472, 1948
26. French JE, Florey HW, Morris BL: The absorption of particles by the lymphatics of the diaphragm. Q J Exp Biol 45:88–103, 1960
27. Coates G, Bush RS, Aspin N: A study of ascites using lymphoscintigraphy with 99m Tc-sulfur colloid. Radiology 107:577–583, 1973
28. Bagley CM, Young RC, Schein PS, Chabner BA, DeVita VT: Ovarian carcinoma metastatic to the diaphragm: Frequently undiagnosed at laparotomy. Am J Obstet Gynecol 116:397–400, 1973
29. Rosenoff SH, DeVita VT, Hubbard S, Young RC: Peritoneoscopy in the staging and follow-up of ovarian cancer. Semin Oncol 2:223–228, 1975
30. Piver MS, Barlow JJ, Lele SB: Incidence of sub-clinical metastasis in Stage I and II ovarian carcinoma. Obstet Gynecol 52:100–104, 1978
31. Feldman GB, Knapp RC, Order SE, Hellman S: The role of lymphatic obstruction in the formation of ascites in a murine ovarian carcinoma. Cancer Res 32:1663–1666, 1972
32. Fisher RI, Young RC: Advances in the staging and treatment of ovarian cancer. Cancer 39:967, 1977
33. Steinberg JJ, Demopoulos RI, Bigelow B: The evaluation of the omentum in ovarian cancer. Gynecol Oncol 2:253, 1975
34. Eichner E, Bove ER: In vivo studies on the lymphatic drainage of the human ovary. Obstet Gynecol 3:287–297, 1954
35. Fuks Z: External radiotherapy of ovarian cancer: Standard approaches and new frontiers. Semin Oncol 2:253–266, 1975
36. Kwaney R, Fuchs WA: Die Lymphographie bei malignen ovarial Tumoren. Fortschr Geb Röntgenstr Nuklearmed 126:564–566, 1977
37. Musumeci R, DePalo G, Kenda R, Tesoro-Tess JD et al: Retroperitoneal metastases from ovarian carcinoma: Reassessment of 365 patients studied with lymphography. AJR 134:449–452, 1980
38. Fuks Z: Patterns of spread of ovarian carcinoma: Relation to therapeutic strategies. In Newman CE, Ford CH, Jordan JA (eds): Ovarian Cancer. Oxford, Pergamon Press, 1980
39. Burghardt E, Pickel H, Stettner H: Management of advanced ovarian cancer. Eur J Gynaecol Oncol 3:155, 1984
40. Buchsbaum HJ, Delgado G, Blessing J et al: Surgical staging of ovarian carcinoma (abstr). Gynecol Oncol 23:253, 1986
41. Barnhill DR, Hoskins WJ, Heller PB et al: The second look surgical reassessment of epithelial ovarian carcinoma. Gynecol Oncol 19:148, 1984
42. Rubin SC, Hoskins WJ, Hakes TB et al: Recurrence after negative second-look laparotomy for ovarian cancer: Analysis of risk factors. Am J Obstet Gynecol 159:1094, 1988
43. Scully RE: Recent progress in ovarian cancer. Hum Pathol 1:73–98, 1970
44. Novak ER, Woodruff JD: Novak's Gynecologic and Obstetric Pathology, p 389. Philadelphia, WB Saunders, 1974
45. Serov SF, Scully RE, Solvin LH: International Histological Classification of Tumors, No. 9: Histological Typing of Ovarian Tumors. Geneva, World Health Organization, 1973

46. International Federation of Gynaecology and Obstetrics: Classification and staging of malignant tumors in the female pelvis. Acta Obstet Gynaecol Scand 50:1–7, 1971
47. Scully RE: Ovarian tumors. Am J Pathol 87:686–720, 1977
48. Nikrui N: Survey of clinical behavior of patients with borderline tumors of the ovary. Gynecol Oncol 12:107–119, 1981
49. Bjorkholm E, Pettersson F, Einhorn N et al: Long term follow-up and prognostic factors in ovarian carcinoma. The Radiumhemmet series 1953–1973. Acta Radiat Oncol 21:413–419, 1982
50. Kottmeier HL: Ovarian cancer with special regard to radiotherapy. Am J Roentgenol Rad Ther Nucl Med 111:417–421, 1971
51. Aure JC, Høeg K, Kolstad P: Clinical and histologic studies of ovarian carcinoma: Long-term follow-up of 900 cases. Obstet Gynecol 37:1–9, 1971
52. Perez CA, Walz BJ, Jacobson PL: Radiation therapy in the management of carcinoma of the ovary. Natl Cancer Inst Monogr 42:119–125, 1975
53. Young RC, Hubbard SP, DeVita VT: The chemotherapy of ovarian carcinoma. Cancer Treat Rev 1:99–110, 1974
54. Smith JP, Rutledge F, Wharton JT: Chemotherapy of ovarian cancer: New approaches to treatment. Cancer 30:1565–1571, 1972
55. Munnell EW, Taylor HC: Ovarian carcinoma: A review of 200 primary and 51 secondary cases. Am J Obstet 58:943, 1949
56. Decker DG, Mussey E, Williams TJ: Grading of gynecologic malignancy: Epithelial ovarian cancer. In Proceedings of the 7th National Cancer Congress, pp 223–231. Philadelphia, JB Lippincott, 1972
57. Day TG, Gallager HS, Rutledge F: Epithelial carcinoma of the ovary: Prognostic importance of histologic grade. Natl Cancer Inst Monogr 42:15–18, 1975
58. Ozols RF, Garvin AJ, Costa J et al: Advanced ovarian cancer: Correlation of histologic grade with response to therapy and survival. Cancer 45:572–581, 1980
59. Dembo AJ, Bush RS, Beale FA: Ovarian carcinoma: Improved survival following abdominopelvic irradiation in patients with a completed pelvic operation. Am J Obstet Gynecol 134:793–800, 1979
60. Dembo AJ, Bush RS: Choice of postoperative therapy based on prognostic factors. Int J Radiat Oncol Biol Phys 8:893–897, 1982
61. Scully RE: World Health Organization classification and nomenclature of ovarian cancer. Natl Cancer Inst Monogr 42:5–7, 1975
62. Colombo N, Sessa C, Landoni F et al: Cisplatin, vinblastine, and bleomycin combination chemotherapy in metastatic granulosa cell tumor of the ovary. Obstet Gynecol 67:265, 1986
63. Perez CA, Bradfield JS: Radiation therapy in the treatment of carcinoma of the ovary. Cancer 29:1027, 1972
64. Fisher RI, Young RC: Chemotherapy of ovarian cancer. Surg Clin North Am 58:143, 1978
65. Sall S, Stone ML: The treatment of ovarian cancer. Prog Clin Cancer 5:249, 1973
66. Kent SN, McKay DG: Primary cancer of the ovary. Am J Obstet Gynecol 80:430–438, 1960
67. Pearse WH, Behrman SJ: Carcinoma of the ovary. Obstet Gynecol 3:32–45, 1954
68. Barber HRK, Graber EA: The PMPO syndrome. Obstet Gynecol 38:921, 1971
69. Flynt JR, Gallup DG: The postmenopausal palpable ovary syndrome: A 14-year review. Milit Med 146:686, 1981
70. Bolandgray A, Mehellati KA, Ardekany MS: Early detection of ovarian malignancy by culdocentesis. J Reprod Med 9:32, 1971
71. Graham JB, Graham RM, Schueller DF: Preclinical detection of ovarian cancer. Cancer 17:414, 1964
72. McGowan L, Stein DB, Miller W: Cul-de-sac aspiration for diagnostic cytology study. Obstet Gynecol 96:413, 1966
73. Rubin SC, Dulaney ED, Markman M et al: Peritoneal cytology as an indicator of disease in patients with residual ovarian carcinoma. Obstet Gynecol 71:851, 1988
74. Samuels BI: Usefulness of ultrasound in patients with ovarian cancer. Semin Oncol 2:229–233, 1975
75. Berkowitz RS, Leavitt T Jr, Knapp RC: Ultrasound directed percutaneous aspiration biopsy of periaortic lymph nodes in cervical carcinoma recurrence. Am J Obstet Gynecol 131:906–908, 1978
76. Parker BR, Castellino RA, Fuks ZY, Bagshaw MA: The role of lymphography in patients with ovarian cancer. Cancer 34:100–105, 1974
77. Schaner EG, Head GL, Kalman MA et al: Whole body computed tomography in the diagnosis of abdominal and thoracic malignancy: Review of 600 cases. Cancer Treat Rep 61:1537–1560, 1977
78. Dunnick NR, Schaner EG, Doppman JL: Detection of subcutaneous metastasis by computed tomography. J Comp Assist Tomogr 2:275–279, 1978
79. Kurman RJ, Norris HJ: Endodermal sinus tumor of the ovary: A clinical and pathologic analysis of 71 cases. Cancer 38:2404–2419, 1976
80. Goldstein DP, Piro AJ: Combination chemotherapy in the treatment of germ cell tumors containing choriocarcinoma in males and females. Surg Gynecol Obstet 134:61–66, 1972
81. DiSaia PJ, Morrow CP, Haverback BJ, Dyce BJ: Carcinoembryonic antigen in cancer of the female reproductive system: Serial plasma values correlated with disease state. Cancer 39:2365–2370, 1977
82. Imamura N, Takahasi T, Lloyd KO et al: Analysis of human ovarian tumor antigens using heterologous antisera: Detection of new antigenic system. Int J Cancer 21:570–577, 1978
83. Dorsett BH, Ioachim HL, Stolbach L et al: Isolation of tumor-specific antibodies from effusions of ovarian carcinoma. Int J Cancer 16:779–786, 1975
84. Bhattacharya M, Barlow JJ: Ovarian Cancer. In Herberman RB, McIntyre KR (eds): Immunodiagnosis of Cancer, pp 632–643, New York, Marcel Dekker, 1979
85. Knauf S, Urbach GI: The development of a double-antibody radioimmunoassay for detecting ovarian tumor-associated antigen fraction OCA in plasma. Am J Obstet Gynecol 131:780–787, 1978
86. Bast RC, Klug TL, St John E et al: A radioimmunoassay using a monoclonal antibody to monitor the course of epithelial ovarian cancer. N Engl J Med 309:883–887, 1983
87. Zurawski VR, Broderick SF, Pickens P et al: Serum CA-125 levels in a group of nonhospitalized women: Relevance for the early detection of ovarian cancer. Obstet Gynecol 69:606, 1987
88. Einhorn N, Bast RC Jr, Knapp RC et al: Preoperative evaluation of serum CA-125 levels in patients with primary epithelial ovarian cancer. Obstet Gynecol 67:414, 1986
89. Malkasian GD Jr, Podratz KC, Stanhope RE et al: CA-125 in gynecologic practice. Am J Obstet 155:515, 1986
90. Barbieri RL, Niloff JM, Bast RC Jr et al: Elevated serum concentrations of CA-125 in patients with advanced endometriosis. Fertil Steril 45:630, 1986
91. Ruibol A, Encabo G, Martinez–Miralles E et al: CA-125 serum levels in non-malignant pathologies. Bull Cancer (Paris) 71:45, 1984
92. Pittaway DE, Foyez JA: Serum CA-125 antigen levels increase during menses. Am J Obstet Gynecol 156:75, 1987
93. Mastropaolo W, Fernandez Z, Miller EL: Pronounced increases in the concentration of an ovarian tumor marker, CA-125, in serum of a healthy subject during menstruation. Clin Chem 32:2110, 1986
94. Halila H, Stennan A, Seppala M: Ovarian cancer antigen CA-125 levels in pelvic inflammatory disease and pregnancy. Cancer 57:1327, 1986
95. International Federation of Gynecology and Obstetrics: Changes in definitions of clinical staging for carcinoma of the cervix and ovary: Am J Obstet Gynecol 156:236, 1987
96. Munnell EW: The changing prognosis and treatment in cancer of the ovary: A report of 235 patients with primary ovarian carcinoma 1952–1961. Am J Obstet Gynecol 100:790, 1968
97. Delclos L, Quinlan EJ: Malignant tumors of the ovary managed with postoperative megavoltage irradiation. Radiology 93:659, 1969
98. Griffiths CT: Surgical resection of tumor bulk in the primary treatment of ovarian carcinoma. Natl Cancer Inst Monogr 42:101, 1975
99. Delgado G, Oram DH, Petrilli EG: Stage III epithelial ovarian cancer: The role of maximal surgical reduction. Gynecol Oncol 18:293, 1984
100. Conte PF, Sertoli MR, Bruzzone M et al: Cisplatin, methotrexate and 5-fluorouracil regimen in the treatment of advanced and recurrent ovarian cancer. Gynecol Oncol 20:23, 1985
101. Posada JG Jr, Marantz AB, Yeung KY et al: The cyclophosphamide, hexamethylmelamine, 5-fluorouracil regimen in the treatment of advanced and recurrent ovarian cancer. Gynecol Oncol 20:23, 1985
102. Hacker NF, Berek JS, Lagasse LD et al: Primary cytoreductive surgery for epithelial ovarian cancer. Obstet Gynecol 61:424, 1983
103. Omura GA, Bundy B, Wilbanks G et al: A randomized trial of cyclophosphamide (C) plus cisplatin (P) with or without Adriamycin (A) in ovarian cancer (abstr). Proc Am Soc Clin Oncol 6:439, 1987
104. Fuks Z, Rizel S, Anteby SO et al: The multimodal approach to the treatment of Stage IV ovarian carcinoma. Rad Oncol Biol Physics 8:903, 1982
105. Dembo AJ: Radiotherapeutic management of ovarian cancer. Semin Oncol 11:238, 1984
106. Chen SS, Bochner R: Assessment of morbidity and mortality in primary cytoreductive surgery for advanced ovarian cancer. Gynecol Oncol 20:190, 1985
107. Blythe JG, Wahl TP: Debulking surgery: Does it increase the quality of survival? Gynecol Oncol 14:396, 1982
108. Ozols RF, Fisher RI, Anderson T, Makuch R, Young RC: Peritoneoscopy in the management of ovarian cancer. Am J Obstet Gynecol 140:611–619, 1981
109. Berek JS, Griffiths CT, Leventhal JM: Laparoscopy for second-look evaluation in ovarian cancer. Obstet Gynecol 58:192–198, 1981
110. Wangenstein OH, Lewis FJ, Tongen L: The "second look" in cancer surgery. Lancet 71:303, 1951
111. Rutledge FN, Burns BC: Chemotherapy for advanced ovarian cancer. Am J Obstet Gynecol 96:761, 1966
112. Smith JP, Rutledge F: Chemotherapy in the treatment of cancer of the ovary. Obstet Gynecol 107:691, 1970
113. Smith JP, Delgado G, Rutledge F: Second look operation in ovarian cancer. Cancer 38:1438, 1976
114. Greco FA, Julian CG, Richardson RL et al: Advanced ovarian cancer: Brief intensive combination chemotherapy and second look operation. Obstet Gynecol 58:199, 1981
115. Berek JS, Hocha NF, Lagasse LD et al: Second look laparotomy in Stage III epithelial ovarian cancer: Clinical variables associated with disease status. Obstet Gynecol 64:14, 1981
116. Hakes TB, Chalas E, Saigo P et al: Randomized trial of cyclophosphamide, doxorubicin and cisplatin (CAP) chemotherapy: 5 versus 10 cycles in Stage III and IV ovarian cancer (abstr). Proc Am Soc Clin Oncol 6:456, 1987
117. Rubin SC, Lewis JL, Jr: Second-look surgery in ovarian carcinoma. CRC Crit Rev Oncol Hematol 8:75, 1988
118. Cain JM, Saigo PE, Pierce VJ et al: A review of second look laparotomy for ovarian cancer. Gynecol Oncol 23:14, 1986
119. Berek JS, Hacker NF, Lagasse LD et al: Second look laparotomy in Stage III epithelial ovarian cancer: Clinical variables associated with disease status. Obstet Gynecol 64:207, 1984

120. Smirz LR, Stehman FB, Ulbright TM et al: Second look laparotomy after chemotherapy in the management of ovarian malignancy. Am J Obstet Gynecol 152:661, 1985

121. Webb MJ, Snyder JA, Williams TJ et al: Second look laparotomy in ovarian cancer. Gynecol Oncol 14:285, 1982

122. Podratz KC, Malkasian GD Jr, Hilton JF, et al: Second look laparotomy in ovarian cancer: Evaluation of pathologic variables. Am J Obstet Gynecol 152(2):230–238, 1985

123. Phibbs GC, Smith JP, Stanhope CR: An analysis of sites of persistent cancer at "second look" laparotomy in patients with ovarian cancer. Am J Obstet Gynecol 147:611, 1983

124. Curry SL, Zembo MM, Nahhas WA et al: Second look laparotomy for ovarian cancer. Gynecol Oncol 11:114, 1981

125. Dauplat J, Ferriere JP, Gorbinet M et al: Second look laparotomy in managing epithelial ovarian carcinoma. Cancer 57:1627, 1986

126. Ballon SC, Protnuf JC, Sikic BI et al: Second look laparotomy in ovarian carcinoma: Precise definition, sensitivity and specificity of the operative procedure. Gynecol Oncol 17:154, 1984

127. Schwartz PE, Smith JP: Second-look operations in ovarian cancer. Am J Obstet Gynecol 138:1124–1130, 1980

128. Creasman WT, Aba-Ghazaleh S, Schmidt HJ: Retroperitoneal metastatic spread of ovarian carcinoma. Gynecol Oncol 6:447, 1978

129. Berek JS, Hacker WF, Lagasse LD et al: Survival of patients following secondary cytoreductive surgery in ovarian cancer. Obstet Gynecol 61:189, 1983

130. Griffiths CT, Parker LM, Fuller AF Jr: Role of cytoreductive surgical treatment in the management of advanced ovarian cancer. Cancer Treat Rep 63:235, 1979

131. Wiltshaw E, Raju KS, Dawson I: The role of cytoreductive surgery in advanced carcinoma of the ovary: An analysis of primary and second surgery. Br J Obstet Gynaecol 92:522, 1985

132. Copeland LJ, Wharton JT, Rutledge FN et al: Role of "third look laparotomy" in the guidance of ovarian cancer treatment. Gynecol Oncol 15:149, 1983

133. Maggino T, Tredese F, Valente S et al: Role of second look laparotomy in multidisciplinary treatment and in the follow up of advanced ovarian cancer. Eur J Gynaecol Oncol 4:26, 1983

134. Luesley DM, Chan KK, Fielding WL et al: Second look laparotomy in the management of epithelial ovarian carcinoma: An evaluation of fifty cases. Obstet Gynecol 64:421, 1984

135. Raju KS, McKinna JA, Barker GH et al: Second look operations in the planned management of advanced ovarian carcinoma. Am J Obstet Gynecol 144:650, 1982

136. Eymer H: Beeinflussung von proliferenden Ovarialtumoren durch Rötgenstrahlen. Strahlen 1:358–361, 1912

137. Fuks Z, Bagshaw MA: The rationale for curative radiotherapy for ovarian carcinoma. Int J Radiat Oncol Biol Phys 1:21–32, 1975

138. Schray MF, Ox RS, Martinez A: Lower abdominal radiotherapy for Stages I, II and selected III epithelial ovarian cancer: 20 years' experience. Gynecol Oncol 15:78–87, 1983

139. Dembo AJ: Radiotherapeutic management of ovarian cancer. Semin Oncol 11:238–250, 1984

140. Dembo AJ: Abdominopelvic radiotherapy in ovarian cancer: A 10-year experience. Cancer 55:2285–2290, 1985

141. Dembo AJ, Bush RS, Beale FA et al: The Princess Margaret study of ovarian carcinoma Stages I, II, and asymptomatic III presentations. Cancer Treat Rep 63:249–254, 1979

142. Dembo AJ: The sequential multiple modality treatment of ovarian cancer. Radiol Oncol 3:187–192, 1985

143. Delclos L, Smith JP: Tumors of the ovary. In Fletcher G (ed): Textbook of Radiotherapy, 2nd Ed, pp 690–702. Philadelphia, Lea & Febiger

144. Perez CA, Korba A, Zivnusk F et al: Cobalt 60 moving strip technique in the management of carcinoma of the ovary: Analysis of tumor control and morbidity. Int J Radiat Oncol Biol Phys 4:379–388, 1978

145. Perez CA, Walz BZ, Jacobson PL: Radiation therapy in the management of carcinoma of the ovary. Natl Cancer Inst Monogr 42:119–125, 1975

146. Hanks G, Bagshaw MA: Megavoltage radiation therapy and lymphangiography in ovarian cancer. Radiology 93:649–654, 1969

147. Delclos L, Barun EJ, Herrera JR et al: Whole abdominal irradiation by cobalt-60 moving strip technique. Radiology 81:632–641, 1963

148. Perez CA, Korba A, Zivnuska F et al: 60Co moving strip technique in the management of carcinoma of the ovary: Analysis of tumor control and morbidity. Int J Radiat Oncol Biol Phys 4:379–388, 1978

149. Glatstein E, Fuks Z, Bagshaw MA: Diaphragmatic treatment in ovarian carcinoma: A new radiotherapeutic technique. Int J Radiat Oncol Biol Phys 2:357–362, 1977

150. Ellis F: Dose–time fractionation: A clinical hypothesis. Clin Radiol 20:1–7, 1969

151. Dixon RL: General equation for the calculation of nominal standard dose. Acta Radiol [Ther] 11:305–311, 1972

152. Orton CG, Ellis F: A simplification in the use of the NSD concept in practical radiotherapy. Br J Radiol 46:529–537, 1973

153. Martinez A: Perspective: The role of radiation therapy in the treatment of epithelial ovarian cancer. In Ballon SC (ed): Gynecologic Oncology: Controversies in Cancer Treatment, pp 300–310. Boston, GK Hall, 1981

154. Martinez A, Schray MF, Hoes AE, Bagshaw MA: Postoperative radiation therapy for epithelial ovarian cancer: The curative role based on a 24-year experience. J Clin Oncol 3:901–922, 1985

155. Schray MF, Cox RS, Martinez A: Lower abdominal radiotherapy for Stages I, II and selected III epithelial ovarian cancer: 20 years' experience. Gynecol Oncol 15:78–87, 1983

156. Fazekas JT, Maier JF: Irradiation of ovarian carcinomas: A prospective comparison of the open-field and moving-strip techniques. Am J Roentgenol Rad Ther Nucl Med 120:118–123, 1974

157. Fuks Z: The role of radiation therapy in the management of ovarian carcinoma. Isr J Med Sci 8:815–828, 1977

158. Smith JP, Rutledge FN, Delclos L: Postoperative treatment of early cancer of the ovary: A random trial between postoperative irradiation and chemotherapy. Natl Cancer Inst Monogr 42:149–153, 1975

159. Brady LW: Advances in the management of gynecologic cancer: Radiation therapy. Cancer 36:661–668, 1975

160. Kjellgren O, Johnsson L: Bone marrow depression in the pelvis after megavoltage irradiation for ovarian carcinoma. Obstet Gynecol 105:849–855, 1969

161. Luxton R: Radiation nephritis. Q J Med 22:215–242, 1953

162. Ingold JA, Reed GB, Kaplan HS et al: Radiation hepatitis. Am J Roentgenol Rad Ther Nucl Med 93:200–205, 1965

163. Hintz BL, Fuks Z, Kempson RL et al: Results of postoperative megavoltage radiotherapy of malignant surface epithelial tumors of the ovary. Radiology 114:695–700, 1975

164. Long RT, Sala JM: Radical surgery combined with radiotherapy in the treatment of advanced ovarian carcinoma. Surg Gynecol Obstet 117:201–204, 1963

165. Kottmeier HL: Carcinoma of the uterine cervix, endometrium and ovary. In Year Book of Cancer, p 293. Chicago, Year Book Medical Publishers, 1962

166. Kjorstad KE, Welander G, Kolstad P: Preoperative irradiation in Stage III carcinoma of the ovary. Acta Obstet Gynecol Scand 56:449–452, 1977

167. Aure JC, Hoeg K, Kolstad P: Radioactive colloidal gold in the treatment of ovarian carcinoma. Acta Radiol [Ther] (Stockh) 10:399–407, 1971

168. Moore DW, Langley II: Routine use of radiogold following operation for ovarian cancer. Am J Obstet Gynecol 98:624–630, 1967

169. Pezner RD, Stevens KR Jr, Tong D, Allen CV: Limited epithelial carcinoma of the ovary treated with curative intent by intraperitoneal installation of radiocolloids. Cancer 42:2563–2671, 1978

170. Bagley CM Jr, Young RC, Canellos GP, DeVita VT: Treatment of ovarian carcinoma: Possibilities for progress, N Engl J Med 287:856–862, 1972

171. Louie KG, Ozols RF, Myers CE et al: Long-term results of a cisplatin-containing combination chemotherapy regimen for the treatment of advanced ovarian carcinoma. J Clin Oncol 4:1579, 1986

172. Schwartz PE, Smith JP: Second-look operations in ovarian cancer. Am J Obstet Gynecol 138:1124–1130, 1980

173. Johnson BL, Fisher RI, Bender RA et al: Hexamethylmelamine in alkylating agent resistant ovarian carcinoma. Cancer 42:2157, 1978

174. Bolis G, D'Incalci M, Belloni C et al: Hexamethylmelamine in ovarian cancer resistant to cyclophosphamide and Adriamycin. Cancer Treat Rep 63:1375, 1979

175. Ozols RF, Young RC: Chemotherapy of ovarian cancer. Semin Oncol 11:251–263, 1984

176. Young RC, Von Hoff DD, Gormley P et al: Cis-dichlorodiammineplatinum(II) for the treatment of advanced ovarian cancer. Cancer Treat Rep 63:1539–1544, 1979

177. Lambert HE, Berry RJ: High-dose cisplatin compared with high-dose cyclophosphamide in the management of advanced epithelial ovarian cancer (FIGO Stages III and IV): Report from the North Thames Cooperative Group. Br Med J 290:889–892, 1985

178. Ozols RF, Ostchega Y, Myers CE et al: High-dose cisplatin in hypertonic saline in refractory ovarian cancer. J Clin Oncol 3:1246–1250, 1985

179. Ozols RF, Corden BJ: High-dose cisplatin in hypertonic saline. Ann Intern Med 100:19–24, 1984

180. Ozols RF, Young RC: High-dose cisplatin therapy in ovarian cancer. Semin Oncol 12:21–30, 1985

181. Bruckner HW, Wallach R: High-dose cisplatin for the treatment of refractory ovarian cancer. Gynecol Oncol 12:64–67, 1984

182. Barker GH, Wiltshaw E: Use of high dose cis-dichlorodiammine platinum-II following failure on previous chemotherapy for advanced carcinoma of the ovary. Br J Obstet Med 88:1192–1199, 1981

183. Levin L, Hryniuk WM: Dose intensity analysis of chemotherapy regimens in ovarian carcinoma. J Clin Oncol 5:756–767, 1987

184. Bolis G, D'Incalci M, Gramellini F et al: Adriamycin in ovarian cancer patients resistant to cyclophosphamide. Eur J Cancer 14:1401, 1978

185. Hubbard SM, Barkes P, Young RC: Adriamycin therapy for advanced ovarian carcinoma after chemotherapy. Cancer Treat Rep 62:1375, 1978

186. Wharton JT, Rutledge F, Smith JP et al: Hexamethylmelamine: An evaluation of its role in the treatment of ovarian cancer. Am J Obstet Gynecol 133:833, 1979

187. Foster BJ, Clagett–Carr K, Marsoni S et al: Role of hexamethylmelamine in the treatment of ovarian cancer: Where is the needle in the haystack? Cancer Treat Rep 70:1003, 1986

188. Wiltshaw E, Evans BD, Jones et al: JM8, successor to cisplatin in advanced ovarian carcinoma. Lancet 1:587, 1983

189. Canetta R, Carter SK: Developing new drugs for ovarian cancer: A challenging task in a changing reality. J Cancer Res Clin Oncol 107:111, 1984

190. Thigpen JT, Vance RB, Balducci L, Khansur T: New drugs and experimental approaches in ovarian cancer treatment. Semin Oncol 11:314, 1984

191. Bruhl P, Gunther V, Hoefer–Janker H et al: Results obtained with fractionated ifosfamide massive-dose treatment in generalized malignant tumors. Int J Clin Pharmacol Biopharmacol 14:29–39, 1976

192. Kuhnle H, Achterrath W, Frischkorn R: Krankheitsorientierte Phase II Studie mit Etoposid (NSC 141540) bei Cisplatin-refraktaren Ovarialkarzinomen. Tumor Diagn Ther 5:152, 1984

193. Hillcoat BL, Campbell JJ, Pepperell R et al: Phase II trail of VP-16-213 in advanced ovarian carcinoma. Gynecol Oncol 22:162, 1985

194. Paccagnella A, Tredese F, Salvagno L et al: Peptichemio in pretreated patients with ovarian cancer. Cancer Treat Rep 69:17, 1985

195. Creech RH, Shah MK, Catalano RB et al: Phase II study of low-dose mitomycin in patients with ovarian cancer previously treated with chemotherapy. Cancer Treat Rep 69:1271, 1985

196. Willocks D, Toppila M, Hudson CN et al: Estrogen and progesterone receptors in human ovarian tumors. Gynecol Oncol 16:246, 1983

197. Wurz H, Wussner E, Citoler P et al: Multiple cytoplasmic steroid hormone receptors in benign and malignant ovarian tumors and in disease-free ovaries. Tumor Diagn Ther 4:15, 1983

198. Ford LC, Berek JS, Lagasse LD et al: Estrogen and progesterone receptors in ovarian neoplasms. Gynecol Oncol 15:299, 1983

199. Geisler H: Megestrol acetate for the palliation of advanced ovarian carcinoma. Obstet Gynecol 61:95, 1983

200. Aabo K, Pedersen AG, Haid I et al: High-dose medroxyprogesterone acetate (MPA) in advanced chemotherapy-resistant ovarian carcinoma: A Phase II study. Cancer Treat Rep 66:407–408, 1982

201. Trope C, Johnsson JE, Sigurdsson K et al: High-dose medroxyprogesterone acetate for the treatment of advanced ovarian carcinoma. Cancer Treat Rep 66:1441–1443, 1982

202. Myers M, Moore GE, Major FJ: Advanced ovarian carcinoma: Response to antiestrogen therapy. Cancer 48:2368–2370, 1981

203. Schwartz P, Kenting G, Maclusky N et al: Tamoxifen therapy for advanced ovarian cancer. Obstet Gynecol 59:583–588, 1982

204. Hamerlynck JVTH, Maskens AP, Mangioni C et al: Phase II trial of medroxyprogesterone acetate in advanced ovarian cancer: An EORTC Gynecological Cancer Cooperative Group study. Gynecol Oncol 22:313, 1985

205. Slevin ML, Harvey VJ, Osborne RJ et al: A Phase II study of tamoxifen in ovarian cancer. Eur J Cancer Clin Oncol 22:309, 1986

206. Shirey DR, Kavanagh JJ, Gershenson DM et al: Tamoxifen therapy of epithelial ovarian cancer. Obstet Gynecol 66:575, 1985

207. Freedman RS, Saul PB, Edwards CL et al: Ethinylestradiol and medroxyprogesterone acetate in patients with epithelial ovarian carcinoma: A Phase II study. Cancer Treat Rep 70:369, 1986

208. Hamburger AW, Salmon SE, Kim MB et al: Direct cloning of human ovarian carcinoma cells in agar. Cancer Res 38:3438–3444, 1978

209. Hanauske AR, Von Hoff DD: The value of the human tumor cloning assay in ovarian cancer. Clin Obstet Gynecol 29:638, 1986

210. Young RC, Chabner BA, Hubbard SP et al: Prospective trial of melphalan (L-PAM) versus combination chemotherapy (Hexa-CAF) in ovarian adenocarcinoma. N Engl J Med 299:1261–1266, 1978

211. Neijt JP, Vanlindert ACM, Vendrijk CPJ et al: Hexa-CAF combination chemotherapy and other multiple drug regimens in advanced ovarian carcinoma: Present and future. Neth J Med 22:28, 1979

212. Vogl SE, Pagano M, Davis T et al: Platinum based combination chemotherapy versus melphalan for advanced ovarian carcinoma. Proc Int Congr Chemother 207:9–13, 1983

213. Delgado G, Smith FP, McLaughlin EF et al: Single agent vs. combination chemotherapy for ovarian cancer. Am J Clin Oncol 8:33–37, 1985

214. Edmonson JH, Fleming TR, Decker DG et al: Different chemotherapeutic sensitivities and host factors affecting prognosis in advanced ovarian carcinoma versus minimal residual disease. Cancer Treat Rep 63:241–247, 1979

215. Williams CJ, Mead GM, Macbeth FR et al: Cisplatin combination chemotherapy versus chlorambucil in advanced ovarian carcinoma: Mature results of a randomized trial. J Clin Oncol 3:1455–1462, 1985

216. Carmo–Pereria J, Costa FO, Henique E: Cis-platin, Adriamycin and hexamethylmelamine vs. cyclophosphamide in advanced ovarian cancer. Cancer Chemother Pharmacol 10:100, 1983

217. Trope C: A prospective randomized trial comparison of melphalan vs. melphalan–Adriamycin in advanced ovarian carcinoma (abstr). Proc Am Soc Clin Oncol 22:469, 1981

218. Decker DG, Fleming TR, Malkasian GD et al: Cyclophosphamide plus cisplatinum in combination: Treatment program for Stage III or IV ovarian carcinoma. Obstet Gynecol 60:481–486, 1982

219. MRC Working Party on Ovarian Cancer: Medical Research Council study on chemotherapy in advanced ovarian cancer. Br J Obstet Gynaecol 88:1174, 1981

220. Carmo–Pereira J, Costa FO, Henriques E et al: Advanced ovarian carcinoma: A prospective and randomized clinical trial of cyclophosphamide versus combination cytotoxic chemotherapy (Hexa-CAF). Cancer 48:1947–1951, 1981

221. Ludwig Institute for Cancer Research: Chemotherapy of advanced ovarian adenocarcinoma: A randomized comparison of combination versus sequential therapy using chlorambucil and cisplatin. Gynecol Oncol 23:1–13, 1986

222. Reimer RR, Hoover R, Fraumeni JF, Young RC: Acute leukemia after alkylating agent therapy in ovarian cancer. N Engl J Med 297:117, 1977

223. Greene MH, Boice JD, Greer BE et al: Acute non-lymphocytic leukemia after therapy with alkylating agents for ovarian cancer. N Engl J Med 307:1416, 1982

224. Weiss GR: Second-line chemotherapy for ovarian cancer. Clin Obstet Gynecol 29:665, 1986

225. Bruntsch U: Sekundare Chemotherapie beim fortgeschrittenen Ovarialkarzinoma: Neue Medikamente. Onkologie 8:410, 1985

226. Kardinal CG, Luce JK: Evaluation of a hexamethylmelamine and 5-fluorouracil combination in the treatment of advanced ovarian carcinoma. Cancer Treat Rep 61:1691, 1977

227. Barlow JJ, Piver MS: High-dose methotrexate plus Cytoxan in ovarian cancer (abstr). Proc Am Assoc Cancer Res 20:361, 1979

228. Briscoe KE, Pasmantier MW, Ohnuma T et al: Cis-dichlorodiammineplatinum (II) and Adriamycin treatment of advanced ovarian cancer. Cancer Treat Rep 62:2027, 1978

229. Bruckner HW, Cohen CJ, Kabakow B et al: Ovarian cancer: Secondary cisplatin regimens and prognostic factors (abstr). Proc Am Assoc Cancer Res 22:469, 1981

230. Neijt JP, ten Bokkel Huinink WW, Hamersma E et al: Combination chemotherapy including cisplatinum in previously treated patients with advanced ovarian carcinoma (abstr). Proc Am Soc Clin Oncol 1:108, 1982

231. Alberts DS, Hilgers RD, Moon TE et al: Combination chemotherapy for alkylator-resistant ovarian carcinoma: A preliminary report of a Southwest Oncology Group trial. Cancer Treat Rep 63:301, 1979

232. Kane R, Harvey H, Andrews T et al: Phase II trial of cyclophosphamide, hexamethylmelamine, Adriamycin and cis-dichlorodiammineplatinum(II) combination chemotherapy in advanced ovarian cancer. Cancer Treat Rep 63:307, 1979

233. Bruckner HW, Cohen CJ, Deppe G et al: Ovarian cancer schedule modification and dosage intensification of cyclophosphamide, hexamethylmelamine, adriamycin, cisplatin regimen (CHAP-II) (abstr). Proc Am Soc Clin Oncol 1:107, 1982

234. Bernath A, Andrews T, Dixon R et al: Long term follow-up of HAP vs. CAP in alkylating agent resistant advanced ovarian carcinoma (abstr). Proc Am Soc Clin Oncol 1:110, 1982

235. Barlow JJ, Piver MS: Second-line efficacy of intermediate high dose methotrexate with citrovorum factor rescue and cyclophosphamide in ovarian cancer. Gynecol Oncol 7:233, 1979

236. Vogl SE, Pagano M, Davis TE et al: Hexamethylmelamine and cisplatin in advanced ovarian cancer after failure of alkylating agent therapy. Cancer Treat Rep 66:1285, 1982

237. Lopez JA, Krikorian JG, Dias SF et al: Cisplatin–hexamethylamine therapy for advanced ovarian cancer. Gynecol Oncol 11:64, 1981

238. Barlow JJ, Lele SB: Etoposide (VP-16) plus cisplatin (DDP): A new active chemotherapeutic combination in patients with Stage III–IV ovarian adenocarcinoma. J Surg Oncol 32:43, 1986

239. De Lena M, Lorusso V, Romito S: Cisplatin plus etoposide as second-line treatment in advanced ovarian carcinoma. Cancer Treat Rep 70:893, 1986

240. Ehrlich CE, Einhorn L, Williams SD et al: Chemotherapy for Stage III–IV epithelial ovarian cancer with cis-dichlorodiammineplatinum(II), Adriamycin, and cyclophosphamide: A preliminary report. Cancer Treat Rep 63:281–288, 1979

241. Parker LM, Griffiths CT, Yankee RA et al: Combination chemotherapy with Adriamycin–cyclophosphamide for advanced ovarian carcinoma. Cancer 46:669–674, 1980

242. Wiltshaw E, Evans B, Rustin G et al: A prospective randomized trial comparing high-dose cisplatin with low-dose cisplatin and chlorambucil in advanced ovarian carcinoma. J Clin Oncol 4:722, 1986

243. Piccart M, Speyer J, Wernz J et al: Advanced epithelial ovarian cancer (OV-CA): Update with impressive survival utilizing cisplatin (DDP) (100 mg/m²/cycle) and cyclophosphamide (CTX) (abstr). Proc Am Soc Clin Oncol 4:117, 1985

244. Neijt JP van der Burg MEL, Vriesendorp R et al: Randomized trial comparing two combination chemotherapy regimens (Hexa-CAF vs. CHAP-5) in advanced ovarian carcinoma. Lancet 2:594–598, 1984

245. Omura G, Blessing JA, Ehrlich CE et al: A randomized trial of cyclophosphamide and doxorubicin with or without cisplatin in advanced ovarian carcinoma. Cancer 57:1725–1730, 1986

246. Neijt JP, ten Bokkel Huinink WW, van der Burg MEL: Randomized trial comparing two combination chemotherapy regimens (CHAP-5 v. CP) in advanced ovarian carcinoma. J Clin Oncol 5:1157–1168, 1987

247. Edmonson JH, McCormack GW, Fleming TR et al: Comparison of cyclophosphamide plus cisplatin versus hexamethylmelamine, cyclophosphamide, doxorubicin, and cisplatin in combination as initial chemotherapy for Stage III and IV ovarian carcinomas. Cancer Treat Rep 69:1243, 1985

248. Omura GA, Bundy B, Wilbanks G et al: A randomized trial of cyclophosphamide (C) plus cisplatin (P) with or without Adriamycin (A) in ovarian carcinoma. Proc Am Soc Clin Oncol 6:A439, 1987

249. Conte PF, Bruzzone M, Chiara S et al: A randomized trial comparing cisplatin plus cyclophosphamide versus cisplatin, doxorubicin, and cyclophosphamide in advanced ovarian cancer. J Clin Oncol 4:965–971, 1986

250. Jakobsen A, Bertelsen K, Sell A et al: Advantage of CAP over CP in terms of survival in advanced ovarian carcinoma (abstr). Proc Am Soc Clin Oncol 4:113, 1985

251. Mayer RJ, Berkowitz RS, Griffiths CT: Central nervous system involvement by ovarian carcinoma: A complication of prolonged survival with metastatic disease. Cancer 41:776, 1978

252. Bast RC, Knapp RC: Immunologic approaches to the management of ovarian carcinoma. Semin Oncol 11:264–274, 1984

253. Hamilton TC, Ozols RF, Longo DL: Biologic therapy for the treatment of malignant common epithelial tumors of the ovary. Cancer 60:2054–2063, 1987

254. Bast RC, Berek JS, Obrist R et al: Intraperitoneal immunotherapy of human ovarian carcinoma with *Corynebacterium parvum* (abstr). Proc Am Soc Clin Oncol 1:38, 1982

255. Mantovani A, Sessa C, Peri G et al: Intraperitoneal administration of *Corynebacterium*

parvum in patients with ascitic ovarian tumors resistant to chemotherapy: Effects on cytotoxicity of tumor-associated macrophages and NK cells. Int J Cancer 27:437–446, 1981

256. Hamilton TC, Young RC, McKoy WM et al: Characterization of a human ovarian carcinoma cell line (NIH:OVCAR-3) with androgen and estrogen receptors. Cancer Res 43:5379–5389, 1983

257. Gudson JP, Homesley HD, Muss HB et al: Chemotherapy of advanced ovarian epithelial carcinoma with melphalan and levamisole: A pilot study of the Gynecologic Oncology Group. Am J Obstet Gynecol 141:65–70, 1981

258. Creasman WT, Yale SA, Blessing JA et al: Chemoimmunotherapy in the management of primary Stage III ovarian cancer. Cancer Treat Rep 63:319, 1979

259. Alberts DS, Moon TE, Stephens RA et al: Randomized study of chemoimmunotherapy for advanced ovarian carcinoma. Cancer Treat Rep 63:325, 1982

260. Steis R, Bookman M, Clark J et al: Intraperitoneal lymphokine activated killer (LAK) cell and interleukin-2 (IL-2) therapy for peritoneal carcinomatosis: Toxicity, efficacy and laboratory results. Proc Am Soc Clin Oncol 6:A984, 1987

261. Pirker R, Fitzgerald DJP, Hamilton TC et al: Anti-transferrin receptor antibody linked to *Pseudomonas exotoxin* as a model immunotoxin in human ovarian carcinoma cell lines. Cancer Res 45:751–757, 1985

262. Pirker R, Fitzgerald DJP, Hamilton TC, et al: Characterization of immunotoxins active against ovarian cancer cell lines. J Clin Invest 76:1261–1267, 1985

263. Shen DW, Fojo A, Chin JE et al: Human multidrug-resistant cell lines: Increased *mdr*-1 expression can precede gene amplification. Science 232:643–645, 1986

264. Fojo A, Hamilton TC, Young RC et al: Multidrug resistance in ovarian cancer. Cancer 60:2075–2080, 1987

265. Juliano RL, Ling V: A surface glycoprotein modulating drug permeability in Chinese hamster ovary cell mutants. Biochim Biophys Acta 455:152–162, 1976

266. Debenham PG, Kartner N, Siminovitch L et al: DNA-mediated transfer of multiple drug resistance and plasma membrane glycoprotein expression. Mol Cell Biol 2:881–889, 1982

267. Roninson IB: Detection and mapping of homologous, repeated and amplified DNA sequences by DNA renaturation in agarose gels. Nucleic Acids Res 11:5413–5432, 1983

268. Riordan JR, Deuchars K, Kartner N et al: Amplification of P-glycoprotein genes in multidrug-resistant mammalian cell lines. Nature 316:817–819, 1985

269. Louie KG, Hamilton TC, Winker MA et al: Adriamycin accumulation and metabolism in Adriamycin-sensitive and resistant human ovarian cancer cell lines. Biochem Pharmacol 35:467–472, 1986

270. Hamilton TC, Masuda H, Young RC, Ozols RF: Modulation of cisplatin cytotoxicity by inhibition of DNA repair in a cisplatin resistant human ovarian cancer cell line 2780^{CP} (abstr). Proc Am Soc Cancer Res 28:291, 1987

271. Rogan AM, Hamilton TC, Young RC et al: Reversal of Adriamycin resistance by verapamil in human ovarian cancer. Science 224:994–998, 1984

272. Ozols RF, Cunnion RE, Klecker RW Jr et al: Verapamil and Adriamycin in the treatment of drug resistant ovarian cancer patients. J Clin Oncol 5:641–647, 1987

273. Meister A: Selective modification of glutathione metabolism. Science 20:472–477, 1983

274. Green JA, Vistica DT, Young RC et al: Potentiation of melphalan cytotoxicity in human ovarian cancer cell lines by glutathione depletion. Cancer Res 44:5427–5431, 1984

275. Ozols RF, Louis KG, Plowman J et al: Enhanced alkylating agent cytotoxicity in human ovarian cancer in vitro and in tumor bearing nude mice by buthionine sulfoximine depletion of glutathione. Biochem Pharmacol 36:147–153, 1987

276. Ozols RF, Hamilton TC, Masuda H, Young RC: The role of thiols in drug resistance. In Woolley PV III, Tew KD (eds): Mechanisms of Drug Resistance in Neoplastic Cells, 289–306 New York, Academic Press, 1988

277. Behrens BC, Hamilton TC, Masuda H et al: Characterization of a cis-diamminedichloroplatinum(II)-resistant human ovarian cancer cell line and its use in evaluation of platinum analogs. Cancer Res 47:414–418, 1987

278. Smith JP, Day TG: Review of ovarian cancer at the University of Texas Center, M.D. Anderson Hospital and Tumor Institute. Am J Obstet Gynecol 135:984–993, 1979

279. Einhorn L, Nilsson BO, Sjorall K: Factors influencing survival in carcinoma of the ovary: Study from a well-defined Swedish population. Cancer 55:2019–2025, 1985

280. Swenerton KD, Hislop TG, Spinelli J et al: Ovarian carcinoma: A multivariate analysis of prognostic factors. Obstet Gynecol 65:265–254, 1985

281. Redman JR, Petroni GR, Saigo PE et al: Prognostic factors in ovarian carcinoma. J Clin Oncol 4:515–523, 1986

282. Young RC, Decker DG, Wharton JT et al: Staging laparotomy in early ovarian cancer. JAMA 250:3072–3076, 1983

283. Webb MJ, Decker DG, Massey et al: Factors influencing survival in Stage I ovarian cancer. Am J Obstet Gynecol 166:222, 1973

284. Hreshchyshyn MW, Park RC, Blessing JA et al: The role of adjuvant therapy in Stage I ovarian cancer. Am J Obstet Gynecol 138:139–145, 1980

285. Young RC, Walton L, Decker D et al: Early stage ovarian cancer: Preliminary results of randomized trials after comprehensive initial staging (abstr). Proc Am Soc Clin Oncol 2:148, 1983

286. Piver SM: Radioactive colloids in the treatment of Stage IA ovarian cancer. Obstet Gynecol 40:42–44, 1972

287. Bush RS: Radiation therapy for patients with ovarian cancer. Strahlentherapie 159:131–137, 1983

288. Smith JP: Treatment of ovarian cancer. In Carter SK, Goldin A, Kuretroi K et al (eds): Advances in Cancer Chemotherapy, pp 493–503. Baltimore, University Park Press, 1978

289. Drouin P, Rutledge FN, Delclos L et al: Comparison of external radiotherapy and chemotherapy in ovarian cancer. Ann R Coll Phys Surg Can 12:61, 1979

290. Delclos L: International Symposium on Combined Modalities Approach on Gynecologic Cancer, Mexico City, May 1983, p 61

291. Einhorn N: The place of adjuvant chemotherapy in early stages. Int J Radiat Oncol Biol Phys 8:257–258, 1982

292. Hacker NF, Berek JS, Burnison CM et al: Whole abdominal radiation salvage therapy for epithelial ovarian cancer. Obstet Gynecol 65:619–623, 1985

293. Belinson JT, McClure M, Ashikaga T, Karakoff IH: Treatment of advanced and recurrent ovarian carcinoma with cyclophosphamide, doxorubicin and cisplatin. Cancer 54:1983–1990, 1984

294. Wharton JT, Edwards CL, Rutledge FN: Long term survival after chemotherapy for advanced epithelial ovarian carcinoma. Am J Obstet Gynecol 148:997–1005, 1984

295. Ozols RF, Young RC: Ovarian Cancer. In Haskell CM (ed): Current Problems in Cancer, Vol 11, pp 59–122. Chicago, Year Book Medical Publishers, 1987

296. Greco FA, Hande KR, Jones HW et al: Advanced ovarian cancer: Long-term follow-up after brief intensive chemotherapy (abstr). Proc Am Soc Clin Oncol 3:166, 1984

297. Hainsworth JD, Malcolm A, Johnson DH: Treatment of minimal residual advanced ovarian carcinoma: Abdominopelvic irradiation following incomplete response to combination chemotherapy. Obstet Gynecol 61:619–623, 1983

298. Dougherty J, Hakes T, Cain J et al: Recurrence pattern of advanced ovarian carcinoma after negative laparotomy (abstr). Proc Am Soc Clin Oncol 4:122, 1985

299. Hintz BL, Fuks Z, Kempson RL et al: Results of postoperative megavoltage radiotherapy of malignant surface epithelial tumors of the ovary. Radiology 114:695–700, 1975

300. Griffiths CT, Grogan RH, Hall TC: Advanced ovarian cancer: Primary treatment with surgery, radiotherapy, and chemotherapy. Cancer 29:1–7, 1972

301. Sigurdson K, Johnsson JE, Trope C: Carcinoma of the ovary in stage III: Effects of postoperative chemotherapy, radiation therapy and repeat laparotomy. Acta Radiat Oncol 21:181–189, 1982

302. Aure JC, Hoeg K, Kolstad P: Clinical and histologic studies of ovarian carcinoma: Long term follow-up of 990 cases. Obstet Gynecol 37:1–9, 1971

303. Delclos L, Quinlan EJ: Malignant tumor of the ovary managed with postoperative megavoltage irradiation. Radiology 93:659–663, 1969

304. Potish R, Adcock L, Brooker D et al: Sequential surgery, radiation therapy and Alkeran in the management of epithelial caricnoma of the ovary. Cancer 45:2754–2758, 1980

305. Nevin JE, Pinzon G, Baggerly TJ et al: The use of intravenous phenylalanine mustard followed by supervoltage irradiation in the treatment of carcinoma of the ovary. Cancer 51:1273–1283, 1984

306. Perez CA, Korba A, Zivnuska F et al: ^{60}Co moving strip technique in the management of carcinoma of the ovary: Analysis of tumor control and morbidity of carcinoma of the ovary: Analysis of tumor control and morbidity. Int J Radiat Oncol Biol Phys 4:379–388, 1978

307. Fuks Z, Rizel S, Anteby SO, Biran S: The multimodal approach to the treatment of stage III ovarian carcinoma. Int J Radiat Oncol Biol Phys 8:903–908, 1982

308. Fuks Z, Rizel S, Biran S: Chemotherapeutic and surgical induction of pathological complete remission and whole abdominal irradiation for consolidation does not enhance the cure of stage III ovarian carcinoma. J Clin Oncol 6:509–516, 1988

309. Neijt JP, ten Bokkel Huinink WW, van der Burg MEL et al: Complete remission at laparotomy: Still gold standard in ovarian cancer? Lancet 1:1028, 1986

310. Coltart RS, Nethersell BW, Brown CH: A pilot study of high dose abdominopelvic radiotherapy following surgery and chemotherapy for Stage III epithelial carcinoma of the ovary. Gynecol Oncol 23:105–110, 1986

311. Piver MS, Barlow JJ, Lee FT, Vongtama V: Sequential therapy for advanced ovarian adenocarcinoma: Operation, chemotherapy, second-look laparotomy and radiation therapy. Am J Obstet Gynecol 122:355–357, 1975

312. Kucera PR, Sheets EE, Micha JP et al: Whole abdominal radiotherapy for patients with minimal residual epithelial ovarian cancer. Presented at the Thirteenth Annual Meeting of the Western Association of Gynecologic Oncologist, San Diego, June 1985

313. Hoskins WJ, Lichter AS, Whittington R et al: Whole abdominal and pelvic irradiation in patients with minimal disease at second-look surgical reassessment for ovarian cancer. Gynecol Oncol 20:271–280, 1985

314. Peters WA, Blasko JC, Bagley CM et al: Salvage therapy with whole-abdominal irradiation in patients with advanced carcinoma of the ovary previously treated by combination chemotherapy. Cancer 58:880–882, 1986

315. Menczer J, Modan M, Brenner et al: Abdominopelvic irradiation for Stage II–IV ovarian carcinoma patients with limited or no residual disease at second-look laparotomy after completion of cisplatin-based combination chemotherpay. Gynecol Oncol 24:149, 1986

316. Young JA, Johnson A, Kroener J et al: Alternating combination chemotherapy for Stages III and IV ovarian carcinoma. J Clin Oncol 2:1317–1320, 1984

317. Dedrick RL, Myers CE, Bungay PM et al: Pharmacokinetic rationale for peritoneal drug administration in the treatment of ovarian cancer. Cancer Treat Rep 62:1, 1978

318. Dedrick RL: Theoretical and experimental bases of intraperitoneal chemotherapy. Semin Oncol 12:1–6, 1985

319. Myers C: The use of intraperitoneal chemotherapy in the treatment of ovarian cancer. Semin Oncol 11:275–284, 1984

320. Jones RB, Myers CE, Guarino AM et al: High volume intraperitoneal chemotherapy ("belly bath") for ovarian cancer. Cancer Chemother Pharmacol 1:161–166, 1978

321. Speyer JL, Collins JM, Dedrick RL et al: Phase I and pharmacologic studies of 5-fluorouracil administered intraperitoneally. Cancer Res 40:567, 1980

322. Ozols RF, Young RC, Speyer JL et al: Phase I and pharmacologic studies of Adriamy-

cin administered intraperitoneally to patients with ovarian cancer. Cancer Res 42:4265, 1982

323. Brenner DE: Intraperitoneal chemotherapy: A review. J Clin Oncol 4:1135–1147, 1986

324. Gyves JW, Ensminger WD, Stetson P et al: Constant intraperitoneal 5-fluorouracil infusion through a totally implanted system. Clin Pharmacol Ther 35:83–89, 1984

325. Howell SB, Pfeifle CL, Wung WE et al: Intraperitoneal chemotherapy with melphalan. Ann Intern Med 101:14–18, 1984

326. Howell SB, Chu BB, Wung WE et al: Long-duration intracavitary infusion of methotrexate with systemic leucovorin protection in patients with malignant effusions. J Clin Invest 67:1161–1170, 1981

327. Howell S, Pfeifle C, Wung W et al: Intraperitoneal cisplatin with systemic thiosulfate protection. Ann Intern Med 97:845–851, 1982

328. Pretorius RG, Hacker NF, Berek JS et al: Pharmacokinetics of IP cisplatin in refractory ovarian carcinoma. Cancer Treat Rep 67:1085–1092, 1983

329. Casper ES, Kelsen DP, Alcock NW et al: IP cisplatin in patients with malignant ascites: Pharmacokinetic evaluation and comparison with the IV route. Cancer Treat Rep 67:235–238, 1983

330. Ozols RF: Intraperitoneal chemotherapy in the management of ovarian cancer. Semin Oncol 12:75–80, 1985

331. Ozols RF, Speyer JL, Jenkins J et al: Phase II trial of 5-FU administered IP to patients with refractory ovarian cancer. Cancer Treat Rep 68:1229–1232, 1984

332. Markman M, Howell SB, Lucas WE et al: Combination intraperitoneal chemotherapy with cisplatin, cytarabine, and doxorubicin for refractory ovarian carcinoma and other malignancies principally confined to the peritoneal cavity. J Clin Oncol 2:1321–1326, 1984

333. ten Bokkel Huinink WW, Dubbelman R, Aartsen E et al: Experimental and clinical results with intraperitoneal cisplatin. Semin Oncol 12:43–46, 1985

334. Cohen CJ: Surgical considerations in ovarian cancer. Semin Oncol 12:53–56, 1985

335. Markman M, Howell S, Cleary S et al: Survival following cisplatin (DDP)-based intraperitoneal chemotherapy for refractory ovarian carcinoma (abstr). Proc Am Soc Clin Oncol 5:113, 1986

336. Markman M, Cleary S, Lucas WE, Howell SB: Intraperitoneal chemotherapy with high-dose cisplatin and cytosine arabinoside for refractory ovarian carcinoma and other malignancies principally involving the peritoneal cavity. J Clin Oncol 3(7):925–931, 1985

337. Zimm S, Cleary S, Lucas W et al: Phase I/pharmacokinetic study of intraperitoneal (IP) cisplatin (DDP) and etoposide (VP-16) (abstr). Proc Am Soc Clin Oncol 5:49, 1986

338. Rutledge FN, Fletcher GH, Smith JP et al: In Clark RL, Howe CD (eds): Cancer Patient Care at M.D. Anderson Hospital and tumor Institute, pp 263–308. Chicago, Year Book Medical Publishers, 1976

339. Stage AH, Grafton WD: Thecomas and granulosa–theca cell tumors of the ovary: An analysis of 51 tumors. Obstet Gynecol 50:21, 1977

340. Diddle AW: Granulosa and thecal-cell ovarian tumors: Prognosis. Cancer 5:215–228, 1952

341. Lusch CJ, Mercurio TM, Runyeon WK: Delayed recurrence and chemotherapy of a granulosa cell tumor. Obstet Gynecol 51:505–507, 1978

342. DiSaia PJ, Saltz A, Kagan AR et al: A temporary response of recurrent granulosa cell tumors to Adriamycin. Obstet Gynecol 52:355–358, 1978

343. Kaye SB, Davies E: Cyclophosphamide, Adriamycin, and cis-platinum for the treatment of advanced granulosa cell tumor, using serum estradiol. Gynecol Oncol 24:261–264, 1986

344. Woodruff JD, Protos P, Peterson WF: Ovarian teratomas. Am J Obstet Gynecol 102:702–715, 1968

345. Jimerson GK, Woodruff JD: Ovarian extraembryoneal teratoma I: Endodermal sinus tumor. Am J Obstet Gynecol 127:73–79, 1977

346. Gallion H, Van Nagell JR, Powell DR et al: Therapy of endodermal sinus tumor of the ovary. Am J Obstet Gynecol 135:447–451, 1979

347. Cangir A, Smith J, VanEys J: Improved prognosis in children with ovarian cancers following modified VAC (vincristine sulfate, dactinomycin and cyclophosphamide) chemotherapy. Cancer 42:1234–1238, 1978

348. Slayton RE, Park RC, Silverberg SG et al: VAC treatment of malignant germ cell tumors of the ovary. Cancer 56:243–248, 1985

349. Williams S, Blessing J, Adcock L, Homesley H: Treatment of ovarian germ cell tumors with cisplatin + vinblastine + bleomycin (PVB). Proc Am Soc Clin Oncol 3:175, 1984

350. Smales E, Peckham MJ: Chemotherapy of germ cell ovarian tumors. Eur J Cancer Clin Oncol 23:469–473, 1987

351. Carlson RW, Sikic BI, Turbow MM, Ballon SC: Combination PVB for malignant germ cell tumors of the ovary. J Clin Oncol 1:546–651, 1983

352. Curry SL, Smith JP, Gallagher HS: Malignant teratoma of the ovary: Prognostic factors and treatment. Am J Obstet Gynecol 131:845–849, 1978

353. Asadourian LA, Taylor HB: Dysgerminoma: An analysis of 105 cases. Obstet Gynecol 33:370–379, 1969

354. Pedowitz P, Felmus LB, Grayzel PM: Dysgerminoma of the ovary. Am J Obstet Gynecol 70:1282–1297, 1955

355. Brody S: Clinical aspects of dysgerminoma of the ovary. Acta Radiol [Ther]56:209–230, 1961

356. Krepart G, Smith JP, Rutledge F, Delclos L: The treatment for dysgerminoma of the ovary. Cancer 41:986–990, 1978

357. Cohen SM, Goldsmith MA: Prolonged chemotherapeutic remission of metastatic ovarian dysgerminoma: Report of a case. Gynecol Oncol 5:299, 1977

358. Goldstein DP, Piro AJ: Combination chemotherapy in the treatment of germ cell tumors containing choriocarcinoma in males and females. Surg Gynecol Obstet 134:61–66, 1972

359. Fanning J, Walker RLA, Shah NR: Mixed germ cell tumor of the ovary with pure choriocarcinoma metastasis. Obstet Gynecol 68:84S, 1986

360. Munnel EW: Primary ovarian cancer associated with pregnancy. Clin Obstet Gynecol 6:983–999, 1963

361. Creasman WT, Rutledge F, Smith JP: Carcinoma of the ovary associated with pregnancy. Obstet Gynecol 38:111, 1971

I. CRAIG HENDERSON

JAY R. HARRIS

DAVID W. KINNE

SAMUEL HELLMAN

CHAPTER 38 *Cancer of the Breast*

In North America, breast cancer is the most common malignancy among women and accounts for 27% of their cancers. Eighteen per cent of the cancer deaths in women are due to breast cancer, but since 1985, lung cancer has equalled or exceeded breast cancer as a cause of cancer death in women.[1] It was estimated that 130,900 new cases of breast cancer would be diagnosed in the United States in 1987 and that 41,300 women would die of breast cancer in that year.

The risk of an individual American woman developing breast cancer over a lifetime exceeds 10%, but this figure is somewhat misleading, because it represents the probability of developing breast cancer in the interval from birth to age 110. The greatest risk is expressed after the age of 65. The cumulative risk for an individual woman before age 70 is about 7%. The risk of dying of breast cancer is about one-third of this (Table 38-1). The relative risk of developing breast cancer for an individual woman in a defined risk group is usually multiplied by the probability of any woman developing breast cancer during a lifetime, and this figure is usually taken as the cumulative risk of that individual's developing breast cancer. However, the observed risk has rarely exceeded 30% in any study. Therefore, a more meaningful calculation to use in counseling women regarding their risk of breast cancer might be a 20-year interval. For example, if a 35-year-old woman with a strong family history of breast cancer is thought to have a relative risk of 2.0, her risk of developing breast cancer by the age of 55 is slightly under 5% and her risk of dying of breast cancer is slightly over 1% (Table 38-1).

ETIOLOGY AND RISK FACTORS

The cause of breast cancer is not known, but epidemiologic evidence points strongly toward three areas: endocrine factors, environment, and genetics (Table 38-2). Breast cancer may be induced by radiation, but this probably is not an important cause of breast cancer in the general population.

ENDOCRINE FACTORS

The age of menarche, menopause, and first pregnancy have been linked to the incidence of breast cancer in numerous studies. Although there is a direct relation between the total duration of menstrual life and the risk of developing breast cancer, the most important interval appears to be the time between menarche and first pregnancy. In one study, women with menarche before the age of 12 had almost a twofold higher incidence of breast cancer than women with menarche occurring after the age of 13.[2] The same investigators observed that a delay in the onset of regular menstrual cycles decreased the risk of breast cancer by one-third to one-half in both the women who had early onset of menarche and those with late onset.[3] Because starvation and strenuous physical activity delay menarche, it is tempting to correlate international differences in the incidence of breast cancer with differences in diet, physical activity, and the onset of menarche.[4] The relative risk of developing breast cancer in women with a natural menopause before age 45 is 0.73 compared with women whose natural menopause occurs be-

TABLE 38-1.   Probability of Eventually Developing and Dying of Breast Cancer*

Age (yr)	Risk of Developing Breast cancer (%)	Risk of Developing Invasive Breast Cancer (%)	Risk of Dying of Breast Cancer (%)
Birth to 110	10.2	9.8	3.6
20 to 30	0.04	0.04	0.00
20 to 40	0.49	0.42	0.09
20 to 110	10.34	9.94	3.05
35 to 45	0.88	0.83	0.14
35 to 55	2.53	2.37	0.56
35 to 110	10.27	9.82	3.56
50 to 60	1.95	1.86	0.33
50 to 70	4.67	4.48	1.04
50 to 110	8.96	8.66	2.75
65 to 75	3.17	3.08	0.43
65 to 85	5.48	5.29	1.01
65 to 110	6.53	6.29	1.53

* Data from Surveillance, Epidemiology, and End Results (SEER): white females. Seidman H, Mushinski MH, Gelb SK et al: Probabilities of eventually developing or dying of cancer: United States, 1985. CA–A Cancer Journal for Clinicians 35:36–56, 1985.

tween the ages of 45 and 54.[5] The relative risk of breast cancer in women with a natural menopause after the age of 55 is 1.48. An artificial menopause before the age of 35 decreases the relative risk to 0.36. Oophorectomy performed between the ages of 35 and 44 reduces the relative risk to between 0.68 and 0.65, but the relative risk of breast cancer is not decreased when ovarian ablation is performed after the age of 50 or in women who have had an early natural menopause.

Nulliparous women have a higher incidence of breast cancer than women who have had one or more pregnancies, but the age of first pregnancy is an even more important determinant. In one study, the risk of developing breast cancer was increased fourfold to fivefold in women whose first pregnancy was after the age of 30 compared with those whose first pregnancy was before the age of 18.[6] It is possible that a first pregnancy after the age of 35 actually increases the risk of breast cancer.[7] It has been observed that prolactin levels in parous women are lower than in nulliparous women,[3] and the observations on the relations between a woman's menstrual history, pregnancy history, and risk of breast cancer suggest that high estrogen and high prolactin levels may promote the development of breast cancer.[3] The

TABLE 38-2.   Risk Factors Associated with Development of Breast Cancer

History of breast cancer
Family history of breast cancer, especially in first-degree relatives
Benign breast "cancer:" atypical hyperplasia
Early menarche, late menopause
Late first pregnancy > no pregnancy
Exogenous estrogens (postmenopausal, prior contraceptives)
Alcohol
Radiation
?Diet

role of progesterone in inhibiting this process is less well understood.[3,8]

The use of estrogens as postmenopausal replacement therapy or in oral contraceptives may be associated with a small increase in the risk of developing breast cancer, but this association is weak compared with the effect of estrogen in inducing or promoting endometrial cancer.[8] The use of small doses of estrogen for short periods as replacement therapy in postmenopausal women appears relatively safe. High daily doses and large cumulative doses of estrogens may result in higher risk, especially in patients who have had an oophorectomy or who have benign breast disease.[9,10] It has been estimated that the risk of developing breast cancer is increased twofold to threefold when estrogens are given for more than 10 years to women who have had an oophorectomy.[9]

There are more than 20 epidemiologic studies of the potential carcinogenic effect of oral contraceptives, and most of these have showed no relation between birth control pills and breast cancer incidence.[8,11] Nevertheless, it is not possible to rule out entirely a promotional effect in at least some patients. Assessment of these studies necessitates consideration of the composition of the oral contraceptive involved, the daily and cumulative doses of the hormone administered, and the latency for the development of breast cancer. The latency period for solid tumors is usually greater than 15 years, and the peak cancer incidence following exposure to a carcinogen occurs in the third decade. The time of exposure to a carcinogen may also be an important consideration in breast cancer epidemiology studies. For example, radiation appears to be carcinogenic for the breast only when exposure occurs at a relatively young age.[12] The only patient groups found to be at increased risk for the development of breast cancer from oral contraceptives are those with exposure prior to a first pregnancy or after the age of 45.[3] In one study, the relative risk of breast cancer was 2.25 after 4 years of oral contraceptive use and 3.52 after 8 years when oral contraceptives were administered prior to the first pregnancy (p = 0.009). These same durations of oral contraceptive use after the first pregnancy resulted in a relative risk of 1.31 and 1.74, respectively (p > 0.30).[2] Although the duration of exposure to oral contraceptives has been the single most important factor in some studies,[2,13] even exposure for more than 15 years did not increase the risk of breast cancer in other studies. Indeed, in one study, there was actually a significant decrease in the incidence of breast cancer with long-term oral contraceptive administration.[14]

ENVIRONMENTAL FACTORS AND DIET

The possibility that environmental factors are important in the etiology of breast cancer is suggested by observations on the incidence of breast cancer in Japanese women who migrate from Japan, where the incidence of breast cancer is low, to North America, where the incidence is high.[15] In a study performed in the San Francisco Bay area during 1969–1971, both Nisei (first-generation U.S. born) and Issei (immigrant) women were found to have an incidence of breast cancer nearly equal to that of the white population in the same area. These data suggest that environmental factors are as important as or more important than genetic considerations.

Diet is an obvious environmental factor, and possible relations between fat or cholesterol intake and steroid hormone metabolism have led to an emphasis on dietary fat as a possible etiologic agent. International studies relating age-adjusted cancer mortality rates and national per-capita fat intake demonstrate a direct correlation.[16] The correlation is stronger in postmenopausal women (r = 0.81) than in premenopausal women (r = 0.66). Laboratory studies provide further evidence of a possible relation between dietary fat and breast cancer.[17] The incidence of mammary cancer in DMBA-challenged rats is much higher among rats fed a diet with 10% to 20% corn oil than in those on a diet with no more than 5% corn oil.

Despite these compelling indirect data, epidemiologic studies correlating dietary fat and the incidence of breast cancer have been inconclusive. In the largest epidemiologic survey, 89,538 nurses between the ages of 34 and 59 were studied.[18] There was no relation between the relative risk of breast cancer and calorie-adjusted total fat, saturated fat, linoleic acid, or cholesterol intake. In fact, the relative risk of developing breast cancer among the women with the highest quintile of total fat intake was 0.85 compared with women in the lowest quintile. However, the difference in fat intake among women in these two extremes was only 25%. Practically, this suggests that women who reduce fat intake in the context of the usual American diet are not likely to reduce their breast cancer risk.

These epidemiologic studies do not rule out the possibility that a greater reduction in fat intake or a reduction in fat intake at an earlier age might have an important effect on breast cancer incidence. Cohort studies in countries where there has been a gradual increase in the incidence of breast cancer demonstrate that the risk is dependent on the year of birth.[19] In Iceland, the incidence of breast cancer increased steadily from 1911 to 1972, but the shape of the breast cancer incidence curves did not change during that period, suggesting that the etiologic or promotional factor important for the increasing incidence of breast cancer was operative well before the age at which the breast cancers were usually diagnosed.

Seventeen cohort or case-control studies on the relation between alcohol intake and breast cancer have been performed, and all but three show an increased risk with use of alcohol. This risk is dose related: a moderate alcohol intake is associated with a 40% to 60% increase in risk.[20,21]

FAMILY HISTORY

Women (and, to a much lesser extent, men) with any family history of breast cancer are at increased risk. However, the relative risk of developing breast cancer in women with a family history in second-degree relatives is about 1.5[22,23] compared with 1.7 to 2.5 among women with a history in first-degree relatives.[22] In some epidemiologic studies, the risk was even greater when two sisters or a mother and one or more sisters had breast cancer,[23,25] but in other studies, no association with the number of cancer-affected first-degree relatives was observed. It has been reported that breast cancer occurring in the premenopausal years or in younger women imparts a higher risk,[23] but this, too, is an inconsistent finding.[22,26] In one study, the risk was greatest in relatives of patients with bilateral breast cancer,[26] whereas in others, it was greatest in relatives of patients with unilateral breast cancer.[23] However, no risk group has been shown to have a lifetime risk in excess of 30%.[26] It is estimated that the probability of a 30-year-old woman developing breast cancer by the age of 70 is 28% if she has two sisters with breast cancer, one bilaterally, and 25% if her mother and sister have breast cancer, one bilaterally.[26]

RADIATION

Radiation is associated with an increased risk of breast cancer in survivors of the atomic bomb blast, in patients given radiation for postpartum mastitis, in women receiving multiple fluoroscopies during therapy for tuberculosis, and in animal models.[12,27] Radiation exposure results in an increased risk after a latency of 10 to 15 years, but there is very little increased risk in women exposed to radiation after the age of 40.[12]

BENIGN BREAST DISEASE

The risk of breast cancer in patients with a history of benign breast disease, especially "fibrocystic disease," has ranged from 1.86 to 2.13.[28] However, the incidence of fibrocystic disease diagnosed on the basis of histologic findings has ranged from 13% to 71% in various studies. "Lumpy breasts," which are often confused with fibrocystic disease, probably occur in more than 85% of patients. As a result, this term and the general category of "benign breast disease" have little practical significance in counseling women regarding their risk of breast cancer.

A retrospective review of more than 10,000 biopsies per-

TABLE 38-3. Patterns of Benign Breast Disease Associated with Increased Risk of Breast Cancer and Association with Family History

Histology	Family History*	No. of Patients	Relative Risk†	p
All patients	—	3303	1.5	<0.0001
	No	2934	1.4	0.0007
	Yes	369	2.5	<0.0001
No proliferative disease	—	1378	0.89	0.51
Proliferative disease	—	1925	1.9	<0.0001
Atypical hyperplasia	—	232	4.4	<0.0001
	No	193	3.5	<0.0001
	Yes	39	8.9	<0.0001

Data from Dupont WD, Page DL: Risk factors for breast cancer in women with proliferative breast disease. N Engl J Med 312:146–151, 1985.
* Cancer in first-degree relative.
† Compared with age-matched population from Third National Cancer Survey.

formed at the Vanderbilt Hospital has led to the conclusion that most of the risk associated with benign breast disease is attributable to the small percentage of patients who have atypical hyperplasia or both atypical hyperplasia and a family history of breast cancer (Table 38-3). In this study, 3303 biopsies were reviewed among the total population. Patients with a family history of breast cancer had a higher incidence of subsequent invasive breast cancer. About one-third of the patients had no evidence of proliferative disease at all, and there was no evidence of an increased risk among this group. Atypical hyperplasia was observed in only 7% of the patients, but their risk of developing breast cancer was increased fourfold. For the 39 patients (about 1% of the total) who had both atypical hyperplasia and a history of breast cancer in a first-degree relative, the risk of subsequent breast cancer was increased ninefold. However, even in this very high-risk group, the observed incidence of breast cancer over 25 years was only about 40%, and less than one-third of these patients eventually died of breast cancer. These data suggest that benign breast disease is rarely an indication for special monitoring and may never be an indication for therapeutic intervention.

NATURAL HISTORY OF BREAST CANCER

The natural history of breast cancer is characterized by a long duration and marked heterogeneity within and between patients. Breast cancer is among the more slowly growing tumors, and as a result, both the preclinical period (before diagnosis) and the clinical phases after initial treatment and metastases are measured in years and decades. Nevertheless, some patients have a very aggressive form of the disease and do poorly. An equal number have such an indolent form of the disease that it is difficult to demonstrate that therapy has any effect at all on survival. During the long clinical phase, there is ample opportunity for clonal mutation and evolution, and it seems probable that almost all breast cancer patients have multiple tumor clones, each with

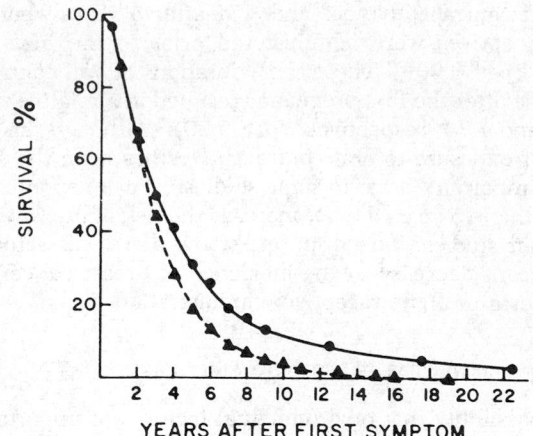

FIG. 38-1. Survival of untreated patients (triangles) seen at the Middlesex Hospital, England, between 1805 and 1933, juxtaposed with survival of patients treated with radical mastectomy (circles) at Johns Hopkins between 1889 and 1931 (Henderson IC, Canellos GP: Cancer of the breast: the past decade. Reprinted by permission of N Engl J Med 302:17–30, 1980)

its own unique growth requirements, growth rates, propensity to metastasize, and sensitivity to drugs.

The long natural history of breast cancer has been emphasized in about a half-dozen studies of patients with untreated breast cancer. Most of the patients in these studies were identified in the late nineteenth and early twentieth century, and then, as now, such patients were self-selected. It therefore cannot be assumed that they are truly representative of the full spectrum of breast cancer patients. All of these series, like the one shown in Figure 38-1, include some patients who lived for two to three decades without any treatment at all. Nevertheless, the median survival for the untreated patients in the Middlesex series was 2.7 years. The survival of patients treated with radical mastectomy by

FIG. 38-2. Relative mortality per year (±SE) of all stages of breast cancer diagnosed in the United States, 1950–1973. (Data from End Results Section, Biometry Branch, National Cancer Institute 1977; Fox M: On the diagnosis and treatment of breast cancer. JAMA 241:489–494, 1979)

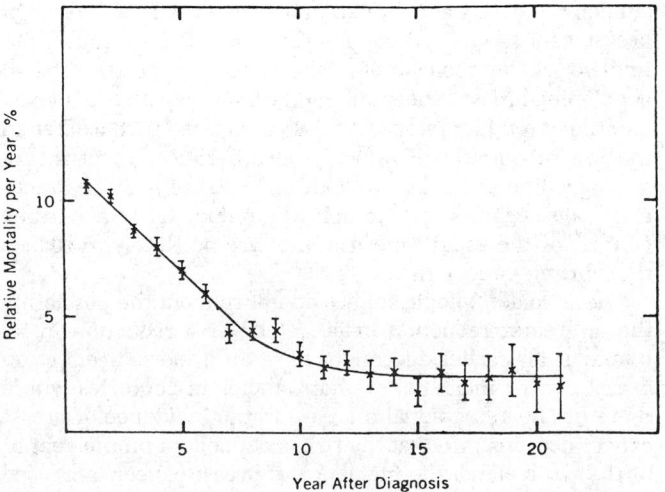

Halsted and his colleagues at Johns Hopkins, also shown in Figure 38-1, is not much different from that of untreated patients. The percentages of patients who ultimately died as a direct result of breast cancer are almost identical in the two series.[29] This comparison undermines the claim that the radical mastectomy is the "proven" therapy for breast cancer.

The heterogeneity of breast cancer is illustrated by an analysis of disease mortality rates in Connecticut between the years 1950 and 1973.[30] The highest mortality rate was observed immediately after diagnosis, and the rate gradually fell during the first decade of follow-up (Fig. 38-2). During the second decade of follow-up, the yearly relative mortality rate for breast cancer remained constant. Maurice Fox has suggested that this Connecticut mortality curve results from superimposition of at least two separate mortality curves from breast cancer populations with uniquely different natural histories (Fig. 38-3). One group, which constituted about 60% of all the patients in the series, had an annual mortality rate of approximately 2.5% per year. Half of these patients died in the first 15 years postmastectomy and the other half between years 15 and 30 (closed circles in Fig. 38-3). The remaining approximately 40% of the patient population had an annual mortality rate of about 25% per year. Most of these patients died within the first decade postmastectomy (open circles in Fig. 38-3). These observations are consistent with the concept that there is both an aggressive form of breast cancer, which contributes most of the observed morbidity and deaths, and an indolent form, which is compatible with long life regardless of the therapy given. Although intuitively one might anticipate that patients with a more indolent form of the disease would be disproportionately represented in an

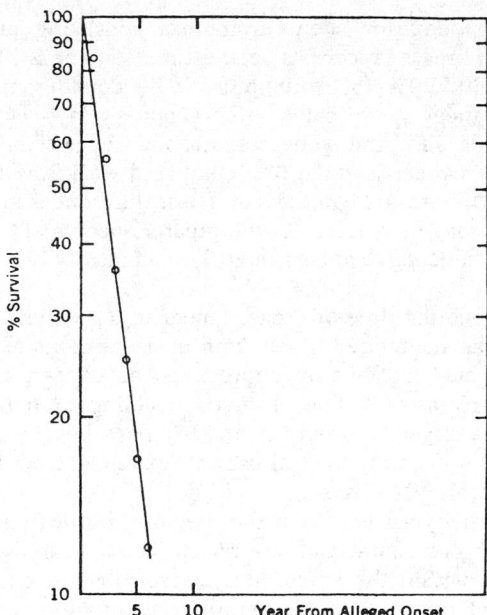

FIG. 38-4. Survival of the untreated patients shown in Fig. 38-1 replotted semilogarithmically.

untreated historical series, such as the one described in Figure 38-1, a semilogarithmic plot of the survival of these patients suggests that these untreated patients were primarily from the group with a mortality rate of about 25% per year (Fig. 38-4). It seems likely that many of the patients being identified in the current era are not represented among historical controls.

The heterogeneity of this disease can also be illustrated by the wide variability in growth rates as measured with labeling indices. The labeling index is a measure of the percentage of cells in a tumor that are undergoing cell division at a single point in time. Patients with high labeling indices are therefore more likely to have rapidly growing cancer than are those with low labeling indices. About 60% of patients have labeling indices less than 4%. The remaining 40% have indices that range from 4% to 41%.[31]

PRECLINICAL EVENTS

Our understanding of the preclinical behavior of breast cancer is dependent on either extrapolation backward from clinical observation or the use of tumor models. Both of these approaches have important limitations. Tumors large enough to be detected and measured in the clinic are likely to have a slower growth rate than microscopic preclinical lesions. Animal model tumors are usually selected because of a high growth fraction, which facilitates laboratory study. However, many human breast cancers have low growth fractions.

The *relative* growth rates of human tumors can be determined from clinical measurements, and these studies suggest that, on average, breast cancer has a lower labeling index, a longer doubling time, and a lower growth fraction than most other human tumors.[32] For example, the mean

FIG. 38-3. Relative survival of patients with a yearly mortality rate of ≤2.5% (*closed circles*) or >2.5% (*open circles*). (Fox M: On the diagnosis and treatment of breast cancer. JAMA 241:489–494, 1979)

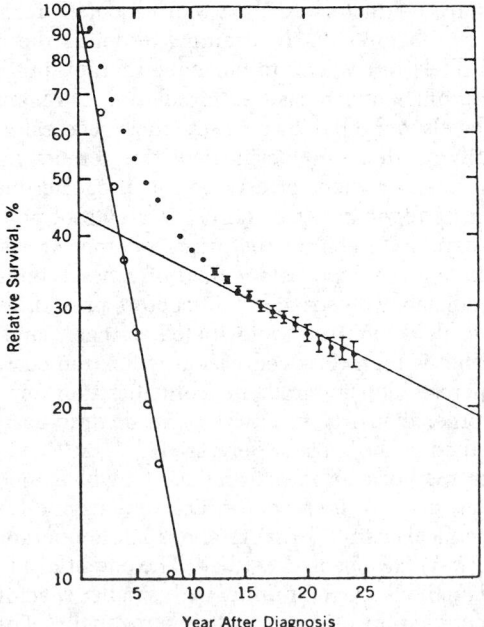

labeling index for adenocarcinomas consisting predominantly of breast cancer has been estimated to be 2.1%, compared with 29% for lymphomas. The doubling time for breast cancer is estimated to be about 83 days, compared with 27 days for embryonal tumors, and the growth fraction of breast cancer is about 6%, compared with 90% for embryonal tumors and lymphomas. These differences in growth fraction may be a factor in the greater success obtained in curing testicular cancers and lymphomas with chemotherapy.

The doubling time of breast cancer in its earliest clinical phases has been determined from measurements of lesions present but not initially appreciated as cancer in serial mammograms.[33-36] The observed doubling time in these studies averaged between 115 and 325 days, but the range of doubling times in individual patients extended from 23 days to more than 940 days.

It is usually assumed that the preclinical growth of breast cancer is logarithmic and continuous. Tumors can usually be palpated within the breast at a size of about 1 cm, and a sphere of this size could contain approximately 10^9 cells. Assuming origin of the cancer in a single-cell mutation, it would take 30 doublings for a malignant cell to produce 10^9 cells, assuming no cell loss during that interval. If all of these assumptions are true, and if one accepts a preclinical doubling time of about 100 days (a value substantially lower than all the mean values obtained in doubling-time measurements of clinically measurable lesions), then the preclinical phase of breast cancer should, on average, exceed 10 years. Even if breast cancer doubling times are actually one-half to one-fourth of that assumed in this illustration, the preclinical phase of breast cancer would still range from 2.5 to 5 years. Of course, these assumptions are all subject to challenge and may seriously underestimate differences in the growth rate of preclinical lesions growing logarithmically compared with clinically detectable lesions in a plateau phase of growth (*i.e.*, Gompertzian growth). It is also possible that the preclinical growth of breast cancer is less than logarithmic or even discontinuous, in which case the preclinical phase would be even longer.

It has recently been suggested that the assumption that preclinical breast cancer growth is logarithmic is inconsistent with observations from large clinical studies. Utilizing data on the interval from initial diagnosis of breast cancer to the appearance of clinically detectable metastases, it has been concluded by mathematical modeling that preclinical breast cancer might be better characterized as having short spurts of logarithmic growth alternating with quiescent periods of little or no growth.[37] To further complicate the issue, it is plausible that growth at various metastatic sites within each patient is asynchronous.

DEFINING PATIENT SUBSETS

The recognition that patients at extremes of the disease spectrum are very different provides a basis for attempting to identify groups of patients likely to benefit uniquely from one or another treatment strategy. However, all such attempts share some limitations, the most important of which is that the spectrum of the disease is continuous. That is, there are no groups of patients uniquely different from all others, and most patients are somewhere in the middle between the two extremes. Well-differentiated tumors slowly merge into moderately well-differentiated tumors. Patients with no evidence of tumor hormone receptors have only a slightly worse prognosis or a slightly lower probability of responding to endocrine therapy than patients with a low-positive receptor value.

A second problem with the use of many subsets is the lack of reproducibility from one observer to the next. In one study, the concordance between two pathologists in defining the cell type (ductal carcinoma not otherwise specified versus nonductal carcinoma) or assigning one of three nuclear grades was little more than might be expected by chance.[38]

In considering the notion of patients "subsets," one must also consider that differences in prognosis between patients in different subsets may be not in the ultimate probability of relapse but rather in the probable time to relapse. This is illustrated in a comparison of the survival of patients without lymph node metastases with that of patients with one lymph node involved.[39] At the end of the first 5 years of observation, the disease-free survival of these two groups of patients was nearly identical, and this was initially taken as evidence that there was no difference in the propensity of these two patient groups to develop distant metastases. However, further follow-up over 12 years demonstrated that the two curves slowly diverged, so that by the end of the 12th year, patients with a single involved node had a significantly higher recurrence rate than those with no lymph node involvement. This observation, once again, underscores the long natural history of the disease.

HORMONE RECEPTORS

It has long been known that only a subset of all patients with breast cancer respond to endocrine therapy and that these patients are characterized by a more indolent form of the disease (see below). Early attempts to define the group of patients likely to respond to hormone therapies utilized endocrine profiles and measured circulating estrogens or androgen levels, or both. However, the most successful method of identifying these endocrine-sensitive tumors has come from the measurement of estrogen or progesterone receptors. The estrogen receptor (ERP) is a cytosol protein that can be identified in either the primary tumor or metastases by incubating the supernatant fluid of a tissue homogenate with a radiolabeled estrogen.[40] Receptors present in the supernatant fluid bind the radiolabeled estrogen, and the unbound label is then removed either by dextran-coated charcoal, sucrose density-gradient centrifugation, or one of several other methods. In practice, the dextran-coated charcoal method is the most widely used.

Newer methods of measuring ERP involve monoclonal antibodies made to the receptor. Both an enzyme-linked immunochemical assay (ERICA) and an immunoradiometric assay (IRMA) have been described. The potential advantages of these methods are their utility with smaller specimens and the demonstration of tumor-cell heterogeneity. The use of these staining techniques also permits an estimate of the percentage of cells with ERP and theoretically permits a better estimate of the maximum cell kill that might be achieved by the use of endocrine therapy. On the other hand, quantification of results is more difficult. At present, there is good correlation between the results of these methods and the bioassay, and it is likely that the techniques utilizing antibodies to ERP or progesterone receptors (PR) will find increasing use.

Approximately two-thirds of all patients have ERP present in their tumor, and about half of the receptor-positive tumors will respond to endocrine therapy. Postmenopausal patients and older patients more frequently have receptor-positive tumors than do younger and premenopausal patients.[40] In general, the incidence of receptor positivity decreases with time, and several studies suggest that a biopsy obtained just before treatment is more predictive of response than a biopsy obtained months or years before. However, receptor status should be measured on all biopsies or mastectomy specimens when feasible. This information has prognostic significance, may influence the selection of an adjuvant therapy, and may be of use in the selection of palliative therapy for metastatic disease in the event that the sites are not easily accessible for biopsy and measurement of receptors.

It is not understood why not all receptor-positive tumors respond to endocrine therapy. It is plausible that many patients have a sufficient number of cells to cause the assay result to be positive but an insufficient number of receptor-positive cells for their death to result in a measurable reduction in the tumor mass. It is also possible that the ER measured in many tumors is not truly functional. Therefore, measurement of the PR has been used as a means of identifying intact ERP. When cancer cells with intact and functioning ERP are exposed to estrogen, the estrogen is transported into the nucleus, where messenger RNA is formed. Among the products of this interaction are additional ERP, PR, and various growth factors[41,42] (Fig. 38-5). Clinical observations appear to confirm the hypothesis that PR are a marker of intact ERP, as tumors with both types of receptors are much more likely to respond to endocrine therapy than are those with ERP alone (see below, Table 38-33).

USE OF RECEPTORS TO DEFINE PROGNOSTIC SUBSETS

Because patients who respond to endocrine therapy are those with the longest disease-free intervals (see below), it is not surprising that patients with ERP or PR are also more likely to have a long disease-free interval. In fact, receptor-positive patients have a longer overall survival and a longer survival from evidence of first metastases than do receptor-negative patients.[43,44] Both ERP status and PR status are predictive of recurrence, and several studies suggest that the PR status has more prognostic value than the ERP status, especially in node-positive patients.[43,45] A multivariate analysis of 1529 patients with Stage II disease demonstrated that the PR had about the same prognostic value as did the presence of histologically involved nodes or tumor size (Table 38-4).

It is tempting to assume that the patient's receptor status is a reflection of the intrinsic growth rate of the tumor. In some studies, receptor-positive patients have had a better short-term prognosis or an improved short-term survival rate. However, the percentages of receptor-positive patients and receptor-negative patients who eventually relapse and die of breast cancer are identical.[46-51] Other investigators have concluded that receptor status is predictive only of the response to endocrine therapy and thus indirectly appears to predict growth rate.[52] In these studies, patients with receptor-positive tumors had an increased overall survival and an increased survival following the appearance of metastases but an insignificant prolongation of the disease-free interval. An improvement in survival was found only among those patients who were both receptor-positive and responsive to endocrine treatment.

Patients without histologically involved lymph nodes have better 10-year disease-free survival and overall survival rates than do node-positive patients. However, 15% to 30% of these patients will relapse, and 12% to 22% will die within 5 years of diagnosis.[53-58] If it were possible to identify those node-negative patients most likely to relapse and die of

FIG. 38-5. Role of estrogen receptor (*ER*) in processing estrogens (*E*) resulting in production of progesterone receptor (*PgR*) and growth factors. (Osborne CK: Receptors. In Harris J, Hellman S, Henderson IC, Kinne DW: [eds]: Breast Diseases, pp 210–232. Philadelphia, JB Lippincott, 1987)

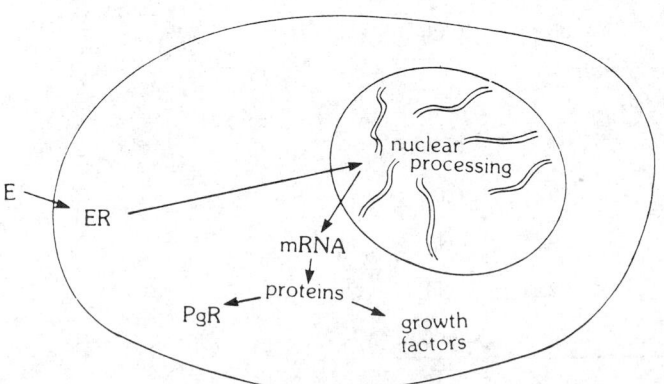

TABLE 38-4. Prognostic Value of Receptors for Disease-Free Survival and Overall Survival in Patients with Stage II Breast Cancer (Multivariate Analysis of 1529 Patients)

Factor	p Value	
	Disease-Free Survival	Overall Survival
Positive nodes	<0.0001	<0.0001
Tumor size	<0.0001	0.0001
Progesterone receptor status	0.0001	0.0001
Endocrine therapy	0.0004	0.0017
Chemotherapy	0.0731	0.0191
Estrogen receptor status	0.1376	0.0017
Age	0.8990	0.0622

McGuire WL, Clark GM, Dressler LG et al: Role of steroid hormone receptors as prognostic factors in primary breast cancer. NCI Monogr 1:19–23, 1986.

breast cancer, they could be considered for treatment with adjuvant chemotherapy, sparing those with the best prognosis from the toxicities of this therapy. Many investigators have tried to use receptor status to identify this poor-prognosis group, but the results are contradictory (Table 38-5). In the Milan study, premenopausal patients without receptors had a significantly poorer survival rate than receptor-positive patients, but survival differences among postmenopausal patients were less obvious.[46] A study performed in the Cleveland area showed that receptor status was more predictive of relapse and death among postmenopausal than premenopausal patients.[47] In the largest of the studies shown in Table 38-5, there was no difference in the relapse rate or the length of survival by receptor status among either premenopausal or postmenopausal women.[59] A similar result has been found by investigators in England, who have demonstrated that the presence of receptors is highly predictive of relapse and survival among node-positive patients but not among node-negative patients.[60] In all of these studies, a substantial portion of the ERP-positive patients relapsed even though the relapse rate among ERP-negative patients was somewhat higher. Collecting these data led to the conclusion that patients who are receptor-negative have a small but significant increase in the risk of early relapse and early death from breast cancer, but that receptor status alone is insufficient to identify the 20% to 30% of node-negative patients at risk of eventually dying of breast cancer.

CLASSIFICATION OF TUMOR TYPES

Histopathologic examination of breast cancer makes available information that establishes the diagnosis of the lesion, aids in determining patient prognosis, and leads to a better understanding of the biology of the disease. This section presents a general overview of the subject, with emphasis on recent contributions that have enhanced our understanding of the nature of breast cancer or that have raised important questions that require resolution.

A number of pathologic classifications of mammary carcinomas are in use. The most commonly used are those presented by the Armed Forces Institute of Pathology (AFIP)[61] and the World Health Organization (WHO).[62] Breast carcinomas are classified as either ductal or lobular, corresponding to the ducts and lobules of the normal breast. However, there is evidence that most tumors arise in the terminal duct section of the breast, regardless of pathologic type.[63]

The frequency of the various histologic types of breast cancer in 1000 cases from NSABP Protocol B-04 is presented in Table 38-6. More than half (52.6%) are pure infiltrating duct lesions, not otherwise specified (NOS).

CARCINOMA IN SITU

Tumors arising from duct epithelium that are confined within the lumen of the ducts or lobules of the breast are

TABLE 38-5. Comparison of Disease-Free and Overall Survival of Patients Without Histologic Node Involvement Who Have Received No Adjuvant Therapy and Are Either Estrogen-Receptor Positive (ER⁺) or Negative (ER⁻)

Study	Patient Population	Total No. of Patients	4–6-Year Disease-Free (%)		p Value
			ER⁺	ER⁻	
Milan (46)	Premenopausal	464	88	59	<0.0001
	Postmenopausal		75	70	0.22
Memorial (59)	Premenopausal	1034	88	83	NS*
	Postmenopausal		84	84	NS
Cleveland (47)	Premenopausal	510	72	72	0.65
	Postmenopausal		80	65	<0.06
			4–6-Year Survival (%)		
Milan (46)	Premenopausal	464	95	77	0.0001
	Postmenopausal		88	79	0.02
Memorial (59)	Premenopausal	1034	92	89	NS
	Postmenopausal		94	92	NS
Cleveland (47)	All Patients	510	87	74	<0.003

* NS = not significant.

TABLE 38-6. Incidence of Histologic Types of Breast Cancer (%)

Pure Tumor Groups	
Infiltrating duct NOS	52.6
Medullary	6.2
Lobular invasive	4.9
Mucinous	2.4
Tubular	1.2
Adenocystic	0.4
Papillary	0.3
Carcinosarcoma	0.1
Paget's Disease	2.3
With intraductal carcinoma	0.2
Infiltrating duct NOS	1.6
Infiltrating duct NOS + tubular	0.4
Infiltrating duct NOS + mucinous	0.1
Combinations with Infiltrating Duct NOS	28.0
+Tubular	16.5
+Lobular invasive	3.3
+Mucinous	1.6
+Lobular invasive + tubular	1.6
+Papillary	1.2
+Adenocystic	1.0
+Tubular + adenocystic	0.8
+Tubular + papillary	0.8
+Mucinous + papillary	0.4
+Adenocystic + mucinous	0.2
+Lobular invasive + adenocystic	0.1
+Lobular invasive + mucinous	0.1
+Lobular invasive + papillary	0.1
+Tubular + mucinous	0.1
+Adenocystic + papillary	0.1
+Lobular invasive + tubular + adenocystic + mucinous	0.1
Other Combinations of Tumor Types Exclusive of NOS	1.6
Tubular + papillary	0.5
Lobular invasive + tubular	0.4
Tubular + mucinous	0.2
Lobular invasive + mucinous	0.1
Tubular + adenocystic	0.1
Adenocystic + mucinous	0.1
Mucinous + papillary	0.1
Lobular invasive + tubular + adenocystic + papillary	0.1

generally referred to as carcinoma in situ. Carcinoma in situ has been classified as either ductal or lobular, depending on the cytologic features and pattern of growth. Both ductal carcinoma in situ (DCIS), also known as intraductal carcinoma or noninvasive ductal carcinoma, and lobular carcinoma in situ (LCIS) are characterized by a proliferation of malignant epithelial cells confined to the mammary ducts or lobules, without light-microscopic evidence of invasion through the basement membrane into the surrounding stroma. The distinction between DCIS and LCIS is usually not difficult, but overlaps exist. The natural history and management of these lesions will be discussed later in this chapter.

INFILTRATING CARCINOMA, NOS

A variety of histologic types of invasive (infiltrating) carcinomas of the breast have been described. Infiltrating ductal carcinomas in which no special histologic features are recognized are designated NOS and are by far the most common ductal tumors, accounting for almost 70% of breast cancers. They are characterized by their stony hardness to palpation.

When transected, a gritty resistance is typically encountered, and the tumor retracts below the cut surface. Histologically, various degrees of fibrotic response and associated DCIS are present. These tumors commonly metastasize to the axillary lymph nodes, and their prognosis is the poorest of the various ductal types.

MEDULLARY CARCINOMA

Medullary carcinomas are circumscribed lesions that can attain large dimensions but demonstrate only low-grade infiltrative properties. They constitute 5% to 7% of all mammary carcinomas and are characterized by poorly differentiated nuclei and infiltration with small lymphocytes and plasma cells. The 5-year survival rate following treatment for medullary carcinoma is better than for NOS ductal carcinomas.

TUBULAR CARCINOMA

A tumor in which tubule formation is conspicuous is known as tubular or well-differentiated carcinoma. Generally, this diagnosis is made only when 75% or more of the tumor is composed of these elements. Axillary metastases are uncommon, and the prognosis is considerably better than for ductal carcinoma, NOS.

MUCINOUS CARCINOMA

Another ductal type, the mucinous or colloid carcinoma, comprises about 3% of all mammary carcinomas and is characterized microscopically by nests and strands of epithelial cells floating in a mucinous matrix. It usually is slow growing and can reach bulky proportions. When the tumor is predominantly mucinous, the prognosis tends to be good.

Other, rarer, types of ductal carcinomas include papillary, adenocystic, and carcinosarcoma or metaplastic duct carcinoma. Of note, in many cases, NOS ductal carcinomas contain small areas of these special types.

INFILTRATING LOBULAR CARCINOMA

Another histologic type of breast cancer is infiltrating lobular carcinoma. It is relatively uncommon, accounting for only 5% to 10% of breast tumors in most series. The clinical presentation is more often an area of ill-defined thickening in the breast, in contrast to the dominant lump characteristic of ductal carcinoma. Microscopically, lobular carcinomas typically are composed of small cells in a linear arrangement ("Indian-filing") with a tendency to grow around ducts and lobules (targetoid growth). Lobular carcinomas are also characterized by a greater proportion of multicentric tumors, either in the same or the opposite breast, when compared with NOS ductal carcinoma. Overall, infiltrating lobular carcinoma has a similar likelihood of axillary nodal involvement and prognosis as infiltrating duct carcinoma. However, the sites of metastases for these two types tend to differ. Ductal carcinomas more characteristically metastasize to bone or to intraparenchymal sites within lung, liver, or brain, whereas lobular carcinomas more often show a predilection for meningeal and serosal surfaces.

PAGET'S DISEASE

Paget's disease of the breast occurs in 1% to 4% of all patients with breast cancer. Clinically, the patient presents with a relatively long history of eczematous changes in the nipple with itching, burning, oozing, bleeding, or some combination of these. The nipple changes are associated with an underlying carcinoma in the breast that can be palpated in about two-thirds of the patients. The subadjacent tumor may be either intraductal or of the invasive duct type. The prognosis is related to the histologic type of the associated tumor. Histologically, the nipple epidermis contains tumor cells singly and in nests. Treatment of Paget's disease is discussed in the section on special problems later in this chapter.

INFLAMMATORY BREAST CARCINOMA

Inflammatory breast cancer is characterized clinically by prominent skin edema, redness and warmth, a visible erysipeloid margin, and induration of the underlying tissue. These criteria in the past were sufficient for the diagnosis. Currently, pathologic corroboration must be obtained. Biopsies of the involved skin reveal cancer cells in the dermal lymphatics. Inflammatory cells rarely are present. The prognosis of patients with inflammatory breast cancer is poor, even if the disease is apparently localized. The management of inflammatory cancer is discussed later in this chapter.

EVALUATION OF BREAST SPECIMENS

In the past, when mastectomy was the standard treatment for breast cancer, it was sufficient for the pathologist to diagnose the disease. Now that breast-conserving treatment is commonly employed, a more extensive evaluation of the resected specimen is critical. The exterior surface of the specimen should be inked to facilitate the assessment of the margins of resection for microscopic tumor involvement. The pathologist should describe the gross appearance of the resected specimen and, after inking, should describe the specimen on cut section, particularly in regard to the greatest dimension of the tumor and the distance from the periphery of the tumor to the closest margin of resection. A tissue sample for measurement of ERP and PR proteins should be obtained in a way that interferes as little as possible with the later evaluation of the margins of resection for tumor involvement. It is important to determine if there is microscopic tumor involvement at the margins of resection. This is best achieved by careful evaluation of permanent sections. One feature of the tumor that should be routinely noted, because it may influence the need for further resection of the primary tumor, is the extent of associated intraductal carcinoma, both in the primary tumor and in the grossly normal adjacent breast tissue.[64]

TUMOR CHARACTERISTICS

A number of morphologic aspects of breast tumors have been evaluated in terms of their relation to prognosis. The most important of these are histologic grade and the presence of lymphatic invasion. Other morphologic features that correlate less consistently with the prognosis include nuclear grade, the presence of necrosis, the frequency of mitoses, and the nature and extent of the cellular reaction of the tumor.

Tumor grading describes the degree of differentiation. The histologic grade of duct carcinoma can be scored by the degree of tubule formation, the size of the nuclei, the degree of nuclear hyperchromatism, and the number of mitoses. Tumors of low-grade malignancy have been designated Grade I and are believed to have the best prognosis. Tumors of high-grade malignancy have been designated Grade III and have the worst prognosis.

Lymphatic invasion refers to the presence of tumor emboli in breast lymphatics. Because tumor cells within an invasive cancer commonly grow in clumps, it is generally best to judge lymphatic invasion in breast tissue adjacent to the tumor. Such invasion is observed in approximately 25% of breast tumors and is associated with a lower likelihood of survival.

The prognostic importance of these morphologic features must be evaluated in relation to stage (the clinical extent of the cancer) and the number of involved axillary nodes, features with well-known prognostic value. It is also important to note that these morphologic features might predict the *pace* of the disease rather than the likelihood of long-term survival. This point is illustrated in the experience of Bloom, Richardson, and Field from the Middlesex and Royal Marsden Hospitals in London.[65] They examined the 20-year results in 1411 patients treated with modified radical mastectomy between 1936 and 1949. Table 38-7 shows the 5- and 15-year survival rates in relation to axillary node involvement and histologic grade, which suggest that histologic grade is a more useful indicator of prognosis at 5 years than it is at 15 years. The likelihood of long-term survival in patients with positive axillary nodes is low regardless of histologic grade. These results suggest that histologic grade is an indicator of the pace of the disease in patients with positive nodes and may be a good indicator of long-term prog-

TABLE 38-7.   Corrected 5- and 15-year Survival by Axillary Nodal Involvement and Tumor Grade

		Nodal Involvement (%)	
	Grade	Negative	Positive
5 Years	1	86	68
	2	68	33
	3	64	19
15 Years	1	49	15
	2	29	11
	3	25	7

Bloom HJG, Field JR: Impact of tumor grade and host resistance on survival of women with breast cancer. Cancer 28:1580–1589, 1971.

nosis in patients with negative axillary nodes. Similar results have been noted by others in regard to histologic and nuclear grade.[66,67]

The level of concordance between different observers in assessing these histologic features can be low. This has been demonstrated in studies by the Eastern Cooperative Oncology Group (ECOG) in the evaluation of specimens for nuclear grade and lymphatic invasion. For example, among three reviewers of nuclear grade, there was complete agreement in only 34% of cases; among five reviewers, there was complete agreement in only 17% of cases.[38] This difficulty in assigning reproducible scores poses a significant practical problem to the use of these histologic features in estimating prognosis.

More recently, investigators have attempted to evaluate biologic aspects of breast tumors in a more quantitative fashion in order to estimate prognosis. These aspects include the determination of ER and PR proteins (ERP, PRP), measurements of tumor-cell kinetics, measurements of DNA content, and the determination of oncogene expression. The ERP and PRP determination has been described earlier in this chapter. The parameter of tumor-cell kinetics that has been studied most extensively is the labeling index, which can be determined by incubating tumor cells with ^{3}H-thymidine and counting the percentage of cells that take up the isotope by autoradiography. Because thymidine is primarily taken up by cells in the DNA synthetic or S phase of the cycle, the labeling index is a measure of the percentage of the cells in this phase and thus a reflection of tumor proliferative activity. More recently, the labeling index has been determined by the use of DNA flow cytometry, which identifies the percentage of cells in each phase of the cell cycle using DNA-specific fluorescent stains. In addition, flow cytometry can determine the degree of abnormality of DNA content (aneuploidy) in the tumor cells.

The labeling index is an important prognostic factor. This is illustrated by the data of Tubiana and colleagues from the Institut Gustave-Roussy.[68] They studied tumor samples from 128 breast cancer patients seen at that institution between 1972 and 1973, 96 of whom had diagnostic axillary dissections. The likelihood of relapse and death was analyzed by the labeling index for the 125 patients evaluable at 10 years. Their results indicate that the index is highly predictive of both relapse and death. Similar findings have been described by Meyer[69] and Silvestrini[70] and their co-workers.

The relation between the labeling index and other prognostic factors was also investigated by Meyer and associates.[69] They found that the index correlated significantly with the histologic features of the tumor but not with tumor size or the number of positive axillary nodes. Tubiana et al. similarly found that the labeling index is not correlated with nodal involvement and that the index was an important prognostic factor independent of clinical and pathologic staging.[68] They found in a multivariate analysis of their results that the index, tumor size, and tumor grade (and not axillary node involvement) were the main independent prognostic factors. Silvestrini and coworkers also did not find any correlation between the labeling index and tumor size or nodal involvement.[70] The index was found to be a highly significant prognostic factor for patients with negative

nodes. All these results indicate that the labeling index correlates with histologic grade and appears to be an important prognostic factor independent of clinical or pathologic staging.

The index is inversely related to the level of steroid hormone receptors (ERP and PRP). At present, the relative prognostic importance of the index and receptors has not been clearly delineated. It is also important to note that the labeling index is not readily obtainable in most institutions. Its determination by autoradiography is tedious, and flow cytometry is not generally available at this time. This limits its utility as a prognostic factor in clinical practice.

More recently, flow cytometry has been used to investigate the relation between aneuploidy and prognosis. Patients with aneuploid tumors have been found to have a worse short-term prognosis than patients with diploid tumors.[71,72] The relation between DNA content, labeling index, and steroid hormone receptors as independent prognostic factors remains to be elucidated. McDivitt and co-workers found that DNA content, S-phase fraction (SPF) as measured by flow cytometry, and ERP were all correlated.[73] It should also be noted that flow cytometry offers the possibility of even more sophisticated characterization of a tumor by the use of monoclonal antibody probes. At present, there are not enough long-term data to support the routine use of these measures of proliferative activity to guide the clinical care of patients.

The most recent attempt to estimate prognosis involves the determination of oncogene expression in breast tumors. The most notable of these studies is by Slamon and colleagues, in which the amplification of the *HER-2/neu* oncogene was correlated with prognosis in 189 patients.[74] Amplification was seen in 35% of cases and was not correlated with ERP, PRP, tumor size, or number of positive axillary nodes. In a multivariate analysis for relapse-free survival, which included the number of positive nodes, *HER-2/neu* amplification, ERP, PRP, tumor size, and patient age, only the number of positive nodes and *HER-2/neu* amplification were statistically significant (both p values = 0.001). Additional studies will be required with more patients and longer follow-up to confirm the results. It is likely, however, that these newer determinations of the biologic aspects of breast tumors will emerge as important predictors of prognosis.

LOCAL SPREAD OF BREAST CANCER

The primary site of breast cancer is described by the quadrant of the breast in which it is found. In one series of 696 cases, 48% of the tumors were located in the upper outer quadrant, 15% in the upper inner quadrant, 11% in the lower outer quadrant, 6% in the lower inner quadrant, and 17% in the central region (designated as within 1 cm of the areola).[75] An additional 3% were termed diffuse because of multifocal origin or involvement of the entire breast. The higher frequency of breast cancer in the upper outer quadrant is thought to be attributable simply to the greater amount of breast tissue in that quadrant. In this series of patients, no differences in survival based on quadrant location were noted. The relation between the location of the primary tumor and prognosis also was examined in another

TABLE 38-8. Five-Year Relapse Rate (%) According to the Location of the Primary and Nodal Status (NSABP)

Location	Negative Nodes	Positive Nodes
UOQ	17 (208)*	63 (239)
UIQ	25 (75)	59 (37)
LIQ	22 (23)	55 (22)
LOQ	26 (46)	70 (44)

* Number of patients in subgroup.

large series from the National Surgical Adjuvant Breast Project (NSABP). Relapse and ultimate survival were related to the pathologic status of the axillary nodes, and there were no significant differences in prognosis by primary tumor location (Table 38-8).[76]

The spread of cancer through the breast has been summarized by Haagensen.[77] This spread occurs by direct infiltration into the breast parenchyma, along mammary ducts, and via breast lymphatics. Direct infiltration tends to occur by ramifying projections that have a characteristic stellate appearance on gross examination. If untreated, direct involvement of overlying skin or deep pectoral fascia is common. Involvement along ducts is observed frequently and may include wide segments of the breast. It is unclear, however, whether this intraductal involvement represents true spread of a primary cancer along previously uninvolved ducts or a "field cancerization" that results in simultaneous transformation along entire lengths of ducts. Spread can also occur by the extensive network of breast lymphatics. Investigators have emphasized lymphatic spread vertically down to the lymphatic plexus in the deep pectoral fascia underlying the breast. In addition, spread to the central subareolar region has been described. These multiple mechanisms of spread emphasize the likelihood of cancer being present in the breast well beyond the palpable primary mass.

A detailed study of the sites of cancer in a breast containing a primary tumor has been performed by Holland et al.[78] They examined 264 mastectomy specimens from patients with clinically unifocal breast cancer measuring 4 cm or less. In only 40% of cases was the cancer in the breast restricted to the primary tumor (Fig. 38-6). The probability

of finding additional foci of cancer decreased as a function of distance from the primary tumor: 41% of the specimens had additional foci of cancer 2 cm or more from the primary tumor, whereas only 11% had additional foci 4 cm or more from the primary tumor. Of the cases with additional foci beyond 2 cm, the additional foci were intraductal in approximately two-thirds of cases.

REGIONAL SPREAD

The most common routes of spread of breast cancer to regional lymph nodes are to the axillary, internal mammary, and supraclavicular lymph node regions. A knowledge of the likelihood of spread to these areas and their significance is critical for planning treatment.

AXILLARY NODE INVOLVEMENT

The axillary lymph node region is the principal site of regional metastases from carcinoma of the breast, and approximately 40% to 50% of patients have evidence of spread to the axillary nodes. The likelihood of axillary nodal involvement appears to be related directly to the size of the primary tumor, as shown in Figure 38-7. Also, although the evidence for this is not clear-cut, most data suggest, that axillary node positivity is slightly more common with tumors located in the lateral portion of the breast than with those in the medial or central portion.

To some extent, the incidence of histologic involvement of axillary nodes is dependent on the extent of the pathologic analysis of the specimen. Pickren was the first to show that a more thorough clearing and sectioning of the axillary specimen resulted in a greater yield of positive nodes.[79] Of 51 specimens analyzed in routine fashion and found to be negative, 11 (22%) showed evidence of involvement on more careful analysis in that study.

Detection of axillary involvement by physical examination has both a high false-positive and a high false-negative rate (Table 38-9). When axillary lymph nodes are palpable, histologic evidence of metastatic disease is not found in approx-

FIG. 38-6. Distribution of tumor foci at different distances from reference tumor and proportions of cases with and without tumor foci around reference tumor. The pathologic size served as reference size.[78]

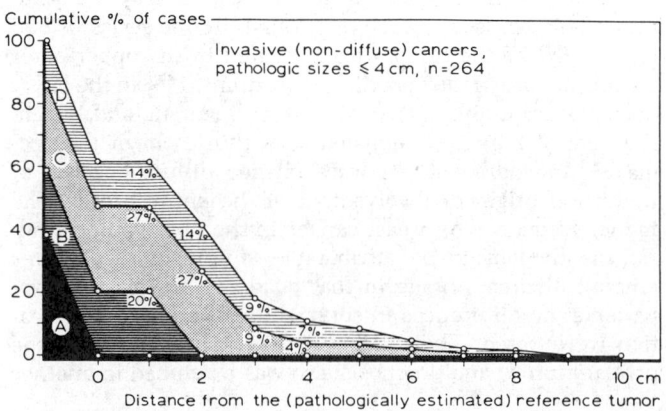

FIG. 38-7. Relation between tumor size and axillary node involvement and recurrence and mortality rates. (Fisher B, Slack NH, Bross ID et al: Cancer of the breast: Size of neoplasm and prognosis. Cancer 24:1071–1080, 1969)

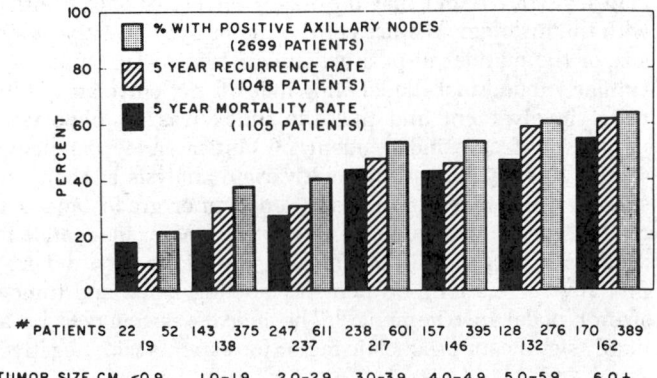

TABLE 38-9.   Accuracy of Physical Examination in Predicting Histologic Involvement of Axillary Nodes

	Series I*	Series 2†	Series 3‡	Series 4§
False-positive (%)	25	24	26	29
False-negative (%)	32	32	27	29

* Butcher H: Radical mastectomy for mammary carcinoma. Ann Surg 170:883–884, 1969.
† Haagensen CD, Cooky E, Miller E et al: Treatment of early mammary carcinoma: A cooperative international study. Ann Surg 170:875–879, 1969.
‡ Schottenfeld D, Nash A, Robbins G, Beattie E: Ten-year results of the treatment of primary operable breast cancer. Cancer 38:1001–1007, 1976.
§ Bucalossi P, Veronesi U, Zingo L, Conti C: Enlarged mastectomy for breast cancer: Review of 1,213 cases. Am J Roentgenol Rad Ther Nucl Med 111:119–122, 1971.

imately 25% of cases. Conversely, when axillary nodes are not palpable, histologic involvement is detected in approximately 30% of cases. These shortcomings of clinical evaluation are of particular importance because histologic involvement of axillary nodes has a high correlation with prognosis. Table 38-10 shows 10-year survival figures according to axillary involvement from six separate series of patients treated with radical mastectomy. Patients with histologically negative axillary nodes have a markedly greater likelihood of survival than patients with histologic involvement. Furthermore, the prognosis is inversely related to the number of involved nodes.[80] At the current level of understanding, the presence and extent of metastases to the axilla represents the single most important prognostic factor for patients with breast cancer.

For the purposes of analysis, the axilla is commonly divided into three levels: proximal—tissue inferior to the lower border of the pectoralis minor muscle (I); middle—tissue directly beneath the pectoralis minor (II); and distal—tissue superior to the pectoralis minor (III). Prognosis is

TABLE 38-11.   Ten-Year Survival (%) Related to Primary Tumor Size (cm) and Level of Axillary Involvement*

	Size of Primary (cm)			
Axillary Status	<2	2–5	>5	Total
Negative	82	65	44	72
Positive				
Proximal only	73	74	39	65
Middle or distal	–†	28	37	31
All	68	51	37	

* Schottenfeld D, Nash AG, Robbins GF et al: Ten-year results of the treatment of primary operable breast carcinoma. Cancer 38:1001–1007, 1976.
† Insufficient data.

related to the level of axillary involvement (Table 38-11). Involvement of the upper level nodes carries a worse prognosis than involvement of proximal level nodes alone. In a series of 182 mastectomy specimens examined by clearing, involvement of nodes at the apex of the axilla was found in 15, and all 15 patients relapsed,[77] indicating the grave prognosis associated with involvement high in the axilla. Also, in general, involvement of upper-level nodes is associated with a high total number of lymph nodes involved; in this group of 15 patients, the mean number of involved nodes was 16.2 (range 4–37). In another study, axillary node involvement and survival were examined in 385 patients to determine whether the total number of involved nodes or the level of axillary involvement was the better indicator of prognosis.[81] For any given number of involved nodes, survival was independent of the level of involvement, and those investigators concluded that prognosis was related more directly to the total number of nodes involved than to the level of involvement.

The distribution of axillary node involvement by level has

TABLE 38-10.   Percent Overall Survival (OS) and Disease-Free Survival (DFS) at 10 Years in Relation to Histologic Involvement of Axillary Lymph Nodes for Patients Treated by Radical Mastectomy

	Series 1 DFS*	Series 2 OS†	Series 3 OS‡	Series 4 DFS§	Series 5 OS¶	Series 6 OS‖
Histologically negative	72	76	72	76	68	76
Histologically positive	25	48	43	24	27	35
1–3 nodes	34	63		36		
≥4 nodes	16	27		14		

* Valagussa P, Bonadonna G, Veronesi U: Patterns of relapse and survival following radical mastectomy. Cancer 41:1170–1178, 1978.
† Haagensen CD: Treatment of curable carcinoma of the breast. Int J Radiat Oncol Biol Phys 2:975–980, 1977.
‡ Schottenfeld D, Nash A, Robbins G, Beattie E: Ten-year results of the treatment of primary operable breast carcinoma. Cancer 38:1001–1007, 1976. (A significant number of patients received postoperative irradiation.)
§ Fisher B, Slack N, Katrych D: Ten-year followup results of patients with carcinoma of the breast in a cooperative clinical trial evaluating surgical adjuvant chemotherapy. Surg Gynecol Obstet 140:528–534, 1975.
¶ Spratt JS, Donegan WL: Cancer of the Breast. Philadelphia, WB Saunders, 1967.
‖ Payne WS, Taylor WF, Khonsari S: Surgical treatment of breast cancer: Trends and factors affecting survival. Arch Surg 101:105–113, 1970.

TABLE 38-12. Five-Year Relapse Rate (%) According to Size of Primary and Axillary Node Involvement

	Size of Primary (cm)		
Axillary Status	<2	2–5	>5
Axillary Nodes Negative			
Fisher et al[84]	12	24	27
Nemoto et al[80]	13	19	25
Valagussa et al[53]	8	24	19
Axillary Nodes Positive			
Fisher et al[84]	50	60	79
Nemoto et al[80]	39	50	65
Valagussa et al[53]	37	64	74

been studied in two large series, with nearly identical results.[82,83] Involvement of level I alone was seen in 54% to 58% of cases; levels I and II in 20% to 22% of cases; and levels I, II, and III in 16% to 22% of cases. Involvement of levels II or III in the absence of involvement of level I ("skip metastases") was seen in only 2% to 4% of cases with nodal involvement. These results indicate that involvement of the axilla is by and large sequential. A level I dissection is therefore highly effective at determining the presence of nodal involvement but will frequently underestimate the extent of involvement.

Prognosis thus is related both to the size of the primary tumor and to axillary node involvement. Whether these two factors independently predict the outcome is addressed in Table 38-12. When axillary nodes are involved, the size of the tumor is still of prognostic value. For example, in the data from Valagussa and colleagues, the 5-year relapse rate was 37% for patients with positive nodes and small (≤2 cm) tumors and 79% for patients with positive nodes and large (>5 cm) tumors.[53] In the data from Fisher and coworkers, this correlation was analyzed further according to the number of positive axillary nodes (1 to 3 or 4 or more).[84] Within each subgroup with positive axillary nodes, the size of the primary tumor was still an independent prognostic factor. When axillary nodes are negative, however, the relation is less clear. The prognosis for patients with small (≤2 cm) tumors and negative nodes is exceptionally good, with a 5-year relapse rate of approximately 10%. For tumors larger than 2 cm, the prognosis is not as good. However, the prognosis for patients with large (>5 cm) tumors and negative nodes is not significantly worse than that of patients with 2- to 5-cm tumors and negative nodes. These data imply that the results of an axillary sampling are of value for prognostic purposes in patients with large primary tumors, because patients with histologically negative axillary nodes do relatively well even without adjuvant therapy. The 30-year results from Adair and associates support these observations: for patients with negative nodes, the 30-year survival rate was 61% when the primary tumor was no larger than 2 cm, 46% when it was 2 cm to 5 cm, and 50% when it was larger than 5 cm.[85] In contrast, for patients with involvement of level I axillary nodes, the 30-year survival rate was 40% when the tumor was no larger than 2 cm, 31% when it was 2 cm to 5 cm, and only 14% when it was larger than 5 cm.

In summary, the axillary nodal region is the principal drainage site for carcinoma of the breast, and a histologic analysis of the axilla provides a useful guide to prognosis. The more practical issue of what, if any, treatment is required for the axillary region will be addressed in later sections.

INTERNAL MAMMARY NODE INVOLVEMENT

The second major site of regional metastases for carcinoma of the breast is in the internal mammary lymph node (IMN) chain, which lies at the anterior ends of the intercostal spaces by the side of the internal thoracic artery. Because of their intrathoracic location and their uncommon clinical presentation, the frequency of internal mammary node involvement was not appreciated as early as was axillary node involvement. One of the first to document this second route of spread was Sampson Handley, who reported his results of internal mammary node biopsy in 1000 patients in 1975 (Table 38-13).[86] These results illustrate the following two points: (1) internal mammary node involvement is more common for inner quadrant or central tumors than for outer quadrant tumors; and (2) axillary lymph node involvement is more likely than is IMN involvement.

In the Handley study, even in patients with inner or central tumors, axillary involvement was more common than IMN involvement (42% versus 28%). Furthermore, if the axillary nodes were uninvolved, IMN involvement was uncommon (8%). Another larger series of patients reported from Italy has confirmed the Handley results.[87] In addition, these authors stressed the importance of primary tumor size in relation to IMN involvement: IMN involvement was seen in 19% of patients with tumors smaller than 5 cm, compared with 37% of patients with tumors larger than 5 cm.

The significance of IMN involvement is similar to that of axillary node involvement. In a large series reported by Veronesi and co-workers, the 10-year rate of disease-free survival was 73% when both the axillary nodes and the IMN were negative, 47% when axillary nodes alone were positive, 52% when the IMN alone were positive, and only 25% when both areas were positive.[88] In practice, however, biopsy of the IMN is associated with greater morbidity than biopsy of axillary nodes and is rarely performed.

SUPRACLAVICULAR NODE INVOLVEMENT

The principal route of spread to the supraclavicular lymph node areas is through the axillary node chain. In one series of

TABLE 38-13. Internal Mammary Node Involvement (%) in Relation to Location of the Primary and Axillary Node Involvement

	Primary Site				
	UIQ	LIQ	Central	UOQ	LOQ
Total	27	33	32	14	13
	67/248	20/61	70/216	54/382	12/93
Axilla not involved	14	6	7	4	5
	20/143	2/36	5/76	7/170	2/40
Axilla involved	45	72	46	22	19
	47/105	18/25	65/140	47/212	10/53

Handley RS: Carcinoma of the breast. Ann R Coll Surg 57:59–66, 1975.

TABLE 38-14. Percentage of Patients with Metastases from Breast Cancer at Various Sites in Three Collected Series

	Series 1 (n = 160)*	Series 2 (n = 43)†	Series 3 (n = 100)‡
Lung	59	65	69
Liver	58	56	65
Bone	44	–	71
Pleura	37	23	51
Adrenals	31	41	49
Kidneys	NR§	14	17
Spleen	14	23	17
Pancreas	–	11	17
Ovaries	9	16	20
Brain	–	9	22
Thyroid	–	–	24
Heart	–	–	11
Diaphragm	–	–	11
Pericardium	5	21	19
Intestine	–		18
Peritoneum	12	9	13
Uterus	–	–	15
Lymph nodes	72	–	76
Skin	34	7	30

* Warren S, Witman EM: Studies on tumor metastases: The distribution of metastases in cancer of the breast. Surg Gynecol Obstet 57:81–1018, 1937.

† Saphillo O, Parker ML: Metastases from primary carcinoma of the breast with special reference to spleen, adrenal glands and ovaries. Arch Surg 42:1003, 1941.

‡ Haagensen CD: Diseases of the Breast. Philadelphia, WB Saunders, 1971.

§ NR = not recorded.

patients undergoing routine supraclavicular dissection, involvement of the region was found in 23 (18%) of the 125 patients who had involvement of axillary nodes but in none of the 149 patients who did not have involvement of axillary nodes.[89] The significance of supraclavicular node involvement was first shown by Halsted, who performed a supraclavicular dissection in 119 patients. Forty-four women (37%) were found to have involvement of these nodes, and only two were free of cancer at 5 years.[90] Supraclavicular node involvement represents a late stage of axillary nodal involvement and carries a grave prognosis.

DISTANT METASTASES

Metastatic spread from carcinoma of the breast can be present in a variety of organs. The likelihood of organ involvement has been studied in a number of autopsy series (Table 38-14).

STAGING

Staging refers to the grouping of patients according to the extent of their disease. It is useful in choosing treatment for individual patients, estimating their prognosis, and comparing the results of different treatment programs. Staging of breast cancer is performed initially on a clinical basis, according to the physical examination as well as laboratory and radiologic evaluation.

The most widely used clinical staging system is the one adopted by both the International Union against Cancer (UICC) and the American Joint Commission on Cancer Staging and End Results Reporting (AJC). It is based on the tumor–nodes–metastases (TNM) system as detailed in the *Manual for Staging of Cancer* (2nd edition, 1983):

T	Primary tumors
T1	Tumor 2 cm or less in its greatest dimension
	a. No fixation to underlying pectoral fascia or muscle
	b. Fixation to underlying pectoral fascia or muscle
T2	Tumor more than 2 cm but not more than 5 cm in its greatest dimension
T3	Tumor more than 5 cm in its greatest dimension
	a. No fixation to underlying pectoral fascia or muscle
	b. Fixation to underlying pectoral fascia or muscle
T4	Tumor of any size with direct extension to chest wall or skin. *Note:* Chest wall includes ribs, intercostal muscles, and serratus anterior muscle, but not pectoral muscle.
	a. Fixation to chest wall
	b. Edema (including peau d'orange), ulceration of the skin of the breast, or satellite skin nodules confined to the same breast
	c. Both of the above
	d. Inflammatory carcinoma

Dimpling of the skin, nipple retraction, or any other skin changes except those in T4b may occur in T1, T2, or T3 without affecting the classification.

N	Regional lymph nodes
N0	No palpable homolateral axillary nodes
N1	Movable homolateral axillary nodes
	a. Nodes not considered to contain growth
	b. Nodes considered to contain growth
N2	Homolateral axillary nodes containing growth and fixed to one another or to other structures
N3	Homolateral supraclavicular or infraclavicular nodes containing growth or edema of the arm.

M	Distant metastasis
M0	No evidence of distant metastasis
M1	Distant metastasis present, including skin involvement beyond the breast area.

Clinical stage grouping

Stage I	T1a or T1b,	N0 or N1a,	M0
Stage II	T0,	N1b,	M0
	T1a or T1b,	N1b,	M0
	T2a or T2b,	N0, N1a, or N1b,	M0
Stage III	T1a or T1b,	N2,	M0
	T2a or T2b,	N2,	M0
	T3a or T3b,	N0, N1 or N2,	M0

Stage IV   T4,   any N,   any M
           any T,   N3,   any M
           any T,   any N,   M1

Another clinical staging system, the Columbia Clinical Classification, (CCC), is at present less widely used but is of historical importance. Like the UICC–AJC system, patients are grouped according to the extent of disease in the primary tumor site, nodal areas, and distant metastases:

Stage A: No skin edema, ulceration, or solid fixation of the tumor to the chest wall. Axillary nodes are not involved clinically.

Stage B: No skin edema, ulceration, or solid fixation of the tumor to the chest wall. Clinically involved nodes, but less than 2.5 cm in transverse diameter and not fixed to overlying skin or deeper structures of the axilla.

Stage C: Any one of the five grave signs of advanced breast carcinoma:
   (1) Edema of the skin of limited extent (involving less than one-third of the skin over the breast)
   (2) Skin ulceration
   (3) Solid fixation of the tumor to the chest wall
   (4) Extensive involvement of axillary lymph nodes (measuring 2.5 cm or more in transverse diameter)
   (5) Fixation of the axillary nodes to overlying skin or deeper structures of the axilla.

Stage D: All other patients with more advanced breast carcinoma, including:
   (1) A combination of any two or more of the five grave signs listed under Stage C
   (2) Extensive edema of the skin (involving more than one-third of the skin over the breast)
   (3) Satellite skin nodules
   (4) Inflammatory type of carcinoma
   (5) Clinically involved supraclavicular lymph nodes
   (6) Internal mammary metastases as evidenced by a parasternal tumor
   (7) Edema of the arm
   (8) Distant metastases.

Both clinical systems are based on the results of surgery in treating breast cancer. The principal points of discrepancy between the UICC–AJC system and the CCC system are the recognition by the UICC–AJC that primary tumor size by itself is of prognostic importance, and the recognition by the CCC that axillary metastases larger than 2.5 cm usually indicate extension beyond the lymph node capsule and therefore a high risk of local recurrence.

As noted before, clinical evaluation of spread to the axilla has a high false-positive and false-negative rate. For this reason, pathologic staging based on histologic study of the axillary specimen is preferable. For the individual patient, prognosis is better determined by pathologic staging than by clinical staging (Table 38-15). For patients who have clinical indications of spread of tumor but negative histologic evaluations, the survival rate (72%) is similar to that of the entire

TABLE 38-15.   Ten-Year Survival (%) According to Clinical and Pathologic Assessment of Axillary Nodes*

Clinical Assessment	Pathologic Assessment		
	N−	N+	All
N0	77	57	71
N1	72	34	44
All	76	48	

* Haagensen CD: Treatment of curable carcinoma of the breast. Int J Radiat Oncol Biol Phys 2:975–980, 1977.

group of patients with histologically negative nodes (76%), not to that of the group with histologically positive nodes (48%).[91] Similarly, if a patient does not have clinical evidence of axillary involvement but microscopic involvement is detected pathologically, the survival rate (57%) is similar to that of the entire group of patients with microscopic involvement (48%).

Pathologic stage is commonly given as Stage I (axillary nodes not involved) or Stage II (axillary nodes involved). Refinements of this simple staging format have been made, such as subdividing Stage II according to the number of positive axillary nodes. Because prognosis is clearly related to the extent of axillary involvement (see Table 38-10), it has become convention to subdivide axillary involvement into one to three nodes positive or more than four nodes positive. Another refinement is based on the recognition that micrometastatic involvement of axillary lymph nodes is not associated with the poor prognosis seen with macrometastatic involvement. A comparison of the significance of these two types of axillary metastases has been the object of recent pathologic study. In one study, occult metastases were demonstrated in the regional lymph nodes by an extended histopathologic technique in 24% of 78 cases of invasive breast cancer that would have been regarded as pathologic Stage I (no nodal metastases) after "routine" pathologic examination.[92] Patients in whom the largest nodal metastases measured 2 mm or less in greatest diameter (micrometastases) were compared with those in whom the lesions were larger than 2 mm (macrometastases). Life-table analysis revealed no significant difference in survival rates of patients with micrometastases and those without nodal metastases, and both of these groups exhibited a significantly greater likelihood of survival than patients with macrometastases. In another study, by Huvos and coworkers from Memorial Hospital in New York City, prognosis also was related to the pathologic extent of axillary nodal involvement.[93] For the 62 patients with no involvement of the axillary nodes, the 8-year survival rate was 82% (51 of 62). When micrometastatic involvement (defined as less than 2 mm) of level I axillary nodes was found, the 8-year survival rate was 94% (17 of 18). In comparison, the survival rate was 62% (28 of 45) for patients with macrometastatic involvement of level I axillary nodes.

Other refinements of the pathologic staging scheme are based on the recognition that extension of metastatic disease beyond the lymph node capsule or involvement of an axillary node larger than 2 cm have been associated with a worse prognosis, independent of the number of nodes involved. These refinements have been included in the Postsurgical Treatment Pathological Classification given by the UICC–AJC in 1977:

Primary tumor (T)

T0   No evidence of primary tumor

T1–4   Same as UICC–AJC classification except for subdivision of T1 into

    i: Tumor less than 0.5 cm

    ii: Tumor 0.5 cm–0.9 cm

    iii: Tumor 1.0 cm–1.9 cm

Nodal involvement (N)

N   No metastatic homolateral axillary nodal involvement

N1   Movable homolateral axillary metastatic nodes not fixed to one another or to other structures

N1a   Lymph nodes with only histologic evidence of metastatic growth

N1b   Gross metastatic carcinoma in lymph nodes

    i: Micrometastatic (smaller than 0.2 cm)

    ii: Metastasis (larger than 0.2 cm) in one to three lymph nodes

    iii: Metastasis to four or more lymph nodes

    iv: Extension of metastasis beyond the lymph node capsule

    v: Any positive node greater than 2 cm in diameter

N2–3   Same as clinical UICC–AJC classification.

SCREENING FOR BREAST CANCER

Screening for cancer represents an important advance in the management of the disease. Two randomized clinical trials have demonstrated a 25% to 30% reduction in breast cancer mortality rates in screened individuals.[94-97] These results are consistent with those obtained in nonrandomized studies.[98-100] The cost : benefit ratio for the use of mammography and its optimal frequency are still a matter of debate.[101-107] However, a randomized controlled clinical trial from Sweden has shown that single view mammography in women 40 years of age or older with repeat screening every 2 or 3 years resulted in an approximately 30% reduction in mortality (Fig. 38-8).[97] These issues are discussed in detail in Chapter 20, section 4.

PRETREATMENT EVALUATION

There is general agreement that the pretreatment evaluation of a patient with breast cancer should include a thorough medical history and physical examination (Table 38-16), chest roentgenogram (postero-anterior and lateral views), complete bloodcount, and liver chemistries. The value of other tests (bone scan, liver scan, and mammogram) has been a matter of controversy.

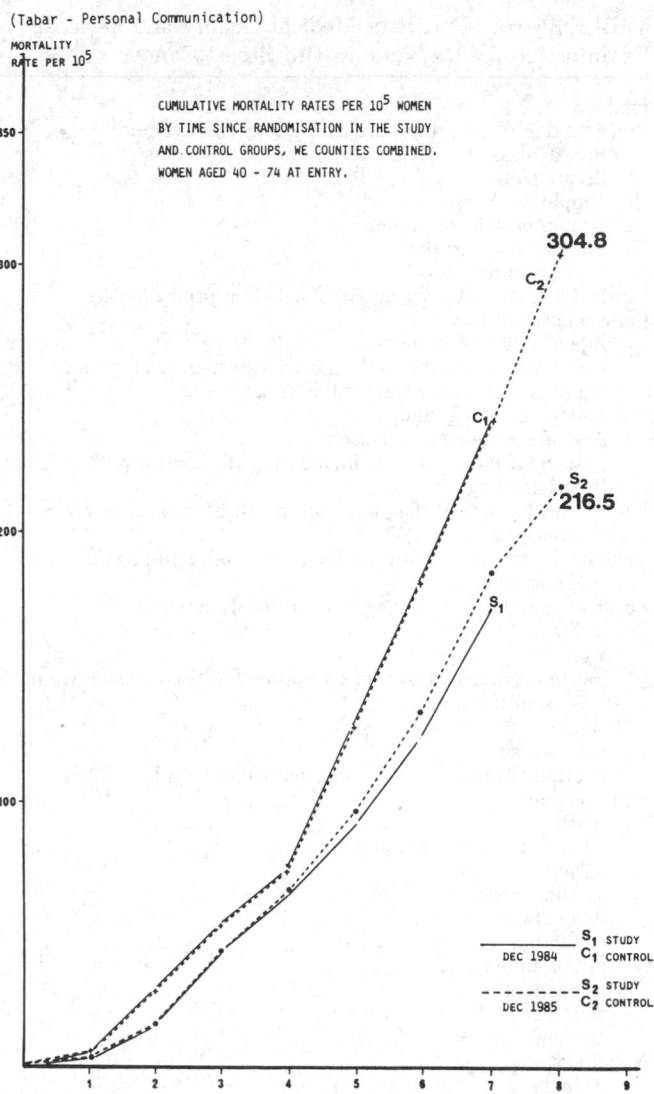

(Tabar - Personal Communication)

CUMULATIVE MORTALITY RATES PER 10⁵ WOMEN BY TIME SINCE RANDOMISATION IN THE STUDY AND CONTROL GROUPS, WE COUNTIES COMBINED. WOMEN AGED 40 - 74 AT ENTRY.

FIG. 38-8. Cumulative mortality rates for screened and control populations. (Tabar L: Unpublished data)

Radionuclide scans are acknowledged to be a sensitive test for early bone metastases. However, the yield of bone scanning in asymptomatic patients with early breast cancer is small. For example, in one study from John Hopkins, only 1 of 64 patients with clinical Stage I or II breast cancer had a positive preoperative bone scan, whereas 25% of patients with Stage III disease had positive scans preoperatively.[108] In another study from the Peter Bent Brigham Hospital, the yield of bone scanning was 0 of 37 in clinical Stage I, 4% in Stage II, and 16% in Stage III.[109] In addition, bone scans can be positive in a number of benign bone conditions, and this can delay treatment and increase patient anxiety. These data suggest that a scan is warranted in Stage III breast cancer, but its usefulness in early stage disease is less certain. Some clinicians claim that a bone scan should be obtained in all patients as a baseline for future comparison, but this justification has not been established.

TABLE 38-16. Pertinent Medical History and Physical Examination for the Patient with Breast Cancer

History
Breast and axillary symptoms: first noted and evolution
    Breast mass
    Breast pain
    Nipple discharge
    Nipple or skin retraction
    Axillary mass or pain
    Arm swelling
Medical history of breast disease, including prior biopsies
Reproductive history
    Age of onset of menses
    Frequency, duration, and regularity of menstrual periods
    Number of pregnancies, children, abortions
    Age at first pregnancy
    Age of onset of menopause
    History of hormone use, including birth control pills
    Breast feeding
Family history: age at diagnosis and death of family members with breast cancer
Review of symptoms, with particular reference to possible metastatic spread
Physical examination (a diagnosis is recommended)
Breast Mass
    size
    location (specified by clock position and the distance from edge of the areola)
    shape
    consistency
    fixation to skin, pectoral muscle or chest wall
Skin changes
    erythema
    edema (note location and extent)
    dimpling
    satellite nodules
Nipple changes
    retraction
    discoloration
    thickening
    reddening
    erosion
Nodal status
    Axillary
        number
        location
        size
        fixation to other nodes or underlying structures
        clinically suspicious or benign
    Infraclavicular fullness
    Supraclavicular nodes or area swelling

The yield of positive pretreatment liver scans is even smaller than that of bone scans. In a series of 234 patients studied with routine preoperative liver scans at the Mt. Sinai Hospital of Cleveland, only 12 (5%) had abnormal scans.[110] Of further interest, eight of these abnormal scans were established as false-positive by further evaluation, so that the ultimate result of the test was only 1% positivity. These findings are not surprising when one considers that metastases larger than 2 cm are required for visualization on liver scans.[111] It generally is recommended that liver scans be reserved for patients with abnormal liver chemistries or hepatomegaly.

It is worth emphasizing that a positive bone or liver scan does not necessarily establish metastatic disease. Both these tests commonly have significant false-positive rates, and the results of a positive scan must be viewed within the context of the total evaluation of the patient. In many cases, histologic confirmation should be obtained before definitive primary therapy is abandoned.

Bilateral mammograms are recommended before a biopsy of a suspicious breast mass to detect any occult lesion that also should be biopsied, either in the ipsilateral or the contralateral breast. The use of mammograms in this setting clearly improves the preoperative diagnostic accuracy, but a negative mammogram in the presence of a suspicious breast mass is not a justification to avoid biopsy. The use of mammography in patients with a positive biopsy is also important, especially in checking the contralateral breast. For patients who will be treated with mastectomy, the detection of additional lesions in the involved breast is of limited value. If a patient is to be treated with conservative surgery and radiation therapy, however, the detection of additional lesions is important, as discovery of multicentric lesions would influence a decision for additional surgery, an altered radiotherapeutic program, or possibly mastectomy. Occult, suspicious areas found on mammography should be removed after preoperative needle localization, which ensures excision of these areas with minimal deformity. When more than one lesion is to be excised, placement of the incisions should be planned to be most cosmetically acceptable if breast preservation is to be done yet without compromise of a possible mastectomy incision.

Newer diagnostic modalities, such as ultrasound, CT scan, and magnetic resonance imaging (MRI) of the breast, have been compared with mammography. None has proved more accurate, and they have the disadvantages of not detecting calcifications, delivering higher radiation doses (CT), and taking more patient time and costing more (CT and MRI).[112]

Radionuclide brain scans and CT scans of the head are both sensitive tests to detect early metastatic involvement. The yield of these studies in a pretreatment setting is very small, however, and they are not recommended in the absence of suspicious signs or symptoms.

An area of growing interest has been the use of biologic markers (see section on markers). A number of substances including carcinoembryonic antigen (CEA), ferritin, and human chorionic gonadotropin (hCG) have been suggested as possible markers. In patients with metastatic breast cancer, 70% have elevated CEA levels, 50% have elevated hCG levels, and 67% have elevated ferritin levels.[113-117] There is preliminary evidence that pretreatment marker concentrations can be a prognostic indicator. In one study, patients with postoperative CEA levels greater than 2.5 ng/ml had a 2-year recurrence rate of 65% compared with 20% for those with normal CEA levels (p <0.001). The use of serial marker determination in the follow-up period also has been suggested as a means for the early detection of recurrence. This field is rapidly evolving, and firm recommendations are not possible at this time. Nevertheless, pretreatment measurements, particularly of CEA, are obtained easily and relatively inexpensively.

SURGICAL MANAGEMENT OF PRIMARY BREAST CANCER

HISTORICAL BACKGROUND

Surgical attempts to provide local–regional control of breast cancer through the end of the 19th century failed uniformly. Patients generally presented with advanced, bulky disease, and various surgeons reported local recurrence rates of 60% to 80%.

In 1894, Halsted published a description of his technique of radical mastectomy, which included excision of a wide margin of skin around the tumor, dissection of thin skin flaps, and en bloc removal of the breast, axillary lymph nodes, and pectoralis major and minor muscles. The local recurrence rate with this technique was 6%.[118] Although most patients later died of distant metastases, the Halsted procedure was recognized as a significant advance and was widely practiced. Indeed, for the first three-quarters of the 20th century, it was the surgical procedure of choice for patients with operable breast carcinoma. Haagensen extended this approach, advocating a wider skin excision which required a skin graft for closure.[119] He also developed the CCC staging system to select patients with lesions more favorable for mastectomy and to classify those with more advanced stages ("grave signs") as inoperable (see section on staging).

The extended radical mastectomy, described by Urban and Baker,[120] added an en bloc dissection of the IMN chain to the radical mastectomy. This operation required an intrapleural dissection with removal of a portion of the sternum and rib cage and closure of the defect with fascia over a chest tube.

In the same time period, other surgeons explored the feasibility of preserving the pectoralis major muscle to improve the cosmetic results. This procedure, termed "modified radical mastectomy," included total mastectomy, axillary dissection, preservation of the pectoralis major muscle, and excision of the pectoralis minor muscle, as described by Patey or later, with preservation of this small muscle, as reported by Auchincloss.[121] This procedure has been the standard surgical approach since the 1970s because of the availability of long-term results showing its effectiveness both in treating multicentric disease in the breast and in treating the axilla. The factors underlying the use of modified radical mastectomy will be discussed below.

MULTICENTRICITY

The reported incidence of multicentric (or multifocal) breast cancer in areas away from the primary tumor in mastectomy specimens ranges from 9% to 75%.[122] This large discrepancy is caused by three factors: differences in the precision of the definition of multicentricity, different techniques of examination, and variations in the extent of the tissue sampling. When sections of breast tissue are taken from each of the three quadrants apart from that containing the primary tumor, high rates of multicentricity have been reported. This was true in a simulated partial mastectomy series of Rosen and colleagues,[123] who reported residual cancer in 56% of patients. In a more recent study of patients with clinically occult (nonpalpable) breast cancers detected by mammography, there was a 44% incidence of multicentricity.[124] When these tumors were microinvasive pathologically, 57% showed multicentricity. In another series of patients from Memorial Hospital who underwent mastectomy for in situ cancers, multicentric disease was present in 60%.[125] Thus, even in the earliest (or nonpalpable) breast cancers treated, occult multicentricity is frequently present.

Lagios and associates[126] examined mastectomy specimens for tumor foci outside a 5-cm radius of the reference tumor, the hypothetical border of a breast quadrant. Multicentricity was found in 20% of cases. This is similar to the findings of Rosen's group of residual tumor in 26% and 38% of cases with reference tumors smaller than and larger than 2 cm, respectively.[123] More recently, Holland and associates examined the mastectomy specimens of patients who would have been considered candidates for breast-sparing procedures and mapped cancer at various distances from the primary tumor.[127] As described elsewhere in this chapter, although most of the cancer was found within the quadrant containing the primary tumor, many patients also had evidence of cancer far from the primary tumor site. In all of these studies, the principal form of breast cancer found in other quadrants was in situ cancer.

The more important question is whether these histologic findings of breast cancer indicate clinical activity, or if they represent "anatomic cancers," with little or no biologic implication. There are few long-term studies of patients with in situ breast cancer treated with biopsy alone. However, the available data for both lobular carcinoma in situ and intraductal carcinoma indicate that over a long period, a significant percentage of these patients will develop invasive breast cancer (see section on in situ cancer).

Additional circumstantial evidence that untreated cancer will progress is that unsuspected cancer is rarely found on autopsies done on elderly women dying of causes other than breast cancer. In a series of 70 patients over the age of 70 years, only four patients (5.7%) had intraductal cancer, one of these with microinvasion.[128] This result contrasts with the much higher incidence of unsuspected prostate cancer found in men at autopsy[129] and suggests that breast cancer is more likely to express itself as a clinical entity during the patient's life.

AXILLARY NODE METASTASES

There are four potential advantages to axillary dissection. First, the procedure provides prognostic information and helps determine the treatment plan. Patients with histologically involved nodes are considered candidates for adjuvant systemic therapy. Accurate staging thus benefits the patient, her family, and physicians.

Second, such dissection is reliable treatment of the axilla: few local recurrences in this area are seen after such dissection in patients with histologically positive nodes.[85,130] If conservative surgery and radiotherapy is the treatment of choice, irradiation of the axilla is unnecessary if complete dissection has been done.

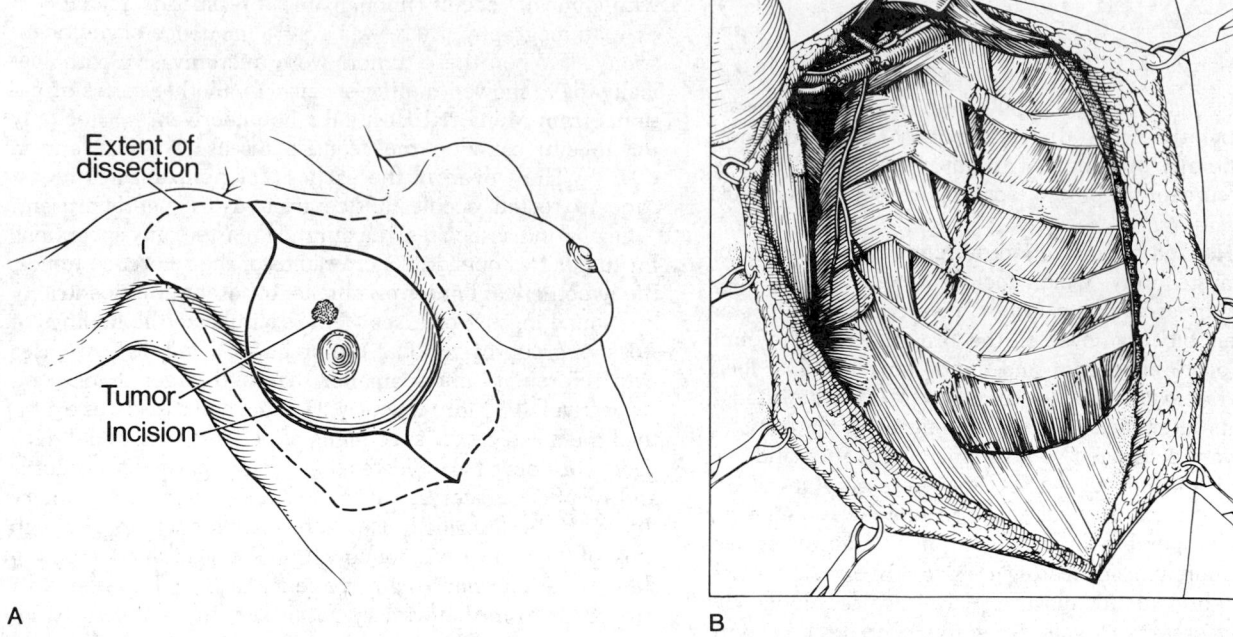

FIG. 38-9. Radical mastectomy. **A.** Outline of vertical incision (*solid lines*) widely encompassing a tumor at the 12:00 axis. Extent of underlying tissue removed is outlined by dotted lines. **B.** Operative field after removal of specimen, showing complete removal of breast, axillary nodes, and both pectoral muscles. Underlying chest wall is shown with intact long thoracic nerve laterally. (Kinne DW. In Harris JR, Hellman S, Henderson IC, Kinne DW [eds]: Breast Diseases, pp 267–268. Philadelphia, JB Lippincott, 1987)

Third, it is possible that axillary dissection improves overall survival. Long-term retrospective studies have shown that many patients with positive nodes are disease free many years after mastectomy, although their prognosis is certainly worse than that of patients with negative nodes.[85,131] However, modern studies suggest that axillary treatment does not greatly affect survival.[132] These studies will be discussed below.

A fourth potential benefit of axillary dissection is palliative. If bulky nodal disease can be excised, patients who eventually succumb to distant metastases may be spared painful lymphedematous extremities caused by tumor involvement of the neurovascular bundle.

LONG-TERM RESULTS WITH MASTECTOMY

Radical mastectomy was once the standard treatment for breast cancer in this country and, as a result, there are many studies using this procedure with long-term results. This en bloc dissection of the breast, all axillary nodes, and both pectoralis muscles is depicted in Figure 38-9. Haagensen reviewed his 50-year personal experience with 1036 patients treated by this procedure.[131] Results were given according to the CCC (see section on staging, above). Local recurrence rates 10 years after radical mastectomy were 3.7% in Stage A disease and 12% in Stage B. Pathologically involved nodes were recovered in 31% of patients with clinical Stage A and 72% of those with Stage B disease. The overall 10-year dis-

ease-free survival rate was 77% for patients with negative nodes and 49% for patients with positive nodes.

Robbins and Berg[133] reported 30-year follow-up on 1458 patients treated at Memorial Hospital with standard radical mastectomy. Thirteen percent of these women survived 30 years free of cancer, 57% died of breast cancer, 24% died of other causes, and 6% were lost to follow-up. As noted before, axillary nodal status was a more important determinant of prognosis than was the size of the primary tumor: patients with tumors smaller than 2 cm and involved nodes did worse than those with large tumors and negative nodes.

The 10-year follow-up of 304 patients treated at Memorial Hospital and classified by the TNM system is reported by Schottenfeld and associates.[130] Eighty-five percent of patients were treated with radical mastectomy and the rest with extended radical, modified radical, or total mastectomy. Thirty-six percent of patients with Stage II or III disease received postoperative radiotherapy. No patient received adjuvant systemic therapy. No local recurrences developed in patients with Stage I disease within 10 years, but recurrence was noted in 6% of those with clinical Stage II or III disease, which is similar to the local recurrence risks reported by Haagensen quoted above.[131] Overall 10-year survival rates were 91% for clinical Stage I, 57% for Stage II, and 34% for Stage III. Overall, patients with clinically negative nodes had a 71% survival rate compared with 48% in patients with positive nodes. As in the Robbins series, the level of axillary metastases was correlated with survival. If the highest axillary node involved was level I, the survival rate was 65%, with a decrease in survival to 30% if levels II and III had metastases. As noted earlier, there is a close correlation between the level of involvement and the total number of nodes harboring metastases.

AXILLARY NODE TREATMENT

The optimal extent of an axillary dissection is not clear. As noted in the section on local spread, skip metastases to the upper levels of axillary nodes are uncommon. The difficulty in interpreting these studies is that they are undertaken in the pathology laboratory on radical or modified radical mastectomy specimens. Although axillary levels were indicated by placement of tags in the operating room, the boundaries between levels are indistinct. Perhaps of more clinical importance is the study by Davies and colleagues at Guy's Hospital[134] comparing clinical examination with a simple axillary node biopsy done in the operating room, with axillary node sampling, and with the completed axillary dissection in the same patients. Axillary node biopsy failed to detect metastases in 42% of patients, and axillary node sampling or excision of nodes in the axillary tail missed 14% of patients with axillary metastases. Even if axillary dissection is considered only a staging procedure, it is apparent that a significant number of patients with involved nodes would not be identified by lesser sampling procedures.

One rationale for a complete dissection is that the upper levels of the axilla are commonly involved when the lower level nodes are involved. An incomplete dissection will therefore underestimate the extent of involvement and will commonly leave involved nodes behind. This is likely to influence the risk of axillary recurrence even if there is no association with an effect on survival. In an analysis of 539 patients with axillary metastases who underwent total axillary dissection, 40% of patients who had involved level I nodes also had positive nodes at higher levels.[82] If a level I and II dissection had been done, 20% would have had involved level III nodes left behind. In another study, 20% of patients with one to three positive lymph nodes in a sampling procedure were found to have four or more involved nodes by complete axillary dissection.[135] This result may have implications for the systemic therapy program undertaken. However, recent studies suggest that a level I and II dissection[136,137] or even a level I dissection alone[138] may adequately stage patients and control disease in the axilla.

The value of treating axillary nodes was examined in a trial performed by the NSABP. The NSABP B-04 trial, begun in 1971, randomized patients with clinically negative axillae to either radical mastectomy, total mastectomy and irradiation of the axillary nodes, or total mastectomy with delayed axillary dissection if nodes became clinically involved. The 10-year results showed no significant differences among the three groups of patients in disease-free or overall survival rates (57%).[132] Forty percent of patients with clinically negative axillary nodes who were treated with radical mastectomy had histologically positive nodes. Assuming that the same percentage of patients undergoing total mastectomy had microscopic involvement of these nodes, it is of interest

that only 18% required delayed axillary dissection because of the development of clinically positive nodes. This finding has been interpreted to mean that not all histologically positive nodes will become biologically active. The results of the NSABP B-04 trial suggest that untreated positive nodes did not serve as a source of further dissemination, leading to a higher rate of distant metastases. There is no support in this study for the concept that nodal metastases in themselves instigate distant metastases. Also of importance is that in the group receiving irradiation to the axilla, these foci were well controlled, with only 3.1% presenting with axillary recurrence.

An analysis of NSABP B-04 trial by Harris and Osteen[139] points out that 35% of patients assigned to treatment by total mastectomy alone actually had a limited axillary dissection. This subgroup of patients required subsequent axillary dissection in fewer instances than did patients who had no nodes removed initially. Furthermore, many patients likely developed axillary metastases at the time of or subsequent to the appearance of distant metastases, thus making axillary dissection unnecessary, and some patients may have had unresectable axillary recurrences. Therefore, the true incidence of axillary failure is unknown. The impact of axillary treatment on survival is also unknown from this study. Because 60% of patients did not have axillary involvement and many of the 40% who did have also had occult distant metastases, the percentage of patients helped by axillary treatment can only be small. It is possible that the trial was simply not large enough to detect a small but clinically significant benefit.

Although providing interesting and important information on the biologic behavior of breast cancer, the NSABP study provides little practical guidance in the management of patients today. With the widespread use of adjuvant systemic therapy for patients with positive axillary nodes, most, if not all, breast cancer patients are advised to undergo axillary dissection as part of the staging. If patients are judged prior to treatment not to be candidates for any systemic therapy— for example, because of advanced age or severe medical illness—this study indicates that either irradiation of the nodes or observation with delayed dissection when they become clinically involved are reasonable options.

MODIFIED RADICAL MASTECTOMY

The modified radical mastectomy, also termed total mastectomy with axillary lymph node dissection and preservation of the pectoralis major muscle, is not as precisely defined or standardized as the radical mastectomy. The pectoralis minor muscle may be excised or divided or left intact, and, more importantly, there may be variation in the extent of axillary lymph node dissection ranging from sampling to full dissection.

One virtue of the modified radical mastectomy is that nearly all patients with operable breast cancers are unquestionable candidates for it. This includes patients with Stages I, II, and III breast cancer not fixed to the pectoralis major muscle or accompanied by bulky axillary lymph node involvement (the latter clinical settings suggesting the advis-

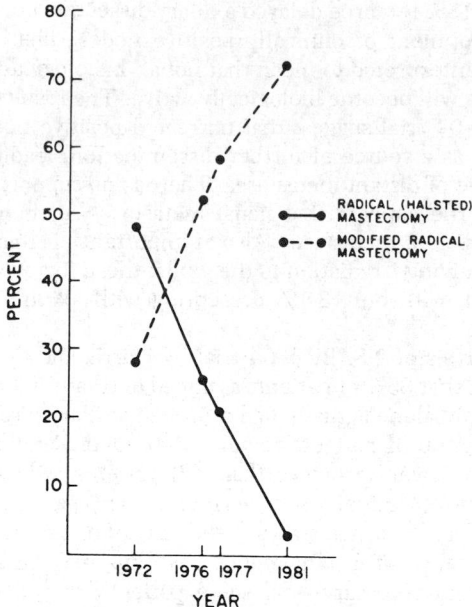

FIG. 38-10. Percentage of patients undergoing Halsted radical mastectomy and modified radical mastectomy in the 1982 National Survey of Cancer of the Breast in the United States. (Wilson RE et al: Trends in operative procedures in the United States, 1972–87, Surg Gynecol Obstet 159:309, 1984)

ability of radical mastectomy). The 1982 National Survey of Carcinoma of the Breast in the United States by the American College of Surgeons,[140] an aggregation of data from several hundred hospitals in the United States, encompassed about one-fifth of the incident cases of breast cancer for that year and is compared with similar surveys conducted in 1972 and 1977 in Figure 38-10. Although breast-sparing procedures were carried out in only 7.2% of cases in this survey, a lag time exists, and it is likely that a higher percentage of breast-conserving operations is being done today. At Memorial Sloan-Kettering Cancer Center, 824 patients with breast cancer were treated by members of the Breast Service in 1986. Sixty-six percent of patients underwent modified radical mastectomy compared with 3% having radical mastectomy. Breast preservation approaches (partial mastectomy, axillary dissection followed by radiation therapy) were performed in 215 patients, or 26%. This represents an increase from 8% of the total number of patients so treated in 1983 and 21% in 1985.

The procedure for modified radical mastectomy is shown in Figure 38-11. The cosmetic difference between this and radical mastectomy, shown in Figure 38-12, is apparent. With a low transverse scar, an intact pectoralis major muscle, and the use of an external prosthesis, more options for clothing are possible with the modified procedure. Also, the breast is easier to reconstruct with intact tissues whereas with a radical mastectomy, a myocutaneous flap is required to fill in the axillary hollow.

The change to modified radical mastectomy was brought about by several factors. Pathologic analysis of axillary nodes indicated that similar numbers were removed in the modified and the radical mastectomy procedures, and retrospec-

tive analysis showed similar overall survival rates for patients treated with either procedure.[141] Of note, a higher local recurrence rate was observed for patients with Stage III disease treated with modified radical mastectomy. This observation was corroborated in a prospective trial by Maddox and colleagues,[142] who noted no differences in overall or disease-free survival in patients undergoing radical or modified radical mastectomies but higher local recurrence rates for patients in the modified operation group who had Stage III lesions. Long follow-up of retrospective series, as reported by the Mayo Clinic,[143] shows nearly identical 10-year survival rates for patients treated by either procedure (approximately 74% for each). These data support the adoption of modified radical mastectomy as the procedure of choice.

Local recurrence after modified radical mastectomy is apparently not influenced by the proximity to the pectoralis major muscle. Patients with a deep margin of 1 mm or less have few local recurrences,[144] suggesting that an intact pectoral fascia is an effective tumor barrier. However, en bloc excision of a small portion of muscle beneath a deep tumor (or a biopsy site of uncertain depth) is useful to ensure an adequate deep margin.[145]

EXTENDED RADICAL MASTECTOMY

Extended radical mastectomy is defined as a standard radical mastectomy plus resection of the internal mammary nodes. Urban reported favorable results with this procedure for selected patients.[146] The survival rate of patients with involved IMN and uninvolved axillary nodes (54%) was identical to that of patients with a positive axilla and a negative internal mammary chain. A prospective randomized trial by Veronesi and Valagussa showed no survival differences between patients treated with radical or extended radical mastectomy.[147] The operation is seldom practiced in this country, accounting for about 1% of all procedures.[140]

However, Lacour and associates recently published 15-year results of patients treated at the Institut Gustave-Roussy with either radical or extended radical mastectomy.[148] For the subset of patients with medial lesions and positive nodes, the overall survival rate was 53% for extended radical mastectomy compared with 28% for radical mastectomy. The small numbers of patients in this subset cast doubt on the significance of this finding.

TOTAL MASTECTOMY

Sometimes referred to as simple mastectomy, this procedure removes the entire breast, including the nipple–areolar complex, but without axillary node dissection or removal of the pectoralis muscles. The operation has four principal indications:

1. Patients with in situ carcinoma (ductal or lobular) with no suspicious axillary lymphadenopathy, among whom metastatic disease to the axillary nodes occurs in less than 1%;
2. Carefully selected patients undergoing prophylactic mastectomy, often of the contralateral breast;

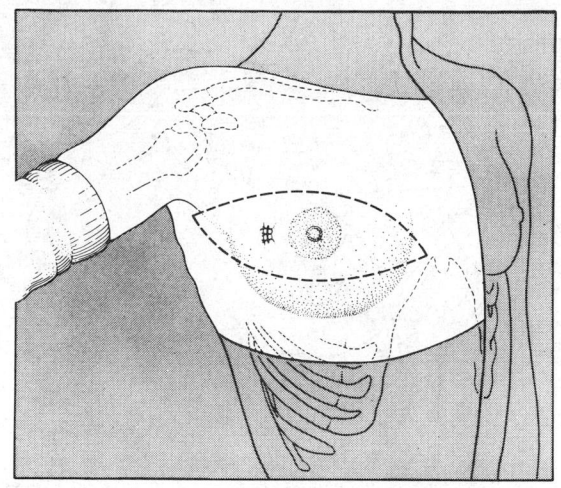

A

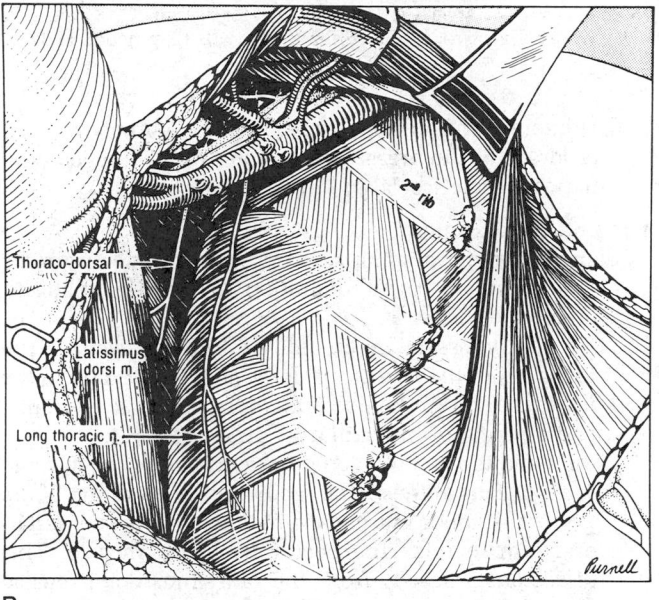

B

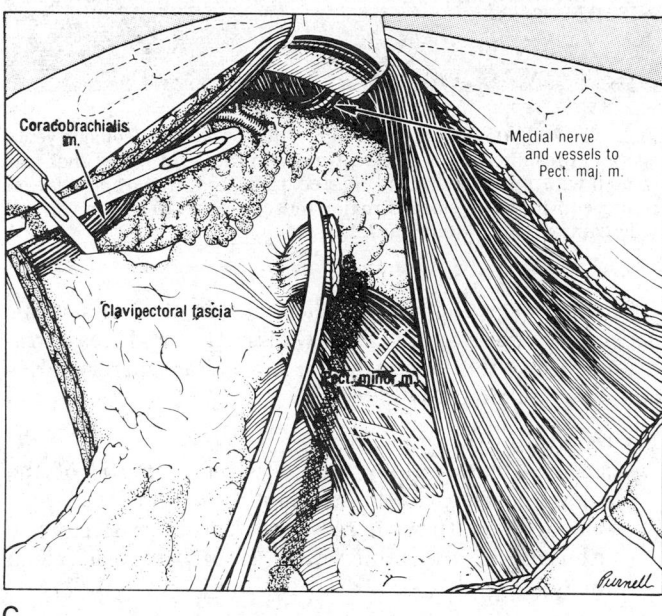

C

FIG. 38-11. Modified radical mastectomy. **A**. Skin incision, transversely placed. **B**. Pectoralis major muscle with intact neuromuscular bundle retracted medially. Pectoralis minor has been divided near coracoid process and will be excised. **C**. Completely dissected axilla, with intact pectoralis major muscle and long thoracic nerve and divided thoracoabdominal bundle (the latter may be preserved in a clinically negative axilla). (Kinne DW: In Harris JR, Hellman S, Henderson IC, Kinne DW [eds]: Breast Diseases, pp 263–266. Philadelphia, JB Lippincott, 1987)

3. Patients who develop breast recurrence after partial mastectomy and axillary dissection (or axillary irradiation), with or without breast irradiation, and who remain free of distant disease ("salvage" mastectomy); and

4. As a palliative procedure in patients with bulky breast tumors and distant metastases in whom local control will be facilitated by removal of the breast.

SUBCUTANEOUS MASTECTOMY

Proposed as a prophylactic and cosmetic procedure, subcutaneous mastectomy involves the removal of the major portion of the breast but spares the nipple–areolar complex. It leaves 10% to 15% of breast tissue behind,[149] and carcinoma has developed in patients after this procedure.[150] Also, the

cosmetic results are frequently unsatisfactory. There is thus very little, if any, indication for this procedure.

BREAST PRESERVATION PROCEDURES

Many attempts have been reported to treat infiltrating breast cancer by excision (partial mastectomy) alone, without treatment of the remaining breast tissue or axilla. As summarized in Table 38-17, the failure rate in the ipsilateral breast is significant, ranging from 25% to 37% within 5 years. These local failure rates are similar to that reported for a subgroup of the NSABP B-06 trial patients treated with segmental mastectomy, axillary dissection, and no further treatment to the breast. In a highly selected series reported by the Cleveland Clinic,[151] a 23% failure rate in the breast and axilla was reported with 15-year follow-up.

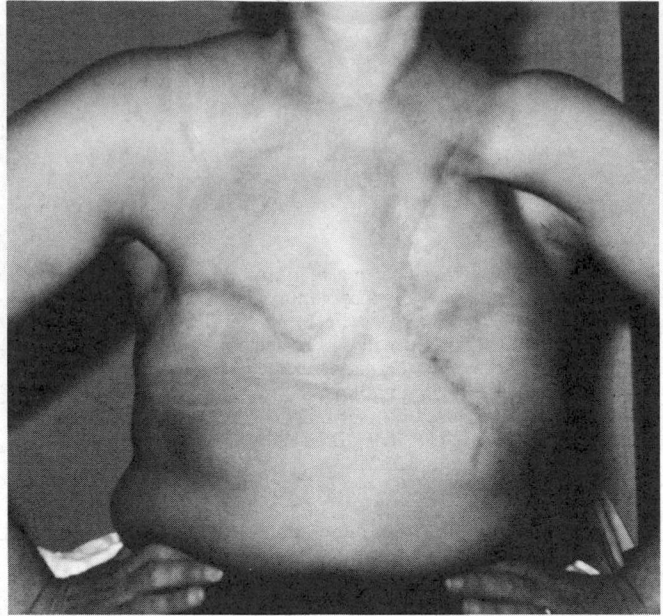

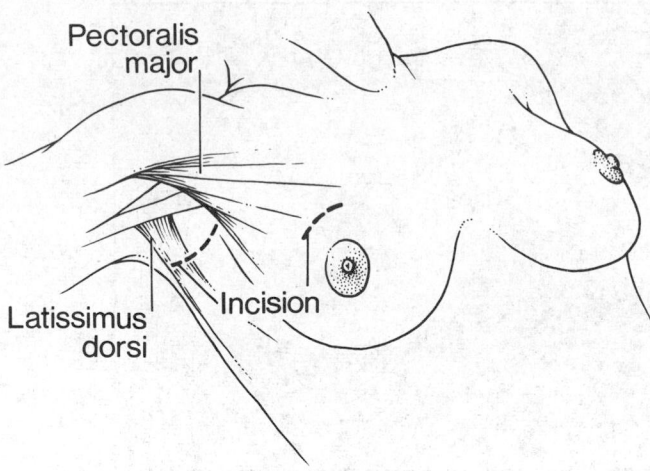

FIG. 38-13. Placement of incisions within skin lines for breast preservation cases. Two incisions are preferable to one when possible. (Kinne DW: In Harris JR, Hellman S, Henderson IC, Kinne DW [eds]: Breast Diseases, p 270. Philadelphia, JB Lippincott, 1987)

FIG. 38-12. Patient had undergone left radical mastectomy years ago and presented with a new primary in the right breast that was treated with modified radical mastectomy. Note transverse scar on right, with intact pectoralis major muscle, compared with vertical scar with axillary hollow on left.

Breast preservation approaches outside of clinical trials consist of tumor excision, axillary dissection, and breast irradiation. The extent of both breast and axillary surgery varies and may be defined as follows:[152]

For removal of the breast tumor:
   Excision (tumorectomy, lumpectomy): removal of the tumor grossly without attention to margins;
   Wide excision (limited resection, partial mastectomy): excision of the tumor with grossly normal, clean margins;

Quadrantectomy: en bloc excision of the tumor within a quadrant of the breast tissue along with the pectoralis major muscle fascia and overlying skin.

For axillary dissection:
   Sampling: removal of an axillary node or nodes from the lower axilla without definition of precise anatomic boundaries;
   Low axillary dissection: en bloc excision of level I of the axilla, from the latissimus dorsi muscle laterally to the lateral border of the pectoralis minor muscle medially, and clearing of the axillary vein superiorly;
   Level I and II dissection: en block excision of the low and mid portions of the axilla, facilitated by elevation of the pectoralis minor muscle and mobilization of the ipsilateral arm to relax the pectoralis major muscle. This dissection proceeds from the latissimus dorsi muscle

TABLE 38-17.   Results of Partial Mastectomy Alone as Treatment for Early Breast Cancer

Institution	Stage	Breast Relapse Rate (%)	Follow-up (yr)
Princess Margaret*	T1–T2, N0	25	5
Royal Marsden†	T1–T2, N0	33	5
Suffolk‡	T1–T2, N0 or N1	37	3
McGill§	T1–T2, N0	28	5
Children's Hospital, San Francisco¶	T1–T2, N0 or N1	28	2

   * Clark RM, Wilkinson RH, Mahoney LJ et al: Breast cancer: A 21 year experience with conservative surgery and radiation. Int J Radiat Oncol Biol Phys 8:967–975, 1982.
   † Montgomery ACV, Greening WP, Levene AL: Clinical study of recurrence rate and survival time of patients with carcinoma of the breast treated by biopsy excision without any other therapy. J R Soc Med 71:339–342, 1978.
   ‡ Tagart REB: Partial mastectomy for breast cancer. Br Med J 2:1268, 1978.
   § Freeman CR, Belliveau NJ, Kim TH et al: Limited surgery with or without radiotherapy for early breast carcinoma. J Can Assoc Radiol 32:125–128, 1981.
   ¶ Lagios MD, Richards VE, Rose MR, Yee E: Segmental mastectomy without radiotherapy: Short-term follow-up. Cancer 52:2173–2179, 1983.

laterally to the medial border of the pectoralis minor muscle medially, with clearing of the axillary vein superiorly;

Full axillary dissection (levels I, II, and III): removal of the entire axillary contents, from the latissimus dorsi muscle laterally to the subclavius muscle (Halsted's ligament) medially, clearing the axillary vein, with preservation of or excision of the pectoralis minor muscle.

Ideal placement of the incisions is shown in Figure 38-13. Although controversy exists, present opinion favors wide excision of the breast tumor in order to achieve complete removal with clear margins, and either a level I and II or a full axillary dissection for adequate staging and axillary treatment.

BREAST RECONSTRUCTION AFTER MASTECTOMY

All women who undergo mastectomy for cancer should be made aware of the possibilities for breast reconstruction.[153-159] Although the attitudes of individual patients toward the psychological and cosmetic effects of the loss of the breast differ greatly, many patients find significant comfort in the possibility of future breast reconstruction.

Prior to undertaking surgery for breast reconstruction, the patient and physician should carefully discuss the expectations and motivation of the patient. It is essential that she have realistic expectations of the cosmetic and sensory differences that will exist in the reconstructed compared with the original breast. It is often helpful to show the prospective patient photographs of typical as well as good and poor results following breast reconstruction.

Considerable flexibility exists as to the timing of breast reconstruction. The breast can be reconstructed at the time of mastectomy, although there is considerably less experience with this technique, and the complication rates are higher.[154,156,160] Most plastic surgeons advocate a delay of 3 to 6 months before the reconstruction procedure. This provides adequate time for resolution of skin changes and contractures and is thought to lead to a more secure blood supply to the skin and soft tissue around any subsequent implants. Longer delays are possible, and many patients have had reconstruction as late as 10 years or more after mastectomy.

There is no evidence that reconstruction either increases the likelihood of local recurrence or makes its detection more difficult. In most cases, the prosthesis used in reconstruction is placed beneath the skin and the pectoralis major muscle, and local recurrence is most likely to develop superficial to this region. Also, in the absence of nodal disease, chest wall recurrence is so rare that most surgeons have abandoned it as an important factor in selecting such patients for breast reconstruction.

TYPES OF BREAST RECONSTRUCTION

Many techniques have been developed for reconstruction of the breast after mastectomy, and decisions for each patient must be made on an individual basis, taking into account the presence of adequate skin coverage, the laxity of the skin on the anterior chest wall, the presence and intact innervation of the pectoralis major muscle, and the contour of the opposite breast. When even slight laxity in the skin over the anterior chest exists, direct implants of inorganic material are the treatment of choice for recreating the breast contour.[153,161-164] Silicone gel implants are the most commonly used, and in a recent survey by Cocke, 310 of 419 patients had this type of prosthesis placed.[155] Also available are inflatable prostheses and polyurethane-coated prostheses with Dacron patches, although the latter are used infrequently.[153] Although contour-form types of prostheses are available, these tend not to be as satisfactory as round prostheses in the majority of patients. Prostheses come in a variety of sizes that can be individualized to the patient.

If the skin of the anterior chest wall is very tight, or if skin changes exist because of radiation, then it is necessary either to use available tissue and a tissue expander[166,167] or to advance both skin and subcutaneous tissue to the area of the breast using one of the various flaps.[154-159] Medially based transverse abdominal flaps can be used to replace or to add skin to the central or lower portion of the mastectomy defect. Perforating branches of the superior epigastric artery enter this flap near the medial aspect of the rectus abdominis sheath.

The latissimus dorsi myocutaneous flap is effective for replacing the bulk lost by removal of the pectoralis major muscle and brings a generous amount of skin to the reconstruction site. Skin in this flap is supplied by musculocutaneous perforating vessels from the latissimus dorsi muscle originating from the thoracodorsal artery. When adequate skin coverage exists and bulk tissue is required to fill the pectoralis major muscle defect, then latissimus dorsi muscle flaps supplied by the thoracodorsal branch of the subscapular artery are useful.

A variety of other types of flaps are possible, including local skin transfer from surrounding tissue, reconstructions that take part of the opposite breast, and the use of distant skin flaps such as elevation of abdominal tubes.[163-165] It is also possible to use a flap of greater omentum pedicled on a single gastroepiploic artery and vein covered with a skin graft.[168,169] Free flap reconstruction is also possible, involving the transfer of composite tissue from a distant area and microvascular anastomoses to nearby vessels, such as the internal mammary chain. The most common donor site is the gluteus maximus.[170,171] Although these flap procedures are more involved, sometimes they represent either the only or the best possible reconstructive approach and offer the additional benefit of obviating the need for a prosthesis. Usually, a satisfactory breast mound can be fashioned from the tissue brought into place. Choosing the exact type of reconstruction to be used requires judgment based on experience and must be determined individually for each patient. It is sometimes necessary to perform a plastic reconstructive procedure, such as reduction mammoplasty, on the remaining breast also because of significant asymmetry that may otherwise exist after reconstruction.

NIPPLE–AREOLAR RECONSTRUCTION

Although the procedures mentioned above can reconstruct the breast mound, reconstruction of the nipple–areolar complex is desired by many women for cosmetic reasons. Preservation of the patient's own nipple–areolar complex is cosmetically superior to other methods for substituting or reconstructing the areola.[153-155,172] However, this procedure has been associated with recurrent cancer in a number of cases[172-174] and should never be done. Another procedure for reconstructing the nipple–areolar complex involves the use of labia minora grafts or grafts of the upper inner thigh skin, where the pigment is darker.[175] A semicircle of these areas can be excised and transferred as full-thickness grafts to the de-epithelialized site on the breast eminence. Nipple prominence can be created by using pursestring sutures at the desired site. Techniques also have been devised for partitioning the nipple on the remaining breast and transplanting one section to the breast eminence on the opposite side.[153-155,176] This produces little cosmetic defect in the remaining breast. It also is possible to simulate the presence of an areola by tattooing the surface of the breast mound, and this method is often satisfactory in creating the appearance of a nipple.

COMPLICATIONS OF RECONSTRUCTIVE PROCEDURES

A variety of complications can attend breast reconstruction.[153-159] The presence of skin changes caused by previous radiation can substantially increase complication rates and may necessitate the use of a myocutaneous flap to provide adequate reconstruction. Other complications include hematoma, infections, soft-tissue ischemia, skin loss, and prosthesis extrusion, all of which are infrequent in experienced hands. A more common problem is capsule formation, in which tight or heavy fibrotic capsules form around breast implants. Secondary procedures may be required to release this capsule.

POSTOPERATIVE RADIOTHERAPY

The first major use of radiotherapy in the primary management of patients with breast cancer was not as definitive treatment but rather as an adjuvant to radical mastectomy. There were two rationales for such prophylactic radiotherapy. The first was that prophylactic radiotherapy could be used to reduce the risk of local–regional tumor recurrence. The risk of local recurrence after mastectomy is 10% to 15% and is related to whether axillary nodes are negative or positive (Table 38-18); it was hoped that postoperative radiotherapy would decrease this risk of local recurrence. This result seemed especially important because these recurrences are often very distressing for afflicted patients, and once clinically manifest, they can be treated effectively in only approximately 50% of patients. The second rationale for postoperative radiotherapy was to improve the likelihood of survival.[177]

It has been well established that radiotherapy after radical mastectomy markedly decreases the risk of local–regional recurrence. At the M. D. Anderson Hospital between 1963 and 1977, 920 patients underwent radiation after radical or modified radical mastectomy. Supraclavicular recurrence was minimal in irradiated patients, and chest wall recurrence was less common than in comparable patients who were not irradiated, particularly for high-risk patients (those with four or more positive nodes) (Table 38-19).

Despite this documented improvement in local–regional disease control, the effect of adjuvant radiation therapy on survival remains uncertain. The survival value of postoperative radiotherapy ideally would be determined by a large, properly conducted, prospective, randomized clinical trial. There are now four trials with published results in which patients have been randomized after radical or modified radical mastectomy to either postoperative radiotherapy or no further treatment (Table 38-20). As indicated in the "comments" column, there are methodologic problems in these trials, particularly the earlier ones. As a group, however, these trials indicate that postoperative radiotherapy decreases local–regional recurrence but does not significantly improve the likelihood of survival.

It is possible that postoperative irradiation is detrimental to survival. This possibility was suggested by Stjernsward, who hypothesized that postoperative radiation increased the mortality rate by suppressing host immunity.[178] More recently, an overview of postoperative radiotherapy has been published by Cuzick and associates.[179] Included in this study were the results from the Manchester trials, the Oslo trials, the Stockholm trial, and an unpublished small trial from Heidelberg. The results of these various trials were combined by the use of a summary logrank statistic (Mantel–Haenzel) obtained by adding together across trials the difference between observed and "expected" deaths. No difference was seen in the summary observed-minus-expected deaths comparing patients treated with and without radiotherapy over the first 10 years after surgery. After 10 years, however, there was a lower rate of survival associated with the use of radiotherapy (p = 0.005). Among patients followed longer than 10 years, 271 of the 683 (40%) who received radiotherapy died compared with 235 of the 691 patients (34%) who did not receive radiotherapy (Fig. 38-14). The overview analysis thus raises the possibility that postoperative irradiation is actually detrimental to survival, although it should be stressed that the technique of radiotherapy used in these older trials is considerably different from that currently used.

At this time, it is clear that postoperative radiation is not of

TABLE 38-18.   Likelihood (%) and Site of First Relapse 5 to 10 Years After Radical Mastectomy According to Status of Axillary Nodes

Site of Relapse	Series 1*		Series 2†	
	Nodes+	Nodes−	Nodes+	Nodes−
Local–regional only	18	6	25	4
Distant only	49	20	43	20
Local–regional and distant	9	2		

* Fisher B, Ravdin RG, Ausman RK et al: Surgical adjunct chemotherapy in cancer of the breast: results of a decade of cooperative investigation. Ann Surg 168:337–356, 1968.

† Valagussa P, Bonadonna G, Veronesi U: Patterns of relapse and survival following radical mastectomy. Cancer 41:1170–1178, 1978.

TABLE 38-19. Incidence of Local-Regional Recurrence After Radical Mastectomy and Postoperative Radiotherapy (M. D. Anderson Hospital)

Site of Irradiation	No. of Positive Axillary Nodes	Recurrence (%)	
		Chest Wall	Supraclavicular Region
Peripheral lymphatics	0	5	1
	1-3	9	2
	≥4	20	1
Peripheral lymphatics and chest wall	0	2	2
	1-3	8	1
	≥4	11	3

value in unselected patients. However, further study will be required to determine whether there are subsets of patients for whom postoperative therapy is beneficial. There is preliminary evidence that patients with inner or central primary tumors and positive axillary nodes are such a subset.[180] In addition, many physicians feel that for high-risk patients, the prevention of local-regional recurrence is sufficient reason to recommend this treatment. As noted above, local-regional recurrence can be highly distressing to a patient and, once manifest, is controlled in only 50% of cases.[181,182]

The above discussion applies to patients who do not receive adjuvant chemotherapy. The use of postoperative radiotherapy also must be considered in the light of adjuvant chemotherapy. It is possible that the chest wall and regional nodes are the site of greatest tumor burden after mastectomy in certain subgroups, such as patients with larger primary tumors or positive axillary nodes. According to the Goldie-Coldman hypothesis, spontaneous mutations of tumor cells to drug resistance may account for failures of chemotherapy. The greater the tumor burden, the more likely it is that drug-resistant cells will emerge.[183] Adjuvant radiation therapy, by decreasing the local tumor burden, therefore might decrease the probability of drug resistance and hence increase the probability of cure.

A few studies have addressed the value of adding radiation therapy to adjuvant chemotherapy.[184-187] Overall, no significant differences in survival rates were seen between those patients randomized to chemotherapy alone and those randomized to chemotherapy and radiotherapy. However, among all patients, local and regional control were significantly improved by the addition of radiation therapy. More recently, the results were published of a randomized trial examining the necessity and effectiveness of postoperative radiotherapy in 510 patients with T1-T2 tumors and pathologically positive nodes or T3 tumors and negative nodes who were treated with adjuvant chemotherapy at the Dana-Farber Cancer Institute in conjunction with the Joint Center for Radiation Therapy (DFCI/JCRT).[188] Patients with four or more positive nodes or at least one positive apical node were randomized to receive either five or ten cycles of cyclophosphamide/Adriamycin (doxorubicin) (CA). Patients with one to three positive nodes, or operable tumors larger than 5 cm and pathologically negative nodes, were randomized to receive eight cycles of either cyclophosphamide-methotrexate-5-fluorouracil (5-FU) (CMF) or methotrexate-5-FU (MF) chemotherapy. Two hundred and six of these patients were subsequently rerandomized to receive either no further treatment or adjuvant radiotherapy. Radiation therapy consisted of 4500 cGy in 5 weeks to the chest wall and appropriate draining lymph nodes. The median follow-up time from chemotherapy randomization was 45 months for patients in the CA arm and 53 months for those in the CMF/MF arm. The crude rate of local failure (chest wall or draining lymph node areas) as the first site of failure for patients randomized to receive chemotherapy only was 14%; for those randomized to receive both chemotherapy and ra-

TABLE 38-20. Results of Randomized Trials of Postoperative Radiotherapy After Radical Mastectomy

Study	No. of Patients	Areas Treated	Follow-up (yr)	Local Control*	Relapse-free Survival*	Survival*	Comments
Manchester I	720	Chest wall + axilla	20-30	+		0	Randomization not strict; orthovoltage
Manchester II	741	Regional lymph nodes	20-30	+		0	
NSABP	RT = 91 control = 235	Regional lymph nodes	5	+	0	0	Randomization not strict; short follow-up
Oslo I	546	Chest wall + regional nodes	>11	+	0	0	Orthovoltage
Oslo II	542	Regional nodes	>11	++	+ Stage II	0	Supervoltage
Stockholm	644	Chest wall + regional nodes	8-14	++	+	0	

* 0 = no significant difference; + = improved with radiotherapy; ++ = greatly improved with radiotherapy.

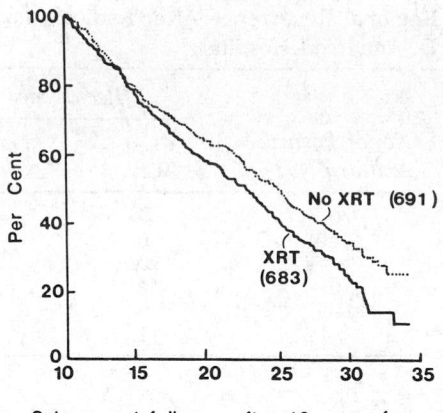

FIG. 38-14. Subsequent survival in patients surviving 10 years in a trial using radical mastectomy. There is a significant difference favoring patients treated with radical mastectomy alone (p = 0.002). Numbers in parentheses are total patients at risk in each arm of trial.[179]

diotherapy, it was 5% (p = 0.03). For patients in the CMF/MF arm, the rate of local failure as the first site of failure was nearly the same for patients randomized to chemotherapy only as for those randomized to adjuvant radiotherapy as well (5% and 2%). For patients in the CA arm, the crude rate of local failure was 20% for patients randomized to receive chemotherapy only and 6% for those randomized to both types of adjuvant treatment (p = 0.03). Moreover, some patients did not actually receive the treatments they were randomized to receive. Among the 43 patients treated with CA who actually received radiotherapy, there was only one local failure, compared with 12 local failures among the 59 patients (20%) who actually did not receive radiotherapy (p = 0.007). No significant difference was seen in disease-free survival or overall survival in either the CA or the CMF/MF arm between patients randomized to receive radiation therapy and those randomized to no further treatment (Fig. 38-15). Taken together, these results suggest that adjuvant chemotherapy alone is not highly effective at preventing local recurrence in patients with four or more positive axillary nodes and that radiation given after chemotherapy significantly reduces local failure as the first site of relapse in these patients. However, none of the available studies provides strong support for a survival benefit for radiotherapy in this setting.

At this time, the use of adjuvant radiotherapy in patients with four or more positive nodes who are treated by adjuvant chemotherapy is a matter of clinical judgment. Many clinicians will judge it useful to add radiotherapy in these patients in order to prevent local recurrence. The results of the DFCI/JCRT trial indicate that radiotherapy can be added at the completion of adjuvant chemotherapy, thus avoiding any possible interference with the administration of the chemotherapy.

CONSERVATIVE SURGERY AND RADIATION THERAPY FOR EARLY BREAST CANCER

The theoretical plan for the use of conservative surgery and radiation therapy is to preserve the breast by resecting only the tumor, leaving behind, in many cases, a subclinical burden of cancer cells. It has been well established that a resection of the tumor without subsequent irradiation results in a 15% to 40% risk of local recurrence.[189-193] Moderate doses of radiation are therefore used to eradicate this residual cancer while preserving an acceptable cosmetic appearance. It is critical to the success of this approach that the conservative resection not leave behind a tumor burden too large to be destroyed completely by the dose of radiation to be employed. Therefore, it is important to identify clinical or pathologic features that indicate when a conservative surgical resection is likely to be associated with a large residual tumor burden.

The recent pathologic study described above by Holland and colleagues from Nijmegen, The Netherlands,[78] is pertinent to the successful application of breast-conserving treatment. They found that 37% of cases showed no residual tumor foci in the breast beyond the primary tumor, 20% showed other tumor foci within 2 cm of the reference tumor, and 43% showed tumor foci further than 2 cm away from the reference tumor. The likelihood of residual tumor foci decreased with increasing distance from the reference tumor. For women with tumors 4 cm or smaller, 61% had tumor foci more than 1 cm away, 41% more than 2 cm away, 18% more than 3 cm away, and 11% more than 4 cm away. This study does not describe the bulk of the residual tumor or which patients are likely to have tumor foci at a great distance from the reference tumor, but it suggests that the residual tumor burden is greater in patients who have exci-

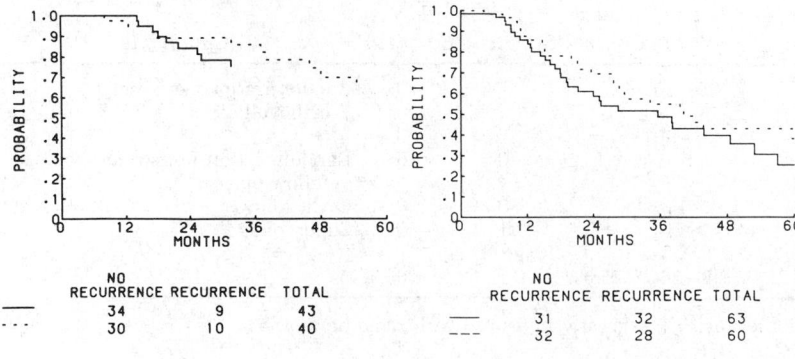

FIG. 38-15. Actuarial relapse-free survival in DFCI–JCRT trial testing value of postoperative radiotherapy (RT) after adjuvant chemotherapy (CT) for moderate-risk patients (*left*) and high-risk patients (*right*). Solid lines indicate patients treated with CT and RT; dotted lines indicate patients treated with CT alone.[188]

sion of the primary tumor with only narrow gross margins than in patients undergoing wider excision, such as quadrantectomy. It also implies that a cosmetically acceptable excision probably will leave behind microscopic disease near the biopsy site in many patients, thus explaining the high rate of local recurrence in the series testing excision only.

RETROSPECTIVE RESULTS

Ten-year results of retrospective studies of conservative surgery and radiotherapy are available from a number of institutions in the United States and Europe.[194-198] The results of the JCRT are representative of these studies and will be discussed in detail.

From July 1968 through December 1980, 525 patients with AJCC clinical Stage I or II carcinoma of the breast were treated at the JCRT. The follow-up was updated and the data were reanalyzed in August 1986. The median follow-up was 74 months, with a range of 33 to 185 months. All of the patients in this series had invasive carcinoma diagnosed by the original hospital pathologist and confirmed by the study pathologists. Nine of the patients had an opposite-breast cancer treated during this period, for a total of 534 breast cancers. The breakdown by TN stages was as follows: T1N0, 248; T1N1, 29; T2N0, 202; and T2N1, 55. The median age of the patients was 52 years, with a range from 25 to 93 years.

The treatment technique at the JCRT has been detailed previously.[199-201] There were some variations in treatment over the years of the study period, and the effect of these variations has been analyzed. Five hundred eight breasts were treated after excisional biopsy and 26 after incisional or needle biopsy. Of the patients treated after excisional biopsy, 411 received supplemental radiation (boost) to the primary site to 6000 cGy or greater. It is important to emphasize that an "excisional biopsy" in this series, for the most part, was simply a gross resection of the tumor without an attempt to obtain microscopically negative margins of resection.

Local recurrence was scored whenever tumor was noted in the treated breast or the skin overlying the breast. Fifty-seven patients had an isolated local recurrence, and two patients had simultaneous local and distant recurrence. The crude incidence of local recurrence thus was 11%. Eight patients had suspected or proven local recurrence after distant recurrence but were censored at the time of distant recurrence. By 10 years, the actuarial probability of local recurrence was 20%, with 23 patients still at risk past that point. The last breast failure was seen 109 months after the start of radiotherapy. When this curve is plotted semilogarithmically as local tumor control over time, a straight line is obtained, implying that the risk of local recurrence is fairly constant for the first 9 years after treatment.

The association between the type of biopsy and the probability of local recurrence was examined. The 10-year probability of local recurrence was 19% for patients treated with excisional biopsy and 43% for patients treated with incisional or needle biopsy (p<0.0001). For the 411 patients treated with excisional biopsy and a boost to the primary site to 6000 cGy or more (now considered optimal treatment) the 10-year probability of local recurrence was 15% (Fig.

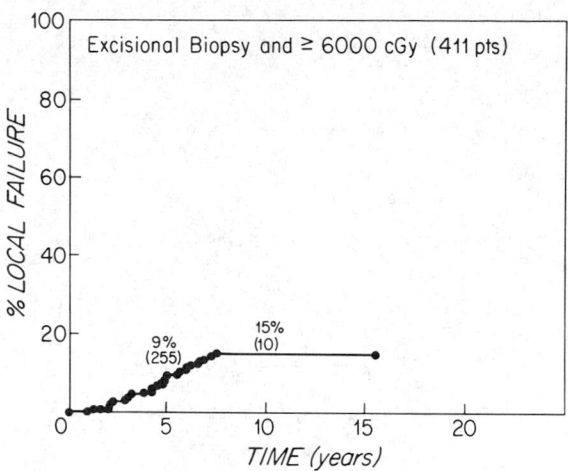

FIG. 38-16. Actuarial risk of breast (or local) failure among 411 patients treated with excisional biopsy and radiotherapy including a boost to the primary site of 6000 cGy or greater (JCRT).

38-16). The use of excisional biopsy facilitates the use of radiation therapy and is now routinely recommended for all patients treated at the JCRT. The optimal extent of the resection beyond the primary tumor into the adjacent grossly normal breast tissue is a more complicated matter (see below).

Local recurrences after breast-conserving treatment can be classified on clinical and pathologic grounds as a true recurrence (TR), a marginal miss (MM), elsewhere in the breast (E), or in skin (S). A TR is one within the borders of the boost or at the site of the primary tumor in the absence of a boost. An MM is a recurrence near the site of the primary tumor but just outside the borders of the boost. An E is a recurrence at least several centimeters from the boosted volume and at a substantial distance from the primary tumor site. An S is a recurrence confined to the skin of the breast without evidence of parenchymal disease. Both TR and MM most likely represent a recurrence of the original cancer as opposed to a new primary tumor in the same breast.

The probability of a TR in the JCRT series for patients treated with radiation therapy after an excisional biopsy of the tumor was 4% at 5 years and 11% at 10 years. The probability of a TR in the 411 patients treated with a boost to the primary site to 6000 cGy or more was compared with that in the 97 patients treated without a boost, although the validity of this comparison is limited by selection bias, because patients thought to be at greater risk for local recurrence more often received a boost. Despite this, patients treated with a boost had a lower probability of a TR (7% at 10 years) than did patients treated without a boost (15% at 10 years; p = 0.19). This result suggests that a boost to the primary site may decrease the likelihood of a true recurrence. The probability of an MM in patients treated with excisional biopsy and radiation therapy including a boost to the primary site was 4% at both 5 and 10 years. The probability of developing either a TR or an MM (*i.e.*, a recurrence of the primary tumor) was 7% at 5 years and 11% at 10 years for patients treated with an excisional biopsy and a boost

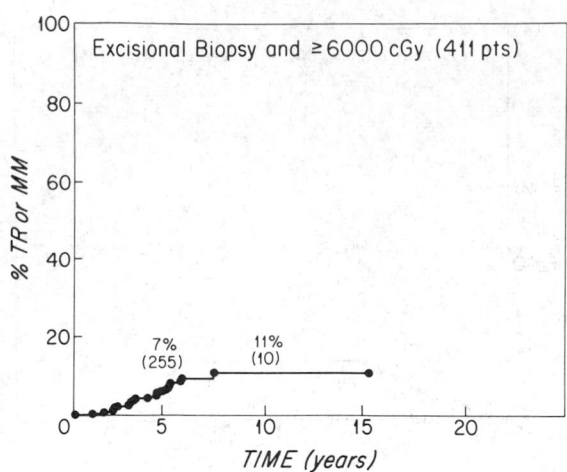

FIG. 38-17. Actuarial risk of a recurrence at (true recurrence, *TR*) or near (marginal miss, *MM*) primary tumor site among 411 patients treated with excisional biopsy and radiotherapy including a boost to the primary site of 6000 cGy or greater (JCRT).

(Fig. 38-17). No TRs or MMs occurred more than 8 years after treatment in the 30 patients followed at least that long.

The probability of a recurrence elsewhere in the treated breast was 1% at 5 years and 7% at 10 years. The time course to this type of recurrence is different from that to TR or MM. TRs and MMs are more common in the first 5 years and less common thereafter, whereas Es are less common in the first 5 years and more common thereafter. The probability of a recurrence elsewhere in the treated breast was greater for patients 49 years of age or younger at the time of diagnosis than in patients 50 or older, but this difference did not reach statistical significance (8% versus 5% at 10 years; p = 0.08).

Skin recurrence was an uncommon event in this series, being seen in only three patients. The 5- and 10-year probability of an S was 0.7%. All three Ss were seen in patients who had pathologically positive axillary nodes on initial presentation. The 5-year probability of an S was 2.5% for node-positive patients compared with 0 for node-negative patients (p = 0.03). These few patients had a rapid downhill course, with distant metastases appearing simultaneously with or soon after the local recurrence. This is very different from the usual course after local recurrence, which will be discussed in more detail below.

Nine women (2%) had bilateral tumors at the time of initial presentation. In the remaining patients, the probability of developing a metachronous opposite breast cancer was 4% at 5 years and 10% at 10 years, similar to that reported after mastectomy.

IMPLICATIONS OF THE JCRT RESULTS

The results obtained from the JCRT illustrate several common findings regarding the use of conservative surgery and radiation therapy. One observation is that the time to local recurrence is protracted: there was a fairly constant risk over a 9-year period. Of note, in a collaborative study of patients treated at the Princess Margaret Hospital, the Institut Curie, and the Marseilles Cancer Institute, a constant risk of local recurrence was observed over a 14-year period.[202] The time to local recurrence after breast-conserving treatment is different from that after mastectomy, in which the majority of recurrences appear within 3 years. In the JCRT series, the site of breast recurrence was different in the first 5 years (when nearly all recurrences were at or near the primary site) than in the second 5 years (when recurrences elsewhere in the treated breast were more common). These observations have implications for the follow-up observation of treated patients, which will be discussed below.

Another important observation is that most local recurrences are at or near the primary site (TR or MM) and likely represent a recurrence of the primary tumor. This observation has also been noted in the NSABP B-06 trial.[193,203,204] Pathologic studies of the primary tumor and the recurrences from both the JCRT[205] and the NSABP[204] indicate that the histologies are identical or similar in nearly all cases. This finding suggests that the techniques of surgery and radiation should emphasize adequate treatment of both the primary tumor and the surrounding area. This observation also provides a rationale for employing a boost to the primary site, a view which is reinforced by pathologic studies such as that of Holland and associates.[78] When patients are treated with excisional biopsy and radiotherapy including a boost to the primary site, recurrences of the primary tumor are rare after 8 years. There are at present very limited long-term data for patients routinely treated without a boost.

A related finding is that recurrences elsewhere in the treated breast are uncommon and are generally seen after a delay of several years. In the JCRT experience, whole-breast irradiation primarily appears to delay the appearance of second tumors in the treated breast. Whether failure elsewhere in the breast is due to multicentric carcinoma or represents a newly developed cancer is unknown. At the JCRT, recurrence elsewhere in the treated breast is viewed as a risk incurred by breast-conserving treatment, just as the appearance of an opposite-breast cancer is a risk incurred by unilateral treatment.

COSMETIC RESULTS

The cosmetic results of conservative surgery and radiotherapy have generally been good to excellent, and most patients have been very satisfied. The cosmetic results of patients treated at the JCRT are typical of other series using modern equipment and currently accepted doses. Measured features included breast edema, retraction, telangiectasia, arm edema, and overall cosmetic appearance as judged by the physician. A series of 239 patients was treated from 1976 to 1980. No patient in this series received chemotherapy. The overall cosmetic results fluctuated during the first 3 years after treatment but then stabilized.[206] At 5 years, the overall cosmetic results were judged excellent (little or no observable change) in 77% of patients, good (minimal but identifiable changes) in 9%, fair (significant results of radiation therapy noted) in 9%, and poor (severe normal-tissue sequelae) in 5% (Fig. 38-18). Moderate or severe retraction was the most common element of a fair or poor result, whereas telangiectasia, breast edema, and arm edema were rarely the cause of a fair or poor result. The cosmetic results were

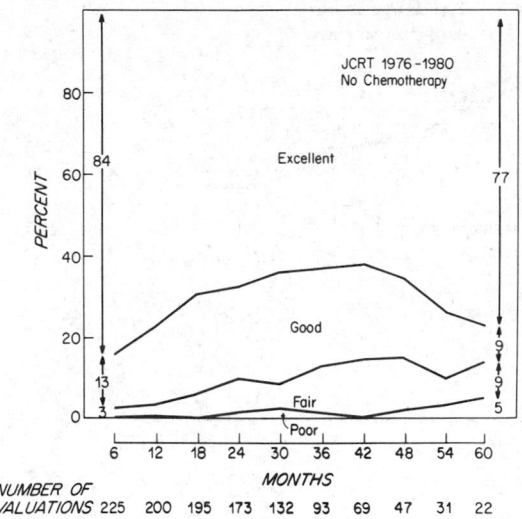

FIG. 38-18. Overall cosmetic results after completion of primary radiation treatment.

somewhat correlated with the dose and technique of radiotherapy, in that poorer cosmetic results were associated with very large implants (more than 100 seeds) and with implant doses exceeding 1800 cGy. Breast and arm edema were more common in patients who underwent axillary dissection.

RANDOMIZED PROSPECTIVE STUDIES OF CONSERVATIVE SURGERY AND RADIATION THERAPY VERSUS MASTECTOMY

The critical issue regarding primary radiation therapy is whether it yields survival rates equal to those achieved with mastectomy. This issue is best addressed by randomized prospective trials in which the treatment arms are well balanced in terms of prognostic features. Since 1970, there have been five prospective randomized trials using modern radiation therapy techniques. One such trial was performed at the National Cancer Institute of Italy in Milan.[207-209] From 1973 to 1980, 701 evaluable patients with primary tumors 2 cm or smaller and clinically uninvolved axillary nodes (T1N0) were entered. Patients were randomized to treatment with either conservative surgery and radiotherapy or radical mastectomy. Conservative surgery consisted of a resection of the entire involved quadrant of the breast (quadrantectomy) and a full axillary dissection. Radiotherapy was then administered to the breast alone through two opposing tangential fields, giving a dose of 5000 cGy in 5 weeks. Another 1000 cGy was then administered to the tumor site using orthovoltage radiation. From 1973 to 1975, patients with involved lymph nodes were further randomized to receive radiotherapy either to the breast alone or to the breast and to the draining lymph node areas as well. After 1975, all patients with involved lymph nodes were treated with 12 cycles of chemotherapy. The two arms of the trial were well balanced with regard to age, tumor size, and axillary nodal status. Microscopically involved axillary nodes were found in 25% of the radical mastectomy group and 27% of the conservatively treated group. Seven patients from the mastectomy group and seven in the quadrantectomy group had developed a local recurrence. Seven additional cases of a second primary cancer in the remnant ipsilateral breast were found in the group that was treated conservatively. The number of deaths in each treatment group since the start of treatment and the relapse-free and overall survival rates were similar between the two groups (Fig. 38-19). Patients with involved axillary nodes had a greater likelihood of relapse-free survival if treated with quadrantectomy and radiotherapy than with mastectomy (72% versus 59% at 10 years; p = 0.03).

The NSABP began a three-arm trial (Protocol B-06) in 1976 comparing mastectomy with segmental mastectomy with or without radiotherapy.[193,203] A total of 1843 evaluable patients with clinical Stage I or II carcinoma whose primary tumors clinically measured no more than 4 cm were entered. One hundred seventy-four patients refused their assigned treatment and were excluded from analysis. All patients underwent axillary dissection. Those with involved lymph nodes received adjuvant chemotherapy. Whereas in the Milan trial an entire quadrant of the breast was removed, segmental mastectomy as performed in the NSABP trial involved resection of the tumor with only enough normal tissue around it to attempt to ensure that the microscopic margins of the specimen were tumor free. It was considered impossible to obtain tumor-free margins in 10% of the patients randomly assigned to segmental mastectomy, and total mastectomy was carried out in these patients. Radiotherapy was delivered to the breast alone with supervoltage equipment using opposed tangential fields (often without wedge filters to compensate for the slope of the breast) to a dose of 5000 to 5300 cGy in 5 to 6 weeks. The regional lymph nodes were not treated, and no boost was given to the tumor site. For the patients who received radiotherapy, the 5-year actuarial incidence of recurrence in the breast was 7%, compared with 32% for patients who did not have radiotherapy (p<0.001).[203] This marked difference was seen both in patients with histologically involved and those with uninvolved lymph nodes. Of note, patients with positive lymph nodes who were treated with segmental mastectomy and adjuvant chemotherapy but without radiotherapy had a greater risk of breast recurrence (38%) than did patients with negative nodes who were treated only with segmental mastectomy (28%). However, patients with positive nodes treated with segmental mastectomy, radiotherapy, and adjuvant chemotherapy had a smaller risk of breast recurrence (4%) than did patients with negative nodes treated with segmental mastectomy and radiotherapy without chemotherapy (9%). This suggests that chemotherapy by itself does little to prevent breast recurrence but that radiotherapy and chemotherapy are additive or synergistic in reducing tumor recurrence in the breast.

Another trial was conducted from 1972 to 1979 at the Institut Gustave-Roussy in Villejuif, France, under the sponsorship of the WHO.[210] This trial included 179 patients with tumors pathologically 2 cm or smaller with either clinically involved or uninvolved lymph nodes. Patients were randomized to receive either modified radical mastectomy or conservative surgery, which consisted of removal of the tumor with a surrounding margin of 2 cm of grossly normal breast

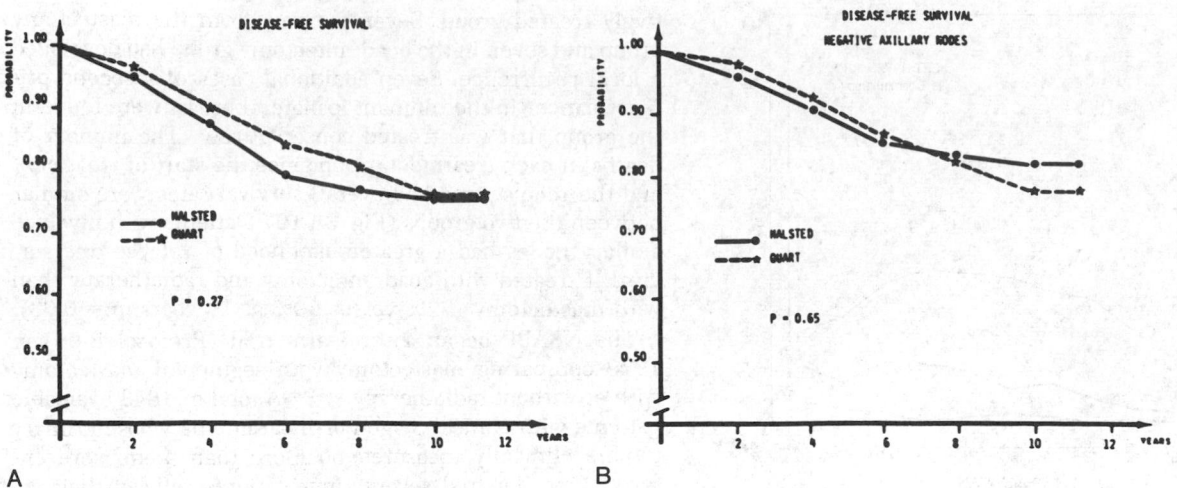

FIG. 38-19. Disease-free survival rates in Milan trial according to type of treatment. **A**. All patients. **B**. Patients with pathologically negative axillary nodes.

tissue ("tumorectomy"). All patients underwent low axillary dissection; if involved lymph nodes were detected, this was extended to a complete axillary dissection. All patients randomized to tumorectomy received breast irradiation. Patients randomized to either mastectomy or tumorectomy who had involved lymph nodes were further randomized to receive postoperative axillary, supraclavicular, and IMN irradiation or no further treatment. Adjuvant chemotherapy was not used. Radiotherapy was given with cobalt-60 to a dose of 4500 cGy in 18 fractions over 1 month, treating the breast four times weekly. A boost of 1500 cGy was given to the tumor bed in six fractions. The total length of irradiation was 6 weeks. With a median follow-up of approximately 10 years, there was no statistically significant difference in local recurrence, freedom from distant metastases, or overall survival rates in the two treatment groups.

The fourth recent prospective randomized trial was begun by the National Cancer Institute of the United States in 1979.[211] By September 1985, 197 patients with clinical Stage I or II cancers had been randomized to receive either modified radical mastectomy or conservative excision, full axillary dissection, and radiotherapy to the breast. Patients with histologically involved nodes also received doxorubicin and cyclophosphamide. With a median follow-up of 32 months, there was no significant difference in outcome between these two groups.

The fifth and most recent trial is one conducted from 1981 to 1986 at Guy's Hospital, London.[212] Patients with tumors smaller than 4 cm in diameter were randomized to treatment with modified radical mastectomy (185 patients) or conservative surgery, axillary clearance, and radiotherapy (214 patients). Patients with positive axillary nodes were subsequently randomized to be watched or to receive 12 cycles of CMF chemotherapy. So far, there are no differences in outcome between the two treatment arms, and the doses of chemotherapy delivered have been the same in both groups.

These randomized prospective trials demonstrate that when adequate treatment techniques are used, there is no significant difference in survival between patients treated with radical surgery and those treated with conservative surgery and radiotherapy. As such, they confirm the evidence of the retrospective trials as to the value of using conservative surgery and radiotherapy for patients with early breast cancer.

COMPLICATIONS

The complications associated with treatment have recently been reviewed elsewhere.[213] Acute complications of radiotherapy for early breast cancer include fatigue and erythema of the skin, occasionally with moist desquamation. However, these are self-limited and resolve within several weeks.

Significant long-term complications are uncommon when good technique is used. At the JCRT, transient or mild complications occurred in a small percentage of patients. The most common were rib fractures (5%), cosmetically (though rarely functionally) significant arm edema (4%),[214] radiation pneumonitis (2%), and, rarely, paresthesias or brachial plexus disorders.[215] Other rare complications were radiation pericarditis (one patient), soft-tissue necrosis (one patient), and occasionally fibrosis of the pectoral muscles.

RADIATION TECHNIQUE AND DOSES

The extent of surgery and the dose of radiation required for local tumor control are complementary: the more extensive the surgical procedure, the less radiation is required for tumor control. The entire breast should be treated with 180 to 200 cGy per day, for a total dose of 4500 to 5000 cGy. Doses exceeding 5000 cGy to the entire breast commonly result in an unacceptable degree of fibrosis and retraction and so should be avoided. It is important to maximize the homogeneity of the dose delivered to the breast. Inhomogeneities above 15% are not advisable, and it is preferable to maintain inhomogeneity below 10%. Bolus (material applied to the skin to circumvent the skin sparing of supervoltage radiation) is not required in the treatment of early breast cancer and should be avoided in most cases.

The question of whether to use a boost to the primary site is controversial. There are a number of reasons to justify routine use of a boost. First, in all reported series, most recurrences are seen at or near the primary site. Second, the data of Holland and colleagues indicate that most of the residual tumor burden after tumor excision is at or near the primary site.[78] Furthermore, excellent long-term local tumor control rates have been demonstrated from institutions in which a boost has been employed.

The principal justification for not using a boost is the report of the NSABP B-06 trial, which demonstrated excellent local tumor control in the absence of a boost.[193,203] However, the follow-up in this trial is still relatively short. In addition, because compensating wedges often were not employed, the actual dose to the site of the primary tumor may have been substantially greater in many cases than the nominal delivered dose of 5000 to 5300 cGy.

The need for a boost should also be considered in relation to the size of the tumor and the extent of the resection. For very small tumors treated with quadrantectomy, a boost is not likely to be of great importance, whereas for larger tumors treated with a gross excision, a boost is more likely to be important to maximize local tumor control. Given the multiplicity of clinical circumstances and the small differences in outcome, it is unlikely that a randomized trial will be useful in settling this issue.

The data from the JCRT have defined the volumes and doses of boost radiation consistent with preserving the cosmetic appearance of the breast. In most situations, this can be achieved using external-beam radiation (electron beam). Late failure at the primary site is rare when a boost is employed. It therefore seems prudent to deliver a modest boost dose (usually 1600 cGy or enough to bring the dose to the primary site to 6000 cGy or more) to the primary site following a local or wide excision of the tumor and 4600 to 5000 cGy to the whole breast.

It is also controversial whether radiation therapy should be delivered to the draining lymph node regions. The preponderance of evidence indicates that such nodal treatment does not have a detectable impact on survival. Nodal treatment will improve tumor control in these areas, but its use must be balanced against the risk of complications, which is related to the dose and techniques of radiotherapy used. It is important to stress that the results achieved in both the Milan and the NSABP trials involved irradiation to the breast alone. In light of their findings, treatment to the breast alone is reasonable in all situations. Treatment of high-risk nodal areas is also reasonable, provided it can be achieved without a significant risk of complications. It is well established that a fully dissected axilla should not be irradiated routinely because of the high risk of developing arm edema.[214,216,217]

FOLLOW-UP OF TREATED PATIENTS

Recurrence in the breast after conservative surgery and radiation therapy has a much better prognosis than a chest-wall recurrence after mastectomy, with approximately 50% of patients being alive and free of distant metastases 5 years later.[202,218] The time to local recurrence is protracted; therefore, treated patients require long-term follow-up to detect such a recurrence promptly. Both physical examination and mammography are critical. One reasonable follow-up program is to obtain mammograms 6 months and 1 year after treatment and then annually thereafter and to perform physical examinations every 4 to 6 months. It is not uncommon for changes in the texture and characteristics of the irradiated breast to continue to take place for 12 to 18 months after treatment, but changes after that time should be regarded with particular suspicion. When warranted, a small open biopsy (1–20 cc of tissue) can be performed safely, with little risk of wound nonhealing, infection, or worsening of the cosmetic outcome.

APPROACH TO THE PATIENT WITH EARLY BREAST CANCER

The preceding pages have discussed extensively the traditional treatment of breast cancer with mastectomy and the preservative approaches combining local excision and radiation therapy. How should one apply these discussions to the individual patient with early breast cancer? Any recommendations given must be considered conditional. The current data have been interpreted, but they are a portion of a continuum that includes both new studies and continued follow-up of earlier series, and it is important to consider the evolutionary nature of these data in the context of improving techniques and increased observation times. As the quality of these techniques improves and the length of follow-up increases, we can come to firmer conclusions as to the appropriate treatment for individual patients.

Analysis of treatment data must include a number of endpoints. The most obvious of these is survival; however, survival data alone do not reveal all the pertinent information. Because the purpose of both mastectomy and preservative management is to eradicate the primary tumor and regional disease, local control is an important endpoint in itself. Even this evaluation must be modified by understanding the consequences for the patient of having a recurrence. It appears that local recurrence after mastectomy has a different outcome than a recurrence following preservative treatment, with the former being more ominous than the latter. A third and very important endpoint is the quality of the functional and cosmetic result, because the purpose of either treatment is to eradicate the disease while allowing the patient to return as closely as possible to her predisease state. Finally, both short- and long-term undesirable consequences of treatment must be considered.

To determine the treatment for an individual patient, one must consider the age of the patient. Whereas younger patients are often more concerned with body image, they also have the longest life expectancy and therefore are potentially most exposed to the long-term complications of treatment. There are also important emotional and physiological considerations, including the woman's feelings about preserving the breast and her body image. Loss of the breast may have devastating psychological consequences; however, selection of breast preservation requires that the woman accept the presence of a potential site of residual or new disease. These considerations must be explored in helping the patient arrive at an appropriate decision. Other considerations that affect the selection of local treatment include breast size, tumor location, number of tumors, and the histologic character of the biopsy. There are no simple answers applicable for all patients. Today, both alternatives must be discussed with the patient; only through this discussion can an informed patient receive information and guidance sufficient to permit her to reach a reasonable decision.

From the available data, it seems clear that both mastectomy and breast preservation utilizing local excision and radiation therapy are acceptable alternatives for the treatment of early breast cancer. Although there are no simple rigid rules to determine which therapy is appropriate for an individual patient, there are some useful guidelines. First among the considerations favoring breast preservation procedures is the patient's desire for such treatment; in the absence of such a desire, there is no incentive. Second, the primary tumor should be small relative to the breast, so that local excision with a negative margin will result in an acceptable cosmetic appearance. Third, there should be a single lesion, as experience in treating patients with multiple lesions in one breast with breast-preserving techniques is limited. There should be no suspicious microcalcifications on the postexcision mammogram, and a review of the excision specimen using an appropriate method to ink the margins should show that these margins are clear of invasive or intraductal disease. Extensive diffuse intraductal disease in a specimen appears to increase the risk of local recurrence, although in studies showing this, resection margins were not always evaluated. It is uncertain whether the presence of extensive intraductal disease will continue to be a factor when carefully reviewed margins are found to be free of such disease. Finally, the patient should understand the requirements of the treatment course, as daily treatments for 5 to 8 weeks require a patient's commitment to such a program.

Considerations that favor mastectomy are in general the converse of those that favor preservative management. For example, some patients have no desire to preserve the affected breast; in fact, some may have a morbid fear of persistent disease lurking within the breast, and such patients are better served by mastectomy. If a cosmetically acceptable incision is not possible, then little is to be gained by preservative treatment. This may be the case when the primary tumor is large relative to the size of the breast and for tumors in certain locations, especially central lesions close to the areola. If there is multifocal disease extending beyond one quadrant, such disease usually cannot be encompassed in a cosmetically acceptable procedure, and the patient is better served by mastectomy. If the excision margins are positive and re-excision still shows disease at the resection margin, mastectomy is preferable. However, if the patient strongly desires preservative treatment, increasing the local radiation dose by means such as interstitial implantation of radioactive material can be considered.

Some women have had breast augmentation procedures with a prosthesis. Such appliances may cause unusual problems for the preservative technique. There is not a large experience in treating patients with a prosthesis, and thus it is difficult to make firm recommendations. A prudent recommendation is to remove the prosthesis, although for some women, this will negate the cosmetic advantage of a preservation technique. Such patients may be better served by mastectomy with appropriate reconstructive procedures.

For individual patients, there are often other considerations. Usually, a frank discussion with the patient and ample time for consideration of the alternatives allows an easy selection. These choices must be made by the patient with the advice, recommendation, and guidance of the physician. The relative importance of each of these considerations will change depending on the accumulated data and the physician's experience with the technical improvements of the various treatment techniques.

The use of adjuvant chemotherapy is discussed separately in this chapter. It may be combined with either mastectomy or preservative management with equal effectiveness and thus should not be a factor in the selection of the primary treatment modality. The timing of chemotherapy relative to the radiation treatment in preservative management is still unresolved. In general, we favor not administering them concomitantly, especially if doxorubicin is a part of the treatment regimen. There are strong reasons to consider giving the adjuvant chemotherapy first in patients at very high risk for distant metastases, the best indicator of which seems to be a large number of positive nodes. This is especially appropriate in patients who have had a good local excision. In patients with only a few positive nodes, the data support the use of chemotherapy following radiation, although some suggest that one cycle may precede the radiation. There are a number of studies in this area that require continued evaluation.

ADJUVANT THERAPY

Screening trials, especially the Health Insurance Plan of Greater New York (HIP) trial described above, have demonstrated conclusively that mastectomy or some other form of local therapy improves the likelihood of survival of some portion of breast cancer patients. Contrary to Halsted's expectations, however, improved local control with more extensive surgery or adjuvant radiotherapy has generally not improved survival. The effects of local therapy are "all or none": either the patient is cured by local treatment, or she dies of distant metastases at about the same time she would have died without local intervention because these metastases were established prior to the time of diagnosis and are outside the scope of even the most extensive local treatment.

These observations on the limitations of local therapy provided the initial rationale for the use of adjuvant systemic therapy (either chemotherapy or endocrine therapy) immediately following local treatment. In addition, it has been shown in animal models that tumors incurable by any form of therapy at a more advanced stage may be cured by surgical excision and adjuvant systemic therapy early after implantation.[219] Breast cancer was the first tumor in which adjuvant therapy was employed, and randomized trials evaluating adjuvant oophorectomy were begun as early as 1948.[220] Although success with adjuvant chemotherapy was first obtained in the treatment of pediatric tumors,[221] it is now firmly established that adjuvant chemotherapy will prolong the survival of premenopausal patients and adjuvant tamoxifen that of postmenopausal patients. These adjuvants to surgery and radiotherapy should now be considered standard treatment for node-positive patients.

ADJUVANT CHEMOTHERAPY

The chemotherapy trials that set today's standards were begun in 1972 and 1973. The first of these was conducted by the NSABP and used a single agent, L-phenylalanine mustard (L-PAM), 0.15 mg/kg orally for 5 days of each 6-week cycle for 2 years. Although less effective than some other agents then available for the treatment of metastatic breast cancer, L-PAM was associated with remarkably little acute toxicity and required no intravenous injections.[222] About 1 year later, the National Cancer Institute of Milan, Italy, initiated a similar trial of CMF. This regimen required intravenous injections on days 1 and 8 of each monthly cycle and oral administration of cyclophosphamide on days 1 through 14. The CMF was given for 1 year and had considerably more acute toxicity, including nausea, vomiting, mucositis, alopecia, leukopenia, and thrombocytopenia.[223] Similar patients were included in these two studies. All patients had operable cancers, including some T3 lesions, and axillary lymph node metastases and were stratified into two groups; those with one to three histologically involved nodes and those with more than four involved nodes. Patients were also stratified by menstrual status as premenopausal or postmenopausal (Milan) or by age (younger than 50 or 50 or older) (NSABP).

The 10-year results from these two trials are summarized in Table 38-21. All treated patients in both studies had a prolongation of disease-free survival, but this was statistically significant only for premenopausal women. Treated premenopausal women also had a statistically significant increase in overall survival. At 10 years, this was 24% for patients treated with L-PAM (p = 0.02) and 14% for patients given CMF (p < 0.02).

Subsequent published trials have more or less confirmed the results of these first studies.[224] In 11 such trials, premenopausal women were randomized to receive either chemotherapy (usually a combination of drugs for at least 6 months) or local therapy alone (mastectomy with or without adjuvant radiotherapy). In all of these trials, the patients who received adjuvant chemotherapy had better disease-free and overall survival rates, and improvement in disease-free survival reached levels of conventional statistical significance in five of the studies. The significant overall survival advantage observed for premenopausal women in the NSABP and Milan trials has now been confirmed in a third trial. In this study by the Danish national trials group, more than 1000 women were randomized to receive either cyclophosphamide as a single agent (130 mg/m² daily for 14 days of each monthly cycle) or CMF in about 75% to 80% of the doses given in the Milan trial. After more than 6 years of follow-up, there is a statistically significant survival advantage for those patients receiving adjuvant CMF and a trend toward improved survival for those receiving cyclophosphamide alone. The follow-up on all of the other published premenopausal studies is shorter than the follow-up of the studies from the NSABP, Milan, and Denmark, and it is reasonable to anticipate that a survival advantage for the treated patients will emerge with additional follow-up of the other trials.

There are also 11 published trials in which postmenopausal women were randomized to receive at least 4 months of adjuvant chemotherapy or local treatment only. In many cases, these were separate studies and not merely strata of larger trials that included both premenopausal and postmenopausal women. There is a trend toward improved disease-free survival in seven of the trials and a trend toward improved survival in three of the trials. However, the disease-free survival advantage reached conventional statistical significance in only three of the trials, and a significant survival advantage has never been observed.[224]

TABLE 38-21.   Ten-Year Results of NSABP and Milan Trials in Which Patients with Histologically Involved Nodes Were Randomized to 1 to 2 Years of Adjuvant Chemotherapy or to Mastectomy Alone

Patient Group	NSABP[222]			Milan[58,223]		
	Control	L-Pam	p	Control	CMF	p
Recurrence-Free at 10 Years (%)						
All patients	29	38	0.06	31	43	0.001
Premenopausal	29	46	0.02	31	48	0.0005
Postmenopausal	28	34	0.49	32	38	0.32
Premenopausal						
1–3 nodes	41	66	0.02	40	61	0.0002
>3 nodes	17	22	0.42	15	26	0.03
Alive at 10 Years (%)						
All patients	41	48	0.30	47	55	0.10
Premenopausal	37	61	0.02	45	59	<0.02
Postmenopausal	43	41	0.80	50	52	0.89
Premenopausal						
1–3 nodes	48	81	0.01	51	68	0.025
>3 nodes	26	35	0.54	30	42	0.29

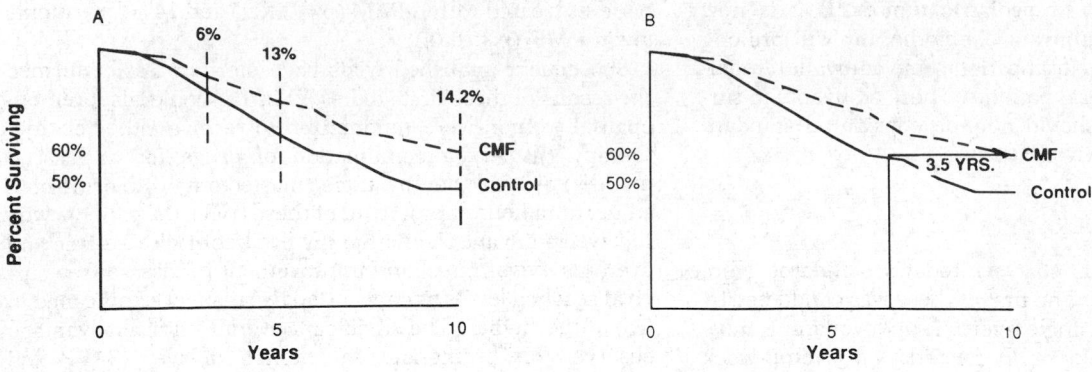

FIG. 38-20. Ten-year survival rate of all premenopausal patients treated in the Milan CMF trial. **A.** Usual way of interpreting survival curves by calculating vertical difference between curves at various time points after entry onto study. **B.** Estimating average survival benefit by calculating difference in the medians of the two curves. Because median has not yet been reached for the treated group in this study, a horizontal at the 60th percentile has been used. (Bonadonna G, Valagussa P, Rossi A et al: Ten-year experience with CMF-based adjuvant chemotherapy in resectable breast cancer. Breast Cancer Res Treat 5:95–115, 1985)

ESTIMATING THE SIZE OF THE BENEFIT

There are several ways in which the benefits of adjuvant chemotherapy in premenopausal women can be expressed. To some clinicians, the fact that the survival difference is statistically significant may be sufficient reason to utilize adjuvant chemotherapy in all node-positive premenopausal women. Others may wish to know the size of the benefit as well. The Kaplan-Meier survival plots for node-positive premenopausal women in the Milan trial are illustrated in Figure 38-20A. These demonstrate an absolute survival difference at 5 years (13%) and 10 years (14.2%) between treated patients and controls. However, it should not be erroneously assumed that only 14% of all treated patients benefited, and it is equally incorrect to conclude that 14% of all patients have been "cured" by adjuvant therapy.

Whereas the absolute survival differences shown in Figure 38-20A provide an estimate of treatment effect in the context of all patients given the treatment, a ratio reduction in mortality rate provides an estimate of benefit for the patients who would have died without therapy. If adjuvant therapy had no effect on patient survival, we would expect the number of deaths in each arm of a randomized study to occur in the same ratio as the number of patients originally randomized to each study arm. If, however, the number of deaths observed is smaller than that expected under the null hypothesis, the ratio of observed to expected deaths (O:E) will be less than 1.0 and will provide some measure of the reduction in mortality rate as a result of therapy. In the Milan trial, the O:E ratio for CMF-treated premenopausal patients was 0.78 and for control patients 1.31. This represents a 40% reduction in the mortality rate during the first 10 years of follow-up.[226]

A third way of expressing the size of the benefit from therapy requires longer follow-up but provides an estimate more consistent with the known biologic effect of systemic therapy. As noted, the effects from mastectomy and local radiotherapy are "all or none": either the patient's tumor is eradicated and the patient is cured, or the patient dies at approximately the time she would have died without treatment. In contrast, the effects of adjuvant systemic therapy are likely to be more variable: some patients may derive several months of additional life as a result of treatment, others may live several decades as a result of therapy, and a few may regain a normal life expectancy (*i.e.*, be "cured") as a result of the therapy. The Kaplan-Meier plots shown in Figure 38-20 are actually a summation of these variable effects. Conventionally, physicians calculate the vertical differences between the two curves (Fig. 38-20A). However, it may be more appropriate to evaluate horizontal differences between the curves, as shown in Figure 38-20B. If this horizontal difference is calculated at the point where 50% of the treated and control patients have died, it would represent a difference in medians. However, this set of data illustrates one of the significant limitations of this method: even after 10 years of follow-up, the median survival of the patients treated with CMF has not been reached. Ideally, the median follow-up of all patients in the study would exceed the median survival of the group with the best survival before a difference in medians is calculated. If the difference illustrated in Figure 38-22B, 3.5 years, were a true difference in medians, it could be interpreted as the average life gained by each treated patient over what she might have had with mastectomy only.

Recently published results from the Milan trial have been expressed as differences in medians. As shown in Table 38-22, the median disease-free survival of all patients randomized to the control arm of the study is 40 months, the median disease-free survival of all patients treated with CMF is 83 months, and the difference in the medians is 43 months. The difference in median disease-free survival for premenopausal women is in excess of 9 years, whereas postmenopausal women treated with one year of CMF had a median prolongation of disease-free survival of only 5 months. The longest benefits accrued to women with one to three positive nodes. Survival data are also shown in Table

TABLE 38-22. Differences in Median Disease-Free Survival and Overall Survival at 12 Years for Patients Randomized to 1 Year of Adjuvant Chemotherapy (CMF) or No Systemic Therapy (Control) in Milan Trial

Patient Group	Disease-Free (mo)			Survival (mo)		
	Control	CMF	Difference	Control	CMF	Difference
All	40	83	43	104	140	36
1–3 positive nodes	63	141	78	130	*	*
≥4 positive nodes	20	44	24	77	82	5
Premenopausal	32	141	109	96	*	*
Postmenopausal	59	64	5	128	113	−15

Modified from Bonadonna G, Valagussa P, Zambetti M et al: Milan adjuvant trials for stage I–II breast cancer. In Salmon SE (ed): Adjuvant Therapy of Cancer V, pp 211–222. New York, Grune & Stratton, 1987.

* Median survival not yet reached for CMF group, and difference in median cannot be calculated.

38-22. The difference in medians for all patients is 3 years; the difference in medians for premenopausal women has still not been reached, and the difference in medians for postmenopausal women is actually a negative value, suggesting a potential detrimental effect of therapy in this group.

ADJUVANT TAMOXIFEN

The first of the adjuvant tamoxifen trials was begun about 3 years after the adjuvant chemotherapy trials just described. Interest in the use of tamoxifen increased when a few studies demonstrated a benefit from adjuvant oophorectomy in premenopausal women and adjuvant chemotherapy failed to prolong the survival of postmenopausal women significantly.

The earliest trial to demonstrate that adjuvant tamoxifen could prolong the survival of patients with early breast cancer was the Nolvadex Adjuvant Therapy Organization (NATO) trial.[227,228] In this British study, node-positive and node-negative patients were randomized to receive either 2 years of tamoxifen following local therapy or local therapy only. At the end of 8 years, the survival advantage for the tamoxifen-treated groups exceeds 10%, and this difference is statistically significant. In this study, the O:E ratio of deaths is 0.86 for tamoxifen-treated patients and 1.14 for the control patients. The reduction of the mortality rate as a result of tamoxifen is estimated to be about 30%.[228] Although more than 1100 patients were enrolled in this trial, only 11% were premenopausal and 45% were node-positive. As a result, the power to detect even moderate to large differences in survival within patient subsets is not great. To circumvent this problem, these data have been analyzed using a Cox model, and in this model, the O:E ratio was similar for all subsets of the trial including premenopausal node-positive patients and postmenopausal patients with or without histologically involved nodes.

Results from nine additional trials in which patients were randomized to either tamoxifen or to no adjuvant systemic therapy have been published.[224] Most or all of the patients in each of these studies were postmenopausal. In each case, tamoxifen treatment resulted in a statistically significant improvement in disease-free survival. However, the overall survival advantage observed in the NATO trial has only recently been confirmed in a second study. In this trial, performed by the Scottish National Trial Group, more than 1300 women were randomized to receive either 5 years of adjuvant tamoxifen or no adjuvant systemic therapy. Unlike most other adjuvant trials, patients in the control group were scheduled to receive tamoxifen as their first systemic therapy after recurrence, and 93% of the patients in the control group were actually treated as planned. At the end of 8 years, there was a 15% survival advantage for the patients given adjuvant tamoxifen. The survival:hazard ratio of the tamoxifen patients was 0.71 compared with the control group (p = 0.002) (Table 38-23). This effect of tamoxifen was evident in all subgroups but was statistically significant only among postmenopausal women and among node-positive patients. All of the premenopausal women entered in this trial were node negative (in contrast to the NATO trial), and the number of deaths observed in the node-negative group, whether postmenopausal or premenopausal, is still considerably

TABLE 38-23. Eight-Year Results of Scottish Trial in which Patients with and without Histologically Involved Nodes Were Randomized to 5 Years of Adjuvant Tamoxifen (TAM) or Tamoxifen as First Systemic Therapy of Recurrence[243]

Patient Group	No. of Patients	Hazard Ratio 5-Year TAM (±95%CI)
Disease-Free Survival		
All patients	1312	0.57*(0.47–0.68)
Survival		
All patients	1312	0.71†(0.58–0.89)
Node negative	751	0.73 (0.51–1.04)
Node positive	456	0.61 (0.46–0.81)
Premenopausal†	242	0.57 (0.27–1.19)
Postmenopausal‡	1070	0.73 (0.59–0.89)

* p < 0.0001.
† p = 0.002.
‡ All premenopausal patients had negative nodes; both node-negative and node-positive postmenopausal patients were included.

fewer than the number of deaths observed in the node-positive group.

A calculation of the differences in median disease-free survival and overall survival rates for patients randomized in the adjuvant tamoxifen trial are shown in Table 38-24. Because so many patients in this study were node negative, the median survivals have not been reached for the entire patient group. However, among the node-positive patients, there was a 53-month difference in the median disease-free survival period of the tamoxifen patients compared with the group who received no adjuvant systemic therapy. The overall survival advantage from adjuvant tamoxifen was 22 months. In this study, survival after recurrence was longer in the control group than in the tamoxifen group.

OVARIAN ABLATION

The first trial of ovarian ablation was begun in 1948, the last in 1965.[224] There were seven of these trials. Some used ovarian radiation and others oophorectomy. Some of the studies included both premenopausal and postmenopausal patients. None of the trials demonstrated a survival benefit from adjuvant oophorectomy at the end of the first 5 years of follow-up, and survival differences at 10 years were not large for most of the studies. As a result, adjuvant ovarian ablation had been abandoned by the time the first adjuvant chemotherapy trials utilizing long courses of chemotherapy were begun in 1972. In retrospect, it is plausible that adjuvant ovarian ablation was abandoned prematurely. The 10- and 15-year results from three of these trials now show larger survival advantages than anticipated. These observations, coupled with the fact that adjuvant chemotherapy appears to benefit premenopausal but not postmenopausal women, have been interpreted by some as evidence that adjuvant chemotherapy is really a form of chemical oophorectomy.[229]

The earliest and largest of the studies conducted in premenopausal women was initiated by the Christie Hospital in 1948. Women were randomized to receive either ovarian ablation or no further therapy after mastectomy.[220] At the end of 10 years, there was a 13% mortality reduction for all patients entered into the trial, a 37% mortality reduction for the node-negative patients, and an 11% mortality reduction for the node-positive patients. These differences were less evident after 15 years of follow-up (Table 38-25).

In a trial conducted in Toronto, Canada, patients under age 45 were randomized to receive ovarian ablation or no further systemic therapy. Those over age 45 were randomized to receive ovarian ablation alone, ovarian ablation plus at least 5 years of prednisone (7.5 mg daily), or no systemic therapy. There were only 150 patients in the group under age 45, and the small survival advantage for patients treated with ovarian ablation alone in this group did not reach statistical significance. However, premenopausal women over age 45 treated with both ovarian radiation and prednisone had a significant disease-free and overall survival advantage that persisted through year 15, at which time 72% of the patients in the treated group were alive compared with 44% in the control group (p = 0.02).[230]

Only one surgical oophorectomy trial has demonstrated a significant survival benefit for treated patients.[231] In this study, half of the patients were node negative, and some of the patients were postmenopausal. At 10 years, 71% of the patients treated with adjuvant oophorectomy were alive compared with 60% of the control group (p < 0.05). A similar trial from Malmö, Sweden, with 20 years of follow-up showed a trend toward improved survival with adjuvant oophorectomy, but this did not reach statistical significance.[232] The median survival of premenopausal women in the treated group was 62 months compared with 53 months in the control group, a difference that was not statistically significant.

OVERVIEW ANALYSIS

It is possible that a survival benefit of scientific or clinical importance may be overlooked even in randomized trials enrolling more than 1000 patients. For example, a mortality reduction of 20% could easily be missed in most of the randomized trials conducted thus far even though a statistically significant mortality reduction of this magnitude represents a large number of lives saved with a disease as common as breast cancer. A smaller but real benefit could also provide impetus for the design of additional clinical trials to develop an apparently promising idea further. However, there are limitations and potential pitfalls in the use of overviews.[233] For example, the greater statistical power may distort and exaggerate a very small benefit and so lead to inappropriate or excessive use of a therapy. The magnitude of a benefit determined in an overview may also be overestimated or

TABLE 38-24.   Differences in Median Disease-Free Survival and Overall Survival for Patients Randomized to 5 Years of Adjuvant Tamoxifen (TAM) or No Systemic Therapy Control Group in Scottish National Trial (8-Year Follow-up Data)

Patient Group	Disease-Free (mo)			Survival (mo)		
	Control	TAM	Difference	Control	TAM	Difference
All	73	*	*	95	*	*
Node negative	*	*	*	*	*	*
Node positive	31	84	53	63	85	22

Modified from Scottish Cancer Trials Office: Adjuvant tamoxifen in the management of operable breast cancer: The Scottish trial. Lancet 2:171–175, 1987.

* Median survival not yet reached for tamoxifen or control group, and difference in medians cannot be calculated.

TABLE 38-25.   Disease-Free Survival and Overall Survival Among Patients Randomized to Ovarian Irradiation or No Systemic Treatment in the Christie Hospital Trial*

Patient Group	Analysis Year	Disease-Free Survival (%)		Overall Survival (%)		p
		Control	Irradiation	Control	Irradiation	
All	10	44	53	48	55	0.07
	15			40	45	NS†
Node negative	10			69	80	0.06
	15	61	64	64	66	NS
Node positive	10			37	44	0.16
	15	24	34	29	36	NS

* Data from Cole MP: A clinical trial of an artificial menopause in carcinoma of the breast. In: Namer M, Lalanne CM (eds): Hormones and breast cancer. Paris: INSERM, 143–150, 1976, and Cole MP: Prophylactic compared with therapeutic x-ray artificial menopause. In Joslin CAF, Gleave EN (eds): The Clinical Management of Advanced Breast Cancer, pp 2–11. Cardiff, Alpha Omega Alpha Publishing, 1970.
† NS = Differences in survival figures not statistically significant.

underestimated. For example, an effect may be overestimated when one large trial with an inordinately large false-positive result contributes most of the weight to the overview estimate. Underestimation may occur when several trials with false-negative results (e.g., from poor patient compliance in utilizing the treatment under study) are summated with the results from more positive trials. The main advantage of an overview thus can also be its weakness, and estimates of benefit obtained in an overview should never be accepted without a careful evaluation of the individual trials that have contributed to it.

Several overview analyses of adjuvant breast trials have now been published. One of these was limited to studies in the published literature.[234] A second attempted to include every trial, published and unpublished, that has been conducted throughout the world.[235] The latter study included patients randomized in trials comparing tamoxifen with no tamoxifen (e.g., tamoxifen versus no systemic therapy, tamoxifen plus chemotherapy versus chemotherapy only) and trials that compared adjuvant chemotherapy with no adjuvant chemotherapy (e.g., chemotherapy versus no systemic therapy, chemotherapy plus tamoxifen versus tamoxifen). This analysis included more than 9000 women randomized in chemotherapy trials and 16,000 women in tamoxifen trials. The estimated reduction in the mortality rate resulting from the use of adjuvant chemotherapy with combination agents was 26 ± 7% in women under the age of 50 and 8 ± 6% in those over the age of 50. The effects of adjuvant tamoxifen were −2 ± 8% in women under age 50 and 20 ± 3% in women over the age of 50. No significant benefit accrued to patients treated with single-agent cytotoxic therapy.

The results of this overview analysis confirm the results of individual trials. Adjuvant chemotherapy is highly effective in premenopausal women and adjuvant tamoxifen in postmenopausal women. Also, adjuvant chemotherapy imparts no significant survival advantage to postmenopausal women, and adjuvant tamoxifen treatment has not yet been proved advantageous for premenopausal women.

NODE-NEGATIVE PATIENTS

Most of the chemotherapy trials just described involved primarily or exclusively patients with histologically involved nodes. In contrast, a large proportion of the patients in the endocrine therapy trials had no lymph node involvement. This is understandable in light of the relative toxicities of the two therapies. Even if the ratio reduction in mortality rate for node-negative and node-positive patients is the same, the absolute differences in mortality rates are likely to be different. Because node-negative patients generally have a better prognosis, the absolute differences in the survival of the treated and untreated patients may be quite small, and in this context, the toxicity of the therapy may easily outweigh the gain. Late toxicity, such as an increased incidence of second tumors, is also a more important consideration in a patient population more likely to live long enough to express the carcinogenic effect of the therapy (see below under toxicity). Because of this, many investigators have tried to identify a "bad prognostic group" among the node-negative patients, anticipating that adjuvant chemotherapy with its attendant toxicities might be more justified, as well as more effective, in patients with high-growth-fraction tumors. Until recently, the lack of ER or PR has been considered a marker of this poor prognosis group. However, a careful analysis of all studies on the prognosis of node-negative patients demonstrates that the 20% to 30% of node-negative patients likely to have recurrences and die of breast cancer in the first decade after diagnosis are not predominantly or exclusively ER-negative patients (see above).

Studies specifically designed to test the efficacy of adjuvant chemotherapy in node-negative patients are of recent vintage.[224] The largest of these trials randomized 457 patients to receive either adjuvant LMF (chlorambucil, methotrexate, and 5-FU) or no systemic treatment. At the end of 7 years, there was no significant difference in the disease-free survival rates of the two groups.[236] A Swiss study using a similar regimen demonstrated a transient effect but no significant long-term improvement in survival.[237] A small Austrian study using a slightly more intensive chemotherapy regimen demonstrated a significant survival benefit without an improvement in the recurrence-free survival rate.[238] This contradiction cannot be fully explained.

The study most frequently cited to support the use of chemotherapy in node-negative patients is the Milan trial in which patients who were both node-negative and ER-negative were randomized to receive either 12 courses of intravenous CMF over a period of 9 months or no systemic treatment.[239] Only 90 patients were enrolled in this trial, and the 5-year mortality rate for the control patients exceeded 35%. There was a significant survival advantage for the patients given adjuvant CMF (p = 0.02), and this was apparent in both premenopausal and postmenopausal women. The number of relapses in the control and treated populations, respectively, was 7 of 27 and 2 of 27 premenopausal patients, and 5 of 18 and 1 of 18 postmenopausal patients.

These results from Milan must be interpreted in the context of two other trials of node-negative patients, each of which has enrolled 500 to 1000 treated patients.[240-242] Although results from these studies have not been published, each has been monitored regularly for evidence of benefit. One of these trials is limited to node-negative, receptor-negative patients. The other stratified patients on the basis of receptor status. Because it is highly unlikely that a significant benefit anywhere near the magnitude of that described in the Milan trial has been observed but not reported, the dramatic results of the Milan trial must be accepted cautiously lest they prove to be an overestimate of the benefit.

Adjuvant systemic therapy is not recommended for node-negative patients at the present time and should not be considered for any patient until it has been reproducibly demonstrated that the survival benefits outweigh both the early and the delayed toxicities.

ENDOCRINE THERAPY IN RECEPTOR-NEGATIVE PATIENTS

In the NATO trial comparing 2 years of adjuvant tamoxifen with no systemic therapy, there was no evidence that the survival benefits for tamoxifen were greater or more significant among receptor-positive than receptor-negative pa-

tients.[227] The ratio of O:E deaths in patients with an ER concentration below and above 5 fmol/mg of cytosol protein was 0.63 and 0.82, respectively. The O:E ratio for patients with receptor levels below and above 30 fmol/mg was 0.76 and 0.71.

The data recently published from the Scottish National Trial appear to confirm the observations from the NATO study (Table 38-26). Patients were divided into groups based on receptor concentrations of 0 to 4, 5 to 19, 20 to 99, and 100 or more fmol/mg.[243] The 3-year disease-free survival rate was higher for the tamoxifen-treated group than for the control group within each subset. The survival:hazard ratio for the total follow-up period was also decreased as a result of tamoxifen treatment for each subgroup. However, this advantage for tamoxifen reached levels of statistical significance only in the group with the highest receptor level. Several other studies evaluating adjuvant tamoxifen have shown a nonsignificant trend toward better survival among ER-negative patients, but two large trials have shown a trend toward decreased survival among the tamoxifen-treated ER-negative patients.[242,244]

Until recently, it was difficult to accept the possibility that tamoxifen might have an effect in receptor-negative patients, as the response rate to endocrine therapy is less than 10% among receptor-negative patients with metastatic disease. However, recent laboratory investigations suggest that estrogen-dependent cells might produce paracrine growth factors that could support the growth of estrogen-independent cells[42] (see below). If so, the eradication of very few receptor-positive, tamoxifen-sensitive cells might affect the growth of a much larger mass of cells.

DURATION OF THERAPY

Perioperative adjuvant chemotherapy trials utilized one or a few doses of chemotherapy during the first week or two after diagnosis and mastectomy. One of these studies demonstrated a statistically significant survival advantage for patients treated with daily doses of intravenous cyclophosphamide.[245] However, the results of this trial have not been confirmed, and other perioperative studies of similar design have not shown such a significant survival benefit.[224]

TABLE 38-26. Correlation of ER Concentration and Disease-Free Survival Benefits from Adjuvant Tamoxifen in the Scottish National Trial (8-Year Report)

ER (fmol/mg)	No. of Patients	Disease-Free (%) at 3 Years		Hazard Ratio Total Follow-up (95% CI)
		Control	Tamoxifen	
All patients	1312	64	79	0.57 (0.47–0.68)
0–4	218	55	66	0.70 (0.47–1.05)
5–19	89	61	72	0.67 (0.36–1.28)
20–99	214	74	86	0.57 (0.33–1.00)
100+	221	61	86	0.35 (0.22–0.57)
Not tested	570	65	80	0.56 (0.43–0.47)

Modified from Scottish Cancer Trials Office. Adjuvant tamoxifen in the management of operable breast cancer: The Scottish trial. Lancet 2:171–175, 1987.

Large survival benefits from adjuvant chemotherapy were first demonstrated with regimens given for 1 to 2 years. A second generation of trials has now been completed in which patients were randomized to two durations of treatment. In the first of these studies, patients were randomized to receive either 15 or 30 weeks of a combination of cyclophosphamide and doxorubicin.[246] With a median follow-up in excess of 5 years and a maximum follow-up in excess of 10 years, there is no survival benefit for patients given the longer course of treatment, and there is a nonsignificant trend toward better survival for patients who received the short course. In Milan, patients were randomized to either 6 or 12 months of CMF,[223,247] and there was a nonsignificant trend toward improved survival with the shorter course of treatment in this study as well. This survival trend in favor of shorter therapy was most evident among the postmenopausal patients, for whom the value of chemotherapy is limited at best. Other studies addressing the issue of optimal therapy duration have randomized patients to intervals of 12 or 6 months, 24 or 6 months, and 2 years or 1 year.[246] None has demonstrated an advantage for the longer treatment.

There are no published results from randomized trials comparing different durations of tamoxifen treatment. Tamoxifen was given for 2 years in one and 5 years in the second trial in which an overall survival advantage was demonstrated. However, the duration of therapy was not the only distinguishing characteristic of these two trials, and it cannot yet be concluded that the optimal duration of adjuvant tamoxifen treatment is known. Until the results from randomized trials specifically designed to address this question are available, it is recommended that tamoxifen be given for at least 2 years and not more than 5 years.

OPTIMAL CHEMOTHERAPY

SINGLE AGENTS VERSUS COMBINATION CHEMOTHERAPY

The results of trials comparing the efficacy of combination chemotherapy with that of a single drug are contradictory.[224] Among premenopausal women, there is a statistically significant survival advantage for patients given combination chemotherapy in two of the studies, a nonsignificant but positive trend in two of the studies, and a nonsignificant negative survival trend in two more studies. The data from a similar number of studies in postmenopausal women are similarly contradictory.

DOXORUBICIN COMBINATIONS

Combination chemotherapy regimens that include doxorubicin have repeatedly induced a higher response in patients with metastatic breast cancer than regimens not including this drug (see below). Several recently reported trials suggest that this may be true in the adjuvant setting as well. In a French trial, patients were randomized to receive either 1 year of adjuvant CMF at conventional doses or one year of AVCF (doxorubicin, vincristine, cyclophosphamide, 5-FU).[249] In the seventh year of follow-up, 58% of the CMF patients and 75% of the AVCF patients were alive (p =

0.015). A trend toward improved disease-free survival rates among postmenopausal women was not statistically significant, but both the disease-free and the overall survival rates of premenopausal women randomized to AVCF were significantly better than those of patients randomized to CMF (p = 0.001). The NSABP randomized receptor-negative patients to receive either PF (L-PAM and 5-FU) or PAF (PF plus doxorubicin). Receptor-positive patients were randomized to the same two combinations with the addition of tamoxifen to each.[250] At the end of 5 years, there was a 20% decrease in the relapse rate and a 15% decrease in the mortality rate among patients receiving the combinations containing doxorubicin. The improvements in the disease-free survival rates were highly significant. The improvement in survival was marginally significant in postmenopausal women but not in premenopausal women.

The Cancer and Leukemia Group B (CALGB) has evaluated the possibility that the introduction of a doxorubicin-containing compound after induction with CMFVP might improve survival.[251] Patients were randomized to receive CMFVP for 14 months or CMFVP for 8 months followed by vinblastine, doxorubicin, thiotepa, and Halotestin (VATH). This trial showed an improvement in the disease-free survival rate that was statistically significant at the time of first analysis and a trend toward improved survival as well.

Conventional CMF has been compared with either CMFP or CMFVP in randomized trials. None of these studies has shown a statistically significant improvement in the overall survival rate, although the authors of these studies have concluded that there may be some advantage for the four- or five-drug regimen for some patient subsets. These conclusions must remain tentative until more data from mature trials are available.

DOSE

In a retrospective analysis of the Milan CMF trial, it was observed that the patients who received more than 85% of the planned dose of CMF had a statistically significant improvement in survival compared with patients who received reduced doses.[223,252] However, only 20% of the patients received full doses of therapy. The survival advantage for patients given the higher doses was seen among both premenopausal and postmenopausal women and has persisted through 10 years of follow-up. Other investigators have performed similar retrospective analyses correlating the dose of chemotherapy with either disease-free or overall survival, and none has found a statistically significant survival advantage for higher doses. Indeed, in some trials, there was not even a trend toward improved disease-free survival among patients who received the higher doses. A retrospective analysis of multiple trials has been reported that shows dose rate to be an important variable in disease-free survival.[253] However, this retrospective analysis is based on many assumptions inconsistent with the general principles of medical oncology practice. In addition, the statistical methodology is probably not appropriate to the data set selected.[254] This analysis therefore cannot be accepted as evidence that dose is an important variable in the use of adjuvant chemotherapy. On the basis of present knowledge, it seems unwise either to escalate or to decrease chemotherapy beyond the limits set by trials in which adjuvant chemotherapy resulted in a significant survival benefit.

CHEMOHORMONAL THERAPY

Many randomized trials have been conducted comparing either chemotherapy alone or endocrine therapy alone with a combination of chemotherapy and endocrine therapy.[224] In spite of this abundance of data, the critical questions regarding the appropriate use of these two modalities cannot yet be fully answered. These questions are:

1. Can all of the benefits of adjuvant chemotherapy be achieved by adjuvant oophorectomy? No published results are available from any trial evaluating the relative efficacy of chemotherapy and oophorectomy (or ovarian radiation) in premenopausal women, and very few randomized trials of this type have been initiated.

2. Is there a benefit from combining endocrine therapy (either tamoxifen or oophorectomy) with chemotherapy in premenopausal women? In one study, there was a nonsignificant trend toward improved survival when oophorectomy was added to CMFP,[242] and in another study, tamoxifen added very little to CMF or CMFP.[255] In NSABP trial B-09, patients who received a combination of PFT (L-PAM, 5-FU, and tamoxifen) had a shorter survival than patients treated with PF alone, but this trend was not statistically significant.

3. Do postmenopausal women who receive a combination of chemotherapy and tamoxifen live longer than those who receive tamoxifen alone? The definitive published trial addressing this issue is the Ludwig III trial.[256] Four hundred sixty-three patients were randomized to receive either daily oral prednisone plus tamoxifen for 12 months (pT), CMFpT for 12 months, or no systemic adjuvant therapy. At the end of 7 years, there is a statistically significant survival advantage for the patients treated with CMFpT compared with either those given pT alone or those randomized to observation (Fig. 38-21). Preliminary results from a somewhat smaller trial comparing 3 years of adjuvant tamoxifen alone with CMFP plus 3 years of tamoxifen has demonstrated a significant increase in the disease-free survival rate among those patients receiving both chemotherapy and endocrine therapy but no overall survival advantage.[257]

4. Is tamoxifen alone as effective as or more effective than chemotherapy in postmenopausal women? Although there are several such studies under way, results have been published from only one.[224,258] At the end of 5 years, the disease-free survival rate of women over age 50 who received tamoxifen was significantly better than that of patients randomized to CMF (p = 0.009), but a small trend in favor of improved survival with tamoxifen alone was not statistically significant. In contrast, women under age 49 who were treated with CMF had a marginally significant improvement in disease-free survival and a highly significant improvement in overall survival compared with women of the same age randomized to treatment with tamoxifen alone.

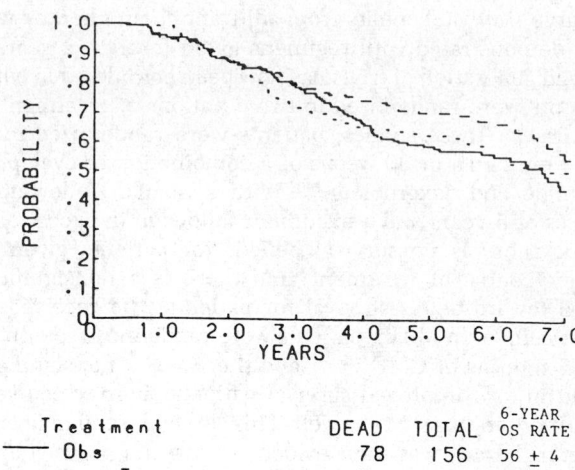

Treatment	DEAD	TOTAL	6-YEAR OS RATE
—— Obs	78	156	56 ± 4
··· p + T	70	153	56 ± 4
— — CMFp + T	56	154	67 ± 4

FIG. 38-21. Overall survival of postmenopausal patients in Ludwig III trial randomized to observation (*Obs*), prednisone plus tamoxifen (*p + T*), or CMFp + T. Three-way comparison, p = 0.12. CMFp + T vs Obs, p = 0.04; CMFp + T vs p + T, p = NS. (Goldhirsch A, Gelber RD: Adjuvant therapy for breast cancer: The Ludwig breast cancer trials 1987. In Salmon SE [ed]: Adjuvant Therapy of Cancer V, pp 297–309. Orlando, Grune & Stratton, 1987)

STANDARD REGIMEN

On the basis of the data currently available, 6 months of CMF should be considered standard adjuvant therapy for premenopausal node-positive patients. Regimens that contain doxorubicin appear to be as effective as CMF-type regimens, but it is plausible that mature data from ongoing trials will demonstrate the superiority of doxorubicin-containing combinations. Postmenopausal women should be treated with adjuvant tamoxifen, especially those who are node-positive and ER-positive. The value of chemotherapy in this group remains to be demonstrated, but the available evidence suggests that chemotherapy, when employed, should be given in combination with adjuvant tamoxifen.

INTEGRATION OF ADJUVANT THERAPY WITH OTHER MODALITIES

The optimal time to initiate adjuvant therapy is not known. It has been suggested that adjuvant chemotherapy be initiated as soon as possible after completion of primary therapy[259] or be given before treatment with mastectomy or radiotherapy.[260] This emphasis on timing is based on theoretical considerations and arises in part from a retrospective analysis of the Scandinavian trial in which patients were randomized to receive six daily doses of intravenous cyclophosphamide or no therapy.[259] The perioperative chemotherapy used in this trial resulted in a survival benefit in all but one of the hospitals contributing patients to the study. In that hospital, therapy was delayed for 2 to 4 weeks compared with the other hospitals, leading to the hypothesis that the time at which chemotherapy is started is important. However, similar retrospective analyses from other studies have not confirmed the observations of the Scandinavian trial. In addition, in a prospective randomized trial conducted to test this hypothesis,[256] in which patients were randomized to receive either no therapy immediately after mastectomy or CMF within 36 hours followed by 6 months of CMFPT or 6 months of CMFPT beginning 25 to 32 days after mastectomy, no significant advantage for early therapy has emerged with a median follow-up of 30 months. However, these results must be considered very preliminary.

Most adjuvant therapy trials have been performed in patients treated with mastectomy or mastectomy plus adjuvant radiotherapy. There are as yet no randomized controlled trials to determine the optimal integration of adjuvant chemotherapy and conservative surgery plus radiotherapy. Although chemotherapy and radiotherapy have been given sequentially and concomitantly, it has not been determined that the use of radiotherapy prior to chemotherapy will compromise the doses of chemotherapy that may be administered or that a compromise in dose is very important (see above). Because short courses of chemotherapy have proved as effective as longer courses, it is reasonable to consider administering all adjuvant chemotherapy after the surgical excision of the breast cancer and before the radiation therapy. However, it has not been shown that this can be done without compromising control of cancer within the breast itself. Uncontrolled trials have shown that chemotherapy may compromise the cosmetic results obtained when conservative surgery and primary radiation are used,[261] and preliminary results suggest that a sequential course of radiotherapy and chemotherapy is preferable to concomitant administration of these two modalities.[262]

TOXICITY

Although the acute toxicities of chemotherapy and the lack of acute toxicity from tamoxifen are well known, the possibility of a second tumor as a result of the therapy awaits further follow-up. The NSABP has reported an 11-fold increase in acute leukemia and a 24-fold increase in acute myelogenous leukemia ($p < 0.01$) within the first 10 years of follow-up after adjuvant therapy with L-PAM.[263] A similarly increased incidence of leukemia has not been observed after the administration of adjuvant CMF,[264] but the database from which this observation has been derived is probably too small to rule out any increased incidence of secondary cancers.[265] Firm evidence regarding the incidence of solid tumors resulting from either adjuvant chemotherapy or adjuvant tamoxifen will require two to three decades of follow-up. The very real possibility of inducing second tumors with adjuvant chemotherapy is readily apparent, as these agents are known to be carcinogens both in the laboratory and in the clinic. However, long-term administration of tamoxifen, a weak estrogen, may also be associated with an increased incidence of second tumors, especially adenocarcinoma. At present, this possibility must remain speculative, although endometrial carcinoma has been observed in patients treated with adjuvant chemotherapy plus tamoxifen.[266]

In spite of the toxicity associated with chemotherapy, the net benefits in overall survival or quality of disease-free survival outweigh the toxic costs. The Ludwig group has addressed this issue by calculation of the average time spent without symptoms or toxicity (TWiST) for postmenopausal women randomized on their trial comparing pT, CMFpT, and observation.[267] In this analysis, a month of TWiST was removed for any month in which a patient experienced even 1 day of subjective treatment toxicity, such as nausea, vomiting, or mucositis. Three months were removed beyond the end of therapy for patients who had alopecia, weight gain, or a local recurrence. The remainder of a patient's lifetime was removed from the analysis if the patient developed distant metastases or a second primary tumor other than a breast cancer. The net TWiST for patients on the three study arms is shown in Table 38-27. During the first years of life, patients under observation had a larger TWiST than patients

TABLE 38-27. Average Time Spent Without Symptoms (of Disease) or Toxicity (from Therapy) (TWiST) among Patients Randomized to Observation Only, Adjuvant Endocrine Therapy with Prednisone and Tamoxifen (p + T), or Adjuvant Chemohormonal Therapy with CMFp + T in Ludwig Breast Cancer Study III

Patient/Treatment Groups	Months from Mastectomy					
	12	24	36	48	60	72
All patients						
Observation	11	19	25	30	31	38*
p + T	9	18	25	31	37	42
CMFp + T	3	13	21	30	37	44*
Estrogen receptor-positive						
Observation	11	20	27	33	38	43
p + T	9	19	27	36	43	49
CMFp + T	3	13	22	30	38	45
Estrogen receptor-negative						
Observation	10	18	23	28	32	35
p + T	8	14	19	23	26	28
CMFp + T	2	11	19	27	34	41

Modified from Gelber RD, Goldhirsch A, Castiglione M et al: Time without Symptoms and Toxicity (TWiST): A quality-of-life-oriented endpoint to evaluate adjuvant therapy. In Salmon SE (ed): Adjuvant Therapy of Cancer, pp 455–465, Orlando, Grune & Stratton, 1987.
* Difference statistically significant. Other differences do not reach conventional levels of statistical significance.

under treatment because of the toxicities from treatment. However, as the disease-free survival benefits began to emerge for the patients receiving adjuvant therapy, these patients began to have a net increase in TWiST compared with the patients under observation. At 72 months of follow-up, the patients given CMFpT had a net TWiST advantage of 6 months compared with controls randomized to observation only. This advantage was statistically significant. Among patients who were ER-positive, however, the greatest TWiST was obtained by patients treated with endocrine therapy alone, whereas for those who were ER-negative, there was actually a loss of TWiST as a result of endocrine therapy. However, these differences among patient subsets defined by receptor status were not statistically significant.

VALUE OF FOLLOW-UP PHYSICAL EXAMINATIONS AND TESTS AFTER PRIMARY TREATMENT

Follow-up of patients with breast cancer is often carried out in an irregular and costly manner. For patients who have been treated for a potentially curable disease, the objectives of follow-up examinations should be oriented principally to the potentially curable diagnoses, that is, early detection of persistent or new breast cancers (in the contralateral breast and, in breast-preservation cases, the ipsilateral breast also) and early detection and treatment of other lesions, such as large-bowel and gynecologic cancers. Bone and other scans, as well as markers such as CEA, do not uniformly detect occult metastases and do not detect curable disease. They are useful in the evaluation of symptomatic patients, but their value in routine follow-up is uncertain.[268]

A considerable proportion of first metastases in breast cancer patients are in the skeletal system. Consequently, the NSABP protocols require radionuclide scans every 6 months for the first 3 postoperative years and yearly thereafter. Recent data from the NSABP indicate that routinely scheduled bone scans to detect metastases in asymptomatic breast cancer patients are relatively unrewarding,[269] as only 52 of 7984 scans (0.06%) detected asymptomatic bone lesions. The average charge for a bone scan is estimated to be $200. Based on a total expenditure of $1.5 million for all scans in this one NSABP clinical trial, the cost of each positive scan in asymptomatic patients thus was approximately $29,000. Pertinent to this issue also is the lack of evidence that the treatment of patients with asymptomatic skeletal metastases improves survival over that obtained when one waits for the appearance of symptoms. As a result of the minimal benefit from such routine scanning, it was recommended that only those asymptomatic patients in the NSABP studies who had positive axillary nodes receive scans at yearly intervals for the first 3 years. Many others, however, would advise these tests for symptomatic patients only.

Most recurrences after mastectomy are symptomatic; in approximately one-third of patients, asymptomatic recurrences are detected on routine follow-up physical examinations.[270,271] Nevertheless, management of chest wall or supraclavicular nodal disease (usually by excision and radiation therapy) may provide significant palliation. Although these patients are seldom curable, avoidance of chest wall ulceration or painful neurovascular involvement of the brachial plexus is of value.

SPECIAL PROBLEMS IN BREAST CANCER MANAGEMENT

DUCTAL CARCINOMA IN SITU

A review of this subject was recently published in the *New England Journal of Medicine* (Schnitt and associates, April 7, 1988), portions of which are abstracted here.

In 1932, Broders defined carcinoma in situ as "a condition in which malignant epithelial cells and their progeny are found in or near positions occupied by their ancestors before the ancestors underwent malignant transformation."[272] In the breast, carcinoma in situ has traditionally been categorized as either lobular or ductal, depending on the cytologic features and the pattern of growth. Ductal carcinoma in situ (DCIS, also known as intraductal carcinoma or noninvasive ductal carcinoma) is characterized by a proliferation of malignant epithelial cells confined to the mammary ducts, without light microscopic evidence of invasion through the basement membrane into the surrounding stroma.

The clinical spectrum of DCIS is broad and includes lesions discovered incidentally during microscopic examination of breast tissue removed because of another abnormality (*e.g.*, a fibroadenoma or an area of fibrocystic change), small foci detected by mammography, palpable but localized masses, and large palpable tumors or large areas of abnormality on mammography. The frequency with which these various patterns of presentation are observed depends on the population under study. In series reported prior to the advent of screening mammography, most patients with DCIS presented with a palpable mass, nipple discharge, or both.[273-275] In contrast, in a recent nationwide study of patients who underwent mammographic screening, 59% of the in situ cancers were detected exclusively by mammography.[99] Thus, small (often less than 1 cm), mammographically detected lesions currently comprise the majority of cases of DCIS at many institutions.

In the past, most patients with DCIS were treated with mastectomy, so the natural history of this lesion could not be studied. The available information on the risk of progression of DCIS to invasive cancer thus is extremely limited. The only studies that have addressed this issue are those in which patients with DCIS were treated with biopsy alone. There are two studies that identified patients with DCIS during histologic review of biopsies originally categorized as benign. One of these, by Page and colleagues, noted subsequent invasive carcinoma in the ipsilateral breast in 7 of 25 patients (28%) at intervals of 3 to 10 years (mean 6.1 years) after the initial biopsy.[276] In the other, by Betsill and colleagues, 8 of 30 patients (27%) developed an invasive carcinoma in the same breast an average of 9.7 years after the initial biopsy showing DCIS, and in nearly all of these patients, the invasive tumor occurred at or near the original biopsy site.[125,277] In both series, the cases of DCIS were all of the micropapillary or cribriform types; neither included examples of comedo-type

DCIS. These studies suggest that some, but not all, patients with DCIS treated with biopsy alone will develop an invasive cancer in the ipsilateral breast, usually in the region of the initial lesion. In these studies, the invasive carcinomas most commonly occurred within 10 years of the initial biopsy.

Insight into the biologic significance of DCIS can also be obtained from studies that indicate that foci of this lesion are frequently detected in the contralateral breast of women with invasive breast cancer. There is, however, a discrepancy between this incidence of contralateral DCIS and the risk of developing a subsequent, clinically evident, opposite-breast cancer. Alpers and Wellings found DCIS in 48% of breasts contralateral to cancer-containing breasts,[278] yet the cumulative risk of opposite-breast cancer has been reported to be only 12.5% at 20 years after diagnosis of the initial tumor.[279] These data also suggest that not all histologically detectable DCIS will progress to clinically significant cancer.

Mastectomy has been the standard form of treatment for DCIS. Although the multicentricity of DCIS and the occasional finding of foci of invasive cancer in breasts removed because of a biopsy diagnosis of DCIS have been used as arguments for mastectomy,[191] the principal rationale for this treatment of DCIS is its demonstrated efficacy: local tumor control and survival rates approaching 100% can be obtained.[273-275]

There are two other treatment options for patients with DCIS: excision combined with radiation therapy and excision alone.[280-284] Both options provide breast preservation, an important goal in terms of the quality of life. The available data indicate that breast-conserving treatment can be associated with reasonably high levels of local tumor control with a significant chance for salvage in the event of local recurrence. Experience with *invasive* breast cancers that have a prominent intraductal component and with pure DCIS has emphasized that the extent of intraductal involvement in the breast is typically not appreciated by palpation and may not even be recognizable at the time of surgery.[285] Therefore, there must be increased reliance on careful mammographic and pathologic evaluation to aid in defining the extent of the DCIS and ensuring that the lesion has been resected if breast-conserving treatment is being considered.

At many institutions, patients with DCIS in whom the lesion has been excised with clearly negative margins are considered candidates for excision and radiotherapy. At some institutions, selected patients with very limited disease are offered the option of treatment with wide excision alone. For example, Lagios and colleagues consider patients for treatment with excision alone if the DCIS is mammographically detected by the presence of microcalcifications, the lesion is 25 mm or smaller, an excision with pathologically negative margins of resection has been performed, a postoperative mammogram reveals no residual calcifications at the biopsy site, the breast is favorable for mammographic and clinical follow-up, and the patient agrees to undergo the careful follow-up required.[191] At the other extreme, in patients with extensive DCIS, mastectomy is recommended.

The need for axillary dissection in patients with DCIS is a matter of debate.[286] Because of the occasional difficulty in identifying foci of stromal invasion, there is a small likelihood of axillary lymph node involvement in patients having DCIS. This likelihood may be related to tumor size.[191] Therefore, in patients with extensive DCIS, it is generally recommended that a lower axillary dissection be performed. In patients with limited DCIS treated using a breast-preserving approach, an axillary dissection is typically not recommended because of the extremely low probability of nodal metastases and because of the desire to reserve this procedure in the event of a local recurrence.

An important consideration in the use of breast-conserving treatment for DCIS is the feasibility and efficacy of salvage in the event of local recurrence. Even with careful selection and treatment, the risk of local recurrence is likely to be greater with breast-conserving treatment than with mastectomy. Of note, approximately 50% of patients who develop a local recurrence after breast-conserving treatment for DCIS will have invasive cancer on relapse.[280-284] Nonetheless, preliminary data suggest that salvage after a local recurrence in patients with DCIS initially treated with excision with or without radiotherapy is highly effective. Salvage for patients initially treated with excision and radiotherapy generally consists of mastectomy, whereas salvage for patients initially treated with excision alone may consist of either excision and radiotherapy or mastectomy. The impact of a recurrence within the breast on survival is an unsettled issue.[132,287,288] In the absence of definitive information on this subject, we believe that the risk of local recurrence should be kept as low as possible, and that patients with DCIS treated with breast-conserving therapy should be monitored carefully to detect such local recurrences promptly. A reasonable follow-up program is physical examination every 4 months and mammograms every 6 months for the first 2 years and annually thereafter.

LOBULAR CARCINOMA IN SITU

In 1941, Foote and Stewart, as well as Muir, called attention to an in situ form of carcinoma of the female breast that apparently arises within the end parts of the lobule, a lesion they designated lobular carcinoma in situ or lobular CIS.[289,290] These in situ carcinomas may develop into, or at least be associated with, either infiltrating lobular or ductal carcinoma, although the frequency or even the absolute certainty of such a progression has been debated.[291-293]

It is virtually impossible to make a diagnosis of lobular carcinoma in situ by clinical examination.[275] In most instances, the signs and symptoms that lead to biopsy are related to benign lesions, such as fibrocystic mastopathy, that have no relation to the lobular carcinoma in situ. Roentgenologic methods (conventional mammography or xeroradiography) are likewise not usually helpful. Lobular carcinoma in situ also cannot be diagnosed by gross pathologic examination, although occasionally and retrospectively, one may gain the impression of an ill-defined area of induration within the breast substance.

The microscopic diagnosis of lobular carcinoma in situ is sometimes difficult because of its similarity to lobular hyperplasias.[294] This dilemma is analogous to that encountered in the differential diagnosis of proliferative or hyperplastic lesions and intraductal carcinomas. Such difficulty and uncertainty frequently are reflected by the designation "atypical" lobular hyperplasia.

In 1967, McDivitt and co-workers from Memorial Hospital (New York) published a report on the long-term follow-up of patients with lobular CIS.[293] Of 40 patients treated with biopsy alone, nine developed infiltrating carcinoma in the ipsilateral breast after 2 to 23 years. The cumulative risk of ipsilateral breast cancer was 10% at 5 years, 15% at 10 years, and 30% at 15 years. Of the 47 evaluable patients, seven subsequently developed contralateral breast cancer at intervals of 1 to 22 years. The cumulative risk of contralateral breast cancer was 5% at 5 years, 10% at 10 years, and 15% at 15 years. Of the subsequent breast cancers detected, approximately half were lobular and half ductal. In 1978, Rosen and associates updated the results at Memorial Hospital and found a similar risk of cancer.[295]

Subsequent reports of the risk of infiltrating cancer with lobular CIS have not indicated figures as high as those reported by McDivitt and colleagues. Wheeler and co-workers studied 25 women with lobular CIS treated with biopsy alone.[296] Only one of these women subsequently developed ipsilateral infiltrating cancer with a mean follow-up for the entire group of 17.5 years. Of this group, three developed contralateral infiltrating cancer. Haagensen and associates reported follow-up on 211 patients with lobular CIS.[297] The cumulative risk at 25 years for ipsilateral breast cancer was 22% and that for contralateral breast cancer was 15%.

The management of lobular CIS is controversial. Rosen and colleagues from Memorial Hospital have recommended ipsilateral mastectomy and generous biopsy of the opposite breast for this condition. In contrast, Haagensen and co-workers have recommended a more conservative approach of periodic follow-up. Those advocating the conservative approach point out that the considerations in the management of lobular CIS are, in effect, similar to those in the management of women at high risk because of family history or prior breast cancer: in all these groups, the risk of breast cancer approaches 1% per year and persists. As discussed above, it is reasonable to adopt a conservative viewpoint on the management of these other high-risk patients. As a result, many surgeons now favor a program of breast self-examination, periodic physician examinations, and mammograms as management of lobular CIS. In selected patients who are particularly anxious about the development of cancer, bilateral total mastectomies and prompt reconstruction is a reasonable approach.

Radiation therapy does not have a role in the management of lobular CIS.

TREATMENT OF LOCALLY ADVANCED BREAST CANCER (STAGE III)

"Locally advanced cancer of the breast" refers to breast carcinomas with significant primary or nodal disease but where distant metastases cannot be documented. This group of cancers has been shown to be poorly controlled by radical surgery alone and also to have a poor prognosis. Any T3b–T4, N2 or N3, M0 lesion now is regarded as locally advanced, inoperable breast cancer. T3a, N0 or N1, M0 cancers are included in the UICC Stage III because of their poor prognosis but generally are considered operable.

Following Halsted's popularization of the radical mastectomy at the turn of the century, the operation was performed without an understanding of which patients benefited from its use. Haagensen and Stout reviewed the records of patients undergoing radical mastectomy at the Presbyterian Hospital between 1915 and 1942 and identified various clinical features that were associated with high local recurrence rates and poor survival.[298] Table 38-28 lists the clinical features that marked a tumor as categorically inoperable by virtue of local recurrence rates greater than 50% and no 5-year clinical cures, and these features form the basis for classifying patients as CCC Class D or inoperable. In addition, those authors identified five "grave signs" that were associated with a somewhat increased likelihood of local recurrence and poor survival (Table 38-29). Although a single grave sign was not necessarily thought to indicate inoperability, in the presence of any two grave signs, 42% of patients developed local recurrence, and only one (2%) was free of disease at 5 years. The presence of a single grave sign forms the basis of CCC Class C, whereas patients with two or more grave signs are included in Class D.

Because of this high incidence of local–regional recurrence with surgical treatment, radiation therapy, either alone or in conjunction with surgery, has come to play a significant role in this stage of the disease. For radiation therapy to be effective in controlling these locally advanced cancers, however, doses greater than those used to treat

TABLE 38-28. Clinical Features of Breast Cancer Associated with Poor Results Following Radical Mastectomy

Clinical Feature	No. of Patients	Local Recurrence (%)	5-Year Clinical Cure (%)
Extensive edema of skin over breast	51	61	0
Satellite nodules	7	57	0
"Inflammatory" carcinoma of the breast	25	60	0
Distant metastases	10	20	0
Parasternal or supraclavicular node metastases	16	56	0
Edema of the arm	4	50	0

Haagensen CD: Diseases of the Breast, rev 2nd Ed., p. 623. Philadelphia, WB Saunders, 1971.

TABLE 38-29. Grave Signs of Breast Cancer

Clinical Feature	No. of Patients	Local Recurrence (%)	5-Year Clinical Cure (%)
Edema of the skin of the breast (less than one-third)	75	32	23
Skin ulceration	14	14	36
Solid fixation of the tumor to the chest wall	20	40	5
Axillary lymph node greater than 2.5 cm	24	13	38
Fixed axillary nodes	8	13	13

Haagensen CD: Diseases of the Breast, rev 2nd Ed., pp. 625–628. Philadelphia, WB Saunders, 1971.

early-stage tumors are required. Whereas 5000 cGy is effective in eradicating microscopic amounts of tumor, doses in excess of 6000 cGy are required for gross tumor. François Baclesse was one of the first to show that tumor control was achievable using sufficiently high radiation doses.[299] In a more recent study, Fletcher and Montague administered 6000 cGy in 8 weeks and obtained local control in 72% of patients with inoperable breast cancers.[300]

In a review from the JCRT, the results of primary radiation therapy in 192 patients with locally advanced cancers (five with bilateral disease) were analyzed.[301] Patients typically received 4500 to 5000 cGy in 5 weeks to the breast and draining lymph nodes. A local boost to areas of gross disease was delivered in 157 patients, using interstitial implantation (124 cases), electrons (6), or photons (27). Excisional biopsy (gross tumor removal) was performed in only 54 of the 197 breasts. Multiagent chemotherapy was given to 53 patients. The median follow-up was 65 months, with a range of 16 to 158 months. The actuarial probability of survival for the entire group was 41% at 5 years and 23% at 10 years. The probability of relapse-free survival was 30% at 5 years and 19% at 10 years. The addition of multiagent chemotherapy was associated with a significantly improved 5-year relapse-free survival (40% versus 26%, p = 0.02) (Fig. 38-22). The 5-year survival rate was 51% for patients who received adjuvant multiagent chemotherapy and 38% for patients who did not (p = 0.16). The actuarial rate of local–regional tumor control (not censored for distant failure) for all patients was 73% at 5 years and 68% at 10 years, and the crude incidence of local–regional control was 78% (153 of 197 breast and nodal groups treated). Local–regional tumor control was influenced principally by the radiation dose. Patients who received 6000 cGy or more to the primary site had a better 5-year rate of control in the breast than did patients who received less than 6000 cGy (83% versus 70%; p = 0.06). Significant complications were seen in 15 patients (8%), including moderate or severe arm edema in six patients and brachial plexopathy in four patients. Cosmetic results at last evaluation were excellent or good in 56% of evaluable patients, fair in 25%, and poor in 19%. These results indicate that high-dose radiation therapy without mastectomy is an effective means of achieving local–regional tumor control in patients with locally advanced breast cancer.

The results from the JCRT emphasize that a number of technical factors are important in achieving a good outcome.

A dose to the primary site greater than 6000 cGy results in better local control. Furthermore, a dose in the range of 7500 cGy may be preferable for patients who have large tumors not amenable to resection.[302] For such patients, the JCRT recommends external-beam radiation to the breast at 180 cGy per day to a total dose of 4500 cGy in 5 weeks, followed by an interstitial implant of the primary site for an additional dose of 3000 cGy. An adequate dose to the axillary nodes is also important. Five thousand cGy in 5 weeks appears to be sufficient for patients without palpable disease in the axilla, whereas for patients with palpable disease, a total dose of 5600 cGy to the axilla is advised. Bolus is another important technical factor: the use of bolus over the entire breast for half or more of the external-beam treatment was associated with a greater degree of breast retraction and telangiectasia and poorer cosmetic results. For this reason, the use of bolus should be limited as much as possible in extent and frequency.

The results of the JCRT study also suggest an improvement in both relapse-free and total survival rates among patients who received multiagent chemotherapy, even though those patients had a worse T–N profile than did patients who were not treated with chemotherapy. These data support other retrospective studies that have shown

FIG. 38-22. Relapse-free survival for patients with Stage III breast cancer treated with conservative surgery and radiation therapy with (*open circles*) or without (*closed circles*) adjuvant CMF or Adriamycin.[298]

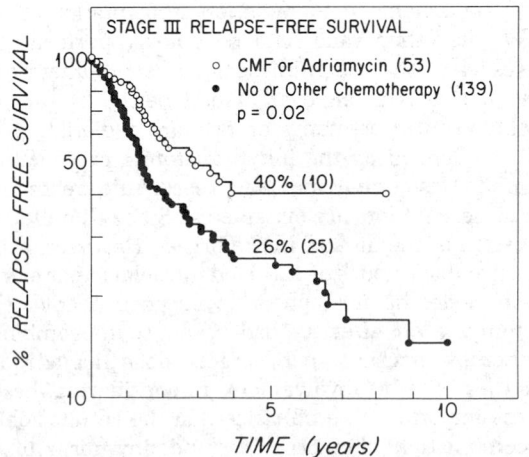

similar results.[303,304] However, in one prospective randomized trial comparing treatment with radiation therapy alone with radiation therapy plus adjuvant systemic therapy, no advantage to the use of adjuvant systemic therapy was noted.[305] This issue requires further prospective analysis.

The relative roles of primary radiation therapy and mastectomy in the treatment of locally advanced breast cancer have been addressed in prospective trials.[306,307] DeLena and colleagues reported rates of local tumor control at 5 years of 75% for patients treated with primary radiotherapy and 82% for patients undergoing mastectomy. No statistically significant differences were seen between the groups in the 5-year rates of either distant disease or overall survival. The probability of disease progression increased at a constant rate over time in both groups, which emphasizes the similarly poor results of both forms of local therapy, even when combined with vigorous systemic therapy. Similar results have been reported by the CALGB.[307] In their study, patients with locally advanced breast cancer were randomized after induction chemotherapy to either modified radical mastectomy or primary radiation therapy, both followed by 2 years of additional chemotherapy. The rates of local relapse, distant metastases, and overall survival were similar in the two groups. The results from these two randomized trials show no advantage for mastectomy over primary radiation therapy in patients with Stage III disease treated with initial chemotherapy.

The benefit of combining mastectomy and postoperative radiation for patients with locally advanced breast cancer has not yet been demonstrated in a prospective study. Retrospective studies of patients treated with a combination of mastectomy and radiation have shown excellent local tumor control at 5 years.[308] The addition of radiation to mastectomy to improve local tumor control must be balanced against a possible increase in the likelihood of complications, such as arm edema.

In considering the options for local treatment, there are a number of factors to be weighed. Primary radiation therapy, which involves 5 to 6 weeks of external-beam irradiation and interstitial implantation, is a time-consuming and technically demanding form of treatment. Furthermore, a breast that has undergone significant cosmetic alteration secondary to the cancer itself is not likely to have a good cosmetic result after treatment. Also, breast masses beyond a certain size are not amenable to radiation implantation. Mastectomy, on the other hand, can be quickly performed and interferes less with the administration of chemotherapy, particularly if this is given over a long period of time. The choice between mastectomy or primary radiation therapy should also depend on the initial anatomic presentation of the disease. Mastectomy may be a reasonable treatment for patients whose tumors are classified as Stage III on the basis of the extent of the disease in the breast. However, patients with fixed axillary nodes or involved infraclavicular or supraclavicular nodes do not appear to be good candidates for mastectomy, even after a good response to combination chemotherapy, because such surgery does not adequately address these sites of involvement. In considering these options, it is important to emphasize that the results achieved using combination chemotherapy and any form of local

treatment are generally poor, with relatively few patients surviving free of systemic relapse beyond 5 years.[306,307] Although mastectomy may be more convenient than radiotherapy, consideration should be given to the psychological and physical effects of mastectomy and to the classic features of "inoperability" in a disease that carries a poor long-term prognosis.

In the absence of definitive data, a reasonable approach is to treat patients who have locally advanced breast cancer with initial combination chemotherapy for 4 to 8 months. If the cosmetic appearance is acceptable at that point, primary radiation therapy is given. However, if the breast tumor appears to be too large for interstitial implantation or the cosmetic appearance is already poor, and if N2 or N3 involvement was not present initially, the policy is to recommend mastectomy. As noted above, the use of postoperative radiation may be considered in this setting in order to optimize local tumor control.

The available data indicate that although locally advanced breast cancer can have a long natural history, systemic relapse and death from breast cancer are eventually observed in the large majority of patients. Substantial improvements in the treatment of locally advanced breast cancer will depend on new developments in systemic therapy.

PAGET'S DISEASE OF THE NIPPLE

Paget's disease of the nipple is characterized clinically by an itchy, eczematoid eruption involving the nipple and pathologically by large cells with pale cytoplasm and prominent irregular nuclei (Paget's cells) in the nipple epidermis. In approximately 60% of patients, an associated breast mass is present. In all cases, either invasive or noninvasive carcinoma is present in the involved breast, sometimes at a considerable distance from the nipple. The relation between the nipple involvement and the underlying malignancy is still a matter of controversy. It has been hypothesized that the nipple involvement represents migration of malignant cells from the underlying carcinoma, or alternatively, that it is an independent process.[309]

The prognosis is related to whether a mass is present. If a mass is present, the prognosis is similar to that in patients with similar masses but without Paget's disease. If a mass is absent, the prognosis is excellent. Nance and associates observed that none of 16 patients without a mass had axillary metastases, whereas axillary metastases were found in 50% when a mass was present.[310] Moreover, none of 21 patients without a mass died of cancer, whereas 18 of 32 with a mass died of cancer within 5 years. Consequently, these authors recommended radical mastectomy for patients with masses and total mastectomy for those without. On the other hand, Maier and coworkers reported that 8 of 56 patients without a mass had positive axillary nodes and advocated radical mastectomy in all patients.[311] At present, total mastectomy and axillary dissection is considered the surgical treatment of Paget's disease, particularly if a mass is present. Breast-preserving surgery, with or without radiotherapy, has been reported in 46 collected cases from the literature.[312] Three local recurrences were seen, indicating that this approach may be acceptable. However, follow-up is short, and the cosmetic results after nipple–areolar excision have not been evaluated.

CARCINOMA OF THE BREAST IN MEN

Carcinoma of the breast occurs infrequently in men, with an estimated incidence about 1% of that in women.[313,314] The average age at diagnosis appears to be about 10 years older for men than for women.[314-317] There have been fewer epidemiologic studies of male breast cancer, but there does appear to be some familial distribution, with very rare families having more than one male with breast cancer.[318,319] Some families with a high likelihood for breast cancer in the women have an occasional male with breast cancer. Male breast cancer appears to be associated with disease that causes hyperestrogenism. For example, bilharzias appear to be associated with the disease.[320] This infection damages the liver and causes hyperestrogenism, and in Egypt, where bilharzias is common, men constitute about 6% of all patients with breast cancer, as opposed to the 1% usually described. There is some evidence that gynecomastia also predisposes to breast cancer in men. There is a significant elevation of the incidence in patients with Klinefelter's syndrome.[321] Whereas earlier reports postulated that the incidence of breast cancer in men with Klinefelter's syndrome was about the same as in women, a recent analysis[322] of 27 reported cases suggested that males with Klinefelter's syndrome have a 3% increased risk of breast cancer.

On pathologic examination, male breast cancer resembles carcinoma of the breast in women with the exception that lobular carcinoma in situ is not seen. Estrogen receptors have been found in as many as 84% of the specimens.[323] Clinically, the disease presents as a unilateral mass, usually firm and painless. There may be abnormality of the nipple, including retraction, crusting or discharge, and ulceration. The tumor is frequently less well defined than in female breast cancer, and, because of the limited breast tissue in men without evidence of lobules, the tumor is frequently closely applied to the pectoral fascia and can involve the muscle itself. Male breast cancer usually presents in a more advanced stage.[315,316] Review of breast cancer cases at the Ellis Fischel State Cancer Hospital revealed a statistically significant difference in stage between male and female breast cancers.[324]

The method of treatment in most reported experience has been mastectomy, usually radical mastectomy because of frequent involvement of the pectoral muscle. Occasionally, if the muscle is not involved extensively, it can be spared. Use of radiation therapy alone for early carcinoma of the male breast has not been reported in significant numbers. It has been used as an adjuvant, both postoperatively following mastectomy, and in advanced cancer.[317] Some authors have advocated routine radiation after modified radical mastectomy except for patients with very small tumors.[325] Lymph node involvement has the same prognostic significance in men as it does in women.

There is some difference of opinion in the literature as to the prognosis. Most authors believe that, although male breast cancer presents in a more advanced stage, within each stage, the prognosis is similar to that in women.[315,316,328] The

Memorial Hospital series, reporting follow-up of 97 male breast cancer patients, showed 80% free of disease 10 years after mastectomy when axillary nodes were histologically negative.[326] This was similar to the data in node-negative female patients. However, male patients with positive nodes had a prognosis much worse than that of women with positive nodes.

The pattern of metastases in men is similar to that in women, with bone (48%), soft-tissue (60%), and various visceral sites predominating.[320] The standard therapy for metastatic disease is orchidectomy, which produces an objective remission rate higher than that of female castration (50%–60%).[327,328] The high response rate most likely reflects the high incidence of ER protein. The responses last 3 to 40 months, with a median duration of 12 months. Further palliation may be obtained by adrenalectomy. A review of the literature by one author identified 17 cases, of which 12 were evaluable.[329] Nine patients objectively responded for 5 months to 5 years.

Hypophysectomy also may palliate advanced disease. A review of the experience with that operation confirmed objective responses in five of eight patients, including three complete remissions.[330] More recent studies report that comparable response rates may be achieved with antiestrogen and other hormonal agents, indicating a shift away from major surgical ablation.[331-333]

The experience with systemic adjuvant therapy in males with positive nodes is anecdotal. The regimen is generally the same combination chemotherapy used in women. In a recent report from the National Cancer Institute, 24 male patients were treated with adjuvant CMF. The 5-year survival rate exceeded 80%, a substantial improvement over that for historical controls.[334]

TREATMENT OF METASTASES

GENERAL PRINCIPLES

Recurrent breast cancer is incurable. This is true whether the site of recurrence is a solitary lesion on the chest wall or multiple foci within the liver and other viscera. The median length of survival after a diagnosis of recurrence is about 2 years, but this span may range from a few months to three decades.[335,336]

There is a role for all of the major modalities in the treatment of breast cancer metastases. Surgery is often used to excise local recurrences, to drain pleural effusions, or to ablate endocrine organs. Radiotherapy may be used alone or in conjunction with surgery to treat locally recurrent disease, and it is the treatment of choice for brain metastases. Radiotherapy is probably also the most effective method of relieving pain from bone lesions. However, when there are multiple sites of disease, and especially when disease involves visceral organs, some form of systemic therapy is usually employed. This may consist of relatively nontoxic endocrine therapies such as tamoxifen, aminoglutethimide, or progestins. Alternatively, symptoms may be relieved with chemotherapy, and most of the cytotoxic agents developed over the

TABLE 38-30. Factors of Importance in Determining When to Treat and Which Therapies to Use for Metastatic Breast Cancer

Patient symptoms
Disease-free interval
Sites of metastases
Menstrual status
Receptor status
Prior therapy
Response to prior therapy
Toxicities of therapy

last 30 years have at least some activity in breast cancer patients.

Patients seeking treatment for breast cancer metastases usually desire palliation of their symptoms, prolongation of survival, or both. The judicious use of the various treatment modalities in sequence may keep a patient symptom-free for many years. Unfortunately, the impact of these therapies on survival is limited. For this reason, this goal is usually of secondary importance in determining when a patient with breast cancer metastases should be treated or which modality to use (Table 38-30).

In making treatment decisions, the presence and nature of the patient's symptoms is the single most important consideration. Patients may live for months or even years with abnormalities on bone scan, elevated tumor markers, or small skin recurrences with almost no symptoms. There is no evidence that earlier treatment with an effective regimen will prolong survival. For example, when patients with metastatic disease are randomized to two regimens, one of which is associated with a significantly higher response rate than the other, and then crossed over to the opposite regimen at the time of progression, there is generally no survival advantage for the group of patients initially treated with the more effective program.[337,338]

The time from first diagnosis of breast cancer to documentation of metastatic disease is referred to as the disease-free interval, and few other pieces of clinical or laboratory data provide as much prognostic information as this figure (Table 38-31). For example, the median survival of patients who relapse in a single site less than 1 year after initial diagnosis is 11 months, whereas the median survival of a similar group of patients with a disease-free interval of more than 5 years is 40 months.[339] The disease-free interval is also an important predictor of the response to endocrine therapy. Patients with an interval in excess of 2 years have a significantly higher probability of responding to endocrine therapy than do those with an interval less than 2 years.[29] Patients who present with metastases but without a prior diagnosis of breast cancer (i.e., with an interval of 0) have a better prognosis than those with a disease-free interval of less than 1 year, presumably because these patients represent a mixed group, some of whom have had long-standing disease that has been indolent and asymptomatic, whereas others have an unusually aggressive form of the disease that metastasizes early.

The number of sites of disease is also an important prognostic indicator, as shown in Table 38-31, and the number and specific sites of disease may strongly influence the type of therapy administered. For example, a patient with a single site of recurrence on the chest wall after a long disease-free interval might appropriately be treated with excision, or radiotherapy, or both. A patient with multiple sites of disease, including a local recurrence, should be treated with some form of systemic therapy. Patients with central nervous system (CNS) and liver metastases are thought to have a particularly dire prognosis. However, CNS metastases may respond dramatically to radiotherapy. Liver metastases are usually treated with chemotherapy, especially if the disease-free interval has been short.

Menstrual status is of help in determining whether the patient is likely to respond to endocrine therapy and if so, which endocrine therapy to use. Postmenopausal women rarely, if ever, respond to oophorectomy, and premenopausal women have not been shown to benefit from estrogens. Postmenopausal women less than 5 years from their last menstrual period are less likely to benefit from any form of endocrine therapy. The ER and PR determinations obtained at the time of the patient's original diagnosis have both prognostic and predictive value after the appearance of metastases: patients without these receptors have a poorer prognosis (see above) and a very low probability of responding to endocrine therapy. However, receptor status may change, and biopsy of a metastatic lesion should be performed for testing whenever possible.

Finally, the toxicity of the therapy must be balanced with a

TABLE 38-31. Effect of Disease-Free Interval and Number of Metastatic Sites on the Median Survival (Months) of Patients from First Recurrence of Breast Cancer

Disease-Free Interval (yr)	Number of Metastatic Sites*				Liver, CNS
	1	2	3	4	
<1	11	7	5	5	5
1–2	16	13	7	6	8
2–5	20	14	12	5	7
>5	40	22	14	21	11

* Excluding patients with liver and central nervous system (CNS) metastases
Modified from Cutler S: Classification of extent of disease in breast cancer. Semin Oncol 1:91–96, 1974.

realistic estimate of the probability of a meaningful response. In controlled trials, even a toxic therapy that induces remission proved more likely to improve the overall quality of a patient's life than a nontoxic therapy that has a low probability of benefit. In one study, patients were randomized to receive either a nontoxic endocrine therapy or a toxic chemotherapy program without regard to usual selection factors such as receptor status or the patient's clinical characteristics.[340] The response rate to the chemotherapy was twice that to the endocrine therapy. Serial evaluation demonstrated that the quality of life associated with the more toxic but more effective chemotherapy was significantly greater than that achieved with the nontoxic but less effective endocrine therapy. Fortunately, there are many situations where the probability of response to two therapies is nearly identical, and in this setting, the less toxic should be used. For example, a 60 year-old postmenopausal woman with a 5-year disease-free interval and a receptor-positive tumor is as likely to respond to endocrine therapy as she is to chemotherapy, and in this circumstance, the nontoxic endocrine therapy is preferred. A patient with a local recurrence on the chest wall and no other site of distant disease 5 years after her mastectomy might more reasonably be treated with local excision alone or radiotherapy alone rather than the more toxic forms of systemic therapy. Similar considerations may be important in selecting radiotherapy fields, choosing among several different types of endocrine therapy, or utilizing a single cytotoxic agent rather than a combination of drugs.

The patient's long-term prognosis is a poor guide to the selection of therapy for patients with metastases. Many physicians feel compelled to treat a patient merely because metastases have been diagnosed and because the patient will eventually die of these metastases. Although it is not necessary to wait until the patient is bedridden to begin treatment, there is no evidence that earlier treatment is better. If the patient is desirous of treatment and is asymptomatic, the physician should consider recommending a new or experimental therapy. A second fallacy of clinical judgment is the use of a nontoxic therapy as a placebo in an asymptomatic patient. Endocrine therapy (*e.g.,* tamoxifen) or radiotherapy are often used in this way. However, the injudicious use of tamoxifen may limit its future value as palliation when a patient is symptomatic, and inappropriate use of radiotherapy may reduce bone marrow reserves and limit the future use of chemotherapy.

INITIAL EVALUATION OF METASTATIC DISEASE AND MONITORING RESPONSE TO THERAPY

Breast cancer may metastasize to almost any site in the body, as evidenced in the autopsy series cited above (see Table 38-14). The symptoms of metastases will usually direct the physician to one site, but a more thorough staging to detect metastases at other sites is recommended. There are several reasons for this. First, the presence of asymptomatic disease in multiple sites or in a visceral organ may suggest the use of systemic therapy rather than a more limited focus on the single symptomatic area. Second, patients frequently develop new symptoms shortly after the initiation of therapy;

documenting these metastases before treatment is begun may discourage premature abandonment of a therapy because of a mistaken assessment that the disease is progressing during therapy. Third, the response to one therapy may influence the choice of future therapies. Finally, documentation of all sites of measurable disease may permit a more accurate assessment of the response to therapy at a later time.

The basic evaluation should encompass the most common sites of metastases. Physical examination should include a careful assessment of regional lymph nodes, the skin overlying the mastectomy site or the irradiated breast, the chest, and the abdomen. Signs of pleural effusions, ascites, and hepatomegaly should be specifically sought. Abnormalities in the blood count may suggest bone metastases. Liver function studies should be obtained for evaluation of potential liver metastases, but liver scans are not recommended as a routine because the frequency of false-positive results exceeds that of true-positive scans in patients without hepatomegaly or abnormal liver function studies.[341] Even though brain metastases are not uncommon in patients with metastatic breast cancer, there is no evidence that a radionuclide brain scan or a CT scan of the head is likely to reveal asymptomatic disease in other than a rare patient.[342]

Serial follow-up bone scans after treatment of the breast primary are no longer recommended in asymptomatic patients without evidence of extraosseous metastases because of the low yield observed in a number of recent studies[343] (see above). A baseline bone scan in a patient with documented metastases at other sites may be of help because of the frequency with which bone metastases appear soon after the initiation of therapy, but these scans must be interpreted very cautiously. Approximately 15% of patients with extraosseous metastases have solitary lesions on such baseline bone scans, and more than a third of these solitary lesions prove to be a benign process.[344] This is especially true when these solitary lesions are in the ribs; as many as 90% of these lesions may be benign.[345] Follow-up bone scans must also be interpreted cautiously, as patients may appear to have increased intensity of radionuclide uptake in responding lesions.[346] It has even been reported that some responding patients develop new abnormalities on bone scan after the initiation of therapy without these representing progressive disease.[347]

Between 50% and 80% of patients with metastatic breast cancer will have elevations of CEA, gross cystic disease protein (GCDP), CA 15-3, casein, ferritin, pregnancy-associated macroglobulin, beta-2-microglobulin, sialytransferase, tissue polypeptide antigen (TPA), or 5-nucleotide phosphodiesterase isoenzyme V (5'-NPD-V).[348,349]

CEA has been studied more extensively than any of the other markers. A serum CEA concentration of more than 3 ng/ml has been observed in 55%, and a CEA greater than 5 ng/ml in 40% to 45%, of patients with metastatic breast cancer.[350,351] Between 69% and 83% of patients who respond to therapy at other sites will also have a fall in CEA,[351,352] although approximately half of these will have a transient early rise in CEA level.[351] CEA is a useful tool for monitoring patients with metastatic breast cancer, although it is difficult to use. A CEA of more than 10 ng/ml almost always reflects metastases. In a rare patient, CEA elevations appear as long as 1.5 years prior to evidence of metastases at specific sites. A falling CEA almost always reflects a response to therapy, and this may be helpful in deciding to persist with therapy in a patient whose response in other sites is ambiguous. Because a rise in CEA may be transient, it cannot be taken as a sign of failure to respond and should not be an indication for discontinuing therapy unless the patient has other good evidence of progressive disease. Finally, a stable or falling CEA in a patient who is responding at other sites might be a basis for continuing therapy if the status of the patient's disease is ambiguous.

GCDP levels may also rise and fall with disease progression or regression, but this marker is abnormal in only 30% of patients with metastatic breast cancer.[353] CA 15-3 is a recently described marker for metastatic breast cancer. This antigen is measured in a bideterminant immunoradiometric assay utilizing two monoclonal antibodies, DF3 and 115 D8. CA 15-3 may be a more sensitive marker of metastatic breast cancer with only a small loss of specificity. A CA 15-3 value of 30 units/ml approximates a CEA of 5 ng/ml. Both CA 15-3 and CEA are abnormally high in most patients with liver metastases, but CA 15-3 is more likely to be abnormal in patients with local recurrences and bone metastases. Preliminary data suggest that changes in CA 15-3 levels accurately reflect disease progression and regression.[350]

USE OF ENDOCRINE THERAPY

Breast cancer is one of the few human tumors very responsive to endocrine therapy. The mechanism of this response is not fully understood. The simplest explanation is that breast cancer growth is directly dependent on a hormone, most likely estrogen.[354,355] However, human breast cancer cell lines have recently been shown to secrete growth factors, such as transforming growth factor (TGF). In estrogen-sensitive cell lines, such as the MCF-7, the secretion of growth factors appears to be controlled by estrogen and mediated through the estrogen receptor.[42] In cell lines without ER, secretion of growth factors appears to be independent of estrogen. These growth factors may stimulate the tumor cell from which they have been secreted (autocrine stimulation) or neighboring cells (paracrine stimulation). It is possible that estrogen may affect the growth of estrogen-independent cells through the release of paracrine growth factors from estrogen-dependent cells. In this way, the destruction of a very small number of estrogen-dependent cells could, theoretically, affect the growth of many estrogen-independent cells as well, and this might account for the apparent benefits from adjuvant tamoxifen given to patients whose tumors are ER-negative (see above).

Simple estrogen dependence does not fully explain the clinical phenomena observed during endocrine therapy. Patients who respond to one type of endocrine therapy are very likely to respond to a second, a third, and on occasion even to a fourth or fifth sequential endocrine maneuver. For example, a postmenopausal woman may respond to the administration of estrogens, have a secondary response to the discontinuance of the estrogen therapy when her tumor regrows after an initial response, and have a tertiary response to major ablative therapy, such as adrenalectomy, after the estrogen withdrawal response. It is difficult to understand why the same tumor responds to both the addition and the removal of estrogens. In addition, breast cancer is responsive to endocrine therapies such as progestins, androgens, and corticosteroids that do not involve estrogens. The "endocrine" therapy most widely used today, tamoxifen, has a cytotoxic effect independent of its ability to block estrogen uptake into tumor cells.[356]

The effects of all forms of endocrine therapy appear to be mediated through receptors, especially the ER. Although about one of three unselected patients will respond to endocrine therapy, the response rate among patients with ER is about twice that (Table 38-32). Patients whose tumors are without ER have a very low probability of responding, less than 10% in most series, whereas patients with a high receptor value have an even greater probability of responding (Table 38-33).[357,358] The receptor value likely reflects the total percentage of tumor cells that are ER positive, and cancer-cell death following endocrine therapy is likely to be greater in patients with higher receptor values. As a result, the durability of response among patients with high receptor values will also be greater.[357]

Patients whose tumors have both ER and PR have a higher response rate to a variety of endocrine therapies than do patients whose tumors have ER without PR (Table 38-33). Because the PR are produced only in cells with functional ER, very few tumors have been found to be ER negative and PR positive. In fact, these few patients may have a false-negative ER assay.[359] However, patients with high ER values are more likely to have PR than those with lower ER values. In one study 40% of tumors were PR positive if the ER was between 3 and 10 fmol/mg, 70% were PR positive if the ER level was 10 to 100 fmol/mg, and 77% were PR positive if the ER exceeded 100 fmol/mg.[496] There may be no advantage in determining both ER and PR values over careful quantification of ER alone.

Receptor information should be combined with other clinical characteristics to select those patients most likely to benefit from endocrine therapy. The clinical characteristics usually associated with endocrine response include a long disease-free interval, usually more than 2 years; disease localized to bone and soft tissues; late premenopausal or late postmenopausal status; and a prior response to endocrine therapy. In one study, 60% of patients with ER and a disease-free interval greater than 10 months responded to endocrine therapy, whereas only 25% of patients who were receptor-positive with a disease-free interval of less than 10 months responded.[360] The response to a second endocrine maneuver was 50% among ER-positive patients who had previously responded to another endocrine maneuver, whereas the response rate was only 30% among the ER-positive patients who had failed the first endocrine therapy.

Choice of Endocrine Therapy

In general, there is little evidence that the response rate or survival benefit from one endocrine therapy is superior to

TABLE 38-32. Endocrine Therapy for Metastatic Breast Cancer: Response (%) and Toxicity (Therapies Listed in Order of Increasing Toxicity)

Endocrine Therapy	Patient Group			Major Toxicities
	Unselected	ERP+	ERP–	
Tamoxifen*	32	54	9	Nausea, hot flashes, "flare," hypercalcemia, thrombocytopenia
Oophorectomy†	33	62	6	Surgical complications, hot flashes
Progestins*	31	(35)§	8	Weight gain, fluid retention, nausea, vaginal bleeding, hotflashes
Aminoglutethimide‡	31	54	6	Lethargy, dizziness/ataxia, rash, Cushingoid symptoms, nausea
LHRH analogues	42	–	–	Hot flashes, nausea, headache
Estrogens*	26	57	9	Nausea and vomiting, fluid retention, incontinence, vaginal bleeding, "flare," hypercalcemia
Androgens*	21	43	8	Masculinization, nausea, weight gain, "flare," hypercalcemia
Adrenalectomy*	32	46	10	Surgical mortality, Addisonian crises, Cushingoid symptoms
Hypophysectomy*	36	–	–	Surgical mortality, Addisonian crises, diabetes insipidus, anosmia

Modified from Henderson IC: Endocrine therapy in metastatic breast cancer. In Harris JR, Hellman S, Henderson IC, Kinne DW (eds): Breast Diseases, pp 398–428. Philadelphia, JB Lippincott, 1987.
* Primarily postmenopausal patients.
† Exclusively premenopausal patients.
‡ Exclusively postmenopausal patients.
§ See text commentary

that achieved with other such therapies.[361] Tamoxifen, oophorectomy, progestins, aminoglutethimide, estrogens, adrenalectomy, and hypophysectomy have been shown to be equivalent in many randomized trials. However, androgen therapy has a lower response rate than estrogens[362] or tamoxifen,[363] and corticosteroids, although they have not been compared with other endocrine therapies in randomized trials, are thought to be less effective on the basis of historical comparisons.

Because most endocrine therapies are equally effective, the choice of a particular one is based primarily on toxicity. The various endocrine therapies are listed in Table 38-32 in order of increasing toxicity, tamoxifen being associated with the least toxicity and adrenalectomy or hypophysectomy with the greatest. Luteinizing-hormone–releasing hormone (LHRH) analogues are still relatively untested forms of endocrine therapy and have not yet been evaluated in randomized trials. Thus, the full range of toxicity is unknown, as is their precise role relative to other forms of endocrine therapy. In premenopausal and postmenopausal patients, tamoxifen is the treatment of choice. Premenopausal patients who respond may later be treated with oophorectomy, then progestins, and finally aminoglutethimide as long as they respond before progression on the previous regimen. Second-

TABLE 38-33. Response to Endocrine Therapy Correlated with Either ER Value or ER and PR Status

ER Value (fmol/mg)	Response Rate (%)*	Frequency PR Positive (%)†	Combined ER/PR Status	Response Rate (%)†
<3	6	9	ER–/PR–	9
3–10		40		
	46		ER+/PR–	32
10–100		70		
>100	81	77	ER+/PR+	71

* McGuire WL, Horwitz KB, Zava DT et al: Progress in endocrinology and metabolism: Hormones in breast cancer: Update 1978. Metabolism 27:487–501, 1978.
† Clark GM, McGuire WL: Progesterone receptors and human breast cancer. Breast Cancer Res Treat 3:157–163, 1983.

ary endocrine therapies in postmenopausal women could be administered in the sequence: progestins, aminoglutethimide, and estrogens.

Tamoxifen

Tamoxifen is usually administered in a dose of 10 mg twice daily. It has been shown in randomized trials that there is no advantage for higher doses of therapy.[364-367] Moreover, long-term administration of very high doses of tamoxifen (*e.g.*, 12 months of 60–100 mg/m² twice daily) has been associated with decreased visual acuity and a retinopathy.[368]

With a dose schedule of 10 mg twice daily, serum tamoxifen levels rise gradually to reach a steady state at about week 16.[369] The half-life of a single dose of tamoxifen is 9 to 12 hours, but the half-life of a chronic dose is 7 days. Circulating plasma levels can be detected 6 weeks after discontinuation of therapy.[369] As a result, the beneficial effects are not likely to be affected if patients miss one or even several doses. Because circulating tamoxifen may result in a false-negative ER determination, at least 6 weeks should elapse after discontinuing tamoxifen before performing a biopsy for receptor determination.

The effectiveness of tamoxifen in premenopausal women has been compared with oophorectomy in two randomized trials.[370,371] In the larger of these studies, there was no difference in the overall response rate to tamoxifen and oophorectomy.[371] The secondary response rate to oophorectomy after tamoxifen treatment was somewhat higher than that to tamoxifen (p = 0.045). The median time to treatment failure, response duration, and survival rate of patients randomized to oophorectomy or tamoxifen were nearly identical. The secondary response rate to oophorectomy following tamoxifen treatment was 33%; to tamoxifen following oophorectomy, 11%.[370] Although there are isolated case reports of patients responding to oophorectomy after tamoxifen failure, the probability of a secondary response to oophorectomy is much higher in patients who have an initial response to tamoxifen. In fact, the initial response to tamoxifen is a better predictor of the response to subsequent oophorectomy than is receptor status.[372]

Tamoxifen is remarkably nontoxic. Less than 10% of patients will experience mild and transient nausea that rarely requires discontinuation of therapy and can sometimes be alleviated if the patient takes tamoxifen before meals. Tamoxifen may cause a transient thrombocytopenia or leukopenia, but this rarely requires treatment or even careful monitoring. Thrombophlebitis has been observed to be increased in 1% to 3% of patients.[373] There is one report of an increased incidence of endometrial carcinoma in patients receiving tamoxifen, but this finding has not yet been confirmed by other observers.[266] A tumor "flare" or hypercalcemia occurs in 4% to 5% of patients (see below).

Ablation Therapy

Adrenalectomy and hypophysectomy are very effective endocrine therapy and were once commonly employed. More recently, these modalities have been abandoned because of the development of treatments with less toxicity. The overall operative mortality rate with these major forms of ablation was about 5%, but in the hands of inexperienced surgeons, it reached to 17% to 25%.[374] In addition, adrenalectomy and hypophysectomy cause permanent endocrine defects that necessitate life-long replacement, usually with corticosteroids.

Ovarian ablation is still commonly used and is considered by many specialists to be the endocrine therapy of choice for premenopausal women. Ablation of ovarian function may be obtained by either surgery or radiation. Although there are no randomized trials comparing these two methods, historical comparisons suggest that the response rates are equivalent.[361] However, the time to response after radiation ablation may be longer than that after surgical oophorectomy. Many patients undergo an inadvertent ovarian ablation when radiation therapy is administered to bone metastases in the pelvis or lumbosacral spine. When these areas are irradiated in a patient who is otherwise a good candidate for endocrine therapy, the patient should be evaluated initially for the response to ovarian ablation before another form of endocrine therapy is employed.

The best responses to ovarian ablation are seen in women over the age of 35 who are either still menstruating or within 1 year of the last menstrual period. Response rates to ovarian ablation in women younger than 35 are usually below 20%.[375,376] The response rate in postmenopausal women is less than 6%, and oophorectomy should never be employed in this group.[375,377,378] The operative mortality rate with surgical oophorectomy is low, usually less than 2% to 3%. In appropriately selected patients, the operative mortality rate is even lower. The principal side effects of this procedure are menopausal symptoms, especially hot flashes.

Aminoglutethimide and Corticosteroids

Corticosteroids are rarely used alone, because the response rate is thought to be lower than that to other forms of endocrine therapy. However, about 25% of patients will respond to corticosteroids.[379] Corticosteroids cause Cushingoid symptoms and osteoporosis when used for long periods of time. However, their value in palliating symptoms such as shortness of breath and bone pain, as well as their ability to improve the patient's overall sense of well-being, should not be overlooked, especially in the terminal phases of the disease.

Aminoglutethimide, given with corticosteroids, is among the more effective and less toxic forms of endocrine therapy. Aminoglutethimide blocks steroid hydroxylation and cleavage enzymes, including cholesterol sidechain cleavage in the initial step of steroidogenesis in the adrenal gland. However, aromatase reactions are more sensitive to the effects of aminoglutethimide.[380] For example, the concentration of aminoglutethimide required to block the conversion of androstenedione to estrone or the conversion of testosterone to estradiol is approximately one-tenth that required to block the cholesterol side chain cleavage. For this reason, it is thought that the principal site of aminoglutethimide action is outside the adrenal gland in fat tissue or within the breast itself.

The standard dose of aminoglutethimide is 250 mg orally

four times per day. Hydrocortisone, 40 mg per day divided into three or four doses, is usually administered with aminoglutethimide. Aminoglutethimide is effective at much lower doses and without hydrocortisone, but dose reduction does not decrease toxicity proportionately.[381] Aminoglutethimide at a dose of 250 mg twice daily will result in the same degree of estrogen suppression as 250 mg four times a day,[382] and this lower dose of aminoglutethimide might be considered an acceptable alternative to 250 mg four times daily. However, neither dose has been specifically approved by the Food and Drug Administration (FDA) for general use in the treatment of breast cancer in the United States.

Aminoglutethimide has been compared with tamoxifen, adrenalectomy, and hypophysectomy in randomized trials. In general, response rates are equivalent, but in several trials, aminoglutethimide plus hydrocortisone appeared to be more effective than tamoxifen in patients with bone metastases.[383,384]

Aminoglutethimide is somewhat more toxic than tamoxifen, oophorectomy, or progestins, although most of the toxicities disappear within 6 weeks of the initiation of therapy.[385] Aminoglutethimide is chemically related to the sedative glutethimide (Doriden), so it is not surprising that approximately one-third of the patients experience lethargy. However, this side-effect can be circumvented by the initial use of a dose of 250 mg twice daily. When this lower dose of aminoglutethimide is given with a full dose of corticosteroids, the patient is likely to experience euphoria, insomnia, and other signs of steroid excess. Approximately one of five patients will develop a rash during the first weeks of aminoglutethimide therapy. This is not an indication for discontinuation of aminoglutethimide, and it can be alleviated by a transient doubling of the steroid dose (e.g., to 80 mg of hydrocortisone a day). Between 2% and 3% of the patients experience Cushingoid symptoms, which can be alleviated by a decrease in the hydrocortisone replacement dose. Addisonian crises are rare among patients who are given any steroid replacement. Patients may have a transient thrombocytopenia or, less commonly, leukopenia. On several occasions, this has been reported to be life threatening. However, in all instances, the thrombocytopenia and leukopenia appeared between weeks two and seven.[386] Monitoring platelet and leukocyte counts during this interval is therefore recommended.

Progestins

This group of compounds was once considered ineffective for the treatment of breast cancer, but more recent studies have shown that both medroxyprogesterone acetate and megestrol acetate are as active as any of the other endocrine therapies commonly used. Although there are no direct comparisons of these two forms of progestational therapy, they appear to be equally effective. Medroxyprogesterone acetate is more frequently used in Europe and megestrol acetate in the United States. Each has been compared in randomized trials with tamoxifen, and there are no differences in the response rates.[361] Although the summary response rate to progestins suggests that these agents are less effective than other endocrine therapies among ER-positive patients (see

Table 38-32), this may reflect the fact that progestins were used as second- or third-line therapy in most of the studies used to calculate this summary response rate. It is premature to conclude that receptor status is unimportant in the selection of patients for the use of progestins.

Although uncontrolled early studies suggested that there might be an advantage to the use of high doses of medroxyprogesterone acetate, this has not been confirmed in randomized trials comparing two doses of this progestin.[361] Moreover, high doses of medroxyprogesterone acetate are associated with more side effects, including an increased incidence of gluteal abscesses, facies lunaris, increased sweating, and fine tremors. There are similar but more recent reports from uncontrolled trials that high doses of megestrol acetate increase the response rate.[387] This remains to be evaluated in controlled trials. In the absence of good evidence for a dose–response correlation, it is recommended that megestrol acetate be administered at a dose of 40 mg four times daily and that medroxyprogesterone acetate be limited to a total dose of 400 mg per day.

The principal toxicity of both of these progestational agents is weight gain, which may occur in 20% to 50% of patients and appears to be dose related.[388] Patients experiencing weight gain may have fluid retention, but it is not certain that fluid is responsible for all of the weight gain. Vaginal bleeding occurs in 5% to 10% of patients either while the patients are taking the progestational agent or when it is discontinued. Somewhat less than 10% of patients experience hot flashes.

Estrogens and Androgens

This group of compounds is rarely used today because estrogens and androgens are more toxic than the other drugs discussed thus far. For example, approximately one-third of patients placed on estrogens will discontinue them because of toxic side-effects, the most important of which are vomiting and fluid retention. Androgens may be associated with a marked improvement in the patient's sense of well-being but are also associated with masculinization, including hoarseness, hirsutism, and acne, in more than 50% of patients. Also, androgens are the endocrine therapy most often associated with "flare" (see below). However, both estrogens and androgens may be useful as third- or fourth-line treatment and are certainly preferable to the major ablative procedures. For example, estrogens might be used in an older patient who has previously responded to tamoxifen and progestational agents. Also, estrogen would be preferred to aminoglutethimide, especially in a patient over age 70, because of the increased frequency of lethargy and CNS effects associated with the latter drug. Androgens are occasionally useful in an older population with congestive heart failure, because androgen use is not accompanied by fluid retention, whereas both progestins and estrogens can exacerbate congestive heart failure.

The estrogens used most frequently are diethylstilbestrol (DES) (5 mg three times daily), ethinyl estradiol (1 mg three times daily), or Premarin (2.5 mg three times daily). The doses of estrogens used for palliation of metastatic breast cancer are usually higher than those commonly used to alleviate postmenopausal symptoms, but the evidence that higher doses of estrogens are more effective than lower doses is weak.[389] It is appropriate to use half doses of estrogen during the first month of therapy, with a gradual increase in dosage as the patient experiences fewer side-effects. There is no evidence that estrogens stimulate tumor growth in premenopausal patients with breast cancer, but estrogens are not effective in these patients.[390] About one-third of patients who respond to estrogens will have a withdrawal response if estrogens are discontinued at the first evidence of tumor regrowth.

Androgens have been shown in randomized trials to be less effective than estrogens.[361] All of the effective androgens tested have masculinizing effects. The androgen most commonly used today is fluoxymesterone (Halotestin) at a dose of 10 mg orally two to four times daily.

LHRH Analogues

The LHRH analogues have only recently been introduced and cannot be considered standard therapies for breast cancer at present. Both buserelin and leuprolide have been used in premenopausal and postmenopausal women.[391-393] Leuprolide has been more extensively tested, and in one study, 12 of 31 (39%) postmenopausal women and 11 of 25 (44%) premenopausal women responded.[392,394] These compounds are associated with minimal toxicity, but premenopausal women develop amenorrhea and postmenopausal symptoms. If further studies show similar response rates with low toxicity, it is possible that these compounds will soon become more widely used for breast cancer therapy, especially in premenopausal women.

Endocrine Therapy Combinations

A variety of endocrine therapies have been utilized in combination. This includes tamoxifen with fluoxymesterone, tamoxifen with DES, tamoxifen with aminoglutethimide, tamoxifen with medroxyprogesterone acetate, and tamoxifen with both aminoglutethimide and danazol. Although there is a trend in a few of these studies toward higher response rates among patients given two or more endocrine therapies, only one study has demonstrated an improvement in the overall survival rate.

Recently, randomized trials have been conducted comparing oophorectomy alone and oophorectomy plus prednisone in premenopausal women and tamoxifen alone versus tamoxifen plus prednisone in postmenopausal women. In both an initial study and a confirmatory study, there was a significant increase in the response rate when prednisone was added to either of the other two forms of endocrine therapy. In one of these two trials, there was a significant improvement in survival as well.[395,396]

Flare

Patients given almost any form of endocrine therapy may experience new symptoms or an exacerbation of old symptoms of their cancers beginning a few hours to a few days after initiation of therapy and subsiding spontaneously within a month. Most commonly, these symptoms consist of a diffuse achiness or increase in pain at sites of known metastases. There may be a transient erythema and slight swelling around skin or soft-tissue lesions. The serum CEA concentration may increase transiently. The most serious side-effect is hypercalcemia. The underlying mechanism for flare is not understood, but patients who experience these side-effects are as likely to go on to respond to endocrine therapy as are patients who do not have such side-effects. Flare has been most frequently observed in patients treated with androgens, tamoxifen, estrogens, and progestins. The incidence of this side-effect ranges from 3% to 9% in various studies.[361] Aminoglutethimide has not been reported to cause flare. However, rare instances of flare have been observed following oophorectomy and adrenalectomy.[397]

USE OF CHEMOTHERAPY

Combination chemotherapy will induce an objective response in approximately two-thirds of patients previously unexposed to chemotherapy, but complete eradication of disease at all sites will occur in less than 20%. The median duration of the response is usually less than 1 year (Table 38-34). The subjective response rate is higher than the objective response rate.[398] The median survival after the first course of chemotherapy is usually in excess of 3 years. However, these "average" figures mask the dramatic response that sometimes occurs: patients bedridden with bone pain not infrequently return to work for periods of several years. Although the numbers of patients with a long but unmaintained remission is small, there are reports of increasing numbers of such patients living almost symptom-free 5 to more than 10 years after completion of a course of chemotherapy.[399-402]

The time to the appearance of a response among breast cancer patients contrasts sharply with experience in patients with lymphomas, testicular cancers, and other tumors especially responsive to combination chemotherapy. The median time to response has ranged from 2 to 3 months in most studies, but this period is dependent in large part on the site of measurable disease. Thus, the median time to the appearance of a response is between 3 and 6 weeks in the skin and

TABLE 38-34.   Response to and Survival after Treatment with Commonly Used Drug Combinations for Metastatic Breast Cancer

Percentage of patients with a response	43–82
Percentage with a complete response	4–27
Time to response (wk)	
Median	7–14
Maximum	72
Duration of response (mo)	
Median	5.3–13
Maximum	180+
Survival of responders (mo)	
Median	14.8–33
Maximum	180+

Modified from Henderson IC: Chemotherapy for advanced disease. In Harris JR, Hellman S, Henderson IC, Kinne DW (eds): Breast Diseases, pp 428–479. Philadelphia, JB Lippincott, 1987.

lymph nodes, 6 and 9 weeks in the lung, about 15 weeks in the liver, and nearly 18 weeks in the bones.[403,404] Practically, this means that a physician should not be discouraged if a response is not immediately apparent and should continue therapy until there is unequivocal evidence of progressive disease (see below regarding duration of chemotherapy). The possibility of disease progression during the first weeks of therapy may be suggested by new lesions on bone scans, increased intensity in old bone scan lesions, and transient elevations of CEA. The possibility of a "flare" following the administration of chemotherapy, similar to that described above for endocrine therapy, has not been carefully studied. However, it is known that some patients may have increased bone pain after chemotherapy begins before having a good response.

Identifying Chemotherapy-Responsive Patients

There are no well-defined clinical characteristics or established tests to identify patients likely to benefit from chemotherapy. This is in contrast to the situation described for endocrine therapy. Patients with metastatic breast cancer who should be treated with chemotherapy include all those who are symptomatic and who have either not responded or are very unlikely to respond to endocrine therapy based on the sites of metastases, disease-free interval, menstrual status, or ER status.

The profile of patients who have the highest response rates to chemotherapy is otherwise quite similar to the profile of patients who respond to endocrine therapy (Table 38-35). Responding patients with a long disease-free interval are more likely to have a durable response. Patients with only a few sites of metastatic disease are more likely to respond and to have a durable response to chemotherapy. Almost all studies have found that patients with a good performance status have a higher response rate than patients who are less than fully ambulatory, an important consideration in the use of historical controls in the evaluation of high- or low-dose chemotherapy regimens. Patients with a good performance status are more likely to tolerate high doses of chemotherapy, and this may erroneously lead to the conclusion that higher doses of drugs are more likely to induce a response.[398] Patients whose disease progresses during chemotherapy have a lower probability of response to a different type of chemotherapy. However, this is not necessarily true for patients who are given a chemotherapy combination after some interval during which they have received no chemotherapy of any type.

Twenty years ago, there were very few chemotherapy agents used routinely for the treatment of breast cancer, and new drugs were introduced earlier in the course of the patient's disease. Phase II studies of new agents are now performed in patients with more advanced disease who have had extensive prior chemotherapy and who have a poor performance status. A comparison of the response to a recently studied new agent with the response to an agent first studied 20 years ago thus may lead to the erroneous conclusion that the current drug is less effective.

Patients who do not respond to endocrine therapy are as likely to respond to chemotherapy as patients who are

TABLE 38-35. Identifying Patients with Metastatic Breast Cancer Most Likely to Benefit from Chemotherapy

Factors Associated with:
Increased Probability of Response
Good performance status
Ambulatory status
Limited number (1–2) of disease sites
Prior hormone therapy
Metastases to lymph nodes
High labelling indices
High thymidine kinase levels
Increased Response Duration or Survival
Good performance status
Disease-free interval
Limited number of disease sites
Prior hormone therapy
Prior response to hormone therapy
Decreased Probability of Response
Bone metastases
Liver metastases
Prior chemotherapy
Prior radiotherapy
Decreased lymphocyte count
Decreased Response Duration or Survival
Prior radiotherapy
Decreased lymphocyte count
Factors Not Associated with Response Rate:
Age
Menopausal status
Dominant disease site
Carcinoembryonic antigen
Receptor status

Modified from Henderson IC: Chemotherapy for advanced disease. In Bonadonna G (ed): Breast Cancer: Diagnosis and Management, pp 274–280. New York, John Wiley & Sons, 1984.

treated with chemotherapy as a primary modality. In a recent trial, patients were randomized to receive chemotherapy alone or tamoxifen alone. Patients who did not respond to the initial therapy were crossed over to the other therapy.[338] The primary response to chemotherapy in this study was 45%, and the secondary response to chemotherapy among those who did not respond to tamoxifen was 35%. The failure to respond to endocrine therapy appeared to have little or no effect on the subsequent response to chemotherapy.

On the basis of in vitro and animal models, one might anticipate that the most responsive patients would be those with the most rapidly growing tumors, possibly receptor-negative tumors. For example, the response to chemotherapy in vitro is twice as high in cell lines with a short doubling time and no ER as in receptor-positive cell lines with a long doubling time.[405] In clinical studies, however, ER status has not proved helpful in selecting chemoresponsive patients.[398] In five of seven studies performed to correlate response to chemotherapy and receptor status, the response rate among patients with receptor-positive tumors was higher than or equal to that in patients with receptor-negative tumors. Other potential markers of patients with high-growth-fraction tumors have been less extensively studied. In one small study, chemotherapy responders were found to have an average labeling index twice as high as that observed in patients who did not respond to chemotherapy.[406] The response rate to chemotherapy of tumors with a high thymidine kinase level was significantly greater than that of tumors with a low level of this enzyme (86% and 13%, respectively; p < 0.001).[407] Although promising, these data are too limited to recommend the use of labeling indices routinely to select patients for chemotherapy.

Active Drugs

Most chemotherapeutic agents active in the treatment of other cancers have at least some activity against breast cancer as well. However, the alkylating agents and the anthracyclines are the main components of most standard regimens. Cyclophosphamide is the most active of these agents, but thiotepa, L-PAM, and chlorambucil are also active. The relative effectiveness of these alkylating agents has never been determined in controlled trials. Cyclophosphamide may be given intravenously or orally. Chlorambucil and L-PAM have less acute toxicity but may be associated with a higher incidence of delayed toxicity, especially late leukemia.[263,408]

The anthracyclines are the most active drugs used as single agents, and doxorubicin has been shown effective against tumors resistant to cyclophosphamide.[409] In some studies, doxorubicin alone has been as active as the drug combinations CFP or CMFVP.[410,411] Although doxorubicin has conventionally been given as an intravenous bolus every 3 weeks, continuous administration over 48 to 96 hours and weekly administration schedules are less cardiotoxic.[412] Although both the continuous and weekly schedules are known to be effective for breast cancer, only the weekly schedule has been shown in a randomized trial to be as effective as a 3-weekly schedule.[413] 4'Epidoxorubicin has been as effective as doxorubicin in a number of randomized trials.[398] Although cardiotoxicity from 4'epidoxorubicin may be less than that from doxorubicin, it is not firmly established that the therapeutic index for 4'epidoxorubicin is really superior.

Although usually incorporated into second-line regimens, there is considerable evidence that mitomycin C and vinblastine are effective against tumors resistant to doxorubicin and cyclophosphamide. The response rate for mitomycin C, shown in Table 38-36, has been determined exclusively in patients refractory to other drugs. Although mitomycin C has recently been included in some first-line regimens, its principal use is still for the treatment of patients refractory to doxorubicin.

Vincristine is frequently used in combination programs for breast cancer, probably because it is not myelosuppressive and so does not compromise the doses of other drugs used in the combination. However, vincristine does cause neurotoxicity, and the incidence of severe neurotoxicity was high in the Phase II studies originally performed to demonstrate that it had any activity.[398] Five randomized trials have shown that vincristine adds nothing to combination chemotherapy. For example, when the regimen CMFP was compared with CMFVP in 427 patients,[414] there was no significant advantage in response rate or survival for patients given CMFVP. Also, doxorubicin alone was compared with the combination of doxorubicin and vincristine in randomized trials that enrolled 109 patients,[415] and the response rate was not sig-

TABLE 38-36. Cytotoxic Drugs Active for Treating Breast Cancer

Drug	Response Rate (%) in Phase II Trials
4'-epidoxorubicin	34
Cyclophosphamide	33
Doxorubicin	32
Thiotepa	29
Methotrexate	28
Elliptinium	27
5-fluorouracil	27
Prednimustine	26
Vindesine	23
Mitomycin C	22
Vinblastine	21
L-Phenylalanine mustard	20
Mitoxantrone	20
Chlorambucil	17
Mitolactol	17

Modified from Henderson IC: Chemotherapy for advanced disease. In Harris JR, Hellman S, Henderson IC (eds): Breast Diseases, pp 428–479. Philadelphia, JB Lippincott, 1987.

nificantly higher for the combination than for patients receiving doxorubicin alone. The use of vincristine for early or metastatic breast cancer is not recommended.

Two other vinca alkaloids are effective. Vinblastine has recently been used as a 5-day continuous infusion, with a response rate of 37% in 106 patients, all of whom were considered refractory to doxorubicin.[416] Studies of bolus infusion of vinblastine are more limited, but the drug is active in this schedule as well. There are no randomized comparisons of the relative efficacy of bolus and continuous-infusion vinblastine. The other active vinca alkaloid, vindesine, has less neurotoxicity than vincristine and causes less myelosuppression than vinblastine. In randomized trials, vindesine has been as active as vinblastine and considerably more active than vincristine.[417,418] However, vindesine has not yet been approved by the FDA for general use in the treatment of metastatic breast cancer.

Other active drugs for breast cancer are listed in Table 38-36. Methotrexate and 5-FU are frequently used in combination, and methotrexate may be given intrathecally or orally to treat carcinomatous meningitis from metastatic breast cancer.[419] Methotrexate is also effective at moderate or high doses with leukovorin rescue, but it has not been demonstrated in controlled trials that there is any therapeutic advantage to the use of higher doses of methotrexate with leukovorin rescue instead of more conventional doses.[420,421] Mitoxantrone and prednimustine are much less toxic but also somewhat less effective than standard agents. Mitolactol has been used in a number of experimental combination programs but has not been shown to be superior to other alkylating agents in controlled trials and may have an unusual degree of tumorgenicity. Elliptinium appears to be very active for breast cancer and has a unique set of side-effects. However, it also does not have a place in the standard treatment of this disease. Several Phase II trials enrolling more than 100 patients failed to show much activity for cisplatin.[398] In one randomized trial, there was no advantage for CAP (49%) compared to CFP (46%).[422] However, two trials have used cisplatin in breast cancer patients not previously exposed to any form of chemotherapy, and in both studies, cisplatin appeared to be active. In one of these trials, cisplatin was used as a single agent,[423] and in the other, cisplatin was compared in a combination, CAP, with a more conventional CMVP.[424] Cisplatin appears to be cross-resistant with the agents most commonly used for breast cancer, and has no established role in the treatment of this disease, but may be an active drug nonetheless.

Drug Combinations

Several randomized trials have been performed to compare the relative efficacy of a single cytotoxic agent and a combination regimen.[398] In most of these studies, the response rate with the combination program was significantly higher, frequently twice as high, as that to the single agent. However, many of these studies were performed to determine if the additional toxicity associated with combination therapy resulted in sufficient benefit to justify its routine use, and the single agents may have been used at less-than-optimal doses. When a very intense program of cyclophosphamide was compared with the combination of CMF plus vinblastine, the efficacy of the two programs was nearly identical,[425] but a lower dose of cyclophosphamide was less effective than CMFVP.[426] Doxorubicin alone has been shown in several studies to be as effective as a combination program. Several randomized trials compared the strategy of sequential single agents with simultaneous use of all the same agents initially. Survival was marginally shorter and the total time spent in remission considerably less for patients treated with sequential single agents.[427,428] None of these studies systematically evaluated the quality of life. The duration of response and length of survival of responders to a single agent are nearly identical to those of responders to a combination. In some instances, the net quality of life may be better with a single agent rather than a combination.

The combinations most frequently utilized for the treatment of metastatic breast cancer are shown in Table 38-37. CMFP represents a truncation of the original Cooper regimen, which utilized CMFVP. As noted above, randomized trials have demonstrated that vincristine adds nothing to the regimen. However, two separate studies have demonstrated that the response rate to CMFP is higher than that to CMF alone. Prednisone may contribute to the efficacy of the regimen because of a direct antitumor effect. However, patients treated with CMFP have significantly less nausea and vomiting and have higher nadir leukocyte counts. As a result, patients treated with CMFP receive higher doses of cyclophosphamide, methotrexate, and 5-FU than patients treated with 5-FU alone.[429,430] The addition of prednisone may cause additional toxicity in some patients, including an increase in the incidence of infection, insomnia, or psychological sequelae. When these symptoms occur, it is advisable to discontinue the prednisone. In the standard CMFP program (Table 38-37), methotrexate and 5-FU are administered together. Attempts to increase the efficacy of CMFP by administering methotrexate and 5-FU sequentially with intervals of 1 to 24 hours have not been universally successful.[396] In conventional CMFP regimens, cyclophosphamide is given orally daily for 14 days. Because cyclophosphamide is effective when administered intravenously, CMF has also been given as an entirely intravenous regimen. However, a recently published randomized trial comparing intravenous CMF with conventional CMF demonstrated both a higher response rate to and a survival advantage for the conventional program.[431]

TABLE 38-37.   Combination Chemotherapy Regimens Commonly Used to Treat Metastatic Breast Cancer

Regimen	Dose (mg/m²)	Route	Day of Cycle Given	Cycle Length (wk)
CMF (P)*†				
Cyclophosphamide	100	PO	1–14	
Methotrexate	40–60	IV	1 + 8	
5-Fluorouracil	600–700	IV	1 + 8	4
(Prednisone)	(40)	(PO)	(1–14)	
CA‡				
Cyclophosphamide	200	PO	3–6	3–4
Adriamycin	40	IV	1	
CAF§¶				
Cyclophosphamide	400–500	IV	1	
Adriamycin	40–50	IV	1	3
5-Fluorouracil	400–500	IV	1 + 8	

* Canellos GP, DeVita V, Gold GL et al: Cyclical combination chemotherapy for advanced breast cancer. Br Med J 1:218–220, 1974.
† Canellos GP, Pocock S, Taylor S et al: Combination chemotherapy for metastatic breast carcinoma. Cancer 38:1882–1886, 1976.
‡ Jones SE, Durie BGM, Salmon SE: Combination chemotherapy with Adriamycin and cyclophosphamide for advanced breast cancer. Cancer 36:90–97, 1975.
§ Bull J, Tormey D, Li SH, et al: A randomized comparative trial of Adriamycin versus methotrexate in combination drug therapy. Cancer 41:1649–1657, 1978.
¶ Smalley R, Carpenter J, Bartolucci A, Vogel C, Krauss S: A comparison of cyclophosphamide, Adriamycin, 5-fluorouracil (CAF) and cyclophosphamide, methotrexate, 5-fluorouracil, vincristine, prednisone (CMFVP) in patients with metastatic breast cancer. Cancer 40:625–632, 1977.

Combination programs that include doxorubicin produce a 15% to 20% higher response rate than identical regimens without doxorubicin.[398] The median duration of response and survival after treatment with a doxorubicin combination is 3 to 6 months longer, but in randomized trials, this difference usually has not been statistically significant. In the largest of these studies, patients were randomized to received CAF, CAFVP, or CMF.[432] Patients treated with CAF and CAFVP had a significantly higher response rate, and the median survival of patients treated with CAF was almost 11 months longer than that of patients treated with CMFVP. However, patients treated with CAFVP had only a 1.5-month prolongation of median survival, and this difference was not significant. In most studies, the doxorubicin combination has been associated with significantly more toxicity, and the rather dramatic alopecia that follows treatment with doxorubicin is unacceptable to many patients. The advantages of a doxorubicin-containing regimen as the initial treatment of patients with metastatic disease must be carefully weighed against the additional toxicity of these regimens and the fact that patients have fewer remaining alternative treatments for palliation at the time of further disease progression.

Secondary and Tertiary Treatments

The probability of a secondary response to chemotherapy among patients whose disease worsens while they are receiving a first combination regimen is between 20% and 35%, depending on whether the previous regimen included doxorubicin. Patients who have been treated with chemotherapy but whose disease progresses after an interval during which chemotherapy was not given (*e.g.*, 6 months or more) have a much higher probability of a secondary response, including a secondary response to the regimen to which they previously responded.

The response to secondary chemotherapy among patients without prior exposure to doxorubicin is approximately 35% (range 17%–54% in 17 separate studies). The median duration of response ranged from 4 to 11.5 months, and the median duration of survival ranged from 7 to 16 months.[398] The response rate to doxorubicin as a single agent in these patients was usually between 30% and 40%. Two combination programs have been reported to have relatively high response rates. One, VATH, has a reported response rate between 45% and 53%, a median duration of response of almost 1 year, and a median survival between 13 and 16 months.[433,434] The second program consists of 5-FU, vincristine (Oncovin), doxorubicin (Adriamycin), and mitomycin C (FOAM). The number of patients treated with this regimen is larger. The reported response rate is 35%, the median duration of response is 7 months, and the median survival is 9 months.[435] Studies of patients already exposed to doxorubicin are more likely to include extensively treated patients with exposure to at least two separate combination programs. The overall response to chemotherapy in these patients is about 21% (range 0–40% in 11 separate studies), with a median survival of 4 to 6 months and a median duration of response of 2 to 8 months.[398] A particularly popular combination for this group of patients includes mitomycin C, 20 mg/m^2 intra-

venously on day one, and vinblastine, 0.5 mg/kg intravenously on days one and twenty-eight, administered on a 6- to 8-week cycle. This regimen is associated with severe myelosuppression, neurologic complications, and pulmonary toxicity.[436] The highest response rate observed in three trials evaluating the combination of mitomycin C and vinblastine was 40%, with a median duration of response of 4 months.[436–438]

No controlled studies have compared the relative efficacy of doxorubicin alone with that of a doxorubicin combination or of mitomycin C alone with that of the combination of mitomycin C and vinblastine as secondary or tertiary treatment. The only goal of therapy in these patients is palliation. The response rate to drug combinations administered in the setting of prior exposure to chemotherapy is unlikely to be much greater than the response to single agents, but the toxicity will almost certainly be greater. In light of this, CMF is recommended as first-line chemotherapy for patients with metastatic disease. Treatment at the time of disease progression should be single-agent doxorubicin, then single-agent mitomycin C, and finally single-agent vinblastine.

Optimal Duration of Therapy

There is no evidence that more than 6 months of chemotherapy is more beneficial than programs that end at about the sixth month. In one study, patients who were stable after 6 months of CMFVP therapy were randomized to continue CMFVP until evidence of disease progression or to stop CMFVP at 6 months.[427] Patients who stopped therapy were frequently retreated with CMFVP at the time of further disease progression, and many had a secondary response. There was a slight trend toward better survival among the patients who stopped CMFVP at the end of the first 6 months of treatment (Figure 38-23). Similar results have been ob-

FIG. 38-23. Effect of duration of therapy on survival. Patients treated with CMFVP who were stable beyond 6 months of therapy were randomized to continue CMFVP beyond 6 months or to discontinue therapy. (Smalley RV, Murphy S, Huguley CM et al: Combination versus sequential five-drug chemotherapy in metastatic carcinoma of the breast. Cancer Res 36:3911–3916, 1976)

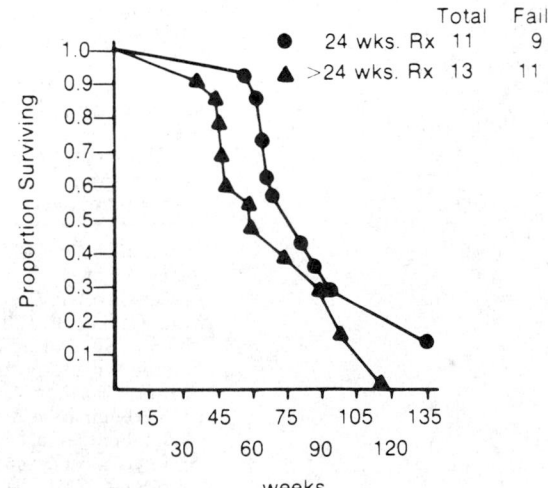

tained in a study of patients with locally advanced breast cancer.[439] In a more recent study, patients were randomized to receive either continuous chemotherapy (CA or CMF) until disease progression or three courses of chemotherapy and observation without treatment until evidence of disease progression.[440] Both objective response rates and quality of life, measured by a linear analogue self-assessment format, were significantly better among the patients randomized to receive chemotherapy continuously, and there was even a marginal survival advantage for the continuous-therapy program.

The optimal duration of chemotherapy is not known; it probably exceeds 3 months but might not exceed 6 months. On the basis of the evidence currently available, it is reasonable to discontinue therapy among patients whose disease is stable after 6 months of chemotherapy.

New Principles in the Use of Chemotherapy

Recent innovations designed to improve the efficacy of combination chemotherapy have included the use of high doses of drugs, alternating regimens, and continuous infusion.

There is undeniably a dose–response effect for most of the drugs used to treat breast cancer, but it has not been demonstrated that the therapeutic index of these agents is increased with higher doses. Most breast cancer dose studies are retrospective. Although patients receiving (or tolerating) a higher dose of drug had a higher response rate, patients with a higher performance status also had a higher response rate. It is likely that patients able to tolerate a higher dose of drug in these studies had a better initial performance status.[398,441,442] A retrospective analysis combining the results of many trials has been performed by Hryniuk and is frequently cited as evidence for a dose–response correlation in the use of chemotherapy for the treatment of breast cancer.[253,443] However, this analysis is based on numerous assumptions, many of which are inconsistent with the general principles of oncologic practice, and the conclusions from this oft-cited reference cannot be accepted as sound evidence of a dose response.[254]

Two randomized trials evaluating dose–response correlations have been performed. In one of these, patients were randomized to either a standard dose or a high dose of CMF.[444] There was no difference in the overall response rate, the median duration of response, or the survival of the two groups. A more recent and larger study randomized patients to standard-dose or low-dose CMF.[445] Patients receiving the standard doses of CMF had a significantly higher response rate and a marginal prolongation of survival.

Very high doses of single agents or drug combinations have been used with autologous bone-marrow transplantation to circumvent dose-limiting myelosuppression.[398] These trials involved from 1 to 16 patients, and the response rates have been as high as 100% with complete response rates between 30% and 100%. Because the number of patients entered in these trials is too small to permit meaningful interpretation, this approach must be considered entirely experimental.

Although dose may eventually be shown to be an important factor in determining the effectiveness of chemotherapy, it has not yet been shown that increasing the drug dose results in much added benefit, nor has it been demonstrated that drug doses can be safely reduced without compromising patient response, quality of life, and survival. Standard regimens are recommended until further evidence emerges from well-designed trials that specifically address these issues.

All tumors eventually develop resistance to these chemotherapeutic agents. Goldie, Coldman, and Gudauskas have hypothesized that the drugs induce resistance and that such resistance occurs very quickly after the first exposure to chemotherapy.[446] One strategy to circumvent this early resistance is the use of alternating, non-cross-resistant regimens. A large number of such trials have been performed,[447] none of which has shown a large advantage for the use of alternating regimens. In one study, more than 300 patients were randomized to receive either CMFP alternating every second cycle with two course of doxorubicin and vincristine.[448] Response to the two programs was almost identical, and both the duration of response and the duration of survival were slightly better for patients randomized to the non-alternating program.

More-frequent administration of drug in an intense dose schedule may result in higher overall response and complete response rates than administration of the same drugs at slightly higher doses intermittently.[411,427,449] In these studies, there was no significant survival advantage for the more intense program. The logical extension of these studies is the continuous administration of drug either for weeks via an implantable pump or for shorter courses using more conventional intravenous therapy in the hospital. Uncontrolled trials using continuous-infusion vinblastine, mitomycin C, doxorubicin, and 5-FU or FUDR suggest an improvement in the therapeutic index with more constant treatment, but none of these studies had appropriate control groups. The data thus are still inadequate to conclude that continuous-infusion therapy is more efficacious than intermittent bolus administration.[398]

Chemotherapy-Endocrine Therapy Combinations

The hypothesis that chemotherapy and endocrine (chemoendocrine) therapy are synergistic depends on the assumption that there are at least two distinctly different clones of cells, one clone responsive to chemotherapy but resistant to hormone therapy and the other resistant to chemotherapy but responsive to hormone therapy. There is abundant evidence that clones of the first type exist, but little evidence for the second.

The first generation of studies evaluating chemoendocrine therapy combinations demonstrated that the response rate to these combinations was consistantly and significantly higher than the response rate to endocrine therapy alone, but only 1 of 12 trials of this type showed a significant improvement in survival for patients receiving the chemoendocrine combination.[398] The response rate to chemoendocrine therapy is also usually higher than the response to chemotherapy alone, but this improvement reached levels of statistical significance in only 4 of 11 of trials designed to address this question. Improvement in the duration of response was marginal, and there was no significant improvement in survival for patients in these studies.[398]

The results from these studies can be illustrated and summarized by a recent large trial performed by the Australian–New Zealand Breast Cancer Trials Group.[338] Patients were randomized to receive either tamoxifen alone, combination chemotherapy with AC (doxorubicin plus cyclophosphamide), or a combination of tamoxifen plus AC (ACT). Patients whose tumors progressed on tamoxifen or AC were immediately crossed over to the other arm of the study. The initial response rates to tamoxifen, AC, and ACT were 22%, 45%, and 51%, respectively (p = <0.001). Because the secondary response to AC among tamoxifen failures is 35%, 43% of the patients randomized to tamoxifen eventually had a response either to tamoxifen alone or to subsequent chemotherapy. Only 6% of the patients whose tumors progressed on AC had a subsequent response to tamoxifen. As a result, the overall response rate of patients randomized to each of these three treatment arms was nearly the same. The median survival was not significantly different: 21 months, 18 months, and 20 months for patients randomized respectively to tamoxifen, AC, or ACT. This study not only failed to show any significant advantage for using chemoendocrine therapy but also suggested an advantage for the initial use of endocrine therapy alone, as more than 20% of the patients randomized to receive initial tamoxifen without chemotherapy had a period in which the symptoms of tumor were palliated without the toxicities of chemotherapy.

Several studies of chemoendocrine therapy have stratified patients by receptor status. In one study, patients were randomized to receive either CAF or CAF plus tamoxifen.[450] Among ER-positive patients, the response rate to CAF was 56% and to CAF plus tamoxifen, 67%. Among ER-negative patients, the response rates were 56% and 62%, respectively (not statistically significant). Receptor status thus does not identify patients more likely to benefit from chemoendocrine therapy.

Combinations of chemotherapy and endocrine therapy are not recommended for the treatment of metastatic breast cancer. Patients who are good candidates for endocrine therapy should be treated with endocrine therapy alone, as these patients may have long-term palliation without the side-effects of therapy. Patients who are not good candidates for endocrine therapy are not likely to derive much benefit from adding tamoxifen or other forms of endocrine therapy to an effective chemotherapy program.

TREATMENT OF SPECIFIC METASTATIC SITES

Breast cancer can, and usually does, metastasize to almost any organ site in the body (see Table 38-14). When multiple sites of disease are involved, systemic therapy should be used. However, in some situations, radiotherapy and, less often, surgery should be employed in addition to or instead of endocrine therapy or chemotherapy.

LOCAL RECURRENCE AFTER MASTECTOMY

Breast cancer recurrent in overlying skin and regional lymph nodes following a mastectomy must be distinguished from a recurrence entirely within breast parenchyma after primary radiation therapy. The natural history and prognosis of the latter is more like that of a new cancer in a contralateral breast and is discussed above in the section on conservative surgery and radiation therapy. Local recurrences after mastectomy are a common problem, occurring in 19% to 27% of patients with histologically involved nodes and in 3% to 8% of patients without node involvement.[218] These local recurrences have the same significance as metastases to distant organs: almost all of these patients will eventually die of breast cancer. Treatment of the isolated metastases will not be curative. On the other hand, many of these patients will live years after the appearance of a local recurrence. Factors predictive of survival are the same as those predictive of survival after recurrence at distant sites. The most important of these factors is the disease-free interval. The median survival of patients with locally recurrent disease is between 2 and 3 years, the 5-year survival rate being less than 35% and the 10-year survival rate less than 25%. The 10-year disease-free survival rate is usually less than 15%. In this context, it may be reasonable to treat some of these patients with local modalities without immediate systemic therapy.

Radiotherapy to the chest wall will result in an initial response rate of 63% to 79%,[218] but one-third to two-thirds of these patients will have a subsequent local recurrence. In a recent series from the JCRT, the actuarial local control rate at 5 years after local radiotherapy was 43%.[451] Local control following radiotherapy will be improved if prior surgery with excision of all apparent disease is possible, if higher doses of radiation therapy are used, or if a boost of radiotherapy is given to areas of gross residual disease.

Systemic therapy may also be useful in inducing regression of local disease. Overall response rates in several recent series are 62% to 85%.[452,453] Endocrine therapy may be as effective as or even more effective than chemotherapy in controlling a local recurrence.[453] This is consistent with the observation from postmastectomy adjuvant therapy trials in which adjuvant tamoxifen appears to be better in reducing local recurrence rates than is adjuvant chemotherapy.

Several other modalities available for the treatment of disease at specific sites include hyperthermia, photoradiation with hematoporphyrin photosensitization, and superficial laser therapy. Hyperthermia has been utilized alone, with radiotherapy, and with chemotherapy. Anecdotal reports concerning all three of these approaches are sometimes impressive and suggest the possibility of local control of disease refractory to more conventional forms of therapy. However, all of these approaches must be considered experimental at present.

When local recurrences accompany distant metastases, systemic therapy should be employed initially and radiotherapy added only if the locally recurrent disease is particularly symptomatic or fails to respond to systemic therapy. On the other hand, if an isolated local recurrence appears after a long disease-free interval and without evidence of distant metastases, initial therapy may consist of excision alone or of excision plus radiation therapy. Several recurrences of this type without evidence of distant metastases should preferentially be treated with radiation therapy.

METASTASES TO THE NERVOUS SYSTEM, SPINE, AND CHOROID

Between 20% and 25% of patients with metastatic breast cancer will eventually develop a problem related to the nervous system: brain metastases, epidural spinal cord compression, carcinomatous meningitis, brachial plexus syndrome, choroidal metastases, or a paraneoplastic syndrome. Breast cancer is one of the two or three most common tumors responsible for metastases at each of these sites. In autopsy series, CNS metastases are observed in 9% to 25% of all breast cancer patients.[349] However, antemortem diagnoses of brain metastases (about 10%) or carcinomatous meningitis (about 5%) are less frequent.[419,454,455]

Radiotherapy plays a central role in the treatment of all types of metastases to the nervous system, and dexamethasone should be administered promptly after the documentation of metastases on CT scan. (Dexamethasone administered prior to the CT scan obscures the diagnosis in occasional patients.) The optimal dose schedule of radiation is a point of some controversy. There is no evidence that either the response rate or the duration of response is significantly different when a high dose of radiation is delivered in multiple fractions over 4 weeks compared with low doses administered in two fractions over 3 to 7 days.[456] However, short high-dose courses of radiation may result in a higher complication rate.[457] Approximately 20% of patients with brain metastases deteriorate rapidly and are unable to complete the course of radiotherapy. However, 50% to 75% of patients who do complete the radiotherapy will have decreased neurologic symptoms, and some patients will remain free of symptoms for years. Dexamethasone should be tapered after the completion of radiation therapy and can be discontinued altogether in more than 50% of patients.

It has not been established that surgical excison of brain metastases has any advantage over radiation therapy alone, especially as radiation is usually administered after surgery. Moreover, brain metastases from breast cancer are often multicentric.[457] Surgery is indicated only when the diagnosis is in doubt or when patients have surgically accessible disease, persistent symptoms, and radioresistant tumors. Concomitant breast cancer metastases to the brain and a meningioma within the brain have been reported.[458] The possibility of meningioma in a breast cancer patient may be suspected on the basis of the CT finding and should lead to surgical exploration.

Until recently, systemic therapy has not been utilized for the treatment of brain metastases of breast cancer because it was assumed that these agents would not cross the blood–brain barrier. However, newer pharmacologic studies have demonstrated that many of the standard drugs utilized to treat breast cancer do indeed cross into the brain. These drugs include cyclophosphamide and 5-FU in conventional doses[459] and methotrexate in high doses.[460] Objective response was observed in 50% of a recent series of 66 patients treated for brain metastases with combination chemotherapy programs that included prednisone.[461] Even tamoxifen has been reported to induce remission of a brain metastasis.[462] However, until comparative studies on the relative efficacy of radiotherapy and systemic therapy have been performed, radiotherapy must be preferred for treatment of brain metastases because of both the high response rate and the very durable responses achieved in some patients.

Carcinomatous meningitis is generally thought to have a dire prognosis; the median survival is 7 months, and the 1-year survival rate is less than 10%.[419,463,464] Because of the diffuse nature of carcinomatous meningitis and the difficulties inherent in delivering radiotherapy to the entire cranial–spinal axis, intrathecal chemotherapy is almost always employed. Methotrexate, thiotepa, and cytosine arabinoside can be utilized; the first two of these agents are especially effective against breast cancer. Recommended regimens include methotrexate, 7 to 12 ml/m^2, twice weekly until neurologic symptoms have subsided. This may be optimally administered through an Ommaya reservoir. Systemic symptoms from methotrexate may be avoided if leukovorin rescue is given as well. When cerebrospinal fluid cytology becomes negative, the frequency of methotrexate administration may be gradually decreased, first to a weekly course and eventually to a single administration every 2 months.[464] Radiotherapy is reserved for symptomatic areas in the brain or spinal cord. However, when cranial nerve palsies are evident, radiation therapy is given to the whole brain because the tumor usually involves the entire subarachnoid space and extends over the convexities of the brain, brainstem, and even throughout the spinal cord. Because radiation therapy to the entire spine would involve more than 40% of bone marrow areas, this is generally not recommended.[464] When both radiotherapy to the CNS and methotrexate are administered, the possibility of a leukoencephalopathy increases.

Choroidal metastases may be the first sign of metastases, occur in 2% to 6% of all patients, and are bilateral in 20% to 50% of those patients who develop choroidal metastases.[465] Radiotherapy will improve visual acuity in 80% to 90% of patients, and complications, such as cataracts or radiation retinitis, are rare. Although there are anecdotal reports of chemotherapy being effective, there is generally no role for either chemotherapy or enucleation when radiation therapy is effective.

Epidural spinal-cord compression causing paralysis and sphincter dysfunction is among the most serious complications from breast metastases and is not an uncommon problem. Compression may occur either from direct encroachment on the spinal cord by expanding tumor or secondary to fractures of the vertebrae. The most common source of tumor growing to compress the spinal canal is metastases to the vertebrae. Because more than two-thirds of patients with breast cancer eventually develop bony metastases and the most common sites of bony metastases are the vertebrae, it is not surprising that this is a frequent problem in the differential diagnosis and management of patients with metastatic breast cancer.

Although radiotherapy remains the most important modality for the prevention of epidural spinal-cord compression, considerable clinical judgment is required to determine when to irradiate and which vertebrae to irradiate. Patients with metastatic breast cancer often have multiple painful areas and multiple abnormalities on bone scan. It is rarely necessary or appropriate to irradiate all of these, especially because large areas of bone marrow may be involved, and subsequent or concomitant chemotherapy will therefore be compromised. The precise nature of the underlying causes of spinal compression should be determined by the use of MRI, CT scans, and myelography. Soft-tissue masses likely to respond rapidly to radiotherapy should be distinguished from compression fractures, which may require surgical stabilization for adequate relief of symptoms or for prevention of paralysis.

When a diagnosis of impending or early epidural spinal-cord compression has been made, dexamethasone should be given first. Radiotherapy to the involved areas (which can be best defined by MRI in a sagittal plane or by myelography) will provide pain relief in two-thirds to three-fourths of patients and will maintain ambulation and sphincter function in more than half.[466] In general, the results of laminectomy plus radiotherapy are no better than the results of radiation therapy alone. However, surgery may be of value in patients with further deterioration after radiation therapy, recurrence in a previously irradiated area, or instability of the vertebral column.[466]

Bone pain in patients with multiple lesions and no evidence of epidural spinal-cord compression should be treated first with systemic therapy. Radiation can then be added to relieve symptoms when systemic therapy is not effective. Chemotherapy and endocrine therapy are not likely to relieve pain when radiation therapy has not been effective. Under these circumstances, other causes of pain or neurologic dysfunction should be sought. Often, compression fracture and other structural abnormalities will persist after treatment of the tumor, and antineoplastic therapy is not likely to provide further relief of these symptoms.

Brachial plexopathy in patients with breast cancer may occur because of tumor infiltration of the brachial plexus or because of radiation damage. A history of radiation treatment, the nature of the symptoms, and their distribution should provide some clues to distinguish between these two causes of plexopathy.[467] Early diagnosis of brachial plexopathy secondary to tumor and prompt administration of radiotherapy may alleviate symptoms before deafferentiation has occurred. When symptoms have advanced before diagnosis, the patient is usually left with permanent disability including permanent intractable pain.

BONE AND BONE MARROW METASTASES AND HYPERCALCEMIA

Because bone metastases are rarely isolated or rarely remain as a single focus for any length of time, the mainstay of treatment is systemic, namely, endocrine therapy or chemotherapy. The response rate of bone lesions in patients with ER-positive tumors or other clinical characteristics predictive of a response to endocrine therapy is nearly equal to the response to chemotherapy in patients refractory to endo-

crine therapy or with receptor-negative tumors. Intensive chemotherapy programs may induce some response in sites of bone disease in 80% to 90% of patients, with a complete response seen in 25% to 50% of patients.[421,468,469]

Radiotherapy is probably more effective than systemic therapy in relieving bone pain but can be applied to only one bone at a time.[470,471] However, the relative effectiveness of these two modalities has never been fully evaluated in randomized controlled trials. The value of radiotherapy or prophylactic surgical fixation in the prevention of fractures has likewise not been evaluated in controlled trials. By convention, prophylactic fixation has been recommended when lesions exceed 2.5 cm, involve 50% of the bone diameter, and invade the bone cortex.[472] Patients with persistent pain 6 to 8 weeks after the completion of radiotherapy should also be evaluated for a possible incomplete or nondisplaced fracture.

Bone-marrow metastases have been found in as many as 55% of patients with bone metastases diagnosed on bone scan or plain films.[473] Marrow metastases are seldom diagnosed by conventional means in patients without bone metastases[474] but may actually be found more frequently when extremely sensitive methods, such as immunocytochemical stains, are used. In one study, 28% of patients with operable breast lesions were found to have occult bone marrow metastases.[475] Bone marrow metastases from breast cancer should be treated with systemic therapy. The choice of endocrine therapy or chemotherapy is made utilizing the criteria described for the selection between these two modalities for other sites of metastases.

Between 5% and 10% of all patients with breast cancer will develop hypercalcemia at some time in the course of their metastatic disease.[476] Not infrequently, hypercalcemia occurs within a few hours to several weeks after the initiation of endocrine therapy. Its management in these patients is similar to the management of this condition in other patients with malignancy.[477] However, when hypercalcemia promptly follows the initiation of endocrine therapy, the endocrine therapy should be continued unless the hypercalcemia is life threatening or exceeds 14 mg/dl. Many of these patients will respond to endocrine therapy despite the hypercalcemia.[361]

PULMONARY METASTASES

Metastases to the lungs may appear as pulmonary nodules, lymphangetic spread, or pleural effusions. Pulmonary nodules are exquisitely sensitive to systemic therapy and may be completely eradicated with chemotherapy in 40% to 80% of patients.[421,468,469] Lymphangetic spread within the lungs has been found in 24% to 34% of patients at autopsy, but an unequivocal antemortem diagnosis is usually made in less than 20% of patients.[478] Although this diagnosis is considered dire, the 1-year survival rate is 80% and the 2-year survival rate is 30% when lymphangetic metastases are the first site of metastatic disease. Because this diagnosis is difficult to document, it is not surprising that it is also difficult to document objective responses to therapy. Systemic therapy is always indicated, and the criteria described above to choose between endocrine therapy and chemotherapy should be applied here as well.

More than 50% of patients with metastatic breast cancer are likely to develop malignant effusions.[479] Pleural effusion, especially when it is an isolated finding, does not carry a bad prognosis. In one series, the median survival of patients who presented with pleural effusion alone was 48 months.[480] Asymptomatic pleural effusions, especially if they are only one manifestation of systemic disease in a patient with multiple other sites, requires no specific therapy. Only 10% of pleural effusions are controlled by the first thoracentesis,[479] and repeated thoracenteses are likely to lead to loculation of fluid and increased difficulty in long-term control. Thoracostomy alone may lead to control of effusion in 20% to 50% of patients, but instillation of agents that induce sclerosis will lead to better control. Although a number of different agents have been shown to be effective, tetracycline is among those that are most readily available and have the least toxicity.[479] The best long-term control will be obtained with talc pleurodesis through a thoracostomy, and this treatment should be considered for patients with a good long-term prognosis who are able to withstand this procedure.[481]

REFERENCES

1. Silverberg E, Lubera J: Cancer Statistics, 1987. CA 37:2–19, 1987
2. Pike MC, Henderson BE, Casagrande JT, Rosario I, Gray GE: Oral contraceptive use and early abortion as risk factors for breast cancer in young women. Br J Cancer, 43:72–76, 1981
3. Henderson BE, Pike MC, Ross RK: Epidemiology and risk factors. In Bonadonna G (ed): Breast Cancer: Diagnosis and Management, pp 15–33. Chichester, John Wiley & Sons, 1984
4. Henderson BE, Ross RK, Judd HL, Krailo MD, Pike MC: Do regular ovulatory cycles increase breast cancer risk? Cancer 56:1206–1208, 1985
5. Thomas DB, Lilienfeld AM: Geographic, reproductive and sociobiological factors. In Stoll B (ed): Risk Factors in Breast Cancer, pp 25–53. Chicago, Wm Heinemann Medical Books, 1976
6. Brinton LA, Hoover R, Fraumeni JF: Reproductive factors in the aetiology of breast cancer. Br J Cancer 47:757–762, 1983
7. Trichopoulos D, Hsieh C, MacMahon B et al: Age at any birth and breast cancer risk. Int J Cancer 31:701–704, 1983
8. Thomas DB: Do hormones cause breast cancer? Cancer 53:595–604, 1984
9. Brinton LA, Hoover RN, Szklo M, Fraumeni JFJ: Menopausal estrogen use and risk of breast cancer. Cancer 47:2517–2522, 1981
10. Ross RK, Paganini–Hill A, Gerkins VR et al: A case-control study of menopausal estrogen therapy and breast cancer. JAMA 243:1635–1639, 1980
11. McPherson K, Drife JO: The pill and breast cancer: Why the uncertainty? Br Med J 293:709–710, 1986
12. Miller AB: Epidemiology and prevention. In Harris JR, Hellman S, Henderson IC, Kinne DW (eds): Breast Diseases, pp 87–102. Philadelphia, JB Lippincott, 1987
13. Meirik O, Adami HO, Christoffersen T, Lund E, Bergstrom R, Bergsho P: Oral contraceptive use and breast cancer in young women. Lancet 2:650–654, 1986
14. Cancer and Steroid Hormone Study of the Centers for Disease Control, the National Institute of Child Health and Human Development: Oral-contraceptive use and the risk of breast cancer. N Engl J Med 315:405–411, 1986
15. Buell P: Changing incidence of breast cancer in Japanese–American women. J Natl Cancer Inst 51:1479–1483, 1973
16. Wynder EL, Rose DP, Cohen LA: Diet and breast cancer in causation and therapy. Cancer 58:1804–1813, 1986
17. Mettlin C: Diet and the epidemiology of human breast cancer. Cancer 53:605–611, 1984
18. Willett WC, Stampfer MJ, Colditz GA, Rosner BA, Hennekens CH, Speizer FE: Dietary fat and risk of breast cancer. N Engl J Med 316:22–28, 1987
19. Bjarnason O, Day N, Snaedal G, Tulinius H: The effect of year of birth on the breast cancer age-incidence curve in Iceland. Int J Cancer 13:689–696, 1974
20. Willett WC, Stampfer MJ, Colditz GA, Rosner BA, Hennekens CH, Speizer FE: Moderate alcohol consumption and the risk of breast cancer. N Engl J Med 316:1174–1180, 1987
21. Schatzkin A, Jones Y, Hoover RN et al: Alcohol consumption and breast cancer in the epidemiologic follow-up study of the First National Health and Nutrition Examination Survey. N Engl J Med 316:1169–1173, 1987
22. Adami H, Hansen J, Jung B, Rimsten A: Characteristics of familial breast cancer in Sweden. Cancer 48:1688–1695, 1981
23. Sattin RW, Rubin GL, Webster LA et al: Family history and the risk of breast cancer. JAMA 253:1908–1913, 1985
24. Dupont WD, Page DL: Risk factors for breast cancer in women with proliferative breast disease. N Engl J Med 312:146–151, 1985
25. Baak JPA, Van Dop H, Kurver PHJ, Hermans J: The value of morphometry to classic prognosticators in breast cancer. Cancer 56:374–382, 1985
26. Anderson DE, Badzioch MD: Risk of familial breast cancer. Cancer 56:383–387, 1985
27. Bailar JC: Screening for early breast cancer: Pros and cons. Cancer 39:2783–2795, 1977
28. Love SM, Gelman RS, Silen W: Fibrocystic "disease" of the breast—A nondisease? N Engl J Med 307:1010–1014, 1982
29. Henderson IC, Canellos GP: Cancer of the breast: The past decade. N Engl J Med 302:17–30; 78–90, 1980
30. Fox MS: On the diagnosis and treatment of breast cancer. JAMA 241:489–494, 1979
31. Silvestrini R, Daidone MG, Gentili C: Biologic characteristics of breast cancer and their clinical relevance. In Bulbrook RD (ed): Commentaries on Research in Breast Disease, Vol 2, pp 1–40. New York, Alan R Liss, 1981
32. Malaise EP, Chavaudra N, Tubiana M: The relationship between growth rate, labelling index and histological type of human solid tumours. Eur J Cancer 9:305–312, 1973
33. von Fournier D, Weber E, Hoeffken W, Bauer M, Kubli F, Barth V: Growth rate of 147 mammary carcinomas. Cancer 45:2198–2207, 1980
34. Heuser L, Spratt JS, Polk HC: Growth rates of primary breast cancers. Cancer 43:1888–1894, 1979
35. Lundgren B: Observations on growth rate of breast carcinomas and its possible implications for lead time. Cancer 40:1722–1725, 1977
36. Gershon-Cohen J, Berger SM, Klickstein HS: Roentgenography of breast cancer moderating concept of "biologic predeterminism." Cancer 16:961–964, 1963
37. Speer JF, Petrosky VE, Retsky MW, Wardwell RH: A stochastic numerical model of breast cancer growth that simulates clinical data. Cancer Res 44:4124–4130, 1984
38. Gilchrist KW, Kalish L, Gould VE et al: Interobserver reproducibility of histopathological features in Stage II breast cancer: An ECOG study. Breast Cancer Res Treat 5:8–10, 1985
39. Rosen PP, Saigo PE, Braun DW et al: Axillary micro- and macrometastases in breast cancer. Ann Surg 194:585–591, 1981
40. Osborne CK: Receptors. In Harris JR, Hellman S, Henderson IC, Kinne DW (eds): Breast Diseases, pp 210–232. Philadelphia, JB Lippincott, 1987
41. Horwitz KB, McGuire WL: Estrogen control of progesterone receptor in human breast cancer: Correlation with nuclear processing of estrogen receptor. J Biol Chem 253:2223–2228, 1978
42. Lippman ME, Dickson RB, Bates S et al: Autocrine and paracrine growth regulation of human breast cancer. Breast Cancer Res Treat 7:59–70, 1986
43. McGuire WL, Clark GM, Dressler LG, Owens MA: Role of steroid hormone receptors as prognostic factors in primary breast cancer. NCI Monogr 1:19–23, 1986
44. Singhakowinta A, Potter H, Buroker T, Samal B, Brooks S, Vaitkevicius V: Estrogen receptor and natural course of breast cancer. Ann Surg 183:84–88, 1976
45. Thorpe SM, Rose C, Rasmussen BB, Mouridsen HT, Bayer T, Keiding N: Prognostic value of steroid hormone receptors: Multivariate analysis of systemically untreated patients with node negative primary breast cancer. Cancer Res 47:6126–6133, 1987
46. Valagussa P, Bignami P, Buzzoni R et al: Are estrogen receptors alone a reliable prognostic factor in node negative breast cancer? In Jones SE, Salmon SE (eds): Adjuvant Therapy of Cancer IV, pp 407–415. Orlando, Grune & Stratton, 1984
47. Crowe JP, Hubay CA, Pearson OH et al: Estrogen receptor status as a prognostic indicator for Stage I breast cancer patients. Breast Cancer Res Treat 2:171–176, 1982
48. Adams HO, Graffman S, Lindgren A, Sallstrom J: Prognostic implication of estrogen receptor content in breast cancer. Breast Cancer Res Treat 5:293–300, 1985
49. Blamey RW, Bishop HM, Blake JRS et al: Relationship between primary breast tumor receptor status and patient survival. Cancer 46:2765–2769, 1980
50. Raemaekers JMM, Beex LVAM, Koenders AJM et al: Disease-free interval and estrogen receptor activity in tumor tissue of patients with primary breast cancer: Analysis after long-term follow-up. Breast Cancer Res Treat 6:123–130, 1985
51. Hahnel R, Woodings T, Vivian AB: Prognostic value of estrogen receptors in primary breast cancer. Cancer 44:671–675, 1979
52. Howell A, Harland RNL, Bramwell VHC et al: Steroid-hormone receptors and survival after first relapse in breast cancer. Lancet 1:588–591, 1984
53. Valagussa P, Bonadonna G, Veronesi U: Patterns of relapse and survival in operable breast carcinoma with positive and negative axillary nodes. Tumori 64:241–258, 1978
54. Fisher B, Slack N, Katrych D, Wolmark N: Ten year follow-up results of patients with carcinoma of the breast in a co-operative clinical trial evaluating surgical adjuvant chemotherapy. Surg Gynecol Obstet 140:528–534, 1975
55. Donegan WL, Skibba JL: Patterns of survival and disease recurrence after mastectomy for carcinoma of the breast. Cancer Treat Symp 2:107–116, 1983
56. Fisher B, Bauer M, Wickerham DL, Redmond CK, Fisher ER: Relation of number of positive axillary nodes to the prognosis of patients with primary breast cancer. Cancer 52:1551–1557, 1983
57. Fisher ER, Sass R, Fisher B: Pathological Findings from the National Surgical Adjuvant Project for Breast Cancers (Protocol No. 4) X: Discriminants for tenth year treatment failure. Cancer 53:712–713, 1984
58. Bonadonna G, Rossi A, Valagusssa P: Adjuvant CMF chemotherapy in operable breast cancer: Ten years later. World J Surg 9:707–713, 1985
59. Butler JA, Bretsky S, Menendez–Botet C, Kinne DW: Estrogen receptor protein of breast cancer as a predictor of recurrence. Cancer 55:1178–1181, 1985

60. Williams MR, Todd JH, Ellis IO et al: Oestrogen receptors in primary and advanced breast cancer: An eight year review of 704 cases. Br J Cancer 55:67–73, 1987
61. McDivitt RW, Stewart FW, Berg JW: Tumors of the Breast. Washington, DC, Armed Forces Institute of Pathology, 1968
62. World Health Organization: Histologic typing of breast tumors. Tumori 68:181, 1982
63. Wellings SR, Jensen HM: On the origin and progression of ductal carcinoma in the human breast. J Natl Cancer Inst 50:1111–1118, 1973
64. Connolly J, Schnitt SJ: Evaluation of breast biopsy specimens in patients considered for treatment by conservative surgery and radiotherapy for early breast cancer. Pathol Annu 23:1–23, 1988
65. Bloom HJG, Field JR: Impact of tumor grade and host resistance on survival of women with breast cancer. Cancer 28:1580–1589, 1971
66. Parl FF, Dupont WD: A retrospective cohort study of histologic risk factors in breast cancer patients. Cancer 50:2410–2416, 1982
67. Rosen PP, Saigo PE, Braun DW Jr, Weathers E, DePalo A: Predictors of recurrence in Stage I (T1 N0 M0) breast carcinoma. Ann Surg 193:15–25, 1981
68. Tubiana M, Pejovic MH, Chavaudra N: Long term prognostic significance of the thymidine labeling index in breast cancer. Int J Cancer 33:441–445, 1984
69. Meyer JS, Freedman E, McCrate MM: Prediction of early course of breast carcinoma by thymidine labeling. Cancer 51:1879–1886, 1983
70. Silvestrini R, Daidone MG, Gasparini G: Cell kinetics as a prognostic marker in node-negative breast cancer. Cancer 56:1982–1987, 1985
71. Hedley DW, Rugg CA, Ng ABP: Influence of cellular DNA content on disease free survival of Stage II breast cancer patients. Cancer Res 44:5395–5398, 1984
72. Coulson PB, Thornthwaite JT, Woolley TW: Prognostic indicators including DNA histogram type, receptor content, and staging related to human breast cancer patient survival. Cancer Res 44:4187–4196, 1984
73. McDivitt RW, Stone KR, Craig B, Palmer JO, Meyer JS, Bauer WC: A proposed classification of breast cancer based on kinetic information. Cancer 57:269–276, 1986
74. Slamon DJ, Clark GM, Wong SG et al: Human breast cancer: Correlation of relapse and survival with amplification of HER-2/neu oncogene. Science 235:177–182, 1987
75. Spratt JS, Donegan WL: Cancer of the breast. Philadelphia, WB Saunders, 1967
76. Fisher B, Slack NH, Ausman RK: Location of breast carcinoma and prognosis. Surg Gynecol Obstet 129:705–716, 1969
77. Haagensen CD: Diseases of the Breast. Philadelphia, WB Saunders, 1971
78. Holland R, Velig SHJ, Mravunac M, Hendriks JHCL: Histologic multifocality of Tis, T1-2 breast carcinomas. Cancer 56:979–990, 1985
79. Pickren JW: Significance of occult metastases. Cancer 14:1266–1271, 1961
80. Nemoto T, Vana J, Bedwani RN et al: Management and survival of female breast cancer. Cancer 45:2917–2924, 1980
81. Smith JA, Gamez–Araujo JJ, Gallager HS, White EC, McBride CM: Carcinoma of the breast. Cancer 39:527–532, 1977
82. Veronesi U, Rilke F, Luini A: Distribution of axillary node metastases by level. Cancer 59:682–687, 1987
83. Rosen PP, Lesser ML, Kinne DW, Beattie EJ: Discontinuous or "skip" metastasis in breast carcinoma. Ann Surg 187:276–283, 1983
84. Fisher B, Slack NH, Bross IDJ: Cancer of the breast: Size of neoplasm and prognosis. Cancer 24:1071–1080, 1969
85. Adair F, Berg J, Joubert L, Robbins GF: Long-term followup of breast cancer patients: The 30-year report. Cancer 33:1145–1150, 1974
86. Handley RS: Carcinoma of the breast. Ann R Coll Surg 57:59–66, 1975
87. Bucalossi P, Veronesi U, Zingo L, Conti C: Enlarged mastectomy for breast cancer: Review of 1,213 cases. Am J Roentgenol Rad Ther Nucl Med 111:119–122, 1971
88. Veronesi U, Cascinelli N, Greco M et al: Prognosis of breast cancer patients after mastectomy and dissection of internal mammary nodes. Ann Surg 202:702–707, 1985
89. Dahl–Iversen E: Recherches sur les Métastases microscopiques des cancers du sein dans les ganglions lymphatiques parasternaux et susclaviculaires. Mem Acad Chin 78:651–652, 1952
90. Halsted WS: The results of radical operations for the cure of cancer of the breast. Ann Surg 46:1–19, 1907
91. Haagensen CD: Treatment of curable carcinoma of the breast. Int J Radiat Oncol Biol Phys 2:975–980, 1977
92. Fisher ER, Swamidoss S, Lee CH: Detection and significance of occult axillary lymph node metastases in patients with invasive breast cancer. Cancer 42:2025–2031, 1978
93. Huvos AG, Hutter RVP, Berg JW: Significance of axillary macrometastases and micrometastases in mammary cancer. Ann Surg 173:44–46, 1971
94. Shapiro S, Strax P, Venet L: Changes in 5 year breast cancer mortality in a breast cancer screening program. Proceedings of the Seventh National Cancer Conference, pp 663–678. Philadelphia, JB Lippincott, 1973
95. Shapiro S, Venet W, Strax P, Venet L, Roeser R: Ten- to fourteen-year effect of screening on breast cancer mortality. J Natl Cancer Inst 69:349–355, 1982
96. Habbema JPF, Van Oortmarssen GJ, VanPutten DJ, Lubbe JT, van der Maas PJ: Age specific reduction in breast cancer mortality for screening: An analysis of the results of the Health Insurance Plan of Greater New York Study. J Natl Cancer Inst 77:317–320, 1986
97. Tabar L, Fagerberg CJG, Gad A et al: Reduction in mortality from breast cancer after mass screening with mammography. Lancet 1:829–832, 1985
98. Verbeek ALM, Hendriks JH, Holland R, Mravunac M, Sturmans F, Day NE: Reduction of breast cancer mortality through mass screening with modern mammography. Lancet 1:1222–1224, 1984
99. Baker LH: Breast Cancer Detection Demonstration Project: Five-year summary report. CA 32:194–225, 1982
100. Seidman H, Gelb SK, Silverberg E, LaVerda N, Lubera JA: Survival experience in the Breast Cancer Detection Demonstration Project. Ca 37:258–290, 1987
101. Bailar JC III: Mammography: A contrary view. Ann Intern Med 84:77–84, 1976
102. Gohagan JK, Darby WP, Spitznagel EL, Monsees BS, Tome AE: Radiogenic breast cancer effects of mammographic screening. J Natl Cancer Inst 77:71–76, 1986
103. Case C: The Breast Cancer Digest, 2nd ed. Washington, DC, US Government Printing Office, 1984
104. Moskowitz M: Breast cancer: Age-specific growth rates and screening strategies. Radiology 161:37–41, 1986
105. Gisvold JJ, Martin JK: Prebiopsy localization of nonpalpable breast lesions. AJR 143:47–481, 1984
106. Meyer VE, Kopans DB, Stomper PC, Lindfors KK: Occult breast abnormalities: Percutaneous preoperative needle localization. Radiology 150:335–337, 1984
107. Poller SR, Mettle E, Bartow SA, Moradian G, Moscowitz M: Occult breast cancer: Prevalence and radiographic detectability. Radiology 163:459–462, 1987
108. Baker ER: The indications for bone scan in the pre-operative assessment of patients with operable breast cancer. Breast Dis 3:43–45, 1977
109. McNeil B, Pace PPD, Gray E: Pre-operative and follow-up bone scans in patients with primary carcinoma of the breast. Surg Gynecol Obstet 147:745–748, 1978
110. Wiener SN, Sachs SH: An assessment of positive liver scanning in patients with breast cancer. Arch Surg 113:126–127, 1970
111. Casta GNA, Benfield J Jr, Yamama H: The reliability of liver scans and function tests in detecting metastases. Surg Gynecol Obstet 124:463–469, 1972
112. Dash N, Lupetin AR, Daffner RH: Magnetic resonance imaging in the diagnosis of breast disease. AJR 146:119–125, 1986
113. Steward AM, Nixon D, Zamcheck N: Carcinoembryonic antigen in breast cancer patients. Cancer 33:1246–1252, 1979
114. Tormey DC, Wastros TT, Ahmann D: Biological markers in breast cancer I: Incidence of abnormalities of CEA, hCG, polyamines and three minor nucleosides. Cancer 35:1095–1100, 1975
115. Tormey DC, Waalkes TP, Semon RM: Biological markers in breast cancer II: Clinical correlation with chorionic gonadotropin. Cancer 39:2391–2396, 1976
116. Marcus DM, Zinbergt N: Measurement of serum ferritin by radioimmunoassay: Results in normal individuals and patients with breast cancer. J Natl Cancer Inst 55:791–795, 1975
117. Waalkes TP, Tormey DC: Biological markers and breast cancer. Semin Oncol 5:434–444, 1978
118. Halsted WS: The results of operations for the cure of cancer of the breast performed at Johns Hopkins Hospital from June, 1889 to January, 1894. Johns Hopkins Hosp Bull 4:497–555, 1894
119. Haagensen CD: Diseases of the Breast, 3rd Ed. Philadelphia, WB Saunders, 1986
120. Urban JA, Baker HW: Radical mastectomy in continuity with en bloc resection of the internal mammary lymph node chain. Cancer 5:992, 1952
121. Auchincloss H: Significance of location and number of axillary metastases in carcinoma of the breast: A justification for a conservative operation. Ann Surg 158:37, 1963
122. Lagios MD, Westdahl PR, Rose MR: The concept and implications of multicentricity in breast carcinoma. Pathol Annu 16:83–102, 1981
123. Rosen PP, Fracchia AA, Urban JA: "Residual" mammary carcinoma following simulated partial mastectomy. Cancer 35:739–747, 1975
124. Schwartz GF, Patchesfsky AS, Feig SA, Shaber GS, Schwartz AB: Multicentricity of non-palpable breast cancer. Cancer 45:2913–2916, 1980
125. Rosen PP, Braun DW, Kinne DW: The clinical significance of pre-invasive breast carcinoma. Cancer 46:919–925, 1980
126. Lagios MD, Richards VE, Rose MR, Yee E: Segmental mastectomy without radiotherapy: short-term follow-up. Cancer 52:2173–2179, 1983
127. Holland R, Solke HJV, Mravunac M: Histologic multifocality of Tis, T1-2 breast carcinomas. Cancer 56:979–990, 1985
128. Kramer WM, Ruch BF Jr: Mammary duct proliferation in the elderly. Cancer 31:130–137, 1973
129. Franks LM: Latent carcinoma of the prostate. J Pathol Bacteriol 68:603–616, 1954
130. Schottenfeld D, Nash A, Robbins G, Beattie E: Ten-year results of the treatment of primary operable breast carcinoma. Cancer 38:1001–1007, 1976
131. Haagensen CD, Bodian C: A personal experience with Halsted's radical mastectomy. Ann Surg 199:143–150, 1984
132. Fisher B, Redmond C, Fisher ER, Bauer M, Wolmark N et al: Ten-year results of a randomized clinical trial comparing radical mastectomy and total mastectomy with or without radiation. N Engl J Med 312:674–681, 1985
133. Robbins GF, Berg J: Curability of patients with invasive breast carcinoma based on a 30-year study. World J Surg 1:284–286, 1977
134. Davies GC, Millis RR, Hayward JL: Assessment of axillary lymph node status. Ann Surg 192:148–151, 1980
135. Danforth DN Jr, Findlay PA, McDonald HD et al: Complete axillary lymph node dissection for Stage I–II carcinoma of the breast. J Clin Oncol 4:655–662, 1986
136. Schwartz GF, Domenico M, D'Ugo MD: Extent of axillary dissection preceding irradiation for carcinoma of the breast. Arch Surg 121:1395–1398, 1986
137. Cady B: Usefulness and technique of axillary dissection in primary breast cancer. J Clin Oncol 4:623–624, 1986
138. Dewar JA, Sarrazin D, Benhamou E: Management of the axilla in conservatively

treated breast cancer: 592 patients treated at Institut Gustave-Roussy. Int J Radiat Oncol Biol Phys 13:475–481, 1987

139. Harris JR, Osteen RT: Patients with early breast cancer benefit from effective axillary treatment. Breast Cancer Res Treat 5:17–21, 1985

140. Wilson RE, Donegan WL, Mettlin C, Smart CR, Murphy GP: The 1982 National Survey of Carcinoma of the Breast in the United States by the American College of Surgeons. Surg Gynecol Obstet 159:309–318, 1984

141. Baker RR, Montague ACW, Childs NJ: A comparison of modified radical mastectomy to radical mastectomy in the treatment of operable breast cancer. Ann Surg 189:553–559, 1979

142. Maddox WA, Carpenter JT, Laws HL: A randomized prospective trial of radical (Halsted) mastectomy versus modified radical mastectomy in 311 breast cancer patients. Ann Surg 198:207–212, 1983

143. Martin JK Jr, van Heerden JA, Taylor W: Is modified radical mastectomy really equivalent to radical mastectomy in treatment of carcinoma of the breast? Cancer 57:510–518, 1986

144. Mentzer SJ, Osteen RT, Wilson RE: Local recurrence and the deep resection margin in carcinoma of the breast. Surg Gynecol Obstet 163:513–517, 1986

145. Kinne DW, DeCosse JJ: Modified radical mastectomy for carcinoma of the breast. Am Surg 48:543–556, 1982

146. Urban JA: Management of operable breast cancer: The surgeon's view. Cancer 42:2066–2077, 1978

147. Veronesi U, Valagussa P: Inefficacy of internal mammary nodes dissection in breast cancer surgery. Cancer 47:170–175, 1981

148. Lacour J, Le MG, Hill C: Is it useful to remove internal mammary nodes in operable breast cancer? Eur J Surg Oncol 13:309–314, 1987

149. Goldman LD, Goldwyn RM: Some anatomical considerations of subcutaneous mastectomy. Plast Reconstr Surg 51:501–505, 1973

150. Goodnought JE, Quagliana JM, Morton DL: Failure of subcutaneous mastectomy to prevent the development of breast cancer. J Surg Oncol 26:198–201, 1984

151. Hermann RE, Esselstyn CB Jr, Crile G Jr: Results of conservative operations for breast cancer. Arch Surg 120:746–751, 1985

152. Harris JR, Hellman S, Kinne DW: Limited surgery and radiotherapy for early breast cancer. N Engl J Med 313:1365–1368, 1985

153. Hohler H: Reconstruction of the female breast after radical mastectomy. In Converse JM (ed): Reconstructive Plastic Surgery, pp 3710–3726. Philadelphia, WB Saunders, 1977

154. Georgiade NG: Reconstructive Breast Surgery. St Louis, CV Mosby, 1976

155. Cocke WM Jr: Breast Reconstruction Following Mastectomy for Carcinoma. Boston, Little, Brown, 1977

156. Hartwell SW Jr, Anderson R, Hall MD: Reconstruction of the breast after mastectomy for cancer. Plast Reconstr Surg 57:152–157, 1976

157. Bostwick J III, Vasconez LO, Jurkiewicz MJ: Breast reconstruction after a radical mastectomy. Plast Reconstr Surg 61:682–693, 1978

158. Lewis JR Jr: Reconstruction of the breasts. Surg Clin North Am 51:429–440, 1971

159. Edgerton MT: Breast reconstruction after radical mastectomy for cancer. South Med J 60:719–723, 1967

160. Watts GT: Restorative prosthetic mammaplasty in mastectomy for carcinoma and benign lesions. Clin Plast Surg 3:177–191, 1976

161. Williams JE: Experience with a late series of Silastic breast implants. Plast Reconstr Surg 49:253–258, 1972

162. Synderman RK, Guthrie RH: Reconstruction of the female breast following radical mastectomy. Plast Reconstr Surg 47:565–567, 1971

163. Bradley SA: Acceptable Plastic Implants. In Simpson DC (ed): Modern Trends in Biomechanics, pp 25–51. London, Butterworths, 1970

164. Rees TD, Guy CL, Coburn RJ: The use of inflatable breast implants. Plast Reconstr Surg 52:609–615, 1973

165. Birnbaum L, Olsen JA: Breast reconstruction following radical mastectomy, using custom designed implants. Plast Reconstr Surg 61:355–363, 1978

166. Radovan C: Tissue expansion in soft-tissue reconstruction. Plast Reconstr Surg 74:482–490, 1984

167. Argenta LC: Reconstruction of the breast by tissue expansion. Clin Plast Surg 11:257–264, 1984

168. Phillips CM: Reconstructive surgery after classical radical mastectomies using omental pedicled grafts and fascia lata. Breast 4:10–18, 1978

169. Arnold PG, Hartrampf CR, Jurkiewicz MJ: One-stage reconstruction of the breast, using the transposed greater omentum (case report). Plast Reconstr Surg 57:520–522, 1976

170. Shaw WW: Breast reconstruction by superior gluteal microvascular free flaps without silicone implants. Plast Reconstr Surg 72:490–499, 1983

171. Bostwick J III: Breast reconstruction after mastectomy. In Harris JR, Hellman S, Henderson IC, Kinne DW (eds): Breast Diseases, pp 668–682. Philadelphia, JB Lippincott, 1987

172. Hohler H: Reconstruction after mastectomy. In Symposium on Neoplastic and Reconstructive Problems of the Female Breast. St Louis, CV Mosby, 1973

173. Allison AB, Howorth MB Jr: Carcinoma in a nipple preserved by heterotopic auto-implantation. N Engl J Med 298:1132, 1978

174. Parry RG, Cochran TC Jr, Wolfort FG: When is there nipple involvement in carcinoma of the breast? Plast Reconstr Surg 59:535–537, 1977

175. Smith J, Payne WS, Carney JA: Involvement of the nipple and areola in carcinoma of the breast. Surg Gynecol Obstet 143:546–548, 1976

176. Adams WM: Labial transplant for correction of lesions of the nipple. Plast Reconstr Surg 4:295–299, 1949

177. Tapley N, Spanos WJ, Fletcher GH: Results in patients with breast cancer treated by radical mastectomy and post-operative irradiation with no adjuvant chemotherapy. Cancer 49:1316–1319, 1982

178. Stjernsward J: Decreased survival correlated to local irradiation in "early" operable breast cancer. Lancet 2:1285–1286, 1974

179. Cuzick J, Stewart H, Peto R et al: Overview of randomized trials comparing radical mastectomy without radiotherapy against simple mastectomy with radiotherapy in breast cancer. Cancer Treat Rep 71:7–14, 1987

180. Host H, Brennhovd IO: The effect of postoperative radiation therapy in breast cancer. Int J Radiat Oncol Biol Phys 2:1061–1067, 1977

181. Chu FCH, Lin FJ, Kim JH: Locally recurrent carcinoma of the breast: Results of radiation therapy. Cancer 37:2677–2681, 1976

182. Zimmerman KW, Montague ED, Fletcher GH: Frequency, anatomic distribution, and management of local recurrences after definite therapy for breast cancer. Cancer 19:67–74, 1966

183. Goldie JH, Coldman AJ: A mathematical model for relating the drug sensitivity of tumors to their spontaneous mutation rate. Cancer Treat Rep 63:1727–1731, 1979

184. Marcial VA, Velez–Garcia E, Moore M: Radiotherapy related adjuvant chemotherapy initiation delay in breast cancer with positive nodes: Does it affect prognosis?—A Southeastern Cancer Study Group Report. Proc ASTRO p 150, 1985

185. Cooper MR, Rhyne AL, Muss HB: A randomized comparative trial of chemotherapy and irradiation therapy for Stage II breast cancer. Cancer 47:2833–2839, 1981

186. Cooper MR, Muss H, Ferree C: A six and one half year follow-up of a randomized adjuvant study of chemotherapy with and without radiation therapy for Stage II breast cancer. Breast Cancer Res Treat 6:169, 1985

187. Ahmann D, O'Fallon J, Scanlon P et al: A preliminary assessment of factors associated with recurrent disease in a surgical adjuvant clinical trial for patients with breast cancer with special emphasis on the aggressiveness of therapy. Am J Clin Oncol 5:371–381, 1982

188. Griem KL, Henderson IC, Gelman R et al: The 5-year results of a randomized trial of adjuvant radiation therapy after chemotherapy in breast cancer treated with mastectomy. J Clin Oncol 5:1546–1555, 1987

189. Crile G: Multicentric breast cancer: The incidence of new cancers in the homolateral breast after partial mastectomy. Cancer 35:475–477, 1975

190. Peters MV: Wedge resection with or without radiation in early breast cancer. J Radiat Oncl Biol Phys 2:1151–1156, 1977

191. Lagios MD, Westdahl PR, Margolin FR, Rose MR: Duct carcinoma-in-situ. Cancer 50:1309–1314, 1982

192. Montgomery ACV, Greening WP, Levene AL: Clinical study of recurrence rate and survival time of patients with carcinoma of the breast treated by biopsy excision without any other therapy. J R Soc Med 71:339–342, 1978

193. Fisher B, Bauer M, Margolese R et al: Five-year results of a randomized clinical trial comparing total mastectomy and segmental mastectomy with or without radiation in the treatment of breast cancer. N Engl J Med 312:666–673, 1985

194. Calle R, Vilcoq JR, Zafrani B, Vielh P, Fourquet A: Local control and survival of breast cancer treated by limited surgery followed by irradiation. Cancer 12:873–878, 1986

195. Kurtz JM, Spitalier JM, Amalric R: Late breast recurrence after lumpectomy and irradiation. Int J Radiat Oncol Biol Phys 9:1191–1194, 1983

196. Clarke DH, Le MG, Sarrazin D et al: Analysis of local–regional relapses in patients with early breast cancers treated by excision and radiotherapy: Experience of the Institut Gustave-Roussy. Int J Radiat Oncol Biol Phys 11:137–145, 1985

197. Clark RM: Alternatives to mastectomy—The Princess Margaret Hospital experience. In Harris JR, Hellman S, Silen W (eds): Conservative Management of Breast Cancer, pp 35–46, Philadelphia, JB Lippincott, 1983

198. Spitalier JM, Gambarelli J, Brandone H: Breast-conserving surgery with radiation therapy for operable mammary carcinoma: A 25-year experience. World J Surg 10:1014–1020, 1986

199. Recht A, Silver B, Schnitt S, Connolly J, Hellman S, Harris JR: Breast relapse following primary radiation therapy for early breast cancer I: Classification, frequency, and salvage. Int J Radiat Oncol Biol Phys 11:1271–1276, 1985

200. Svensson GK, Bjarngard BE, Larson RD, Levene MB: A modified three-field technique for breast treatment. Int J Radiat Oncol Biol Phys 6:689–694, 1980

201. Siddon RL, Buck BA, Harris JR, Svensson GK: Three field corner technique for breast irradiation using tangential field corner blocks. Int J Radiat Oncol Biol Phys 9:583–588, 1983

202. Harris JR, Recht A, Amalric A et al: Time course and prognosis of local recurrence following primary radiation therapy for early breast cancer. J Clin Oncol 2:37–41, 1984

203. Fisher B, Wolmark N: Conservative surgery: The American experience. Semin Oncol 13:425–433, 1986

204. Fisher ER, Sass R, Fisher B, Gregorio R, Brown R, Wickerham L: Pathologic findings from the National Surgical Adjuvant Breast Project (Protocol 6). II: Relation of local breast recurrence to multicentricity. Cancer 57:1717–1724, 1986

205. Schnitt S, Connolly J, Recht A, Silver B, Harris JR: Breast relapse following primary radiation therapy for early breast cancer II: Detection, pathologic features, and prognostic significance. Int J Radiat Oncol Biol Phys 11:1277–1284, 1985

206. Beadle GF, Silver B, Botnick L, Hellman S, Harris JR: Cosmetic results following primary radiation therapy for early breast cancer. Cancer 54:2911–2918, 1984

207. Veronesi U, Saccozzi R, DelVecchio M et al: Comparing radical mastectomy with

quadrantectomy, axillary dissection and radiotherapy in patients with small cancers of the breast. N Engl J Med 305:6–11, 1981

208. Veronesi U: Randomized trials comparing conservation techniques with conventional surgery: An overview. In Tobias JS, Peckham MJ (eds): Primary Management of Breast Cancer: Alternatives to Mastectomy, pp 131–152. London, Edward Arnold Publishers, 1985

209. Veronesi U, Zucali R, Luini A: Local control and survival in early breast cancer: The Milan trial. Int J Radiat Oncol Biol Phys 12:717–720, 1986

210. Sarrazin D, Le M, Contesso G et al: Conservative treatment versus mastectomy in breast cancer: 10 year results of a randomized trial. Proc ESTRO p 249, 1987

211. Findlay P, Lippman M, Danforth D: A randomized trial comparing mastectomy to radiotherapy in the treatment of stage I–II breast cancer: A preliminary report. Proc Am Soc Clin Oncol 5:63, 1986

212. Habibollahi F, Fentiman IB, Chaudary MA: Conservation treatment of operable breast cancer. Proc Am Soc Clin Oncol 6:59, 1987

213. Recht A, Connolly JL, Schnitt SJ et al: Conservative surgery and radiation therapy for early breast cancer: Results, controversies, and unsolved problems. Semin Oncol 13:434–449, 1986

214. Larson D, Weinstein M, Goldberg I et al: Edema of the arm as a function of the extent of axillary surgery in patients with stage I–II carcinoma of the breast treated with primary radiotherapy. Int J Radiat Oncol Biol Phys 12:1575–1582, 1986

215. Salner AL, Botnick LE, Herzog AG et al: Reversible brachial plexopathy following primary radiation therapy for breast cancer. Cancer Treat Rep 65:797–802, 1981

216. Kissin MW, della Rovere GQ, Easton D, Westbury G: Risk of lymphoedema following treatment of breast cancer. Br J Surg 73:580–584, 1986

217. Mazeron JJ, Otmezguine Y, Huaro J, Pierquin B: Conservative treatment of breast cancer: Results of management of axillary lymph node area in 3353 patients. Lancet 1:1387, 1985

218. Recht A, Hayes DF: Specific sites and emergencies: Local recurrence. In: Harris JR, Hellman S, Henderson IC, Kinne DW (eds): Breast Diseases, pp 508–524. Philadelphia, JB Lippincott, 1987

219. Skipper HE: Kinetics of mammary tumor cell growth and implications for therapy. Cancer 28:1479–1499, 1971

220. Cole MP: A clinical trial of an artificial menopause in carcinoma of the breast. Inserm 55:143–150, 1975

221. Frei EF I: Selected considerations regarding chemotherapy as adjuvant in cancer treatment. Cancer Chemother Rep 50:1–8, 1966

222. Fisher B, Fisher ER, Redmond C: Ten year results from the NSABP clinical trial evaluating the use of L-phenylalanine mustard (L-PAM) in the management of primary breast cancer. J Clin Oncol 4:929–941, 1986

223. Bonadonna G, Valagussa P, Rossi A et al: Ten-year experience with CMF-based adjuvant chemotherapy in resectable breast cancer. Breast Cancer Res Treat 5:95–115, 1985

224. Henderson IC: Adjuvant systemic therapy for early breast cancer. Curr Probl Cancer 11:125–207, 1987

225. Brincker H, Rose C, Rank F et al: Evidence of a castration-mediated effect of adjuvant cytotoxic chemotherapy in premenopausal breast cancer. J Clin Oncol 5:1771–1778, 1987

226. Bonadonna G, Valagussa P, Tancini G et al: Current status of Milan adjuvant chemotherapy trials for node-positive and node-negative breast cancer. NCI Monogr 1:45–49, 1986

227. Nolvadex Adjuvant Trial Organisation: Controlled trial of tamoxifen as single adjuvant agent in management of early breast cancer: Analysis at six years. Lancet 1:836–839, 1985

228. Baum M, Wilson AJ, Ebbs SR: The role of adjuvant endocrine therapy in primary breast cancer. In Salmon SE (ed): Adjuvant Therapy of Cancer V, pp 377–390. Orlando, Grune & Stratton, 1987

229. Padmanabhan N, Howell A, Rubens RD: Mechanism of action of adjuvant chemotherapy in early breast cancer. Lancet 2:411–414, 1986

230. Meakin JW, Allt WEC, Beale FA et al: Ovarian irradiation and prednisone following surgery and radiotherapy for carcinoma of the breast. Breast Cancer Res Treat 3:s45–s48, 1983

231. Bryant AJ, Weir JA: Prophylactic oophorectomy in operable instances of carcinoma of the breast. Surg Gynecol Obstet 153:660–664, 1981

232. Tengrup I, Nittby LT, Landberg T: Prophylactic oophorectomy in the treatment of carcinoma of the breast. Surg Gynecol Obstet 162:209–214, 1986

233. Gelber RD, Goldhirsch A: The concept of an overview of cancer clinical trials with special emphasis on early breast cancer. J Clin Oncol 4:1696–1703, 1986

234. Himel HN, Liberati A, Gelber RD, Chalmers TC: Adjuvant chemotherapy for breast cancer: A pooled estimate based on published randomized control trials. JAMA 256:1148–1159, 1986

235. Early Breast Cancer Trialists Collaborative Group: The effects of adjuvant tamoxifen and of cytotoxic therapy on mortality in early breast cancer: An overview of 70 randomized trials among 30,000 women. N Engl J Med (in press)

236. Morrison JM, Howell A, Grieve RJ et al: The West Midlands Oncology Association Trials of adjuvant chemotherapy for operable breast cancer. In Jones SE, Salmon SE (eds): Adjuvant Therapy of Cancer IV, pp 253–259. Orlando, Grune & Stratton, 1984

237. Senn HJ, Barett–Mahler R: Update of Swiss adjuvant trials with LMF and CMF in operable breast cancer. In Salmon SE (ed): Adjuvant Therapy of Cancer V, pp 243–252. Orlando, Grune & Stratton, 1987

238. Jakesz R, Kolb R, Reiner G et al: Adjuvant chemotherapy in node-negative breast cancer patients. In Salmon SE (ed): Adjuvant Therapy of Cancer V, pp 223–231. Orlando, Grune & Stratton, 1987

239. Bonadonna G, Valagussa P, Zambetti M, Bozzoni R, Moliterni A: Milan adjuvant trials for stage I–II breast cancer. In Salmon SE (ed): Adjuvant Therapy of Cancer VI, pp 211–221. Orlando, Grune & Stratton, 1987

240. Fisher B, Redmond C, Fisher ER, Wolmark N: Systemic adjuvant therapy in treatment of primary operable breast cancer: National Surgical Adjuvant Breast and Bowel Project experience. NCI Monogr 1:35–43, 1986

241. Carbone PP: Multiple trials of adjuvant chemohormonal therapy in the treatment of breast cancer: Preliminary results — The ECOG experience. Breast Cancer Res Treat 3:35–38, 1983

242. Goldhirsch A, Gelber R: Adjuvant treatment for early breast cancer: The Ludwig Breast Cancer studies. NCI Monogr 1:55–70, 1986

243. Scottish Cancer Trials Office: Adjuvant tamoxifen in the management of operable breast cancer: The Scottish trial. Lancet 2:171–175, 1987

244. Pritchard KI, Meakin JW, Boyd NF et al: A randomized trial of adjuvant tamoxifen in postmenopausal women with axillary node positive breast cancer. In Jones SE, Salmon SE (eds): Adjuvant Therapy of Cancer IV, pp 339–347. Orlando, Grune & Stratton, 1984

245. Nissen–Meyer R, Host H, Kjellgren K, Mansson B, Norin T: Neoadjuvant chemotherapy in breast cancer: As single perioperative treatment and with supplementary long-term chemotherapy. In: Salmon SE (ed): Adjuvant Chemotherapy for Cancer V, pp 253–261. Orlando, Grune & Stratton, 1987

246. Henderson IC, Gelman RS, Harris JR, Canellos GP: Duration of therapy in adjuvant chemotherapy trials. NCI Monogr 1:95–98, 1986

247. Tancini G, Bonadonna G, Valagussa P, Marchini S, Veronesi U: Adjuvant CMF in breast cancer: Comparative 5-year results of 12 versus 6 cycles. J Clin Oncol 1:2–10, 1983

248. Osborne CK, Rivkin SE, McDivitt RW et al: Adjuvant therapy of breast cancer: Southwest Oncology Group studies. NCI Monogr 1:71–74, 1986

249. Mathe G, Plagne R, Morice V, Misset JL: Consistencies and variations of observations during serial analyses of a trial of adjuvant chemotherapy in breast cancer. In Salmon SE (ed): Adjuvant Chemotherapy for Cancer V, pp 271–280. Orlando, Grune & Stratton, 1987

250. Fisher B, Redmond CK, Wolmark N: Long term results from NSABP trials of adjuvant therapy for breast cancer. In Salmon SE (ed): Adjuvant Therapy of Cancer V, pp 283–295. Orlando, Grune & Stratton, 1987

251. Perloff M, Norton L, Korzun A et al: Advantage of an Adriamycin (A) combination plus Halotestin (H) after initial cyclophosphamide, methotrexate, 5-fluorouracil, vincristine and prednisone (CMFVP) for adjuvant therapy of node-positive Stage II breast cancer (abstract). Proc Am Soc Clin Oncol 5:70, 1986

252. Bonadonna G, Valagussa P: Dose–response effect of adjuvant chemotherapy in breast cancer. N Engl J Med 304:10–15, 1981

253. Hryniuk W, Levine MN: Analysis of dose intensity for adjuvant chemotherapy trials in Stage II breast cancer. J Clin Oncol 4:1162–1170, 1986

254. Henderson IC, Gelman RS: A reanalysis of dose intensity for adjuvant chemotherapy trials in Stage II breast cancer. SAKK Bull 1:10–12, 1987

255. Tormey DC, Gray R, Taylor IV SG, Knuiman M, Olson JE, Cummings FJ: Postoperative chemotherapy and chemohormonal therapy in women with node-positive breast cancer. NCI Monogr 1:75–80, 1986

256. Goldhirsch A, Gelber RD: Adjuvant therapy for breast cancer: The Ludwig Breast Cancer Trials 1987. In Salmon SE (ed): Adjuvant Therapy of Cancer V, pp 297–309. Orlando, Grune & Stratton, 1987

257. Hubay CA, Pearson OH, Gordon NH et al: Randomized trial of endocrine versus endocrine plus cytotoxic chemotherapy in women with Stage II, estrogen receptor positive breast cancer (abstract). Proc Am Soc Clin Oncol 5:63, 1986

258. Kaufmann M, Jonat W, Caffier H et al: Adjuvant systemic risk adapted cytotoxic plus/minus tamoxifen therapy in women with node positive breast cancer. In Salmon SE (ed): Adjuvant Therapy of Cancer V, pp 337–346. Orlando, Grune & Stratton, 1987

259. Nissen–Meyer R, Kjellgren K, Mansson B: Adjuvant chemotherapy in breast cancer. Recent Results Cancer Res 80:142–148, 1982

260. Ragaz J: Emerging modalities for adjuvant therapy of breast cancer: Neoadjuvant chemotherapy. NCI Monogr 1:145–152, 1986

261. Beadle G, Come S, Henderson IC et al: The effect of timing of primary breast irradiation and chemotherapy on the cosmetic results. Int J Radiat Oncol Biol Phys 10(suppl 2):77, 1984

262. Gore SM, Come SE, Griem K et al: Influence of the sequencing of chemotherapy and radiation therapy in node-negative breast cancer patients treated by conservative surgery and radiation therapy. In Salmon SE (ed): Adjuvant Therapy of Cancer V, pp 365–373. Orlando, Grune & Stratton, 1987

263. Fisher B, Rockette H, Fisher ER, Wickerham DL, Redmond C, Brown A: Leukemia in breast cancer patients following adjuvant chemotherapy or postoperative radiation: The NSABP experience. J Clin Oncol 3:1640–1658, 1985

264. Valagussa P, Tancini G, Bonadonna G: Second malignancies after CMF for resectable breast cancer. J Clin Oncol 5:1138–1142, 1987

265. Henderson IC, Gelman R: Second malignancies from adjuvant chemotherapy? Too soon to tell. J Clin Oncol 5:1135–1137, 1987

266. Killackey MA, Hakes TB, Pierce VK: Endometrial adenocarcinoma in breast cancer patients receiving antiestrogens. Cancer Treat Rep 69:237–238, 1985

267. Gelber RD, Goldhirsch A, Castiglione M, Price K, Isley M, Coates A: Time without Symptoms and Toxicity (TWiST): A quality-of-life-oriented endpoint to evaluate adjuvant therapy. In Salmon SE (ed): Adjuvant Therapy of Cancer V, pp 455–465. Orlando, Grune & Stratton, 1987

268. Horton J: Follow-up of breast cancer patients. Cancer 53:790–797, 1984

269. Wickerham L, Fisher B, Cronin W, Members of the NSABP Committee for Treatment Failure Criteria: The efficacy of bone scanning in the follow-up of patients with operable breast cancer. Breast Cancer Res Treat 1:24–84, 1983

270. Tomin R, Donegan WL: Screening for recurrent breast cancer—Its effectiveness and prognostic value. J Clin Oncol 5:62–67, 1987

271. Marrazzo A, Solina G, Puccia V: Evaluation of routine follow-up after surgery for breast carcinoma. J Surg Oncol 32:179–181, 1986

272. Broders AC: Carcinoma in situ contrasted with benign penetrating epithelium. JAMA 99:1670–1674, 1932

273. Ashikari R, Huvos AG, Snyder RE: Prospective study of noninfiltrating carcinoma of the breast. Cancer 39:435–439, 1977

274. Sunshine JA, Moseley HS, Fletcher WS, Krippaehne WW: Breast carcinoma in situ: A retrospective review of 112 cases with a minimum 10 year follow-up. Am J Surg 150:44–50, 1985

275. Farrow JH: The James Ewing Lecture: Current concepts in the detection and treatment of the earliest of the early breast cancers. Cancer 25:468–477, 1970

276. Page DL, Dupont WD, Rogers LW, Landenberger M: Intraductal carcinoma of the breast: Follow-up after biopsy only. Cancer 49:751–758, 1982

277. Betsill WL, Rosen PP, Lieberman PH, Robbins GF: Intraductal carcinoma: Long-term follow-up after treatment by biopsy alone. JAMA 239:1863–1867, 1978

278. Alpers CE, Wellings SR: The prevalence of carcinoma in situ in normal and cancer associated breasts. Hum Pathol 16:796–807, 1985

279. Robbins GF, Berg JW: Bilateral primary breast cancers: A prospective clinicopathological study. Cancer 17:1501–1527, 1964

280. Recht A, Danoff BS, Solin LJ: Intraductal carcinoma of the breast: Results of treatment with excisional biopsy and irradiation. J Clin Oncol 3:1339–1343, 1985

281. Zafrani B, Fourquet A, Vilcoq JR, Legal M, Calle R: Conservative management of intraductal breast carcinoma with tumorectomy and radiation therapy. Cancer 57:1299–1301, 1986

282. Montague ED: Conservation surgery and radiation therapy in the treatment of operable breast cancer. Cancer 53:700–704, 1984

283. Fisher ER, Saas R, Fisher B, Wickerham L, Paik SM: Pathologic findings from the National Surgical Adjuvant Breast Project (Protocol 6) I: Intraductal carcinoma (DCIS). Cancer 57:197–208, 1986

284. Lagios MD: Human breast precancer: Current status. Cancer Surv 2:383–402, 1983 (Updated by personal communication, 1987.)

285. Harris JR, Connolly JL, Schnitt SJ et al: The use of pathologic features in selecting the extent of surgical resection necessary for breast cancer patients treated by primary radiation therapy. Ann Surg 201:164–169, 1985

286. Silverstein MJ, Rosser RJ, Gierson ED: Axillary lymph node dissection for intraductal breast carcinoma: Is it indicated? Cancer 59:1819–1824, 1987

287. Fisher B: Breast cancer management: Alternatives to radical mastectomy. N Engl J Med 301:326–328, 1979

288. Hellman S, Harris JR: The appropriate breast cancer paradigm. Cancer Res 47:339–342, 1987

289. Foote FW Jr, Stewart FW: Lobular carcinoma in situ: A rare form of mammary cancer. Am J Pathol 17:491–496, 1941

290. Muir R: The evolution of carcinoma of the mamma. J Pathol Bacteriol 52:155, 1941

291. Benfield JR, Jacobson M, Warner NE: In situ lobular carcinoma of the breast. Arch Surg 91:130, 1965

292. Newman W: Lobular carcinoma of the female breast: Report of 73 cases. Ann Surg 164:305, 1966

293. McDivitt RW, Hutter RVP, Foote FW Jr: In situ lobular carcinoma: A prospective follow-up study indicating cumulative patient risks. JAMA 201:96–100, 1967

294. Stewart FW: Tumors of the Breast: Atlas of Tumor Pathology. Washington, DC, Armed Forces Institute of Pathology, 1950

295. Rosen P, Lieberman P, Braun D, Kosloff C, Adair F: Lobular carcinoma in situ of the breast. Am J Surg Pathol 2:225–251, 1978

296. Wheeler JE, Interline HT, Roseman JM: Lobular carcinoma-in situ of the breast: Long-term follow-up. Cancer 34:554–563, 1974

297. Haagensen CD, Lane N, Lattes R, Bodian C: Lobular neoplasia (so-called lobular carcinoma in situ) of the breast. Cancer 42:737–769, 1978

298. Haagensen CD, Stout AP: Carcinoma of the breast: Criteria of operability. Ann Surg 118:859–870, 1932

299. Baclesse FL: Roentgen therapy as the sole method of treatment of cancer of the breast. Am J Roentgenol Rad Ther Nucl Med 62:311–319, 1949

300. Fletcher GH, Montague ED: Radical irradiation of advanced breast cancer. Am J Roentgenol Rad Ther Nucl Med 93:573–584, 1965

301. Sheldon T, Hayes DF, Cady B et al: Primary radiation therapy for locally advanced breast cancer. Cancer 60:1219–1225, 1987

302. Arriagada R, Mouriesse H, Sarrazin D, Clark RM, Doboer G: Radiotherapy alone in breast cancer I: Analysis of tumor parameters, tumor dose and local control: The experience of the Gustave-Roussy Institute and the Princess Margaret Hospital. Int J Radiat Oncol Biol Phys 11:1751–1757, 1985

303. De Lena M, Varini M, Zucali R et al: Multimodal treatment for locally advanced breast cancer: Results of chemotherapy–radiotherapy versus chemotherapy–surgery. Cancer Clin Trials 4:229–236, 1981

304. Rubens RD, Sexton S, Tong D, Winter PJ, Knight RK, Hayward JL: Combined chemotherapy and radiotherapy for locally advanced breast cancer. Eur J Cancer 16:351–356, 1980

305. Schaake–Koning C, van der Linden EH, Hart G, Engelsman E: Adjuvant chemo- and hormonal therapy in locally advanced breast cancer: A randomized clinical study. Int J Radiat Oncol Biol Phys 11:1759–1763, 1985

306. Valagussa P, Zambetti M, Bignami P et al: T3b–T4 breast cancer: Factors affecting results in combined modality treatments. Clin Exp Metastasis 1:191–202, 1983

307. Perloff M, Korzun A, Chu F, Lesnick G: Combination chemotherapy (CT) with surgery (S) or radiotherapy (RT) for Stage III breast carcinoma (abstract). Proc Am Soc Clin Oncol 4:60, 1985

308. Balawajder I, Antich PP, Boland J: An analysis of the role of radiotherapy alone and in combination with chemotherapy and surgery in the management of advanced breast carcinoma. Cancer 51:574–580, 1983

309. Paone JF, Baker RR: Pathogenesis and treatment of Paget's disease of the breast. Cancer 48:825–829, 1981

310. Nance FC, DeLoach DH, Welsh RA: Paget's disease of the breast. Ann Surg 171:864–874, 1970

311. Maier WP, Rosemond GP, Harasym EL: Paget's disease in the female breast. Surg Gynecol Obstet 128:1253–1263, 1969

312. Osteen RT: Paget's disease of the nipple. In Harris JR, Hellman S, Henderson IC, Linne DW (eds): Breast Diseases, pp 589–595. Philadelphia, JB Lippincott, 1987

313. Treves N, Holleb AI: Cancer of the male breast: A report of 146 cases. Cancer 8:1239–1250, 1955

314. Haagensen CD: Carcinoma of the male breast. In Diseases of the Breast, 2nd Ed, pp 779–792. Philadelphia, WB Saunders, 1971

315. Langlands AO, Maclean N, Ken GR: Carcinoma of the male breast: Report of a series of 88 cases. Clin Radiol 27:21–25, 1976

316. Donegan WL, Perez–Mesa C: Carcinoma of the male breast. Arch Surg 106:273–279, 1973

317. Roswit B, Edlis H: Carcinoma of the male breast: A thirty-year experience and literature review. Int J Radiat Oncol Biol Phys 4:711–715, 1978

318. Anderson DE: Genetic considerations in breast cancer. In Breast Cancer: Early and Late, pp 27–36. Chicago, Year Book Medical Publishers, 1970

319. Everson RB, Li FP, Fraumeni JF: Familial male breast cancer. Lancet 1:9–12, 1976

320. El-Gazayerli MM, Abel-Aziz AS: On biharziasis and male breast cancer in Egypt. Br J Cancer 17:566–571, 1963

321. Harnden DG, Maclean N, Langlands AO: Carcinoma of the male breast and Klinefelter's syndrome. J Med Genet 8:460–461, 1971

322. Evans DB, Crichlow RW: Carcinoma of the male breast and Klinefelter's syndrome: Is there an association? Cancer 37:246–251, 1987

323. Gupta N, Cohen JL, Rosenbaum C: Estrogen receptors in male breast cancer. Cancer 46:1781–1784, 1980

324. Yap HY, Tashima CK, Blumenschein GR: Male breast cancer: A natural history study. Cancer 44:748–754, 1979

325. Robinson R, Montague ED: Treatment results in males with breast cancer. Cancer 49:403–406, 1982

326. Heller KS, Rosen PP, Schottenfeld D: Male breast cancer: A clinicopathologic study of 97 cases. Ann Surg 188:60–65, 1978

327. Treves N: Treatment of cancer of the male breast by ablative surgery and hormonal therapy: An analysis of 42 patients. Cancer 12:820–832, 1959

328. Holleb A, Freeman HP, Farrow JH: Cancer of the male breast. NY State J Med 68:544–553, 1968

329. Li MC, Janelli DE, Kelly EJ: Metastatic carcinoma of the male breast treated with bilateral adrenalectomy and chemotherapy. Cancer 25:678–681, 1970

330. Kennedy BJ, Kiang DT: Hypophysectomy in the treatment of advanced cancer of the male breast. Cancer 29:1606–1612, 1972

331. Patterson JS, Battersby LA, Bach BK: Use of tamoxifen in advanced male breast cancer. Cancer Treat Rep 64:801–804, 1980

332. Lopez M, DiLauro L, Lazzaro B: Hormonal treatment of disseminated male breast cancer. Oncology 42:345–349, 1985

333. Bezwoda WR, Hesdorffer C, Dansey R: Breast cancer in men: Clinical features, hormone receptor status, and response to therapy. Cancer 60:1337–1340, 1987

334. Bagley CS, Wesley MN, Young RC, Lippman ME: Adjuvant chemotherapy in males with cancer of the breast. Am J Clin Oncol 10:55–60, 1987

335. Paterson AHG, Lees AW, Hanson J, Szafran O, Cornish F: Impact of chemotherapy on survival in metastatic breast cancer. Lancet 2:312, 1980

336. Fey MF, Brunner KW, Sonntag RW: Prognostic factors in metastatic breast cancer. Cancer Clin Trials 4:237–247, 1981

337. Cavilli F, Beer M, Martz G et al: Concurrent or sequential use of cytotoxic chemotherapy and hormone treatment in advanced breast cancer: Report of the Swiss Group for Clinical Cancer Research. Br Med J 286:5–8, 1983

338. Australian and New Zealand Breast Cancer Trials Group: A randomized trial in postmenopausal patients with advanced breast cancer comparing endocrine and cytotoxic therapy given sequentially or in combination. J Clin Oncol 4:186–193, 1986

339. Cutler S: Classification of extent of disease in breast cancer. Semin Oncol 1:91–96, 1974

340. Baum M, Priestman T, West RR, Jones EM: A comparison of subjective responses in a trial comparing endocrine with cytotoxic treatment in advanced carcinoma of the breast. In Mouridsen HT, Palshof T (eds): Breast Cancer—Experimental and Clinical Aspects, pp 223–226. Oxford, Pergamon Press, 1980

341. Sears HF, Gerber FH, Sturtz DL, Fouty WJ: Liver scan and carcinoma of the breast. Surg Gynecol Obstet 140:409–411, 1975

342. Muss HB, White DR, Cowan RJ: Brain scanning in patients with recurrent breast cancer. Cancer 38:1574–1576, 1976

343. Pedrazzini A, Gelber R, Isley M, Castiglione M, Goldhirsch A: First repeated bone scan in the observation of patients with operable breast cancer. J Clin Oncol 4:389–394, 1986

344. Corcoran RJ, Thrall JH, Kyle RW, Kaminski RJ, Johnson MC: Solitary abnormalities

in bone scans of patients with extraosseous malignancies. Radiology 121:663–667, 1976

345. Tumeh SS, Beadle G, Kaplan WD: Clinical significance of solitary rib lesions in patients with extraskeletal malignancy. J Nucl Med 26:1140–1143, 1985

346. Gillespie PJ, Alexander JL, Edelstyn GA: Changes in 87m-Sr concentrations in skeletal metastases in patients responding to cyclical combination chemotherapy for advanced breast cancer. J Nucl Med 16:191–193, 1975

347. Rossleigh MA, Lovegrove FTA, Reynolds PM, Byrne MJ: Serial bone scans in the assessment of response to therapy in advanced breast carcinoma. Clin Nucl Med 7:397–402, 1982

348. Buckman R, Coombes RC, Dearnaley DP, Gore M, Gusterson B, Neville AM: Some clinical uses of biological markers. In Bonadonna G (ed): Breast Cancer: Diagnosis and Management, pp 109–126. Chichester, Wiley & Sons, 1984

349. Smith IE: Recurrent disease. In Harris JR, Hellman S, Henderson IC, Kinne DW (eds): Breast Diseases, pp 369–384. Philadelphia, JB Lippincott Company, 1987

350. Hayes DF, Zurawski VR Jr, Kufe DW: Comparison of circulating CA 15-3 and carcinoembryonic antigen levels in patients with breast cancer. J Clin Oncol 4:1542–1550, 1986

351. Loprinzi CL, Tormey DC, Rasmussen P et al: Prospective evaluation of carcinoembryonic antigen levels and alternating chemotherapeutic regimens in metastatic breast cancer. J Clin Oncol 4:46–56, 1986

352. Mughal AW, Hortobagyi GN, Fritsche HA, Buzdar AU, Yap H, Blumenschein GR: Serial plasma carcinoembryonic antigen measurements during treatment of metastatic breast cancer. JAMA 249:1881–1886, 1983

353. Haagensen DE Jr, Mazoujian G, Holder WD Jr, Kister SJ, Wells SA Jr: Evaluation of a breast cyst fluid protein detectable in the plasma of breast carcinoma patients. Ann Surg 185:279–285, 1977

354. Welsch CW: Host factors affecting the growth in carcinogen-induced rat mammary carcinomas: A review and tribute to Charles Brenton Huggins. Cancer Res 45:3415–3443, 1985

355. Aitken SC, Lippman ME: Effect of estrogens and antiestrogens on growth-regulatory enzymes in human breast cancer cells in tissue culture. Cancer Res 45:1611–1620, 1985

356. Lippman M, Bolan G, Huff K: Interactions of antiestrogens with human breast cancer in long-term tissue culture. Cancer Treat 60:1421–1429, 1976

357. Campbell FC, Elston CW, Blamey RW et al: Quantitative oestradiol receptor values in primary breast cancer and response of metastases to endocrine therapy. Lancet 2:1317–1319, 1981

358. Allegra J, Lippman M, Thompson E et al: Estrogen receptor status: An important variable in predicting response to endocrine therapy in metastatic breast cancer. Eur J Cancer 16:323–331, 1980

359. Kiang DT, Kollander R: Breast cancers negative for estrogen receptor but positive for progesterone receptor: A true entity? J Clin Oncol 25:662–666, 1987

360. Byar D, Sears M, McGuire W: Relationship between estrogen receptor values and clinical data in predicting the response to endocrine therapy for patients with advanced breast cancer. Eur J Cancer 15:299–310, 1979

361. Henderson IC: Endocrine therapy of metastatic breast cancer. In Harris JR, Hellman S, Henderson IC, Kinne DW (eds): Breast Diseases, pp 398–428. Philadelphia, JB Lippincott, 1987

362. Cooperative Breast Cancer Group: Results of studies of the Cooperative Breast Cancer Group—1961–63. Cancer Chemother Rep 41:1–24, 1964

363. Westerberg H: Tamoxifen and fluoxymesterone in advanced breast cancer: A controlled clinical trial. Cancer Treat Rep 64:117–121, 1980

364. Ward HWC: Anti-oestrogen therapy for breast cancer: A trial of tamoxifen at two dose levels. Br Med J 1:13–14, 1973

365. Tormey DC, Lippman ME, Edwards BK, Cassidy JG: Evaluation of tamoxifen doses with and without fluoxymesterone in advanced breast cancer. Ann Intern Med 98:139–144, 1983

366. Rose C, Theilade K, Boesen E et al: Treatment of advanced breast cancer with tamoxifen. Breast Cancer Res Treat 2:395–400, 1982

367. Bratherton DG, Brown CH, Buchanan R et al: A comparison of two doses of tamoxifen (Nolvadex) in postmenopausal women with advanced breast cancer: 10 mg BD versus 20 mg BD. Br J Cancer 50:199–205, 1984

368. Kaiser–Kupfer MI, Lippman ME: Tamoxifen retinopathy. Cancer Treat Rep 62:315–320, 1978

369. Fabian C, Sternson L, El-Serafi M, Cain L, Hearne E: Clinical pharmacology of tamoxifen in patients with breast cancer: Correlation with clinical data. Cancer 48:876–882, 1981

370. Ingle JN, Krook JE, Green SJ et al: Randomized trial of bilateral oophorectomy versus tamoxifen in premenopausal women with metastatic breast cancer. J Clin Oncol 4:178–185, 1986

371. Buchanan RB, Blamey RW, Durrant KR et al: A randomized comparison of tamoxifen with surgical oophorectomy in premenopausal patients with advanced breast cancer. J Clin Oncol 4:1326–1330, 1986

372. Pritchard K, Meakin JW, Sawka C et al: The role and mechanism of action of tamoxifen in premenopausal women with metastatic carcinoma of the breast: An update (abstract). Proc Am Soc Clin Oncol 4:54, 1985

373. Lipton A, Harvey HA, Hamilton RW: Venous thrombosis as a side effect of tamoxifen treatment. Cancer Treat Rep 68:887–889, 1984

374. Robin PE, Dalton GA: The role of major endocrine ablation. In: Stoll BA (ed): Breast Cancer—Early & Late, pp 147–156. Chicago, Year Book Med Publishers, 1977

375. Dao TL: Ablation therapy for hormone-dependent tumors. Annu Rev Med 23:1–18, 1972

376. Fracchia AA, Farrow JH, DePalo AJ, Connolly DP, Huvos AG: Castration for primary inoperable or recurrent breast carcinoma. Surg Gynecol Obstet 128:1226–1234, 1969

377. Veronesi U, Pizzocaro G, Rossi A: Oophorectomy for advanced carcinoma of the breast. Surg Gynecol Obstet 141:569–570, 1975

378. Fitzpatrick PJ, Garrett PG: Metastatic breast cancer: Ovarian ablation with lower half-body irradiation. Int J Radiat Oncol Biol Phys 7:1523–1526, 1981

379. Stuart–Harris RC, Smith IE: Aminoglutethimide in the treatment of advanced breast cancer. Cancer Treat Rev 11:189–204, 1984

380. Santen RJ, Samojlik E, Worgul TJ: Aminoglutethimide. In Santen RJ, Henderson IC (eds): A Comprehensive Guide to the Therapeutic Use of Aminoglutethimide, pp 101–160, Basel, S Karger, 1982

381. Stuart-Harris R, Bozek T, Gazet JC et al: Low-dose aminoglutethimide in treatment of advanced breast cancer. Lancet 2:604–607, 1984

382. Santen RJ, Boucher AE, Santner SJ, Henderson IC, Harvey H, Lipton A: Inhibition of aromatase as treatment of breast carcinoma in postmenopausal women. J Lab Clin Med 109:278–289, 1987

383. Lipton A, Harvey HA, Santen RJ et al: Randomized trial of aminoglutethimide versus tamoxifen in metastatic breast cancer. Cancer Res 42:3434s–3436s, 1982

384. Smith IE, Harris AL, Morgan M, Gazet JC, McKinna JA: Tamoxifen versus aminoglutethimide versus combined tamoxifen and aminoglutethimide in the treatment of advanced breast carcinoma. Cancer Res 42:3430s–3433s, 1982

385. Santen RJ, Worgul TJ, Samojlik E et al: A randomized trial comparing surgical adrenalectomy with aminoglutethimide plus hydrocortisone in women with advanced breast cancer. N Engl J Med 305:545–551, 1981

386. Messeih AA, LiptonA, Santen RJ et al: Aminoglutethimide-induced hematologic toxicity: Worldwide experience. Cancer Treat Rep 69:1003–1004, 1985

387. Tchekmedyian NS, Tait N, Aisner J: Phase I/II trial of high-dose (HD) megestrol acetate (MA) in breast cancer (abstract). Proc Am Soc Clin Oncol 5:72, 1986

388. Hortobagyi GN, Buzdar AU, Frye D et al: Oral medroxyprogesterone acetate in the treatment of metastatic breast cancer. Breast Cancer Res Treat 5:321–326, 1985

389. Carter AC, Sedransk N, Kelley RM, Ansfield FJ, Ravdin RG, Potter NR: Diethylstilbestrol: Recommended dosages for different categories of breast cancer patients—Report of the Cooperative Breast Cancer Group. JAMA 237:2079–2085, 1977

390. Kennedy BJ: Massive estrogen administration in premenopausal women with metastatic breast cancer. Cancer 15:641–648, 1962

391. Klijn JGM, deJong FH: Treatment with a luteinising-hormone–releasing-hormone analogue. Lancet 1:1213–1216, 1982

392. Harvey HA, Lipton A, Santen RJ et al: Phase II study of a gonadotropin-releasing hormone analogue (leuprolide) in postmenopausal advanced breast cancer patients (abstract). Proc Am Soc Clin Oncol 2:444, 1981

393. Nagasawa H: Prolactin and human breast cancer: A review. Eur J Cancer 15:267–279, 1979

394. Harvey HA, Lipton A, Max DT et al: Medical castration produced by the GnRH analogue leuprolide to treat metastatic breast cancer. J Clin Oncol 3:1068–1072, 1985

395. Rubens RD, Knight RK: The contribution of prednisone (P) to primary endocrine therapy (PET) in advanced breast cancer (abstract). Proc Am Soc Clin Oncol 4:53, 1985

396. Stewart JF, Rubens RD, King RJB et al: Contribution of prednisolone to the primary endocrine treatment of advanced breast cancer. Eur J Cancer Clin Oncol 18:1307–1314, 1982

397. Wilson RE, Jessiman AG, Moore FD: Severe exacerbation of cancer of the breast after oophorectomy and adrenalectomy: Report of four cases. N Engl J Med 258:312–317, 1958

398. Henderson IC: Chemotherapy for advanced disease. In Harris JR, Hellman S, Henderson IC, Kinne DW (eds): Breast Diseases, pp 428–479. Philadelphia, JB Lippincott, 1987

399. Nemoto T: Metastatic breast cancer: Prolonged complete response or possible cure by chemotherapy (abstract). Proc Am Soc Clin Oncol 2:110, 1983

400. Legha SS, Buzdar AU, Smith TL et al: Complete remissions in metastatic breast cancer treated with combination drug therapy. Ann Intern Med 91:847–852, 1979

401. Decker DA, Ahmann DL, Bisel HF, Edmonson JH, Hahn RG, O'Fallon J: Complete responders to chemotherapy in metastatic breast cancer. JAMA 242:2075–2079, 1979

402. Abramowitz JW: Long term complete remissions from chemotherapy +/− hormonal therapy in breast cancer patients (abstract). Proc Am Soc Clin Oncol 1:76, 1982

403. Mattson W, Arwidi A, von Eyben F, Lindholm C: Phase II study of combined vincristine, Adriamycin, cyclophosphamide, and methotrexate with citrovorum factor rescue in metastatic breast cancer. Cancer Treat Rep 61:1527–1531, 1977

404. Henderson IC, Gelman RS, Canellos GP, Frei EI: Time to first response (IMP), partial response (PR), and complete response (CR) in breast cancer (BC) patients (PTS) treated with intensive chemotherapy (abstract). Proc Am Soc Clin Oncol 22:445, 1981

405. Franco LA, Shafie SM: Estrogen receptor status, doubling time and sensitivity of breast carcinoma cells to Adriamycin in tissue culture (abstract). Proc Am Assoc Cancer Res 22:5, 1981

406. Sulkes A, Livingston RB, Murphy WK: Tritiated thymidine labeling index and response in human breast cancer. J Natl Cancer Inst 62:513–515, 1979

407. Zhang HJ, Kennedy BJ, Kiang DT: Thymidine kinase as a predictor of response to chemotherapy in advanced breast cancer. Breast Cancer Res Treat 4:221–225, 1984

408. Lerner HJ: Acute myelogenous leukemia in patients receiving chlorambucil as long-term adjuvant chemotherapy for Stage II breast cancer. Cancer Treat Rep 62:1135–1138, 1978

409. Brambilla C, DeLena M, Rossi A, Valagussa P, Bonadonna G: Response and survival in advanced breast cancer after two non-cross-resistant combinations. Br Med J 1:801–804, 1976

410. Ahmann D, Bisel H, Eagan R, Edmonson J, Hahn R: Controlled evaluation of Adriamycin (NSC-123127) in patients with disseminated breast cancer. Cancer Chemother Rep 58:877–882, 1974

411. Hoogstraten B, George SL, Samal B et al: Combination chemotherapy and Adriamycin in patients with advanced breast cancer. Cancer 38:13–20, 1976

412. Legha SS, Benjamin RS, Mackay B et al: Adriamycin therapy by continuous intravenous infusion in patients with metastatic breast cancer. Cancer 49:1762–1766, 1982

413. Jain K, Wittes R, Benedetto P et al: A randomized comparison of weekly (arm I) vs. monthly (arm II) doxorubicin(DOX) in combination with mitomycin C (MMC) in advanced breast cancer (abstract). Proc Am Soc Clin Oncol 2:109, 1983

414. Segaloff A, Carter AC, Escher GC, Ansfield FJ, Talley RW: An evaluation of the effect of vincristine added to cyclosphosphamide, 5-fluorouracil, methotrexate, and prednisone in advanced breast cancer. Breast Cancer Res Treat 5:311–319, 1985

415. Steiner R, Stewart JF, Rubens RD: Results of endocrine therapy do not predict response to chemotherapy in advanced breast cancer. Eur J Cancer Clin Oncol 19:1559–1563, 1983

416. Fraschini G, Yap HY, Hortobagyi GN, Buzdar A, Blumenschein G: Five-day continuous-infusion vinblastine in the treatment of breast cancer. Cancer 56:225–229, 1985

417. Yap HY, Blumenschein GR, Hortobagyi GN, Buzdar A, Bodey GP: A randomized comparative study of vinblastine (VLB), vindesine (VDS) and vincristine (VCR) in patients (PTS) with refractory metastatic breast cancer (abstract). Proc Am Soc Clin Oncol 22:441, 1981

418. Smith IE, Powles TJ, Coombes RC et al: A control randomized trial comparing vindesine and Adriamycin with vincristine and Adriamycin in the treatment of advanced breast carcinoma. In Brade W, Nagel GA, Seeber S (eds): Proceedings of the International Vinca Alkaloid Symposium—Vindesine, pp 185–194. Karger Basel, Frankfurt, 1980

419. Yap HY, Yap BS, Rasmussen S, Levens ME, Hortobagyi GN, Blumenschein GR: Treatment for meningeal carcinomatosis in breast cancer. Cancer 49:219–222, 1982

420. Yap HY, Blumenschein GR, Yap BS et al: High-dose methotrexate for advanced breast cancer. Cancer Treat Rep 63:757–761, 1979

421. Henderson IC, Gelman R, Canellos GP, Frei E: Prolonged disease-free survival in advanced breast cancer treated with "super-CMF" Adriamycin: An alternating regimen employing high-dose methotrexate with citrovorum factor rescue. Cancer Treat Rep 65:67–75, 1981

422. Creagan ET, Green ST, Ahmann DL, Ingle JN, Edmonson JH, Marschke RF: A Phase III clinical trial comparing the combination cyclophosphamide, Adriamycin, cisplatin with cyclophosphamide, 5-fluorouracil, prednisone in patients with advanced breast cancer. J Clin Oncol 2:1260–1265, 1984

423. Sledge GW Jr, Loehrer PJ Sr, Roth BJ, Einhorn LH: Cisplatin as first-line therapy for metastatic breast cancer (abstract). Proc Am Soc Clin Oncol 6:53, 1987

424. Kolaric K, Roth A, Vukas D, Cervek J: CAP (cyclophosphamide, Adriamycin, platinum) vs CMFVP (cyclophosphamide, methotrexate, 5-fluorouracil, vincristine, prednisolone) combination chemotherapy in untreated metastatic breast cancer: A preliminary report of a controlled clinical study. Cancer Chemother Pharmacol 13:142–144, 1984

425. Rubens RD, Knight R, Hayward JL: Chemotherapy of advanced breast cancer: A controlled randomized trial of cyclophosphamide versus a four-drug combination. Br J Cancer 32:730–736, 1975

426. Mouridsen HT, Palshof T, Brahm M, Rahbek I: Evaluation of single-drug versus multiple-drug chemotherapy in the treatment of advanced breast cancer. Cancer Treat Rep 61:47–50, 1977

427. Smalley RV, Murphy S, Huguley CM, Bartolucci AA: Combination versus sequential five-drug chemotherapy in metastatic carcinoma of the breast. Cancer Res 36:3911–3916, 1976

428. Chlebowski R, Irwin LE, Pugh RP et al: Survival of patients with metastatic breast cancer treated with either combination or sequential chemotherapy. Cancer Res 39:4503–4506, 1979

429. Tormey DC, Gelman R, Band PR et al: Comparison of induction chemotherapies for metastatic breast cancer. Cancer 50:1235–1244, 1982

430. Ramirez G, Klotz J, Strawitz JG et al: Combination chemotherapy in breast cancer: A randomized study of 4 versus 5 drugs. Oncology 32:101–108, 1975

431. Englesman E, Rubens RD, Klijn JGM, Wildiers J, Rotmensz N, Sylvester R: Comparison of "classical CMF" with a three-weekly intravenous CMF schedule in postmenopausal patients with advanced breast cancer: An EORTC study (Trial 10808). Proc 4th EORTC Breast Cancer Working Conf 1987, p 1

432. Aisner J, Weinberg V, Perloff M et al: Chemotherapy versus chemoimmunotherapy (CAF v CAFVP v CMF each plus/minus MER) for metastatic carcinoma of the breast: A CALGB study. J Clin Oncol 5:1523–1533, 1987

433. Hart R, Perloff M, Holland J: One-day VATH (vinblastine, Adriamycin, thiotepa, and Halotestin) therapy for advanced breast cancer refractory to chemotherapy. Cancer 48:1522–1527, 1981

434. Perloff M, Hart R, Holland J: Vinblastine, Adriamycin, thiotepa, and Halotestin (VATH). Cancer 42:2534–2537, 1978

435. Friedman MA, Marcus FS, Cassidy MJ et al: 5-Fluorouracil + Oncovin + Adriamycin + mitomycin C (FOAM): An effective program for breast cancer, even for disease refractory to previous chemotherapy. Cancer 52:193–197, 1983

436. Konits P, Aisner J, VanEcho D, Lichtenfeld K, Wiernik P: Mitomycin C and vinblastine chemotherapy for advanced breast cancer. Cancer 48:1295–1298, 1981

437. Denefrio JM, East DR, Troner MB, Vogel CL: Phase II study of mitomycin C and vinblastine in women with advanced breast cancer refractory to standard cytotoxic therapy. Cancer Treat Rep 62:2113–2115, 1978

438. Garewal HS, Brooks RJ, Jones SE, Miller TP: Treatment of advanced breast cancer with mitomycin C combined with vinblastine or vindesine. J Clin Oncol 1:772–775, 1983

439. De Lena M, Zucali R, Viganotti G, Valagussa P, Bonadonna G: Combined chemotherapy–radiotherapy approach in locally advanced (T3b–T4) breast cancer. Cancer Chemother Pharmacol 1:53–59, 1978

440. Coates A, Gebski V, Bishop JF et al: Improving the quality of life during chemotherapy for advanced breast cancer. N Engl J Med 317:1490–1495, 1987

441. Bonadonna G, Valagussa P: Dose–response effect of CMF in breast cancer (abstract). Proc Am Soc Clin Oncol 21:413, 1980

442. Brufman G, Sulkes A, Fuks Z, Biran S: Cytoxan, methotrexate and 5-fluorouracil (CMF) chemotherapy (CHTX) in metastatic breast cancer (MBC): The influence of dose levels (DL) and performance status (PS) upon response rates and survival (abstract). Proc Am Soc Clin Oncol 2:103, 1983

443. Hryniuk W, Bush H: The importance of dose intensity in chemotherapy of metastatic breast cancer. J Clin Oncol 2:1281–1288, 1984

444. Hortobagyi GN, Buzdar AU, Bodey GP et al: High-dose induction chemotherapy of metastatic breast cancer in protected environment: A prospective randomized study. J Clin Oncol 5:178–184, 1987

445. Tannock IF, Boyd NF, Perrault DJ: Randomized trial of two doses of CMF chemotherapy for metastatic breast cancer (abstract). Proc Am Soc Clin Oncol 6:50, 1987

446. Goldie JH, Coldman AJ, Gudauskas GA: Rationale for the use of alternating non-cross-resistant chemotherapy. Cancer Treat Rep 66:439–449, 1982

447. Henderson IC, Hayes DF, Come S, Harris J, Canellos G: New agents and new medical treatments for advanced breast cancer. Semin Oncol 14:34–64, 1987

448. Tormey D, Gelman R, Falkson G: Prospective evaluation of rotating chemotherapy in advanced breast cancer. Am J Clin Oncol 6:1–18, 1983

449. Tormey DC, Weinberg VE, Leone LA et al: A comparison of intermittent vs. continuous and of Adriamycin vs. methotrexate 5-drug chemotherapy for advanced breast cancer. Am J Clin Oncol 7:231–239, 1984

450. Perry MC, Kardinal CG, Korzun AH et al: Chemohormonal therapy in advanced carcinoma of the breast: Cancer and Leukemia Group B protocol 8081. J Clin Oncol 5:1534–1545, 1987

451. Aberizk WJ, Silver B, Henderson IC, Cady B, Harris JR: The use of radiotherapy for treatment of isolated locroregional recurrence of breast carcinoma after mastectomy. Cancer 58:1214–1218, 1986

452. Hoogstraten B, Gad-El-Mawla N, Maloney TR et al: Combined modality therapy for first recurrence of breast cancer: A Southwest Oncology Group study. Cancer 54:2248–2256, 1984

453. Beck TM, Hart NE, Woodard DA, Smith CE: Local or regionally recurrent carcinoma of the breast: Results of therapy in 121 patients. J Clin Oncol 1:400–405, 1983

454. Tsukada Y, Fouad A, Pickren JW, Lane WW: Central nervous system metastasis from breast carcinoma. Autopsy study. Cancer 52:2349–2354, 1983

455. DiStefano A, Yap HY, Hortobagyi GN, Blumenschein GR: The natural history of breast cancer patients with brain metastases. Cancer 44:1913–1918, 1979

456. Borgelt B, Gelber R, Kramer S et al: The palliation of brain metastases: Final results of the first two studies by the Radiation Therapy Oncology Group. Int J Radiat Oncol Biol Phys 6:1–9, 1980

457. Glass JP, Foley KM: Specific sites of metastatic disease and emergencies: Brain metastases in patients with breast cancer. In Harris JR, Hellman S, Henderson IC, Kinne DW (eds): Breast Diseases, pp 480–487. Philadelphia, JB Lippincott, 1987

458. Burns PE, Jha N, Bain GO: Association of breast cancer with meningioma: A report of five cases. Cancer 58:1537–1539, 1986

459. Ushio Y, Posner JB, Sharpiro WR: Chemotherapy of experimental meningeal carcinomatosis. Cancer Res 37:1232–1237, 1977

460. Bertino JR: Toward improved selectivity in cancer chemotherapy: The Richard and Hinda Rosenthal Foundation Award Lecture. Cancer Res 39:293–304, 1979

461. Rosner D, Nemoto T, Lane WW: Chemotherapy induces regression of brain metastases in breast carcinoma. Cancer 58:832–839, 1986

462. Carey RW, Davis JM, Zervas NT: Tamoxifen-induced regression of cerebral metastases in breast carcinoma. Cancer Treat Rep 65:793–795, 1981

463. Smith DB, Howell A, Harris M, Bramwell VHC, Sellwood RA: Carcinomatous meningitis associated with infiltrating lobular carcinoma of the breast. Eur J Surg Oncol 11:33–36, 1985

464. Glass JP, Foley KM: Specific sites of metastatic disease and emergencies: Carcinomatous meningitis. In Harris JR, Hellman S, Henderson IC, Kinne DW (eds): Breast Diseases, pp 497–505. Philadelphia, JB Lippincott, 1987

465. Rose MA, Feldman EL: Specific sites of metastatic disease and emergencies: Choroidal metastases from breast cancer. In Harris JR, Hellman S, Henderson IC, Kinne DW (eds): Breast Diseases, pp 506–508. Philadelphia, JB Lippincott, 1987

466. Stillman M, Foley KM: Specific sites of metastatic disease and emergencies: Breast cancer and epidural spinal cord compression: Diagnostic and therapeutic strategies. In Harris JR, Hellman S, Henderson IC, Kinne DW (eds): Breast Diseases, pp 488–497. Philadelphia, JB Lippincott, 1987

467. Foley KM: Specific sites of metastatic disease and emergencies: Brachial plexopathy in patients with breast cancer. In Harris JR, Hellman S, Henderson IC, Kinne DW (eds): Breast Diseases, pp 532–538. Philadelphia, JB Lippincott, 1987

468. Israel L, Breau JL, Aguilera J: High-dose cyclophosphamide and high-dose 5-fluorouracil: A new first-line regimen for advanced breast cancer. Cancer 53:1655–1659, 1984

469. Tormey DC, Kline JC, Palta M, Davis TE, Love RR, Carbone PP: Short term high density systemic therapy for metastatic breast cancer. Breast Cancer Res Treat 5:177–188, 1985

470. Cheng DS, Seitz CB, Eyre HJ: Nonoperative management of femoral, humeral, and acetabular metastases in patients with breast carcinoma. Cancer 45:1533–1537, 1980

471. Tong D, Gillick L, Hendrickson FR: The palliation of symptomatic osseous metastases: The final results of the study by the Radiation Therapy Oncology Group. Cancer 50:893–899, 1982

472. Cornell CN, Lane JM: Specific sites of metastatic disease and emergencies: Management of pathologic fractures. In Harris JR, Hellman S, Henderson IC, Kinne DW (eds): Breast Diseases, pp 525–532. Philadelphia, JB Lippincott, 1987

473. Ingle JN, Tormey DC, Tan HK: The bone marrow examination in breast cancer. Cancer 41:670–674, 1978

474. Come SE, Schnipper LE: Specific sites of metastatic disease and emergencies. In Harris JR, Hellman S, Henderson IC, Kinne DW (eds): Breast Diseases, pp 557–562. Philadelphia, JB Lippincott, 1987

475. Redding WH, Monaghan P, Imrie SF et al: Detection of micrometastases in patients with primary breast cancer. Lancet 2:1271–1273, 1983

476. Kennedy BJ, Tibbetts DM, Nathanson IT, Aub JC: Hypercalcemia: A complication of hormone therapy of advanced breast cancer. Cancer Res 13:445–459, 1953

477. Henderson IC: Hypercalcemia of malignant disease. In: Brain MC, Carbone PP (eds): Current Therapy in Hematology–Oncology 1985–86, pp 254–257. Philadelphia, BC Decker, 1985

478. Henner WD: Specific sites of metastatic disease and emergencies: Lymphangetic spread of carcinoma of the breast. In Harris JR, Hellman S, Henderson IC, Kinne DW (eds): Breast Diseases, pp 538–540. Philadelphia, JB Lippincott, 1987

479. Henner WD: Specific sites of metastatic disease and emergencies: Malignant effusions in breast cancer. In Harris JR, Hellman S, Henderson IC, Kinne DW (eds): Breast Diseases, pp 540–547. Philadelphia, JB Lippincott, 1987

480. Poe RH, Qazi R, Israel RH, Wicks CM, Rubins JM: Survival of patients with pleural involvement by breast carcinoma. Am J Clin Oncol 6:523–527, 1983

481. Fentiman IA, Rubens RD, Hayward JL: Control of pleural effusions in patients with breast cancer. Cancer 52:737–739, 1983

482. Butcher H: Radical mastectomy for mammary carcinoma. Ann Surg 170:883–884, 1969

483. Haagensen CD, Cooley E, Miller E et al: Treatment of early mammary carcinoma: A cooperative international study. Ann Surg 170:875–879, 1969

484. Valagussa P, Bonadonna G, Veronesi U: Patterns of relapse and survival following radical mastectomy. Cancer 41:1170–1178, 1978

485. Fisher B, Slack N, Katrych D: Ten-year followup results of patients with carcinoma of the breast in a cooperative clinical trial evaluating surgical adjuvant chemotherapy. Surg Gynecol Obstet 140:528–534, 1975

486. Payne WS, Taylor WF, Khonsari S: Surgical treatment of breast cancer: Trends and factors affecting survival. Arch Surg 101:105–113, 1970

487. Warren S, Witman EM: Studies on tumor metastases: The distribution of metastases in cancer of the breast. Surg Gynecol Obstet 57:81–85, 1937

488. Saphir O, Parker ML: Metastases of primary carcinoma of the breast with special reference to spleen, adrenal glands and ovaries. Arch Surg 42:1003–1018, 1941

489. Clark RM, Wilkinson RH, Mahoney LJ et al: Breast cancer: A 21 year experience with conservative surgery and radiation. Int J Radiat Oncol Biol Phys 8:967–975, 1982

490. Davis HL, Wiseley AN, Ramirez G, Ansfield FJ: Hypercalcemia complicating breast cancer. Oncology 28:126–137, 1973

491. Freeman CR, Belliveau NJ, Kim TH et al: Limited surgery with or without radiotherapy for early breast carcinoma. J Can Assoc Radiol 32:125–128, 1981

492. Fisher B, Ravdin RG, Ausman RK, Slack NH, Moore GE, Noer RJ: Surgical adjuvant chemotherapy in cancer of the breast: Results of a decade of cooperative investigation. Ann Surg 168:337–356, 1968

493. Baum M, Wilson AJ, Ebbs SR: The role of adjuvant endocrine therapy in primary breast cancer. In Salmon SE (ed): Adjuvant Therapy of Cancer V, pp 377–390. Orlando, Grune & Stratton, 1987

494. Cole MP: Prophylactic compared with therapeutic X-ray artificial menopause. In Joslin CAF, Gleave EN (eds): The Clinical Management of Advanced Breast Cancer: 2nd Tenovous Workshop, pp 2–11. Cardiff, Wales, Alpha Omega Alpha Publishing, 1970

495. McGuire WL, Horwitz KB, Zava DT, Garola RE, Chamness GC: Progress in endocrinology and metabolism: Hormones in breast cancer: Update 1978. Metabolism 27:487–501, 1978

496. Clark GM, McGuire WL: Progesterone receptors and human breast cancer. Breast Cancer Res Treat 3:157–163, 1983

497. Canellos GP, Devita V, Gold GL et al: Cyclical combination chemotherapy for advanced breast carcinoma. Br Med J 1:218–220, 1974

498. Canellos GP, Pocock S, Taylor S et al: Combination chemotherapy for metastatic breast carcinoma. Cancer 38:1882–1886, 1976

499. Jones SE, Durie BGM, Salmon SE: Combination chemotherapy with Adriamycin and cyclophosphamide for advanced breast cancer. Cancer 36:90–97, 1975

500. Bull J, Tormey D, Li SH et al: A randomized comparative trial of Adriamycin versus methotrexate in combination drug therapy. Cancer 41:1649–1657, 1978

501. Tranum B, Hoogstraten B, Kennedy A et al: Adriamycin in combination for the treatment of breast cancer. Cancer 41:2078–2083, 1978

502. Smalley R, Carpenter J, Bartolucci A, Vogel C, Krauss S: A comparison of cyclophosphamide, Adriamycin, 5-fluorouracil (CAF) and cyclophosphamide, methotrexate, 5-fluorouracil, vincristine, prednisone (CMFVP) in patients with metastatic breast cancer. Cancer 40:625–632, 1977

Index

Index

Page numbers in *italics* indicate figures; page numbers followed by *t* indicate tabular material.

1

antidepressants and, 2078
butyrophenones and, 2078
phenothiazines and, 2078
steroids and, 2078
non-opioid, in pain management,
2071, 2072t
opioid, 2071–2077, 2073t
combination of, 2075–2076
complications with, 2077
drug tolerance and, 2076–2077
equianalgesic dose and route of,
2074, 2074t
regular administration of,
2074–2075
route of administration and, 2075
side-effects and, 2076
specific drugs for specific types of
pain and, 2071–2073, 2073
Anaplastic carcinoma
of salivary glands, 575
of thyroid gland, 1273
management of, 1283–1284, 1284t
Androgens, breast cancer metastases
and, 1251–1252
Anemia
myeloma and, 1859, 1880
paraneoplastic, 1917–1918
pernicious, upper gastrointestinal
endoscopy and, 431
Anesthetics
in pain management, 2079t,
2080–2082
autonomic nerve block and, 2082,
2083
epidural and intrathecal neurolytic
blocks and, 2081–2082
epidural infusions and local anesthetics and, 2081
neuroadenolysis of pituitary and,
2082
nitrous oxide and, 2082
peripheral nerve blocks and, 2081
trigger point injections and, 2081
for surgery, 237–238, 238t
Aneurysmal bone cyst, 1440–1441,
1442
Angiography
anthracycline-induced cardiomyopathy and, 2158–2159
bone tumors and, 1424, 1425
skeletal metastases and, 2304,
2306
staging and, 1426, 2306
pulmonary, staging of lung cancer by,
627
Angioinfarction, in renal cell carcinoma, metastatic,
991–992
Angiosarcomas, unique features of,
1364

Animal studies
anal region cancer and, 966
transgenic animals and
gene transfer and, 41–42, 42
oncogenes in, 57
ANLL. See Leukemia, acute
nonlymphocytic
Anorectal melanoma, 976
Anorexia, paraneoplastic, 1930–1931
Anthracyclines, 376, 376–380
analogues of, 379, 379–380
cardiomyopathy induced by,
2156–2160
clinical assessment and monitoring
of, 2158–2159
histopathology of, 2156–2157
incidence and prognosis of, 2157
management of, 2160
mechanisms of action and, 2157
prevention of, 2159–2160
risk factors for, 2157–2158
clinical pharmacology and pharmacokinetics of, 378
dose and scheduling of, 379
electrocardiogram changes and
arrhythmias and, 2153
extravasation and, 2388
mechanism of action of, 377–378,
378
myocardial ischemia and infarction
induced by, 2155
pericarditis induced by, 2154
toxicity of, 378–379
Antibacterial agents. See also specific
agents
prophylactic, 2126
Antibiotic therapy, 375–382. See also
specific drugs
adjuncts to, infection and, 2100–2101
empiric, infection and, 2093–2095,
2094, 2095–2101t, 2100
septicemia and, 2104, 2106
Antibodies, monoclonal. See Immunology, monoclonal antibodies
and
Anticancer drugs. See Chemotherapeutic agents; Chemotherapy;
specific drugs
Anticonvulsants, as adjuvant analgesic
drugs, 2077
Antidepressants, as adjuvant analgesic
drugs, 2078
Antidiuretic hormone. See Syndrome of
inappropriate secretion of
antidiuretic hormone
Antiemetic agents, 2138–2142, 2139t
combinations of, 2140t, 2142
Antifolates, 350–351, 354–359, 358.
See also Chemotherapeutic
agents; Chemotherapy; specific drugs

clinical pharmacology and pharmacokinetics of, 354–355
dose adjustment and, 355–358, 358t,
359
mechanism of action of, 350–351,
354, 358
toxicity of, 358–359
Antifungal therapy
empiric, neutropenia with unexplained fever and,
2102–2103, 2105
prophylactic, 2126–2127
Antigens
blood group, colorectal cancer staging and, 917
carcinoembryonic. See Carcinoembryonic antigen
of Epstein-Barr virus, 161
tumor, 306–307
Antimetabolites. See specific drugs and
drug types
Antineoplastic agents. See Chemotherapeutic agents;
Chemotherapy; specific
drugs
Antioncogene, lost in retinoblastoma,
2416–2417
Antiparasitic agents, prophylactic, 2127
Antisense RNA, inhibition of oncogene
expression by, 2424,
2424–2425
Antitumor drugs. See Chemotherapeu-
tic agents; Chemotherapy;
specific drugs
Antiviral agents. See also specific drugs
prophylactic, 2127
Anxiety, in cancer patients, 2196, 2199
AP-1, 40
Apheresis, 2055
Apocrine carcinoma, of skin, 1478
Appendicitis, as surgical emergency,
2006, 2007–2008
Ara-C. See Cytosine arabinoside
Arginine vasopressin (AVP), ectopic
production of, diagnosis of,
SIADH syndrome and,
1903t, 1903–1904
Arousal, sexual, problems of,
2209–2211
Arrhythmias, chemotherapy and, 2153
Arterial supply, to large bowel, 897,
897
Arthritis, as paraneoplastic syndrome,
1933
Aryepiglottic fold, laryngeal cancer
and, 535–536
Arytenoid, laryngeal cancer and,
535–536
Asbestos, carcinogenesis and, 145–146,
1401

tumors with systemic features and, 1306

tumors without systemic features and, 1305t, 1305–1306

colorectal, 952

diagnosis of, 1308–1309

of esophagus, 759

pathology of, 1303–1305, 1304t

prognosis in, 1309t, 1309–1310

of small intestine, 890

of thymus, 718–719

treatment of, 1312–1314, 1313t

carcinoid syndrome and, 1310t, 1310–1312, *1311, 1312*

Carcinoma. *See specific sites and types of carcinomas*

Carcinoma in situ

of bladder, treatment of, 1011–1012

of breast, 1204–1205

ductal, 1240–1241

lobular, 1241–1242

vaginal, treatment of, 1111

of vocal cords, treatment of, 538

Carcinosarcoma, of esophagus, 758

Cardiac irradiation, as risk factor for anthracycline-induced cardiomyopathy, 2157–2158

Cardiac status, physiologic staging of lung cancer and, 629–630

Cardiac toxicity, cancer therapy and, 2153–2160. *See also specific effects*

acute and subacute effects and, 2153

Cardiomyopathy

anthracycline, 2156–2160

clinical assessment and monitoring of, 2158–2159

histopathology of, 2156–2157

incidence and prognosis of, 2157

management of, 2160

mechanisms of action and, 2157

prevention of, 2159–2160

risk factors for, 2157–2158

anticancer drugs inducing, 2160

Cardioprotective agents, anthracycline-induced cardiomyopathy and, 2160

Cardiopulmonary manifestations, pathology of acute leukemia and, 1816

Cardiovascular system

disuse syndrome and, rehabilitation and, 2338–2339

infections of, 2116

Carotenoids, cancer risk and, 169–170

Carotid body tumors. *See* Chemodectomas

Case-control studies, epidemiological, 211

Catheters

bacteremia associated with, 2103–2104

care of, 2379–2381

central venous, 2378–2379

indwelling, 2379

superior vena cava syndrome induced by, 1975

Causality, determining, epidemiology and, 216

cDNA cloning, 34

CEA. *See* Carcinoembryonic antigen

Cecal cancer, surgical treatment of, 920, *921*

Celioscopy. *See* Peritoneoscopy

Cell(s)

destruction of, immune effector mechanisms resulting in, 302–304, 304t

embryonic, tumors originating in, karyotypes of, 89–90

hypoxic. *See* Hypoxia

of immune system, 302, 303t

lymphoid, identification of, 1744–1747, 1745t, *1746, 1747*

proliferation of, 3–13

diagnosis and, 9

flow cytometry and, 9

during division cycle, radiation and, 261–262

in human tumors, 3–5

cell kinetics and, 5–7, 5–9, 8t

preclinical growth and, 3–5, *4*

tumor doubling times and, 3, *4*, 4t

prognosis and, 9–10, 10t

treatment and, 10–12

cycle-dependence of therapy and, 10–11, *11*

scheduling of chemotherapy and, 11–12, *12*

scheduling of radiotherapy and, 12

survival of, radiation therapy and, 254–263, *256–257*

importance of oxygen and, 257–261, *259, 260,* 260t, 261t

pharmacologic modification of radiation effects and, *262, 262–263, 263*

repair of radiation damage and, 256–257, *258,* 258t, *259*

survival curves and, 255–256, *258,* 258t

variable radiation response during division cycle and, 261t, 261–262

Cell biology. *See* Molecular cell biology

Cell cycle parameters, colorectal cancer staging and, 916

Cell killing, hypoxia and. *See* Hypoxia

Cell kinetics, of human tumors, 5–7, 5–9

basic concepts in, 5, 5–6

flow cytometry and, 7, 7–8

kinetic properties of tumors and, 8t, 8–9

tritiated thymidine and autoradiography and, *6, 6–7*

Cell sensitizers

hypoxic, 261

nonhypoxic, radiosensitization by, 2443–2444

Cellular immunity, impaired, infection and, 2089–2090

Cellulitis, perirectal, 2119–2120

Central nervous system. *See also* Brain; Brain cancer; Central nervous system tumors; Intracranial tumors; Spinal cord

breast cancer metastases to, 1259–1260

infections of, 2122–2124

leukemia and, in children, 1674

preventive therapy and

in acute lymphoblastic leukemia, in children, 1679

in non-Hodgkin's lymphoma, in children, 1691–1692

relapse and, in acute lymphoblastic leukemia, in children, 1681

Central nervous system tumors, 448–450, 1557–1608. *See also* Brain cancer; Intracranial tumors; Spinal cord tumors; *specific tumors*

anatomy and clinical considerations with, 1559–1567, *1560, 1561*

focal infratentorial syndromes and, 1563–1566, 1564t, 1565t

intracranial tumors and, 1560, 1562t, 1562–1563

spinal axis and, 1566–1567

of brain, radiology and, 448–450, *449–451*

chemotherapy and, 1578–1579

regional drug delivery and, 1579

classification and treatment by anatomical location, 1579–1608

epidemiology of, 1558–1559

chemical causes and, 1558–1559

genetics and, 1558

irradiation, chemotherapy, and immunosuppression and, 1559

trauma and, 1559

viral causes and, 1559

incidence and classification of, 1557–1558, 1558t, 1559t

Chemotherapy, in gastric cancer (continued)
  single-agent, 791t, 791–793
  in germ cell tumors, in childhood, 1643
  in gestational trophoblastic disease, long-term complications of, 1152
  gonadal dysfunction induced by
    in adult men, 2170–2172, 2171, 2171t, 2172, 2172t
    in adult women, 2172–2173, 2173t
    in children, 2173–2174
    counseling and, 2178, 2178t
    in female children, 2174
    genetic concerns and, 2175–2176
    in male children, 2173
    pregnancy outcomes and, 2176–2178, 2177t
    techniques to protect fertility and, 2175
  in head and neck cancer, 495–497
    adjuvant, 502
    combination, for advanced disease, 497, 498t
    single-agent, for advanced disease, 496t, 496–497
  hematuria induced by, 2016–2018
  hepatic metastases and
    intrahepatic, through implantable pump, toxicity of, 2289–2292, 2290t
    regional, 2287–2289, 2288t, 2289t
      local tumor destruction plus, 2294–2295
    systemic, 2285–2287, 2287t
  in hepatic tumors, primary, in childhood, 1640
  in hepatocellular carcinoma, 849–853
    chemoradiation and, 852
    combination, 850t, 851t, 852
    determination of tumor response and, 849
    hepatic artery infusion and, 852–853
    single-agent, 849, 850t
    status of, 852
  hexamethylmelamine in, 385, 385
  in Hodgkin's disease, 1716–1721, 1717, 1718t, 1719, 1719t, 1720, 1721–1725t, 1723–1731
    advanced, selection of treatment for, 1729
    early-stage, 1731
    impact of dose intensity on outcome of, 1726–1728, 1727t, 1728, 1728t
    new drugs and biologics in, 1733, 1733t

  radiation combined with, in stages I, II, and III disease, 1733, 1733–1734
  salvage, for advanced disease, 1729–1731, 1730t
  hyperthermia combined with, 2428, 2428–2429
  ifosfamide in, 371
  impact of, 296, 296–298, 297t
  induction, 287
    adjuvant therapy and, in head and neck cancer, 502
    in head and neck cancer, 499–502, 501t
  in initial treatment, 287–288
    adjuvant chemotherapy and, 288
    induction chemotherapy and, 287
    primary chemotherapy and, 288
  in insulinomas, 1328–1329
  for in-transit metastases of cutaneous melanoma, 1514
  intra-arterial, 466–467, 467
  intravenous, 2370, 2371–2377t, 2375, 2377–2388
    catheter care and, 2379–2381
    central venous catheters and, 2378–2379
    complications of, 2384–2386
    cytapheresis and, 2384
    extravasation and, 2386t, 2386–2388
    implantable vascular access devices and, 2382, 2382–2383
    intraperitoneal administration and, 2383–2384
    intrathecal therapy and, 2384
    nurses' knowledge and skills and, 2375, 2377
    portable infusion pumps and, 2381, 2381–2382
    technique and, 2377–2378, 2378, 2379
  in lung cancer
    adjuvant, postoperative, 654–655
    neoadjuvant, 656t, 656–657
      regimens and toxicity of, 657, 657t
    non-small cell
      cisplatin-combination, outpatient regimens for, 663, 664t
      combination
        responses to, 661, 661t, 662t
        supportive care versus, 663
      neoadjuvant therapy with, 656t, 656–657
      new drugs with potential for, 660–661
      patient selection for, 660
      prognostic factors in patient selection for, 663–665

  radiotherapy combined with, 665
    risk:benefit ratio and, 665
    single-agent, response to, 660, 661t
    single-agent versus combination, 662–663
    toxicities and, 665
  radiation therapy combined with, 655
  small cell, 669, 669t
    combination, 669–676, 670, 671t–675t
  melphalan in, 371–372
  in mesothelioma, 1411–1412
    combination, 1411t, 1411–1412, 1412t
    intracavitary delivery and, 1412
    single-agent, 1410t, 1411
  metastatic melanoma at distant sites and, 1521–1523
    combination, 1523
    high-dose, 1523
    single-agent, 1522t, 1522–1523
  mithramycin in, 382
  mitomycin C in, 380–381
    clinical pharmacology of, 380
    structure and mechanism of action of, 380, 381
    toxicity of, 380–381
  modifications of, recurrence of malignant disease and, bone marrow transplantation and, 2485–2486
  in myeloma
    combination regimens of, 1875–1876, 1876t
    high-dose, alone or with bone marrow transplantation, 1876–1877
    induction, magnitude of cell kill with, 1873
    multiagent combination, 1869–1873, 1870t, 1871, 1872t
    remission-induction, 1869–1873
  myocardial ischemia and infarction induced by, 2155–2156
    management of, 2155–2156
  in neuroblastoma, 1630
  nitrogen mustard in, 369
  nitrosurea in, 372, 372–373
  in non-Hodgkin's lymphoma, in children, 1688–1689, 1690t, 1691
  oral complications of, 2146, 2146–2152
    direct stomatotoxicity and, 2147, 2147–2148, 2148, 2148t, 2149t

Vol. 1: pp. 1–1268; Vol. 2: pp. 1269–2490

radiology and, 458, 460
relative therapeutic effectiveness and, 831
surgical treatment of, 812–819
bypass procedures and, 817–819, 819, 820
preoperative biliary decompression for obstructive jaundice and, 812–813, 813t
resection and, 813–817
and, extended, 815
incision and evaluation and, 813–814
pancreaticoduodenectomy and, 814, 814
reconstruction and, 814–815, 815
results of, 816, 816–817
upper gastrointestinal endoscopy and, 431–433
jaundiced patients and, 431–433, 432, 432t
pancreatic duct cytology and tumor antigens and, 433
Pancreatic islet cell tumors. See Islet cell tumors
Pancreaticoduodenectomy, in pancreatic cancer, 814, 814
Pancreatitis, 2006
Papillary adenocarcinoma, of thyroid gland, 1271
Papillary cystadenoma lymphomatosum, 575
Papilloma
of choroid plexus, 1605–1606
chemotherapy for, 1606
clinical and pathologic considerations and, 1605–1606
radiation therapy for, 1606
surgery for, 1606
inverting
of paranasal sinuses, 563
results of treatment of, 567–568
squamous cell, of esophagus, 726
Papillomaviruses, carcinogenesis and, 155–160
biology of papillomavirus infection and, 155, 156t
epidermodysplasia verruciformis and, 158
genital carcinomas and, 158–160
genomic organization and, 155–157, 157, 157t
Papulosis, lymphomatoid, 1803
Paracentesis, ascites and, 2329
Parameningeal rhabdomyosarcomas, in childhood, treatment of, 1653
Paranasal sinus cancer, 560–570
anatomy and, 560–561

lymphatics and, 561
clinical picture in, 564
diagnosis and staging of, 564–565
pathology of, 561–562
patterns of spread of, 562–563
treatment of, 566–567
combined modalities in, 567
complications of, 569–570
irradiation technique and, 567
management of recurrence and, 567
results of, 567–569
selection of modality for, 566, 567
surgical, 566–567
Paraneoplastic syndromes, 1896–1933
amylase elevation as, 1931
amyloidosis as, 1932
arthritis polymyalgia rheumatica as, 1933
endocrinologic manifestations and, 1897–1899t, 1897–1910
ACTH/Cushing's syndrome and, 1898–1902
calcitonin and, 1906–1907
chromogranin A and, 1907
human placental and pituitary glycoprotein hormones and their subunits and, 1907–1909
human placental lactogen, growth hormone, growth hormone-releasing hormone, prolactin, and thyrotropic substance and, 1909
hypercalcemia and, 1905–1906
hypocalcemia and, 1906
hypoglycemia and, 1909–1910
hypophosphatemic osteomalacia associated with benign mesenchymal tumors and, 1906
neurogastrointestinal peptides and, 1910
syndrome of inappropriate secretion of antidiuretic hormone and, 1902–1905
etiology and pathogenesis of, 1897
fever as, 1931
gastrointestinal manifestations and, 1928–1931
anorexia, cachexia, and taste abnormalities and, 1930–1931
hepatopathy and, 1930
protein-losing enteropathies and, 1928, 1930
hematologic manifestations and, 1916–1923
anemia and, 1917–1918
eosinophilia and basophilia and, 1919

erythrocytosis and, 1916–1917
granulocytopenia and, 1919
granulocytosis associated with non-hematologic malignancies and, 1918–1919
hypercoagulable state and, 1920–1923
thrombocytopenia and, 1919–1920
thrombocytosis and, 1919
hyperlipidemia as, 1931
hypertension-hypotension as, 1931
hypertrophic pulmonary osteoarthropathy as, 1931–1932
involving skin, 1924–1928
evaluation of, 1924–1928
lactic acidosis as, 1931
lung cancer and, 611–612, 613t
neurologic manifestations and, 1910–1916, 1911–1913t
myeloma and, 1879
remote effects
involving spinal cord and, 1914
on cerebrum and cranial nerves and, 1911, 1914
on muscle and neuromuscular function and, 1915–1916
on peripheral nervous system and, 1914–1915
occult primary malignancy and, 1949
palmar fasciitis and arthritis as, 1933
renal manifestations and, 1923t, 1923–1924
glomerular lesions of indirect cause and, 1923–1924
systemic lupus erythematosus as, 1933
Parasaggital meningiomas, surgical treatment of, 1590–1591, 1591
Parathyroid gland
in multiple endocrine neoplasia, type I, 1330, 1330t
cancer of, 1284–1285, 1285t
Parenteral chemotherapy. See Chemotherapy, intravenous
Parenteral nutrition, 2037–2039
calories in, 2037–2038
metabolic complications and monitoring, 2039
minerals in, 2035
protein in, 2037
solutions for, 2037, 2037t
venous access for, 2037
vitamins in, 2038t, 2038–2039
Parosteal osteosarcoma. See Osteosarcoma, parosteal
Parotid gland. See Salivary gland cancer
Particle beam radiation therapy. See Radiation therapy, particle beam

ISBN 0-397-50843-3

90000

9 780397 508433